Manual of CLINICAL MICROBIOLOGY

7*th* EDITION

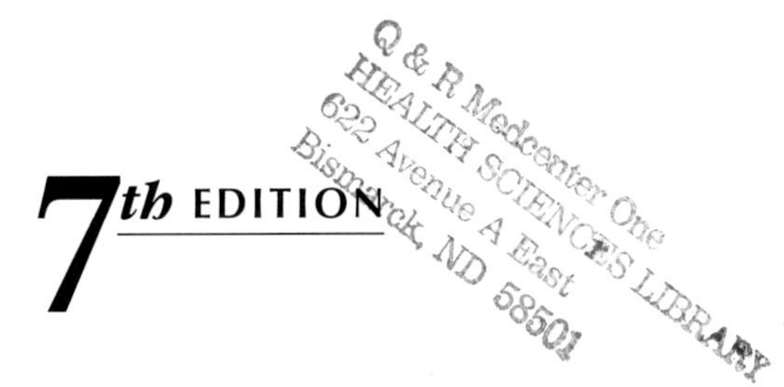

7th EDITION

Manual of CLINICAL MICROBIOLOGY

EDITOR IN CHIEF

Patrick R. Murray
Departments of Pathology and Medicine
Washington University School of Medicine
St. Louis, Missouri

EDITORS

Ellen Jo Baron
Department of Medicine
Stanford University School of Medicine, and
Clinical Microbiology/Virology Laboratory
Stanford, California

Michael A. Pfaller
Department of Pathology
University of Iowa College of Medicine
Iowa City, Iowa

Fred C. Tenover
Hospital Infections Program
Centers for Disease Control and Prevention
Atlanta, Georgia

Robert H. Yolken
Department of Pediatrics, Stanley Division
of Developmental Neurovirology
Johns Hopkins Hospital
Baltimore, Maryland

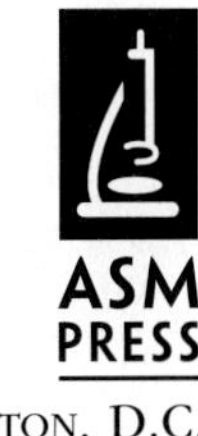

ASM PRESS
Washington, D.C.

1325 Massachusetts Avenue, N.W.
Washington, DC 20005

Library of Congress Cataloging-in-Publication Data

Manual of clinical microbiology/editor in chief, Patrick R. Murray: editors. Ellen Jo Baron . . . [et al.].—7th ed.
p. cm.
Includes index.
ISBN 1-55581-126-4 (hardcover)
1. Medical microbiology—Handbooks, manuals, etc. 2. Diagnostic microbiology—Handbooks, manuals, etc. I. Murray, Patrick R. II. American Society for Microbiology.
QR46.M425 1999
616'.01—dc21

98-46075
CIP

10 9 8 7 6 5 4 3 2 1

Printed in the United States of America

Fred C. Tenover's role as an editor of this book was carried out completely in his private capacity and his contribution as an editor in no way reflects official support or endorsement by the Centers for Disease Control and Prevention.

Contents

SECTION V
VIROLOGY / 832
VOLUME EDITOR: ROBERT H. YOLKEN
SECTION EDITORS: DAVID A. LENNETTE, THOMAS F. SMITH, AND JOSEPH L. WANER

Editorial Board

Contributors

SHARON ABBOTT
Microbial Diseases Laboratory, California State Department of Health Services, 2151 Berkeley Way, Berkeley, CA 94704

STOJANKA ALEKSIC
Division of Bacteriology, Institute of Hygiene, Marckmannstrasse 129a, D-20539 Hamburg, Germany

ANNIKA ALLARD
Department of Virology, Umeå University, S-901 85 Umeå, Sweden

STEPHEN D. ALLEN
Department of Pathology and Laboratory Medicine, Indiana University School of Medicine, Indianapolis, IN 46202-5283

MARTIN ALTWEGG
Department of Medical Microbiology, University of Zürich, Gloriastrasse 30, CH-8028 Zürich, Switzerland

ROBERT D. ARBEIT
Research Service, Veterans Affairs Medical Center, Boston, MA 02130, and Departments of Medicine and Microbiology, Boston University School of Medicine, Boston, MA 02118

ANN M. ARVIN
Department of Pediatric Infectious Diseases, Stanford Medical Center, Stanford, CA 94305

LAWRENCE R. ASH
Department of Epidemiology, School of Public Health, University of California, Los Angeles, CA 90095-1772

DAVID M. ASHER
Laboratory of Method Development, Division of Viral Products, Office of Vaccine Research and Review, Center for Biologics Evaluation and Review, U.S. Food and Drug Administration, Bethesda, MD 20892-0001

TAMMY L. BANNERMAN
Department of Pathology and School of Allied Medical Professions, The Ohio State University, Columbus, OH 43210-1234

ELLEN JO BARON
Department of Medicine, Stanford University School of Medicine, and Clinical Microbiology/Virology Laboratory, Stanford Hospital and Clinics, Stanford, CA 94305-5250

JAMES BEEBE
Laboratory and Radiation Services Division, Colorado Department of Public Health and Environment, Denver, CO 80217

D. BEIGHTON
Joint Microbiology Research Unit, King's College School of Medicine and Dentistry, London, England

KATHRYN A. BERNARD
Special Bacteriology Section, Federal Laboratories for Health Canada, Winnipeg, Manitoba R3E 3P6, Canada

JOHN BESSER
Public Health Laboratory Division, Minnesota Department of Health, Minneapolis, MN 55440

JACQUES BILLE
Centre National de Référence Listeria, Institut de Microbiologie, Rue du Bugnon, CH-1011 Lausanne, Switzerland

JOCHEN BOCKEMÜHL
Division of Bacteriology, Institute of Hygiene, Marckmannstrasse 129a, D-20539 Hamburg, Germany

CHERYL A. BOPP
Foodborne and Diarrheal Diseases Laboratory Section, Foodborne and Diarrheal Diseases Branch, Division of Bacterial and Mycotic Diseases, National Center for Infectious Diseases, Centers for Disease Control and Prevention, Atlanta, GA 30333

SANDRA L. BRAGG
Meningitis and Special Pathogens Branch, Division of Bacterial and Mycotic Diseases, National Center for Infectious Diseases, Centers for Disease Control and Prevention, Atlanta, GA 30333

FRANCES W. BRENNER
Foodborne and Diarrheal Diseases Laboratory Section, Foodborne and Diarrheal Diseases Branch, Division of Bacterial and Mycotic Diseases, National Center for Infectious Diseases, Centers for Disease Control and Prevention, Atlanta, GA 30333

JUNE M. BROWN
Meningitis and Special Pathogens Branch, Division of Bacterial and Mycotic Diseases, National Center for Infectious Diseases, Centers for Disease Control and Prevention, Atlanta, GA 30333

DAVID A. BRUCKNER
Department of Pathology and Laboratory Medicine, UCLA Medical Center, Los Angeles, CA 90095-1713

WILLY BURGDORFER
Rocky Mountain Laboratories, National Institute of Allergy and Infectious Diseases, National Institutes of Health, Hamilton, MT 59840

JOSEPH M. CAMPOS
Department of Laboratory Medicine, Children's National Medical Center, Washington, DC 20010, and Departments of Pediatrics, Pathology, and Microbiology/Immunology, George Washington University Medical Center, Washington, DC 20037

ELIZABETH U. CANNING
Imperial College of Science, Technology and Medicine, Ascot, Berks LS5 7PY, United Kingdom

KIMBERLE C. CHAPIN
Department of Laboratory Medicine, Lahey Clinic, 41 Mall Road, Burlington, MA 01805-0001

MAX A. CHERNESKY
McMaster Regional Virology and Chlamydiology Laboratory, Department of Pathology and Molecular Medicine, and Department of Pediatrics, McMaster University and St. Joseph's Hospital, 50 Charlton Avenue East, Hamilton, Ontario, Canada L8N 4A6

MARY L. CHRISTENSEN
Department of Pathology, Northwestern University Medical School, Chicago, IL 60611, and Virology Laboratory, Department of Pathology, The Children's Memorial Hospital, Chicago, IL 60614

DIANE M. CITRON
R. M. Alden Research Laboratory, Santa Monica Hospital, 1250 16th Street, Santa Monica, CA 90404

PATRICE COURVALIN
Unité des Agents Antibactériens, Institut Pasteur, 75724 Paris, France

NANCY J. COX
Influenza Branch, Division of Viral and Rickettsial Diseases, National Center for Infectious Diseases, Centers for Disease Control and Prevention, Atlanta, GA 30333

EDWARD P. DESMOND
Microbial Diseases Laboratory, California Department of Health Services, Berkeley, CA 94704

CHARLENE S. DEZZUTTI
Retrovirus Diseases Branch, Division of AIDS, STD, TB and Laboratory Research, Centers for Disease Control and Prevention, Atlanta, GA 30333

JULES L. DIENSTAG
Harvard Medical School and Massachusetts General Hospital, Boston, MA 02114

DENNIS M. DIXON
Division of Microbiology and Infectious Diseases, National Institute of Allergy and Infectious Diseases, National Institutes of Health, Bethesda, MD 20892

J. STEPHEN DUMLER
Department of Pathology, The Johns Hopkins University School of Medicine, The Johns Hopkins Hospital, Baltimore, MD 21287

CHRISTOPHER L. EMERY
Department of Pathology and Laboratory Medicine, Indiana University School of Medicine, Indianapolis, IN 46202-5283

ANA ESPINEL-INGROFF
Medical Mycology Research Laboratory, Division of Infectious Diseases, Medical College of Virginia of Virginia Commonwealth University, Richmond, VA 23298-0049

JOSEPH J. ESPOSITO
Division of Viral and Rickettsial Diseases, Centers for Disease Control and Prevention, Atlanta, GA 30333

RICHARD R. FACKLAM
Streptococcus Laboratory, Respiratory Diseases Branch, Division of Bacterial and Mycotic Diseases, Centers for Disease Control and Prevention, Atlanta, GA 30333

J. J. FARMER III
Enteric Reference Laboratory, Foodborne and Diarrheal Diseases Laboratory Section, Division of Bacterial and Mycotic Diseases, National Center for Infectious Diseases, Centers for Disease Control and Prevention, Atlanta, GA 30333

MARY JANE FERRARO
Clinical Microbiology Laboratory, Massachusetts General Hospital, and Departments of Pathology and Medicine, Harvard Medical School, Boston, MA 02114

SYDNEY M. FINEGOLD
Medical Service, VA Medical Center West Los Angeles, UCLA School of Medicine, Los Angeles, CA 90073

JAMES G. FOX
Division of Comparative Medicine, Massachusetts Institute of Technology, Cambridge, MA 02139

RENO FREI
Bacteriology Laboratory, University Hospitals, Basel, Switzerland

THOMAS R. FRITSCHE
Department of Laboratory Medicine, University of Washington, Seattle, WA 98185-7110

ROBERT A. FROMTLING
Merck Research Laboratories, Rahway, NJ 07065-0900

GUIDO FUNKE
Department of Medical Microbiology, Gärtner and Colleagues Laboratories, D-88250 Weingarten, Germany

LYNNE S. GARCIA
Department of Pathology and Laboratory Medicine, UCLA Medical Center, Los Angeles, CA 90095-1713

ANNE A. GERSHON
Department of Pediatrics, Columbia University College of Physicians and Surgeons, New York, NY 10032

PETER H. GILLIGAN
Clinical Microbiology-Immunology Laboratories, University of North Carolina Hospitals, and Department of Microbiology-Immunology and Pathology, University of North Carolina School of Medicine, Chapel Hill, NC 27514

PATRICK A. D. GRIMONT
Unité des Entérobactéries, Institut Pasteur, 75724 Paris Cedex 15, France

W. KEITH HADLEY
Department of Laboratory Medicine, University of California, San Francisco, and San Francisco General Hospital, San Francisco, CA 94110

KEVIN C. HAZEN
Department of Pathology, University of Virginia Health Sciences Center, Charlottesville, VA 22908

DAVID W. HECHT
Division of Infectious Diseases and Department of Microbiology and Immunology, Loyola University Medical Center, Maywood, IL 60153

JOHN C. HIERHOLZER
Respiratory and Enteric Viruses Branch, Division of Viral and Rickettsial Diseases, Center for Infectious Diseases, Centers for Disease Control and Prevention, Atlanta, GA 30333

SHARON L. HILLIER
Department of Obstetrics, Gynecology, and Reproductive Sciences, University of Pittsburgh/Magee-Womens Hospital, Pittsburgh, PA 15213

JANET A. HINDLER
Clinical Microbiology Laboratory, UCLA Medical Center, Los Angeles, CA 90024

RICHARD L. HODINKA
Division of Immunologic and Infectious Diseases, University of Pennsylvania School of Medicine, and Clinical Virology Laboratory, Children's Hospital of Philadelphia, Philadelphia, PA 19104

F. BLAINE HOLLINGER
Baylor College of Medicine, Houston, TX 77030

DANNIE G. HOLLIS
Division of Bacterial Diseases, Centers for Disease Control and Prevention, Atlanta, GA 30333

BARRY HOLMES
National Collection of Type Cultures, Central Public Health Laboratory, London NW9 5HT, England

HARVEY T. HOLMES
Microbiology Laboratories, St. Joseph Mercy Hospital, Pontiac, MI 48053

JÖRG E. HOPPE
Section of Bacteriology, University Children's Hospital, Hoppe-Seyler-Strasse 3, D-72076 Tübingen, Germany

CLARK B. INDERLIED
Clinical and Molecular Microbiology Laboratory, Department of Pathology and Laboratory Medicine, Childrens Hospital Los Angeles, and Department of Pathology, University of Southern California, Los Angeles, CA 90027

PETER B. JAHRLING
U.S. Army Medical Research Institute of Infectious Diseases, Fort Detrick, Frederick, MD 21702-5011

J. MICHAEL JANDA
Enterics and Special Pathogens Section, Microbial Diseases Laboratory, California Department of Health Services, 2151 Berkeley Way, Berkeley, CA 94704-1011

JAMES H. JORGENSEN
Department of Pathology, The University of Texas Health Science Center, San Antonio, TX 78284-7750

HANNELE R. JOUSIMIES-SOMER
Anaerobe Reference Laboratory, National Public Health Institute, 00300 Helsinki, Finland

JULIUS KANE
Sunnybrook-Dynacare Laboratories, Toronto, Ontario, Canada M4N 3N5, and Department of Laboratory Medicine and Pathobiology, University of Toronto, Toronto, Ontario, Canada M5G 1L5

ARNOLD F. KAUFMANN
Meningitis and Special Pathogens Branch, Division of Bacterial and Mycotic Diseases, National Center for Infectious Diseases, Centers for Disease Control and Prevention, Atlanta, GA 30333

MICHAEL J. KENNEDY
Animal Health Discovery Research, Veterinary Infectious Diseases, Pharmacia and Upjohn, Kalamazoo, MI 49001

DEANNA L. KISKA
Department of Clinical Pathology, SUNY Health Science Center, Syracuse, NY 13210

NANCY B. KIVIAT
Department of Pathology, University of Washington, Seattle, WA 98104

WESLEY E. KLOOS
Department of Genetics, North Carolina State University, Raleigh, NC 27695-7614

JOAN S. KNAPP
Division of AIDS, STD, and TB Laboratory Branch, National Center for Infectious Diseases, Centers for Disease Control and Prevention, Atlanta, GA 30333

EMILY H. KOUMANS
Division of STD Prevention, Centers for Disease Control and Prevention, Atlanta, GA 30333

JAIME A. LABARCA
Internal Medicine Department, Facultad de Medicina, Pontificia Universidad Católica de Chile, Santiago, Chile

RENU B. LAL
Retrovirus Diseases Branch, Division of AIDS, STD, TB and Laboratory Research, Centers for Disease Control and Prevention, Atlanta, GA 30333

MARIE L. LANDRY
Department of Laboratory Medicine, Yale University School of Medicine, New Haven, CT 06510; Clinical Virology Laboratory, Yale New Haven Hospital, New Haven, CT 06504; and Virology Reference Laboratory, VA Connecticut, West Haven, CT 06516

DAVISE H. LARONE
Clinical Microbiology, The New York Hospital-Cornell Medical Center, 525 East 68th Street, New York, NY 10021

SANDRA A. LARSEN
330 Pine Valley Drive, Marietta, GA 30067

PHILIP LaRUSSA
Department of Pediatrics, Columbia University College of Physicians and Surgeons, New York, NY 10032

TSAI-LING LAUDERDALE
Department of Pathology, University of South Alabama Hospitals, Mobile, AL 36617

AMY L. LEBER
Clinical Microbiology, UCLA Medical Center, Los Angeles, CA 90049

DAVID A. LENNETTE
Virolab, Inc., 1204 Tenth Street, Berkeley, CA 94710-1509

EVELYNE T. LENNETTE
Virolab, Inc., 1204 Tenth Street, Berkeley, CA 94710

NIALL A. LOGAN
Department of Biological Sciences, Glasgow Caledonian University, Cowcaddens Road, Glasgow G4 0BA, United Kingdom

VLADIMIR N. LOPAREV
Division of Viral and Rickettsial Diseases, Centers for Disease Control and Prevention, Atlanta, GA 30333

JAMES D. MACLOWRY
Department of Pathology, Oregon Health Sciences University, Portland, OR 97201

JAMES B. MAHONY
McMaster Regional Virology and Chlamydiology Laboratory and Department of Pathology and Molecular Medicine, McMaster University and St. Joseph's Hospital, 50 Charlton Avenue East, Hamilton, Ontario, Canada L8N 4A6

EUGENE O. MAJOR
Laboratory of Molecular Medicine and Neurosciences, National Institute of Neurological Disorders and Stroke, Bethesda, MD 20892

THOMAS J. MARRIE
Departments of Medicine and Microbiology, Dalhousie University and Queen Elizabeth Health Sciences Centre, Halifax, Nova Scotia B3H 2Y9, Canada

JAMES B. MCAULEY
Field Services Branch, Division of Tuberculosis Elimination, National Center for HIV, STD, and Tuberculosis Elimination, Centers for Disease Control and Prevention, Atlanta, GA 30341, and Rush Children's Hospital, Chicago, IL 60612

MICHAEL R. MCGINNIS
Center for Tropical Diseases, Department of Pathology, University of Texas Medical Branch at Galveston, Galveston, TX 77555

JOHN E. MCGOWAN, JR.
Department of Epidemiology, Rollins School of Public Health, Emory University, Atlanta, GA 30322

MICHAEL M. MCNEIL
Meningitis and Special Pathogens Branch, Division of Bacterial and Mycotic Diseases, National Center for Infectious Diseases, Centers for Disease Control and Prevention, Atlanta, GA 30333

JOSEPH L. MELNICK
Baylor College of Medicine, Houston, TX 77030-3498

WILLIAM G. MERZ
Microbiology Division, Department of Pathology, The Johns Hopkins University, Baltimore, MD 21287-7093

BEVERLY G. METCHOCK
Diagnostic Mycobacteriology Section, Division of AIDS, STD, and TB Laboratory Research, National Center for Infectious Diseases, Centers for Disease Control and Prevention, Atlanta, GA 30333

J. MICHAEL MILLER
Hospital Environment Branch, Hospital Infections Program, National Center for Infectious Diseases, Centers for Disease Control and Prevention, Atlanta, GA 30333

THOMAS G. MITCHELL
Department of Microbiology and Immunology, Duke University Medical Center, Durham, NC 27710

ROBERT C. MOELLERING, JR.
Department of Medicine, Beth Israel Deaconess Medical Center, Harvard Medical School, Boston, MA 02215

BERNARD J. MONCLA
Department of Microbiology and Biochemistry, School of Dental Medicine, University of Pittsburgh, Pittsburgh, PA 15261

PATRICK R. MURRAY
Departments of Pathology and Medicine, Washington University School of Medicine, St. Louis, MO 63110

MONICA MUSIANI
Department of Clinical Experimental Medicine, Division of Microbiology, University of Bologna, 40138 Bologna, Italy

REINIER MUTTERS
Institute of Medical Microbiology and Hospital Hygiene, Philipps University, D-35037 Marburg, Germany

IRVING NACHAMKIN
Department of Pathology and Laboratory Medicine, University of Pennsylvania School of Medicine, Philadelphia, PA 19104-4283

VALERIE L. NG
Department of Laboratory Medicine, University of California, San Francisco, and San Francisco General Hospital, San Francisco, CA 94110

PHUC NGUYEN-DINH
Division of Parasitic Diseases, Centers for Disease Control and Prevention, 4770 Buford Highway, Chamblee, GA 30341

FREDERICK S. NOLTE
Emory University Hospital and Department of Pathology and Laboratory Medicine, Emory University School of Medicine, Atlanta, GA 30322

STEVEN J. NORRIS
Department of Pathology and Laboratory Medicine, University of Texas Medical School at Houston, Houston, TX 77225

SUSAN M. NOVAK
Clinical Microbiology, Kaiser Permanente Regional Reference Laboratory, Southern California Permanente Medical Group, North Hollywood, CA 91605

CAROLINE M. O'HARA
Diagnostic Microbiology Section, Hospital Infections Program, National Center for Infectious Diseases, Centers for Disease Control and Prevention, Atlanta, GA 30333

THOMAS C. ORIHEL
Department of Tropical Medicine, School of Public Health and Tropical Medicine, Tulane University, New Orleans, LA 70112

YNES R. ORTEGA
Department of Veterinary Science and Microbiology, University of Arizona, Tucson, AZ 85721

ARVIND A. PADHYE
Mycotic Diseases Branch, Division of Bacterial and Mycotic Diseases, National Center for Infectious Diseases, Centers for Disease Control and Prevention, Atlanta, GA 30333

JOSEPHINE C. PALMER
MDS Laboratories, 100 International Boulevard, Etobicoke, Ontario M9W 6J6, Canada

GREGORY J. PALUMBO
Department of Microbiology and Immunology, University of Oklahoma Health Sciences Center, Oklahoma City, OK 73104

LESTER PASARELL
Department of Pathology, University of Texas Medical Branch, Galveston, TX 77555

JOANNE L. PATTON
Division of Viral and Rickettsial Diseases, National Center for Infectious Diseases, Centers for Disease Control and Prevention, Atlanta, GA 30333

DAVID W. PERSING
Division of Clinical Microbiology, Department of Laboratory Medicine and Pathology, Mayo Clinic, Rochester, MN 55905

LANCE R. PETERSON
Clinical Microbiology Laboratory, Northwestern Memorial Hospital, Chicago, IL 60611

MARTIN PETRIC
Division of Microbiology, The Hospital for Sick Children, Toronto, Ontario M5G 1X8, Canada

MICHAEL A. PFALLER
Medical Microbiology Division, Department of Pathology, University of Iowa College of Medicine, Iowa City, IA 52242

M. JOHN PICKETT
Department of Microbiology and Molecular Genetics, University of California, Los Angeles, CA 90024

VICTORIA POPE
Division of AIDS, STD, and TB Laboratory Research, Centers for Disease Control and Prevention, Atlanta, GA 30333

CHARLES G. PROBER
Department of Pediatric Infectious Diseases, Stanford Medical Center, Stanford, CA 94305

RICHARD QUINTILIANI, JR.
Department of Microbiology and Immunology, Georgetown University, Washington, DC 20007

DIDIER RAOULT
Unité des Rickettsies, CNRS EJP 0054, Faculté de Médicine, Université de la Méditerranée, Marseille, France

J. KAMILE RASHEED
Hospital Infections Program, National Center for Infectious Diseases, Centers for Disease Control and Prevention, Atlanta, GA 30333

BARBARA S. REISNER
Department of Pathology, University of Texas Medical Branch, Galveston, TX 77555-0740

JUDITH C. RHODES
Department of Pathology and Laboratory Medicine, University of Cincinnati, and Clinical Microbiology, Health Alliance of Greater Cincinnati, Cincinnati, OH 45267-0529

MALCOLM D. RICHARDSON
Regional Mycology Reference Laboratory, Department of Dermatology, University of Glasgow and West Glasgow Hospitals University NHS Trust, Glasgow, United Kingdom

GLENN D. ROBERTS
Division of Clinical Microbiology, Mayo Clinic and Mayo Foundation, Rochester, MN 55905

JOCELYNE ROCOURT
Centre National de Référence Listeria, Institut Pasteur, 28, rue du Docteur Roux, F-75724 Paris Cédex 15, France

ARNE C. RODLOFF
Institut für Medizinische Mikrobiologie und Infektionsepidemiologie, University of Leipzig, D-04103 Leipzig, Germany

WILLIAM O. ROGERS
Malaria Program, Naval Medical Research Institute, Rockville, MD 20852

SUSAN L. ROPP
Division of Viral and Rickettsial Diseases, Centers for Disease Control and Prevention, Atlanta, GA 30333

PATRICIA A. ROSA
Rocky Mountain Laboratories, National Institute of Allergy and Infectious Diseases, National Institutes of Health, Hamilton, MT 59840

HARLEY A. ROTBART
Departments of Pediatrics and Microbiology, University of Colorado School of Medicine, Denver, CO 80262

KATHRYN L. RUOFF
Microbiology Laboratories, Massachusetts General Hospital, Boston, MA 02114, and Department of Pathology, Harvard Medical School, Boston, MA 02114

DANIEL F. SAHM
MRL Pharmaceutical Services, Herndon, VA 20171

MAX SALFINGER
Clinical Mycobacteriology Laboratory, Wadsworth Center, New York State Department of Health, and Department of Medicine, Albany Medical College, Albany, NY 12201-0509

IRA F. SALKIN
Wadsworth Center, New York State Department of Health, Albany, NY 12201

AIMO A. SALMI
Department of Virology, University of Turku, Kiinamyllynkatu 13, FIN-20520 Turku, Finland

JULIUS SCHACHTER
Chlamydia Research Laboratory, University of California, San Francisco, San Francisco, CA 94143

WILEY A. SCHELL
Medical Mycology Research Center, Department of Medicine, Division of Infectious Diseases and International Health, Duke University Medical Center, and Pathology and Laboratory Medicine, Veterans Affairs Medical Center, Durham, NC 27710

PAUL C. SCHRECKENBERGER
Division of Clinical Pathology, University of Illinois College of Medicine at Chicago, 840 S. Wood Street, Chicago, IL 60612

JÖRG SCHÜPBACH
Swiss National Center for Retroviruses, University of Zurich, Gloriastrasse 30, CH-8028 Zurich, Switzerland

TOM G. SCHWAN
Rocky Mountain Laboratories, National Institute of Allergy and Infectious Diseases, National Institutes of Health, Hamilton, MT 59840

W. EVAN SECOR
Division of Parasitic Diseases, Centers for Disease Control and Prevention, 4770 Buford Highway, Chamblee, GA 30341

DAVID L. SEWELL
Pathology and Laboratory Medicine Service, Veterans Affairs Medical Center, and Department of Pathology, Oregon Health Sciences University, Portland, OR 97201

GILLIAN S. SHANKLAND
Regional Mycology Reference Laboratory, Department of Dermatology, University of Glasgow and West Glasgow Hospitals University NHS Trust, Glasgow, United Kingdom

DANIEL S. SHAPIRO
Clinical Microbiology Immunology Laboratory, Boston Medical Center, Boston University School of Medicine, Boston, MA 02118-2520

SUSAN E. SHARP
Department of Clinical Microbiology, Mount Sinai Medical Center, Miami Beach, FL 33140

ROBYN Y. SHIMIZU
Department of Pathology and Laboratory Medicine, UCLA Medical Center, Los Angeles, CA 90095-1713

JEAN A. SIDERS
Department of Pathology and Laboratory Medicine, Indiana University School of Medicine, Indianapolis, IN 46202-5283

LYNNE SIGLER
University of Alberta Microfungus Collection and Herbarium, Devonian Botanic Garden, and Department of Medical Microbiology and Immunology, University of Alberta, Edmonton, Alberta, Canada T6G 2E1

LEONARD N. SLATER
Department of Medicine, University of Oklahoma Health Sciences Center and Veterans Affairs Medical Center, Oklahoma City, OK 73104

JEAN S. SMITH
Rabies Laboratory, Viral and Rickettsial Zoonoses Branch, Division of Viral and Rickettsial Diseases, National Center for Infectious Diseases, Centers for Disease Control and Prevention, Atlanta, GA 30333

THOMAS F. SMITH
Division of Clinical Microbiology, Mayo Clinic, Rochester, MN 55905

WALTER E. STAMM
University of Washington Medical Center, Seattle, WA 98195

JACK T. STAPLETON
Department of Internal Medicine, University of Iowa College of Medicine, and The Iowa City Veterans Affairs Medical Center, Iowa City, IA 52242

SHARON P. STEINBERG
Department of Pediatrics, Columbia University College of Physicians and Surgeons, New York, NY 10032

JOHN A. STEWART
Division of Viral and Rickettsial Diseases, National Center for Infectious Diseases, Centers for Disease Control and Prevention, Atlanta, GA 30333

NANCY A. STROCKBINE
Foodborne and Diarrheal Diseases Laboratory Section, Foodborne and Diarrheal Diseases Branch, Division of Bacterial and Mycotic Diseases, National Center for Infectious Diseases, Centers for Disease Control and Prevention, Atlanta, GA 30333

PAULA H. SUMMANEN
Research Service, VA Medical Center West Los Angeles, Los Angeles, CA 90073

RICHARD C. SUMMERBELL
Ontario Ministry of Health, Toronto, Ontario, Canada M9P 3T1, and Department of Laboratory Medicine and Pathology, University of Toronto, Toronto, Ontario, Canada M5G 1L5

BALA SWAMINATHAN
Division of Bacterial and Mycotic Diseases, Centers for Disease Control and Prevention, Atlanta, GA 30333

JANA M. SWENSON
Hospital Infections Program, Centers for Disease Control and Prevention, Atlanta, GA 30333

ELLA M. SWIERKOSZ
Departments of Pathology and Pediatrics, St. Louis University School of Medicine, St. Louis, MO 63104

YI-WEI TANG
Department of Medicine, Division of Infectious Diseases, Department of Pathology, Vanderbilt University School of Medicine, Nashville, TN 37232

DAVID TAYLOR-ROBINSON
Imperial College School of Medicine at St. Mary's Jeferiss Research Trust Laboratories, Praed Street, London W2 1PG, United Kingdom

LÚCIA MARTINS TEIXEIRA
Instituto de Microbiologia, Universidade Federal do Rio de Janeiro, Rio de Janeiro 21941, Brazil

FRED C. TENOVER
Hospital Infections Program, National Center for Infectious Diseases, Centers for Disease Control and Prevention, Atlanta, GA 30333

RICHARD B. THOMSON, JR.
Northwestern University Medical School and Evanston Northwestern Healthcare, Evanston Hospital, 2650 Ridge Avenue, Evanston, IL 60201-1783

JOHN R. TICEHURST
Microbiology Branch, Division of Clinical Laboratory Services, Office of Device Evaluation, Center for Devices and Radiological Health, U.S. Food and Drug Administration, Rockville, MD 20850-4015, and Medical Microbiology Division, Department of Pathology, The Johns Hopkins University School of Medicine, Baltimore, MD 21287-7093

DAVID L. TISON
Clinical Microbiology Laboratory, MultiCare Medical Center, Tacoma, WA 98415

DEBRA A. TRISTRAM
ECU Department of Pediatrics, Greenville, NC 27858

THEODORE F. TSAI
Centers for Disease Control and Prevention, Ft. Collins, CO 80522

PETER C. B. TURNBULL
Centre for Applied Microbiology and Research, Porton Down, Salisbury SP4 0JG, United Kingdom

JOHN D. TURNIDGE
Microbiology and Infectious Diseases, Women's and Children's Hospital, North Adelaide 5006, Australia

JAMES VERSALOVIC
Department of Pathology, Massachusetts General Hospital, Boston, MA 02114

GOVINDA S. VISVESVARA
Division of Parasitic Diseases, Center for Infectious Diseases, Centers for Disease Control and Prevention, 4770 Buford Highway NE, Atlanta, GA 30341-3724

ALEXANDER VON GRAEVENITZ
Department of Medical Microbiology, University of Zurich, Gloriastrasse 32, CH-8028 Zurich, Switzerland

ANDREAS VOSS
Department of Medical Microbiology, University Hospital St. Radboud, 6500 HB Nijmegen, The Netherlands

GÖRAN WADELL
Department of Virology, Umeå University, S-901 85 Umeå, Sweden

KEN B. WAITES
Departments of Pathology and Microbiology, University of Alabama at Birmingham Schools of Medicine and Dentistry, Birmingham, AL 35233-7331

DAVID H. WALKER
Department of Pathology, University of Texas Medical Branch, Galveston, TX 77555-0609

RICHARD J. WALLACE, JR.
Department of Microbiology, The University of Texas Health Center at Tyler, Tyler, TX 75708

THOMAS J. WALSH
Infectious Diseases Section, National Cancer Institute, Bethesda, MD 20892

JOSEPH L. WANER
Pediatric Infectious Diseases, University of Oklahoma Health Sciences Center, Oklahoma City, OK 73190

NANCY G. WARREN
Laboratory Corporation of America, 1447 York Court, Burlington, NC 27215

JOHN A. WASHINGTON
Section of Microbiology, The Cleveland Clinic Foundation, Cleveland, OH 44195

RAINER WEBER
Division of Infectious Diseases and Hospital Epidemiology, Department of Internal Medicine, University Hospital, CH-8091 Zurich, Switzerland

DAVID F. WELCH
Laboratory Corporation of America and Department of Pathology, University of Texas Southwestern Medical Center, Dallas, TX 75230

ROBERT C. WELLIVER
Department of Pediatrics, Division of Infectious Diseases, State University of New York, Buffalo, NY 14222-2006

JOY G. WELLS
Foodborne and Diarrheal Diseases Laboratory Section, Foodborne and Diarrheal Diseases Branch, Division of Bacterial and Mycotic Diseases, National Center for Infectious Diseases, Centers for Disease Control and Prevention, Atlanta, GA 30333

ROBBIN S. WEYANT
Meningitis and Special Pathogens Branch, Division of Bacterial and Mycotic Diseases, National Center for Infectious Diseases, Centers for Disease Control and Prevention, Atlanta, GA 30333

R. A. WHILEY
Department of Oral Microbiology, St. Bartholomew's and the Royal London School of Medicine and Dentistry, London, England

THEODORE WHITE
Seattle Biomedical Research Institute, Seattle, WA 98109-1651

SUSAN WHITTIER
Clinical Microbiology Service, Columbia Presbyterian Medical Center, New York, NY 10032-3784

ANDREAS F. WIDMER
Division of Clinical Epidemiology, University Hospitals, Basel, Switzerland

JUDITH C. WILBER
Chiron Corporation, 4560 Horton Street, Emeryville, CA 94608, and Laboratory Medicine, University of California, San Francisco, San Francisco, CA 94143

MARIANNA WILSON
Biology and Diagnostics Branch, Division of Parasitic Diseases, National Center for Infectious Diseases, Centers for Disease Control and Prevention, Atlanta, GA 30341

WASHINGTON C. WINN, JR.
Department of Pathology and Laboratory Medicine, University of Vermont College of Medicine, Fletcher Allen Health Care, Burlington, VT 05401

JANE D. WONG
Microbial Diseases Laboratory, State of California Department of Health Services, 2151 Berkeley Way, Berkeley, CA 94704

GAIL L. WOODS
Department of Pathology, University of Texas Medical Branch, Galveston, TX 77555-0740

JINHUA XIANG
Division of Infectious Diseases, Department of Internal Medicine, University of Iowa College of Medicine, Iowa City, IA 52242

JOSEPH D. C. YAO
Mayo Clinic—Jacksonville, Jacksonville, FL 32224

ROBERT H. YOLKEN
Department of Pediatrics, Stanley Division of Developmental Neurovirology, Johns Hopkins University, Baltimore, MD 21205-2180

MARIALUISA ZERBINI
Department of Clinical Experimental Medicine, Division of Microbiology, University of Bologna, 40138 Bologna, Italy

THEDI ZIEGLER
Department of Medical Microbiology, University of Oulu, Kajaanintie 46E, FIN-90220 Oulu, Finland

Acknowledgment of Previous Contributors

The *Manual of Clinical Microbiology* is by its nature a continuously revised work which refines and extends the contributions of authors of previous editions. Since its first edition in 1970, more than 500 authors have contributed to this important reference work. The American Society for Microbiology and its Publications Board would like to acknowledge the contributions of all of these authors over the life of this Manual.

Preface

Five years ago we were asked to assume responsibility for the sixth edition of the *Manual of Clinical Microbiology*. Despite our reservations and anxieties, we accepted this challenge and were pleased with the final product. We had endeavored to produce a reference book that could serve clinical microbiologists, infectious disease specialists, medical technologists, pathologists, clinicians, teachers, and their students. Obviously, there are both hits and misses with any project of this magnitude, but most of the shortcomings were the result of our decisions rather than the mistakes of our editors or authors. For that we were thankful but also realized that our challenge for the seventh edition was to continue the process of producing the most useful reference text in the area of clinical microbiology. To achieve that goal, we have made many small changes and two major changes. In an effort to make this Manual more relevant to the non-U.S. readership, we have enlisted the talents of foreign editors and authors. We believe that their perspective has enhanced this edition. We have also reorganized the Manual by consolidating the laboratory management, infection control, and diagnostic technology sections; added a series of algorithm chapters to fuse a bridge between specimen processing and organism identification; and reintroduced the Reagent, Stains, and Media section. The goal of this reorganization is to make the Manual more "user-friendly," which we hope has been accomplished.

These changes placed enormous demands on the scientific skills, patience, and persistence of our editors. We thank them for their success in accomplishing their daunting assignments. The success of a multiauthored textbook also requires that each chapter conform to a rigid format. To ensure the uniform presentation of chapters, authors must sacrifice their individual styles and accept the demands of the editorial board. For their willingness to accept these restrictions and for their tremendous work in preparing the individual chapters, we thank our authors. Finally, we would be remiss if we neglected the staff at ASM. They have made every step of producing the seventh edition of the Manual move seamlessly. Special thanks should be extended to Jeff Holtmeier, Director of ASM Press, and Susan Birch, Production Manager and miracle worker. Without their efforts, this Manual would never be published.

We hope the readership will share our belief that the *Manual of Clinical Microbiology* remains a useful resource. Please let us know if we have satisfied your expectations.

PATRICK R. MURRAY
ELLEN JO BARON
MICHAEL A. PFALLER
FRED C. TENOVER
ROBERT H. YOLKEN

GENERAL ISSUES IN CLINICAL MICROBIOLOGY

I

VOLUME EDITOR
PATRICK R. MURRAY

SECTION EDITOR
BETTY ANN FORBES

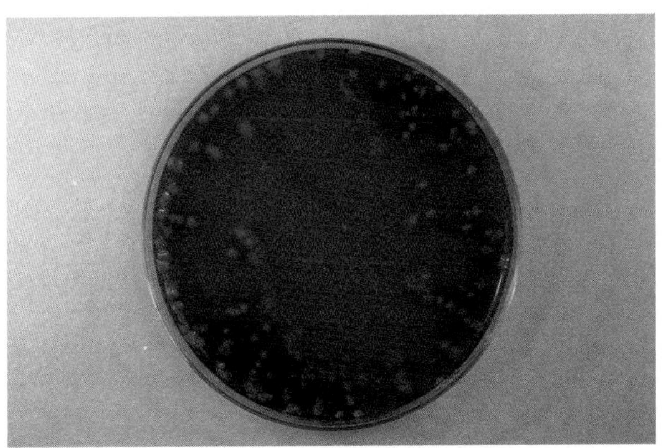

Urine cultured on blood agar with *Esherichia coli* inhibited by antibiotics in the specimen.

Introduction to the Seventh Edition of the *Manual of Clinical Microbiology*

PATRICK R. MURRAY

1

In 1970, the first edition of the *Manual of Clinical Microbiology* (MCM) was published by the American Society for Microbiology. Nineteen editors and 98 authors presented, in 77 chapters and 727 pages of text, a state-of-the-art description of clinical microbiology. In 1995, 20 editors and 205 authors were responsible for MCM6. The Manual had expanded to 123 chapters and 1,482 pages of text. During that 25-year period, new organisms and diseases were discovered; old organisms were subdivided, named, and renamed; testing methods such as enzyme immunoassays, gene amplification, and computerized identification and antimicrobial susceptibility testing were discovered and integrated into routine diagnostics; and the economics of the health care industry were radically changed. The evolution of clinical microbiology has continued. In MCM7, the five volume editors have remained, but 6 of the 15 section editors are new. Likewise, many of the more than 200 authors prepared chapters for the Manual for the first time. The Manual has now expanded to 130 chapters and 1,773 pages of text. Despite the many changes in clinical microbiology, the fundamental philosophy of the Manual has remained the same. As stated in the introduction to the sixth edition, the Manual "is intended to guide clinical microbiologists in the selection, performance, and interpretation of laboratory procedures for diagnostic and therapeutic applications. It is a reference source defining not only what is done in clinical microbiology laboratories but also what these activities signify."

As would be expected, changes have been introduced into this edition. New editors and authors were selected to ensure a fresh infusion of knowledge and perspective. It was particularly important to select editors and authors without regard to geographic boundaries because the audience of the Manual is international. MCM7 was also reorganized in subtle ways to make it more useful for the readership.

MCM7 is organized in nine sections. General issues in clinical microbiology, infection control principles, and diagnostic methods are presented in 13 chapters in the first three sections. This is a reduction from four sections with 19 chapters in the sixth edition. Additionally, four chapters on specimen processing were reorganized into a single chapter in the current edition. The "organism" sections (sections IV to VII) were reorganized, with some chapters consolidated and others expanded into additional chapters. However, the most significant change in these sections was the inclusion of nine "algorithm" chapters (chapters 15, 20, 26, 45, 49, 55, 62, 94, and 104). These chapters are designed to guide clinical microbiologists from preliminary information about an organism (e.g., microscopic or macroscopic appearance, preliminary biochemical test results) to definitive test procedures (e.g., phenotypic tests, molecular diagnostic tests, immunological tests). Section VIII, with 13 chapters, is a comprehensive summary of susceptibility tests and antimicrobial agents for bacterial, mycobacterial, viral, fungal, and parasitic infections. New features in this section include the discussion of new therapeutic agents, testing methods, and the use of computerized expert systems to verify the test results. Finally, in section IX the Manual has reintroduced chapters for reagents, stains, and media. Although this section was eliminated from the sixth edition because the editors felt that this information was available in other reference texts, many microbiologists thought that this was a serious omission. This material has been reorganized in the seventh edition in a manner that should be unique and useful for the day-to-day practice of clinical microbiology.

With the many changes in editors, authors, subject matter, and presentation, we believe that we have maintained the tradition of MCM and improved from the foundation of the last six editions. We hope that the readership will find this text useful, accurate, and timely.

Laboratory Management*

DAVID L. SEWELL AND JAMES D. MacLOWRY

2

The rapidity and extent of change that has occurred in the health care delivery system in the United States and elsewhere in the last decade have been nothing short of remarkable. For better or worse, microbiology laboratories are part of this change. It is now imperative that laboratory directors obtain the management skills necessary to participate and survive in this new and changing environment. If they don't someone else will usurp their responsibilities.

This chapter is an attempt to expose the reader to the various management concepts and techniques being used today and more importantly to stimulate the reader to pursue additional information in this area. The chapter is presented in six parts: (i) basic management concepts, (ii) determination and management of laboratory costs, (iii) analysis of laboratory activities, (iv) quality assessment and control, (v) issues affecting laboratory management, and (vi) regulatory issues affecting the microbiology laboratory.

The section on management concepts provides an overview of the elements of management such as human resources, the planning and implementation of goals, and the control and improvement of the laboratory process. Facets of managing laboratory costs are reviewed in the second section through a discussion of budgeting, cost accounting, determination of direct and indirect costs, and pricing strategies. The third section outlines approaches to cost containment in the microbiology laboratory. These approaches vary from changing the operation of the laboratory to managing test utilization and include specific suggestions for reducing test costs. The final three sections deal with laboratory regulatory issues, basic quality assessment and control concepts, and other more global issues such as health care practices and workforce changes that are affecting microbiology laboratories.

Our intent is not to provide an exhaustive review of all aspects of laboratory management but rather to provoke a discussion of the issues and problems facing the microbiology laboratory today. The laboratory cannot stand alone but must be an active, integrated participant in today's health care delivery system. The key terms and acronyms used in this chapter are presented in Table 1.

* This chapter contains information presented in chapter 5 by David L. Sewell and Ron B. Schifman and chapter 6 by John E. McGowan, Jr., and James D. MacLowry in the sixth edition of this Manual.

BASIC MANAGEMENT CONCEPTS

Management Functions

Management is the act, manner, or practice of managing, supervising, or controlling. The science of management in the United States began in the late 1800s and has evolved dramatically over the years, with increased recognition of the importance of the employees for the achievement of the organization's goals and missions.

Traditional management principles espouse a classic pyramid form of management, with the top management personnel managing the "supervisors" who in turn manage the employees producing the product. Communication in the form of directives from top to bottom is one way. Management believes that quality control inspectors ensure quality, that the management process can be optimized by experts, that employees are a commodity which is motivated by fear and reward, and that profits are made by keeping revenues high and costs low (54).

Juran and Deming introduced a system of management based on the quality of the product. The Juran system (28, 29) is based on quality planning (determining the needs of the customer), quality control (evaluating actual product performance), and quality improvement (identifying problems and the solutions). Deming, as described by DeAguayo (15), believed that quality is determined and controlled by the employees, that the manufacturing process can always be improved, that employees are not motivated by fear and rewards (such motivation actually destroys teamwork and cooperation), and that profits are generated by loyal customers. These management concepts form the basic philosophy found in many organizations today.

Coupled with this evolution of management theory is the transition from an industrial economy to a highly competitive service economy in which the organization or producer must meet the customer's expectations with regard to the product as well as other needs. In the service industry, which includes the laboratory, the classic pyramid structure is inverted (Fig. 1). Because client services and the employees who produce the product often interact directly with the customer, they are critical elements in this management structure and give input to the director. The customer's needs are or should be the driving force in this arrangement. In the 1990s, the U.S. health care industry has struggled to

TABLE 1 Key terms and acronyms

ABN: Advanced beneficiary notice
A 1998 HCFA initiative which requires that patients be notified in writing that a test will not be reimbursed by HCFA and that the patient agrees to be billed directly for the test.
CAP: College of American Pathologists
CLIA 88: Clinical Laboratory Improvement Amendments 1988
Applies to laboratories licensed for interstate commerce and/or certified to receive reimbursement from Medicare and Medicaid.
CQI: Continuous quality improvement
A proactive managerial concept that promotes ongoing QI and customer satisfaction. Resolves identified problems and seeks improvement where no problems exist.
DHHS: U.S. Department of Health and Human Services
DRG: Diagnosis-related groups
System of reimbursement for inpatient health care costs.
FDA: U.S. Food and Drug Administration
FTE: Full-time equivalent
Employee who works at least 40 hours per week.
Gatekeeper:
A health care provider who assesses the need for complex testing and provides the least expensive method to diagnose a patient's condition.
HCFA: Health Care Financing Administration
JCAHO: Joint Commission on Accreditation of Healthcare Organizations
OIG: Office of the Inspector General
OSHA: Occupational Safety and Health Administration
PPM: Provider-performed microscopy
Microscopic tests (e.g., wet mounts and KOH), defined by HCFA, that can be performed by physician and nonphysician personnel and that are not subject to routine biennial inspection.
QA: Quality assurance
A planned and systematic process for evaluating and monitoring the quality and appropriateness of patient care, focusing on problem finding.
QC: Quality control
A system for detecting and correcting analytical errors by establishing performance limits.
QI: Quality improvement
A system for identifying processes that can be used to improve performance and customer satisfaction.
TQM: Total quality management
A system of managerial programs (team, plans, and improvement management) that provide the processes by which CQI can be implemented and maintained.
Waived tests
Tests that use simple and accurate methodologies, that pose no reasonable risk of harm if performed incorrectly, or that are approved for home use. Laboratories performing waived tests are not inspected routinely, nor are they required to meet certain other CLIA 88 requirements.

meet its customers' demand for high-quality products and service at a reduced cost.

What is the role of management in this process? Simply stated, management attempts to coordinate the actions of the employees to accomplish the goals and mission of the organization. Whether the organization is a for-profit or a not-for-profit medical center or a microbiology laboratory, the management team is responsible for the operation of the unit which includes human resources management, planning and implementation of goals and priorities, and control and improvement of the overall process. Although the attempt is made to manage laboratories by business techniques used in the non-health-care environments, management of laboratories is often more complicated. The laboratory not only produces, interprets, and reports test results to its customers but in many situations it also provides research and teaching services. In addition, the laboratory is responsible for meeting the needs of the patients and the medical staff, as well as the goals, objectives, and missions of the hospital or medical center and the corporate organization. In this process, the laboratory becomes an integral part of patient care.

Hardwick and Morrison (23) described the basic elements of management as ideas, things, and people. The tasks associated with these elements are listed in Table 2. To accomplish these tasks, the laboratory manager must be (i) a visionary and strategist, recognizing opportunities for growth and progress; (ii) a teacher, guiding others to identify and solve problems; (iii) a leader, providing a clear course of action and inspiring the employees' commitment to the objectives of the laboratory and the larger organization; and (iv) a problem solver (1).

Human Resources Management

Today, most laboratory managers recognize that employees are the key element in the success or failure of an organization. To effectively understand human behavior and manage people, managers need to understand and incorporate the following elements into their managerial skills: (i) motivation, (ii) perception (how a person reacts to a stimulus), (iii) communication, (iv) leadership versus managership, (v) group dynamics, and (vi) morale (55). The management of people relies on motivation and listening, delegation, and supervision.

Appropriate motivation encourages employees to work at a high level of performance and stimulates creativity. Systems that judge, punish, or reward above- or below-average performance do not motivate over the long term, especially in laboratories staffed with highly trained personnel. Persuasion and the use of professional guidelines achieve far better results in this environment. Generally, people are motivated by leaders who understand and appreciate the diversity of people's talents and skills and who allow people to do what is required of them (16). A motivational leader possesses the following attributes:

Has integrity and fairness
Promotes heterogeneity and diversity
Finds competence, skills, and talents in others
Is open to contrary opinions
Communicates easily at all levels
Leads through serving
Understands the organization and its mission
Is visionary and able to see the broad picture
Is a spokesperson and diplomat
Can present the organization's culture
Tells why rather than how

The good manager is also able to delegate tasks and responsibilities at the level where they can best be accomplished. Supervision ensures that the organizational goals are met and that policies are followed. Leadership in the health care arena is often more difficult than leadership in other businesses because managers must interact with

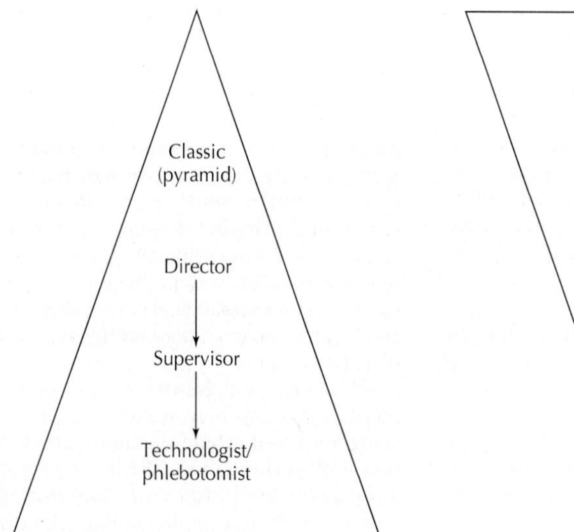

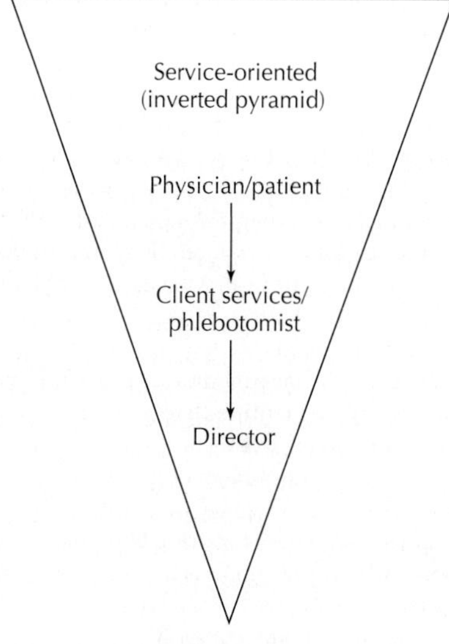

FIGURE 1 Information transfer in classic versus service-oriented management structures in the clinical laboratory. Adapted from Fig. 1.8 of Travers and McClatchey (54).

independent, autonomous, and highly skilled health care practitioners.

Planning and Implementation

In today's rapidly changing health care environment, management must accept change as an integral part of its function and prepare plans to accommodate change. These plans may include (i) the business plan (which details the laboratory's mission, goals, and objectives), (ii) the marketing plan (which describes customers, test products, and services), (iii) the operation plan (which describes facilities, equipment, capacity, etc.), (iv) the staffing plan (which describes workload and staffing requirements), and (v) the financial plan (which describes needs for capital, financial resources, budget, and reimbursement structure) (56).

Juran (28) described the planning process as follows:

Identify the customers (patients, physician, third-party payer) and their needs

Develop a product that meets the needs of the customer and the laboratory

Develop and optimize the process to produce the product (procedures and work flow)

Transfer the process to the operating personnel (training and implementation)

Establish a measurement system (evaluate the process)

The budget is a critical element of the laboratory's planning process as a consequence of the laboratory's shift from a revenue-generating center to a cost center within the organization. It is imperative that laboratory managers inform their customers and other managers within the organization of the value of the new procedures and technologies, provide the data to substantiate the fiscal soundness of the laboratory's plan, and negotiate an adequate budget to secure the necessary personnel, equipment, and supplies to meet its goals and the needs of its customers. This is often a difficult, if not impossible, task because of the inadequate cost-accounting methods used by most health care organizations.

Control

After the plan is implemented, management must monitor or evaluate the overall process and product performance,

TABLE 2 Tasks associated with management[a]

	Management		
Elements	Ideas	Things	People
Tasks	Conceptual thinking	Administration	Leadership
Functions	Analyze problems Gather facts, ascertain causes, develop alternatives	Make decisions Establish conclusions	Communicate Ensure understanding
Activities	Set objectives Define performance standards Develop strategies Prepare budgets	Study work flow and tasks Establish organizational structure Select and schedule staff	Monitor performance against standards
Action items	Plan	Organize and staff	Direct; control

[a] Adapted from Fig. 1.1 of Hardwick and Morrison (23).

compare the results to the initial goals and expectations, and explore possible alternatives. This generally means analyzing the preanalytic phase (prior to testing a specimen), the analytic phase (test procedure performed in the laboratory), and the postanalytic phase (after the test results leave the laboratory) of the test or product for problems. For the preanalytic phase, the laboratory provides the customer (e.g., the health care provider) with information about specimen collection and transportation, interpretation of results, and test utilization. Producing quality test results during the analytic phase is dependent upon employment of qualified staff, use of written procedures, and availability of adequate resources such as space, supplies, and equipment. To ensure the accuracy of the test results, all methods are verified and appropriate controls are used during the analysis of the patient's specimen. During the postanalytic phase, management reviews the accuracy of the released result and its interpretation, its integration into the patient's record, and if appropriate, the clinical relevance of the test. If the review of these processes reveals problems affecting patient care or inefficiencies, a quality assurance (QA) plan can be instituted. The QA plan should define the problem, propose changes to correct the problem, and monitor the correction process. The goal of the QA process should be a quick resolution of the problem.

Improvement

Quality improvement (QI) is a management tool used to define the customer's expectations, to describe and evaluate the processes used to provide service, and to continuously improve these processes and outcomes (31). QI should focus on the customer's needs rather than process problems and should rely on training and prevention to improve service. The laboratory's customers include the patient, the health care provider, the third-party payers, and other individuals or organizations who interact with the laboratory (61). After identifying the customer's needs and expectations, management describes the process that serves the customer, gathers data on how the process works, identifies areas for improvement based upon the customer's expectations, and implements solutions. Because the customer's and organization's needs change, the laboratory must continuously monitor and improve this process.

DETERMINATION AND MANAGEMENT OF LABORATORY COSTS

Budget

The budget statement for the laboratory or a section of laboratory can be viewed as the primary document which summarizes the fiscal management of the laboratory. The budget can be a very deceptive document in that it can create rigid guidelines for the activities of the laboratory or can be used in a more general way with the expectation that only certain predetermined goals be reached each fiscal year. Aspects of the budget which may be critical to the laboratory have to do with who creates the document, who controls the elements therein, how the ongoing process is monitored, who is actually responsible for meeting the goals of the document, how the budget is integrated into the whole organization's budget, if at all, and how the budget is viewed by the organization as a whole. A few features of the budgetary process and the integration of cost-accounting and pricing strategies for the department will be discussed in more detail. This will not be an exhaustive discussion on cost-accounting methods but rather an attempt to point out certain pitfalls that are obvious to individuals who have worked extensively with this process and that may not be quite so obvious to someone who is new to the budget process.

For many laboratories the budgeting process and final document may be imposed by individuals who are outside of the activities of the laboratory but who may have organizational responsibility to "administer the lab." One previously acceptable but now counterproductive consequence of this administrative budgetary oversight rewarded the administrator by increasing the gross revenues assigned to a particular activity. This philosophy rewarded unnecessary utilization of laboratory activities in the past but now may produce unrealistic pricing strategies which have to be corrected by deep discounts if the laboratory is to be competitive in the market. Another frequently used strategy is "reduction of costs" by making across-the-board decreases in the fiscal resources available to the laboratory. Under these circumstances it is not uncommon that each year a laboratory will be given another cost reduction "goal" that must be reached. Since the majority of laboratory costs are for labor, it becomes obvious that personnel must be reduced, and this often can be done only by reducing the services provided. Another less obvious consequence of budgeting from "on high" is the difficulty in justifying expenditures in the laboratory, which in the long run may be detrimental, from both quality and fiscal standpoints, to the organization as a whole. Many institutions do not recognize the interconnections of activities in different parts of the system. Such recognition is necessary so that costs can be viewed more globally rather than as being related to just one department. For example, it is possible that rearranging scheduling in the laboratory, and perhaps increasing some cost in doing so, provides laboratory results for inpatients earlier in the day and encourages earlier discharges or that, in the outpatient setting, performing more testing on-site at a greater cost permits clinicians to run their practices more efficiently. Point-of-care testing, which is more expensive than centralized testing, may be more efficient in the long run if it is used judiciously and creatively. Although these practices are more costly for the laboratory, they may provide overall savings to the institution.

Control of the budget is critical to efficient laboratory activity because repeated personnel reductions made to meet decreased budgeting goals make it virtually impossible for the laboratory to develop a strategy to integrate their activities with organizational needs and goals. For some organizations, the direct labor costs, the direct reagent costs, and the depreciation or reagent rental expenses associated with the test may be the only concerns in deriving the total direct cost of the test, but this omits significant indirect costs which are often more difficult to identify. These indirect costs, such as space rental, utilities, insurance, and administrative salaries, occur at many organizational levels, including the specific laboratory section, the laboratory, and the institution as a whole. The laboratory rarely has an opportunity to help determine or have input into the institutional indirect costs which may be allocated directly to each test. Many budgets do not include these indirect costs, and they may not need to be included in the budgets, but they are critical when pricing strategies are used to determine competitive fees.

Superficially, it would appear that revenues could be easily defined, but in fact, for many institutions they are not. Depending on the part of the country being considered and the number of Medicare and Medicaid patients being treated, many inpatients are covered under a Diagnosis-Related Group (DRG) global payment for their hospitalization. These payments are not broken down into each of the services provided, and it is difficult to be certain of the revenue generated by the laboratory unless the institution arbitrarily allocates some percentage of the total DRG payments as revenue to the laboratory. Other managed care payers may have more complex allocations of money for laboratory activities for inpatients, and the institution may or may not make the effort to allocate those revenues back to the laboratories. It is often easier for the institution to first determine globally what the history of payment is for certain health care providers. This percentage of collection of the gross revenues is assigned back to the laboratory, and that constitutes the net revenue from that payer. This net revenue is then compared with the laboratory cost to determine whether or not there is a profit, if it is a for-profit institution, or a revenue margin, if it is a not-for-profit institution. These allocations back to the laboratory may have little to do with the revenues designated for laboratory activities by a particular payer. One consequence of this inadequacy of fiscal management is that the laboratory never really knows whether it is doing well or poorly in terms of compensation. If the institution has an expected target for a revenue margin, the laboratory may be viewed negatively when, in fact, the revenues may have been much greater than allocated, or vice versa.

Continued efforts at decreasing costs usually mean decreasing labor costs. Generally, most laboratory directors object to decreasing their labor costs because they feel that the productivity of their personnel is appropriate or the most that can be obtained from the system and that the quality of the work is satisfactory. However, each organization can benefit considerably from looking critically at those things which it does and the ways in which they are done. Microbiology has for many years been relatively unrestricted in terms of the tests which it has offered to clinicians. In the fee-for-service arena, microbiology was rewarded for doing more rather than less work. Readjusting the workload, such that clinically relevant testing is encouraged and nonrelevant testing is either discouraged or not done, can reduce labor costs with no sacrifice of quality. One could argue that the quality of patient care may increase as the clinicians are presented with fewer data and more clinically appropriate information.

It is difficult to document whether test quality is affected by altering the skill mix of the laboratory personnel. The interest in developing more appropriate skill mixes has to do with trying to match individuals' experience and educational background with the tasks which they are performing. This is a laudable goal, but there is a line which can easily be overstepped. Evaluation of the accuracy of test results is extremely difficult and relies very heavily on proficiency testing, which many have argued may not be the most reliable way of gauging accuracy.

Another area which may suffer from reductions in numbers of personnel and which may be more quantitative than qualitative has to do with the availability of services. This includes both the menu of tests offered by a given laboratory and the turnaround times which can be provided by a laboratory. The need to reduce labor costs often translates quickly into reducing hours of service. When that happens, the unavailability of service to the clinicians can have patient care consequences, although they are usually difficult to document. Another area germane to the cutting of labor costs is deciding whether or not one should either perform the test in-house or send it out. These so-called make-buy decisions are actually very critical to most laboratories' functions and are probably underused. As will be discussed shortly, many of these decisions are predicated on the test volume coming to the laboratory, and the whole issue of laboratory consolidation, particularly in microbiology, will be addressed.

Cost Accounting

Cost-accounting systems make it possible to respond to budgetary needs, and there are a variety of options available to a laboratory director. There are the more traditional cost-accounting systems, which look rather globally at the costs incurred for a whole section and determine the cost per test by averaging the cost versus the productive results in determining a unit cost. In these systems it is difficult to account for a number of nontesting activities such as continuing education, proficiency testing, teaching, and administrative activities such as updating of manuals. Other more focused cost-accounting methods, such as activity-based cost accounting, can help one determine the cost involved with each activity of the laboratory, but this type of a system comes at a high price in terms of the amount of data which must be collected, stored, and manipulated in order to produce good decisions. Each institution needs to determine its specific needs, how best they can be served, and whether complex cost-accounting methods are worth it either fiscally or intellectually. There are different approaches to obtaining the information which should be kept for each laboratory activity and also how those activities are defined, but it is not the purpose of this discussion to go into great detail about those approaches. A concise, laboratory-oriented guideline for cost accounting is available and should be part of each laboratory's library (43).

Laboratory Costs

In discussions of direct costs, the decision as to what constitutes the direct cost must be made. It does not make too much difference exactly how one laboratory defines its direct costs and indirect costs, but it is essential that the particular components are accounted for and that they not be ignored. Generally, for direct costs, the cost of labor including benefits, supplies and reagents, and also some allocation for instrument depreciation, maintenance, rental, or lease costs would be considered part of the direct cost because they can be referred back directly to testing activities. If one is involved in a reagent rental or a lease program, a specific termination clause should be included in the contract so that the contract can be canceled on short notice either to upgrade to another instrument or to change the configuration of testing. Some contracts do not allow this flexibility, and the institution may suffer because of monies being committed unnecessarily to a specific instrument.

The indirect cost will generally include all other expenses necessary to do business and are generally not directly related to a specific instrument or test. In this category there can be a number of sources for indirect costs that can come from the section where the test is being done, from the laboratory itself, or from the institution as a whole. Usually, these indirect costs are difficult to obtain and document or are part of an institutional formula which assigns some fraction of the direct cost as an indirect cost. These assignments may or may not be based on a reality that is appropriate for the laboratory.

Across-the-board cutting of labor costs is not useful for cost control. The analysis of these different components requires a certain amount of experience and creative thoughtfulness as to how specific costs can be controlled or decreased. For example, significant reductions in labor costs can be achieved by readjusting the skill levels required for different processes. In this way personnel can be utilized much more effectively rather than insisting that all testing in all parts of the laboratory be performed by a medical technologist. On the other hand, labor expense such as overtime is sometimes ignored because it is considered part of the incentive for working in a particular area. Under such circumstances, it is absolutely essential that one look at the possibility of creatively revising schedules, having staff arrive earlier or later, or including as part of a 5-day work week either Saturdays or Sundays in order to decrease overtime. Some administrators are concerned about adding more personnel and would rather pay much more expensive overtime than add another full-time equivalent (FTE) or part of an FTE. Other institutions use compensatory time as a way to reduce overtime costs, but unless it is used sparingly, it can be a self-defeating maneuver. Positions must be covered, and therefore, there will have to be an expense for covering that compensatory time. Some institutions may use part-time personnel at levels of part time such that they are not required to pay for benefits or they pay for reduced levels of benefits. It is hard to know whether or not this is an appropriate solution. It should be noted that the more part-time people used, the more need there is for increased training. Also, the use of temporary personnel gives the laboratory administration flexibility if there is the potential for laboratory consolidation moves in the future. If bargaining units are involved, there would be an opportunity for less severance pay. It should be noted that these attempts at reducing labor costs are often associated with increasing turnover of personnel and probably personnel with lower levels of expertise in some of the areas that are more difficult to staff, such as mycology, mycobacteriology, and virology.

Pricing Strategies

A brief comment about pricing strategies is relevant. In the present environment with DRG-related compensation, some laboratories have tended to feel that there is less of a need to be concerned with the fee schedules that they develop. This may be a myopic view of reality in that laboratories are trying harder to develop more outpatient activities, and at least for the present time and perhaps for the near future, those visits will not be covered by outpatient DRGs, although this has been talked about for some time. Therefore, the fee schedules for laboratory testing must accomplish at least two things. First, they must be well based in the cost reality of the laboratory, and second, they must be competitive in the marketplace. Some laboratories have felt that because they have done some client's business for a long time, they are immune to the possibility of losing that business. This assumption has been proven again and again to be wrong, in that loyalty in the marketplace is in very short supply at the present time. Therefore, each laboratory must be cognizant of its place in the competitive market. Others have suggested that searching for the lowest cost would mean that quality would be sacrificed, but painfully little information is available to document this. The large reference laboratories have resources that permit the development of sophisticated quality control systems. Even though many reference laboratories have gone through episodes of embarrassment related to inappropriate billing, resulting in staggering fines by the federal government and probably by private insurers as time goes on, it does not necessarily follow that the quality of their work is less than that of the local community hospital. One general observation which would seem to be obvious is that it does not make sense to price laboratory tests below the prices on established fee schedules. Laboratories are not philanthropies. Also, laboratory personnel are well advised to be cognizant of the way in which the fiscal services department in their organization may be attempting to or in fact are applying fees to their tests. It has happened in many cases that specific formulae are used to develop fees which have priced the laboratory out of the marketplace, but the laboratory may have been unaware that this particular practice had occurred. It is therefore necessary to work constantly with fiscal services to make sure that both are working together. It must be realized that fiscal services are often under great pressure to at least try to increase the gross revenues to an organization, and this is sometimes done in counterproductive ways.

ANALYSIS OF LABORATORY ACTIVITIES

Management Techniques

The primary goal of the clinical microbiology laboratory is to provide accurate diagnostic testing and high-quality service at the lowest cost for its customers. Achieving this goal requires a detailed analysis of the laboratory's processes and products. Management must, as a first step, critically define the laboratory's goals. These goals may include reduction of reagent and labor costs, reduction of length of stay for patients, improvement of productivity, improvement of turnaround times for tests, improvement of the quality of specimens submitted, and improvement of the clinical relevance of test results. It is easier to achieve a goal that is clearly and concisely defined.

After the laboratory's goals have been defined, the method or approach to changing the laboratory's operations must be decided. There are four broad approaches to change: (i) reengineering, (ii) downsizing or reorganizing, (iii) process improvement, and (iv) systems analysis (7, 30, 38, 57). The method or methods used are dictated, to some extent, by the degree and rapidity of change deemed necessary by the organization.

Reengineering is a concept that promotes a radical rethinking and redesign of the systems and processes used to produce, deliver, and support patient care. In other words, reengineering means "starting over" and developing an entirely new system, not incrementally changing the current organization. The employees must be involved in the process, and results are expected within 1 to 4 years. Generally, reengineering involves the entire laboratory (optimally, the entire organization) and critically rethinks how health care is produced and delivered. Automation, point-of-care testing, computerization, and elimination of traditional laboratory sections are all part of the process.

Downsizing or reorganizing is often considered a part of reengineering, but the approaches to achieving each one are quite different. While reengineering seeks to improve the overall quality of services, downsizing and reorganizing are usually focused on reducing costs, primarily by laying off employees. The goal of management is a quick reduction of costs, and at times this is done without a critical evaluation of the impact on the quality of services produced. It is hoped that this approach is reserved only for the management of crisis situations.

Process improvement (total quality management [TQM] or continuous quality improvement [CQI]) is now a regulatory and accreditation mandate by the Joint Commission on Accreditation of Healthcare Organizations (JCAHO) and the College of American Pathologists (CAP). It is a systematic, objective approach to improving patient care and uses a bottom-up or team approach to achieve improvement in services. The approach focuses on resource use, employee education to reduce errors and minimize delays, adaptation to customer's needs, and efficient use of employees to improve customer satisfaction and reduce costs. Because process improvement examines the performance of processes (not the performance of people) to increase customer satisfaction, it often involves multidisciplinary teams and is a continuous, ongoing exercise. CQI focuses on outcome measurements that affect patient care and seeks to incrementally change the process in order to improve outcome and reduce costs. The analysis phase identifies the customers, the resources, the inputs and outputs of each laboratory activity, how activities are interrelated, and whether the activity improves customer satisfaction and outcome. The process improvement change is introduced and the process is monitored to determine whether the change produced the desired result. Thus, CQI involves continuous cycles of improvement which are built into the daily activities of the laboratory and organization. The length of time required to affect change by this method is a problem in the rapidly changing health care industry today.

The systems analysis approach focuses on improving the productivity and efficiency of the organization and reducing costs by analyzing the four basic elements of a laboratory's operation: (i) equipment and technology, (ii) human resources, (iii) reagents and supplies, and (iv) space (57). Laboratory work flow is composed of these four interrelated elements and can be analyzed by breaking the process into three components: (i) preanalytic (prelaboratory) phase, (ii) analytic (laboratory) phase, and (iii) postanalytic (postlaboratory) phase (57, 67).

The prelaboratory or preanalytic phase includes all processes prior to testing of the specimen in the laboratory. The productivity and efficiency of this aspect of laboratory operations can be improved by developing criteria for test selection and utilization through consultation with the involved health care providers (critical pathways); optimization of the collection, transport, and storage of specimens; definition of specimen acceptability; and definition of the tests that are offered. Strategies for controlling test utilization are the most effective means of controlling inappropriate test requests.

The laboratory or analytic phase is generally focused on reducing turnaround time (TAT) and test costs. Batch processing may negatively affect patient care by causing delays, and better service is obtained with continuous processing. However, this may not be cost-effective. Newer state-of-the-art equipment and technology must be evaluated as to whether it will reduce laboratory reagent and labor costs, reduce TAT, and significantly improve patient care (i.e., whether it will reduce the length of stay and improve test sensitivity and specificity and whether it is clinically relevant). Some questions that must be addressed prior to purchase or implementation include the cost per test, space and staffing requirements, maintenance, and customer needs. Also, the microbiology tests to be performed (i.e., organism workup, identification, and antimicrobial susceptibility testing) need to be defined for the specimen type and body site to improve the medical relevance of the information produced (67).

The postlaboratory or postanalytic phase involves the review and reporting of test results. Efficiencies in TAT and ease of access are accomplished with computerized reporting in which abnormal results are highlighted and an interpretation of the results may be provided. Feedback to ordering physicians or other health care providers on the cost of their overall laboratory utilization may help reduce excessive or inappropriate test requests.

Because labor accounts for 60 to 80% of all direct laboratory costs, increased attention is being focused on improving employee productivity. In general productivity is most influenced by the work methods and processes, the position description, the facilities layout, personnel scheduling, and material flows (58). Productivity can be improved by increasing the number of tests performed per individual, decreasing the effort necessary to produce the test, and increasing the quality of the test or service with the same effort. Often, productivity improvement is achieved by simply reducing the number of staff. However, other methods, such as changing the staffing mix, consolidating supervisory positions, scheduling more efficiently, eliminating unnecessary and labor-intensive tests, prioritizing or consolidating testing, removing overlapping functions, and providing employee incentives, are available to increase productivity.

Test Utilization Management

In this era of reduced reimbursement for health care services of all types, the laboratory should attempt to manage test utilization to improve patient care practices through the appropriate use of laboratory testing, to improve laboratory efficiency, and to reduce both laboratory and other patient care costs (46, 59, 60, 63). One means of controlling test utilization is the establishment of a "gatekeeper," who in the larger organization is usually the patient's primary care physician. However, as part of its function the gatekeeper should ensure participation of the laboratory to ensure the use of the least expensive and most clinically relevant test necessary to appropriately manage the patient. In some instances, the laboratory's gatekeeping function becomes adversarial, with the laboratory denying a test request and the clinician demanding that the test be performed. A preferred approach is the development of a consensus between the medical staff and the laboratory as to the appropriate clinical practice guidelines that should commonly be followed on the basis of the severity and acuteness of the disease process. It is important to remember that the education involved in this process must be bidirectional. The laboratory must comprehend the needs of the medical staff, and the medical staff in turn must understand the laboratory's need to reduce costs without decreasing the quality of testing. This process requires commitment by both groups and is only beginning to be adopted by organizations.

An often tried but difficult to achieve method of cost reduction is modifying the test ordering pattern of health care providers. Patterns vary with the clinician's age, fiscal incentives, experience, site of training, degree of risk aversion (fear of malpractice claims), and type of organization (14). It is generally believed that most physicians will change their test ordering patterns when they are provided with information on practice patterns and patient outcomes, but this information is not available in most organizations. The most effective approaches to modifying test utilization are (i) clinical and financial feedback, (ii) education by local experts, and (iii) rationing of care and testing (59, 63). The clinical and financial feedback method informs the physician of his or her test utilization pattern compared to the patterns of his or her peers, the cost of that testing, and the reimbursement received by the hospital. The education approach involves lectures, discussions, written material (e.g., clinical pathways and guidelines or standard protocols), and interpretive laboratory reporting that provides clinically useful information and that addresses the clinical relevance of a particular test. To be effective, the education must be continuous and must originate from clinical opinion leaders in the organization or community. Lastly, for the rationing of patient care or testing to be successful, it must be physician directed and consensus among the members of this group must be achieved.

Approaches to Cost Containment in the Clinical Microbiology Laboratory

The following discussion of cost reduction in the clinical microbiology laboratory is not meant to be all inclusive or a mandate for all laboratories. Rather, it is meant to stimulate discussion between clinicians and the clinical microbiologist for the implementation of cost-effective, clinically relevant policies. Cost-containment policies will not be identical for all laboratories because they are affected by the patient mix, the needs of the customers, and the form of reimbursement. McLaughlin (33) has published a 10-point plan for the "implementation of cost-effective, clinically relevant diagnostic microbiology policies" that clearly identifies the process that should be followed. A modified version follows:

1. Base changes on published data and opinions of respected experts.
2. Supplement the changes with in-house data when possible.
3. Secure support for the changes from the infectious diseases service.
4. Discuss in advance the changes with the affected groups or the most influential users in the groups.
5. Educate potential users who will be affected by the changes.
6. Announce the proposed changes by a means that will reach most users.
7. Educate technologists who will implement the changes.
8. Revise laboratory procedure manuals.
9. Provide users with a mechanism to override the changes in special situations.
10. Provide explanations to users who are uninformed or who are opposed to the changes.

All major changes are difficult, are not made and accepted quickly, require a collaborative effort between the laboratory and medical staff, and must have the overall support of the organization's administration (5, 63). It is important to emphasize to the customer that the change will improve the overall quality of patient care and is not only a cost reduction for the laboratory. Areas of operations in the clinical microbiology laboratory that may provide some cost containment or reduction include (i) automation, (ii) alternative technology or methods, (iii) specimen acceptability, (iv) extent of specimen workup and organism identification, and (v) limiting of diagnostic tests for a single diagnosis. Cost reduction from volume aggregation by consolidation or merger of laboratories is discussed elsewhere in this chapter.

Automation

Automation is generally thought to be the process that reduces the laboratory's labor costs. In fact, automation tends to redistribute the workload and minimize future staff increases but may not result in an absolute reduction of staffing (57). The most efficient use of automation occurs when it is interfaced with the laboratory or hospital computer. For automation to be effective, there must be sufficient volume to support its use, the automation must support the pattern of demand and laboratory practice, and in most cases, the automation must replace a traditional test method, not add to the test menu. Although the clinical microbiology laboratory remains highly labor intensive, automated or semiautomated instruments are available for blood cultures, mycobacterial cultures and susceptibility testing, bacterial susceptibility testing and identification, specimen plating, and immunological or serological testing. However, cost economies can be realized only with volume testing.

Alternative Technology or Methods

Traditional methods and procedures should be compared to alternative methods that may provide better diagnostic results, that may be less expensive, and that may provide more specific information. As an example, laboratories might initially test stool specimens submitted for ovum and parasite (O&P) examinations only for *Giardia* and *Cryptosporidium* by an immunoassay. The need for additional testing would be based on the results of the initial test. Also, the laboratory might evaluate the use of a dipstick method (not currently approved by the U.S. Food and Drug Administration) as a replacement for the traditional microscopic diagnosis of malaria (45). Many moderate- to low-volume laboratories have switched to the use of the traditional disk diffusion method for antimicrobial susceptibility testing instead of the use of instrumented systems because of cost savings. Whenever an alternative method is considered, the cost of changing test methods must be assessed in light of the impact on patient care. For example, the use of nucleic acid-based amplification techniques for the diagnosis of tuberculosis may decrease the time to the detection of a positive specimen but will significantly increase the cost for the detection of each new case (18). For laboratories that serve a population with a low prevalence of disease, the increased cost may not be justified.

Specimen Acceptability

The laboratory can improve the quality of test results and reduce costs by accepting only specimens that are properly collected, transported, and labeled and that are appropriate for the laboratory diagnosis of an infectious disease. The following discussion identifies some general areas of specimen processing where modification of traditional procedures can improve the clinical relevance of microbiological test results, reduce costs, and reduce unnecessary work. Specific information is found in the references (21, 51, 66) (see also chapter 4).

Blood Cultures

Significant data exist regarding the appropriate number of blood samples for cultures collected per septic episode, the volume of blood cultured, and the necessity for including an anaerobic blood bottle in the set. As a general rule, no more than two or three blood samples should be submitted for culture per septic episode, with each sample for culture consisting of 20 to 30 ml of blood. Additional samples may need to be cultured for a patient with culture-negative endocarditis or to recover a fastidious microorganism. An anaerobic blood bottle may not be routinely required for each set of specimens, but this should be assessed by each laboratory.

Most bacterial pathogens are recovered from blood cultures within 5 days (67). Bacteremia caused by *Mycobacterium avium* complex can be detected in 85 to 90% of patients with one blood culture, and *M. avium* complex organisms are recovered from nearly 100% of patients with two blood cultures (53, 68). Aerobic blood cultures are adequate for the recovery of most common *Candida* species, but other methods are necessary for the recovery of the filamentous fungi (67). One approach to reducing patient care costs is to decrease the rate of blood culture contamination by use of a dedicated team for blood collections and to track the contamination rate for each team member.

CSF Specimens

Many bacterial antigen tests are marketed because a rapid and accurate diagnosis of bacterial meningitis is essential for the patient's survival. In general, these tests have not proven to be cost-effective and should not be performed. If they are used at all, the tests should be performed only when the cell count in cerebrospinal fluid (CSF) is abnormal and the Gram stain is negative.

Because tuberculous meningitis is rare in the United States, cultures of CSF for *Mycobacterium tuberculosis* should be performed only when the cell count in CSF and the CSF protein and glucose levels are consistent with meningitis (2). In addition, the laboratory should require 7 to 20 ml of CSF to optimize the recovery of *M. tuberculosis*.

Neurosyphilis is also infrequently diagnosed in the United States. Therefore, most Venereal Disease Research Laboratory tests should be performed with CSF only when the patient has documented *Treponema pallidum* infection (e.g., a positive serum rapid plasma reagin or fluorescent treponemal antibody absorption test or a positive dark-field examination of an appropriate lesion) and the patient's CSF has abnormalities consistent with neurosyphilis (3). These screening approaches can significantly decrease the number of inappropriate tests performed for the diagnosis of neurosyphilis and tuberculous meningitis.

Stool Cultures and O&P Examinations

It is now accepted laboratory practice to reject for culture and O&P examination stool specimens collected after the patient has been hospitalized for 3 or 4 days (26). The yield from these specimens is minimal and on the basis of a recent survey, it is estimated that the health care system in the United States could save between $27 million and $73 million per year if this practice was implemented in all laboratories (37). The appropriate number of specimens required to detect pathogens in stool specimens is somewhat more controversial. Valenstein et al. (64) currently recommend the use of one or two specimens for the detection of bacterial pathogens and two or three specimens for the detection of stool parasites in a routine workup. Other recommendations include the use of methods that detect specific parasites such as *Giardia*, *Cryptosporidium*, and *Entamoeba histolytica* in place of the traditional method of concentration and microscopy. If the results of these initial tests are negative, a decision for ordering a complete O&P workup would be determined (26).

For the detection of *Clostridium difficile* disease by a toxin assay, Hines and Nachamkin (26) suggest that testing of two or three specimens obtained over several days is adequate. The second or third specimen would be tested only after the prior specimens are determined to be negative. Almost by definition, testing of formed stool specimens is unacceptable in the management of diarrhea, regardless of whether the etiologic agent sought is a parasite or a bacterium (including *C. difficile*). However, formed stools may be cultured in order to identify individuals who may be carriers.

Respiratory Cultures

Screening of sputum specimens by Gram staining and rejection of specimens on the basis of the relative proportion of leukocytes and squamous epithelial cells is a routine and accepted practice (6, 39). More controversial is the use of a similar approach for the screening of respiratory secretions collected by endotracheal suction. Morris et al. (35) recommended that specimens collected by endotracheal suction should be rejected if more than 10 epithelial cells/low-power field are observed or if no bacteria are seen on the Gram-stained smear. Generally, no more than one sputum specimen should be cultured per 24 to 48 h (67).

Wound, Tissue, and Body Fluid Cultures

The medium inoculated and the length of incubation should be based on the type of specimen submitted and the pathogen(s) sought. Most fungal isolates, with the exception of the dimorphic fungi, are recovered from routine fungal cultures within 14 days (36). The routine use of broth medium for cultures of wound specimens primarily recovers contaminants and does not generally produce clinically useful information (17, 36, 52). However, a broth medium should be inoculated for tissue, CSF from patients with a CSF shunt, and continuous ambulatory peritoneal dialysis fluid specimens (34, 36).

Extent of Specimen Workup and Organism Identification

Should all isolates or only clinically relevant isolates recovered from a specimen be identified and have antimicrobial susceptibilities performed? Clinical microbiologists have struggled when attempting to define the extent of the workup that should be performed with a specimen. Generally, the past approach of a more complete workup of these isolates has contributed to our understanding of the disease process, provided the evidence for the nosocomial spread of organisms within the hospital, and led to the discovery of "new" pathogens and emerging antimicrobial resistance. However, given our current limited resources and cost-containment dictates, the clinician and clinical microbiologist must now determine the clinical importance of the test results produced. Although there are few published data on this topic, a great need exists to achieve a consensus between the laboratory and health care providers.

In determining the extent of the workup, the following factors should be considered: (i) the immune status of the patient, (ii) the severity of the disease, (iii) the type of specimen submitted, (iv) the etiologic agents sought, and (v) the clinical management of the patient. For example, tissue obtained from organ transplantation patients should be more thoroughly evaluated than a clean-catch urine sample submitted from an outpatient with uncomplicated cystitis. The laboratory's goal is to minimize the expenditure of resources producing results of questionable or easily predictable medical value in order to maximize the effort expended on more clinically relevant specimens.

Factors that need to be defined for the different specimen types include (i) the number of different organisms worked up per specimen, (ii) the organisms that require a susceptibility test, (iii) the method of identification, (iv) the testing of replicate specimens from the same patient, and (v) the frequency of repeat susceptibility tests with organisms recovered in subsequent specimens. In general, there is little need to identify or perform susceptibility tests on greater than two gram-negative rods recovered from sputum, two predominant bacteria recovered from a clean-catch urine specimen, or multiple isolates recovered from superficial wounds. Duplicate specimens such as urine, sputum, and stool probably should not be cultured or tested for *C. difficile* received within 72 h if the initial specimen is positive. Spot tests (e.g., indole, oxidase, and catalase tests), pigment, colony morphology, and odor can be used to categorize or presumptively identify isolates recovered from nonsterile sites such as sputum, urine, or superficial wounds (4, 25). Organisms of little clinical relevance in the disease process should not be further identified without consultation with the laboratory director (9). For example, *Haemophilus* spp., *Corynebacterium* spp., and gram-negative rods recovered from throat specimen cultures are not usually associated with pharyngitis and should not be identified. Other considerations include limiting the identification of yeasts and anaerobic gram-positive cocci from most body sources, eliminating the serotyping of *Salmonella* isolates (these should be submitted to the state health laboratory), and reporting of coagulase-negative staphylococci from urine or a single blood bottle without further identification. Because outpatients are generally treated empirically, the susceptibilities of urine isolates of *Escherichia coli*, *Proteus* spp., *Klebsiella* spp., and *Enterococcus* spp., respiratory isolates of *Haemophilus* spp., and genital isolates of *Neisseria gonorrhoeae* are not usually determined. Laboratories may save these isolates for up to 7 days in the event that a workup is required.

Limiting of Diagnostic Tests for a Single Diagnosis

Often, multiple laboratory tests can be used to diagnose an infectious disease (e.g., *Legionella* pneumonia). Commercially available diagnostic tests for *Legionella* pneumonia include the direct fluorescent-antibody test, a test for the detection of antigen in urine, serology, and culture. Should all of these tests be offered and performed by the clinical laboratory? Probably not. The laboratory needs to assess the clinical value of the test with input from clinicians and determine the test sensitivity, specificity, and predictive value for the patient population being served. On the basis of these data, one or possibly two tests can be selected for routine use and the other tests can be made available on a restricted basis from a reference laboratory.

QUALITY ASSESSMENT AND CONTROL

Basic Quality Assessment Concepts

In 1980, JCAHO established the QA standard for hospitals (10, 11, 22). This standard emphasizes the identification and resolution of problems through a coordinated hospital-wide program based upon changing behavior through investigation of problems by the following 10-step process:

1. Assign responsibility.
2. Define the scope of care.
3. Identify important aspects of care.
4. Identify indicators related to outcome of care.
5. Set thresholds to be measured.
6. Collect the data.
7. Evaluate the care
8. Take action to resolve identified problems.
9. Assess actions and document improvement.
10. Communicate information to the hospital's QA program.

In general, QA attempts to identify, monitor, evaluate, and improve practices related to patient care. In the past, QA focused on problem finding. Now the focus of quality care has shifted to quality assessment and QI which, in addition to problem identification, emphasizes methods for improving practices. As these quality management concepts matured, the emphasis in the 1990s has shifted toward satisfying the needs of the customers through CQI.

CQI is both an organizational philosophy and a systematic process that promotes patient outcome enhancement by measuring customer satisfaction (44). CQI identifies problems that need immediate resolution and seeks to improve processes that are not current problems but that may improve customer satisfaction. Overall, CQI is one approach to managing resources in the constantly changing health care environment.

TQM is a system of managerial programs that includes (i) team management, (ii) plans management, and (iii) improvement management (44). These programs provide the processes by which CQI can be implemented and maintained. All three TQM programs are interrelated, and the success of this approach depends upon the sharing of information by the three programs.

The team management program emphasizes team decision making through leadership skills, education, and delegation of responsibility. This program assesses morale, work attitude, and decision-making skills; provides the support needed to improve these attitudes and skills; and monitors the team's success in these areas. The goal of the team management program is the continuous improvement of employee decision making, which enhances external customer satisfaction. Thus, the importance of the role and needs of the employee (internal customer) in achieving CQI is recognized. The team management program, if successful, must provide employees with team skills training that may include conflict resolution, motivation, empowerment, opportunity identification, customer-oriented planning, and decision making.

The plans management program strives to improve the organizational process through anticipatory planning consisting of four phases:

Phase 1: Organizational direction
: Based on current and future customer needs identified through analysis of data.

Phase 2: Strategic prioritization
: Prioritize goals based on available resources, analysis of the organization's strengths and weaknesses, and external market opportunities. May prioritize by short-, medium-, or long-range goals.

Phase 3: Action planning
: Implement the priorities by identifying the goal objectives and tasks and assigning these items to an individual(s).

Phase 4: Action follow-up
: Evaluate the actions in improving customer satisfaction and correct the actions when necessary.

The improvement management program achieves CQI through ongoing quality surveillance and identification of current problems as well as processes that will improve customer satisfaction. This program is similar to the older QA and QI programs. The program identifies quality indicators or monitors (e.g., specimen acceptability, appropriateness of test utilization, accuracy and timeliness of reports, and customer perceptions); collects and evaluates the data; takes appropriate action to improve the process; and lastly, assesses the effectiveness of the action (47, 50). Many of these processes involve areas outside of the laboratory and require cooperation among the affected groups in order to achieve the desired improvement. The first critical step of the improvement management program is to reach a consensus among the customers as to the importance of the monitors or indicators selected. Clark (12) has identified six alternative improvement approaches. The success of a CQI program rests upon the commitment of the organization's leadership to the concept and to providing the necessary resources to implement the program.

Basic QC Concepts and Guidelines

Quality control (QC) is a concept that includes evaluating product performance, comparing this performance to stated goals, and taking action when the product fails. In the microbiology laboratory, the accuracy of the test information is dependent upon the specimen quality; the correlation of the test method with clinical data; the performance of test procedures, personnel, media, reagents, and instruments; and the method for the reporting of results. The QC program is designed to continuously monitor these elements, identify problems in test performance or the test process, and correct the problem. Documentation is the cornerstone of a QC program, and all methods, policies, test results, and corrective actions must be recorded. As a minimum, microbiology QC programs should address the following elements:

- Test methods and procedures
- Verification and validation of tests
- Content of procedure manuals
- Content and storage of records and reports
- Competency of personnel
- Proficiency testing

Test Methods and Procedures

A QC program monitors, evaluates, and documents the performance of all aspects of a test procedure. This includes the quality of the specimen; the performance of reagents, media, and instruments; and a review of the test results for errors. Appropriately collected and transported specimens are essential for quality microbiology results. Processing of unsuitable specimens may produce misleading results. The laboratory must specify for the customer (i.e., the health care provider) the appropriate techniques for the collection and transportation of specimens as well as the volume and number of specimens necessary to ensure the reliability of the test result (51) (see chapter 4). Elements of the collection process that can be monitored include volume (e.g., CSF submitted for multiple cultures and blood submitted for culture); number of specimens (e.g., stool specimens for diarrheal pathogens); quality of specimens (e.g., sputum); and rates of contamination of blood, body fluid, and urine specimens (48). The laboratory should monitor the quality of specimens received and be proactive in improving performance.

Reagents, supplies, and stains are labeled to indicate identity, concentration, storage requirements, preparation and expiration dates, and, if applicable, the type of safety hazard associated with their use. In general, negative and positive controls are required for qualitative tests (e.g., catalase and oxidase tests), and two controls with different titers or concentrations are necessary for quantitative tests (e.g., serology). The QC strains, frequency of testing, and expected results can be found in other references (27, 49, 50).

Commercially prepared media whose quality is controlled by the manufacturer and listed in the National Committee on Clinical Laboratory Standards (NCCLS) publication M22-A2 (41) are exempt from QC testing by the user except to verify that the media are not dehydrated, hemolyzed, cracked, contaminated, or filled improperly. The manufacturers' quality assurance procedures are listed in publication M22-A2 (41).

Equipment maintenance and function checks are performed and documented as specified by the manufacturer or as established by the user to guarantee accurate test results. These records are retained for the life of the equipment.

The quality and medical relevance of the microbial test information are dependent upon the timeliness and accuracy of the reports. The laboratory should establish clinically useful TATs for critical tests such as body fluid smears, acid-fast bacillus smears, and cultures (50) through consensus of those involved in patient management. When possible, TAT begins with the collection of the specimen and ends when the result is used for patient care. The final report is checked for clerical and computer errors by comparison to the laboratory work card and instrument logs. When an error is detected after the final report is released, the revised report should provide the correct information but must not delete the original error. Clinically significant changes in the test result in the report should be conveyed immediately to the physician. When an error is found, policies and procedures should be modified, if warranted, to prevent recurrences.

Verification and Validation of Tests

New test methods of high complexity must be verified for accuracy and precision before they are used for testing of samples from patients, and the laboratory must validate existing methods (19, 20, 40). Verification demonstrates that the laboratory can reproduce the manufacturer's claims or that the new method compares favorably with an accepted reference method. Several examples of verification methods for selected microbiology tests are available (19, 20). Validation of an existing test documents that the test performs satisfactorily on the basis of QC data, proficiency testing, and correlation with clinical data.

Content of Procedure Manuals

The laboratory's policy and procedure manual must contain all material relevant to the operation of the laboratory and production of patients' test results. The procedure's format, where appropriate, should generally adhere to the recommendations specified in NCCLS publication GP2-A3 (42). All original procedures and revisions must be dated, approved, and signed by the current laboratory director. The manual should be readily available to the staff and should be reviewed annually. Manuals for procedures that are no longer in use must be retained for at least 2 years.

Content and Storage of Records and Reports

The laboratory must maintain sufficient records to document all aspects of testing performed on a patient's specimen. The test requisition should contain the patient's name or identifier, the date of collection of the specimen, the date that the specimen was received in the laboratory, the name of the test requester, and the test requested. The procedures performed on the specimen, the personnel performing the test, communication with the requester, and the results obtained should be documented. The final test report also contains the name and address of the laboratory performing the test, appropriate reference ranges, and test interpretation. All records and reports are retained for at least 2 years.

Competency of Personnel

The Clinical Laboratory Improvement Amendments of 1988 (CLIA 88) define the personnel requirements for microbiology laboratories on the basis of a complexity test model (24). Because CLIA 88 reduced the educational requirements for laboratory personnel, annual documentation of the competency of personnel to perform microbiology tests is required, regardless of the individual's experience and education. For most individuals, this documentation process is a time-consuming exercise that does not materially improve the quality of the test results produced. Written training methods are advised for new employees and for the retraining of other employees (20, 44). The competency of experienced microbiologists may be verified by review of work cards, interpretation of unknowns, the use of proficiency samples, or a written examination. The competency information, the annual performance appraisal, past training and certification, and continuing education experiences should be retained in the individual's personnel folder.

Proficiency Testing

All microbiology laboratories must participate in an external proficiency testing program that is approved by the U.S. Department of Health and Human Services and that reflects the laboratory's specialty and level of expertise (24). Some of the approved programs are listed elsewhere (48). Sanctions may be imposed on laboratories that fail to submit correct responses for at least 80% of the test samples for two of three testing events.

ISSUES AFFECTING LABORATORY MANAGEMENT

Health Care Practices

The remarkable changes which have occurred in our health care delivery system in the last decade and particularly in the last 5 years need no specific documentation. It is necessary to reduce the increasing cost of health care, which presently uses approximately one-seventh of the gross national product. The attempts which are being made to alter the delivery of health care, the reimbursement for health care, the extent of health care, and the quality of health care have created many varied initiatives and have also opened the floodgates to discussions which would have been thought impossible not long ago. For example, serious controversy exists regarding the utilization of limited health care resources, and in some states, such as Oregon, there have been legislative initiatives to expand health care to more state citizens. With fixed fiscal resources, legislative solutions which, in fact, ration clinical services have been tendered (8). The restriction of services, particularly for individuals in the Medicare population who are approaching the ends of their lives, engenders active and heated discussion which has become admixed with such initiatives as that related to physician-assisted suicide for terminally ill patients, which has been passed twice by the voters of Oregon. Although many controversies need to be explored further, those which affect the laboratory most significantly have to do with the decrease in fiscal resources. There exists the conundrum that with decreasing resources it is hoped that there can be increasing productivity without any compromise in quality. Little information is available as to exactly how successful are the resolutions of these competing forces. Health care systems are merging and consolidating, and the numbers of laboratories in physicians' offices and hospitals are decreasing. There is considerable concern that patient care will be compromised as specimens are transported to centralized institutional or commercial laboratories, but often, these concerns are mainly focused on the loss of jobs and changes from traditional patterns of behavior.

In the area of clinical microbiology there have been attempts to reduce costs by performing more clinically relevant activities. Doing fewer cultures may reduce costs, but as the volume decreases the unit cost increases, and therefore, performing only those tests which are clinically relevant may somewhat miss the point in cost reduction. Whereas it is obvious in clinical chemistry and hematology that increased volume is associated with decreased costs because automated instrumentation can be used more efficiently, similar changes are not quite so obvious in clinical microbiology. A few general statements about changing patterns of practice are necessary. First, whether the laboratory community agrees or not, there will be continuing pressure to reduce laboratory services, which will decrease the test volume for any given entity. Second, the reduction in testing is not necessarily a malevolent product of this process, since it must be remembered that we are leaving an era where excessive and often unnecessary testing was fiscally rewarded. Now we are in a milieu where it becomes critical for the clinical microbiology laboratory to perform relevant testing while maintaining appropriate quality. Third, there is a great interest in using new technological methods to solve old problems. The mere fact that something can be done by one of these new approaches does not mean that it should be done that way or that it is most cost-effective to do it that way. Some molecular techniques are touted to have extraordinary specificity, and some have even greater sensitivity than traditional methods, but at least at the present time, their costs may well preclude their routine use. Finally, the laboratory must try to find a better way to integrate its activities both into the institution's administrative needs and into the clinical care needs of the patients. It must be accepted that patients now are viewed as customers or covered lives and that all of the marketing initiatives that go along with that philosophy must be understood by the laboratory.

Consolidation of clinical microbiology laboratories will be discussed from the standpoint of a general conceptual framework as well as personal experience. Consolidation has obvious advantages, some of which are not quite so obvious, and a number of potential detractions. First, in terms of the advantages of consolidation, it should be mentioned that the aggregation of volume must be of paramount consideration. The question of how the bringing together of a larger volume of culture specimens helps the laboratory become more efficient has been raised. The ability to consider multiple diagnostic approaches including potential instrumentation which would otherwise be too costly is only one concern. More important is the opportunity of decreasing reagent costs, increasing the skill of personnel, and enhancing the efficiency of personnel by working with a larger volume of material. Although the technologist or microbiologist who works with a wide variety of culture specimens as a daily occurrence may find it somewhat more interesting, the ability to concentrate on different specimen types for blocks of time can create a more efficient work flow. Second, and equally important, consolidation allows a focusing and concentration of intellectual resources in one area. We are fast approaching the time when each laboratory will not be expected to have internal to its workforce the expertise needed to provide a high quality of work in all the diverse areas of clinical microbiology. The attempts to maintain this type of a workforce, particularly one that works with small volumes of specimens, as in mycology, mycobacteriology, or virology, often establish very inefficient work patterns and encourage the evolution of inefficient performance by these expert individuals. This focusing of expert resources occurs both at the bench and at the management level. It is becoming much more difficult to make the argument that a medium-sized city can justify having more than one centralized community clinical microbiology laboratory. Many object to this vision, but reality has a way of overcoming wishful thinking. It makes little sense to have these highly trained expert individuals processing specimens when they could be spending their time in the actual evaluation of problem organisms or helping the providers understand the meaning of test results. A third advantage of a consolidated laboratory is that it helps the member organizations develop similar practice patterns for use of the laboratory. These practice patterns should extend to the use of pharmaceutical agents as well, and the more rational interaction between institutions as they use some of these expensive agents not only will decrease operation costs but, more importantly, can also increase the quality of care at each of the institutions. A fourth advantage is that laboratory services performed by more qualified individuals can be made available over longer time frames. As mentioned earlier, there is a tendency to look for cost savings by making personnel reductions, and one of the first things that happens is that service availability decreases. With the consolidated laboratory, particularly with creative scheduling, considerable expertise can be made available at all times or at least can quickly be obtained at unusual times. A final general advantage to the consolidation of laboratories is the ability to more constructively interact with the providers in terms of helping both in the definition of appropriate specimens and in the interpretation of the results from those specimens. There is great pressure for health care delivery systems to use individuals, both physicians and nonphysicians, who are much more generalist in their training and experience and who are therefore realistically less able to keep up with all of the nuances and changes which keep occurring in terms of both the diagnostic statements and the therapeutic consequences which are inherent in the clinical microbiology results. The training of physician and nonphysician practitioners, although hoping to create a better clinical environment for the patient at a lower cost, cannot realistically be expected to necessarily increase the quality of care for the patient. It would seem that the laboratory has an opportunity to play a critical role in helping these providers by pooling laboratory expertise and providing higher-quality laboratory services. Some have suggested that specialists, such as infectious disease specialists, will suffer as the laboratory assumes a more proactive role in this interaction with the providers. It is not at all obvious that this will be the case. Infectious disease specialists are under great pressure to decrease their training programs, just as is the case with most specialists. As a consequence, it would seem to be necessary to use those expert individuals in complex clinical situations rather than assume that each unusual organism or strange antibiogram necessarily demands their attention.

Consolidation of laboratories, particularly the clinical microbiology laboratory, is something which is occurring in some geographic areas but which must occur in most areas. The cost of individual microbiology laboratories will not be tolerated by the health care delivery system, but it is also important that some of the drawbacks be identified. In our experience, the first and most important problem to be overcome is that of trust between different institutions. Each institution has its own tradition, and usually associated with that tradition is a certain understanding, rightly or wrongly, of how other institutions have acted. The tendency to be competitive rather than cooperative is powerful, and the ability to remember anecdotes which place potential partners in a negative light occurs frequently. Laboratory directors must react with each other in a way which creates and fosters professionalism and educational opportunities rather than in a way which detracts from these necessary ventures. The consolidation can occur as a consequence of the coming together of parties with a strong will and cooperative vision, or it can occur when a large group comes in and imposes the consolidation on laboratories. When consolidation happens, there usually is great dislocation, but it must be said in all candor that the ensuing consolidation may not create the clinical havoc that most of the participants predict. Consolidation can and in fact must create a better quality of care than the original situation provided. Second, an almost trivial but very important aspect of consolidation has to do with how an infrastructure is created to allow the movement of specimens from one point to another. The cost of creating this infrastructure can be considerable, and in any evaluation of a merger or consolidation, it must be considered very seriously. The more institutions which can participate in the courier or transfer service, the greater will be the ability to distribute the transportation costs over a wider base and the smaller will be the cost added to each test. There needs to be retention of some of the "stat" functions at each institution, but these should be kept to a minimum, with the majority of testing being done at the centralized laboratory. Third, a considerable problem of consolidation has to do with the general area of information exchange. Most institutions are not apt to have similar laboratory information systems, and even if they do have similar systems, they may have different file structures which make the interface between them cumbersome. The goal must be to have an integrated laboratory information system between various components of a network, but this initially may create a cost which is considerable. The cost needs to be clearly identified and then appropriately amortized over the time necessary to get a more cost-effective interaction. Fourth, during consolidation there will of necessity be a reduction in personnel. It makes no sense to consolidate and keep all existing positions. If a consolidation is structured such that there is not a reduction of personnel, then one needs to look very seriously at what is being accomplished or who is designing the system. Another cost of consolidation relates to the severance packages which may be necessary as part of the consolidation, particularly if bargaining units are involved, and this particular expense needs to be calculated into the merger.

Technology

The general area of technology change deserves a few comments. First, in most laboratories which have various types of semiautomated or automated instruments, it is usually safe to say that the excess capacity of those instruments is considerable. The ability to consolidate this excess capacity is a real efficiency, and the ability to decrease the cost of the reagents represents further savings. Some of these instruments require more sophisticated expertise which can best be made available at a central facility rather than at each local facility. It is difficult, at the present time, to know exactly where diagnostic microbiology will be moving in the next few years, although many soothsayers feel very strongly that the area of molecular diagnostics will replace more traditional means. It is obvious that in the area of molecular diagnostics there will be opportunities for more sophisticated diagnoses, but with the very considerable pressure on cost containment, it is not clear that these methodologies will be as useful as the most active proponents of them would suggest. Unless the costs of doing some of these molecular diagnostic procedures fall considerably and approach the costs of the manual or simple automated procedures, they will continue to remain oddities on the outside of the general practice and be confined to a few reference laboratories. The ability to use robotics-based techniques is predicated upon the testing of large volumes, and it is only when some very large volume laboratories in microbiology exist can these more sophisticated, newer technologies be applied to the routine testing of specimens.

An area which has been given very little attention through the course of traditional microbiological examinations has to do with an evaluation of the host response to various agents and the ability to predict more accurately what the host response might be. It is entirely possible that these procedures, which probably would be predominately immunological or perhaps cytometric, will over the course of time replace our more standard approach to the evaluation of specific organisms with an evaluation of the host response to organisms.

Workforce Issues

The final concern in this section has to do with workforce issues. The greatest cost for all laboratories is labor, and therefore, the desire to decrease labor requirements receives much attention. Often, this attention is misdirected in terms of global reductions in labor costs with perhaps some kind of hoped for increased efficiency. Visits to numerous laboratories quickly demonstrate that productivity is a considerable variable, and when this is pointed out, each laboratory defends its traditional productivity. In general, it may be safe to say that the levels of productivity are traditional in that individuals have worked in a certain environment with certain expectations of them for a long time, and that is considered their level of productivity. Attempts to change this perception are met with great resistance, because individuals are apt to stay in an environment where they are not being pushed as hard as they might be, and as they become entrenched they adopt that level of workload as their output standard. There are, unfortunately, few published productivity benchmarks which a manager can use to counsel employees. Slow employees often fall back on the explanation that they are more careful and more accurate than more rapid colleagues. If a bargaining unit is involved, it may be even more difficult to alter traditional productivity expectations unless there is specific documentation of what is expected. In the long run, the attempt to document expectations is probably to everyone's advantage and should be considered more than just an inconvenience but as an adjunct to contract guidelines. In general, it is safe to say that most laboratory managers have not been effective in clearly defining expectations for both their supervisory and technical personnel. A corollary to decreasing FTEs is the popular concept of defining skill mix needs. In general, this is intended to have individuals with various levels of training doing activities which are commensurate with that training. The smaller the laboratory, the more difficult it is to realize any efficiencies in this realm, since the use of individuals who have only a high school diploma or perhaps an associate degree, as opposed to a medical technologist or microbiologist, decreases considerably the flexibility within the whole laboratory environment. The consequence is that highly trained medical technologists and microbiologists end up performing a number of tasks, particularly in the processing arena, which do not require their levels of skill. The laboratory, in general, is struggling with this concept of skill mix in that it becomes very difficult at times to clearly define a line between expectations based on educational background. Some individuals with a very modest educational background who are well motivated and have had good on-the-job training are able to easily perform many tasks otherwise assigned to a medical technologist or a microbiology specialist. The tendency to try to use less trained individuals in more areas of the laboratory may have quality ramifications, but often, this is difficult to document. The use of proficiency testing to document this is probably inadequate, in that the more highly trained individual may be given the proficiency test specimen for evaluation when, in fact, the less trained individual may handle more of the routine specimens.

Another area of considerable interest is that of cross-training of personnel to do a number of functions either within the laboratory or between the laboratory and other departments such as radiology and perhaps electrocardiography. The advantages of cross-training usually are more obvious in smaller, more rural hospitals, where a case can be made for the necessity of clearly defining and training individuals in this way. It is interesting that in a larger laboratory there is often a great deal of resistance on the part of the medical technologists to perform tasks in areas other than those for which they have had most of their training. The reading of a Gram smear by anyone other than a microbiologically trained technologist is met with resistance, and on the other hand, the microbiologist may not be able to adequately function in other areas of the laboratory. This is not to say that in appropriate circumstances both cross-training and evaluation of skill mix needs are not appropriate goals for the manager. However, the situations for which these techniques are used need to be very carefully defined, and appropriate training programs must be implemented. As mentioned earlier, the primary driver for evaluating workforce issues is the decrease in economic resources available to each department.

Each laboratory must establish its own policies regarding the more optimal use of its facilities, and this is sometimes done in concert with the infectious disease specialist or the medical board of the hospital in order to try to decrease repetitive cultures, overculturing, inappropriate culturing, and inpatient parasitological tests and to address the myriad of other suggestions which have been made regarding decreases in the number of nonrelevant diagnostic procedures. It should be noted that these maneuvers decrease the workload in the laboratory at the same time that there is decreased funding. It should also be noted that the double-digit increase in workload that most laboratories felt for many years has generally fallen off in the last few years. These are even greater incentives to try to look at the areas of efficiency in the evaluation of specimens within the laboratory as well as to seriously consider the merging of laboratory facilities such that one can make a rational case for a more effective high-quality laboratory.

There is much anguish over the decrease in fiscal resources, with the assumption generally being made that the previous professional economic milieu was somehow rather ideal and necessary for quality patient care. There is no information that in fact this was the case, and constructive review of procedures, processes, and employee utilization may contribute significantly to more relevant, high-quality, and less costly care. However, there is the hazard that as economic resources are further diminished there will come a point that it is not possible to sustain quality. It is incumbent on the laboratory director to make a documentable case, as the patient advocate, against negative alterations in quality. It has been suggested that many of the initial savings have been wrung out of the health care system by the managed care initiative and that the continued insistence on the part of some health systems to maintain high profit margins is not consonant with good care or legal activities.

The continuing constraining effect of the federal bureaucracy on laboratory care is of considerable interest and must be evaluated critically by all of us. It has been suggested by some inside and outside the federal government that the ultimate goal of the continued reduction in payments and the increasing burdensome bureaucracy of regulations is to get the health delivery systems to basically give up and not try to get compensation from the federal government because it will become too expensive to do so. This may be overly cynical, but the continued exercise of control and micromanagement by individuals who have little understanding of the laboratory, who use the words "quality management" with reckless abandon, and who have managed to develop another cottage industry which provides them with financial security does nothing demonstrable to aid in patient care.

REGULATORY ISSUES AFFECTING THE MICROBIOLOGY LABORATORY

The continued proliferation of government regulations related to the laboratory is an ongoing concern to all laboratory managers. The general structure of regulatory oversight for the clinical laboratory was described in detail in the sixth edition of the *Manual of Clinical Microbiology* (32). Specific reiteration of the role of the federal government is redundant, and only updates of relevant regulations will be included here. Regular and timely updates are available in the *National Intelligence Report* (65), and laboratory managers are encouraged to follow these brief synopses, which are published twice monthly. That source has proven to be a reliable, concise, annotated resource of existing and impending regulatory change.

With regard to CLIA 88, changes for the clinical microbiology laboratory have been relatively minimal and controlled. In the category of waived testing, a number of kits are now approved for group A streptococcal antigen detection, for the detection of *Helicobacter pylori* in gastric biopsy materials, and for the detection of *H. pylori* antibody in blood. The other waived test changes relate to other areas of the clinical laboratory. The category of microscopy testing, which had been called "physician-performed microscopy," has been changed in name to "provider-performed microscopy" (PPM) in order to more accurately define some of the individuals who perform this test. It should be noted, however, that Gram staining may not be performed by those with this particular license and that attempts to add Gram staining to the tests that can be performed by individuals with this license have, so far, not met with success. In discussing Gram stains, it should be noted that for those with the moderate-complexity license, only Gram stains related to male and female genital specimens are considered appropriate; Gram staining of all other clinical specimens is considered to be of high complexity. The fact that there is an incongruity here, in that most laboratories would not attempt to rule out the diagnosis of gonorrhea based on the Gram-staining result for a female genital specimen, has not persuaded the rule makers to change that particular anomaly. It is hoped that this can be changed in the future and that only Gram smears of the male urethral discharge be allowed to be used to diagnose gonorrhea. The regulatory consequences are considerable for performing Gram smears on specimens other than genital specimens since a high-complexity license is required, which necessitates very specific training in terms of the directorship and the experience of individuals performing these tests. It would probably not be possible for the vast majority of small clinic or physician office laboratories to perform at a high-complexity level.

One very disturbing aspect of the regulatory initiative is that the CLIA certificate fees were increased considerably in 1998. When the U.S. Congress passed the original CLIA 88 law, it did not provide monies to fund this initiative, and therefore, it was a program which was to be self-sustaining by the fees which were generated from its activities. The Health Care Finance Administration (HCFA) maintained that it was no longer able to support the program with the existing fee structure and raised the fees as of 1 January 1998. These fees are levied biennially, and the increase for waived and low-volume laboratories, that is, fewer than 10,000 tests per year, increased from $100 to $150. The PPM fee increased from $150 to $200, and all other laboratories had a fee increase dependent upon their volume. For example, for the laboratory with an annual test volume of 10,000 to 25,000, the fee increased from $100 to $430. For the laboratory which performs more than 1 million tests per annum, the fee increased from $600 to $7,940. The increase in cost per test was much less for the higher-volume laboratories, but these increases probably represent only the first step in a fee escalation process.

Another new government initiative, which was promulgated in February 1997 from the Office of the Inspector General of the U.S. Department of Health and Human Services, was entitled the Model Compliance Plan for Clinical Laboratories. This initiative attempts to decrease the fraud and abuse which have occurred in the Medicare and Medicaid programs. It is not entirely clear how all laboratories are going to respond to these requests, but it is fairly obvious that the laboratory must take seriously this new and costly initiative. The initiative itself contains a number of elements which include standards of conduct for the employees, the distribution of compliance policies regarding potential fraud, the designation of a compliance officer who has specific charge for the program, the education and training of employees under the terms of this compliance initiative, auditing of compliance monitoring, the development of codes for illegal activities, investigation and resolution of specific personnel problems, adherence to compliance as an element of evaluating supervisors and managers, the establishment of policies of nonemployment of sanctioned individuals who have been involved with Medicare abuse, establishment of a hotline to receive complaints, procedures to protect the anonymity of complaints regarding potential fraud, and the adoption of requirements for record creation and retention (62). This new mandate is not specifically focused on activities in the microbiology laboratory but is more concerned with problems of billing, particularly those related to high-volume chemistry and hematology testing and the use of inappropriate panels. However, each section of the laboratory must be in compliance with these regulations. The U.S. Department of Health and Human Services is specifically not putting out an example of what is intended in each of these areas and is forcing each laboratory to develop its own plan. It is not entirely clear how a laboratory will know whether its plan sufficiently complies with the overall initiative. Apparently, the laboratory compliance plan will be modified to some degree as a consequence of changes that have occurred in HCFA's new requirements regarding billing for automated multichannel tests. Exactly what modification will be made is not entirely clear, and the extent of the modification is equally unclear at the present time. The whole compliance plan initiative has generated a tremendous amount of resistance from the laboratory and medical communities because they see it as bringing considerable increases in costs with no hope of reimbursement but little opportunity to alter the fraud and abuse that have occurred.

HCFA ruled that, as of 1 April 1998, all medical and nonmedical providers must provide a code of medical necessity for each laboratory test ordered and that no Medicare reimbursement would be provided for those tests without an appropriate code. The diagnostic code, an International Classification of Diseases, 9th revision, code, must document the appropriate medical necessity for each test. However, HCFA has not made available the acceptable codes for each test. This rather draconian invention to reduce the amount of chemistry and hematology testing applies to all laboratory tests. Originally, HCFA wanted the laboratories to be responsible for assigning the codes, but it quickly became clear that accurate coding would not be possible because the laboratory was not in a position to determine the necessity of a test. It should be noted that screening tests are not reimbursed by HCFA, but there are no definitive guidelines as to when a test moves from diagnosis, to monitoring for recurrence, to screening for future infections. Also, this requirement applied only to outpatient billing, since the inpatient is covered under a lump-sum payment determined by the DRG code assigned for the hospitalization. If outpatient DRG payments are developed, then much of this extraordinary problem will disappear. Although only HCFA is using this payment mechanism for Medicare recipients, it is anticipated that Medicare and many other third-party payers will follow.

Another, perhaps more complicated, initiative was also introduced as part of these changes, and that was the Advanced Beneficiary Notice (ABN), which requires that the patient be notified in writing when a test which will not be reimbursed by HCFA is performed. It also requires the Medicare patient to agree to be billed directly by the laboratory or institution. The philosophy behind this innovation was that if a test is deemed by HCFA not to be of medical necessity (not reimbursable), then the patients should have the opportunity to decide whether they want the test performed and work that out with the ordering provider. Not having clear directions as to what constitutes HCFA-determined medical necessity creates much misunderstanding between the patient and provider and may encourage laboratories not to bill in order to maintain good customer service relations. This may be the main reason behind this initiative. Both the medical necessity code and ABN activities were part of the compliance plan initiative to reduce fraud and abuse.

One question which is raised with some frequency by conscientious laboratorians is, "How will anyone find out if we are not adhering strictly to the rules and the letter of the law and all of these multiple layers of HCFA and OSHA [Occupational Safety and Health Administration] regulations?" There are probably two answers to this plaintive question. First, most of the violations or the inadvertent failure to adhere to the regulations will, in fact, go unnoticed during the various inspection processes. The second answer is that most violations come to light as a consequence of disgruntled employees making a complaint to the appropriate government agency. In areas where there is fraud in billing, the employee has an opportunity to recover extraordinary amounts of money as a certain percentage of whatever settlement is levied against the offender. Under the provisions of the Federal False Claims Act, individuals who not only point out but who are also able to document fraudulent claims are able to share in a significant percentage of the judgment. Recently, a federal judge in Houston, Texas, ruled that this particular provision was unconstitutional and stated that the U.S. Congress lacks the power to authorize private citizens who are not personally injured by a defendant's action to perform a function which is normally delegated to the executive branch. It will be interesting to see how this challenge to the provision is resolved in that it has been the pivotal instrument used by the government against billing fraud.

Accreditation and Licensure of Laboratories

The main changes in the area of accreditation and licensure of laboratories relate to some additional states being given previously nonexistent inspection and licensure authority from HCFA, with this authority being dependent upon the state adopting regulations which are at least as stringent as the federal regulations. What this means from a practical standpoint is that the state instead of HCFA can serve as the inspection authority and that different states may pursue this inspection activity depending on the financial resources available to them or what they feel to be the adequacy of the inspection by agencies such as JCAHO or CAP.

It should also be noted that each state has its own requirements for notification of infectious diseases, and although this list does not change frequently, it is incumbent upon the laboratory director to make sure that the laboratory is in compliance with these state regulations. It might be mentioned that on occasion the state department of health will make certain demands on a laboratory in terms of reporting organisms or providing material to them in order to satisfy certain requirements of the federal government or because of collaborative investigative work. The laboratory is not necessarily obligated to respond to these demands, although the state may sometimes make it appear as if it is a mandated function. It is appropriate for the laboratory director to press the state requester for specific documentation of why additional reporting, evaluation of laboratory records, provision of selected organisms, or other general intrusions into laboratory activity are in fact necessary. Also, it should be noted that these invitations to participation usually are done without funding by the state, and unless the laboratory wishes to do this as a general response of collegiality, it need not be viewed as a necessary response unless there is a sufficient legal mandate.

It was noted (32) that there is a continued expanding

of guidelines, which was referred to as "guideline creep." This has not abated, and federal, state, and accrediting agencies have been guilty of encouraging the proliferation of either guidelines or documentation requirements which are often couched in terms having to do with the improvement of clinical outcomes, the protection of workers, or the protection of the public at large, but often, little documentation is available to support this claim. Some of these can be resisted or, more importantly, can be evaluated in terms of satisfying the spirit of the law or recommendation in the context of a particular laboratory situation. At times there is a slavish adherence to regulations when, in fact, a well-documented common-sense approach would benefit both the laboratory and the patients much more adequately, and usually, the accrediting agencies are quite willing to accept a well thought out, reasonable response to these increasing guidelines. It must be remembered that most of these guidelines are attempts to improve quality, but often then are promulgated by individuals who are unfamiliar with their implementation and necessity and proceed from the need for information which may serve their own political territorial needs. It is quite appropriate to resist these capricious and arbitrary requests as long as the general spirit in which they are made can be met.

In conclusion, the regulatory initiatives can be viewed as burdensome, frequently misdirected, inadequately documented as to their utility, and generally causing a high level of frustration. However, it needs to be emphasized that these regulatory initiatives are created in the context of the legislative process and that all of us as laboratory directors have an opportunity to provide input into that process. Frequently, there is concern that individual voices will not be heard, but in fact, the government takes very seriously the responses to the proposed regulations. The advantage of being current by using references such as the *National Intelligence Report* (65) or the Statline from CAP (13) allows one to know when to look at the *Federal Register* to make comments. There is a tendency for laboratory directors to allow their professional societies such as the American Society for Microbiology, CAP, the American Society of Clinical Pathologists, and the Clinical Laboratory Management Association to make specific statements of objection or a suggestion for rule making. This is useful, but each laboratory director should try to take time to look at the proposed regulations and, if he or she feels that these regulations are inadequate or inappropriate, should respond directly to whatever agency is identified in the *Federal Register* within the appropriate time frame. A lack of response to these regulations will permit their imposition, and there then should be no complaint if an attempt has not been made to temper the rule making. This situation is analogous to that of individuals being told not to complain about the type of government which they must live under if they do not vote. These rule makings are frequently very complex, and many individuals are quick to comment that the devil is in the details, but in this situation, the devil is probably inappropriately maligned. What is in the details are the desires of special-interest groups or very vocal individuals or just plain incompetence or ignorance. Although many of the rule makers will claim that they have laboratory experience, this experience may be antiquated, inappropriate, limited, or irrelevant. Much of the rule making is done in a very carefully reasoned and competent fashion and in an attempt to follow the spirit of the usually very vague legislation which prompts the rule making. It is our task and necessary responsibility to help the rule makers promulgate initiatives that will be to the benefit of the patient, that are consonant with patient advocacy, and that can be documented to have relevance to clinical laboratory activities.

REFERENCES

1. **Albrecht, K.** 1988. Successful management by objectives, p. 1–40. Prentice-Hall Press, New York, N.Y.
2. **Albright, R. E., C. B. Graham III, R. H. Christianson, W. A. Schell, M. C. Bledsoe, J. L. Emlet, T. P. Mears, L. B. Reller, and K. A. Schneider.** 1991. Issues in cerebrospinal fluid management: acid-fast bacillus smear and culture. *Am. J. Clin. Pathol.* **95:**418–423.
3. **Albright, R. E., Jr., R. H. Christianson, J. L. Emlet, C. B. Graham III, E. G. Estevez, M. L. Wilson, L. B. Reller, and K. A. Schneider.** 1991. Issues in cerebrospinal fluid management: CSF venereal disease research laboratory testing. *Am. J. Clin. Pathol.* **95:**397–401.
4. **Bale, M. J., S. M. McLaws, and J. M. Matsen.** 1985. The spot indole test for identification of swarming *Proteus*. *Am. J. Clin. Pathol.* **83:**87–90.
5. **Baron, E. J., D. Francis, and K. M. Peddecord.** 1996. Infectious disease physicians rate microbiology services and practices. *J. Clin. Microbiol.* **34:**496–500.
6. **Bartlett, R. C.** 1974. *Medical Microbiology: Quality, Cost and Clinical Relevance*. John Wiley & Sons, Inc., New York, N.Y.
7. **Bergman, R.** 1994. Reengineering health care. *Hosp. Health Net.* **68:**28–36.
8. **Bodenheimer, T.** 1997. The Oregon health plan—lessons for the nation. *N. Engl. J. Med.* **337:**651–655, 720–723.
9. **Carroll, K., and L. Reimer.** 1996. Microbiology and laboratory diagnosis of upper respiratory tract infections. *Clin. Infect. Dis.* **23:**442–448.
10. **Clark, G. B.** 1990. Quality assurance, an administrative means to a managerial end. Part I. A historical review. *Clin. Lab. Management Rev.* **17:**7–15.
11. **Clark, G. B.** 1990. Quality assurance, an administrative means to a managerial end. Part II. The JCAHO ten step process selecting indicators of quality. *Clin. Lab. Management Rev.* **17:**224–257.
12. **Clark, G. B.** 1995. *Systematic Quality Management*. American Society for Clinical Pathologists Press, Chicago, Ill.
13. **College of American Pathologists.** *Statline*. College of American Pathologists, Washington, D.C.
14. **Daniels, M., and S. A. Schroeder.** 1977. Variation among physicians in use of laboratory tests: relation to clinical productivity and outcomes of care. *Med. Care* **15:**482–487.
15. **DeAguayo, R.** 1990. Deming: the American who taught the Japanese about quality, p. 1–60. Simon & Schuster, New York, N.Y.
16. **DePree, M.** 1989. *Leadership Is an Art*. Bantam/Doubleday/Dell Publishing Group, New York, N.Y.
17. **Derby, P., R. Davies, and S. Oliver.** 1997. The value of including broth cultures as part of a routine culture protocol. *J. Clin. Microbiol.* **35:**1101–1102.
18. **Doern, G. V.** 1996. Diagnostic mycobacteriology: where are we today? *J. Clin. Microbiol.* **34:**1873–1876.
19. **Elder, B. L.** 1997. Verification and validation of procedures in the clinical microbiology laboratory. *Clin. Microbiol. Newsl.* **19:**153–156.
20. **Elder, B. L., S. A. Hanson, J. A. Kellogg, F. J. Marsk, and R. J. Zabransky.** 1997. *Cumitech 31: Verification and Validation of Procedures in the Clinical Microbiology Laboratory*. Coordinating ed., B. W. McCurdy. American Society for Microbiology, Washington, D.C.
21. **Forbes, B. A., and P. A. Granato.** 1995. Processing specimens for bacteria, p. 265–281. *In* P. R. Murray, E. F. Barron, M. A. Pfaller, F. C. Tenover, and R. H. Yolken (ed.),

Manual of Clinical Microbiology, 6th ed. American Society for Microbiology, Washington, D.C.

22. **Fromberg, R.** 1988. *The Joint Commission Guide to Quality Assurance*. Joint Commission on Accreditation of Healthcare Organizations, Chicago, Ill.
23. **Hardwick, D. F., and J. I. Morrison.** 1990. *Directing the Clinical Laboratory*. Field and Word, Inc., New York, N.Y.
24. **Health Care Financing Administration.** 1992. Clinical Laboratory Improvement Amendments of 1988; final rule. *Fed. Regist.* **57:**7137–7186.
25. **Hicks, M. J., and K. J. Ryan.** 1976. Simplified scheme for identification of prompt lactose-fermenting members of the *Enterobacteriaceae*. *J. Clin. Microbiol.* **4:**511–514.
26. **Hines, J., and I. Nachamkin.** 1996. Effective use of the clinical microbiology laboratory for diagnosing diarrheal diseases. *Clin. Infect. Dis.* **23:**1292–1301.
27. **Isenberg, H. D. (ed.).** 1995. *Guide to Regulatory Requirements*. American Society for Microbiology, Washington, D.C.
28. **Juran, J. M.** 1988. Company wide planning for quality, p. 1–51. *In* J. M. Juran and F. M. Gryna (ed.), *Juran's Quality Control Handbook*, 4th ed. McGraw-Hill Book Company, New York, N.Y.
29. **Juran, J. M.** 1989. *Juran on Leadership for Quality: an Executive Handbook*, p. 1–80. Collier MacMillan, New York, N.Y.
30. **LaRocco, M.** 1995. Quality and productivity in the microbiology laboratory: continuous quality improvement. *Clin. Microbiol. Newsl.* **17:**129–131.
31. **Lepoff, R., and P. Romfh.** 1997. Quality management as the basis for cost management, p. 57–75. *In* E. M. Travers (ed.), *Clinical Laboratory Management*. The Williams & Wilkins Co., Baltimore, Md.
32. **McGowan, J. E., and J. D. MacLowry.** 1995. Addressing regulatory issues in the clinical microbiology laboratory, p. 67–74. In P. R. Murray, E. F. Barron, M. A. Pfaller, F. C. Tenover, and R. H. Yolken (ed.), *Manual of Clinical Microbiology*, 6th ed. American Society for Microbiology, Washington, D.C.
33. **McLaughlin, J.** 1995. The implementation of cost-effective, clinically relevant diagnostic microbiology policies: the approach. *Clin. Microbiol. Newsl.* **17:**70–71.
34. **Meredith, F. T., H. K. Phillips, and L. B. Reller.** 1997. Clinical utility of broth cultures of cerebrospinal fluid from patients at risk for shunt infections. *J. Clin. Microbiol.* **35:**3109–3111.
35. **Morris, A. J., D. C. Tanner, and L. B. Reller.** 1993. Rejection criteria for endotracheal aspirates from adults. *J. Clin. Microbiol.* **31:**1027–1029.
36. **Morris, A. J., S. J. Wilson, C. E. Marx, M. L. Wilson, S. Mirrett, and L. B. Reller.** 1995. Clinical impact of bacteria and fungi recovered only from broth culture. *J. Clin. Microbiol.* **33:**161–165.
37. **Morris, A. J., P. R. Murray, and L. B. Reller.** 1996. Contemporary testing for enteric pathogens: the potential for cost, time, and health care savings. *J. Clin. Microbiol.* **34:**1776–1778.
38. **Mortensen, J. E.** 1995. Quality and productivity in the microbiology laboratory: reengineering. *Clin. Microbiol. Newsl.* **17:**131–133.
39. **Murray, P. R., and J. A. Washington II.** 1975. Microscopic and bacteriologic analysis of expectorated sputum. *Mayo Clin. Proc.* **50:**339–334.
40. **National Committee on Clinical Laboratory Standards.** 1995. *Training Verification for Laboratory Personnel*. Publication GP21-A. National Committee for Clinical Laboratory Standards, Wayne, Pa.
41. **National Committee for Clinical Laboratory Standards.** 1996. *Quality Assurance for Commercially Prepared Microbiological Culture Media*. Publication M22-A2. National Committee for Clinical Laboratory Standards, Wayne, Pa.
42. **National Committee for Clinical Laboratory Standards.** 1996. *Clinical Laboratory Procedure Manuals*. Publication GP2-A3. National Committee for Clinical Laboratory Standards, Wayne, Pa.
43. **National Committee for Clinical Laboratory Standards.** 1996. *Cost Accounting in the Clinical Laboratory*. Tentative guideline GP11-T. National Committee for Clinical Laboratory Standards, Wayne, Pa.
44. **National Committee for Clinical Laboratory Standards.** 1997. *Continuous Quality Improvement: Essential Management Approaches and Their Use in Proficiency Testing*. Publication GP22-P. National Committee for Clinical Laboratory Standards, Wayne, Pa.
45. **Palmer, C. J., J. F. Lindo, W. I. Klaskala, J. A. Quesada, R. Kaminsky, M. K. Brum, and A. L. Ager.** 1998. Evaluation of the OptiMAL test for rapid diagnosis of *Plasmodium vivax* and *Plasmodium falciparum* malaria. *J. Clin. Microbiol.* **36:**203–206.
46. **Robinson, A.** 1994. Rationale for cost-effective laboratory medicine. *Clin. Microbiol. Rev.* **7:**185–199.
47. **Schifman, R. B.** 1994. Quality control and quality assurance, p. 1313–1334. *In* K. D. McClatchey (ed.), *Clinical Laboratory Medicine*. The Williams & Wilkins Co., Baltimore, Md.
48. **Sewell, D. L.** 1998. Quality assessment and control, p. 731–743. *In* H. D. Isenberg (ed.), *Essential Procedures in Clinical Microbiology*. American Society for Microbiology, Washington, D.C.
49. **Sewell, D. L.** 1992. Quality control, p. 13.2.1–13.2.35. *In* H. D. Isenberg (ed.), *Clinical Microbiology Procedures Handbook*, vol. 2. American Society for Microbiology, Washington, D.C.
50. **Sewell, D. L., and R. B. Schifman.** 1995. Quality assurance: quality improvement, quality control, and test validation, p. 55–66. *In* P. R. Murray, E. F. Barron, M. A. Pfaller, F. C. Tenover, and R. H. Yolken (ed.), *Manual of Clinical Microbiology*, 6th ed. American Society for Microbiology, Washington, D.C.
51. **Shea, Y. R.** 1992. Specimen collection and transport, p. 1.1.1–1.1.30. *In* H. D. Isenberg (ed.), *Clinical Microbiology Procedures Handbook*, vol. 1. American Society for Microbiology, Washington, D.C.
52. **Silletti, R. P., E. Ailey, S. Sun, and D. Tang.** 1997. Microbiologic and clinical value of primary broth cultures of wound specimens collected with swabs. *J. Clin. Microbiol.* **35:**2003–2006.
53. **Stone, B. L., D. L. Cohn, M. S. Kane, M. V. Hildred, M. L. Wilson, and R. R. Reves.** 1994. Utility of paired blood cultures and smears in the diagnosis of disseminated *Mycobacterium avium* complex infection in AIDS patients. *J. Clin. Microbiol.* **32:**841–842.
54. **Travers, E. M., and K. D. McClatchey.** 1994. Laboratory management, p. 3–33. *In* K. D. McClatchey (ed.), *Clinical Laboratory Medicine*. The Williams & Wilkins Co., Baltimore, Md.
55. **Travers, E. M.** 1997. Human resource management, p. 121–139. *In* E. M. Travers (ed.), *Clinical Laboratory Management*. The Williams & Wilkins Co., Baltimore, Md.
56. **Travers, E. M.** 1997. The business plan and strategic planning process, p. 101–119. *In* E. M. Travers (ed.), *Clinical Laboratory Management*. The Williams & Wilkins Co., Baltimore, Md.
57. **Travers, E. M.** 1997. Changing operations to improve productivity and reduce costs, p. 435–486. *In* E. M. Travers (ed.), *Clinical Laboratory Management*. The Williams & Wilkins Co., Baltimore, Md.

58. **Travers, E. M.** 1997. Improving productivity and efficiency in laboratories, p. 397–410. *In* E. M. Travers (ed.), *Clinical Laboratory Management*. The Williams & Wilkins Co., Baltimore, Md.
59. **Travers, E. M.** 1997. Controlling test utilization and appropriateness, p. 669–687. *In* E. M. Travers (ed.), *Clinical Laboratory Management*. The Williams & Wilkins Co., Baltimore, Md.
60. **Travers, E. M.** 1997. Methods to manage test utilization and ensure good medical practice, p. 689–714. *In* E. M. Travers (ed.), *Clinical Laboratory Management*. The Williams & Wilkins Co., Baltimore, Md.
61. **Umiker, W.** 1991. *The Customer Orientated Laboratory*. American Society of Clinical Pathologists, Chicago, Ill.
62. **U.S. Department of Health and Human Services.** 1997. Model compliance plan for clinical laboratories, January 24. Office of the Inspector General, U.S. Department of Health and Human Services, Washington, D.C.
63. **Valenstein, P.** 1996. Managing physician use of laboratory tests. *Clin. Lab. Med.* **16:**749–771.
64. **Valenstein, P., M. Pfaller, and M. Yungbluth.** 1996. The use and abuse of routine stool microbiology: a College of American Pathologists Q-probe study of 601 institutions. *Arch. Pathol. Lab. Med.* **120:**206–211.
65. **Washington G2 Reports.** *National Intelligence Report*. Washington G2 Reports, Washington, D.C.
66. **Wilson, M. L.** 1996. General principles of specimen collection and transport. *Clin. Infect. Dis.* **22:**766–777.
67. **Wilson, M. L.** 1997. Clinically relevant, cost-effective clinical microbiology. *Am. J. Clin. Pathol.* **107:**154–167.
68. **Yagupsky, P., and M. Menegus.** 1990. Cumulative positivity rates of multiple blood cultures for *Mycobacterium avium-intracellulare* and *Cryptococcus neoformans* in patients with the acquired immunodeficiency syndrome. *Arch. Pathol. Lab. Med.* **114:**923–925.

Commensal and Pathogenic Microorganisms of Humans*

SUSAN E. SHARP

3

The microbes that normally live in or on humans usually cause no ill effects to their host; however, the majority of pathogens responsible for human disease are also derived from these organisms. To comprehend the complexity of the relationships which develop between humans and their microbes, an understanding of some basic terms is first necessary. A pathogen is defined as any disease-producing microorganism, while a commensal is defined as an organism living on or within another organism that derives benefit from that organism without causing it injury. So which of these then defines an infecting organism? Although infection of a host by an organism is necessary for the production of disease, it does not always result in disease. Colonization of the host is also an infection, but it is one in which the host and organism evolve a commensal relationship without the development of disease. Thus, the answer is that both pathogenic and commensal organisms can be involved in the establishment of infection, and the disease process that may or may not develop is determined by the intricate interactions between the infecting organism and the host in which the infection has taken place.

The essential feature of an infection is the successful multiplication of a microbe on or within a host, and the term infectious disease applies when signs and symptoms result from this infection. Pathogenicity refers to the ability of an organism to cause disease, and virulence provides a quantitative measure of this property. Virulence factors refer to the properties that enable a microorganism to establish itself on or within a host and enhance its potential to cause disease. Virulence is not generally attributable to a single discrete factor but depends on several parameters related to the organism, the host, and their interaction. Virulence encompasses two general features of a pathogenic microorganism: its infectivity (ability to initiate an infection) and the severity of the condition produced. Highly virulent, moderately virulent, or avirulent strains may occur within a single species of organism. If host defenses are adequate, a person may be infected with a potential disease-causing microorganism for a prolonged period without the development of any signs or symptoms of disease. This is called asymptomatic carriage or asymptomatic infection. It should be emphasized that host factors will greatly influence whether infection results in colonization or disease.

Organisms of the normal flora (also known as commensal, colonizing, or endogenous organisms) become established in and on a host early in life and persist throughout life. Environmental factors, host characteristics, and microbial properties are all factors that determine whether exposure to a microbe will result in it becoming a colonizing part of the normal flora. Once established, a mutually beneficial relationship develops among the commensals as well as with the host. If the normal balance of these organisms is disrupted, as when host defense mechanisms are compromised, or if endogenous organisms are introduced into normally sterile body sites, they may then become pathogenic and cause disease. Other sources of pathogenic organisms are those from exogenous sources. These organisms enter the body through one of three routes: ingestion, inhalation, or direct penetration. Certain of these organisms will always be associated with pathogenicity, while others appear to cause disease only under certain circumstances. For example, a strict pathogen is always associated with disease, while principal pathogens are those which regularly cause disease in some proportion of healthy individuals. Opportunistic pathogens do not usually cause disease in people with intact defense systems yet are capable of devastating disease in immunocompromised individuals. The facultative pathogens exist between the two extremes of strict and opportunistic pathogens and comprise the majority of organisms found in the body. The capacity of some microorganisms but not others to cause disease reflects fundamental differences in their virulence capabilities. Tables 1 and 2 outline the most common organisms that are found as commensals and pathogens, respectively, in humans.

The current view is that a microbial pathogen is a highly adapted organism that follows an intricate strategy for survival. This chapter will focus on the complex issue of host-microbe interactions and the steps that are necessary for the development of disease.

COMPLEX NATURE BETWEEN HOST AND ORGANISM

The human body contains thousands of species of bacteria, viruses, fungi, and protozoa, and the interaction between the host and these microorganisms plays a critical role in the

* This chapter contains information presented in chapter 2 by Henry D. Isenberg and Richard F. D'Amato in the sixth edition of this Manual.

TABLE 1 Most common commensal organisms and sites

Body site	Organisms
Respiratory tract	
Aerobic bacteria	*Streptococcus pyogenes* (and other beta-hemolytic *Streptococcus*), *Streptococcus pneumoniae*, *Staphylococcus aureus*, coagulase-negative *Staphylococcus*, *Neisseria*, *Haemophilus*, *Moraxella*, *Corynebacterium*, *Stomatococcus*, enteric organisms, *Micrococcus*, *Lactobacillus*, *Mycoplasma*
Anaerobic bacteria	*Veillonella*, *Peptostreptococcus*, *Fusobacterium*, *Porphyromonas*, *Bacteroides*, *Prevotella*, *Actinomyces*, *Eubacterium*, *Bifidobacterium*, *Propionibacterium*
Fungi	*Candida* spp.
Parasites	*Entamoeba gingivalis*, *Trichomonas tenax*
Gastrointestinal tract	
Aerobic bacteria	*Lactobacillus*, *Enterococcus*, enteric organisms, *Corynebacterium*, *Streptococcus*, *Staphylococcus*
Anaerobic bacteria	*Bacteroides*, *Prevotella*, *Porphyromonas*, *Eubacterium*, *Fusobacterium*, *Peptostreptococcus*, *Clostridium*, *Bifidobacterium*, *Veillonella*, *Propionibacterium*, *Actinomyces*, *Mobiluncus*
Parasites	*Iodamoeba butschlii*, *Entamoeba coli*, *Entamoeba hartmanni*, *Endolimax nana*, *Chilomastix mesnili*, *Trichomonas hominis*
Viruses	Enteroviruses
Genital-urinary tract	
Aerobic bacteria	*Corynebacterium*, *Lactobacillus*, *Staphylococcus*, *Streptococcus*, nonpathogenic *Neisseria*, *Mycoplasma*, *Ureaplasma*, *Gardnerella vaginalis*, enteric organisms, *Acinetobacter*, *Capnocytophaga*, *Enterococcus*
Anaerobic bacteria	*Bacteroides*, *Porphyromonas*, *Prevotella*, *Fusobacterium*, *Mobiluncus*, *Peptostreptococcus*, *Propionibacterium*, *Actinomyces*, *Bifidobacterium*
Viruses	Adenovirus
Fungi	*Candida* spp.
Skin, ear, eye	
Aerobic bacteria	*Corynebacterium*, *Staphylococcus*, *Micrococcus*, nonpathogenic *Neisseria*, *Acinetobacter*, *Aerococcus*
Anaerobic bacteria	*Propionibacterium*, *Clostridium*, *Peptostreptococcus*
Fungi	*Candida*, *Absidia*, *Mucor*, *Malassezia*

host's survival. The normal population of these endogenous organisms participates in the metabolism of the host's food products and the production of essential growth factors, while it protects against infections with highly virulent microorganisms. The host does not carry all of these organisms all of the time, but at any one time, the host will possess a spectrum of species and strains. However, the line of demarcation of what constitutes the normal flora is often not clear. An important distinction exists between colonization with a pathogenic organism and the disease state produced by that organism. Although colonization is necessary for infection to take place, not all colonized persons will develop disease. Our normal microbial flora halts the proliferation of pathogenic organisms by a variety of methods including competition for nutrients or receptors on hosts cells, production of bacteriocins, and stimulation of the immune response. Thus, the pathogenic organisms residing in or on the body are, to an extent, controlled by our normal commensal organisms.

The establishment of disease relies on the ability of a microorganism to enter the host or to be introduced into a sterile area of the body and initiate infection. The first step of infection depends on the ability of the organism to attach to and survive within the host. Some pathogens will attach to superficial epithelial cells without invasion of subcutaneous tissues. In such cases, the toxins produced by the organisms are usually responsible for their associated pathology. Other organisms will also attach to epithelial cells but will subsequently penetrate this barrier, multiply in the subepithelium, and eventually gain access to the bloodstream, causing widespread dissemination of infection. Whether it is a primary or an opportunistic pathogen, an organism must be capable of entering a host, finding a unique niche, somehow avoiding or subverting the host's normal defenses, and multiplying in that setting. The capacity to reach a unique host niche free from microbial competition and safe from host defense mechanisms sets the foundation for the expression of specific determinants (virulence factors) that permit pathogens to establish themselves within a host and to be transmitted to new hosts.

Of the numerous microorganisms to which humans are exposed, very few actually succeed in causing disease. The ability to produce disease is determined by the organism's virulence properties, as well as by specific factors of the host. When first encountering its host, a successful pathogen must adapt dramatically to its changed environment. The transition from an external to an internal environment or from one host to a new host must be accomplished through substantial genetic regulatory events and the production of a variety of virulence factors by the infecting organism. The virulence factors involved in initially gaining access to the host involve the microbe's motility, chemotactic properties, and adhesive structures that mediate binding to host cells. Next, the pathogen must have mechanisms that allow it to survive its host's defenses. These mechanisms include avoidance (via antiphagocytic capsules, sialylation of cell envelopes, and immunoglobulin-covered cell membranes), subversion (via utilization of the host's enzymes for pathogenic processes, iron sequestering mechanisms, antigenic variation, and intracellular invasion and survival), and circumvention (via the production of enzymes and toxins and attachment to alternative cellular receptors). If the pathogen has been successful in initiating an infection, three possible outcomes exist: (i) a state of relative equilibrium develops, with the host establishing a chronic infection which may or may not be associated with significant morbidity;

TABLE 2 Most common pathogenic organisms and sites

Body site	Organisms	Body site	Organisms
Blood		Ear	
Aerobic bacteria	Coagulase-negative *Staphylococcus*, *Staphylococcus aureus*, *Streptococcus pneumoniae*, *Enterococcus*, enteric organisms, *Pseudomonas*, *Haemophilus influenzae*	Aerobic bacteria	*Streptococcus pneumoniae*, *Haemophilus influenzae*, *Moraxella catarrhalis*, *Pseudomonas aeruginosa*
Anaerobic bacteria	*Bacteroides fragilis*	Fungi	*Aspergillus*, *Candida* spp.
Fungi	*Candida albicans*	Viruses	Respiratory syncytial virus, influenza virus, enterovirus, rhinovirus
Viruses	Human immunodeficiency virus, hepatitis B virus, hepatitis A virus, cytomegalovirus	Eye	
Central nervous system		Aerobic bacteria	*Streptococcus pneumoniae*, *Staphylococcus aureus*, coagulase-negative *Staphylococcus*, *Haemophilus influenzae*, subsp. *aegypticus*, *Neisseria gonorrhoeae*, *Pseudomonas*, *Moraxella catarrhalis*, *Bacillus*, *Chlamydia trachomatis*
Aerobic bacteria	*Streptococcus pneumoniae*, *Haemophilus influenzae*, *Neisseria meningitidis*, *Streptococcus agalactiae*, coagulase-negative *Staphylococcus*, *Staphylococcus aureus*, *Listeria monocytogenes*, *Escherichia coli*, *Mycobacterium tuberculosis*, *Nocardia*, *Treponema pallidum*, *Borrelia*, *Leptospira*	Parasites	*Acanthamoeba* spp.
		Viruses	Adenovirus, cytomegalovirus
		Stomach	
		Aerobic bacteria	*Helicobacter pylori*
Fungi	*Candida albicans*, *Cryptococcus neoformans*, *Histoplasma capsulatum*, *Coccidioides immitis*	Intestine	
Viruses	Enteroviruses, herpes simplex virus, arboviruses, mumps virus, human immunodeficiency virus	Aerobic bacteria	*Campylobacter*, *Salmonella*, *Shigella*, *Vibrio*, *Staphylococcus aureus*, *Bacillus cereus*, *Yersinia*, *Escherichia coli*, *Edwardsiella*, *Aeromonas*
Parasites	*Naegleria fowleri*, *Acanthamoeba* spp.	Anaerobic bacteria	*Clostridium*, *Bacteroides*
Upper respiratory tract		Parasites	*Giardia lamblia*, hookworms, tapeworms, *Blastocystis hominis*, *Trichuris trichiura*, *Ascaris lumbricoides*, *Clonorchis sinensis*, *Strongyloides stercoralis*, *Enterobius vermicularis*, *Entamoeba histolytica*, *Cryptosporidium parvum*, *Dientamoeba fragilis*, *Microsporidium*, *Cyclospora*, *Balantidium*, *Isospora*
Aerobic bacteria	*Streptococcus pyogenes*, *Arcanobacterium haemolyticum*, *Chlamydia pneumoniae*, *Neisseria gonorrhoeae*, *Corynebacterium diphtheriae*, *Mycoplasma pneumoniae*		
Fungi	*Candida* spp.		
Viruses	Rhinovirus, coronavirus, herpes simplex virus, Epstein-Barr virus, adenovirus, coxsackievirus A, parainfluenza viruses	Viruses	Rotavirus, Norwalk viruses, adenovirus, astrovirus, coronavirus
		Genital	
Lower respiratory tract		Aerobic bacteria	*Neisseria gonorrhoeae*, *Chlamydia trachomatis*, *Mycoplasma*, *Ureaplasma*, *Treponema pallidum*, *Haemophilus ducreyi*, *Calymmatobacterium*
Aerobic bacteria	*Staphylococcus aureus*, *Streptococcus pneumoniae*, *Haemophilus influenzae*, *Moraxella catarrhalis*, *Klebsiella pneumoniae*, *Escherichia coli*, *Pseudomonas aeruginosa*, *Legionella*, *Mycobacterium tuberculosis*, *Nocardia*, *Mycoplasma pneumoniae*, *Chlamydia pneumoniae*, *Bordetella pertussis*, *Chlamydia trachomatis*, *Chlamydia psittaci*	Anaerobic bacteria	*Actinomyces*, *Bacteroides*, *Fusobacterium*, *Clostridium*, *Mobiluncus*
		Fungi	*Candida* spp.
		Parasites	*Trichomonas vaginalis*
		Viruses	Herpes simplex virus, papillomavirus
Anaerobic bacteria	Mixed anaerobes		
Viruses	Respiratory syncytial virus, parainfluenza viruses, influenza virus, rhinovirus, adenovirus, coxsackievirus A		
Fungi	*Pneumocystis carinii*, *Histoplasma*, *Blastomyces*, *Coccidioides*, *Cryptococcus*		

(Continued on next page)

TABLE 2 Most common pathogenic organisms and sites (*Continued*)

Body site	Organisms	Body site	Organisms
Skin and soft tissue		Bone and joint	
Aerobic bacteria	*Streptococcus pyogenes*, *Staphylococcus aureus*, coagulase-negative *Staphylococcus*, *Pseudomonas aeruginosa*, *Haemophilus influenzae*, enteric organisms, *Mycobacterium*, *Nocardia*, *Vibrio vulnificus*, *Francisella*, *Erysipelothrix*, *Bartonella*, *Treponema*	Aerobic bacteria	*Staphylococcus aureus*, *Neisseria gonorrhoeae*, *Streptococcus*, *Haemophilus influenzae*, enteric organisms, *Pseudomonas*, coagulase-negative *Staphylococcus*, *Mycobacterium*
		Fungi	*Sporothrix schenckii*, *Coccidioides*, *Candida* spp.
		Viruses	Rubella virus, hepatitis B virus, mumps virus, parvovirus B19
Anaerobic bacteria	*Clostridium perfringens*, *Bacteroides fragilis*, *Peptostreptococcus*		
Fungi	*Candida* spp., *Malassezia furfur*, *Epidermophyton*, *Microsporum*, *Trichophyton*, *Sporothrix schenckii*, *Aspergillus*, *Blastomyces*	Urinary tract	
		Aerobic bacteria	*Escherichia coli*, *Proteus mirabilis*, *Klebsiella*, *Enterobacter*, *Pseudomonas*, *Enterococcus*, *Staphylococcus saprophyticus*, *Staphylococcus aureus*, *Ureaplasma*, *Mycobacterium tuberculosis*, *Neisseria gonorrhoeae*
Parasites	*Onchocerca*, *Mansonella*, *Leishmania*		
Viruses	Herpes simplex virus, varicella-zoster virus, coxsackie virus A, papillomavirus		
		Fungi	*Candida* spp.
		Parasites	*Schistosoma haematobium*
		Viruses	Cytomegalovirus, adenovirus

(ii) host defense mechanisms supervene and the infectious organism is cleared; and less commonly, (iii) the organism proliferates and produces toxic products, resulting in a wide range of signs and symptoms of disease, including death. The host involved in the first two more common scenarios is most often asymptomatic or exhibits only subclinical signs but is generally better off for its encounter with the infecting organism (e.g., because of the development of specific immunity).

The eventual outcome of infection involves a wide array of interactions between the host and the organism. The concept that a few virulence factors are sufficient to explain why one organism can cause disease and another one cannot oversimplifies the complex nature of the interaction between a microbe and its host. We must consider how a cause-and-effect relationship is established between an organism and the disease that it causes and between a particular trait of an organism and its virulence. A review of Koch's postulates, guidelines for determining whether a microorganism is the cause of disease, implies that virulence is a trait that resides entirely in the organism and is independent of the host. It is now quite clear that the attributes of the human host are at least as important as the traits of the microorganism. Normal host defenses pose the most difficult set of obstacles to the arriving pathogen. The primary host defenses that are most effective against the initial assault by infecting organisms include anatomic barriers such as intact skin, ciliated cells in the respiratory and alimentary canals, and the flow of substance through the respiratory and alimentary tracts. Any breaks in the skin or mucosal surfaces can lead to local proliferation of organisms and the potential onset of infection. Host physiologic factors that inhibit microbial growth and minimize the chance for infection include the accumulation of fatty acids in the skin, high or low pH and oxygen tensions, and biological enzymes and acids. The normal flora of the host also inhibits the proliferation of pathogens by competing for nutrients or cell membrane binding sites and by producing substances that destroy invading organisms. Secondary host defenses include naturally occurring substances such as complement, lysozyme, opsonin in plasma, and other body secretions, phagocytosis by neutrophils and macrophages, the production of antibodies, and cell-mediated immune responses. Obviously, any defects in the host's humoral or cellular immune defenses will increase the susceptibility of a host to infection. Other factors that affect host resistance to infection and/or disease include age (with those at the extremes of age, i.e., very young and very old people, being more susceptible to disease); the presence of chronic or debilitating diseases; the use of therapeutic agents, alcohol, and illicit drugs; traumatic, physical, or emotional stress; and the presence of foreign material at the site of infection. Diet is also an important host factor in resistance to disease. Malnutrition has a profound impact on certain host defense systems, the most consistent being the inhibition of cell-mediated immunity due primarily to a lack of mature functionally differentiated T lymphocytes. Although B cells and immunoglobulin levels are normal in malnourished individuals, these individuals show a diminished production of those antibodies that depend on T cells to help initiate the B-cell response and show a decrease in the switch from immunoglobulin M (IgM) to IgG production that is likewise T-cell dependent. Other abnormalities of the immune system associated with malnutrition are the decrease in secretory IgA (sIgA) production and the depression of the complement system (9). Small defects in individual defense mechanisms may be unimportant alone, but together they can make the difference between asymptomatic infection and severe disease.

Before discussing individual virulence factors, we must realize how our understanding of pathogenic organisms and mechanisms of disease has changed over the years. The most revolutionary advance in biomedical science since the time of Koch and his postulates is the discovery of nucleic acids as a source of genetic information and as the basis for the precise characterization of an organism. The ability to detect and manipulate these nucleic acids has created a powerful means for identifying previously unknown microbial pathogens and for studying the host-microbe relationship. Fredricks and Relman (6) offer new guidelines for the establishment of causal relationships between microbes and disease on the basis of nucleic acid technology. These more sophisticated techniques now enable us to recognize the roles played in diseases by microbes that were not even known to be infectious at one time.

In summary, a wide variety of microorganisms are able to enter, survive, and multiply within their hosts by evolving an almost endless collection of adaptations and virulence factors that allow them to overcome or avoid host defenses. It is the complex interactions of these organisms with the host's defense mechanisms that determine the outcome of the infective process. Many of these mechanisms and interactions will be discussed in this chapter.

VIRULENCE FACTORS

Microbial virulence factors that influence an organism's outcome upon entering a host include those that promote adherence and binding to cells and surfaces, force phagocytosis of organisms by nonphagocytic cells, acquire and utilize host resources, and prevent phagocytic uptake. Additional factors include those that reduce complement activation, render them resistant to serum, destroy phagocytes and tissues, and allow modulation and evasion of the immune system. With an understanding of these mechanisms, one can begin to comprehend the complexity of the host-microbe interaction that may or may not lead to disease.

Attachment

Most infections are initiated by the attachment of the microbe to host tissues, followed by microbial replication in order to establish colonization. This attachment can be relatively nonspecific or can require the interaction between structures on the microbial surface and specific receptors on host cells. Two common elements are used by microbes for adherence: pili and adhesins. A pilus is a rod-shaped protein structure that extends outward from the microbial surface to establish contact between its surface and the surface of the host cell. Binding of a pilus to its host target cell can be quite specific, and the availability of suitable receptors will often determine what body site is infected with the organism. Bacterial adherence can also be accomplished by a process involving bacterial cell surface structures known as adhesins and complementary receptors on the surfaces of host cells. Adhesins are the proteins that promote the tighter binding of bacteria to host cells following initial binding via pili. The mechanism used by a microorganism to adhere to a host cell dictates its ability to enter the cell and set into motion a number of physiologic events. An elegant example of microbial attachment followed by a sequence of pathological effects is that of enteropathogenic *Escherichia coli* (EPEC). Following initial adhesion, intracellular calcium levels increase, activating actin-severing enzymes and protein kinases, which then lead to vesiculation and disruption of the microvilli. The bacteria are then able to attach to the epithelium in a more intimate fashion, allowing maximal activation of protein kinases. This results in major changes to the cytoskeleton and alterations in the permeability of the membrane to ions. Changes in ion permeation result in ion secretion and reduction in absorption, resulting in the secretory diarrhea that is the hallmark of this disease. It has been found that a majority of EPEC isolates contain a large plasmid that codes for its adhesive properties (1).

As well as binding to receptors on the host cell surface, some bacteria also form dense, multiorganism layers, called biofilms, in which the first layer of bacteria attaches directly to the surface of the host cells and other layers of bacteria are attached to this basal layer by a polysaccharide matrix. Biofilms have been detected in the vaginal tract, the mouth, and the intestines, and in fact, the resident microflora of these sites may largely be organized into biofilms. These dense mats of organisms may help explain the barrier function of these sites in protection of the host. However, the formation of biofilms may also be the prelude to disease. For example, dental plaque is a biofilm that is known to cause disease, and *Pseudomonas aeruginosa* has been shown to establish pathogenic biofilms in the lungs of cystic fibrosis patients. Indeed, hospital-acquired infections in patients with indwelling urinary or venous catheters are generally preceded by the formation of a biofilm on the interior wall of the catheter. Organisms within biofilms are more resistant to antibiotics than individual bacteria and are partially protected from phagocytes as well. Biofilm formation on embedded plastic devices provides yet another example of the iatrogenic activities that continue to create new niches that microorganisms can exploit.

After successfully adhering to the host and initiating infection, an organism must successfully survive and multiply within its host. To help achieve this goal, organisms have developed the ability to produce a variety of substances that allow them to neutralize host defense mechanisms. Collectively, these substances are termed "aggressins" and comprise capsules and extracellular slime substances, surface proteins, carbohydrates, enzymes, toxins, and various other molecules. Some aggressins act after phagocytosis of the organism has taken place either by inhibiting phagosome-lysosome fusion or by producing enzymes such as catalase and superoxide dismutase, which inhibit the organism's destruction by the myeloperoxidase system of the phagocyte. Survival inside phagocytes also protects the organisms from destruction by specific antibodies and complement components of the host. Many of these virulence factors will be further detailed on the pages that follow, with examples given in Table 3.

Motility

Some mucosal surfaces are protected from microbial colonization because they are constantly being washed with fast-moving fluids. In such cases, organisms that can move directionally toward a mucosal surface will have a better chance of contacting host surfaces than nonmotile organisms. Although motility due to flagella and directional swimming (chemotaxis) are appealing candidates for virulence factors, in only a few cases has motility been proven to be essential for virulence (17).

Resistance to Serum

Resistance to the lytic effects of complement is almost a universal requirement for pathogens that traverse mucosal or skin barriers but remain in the extracellular environment. The lytic effect of serum on gram-negative organisms is complement mediated and can be initiated by the classical or alternative pathway. One of the principal targets of complement is the lipopolysaccharide (LPS) layer of gram-negative bacteria. Certain pathogens, called "serum resistant," have evolved defense mechanisms that allow them to negate the detrimental effects of complement. Serum resistance can

TABLE 3 Examples of virulence factors

Virulence factor	Examples	Effect(s)
Attachment	Pili of *Neisseria gonorrhoeae*	Allows for nonspecific attachment and penetration into host cell
	Adhesins of EPEC	Interaction of specific receptors between host and organism
	Staphylococcus species and catheter-related biofilms	Allows more resistance to antimicrobial agents
Aggressins	LPS (endotoxin) of gram-negative bacilli	Blunts inflammatory response allowing establishment
	Serum resistance of gram-negative bacilli	Failure to bind and activate complement
	Capsules of *Cryptococcus neoformans*	Decreases phagocytosis by polymorphonuclear cells
	Enzymes: hyaluronidase, protease, DNase, elastinase, collagenase, and phospholipase	Destroys structural barriers and facilitates invasion and spread in tissue by organisms
	Siderophores of *Haemophilus influenzae*	Utilizes biological heme complexes for essential iron
	Toxins of *Vibrio cholerae*	Responsible for profuse diarrhea
	Superantigens of *Staphylococcus aureus*	Massive release of cytokines leading to systemic symptoms
Antigenic variation	Hemagglutinin and neuraminidase of influenza viruses	Evades herd immunity by periodically changing antigenic types
	Protein A of *Staphylococcus aureus*	Binds to Fc portion of immunoglobulins, prevents recognition by immune system
Intracellular residence	pH modulation of phagolysosome by *Histoplasma capsulatum*	Intraphagocytic survival of *Histoplasma capsulatum*
	Listeriolysin of *Listeria monocytogenes*	Dissolves phagolysosomal membrane prior to lysosomal enzyme damage to bacterium

occur by several mechanisms: (i) failure to bind and activate complement, (ii) shedding of the surface molecules that activate the complement system, (iii) interruption of the complement cascade before the formation of C5b-C9, and (iv) enhancement of the formation of nonlytic complexes. Many of the microbes that are able to cause systemic infections are serum resistant, indicating the importance of this trait.

Capsules

A capsule is a loose, relatively unstructured network of polymers that covers the surface of an organism. Most of the well-studied capsules are composed of polysaccharides, but capsules can also be made of proteins or protein-carbohydrate mixtures. The role of capsules in microbial virulence is to protect the organism from the host inflammatory response of complement activation and phagocyte-mediated destruction. Although the host will normally make antibodies directed against the bacterial capsule, some bacteria are able to subvert this type of protective host response by having capsules that resemble host polysaccharides.

Cryptococcus neoformans is an encapsulated pathogenic fungus. The mechanism by which the capsule of *C. neoformans* enables the organism to evade host defenses is the presentation of a surface not recognized by phagocytes. Although the capsule of *C. neoformans* is a potent activator of the alternative complement pathway, in cryptococcal sepsis, massive activation of complement by capsular polysaccharides can lead to marked depletion of serum complement components and the subsequent loss of serum opsonic capacity. Other immunosuppressive effects that have been attributed to the presence of capsules include down-regulation of cytokine secretion, inhibition of leukocyte accumulation, induction of suppressor T cells and suppressor factors, inhibition of antigen presentation, and inhibition of lymphoproliferation.

Intracellular Residence

Invasive organisms penetrate anatomic barriers and either enter cells or pass through them to disseminate within the body. To survive under these conditions, organisms have developed special virulence factors that enable them to avoid or disarm host phagocytes. One such antiphagocytic strategy prevents the migration of phagocytes to the site where organisms are growing or limits their effectiveness once there. Some microbes are capable of producing toxic proteins that kill phagocytes once they have arrived, while other microbes have developed the ability to survive after phagocytosis by polymorphonuclear cells, monocytes, or macrophages. Strategies for surviving phagocytosis include escaping from the phagosome before it merges with the lysosome, preventing phagosome-lysosome fusion from occurring, or after fusion, enzymatically dissolving the phagolysosome membrane and escaping. *Toxoplasma gondii* is a classic example of an organism that is a successful intracellular parasite. After entry *T. gondii* resides within a phagosome vacuole that is permanently made incapable of fusion with other intracellular organelles, including lysosomes. The parasite's survival within this vacuole depends on maintaining the appropriate pH, excluding lysosomal contents, and turning on specific mechanisms necessary for nutrient acquisition while it is contained inside the vacuole (18).

Long-term survival within macrophages after the resolution of initial disease is responsible for the late reactivation of *Histoplasma capsulatum* infection when host immunity is compromised. Intracellular parasitism by *H. capsulatum* yeast cells and microconidia begins with attachment via specific receptors to human macrophages followed by rapid phagocytosis. Intracellular *H. capsulatum* yeasts have evolved mechanisms that allow them to survive in the presence of products of the respiratory burst while living and growing inside of phagocytes. A key virulence factor for the survival of intracellular *H. capsulatum* may be its ability to modulate the phagolysosomal pH. Lysosomal hydrolases require acidic pH for activity, and resistance of the yeasts to phagolysosomal destruction by those hydrolases stems from their ability to keep an elevated pH (3). Possible mechanisms used by *H. capsulatum* to alter the pH of phagolysosomes include active buffering of the compartment or modification of the proton pump in the compartment's membrane.

Enzymes

Many pathogenic organisms produce enzymes such as hyaluronidase, proteases, DNases, collagenase, elastinase, and phospholipases which are capable of hydrolyzing host tissues and disrupting the cellular structure. Although not normally considered classic exotoxins, these enzymes can destroy host cells as effectively as exotoxins and are frequently sufficient to initiate clinical disease. For example, *Aspergillus* species secrete a variety of proteases which function as virulence factors by degrading the structural barriers of the host, thereby facilitating the invasion of tissues (12). Other examples are the hyaluronidase and gelatinase enzymes that have been long associated with virulent enterococci. Hyaluronidase-producing enterococci have been implicated as the cause of periodontal disease due to their disruption of the intercellular cementing substances of the epithelium (16). Studies of hyaluronidase in other microorganisms describe it as a spreading factor in *Ancylostoma duodenale* cutaneous larva migrans (8) and as an important factor in the dissemination of *Treponema pallidum* (5).

Organisms attempting to establish themselves in a host must avoid being trapped in the mucin layer of the host's surfaces. The stickiness of the mucin layer is caused in part by sIgA molecules which specifically prevent organism attachment. sIgA proteases are microbial enzymes that cleave sIgA molecules, and although their role is not yet fully defined, it is suggested that these enzymes play an important part in the colonization of mucosal surfaces by invading organisms (17).

Iron Acquisition Mechanisms

Although the human body contains a plentiful supply of iron, the majority of this iron is not easily accessible to microorganisms. The concentration of usable iron is particularly low in the human body because lactoferrin, transferrin, ferritin, and hemin bind most of the available iron, and the amount of free iron remaining is far below the level required to support microbial growth (17). Thus, microorganisms have evolved a number of mechanisms for the acquisition of iron from their environments (13). Microorganisms produce siderophores which chelate iron with a very high affinity and which compete effectively with transferrin and lactoferrin to mobilize iron for microbial use. Although siderophore-based iron acquisition has been shown to contribute to the virulence of some pathogens, mutations that eliminate specific siderophore production or uptake do not always decrease virulence. This could explain why microorganisms often have more than one iron-sequestering system. In addition, some microbial species can utilize host iron complexes directly without the production of siderophores. For example, *Neisseria* species possess specific receptors for transferrin and can remove iron from transferrin at the cell surface; *Yersinia pestis* can use heme as a sole source of iron; *Vibrio vulnificus* can utilize iron from the hemoglobin-haptoglobin complex; and *Haemophilus influenzae* can utilize hemoglobin, hemoglobin-haptoglobin, heme-hemopexin, and heme-albumin complexes as iron sources. Another mechanism for iron acquisition is the production of hemolysins, which act to release iron complexed to intracellular heme and hemoglobin.

Exotoxins

Disease is frequently the result of the production of microbial toxins, which generally fall into two groups: exotoxins and endotoxins. Exotoxins are toxic microbial proteins that are usually heat labile and that are excreted into the surrounding environment during exponential growth of the organisms, while endotoxins, also known as LPSs, are embedded in the outer membranes of gram-negative bacteria. Another term commonly used for some microbial toxic products are enterotoxins, which are proteins that cause enteric symptoms such as diarrhea or vomiting.

Exotoxins are produced by a variety of organisms, including gram-positive and gram-negative bacteria, and can cause disease through several different mechanisms. First, exotoxins can be produced in food and consumed along with the food. Disease produced by these exotoxins is generally self-limiting because the bacteria do not remain in the body, thus eliminating the source of the exotoxin. Second, bacteria growing in a wound or tissue produce exotoxins that cause damage to the surrounding tissues of the host, contributing to the spread of infection. Third, bacteria can colonize a wound or mucosal surface and produce exotoxins which enter the bloodstream and affect distant organs and tissues. The toxins that attack a variety of different cell types are called cytotoxins, whereas those that attack specific cell types are designated by the cell type or organ affected, such as a neurotoxins, leukotoxin, or hepatotoxin. Exotoxins can also be named for the species of bacteria that produces them or for the disease with which they are associated, such as cholera toxin, Shiga toxin, diphtheria toxin, and tetanus toxin. Toxins are also named on the basis of their activities, for example, adenylate cyclase and lecithinase, while others are simply given letter designations, such as *P. aeruginosa* exotoxin A.

Three general types of exotoxins have been described on the basis of their structure and activities. The first type is known as the A-B toxin, which is so designated because the portion of the toxin that binds to a host cell receptor (portion B) is separate from the portion that mediates the enzyme activity responsible for its toxicity (portion A). Two structural types of A-B toxins exist. The simplest kind is synthesized as a single protein with a disulfide bond. A more complex type of A-B toxin has a binding portion (portion B) that is composed of multiple subunits but that is still attached to the A portion by a disulfide bond. The disulfide bonds are broken when the B portion binds to a specific host cell surface molecule and the A portion is taken into the host cell. Thus, the B portion of the molecule determines the host cell specificity of the toxin. For example, if the B portion binds specifically to cell receptors found only on the surface of neurons, the toxins will be a specific neurotoxin. Generally speaking, without this cell receptor specificity, the A portion of these toxins could kill many cell types if they were to gain entry into the cells. Once having entered the host cell, the A portion becomes enzymatically active and exerts its toxic effect. The A portion of most exotoxins affects the cyclic AMP (cAMP) levels in the host cell by ribosylating the protein that controls cAMP. Processes or compounds that affect the cAMP levels in the cell cause a variety of metabolic effects, including the loss of control of ion flow, which results in the loss of water from the host tissue into the lumen of the intestine, causing diarrhea. Other toxins have A portions that cleave host cell rRNA, thereby shutting down protein synthesis.

A second type of exotoxin, called membrane-disrupting toxins, lyse host cells by disrupting the integrity of their plasma membranes. There are two types of membrane-disrupting toxins. One is a protein that inserts itself into the host cell membrane by using cholesterol as a receptor and forms channels or pores, allowing cytoplasmic contents to leak out and water to enter. The second type of membrane-disrupting exotoxin is phospholipases. These enzymes remove the charged head group from the phospholipids of the cell membrane, which destabilizes the membrane and causes cell lysis. These enzymes are appropriately referred to as cytotoxins.

In recent years, a significant amount of information has been generated about the third group of microbial exotoxins, those known as superantigens (11). Normally, antigen-presenting cells (APCs) process antigens by cleaving them into peptides and displaying one of the resulting peptides along with major histocompatibility complex (MHC) proteins on its surface. Only a few T cells will have the receptors that recognize this particular MHC-peptide complex, so only a few T cells will be stimulated. Superantigens, however, are not processed inside of APCs but indiscriminately bind directly to MHC receptors on the APC surface. For example, a conventional antigen can interact with 0.0001 to 0.000001% of a host's T cells, while superantigens are capable of interaction with as many as 5 to 20% of T cells. This binding of superantigens triggers cell activation, differentiation, proliferation, and the excessive release of inflammatory cytokines. These cytokins give rise to a variety of symptoms including nausea, vomiting, malaise, fever, and shock. Although a number of gram-negative and gram-positive bacteria have been shown to produce superantigens, the pathogenic role of superantigens in human disease is best defined by staphylococcal and streptococcal toxic shock syndrome (TSS). Staphylococcal TSS is a severe multisystem disorder characterized by fever, rash, hypotension, and multiple organ failure. In its most severe form, streptococcal TSS manifestations include shock, multiple organ failure, soft tissue destruction, capillary leakage, and necrotizing fasciitis and can lead to death in 30% of patients (19, 20). It is believed that infection with certain organisms that produce superantigens can also trigger autoimmunity (10). This may be done by superantigens indiscriminately activating cells that lead to polyclonal activation of B cells and the generation of autoantibodies (7). Several autoimmune disorders, including rheumatic heart disease, rheumatoid arthritis, multiple sclerosis, and Graves' disease, have been linked to superantigens. Several groups have also hypothesized that superantigens of some strains of *Streptococcus pyogenes* and *Staphylococcus aureus* induce the release of cytokines that can alter infant sleep patterns, induce deep sleep, and result in failure of the infant to breath properly, leading to sudden infant death syndrome (2, 14).

It has been proposed that superantigens also allow microorganisms to avert the effects of the immune system by at least three mechanisms. First, the ability to induce superantigen-dependent cellular cytotoxicity may render T cells anergic and incapable of responding to the pathogen. Second, the ability of superantigens to cause the overproduction of inflammatory cytokines may allow them to specifically kill T cells that have receptors for that superantigen. Lastly, the generation of a nonspecific immune response by the superantigen directs attention away from what would have been a specific response to the pathogen. Inasmuch as cytokines play a pivotal role in mediating the pathogenesis of TSS, host genetic factors that regulate cytokine responses to superantigens and environmental factors such as coinfection, stress, or hormonal changes in the host are equally as important.

Endotoxins

Endotoxin is the LPS component of the outer membrane of gram-negative bacteria. Its toxic lipid portion (lipid A) is embedded in the outer membrane, with its core antigen extending outward from the bacterial surface. Endotoxins are heat stable, destroyed by formaldehyde, and relatively less toxic than many exotoxins. Lipid A exerts its effects when bacteria lyse by binding to plasma proteins and then interacting with receptors on monocytes, macrophages, and other host cells, thereby forcing the production of cytokines and the activation of the complement and coagulation cascades. The result of these events is an increase in temperature, a decrease in blood pressure, damage to vessel walls, disseminated intravascular coagulation, and a decrease in blood flow to essential organs such as the lung, kidney, and brain, leading to organ failure. Also, activation of the coagulation cascade leads to insufficiency of clotting components, resulting in hemorrhage and further organ damage. Superantigens can also greatly enhance the host's susceptibility to endotoxic shock by acting synergistically with endotoxin to further augment the release of inflammatory cytokines that are lethal to cells of the immune system (11).

Antigenic Variation

Certain bacteria, viruses, and protozoa are unusually adept at evading the host's immune response by changing their surface antigens (15). Bacteria growing in the body are constantly losing and reforming pili. This continual pilus replacement provides the bacteria a way of evading the host's immune response. Once the host begins to produce antibody to a particular type of pilus, that pilus type is no longer useful to the bacterium. Replacing one type of pilus with another renders the host's antibody response useless. For example, *Neisseria gonorrhoeae* will intermittently produce pili as well as vary the antigenic type of pilus produced often enough so that the host cannot mount a successful antibody response in order to prevent colonization. In addition to the changes in the antigenicity of pilin, the outer membrane proteins of the gonococcus also undergo antigenic variation. Thus, the surfaces of these organisms display a highly variable antigenic profile to their host's immune system. The tendency of influenza to reappear in a population on a regular basis is partly due to the ability of influenza viruses to undergo antigenic variation. A minor change in its surface proteins, i.e., hemagglutinin and neuraminidase, that occurs every 2 to 3 years is called "antigenic drift," while major changes, called "antigenic shifts," are associated with outbreaks of clinically severe influenza which occur approximately every 10 years. *Trypanosoma brucei* organisms, the protozoal parasites that cause African sleeping sickness, are covered with thick protein coats which undergo antigenic change during infection. These parasites have several hundred genes that encode different antigenic surface types but express only one antigenic type at a time. When antibody against one type of antigen is made by the host, the level of parasitemia drops, only to rebound with a new antigenic type, resulting in several waves of parasitemia. Another way that organisms can evade the host's antibody response is to vary their surface proteins so that they are mistaken for a part of the host itself. Organisms can also coat themselves with host proteins to accomplish this same result. An interesting example of this type of defense is the protein A of *S. aureus* that binds to the Fc portion of antibodies, thus coating the bacteria with host antibody, which prevents recognition of the bacteria by the immune system. It is conceivable that microbial binding of lactoferrin, transferrin, and other host iron-binding proteins serves a dual function, one as a protective coat and the other as a source of iron acquisition (17).

REGULATION OF VIRULENCE

The human body presents incoming microorganisms with a variety of ecological niches, all of which provide opportunities for colonization if the organism can adapt rapidly enough to take advantage of its new surroundings. Pathogens entering the human body must quickly adapt to changes in temperature, pH, osmotic strength, oxygen availability, and nutrient concentrations. For effective microbial pathogenesis, an organism must sense its environment accurately and respond with appropriate alterations in its expression of virulence. The ability to produce virulence factors in the amounts that are needed and when they are needed and to stop producing factors that are no longer appropriate is one of the most important characteristics of a successful pathogen. The production of virulence factors is controlled by regulatory mechanisms that fall into three categories. First are mechanisms that increase the number of copies of the gene (gene amplification) or that affect genetic structure (gene rearrangements, gene replacements, and gene mutations). Second are mechanisms that affect the number of transcripts made from a particular gene (transcriptional regulation), and third are those that determine the amount of gene product made from each transcript (posttranscriptional regulation). It is not uncommon for more than one regulatory strategy to be used to control a set of virulence genes, which can allow the organism to respond to combinations of environmental signals.

Gene rearrangements, replacements, and mutations involve changes in the structure of a gene itself. The new version of the protein produced from the altered gene is no longer recognized by antibodies directed against the original protein. This type of switching allows for antigenic variation which helps the organisms evade the host's antibody response. Similar results could be achieved by spontaneous mutation; however, the rate of spontaneous mutation in a gene is usually too low to allow the organism to respond rapidly to environmental conditions and may not have the desired effect of making a new protein that is functional but antigenically different from the original one. The advantage of the gene replacement strategy is that the organism is able to shift between mutant forms of the gene that are all functional yet antigenically distinct.

Transcriptional regulation controls the number of transcripts made from a genetic sequence via mechanisms of gene organization, transcriptional activation, and transcriptional repression.

Gene organization. Virulence genes can be transcribed as a part of a single transcript (or operon) that is controlled by a single promoter or as a part of a regulon whose genes are located in different areas but have the same promoter region and respond in the same way to the same regulatory protein. Conversely, a set of genes that respond to the same signal but that do not respond in the same way is called a stimulon. The advantage of the regulon and stimulon systems is that a gene located anywhere on the chromosome or even on an extrachromosomal element can be part of the assault arsenal as long as it has the appropriate type of promoter region.

Transcriptional activation. For a gene to be transcribed, RNA polymerase must bind to the promoter and produce the form of DNA that allows mRNA synthesis to proceed. Transcriptional activators are the proteins that facilitate the binding of RNA polymerases to the promoter region and that also act to increase the number of transcripts made from a gene. In many cases, regulation of virulence genes appears to involve a cascade of activators, which has the advantage of enabling the organism to modulate its response to a particular stimulus in a more efficient way than if all of the genes were controlled by a single activator.

Transcriptional repression. Transcriptional repressors are the opposite of transcriptional activators and act by preventing transcription. Repressors act either by binding to the promoter, thus preventing RNA polymerase from binding to the promoter, or by binding downstream of RNA polymerase, preventing the bound RNA polymerase from starting transcription. Transcriptional activators and repressors have active and inactive forms, and usually the shift from one to the other is accomplished by the binding of a ligand. For example, iron is an important regulator of many virulence genes, and in some cases high levels of virulence gene expression are seen only when iron concentrations are low.

The step after transcription is translation, and posttranscriptional regulation is of considerable importance in controlling the levels of active virulence factors. It is noteworthy that regulation at the posttranscriptional level does not preclude regulation at transcriptional and other levels and that the production of a single virulence factor is often regulated at multiple levels. Also, the form of the protein translated from mRNA may not be in an active state, and this allows yet another level of regulation, that of posttranslational activation. Many virulence factors undergo a posttranslational processing in which the protein is cleaved or covalently modified to become activated. Thus, it is apparent that the synthesis of many microbial virulence factors is tightly controlled by multiple regulatory systems.

Pathogenicity is not a microbial trait that has appeared by chance. Instead, particular microbial strains and species have evolved to carry very specific arrays of virulence-associated genes. Although periodic selection of mutant clones may play a role in the evolution of pathogenesis, it does not explain many of the differences between pathogenic and nonpathogenic organisms of the same species. A number of separate observations also indicate that microbes frequently carry virulence genes and regulators of virulence genes on mobile genetic elements. Bacteriophages, transposons, and extrachromosomal elements such as plasmids are supplements to the genome that allow a microbe to maintain the integrity of its chromosome and yet increase its genetic diversity. Thus, acquisition of an adhesin, toxin, or serum resistance factor might lead a nonpathogenic organism to cause disease in a host in which it previously could not. Recently, investigators have seen that many bacterial pathogens carry large inserts of DNA, called pathogenicity islands, that are not found in nonpathogenic members of the species (4). For instance, uropathogenic *E. coli* and enteropathogenic *E. coli* possess large fragments of DNA which include a number of virulence genes that are absent from commensal *E. coli* strains. Interestingly, the DNA compositions of these genetic inserts differ markedly from the DNA composition normally found within the genomes of these organisms. This difference in DNA suggests that the pathogenicity islands are alien to the host chromosome, perhaps being derived from recombinations of horizontally transmitted mobile genetic elements (4).

Thus, the regulation of a number of virulence determinants by environmental substances appears to be complex and to require more than one regulatory factor. Additional regulatory proteins may be needed to provide the fine-tuning necessary for the precise regulation of individual virulence genes in response to environmental signals. It is very apparent that studies of microbial pathogenicity at the molecular level have made substantial contributions to our understanding of the epidemiology, clinical manifestations, diagnosis, and immunoprophylaxis of infectious diseases. Further studies of the interactions of environmental factors on virulence gene expression will lead to a better understanding of the adaptive responses of organisms to the complex environments of their hosts.

CONCLUSIONS

The distinction between the commensal population and the organisms most commonly associated with disease in humans is very subtle. As discussed in this chapter, the definition of normal flora or pathogen is one that is derived from the resultant complex interaction between an organism and its host.

REFERENCES

1. **Baldini, M. M., J. B. Kaper, M. M. Levine, D. C. A. Candy, and H. W. Moon.** 1983. Plasmid-mediated adhesion of enteropathogenic *Escherichia coli*. *J. Pediatr. Gastroenterol. Nutr.* **2:**534–538.
2. **Blackwell, C. C., A. T. Saadi, M. W. Raza, D. M. Weir, and A. Busuttil.** 1993. The potential role of bacterial toxins in sudden infant death syndrome (SIDS). *Int. J. Legal Med.* **105:**333–338.
3. **Eissenberg, L. G., P. H. Schlesinger, and W. E. Goldman.** 1988. Phagosome-lysosome fusion in P388D1 macrophages infected with *Histoplasma capsulatum*. *J. Leukocyte Biol.* **43:** 483–491.
4. **Falkow, S.** 1997. What is a pathogen? Developing a definition of a pathogen requires looking closely at the many complicated relationships that exist among organisms. *ASM News* **7:**359–365.
5. **Fitzgerald, T. J., and L. A. Repesh.** 1987. The hyaluronidase associated with *Treponema pallidum* facilitates treponemal dissemination. *Infect. Immun.* **55:**1023–1028.
6. **Fredricks, D. N., and D. A. Relman.** 1996. Sequence-based identification of microbial pathogens: a reconsideration of Koch's postulates. *Clin. Microbiol. Rev.* **9:**18–33.
7. **Friedman, S. M., D. N. Posnett, J. R. Tumang, B. C. Cole, and M. K. Crow.** 1991. A potential role for microbial superantigens in the pathogenesis of systemic autoimmune disease. *Arthritis Rheum.* **34:**468–480.
8. **Hortez, P. J., S. Narasimhan, J. Haggerty, L. Milstone, V. Bhopale, G. A. Schad, and F. F. Richards.** 1992. Hyaluronidase from infective *Ancylostoma* hookworm larvae and its possible function as a virulence factor in tissue invasion and in cutaneous larva migrans. *Infect. Immun.* **60:** 1018–1023.
9. **Knutton, S. M., M. Baldini, J. B. Kaper, and A. S. McNeish.** 1987. Role of plasmid-encoded adherence factors in adhesion of enteropathogenic *Escherichia coli* to HEp-2 cells. *Infect. Immun.* **55:**78–85.
10. **Kotb, M.** 1994. Infection and autoimmunity: a story of the host, the pathogen, and the co-pathogen. *Clin. Immunol. Immunopathol.* **74:**10–22.
11. **Kotb, M.** 1995. Bacterial pyrogenic exotoxins as superantigens. *Clin. Microbiol. Rev.* **8:**411–426.
12. **Kothary, M. H., T. Chase, Jr., and J. D. Macmillan.** 1984. Correlation of elastase production by some strains of *Aspergillus fumigatus* with ability to cause pulmonary invasive aspergillosis in mice. *Infect. Immun.* **43:**320–325.
13. **Litwin, C. M., and S. B. Calderwood.** 1993. Role of iron in regulation of virulence genes. *Clin. Microbiol. Rev.* **6:** 137–149.
14. **Morris, J. A., D. Harran, and A. Smith.** 1987. Hypothesis: common bacterial toxins are a possible cause of the sudden infant death syndrome. *Med. Hypotheses* **22:**211–222.
15. **Plant, A.** 1993. Microbial subversion of host defenses, p. 154–161. *In* M. Schaechter, G. Medoff, and B. I. Eisenstein (ed.), *Mechanisms of Microbial Disease*. The Williams & Wilkins Co., Baltimore, Md.
16. **Rosan, B., and N. B. Williams.** 1964. Hyaluronidase production by oral enterococci. *Arch. Oral Biol.* **9:**291–298.
17. **Salyers, A. A., and D. D. Whitt.** 1994. Virulence factors that promote colonization, p. 30–46. *In* A. A. Salyers and D. D. Whitt (ed.), *Bacterial Pathogenesis: A Molecular Approach*. ASM Press, Washington, D.C.
18. **Schaechter, M., and B. I. Eisenstein.** 1993. Genetics of bacteria, p. 57–76. *In* M. Schaechter, G. Medoff, and B. I. Eisenstein (ed.), *Mechanisms of Microbial Disease*. The Williams & Wilkins Co., Baltimore, Md.
19. **Stevens, D. L.** 1992. Invasive group A *Streptococcus* infections. *Clin. Infect. Dis.* **14:**2–13.
20. **Working Group on Severe Streptococcal Infections.** 1993. Defining the group A streptococcal toxic shock syndrome. Rationale and consensus definition. *JAMA* **269:** 390–391.

Specimen Collection, Transport, and Storage

J. MICHAEL MILLER AND HARVEY T. HOLMES

4

In terms of the effectiveness of the laboratory, nothing is more important than the appropriate selection, collection, and transportation of a specimen. When specimen collection and management are not priorities, the laboratory can contribute little to patient care. Consequently, all members of the medical staff involved in this process must understand the critical nature of maintaining specimen quality throughout the total testing process. It is the responsibility of the laboratory to provide this information in a form that can be easily incorporated into each department's nursing manual, which should include specific criteria for safety and for specimen selection, collection, transportation, acceptability, and labeling. This chapter provides practical guidelines for the proper collection and handling of specimens destined for analysis in the clinical microbiology laboratory.

SAFETY

Biosafety at the laboratory bench is of primary concern to laboratorians. Health care workers may be unaware of the potential etiologic agent(s) residing in the specimen being transported to the laboratory. Policies that are designed to protect the laboratory worker and other personnel from accidental exposure to these agents must be in place. Most microbiology laboratory texts, including this one, have sections on laboratory safety procedures, and the laboratory procedure manual should contain safety information related to specimen management. Specific reference material on biosafety should be available in every microbiology laboratory. The reference materials available in the laboratory could include *Biosafety in Microbiological and Biomedical Laboratories*, 3rd ed. (50), and *Biosafety in the Laboratory: Prudent Practices for the Handling and Disposal of Infectious Materials* (40b).

Directly related policies for safety in specimen management include the following:

1. All specimen collection procedures must be performed while wearing gloves, a laboratory coat, and, where appropriate, masks and/or goggles (38).
2. All primary specimen containers should be leak-proof and should be transported within a sealable, leak-proof plastic bag having a separate compartment for paperwork (39).
3. Never transport syringes with needles to the laboratory. Instead, the contents should be transferred to a sterile tube or the needle should be removed with a protective device, and the syringe should be recapped and placed in a sealable, leak-proof plastic bag (45).
4. Do not transport leaking specimen containers to the laboratory or process them. Notify the physician of the leaking container and explain the potential compromised nature of the results if processing is continued and ask for a repeat specimen. If a new specimen is submitted, autoclave and discard the leaking one (35).

SELECTION AND COLLECTION OF THE SPECIMEN

Before a specimen is collected for analysis, the specimen or the collection site must be selected and must represent the active disease process. Even careful collection methods will produce a specimen of little clinical value if it is not selected and taken from a site where organisms are active. Some of the common sites of infection where a ready source of contamination resides include the bladder, where urethral organisms and those from the perineum may easily contaminate the urine specimen; blood, which is often contaminated by commensal flora from the venipuncture site; the endometrium, which may contain unrelated vaginal flora; fistulas, which may contain organisms from the gastrointestinal tract; the middle ear, which will be contaminated with external ear canal flora if a swab is used to collect the specimen; the nasal sinus, which may contain nasopharyngeal flora; and sites of subcutaneous infections and superficial wounds, which are commonly contaminated by skin and mucous membrane flora. In addition, methods for collecting specimens for viral culture differ from those used to collect specimens for bacterial culture.

Some general specimen selection and collection guidelines should include the following:

1. Avoid contamination from indigenous flora, whenever possible, to ensure a sample representative of the infectious process (6, 35, 45). There are many sites of infection where the specimen may contain an etiologic agent whose presence in a healthy host would otherwise be considered normal flora. This "background noise" of normal flora (i.e., from skin, membranes, and the respiratory tract) could interfere with the interpretation of culture results as well as overgrow and obscure the true agent of disease.

TABLE 1 Suitability of various clinical materials for anaerobic culture

Acceptable material	Unacceptable material
Aspirate (by needle and syringe)	Bronchoalveolar washing not protected
Bartholin's gland	Cervical
Bile	Endocervical swab, contaminated
Blood	Endotracheal aspirate
Bone marrow	Lochia
Bronchoscopic, protected brush	Nasopharyngeal swab
Culdocentesis	Perineum
Fallopian tube	Prostatic or seminal fluid
IUD,[a] for *Actinomyces* spp.	Sputum, expectorated
Ovary	Sputum, induced
Placenta, via cesarean delivery	Stool[b] or rectal samples
Sinus aspirate	Throat swab
Stool, for *Clostridium difficile*	Tracheostomy aspirate
Surgery, swab	Urethral
Surgery, tissue	Urine, from bladder or catheter
Transtracheal aspirate	Urine, voided
Urine, suprapubic aspirate	Vaginal or vulval swab
Uterus, endometrial aspirate	

[a] IUD, intrauterine device.

[b] There are a few exceptions, i.e., botulism (especially infant botulism), *Clostridium perfringens* food-borne disease, and *Clostridium difficile* antibiotic-associated pseudomembranous colitis; some maladsorption syndromes may require detection of overcolonization of the upper intestine.

2. Select the correct anatomic site from which to obtain the specimen, and collect the specimen by the proper technique and with the proper supplies, as indicated in the tables.

3. For selecting appropriate sites for samples for anaerobic culture, refer to Table 1, biopsy or needle aspirates are the specimens of choice, while anaerobic swabs are the least desirable (24, 35). Never refrigerate specimens for anaerobic culture but, rather, maintain them at room temperature (20).

4. Collect adequate volumes; insufficient material may yield false-negative results.

5. Label each specimen with the patient's name, identification number, source, specific site, date, time of collection, and the initials of the collector (13).

6. Place the specimen in a container designed to promote the survival of suspected agents and to eliminate leakage and potential safety hazards

TABLE 3 Specimens to be discouraged due to questionable microbial information

Specimen type	Alternative or comment
Burns, wounds (swabs)	Submit tissue or aspirate.
Colostomy discharge	Do not process.
Decubiti (swabs)	Submit tissue or aspirate.
Foley catheter tip	Do not process.
Gangrenous lesion (swab)	Submit tissue or aspirate.
Gastric aspirates of newborns	Do not process.
Lochia	Do not process.
Periodontal lesion (swab)	Submit tissue or aspirate.
Perirectal abscess (swabs)	Submit tissue or aspirate.
Varicose ulcer (swab)	Submit tissue or aspirate.
Vomitus	Do not process.

VIRUS, RICKETTSIA, CHLAMYDIA, AND MYCOPLASMA TRANSPORT

Methods and media used for bacterial transport are inappropriate for virus and chlamydia transport. Viral transport media (VTM) are designed to prevent drying, maintain viral viability during transport, and prevent the overgrowth of contaminating bacteria. Many of the formulations contain either Eagle's minimum essential medium or Hank's balanced salt solution, along with fetal bovine serum (FBS) or

TABLE 2 Storage conditions for various transport systems and suspected bacterial agents[a]

Preservative[a]	Held at 4°C	Held at 25°C
No preservative	Autopsy tissue, bronchial wash, catheter, i.v., CSF, lung biopsy, pericardial fluid, sputum, urine (all)	CSF (bacterial agents), synovial fluid
Anaerobic transport		Abdominal fluid, amniotic fluid, anaerobic cultures, aspirates, bile, cul-de-sac, deep lesion material, IUD for *Actinomyces* spp., lung aspirate, placenta (cesarean delivery), sinus aspirate, tissue (surgery), transtracheal aspirate, urine (suprapubic aspirate)
Direct inoculation of media		Corneal scraping, blood cultures, RL or BG plates for *Bordetella* spp., JEMBEC plates for *Neisseria gonorrhoeae*, vitreous humor
Aerobic transport media[b]	Burn wound biopsy, *Campylobacter* spp., ear (external), *Shigella* spp., *Vibrio* spp., *Yersinia* spp.	Bone marrow, *Bordetella* spp., cervix, conjunctiva, *Corynebacterium* spp., ear (internal), genital cultures, nasopharynx, *Neisseria* spp., *Salmonella* spp., upper respiratory cultures

[a] Abbreviations: BG, Bordet-Gengou medium; CSF, cerebrospinal fluid; IUD, intrauterine device; i.v., intravenous; JEMBEC, John E. Martin Biological Environmental Chamber; RL, Regan-Lowe medium.

[b] Stuart's medium, charcoal-impregnated swabs originally formulated for *N. gonorrhoeae* transport; Amies medium, modified Stuart's medium but incorporates charcoal in medium instead of swab; Cary-Blair medium, similar to Stuart's medium but modified for fecal specimens, with the pH increased from 7.4 to 8.4.

bovine serum albumin (BSA). VTM may be prepared in-house or purchased commercially. There is little evidence in the literature that one VTM is better than another. However, in virtually all cases in which a specimen is submitted for viral analysis, the specimen should be selected and collected in a manner that reflects the target organ which may often be typified by the classic symptoms of the viral disease (25).

Liquid-based transport systems contain a protein (BSA, gelatin, or FBS) and a combination of antimicrobial agents in a buffered solution. Viruses are not inhibited by antibacterial drugs. Tissue for viral analysis may also be placed into this type of medium. A buffered sucrose-containing transport system (2-SP) may be used for virus and for chlamydia transport. The antimicrobial agents present in the 2-SP are not inhibitory to *Chlamydia* spp.

A transport system containing human newborn foreskin fibroblasts is commercially available and is useful for the recovery and early detection of cytomegalovirus and herpes simplex virus. Because of the cells, however, this system has a limited shelf life and is useful only for viruses that grow in fibroblasts.

If specimens arrive in the laboratory in Stuart's or Amies bacterial transport systems, the swabs may be transferred into one of the liquid VTM systems.

Rickettsial recovery seems to be enhanced if glutamate is present in a sodium-free, buffered salt solution. A sucrose-phosphate-glutamate transport medium containing BSA is often used to transport rickettsiae, mycoplasmas, and chlamydiae (25). Manufacturers of probes, amplification systems, or enzyme immunoassay (EIA) antigen detection systems often recommend or supply specific transport media and swabs for the collection and transport of specimens for testing in their systems.

TRANSPORTATION

1. All specimens must be *promptly* transported to the laboratory, preferably within 2 h (24). If processing is delayed, specimens used for the detection of bacterial agents may be stored under the conditions specified in Table 2.

2. In general, do not store specimens for bacterial culture for more than 24 h. Viruses, however, usually remain stable for 2 to 3 days at 4°C (25, 26).

3. Optimal transport of clinical specimens, including specimens for anaerobic culture, depends primarily on the volume of material obtained. Submit small amounts within 15 to 30 min of collection; biopsy tissue may be maintained for up to 20 to 24 h if it is stored at 25°C in an anaerobic transport system (24).

4. Environmentally sensitive organisms include *Shigella* spp. (process immediately), *Neisseria gonorrhoeae*, *Neisseria meningitidis*, and *Haemophilus influenzae* (which is sensitive to cold temperatures). Never refrigerate spinal fluid, genital, eye, or internal ear specimens (35).

5. Transportation of clinical specimens and transportation of infectious substances from one health care facility or laboratory to another, regardless of the distance, require strict attention to specimen packaging and labeling instructions (25, 38, 39). Materials for transport must be labeled properly, packaged, and protected during transport; the courier vehicles must also be marked and designated as carrying biologic agents. U.S. Department of Transportation regulations are available on the Internet (www.dot.gov). The definition of "clinical specimen" and "infectious substance" will have a direct impact on transportation methods.

SPECIMEN ACCEPTABILITY OR REJECTION CRITERIA

At times, specimens arriving in the laboratory may be improperly selected, collected, or transported. This is essentially the equivalent of a specimen being out of control. This out-of-control process must receive the same attention as does an out-of-control identification or susceptibility test; there must be a corrective action. Processing and reporting of results for these specimens to the physician may provide misleading information that can lead to misdiagnosis

TABLE 4 Specimen management of sterile body fluids[a]

Fluid	Collection container	Concentration	Stain	Comment
Amniotic	Anaerobic tube	No	Gram stain	
Culdocentesis	Anaerobic tube	No	Gram stain	
Dialysis effluent	Isolator tube, urine cup, or Bx2	Centrifuge or filter	Gram stain or AO (low detection rate)	<100 leukocytes is normal Use one-third of filter for one of three media
Pericardial	B and/or anaerobic tube	Cytospin preparation from tube	Gram stain from cytospin	Few leukocytes in normal fluid
Peritoneal (ascites)	Bx2 (10 ml) + anaerobic tube	Cytospin preparation from tube	Gram stain from cytospin	<300 leukocytes/ml is normal
Pleural (effusion, transudate, thoracentesis, empyema)	Anaerobic tube	Cytospin preparation from tube	Gram stain from cytospin	>5 ml needed for fungi; none to a few leukocytes is normal; many leukocytes are found with empyema
Synovial	B + anaerobic tube	Cytospin from tube	Gram stain from cytospin	A few leukocytes is normal

[a] The information in this table is from reference 4. Abbreviations: B, blood culture bottle; Bx2, aerobic and anaerobic blood bottles; AO, acridine orange stain. Cultures and stains can be done from any cytospin sediment.

TABLE 5 Bacteriology and mycology specimen collection guidelines

Specimen type (reference)	Collection		Time and temp		Replica limits	Comments
	Guidelines	Device and/or minimum vol	Transport[b]	Storage		
Abscess (46)	Remove surface exudate by wiping with sterile saline or 70% EtOH.					Tissue or fluid is always superior to a swab specimen. If swabs must be used, collect two, one for culture and one for Gram staining. Preserve them with Stuart's or Amies medium.
Open	Aspirate if possible or pass a swab deep into the lesion and firmly sample the lesion's advancing edge.	Swab transport system	≤2 h, RT	≤24 h, RT	1/day/source	A sample of the base of the lesion and a sample of the abscess wall are most productive.
Closed	Aspirate abscess wall material with needle and syringe. Aseptically transfer *all* material into anaerobic transport device.	Anaerobic transport system, ≥1 ml	≤2 h, RT	≤24 h, RT	1/day/source	Sampling of surface area can introduce colonizing bacteria not involved in the infectious process.
Bite wound (14, 18, 46)	See Abscess.					Do not culture animal bite wounds ≤12 h old (agents are usually not recovered) unless they are on the face or hand or unless signs of infection are present.
Blood culture (15, 31, 33, 42, 43)	Disinfection of culture bottle: apply 70% isopropyl alcohol to rubber stoppers and wait 1 min.	Bacteria: blood culture vials Adult, 10 to 20 ml/set Higher volume most productive	≤2 h, RT	≤24 h, RT or per instructions	3 sets in 24 h	Acute sepsis: 2 to 3 sets from separate sites, all within 10 min Endocarditis, acute: 3 sets from 3 separate sites, over 1–2 h Endocarditis, subacute: 3 sets from 3 separate sites, taken ≥15 min apart. If negative at 24 h, obtain 3 more sets.
	Palpate for the vein first.					Fever of unknown origin: 2 to 3 sets from separate sites ≥1 h apart. If negative at 24 h, obtain 2 to 3 more sets.

	Disinfection of venipuncture site: 1. Cleanse site with 70% alcohol. 2. Swab concentrically, starting at the center, with an iodine preparation. 3. Allow the iodine to dry. 4. *Do not palpate vein at this point.* 5. Collect blood. 6. After venipuncture, remove iodine from the skin with alcohol.	Infant, 1–10 ml/set Fungi: 1. Biphasic culture 2. Lysis-centrifugation				Some data indicate that an additional aerobic bottle or fungal bottle is more productive than the anaerobic bottle.
Bone marrow	Prepare puncture side as for surgical incision.	Inoculate blood culture bottle or a lysis-centrifugation tube	≤24 h, RT if in culture bottle or tube	≤24 h, RT	1/day	Small volumes of bone marrow may be inoculated directly onto culture media.
Burn	Clean and debride the burn wound prior to specimen collection.	Tissue is placed into a screw-cap container Swab exudate	≤2 h, RT	≤24 h, RT	1/day/source	A 3- to 4-mm-punch biopsy specimen is optimum when quantitative cultures are ordered. Process for aerobic culture only. Quantitative culture may or may not be valuable. Cultures of surface samples of burns may be misleading.
Catheter: i.v. (17, 30, 32)	1. Cleanse the skin around the catheter site with alcohol. 2. Aseptically remove catheter and clip 5 cm of the distal tip of the catheter directly into a sterile tube. 3. Transport directly to microbiology laboratory to prevent drying.	Sterile screw-cap tube or cup	≤15 min, RT	≤24 h, 4°C	None	Acceptable i.v. catheters for semiquantitative culture (Maki method): central, CVP, Hickman, Broviac, peripheral, arterial, umbilical, hyperalimentation, Swan-Ganz.

(Continued on next page)

TABLE 5 Bacteriology and mycology specimen collection guidelines (*Continued*)

Specimen type (reference)	Collection		Time and temp		Replica limits	Comments
	Guidelines	Device and/or minimum vol	Transport[b]	Storage		
Foley (35)	Do *not* culture since growth represents distal urethral flora.					Not acceptable for culture.
Cellulitis (46, 48)	1. Cleanse site by wiping with sterile saline or 70% alcohol. 2. Aspirate the area of maximum inflammation (commonly the center rather than the leading edge) with a fine needle and syringe. 3. Draw small amount of sterile saline into syringe and aspirate into sterile screw-cap tube.	Sterile tube (syringe transport not recommended)	≤15 min, RT	≤24 h, RT	None	Yield of potential pathogens is only 25 to 35%.
CSF (19, 41, 49)	1. Disinfect site with 2% iodine tincture. 2. Insert a needle with stylet at L3–L4, L4–L5, or L5–S1 interspace. 3. Upon reaching the subarachnoid space, remove the stylet and collect 1 to 2 ml of fluid into each of 3 leak-proof tubes.	Sterile screw-cap tube Minimum amt required: Bacteria, ≥1 ml Fungi, ≥2 ml AFB, ≥2 ml Virus, ≥1 ml on ice (see Table 8)	Bacteria: never refrigerate; ≤15 min, RT	≤24 h, RT	None	Obtain blood for culture also. If only 1 tube of CSF is collected, it should be submitted to microbiology first; otherwise submit tube 2. Aspirate of brain abscess or a biopsy may be necessary to detect anaerobic bacteria or parasites.

Decubitus ulcer (46)	A swab is not the specimen of choice (see comments). 1. Cleanse surface with sterile saline. 2. If a sample biopsy is not available, vigorously swab the base of the lesion. 3. Place swab in appropriate transport system.	Swab transport (aerobic) or anaerobic system (for tissue)	≤2 h, RT	≤24 h, RT	1/day/source	Since a decubitus ulcer swab provides little clinical information, its collection should be discouraged. A tissue biopsy sample or a needle aspirate is the specimen of choice.
Dental culture: gingival, periodontal, periapical, Vincent's stomatitis	1. Carefully cleanse gingival margin and supragingival tooth surface to remove saliva, debris, and plaque. 2. Using a periodontal scaler, carefully remove subgingival lesion material and transfer it to an anaerobic transport system. 3. Prepare for staining smears that have been collected in the same fashion. See comments.	Anaerobic transport system	≤2 h, RT	≤24 h, RT	1/day	Periodontal lesions should be processed only by laboratories equipped to provide specialized techniques for the detection and enumeration of specific agents.

(Continued on next page)

TABLE 5 Bacteriology and mycology specimen collection guidelines (*Continued*)

Specimen type (reference)	Collection		Time and temp		Replica limits	Comments
	Guidelines	Device and/or minimum vol	Transport[b]	Storage		
Ear						
Inner (2)	Tympanocentesis reserved for complicated, recurrent, or chronic persistent otitis media. 1. For intact ear drum, clean ear canal with soap solution and collect fluid via syringe aspiration technique. 2. For ruptured ear drum, collect fluid on flexible-shaft swab via an auditory speculum.	Sterile tube, swab transport medium, or anaerobic system	≤2 h, RT	≤24 h, RT	1/day/source	Results for throat or nasopharyngeal swab cultures are not predictive of agents responsible for otitis media and should not be submitted for that purpose.
Outer (2)	1. Use moistened swab to remove any debris or crust from the ear canal. 2. Obtain a sample by firmly rotating swab in the outer canal.	Swab transport	≤2 h, RT	≤24 h, 4°C	1/day/source	For otitis externa, *vigorous* swabbing is required since surface swabbing may miss streptococcal cellulitis.
Eye						
Conjunctiva (1, 27)	1. Sample both eyes with separate swabs (premoistened with sterile saline) by rolling over each conjunctiva. 2. Inoculate medium at time of collection. 3. Smear swabs onto 2 slides for staining.	Direct culture inoculation: BAP and CHOC or swab transport	Plates: ≤15 min, RT Swabs: ≤2 h, RT	≤24 h, RT	None	If possible, sample both conjunctiva, even if only one is infected, to determine indigenous microflora. The uninfected eye can serve as a control with which to compare the agents isolated from the infected eye. If cost prohibits this approach, rely on the Gram stain to assist in interpretation of culture.

Corneal scrapings (1, 27)	1. Obtain conjunctival swab specimens as described above. 2. Instill 2 drops of local anesthetic. 3. Using sterile spatula, scrape ulcers or lesions, and inoculate scraping directly onto medium. 4. Apply remaining material to 2 clean glass slides for staining.	Direct culture inoculation: BHI with 10% sheep blood, CHOC, and inhibitory mold agar	≤15 min, RT	≤24 h, RT	None	It is recommended that swabs for culture be taken prior to anesthetic application, whereas corneal scrapings can be obtained afterward.
Fluid or aspirates	Prepare eye for needle aspiration of fluid.	Sterile screw-cap tube or direct inoculation of small amount of fluid onto media	≤15 min, RT	≤24 h, RT	1/day	Include fungal media. Anesthetics may be inhibitory to some etiologic agents.
Feces						
Routine culture (44)	Pass directly into a clean, dry container. Transport the specimen to microbiology laboratory within 1 h of collection or transfer a visible portion on a swab to a transport system such as Stuart's or Amies.	Clean, leak-proof, wide-mouth container or use a swab transport system; ≥2 g	Unpreserved: ≤1 h, RT	≤24 h, 4°C	1/day	Do not perform routine stool cultures for patients whose length of stay was >3 days and the admitting diagnosis was not gastroenteritis. Culture and toxin tests for *Clostridium difficile* should be considered for these patients.
			Swab transport system; ≤24 h, RT	≤48 h, RT or 4°C		Swabs for routine pathogens are not recommended except for infants and patients with active diarrhea (see Rectal swabs).
C. difficile (3, 28, 44)	Pass liquid or soft stool directly into a clean, dry container. Soft stool is defined as stool assuming the shape of its container. Swab specimen not recommended for toxin testing.	Sterile, leak-proof, wide-mouth container; ≥5 ml	≤1 h, RT 1–24 h, 4°C >24 h, −20°C	2 days, 4°C for culture 3 days, 4°C or longer at −70°C for toxin test	1/2 day	Patients should be passing ≥5 liquid or soft stools per 24 h. Testing of formed or hard stool is often unproductive and may indicate only commensal carriage. Freezing at −20°C facilitates rapid loss of cytotoxin activity.

(Continued on next page)

TABLE 5 Bacteriology and mycology specimen collection guidelines (*Continued*)

Specimen type (reference)	Collection		Time and temp		Replica limits	Comments
	Guidelines	Device and/or minimum vol	Transport[b]	Storage		
E. coli O157:H7 (44)	Pass liquid or bloody stool into a clean, dry container.	Sterile, leak-proof, wide-mouth container or use swab transport system; >2 ml	Unpreserved: ≤1 h, RT Swab transport system: ≤24 h, RT or 4°C	≤24 h, 4°C ≤48 h, RT	1/day	Bloody or liquid stools collected within 6 days of onset among patients with abdominal cramps have the highest yield.
Leukocytes (22) (not recommended)	Pass feces directly into a clean, dry container. Transport to microbiology laboratory within 1 h of collection, or transfer to ova and parasite transport system (10% Formalin or PVA).	Sterile, leak-proof, wide-mouth container or 10% Formalin and/or PVA; >2 ml	Unpreserved: ≤1 h, RT Formalin/PVA: indefinite, RT	≤24 h, 4°C Indefinite, RT	1/day	This procedure should be discouraged because it often provides results of little clinical value and could be misleading. A Gram stain or a simple methylene blue stain may be used to visualize leukocytes. Commercial detection methods are also available.
Rectal swab	1. Carefully insert a swab ≈1 in. beyond the anal sphincter. 2. Gently rotate the swab to sample the anal crypts. 3. Feces should be visible on the swab for detection of diarrheal pathogens.	Swab transport	≤2 h, RT	≤24 h, RT	1/day	Reserved for detecting *Neisseria gonorrhoeae*, *Shigella*, *Campylobacter*, and herpes simplex virus and anal carriage of group B *Streptococcus* or for patients unable to pass a specimen.
Fistulas	See Abscess.					
Fluids: abdominal, amniotic, ascites, bile, joint, paracentesis, pericardial, peritoneal, pleural, synovial, thoracentesis	1. Disinfect overlying skin with 2% iodine tincture. 2. Obtain specimen via percutaneous needle aspiration or surgery. 3. Transport immediately to laboratory.	Blood culture bottle for bacteria and yeast or sterile screw-cap tube or anaerobic transport system Bacteria, ≥1 ml	≤15 min, RT	≤24 h, RT Pericardial fluid and fluids for fungal cultures, ≤24 h, 4°C	None	Amniotic and culdocentesis fluids should be transported in an anaerobic system and need not be centrifuged prior to Gram staining. Other fluids are best examined by Gram staining of a cytocentrifuged preparation (see Table 4).

	4. Always submit as much fluid as possible; *never* submit a swab dipped in fluid.	Fungi, ≥10 ml Mycobacteria, ≥10 ml				
Gangrenous tissue	See Abscess.					Discourage sampling of surface or superficial tissue; tissue biopsy or aspirates are preferred.
Gastric: wash or lavage (7)	Collect in early morning before patients eat and while they are still in bed. 1. Introduce a nasogastric tube orally or nasally to the stomach. 2. Perform lavage with 25 to 50 ml of chilled, sterile, distilled water. 3. Recover sample and place in a leak-proof, sterile container. 4. Before removing the tube, release suction and clamp it.	Sterile, leak-proof container	≤15 min, RT or neutralize within 1 h of collection	≤24 h, 4°C	1/day	The specimen must be processed promptly, since mycobacteria die rapidly in gastric washings. Neutralize each 35 to 50 ml of gastric washing with 1.5 ml of 40% anhydrous Na_2HPO_4.
Genital: female Amniotic (51)	1. Aspirate via amniocentesis, cesarean delivery, or intrauterine catheter. 2. Transfer fluid to anaerobic transport system.	Anaerobic transport system, ≥1 ml	≤15 min, RT	≤24 h, RT	None	Swabbing or aspiration of vaginal membrane is *not* acceptable because of the potential for culture contamination by commensal vaginal flora.
Bartholin	1. Disinfect skin with iodine preparation. 2. Aspirate fluid from ducts.	Anaerobic transport system, ≥1 ml	≤2 h, RT	≤24 h, RT	1/day	

(Continued on next page)

TABLE 5 Bacteriology and mycology specimen collection guidelines (*Continued*)

Specimen type (reference)	Collection		Time and temp		Replica limits	Comments
	Guidelines	Device and/or minimum vol	Transport[b]	Storage		
Cervix (16)	1. Visualize the cervix using a speculum without lubricant. 2. Remove mucus and secretions from the cervix with swab and discard the swab. 3. Firmly yet gently sample the endocervical canal with a newly obtained sterile swab.	Swab transport	≤2 h, RT	≤24 h, RT	1/day	See text on collection and transport needs for virus and chlamydia. *Neisseria gonorrhoeae* is found in exudates, whereas chlamydia infect specific cells.
Cul-de-sac	Submit aspirate or fluid.	Anaerobic transport system, >1 ml	≤2 h, RT	≤24 h, RT	1/day	
Endometrial	1. Collect transcervical aspirate via a telescoping catheter. 2. Transfer entire amount to anaerobic transport system.	Anaerobic transport system, ≥1 ml	≤2 h, RT	≤24 h, RT	1/day	
Products of conception	1. Submit a portion of tissue in a sterile container. 2. If obtained by cesarean delivery, immediately transfer to an anaerobic transport system.	Sterile tube or anaerobic transport system	≤2 h, RT	≤24 h, RT	1/day	Do not process lochia. Culture of this specimen may or may not provide clinically relevant results, and such results could be misleading.
Urethral (16)	Collect 1 h after patient has urinated. 1. Remove exudate from the urethral orifice. 2. Collect discharge material on a swab by massaging the urethra against the pubic symphysis through the vagina.	Swab transport	≤2 h, RT	≤24 h, RT	1/day	If no discharge can be obtained, wash the external urethra with Betadine soap and rinse with water. Insert a urethrogenital swab 2 to 4 cm into the urethra and rotate the swab for 2 s.

Vaginal (16)	1. Wipe away excessive amount of secretion or discharge. 2. Obtain secretions from the mucosal membrane of the vaginal vault with a sterile swab or pipette. 3. If a smear is also requested, use a second swab.	Swab transport	≤2 h, RT	≤24 h, RT	1/day	For intrauterine devices, place entire device into a sterile container and submit at RT. A Gram stain is recommended for confirmation of bacterial vaginosis. Cultures are often inaccurate and misleading.
Genital: female or male, lesion	1. Clean the lesion with sterile saline and remove lesion's surface with a sterile scalpel blade. 2. Allow transudate to accumulate. 3. While pressing the base of the lesion, *firmly* sample exudate with a sterile swab.	Swab transport	≤2 h, RT	≤24 h, RT	1/day	For dark-field examination to rule out syphilis, touch a glass slide to the transudate, add coverslip, and transport immediately to the laboratory in a humidified chamber (petri dish with moist gauze). Specimens for syphilis are not submitted for culture.
Genital: male						
Prostate (45)	1. Cleanse the glans with soap and water. 2. Massage prostate through rectum. 3. Collect fluid on a sterile swab or in a sterile tube.	Swab transport or sterile tube	≤2 h, RT	≤24 h, RT	1/day	More relevant results may occur by adding urine specimens obtained immediately before and after massage to indicate urethral and bladder organisms. Ejaculate may also be cultured.
Urethra	Insert a urethrogenital swab 2 to 4 cm into the urethral lumen, rotate swab, and leave it in place for at least 2 s to facilitate absorption.	Swab transport	≤2 h, RT	≤24 h, RT	1/day	
Hair, dermatophytosis (21)	1. With forceps, collect at least 10 to 12 affected hairs with the base of shaft intact. 2. Place in a clean tube or container.	Clean container, 10 hairs	≤24 h, RT		1/day/site	Collect scalp scales, if present, along with scrapings of active borders of lesions. Note any antifungal therapy taken recently.

(*Continued on next page*)

TABLE 5 Bacteriology and mycology specimen collection guidelines (*Continued*)

Specimen type (reference)	Collection		Time and temp		Replica limits	Comments
	Guidelines	Device and/or minimum vol	Transport[b]	Storage		
Nail, dermatophytosis (21)	1. Wipe nail with 70% alcohol using gauze (not cotton). 2. Clip away a generous portion of the affected area and collect material or debris from *under* the nail. 3. Place material in a clean container.	Clean container Enough scrapings to cover the head of a thumbtack	≤24 h, RT		1/day	
Pilonidal cyst	See Abscess.					
Respiratory, lower Bronchoalveolar lavage, bronchial brush or wash, tracheal aspirate	1. Place aspirate or washing into a sputum trap. 2. Place brush into a sterile container with saline.	Sterile container, >1 ml	≤2 h, RT	≤24 h, 4°C	1/day	A total of 40 to 80 ml of fluid is needed for quantitative analysis. For quantitative analysis of brushings, place brush into 0.5 ml of Trypticase soy broth.
Sputum, expectorate (5)	1. Collect specimen under the direct supervision of a nurse or physician. 2. Have patient rinse or gargle with water to remove superficial flora. 3. Instruct patient to cough deeply to produce a lower respiratory specimen (not postnasal fluid). Collect in a sterile container.	Sterile container, >1 ml Minimum amounts: Bacteria, >1 ml Fungi, 3–5 ml Mycobacteria, 5–10 ml Parasites, 3–5 ml	≤2 h, RT	≤24 h, 4°C	1/day	For pediatric patients unable to produce a specimen, a respiratory therapist should collect a specimen via suction. The best specimen should have ≤10 squamous cells/×100 field.

Sputum, induced (5)	1. Have patient rinse mouth with water after brushing gums and tongue. 2. With the aid of a nebulizer, have patients inhale ≈25 ml of 3 to 10% sterile saline. 3. Collect the induced sputum into a sterile container.	Sterile container	≤2 h, RT	≤24 h, RT	1/day	*Histoplasma capsulatum* and *Blastomyces dermatitidis* survive for only short periods of time once a specimen is obtained. Fungal recovery is primarily for *Cryptococcus* and some filamentous fungi; other yeasts rarely cause lower respiratory tract infection.
Respiratory, upper						
Oral	1. Remove oral secretions and debris from the surface of lesion with a swab and then discard. 2. Using a second swab, vigorously sample the lesion, avoiding any areas of normal tissue.	Swab transport	≤2 h, RT	≤24 h, RT	1/day	Discourage sampling of superficial tissue for bacterial evaluation. Tissue biopsy specimens or needle aspirates are the specimens of choice.
Nasal	1. Insert a swab, premoistened with sterile saline, ≈2 cm into the nares. 2. Rotate the swab against the nasal mucosa.	Swab transport	≤2 h, RT	≤24 h, RT	1/day	Anterior nose cultures are reserved for detecting staphylococcal and streptococcal carriers or for nasal lesions. A nasal speculum may be appropriate.
Nasopharynx (2)	1. Gently insert a calcium alginate swab into the posterior nasopharynx via the nose. 2. Rotate swab slowly for 5 s to absorb secretions. 3. Remove swab and inoculate medium at the bedside or examination table or place swab in transport medium.	Direct media inoculation or swab transport	Plates: ≤15 min, RT Swabs: ≤2 h, RT	≤24 h, RT	1/day	

(Continued on next page)

TABLE 5 Bacteriology and mycology specimen collection guidelines (*Continued*)

Specimen type (reference)	Collection		Time and temp		Replica limits	Comments
	Guidelines	Device and/or minimum vol	Transport[b]	Storage		
Throat	1. Depress tongue with a tongue depressor. 2. Sample the posterior pharynx, tonsils, and inflamed areas with a sterile swab.	Swab transport	≤2 h, RT	≤24 h, RT	1/day	Throat swab cultures are contraindicated for patients with an inflamed epiglottis. Swabs for *Neisseria gonorrhoeae* should be placed into charcoal-containing transport medium and plated ≤12 h after collection. JEMBEC, Biobags, and the GonoPak are better for transport at RT.
Skin, dermatophytosis (21)	1. Cleanse the affected area with 70% alcohol. 2. Gently scrape the surface of the skin at the active margin of the lesion. *Do not draw blood.* 3. Place sample in clean container or between 2 clean, glass slides.	Clean container, enough scrapings to cover the head of a thumbtack	≤24 h, RT		1/day/site	If the specimen is submitted between glass slides, tape the slides together and submit them in an envelope.
Tissue	1. Submit in a sterile container. 2. For small samples, add several drops of sterile saline to keep moist. 3. *Do not allow tissue to dry out.*	Anaerobic transport system or sterile, screw-cap jar. Saline may need to be added.	≤15 min, RT	≤24 h, RT	None	Always submit as much tissue as possible. If possible, save an amount of surgical tissue at −70°C in case further studies are needed. Never submit a swab that has simply been rubbed over the surface. For quantitative study, a sample of 2 by 1 cm, i.e., about 500 mg, is appropriate. Some *Legionella* may be inhibited by saline.
Urine						
Female, midstream (12)	1. Thoroughly cleanse the urethral area with soap and water. 2. Rinse area with wet gauze pads. 3. While holding the labia apart, begin voiding.	Sterile, wide-mouth container, ≥1 ml, or urine transport kit	Unpreserved: ≤2 h, RT Preserved: ≤24 h, RT	≤24 h, 4°C	1/day	Chlamydial antigen detection in urine from women may be unproductive (36). Urine is toxic to cell lines and is therefore not the specimen of choice for chlamydial culture.

	4. After several milliliters has passed, collect a midstream portion without stopping the flow of urine.					The midstream portion is used for bacterial culture.
Male, midstream (12)	1. Cleanse the glans with soap and water. 2. Rinse with wet gauze pads. 3. While holding the foreskin retracted, begin voiding. 4. After several milliliters has passed, collect a midstream portion without stopping the flow of urine.	Sterile, wide-mouth container, ≥1 ml, or urine transport kit	Unpreserved: ≤2 h, RT Preserved: ≤24 h, RT	≤24 h, 4°C	1/day	First part of urine stream is used for probe tests and antigen tests for chlamydia. Wait 2 h after the last micturition. The midstream portion is used for culture.
Straight catheter (12)	1. Thoroughly cleanse the urethral area with soap and water. 2. Rinse area with wet gauze pads. 3. Aseptically, insert a catheter into the bladder. 4. After allowing ≈15 ml to pass, collect urine to be submitted in a sterile container.	Sterile, leak-proof container	Unpreserved: ≤2 h, RT Preserved: ≤24 h, RT	≤24 h, 4°C	1/day	The procedure may introduce urethral flora into the bladder and increase the risk of iatrogenic infection.
Indwelling catheter (45)	1. Disinfect the catheter collection port with 70% alcohol. 2. Use needle and syringe to aseptically collect 5 to 10 ml of urine. 3. Transfer to a sterile tube or container.	Sterile leak-proof container	Unpreserved: ≤2 h, RT Preserved: ≤24 h, RT	≤24 h, 4°C	1/day	
Wound	See Abscess.					

[a] Abbreviations: AFB, acid-fast bacilli; BAP, blood agar plate; BHI, brain heart infusion; CHOC, chocolate agar; CSF, cerebrospinal fluid; CVP, central venous pressure; EtOH, ethanol; i.v., intravenous; PVA, polyvinyl alcohol fixative; RT, room temperature.

[b] All specimens are to be transported in leak-proof plastic bags having a separate compartment for the requisition.

TABLE 6 Specimen management for infrequently encountered organisms[a]

Organism	Specimen of choice	Transport issues	Comment
Bartonella sp. *Afipia* sp. (cat scratch fever)	Blood, tissue, lymph node aspirate	1 wk, 4°C; indefinitely, −70°C	May see organisms in or on erythrocytes with Giemsa stain. Use Warthin-Starry silver stain for tissue. SPS is toxic.
Borrelia burgdorferi (Lyme disease)	Skin biopsy at lesion periphery, blood, CSF	Keep tissue moist and sterile; hand carry to laboratory if possible	Consider serology in addition to culture. Culture yield is low. Warthin-Starry silver stain for tissue. AO, FA, Giemsa for blood and CSF.
Borrelia sp. (relapsing fever)	Blood smear (blood)	Hand carry to laboratory if possible	Use direct wet mount in saline or use dark-field microscopy. Stain with Wright's or Giemsa stain. Blood culture is unreliable.
Brucella sp.[b]	Blood, bone marrow	Transport at room temperature; pediatric lysis-centrifugation tube helpful	Routine blood culture bottles are useful if held 30 days. Joint fluid culture in arthritis. Notify laboratory with suspicion of *Brucella*.
Calymmatobacterium (granuloma inguinale; donovanosis)	Tissue, subsurface scrapings	Transport at room temperature	Mostly a tropical disease. Stain with Wright's or Giemsa stain. Epithelium alone is inadequate. Culture is nonproductive.
Coxiella (Q fever),[b] *Rickettsia* (spotted fevers; typhus)	Serum, tissue (blood)	Blood and tissue are frozen at −70°C until shipped	Refer isolation to reference laboratory. Serologic diagnosis is preferred.
Ehrlichia sp.	Blood smear, skin biopsy, blood (with heparin or EDTA anticoagulant), CSF, serum	Material for culture sent on ice; keep tissue moist and sterile; hold at 4 to 20°C until tested or at −70°C for shipment; transport on ice or frozen for PCR test.	Serologic diagnosis preferred. Mix smear in methanol. Tissue stained with FA or Gimenez stain. Refer isolation to reference laboratory. CSF for direct examination and PCR.
Francisella sp. (tularemia)[b]	Lymph node aspirate, scrapings, lesion biopsy specimen, blood, sputum	Rapid transport to laboratory or freeze; ship on dry ice	Send to reference laboratory. Serology helpful. Gram stain of tissue is not productive. IFA available. Culture effective 10% of the time
Leptospira sp.	Serum, blood (with heparin or sodium oxalate anticoagulant), CSF (1st wk), urine (after 1st wk)	Blood, <1 h; urine, <1 h or dilute 1:10 in 1% bovine serum albumin and store at 4 to 20°C	Serology most helpful. Acidic urine is detrimental. Dark-field microscopy and direct FA available. Warthin-Starry silver stain for tissue.
Streptobacillus sp. (rat bite fever; Haverhill fever)	Blood, aspirates of joint fluid	High-volume bottle preferred	Do not refrigerate. Requires blood, serum, or ascitic fluid for growth. SPS is inhibitory. AO staining is helpful.

[a] The information presented in this table is from previous reports (4, 25). Abbreviations: AO, acridine orange stain; FA, fluorescent-antibody stain; IFA, indirect fluorescent-antibody stain; CSF, cerebrospinal fluid; SPS, sodium polyanethol sulfonate.

[b] Laboratory safety hazard.

TABLE 7 Specimen guide for virus isolation[a]

Clinical syndrome	Associated viruses	Specimens for virus isolation: THR	LES	URN	CSF	FEC	Other specimens	Usefulness of serology	Other agents to consider
Cardiac	Enterovirus[b]	X				X	Heart tissue or fluid	Yes	Enterovirus[c,d]
CNS infection	Enteroviruses	X			X	X	Rectal swab	No	Arbovirus[d,e]
	HSV	X			PCR		Brain biopsy	No	HIV[d,f]
	Mumps virus[b]	X		X	X		Saliva	Paired sera	Measles virus[d]
									Rabies virus[d,f]
									Lymphocytic choriomeningitis virus[d]
Congenital or neonatal	CMV[b]	X		X			Buffy coat	IgM	Hepatitis B virus
	Enteroviruses[b]	X	X	X	X	X	Rectal swab	No	HIV[d,f]
	HSV[b]	X	X	X	PCR		Lesion → DFA	IgM	Parvovirus B-19[d]
	Varicella-zoster virus[b]	X	X						Virus causing rubella[d]
Gastrointestinal	Adenoviruses 40/41[f]					X	Rectal swab	No	Norwalk virus[f]
	CMV[b]						Biopsy for culture	No	
	Rotavirus[f]					X	Rectal swab	No	
Genital	HSV[b]		X				Cervix or vulva	No	CMV[b]
	Mumps virus[b] (orchitis)	X		X			Saliva	Paired sera	Human papillomavirus[f]
Mononucleosis, fever of unknown origin	EBV[d]						Buffy coat	Yes	Dengue virus[d]
	CMV[b]	X		X				IgM	Hepatitis viruses A to E[d,f]
									Parvovirus B-19[d]
Ocular	Adenovirus[b]	X					Conjunctival	No	Enterovirus[b]
	HSV[b]	X					Conjunctival	No	CMV[b]
Rash, maculopapular	Enteroviruses[b]	X		X		X	Rectal swab	No	Human herpesvirus 6[d]
	Virus causing measles/rubeola[d]	X		X			Respiratory secretions	Paired sera	Parvovirus B-19[d]
									Rubella[d]
Rash, vesicular	Enteroviruses[b]		X					No	
	Herpes simplex virus[b,f]		X					No	
	Varicella-zoster virus[b]		X					Paired sera	
Respiratory infection	Adenovirus[b]	X					Nasopharynx	No	CMV[b] (in bronchoalveolar lavages); hantavirus[d]
	Enteroviruses[b]	X					Nasopharynx	No	
	Influenza virus[b,f]	X					Nasopharynx	No	
	Parainfluenza virus[b]	X					Nasopharynx	No	
	Respiratory syncytial virus[f]	X					Nasopharynx	No	
	Rhinovirus[b]	X					Nasopharynx	No	

[a] Abbreviations: CSF, cerebrospinal fluid; DFA, direct fluorescent-antibody assay; EBV, Epstein-Barr virus; HIV, human immunodeficiency virus; HSV, herpes simplex virus; IgM, immunoglobulin M; LES, lesion; THR, throat; URN, urine.

[b] Virus isolation is the method of choice for diagnosis.

[c] Enterovirus includes the historical designation of echovirus and Coxsackievirus types A and B.

[d] Serology is the method of choice for diagnosis.

[e] Includes western equine, eastern equine, St. Louis, and California encephalitis.

[f] Antigen detection and nucleic acid detection are the available methods.

[g] Includes coxsackievirus types A and B, echovirus, and enterovirus.

TABLE 8 Virology specimen collection guidelines[a]

Specimen type (references)	Collection		Transport time and temp	Replica limits	Comments
	Guidelines	Device and minimum vol			
For virus specimen selection guidelines, refer to Table 7 (8, 9, 26)	In general, specimens for virus isolation should be collected within 4 days after onset of illness because virus shedding decreases rapidly after that time. With only a *rare* exception, cultures for virus are not worthwhile for specimens collected more than 7 days after the onset of illness.	Except for body fluids (BAL, CSF, urine, blood), place all viral specimens in VT.	Most viruses remain stable at 4°C for 2–3 days and almost indefinitely at −70°C. *Do not freeze at −20°C.*		To ensure proper evaluation, the following information should accompany the specimen: 1. Date of illness onset 2. Date and time specimen collected 3. Admitting diagnosis Collection of acute- and convalescent-phase sera should always be considered.
Blood (8, 26)	1. Cleanse venipuncture site with 70% isopropyl alcohol. 2. Then swab concentrically, starting at the site, with 2% iodine tincture. 3. Allow the iodine to dry (≈1 min). 4. *Do not palpate the vein at this point.* 5. Collect 8 to 10 ml in anticoagulant tube (viral transport *not* required). 6. After venipuncture, remove iodine from the skin with alcohol.	Tube containing citrate, EDTA, or heparin; 8 to 10 ml/tube. You may need to draw ≥2 tubes of blood from patients who are leukopenic.	Submit at RT.	None	Commonly isolated: CMV and HSV. Less frequently isolated: arboviruses, arena viruses, EBV, HIV-1, enterovirus (newborn). Collect blood during the early, acute phase of infection. For specimens requiring cell separation, maintain at RT. *Do not refrigerate.*
CSF (10, 41)	1. Disinfect site with 2% iodine tincture. 2. Insert a needle with stylet at L3–L4, L4–L5, or L5–S1 interspace. 3. Upon reaching the subarachnoid space, remove the stylet and collect 2 to 5 ml in a sterile leak-proof tube (VT not required).	Sterile, screw-cap tube, 1.0 ml	Submit immediately (<15 min) at 4°C on ice. Can be stored at 4°C for up to 72 h.	None	Frequently isolated: coxsackievirus (some), echovirus, enterovirus, mumps virus Less frequently isolated: arboviruses, HSV, lymphocytic choriomeningitis virus, rabies virus

Cervical or vaginal swab[b] (8, 26)	1. If lesions are present, swab vigorously. Place swab in VT. 2. If lesions are not present, remove mucus from the cervix with a swab and discard the swab. 3. Firmly sample the endocervix (≈1 cm into cervical canal) with a fresh swab by rotating the swab for 5 s. 4. Place swab into VT. 5. Carry out a vulvar sweep using a second swab; place both swabs in the same transport tube.	Swab[b]	Immediately place swab in VT. Submit at 4°C.	1/day/source	Frequently isolated: HSV, CMV Noncultivable: papillomavirus, virus causing molluscum contagiosum Although cervical swabs are the specimen of choice when monitoring pregnant women who have a past history of genital HSV infection, recovery of HSV may be increased by sampling the vulva.
Conjunctiva swab[b] (8, 26)	1. Collect material from the lower conjunctiva with flexible, fine-shafted swab moistened with sterile saline. 2. Place swab in VT.	Swab[b]	Immediately place swab in VT. Submit at 4°C.	None	Frequently isolated: adenovirus; coxsackievirus A (some), CMV, HSV, enterovirus (including type 70), Newcastle disease virus
Feces (11, 23)	1. Pass directly into a clean, dry container. 2. Add sufficient VT to prevent drying. 3. Or transfer 2 to 4 g of stool to a sterile, leak-proof container and transport immediately to the laboratory.	Sterile, leak-proof, wide-mouth container; ≥2 g	Transfer to 8–10 ml of VT. Submit at 4°C.	1/day	Frequently isolated: adenoviruses, enteroviruses Less frequently isolated: rotavirus; rotavirus antigen is detected by EIA.
Nasal swab[b] (8, 26)	1. Pass a flexible, fine-shafted swab into the nostril. 2. Rotate slowly for 5 s to absorb secretions. 3. Remove swab and place in VT. 4. Repeat for the other nostril using a fresh swab. Place both swabs into the same transport tube.	Swab[b]	Immediately place swab in VT. Submit at 4°C.	1/day	Frequently isolated: influenza virus, parainfluenza virus, rhinovirus (limited); RSV (nasopharyngeal swab is preferred) Influenza A virus and RSV are usually detected by antigen assay (ELISA, EIA).

(Continued on next page)

TABLE 8 Virology specimen collection guidelines[a] (*Continued*)

Specimen type (references)	Collection		Transport time and temp	Replica limits	Comments
	Guidelines	Device and minimum vol			
Nasopharynx Aspirate or wash (8, 26)	1. Pass appropriately sized tubing or catheter into the nasopharynx. 2. Aspirate material with a small syringe. 3. If material cannot be aspirated, tilt patient's head back about 70° and instill 3 to 7 ml of sterile saline or VT until it occludes the nostril. 4. Reaspirate. If <2 ml is recovered, deposit aspirate into VT. If >2 ml is recovered, no VT required. 5. Immediately place specimen at 4°C.	Viral transport tube	Immediately place 8 to 10 ml in VT. Submit at 4°C.	1/day	Frequently isolated: influenza virus, parainfluenza virus, rhinovirus (limited), RSV Influenza A virus and RSV may be detected by antigen assay. Turnaround time for influenza virus shell vial culture: 24 to 48 h.
Swab[b] (8, 26)	1. Pass a flexible, fine-shafted swab into the nasopharynx. 2. Allow secretions to absorb for 5 s and then carefully remove swab and place it in VT. 3. Repeat for other nostril using a fresh swab. Place both swabs into the same transport tube.	Swab[b]	Immediately place swab in VT. Submit at 4°C.	1/day	Frequently isolated: influenza virus, parainfluenza virus, rhinovirus (limited), RSV
Oral swab[b]	1. Firmly sample the base of a lesion(s) with a swab. 2. Place swab in VT.	Swab[b]	Immediately place swab in VT. Submit at 4°C.	1/day	Frequently isolated: enterovirus (some), HSV
Rash Maculopapular (8, 26)	1. Gently cleanse area with sterile saline. 2. Disrupt the lesion's surface and firmly sample its base with a swab moistened with sterile saline. 3. Place swab in VT.	Swab[b]	Immediately place swab in VT. Submit at 4°C.	1/day/source	Frequently isolated: adenovirus, enterovirus, virus causing rubella, measles virus (rubeola) Less frequently isolated: poxviruses Noncultivable: parvovirus B-19
Vesicular (8, 26)	1. Sample only *fresh* vesicles, because older crusted vesicles may not contain viable virus.	Swab[b]	Immediately place swab in VT.	1/day/source	Frequently isolated: enterovirus (some), echovirus, HSV, VZV Less frequently isolated: poxviruses

	2. Cleanse area with sterile saline. 3. Carefully open the vesicle with a needle or a scalpel blade. 4. With swab, collect fluid and cellular material by vigorously sampling the base of the lesion. 5. Place in VT.		Submit at 4°C.		The preferred specimen for VZV is a vesicle; aspirate is placed in 1 ml of VT.
Throat swab[b]	1. Using a tongue depressor, depress the tongue to prevent contamination with saliva. 2. Firmly sample the posterior pharynx, tonsils, and inflamed areas with a sterile swab. 3. Place swab in VT.	Swab[b]	Immediately place swab in VT. Submit at 4°C.	1/day	Frequently isolated: adenovirus, CMV, enterovirus, HSV, influenza A and B viruses, measles virus, mumps virus, parainfluenza virus Less frequently isolated: RSV
Tissue (8, 26)	1. Obtain samples from areas directly adjacent to affected tissue. 2. Place specimen into a sterile vial containing VT.	VT	Submit at 4°C.	None	Always submit as much tissue as possible. *Never* submit a swab that has simply been rubbed over the surface. See Table 7.
Urethral swab[b]	Patient should not have urinated ≤1 h prior to collection. 1. Express and discard any exudate. 2. Carefully insert flexible, fine-shafted swab 4 cm into urethra. 3. Rotate swab 2 to 3 times to obtain an adequate number of cells. 4. Remove swab and place in VT.	Swab[b]	Immediately place swab in VT. Submit at 4°C.	1/day	Frequently isolated: CMV, HSV
Urine	Refer to Table 5 for specific guidelines for urine collection. Collect 5 ml of midstream, clean, voided urine in a sterile container (VT not required).	Sterile container, 5 ml	Submit at 4°C.	1/day	Frequently isolated: adenovirus, CMV, HSV, mumps virus Less frequently isolated: polyomavirus (JC virus), virus causing rubella Two or three specimens on successive days will maximize recovery of CMV.

[a] Abbreviations: BAL, bronchoalveolar lavage; CMV, cytomegalovirus; CSF, cerebrospinal fluid; EBV, Epstein-Barr virus; ELISA, enzyme-linked immunosorbent assay; HIV-1, human immunodeficiency virus type 1; HSV, herpes simplex virus; RSV, respiratory syncytial virus; RT, room temperature; VT, viral transport medium; VZV, varicella-zoster virus.

[b] Swab: dacron-, rayon-, or cotton-tipped swabs with plastic or aluminum shafts are acceptable; calcium alginate swabs or swabs with wooden shafts are not acceptable.

TABLE 9 Parasitology: anatomical site containing diagnostic stage[a]

Parasite	Site of diagnostic state									
	BLD	CNS	EYE	GI	L/S	LUNG	LN	MUS	Skin	Other
Acanthamoeba spp.		X	X						X (rare)	
Ascaris, larvae						X				
Babesia spp.	RBC									
Balamuthia mandrillaris		X							X	
Cryptosporidium parvum				X		X				
Cyclospora sp.				X						
Echinococcus spp.		X			X	X				
Entamoeba histolytica				X	X					
Fasciola hepatica				X	X					Bile duct
Hartmanella spp.		X								
Hookworm, larvae						X				
Leishmania donovani	WBC				X		X			Bone marrow
Leishmania spp.[b]									X	
Loa loa			X							Calabar swellings
Microfilariae	Plasma						X[c]		X[d]	
Microsporidia			X	X		X		X		Urogenital
Naegleria spp.		X[e]	X							
Onchocerca volvulus								X	X[d]	
Opisthorchis sinensis[f]				X	X					
Paragonimus westermanii				X		X				
Plasmodium spp.	RBC									
Schistosoma spp.				X						Urogenital
Strongyloides larvae				X		X				
Taenia solium		X[g]	X[g]	X				X[g]		
Toxoplasma gondii	WBC	X			X		X			
Trichinella spiralis								X		
Trichomonas vaginalis										Urogenital
Trypanosoma cruzi	Plasma						X	X		Heart
Trypanosoma spp.[h]	Plasma	X					X			

[a] Abbreviations: BLD, blood; B marrow, bone marrow; CNS, central nervous system; GI, gastrointestinal tract; LN, lymph node; L/S, liver/spleen; MUS, muscle; RBC, erythrocyte; WBC, leukocyte.
[b] Includes *L. tropica*, *L. mexicana* complex, and *L. brazilensis* complex.
[c] *Wuchereria bancrofti* and *Brugia malayi*.
[d] Skin snips for *Mansonella streptocerca* and *Onchocerca volvulus*.
[e] *Naegleria fowleri*.
[f] *Clonorchis sinensis*.
[g] Cysticerci.
[h] Includes: *T. brucei gambiense* and *I. brucei rhodesiense*.

TABLE 10 Parasitology specimen collection guidelines[a]

Specimen type (references)	Collection: Guidelines	Collection: Device	Collection: Preservative	Collection: Minimum vol	Collection: Replica limits	Transport time and temp	Comments
Blood Direct smear (37, 40)	1. Warm the patient's hands by covering them with a hot moist towel, immersing them under warm water, or rubbing them together briskly. 2. Disinfect the palmar surface of the tip of the middle or ring finger with gauze soaked with 70% alcohol (do not use cotton because it may introduce artifacts). 3. Allow alcohol to *dry completely*, because residual alcohol will not permit drop to "round up" and may also fix the erythrocytes, rendering the thick smear unsuitable for staining. 4. Puncture the palmar area with a sterile, disposable lancet, resulting in free-flowing blood.	*Wear gloves when preparing thin/thick films.* Thin smear preparation: 1. Place one drop of blood near one end of a slide. 2. Hold another slide at a 45° angle and draw it into the drop of blood. 3. Allow the blood to spread the width of the slide and then rapidly push the spreader slide to the opposite end, producing a feathered smear. 4. Label slide, dry at RT, and stain as soon as visibly dry. Thick smear preparation: 1. Touch a slide to a drop of blood (rounded up on the finger). 2. Rotate the slide to form a circular film about the size of a nickel. For blood without anticoagulant, stir blood for 20 to 30 s to prevent the formation of a fibrin clot.				Malaria: stat Other: ≤2 h, RT	Optimal times to obtain samples for smears: *Babesia* spp.: any time *Brugia malayi*: ≈midnight *Leishmania donovani*: any time *Loa loa*: ≈noon *Mansonella ozzardi*: day or night *Mansonella perstans*: night better than day *Plasmodium* spp.[b]: between chills *Trypanosoma cruzi*: acute stage *Trypanosoma brucei gambiense*[c]: acute *Trypanosoma brucei rhodesiense*[c]: acute *Wuchereria bancrofti*[b]: ≈midnight
Venipuncture (40)	1. For buffy coat concentration of filariasis, trypanosomiasis, and to a lesser extent, leishmaniasis, collect 10 ml of whole blood with heparin (0.002 g/10 ml of blood). 2. Submit directly (≤15 min) to the laboratory at RT. 3. Thick/thin smears should be obtained via finger puncture; see above.	Vacutainer	Heparin: filariasis, *Trypanosoma* EDTA: malaria (see comment)	≥10 ml	1/day	≤15 min, RT	Common parasites: *Leishmania donovani*, *Trypanosoma* spp., microfilariae Venipuncture for malaria is common but is *not* recommended because smears must be made within 1 h to detect stippling. However, this approach is common, and personnel learn to identify species with or without stippling.
CSF, CNS	See Table 5, CSF, for specific guidelines for obtaining a CSF specimen.	Sterile tube	None	≥1 ml	None	≤15 min, RT	Common parasites: *Acanthamoeba* spp., *Balamuthia mandrillaris*, *Echinococcus*, larval cestodes, microsporidia, *Naegleria fowleri*, *Taenia solium*, *Toxoplasma gondii*, *Trypanosoma* spp.

(Continued on next page)

TABLE 10 Parasitology specimen collection guidelines[a] (*Continued*)

Specimen type (references)	Collection					Transport time and temp	Comments
	Guidelines	Device	Preservative	Minimum vol	Replica limits		
Duodenal aspirate	1. Obtain a specimen via nasogastric intubation or with a string test (Entero-Test capsule). 2. Place aspirate into a sterile centrifuge tube and transport it directly (≤15 min) to the laboratory since specimens must be examined within 1 h of collection.	Sterile centrifuge tube	None	≥2 ml	None	≤15 min, RT	Common parasites: *Clonorchis sinensis* (eggs), *Cryptosporidium parvum* (oocyst), *Giardia lamblia* (trophozoite), *Isospora belli* (oocyst), *Strongyloides* spp. (larvae)
Eye, corneal scraping for *Acanthamoeba* (1, 27)	1. Instill 2 drops of local anesthetic into the conjunctival sac and/or onto the corneal epithelium. 2. Using a sterile spatula, scrape ulcers or lesions and either inoculate a nonnutrient agar plate directly or place scraping into Page's saline and transport to laboratory. 3. Apply remaining material to 2 clean glass slides for staining and fix immediately with 95% ethanol (cysts may become airborne when allowed to air dry).	Direct inoculation of nonnutrient agar coated with bacterial overlay or Page's amoeba saline	Page's amoeba saline	None	None	≤15 min, RT	Common parasites: *Acanthamoeba* spp., *Naegleria* spp. Contact lenses, lens cases, and all opened solutions can be cultured.
Feces							
Preserved (34, 40a)	1. Pass directly into a clean, dry container. 2. Specimens that cannot be examined within the recommended time must be transferred to an appropriate preservative (FOR, MIF, SAF, PVA). Mix well and allow to stand at RT for 30 min for adequate fixation. 3. For unpreserved specimens, the transport times must correspond to the recommendations provided below. 4. Submit 3 specimens over 7 to 10 days, because shedding may be intermittent.	Sterile, leak-proof, wide-mouth container	FOR + PVA, MIF + PVA, SAF, or other one-vial system Hold at RT for 30 min for fixation.	1 part feces to 3 parts fixative	1/day	Indefinite, RT	Common parasites: helminths, protozoa Unacceptable stool specimen: 1. Contaminated with urine or water (e.g., from diapers). 2. Nonpuncturable or dried specimen. 3. Specimens having bismuth, barium, magnesium, mineral oil, or gallbladder dye. The general waiting period necessary to allow these substances to clear is 7 days; for gallbladder dye, however, 21 days may be required.

Unpreserved (34, 40a)	Parasite: / Cyclical peak: *Ascaris lumbricoides* — Constant *Dientamoeba fragilis* — Irregular *Diphyllobothrium latum* — Irregular *Entamoeba histolytica* — 7–10 days *Giardia lamblia* — 3–7 days Hookworm — Constant *Trichuris trichiura* — Constant *Schistosoma* spp. — Irregular	Sterile, leak-proof wide-mouth container	None[d]	5 g	1/day	Liquid: ≤30 min, RT Semisolid: ≤1 h, RT Formed: ≤24 h, 4°C	
Pinworm paddle (40a)	1. Gently press the paddle's sticky side against several areas of the perianal region while spreading open the perianal folds. 2. Place the paddle into the transport container and tighten the cap. 3. Daily consecutive specimens (≥6) should be obtained before the patient is considered infection-free.	Pinworm paddle kit	None	None	1/day	≤24 h, RT	Common parasites: *Enterobius vermicularis*, *Taenia* spp. Specimens are best obtained at 10 to 11 p.m. or upon waking and before a bowel movement or bath. Wash hands after collection.
Skin snip (47)	1. A sharp razor blade may be used to obtain a sample of skin; the sample may be so superficial that no bleeding occurs. 2. Alternatively, a needle may be used to raise the skin and the skin below the needle is removed with a scalpel. 3. Any body location is satisfactory, but the middorsal region just to one side of the midline is frequently selected. 4. Place the skin snip into a tube containing 0.2 to 0.4 ml of saline.	Sterile tube	Sterile saline	None	None	≤15 min, RT	Common parasites: *Mansonella streptocerca*, *Onchocerca volvulus*

(Continued on next page)

TABLE 10 Parasitology specimen collection guidelines[a] (*Continued*)

Specimen type (references)	Collection					Transport time and temp	Comments
	Guidelines	Device	Preservative	Minimum vol	Replica limits		
Skin ulcer (29)	1. Obtain scrapings or biopsy specimens of the active margin of cutaneous or mucocutaneous ulcers. A punch biopsy specimen is recommended. 2. Place the sample in a sterile tube containing enough sterile saline to keep it moist.	Sterile tube	Sterile saline	None	1/day/site	≤15 min, RT	Common parasites: *Acanthamoeba* spp., *Entamoeba histolytica*, *Leishmania* spp. If cultures will be used for *Leishmania* spp., the specimen must not be contaminated with bacteria.
Urine *Schistosoma* (47)	Peak egg excretion occurs between noon and 3 p.m. 1. Collect *midday* urine specimen in a sterile container. 2. For patients with hematuria, eggs are associated with the terminal (last-voided) portion of the specimen containing mucus and blood.	Sterile, leak-proof container	None	Entire voided midday urine	1/day	≤2 h, RT	Parasites: *Schistosoma haematobium*, *Strongyloides stercoralis*, *Trichomonas vaginalis*, *Wuchereria bancrofti*
Trichomonas	Trophozoites may be found in the urine of both sexes. 1. For males, prostatic massage may be useful. 2. Collect first-voided urine in a sterile container. 3. Transport to the laboratory in <1 h at RT. If transportation will be delayed, centrifuge at 500 × *g* for 5 min, remove supernatant, overlay sediment with 0.2 ml of sterile saline, and transport at RT. 4. The sediment may also be smeared onto a microscope slide, air dried, and stained (Papanicolaou stain).	Sterile, leak-proof container	None	Entire void	1/day	≤1 h, RT Do not refrigerate	Specimens must be held at RT and processed within 1 h of collection. Alternatively, the centrifuged pellet may be adsorbed onto a Dacron swab and transported in Amies medium, in which the organisms remain viable for ≈24 h. *Do not use calcium alginate swabs*. New, commercial "pouch" methods that accomplish transport and culture are available. Papanicolaou smears may be difficult to interpret for *Trichomonas*.

Urogenital: penile, urethral, and vaginal	1. Collect discharge material with sterile swab or speculum. 2. Place specimen in 0.5 ml of sterile saline and transport directly to the laboratory (≤1 h) at RT. 3. If transport is delayed, place swab in Amies transport medium, which will maintain *Trichomonas* viability for 24 h at RT.	Sterile tube or swab transport medium Commercial pouch	Saline or Amies medium		1 day	Saline: ≤1 h at RT Amies: ≤24 h at RT	Parasites: *Enterobius vermicularis*, *Trichomonas vaginalis*. Discharge material may also be smeared onto microscope slide with 1 to 2 drops of saline and air dried.
Worm or object (34, 47)	1. Rinse debris from worm, proglottid, or object and place in saline or water. 2. Transport to laboratory. Identification may require relaxation of worm (warm at 56°C for 1 h) and clearing (immersion in carbolxylene overnight). 3. When multiple worms or objects are present, some may be placed in 10% formalin.	Clean container	Saline or water	Entire worm or object	None	≤24 h at RT	Parasites: *Ascaris lumbricoides*, *Enterobius vermicularis*, *Taenia* proglottids. Do not wrap in toilet paper because worms may dry out.

[a] Abbreviations: CNS, central nervous system; CSF, cerebrospinal fluid; FOR, 10% formalin; MIF, merthiolate-iodine-formalin; PVA, polyvinyl alcohol; RT, room temperature; SAF, sodium acetate-formalin.

[b] Additional samples for smears obtained 6, 12, or 24 h after admission may be necessary.

[c] Cerebrospinal fluid is the specimen of choice for patients infected for >6 months.

[d] Potentially infectious agents: *Cryptosporidium* oocysts, *Enterobious* eggs, enteric bacterial pathogens (*Campylobacter* spp., *Salmonella* spp., *Shigella* spp.), *Hymenolepis nana* eggs, protozoan cysts, *Taenia solium* eggs, *Strongyloides* larvae, microsporidian spores, and bloodborne parasites and viruses (hepatitis viruses A to E, human immunodeficiency virus).

and inappropriate therapy. Consequently, the laboratory must adhere to a strict policy of specimen acceptance and rejection.

Listed below are several examples of situations in which specific laboratory policies must be formulated and enforced to ensure specimen quality:

1. No label. Do not process. Contact the submitting physician or nurse. For specimens obtained by noninvasive means (urine, sputum, or throat specimens), have a new specimen submitted. For specimens obtained by invasive procedures (needle aspirates, body fluids, or tissues), process the specimen only after consulting with the physician who obtained the specimen. Note the problem on the report, and document the corrective action taken.

2. Prolonged transport. Do not process. Alert the submitter and request a repeat specimen. Note the problem on the patient's report: "Received after prolonged delay."

3. Improper or leaking container. Do not process. Call the submitter and request a repeat specimen. Note the problem on the patient's report and the corrective action taken.

4. Specimen unsuitable for request (i.e., anaerobic request from aerobic transport). Do not process. Contact the submitter, clarify the test request, and indicate the discrepancy. Request a proper specimen for the test requested.

5. Duplicate specimens on the same day for the same test request (except blood). Do not process. Place the specimen in the proper preservative at the correct storage temperature. Call the submitter and indicate the duplication. Note the problem on the report.

There may be instances in which a given specimen must be processed even though quality has been compromised, e.g., a difficult or unusual case or an infectious disease consult. Table 3 lists specimens that provide little, if any, clinical information; processing of these specimens should be discouraged.

Sterile body fluids may represent serious or life-threatening illness and must be handled quickly and appropriately. The decision of whether to centrifuge the fluid or to culture the specimen on agar media or in blood culture bottles must be incorporated into the laboratory protocol. Table 4 lists some management suggestions for handling sterile body fluids (4).

SPECIMEN MANAGEMENT

Tables 5 through 10 document the salient features of specimen management for the commonly received requests in most clinical microbiology laboratories including bacteriology, mycology, virology, and parasitology.

Specimens for *Mycoplasma* and *Ureaplasma*

Specimens for *Mycoplasma pneumoniae* are usually of respiratory origin, although specimens such as blood and other body fluids may be submitted. Carefully taken throat swabs and early morning sputum specimens are both valuable for the detection of *M. pneumoniae* from the respiratory tract. It is important for throat specimens that the affected area be firmly swabbed to obtain mucosal cells. The swab is immersed and agitated in transport medium, and then the fluid is expressed from the swab and the swab is removed and discarded prior to transport. Specimens may be transported and stored in either mycoplasma growth medium, nutrient broth enriched with serum, or serum-enriched sucrose-phosphate transport medium (2-SP). The 2-SP medium may also be used for transport of specimens for *Chlamydia* isolation. Specimens may be held at 4°C for up to 24 h, although ideally, specimens should be cultured within 6 h. Long-term storage should be at −70°C.

Regarding genital mycoplasmas, both *Ureaplasma urealyticum* and *Mycoplasma hominis* may be isolated from the urogenital tract. For males, urethral swabs are commonly submitted. Vaginal, cervical, or urethral swabs may be submitted from women, although the mollicutes are not usually associated with vaginitis. Urine may also be submitted for analysis, but this specimen yields fewer organisms than swabs. Transport and storage conditions are the same as those described for *M. pneumoniae*.

REFERENCES

1. **Baker, A. S., B. Paton, and J. Haaf.** 1989. Ocular infections: clinical and laboratory considerations. *Clin. Microbiol. Newsl.* **11**:97–101.
2. **Bannatyne, R. M., C. Clausen, and L. R. McCarthy.** 1979. *Cumitech 10, Laboratory Diagnosis of Upper Respiratory Tract Infections*. Coordinating ed., I. B. R. Duncan. American Society for Microbiology, Washington, D.C.
3. **Bannister, E. R.** 1993. *Clostridium difficile* and toxin detection. *Clin. Microbiol. Newsl.* **15**:121–123.
4. **Baron, E. J.** 1994. *Bailey and Scott's Diagnostic Microbiology*, 9th ed. The C. V. Mosby Co., St. Louis, Mo.
5. **Bartlett, J. G., K. J. Ryan, T. F. Smith, and W. R. Wilson.** 1987. *Cumitech 7A, Laboratory Diagnosis of Lower Respiratory Tract Infections*. Coordinating ed., J. A. Washington II. American Society for Microbiology, Washington, D.C.
6. **Bartlett, R. C.** 1985. Quality control, p. 14–23. *In* E. H. Lennette, A. Balows, W. J. Hausler, Jr., and H. J. Shadomy (ed.), *Manual of Clinical Microbiology*, 4th ed. American Society for Microbiology, Washington, D.C.
7. **Carr, D. T., A. G. Karlson, and G. G. Stillwell.** 1967. A comparison of cultures of induced sputum and gastric washings in the diagnosis of tuberculosis. *Mayo Clin. Proc.* **42**:23–25.
8. **Chernesky, M. A., C. G. Ray, and T. F. Smith.** 1982. *Cumitech 15, Laboratory Diagnosis of Viral Infections*. Coordinating ed., W. L. Drew. American Society for Microbiology, Washington, D.C.
9. **Cherry, J. D., and M. J. Miller.** 1992. Use of the virology laboratory, p. 2363–2369. *In* R. D. Feigin and J. D. Cherry (ed.), *Textbook of Pediatric Infectious Diseases*, 3rd ed. The W. B. Saunders Co., Philadelphia, Pa.
10. **Chonmaitree, T., C. D. Baldwin, and H. L. Lucia.** 1989. Role of the virology laboratory in diagnosis and management of patients with central nervous system disease. *Clin. Microbiol. Rev.* **2**:1–14.
11. **Christensen, M. L.** 1989. Human viral gastroenteritis. *Clin. Microbiol. Rev.* **2**:51–89.
12. **Clarridge, J. E., M. T. Pezzlo, and K. L. Vosti.** 1987. *Cumitech 2A, Laboratory Diagnosis of Urinary Tract Infections*. Coordinating ed., A. S. Weissfeld. American Society for Microbiology, Washington, D.C.
13. **Cook, J. H., and M. Pezzlo.** 1992. Specimen receipt and accessioning. Section 1. Aerobic bacteriology, p. 1.2.1–1.2.4. *In* H. D. Isenberg (ed. in chief), *Clinical Microbiology Procedures Handbook*. American Society for Microbiology, Washington, D.C.
14. **Edwards, M. S.** 1992. Infections due to human and animal bites, p. 2234–2345. *In* R. D. Feigin and J. D. Cherry (ed.), *Textbook of Pediatric Infectious Diseases*, 3rd ed. The W. B. Sanders Co., Philadelphia, Pa.
15. **Ellis, C. J.** 1991. The use and abuse of blood cultures. *Infect. Dis. Newsl.* **10**:27–30.
16. **Eschenbach, D., H. M. Pollock, and J. Schachter.** 1983. *Cumitech 17, Laboratory Diagnosis of Female Genital Tract*

Infections. Coordinating ed., S. J. Rubin. American Society for Microbiology, Washington, D.C.

17. **Goldmann, D. A., and G. B. Pier.** 1993. Pathogenesis of infections related to intravascular catheterization. *Clin. Microbiol. Rev.* **6:**176–187.
18. **Goldstein, E. J. C.** 1989. Bite infections, p. 455–463. *In* S. W. Finegold and W. L. George (ed.), *Anaerobic Infections in Humans*. Academic Press, Inc., San Diego, Calif.
19. **Gray, L. D., and D. P. Fedorko.** 1992. Laboratory diagnosis of bacterial meningitis. *Clin. Microbiol. Rev.* **5:**130–145.
20. **Hagen, J. C., W. S. Wood, and T. Hashimoto.** 1977. Effect of temperature on survival of *Bacteroides fragilis* subsp. *fragilis* and *Escherichia coli* in pus. *J. Clin. Microbiol.* **6:**567–570.
21. **Haley, L. D., J. Trandel, and M. B. Coyle.** 1980. *Cumitech 11, Practical Methods for Culture and Identification of Fungi in the Clinical Microbiology Laboratory*. Coordinating ed., J. C. Sherris. American Society for Microbiology, Washington, D.C.
22. **Harris, J. C., H. L. DuPont, and R. B. Hornick.** 1972. Fecal leukocytes in diarrheal illness. *Ann. Intern. Med.* **76:** 697–703.
23. **Hedberg, C. W., and M. T. Osterholm.** 1993. Outbreaks of foodborne and waterborne viral gastroenteritis. *Clin. Microbiol. Rev.* **6:**199–207.
24. **Holden, J.** 1992. Collection and transport of clinical specimens for anaerobic culture, 2.2.1–2.2.6. *In* H. D. Isenberg (ed. in chief), *Clinical Microbiology Procedures Handbook*. American Society for Microbiology, Washington, D.C.
25. **Isenberg, H. D. (ed. in chief).** 1994. *Clinical Microbiology Procedures Handbook*, vol. 1 and 2. American Society for Microbiology, Washington, D.C.
26. **Johnson, F. B.** 1990. Transport of viral specimens. *Clin. Microbiol. Rev.* **3:**120–131.
27. **Jones, D. B., T. J. Liesegang, and N. M. Robinson.** 1981. *Cumitech 13, Laboratory Diagnosis of Ocular Infections*. Coordinating ed., J. A. Washington II. American Society for Microbiology, Washington, D.C.
28. **Knoop, F. C., M. Owens, and I. C. Crocker.** 1993. *Clostridium difficile*: clinical disease and diagnosis. *Clin. Microbiol. Rev.* **6:**251–258.
29. **Krogstad, D. J., G. S. Visvesvara, K. W. Walls, and J. W. Smith.** 1991. Blood and tissue protozoa, p. 727–750. *In* A. Balows, W. J. Hausler, Jr., K. L. Herrmann, H. D. Isenberg, and H. J. Shadomy (ed.), *Manual of Clinical Microbiology*, 5th ed. American Society for Microbiology, Washington, D.C.
30. **Linares, J., A. Sitges-Serra, J. Garau, J. L. Perez, and R. Martin.** 1985. Pathogenesis of catheter sepsis: prospective study with quantitative and semiquantitative cultures of catheter hub and segments. *J. Clin. Microbiol.* **21:**357–360.
31. **MacLowry, J. D., P. R. Murray, and L. B. Reller.** 1982. *Cumitech 1A, Blood Cultures II*. Coordinating ed., J. A. Washington II. American Society for Microbiology, Washington, D.C.
32. **Maki, D. G.** 1980. Sepsis associated with infusion therapy, p. 207–253. *In* S. Karan (ed.), *Controversies in Surgical Sepsis*. Praeger, New York, N.Y.
33. **Mattia, A. R.** 1993. FDA review criteria for blood culture systems. *Clin. Microbiol. Newsl.* **15:**132–136.
34. **Melvin, D. M., and M. M. Brooke.** 1982. *Laboratory Procedures for the Diagnosis of Intestinal Parasites*, 3rd ed. HHS publication no. (CDC) 82-8282. U.S. Department of Health and Human Services, Washington, D.C.
35. **Miller, J. M.** 1996. *A Guide to Specimen Management in Clinical Microbiology*. ASM Press, Washington, D.C.
36. **Murray, P. R., E. J. Baron, M. A. Pfaller, F. C. Tenover, and R. H Yolken (ed.).** 1995. *Manual of Clinical Microbiology*, 6th ed. American Society for Microbiology, Washington, D.C.
37. **Nanduri, J., and J. W. Kazura.** 1989. Clinical and laboratory aspects of filariasis. *Clin. Microbiol. Rev.* **2:**39–47.
38. **National Committee for Clinical Laboratory Standards.** 1989. *Guidelines for Laboratory Safety*, p. 11–16. CAP Environment, Safety, and Health Committee. National Committee for Clinical Laboratory Standards, Wayne, Pa.
39. **National Committee for Clinical Laboratory Standards.** 1991. Tentative standard M29-T2. *Protection of Laboratory Workers from Infectious Disease Transmitted by Blood, Body Fluid, and Tissue*, vol. 11, no. 14, p. 28–29. National Committee for Clinical Laboratory Standards, Wayne, Pa.
40. **National Committee for Clinical Laboratory Standards.** 1992. Tentative standard M15-T. *Slide Preparation and Staining of Blood Films for the Laboratory Diagnosis of Parasitic Diseases*, vol. 12, no. 15. National Committee for Clinical Laboratory Standards, Wayne, Pa.

40a. **National Committee for Clinical Laboratory Standards.** 1997. Approved standard M28-A. *Procedures for the Recovery and Identification of Parasites from the Intestinal Tract*. National Committee for Clinical Laboratory Standards, Wayne, Pa.

40b. **National Research Council.** 1989. *Biosafety in the Laboratory: Prudent Practices for the Handling and Disposal of Infectious Materials*. National Academy Press, Washington, D.C.

41. **Ray, C. G., B. L. Wasilauskas, and R. Zabransky.** 1982. *Cumitech 14, Laboratory Diagnosis of Central Nervous System Infections*. Coordinating ed., L. R. McCarty. American Society for Microbiology, Washington, D.C.
42. **Riley, J. A., and M. P. Weinstein.** 1991. Laboratory diagnosis of bacteremia and endocarditis. *Infect. Dis. Newsl.* **10:**4–6.
43. **Ryan, M. R., and P. R. Murray.** 1993. Historical evolution of automated blood culture systems. *Clin. Microbiol. Newsl.* **15:**105–108.
44. **Sack, R. B., R. C. Tilton, and A. S. Weissfeld.** 1980. *Cumitech 12, Laboratory Diagnosis of Bacterial Diarrhea*. Coordinating ed., S. J. Rubin. American Society for Microbiology, Washington, D.C.
45. **Shea, Y. R.** 1992. Specimen collection and transport. Section 1. Aerobic bacteriology, p. 1.1.1–1.1.30. *In* H. D. Isenberg (ed. in chief), *Clinical Microbiology Procedures Handbook*. American Society for Microbiology, Washington, D.C.
46. **Simor, A. E., F. J. Roberts, and J. A. Smith.** 1988. *Cumitech 23, Infections of the Skin and Subcutaneous Tissues*. Coordinating ed., J. A. Smith. American Society for Microbiology, Washington, D.C.
47. **Smith, J. W., and M. S. Bartlett.** 1991. Diagnostic parasitology: introduction and methods, p. 701–726. *In* A. Balows, W. J. Hausler, Jr., K. L. Herrmann, H. D. Isenberg, and H. J. Shadomy (ed.), *Manual of Clinical Microbiology*, 5th ed. American Society for Microbiology, Washington, D.C.
48. **Swartz, M. N.** 1990. Cellulitis and superficial infections, p. 796–807. *In* G. L. Mandell (ed.), *Principles and Practices of Infectious Diseases*, 3rd ed. Churchill Livingstone, London, United Kingdom.
49. **Tunkel, A. R., and W. M. Scheld.** 1993. Pathogenesis and pathophysiology of bacterial meningitis. *Clin. Microbiol. Rev.* **6:**118–136.
50. **U.S. Department of Health and Human Services.** 1993. *Biosafety in Microbiological and Biomedical Laboratories*, 3rd ed. HHS publication no. (CDC) 93-8395. U.S. Department of Health and Human Services, Washington, D.C.
51. **Van Enk, R. A., and K. D. Thompson.** 1990. Microbiologic analysis of amniotic fluid. *Clin. Microbiol. Newsl.* **12:** 169–172.

Specimen Processing*

BARBARA S. REISNER, GAIL L. WOODS, RICHARD B. THOMSON, JR., DAVISE H. LARONE, LYNNE S. GARCIA, AND ROBYN Y. SHIMIZU

5

Appropriate specimen collection and handling are key to the diagnosis of infectious diseases. Guidelines for specimen collection and transport are discussed in the previous chapter. It is the laboratory's responsibility to provide instructions for appropriate collection and transport of specimens. This often is achieved through publication of a laboratory manual. The laboratory also should provide training when necessary, and changes in laboratory policies and procedures must be communicated in a timely fashion.

Upon arrival of a specimen in the laboratory, the time and date of receipt should be recorded on the requisition. Many laboratories employ a time stamp device for this purpose. At this time, the specimen and requisition should be examined to ensure that all criteria for acceptance are fulfilled. Minimum criteria for an acceptable specimen should be established, along with guidelines for rejecting specimens that do not meet these criteria. Some circumstances in which specimens should be rejected for culture are listed in Table 1. When specimens are rejected, the health care provider must be notified of the reason in a timely fashion so that another specimen may be properly submitted.

The requisition and specimen label should include the following information: patient name, age, and sex; hospital number and location or address; ordering physician's name; specimen source; date and time of collection; and procedure(s) requested. If the information is incomplete, the laboratory should ask a responsible person to provide the missing information before processing the specimen further. If a specimen is mislabeled, the sample should be re-collected. Relabelling of a specimen should be allowed only for difficult-to-collect specimens, such as tissue obtained during a surgical procedure or cerebrospinal fluid (CSF); these exceptions must be documented by the laboratory.

All patient specimens should be presumed to contain transmissible agents and therefore should be handled with standard precautions. Standard precautions are equivalent to what had previously been termed universal precautions (40) and are designed to reduce the risk of transmission of microorganisms from both recognized and unrecognized sources of infection. In most clinical laboratories, a special area is designated for processing clinical samples for culture. Ideally all specimen processing, but at a minimum processing of respiratory secretions and specimens submitted for the detection of mycobacteria or fungi, should be performed in a class II biological safety cabinet. Gloves always should be worn, and an impermeable gown, mask, and protective eyewear (or a plastic shield) must be used in situations in which there is a risk of splashes or droplet formation.

When making decisions about which procedures, media, and direct-detection methods will be used routinely for the timely and cost-effective laboratory diagnosis of infectious diseases, special consideration must be given to the type of patient population served by the laboratory, the incidence of certain diseases in a particular geographic area of the country, and pertinent patient history and/or current therapeutic regimens.

The remainder of this chapter contains specific guidelines for handling specimens received for microbiological evaluation. This information is divided into four subsections: bacteriology, virology, mycology, and parasitology. Each subsection is organized by specimen type and includes recommendations for processing, direct-detection procedures, and cultivation of microorganisms from that specimen.

BACTERIOLOGY

General Considerations

Successful laboratory diagnosis of bacterial infection depends on many factors. Proper specimen selection, collection, and transport are critical to ensure that the specimen is representative of the disease process with minimal contamination from the microorganisms present in adjacent tissues. It is the laboratory's responsibility to reject specimens that have not been properly collected and transported. Upon receipt of a specimen in the laboratory, the processing procedures, media, and incubation conditions must be carefully selected based on the specimen type.

The enormous array of organisms capable of causing infection challenges the microbiologist to create a rational approach to processing all specimen types. Certain specimens require some form of initial treatment prior to inoculation, such as dilution, concentration, homogenization, or decontamination. Most specimens submitted for detection

* This chapter contains information presented in chapter 21 by Betty A. Forbes and Paul A. Granato, chapter 60 by William G. Merz and Glenn D. Roberts, chapter 70 by David A. Lennette, and chapter 102 by Lynne S. Garcia, Sandra Bullock-Iacullo, Josephine Palmer, and Robyn Y. Shimizu in the sixth edition of this Manual.

TABLE 1 Criteria for specimen rejection

Improper transport temperature
Improper transport medium
Prolonged transport time
Unlabeled or mislabeled specimen
Leaking specimen
Cracked or broken container
Obvious contamination of specimen
Dried-out specimen on swab
Inappropriate specimen for a given test
Specimen received in fixative
Inadequate volume
Duplicate specimens (except for blood culture) in a 24-h period

of bacteria should be examined directly with the Gram stain; and if mycobacteria are suspected, a stain for acid-fast bacilli (AFB) also should be performed. Other techniques for directly examining specimens, such as direct fluorescent-antibody (DFA) stains, enzyme immunoassays (EIA), and DNA hybridization or amplification assays, are used only in selected situations. A combination of medium types generally is used for the isolation of bacteria. These may include enriched, nonselective, selective, or differential media. Most routine cultures are incubated at 35 to 37°C; however, some organisms have optimal temperatures above or below this range. A variety of atmospheric conditions, including ambient, CO_2-enriched, microaerophilic, and anaerobic, may be required.

The purpose of this section is to discuss laboratory protocols recommended for processing specimens for recovery of bacteria. These recommendations are neither all-inclusive nor applicable to all laboratory settings. Suggested primary plating media for aerobic and anaerobic bacterial culture are summarized in Table 2.

Blood

Blood is one of the most important specimens received by the laboratory. It may be submitted to aid in identifying bacteria and fungi responsible for many conditions including bacteremia, sepsis, infections of native and prosthetic valves, suppurative thrombophlebitis, and infections or vascular grafts. Because a wide variety of microorganisms can be involved in bloodstream-related infections, the methods used to recover organisms from the blood should be capable of supporting a range of microorganisms. Fortunately, there have been many improvements in the media and technology for culturing blood during the past decade, resulting in highly reliable manual and automated systems.

Specimen Number, Timing, and Volume

For adult patients, two sets of cultures should be collected per febrile episode to help distinguish probable pathogens from possible contaminants (51), especially when considering the significance of coagulase-negative staphylococci, corynebacteria, viridans streptococci, and *Bacillus* spp. In general, contaminants are more likely to be recovered from a single set of cultures whereas pathogens typically are recovered from more than one set. No more than four sets should be submitted in a 24-h period. This limit allows for the evaluation of two febrile episodes per day with two blood culture sets submitted per episode. Greater numbers of cultures are not necessary, based on data from several studies which showed that more than 95% of bacteremias are detected with the first two to three cultures (120, 122).

Blood specimens should be collected before antimicrobial agents are administered, although there are media available which contain substances designed to minimize the effect of these agents on bacterial growth. Optimally, the specimen should be collected just before a fever spike; however, practically, the specimen should be collected immediately after the spike. The total volume of blood cultured is one of the most important factors in the recovery of the bacterial pathogen. In one study, increasing the volume of blood cultured over a 24-h period from 40 to 60 ml increased the recovery by 10% (55). For adults, 20 to 30 ml of blood should be collected per venipuncture (67, 126). Less blood is required for children, because there are more microorganisms per milliliter of blood (82, 94, 114). A 1:5 to 1:10 blood-to-broth ratio has been shown to increase microbial recovery (3, 98), probably by diluting inhibitory substances. Most blood culture systems specify the volume of blood necessary for optimal recovery. Blood cultures should not be rejected for inadequate volume except when using the Isolator system (Wampole Laboratories, Cranbury, N.J.), which contains factors that inhibit the growth of microorganisms if the minimum blood volume is not present. Periodically, blood culture volumes should be monitored to identify opportunities for educating the health care providers about optimal blood culture techniques.

Initial Processing

Initial processing of a blood specimen depends on the culture system used. Specimens submitted in blood culture vials should be held at room temperature until they can be appropriately processed. For some continuously monitoring systems, bottles may have to be vented with a needle or an attachment placed on top for pressure detection. For the Septi-Chek (Becton Dickinson Microbiology Systems, Cockeysville, Md.), a paddle is attached and the bottles are inverted to inoculate the agar on the paddle prior to incubation. Isolator tubes must be centrifuged at 3,000 × *g* for 30 min within 16 h of receipt. The supernatant is discarded, and the pellet is used to inoculate the media.

Direct Methods

Direct Gram staining of a blood specimen is not recommended due to the inability of this procedure to detect the small numbers of organisms generally present in the bloodstream (<10 cfu/ml) (94, 123). Gram stain of the broth from positive cultures or colonies on a solid medium (either agar plates or paddle for Septi-Chek) should be performed as soon as growth is detected. The Gram stain report should be descriptive enough to allow the appropriate selection of antibiotics. For example, the arrangement of gram-positive cocci should be described, i.e., pairs, clusters, or chains; and gram-negative bacilli should be described as small or coccobacillary when appropriate.

A 2-h tube coagulase test can be performed directly on a positive broth culture to rapidly identify suspected *Staphylococcus aureus* (63). Data from various studies have demonstrated that some commercial identification kits are capable of identifying gram-negative organisms, using the broth from a positive blood culture as the inoculum (2, 9, 100).

Culture Systems

Conventional broth blood culture systems that use nutritionally enriched liquid media recover most bacteria, including anaerobes. Traditionally two bottles are inoculated; one is vented to ensure the recovery of strict aerobes. Bottles are examined daily for evidence of growth, indicated by

TABLE 2 Recommendations for Gram stain and plating media for microbiology specimens (except blood)

Specimen or organism	Gram stain	Aerobic media[a]	Anaerobic media[b]	Comments
Body cavity fluids				Blood culture bottles can be used to incubate large-volume specimens
CSF (routine)	x	B C		
CSF (shunt)	x	B C Th		
Pericardial	x	B C	BBA	
Pleural	x	B C	BBA	
Peritoneal	x	B C Mac	BBA LKV BBE CNA	
CAPD	x	B C Th	BBA	
Synovial	x	B C		
Bone marrow	x	B C	BBA	
Catheter tip		B		
Ear external fluid		B Mac		
	x	B C	BBA	
Eye	x	B C		
Gastrointestinal tract				
Feces		B Mac HE Ca		
Rectal swab		B Mac HE Ca EB		
Genitourinary tract				
Vagina/cervix		B TM		
Urethra/penis	x	TM		
Other	x	B C Mac TM	BBA LKV BBE CNA	
Lower respiratory tract				
Sputum	x	B C Mac		
Tracheal aspirate	x	B C Mac		
Bronchoalveolar lavage fluid	x	B C Mac	BBA LKV BBE CNA	Protected bronchoscope required for anaerobic culture
Bronchoalveolar brushing, washing	x	B C Mac		
Tissue	x	B C Mac Th	BBA LKV BBE CNA	
Upper respiratory tract				
Nose		B C		
Throat		B or SSA		Add chocolate agar for epiglottitis
Urine		B Mac		
Wound or abscess				
Swab	x	B C Mac	BBA LKV BBE CNA	
Aspirate	x	B C Mac	BBA LKV BBE CNA	
Bordetella pertussis and *B. parapertussis*		Regan Lowe		
Brucella spp.		B C		
Corynebacterium diphtheriae		cystine-tellurite or Loeffler's serum		
Clostridium difficile		CCFA		
E. coli O157		sorbitol-Mac		
Francisella tularensis		C or BCYE		
Group B *Streptococcus*		LIM broth		
Haemophilus ducreyi		C + vancomycin		
Legionella		BCYE		
Neisseria gonorrhoeae		TM		
Vibrio		TCBS		
Yersinia		CIN		

[a] B, blood agar; C, chocolate blood agar; Mac, MacConkey agar; Th, thioglycolate broth; Ca, Campylobacter agar; HE, Hektoen enteric; EB, enrichment broth; SSA, group A *Streptococcus* selective agar; TM, Thayer-Martin; BCYE, buffered charcoal yeast extract; TCBS, thiosulfate citrate bile salt sucrose; CIN, cefsulodin-irgasan-novobiocin; BBA, Brucella blood agar; LKV, laked blood with kanamycin and vancomycin; BBE, *Bacteroides* bile esculin; CNA, anaerobic colistin-nalidixic acid; CCFA, cycloserine-cefoxitin-fructose agar; CAPD, fluid from chronic ambulatory peritoneal dialysis.

[b] Set up anaerobic culture upon request, if specimen is collected appropriately.

turbidity, hemolysis, gas production, or the presence of colonies. Subculture of the contents of the aerobic bottle after 6 to 18 h of incubation is required. Routine subculture of the anaerobic bottles is not necessary (75, 81). These systems have the advantage of being inexpensive with regard to reagents, but they are relatively labor-intensive.

The biphasic Septi-Chek is a manual method that involves a bottle containing broth to which an agar paddle is attached. The agar is inoculated by inverting the bottle until the broth comes in contact with the agar medium. The agar and the broth are then visually inspected for evidence of growth. This system performs well with regard to recovery of aerobic and facultative bacteria (anaerobes are recovered with a separate bottle with no paddle attached), and it is less labor-intensive than the conventional systems. Additionally, colonies are immediately available for identification and susceptibility testing.

The Isolator lysis centrifugation system is another commercially available manual blood culture method. This system consists of a tube containing the anticoagulant EDTA and the lysing agent saponin. After the tube is inoculated with blood, it is centrifuged and the resulting pellet is plated onto agar media. This system has been shown to effectively recover aerobic and facultatively anaerobic bacteria and fungi; however, it does not perform as well as other systems with regard to the recovery of *Streptococcus pneumoniae*, other streptococci, *Pseudomonas aeruginosa*, and anaerobes (123). The main disadvantages of this system are that it is labor-intensive and, because of the increased manipulation during processing, can be subject to higher rates of contamination.

The fully automated continuously monitoring blood culture systems are the newest type of systems developed for the detection of bacteria and fungi in blood (see references 94 and 127 for comprehensive reviews). The systems available in the United States are the BacT/Alert (Organon Teknika Corp., Durham, N.C.), BACTEC 9000 (Becton Dickinson Microbiology Systems), and ESP (Accumed International Inc., Westlake, Ohio). The systems are alike in that the culture bottles are incubated in an instrument, where they are continuously monitored (typically at 10-min intervals) for the production and/or consumption of gas. The data collected are transmitted to a computer and analyzed to allow rapid detection of microbial growth. Each system utilizes a noninvasive method (e.g., colorimetric, fluorescent, or manometric methods for detecting CO_2 or other gases) to monitor growth. The systems offer a variety of media, including those for the recovery of aerobes or anaerobes, those for use with patients taking antibiotics, and those for use with pediatric patients. Most systems and available media have been extensively evaluated, and in general, the data from these studies indicate that these systems are a reliable and rapid alternative to conventional systems for the detection of bacteria and yeast in blood.

Incubation Conditions

All bacterial blood cultures should be incubated at 35°C. Manual blood culture systems should be incubated for 7 days. Manual broth-only systems should include a terminal subculture of the aerobic bottle on the final day. For automated systems, data from several studies have shown that incubation for 5 days is sufficient to recover most bacteria. Moreover, by limiting the incubation time in this way, fewer contaminants are recovered. Terminal subculture of automated blood culture bottles is unnecessary (94). When subculturing positive blood culture vials, the aerobic media used should be selected based on the organism seen in the Gram-stained smear. Anaerobic media and culture conditions should be used if the morphology of the organism seen in the Gram-stained smear is suggestive of an anaerobic organism or if the organism is recovered from an anaerobic blood bottle only.

Special Considerations

Anaerobes

Anaerobes have always accounted for a relatively small percentage of organisms recovered from blood. Over the past several years, some investigators have noted a decline in anaerobic bloodstream infections (22, 56, 76). However, this is not the case in all hospitals (17, 18); therefore, laboratories should review their own data when deciding whether to include an anaerobic culture as part of the routine workup of blood specimens. Neither the Septi-Chek system nor the Isolator system is optimal for recovering anaerobes. The anaerobic media available for use with the automated systems appear to perform adequately, although the capabilities of these instruments to detect anaerobes have not been rigorously assessed (94).

Fastidious Bacteria

Various bacteria capable of causing bloodstream infection may not be recovered by routine blood culture procedures. Brucellae will grow in routine blood culture media; and although these organisms may be recovered in as few as 3 days, it is recommended that cultures be held for 21 days, and in some cases a terminal subculture is necessary (4, 132). The HACEK group of bacteria (i.e., *Haemophilus aphrophilus*, *Actinobacillus actinomycetemcomitans*, *Cardiobacterium hominis*, *Eikenella corrodens*, and *Kingella kingae*), associated with bacterial endocarditis, also are recovered from routine media; however, up to 14 days of incubation and terminal subculture of the broth may be useful. When the clinical history is suggestive of infection with *Francisella*, positive blood cultures should be subcultured to BCYE agar in addition to the standard agar media and all manipulations of the culture should be conducted in a laminar-flow hood with biosafety level 3 practices. *Leptospira* species are not recovered with routine media; 1 or 2 drops of blood, collected during the first week of illness, should be inoculated to a semisolid medium such as Fletcher's Ellinghausen-McCullough/Johnson-Harris, or Polysorbate 80 (48). Cultures should be incubated at room temperature for up to 6 weeks.

Recovery of *Bartonella henselae* from blood is difficult, but it is possible with some blood culture systems. With the Isolator system, processed blood should be plated to an enriched blood or chocolate blood agar growth medium (as freshly prepared as possible) and incubated at 35°C under conditions of elevated CO_2 and humidity for up to 4 weeks. With the Septi-Chek system, growth may be achieved after incubation for at least 40 days. In broth-only systems, the organisms may be observed by staining a smear of the broth with acridine orange; however, the organism does not produce turbidity or enough CO_2 to be detected by using instrumentation.

Mycobacteria

Mycobacteremia has become more frequent during the past several years as a result of the epidemic of infection with human immunodeficiency virus (HIV). These organisms generally are not recovered by routine blood culture practices. Methods that may be used to isolate mycobacteria from blood include lysis centrifugation followed by inoculation of the blood pellet to a solid medium (i.e., Middlebrook 7H11 or 7H10 or Lowenstein Jensen) or to the BACTEC 12B medium and/or the ESPII medium or direct inoculation of the BACTEC 13A medium. Generally, two blood cultures per week are adequate for diagnosing mycobacteremia (131). Cultures should be held for at least 6 weeks.

Catheter Tips

Culture of catheter tips is performed to determine the source of a bacteremia. The most commonly used technique is the semiquantitative method (59), in which a 5-cm segment of the distal portion of the catheter is rolled across a blood agar plate four times. Cultures yielding organisms present at >15 colonies are considered to be significant, potentially indicating a catheter-related infection.

Many other techniques have been described for the identification of catheter-related infections. Recently, a meta-analysis of data reported in the scientific literature concerning the use of three types of catheter segment cultures (qualitative, semiquantitative, and quantitative) and three blood culture methods (unpaired qualitative catheter blood culture, unpaired quantitative catheter blood culture, and paired quantitative catheter blood culture) was performed (103) to determine the sensitivity, specificity, accuracy, and overall cost-effectiveness of each method. Based on this analysis, a quantitative catheter segment culture was the most accurate method and a single quantitative culture of blood aspirated from the catheter was associated with the lowest expense to the entire hospital. At this time, the optimal laboratory method for assessing catheter-related infections has not been determined. Because the most serious manifestation of these infections is bacteremia, ordinary blood cultures may be the best way to determine which patients require therapy (93).

Sterile Body Fluids

Cerebrospinal Fluid

CSF is collected for the diagnosis of meningitis. Bacterial meningitis is divided into acute and chronic clinical syndromes. Acute meningitis, with onset of symptoms within the previous 24 h, is usually caused by pyogenic bacteria. The most likely pathogen varies according to the age of the individual (102) and whether the disease is community or nosocomially acquired. Bacteria typically causing chronic meningitis, with symptoms persisting for at least 4 weeks, include *Mycobacterium tuberculosis*, *Treponema pallidum*, *Brucella* spp., *Leptospira interrogans*, and *Borrelia burgdorferi*.

CSF usually is obtained by lumbar spinal puncture. Each bacteriologic procedure requires at least 0.5 ml of CSF, although larger volumes are preferred. The specimen should be transported to the laboratory promptly and processed as soon as possible. If a delay in processing is unavoidable, the specimen should be held at room temperature.

If more than 1.0 ml of CSF is received, it should be concentrated by centrifugation at a minimum of 1,500 × *g* for 15 min. The supernatant is decanted into a sterile tube, leaving 0.5 ml of sediment and fluid. This is thoroughly mixed and used to prepare a smear for direct examination and to inoculate media for culture. Alternatively, an aliquot of the original specimen can be used to make a cytocentrifuged preparation.

A Gram stain should be performed on all CSF specimens as soon as they are received in the laboratory. Results, including a description and quantitation of both microorganisms and cellular elements present in the specimen, should be reported to the requesting physician. Rapid tests for bacterial antigens of group B streptococci, *S. pneumoniae*, some serotypes of *Neisseria meningitidis*, *Escherichia coli* (K1 capsular antigen cross-reacts with that of *N. meningitidis* type B), and *Haemophilus influenzae* type b may be performed on the supernatant of a centrifuged specimen or the original specimen. Data from several studies indicate that the sensitivity of these tests is less than or equal to that of Gram staining (31, 85), except in cases of partially treated meningitis, where the antigen tests may be more sensitive (7, 62). In addition, it has been shown that the results of these tests have very little effect on the care of the patient (31, 62, 85). For these reasons and because the rapid bacterial antigen tests are much more expensive and more labor-intensive than the Gram stain, many laboratories no longer offer these tests or strictly limit their use (e.g., to CSF specimens containing >50 leukocytes [52, 74, 115]) or require consultation between the clinician and the clinical microbiologist.

Cultivation of a CSF specimen should include media and incubation conditions appropriate to recover fastidious organisms. Broth cultures traditionally have been included among the media inoculated; however, data from a few studies indicate that the results of broth cultures contribute very little to the management of the patient and may be necessary only when culturing specimens collected from patients with a CSF shunt (73, 113).

Special Considerations

Anaerobes

Anaerobic bacteria very rarely cause meningitis; therefore, routine anaerobic culture of CSF is not required. Anaerobes commonly are involved in brain abscess formation, subdural empyema, and epidural abscess; however, CSF examination is not likely to be helpful diagnostically in these cases.

Mycobacteria

With the exception of specimens from patients with AIDS, processing CSF for mycobacteria is indicated only for samples with pleocytosis or abnormal glucose or protein levels. Because the number of mycobacteria present in CSF is small, a large volume of specimen (3 to 5 ml optimal) is necessary to maximize recovery of the organism in culture. The fluid is centrifuged at 3,000 to 3,600 × *g* for 30 min, the supernatant is decanted, and the sediment is thoroughly mixed on a vortex mixer and used to prepare smears for staining for AFB and to inoculate appropriate media, which should include a liquid medium. Cultures should be incubated at 35°C in the presence of 8% CO_2 for at least 6 weeks. Given the low sensitivity of the AFB smear for this specimen type, individual laboratories may want to review their own data to determine the need for routinely performing a direct smear on CSF.

Leptospires

Leptospires can be recovered from the CSF during the first 10 days of illness. The specimen should be collected before antibiotic treatment and while the patient is febrile. For the direct detection of leptospires, the specimen is centrifuged at 1,500 × *g* for 30 min and the sediment is used to prepare a wet mount for dark-field microscopy. Leptospires can be recovered in culture with a semisolid medium such as Fletcher's, Ellinghausen-McCullough/Johnson-Harris, or Polysorbate 80. An inoculum of 0.5 ml is recommended. Cultures should be incubated at room temperature for up to 6 weeks.

Other Body Fluids

Specimens include pericardial, pleural, peritoneal, and synovial fluids. For optimal microbiological analysis, it is essential that fluid, rather than a fluid-saturated swab, be submitted. A volume of 1 to 5 ml is adequate for the isolation of most organisms (129). For diagnosing peritonitis associated with chronic ambulatory peritoneal dialysis, collection of at least 50 ml of fluid may improve recovery of the responsible pathogen (20). Body fluids should be directly inoculated into a blood culture bottle or sterile, anaerobic container at the bedside and transported promptly to the laboratory.

In the laboratory, volumes greater than 1.0 ml should be centrifuged at a minimum of 1,500 × *g* for 15 min. The supernatant is removed, leaving about 0.5 ml, in which the sediment is mixed. The resuspended sediment is used to prepare smears for Gram staining and to inoculate media. If cytocentrifugation is used to prepare a smear, approximately 0.5 ml is removed prior to centrifugation for this purpose. Uncentrifuged fluids may also be directly inoculated to a blood culture bottle in the laboratory, reserving a small volume (0.5 to 1 ml) for Gram staining.

Solid media used for culture of body fluid specimens should be selected to allow recovery of fastidious organisms. Inoculating a liquid medium may be necessary only when culturing dialysate from patients undergoing chronic ambulatory peritoneal dialysis (73, 74), where the number of organisms present in the specimen can be as small as 1 CFU/ml. The need for a liquid culture for other types of fluids should be determined by each laboratory. Cultures should be incubated at 35°C in the presence of CO_2.

Special Considerations

Processing body fluids for mycobacteria differs from that for other bacteria in that the specimen is centrifuged at 3,000 to 3,600 × *g* for 30 min. The supernatant is decanted, and the sediment is used to prepare a smear for staining for AFB and inoculation of appropriate media. Cultures for mycobacteria are incubated at 35°C with 8% CO_2 and are held for at least 6 weeks.

Body fluids may be submitted in tubes containing anticoagulating agents. However, because certain anticoagulants, including heparin, sodium citrate, and EDTA, are inhibitory to some organisms (23, 96), this practice is not recommended. If the laboratory chooses to process a fluid submitted in an anticoagulant, the ordering physician must be informed about the limitations of the result.

Ear

Two types of ear specimens are generally received by the laboratory, i.e., swab specimens for the diagnosis of otitis externa and middle ear fluid for the diagnosis of otitis media. The potential pathogens at these two sites differ. *P. aeruginosa* is a frequent cause of otitis externa. Other aerobic organisms may also be involved, but anaerobes are not; therefore, anaerobic culture is not necessary. Organisms derived from the respiratory flora, including *S. pneumoniae, H. influenzae*, and *Moraxella catarrhalis*, as well as *S. aureus* and gram-negative bacilli, are potential causes of otitis media, and the media inoculated and incubation conditions should allow the recovery of these pathogens. Anaerobic bacteria can be involved in these middle ear infections; therefore, anaerobic culture should be performed upon request. Direct examination of a smear of the middle ear fluid with the Gram stain may be performed if an adequate volume is submitted. Direct examination of other types of ear specimens is not commonly performed.

Eye

Several types of specimens may be collected for the microbiological analysis of eye infections, including conjunctival specimens obtained with a swab or sterile spatula for the diagnosis of conjunctivitis, corneal scrapings collected with a sterile spatula for the diagnosis of keratitis, vitreous fluid for the diagnosis of endophthalmitis, and purulent material for the diagnosis of cellulitis. Because the volume of specimen obtained in many cases of ocular infections is small, it is recommended that inoculation of media and preparation of smears for direct examination be performed at the patient's bedside.

Direct examination of smears is important for rapid diagnosis of eye infections and should include a Gram stain for detection of bacteria. To detect *Chlamydia trachomatis* directly in a conjunctival specimen, several methods are available. A Giemsa stain of conjunctival scrapings may be examined for the presence of epithelial cells containing basophilic intracytoplasmic inclusions. However, monoclonal antibodies for use in DFA are preferred because they are more sensitive and specific than the Giemsa stain. For optimal results with these DFA tests, the collection kit provided by the manufacturer should be used and the specimen should contain at least 10 columnar or metaplastic squamous cells. A commercial EIA (Chlamydiazyme; Abbott Laboratories, Abbott Park, Ill.) and a nucleic acid probe assay (Pace; Gen-Probe Incorporated, San Diego, Calif.) are also available for detection of *C. trachomatis* in conjunctival specimens.

Whether inoculated at the bedside or in the laboratory, the media for routine bacterial culture of eye specimens should include an enriched medium for the recovery of fastidious organisms such as *S. pneumoniae, H. influenzae*, and *Neisseria* spp., and the selected media should be incubated in the presence of CO_2.

For isolation of *C. trachomatis*, cell culture is required. The specimen should be collected in 2-sucrose-phosphate or sucrose-glutamate-phosphate containing antimicrobial agents (usually gentamicin, vancomycin, and nystatin or amphotericin B; penicillin should not be used) to inhibit the overgrowth of bacteria and fungi. Swabs with wooden shafts should be avoided because the wood may be toxic to the organism. Specimens should be refrigerated until processed or stored at −70°C for delays longer than 48 h. In the laboratory, the specimen is vigorously shaken in the presence of glass beads to disrupt somatic cells. A portion of the inoculum is then centrifuged onto a monolayer of cycloheximide-treated McCoy or buffalo green monkey cells at 3,000 × *g* for 1 h.

Gastrointestinal Tract

Feces and in some cases rectal swabs are submitted to the laboratory primarily to determine the etiologic agent of infectious diarrhea or food poisoning. Feces should be collected in a clean container with a tight lid and should not be contaminated with urine, barium, or toilet paper. Rectal swabs should be placed in a tube transport system containing modified Stuart's medium.

It is becoming standard practice to reject stool specimens for routine bacterial culture from patients who have been hospitalized longer than 3 days, based on data from studies indicating that it is not cost-effective (74, 95). Diarrhea that develops in the hospital is not likely to be due to food-borne pathogens; for such patients, examination for the toxins produced by *Clostridium difficile* is recommended.

For "routine" stool culture, the media inoculated should allow the detection of *Salmonella, Shigella,* and *Campylobacter* spp. at a minimum. Usually this consists of a selective and differential medium such as MacConkey agar, a more selective medium such as Hektoen enteric or xylose-lysine-desoxycholate agar, and a medium for growth of *Campylobacter* spp., such as campylobacter agar with 10% sheep blood. Enrichment broth media that enhance the recovery of *Salmonella* and *Shigella* spp. are available; however, for optimal use, subcultures to an agar medium must be performed in as little as 6 to 8 h for Gram Negative (GN) broth and 12 to 18 h for Selenite F broth, to prevent overgrowth with normal flora. Special enrichment broths are available for *Campylobacter* spp.; however, their routine use is not indicated. Media for the recovery of *Salmonella* and *Shigella* spp. are incubated in air at 35°C for 2 days. Media for the recovery of *Campylobacter* spp. are incubated in a microaerophilic environment at 42°C for up to 3 days.

Special Considerations

The prevalence of gastroenteritis caused by *Aeromonas* spp., *Plesiomonas* spp., *Vibrio* spp., and *Yersinia enterocolitica* is sufficiently low in most parts of the United States that cultures for these organisms generally are performed upon request only. Media routinely used to culture for enteric pathogens are sufficient to recover *Aeromonas* and *Plesiomonas* spp., although the use of blood agar may be helpful in detecting the hemolytic *Aeromonas* spp. Selective media for these organisms are also available. *Vibrio* spp. and *Y. enterocolitica* will also grow on routine stool culture media, but the selective medium thiosulfate citrate bile salts sucrose (TCBS) agar should be inoculated for optimal recovery of *Vibrio* spp. and cefsulodin-irgasan-novobiocin (CIN) agar should be inoculated and incubated at room temperature for the optimal recovery of *Y. enterocolitica.*

Enterohemorrhagic *E. coli*

The prevalence of enterohemorrhagic *E. coli*-associated enterocolitis varies in different parts of the United States, and in many areas of the country it is so low that laboratories culture for it upon request only. However, in 1993, the Council of State and Territorial Epidemiologists recommended that bloody stools be routinely cultured for this organism (19). To detect enterohemorrhagic *E. coli*, the stool specimen is inoculated onto sorbitol-MacConkey agar (containing 1% D-sorbitol instead of lactose), a medium that differentiates isolates of enterohemorrhagic *E. coli*, which do not ferment sorbitol, from almost all other *E. coli* isolates, which are sorbitol fermentation positive. In addition, stool filtrates can be tested for toxin production in Vero cells or by a commercial EIA (Premier E. coli O157; Meridian Diagnostics Inc., Cincinnati, Ohio).

Clostridium difficile

Diseases associated with *C. difficile*, such as pseudomembranous colitis and antibiotic-associated diarrhea, are caused by the toxins produced by the organism, and are diagnosed by detecting toxins in feces. The reference method for detection of the cytotoxin is cell culture assay. To extract toxin, the stool specimen is clarified by centrifugation at 2,000 × *g* for 20 min or 10,000 × *g* for 10 min and filtered through a 0.45-μm-pore-size membrane filter. Serial dilutions of the filtrate are prepared and inoculated to monolayers of human diploid lung fibroblasts. Alternatively, toxin may be detected in stool samples by one of many commercial EIAs. The EIA methods are less sensitive than cell culture but provide results within a few hours. A latex agglutination test, which detects glutamate dehydrogenase produced by the organism, is available; however, this enzyme is not found exclusively in toxin-producing isolates of *C. difficile*, and cross-reactivity with other bacterial species occurs (57, 69).

For epidemiologic purposes, stool or rectal swabs placed in an anaerobic transport system may be cultured anaerobically to isolate *C. difficile*. The sample is inoculated to a selective medium such as cycloserine-cefoxitin-fructose agar (CCFA), and incubated anaerobically for 48 h. Isolates identified as *C. difficile* must be tested for toxin production to determine the association of the organism with disease.

Staphylococcus aureus and *Bacillus cereus*

Stool specimens or gastric contents collected from persons with short-incubation food poisoning should be evaluated for *S. aureus* and *B. cereus*. Specimens should be examined by Gram stain, and because both of these organisms may be present normally in food, quantitative cultures must be performed. A series of dilutions (10^{-1} to 10^{-5}) of the specimen are prepared in buffered gelatin diluent, and 0.1-ml samples of the undiluted specimen and each of the dilutions are plated onto colistin nalidixic-acid or phenylethyl alcohol blood agar. The presence of 10^5 CFU or more of *S. aureus* or *B. cereus* per g of specimen is of potential significance (11, 68).

Clostridium botulinum

The clinical diagnoses of food-borne botulism and infant botulism may be confirmed by detecting botulinal toxin, *C. botulinum*, or both in feces. Optimally, 25 to 50 ml of stool, 15 to 20 ml of serum, and a sample of the suspect food should be collected. Most clinical laboratories are not properly equipped to process specimens from persons with suspected botulism. In the United States when a case of botulism is suspected, investigators at the Centers for Disease Control and Prevention (CDC) should be notified to ensure appropriate diagnosis, treatment, and investigation of the potential outbreak.

Mycobacteria

With regard to mycobacterial culture, stool specimens usually are submitted for isolation of *Mycobacterium avium* complex (primarily in patients with AIDS). Processing the specimen (1 to 2 g of formed stool or 5 ml of liquid stool) involves decontamination, concentration, preparation of smears, and inoculation of appropriate media. Gastric aspirates representing swallowed sputum are occasionally submitted for mycobacterial culture from infants, young children, and persons who are obtunded. These should be obtained in the early morning before the patient eats and are collected in a container containing sodium carbonate to neutralize the pH.

Genital Tract

Genital tract specimens are sent to the laboratory to determine the cause of various clinical syndromes, including vulvovaginitis, bacterial vaginosis, genital ulcers, urethritis, cervicitis, endometritis, salpingitis, and ovarian abscess in females and urethritis, epididymitis, prostatitis, and genital ulcers in males. Many specimens are contaminated with the normal microbiota of the genital tract or skin; therefore, the microbiologist must be able to differentiate the normal flora from organisms that are potential pathogens. Certain organisms such as *Neisseria gonorrhoeae*, *C. trachomatis*, and *Haemophilus ducreyi* are always pathogenic, while other organisms such as the *Enterobacteriaceae*, *S. aureus*, and group B *Streptococcus* are pathogenic only in certain clinical situations.

A direct Gram stain should be performed on any aspirated material. Gram stains of other specimens may be useful in only a few situations. For example, the presence of gram-negative diplococci within polymorphonuclear leukocytes in urethral discharge from males is sufficient for the presumptive diagnosis of gonorrhea. A decreased ratio of lactobacilli to *Gardnerella* spp., *Bacteroides* spp., and curved, gram-variable bacilli in a Gram-stained smear of a vaginal specimen can be useful for the diagnosis of vaginosis (79).

A wet mount preparation of vaginal secretions is a rapid and simple method for determining the etiologic agent of bacterial vaginosis as well as vulvovaginitis. For optimal results, the wet mount should be prepared and examined within 1 to 2 h of specimen collection. If *Trichomonas* is suspected, the specimen must be examined immediately because motility is lost rapidly. To prepare the wet mount, a sample of the discharge is mixed with saline and a portion of the mixture is placed on a glass slide, covered with a coverslip, and examined under low and high power for the presence of clue cells (epithelial cells covered with small coccobacillary bacteria), consistent with the diagnosis of vaginosis; pseudohyphae, suggestive of vaginal candidiasis; and motile trichomonads. Two other diagnostic tests performed in conjunction with the wet mount are vaginal pH and the "whiff test." The vaginal pH is usually $\leq$4.5 in the absence of infection and in women with vulvovaginal candidiasis but >4.5 in those with bacterial vaginosis or trichomoniasis. A positive whiff test (i.e., generation of a pungent, fishy odor upon addition of 10% potassium hydroxide to the specimen) is associated predominantly with bacterial vaginosis but occasionally occurs with trichomoniasis.

Direct examination by dark-field microscopy or DFA (reagents are available from the CDC) is required for the detection of *T. pallidum* in tissues and tissue exudates. For dark-field microscopy, the specimen should be examined within 20 min of collection to ensure retention of motility. The test requires a microscope with a dark-field condenser and well-trained and experienced personnel who are able to recognize *T. pallidum* spirochetes based on the tightness and regularity of the spirals and on its characteristic corkscrew movement. The DFA, on the other hand, is performed on air-dried specimens, including tissues, body fluids, secretions, and lesion exudates, and is specific for *T. pallidum*, making it easier to interpret.

Both EIA and the DFA test are commercially available for the direct detection of *C. trachomatis* in genital specimens. If these kits are used, the specimen must be collected by using the procedures and collection kits recommended by the manufacturer.

Nucleic acid probe and amplification methods are commercially available for direct detection of *N. gonorrhoeae* and *C. trachomatis* in endocervical and urethral specimens, and recently a combination probe assay, the Affirm VPIII microbial identification test (Becton Dickinson), has been introduced for the detection of *Candida* spp., *Gardnerella vaginalis*, and *Trichomonas vaginalis* in vaginal secretions. As with the immunoassays, the specimen must be collected by using the procedures and collection kits recommended by the manufacturer.

The optimal culture medium and incubation conditions for genital specimens depend on the source and the organisms likely to cause disease at that site. Tissues and aspirates should be plated to media capable of recovering fastidious organisms. Specimens from the cervix, vagina, and urethra should at a minimum be evaluated for *N. gonorrhoeae* and *C. trachomatis* by culture or a direct detection method. Culture is currently the only acceptable diagnostic procedure in a medical-legal case. The optimal approach for isolation of *N. gonorrhoeae* is direct inoculation of a selective agar medium, such as modified Thayer-Martin medium, at the patient's bedside, with transport to the laboratory in a CO_2-containing environment. Alternatively, the swab specimen (cotton swabs should be avoided because they may be toxic) can be placed in a transport system containing Stuart's or Amies medium and delivered to the laboratory within 24 h. If a delay in transport cannot be avoided, the swab should be left at room temperature, never refrigerated. For recovery of *C. trachomatis*, the specimen should be collected and placed in liquid transport medium as described previously. Specimens should be transported to the laboratory without delay, where they are inoculated to cells by using the shell vial technique.

Special Considerations

Group B *Streptococcus* spp.

It is important to isolate and identify group B streptococci in vaginal and perineal specimens from obstetric patients because this organism may cause severe sepsis and/or meningitis in neonates. For optimal recovery of group B streptococci, the procedures outlined by the CDC (101) should be followed; a swab specimen of the vaginal introitus and anorectum is collected and inoculated into an enrichment broth such as LIM broth or comparable medium (refer to chapter 17). This broth is incubated at 35°C and subcultured to a blood agar plate after overnight incubation.

Haemophilus ducreyi

If infection with *H. ducreyi* is suspected, material from the base of the ulcer is collected and held at room temperature until processed. One swab is used to prepare a smear for Gram staining. The presence of many small pleomorphic gram-negative bacilli and coccobacilli arranged in chains and groups suggests *H. ducreyi*. Recovery of the organisms by culturing on an enriched medium such as chocolate agar supplemented with IsoVitaleX (Becton Dickinson Microbiology Systems) is necessary to confirm the diagnosis.

Actinomyces spp.

Actinomyces spp. may cause pelvic inflammatory disease in women who use intrauterine contraceptive devices. An IUD submitted for culture should be placed in a sterile liquid medium and vortexed, and the liquid is used to inoculate the culture medium. Cultures for *Actinomyces* spp. should be incubated anaerobically and held for 14 days.

Lower Respiratory Tract

Specimens from the lower respiratory tract are submitted primarily to determine the etiologic agent of pneumonia. The most common respiratory specimen received in the laboratory is sputum, expectorated or induced. Other types of specimens included in this category are tracheal aspirates, transtracheal aspirates, bronchial washes, bronchial brushings, and bronchoalveolar lavage fluids.

Lower respiratory tract specimens should be delivered promptly to the laboratory; however, if delays in transport or processing are unavoidable, the specimen should be refrigerated. In general, expectorated sputa and tracheal aspirates should be screened microscopically before processing to determine whether they are representative of lower respiratory secretions or saliva. This is accomplished by examining a Gram-stained smear prepared from the purulent portion of the specimen under low-power magnification to determine the number of squamous epithelial cells and/or neutrophils present. There are many ways that this information may be used to assess the quality of the specimen (72). A simple screening method involves assessment of the squamous epithelial cells only: >10 squamous epithelial cells per low-power field indicates that the specimen is contaminated with saliva and hence is not acceptable for culture. This criterion is particularly useful when evaluating specimens from neutropenic patients, because the presence of neutrophils is not required for a specimen to be acceptable. Expectorated sputa for detection of *Mycoplasma pneumoniae*, *Legionella* spp., and mycobacteria do not have to be screened for adequacy (34, 43).

For all acceptable lower respiratory tract specimens, a smear should be stained with Gram stain and examined under oil immersion to determine the relative numbers of organisms present. Any intracellular organisms should be reported. With regard to culture, the use of both selective and nonselective media is recommended. In addition, a medium capable of recovering *Haemophilus* spp. should be inoculated. Cultures are incubated at 35°C in the presence of 5% CO_2.

Special Considerations

Bronchoalveolar Lavage Fluid and Bronchial Brush Specimens

It is recommended that bronchoalveolar lavage fluid and bronchial brush specimens from patients with suspected ventilator-associated pneumonia be cultured quantitatively to optimally evaluate the significance of the organisms recovered (5, 14, 99). Bronchial brush specimens, which contain approximately 0.01 to 0.001 ml of secretions, are placed in 1 ml of sterile saline or broth immediately after collection, and the sample is promptly transported to the laboratory. In the laboratory, the specimen is first agitated on a vortex mixer; a smear for direct evaluation is prepared by cytocentrifugation and stained with the Gram stain, and 0.01 ml of the specimen is plated to appropriate media by using a pipette or calibrated loop. Colony counts of more than 1,000 organisms/ml of broth (corresponding to 10^6 CFU/ml of original specimen) appear to correlate with infection. During bronchoalveolar lavage, 10 to 100 ml of fluid is collected. A portion of this sample is transported to the laboratory, where a smear is prepared by cytocentrifugation and Gram stained. The Gram stain report should include a statement regarding the presence or absence of intracellular organisms. In a few studies, the observation of >7% cells containing intracellular organisms correlated with ventilator-associated pneumonia (1, 65). A 0.001-ml aliquot of the specimen is inoculated onto agar media, and the recovery of 10,000 colonies or more of a specific organism per ml of fluid correlates with pneumonia.

Legionella spp.

Legionella spp. are not an uncommon cause of community-acquired or nosocomial pneumonia. Legionellosis can be diagnosed by culture, by detection of antigens in the urine, or by serologic testing. Culture is preferred because, unlike the other methods, it is not limited to detection of certain species or serotypes. Before culture, respiratory samples should be diluted 10-fold in a bacteriologic broth such as tryptic soy broth or sterile water to dilute inhibitory substances that may be present in the specimen. Because legionellae grow slowly, optimal isolation from highly contaminated specimens, such as sputa or tracheal aspirates, is achieved by decontaminating the specimens with acid before plating (119). The specimen is diluted 1:10 in KCl-HCl buffer (pH 2.2) and incubated for 4 min at room temperature. It is important not to incubate the specimen for longer than 4 min because legionellae may slowly become inactivated by the acid. Specimens then are inoculated to buffered charcoal yeast extract agar with and without antimicrobial agents (e.g., vancomycin, polymyxin B, and anisomycin). The cultures are incubated in humidified air at 35°C for a minimum of 5 days.

Mycoplasma pneumoniae

M. pneumoniae is a major cause of primary atypical pneumonia. Because mycoplasmas are fastidious and grow very slowly, a definitive diagnosis often is based on the results of serologic tests. When culture is required, the specimen of choice is a throat swab; however, sputa or other respiratory specimens are also acceptable. The specimen should be placed immediately into a transport medium containing protein, such as albumin, and penicillin to reduce the growth of contaminating organisms. Specimens may be stored in the transport medium for up to 48 h at 4°C or frozen for longer periods at −70°C. Chapter 56 contains a complete discussion of the optimal methods for processing specimens for mycoplasma culture.

Burkholderia cepacia

Burkholderia (formerly *Pseudomonas*) *cepacia* is an important respiratory pathogen in persons with cystic fibrosis. This organism grows well on routine media; however, selective media such as PC (for *Pseudomonas cepacia*) and OFPBL (oxidative-fermentative-polymyxin B-bacitracin-lactose) agars are useful for its optimal recovery from respiratory secretions.

Chlamydia spp.

Chlamydiae are also an important cause of respiratory illnesses. *C. trachomatis* can cause serious respiratory disease in infants. *Chlamydia pneumoniae* causes illness in all age groups, but the most severe disease generally occurs in young children and the elderly. *Chlamydia psittaci* is primarily an animal pathogen but occasionally causes disease in humans. Specimens for detection of chlamydiae are collected in a medium that contains selected antimicrobial agents (generally aminoglycosides and antifungal agents). To maintain the viability of chlamydiae, the specimen should be transported to the laboratory immediately, where it is inoculated into McCoy or buffalo green monkey cells by the shell vial technique. For delays in processing of up to 48 h, the specimen may be stored in the refrigerator; for longer delays, the specimen should be stored at −70°C or colder. Chapter 57 contains a complete discussion of the optimal methods for recovery of *Chlamydia* spp. from clinical specimens.

Nocardia spp.

Nocardia spp. can be important respiratory tract pathogens. Specimens for culture should be transported promptly to the laboratory; however, for short delays, storage at 4°C is acceptable. Direct examination of a Gram-stained smear of the specimen may reveal thin, beaded, gram-positive organisms that are branching, filamentous, or coccobacillary in appearance. These organisms also are partially acid fast. There are no specific media for the recovery of *Nocardia*; these organisms grow on Sabouraud dextrose agar with heart infusion supplementation, brain heart infusion agar, sheep blood agar, or tryptic soy agar. They may also survive mycobacterial decontamination procedures and be recovered on media designed for mycobacterial culture. For heavily contaminated specimens such as sputa, selective buffered charcoal yeast extract agar is recommended. Cultures are incubated for up to 3 weeks at temperatures ranging from 25 to 37°C, but 37°C is optimal.

Mycobacteria

To recover mycobacteria from contaminated respiratory tract specimens, the specimen must first be decontaminated and concentrated. A discussion of the commonly used decontamination methods and references for step-by-step instructions are included in chapter 25. A smear prepared from the concentrated specimen is stained for AFB. Fluorescent stains containing rhodamine and/or auramine are recommended for optimal sensitivity. Commercial nucleic acid amplification methods capable of detecting *M. tuberculosis* complex are available for use on acid-fast smear-positive specimens. For culture, specimens are inoculated into at least one liquid medium and one solid medium and incubated at a minimum of 6 weeks at 35°C in 8% CO_2.

Upper Respiratory Tract

Nasopharynx

Nasopharyngeal aspirates, washings, and swab specimens are useful for the diagnosis of pertussis, diphtheria, and chlamydia infections, as well as for the identification of carriers of *N. meningitidis* or *S. aureus*. Nasopharyngeal cultures have no utility in the diagnosis of otitis media; however, they may have epidemiologic value for monitoring the antibiotic susceptibility of *S. pneumoniae* in children (12, 29).

Bordetella spp.

The preferred specimen for the recovery of *Bordetella pertussis* is nasopharyngeal cells collected with a small-tipped calcium alginate or Dacron swab. Rayon or cotton swabs should not be used because they may contain fatty acids that are toxic to the organism. Optimally, media should be inoculated at the bedside; however if this is not feasible, the swab specimen may be transported to the laboratory in special transport medium. For delays in transport of <2 h, a 1% Casamino Acids solution is suitable. For delays of up to 24 h, Amies medium with charcoal can be used. If the transport time is >24 h, for example when specimens are sent to reference laboratories for culture, Regan-Lowe transport medium should be used.

Direct examination of the nasopharyngeal specimen for *B. pertussis* is performed by a DFA procedure. Depending on the antibodies used, these assays may or may not distinguish between *B. pertussis* and *Bordetella parapertussis*. In general, the DFA test has relatively low sensitivity and specificity for the diagnosis of pertussis and should be performed only as a supplement to, not a replacement for, culture.

The preferred medium for culture of *B. pertussis* is Regan-Lowe charcoal agar containing 10% horse blood and cephalexin. Because a few strains of *B. pertussis* will not grow in the presence of cephalexin, the use of Regan-Lowe media with and without cephalexin is recommended for optimal recovery. At the bedside, the specimen is inoculated onto one-third of the agar surface; when the agar is received in the laboratory, the inoculum is streaked further for isolation. Cultures are incubated at 35°C for 5 to 7 days in a humid atmosphere without CO_2.

PCR may be the most sensitive test method for detecting *B. pertussis*. Dacron swabs are preferred for PCR tests, because cotton and alginate fibers may interfere with the reaction. Refer to chapter 40 for additional information about specimen collection, transport, and processing for *B. pertussis*.

Corynebacterium diphtheriae

For the optimal recovery of *Corynebacterium diphtheriae*, both nasopharyngeal and throat specimens should be submitted for culture. When specimens are processed for culture without delay, no special transport medium or conditions are required. For transport to a reference laboratory, it has been recommended that the specimen be sent dry in a container with desiccant (16). Alternatively, the specimen may be placed in Stuart's or Amies transport medium or plated on Loeffler's serum or tellurite medium and preincubated overnight at 35°C in 5% CO_2.

Smears of specimens for diagnosis of diphtheria may be stained with the Gram stain and examined for pleomorphic gram-positive rods. Alternatively, smears may be stained with Loeffler's methylene blue stain and examined for pleomorphic beaded rods with swollen ends and reddish-purple metachromatic granules. The presence of organisms with the described morphology by either staining method is consistent with but not specific for *C. diphtheriae*. The specimen should be plated onto Loeffler's serum medium or medium containing potassium tellurite for the recovery of *C. diphtheriae*. Cultures should be incubated for 2 days at 35°C in 5% CO_2.

Chlamydia pneumoniae

Infections with *C. pneumoniae* are often diagnosed serologically; however, when culture is required, a nasopharyngeal swab specimen is optimal. Culture is performed as described above for lower respiratory tract specimens.

Staphylococcus aureus

To identify carriers of *S. aureus*, nasal secretions are collected from the anterior nares with a polyester-tipped swab, which is placed in a tube transport system and promptly delivered to the laboratory. The specimen is plated onto 5% sheep blood agar, an agar medium selective for gram-positive organisms (i.e., colistin-nalidixic acid agar or phenylethyl alcohol agar), or mannitol salt agar, a medium selective for staphylococci and helpful in differentiating coagulase-positive from coagulase-negative species. Cultures are incubated at 35°C for 2 days.

Neisseria meningitidis

To identify carriers of *N. meningitidis*, a nasopharyngeal swab specimen is collected and transported to the laboratory in Amies or Stuart's medium; alternatively, the specimen may be plated directly onto medium and transported in a CO_2-containing system. A Gram-stained smear is not useful because *N. meningitidis* cannot be distinguished morphologically from commensal neisseriae in the upper respiratory tract. Specimens should be inoculated onto an enriched medium such as blood or chocolate agar; modified Thayer-Martin, Martin-Lewis, or New York City medium may be used as well. The cultures are incubated in a humidified atmosphere at 35°C in the presence of 5% CO_2 for 72 h.

Throat

Throat swab specimens most commonly are collected to diagnose group A streptococcal pharyngitis. Throat swabs received in the clinical laboratory for routine bacterial culture should be evaluated only for this agent. Swab specimens should be placed in a tube transport system containing modified Stuart's medium, delivered promptly to the laboratory, or refrigerated for a short time if a delay in transport is unavoidable.

Many rapid direct tests for group A streptococci are commercially available, including EIA, optical immunoassay, and nucleic acid-based assays. The reported sensitivities of the EIAs vary between 60 and 95% (12) but can be as low as 31% (121). The sensitivity of the optical immunoassay also varies, but some reports suggest that it is higher than that of EIA (33, 37). In general, the nucleic acid-based test has a sensitivity of >90% (35, 36). The specificity of all the direct tests generally is very high, between 95 and 100% (8, 12). When a rapid, direct test is requested, two throat swabs should be collected. If the direct test is positive, the second swab may be discarded; but if the direct test is negative, the second swab must be cultured, because the sensitivity of the direct tests is <100%.

To culture group A streptococci, either blood agar or selective blood agar may be used. The use of selective agar makes the organism easier to visualize but may delay its growth. Cultures should be incubated for 48 h at 35°C in an environment with reduced oxygen tension, achieved by incubating the cultures anaerobically, in 5 to 10% CO_2, or in air with a coverslip placed over the primary inoculum (12, 50). These culture conditions may also allow the recovery of group C and G streptococci, organisms which may cause pharyngitis but do not cause the serious sequelae associated with group A streptococci.

Special Considerations

Epiglottitis

Throat swabs may be helpful in determining the etiologic agent of epiglottitis, a rapidly progressing cellulitis with the potential to cause obstruction of the airway (almost always due to *H. influenzae* type b but occasionally due to *S. aureus* or *S. pneumoniae*). The specimen should be collected only by a physician in a setting where intubation of the patient may be performed immediately, if necessary. Specimens should be plated to an enriched medium and incubated at 35°C in the presence of 5 to 10% CO_2 for 72 h. Alternatively, the etiologic agent of epiglottitis may be determined by using blood cultures.

Diphtheria

Culture of throat specimens is important in the diagnosis of diphtheria. Direct evaluation of the specimen and culture should be performed as described above for nasopharyngeal specimens.

Arcanobacterium haemolyticum

A. haemolyticum may cause pharyngitis and peritonsillar abscess. The organism will be recovered on the selective media used to recover group A *Streptococcus* spp. Incubation of plates for up to 72 h may be required for optimal recovery.

Neisseria gonorrhoeae

To detect *N. gonorrhoeae* in the throat, the swab specimen should be inoculated at the bedside or transported promptly and inoculated as soon as possible onto a selective medium, such as modified Thayer-Martin agar. Cultures are incubated at 35°C in the presence of 5 to 10% CO_2 for 72 h.

Other Specimens

Vincent's angina is an acute necrotizing ulcerative tonsilitis that may be caused by *Fusobacterium* spp., *Borrelia vincentii*, and other anaerobes. This condition usually occurs in adults who practice poor mouth hygiene or have serious systemic disease. The laboratory diagnosis is made by direct examination of a smear of a swab specimen collected from the ulcerated lesion and stained with diluted carbol fuchsin (Ziehl-Neelson stain diluted 1:10 with water) or Gram stain. The presence of many spirochetes, fusiform bacilli, and polymorphonuclear leukocytes is presumptive evidence of this disease. Cultures of the involved area usually are not helpful because many species of anaerobes are present in the oral cavity; however, blood cultures should be collected because the illness commonly is accompanied by sepsis.

Tissues

Tissue specimens obtained surgically are procured at great expense and considerable risk to the patient; therefore, for optimal evaluation, enough material should be collected to allow both histopathologic and microbiologic examination of the specimen. The histopathology of the lesion serves to differentiate between infection and malignancy and also to distinguish between acute and chronic infectious processes. In chronic lesions, the differential diagnosis includes disease due to actinomycetes, brucellae, mycobacteria, and fungi, any one of which may be present only in small numbers, emphasizing the need to obtain adequate samples for examination and culture. Swabs are rarely adequate, and their use should be discouraged.

Following collection, tissues should be placed in a sterile container and transported rapidly to the laboratory to prevent drying. Upon receipt, the specimen is placed in a small amount of sterile medium or sterile saline and homogenized. This can be accomplished by mincing with a sterile scalpel, grinding with a mortar and pestle or tissue grinder, or using a stomacher. The resulting homogenate is used to prepare smears for Gram stain or other stains as indicated by the clinical picture and to inoculate culture media. The Gram stain should be examined for the presence of microorganisms, leukocytes, and squamous epithelial cells (suggestive of surface contamination). For routine culture, tissue should be inoculated to a liquid medium (94, 95) and an enriched agar medium is used to recover fastidious organisms. Cultures are incubated at 35°C in the presence of 5 to 10% CO_2.

Special Considerations

Bone Marrow

Bone marrow aspirates are optimally submitted to the microbiology laboratory by using the collection tubes for the lysis centrifugation blood culture system. The pediatric tubes should be used when less than 7 ml is collected. Bone marrow may also be submitted in a sterile container or con-

tainers containing anticoagulants. However, because certain anticoagulants, such as heparin, sodium citrate, and EDTA, have been shown to be inhibitory to some organisms (23, 96), the use of anticoagulants is not recommended. If the laboratory chooses to process a specimen containing an anticoagulant, the ordering physician must be informed about the limitations of the results.

Quantitative Tissue Culture

Tissue from a traumatic wound or thermal injury may be submitted for quantitative culture, with results of $\geq 10^5$ CFU/ml being used to predict the likelihood of the development of wound-related sepsis. The utility of this procedure has been questioned for two reasons: (i) the lack of reproducible results (130) and (ii) the low positive predictive value compared to histologic examination of tissue (64). To perform a quantitative culture, a portion of the specimen is weighed and homogenized in saline and the homogenized suspension is used to prepare serial dilutions of the specimen for culture. Detailed procedures for quantitative tissue culture are given elsewhere (112).

Helicobacter pylori

Gastric biopsy specimens or brushings may be submitted for the detection of *H. pylori*, an important cause of gastritis and peptic ulcer disease. The organism can be observed in tissue sections by using Giemsa, hematoxylin and eosin, or the Warthin-Starry silver stain. In addition, organisms can be visualized in touch preparations of minced tissue, stained with the Gram stain. The urease test is an indirect method of diagnosing *H. pylori* gastritis or peptic ulcer disease. The organism produces large amounts of this enzyme, which can be detected by inoculating urea broth or media with a portion of the homogenized tissue. Alternatively, a piece of tissue can be placed directly into a commercially available test kit. The urease test may be positive in as little as 15 min, but it should be held for 24 h before a negative report is issued. To recover *H. pylori* in culture, the biopsy specimen is homogenized in 0.9% saline and inoculated onto chocolate, brain heart infusion, or brucella agar supplemented with horse or rabbit blood. The optimal agar medium for recovery of *H. pylori* has not yet been determined. The cultures are incubated at 35°C in a microaerophilic, humid environment for 7 days.

Bartonella spp.

B. henselae is one agent of cat scratch disease and bacillary angiomatosis. Because culture of this organism is very difficult, diagnosis is most often made by clinical manifestations and exclusion of other diseases or by serologic analysis. The organism may be observed in sections of fixed tissue specimens stained with the Warthin-Starry silver stain or a tissue Gram stain. It is very occasionally recovered by inoculating the specimen onto freshly prepared heart infusion agar containing 5 to 10% defibrinated rabbit or horse blood, chocolate agar, or sheep blood agar. The plates are incubated in high humidity at 35°C for up to 1 month.

Other Organisms

Legionella spp., *Nocardia* spp., *C. diphtheriae*, and mycobacteria are all potential pathogens in diseased tissue. These organisms may be recovered by methods described above.

Urine

Acceptable methods of urine collection include midstream clean catch (preferably a first-voided morning specimen), catheterization, and suprapubic aspiration. Foley catheter tips should not be accepted for culture because they almost always are contaminated with urethral organisms. Most commonly, the midstream flow of a clean-catch urine specimen is collected. All urine specimens should be transported promptly to the laboratory and processed within 2 h of collection. If a delay in transport or processing cannot be avoided, specimens may be refrigerated for up to 24 h. Collection kits containing preservatives to maintain the bacterial population stable for 24 h at room temperature are commercially available, but they offer no advantage over refrigeration.

The urinary tract above the urethra is sterile in healthy humans, but the urethra normally is colonized with many different bacteria, and so urine specimens collected by a noninvasive method become contaminated during passage. Commensal bacteria are differentiated from potential pathogens by quantitative cultures of urine (47). Originally, growth of 10^5 or more CFU/ml was considered highly indicative of infection, but this criterion has been modified for different situations. For example, in young, sexually active women with acute urethral syndrome, as little as 10^2 CFU/ml is considered significant in the presence of concomitant pyuria (111). True urinary infections associated with fewer than 10^5 CFU/ml may occur in infants and children, in males, and in persons who are catheterized, have recently been treated with antimicrobial agents, drink large amounts of fluids, have symptoms and concomitant pyuria, have urinary obstruction, or have pyelonephritis acquired from hematogenous spread.

Direct examination of urine is possible by many methods, which may be used as a screening test to quickly identify samples that most probably will not yield clinically significant organisms. These screening methods correlate well when growth of 10^5 CFU/ml or greater is the reference, but they compare less favorably in the presence of lower colony counts (87). Screening urine specimens by staining with the Gram stain is rapid and economical with regard to reagents but is very time-consuming. Finding one or more organisms per oil immersion field in a smear prepared from an uncentrifuged specimen correlates well with growth of 10^5 CFU/ml or greater (47). Commercially available dipstick tests that combine nitrate reductase (an enzyme produced by most gram-negative bacilli that cause urinary tract infections) and leukocyte esterase (an enzyme produced by neutrophils) are rapid, inexpensive, and simple to perform, but their sensitivity is low (87).

Several automated urine-screening systems are commercially available. With the FiltraCheck-UTI colorimetric filtration system (Meridian Diagnostics Inc.), urine is forced through a filter paper that retains cells and then a stain is passed through the filter. The intensity of the resulting color correlates with the number of particles adherent to the filter. This system provides rapid results and detects over 90% of all positive samples, but it may yield false-negative results with gram-positive organisms and *P. aeruginosa* (87, 104).

The UTI screen Bacterial ATP Assay (Coral Biotechnology, San Diego, Calif.) is a bioluminescent system based on the reaction of ATP with luciferin and luciferase, which produces light. By selectively releasing ATP from bacteria alone, the number of CFU per milliliter of urine is estimated with a luminometer. This procedure requires an incubation step, and results are not available for a few hours. This method has a sensitivity equal to that of other screening methods, but it appears to have a higher specificity than either the dipstick or the filter method (88).

The Urine ID card (bioMérieux Vitek, Inc., Hazelwood, Mo.) uses electro-optics to detect, quantitate, and identify organisms present in a urine specimen by measuring changes in the color or turbidity of a broth medium. Results are available within 1 to 13 h after inoculation of the urine sample.

Quantitative bacterial culture of a urine specimen is accomplished by inoculating appropriate media, often blood and MacConkey agars, with a measured amount of urine, most commonly via a plastic or wire calibrated loop designed to deliver a known volume. A 0.001-ml loop is used to inoculate all urine specimens, except those collected from women with suspected acute urethral syndrome and suprapubic aspirates, which are inoculated with a 0.01-ml loop. The loop is inserted vertically into the well-mixed specimen, and the loopful of urine removed is spread over the surface of the agar plate by streaking from top to bottom in a vertical line and again from top to bottom perpendicular to the line in a back-and-forth fashion. Urine cultures are incubated at 35°C in the presence of 5 to 10% CO_2.

Special Considerations

Leptospires

L. interrogans may be recovered from urine after the first week of illness and for several months thereafter. Urine should be processed as soon as possible after collection, because acidity may harm the organisms. If a delay in processing is expected, the urine should be diluted 1:10 in 1% bovine serum albumin and stored at 5 to 20°C. Both undiluted urine and urine diluted 1:10, 1:100, and 1:1,000 in sterile buffered saline should be inoculated to Fletcher's, Ellinghausen-McCullough/Johnson-Harris, or Polysorbate 80 medium with and without neomycin (48). Cultures are incubated at room temperature for at least 6 weeks.

Mycobacteria

Mycobacteria can be recovered from urine by procedures discussed above.

Bacterial Antigen Testing

Many commercial bacterial antigen-testing kits developed for the purpose of diagnosing bacterial meningitis include procedures for use on urine specimens. In general, these kits should not be used with urine specimens for the diagnosis of bacterial meningitis and their use with CSF should be limited, as discussed above. Importantly, the Food and Drug Administration recently issued a product alert specifically cautioning against the use the group B *Streptococcus* antigen kits with urine specimens because of the risk of both false-positive and false-negative results (25).

A radioimmunoassay and an EIA are commercially available for detection of the *Legionella pneumophila* serogroup 1 antigen in urine. The antigen may be detectable in urine for months following an infection. These assays have sensitivities of 80% or greater when performed on concentrated urine and specificities of >98% (13, 21, 32, 49). The drawback of both assays is that one *L. pneumophila* serogroup is detected.

Recently, a nucleic acid amplification assay has become commercially available for the detection of *N. gonorrhoeae* and *C. trachomatis* in urine samples from both males and females. Specimens are collected in a sterile container without preservative. The only special sample requirements are that the patient not urinate for 1 h prior to sample collection and the specimen be refrigerated until processed. These assays promise to simplify the medical procedures required to diagnose these sexually transmitted diseases.

Wounds and Abscesses

Ideally, purulent material is aspirated with a needle and syringe, transferred to a sterile container, and promptly delivered to the laboratory. If an aspirate cannot be obtained, swab specimens of exudate collected from the deep portion of the lesion are acceptable. A minimum of two swab specimens should be collected, one for culture and the other for preparation of smears for staining. All swabs may be placed in tube transport systems containing modified Stuart's medium. For the recovery of anaerobes, the use of swabs should be discouraged. However, if swabs are submitted, they must be placed in an anaerobic transport system. Specimens should be transported promptly to the laboratory. If a delay in processing is unavoidable, specimens may be stored in the refrigerator, except those for recovery of anaerobes, which should be maintained at room temperature. Processing specimens involves preparation of a smear for Gram stain examination and inoculation of appropriate media for culture. When swab specimens are processed, it is not necessary to inoculate a broth medium, because organisms recovered from broth cultures of swab specimens are rarely significant (74, 106).

VIROLOGY

General Considerations

Processing specimens for the detection of virus, viral components, or virus-specific antibody assumes appropriate selection, collection, and transport of clinical specimens based on suspected viral etiologies (45). Although processing concepts are similar to those used in bacteriology, important differences exist between viruses and bacteria, necessitating changes in processing procedures. Unlike most bacteria, viruses are capable of persistence in presumably sterile tissues and subclinical reactivation. Latent virus is the rule following most, if not all, DNA virus infections. Consequently, detection of viral nucleic acid in specimens such as blood may not be a significant finding. Tests are selected based on the predictive values of positive and negative results, in addition to the sensitivity of various methods. All viruses are strict intracellular pathogens which do not grow on or in artificial agar or broth media, respectively. The use of living cells in culture is required for virus isolation. Individual virions are beyond the resolution of conventional light microscopes. Because of the expense and time involved in electron microscopy, conventional microscopy using stains to detect viral antigen or aggregates of viral components is used. Common stains include fluorochrome-labeled antibody to detect viral antigen, and hematoxylin and eosin, Giemsa, or Papanicolaou to detect aggregates of viral components.

The laboratory diagnosis of viral infections is accomplished by (i) visualizing virus by electron microscopy, (ii) detecting cytologic or histologic evidence of virus replication, (iii) detecting viral antigen, (iv) detecting viral nucleic acid, (v) isolating and identifying virus in cell culture, and (vi) demonstrating serum antibody to a specific virus. Proper use of the many tests available for viral disease diagnosis requires deliberate test selection and efficient and timely processing. Test selection is based on likely etiologies, sensitivity of method, turnaround time needed for a particular clinical situation, and cost. Efficient and timely processing includes the use of precautions which protect personnel from laboratory-acquired infection and prevent cross-contamination of specimens or culture tubes. This section describes guidelines and specific recommendations for processing viral specimens based on specimen type, suspected etiologies, and clinical syndromes. In addition, an overview of methods unique to virus detection, such as cell culture, is provided.

Methods Used for Virus Detection

Electron Microscopy

Viruses range in size from approximately 20 to 500 nm, generally below the lower limits of detection by conventional bright-field microscopes. Before the advent of cell culture and the commercial availability of antibodies for antigen detection, viruses were detected best by electron microscopy (EM). Although the need for EM as a routine clinical virology procedure no longer exists, it can be useful for the laboratory diagnosis of viral disease in situations where methods for detection of suspected virus are not readily available, including (i) noncultivable virus (e.g., Norwalk viruses and other agents of gastroenteritis), (ii) necessity for rapid detection for public health reasons (e.g., Ebola and other hemorrhagic viruses), (iii) a syndrome that represents the appearance of an emerging virus (e.g., Sin Nombre virus and other hantaviruses), and (iv) cases when the virus in a lesion or isolated in cell culture is best identified by characteristic morphology (e.g., poxviruses [Orf virus] causing Orf). The reader is referred to a comprehensive description of methods and viral morphologies (70).

Cytology and Histology

The presence of virus in clinical material can be recognized by its characteristic cytologic and histologic appearances (Table 3). In addition to tissue reactions suggestive of viral invasion, cells infected with virus may show inclusions, i.e., cytoplasmic or nuclear clusters of virus or viral components, that are indicative of a particular virus. Papanicolaou and Giemsa stains are used for cytologic preparations, whereas the hematoxylin and eosin stain is preferred for staining sections of tissue.

The Tzanck preparation is a useful cytologic technique for detecting herpes simplex virus (HSV) or varicella-zoster virus (VZV) in cutaneous vesicles. The smear, containing epithelial cells from the base of the ulcer, is stained and examined for virus and cellular changes pathognomonic of herpesvirus infection. Traditionally, Giemsa or Papanicolaou stain has been used. More recently, immunofluorescent staining with HSV- or VZV-fluorescein isothiocyanate conjugates has been shown to be more sensitive than dye-based stains (30).

Antigen Detection

The mainstay of viral diagnosis in many clinical laboratories is antigen detection by fluorescent-antibody or EIA procedures. A thorough explanation of immunoassays can be found in chapter 12 and in reference 116. Fluorescent-antibody techniques perform best when specimens contain numerous host cells, since infection by virus is detected and confirmed by the characteristic pattern of staining of viral antigen within cells. In addition, the insensitivity of fluorescent-antibody staining requires relatively large quantities of virus to ensure a positive result. Fixation of smears for fluorescent-antibody staining is accomplished with air-dried slides by immersion in room temperature acetone for 5 min. Fixation by other means, e.g., methanol, should be undertaken only after evaluation to ensure that the reactivity of antigens to be detected is not destroyed or diminished.

TABLE 3 Virus-induced changes in clinical specimens

Virus	Virus-induced changes
HSV	Intranuclear "ground glass" inclusion (early), eosinophilic with "halo" (late); multinucleated giant cells
VZV	Same as for HSV
CMV	Intranuclear (Cowdry A) and intracytoplasmic (basophilic) inclusions; enlarged cells
Adenovirus	Amphophilic or basophilic intranuclear inclusion; mature inclusion called "smudge" cell
Parvovirus B19	Nuclear inclusions in erythroid precursor cell in bone marrow or liver (fetus)
Measles virus	Multinucleated syncytial cell (giant cell); intranuclear and intracytoplasmic inclusions
RSV	Rare, pink intracytoplasmic inclusions
Rabies virus	Eosinophilic, intracytoplasmic neuronal inclusion (Negri body)
Human papillomavirus	Perinuclear vacuolization and nuclear enlargement, referred to as koilocytosis
Molluscum contagiosum virus	Eosinophilic inclusions filling cytoplasm
JC virus (polyomavirus)	Enlarged, amphophilic oligodendroglial nuclei

EIAs are performed in a membrane or reaction vessel format. The membrane assays have been adopted for ease of use in stat laboratories or nonlaboratory settings. Assays that are formatted for a reaction vessel, such as a microtiter well, can be automated, resulting in minimum costs for batch testing. As with fluorescent-antibody assays, the sensitivity is lower than that of cell culture or other techniques that incorporate amplification of virus before detection.

When deciding between fluorescent-antibody or EIA format, one must consider the resolution of weak or indeterminant results. Weak fluorescence reactions can more easily be labeled as positive or negative based on fluorescence morphology and intensity. Indeterminant enzyme results should not be resolved without testing by another method or testing a subsequent specimen.

Molecular Detection

Detection of viral genome is rapid, sensitive, and applicable to viruses that cannot be detected by cell culture. Nucleic acid probes are useful in settings where sufficient virus is present to allow detection without amplification, such as human papillomavirus in cutaneous biopsy specimens. Amplification of genomes by PCR, reverse transcriptase PCR (RT-PCR), ligase chain reaction, and related techniques and subsequent detection by gel electrophoresis and/or probing provides sensitivities similar to or exceeding culture (86). The ability of molecular detection tests to detect the viral genome of latent, nonreplicating virus introduces the problem of the detection test being too sensitive. Validation of molecular tests, especially with the herpes group viruses, requires calculation of predictive values for clinical disease.

Cell Culture

Viruses require living host cells for multiplication and spread. Cells are established in culture by gently disrupting tissue by enzymatic digestion or mincing, and growing in culture. Host cells originate as a few cells and grow into a monolayer on the sides of glass or plastic test tubes or flasks. These are referred to as adherent cell cultures. A cell culture becomes a cell line once it has been passed or subcultured in vitro. Cell lines are classified as primary, low-passage, or continuous. Primary cell lines, such as primary rhesus monkey kidney cells, are those which can be passed up to 10 to 15 times in culture but which have decreased receptivity to viral infection after only a few passages. Low-passage, also called established, cell lines are those which remain viable and virus sensitive through 20 to 50 passages. Human diploid fibroblast cells, such as lung fibroblasts, are common low-passage cells. Continuous cell lines, usually derived from human cancers or transformed in vitro, can be passed and remain sensitive to infection by some viruses indefinitely. Unfortunately, most viruses do not grow well in continuous cell lines. Several different cell lines are used for the growth and detection of viruses (Table 4) (10).

Cell cultures are kept moist and supplied with nutrients by keeping them continuously immersed in cell culture medium. Two kinds of media, growth medium and maintenance medium, are used for cell culture. Both are prepared with a minimal medium containing a balanced salt solution, amino acids, vitamins, a pH buffering system, and antimicrobial agents. Eagle's minimal essential medium, RPMI 1640, and Dulbecco's medium are examples of commercially available minimal media. All are supplemented with a balanced salt solution, such as Earle's or Hank's balanced salt solutions, and all have a bicarbonate buffering system to counteract acidification of the growth medium caused by the metabolism of growing cells, production of CO_2, and acidification of the liquid growth medium in a closed tube. Phenol red, a pH indicator that is red at physiologic pH, yellow at acidic pH, and purple at alkaline pH, is added to monitor adverse pH changes (10). Antimicrobial agents are added to prevent bacterial contamination. The usual antimicrobial agents are vancomycin (10 μg/ml), gentamicin (20 μg/ml), and amphotericin B (2.5 μg/ml). Other antimicrobial agent combinations are used but are less active against the many resistant microorganisms encountered today (27).

Growth medium is a serum-rich (10% fetal, newborn, or agammaglobulinemic calf serum) medium designed to support rapid cell growth. This medium is used for initiating growth of cells in a tube when cell cultures are being prepared in-house or for feeding tubes of purchased cell cultures

TABLE 4 Cells used for virus isolation

Type of cell[a]	Animal and tissue of origin	Viruses isolated[b]
Primary cell lines		
African green monkey	Kidney	HSV, mumps virus, RSV, rubella virus, VZV
CBMC, PBMC	Human	HIV-1, HIV-2, HTLV-1, HTLV-2, HHV-6
Embryonic kidney, lung	Human	Adenoviruses, BK, mumps virus
Rabbit	Kidney	HSV
Rhesus or cynomolgus monkey	Kidney	ECHO, polioviruses, coxsackievirus groups A and B, mumps virus, reoviruses, influenza virus, measles virus, parainfluenza virus, RSV
Low-passage/finite cell lines		
Foreskin fibroblasts	Human	CMV, HSV
Lung fibroblasts	Human, embryo	Coronaviruses, CMV, rhinoviruses, VZV
WI-38, MRC-5	Human fetal lung	Adenoviruses, CMV, polioviruses, coxsackievirus group B, enteroviruses (types 68–71), RSV, rhinoviruses
Continuous cell lines		
293	Human kidney	Adenoviruses (types 5, 40, and 41)
A549	Human lung	Adenoviruses (types 1–39), HSV
BGMK	Buffalo green monkey	Polioviruses, coxsackievirus groups, reoviruses
HeLa	Human cervix	Poxviruses, reoviruses, RSV, rhinoviruses, coxsackievirus groups A and B
HEp-2	Human larynx	Adenoviruses, RSV
MDCK	Canine kidney	Influenza virus, parainfluenza virus
Mink lung	Mink	HSV
RD	Human rhabdomyosarcoma	Coronaviruses, coxsackievirus group A, polioviruses, enteroviruses (types 68–71)
RK_{13}	Rabbit kidney	Rubella virus, poxviruses
Vero, CV-1	African green monkey	HSV, measles virus, poxviruses, BK, rubella virus, RSV, parainfluenza virus

[a] CBMC, cord blood mononuclear cells; PBMC, peripheral blood mononuclear cells.
[b] BK, human polyomavirus BK; ECHO, enteric cytopathic human orphan viruses; NDV, Newcastle disease virus.

that have incomplete cell monolayers. Feeding refers to the removal of old medium followed by the addition of fresh culture medium.

Maintenance medium is similar to growth medium but contains less (0 to 2%) serum and is used to keep cells in a steady state of metabolism. Fetal, newborn, or agammaglobulinemic calf serum is used to avoid inhibitors, such as specific antibody, and to be free of mycoplasmas present in serum from older animals.

Conventional Cell Culture

Cell culture methods used to detect virus include conventional cell culture, rapid shell vial methods, or an enzyme-linked virus-inducible system called ELVIS (BioWhittaker, Walkersville, Md.).

Conventional cell culture tubes are inoculated with up to 0.25 ml of specimen, depending on the specimen toxicity. In general, the more specimen that can be inoculated, the more likely it is that a virus will be detected. Some viruses, such as reoviruses and rotaviruses, which are difficult to isolate in cell culture from clinical specimens, may have their infectivities greatly enhanced by treatment with proteolytic enzymes, notably trypsin (15, 109). Similarly, the growth of influenza viruses may be enhanced by trypsin (117). Laboratories that wish to use proteolytic methods for the biologic enhancement of infectivity should adopt two simple procedures (54): (i) trypsin (0.01 mg/ml) should be added to processed stool extracts or respiratory specimens, and (ii) serum-free cell culture maintenance medium containing 0.5% bovine serum albumin and 5 mg of trypsin per liter should be used with cell cultures inoculated with the trypsin-treated specimens.

Inoculated cell cultures should be incubated immediately at 35 to 37°C. After allowing virus to adsorb to the cell monolayer for 12 to 24 h, it is common practice to remove the remaining inoculum and culture medium and replace it with fresh maintenance medium. This avoids most inoculum-induced cell culture toxicity and improves virus recovery. Incubation should be continued for 5 to 28 days depending on the viruses suspected. Maintenance medium should be changed periodically (usually once or twice weekly) to provide fresh nutrients to the cells.

Cell cultures generally are incubated on a roller drum which holds the culture tubes tilted (5 to 7°) while they slowly revolve (0.5 to 1 rpm) at 35 to 37°C. Virus-infected cell cultures undergo disruption of cell function and cell death, resulting in morphologic alterations called cytopathic effect (CPE). The presence of a specific virus is signaled by characteristic CPE occurring in specified cell cultures after predictable lengths of incubation.

Blind passage is used to detect viruses which may not produce CPE in the initial culture tube but will produce CPE when the inoculum is passed to a second tube. Cell cultures that show nonspecific or ambiguous CPE are also passed to additional cell culture tubes. Toxicity, which causes ambiguous CPE, usually is diluted during passage and does not appear in the second cell culture tube. In both instances, passage is performed by scraping the monolayer off the sides of the tube with a pipette or disrupting the monolayer by vortexing with sterile glass beads added to the culture tube, followed by inoculating 0.25 ml of the resulting suspension into new cell cultures. Blind passage is less frequently used today because the added time and expense do not justify the detection of a few additional isolates.

Rapid Shell Vial (Spin Amplification) Cell Culture

The shell vial culture is a rapid modification of conventional cell culture in which the infected cell monolayer is stained for viral antigens found soon after infection, before the development of CPE. Viruses which normally take days or weeks to produce CPE can be detected within 1 to 2 days. Shell vial culture tubes (i.e., 15- by 45-mm 1-dram vials) may be prepared in-house by adding a round coverslip to the bottom, covering this with growth medium, and adding appropriate cells forming a cell monolayer on top of the coverslip (105) or purchased with the monolayer already formed. Shell vials should be used 5 to 9 days after cells have been inoculated. Specimens are inoculated onto the shell vial cell monolayer by the following procedure. (i) Maintenance medium is aspirated from the shell vial. (ii) The shell vial is inoculated with 0.1 to 0.25 ml of specimen. All specimens are inoculated before the controls are inoculated, and the negative control is inoculated before the positive control. (iii) The vials are capped and centrifuged at 700 × g for 40 min at 35°C. Low-speed centrifugation enhances viral infectivity by a poorly understood mechanism (42). (iv) Maintenance medium (2 ml) is added to each shell vial. The vials are recapped and incubated at 35 to 37°C for 24 to 48 h (depending on the virus). (v) Coverslips are stained with virus-specific immunofluorescent conjugates. The presence of typical fluorescing inclusions confirms the presence of virus.

The shell vial culture technique can be used to detect several viruses which grow in conventional cell culture. It is best used for viruses which require relatively long periods of incubation before producing CPE, such as cytomegalovirus (CMV) and VZV. The advantage of shell vial cultures is speed; most viruses are detected within 24 h. Disadvantages are that only one type of virus can be detected per shell vial, and that for certain viruses (e.g., HSV, adenovirus, and influenza virus) the technique is not as sensitive as cell culture.

Cell Culture with an Enzyme-Linked Detection System

The ELVIS system uses cell culture with a cloned β-galactosidase gene that is expressed only when cells are infected with HSV (110). Following inoculation of specimen and overnight incubation, growth of virus results in production of the β-galactosidase enzyme by the infected cells. β-Galactosidase serves as the "reporter" molecule. When cells are fixed and stained for galactosidase activity, positive staining indicates the presence of virus and no staining indicates no virus.

Serologic Testing

Serologic testing was the primary means of the laboratory diagnosis of viral infections until the mid-1970s. After that time, culture and detection of viral antigen and, more recently, molecular detection became widely available. Viral serologic testing is now used primarily to determine immune status and to diagnose infections in situations where the virus cannot be cultivated in cell culture or detected by immunoassay.

During most viral infections, immunoglobulin M (IgM) antibody is detectable within 3 to 5 days of onset of disease and persists for 1 to 4 months. IgG antibody appears concurrently or a few days later and, as a rule, is detectable for the life of the patient. If a patient is infected by an antigenically similar virus or the original strain has remained latent and reactivates at a later time, these virus-specific IgG and IgM antibody levels may rise again. The secondary IgM response may be difficult to detect; however, a significant (fourfold or equivalent) rise in the IgG titer is readily apparent in an immune competent patient.

An immune status test indicates whether a patient has been infected by a particular virus in the past. A positive result with a virus-specific IgG test signifies past infection. Some immune status tests measure both IgG and IgM to detect recent or active infections.

To help diagnose active disease, two approaches are helpful: (i) detection of virus-specific IgM in an acute-phase specimen and (ii) detection of a fourfold or equivalent rise in antibody titer between acute- and convalescent-phase sera. The convalescent-phase specimen generally is collected 2 to 3 weeks after the acute-phase specimen; however, with some diseases, 6 to 12 weeks or more may be necessary before seroconversion is detected. If a single post-acute-phase serum sample, collected between the acute and convalescent times, or a later convalescent-phase specimen is all that is available for testing, an extremely high, virus-specific IgG titer may be suggestive of infection. The exact titer specific for active disease, if known at all, varies with each testing method and virus. In general, titers high enough to be diagnostic are unusual and testing of single specimens should not be performed. A reasonable policy would be to include IgM tests, where available, and to perform IgG testing only on paired acute- and convalescent-phase specimens. IgG testing need not be performed on the acute-phase specimen until receipt of the convalescent-phase specimen. This eliminates useless testing of single specimens in those instances where a second sample is never collected or submitted for analysis.

Processing Specimens for Detection of Virus

Specimens should be processed as soon as possible following receipt by the laboratory. This may be done by combining all microbiology processing responsibilities, since laboratories commonly process bacteriology specimens 7 days per week. When delays occur, specimens should be stored at 4°C. Specimens collected with a swab and small volumes of fluid should be held in viral transport medium (VTM). Tissues should be minced and stored in VTM. If tissues cannot be minced, they should be kept moist during refrigeration. Large volumes of fluid which have not been added to VTM should be diluted in VTM (1:5) before storage.

In general, specimens should be processed in a biologic safety cabinet. This protects specimens from environmental contamination and diminishes the possibility of cross-contamination among patient specimens. Viruses are easily aerosolized, and contamination of one specimen with another can readily occur. The downward flow of air in a biologic safety cabinet helps clear aerosols. In addition, to diminish the chance of cross-contamination, tops or lids from separate specimens should never be opened at the same time. If processing cannot be performed in a biologic safety cabinet, simple manipulations can be safely accomplished behind a protective Plexiglas barrier shield on the countertop. Vortexing, pipetting, and centrifugation can all create dangerous aerosols. Vortexing can be done in a tightly capped tube behind a shield, but after vortexing, the tube should be opened in a safety cabinet, as should tubes following centrifugation. Pipetting also must be performed behind a protective shield, with pipettes being discarded into a disinfectant fluid, ensuring that the disinfectant reaches the inside of the pipette. Discarding the pipette into a leakproof biosafety bag is an acceptable alternative.

VTM or fluid specimens not in transport medium should be vortexed just before inoculation to break up aggregates of specimen and resuspend the inoculum. Addition of sterile glass beads to the transport medium helps with this process during vortexing. Grossly contaminated or potentially toxic specimens, such as minced or ground tissue, can be centrifuged (1,000 × *g* for 15 min), and the virus-containing supernatant can be used as inoculum. If the specimen volume is insufficient for all tests needed, it should be diluted with VTM. Excess specimen should be saved at 4°C in case additional tests are needed. Cell cultures contaminated with bacteria can be reprocessed with antibiotic-containing VTM or can be filtered with a 0.22-μm-pore-size filter and the filtrate can be recultured.

Blood (Whole Blood)

Blood specimens are used most often for the detection of CMV, HIV, and hepatitis C virus (HCV) and less commonly for other viruses. Leukocytes (CMV) and plasma (HIV and HCV) are components of whole blood used for detection of virus. The volume of blood and timing of blood collection necessary for optimal viral detection have not been extensively studied. In general, collection of the specimen early in the course of disease and before administration of specific antiviral agents is preferred. For the CMV antigenemia and HIV viral load RT-PCR assays, antigen and genome, respectively, are quantitated sequentially for prognostic information. Blood should be processed only for the viral agents specifically requested.

Direct detection of CMV is accomplished by a CMV antigenemia assay (lower matrix protein pp65). Kit procedures should be followed closely. In general, processing blood for an antigenemia assay includes: (i) leukocyte isolation from peripheral blood in which a sufficient volume of anticoagulated blood (EDTA or heparin), usually 5 to 10 ml, is collected to provide leukocytes for smear preparation (a larger blood volume will be necessary if the patient is severely neutropenic); (ii) counting cells and preparing a suspension of leukocytes containing 2×10^6 cells/ml (hematology cell counting instrumentation can be used to provide the initial count needed to determine dilution); and (iii) preparation of smears in which each smear should contain 200,000 leukocytes (smears can be made with the Cytospin [Shandon, Pittsburgh, Pa.]).

The RT-PCR test is used as a surrogate measure of HIV in serum. Blood should be collected in tubes containing anticoagulant which is specified by the method used. Plasma for use with the Amplicor HIV Monitor test (Roche Assay; Roche Diagnostics Systems, Inc., Branchburg, N.J.) must be separated within 6 h and refrigerated (4°C) for up to 1 week or frozen (<−20°C) for longer periods to prevent RNA degradation. Repeat freeze-and-thaw cycles should be avoided. Further processing is based on the assay being used. Other methods for measuring HIV RNA include the branched DNA (BDNA) sigma amplification assay (Chiron Corp., Emeryville, Calif.), Digene HIV RNA test (Digene Corp., Silver Spring, Md.), and nucleic acid sequence-based assay (NASBA) for HIV-1 RNA (Organon Teknika Corp.).

The RT-PCR test is also used to detect HCV in blood. Procedures mentioned above to prevent RNA degradation should be followed. Blood is processed by following the specific instructions dictated by the assay method.

Isolation of virus from blood by cell culture is seldom needed, with the exception of CMV disease. For the detection of CMV, leukocytes are fractionated and inoculated to diploid fibroblast cells. The use of two or three cell culture tubes with different inoculum volumes is recommended to enhance detection without toxicity, e.g., 0.25 ml in one tube and 0.1 ml in a second tube. Following adsorption for a few hours to overnight, a wash is necessary to remove toxic leukocytes from the cell monolayer. Low titers of virus and the slow growth of CMV mandate 2 to 4 weeks of incubation to ensure detection. This prolonged incubation time encourages the use of the rapid shell vial in place of cell culture for clinically useful information. Shell vial cell cultures also should be inoculated with leukocyte-rich fractions.

Leukocytes were originally added to cell culture by harvesting the buffy coat after concentration by centrifugation. This method was found to be inferior to leukocyte concentration by density gradient centrifugation and sedimentation with Ficoll-paque/Macrodex (41). Other density gradient methods have been used, including those with Plasmagel, LeucoPREP, Sepracell-MN, Mono-Poly resolving medium, and Polymorphprep. However, leukocyte preparation with Polymorphprep, a mixture of sodium metrizoate and dextran, is one of the best, since mononuclear and polymorphonuclear cells are isolated from erythrocytes in a one-step procedure (83, 108, 128). A 3- to 5-ml volume of anticoagulated blood is optimal (2 ml for pediatric patients); EDTA, citrate, or heparin anticoagulant-containing tubes can be used. Specimens should be processed immediately; when a delay is unavoidable, the specimens should be held at refrigeration temperature (4°C). In addition, processing must occur within 12 to 24 h. Before processing, the blood specimen and all reagents are allowed to come to room temperature. After the blood specimen is mixed well by being inverted five times, it is transferred to a sterile conical centrifuge tube and centrifuged at 500 × *g* for 10 min at room temperature (18 to 22°C). After removal of plasma, the remaining cells are diluted 1:1 with 0.9% NaCl. Polymorphprep (3.5 ml; Robbins Scientific, Sunnyvale, Calif.) is added to a 15-ml conical centrifuge tube, and the entire volume of diluted blood cells is carefully layered over the Polymorphprep in the centrifuge tube. After centrifugation of the tube containing blood and Polymorphprep at 450 to 500 × *g* for 30 min at room temperature (18 to 22°C), two leukocyte bands should be visible after centrifugation. The top band at the blood sample/Polymorphprep interface consists of mononuclear cells. The lower band contains polymorphonuclear cells. Erythrocytes are pelleted at the bottom of the tube. The mononuclear and polymorphonuclear bands are collected and transferred to a centrifuge tube, washed twice, and resuspended in Eagle's minimal essential medium–2% fetal bovine serum. The specimen is ready for inoculation into conventional or rapid shell vial cell culture.

Blood for CMV isolation or antigenemia staining should be fractionated and inoculated as soon as possible after collection. Processing delays result in a decrease in CMV detection by cell culture or the number of CMV inclusions quantitated in the antigenemia assay. Unfractionated blood or isolated leukocytes can be refrigerated for 24 h without excessive loss of sensitivity (53). Scheduling specimen collection during the hours most convenient for processing helps avoid viral loss during holding times.

Blood may be used for the detection of other viruses. Serum is a suitable specimen for isolation of enteroviruses from perinatally infected infants (90) and for isolation of some arboviruses, such as dengue virus (38). Blood clots are used for the recovery of Colorado tick fever virus (54). In addition, human herpesvirus 6 disease in transplant recipients can be detected by conventional or shell vial cell cultures or PCR (107).

Central Nervous System

CSF and brain tissue specimens are used to detect disease caused by arboviruses, enteroviruses, HSV, CMV, VZV, JC polyomavirus, HIV, and other, less commonly encountered viruses (Table 5). The availability of PCR in clinical laboratories has revolutionized the detection of neurotropic viruses and necessitated the selective use of expensive laboratory testing (92).

Molecular detection by PCR and RT-PCR requires CSF or fresh (unfixed) biopsy tissue. A minimum of 1 ml of CSF should be refrigerated for short-term storage (24 to 48 h) at 4°C or frozen at <-20°C for longer periods. Processing prior to DNA extraction and PCR testing requires centrifugation (30 min at 10,000 × *g* in a microcentrifuge). Tissue should be frozen at <-20°C immediately. Brain tissue for electron microscopy (especially JC virus detection) should be fixed immediately in glutaraldehyde. Cell culture is recommended only for enterovirus detection and then only if RT-PCR is unavailable. CSF (0.1 to 0.25 ml) or minced tissue is inoculated into primary monkey kidney and diploid fibroblast cell lines. Incubation at 35 to 37°C for 7 to 10 days is required.

Eye

Many viruses cause conjunctivitis, keratoconjunctivitis, or chorioretinitis, in addition to the pathologic changes induced by congenital rubella syndrome (Table 6). Adenoviruses, HSV, and VZV are detected most rapidly by fluorescent-antibody staining (124). Material collected by conjunctival or corneal scraping is applied to a small area of a clean glass slide. Smears should be transported to the laboratory immediately for acetone fixation. CMV should be detected by rapid shell vial culture. Conventional cell cultures with HEp-2 cells, or an equivalent continuous line, to detect adenoviruses and human diploid fibroblast cells to detect HSV, VZV, and CMV are recommended as backup for specimens with negative fluorescence staining or as the sole avenue for detection. The HEp-2 cells are incubated at 35 to 37°C for 7 to 10 days, whereas the fibroblast cells require 3 to 5 days incubation for HSV and 2 to 4 weeks for CMV and VZV.

Respiratory Tract

Respiratory viruses are detected by testing respiratory tract mucous membrane secretions containing virus-infected epithelial cells. Such specimens are collected by swabbing the throat or nasopharynx, washing the nasopharynx, collecting expectorated sputum, washing the trachea or bronchial airways, or lavaging the distal bronchi and alveoli. Of the noninvasive tests, throat swabs are acceptable for viral culture but nasopharyngeal swabs or washes are preferred for direct detection tests (direct fluorescent-antibody [DFA] staining and EIA). Viral etiologies are numerous, and selection of a method for detection depends on cost, turnaround time, and the technology available (Table 7). Laboratory tests must be guided by clinical information such as age of patient (pediatric or adult), severity of illness, and immune system competency (underlying diseases, neutropenia, etc.). Pediatric patients generally require a rapid, nonculture respiratory syncytial virus (RSV) test (DFA, EIA). Hospitalized individuals with negative rapid RSV test results benefit from

TABLE 5 Methods for detection of viruses in central nervous system specimens[a]

Disease	Virus	Suggested methods for laboratory diagnosis
Meningitis	Enteroviruses	RT-PCR or cell culture
	HSV	PCR, cell culture
	Lymphocytic choriomeningitis virus	Serology, animal inoculation (mice)
	Mumps virus	Serology, cell culture
	Other herpesviruses	PCR
Encephalitis	HSV	PCR or cell culture
	Mumps virus	Serology, cell culture
	Arboviruses (alphaviruses, flaviviruses, bunyaviruses)	Serology, PCR, virus isolation
	Rabies virus	Histopathology, FA staining
	Enterovirus	RT-PCR or cell culture
	Many hemorrhagic fever viruses	Antigen or antibody detection in serum, RT-PCR, virus isolation, EM
	Other herpesviruses	PCR, serology
Postinfectious encephalomyelitis	Measles virus	Autoimmune pathogenesis, serodiagnosis or clinical evidence of past infection
	VZV	
	Rubella virus	
	Mumps virus	
Subacute sclerosing panencephalitis	Measles virus	Histopathology, immunohistochemical staining, EM
Progressive multifocal leukoencephalopathy	JC virus (polyomavirus)	Histopathology, immunohistochemical staining, EM, PCR
AIDS encephalopathy	HIV	Histopathology, immunohistochemistry, EM
Tropical spastic paraparesis	HTLV-1	Serology, detection of viral antigen and genome, virus isolation
Subacute spongiform encephalopathy	Prions	Histopathology

[a] EM, electron microscopy; FA, fluorescent antibody.

TABLE 6 Methods for detection of viruses encountered in eye specimens[a]

Disease	Virus	Suggested methods for laboratory diagnosis
Conjunctivitis	Adenoviruses	Cell culture, FA staining
	Enteroviruses	Cell culture
	Measles virus	Serology, cell culture
	Rubella virus	Serology
	Dengue virus	Serology, PCR
	Hemorrhagic fever viruses	Antigen or antibody detection in serum, RT-PCR, virus isolation, EM
Keratoconjunctivitis	Adenoviruses	Cell culture, FA staining
	HSV	Cell culture, FA staining
	VZV	FA staining, cell culture
Chorioretinitis	CMV	Cell culture
Congenital rubella syndrome	Rubella virus	Serology

[a] FA, fluorescent antibody; EM, electron microscopy.

cell culture to detect other respiratory viruses, especially influenza and parainfluenza viruses. During the influenza "season," hospitalized adults should be tested for influenza A and B viruses and other respiratory viruses including adenoviruses, RSV, and parainfluenza virus. Unusual exposures or travel history can suggest less commonly encountered viruses, such as Sin Nombre virus.

RSV, influenza virus, parainfluenza virus, and adenoviruses can be detected rapidly by DFA staining or EIA. Smears of cellular secretions are prepared for DFA staining by cytocentrifugation or from centrifugation pellets (1,000 × *g* for 10 min). The sensitivity of DFA staining or EIA approaches that of culture in young, nonimmune patients (71). The sensitivity of DFA staining or EIA in older patients depends on the type of specimen (throat swab, sputum, washes or lavage collected during bronchoscopy) and the timing of specimen collection. Generally, the earlier in the course of disease the specimen is collected, the more likely it is that virus will be detected. Fluorescent staining requires experience in interpretation. Backup cell culture is useful when first using DFA staining to confirm the accuracy of positive and negative results. Adherence to manufacturers' instructions is mandatory for all direct enzyme tests.

Cell culture is standard for comprehensive detection of most viruses (Table 4). All cell cultures are incubated at 35 to 37°C for at least 7 to 10 days. Less commonly encountered viruses, such as Sin Nombre virus, may require unique diagnostic approaches. Electron microscopy has been used for the rapid detection of Sin Nombre virus (133).

Immunocompromised hosts are susceptible to primary or reactivation disease caused by CMV. CMV is readily de-

TABLE 7 Methods for detection of viruses in respiratory tract specimens[a]

Disease	Viruses	Suggested methods for laboratory diagnosis
Rhinitis	Rhinoviruses	Cell culture (30°C)
	Coronaviruses	EM
	RSV	FA stain, EIA, cell culture
	Influenza viruses	FA stain, EIA, cell culture
	Adenoviruses	FA stain, cell culture
	Enteroviruses	Cell culture
Pharyngitis	Parainfluenza viruses	FA stain, cell culture
	Influenza viruses	FA stain, EIA, cell culture
	HSV	Cell culture
	Epstein-Barr virus	Serology
	CMV	Cell culture
	Most viruses causing rhinitis	Cell culture, EM
Laryngotracheobronchitis	Parainfluenza viruses	FA stain, cell culture
	Influenza viruses	FA stain, EIA, cell culture
	RSV	FA stain, EIA, cell culture
Bronchitis/bronchiolitis	RSV	FA stain, EIA
	Parainfluenza viruses	FA stain, cell culture
	Influenza viruses	FA stain, EIA, cell culture
Pneumonia	Influenza	FA stain, EIA, cell culture
	RSV	FA stain, EIA, cell culture
	Parainfluenza viruses	FA stain, cell culture
	Adenoviruses	FA stain, cell culture
	CMV	Histopathology, cell culture
	Measles virus	Serology, FA stain, cell culture
	VZV	FA stain, cell culture
	Sin Nombre virus	Serology, EM, PCR

[a] FA, fluorescent antibody; EM, electron microscopy.

tected in respiratory secretions by the rapid shell vial assay. However, asymptomatic reactivation of latent virus is a common cause of positive viral culture and provides poor predictive value for symptomatic CMV disease (39).

Semen

Recovery of viruses other than CMV from semen is uncommon. Semen is often toxic to cell cultures. Special processing is required to reduce toxicity and enhance CMV recovery (54). (i) Semen is diluted 1:2 in VTM. (ii) The diluted semen is transferred to a 1.5-ml microcentrifuge tube and centrifuged for 5 min at high speed in a compatible microcentrifuge system. (iii) The supernatant fraction is removed and discarded. The pellet is suspended in 1 ml of VTM and mixed by vortexing. (iv) The sample is inoculated in 0.2-ml amounts into diploid fibroblast shell vial or conventional cell cultures.

Serum for Serologic Testing

Acute- and convalescent-phase serum specimens are separated from clotted blood by centrifugation (1,000 $\times$ g for 10 min) and refrigerated (4°C) for short-term (24- to 48-h) storage or frozen (< -20°C) for longer periods. Tubes should be tightly capped and not placed in a "frost-free" freezer which repeatedly warms and cools to prevent build-up of ice, since IgM antibody in serum may aggregate with repeat freezing and thawing. This risk is minimized by freezing small-volume aliquots.

Skin and Vesicles

Many viruses cause pathologic changes in the dermis. Detection tests are based on the virus or viruses suspected of causing a particular rash. Maculopapular exanthems caused by viruses do not result in virus being shed from the lesions. Many such rashes are, in fact, the result of a systemic viral infection and appear because of a hypersensitivity response to the virus growing in the capillary endothelium. In fact, diagnosis may be accomplished best by testing specimens from other sites, e.g., throat, rectal swab.

Vesicular lesions contain clear fluid from which virus is readily detected. A Tzanck preparation, using DFA staining, is the preferred method for detecting VZV (30). Smears can be prepared for staining by carefully removing the top of the skin vesicle with the needle on a tuberculin syringe, gently soaking up excess fluid with sterile gauze, and pressing a clean glass slide against the base of the lesion. Conventional cell culture is rapid, sensitive, and inexpensive for the detection of HSV, with nearly 100% of positive specimens being detected within 48 h. A Tzanck preparation for HSV is less sensitive and more labor-intensive than culture; it should be reserved for special situations where rapid detection is clinically warranted. Systemic enterovirus disease resulting in vesicle formation may be diagnosed by culturing vesicle fluid in primary monkey kidney and human diploid fibroblast cells; throat, rectal, and, in some clinical presentations, CSF specimens are also useful.

Pustular and nodular lesions are caused by viruses that grow poorly or not at all in cell culture. If clinical diagnosis is not possible, biopsy of the dermis and DNA probing will detect the genotype of papillomaviruses; biopsy, formalin fixation, and hematoxylin and eosin staining will detect the characteristic histopathologic findings of molluscum contagiosum virus infection; and electron microscopy of biopsy material will detect Orf virus.

Stool

Viral gastroenteritis is a common disease, and many viruses can be detected in the feces. Which viruses are true etiologic agents of gastroenteritis and which cause silent infection is unclear. Electron microscopy has been used to detect and establish an etiologic role for rotaviruses, enteric adenoviruses, caliciviruses, astroviruses, and Norwalk-like viruses (84). Due to the self-limited nature of viral gastroenteritis, laboratory confirmation of disease typically is needed only with childhood rotavirus and enteric adenovirus (serotypes 40 and 41) infection and with outbreak investigations of Norwalk and Norwalk-like viral agents. Detection of rotaviruses and adenoviruses is required for isolation and cohorting of patients during hospitalization. For Norwalk-like agents, detection is carried out for epidemiologic reasons.

Rotaviruses are readily and easily detected by one of the many commercially available EIAs. Both the membrane and conventional (well or tube) formats are acceptable. The membrane formats are better for rapid, single or small-batch testing. Conventional formats are more economical with large batches of specimens. Stool, rectal swabs, and specimens in diapers can be used for testing. If saline must be added to wash the specimen from a swab or diaper, only a small amount should be used because dilution decreases the test sensitivity. Specimens should be refrigerated (4°C) if a delay will occur before testing. Instructions provided with the specific kit should be closely followed.

Enteric adenoviruses belonging to serotypes 40 and 41 also can be detected by EIA. Stool processing is similar to methods used for rotavirus detection.

Electron microscopy is needed for detection of Norwalk-like viruses, caliciviruses, and astroviruses. Stool should be stored at refrigeration temperature (4°C) until testing.

Tissue

Biopsy of tissue may be necessary for diagnosis of myocarditis caused by certain enteroviruses (especially coxsackie B viruses), gastrointestinal and myocardial infection by CMV, and Kaposi's sarcoma-associated herpesvirus (HHV-8) (26). Viruses in autopsy tissues can be detected by cell culture or nonculture methods. A portion of tissue is minced and emulsified in VTM and then stored at 4°C until appropriate tests have been selected. A similar portion of fresh tissue should be frozen (≤ -20°C) for electron microscopy or molecular detection as deemed necessary following histopathologic examination.

Enteroviruses should be detected in myocardial tissue by RT-PCR and should be frozen (< -20°C) until testing takes place. Cell culture for enterovirus is less frequently positive.

Gently minced or ground tissue should be cultured for CMV by the rapid shell vial technique. Cell culture is equally sensitive but requires extended incubation (2 to 4 weeks).

Detection and identification of Kaposi's lesions by histopathologic testing are evidence of the presence of HHV-8, which can be confirmed by cell culture or electron microscopy.

Urine and Other Genitourinary Tract Specimens

Genital herpes, genital warts, molluscum contagiosum, and acute hemorrhagic cystitis caused by adenovirus or BK polyomavirus are notable viral diseases of the genitourinary tract (Table 8). In newborns, detection of CMV in urine before the age of approximately 7 days confirms congenital acquisition of the virus. Other viruses, such as HIV-1 and -2, human T-cell leukemia virus type 1 (HTLV-1) and HTLV-2, HBV, HCV, JC virus, and CMV, may be present in semen and shed in urine, but their clinical significance is determined by testing other specimens. Dilution of urine specimens (1:2 in VTM containing antibiotics) is required to inhibit contaminating bacteria and buffer excessively acidic specimens; these specimens are held at refrigeration temperature (4°C) until used for cell culture inoculation. Alternatively, urine can be neutralized with a few drops of sodium bicarbonate solution (7.5%) and filtered (0.2-μm-pore-size filter) to remove bacteria. Swabs of vesicular lesions are emulsified in VTM and held at 4°C until culturing.

HSV can be detected by conventional cell culture, using diploid lung fibroblasts or equivalent cell lines, or by the enzyme-linked cell culture system. A conventional cell culture is incubated at 35 to 37°C for 3 to 5 days. The ELVIS is incubated and stained after 16 to 24 h (110).

TABLE 8 Methods for detection of viruses in urine and other genitourinary tract specimens[a]

Disease	Virus	Suggested methods for laboratory diagnosis
Urinary tract		
Urethritis	HSV	Cell culture
	Adenovirus	Cell culture
Acute hemorrhagic cystitis	Adenovirus	Cell culture
	BK virus (polyomavirus)	Cell culture (shell vial)
Nephropathy	CMV	Cell culture, cytology (urine)
	Hantaviruses	Serology, RT-PCR
Genital tract		
Genital herpes	HSV	Cell culture, FA (Tzanck preparation)
Genital warts	Human papillomaviruses	Histopathology (DNA probe)
Molluscum contagiosum	Molluscum contagiosum virus	Histopathology
Cervicitis	Adenovirus	Cell culture

[a] FA, fluorescent antibody.

TABLE 9 Etiologies of viral hepatitis and suggested diagnostic tests[a]

Disease	Virus	Suggested methods for laboratory diagnosis
Hepatitis A	Enterovirus 72	Serology
Hepatitis B	Hepadnavirus	Serology, antigen detection
Hepatitis C	Flavivirus	Serology, RT-PCR
Hepatitis D	HDV (delta agent)	Serology
Hepatitis E	Calicivirus-like	Serology
Hepatitis G	Flavivirus	None currently available
Hepatitis secondary to infection at another site	Epstein-Barr virus	Serology
	CMV	Serology, cell culture
Infection of liver or fetus	Parvovirus B19	PCR (amniotic fluid), histopathology (liver)

Papillomavirus genotypes and molluscum contagiosum virus are detected as described above for skin and vesicular specimens. Adenoviruses are detected by conventional cell culture, and BK viruses are detected by rapid shell vial cell culture (61). In general, CMV in urine from newborns is plentiful and easily detected by rapid shell vial culture.

Specimens from Patients with Hemorrhagic Fevers

More than a dozen major hemorrhagic fevers, caused by a variety of unrelated viruses, have been described. The African filovirus hemorrhagic fevers have the highest case-fatality rate, but dengue hemorrhagic fever, Hantaan hemorrhagic nephropathy, yellow fever, Rift Valley fever, and Lassa fever are the most prevalent worldwide. Serologic diagnosis, rapid electron microscopic identification of virus, and PCR are suggested diagnostic tests. Working with specimens containing African filoviruses, Lassa fever virus, and other hemorrhagic viruses represents a significant biohazard; therefore, the recommended precautions regarding laboratory testing must be followed (118).

Specimens from Patients with Hepatitis

Disease or asymptomatic carriage caused by HAV, HBV, HCV, HDV, HEV, and HGV is detected by serologic testing, antigen detection, or PCR (Table 9). HFV and hepatitis GB (GBV-A and GBV-B) viruses have been reported, but further investigation is required to confirm their association with human disease.

Specimens from Pregnant or Peripartum Women (TORCH Testing)

Organisms that may cause peripartum disease of the newborn include *Treponema pallidum*, *Toxoplasma gondii*, rubella virus, CMV, HSV, HIV, HBV, VZV, and enteroviruses. Although routine testing for all agents is rarely necessary, testing for individual agents in pregnant patients and newborns is needed in specific clinical situations. Table 10 suggests processing strategies for individual viruses.

MYCOLOGY

General Considerations

The first step taken in the laboratory toward diagnosis of fungal infections is often direct microscopic examination and/or direct antigen detection performed on select specimens (discussed in chapter 94). Cultures are performed on all acceptable specimens regardless of whether fungal elements are observed on direct examination, since culture is more sensitive than direct microscopic examination and is necessary to confirm the direct findings and identify the organisms in positive specimens. The pretreatment that is

TABLE 10 Etiologies of viral disease in the newborn and suggested diagnostic tests[a]

Virus	Specimen	Suggested method(s) for laboratory diagnosis
Rubella virus	Serum	Serology
CMV	Urine	Cell culture (shell vial)
	Tissue	Cell culture (shell vial), histopathology
HSV	Cutaneous lesion	Cell culture
	CSF	PCR, cell culture
HIV	Blood, tissue	RT-PCR, cell culture
	Serum	Serology
HBV (hepadnavirus)	Blood	PCR, serology
VZV	Cutaneous lesion	FA (Tzanck preparation)
	Tissue, fluid, or secretions	Cell culture (shell vial)
Enteroviruses	Cutaneous lesion, tissue	Cell culture, RT-PCR

[a] FA, fluorescent antibody.

TABLE 11 Pretreatment of clinical specimens prior to plating for fungi

Specimen	Pretreatment	Comments
Blood	Lysis and centrifugation (30 min) at 3,000 × *g*, 35° fixed-angle rotor, or 2,400–3,000 × *g*, swinging bucket	Method of choice and necessary for isolation of *H. capsulatum*
Body fluids	Filtration or centrifugation at 2,000 × *g* for 10 min	Necessary for optimal recovery; used on all specimens >2 ml
Urine	Centrifugation at 2,000 × *g* for 10 min	Necessary for optimal recovery, especially for agents of systemic or disseminated mycoses
Respiratory secretions	Liquefication with mucolytic agent	Necessary (with centrifugation) on induced sputum specimens for *P. carinii*. Optional for other mycoses; centrifugation may improve yield but also increases numbers of interfering organisms, e.g., bacteria and colonizing yeasts
Exudates, pus, drainage	Washing, centrifugation, and crushing of granules	Recommended if granules are present
Tissue	Mincing or grinding	Necessary for optimal recovery of all fungi; specimens must be cut into small pieces if a zygomycete is suspected or ground if *H. capsulatum* is suspected
Nails	Cutting into small pieces	Necessary for optimal recovery of fungi

advised for culture of designated specimens (Table 11) should usually be carried out before direct microscopic examination.

Pretreatment of certain specimens for fungus culture is required to optimize the recovery of the etiologic agents. Procedures that concentrate the fungi (centrifugation), liberate them from cells (blood cell lysis), or increase the surface area of the specimen (maceration or mincing) can be extremely beneficial when applied to appropriate specimens. This can be especially appreciated when realizing that there are generally fewer fungal cells at the site of an infection than there are bacterial cells in a bacterial infection. Because of the anticipated low organism count, an adequate specimen should consist of enough material to inoculate ~0.5 ml onto several agar surfaces.

Media for Primary Isolation

A large variety of media are appropriate for primary isolation of fungi (Table 12). No one medium is best for all types of specimens or for all medically important fungi, and so ordinarily a few appropriate media must be inoculated. Although the choice of media often depends on availability, cost, and personal preference, it is still imperative that certain requirements be met. A medium that supports fungi while inhibiting bacteria must be used with any specimen that might contain bacterial flora. The most commonly used media are brain heart infusion (BHI) plus antibiotics, Sabhi agar plus antibiotics, or inhibitory mold agar (IMA). The antibiotics that have traditionally been added, alone or in various combinations to mycology media to inhibit bacteria are chloramphenicol (≥16 μg/ml), gentamicin (5 to 100 μg/ml), penicillin (20 U/ml), and streptomycin (40 μg/ml). Ciprofloxacin (5 μg/ml) has also been used with success. The antibacterial agents will inhibit *Nocardia* spp; therefore, if this organism is suspected, medium free of antibacterial agents must be used. *Nocardia*, although often handled in mycology, is a filamentous bacterium and is further discussed in chapter 24.

Cycloheximide, a eukaryotic protein synthesis inhibitor, should be used in one medium, particularly if there is a possibility of fungal contamination of the specimen, e.g., hair, skin, or nails. The cycloheximide is usually added to Sabouraud's dextrose agar (SDA) or Sabhi agar in combination with an antibacterial agent, most commonly chloramphenicol. The intended function of cycloheximide (0.5 mg/ml) is to inhibit or completely prevent the proliferation of rapidly growing fungi that are commonly considered contaminants in order to prevent their overgrowth of significant pathogens that may also be present in the specimen. While inhibiting true saprobes, cycloheximide inhibits many strains of opportunistic fungi and known pathogens such as *Pseudallescheria boydii*, *Cryptococcus neoformans*, *Trichosporon beigelii*, some species of *Candida* and *Aspergillus*, and most zygomycetes. For this reason, at least one medium without cycloheximide must be included in the battery of media used.

For many years, it has been traditional to use SDA without antifungal or antibacterial agents as the basic primary medium for isolation of fungi. This is now being discouraged in favor of one of the more enriched and antibacterial media, e.g., Sabhi plus antibacterial agents or IMA. Of the SDA formulations, Emmons' modification, containing 2% dextrose and having a pH near neutral, is recommended.

For specimens that may contain fastidious thermally dimorphic fungi, BHI agar, preferably augmented with antibacterial agents, has customarily been included in the battery to ensure maximum recovery. The addition of 5 to 10% sheep blood improves the yield slightly, but organisms must be subcultured to a blood-free medium to induce conidiation. To isolate a dimorphic fungus from a heavily contaminated specimen, yeast extract phosphate medium with ammonium hydroxide is the optimal medium.

TABLE 12 Media for primary isolation of fungi

Type of medium[a]	Additive	Uses and comments
Without antibacterial or antifungal agents		
SDA	None	Classic pigment and colony formation
BHI agar	Sheep blood optional	Cultivation of all fungi including the fastidious dimorphics; blood inhibits conidiation
Sabhi agar	Sheep blood optional	Cultivation of all fungi including the fastidious dimorphics; blood inhibits conidiation
PDA or PFA	None	Production of conidia and fruiting bodies
Any of the above	Olive oil on surface	Cultivation of *Malassezia furfur*
With antibacterial agent(s)		
SDA, BHI agar, or Sabhi plus	Separate or in combination: chloramphenicol, ciprofloxacin, gentamicin, penicillin, streptomycin	Inhibition of bacteria while allowing most fungi to grow; BHI agar, Sabhi, and IMA are more enriched than SDA and better support the growth of the more fastidious fungi
IMA	Contains chloramphenicol	
With antibacterial and antifungal agents		
Mycosel or Mycobiotic agar	SDA with chloramphenicol and cycloheximide	Inhibition of bacteria and many saprobic and rapidly growing fungi that may overgrow the pathogens, but some opportunistic and true pathogens may also be inhibited
BHI agar or Sabhi	Any antibacterial agent in previous group plus cycloheximide	As above
Selective for dimorphic fungi		
Yeast extract phosphate medium	Add ammonia to surface	Inhibition of bacteria, yeasts, and many molds and enhancement of slow-growing dimorphic fungi
For dermatophytes		
DTM	Chloramphenicol, gentamicin, cycloheximide, with phenol red	Both are meant to isolate dermatophytes and show a color change of the medium; DIM appears to be more successful
DIM	Penicillin, streptomycin, cycloheximide, with bromcresol purple	
Selective and differential for yeasts		
CHROM agar Candida Albicans ID	Antimicrobial agents and chromogenic substrates	Isolation of yeasts with color development in colonies allows for presumptive identification of some common species of *Candida*

[a] SDA, Sabouraud dextrose agar; PDA, potato dextrose agar; PFA, potato flake agar; IMA, inhibitory mold agar; DTM, dermatophyte test medium; DIM, dermatophyte identification medium.

Two relatively new chromogenic media, CHROMagar Candida (Hardy Diagnostics, Santa Maria, Calif.) and Candida ID (bioMérieux), designed for the isolation and presumptive identification of *Candida* spp. have shown high sensitivities and specificities. They facilitate the detection of mixed yeast cultures and allow the direct presumptive identification of some common *Candida* species. This can play an important role in detecting the more fluconazole-resistant *Candida* species that might be mixed with *C. albicans* (6, 80, 89).

Additional specialized media for the recovery of specific fungi may be used, e.g., media containing substrates (L-dopa, caffeic acid, etc.) for detection of *Cryptococcus neoformans* by its phenol oxidase activity, media containing or overlaid with a source of long-chain fatty acids (e.g., olive oil) for the recovery of *Malassezia furfur*, or dermatophyte test medium (DTM) or dermatophyte identification medium (DIM) specifically formulated for the culture and isolation of dermatophytes (97). Refer to chapter 130 for more detailed information on media.

Specimens should be cultured in a certified, laminar-flow biologic safety cabinet. Petri dishes, screw-cap tubes, or screw-cap flat bottles may be selected for isolation media. Plates provide a larger surface area and ease in isolating and reaching colonies, but they may be perceived as more hazardous to handle. If plates are used, dehydration can be deterred by using a high volume (40 ml) of medium and surrounding the plate with a shrink seal or air-permeable tape. The seal or tape also serves to prevent unintentional opening. Placing a pan of water in the incubator will help maintain humidity. When *Coccidioides immitis* is suspected, as a safety measure plates should not be used.

If tubes are used, they should have as large a diameter as is reasonably possible. Most commercially prepared fungal media are available as slants in 20-mm-diameter tubes and in small bottles or flasks. Screw-caps must be kept partially loosened to ensure proper aeration, or else growth will be either inhibited or very abnormal, and this will lead to erroneous or delayed results. Slants should be incubated horizontally (on an AFB culture rack) for at least 24 h after inoculation to ensure that the inoculum remains spread over the whole surface area of the agar; the slants can then be placed upright.

Pretreatment and Culture Guidelines

When a properly collected, labelled, and transported specimen (see chapter 4) reaches the mycology laboratory, it should be processed as soon as possible. If delay is unavoidable, most specimens can be stored at 4°C, but there are definite exceptions, as specified below. The specimen must be grossly examined for caseous, purulent, bloody, and necrotic material. Those are the portions of the specimen from which material should be taken for microscopic examination and culture. Refer to Table 2 for categories of fungal culture media.

Blood

The most sensitive method for isolating fungi from blood specimens is lysis-centrifugation, commercially available as the Isolator System. The Isolator tube contains saponin, which lyses leukocytes and erythrocytes, releasing intracellular fungi, which are then concentrated by centrifugation. The sediment should be streaked onto enriched media, e.g., IMA, BHI, or sheep blood agar. Cycloheximide must not be included in the media because it inhibits certain fungi that are pathogenic in the blood. An antibacterial medium should also be inoculated if a mixed infection with bacteria is a possibility. Optimally, the Isolator tube should be processed within 16 h of blood collection; until processing, the tube should be maintained at room temperature.

Recent studies have shown that some of the special enhanced broth bottles used in the blood culture systems that feature continuous shaking and monitoring have improved the automated detection of fungemia with a 7-day protocol (18, 46). If unenhanced basic broth is used, terminal subculturing may be required. If a laboratory is using a noncontinuous shaking broth system, it is recommended that the bottles for fungal culture be agitated throughout the incubation period rather than for only the first 24 h, as is the usual procedure for bacteria (91). Certain fungi, however, are reliably recovered only by the lysis-centrifugation method. This is especially true for *Histoplasma capsulatum* but can pertain to other fungi as well (18, 46, 58).

Bone Marrow

Heparinized bone marrow aspirates may be inoculated at the bedside directly onto enriched media as recommended for blood cultures (see above). The total inoculum should consist of at least 0.5 ml. The pediatric Isolator 1.5 system is suitable for this small-volume specimen, and its lysing capabilities can enhance fungal cultivation. If delay in plating is unavoidable, the tube can be held for up to 16 h at room temperature. Blood culture bottles are not recommended because the broths do not support the growth of *H. capsulatum*, an organism that must often be considered when culturing bone marrow.

Normally Sterile Body Fluids

Normally sterile body fluids include CSF; pericardial, peritoneal, and synovial fluids; and vitreous humor. If the specimen consists of more than 2 ml, it requires centrifugation at 2,000 × *g* for 10 min; 1 to 2 ml of the sediment is inoculated onto medium surfaces (at least one being cycloheximide free). Low-volume specimens (less than 2 ml) are inoculated directly onto the medium. Alternatively, specimens can be filtered through a membrane filter, which is then placed (particle side down) on the surface of a medium that does not contain cycloheximide. The filter can be periodically moved to another area of the medium, and the previous location can be examined for growth. Any clotted material present in a specimen should be minced with a sterile scalpel before being processed.

Tissue

Tissue specimens should be minced or ground before plating. If the suspected etiologic fungal agent in a tissue sample is unknown or thought to be a zygomycete, it is advisable to cut the specimen with a scalpel into 1-mm pieces; grinding or homogenization of the specimen can be detrimental to the hyphae of zygomycetes and prevent their growth on culture. If *H. capsulatum* is suspected, subsequent grinding of the specimen may be required. Fragments and/or homogenates of tissue are inoculated onto an uninhibitory enriched medium and an antibacterial medium; a medium with cycloheximide should be included if fungal contamination is a possibility. The tissue is submerged slightly into the agar surfaces.

Exudates, Pus, and Drainage Specimens

Exudates, pus, and drainage specimens should be examined for granules under a dissecting microscope. If no granules are seen, a smear is prepared and the specimen is inoculated directly onto isolation media. If granules are present, a portion of the specimen is teased apart and crushed between two glass slides; each slide is examined microscopically for fungal elements. The remainder of the specimen should be washed in sterile distilled water, and the granules should be crushed with a sterile glass or plastic rod. For fungal culture, the crushed granular material is inoculated onto antibacterial media with and without cycloheximide; if the granules are bacterial, they are plated accordingly.

External Eye Specimens

Specimens from patients with presumed mycotic keratitis should be obtained by an ophthalmologist and inoculated directly onto the medium and an alcohol-cleaned, flamed slide. Corneal scrapings are transferred from the surgical instrument to a noninhibitory agar plate by making a series of C- or X-shaped cuts on the medium. Inoculated plates are maintained at room temperature if transport to the laboratory may be delayed.

Respiratory Secretions

Care should be taken to culture the most bloody, purulent, or mucus-laden portions of the respiratory specimen directly onto antibacterial media with and without cycloheximide. Very viscous specimens can be liquefied with a dash of crystalline *N*-acetyl-L-cysteine, but sodium hydroxide (used for decontamination of cultures for mycobacteria) must not be used because it inhibits the growth of many fungi. Centrifugation of respiratory specimens has not been shown to increase the isolation of fungi; it is more likely to result in overgrowth by bacteria.

Upper Respiratory Tract

Oropharyngeal candidiasis is readily diagnosed by smear and/or culture on routine mycology agar. Antibacterial medium should be used to avoid overgrowth of culture by members of the normal oral bacterial flora.

Urine

Urine samples (10 to 50 ml) are centrifuged, and the sediment is inoculated onto antibacterial media with and without cycloheximide. If quantitation is required, uncentrifuged urine can be streaked with a calibrated loop onto a plate of noninhibitory medium. The quantity of yeasts in a urine sample does not appear to have the same interpretative value as that of bacteria. The persistence of yeast in several carefully collected midstream urine samples and the clinical picture of the patient in whom candiduria of any count develops are the most important factors in interpreting its significance (24). In the severely ill, predisposed patient, candiduria may be an early indication of disseminated candidiasis.

Vaginal Secretions

Clinical characteristics along with direct microscopic examination of vaginal secretions are better than culture for the diagnosis of vaginal candidiasis. Since yeast cells are part of the normal vaginal flora in up to 20% of healthy women, growing *Candida* on culture without considering other factors may be meaningless or misleading. However, cultures may be helpful in monitoring therapy, managing individuals with chronic recurring disease, or determining the etiology of infectious vaginitis when other tests have been unrewarding. Antibacterial media with and without cycloheximide should be inoculated.

Stool Specimens

It is not advised to culture stool specimens for fungi, because positive results may be misleading. Up to 40% of healthy individuals and up to 75% of immunocompromised patients are colonized with yeasts without disease. Biopsy specimens of pathologic tissue are preferred for the diagnosis of many fungal infections of the gastrointestinal tract.

Hair, Skin, and Nails

Hair fragments and skin scrapings are placed directly on the agar surface. Nails yield the best culture results if they are cut into smaller pieces with a scalpel before culturing. It helps to inoculate these specimens onto the agar by applying light pressure to submerge them slightly under the agar surface to ensure complete contact of the specimen with the medium. In an effort to isolate dermatophytes, a medium containing an antibacterial agent(s) and cycloheximide should be inoculated. If the specimen must be stored before culturing, it should be held at room temperature; a few dermatophytes do not tolerate refrigeration.

Incubation

All cultures should be incubated at ≤30°C (the incubator should be at 29°C to allow for ± 1°C); this temperature is optimal for most medically important fungi. If a 30°C incubator is not available, cultures should be incubated at room temperature (~25°C). Routine incubation is continued for 4 weeks. When *H. capsulatum* or *Blastomyces dermatitidis* is suspected, 6 to 8 weeks of incubation may be required for growth. Specimens that are being screened primarily for yeasts, e.g., oropharyngeal and vaginal cultures, need be incubated for only 7 days. Cultures should be examined at least every 2 or 3 days for the first 2 weeks and weekly thereafter.

PARASITOLOGY

General Considerations

Diagnostic parasitology generally includes laboratory procedures that are designed to detect organisms within clinical specimens by using morphologic criteria rather than culture, biochemical tests, and/or physical growth characteristics (Table 13). Many clinical specimens, such as those from the intestinal tract, contain multiple artifacts that complicate the differentiation of parasites from surrounding debris. Final identification is often based on microscopic examination of stained preparations (Tables 14 and 15).

Specimen preparation generally includes a concentration procedure, all of which are designed to increase the chances of finding the organism(s). Microscopic examination requires review of the prepared clinical specimen under multiple magnifications, including oil immersion (magnification × 1,000).

Protozoa are quite small and tend to range from 1.5 μm (microsporidia) to ~80 μm (*Balantidium coli*, a ciliate). Some organisms are intracellular and require multiple isolation and staining methods for identification. Helminth infections are usually diagnosed by finding eggs, larvae, and/or adult worms in various clinical specimens, primarily those from the intestinal tract. Identification to the species level may require microscopic examination of the specimen. The recovery and identification of blood parasites can require concentration, culture, and microscopy. Confirmation of suspected parasitic infections depends on the proper collection, processing, and examination of clinical specimens; multiple specimens must often be submitted and examined to find and confirm the suspected organism(s).

Direct Detection by Routine Methods

Intestinal Tract Specimens

The most common specimen submitted to the diagnostic parasitology laboratory is the stool specimen. The most widely used procedure for specimen processing is the ova and parasite examination (O&P), which consists of three separate protocols: the direct wet mount, the concentration, and the permanent stained smear (28, 44, 60, 66, 77). The direct wet mount requires fresh stool, is designed to allow the detection of motile protozoan trophozoites, and is examined microscopically at low and high dry magnifications (×100, entire 22- by 22-mm coverslip; ×400, one-third to one-half of a 22- by 22-mm coverslip). However, due to potential problems with the lag time between the time of specimen passage and receipt in the laboratory, the direct wet examination has been eliminated from the routine O&P under the circumstances of receipt of specimens collected in stool preservatives; if specimens are received in the laboratory in stool collection preservatives, the direct wet preparation is not performed.

The second part of the O&P is the concentration, which is designed to facilitate the recovery of protozoan cysts, coccidian oocysts, microsporidial spores, and helminth eggs and larvae. Both flotation (zinc sulfate) and sedimentation methods are available, the most common procedure being the formalin-ethyl acetate sedimentation method (formerly called the formalin-ether method). The concentrated speci-

TABLE 13 Body sites and possible parasites recovered[a]

Site	Parasites
Blood	
Erythroyctes	*Plasmodium* spp. *Babesia* spp.
Leukocytes	*Leishmania donovani*, *Toxoplasma gondii*
Whole blood/plasma	*Trypanosoma* spp., microfilariae
Bone marrow	*Leishmania donovani*
Central nervous system	*Taenia solium* (cysticerci), *Echinococcus* spp., *Naegleria fowleri*, *Acanthamoeba* spp., *Balamuthia mandrillaris*, *Toxoplasma gondii*, microsporidia, *Trypanosoma* spp.
Liver, spleen	*Echinococcus* spp., *Entamoeba histolytica*, *Leishmania donovani*, microsporidia
Lungs	*Cryptosporidium* spp.,[b] *Echinococcus* spp., *Paragonimus* spp., microsporidia
Muscle	*Taenia solium* (cysticerci), *Trichinella spiralis*, *Onchocerca volvulus* (nodules), *Trypanosoma cruzi*, microsporidia
Cutaneous ulcers	*Leishmania* spp., *Acanthamoeba* spp.
Intestinal tract	*Entamoeba histolytica*, *Entamoeba dispar*, *Entamoeba coli*, *Entamoeba hartmanni*, *Endolimax nana*, *Iodamoeba bütschlii*, *Blastocystis hominis*, *Giardia lamblia*, *Chilomastix mesnili*, *Dientamoeba fragilis*, *Trichomonas hominis*, *Balantidium coli*, *Cryptosporidium parvum*, *Isospora belli*, microsporidia, *Ascaris lumbricoides*, *Enterobius vermicularis*, hookworm, *Strongyloides stercoralis*, *Trichuris trichiura*, *Hymenolepis nana*, *Hymenolepis diminuta*, *Taenia saginata*, *Taenia solium*, *Diphyllobothrium latum*, *Clonorchis sinensis*, (*Opisthorchis*), *Paragonimus westermani*, *Schistosoma* spp., *Fasciolopsis buski*, *Fasciola hepatica*, *Metagonimus yokogawai*, *Heterophyes heterophyes*
Skin	*Leishmania* spp., *Onchocerca volvulus*, microfilariae
Urogenital system	*Trichomonas vaginalis*, *Schistosoma* spp., microsporidia
Eye	*Acanthamoeba* spp., *Toxoplasma gondii*, *Loa loa*, microsporidia

[a] Parasites include trophozoites, cysts, oocysts, spores, adults, larvae, eggs, amastigotes, and trypomastigotes. The table does not include every possible parasite that could be found in a particular body site. However, the most likely organisms are listed.

[b] Disseminated in severely immunosuppressed individuals.

men is examined as a wet preparation, with or without iodine, using low and high dry magnifications (×100 and ×400) as indicated for the direct wet examination.

The third part of the O&P is the permanent stained smear, which is designed to facilitate the identification of intestinal protozoa (Table 14). Several staining methods are available, the two most common being the Wheatley modification of the Gomori tissue trichrome method and the iron-hematoxylin staining method. This part of the O&P is critical for the confirmation of suspicious objects seen in the wet examination and identification of protozoa that might not have been seen in the wet preparation (28, 44, 60, 66, 77). This is the most important procedure performed for the identification of intestinal protozoan infections; the permanent-stained smears are examined with oil immersion objectives (600× for screening, 1,000× for final review of ≥300 oil immersion fields).

Other specimens from the intestinal tract, such as duodenal aspirates or drainage, mucus from the Entero-Test Capsule technique, and sigmoidoscopy material, can also be examined as wet preparations and as permanent stained smears after processing with either trichrome or iron-hematoxylin stain.

Urogenital Tract Specimens

The identification of *Trichomonas vaginalis* is usually based on the examination of wet preparations of vaginal and urethral discharges and prostatic secretions or urine sediment (Table 14). Multiple specimens may have to be examined to detect the organisms. These specimens are diluted with a drop of saline and examined under low power (×100) and reduced illumination for the presence of actively motile organisms; as the jerky motility begins to diminish, it may be possible to observe the undulating membrane, particularly under high dry power (×400) (28). Culture systems (In-Pouch TV; BioMed Diagnostics, San Jose, Calif.; and Empyrean Diagnostics, Inc., Mountain View, Calif.) that allow direct inoculation, transport, culture, and microscopic examination are available commercially (28). Stained smears such as Papanicolaou or Giemsa can be used but are usually not necessary for the identification of this organism and can be difficult to interpret. If a dry smear is received by the laboratory, it can be fixed with absolute methanol and stained with Giemsa stain; this approach is not optimal, but the smear can be examined and may confirm a positive infection. Many times, the number of false-positive and false-negative results reported on the basis of stained smears strongly suggests the value of confirmation by observation of motile organisms from the direct mount, from appropriate culture media, or from direct detection using monoclonal antibodies.

Examination of urinary sediment may be indicated for certain filarial infections. Administration of the drug diethylcarbamazine (Hetrazan) has been reported to enhance the recovery of microfilariae from the urine. The triple-concentration technique is recommended for the recovery of mi-

TABLE 14 Body site, specimen and procedures, recommended stain(s) and relevant parasites, and additional information

Body site	Specimen and procedures[a]	Recommended stains and relevant parasites[a]	Additional information
Blood	Whole or anticoagulated blood. Fresh blood preferred but may not be practical for many laboratories. If anticoagulant is used, EDTA is preferred (purple top). Common: thin and thick blood films. Less common: various concentrations, QBC microhematocrit tube, ParaSight F, and PCR.	Giemsa (all blood parasites); hematoxylin-based stain (microfilariae [sheathed]). NOTE: The QBC tube has also been recommended as a screening method for blood parasites (hematocrit tube contains acridine orange) and has been used for malaria, *Babesia*, trypanosomes, leishmaniae, and microfilariae.	Most drawings and organism descriptions of blood parasites are based on Giemsa-stained blood films. Although Wright's stain (or Wright-Giemsa combination stain) will work, stippling in malaria may not be visible and the organism colors will not match the descriptions. However, with other stains (those listed above, in addition to some of the "quick" blood stains), the organisms should be visible on the blood film. The use of blood collected with anticoagulant (rather than fresh) has direct relevance to the morphology of malaria organisms seen in peripheral blood films. If the blood smears are prepared after more than 1 h, stippling may not be visible. Also, if blood is held at room temperature (with the stopper removed), the male microgametocyte may exflagellate and fertilize the female macrogametocyte, and development continues within the tube of blood (as it would in the mosquito host). The ookinete may actually resemble *Plasmodium falciparum* gametocytes.
Bone marrow	Aspirate. Common: thin and thick films. Less common: cultures (leishmaniae, trypanosomes) and PCR.	Giemsa (all blood parasites).	See comments listed above for blood.
Central nervous system	Spinal fluid, brain biopsy specimen. Common: CSF (wet examination, stained smears), brain biopsy (touch or squash preparations, stained). Less common: cultures (free-living amebae), EM.	Giemsa (trypanosomes, *Toxoplasma gondii*); Giemsa, Trichrome, or Calcofluor (amebae [*Naegleria*, *Acanthamoeba*, *Balamuthia*]); Giemsa, acid-fast, PAS, modified Trichrome, silver methenamine (microsporidia); hematoxylin and eosin, routine histology (larval cestodes).	If CSF is received (with no suspect organism suggested), Giemsa would be the best choice; however, Calcofluor is also recommended as a second stain (amebic cysts, microsporidia). If brain biopsy material is received (particularly from an immunocompromised patient), EM studies may be required to identify microsporidia to the genus or species levels; however, modified Trichrome and/or Calcofluor methods can be used to visualize the spores. Culture would be recommended for the free-living amebae (exception: *Balamuthia* will not grow in the routine agar/bacterial overlay method).
Cutaneous ulcers	Aspirate, biopsy. Common: aspirate (stained smears), biopsy (touch or squash preparations, stained). Less common: cultures (leishmaniae, free-living amebae), PCR.	Giemsa (leishmaniae); hematoxylin and eosin, routine histology (*Acanthamoeba* spp., *Entamoeba histolytica*).	Most likely causative agent would be leishmaniae, all of which would stain with Giemsa. Hematoxylin and eosin (routine histology) could also be used to identify these organisms. In the immunocompromised patient, skin ulcers have been documented where the causative agents were amebae. Certainly, in some parts of the world, leishmaniae would be a likely cause (particularly in AIDS patients).

(Continued on next page)

TABLE 14 Body site, specimen and procedures, recommended stain(s) and relevant parasites, and additional information (*Continued*)

Body site	Specimen and procedures[a]	Recommended stains and relevant parasites[a]	Additional information
Eye	Biopsy, scrapings, contact lens, lens solution. Common: stained smears. Less common: Cultures (free-living amebae, *Toxoplasma gondii*), EM.	Calcofluor, cysts only (amebae [*Acanthamoeba*]); Giemsa, trophozoites, cysts (Amebae); hematoxylin and eosin, routine histology (cysticerci, *Loa loa*, *Toxoplasma gondii*); silver methenamine stain, PAS, acid-fast, EM (microsporidia).	Some free-living amebae (most commonly *Acanthamoeba*) have been implicated as a cause of keratitis. Although Calcofluor will stain the cyst walls, it will not stain the trophozoites. Therefore, in suspect cases of amebic keratitis, both stains should be used. Hematoxylin and eosin (routine histology) can be used to detect and confirm cysticercosis. The adult worm of *Loa loa*, when removed from the eye, can be stained with a hematoxylin-based stain (Delafield's) or can be stained and examined by routine histology. *Toxoplasma* infection could be diagnosed from routine histology and/or serology results. Microsporidia confirmation to the genus or species levels may require EM studies; however, the spores could be found by routine light microscopy with modified Trichrome and/or Calcofluor stains.
Intestinal tract	Stool, sigmoidoscopy material, duodenal contents. Common: direct wet smear, concentration, and permanent stained smear, modified acid-fast stains. Less common: modified Trichrome stains, immunoassays on specimen, EM.	Trichrome or iron hematoxylin (intestinal protozoa); modified trichrome (microsporidia); modified acid-fast (*Cryptosporidium parvum*, *Cyclospora cayetanensis*) monoclonal reagents, e.g., EIA, FA (*Entamoeba histolytica*, *Giardia lamblia* *Cryptosporidium parvum*, microsporidia [experimental]).	Although Trichrome or iron hematoxylin stains can be used on almost all specimens from the intestinal tract, actual worm segments (tapeworm proglottids) can be stained with special stains. However, after routine dehydration through alcohols and xylenes (or xylene substitutes), the branched uterine structure will be visible, allowing identification of the proglottid to the species level. Immunoassay detection kits are also available for the identification of *Giardia lamblia*, *Entamoeba histolytica*, *Entamoeba dispar*, and *Cryptosporidium parvum*. Microsporidia confirmation to the genus or species levels may require EM studies; however, modified Trichrome and/or Calcofluor stains can be used to confirm the presence of spores.
	Anal impression smear.	No stain, cellulose tape.	Four to six consecutive negative tapes required to "rule out" infection.
	Adult worm or worm segments.	Carmine stains (rarely used).	Proglottids can usually be identified to the species level without using tissue stains.
	Biopsy.	Hematoxylin and eosin, routine histology (*Entamoeba histolytica*, *Cryptosporidium parvum*, *Cyclospora cayetanensis*, *Isospora belli*, *Giardia lamblia*, microsporidia).	Special stains may be helpful in the identification of microsporidia: tissue Gram stains, silver stains, PAS, and Giemsa.
Liver and spleen	Aspirates, biopsy. Common: touch and squash preparations, stain. Less common: cultures, EM, PCR.	Giemsa (leishmaniae); hematoxylin and eosin, routine histology.	Aspirates and/or touch preparations from biopsy material can be routinely stained with Giemsa stain. This will allow the identification of the leishmania. There are definite risks associated with spleen aspirates and/or biopsy. Other parasites, such as larval cestodes, trematodes, amebae, or microsporidia, could be seen and identified from routine histologic staining.

(*Continued on next page*)

TABLE 14 *(Continued)*

Body site	Specimen and procedures[a]	Recommended stains and relevant parasites[a]	Additional information
Lungs	Sputum, induced sputum, bronchoalveolar lavage, transbronchial aspirate, tracheobronchial aspirate, brush biopsy, open-lung biopsy. Common: stained smears. Less common: special stains, culture, EM, PCR.	Modified acid-fast stains (*Cryptosporidium parvum*); hematoxylin and eosin, routine histology (*Strongyloides stercoralis*, *Paragonimus* spp., amebae); silver methenamine stain, PAS, acid-fast, tissue Gram stains, modified Trichrome, EM (microsporidia).	There are also monoclonal reagents (FA) available for the diagnosis of pulmonary cryptosporidiosis. Routine histologic procedures would allow the identification of any of the helminths or helminth eggs present in the lung. Disseminated microsporidiosis is now well documented, with organisms being found in many different respiratory specimens.
Muscle	Biopsy. Common: touch and squash preparations. Less common: Special stains, EM, PCR.	Hematoxylin and eosin, routine histology (*Trichinella spiralis*, cysticerci); silver methenamine stain, PAS, acid-fast, tissue Gram stains, EM (microsporidia).	If *Trypanosoma cruzi* were present in the striated muscle, the organisms could be identified from routine histology preparations. Microsporidia confirmation to the genus or species levels may require EM studies; however, modified Trichrome and/or Calcofluor stains could be used to confirm the presence of spores.
Skin	Aspirates, skin snip, scrapings, biopsy. Common: wet examination, stained smear. Less common: special stains, EM.	See Cutaneous ulcer (above). Hematoxylin and eosin, routine histology (*Onchocerca volvulus*, *Dipetalonema streptocerca*, leishmaniae, *Acanthamoeba* spp., *Entamoeba histolytica*, microsporidia).	Any of the potential parasites present could be identified by routine histology procedures and routine stains.
Urogenital system	Vaginal discharge, urethral discharge, prostatic secretions, urine. Common: stained smears. Less common: culture, EM, biopsy.	Giemsa, immunoassay reagents (FA) (*Trichomonas vaginalis*); Delafield's hematoxylin (microfilariae); modified Trichrome (microsporidia); hematoxylin and eosin, routine histology (*Schistosoma haematobium*, microfilariae); PAS, acid-fast, tissue Gram stains, EM (microsporidia)	Although *T. vaginalis* is probably the most common parasite identified, there are others to consider, the most recently implicated organisms being in the microsporidia group. Microfilariae could also be recovered and stained.

[a] EM, electron microscopy; FA, fluorescent antibody; GAE, granulomatous amebic encephalitis; GI, gastrointestinal; PAM, primary amebic meningoencephalitis; PAS, periodic acid-Schiff stain.

TABLE 15 Examination of tissue and aspirated body fluids

Parasite	Disease(s)[a]	Appropriate test(s)[a]	Positive result and additional information
Protozoa (free-living)			
Naegleria fowleri	PAM	Wet exam of CSF (not in counting chamber) Stained preparation of CSF sediment Culture	Trophozoites present and identified. Cultures may be positive when stained smears are negative.
Acanthamoeba spp.	Amebic keratitis, chronic meningoencephalitis (GAE)	Culture/stained smears Calcofluor (cysts only) Biopsy/routine histology	Trophozoites and/or cysts present and identified. Cultures may be positive when stained smears are negative.
Balamuthia mandrillaris	Chronic meningoencephalitis (GAE)	Calcofluor (cysts only) Stained smears Biopsy/routine histology	Trophozoites and/or cysts present and identified. Culture not appropriate.
Protozoa (intestinal)			
Entamoeba histolytica	Amebiasis	Biopsy/routine histology Liver abscess aspirate	Trophozoites present and identified. Immunoassay reagents available for confirmation of *E. histolytica*.
Giardia lamblia	Giardiasis	Duodenal aspirate Duodenal biopsy/routine histology Entero-Test capsule EIA, FA	Trophozoites and/or cysts present and identified. Immunoassay reagents can be used on duodenal aspirate specimens.
Cryptosporidium parvum	Cryptosporidiosis	Duodenal scraping Duodenal biopsy Stain Routine histology Other tissue biopsy Routine histology Squash preparation Sputum (modified AFB stains)	Identification of organisms in microvillus border or in other tissues (lung and gallbladder have also been involved).
Microsporidia *Nosema* spp. *Encephalitozoon* spp. *Enterocytozoon bieneusi* *Pleistophora* spp. *Trachipleistophora hominis* *Vittaforma corneae* "Microsporidium" spp.	Microsporidiosis	Routine histology (fair); acid fast, PAS, tissue Gram stains, modified Trichrome, Giemsa stains recommended (spores); animal inoculation not recommended due to latent animal infections; EM may be necessary to confirm identification to the species level	These organisms (spores) have been found as insect or other animal parasites; the most common route of infection is probably ingestion (inhalation and direct inoculation into the eye have also been documented). Human cases involve GI tract, muscle, CSF (AIDS); other body sites have also been documented. Disseminated infections seen in AIDS patients with CD4 count of <50. PCR has been used but is not routinely available in most laboratories.

(Continued on next page)

TABLE 15 (*Continued*)

Parasite	Disease(s)[a]	Appropriate test(s)[a]	Positive result and additional information
Protozoa (blood or tissue)			
Leishmania spp. (cutaneous lesions)	Cutaneous leishmaniasis	Material from under bed of ulcer Smear Culture Animal inoculation Punch biopsy Routine histology Squash preparation Culture Animal inoculation	Amastigotes recovered in macrophages of skin, or from animal inoculation; other stages recovered in culture. PCR has also been used but is not routinely available in most laboratories.
Leishmania spp. (mucocutaneous lesions)	Mucocutaneous leishmaniasis	As listed for Cutaneous Leishmaniasis	Amastigotes recovered in macrophages of skin and mucous membranes, or from animal inoculation of animals; other stages recovered in culture. PCR has also been used but is not routinely available in most laboratories.
Leishmania spp. (visceral)	Visceral leishmaniasis (kala azar)	Buffy coat Stain Culture Animal inoculation Bone marrow Stain Culture Animal inoculation Liver or spleen biopsy Routine histology Stain Culture Animal inoculation	Amastigotes recovered in cells of reticuloendothelial system. PCR has also been used but is not routinely available in most laboratories.
Toxoplasma gondii	Toxoplasmosis	Lymph node biopsy Routine histology Tissue culture isolation Animal inoculation Serology	Identification of organisms plus appropriate serologic test results.
Helminths			
Larvae (*Ascaris lumbricoides*, *Strongyloides stercoralis*)	"Pneumonia"	Sputum Wet examination Stained smear	This is an incidental finding but has been reported in severe infections, particularly in immunocompromised patients.
Eggs (*Paragonimus* spp.)	Paragonimiasis	Sputum Wet examination Routine stool exam	Eggs will be coughed up and will appear as "iron filings"; eggs could also be found in stool.
Hooklets (*Echinococcus*)	Hydatid disease	Sputum	Rare finding, but hooklets can be found when the hydatid cyst is in the lungs.

(*Continued on next page*)

TABLE 15 Examination of tissue and aspirated body fluids (*Continued*)

Parasite	Disease(s)[a]	Appropriate test(s)[a]	Positive result and additional information
Onchocerca volvulus *Mansonella streptocerca*	Onchocerciasis	Skin	Skin snips examined in saline; microfilariae may be present.
Schistosoma spp.	Schistosomiasis	Rectal valve biopsy Bladder biopsy Routine stool and urine examinations Hatching technique	Eggs present and identified. In any case of suspected schistosomiasis, spot urine samples, 24-h urine samples, and stool specimens should be submitted (all of which should be fresh—collected with no preservatives).

[a] EM, electron microscopy; FA, fluorescent antibody; GAE, granulomatous amebic encephalitis; GI, gastrointestinal; PAM, primary amebic meningoencephalitis; PAS, Periodic acid-Schiff stain.

crofilariae. The membrane filtration technique can also be used with urine for the recovery of microfilariae. A membrane filter technique for the recovery of *Schistosoma haematobium* eggs has also been useful (28).

Sputum

Although not one of the more common specimens for examination for parasites, expectorated sputum may be submitted. Organisms in sputum that may be detected and may cause pneumonia, pneumonitis, or Loeffler's syndrome include the migrating larval stages of *Ascaris lumbricoides*, *Strongyloides stercoralis*, and hookworm; the eggs of *Paragonimus westermani; Echinococcus granulosus* hooklets; the protozoa *Entamoeba histolytica*, *Entamoeba gingivalis*, *Trichomonas tenax*, *Cryptosporidium parvum*; and possibly the microsporidia. In a *Paragonimus* infection, the sputum may be viscous and tinged with brownish flecks, which are clusters of eggs ("iron filings"), and may be streaked with blood. Sputum is usually examined as a wet mount (saline or iodine), under low and high dry power (×100 and ×400) (28). The specimen is not concentrated before preparation of the wet mount. If the sputum is thick, an equal amount of 3% sodium hydroxide (NaOH) (or undiluted chlorine bleach) can be added; the specimen is thoroughly mixed and then centrifuged. NaOH should not be used if one is looking for *Entamoeba* spp. or *T. tenax*. After centrifugation, the supernatant fluid is discarded and the sediment can be examined as a wet mount with saline or iodine. If examination has to be delayed for any reason, the sputum should be fixed in 5 or 10% formalin to preserve helminth eggs or larvae or in polyvinyl alcohol fixative to be stained later for protozoa.

Aspirates

The examination of aspirated material for the diagnosis of parasitic infections may be extremely valuable, particularly when routine testing methods have failed to demonstrate organisms (Table 15) (28). These types of specimens should be transported to the laboratory immediately after collection. Aspirates include liquid specimens collected from a variety of sites where organisms might be found. Aspirates most commonly processed in the parasitology laboratory include fine-needle and duodenal aspirates. Fluid specimens collected by bronchoscopy include bronchoalveolar lavage fluid and bronchial washings.

Fine-needle aspirates may be submitted for slide preparation and/or culture. Aspirates of cysts and abscesses for amebae may require concentration by centrifugation, digestion, microscopic examination for motile organisms in direct preparations, and cultures and microscopic evaluation of stained preparations.

Bone marrow aspirates for *Leishmania* amastigotes, *Trypanosoma cruzi* amastigotes, or *Plasmodium* spp. require Giemsa staining. Examination of these specimens may confirm an infection that has been missed by examination of routine blood films (28, 78).

Biopsy Specimens

Biopsy specimens are recommended for the diagnosis of tissue parasites (Table 15). The following procedures may be used for this purpose in addition to standard histologic preparations: impression smears and teased and squash preparations of biopsy tissue from the skin, muscles, corneas, intestines, liver, lungs, and brain. Tissue to be examined by permanent sections or electron microscopy should be fixed as specified by the laboratories that will process the tissue. In certain cases, a biopsy specimen may be the only means of confirming a suspected parasitic infection. Specimens that are going to be examined as fresh material rather than as tissue sections should be kept moist in saline and submitted to the laboratory immediately.

Success in detection of parasites in tissue depends in part on specimen collection and having sufficient material to perform the recommended diagnostic procedures. Biopsy specimens are usually quite small and may not be representative of the diseased tissue. Multiple tissue samples will often improve the diagnostic results. To optimize the yield from any tissue specimen, all areas should be examined by as many procedures as possible. Tissues are obtained from invasive procedures, many of which are very expensive and lengthy; consequently, these specimens deserve the most comprehensive procedures possible.

Tissue submitted in a sterile container on a sterile sponge dampened with saline may be used for cultures of protozoa after mounts for direct examination or impression smears for staining have been prepared. If cultures for parasites are to be made, sterile slides should be used for smear and mount preparation.

Blood

Depending on the life cycle, a number of parasites may be recovered in a blood specimen, either whole blood, buffy coat preparations, or various types of concentrations (Table 13) (28, 44, 78). Although some organisms may be motile in fresh, whole blood, species identification will normally be accomplished from the examination of permanent stained blood films, both thick and thin. Blood films can be prepared from fresh, whole blood collected with no anticoagulants, anticoagulated blood, or sediment from the various concentration procedures. The recommended stain of choice is Giemsa stain; however, the parasites can also be seen on blood films stained with Wright's stain. Delafield's hematoxylin stain is often used to stain the microfilarial sheath, since in some cases Giemsa stain does not provide sufficient stain intensity to allow the differentiation of the microfilariae based on the presence or absence of the sheath.

Thin Blood Films

In any examination of thin blood films for parasitic organisms, the initial screen should be carried out with the low-power objective (10×) of a microscope (28, 44, 78). Microfilariae may be missed if the entire thin film is not examined. Microfilariae are rarely present in large numbers, and frequently only a few organisms occur in each thin-film preparation. Microfilariae are commonly found at the edges or the feathered end of the film because they are carried to these sites during the process of spreading the blood. The feathered end of the film, where the erythrocytes are drawn out into one single, distinctive layer of cells, should be examined for the presence of malaria parasites and trypanosomes. In these areas, the morphology and size of the infected erythrocytes are most clearly seen.

Depending on the training and experience of the microscopist, examination of the thin film usually takes 15 to 20 min (≥300 oil immersion fields) for the film at a magnification of ×1,000. Although some people use a 50× or 60× oil immersion objective to screen stained blood films, there is some concern that small parasites such as plasmodia, *Babesia* spp., or *Leishmania donovani* may be missed at this lower total magnification (×500 or ×600) compared with the ×1,000 total magnification obtained with the more traditional 100× oil immersion objective. Because people tend to scan blood films at different rates, it is important to examine a minimum number of fields. If something suspicious has been seen in the thick film, the number of fields examined on the film is often considerably more than 300. The request for blood film examination should always be considered a STAT procedure, with all reports (negative as well as positive) being reported by telephone to the physician as soon as possible. If the results are positive, appropriate governmental agencies (local, state, and federal) should be notified within a reasonable time frame in accordance with guidelines and laws.

Both malaria and *Babesia* infections have been missed with automated differential instruments, and therapy was delayed (28). These instruments are not designed to detect intracellular blood parasites, and the inability of the automated systems to discriminate between uninfected erythrocytes and those infected with parasites may pose serious diagnostic problems.

Thick Blood Films

In the preparation of a thick blood film, the greatest concentration of blood cells will be in the center of the film (28, 44, 78). The examination should be performed at low magnification to detect microfilariae more readily. Examination of a thick film usually requires 5 to 10 min (approximately 100 oil immersion fields). The search for malarial organisms and trypanosomes is best done under oil immersion (total magnification, ×1,000). Intact erythrocytes are frequently seen at the very periphery of the thick film; such cells, if infected, may prove useful in the diagnosis of malaria, since they may demonstrate the characteristic morphology necessary to identify the organisms to the species level.

Blood Stains

For accurate identification of blood parasites, a laboratory should develop proficiency in the use of at least one good staining method. It is better to select one method that will provide reproducible results than to use several on a hit-or-miss basis. Blood films should be stained as soon as possible, since prolonged storage may result in stain retention. Failure to stain positive malarial smears within a month may result in failure to demonstrate typical staining characteristics for individual species.

The most common stains are of two types. Wright's stain has the fixative in combination with the staining solution, so that both fixation and staining occur at the same time; therefore, the thick film must be laked before staining. Since the fixative and stain are separate in Giemsa stain, the thin film must be fixed with absolute methanol before being stained (28, 44, 60, 78).

Buffy Coat Films

L. donovani, trypanosomes, and *H. capsulatum* (a fungus with intracellular elements resembling those of *L. donovani*) are occasionally detected in the peripheral blood. The parasite or fungus will be found in the large mononuclear cells in the buffy coat (a layer of leukocytes resulting from centrifugation of whole citrated blood). The nuclear material will stain dark red-purple, and the cytoplasm will be light blue (*L. donovani*). *H. capsulatum* will appear as a large dot of nuclear material (dark red-purple) surrounded by a clear halo area. Trypanosomes in the peripheral blood will also concentrate with the buffy coat cells.

QBC Microhematocrit Centrifugation Method

Microhematocrit centrifugation with use of the QBC malaria tube (glass capillary tube and closely fitting plastic insert; CBC malaria blood tubes; Becton Dickinson, Tropical Disease Diagnostics, Sparks, Md.) has been used for the detection of blood parasites (28). At the end of centrifugation of 50 to 60 μl of capillary or venous blood (5 min in a QBC centrifuge at 14,387 × g), parasites or erythrocytes containing parasites are concentrated into a small, 1- to 2-mm region near the top of the erythrocyte column and are held close to the wall of the tube by the plastic float, thereby making them readily visible by microscopy. Tubes precoated with acridine orange provide a stain which induces fluorescence in the parasites. This method automatically prepares a concentrated smear, which represents the distance between the float and the walls of the tube. Once the tube is placed into the plastic holder (Paraviewer) and immersion oil is applied to the top of the hematocrit tube (no coverslip is necessary), the tube is examined with a 40× to 60× oil immersion objective (which must have a working distance of 0.3 mm or greater).

ParaSight F Test

A new *Plasmodium falciparum* antigen detection system, the ParaSight F test (Becton Dickinson), has been found to be very effective in field trials. This procedure is based on an antigen capture approach and has been incorporated in a dipstick format; the entire test takes approximately 10 min. Unfortunately, this kit is not yet available within the United States, but it has proven to be very useful in other parts of the world (28).

Knott Concentration

The Knott concentration procedure is used primarily to detect the presence of microfilariae in the blood, especially when a light infection is suspected (28, 44). The disadvantage of the procedure is that the microfilariae are killed by the formalin and are therefore not seen as motile organisms.

Membrane Filtration Technique

The membrane filtration technique involving Nuclepore filters has proved highly efficient in demonstrating filarial infections when microfilaremias are of low density. It has also been successfully used in field surveys (28, 44).

Culture Methods

Very few clinical laboratories offer specific culture techniques for parasites. The methods for in vitro culture are often complex, while quality control is difficult and not really feasible for the routine diagnostic laboratory (28, 44). In certain institutions, some techniques may be available, particularly where consultative services are provided and for research purposes (Table 16).

Few parasites can be routinely cultured, and the only procedures that are in general use are for *Entamoeba histolytica*, *Naegleria fowleri*, *Acanthamoeba* spp., *Trichomonas vaginalis*, *Toxoplasma gondii*, *Trypanosoma cruzi*, and the leishmanias. These procedures are usually available only on special request and after consultation with the laboratory.

Cultures of parasites grown in association with an unknown microbiota are referred to as xenic cultures. A good example of this type of culture would be stool specimens cultured for *E. histolytica*. If the parasites are grown with a single known bacterium, the culture is referred to as monoxenic. An example of this type of culture would be clinical specimens (corneal biopsy specimens) cultured with *Escherichia coli* as a means of recovering species of *Acanthamoeba* and *Naegleria*. If parasites are grown as pure culture without any bacterial associate, the culture is referred to as axenic. An example of this type of culture would be the use of media for the isolation of *Leishmania* spp. or *T. cruzi*.

Animal Inoculation and Xenodiagnosis

Most routine clinical laboratories do not have the animal care facilities necessary to provide animal inoculation capabilities for the diagnosis of parasitic infections. Host specificity for many animal parasite species is a well-known fact and will limit the types of animals available for these procedures. In certain suspect infections, animal inoculation may be requested and can be very helpful in making the diagnosis, although animal inoculation certainly does not take the place of other, more routine procedures (28).

Xenodiagnosis is a technique that uses the arthropod host as an indicator of infection. Uninfected reduviid bugs are allowed to feed on the blood of a patient who is suspected of having Chagas' disease (*T. cruzi* infection). After 30 to 60 days, feces from the bugs are examined over a 3-month time frame for the presence of developmental stages of the parasite, which are found in the hindgut of the vector. This type of procedure is used primarily in South America for field work, and the appropriate bugs are raised in various laboratories specifically for this purpose.

Antigen and Antibody Detection

Human parasites can be divided into two groups: (i) those that multiply within the host (e.g., protozoa) and (ii) those that mature within the host but never multiply (e.g., schistosomes and *Ascaris* spp.). Infections caused by protozoa that multiply within the host are similar to infections caused by bacterial, fungal, or viral organisms. There is continuous antigenic stimulation of the host immune system as the infection progresses. In these instances, there is usually a positive correlation between clinical symptoms and serologic test results.

Some helminths migrate through the body and pass through a number of developmental stages before becoming mature adults. With rare exceptions, these infections have been difficult to confirm serologically, possibly because of a limited antigenic response by the host or failure to use the appropriate antigen in the test system. Most antigens used in serologic procedures are heterogeneous mixtures that are not well defined. The use of such antigens may result in cross-reactions or inadequate sensitivity.

Even though parasites and their by-products are immunogenic for the host, the host immune response is usually not protective. Any immunity that does develop is usually species specific and even strain or stage specific.

Historically, diagnostic parasitology procedures have been based on the demonstration of the organisms (e.g., trophozoites, cysts, eggs, larvae, and adults) in tissue, body fluids, or fecal specimens. These procedures are very labor-intensive, require a skilled microscopist to identify the organisms, and have limited sensitivity. Alternative methods for the detection of infections have been investigated for years and include antibody, antigen, and nucleic acid detection. In many instances, serologic methods would be more practical, especially in cases in which invasive procedures must be used to obtain the specimen for diagnostic workup. However, even with the most sophisticated technology, few serologic tests for parasitic infections can be used to confirm an infection or predict the disease outcome. Interpretation of test results may also present problems, particularly when one is dealing with patients from areas of endemic infection, who may have higher baseline titers than do patients from other areas, in whom a low titer may actually be significant. Some titers may reflect exposure rather than actual disease.

Although serologic procedures have been available for many years, they are not routinely offered by most clinical laboratories for the reasons mentioned above (sensitivity, specificity, and interpretation). Standard techniques that have been used include complement fixation, indirect hemagglutination, indirect fluorescent antibody, soluble-antigen fluorescent antibody, bentonite flocculation, latex agglutination, double diffusion, counterelectrophoresis, immunoelectrophoresis, radioimmunoassay, and intradermal tests. An excellent review of these procedures, the rationale for their use, and their advantages and limitations is that by Wilson (126).

The CDC offers a number of serologic procedures for diagnostic purposes, some of which are not available elsewhere. Because regulations as to submission of specimens

TABLE 16 Parasites and appropriate culture media

Parasite	Quality control organism	Medium	Comments
Intestinal amebae	*E. histolytica* ATCC 30925 (HU-1; CDC), ATCC 30015 (HK-9), ATCC 30042 (Laredo strain, 25°C)	Balamuth's aqueous egg yolk infusion	May need to subculture to confirm positive culture; with rice flour, used to culture *B. coli*
		Boeck and Drbohlav's Locke-egg-serum (LES)	Sterile rice powder added before inoculation
		TY1-S-33 (*E. histolytica*)	Some lots of components may actually inhibit growth
		TYSGM-9 (*E. histolytica*)	Relatively complex
Free-living amebae	*A. castellanii* ATCC 30010 *N. fowleri* ATCC 30215	*Acanthamoeba* or *Naegleria*	Nonnutrient agar with bacterial overlay
		Balamuthia not recovered with this culture system	Nonnutrient agar with bacterial overlay
Flagellates			
Trichomonas vaginalis	*T. vaginalis* ATCC 30001	Lash's casein hydrolysate-serum pouch methods (collection and culture)	Specimen must not be refrigerated
		Cysteine-peptone-liver-maltose (CPLM)	Use as long as amber zone indicates an anaerobic condition persists
		Diamond's Trypticase-yeast extract-maltose	Has been used for many years
Blood and tissue flagellates			
Trypanosoma spp. *Leishmania* spp.	*L. mexicana* ATCC 30883, *T. cruzi* ATCC 30160	NNN (trypanosomes, leishmaniae)	Fresh, defibrinated rabbit blood best
		NNN (Offutt's) (leishmaniae)	
		Evan's modified Tobie's medium (leishmaniae, *T. cruzi*)	NaCl is in overlay, not agar; contains beef extract
		NIH (trypanosomes, leishmaniae)	Contains infused dry beef; overlay is Locke's solution
		NNNN (trypanosomes, leishmaniae)	Contains blood sugar base, Locke's overlay
		Yaeger's LIT (*T. cruzi*)	Contains hemin
		USAMRU blood agar (leishmaniae)	Useful for isolation of *L. braziliensis* complex
		Schneider's *Drosophila* medium; (liquid) (trypanosomes, leishmaniae)	30% (vol/vol) fetal calf serum; used for routine culture maintenance
Toxoplasma gondii		Tissue culture	Buffy coat cells, human foreskin fibroblast monolayers (tubes, shell vials)

may vary from state to state, each laboratory should check with its own county or state health department of public health for the appropriate instructions. Additional information on procedures, availability of skin test antigens, and interpretation of test results may be obtained directly from the CDC by contacting

Serology Unit Parasitology Diseases Branch
Building 4, Room 1009
Mail Stop F13
Centers for Disease Control and Prevention
4770 Buford Highway
Atlanta, GA 300341

Serology (770) 488-7760
Chagas' Disease and Leishmaniasis (770) 488-4474
Malaria (770) 488-7765.

Progress has been made in the development and application of molecular methods for diagnostic purposes including the use of purified or recombinant antigens and nucleic acid probes. The detection of parasite-specific antigen is more indicative of current disease. Many of the assays were originally developed with polyclonal antibodies which were targeted to unpurified antigens that markedly decreased the sensitivity and specificity of the tests. Immunoassays are generally simple to perform and allow a large number of tests to be performed at one time, thereby reducing overall costs. A major disadvantage of antigen detection in stool specimens is that the method can detect only one or two pathogens at one time. One still must perform a routine O&P to detect other parasitic pathogens. The current commercially available antigen tests (DFA, EIA, or indirect fluorescent antibody) have excellent sensitivity and specificity compared to routine microscopy.

Nucleic acid-based diagnostic tests for parasitology are primarily available only in specialized research or reference centers. PCR and other nucleic acid probe tests have been reported for almost all species of parasites. The only nucleic acid-based probe test commercially available is for the detection of *T. vaginalis*. As the costs of these tests decrease and the various steps necessary to perform the tests become automated, there will be increasing demand for commercially available reagents.

REFERENCES

1. **Allen, R. M., W. R. Dunn, and A. H. Limper.** 1994. Diagnosing ventilator-associated pneumonia: the role of bronchoscopy. *Mayo Clin. Proc.* **69:**962–968.
2. **Applebaum, P. D., S. F. Schick, and J. A. Kellogg.** 1980. Evaluation of four hour Micro-ID technique for direct identification of oxidase-negative, gram negative rods from blood cultures. *J. Clin. Microbiol.* **12:**533–537.
3. **Auckenthaler, R., D. M. Ilstrup, and J. A. Washington II.** 1982. Comparison of recovery of organisms from blood cultures diluted 10% (volume/volume) and 20% (volume/volume). *J. Clin Microbiol.* **15:**860–864.
4. **Bannatyne, R. M., M. C. Jackson, and S. Memish.** 1997. Rapid diagnosis of *Brucella* bacteremia by using the BACTEC 9240 system. *J. Clin. Microbiol.* **35:**2673–2674.
5. **Baselski, V. S., M. El-Torky, J. J. Coalson, and J. P. Griffin.** 1992. The standardization of criteria for processing and interpreting laboratory specimens in patients with suspected ventilator-associated pneumonia. *Chest* **102:** 571S–579S.
6. **Baumgartner, C., A. M. Freydiere, and Y. Gille.** 1996. Direct identification and recognition of yeast species from clinical material by using Albicans ID and CHROMagar Candida plates. *J. Clin. Microbiol.* **34:**454–456.
7. **Bhisitkul, D. M., A. E. Hogan, and R. R. Tanz.** 1994. The role of bacterial antigen detection tests in the diagnosis of bacterial meningitis. *Pediatr. Emerg. Care.* **10:** 67–71.
8. **Bisno, A. L., M. A., Gerber, J. M, Gwaltney, E. L., Kaplan, and R. H. Schwartz.** 1997. Diagnosis and management of group A streptococcal pharyngitis: a practice guideline. *Clin. Infect. Dis.* **25:**574–583.
9. **Blazevic, D. J., C. M. Trombley, and M. E. Lund.** 1976. Inoculation of API-20E from positive blood cultures. *J. Clin. Microbiol.* **4:**522–523.
10. **Brando, L. V. J.** 1995. Cell culture systems, p. 158–165. *In* P. R. Murray, E. J. Baron, M. A. Pfaller, F. C. Tenover, and R. H. Yolken (ed.), *Manual of Clinical Microbiology*, 6th ed. ASM Press, Washington, D.C.
11. **Bryan, F. L.** 1995. Procedures to use during outbreaks of food-borne disease. p. 209–226. In P. R. Murray E. J. Baron, M. A. Pfaller, F. C. Tenover, and R. H. Yolken (ed.), *Manual of Clinical Microbiology*, 6th ed. ASM Press, Washington, D.C.
12. **Carroll, K., and L. Reimer.** 1996. Microbiology and laboratory diagnosis of upper respiratory tract infections. *Clin. Infect. Dis.* **23:**4442–4448.
13. **Chang, F. T. J. E. Stout, and V. L. Yu.** 1996. Assessment of enzyme immunoassay versus radioimmunoassay for detection of *Legionella pneumophila* serogroup 1 antigen in frozen urine specimens. *J. Clin. Microbiol.* **34:**2628–2629.
14. **Chastre, J., J. Fagon, M. Bornet-Lecso, S. Calvat, M. Dombret, R. Al Khani, F. Basset, and C. Gilbert.** 1995. Evaluation of bronchoscopic techniques for the diagnosis of nosocomial pneumonia. *Am. J. Respir. Crit. Care Med.* **152:**231–240.
15. **Clark, S. M., J. R. Roth, M. L. Clark, B. B. Barnette, and R. S. Spendlove.** 1981. Trypsin enhancement of rotovirus infectivity: mechanisms of enhancement. *J. Virol.* **39:**816–822.
16. **Clarridge, J. E., and C. A. Spiegel.** 1995. *Corynebacterium* and miscellaneous irregular gram-positive rods, *Erysipelothrix*, and *Gardnerella*. p. 357–378. In. P. R. Murray, E. J. Baron, M. A. Pfaller, F. C. Tenover, and R. H. Yolken (ed.), *Manual of Clinical Microbiology*, 6th ed. ASM Press, Washington, D.C.
17. **Cockerill, F. R., G. S. Reed, J. G. Hughes, C. A. Torgerson, E. A. Vetter, W. S. Harmsen, J. C. Dale, G. D. Roberts, D. M. Ilstrup, and N. K. Henry.** 1997. Clinical comparison of BACTEC 9240 Plus Aerobic/F resin bottles and the ISOLATOR aerobic culture system for detection of bloodstream infections. *J. Clin. Microbiol.* **35:** 1469–1472.
18. **Cockerill, F. R., J. G. Hughes, E. A. Vetter, R. A. Mueller, A. L. Weaver, D. M. Ilstrup, J. E. Rosenblatt, and W. R. Wilson.** 1997. Analysis of 281,797 consecutive blood cultures performed over an eight-year period: trends in microorganisms isolated and the value of anaerobic culture of blood. *Clin. Infect. Dis.* **24:**403–418.
19. **Council of State and Territorial Epidemiologists.** 1993. CSTE Position Statement 4. *National Surveillance of* Escherichia coli *O157:H7*. Council of State and Territorial Epidemiologists, Atlanta, Ga.
20. **Dawson, M. S., A. M. Harford, B. K. Garner, D. A. Sica, D. M. Landwehr, and H. P. Dalton.** 1985. Total volume culture technique for the isolation of microorganisms from continuous ambulatory peritoneal dialysis patients with peritonitis. *J. Clin. Microbiol.* **22:**391–394.
21. **Dominguez, J. A., L. Matas, F. M. Manterola, R. Blavia,**

N. Sopena, F. J. Belda, E. Padilla, M. Gimenez, M. Sabria, J. Morera, and V. Ausina. 1997. Comparison of radioimmunoassay and enzyme immunoassay kits for detection of *Legionella pneumophila* serogroup 1 antigen in both concentrated and nonconcentrated urine samples. *J. Clin. Microbiol.* **35:**1627–1629.

22. **Dorsher, C. W., J. E. Rosenblatt, and W. R. Wilson.** 1990. Anaerobic bacteremia: decreasing rate over a 15 year period. *Rev. Infect. Dis.* **13:**633–636.
23. **Evans, G. L, T. Cekoric, and R. L. Searcy.** 1968. Comparative effects of anticoagulants on bacterial growth in experimental blood cultures. *Am. J. Med. Technol.* **34:** 103–112.
24. **Fisher, J. F., C. L. Newman, and J. D. Sobel.** 1995. Yeast in the urine: solutions for a budding problem. *Clin. Infect. Dis.* **20:**183–189.
25. **Food and Drug Administration.** 1997. *FDA Safety Alert: Risks of Devices for Direct Detection of Group B Streptococcal Antigen.* Food and Drug Administration, Rockville, Md.
26. **Foreman, K., J. Friborg, W. Kong, C. Woffendin, P. Polverini, B. Nickoloff, and G. Nabel.** 1997. Propagation of a human Herpesvirus from AIDS-associated Kaposi's sarcoma. *N. Engl. J. Med.* **363:**163–171.
27. **Forrer, C. B., A. L. Blahy, A. L. Malatico, J. M. Campos, and H. M. Friedman.** 1982. Comparison of vancomycin and penicillin for virus isolation. *J. Clin. Microbiol.* **16:** 295–298.
28. **Garcia, L. S., and D. A. Bruckner.** 1997. *Diagnostic Medical Parasitology,* 3rd ed. ASM Press, Washington, D.C.
29. **Gehanno, P., G. Lenoir, B. Barry, J. Bons, I. Boucot, and P. Berche.** 1996. Evaluation of nasopharyngeal cultures for bacteriologic assessment of acute otitis media in children. *Pediatr. Infect. Dis. J.* **15:**329–332.
30. **Gleaves, C., C. Lee, C. Bustamante, and J. Meyers.** 1988. Use of murine monoclonal antibodies for laboratory diagnosis of varicella-zoster virus infection. *J. Clin. Microbiol.* **26:**1623–1625.
31. **Granoff, D. M., T. V. Murphy, D. L. Ingram, and L. Cates.** 1986. Use of rapidly generated results in patient management. *Diagn Microbiol. Infect. Dis.* **4:**157S–166S.
32. **Hackman, B. A., J. F. Plouffe, R. F. Benson, B. S. Fields, and R. F. Breiman.** 1996. Comparison of Binax Legionella urinary antigen EIA kit with Binax RIA urinary antigen kit for detection of *Legionella pneumophila* serogroup 1 antigen. *J. Clin. Microbiol.* **34:**1579–1580.
33. **Harbeck, R. J., J. Teague, G. R. Crossen, D. M. Maul, and P. L. Childers.** 1993. Novel, rapid optical immunoassay technique for detection of group A streptococci from pharyngeal specimens: comparison with standard culture methods. *J. Clin. Microbiol.* **31:**839–844.
34. **Havlik, D., and G. L. Woods.** 1995. Screening sputum specimens submitted for mycobacterial culture. *Lab. Med.* **26:**411–413.
35. **Heelen, J. S., S. Wilbur, G. Depetris, and C. Letournou.** 1996. Rapid antigen testing for group A streptococcus by DNA probe. *Diagn. Microbiol. Infect. Dis.* **24:**65–69.
36. **Heiter, B. J., and P. P. Bourbeau.** 1993. Comparison of the Gen-Probe group A streptococcus direct test with culture and a rapid streptococcal antigen detection assay for diagnosis of streptococcal pharyngitis. *J. Clin. Microbiol.* **31:**2070–2073.
37. **Heiter, B. J., and P. P. Bourbeau.** 1995. Comparison of two rapid streptococcal antigen detection assays with culture for diagnosis of streptococcal pharyngitis. *J. Clin. Microbiol.* **33:**1408–1410.
38. **Henchal, E., and R. Putnak.** 1990. The dengue viruses. *Clin. Microbiol. Rev.* **3:**376–396.
39. **Hodinka, R.** 1997. Laboratory diagnosis of herpesvirus infections. *Semin. Pediatr. Infect. Dis.* **8:**178–187.
40. **Hospital Infection Control Practices Committee.** 1996. Guideline for isolation precautions in hospitals. II. Recommendations for isolation precautions in hospitals. *Am. J. Infect. Control* **24:**32–52.
41. **Howell, C., M. Miller, and W. Martin.** 1979. Comparison of rates of virus isolation from leukocyte populations separated from blood by conventional and Ficoll-plaque/Macrodex methods. *J. Clin. Microbiol.* **10:** 533–537.
42. **Hughes, J. H.** 1993. Physical and chemical methods for enhancing rapid detection of viruses and other agents. *Clin. Microbiol. Rev.* **6:**150–175.
43. **Ingram, J. G., and J. F. Plouffe.** 1994. Danger of sputum purulence screen in culture *Legionella* species. *J. Clin. Microbiol.* **32:**209.
44. **Isenberg, H. D. (ed.).** 1992. *Clinical Microbiology Procedures Handbook,* vol. 1 and 2. American Society for Microbiology, Washington, D.C.
45. **Johnson, B.** 1990. Transport of viral specimens. *Clin. Microbiol. Rev.* **3:**120–131.
46. **Jorgensen, J. H., S. Mirrett, L. C., McDonald, P. R. Murray, M. P. Weinstein, J. Fune, C. W. Trippy, M. Masterson, and L. B. Reller.** 1997. Controlled clinical laboratory comparison of BACTEC Plus Aerobic/F resin medium with BacT/Alert aerobic FAN medium for detection of bacteremia and fungemia. *J. Clin. Microbiol.* **35:** 53–58.
47. **Kass, E. H.** 1956. Asymptomatic infections of the urinary tract. *Trans. Assoc. Am. Physicians* **69:**56–63.
48. **Kaufmann, A. F., and R. S. Weyant.** 1995. *Leptospiraceae,* p. 621–625. *In* P. R. Murray, E. J. Baron, M. J. Pfaller, F. C. Tenover, and R. H. Yolken (ed.), *Manual of Clinical Microbiology,* 6th ed. ASM Press, Washington, D.C.
49. **Kazandjian, D., R. Chiew, and G. L. Gilbert.** 1997. Rapid diagnosis of *Legionella pneumophila* serogroup 1 infection with the Binax enzyme immunoassay urinary antigen test. *J. Clin. Microbiol.* **35:**954–956.
50. **Kellog, J. A.** 1990. Suitability of throat culture procedures for detection of group A streptococci and as reference standards for evaluation of streptococcal antigen detection kits. *J. Clin. Microbiol.* **28:**165–169.
51. **Kellog, J. A., F. L. Ferrentino, J. Liss, S. L. Shapiro, and D. A. Bankert.** 1994. Justification and implementation of a policy requiring two blood cultures when one is ordered. *Lab. Med.* **25:**323–330.
52. **Kiska, D. L., M. C. Jones, M. E. Mangum, D. Orkiszewski, and P. H. Gilligan.** 1995. Quality assurance study of bacterial antigen testing of cerebrospinal fluid. *J. Clin. Microbiol.* **33:**1141–1144.
53. **Landry, M. L., D. Ferguson, S. Cohen, K. Huber, and P. Wetherill.** 1995. Effect of delayed specimen processing on cytomegalovirus antigenemia test results. *J. Clin. Microbiol.* **33:**257–259.
54. **Lennette, D. A.** 1995. Collection and preparation of specimens for virology examination, p. 868–875. *In* P. R. Murray, E. J. Baron, M. A. Pfaller, F. C. Tenover, and R. H. Yolken (ed.), *Manual of Clinical Microbiology,* 6th ed. ASM Press, Washington, D.C.
55. **Li, J., J. J. Plorde, and L. G. Carlson.** 1994. Effects of volume and periodicity on blood cultures. *J. Clin. Microbiol.* **32:**2829–2831.
56. **Lombardi, D. P., and N. C. Engleberg.** 1992. Anaerobic bacteremia: incidence, patient characteristics, and clinical significance. *Am. J. Med.* **92:**53–60.
57. **Lyerly, D. M., and T. D. Wilkins.** 1986. Commercial latex test for *Clostridium difficile* toxin A does not detect toxin A. *J. Clin. Microbiol.* **23:**622–623.
58. **Lyon, R., and G. Woods.** 1995. Comparison of the

BacT/Alert and ISOLATOR blood culture systems for recovery of fungi. *Am. J. Clin. Pathol.* **103:**660–662.

59. **Maki, D. G., C. E. Weise, and H. W. Sarafin.** 1977. A semiquantitative culture method for identifying intravenous-catheter-related infection. *N. Engl. J. Med.* **296:** 1305–1309.
60. **Markell, E. K., M. Voge, and D. T. John.** 1992. *Medical Parasitology*, 7th ed. The W. B. Saunders Co., Philadelphia, Pa.
61. **Marshall, W. F., A. Telenti, J. Proper, A. J., Aksamit, and T. F. Smith.** 1990. Rapid detection of polyomavirus BK by a shell vial cell culture assay. *J. Clin. Microbiol.* **28:**1613–1615.
62. **Maxson, S., M. J. Lewno, and G. E. Schutze.** 1994. Clinical usefulness of cerebrospinal fluid bacterial antigen studies. *J. Pediatr.* **125:**235–238.
63. **McDonald, C. L., and K. Chapin.** 1995. Rapid identification of *Staphylococcus aureus* from blood culture bottles by a classic 2-hour tube coagulase test. *J. Clin. Microbiol.* **33:**50–52.
64. **McManus, A. T., S. H. Kim, W. F. McManus, A. D. Mason, and B. A. Pruitt.** 1987. Comparison of quantitative microbiology and histopathology in divided burn-wound biopsy specimens. *Arch. Surg.* **122:**74–76.
65. **Meduri, G. U., and J. Chastre.** 1992. The standardization of bronchoscopic techniques for ventilator-associated pneumonia. *Infect. Control Hosp. Epidemiol.* **13:**640–649.
66. **Melvin, D. M., and M. M. Brooke.** 1985. *Laboratory Procedures for the Diagnosis of Intestinal Parasites*, p. 163–189. U.S. Department of Health, Education, and Welfare publication. (CDC) 85-8282. U.S. Government Printing Office, Washington, D.C.
67. **Mermel, L. A., and D. G. Maki.** 1993. Detection of bacteremia in adults: consequences of culturing an inadequate volume of blood. *Ann. Intern. Med.* **119:**270–272.
68. **Messer, J. W., T. F. Midura, and J. T. Peeler.** 1993. Sampling plans, sample collection, shipment, and preparation for analysis, p. 25–49 *In* C. Vanderzaant and D. Splittstoesser (ed.), *Compendium of Methods for the Microbiological Examination of Foods*, 3rd ed. American Public Health Association, Washington, D.C.
69. **Miles, B. L., J. A. Siders, and S. D. Allen.** 1988. Evaluation of a commercial latex test for *Clostridium difficile* for reactivity with *C. difficile* and cross-reactions with other bacteria. *J. Clin. Microbiol.* **26:**2452–2455.
70. **Miller, S.** 1988. Diagnostic virology by electron microscopy. *ASM News* **54:**475–485.
71. **Minnich, L., T. Smith, and C. Ray.** 1988. *Cumitech 24, Rapid Detection of Viruses by Immunofluorescence*. Coordinating ed., S. Spector. American Society for Microbiology, Washington, D.C.
72. **Morin, S., J. Tetrault, L. James, J. E. Hoppe-Bauer, and M. Pezzlo.** 1992. Specimen acceptability: evaluation of specimen quality, p. 1.3.1–1.3.6. *In* H. D. Isenberg (ed.), *Clinical Microbiology Procedures Handbook*. American Society for Microbiology, Washington, D.C.
73. **Morris, A. J., S. J. Wilson, C. E. Marx, M. L. Wilson, S. Mirrett, and L. B. Reller.** 1995. Clinical impact of bacteria and fungi recovered only from broth cultures. *J. Clin. Microbiol.* **33:**161–165.
74. **Morris, A. J., L. K. Smith, S. Mirrett, and L. B. Reller.** 1996. Cost and time savings following introduction of rejection criteria for clinical specimens. *J. Clin. Microbiol.* **34:**355–357.
75. **Murray, P. R., and J. E. Sondag.** 1978. Evaluation of routine subcultures of macroscopically negative blood cultures for detection of anaerobes. *J. Clin. Microbiol.* **8:** 427–430.
76. **Murray, P. R., P. Traynor, and H. Hopson.** 1992. Critical assessment of blood culture techniques: analysis of recovery of obligate and facultative anaerobes, strict aerobic bacteria, and fungi in aerobic and anaerobic blood culture bottles. *J. Clin. Microbiol.* **30:**1462–1468.
77. **National Committee for Clinical Laboratory Standards.** 1993. *Procedures for the Recovery and Identification of Parasites from the Intestinal Tract*. Approved guideline M28-A. National Committee for Clinical Laboratory Standards, Villanova, Pa.
78. **National Committee for Clinical Laboratory Standards.** 1990. *Use of Blood Film Examination of Parasites*. Tentative guideline M15-T. National Committee for Clinical Laboratory Standards, Villanova, Pa.
79. **Nugent, R. P., M. A. Krohn, and S. L. Hillier.** 1991. Reliability of diagnosing bacterial vaginosis is improved by a standardized method of Gram stain interpretation. *J. Clin. Microbiol.* **29:**297–301.
80. **Odds, F. C., and R. Bernearts.** 1994. CHROMagar Candida, a new differential isolation medium for presumptive identification of clinically important *Candida* species. *J. Clin. Microbiol.* **32:**1923–1929.
81. **Paisley, J. W., J. E. Rosenblatt, M. Hall, and J. A. Washington.** 1978. Evaluation of a routine anaerobic subculture of blood cultures for detection of anaerobic bacteremia. *J. Clin. Microbiol.* **8:**764–766.
82. **Paisley, J. W., and B. A. Lauer.** 1994. Pediatric blood cultures. *Clin. Lab. Med.* **14:**17–30.
83. **Paya, C. V., A. D. Wold, and T. S. Smith.** 1988. Detection of cytomegalovirus from blood leukocytes separated by Separecell-MN and Ficoll-paque/Macrodex methods. *J. Clin. Microbiol.* **26:**2031–2033.
84. **Payne, C., C. G. Ray, V. Borduin, L. Minnich, and M. Lebowitz.** 1986. An eight-year study of the viral agents of acute gastroenteritis in humans: ultrastructural observations and seasonal distribution with a major emphasis on coronavirus-like particles. *Diagn. Microbiol. Infect. Dis.* **5:**39–54.
85. **Perkins, J. D., S. Mirrett, and L. B. Reller.** 1995. Rapid bacterial antigen detection is not clinically useful. *J. Clin. Microbiol.* **33:**1486–1491.
86. **Persing, D. H., T. F. Smith, F. C. Tenover, and T. J. White (ed.).** 1993. *Diagnostic Molecular Microbiology: Principles and Applications*, p. 309–414. American Society for Microbiology, Washington, D.C.
87. **Pezzlo, M.** 1988. Detection of urinary tract infections by rapid methods. *Clin. Microbiol. Rev.* **1:**268–280.
88. **Pezzlo, M. T., V. Ige, A. P. Woolard, E. M. Peterson, and L. M. de la Maza.** 1989. Rapid bioluminescence method for bacteriuria screening. *J. Clin. Microbiol.* **27:** 716–720.
89. **Pfaller, M. A., A. Houston, and S. Coffmann.** 1996. Application of CHROMagar Candida for rapid screening of clinical specimens for *Candida albicans*, *Candida tropicalis*, *Candida krusei*, and *Candida (Torulopsis) glabrata*. *J. Clin. Microbiol.* **34:**58–61.
90. **Prather, S., J. Jenista, and M. Menegus.** 1984. The isolation of nonpolio enteroviruses from serum. *Diagn. Microbiol. Infect. Dis.* **2:**353–357.
91. **Prevost-Smith, E., and N. Hutton.** 1994. Improved detection of *Cryptococcus neoformans* in the BACTEC NR 660 blood culture system. *Am. J. Clin. Pathol.* **102:** 741–745.
92. **Read, S., K. Jeffery, and M. Bangham.** 1997. Aseptic meningitis and encephalitis: the role of PCR in the diagnostic laboratory. *J. Clin. Microbiol.* **35:**691–696.
93. **Reimer, L. G.** 1994. Catheter-related infections and blood cultures. *Clin. Lab. Med.* **14:**51–58.
94. **Reimer, L. G., M. L. Wilson, and M. P. Weinstein.** 1997.

Update on detection of bacteremia and fungemia. *Clin. Microbiol. Rev.* **10:**444–465.
95. **Rohner, P., D. Pittet, B. Pepey, T. Nije-Kinge, and R. Auckenthaler.** 1997. Etiological agents of infectious diarrhea: implications for requests for microbial culture. *J. Clin. Microbiol.* **35:**1427–1432.
96. **Rosett, W., and G. R. Hodges.** 1980. Antimicrobial activity of heparin. *J. Clin. Microbiol.* **11:**30–34.
97. **Salkin, I. F., A. A. Padhye, and M. E. Kemna.** 1997. A new medium for the presumptive identification of dermatophytes. *J. Clin. Microbiol.* **35:**2660–2662.
98. **Salventi, J. F., T. A. Davies, E. L. Randall, S. Whitaker, and J. R. Waters.** 1979. Effect of blood dilution on recovery of organisms from clinical blood cultures in medium containing sodium polyanethol sulfonate. *J. Clin. Microbiol.* **9:**248–252.
99. **Sanchez-Nieto, J. M., and A. C. Alcaraz.** 1995. The role of bronchoalveolar lavage in the diagnosis of bacterial pneumonia. *Eur. J. Clin. Microbiol. Infect. Dis.* **14:** 839–850.
100. **Schifman, R. B., and K. J. Ryan.** 1982. Rapid automated identification of gram-negative bacilli from blood cultures with the AutoMicrobic system. *J. Clin. Microbiol.* **15:** 260–264.
101. **Schuchat, A., C. Whitney, and K. Zangwill.** 1996. Prevention of perinatal group B streptococcal disease: a public health perspective. *Morbid. Mortal. Weekly Rep.* **45:** RR-7:1–24.
102. **Schuchat, A., K. Robinson, J. D. Wenger, L. H. Harrison, M. Farley, A. L. Reingold, L. Lefkowitz, and B. A. Perkins.** 1997. Bacterial meningitis in the United States in 1995. *N. Engl. J. Med.* **337:**970–976.
103. **Seigman-Igra, Y., A. M. Anglim, D. E. Shapiro, K. A. Adal, B. A. Strain, and B. M. Farr.** 1997. Diagnosis of vascular catheter-related bloodstream infection: a meta-analysis. *J. Clin. Microbiol.* **35:**928–936.
104. **Shaw, K. N., and K. L. McGowan.** 1997. Evaluation of a rapid screening filter test for urinary tract infection in children. *Pediatr. Infect. Dis. J.* **16:**283–287.
105. **Shuster, E., J. Beneke, G. Tegtmeier, G. Pearson, C. Gleaves, A. Wold, and T. Smith.** 1985. Monoclonal antibody for rapid laboratory detection of cytomegalovirus infections: characterization and diagnostic application. *Mayo Clin. Proc.* **60:**577–585.
106. **Silletti, R. P., E. Ailey, S. Sun, and D. Tang.** 1997. Microbiologic and clinical value of primary broth cultures of wound specimens collected with swabs. *J. Clin. Microbiol.* **35:**2003–2006.
107. **Singh, N., and D. R. Carrigan.** 1996. Human herpesvirus 6 in transplantation: an emerging pathogen. *Ann. Intern. Med.* **124:**1065–1071.
108. **Slifkin, M., and R. Cumbie.** 1992. Comparison of the Histopaque-1119 method with the Plasmagel method for separation of blood leukocytes for cytomegalovirus isolation. *J. Clin. Microbiol.* **30:**2722–2724.
109. **Spendlove, R. S., M. E. McClain, and E. H. Lennette.** 1970. Enhancement of reovirus infectivity by extracellular removal or alterations of the virus capsid by proteolytic enzymes. *J. Gen. Virol.* **8:**83–94.
110. **Stabell, E. C., S. R. O'Rourke, G. A. Storch, and P. D. Olivo.** 1993. Evaluation of a genetically engineered cell line and a histochemical B-galactosidase assay to detect herpes simplex virus in clinical specimens. *J. Clin. Microbiol.* **31:**2796–2798.
111. **Stamm, W. E, G. W. Counts, K. R. Running S. Fihn, M. Turck, and K. K. Holmes.** 1982. Diagnosis of coliform infection in acutely dysuric women. *N. Engl. J. Med.* **307:** 463–468.
112. **Strain, B.** 1992. Quantitative bacteriology: tissues and aspirates, p. 1.16a.1–16a.4. *In* H. D. Isenberg (ed.), *Clinical Microbiology Procedures Handbook*. American Society for Microbiology, Washington, D.C.
113. **Sturgis, C. D., L. R. Peterson, and J. R. Warren.** 1997. Cerebrospinal fluid broth culture isolates, their significance for antibiotic treatment. *Am J. Clin. Pathol.* **108:** 217–221.
114. **Szymszak, E. G., J. T. Barr, W. A. Durbin, and D. A. Goldmann.** 1979. Evaluation of blood culture procedures in a pediatric hospital. *J. Clin. Microbiol.* **9:**88–92.
115. **Thomas, J. G.** 1994. Routine CSF antigen detection for agents associated with bacterial meningitis: another point of view. *Clin. Microbiol. Newsl.* **16:**89–95.
116. **Thomson, R. B.** 1994. Laboratory methods in basic virology, p. 655–677. *In* E. J. Baron, L. R. Peterson, and S. M. Finegold (ed.), *Bailey and Scott's Diagnostic Microbiology*. Mosby-Year Book, Inc., St. Louis, Mo.
117. **Tobita, K., A. Sugiura, C. Enomoto, and M. Furuyama.** 1975. Plaque assay and primary isolation of influenza A viruses in an established line of canine kidney cells (MDCK) in the presence of trypsin. *Med. Microbiol. Immunol.* **162:**9–14.
118. **U.S. Department of Health and Human Services.** 1988. Management of patients with suspected viral hemorrhagic fever. *Morbid Mortal. Weekly Rep.* **37**(no. S-3).
119. **Ward, K. W.** 1992. Processing and interpretation of specimens for *Legionella* spp. 1. *Legionella* specimen processing, p. 1.12.1–1.12.8. *In* H. D. Isenberg (ed.), *Clinical Microbiology Procedures Handbook*. American Society for Microbiology, Washington, D.C.
120. **Washington, J. A. II.** 1975. Blood cultures: principles and techniques. *Mayo Clin. Proc.* **50:**91–98.
121. **Wegner, D. L., D. L Witte, and R. D. Schrantz.** 1992. Insensitivity of rapid antigen detection methods and single blood agar plate culture for diagnosing streptococcal pharyngitis. *JAMA* **267:**695–697.
122. **Weinstein, M. P., L. B. Reller, J. R. Murphy, and K. A. Lichtenstein.** 1983. The clinical significance of positive blood cultures: a comprehensive analysis of 500 episodes of bacteremia and fungemia in adults. I. Laboratory and epidemiologic observations. *Rev. Infect. Dis.* **5:**35–53.
123. **Weinstein, M. P.** 1996. Current blood culture methods and systems: clinical concepts, technology and interpretation of results. *Clin. Infect. Dis.* **23:**40–46.
124. **Wiley, L., D. Springer, R. Kowalski, R. Arffa, M. Roat, R. Thoft, and J. Gordon.** 1988. Rapid diagnostic test for ocular adenovirus. *Ophthalmology* **95:**431–433.
125. **Wilson, M., P. Schantz, and N. Pieniazek.** 1995. Diagnosis of parasitic infections: immunologic and molecular methods, p. 1159–1170. *In* P. R. Murray, E. J. Baron, M. A. Pfaller, F. C. Tenover, and R. H. Yolken (ed.), *Manual of Clinical Microbiology*, 6th ed. ASM Press, Washington, D.C.
126. **Wilson, M. L., and M. P. Weinstein.** 1994. General principles in the laboratory detection of bacteremia and fungemia. *Clin. Lab. Med.* **14:**69–82.
127. **Wilson, M. L.** 1996. Continuously monitoring blood culture systems: an update. ASCP Check Sample **39:** 129–144.
128. **Woods, G. L., and M. R. Profitt.** 1987. Comparison of Plasmagel with LeucoPREP Macrodex methods for separation of leukocytes for virus isolation. *Diagn. Microbiol. Infect. Dis.* **8:**123–126.
129. **Woods, G. L.** 1996. Specimen collection and handling for diagnosis of infectious diseases, p. 1311–1331. *In* J. B. Henry (ed.), *Clinical Diagnosis and Management by Laboratory Methods*, 19th ed. The W. B. Saunders Co., Philadelphia, Pa.
130. **Woolfrey, B. F., J. M. Fox, and C. O. Quall.** 1981. An evaluation of burn wound quantitative microbiology. I.

Quantitative eschar cultures. *Am. J. Clin. Pathol.* **75:** 532–537.

131. **Yagupsky, P., and M. A. Menegus.** 1990. Cumulative positivity rates of multiple blood cultures for *Mycobacterium avium-intracellulare* and *Cryptococcus neoformans* in patients with the acquired immunodeficiency syndrome. *Arch. Pathol. Lab. Med.* **114:**923–925.
132. **Yagupsky, P., N. Peled, J. Press, O. Abramson, and M. Abu-rashid.** 1997. Comparison of BACTEC 9240 peds plus medium and Isolator 1.5 microbial tube for detection of *Brucella melitensis* from blood cultures. *J. Clin. Microbiol.* **35:**1382–1384.
133. **Zaki, S., P. Greer, L. Coffield, C. Goldsmith, K. Nolte, K. Foucar, R. Feddersen, R. Zumwalt, G. Miller, A. Khan, P. Rollin, T. Ksiazek, S. Nichol, B. Mahy, and C. Peters.** 1995. Hantavirus pulmonary syndrome pathogenesis of an emerging infectious disease. *Am. J. Pathol.* **146:**552–571.

THE CLINICAL MICROBIOLOGY LABORATORY IN INFECTION CONTROL AND PREVENTION

II

VOLUME EDITOR
MICHAEL A. PFALLER

SECTION EDITOR
RICHARD P. WENZEL

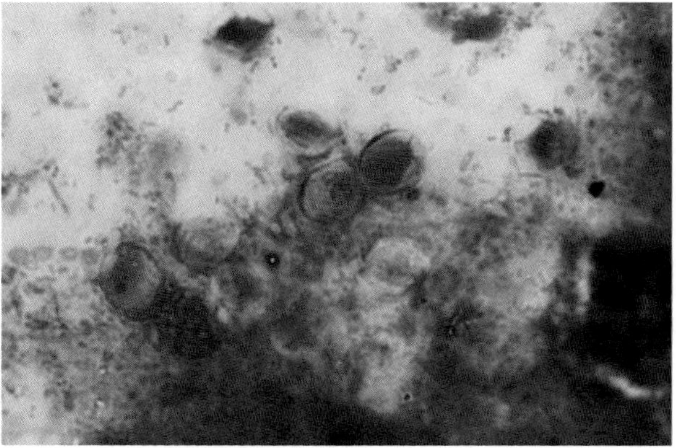

Cyclospora cayetanensis isolated in foodborne outbreak. Acid-fast stain.

Infection Control Epidemiology and Clinical Microbiology

JOHN E. McGOWAN, JR., AND BEVERLY G. METCHOCK

6

Nosocomial infections (those acquired in a hospital or other health care facility) remain an important problem today. Dealing effectively with such infections in a health care institution (HCI) requires the identification of cases and their etiology, comparison of current attack rates of infection with usual baselines, characterization of epidemiologic features of the infections, development and implementation of control measures, and continuing follow-up surveillance to determine the success of the control measures. The microbiology laboratory has important responsibilities related to each step in this process. This chapter describes some of the basic epidemiologic concepts underlying the control of both epidemic and endemic nosocomial infections and the relationship of these to the microbiology laboratory. Table 1 provides relevant definitions.

INFECTION CONTROL EPIDEMIOLOGY AND ITS METHODS

Epidemiology is the study of the occurrence, distribution, and determinants of disease (or health) in a specific human population (8). Hospital epidemiology involves the study of these three features in patients at an HCI. A specific aspect of hospital epidemiology concerns nosocomial infections and their determinants. By describing and defining occurrences of nosocomial infections and identifying reservoirs and sources, routes of transmission, likely victims, and associated factors, an infection control epidemiologist can develop procedures for the control and prevention of these infections (18).

Nosocomial infections are those which develop within an HCI or are produced by organisms acquired during a stay in such a facility. Such infections may involve health care workers and visitors as well as patients (12, 28).

EPIDEMIC VERSUS ENDEMIC OCCURRENCE

Infection control epidemiology focuses both on the epidemic occurrence of nosocomial infections and on baseline, or endemic, levels of disease in an attempt to minimize the occurrence of each. Epidemics or outbreaks of infection are a major focus of concern for infection control programs. The need for HCI infection control programs arose from staphylococcal epidemics from 1950 to 1970, and outbreaks still justify infection control efforts today.

Infections that occur as part of an epidemic often are amenable to control measures, so all clusters of infection should be considered within the scope of infection control activities (2). What defines an HCI outbreak (epidemic)? Many answers have been proposed, but one with general applicability defines an HCI outbreak as the occurrence of a larger-than-expected number of cases of a specific infection acquired in an institution (2). Usually, the cases occur in a brief interval and involve a specific patient population. By this definition, the baseline rate of occurrence of infections determines the presence or absence of an outbreak.

Classically, sharp and unexpected increases in the number of cases make recognition easy (13). However, this is not always the case. For example, even one case of infection due to a strain of *Staphylococcus aureus* with reduced susceptibility to vancomycin is of importance, because no such strains had been reported until 1997 (4). Thus, one case of infection due to a vancomycin-resistant *S. aureus* strain may well be defined as an outbreak. On the other hand, several cases of nosocomial infections due to *Escherichia coli* may not be considered an outbreak if the isolates all have the susceptibility pattern and biochemical reactions characteristic of most strains found in the HCI and if cases of infection due to this organism are encountered frequently at the institution. In addition, increasing infection occurrence may represent changes in the number of patients being cared for at an HCI or changes in the patient population that reflect changes in average host susceptibility. Thus, not every cluster of cases represents an outbreak. When outbreaks occur, the organisms associated with them vary greatly from location to location. For example, outbreaks in larger hospitals may be "uncharacteristic" of epidemic organisms in small community hospitals (9).

Outbreaks are not frequent occurrences in HCIs in the United States at this time (2). Equally important and occupying much of the attention of hospital epidemiologists is attempting to minimize baseline, usual, or endemic nosocomial infections. Endemic infections constitute the majority of preventable nosocomial infections (6). Most infection prevention techniques rely on controlling exogenous spread from one person or environmental source to a susceptible patient. Nosocomial infections remain unavoidable when they arise from the patient's endogenous flora, so total prevention of such infections still is an unattainable goal. Nevertheless, many can be prevented, and the focus of a

TABLE 1 Definitions

Terms	Definition
Case-control study	Study in which a group of patients who have an outcome of interest (in this case, nosocomial infection) is compared with a control (comparison) group of patients who do not have the attribute; the proportions of patients with given characteristics (attributes or exposures) of interest in the two groups are compared in order to identify differences that might suggest why infection occurred
Cohort study	Study in which subjects are classified as to the presence or absence of some item of interest (exposure), and then members of both groups (those with and those without the feature) are monitored during their HCI stay to determine which develop the outcome of interest (in this case, nosocomial infection); the aim is to identify exposures that vary between subjects developing and those remaining free of nosocomial infection to help identify associated factors that might suggest why infection occurred
HCI	Facility that is part of an integrated health care system, such as an acute-care hospital, extended-care facility, ambulatory surgical center, or ambulatory care clinic
Incidence rate	Ratio of the number of new cases of an entity (in this case, nosocomial infection) occurring in a specified population at risk of infection in a defined time period (the numerator) to the number of persons in the population at risk (the denominator)
Interventional study	Study in which the investigators assign the exposure of given study participants to the subject of interest (usually an intervention or procedure); monitoring of patient clinical courses to identify the occurrence of the end point of interest (in this case, infection) in each group then allows an inference to be made about the value of the exposure
Nosocomial infection	Infection that was not present or incubating at the time of admission to a health care facility or, more broadly, infection acquired during an interaction in a hospital or other health care facility
Observational study	Study that reviews and monitors the natural course of events without intervening in the process
Prevalence rate	Total number of cases of nosocomial infection in the defined population at risk at one point in time (point prevalence) or in a given interval (period prevalence)
Reservoir	Place in which an organism maintains its presence in the setting of interest (in this case, the health care system or hospital)
Source	Place from which the infectious agent directly contacts its victim

hospital infection control program should be the identification of preventable infections, determination of why they occur, and minimization of their occurrence (6). The study of endemic infections by epidemiologic techniques discussed below provides the means to identify control and prevention measures that can have a measurable impact.

STEPS IN EPIDEMIOLOGIC EVALUATION

The fundamental approach to dealing with an HCI problem of nosocomial infection, whether epidemic or endemic, involves several steps and phases. The laboratory has a role in virtually all of these activities (Table 2). Seven steps are considered (2, 16–18).

Problem Recognition

The initial step of realizing that a problem exists and defining its features perhaps is the most important action to be taken. Infection control personnel may become aware of the problem through their contact with and surveillance of clinical services. On occasion, however, the laboratory, a follow-up clinic, or even another HCI in the area provides the first report. When a question arises about an endemic cross-infection problem or when an outbreak is clearly occurring, the investigators must begin by establishing a definition of a case. Even a rough case definition will allow initial control measures to be taken, ensure that all persons involved agree on the nature of the problem, and help the laboratory to begin examining microbiologic aspects. This step will prevent problems such as an investigation of presumed staphylococcal toxic shock syndrome that turns out to be streptococcal scarlet fever, or vice versa. It will also allow personnel to confirm that they are dealing with potentially preventable infections rather than wasting time and effort characterizing issues that cannot be changed (2).

Certain situations or types of infection are so dramatic or uncommon that even a single case may be recognized as a problem requiring immediate attention. For example, group A streptococcal infections in surgical or obstetric patients are rare enough at this time that the occurrence of one such case would almost surely trigger an investigation by an infection control team.

Case Finding and Surveillance

Once a case definition has been made, attempts to identify all possible cases can begin. This effort at complete case finding is crucial because the more cases that are available for analysis, the better the chance of determining the process involved. Case finding has three major aspects.

TABLE 2 Steps in investigating an HCI outbreak and the role of the laboratory in each step[a]

Investigative step	Laboratory participation
1. Recognize the problem. a. Case definition b. Verification of clinical entity	1. Laboratory should be a surveillance and early-warning system. a. Microbiologic confirmation
2. Complete case finding. a. Reliability of reporting b. Completeness of reporting c. Obtain additional data	2. Characterize isolates accurately and store isolates. a. Search database for other cases and review laboratory methods b. Review and validate demographics c. Perform new testing as needed
3. Is this unusual? a. Calculate attack rate b. Compare with baseline rates c. Epidemic = higher-than-usual rate	3. Provide archival data on occurrence.
4. Characterize the outbreak. a. Patient demography b. Location c. Time	4. Is this one strain or many? a. Type isolates if necessary (see chapter 7)
5. Form hypotheses about causes. a. Modes of spread b. Reservoirs c. Vectors	5. Do supplementary studies as needed in: a. Personnel or patients b. Environment c. Other problem-focused testing
6. Initiate control measures.	6. Initiate laboratory procedural changes if needed.
7. Do follow-up surveillance to ensure that control measures are effective.	7. Maintain laboratory as a surveillance and early-warning system.

[a] Adapted in part from references 2, 16, 17, and 18.

Reliability

The first activity is ascertaining the reliability of both clinical and laboratory information. Can the clinical staff identify a case of the entity under investigation? Does the laboratory have experience in recognizing the microbiologic entity being considered? This is the stage at which "pseudo-outbreaks" or "pseudoproblems" (see below) need to be weeded out.

Universality

Next, the completeness of the reporting of cases must be considered (2). Most nosocomial infections manifest themselves while the afflicted patient is still in the HCI. Some appear only after the patient has been discharged. For example, studies have shown that one-half or more of all surgical wound infections are manifested after the patient has left the hospital (25). Conversely, some infections with an onset during the patient's stay at the institution were acquired in the community and were incubating during the period after admission. In addition, laboratory records may not include basic demographic information needed to identify a problem. Thus, laboratory data alone cannot be used to identify nosocomial infections; surveillance programs must use other sources of data as well. In investigations of outbreaks or changes in patterns of endemic infection, new systematic and rigorously applied surveillance may be needed to recognize subtle but important changes in patterns of infection, especially when polymicrobial etiology is present (2). Later, personnel must decide whether the surveillance steps that were added should be discontinued or continued to recognize future episodes earlier.

Information Collected

When an intense search for all cases is completed, the completeness of the information obtained about each case must be reviewed. For example, infections with an onset during an HCI stay sometimes have been acquired in the community and have been incubating during the period since HCI admission. Thus, not all infections with an onset during an HCI stay are nosocomial. This fact is a major reason why laboratory data alone cannot be used to define nosocomial infections and why surveillance programs for these infections must draw on other sources of data as well. Likewise, laboratory records may lack basic demographic information. For example, at Grady Memorial Hospital, our laboratory requisition records the ward on which the inpatient is found but not the clinical service of the patient. Thus, our laboratory would be unlikely to recognize a service-specific outbreak or endemic infection problem. Likewise, it may be important to trace a patient's travels in the hospital (initial room at admission, location at which the specimen was collected, location of the patient when the report on the specimen was issued, and so forth). Many laboratory information systems are unable to do this. Unless such tracking is appreciated through a comparison of rates at the instituion with benchmark rates from other sites, an outbreak or infection control problem may not be recognized. National and other surveillance programs provide in the medical literature on a periodic basis data that can be used for such benchmark procedures (3).

Defining Occurrence

When as many cases as possible have been identified, the question of whether an episode meets the definition of an epidemic can be considered. This step requires two actions.

Rate of Occurrence

First, an attack rate must be calculated. Usual measures of infection occurrence in nosocomial infection studies are incidence or prevalence rates (7). The incidence rate is the ratio of the number of new cases of an entity (in this case, nosocomial infection) occurring in a specified population at risk of infection in a defined time period (the numerator) to the number of persons in the population (the denominator). In contrast, the prevalence rate is the total number of cases of nosocomial infection in the defined population at risk at one point in time (point prevalence) or in a given interval (period prevalence). In each of these definitions, the number of episodes of interest (here, nosocomial infection) is the numerator of a fraction in which the denominator is the number of persons at risk for the occurrence of the numerator event. This fraction can be adjusted for a specific characteristic of interest. For example, in a study of the occurrence of infections associated with intravascular catheters, the denominator might be the number of days such a catheter was in place or the number of patients in whom a catheter was present, depending on the focus of the study.

Comparison with Baseline

After these calculations are completed, the attack rate for current cases should be compared with the usual, baseline occurrence of the entity at the institution. The presence of an attack rate that is higher than usual confirms that an outbreak is occurring. Note that situations in which no clear increase in a high number of cases is noted from surveillance data may exist. In such situations, rates of infection may have been excessive for extended periods, so that baseline infection rates themselves constitute a problem worthy of attention (6).

Characterizing the Episode

Description of Features

Framing the problem in terms of location, time, persons, procedures, instruments, or other features is the next step in the systematic approach (2). The time course of an infection often is shown in the form of an epidemic curve, which is a graph of the number of cases of disease in relation to the time of onset of the nosocomial infection. This graph allows a comparison of periods before the episode in question (baseline periods) with the time at which the problem appeared. Such an observation may be all that is needed to determine if an outbreak exists (see below). In addition, the characteristics of the curve itself often suggest the means by which the organism has been spread (2). Among the time trends to consider are secular (long-term) patterns, seasonal changes (important for some organisms), and acute changes from the baseline (clustering) (18). Location within the HCI also should be evaluated, and such an analysis also can suggest the mode of spread of the organism. For example, HCI-acquired cases of tuberculosis in patients widely spread throughout the institution may suggest an airborne mode of transmission through the heating-cooling system of the HCI. Finally, evaluation of the demographic and clinical characteristics of the infected patients (evaluation of persons) may allow the discovery of common features of the infected patients not shared with those without infection. Age, gender, type of underlying disease, prior therapy, and other factors may be relevant or irrelevant in different situations. Any host factor that can influence the development of disease must be considered; those that are found to increase the chance of infection are defined as risk factors (7, 15).

In the presence of enough cases, a description of epidemiologic patterns may allow the problem to be understood. However, determining the important factors often requires the use of some of the analytic techniques of epidemiology that are used in other kinds of biomedical research as well. Analytic studies can be observational or interventional. These methods more often than not involve the use of appropriate control groups.

Observational Studies

Observational studies review and monitor the natural course of events and are the type most frequently used in investigations of clusters of hospital infections (10). Observational studies commonly are of two different types: case-control and cohort. In a case-control study, a group of patients who have a nosocomial infection of interest are compared with a control (comparison) group of patients who do not have that nosocomial infection. The proportions of patients with the attribute or exposure of interest in the two groups are compared in order to identify differences that might suggest why infection occurred. Case-control studies are relatively inexpensive, quick, and reproducible compared to other options (7). This technique is used most frequently for acute investigations, such as suspected hospital outbreaks. Disadvantages of case-control studies include difficulties in choosing an appropriate control group and ruling out confounding variables. The cohort study takes a different approach. Subjects are classified as to the presence or absence of some study feature of interest, and then members of both groups (those with and those without the feature) are monitored during their HCI stay to determine which develop a nosocomial infection. The aim is to identify study characteristics that vary between subjects developing and those remaining free of a nosocomial infection. Cohort studies can be retrospective (the outcome of interest has already occurred when the study is begun) or prospective (the outcome has not yet occurred when the study is begun, so a period of follow-up is involved). An advantage of cohort studies is that they permit direct estimation of the infection risk associated with a particular exposure, which cannot be done with case-control studies. On the other hand, cohort studies usually are more difficult to manage and more expensive and take longer to complete than case-control studies (2). Thus, each of these types of studies has benefits and drawbacks in terms of practicality in the HCI setting, cost, and the type of results that can be obtained.

Interventional Analytic Studies

Clinical trials, or interventional studies, also can be conducted as part of infection control epidemiology. In such studies, the investigators assign the exposure of given study participants to the subject of interest. Thus, patients in one group may receive therapy through a new type of intravascular catheter, while others receive it through a current standard catheter, with the choice of catheter for each patient being left to random chance. Monitoring of patient clinical courses to identify the occurrence of infection in each group then allows an inference to be made about the value of the intervention (here, of the catheter) as a preventive measure. Since observational studies provide no control over the interactions of different factors, it is often difficult to sort out the effect of interest from other background influences (confounders). Interventional studies offer the opportunity to make this discrimination. However, this study method requires a willing population, informed consent, and resources of time and personnel to maintain the strict control needed to conduct an appropriate evaluation (10, 23).

Developing and Testing Hypotheses

Forming postulates about the reasons for the outbreak, the reservoir of the organisms, and the mode of spread of the organisms to the patient is the goal of the next step in the process. Establishing these characteristics may require making decisions about factors causing the episode. In developing hypotheses, the medical literature is often a good place to start: other institutions may have had similar problems with a given organism and identified the reservoir and mode of spread.

Reservoir, Source, and Mode of Spread

The reservoir of an infecting agent is the place in which the organism maintains its presence in the hospital setting. The source is the place from which the infectious agent directly contacts its victim. Reservoir and source may be identical or may differ. For example, in an outbreak of *Pseudomonas aeruginosa* infections in dialysis outpatients at Grady Memorial Hospital, the source of transmission to patients was the small pour bottles of iodophor antiseptic in the dialysis unit, but the reservoir of the organisms was contaminated stocks of antiseptic that were received from the manufacturer and that were already colonized with the organisms (20).

Mode of spread is the means by which an organism moves from the source to the infection victim. There are several important modes of spread; only some are relevant to nosocomial transmission (Table 3) (2). The most common mode of spread of infectious agents in HCIs is from person to person on the hands of personnel. This mode exemplifies indirect contact through the participation of an intermediary, in this case, a health care worker. Other indirect modes of spread include instruments (e.g., an endoscope used on one patient, inadequately decontaminated, and then used on another patient). Direct contact between the person or environmental object containing the infecting organism and the person who acquires the organism also is involved in hospital infection, and droplet transmission directly to a victim is possible as well. A special case of contact spread is so-called common-vehicle spread, in which more than one person acquires the same organism(s) from a single source. Airborne transmission of infections, such as tuberculosis and measles, is of concern in a modern hospital, whereas vector-borne spread is rare for nosocomial infections. The distinction between direct droplet spread and airborne transmission is one of distance: droplet spread occurs by travel of droplets within a short distance, whereas airborne particles or droplet nuclei may be transmitted far beyond the physical presence of the source patient. In the HCI setting, organisms may have more than one mode of spread. For example, *Salmonella* infection may be food borne, may contaminate a gastrointestinal endoscope, or may be transmitted by fecal contamination of hands of health care workers or patients (27). The versatility of methods for spread often complicates the investigation of HCI infection episodes.

TABLE 3 Modes of spread, with examples from nosocomial infection[a]

Type of spread	Example
Indirect contact	Patient to patient on hands of health care workers; patient to patient on inadequately disinfected endoscope
Direct contact	Contaminated iodophor; contaminated food
Droplet contact	Measles
Airborne	Tuberculosis
Endogenous	Cytomegalovirus reactivation in transplant patient; mother colonized with group B streptococcus becomes infected at time of delivery
Vector borne	Rare in hospital setting in developed countries

[a] Adapted in part from references 7 and 8.

The need to distinguish the reservoirs of infection and the transmission characteristics for an episode underlies one of the major differences between the epidemiologist and the clinician in the use of microbiologic data. Colonization is the presence of a microorganism that is not associated with clinical illness. In contrast, in an infection, an organism produces illness. The clinician is concerned with patient welfare and so usually disregards positive cultures or other microbiologic data indicating colonization rather than infection. To the epidemiologist, however, colonization and infection can be equally helpful in tracking the movement of an organism from one HCI area to another (18).

Chance, Bias, and Confounding

Testing epidemiologic hypotheses involves deciding whether there is an association between a particular risk factor and the occurrence of nosocomial infection. One characteristic of a causal association is that a change in the frequency or quantity of exposure leads to a corresponding change in the occurrence of hospital infection (10). Associations indicate only that there is a statistical link (either positive or negative) between the presence of exposure and the occurrence of infection. This apparent connection, however, may exist only because of chance association, bias, or confounding (10). Chance association can exist when a study population provides results unlike that of an entire population. Random variation from usual behavior can produce results that appear to provide a link when there is none and can suggest a lack of association when one truly exists as well. Statistical methods to estimate the probability of either of these two incorrect interpretations of epidemiologic data have been developed (23). A second factor that can interfere with the recognition of associations is bias. Bias is a systematic error in the ways in which study subjects were chosen, information was obtained from or about the subjects, or study data were reported. Errors often occur in data collection or transcription. Epidemiologic bias is present when the errors apply differently to subjects with infection and those without or to subjects with the exposure of interest and those without. Even when systematic errors in collection or reporting of data apply equally to each study group, the result is underestimation of the degree of association between exposure and infection occurrence. Efforts to avoid bias need to be considered at the time of study design as well as at the time of analysis. The third risk in determining associations is confounding. Confounding is present when an apparent association or lack of association is really due to the impact of a third factor that is associated with both exposure and infection occurrence but is independent of each (8, 10).

Establishing Causation

Even when chance, bias, and confounding can be ruled out, the presence of a valid association does not demonstrate a cause-and-effect relationship between exposure and occurrence of infection. It is, however, one of the features of an episode that allows a judgment by the epidemiologist as to whether a causal relationship exists. Causation remains a matter of belief or judgment based on available evidence. Unfortunately, in a field as complicated as infection control epidemiology, it is often difficult to define a clear causal relationship from observational studies. For example, nosocomial pneumonia may be associated with recent chest surgery, and this link may persist after chance, bias, and confounding are examined and ruled out. However, the association merely indicates that something related to the surgery increases the risk of pneumonia, not that the surgery itself causes the infection (15). In these situations, other evidence, such as the results of experimental studies (clinical trials), often is needed to establish a causal link. Thus, observational studies can be of great value in identifying the exposures, control methods, or equipment for which clinical trials that are likely to show causation may be designed.

Control Activities

Defining the reservoir, mode of spread, and associated risk factors usually suggests certain control measures that can be taken to slow or stop the progress of the epidemic or other problem under study (15). For example, if the data suggest that the air-conditioning system of the operating suite is contaminated with the problem organism, the actions needed to minimize this problem focus on improving air cleanliness rather than on hand washing. Actions needed to control an outbreak can be based on the conclusions of an analysis. At this point, new steps should be implemented, and any control efforts made earlier in the investigation should be revised as needed.

Infection control measures for the HCI usually focus on altering or removing one of the three elements requisite for infection: a pathogenic microorganism, a susceptible victim, and a mode of transmission of the organism to its victim (2). This situation explains the need for the development and testing of hypotheses in the steps described above. The epidemiologic investigation attempts not only to characterize the nature of any and all of these determinants but also to decide which factor(s) it will be most practical to alter.

Follow-Up Surveillance

New data must be collected to make sure that the control measures achieved the desired effect. In this step, the laboratory retains a prominent role as a potential early-warning system for recurrent cases if control measures are ineffective.

ROLE OF THE LABORATORY IN EPIDEMIOLOGIC EVALUATIONS

The laboratory has an important role in each aspect of epidemiologic investigation listed in Table 2 (18, 21).

Organism Identification

Perhaps the most important role for the laboratory is accurate identification and susceptibility testing of organisms causing nosocomial infection. The initial step of realizing that a problem exists and defining it precisely is crucial. The spectrum of organisms important in the health care setting has changed dramatically in the recent past (21). Still, most of the organisms causing outbreaks or special problems of endemic nosocomial infection can be identified with techniques routinely available in the hospital laboratory. Thus, laboratory workers must be taught to recognize the findings or situations that may indicate an infection control problem and to report any of these events in a timely fashion. Examples of such problems include any isolation of *Neisseria meningitidis* to which exposure in the HCI might have occurred; *Salmonella* isolates from nursery patients; positive smears or cultures for *Mycobacterium tuberculosis* from any patient or employee; organisms resistant to an unusual number of antimicrobial agents; and an unusual number of a given organism appearing on a given HCI unit or in an intensive-care unit (14). Results can be brought to the attention of infection control colleagues by telephone or by pager if the matter is urgent. Otherwise, a mention during the daily visit of the infection control staff to the laboratory usually suffices.

Identification of the etiology of an infection problem can depend on the extent to which the laboratory characterizes the organism(s) in question both routinely and in special outbreak circumstances. Fortunately, technologic developments in the laboratory have increased the ability to keep pace with the changes in etiology and resistance to antimicrobial agents of HCI pathogens (18). How these tests, especially those performed rapidly, can be of value in infection control settings depends on their specificity, sensitivity, and other characteristics in conjunction with the setting at hand. The use of such tests instead of more traditional microbiologic procedures should be determined by the clinical microbiologist after consultation with appropriate clinicians and the infection control team (21).

The microbiologist must ascertain whether the laboratory has sufficient experience and expertise to recognize the microbiologic entity under investigation. Some HCIs do not have the resources to identify certain organisms to the species level in routine practice. For epidemiologic investigations, these institutions may have to begin to identify relevant isolates to the species level or to retrieve relevant isolates for identification as circumstances demand. For example, if the laboratory does not identify the individual species of *Klebsiella* but instead groups them as *Klebsiella* species, then the infection control program will not recognize increased rates of nosocomial infection caused by a particular species of this organism. At a minimum, the laboratory should be capable of identifying gram-positive cocci and gram-negative aerobic bacilli to the species level when special or recurring cross-infection problems make this necessary (17). The use of commercial identification and antimicrobial susceptibility testing systems offers several advantages in accomplishing this goal, as long as their potential drawbacks are kept in mind as well. Newer methods allow the performance of a wider variety of tests than could be accomplished with manual methods. These resources could permit the processing on-site of specimens that otherwise would have to be referred. This ability could have advantages during hospital or other HCI outbreaks. However, these systems may misclassify organisms or misestimate the frequency with which resistant isolates are found. The combination of these problems could cause difficulty in deciding on the appropriate steps for the control of a true problem (21).

Identification of resistant isolates has been complicated by new patterns of antimicrobial resistance in nosocomial organisms. For example, clinical laboratories have continued to experience problems in the detection of low to moderate levels of vancomycin resistance in enterococci in several geographic areas (22). Making sure that newly reported resistance patterns in nosocomial pathogens can be accurately detected is a keystone of laboratory efforts in infection control.

Storage of Data and Isolates

Archival information must be maintained by the laboratory to establish the baseline frequency with which organisms of episodic or continuing interest cause infections. The microbiologist periodically should assess which data will be saved after consultation with infection control personnel. Ironically, archival information required for epidemiologic investigations may be more difficult to retrieve now than before the advent of electronic data processing systems, as information on biochemical reactions and other data, traditionally saved on laboratory worksheets, may not be part of the records maintained on a modern laboratory information system (18). Saving the information for 6 months seems to be a minimum requirement.

Retrospective testing of strains is possible only when isolates of possible epidemiologic importance have been saved systematically by the laboratory. The resources to do this vary markedly from HCI to HCI, so it may well be that prior isolates are not always available when further testing is needed. Decisions about the period for which isolates should be saved routinely and in special investigative situations should be discussed with infection control personnel on a regular and routine basis (18). The source of an isolate is an important factor in making such a decision; for example, isolates from blood may be kept longer than those from urine specimens. Likewise, the organism will influence this decision; for example, it is more desirable to store isolates of M. *tuberculosis* than most routine isolates of *E. coli*, as special laboratory studies often are quite helpful in resolving episodes of nosocomial tuberculosis in HCIs (19).

Timely Reporting

A crucial responsibility of the laboratory is to serve as an early-warning system for infection control problems (18). Whenever it is apparent that a problem exists, all relevant organisms should be reported to infection control personnel as soon as their isolation is recognized. At this point, arrangements should be made to save all potentially relevant organisms, at least for the duration of the investigation and perhaps longer, if storage facilities allow.

Periodic summaries of microbiologic test results may be useful to the infection control team as well as to clinicians. Just as microbiologists summarize data such as susceptibility profiles on a periodic basis for patient care, they may wish to summarize information and trends about HCI isolates as well. For both of these ends, timeliness in reporting is important.

Supplementary Studies

On rare occasions, solving an infection control problem may require processing of supplementary cultures from patients, personnel, or the environment. Special techniques for culturing, immunologic testing, or genetic testing may be required to accomplish such projects (2). For example, reliable detection of *Salmonella* carriage may require the enhancement of growth by use of selective media. Likewise, new genetic techniques may enhance the sensitivity of methods for detecting nosocomial pathogens (26). The laboratory must make a careful assessment of the sites to be cultured and of the supplies and techniques to be used (17).

Surveillance cultures of the hospital environment and personnel once were advocated on a routine basis. During the 1970s, studies found these programs to be of minimal value in infection control; by 1980, most institutions took the approach that routine environmental culturing should be severely limited (17). During the past decade, limiting cultures of the environment has become even more imperative because of changes in the economics of health care in the United States. Fortunately, further studies have supported this selective approach (24). For example, a study from Hungary found that surveillance cultures are of limited value in predicting infection or identifying the causative organisms of fever (5). However, in specific areas or regions, routine checks on the adequacy of sterilizer function, culturing of dialysis infusion solutions and the water used to prepare them, and culturing of infant formula and some other products prepared in the hospital and periodic checks on the effectiveness of disinfection of certain equipment that directly contacts tissues other than skin may help prevent infections from these sources; such checks may be mandated by local regulations (17). In the absence of an epidemic or regulatory fiat, sampling should be minimal; microbiologists and infection control personnel should be firm in not conducting indiscriminate routine microbiologic sampling and testing (17). Close communication between epidermiologists and microbiologists about the need for such cultures continues to be essential to avoid wasting valuable resources.

On occasion it is important to identify not only patients but also personnel who may be colonized with the strain being studied. Likewise, special approaches may be required for the processing of environmental cultures to help determine or confirm the mode of spread. These personnel or environmental cultures should be considered one of the costs of the infection control program of the HCI and should not be billed to the individual patients affected by the problem strain. Specific culture and other test techniques for a wide variety of inanimate items and substances have been described (17). Identifying periodically the most likely organisms or problems occurring in a given setting and planning in advance for difficulties with them may be the key to a rapid and effective response when a problem does arise (21).

Typing: Establishing Microbiologic Similarity or Difference

Determining the features of an epidemiologic problem or testing certain hypotheses about reservoir or mode of spread often requires a laboratory to define whether the outbreak strains are related or not related to each other. Such a determination involves conducting microbiologic studies to establish similarities or differences among isolates. To achieve this, a number of typing systems have been designed to determine organism similarity or difference; this aspect is discussed in detail in chapter 7 of this Manual.

POTENTIAL PROBLEMS RELATED TO LABORATORY ACTIVITIES IN EPIDEMIOLOGIC INVESTIGATIONS

The importance of the laboratory role in epidemiology is demonstrated by the success of investigations in which laboratory work is appropriate. It is equally well emphasized when laboratory problems lead to difficulties in characterizing a problem or potential problem in an HCI. Some of the most common problems in laboratory support for epidemiologic activities are considered below (18).

Misdiagnosis of Outbreak ("Pseudo-Outbreak")

On occasion, the existence of an epidemic is postulated when none is actually present (21). These episodes occur when there is a clustering of apparent infections but infection is not actually present or when the pattern of actual infections gives a false appearance of clustering.

Spurious outbreaks of nosocomial infection have been traced to a variety of sources (Table 4). For example, an increase in blood cultures that yielded rapidly growing mycobacteria for patients with human immunodeficiency virus was found to be associated with extrinsic contamination of the cultures in the laboratory (1). A source of pseudo-outbreaks that has special importance to the laboratory is problems with instrumentation. For example, an episode of cross-contamination leading to false-positive cultures of *Nocardia asteroides* arose from instrument motor drive misalignment, inadequate sterilization, and contamination of blood culture vials in a BACTEC 460 TB system (11).

Pseudo-outbreaks can take a considerable amount of time to identify. On occasion someone in a laboratory finds a problem in a technique or procedure that brings a pseudo-outbreak to light. Usually, however, a clinician recognizes these problems by noting a great disparity between the patient's clinical status and the laboratory results.

Inadequate Quality Control

Organisms associated with infection control problems usually are isolated at different times. Thus, laboratory characterization procedures often will be performed at different times. The results of many laboratory tests used for infection control (e.g., identification, susceptibility testing, and typing procedures) can vary from day to day and batch to batch. The need for control of these types of variation in media, reagents, and so forth is especially important. For example, in some cases one may need to go back and identify or type isolates recovered at a different time on the same media to remove confounding variables of the testing process.

Needles Culturing, Organism Identification, or Susceptibility Testing

The overuse of supplementary culturing wastes valuable laboratory resources. It is important for laboratories to avoid the excessive use of environmental cultures, personnel cultures, organism identification, and susceptibility testing. For example, if a laboratory uses 20 different antibiotics to define susceptibility patterns, there is a high likelihood that organisms that actually are part of the outbreak will be identified as different by at least one tested drug and thus considered unrelated.

TABLE 4 Sources of pseudo-outbreaks of nosocomial infection[a]

A. Related to clinician or clinical entity
   1. Incorrect diagnosis of clinical entity
   2. Positive cultures represent colonization rather than infection
   3. Failure to distinguish community-acquired from nosocomial cases
B. Related to laboratory
   1. Contamination during specimen collection
   2. Contamination during specimen transport
   3. Contamination during laboratory processing
      a. Media, solutions, or other reagents
      b. Equipment or instrumentation
   4. Use of inadequate method or technique
C. Related to case finding
   1. Increased surveillance efficiency
   2. Improved laboratory techniques for identification
D. Related to chance clustering

[a] Adapted in part from references 16 and 17.

Overuse or Overinterpretation of Typing Techniques

Typing procedures represent a great advance in the ability to characterize an outbreak. Nevertheless, certain problems still are associated with their use. Interpretation is a potential pitfall; on occasion, typing is interpreted to show that organisms are identical. In reality, however, these procedures rarely can prove that organisms are identical. Instead, they usually show only that organisms are not different by the typing methods used. This considerable distinction focuses attention on the possibility that similar reactions can be obtained by chance alone.

One must be selective in the use of typing systems, even when an outbreak occurs. Basic infection control measures can resolve some problems without additional microbiologic data or epidemiologic investigation (2). In other situations, simple marker systems, such as biotyping and antibiotic resistance patterns, provide sufficient data so that no further testing is needed. The use of more complicated and/or less readily available typing systems should be reserved for situations in which control measures fail or in which organism or infection occurrence is being studied for academic reasons. Dealing with these aspects of typing is described in detail in chapter 7 of this Manual.

CONCLUSION

Epidemiologic methods permit the efficient evaluation of many different aspects of nosocomial infection control as well as the study of other aspects of care in the health care setting. The steps of an epidemiologic assessment are aimed at prevention and control efforts and allow the assessment of the most efficient as well as the most effective ways to achieve these efforts. The laboratory plays a major role in epidemiologic attempts to deal with an endemic nosocomial infection and faces exceptional demands for service at the beginning of and throughout a period of epidemiologic study. These activities are essential in the fight against outbreaks of HCI infection. An understanding of the usual methods and approaches of the epidemiologist can help the clinical microbiologist provide more effective support for hospital infection control activities. The investigations must be carried out rapidly and effectively yet must be as efficient and cost-effective as possible. For all these attributes to be blended, the microbiologist must prepare in advance for the various diagnostic tasks, whether performed on-site or by referral to other laboratories. After the investigations begin, it is too late to initiate a plan for a laboratory response; contingency plans must be available for dealing with the types of cross-infection problems that have occurred most often in the past in the institution. This strategy allows exceptional requests to be dealt with smoothly and accurately. Fortunately, the past decade has brought improvements in epidemiologic methods and in laboratory procedures to aid in infection control efforts. Regular and frequent communication between the microbiologist and infection control personnel is the best strategy for success.

REFERENCES

1. **Ashford, D. A., S. Kellerman, M. Yakrus, S. Brim, R. C. Good, L. Finelli, W. R. Jarvis, and M. M. McNeil.** 1997. Pseudo-outbreak of septicemia due to rapidly growing mycobacteria associated with extrinsic contamination of culture supplement. *J. Clin. Microbiol.* **35:**2040–2042.
2. **Beck-Sague, C., W. R. Jarvis, and W. J. Martone.** 1997. Outbreak investigations. *Infect. Control Hosp. Epidemiol.* **18:**138–145.
3. **Centers for Disease Control and Prevention.** 1996. National Nosocomial Infections Surveillance (NNIS) report. Data summary from October, 1986 to April, 1996, issued May, 1996. *Am. J. Infect. Control* **24:**380–388.
4. **Centers for Disease Control and Prevention.** 1997. Update: *Staphylococcus aureus* with reduced susceptibility to vancomycin—United States, 1997. *JAMA* **278:** 1145–1146.
5. **Czirok, E., G. Y. Prinz, R. Denes, P. Remeny, and A. Herendi.** 1997. Value of surveillance cultures in a bone marrow transplantation unit. *J. Med. Microbiol.* **46:** 785–791.
6. **Dixon, R. E.** 1992. Investigation of endemic and epidemic nosocomial infections, p. 109–133. *In* J. V. Bennett and P. S. Brachman (ed.), *Hospital Infections*, 3rd ed. Little, Brown & Co., Boston, Mass.
7. **Freeman, J.** 1996. Quantitative epidemiology. *Infect. Control Hosp. Epidemiol.* **17:**249–255.
8. **Greenberg, R. S., S. R. Daniels, W. D. Flanders, J. W. Eley, and J. R. Boring.** 1993. *Medical Epidemiology*. Appleton & Lange, Norwalk, Conn.
9. **Haley, R. W., J. H. Tenney, J. O. Lindsey, J. S. Garner, and J. V. Bennett.** 1985. How frequent are outbreaks of nosocomial infection in community hospitals? *Infect. Control* **6:**233–236.
10. **Hennekens, C. H., and J. E. Buring.** 1987. *Epidemiology in Medicine*. Little, Brown & Co., Boston, Mass.
11. **Louie, L., M. Louie, and A. E. Simor.** 1997. Investigation of a pseudo-outbreak of *Nocardia asteroides* infection by pulsed-field gel electrophoresis and randomly amplified polymorphic DNA PCR. *J. Clin. Microbiol.* **35:**1582–1584.
12. **Mayhall, C. G. (ed.).** 1996. *Hospital Epidemiology and Infection Control*. The Williams & Wilkins Co., Baltimore, Md.
13. **McGowan, J. E., Jr.** 1991. Abrupt changes in antibiotic resistance. *J. Hosp. Infect.* **18:(Suppl. A):**202–210.
14. **McGowan, J. E., Jr.** 1991. Communication with hospital staff, p. 151–158. *In* A. Balows, W. J. Hausler, Jr., K. L. Herrmann, H. D. Isenberg, and H. J. Shadomy (ed.), *Manual of Clinical Microbiology*, 5th ed. American Society for Microbiology, Washington, D.C.
15. **McGowan, J. E., Jr.** 1996. Risk factors and nosocomial infection control, p. 225–235. *In* A. M. Emmerson and G. Ayliffe (ed.), *Balliere's Clinical Infectious Diseases*, vol. 3. Balliere-Tindall, London, England.
16. **McGowan, J. E., Jr., and B. G. Metchock.** 1995. Infection control epidemiology and clinical microbiology, p. 182–189. *In* P. R. Murray, E. J. Baron, M. A. Pfaller, F. C. Tenover, and R. H. Yolken (ed.), *Manual of Clinical Microbiology*, 6th ed. American Society for Microbiology, Washington, D.C.
17. **McGowan, J. E., Jr., and R. A. Weinstein.** 1998. The role of the laboratory in control of nosocomial infection, p. 143–164. *In* J. V. Bennett and P. S. Brachman (ed.), *Hospital Infections*, 4th ed. Little, Brown & Co, Boston, Mass.
18. **McGowan, J. E., Jr., and B. G. Metchock.** 1996. Basic microbiology support for hospital epidemiology. *Infect. Control Hosp. Epidemiol.* **17:**298–303.
19. **Michele, T. M., W. A. Cronin, N. M. H. Graham, D. M. Dwyer, D. S. Pope, S. Harrington, R. E. Chaisson, and W. R. Bishai.** 1997. Transmission of *Mycobacterium tuberculosis* by a fiberoptic bronchoscope. Identification by DNA fingerprinting. *JAMA* **278:**1093–1095.
20. **Parrott, P. L., P. M. Terry, E. N. Whitworth, L. W. Frawley, R. S. Coble, I. K. Wachsmuth, and J. E. McGowan, Jr.** 1982. *Pseudomonas aeruginosa* peritonitis associated with a contaminated poloxamer-iodine solution. *Lancet* **ii:**683–685.
21. **Pfaller, M. A., and L. A. Herwaldt.** 1997. The clinical microbiology laboratory and infection control: emerging pathogens, antimicrobial resistance, and new technology. *Clin. Infect. Dis.* **25:**858–870.
22. **Rosenberg, J., F. C. Tenover, J. Wong, W. Jarvis, and D. J. Vugia.** 1997. Are clinical laboratories in California accurately reporting vancomycin-resistant enterococci? *J. Clin. Microbiol.* **35:**2526–2530.
23. **Rothman, K. J.** 1986. *Modern Epidemiology*. Little, Brown & Co., Boston, Mass.
24. **Rutala, W. A., and D. J. Weber.** 1995. Environmental interventions to control nosocomial infections. *Infect. Control Hosp. Epidemiol.* **16:**442–443.
25. **Sands, K., G. Vineyard, and R. Platt.** 1996. Surgical site infections occurring after hospital discharge. *J. Infect. Dis.* **173:**963–970.
26. **Satake, S., N. Clarke, D. Rimland, F. S. Nolte, and F. C. Tenover.** 1997. Detection of vancomycin-resistant enterococci in fecal samples by PCR. *J. Clin. Microbiol.* **35:** 2325–2330.
27. **Wall, P. G.** 1996. Outbreaks of salmonellosis in hospitals in England and Wales: 1992–1994. *J. Hosp. Infect.* **33:** 181–190.
28. **Wenzel, R. P. (ed.).** 1997. *Prevention and Control of Nosocomial Infections*, 3rd ed. The Williams & Wilkins Co., Baltimore, Md.

Laboratory Procedures for the Epidemiologic Analysis of Microorganisms

ROBERT D. ARBEIT

7

INTRODUCTION

A considerable portion of this Manual is directed toward the process of identifying the genus and species of microorganisms (bacteria, mycobacteria, and fungi) isolated from clinical specimens. The focus of this chapter is the process of analyzing multiple isolates within a given species to determine whether they represent a single strain or multiple different strains. Such analyses are useful in several different clinical settings. Infection control practitioners increasingly solicit laboratory support to complement intensive epidemiologic investigations as well as to help determine whether to initiate such investigations or how to focus them. Clinicians may request that isolates from an individual patient be examined to help determine whether a set of isolates represents a single infecting strain or mutiple contaminants or whether a series of isolates obtained over time represents the relapse of an infection due to a single strain or separate episodes of disease due to different strains. In research settings, the detailed analysis of multiple isolates can contribute to the development of new insights into both the epidemiology and the pathogenesis of infection.

Strong basic clinical microbiology practices are prerequisites to further typing studies. The technologists at the bench are often the first to detect a cluster of isolates based on a distinctive colonial morphology or biotype or the increased prevalence of a particular species. Their observations should be encouraged and pursued by laboratory supervisors and directors. The identification of isolates to the species level and antimicrobial susceptibility testing should be completed promptly and accurately. Contemporary computer systems can greatly facilitate access to these laboratory reports and can often be programmed to alert hospital staff to the appearance of a new species or antibiotic susceptibility pattern and to provide basic routine epidemiologic analyses. Frequent, open communication between the laboratory, infection control practitioners, and infectious diseases clinicians is obviously critical. With the increasing sophistication and complexity of microbial typing studies, an active collaboration is required in order to interpret the results appropriately and to apply them effectively in the clinical realm.

Theoretical Considerations

The central hypothesis motivating typing studies is that a series of isolates obtained from an epidemiologic cluster or during the course of an infection in a single patient are clonally related, that is, are directly descended from a common precursor. Generations of microbiologists have observed that epidemiologically unrelated isolates of the same species often differ in multiple characteristics. Typing systems are based on the premise that clonally related isolates will share characteristics by which they can be differentiated from unrelated isolates. In this chapter, the term "isolate" will be used to refer to a pure culture derived from a single colony, which is presumed to arise from a single organism. A "strain" is a set of isolates which, as analyzed by a typing system, are indistinguishable from each other and which can be differentiated from other isolates; such isolates are thereby inferred to be clonally related to each other. (A single isolate with a distinctive characteristic[s] may also represent a strain.) The utility of a particular characteristic for typing is related to its stability within a strain and its diversity within the species. Note that the definition of a strain is operationally dependent on the resolution of the typing system, and as discussed further below, clonality is more usefully considered a relative concept rather than an absolute condition (48).

There is generally substantial genetic diversity within microbial species, and isolates are typically distributed among many genetically diverging lineages. This evolutionary divergence reflects the accumulation of random, nonlethal mutations, including single-base-pair substitutions, the deletion of individual genes, or even the acquisition of DNA from other microbial species. With the development of highly sensitive molecular techniques, subtle alterations can be precisely detected and the mechanisms underlying complex variations can be resolved.

Nevertheless, the analysis of clinically relevant isolates remains a substantial challenge. Because of the powerful selective pressure on critical microbial genetic elements, such as virulence factors and antimicrobial resistance determinants, the human pathogens within a species may represent only a subset of the genotypes within the species as a whole, which can include clinical, commensal, animal, and environmental strains. For example, the genetic diversity among invasive isolates of *Escherichia coli* cultured from patients with pyelonephritis or bacteremia is relatively limited compared to that among isolates colonizing the intestinal tract (136). The pathogenic isolates are characterized by virulence factors that enhance colonization, persistence, and invasion at the infecting site; such virulence determinants are absent from most commensal (i.e., fecal) isolates (12, 13, 89).

Furthermore, particular bacterial lineages characterized by unique concatenations of virulence genes or variants (alleles) of such genes may emerge and disseminate relatively rapidly, causing clinically and epidemiologically important increases in the frequency and severity of particular infections (106). Examples of this include the *Streptococcus pyogenes* isolates associated with toxic shock-like syndrome, antibiotic-resistant *Streptococcus pneumoniae*, and *E. coli* O157:H7. In some instances an existing but unappreciated pathogen will emerge in association with a new opportunistic niche, such as the epidemic of vaginal toxic shock syndrome associated with new classes of tampons (106). Although precise identification of such lineages requires specific studies with the tools of population genetics, the critical implication of this issue for strain typing is that it may be very difficult to differentiate among epidemiologically unrelated isolates of such pathogens that have emerged. *Clostridium difficile* strains associated with geographically and temporally diverse nosocomial outbreaks are often closely related genetically (129). Isolates of methicillin-resistant *Staphylococcus aureus* (MRSA) from diverse geographic locations appear to be derived from one or a very few precursor strains and, consequently, are genetically restricted compared to the genetic diversity among methicillin-susceptible *S. aureus* isolates (74, 107). Thus, the most clinically relevant isolates—those with increased virulence or resistance—are often the most difficult to differentiate unambiguously.

Criteria for Evaluating Typing Systems

There is no "gold standard" by which to judge a typing method or consistently define true-positive or true-negative results. Consequently, the terminology usually used to describe the operating characteristics of laboratory tests (e.g., sensitivity and specificity) is not strictly applicable, and the results of a typing system must be considered relative to the available epidemiologic data or to the results of other systems. Several criteria are useful in evaluating typing systems (Table 1). Typeability refers to the ability to obtain an unambiguous, positive result for each isolate analyzed; nontypeable isolates are those that give either a null or an uninterpretable result. Reproducibility refers to the ability of a technique to yield the same result when the same strain is tested repeatedly. Reproducibility is influenced by both technical and biologic factors; the former may be reflected in run-to-run variations among replicate aliquots of a single isolate. In addition, biologic variation in the bacterial characteristic being examined may produce differences among independent isolates representing the same strain. Discriminatory power refers to the ability to differentiate among unrelated strains. Ideally, each unrelated isolate is detected as unique. In practice, a technique is statistically useful when the most commonly detected type represents less than 5% of the population (64, 65). For techniques that assess multiple individual characteristics (e.g., bacteriophage typing and electrophoretic methods), discriminatory power typically diminishes as reproducibility decreases, since unrelated strains must differ for a greater number of component characteristics in order to be reliably differentiated (64).

The classic strain typing techniques—biotyping, antibiotic susceptibility pattern determination, serotyping, and bacteriophage typing—were based on the presence or absence of metabolic or biologic activities as expressed by whole organisms. Interpretation of such results is relatively straightforward. More recently, electrophoretic analysis of molecular subcomponents (e.g., proteins, metabolic enzymes, plasmid DNA, chromosomal DNA, and DNA produced by PCR) has been shown to be a powerful tool for differentiating strains. Electrophoretic results are typically patterns of "bands," each band representing a discrete bacterial product or DNA fragment. Such patterns may be extremely complex, subject to considerable technical variation, and, thus, difficult to analyze by using logical, objective, readily applied criteria. Consequently, ease of interpretation has become an important criterion for evaluating typing systems. Ease of performance is also critical. To be widely useful a typing method should be applicable to a broad range of microorganisms as well as inexpensive and technically accessible, requiring neither special expertise, expensive equipment, nor restricted reagents. Results should be available rapidly enough to be relevant to patient management or infection control. At this time no single typing system is optimal by all of these criteria and no one approach is preferred for all clinical settings or infecting species.

Over the past decade with the application of numerous DNA-based techniques there have been literally hundreds of reports describing bacterial strain typing systems. Many systems are proposed or applied without adequate knowledge of their effectiveness for a broad sample of isolates. It is clearly insufficient to evaluate a typing system by comparing the results for a single, well-defined outbreak with a handful of epidemiologically unrelated "control" strains. Almost any system will have sufficient reproducibility and discriminatory power to indicate that the outbreak isolates are more similar to each other than to a few random unrelated isolates. In the absence of a gold standard, two typing systems can be formally compared only if both have been applied to the same set of isolates. Thus, rigorous evaluation of a typing method involves analyses of adequate numbers of epidemic and sporadic isolates and comparison of the results directly with those obtained by previously well-studied approaches. A meaningful assessment of reproducibility requires examination of sets of isolates whose relatedness has been unequivocally established on the basis of clinical and epidermiologic data. Determination of discriminatory power involves analyses of sets of clinically significant, epidemiologically unrelated isolates; it is particularly informative to examine such isolates that have proven to be indistinguishable by other techniques.

Classification of Typing Methods

A convenient basis for classifying typing systems is to divide them into phenotypic techniques—those that detect characteristics expressed by the microorganisms—and genotypic techniques—those that involve direct DNA-based analyses of chromosomal or extrachromosomal genetic elements.

TABLE 1 Criteria for evaluating typing systems

Typeability	Ease of interpretation
Reproducibility	Ease of performance
Discriminatory power	

PHENOTYPIC TECHNIQUES

Typing methods that assess phenotypic differences (Table 2) are inherently limited by the capacity of microorganisms to alter the expression of the underlying genes (166). Such changes may occur unpredictably or in response to various

TABLE 2 Characteristics of phenotypic typing systems[a]

Typing system	Proportion of strains typeable	Reproducibility	Discriminatory power	Ease of interpretation	Ease of performance
Biotyping	All	Poor	Poor	Excellent	Excellent
Antimicrobial susceptibilities	All	Fair	Poor	Excellent	Excellent
Serotyping	Most	Good	Fair	Good	Fair
Bacteriophage typing	Most	Fair	Fair	Fair	Poor
MLEE	All	Excellent	Good	Excellent	Good

[a] These judgments represent the views of the author; many systems remain incompletely evaluated, and characteristics may vary as the systems are applied to different species. See the text for details.

environmental stimuli (100). In addition, point mutations representing a single nucleotide in the entire chromosome can result in the abnormal regulation or function of the gene responsible for a particular phenotype. Thus, isolates that represent the same strain and that are genetically indistinguishable (or almost so) can vary in the phenotype detected. Some phenotypic approaches, such as serotyping and bacteriophage typing, require specific reagents for the detection of individual types. Since the available materials may not be appropriate for all strains, a relatively large fraction of strains may give a null phenotype and, consequently, be nontypeable.

The problems associated with many of the phenotypic techniques stimulated the development and refinement of DNA-based typing methods. At this time DNA-based approaches have emerged as the preferred methods for the strain typing of most common bacterial pathogens in both reference and clinical laboratories (151). Consequently, only selected phenotypic techniques will be considered in this chapter; the reader is referred to published reviews for more complete coverage of these approaches (5, 90).

Biotyping

Biotyping refers to the pattern of metabolic activities expressed by an isolate and may include specific biochemical reactions, colonial morphology, and environmental tolerances (e.g., the ability to grow on certain media or at extremes of pH or temperature). Such characteristics have classically been used for taxonomy. In most clinical microbiology laboratories biotyping is now routinely and reliably performed with automated systems designed for species identification. The detection of multiple isolates of an unusual species can effectively detect an outbreak (85), and occasionally, epidemic strains of common bacterial species will exhibit distinctive biotypes (117). In general, however, biotyping has only limited ability to differentiate among strains within a species, and consequently, the technique has relatively poor discriminatory power.

Although variations in gene expression are the most common cause for isolates that represent the same strain to differ in one or more biochemical reactions, random mutations may also confound the interpretation of these data. One instructive example involves two colonies of *Klebsiella* that were isolated from the same urine sample and that differed only in their ability to produce indole from tryptophan (87). Since that metabolic reaction is the basis for differentiating *Klebsiella oxytoca* (indole positive) from *Klebsiella pneumoniae* (indole negative), the two isolates were considered different species. However, on detailed examination the isolates were otherwise phenotypically and genotypically identical, suggesting that they were simply variants derived from a single clone. Although this is an extreme example, it illustrates not only the limited utility of biotyping in epidemiologic studies but also the hazard of making any identification system critically dependent upon a single characteristic.

Antimicrobial Susceptibility Testing

Clinical microbiology laboratories routinely test most bacterial isolates for susceptibility to a panel of antimicrobial agents. Both manual and automated methods are widely available, rigorously quality controlled, typically easily performed, and relatively inexpensive. These data are readily available to clinicians and infection control practitioners. The identification of a new or unusual pattern of antibiotic resistance among isolates cultured from multiple patients is often the first indication of an outbreak (31).

For detailed epidemiologic studies, however, antibiotic susceptibility testing has relatively limited utility not only because of phenotypic variation but also because antibiotic resistance is under extraordinary selective pressure in contemporary hospitals. There are multiple genetic mechanisms by which a given strain can become abruptly resistant to a particular antibiotic. These include spontaneous point mutations (e.g., quinolone resistance in *Staphylococcus aureus* [55]) and the acquisition of specific resistance genes via plasmids and transposons from other strains or even other species (e.g., the transfer of aminoglycoside-modifying enzymes among members of the family *Enterobacteriaceae* [96] or pathways mediating vancomycin resistance among enterococci [30]). Since a single plasmid or compound transposon can carry multiple resistance determinants, resistance to multiple antimicrobial agents may be acquired simultaneously. On the other hand, in the absence of specific selective pressure, such elements may be lost (48, 96, 101). As a consequence of these various genetic mechanisms, different strains may develop similar resistance patterns, and, conversely, the susceptibility patterns of sequential clinical isolates representing the same strain may differ for one or more antibiotics (101, 150).

Serotyping

Serologic typing (serotyping) is based on the long-standing observation that microorganisms of the same species can differ in the antigenic determinants expressed on the cell surface. Multiple surface constituents exhibit such antigenic variation, including lipopolysaccharides, capsular polysaccharides, membrane proteins, and extracellular organelles (e.g., flagella and fimbriae). Serotyping has been applied to numerous species and has been one of the classic tools for epidemiologic studies. Some distinct virulence factors and related clinical syndromes are linked to particular serotypes within a species. For example, infection with *E. coli* O157:H7 isolates is associated with the hemolytic-uremic syndrome (168). In general, however, the utility of serotyping is limited by the relatively poor discriminatory power of the technique and the relatively high frequency of nontypeable isolates. At this time, serotyping remains a key method for typing isolates of *Salmonella*, *Shigella*, and pneumococci (151). Even for these species, DNA-based approaches are increasingly being used because of their increased discriminatory power as well as the difficulty of maintaining extensive stocks of typing sera (e.g., >2,200 antisera are required for definitive *Salmonella* typing).

Bacteriophage Typing

Among species for which numerous lytic bacteriophages (i.e., viruses capable of infecting and lysing bacterial cells) have been identified, strains can be characterized by their patterns of resistance or susceptibility to a standard set of phages. Until relatively recently, phage typing was the authoritative system for differentiating strains of *S. aureus* (25). However, because of the technical demands of this approach and its relatively poor reproducibility, DNA-based techniques are now the strain typing methods of choice for staphylococci (16, 151).

MLEE

In multilocus enzyme electrophoresis (MLEE), isolates are analyzed for differences in the electrophoretic mobilities of a set of metabolic enzymes (135). MLEE data are suitable for rigorous mathematical analysis and can be used to describe the genetic diversity and structure of a bacterial population, which can be represented graphically as a dendrogram (135). By this approach, comprehensive population analyses have been performed for several species of pathogenic bacteria (137), although such studies are increasingly performed by DNA sequencing (106). As a strain typing technique, MLEE is only moderately discriminatory.

GENOTYPIC TECHNIQUES

With the wide dissemination of the tools for analyzing DNA, almost every technique has been applied to strain typing (Table 3). Nevertheless, no approach yet combines reproducibility and discriminatory power with speed and simplicity. In addition, there remain substantial complexities in interpreting the results of these methods and effectively applying them to epidemiologic studies. Additional detailed background regarding the technical aspects of several of these methods is presented in chapter 13.

Plasmid Analyses

Typing systems based on plasmid analyses suffer from significant limitations inherent in the fact that plasmids are mobile, extrachromosomal elements and are not part of the chromosomal genotype that defines the host strain. Plasmids can be spontaneously lost from or readily acquired by a host strain; consequently, epidemiologically related isolates can exhibit different plasmid profiles (101). Since many plasmids carry antibiotic resistance determinants contained within mobile genetic elements (transposons) which can be readily acquired or deleted, the DNA compositions of plasmids can change rapidly (10, 84, 152). Furthermore, the strong selective pressure for nosocomial organisms to express antibiotic resistance may cause such plasmids to spread rapidly among strains and even among different species and to persist for prolonged periods within an institution (10, 69, 172). Plasmids may also be involved in the spread of virulence factors and may be selected for on that basis. For example, among enterotoxigenic and enteroinvasive *E. coli* isolates, the pathogenic toxins, adhesins, and invasins are often plasmid associated (96). Many clinical isolates lack plasmids and are therefore nontypeable (117); others carry only one or two plasmids, a situation which provides relatively poor discriminatory power. Despite these limitations, plasmid analyses have proven useful in numerous investigations (for reviews, see references 69, 96, 131, and 166) and may be quite effective in evaluating isolates obtained in a restricted time and place, for example, acute outbreaks within a single hospital.

Plasmid profile analysis was among the earliest DNA-based techniques applied to epidemiologic studies (96). The number and sizes of the plasmids carried by an isolate can be determined by preparing a plasmid extract and subjecting it to routine agarose gel electrophoresis. However, the reproducibilities of such profiles are confounded by the fact that a plasmid can exist in different molecular forms (i.e., supercoiled [closed circle], nicked [open circle], and linear), each of which migrates differently during agarose gel electrophoresis. Thus, in different preparations, each individual plasmid can be represented by a variable number of bands. Both the reproducibility and the discriminatory power of plasmid analyses can be substantially improved by digesting the plasmids with restriction enzymes (discussed below) and then electrophoretically analyzing the number and size of the resulting restriction fragments (96). This procedure—often referred to as restriction enzyme analysis of plasmids—is now the method of choice for plasmid studies (15, 31, 152); it is technically simple, requires only modest

TABLE 3 Characteristics of genotypic typing systems[a]

Typing system	Proportion of strains typeable	Reproducibility	Discriminatory power	Ease of interpretation	Ease of performance
Plasmid restriction digests	Most	Good	Good	Good	Excellent
REA	All	Good	Good	Poor	Excellent
Ribotyping	All	Excellent	Fair	Good	Good
PFGE	All	Excellent	Excellent	Excellent	Good
Restriction digests of PCR products	All	Excellent	Good	Excellent	Good
PCR based on repeated sequences	All	Good	Good	Good	Good
AP-PCR	All	Fair	Good	Fair	Good
Nucleotide sequence analysis	All	Excellent	Excellent	Excellent	Fair

[a] These judgments represent the views of the author; many systems remain incompletely evaluated, and characteristics may vary as the systems are applied to different species. See the text for details.

specialized equipment, and can be performed relatively quickly.

Plasmid analysis (with or without restriction digestion) remains a simple and effective approach for strain typing of staphylococci (both *S. aureus* and coagulase-negative species) and several species of the family *Enterobacteriaceae* (viz., *Klebsiella*, *Enterobacter*, and *Serratia*).

REA of Chromosomal DNA

A restriction endonuclease enzymatically cuts ("digests") DNA at a specific ("restricted") nucleotide recognition sequence. The number and sizes of the restriction fragments generated by digesting a given piece of DNA are influenced by both the recognition sequence of the enzyme and the composition of the DNA. Thus, an enzyme whose recognition sequence is composed of only guanine and cytosine will cut DNA with a low G+C content less frequently and, consequently, will generate fewer and larger restriction fragments than an enzyme recognizing sequences of only adenine and thymine. An enzyme that recognizes a sequence of 6 bp (a "6-bp cutter") typically has more recognition sites than an 8-bp cutter, will digest DNA more frequently, and, consequently, will generate more and smaller restriction fragments.

In conventional restriction enzyme analysis (REA), bacterial DNA is digested with endonucleases that have relatively frequent restriction sites, thereby generating hundreds of fragments ranging from ~0.5 to 50 kb in length. Such fragments can be separated by size by constant-field agarose gel electrophoresis, and the pattern can be detected by staining the gel with ethidium bromide and examining it under UV light (Fig. 1). Different strains of the same bacterial species have different REA profiles because of variations in their DNA sequences that alter the number and distribution of restriction sites. All isolates are typeable by REA; however, the utility of the technique is sharply limited by the difficulty of comparing the complex profiles, which consist of hundreds of bands that may be unresolved and overlapping (19, 39, 113). At this time, REA remains a recommended typing method only for *C. difficile* (38, 71, 151).

Southern Blot Analysis of RFLPs

REA patterns are complex because the ethidium bromide stain detects all of the hundreds of fragments generated by the restriction enzymes used. In contrast, Southern blot analyses detect only the particular restriction fragments associated with specific chromosomal loci. Southern blots, named after the investigator who first described the technique (140), are prepared by digesting bacterial DNA, separating the restriction fragments by agarose gel electrophoresis, and then transferring ("blotting") the fragments onto a nitrocellulose or nylon membrane. The fragment(s) containing specific sequences (loci) is then detected by using a labeled piece of homologous DNA as a probe. Under the

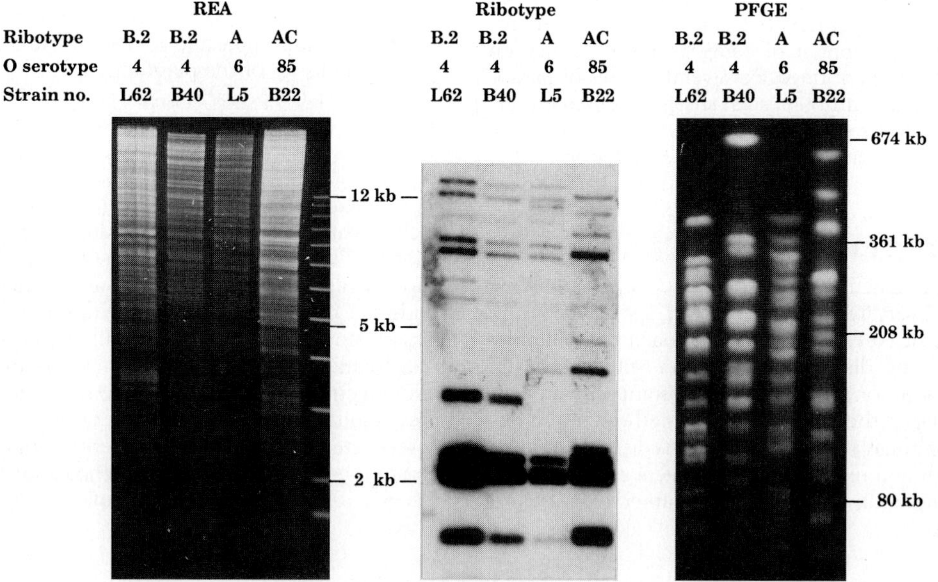

FIGURE 1 Bloodstream isolates of *E. coli* cultured from four epidemiologically unrelated patients from Long Beach, Calif. (isolates L62 and L5), and Boston, Mass. (isolates B40 and B22), compared by three genotypic typing systems: REA, ribotyping, and PFGE. Isolates L62 and B40, from two geographically diverse sites, were indistinguishable by REA and ribotyping analysis of an *Eco*RI restriction digest; however, these isolates were distinctly different by PFGE analysis of an *Xba*I digest. Isolate L5 had some similarities to both L62 and B40 by REA and ribotyping but differed by PFGE; isolate B22 was different by all three techniques. The isolates were also analyzed phenotypically. Biotyping by 30 biochemical tests (Vitek, Hazelwood, Mo.) indicated that the results of only 4 tests differed among the isolates, with three different overall patterns detected. Two isolates (L5 and L62) had the same biotype; the biotypes of strains B40 and B22 differed from that biotype by two and three tests, respectively. Of 18 antibiotics evaluated, isolates B22 and L62 were resistant only to tetracycline, whereas isolates B40 and L5 were sensitive to all antibiotics tested. The O serotypes are listed above each strain (serotyping was performed by Richard Wilson, Pennsylvania State University, State College). This figure appeared previously (90).

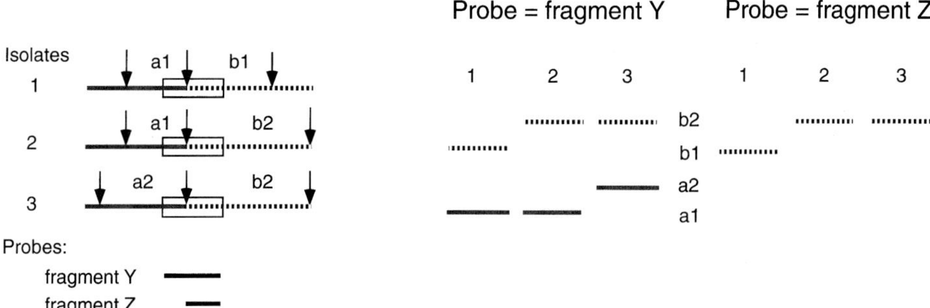

FIGURE 2 Correlation between variations in restriction sites and variations in the RFLPs detected by Southern blot analysis. As depicted, restriction enzyme A has an invariant internal restriction site within the gene (or locus) of interest and variable ("polymorphic") restriction sites to the sides ("flanks") of the gene. Fragment Y is wholly internal to the gene of interest and spans the conserved internal restriction site. A Southern blot prepared from a digest with enzyme A and probed with fragment Y will demonstrate the RFLPs shown. Fragment a is constant between isolates 1 and 2 and polymorphic between isolates 2 and 3; conversely, fragment b is polymorphic between isolates 1 and 2 and constant between isolates 2 and 3. This situation is analogous to the RFLPs described for the *mec* locus of MRSA as described in detail by Kreiswirth et al. (74). If the same blot is probed with fragment Z which is wholly to the right of the conserved internal restriction site, then only fragment b is detected. This situation is analogous to the methodology used to detect IS*6110* elements in *M. tuberculosis* described by van Embden et al. (160). The locus shown in this diagram would represent a single IS element; since isolates of *M. tuberculosis* typically have multiple copies of the IS element, the appearance of the blots is as depicted in Fig. 3.

appropriate conditions, the probe binds ("hybridizes") by complementary base pair matching only to those fragments containing identical or nearly identical nucleotide sequences. Variations in the number and size of the fragments detected are referred to as restriction fragment length polymorphisms (RFLPs) and reflect variations in both the number of loci that are homologous to the probe and the location of restriction sites within or flanking those loci (Fig. 2). All strains carrying loci homologous to the probe are typeable, and the results are, in general, highly reproducible. The discriminatory power of an analysis is directly related to the frequency with which the fragments detected vary in number and/or in size. Thus, the choice of probes is a critical consideration.

Although Southern blot analyses have generally been performed by research laboratories, the procedure has been simplified as a result of technical refinements and the existence of commercially available materials, such that only moderate levels of expertise and specialized equipment are required. The preparation of probes has classically involved the isolation of cloned DNA fragments and labeling of these fragments with radioisotopes; however, the process has been substantially simplified by the use of PCR (discussed below) to generate probes and the development of reliable nonradioactive detection systems (60).

Ribotyping refers to a Southern blot analysis in which strains are characterized for the RFLPs associated with the ribosomal operon(s) (145). Operons are clusters of genes which share related functions and which are often coordinately regulated; the ribosomal operons comprise nucleotide sequences coding for 16S rRNA and 25S rRNA, as well as one or more RNAs. Ribosomal sequences are highly conserved, and probes prepared from isolated *E. coli* rRNA (145) or a cloned ribosomal operon (*rrn*) (12) hybridize to the chromosomal ribosomal operons of a wide range of bacterial species. All bacteria carry these operons and are therefore typeable. In general, ribotypes are stable and reproducible, with isolates from an outbreak typically having the same ribotype (124, 150).

For organisms with multiple (five to seven) ribosomal operons, such as *E. coli*, *Klebsiella*, *Haemophilus*, and *Staphylococcus*, ribotype patterns commonly have 10 to 15 bands and have moderate discriminatory power (Fig. 1). Nevertheless, epidemiologically unrelated isolates not infrequently demonstrate the same pattern, limiting the utility of the method (12, 121, 150). For example, ~20% of 188 bloodstream isolates of *E. coli* from each of three geographically dispersed sites (Massachusetts, California, and Kenya) represented the same ribotype (93), although another genotypic technique (i.e., pulsed-field gel electrophoresis; discussed below) generally resolved each isolate as a distinct strain (Fig. 1). Isolates of this ribotype typically expressed adhesin and hemolysin virulence factors; as discussed above, virulent genotypes are frequently overrepresented among collections of bacterial pathogens. For bacterial species with only a single ribosomal operon, such as mycobacteria, ribotyping typically detects only one or two bands and has limited utility for epidemiologic studies (9).

The discriminatory power of ribotyping is comparable to or slightly less than that of MLEE. In studies with isolates of *E. coli*, *S. aureus*, and *H. influenzae* type b, both techniques assigned isolates to the same or closely related genotypes (12, 150). Such consistent, congruent results from two methods that are technically very different strongly support the hypothesis that the variations in both methods reflect the diverging genetic lineages that are characteristic of the bacterial populations. Because of its limited discriminatory power and relative technical complexity, ribotyping is not currently the preferred strain typing method for any common bacterial pathogen (151). However, a recently developed automated ribotyping system (RiboPrinter Microbial Characterization System; DuPont, Wilmington, Del.) offers the potential for increased throughput with modest laboratory effort as well as computerized analysis, permitting the development of standardized databases. For reference laboratories, such a system may prove to be useful and reliable for the screening of isolates prior to the application of a more discriminatory but labor-intensive strain typing method (119).

Southern blot analyses in which insertion sequences (ISs) and transposons are used as probes have proven to be reproducible and highly discriminatory methods for strain identification (47, 74, 77, 142). These mobile genetic elements are typically present as multiple copies positioned at different chromosomal loci (84). The number and locations of IS elements and, consequently, the RFLP(s) detected can vary appreciably among different bacterial strains. For example, an outbreak strain of multidrug resistant (MDR) *Mycobacterium tuberculosis* was readily differentiated from other sporadic MDR *M. tuberculosis* strains by Southern blot analysis of IS*6110*, an IS present in multiple copies within the *M. tuberculosis* genome (47). This approach is the method of choice for epidemiologic studies of *M. tuberculosis* (Fig. 3), although its discriminatory power is relatively poor for those strains that have only a few copies of the IS element. To facilitate comparison of the results of different studies, multiple independent laboratories have agreed to use a specific restriction enzyme to digest the chromosomal DNA and a specific subfragment of the IS to probe the Southern blots (160). By standardizing these technical variables, using internal molecular weight markers or reference strains, and applying computerized scanners and pattern analysis, it is possible to develop large databases of strain types (171).

The ease of interpreting Southern blots can be directly affected by the choice of enzymes for preparing the chromosomal DNA digest and the choice of probes. For example, the IS*6110* blots of *M. tuberculosis* isolates are typically easier to interpret than the ribotype blots of *E. coli*. In the analysis of the IS elements, essentially every band detected for a given isolate is of equal intensity; in contrast, in the ribotype blots, there is considerable variability among the bands detected for each isolate (compare Fig. 1 with Fig. 3) (58). The restriction enzyme and probe used in the IS analysis were selected such that each band detected includes all of the sequences in the probe and thus hybridizes efficiently and consistently with the probe (160). In the ribotype blots shown, the restriction enzyme used (*Eco*RI) cuts at several variable sites within the ribosomal operons, generating some restriction fragments that have only short sequences homologous to the probe and consequently that are detected with only a weak signal relative to those fragments that have more extensive homologous sequences. Part of such variability can be eliminated by choosing a restriction enzyme (e.g., *Bam*HI) that typically cuts only outside the ribosomal operons, so that the entire operon is present on a single fragment. With that modification, all of the fragments detected generate a strong, consistent signal; however, the absolute number of fragments detected decreases, and there is a concomitant decrease in the discriminatory power of the method (6). Thus, defining the optimal strategy for a Southern blot analysis can require considerable thought and effort.

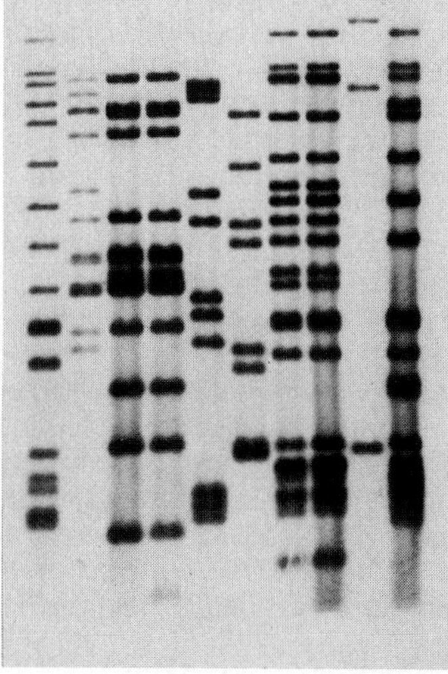

FIGURE 3 Southern blot of RFLPs associated with IS*6110* among isolates of *M. tuberculosis*. The blot was prepared as described by van Embden et al. (160) from whole chromosomal DNA digested with *Pvu*II and probed with a fragment wholly internal to IS*6110* and to the right of a conserved interval *Pvu*II site. Thus, each fragment represents a separate copy of the IS element. Because each fragment carries the same DNA sequences homologous to the probe, each fragment within an isolate is detected with similar intensity. Variations in intensities among different isolates reflect different quantities of DNA. Isolates with indistinguishable RFLP patterns are designated the same type; isolates with different patterns are designated different types. The Southern blot was generously provided by Barry Kreiswirth, Tuberculosis Center, Public Health Research Institute, New York, N.Y.

PFGE of Chromosomal DNA

As noted above, a major limitation of REA with enzymes with relatively frequent recognition sites is the difficulty of analyzing the resulting patterns composed of large numbers of overlapping, poorly resolved restriction fragments. If the bacterial genome is digested with enzymes with relatively few restriction sites, then considerably fewer, but much larger, restriction fragments are generated. Until relatively recently, the characterization of large DNA fragments was limited by two major factors. First, DNA fragments of ≥25 kb are separated poorly or not at all by conventional agarose gel electrophoresis; second, DNA prepared in solution is spontaneously sheared into random fragments typically of ≤100 kb. Pulsed-field gel electrophoresis (PFGE), developed by Schwartz and Cantor in 1984 (134), is a variation of agarose gel electrophoresis in which the orientation of the electric field across the gel is changed periodically ("pulsed") rather than being kept constant as in conventional agarose gel electrophoresis used for the REA and Southern blot studies described above. For technical reasons (23), this critical modification enables DNA fragments as large as megabases to be separated effectively by size. Suitable unsheared DNA is obtained by embedding intact organisms in agarose plugs ("inserts") and enzymatically lysing the cell wall and digesting the cellular proteins. The isolated genomes are then digested in situ with restriction enzymes that have few recognition sites (6, 92). PFGE analysis of such digests provides a chromosomal restriction profile typically composed of 5 to 20 distinct, well-resolved fragments ranging from approximately 10 to 800 kb (Fig. 1). All bacterial isolates are theoretically typeable by PFGE, and the results are highly reproducible. The relative simplicity of the restriction profiles greatly facilitates the analysis and comparison of multiple isolates.

PFGE has been applied to a wide range of organisms (92)

and has proven to be highly discriminatory and reproducible, with performance comparable or superior to that of other available techniques (Fig. 1) (6, 9, 103, 121, 123, 150). At this time, PFGE is the strain typing method of choice for many commonly encountered bacterial pathogens, including staphylococci, enterococci, members of the family *Enterobacteriaceae*, *Pseudomonas aeruginosa* and other gram-negative rods, and nontuberculous mycobacteria. However, as mentioned above, some pathogens, such as methicillin-resistant *S. aureus*, *H. influenzae* type b, and *E. coli* O157:H7, represent genetically restricted subsets of strains within a species (74, 109, 168), and consequently, epidemiologically unrelated isolates may have very similar genotypes and may be indistinguishable by PFGE, as well as by other typing methods (26, 150).

PFGE has two notable limitations. First, because of the need to diffuse all buffers and enzymes into the agarose insert, the preparation of suitable DNA involves several extended incubations and takes from 2 to 4 days (92). This effort is partially offset by the fact that DNA in agarose is stable for years at 4°C and can easily be released into solution for use in other protocols. Recently, substantially shorter protocols have been reported for staphylococci and enterococci (16, 79) and may be feasible for additional species. Second, PFGE requires relatively expensive, specialized equipment (23).

Typing Systems Applying PCR

PCR is increasingly being applied to the detection of infectious agents (116). The essential feature of PCR is the ability to replicate ("amplify") rapidly and exponentially a particular DNA sequence (the "template"). The basic procedure involves several distinct components. (i) The template should represent a relatively small fragment of DNA, typically 0.5 to 2.0 kb, because larger target sequences are more difficult to amplify efficiently. Only minute quantities of the template need be present; theoretically, even a single copy is detectable. (ii) Two small oligonucleotides (termed "primers"), corresponding to sequences at opposite ends of the template, define the sites at which replication is initiated. The primers should be long enough to define those sites uniquely; on the basis of statistical calculations, 18 to 20 bp is typically sufficient. A cycle of replication involves denaturation of the double-stranded DNA template, binding of the primers to each strand of the template, and then synthesis ("polymerization") of the complementary strand. (iii) A rapid, self-contained "chain reaction" is achieved by using thermostable DNA polymerases and programmable thermocyclers. An entire procedure, consisting of 20 to 30 cycles, can be conducted in a small, closed container (e.g., a microcentrifuge tube) and within a few hours will generate sufficient product ("amplicon") to be visualized and sized directly in an agarose or polyacrylamide gel.

PCR can be readily performed with commercially available reagents and thermocyclers. Since contamination with even a single copy of target DNA can produce a false-positive result, many experienced workers recommend having two physically separate work areas—one for preparing the samples and the other for performing the reactions. For diagnostic purposes, the basic procedure described above can be used directly to detect the presence of the target sequences within a sample (chapter 13). Numerous variations have been proposed to provide additional information to distinguish different strains, and the development of new applications of PCR for molecular strain typing is a very active area of investigation.

Restriction Digestion of PCR Products

In the most direct modification, the PCR product is digested with a restriction endonuclease and the resulting restriction fragments are analyzed for polymorphisms by electrophoresis. This approach has been successfully used to type strains of both fungi and bacteria, including *Cryptococcus neoformans*, *S. aureus*, *Helicobacter pylori*, mycobacteria, and *Rochalimaea* (54, 94, 148, 163). The restriction digests are highly reproducible; however, the discriminatory power of the approach varies substantially for different species, loci, and restriction enzymes. In some instances, the digest patterns are species specific but do not identify individual strains (148), whereas in other analyses, the approach appears to be moderately discriminatory (54). Strain differentiation can be increased by evaluating digests prepared with several different restriction enzymes (94) or by using new techniques to obtain substantially larger PCR products and thus to have more restriction sites available for analysis (139).

Since a highly homogeneous PCR product is required to obtain distinct restriction fragments, some investigators have used nested PCR (54). This procedure involves a second set of primers representing sequences located inside ("nested" within) the target sequences of the initial primers. The second set of primers is added to the reaction mixture after approximately half the cycles, at which time numerous copies of the fragment specified by the initial primers have been produced. Consequently, the subfragment defined by the nested primers is amplified very rapidly. In contrast, any extraneous fragments, i.e., those generated by unanticipated binding of the first set of primers to sites other than the intended target, will not have sequences homologous to the nested primers and will not be replicated further. Thus, the final amplicon is highly enriched for the nested subfragment; this protocol obviously requires more reagents and technical effort than the routine procedure.

AP-PCR

The arbitrarily primed PCR (AP-PCR) variation, also referred to as the randomly amplified polymorphic DNA (RAPD) assay, is based on the observation that short primers (typically 10 bp) whose sequence is not directed to any known genetic locus will nevertheless hybridize at random chromosomal sites with sufficient affinity to permit the initiation of polymerization. If two such sites are located within a few kilobases of each other on opposite DNA strands and in the proper orientation, then amplification of the intervening fragment will occur (167, 170). The number and locations of these random sites will vary among different strains, and thus, the number and sizes of the fragments detected by electrophoresis of the amplicon will also vary. The approach is attractive because it is conceptually simple and theoretically suitable for use with any organism, although the identification of a suitable primer(s) may require considerable effort (80). Numerous reports have described the application of AP-PCR to the strain typing of multiple different species of bacteria and fungi (1, 14, 21, 34, 73, 78, 110, 125, 130, 159).

In practice, however, there are significant problems in achieving reproducible, discriminatory results by AP-PCR. Compared with PCR with conventional site-specific primers, the reaction conditions (e.g., the hybridization temperature) used in AP-PCR are typically less stringent in order to facilitate the initiation of the polymerization reaction at sites having one or more sequence mismatches. However, polymerization is initiated with various efficiencies at such sites, and the final quantities of DNA produced may vary widely among the different fragments amplified from a given isolate. Consequently, when the products of the reaction are visualized by ethidium bromide staining, the individual bands produced for that isolate may vary widely in intensity.

Such variation is inherent in AP-PCR, is almost always present, and introduces several specific problems. First, it can be quite difficult to compare and interpret patterns whose bands demonstrate such differences in intensity (130). Second, because some of the products may represent relatively inefficient reactions, the actual fragments generated from a particular isolate may vary substantially among different amplification reactions due to minor variations in technical factors such as temperature, Mg^{2+} concentration, and source of polymerase (80, 122). An additional factor impairing the reproducibility of AP-PCR in some instances may be the amplification of fragments encoded by cryptic prophages or plasmids, which may be gained or lost unpredictably (161).

Decreased reproducibility directly compromises discriminatory power (64) and greatly impedes comparison of results among different laboratories. Both of these problems have been observed in two large studies in which sets of isolates were analyzed by AP-PCR in multiple laboratories (157). In general, AP-PCR has proven to be less discriminatory than PFGE (130)

Some reports indicate that reproducibility can be increased by using defined concentrations of purified DNA (155) and that the discriminatory power of the technique can be increased by performing multiple amplifications with different primers (143). Although PCR itself is rapid, such efforts substantially increase the time and effort required to implement the procedure.

rep-PCR

As initially described, PCR based on repetitive chromosomal sequences (rep-PCR) uses primers based on short extragenic repetitive sequences which have been identified for many members of the family *Enterobacteriaceae* and for some gram-positive bacteria, as well as for fungi (156, 162, 173). Such sequences are typically present at many sites around the bacterial chromosome; when two sequences are located near enough to each other (e.g., within a few kilobases), then the DNA fragment between those sites (referred to as an "interrepeat" fragment) is effectively amplified. Since the number and locations of the repetitive sequences are quite variable, the number and size of the interrepeat fragments generated can similarly vary from strain to strain. The initial reports suggested that this technique has good reproducibility and moderate discriminatory power. For example, in an analysis of 29 epidemiologically unrelated isolates of *Citrobacter diversus*, 16 rep-PCR profiles were detected among isolates representing 14 MLEE types (173).

The same strategy has been applied with other sequences represented repeatedly at diverse chromosomal sites, including sequences related to ribosomal operons (139), insertion elements (41), and the Shine-Dalgarno ribosomal binding site (41). Species-specific polymorphic repetitive elements have also been identified. For example, PCR with repetitive sequences present in M. *tuberculosis* has proven to be useful for typing those M. *tuberculosis* isolates for which IS*6110* analysis is poorly discriminatory because fewer than five copies are present (50).

Although some amplicons generated by PCR based on repetitive sequences demonstrate very crisp, distinct fragments, more commonly there is considerable variability in the intensities of the fragments generated; similar to that typical of AP-PCR systems. Plikaytis et al. (120) performed a highly informative experiment to determine the nature of the fragments generated in their system, which used two primers, one derived from IS*6110* and the other derived from a tandem repeat element widely dispersed in the M. *tuberculosis* genome. A Southern blot was prepared from the agarose gel resolving the amplified fragments and was probed with a portion of IS*6110* that should have been present in all products generated if the system performed as predicted. In fact, a large proportion of the fragments apparent in the gel were not detected on the Southern blot. The investigators concluded that such fragments, which included some of the most prominent products visible in the ethidium bromide-stained gel, were generated as a result of "mispriming"; that is, they were randomly amplified. To the extent that the PCR amplicons produced with primers directed at repetitive sequences actually represent arbitrary priming, then the reproducibility of the approach is likely to suffer the same limitations that characterize AP-PCR (158).

Collier et al. (40) directly compared PFGE, PCR typing with rRNA-directed primers, and PCR with arbitrary primers for analyzing well-characterized isolates of C. *difficile*. "PCR ribotyping" proved to be more reproducible and discriminatory than AP-PCR and nearly as discriminatory as PFGE. The results of AP-PCR and PFGE were poorly concordant, suggesting that artifactual variation was affecting the AP-PCR patterns. In contrast, PCR ribotyping and PFGE gave highly concordant results, suggesting that both techniques were similarly detecting underlying genomic diversity. If these results can be reproduced in other laboratories, PCR ribotyping may become the method of choice for the strain typing of C. *difficile*.

PCR-Based Detection of Restriction Sites

The most recent adaptations of PCR to molecular strain typing are directed toward the detection of restriction sites. In amplified restriction fragment length polymorphism (AFLP) analysis, whole-cell DNA is digested with a relatively frequently cutting restriction enzyme and then specific oligonucleotide linkers that match the digested ends of the fragment are ligated to the fragments (165). By using primers that are directed toward the linker and the restriction sequence plus additional arbitrary sequences extending into the restriction fragment, it is possible to selectively amplify a random subset of fragments without prior knowledge of particular target nucleotide sequences. The number of fragments generated can vary substantially on the basis of the choice of primers and the amplification conditions. Initial reports describe 30 to 100 fragments ranging from 80 to 550 bp and claim high discriminatory power (68, 165). As might be expected, some of the variable fragments represent plasmid-associated sequences sequences present on episomal plasmids (72).

Infrequent-restriction-site PCR (IRS-PCR) is designed to detect variations in the number and location of infrequently cutting restriction sites (98); such variations are at least partially responsible for the discriminatory power demonstrated by PFGE. Template DNA is digested with both one infrequently cutting and one frequently cutting restriction enzyme and is then ligated to two pairs of linkers, one pair directed toward each restriction site. Amplification proceeds with two primers, one directed toward each linker. The amplicon is a set of fragments each representing the sequences on one flank of a different infrequent restriction site. The initial report suggests that the specificities of the linkers and primers make this approach relatively stable to minor variations in PCR conditions.

Additional detailed evaluations of the discriminatory powers and reproducibilities of these new approaches should be forthcoming. The major challenges will be to develop protocols that can be applied to multiple different bacterial species and to avoid the problems of reproducibility that have been associated with AP-PCR.

Nucleotide Sequence Analysis

Cloning and sequencing of a particular locus in even a single isolate once represented a substantial technical effort. Two developments have made it feasible to compare multiple isolates by sequencing each one at the same locus: (i) PCR, which enables a known DNA segment to be rapidly amplified and isolated; and (ii) automated sequencers, which can typically sequence 500 bp in a single run. This approach has been used to analyze the natural variation within bacterial populations and clearly provides highly reliable and objective data suitable for subsequent quantitative analyses (46).

PCR-based sequence analysis of bacterial rRNA genes has been used to detect and identify bacterial pathogens that cannot be recovered from infected tissues by culture techniques. Because certain ribosomal sequences are highly conserved across the bacterial kingdom, primers that will amplify ribosomal sequences from essentially any bacterium can be defined. By sequencing the amplified product and analyzing the relatively variable areas within the ribosomal operon, the family, genus, and species of the infecting organism can be identified. This approach has successfully detected bacteria corresponding to an unusual gram-positive actinomycete in the tissues of patients with Whipple's disease (126) and a new *Mycobacterium* species causing disseminated disease in patients with AIDS (27).

A particularly attractive advantage of nucleotide sequences is that the data are precise and extensive databases can be shared with relative ease, thus facilitating comparative analyses. For example, sequence analysis of the *rpoB* chromosomal locus of multiple *M. tuberculosis* isolates has identified the distribution of different point mutations that result in rifampin resistance (147). The combination of IS*6110* Southern blot analysis and nucleotide sequencing of antibiotic resistance loci was applied to a large collection of MDR *M. tuberculosis* isolates (20). The analysis resolved the origin, spread, and molecular evolution of an extended lineage comprising more than a dozen related IS*6110* types and multiple different drug resistance phenotypes. Nucleotide sequencing has also been used to analyze an outbreak of *S. pyogenes* invasive disease (108).

Although nucleotide sequencing may emerge as the strain typing method of choice for reference laboratories (105), several critical issues are unresolved. First, loci with sufficient sequence variability to permit epidemiologically useful strain differentiation must be identified for each bacterial species. In particular, the loci must be present in all isolates and have sufficient sequence variability within a span that is practical for repeated sequencing with multiple isolates. Furthermore, it is not clear if sequencing at a single locus will provide reliable, unambiguous strain identification (24, 46). Finally, automated sequencers remain prohibitively expensive for most settings.

MOLECULAR TYPING OF SPECIFIC ORGANISMS

In practice, the majority of hospital-based epidemiologic analyses involve a relatively limited set of organisms. Virtually every method described has been applied to these species, and a consideration of all available reports is outside the scope of this review. A recent position paper by the Society of Hospital Epidemiologists of America has identified the preferred techniques for common bacterial pathogens (151) (Table 4). This section will focus on those recommendations and will emphasize the use of the two most commonly cited approaches—PFGE and PCR-based techniques.

TABLE 4 Preferred strain typing techniques for common bacterial pathogens[a]

Species	Reference method	Alternative methods
Staphylococcus aureus	PFGE	AP-PCR, plasmid analysis[b]
Coagulase-negative staphylococci	PFGE	
Streptococcus pneumoniae	PFGE	Serotyping
Enterococci	PFGE	AP-PCR
Escherichia coli,[c] *Citrobacter, Proteus, Providencia*	PFGE	AP-PCR
Klebsiella, Enterobacter, Serratia	PFGE	Plasmid analysis
Salmonella, Shigella	Serotyping	PFGE
Pseudomonas aeruginosa	PFGE	
Clostridium difficile	rep-PCR, AP-PCR	REA, PFGE[d]
Myocbacterium tuberculosis	IS*6110* RFLP	rep-PCR
Mycobacteria other than *M. tuberculosis*	PFGE	

[a] The table is adapted from Tenover et al. (151); the judgments represent the views of the author. Abbreviations: IS*6110* RFLP, RFLPs detected on Southern blots probed with IS*6110*; rep-PCR, PCR with primers directed toward repetitive chromosomal elements (e.g., ribosomal sequences and repetitive oligonucleotide sequences). The other abbreviations are defined in the text.

[b] Plasmid analysis may include restriction digestion of plasmids.

[c] *E. coli* O157:H7 must be identified by serotyping.

[d] Many isolates of *C. difficile* are nontypeable by PFGE due to DNA degradation.

S. aureus

Because of their virulence, their frequent association with nosocomial outbreaks, and the emergence of MDR strains, isolates of *S. aureus* have been the subject of numerous epidemiologic studies and have been examined by essentially all of the available typing techniques (4). PFGE has been reported to be the most discriminatory method available, particularly for MRSA, and is the preferred reference method (15, 66, 123, 132, 144). Plasmid restriction digests have frequently proven to be useful (15, 31, 118). A multicenter study of AP-PCR suggests that it has good discriminatory power, although there are problems with reproducibility and interpretation (157).

Tenover et al. (150) examined 59 isolates of *S. aureus*, including methicillin-susceptible and -resistant strains, using 14 different methods. The study set contained 29 isolates representing four distinct, previously established outbreaks, plus additional epidemiologically related and unrelated isolates. This is the largest available analysis of a substantial set of isolates (of any species) evaluated by multiple techniques, and it represents a paradigm for both the insights and the complexities associated with such an investigation. In this study, PFGE detected essentially all outbreak isolates, but it failed to discriminate an appreciable number of control strains. This result may reflect a subtle bias in that the control isolates were often selected to have the same bacteriophage type as the outbreak strain; however, epidemiologically unrelated isolates representing the same phage type are more likely to be genetically related than truly random isolates (25). In contrast, plasmid analysis, which is independent of the host strain genome, was highly effective at differentiating the outbreak strains from the controls, but it was less consistent at detecting the outbreak isolates. Taken together, these data suggest that in particularly complex or ambiguous situations a combination of techniques that assess qualitatively different characteristics may be of value.

Coagulase-Negative Staphylococci

PFGE is the recommended strain typing technique for *Staphylococcus epidermidis* and other coagulase-negative staphylococci (52, 63). Plasmid analyses have also been very effective (11, 32); however, plasmid variability can be appreciable (10, 101). Although phenotypic studies have generally demonstrated extensive variation among *S. epidermidis* isolates, recent genotypic analyses suggest that, as for other pathogens, clinically significant isolates may represent a genetically restricted subset of the species. Specifically, the same ribotypes have been detected among geographically distant isolates, and a study of isolates cultured from the bloodstreams of infants treated in a neonatal intensive care unit demonstrated endemic persistence of the same PFGE types (63). These observations suggest that certain lineages or genotypes of *S. epidermidis* may have greater pathogenicity, perhaps related to such virulence factors as surface adhesions (154).

Enterococci

PFGE has emerged as the method of choice for analyzing isolates of the genus *Enterococcus* (44, 103, 104, 115).

E. coli and Other Members of the Family *Enterobacteriaceae*

PFGE is the most effective method for differentiating among isolates of *E. coli* and has proven to be appreciably more discriminatory than MLEE or ribotyping (6). Nevertheless, some epidemiologically unrelated isolates representing the same genetic lineage as defined by complete serotyping will have indistinguishable PFGE profiles (26, 114, 175). Although the data are limited, PFGE also appears to be highly effective for typing other members of the family *Enterobacteriaceae*, such as *Klebsiella* (87) and *Enterobacter* (61).

Alternative techniques for strain typing of the *Enterobacteriaceae* include plasmid analysis, rep-PCR, and AP-PCR (96, 131).

Serotyping remains the primary basis for characterizing *Salmonella* and *Shigella* isolates and appears to be reasonably well correlated with distinct genetic lineages (18). PFGE is a useful alternative technique (17), although reliably differentiating among epidemiologically unrelated isolates of the same serotype is often difficult, reflecting restricted genetic diversity (153).

Pseudomonas and Other Aerobic Gram-Negative Rods

PFGE has been demonstrated to be highly effective for analyzing isolates of *Pseudomonas aeruginosa*, *Pseudomonas cepacia*, and *Acinetobacter* (3, 28, 56, 57, 121, 169).

C. difficile

At this time, the application of PFGE to clinical isolates of *C. difficile* appears to be hindered by an unusual technical problem that has not been encountered with other microbial species. For 10 to 40% of nosocomial isolates of *C. difficile*, the standard protocol for in situ lysis in agarose yields genomic DNA that is partially degraded and, consequently, that is not suitable for PFGE analysis (76). Among those isolates that can be analyzed by PFGE, the discriminatory power of the technique is comparable to that of routine REA; both methods are superior to ribotyping.

Currently, PCR-based methods including AP-PCR and rep-PCR are the methods of choice for typing *C. difficile* (40). Routine REA of chromosomal DNA has also been effective at deciphering epidemiologic relationships among *C. difficile* isolates (37, 42, 71). However, interpretation of the complex patterns detected by this method requires experience, and comparison of large numbers of strains is often difficult (76).

Mycobacteria

With the resurgence of tuberculosis associated with the human immunodeficiency virus (HIV) pandemic and the development of outbreaks due to MDR strains, the typing of *M. tuberculosis* has become an urgent issue. As noted above, the current method of choice is Southern blot analysis of the RFLPs associated with IS*6110* (160). A major limitation of this system is that the preparation of suitable DNA requires the handling of high concentrations of this pathogen and, consequently, requires more stringent containment facilities than those required for handling routine bacterial isolates (127). Alternative approaches by PCR-based methods may bypass this problem (120). PFGE is also effective for typing isolates of the *M. tuberculosis* complex (75, 174).

PFGE has successfully been used to analyze isolates of many different nontuberculous mycobacterial species, including the *M. avium* complex (MAC), *M. gordonae*, and *M. fortuitum* (9, 33, 97). For MAC isolates in particular, PFGE provides excellent discriminatory power (9, 138, 164). The IRS-PCR technique was initially applied to MAC isolates and provided excellent results (98). Isolates of *M. avium* typically carry multiple polymorphic copies of IS*1245*, which have been used for typing in conjunction with Southern blot analysis or PCR (59).

APPLICATION OF MICROBIAL TYPING SYSTEMS

Most requests for microbial typing reflect one apparently simple question: "Are these isolates the same or different?" As noted above, the implicit assumptions are that epidemiologically related isolates represent the clonal expansion of a single precursor, that such clonal isolates will be of the same type, and that unrelated isolates will have different types. A constructive response to this ingenuous question requires an appreciation of the complexities inherent both in microbial biology and in obtaining and interpreting typing data.

Factors Complicating Interpretation of Strain Typing Data

As emphasized above, natural biologic variation provides the basis for all strain typing systems; however, such variation can also complicate the interpretation of strain typing data. In any typing system, a change(s) that can be attributed to a single genetic event (e.g., a difference in a single metabolic enzyme [87] or the shift of a single band on an electrophoretic gel) is not a reliable basis for concluding that two isolates represent different strains, that is, are epidemiologically unrelated (92). Such variations may be present, albeit infrequently, by both Southern blotting and PFGE analysis of multiple isolates from the same or sequential cultures of blood from individual patients (8, 9). Although such isolates are not strict "clones," they are so closely related both epidemiologically and genetically that they are presumed to be recently derived from a common precursor. These observations reinforce the fact that clonality is a relative concept (48). In studies examining isolates collected over an extended interval and/or from multiple patients, epidemiologically related isolates of the same strain are relatively likely to demonstrate minor typing differences due to phenotypic variation or actual genotypic alterations, for example, changes in plasmid or phage content or sequence mutations altering restriction sites (150).

Both biologic and technical variabilities directly limit the reproducibilities of molecular typing methods, which in turn limit their discriminatory powers (64). That is, if isolates known to represent the same strain can differ to a certain degree (e.g., a single band shift), then random isolates demonstrating such differences cannot be reliably designated different strains. The interpretation of molecular typing data must explicitly address these ambiguities.

Finally, the nature of the typing data itself may create difficulties. The most widely used genotypic typing systems are based on the detection of RFLPs (e.g., plasmid digests, Southern blot analyses, and PFGE) or simply polymorphisms within amplicons (e.g., AP-PCR). In these systems, an isolate is represented by a pattern of fragments—a "fingerprint"—which is affected by variations in the underlying DNA as well as by technical variations in the method, such as amplification or electrophoresis conditions. A comparison of two patterns involves a series of judgments, some of which are relatively objective (e.g., are the same number of fragments present?), while others are more subjective and inherently imprecise (e.g., are two corresponding fragments the same size?). The comparisons can be made more reliable and consistent by using reference standards, strict criteria, and computer imaging, although such procedures may entail considerable effort and expense (171). The different approaches to interpreting typing data also seek to minimize the limitations of typing systems based on DNA fragments. However, as discussed below, some methods for interpretation may obscure or misrepresent the actual results and thus create new problems.

Interpretation of Typing Results

The most common goal of molecular strain typing is to define the genotypic relationships among a set of isolates and thereby infer their epidemiologic relationships. One approach to reconciling the limitations inherent in molecular typing with the need for clinically and epidemiologically useful reports is to associate different classes of genetic relatedness with different probabilities of clinical and epidemiologic relatedness (149). This method, which is considered in detail below, was specifically developed for the analysis of PFGE profiles, on which the impacts of specific particular genetic events can be predicted. The approach is readily applied to Southern blot analysis but not to AP-PCR.

The interpretation of typing data can be further facilitated by (i) restricting the analysis to a discrete set of isolates (typically ≤30) and (ii) identifying an "index isolate" to serve as a starting point for the analysis. Limiting the number of isolates effectively limits the number of comparisons and is almost essential in the absence of computer imaging systems, although with experience sets of up to 75 isolates can be evaluated manually (58, 86). The index isolate (or strain) serves as a meaningful starting point for the analysis and can be defined on the basis of epidemiologic data (e.g., the first case in a putative outbreak), clinical data (e.g., the initial isolate from a patient with multiple episodes of infection), or even the strain typing data themselves (e.g., the modal or most common strain type in the set).

The analysis then proceeds by comparing the typing pattern for each isolate in the set with the pattern for the index isolate. For the purposes of this discussion, the isolates being examined will be assumed to represent a putative outbreak. The index isolate will be defined as an isolate representing the most common (or modal) typing profile detected within the set; such isolates would typically be considered collectively to represent the outbreak strain. The goal of the interpretative process is to use the typing data to predict the clinical and epidemiologic relationships among isolates (Table 5).

Multiple isolates representing a single type are most appropriately designated "indistinguishable." This description emphasizes that the analysis is critically dependent on the particular typing system used and that an alternative typing system might resolve differences, albeit typically minor. Strictly defined, a clone is "one or more genetically identical organisms descended from a single common ancestor" (2).

TABLE 5 Criteria for interpreting genotypic strain typing patterns among a set of isolates (typically ≤30) collected to evaluate a putative outbreak[a]

Category	No. of genetic differences compared with outbreak strain[b]	No. of fragment differences compared with outbreak strain in PFGE analysis[c]	Inferred relationship between isolate and outbreak strain
Indistinguishable[c]	0	0	Isolate represents the outbreak strain
Closely related	1	2–3	Isolate probably represents the outbreak strain
Possibly related	2	4–6	Isolate possibly represents the outbreak strain
Different	≥3	≥7	Isolate is different from the outbreak strain

[a] Adapted from Tenover et al. (149). These criteria are most appropriate for genomic analyses performed by gel electrophoresis (e.g., PFGE, ribotyping, and Southern blot analysis).

[b] Presumes that there is a single most common (modal) genotype which represents the putative outbreak strain. In other contexts, an "index isolate" may be designated as the internal referent. See text for details.

[c] See Fig. 4 for examples. The specific pattern changes that can result from a single genetic event will vary with the typing technique.

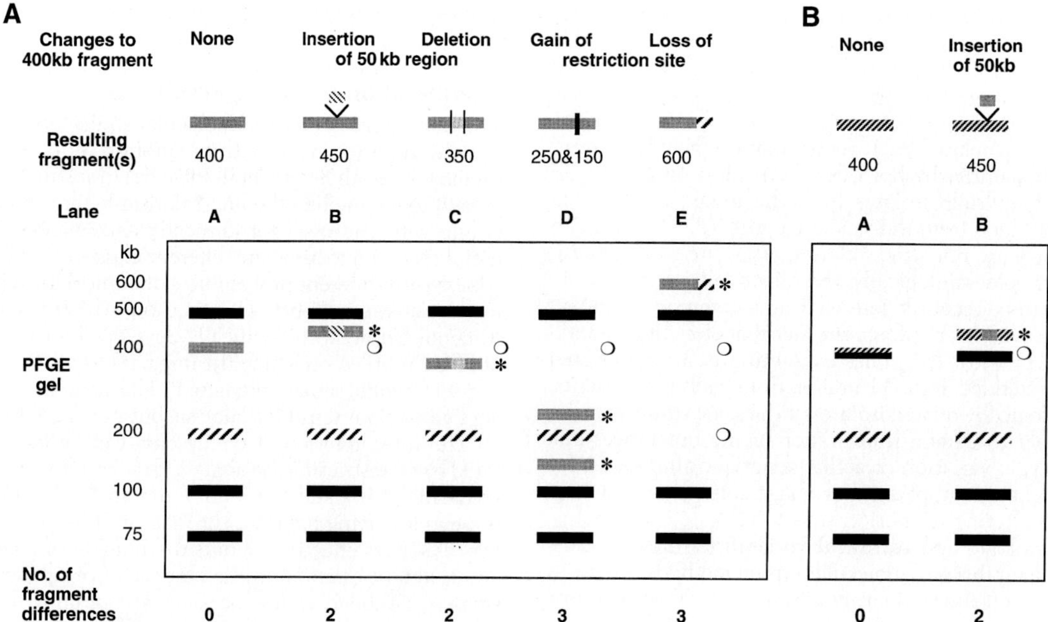

FIGURE 4 (A) Schematic diagram depicting the changes in the PFGE pattern of an isolate as a result of different classes of single genetic events. Lane A, index (outbreak) pattern; lane B, insertion of 50 kb of DNA into a 400-kb fragment; lane C, deletion of 50 kb of DNA from a 400-kb fragment; lane D, gain of a restriction site within the 400-kb fragment; lane E, loss of a restriction site between the 400- and 200-kb fragments. Open circles, fragments present in the index pattern and missing from the comparison isolate as a consequence of the genetic event; asterisks, fragments absent from the index pattern and present only after the genetic event. The number of fragment differences represents the total number of fragments present in either the index or the comparison isolate, but not in both. (B) Schematic diagram depicting a change in a PFGE pattern that appears to represent the addition of an entire restriction fragment. Lane A, an index isolate for which two restriction fragments are essentially the same size (~400 kb) and therefore comigrate; lane B, the comparison isolate which appears to have an entire new 450-kb fragment, but in fact the change in the pattern reflects the simple shift of one of the comigrating 400-kb fragments due to the insertion of 50 kb of DNA. On reflection, it is implausible to postulate the insertion or duplication of a large DNA region that is precisely flanked by restriction sites. This example also emphasizes the fact that comigrating fragments in different isolates need not represent the same DNA sequences. This figure appeared previously (4).

No typing method confirms that the entire genomes of two organisms are identical. Nevertheless, for highly discriminatory methods that consistently distinguish among epidemiologically unrelated isolates, the observation that two isolates represent the same type strongly suggests that they are both genetically and epidemiologically related (6).

Isolates whose typing profiles differ from that of the outbreak strain by a single genetic event are considered "closely related" genetically and "probably part of the outbreak" for clinical or epidemiologic purposes. Figure 4 illustrates examples of the effect of single genetic events on PFGE profiles. These designations emphasize that this level of genetic variability is not uncommon among clinically and epidemiologically related isolates derived from a common precursor. Isolates whose profiles differ from that of the outbreak stain by two genetic events are considered "possibly related" genetically and "possibly part of the outbreak." This represents an equivocal or borderline category; additional genotypic or epidemiologic data may be required to resolve the relationships among these isolates. Isolates whose profiles differ by three or more genetic events are considered genetically "different" and not part of the outbreak. The final decision about whether to include closely and possibly related isolates in the epidemiologic case definition of the outbreak represents the integration of the molecular and clinical analyses.

Potential Problems in Interpreting Typing Data

Although the approach described above can be highly effective, the process of multiple comparisons can create awkward assignments. For example, two different "possibly related" genotypes might differ from each other by more than three genetic events and thus appear to have diverged into different strains. Additional problems can arise in the absence of an index isolate or type; for example, a given isolate might be related to isolates representing distinctly different types.

Such logical confounds can also complicate other methods of analysis. In many typing systems, isolates are assigned different types if they differ in some specified manner (e.g., two or more different antibiotic susceptibilities or bacteriophage reactions or three or more band shifts on a Southern blot analysis). Isolates that differ but that do not differ sufficiently to be designated distinct types are typically designated a subtype of the most similar type. This process is also potentially problematic. For example, an isolate might represent a subtype of either of two different types; con-

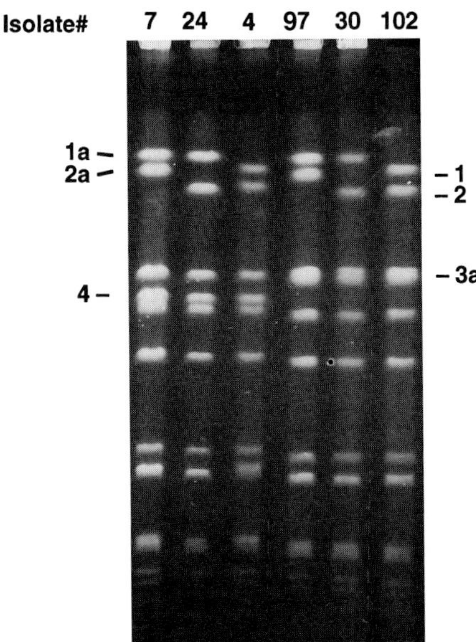

FIGURE 5 How many strains? Analysis of MRSA isolates by PFGE of *Sma*I restriction digests. All isolates were obtained from a single hospital over the course of 1 year; each pattern shown was represented by 1 to 13 isolates among more than 75 isolates examined. The set of isolates explicitly illustrates the difficulty of unambiguously designating types and subtypes, because most pairs of isolates differ by only one or two bands, but two pairs (isolates 4 and 97 and isolates 7 and 102) differ by three bands. In addition, Southern blot analyses (data not shown) indicate that the bands designated 1, 2, and 4 shift to bands 1a, 2a, and 3a, respectively, due to the insertion of three different lysogenic bacteriophages. Thus, all six isolates have indistinguishable *Sma*I restriction fragments with respect to chromosomal DNA but differ by the presence or absence of three different lysogenic bacteriophages. All isolates for which results are presented here were run in a single gel (4a).

versely, two subtypes of a particular type might differ sufficiently from each other to define distinct types (Fig. 5). While the approach to interpretation described above does not avoid all of these problems, the identification of an index isolate and the application of defined categories help make such complexities in the typing data more explicit and facilitate collaboration between the typing laboratory and the epidemiologist or clinician.

In some reports, complex typing data have been analyzed by numerical and graphical methods (e.g., with Dice coefficients and by use of dendrograms) developed for the study of evolutionary and population genetics. These powerful computational techniques require data sets that meet certain critical assumptions; in particular, each isolate must be described with respect to multiple distinct characteristics that vary independently. The most robust data for such analyses are nucleotide sequences, in which each nucleotide position is a characteristic and each substitution is an allelic variant (45). MLEE data are also suitable (5, 135).

RFLP data sets typically do not satisfy these requirements. Each restriction fragment does not represent a separate, distinct characteristic; rather, it is defined by two restriction sites, each comprising 4, 6, or 8 nucleotides. In the simplest situation—an analysis of fragments associated with a single, well-defined chromosomal locus in which one restriction site is highly conserved and essentially invariant—the relationships among distinct polymorphisms can be resolved, as described by Kreiswirth et al. (74) for a set of six RFLP classes detected in association with the *mec* locus of MRSA. However, the quantitative analysis of more complex Southern blots (e.g., ribotypes or IS elements present at multiple loci) is highly problematic, because variations in the RFLP profile cannot be attributed to specific individual restriction sites. For PFGE profiles, which represent the entire circular chromosome, the creation or loss of a single restriction site affects two fragments. Moreover, fragments of the same molecular size cannot be assumed to represent the same chromosomal region; this can be determined only by preparing PFGE-based Southern blots and physically mapping specific loci (7, 26, 114). Conversely, restriction fragments of different sizes may represent the same chromosomal DNA and may differ due to the insertion or deletion of extrachromosomal DNA, such as bacteriophage DNA (Fig. 5) (7, 35, 81). For obvious reasons, the variations in amplicons generated by AP-PCR are even less suitable for analysis.

The Dice coefficient quantitates the similarity between two items (in Dice's examples, different species; here, different isolates) and is expressed algebraically as $2 \cdot n/(a + b)$, where a and b are the number of characteristics (here, restriction fragments) assessed for each of the two items, and n is the number of characteristics that both items have in common (43). Dice's approach offers a consistent system for enumerating the differences between the two profiles (Fig. 4). For two isolates whose complex restriction fragment profiles differ only minimally, the assumption that all shared elements of the profile represent the same DNA is likely sound and the resulting coefficients are conceptually valid. Thus, isolates whose RFLP patterns are highly similar as indicated by a Dice coefficient of ≥ 0.90 are likely to be related genetically and thus possibly epidemiologically. Because Dice coefficients represent a numerical result readily manipulated by digital computers, they can facilitate the application of computer imaging and analysis systems to the screening of RFLP databases and the finding of potentially related isolates (20, 171). Typically, such putative matches must be confirmed by visual examination of the original patterns or direct side-by-side comparisons.

For RFLP patterns that demonstrate more than minimal divergence, the assumption that two fragments with similar positions represent the same DNA is not appropriate for the reasons discussed above and the coefficients are considerably less meaningful, although the apparent quantitative precision confers an air of accuracy. Thus, the analysis of sizable collections of RFLP patterns from diverse isolates by means of a matrix of Dice coefficients, the application of numerical methods, and the construction of graphical representations (e.g., dendrograms) is questionable.

Two recent studies have examined the relationships defined among sets of isolates as determined by PFGE and AP-PCR (17a, 36). In both reports, isolates that were indistinguishable or very closely related by one method were typically also closely related by the other method. This is consistent with the basic concept that DNA typing systems identify specific genotypes or genetic lineages. Overall, however, dendrograms based on the different DNA typing systems gave substantially different results; that is, the relative genetic distance (relatedness) among different genotypes varied greatly between the two systems. Mathiesen et al. (95) analyzed *Borrelia burgdorferi* isolates using both PFGE and nucleotide sequencing. Isolates that were closely related by PFGE were typically closely related by sequencing, but the two approaches correlated poorly for more distantly related isolates. In contrast, dendrograms based on nucleotide sequences at different loci are typically highly congruent (146). Taken together these observations strongly suggest that DNA fragment data are not suitable for quantitating genetic relatedness among diverse isolates.

Detection of Outbreaks

Typing methods have been widely applied in epidemiologic studies of transmissible bacterial infections. However, since true-positive and true-negative results typically cannot be established, the performance of a typing method is surprisingly difficult to express quantitatively. Nevertheless, the basic principles used in considering the performance of other laboratory tests remain relevant (67). In particular, the concept of "prior probability" is directly applicable—that is, the reliability of typing results indicating that isolates represent the same strain is directly influenced by the likelihood that the isolates were epidemiologically related independent of the results of typing.

Epidemiologic investigations are typically triggered by an increase in the prevalence of infection due to a particular bacterial species, by isolating the same species from a cluster of patients, or by noting multiple isolates with a distinctive biotype or antibiotic susceptibility pattern. Thus, basic infection control surveillance and routine laboratory evaluation of isolates are practical epidemiologic screening tools. Such putative outbreaks are best established by detailed epidemiologic investigation, with molecular typing studies serving to verify that the isolates represent a single strain. In this setting, strain typing is being used to confirm a strong clinical and epidemiologic hypothesis. Since there is a high prior probability that an outbreak has been defined, even a moderately reproducible and discriminatory method is likely to provide useful confirmatory data. This process was well demonstrated in an investigation of a nosocomial outbreak of *S. aureus* (31). The outbreak was initially suspected due to the increased frequency of *S. aureus* isolates with a distinctive antibiotic susceptibility pattern; the source of the outbreak, a respiratory therapist with chronic sinusitis, was identified by case-control analysis and was clearly confirmed by examining plasmid restriction digests. The molecular analysis proved to be particularly useful as the outbreak extended in time and the antibiotic susceptibility pattern of the strain changed.

However, to the extent that the typing results become a primary factor in defining the outbreak, then the limitations and vagaries of microbial typing may become critical and must be appreciated. This circumstance is illustrated in a study by Tenover et al. (150), in which epidemic and nonepidemic isolates of *S. aureus* were reanalyzed by multiple different typing methods. One outbreak in the data set was represented by four isolates of methicillin-susceptible *S. aureus* related to a contaminated anesthetic; the isolates were "originally classified by bacteriophage typing as being part of the outbreak." Three isolates from the cluster were identical by 11 additional typing methods. However, the fourth isolate represented a different strain by plasmid restriction digests, PCR-based RFLPs, and PFGE. Thus, in the absence of rigorous epidemiologic data, a less discriminatory typing method resulted in the fourth isolate being erroneously assigned to the outbreak.

The key concepts in these examples are that epidemiologic conclusions should be based on both epidemiologic and molecular typing data. To the extent that strain typing alone is used to identify putative clusters, then the prior probability of an outbreak is relatively low (i.e., the hypothesis motivating the typing is relatively weak) and, consequently, misleading (false-positive) results are more likely.

Typing techniques that are both discriminatory and reproducible can be effectively used to screen putative outbreaks to determine whether a detailed epidemiologic study is indicated. In that context, typing results indicating that a putative cluster represents multiple different strains are sufficient to rule out the presence of an outbreak. Although ribotyping has only moderate discriminatory power, a recently developed rapid, automated ribotyping system may be suitable for use as a screening method, particularly in conjunction with a second, more discriminatory technique such as PFGE (119). The value of performing confirmatory molecular typing studies has been dramatically demonstrated in situations in which the epidemiologic hypothesis was incorrect (15, 99) or ambiguous (22, 111); in each of these instances, molecular analyses served to redirect the infection control efforts.

Recent reports also indicate that, when properly applied, highly discriminatory typing methods can expand traditional concepts of nosocomial epidemiology. Classically, acute outbreaks due to a single strain are distinguished from sporadic, unrelated infections (15, 31). In contrast, several studies of nosocomial isolates representing either acute clusters or ongoing endemic persistence have documented the concurrent presence of multiple distinct strains of the same species in the hospital (49, 53, 82, 88, 111, 112, 133). These experiences emphasize the value of careful strain typing in facilitating the analysis of complex epidemiologic processes.

Distinguishing Relapse from Reinfection

In addition to assisting in epidemiologic investigations, bacterial typing can contribute to the diagnosis and management of infection in the individual patient. The analysis of multiple isolates cultured from sequential episodes of infection in an individual patient can distinguish a relapsing infection due to a single strain from reinfection due to a new strain and, thus, may help define the pathophysiology of the infection (70, 83, 88, 90, 91). The identification of a reinfection may indicate that a patient is predisposed to the particular infection due to a host defense defect (89). Culturing of the same strain from a patient during separate episodes of infection suggests relapse, possibly arising from a residual focus of infection or from a site of persistent colonization (91).

Clonality of Acute Infection

Examination of multiple different isolates of the same species cultured from a patient can be useful in evaluating the presence of infection. For example, in a patient with a prosthetic valve or cerebrospinal fluid shunt, an analysis of multiple bloodstream isolates of *S. epidermidis* indicating that the isolates represented a single strain would suggest a true bacteremia, whereas the detection of multiple different strains would be more compatible with independent skin contaminants (11). Molecular typing of *S. epidermidis* isolates from the skin and eyes of patients with acute postoperative endophthalmitis has implicated the patients' external tissues as the most common source of the infecting organisms (141). These interpretations are based on the assumption that acute infections due to a single species represent invasion and proliferation of a single strain (128), a hypothesis that has been formally confirmed for some other acute infections, such as bacteremic pyelonephritis (6).

In contrast, recent molecular analyses of disseminated M. *avium* infection among HIV-infected patients indicated that 15 to 25% concurrently have invasive disease caused by two distinctly different strains (9, 138). Polyclonal infection and colonization have also been demonstrated with subsets of patients infected or colonized with other pathogens, including *S. aureus* in hospitalized patients (88), *P. aeruginosa* in patients with cystic fibrosis (29), and *H. pylori* in patients with gastritis (51). A provocative report by Hartstein et al. (62) suggests that *Enterobacter cloacae* may frequently cause polyclonal nosocomial infection. These results suggest that different infections may have different mechanisms of pathogenesis and progression.

IMPLEMENTING A MOLECULAR EPIDEMIOLOGY LABORATORY

As the principles and practice of molecular epidemiology have become more clearly defined, many clinical laboratories faced with the need for strain typing have considered adopting molecular procedures. The ideal technique would meet multiple criteria: (i) Since clinical laboratories must be prepared to analyze isolates of virtually any species, the method should be applicable to as broad a range of organisms as possible. (ii) The method should have excellent reproducibility and discriminatory power. The results should also be reasonably easy to interpret without extensive prior experience or expertise. (iii) The feasibility and utility of an approach should have been demonstrated in multiple independent laboratories. Choosing a widely used method also facilitates obtaining consultation and assistance in the event of difficulties. (iv) A rapid turnaround time is highly desirable. (v) Cost considerations include both the initial capital equipment investment and the recurrent expense of reagents and labor. Although no strain typing system is ideal, PFGE and various PCR-based techniques are considered the two most practical and effective approaches. In the future, the full potential of nucleotide sequence analysis may be realized, but the cost of automated equipment (~$60,000) now sharply limits its dissemination.

The utility and reproducibility of PFGE have been confirmed in numerous laboratories; all the necessary reagents are commercially available, and the technical parameters are well described. Genomic restriction digests of many different microbial species can be analyzed by PFGE with only minor alterations in the procedure (102, 149). For example, different species may require additional enzymes for cell lysis, alternative restriction endonucleases for DNA digestion, or various pulsing conditions to resolve restriction fragments spanning different size ranges (23, 92). Specialized equipment is required, including an appropriately configured gel box, a programmable controller, a power supply, and a unit for cooling and recirculating the electrophoresis buffer; a UV transilluminator is also necessary. Systems of coordinated components are available from commercial suppliers for $7,000 to $20,000 (23). With the development of commercially available aids to facilitate the procedure, the technical sophistication required to implement this approach is within the reach of most clinical laboratories. Labor and material costs are estimated at ~$40 per isolate.

The power and flexibility of PCR have made it a revolutionary tool in contemporary molecular biology. However, the potential speed and ease of the method must be tempered by the need to prepare samples with great care to avoid cross-contamination. Although different primers may be required for each species, custom-prepared oligonucleotides are now commercially available on immediate request. Analysis of restriction digests of amplified fragments is the most reproducible and interpretable PCR-based approach; however, at this time, specific primers and protocols providing highly discriminatory typing have been defined and validated for only a few species. As discussed in detail above, the reproducibility and the ease of interpreting the results of AP-PCR are problematic. New approaches aimed at detecting restriction sites (e.g., AFLP and IRS-PCR) are promising, but the need for linkers and ligations is associated with both increased cost and increased technical effort. PCR can readily be performed with commercially available thermocyclers (cost, $3,000 to $7,000) and reagents; a routine gel electrophoresis system and UV transilluminator are also required. Labor and material costs are estimated at ~$20 to 25 per isolate.

Technical Aspects of Microbial Typing

Regardless of the method used, certain issues are routinely encountered in operating a typing laboratory. A clear, concise system for uniquely identifying every isolate is required, together with a log for recording the date, source (hospital, laboratory, patient, specimen, subculture, etc.), and other pertinent information. The routine clinical specimen numbers are likely to be insufficient for a typing laboratory, since the isolate identification system needs to include provision for processing multiple isolates from a single specimen or multiple different subcultures derived from the same colony. A mix-up among isolates is a potential and relatively common cause of disagreement between the typing results and the clinical epidemiology; such problems may also become apparent as logical inconsistencies between the results of two independent typing methods (76). Therefore, the isolate register should unambiguously identify repeated, independent samples representing the same initial organism. Finally, isolates may be provided by other institutions, either for primary analysis or for comparison.

With notable exceptions (160), there has been little formal concurrence about methodology, interpretation, or quality control in microbial typing. Pending such guidelines, one approach to monitoring the processing of isolates is analysis of isolates of a particular species in batches by using species-specific reference strains as concurrent internal controls. For electrophoretic typing methods, molecular weight standards or precisely characterized digests of reference strains (149) are available. Since there is no gold standard typing method, it is occasionally very useful to have the capability of analyzing isolates by two distinct methods so that the results of one system can be compared to those of the other.

Final Considerations

The application of molecular techniques to microbial typing has provided a powerful set of new tools that can facilitate both epidemiologic investigations and patient management. Typing data are most appropriately evaluated in the context of hypotheses and questions thoughtfully developed by the clinician or epidemiologist and thus are used to augment rather than replace those analyses. Ideally, typing is performed independently by the laboratory to avoid any bias, but the results are considered collaboratively to ensure that both the potential insights and the unavoidable ambiguities are clearly appreciated. The manner in which the typing results are interpreted and applied is as important as the particular method used.

REFERENCES

1. **Akopyanz, N., N. O. Bukanov, T. U. Westblom, S. Kresovich, and D. E. Berg.** 1992. DNA diversity among clinical isolates of *Helicobacter pylori* detected by PCR-based RAPD fingerprinting. *Nucleic Acids Res.* **20:** 5137–5142.
2. **American Heritage Dictionary of the English Language.** 1992. *American Heritage Dictionary of the English Language*, 3rd ed. Houghton Mifflin Company, Boston, Mass.
3. **Anderson, D. J., J. S. Kuhns, M. L. Vasil, D. N. Gerding, and E. N. Janoff.** 1991. DNA fingerprinting by pulsed field gel electrophoresis and ribotyping to distinguish *Pseudomonas cepacia* isolates from a nosocomial outbreak. *J. Clin. Microbiol.* **29:**648–649.
4. **Arbeit, R.** 1997. Laboratory procedures for epidemiologic analysis, p. 253–286. *In* K. Crossley and G. Archer (ed.), *The Staphylococci in Human Disease*. Churchill Livingstone, New York, N.Y.

4a. **Arbeit, R. D.** Unpublished data.

5. **Arbeit, R. D.** 1995. Laboratory procedures for the epidemiologic analysis of microorganisms, p. 190–208. *In* P. R. Murray, E. J. Baron, M. A. Pfaller, F. C. Tenover, and R. H. Yolken (ed.), *Manual of Clinical Microbiology*, 6th ed. American Society for Microbiology, Washington, D.C.
6. **Arbeit, R. D., M. Arthur, R. D. Dunn, C. Kim, R. K. Selander, and R. Goldstein.** 1990. Resolution of recent evolutionary divergence among *Escherichia coli* from related lineages: the application of pulsed field electrophoresis to molecular epidemiology. *J. Infect. Dis.* **161:** 230–235.
7. **Arbeit, R. D., B. Kreiswirth, J. N. Maslow, T. Morris, and K. Murray-Leisure.** Unpublished data.
8. **Arbeit, R. D., and J. N. Maslow.** Unpublished data.
9. **Arbeit, R. D., A. Slutsky, T. W. Barber, J. N. Maslow, S. Niemczyk, J. O. Falkinham III, G. T. O'Conner, and C. F. von Reyn.** 1993. Genetic diversity among strains of *Mycobacterium avium* causing monoclonal and polyclonal bacteremia in patients with AIDS. *J. Infect. Dis.* **167:** 1384–1390.
10. **Archer, G. L., D. R. Dietrick, and J. L. Johnston.** 1985. Molecular epidemiology of transmissible gentamicin resistance among coagulase-negative staphylococci in a cardiac surgery unit. *J. Infect. Dis.* **151:**243–251.
11. **Archer, G. L., A. W. Karchmer, N. Vishniavsky, and J. L. Johnston.** 1984. Plasmid-pattern analysis for the differentiation of infecting from non-infecting *Staphylococcus epidermidis*. *J. Infect. Dis.* **149:**913–920.
12. **Arthur, M., R. D. Arbeit, C. Kim, P. Beltran, H. Crowe, S. Steinbach, C. Campanelli, R. A. Wilson, R. K. Selander, and R. Goldstein.** 1990. Restriction fragment length polymorphisms among uropathogenic *Escherichia coli* isolates: *pap*-related sequences compared with *rrn* operons. *Infect. Immun.* **58:**471–479.
13. **Arthur, M., C. E. Johnson, R. H. Rubin, R. D. Arbeit, C. Campanelli, C. Kim, S. Steinbach, M. Agarwal, R. Wilkinson, and R. Goldstein.** 1989. Molecular epidemiology of adhesin and hemolysin virulence factors among uropathogenic *Escherichia coli*. *Infect. Immun.* **57:** 303–313.
14. **Aufauvre-Brown, A., J. Cohen, and D. W. Holden.** 1992. Use of randomly amplified polymorphic DNA markers to distinguish isolates of *Aspergillus fumigatus*. *J. Clin. Microbiol.* **30:**2991–2993.
15. **Back, N. A., C. C. Linnemann, Jr., M. A. Pfaller, J. L. Staneck, and V. Morthland.** 1993. Recurrent epidemics caused by a single strain of erythromycin-resistant *Staphylococcus aureus:* the importance of molecular epidemiology. *JAMA* **270:**1329–1333.
16. **Bannerman, T. L., G. A. Hancock, F. C. Tenover, and J. M. Miller.** 1995. Pulsed-field gel electrophoresis as a replacement for bacteriophage typing of *Staphylococcus aureus*. *J. Clin. Microbiol.* **33:**551–555.
17. **Baquar, N., A. Burnens, and J. Stanley.** 1994. Comparative evaluation of molecular typing strains from a national epidemic due to *Salmonella brandenburg* by rRNA gene and IS*200* probes and pulsed-field gel electrophoresis. *J. Clin. Microbiol.* **32:**1876–1880.

17a. **Barbier, N., P. Saulnier, E. Chachaty, S. Dumontier, and A. Andremont.** 1996. Random amplified polymorphic DNA typing versus pulsed-field gel electrophoresis for epidemiological typing of vancomycin-resistant enterococci. *J. Clin. Microbiol.* **34:**1096–1099.

18. **Beltran, P., J. M. Musser, R. Helmuth, J. J. Farmer III, W. M. Frerichs, I. K. Wachsmuth, K. Ferris, A. C. McWhorter, J. C. Wells, A. Cravioto, and R. K. Selander.** 1988. Toward a population genetic analysis of *Salmonella:* genetic diversity and relationships among strains of serotypes *S. choleraesuis, S. derby, S. dublin, S. enteritidis, S. heidelberg, S. infantis, S. newport, S. typhimurium*. *Proc. Natl. Acad. Sci. USA* **85:**7753–7757.
19. **Bialkowska-Hobrazanska, H., D. Jaskot, and O. Hammerberg.** 1990. Evaluation of restriction endonuclease fingerprinting of chromosomal DNA and plasmid profile analysis for characterization of multiresistant coagulase-negative staphylococci in bacteremic neonates. *J. Clin. Microbiol.* **28:**269–275.
20. **Bifani, P. J., B. B. Plikaytis, V. Kapur, K. Stockbauer, X. Pan, M. L. Lutfey, S. L. Moghazeh, W. Eisner, T. M. Daniel, M. H. Kaplan, J. T. Crawford, J. M. Musser, and B. N. Kreiswirth.** 1996. Origin and interstate spread of a New York City multidrug-resistant Mycobacterium tuberculosis clone family. *JAMA* **275:**452–457.
21. **Bingen, E., C. Boissinot, P. Desjardins, H. Cave, N. Brahimi, N. Lambert-Zechovsky, E. Denamur, P. Blot, and J. Elion.** 1993. Arbitrarily primed polymerase chain reaction provides rapid differentiation of *Proteus mirabilis* isolates from a pediatric hospital. *J. Clin. Microbiol.* **31:** 1055–1059.
22. **Bingen, E., E. Denamur, N. Lambert-Zechovsky, N. Brahimi, M. El Lakany, and J. Elion.** 1992. Rapid genotyping shows the absence of cross-contamination in *Enterobacter cloacae* nosocomial infections. *J. Hosp. Infect.* **21:**95–101.
23. **Birren, B., and E. Lai.** 1993. *Pulsed Field Gel Electrophoresis: A Practical Guide*. Academic Press, Inc., San Diego, Calif.
24. **Bisercic, M., J. Y. Feutrier, and P. R. Reeves.** 1991. Nucleotide sequences of the *gnd* genes from nine natural isolates of *Escherichia coli:* evidence of intragenic recombination as a contributing factor in the evolution of the polymorphic *gnd* locus. *J. Bacteriol.* **173:**3894–3900.
25. **Blair, J. E., and R. E. O. Williams.** 1961. Phage typing of staphylococci. *Bull. W. H. O.* **24:**771–784.
26. **Böhm, H., and H. Karch.** 1992. DNA fingerprinting of *Escherichia coli* O157:H7 strains by pulsed-field gel electrophoresis. *J. Clin. Microbiol.* **30:**2169–2172.
27. **Böttger, E. C., A. Teske, P. Kirschner, S. Bost, H. R. Chang, V. Beer, and B. Hirschel.** 1992. Disseminated "*Mycobacterium genavense*" infection in patients with AIDS. *Lancet* **340:**76–80.
28. **Boukadida, J., M. de Montalembert, J.-L. Gaillard, J. Gobin, F. Grimont, D. Girault, M. Véron, and P. Berche.** 1991. Outbreak of gut colonization by *Pseudomonas aeruginosa* in immunocompromised children undergoing total digestive decontamination: analysis by pulsed-field electrophoresis. *J. Clin. Microbiol.* **29:**2068–2071.
29. **Boukadida, J., M. de Montalembert, G. Lenoir, P. Scheinmann, M. Véron, and P. Berche.** 1993. Molecular

epidemiology of chronic pulmonary colonisation by *Pseudomonas aeruginosa* in cystic fibrosis. *J. Med. Microbiol.* **38**:29–33.

30. **Boyce, J. M.** 1997. Vancomycin-resistant enterococcus. Detection, epidemiology, and control measures. *Infect. Dis. Clin. N. Am.* **11**:367–384.
31. **Boyce, J. M., S. M. Opal, G. Potter-Bynoe, and A. A. Medeiros.** 1993. Spread of methicillin-resistant *Staphylococcus aureus* in a hospital after exposure to a health care worker with chronic sinusitis. *Clin. Infect. Dis.* **17**: 496–504.
32. **Boyce, J. M., G. Potter-Bynoe, S. M. Opal, L. Dziobek, and A. A. Medeiros.** 1989. A common-source outbreak of *Staphylococcus epidermidis* infections among patients undergoing cardiac surgery. *J. Infect. Dis.* **161**:493–499.
33. **Burns, D. N., R. J. Wallace, Jr., M. E. Schultz, Y. Zhang, S. Q. Zubairi, Y. Pang, C. L. Gibert, B. A. Brown, E. S. Noel, and F. M. Gordin.** 1991. Nosocomial outbreak of respiratory tract colonization with *Mycobacterium fortuitum*: demonstration of the usefulness of pulsed-field gel electrophoresis in an epidemiologic investigation. *Am. Rev. Respir. Dis.* **144**:1153–1159.
34. **Caetano-Anollés, G., B. J. Bassam, and P. M. Gresshoff.** 1992. Primer-template interactions during DNA amplification fingerprinting with single arbitrary oligonucleotides. *Mol. Gen. Genet.* **235**:157–165.
35. **Carles-Nurit, M. J., B. Christophle, S. Broche, A. Gouby, N. Bouziges, and M. Ramuz.** 1992. DNA polymorphisms in methicillin-susceptible and methicillin-resistant strains of *Staphylococcus aureus*. *J. Clin. Microbiol.* **30**:2092–2096.
36. **Chachaty, E., P. Saulnier, A. Martin, N. Mario, and A. Andremont.** 1994. Comparison of ribotyping, pulsed-field gel electrophoresis and random amplified polymorphic DNA for typing *Clostridium difficile* strains. *FEMS Microbiol. Lett.* **122**:61–68.
37. **Clabots, C. R., S. Johnson, K. M. Bettin, P. A. Mathie, M. E. Mulligan, D. R. Schaberg, L. R. Peterson, and D. N. Gerding.** 1993. Development of a rapid and efficient restriction endonuclease analysis typing system for *Clostridium difficile* and correlation with other typing systems. *J. Clin. Microbiol.* **31**:1870–1875.
38. **Clabots, C. R., S. Johnson, M. M. Olson, L. R. Peterson, and D. N. Gerding.** 1992. Acquisition of *Clostridium difficile* by hospitalized patients: evidence for colonized new admissions as a source of infection. *J. Infect. Dis.* **166**: 561–567.
39. **Cleary, P. P., E. L. Kaplan, C. Livdahl, and S. Skjold.** 1988. DNA fingerprints of *Streptococcus pyogenes* are M type specific. *J. Infect. Dis.* **158**:1317–1323.
40. **Collier, M. C., F. Stock, P. C. De Girolami, M. H. Samore, and C. P. Cartwright.** 1996. Comparison of PCR-based approaches to molecular epidemiologic analysis of *Clostridium difficile*. *J. Clin. Microbiol.* **34**:1153–1157.
41. **Cuny, C., and W. Witte.** 1996. Typing of *Staphylococcus aureus* by PCR for DNA sequences flanked by transposon Tn*916* target region and ribosomal binding site. *J. Clin. Microbiol.* **34**:1502–1505.
42. **Devlin, H. R., W. Au, L. Foux, and W. C. Bradbury.** 1987. Restriction endonuclease analysis of nosocomial isolates of *Clostridium difficile*. *J. Clin. Microbiol.* **25**: 2168–2172.
43. **Dice, L.** 1945. Measures of the amount of ecologic association between species. *Ecology* **26**:297–302.
44. **Donabedian, S. M., J. W. Chow, J. M. Boyce, R. E. McCabe, S. M. Markowitz, P. E. Coudron, A. Kuritza, C. L. Pierson, and M. J. Zervos.** 1992. Molecular typing of ampicillin-resistant, non-β-lactamase-producing *Enterococcus faecium* isolates from diverse geographic areas. *J. Clin. Microbiol.* **30**:2757–2761.
45. **Doolittle, R. F. (ed.).** 1990. Molecular evolution: computer analysis of protein and nucleic acid sequences. *Methods Enzymol.* **183**.
46. **DuBose, R. F., D. E. Dykhuizen, and D. L. Hartl.** 1988. Genetic exchange among natural isolates of bacteria: recombination within the *phoA* gene of *Escherichia coli*. *Proc. Natl. Acad. Sci. USA* **85**:7036–7040.
47. **Edlin, B. R., J. I. Tokars, M. H. Grieco, J. T. Crawford, J. Williams, E. M. Sordillo, K. R. Ong, J. O. Kilburn, S. W. Dooley, K. G. Castro, W. R. Jarvis, and S. D. Holmberg.** 1992. An outbreak of multidrug-resistant tuberculosis among hospitalized patients with the acquired immunodeficiency syndrome. *N. Engl. J. Med.* **326**: 1514–1521.
48. **Eisenstein, B. I.** 1990. New molecular techniques for microbial epidemiology and the diagnosis of infectious diseases. *J. Infect. Dis.* **161**:595–602.
49. **el-Adhami, W., L. Roberts, A. Vickery, B. Inglis, A. Gibbs, and P. R. Stewart.** 1991. Epidemiological analysis of a methicillin-resistant *Staphylococcus aureus* outbreak using restriction fragment length polymorphisms of genomic DNA. *J. Gen. Microbiol.* **137**:2713–2720.
50. **Friedman, C., M. Stoeckle, W. Johnson, and L. Riley.** 1995. Double-repetitive-element PCR method for subtyping *Mycobacterium tuberculosis* clinical isolates. *J. Clin. Microbiol.* **33**:1383–1384.
51. **Fujimoto, S., B. Marshall, and M. J. Blaser.** 1994. PCR-based restriction fragment length polymorphism typing of *Helicobacter pylori*. *J. Clin. Microbiol.* **32**:331–334.
52. **Goering, R. V., and M. A. Winters.** 1992. Rapid method for epidemiological evaluation of gram-positive cocci by field inversion gel electrophoresis. *J. Clin. Microbiol.* **30**: 577–580.
53. **Goetz, M. B., M. E. Mulligan, R. Kwok, H. O'Brien, C. Caballes, and J. P. Garcia.** 1992. Management and epidemiologic analyses of an outbreak due to methicillin-resistant *Staphylococcus aureus*. *Am. J. Med.* **92**:607–614.
54. **Goh, S.-H., S. K. Byrne, J. L. Zhang, and A. W. Chow.** 1992. Molecular typing of *Staphylococcus aureus* on the basis of coagulase gene polymorphisms. *J. Clin. Microbiol.* **30**:1642–1645.
55. **Goswitz, J. J., K. E. Willard, C. E. Fashing, and L. R. Peterson.** 1992. Detection of *gyrA* gene mutations associated with ciprofloxacin resistance in methicillin-resistant *Staphylococcus aureus*: analysis by polymerase chain reaction and automated direct DNA sequencing. *Antimicrob. Agents Chemother.* **36**:1166–1169.
56. **Gouby, A., M.-J. Carles-Nurit, N. Bouziges, G. Bourg, R. Mesnard, and P. J. M. Bouvet.** 1992. Use of pulsed-field gel electrophoresis for investigation of hospital outbreaks of *Acinetobacter baumannii*. *J. Clin. Microbiol.* **30**: 1588–1591.
57. **Grothues, D., U. Koopman, H. von der Hardt, and B. Tümmler.** 1988. Genome fingerprinting of *Pseudomonas aeruginosa* indicates colonization of cystic fibrosis siblings with closely related isolates. *J. Clin. Microbiol.* **26**: 1973–1977.
58. **Grundmann, H., C. Schneider, D. Hartung, F. D. Daschner, and T. L. Pitt.** 1995. Discriminatory power of three DNA-based typing techniques for *Pseudomonas aeruginosa*. *J. Clin. Microbiol.* **33**:528–534.
59. **Guerrero, C., C. Bernasconi, D. Burki, T. Bodmer, and A. Telenti.** 1995. A novel insertion element from *Mycobacterium avium*, IS *1245*, is a specific target for analysis of strain relatedness. *J. Clin. Microbiol.* **33**:304–307.
60. **Gustaferro, C. A.** 1993. Chemiluminescent ribotyping, p. 584–589. *In* D. H. Persing, T. F. Smith, F. C. Tenover,

and T. J. White (ed.), *Diagnostic Molecular Microbiology: Principles and Applications*. American Society for Microbiology, Washington, D.C.

61. **Haertl, R, and G. Bandlow.** 1993. Epidemiological fingerprinting of *Enterobacter cloacae* by small-fragment restriction endonuclease analysis and pulsed-field gel electrophoresis of genomic restriction fragments. *J. Clin. Microbiol.* **31:**128–133.
62. **Hartstein, A. I., P. Chetchotisakd, C. L. Phelps, and A. M. Le Monte.** 1995. Typing of sequential bacterial isolates by pulsed-field gel electrophoresis. *Diagn. Microbiol. Infect. Dis.* **22:**309–314.
63. **Huebner, J., G. B. Pier, J. N. Maslow, E. Muller, H. Shiro, M. Parent, A. Kropec, R. D. Arbeit, and D. A. Goldmann.** 1994. Endemic nosocomial transmission of *Staphylococcus epidermidis* bacteremia strains in a neonatal ICU over a 10-year period. *J. Infect. Dis.* **169:**526–531.
64. **Hunter, P. R.** 1990. Reproducibility and indices of discriminatory power of microbial typing methods. *J. Clin. Microbiol.* **28:**1903–1905.
65. **Hunter, P. R., and M. A. Gaston.** 1988. Numerical index of the discriminatory ability of typing systems: an application of Simpson's index of diversity. *J. Clin. Microbiol.* **26:**2465–2466.
66. **Ichiyama, S., M. Ohta, K. Shimokata, N. Kato, and J. Takeuchi.** 1991. Genomic DNA fingerprinting by pulsed-field gel electrophoresis as an epidemiological marker for study of nosocomial infections caused by methicillin-resistant *Staphylococcus aureus*. *J. Clin. Microbiol.* **29:**2690–2695.
67. **Ingelfinger, J. A., F. Mosteller, L. A. Thibodeau, and J. H. Ware.** 1983. *Biostatistics in Clinical Medicine*. Macmillan Publishing Co., Inc., New York, N.Y.
68. **Janssen, P., R. Coopman, G. Huys, J. Swings, M. Bleeker, P. Vos, M. Zabeau, and K. Kersters.** 1996. Evaluation of the DNA fingerprinting method AFLP as a new tool in bacterial taxonomy. *Microbiology* **142:** 1881–1893.
69. **John, J. F., Jr., and J. A. Twitty.** 1986. Plasmids as epidemiologic markers in nosocomial gram-negative bacilli: experience at a university and review of the literature. *Rev. Infect. Dis.* **8:**693–704.
70. **Johnson, C. E., J. N. Maslow, D. C. Fattlar, K. S. Adams, and R. D. Arbeit.** 1993. The role of bacterial adhesins in the outcome of childhood urinary tract infections. *Am. J. Dis. Child.* **147:**1090–1093.
71. **Johnson, S., C. R. Clabots, F. V. Linn, M. M. Olson, L. R. Peterson, and D. N. Gerding.** 1990. Nosocomial *Clostridium difficile* colonisation and disease. *Lancet* **336:** 97–100.
72. **Keim, P., A. Kalif, J. Schupp, K. Hill, S. E. Travis, K. Richmond, D. M. Adair, M. Hugh-Jones, C. R. Kuske, and P. Jackson.** 1997. Molecular evolution and diversity in *Bacillus anthracis* as detected by amplified fragment length polymorphism markers. *J. Bacteriol.* **179:**818–824.
73. **Kersulyte, D., J. P. Woods, E. J. Keath, W. E. Goldman, and D. E. Berg.** 1992. Diversity among clinical isolates of *Histoplasma capsulatum* detected by polymerase chain reaction with arbitrary primers. *J. Bacteriol.* **174:** 7075–7079.
74. **Kreiswirth, B., J. Kornblum, R. D. Arbeit, W. Eisner, J. N. Maslow, A. McGeer, D. E. Low, and R. P. Novick.** 1993. Evidence for a clonal origin of methicillin resistance in *Staphylococcus aureus*. *Science* **259:**227–230.
75. **Kristjánsson, M., P. Green, H. L. Manning, A. M. Slutsky, S. M. Brecher, C. F. von Reyn, R. D. Arbeit, and J. N. Maslow.** 1993. Molecular confirmation of Bacillus Calmette-Guérin (BCG) as the cause of pulmonary infection following urinary tract instillation. *Clin. Infect. Dis.* **17:**228–230.
76. **Kristjánsson, M., M. H. Samore, D. N. Gerding, P. C. DeGirolami, K. M. Bettin, A. W. Karchmer, and R. D. Arbeit.** 1994. Comparison of restriction endonuclease analysis, ribotyping, and pulsed field gel electrophoresis for molecular differentiation of *Clostridium difficile* strains. *J. Clin. Microbiol.* **32:**1963–1969.
77. **Lawrence, J. G., D. E. Dykhuizen, R. F. DuBose, and D. L. Hartl.** 1989. Phylogenetic analysis using insertion sequence fingerprinting in *Escherichia coli*. *Mol. Biol. Evol.* **6:**1–14.
78. **Lehmann, P. F., D. Lin, and B. A. Lasker.** 1992. Genotypic identification and characterization of species and strains within the genus *Candida* by using random amplified polymorphic DNA. *J. Clin. Microbiol.* **30:** 3249–3254.
79. **Leonard, R., and K. Carroll.** 1997. Rapid lysis of gram-positive cocci for pulsed-field gel electrophoresis using achromopeptidase. *Diagn. Mol. Pathol.* **6:**288–291.
80. **Lin, A. W., M. A. Usera, T. J. Barrett, and R. A. Goldsby.** 1996. Application of random amplified polymorphic DNA analysis to differentiate strains of Salmonella enteritidis. *J. Clin. Microbiol.* **34:**870–876.
81. **Lina, B., M. Bes, F. Vandenesch, T. Greenland, J. Etienne, and J. Fleurette.** 1993. Role of bacteriophages in genomic variability of related coagulase-negative staphylococci. *FEMS Microbiol. Lett.* **109:**273–278.
82. **Linnemann, C. C., Jr., P. Moore, J. L. Staneck, and M. A. Pfaller.** 1991. Reemergence of epidemic methicillin-resistant *Staphylococcus aureus* in a general hospital associated with changing staphylococcal strains. *Am. J. Med.* **91**(Suppl. 3B):238S-244S.
83. **LiPuma, J., T. Stull, S. Dasen, K. Pidcock, D. Kaye, and O. Korzeniowski.** 1989. DNA polymorphisms among *Escherichia coli* isolated from bacteruric women. *J. Infect. Dis.* **159:**526–532.
84. **Lupski, J. R.** 1987. Molecular mechanisms for transposition of drug-resistance genes and other movable genetic elements. *Rev. Infect. Dis.* **9:**357–368.
85. **Maki, D. G., F. S. Rhame, D. C. Mackel, and J. V. Bennett.** 1976. Nationwide epidemic of septicemia caused by contaminated intravenous products. I. Epidemiologic and clinical features. *Am. J. Med.* **60:**471–485.
86. **Maslow, J., S. Brecher, J. Gunn, A. Durbin, M. Barlow, and R. Arbeit.** 1995. Persistence and variation of methicillin-resistant Staphylococcus aureus strains among individual patients over extended periods of time. *Eur. J. Clin. Microbiol. Infect. Dis.* **14:**282–290.
87. **Maslow, J. N., S. Brecher, K. S. Adams, A. Durbin, S. Loring, and R. D. Arbeit.** 1993. Relationship between indole production and the differentiation of *Klebsiella* species: indole-positive and -negative isolates of *Klebsiella* determined to be clonal. *J. Clin. Microbiol.* **31:** 2000–2003.
88. **Maslow, J. N., S. Brecher, A. Durbin, J. Gunn, M. Barlow, and R. D. Arbeit.** 1993. Diversity among strains of methicillin-resistant *Staphylococcus aureus* (MRSA) from patients with long-term colonization, abstr. 143. *In Abstracts of the Annual Meeting of the Infectious Diseases Society of America*.
89. **Maslow, J. N., M. E. Mulligan, K. S. Adams, J. C. Justis, and R. D. Arbeit.** 1993. Bacterial adhesins and host factors in the development and outcome of *Escherichia coli* bacteremia. *Clin. Infect. Dis.* **17:**89–97.
90. **Maslow, J. N., M. E. Mulligan, and R. D. Arbeit.** 1993. Molecular epidemiology: the application of contemporary techniques to typing bacteria. *Clin. Infect. Dis.* **17:** 153–164.

91. **Maslow, J. N., M. E. Mulligan, and R. D. Arbeit.** 1994. Recurrent *Escherichia coli* bacteremia. *J. Clin. Microbiol.* **32:**710–714.
92. **Maslow, J. N., A. M. Slutsky, and R. D. Arbeit.** 1993. The application of pulsed field gel electrophoresis to molecular epidemiology, p. 563–572. *In* D. H. Persing, T. F. Smith, F. C. Tenover, and T. J. White (ed.), *Diagnostic Molecular Microbiology: Principles and Applications*. American Society for Microbiology, Washington, D.C.
93. **Maslow, J. N., T. Whittam, R. A. Wilson, M. E. Mulligan, C. Gilks, K. S. Adams, and R. D. Arbeit.** 1995. Clonal relationship among bloodstream isolates of *Escherichia coli*. *Infect. Immun.* **63:**2409–2417.
94. **Matar, G. M., B. Swaminathan, S. B. Hunter, L. N. Slater, and D. F. Welch.** 1993. Polymerase chain reaction-based restriction fragment length polymorphism analysis of a fragment of the ribosomal operon from *Rochalimaea* species for subtyping. *J. Clin. Microbiol.* **31:** 1730–1734.
95. **Mathiesen, D. A., J. H. Oliver, Jr., C. P. Kolbert, E. D. Tullson, B. J. Johnson, G. L. Campbell, P. D. Mitchell, K. D. Reed, S. R. R. Telford, J. F. Anderson, R. S. Lane, and D. H. Persing.** 1997. Genetic heterogeneity of Borrelia burgdorferi in the United States. *J. Infect. Dis.* **175:**98–107.
96. **Mayer, L. W.** 1988. Use of plasmid profiles in epidemiologic surveillance of disease outbreaks and in tracing the transmission of antibiotic resistance. *Clin. Microbiol. Rev.* **1:**228–243.
97. **Mazurek, G. H., S. Hartman, Y. Zhang, B. A. Brown, J. S. R. Hector, D. Murphy, and R. J. Wallace, Jr.** 1993. Large DNA restriction fragment polymorphism in the *Mycobacterium avium-M. intracellulare* complex: a potential epidemiologic tool. *J. Clin. Microbiol.* **31:**390–394.
98. **Mazurek, G. H., V. Reddy, B. J. Marston, W. H. Haas, and J. T. Crawford.** 1996. DNA fingerprinting by infrequent-restriction-site amplification. *J. Clin. Microbiol.* **34:**2386–2390.
99. **McGeer, A., D. E. Low, J. Penner, J. Ng, C. Goldman, and A. E. Simor.** 1990. Use of molecular typing to study the epidemiology of *Serratia marcescens*. *J. Clin. Microbiol.* **28:**55–58.
100. **Mekalanos, J. J.** 1992. Environmental signals controlling expression of virulence determinants in bacteria. *J. Bacteriol.* **174:**1–7.
101. **Mickelsen, P. A., J. J. Plorde, K. P. Gordon, C. Hargiss, J. McClure, F. D. Schoenknecht, F. Condie, F. C. Tenover, and L. S. Tompkins.** 1985. Instability of antibiotic resistance in a strain of *Staphylococcus epidermidis* isolated from an outbreak of prosthetic valve endocarditis. *J. Infect. Dis.* **152:**50–58.
102. **Morris, T., S. Brecher, D. Fitzsimmons, A. Durbin, R. Arbeit, and J. Maslow.** 1995. A pseudoepidemic of septic arthritis. *Infect. Control Hosp. Epidemiol.* **16:**82–87.
103. **Murray, B. E., K. V. Singh, J. D. Heath, B. R. Sharma, and G. M. Weinstock.** 1990. Comparison of genomic DNAs of different enterococcal isolates using restriction endonucleases with infrequent recognition sites. *J. Clin. Microbiol.* **28:**2059–2063.
104. **Murray, B. E., K. V. Singh, S. M. Markowitz, H. A. Lopardo, J. Evans Patterson, M. J. Zervos, E. Rubeglio, G. M. Eliopoulos, L. B. Rice, F. W. Goldstein, S. G. Jenkins, G. M. Caputo, R. Nasnas, L. S. Moore, E. S. Wong, and G. Weinstock.** 1991. Evidence for clonal spread of a single strain of β-lactamase-producing *Enterococcus (Streptococcus) faecalis* to six hospitals in five states. *J. Infect. Dis.* **163:**780–785.
105. **Musser, J.** 1993. Multilocus enzyme electrophoresis "real time" DNA sequence analysis of nosocomial outbreaks, session 2. *In Program and Abstracts of the 33rd Interscience Conference on Antimicrobial Agents and Chemotherapy*. American Society for Microbiology, Washington, D.C.
106. **Musser, J. M.** 1996. Molecular population genetic analysis of emerged bacterial pathogens: selected insights. *Emerg. Infect. Dis.* **2:**1–17.
107. **Musser, J. M., and V. Kapur.** 1992. Clonal analysis of methicillin-resistant *Staphylococcus aureus* strains from intercontinental sources: association of the *mec* gene with divergent phylogenetic lineages implies dissemination by horizontal transfer and recombination. *J. Clin. Microbiol.* **30:**2058–2063.
108. **Musser, J. M., V. Kapur, J. E. Peters, C. W. Hendrix, D. Drehner, G. D. Gackstetter, D. R. Skalka, P. L. Fort, J. T. Maffei, L. L. Li, et al.** 1994. Real-time molecular epidemiologic analysis of an outbreak of Streptococcus pyogenes invasive disease in US Air Force trainees. *Arch. Pathol. Lab. Med.* **118:**128–133.
109. **Musser, J. M., J. S. Kroll, E. R. Moxon, and R. K. Selander.** 1988. Evolutionary genetics of the encapsulated strains of *Haemophilus influenzae*. *Proc. Natl. Acad. Sci. USA* **85:**7758–7762.
110. **Myers, L. E., S. V. P. S. Silva, J. D. Procunier, and P. B. Little.** 1993. Genomic fingerprinting of "Haemophilus somnus" isolates by using a random-amplified polymorphic DNA assay. *J. Clin. Microbiol.* **31:**512–517.
111. **Nicolle, L. E., H. Bialkowska-Hobrzanska, L. Romance, V. S. Harry, and S. Parker.** 1992. Clonal diversity of methicillin-resistant *Staphylococcus aureus* in an acute-care institution. *Infect. Control Hosp. Epidemiol.* **13:** 33–37.
112. **Noel, G. J., B. N. Kreiswirth, P. J. Edelson, M. Nesin, S. Projan, W. Eisner, D. J. Bauer, H. de Lencastre, A. M. sa Figueiredo, and A. Tomasz.** 1992. Multiple methicillin-resistant *Staphylococcus aureus* strains as a cause for a single outbreak of severe disease in hospitalized neonates. *Pediatr. Infect. Dis. J.* **11:**184–188.
113. **Ogle, J. W., J. M. Janda, D. E. Woods, and M. L. Vasil.** 1987. Characterization and use of a DNA probe as an epidemiological marker for *Pseudomonas aeruginosa*. *J. Infect. Dis.* **155:**119–126.
114. **Ott, M., L. Bender, G. Blum, M. Schmittroth, M. Achtman, H. Tschäpe, and J. Hacker.** 1991. Virulence patterns and long-range genetic mapping of extraintestinal *Escherichia coli* K1, K5, and K100 isolates: use of pulsed-field gel electrophoresis. *Infect. Immun.* **59:**2664–2672.
115. **Patterson, J. E., A. Wanger, K. K. Zscheck, M. J. Zervos, and B. E. Murray.** 1990. Molecular epidemiology of β-lactamase-producing enterococci. *Antimicrob. Agents Chemother.* **34:**302–305.
116. **Persing, D. H.** 1993. In vitro nucleic acid amplifications techniques, p. 51–87. *In* D. H. Persing, T. F. Smith, F. C. Tenover, and T. J. White (ed.), *Diagnostic Molecular Microbiology: Principles and Applications*. American Society for Microbiology, Washington, D.C.
117. **Pfaller, M. A.** 1991. Typing methods for epidemiologic investigation, p. 171–182. *In* A. Balows, W. J. Hausler, Jr., K. L. Herrmann, H. D. Isenberg, and H. J. Shadomy (ed.), *Manual of Clinical Microbiology*, 5th ed. American Society for Microbiology, Washington, D.C.
118. **Pfaller, M. A., D. S. Wakefield, R. Hollis, M. Fredrickson, E. Evans, and R. M. Massanari.** 1991. The clinical microbiology laboratory as an aid in infection control: the application of molecular techniques in epidemiologic studies of methicillin-resistant *Staphylococcus aureus*. *Diagn. Microbiol. Infect. Dis.* **14:**209–217.
119. **Pfaller, M. A., C. Wendt, R. J. Hollis, R. P. Wenzel, S. J. Fritschel, J. J. Neubauer, and L. A. Herwaldt.** 1996. Comparative evaluation of an automated ribotyping sys-

tem versus pulsed-field gel electrophoresis for epidemiological typing of clinical isolates of Escherichia coli and Pseudomonas aeruginosa from patients with recurrent gram-negative bacteremia. *Diagn. Microbiol. Infect. Dis.* **25:**1–8.

120. **Plikaytis, B., J. Marden, C. Woodley, W. Butler, J. Crawford, and T. Shinnick.** 1993. Multiplex PCR specific for multidrug-resistant *Mycobacterium tuberculosis* strain W, abstr. T19. *In Abstracts of the Conference on Molecular Diagnostics and Therapeutics*. American Society for Microbiology, Washington, D.C.
121. **Poh, C. L., C. C. Yeo, and L. Tay.** 1992. Genome fingerprinting by pulsed-field gel electrophoresis and ribotyping to differentiate *Pseudomonas aeruginosa* serotype O11 strains. *Eur. J. Clin. Microbiol. Infect. Dis.* **11:**817–822.
122. **Power, E. G.** 1996. RAPD typing in microbiology—a technical review. *J. Hosp. Infect.* **34:**247–265.
123. **Prevost, G., B. Jaulhac, and Y. Piemont.** 1992. DNA fingerprinting by pulsed-field gel electrophoresis is more effective than ribotyping in distinguishing among methicillin-resistant *Staphylococcus aureus* isolates. *J. Clin. Microbiol.* **30:**967–973.
124. **Rabkin, C. S., W. R. Jarvis, R. L. Anderson, J. Govan, J. Klinger, J. LiPuma, W. J. Martone, H. Monteil, C. Richard, S. Shigeta, A. Sosa, T. Stull, J. Swenson, and D. Woods.** 1989. *Pseudomonas cepacia* typing systems: collaborative study to assess their potential in epidemiologic investigations. *Rev. Infect. Dis.* **11:**600–607.
125. **Ralph, D., M. McClelland, J. Welsh, G. Baranton, and P. Perolat.** 1993. *Leptospira* species categorized by arbitrarily primed polymerase chain reaction (PCR) and by mapped restriction polymorphisms in PCR-amplified rRNA genes. *J. Bacteriol.* **175:**973–981.
126. **Relman, D. A., T. M. Schmidt, R. P. MacDermott, and S. Falkow.** 1992. Identification of the uncultured bacillus of Whipple's disease. *N. Engl. J. Med.* **327:**293–301.
127. **Richardson, J. H., and W. E. Barkley (ed.).** 1988. *Biosafety in Microbiological and Biomedical Laboratories (CDC-NIH)*. HHS publication no. (NIH) 88–8395. U.S. Government Printing Office, Washington, D.C.
128. **Rubin, L. G.** 1987. Bacterial colonization and infection resulting from multiplication of a single organism. *Rev. Infect. Dis.* **9:**488–493.
129. **Samore, M., G. Killgore, S. Johnson, R. Goodman, J. Shim, L. Venkataraman, S. Sambol, P. DeGirolami, F. Tenover, R. Arbeit, and D. Gerding.** 1997. Multicenter typing comparison of sporadic and outbreak *Clostridium difficile* isolates from geographically diverse hospitals. *J. Infect. Dis.* **176:**1233–1238.
130. **Saulnier, P., C. Bourneix, G. Prévost, and A. Andremont.** 1993. Random amplified polymorphic DNA assay is less discriminant than pulsed-field gel electrophoresis for typing strains of methicillin-resistant *Staphylococcus aureus*. *J. Clin. Microbiol.* **31:**982–985.
131. **Schaberg, D. R., and M. Zervos.** 1986. Plasmid analysis in the study of the epidemiology of nosocomial gram-positive cocci. *Rev. Infect. Dis.* **8:**705–712.
132. **Schlichting, C., C. Branger, J.-M. Fournier, W. Witte, A. Boutonnier, C. Wolz, P. Goullet, and G. Döring.** 1993. Typing of *Staphylococcus aureus* by pulsed-field gel electrophoresis, zymotyping, capsular typing, and phage typing: resolution of clonal relationships. *J. Clin. Microbiol.* **31:**227–232.
133. **Schoonmaker, D., T. Heimberger, and G. Birkhead.** 1992. Comparison of ribotyping and restriction enzyme analysis using pulsed-field gel electrophoresis for distinguishing *Legionella pneumophila* isolates obtained during a nosocomial outbreak. *J. Clin. Microbiol.* **30:**1491–1498.
134. **Schwartz, D. C., and C. R. Cantor.** 1984. Separation of yeast chromosome-sized DNAs by pulsed field gradient gel electrophoresis. *Cell* **37:**67–75.
135. **Selander, R. K., D. A. Caugant, H. Ochman, J. M. Musser, M. N. Gilmour, and T. S. Whittam.** 1986. Methods of multilocus enzyme electrophoresis for bacterial population genetics and systematics. *Appl. Environ. Microbiol.* **51:**873–884.
136. **Selander, R. K., D. A. Caugant, and T. S. Whittam.** 1987. Genetic structure and variation in natural populations of *Escherichia coli*, p. 1625–1648. *In* F. C. Neidhardt, K. L. Ingraham, B. Magasanik, K. B. Low, M. Schaechter, and H. E. Umbarger (ed.), Escherichia coli *and* Salmonella typhimurium: *Cellular and Molecular Biology*. American Society for Microbiology, Washington, D.C.
137. **Selander, R. K., J. M. Musser, D. A. Caugant, M. N. Gilmour, and T. S. Whittam.** 1987. Population genetics of pathogenic bacteria. *Microb. Pathog.* **3:**1–7.
138. **Slutsky, A. M., R. D. Arbeit, T. W. Barber, J. Rich, C. F. von Reyn, W. Pieciak, M. A. Barlow, and J. N. Maslow.** 1994. Polyclonal infection due to *Mycobacterium avium* complex in patients with AIDS detected by pulsed field gel electrophoresis of sequential clinical isolates. *J. Clin. Microbiol.* **32:**1773–1778.
139. **Smith-Vaughan, H. C., K. S. Sriprakash, J. D. Mathews, and D. J. Kemp.** 1995. Long PCR-ribotyping of nontypeable *Haemophilus influenzae*. *J. Clin. Microbiol.* **33:**1192–1195.
140. **Southern, E. M.** 1975. Detection of specific sequences among DNA fragments separated by gel electrophoresis. *J. Mol. Biol.* **98:**503–517.
141. **Speaker, M. G., F. A. Milch, M. K. Shah, W. Eisner, and B. N. Kreiswirth.** 1991. Role of external bacterial flora in the pathogenesis of acute postoperative endophthalmitis. *Ophthalmology* **98:**639–650.
142. **Stanley, J., N. Baquar, and E. J. Threlfall.** 1993. Genotypes and phylogenetic relationships of *Salmonella typhimurium* are defined by molecular fingerprinting of IS*200* and 16S *rrn* loci. *J. Gen. Microbiol.* **139:**1133–1140.
143. **Struelens, M. J., R. Bax, A. Deplano, W. G. V. Quint, and A. van Belkum.** 1993. Concordant clonal delineation of methicillin-resistant *Staphylococcus aureus* by macrorestriction analysis and polymerase chain reaction genome fingerprinting. *J. Clin. Microbiol.* **31:**1964–1970.
144. **Struelens, M. J., A. Deplano, C. Godard, N. Maes, and E. Serruys.** 1992. Epidemiologic typing and delineation of genetic relatedness of methicillin-resistant *Staphylococcus aureus* by macrorestriction analysis of genomic DNA by using pulsed-field gel electrophoresis. *J. Clin. Microbiol.* **30:**2599–2605.
145. **Stull, T. L., J. J. LiPuma, and T. D. Edlind.** 1988. A broad-spectrum probe for molecular epidemiology of bacteria: ribosomal RNA. *J. Infect. Dis.* **157:**280–286.
146. **Swanson, D. S., V. Kapur, K. Stockbauer, X. Pan, R. Frothingham, and J. M. Musser.** 1997. Subspecific differentation of *Mycobacterium avium* complex strains by automated sequencing of a region of the gene (*hsp65*) encoding a 65-kilodalton heat shock protein. *Int. J. Syst. Bacteriol.* **47:**414–419.
147. **Telenti, A., P. Imboden, F. Marchesi, D. Lowrie, S. Cole, M. J. Colston, L. Matter, K. Schopfer, and T. Bodmer.** 1993. Detection of rifampicin-resistance mutations in *Mycobacterium tuberculosis*. *Lancet* **341:**647–650.
148. **Telenti, A., F. Marchesi, M. Balz, F. Bally, E. C. Böttger, and T. Bodmer.** 1993. Rapid identification of mycobacteria to the species level by polymerase chain reaction and restriction enzyme analysis. *J. Clin. Microbiol.* **31:** 175–178.
149. **Tenover, F., R. Arbeit, R. Goering, P. Mickelsen, B. Murray, D. Persing, and B. Swaminathan.** 1995. Inter-

preting chromosomal DNA restriction patterns produced by pulsed-field gel electrophoresis: criteria for bacterial strain typing. *J. Clin. Microbiol.* **33:**2233–2239.

150. **Tenover, F. C., R. Arbeit, G. Archer, J. Biddle, S. Byrne, R. Goering, G. Hancock, G. A. Hébert, B. Hill, R. Hollis, W. R. Jarvis, B. Kreiswirth, W. Eisner, J. Maslow, L. K. McDougal, J. M. Miller, M. Mulligan, and M. A. Pfaller.** 1994. Comparison of traditional and molecular methods of typing isolates of *Staphylococcus aureus*. *J. Clin. Microbiol.* **32:**407–415.

151. **Tenover, F. C., R. D. Arbeit, and R. V. Goering.** 1997. How to select and interpret molecular strain typing methods for epidemiological studies of bacterial infections: a review for healthcare epidemiologists. Molecular Typing Working Group of the Society for Healthcare Epidemiology of America. *Infect. Control. Hosp. Epidermiol.* **18:** 426–439.

152. **Thal, L. A., J. W. Chow, J. Evans Patterson, M. B. Perri, S. Donabedian, D. B. Clewell, and M. J. Zervos.** 1993. Molecular characterization of highly gentamicin-resistant *Enterococcus faecalis* isolates lacking high-level streptomycin resistance. *Antimicrob. Agents Chemother.* **37:**134–137.

153. **Thong, K. L., Y. F. Ngeow, M. Altwegg, P. Navaratnam, and T. Pang.** 1995. Molecular analysis of *Salmonella enteritidis* by pulsed-field gel electrophoresis and ribotyping. *J. Clin. Microbiol.* **33:**1070–1074.

154. **Tojo, M., J. Yamashita, D. A. Goldmann, and G. B. Pier.** 1988. Isolation and characterization of a capsular polysaccharide adhesin from *Staphylococcus epidermidis*. *J. Infect. Dis.* **157:**713–722.

155. **van Belkum, A., R. Bax, P. Peerbooms, W. H. F. Goessens, N. van Leeuwen, and W. G. V. Quint.** 1993. Comparison of phage typing and DNA fingerprinting by polymerase chain reaction for discrimination of methicillin-resistant *Staphylococcus aureus* strains. *J. Clin. Microbiol.* **31:**798–803.

156. **van Belkum, A., J. De Jonckheere, and W. G. V. Quint.** 1992. Genotyping *Naegleria* spp. and *Naegleria fowleri* isolates by interrepeat polymerase chain reaction. *J. Clin. Microbiol.* **30:**2595–2598.

157. **van Belkum, A., J. Kluytmans, W. van Leewen, R. Bax, and Q. Wim.** 1995. Multicenter evaluation of arbitrarily primed PCR for typing of *Staphylococcus aureus* strains. *J. Clin. Microbiol.* **33:**1537–1547.

158. **van Belkum, A., M. Sluijuter, R. de Groot, H. Verbrugh, and P. W. Hermans.** 1996. Novel BOX repeat PCR assay for high-resolution typing of *Streptococcus pneumoniae* strains. *J. Clin. Microbiol.* **34:**1176–1179.

159. **van Belkum, A., M. Struelens, and W. Quint.** 1993. Typing of *Legionella pneumophila* strains by polymerase chain reaction-mediated DNA fingerprinting. *J. Clin. Microbiol.* **31:**2198–2200.

160. **van Embden, J. D. A., M. D. Cave, J. T. Crawford, J. W. Dale, K. D. Eisenach, B. Gicquel, P. Hermans, C. Martin, R. McAdam, T. M. Shinnick, and P. M. Small.** 1993. Strain identification of *Mycobacterium tuberculosis* by DNA fingerprinting: recommendations for a standardized methodology. *J. Clin. Microbiol.* **31:**406–409.

161. **van Leeuwen, W., M. Sijmons, J. Sluijs, H. Verbrugh, and A. van Belkum.** 1996. On the nature and use of randomly amplified DNA from *Staphylococcus aureus*. *J. Clin. Microbiol.* **34:**2770–2777.

162. **Versalovic, J., T. Koeuth, and J. R. Lupski.** 1991. Distribution of repetitive DNA sequences in eubacteria and application to fingerprinting of bacterial genomes. *Nucleic Acids Res.* **19:**6823–6831.

163. **Vilgalys, R., and M. Hester.** 1990. Rapid genetic identification and mapping of enzymatically amplified ribosomal DNA from several *Cryptococcus* species. *J. Bacteriol.* **172:** 4238–4246.

164. **von Reyn, C. F., J. N. Maslow, T. W. Barber, J. O. Falkinham III, and R. D. Arbeit.** 1994. Persistent colonization of potable water as a source of *Mycobacterium avium* infection in AIDS. *Lancet* **343:**1137–1141.

165. **Vos, P., R. Hogers, M. Bleeker, M. Reijans, T. van de Lee, M. Hornes, A. Frijters, J. Pot, J. Peleman, M. Kuiper, et al.** 1995. AFLP: a new technique for DNA fingerprinting. *Nucleic Acids Res.* **23:**4407–4414.

166. **Wachsmuth, K.** 1985. Genotypic approaches to the diagnosis of bacterial infections: plasmid analyses and gene probes. *Infect. Control* **6:**100–109.

167. **Welsh, J., and M. McClelland.** 1990. Fingerprinting genomes using PCR with arbitrary primers. *Nucleic Acids Res.* **18:**7213–7218.

168. **Whittam, T. S., I. K. Wachsmuth, and R. A. Wilson.** 1988. Genetic evidence of clonal descent of *Escherichia coli* O157:H7 associated with hemorrhagic colitis and hemolytic uremic syndrome. *J. Infect. Dis.* **157:**1124–1133.

169. **Widmer, A. F., R. P. Wenzel, A. Trilla, M. J. Bale, R. N. Jones, and B. N. Doebbeling.** 1993. Outbreak of *Pseudomonas aeruginosa* infections in a surgical intensive care unit: probable transmission via hands of a health care worker. *Clin. Infect. Dis.* **16:**372–376.

170. **Williams, J. G. K., A. R. Kubelik, K. J. Livak, J. A. Rafalski, and S. V. Tingey.** 1990. DNA polymorphisms amplified by arbitrary primers are useful as genetic markers. *Nucleic Acids Res.* **18:**6531–6535.

171. **Woelffer, G. B., W. Z. Bradford, A. Paz, and P. M. Small.** 1996. A computer-assisted molecular epidemiologic approach to confronting the reemergence of tuberculosis. *Am. J. Med. Sci.* **311:**17–22.

172. **Woodford, N., D. Morrison, A. P. Johnson, V. Briant, R. C. George, and B. Cookson.** 1993. Application of DNA probes for rRNA and *vanA* genes to investigation of a nosocomial cluster of vancomycin-resistant enterococci. *J. Clin. Microbiol.* **31:**653–658.

173. **Woods, C. R., Jr., J. Versalovic, T. Koeuth, and J. R. Lupski.** 1992. Analysis of relationships among isolates of *Citrobacter diversus* by using DNA fingerprints generated by repetitive sequence-based primers in the polymerase chain reaction. *J. Clin. Microbiol.* **30:**2921–2929.

174. **Zhang, Y., G. H. Mazurek, M. D. Cave, K. D. Eisenach, Y. Pang, D. T. Murphy, and R. J. Wallace, Jr.** 1992. DNA polymorphisms in strains of *Mycobacterium tuberculosis* analyzed by pulsed-field gel electrophoresis: a tool for epidemiology. *J. Clin. Microbiol.* **30:**1551–1556.

175. **Zingler, G., M. Ott, G. Blum, U. Falkenhagen, G. Naumann, W. Sokolowska-Köhler, and J. Hacker.** 1992. Clonal analysis of *Escherichia coli* serotype O6 strains from urinary tract infections. *Microb. Pathog.* **12:**299–310.

Decontamination, Disinfection, and Sterilization*

ANDREAS F. WIDMER AND RENO FREI

8

Decontamination, disinfection, and sterilization are basic components of any infection control program. Patients expect that any reusable instrument or device used for diagnosis of their illness or for treatment has undergone a process to eliminate any risks for cross-infection. However, many failures of adequate reprocessing have been reported in the literature (12, 76, 126). The basics of the technologies—chemicals for disinfection, heat for sterilization—go well back to the 19th century with Koch, Pasteur, and Lister. However, the principles had already been referenced in the Bible, as the following example shows: "Or if a person touches anything ceremonially unclean—whether the carcasses of unclean wild animals or of unclean livestock or of unclean creatures that move along the ground—even though he is unaware of it, he has become unclean and is guilty" (Lev. 5:2). The burning of victims of the plague in Venice in the 16th century is among the many reports of the use of heat to kill microorganisms to limit the spread of infectious diseases. In addition, much information on disinfection came from the preservation technology used to retard the decay of food.

Long before the introduction of routine antimicrobial prophylaxis, the incidence of postoperative site infection could be limited to <5% if the surgical site was adequately disinfected, strict asepsis was used throughout the procedure, and sterile items were used (37). In the past, surgeons relied predominantly on the knowledge of the operating room nurses who were responsible for adequate reprocessing of surgical instruments and reusable items. The availability and widespread use of disposable or single-use items transferred part of the responsibility of reprocessing from nursing to industry and managers, because the tasks of the central sterilization staff were primarily purchasing, storage, and rapid turnaround. Detailed know-how regarding disinfection and sterilization procedures was no longer necessary in hospitals. Expensive electronic items for computer-assisted surgery, the cost of single-use items, environmental concerns, and new low-temperature sterilization technology (e.g., plasma sterilization) were reasons for the return of reprocessing of multiple-use items. In addition, expensive devices for minimally invasive surgery (e.g., video-assisted surgery) and use of endoscopes challenged reprocessing technologies because most items are heat labile, have narrow lumens, and are difficult to disassemble and clean of proteins and debris. Not surprisingly, there are dozens of reports of transmission of nosocomial pathogens from contaminated endoscopes (26, 148, 178). Until recently, it was very difficult to prove a causal relationship between a contaminated device and a subsequent nosocomial infection. However, state-of-the-art clinical epidemiology supported by molecular typing tools such as pulsed-field gel electrophoresis and, in some cases, genome sequencing are available, and these are powerful tools that can be used to ultimately prove a causal relationship between the use of reprocessed but still contaminated devices and cross-infection between patients. These tools provided the scientific background required to identify the limitations of the available methods and to improve the reprocessing technologies. Reprocessing starts with the purchase of items and devices on the basis of a list that provides ample information about the disassembly, cleaning, and disinfection or sterilization of those items or devices. Items and devices that do not meet the basic prerequisites should *not* be purchased. The Food and Drug Administration (FDA) today has in place a set of requirements demanding the inclusion of detailed information on reprocessing and a telephone number (hotline) of the manufacturer. However, before purchase it is prudent to ask specific information about the methods of reprocessing the reusable devices. Most of the available disinfectants were introduced into the market more than 20 years ago, and only one new technology for sterilization has been developed during this time. The limited resources available for research on reprocessing explain in part the lack of sound scientific data. Therefore, it is unlikely that major breakthroughs will occur within the next several years, and the standardization and optimized application of the current knowledge rather than the development of newer technologies will be key issues in the near future.

PRINCIPLES ON TERMINOLOGY, DEFINITIONS, AND CLASSIFICATION OF MEDICAL DEVICES

Background

There is no uniform terminology for disinfection and sterilization, and many problems arise, since health care profession-

* This chapter contains information presented in chapter 8 by Frederic John Marsik and Gerald A. Denys and chapter 19 by William A. Rutala in the sixth edition of this Manual.

als do not use the same definitions for similar or identical terms. Most terms are ill-defined even within the United States or Europe. In addition, the testing procedures for disinfectants are not as far advanced and well-defined as MIC testing based on the recommendations of the National Committee for Clinical Laboratory Standards. Furthermore, considerable differences exist between the European Union and the United States. For example, liquid sterilization is not considered an appropriate method for sterilization because the process cannot be adequately monitored and validated at this time, whereas it is possible for autoclaving. Similar to the case when choosing antimicrobial agents for the treatment of infectious diseases, the choice of the optimal liquid chemical germicide or sterilization process depends on a variety of factors, and no single germicide or process is adequate in all circumstances. The principal goal is to reduce the numbers of microorganisms on the device to a level that is insufficient to transmit infection with a considerable safety margin. The most conservative approach would be to reprocess all items and devices with overkill sterilization. Obviously, not all items must undergo the most vigorous process to eliminate any microorganisms because some items are intended to be used at a nonsterile body site that does not require an overkill sterilization process. For example, a blood pressure cuff that comes into contact only with intact skin does not require sterilization before use between patients. In contrast, only sterilization will provide adequate safety to eliminate any risk of infection if the device comes into contact with a normally sterile body site such as an orthopedic implant. The minimum infectious dose required to trigger an infection, the severity of the disease in case of an infection, the feasibility, and, last but not least, human and financial resources are among the factors that ultimately determine the optimum reprocessing method. The optimum choice can also be the use of disposable or single-use items instead of reusable devices, because reprocessing may be more expensive or does not provide the desired level of safety. This may specifically apply to the reprocessing of items that may have been in contact with the neural tissue of a patient suffering from any form of Creutzfeldt-Jakob disease (CJD) (184). The most recent research has led to isolation of the infecting agent not only from neural tissue and cerebrospinal fluid but also from tonsils and other tissues, indicating that bovine spongiform encephalopathy can be transmitted from animals to humans as new-variant CJD (nvCJD) (94, 104). In addition, current knowledge about prions indicates that the sterilization procedures used to eliminate microorganisms do not provide the desired level of safety for the elimination of prions.

Therefore, a classification of devices is needed to better define the appropriate method for disinfection and/or sterilization. This classification should balance the potential risks for transmission of infection and the resources available to achieve the necessary or desired level of antimicrobial killing. The most commonly used classification was proposed by Earle H. Spaulding in 1968 (179). He proposed three categories: critical, semicritical, and noncritical (Table 1). This classification has been used by the Centers for Disease Control and Prevention (CDC) in *Guidelines for Handwashing and Hospital Environment Control* (47a) and by FDA for approval of sterilants and high-level disinfectants (see http://www.fda.gov/cdrh/index.html) and is used by most infection control professionals worldwide. The three classes of devices will guide infection control professionals in selecting the appropriate method for reprocessing. However, this simple classification will not work perfectly for all devices. Even the definition of sterilization as the absence of any viable microorganisms must be revised with the novel concept of proteinaceous infectious agents as the cause of nvCJD promulgated by the 1997 Nobel Prize winner Stanley Prusiner. However, the prevalence of CJD is 1 in 10^6 population, and even with nvCJD in Europe, there is no need for major

TABLE 1 Spaulding classification of devices

Clinical device	Definition	Example	Infectious risk	Reprocessing procedure	
				FDA classification	EPA classification
Critical device	A medical device that is intended to enter a normally sterile environment, sterile tissue, or the vasculature	Surgical instruments	High	Sterilization by steam, plasma, or ethylene oxide; liquid sterilization acceptable if no other methods feasible	Sterilant or disinfectant
Semicritical device	A medical device that is intended to come into contact with mucous membranes or minor skin breaches	Flexible endoscope	High, intermediate	Sterilization desirable; high-level disinfection acceptable	Sterilant or disinfectant
Noncritical device	A medical device that comes into contact with intact skin	Blood pressure cuff, electrocardiogram electrodes	Low	Intermediate or low level	Hospital disinfectant with label claim for tuberculocidal activity
Medical equipment	A device or a component of a device that does not typically come in direct contact with the patient	Examination table	Low	Low-level disinfection, sanitizer	Hospital disinfectant without label claim for tuberculocidal activity but for virucidal activity against HIV

changes in the current guidelines for general surgery. However, it is likely that policies for the reprocessing of items and devices that have been used in a neurosurgical procedure or that have been in contact with cerebrospinal fluid or tissue might be revised. The French approach is based on the concept of universal precautions for blood-borne pathogens: all patients undergoing a neurosurgical procedure are potential carriers of prions, and therefore, all necessary precautions should be implemented for all neurosurgical patients. However, no case of nvCJD has yet been diagnosed in the United States, even though the clinical presentation of nvCJD has recently been published (205, 206). In addition, documented transmission by adequately reprocessed items or devices has not been observed in the last decade. CDC will publish guidelines on this topic, but the nvCJD issue was not included in its 1997 draft. Ongoing research will likely influence the guidelines as the latest information becomes available. The reader should check the CDC home page for CDC's latest update.

Surprisingly little is known about the target of action of disinfectants. Most modes of action are ill-defined. Generally, disinfectants kill as a result of effects on multiple targets, but the mechanisms, including the problem of the emergence of resistance, remain to be elucidated. Discussion of the presumed or established modes of antimicrobial action of disinfectants are beyond the scope of this chapter but are reviewed in detail by Block (29) and Russell et al. (156). Basic information is provided below in the sections dealing with the various disinfectants.

Definition and Classification of Devices

FDA has defined medical devices as follows (as defined by the Food, Drug, and Cosmetic Act [FD&C Act]): an instrument, apparatus, implement, machine, contrivance, implant, in vitro reagent, or other similar or related article, including any component, part, or accessory, which is

1. recognized in the official National Formulary, the United States Pharmacopeia, or any supplement to them;
2. intended for use in the diagnosis of disease or other conditions or in the cure, mitigation, treatment, or prevention of disease, in humans or animals; or
3. intended to affect the structure or any function of the body of humans or other animals and which does not achieve its primary intended purposes through chemical action within or on the body of humans or other animals and which is not dependent upon being metabolized for the achievement of any of its principal intended purposes.

FDA uses three different levels to classify devices on the basis of a risk analysis (Table 2). These levels regulate the requirements that apply to the device and that the company must adhere to before it is able to legally market a device (Table 1). The premarket notification [510(k)] review determines whether a device is substantially equivalent to an earlier, legally marketed device. A manufacturer must submit a 510(k) application and receive clearance before it can legally market the device.

The Spaulding classification has been retained because it is simple, easy to understand, and applies to the majority of devices. However, this clear-cut classification has limitations with newer technologies such as minimal invasive surgery, computer-assisted surgery, and endoscopy-guided surgery. Therefore, these special cases require more sophisticated approaches, as discussed below.

Classification of Devices for Reprocessing

Critical Items

Items are classified as "critical items" if they enter normally sterile parts of the human body, such as surgical instruments used during an operation, implants, or monitoring devices used during an operation (Table 1). Items classified as critical carry the highest risk for the patient. Therefore, sterilization is the preferred method for reprocessing, and autoclaving is the method of choice, if it is feasible. However, some items and devices are heat labile and do not tolerate heat. Alternative methods such as ethylene oxide sterilization and sterilization with plasma require prolonged times, and these methods do not have FDA clearance for use with small dead-end lumens, which are difficult to sterilize. Liquid sterilization with, for example, a glutaraldehyde-based formulation or peracetic acid is acceptable if sterilization by one of the methods mentioned above is not feasible and the formulation and/or automated device has been cleared by FDA.

Semicritical Items

Semicritical objects come into contact with mucous membranes or skin that is not intact and should be free of microorganisms except spores. Intact mucous membranes generally resist bacterial spores but are susceptible to other microorganisms such as vegetative bacteria (e.g., *Mycobacterium tuberculosis*) or viruses (e.g., human immunodeficiency virus [HIV] and cytomegalovirus). Typical examples are anesthesia equipment, respiratory equipment, and endoscopes. The appropriate process is the use of a high-level disinfectant such as glutaraldehyde, stabilized hydrogen peroxide, peracetic acid, and chlorine compounds. Chlorine compounds, however, corrode items and therefore are rarely used to disinfect devices.

Noncritical Items

Noncritical items come into contact with intact skin only. Intact skin is a very effective barrier against microorganisms, and therefore, there is no need for sterilization of such items and devices. Examples are bedside tables, crutches, stetho-

TABLE 2 Classification of devices

Classification	FDA regulation	Premarket requirements by FDA	Examples
Class I	Least regulated, requires fewest regulations	None	Band-Aid, tongue depressor
Class II	Must meet federal performance standards	Premarket notification [510(k)]	Sterilizers, gowns, drapes, scrub sponges
Class III	Implanted and life-supporting or life-sustaining devices are required to have FDA approval for safety and effectiveness	Premarket approval	Artificial hearts

scopes, furniture, and floors. They pose a very small risk for the direct transmission of pathogens and can usually be cleaned at the bedside or where they have been used. Noncritical devices can contribute to the transmission of pathogens by the indirect route. Contamination of the environment near patients colonized or infected with vancomycin-resistant enterococci is observed in up to 60% of samples obtained from such environments. The hands of health care workers (HCWs) may subsequently be contaminated by touching these surfaces and may thereby spread the pathogens to devices or patients. Therefore, it is very important to disinfect noncritical items if contamination by a multidrug-resistant pathogen is likely. An example is the stethoscope, which can be disinfected by wiping the surface of the membrane with alcohol. Low-level disinfectants may be used to process noncritical items.

DECONTAMINATION AND CLEANING

In Europe, the cleaning process used to remove organic material, protein, and fat is called "decontamination." In the United States, this term applies to a process that ensures that an item is "safe to handle" by an HCW without protective attire. This may be simple, manual cleaning but may also include a disinfection and even a sterilization process. In Europe, decontamination basically means cleaning. In the United States the term describes a cleaning step and any additional step required to eliminate any risk of infection to the HCW during handling. However, cleaning is always part of the decontamination process on both continents. In this chapter, the term will be used to describe the removal of debris, blood, and proteins and the bulk of microorganisms which usually, but not necessarily, renders the device "safe to handle" by the HCW without protective attire. Physical or chemical cleaning, manually or by sonication or with washers, is always the primary step in any reprocessing cycle. It is intended to remove debris, blood, and proteins. All sterilization techniques other than steaming have been shown to fail in 1 to 40% of sterilization cycles if residual proteins and/or salts are not removed by a proper cleaning process (10, 11). Other processes such as high-level disinfection and/or sterilization may follow this cleaning process. The U.S. term "decontamination" applies to the safety of handling of the device by HCWs and not necessarily to the device itself. In Europe, the term most frequently applies only to the device and is used as a synonym for the U.S. term "cleaning." Cleaning is extremely effective in removing microorganisms. Studies with endoscopes have shown reductions of >99.99% or 4 logs for viruses (88, 90) and vegetative bacteria. In addition, the activities of disinfectants can be reduced if proteins and debris limit the activity and/or access of the compound to the microorganisms on the surface of the device. In the United States cleaning is frequently performed manually with water and a detergent. In Europe, many countries rely on washers-disinfectors. They rinse items with cold water, followed by rinsing with warm water and a detergent. The cycle is completed with hot water at ≥90°C. Items such as bedpans and urinals can be cleaned and disinfected by putting the items into a machine, pushing a button, and removing them after a 2- to 5-min procedure. For noncritical devices such as floors, manual cleaning with a bucket containing water and a detergent is almost as effective as cleaning with disinfecting agents. Therefore, a large biological burden should always be reduced before attempting to disinfect and/or sterilize a device. An infectious disease analogy is the physical removal of an abscess by surgery before optimal antimicrobial therapy will be effective. As is the case in the process involving antibiotics, killing of microorganisms by disinfection or sterilization is a kinetic process requiring prolonged exposure times if large inocula are present. The presence of proteins, blood, and debris after cleaning renders any following disinfection or sterilization process futile.

DISINFECTION

Principles and Antimicrobial Activities of Compounds

Comprehensive, scientifically sound criteria for the evaluation of chemical germicides help to ensure that these agents are safe and effective for their intended use. Therefore, data on antimicrobial activity should ensure that the compounds adequately kill the expected microorganisms on a device or on the skin. MIC data are of little help since the goal of disinfection is to kill rather than inhibit the growth of microorganisms. One important issue on the testing of disinfectants is the fact that almost all compounds need to be inactivated before they are incubated in media or plated, a similar problem as with the carryover effect with minimal bactericidal concentration and killing curve studies. For example, bacteria do not grow in the presence of very low concentrations of a disinfectant (inhibitory effect). However, if the compound is inactivated, bacterial growth can be demonstrated. The effect is inhibition only, not killing. The patient may be exposed to a large inoculum because body fluids might dilute and inactivate the compound, releasing vital vegetative bacteria. Therefore, a laboratory testing disinfectants should be familiar with these special methods. It should always present data from dilution experiments to demonstrate the optimal dilutions and concentrations of the inactivating compounds.

In contrast to sterilization, killing curves for disinfectants are not linear, and the rate of log killing decreases at lower inoculum concentrations (as numbers of CFU per milliliter). Therefore, a 3-log killing is more easily achieved with disinfectants if the inoculum is large, e.g., 10^8 CFU, but is rather difficult with an inoculum of 10^4 CFU. As for antibiotics, there is also a lag of regrowth (postantibiotic effect) after bacteria are exposed to a disinfectant. This postexposure effect has recently been quantified for a variety of disinfectants. Alcohols in general have little, if any, postexposure effect, but chlorhexidine delays regrowth after exposure for more than 2 h, and chloramine delays regrowth even for more than 4 h. Disinfectants differ in their spectra of antimicrobial activity, and their use relates to the Spaulding classification (Table 1 and Fig. 1). In the last decade, bloodborne viruses have received considerable attention, and disinfection of virus-contaminated devices and spills is critical to protecting HCWs. Initially, hepatitis B virus (HBV) was considered to be difficult to eradicate with disinfectants, but several studies showed that even low-level disinfectants are able to kill HBV, hepatitis C virus (HCV), and HIV (31, 108, 143).

Before a disinfectant for critical or semicritical devices can be legally marketed, FDA must grant marketing clearance by

1. issuance of an order in response to a section 510(k) submission which exempts the device from the FD&C Act's premarket approval requirements, or
2. approval of a premarket approval application. In

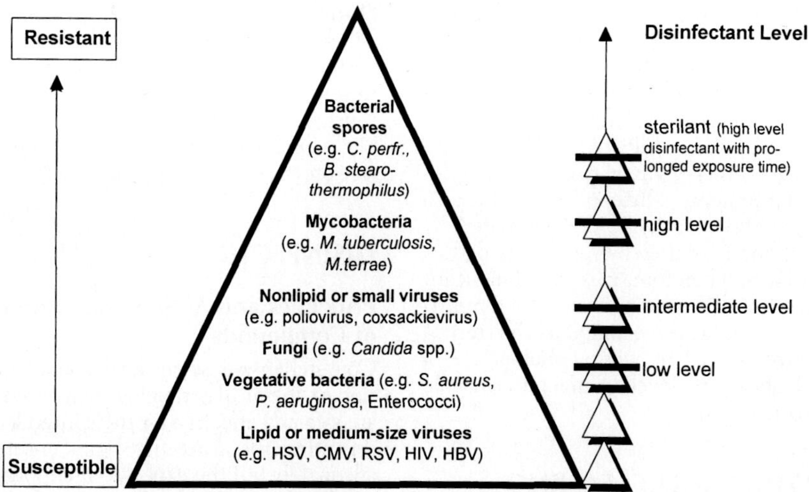

FIGURE 1 Increasing order of resistance of microorganisms to disinfectants. CMV, cytomegalovirus; RSV, respiratory syncytial virus; the other abbreviations are defined in the text.

granting marketing clearance by issuance of a section 510(k) order exempting a liquid chemical germicide from premarket approval, FDA must find the device to be "substantially equivalent," as the term is defined in section 21 of the U.S. Code.

The microbicidal efficacy testing of liquid chemical sterilants and high-level disinfectants is based on a three-tier approach that includes the following:

1. potency testing, which incorporates Environmental Protection Agency (EPA) test requirements for the registration of germicides, such as the Association of Official Analytical Chemists (AOAC) sporocidal test, tuberculocidal test, etc., and FDA-recommended tests, such as total killing or endpoint analysis and comparison of the survivor curve to the predicted curve;
2. simulated use testing with medical devices contaminated with an organic load and the appropriate test microorganisms for the level of disinfection being claimed; the conditions of the artificially contaminated devices represent worst-case postcleaning conditions prior to exposure to the germicide; and
3. "in-use" testing with clinically used medical devices; in-use testing incorporates cleaning of the devices according to the operating procedures of the facility prior to exposure to the germicide.

There is still controversy about the optimal test procedure that should be used to ensure that the germicide achieves the desired log killing. Lipid-enveloped viruses such as HIV and most vegetative bacteria are destroyed even by a low-level disinfectant (Fig. 1). Non-lipid-enveloped or small viruses such as poliovirus can challenge many disinfectants, including alcohol. For example, isopropyl alcohol has little activity against poliovirus. In contrast, >90% ethanol is very active against these viruses (180). Of the vegetative bacteria, nontuberculous mycobacteria are most resistant to many disinfectants. Therefore, FDA includes a tuberculocidal test in its test procedures. This test does not allow for cleaning, uses 2% horse serum as the proteinaceous load, and is performed with an extremely large number of microorganisms (10^5 to 10^6 CFU). Therefore, devices must be exposed to disinfectants for extended immersion times (>45 min) and at elevated temperatures (≥25°C). In the absence of cleaning and the presence of proteinaceous materials with large microbial loads, immersion in 2.4% alkaline glutaraldehyde for 45 min at 25°C is frequently required for complete tuberculocidal killing.

However, Rutala and Weber (164a) conclusively demonstrated that proper cleaning eradicates at least 4 logs of microorganisms. In another study, the cleaning of bronchoscopes before disinfection removed all detectable contaminants, with up to an 8-log reduction of viral load (89). Therefore, Rutala and Weber (164a) recommended that FDA reconsider its procedures regarding testing for activity against mycobacteria. They propose the following: A standardized cleaning protocol and then a 20-min immersion at 20°C with an FDA-cleared disinfectant will be sufficient to achieve high-level disinfection. However, it must be reiterated that disinfection or sterilization without an antecedent proper cleaning and removal of any debris is a major failure in the decontamination process, and even the use of disinfectants with the highest level of safety is no substitute for appropriate training of HCWs to avoid human errors. Many factors should be considered before one makes a final decision as to the specific disinfectant to be used. The concentration of the disinfectant should be checked regularly if it is diluted at the place of use, even if it is diluted with an electronically monitored dilution device. Failures of the valve or other critical parts of the device can result in an insufficient final concentration that usually cannot be detected by visual inspection or the odor of the disinfectant.

Definition and Terms (Adapted from Definitions of FDA and EPA)

Definitions vary worldwide, and even EPA and FDA do not use identical terminologies (Table 3). Therefore, it is very important to take this fact into account before evaluating publications from different countries or classifications from different agencies. Since FDA regulates the most critical part of disinfection and sterilization, the definitions from FDA are used throughout the chapter unless stated otherwise. The most important definitions are summarized in Table 3. Other important terms adapted from FDA are given below.

Germicide: an agent that destroys microorganisms. Other

TABLE 3 Definitions and terms

Term	Standard	Technical-microbiological log CFU reduction	Comment
Sterilization	A (closely monitored) validated process used to render a product free of all forms of viable microorganisms, including all bacterial endospores	A $\geq 10^6$ log CFU reduction of the most resistant spores for the sterilization process studied, achieved at the half-time of the regular cycle (ISO 14937)	Prions require an adapted definition because of their high level of resistance to any form of sterilization
Disinfection	Elimination of most if not all pathogenic microorganisms excluding spores	There is not a clear-cut defined reduction level. A minimum estimate is $\geq 10^3$ log CFU reduction of microorganisms excluding spores, common are 4–5 logs for devices. These are estimates because there is no international standardization.	Some high-level disinfectants achieve levels of microbial reduction including reduction of spores similar to levels achieved by sterilization if long incubation times and/or temperatures of >25°C are applied. This is called liquid sterilization by sterilants.
Decontamination	Reduction of pathogenic microorganisms to a level where items are "safe to handle" without protective attire	Elimination of debris and proteins by cleaning and/or disinfection or sterilization process. In Europe, it is restricted to cleaning only, which achieves a minimum of ≥ 1 log CFU. Most cleaning processes achieve 3–5 log CFU reductions. These are estimates because there is no international standardization.	Manual and/or mechanical cleaning with water and detergents or enzymes. It is a prerequisite before disinfection or sterilization. In Europe, this term is used for cleaning of the items. In the United States it defines an item to be "safe to handle." It may include a cleaning process, but it may also include a disinfection or even a sterilization process. The U.S. term decontamination refers to the HCW's safety. In Europe, the term is used for the item only.
Antisepsis	*Patient related*: disinfection of living tissue or skin	Preoperative skin preparation with an alcohol-based iodine compound	Antiseptic agents are handled as drugs by FDA.
	HCW related: Reduction or removal of transient microbiologic flora	Hand washing (scrub): reduction of ≥ 1 log CFU Hand disinfection (rub-in): reduction of ≥ 2.5 log CFU	

terms with the suffix -cide (e.g., virucide, fungicide, bactericide, sporicide, and tuberculocide) relate to the killing of the microorganisms identified by the prefix.

Sterilant (chemical): a chemical germicide which achieves sterilization. Only limited data are available to validate the fact that liquid chemical germicides can achieve a defined sterility assurance level (SAL). Liquid chemical germicide sterilization is acceptable only for critical devices that are heat labile or that are otherwise unable to be sterilized by all other sterilization methods that can be biologically monitored.

High-level disinfectant: a germicide that kills all microbial pathogens except large numbers of bacterial endospores when used according to the labeling.

Intermediate-level disinfectant: a germicide that kills all microbial pathogens except bacterial endospores when used according to the labeling.

Low-level disinfectant: a germicide that kills most vegetative bacteria and lipid-enveloped or medium-size viruses when used according to the labeling.

Minimum effective concentration: the minimum effective concentration of a liquid chemical germicide which still achieves the claimed microbicidal activity. Reporting of MICs of disinfectants is not useful, but these reports continue to be published.

Cleaning (or precleaning): the removal of foreign material, e.g., organic or inorganic contaminants, from medical devices as part of a decontamination process.

Guidelines for Choosing a Disinfectant

Several factors should be included in an evaluation of a disinfectant. A prerequisite for a disinfectant is its effectiveness against the expected spectrum of pathogens (Tables 4 and 5). Data on disinfectants should be reviewed, although this process has been performed by EPA or FDA, before registering or clearing the disinfectant. The data required to pass the tests by these agencies include the following: the AOAC tuberculocidal test for a claim of tuberculosis; the AOAC fungicidal test; the AOAC use-dilution tests for *Staphylococcus aureus*, *Staphylococcus choleraesuis*, and *Pseudomonas aeruginosa*; and EPA virucidal tests for viruses including poliovirus type 2 and herpes simplex virus. In Eu-

TABLE 4 Overview of common disinfectants[a]

Germicide	Use dilution	Level of disinfection	Active against: Bacteria	Lipophilic viruses	Fungi	Small or hydrophilic viruses	*M. tuberculosis*	Bacterial spores	Important characteristics: Shelf life, >1 wk	Corrosive or deleterious effect	Residue	Inactivated by organic matter	Skin irritant	Eye irritant	Respiratory irritant	Toxic	Environmental concerns	Typical application in hospitals
Glutaraldehyde	2–3.2%	High/CS	+	+	+	+	+	+	+	–	+	–	+	+	+	+	–	Endoscopes
Hydrogen peroxide	3–25%	High/CS	+	+	+	+	+	±	+	±	–	±	+	+	–	+	–	Contact lenses
Chlorine	100–1,000 ppm free chlorine	High	+	+	+	+	+	±	+	+	+	+	+	+	+	+	±	Selected semicritical devices
Isopropyl alcohol	60–95%	Int	+	+	+	±	+	–	+	±	–	±	±	+	–	+	–	Small area surfaces
Glucoprotamine[b]	4%	Int	+	+	+	+	+	–	+	–	–	–	+	+	–	–	–	Diagnostic instruments
Phenolic compounds	0.4–5% aqueous	Int	+	+	+	±	+	–	+	–	+	–	+	+	–	+	+	Surgical instruments
Iodophors	30–50 ppm free iodine	Int	+	+	+	+	±	–	+	±	+	+	±	+	–	+	–	Medical equipment
Quaternary ammonium compounds	0.4–1.6% aqueous	Low	±	+	±	–	–	–	+	–	+	+	+	+	–	+	–	Disinfection in food preparation areas and floors

[a]Adapted from references 19, 29, 155, 157, 186, and 200. Abbreviations: Int, intermediate; CS, chemical sterilant; +, yes; −, no; ±, variable results. The efficacies of the disinfectants are based on exposure times of less than 30 min at room temperature. Spores require prolonged exposure times (up to 10 h) unless they are used with a machine at higher temperatures.
[b]Not available in the United States.

rope, disinfectants should have been tested by the methods defined by an established or proposed European Norm (EN) such as EN 1499 or EN 1500. In addition to the activity of the disinfectant, its compatibility with devices should be reviewed in detail; this should include a review of data on devices that have been immersed for longer than the recommended times. Instruments can be forgotten after immersion, and this mistake should not necessarily result in irreparable damage to the device. Other issues are toxicity, odor, compatibility with other compounds, and residual activity. In addition to scientific data, knowledge of the hands-on experience of other health care professionals at different institutions help to avoid simple but sometimes cumbersome problems such as interactions with detergents, unexpected coloring, or odors. At the authors' institution, a change to the color of a disinfectant made the otherwise identical disinfectant "not acceptable" to HCWs. Therefore, it is prudent not to switch frequently to other disinfectants with similar or identical active compounds unless there is scientific evidence for improved activity or faster action. An up-

TABLE 5 Overview of common antiseptic compounds[a]

Compound	Antiseptic effect on: Gram-positive bacteria	Gram-negative bacteria	Viruses	Fungi	*M. tuberculosis*	Rapidity of action	Residual activity	Typical conc (%)	Affected by organic matter	Safety for humans
Alcohols	+ + +	+ + +	+ +[b]	+ + +	+ + +	15–30 s	None	70–95	?[c]	Drying, flammable
Chlorhexidine	+ + +	+ +	+ +	+	+ +	Minutes	+ + +	4, 2, and 0.5 in alcohol	Minimally	Ototoxicity, keratitis
Iodophors	+ + +	+ +	+ +	+ +	+ +	Minutes	+	10%, 7.5%, 2, 0.5	Yes	Skin irritation
Octenidine[d]	+ + +	+ + +	+ +	+ +	No data	Minutes	+ + +	0.1	Minimally	Limited experience
PCMX	+ +	+	+	+	+	Minutes	+ +	0.5–3.75	Minimally	Limited data
Triclosan	+ +	+ +	No data	±	+	Minutes	+ + +	0.3–1.0	Minimally	Limited data

[a] Adapted from references 115 and 157. Symbols: ±, poor; +, fair; + +, good; + + +, excellent.
[b] Ethanol at >95% is highly effective against viruses; isopropanol has limited effectiveness against small or non-lipid-enveloped viruses.
[c] Conflicting data.
[d] Not available in the United States.

TABLE 6 Disinfectants registered by EPA or cleared by FDA

Agency	Disinfectant	Internet address for updated list
FDA	Liquid disinfectants (sterilants and high-level disinfectants)	http://www.fda.gov/cdrh/ode/germlab.html
EPA	Disinfectant with claim of action against M. *tuberculosis*: (intermediate-level disinfectants)	http://ace.ace.orst.edu/info/nain/lstbpgts.htm
EPA	Disinfectant with claim of action against HIV but not M. *tuberculosis* (low-level disinfectants)	http://ace.ace.orst.edu/info/nain/lstcpgts.htm

dated list of low-level and intermediate-level disinfectants registered by EPA or high-level disinfectants and sterilants cleared by FDA is given in Table 6.

In Europe, most disinfectants are registered by individual countries. A recent German publication (*Desinfektionsmittel-Liste der Deutschen Gesellschaft für Hygiene und Mikrobiologie*, 17 September 1997) provides an excellent review of disinfectants, including the exposure times required to achieve the desired level of killing. Its criteria for disinfectants for use with devices require documentation of a 5-log killing for bacteria and a 4-log killing for viruses. These data must be generated by an institution independent of the manufacturer. Some products that are on the European market have not yet been registered by EPA or cleared by FDA. Unfortunately, the disinfectants that have been registered, approved, or cleared by a European country cannot yet be accessed on the Internet. In addition, controversies among the European countries remain even after the ENs have been accepted by countries of the European Union.

Regulation and Legal Aspects of Chemical Germicides

Until 1996, two government agencies regulated chemical germicides in the health care setting: EPA and FDA. With the passage of the Food Quality Protection Act of 1996 (FQPA), liquid chemical germicides intended for use in the processing of critical and semicritical devices were exempted from regulation under the federal Insecticide, Fungicide, and Rodenticide Act (FIFRA). Under FQPA, the term "pesticide" does not include liquid chemical sterilant products (including any products with sterilant or subordinate disinfectant claims) for use on a critical or semicritical device, as defined in Section 201 of the FD&C Act (21 U.S. Code 321). Today, sterilants and high-level disinfectants and their affected claims are no longer regulated by EPA but are solely under the regulatory authority of FDA. FDA now has regulatory jurisdiction over liquid chemical sterilants and high-level disinfectants intended for use in the processing of reusable critical and semicritical medical devices under authority of the FD&C Act.

In July 1995, FDA recommended that liquid chemical sterilants be classified as class II devices (special controls) and that general-purpose disinfectants be classified as class I devices (general controls) and be exempted from the premarket notification procedures [section 510(k) of the FD& C Act]. Regulatory authority over general-purpose disinfectants was not affected by FQPA. Therefore, the dual regulatory requirements for these germicides will continue until the rule-making process for the classification of germicides is completed. The reader is referred to the FDA home page (http://www.fda.gov) for an update on these regulations because many changes were expected in 1998. Professionals in the health care setting were additionally challenged because EPA, FDA, and CDC did not use uniform terminologies for disinfectants.

A Memorandum of Understanding (MOU) was signed between EPA and FDA on 4 June 1993 and was amended on 20 June 1994. Under the MOU, FDA was given primary jurisdiction over liquid chemical sterilants and/or high-level disinfectants intended for use in the reprocessing of critical and semicritical devices, and EPA was given primary jurisdiction over the general-purpose disinfectants intended for use in the reprocessing of noncritical devices and medical equipment surfaces. The MOU calls for both EPA and FDA to initiate a rule-making process to give each agency sole jurisdiction over its designated products. EPA is responsible for low- to medium-level disinfectants including products used in environmental sanitation or disinfectants. It is important to know that EPA classifies microorganisms as "pests" under FIFRA. The agency bases registration decisions on its evaluation of required test data concerning the chemistry, effectiveness, and toxicity of the product. EPA relies on the manufacturer's data only, and independent testing is not required. Another agency is involved in this business: the Occupational Safety and Health Administration (OSHA). It regulates the use of ethylene oxide (see Sterilization), and for some disinfectants—such as formaldehyde—OSHA established an employee exposure standard of 0.75 ppm as an 8-h time-weighted average. Therefore, one should be familiar with terms such as the permissible exposure limit and short-term exposure limit before making recommendations for ethylene oxide sterilization or disinfection when maximal exposure is regulated by OSHA. The legal problems on reprocessing of single-use devices are beyond the scope of this chapter. Current FDA policy states that the responsibility for the safety and performance of reprocessed single-use devices lies in the hands of the reprocessor, not the original manufacturer. The "good manufacturing practices" guidelines (see http://www.fda.gov/cdrh/fr1007ap.pdf for details) indicate that the reprocessor of a single-use item should introduce this reprocessed item to the market as a new product. Therefore, the reprocessor is responsible not only for the sterility and the absence of toxic substances such as endotoxins or residual ethylene oxide but also for the product's integrity and for ensuring that the material's composition is almost identical to that of a new product. Most hospitals cannot afford to generate appropriate data on the quality and performance of reprocessed single-use items. In addition, a manufacturer can change, for example, an additive to a single-use catheter that would require a reprocessor of single-use devices to redo all analyses for the mixture of the catheter before it could be legally marketed after reprocessing. A pro and con session at the Annual Meeting of the Society of Healthcare Epidemiology of America 1997 was unable to provide appropriate guidance on this hot topic issue, as was the case for the same topic at European meetings. However, the reprocessing of single-use items is performed (sometimes illegally) in many countries throughout the world and may be an important component in the provision of access to state-of-the-art health care in times of limited resources. In the authors' personal opinions, the new reprocessing technologies that use a washer-disinfector coupled with a highly effective low-temperature sterilizer (e.g., the Sterrad 100S plasma sterilizer) are able to provide sufficient levels of safety to ensure the absence of viable microorganisms even in narrow lumens such as cardiac catheters. Infection control professionals will be able to provide the desired level of safety in terms of microbiologic and toxicologic safety. Some institutions resterilize items that have not been used on patients but that, for instance, have been dropped and the package has been damaged. Even this simple approach, however, creates some risks for the device as a result of the reprocessing. FDA published an alert regarding an ethylene oxide-sterilized implant that had been resterilized with steam. The quality of the implant has been impaired by this reprocessing method (see http://www.fda.gov/cdrh/steamst.html for details). However, unresolved issues are quality, product integrity, and the performance of the frequently plastic or rubber products after reprocessing. The legal aspects and the appropriate sterilization process should be regulated, for example, by FDA before one considers the reprocessing of single-use items. Health authorities in Canada have published guidelines on the reprocessing of single-use items that can be done legally (44). It is hoped that manufacturers will bring to the market similar reusable devices that are designed today as single-use items. An additional problem to be considered are medical devices that are rented or leased from third parties and that may not be properly cleaned, disinfected, and/or sterilized prior to delivery to the health care facility. This may also apply when health care facilities exchange equipment with other institutions. An alert has been issued by FDA because outsourcing of reprocessing does not transfer full responsibility to the reprocessor (see full text at http://www.fda.gov/medwatch/safety/1997/device.htm).

The European Committee for Standardization (CEN) has appointed technical committees (TCs) to define standards for the testing of chemical germicides. Once established, the European Union will accept products that will have met the required efficacy on the basis of the microbiological tests recommended by TCs. At present, some European countries continue to rely on their local standards and will do so until CEN has standardized the process. However, many countries such as the United Kingdom do not have a standard test for instrument disinfectants (20).

Disinfection by Heat Versus Immersion in Germicides

Disinfection by heat—sometimes called pasteurization—is an important tool in Europe and has replaced disinfection with germicides for many applications. The advantages are obvious: automation of the process, monitoring and documentation of the process similar to that for sterilization, lack of emergence of resistance, and, probably, a lower cost per load compared to the cost of germicides. However, there are some obstacles to thermal disinfection: the costs for the purchase and installation of the equipment are much higher than those when a germicide is used and considerable power is needed to heat the water. Vegetative bacteria are killed within seconds at temperatures of >80 to 85°C. The current German recommendation (Bundesseuchengesetz) for manufacturers of washers-disinfectors for thermal disinfection of devices is 10 min at 92°C, a process that kills all vegetative bacteria and viruses including HBV. In the United Kingdom, the Department of Health requires 65°C for 10 min, 71°C for 3 min, or 80°C for 1 min (36). Non-spore-forming microorganisms such as enterococci have been shown to resist temperatures of up to 71°C for 10 min, challenging these recommendations (36). In the United States, this hot-water pasteurization is generally performed at 77°C for 30 min (86), but few scientific data support a certain higher or lower temperature. Studies by Gurevich et al. (86) indicate that pasteurization with a germicide is more effective than pasteurization without a germicide. However, the washer includes a cleaning process with an average reduction of 4 logs coupled with heat disinfection (5-log killing), resulting in a total reduction of 8 to 9 logs. This surpasses any international requirements for high-level disinfection. Data on the effectiveness of these machines have been summarized in local reports, but most have not been published in peer-reviewed journals. Washers-disinfectors such as the AMSCO Reliance 430 achieved an inactivation factor of >5 logs (80, 99). At the authors' institution, thermal disinfection has almost completely replaced germicide-based disinfection because it is safer and less expensive once the equipment has been purchased (176). In conclusion, thermal disinfection of devices with a washer-disinfector is an excellent alternative to germicide-based immersion. The decision regarding the basic concept of disinfection should balance the availability and the expense of the equipment, the savings achieved in terms of working hours and the storage and distribution of disinfectants, HCW safety, and the greater risks for human errors.

Overview of Commonly Used Disinfectants for Devices

Glutaraldehyde

Glutaraldehyde and formaldehyde are the most extensively studied aldehydes among several others that exhibit biocidal activity, including glyoxal, ortho-phthalaldehyde, succinaldehyde, and benzaldehydes. Extensive reviews may be found elsewhere (17, 154, 157). In commercially available products, glutaraldehyde is the predominant aldehyde. Because of its potent and broad-spectrum microbicidal activities as well as its noncorrosive properties, glutaraldehyde is often accepted as the high-level disinfectant and chemical sterilant of choice. Accordingly, the use of glutaraldehyde-based solutions is widespread in health care facilities. The mechanism by which glutaraldehyde inactivates microorganisms seems to be complex and related to the alkylation of the sulfhydryl, hydroxyl, carboxy, and amino groups of microorganisms. Several target sites for the action are known, such as cell wall and membrane components, nucleic acids, as well as enzymes and other proteins. The biocidal activities of glutaraldehyde solutions are dependent on a variety of variables, such as pH, temperature, glutaraldehyde concentration at the time of use, the presence of inorganic ions, and the age of the solution (17). Aqueous solutions of glutaraldehyde are usually acidic and are not sporicidal in this form. Therefore, they need to be activated by the addition of an alkalinazing agent. These activated solutions, however, rapidly lose their activity due to polymerization of the glutaraldehyde molecules at an alkaline pH. Therefore, the shelf life of such solutions is limited to 14 days unless other recommendations of the manufacturer are listed. To overcome this problem, novel formulations that have longer shelf lives but whose microbicidal potencies are maintained have been developed. The activities of disinfectants increase as the temperature is raised. Among eight disinfectants tested, glutaraldehyde was found to be the chemical most affected by temperature (74).

A standard 2% aqueous solution of glutaraldehyde buffered to pH 7.5 to 8.5 is bactericidal, tuberculocidal, sporicidal, fungicidal, and virucidal. It rapidly kills both gram-negative and gram-positive vegetative bacteria. To inactivate spores and mycobacteria, longer exposure times are required. Spores of *Bacillus* and *Clostridium* spp. are generally destroyed by 2% glutaraldehyde in 3 h, whereas spores of *Clostridium difficile* are more rapidly eliminated (163). The mycobactericidal activity has been questioned by several investigators. Against *M. tuberculosis*, Rubbo et al. (153) demonstrated that glutaraldehyde has a slow action in comparison with alcohols, formaldehyde, iodine, and phenol. Ascenzi et al. (18) found in the quantitative suspension test that 2% glutaraldehyde killed only 2 to 3 logs of *M. tuberculosis* in 20 min at 20°C. Similarly, Collins (52) reported that a standardized suspension of *M. tuberculosis* could not be completely inactivated within 10 min. *Mycobacterium avium*, *Mycobacterium intracellulare*, and *Mycobacterium gordonae* were more resistant to inactivation than *M. tuberculosis* (51). These and other data suggest that 20 min (at 20°C) is the minimum exposure time needed to reliably inactivate tuberculous and nontuberculous mycobacteria by 2% glutaraldehyde, provided that the contaminated item has been cleaned prior to disinfection (98, 157). Recently, glutaraldehyde-resistant mycobacteria have been isolated from endoscope washers-disinfectors (82) (see section on endoscopes below). The virucidal activity of glutaraldehyde also extends to the nonenveloped (hydrophilic) viruses, which are generally more resistant to disinfectants than the enveloped (lipophilic) viruses. Numerous viruses were documented to be inactivated, including HIV, hepatitis A virus, HBV, poliovirus type 1, coxsackievirus type B, yellow fever virus, and rotavirus (17, 106).

Glutaraldehyde is noncorrosive to metal and does not damage rubber and plastic equipment. It retains activity in the presence of organic matter. Glutaraldehyde-based formulations are used most commonly for high-level disinfection of medical equipment such as endoscopes, transducers, dialysis systems, and anesthesia and respiratory therapy equipment (157). Due to dilution, glutaraldehyde concentrations commonly decline during use in manual and automatic baths used for endoscopes (128). Test strips are available to ensure that the glutaraldehyde concentration has not fallen below 1 to 1.5%. Glutaraldehyde vapor at the level of 0.2 ppm is irritating to the eyes, throat, and nose. In HCWs exposed to glutaraldehyde, allergic contact dermatitis, asthma, rhinitis, and epistaxis have been observed. Measures that may minimize employee exposure include use of tight-fitting lids on immersion baths, improved ventilation, ducted exhaust hoods or ductless fume hoods to absorb glutaraldehyde vapor, personal protective equipment, and appropriate automated machines for endoscope disinfection (157). Inadequate rinsing of colonoscopes after immersion in glutaraldehyde may result in proctocolitis (60). In addition, keratopathy caused by ophthalmic instruments that were not properly rinsed after soaking has been reported.

Formaldehyde

Formaldehyde and its condensates have been reviewed in depth elsewhere (149). Formaldehyde in aqueous solutions or as a gas has been used as a disinfectant and sterilant for many decades. Its use in the health care setting, however, has sharply decreased for several reasons. The irritating vapors and pungent odor produced by formaldehyde are apparent at very low levels (<1 ppm). In addition, allergy to formaldehyde is not uncommon. The strongest impact on banning of formaldehyde for sterilization and disinfection processes was the actions of agencies of the U.S. federal government, such as OSHA, and the Health and Safety Executive of the United Kingdom. They indicated that the inhalation of formaldehyde vapors may pose a carcinogenic risk. OSHA limits an 8-h time-weighted average exposure to a concentration of 0.75 ppm in the workplace. Elevated levels of occupational exposures have been found among workers in dialysis units and gross anatomy laboratories (6). For these reasons, the use of formaldehyde and formaldehyde-releasing agents in hospitals is very limited, despite its broad-spectrum microbicidal activity. The 37% (by weight) water-based solution called formalin is used to preserve anatomical, surgical, and biopsy specimens as well as for embalming purposes. Formaldehyde has been used for the disinfection of hemodialysis equipment and water dialysate distribution systems. Other disinfectants, such as chlorines, glutaraldehydes, hydrogen peroxide, and peracetic acid, may replace formaldehyde for the reprocessing of dialysis systems. Paraformaldehyde vaporized by heat is still used for the gaseous decontamination of biological safety cabinets.

Chlorine and Chlorine-Releasing Compounds

Among the large number of chlorine compounds commercially available, hypochlorites are the most widely used disinfectants. Hypochlorite has been used for more than a century and remains an important disinfectant. Rutala and Weber (165) recently published an extensive review on the use of inorganic hypochlorite in health care facilities. Aqueous solutions of sodium hypochlorite are usually called household bleach. Bleach commonly contains 5.25% sodium hypochlorite or 52,500 ppm available chlorine; a 1:10 dilution of bleach provides about 5,000 ppm available chlorine. Alternative chlorine-releasing compounds frequently used in health care facilities include chloramine T, sodium dichloroisocyanurate tablets, and demand-release chlorine dioxide. Demand-release chlorine dioxide is an extremely reactive compound and, consequently, is prepared at the point of use. It is largely used in the chlorination of potable water, swimming pools, and wastewater. Due to its hazardous nature, chlorine gas is rarely used as a disinfectant. In aqueous solution all chlorine compounds release hypochlorous acid, which is considered to be the active compound. The mechanism of microbicidal action of hypochlorous acid has not been fully elucidated. Inhibition of some key enzymatic reactions within the cell and denaturation of proteins play major roles in killing. Lowering of the pH or an increase in the temperature or concentration increases its antimicrobial efficacy. Chlorine compounds have broad antimicrobial spectra that include bacterial spores and *M. tuberculosis* at higher concentrations. Therefore, hypochlorite can be used as a high-level disinfectant for semicritical items. Hypochlorite is fast acting, nonstaining, nonflammable, and inexpensive. However, its use is limited by its corrosive effects, inactivation by organic matter, and relative instability. Although exposure to sodium hypochlorite through direct contact may result in tissue injury, the incidence of injury due to hypochlorite use in health care facilities is extremely low (165). Inhalation of chlorine gas may cause irritation of the respiratory tract, resulting in cough, dyspnea, and pulmonary edema or chemical pneumonitis. Since the potential carcinogens trihalomethanes have been detected in chlorine-treated waters, potential health concerns regarding chlorination of water supplies have been raised. High levels of trihalomethanes were found during continuous hyperchlorination of hospital water when the levels of chlorine in hot water exceeded 4 mg/liter (92). The potential hazards and significant benefits of chlorine use have recently been discussed elsewhere (103).

Available chlorine concentrations of 100 ppm for contact times of 10 min very effectively inactivate vegetative bacteria and viruses. In suspension tests, significant inactivation of both enveloped and nonenveloped viruses, including HIV, hepatitis A virus, HBV, herpes simplex virus types 1 and 2, poliovirus, coxsackievirus, and rotavirus, has been established (165). In general, endospore-forming bacteria, mycobacteria, fungi, and protozoa are less susceptible, and higher concentrations of chlorine (1,000 ppm) are required to completely destroy these germs. A concentration of 100 ppm eliminated 99.9% of *Bacillus subtilis* endospores in 5 min (199). In a *C. difficile* outbreak, the use of sodium hypochlorite solutions (500 and 1,600 ppm) to decontaminate environmental surfaces was associated with both reductions in the levels of surface contamination (79 and 98%, respectively) and control of the outbreak (101). Chloramine T and sodium dichloroisocyanurate seem to have less sporicidal action than sodium hypochlorite. Hypochlorites and other chlorine compounds are substantially inactivated in the presence of blood or other organic matter. Consequently, items used for patient care and environmental surfaces must be cleaned before the disinfectant is used. The presence of a biofilm (e.g., in the pipes of a water distribution system) significantly reduces the efficacies of chlorines as well. In addition, the free available chlorine levels in solutions of opened containers can decay to 40 to 50% of the original concentration within 1 month. Therefore, concentrations higher than those established in laboratory experiments should be used in practice. The following conditions of chlorine use favor the stability of available chlorine: use at room temperature, use of diluted solutions, use of solutions in an alkaline pH range, and storage in closed opaque containers.

Depending on the concentrations employed, sodium hypochlorite is used in hospitals as a high-level disinfectant for selected semicritical devices (e.g., dental equipment and mannequins used for cardiopulmonary resuscitation training) and as a low-level disinfectant for environmental surfaces. CDC recommends use of a 1:100 dilution (5,000 ppm) to decontaminate environmental spills of blood and certain other body fluids (45). Because chlorine can be inactivated by blood and other organic material, the use of a full-strength solution is safer, unless the surface is cleaned prior to disinfection (68). Household bleach is also an appropriate laboratory disinfectant for tabletops, incubators, and laboratory spills. For drug addicts, CDC recommends the use of bleach to disinfect syringes before reuse of the syringe if no sterile disposable syringes are available (47). Chlorines at low concentrations (usually approximately 0.5 ppm free chlorine) are used in the chlorination of drinking water. Hyperchlorination of institutional water systems contaminated with *Legionella pneumophila* has been successfully used to control epidemic nosocomial legionellosis (92). However, corrosion damage to the water distribution system occurs and represents a long-term problem (92). Stabilized solutions of chlorine dioxide appear to be more efficacious than chlorine for the control of legionella (87). This compound also has a reputed lower level of toxicity.

Hydrogen Peroxide

Hydrogen peroxide is a strong oxidizer that is used for high-level disinfection and sterilization. It produces destructive hydroxyl free radicals which can attack membrane lipids, DNA, and other essential cell components (30). Although the catalase produced by anaerobic and some aerobic bacteria may protect cells from hydrogen peroxide, this defense is overwhelmed by the concentrations used for disinfection (30). Generally, a 3% hydrogen peroxide solution is rapidly bactericidal. It is less rapid in its action against organisms with high cellular catalase activity (e.g., *S. aureus*, *Serratia marcescens*) and especially bacterial spores. Surprisingly, 3% hydrogen peroxide was ineffective against vancomycin-resistant enterococci in a recent study (175). Use of a 3% solution for 150 min was shown to destroy 10^6 spores in six of seven exposure trials, whereas use of a 10% concentration and a 60-min exposure time was always successful (193). *Bacillus subtilis* spores were killed by concentration of 17.7 and 35.4% in 9.4 and 2.3 min, respectively (117). In a recent investigation, 10% hydrogen peroxide was the most active chemical disinfectant against *B. subtilis* spores among seven liquid agents tested (169). In contrast, other investigators found that the sporicidal activity of hydrogen peroxide was lower than those of peracetic acid and chlorine (8). Killing of spores is greatly enhanced by increased concentration or temperature. Hydrogen peroxide also acts synergistically against spores with ultrasonic energy, UV radiation, and some chemical agents such as peracetic acid. Martin et al. (125) have demonstrated that 0.3% hydrogen peroxide is able to inactivate HIV in 10 min. A 3% concentration inactivated rhinovirus in 6 to 8 min at 37°C (130), whereas up to 6% was ineffective against poliovirus in 1 min (186). Hydrogen peroxide has low levels of toxicity to humans and the environment. It is neither carcinogenic nor mutagenic. Concentrated solutions may irritate the eyes, skin, and mucous membranes. Hydrogen peroxide can be easily destroyed by heat or the enzymes catalase and peroxidase to give the innocuous end products oxygen and water. Therefore, it is environmentally safe. Only limited data on the use of stabilized hydrogen peroxide in health care have been published in the scientific literature. Stabilized 6% solutions can be used for high-level disinfection of semicritical items, considering the corrosive effects of hydrogen peroxide on copper, zinc, and brass (157). It has been demonstrated that 6% hydrogen peroxide was significantly more effective than 2% glutaraldehyde in the disinfection of flexible endoscopes. Sattar et al. (174) recently evaluated a 7.5% commercially available hydrogen peroxide solution using a soaking time of only 10 min at room temperature. Nevertheless, hydrogen peroxide is not widely used for endoscope disinfection because of concerns that it may be harmful to the endoscopes. Moreover, cases of pseudomembrane-like enterocolitis (pseudolipomatosis) have been associated with exposure to residual hydrogen peroxide in endoscopes (167). Concentrations of 3 to 6% have been used for the disinfection of ventilators, soft contact lenses (3% for 2 to 3 h), and tonometer biprisms (119, 157). Corneal damage after the use of hydrogen peroxide-disinfected tonometer tips that were improperly rinsed has been reported (118). Controversy exists surrounding both the beneficial and the harmful effects of the use of hydrogen peroxide as an antiseptic for wound cleansing and dental regimens (119). Vaporized hydrogen peroxide is also used for low-temperature sterilization (see below).

Peracetic Acid

Peracetic acid or peroxyacetic acid is a germicidal agent that is even more potent than hydrogen peroxide. In comparison to other disinfectants, it was the most active agent in several in vitro studies (7, 8, 123, 170). Concentrations of ≤1% are sporicidal even at low temperatures. Accordingly, it is listed as a high-level disinfectant and chemical sterilant by FDA. The mechanism of action of peracetic acid has not been clearly elucidated, but it is likely to function much as hydrogen peroxide and other oxidizing agents. Synergistic sporicidal effects of peracetic acid with alcohols have been observed. Peracetic acid remains effective in the presence of organic matter. Although at low concentrations it is considerably less stable than hydrogen peroxide, preparations with appropriate stability have been developed and are commercially available. Peracetic acid is corrosive to plain steel, galvanized iron, copper, brass, and bronze. Additionally, it will attack natural and synthetic rubbers. Its powerful germicidal activity and its lack of environmentally problematic or toxic residues make peracetic acid very attractive for use in health care settings. It is used in combination with hydrogen peroxide to disinfect hemodialyzers in many hospitals. However, concerns about the potential toxicity of the combination of peracetic and acetic acids to hemodialysis patients have been raised (91). Feldman et al. (67) recently reported that dialysis in freestanding facilities that reprocess dialyzers with peracetic and acetic acids was associated with higher rates of mortality than treatment in facilities that do not reprocess dialyzers or that use formaldehyde. It is not known if the higher death rate arose from the direct toxicity of peracetic and acetic acids or other factors related to the patients and facilities. The use of peracetic acid for chemical sterilization of instruments and endoscopes is discussed below. Recently, a new formulation that contains 0.35% peracetic acid and that demonstrated rapid sporicidal and mycobactericidal activities has been introduced (50).

Alcohols

For centuries, the alcohols have been appreciated for their antimicrobial properties. For infection control purposes, ethyl alcohol (ethanol) and isopropyl alcohol (isopropanol) are the alcoholic solutions most often used. Their antimicrobial efficacies are enhanced in the presence of water, with optimal concentrations being from 60 to 90%, by volume. The exact mechanism by which alcohols destroy microorganisms is not fully understood. The most plausible explanation for the antimicrobial action is coagulation (denaturation) of proteins, e.g., of enzymatic proteins, leading to the loss of specific cellular functions (114). Ethyl and isopropyl alcohols at appropriate concentrations have broad spectra of antimicrobial activity that includes vegetative bacteria, fungi, and viruses. However, they generally do not destroy bacterial spores. Fatal infections due to *Clostridium* spp. were observed when alcohol was used for sterilization of surgical instruments. Against vegetative bacteria, such as *S. aureus*, *Streptococcus pyogenes*, members of the family *Enterobacteriaceae*, and *P. aeruginosa*, alcohols are rapidly bactericidal. These germs were killed by 70 to 80% ethyl alcohol in 10 to 90 s in suspension tests. (151). Isopropyl alcohol was found to be slightly more bactericidal than ethyl alcohol (114). In a recent study, isopropyl alcohol was highly effective against vancomycin-resistant enterococci, in contrast to hydrogen peroxide, which was ineffective against all eight strains tested (175). Isopropyl alcohol has also been demonstrated to have excellent activity against mycobacteria including *M. tuberculosis* and fungi, such as *Candida* spp., *Cryptococcus neoformans*, *Blastomyces dermatitidis*, *Coccidioides immitis*, *Histoplasma capsulatum*, *Aspergillus niger*, and dermatophytes. Controversial data on the antiviral activity of alcohols have been reported. While both ethyl and isopropyl alcohols are able to inactivate most viruses with a lipid envelope (e.g., influenza virus, herpes simplex virus, and adenovirus), several investigators found that isopropyl alcohol had less virucidal activity against naked, nonenveloped viruses (22, 106). In experiments by Klein and DeForest (106), propan-2-ol even at 95% could not inactivate the nonenveloped viruses poliovirus type 1 and coxsackievirus type B in 10 min. In contrast, these enteroviruses were inactivated by 70% ethanol (106). Against hepatitis A virus, however, 70% ethanol and 45% propan-2-ol were not effective when their activities were assessed on stainless-steel disks contaminated with fecally suspended virus. Among 20 disinfectants tested, only 3 were able to reduce the titer of hepatitis A virus by greater than 99.9% in 1 min (2% glutaraldehyde, sodium hypochlorite with >5,000 ppm free chlorine, and a quaternary ammonium formulation containing 23% HCl) (127). Experiments by Bond et al. (31) and Kobayashi et al. (108) demonstrated that treatment of human plasma containing high-titer HBV with propan-2-ol (70% for 10 min) or ethanol (80% for 2 min) was effective when treatment was tested by inoculation of the treated plasma into susceptible chimpanzees. In a suspension test, 40% propanol was able to reduce the rotavirus titer by at least 4 logs in 1 min (110). HIV is readily inactivated by both ethyl and isopropyl alcohols. Martin et al. (125) found that 15% ethyl alcohol and 35% isopropyl alcohol were effective in a suspension test. More recently, high titers of HIV in suspension have been shown to be rapidly inactivated by 70% ethanol, independent of the protein load. However, the rate of inactivation decreased when virus was dried onto a glass surface and high levels of protein were present (187). Alcohols cannot penetrate protein-rich materials. Therefore, a spray or a wipe with alcohol cannot be guaranteed to disinfect a surface contaminated with blood or other body fluids without preliminary cleaning. The antiviral activities of alcoholic agents found in vitro were confirmed by studies with artificially contaminated hands or fingertips. As an example, both 70% propanol and 70% ethanol reduced the release of rotavirus from the contaminated fingertips by 2.7 logs. In comparison, the mean log reductions obtained with liquid soap and an aqueous solution of chlorhexidine gluconate were 0.9 and 0.7, respectively, which are 100 times less than the reductions achieved with the alcohols (15).

Alcohols possess many qualities that make them suitable both for antisepsis of skin and for disinfection of equipment. They are fast acting, hardly toxic with topical application, nonstaining, and nonallergenic and readily evaporate. The rapid evaporation is advantageous for most disinfection and antisepsis procedures. The uptake of alcohol by intact skin and the lungs when alcohol is used on the skin surface is so small that health concerns are not justified. Alcohols have better wetting properties than water due to their lower surface tensions. This represents an important feature for skin antisepsis, along with their cleansing and degreasing actions. Repeated application of alcoholic antiseptics, however, may cause drying and irritation of the skin. Therefore, commercial preparations for hand disinfection should contain refatting agents and emollients. The use of alcohols for antisepsis of hands and skin is further discussed below. Alcohols are also excellent for intermediate-level and low-level disinfection of small and clean surfaces of objects, equipment, and environment (e.g., rubber stoppers of medication vials, stethoscopes, and medication preparation areas). After prolonged and repeated use, alcohols may damage rubber and certain plastic items as well as the shellac mountings of lensed instruments (157). Alcoholic formulations used prior to invasive procedures should be free of spores, a process that is achieved in commercial products by filtration. Since alcohols are flammable, one should consider the flame point. They must not be used on larger surfaces, particularly in closed, poorly ventilated areas.

Phenolics

Since the pioneering use of phenol (carbolic acid) as an antiseptic by Lister, a large number of phenol derivatives or phenolics have been developed and marketed. Today, phenolics make up one of the major classes of disinfectants used in hospitals. Phenol derivatives originate when a functional group (e.g., alkyl, benzyl, phenyl, amyl, or chloro) replaces one of the hydrogen atoms on the aromatic ring. The three phenolics most commonly found as constituents of disinfectants are *o*-phenylphenol, *o*-benzyl-*p*-chlorophenol, and *p*-*tert*-amylphenol. The addition of detergents to the basic formulation results in products with excellent detergent properties that clean, dissolve proteins, and disinfect in one step. Phenolics at higher concentrations act as a gross protoplasmic poison, penetrating and disrupting the bacterial cell wall and precipitating the cell proteins (137). Lower concentrations of these compounds inactivate cellular enzyme systems and cause leakage of essential metabolites from the cell. Phenol compounds at concentrations of 2 to 5% are generally considered bactericidal, tuberculocidal, fungicidal, and virucidal against lipophilic viruses (137). However, the manufacturers' efficacy claims against microorganisms have generally not been verified by independent laboratories or EPA (157). A collaborative study by Rutala and Cole (160) documented the fact that randomly selected EPA-registered phenolic detergents and quaternary ammonium compounds do not consistently meet the manufacturers' bactericidal label claims. By the AOAC use-dilution method, the phenolics tested at the recommended use dilution failed against *P. aeruginosa* in 33 to 78% of the laboratories. However, extreme variability of test results has been observed among laboratories testing identical products (160). Phenolics at the use dilutions are not lethal to bacterial spores. A 2% phenolic was shown to kill a wide spectrum of clinically important fungi except *Aspergillus fumigatus* (185). Klein and DeForest (106) found that 12% *o*-phenylphenol was effective only against lipophilic viruses, although 5% phenol inactivated both lipophilic and hydrophilic viruses. Similarly, other investigators demonstrated little or no virucidal effect of a phenolic against coxsackievirus type B4, echovirus type 11, or poliovirus type 1 (136). Martin et al. (125) showed that a 0.5% commercial phenolic formulation (2.8% *o*-phenylphenol and 2.7% *o*-benzyl-*p*-chlorophenol) inactivated HIV. In contrast, another commercial product containing phenolics at a final concentration of 1% failed to completely inactivate cell-associated HIV suspended in blood (62). A phenol-based preparation (14.7% phenol diluted 1:256 in tap water) produced a reduction in rotavirus similar to that achieved with a bleach dilution (800 ppm available chlorine) (173). In a further experiment, both the phenolic and the bleach were able to interrupt the transfer of virus from disks to fingerpads (173). Phenolic compounds are tolerant of anionic and organic matter. They are assimilated by porous materials and leave a residual film. The residual films may cause irritation to the skin and tissues. Depigmentation of the skin caused by preparations containing *p*-*tert*-butylphenol and *p*-*tert*-amylphenol has been reported. Phenolic germicidal detergent solutions may be used for intermediate-level and low-level disinfection of surgical instruments and noncritical patient care items with smooth and hard surfaces. These compounds are also appropriate for the decontamination of the hospital environment, including laboratory surfaces. Their use in nurseries should be prohibited since hyperbilirubinemia has occurred in phenol-exposed infants (201). Infant bassinets and incubators should not be disinfected with phenols (157).

Quaternary Ammonium Compounds

A wide variety of quaternary ammonium compounds (quats) exhibiting antimicrobial activity have been introduced in the past decade. Some of the compounds used in health care settings are benzalkonium chloride, alkyldimethylbenzyl ammonium chloride, and didecyldimethyl ammonium chloride. Quats are cationic surface-active detergents. Their biocidal actions appear to result from the disruption of the cell membrane, inactivation of enzymes, and denaturation of cell proteins (131). Quats are nonstaining, odorless, noncorrosive, and relatively nontoxic. However, they have a limited antimicrobial spectrum. Products sold as hospital disinfectants are not sporicidal and are generally not tuberculocidal or virucidal against hydrophilic viruses. Scientific investigations by the AOAC use-dilution method have failed to reproduce the bactericidal and tuberculocidal claims made by manufacturers of quats (161). Manufacturers' label claims and results from in-house evaluations not verified by an independent laboratory should be considered questionable. The overestimation of the germicidal activity may be related to incomplete inactivation of the compounds tested. In this case, the bacteriostatic (inhibitory) activity rather than the bactericidal activity is measured (131). Several outbreaks of infections associated with in-use contamination of quat solutions have been reported. In those solutions, gram-negative bacteria such as *Pseudomonas* spp. (69) and *S. marcescens* (63, 135) were found to survive or grow. The contaminated solutions were used for antisepsis on skin and tissue as well as for disinfection of patient care supplies or equipment (i.e., cardiac catheters and cystoscopes). Organic matter, anionic detergents (soaps), and materials such as cotton and gauze pads can reduce the microbicidal activities of quats. Quaternary ammonium germicidal detergent solutions are excellent cleaning agents. Therefore, they are preferred agents for the cleaning of floors. On the basis of their limited antimicrobial spectra, their use in hospitals should be restricted to ordinary environmental sanitation of noncritical surfaces such as floors, furniture, and walls (157).

Other Germicides of Interest

The novel antimicrobial compound *glucoprotamine* is the conversion product of L-glutamic acid and cocopropylene-1,3-diamine. It has been demonstrated to possess a broad antimicrobial spectrum that includes vegetative bacteria, mycobacteria, fungi, and enveloped viruses (58). A clinical study examining used specula from a gynecologic clinic demonstrated the product's >6 log killing of vegetative bacteria excluding spores (unpublished data from the authors' institution). Results from the manufacturer's data sheets indicate good compatibility of the compound with humans and the environment as well as various materials. A commercial product is available in Europe for disinfection of instruments.

Peroxygen compounds have been claimed to be effective against a wide variety of microorganisms including bacterial spores. A 1% concentration of a new commercial formulation containing peroxygen achieved a 10^5-fold killing of *B.*

TABLE 7 Outbreaks and pseudo-outbreaks associated with contaminated endoscopes

Microorganisms	No. of cases	No. of deaths	Yr of publication	Problem identified	Type of outbreak	Reference
HCV	2	0	1997	Cleaning, immersion	Disease	39
M. tuberculosis	2	0	1997	Cleaning, immersion	Disease	133
M. tuberculosis (multidrug resistant)	5	1	1997	Cleaning, immersion	Disease	3
M. xenopi	>49	?	1997	Use of tap water to rinse; cases occurred from 1987 to 1993; inappropriate microbiological technique for *M. xenopi*	Disease	61a
P. aeruginosa	23	0	1996	Failure of washer-disinfector	Pseudo-outbreak	27
Nontuberculous mycobacteria	4	0	1992	Failure of washer-disinfector	Pseudo-outbreak	
Multiple microorganisms	377	7	1993	Cleaning, immersion, use of tap water, design errors of washer-disinfector	Disease	Review 178

subtilis in 2 to 3 h in the absence of blood, but killing was poor in the presence of blood (50). Griffiths et al. (82) have found that peroxygen has poor mycobactericidal activity. Likewise, concentrations of 2.3 and 4% and exposure times ranging between 30 and 120 min were not able to inactivate mycobacteria in another study (38).

Superoxidized water is prepared by mixing a small amount of NaCl with tap water in an electrolyzer. Preliminary data indicate that this solution has powerful bactericidal activity, although further studies are needed to explore the use of this new, low-cost germicide in clinical settings (183).

Metals such as *copper* and *silver* ions have been demonstrated to inactivate a wide variety of microorganisms (168). Although further work is required, they could be used for disinfection of water or medical devices.

The number of germicidal agents is too large to be covered in this overview. A more comprehensive review may be found in two renowned references (29, 156). Guidelines for the selection and use of disinfectants and recommendations on the preferred method for disinfection and sterilization of patient care items have been recently published by Rutala (157, 158).

Specific Issues

Endoscopes

The shortcomings encountered with the reprocessing of endoscopes are well known, but outbreaks and even outbreaks with deaths continue to be reported. It is probably the most challenging issue in reprocessing for infection control professionals. Flexible endoscopes have an intricate design and have sophisticated small parts that are difficult to clean, but cleaning is a prerequisite for any disinfection process. A large study in several U.S. centers found that 78% of the facilities failed to sterilize all biopsy forceps. In addition, a total of 23.9% of the cultures of specimens from the internal channels of 71 gastrointestinal endoscopes grew $\geq 10^6$ CFU bacteria (102). These specimens were obtained after the completion of all disinfection and sterilization procedures, and the device had been deemed ready for use on the next patient. Up to 40% of the institutions do not follow published guidelines for endoscope disinfection, thus explaining the frequency of outbreaks (Table 7) (65, 78, 159). The inherent problem of human errors in manual reprocessing promoted the use of automated washers-disinfectors specifically for endoscopes. They rinse the instruments, clean them in several steps, and run a full-cycle disinfection process. In addition, the time of exposure to disinfectants is given by the machine and cannot be shortened, as it can with manual reprocessing in a busy endoscopy unit. However, none of the current machines fulfill all demands of infection control professionals. In a study with endoscope washers, microbiologic cultures demonstrated growth of gram-negative bacteria and/or mycobacteria in 27% of cultures for specimens obtained before the final alcohol rinse and in 10% of cultures for specimens obtained thereafter. In the same study with specimens obtained at the same times described above, 37 and 27% of manually disinfected endoscopes remained contaminated, respectively (70). In 1992, 835 Olympus endoscope washers were recalled: the design of the device allowed colonization by water-borne organisms such as *Pseudomonas* spp. in the internal tanks and tubing (recall no. Z-039/040-2 by FDA [www.fda.gov]). Therefore, extensive review of the current marketed products is crucial before choosing an endoscope washer. The quality of the machine and not the price at purchase should guide the final decision. These machines are designed to run for several years, and even an expensive machine but one with an excellent design will pay off by preventing cross-contamination over the years that it is in use.

Problems related to contamination of endoscope washers do not apply to disinfectors that use peracetic acid, such as the STERIS SYSTEM 1. However, this machine requires sufficient manual cleaning before using and has the risks for human error mentioned above (35). Newer washers-disinfectors should at least continuously monitor the pressure in all channels to detect debris blocking the channels, provide adapters for all kinds of endoscopes, use an appropriate disinfection process with an FDA-cleared disinfectant, use filtered water or sterile water for rinsing, and have a built-in automatic disinfection process. Ample data indicate that a sufficient level of safety can be achieved even with manual disinfection of endoscopes if the guidelines are strictly followed (126). A minimum requirement for an institution is to provide sufficient training for the HCW responsible for endoscope reprocessing. It should include written instructions concerning cleaning, use of disinfectants, immersion times with special attention to all channels, and a system for basic quality assurance. In Germany, routine microbiologic testing of disinfected endoscopes is recommended every 3 to 4 months. The most frequent causes of contamination of endoscopes with pathogens after reprocessing are inadequate cleaning or incomplete immersion of the endoscope and blocked channels. Immersion for ≥20 min in ≥2% glutaraldehyde is required to disinfect endoscopes belonging to the semicritical items. This exposure time and the concentration of glutaraldehyde are sufficient to kill ≥3 logs of mycobacteria, the most resistant vegetative bacteria. However, there are reports of glutaraldehyde-resistant mycobacteria, requiring that more stringent guidelines be used to monitor the effectiveness of the disinfection process (82). The glutaraldehyde concentration decreased by more than 50% after 2 weeks in a commercial cleaner-disinfector, promoting the emergence of resistant bacteria (188). Higher concentrations of glutaraldehyde (3.2% instead of 2%) appear to be safe for endoscopes and achieve the required ≥3-log killing with a higher margin of safety than those achieved with the standard concentration (5). Information on this topic is regularly published by the American Association of Practitioners of Infection Control (126, 157). The debate on sterilization versus high-level disinfection of endoscopes continues (134). However, it is a fact that epidemics caused by contaminated endoscopes are ongoing, despite publications assuring the appropriateness of high-level disinfection. The problem—in the authors' personal opinions—is based on the fact that an extreme safety margin has been introduced for steam sterilization, allowing even multiple errors in reprocessing. The HCW might believe that this is true for disinfection of endoscopes as well. However, high-level disinfection of endoscopes lacks an adequate safety margin. A single error by an HCW may result in the transmission of an infection by a contaminated endoscope. Therefore, only HCWs with adequate training should be responsible for this reprocessing. In addition, ongoing quality assurance is necessary to minimize the risk for cross-infection.

Dental Equipment

Dental patients and HCWs may be exposed to a variety of microorganisms by dental instruments or by direct contact with blood or respiratory secretions. Therefore, blood-borne and airborne pathogens are of concern. The most likely mode of transmission is droplets from infected patients. Typical microorganisms include cytomegalovirus, HBV, HCV, herpes simplex virus types 1 and 2, HIV, and *M. tuberculosis*. Staphylococci and streptococci are commonly isolated but are rarely involved in infections. Pathogens may be transmitted by direct contact with blood, oral fluids, or other secretions; indirect contact with contaminated instruments, operatory equipment, or environmental surfaces; or contact with airborne contaminants present in droplets. Current recommendations are summarized in a report published by CDC in 1993 (46) and a publication of the American Dental Association (1). Several issues are outlined: use of gloves during procedures, hand disinfection or hand washing between patients, use of a surgical mask and protective eyeware when splashing is likely, and the use of laboratory coats. Critical and semicritical instruments should be sterilized and packaged prior to sterilization if they are not used immediately. The adequacy of sterilization cycles should be verified by the periodic use (e.g., at least weekly) of biologic indicators. This recommendation is rarely followed in Europe (84). Routine between-patient sterilization is recommended for all high-speed dental handheld pieces. Handheld pieces that cannot be heat sterilized should be retrofitted to attain heat tolerance or, if this is not feasible, should not be used. Alcohol (70 to 80%) is preferred in Europe for uncovered operating surfaces because of its rapid action (within seconds) and evaporation, but other EPA-registered disinfectants can be used as well. *Legionella* spp. can contaminate air-water syringes and high-speed outlets: In one study, 25% of the water samples were contaminated (48). In addition, more than 6% of samples from workbenches, air turbine handheld pieces, holders, suction units, forceps, and dental mirrors were found by PCR to be positive for HCV, indicating extensive HCV contamination of dental surgeries after treatment of HCV-positive patients (141). Therefore, infection control issues, particularly with regard to HCV and HBV, may be more important in dentistry than has been appreciated in the past 10 years.

Disinfectants for Living Tissue

Compounds that disinfect living tissue are frequently called antiseptic agents. They must meet many more requirements than compounds used for disinfection of, for example, floors. In addition, some of the agents are considered drugs and, thus, are regulated by FDA. Several agents are commercially available. Their antimicrobial spectra are summarized in Table 5. The choice of the agent not only should be based on their desired effect but should also include consideration of side effects, similar to the case for antibiotics. An example is the observation of anaphylactic shock after the application of chlorhexidine onto patients (64, 139). However, side effects are rare, and most agents on the market have excellent safety profiles. Nevertheless, the potential for side effects should be kept in mind when antiseptic agents are used.

Hygienic Hand Washing and Hand Disinfection

The most important issue is not hand washing, hand disinfection, or the choice of the disinfectant but the need to motivate the HCW to perform the simple procedure when necessary. Indications for hand washing or disinfection were classified in a hierarchical order by CDC in 1985 (http://www.cdc.gov.ncidod/hip/guide/handwash.htm) and by professional organizations (115). Microorganisms on the hands can be classified into three groups (142): transient flora, which are contaminants taken up from the environment; resident flora, which are permanent microorganisms on the skin; and infectious flora, which are pathogens that cause infections.

The goal of hand washing or hand disinfection outside the operating room is to eliminate the transient flora. Long-term reduction is not desirable, because it may alter the resident flora. The surgical hand scrub or hand disinfection aims to eliminate both transient and resident flora. Hand washing or hand disinfection represents the single most important procedure for infection control (115). The density of resident bacteria on the skin ranges between 10^2 and 10^3 CFU/cm^2. These resident bacteria limit colonization with more pathogenic microorganisms. The pathogenicity is low, and infections with these bacteria usually require some physical alteration of the host immunity such as placement of an implant or any foreign body. This function is called colonization resistance. HCWs can acquire pathogens from patients during their daily work and can transmit them to susceptible patients. Multiple epidemics have been traced to contaminated hands of HCWs (34, 166, 172, 198, 204).

Most of the resident flora are found on the uppermost level of the stratum corneum. HCWs' hands are frequently contaminated by direct contact while caring for a patient or indirect contact while touching a contaminated surface or device. Several studies indicated that pathogens can be found on the hands of HCWs, such as *S. aureus* in ≥18% of HCWs (113, 147), and one can find *Klebsiella pneumoniae* (2), *Acinetobacter* spp., *Enterobacter* spp., or *Candida* spp. in more than 20% of HCWs. Therefore, CDC has set a high priority for hand washing and has issued specific recommendations. Most research was guided by problems concerning effectiveness and compliance with hand washing (9, 59, 129). Most studies have proved that hand disinfection is much more effective at killing bacteria and most viruses than hand washing with a medicated soap (23, 152). However, no sound epidemiologic data have demonstrated that a certain level of killing is needed to have an impact on the incidence of nosocomial infection. The level of compliance with hand-washing procedures does not exceed 40% even under controlled study conditions (81, 111). Interventions against the bacterial load of the skin should balance two goals: protection of the skin with its resident flora and killing of the transient flora. Intact skin on HCWs' hands helps to protect both patients and HCWs from getting or transmitting nosocomial infections. Therefore, any recommendation for hand washing or hand disinfection should include some advice for skin care, for example, by making a skin care product available free of charge for HCWs. Compliance with hand-washing procedures also depends on the time necessary to perform an adequate hand washing and the time available. Hand washing for 15 and 30 s achieves levels of microbial killing of 0.6 to 1.1 and 1.8 to 2.8 logs, respectively (150). However, hand washing for less than 10 s is common in clinical practice (112). A mathematical model estimated that the time required to perform hand disinfection is only 26% of that required to perform regular hand washing (195). This model was subsequently tested in a tertiary-care center, and similar time savings were observed (190). In addition, hand disinfection achieves a much higher level of microbial killing than hand washing does (194). These in vitro and experimental data have also been supported in a crossover clinical trial with surgeons (197). In addition, sinks are expensive and cannot be installed at locations that are as convenient for HCWs as disinfectant dispensers. HCWs can even contaminate the faucets, as was recently observed during a shigella outbreak (132). Therefore, health care institutions in northern Europe have replaced hand washing with hand disinfection for many indications for which hand washing was previously the standard of care. At the authors' institution, hand disinfection replaced hand washing for >90% of opportunities for hand washing, provided that the hands were not visibly soiled. An alcohol dispenser is available between all beds and at each nurse's desk, and two are available at each bed in intensive care units. A database of the 4,500 HCWs did not identify a single case of documented allergy to the commercial alcohol compound in use, resulting in an incidence density of <1:45,000 person-years. An outstanding review of the use of alcohol for hand disinfection has been written by Rotter (150).

Surgical Hand Washing (Scrub) or Surgical Hand Disinfection

The objective of the surgical scrub is to eliminate the transient flora and most of the resident flora. The rationale is to limit bacterial exposure of the surgeon's skin in case the surgical glove is punctured or torn. Tiny holes are observed in ≥30% of surgeons' gloves after an operation, even when high-quality gloves are used. In a large study, the incidence of surgical site infection (SSI) after clean surgery was related to punctures in the surgeon's gloves: the incidence of SSI was three times higher if a puncture of the surgeon's gloves was observed than if intact gloves were noted after the procedure (1.7 versus 5.7%) (55). An experimental study demonstrated that the level of bacterial leakage through pinholes ranged between 10^3 and 10^4 CFU (71). In contrast to the hygienic hand wash, a long-term antimicrobial effect is required after washing or disinfection to limit bacterial regrowth below the gloves (73). Therefore, agents with a prolonged postexposure effect are preferred. Chlorhexidine is one of the most frequently used agents. However, no controlled clinical trials have demonstrated that it has an impact on the incidence of SSIs. Given the low frequency of transmission of blood-borne pathogens, such a study will never be completed (39). Alcoholic preparations are also more effective than any medicated soap for the surgical scrub (150). In addition, they do not alter the skin as much as chlorhexidine washes do (197). Therefore, the presurgical scrub has been replaced in many European countries by the alcoholic rub. The antimicrobial efficacy was also much better in a clinical trial in the operating room. The alcoholic compound killed bacteria significantly better than the standard scrub with a chlorhexidine soap did (197). Brushes may harm more than they contribute to cleaning: their use should be restricted to cleaning the fingernails.

Presurgical Skin Disinfection

The aim of skin disinfection is the rapid removal and killing of the skin flora at the site of a planned surgical incision. FDA defines a skin disinfectant as a "fast-acting, broad-spectrum and persistent antiseptic-containing preparation that significantly reduces the number of microorganisms on intact skin" (14). Alcohols are well suited for this purpose, but they lack long-term effects. Therefore, iodine is frequently added for this purpose (75). However, for a short-term procedure, alcoholic preparations frequently suffice for skin preparation. Alcohols used for presurgical skin preparation must be sterile, which is usually achieved by filtration or, in some countries, by adding 0.5% hydrogen peroxide to ethanol (151). Spores are usually not of concern, but preoperative skin preparation before amputation of a malperfused leg might be done with an agent with activity against spores (151). Antiseptics should be applied with pressure since friction increases the antibacterial effect: alcohol applied without friction reduces bacterial counts by 1.0 to 1.2 log CFU compared to 1.9 to 3.0 log CFU with friction. In comparison, alcoholic sprays have little antimicrobial effect and produce potentially explosive vapors (121). An extensive review was published by FDA in 1994 (14). Only iodine products in alcohol were listed as category I (generally recognized as safe and effective).

Common Antiseptic Compounds

Alcoholic Compounds

The reader is referred to the earlier section on alcoholic compounds. Alcohol is the most important skin disinfectant. Alcohols used for skin disinfection prior to invasive procedures should generally be free of spores to avoid any contamination. Although the risk of infection is minimal, the low additional cost for a spore-free product is justified.

Chlorhexidine

Chlorhexidine gluconate, a cationic bisbiguanide, has been widely recognized as an effective and safe antiseptic for more than 30 years (57, 146). Its most common formulation is a 4% aqueous solution in a detergent base. The antimicrobial spectrum includes vegetative bacteria, fungi, and viruses. Bactericidal concentrations cause destruction of the bacterial cell membrane, leading to leakage of cellular constituents and coagulation of cell contents (57). Chlorhexidine has been demonstrated to be bactericidal against both gram-positive and gram-negative bacteria. However, Stickler and Thomas (181) found chlorhexidine-resistant bacteria after extensive and long-term use of chlorhexidine prior to bladder catheterization. A recent report documented microbial contamination of 0.02 and 0.05% chlorhexidine gluconate solutions manufactured in a hospital (138). The chlorhexidine resistance of vegetative bacteria appears to be limited to certain gram-negative bacilli (such as *P. aeruginosa, Burkholderia [Pseudomonas] cepacia, Proteus mirabilis*, and *S. marcescens*) (181). In addition to its rapid bactericidal action, chlorhexidine gluconate provides a persistent antimicrobial action that prevents the regrowth of microorganisms. This effect is desirable when a sustained reduction in microbial flora reduces infection risk (e.g., during surgical procedures). Chlorhexidine has little activity against bacterial and fungal spores except at high temperatures. Mycobacteria are inhibited but are not killed by aqueous solutions. Yeasts and dermatophytes are usually sensitive, although the fungicidal action varies with the species (57). Chlorhexidine was effective against lipophilic viruses (e.g., HIV, influenzavirus, and herpes simplex virus types 1 and 2). Other viruses, such as poliovirus, coxsackievirus, and rotavirus, were not inactivated (57). The antimicrobial activity of chlorhexidine is little affected by blood and other organic material, in contrast to povidone-iodine (120). However, inorganic anions and organic anions such as soaps are incompatible with chlorhexidine. Its activity is also reduced at an extreme acidic or alkaline pH and in the presence of anionic- and nonionic-based moisturizers and detergents. Chlorhexidine absorbed onto the fibers of cotton and certain other fabrics usually resists removal by washing. If a hypochlorite (bleach) is used during the washing procedure, a brown stain may develop (57). Long-term experience with the use of chlorhexidine has demonstrated that the incidence of hypersensitivity and skin irritation is low. However, severe allergic reactions including anaphylaxis have been reported (64, 140, 202). Although cytotoxicity has been observed in exposed fibroblasts, no deleterious effects on wound healing were found in vivo. There is no evidence that chlorhexidine gluconate is toxic if it is absorbed through the skin. However, ototoxicity can occur when chlorhexidine is instilled into the middle ear during surgery. High concentrations and preparations containing other compounds (e.g., alcohols and surfactants) may cause eye damage (182). Chlorhexidine formulations are extensively used for surgical hand disinfection and hygienic hand disinfection. This topic was discussed above. Other applications include preoperative whole-body disinfection, antisepsis in obstetrics and gynecology, management of burns, wound antisepsis, as well as prevention and treatment of oral disease (plaque control, pre- and postoperative mouthwash, oral hygiene) (57, 146). When chlorhexidine is used orally, its bitter taste must be masked, and tooth staining usually occurs. Chlorhexidine alcoholic preparations have been demonstrated in numerous studies to have superior antimicrobial activity compared with those of detergent-based formulations (116). Despite the documented superiority of alcoholic solutions, they are widely used in only some European countries.

Iodophors

The previously used aqueous iodine and tincture have largely been replaced by the iodophors. The risk of side effects from the use of these compounds, such as staining, irritation of tissue, and resorption, is lower than that from the use of aqueous iodine. Iodophors are chemical complexes with iodine bound to a carrier such as polyvinylpyrrolidone (povidone, PVP) or ethoxylated nonionic detergents (poloxamers). These complexes gradually release small amounts of free microbicidal iodine. The most commonly used iodophor is povidone-iodine. Its preparations generally contain 1 to 10% povidone-iodine, which is equivalent to 0.1 to 1.0% available iodine. The active species appears to be free molecular iodine (I_2). A paradoxical effect of dilution on the activity of povidone-iodine has been observed. As the degree of dilution increases, bactericidal activity increases up to a maximum and then falls (79). Commercial povidone-iodine solutions at dilutions of 1:2 to 1:100 killed *S. aureus* and *Mycobacterium chelonae* more rapidly than the stock solutions did (24). *S. aureus* survived a 2-min exposure to full-strength povidone-iodine solution, but it did not survive a 15-s exposure to a 1:100 dilution of the iodophor (24). Thus, iodophors must be used at the dilution stated by the manufacturer. The exact mechanism by which iodine destroys microorganisms is not known. It has been postulated that iodine reacts with amino acids and fatty acids of microorganisms, resulting in the destruction of cell structures and enzymes (79). Depending on the concentration of free iodine and other factors, iodophors exhibit a broad range of microbicidal activity. Commercial preparations have been shown to be bactericidal, mycobactericidal, fungicidal, and virucidal but not sporicidal at their dilution recommended for use. Prolonged contact times are required to inactivate certain fungi and bacterial spores (157). However, reports on intrinsic contamination of povidone-iodine and poloxamer-iodine solutions with *B. cepacia* or *P. aeruginosa*, which caused pseudobacteremia and peritonitis, have questioned the killing actions of iodophors (25, 53). *B. cepacia* was found to survive for up to 68 weeks in a contaminated povidone-iodine antiseptic solution (13). The most likely explanation for the prolonged survival of microorganisms in iodophor solutions is mechanical protection of microorganisms by organic and inorganic material and possibly by biofilm formation. Unlike iodine, iodophors are relatively free of toxic effects, do not cause irritability, and do not corrode metal surfaces (79). They have little if any residual effect. However, for a limited time they may have a residual bactericidal activity on the skin surface, because free iodine diffuses not only into deep regions but also back to the skin surface (79). The antimicrobial efficacy of iodophors is reduced in the presence of organic material such as blood. A body surface treated with an iodine or iodophor solution may absorb free iodine. Consequently, increased serum iodine levels (and serum iodide levels) were found, especially when large areas were treated for a long period (79). For this reason, hyperthyroidism and other disorders of thyroid functions are contraindications for the use of iodine-containing preparations. Likewise, iodophors should be applied neither to pregnant and nursing women nor to newborns and infants (41). Because severe local and systemic allergic reactions have been observed, iodophors must not be used in patients with allergies to these preparations or iodine (192). Iodophors are widely used for antisepsis of skin, mucous membranes, and wounds. A 2.5% ophthalmic solution of povidone-iodine was shown to be more effective and less toxic than silver nitrate or erythromycin ointment used as prophylaxis against neonatal conjunctivitis (ophthalmia neonatorum) (97). In some countries, povidone-iodine alcoholic solutions are successfully used for skin antisepsis prior to invasive procedures (16). Iodophors containing higher concentrations of free iodine may be used for disinfection of medical equipment (157). Disinfectants for antisepsis are not suitable as hard-surface disinfectants since the concentrations of these disinfectants are usually lower (157).

Octenidine and Others

Octenidine dihydrochloride is a newly developed bispyridine compound, which has been shown to be an effective and safe antiseptic agent. The 0.1% commercial formulation compared favorably with other antiseptics with respect to antimicrobial activity and toxicologic properties. It rapidly killed both gram-positive and gram-negative bacteria as well as fungi in vitro and in vivo (77, 177). Octenidine was virucidal against HIV, HBV, and herpes simplex virus. Similar to chlorhexidine, it has a marked residual effect. No toxicologic problems have been found when the 0.1% formulation was applied according to the manufacturer's recommendations. The colorless solution has proved to be useful as an antiseptic for mucous membranes of the female and male genitals and the oral cavity (21). However, its bad taste severely limits its oral application. Octenidine is not registered for use in the United States. *Triclosan* (irgasan DP-300) and *chloroxylenol* (PCMX) are common antimicrobial ingredients of hand-washing products. They have good activities against gram-positive organisms but lower levels of activity against gram-negative bacteria, *M. tuberculosis*, and fungi. Both agents are less effective than the antiseptics mentioned above. A 0.3% triclosan formulation was shown to be less effective than 2% chlorhexidine gluconate in reducing hand flora (111). Both triclosan and PCMX produce a sustained residual activity. Their actions are only minimally reduced by organic matter. However, nonionic surfactants may neutralize PCMX.

STERILIZATION

Principles, Definitions, and Terms

As outlined in Table 3, sterilization is not a relative term but defines the complete absence of any viable microorganisms including spores. However, this absence cannot be proved with current microbiologic techniques (100). Therefore, sterilization can be defined as a closely monitored, validated process used to render a product free of all forms of viable microorganisms, including all bacterial endospores. Therefore, manufacturers of sterilization systems developed a worst-case scenario that allows quantification of the process (log killing) and estimates the probability of process failure. A high degree of conservatism and safety margins have been included for testing purposes. It assumes that items are heavily contaminated with large numbers of spores, soil, and proteins, a scenario that is considered a critical failure of the reprocessing cycle in clinical practice.

The following definitions are based on those of FDA and are required to understand, review, and evaluate data on sterilization. More data on and recommendations for sterilization are provided in reference books such as those by Block (29) and Reichert and Young (147a). The basic prerequisite for any disinfection or sterilization process is reiterated because of its critical importance for adequate reprocessing: Any device undergoing sterilization *must undergo an appropriate cleaning process*. A manufacturer must demonstrate that the sterilizer is effective against a wide range of clinically important microorganisms before being cleared by FDA. In addition, proof of efficacy must be performed with organisms (usually bacterial spores) that have been shown to be the most resistant to the new technology. A validated and reliable biologic indicator must be developed, and studies must establish that sterility will be consistently achieved when critical process parameters operate within a defined range. This assures the operator that as long as there is no operational error or equipment failure, sterility is achieved. The most important terms for sterilization are listed to better understand the literature (these definitions are adapted from those of FDA).

Validation: a documented program which provides a high degree of assurance that a specific process will consistently meet its predetermined specifications and quality attributes.

D value (decimal reduction value): the time required to kill 90% (one logarithmic cycle) of a specified population of microorganisms. For calculation purposes it is assumed that the killing rate follows first-order kinetics.

F value: the F value defines the time (in minutes) required to kill all the spores in suspension at a temperature of 121°C (250°F) or 132°C (270°F) in the United States (134°C in Europe). The different temperatures used in the United States and Europe are probably guided by temperatures of 121°C (250°F) and 132°C (270°F) (in the United States) or 3 atm of pressure resulting in 134°C (in Europe).

Sterility assurance level (SAL): the expected probability that a microorganism is surviving on each individual product after exposure to a validated sterilization process. SAL is expressed as 10^{-n}, where *n* is the level of probability that survivors exist. The Norm ISO 14937 requires a reduction of 10^{-6} CFU of spores at half of the normal cycle to meet the standard established by the norm. This value is part of the European sterilization definition according to EN 556.

Bioburden: the number and types of viable microorganisms on a medical device prior to exposure to a cleaning and/or microbicidal process.

The killing curves show a linear decrease in the numbers of CFU on a semilogarithmic scale. Therefore, the required killing is easily computed by drawing a line between measurements of microbial killing. Commercially available spores provide evidence of killing of $\geq 10^6$ CFU if no growth can be detected after an appropriate incubation. The customer of a sterilizer can expect this level of performance if the device has been cleared by FDA and is operated according to the manufacturer's instructions. Several sources of data have been reviewed in detail and should be read before evaluating a large sterilizer (65, 100, 122, 158, 203). In Europe, EN 550, EN 554, and EN 285 define the standards for steam and ethylene oxide sterilization.

Monitoring

Any sterilization process must be monitored by mechanical, physical, chemical, and facultatively biologic methods. It includes temperature, pressure, and other methods depending on the sterilization method. Before routine use the performance of the machine should be validated with the most difficult load used at the institution to ensure the safety of the process. In addition, a printout of the physical parameters used during sterilization should be kept for documentation purposes. Temperature and pressure are routinely recorded in today's sterilizers and are printed out at the end of the sterilization process. In addition, chemical indicators stacked on the tested items change their color if they were exposed to the adequate temperatures and exposure times. Their use is inexpensive and convenient, and they immediately indicate that the item has been exposed to the sterilization process. However, there is no perfect chemical indicator: Some are too sensitive, resulting in false-positive results (162, 164). They may cause an unnecessary recall of adequately sterilized items. Less sensitive chemical indicators do not indicate small deviations in the process. However, good clinical indicators are able to identify a failure of the sterilizer.

The Bowie-Dick test originated in 1963, when Bowie and Dick determined that if residual air remained in a sterilizer after the vacuum phase and there was only one package in the chamber, the air would concentrate in that package (32, 33). A satisfactory test indicates that steam penetration and air removal had occurred. It does not provide information about the sterilization process.

Biologic indicators are recognized as being the closest to ideal monitors of the sterilization process. Most organizations such as CDC and the Joint Commission on Accreditation of Healthcare Organizations (JCAHO) recommend the use of biologic indicators at least weekly. For flash sterilization, the Attest Rapid Readout biologic indicator detects the presence of a spore-associated enzyme, α-D-glucosidase, and permits an assessment of sterilization effectiveness within 60 min (189). An important question is whether or not a load can be distributed before a biologic indicator proves adequate sterilization. This is also called parametric release. The JCAHO standard allows the use of appropriate chemical indicators without routine use of a biologic indicator. A common approach is to use the sterilized items on the basis of physical and chemical documentation of an adequate sterilization process and not to await the culture results for the biologic indicators. A recent study showed the usefulness of routine biologic indicators for monitoring: The biologic indicators detected a failure of steam sterilization before nosocomial infections were recorded, supporting the current practice (43). In Europe, routine use of biologic indicators is not required if the sterilizer has undergone testing by a validation procedure used for industrial steam sterilization (EN 285, EN 550, EN 554, and EN 556). Most sterilizers in European hospitals probably do not meet these very strict requirements, and consequently, biologic indicators are regularly used. However, these new standards will be implemented for steam sterilization validation in health care organizations because they are already mandated for industrial steam sterilization validation, but the associated expenses are part of an ongoing dispute. The future is likely parametric release with regular validation and/or commissions of the equipment. Legal aspects will probably determine the outcome of this discussion, and lawyers are likely to accept nothing but a zero risk. However, the goal of a zero risk for contamination in central sterilization services will likely contribute to excessive health care costs. Therefore, standards for sterilization should exclude a risk for contamination after the reprocessing cycle but should avoid steps that are performed only for legal reasons.

Packaging, Loading, and Storage

Once items are clean, dry, and inspected, instruments and devices must be wrapped and packaged before sterilization. Wrappers should allow penetration of steam or gas but should serve as a barrier against recontamination after sterilization. For steam, only muslin has limitations, and handling of items made of muslin leads to contamination (196). For gas sterilization, only wrappers approved for use in the sterilization process should be used. Items should be labeled with information, including details of the reprocessing cycle and an expiration date.

Steam Sterilization

The most reliable method of sterilization is one that uses saturated steam under pressure. It is inexpensive, nontoxic, and very reliable, penetrates fabrics, and has an inherent safety margin much higher than that of any other sterilization technique. Therefore, it should be used whenever possible. Pressurized steam destroys microorganisms by irreversible coagulation and denaturation of enzymes and proteins. The pressure allows one to achieve dry 100% saturated steam, without water in the form of a fine mist. Dry air does not provide steam for condensation, and the heat transfer to objects is slowed down. Obviously, this technique cannot be used for plastic, rubber, or objects that are sensitive to heat or moisture, limiting the use of this method for many devices and instruments. The process of sterilization has several cycles: conditioning, exposure, and drying cycle. Common cycles for prevacuum or flash-pressure pulsing steam sterilizers are 121°C for 15 min (121°C for 30 min in a gravity-displacement sterilizer) and 132°C for 4 mins (FDA addendum to the Sterilizer Guidance, 19 September, 1995). The machine should provide this temperature anywhere in the chamber within a narrow margin (0 to +3°C on the basis of EN 554). Several types of autoclaves are available: gravity-displacement steam sterilization, prevacuum steam sterilization, and steam flash-pressure pulsing steam sterilization autoclaves. The problem with gravity-displacement steam sterilization is the unpredictable performance of the sterilization process (54). Insufficient air removal before the addition of steam at the correct temperature is much more likely with gravity-displacement autoclaves than with the more sophisticated systems. The prevacuum sterilizer resolved part of the problem and cut the cycle time by half. However, the effectiveness of sterilization can be compromised by small leaks (1 to 10 mm Hg/min) in the sterilizer (100). The most current technology is the steam flash-pressure pulsing steam sterilization technique because air leaks do not decrease the effectiveness of the process. It almost eliminates the most important remaining risk in steam sterilization: air in the chamber (54). The steam flash-pressure pulsing steam sterilization system has been found to be most useful for general use, since it reduces the thermal lag upon heating of the load to the desired exposure temperature. Detailed reviews including all details on requirements, monitoring, and maintenance of a large steam sterilizer have been published (100, 105, 203) and are included in EN 285.

A hot topic is flash sterilization, an emergency process used, for example, after a surgical instrument is dropped but needs to be immediately available during a procedure (122). It exposes unwrapped devices to pressurized steam for 3 min, usually in the operating room area, sometimes without a biologic indicator. In addition, the autoclaves are gravity-displacement sterilizers that have the problems mentioned above. Flash sterilization is sometimes performed by HCWs without appropriate training. Therefore, several investigators have advocated that this method be strictly limited to emergency situations when no other device from the institution's central sterilization service is available. It is not intended to replace routine regular sterilization because of ease of use and speed (66). As outlined above, the cleaning process may not be observed, which is a prerequisite for an appropriate reprocessing cycle with steam sterilization, and lack of protective packaging can render the device unsterile even after a successful sterilization. In addition, even properly wrapped sterile items can become contaminated if they are transported several times (196).

Three parameters are critical to ensuring steam sterilization: time of exposure to steam, temperature, and moisture. The D value determines the time frame required to achieve killing of 10^6 CFU of spores most resistant to the sterilization process under study. The temperature is critical for the process: The temperature of any device or instrument must reach the desired temperature, which is not necessarily identical to the gauge display of the autoclave. A drop of only 1.7°C (3°F) results in a 48% increase in the time required to sterilize an item. Pressurized steam allows quick energy transfer to the sterilizer load and, probably, the more rapid denaturation and coagulation of proteins. Without moisture, a temperature of 160°C is required for dry heat sterilization. Therefore, residual air interferes with the sterilization process. Unlike time and temperature, the moisture condition in the autoclave cannot be directly determined. The amount of air within the sterilizer can be estimated by comparing the chamber pressure with the saturated steam pressure calculated from the average chamber temperature. A measured pressure greater than the calculated saturated pressure indicates the presence of residual air in the chamber. Such monitoring devices are common in the United Kingdom.

Ethylene Oxide Gas

Temperature- and/or pressure-sensitive items were traditionally sterilized with ethylene oxide in a standard gas sterilizer that used Freon as a carrier gas. As of 1 January 1996, however, the Clean Air Act banned the use of chlorofluorocarbons as sterilant gases, calling for the use of alternatives for heat-sensitive items and devices. Alternatives are ethylene oxide sterilizers that use 100% ethylene oxide or sterilizers that use other technologies. Ethylene oxide is flammable, explosive, and carcinogenic to laboratory animals, and it requires the use of additional safety precautions. Nitrogen gas is added to remove air from the chamber or the chamber is evacuated. Items to be sterilized are usually exposed to ethylene oxide at a temperature of 55°C (130°F). They are then aerated for approximately 12 h to remove any traces of the gas. The total process takes >16 h. Ethylene oxide inactivates all microorganisms including spores, probably by an alkylation process. *B. subtilis* has among the most resistant bacterial spores and therefore is used as a biologic monitor. Ethylene oxide is useful only as a surface sterilizer. It is unable to reach blocked-off surfaces. The use of ethylene oxide requires the careful and simultaneous control of six variable but interdependent parameters: gas concentration, vacuum, pressure, temperature, relative humidity, and time of exposure. The gas concentration cannot be measured online, limiting the extent of monitoring. Therefore, validation of the concentration is recommended. Another issue is the toxic residues trapped in the wrapper or the items. Polyvinyl chloride (PVC) and polyurethane are examples of very strong absorbers of ethylene oxide. They require long periods to dissipate the oxide. The wrapper itself should be a barrier against recontamination after sterilization, but it also serves as a potential barrier to the access of ethylene oxide to the item. Therefore, only materials with documented ethylene oxide penetration and dissipation properties should be used. The future of ethylene oxide in sterilization is limited, mainly due to environmental concerns surrounding its toxicity. However, plasma sterilization can only partially replace sterilization with ethylene oxide. No currently available technology could completely replace ethylene oxide. In addition, sterilization with ethylene oxide does not fail as frequently as sterilization with plasma in the presence of residual proteins and/or salts (10, 11, 42).

Plasma Sterilization

Plasma describes any gas that consists of electrons, ions, or neutral particles. The formation of a low-temperature plasma requires a closed chamber, a deep vacuum, and a chemical precursor from which to derive the plasma. In addition, a source of electromagnetic energy, such as radiofrequency energy, creates an electromagnetic field that generates the plasma. The electromagnetic field interacts with the chemical (hydrogen peroxide or a mixture with peracetic acid) and induces the plasma. The resulting free radicals, the chemical precursors, and the UV radiation are among the postulated reactions that rapidly destroy vegetative microorganisms including spores. At the time of this writing, two plasma sterilizers are commercially available and cleared by FDA: the Sterrad 100 sterilizer and the Plazlyte sterilizer.

Sterrad 100S Sterilizer

The Sterrad 100 sterilizer was the first machine available for health care facilities and has been on the market in Europe since 1990 and in the United States since 1993. Several steps run automatically during a sterilization cycle: medical instruments are placed in the sterilization chamber under a strong vacuum. A solution of 59% hydrogen peroxide and water from a cassette is automatically injected into the sterilization chamber. The solution vaporizes and diffuses throughout the chamber, surrounding the items to be sterilized. Radio-frequency energy is applied to create an electrical field, which in turn initiates the generation of the low-temperature plasma, inducing free radicals. The combination of the diffusion pretreatment and plasma phases acts to sterilize the item while eliminating harmful residuals. The radio-frequency energy is turned off, the vacuum is released, and the chamber is filled with filtered air, returning it to normal atmospheric pressure. In August 1997, the Sterrad 100 System was cleared for use in the sterilization of surgical instruments containing longer and narrower lumens, such as those used in urologic, laparoscopic, and arthroscopic procedures including single stainless steel lumens ≥3 and <400 mm in length. Important restrictions are (i) materials that absorb too much hydrogen peroxide such as cellulosics and some nylons, e.g., from connectors, cables, and insulators; (ii) materials that catalytically decompose hydrogen peroxide such as copper and nickel alloys from electrical wire, solder, and surgical instruments; and (iii) materials that react with hydrogen peroxide such as organic dyes (colored anodized aluminum) and organic sulfides (M_2oS of solid lubricant in endoscopic devices). Training of the operators is critical: Up to 30% of the sterilization cycles were automatically canceled after installation of the sterilizer at the authors' institution because the operators did not comply with the loading instructions. Today, between 1 and 5% of the cycles are canceled, and the Sterrad 100S sterilizer appears to be less prone to minimal deviations from optimal loading.

Abtox Plazlyte Sterilizer

Two agents are used for the Abtox Plazlyte sterilizer. First, a solution containing 5% peracetic acid and 22% hydrogen peroxide is injected into the chamber under vacuum and is vaporized. A second agent, PlazGas, a gas mixture consisting of argon, oxygen, and hydrogen, is added after evacuation and is exposed to an electromagnetic field to form a low-temperature gas plasma. The system was cleared by FDA in December 1994 for use with an exposure time of 3 h at 40°C, resulting in a total cycle time of 4.5 h. The system must be permanently located and must have ventilation to the exterior of the building to allow the removal of the vaporized peracetic acid directly into the atmosphere, and it requires the storage of large, high-pressure gas cylinders. A recent peer-reviewed evaluation demonstrated major deficiencies even for vegetative microorganisms if the system is challenged with proteins and/or salts (42). OSHA has established 8-h time-weighted average worker exposure limits of 10 and 1 ppm for acetic acid and hydrogen peroxide, respectively. In addition, a recent alert (13 April 1998) by FDA calls for caution when using this device. The AbTox Plazlyte Sterilization System should not be used to sterilize any ophthalmic, brass, copper, zinc, or soldered device. In addition, FDA has not cleared the safety, performance, or instructions for use of the AbTox Plazlyte Sterilization System (see http://www.fda.gov/cdrh/abtox.html for details).

Liquid Sterilization

The STERIS SYSTEM 1 was cleared by FDA for marketing in the United States in 1988. The machine is designed for liquid sterilization with peracetic acid for immersible devices including flexible endoscopes. The machine does not clean the device. The process takes approximately 30 min at ≈50°C. The items can be used immediately upon completion without aeration. The sterilant concentrate contains 35% liquid peracetic acid and buffering, anticorrosion, wetting, and surface-active agents. Peracetic acid is automatically diluted within the processor with sterile filtered water, and the items are exposed for 12 min. Clinical studies have been performed with bronchoscopes, hysteroscopes, colonoscopes, and rigid endoscopes (35, 191). Independent efficacy tests demonstrated some failures with spores, but outbreaks have not been associated with the use of the STERIS SYSTEM 1 (35). Peracetic acid is an FDA-cleared sterilant and is sporicidal (95, 96). It was the only available cleared sterilizer system for endoscopes with a rapid turnaround time before the Sterrad 100 plasma sterilizer was cleared for this application by FDA. The STERIS SYSTEM 1 is not considered a sterilizer in Europe (56), lacking an appropriate physical and biologic monitoring system as required by EN. However, a recent study demonstrated that commercially available spores can be used for monitoring (109). False-positive test strips were identified from improper clip use (85). Exposure time and temperature are monitored electronically, and conductivity is used as a surrogate marker for peracetic acid concentration. On occasion, the machine has been known to complete its cycle normally and print a concentration of peracetic acid in the normal range even when it is run intentionally without peracetic acid (124). The cost of purchasing and using the equipment is considerably greater than the cost of purchasing and using high-level disinfection with glutaraldehyde (72). The current problems with endoscopes require improved safety margins that can probably be met by using the STERIS SYSTEM 1, but newer technologies such as plasma sterilizers may be more appropriate for this application. It must be reiterated that none of the non-steam sterilizers is able to meet sterilization requirements if there is residual debris and/or proteins on the items.

Other Sterilization Techniques

Cobalt 60 is the most common compound used for the commercial sterilization of single-use items. In this process, ionic energy is converted to thermal energy, killing microorganisms and their spores in the process. Design, quality control, and experience rely on experts from industry since this technology is rarely used in hospitals.

Issues on Bovine Spongiform Encephalopathy

CJD has been identified in all developed countries and is thought to occur worldwide. CJD is not a reportable illness in the United States. However, the incidence of CJD is estimated to be about 1 case per 10^6 persons per year, similar to rates in European countries. Most cases of CJD are sporadic: <10% of CJD cases may be related to a genetic autosomal dominant predisposition, and few nosocomial cases are related to contact with contaminated tissue. nvCJD has brought about a major medical and economic crisis in Europe (40, 104, 145). The new disease is probably transmitted by eating bovine spongiform encephalopathy agent-contaminated meat (93, 145). The United Kingdom discontinued selling T-bone steaks in 1998 because of concerns over nvCJD transmission. The disease occurred in the mid-1980s in the United Kingdom because the meat of carcasses for slaughterhouses did not undergo a solvent extraction that may have previously removed the agent, which is solvent sensitive. In addition, it is speculated that the animal food was no longer sterilized at 134°C for 30 min but was pasteurized before being fed to animals. nvCJD has a clinical presentation different from that of CJD and occurs at a much younger age (49, 104). The new agent is not a classic microorganism but an altered prion protein, based on strong evidence from studies by Prusiner (144) and Aguzzi and colleagues (4, 28, 171). Previously, problems with reprocessing were limited to invasive instruments that came into contact with neural tissue, predominantly instruments used in neurosurgery. However, the detection of the prion agent in lymphoid tissue and tonsils challenges its restriction to neural tissue (104). The latest update indicates the potential of transmission of the bovine spongiform encephalopathy agent by B cells (107). nvCJD is highly lymphotropic, making any instruments used in lymphoid tissues at risk for contamination with prions (107). Many approaches have been recommended, but none of them can fulfill the SAL as required for microorganisms. Therefore, the reader is referred to the home pages of CDC, FDA, and the World Health Organization to obtain the most recent update on this topic. Several methods have been shown not to be sufficient for sterilization of prion-contaminated items, including dry heat (160°C for 24 hours), formaldehyde sterilization, and standard steam sterilization (61). The minimum requirements for decontamination procedures and precautions for materials potentially contaminated with the agent that causes CJD are unknown. Limited scientific information provides the basis for CDC's recommendations (see http://www.cdc.gov/ncidod/diseases/hip/cjd.htm):

- Steam autoclave for 1 to 1.5 h at 132 to 134°C.
- Immerse in 1 N sodium hydroxide for 1 h at room temperature.
- Immerse in sodium hypochlorite 0.5% (at least 2% free chlorine) for 2 h at room temperature.

Several European countries use different approaches for category I tissue and body fluids. In The Netherlands, potentially contaminated items undergo six consecutive standard cycles (3 min at 134°C, for a total of 18 min) for steam sterilization, in France items are treated for 30 min at 134°C, and in Switzerland items are treated for 18 min at 134°C, highlighting the uncertainty of the optimal approach (100). High-risk patients are CJD patients and their family members, patients with a medical history of treatment with pituitary extracts, and cornea transplant patients. In addition, items should be considered prion contaminated if a brain biopsy for the diagnosis of CJD is requested. An excellent review was published in late 1996 (61). However, given the latest data, the appropriate reprocessing approach remains unknown (4). The level of knowledge about this situation is similar to that about the HIV epidemic in 1982 to 1984, when nobody was aware of the extent of the epidemic. It is hoped that the nvCJD will never become even remotely as epidemic as HIV, but today's knowledge is insufficient for evidence-based guidelines.

REFERENCES

1. **ADA Council on Scientific Affairs and ADA Council on Dental Practice.** 1996. Infection control recommendations for the dental office and the dental laboratory. *J. Am. Dent. Assoc.* **127:**672–680.
2. **Adams, B. G., and T. J. Marrie.** 1982. Hand carriage of aerobic gram-negative rods may not be transient. *J. Hyg. (London)* **89:**33–46.
3. **Agerton, T., S. Valway, B. Gore, C. Pozsik, B. Plikaytis, C. Woodley, and I. Onorato.** 1997. Transmission of a highly drug-resistant strain (strain W1) of *Mycobacterium tuberculosis*. Community outbreak and nosocomial transmission via a contaminated bronchoscope. *JAMA* **278:**1073–1077.
4. **Aguzzi, A., and C. Weissmann.** 1998. Spongiform encephalopathies. The prion's perplexing persistence. *Nature* **392:**763–764.
5. **Akamatsu, T., K. Tabata, M. Hironaga, and M. Uyeda.** 1997. Evaluation of the efficacy of a 3.2% glutaraldehyde product for disinfection of fibreoptic endoscopes with an automatic machine. *J. Hosp. Infect.* **35:**47–57.
6. **Akbar-Khanzadeh, F., M. U. Vaquerano, M. Akbar-Khanzadeh, and M. S. Bisesi.** 1994. Formaldehyde exposure, acute pulmonary response, and exposure control options in a gross anatomy laboratory. *Am. J. Ind. Med.* **26:** 61–75.
7. **Alasri, A., C. Roques, G. Michel, C. Cabassud, and P. Aptel.** 1992. Bactericidal properties of peracetic acid and hydrogen peroxide, alone and in combination, and chlorine and formaldehyde against bacterial water strains. *Can. J. Microbiol.* **38:**635–642.
8. **Alasri, A., M. Valverde, C. Roques, G. Michel, C. Cabassud, and P. Aptel.** 1993. Sporocidal properties of peracetic acid and hydrogen peroxide, alone and in combination, in comparison with chlorine and formaldehyde for ultrafiltration membrane disinfection. *Can. J. Microbiol.* **39:**52–60.
9. **Albert, R. K., and F. Condie.** 1981. Hand-washing patterns in medical intensive care units. *N. Engl. J. Med.* **304:**1465–1466.
10. **Alfa, M. J., P. DeGagne, and N. Olson.** 1997. Bacterial killing ability of 10% ethylene oxide plus 90% hydrochlorofluorocarbon sterilizing gas. *Infect. Control. Hosp. Epidemiol.* **18:**641–645.
11. **Alfa, M. J., P. DeGagne, N. Olson, and T. Puchalski.** 1996. Comparison of ion plasma, vaporized hydrogen peroxide, and 100% ethylene oxide sterilizers to the 12/88 ethylene oxide gas sterilizer. *Infect. Control Hosp. Epidemiol.* **17:**92–100.
12. **Alvarado, C. J., S. M. Stolz, and D. G. Maki.** 1991. Nosocomial infections from contaminated endoscopes: a flawed automated endoscope washer. An investigation using molecular epidemiology. *Am. J. Med.* **91:** 272S–280S.
13. **Anderson, R. L., R. W. Vess, A. L. Panlilio, and M. S. Favero.** 1990. Prolonged survival of *Pseudomonas cepacia* in commercially manufactured povidone-iodine. *Appl. Environ. Microbiol.* **56:**3598–3600.
14. **Anonymous.** 1997. Tentative final monograph for health-care antiseptic drug products. *Fed. Regist.* **59:** 31401–31452.
15. **Ansari, S. A., S. A. Sattar, V. S. Springthorpe, G. A. Wells, and W. Tostowaryk.** 1989. In vivo protocol for testing efficacy of hand-washing agents against viruses and bacteria: experiments with rotavirus and *Escherichia coli*. *Appl. Environ. Microbiol.* **55:**3113–3118.
16. **Arata, T., T. Murakami, and Y. Hirai.** 1993. Evaluation of povidone-iodine alcoholic solution for operative site disinfection. *Postgrad. Med. J.* **69**(Suppl. 3)**:**S93–S96.
17. **Ascenzi, J. M.** 1996. Glutaraldehyde-based disinfectants, p. 111–132. *In* J. P. Ascenzi (ed.), *Handbook of Disinfectants and Antiseptics*. Marcel Dekker, Inc., New York, N.Y.
18. **Ascenzi, J. M., R. J. Ezzell, and T. M. Wendt.** 1987. A more accurate method for measurement of tuberculocidal activity of disinfectants. *Appl. Environ. Microbiol.* **53:** 2189–2192.
19. **Ayliffe, G. A., J. R. Babb, and C. R. Bradley.** 1986. Disinfection of endoscopes. *J. Hosp. Infect.* **7:**296–299.
20. **Babb, J. R., and C. R. Bradley.** 1995. Endoscope decontamination: where do we go from here? *J. Hosp. Infect.* **30**(Suppl.)**:**543–551.
21. **Beiswanger, B. B., M. E. Mallatt, M. S. Mau, R. D. Jackson, and D. K. Hennon.** 1990. The clinical effects of a mouthrinse containing 0.1% octenidine. *J. Dent. Res.* **69:**454–457.
22. **Bellamy, K.** 1995. A review of the test methods used to establish virucidal activity. *J. Hosp. Infect.* **30**(Suppl.)**:** 389–396.
23. **Bellamy, K., R. Alcock, J. R. Babb, J. G. Davies, and G. A. Ayliffe.** 1993. A test for the assessment of 'hygienic' hand disinfection using rotavirus. *J. Hosp. Infect.* **24:** 201–210.
24. **Berkelman, R. L., B. W. Holland, and R. L. Anderson.** 1982. Increased bactericidal activity of dilute preparations of povidone-iodine solutions. *J. Clin. Microbiol.* **15:** 635–639.
25. **Berkelman, R. L., S. Lewin, J. R. Allen, R. L. Anderson, L. D. Budnick, S. Shapiro, S. M. Friedman, P. Nicholas, R. S. Holzman, and R. W. Haley.** 1981. Pseudobacteremia attributed to contamination of povidone-iodine with *Pseudomonas cepacia*. *Ann. Intern. Med.* **95:**32–36.
26. **Biron, F., B. Verrier, and D. Peyramond.** 1997. Transmission of the human immunodeficiency virus and the hepatitis C virus. *N. Engl. J. Med.* **337:**348–349.
27. **Blanc, D. S., T. Parret, B. Janin, P. Raselli, and P. Francioli.** 1997. Nosocomial infections and pseudoinfections from contaminated bronchoscopes: two-year follow up using molecular markers. *Infect. Control Hosp. Epidemiol.* **18:**134–136.
28. **Blattler, T., S. Brandner, A. J. Raeber, M. A. Klein, T. Voigtlander, C. Weissmann, and A. Aguzzi.** 1997. PrP-expressing tissue required for transfer of scrapie infectivity from spleen to brain. *Nature* **389:**69–73.
29. **Block, S. S. (ed.).** 1991. *Disinfection, Sterilization and Preservation*. Lea & Febiger, Philadelphia, Pa.
30. **Block, S. S.** 1991. Hydrogen peroxide, p. 167–181. *In* S.

S. Block (ed.), *Disinfection, Sterilization and Preservation*. Lea & Febiger, Philadelphia, Pa.

31. **Bond, W. W., M. S. Favero, N. J. Petersen, and J. W. Ebert.** 1983. Inactivation of hepatitis B virus by intermediate-to-high-level disinfectant chemicals. *J. Clin. Microbiol.* **18:**535–538.
32. **Bowie, J. H.** 1974. Bowie and Dick test. *Lancet* **i:**1233.
33. **Bowie, J. H., M. H. Kennedy, and I. Robertson.** 1975. Improved Bowie and Dick test. *Lancet* **i:**1135.
34. **Boyce, J. M., G. Potter-Bynoe, S. M. Opal, L. Dziobek, and A. A. Medeiros.** 1990. A common-source outbreak of *Staphylococcus epidermidis* infections among patients undergoing cardiac surgery. *J. Infect. Dis.* **161:**493–499.
35. **Bradley, C. R., J. R. Babb, and G. A. Ayliffe.** 1995. Evaluation of the Steris System 1 peracetic acid endoscope processor. *J. Hosp. Infect.* **29:**143–151.
36. **Bradley, C. R., and A. P. Fraise.** 1996. Heat and chemical resistance of enterococci. *J. Hosp. Infect.* **34:**191–196.
37. **Brewer, G. E.** 1915. Studies in aseptic technique. *JAMA* **64:**1369–1372.
38. **Broadley, S. J., J. R. Furr, P. A. Jenkins, and A. D. Russell.** 1993. Antimycobacterial activity of 'Virkon'. *J. Hosp. Infect.* **23:**189–197.
39. **Bronowicki, J. P., V. Venard, C. Botte, N. Monhoven, I. Gastin, L. Chone, H. Hudziak, B. Rhin, C. Delanoe, A. LeFaou, M. A. Bigard, and P. Gaucher.** 1997. Patient-to-patient transmission of hepatitis C virus during colonoscopy. *N. Engl. J. Med.* **337:**237–240.
40. **Bruce, M. E., R. G. Will, J. W. Ironside, I. McConnell, D. Drummond, A. Suttie, L. McCardle, A. Chree, J. Hope, C. Birkett, S. Cousens, H. Fraser, and C. J. Bostock.** 1997. Transmissions to mice indicate that 'new variant' CJD is caused by the BSE agent. *Nature* **389:** 498–501.
41. **Bryant, W. P., and D. Zimmerman.** 1995. Iodine-induced hyperthyroidism in a newborn. *Pediatrics* **95:** 434–436.
42. **Bryce, E. A., E. Chia, G. Logelin, and J. A. Smith.** 1997. An evaluation of the AbTox plazlyte sterilization system. *Infect. Control Hosp. Epidemiol.* **18:**646–653.
43. **Bryce, E. A., F. J. Roberts, B. Clements, and S. MacLean.** 1997. When the biological indicator is positive: investigating autoclave failures. *Infect. Control Hosp. Epidemiol.* **18:**654–656.
44. **Canadian Healthcare Association.** 1996. *The Reuse of Single-Use Medical Devices: Guidelines for Healthcare Facilities*, p. 1–127. CHA Press, Ottawa, Ontario, Canada.
45. **Centers for Disease Control.** 1989. Guidelines for prevention of transmission of human immunodeficiency virus and hepatitis B virus to health-care and public-safety workers. *Morbid. Mortal. Weekly Rep.* **38**(Suppl. 6)**:**1–37.
46. **Centers for Disease Control and Prevention.** 1993. Recommended infection-control practices for dentistry. *Morbid. Mortal. Weekly Rep.* **42:**1–12.
47. **Centers for Disease Control and Prevention.** 1996. Community-level prevention of human immunodeficiency virus infection among high-risk populations: the AIDS community demonstration projects. *Morbid. Mortal. Weekly Rep.* **45**(No. RR6)**:**1–31.

47a. **Centers for Disease Control and Prevention.** 1985. *Guidelines for Handwashing and Hospital Environment Control.* Centers for Disease Control and Prevention, Atlanta, Ga.

48. **Challacombe, S. J., and L. L. Fernandes.** 1995. Detecting *Legionella pneumophila* in water systems: a comparison of various dental units. *J. Am. Dent. Assoc.* **126:**603–608.
49. **Chazot, G., E. Broussolle, C. Lapras, T. Blattler, A. Aguzzi, and N. Kopp.** 1996. New variant of Creutzfeldt-Jacob disease in a 26-year-old French man. *Lancet* **347:** 1181.
50. **Coates, D.** 1996. Sporicidal activity of sodium dichloroisocyanurate, peroxygen and glutaraldehyde disinfectants against Bacillus subtilis. *J. Hosp. Infect.* **32:**283–294.
51. **Collins, F. M.** 1986. Bactericidal activity of alkaline glutaraldehyde solution against a number of atypical mycobacterial species. *J. Appl. Bacteriol.* **61:**247–251.
52. **Collins, F. M.** 1986. Kinetics of the tuberculocidal response by alkaline glutaraldehyde in solution and on an inert surface. *J. Appl. Bacteriol.* **61:**87–93.
53. **Craven, D. E., B. Moody, M. G. Connolly, N. R. Kollisch, K. D. Stottmeier, and W. R. McCabe.** 1981. Pseudobacteremia caused by povidone-iodine solution contaminated with *Pseudomonas cepacia*. *N. Engl. J. Med.* **305:**621–623.
54. **Crow, S.** 1993. Steam sterilizers: an evolution in design. *Infect. Control Hosp. Epidemiol.* **14:**488–490.
55. **Cruse, P. J., and R. Foord.** 1973. A five-year prospective study of 23,649 surgical wounds. *Arch. Surg.* **107:** 206–210.
56. **Daschner, F.** 1994. STERIS SYSTEM 1 in Germany. *Infect. Control Hosp. Epidemiol.* **15:**294–296.
57. **Denton, G. E.** 1991. Chlorhexidine, p. 274–289. *In* S. S. Block (ed.), *Disinfection, Sterilization and Preservation*. Lea & Febiger, Philadelphia, Pa.
58. **Disch, K.** 1994. Glucoprotamine—a new antimicrobial substance. *Zentbl. Hyg. Umweltmed.* **195:**357–365.
59. **Doebbeling, B. N., G. L. Stanley, C. T. Sheetz, M. A. Pfaller, A. K. Houston, L. Annis, N. Li, and R. P. Wenzel.** 1992. Comparative efficacy of alternative hand-washing agents in reducing nosocomial infections in intensive care units. *N. Engl. J. Med.* **327:**88–93.
60. **Dolce, P., M. Gourdeau, N. April, and P. M. Bernard.** 1995. Outbreak of glutaraldehyde-induced proctocolitis. *Am. J. Infect. Control* **23:**34–39.
61. **Dormont, D.** 1996. How to limit the spread of Creutzfeldt-Jakob disease. *Infect. Control Hosp. Epidemiol.* **17:** 521–528.

61a. **Dorozynski, A.** 1997. Poor sterilization of instruments leads to infection outbreak in Paris. *BMJ* **315:**699.

62. **Druce, J. D., D. Jardine, S. A. Locarnini, and C. J. Birch.** 1995. Susceptibility of HIV to inactivation by disinfectants and ultraviolet light. *J. Hosp. Infect.* **30:** 167–180.
63. **Ehrenkranz, N. J., E. A. Bolyard, M. Wiener, et al.** 1980. Antibiotic-sensitive *Serratia marcescens* infections complicating cardiopulmonary operations: contaminated disinfectant as a reservoir. *Lancet* **ii:**1289–1292.
64. **Evans, R. J.** 1992. Acute anaphylaxis due to topical chlorhexidine acetate. *Br. Med. J.* **304:**686.
65. **Favero, M. S.** 1991. Strategies for disinfection and sterilization of endoscopes: the gap between basic principles and actual practice. *Infect. Control Hosp. Epidemiol.* **12:** 279–281.
66. **Favero, M. S., and F. A. Manian.** 1993. Is eliminating flash sterilization practical? *Infect. Control Hosp. Epidemiol.* **14:**479–480.
67. **Feldman, H. I., M. Kinosian, W. B. Bilker, C. Simmons, J. H. Holmes, M. V. Pauly, and J. J. Escarce.** 1996. Effect of dialyzer reuse on survival of patients treated with hemodialysis. *JAMA* **276:**1724.
68. **Flynn, N., S. Jain, E. M. Keddie, J. R. Carlson, M. B. Jennings, H. W. Haverkos, N. Nassar, R. Anderson, S. Cohen, and D. Goldberg.** 1994. In vitro activity of readily available household materials against HIV-1: is bleach enough? *J. Acquired Immune. Defic. Syndr.* **7:**747–753.
69. **Frank, M. J., and W. Schaffner.** 1976. Contaminated aqueous benzalkonium chloride. An unnecessary hospital infection hazard. *JAMA* **236:**2418–2419.

70. **Fraser, V. J., G. Zuckerman, R. E. Clouse, S. O'Rourke, M. Jones, J. Klasner, and P. Murray.** 1993. A prospective randomized trial comparing manual and automated endoscope disinfection methods. *Infect. Control Hosp. Epidemiol.* **14:**383–389.
71. **Furuhashi, M., and T. Miyamae.** 1979. Effect of preoperative hand scrubbing and influence of pinholes appearing in surgical rubber gloves during operation. *Bull. Tokyo Med. Dent. Univ.* **26:**73–80.
72. **Fuselier, H. A. J., and C. Mason.** 1997. Liquid sterilization versus high level disinfection in the urologic office. *Urology* **50:**337–340.
73. **Fuursted, K., A. Hjort, and L. Knudsen.** 1997. Evaluation of bactericidal activity and lag of regrowth (postantibiotic effect) of five antiseptics on nine bacterial pathogens. *J. Antimicrob. Chemother.* **40:**221–226.
74. **Gelinas, P., J. Goulet, G. M. Tastayre, and G. A. Picard.** 1991. Effect of temperature and contact time on the activity of eight disinfectants—a classification. *J. Food Prot.* **47:**841–847.
75. **Georgiade, G., R. Riefkohl, N. Georgiade, R. Georgiade, and M. F. Wildman.** 1985. Efficacy of povidone-iodine in pre-operative skin preparation. *J. Hosp. Infect.* **6**(Suppl. A) **:**67–71.
76. **Gerding, D. N., S. Johnson, L. R. Peterson, M. E. Mulligan, and J. Silva, Jr.** 1995. Clostridium difficile-associated diarrhea and colitis. *Infect. Control Hosp. Epidemiol.* **16:**459–477.
77. **Ghannoum, M. A., K. A. Elteen, M. Ellabib, and P. A. Whittaker.** 1990. Antimycotic effects of octenidine and pirtenidine. *J. Antimicrob. Chemother.* **25:**237–245.
78. **Gorse, G. J., and R. L. Messner.** 1991. Infection control practices in gastrointestinal endoscopy in the United States: a national survey. *Infect. Control Hosp. Epidemiol.* **12:**289–296.
79. **Gottardi, W.** 1991. Iodine and iodine compounds, p. 152–166. *In* S. S. Block (ed.), *Disinfection, Sterilization and Preservation.* Lea & Febiger, Philadelphia, Pa.
80. **Graham, G. S.** 1997. Decontamination: scientific principles, p. 1–9. *In* M. Reichert and J. H. Young (ed.), *Sterilization Technology.* Aspen Publications, Gaithersburg, Md.
81. **Graham, M.** 1990. Frequency and duration of handwashing in an intensive care unit. *Am. J. Infect. Control* **18:**77–81.
82. **Griffiths, P. A., J. R. Babb, C. R. Bradley, and A. P. Fraise.** 1997. Glutaraldehyde-resistant *Mycobacterium chelonae* from endoscope washer disinfectors. *J. Appl. Microbiol.* **82:**519–526.
83. **Gubler, J. G., M. Salfinger, and A. von Graevenitz.** 1992. Pseudoepidemic of nontuberculous mycobacteria due to a contaminated bronchoscope cleaning machine. Report of an outbreak and review of the literature. *Chest* **101:**1245–1249.
84. **Gurevich, I., R. Dubin, and B. A. Cunha.** 1996. Dental instrument and device sterilization and disinfection practices. *J. Hosp. Infect.* **32:**295–304.
85. **Gurevich, I., S. M. Qadri, and B. A. Cunha.** 1993. False-positive results of spore tests from improper clip use with the STERIS chemical sterilant system. *Am. J. Infect. Control* **21:**42–43.
86. **Gurevich, I., P. Tafuro, P. Ristuccia, J. Herrmann, A. R. Young, and B. A. Cunha.** 1983. Disinfection of respirator tubing: a comparison of chemical versus hot water machine-assisted processing. *J. Hosp. Infect.* **4:**199–208.
87. **Hamilton, E., D. V. Seal, and J. Hay.** 1996. Comparison of chlorine and chlorine dioxide disinfection for control of Legionella in a hospital potable water supply. *J. Hosp. Infect.* **32:**156–160.
88. **Hanson, P. J., J. Bennett, D. J. Jeffries, and J. V. Collins.** 1994. Enteroviruses, endoscopy and infection control: an applied study. *J. Hosp. Infect.* **27:**61–67.
89. **Hanson, P. J., D. Gor, J. R. Clarke, M. V. Chadwick, B. Gazzard, D. J. Jeffries, H. Gaya, and J. V. Collins.** 1991. Recovery of the human immunodeficiency virus from fibreoptic bronchoscopes. *Thorax* **46:**410–412.
90. **Hanson, P. J., D. J. Jeffries, and J. V. Collins.** 1991. Viral transmission and fibreoptic endoscopy. *J. Hosp. Infect.* **18**(Suppl. A)**:**136–140.
91. **Held, P. J., R. A. Wolfe, D. S. Gaylin, F. K. Port, N. W. Levin, and M. N. Turenne.** 1994. Analysis of the association of dialyzer reuse practices and patient outcomes. *Am. J. Kidney Dis.* **23:**692–708.
92. **Helms, C. M., R. M. Massanari, R. P. Wenzel, M. A. Pfaller, N. P. Moyer, and N. Hall.** 1988. Legionnaires' disease associated with a hospital water system. A five-year progress report on continuous hyperchlorination. *JAMA* **259:**2423–2427.
93. **Hill, A. F., M. Desbruslais, S. Joiner, K. C. Sidle, I. Gowland, J. Collinge, L. J. Doey, and P. Lantos.** 1997. The same prion strain causes vCJD and BSE. *Nature* **389:**448–450.
94. **Hill, A. F., M. Zeidler, J. Ironside, and J. Collinge.** 1997. Diagnosis of new variant Creutzfeldt-Jakob disease by tonsil biopsy. *Lancet* **349:**99–100.
95. **Holton, J., and N. Shetty.** 1997. In-use stability of Nu-Cidex. *J. Hosp. Infect.* **35:**245–248.
96. **Hussaini, S. N., and K. R. Ruby.** 1976. Sporicidal activity of peracetic acid against B. anthracis spores. *Vet. Rec.* **98:**257–259.
97. **Isenberg, S. J., L. Apt, and M. Wood.** 1995. A controlled trial of povidone-iodine as prophylaxis against ophthalmia neonatorum. *N. Engl. J. Med.* **332:**562–566.
98. **Jackson, J., J. E. Leggett, D. A. Wilson, and D. N. Gilbert.** 1996. *Mycobacterium gordonae* in fiberoptic bronchoscopes. *Am. J. Infect. Control* **24:**19–23.
99. **Jette, L. P., and N. G. Lambert.** 1988. Evaluation of two hot water washer disinfectors for medical instruments. *Infect. Control Hosp. Epidemiol.* **9:**194–199.
100. **Joslyn, L. J.** 1991. Sterilization by heat, p. 495–526. *In* S. S. Block (ed.), *Disinfection, Sterilization and Preservation.* Lea & Febiger, Philadelphia, Pa.
101. **Kaatz, G. W., S. D. Gitlin, D. R. Schaberg, K. H. Wilson, C. A. Kauffman, S. M. Seo, and R. Fekety.** 1988. Acquisition of *Clostridium difficile* from the hospital environment. *Am. J. Epidemiol.* **127:**1289–1293.
102. **Kaczmarek, R. G., R. M. J. Moore, J. McCrohan, D. A. Goldmann, C. Reynolds, C. Caquelin, and E. Israel.** 1992. Multi-state investigation of the actual disinfection/sterilization of endoscopes in health care facilities. *Am. J. Med.* **92:**257–261.
103. **Karol, M. H.** 1995. Toxicologic principles do not support the banning of chlorine. A Society of Toxicology position paper. *Fundam. Appl. Toxicol.* **24:**1–2.
104. **Kawashima, T., H. Furukawa, K. Doh-ura, and T. Iwaki.** 1997. Diagnosis of new variant Creutzfeldt-Jakob disease by tonsil biopsy. *Lancet* **350:**68–69.
105. **Keene, J. H.** 1996. Sterilization and pasteurization, p. 937–946. *In* C. G. Mayhall (ed.), *Hospital Epidemiology and Infection Control.* The Williams & Wilkins Co., Baltimore, Md.
106. **Klein, M., and A. DeForest.** 1963. The inactivation of viruses by germicides. *Chem. Specialists Manufact. Assoc. Proc.* **49:**116–118.
107. **Klein, M. A., R. Frigg, E. Flechsig, A. J. Raeber, U. Kalinke, H. Bluethman, F. Bootz, J. Suter, R. M. Zinkernagel, and A. Aguzzi.** 1997. A crucial role for B cells in neuroinvasive scrapie. *Nature* **390:**687.
108. **Kobayashi, H., M. Tsuzuki, K. Koshimizu, H. Toyama,**

N. Yoshihara, T. Shikata, K. Abe, K. Mizuno, N. Otomo, and T. Oda. 1984. Susceptibility of hepatitis B virus to disinfectants or heat. *J. Clin. Microbiol.* **20:** 214–216.

109. **Kralovic, R. C.** 1993. Use of biological indicators designed for steam or ethylene oxide to monitor a liquid chemical sterilization process. *Infect. Control Hosp. Epidemiol.* **14:**313–319.
110. **Kurtz, J. B., T. W. Lee, and A. J. Parsons.** 1980. The action of alcohols on rotavirus, astrovirus and enterovirus. *J. Hosp. Infect.* **1:**321–325.
111. **Larson, E., K. Mayur, and B. A. Laughon.** 1989. Influence of two handwashing frequencies on reduction in colonizing flora with three handwashing products used by health care personnel. *Am. J. Infect. Control* **17:**83–88.
112. **Larson, E., A. McGeer, Z. A. Quraishi, D. Krenzischek, B. J. Parsons, J. Holdford, and W. J. Hierholzer.** 1991. Effect of an automated sink on handwashing practices and attitudes in high-risk units. *Infect. Control Hosp. Epidemiol.* **12:**422–428.
113. **Larson, E., K. J. McGinley, G. L. Grove, J. J. Leyden, and G. H. Talbot.** 1986. Physiologic, microbiologic, and seasonal effects of handwashing on the skin of health care personnel. *Am. J. Infect. Control* **14:**51–59.
114. **Larson, E. L.** 1991. Alcohols, p. 191–203. *In* S. S. Block (ed.), *Disinfection, Sterilization and Preservation.* Lea & Febiger, Philadelphia, Pa.
115. **Larson, E. L.** 1995. APIC guideline for handwashing and hand antisepsis in health care settings. *Am. J. Infect. Control* **23:**251–269.
116. **Larson, E. L., A. M. Butz, D. L. Gullette, and B. A. Laughon.** 1990. Alcohol for surgical scrubbing? *Infect. Control Hosp. Epidemiol.* **11:**139–143.
117. **Leaper, S.** 1984. Influence of temperature on the synergistic sporicidal effect of peracetic acid plus hydrogen peroxide in *Bacillus subtilis* SA22 (NCA 72-52). *Food Microbiol.* **1:**199–203.
118. **Levenson, J. E.** 1989. Corneal damage from improperly cleaned tonometer tips. *Arch. Ophthalmol.* **107:**1117.
119. **Lever, A. M., and S. V. W. Sutton.** 1996. Antimicrobial effects of hydrogen peroxide as an antiseptic and disinfectant, p. 159–176. *In* J. P. Ascenzi (ed.), *Handbook of Disinfectants and Antiseptics.* Marcel Dekker, Inc., New York, N.Y.
120. **Lowbury, E. J., and H. A. Lilly.** 1974. The effect of blood on disinfection of surgeons' hands. *Br. J. Surg.* **61:** 19–21.
121. **Lowbury, E. J., H. A. Lilly, and J. P. Bull.** 1964. Methods for disinfection of operation sites. *Br. Med. J.* **2:** 531–533.
122. **Maki, D. G., and C. A. Hassemer.** 1987. Flash sterilization: carefully measured haste. *Infect. Control* **8:**307–310.
123. **Malchesky, P. S.** 1993. Peracetic acid and its application to medical instrument sterilization. *Artif. Organs* **17:** 147–152.
124. **Mannion, P. T.** 1995. The use of peracetic acid for the reprocessing of flexible endoscopes and rigid cystoscopes and laparoscopes. *J. Hosp. Infect.* **29:**313–315.
125. **Martin, L. S., J. S. McDougal, and S. L. Loskoski.** 1985. Disinfection and inactivation of the human T lymphotropic virus type III/lymphadenopathy-associated virus. *J. Infect. Dis.* **152:**400–403.
126. **Martin, M. A., and M. Reichelderfer.** 1994. APIC guidelines for infection prevention and control in flexible endoscopy. Association for Professionals in Infection Control and Epidemiology, Inc. 1991, 1992, and 1993 APIC Guidelines Committee. *Am. J. Infect. Control* **22:**19–38.
127. **Mbithi, J. N., V. S. Springthorpe, and S. A. Sattar.** 1990. Chemical disinfection of hepatitis A virus on environmental surfaces. *Appl. Environ. Microbiol.* **56:**3601–3604.
128. **Mbithi, J. N., V. S. Springthorpe, S. A. Sattar, and M. Pacquette.** 1993. Bactericidal, virucidal, and mycobactericidal activities of reused alkaline glutaraldehyde in an endoscopy unit. *J. Clin. Microbiol.* **31:**2988–2995.
129. **Meengs, M. R., B. K. Giles, C. D. Chisholm, W. H. Cordell, and D. R. Nelson.** 1994. Hand washing frequency in an emergency department. *Ann. Emerg. Med.* **23:**1307–1312.
130. **Mentel, R., and J. Schmidt.** 1973. Investigations on rhinovirus inactivation by hydrogen peroxide. *Acta Virol.* **17:**351–354.
131. **Merianos, J. J.** 1991. Quaternary ammonium antimicrobial compounds, p. 225–255. *In* S. S. Block (ed.), *Disinfection, Sterilization and Preservation.* Lea & Febiger, Philadelphia, Pa.
132. **Mermel, L. A., S. L. Josephson, J. Dempsey, S. Parenteau, C. Perry, and N. Magill.** 1997. Outbreak of *Shigella sonnei* in a clinical microbiology laboratory. *J. Clin. Microbiol.* **35:**3163–3165.
133. **Michele, T. M., W. A. Cronin, N. M. Graham, D. M. Dwyer, D. S. Pope, S. Harrington, R. E. Chaisson, and W. R. Bishai.** 1997. Transmission of *Mycobacterium tuberculosis* by a fiberoptic bronchoscope. Identification by DNA fingerprinting. *JAMA* **278:**1093–1095.
134. **Muscarella, L. F.** 1996. High-level disinfection or "sterilization" of endoscopes? *Infect. Control Hosp. Epidemiol.* **17:**183–187.
135. **Nakashima, A. K., A. K. Highsmith, and W. J. Martone.** 1987. Survival of *Serratia marcescens* in benzalkonium chloride and in multiple-dose medication vials: relationship to epidemic septic arthritis. *J. Clin. Microbiol.* **25:** 1019–1021.
136. **Narang, H. K., and A. A. Codd.** 1983. Action of commonly used disinfectants against enteroviruses. *J. Hosp. Infect.* **4:**209–212.
137. **O'Connor, D. O., and J. R. Rubino.** 1991. Phenolic compounds, p. 204–224. *In* S. S. Block (ed.), *Disinfection, Sterilization and Preservation.* Lea & Febiger, Philadelphia, Pa.
138. **Oie, S., and A. Kamiya.** 1996. Microbial contamination of antiseptics and disinfectants. *Am. J. Infect. Control* **24:** 389–395.
139. **Parker, F., and S. Foran.** 1995. Chlorhexidine catheter lubricant anaphylaxis. *Anaesth. Intensive Care* **23:**126.
140. **Peutrell, J. M.** 1992. Anaphylactoid reaction to topical chlorhexidine during anaesthesia. *Anaesthesia* **47:**1013.
141. **Piazza, M., G. Borgia, L. Picciotto, S. Nappa, S. Cicciarello, and R. Orlando.** 1995. Detection of hepatitis C virus-RNA by polymerase chain reaction in dental surgeries. *J. Med. Virol.* **45:**40–42.
142. **Price, P. B.** 1938. The bacteriology of normal skin; a new quantitative test applied to a study of the bacterial flora and the disinfectant action of mechanical cleansing. *J. Infect. Dis.* **63:**301–318.
143. **Prince, D. L., H. N. Prince, O. Thraenhart, E. Muchmore, E. Bonder, and J. Pugh.** 1993. Methodological approaches to disinfection of human hepatitis B virus. *J. Clin. Microbiol.* **31:**3296–3304.
144. **Prusiner, S. B.** 1982. Novel proteinaceous infectious particles cause scrapie. *Science* **216:**136–144.
145. **Prusiner, S. B.** 1997. Prion diseases and the BSE crisis. *Science* **278:**245–251.
146. **Ranganathan, N. S.** 1996. Chlorhexidine, p. 235–264. *In* J. P. Ascenzi (ed.), *Handbook of Disinfectants and Antiseptics.* Marcel Dekker, Inc., New York, N.Y.
147. **Reagan, D. R., B. N. Doebbeling, M. A. Pfaller, C. T. Sheetz, A. K. Houston, R. J. Hollis, and R. P. Wenzel.**

1991. Elimination of coincident *Staphylococcus aureus* nasal and hand carriage with intranasal application of mupirocin calcium ointment. *Ann. Intern. Med.* **114:** 101–106.

147a. **Reichert, M., and J. H. Young.** 1997. *Sterilization Technology for the Health Care Facility*, 2nd ed. Aspen Publishers, Inc., Gaithersburg, Md.

148. **Roosendaal, R., E. J. Kuipers, A. J. van den Brule, A. S. Pena, A. M. Uyterlinde, J. M. Walboomers, S. G. Meuwissen, and J. de Graaff.** 1994. Importance of the fiberoptic endoscope cleaning procedure for detection of *Helicobacter pylori* in gastric biopsy specimens by PCR. *J. Clin. Microbiol.* **32:**1123–1126.

149. **Rossmoore, H. W., and M. Sondossi.** 1988. Applications and mode of action of formaldehyde condensate biocides. *Adv. Appl. Microbiol.* **33:**223–277.

150. **Rotter, M. L.** 1996. Hand washing and hand disinfection, p. 1052–1068. *In* C. G. Mayhall (ed.), *Hospital Epidemiology and Infection Control.* The Williams & Wilkins Co., Baltimore, Md.

151. **Rotter, M. L.** 1996. Alcohols for antisepsis of hands and skin, p. 177–234. *In* J. P. Ascenzi (ed.), *Handbook of Disinfectants and Antiseptics.* Marcel Dekker, Inc., New York, N.Y.

152. **Rotter, M. L., W. Koller, G. Wewalka, H. P. Werner, G. A. Ayliffe, and J. R. Babb.** 1986. Evaluation of procedures for hygienic hand-disinfection: controlled parallel experiments on the Vienna test model. *J. Hyg. (London)* **96:**27–37.

153. **Rubbo, S. D., J. F. Gardner, and R. L. Webb.** 1967. Biocidal activities of glutaraldehyde and related compounds. *J. Appl. Bacteriol.* **30:**78–87.

154. **Russell, A. D.** 1994. Glutaraldehyde: current status and uses. *Infect. Control Hosp. Epidemiol.* **15:**724–733.

155. **Russell, A. D., and M. J. Day.** 1993. Antibacterial activity of chlorhexidine. *J. Hosp. Infect.* **25:**229–238.

156. **Russell, A. D., W. B. Hugo, and G. A. J. Ayliffe.** 1992. *Principles and Practice of Disinfection, Preservation and Sterilization.* Blackwell Scientific Publications, London, United Kingdom.

157. **Rutala, W. A.** 1996. APIC guideline for selection and use of disinfectants. 1994, 1995, and 1996 APIC Guidelines Committee. Association for Professionals in Infection Control and Epidemiology, Inc. *Am. J. Infect. Control* **24:** 313–342.

158. **Rutala, W. A.** 1996. Disinfection and sterilization of patient-care items. *Infect. Control Hosp. Epidemiol.* **17:** 377–384.

159. **Rutala, W. A., E. P. Clontz, D. J. Weber, and K. K. Hoffman.** 1991. Disinfection practices for endoscopes and other semicritical items. *Infect. Control Hosp. Epidemiol.* **12:**282–288.

160. **Rutala, W. A., and E. C. Cole.** 1987. Ineffectiveness of hospital disinfectants against bacteria: a collaborative study. *Infect. Control* **8:**501–506.

161. **Rutala, W. A., E. C. Cole, N. S. Wannamaker, and D. J. Weber.** 1991. Inactivation of *Mycobacterium tuberculosis* and *Mycobacterium bovis* by 14 hospital disinfectants. *Am. J. Med.* **91:**267S–271S.

162. **Rutala, W. A., M. F. Gergen, and D. J. Weber.** 1993. Evaluation of a rapid readout biological indicator for flash sterilization with three biological indicators and three chemical indicators. *Infect. Control Hosp. Epidemiol.* **14:** 390–394.

163. **Rutala, W. A., M. F. Gergen, and D. J. Weber.** 1993. Inactivation of *Clostridium difficile* spores by disinfectants. *Infect. Control Hosp. Epidemiol.* **14:**36–39.

164. **Rutala, W. A., S. M. Jones, and D. J. Weber.** 1996. Comparison of a rapid readout biological indicator for steam sterilization with four conventional biological indicators and five chemical indicators. *Infect. Control Hosp. Epidemiol.* **17:**423–428.

164a. **Rutala, W. A., and D. J. Weber.** 1985. FDA labelling requirements for disinfection of endoscopes: a counterpoint. *Infect. Control Hosp. Epidemiol.* **16:**231–235.

165. **Rutala, W. A., and D. J. Weber.** 1997. Uses of inorganic hypochlorite (bleach) in health-care facilities. *Clin. Microbiol. Rev.* **10:**597–610.

166. **Rutala, W. A., D. J. Weber, C. A. Thomann, J. F. John, S. M. Saviteer, and F. A. Sarubbi.** 1988. An outbreak of *Pseudomonas cepacia* bacteremia associated with a contaminated intra-aortic balloon pump. *J. Thorac. Cardiovasc. Surg.* **96:**157–161.

167. **Ryan, C. K., and G. D. Potter.** 1995. Disinfectant colitis. Rinse as well as you wash. *J. Clin. Gastroenterol.* **21:**6–9.

168. **Sagripanti, J. L.** 1992. Metal-based formulations with high microbicidal activity. *Appl. Environ. Microbiol.* **58:** 3157–3162.

169. **Sagripanti, J. L., and A. Bonifacino.** 1996. Comparative sporicidal effect of liquid chemical germicides on three medical devices contaminated with spores of *Bacillus subtilis. Am. J. Infect. Control* **24:**364–371.

170. **Sagripanti, J. L., C. A. Eklund, P. A. Trost, K. C. Jinneman, C. J. Abeyta, C. A. Kaysner, and W. E. Hill.** 1997. Comparative sensitivity of 13 species of pathogenic bacteria to seven chemical germicides. *Am. J. Infect. Control* **25:**335–339.

171. **Sailer, A., H. Bueler, M. Fischer, A. Aguzzi, and C. Weissmann.** 1994. No propagation of prions in mice devoid of PrP. *Cell* **77:**967–968.

172. **Samore, M. H., L. Venkataraman, P. C. DeGirolami, R. D. Arbeit, and A. W. Karchmer.** 1996. Clinical and molecular epidemiology of sporadic and clustered cases of nosocomial *Clostridium difficile* diarrhea. *Am. J. Med.* **100:** 32–40.

173. **Sattar, S. A., H. Jacobsen, H. Rahman, T. M. Cusack, and J. R. Rubino.** 1994. Interruption of rotavirus spread through chemical disinfection. *Infect. Control Hosp. Epidemiol.* **15:**751–756.

174. **Sattar, S. A., Y. E. Taylor, M. Paquette, and J. Rubino.** 1996. In-hospital evaluation of 7.5% hydrogen peroxide as a disinfectant for flexible endoscopes. *Can. J. Infect Control* **11:**51–54.

175. **Saurina, G., D. Landman, and J. M. Quale.** 1997. Activity of disinfectants against vancomycin-resistant *Enterococcus faecium. Infect. Control Hosp. Epidemiol.* **18:** 345–347.

176. **Scherrer, M., and K. Kümmerer.** 1997. Manual and automated processing of medical instruments—environmental and economic aspects. *Central Services* **5:**183–194.

177. **Sedlock, D. M., and D. M. Bailey.** 1985. Microbial activity of octenidine hydrochloride, a new alkanediylbis[pyridine] germicidal agent. *Antimicrob. Agents Chemother.* **28:** 786–790.

178. **Spach, D. H., F. E. Silverstein, and W. E. Stamm.** 1993. Transmission of infection by gastrointestinal endoscopy and bronchoscopy. *Ann. Intern. Med.* **118:**117–128.

179. **Spaulding, E. H.** 1968. Chemical disinfection of medical and surgical materials, p. 517–531. *In* S. S. Block (ed.), *Disinfection, Sterilization and Preservation.* Lea & Febiger, Philadelphia, Pa.

180. **Steinmann, J., R. Nehrkorn, A. Meyer, and K. Becker.** 1995. Two in-vivo protocols for testing virucidal efficacy of handwashing and hand disinfection. *Zentbl. Hyg. Umweltmed.* **196:**425–436.

181. **Stickler, D. J., and B. Thomas.** 1980. Antiseptic and antibiotic resistance in gram-negative bacteria causing urinary tract infection. *J. Clin. Pathol.* **33:**288–296.

182. **Tabor, E., D. C. Bostwick, and C. C. Evans.** 1989. Corneal damage due to eye contact with chlorhexidine gluconate. *JAMA* **261:**557–558.

183. **Tanaka, H., Y. Hirakata, M. Kaku, R. Yoshida, H. Takemura, R. Mizukane, K. Ishida, K. Tomono, H. Koga, S. Kohno, and S. Kamihira.** 1996. Antimicrobial activity of superoxidized water. *J. Hosp. Infect.* **34:**43–49.

184. **Taylor, D. M., H. Fraser, I. McConnell, D. A. Brown, K. L. Brown, K. A. Lamza, and G. R. Smith.** 1994. Decontamination studies with the agents of bovine spongiform encephalopathy and scrapie. *Arch. Virol.* **139:** 313–326.

185. **Terleckyj, B., and D. A. Axler.** 1987. Quantitative neutralization assay of fungicidal activity of disinfectants. *Antimicrob. Agents Chemother.* **31:**794–798.

186. **Tyler, R., G. A. Ayliffe, and C. Bradley.** 1990. Virucidal activity of disinfectants: studies with the poliovirus. *J. Hosp. Infect.* **15:**339–345.

187. **van Bueren, J., D. P. Larkin, and R. A. Simpson.** 1994. Inactivation of human immunodeficiency virus type 1 by alcohols. *J. Hosp. Infect.* **28:**137–148.

188. **Van Klingeren, B., and W. Pullen.** 1993. Glutaraldehyde resistant mycobacteria from endoscope washers. *J. Hosp. Infect.* **25:**147–149.

189. **Vesley, D., M. A. Nellis, and P. B. Allwood.** 1995. Evaluation of a rapid readout biological indicator for 121 degrees C gravity and 132 degrees C vacuum-assisted steam sterilization cycles. *Infect. Control Hosp. Epidemiol.* **16:** 281–286.

190. **Voss, A., and A. F. Widmer.** 1997. No time for handwashing? Handwashing versus alcoholic rub: can we afford 100% compliance? *Infect. Control Hosp. Epidemiol.* **18:** 205–208.

191. **Wallace, J., P. M. Agee, and D. M. Demicco.** 1995. Liquid chemical sterilization using peracetic acid. An alternative approach to endoscope processing. *ASAIO J.* **41:** 151–154.

192. **Waran, K. D., and R. A. Munsick.** 1995. Anaphylaxis from povidone-iodine. *Lancet* **345:**1506.

193. **Wardle, M. D., and G. M. Renninger.** 1975. Bactericidal effect of hydrogen peroxide on spacecraft isolates. *Appl. Microbiol.* **30:**710–711.

194. **Wewalka, G., M. Rotter, W. Koller, and G. Stanek.** 1977. Comparison of efficacy of 14 procedures for the hygienic disinfection of hands. *Zentbl. Bakteriol. Parasitenkd. Infektionskr. Hyg. Abt. 1 Orig. Reihe B* **165:** 242–249.

195. **Widmer, A. F.** 1994. Infection control and prevention strategies in the ICU. *Intensive Care. Med.* **20**(Suppl. 4)**:** S7–S11.

196. **Widmer, A. F., A. Houston, E. Bollinger, and R. P. Wenzel.** 1992. A new standard for sterility testing for autoclaved surgical trays. *J. Hosp. Infect.* **21:**253–260.

197. **Widmer, A. F., M. Perschmann, T. C. Gasser, and R. Frei.** 1994. Alcohol (ALC) vs chlorhexidinegluconate (CHG) for preoperative hand scrub: a randomized crossover clinical trial, abstr. J180, p. 187. *In Program and Abstracts of the 34th Interscience Conference on Antimicrobial Agents and Chemotherapy.* American Society for Microbiology, Washington, D.C.

198. **Widmer, A. F., R. P. Wenzel, A. Trilla, M. J. Bale, R. N. Jones, and B. N. Doebbeling.** 1993. Outbreak of *Pseudomonas aeruginosa* infections in a surgical intensive care unit: probable transmission via hands of a health care worker. *Clin. Infect. Dis.* **16:**372–376.

199. **Williams, N. D., and A. D. Russell.** 1991. The effects of some halogen-containing compounds on *Bacillus subtilis* endospores. *J. Appl. Bacteriol.* **70:**427–436.

200. **World Health Organization.** 1983. *Laboratory Safety Manual.* World Health Organization, Geneva, Switzerland.

201. **Wysowski, D. K., J. W. Flynt, M. Goldfield, R. Altman, and A. T. Davis.** 1978. Epidemic neonatal hyperbilirubinemia and use of a phenolic disinfectant detergent. *Pediatrics* **61:**165–170.

202. **Yong, D., F. C. Parker, and S. M. Foran.** 1995. Severe allergic reactions and intraurethral chlorhexidine gluconate. *Med. J. Aust.* **162:**257–258.

203. **Young, J. H.** 1997. Steam sterilization: scientific principles, p. 124–133. *In* M. Reichert and J. H. Young (ed.), *Sterilization Technology.* Aspen Publications, Gaithersburg, Md.

204. **Zaidi, M., J. Sifuentes, M. Bobadilla, D. Moncada, and S. Ponce de León.** 1989. Epidemic of *Serratia marcescens* bacteremia and meningitis in a neonatal unit in Mexico City. *Infect. Control Hosp. Epidemiol.* **10:**14–20.

205. **Zeidler, M., E. C. Johnstone, R. W. Bamber, C. M. Dickens, C. J. Fisher, A. F. Francis, R. Goldbeck, R. Higgo, E. C. Johnson-Sabine, G. J. Lodge, P. McGarry, S. Mitchell, L. Tarlo, M. Turner, P. Ryley, and R. G. Will.** 1997. New variant Creutzfeldt-Jakob disease: psychiatric features. *Lancet* **350:**908–910.

206. **Zeidler, M., G. E. Stewart, C. R. Barraclough, D. E. Bateman, D. Bates, D. J. Burn, A. C. Colchester, W. Durward, N. A. Fletcher, S. A. Hawkins, J. M. Mackenzie, and R. G. Will.** 1997. New variant Creutzfeldt-Jakob disease: neurological features and diagnostic tests. *Lancet* **350:**903–907.

Prevention and Control of Laboratory-Acquired Infections

ANDREAS VOSS

9

Laboratories in the United States employ approximately 500,000 laboratory workers (LWs) who are at occupational risk of exposure to microbiological pathogens that may cause inapparent to life-threatening infections (63). Laboratory-acquired infections (LAIs) are defined as all infections acquired through laboratory activities, regardless of their clinical or subclinical manifestation (66). The actual risk of LAIs is difficult to estimate, since no regional or national reporting systems are in place. Furthermore, LAIs may be underreported even on a local level due to atypical or subclinical manifestations of infections or the LW's fear of embarrassment. Data on LAIs were collected and published as early as 1949, and reviews of the incidence, consequences, and control of LAIs, such as those of Pike (58) in 1979, stimulated the development of laboratory safety programs. Despite these early guidelines, LAIs still occurred, probably due to a lack of instructions and/or poor compliance with safe laboratory practices, as examples in this chapter will prove.

The emergence (or reemergence) of human immunodeficiency virus (HIV), hantavirus, hepatitis C virus, and multidrug-resistant *Mycobacterium tuberculosis* has not only renewed the interest in biosafety measures but has also probably enhanced compliance with those measures. Strategies for the prevention and management of LAIs should be aimed at containing the biohazardous agents and educating LWs about the occupational risks. In general, biosafety programs include recommendations on work practices, laboratory design, personal protective equipment, and safety devices. Adherence to these biosafety guidelines can reduce the risk of exposure and consequent LAIs.

The body of literature on "biosafety" is enormous and includes recent reviews (61–63), as well as excellent publications from the Centers for Disease Control and Prevention (CDC) (22) and the Occupational Safety and Health Administration (OSHA), which can be found on the respective web sites (http://www.cdc.gov/od/ohs/biosfty/bmbl/ and http://www.osha-sk.gov). In addition to CDC and OSHA, other agencies issuing guidelines or rules regarding laboratory safety are the National Institute of Occupational Safety and Health, the National Institutes of Health (NIH), the National Committee for Clinical Laboratory Standards, the College of American Pathologists, and the Joint Commission on Accreditation of Healthcare Organizations. In this chapter the basic principles of laboratory safety will be described, and examples of specific LAIs and their prevention will be given.

LABORATORY-ACQUIRED INFECTION SURVEYS

Sulkin and Pike (66) were the first to study LAIs systematically. By 1976 Pike (57) published the results of a comprehensive review of the incidence, outcome, and prevention of LAIs after analyzing close to 4,000 cases of LAIs gathered through literature reviews, mail surveys, and personal communications. Despite identifying the major pathogens of LAIs and recognizing that aerosols are the primary route of transmission, Pike's data could not provide information about the denominators to be used to estimate actual risks (63).

Most LAIs (43%) were caused by bacteria, followed by viruses (27%) and rickettsiae (15%) (57). Brucellosis, typhoid fever, and Q fever were the most frequently reported infections (Table 1). The overall mortality rate among more than 3,900 reported cases of LAIs was 4.2%, with the highest mortality rate (7.8%) occurring among LWs with chlamydial infections. These fatalities originated from cases of psittacosis that occurred prior to 1955, at a time when LWs had just begun to implement the use of safe work practices and equipment. Furthermore, Pike (57) pointed out that 97% of the brucellosis and typhoid fever cases were reported before 1955 and that 10 of the 159 agents identified as pathogens responsible for LAIs caused more than 50% of the cases of LAIs. Thirty-six percent of all viral LAIs were caused by a hepatitis virus and Venezuelan equine encephalitis virus, with half of the cases due to the latter agent being reported in only four laboratories. More than 50% of the fungal infections were caused by two pathogens: *Histoplasma capsulatum* and *Coccidioides immitis*. Among cases of LAIs due to rickettsial and parasitic agents, 50 and 24% of the infections were caused by *Coxiella burnetii* and *Toxoplasma gondii*, respectively. After 1955, the relative frequency of fungal and especially viral LAIs increased, whereas bacterial, chlamydial, and rickettsial infections notably decreased (44, 58).

During the 1980s, the most frequently found pathogens in a series of surveys (29–31, 40, 58, 68) were *M. tuberculosis*, *Salmonella* species, *Shigella* species, hepatitis B virus, and hepatitis non-A, non-B virus. Jacobson et al. (40) described an annual incidence of LAIs of approximately 3 per 1,000

TABLE 1 Most frequently reported laboratory-acquired infections in the world and the United States[a]

Infection	Total no. (%) of cases reported for the following[b]:	
	United States and world (1976)	United States (1969)
Brucellosis	423 (10.8)	274 (9.4)
Q fever	278 (7.1)	184 (6.3)
Typhoid fever	256 (6.5)	292 (10.0)
Hepatitis	234 (6.0)	126 (4.3)
Tularemia	225 (5.7)	129 (4.4)
Tuberculosis	176 (4.5)	174 (6.0)
Dermatomycosis	161 (4.1)	84 (2.9)
Venezuelan equine encephalitis	141 (3.6)	118 (4.1)
Typhus	124 (3.2)	82 (2.8)
Psittacosis	116 (3.0)	70 (2.4)
Coccidioidomycosis	93 (2.4)	108 (3.7)
Leptospirosis	87 (2.2)	43 (1.5)
Streptococcal infection	78 (2.0)	67 (2.3)
Histoplasmosis	71 (1.8)	81 (2.8)
Shigellosis	58 (1.5)	54 (1.9)
Salmonellosis	48 (1.2)	54 (1.9)

[a] Adapted from Sewell (63).

[b] Entries in the column of data for the United States may be larger than the corresponding entries in the column of data for the world and the United States due to shifts in the numbers of various LAIs over time.

employees in hospital laboratories. The risk of acquiring specific infections seems to differ among the different types of laboratories. LWs in pathology laboratories had a greater risk of contracting tuberculosis, whereas the microbiology laboratory staff had a greater risk of contracting gastrointestinal infections, such as salmonellosis and shigellosis (29, 30, 36, 58, 68). Furthermore, a three times greater number of LAIs occurred in laboratories with fewer than 25 employees, possibly reflecting the fact that these LWs have less experience in the handling of hazardous agents. In one of the most recent reviews of 58 publications published between 1980 and 1991, Harding and Lieberman (35) reported 375 infections or seroconversions, resulting in 23 fatalities. Forty-three percent (n = 162) of all LAIs were due to rickettsia, with *C. burnetii* accounting for 95% of these infections. Three-fourths of the viral infections (n = 119) were caused by arbo- and hantaviruses. *Salmonella typhi*, *Brucella melitensis*, and *Chlamydia* species were the most frequent causes of bacterial LAIs.

EXPOSURE RESULTING IN LAIs

The most common types of exposure resulting in LAIs are inhalation, ingestion, inoculation, and contamination of skin and mucous membranes (Table 2). About two-thirds of all LAIs result from direct work with the infectious agent (57). Laboratory accidents were the second greatest source of LAIs, with approximately 70% of the accidents caused by splashes or sprays, needlesticks, and cuts.

Inhalation

Various procedures in the laboratory, such as mixing, vortexing, grinding, blending, and flaming of a loop, may generate aerosols. After being discharged into the air, droplets may fall onto surfaces or evaporate, leaving droplet nuclei (≤5 μm) that remain suspended in the air and that are able to reach the alveoli of the lungs when inhaled (26). Aside from typically airborne pathogens, such as *M. tuberculosis*, airborne transmission of organisms that do not naturally follow this route may take place in the laboratory. Manipulations of severely contaminated or large volumes of fluids may lead to inhalation of an increased inoculum and an increased probability of infection, respectively.

Ingestion

Ingestion may occur through subconscious hand-to-mouth actions, by placing contaminated articles (e.g., pencils) or fingers (e.g., by biting the fingernails) in the mouth. Food consumption at the workplace or lack of hand disinfection before eating and smoking may be other causes. Furthermore, 13% of all accidental LAIs are associated with mouth pipetting, indicating that LWs still neglect basic safety techniques (57).

Inoculation

Parenteral inoculation of infectious materials through accidents with needles, blades, and broken glassware is one of the leading causes of LAIs, with needlesticks and cuts alone accounting for 25.2 and 15.9% of all types of accidents resulting in infections, respectively (21, 57). Needles and sharp objects used by LWs need to be disposed of in appropriate containers in order to reduce their own risk of injury as well as that of personnel who handle waste.

Contamination of Skin and Mucous Membranes

Splashes onto the mucous membranes of the eyes, nasal cavity, and mouth and hand-to-face actions may lead to the transmission of pathogenic microorganisms. Hand washing

TABLE 2 Routes of exposure associated with LAIs[a]

Route	Laboratory practices and/or accidents
Inhalation	Procedures that produce aerosols: • Centrifugation • Spillage and splashes • Mixing, vortexing, grinding, blending, sonicating • Separating two surfaces enclosing a fluid (opening)
Ingestion	• Mouth pipetting • Splashes into mouth • Eating, drinking, smoking, placing fingers in the mouth (e.g., nail biting) • Leaking contaminated items (labels, pens)
Inoculation	• Needlesticks • Cuts from sharp objects (e.g., blades or broken glassware) • Animal and insect bites and scratches
Percutaneous or mucosal penetration	• Spills and splashes • Contact with contaminated surfaces and items • Transfer by hand-to-face actions

[a] Adapted from Sewell (63) and Berrouane (9).

and disinfection remain the major means of preventing LAIs.

Intact skin is an efficient barrier against most infectious agents; however, small lesions are frequent and may serve as points of entry. This route of exposure should not be underestimated, especially since Levy et al. (43) found that accidental blood-skin contact may occur between 2 and 10 times a day in LWs.

SPECIFIC LAIs AND AGENTS OF LAIs

Bacteria

Brucellosis

As shown in Table 1, brucellosis is the most frequently reported bacterial LAI. Human infections may be caused by *B. melitensis*, *B. abortus*, *B. canis*, or *B. suis* (70). All *Brucella* species are highly contagious when handled in the laboratory, frequently causing small epidemics among laboratory technicians (32, 45, 65) or their families (16). Martin-Mazuelos et al. (45) and Gruner et al. (32) reported on four and five microbiology technicians with laboratory-acquired *B. melitensis* infections, respectively (Table 3). Infections may occur when LWs do not expect this pathogen and neglect to take appropriate safety measures. Biochemical misidentification of a *Brucella* species as a *Moraxella* species, with the consequent mishandling, was shown to be another reason for laboratory-acquired brucellosis (5). Therefore, it seems prudent that clinicians should alert the laboratory when brucellosis is suspected. Furthermore, clinical specimens should be handled according to the most stringent safety measures (biosafety level 3 [BSL-3]) since the infection can be transmitted by aerosols (52).

B. pseudomallei

Burkholderia pseudomallei (formerly *Pseudomonas pseudomallei*) is the causative agent of melioidosis. In humans, the infection typically produces subclinical disease and an asymptomatic carrier state. Even though clinical illness rarely occurs, it may be associated with a lethal outcome (3). Consequently, LWs need to be trained to handle this bacterium by safe work procedures and with adequate laboratory facilities. To prevent LAIs, special precautions (BSL-2) should be used, including prohibition of the "sniff" test and the use of centrifugation cups and biological safety cabinets (BSCs) for the processing of sputum, subculturing of stock strains, preparation of antigen, and research studies (3).

F. tularensis

In the survey published by Pike in 1976 (57), infections due to *Francisella tularensis* were the third most common bacterial LAIs. Most of the cases occurred in LWs in tularemia research laboratories, probably due to the transmission of infectious aerosols produced during the processing of cultures.

Leptospira

LAIs associated with *Leptospira* species are mainly due to accidental parenteral exposure (27, 69). Since animals are the natural host of *Leptospira*, LWs involved in animal care or research are at higher risk of infection (23, 47).

M. tuberculosis

The *M. tuberculosis* complex includes three human pathogens: *M. tuberculosis*, *M. bovis*, and *M. africanum*. In the hospital, administrative controls, such as patient screening and risk assessment, followed by prompt isolation and appropriate therapy, are the most important components of tuberculosis prevention (11, 12). Among LWs, the risk of exposure to species of the *M. tuberculosis* complex is especially high in anatomic pathology laboratories (morgue, frozen section suite) and is increased in general clinical laboratories and mycobacteriological laboratories (48). Since the source of laboratory-acquired tuberculosis is often unclear, occupational transmission is difficult to prove. Due to its known characteristics, Mazurek et al. (46) genotypically proved the transmission of the reference strain *M. tuberculosis* Erdman using DNA fingerprinting (Table 3). Generally, LAIs with *M. tuberculosis* cause pulmonary infections, but other body sites may be involved. Shireman et al. (64) described a case of granulomatous endometrial tuberculosis that was probably due to respiratory tract exposure as a result of a faulty exhaust hood.

Recently, CDC (15a) published regulatory guidelines entitled "Goals for Working Safely with Mycobacterium tuberculosis." A copy of these draft guidelines may be obtained from the American Society for Microbiology (ASM) via http://www.asmusa.org/pasrc/regulat.htm. ASM specifically questions CDC's advice to apply BSL-3 and respirators in all tuberculosis laboratory operations, providing virtually no stratification of safety standards for different risks and/or settings. At least among health care workers (HCWs) the tuberculin skin test conversion rates did not differ between hospitals in which surgical masks or disposable particulate respirators were used (24), suggesting that respirators certainly are not indicated for all laboratory activities. Still, since the infectious dose of *M. tuberculosis* is very low (26), all activities that may produce aerosols (e.g., opening of test tubes containing cultures) should be done in a biological safety cabinet. Next to ASM and CDC, OSHA issued mandatory guidelines regarding tuberculosis exposure (51). A new OSHA standard is currently under development and will be released in 1998.

N. meningitidis

Recently, Guibourdenche et al. (33) proved the transmission of *Neisseria meningitidis* using serotyping, outer membrane protein characterization, and enzyme electrophoresis to confirm the identities of the clinical isolates from two laboratory technicians infected with laboratory strains (Table 3).

Salmonella, *Shigella*, and Other Stool Pathogens

Salmonellosis and shigellosis are the most commonly reported laboratory-acquired gastrointestinal infections (17, 31, 40, 57, 58). Infections occur from ingestion or, on rare occasions, from inoculation of the stool pathogens from clinical specimens, as well as from the handling of proficiency test strains (39). Chronic nail-biters may be at risk, as shown among HCWs in a nursery for newborns (7). The incidences of salmonellosis and shigellosis in Great Britain are reported to be 0.137 and 0.322 infections per 1,000 LWs, respectively (63), but these infections are probably vastly underreported. In a comparison of LWs from clinical laboratories with those from microbiological laboratories, the latter group had an approximately eightfold higher incidence of laboratory-acquired shigellosis (40). The most serious gastrointestinal infections acquired in the laboratory are probably due to *S. typhi*. A case of laboratory-acquired typhoid fever has been described in a situation in which no obvious breakdown of laboratory safety techniques could be detected

TABLE 3 Examples of bacterial, fungal, parasitic, chlamydial, rickettsial, and viral LAIs reported between 1990 and 1996

Pathogen (infection)	Reference	Comment
Bacteria		
B. melitensis (brucellosis)	Martin-Mazuelos et al. (45)	Outbreak involving four technicians
	Gruner et al. (32)	Outbreak involving five technicians
	Batchelor et al. (5)	Infection due to misidentification
Leptospira species (leptospirosis)	Waitkins (69)	Accidental parenteral exposure
	Gilks et al. (27)	Accidental parenteral exposure
M. tuberculosis (tuberculosis)	Mazurek et al. (46)	LAI proven by DNA fingerprinting
	Muller (48)	Higher risk in laboratories
	Shireman (64)	Endometrial tuberculosis
N. meningitidis (meningitis)	Guibourdenche et al. (33)	Transmission confirmed by typing
	Paradis and Grimard (54)	Invasive infection in LW
Salmonella or *Shigella*	Beers et al. (7)	Nail biters were found to be at higher risk
	Holmes et al. (39)	Handling of strains for proficiency testing
S. typhi (typhoid fever)	Ashdown and Cassidy (2)	No obvious breakdown in safety techniques
E. coli O157:H7	Burnens et al. (13)	Proven by toxin type and plasmid profile analyses
C. jejuni	Penner et al. (55)	Transmission confirmed by typing
Fungi		
Penicillium marneffei	Hilmarsdottir et al. (38)	In an HCW with AIDS
S. schenckii (sporotrichosis)	Cooper et al. (18)	In the absence of apparent trauma
B. dermatitidis, *H. capsulatum*, and *C. immitis*	Baum and Lerner (6) and Collins (17)	Transmission by inhalation
Protozoa		
Trypanosoma brucei gambiense	Receveur et al. (59)	Trypanosomiasis
T. gondii	Herwaldt and Juranek (37)	Most common protozoal LAI
Chlamydia		
C. trachomatis	Bernstein et al. (8)	Pneumonitis, lymphadenitis
Rickettsia		
C. burnetii	Hamadeh et al. (34)	Q-fever epidemics by aerosol transmission
R. rickettsii	Oster et al. (53)	Rocky Mountain spotted fever due to aerosol transmission
Viruses		
Blood-borne pathogens	Jacobson et al. (40)	Despite considerable risk, no attention
	Levy et al. (43)	Due to exposure to HBV-contaminated blood
	Favero and Bond (20)	No evidence of aerosol transmission
Hemorrhagic fever (e.g., Sabia virus)	Gonzales et al. (28) and Barry et al. (4)	Two LAIs caused by strain that caused fatal cases in São Paulo, Brazil, 1990
	Gandsman et al. (25) and Ryder and Gandsman (60)	Scientist exposure while purifying the virus from tissue culture
Arenavirus	Vasconcelos et al. (67)	Transmission through aerosols

(2). In addition to the transmission to or among LWs, cases of typhoid fever may occur among people outside the laboratory (10). Since the infectious dose of *S. typhi* is smaller than that of most enteric pathogens, handling of specimens containing this pathogen might bear a higher risk of an LAI.

As with *S. typhi*, Burnens et al. (13) suggested that the infecting dose of *Escherichia coli* O157:H7 is low since they found no break in preventive measures preceding a case of LAI caused by this microorganism. Some authorities in the United Kingdom advise that evaluations of the immunization histories of staff working in the microbiological laboratory with regard to their immunity to *S. typhi* be performed and recommend a course of typhoid vaccine (56).

Despite causing frequent problems in the hospital, *Clostridium difficile* has not been reported to be a cause of LAIs. Penner et al. (55) used different typing techniques to confirm a laboratory-acquired case of *Campylobacter jejuni* enteritis caused by a frequently passaged laboratory strain.

Chlamydial Infections

To date, only sporadic laboratory cases of chlamydial infections due to *Chlamydia psittaci* and *Chlamydia trachomatis* have been reported (8, 17). Prior to the 1960s these infections used to be common and were associated with a high mortality rate (57).

Fungal Infections

Laboratory-acquired fungal infections most commonly originate from inhalation of spores or conidia of *Blastomyces dermatitidis* (6, 17), *H. capsulatum* (17, 49), and *C. immitis* (17). These fungal pathogens, as well as *Sporothrix schenckii*, may furthermore lead to cutaneous LAIs after accidental inoculation (17, 18, 42, 57). Cooper et al. (18) reported a case of laboratory-acquired sporotrichosis associated with research activities (Table 3). Since no apparent trauma or other predisposing factors were known, the investigators suggested the possibility that *S. schenckii* (at least under laboratory conditions) can invade intact, healthy skin.

Despite ranking high on the list of LAI-associated fungal pathogens (Table 1), dermatophytes are not usually seen among LWs of clinical laboratories but are seen among those of animal facilities.

Parasitic Infections

Only a small part (~3%) of all LAIs are caused by protozoal agents. *T. gondii* is the most frequently observed agent of parasitic LAIs. Other common laboratory-acquired parasitic infections are malaria, leishmaniasis, and trypanosomiasis (37, 59). The majority of these cases occur among LWs of animal research facilities. Needlestick injuries were the major source in cases in which an accident could be recalled. Usually, accidents or breaks in laboratory safety measures were not recalled.

Rickettsial Infections

Q fever is the second most commonly reported LAI in the world and in the United States (Table 1). LWs in animal research facilities are particularly at risk, since research animals such as sheep may be asymptomatic carriers of *C. burnetii*. As shown with *Brucella* species, aerosol transmission of *C. burnetii* may cause small Q-fever epidemics among LWs of the same facility (34). Furthermore, multiple cases of laboratory-acquired Rocky Mountain spotted fever due to aerosol transmission of *Rickettsia rickettsii* have been reported (53).

Viral Infections Caused by Blood-Borne Pathogens

Despite the considerable risk of contraction of the hepatitis B virus (HBV) by LWs (20, 40, 43) and the consequential morbidity and mortality from HBV infections among health care workers, it required the advent of the HIV and AIDS epidemic to increase the general attention of HCWs to the risk of blood-borne transmission of viral pathogens. In 1994, a total of 32 laboratory technicians were reported by CDC to have documented ($n = 17$) and possible ($n = 15$) cases of HIV infection as a result of occupational transmission (14). Percutaneous exposure was the leading cause in these cases, but nevertheless, transmissions after mucocutaneous contact were reported.

Parenteral inoculation, percutaneous contact in the presence of skin lesions, and exposure of mucous membranes present a high risk of HIV transmission. So far, no evidence of aerosol HIV transmission exists (20). Evans et al. (19) assessed the risk for occupational exposures to biohazardous agents found in blood by taking environmental samples from a total of 10 clinical and research laboratories. HBV surface antigen was found in 31 of the 800 environmental samples from 11 workstations in three laboratories.

Environmental contamination arises as a result of several factors, such as high workloads, inappropriate behavior, and flawed laboratory techniques. Therefore, a multifactorial approach is necessary to prevent or minimize viral and blood-borne LAIs. Guidelines for prevention of blood-borne infections are in general alike for most of the so-called blood-borne pathogens, such as hepatitis B, C, and D viruses and HIV. Avoidance of unprotected contact with infectious materials (blood, semen, saliva, tears, urine, cerebrospinal fluid, breast milk, and other excretions or secretions) by the use of BSL-2 practices and containment equipment is the most important means of prevention. For further regulations regarding occupational exposure to blood-borne pathogens, OSHA's rules should be consulted (1, 50). A high educational level and vaccination against hepatitis B are major players in the prevention of LAIs caused by blood-borne pathogens.

Hemorrhagic Fever

Arenavirus was isolated from a single patient with fatal hemorrhagic fever in the state of São Paulo, Brazil, in 1990. A serologically proven LAI transmitted by aerosols was described by Vasconcelos et al. (67) in an LW with symptoms of hemorrhagic fever (Table 3). Attempts to isolate the virus from the patient did not succeed. Several other cases of laboratory-acquired hemorrhagic fever due to Sabia virus have been reported (25, 28, 60). In general, arboviruses are assigned to BSL-1 to BSL-4, depending on their mode of transmission and the consequent severity and/or frequency of LAIs. The most virulent agents, such as Ebola, Lassa, and Marburg viruses, as well as the viruses associated with tick-borne encephalitis, should be handled at BSL-4 facilities. In 1993, the Subcommittee on Arbovirus Laboratory Safety of the American Society of Tropical Medicine and Hygiene developed and published further recommendations (15).

LWs are exposed to a wide variety of other viral agents, which are described in further detail in the review by Sewell (63).

BIOSAFETY AND INFECTION CONTROL IN THE MICROBIOLOGY LABORATORY

Containment of hazardous agents is achieved by adherence to strict standard laboratory practices and techniques, supplemented by primary (safety equipment) and secondary (facility design) barriers. Laboratory personnel need to be aware of the potential hazards of infectious agents and materials. The practices and procedures used to eliminate the risk of LAIs should be described in a laboratory manual.

Biological Safety Cabinets and Other Primary Barriers

BSCs provide protection for personnel, the product, and the environment by minimizing exposures to hazardous biological materials. Class I and II BSCs offer significant levels of protection to laboratory personnel and to the environment. The class I BSC has a negative pressure, is ventilated, and is usually operated with an open front. It is designed for general microbiological research with agents of low to moderate risk. Class II cabinets include HEPA-filtered vertical laminar airflow and protect against external contamination with the materials handled inside the BSC. Depending on their inlet flow velocity and the percentage of air that is HEPA filtered and recirculated, class II BSCs are also differentiated into type A and type B class II BSCs. Generally, class IIA BSCs are used for microbiological procedures requiring BSL-2 or BSL-3. Class III BSCs are totally enclosed cabinets with a gas-tight construction and provide the highest possible level of protection to personnel and the environment, thereby being suitable for work requiring BSL-3 or BSL-4 (22).

Additional detailed information on BSC construction, certification procedures, instructions for decontamination, and levels of containment for microorganisms can be found in the literature (22, 41) or on the Web sites of OSHA, NIH, and CDC (e.g., www.cdc.gov/od/ohs/biosfty/bmbl/bmbl-1.htm). Personal protection items such as goggles, respirators, face shields, gloves, and gowns are frequently used in combination with BSCs. Additional equipment used to contain infectious splashes or aerosols includes safety centrifuge cups, which prevent the release of infectious agents that can be transmitted during centrifugation.

Biosafety Levels

In an effort to diminish the risk of LAIs, a system for categorizing infectious agents into groups on the basis of the mode of transmission, availability of preventive measures and antimicrobial treatment, and the type and seriousness of a possible infection was formulated. In regard to the different groups and categories, guidelines that describe appropriate containment equipment, facilities, and procedures to be used by LWs were developed. These guidelines are referred to as biosafety levels (BSLs). In general, four BSLs are described and these consist of the use of combinations of primary and secondary barriers for particular microbiological practices. Each BSL is designed to ensure the safety of personnel and the environment during work with specific infectious agents. With class 1 agents, hazards are minimal; class 4 agents require maximum containment. Detailed information on BSLs recommended for specific bacterial, fungal, parasitic, and viral agents can be found in the Agent Summary Statements in *Laboratory Safety: Principles and Practices* (22) or at the CDC Web site on Biosafety in Microbiological and Biomedical Laboratories at www.cdc.gov/od/ohs/biosfty/bmbl/bmbl-1.htm (section VII). Categorization of the various organisms is especially based on the likelihood of their transmission. When working with known organisms, such as in the research setting, the implementation of the appropriate practices for each BSL may be simple. Application of the correct BSL in the clinical laboratory remains difficult, since the infectious nature of the clinical material is typically unknown.

BSL-1 describes the lowest level of containment or microbiological safety and is entirely based on standard laboratory practices. It is recommended for work with microorganisms that are not known to cause infections in healthy adults, such as *Bacillus subtilis*.

BSL-2 practices are generally applied in bacteriology laboratories during work with agents (e.g., *Salmonella* species) associated with human diseases of various severities. The pathogens may be transmitted by accidental ingestion, percutaneous exposure, or mucous membrane exposure. When standard microbiological practices are applied, the agents may be handled on open benches, especially if primary barriers such as face protection, gowns, and gloves are used when appropriate. BSCs and safety centrifuge cups should be used when exposure to infectious splashes and aerosols is expected.

BSL-3 recommendations are aimed at the containment of hazardous microorganisms primarily transmitted by aerosols, such as *M. tuberculosis* or *C. burnetii*. BSL-3 makes use of stringent practices as well as primary and secondary safety equipment, including specific requirements for the facility, such as a suitable ventilation system. All microorganisms of BSL-3 need to be processed in a BSC.

BSL-4 applies to agents causing life-threatening or untreatable diseases that can affect the laboratory worker via aerosols (e.g., hemorrhagic fever viruses). Manipulations are generally performed in a class III BSC or by personnel wearing full-body, air-supplied, positive-pressure suits. The facility itself is totally isolated from other laboratories and includes a specialized ventilation and waste management system. A summary of the recommended BSLs for infectious agents is given in Table 4.

Biosafety Practices

In the United States biosafety-related issues in microbiology laboratories are regulated by federal agencies, the states, and local jurisdictions. The guidelines published by OSHA (including the National Institute for Occupational Safety and Health), the Environmental Protection Agency, CDC, NIH, and the Joint Commission on Accreditation of Healthcare Organizations are not mandated by law but must be seen as "standards of practice."

To ensure biosafety in the individual laboratory, programs should be implemented and documented in writing, and LWs should be trained in order to perceive and follow up on these guidelines. The safety program should include LAI surveillance (including surveillance for HBV, HIV, and *M. tuberculosis* infections), vaccination plans, and guidelines that restrict the duties of highly susceptible LWs (e.g., during pregnancy).

The standard laboratory practices that are of utmost importance for the prevention of LAIs are listed in Table 5. Application of CDC's universal precautions to the laboratory area would require that all blood and blood-contaminated specimens be considered "infected." Sharp objects and needles should be used and deposited according to the guidelines, and hands should be disinfected whenever necessary.

Decontamination and Waste Disposal

Decontamination procedures and waste disposal management are described in detail in chapter 8 of this Manual. Nevertheless, a few infection control and biosafety guidelines are mentioned here, since improper waste disposal can be a main source of laboratory accidents.

TABLE 4 Summary of recommended BSLs for infectious agents[a]

BSL	Agents	Practices and techniques	Safety equipment	Facilities
1	No disease in healthy adults (e.g., *B. subtilis*)	Standard microbiological practices	None required. Laboratory clothing recommended. Protection of skin lesions and eyes if indicated.	Open bench top resistant and impervious to water. Sink required.
2	Associated with human disease. Transmission generally *not* via aerosols (e.g., *Salmonella* spp.)	BSL-1 plus: • Limited access • Biohazard label • "Sharp" object precautions • Biosafety manual (including waste decontamination, immunization policies, training)	Class I or II BSC or other containment devices if infectious aerosols or splashes may occur. Appropriate PPE[b]	BSL-1 plus: • Autoclave • Eyewash facility
3	Serious or lethal consequences. Potential for aerosol transmission (e.g., *M. tuberculosis*)	BSL-2 plus: • Controlled access • Decontamination of all waste and clothing • Baseline serum sample	Class I or II BSC or other containment devices for *all* procedures. Appropriate PPE	BSL-2 plus: • Negative air flow • Air exhaust to outside • Self-closing, double doors
4	Life-threatening. Transmission by aerosol or unknown risk of transmission (e.g., Ebola virus)	BSL-3 plus: • Facility-specific clothing • Shower on exit • Decontamination of all materials on exit	Class III or class II BSC in combination with full-body, air-supplied, positive-pressure suit for all procedures	BSL-3 plus separate building and special engineering and design features

[a] Adapted from references 9, 22, and 63.
[b] PPE, personal protective equipment (e.g., lab clothing, gloves, and face or respiratory protection).

As a general rule, laboratories should have in writing procedures for waste management, accidents, and spills with infectious agents and, moreover, should ensure that LWs are familiar with these guidelines. Potentially infectious waste should be separated immediately at the time of production and should be disposed of in sturdy bags marked with biohazard logos. Puncture-resistant, leak-proof containers should be used when disposing of any kind of sharp object. Furthermore, tuberculocidal disinfectants should be used for regular decontamination of work surfaces and equipment, and antibacterial soaps or alcoholic hand rubs should be used for hand disinfection.

TABLE 5 Standard microbiological biosafety practices

Employ constant precautions in handling blood and body fluid (universal precautions).
Deposit sharp objects in special, puncture-resistant containers.
Comply with hand disinfection procedures by using alcoholic hand rubs or medicated soaps.
No eating, drinking, or smoking should be allowed in the laboratory. Food may not be stored in refrigerators used for clinical specimens.
Use disposable plastic pipettes and avoid mouth pipetting by using proper mechanical pipetting devices.
Work surfaces should be decontaminated daily and after spills.
Wear appropriate personal protective equipment during laboratory work and remove it before leaving the laboratory area.
Well-fitting (latex) gloves must be provided in order to increase compliance with glove use.
Face shields or masks and eye protection should be worn when splashes of blood or body fluids are possible.
Use containment equipment for all laboratory procedures that generate large amounts of aerosols or splashes.

REFERENCES

1. **Anonymous.** 1993. OSHA's bloodborne pathogens standard: analysis and recommendations. *Health Devices* **22:** 35–92.
2. **Ashdown, L., and J. Cassidy.** 1991. Successive Salmonella give and Salmonella typhi infections, laboratory-acquired. *Pathology* **23:**233–234.
3. **Ashdown, L. R.** 1992. Melioidosis and safety in the clinical laboratory. *J. Hosp. Infect.* **21:**301–306.
4. **Barry, M., M. Russi, L. Armstrong, D. Geller, R. Tesh, L. Dembry, J. P. Gonzalez, A. S. Khan, and C. J. Peters.** 1995. Brief report: treatment of a laboratory-acquired Sabia virus infection. *N. Engl. J. Med.* **333:**294–296.
5. **Batchelor, B. I., R. J. Brindle, G. F. Gilks, and J. B. Selkon.** 1992. Biochemical mis-identification of Brucella melitensis and subsequent laboratory-acquired infections. *J. Hosp. Infect.* **22:**159–162.
6. **Baum, G. L., and P. I. Lerner.** 1971. Primary pulmonary blastomycosis: a laboratory-acquired infection. *Ann. Intern. Med.* **73:**263–265.
7. **Beers, L. M., T. L. Burke, and D. B. Martin.** 1989. Shigellosis occurring in newborn nursery staff. *Infect. Control* **10:** 147–149.
8. **Bernstein, D. L., T. Hubbard, W. M. Wenman, B. L. Johnson, K. K. Holmes, H. Liebhaber, J. Schachter, R. Barnes, and M. A. Lovett.** 1984. Mediastinal and supraclavicular lymphadenitis and pneumonitis due to Chlamydia trachomatis serovars L1 and L2. *N. Engl. J. Med.* **311:** 1543–1546.
9. **Berrouane, Y.** 1997. Laboratory-acquired infections, p. 607–618. *In* R. P. Wenzel (ed.), *Prevention and Control of*

Nosocomial Infections. The Williams & Wilkins Co., Baltimore, Md.

10. **Blaser, M. J., and R. A. Feldman.** 1981. Acquisition of typhoid fever from proficiency-testing specimens. *N. Engl. J. Med.* **303:**1481.
11. **Blumberg, H. M.** 1997. Tuberculosis and infection control. *Infect. Control Hosp. Epidemiol.* **18:**538–541.
12. **Blumberg, H. M., D. L. Watkins, J. D. Berschling, et al.** 1995. Preventing the nosocomial transmission of tuberculosis. *Ann. Intern. Med.* **122:**658–663.
13. **Burnens, A. P., R. Zbinden, L. Kaempf, I. Heinzer, and J. Nicolet.** 1993. A case of laboratory acquired infection with Escherichia coli O157:H7. *Int. J. Med. Microbiol. Virol. Parasitol. Infect. Dis.* **279:**512–517.
14. **Centers for Disease Control and Prevention.** 1994. *HIV/AIDS Surveillance Report*. Report 5. Centers for Disease Control and Prevention, Atlanta, Ga.
15. **Centers for Disease Control and Prevention.** 1994. Laboratory management of agents associated with hantavirus pulmonary syndrome: interim biosafety guidelines. *Morbid. Mortal. Weekly Rep.* **43:**1–7.

15a. **Centers for Disease Control and Prevention.** 1997. Goals for working safely with Mycobacterium tuberculosis. *Fed. Regist.*

16. **Chusid, M. J., S. K. Russler, B. A. Mohr, D. A. Margolis, C. A. Hillery, and K. C. Kehl.** 1993. Unsuspected brucellosis diagnosed in a child as a result of an outbreak of laboratory-acquired brucellosis. *Pediatr. Infect. Dis. J.* **12:** 1031–1033.
17. **Collins, C. H.** 1993. *Laboratory-Acquired Infections: History, Incidence, Causes, and Prevention*. Butterworth-Heinemann Ltd., Oxford, United Kingdom.
18. **Cooper, C. R., D. M. Dixon, and I. F. Salkin.** 1992. Laboratory-acquired sporotrichosis. *J. Med. Vet. Mycol.* **30:** 169–171.
19. **Evans, M. R., D. K. Henderson, and J. E. Bennett.** 1990. Potential for laboratory exposures to biohazardous agents found in blood. *Am. J. Public Health* **80:**423–427. (Erratum, **80:**658.)
20. **Favero, M., and W. W. Bond.** 1995. Transmission and control of laboratory-acquired hepatitis infection, p. 19–32. *In* D. O. Fleming, J. H. Richardson, J. J. Tulis, and D. Vesley (ed.), *Laboratory Safety: Principles and Practices*. American Society for Microbiology, Washington, D.C.
21. **Fleming, D. O.** 1995. Laboratory biosafety practices, p. 203–218. *In* D. O. Fleming, J. H. Richardson, J. J. Tulis, and D. Vesley (ed.), *Laboratory Safety: Principles and Practices*. American Society for Microbiology, Washington, D.C.
22. **Fleming, D. O., J. H. Richardson, J. J. Tulis, and D. Vesley (ed.).** 1995. *Laboratory Safety: Principles and Practices*, 2nd ed. American Society for Microbiology, Washington, D.C.
23. **Fox, J. G., and N. S. Lipman.** 1991. Infections transmitted by large and small laboratory animals. *Infect. Dis. Clin. N. Am.* **5:**131–163.
24. **Fridkin, S. K., L. Manangan, E. Boylard, The Society for Healthcare Epidemiology of America, and W. R. Jarvis.** 1995. SHEA-CDC TB survey. Part II. Efficacy of TB infection control programs at member hospitals 1992. *Infect. Control Hosp. Epidemiol.* **16:**135–146.
25. **Gandsman, E. J., H. G. Aaslestad, T. C. Ouimet, and W. D. Rupp.** 1997. Sabia virus incident at Yale University. *Am. Ind. Hyg. Assoc. J.* **58:**51–53.
26. **Gilchrist, M. J. R.** 1995. Biosafety precautions for airborne pathogens, p. 67–76. *In* D. O. Fleming, J. H. Richardson, J. J. Tulis, and D. Vesley (ed.), *Laboratory Safety: Principles and Practices*. American Society for Microbiology, Washington, D.C.
27. **Gilks, G. F., H. P. Lambert, E. S. Broughton, and C. C. Baker.** 1988. Failure of penicillin prophylaxis in laboratory acquired leptospirosis. *Postgrad. Med. J.* **64:**236–238.
28. **Gonzalez, J. P., M. D. Bowen, S. T. Nichol, and H. R. Rico.** 1996. Genetic characterization and phylogeny of Sabia virus, an emergent pathogen in Brazil. *Virology* **221:** 318–324.
29. **Grist, N. R., and J. A. N. Emslie.** 1987. Infections in British clinical laboratories, 1984–85. *J. Clin. Pathol.* **40:** 826–829.
30. **Grist, N. R., and J. A. N. Emslie.** 1989. Infections in British clinical laboratories, 1986–87. *J. Clin. Pathol.* **42:** 677–681.
31. **Grist, N. R., and J. A. N. Emslie.** 1991. Infections in British clinical laboratories, 1988–89. *J. Clin. Pathol.* **44:** 667–669.
32. **Gruner, E., E. Bernasconi, R. L. Galeazzi, D. Buhl, R. Heinzle, and D. Nadal.** 1994. Brucellosis: an occupational hazard for medical laboratory personnel. Report of five cases. *Infection* **22:**33–36.
33. **Guibourdenche, M., J. P. Darchis, A. Boisivon, E. Collatz, and J. Y. Riou.** 1994. Enzyme electrophoresis, sero- and subtyping, and outer membrane protein characterization of two *Neisseria meningitidis* strains involved in laboratory-acquired infections. *J. Clin. Microbiol.* **32:**701–704.
34. **Hamadeh, G. N., B. W. Turner, W. Trible, B. J. Hoffmann, and R. M. Anderson.** 1992. Laboratory outbreak of Q-fever. *J. Fam. Pract.* **35:**683–685.
35. **Harding, L., and D. F. Lieberman.** 1995. Epidemiology of laboratory-associated infections, p. 7–15. *In* D. O. Fleming, J. H. Richardson, J. J. Tulis, and D. Vesley (ed.), *Laboratory Safety: Principles and Practices*. American Society for Microbiology, Washington, D.C.
36. **Harrington, J. M., and H. S. Shannon.** 1976. Incidence of tuberculosis, hepatitis, brucellosis and shigellosis in British medical laboratory workers. *Br. Med. J.* **1:**759–762.
37. **Herwaldt, B. L., and D. D. Juranek.** 1993. Laboratory-acquired malaria, leishmaniasis, trypanosomiasis, and toxoplasmosis. *Am. J. Trop. Med. Hyg.* **48:**313–323.
38. **Hilmarsdottir, I., A. Coutellier, J. Elbaz, J. M. Klein, A. Datry, E. Gueho, and S. Herson.** 1994. A French case of laboratory-acquired disseminated *Penicillium marneffei* infection in a patient with AIDS. *Clin. Infect. Dis.* **19:** 357–358. (Letter.)
39. **Holmes, M. B., D. L. Johnson, N. J. Fiumara, and W. M. McCormack.** 1980. Acquisition of typhoid fever from proficiency-testing specimens. *N. Engl. J. Med.* **303:** 519–521.
40. **Jacobson, J. T., R. B. Orlob, and J. L. Clayton.** 1985. Infections acquired in clinical laboratories in Utah. *J. Clin. Microbiol.* **21:**486–489.
41. **Kruse, R. H., W. H. Puckett, and J. H. Richardson.** 1991. Biological safety cabinetry. *Clin. Microbiol. Rev.* **4:** 207–241.
42. **Larson, D. M., M. R. Eckman, C. L. Alber, and V. G. Goldschmidt.** 1983. Primary cutaneous (inoculation) blastomycosis: an occupational hazard to pathologists. *Am. J. Clin. Pathol.* **79:**253–255.
43. **Levy, B. S., J. C. Harris, J. L. Smith, et al.** 1977. Hepatitis B in ward and clinical laboratory employees of a general hospital. *Am. J. Epidemiol.* **106:**330–335.
44. **Mackel, D. C., and J. E. Forney.** 1986. Overview of the epidemiology of laboratory-acquired infections, p. 37–42. *In* B. M. Miller, J. H. Groschel, J. H. Richardson, D. Vesley, J. R. Songer, R. D. Housewright, and W. E. Barkley (ed.), *Laboratory Safety: Principles and Practices*. American Society for Microbiology, Washington, D.C.
45. **Martin-Mazuelos, E., M. C. Nogales, C. Florez, M. J. Gomez, F. Lozano, and A. Sanchez.** 1994. Outbreak of

Brucella melitensis among microbiology laboratory workers. *J. Clin. Microbiol.* **32:**2035–2036.

46. **Mazurek, G. H., M. D. Cave, K. D. Eisenach, R. J. Wallace, Jr., J. H. Bates, and J. T. Crawford.** 1991. Chromosomal DNA fingerprint patterns produced with IS*6110* as strain-specific markers for epidemiologic study of tuberculosis. *J. Clin. Microbiol.* **29:**2030–2033.
47. **Miller, C. D., J. R. Songer, and J. F. Sullivan.** 1987. A twenty-five year review of laboratory-acquired human infections at the National Animal Disease Center. *Am. Ind. Hyg. Assoc. J.* **48:**271–275.
48. **Muller, H. E.** 1988. Laboratory-acquired mycobacterial infection. *Lancet* **ii:**331.
49. **Murray, J. F., and D. H. Howard.** 1964. Laboratory-acquired histoplasmosis. *Am. Rev. Respir. Dis.* **89:**631–640.
50. **Occupational Safety and Health Administration.** 1991. Occupational exposure to bloodborne pathogens: final rule. *Fed. Regist.* **56:**64003–64182.
51. **Occupational Safety and Health Administration.** 1993. Draft guidelines for preventing the transmission of tuberculosis in healthcare facilities. *Fed. Regist.* **58:**52810–52854.
52. **Olle-Goig, J., and J. C. Canela-Soler.** 1987. An outbreak of *Brucella melitensis* infection by airborne transmission among laboratory workers. *Am. J. Public Health* **77:** 335–338.
53. **Oster, C. N., D. S. Burke, R. H. Kenyon, M. S. Ascher, P. Harber, and C. E. Pedersen.** 1977. Laboratory-acquired Rocky Mountain spotted fever. The hazard of aerosol transmission. *N. Engl. J. Med.* **297:**859–863.
54. **Paradis, J. F., and D. Grimard.** 1994. Laboratory-acquired invasive meningococcus—Quebec. *Can. Communicable Dis. Rep.* **20:**12–14.
55. **Penner, J. L., J. N. Hennessy, S. D. Mills, and W. C. Bradbury.** 1983. Application of serotyping and chromosomal restriction endonuclease digest analysis in investigating a laboratory-acquired case of *Campylobacter jejuni*. *J. Clin. Microbiol.* **18:**1427–1428.
56. **Philipott, J., and J. Casewell.** 1994. *Hospital Infection Control.* Saunders, London, United Kingdom.
57. **Pike, R. M.** 1976. Laboratory-associated infections. Summary and analysis of 3921 cases. *Health Lab. Sci.* **13:** 105–114.
58. **Pike, R. M.** 1979. Laboratory-associated infections: incidence, fatalities, causes and prevention. *Annu. Rev. Microbiol.* **33:**41–66.
59. **Receveur, M. C., M. LeBras, and P. Vincendeau.** 1993. Laboratory-acquired Gambian trypanosomiasis. *N. Engl. J. Med.* **329:**209–210. (Letter.)
60. **Ryder, R. W., and E. J. Gandsman.** 1995. Laboratory-acquired Sabia virus infection. *N. Engl. J. Med.* **333:**1716. (Letter.)
61. **Sepkowitz, K. A.** 1996. Occupational acquired infections in health care workers. Part I. *Ann. Intern. Med.* **125:** 826–834.
62. **Sepkowitz, K. A.** 1996. Occupationally acquired infections in health care workers. Part II. *Ann. Intern. Med.* **125:**917–928.
63. **Sewell, D. L.** 1995. Laboratory-associated infections and biosafety. *Clin. Microbiol. Rev.* **8:**389–405.
64. **Shireman, P. K.** 1992. Endometrial tuberculosis acquired by a health care worker in a clinical laboratory. *Arch. Pathol. Lab. Med.* **116:**521–523.
65. **Staszkiewicz, J., C. M. Lewis, J. Colville, M. Zervos, and J. Band.** 1997. Outbreak of *Brucella melitensis* among microbiology laboratory workers in a community hospital. *J. Clin. Microbiol.* **29:**287–290.
66. **Sulkin, S. E., and R. M. Pike.** 1951. Laboratory-acquired infections. *JAMA* **147:**1740–1745.
67. **Vasconcelos, P. F., R. A. Travassos-da, S. G. Rodrigues, R. Tesh, R. J. Travassos-da, and R. E. Travassosda.** 1993. Laboratory-acquired human infection with SP H 114202 virus (Arenavirus: Arenaviridae family): clinical and laboratory aspects. *Rev. Inst. Med. Trop. Sao Paulo* **35:** 521–525.
68. **Vesley, D., and H. M. Hartman.** 1988. Laboratory-acquired infections and injuries in clinical laboratories: a 1986 survey. *Am. J. Public Health* **78:**1213–1215.
69. **Waitkins, R. A.** 1985. Update on leptospirosis. *Br. Med. J.* **290:**1502–1503.
70. **Young, E. J.** 1983. Human brucellosis. *Rev. Infect. Dis.* **5:** 821–842.

Investigation of Foodborne and Waterborne Disease Outbreaks*

BALA SWAMINATHAN, JAMES BEEBE, AND JOHN BESSER

10

Each year, as many as 80 million persons in the United States are afflicted by foodborne infections caused by bacteria, viruses, and parasites. These cases result in approximately 800,000 hospitalizations, 9,000 deaths, and an estimated cost of 7 to 17 billion dollars. Worldwide, there are an estimated 1.5 billion cases and over 3 million deaths per year (3, 19, 22, 29, 33). Although most foodborne infections resolve after a few days with or without medical intervention, some progress to more severe sequelae such as septicemia, meningitis, meningoencephalitis, hemolytic-uremic syndrome, reactive arthritis, and Guillain-Barré syndrome.

Waterborne diseases are a major public health problem globally, with as many as 13 million cases of infections and parasitic diseases being attributed to contaminated water. Diarrheal diseases attributable to contaminated water are estimated to cause the death of 2 million children worldwide each year. The seventh pandemic of cholera started in Indonesia in 1961, reached South America in 1991, and was responsible for more than 1,000,000 cases and 10,000 deaths in the Americas by 1995 (20). Major outbreaks of cryptosporidiosis have been reported in the United States, the United Kingdom, and Canada in the 1990s (20).

Food and water safety are complex issues that depend on a number of interrelated environmental, cultural, and socioeconomic factors. Thus, prevention of these diseases is a multifactorial process, without simple or universal solutions. For most foodborne and waterborne pathogens, vaccines are not available. Education of consumers and food handlers about basic principles of safe food handling is an important aspect of prevention but is insufficient by itself. The general strategy of prevention of foodborne and waterborne diseases is to understand the mechanisms by which contamination and disease transmission occur and to institute appropriate prevention measures. Therefore, investigation of foodborne and waterborne disease outbreaks offers an excellent opportunity to accomplish this objective.

This chapter provides a framework for investigation of foodborne and waterborne disease outbreaks. General principles and strategies of investigation, design of the investigation team, sample selection criteria, and the role of rapid diagnostic methods and molecular subtyping methods are discussed. Details of clinical specimen collection, transport to the laboratory, and analytical methods can be found in other chapters of this Manual. The details of food and environmental sample collection and analysis will vary for each pathogen and are available from excellent published sources such as the *Bacteriological Analytical Manual* (25), *Compendium of Methods for the Microbiological Examination of Foods* (34), *Official Methods of Analysis of AOAC International* (1), and *Standard Methods for the Examination of Dairy Products* (27). Information on analysis of water samples may be found in the manual on *Standard Methods for the Examination of Water and Wastewater* and its supplement (15, 17).

DEFINITION OF A FOODBORNE OR WATERBORNE DISEASE OUTBREAK

A fundamental goal of epidemiologic investigations is to understand the nature and causes of diseases in populations and to develop strategies to control their occurrence. When the observed rate of disease is higher than expected and cases are unusually close together in time and/or space or within the same demographic group, that group of cases is considered an outbreak (29). A foodborne disease outbreak is defined as the occurrence of two or more cases of a similar illness resulting from the ingestion of a common food (11). A waterborne disease outbreak is defined as the occurrence of two or more cases of similar illness after ingestion of drinking water from a common source or after exposure to water used for recreational purposes (12). Outbreaks caused by contamination of water or ice at the point of use (e.g., contaminated serving containers) are not considered waterborne disease outbreaks but are reported as foodborne disease outbreaks.

RATIONALE FOR INVESTIGATING FOODBORNE DISEASE OUTBREAKS

Foodborne disease continues to be a significant public health problem. From 1988 to 1992, 1,001 foodborne disease outbreaks of known etiology and involving 36,890 ill persons were reported to the U.S. Centers for Disease Control and Prevention (CDC) (11). It is believed that reported cases represent only a very small fraction of the true incidence. Investigations of foodborne disease outbreaks provide information on the sources and modalities of food contamination that causes outbreaks and sporadic disease, which

* This chapter contains information presented in chapter 18 by Frank L. Bryan in the sixth edition of this Manual.

ultimately helps to improve food safety. Investigations may uncover specific occurrences of food contamination or may reveal intrinsic problems in food production, processing, storage, distribution, or preparation. Specific control strategies developed as a result of these investigations may be as simple as removing products from distribution or increasing public awareness of safe food-handling practices. Problems uncovered in food delivery systems may result in more extensive control measures, such as processing or regulatory changes.

RATIONALE FOR INVESTIGATING WATERBORNE DISEASE OUTBREAKS

In the United States, 30 outbreaks associated with drinking water and 26 outbreaks associated with recreational water were reported in 1993 to 1994. *Giardia lamblia* and *Cryptosporidium parvum* were responsible for 33% of the drinking-water-associated outbreaks and 70% of the gastroenteritis outbreaks associated with recreational water use (20). Other pathogens associated with drinking-water-related outbreaks were *Campylobacter jejuni, Shigella sonnei, S. flexneri*, and *Vibrio cholerae* non-O1, while those associated with recreational water (lakes) were *S. sonnei, S. flexneri*, and *Escherichia coli* O157:H7 (12). In 1998, two *E. coli* O157:H7 outbreaks associated with recreational water use received much attention: one was caused by fecal contamination of a children's pool at a water theme park in a major city in the southeastern United States, and the other outbreak, in a northwestern town, was associated with unchlorinated municipal water for which the source was a natural spring (14a). Also, a large outbreak of leptospirosis among athletes participating in triathlon events in the midwestern United States was associated with swimming in a contaminated lake (14).

Since 1971, CDC, the U.S. Environmental Protection Agency, and the Council of State and Territorial Epidemiologists have maintained a collaborative surveillance system for waterborne disease outbreaks. Information gathered through this surveillance is useful for evaluating the adequacy of current technologies to provide safe drinking and recreational water. The objectives of the surveillance are (i) to characterize the epidemiology of the outbreaks, (ii) to identify the etiologic agents of the outbreaks and determine why the outbreaks occurred, and (iii) to collaborate with local, state, federal, and international agencies on initiatives to prevent future occurrences of waterborne disease outbreaks.

FEATURES OF OUTBREAKS AND OUTBREAK INVESTIGATIONS

Foodborne and waterborne disease outbreaks are detected either by surveillance programs monitoring conditions such as salmonellosis, campylobacteriosis, or listeriosis or as a result of self-reporting by consumers or clinicians. The causative etiologic agent is usually known in outbreaks detected by surveillance but often must be determined in outbreaks detected by self-reporting. When the agent is initially unknown, investigators rely on a combination of clinical features of the illness, available laboratory data, and other epidemiologic findings to establish presumptive causation.

Of the 1,001 reported foodborne disease outbreaks of known etiology described above, 796 (79.5%) were caused by bacteria, 143 (14.3%) were caused by chemicals, 17 (1.7%) were caused by parasites, and 45 (4.5%) were caused by viruses (11). However, outbreaks of known etiology constitute less than half of the total number of outbreaks reported to CDC each year (4, 24). A significant proportion of outbreaks may be caused by viruses or other organisms for which routine diagnostic methods are not readily available. The most common causes of foodborne disease outbreaks, their clinical symptoms and onset time, and recommended confirmation guidelines are summarized in Table 1.

Of 30 waterborne disease outbreaks reported in the United States in 1993 to 1994, 22 (73.3%) were known or suspected to be associated with infectious agents and 8 (26.7%) were associated with chemical contaminants. Of the waterborne disease outbreaks associated with contaminated drinking water, 33.3% were caused by parasitic protozoa (*G. lamblia* or *C. parvum*), 23.3% were caused by bacteria, 26.7% were caused by chemicals, and 16.7% had an unknown etiology. Of recreational water-associated outbreaks, 71.5% were caused by *G. lamblia* and *C. parvum* and 28.5% were caused by *E. coli* O157:H7 and *Shigella* spp.

The foodborne and waterborne diseases that were designated as notifiable at the national level in the United States in 1996 are listed in Table 2. A notifiable disease is one for which regular, frequent, and timely information about individual cases is considered necessary for the prevention and control of the disease (13). Public health officials at state health departments and CDC collaborate in determining which diseases should be notifiable. The Council of State and Territorial Epidemiologists, with input from CDC, makes recommendations annually for additions to and deletions from the list of nationally notifiable diseases. However, reporting of nationally notifiable diseases to CDC by states is voluntary; reporting is currently mandated only at the state level.

The magnitude of foodborne disease outbreaks may range from a small outbreak of only two cases to one that is multinational in scope and involves thousands of cases. Among the largest foodborne disease outbreaks ever recorded are the nationwide U.S. ice-cream-associated salmonellosis outbreak in 1995 (estimated at 224,000 cases) (23), the Midwestern U.S. salmonellosis outbreak caused by contaminated pasteurized milk in 1985 (an estimated 198,000 cases) (30), and the *E. coli* O157:H7 outbreak among schoolchildren in Japan in 1996 (more than 6,000 cases) (36). The centralization of food production and globalization of food distribution have greatly increased the chances for large outbreaks of foodborne disease. Similarly, waterborne disease outbreaks may affect as few as two persons or as many as several hundred persons depending on how widely the contaminated water is distributed. The outbreak of cryptosporidiosis in Milwaukee, Wis., which resulted in illness in more than 400,000 persons in 1985, was the largest documented waterborne disease outbreak in the United States. An estimated 4,400 persons were hospitalized. The outbreak was associated with water from Lake Michigan that had been filtered and chlorinated. Deterioration in lake water quality and decreased effectiveness of the coagulation-filtration process led to an increase in the turbidity of the treated water and to inadequate removal of *C. parvum* oocysts (12).

The scope of investigations may be narrowly focused on specific disease clusters or may involve broader investigations into the causes of sporadic disease in the population. For example, a large investigation identified eggs as the most important source of *Salmonella* serotype Enteritidis infections (32). Other investigations revealed that most sporadic cases of *Campylobacter jejuni* and *C. coli* infections during

TABLE 1 Guidelines for confirmation of foodborne disease outbreaks[a]

Etiologic agent	Incubation period	Clinical syndrome	Confirmation
Bacterial			
Bacillus cereus			
Vomiting toxin	1–6 h	Vomiting, occasional diarrhea; fever uncommon	Isolation of organism from stool of two or more ill persons and not from stool of controls OR Isolation of ≥10^5 organisms/g from epidemiologically implicated food, provided the specimen is properly handled
Diarrheal toxin	6–24 h	Diarrhea, abdominal cramps, and vomiting in some patients; fever uncommon	Isolation of organism from stool of two or more ill persons and not from stool of controls OR Isolation of ≥10^5 organisms/g from epidemiologically implicated food, provided the specimen is properly handled
Brucella	Several days to several months, usually >30 days	Weakness, fever, headache, sweats, chills, arthralgia, weight loss, splenomegaly	Two or more ill persons and isolation of organism in culture of blood or bone marrow, greater than fourfold increase in standard agglutination titer (SAT) over several weeks, or single SAT titer of >1:160 in a person with compatible clinical symptoms and history of exposure
Campylobacter	2–10 days, usually 2–5 days	Diarrhea (often bloody), abdominal pain, fever	Isolation of organism from clinical specimens from two or more ill persons OR Isolation of organism from epidemiologically implicated food
Clostridium botulinum	2 h–8 days, usually 12–48 h	Illness of variable severity; common symptoms are diplopia, blurred vision, and bulbar weakness; paralysis, which is usually descending and bilateral, may progress rapidly	Detection of botulinal toxin in serum, stool, gastric contents, or implicated food OR Isolation of organism from stool or intestine
Clostridium perfringens	6–24 h	Diarrhea, abdominal cramps; vomiting and fever uncommon	Isolation of ≥10^6 organisms/g in stool of two or more ill persons, provided the specimen is properly handled OR Demonstration of enterotoxin in the stool of two or more ill persons OR Isolation of ≥10^5 organisms/g from epidemiologically implicated food, provided the specimen is properly handled

(*Continued on next page*)

TABLE 1 *(Continued)*

Etiologic agent	Incubation period	Clinical syndrome	Confirmation
Escherichia coli			
Enterohemorrhagic (*E. coli* O157:H7 and other serotypes that produce Shiga toxins) (EHEC)	1–10 days, usually 4–5 days; approximately 6% go on to develop hemolytic-uremic syndrome (HUS) (children) or thrombotic thrombocytopenic purpura (TTP) (adults)	Diarrhea (often bloody), abdominal cramps (often severe), little or no fever. Acute renal failure in HUS or TTP	Isolation of *E. coli* O157:H7 or other Shiga toxin-producing *E. coli* from clinical specimen of two or more ill persons OR Isolation of *E. coli* O157:H7 or other Shiga toxin-producing *E. coli* from epidemiologically implicated food
Enterotoxigenic *E. coli* (ETEC)	6–48 h	Diarrhea, abdominal cramps, nausea; vomiting and fever less common	Isolation of organisms of same serotype, which are demonstrated to produce heat-stable (ST) and/or heat-labile (LT) enterotoxin, from stool of two or more ill persons
Enteropathogenic *E. coli* (EPEC)	Variable	Diarrhea, fever, abdominal cramps	Isolation of the same enteropathogenic serotype from stool of two or more ill persons
Enteroinvasive *E. coli* (EIEC)	Variable	Diarrhea (may be bloody), fever, abdominal cramps	Isolation of the same enteroinvasive serotype from stool of two or more ill persons
Listeria monocytogenes			
Invasive disease	2–6 wk	Meningitis, meningoencephalitis, neonatal sepsis, abortions, stillbirths	Isolation of organism from blood or cerebrospinal fluid of two or more patients and the same serotype and subtype of organism from implicated food(s)
Diarrheal disease	9–32 h	Diarrhea, abdominal cramps, fever	Isolation of organism of same serotype from stool of two or more ill persons exposed to food that is epidemiologically implicated or from which an organism of the same serotype has been isolated
Nontyphoidal salmonellosis	6 h–10 days, usually 6–48 h	Diarrhea, often with fever and abdominal cramps	Isolation of organism of same serotype and subtype from clinical specimens from two or more ill persons OR Isolation of organism from epidemiologically implicated food
Salmonella serotype typhi	3–60 days, usually 7–14 days	Fever, anorexia, malaise, headache, and myalgia; sometimes diarrhea and constipation	Isolation of organism of the same serotype from clinical specimens from two or more ill persons OR Isolation of organism from epidemiologically implicated food
Shigella	12 h–6 days, usually 2–4 days	Diarrhea (often bloody), frequently accompanied by fever and abdominal cramps	Isolation of organism of same serotype from clinical specimens from two or more ill persons OR Isolation of organism from epidemiologically implicated food
Staphylococcus aureus	30 min–8 h, usually 2–4 h	Vomiting, diarrhea	Isolation of organism of same phage type/molecular subtype from stool or vomitus of two or more ill persons OR Detection of same serotype of enterotoxin in epidemiologically implicated food

(Continued on next page)

TABLE 1 Guidelines for confirmation of foodborne disease outbreaks[a] (*Continued*)

Etiologic agent	Incubation period	Clinical syndrome	Confirmation
Streptococcus group A	1–4 days	Fever, pharyngitis, scarlet fever, upper respiratory infection	Isolation of organism of same M or T type from throats of two or more ill persons OR Isolation of organism of same M or T type from epidemiologically implicated food
Vibrio cholerae			
O1 or O139	1–5 days	Watery diarrhea, often accompanied by vomiting	Isolation of toxigenic organism from stool or vomitus of two or more ill persons OR Significant rise in vibriocidal, bacterial agglutination, or antitoxin antibodies in acute- and early convalescent-phase sera among persons not recently immunized OR Isolation of toxigenic organism from epidemiologically implicated food
Non-O1 and non-O139	1–5 days	Watery diarrhea	Isolation of toxigenic organism from stool or vomitus of two or more ill persons OR Significant rise in vibriocidal, bacterial agglutination, or antitoxin antibodies in acute- and early convalescent-phase sera among persons not recently immunized OR Isolation of toxigenic organism from epidemiologically implicated food
Vibrio parahemolyticus	4–30 h	Diarrhea	Isolation of Kanagawa-positive organism from stool of two or more ill persons OR Isolation of $\geq 10^5$ Kanagawa-positive organisms/g from epidemiologically implicated food, provided the specimen is properly handled
Yersinia enterocolitica	1–10 days, usually 4–6 days	Diarrhea, abdominal pain (often severe)	Isolation of organism from clinical specimens of two or more ill persons OR Isolation of pathogenic strain or organism from epidemiologically implicated food
Chemical			
Marine toxins			
Ciguatoxin	1–48 h, usually 2–8 h	Usually gastrointestinal symptoms followed by neurologic symptoms (including paresthesia of lips, tongue, throat, or extremities) and reversal of hot and cold sensation	Demonstration of ciguatoxin in epidemiologically implicated fish OR Clinical syndrome among persons who have eaten a type of fish previously associated with ciguatera fish poisoning (e.g., snapper, grouper, or barracuda)

(*Continued on next page*)

TABLE 1 (*Continued*)

Etiologic agent	Incubation period	Clinical syndrome	Confirmation
Scombroid toxin (histamine)	1 min–3 h, usually less than 1 h	Flushing, dizziness, burning of mouth and throat, headache, gastrointestinal symptoms, urticaria, and generalized pruritus	Demonstration of histamine in epidemiologically implicated food OR Clinical syndrome among persons who have eaten a type of fish previously associated with histamine fish poisoning (e.g., mahimahi or fish of order Scombroidei)
Paralytic or neurotoxic shellfish poison	30 min–3 h	Paresthesia of lips, mouth, or face, and extremities; intestinal symptoms or weakness, including respiratory difficulty	Detection of toxin in epidemiologically implicated food OR Detection of large numbers of shellfish-poisoning-associated species of dinoflagellates in water from which epidemiologically implicated mollusks were gathered Demonstration of tetrodotoxin in epidemiologically implicated fish
Puffer fish, tetrodotoxin	10 min–3 h, usually 10–45 min	Paresthesia of lips, tongue, face, or extremities, often following numbness; loss of proprioception or "floating" sensations	Demonstration of tetrodotoxin in epidemiologically implicated fish OR Clinical syndrome among persons who ate puffer fish
Heavy metals (antimony, cadmium, copper, iron, tin, zinc)	5 min–8 h, usually less than 1 h	Vomiting, often a metallic taste	Demonstration of high concentration of metal in epidemiologically implicated food
Monosodium glutamate (MSG)	3 min–2 h, usually less than 1 h	Burning sensation in chest, neck, abdomen, or extremities; sensation of lightness and pressure over face or heavy feeling in chest	Clinical syndrome among persons who have eaten food containing MSG (usually ≥1.5 g of MSG)
Mushroom toxins			
Shorter-acting toxins (Muscimol, muscarine, psilocybin, Coprine [produced by *Coprinus atramentarius*], ibotenic acid)	2 h	Usually vomiting and diarrhea; other symptoms (confusion and visual disturbance [muscimol, ibotenic acid], salivation and diaphoresis [muscarine], hallucinations [psilocybin], disulfiram-like reaction [C. *artementaris*]) differ with toxin	Clinical syndrome among persons who have eaten mushroom identified as toxic type OR Demonstration of toxin in epidemiologically implicated mushroom or mushroom-containing food
Longer-acting toxin (e.g., *Amanita* spp.)	6–24 h	Diarrhea and abdominal cramps for 24 h followed by hepatic and renal failure	Clinical syndrome among persons who have eaten mushroom identified as toxic type OR Demonstration of toxin in epidemiologically implicated mushrooms or mushroom-containing food

(*Continued on next page*)

TABLE 1 Guidelines for confirmation of foodborne disease outbreaks[a] (*Continued*)

Etiologic agent	Incubation period	Clinical syndrome	Confirmation
Parasitic			
Cryptosporidium parvum	2–28 days, median 7 days	Diarrhea, nausea, vomiting, fever	Demonstration of organism or antigen in stool or in small-bowel biopsy specimens from two or more ill persons OR Demonstration of organism in epidemiologically implicated food
Cyclospora cayetanensis	1–11 days, median 7 days	Fatigue, protracted diarrhea, often relapsing	Demonstration of organism in stool of two or more ill persons
Giardia lamblia	3–25 days, median 7 days	Diarrhea, gas, cramps, nausea, fatigue	Two or more ill persons and detection of antigen in stool or demonstration of organism in stool, duodenal contents, or small-bowel biopsy specimen
Trichinella spp.	1–2 days for intestinal phase; 2–4 wk for systemic phase	Fever, myalgia, periorbital edema, high eosinophil count	Two or more ill persons and positive serologic test or demonstration of larvae in muscle biopsy specimen OR Demonstration of larvae in epidemiologically implicated meat
Viral			
Hepatitis A	15–50 days, median 28 days	Jaundice, dark urine, fatigue, anorexia, nausea	Detection of IgM anti-hepatitis A virus in serum from two or more persons who consumed epidemiologically implicated food
Norwalk family of viruses, small round-structured viruses (NLV)	15–77 h, usually 24–48 h	Vomiting, cramps, diarrhea, headache	More than fourfold rise in antibody titer to Norwalk virus or Norwalk-like virus in acute- and convalescent-phase sera in most serum pairs OR Visualization of small, round-structured viruses that react with patient's convalescent-phase sera but not acute-phase sera by immunoelectron microscopy (assays based on molecular diagnostic techniques [e.g., PCR, probes, or assays for antigen and antibodies from expressed antigen] are available in reference laboratories)
Astrovirus, calicivirus, others	15–77 h, usually 24–48 h	Vomiting, cramps, diarrhea, headache	Visualization of small, round viruses that react with patient's convalescent-phase sera but not acute-phase sera by immunoelectron microscopy (assays based on molecular diagnostics [e.g., PCR, probes, or assays for antigen and antibodies from expressed antigen] are available in reference laboratories)

[a] Data from reference 11.

TABLE 2 Foodborne and waterborne diseases designated as notifiable in the United States as of 1996[a]

Botulism
Brucellosis
Cholera
Cryptosporidiosis
E. coli O157:H7 infection
Hemolytic-uremic syndrome (postdiarrheal)
Hepatitis A
Salmonellosis
Shigellosis
Trichinosis
Typhoid fever

[a] Data from reference 13.

the summer months appear to be associated with handling and eating undercooked poultry, while the relatively infrequent outbreaks due to *C. jejuni* and *C. coli* during spring and fall are caused by the consumption of unpasteurized milk or untreated surface water (29).

Successful epidemiologic and laboratory investigations of these outbreaks require extensive coordination between multiple public health and food regulatory agencies at the federal, state, county, and city levels. Since foodborne and waterborne disease outbreaks often have important political, social, and economic consequences, a coherent public message is another hallmark of the well-managed investigation.

Foodborne outbreak investigations frequently begin with establishment of a precise definition of illness to classify persons as ill or not ill and to help investigators identify additional related cases. These investigations usually involve either a retrospective cohort design or a case-control study design. A retrospective cohort design is the technique of choice when one is faced with an acute outbreak in a well-defined population, and it relies on historical exposure data. The classic example of a retrospective cohort study is the typical "church supper" outbreak, where all or a representative sample of participants are interviewed by the investigators about foods (exposures) they may have eaten at the supper and rates of illness are compared between those who did and those who did not eat a certain food.

However, when the population at risk is not well defined, as would occur with a food distributed throughout a wide geographic area, the scientifically appropriate way to analyze the problem is to use case-control methodology. In a case-control study, people with the illness being investigated (cases) are compared to people without the illness (controls). Relevant food exposure histories are collected from cases and controls. Often a "matched" case-control study will be performed to take into account the variability in food consumption patterns attributable to age, sex, and geographic location. In a matched case-control study, for each case one to three controls of the same sex and similar age are selected randomly from the same community or geographic area as the corresponding case. The data from interviews of cases and controls are then statistically analyzed to identify any foods or other exposures that are significantly associated with illness. After identification of the probable cause of the outbreak by the case-control study, microbiological confirmation of the epidemiologic association is obtained by analyzing appropriate human or food samples for etiologic agents. The isolates may then be further analyzed for antimicrobial susceptibility profile, molecular subtype, virulence factors, or other markers. Thus, careful epidemiologic investigation combined with targeted microbiologic analysis is most likely to yield relevant information. Broad microbiological sampling of foods and food workers without epidemiologic investigation rarely identifies the correct cause of outbreaks. Also, public health interventions can frequently be initiated before microbiological confirmation is obtained if the statistical association between illness and exposure is strong and confounding factors or effect modifiers have been considered.

TEAM APPROACH TO INVESTIGATIONS—GENERAL PRINCIPLES

As information accumulates indicating that a foodborne disease outbreak has occurred, the following should be done: (i) a team of qualified individuals must be recruited to conduct the investigation; (ii) a team leader must be appointed; (iii) lines of communication must be established between team members and, as appropriate, the health care community affected, the public, and, in some cases, the media; (iv) team members must be assigned their individual responsibilities; and (v) a system must be established for data collection, retrieval, and analysis, including laboratory information, which allows updating of this information on a daily or more frequent basis (9, 10, 35).

In the early stages of an investigation, it may be determined that the outbreak is over; that is, a food vehicle was consumed and is no longer on the market, or factors responsible for contamination of drinking or recreational water no longer existed, and no more cases are expected. On the other hand, it may be obvious that the outbreak and exposure to the contaminated food or water are still occurring and that more cases of illness are to be expected. In the latter case, the team must be formed rapidly and all the team members must be informed of the nature of the outbreak and their responsibilities to ensure that they can all contribute in a timely fashion. For example, laboratory team members must know as soon as possible which disease agents are suspected so that bacteriologic media can be prepared and analysts can arrange for conduction of specimen testing.

Investigations of foodborne and waterborne disease outbreaks are often supervised by local public health authorities with jurisdictional responsibility for a city- or a countywide area. Larger outbreaks with a multijurisdictional or statewide impact will call for leadership at the state government level. Outbreaks with a national impact will require federal leadership. In most circumstances, three key professional groups—epidemiologists, sanitarians, and laboratorians—will form the team. However, depending on the nature of the outbreak, other team members, including other public health officials, health care physicians, and representatives from food regulatory agencies and/or the Environmental Protection Agency, may be recruited. Outbreaks with national and/or international impact will require the participation of epidemiologists and laboratory scientists from the federal organization charged with responsibility for epidemiology and surveillance of infectious diseases at the national level. In the United States, the CDC is charged with this responsibility. Persons with expertise in biostatistics, environmental microbiology, and engineering should be included on the investigative team as appropriate. In the investigation of outbreaks which attract attention from electronic and print media, the presence of an experienced and knowledgeable information officer who can respond to inquiries from the media and the public can be invaluable (21).

Unusual clusters of illness indicating potential outbreaks are detected by physicians, laboratorians, or local, state, or federal health agencies. The factors that led to the recognition of the Milwaukee outbreak of cryptosporidiosis included widespread absenteeism among hospital employees, students, and schoolteachers; an increased number of emergency room visits for diarrheal illness; and a citywide shortage of antidiarrheal drugs. Regardless of how or where the information appears, when there is sufficient evidence that an outbreak has occurred, it is essential that a team be assembled as soon as possible and a team leader be appointed to direct the activities of the team. Often an experienced epidemiologist with primary investigative authority will be appointed as the team leader. The team leader will direct team members to collect, codify, and analyze incoming outbreak information; form a hypothesis; dispatch sample collectors and oversee their activities; provide information to the health care community, the public, and the media regarding the outbreak investigation; and devise intervention strategies. All team members must understand that the resources available to the investigation must be used at the direction of the team leader and that information provided to the team leader must be accurate and concise. The intensity of activity that arises in performing all these functions often strains communications. Laboratorians, who usually operate at a distance from the team command center, should be proactive, seeking contact with the team leader or the team member responsible for collection of samples for laboratory testing.

ROLE OF TEAM MEMBERS

Successful investigations of outbreaks occur when a group of dedicated, experienced professionals is assembled and is provided with the tools to conduct the investigative work. A prototype team—consisting of an epidemiologist, a sanitarian, and a laboratorian—will rely on the expertise and contribution of each team member and their respective organizations for the desired outcome: determination of the cause, rapid resolution of the outbreak, and prevention of future outbreaks.

Epidemiologists are responsible for the collection and analysis of information to determine the cause of the outbreak. Epidemiologists receive disease case reports, laboratory reports, and observations from health care physicians and often detect outbreaks by analyzing this information. They contact ill persons and administer questionnaires to define the illness with respect to the time of occurrence, location, and associated food consumption. Their preliminary analysis is often designed to determine attack rates or risk factors and to evaluate exposures for a statistical association with illness. Consideration of incubation times and the clinical signs and symptoms leads to the development of a hypothesis including the suspected agent and means of transmission (6).

Sanitarians are charged with examination and analysis of food preparation and processing methods in a search for deviations from standard operating procedures that may have resulted in contamination of food and subsequent illness. Sanitarians are trained in good manufacturing practice (GMP) inspections and hazard analysis critical control points (HACCP) investigative techniques, which are used to identify such food-processing and food preparation problems as cross-contamination of raw foods with cooked foods and improper cooking and/or holding temperatures (7, 28, 31). Sanitarians receive consumer complaints regarding restaurants and other food service establishments and food products provided by retail vendors, and after review and analysis of complaint information, they decide whether sufficient information has accumulated to warrant the initiation of a formal investigation. More detailed descriptions of the typical procedures used by both epidemiologists and sanitarians during investigations of foodborne disease outbreaks can be found elsewhere (8–10, 35).

Laboratorians are responsible for providing analytical information obtained by testing human specimens, food samples, and other appropriate specimens (water, animal, and environmental samples) to detect agents of illness or their toxins. This information provides independent confirmation of the epidemiologic hypothesis developed by the team during the early stages of the investigation. Clinical laboratory microbiologists play a pivotal role in the process of outbreak investigation by recovering the etiologic agents of diarrheal illness and forwarding the isolates to public health laboratories. To detect outbreaks in a timely fashion, culture methods must be effective and viable isolates must be referred expeditiously to the appropriate (city, county, or state) public health laboratory. Clinical laboratorians may also receive food samples for analysis. However, unless trained and equipped to perform accurate microbiological analyses on food, clinical microbiologists are advised to contact the public health laboratory and arrange for the transfer of food samples. Improvised culture techniques and attempts to adapt clinical microbiology culture methods to food analysis are rarely successful and can result in the loss of critical food samples to the investigative process.

Public health laboratory microbiologists provide investigation team members with up-to-date information on the selection, collection, preservation, and transport of human specimens and food samples; conduct laboratory analyses on food and human specimens by standardized and validated methods; and provide interpretations of laboratory data. Routine public health laboratory epidemiologic typing of pathogens, by conventional methods such as serotyping of *Salmonella* or by molecular methods such as pulsed-field gel electrophoresis typing of genomic DNA restriction digests, has been demonstrated to be effective for the recognition of outbreaks undetected by routine surveillance methods, such as disease case reporting (5).

INVESTIGATION STRATEGY

The investigation team leader, in concert with team members, collects and analyzes information from outbreak victims and health care providers. It is often necessary for the team to devise a case definition for the illness and to disseminate this information to health care providers to increase the likelihood of detection of cases. Analysis of data is initially directed toward describing the outbreak in terms of time, place, and person. Time may refer to illness onset, and place may refer to a restaurant patronized by all the victims. Person factors include demographic characteristics, such as age, gender, race, or ethnicity, or other determinants such as belonging to an organization or eating the same foods. Initially, a small subset of ill persons may be intensively interviewed in an open-ended fashion to discern frequent exposures among ill persons and to generate hypotheses which may then be tested in an epidemiologic study by using a questionnaire developed for the investigation. Team members may then query outbreak victims by using this study questionnaire. The questionnaire allows a consistent and detailed description of the signs and symptoms of illness, a history of food consumption for three or more days before the onset of illness, and other items, which can be entered into a computerized database or analyzed manually. These data can be analyzed for such parameters as attack rate by factors of interest such as age or a particular food item, average incubation time, and other key elements. Using these data, the team leader, with counsel from experienced team members, will implicate the suspected agent and the food vehicle responsible for the outbreak.

The probable agent and food vehicle will guide team members in the selection of food samples and clinical specimens. Since each outbreak is different, the team will invariably tailor these efforts to the availability of materials. Early retrieval of food samples, as close to the time of the suspect meal or event, is highly desirable, although food is often consumed or discarded before investigators are aware of the outbreak. Recovery of food from a suspect meal may be available only if victims have retained and refrigerated or frozen uneaten portions.

The suspect agent may lead investigators to examine the site where foods were grown, harvested, processed, prepared, stored, or served and to interview food service workers. These inspections and interviews can identify outbreak sources such as a worker with diarrhea who failed to perform adequate hand washing (*Shigella*, viral gastroenteritis) or who worked with a hand lesion (*Staphylococcus aureus*). Cross-contamination between raw meat or poultry and an uncooked food such as a salad may be suspected (*Campylobacter*, *E. coli* O157:H7, *Salmonella*, *Yersinia*).

It is recommended that any suspect food be secured by investigators as soon as possible, even before attack rates for suspect foods are calculated, because once discarded, food samples cannot be used in a confirming laboratory test which may help to corroborate the epidemiologically identified source of the outbreak. A public health laboratory can receive and store a number of food samples while team members continue to collect and analyze information and eventually implicate a food which will direct laboratory testing. For example, with family permission, the entire contents of a refrigerator of a probable botulism case can be secured while medical examination and clinical laboratory tests are conducted to rule out botulism. In some instances, it may be desirable to swab surfaces of food-processing or food preparation equipment or surfaces.

Investigations are often aided by the use of a name or code for the site being investigated. This can be the name of a food product or a food service establishment. This simple strategy facilitates communications, laboratory test requests, and the grouping of information at investigation team headquarters. In the event that team members are dealing with more than one outbreak at the same time, the use of an outbreak name avoids confusion.

CLINICAL AND FOOD SAMPLES: SPECIMEN SELECTION CRITERIA

The ability to detect the etiologic agent of foodborne infection in specimens obtained from ill persons is dependent on two major factors: (i) the availability of appropriate validated diagnostic tests for the pathogen and (ii) collection of appropriate specimens in a timely and appropriate manner. Fecal specimens collected from ill persons often do not yield a pathogen because they were collected at an inappropriate time (for example, after initiation of treatment with antimicrobial agents) or were collected or handled inappropriately. Detailed recommendations for collection of laboratory specimens associated with gastroenteritis outbreaks have been published by CDC (26). Instructions for collection of stool specimens from ill persons for foodborne disease outbreak investigations are summarized in Table 3, which is adapted from the CDC recommendations.

The isolation of diarrheal pathogens from foods presents greater challenges than their isolation from acutely ill patients. Both false-positive (organisms isolated which are not responsible for the observed illness) and false-negative (organisms not found that are responsible for the observed illness) results are potential problems with food testing. The organism that caused an outbreak may be present in very small numbers or may be sublethally stressed or injured. Therefore, food samples from outbreaks must be examined with the greatest care. Samples must often be processed simultaneously by multiple methods to increase the probability of isolating the pathogen.

It is not known at the time of microbiological examination whether the pathogen is present at very low or very high levels. A homogenate or suspension of the food sample may be directly plated on appropriate selective enrichment media; if the pathogen is present at a high concentration, this will be the most rapid means of isolating it. At the same time, the food sample must be enriched in a suitable selective enrichment medium for 24 to 48 h and then plated on selective plating media to enhance the probability of isolating the pathogen even if it is present at very low levels. Selective enrichment methods used by the food regulatory agencies are generally capable of yielding a positive result if the target pathogen is present at a level equal to or greater than 1 cell per 25 g of food. The sensitivity of the selective enrichment method can be increased beyond this level by culturing a larger sample or multiple samples of food (450 g of food in 4,050 ml of enrichment medium).

Sublethally injured bacteria are usually sensitive to the selective agents (such as bile salts, dyes, antimicrobial agents, potassium tellurite, sodium selenite, etc.) that are commonly used in selective enrichment media, and they may not grow if the sample is placed directly in selective enrichment media. Protocols for isolation of pathogenic bacteria from foods often include a preenrichment in a nonselective nutritionally complete medium to allow the injured cells to repair their damage before they are exposed to the selective enrichment medium (25, 34). This is particularly important for isolation of pathogenic bacteria from foods which have been preserved by heating, freezing, drying, or addition of acids and other chemicals. Because preenrichment media do not contain selective chemicals, nonpathogenic contaminants may overgrow the pathogen if preenrichment is allowed to proceed for extended periods.

RAPID METHODS FOR DETECTION OF FOODBORNE AND WATERBORNE PATHOGENS AND THEIR TOXINS

The conclusions reached after epidemiologic investigations of outbreaks are significantly strengthened if the results of microbiological investigations support epidemiologic findings. This is particularly true when a common source such as a particular food item is implicated as the outbreak vehicle. Isolation of the pathogenic microorganism and further characterization of it below the species level by methods such as serotyping or molecular subtyping may provide crucial corroborating evidence. Isolates are also required for antimicrobial susceptibility testing, which not only provides epidemiologic markers but also may be critical for the design

TABLE 3 General instructions for collecting, storing, and transporting stool specimens

Procedure	Instructions regarding specimens to be tested for:		
	Viruses	Bacteria	Parasites
Collection			
When to collect	Within 48 h after onset of illness.	During period of active diarrhea (preferably as soon as possible).	Any time after onset of illness (preferably as soon as possible).
How much to collect	As much stool sample as possible from each of 10 ill persons (a minimum of 10 ml of stool from each); samples may also be obtained from 10 controls.	Two rectal swabs or swabs of each stool from each of 10 ill persons; samples may also be obtained from 10 controls. Also, whole stools may be collected. When testing food handlers or other individuals in a potential chain of transmission, stool cultures should be taken and tested until there are a minimum of two consecutive negative stools collected not less than 24 h apart.	A fresh stool sample from each of 10 ill persons; samples may also be obtained from 10 controls. At least three specimens collected 48 h or more apart should be obtained from each patient.
Method of collection	Place fresh specimens (liquid preferable), unmixed with urine, in clean, dry containers.	For rectal swabs, moisten each of two swabs in an appropriate transport medium (Cary-Blair, Stuart, Amies, etc.; buffered glycerol-saline is suitable for *E. coli*, *Salmonella*, *Shigella*, and *Y. enterocolitica* but not for *Campylobacter* and *Vibrio*) and then insert sequentially in rectum and gently rotate. Place both swabs into the same Cary-Blair medium tube. Break off top portions of swab sticks and discard.	Collect a bulk stool specimen, unmixed with urine, in a clean container. Place a portion of each stool sample into 10% formalin and polyvinyl alcohol preservatives (or other commercial preservative) at a ratio of 1 part stool to 3 parts preservative. Mix well. A portion of the unpreserved stool may be saved for antigen testing or PCR testing.
Storage	Immediately refrigerate at 4°C. Specimens for electron microscopic examination should not be frozen. A portion of each stool specimen may be stored frozen at −15°C or lower for antigen or PCR testing.	Immediately refrigerate at 4°C if testing is to be done within 48 h after collection. If testing is to be done after 48 h, store samples frozen at −70°C. (Same recommendations apply for whole stools.) A portion of each stool specimen may be stored frozen at −15°C or lower for antigen or PCR testing.	Store at room temperature or refrigerate at 4°C. DO NOT FREEZE. Store unpreserved stool specimen frozen at −15°C or lower for antigen or PCR testing.
Transportation to testing laboratory[a]	Keep refrigerated. Place bagged and sealed specimens on ice or frozen refrigerant packs in an insulated box. Send by overnight mail. DO NOT FREEZE. Send frozen specimens on dry ice for antigen or PCR testing.	Refrigerate as instructed for viral specimens. Place bagged and sealed frozen specimens on dry ice in an insulated box and send by overnight mail.	Refrigerate preserved stool as instructed for viral specimens. For room temperature specimens, mail in waterproof containers. For antigen and/or PCR testing, place bagged and sealed frozen specimens on dry ice in an insulated box and send by overnight mail.

[a] Label each specimen with a waterproof marker. Pack samples in sealed, waterproof containers. Batch the collection and send by overnight mail to arrive in the testing laboratory on a weekday during business hours, unless other arrangements have been made with the testing laboratory in advance. Give the testing laboratory as much advance notice as possible so that testing can begin as soon as samples arrive.

of strategies to reduce transmission and protect contacts. Therefore, rapid detection methods which do not involve pathogen isolation are useful only for rapidly screening specimens so that the specimens needed for additional work-up are identified and negative specimens are eliminated. Rapid tests used in this manner should have high sensitivity, since specimens giving false-negative results are lost to follow-up. Specificity is less critical, since positive results are confirmed by culture.

In the United States, methods used in microbiological analysis of foods are validated by the Association of Official Analytical Chemists (AOAC) International (2). AOAC International official methods result from collaborative studies in which experienced, competent analysts work independently in different laboratories, using a specific test method to analyze homogeneous test samples for a pathogenic microorganism or chemical agent. Approved official methods are initially granted First Action status; a method may be given Final Action status, the highest level of sanction of AOAC International, 3 years after it is granted First Action status. AOAC International also offers a peer-verified methods program and a test kit performance-testing program. These are less rigorous than the collaborative studies; consequently, methods and test kits certified by these programs do not enjoy official status (2).

Several rapid detection methods for pathogens in foods are available. An exhaustive list of rapid food-testing methods has been compiled by Feng (18). Table 4 lists a selection of these tests. Table 5 lists some of the commercially available tests for rapid detection of parasitic organisms in stool specimens.

MOLECULAR EPIDEMIOLOGIC METHODS

Molecular subtyping of the microorganism isolated from suspected food samples provides confirmation of epidemiologic associations. In some instances, results of molecular subtyping provide additional essential information to improve the precision of epidemiologic analyses, may suggest association of food items that were not previously considered in the questionnaires administered to cases and controls, and can help to link geographically disparate cases or clusters of illness to the outbreak under investigation. Furthermore, molecular subtyping is extremely valuable in tracing the source of contamination of the implicated food.

Other chapters in this manual provide detailed descriptions of molecular subtyping protocols and suggest approaches for interpretation of results. Table 6 provides information on phenotypic and molecular subtyping methods that are useful for characterizing foodborne pathogens to aid in outbreak investigations.

TABLE 4 Commercial tests for rapid detection and identification of foodborne pathogenic bacteria and their toxins in foods[a]

Bacteria or toxin	Commercial assay	Manufacturer	Format of assay[b]	Comments
Bacillus cereus diarrheal toxin	TECRA	TECRA	ELISA	
	BCET	Oxoid-Unipath	RPLA	
Botulinal toxins	ELCA-ELISA	Elcatech	Amplified ELISA	
Campylobacter jejuni, *C. coli*	Campyslide	Becton-Dickinson	Latex agglutination	
	Meritec-Campy	Meridian	Latex agglutination	
	Microscreen	Mercia	Latex agglutination	
	VIDAS	bioMérieux	Automated ELISA	
Clostridium perfringens enterotoxin	PET	Oxoid-Unipath	RPLA	
Escherichia coli O157:H7	RIM	Remel	Latex agglutination	Facilitates identification only
	E. coli O157	Oxoid-Unipath	Latex agglutination	Facilitates identification only
	Prolex	Pro Labs	Latex agglutination	Facilitates identification only
	EcolexO157	Orion Diagnostics	Latex agglutination	Facilitates identification only
	PetrifilmHEC	3M	Immunoblot	
	EZ COLI	Difco	Tube EIA	
	Dynabeads	Dynal	Immunomagnetic beads	
	EHEC-TEK	Organon-Teknika	ELISA	
	Assurance	Biocontrol	ELISA	
	HECO157	3M Canada	ELISA	
	TECRA	TECRA	ELISA	
	E. coli O157	LMD Lab.	ELISA	
	VIP	Biocontrol	Immunoblot	
	Reveal	Neogen	Immunoblot	
	NOW	Binax	Immunoblot	
	VIDAS	bioMérieux	Automated ELISA	

(Continued on next page)

TABLE 4 Commercial tests for rapid detection and identification of foodborne pathogenic bacteria and their toxins in foods[a] (*Continued*)

Bacteria or toxin	Commercial assay	Manufacturer	Format of assay[b]	Comments
Shiga toxins	VEROTEST	Microcarb	ELISA	
	Premier EHEC	Meridian	ELISA	
	Verotox-F	Denka Seiken	RPLA	
Listeria	Listeria-TEK	Organon Teknika	ELISA	
	TECRA	TECRA	ELISA	
	Assurance	Biocontrol	ELISA	
	Listertest	Vicam	Immunobeads	
	VIP	Biocontrol	Immunoprecipitation	
	Clearview	Unipath	Immunoprecipitation	
	RAPIDTEST	Unipath	Immunoprecipitation	
	VIDAS	bioMérieux	ELISA	
	OPUS	TECRA	ELISA	
Salmonella	Bactigen	Wampole Labs	Latex agglutination	Facilitates identification only
	Spectate	Rhone-Poulenc	Latex agglutination	Facilitates identification only
	Microscreen	Mercia	Latex agglutination	Facilitates identification only
	Wellcolex	Laboratoire Wellcome	Latex agglutination	Facilitates identification only
	Serobact	Remel	Latex agglutination	Facilitates identification only
	RAPIDTEST	Unipath	Latex agglutination	Facilitates identification only
	Dynabeads	Dynal	Immunomagnetic beads	
	Screen	VICAM	Immunomagnetic beads	
	CHECKPOINT	KPL	Immunoblot	
	1–2 test	Biocontrol	Motility-based immunoprecipitation	
	SalmonellaTEK	Organon Teknika	ELISA	
	TECRA	TECRA	ELISA	
	EQUATE	Binax	ELISA	
	BacTrace	KPL	ELISA	
	LOCATE	Rhone-Poulenc	ELISA	
	Assurance	Biocontrol	ELISA	
	Salmonella	GEM Biomedical	ELISA	
	VIDAS	bioMérieux	Automated ELISA	
	OPUS	TECRA	ELISA	
	PATH-STIK	LUMAC	Immunoprecipitation	
	Reveal	Neogen	Immunoprecipitation	
	Clearview	Unipath	Immunoprecipitation	
	UNIQUE	TECRA	Capture ELISA	
Shigella	Bactigen	Wampole Labs	Latex agglutination	Facilitates identification only
	Wellcolex	Laboratoire Wellcome	Latex agglutination	Facilitates identification only
Staphylococcus aureus enterotoxins	Staphyloslide	Becton-Dickinson	Latex agglutination	
	AureusTest	Trisum	Latex agglutination	
	SET-EIA	Toxin Technology	ELISA	
	SET-RPLA	Unipath	RPLA	
	TECRA	TECRA	ELISA	
	RIDASCREEN	R-Biopharm	ELISA	
	VIDAS	bioMérieux	Automated ELISA	
	OPUS	TECRA	ELISA	
Vibrio cholerae	choleraSMART	New Horizon	Immunoprecipitation	
	bengalSMART	New Horizon	Immunoprecipitation	
Cholera toxin and heat-labile enterotoxin of *E. coli*	VET-RPLA	Unipath	RPLA	

[a] Data from reference 18.
[b] ELISA, enzyme-linked immunosorbent assay; RPLA, reversed passive latex agglutination; EIA, enzyme immunoassay.

TABLE 5 Rapid commercial methods for detection of foodborne and waterborne parasites

Target parasite	Commercial test	Assay format[a]	Manufacturer
Cryptosporidium parvum	ProSpecT assay	Direct antigen test	Alexon, Sunnyvale, Calif.
	Crypto/*Giardia* IF kit	DFA	TechLab, Blacksburg, Va.
	Crypto test	Enzyme immunoassay	TechLab
	Merifluor	DFA	Meridian Diagnostics, Cincinnati, Ohio
	RIM *Cryptosporidium* antigen detection	Microwell enzyme immunoassay	Remel, Lenexa, Kans.
Giardia lamblia	ProSpecT assay	Direct antigen test	Alexon
	Merifluor	DFA	Meridian Diagnostics
	Premier	ELISA	Meridian Diagnostics
	RIM *Giardia* antigen detection	Microwell enzyme immunoassay	Remel
	Prospect *Giardia* rapid assay	Membrane-based enzyme immunoassay	Remel
	Giardia test	Enzyme immunoassay	TechLab

[a] DFA, direct fluorescent-antibody assay; ELISA, enzyme-linked immunosorbent assay.

TABLE 6 Subtyping methods for foodborne pathogens

Pathogen	Phenotypic subtyping method(s)	Molecular subtyping methods[a]	Restriction enzyme for RFLP	Comments
Bacillus cereus	Serotyping	RFLP/PFGE	*Sma*I	
Campylobacter jejuni, *C. coli*	Serotyping	*flaA* RFLP, RFLP/PFGE	*Dde*I, *Sma*I[b]	
Clostridium botulinum	Toxin typing	RFLP/PFGE	*Mlu*I, *Sma*I, *Xho*I	Nuclease activity of isolates may present problems
Clostridium perfringens	Serotyping	RFLP/PFGE	*Sma*I	
E. coli O157	Serotyping, phage typing	RFLP/PFGE	*Xba*I, *Avr*II (*Bln*I)	
Listeria monocytogenes	Serotyping, phage typing	RFLP/MRA, RFLP/PFGE, RAPD	*Hha*I, *Apa*I, *Asc*I, *Sma*I	Methods are being standardized by a WHO-sponsored international group
Salmonella serovar typhimurium	Phage typing, antimicrobial susceptibility	RFLP/PFGE	*Xba*I, *Avr*II (*Bln*I)	Antimicrobial susceptibility and phage typing required for identification of DT 104
Salmonella serovar enteritidis	Phage typing	Plasmid profiles, ribotyping, RFLP/PFGE, RAPD	*Sph*I, *Pst*I, *Sma*I, *Xba*I, *Bln*I (*Avr*II)	No single molecular method has adequate discriminating ability
Other nontyphoidal salmonellae	Phage typing, if available	RFLP/PFGE, RAPD	*Xba*I, *Avr*II (*Bln*I)	Some strains may not be typeable by PFGE
Shigella spp.		RFLP/PFGE	*Xba*I	
Yersinia enterocolitica	Serotyping	RFLP/PFGE	*Xba*I, *Sma*I	
Cryptosporidium parvum		MLEE, RAPD, RFLP/repetitive DNA, Differential PCR/18S rRNA + ITS, RFLP/DHFR-TS, PCR/DNA sequence analysis (TRAP-C2)	*Hinf*I, *Rsa*I	
Caliciviruses		PCR/DNA sequence analysis		

[a] MLEE, multilocus enzyme electrophoresis; RAPD, random amplified polymorphic DNA; RFLP, restriction fragment length polymorphism; MRA, microrestriction analysis; ITS, internally transcribed spacer; DHFR-TS, dihydrofolate reductase-thymidilate synthase; PFGE, pulsed-field gel electrophoresis; TRAP-C2, thrombospondin-related adhesin protein.

[b] *Dde*I used for *flaA* RFLP; *Sma*I used for RFLP/PFGE.

COMMUNICATION

Investigation team members, especially public health laboratorians, are often separated from other team members by considerable distances during the entire course of an investigation. Face-to-face exchanges among all team members regarding the progress of the investigation can be rare, and so other avenues of communication must be used. Daily updates to all team members by the team leader ensures that all actions are directed toward proof of the hypothesis—which can change, especially during the earliest phase of investigations, when reported cases are fewest and information is fragmentary and sometimes contradictory. Telephone, voice mail, electronic bulletins, and e-mail can all be of value, as long as all team members receive a comprehensive interim report and are made aware of shifts in the direction of activities. A telephone bridge conference can be the most effective means to interactively conduct updates and allow all team members to contribute and receive information.

Laboratorians, especially, may be isolated from the details of the developing investigation due to the intensity of activities at team command centers. It is recommended that laboratory supervisors assume the role of primary team liaison and remain in daily contact with the investigation team leader or his or her designee. The laboratory team member should inform the team leader of the following: (i) laboratory capability, that is, the type of testing the laboratory can perform in support of the investigation; (ii) laboratory capacity, that is, the number of tests that the laboratory can perform with existing staff and supplies; (iii) specific information on the selection, collection, storage, and transport of samples; and (iv) the time when results will be available to the team.

The laboratory personnel should know who is authorized to order tests and to whom the results should be reported. If the team effort is not properly coordinated, contradictory messages may be received by the laboratory, and labor and supplies may be wasted in bacteriologic medium preparation or other activities. After a food has been epidemiologically implicated, the laboratory team member should advise the team leader of the value of the requested tests based on the condition of specimens, delays in collection, suboptimal or improper storage, or transport time or conditions. If a bacterial agent has been recovered by hospital or reference laboratories, the team leader should be advised about the importance of referral of these culture isolates to the public health laboratory for confirmation testing and epidemiologic typing.

To ensure that misinformation is not spread and public confidence is not eroded during an investigation, all requests for information, whether from the public or the media, should be referred to the team leader or the public relations designee. Team members should not act independently but should relay information to the team leader and allow team judgment to prevail in decisions about release of information.

DOCUMENTATION

The actions of local health authorities, including sanitarians, epidemiologists, and environmental health specialists, can be facilitated by the compilation and dissemination of a set of written procedures to be used in the event of a foodborne disease outbreak. This document should include the following: (i) the procedure for collection of complaint data and a standardized format for recording food-related complaints; (ii) a set of guidelines for the initiation of an investigation based on evaluation of epidemiologic data; (iii) a set of instructions for the collection, storage, and transport of human specimens and food samples, as well as a list of laboratory tests available from the central public health laboratory; and (iv) an up-to-date list of the principal public health contacts, including phone and fax numbers and e-mail addresses. This compendium of information will save valuable time in the early stages of an outbreak investigation, when data are being collected, the investigation team is being assembled, and a communication network is being formed. Examples of standardized forms and procedures are available from the International Association of Milk, Food and Environmental Sanitarians (9).

The investigation team will typically establish a computerized database for the retrieval and analysis of data. EPI-INFO, a software package made available by CDC, is frequently used for this function (16). Although small outbreaks with few cases can be managed with manual recording and analysis, larger outbreaks will require computerized management of data. Effective management of a growing database requires daily, even hourly, updates. This is especially true of spreading outbreaks, such as hepatitis A virus infections caused by an infected food worker, in which rapid identification of cases and institution of interventions is essential to limit the extent of the outbreak.

The laboratory is advised to begin a file when it is notified of a possible outbreak. This file can be a simple one-page form for collection of the following information: (i) the name and phone number of the investigation team leader or the team's laboratory liaison, (ii) the suspected agent(s), (iii) the number of samples to be submitted, and (iv) the mode of transport (team member, courier, bus line, etc.) and estimated time of arrival of the samples. Laboratory personnel who will perform the testing should be informed to allow them to reschedule routine workloads, order the preparation of bacteriologic media, and check on the availability of supplies. Bacteriologic media can be prepared in advance of receipt of specimens, but since culture procedures for food often require many units of freshly prepared media for each sample, the laboratory team contact is advised to make certain of the number of samples to be submitted before the preparation of media begins. A requisition or food collection form should accompany each specimen or set of specimens. For food samples, this document should provide a description of each sample, including the quantity, method of collection, time and date of collection, name of the collector, analyses requested, and the agency or individual to whom the report should be sent. Each food sample should be marked at a minimum with the date and time of collection and a unique collection number, which is also recorded or preprinted on the request form. Written procedures and published reference works for the collection, transport, and analysis of food samples should be available and should be consulted in the performance of the laboratory analysis of food. The laboratory procedure manual should be consulted in the analysis of human specimens. Human specimens should be marked with the patient's name or another appropriate identifier and the date and time of collection and should be individually packaged or attached to a test request form which clearly records the patient's name; the name, address, and phone number of the health care provider; and the tests requested. Recording of the outbreak name or code (example: "Joe's Restaurant") on both the food and human test request forms facilitates the laboratory's effort to compile outbreak information in a useful format for the investigation team. Human-specimen testing is subject to the regulations of the Clinical Laboratory Improvement Act (CLIA), including such quality control requirements as performance of diagnostic bacteriologic cultures and other tests according to written procedures and adherence to written specimen rejection criteria.

Reporting of the results of laboratory tests should be tailored to the needs of the investigation team. The generation of line lists of results of human testing, simply detailing patient identifier and test result, speeds the review of data by the team and facilitates decision-making. Fax transmissions of results are quite acceptable and favored over telephone reporting of a large number of test results. Test results for food analysis, which typically take longer to complete but are fewer in number, can be telephoned. Final hard copy reports can be mailed or electronically transmitted depending on the laboratory's capabilities.

REFERENCES

1. **Andrews, W. H.** 1995. Microbiological methods, p. 1–119. *In* P. Cunnif (ed.), *Official Methods of Analysis of AOAC International*, 16th ed., vol. 1. AOAC International, Gaithersburg, Md.
2. **Andrews, W. H.** 1996. AOAC International's three validation programs for methods used in the microbiological analysis of foods. *Trends Food Sci. Technol.* **7:**147–151.
3. **Anonymous.** 1997. *Food Safety from Farm to Table: a National Food-Safety Initiative.* A report to the President. Department of Health and Human Services, U.S. Department of Agriculture and U.S. Environmental Protection Agency, Washington, D.C.
4. **Bean, N. H., P. M. Griffin, J. S. Goulding, and C. B. Ivey.** 1990. Foodborne disease outbreaks, 5-year summary, 1983–1987. *Morbid. Mortal. Weekly Rep.* **39**(SS01): 15–23.
5. **Bender, J. B., C. W. Hedberg, J. M. Besser, D. J. Boxrud, K. L. MacDonald, and M. T. Osterholm.** 1997. Surveillance for *Escherichia coli* O157:H7 infections in Minnesota by molecular typing. *N. Engl. J. Med.* **337:**388–394.
6. **Benenson, A. A. (ed.).** 1990. *Control of Communicable Diseases in Man*, 15th ed. American Public Health Association, Washington, D.C.
7. **Bryan, F. L.** 1990. Hazard Analysis Critical Control Point (HACCP) concept. *Dairy Food Environ. Sanit.* **10:** 416–418.
8. **Bryan, F. L.** 1995. Procedures to use during outbreaks of food-borne disease, p. 209–226. In P. R. Murray, E. J. Baron, M. A. Pfaller, F. C. Tenover, and R. H. Yolken (ed.), *Manual of Clinical Microbiology*, 6th ed. ASM Press, Washington, D.C.
9. **Bryan, F. L., H. W. Anderson, O. D. Cook, J. Guzewich, K. H. Lewis, R. C. Swanson, and E. C. D. Todd.** 1989. *Procedures To Investigate Foodborne Illness.* International Association of Milk, Food and Environmental Sanitarians, Ames, Iowa.
10. **Centers for Disease Control and Prevention.** 1990. Guidelines for investigating clusters of health events. *Morbid. Mortal. Weekly Rep.* **39**(RR-11)**:**1–23.
11. **Centers for Disease Control and Prevention.** 1996. CDC Surveillance Summaries: Surveillance for Foodborne-Disease Outbreaks-United States, 1988–1992. *Morbid. Mortal. Weekly Rep.* **45**(SS-5)**:**66.
12. **Centers for Disease Control and Prevention.** 1996. CDC surveillance summaries: surveillance for waterborne-disease outbreaks—United States, 1993–1994. *Morbid. Mortal. Weekly Rep.* **45**(SS-1)**:**40.
13. **Centers for Disease Control and Prevention.** 1996. Summary of notifiable diseases, United States, 1996. *Morbid. Mortal. Weekly Rep.* **45**(53)**:**1–103.
14. **Centers for Disease Control and Prevention.** 1998. Outbreak of acute febrile illness among athletes participating in triathlons—Wisconsin and Illinois, 1998. *Morbid. Mortal. Weekly Rep.* **47:**585–588.

14a. **Centers for Disease Control and Prevention.** Unpublished data.

15. **Clesceri, L. S., A. D. Eaton, and A. E. Greenberg (ed.).** 1996. *Standard Methods for the Examination of Water and Wastewater*; 19th ed. suppl. American Public Health Association, Washington, D.C.
16. **Dean, A. G., J. A. Dean, D. Coulombier, et al.** 1994. *EPI-INFO: a Word Processing, Database, and Statistics Program for Epidemiology on Microcomputers*, version 6. Centers for Disease Control and Prevention, Atlanta, Ga.
17. **Eaton, A. D., L. S. Clesceri, and A. E. Greenberg (ed.).** 1995. *Standard Methods for the Examination of Water and Wastewater*, 19th ed. American Public Health Association, Washington, D.C.
18. **Feng, P.** 1996. Emergence of rapid methods for identifying microbial pathogens in foods. *J. AOAC Int.* **79:**809–812.
19. **Foegeding, P. M., T. Roberts, J. Bennett, F. L. Bryan, D. O. Cliver, M. P. Doyle, R. F. Eden, R. S. Flowers, C. T. Foreman, B. Lorber, J. M. Madden, J. B. Rose, J. L. Smith, E. C. D. Todd, and M. M. Wekell.** 1994. *Foodborne Pathogens: Risks and Consequences.* Task Force report 122, Sept. 1994. Council for Agricultural Science and Technology, Ames, Iowa.
20. **Ford, T. E., and R. R. Colwell (ed.).** 1996. *A Global Decline in Microbiological Safety of Water: a Call for Action.* Report based on the American Academy of Microbiology colloquium, 4 to 6 April 1995, Guayaquil, Ecuador. American Society for Microbiology, Washington, D.C.
21. **Gregg, M. B., and J. Parsonnet.** 1997. The principles of an epidemic field investigation, p. 537–546. *In* R. Detels, W. W. Holland, J. McEwen, and G. S. Omenn (ed.), *Oxford Textbook of Public Health*, 2nd ed., vol 2. Oxford University Press, London, United Kingdom.
22. **Helmick, C. G., P. M. Griffin, D. G. Addiss, R. V. Tauxe, and D. D. Juranek.** 1994. Infectious diarrheas, p. 85–123. *In* J. E. Everhart (ed.), *Digestive Diseases in the United States: Epidemiology and Impact.* NIH publication 94-1447. U.S. Department of Health and Human Services, Public Health Service, National Institutes of Health, Bethesda, Md.
23. **Hennessy, T. W., C. W. Hedberg, L. Slutsker, K. White, J. Besser-Wiek, M. Moen, J. Feldman, W. Coleman, L. Edmonson, K. MacDonald, M. Osterholm, and the Investigation Team.** 1996. A multistate outbreak of *Salmonella enteritidis* infections associated with the consumption of Schwan's ice cream. *N. Engl. J. Med.* **334:**1281–1286.
24. **Hughes, J. M., and F. J. Angulo.** 1996. Foodborne diseases, p. 344–347. *In* J. W. Hurst, J. A. Shulman, and D. S. Stephens (ed.), *Medicine for the Practicing Physician*, 4th ed. Appleton & Lange, Stamford, Conn.
25. **Jackson, G. J. (ed.).** 1992. *Bacteriological Analytical Manual.* AOAC International, Arlington, Va.
26. **Lew, J. F., C. W. LeBaron, R. I. Glass, T. Torok, P. M. Griffin, J. G. Wells, D. D. Juranek, and S. P. Wahlquist.** 1990. Recommendations for collection of laboratory specimens associated with outbreaks of gastroenteritis. *Morbid. Mortal. Weekly Rep.* **39**(RR-14)**:**1–13.
27. **Marshall, R. T. (ed.).** 1993. *Standard Methods for the Examination of Dairy Products*, 16th ed. American Public Health Association, Washington, D.C.
28. **McIntyre, C. R.** 1991. Hazard analysis critical control point (HACCP) identification. *Dairy Food Environ. Sanit.* **11:**73–81.
29. **Potter, M. E., and R. V. Tauxe.** 1997. Epidemiology of

foodborne diseases: tools and applications. *Rapp. Trimest. Stat. Sanit. Mond.* **50:**24–29.

30. **Ryan, C. A., M. T. Nickels, N. T. Hargrett-Bean, M. E. Potter, T. Endo, L. Mayer, C. W. Langkop, C. Gibson, R. C. McDonald, R. T. Kenney, N. D. Puhr, P. J. McDonnell, R. J. Martin, M. L. Cohen, and P. A. Blake.** 1987. Massive outbreak of antimicrobial-resistant salmonellosis traced to pasteurized milk. *JAMA* **258:**3269–3274.
31. **Snyder, O. P.** 1991. HACCP in the retail food industry. *Dairy Food Environ. Sanit.* **11:**73–81.
32. **Tauxe, R. V.** 1989. The role of epidemiology in the detection and prevention of foodborne disease, p. 40–46. *In Issues in Food Safety. Proceedings of a Joint Meeting of the Toxicology Forum and the Chinese Academy of Preventive Medicine.* Beijing, 16 to 20 October 1988. Toxicology Forum, Washington, D.C.
33. **Tauxe, R. V.** 1997. Emerging foodborne diseases: an evolving public health challenge. *Emerging Infect. Dis.* **3:**425–434.
34. **Vanderzant, C., and D. Splittstoesser (ed.).** 1993. *Compendium of Methods for the Microbiological Examination of Foods.* American Public Health Association, Washington, D.C.
35. **Veek, M. E., I. Weitzman, R. C. Swanson, and J. P. Lucas.** 1993. Investigation of foodborne illness outbreaks, p. 747–761. *In* C. Vanderzant and D. F. Splittstoesser (ed.), *Compendium of Methods for the Microbiological Examination of Foods.* American Public Health Association, Washington, D.C.
36. **Watanabe, H., A. Wada, Y. Inagaki, K. Itoh, and K. Tamura.** 1996. Outbreaks of enterohemorrhagic *Escherichia coli* O157:H7 infection by two different genotypes in Japan, 1996. *Lancet* **348:**831–832.

DIAGNOSTIC TECHNOLOGIES IN CLINICAL MICROBIOLOGY

VOLUME EDITOR
FRED C. TENOVER

SECTION EDITOR
GARY V. DOERN

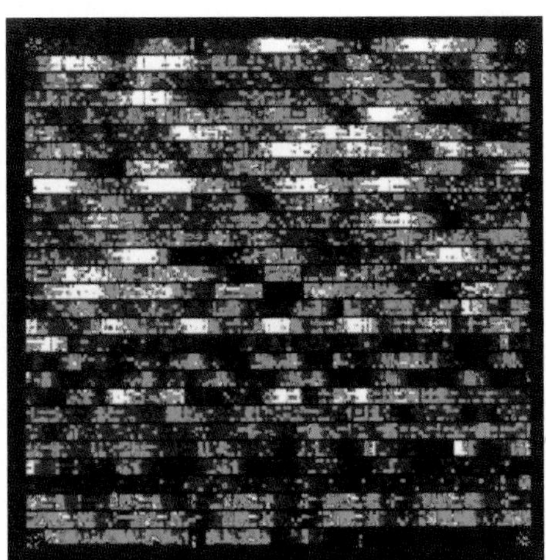

GeneChip analysis for detection of mutations associated with HIV drug resistance *(photograph courtesy of John W. Wilson, Paul N. Rys, and David H. Persing).*

Manual and Automated Systems for Microbial Identification

J. MICHAEL MILLER AND CAROLINE M. O'HARA

11

Gaining and maintaining expertise in identifying clinically important microbes has been the goal of clinical laboratorians for decades. From the early years of diagnostic methods in microbiology up to the 1960s, when advances in microbial identification began to emerge, skill in interpretive judgement and the use of tubed and plated media were the basis of identification. Organisms were identified by what we now refer to as conventional procedures, which include reactions in tubed media and observation of physical characteristics, such as colony morphology and odor, coupled with the results of the Gram stain, agglutination tests, and antimicrobial susceptibility profiles. These conventional procedures eventually defined the genera and species of bacteria and yeasts and became the reference method by which we confirm isolates.

The next step in the evolution of identification methods simply miniaturized commonly used biochemical reactions into a more convenient format (5). Later, a systems approach became the industry standard, and it remains the basis upon which most currently used substrate profile systems rely. In a system-dependent methodology, a set of substrates is carefully selected that will allow a positive- and negative-reaction pattern to emerge, creating a metabolic profile to be compared with an established database profile. In many systems, different sets of substrates are necessary to identify rapidly growing members of the family *Enterobacteriaceae*, slower-growing gram-negative non-*Enterobacteriaceae*, gram-positive cocci, gram-negative cocci, and anaerobes. Yeasts require yet another profile set.

Biochemical profiles are determined by the reactions of individual organisms with each of the substrates in the system. The accuracy of the reactions is dependent upon the user's following the directions of the manufacturer regarding inoculum preparation, inoculum density, incubation conditions, and test interpretation. Most systems rely upon pH changes resulting from utilization of substrate, enzymatic reactions that allow the release of a chromogenic or fluorogenic compound, tetrazolium-based indicators of metabolic activity in the presence of a variety of carbon sources, detection of volatile or nonvolatile acids, or recognition of visible growth (Table 1). Additional tests for microbial identification that use other means of detecting a positive response for a given substrate may also be included.

Although no formal definition of "rapid" exists for describing the time required for results to be generated, most microbiologists expect rapid systems to provide usable results within 2 to 4 h of incubation. Clearly, the generation times of microbes (usually 30 min or longer) will not allow growth-dependent methods to generate detectable biochemical responses within this time. To overcome the problem of generation times, manufacturers of rapid systems utilize novel substrates on which performed enzymes, produced by the organisms to be tested, may react to elicit responses detectable within 2 to 4 h.

CRITERIA FOR SELECTING A SYSTEM

The laboratorian must consider several issues when selecting a system to be used in the laboratory, especially when the equipment will probably provide both organism identification and antimicrobial susceptibility test results. Because the cost of some instrument-based systems may exceed $100,000, purchase of these identification systems represents a significant capital expenditure and a long-term commitment to that technology. Supervisors and managers in the laboratory should make such major decisions carefully and with expert consultation. Before the first technical representative is seen in the laboratory, several important questions must be answered.

1. Why do I need a new system? Can I justify it as a benefit to the laboratory or the hospital?
2. Will management support the need for a new system? Is funding available?
3. Do I truly need a "rapid" system? Will earlier results actually get to physicians or patient records and affect patient care?
4. On what will I base my final decision? What questions do I need to have answered about the system?
5. Should I buy the system outright or negotiate for a reagent rental contract?

Once these questions are answered, the next step is to begin the search for the right instrument or system to meet the needs of the laboratory and the medical staff. As a general rule, it is best not to be the first to purchase a new system without having seen in the peer-reviewed literature the results of evaluations performed by reputable clinical laboratories. If microbiology journals are unavailable, ask the representative to supply you with articles about the ability of the system to correctly identify the range of isolates usually seen

TABLE 1 Basis of identification system reactivity

System reactivity	Need for growth	Analyte	Indicator of positive result	Examples of system
pH-based reactions (mostly 15–24 h)	Y	Carbohydrate utilization	Color change due to pH indicator; carbohydrate utilization = acidic pH; protein utilization or release of nitrogen-containing products = alkaline pH	API; Crystal; Vitek cards; MicroScan conventional panels
Enzyme profile (mostly 2–4 h)	N	Preformed enzymes	Color change due to chromogen/fluorogen release when colorless complex is hydrolyzed by an appropriate enzyme	MicroScan rapid panels; IDS (Remel)
Carbon source utilization	Y	Organic products	Color change as a result of metabolic activity transferring electrons to colorless tetrazolium-labeled carbon sources and converting the dye to purple	Biolog
Volatile or nonvolatile acid detection	Y	Cellular fatty acids	Chromatographic tracing based on detection of end products which are then compared to a library of known patterns	MIDI
Visual detection of growth	Y	Various substrates	Turbidity due to growth of organism in the presence of a substrate	Yeast identification

in your laboratory. During conversations and demonstrations, make sure the following questions are answered.

1. Technical applications
   a. Do I like the overall quality of the system?
   b. How accurate are the identification and antimicrobial susceptibility test results? (get documentation to prove it).
   c. What is the turnaround time for a completed test?
   d. What is the cost per test including the instrument, consumables, and technologist time? What is the cost of quality control testing?
   e. What is the shelf life of the test kits? What are their storage requirements, and do I have adequate space for storage?
   f. Are epidemiology programs available with the software? Can the pharmacy be linked to the system?
   g. Are the printed reports usable?
   h. Who else in this geographic area uses this system?
   i. Do I trust this system to give me accurate results?
2. Manufacturer issues
   a. Can the system be interfaced with our current laboratory computer system? One-way or two-way interface?
   b. Is there technical and mechanical service from the company on weekends and holidays?
   c. Is the system expandable?
   d. How much training time is required/suggested by the manufacturer?
   e. What service contracts are recommended? Cost?
   f. How much bench space is required? How much does the system weigh, and will this pose an engineering or structural problem in my lab? Are special electrical outlets or communication lines required?
   g. Is the instrument protected from brownout?
   h. How are software updates handled? Are they free?
   i. Can I trade in my current system?
3. Personnel issues
   a. How much technologist time is required for test setup? For test completion? For quality control?
   b. Is the system usable by all shifts?

It is often helpful to visit other laboratories similar to yours that are now using the system and talk with the users. Ask if they like the system; would they buy it again; how much downtime have they experienced, and whether the service from the manufacturer has been acceptable. Discuss the issues of serviceability and the mechanical reliability of the test system.

Select a system that has been fully evaluated and whose accuracy exceeds 90% in its overall ability to identify common and uncommon bacteria normally seen in your hospital or laboratory. Commonly isolated organisms should be identified with at least 95% accuracy compared with conventional methods. Do not place unwarranted expectations on the system being considered. Some systems may be unable to accurately identify the more fastidious isolates even though these isolates may be listed in the manufacturer's database.

The accuracy of antimicrobial susceptibility testing for combination panels is as important as the accuracy of identification, perhaps more so. Because of the complexities of drug-microbe interactions and the novel resistance mechanisms that appear to be emerging, consultation may be necessary to be assured of the accuracy of susceptibility test results of a commercial system. Section VIII of this manual discusses the issues involved in susceptibility testing.

EVALUATING AN INSTRUMENT OR SYSTEM

Anytime an identification system is added to the laboratory, it is necessary to document that the system performs as described by the manufacturer. The first evidence of acceptable performance should be found in published reports by other laboratories that have evaluated the system in a sound, scientific manner (7). These reports should be read carefully, with particular attention to data that support the conclusions of the paper. Simply reading and accepting the abstract from these published studies may be misleading, especially if the study protocol was poorly conceived (6). Microbiologists who evaluate instruments against a "gold standard" or compare one system performance against another must be precise in experimental design, or the resulting data interpretation could be misleading (3, 6). Because current taxonomic definitions are linked to conventional biochemicals, the results of conventional biochemical testing are usually considered the gold standard against which a system should be measured for determining its overall accuracy. To use another commercial product as a gold standard may be acceptable when introducing a new product into a local laboratory, but such a comparison will not reveal the true accuracy of the system since all commercial products have some drawbacks or weaknesses.

The next evidence of acceptable performance by a new identification instrument should be in-laboratory verification of performance by the purchasing laboratory. The Clinical Laboratory Improvement Amendments of 1988 (CLIA '88) (4) specify the following conditions for systems placed into service after 1 September 1992:

> Prior to reporting patient test results, the laboratory must verify or establish, for each method, the performance specifications for the following performance characteristics: accuracy; precision; analytical sensitivity and specificity, if applicable; . . .

Because identification systems provide qualitative information, only accuracy should be addressed. CLIA does not specify how the accuracy verification process is to be done. Each laboratory is responsible for devising its own verification protocol, and verification must be done whether the laboratory is first introducing a new system or is replacing an old system with a new one.

Clearly, smaller laboratories will have fewer resources to verify an identification system than will larger laboratories. Laboratory size, however, has no bearing on the need to ensure the accuracy of laboratory identification methods and of the work performed by a laboratory in support of patient care. It is unreasonable to require that every laboratory reverify what has already been done by the manufacturer and by other laboratories that have published data on the accuracy of a system. A true establishment or verification of accuracy requires exhaustive testing of hundreds of strains. The role of verification by the purchasing laboratory should be to ensure that the personnel using the system can make it perform at the levels of accuracy already documented by the manufacturer and published in the literature.

The laboratorian should expect a level of 95% agreement with the existing system or reference method and accept, in the final analysis, no less than 90% agreement. This takes into account the fact that the new system may be more accurate than the old one. One should try to keep the total cost of verification within a range of $250 to $1,000 depending upon the size of the laboratory. In fact, one may negotiate with the manufacturer that the final purchase of a system be dependent upon successful verification of the system's accuracy and that the manufacturer assist in the process by providing stock strains for that purpose. Verification protocols for identification systems will vary but may be structured around one of the following suggestions:

1. Test the quality control organisms PLUS achieve >90.0% agreement for 1 week of consecutive parallel testing (a minimum of 50 strains) by the existing method. Discrepancies must be arbitrated by a reference laboratory.
2. Test the quality control organisms PLUS two or three known reference strains (stock cultures) of each commonly isolated organism in up to 50 tests (small laboratories) or 100 tests (large laboratories).
3. Test the quality control organisms PLUS ensure that 20 to 50 organism identifications (12 to 15 different species) agree in concurrent testing with the current method or with the results of reference laboratory testing of split samples.

As of early 1998, the Food and Drug Administration (FDA) no longer does premarket [510(K)] evaluations to "clear" automated or manual phenotypic identification systems nor do they receive or approve quality control protocols from these devices to meet CLIA requirements. Laboratorians must be aware that the identification component of the new or modified system that they are using is not "FDA cleared" because this approval is no longer required. This makes it even more important for laboratorians to search the literature for valid evaluations of their chosen instrument and to conduct their own in-house validation to make sure the instrument meets the claims of the manufacturer regarding identification. Devices and methods incorporating probes, nucleic acid amplification, and other genetic methods, as well as the susceptibility test component of commercial instruments, will continue to be reviewed by FDA for clearance.

System Construction

Microbial identification systems are considered either manual or automated. Manual methods offer the advantages of using the analytical skills of the technologists for reading and interpreting the tests, whereas automated systems offer a hands-off approach allowing more technologist time for other duties. For all systems, the backbone of accuracy is the strength and utility of the database. Databases are constructed by using known, clinically relevant strains and include the type strains of most taxa. In some cases, before an organism is added to the database, it is evaluated by cluster analysis to confirm its relationship to other strains in the same taxon.

The number of species included in a database may vary from 200 to as many as 1,200 if the system is to be used not only in clinical but also in environmental and research settings. For most commercial systems, database maintenance is a continuous process and software upgrades incorporating major taxonomic changes are provided by the manufacturer at intervals of up to every 4 years. Some systems may allow users to make minor changes at their local workstation.

System identifications are supported by algorithm-based decision-making that is generally available through a computer. Occasionally these identifications are compiled into a preprinted index, which is used to manually convert the organism's biochemical profile number into an identification. Bayes's theorem, or modifications of it, is often the basis of algorithm construction from data matrices.

Bayes's theorem is one of the statistical methods used by manufacturers to arrive at a certain taxon based on the reaction profile produced by the unknown clinical isolate (8). Bayes's theorem allows us to consider two important issues in order to arrive at an accurate conclusion: (i) $P(t_i/R)$ is the probability that an organism exhibiting test pattern R belongs to taxon t_i and (ii) $P(R/t_i)$ is the probability that members of taxon t_i will exhibit test pattern R. Before testing, we make the assumption that an unknown isolate has an equal chance of being any taxon and that each test used to identify the isolate is independent of all other tests. In this case, Bayes's theorem can be written as

$$P(t_i/R) = \frac{P(R/t_i)}{\sum_i P(R/t_i)}$$

By observing reference identification charts derived by conventional biochemical tests, we know the expected pattern of the population of taxon t_i (e.g., *Escherichia coli* is indole positive and citrate negative). R in the formula is the test pattern composed of $R_1, R_2, \ldots R_n$, where R_1 is the

TABLE 2 Summary of identification systems available in 1997

System	Manufacturer	Organisms targeted	Storage temp (°C)	No. of tests	Incubation	Automated
AN	Biolog	Anaerobes	2–8	95	4–16 h; aerobic	No
ANI	bioMérieux Vitek	Anaerobes	2–8	28	4 h; aerobic	Fill only[a]
API An-IDENT	bioMérieux Vitek	Anaerobes	2–8	28	4 h; aerobic	No
API 20A	bioMérieux Vitek	Anaerobes	2–8	21	24 h; anaerobic	No
API 20C AUX	bioMérieux Vitek	Yeasts	2–8	20	48–72 h	No
API 20E	bioMérieux Vitek	*Enterobacteriaceae* and nonfermenting gram-negative bacteria	2–8	21	24–48 h	No
API 20 Strep (Rapid STREP)	bioMérieux Vitek	Streptococci and enterococci	2–8	20	4–24 h	No
API Coryne (Rapid CORYNE)	bioMérieux Vitek	Corynebacteria and coryne-like organisms	2–8	20	24 h	No
API 20 NE (API NFT)	bioMérieux Vitek	Gram-negative non-*Enterobacteriaceae*	2–8	20	24–48 h	No
API Rapid 20E (Rapid E)	bioMérieux Vitek	*Enterobacteriaceae*	2–8	21	4 h	No
API Staph (STAPH-Trac)	bioMérieux Vitek	Staphylococci and micrococci	2–8	20	24 h	No
Crystal Anaerobe	BDMS[b]	Anaerobes	2–8	29	4 h	No
Crystal E/NF	BDMS	*Enterobacteriaceae*, some gram-negative nonfermenters	2–8	30	18–20 h	No
Crystal Gram-Positive	BDMS	Gram-positive cocci and bacilli	2–8	29	18–24 h	No
Crystal MRSA ID	BDMS	Methicillin-resistant *Staphylococcus aureus*	2–25	1	4 h	No
Crystal *Neisseria/Haemophilus*	BDMS	*Neisseria*, *Haemophilus*, *Moraxella*, *Gardnerella* spp., other fastidious pathogens	2–8	29	4 h	No
Crystal Rapid Gram-Positive	BDMS	Gram-positive cocci and bacilli	2–8	29	4 h	No
Crystal Rapid Stool/Enteric	BDMS	Gram-negative stool pathogens	2–8	30	3 h	No
Enterotube II	BDMS	*Enterobacteriaceae*	2–8	15	18–24 h	No
EPS (Enteric Pathogen Screen)	bioMérieux Vitek	*Edwardsiella*, *Salmonella*, *Shigella*, *Yersinia* spp.	2–8	10	4–8 h	Fill only
Fox Extra GNI	Medical Specialties, Inc.	Enteric and nonenteric gram-negative bacteria	−20 to −40	33	18–24 h	No
GN Microplate	Biolog	Aerobic gram-negative bacteria	2–8	95	4–24 h	Reader only[c]
GNI	bioMérieux Vitek	*Enterobacteriaceae* and other nonfermenting bacteria	2–8	29	2–18 h	Yes
GNI+	bioMérieux Vitek	*Enterobacteriaceae* and other nonfermenting bacteria	2–8	28	2–12 h	Yes
GP Microplate	Biolog	Most gram-positive cocci and bacilli	2–8	95	4–24 h	Reader only
GPI	bioMérieux Vitek	Gram-positive cocci and bacilli	2–8	29	2–15 h	Yes
ID 32 Staph	bioMérieux Vitek	Staphylococci	2–8	26	24 h	No
ID Tri-Panel	BDMS/Difco	Gram-negative and gram-positive bacteria	−70 to −20	30	16–20 h; 40–44 h	Reader only
Micro-ID	IDS[d]	*Enterobacteriaceae*	2–8	15	4 h	No

Minitek	BDMS	Anaerobes, *Enterobacteriaceae*, gram-positive bacteria, *Neisseria* spp., nonfermenters, and yeasts	2–25	4–21 depending on need	4 h for *Enterobacteriaceae* and *Neisseria* spp.; 72 h for yeasts	No
NEG ID Type 2	Dade MicroScan	*Enterobacteriaceae*, other fermenting and nonfermenting bacteria	2–8	36	15–42 h	Yes
Neisseria Enzyme Test	Remel	*Neisseria*, *Moraxella* spp.	2–8	3	30 min	No
NHI	bioMérieux Vitek	*Neisseria*, *Haemophilus* spp.	2–8	15	4 h	No
Oxi/Ferm II	BDMS	Gram-negative, oxidase-positive glucose fermenters and nonfermenters	2–8	9	24–48 h	No
Pos ID	Dade MicroScan	Gram-positive cocci and *Listeria* spp.	2–30	27	18–48 h	Yes
quadFERM +	bioMérieux Vitek	*Neisseria* spp., *Moraxella catarrhalis*	2–8	4	2 h	No
RapID ANA II	Innovative Diagnostics (IDS)	Anaerobes	2–8	18	4–6 h; aerobic	No
Rapid Anaerobe	Dade MicroScan	Anaerobes	2–8	24	4 h; aerobic	Yes
RapID CB Plus	IDS	Coryneform bacilli	2–8	18	4 h	No
RAPIDEC STAPH	bioMérieux Vitek	Staphylococci	2–8	4	2 h	No
Rapid HNID	Dade MicroScan	*Neisseria*, *Haemophilus*, *Moraxella catarrhalis*, *Gardnerella vaginalis*	2–8	18	4 h	Yes
Rapid NEG ID Type 2	Dade MicroScan	*Enterobacteriaceae*, other fermenting and nonfermenting bacteria	2–8	36	2 h	Yes
Rapid NEG ID Type 3	Dade MicroScan	*Enterobacteriaceae*, other fermenting and nonfermenting bacteria	2–8	36	2.5 h	Yes
RapID NF Plus	IDS	Nonfermenting gram-negative bacteria	2–8	17	4 h	No
RapID NH	IDS	*Neisseriaceae*, *Haemophilus* spp., and other gram-negative bacteria	2–8	13	4 h; 1 h for gonococci	No
RapID onE	IDS	*Enterobacteriaceae* and other oxidase-negative bacteria	2–8	19	4 h	No
Rapid POS ID	Dade MicroScan	Gram-positive cocci and *Listeria* spp.	2–8	34	2 h	Yes
RapID SS/u	IDS	Common urinary tract pathogens	2–8	11	2 h	No
RapID STR	IDS	Streptococci	2–8	14	4 h	No
Rapid Yeast ID	Dade MicroScan	Yeast	2–8	27	4 h	Yes
RapID Yeast Plus	IDS	Yeast and yeast-like organisms	2–8	18	4 h	No
r/b Enteric Differential System	Remel	*Enterobacteriaceae*	2–8	15	18–24 h	No
Sensititre AP 80	AccuMed International, Inc.	*Enterobacteriaceae* and nonfermenting gram-negative bacteria	RT[e]	32	5–18 h	Yes
UID/UID-3	bioMérieux Vitek	Urinary tract pathogens directly from urine	2–8	9	1–13 h	Yes
Uni-N/F-Tek	Remel	Gram-negative, fermenting and nonfermenting bacteria	2–8	18	24–48 h	No
Uni-Yeast Tek	Remel	Yeasts	2–8	13	24 h–6 days	No
YBC	bioMérieux Vitek	Yeasts	2–8	26	24–48 h	Yes
YT	Biolog	Yeasts	2–8	94	24–72 h	No

[a] Strips are filled automatically but read visually.
[b] Becton Dickinson Microbiology Systems.
[c] Plates are filled manually, but the system has an automated reading device.
[d] IDS products now owned by Remel.
[e] Room temperature.

TABLE 3 Comparison of features of automated identification systems[a]

Feature	Value for automated identification system:						
	Vitek	autoSCAN-4	Walk/Away	Sensititre	Biolog	MIS	AutoSceptor
Capacity of system	32/60/120	Unlimited	40/96	92	Unlimited	60	Unlimited
No. of species in database/no. of substrates[b]							
GN	116 (29)	112 (35)	139 (35[c], 36[d])	147 (32)	566 (95)	480 (NA)[e]	78 (24)
GP	50 (29)	49 (29)	49 (29[c], 34[d])	No	246 (95)	240 (NA)	No
ANA	No	58 (25)	54 (25)	No	No	815 (NA)	No
FAS	No	21 (18)	20 (18)	No	No	50 (NA)	No
ENV	No	No	No	No	No	300 (NA)	No
Yeasts	36 (26)	40 (27)	42 (27)	No	Included in GN	194 (NA)	No
Myco	No	No	No	No	No	28 (NA)	No
Inoculation	Automated	Manual	Manual	Automated	Manual	Automated	Automated
Incubation	On-line	Off-line	On-line	On-line	Off-line	On-line	Off-line
GN	2–18 h	24 or 48 h	2 or 15–42 h	5 or 18 h	4 or 16 h	30 min	18–24 h
GP	2–15 h	24 or 48 h	2 or 15–42 h		4 or 16 h	30 min	
ANA	N/A	4 h	4 h			30 min	
ENV	N/A				4 or 16 h	30 min	
Yeast	24 or 48 h	4 h	4 h			30 min	
Myco	NA					30 min	
Manual reagent addition	No	Yes	No	No	No	No	Yes
Additional tests required before incubation	Yes	Yes	Yes	No	No	No	Yes
Storage temp	4°C	RT[f], 4°C[g]	RT[f], 4°C[g]	RT	4°C	RT	RT
Other features							
Susceptibility testing	Yes	Yes	Yes	Yes	No	No	Yes
Urine screen/identification	Yes	No	No	No	No	No	Yes
DMS[h]	Yes	Yes	Yes	Yes	Yes	Yes	Yes
Computer interface	Yes	Yes	Yes	Yes	No	Yes	Yes
List price	$39,500/$67,500/ $84,500	$45,900	$85,000/$125,000	$42,500	$31,412	$45,000	—[i]

[a] Modified from reference 7 and updated in 1997.
[b] Number of groups, genera, or species identified; GN, aerobic gram-negative bacilli; GP, aerobic gram-positive cocci; ANA, anaerobic bacteria; FAS, fastidious bacteria; ENV, environmental bacteria/species; Myco, mycobacteria.
[c] Conventional identification panel.
[d] Fluorogenic identification panel.
[e] NA, not applicable.
[f] RT, room temperature.
[g] All rapid identification panels.
[h] DMS, Data Management System.
[i] AutoSceptor hardware is no longer available for purchase; however, all disposables and panels are still available to current owners of the system.

TABLE 4 Database entries of the *Enterobacteriaceae* (human isolates)

Species	API 20E v. 10.1[a]	BBL Crystal v. 3.0	IDS RapID onE v. 1.93	Vitek		MicroScan		Biolog v. 3.5	Midi v. 3.9
				GNI v. R5.03	GNI + v. R5.03	Conv. v. 20.55	Rapid v. 20.55		
Budvicia aquatica					×			×	
Buttiauxella agrestis								×	
Cedecea davisae	×	×	×	×	×	×	#[b]	×	×
Cedecea lapagei	×	×	×	×	×	×	#	×	×
Cedecea neteri	×	×	×			×	#	×	×
Cedecea sp. 3	×		×			×	#		
Cedecea sp. 5	×		×			×	#		
Citrobacter amalonaticus	×	×	×	×	×	×	× (*diversus*)	×	×
Citrobacter braakii					×				
Citrobacter farmeri					×				
Citrobacter freundii	×	×	×	×	× (group)	×	×	× (group)	×
Citrobacter koseri	× (*diversus*)	×	× (*diversus*)	×	×	×	× (*amalonaticus*)	×	×
Citrobacter sedlakii					× (group)				
Citrobacter sp. 10					× (group)				
Citrobacter sp. 11					× (group)				
Citrobacter werkmanii					× (group)				
Citrobacter youngae					× (*freundii*)				
Edwardsiella hoshinae	×	×	×		×			×	×
Edwardsiella tarda	×	×	×	×	×	×	×	×	×
Enterobacter agglomerans group	× (four types)		×			×	×	×	×
Enterobacter amnigenus group 1			×	× (1 and 2)	×	×	×	× (1 and 2)	×
Enterobacter amnigenus group 2			×	× (1 and 2)	×	×	×	× (1 and 2)	×
Enterobacter aerogenes	×	×	×	×	×	×	×	×	×
Enterobacter asburiae	×	×	×	×	× (*cloacae*)	×	×	×	×
Enterobacter cancerogenus	×[c]	×[c]	×[c]	×[c]	×	×[c]	×[c]	×[c]	×
Enterobacter cloacae	×	×	×	×	×	×	×	×	×
Enterobacter gergoviae	×	×	×	×	×	×	×	×	×
Enterobacter hormaechei				×	×			×	
Enterobacter intermedium	×		×	×	×	×	×	×	×
Enterobacter sakazakii	×	×	×	×	×	×	×	×	×
Escherichia coli	×	×	×	×	×	×	×	×	×
Escherichia fergusonii	×	×	×	×	×	×	×	×	×
Escherichia hermannii	×	×	×	×	×	×	×	×	×
Escherichia vulneris	×	×	×	×	×	×	×	×	×
Ewingella americana	×	×	×	×	×	×	×	×	
Hafnia alvei	×	×	×	×	×	×	×	×	×
Klebsiella ornithinolytica	× (group 47)	×	×		×	×	×	×	
Klebsiella oxytoca	×	×	×	× (*pneumoniae*)	× (*pneumoniae*)	×	×	×	×
Klebsiella ozaenae	×	×	×	×	×	×	×	×	×
Klebsiella planticola			×					×	×
Klebsiella pneumoniae	×	×	×	× (*oxytoca*)	× (*oxytoca*)	×	×	×	×
Klebsiella rhinoscleromatis	×	×	×	×	×	×	×	×	×

(*Continued on next page*)

TABLE 4 Database entries of the *Enterobacteriaceae* (human isolates) (*Continued*)

Species	API 20E v. 10.1[a]	BBL Crystal v. 3.0	IDS RapID onE v. 1.93	Vitek		MicroScan		Biolog v. 3.5	Midi v. 3.9
				GNI v. R5.03	GNI+ v. R5.03	Conv. v. 20.55	Rapid v. 20.55		
Klebsiella terrigena								×	×
Kluyvera ascorbata	#	×	×	#	#	×	#	×	×
Kluyvera cryocrescens	#	×	×	#	#	×	#	×	×
Leclercia adecarboxylata	×	×	×	×	×	×	×	×	×
Leminorella grimontii			×			#	#	×	×
Leminorella richardii			×			#	#	×	×
Moellerella wisconsensis	×	×	×		×	×	×	×	
Morganella morganii	×	×	×	×	×	×	×	×	×
Pantoea dispersa								×	
Pantoea agglomerans	× (*E. agglomerans*)	×		×	×			×	× (*E. agglomerans*)
Pragia fontium								×	
Proteus mirabilis	×	×	×	×	×	×	×	×	×
Proteus penneri	×	×	×	× (*vulgaris*)	× (*vulgaris*)	×	×	× (*vulgaris*)	×
Proteus vulgaris	×	×	× (two groups)	× (*penneri*)	× (*penneri*)	×	×	× (*penneri*)	×
Providencia alcalifaciens	×	×	×	×	×	×	× (*rustigianii*)	×	×
Providencia rettgeri	×	×	×	×	×	×	×	×	×
Providencia rustigianii		×	×			×	× (*alcalifaciens*)	×	×
Providencia stuartii	×	×	×	×	×	×	×	×	×
Rahnella aquatilis		×	×		×			×	×
Salmonella spp.	× (eight groups)	× (five groups)	× (three groups)	× (five groups)	× (three groups)	× (five groups)	× (five groups)	× (eight groups)	×
Serratia ficaria		×							
Serratia fonticola	×	×		×	×	×	×	×	
Serratia liquefaciens	×	×	×	×	×	×	×	×	×
Serratia marcescens	×	×	×	×	×	×	×	×	×
Serratia odorifera group 1	×	×	×	× (1 and 2)	× (1 and 2)	×	×	× (1 and 2)	×
Serratia odorifera group 2	×	×	×	× (1 and 2)	× (1 and 2)	×	×	× (1 and 2)	×
Serratia plymuthica	×	×	×	×	×	×	×	×	×
Serratia rubidaea	×	×	×	×	×	×	×	×	×
Shigella sp.	× (four spp.)	× (three spp.)	× (two spp.)	× (four spp.)	× (three spp.)	× (two spp.)	× (two spp.)	× (four spp.)	×
Tatumella ptyseos		×	×			×		×	
Trabulsiella guamensis								×	×
Yersinia pseudotuberculosis	×	×	×	×	×	×	×	×	
Yersinia enterocolitica	×	× "group"	×	×	×	× "group"	× "group"	×	
Yersinia frederiksenii	×	× "group"	×	×	×			×	
Yersinia intermedia	×	× "group"	×	×	×			×	
Yersinia kristensenii	×	× "group"	×	×	×			×	
Yersinia pestis	×			×	×	×		×	
Yersinia ruckeri	×					×	×	×	
Yokenella regensburgei	× (*Koserella*)	×	× (*Koserella*)		×	×	× (*Koserella*)		

[a] Software version. [b] #, Genus-only designation. [c] Reported as *Enterobacter taylorae*.

result for test 1, R_2 is the result for test 2, etc., for a given taxon. We can then incorporate the percentages (likelihoods that t_i will exhibit R_1, etc.) into Bayes's theorem to arrive at an accurate taxon.

Clinical microbiologists must not, however, become dependent upon these likelihoods and percentages when interpretive judgement would suggest an alternative taxonomic conclusion. Bacteria often tend to stretch the rules of nomenclature when isolated from clinical specimens, and they may not react as expected in a commercial system even though a legitimate result is produced (e.g., lactose-positive *Salmonella* spp. or H_2S-positive *E. coli*). The result from the most reliable system can be misleading! In these cases, a backup method of identification must be used. D'Amato et al. have described how the systems use the database profiles and probability matrices to arrive at an identification of an unknown taxon (1, 2).

Commercial manufacturers of identification systems rely heavily on input from their clients and customers. Laboratorians are encouraged to communicate with the product manufacturer about problems such as unusual organism identifications that develop when a method or system is being used. Manufacturers depend on customer satisfaction, and most are willing to assist in problem-solving or in projects that could add strength to their system. These companies, like their users, are clearly interested in the highest quality of cost-effective patient care. Tables 2 through 4 provide a summary of available identification systems and compare the salient features offered by the automated and nonautomated organism identification methods.

LIMITATIONS OF THE SYSTEMS

The databases of microbial identification systems must be frequently revised to accommodate newly named species. For example, if a physician requested that specimens from children with chronic otitis media be screened for the presence of *Alloiococcus* species and that organism was not present in the system's database, it would be necessary to explain that such screening could not be done routinely with the instrumentation in the laboratory and would require additional testing methods. Laboratorians must be aware that the accuracy of their system is limited only to the claims of the manufacturer for the version of the database currently in the instrument and that it may be outdated.

These limitations must be understood by the laboratorian, whose job it is to inform the physician why the laboratory may be unable to accommodate an analytic request or why the results may be delayed or even inaccurate.

The laboratory procedure manual must stipulate the action to take when a result is questionable either because of the unusual biochemical profile of the organism or because an unexpected susceptibility profile appeared. A backup method must be used to achieve an accurate identification profile. Otherwise the isolate should be sent to a reference laboratory for analysis.

The biochemical properties of closely related species may make it difficult or impossible for the algorithms of the identification process to separate these organisms accurately. For example, accurate identification of all of the newly recognized *Citrobacter* species may not be possible for some of the systems. In this case, the effect on patient outcome of the inability of a system to recognize *C. werkmanii* may be negligible, and a simple report of "*Citrobacter* species" may provide adequate data for patient management.

Consequently, laboratorians must pay attention to the manufacturer's communications about products, such as letters, notices, or test exclusions regarding the accuracy of their methods, as well as the published literature describing the potential problems encountered by others using these identification systems.

REFERENCES

1. **D'Amato, R. F., E. J. Bottone, and D. Amsterdam.** 1991. Substrate profile systems for the identification of bacteria and yeasts by rapid and automated approaches, p. 128–136. *In* A. Balows, W. J. Hausler, Jr., K. L. Herrmann, H. D. Isenberg, and H. J. Shadomy (ed.), *Manual of Clinical Microbiology*, 5th ed. American Society for Microbiology, Washington, D.C.
2. **D'Amato, R. F., B. Holmes, and E. J. Bottone.** 1981. The systems approach to diagnostic microbiology. *Crit. Rev. Microbiol.* **9:**1–44.
3. **Edberg, S. C., and L. S. Konowe.** 1982. A systematic means to conduct a microbiology evaluation, p. 268–299. *In* V. Lorian (ed.), *Significance of Medical Microbiology in the Care of Patients*, 2nd ed. The Williams & Wilkins Co., Baltimore, Md.
4. **Federal Register.** 1992. Clinical Laboratory Improvement Amendments of 1988; final rule. *Fed. Regist.* **57:**7164.
5. **Hartman, P. A.** 1968. *Miniaturized Microbiological Methods*. Academic Press, Inc., New York, N.Y.
6. **Miller, J. M.** 1991. Guest commentary: evaluating biochemical identification systems. *J. Clin. Microbiol.* **29:** 1559–1561.
7. **Stager, C. E., and J. R. Davis.** 1992. Automated systems for identification of microorganisms. *Clin. Microbiol. Rev.* **5:**302–327.
8. **Willcox, W. R., S. P. Lapage, S. Bascomb, and M. A. Curtis.** 1973. Identification of bacteria by computer: theory and programming. *J. Gen. Microbiol.* **77:**317–330.

Immunoassays for the Diagnosis of Infectious Diseases*

JAMES B. MAHONY AND MAX A. CHERNESKY

12

Immunoassays by definition are procedures which measure antigens or antibodies to determine whether patients are infected or immunologically responding to infection or immunization. The more traditional assays, such as hemagglutination inhibition, neutralization, or complement fixation, which have played important roles in diagnosis and which have enhanced understanding of the natural history of disease, are described in detail elsewhere (7, 15, 19). This chapter will describe immunoassays in greater use at the present time for the diagnosis of infectious diseases.

The diagnosis of infectious diseases with immunoassays involves two general approaches: testing for specific microbial antigens or testing for microbial antigen-specific antibodies. Antigen tests can be applied for the direct detection of microorganisms in a clinical specimen or for identification of a given agent after it has been cultivated. Antibody assays can be used to measure any antibody response regardless of immunoglobulin class or to detect class-specific antibody. Immunoglobulin M (IgM) antibodies appear earlier during infection, whereas IgG antibodies appear later, generally reaching peak levels in serum 4 to 6 weeks after infection and often persisting for life. Because the IgM antibody response is transient, the presence of this antibody indicates recent infection, and determination of specific IgM antibody and thus diagnosis of infection can be made with a single serum specimen. IgM antibody responses, however, do not occur solely during primary infections and in some cases may persist for long periods of time. Persistence of IgM may also depend on the infectious agent. Thus, the suitability of IgM antibody testing needs to be evaluated for each infectious agent.

For immunodiagnostic tests measuring IgG antibody, paired sera are required: one taken during the acute phase of the disease (preferably within 5 to 7 days of the onset of symptoms) and one taken during convalescence (3 to 4 weeks later). A fourfold or greater increase in IgG antibody titer is considered evidence of recent or current infection.

Other classes of immunoglobulins offer variable diagnostic opportunities. Serum IgA antibodies vary greatly as to when they first appear and how long they persist and are not routinely used for immunodiagnosis. Serum IgE antibodies may be elevated in parasitic infections but are not specifically associated with other infectious agents. The diagnostic role of IgD has not been determined.

Immunoassays may be constructed as liquid-phase immunoassays (LPIA) or solid-phase immunoassays (SPIA). LPIA were popularized in the field of chemistry but have not been extensively explored for microbiology. Most LPIA are competitive between the assayed sample and the labelled sample. After determination of the fraction of a labelled sample bound by antigen or antibody, the concentration of the sample can be calculated by comparison with results for appropriate standards. In the absence of a solid phase to separate labelled and unlabelled samples, the procedure depends upon a change in the specific enzyme activity when antibody-antigen complexes form.

SPIA for the detection of antigens or antibodies use as reaction indicators a radioactive label for a radioimmunoassay (RIA), an enzyme which will react with a substrate in an enzyme immunoassay (EIA), or a fluorescent dye for a fluorescence immunoassay. The substrate to be acted on by an enzyme may be fluorescent, radioactive, chemiluminescent, or chromogenic.

The first EIA was described by Engvall and Perlman in 1971 (11). They used the method of Nakane and Pierce (32) to conjugate the enzyme horseradish peroxidase (HRP) to an immunoglobulin preparation and used this enzyme conjugate for the detection of specific immunoglobulin in plastic microtiter plates. They termed this solid-phase assay an enzyme-linked immunosorbent assay. An improved one-step method of conjugation was subsequently described and has been used widely. Early solid-phase EIAs were less sensitive than corresponding RIAs, but gradual improvements in enzyme-labelling techniques have increased the sensitivity of the former and made these two types of assays comparable for detecting a number of antigens and antibodies.

SPIA COMPONENTS

Solid Phases

A number of surfaces can be used for SPIA: plastic, polyvinyl chloride, nitrocellulose, agarose, glass, cellulose, polyacrylamide, and dextran. Plastic is the most popular solid phase, especially with the frequent use of 96-well microtiter plates. These plates can also be purchased as 8- or 12-well individual strips for testing a small number of samples. Plastic beads

* This chapter contains information presented in chapter 11 by John E. Herrmann in the sixth edition of this Manual.

are also popular, especially with some commercial companies. Most antigens and antibodies are bound through hydrophobic interactions. Proteins generally are used at a concentration of 1 to 50 μg/ml. A high-pH (9.6) carbonate coating buffer is often used as the diluent; however, the optimal buffer needs to be determined experimentally for each system. In addition to passive absorption, immunoreactants can be coupled covalently by a variety of methods.

Absorption depends on the concentration and type of antigen, surface characteristics of the plastic, time, and temperature. Several studies have shown that the use of too much antigen may actually result in the stacking of several layers of antigen, which results in a protein-plastic layer that is subsequently covered by a second layer formed by protein-protein interactions. To avoid this problem, at least three washes, preferably more, need to be performed between assay steps. Both the isoelectric point and the chemical composition of the antigen may affect its ability to adhere to the solid phase. Lipid antigens may pose difficulties in obtaining reproducible coating of the wells of the solid phase. It is critical with these types of antigens that several plates be screened for optimal coating. In addition, the physical characteristics of 96-well microtiter plates have important variables such as an "edge effect," in which the perimeter wells of plates may absorb more protein than the inner wells, thereby causing an assay bias. Different plates from several manufacturers should be screened for this effect when an assay is set up. When a new lot of plates is used, they should be reevaluated to ensure that none of the assay parameters need to be modified. Coated plates generally are stable for a few weeks to several months, depending on conditions. Most antigens have the greatest stability when desiccated in a foil pack. Commercial kits usually have plates packaged in this way, providing a longer shelf life. For in-house assays in which stable packaging may be more difficult to achieve, the integrity of the solid phase should be closely monitored. A procedure which should be done at all times is to wash stored plates prior to use so as to remove any free antigen that may have desorbed during storage.

Conjugates

Depending on the assay, an EIA must contain either an antibody or an antigen conjugated with an enzyme. The desirable properties of such an enzyme include a high turnover rate, stability, low cost, ease of conjugation, lack of endogenous enzyme in the patient sample, easy detection, and compatibility with the standard conditions used. The most popular enzymes are alkaline phosphatase (AP) and HRP. A variety of other enzymes are also available, but they are not used as frequently; they include β-galactosidase, glucose oxidase, urease, and carbonic anhydrase, which are primarily used in immunohistochemistry and for assays with a fluorometric or other end point (22).

There are a number of choices available for an antibody conjugate: crude polyclonal antibodies, IgG fractions, $F(ab')_2$ fragments of polyclonal antibodies, affinity-purified polyclonal antibodies, or monoclonal antibodies. It is best to screen several antibody preparations and choose the conjugate that provides optimal results for the lowest cost. The least purified antibodies, such as crude polyclonal antibodies, are inexpensive, but they frequently give high background levels. This problem often can be alleviated with the use of an IgG fraction of the same antisera. If one is performing an IgM assay or using an antigen source containing Fc receptors, the use of $F(ab')_2$ fragments may significantly improve results. Overall, affinity-purified antibodies often give the best results, with high detectability and low background levels. In addition, they are available from several commercial companies and are relatively inexpensive. AP-conjugated affinity-purified antibodies are generally more expensive than HRP conjugates. Monoclonal antibodies are the most expensive, but some assays require the specificity that they offer. In choosing the proper dilution of an antibody conjugate, one can run a checkerboard titration with high- and low-positive standards along with buffer alone. The optimal conjugate dilution is one in which the absorbance of the high-positive control is 1.0 or greater, coupled with background levels of less than 0.1 absorbance unit.

Enzyme-Antibody Conjugation

Excellent-quality enzyme-labelled antibodies of various specificities are available from several commercial sources. However, in some circumstances it may be necessary to label antibodies in the laboratory. The procedure begins with enrichment of the antibodies from serum or ascites fluid. This initial step is required so that proteins other than antibodies will not be labelled and give false-positive results. Antibody enrichment is conveniently performed with ammonium sulfate fractionation, ion-exchange chromatography, or protein A columns. The second step is coupling of the enzyme to the antibody. Several methods, including periodate oxidation and glutaraldehyde procedures, are widely used (3, 32). The conditions used ordinarily result in optimum labelling of the antibody. Blocking solutions and wash buffers containing detergent are required to decrease nonspecific color intensity in EIA procedures. When the concentration of protein in the coating solution is suboptimal for the saturation of plate well binding sites, an immunologically irrelevant protein is used to occupy (block) the remaining plate surface. Buffers containing bovine serum albumin or gelatin are commonly used for this purpose. To prevent nonimmunological interactions in the plate wells, all subsequent reagents are added in buffers containing detergent (usually 0.1% Tween 20). In addition, all washing steps between reagent additions are also done with buffers containing Tween 20.

Substrates

When choosing a substrate for an enzyme conjugate, one should consider several factors. First, the substrate must produce a measurable soluble reaction product. For most EIAs, this is a colored reaction product, although fluorescent substrates can be used. Other variables to consider include sensitivity, background absorbance, stability of the compound, toxicity, and cost. Toxicity is a particular concern, since a number of substrates are suggested to be potentially carcinogenic. If the color will be monitored spectrophotometrically, the maximum wavelength of the absorbance is also a factor, since readers generally come with a limited number of filters.

A variety of substrates are available for HRP. The enzyme reduces hydrogen peroxide (H_2O_2) and oxidizes a second substrate, which produces a colored reaction product; thus, H_2O_2 is always required along with another substrate. The most popular substrates include *o*-phenylenediamine, 5-aminosalicylic acid, 2,2-asinodi-(3-ethylbenz-*o*-thiazoline-6-sulfonate, and 3,3′,5,5′-tetramethylbenzidine. Although various studies have shown some substrates to be preferable to others, generally they all perform adequately in most assays. When a new procedure is set up, several substrates may be evaluated to determine the optimal compound. Regardless of the secondary substrate used, the most critical variable in catalyzing HRP is the H_2O_2 concentration. H_2O_2 is usually kept as a 30% solution; however, it has limited stability and may account for significant interassay variability.

For AP, the most popular substrate is *p*-nitrophenyl phosphate, which absorbs strongly at 405 nm. *p*-Nitrophenyl phosphate is generally dissolved in a high-pH diethanolamine buffer with magnesium added. The use of phosphate-buffered saline (PBS) as a wash buffer in AP-based EIAs may result in low optical density (OD) values. Phosphate is a potent inhibitor of AP, so any phosphate left in the plate wells after washing may cause inhibition of the enzyme reaction. Although many laboratories report few problems with the use of PBS as the wash buffer in AP-catalyzed EIAs, it is a variable to consider if the color reaction does not develop sufficiently. One can substitute a Tris buffer for PBS, as Tris may actually increase AP activity.

Assay Enhancement

Bacterial Proteins

The immunoglobulin-binding properties of protein A make this molecule useful as a developing reagent in EIAs. Protein A covalently bound to enzymes is available from several commercial sources and can substitute for enzyme-labelled secondary antibodies in EIAs. Protein A binds poorly to human IgG3 and some immunoglobulins from other mammals. Protein G, a cell wall constituent of some *Streptococcus* strains, exhibits high-affinity interactions with these immunoglobulins (44). Protein G is used in EIAs much like protein A and is available in a genetically engineered form designed to reduce nonspecific interactions. It is also used to detect IgA and IgM responses to microbial antigens. In this method, IgG is removed from sera by use of protein G coupled to agarose. The residual antibodies are then incubated with the target antigen. The use of enzyme-labelled secondary antibodies that recognize the heavy chain of IgM or IgA allows the resolution of immune responses of these isotypes.

Avidin-Biotin

The strong interaction between avidin, an egg white protein, and biotin, a low-molecular-weight vitamin, has been used to amplify the sensitivity of EIAs. Each of the four subunits of avidin contains a site that interacts with the ureido ring of biotin. The remaining valeric acid side chain of the biotin molecule can be chemically modified to generate reactive groups without altering avidin interactions. The length of the spacer between the ureido group and the chemically reactive group is sufficient in several commercially available forms of biotin to allow attachment of the biotin to antibodies or enzyme and still permit interactions with avidin. Avidin itself may be covalently linked to enzyme reporter molecules by several available methods. Streptavidin from *Streptomyces avidinii* has a lower isoelectric point and is used more widely than egg white avidin because of lower background intensity. Use of avidin-biotin interactions in EIAs is accomplished in two different ways. The first method makes use of a biotinylated secondary antibody. Avidin-enzyme conjugates are then used to detect the bound biotinylated antibody. The increase in sensitivity over that of standard EIA methods results from a pyramid-like enhancement of reporter group molecules. The other major format of avidin-biotin EIAs takes advantage of the multivalency of avidin. Unconjugated avidin serves as a bridge between a biotinylated antibody and biotin-enzyme conjugates. Alternatively, complexes of avidin and biotinylated enzyme can be used to detect the biotinylated antibody (see the discussion of antigen detection assays below).

Chemiluminescent Substrates

The cyclic hydrazide luminol (5-amino-2,3-dihydro-1,4-phthalazinedione) can be used directly as a label (for example, for avidin) in SPIA or as a substrate to interact with peroxidase enzyme. Oxidation of luminol to a chemiluminescent product is catalyzed by free iron ions or chelated iron in peroxidase. An electronically excited aminophthalate anion decay provides an enhanced signal. Peroxidase conjugated to antibody may act more effectively on luminol than on chromogenic substrates because conjugation of peroxidase may destroy substantial amounts of enzyme activity but still allow the large heme (iron) donation needed to allow luminol oxidation to take place in a chemiluminescence test.

Radioactive Isotopes

Although the use of isotopes for diagnostic tests has fallen from popularity, the principles are worth discussing. The use of a radioactive conjugate in an SPIA may result in a more sensitive assay based on the kinetics of reaction of the components in the assay. The most commonly used isotope is ^{125}I, which is a weak gamma ray emitter with a half-life of 60 days. ^{125}I can be incorporated effectively into protein molecules of high specific activity by several methods without markedly affecting the immunological activity and specificity of the proteins. The most commonly used conjugation procedure is the chloramine-T method of Hunter and Greenwood (18).

Because the activity of labelled immunoglobulin preparations decreases continuously due to radioactive decay, frequent standardization is necessary.

RIAs can be used to measure antibodies from all body fluids. Nonspecific inhibitors of hemagglutination and anticomplementary factors, which seriously affect some serological antibody tests, do not interfere with the RIA. The expression of a serum antibody concentration with an endpoint titer is the most commonly used method of expressing RIA results. The specimens are tested in several serial dilutions, and the titer is interpolated from the counts per minute-serum dilution curve as the highest dilution at which the counts per minute of the test specimen is 2.1 times higher than the counts per minute of the negative control at the same dilution.

SPIA Readout Measurements

Each SPIA has characteristic methods for measuring and interpreting the reaction. The color development can be monitored visually for a qualitative result. For quantitative readings or a more sensitive qualitative assessment, a spectrophotometer can be used. The spectrophotometer can be interfaced with a microcomputer equipped with a data reduction package for direct calculation of results.

It is adequate for most assays to use air as a blank for OD measurements. However, some investigators prefer to use a well containing either substrate or substrate-antibody conjugate alone as a blank. If this procedure is used, it is important to document the absolute absorbance of the well used as a blank. An OD value much higher than 0.1 may indicate a deterioration in some of the assay components. For reporting the analyte in an absolute amount per milliliter, a reference preparation is used as the source of calibration. A number of these preparations are available from commercial companies, professional organizations, and government agencies. Instead of the use of a valuable reference preparation, a test can be calibrated against a standard and used for regular assays. A dose-response curve, consisting of the concentration of the reference preparation plotted against its absorbance, is made. When making this curve, one must carefully evaluate the characteristics of the data. Although a standard curve can often be constructed by simply plotting the absorbance against the log concentration and performing linear regression, this procedure may not be the best treatment for all systems. A variety of computer software packages (e.g., SAS or SPSS) offer a range of curve-fitting techniques for evaluating EIA data.

One common method of expressing data is to determine the mean absorbance of samples from normal individuals and report patient samples as positive when they are 2 or 3 standard deviations above this value. Although this method requires testing only one dilution of a patient sample, a number of problems can arise. From a statistical point of view, it may not be correct to apply a mean and a standard deviation to these types of data, as they are often not normally distributed and there may be an insufficient sample size to apply nonparametric statistics. The greatest problem with the use of absolute absorbance values is the poor reproducibility of results. To deal with this problem, one can use an adjusted absorbance value, in which the patient value is presented as a ratio or as a percentage of a positive control value. These methods are simple and incorporate an internal control but must be carefully standardized. It is important to monitor the level of absolute absorbance values to ensure that they are relatively constant from day to day and within the linear range of the assay. One can use a reference pool of sera with assigned arbitrary units to establish a dose-response curve and then determine patient values from the curve. In addition to extrapolating the values directly from the curve, some investigators have suggested determining the ratio of the area under the dose-response curve of the test serum and the reference serum. These techniques offer much improved reproducibility and a quantitative answer, but the required calculations are more time-consuming and may necessitate several dilutions of patient sera to obtain a value falling on the linear portion of the curve. Use of a microcomputer interfaced with the reader greatly simplifies the calculations.

Controls and Standardization

The basic controls in all assays should include a buffer, a negative sample, and low- and high-positive samples. Initially, one should assess the background absorbance of all reagents alone. One important control is to assess the binding of patient sera to the uncoated solid-phase material. In a minority of samples, significant binding to the solid phase occurs even when it is coated with a nonspecific protein. Such binding may be a problem, especially in IgM assays, and may require testing all samples in both coated and uncoated wells, with subtraction of the OD reading for the uncoated wells. Whenever reagents from new suppliers are used, comparative studies for equivalency should be performed. There can be significant variability within different lots of plates and the conjugate, and one can never assume that the assay parameters will remain unchanged. Factors such as alterations in room temperature and the quality of water can also significantly affect day-to-day variability in assays. For these reasons, reliance on standard curves will yield more reproducible results.

The absorbance in PBS control wells should be less than 0.1 (optimally less than 0.05) OD unit. If the absorbance is higher, the most likely reason is either inadequate washing or a problem with the enzyme conjugate. It may be important to increase the number and efficiency of the wash steps. If this action is not effective, the dilution and purity of the enzyme conjugate should be evaluated. If the conjugate cannot be diluted further without affecting the sensitivity of the assay, one should look for either a higher-avidity or an affinity-purified conjugate. Another way to deal with the problem is to add normal serum (1 to 5%) of the same species as the conjugate to the conjugate dilution buffer. In addition, the use of 1 to 5% bovine serum albumin or another nonspecific protein to bind nonreactive sites on the solid phase may correct the problem. Another problem—a high absorbance (>0.2 OD unit) of a negative patient sample—can be dealt with in the same manner as for the PBS control.

An unexpected decrease in the amount of an analyte at the high end of the dose-response curve (hook effect), resulting in a gross underestimation of the analyte, may be a problem in sandwich immunoassays with patient samples that contain an extremely high level of an analyte. The patient samples will give a low to moderately high result when the standard assay dilution is used. Upon further dilution of the sample, the result will either be out-of-range high or, if it is diluted enough, extremely elevated. Therefore, if the laboratory ran the sample only at the routine dilution, significant underestimation of the value would be reported. This problem may arise from low-affinity antibody, inadequate washing, or suboptimal concentrations of labelled antibody. Adequate washing should be performed between all steps, especially following the addition of each antibody. When one is performing new kit evaluations, testing specimens with high levels of the analyte is important, as the frequency of the hook effect with different kits may be variable.

Heterophile antibodies may interfere with sandwich EIAs. These antibodies can be directed to several different species (e.g., sheep, goat, mouse, and rabbit). Their presence can have a variable effect on SPIA. If the analyte is not present, a false-positive result may arise from the heterophile antibody cross-linking the two antibodies of the sandwich. As monoclonal antibody-based assays are often used for diagnostically important analytes, erroneous results can cause significant problems in patient care. The addition of nonimmune immunoglobulin from the appropriate species will eliminate this interference; however, the amount and source of the normal serum may be crucial.

By use of a systematic approach with some or all of these tactics, the majority of background problems can be solved.

ANTIGEN DETECTION ASSAYS

Most SPIA for the detection of antigen use one of three methods: competitive, direct (double-antibody sandwich method), or indirect (double-antibody sandwich-antiglobulin method). In competitive assays, labelled antigen is mixed with the test sample that may contain antigen, and they compete for a limited amount of antibody attached to the solid phase. A negative control sample containing only labelled antigen is included. Unbound antigen is washed away, and the difference in indicator activity between the specimen and the control is measured. The detector antibody can be labelled with enzyme, ^{125}I, or biotin, and the solid phase can be beads, plates, or tubes.

A direct SPIA for detection of antigen involves adding the clinical specimen to a capture antibody attached to the solid phase. Unbound antigen is washed away before the

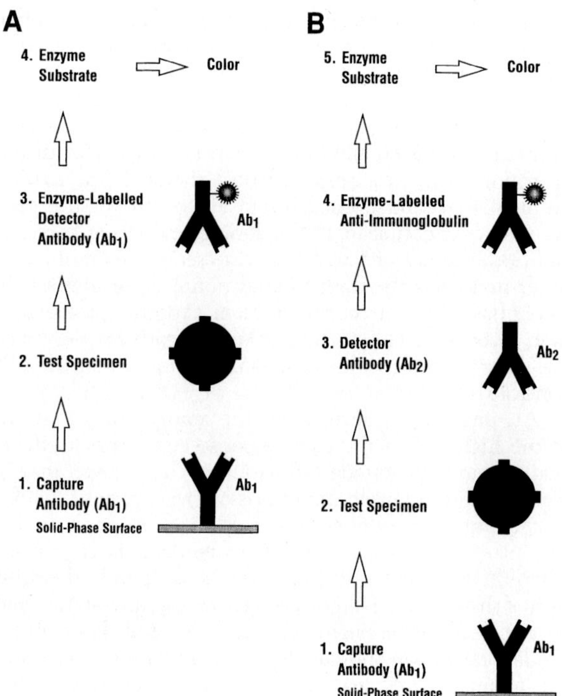

FIGURE 1 Antigen detection with direct (A) and indirect (B) EIAs. Specific capture antibody directed against the antigen being sought in a clinical specimen is bound to wells of microtiter plates. For the direct test, a specimen is added, followed by an enzyme-labelled DA and substrate. For the indirect test, a specimen is added, followed by an unlabeled DA, an enzyme-labelled anti-species IgG antibody, and substrate. A positive specimen is indicated by color development.

addition of a labelled detector antibody (DA). The DA is measured, and the more labelled substrate that is detected, the more antigen that is present in the sample (Fig. 1A). Assays with a combination of polyclonal capture and monoclonal detector antibodies usually provide the best performance. Sandwich assays have been developed for a number of microorganisms, including rotavirus (5), influenza virus (42), respiratory syncytial virus (23), astrovirus (16), *Legionella pneumophila* (1), and *Chlamydia trachomatis* (6), and several are now available as commercial kits.

The indirect test is similar to the direct test in that it uses a capture antibody and a DA, but the DA is not labelled. Instead, a third indicator antibody, which is an anti-immunoglobulin antibody raised in a different animal, is labelled; the remainder of the assay is similar to the direct assay (Fig. 1B). This approach has become the most popular because of the availability of indicator antibody conjugates from commercial sources. The indirect test provides some amplification of binding reactions. Their use may create some problems, however, as they are very sensitive and antispecies antisera may cross-react nonspecifically.

The immunodot assay (IDA) for antigen is similar to Western blotting for antibody, as both use nitrocellulose membranes. In the IDA, antigen in a clinical specimen is detected by dotting the specimen onto nitrocellulose and reacting the strip with antibody in either a direct or an indirect format. The IDA has been used to detect human immunodeficiency virus (HIV) following amplification of virus in H9 cell cultures (2) and to detect rotavirus antigen in stool specimens. A modification of the IDA called the immune complex dot assay, in which antigen is allowed to react with specific antibody and the antigen-antibody complex is spotted onto nitrocellulose and detected with colloidal gold-labelled antispecies antibody, has been described (46). The immune complex dot assay was more sensitive than the IDA for detecting rotavirus antigen in stool specimens (47).

Other antigen detection immunoassays include immunofluorescence, immunoelectron microscopy (IEM), and immunohistochemical staining. In immunofluorescence tests for microbial antigens, cells from clinical specimens, e.g., sputum, nasal washings, and bronchoalveolar lavage, are washed with PBS to remove mucus and placed onto glass slides. The specimens are fixed and then tested for the presence of a specific antigen by incubation with a fluorescein-labelled antibody in a direct test (Fig. 2A) or with a specific antibody and then fluorescein-labelled anti-immunoglobulin antibody in an indirect test (Fig. 2B). Direct or indirect immunofluorescence tests have been developed for many microorganisms, including *Treponema pallidum* (17) and *C. trachomatis* (37). More than one antigen or microbial species can be detected in a given specimen if the specific antibodies are labelled with different fluorescent dyes, such as fluorescein and rhodamine, that appear as different colors under fluorescent light. Alternatively, multiple antigens can be detected by an indirect approach with a panel of different primary antibodies and a fluorescein isothiocyanate-labelled anti-immunoglobulin provided that replicate specimen preparations are possible. This approach is widely used in virology laboratories for the detection of respiratory viruses in nasopharyngeal specimens (14).

IEM has been used for the detection of both bacterial and viral antigens. Solid tissue specimens can be embedded in plastic (Epon or Araldite), and thin sections can be cut with an ultramicrotome. Sections are placed onto electron microscope grids, which are then stained sequentially with specific antisera and colloidal gold-labelled anti-immuno-

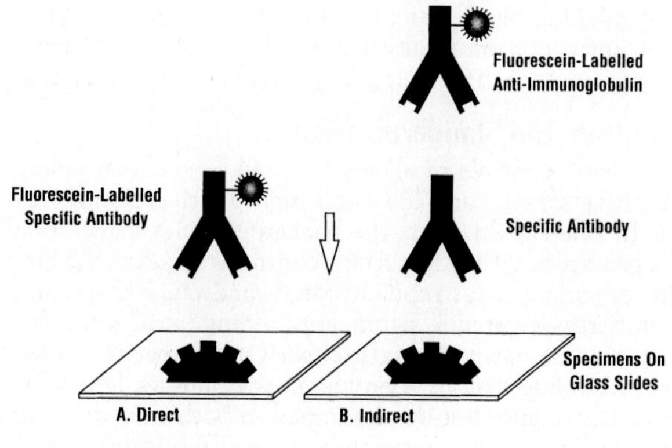

FIGURE 2 Detection of specific antigen with direct (A) and indirect (B) immunofluorescence assays. Cells from clinical specimens (e.g., nasopharyngeal swabs) are washed, deposited onto glass microscope slides, and fixed. Fluorescein-labelled antibodies to specific microorganism epitopes or unlabelled primary antibodies (as a negative control) followed by fluorescein isothiocyanate-labelled secondary anti-species IgG antibodies are added. Bound antibodies are visualized with a fluorescence microscope. Monoclonal antibodies are often used, giving more specific staining.

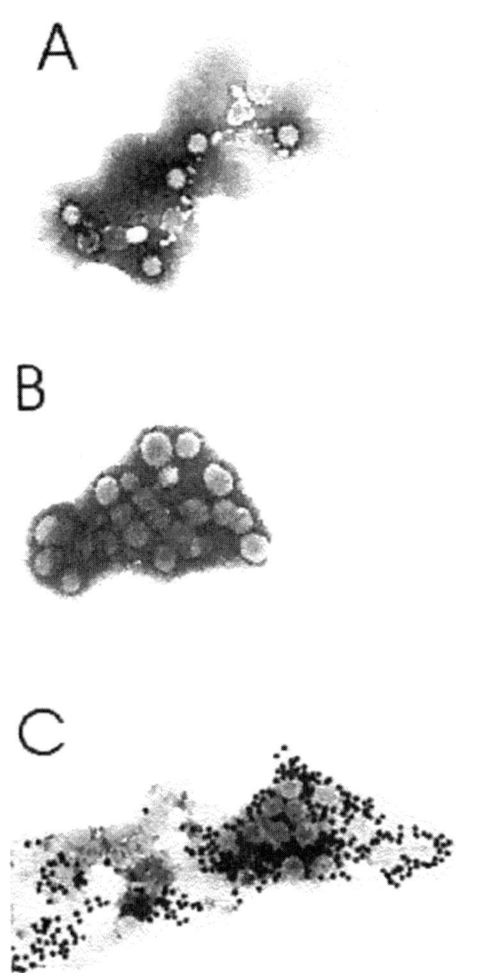

FIGURE 3 Detection of rotaviruses by IEM. (A) Rotavirus was detected in stool specimens by direct electron microscopy without antibody. (B) IEM was performed with antirotavirus antibody, causing aggregation of the virus particles. (C) IEM was performed with colloidal gold-labelled DA to enhance staining and identification in a solid-phase IEM format. Magnification, ×59,500.

globulin antibody by being floated on reagent drops placed on a Parafilm sheet. IEM has been used to investigate bacterial morphology or to confirm an association of new or unusual bacteria with a clinical presentation, e.g., *Borrelia burgdorferi* and Lyme disease (33). The technique has also been used to detect numerous viruses in a wide range of clinical specimens, including tissue, cerebrospinal fluid, urine, and vesicle fluid (27). Rotaviruses can be detected directly in stool specimens by IEM (44) (Fig. 3) and even typed with type-specific monoclonal antibodies. Solid-phase IEM uses antibody coated electron microscope grids for virus capture and has been used to detect polyomavirus BK in urine specimens and rotavirus antigen in stool specimens (27, 45).

The immunohistochemical staining technique involves several steps, including (i) histological preparation of paraffin sections on glass slides, (ii) deparaffinization of tissue with xylol and graded alcohols, (iii) replacement of alcohols with buffer, (iv) limited proteolysis of tissue, (v) reaction of tissue with specific antibodies (either monoclonal antibodies or polyclonal antisera, usually adsorbed to remove tissue cross-reactivity), and (vi) addition of enzyme-labelled antispecies antibody and appropriate substrate. The most widely used enzymes are AP and HRP. AP–anti-AP (APAAP) uses preformed enzyme-antibody complexes to increase the intensity of staining (9). Another modification, called the ABC method, uses biotinylated antispecies IgG antibody and reformed avidin-biotin complexes to increase staining intensity (12). APAAP and ABC reagents are available from several commercial suppliers. These methods have been used successfully to identify viruses or bacteria in tissues from patients with unique clinical presentations, including HIV in neuroblastoma cells (41), *C. trachomatis* in endometrial tissue (25), and *Chlamydia pneumoniae* and cytomegalovirus (CMV) in carotid endarterectomy specimens in patients with coronary heart disease (8).

Agglutination tests for detecting antigens use antibody-coated latex particles, which are stable for long periods of time. These rapid assays require only 15 to 30 min for completion and are simple to perform. Polystyrene beads of uniform size (generally, 1 to 5 μm) and coated with a specific antibody are mixed with a test specimen, and the suspension is examined for visible evidence of clumping. Antibody can be bound to latex beads by passive adsorption or covalent linkage by a variety of methods (38). Agglutination assays can be performed with tubes or slides. The reactions can also be recorded photometrically. Latex agglutination tests have found the widest application in detecting soluble antigens in urine, cerebrospinal fluid, and serum from patients with infections due to *Haemophilus influenzae*, *Streptococcus pneumoniae*, group A and B streptococci, *Neisseria meningitidis*, and group B and *Cryptococcus neoformans*.

The major problem to date with the use of agglutination tests for direct detection of viruses is their lack of sensitivity. EIA techniques amplify antigen-antibody reactions because of substrate turnover. In theory, one enzyme molecule can be detected; hence, one antibody molecule and one molecule of analyte can also be detected. Agglutination reactions are not amplified but are based on antigen-antibody reactions forming visible complexes. This complex formation requires a larger number of antigen and antibody molecules than would be required for EIAs; thus, the sensitivity is lower. The sensitivity of an agglutination test may be satisfactory for diagnosing some bacterial infections, but the test may not be as useful for detecting viral infections, which have a much lower antigenic mass. For example, several commercial latex agglutination tests for the diagnosis of rotavirus infection are available for testing fecal samples, but they are less sensitive than EIAs (30).

ANTIBODY DETECTION ASSAYS

Principles of Antibody Detection

In competitive assays, human antibody against a viral antigen(s) can be measured by combining the sample with a predetermined amount of conjugated antibody directed against the same viral antigen(s) and incubating the mixture with the antigen-coated solid phase. Specific antibody, if present in the sample, will compete with the conjugated antibody for binding sites on the solid phase and lead to a reduction in the signal (Fig. 4B). The signal generated will be inversely proportional to the amount of antibody in the sample.

Antibodies against the antigens of interest can be prepared from animals or purified from human serum. Alternatively, specific monoclonal antibodies can be developed.

The antibodies must be purified, conjugated with the appropriate label (fluorochrome, enzyme, lanthanide, or radioisotope), and rigorously evaluated before use. An important aspect of conjugate evaluation involves the serial titration of the conjugate against serial dilutions of antigen to measure activity and define the titration curve of the conjugate across several antigen concentrations. Each conjugate titration curve will exhibit a point at which the next dilution of conjugate will exhibit a substantial drop in the signal. Several conjugate-antigen dilution pairs that meet the basic criteria should be selected and then further characterized with respect to sensitivity by use of preparations containing known amounts of antigen-specific antibody. The goal is to select the conjugate-antigen pair that contains the highest dilutions of conjugate and antigen which will permit the generation of a high signal, exhibit a substantial reduction in the signal in the presence of sample antibody, and allow the measurement of small amounts of sample antibody against important antigenic determinants.

Competitive assays are based on a limiting-reagent concept in which solid-phase antigen and conjugate concentrations are minimized so that even small quantities of sample antibody can effectively block the binding of the conjugate. An advantage of the use of the competitive format for antibody measurement is the relative ease with which highly specific antibodies, especially monoclonal antibodies, can be purified and conjugated. In general, antibodies are easier to purify than antigens, and since the specificity of a test is conveyed by the conjugate, a relatively impure antigen can be used on the solid phase. Competitive assays are generally more sensitive than indirect assays. Competitive RIAs and EIAs have been used to measure antibody to hepatitis B core antigen. An assay for antibody to hepatitis B core antigen has been commercialized by Abbott Diagnostics and has been used extensively in clinical laboratories for over 20 years (31, 35).

Either direct or indirect approaches may be used to construct a SPIA to measure antibodies in patient specimens (Fig. 4). The solid phase is usually coated with either antigen(s) or anti-immunoglobulin antibodies (anti-total or anti-class, i.e., anti-IgG, -IgM, -IgA, and so forth). If the solid phase is coated with antigen, all classes of antibodies in the specimen will be captured. A conjugated antispecies DA can then be used to detect all antibody classes trapped, or the DA can be specific for a class, such as anti-human IgM or IgG antibody. This approach usually requires the preadsorption of the specimen with anti-rheumatoid factor (RF) antibody or aggregated IgG to eliminate RF interference (described in more detail below). When antispecies antibodies are used on the solid phase, they are usually anti-IgM antibodies. This approach will capture only IgM, which will be available for the detector reagent (which can be enzyme-labelled antigen) to act on an added substrate. Alternatively, at this stage an unlabelled antigen is added and detected by a virus-specific DA (which may be labelled for a direct assay) or followed by a labelled antispecies antibody.

A further modification of the antibody class capture assay, and one that will permit the measurement of antigen-specific IgG, involves the use of labelled antigen and a solid phase coated with RF IgM. A sample containing antigen-specific IgG is mixed with a labelled conjugate and incubated with the solid-phase coated with RF IgM. Only antigen-specific IgG complexed with the labelled antigen is bound by RF IgM; therefore, only a single incubation step is required. Antigen quality, as well as the quality of RF IgM coating the solid phase, must be carefully assessed.

These techniques have been widely used to measure specific antiviral antibody and require only a few reagents. They are easy to perform and provide objective quantifiable results. This format has allowed commercial companies to develop automated instrumentation with increased throughput for processing several hundred specimens per day.

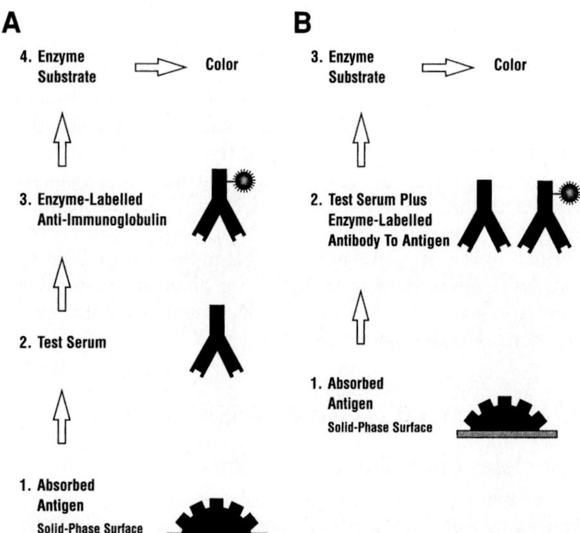

FIGURE 4 Detection of antibody by competitive and noncompetitive EIAs. Wells of microtiter plates are first coated with specific antigen. In the noncompetitive well (A), serum is added and specific antibody is detected with enzyme-labelled anti-species immunoglobulin antibody and substrate. In the competitive well (B), serum and an enzyme-labelled antibody are added together so that specific serum antibody will compete against the labelled antibody. A positive specimen is indicated by a reduction or the lack of color in the well following the addition of substrate.

IgM Measurement

The most common assays for IgM use a standard indirect SPIA with the antigen immobilized and an IgM-specific secondary DA. As mentioned above, false-positivity is common due to the presence of IgM RF in the patient sample. False-negativity can also occur from competitive inhibition of IgM binding in the presence of high levels of specific IgG. One way to approach these problems is to use an isolated IgM preparation from the patient sample, thereby removing IgG, which acts as a substrate for IgM RF and competes with specific IgM for binding to the antigen. Alternatively, one can remove all of the IgG with the addition of a precipitating anti-IgG antibody. Another approach is to remove RF by use of an aggregated IgG preparation, such as RF sorbent (Behringwerke) or Gullsorb (Gull Laboratories) (48).

The use of an IgM capture assay eliminates inherent interference problems (Fig. 5). In this procedure, a polyclonal anti-IgM antibody is bound to the solid phase. Upon incubation of the patient sample, all IgM will be captured on the plate. The test antigen is then added, binding any specific IgM present on the plate. An enzyme-labelled secondary antibody is then added, and the reaction is completed. This assay obviates the problems with false-negative results due to competitive inhibition with IgM, as all of the IgG in the patient sample is washed away in the first step. False-positive

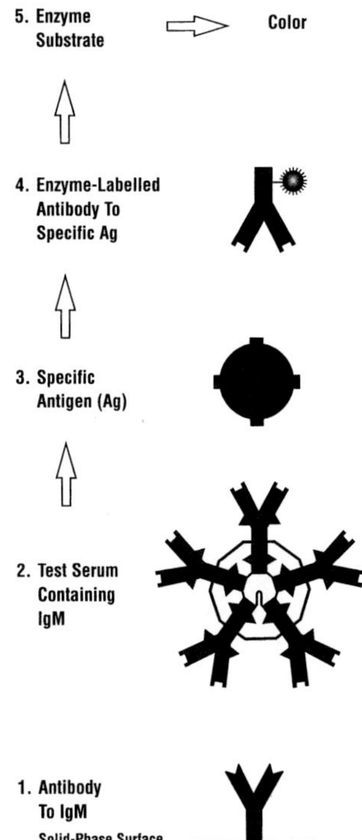

FIGURE 5 Detection of specific IgM antibody with an IgM capture EIA. Wells of microtiter plates coated with anti-human IgM antibody are reacted with serum specimens to capture specimen IgM antibody. Viral antigen, enzyme-labelled antiviral antibody, and substrate are added sequentially to detect specific antiviral IgM antibody.

results, however, may still occur as a result of bound IgM RF either reacting with the IgG conjugate or binding to any antigen-specific IgG in the sample. One way to avoid the problem with conjugate binding is to use $F(ab')_2$-conjugated antibodies. Alternatively, the assay can be modified to a direct technique by use of an enzyme-labelled antigen in the second step, thus eliminating any immunoglobulin that could bind RF. Even with these modifications, problems can still occur with borderline and low-positive IgM results.

Immunoblotting

Immunoblotting or Western blotting has been used to detect specific antibodies to a number of viruses. Viral proteins are separated by polyacrylamide gel electrophoresis, transblotted to nitrocellulose or nylon membranes, and then reacted with clinical specimens. Sera are usually immunoblotted, but saliva or urine can also be tested (Fig. 6). Recombinant immunoblot assays (RIBA) use recombinant proteins expressed in prokaryotic or eukaryotic expression systems instead of viral polypeptides in the form of purified viral antigens prepared from infected cell cultures. Western blotting and RIBA have been successfully commercialized, and supplementary or confirmatory kits are available for detecting antibodies to a number of viruses, including HIV type 1, human T-cell leukemia virus type 1, and hepatitis C virus. These assays can also be used for typing herpes simplex virus and HIV antibodies (21).

Radioimmunoprecipitation Assays

In radioimmunoprecipitation assays, specific antiviral antibodies are detected by immunoprecipitation of radiolabeled viral proteins followed by either scintillation counting of washed precipitates or immune complex dissociation, polyacrylamide gel electrophoresis, and autoradiography to identify specific proteins. This method has not had widespread application in virology but is used for confirming hepatitis C virus antibody and in place of Western blotting as a confirmatory test for HIV.

Immunofluorescence Assays

Both direct and indirect fluorescent-antibody techniques have been used for the detection of antimicrobial antibodies. To test for antibodies in a patient's serum, microbial

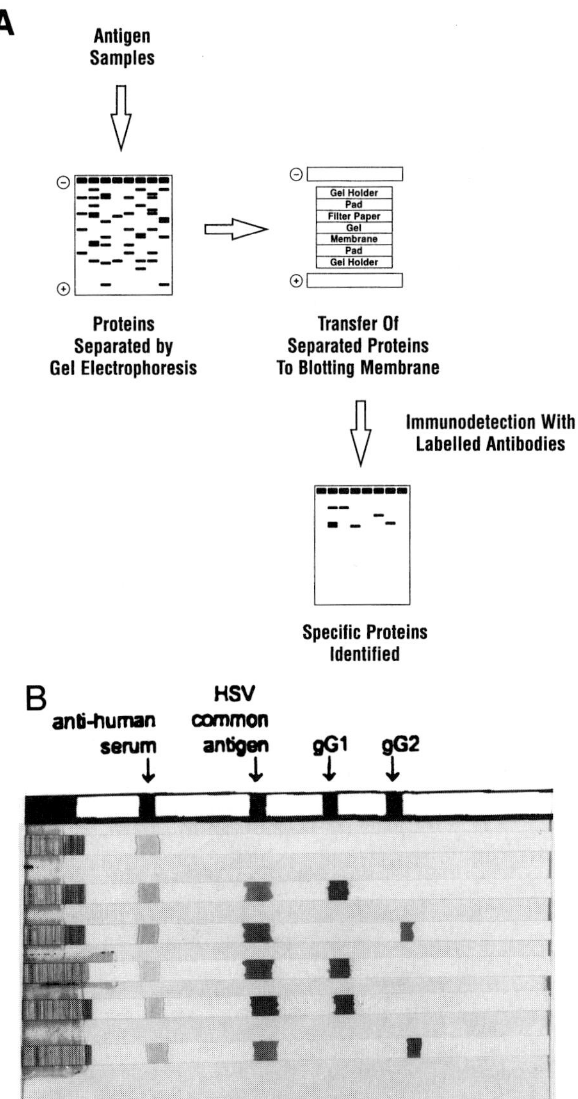

FIGURE 6 Detection of antimicrobial antibodies by immunoblotting. (A) Bacterial or viral antigens are separated by sodium dodecyl sulfate-polyacrylamide gel electrophoresis and transblotted to a sheet of nitrocellulose or nylon by capillary action (or electrophoretically). Strips containing separated polypeptides are reacted with serum specimens, and bound antibody is detected with enzyme-labelled anti-species IgG antibody and substrate. (B) RIBA for the detection of herpes simplex virus (HSV) type 1- and 2-specific antibodies.

antigens are dried onto multiwell glass slides and fixed with acetone or methanol. Dilutions of test sera are incubated with the antigens, the slides are washed, and fluorescein-labelled anti-immunoglobulin antibodies are added. The slides are washed again and air dried, and a coverslip is mounted on a few drops of buffered glycerol. The slides are examined under a fluorescence microscope together with appropriate positive and negative controls. Fluorescent-antibody techniques have been used for detecting antibodies to many microorganisms, such as *C. trachomatis* (43), HIV (26), and *L. pneumophila* (1). The approach has also been popular for the serodiagnosis of several parasitic diseases, including malaria, leishmaniasis, African trypanosomiasis, pneumocystis, toxoplasmosis, and schistosomiasis. Antibody levels resulting from these infections are often high, and because of the chronic nature of many parasitic diseases, detection of antibodies of any immunoglobulin class in a single serum specimen can be presumptive evidence of an active infection.

The solid-phase fluorescence immunoassay is similar in principle to other fluorescent-antibody techniques, except that fluorescence is measured by a fluorometer rather than by a fluorescence microscope. The most common use of this assay in clinical laboratories is the FIAX system from BioWhittaker, Inc. (Walkersville, Md.). In FIAX assays, microbial antigens are immobilized on nitrocellulose disks attached to plastic strips rather than on glass microscope slides. The FIAX sampling strips are immersed in the serum samples to be tested, and specific antibodies, if present, bind to the antigens on the strips. The strips are transferred to a solution of fluorescein-labelled anti-human IgG antibody, which binds to the IgG antibodies complexed to the antigens. The amount of bound, labelled antibody is determined with a fluorometer, which quantitates the fluorescence signal emitted. FIAX tests for detecting antibodies to CMV, Epstein-Barr virus, and measles, mumps, rubella, herpes simplex, and varicella viruses, *Toxoplasma gondii*, *Mycoplasma pneumoniae* (IgG and IgM), *B. burgdorferi* (IgG and IgM), and *Helicobacter pylori* have been commercially available for over 10 years; however, these tests are seeing less use in clinical laboratories, giving way to microtiter plate EIAs, which afford greater throughput.

Agglutination Assays

Passive hemagglutination (PHA) and hemagglutination inhibition (HAI) are modified agglutination assays that have been used extensively for measuring antibodies to viruses. HAI has been the preferred serological test for measuring antibodies to viruses, such as rubella, influenza, respiratory syncytial, and parainfluenza viruses (39). Commercial HAI kits for rubella virus were popular in the 1980s but have now been replaced by EIAs (24). In the PHA test, erythrocytes coated with viral antigens agglutinate in the presence of specific antibodies. PHA has been used for rubella virus immunity screening (28). In the HAI antibody test, sera are reacted with a predetermined amount of virus (usually four hemagglutination units). The presence of antibodies prevents the virus from agglutinating the erythrocytes. The test is usually performed with microtiter plates and serum dilutions. The antibody titer is read as the last dilution showing no visible agglutination.

ELISPOT Test

The enzyme-linked immunosorbent spot (ELISPOT) test is an adaptation of EIA technology for the detection and enumeration of B lymphocytes producing antibody to a specific antigen. Peripheral blood cells are collected, counted, and placed into wells of microtiter plates coated with antigens. The plates are incubated for 4 h at 37°C, washed, and reacted with anti-immunoglobulin antibody followed by an AP-labelled secondary anti-species IgG antibody and 5-bromo-4-chloro-3-indolylphosphate substrate. Antibody spots are counted over a light source. ELISPOT has been used to assess immune responsiveness to potential *Plasmodium falciparum* vaccine candidate antigens (13) and for the diagnosis of HIV perinatal infections (34).

RAPID ASSAYS

Rapid assay formats have been developed for the detection of both antibodies and antigens in clinical specimens. Interest in rapid antigen detection assays remains high because these tests are simple to perform, require less technologist training than culturing, and can provide a result in 15 to 20 min, allowing on-the-spot treatment of patients. These single-use, disposable assays can take the form of either an immunochromatographic line immunoassay or an EIA contained in a disposable cartridge. The line immunoassay uses colloidal gold-labelled antibody as the DA and takes advantage of capillary flow to move antigens toward the DA. The DA is immobilized on a paper strip and also migrates in the fluid phase after the specimen "wets" the paper strip. A control reagent (an antispecies antibody when serum antibody is being measured) also labelled with gold is positioned as a horizontal bar to show a negative sign for a negative specimen and a crossed bar for a positive specimen. The vertical bar for a positive specimen results from capture of the colloidal gold-labelled reagent with immobilized antispecies antibody. Commercial line immunoassays have been developed for the detection of a number of antibodies and antigens, including HIV antibody and *C. trachomatis* antigen.

Dengue virus infection was recently diagnosed by immunochromatographic assays detecting serum IgG and IgM anti-dengue virus antibodies (40). Rapid cartridge assays generally use 2- to 3-cm plastic wafers containing absorbent pads to collect liquid reagents that are added by dropper or pipette. This format has been used successfully for both antibodies and antigens. These assays usually involve three or four pipetting steps and provide an answer in about 15 min. The rapid chlamydia tests are generally less sensitive than microtiter plate EIAs and culturing and have found limited use in clinical settings (36). Other commercially available rapid tests have appeared for influenza virus (42), respiratory sycytial virus (10), and HIV (20, 29) antibodies. Rapid tests for antibody have proven more useful than rapid antigen assays in the clinical laboratory because they have sensitivities approaching those of conventional EIAs.

EVALUATION OF ASSAY PERFORMANCE

The performance of a particular immunoassay can be evaluated by calculating its sensitivity, specificity, and predictive values. The sensitivity of a test refers to the percentage of persons who have a disease and who show a positive test result. Negative results in persons who have the disease are referred to as false-negatives, which reduce the sensitivity of the test. The specificity of a test refers to the percentage of persons who do not have a disease and who show a negative test result. Positive results in persons who do not have the disease are referred to as false-positives, which reduce the specificity of the test. Sensitivity can also be used to

$$\% \text{ Sensitivity} = \frac{\text{true positives}}{\text{true positives} + \text{false negatives}} \times 100$$

$$\% \text{ Specificity} = \frac{\text{true negatives}}{\text{false positives} + \text{true negatives}} \times 100$$

$$\% \text{ Positive predictive value} = \frac{\text{true positives}}{\text{true positives} + \text{false positives}} \times 100$$

$$\% \text{ Negative predictive value} = \frac{\text{true negatives}}{\text{true negatives} + \text{false negatives}} \times 100$$

FIGURE 7 Calculation of the sensitivity, specificity, and predictive values of a diagnostic test.

refer to the minimum amount of a particular antigen or antibody that can be detected by a given test. This sensitivity is referred to as the analytical sensitivity, while the former can be thought of as the diagnostic or clinical sensitivity. The term specificity used with regard to antibodies can also refer to the ability of the assay to distinguish the target antigen from other antigens. The predictive value of a test indicates the probability that the test will correctly indicate the presence or absence of the disease state. The predictive value of a positive test, or the positive predictive value, is the proportion of individuals who show a positive test result and who are truly positive or have disease. The predictive value of a negative test, or the negative predictive value, is the proportion of individuals who show a negative test result and who are truly negative or do not have disease. Predictive values are influenced by the prevalence of infection in any population. The methods of calculating sensitivity, specificity, and predictive values are shown in Fig. 7.

In clinical evaluations of new diagnostic tests, the determination of the true status of a given individual (positive or negative) may be based on clinical criteria alone or, more often, on the results of one or more other reference diagnostic tests. The standard against which the new test is evaluated is referred to as the gold standard or reference standard. The sensitivity, specificity, and predictive values of immunoassays are calculated as percentages, with a perfect test having a sensitivity and a specificity of 100%. The suitability of a given test for a given infection must take into consideration several factors, such as performance (sensitivity and specificity), cost, and test turnaround time.

False-Negative Results

Antibody EIAs can yield false-negative results for various reasons. Competition between IgG and IgM antibodies can cause false-negative IgM results if the amount of solid-phase antigen is limiting and IgG outcompetes IgM for antigen-binding sites. False-negative results have been observed with some sera when total antibody is measured by latex agglutination assays. Sera containing a high level of specific antibody can demonstrate a "prozone" or hook effect, testing negative at low serum dilutions but testing positive at higher dilutions (3, 38). This situation has been observed for some commercially available latex agglutination tests, and laboratories using these assays may need to test at more than a single screening dilution to eliminate false-negatives. A "clinical" false-negative antibody result can occur if the specimen is collected at an inappropriate time relative to the time of onset of infection. For example, following infection with rubella virus, IgM antibody usually appears within 3 to 5 days and all sera collected by day 5 following infection will be positive for IgM antibody (4). Serum collected from an infected patient prior to the appearance of IgM antibody will test negative in an IgM assay. Knowledge of the natural history of infection and immune response to a particular virus is therefore important, and an accurate diagnosis may be predicated upon the collection of specimens at specific times to avoid false-negative results.

False-Positive Results

Antibody EIAs can result in false-positive results for various reasons. RF, an IgM anti-immunoglobulin antibody, will cause false-positive IgM results for sera containing IgG antibody in an EIA with a solid-phase antigen. For example, sera containing RF and rubella virus IgG antibody have produced false-positive results when tested for rubella virus IgM antibody, since RF (IgM antibody) binds to bound rubella virus IgG antibody, which in turn binds to the IgM conjugate. False-positives due to RF have been reported for parvovirus B19, CMV, and papovavirus BK IgM assays. RF interference can be avoided by removal of IgG antibody from the specimens (48) or by use of an IgM capture EIA format (as noted above).

Antibody cross-reactivity can be a major cause of false-positive results in immunoassays for antigen. Antigen-specific DA may have to be enriched by removing cross-reactive antibody. This procedure is done by adsorbing the serum with other antigens that have been found to be cross-reactive to remove the offending antibody. An alternative approach to removing cross-reactive antibody is to purify the desired antibody by adsorption and elution with columns containing immobilized antigen. Affinity chromatography can be done with antigen coupled to cyanogen bromide-activated Sepharose 4B, agarose, or other substrates. When assays generate false-positives, especially in populations of low prevalence, confirmatory or supplementary testing may be required. This has been the case for *C. trachomatis* antigen EIAs.

Laboratory results are subject to error. Factors contributing to erroneous results can be manifested as human and instrument errors. Mistakes can be made at several levels of specimen processing, including labelling at the time of collection, transport to the laboratory, and after receipt in the laboratory. Every time a specimen is handled, there is a chance for specimens to be mixed up. Manual assays are subject to operator error or error introduced by any equipment used in the assays. Errors can be made at the time of reporting, during manual computer entry, or as a result of a specimen or clerical mix-up. For these reasons, clinicians should interpret all laboratory findings in conjunction with clinical findings and history taking and not view laboratory results on their own. Laboratory findings that are not consistent with clinical findings or physician suspicion (pretest probability) should be viewed with caution and warrant consultation with the laboratory staff.

QUALITY CONTROL

Quality control is important because of the complexity and sensitivity of immunoassays. Exacting control standards are needed to ensure accurate and precise test results. Critical elements of a control program are standardization of the serochemistry, continuous monitoring of the test processes, and pretest inspection of test specimens.

Optimum antigen-antibody concentrations are established by conventional block titrations with reference specimens. From these experiments, the test reagent concentrations for the maximum specific reactivity and the minimum nonspecific signal are established. Test protocols are further validated by testing of known positive and presumed normal specimens from the target diagnostic population. From these developmental studies, the test findings that correctly differentiate reactive-positive specimens from nonreactive-negative specimens are identified. The cutoff value is expressed as (i) a fixed absorbance value determined on the basis of the experience of the test developer, (ii) an absorbance value that is a multiplier of a number of standard deviations above the negative population absorbance value, (iii) a fraction or percentage of a known positive reference value, or (iv) a combination of these. In each case, specimens with absorbance values higher than the cutoff value are reactive or positive, and those with values lower than the cutoff value are nonreactive or negative. Some manufacturers establish a "grey or equivocal" zone, which is neither positive nor negative. This approach complicates test interpretation and patient management and is therefore not recommended.

The equipment manuals provided by manufacturers must be consulted for performance characteristics, calibration specifications, and operating procedures of all instruments used with EIA tests. Pipetting devices, plate washers, and well readers must be calibrated, and schedules for calibration checks and routine maintenance must be established and recorded. Special attention must be paid to pipetting devices. Accuracy for these devices is maximized by ensuring correct fit of the tips to the device barrel, prewetting tips, and keeping volume delivery below a reagent level so as not to contaminate the pipette. Washers, like reagent delivery devices, must perform exactly as specified. Vacuum and fluid delivery must be set for and matched to the plate test wells. A simple measure of wash efficiency is a plate-to-plate inspection for residual wash fluid. Either excess residual fluid or excessive aspiration in wash cycles and thus excessive drying may adversely affect test reactivity. Since all EIA reactions are temperature and time sensitive, technical protocols must include clocks and thermometers as standard monitoring devices to ensure compliance with the parameters established for each test.

Each EIA run should include controls from the reagent manufacturer, a set prepared in-house or obtained from other sources (external or supplemental controls), and, whenever possible, a set of primary standards from a recognized reference laboratory. This set is used initially and at appropriate intervals to ensure the optimum level of reactivity in consensus with other laboratories. The control set provided by the manufacturer describes the optimum performance characteristics of the test. The results obtained with this control set, however, apply only to the potency of the reagents in the set in use. Variations in reagents (kit to kit or lot to lot) are monitored with the external control set, which should consist of multiple (duplicate or triplicate) high- and mid-range-reactive specimens or specimen pools and a nonreactive specimen or specimen pool. This external control thus serves not only to detect immediate failure but also to monitor both excessive run-to-run variations and long-term trends. Values obtained at each test run are efficiently monitored by charts that show, for example, nonreactivity or background reactivity as well as specific reactivity over time.

REFERENCES

1. **Bibb, W. F., P. M. Arnow, L. Thacker, and R. M. McKiney.** 1984. Detection of soluble *Legionella pneumophila* antigens in serum and urine specimens by enzyme-linked immunosorbent assay with monoclonal and polyclonal antibodies. *J. Clin. Microbiol.* **20:**478–482.
2. **Blumberg, R. S., K. L. Hartshorn, B. Ardman, J. C. Kaplan, T. Paradis, H. Vogt, M. S. Hirsch, and R. T. Schooley.** 1987. Dot immunobinding assay for detection of human immunodeficiency virus-associated antigens. *J. Clin. Microbiol.* **25:**1989–1992.
3. **Carpenter, A. B.** 1997. Enzyme-linked immunoassays, p. 20–29. *In* N. R. Rose, E. C. de Macario, J. D. Folds, H. C. Lane, and R. M. Nakamura (ed.), *Manual of Clinical Laboratory Immunology*, 5th ed. ASM Press, Washington, D.C.
4. **Chernesky, M., L. Wyman, J. Mahony, S. Castriciano, J. T. Unger, J. W. Safford, and P. S. Metzel.** 1984. Clinical evaluation of the sensitivity and specificity of a commercially available enzyme immunoassay for detection of rubella virus-specific immunoglobulin M. *J. Clin. Microbiol.* **20:**400–404.
5. **Chernesky, M., S. Castriciano, J. Mahony, and D. DeLong.** 1985. Examination of the Rotazyme II enzyme immunoassay for the diagnosis of rotavirus gastroenteritis. *J. Clin. Microbiol.* **22:**462–464.
6. **Chernesky, M., D. Jang, J. Sellors, P. Coleman, J. Bodner, I. Hrusovsky, S. Chong, and J. Mahony.** 1995. Detection of *Chlamydia trachomatis* antigens in male urethral swabs and urines with a microparticle enzyme immunoassay. *Sex. Transm. Dis.* **22:**55–59.
7. **Chernesky, M. A.** 1996. Traditional serological tests, p. 107–123. *In* B. W. J. Mahy and H. O. Kangro (ed.), *Virology Methods Manual*. Academic Press Ltd., London, England.
8. **Chiu, B., E. Viira, W. Tucker, and I. W. Fong.** 1997. *Chlamydia pneumoniae*, cytomegalovirus, and herpes simplex virus in atherosclerosis of the carotid artery. *Circulation* **96:**2144–2148.
9. **Cordell, J. L., B. Falini, W. N. Erber, A. K. Ghosh, A. Abdulazia, Z. MacDonald, K. A. F. Pulford, H. Stein, and D. Y. Mason.** 1984. Immunoenzymatic labelling of monoclonal antibodies using immune complexes of alkaline phosphatase and monoclonal anti-alkaline phosphatase (APAAP complexes). *J. Histochem. Cytochem.* **32:**219–229.
10. **Englund, J. A., P. A. Piedra, A. Jewell, K. Patel, B. B. Baxter, and E. Whimbey.** 1996. Rapid diagnosis of respiratory syncytial virus infections in immunocompromised adults. *J. Clin. Microbiol.* **34:**1649–1653.
11. **Engvall, E., and P. Perlman.** 1971. Enzyme-linked immunosorbent assay (ELISA). Quantitative assay of immunoglobulin G. *Immunochemistry* **8:**871–874.
12. **Eriksen, K., T. Landsverk, B. Gondrosen, and J. Vormeland.** 1990. Immuno-histochemical and -cytochemical evidence suggesting the presence of Campylobacer jejuni and Campylobacer coli in cases of porcine intestinal adenomatosis. *Acta Vet. Scand.* **31:**445–451.
13. **Fievet, N., C. Chougnet, B. Dubois, and P. Deloron.** 1993. Quantification of antibody-secreting lymphocytes that react with Pf155/RESA from *Plasmodium falciparum*:

an ELISPOT assay for field studies. *Clin. Exp. Immunol.* **91:**63–67.

14. **Grandien, M., C. A. Pettersson, P. S. Gardner, A. Linde, and A. Stanton.** 1985. Rapid viral diagnosis of acute respiratory infections: comparison of enzyme-linked immunosorbent assay and the immunofluorescence technique for detection of viral antigens in nasopharyngeal secretions. *J. Clin. Microbiol.* **22:**757–760.
15. **Herrmann, J. E.** 1995. Immunoassays for the diagnosis of infectious diseases, p. 110–122. *In* P. R. Murray, E. J. Baron, M. A. Pfaller, F. C. Tenover, and R. H. Yolken (ed.), *Manual of Clinical Microbiology*, 6th ed. ASM Press, Washington, D.C.
16. **Herrmann, J. E., N. A. Nowak, D. M. Perron-Henry, R. W. Hudson, W. D. Cubitt, and N. R. Blacklow.** 1990. Diagnosis of astrovirus gastroenteritis by antigen detection with monoclonal antibodies. *J. Infect. Dis.* **161:**180–184.
17. **Hook, E. W., III, R. E. Roddy, S. A. Lukehart, J. Hom, K. K. Holmes, and M. R. Tam.** 1985. Detection of *Treponema pallidum* in lesion exudate with a pathogen-specific monoclonal antibody. *J. Clin. Microbiol.* **22:**241–244.
18. **Hunter, W. M., and F. C. Greenwood.** 1962. Preparation of iodine-131 labelled human growth hormone of high specific activity. *Nature* **194:**495–496.
19. **Kasakara, Y.** 1997. Agglutination immunoassays, p. 7–12. *In* N. R. Rose, E. C. de Macario, J. D. Folds, H. C. Lane, and R. M. Nakamura (ed.), *Manual of Clinical Laboratory Immunology*, 5th ed. ASM Press, Washington, D.C.
20. **Kassler, W. J., B. A. Dillon, C. Haley, W. K. Jones, and A. Goldman.** 1997. On-site rapid HIV testing with same-day results and counseling. *AIDS* **11:**1045–1051.
21. **Kline, R. L., D. McNairn, M. Holodniy, L. Mole, D. Margolis, W. Blattner, and T. C. Quinn.** 1996. Evaluation of Chiron HIV-1/HIV-2 recombinant immunoblot assay. *J. Clin. Microbiol.* **43:**2650–2653.
22. **Kricka, L. J.** 1997. Chemiluminescence immunoassays, p. 49–53. *In* N. R. Rose, E. C. de Macario, J. D. Folds, H. C. Lane, and R. M. Nakamura (ed.), *Manual of Clinical Laboratory Immunology*, 5th ed. ASM Press, Washington, D.C.
23. **Lauer, B. A., H. A. Masters, C. G. Wren, and M. J. Levin.** 1985. Rapid detection of respiratory syncytial virus in nasopharyngeal secretions by enzyme-linked immunosorbent assay. *J. Clin. Microbiol.* **22:**782–785.
24. **Mahony, J., S. Castriciano, and M. Chernesky.** 1987. Cost and performance analysis of haemagglutination inhibition, passive haemagglutination, radial haemolysis, and enzyme immunoassay for measuring rubella antibody. *J. Virol. Methods* **18:**133–142.
25. **Mahony, J., J. Sellors, and M. Chernesky.** 1987. Detection of chlamydial inclusions in cell culture or biopsy tissue by alkaline phosphatase–anti-alkaline phosphatase staining. *J. Clin. Microbiol.* **25:**1864–1867.
26. **Mahony, J., K. Rosenthal, M. Chernesky, S. Castriciano, E. Scheid, M. Blajchman, and D. Harnish.** 1989. Agreement study between two laboratories of immunofluorescence as a confirmatory test for human immunodeficiency virus type 1 antibody screening. *J. Clin. Microbiol.* **27:**1234–1237.
27. **Mahony, J., and M. Chernesky.** 1991. Negative staining in the detection of viruses in clinical specimens. *Micron Microsc. Acta* **22:**449–460.
28. **Mahony, J. B., and M. A. Chernesky.** 1997. Rubella virus, p. 693–699. *In* N. R. Rose, E. C. de Macario, J. D. Folds, H. C. Lane, and R. M. Nakamura (ed.), *Manual of Clinical Laboratory Immunology*, 5th ed. ASM Press, Washington, D.C.
29. **McKenna, S. L., G. K. Muyinda, D. Roth, M. Mwali, N. Ng'andu, A. Myrick, C. Luo, F. H. Priddy, V. M. Hall, A. A. von Lieven, J. R. Sabatino, K. Mark, and S. A. Allen.** 1997. Rapid HIV testing and counseling for voluntary testing centers in Africa. *AIDS* **11**(Suppl. 1)**:**S103–S110.
30. **Morinet, F., F. Ferchal, R. Colimon, and Y. Perol.** 1984. Comparison of six methods for detecting human rotavirus in stools. *Eur. J. Clin. Microbiol.* **3:**136.
31. **Mushahwar, I. K., L. R. Overby, G. Frosner, F. Deinhardt, and C. M. Ling.** 1978. Prevalence of hepatitis B e antigen and its antibody as detected by radioimmunoassays. *J. Med. Virol.* **2:**77–87.
32. **Nakane, P. K., and G. B. Pierce, Jr.** 1966. Enzyme-labelled antibodies: preparation and application for the localization of antigens. *J. Histochem. Cytochem.* **14:**929–931.
33. **Nanagara, R., P. H. Duray, and H. R. Schumacher Jr.** 1996. Ultrastructural demonstration of spirochetal antigens in synovial fluid and synovial membrane in chronic Lyme disease: possible factors contributing to persistence of organisms. *Hum. Pathol.* **27:**1025–1034.
34. **Palomba, E., V. Gay, C. Gabiano, L. Perugini, and P. A. Tovo.** 1990. *In-vitro* production of HIV-1 specific antibody for diagnosis of perinatal infection. *Lancet* **336:**940–941.
35. **Perrillo, R. P., K. H. Chau, L. R. Overby, and R. H. Decker.** 1983. Anti-hepatitis B core immunoglobulin M in the serologic evaluation of hepatitis B virus infection and simultaneous infection with type B, delta agent, and non-A non-B viruses. *Gastroenterology* **85:**163–167.
36. **Sellors, J., J. Mahony, D. Jang, L. Pickard, S. Castriciano, S. Landis, I. Stewart, W. Seidelman, I. Cunningham, and M. Chernesky.** 1991. Rapid, on-site diagnosis of chlamydial urethritis in men by detection of antigens in urethral swabs and urine. *J. Clin. Microbiol.* **29:**407–409.
37. **Tam, M. R., W. E. Stamm, H. H. Handsfield, R. Stephens, C. C. Kuo, K. Holmes, K. Ditzenberg, M. Krieger, and R. C. Nowinski.** 1984. Culture-independent diagnosis of *Chlamydia trachomatis* using monoclonal antibodies. *N. Engl. J. Med.* **310:**1146–1150.
38. **Tijssen, P.** 1985. *Practice and Theory of Enzyme Immunoassays*. Elsevier Science Publishers, Amsterdam, The Netherlands.
39. **Vaananen, P., V. M. Haiva, P. Koskela, and O. Meurman.** 1985. Comparison of a simple latex agglutination test with hemolysis-in-gel, hemagglutination inhibition, and radioimmunoassay for detection of rubella virus antibodies. *J. Clin. Microbiol.* **21:**793–795.
40. **Vaughn, D. W., A. Nisalak, S. Kalayanarooj, T. Solomon, N. M. Dung, A. Cuzzubbo, and P. L. Devine.** 1998. Evaluation of a rapid immunochromatographic test for diagnosis of dengue virus infection. *J. Clin. Microbiol.* **36:**234–238.
41. **Vesanen, M., T. Linna, and A. Vaheri.** 1991. Persistent inapparent HIV-1 infection of human neuroblastoma cells. *Arch. Virol.* **120:**253–261.
42. **Waner, J. L., S. J. Todd, J. Shalaby, P. Murphy, and L. V. Wall.** 1991. Comparison of Directigen FLU-A with viral isolation and direct immunofluorescence for the rapid detection and identification of influenza A virus. *J. Clin. Microbiol.* **29:**470–482.
43. **Wang, S. P., J. T. Grayston, E. R. Alexander, and K. K. Holmes.** 1975. Simplified microimmunofluorescence test with trachoma lymphogranuloma venereum (*Chlamydia trachomatis*) antigens for use as a screening test for antibody. *J. Clin. Microbiol.* **1:**250–255.
44. **Widjojoatmodjo, M. N., A. C. Fluit, R. Torensma, and J. Verhoef.** 1993. Comparison of immunomagnetic beads coated with protein A, protein G, or goat anti-mouse immunoglobulins. Applications in enzyme immunoassays and

immunomagnetic separations. *J. Immunol. Methods* **165:** 11–19.

45. **Wu, B., J. Mahony, and M. Chernesky.** 1989. Comparison of three protein A-gold immune electron microscopy methods for detecting rotaviruses. *J. Virol. Methods* **25:**109–118.
46. **Wu, B., J. Mahony, G. Simon, and M. Chernesky.** 1990. Sensitive solid-phase immune electron microscopy double-antibody technique with gold-immunoglobulin G complexes for detecting rotavirus in cell culture and feces. *J. Clin. Microbiol.* **28:**864–868.
47. **Wu, B., J. B. Mahony, and M. A. Chernesky.** 1990. A new immune complex dot assay for detection of rotavirus antigen in faeces. *J. Virol. Methods* **29:**157–166.
48. **Zapata, M., J. Mahony, and M. Chernesky.** 1984. Measurement of BK papovavirus IgG and IgM by radioimmunoassay (RIA). *J. Med. Virol.* **14:**101–114.

Molecular Detection and Identification of Microorganisms*

YI-WEI TANG AND DAVID H. PERSING

13

Since publication of the sixth edition of this Manual, significant changes have occurred in the practice of molecular microbiology. This chapter reviews the underlying principles of hybridization and amplification of nucleic acids, as well as the application of these techniques to the detection and characterization of pathogens.

Generally speaking, molecular microbiology also encompasses molecular typing methods such as plasmid analysis, fingerprinting, and ribotyping. These techniques have been widely applied in epidemiological investigations and nosocomial infection surveillance studies (for a review, see reference 258). Chapter 7 is intended to cover these techniques in detail. The present chapter will highlight practical issues surrounding molecular diagnostics and will emphasize automation, postamplification detection, and current applications. This chapter is not intended to provide specific step-by-step instructions for molecular diagnostic procedures. The reader is referred to protocols of the commercially available systems and other sources for more detailed descriptions of these procedures and their applications (78, 203, 204).

MOLECULAR DIAGNOSTICS: AN INTRODUCTION

A fundamental principle of diagnostic microbiology is improvement of patient care through the rapid detection and characterization of specific pathogens. Over the past century, the identification of microorganisms has relied principally upon phenotypic characteristics such as morphology and biochemical characterization. However, in some cases, growth-based systems are often time-consuming, expensive, or simply unavailable. Advances in molecular biology over the past 10 years have opened a new frontier for the genotypic identification and characterization of microorganisms. These developments are beginning to affect many areas of patient management (205, 252).

DNA hybridization studies were first used to demonstrate relatedness among bacteria. This understanding of nucleic acid hybridization chemistry made possible nucleic acid probe technology (68, 74, 103, 109, 142, 156, 225, 247). Nucleic acid probes have been used to detect antimicrobial resistance genes or the presence of fastidious microorganisms like mycobacteria and legionella (74, 222). Like phenotypic parameters, however, hybridization methods may be limited by microbial recovery and growth. Nucleic acid amplification technology has opened new avenues for the detection, identification, and characterization of pathogenic organisms in the clinical microbiology laboratory (80, 205, 252, 271, 283). Growth in vitro is no longer always necessary for microbial identification (105, 177).

Nucleic acid amplification techniques fall into three general categories: (i) target amplification systems, which use PCR, transcription-mediated amplification (TMA) and similar technologies, or strand displacement (SDA); (ii) probe amplification systems, which include those involving $Q\beta$ replicase ($Q\beta R$) or thermostable DNA ligase (LCR); and (iii) signal amplification, in which the signal generated from each probe molecule is increased by using compound probes or branched-probe technology (Table 1). Examples of each category will be discussed separately below; however, they all share certain advantages over traditional methods, particularly for the detection of fastidious organisms.

Molecular applications enhance the speed, sensitivity, and sometimes the specificity of an etiologic diagnosis. The promise of these techniques is the replacement of biological amplification—growth in culture—by enzymatic amplification of specific nucleic acid sequences. During the last decade, the advantages of diagnostic molecular techniques have been so widely publicized that increasing pressure has been placed on clinical microbiology laboratories to use these techniques for the detection of many infectious agents, especially those for which commercial test kits are available.

However, before introducing molecular techniques in the diagnostic laboratory, three strategic questions must be addressed. First, which organisms need a test better than those offered by traditional methods? Second, which clinical specimens should be tested? Third, do the available molecular tests fulfill the required criteria of high sensitivity and specificity, speed, simplicity, and clinical relevance? In general, molecular diagnostic techniques are indicated for the detection of organisms that cannot be grown in vitro or for which current culture techniques are too insensitive, too costly, or too time-consuming.

As more experience has been gained in the use of molecular methods, additional limitations have also become apparent. The most serious challenge is prevention of contamination of negative specimens from either template

* This chapter contains information presented in chapter 13 by Raymond P. Podzorski and David H. Persing in the sixth edition of this Manual.

TABLE 1 Nucleic acid amplification methods

Amplification method	Amplification category	Manufacturer or license holder	Enzyme(s) used	Temp requirement	Nucleic acid target	Key reference(s)
PCR	Target	Roche Molecular System, Inc., Branchburg, N.J.	*Taq* DNA polymerase	Thermal cycler	DNA (RNA)	184, 228
TMA	Target	Gen-Probe, Inc., San Diego, Calif.	RT, RNA *pol*, RNase H	Isothermal	RNA and DNA	147
NASBA	Target	Organon-Teknika Corp., Durham, N.C.	RT, RNA *pol*, RNase H	Isothermal	RNA and DNA	56, 107
SDA	Target	Becton-Dickinson & Co., Rutherford, N.J.	Restrictive endonucleonase, DNA polymerase	Isothermal	DNA	274, 275
QβR	Probe	Vysis, Inc., Naperville, Ill.	Qβ replicase	Isothermal	DNA and RNA	145
LCR	Probe	Abbott Laboratories, Abbott Park, Ill.	DNA ligase	Thermal cycler	DNA	291
bDNA	Signal	Chiron Corp., Emeryville, Calif.	None	Isothermal	DNA and RNA	262

carryover or cross contamination from positive controls and/or specimens prepared in parallel. Due to the amplification capacity of PCR, contamination of a given sample with immeasurably small amounts of exogenous template nucleic acids can create false-positive results. Cross-reactivity can also become a concern. For example, primers targeting the immediate-early 1 gene of human cytomegalovirus (CMV) also amplified *Escherichia coli* 23S rRNA or DNA (137), demonstrating that even totally unrelated organisms can compete and cross amplify in PCR. Cross-reactivity between *Toxoplasma gondii* and *Nocardia asteroides* may also lead to false-positive results in some systems, and misdiagnosis of a cerebral *Nocardia* infection has been reported (171). Thus, clinical validation is essential for these assays, especially those that are user developed.

A variety of factors may also produce false-negative results. For example, inhibitors of enzymes used in amplification tests may be present; such inhibitors can be detected by spiking a small amount of nucleic acid target into the specimen (181). Routine quality control measures may be as complex as introducing into each reaction mixture a control template engineered to produce a product of a different size or as simple as diluting the specimen to minimize the effects of inhibitors. When inhibition is suspected, the lysis and nucleic acid extraction method should be scrutinized because assay performance can be affected.

One disadvantage of molecular diagnostic kits and many user-developed tests is that they are narrow in scope. Current organism-specific nucleic acid detection methods assume that the physician or laboratorian knows which pathogen is causing the disease—an assumption which, if true, makes the test useful only as an expensive confirmation for the clinical diagnosis. For example, a test specific for the agent of human granulocytic ehrlichiosis (HGE) may produce a negative result if the infection is due to *Ehrlichia chaffeensis*, a potentially common cause of the same disease (77, 143). Multiple infections may be a particular problem for nucleic acid detection methods because coinfection will not be detected unless the laboratory is specifically instructed to look for multiple organisms, such as herpes simplex virus and human herpesvirus 6 in the cerebrospinal fluid (CSF) (253). In the future, the most useful molecular diagnostic tests will be those that can simultaneously test for more than one organism. Multiplex PCR, which uses multiple primers within a single reaction tube to amplify nucleic acid fragments from different organisms, may be used to solve this problem (see below).

The final drawback of nucleic acid amplification techniques is their expense. The costs of reagents, patent royalties, equipment, and the space needed to separate preamplification from postamplification procedures have hindered the introduction of molecular methods in many clinical laboratories. For the immediate future, amplification techniques probably will not be used for the diagnosis of infections when conventional methods are sufficient. These include common bacterial infections of the urinary tract, upper respiratory tract, and soft tissues. On the other hand, molecular diagnosis may have a significant benefit when applied to selected sites (such as the central nervous system) or for organisms (e.g., *Legionella*) for which conventional means are inefficient, unreliable, or simply unavailable. As molecular techniques become more efficient and more widespread, resulting in lower costs per unit, molecular diagnostics will likely have a broader impact on the diagnosis of infectious diseases.

NUCLEIC ACID PROBES

The principle of nucleic acid probe technology is straightforward. Genomic sequences specific for a particular group of infectious agents are selected, cloned, synthesized, and used as probes. Probes hybridize with DNA or RNA targets in the clinical specimen. Nucleic acid probes can bind with high specificity to complementary sequences of a target nucleic acid and are capable of identifying organisms at, above, and below the species level. Probes labeled with enzymes, antigenic or chemiluminescent moieties, or radioisotopes are readily detectable by automated systems. The sensitivity of the method varies directly with the size and composition of the probe as well as the nature of the original specimen. Identification of organisms in pure culture is generally more straightforward than detection of organisms in clinical specimens, since competing background nucleic acids are not present. A number of commercially prepared DNA probes for the identification of infectious agents have been described (74, 103, 109, 142, 156).

Three DNA probe hybridization formats have been commonly used: liquid-phase, solid-phase, and in situ hybridization. The liquid-phase format has the fastest rate of hybridization (167, 280). The key to successful solution-phase hybridization is use of a single-stranded probe which does not hybridize with itself. The leading method in routine use for detecting hybridization in solution is the hybridization protection assay (HPA) (8). A probe labeled with an acridinium ester and the target are incubated together followed by alkaline hydrolysis, and the binding of the probe to the target is measured without further separation steps (8). In a positive sample, the bound probe is protected from alkaline hydrolysis and, upon the addition of peroxides, emits detectable light. The assay can be performed in a few hours and does not require removal of excess unbound single-stranded DNA or isolation of probe-bound double-stranded DNA complexes (212). A simple and convenient detection system, HPA is also used to detect amplified DNA products in commercially available amplification systems developed by Gen-Probe Inc. (2, 151).

Solid-phase hybridization is used in research and in many clinical laboratories (94, 257). Nucleic acid-bound nylon membranes or nitrocellulose are hybridized with a nucleic acid probe in solution. Unbound probes are washed away, and the bound probe is detected by means of fluorescent, luminescent, radioactive, or enzymatically active moieties incorporated into the probe. Various techniques are used to detect DNA or RNA targets in clinical specimens. Southern blotting is a solid-phase hybridization assay that allows determination of the sizes of DNA fragments electrophoretically separated on a gel prior to binding by the reporter probe (245, 257). A Northern blot is similar except that the reporter probe detects bound RNA instead of DNA fragments (257). Solid-phase hybridization can also be used for detecting and verifying amplified DNA fragments (124, 203, 204). The length and complexity of the assays, however, limit their application in clinical practice.

In situ hybridization assays use whole cells or tissue sections affixed to microscope slides. The nucleic acid in the target tissue is hybridized to nucleic acid probes by the same general principles used for solid-phase hybridization (112, 248). In clinical settings, formalin-fixed, paraffin-embedded tissue sections are the most common target tissue used. The sensitivity of in situ hybridization is limited by the accessibility of target nucleic acids within the cell. Probes of less than 300 bp favor tissue penetration (112, 248). At present, the detection and typing of human papillomavirus (HPV) by colorimetric in situ hybridization is the most common diagnostic application (14, 41). Commercial systems are available from Digene Diagnostics, Inc., and other suppliers.

Nucleic acid probes have been used routinely in many clinical mycobacteria laboratories for the identification of mycobacteria species (74). These DNA probe techniques have proven to be rapid, sensitive, and specific and require only small inocula. Most laboratories use these probes in conjunction with radiometric or fluorometric systems for the detection of mycobacteria, with a biologically amplified specimen used for probing (57, 208). This technique has had a positive effect on patient management by providing a rapid and accurate diagnosis. However, these probes are expensive and are priced on a per-species basis.

In clinical specimens, DNA probes may have a particular advantage in detecting pathogens for which reliable culture systems are not practical. This is true of certain viruses such as HPV, hepatitis B virus (HBV), and Epstein-Barr virus (6, 142, 238). Culture confirmation probes for *Histoplasma capsulatum*, *Blastomyces dermatiditis*, *Coccidioides immitis*, and *Cryptococcus neoformans* present distinct advantages over conventional means of identification (109, 247). DNA probes have also been applied to the detection of parasites (225). Gen-Probe Inc. and Digene Diagnostics, Inc., are manufacturing several direct detection and culture identification nucleic probes which have been approved by the U.S. Food and Drug Administration (FDA) (Table 2). Although these commercial products are more expensive than conventional approaches, the decrease in turnaround time has the potential to improve patient outcome and reduce overall health care costs. Procedures for the use of DNA probes are now well standardized, and the advent of synthetic short oligonucleotide DNA probes has shortened the time required for these assays owing largely to faster kinetics of hybridization. Probing of clinical specimens, however, is in most cases limited by poor sensitivity. The nucleic acid amplification methods described below address this problem.

SIGNAL AMPLIFICATION TECHNIQUES

Signal amplification methods (85) are designed to strengthen the signal by increasing the concentration of label (radioisotopes, enzymes, fluorochromes, etc.) attached to the target nucleic acid. Multiple enzymes, multiple probes, two-tiered probes, and multiple probes and enzymes have been used to enhance target detection (285).

Unlike procedures which increase the concentration of the probe or target, signal amplification increases the signal generated by a fixed amount of probe hybridized to a fixed amount of specific target. The fact that signal amplification procedures do not involve a nucleic acid target or probe amplification is a theoretical advantage because of the lower susceptibility to contamination problems inherent in enzyme-catalyzed nucleic acid amplification. The sensitivities of signal amplification techniques, however, compared to those of target nucleic acid amplification techniques may be a limiting factor (262). Another limitation of signal amplification is background noise due to nonspecific binding of reporter probes (123).

One example of signal amplification is the Digene Hybrid Capture System, which is a solution hybridization antibody capture assay that uses chemiluminescent detection (162, 183). Specimens containing the target DNA hybridize with a specific RNA probe. The resultant RNA-DNA hybrids are captured onto the surface of a tube coated with antibodies specific for RNA-DNA hybrids. Immobilized hybrids are then reacted with antibodies specific for the RNA-DNA hybrids. Signal amplification occurs at this step because multiple antibodies bind to a single target sequence. The enzyme-conjugated antibodies are then detected with a chemiluminescent substrate. As the substrate is cleaved by the bound enzyme, it emits light which is measured on a luminometer (Fig. 1). The intensity of the emitted light is proportional to the concentration of target DNA in the specimen. This system is widely used to determine HPV infection and viral types in cervical swabs or fresh cervical biopsy specimens (162, 183). A recently developed SHARP signal system, similar in principle to the Digene Hybrid Capture assay described above, has been used for the quantitation of biotinylated amplified DNA products (see below).

Developed and manufactured by Chiron Corp., the branched DNA (bDNA) probe technique is the most widely used signal amplification method. The technique uses a branched multiple probe-enzyme complex to increase the signal in proportion to the amount of target in the reaction mixture (262). The system consists of a series of primary

TABLE 2 Commercially available nucleic acid probes for detection of microbial pathogens[a]

Manufacturer	Primary application	Organism detected	Additional comments
Gen-Probe	Direct detection in clinical samples	*Chlamydia trachomatis* Group A streptococci *Mycobacterium tuberculosis* *Neisseria gonorrhoeae*	Customer service: 1-800-523-5001
Gen-Probe	Culture confirmatory assays	*Blastomyces dermatitidis* *Campylobacter* spp. *Coccidioides immitis* Enterococci Group A streptococci Group B streptococci *Haemophilus influenzae* *Histoplasma capsulatum* *Listeria monocytogenes* *Mycobacterium avium* *Mycobacterium avium* complex *Mycobacterium gordonae* *Mycobacterium intracellulare* *Mycobacterium kansasii* *Mycobacterium tuberculosis* complex *Neisseria gonorrhoeae* *Staphylococcus aureus* *Streptococcus pneumoniae*	Includes *Campylobacter jejuni*, *Campylobacter coli*, and *Campylobacter lari*
Digene	Direct detection in clinical samples	Human papillomavirus	Customer service: 1-800-344-3631
Digene	Typing of isolates detected by the viral Pap test	Human papillomavirus	

[a] All tests listed here have been cleared by FDA.

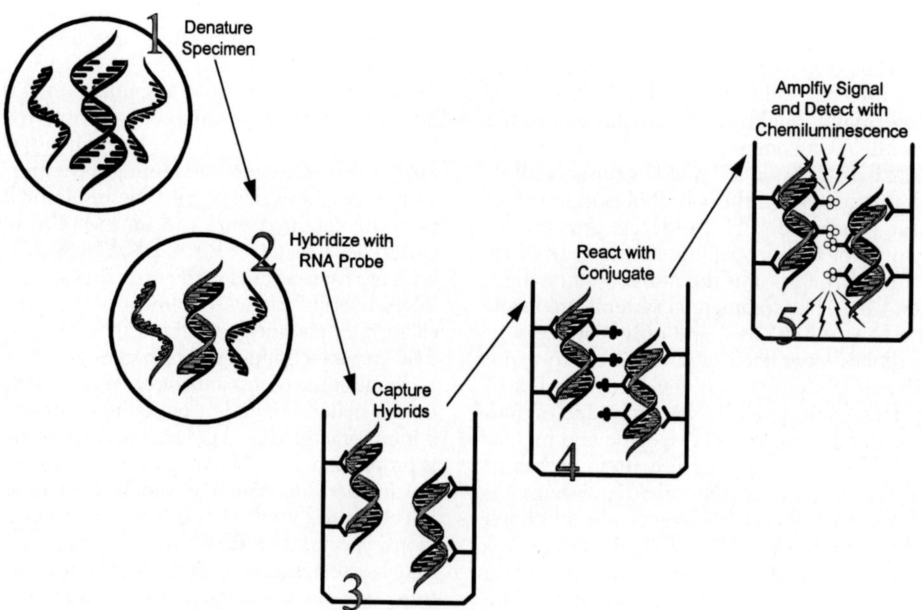

FIGURE 1 Digene hybrid capture system. The system is a signal amplification technology for the detection and quantitation of viral DNA. The patient's specimen is denatured (step 1) and then hybridized with an RNA probe (step 2). If the target nucleic acid is present, the resulting RNA-DNA hybrid is captured by an antibody specific for RNA-DNA hybrids (step 3). Multiple alkaline-phosphatase conjugates bind to the hybrid amplifying the signal (step 4). A chemiluminescent substrate emits light which is measured with a luminometer (step 5).

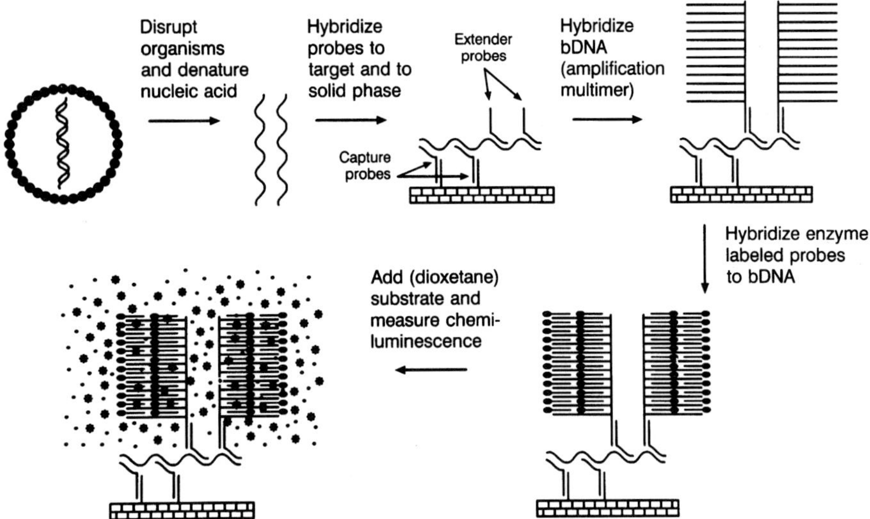

FIGURE 2 bDNA-based signal amplification. Target nucleic acid is released by disruption and is captured onto a solid surface via multiple contiguous capture probes. Contiguous extended probes hybridize with adjacent target sequences and contain additional sequences homologous to the branched amplification multimer. Enzyme-labeled oligonucleotides bind to the bDNA by homologous base pairing, and the enzyme-probe complex is measured by detection of chemiluminescence. All hybridization reactions occur simultaneously.

probes, a novel branched secondary probe, and short enzyme-labeled tertiary probes (Fig. 2). Multiple specific synthetic oligonucleotides hybridize to the target and capture it onto a solid surface. Synthetic, enzyme-conjugated, branched oligonucleotide probes (bDNA amplifiers) are then added. Hybridization occurs between the amplifiers and the immobilized targets. By the bDNA technique, it is relatively easy to attach 60 to 300 enzyme molecules to each target sequence. A chemiluminescent substrate is added, and light emission may then be quantified.

In bDNA assays, all hybridization reactions occur simultaneously, and the observed signal is proportional to the amount of target DNA. Target DNA can be quantified from a standard curve. Because the target molecules themselves are not amplified during the process, the process is less likely to have the contamination problems associated with enzymatic nucleic acid amplification methods. The bDNA method is also highly reproducible and represents an excellent method for quantitation and therapeutic response monitoring (36, 70, 71, 117, 173, 196, 221). A separate section below deals with this particularly important issue. The principal disadvantage is that the bDNA assay is currently less sensitive than enzymatic amplification techniques, with a practical detection limit of 5×10^2 to 2×10^5 nucleic acid target molecules, depending on the test. As for most techniques, the specificity of the bDNA assay may decline as higher sensitivity is sought. Recent advances in sample concentration and nucleotide chemistry may help to circumvent some of these problems.

TARGET AND PROBE AMPLIFICATION TECHNIQUES

PCR

PCR has dramatically changed the way that we detect and characterize nucleic acids (184, 228). First described in 1985, PCR has become a technological milestone in the field of biotechnology, and its inventor, Kary B. Mullis, was awarded the Nobel Prize for Medicine in 1993. The PCR process was reportedly conceived by Mullis on a moonlit drive through the California mountains, and he has described the developmental process of PCR as being interwoven with romance, intrigue, corporate politics, and legal entanglements (184).

Although other strategies are in use, PCR and PCR-derived techniques are the best-developed and the most widely used methods of nucleic acid amplification. PCR is based on the ability of DNA polymerase to copy a strand of DNA. The enzyme initiates elongation at the 3′ end of a short (primer) sequence bound to a longer (target) strand of DNA. When two primers bind to complementary strands of target DNA, the sequence between the two primer binding sites is amplified exponentially with each cycle of PCR (184, 228). Each cycle consists of three steps: (i) a DNA denaturation step, in which the double strands of the target DNA are separated; (ii) a primer annealing step, in which primers anneal to their complementary amplification target sequences at a lower temperature; and (iii) an extension reaction step, in which DNA polymerase extends the target sequences between the primers. At the end of each cycle, which consists of the three steps described above, the PCR products are theoretically doubled (Fig. 3). The whole procedure is carried out in a programmable thermal cycler. Generally, 30 to 50 thermal cycles result in a detectable amount of a target sequence originally presented in less than 100 copies (283).

PCR techniques are widely used because of their simplicity and flexibility. In 1992, Roche Diagnostics Systems Inc. purchased the patent rights to the PCR from Cetus Corp. for the sum of approximately \$300 million, with the goal of developing PCR-based kits for the diagnosis of genetic and infectious diseases. Semiautomated and automated systems for detection and/or quantitation of several organisms

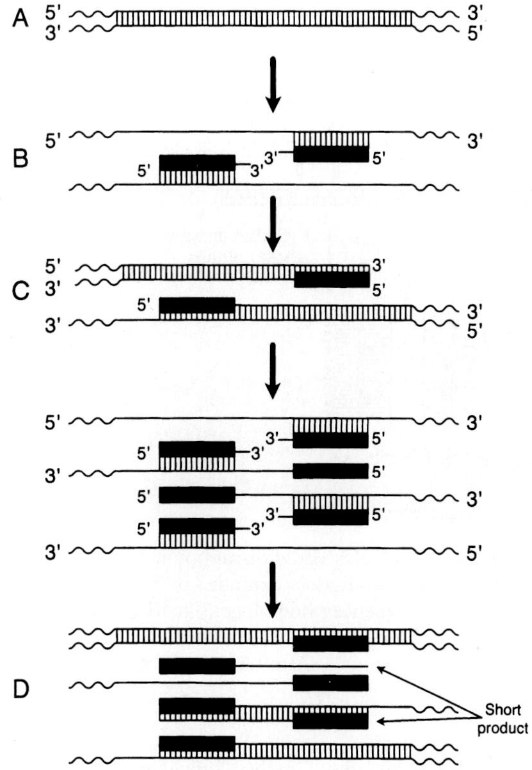

FIGURE 3 PCR. (A) In the first cycle, a double-stranded DNA target sequence is used as a template. (B) These two strands are separated by heat denaturation, and the synthetic oligonucleotide primers (solid bars) anneal to their respective recognition sequences in the $5' \rightarrow 3'$ orientation. Note that the $3'$ ends of the primers are facing each other. (C) A thermostable DNA polymerase initiates synthesis at the $3'$ ends of the primers. Extension of the primer via DNA synthesis results in new primer-binding sites. The net result after one round of synthesis is two "ragged" copies of the original target DNA molecule. (D) In the second cycle, each of the four DNA strands in panel C anneals to primers (present in excess) to initiate a new round of DNA synthesis. Of the eight single-stranded products, two are of a length defined by the distance between and including the primer-annealing sites; these "short products" accumulate exponentially in subsequent cycles.

have now been manufactured by Roche (Table 3). These organisms include human immunodeficiency virus (HIV) type 1 (HIV-1), hepatitis C virus (HCV), CMV, human T-cell lymphotropic virus type I/II (HTLV-I/II) (270), enterovirus (138, 294), *Chlamydia trachomatis* (160, 198, 214), *Neisseria gonorrhoeae* (119), and *Mycobacterium tuberculosis* (16, 39, 287). In addition, numerous user-developed PCR-based DNA amplification techniques have been developed and applied to the detection of microbial pathogens (32, 72, 149, 155, 235, 268), identification of clinical isolates (37, 233, 259, 298), and strain subtyping (9, 104, 118, 139).

RT-PCR

Reverse transcriptase (RT)-PCR was developed to amplify RNA targets. In this process, RNA targets are first converted to complementary DNA (cDNA) by RT and are then amplified by PCR. RT-PCR has played an important role in detecting RNA virus infections and *Mycobacterium* species and in determining the effectiveness of antimicrobial therapy (23, 130, 229). Conventional RT cannot tolerate the higher temperatures of PCR, which may limit the specificity of primer annealing. Thermostable DNA polymerase derived from *Thermus thermophilus* and its cousins derived from other organisms have efficient reverse transcription activity. These enzymes can be used to amplify RNA targets without the need for a separate reverse transcription step (186, 296). The elevated reaction temperature increases the stringency of primer hybridization and avoids the formation of RNA secondary structure, which can prevent primer binding or elongation, or both. The reactions are then more specific and efficient than previous protocols with avian myeloblastosis virus RT. Commercial kits which use this single-enzyme technology are now available for the detection of HIV. Quantitative RT-PCR assays for HIV RNA have now become exceedingly popular (see below).

Nested PCR

Designed mainly to increase sensitivity, nested PCR uses two sets of amplification primers (113). One set is used for first-round amplification which consists of 15 to 30 cycles. The products of the first reaction are then subjected to a second round of amplification with another set of primers specific for a sequence within the product of the first primer pair (113, 235). Nested PCR has high sensitivity due to the high total cycle number and is theoretically more specific than amplification with the same number of cycles with a single primer set, because the DNA product from the first round of amplification must contain hybridization sites for the second primer pair; thus, amplification by the second primer set verifies the specificity of the first-round product. The major disadvantage of nested amplification is the high probability of contamination during the transfer of first-round products to a second tube. This can be avoided either by physically separating the two amplification mixtures with a layer of wax or oil (282) or by designing single-tube amplification protocols.

Multiplex PCR

Multiplex PCR is an amplification reaction in which two or more sets of primers specific for different targets are introduced in the same tube. More than one target sequence in a specimen can be amplified at the same time (44). The primers used in multiplex reactions must be designed carefully to have similar annealing temperatures and to lack complementarity. Extensive empirical testing is often needed. Coamplification of multiple targets can be used for different purposes. For diagnostic purposes, multiplex PCR can be used for the detection of internal controls, as well as for the detection of multiple pathogens from a single specimen (15, 100, 224). Quantitative competitive PCR, a variation of multiplex PCR, can be used to quantify the amount of target sequence in a specimen (210, 293). Multiplex PCR assays play a larger role in human and cancer genetics, in which target nucleic acid quantity is not limiting. However, the development of multiplex PCR assays for the detection of infectious organisms is more complicated and often results in lower sensitivity. The use of specialized enzymes may help to overcome some of these limitations (20).

Arbitrarily Primed PCR

Originally developed by Welsh and McClelland in 1990 (279), arbitrarily primed PCR (AP-PCR), also referred to

TABLE 3 Commercially available amplification techniques for detection of microbial pathogens[a]

Company	Organism detected	Trademark or name	Specimen processing	Basic method	Detection system	Contamination potential	Analytical sensitivity or testing range	Clinical sensitivity (%)	Clinical specificity (%)	Primary application	Regulatory status	Additional comments/ information
Roche	HIV-1	Amplicor	Chaotrope lysis-alcohol precipitation	PCR	EIA	Low to moderate	<100 copies/ml[b]	>99[b]	No claims	Confirmatory testing		Customer service: 1-800-526-1247
Roche	HIV-1	Monitor		Quantitative PCR	EIA	Low to moderate	400–750,000 copies/ml[c]	NA[d]	No claims	Quantitation during therapy	FDA cleared	
Roche	HCV	Amplicor		PCR	EIA	Low to moderate	<200 copies/ml[b]	98%[b]	No claims	Confirmatory testing		
Roche	HCV	Monitor		Quantitative PCR	EIA	Low to moderate	200–10^7 copies/ml[b]	NA	No claims	Quantitation during therapy		
Roche	*M. tuberculosis*	Amplicor		PCR	EIA	Low to moderate	≥20 organisms/ reaction[c]	88.9–100[c]	100[c]	Smear-positive and untreated patients only	FDA cleared	Has been used on BACTEC broth culture
Roche	*C. trachomatis*	Amplicor		PCR	EIA	Low to moderate	10–20 elementary bodies/ reaction[c]	93.2[c]	98.4[c]	Monitoring and confirmatory testing	FDA cleared	
Roche	*N. gonorrhoeae*	Amplicor		PCR	EIA	Low to moderate	No claims	No claims	No claims	Monitoring and confirmatory testing		
Roche	CMV	Amplicor		PCR	EIA	Low to moderate	No claims	No claims	No claims	Confirmatory testing		
Roche	CMV	Monitor		Quantitative PCR	EIA	Low to moderate	No claims	NA	No claims	Quantitation and monitoring		
Roche	HTLV-I/II	Amplicor		PCR	EIA	Low to moderate	No claims	No claims	No claims	Monitoring and confirmatory testing		
Roche	Enterovirus	Amplicor		PCR	EIA	Low to moderate	No claims	No claims	No claims	Monitoring and confirmatory testing		
Organon-Teknika	HIV-1	HIV-1 QL	Silica	NASBA	ECL[e]	Moderate	80 copies/ml[c]	>99[c]	>99[c]	Confirmatory testing		Customer service: 1-800-682-2666
Organon-Teknika	HIV-1	HIV-1 QT		Quantitative NASBA	ECL	Moderate	200–10^6 copies/ml[c]	NA	>99[c]	Quantitation during therapy		

(*Continued on next page*)

TABLE 3 Commercially available amplification techniques for detection of microbial pathogens[a] (*Continued*)

Company	Organism detected	Trademark or name	Specimen processing	Basic method	Detection system	Contamination potential	Analytical sensitivity or testing range	Clinical sensitivity (%)	Clinical specificity (%)	Primary application	Regulatory status	Additional comments/ information
Chiron	HIV-1	Quantiplex	Detergent lysis	Quantitative bDNA assay	EIA	Low	500–800,000 copies/ml[c]	NA	95[c]	Quantitation during therapy		Customer service: 1-800-653-1353
Chiron	HCV	Quantiplex		Quantitative bDNA assay	EIA	Low	200,000–120 $\times 10^6$ copies/ml[c]	NA	98[c]	Quantitation during therapy		
Chiron	Hepatitis B virus	Quantiplex		Quantitative bDNA assay	EIA	Low	0.7 $\times 10^6$–5,000 $\times 10^6$ copies/ml[c]	NA	98[c]	Quantitation and monitoring		
GenProbe	*M. tuberculosis*	MTD	TIGRIS	TMA	HPA-ECL[f]	Moderate	Unknown	95.5[c]	100[c]	Smear-positive and untreated patients only	FDA cleared	Customer service: 1-800-523-5001
GenProbe	*C. trachomatis*	AMP		TMA	HPA-ECL	Moderate	Unknown	86.7–99.2[c]	>99[c]	Monitoring and confirmatory testing	FDA cleared	Sensitivity varies by sex and specimen source
Abbott	*C. trachomatis*	LCX	Phenol-chloroform	LCR	EIA	Low to moderate	Unknown	>95[b]	>99[b]	Monitoring and confirmatory testing	FDA cleared	Customer service: 1-800-527-1869
Abbott	*N. gonorrhoeae*	LCX		LCR	EIA	Low to moderate	Unknown	>95[b]	>99[b]	Monitoring and confirmatory testing	FDA cleared	

[a] Modified from *Clinical Chemistry* (252), with permission of the publisher.
[b] Based on the experience of Mayo Clinic.
[c] Based on manufacturer's claim.
[d] NA, not applicable (used to test seropositive patients only).
[e] ECL, enhanced chemiluminescence
[f] HPA-ECL, hybridization protection assay-ECL.

as the randomly amplified polymorphic DNA assay, involves the use of a single short (usually 10- to 15-base), arbitrarily chosen primer to amplify genomic DNA under low-stringency conditions. Only regions flanked by primer binding sites on complementary strands will be amplified. AP-PCR has been used to differentiate strains of various species, various serotypes within species, and various subtypes within a serotype (104, 164, 263, 289). It is therefore useful for determining whether two isolates of the same species are epidemiologically related. AP-PCR is probably the simplest DNA-based subtyping method developed to date. However, this method requires a temperature-cycling instrument, and the reproducibility of this technique between runs and among laboratories has been questioned (see chapter 6).

Broad-Range PCR

Another important technical modification that has been developed is the broad-range PCR. This application uses conserved sequences within phylogenetically informative genetic targets to diagnose infection. Novel, fastidious, or uncultivated pathogens have been identified directly from infected human tissue or blood by this method (62, 218–220, 249, 281). A universal primer set designed to target herpesvirus DNA polymerases may be useful for diagnosing herpesvirus infection (265). Broad-range rRNA PCR techniques offer the possibility of rapid bacterial identification with a single pair of primers targeting a bacterial small-subunit (16S) rRNA gene (106, 140, 180, 188, 206). The major obstacles to the implementation of rapid, automated rRNA gene-based bacterial identification systems are background contamination and cost.

Transcription-Based Amplification

Described in 1989 by Kwoh et al. (147), transcription-based amplification begins with synthesis of a DNA molecule complementary to the target nucleic acid (usually RNA). This is followed by in vitro transcription with the newly synthesized cDNA as a template. Variations on this process are referred to as self-sustaining sequence replication (3SR), nucleic acid sequence-based amplification (NASBA), or TMA (56, 107). In one version of transcription-based amplification, three enzymes, RT, RNase H, and T7 DNA-dependent RNA polymerase, are used in the reaction. Amplification steps involve the formation of cDNAs from the target RNA with primers containing an RNA polymerase-binding site. RNase H then degrades the initial strand of target RNA in the RNA-DNA hybrid after it has served as template for the first primer. The second primer binds to the newly formed cDNA and is extended, resulting in the formation of double-stranded cDNAs with one or both strands capable of serving as transcription templates for RNA polymerase (Fig. 4).

TMA involves several enzymes and a complex series of reactions which all take place simultaneously at the same temperature and in the same buffer. The advantages of TMA include its very rapid kinetics and the lack of a requirement for a thermocycler. Isothermal conditions in a single tube with a rapidly degradable product (RNA) help minimize (but may not eliminate) contamination risks (107). TMA is very useful for amplifying single-stranded RNA targets without RNA isolation or DNase pretreatment, which are required in RT-PCR. Amplification of RNA not only makes it possible to detect RNA viruses but also increases the sensitivity of detecting bacterial and fungal pathogens by using high-copy-number RNA targets (56). A TMA-based system manufactured by GenProbe Inc. has been used to detect *M. tuberculosis* in smear-positive sputum specimens and to

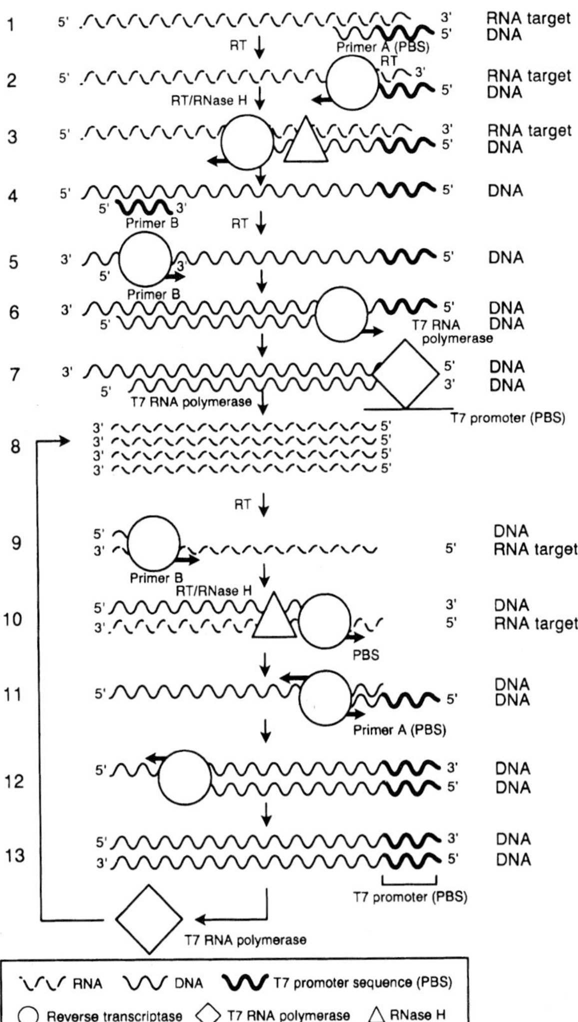

FIGURE 4 TMA. The initial steps in the reaction involve the formation of cDNAs from the target RNA by using oligonucleotide primers with a T7 binding site. The RNase H in the reaction degrades the initial strands of target RNA in the RNA-DNA hybrids after they have served as templates for the initial primer. The second T7-containing primer then primes the initial single-stranded cDNAs, resulting in the formation of double-stranded cDNAs with one strand capable of serving as the transcription template for T7 RNA polymerase. This results in the synthesis of numerous copies of antisense RNA. These antisense RNAs serve as templates for one of the T7-containing oligonucleotide primers. After a round of priming, DNA polymerization by RT, RNase H degradation of the RNA-DNA hybrid, priming, and extension of the newly formed cDNA strand by the other T7-containing oligonucleotide primer, numerous copies of double-stranded cDNA are formed again. At this stage of the reaction, both strands of the cDNA are capable of serving as transcription templates for T7 polymerase. These cDNAs can yield either sense or antisense RNAs, which then reenter the cycle of priming, DNA polymerization by RT, RNase H degradation of the RNA-DNA hybrid, priming, and extension of the newly formed cDNA strand by the other T7-containing oligonucleotide primer with the subsequent formation of additional double-stranded cDNAs that can serve as templates for either sense or antisense RNA synthesis.

detect *C. trachomatis* infection. A NASBA system is commercially available from Organon-Teknika Corp. for the detection and quantitation of HIV-1 infection (221, 264, 267) (Table 3).

LCR

Given the patent restrictions on PCR and the expanding interest in nucleic acid-based diagnosis, alternative amplification methods are hotly sought after by both microbiologists and industry. LCR is one of the most successful alternatives. Also called ligase amplification reaction, LCR is a probe amplification technique that was first described in 1989 by Wu and Wallace (291). Successful ligation relies on contiguous positioning and correct base pairing of the 3′ and 5′ ends of oligonucleotide probes on a target DNA molecule. In this process, probes are annealed to template molecules in a head-to-tail fashion, with the 3′ end of one probe abutting the 5′ end of the second probe. DNA ligase then joins the adjacent 3′ and 5′ ends to form a duplicate of one strand of the target. A second primer set, complementary to the first, then uses this duplicated strand (as well as the original target) as a template for ligation. Repeating the process results in exponential accumulation of ligation products, which can be detected via functional groups attached to the probes (234). A variation on LCR, which uses limited extension of template nucleotides by DNA polymerase followed by ligation, is incorporated into assays manufactured by Abbott Laboratories. Inclusion of this template extension step, however limited, led to PCR patent infringement lawsuits, resulting in the unofficial renaming of LCR as the "litigation chain reaction."

As for PCR, the use of thermostable DNA ligase greatly simplifies this technique and increases specificity by avoiding the problem of blunt-end ligation at low annealing temperature (11). Although convenient and readily automated, one potential drawback of LCR is the difficult inactivation of postamplification products. The nature of the technique does not allow the most widely used contamination control methods to be applied. The inclusion of a detection system within the same reaction tube would significantly decrease the possibility of contamination which is associated with the opening of reaction tubes, and current assays based on LCR do not appear to be especially prone to contamination problems. A combination LCR kit for the detection of both *C. trachomatis* and *N. gonorrhoea* is now commercially available from Abbott Laboratories (46, 47) (Table 3).

Practical information about current commercially available amplification techniques for the detection of microbial pathogens is summarized in Table 3.

POSTAMPLIFICATION DETECTION AND ANALYSIS

Gel Electrophoresis

After target amplification, the conventional method of product detection is the use of agarose gel electrophoresis following ethdium bromide staining. Several other techniques have been developed not only to "visualize" the products but to enhance both sensitivity and specificity as well. A probe-based DNA detection system has the advantage of providing sequence specificity and increased sensitivity. After routine agarose gel electrophoresis, the DNA is transferred to a solid phase, e.g., nitrocellulose or nylon membrane, and is identified by hybridization to a specific probe. Membranes with bound radiolabeled or fluorescein-labeled probes are exposed to X-ray film, and the hybridization products appear as dark bands. Enzyme-labeled probes may be visualized through either light or color production. This technique, although still an important research and confirmatory testing tool, is being replaced by other simpler and faster systems which are described in the following sections.

Single-strand conformational polymorphism (SSCP) analysis, described by Orita et al. (194), is used to expand the information content of the DNA fragments visualized on the gel. DNA is subjected to PCR with primers that flank a region of suspected polymorphism. Variations in the physical conformation of the PCR products are reflected in differential gel migration, which is not directly proportional to molecular weight. This technique is sensitive enough to detect all single nucleotide substitutions. One area in which it may eventually prove to be of value is in the detection of mutations related to resistance mechanisms. SSCP analysis and variations on the technique have been used successfully to examine the genes contributing to multidrug resistance of *M. tuberculosis* (88, 256). Given the recent drop in the cost of doing DNA sequencing, SSCP will probably fall out of favor.

In postamplification restriction fragment length polymorphism (RFLP) analysis, amplified DNA fragments are cleaved with a restriction endonuclease, separated by gel electrophoresis, and then transferred to a nitrocellulose or a nylon membrane. A fragment(s) containing specific sequences may then be detected by using a labeled complementary oligonucleotide as a probe. Variations in the number and sizes of the fragments detected are referred to as RFLPs and reflect variations in both the number of loci that are homologous to the probe and the location of restriction sites within or flanking those loci (266). Again, for short products, direct sequencing will probably become the favored analytical method (see below).

Colorimetric Microtiter Plate Systems

Many current PCR applications such as the analysis of microorganisms in biological samples and the detection of specific gene mutations require precise verification of PCR product specificity. Conventional detection techniques, such as Southern blotting following hybridization, are too lengthy and labor intensive. A more practical approach for the routine diagnostic setting is colorimetric detection in the wells of a microtiter plate (MTP). In this system, which is somewhat similar to an enzyme immunoassay system, amplified DNA is captured on the well of an MTP by a complementary oligonucleotide capture probe which is previously attached to the plastic surface. Detection is accomplished by a color change that takes place after the addition of an enzyme conjugate and appropriate substrate.

Colorimetric MTP systems use a sequence-specific capture probe. They can be adapted to many protocols by varying the sequence of the capture probe to correspond to the desired target sequence. The system provides three technical advantages compared to traditional methods. First, its sensitivity for the detection of PCR products is 10- to 100-fold greater than that of staining of agarose gels. Second, the use of a capture probe proves the specificity of the PCR product. Third, the use of an MTP system affords rapid analysis of multiple reactions simultaneously when combined with a 96-well thermocycler. In the clinical setting, colorimetric MTP systems require less than 4 h for amplification product identification, thereby providing a much promised rapid result (250).

Several formats are commercially available. In one format, amplification of the target is performed with the biotinylated primers included in the system. The amplified product is denatured and transferred directly to the MTP, which is precoated with a sequence-specific capture probe. After hybridization, the unbound amplification products are washed away and a streptavidin-enzyme conjugate is added, followed by enzymatic colorimetric detection. Several manufacturers have adopted this format for analysis of the products of nucleic acid amplification (83, 160).

Another MTP system for the detection of nucleic acid previously amplified by PCR was described recently (166). An anti-double-stranded DNA antibody exclusively recognizes the hybridization product resulting from the reaction between the target DNA and a DNA probe. The final product is revealed colorimetrically (166). The system increases the sensitivity of the previous PCR by including enzymatic reactions. The hybridization between specific probe and PCR-amplified target DNA, as well as the formation of target DNA-probe hybrids and anti-double-stranded DNA antibody complex, enhances the specificity as well. A recently developed and manufactured PCR enzyme-linked immunosorbent assay kit from Boehringer Mannheim, which uses digoxigenin-dUTP incorporated into the PCR product, also allows the precise characterization and quantitation of PCR products (211).

Chemiluminescence

Advances in chemiluminescent labeling have significantly improved the sensitivity of nonisotopic DNA probe tests (102). Biotin- and digoxigenin-labeled probe systems and enzyme-activated chemiluminescence systems are at least as sensitive as isotopic methods. In addition to the long shelf lives of these products, this detection time is measured in minutes rather than the hours or days required for routine radioisotopic procedures. In molecular microbiology laboratories, all these characteristics have significantly improved turnaround times, reduced start-up costs, and eliminated many of the regulatory hurdles facing laboratories that offer nucleic acid-based tests. A luminol-based chemiluminescence detection system is commercially available from Amersham (102).

A recently developed assay, the OPCR System from Perkin-Elmer Instruments, uses the analytical capabilities of an electrically initiated chemiluminescence reaction (electrochemiluminescence) to provide sensitive and reproducible DNA quantitation at the attomole level. In contrast to commonly applied acridinium esters (8), the high stability of ruthenium bipyridyl labels allows their incorporation during oligonucleotide synthesis (136). The initial amount of specific amplification products can be quantified by measuring integrated light intensity. Although the practical impact of this theoretical advantage remains to be determined, this system can be easily automated and provides linear responses over more than 3 orders of magnitude, which corresponds to a dynamic range of at least 4 logs of initial copy numbers (272).

Direct Amplification Product Sequencing

Direct sequencing offers a simple, rapid, and accurate means of analysis of amplification products. The PCR sequencing system combines PCR and dideoxynucleotide chain termination methods to determine DNA sequences directly from crude clinical materials (125). As described in the previous section, broad-range PCR amplifies conserved regions of a wide range of organisms (140, 220). The amplification product sequence is first determined, and then a DNA sequence-based phylogenetic analysis is performed and is used to identify the pathogen specifically (76). Because it is now possible for one individual to sequence tens of thousands of base pairs in a single 8-h day, the technology is amenable to automation, and many diagnostic distinctions are possible at the single-nucleotide level. The role of sequencing will likely increase substantially in the clinical microbiology laboratory of the future.

Current sequencing technologies are based on one of two approaches: (i) electrophoretic separation based on polyacrylamide slab gels or glass capillaries and (ii) solid-phase sequencing by matrix hybridization. Electrophoretic separation technology is dominated by fluorescent dye terminator chemistry and laser scanning in a polyacrylamide slab gel electrophoresis format. Sequencing by this approach is performed with instruments made by several manufacturers. Recent application of capillary electrophoresis techniques to the separation of PCR amplification products and dideoxy chain termination products has eliminated two labor-intensive steps: the preparation of polyacrylamide gels and the loading of individual samples (89). Another advantage of this type of system is its use of a closed collection chamber, which helps reduce problems with amplification product contamination. Another recently developed approach is matrix hybridization (93, 290), which uses hundreds or thousands of oligonucleotide probes on a solid substrate to carry out multiple hybridization reactions simultaneously (see below).

Direct sequencing of amplicons provides not only accurate identification of organisms but also a high-resolution method for studying organism variation, molecular epidemiology, drug resistance, and virulence factors. Sequence analysis has been an important tool for classifying certain viruses and evaluating strain relatedness (18, 182, 241, 297). Several putative point source outbreaks of bacterial infections have been investigated by DNA sequence-based approaches (185). Sequence-determined mutations in the precore region of the HBV genome are associated with the occurrence of fulminant hepatitis (152, 157). Mutations in the HIV genome are associated with drug resistance (144).

Matrix Hybridization

Matrix hybridization is accomplished by attaching or synthesizing hundreds or thousands of oligonucleotides to a solid support. A labeled amplification product for a designated target is then hybridized to the probes, giving rise to specific hybridization signals within various loci of the matrix. Reading of the pattern generated by the hybridization reactions allows extensive analysis of the amplification product; if enough probes are used, the sequence of the amplified target can be determined by computer analysis of the hybridization signal pattern, in light of the DNA sequences of the individual probes at each position in the matrix. A number of manufacturers in the United States and abroad currently claim to be developing hybridization matrices.

Perhaps the most elegant and complex approach to matrix hybridization takes advantage of semiconductor industry technology and its ability to fabricate complex structures on silicon chips (93, 200). This system uses light to direct the synthesis of small fragments of DNA on a glass wafer (93, 158). On a silica substrate 15 mm across, an array of hundreds or thousands of individual sites can be established. At each site, specific oligonucleotide probes are built up, one nucleotide at a time, by photo-activated chemical synthesis. The chip is incubated with the amplified DNA products, which are tagged with a fluorescent marker in a flow

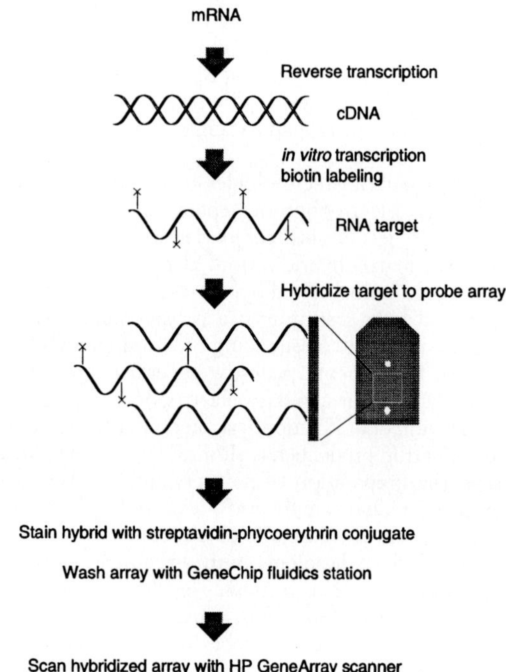

FIGURE 5 Example of DNA chip technology. The GeneChip expression analysis process involves the isolation of mRNA transcripts, creation of cDNA, transcription of biotinylated RNA target, hybridization of the target to an array, and staining of the hybrid with phycoerythrin-streptavidin complex. The array is then washed by the GeneChip fluidics station and scanned with a Hewlett-Packard (HP) GeneArray scanner. Fluorescence hybridization intensity data collected by the scanner are analyzed and displayed as relative mRNA expression level information with GeneChip software.

cell (Fig. 5). After hybridization, a scanning laser confocal fluorescence microscope evaluates the surface fluorescence intensity on the chip. The confocal aspect of the microscope detects only the fluorescence on the surface of the chip, thus helping to avoid background fluorescence problems. Automated scanning by the microscope produces an image of the entire surface of the chip in a few minutes (93, 158), and software carries out automated data analysis of the fluorescent image.

One advantage of matrix hybridization is the ability to resolve complex mixtures of amplified sequences. Imagine an infectious disease chip with DNA probes for hundreds or thousands of specific microbial targets. Conceivably, such a chip could comprise all of the known sequences of bacterial drug resistance genes; if bacterial RNA from a colony was incubated with the chip, the RNA could be simultaneously sequenced and its level measured to account for gene expression differences. Efforts have been sought to build an entire "molecular laboratory as a microdevice" by putting PCR, along with all the other steps of sample preparation and signal detection, on a small semiconductor DNA chip (193).

The first commercial matrix hybridization system, available now, is a test that can identify HIV-1 genome mutations known to be associated with drug resistance (144). A customized chip that represented the last 18 bases of *gag*, all 297 bases of *pol*, and the first 123 bases of the RT gene was designed (144). The chip has 18,495 sites or so-called features probing the HIV-1 genome on the surface. Given the same small aliquot of plasma, one can discover not only whether a subject has HIV-1 infection but also whether the virus genomes carry mutations that make the infection resistant to therapy. Chips that facilitate pharmacogenetic analysis are also being manufactured, and these may someday be used to guide the administration of antibiotics, antiviral agents, and anticancer agents.

The main drawbacks of the gene chip system include the complexity of fabricating the chips and test cost. The presence of multiple probes on one chip is a challenge for hybridization conditions, since the optimal conditions for one probe might be quite different from those for another probe. A careful performance evaluation, including evaluations of sensitivity, specificity, and reproducibility, should be carried out before wide application of these chips can be considered in diagnostic molecular microbiology.

AMPLIFICATION PRODUCT INACTIVATION

Amplification product contamination is one of the greatest impediments to the routine use of nucleic acid amplification in the clinical microbiology laboratory. Because a single molecule of template DNA can be amplified many millionfold and previously amplified material already contains primer sequences on each end, amplification products can be considered analogous to infectious agents that can "infect" amplification reactions. It is critical to take precautions to minimize contamination and inactivate the "infectivity" of the products. Specific steps should be taken to inactivate the amplified nucleic acids so that if a carryover event does occur, the nucleic acid cannot be reamplified (191, 227). This is of greatest importance for user-developed protocols.

Inactivation procedures are an important component of all enzyme-catalyzed nucleic acid amplification methods (191). Several inactivation procedures have been applied to prevent false-positive results due to the carryover of amplified DNA or RNA targets (227). They can be divided into two general approaches: pre- and postamplification. Theoretically, the short amplification products associated with LCR or SDA may be more difficult to inactivate than the longer products from the other methods. RNA product contamination may prove to be simpler to control because of the inherent lability of RNA compared to that of DNA; however, significant contamination problems with RNA targets have been reported. Current techniques for amplicon inactivation are summarized in Table 4. This section focuses on the methods most commonly used in the diagnostic microbiology laboratories.

UNG

One effective preamplification decontamination procedure involves modification of PCR-amplified DNA during amplification. This method allows products of previous reactions to be destroyed selectively prior to amplification of unmodified target DNA. Uracil-*N*-glycosylase (UNG) is one of several enzymes of the excision repair system used by many bacteria to remove inappropriate bases from damaged DNA (99, 161). The function of UNG is to recognize and cleave uracil residues that arise in DNA as a result of spontaneous deamination of cytosine. In a UNG-based decontamination system, dUTP replaces TTP in the PCR mixture and results in amplified DNA with deoxyuracil residues in place of thymidine residues (161). Amplified DNA with dUTP is chemically distinct from target DNA. UNG is added to the reaction mixture prior to PCR, and the mixture is incubated

TABLE 4 Methods used for amplification product inactivation

Method	Clinical application	Optimum conditions	Advantage	Disadvantage	Key reference(s)
UV light irradiation	Reagent inactivation	Higher A+T content; length, >300 bp	Inexpensive; no additional protocol needed	Dependent on distance from light source	51, 141, 231
UNG	Preinactivation	Higher A+T content; length, >150 bp	Easy to perform; no additional instrument required	May interfere with amplification efficiency; polymerase intolerance	99, 161
Photochemical cross-linkers	Postinactivation	Higher A+T content; length, >100 bp	Simple and powerful	Additional instruments needed; some protocols may not tolerate addition of isopsoralen	52, 126
Selective primer cleavage			No requirement on product size and G+C content; no effects on amplicon analysis	Potential contamination due to reagent addition	273
Hydroxylamine treatment		Higher G+C content; length, >250 bp	Effective on short and G+C-rich amplicons	Potential contamination due to reagent addition; may have effects on amplicon analysis	10

briefly at room temperature and then at a higher temperature. If uracil-containing DNA is present in the preamplification mixture, the UNG cleaves the modified DNA at the uracil residues and destroys its template activity. Target DNA is unaffected following this treatment.

Although UNG-based inactivation systems have been reported to work very efficiently, there are some important considerations. Similar to UV inactivation, the efficacy of UNG decontamination most likely depends on the length and G+C content of the amplification product. One study recommended that UNG should not be used on amplification products of less than 100 bp, and for maximum UNG efficiency, amplification products should be 150 bp or more in length (84). Thus, it follows that the UNG system should be optimized for maximum efficiency for each application. It has also been found that partial dUTP substitution in amplified DNA can interfere with the hybridization of oligonucleotide reporter probes, decreasing the sensitivity of the assay (38). The magnitude of the decrease in signal appears to be proportional to both the dUTP concentration in the reaction mixture and the number of thymidylate residues in the probe binding site. In addition, it has been reported that some polymerases do not tolerate the substitution of dUTP for TTP (242). This fact must be taken into consideration when DNA polymerases other than AmpliTaq are used in a PCR-based system with a UNG-based inactivation procedure.

Photochemical Cross-Linkers

Photochemical inactivation is a simple and powerful method for postamplification decontamination of PCR products. Photochemical cross-linkers derived from psoralens and isopsoralens are being evaluated as postamplification inactivation agents (52). These furocoumarin compounds represent a class of planar tricyclic reagents known to intercalate between base pairs, thereby inactivating DNA amplicons (50). Isopsoralen derivatives have the greatest potential use in clinical laboratories because (unlike psoralen) they do not cross-link the strands of a double-stranded DNA molecule. This allows probe-based detection systems to be used following isopsoralen inactivation (84, 126, 253). Psoralen derivatives may be most useful when they are incorporated in a preamplification decontamination scheme. Like all inactivation systems, protocols based on psoralen and isopsoralen derivatives have certain limitations. The isopsoralen concentration and the time of UV light exposure must be optimized empirically for each amplification product; some reactions appear to be severely inhibited by isopsoralen addition. Short and GC-rich products are difficult to decontaminate. As with UNG, amplicons should be more than 100 bp for reliable inactivation (84, 227). Photochemical cross-linking can be used with dUTP incorporation, so both methods described above are not mutually exclusive (227).

Topical Inactivation

Methods for eliminating amplification product "spills" and for routine maintenance of work areas include topical application of dilute bleach to the contaminated areas and the working surfaces. This method, when combined with a routine cleaning of the laboratory, can greatly reduce problems associated with contamination. UV light exposure is also effective at eliminating amplified templates, but its effectiveness is limited by distance. UV light sources installed inside "dead-air boxes" are probably more effective at eliminating contamination (see below).

Other Sources of Contamination

Amplification products are not the only source of nucleic acid contamination. Genomic DNA from microbial sources, especially if amplified by cultures, can also contaminate the environment and presumably clinical samples as well. Examples of contamination associated with processing of samples in areas used for culturing of target organisms have been described (203, 204). Carryover from specimen to specimen by aerosolization can also occur, and this may become a special problem in so-called ultrasensitive assays.

CURRENT APPLICATIONS OF MOLECULAR DIAGNOSTICS

Detecting Unculturable, Slowly Growing Microorganisms

In selected situations, the primary isolation of an organism and the use of specific media and culture conditions may be replaced by molecular microbiology. Microbial DNA or RNA extracted from a clinical specimen may be analyzed for the presence of various organism-specific nucleic acid sequences regardless of the physiologic requirements or viability of the organism (87, 180, 237). For example, the inability to culture and analyze the principal etiologic agent of non-A, non-B hepatitis (HCV) limited medical advances in this area. Using various molecular methods, investigators have been able to isolate HCV nucleic acid (48). Analysis and cloning of the HCV genome have provided the viral antigens necessary for the development of specific serologic tests (1, 4). Currently, RT-PCR allows the identification, quantitation, and sequence analysis of the HCV genome in infected individuals (187, 296).

Some organisms, although they are not difficult to culture, are infrequently encountered and require special media for isolation. In these instances, culture may not be cost-effective for smaller laboratories since reagents may expire prior to their use. In these instances, samples for culture may be sent to reference laboratories for the sake of economy. Fragile organisms may die in transit or may become overgrown by contaminating bacteria, thereby making the subsequent culture useless. If molecular microbiology facilities are not available in community laboratories, nucleic acids extracted by the use of commercially available kits may be sent to regional reference facilities. Alternatively, if molecular facilities are available, PCR primers and probes for relatively rare microorganisms may be maintained frozen at −70°C for extended periods and used when needed. This eliminates the need for special culture media and circumvents problems related to specimen transit. As molecular techniques become more widely available and increasingly automated, this can extend the spectrum of rapid and cost-effective clinical microbiology tests available to smaller laboratories.

Identifying Unusual Bacteria by 16S rRNA Gene Sequencing

Nucleotide sequence analysis of the small-subunit (16S) bacterial rRNA gene has greatly expanded our understanding of phylogenetic relationships among members of the bacterial kingdom (288). rRNA molecules contain several functionally different regions, some of which have conserved sequences and others of which are highly varied. These imprints, or molecular signatures, form the basis for identifying microorganisms. The 16S rRNA sequence of a species is a stable genotypic feature which may be useful for the identification of microbes at the genus or species level (288). Direct 16S rRNA gene sequence determination provides identifying information and objective results independent of phenotypic characteristics, which form the basis of a rapid identification system.

This approach also allows characterization of previously unrecognized species. One intriguing application of 16S rRNA sequencing is the identification of novel pathogens prior to the availability of in vitro culture methods. In 1990, a patient infected with HIV-1 died of an overwhelming infection with an acid-fast microorganism (now known as *Mycobacterium genavense*) which, at the time, could not be propagated in vitro (121). While biochemical analysis and characterization were impossible, analysis of the 16S rRNA sequences present in patient tissue successfully characterized the organism from the decedent and several other AIDS patients (27). Armed with the knowledge that the organism was a mycobacterium species, *M. genavense* was later cultivated on mycobacterial growth medium (62).

Tropheryma whippelii, the causative agent of Whipple's disease (215, 220, 269), is another unculturable microbe which was initially identified by PCR with broad-range primers and sequence analysis of 16S rRNA genes. Because of the inability of this organism to grow on conventional media and the lack of a serologic test, the diagnosis of Whipple's disease is usually based on clinical and biopsy findings in which small-bowel biopsy specimens reveal characteristic foamy histiocytes which fill the lamina propria. The definitive diagnosis is made by the identification of non-acid-fast, periodic acid-Schiff-positive, diastase-resistant bacillary forms within the histiocytes. Extraintestinal Whipple's disease, principally arthritis and central nervous system involvement, may be missed entirely unless there is a high index of suspicion. Advances in the molecular detection of *T. whippelii* have resolved this dilemma (215, 220, 269). Other novel bacterial pathogens have been identified and/or classified by 16S rRNA gene sequencing (Table 5).

TABLE 5 Human bacterial pathogens recently identified or characterized by 16S rRNA gene sequencing

Organism	Reference(s)
Actinobaculum suis	153
Actinomyces europaeus	98
Alpha-2 *Proterobacterium*	22
Bartonella bacilliformis	28
Bartonella elizabethae	29
Bartonella henselae	17, 29, 35
Bartonella quntana	168, 218
Bordetella holmesii	249, 281
Ehrlichia canis	202
Ehrlichia chaffeensis	77, 143
Ehrlichia microti (HGE agent)	45, 223
Facklamia hominis	55
Gordona terrae	75
Haemophilus parainfluenzae	110
Mycobacterium genavense	27, 108, 140
Mycobacterium shimoidei	116
Mycobacterium triplex	92
Rickettsia felis (ELB agent)	120, 236
Tropheryma whippelii	215, 220, 269

The DNA sequencing procedure involves extraction of nucleic acids, PCR-mediated amplification of a 16S rRNA gene fragment, sequence determination, and computer-aided analysis (Fig. 6). At present, the time and effort associated with data analysis and the cost are major limitations. The capital investment is high, particularly for automated analysis. To make 16S rRNA gene sequence analysis a routine tool, appropriate software needs to be developed, including programs that can cope with sequencing errors. In addition, the rRNA sequence database must be expanded to include more clinically relevant isolates, and its quality

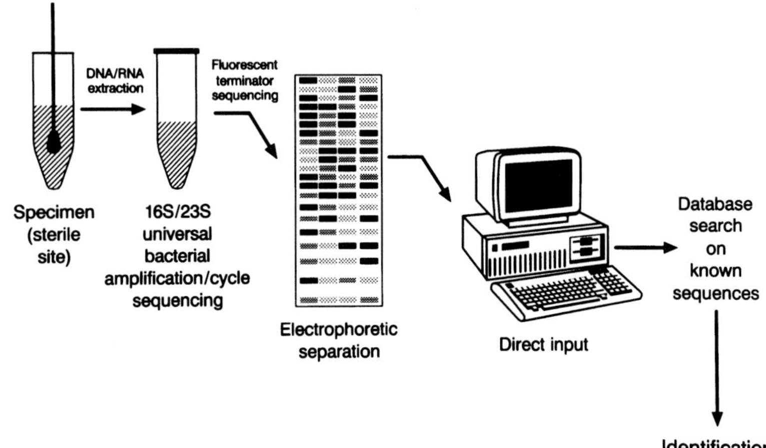

FIGURE 6 Nucleic acid sequence-based microbial identification. Broad-range or universal primers are used in a target amplification protocol for amplification of 16S or 23S rRNA gene sequences. An automated sequencer determines the composition of the intervening nucleotides and directly enters the sequence data into a computerized workstation. Database analysis creates a hierarchical cluster of related sequences and then generates a list of related or identical organisms.

control standards must improve. Perkin-Elmer Biosynthesis and MIDI systems have jointly developed a 16S rRNA gene sequence database from more than 1,200 American Type Culture Collection prototype bacterial strains. Their microbial identification system based on 16S rRNA sequence information is now commercially available (251). With improved automation and decreased cost, both of which are likely in the next few years, such systems may become established in many clinical microbiology laboratories.

Prognostication by Subtyping of Microorganisms

Subtyping by amplification-based techniques has important implications for infectious disease prognosis and therapy. It has been described that pathogenic diversity exists between *cagA*-positive and *cagA*-negative *Helicobacter pylori* strains. Infection with a *cagA*-positive strain increases the risk for the development of gastric ulcer and gastric cancer (21, 61). In dermatophyte infections, distinct ecological niches of the pathogens have prognostic value. The anthropophilic dermatophytes tend to cause chronic infections and may be difficult to treat, whereas zoophilic and geophilic isolates cause inflammatory lesions that may heal spontaneously (278).

Subtyping of viral infections may also have prognostic value. Group A respiratory syncytial virus (RSV) infection results in greater disease severity than group B RSV infection among hospitalized infants (276). HPV is a common cause of dysplasia, intraepithelial neoplasia, and carcinoma in the female genital tract. Certain types, such as types 16 and 18, are associated with a high risk of progressive neoplasia, while types 6 and 11 are "low-risk" subtypes (97, 216). DNA hybridization assays are used to determine HPV infection and viral types in cervical swabs or biopsy specimens. This provides helpful information for use in patient assessment and treatment (162, 183). Different HCV genotypes have distinct profiles of pathogenicity, infectivity, and response to antiviral therapy (49). Specific primer sets for detection of the 5′ untranslated or NS5 regions are designed to allow differentiation of genotypes (172). Using PCR followed by automated sequencing, several studies have revealed that the most common genotypes of HCV in the United States and Western Europe are 1a and 1b, while other genotypes, including 2a, 2b, 3, 4, 5, and 6, have their own distinct global distributions and prognostic significance (295, 297). In the United States, infection with type 1b is associated with a longer duration of infection, which perhaps explains the finding in some studies of an overrepresentation of this subtype in patients with liver cancer (297).

Disease Monitoring by Organism Quantitation

In recent years, there has been growing demand for the quantitation of nucleic acid targets (63, 217); at the Mayo Clinic, for instance, virus quantitation now comprises 60% of the molecular diagnostic test volume. Viral load data are used to monitor therapeutic response and provide prognostic information for patients infected with HIV (36, 71, 173, 196, 221, 267) and less definitively for those infected with HCV (70, 128) and HBV (117). Plasma HIV load is an early and accurate marker of disease progression (173, 174). This may result in better prediction of disease progression and outcome and may be useful for determining the need for the initiation or modification of antiviral therapy. Quantitation of viral load is based primarily on (i) target amplification, which includes both PCR- and NASBA-based techniques, and (ii) bDNA-based signal amplification. Kit-based technologies make it possible for many laboratories to carry out quantitative analyses. To date, only the PCR-based methods have received FDA approval.

The task of quantitative amplification was and still is problematic. This is because the amplification techniques yield products in an exponential manner until a plateau is reached; any factor interfering with the exponential nature of the amplification process would thereby affect the result of the quantitative assay. To overcome this problem, a competitive RT-PCR has been developed on the basis of coamplification of an internal competitor with the target sequence (13). This approach forms the basis of the Amplicor Monitor kits manufactured by Roche. These kits are now widely used for HIV-1 and HCV quantitation. Another quantitation technique based on NASBA also uses an internal competitor; this test was developed by Organon-Teknika to determine the level of HIV-1 RNA and includes an automated sample preparation system (267). The NASBA-based system is pending FDA approval.

The bDNA technology, with sensitivity derived from signal amplification, is also used to quantify cell-free HIV-1 genomic RNA in serum (36, 71, 196, 221). Currently, the manufacturer's claim for the bDNA detection threshold for HIV-1 RNA in plasma or serum is 5×10^2 molecules per ml (36). Manufactured by Chiron, the bDNA technology is also developed for quantitation of HCV and HBV in plasma or serum specimens to monitor the efficacy of antiviral chemotherapy (70, 117).

Genotypic Approaches to Detection of Antimicrobial Drug Resistance

Antimicrobial susceptibility testing is one of the most important tasks in the clinical microbiology laboratory. It provides an in vitro estimate of the probability that an infection will respond to therapy in vitro. Molecular techniques are starting to play a role in the rapid detection of resistance. In some cases, such techniques offer the opportunity to reduce the time required for institution of definitive therapy, thus reducing the use of inappropriate antibiotics. Rapid detection may also allow early recognition of carriers infected with resistant organisms and appropriate implementation of isolation, epidemiological investigation, and integrated infection control practices. There is considerable interest in the application of molecular methods directly to clinical specimens to provide a more rapid means of identification of resistance (40, 209), resulting in improved patient outcome and reductions in overall costs (see chapter 122).

Application of molecular techniques to the problem of drug resistance depends on knowing the genotypic basis for that resistance. For organisms with resistance mechanisms of unknown genotypes, conventional susceptibility testing remains essential. Some drug resistance is due to multiple mechanisms. Under certain circumstances, a single organism type may express its antimicrobial resistance by expressing different genes. This presents a tremendous challenge to the determination of bacterial drug resistance by molecular techniques except in certain instances. It is important to determine the degree of consistency with which each gene that encodes for a resistance mechanism is expressed by the organism. For *mecA*-containing *Staphylococcus aureus*, almost all strains which possess the gene express the resistance to methicillin. This is not the case for coagulase-negative staphylococci, in which resistance can be induced by propagation of isolates in progressively higher concentrations of oxacillin.

Because of the great variety of bacterial genes encoding drug resistance and the added complexity of differential expression, a universal genotypic approach to the detection of drug resistance would have been unthinkable only a few years ago. However, with the advent of matrix hybridization, the landscape has now changed. Already, "sequencing chips" are being developed for the simultaneous identification and genotypic determination of drug resistance for *M. tuberculosis*. Under discussion are "universal drug resistance" chips which contain oligonucleotide arrays specific for all of the known bacterial drug resistance genes on a single chip. To address the concern about expression, such chips may be designed to detect DNA or RNA; the advantages to the detection of RNA expression from a bacterial isolate may be augmented by the ability to detect structural mutations indirectly via the expression of mRNA. Clearly, the advent of these technologies makes it possible to imagine numerous diagnostic applications in the future.

Evaluating Epidemic and Nosocomial Infections

Investigation and control of nosocomial infections are complex activities. The efforts of both the microbiologist and the hospital epidemiologist are facilitated by the availability of new molecular typing techniques. Molecular diagnostic techniques have been successful in the investigation and control of classical and emerging nosocomial pathogens (see chapters 6 and 7).

The ability to characterize organisms suspected of causing a community disease outbreak is critical to public health efforts. Identification must be rapid and unambiguous. Several recent contributions to clinical and hospital epidemiology have depended on PCR, and many putative epidemics have been investigated by other molecular techniques. Examples include investigation of clustered cases of invasive disease (due to *Streptococcus pyogenes*) in Air Force recruits (185), a cluster of lymphogranuloma venereum cases caused by *C. trachomatis* serovar L1 in homosexual men (12), and an outbreak of *E. coli* O157:H7 due to contaminated deer jerky (134).

So-called broad-range PCR techniques can also identify novel agents as the cause of epidemics. In May 1993, a mysterious outbreak was reported in the southwestern United States. Patients had unexplained adult respiratory distress syndrome or acute bilateral pulmonary interstitial infiltrates, with a case fatality rate of 75%. Preliminary serologic studies found antibodies in patients' sera in patterns suggesting cross-reactivity (but not identity) with previously known hantaviruses (43). Genome sequence analysis of available hantavirus strains identified regions of sequence conservation within the G2 protein-coding region of the M segment of the hantavirus genome (7, 254). Deoxyoligonucleotide primers were designed for the detection of the hantavirus genome by a broad-range nested RT-PCR assay. This assay generated hantavirus-specific amplicons from the RNA of patients as well as deer mice from the outbreak area. Within months, molecular epidemiological techniques showed the agent to be a new hantavirus species and provided a direct genetic link between infection in patients and rodents (190).

SPECIMEN PROCESSING FOR MOLECULAR DIAGNOSTICS

Good specimen quality and good specimen preparation are as critical for molecular diagnostics as they are in other areas of the microbiology laboratory. Specimen preparation comprises efficient target recovery, establishment of the integrity of the nucleic acid target, optimal removal of amplification inhibitors, elimination of components which affect other enzymatic substrates (e.g., metals), and sterilization of potentially hazardous organisms. Nucleic acid specimen preparation should concentrate the target into a small volume and place the target into an aqueous environment compatible with amplification.

In general, it is preferred that specimens received for molecular diagnostics be handled in a manner consistent with standard tissue culture techniques (203, 271). Specimens should be processed in a timely manner or stored at −80°C until processing; whole blood specimens, however, should be frozen only after component fractionation. The type of processing varies with target and specimen sources. However, many specimens can be handled by relatively simple processing procedures. For some specimens other than blood and urine, boiling of the sample followed by concentration is sufficient to make the organisms' nucleic acids accessible. For urine specimens, treatment of sediment with proteinase K followed by heating has been used for DNA amplification. However, sample boiling may lead to an unacceptable rate of inhibition in some cases. Some specimens, such as CSF, contain undefined inhibitors of the PCR, reducing the efficiency of amplification, so that a nucleic acid extraction step must be used (179).

Extraction of nucleic acids from biological materials is one of the most important steps performed in molecular microbiology. Conventional methods for extracting nucleic acids from clinical specimens involve proteinase K digestion followed by multiple phenol and chloroform-isoamyl alcohol (24:1) extractions. The resulting nucleic acids are precipitated in the presence of salts and ethanol. The DNA pellet is washed with cold 70% ethanol to remove any contaminants, dried, and dissolved in a suitable buffer system for the ensuing procedures. Phenol and chloroform are hazardous, and conventional methods require considerable specimen manipulation. Several procedures other than standard phenol-chloroform extraction have been used for nucleic acid extraction. These include ethanol precipitation (82–84, 203), use of diatom or glass matrices (26, 203), and pelleting and cell lysis (203, 246). Quick, efficient commercial kits are now available for DNA and RNA extraction (271). The following sections describe the approaches that have been used for various sample types. Automated extraction, which is a direct spin-off of the large-scale genomic sequencing efforts of the human genome project, is now being explored for microbiology laboratories and may provide a critical link in the establishment of inexpensive, automated nucleic acid-based tests.

Blood Specimens

Blood specimens can be divided into several categories: plasma, serum, whole blood, and leukocytes. Furthermore, there is a choice of anticoagulants if the specimen is plasma: EDTA, heparin, citrate, or oxalate. Heparin inhibits the activities of both RT and DNA polymerase and should not be used for specimen preparations used for molecular diagnostics (19). Whole-blood specimens have been used for nucleic acid detection for several organisms, including *Ehrlichia chaffeensis* (5), *Campylobacter fetus* (197), *Treponema pallidum* (284), *Plasmodium vivax* (133), and *Babesia microti* (207). Various procedures for inactivation of inhibitors in whole-blood specimens have been described (5, 133, 170, 197, 207, 284). Blood leukocytes, a preferred specimen for intracellular virus detection, can be obtained through Ficoll-Hypaque gradient centrifugation. The nucleic acids are then isolated by lysing the purified leukocytes with detergent and digestion with proteinase K or detergent alone (3, 24, 58).

Serum or plasma specimens make up approximately 60% of specimens submitted to many molecular microbiology laboratories. Several standard nucleic acid isolation procedures have been successful in obtaining amplifiable DNA following disruption of capsid by detergents, proteinases, or both (150, 277). Both phenol-chloroform extraction and DNA adsorption to silica matrices have been used (25, 169, 292). Extraction with phenol and phenol-chloroform followed by ethanol precipitation has been applied to the isolation of viral target RNA from serum and plasma (34, 277). In general, conventional guanidinium isothiocyanate or cesium chloride gradient procedures are too difficult or hazardous for routine diagnostic use. There is great need to improve on RNA target extraction techniques and to develop ways to stabilize the capsids or the RNA itself in the specimen during collection and transport. The specimen should be processed promptly or stored at −80°C. Whole blood from which RNA is to be extracted should remain at 4 to 6°C. Room temperature storage of serum results in a substantial decrease in the level of HCV RNA detected, and repeated freezing and thawing causes a moderate reduction in viral titer. Minor effects of freeze-thawing have also been noted for HIV (59). In general, viral RNA appears to be more stable inside intact virions than in pure form, so repeat testing of specimens is best done for reextracted samples.

CSF

CSF specimens are now commonly used in various molecular diagnostic tests. Amplification of pathogen-specific nucleic acids from CSF has considerably improved the diagnosis of several acute, subacute, and chronic viral infections of the central nervous system. One advantage of using CSF specimens for molecular diagnosis is the uniformity of the samples. Like serum, CSF should be easily adaptable to automated processing. In HSV encephalitis or meningitis, PCR has become the method of choice for rapid, noninvasive diagnosis (179, 253, 255). Small volumes ($<10\ \mu l$) of CSF have been used successfully in PCR-based assays without DNA extraction. At the Mayo Clinic, however, chaotropic lysis methods are used routinely for the extraction of DNA and RNA from CSF specimens to inactivate nucleases, to remove nonspecific inhibitors, and to concentrate nucleic acids (84, 179, 227, 253).

Urine Specimens

Urine specimens can be used in the molecular microbiology laboratory, especially for the detection of sexually transmitted pathogens, such as *C. trachomatis* and *N. gonorrhoeae* (46, 198, 214, 243). Numerous lysis and nucleic acid extraction procedures for use with urine specimens have been reported (26, 33, 101, 154, 226). These procedures, which are similar to those outlined above for CSF, require evaluation for their efficacy in removing amplification inhibitors.

Sputum Specimens

Sputum is the most important specimen source for the diagnosis of tuberculosis. A quick, sensitive, and safe method of lysis and extraction of nucleic acid from sputum is an important goal of molecular diagnostics. Because acidic polysaccharides in sputum are known to inhibit DNA polymerases, successful sputum preparation must separate the nucleic acids from the inhibitors. Phenol-chloroform extraction of DNA followed by ethanol precipitation has been used with sputum specimens (27, 60). The use of silica matrices that bind to DNA followed by repetitive washing with detergents has also yielded amplifiable DNA from sputum specimens (246).

It has been considered that DNA extracted from dead mycobacterial pathogens in sputum may not be associated with active disease, particularly when the patient is on therapy. Extraction of RNA from sputum has been recommend as a solution to this problem. However, because of the fragility of RNA molecules, specimen processing is difficult (69). Treatment of the sputum sample with the mucolytic agent Sputolysin and incubation of the sample with equal volumes of sodium hydroxide containing phenolphthalein before RNA extraction seem to be effective preextraction steps (130). Direct ethanol fixation followed by nucleic acid extraction has also been described. In general, the challenges of sample processing appear to be responsible for the still wide disparity in the sensitivities of amplification methods relative to that of culture for the detection of *M. tuberculosis*.

Fecal Specimens

Fecal specimens remain the most difficult clinical samples for DNA extraction and amplification. A variety of stool components inhibit DNA amplification. Resolution of this problem would render PCR a valuable diagnostic tool for enteric pathogens since many are present in feces but are not readily culturable (181, 261). Despite the very high concentration of enteropathogenic bacteria in stools, it has always been difficult to use PCR to detect these microorganisms because of inhibitors and the genetic complexity of fecal material. One study demonstrated that even after the spiking of feces with 8×10^7 *H. pylori* cells per g, the pathogen remained undetectable by PCR (181).

Several efforts have been made to remove inhibitory components from stool specimens during processing. These include phenol-chloroform extraction (30, 95), treatment with Chelex 100 followed by solvent extraction (66, 127), immunomagnetic extraction (81, 163, 240), treatment with hexadecyltrimethylammonium bromide followed by a phenol-chloroform extraction (122), and purification of nucleic acids with silica particles in the presence of guanidium thiocyanate. Other studies suggest that amplification inhibition can be overcome to a great extent simply by increasing the concentration of bovine serum albumin in the PCR master mixture (146). Recent work by Monteiro and coworkers (181) characterized the inhibitory components in feces as complex polysaccharides possibly originating from vegetable material in the diet. The inhibitor was successfully removed by using a modified QIAamp tissue method including the passing of specimens through an Ultrogel AcA44 column (181). In the end, target-specific capture methods may win out in the analysis of fecal material.

Other Specimens

In addition to those described above, other specimen types can and have been used for molecular diagnostic testing. A quantitative PCR technique was used for the detection of human herpesviruses 6 and 7 in lymph nodes (239). Gastric biopsy tissue was adapted for *H. pylori* DNA detection by PCR following colorimetric hybridization (149). Synovial fluids are good specimens for use in the detection of *Borrelia burgdorferi* by PCR (192). A simple and quick extraction procedure has been used for the detection of *C. trachomatis* in endocervical swabs (135, 160). Detection and differentiation of organisms retained in formalin-fixed and paraffin-embedded tissues have some value in anatomic pathology, especially for slowly growing mycobacteria and difficult-to-differentiate fungi (105, 114, 213). Theoretically, the stability of nucleic acids makes it possible to detect most microorganisms in formalin-fixed, paraffin-embedded tissue sections. Special processing, including limited fixation time, may be needed to obtain good-quality DNA for amplification from this source, however. In addition, a small target length (less than 250 bp) is recommended for test sensitivity, since the fixation and embedding steps might break nucleic acid chains (105).

QUALITY ASSURANCE AND QUALITY CONTROL

Quality assurance programs constitute an integral part of any diagnostic laboratory and can account for 15 to 25% of the laboratory's consumable supply costs (42). Because of the requisite sensitivity of nucleic acid amplification procedures, quality assurance programs in molecular microbiology are more complicated and expensive than those used in other laboratories; at the same time, their implementation is of the utmost importance.

Cross-Contamination Prevention

The requirements of a molecular microbiology laboratory facility depend on the type and number of procedures performed in the facility. The laboratory must accommodate four separate functions: reagent preparation, sample processing, reaction setup, and postamplification detection and analysis. The ideal molecular microbiology laboratory will have a separate room for each function. However, laboratories with limited space can separate these functions by establishing separate workstations in less space and within one or a few rooms. In the ideal facility, each room is designed to isolate potentially contaminating aerosols and nucleic acids bound to particulate material by using controlled airflow, two-door vestibule-type entrances with magnetic interlocks, and UV light fixtures installed in the overhead lighting and in "dead-air boxes" used as workspaces (79). Each workstation should have dedicated supplies and equipment. Laboratory work surfaces should be smooth and unobstructed and should be constructed to withstand regular cleaning with diluted bleach and/or shortwave UV radiation. All laboratory coats, sleeves, gloves, masks, shoe covers, and caps should be clearly marked for each area, preferably by color coding.

To further reduce the possibility of cross contamination, the concept of unidirectional work flow is integrated with physical separation of the major work areas. Specimens should be received and accessioned in an area of the facility that is isolated from any areas of the laboratory used for cultivation of the target organism. Each phase of the testing process proceeds from the reagent preparation area to specimen preparation, then to amplification, and finally, to the detection areas. This one-way work flow policy is applied to laboratory workers, directors, specimens, and work cards. "Reverse personnel flow" should be minimized by careful planning. Performance of several tasks at the same time and place should be discouraged whenever possible. It should be made clear at the outset that these recommendations apply mainly to user-developed tests and large reference laboratories and not to laboratories that presumably use commercially prepared kits. Contamination control will also lessen the need for "four rooms" as a concept.

Routine Preventive Measures

Especially for user-developed (so-called home-brewed) assays, amplification product buildup in laboratory reagents, glassware, instruments, autoclaves, and ventilation systems may be a serious problem (148). Bench-top work areas should be covered with plastic-backed absorbent paper that is changed for each run. Disposable gloves should be worn at all times and should be changed as needed. Use of aerosol-resistant filter tips and positive-displacement pipettes is strongly encouraged. A low-copy-number (10 to 50 copies per reaction mixture) positive control, several negative controls, and reagent controls (no target DNA) should be included with every amplification in order to detect contamination if it occurs.

Regular quality control activities in the laboratory should include pipettor calibration and temperature and ramp time monitoring of the thermal cycler. A daily-task checklist includes checking and recording temperatures in all water baths, heat blocks, and incubators and making a fresh 10% bleach solution for cleaning. After completion of each assay, all pipettors, instruments, and work surfaces should be decontaminated by UV irradiation and should be wiped clean with 10% bleach and 70% alcohol.

Another way of preventing cross contamination is adoption of a closed-vessel system. As soon as processed specimens are loaded into a tube or chamber, the tube or chamber will go through all amplification and detection procedures and will never be opened again. By eliminating the handling of amplification products in an open environment, the false-positive results due to product carryover can be avoided. An automated system for PCR amplification and detection that combats false-positive results has been described (91). The system uses a single vessel (PCR pouch) for both PCR amplification and the subsequent detection of PCR products, eliminating the need to handle PCR products in an open environment and the risk of product carryover. All of the major diagnostic system manufacturers are developing and evaluating similar sealed automated systems.

Proficiency Testing

The proficiency test provides an excellent means of determining test variability among laboratories (external proficiency tests) and within laboratories (internal proficiency tests). Proficiency testing is extremely important for molecular diagnostic laboratories since PCR diagnosis remains largely unregulated. Different laboratories use different primer sets, protocols, and standards to detect the same pathogen, producing different rates of false-positive and false-negative results. For designated approved vendors, the College of American Pathologists (CAP) has offered an ungraded infectious disease survey over the past 2 years. The survey has included HIV-1, HCV, HSV, *M. tuberculosis*, *C. trachomatis*, and *N. gonorrhoeae* for detection by PCR-based molecular techniques. *B. burgdorferi* and CMV will be offered in future infectious disease surveys. Starting in 1998, two test sets which consist of three mailings each have been offered to the molecular microbiology survey for testing by nucleic acid amplification techniques. The HC6 set includes five swab challenges for testing *C. trachomatis* and/or *N. gonorrhoeae*, and the HIV/HV2 set consists of five 0.5- or 2.5-ml plasma specimens for the quantitative and/or qualitative detection of HIV-1. Similar to the proficiency testing in other laboratories, test results should be returned within 10 working days after receipt of the specimens.

Internal proficiency testing is also an important part of molecular microbiology. Some form of internal testing program is required under the regulations of the Clinical Laboratory Improvement Act of 1988 (53). Internal proficiency testing can be started by using leftover microbiology survey materials from CAP or samples exchanged with other laboratories. The quality control technologist or supervisor should integrate these samples blindly within the routine laboratory workload. Such internal programs are often the first to identify problems; additional attention can be paid to tests or sample types that consistently fail internal programs.

INTERPRETATION OF RESULTS

It is important to remember that molecular diagnostic techniques and their results may mean different things in comparison with conventional culture and serology and their results. A culture positive for an organism clearly demonstrates the viability of the organism, while a rise in titer of antibody to a specific organism strongly suggests a response to infection. A nucleic acid probe or amplification procedure, on the other hand, determines whether specific sequences of nucleic acids, DNA or RNA, from a particular organism are present in the specimen. Therefore, special attention should be paid to the interpretation of the results of molecular diagnostic techniques.

Dead Versus Live Pathogens

Because dead organisms may contain amplifiable DNA, a positive result obtained by a molecular technique does not necessarily demonstrate that viable organisms are present in a particular specimen. In tuberculosis, nonviable organisms apparently remain intact in the lung for a long time, resulting in difficulties in evaluating the effect of therapy. This "dead cell" objection might be overcome by shifting the target of the assay from DNA molecules to mRNA (165). mRNAs generally have much shorter half-lives than rRNA and DNA and would tend to reflect more accurately the viability of the organisms in a specimen than would the presence of amplifiable DNA. A single-tube, nested, RT-PCR for the detection of viable *M. tuberculosis* has recently been reported (130). Targeting a short-half-life mRNA molecule may also provide a rapid means of determination of antibiotic resistance, although at the cost of more difficult sample processing (69). For now, however, amplification-based tests cannot be used to monitor the treatment of mycobacterial infection.

Presence of Nucleic Acid Versus Disease

Amplification of certain organisms' nucleic acid sequences from nonsterile specimens may be consistent with contamination, colonization, or infection. Identification of certain nucleic acid sequences in patients can prove that the patient carries the genome of a specific organism, but it may not prove that the organism is responsible for the disease in question. Although this does not necessarily mean that the patient suffers from a disease associated with this particular organism, the presumption of causality is strengthened if other symptoms are also identified (48, 190, 220, 253). For example, detection of the HSV-1 genome from CSF is generally consistent with infection and active disease; however, there is no definitive means by which to decide if the patient suffers from primary infection or reactivation. It is also possible that another cause of encephalitis is present as well. In some cases, symptoms may occur only after several years or not at all, and it is yet to be determined whether the positive signal in the sensitive PCR should be a cautionary sign for closer follow-up or, alternatively, a sign for initiating preventive measures. The presence of hepatitis G virus RNA in plasma is perhaps an example of an active, persistent viremia in search of a disease (232, 260).

Causal or Casual? Modification of Koch's Postulates

The ability to detect and manipulate nucleic acid molecules in microorganisms has created a powerful means for identifying previously unknown microbial pathogens and for studying the host-parasite relationship (86). There are and probably always will be circumstances in which an organism resists cultivation; in this setting, genotypic methods may be the only method for the identification of the microbial pathogens, thereby providing convincing evidence of disease association or causation. However, in many cases described above, a causal relationship cannot be firmly established on the basis of Koch's postulates (96), especially for those agents that cannot be cultivated in the laboratory. Instead, various forms of evidence taken collectively provide a basis for assessing causation. Koch's postulates for determining the causal relationship between a microorganism and a disease have been modified by many investigators working outside the traditional infectious disease paradigm (96), but they might need to be modified again to incorporate newly developed molecular technology. A revision to Koch's postulates has been proposed to determine whether pathogen-specific nucleic acid sequences are necessary for a particular disease to occur (96). The preliminary guidelines have been listed elsewhere (204).

In general, it is important to keep in mind the distinction between "necessary" and "both necessary and sufficient." A good example is HPV, for which there is increasing evidence for an important role in the development of cervical and other epithelial cancers. However, while HPV may be necessary for the development of perhaps 90% of cervical cancer cases, most cases of HPV infection do not lead to cervical cancer. Thus, although HPV is an important cofactor, it does not in itself "cause" cervical cancer.

FUTURE DIRECTIONS

Automation

Increased workloads in clinical microbiology laboratories have led to a search for more automated procedures. In the past several decades, clinical chemistry laboratories have developed extensive automation. With the emergence of molecular techniques, expansion of automation in clinical microbiology is now within the realm of possibility (286). The biochemical methods used for the specific identification of infectious agents at the nucleic acid level represent a legitimate synthesis of clinical chemistry and clinical microbiology techniques.

Automation in molecular diagnostics is divided into three areas: specimen processing, nucleic acid amplification, and amplification product detection and quantitation. Automation of detection has been achieved by several companies. One such example is the Abbott LCX system for the detection of LCR amplification products from both *C. trachomatis* and *N. gonorrhoeae* in clinical specimens. COBAS Amplicor, a Roche-developed system with automated amplification and detection steps, yields results 5 h after extracted specimens are loaded (73, 132). This system is now in widespread use in Europe and is under clinical investigation in the United States. Matrix hybridization provides another good example of automated amplification product detection (93, 158).

To a great extent, the future of molecular microbiology will depend on automation of sample processing. Since the targets in molecular diagnostics are nucleic acids, the highly automated instruments used in clinical chemistry should be adaptable for molecular microbiology laboratories. Among specimens sent to molecular microbiology at the Mayo Clinic, up to 60% are serum or plasma specimens and 15 to 20% are CSF specimens. The uniformity of these specimens should facilitate the development of automated systems for sample processing.

All of the major diagnostic companies are developing fully automated systems for molecular diagnostics. The test volumes and turnaround times for these systems are quite variable. For example, the TIGRIS system developed by Gen-Probe can reportedly process 500 tests in an 8-h shift, and the VITROS system developed by Johnson & Johnson can detect the presence of an infectious agent in less than 2 h (91). Automated systems should be constructed as sealed systems, thereby nearly eliminating aerosolization and contamination of amplification products. With the development of more user-friendly and automated systems, the expansion of these technologies to smaller institutions and hospitals may occur.

"One Stone for Many Birds"

Molecular screening of at-risk populations for a group of possible pathogens is an exciting area of development in molecular microbiology. For example, numerous etiologic agents cause debilitating gastroenteritis in immunosuppressed patient populations. These include mycobacteria (e.g., *M. avium* complex and *M. genavense*), parasites (e.g., *Cryptosporidium*, *Microsporidium*), viruses (e.g., rotavirus, and the Norwalk agent), and typical bacterial pathogens (*E. coli* variants, *Salmonella*, *Shigella*, and *Campylobacter*). Traditionally, different methods of detection are used for each group of pathogens. This requires special media, equipment, and expensive facilities for the culture of mycobacteria, expertise in the identification of parasites and ova in stool preparations, virology facilities, and special media for bacterial enteric pathogens. Although these tests are individually inexpensive, comprehensive workup for enteric pathogens is quite costly.

Molecular techniques can screen a patient population for panels of probable pathogens. Nucleic acids extracted from the stools of patients with gastroenteritis may be probed for organism- or group-specific nucleic acids. The development of multiplex PCR assays for urethritis or genital ulcerative diseases has been pursued by several diagnostic system manufacturers (195). The application of such assays could play a significant role in the control of many sexually transmitted diseases in the future. In this manner, a single test may be used to identify the etiologic agent of disease from among numerous possibilities (106). The application of these tests could be used to reduce the numbers of cultures that are performed.

Multiplex PCR uses numerous primers within a single reaction tube in order to amplify nucleic acid fragments from different targets. Specific nucleic acid amplification should occur if the appropriate target DNA is present in the sample tested (15, 100, 130, 224). Detection may then be accomplished with a nucleic acid probe, by a colorimetric reaction, or by matrix hybridization. This technology is limited by the number of primers which can be included in a single reaction, the primer-primer interference, and nonspecific nucleic acid amplification. However, use of certain polymerases such as TaqGold may facilitate the development of multiplex assays that are truly useful in a panel format (20).

Detection of Infection-Related Host Factor(s)

Host immunogenetic factors may influence the risk of becoming infected with certain pathogens, as well as the rate of disease progression once one is infected. Individuals deficient in the terminal components of the complement cascade, the membrane attachment complex, are predisposed to recurrent systemic *Neisseria* infections (90). Mutations in the gamma interferon receptor predispose patients to severe disseminated atypical mycobacterial infections (189) and fatal infection with *Mycobacterium bovis* bacillus Calmette-Guérin, the most widely used tuberculosis vaccine (131).

Genetic polymorphism has been described in the cytochrome P-450 system, which can markedly affect drug kinetics (64, 175). Advances in molecular genetics have elucidated the molecular basis for several of these polymorphisms, allowing the development of PCR-based genotyping assays (67, 115, 129). Determination of cytochrome P-450 patterns will allow prediction of each individual's metabolic capacity and, consequently, the most appropriate drug dosage for that individual. This approach is particularly helpful in establishing HIV treatment regimens, since early, maximal, prolonged combination therapy is necessary (54, 111, 201).

A major effort in HIV research in recent years has been to discover the underlying mechanisms that allow some long-term survivors to resist disease 10 to 20 years after HIV-1 infection or to allow some highly exposed individuals to remain uninfected. Recent studies revealed that entry of HIV-1 into human cells requires CD4 and a coreceptor such as CC-chemokine receptor 5 (CCR-5) and CCR-2. CCR-5 is a common coreceptor for macrophage-tropic, non-syncytium-inducing HIV-1 strains that predominate during initial infection. Recently, an internal 32-bp deletion in the human *CCR-5* gene has been identified to be associated with resistance to HIV-1 infection both in vitro and in vivo (65, 159, 199, 230). Heterozygosity for the *CCR-5Δ32* deletion does not protect children from infection by the maternal virus but substantially reduces the progression of the disease in HIV-1-infected children (178). It has been reported recently that a point mutation in *CCR-2* that, when considered with the deletion in *CCR-5*, explains the ability of about 25% of long-term survivors to avoid progressive infection (244). Genetic polymorphism of human genes also restricts the entry, multiplication, and survival of malarial parasites and is associated with resistance to malarial infection (176). Similarly, the absence of an erythrocyte antigen among inbred human subpopulations appears to confer absolute resistance to parvovirus B19 infection (31). If infections, especially chronic infections, can be viewed as horizontally acquired genetic diseases, it makes perfect sense to view the pathogen and the host as an integrated system. Accordingly, detection of host factors by genetic methods may become an increasingly important role of clinical microbiology laboratories in the future.

REFERENCES

1. **Aach, R. D., C. E. Stevens, F. B. Hollinger, J. W. Mosley, D. A. Peterson, P. E. Taylor, R. G. Johnson, L. H. Barbosa, and G. J. Nemo.** 1991. Hepatitis C virus infection in post-transfusion hepatitis. An analysis with first- and second-generation assays. *N. Engl. J. Med.* **325:** 1325–1329.
2. **Abe, C., K. Hirano, M. Wada, Y. Kazumi, M. Takahashi, Y. Fukasawa, T. Yoshimura, C. Miyagi, and S. Goto.** 1993. Detection of *Mycobacterium tuberculosis* in clinical specimens by polymerase chain reaction and Gen-Probe Amplified Mycobacterium Tuberculosis Direct Test. *J. Clin. Microbiol.* **31:**3270–3274.
3. **Albert, J., and E. M. Fenyo.** 1990. Simple, sensitive, and specific detection of human immunodeficiency virus type 1 in clinical specimens by polymerase chain reaction with nested primers. *J. Clin. Microbiol.* **28:**1560–1564.
4. **Alter, H. J., R. H. Purcell, J. W. Shih, J. C. Melpolder, M. Houghton, Q. L. Choo, and G. Kuo.** 1989. Detection of antibody to hepatitis C virus in prospectively followed transfusion recipients with acute and chronic non-A, non-B hepatitis. *N. Engl. J. Med.* **321:**1494–1500.
5. **Anderson, B. E., J. W. Sumner, J. E. Dawson, T. Tzianabos, C. R. Greene, J. G. Olson, D. B. Fishbein, M. Olsen-Rasmussen, B. P. Holloway, and E. H. George.** 1992. Detection of the etiologic agent of human ehrlichiosis by polymerase chain reaction. *J. Clin. Microbiol.* **30:**775–780.
6. **Andiman, W., L. Gradoville, L. Heston, R. Neydorff, M. E. Savage, G. Kitchingman, D. Shedd, and G. Miller.** 1983. Use of cloned probes to detect Epstein-Barr viral DNA in tissues of patients with neoplastic and lymphoproliferative diseases. *J. Infect. Dis.* **148:**967–977.
7. **Arikawa, J., H. F. Lapenotiere, L. Iacono-Connors, M. L. Wang, and C. S. Schmaljohn.** 1990. Coding properties of the S and the M genome segments of Sapporo rat virus: comparison to other causative agents of hemorrhagic fever with renal syndrome. *Virology* **176:**114–125.
8. **Arnold, L. J., Jr., P. W. Hammond, W. A. Wiese, and N. C. Nelson.** 1989. Assay formats involving acridinium-ester-labeled DNA probes. *Clin. Chem.* **35:**1588–1594.
9. **Arola, A., J. Santti, O. Ruuskanen, P. Halonen, and T. Hyypia.** 1996. Identification of enteroviruses in clinical specimens by competitive PCR followed by genetic typing using sequence analysis. *J. Clin. Microbiol.* **34:**313–318.
10. **Aslanzadeh, J.** 1993. Application of hydroxylamine hydrochloride for post-PCR sterilization. *Mol. Cell. Probes* **7:**145–150.
11. **Barany, F.** 1991. Genetic disease detection and DNA amplification using cloned thermostable ligase. *Proc. Natl. Acad. Sci. USA* **88:**189–193.
12. **Bauwens, J. E., M. F. Lampe, R. J. Suchland, K. Wong, and W. E. Stamm.** 1995. Infection with *Chlamydia trachomatis* lymphogranuloma venereum serovar L1 in homosexual men with proctitis: molecular analysis of an unusual case cluster. *Clin. Infect. Dis.* **20:**576–581.
13. **Becker-Andre, M., and K. Hahlbrock.** 1989. Absolute mRNA quantification using the polymerase chain reaction (PCR). A novel approach by a PCR aided transcript titration assay (PATTY). *Nucleic Acids Res.* **17:** 9437–9446.
14. **Beckmann, A. M., D. Myerson, J. R. Daling, N. B. Kiviat, C. M. Fenoglio, and J. K. McDougall.** 1985. Detection and localization of human papillomavirus DNA in human genital condylomas by in situ hybridization with biotinylated probes. *J. Med. Virol.* **16:**265–273.
15. **Bej, A. K., M. H. Mahbubani, R. Miller, J. L. DiCesare, L. Haff, and R. M. Atlas.** 1990. Multiplex PCR amplification and immobilized capture probes for detection of bacterial pathogens and indicators in water. *Mol. Cell. Probes* **4:**353–365.
16. **Bergmann, J. S., and G. L. Woods.** 1996. Clinical evaluation of the Roche AMPLICOR PCR *Mycobacterium tuberculosis* test for detection of *M. tuberculosis* in respiratory specimens. *J. Clin. Microbiol.* **34:**1083–1085.
17. **Bergmans, A. M., J. F. Schellekens, J. D. van Embden, and L. M. Schouls.** 1996. Predominance of two *Bartonella henselae* variants among cat-scratch disease patients in the Netherlands. *J. Clin. Microbiol.* **34:**254–260.
18. **Bernard, H. U., S. Y. Chan, M. M. Manos, C. K. Ong, L. L. Villa, H. Delius, C. L. Peyton, H. M. Bauer, and C. M. Wheeler.** 1994. Identification and assessment of known and novel human papillomaviruses by polymerase chain reaction amplification, restriction fragment length polymorphisms, nucleotide sequence, and phylogenetic algorithms. *J. Infect. Dis.* **170:**1077–1085.
19. **Beutler, E., T. Gelbart, and W. Kuhl.** 1990. Interference of heparin with the polymerase chain reaction. *BioTechniques* **9:**166.
20. **Birch, D. E., L. Kolmodin, W. J. Laird, N. McKinney, J. Wong, K. K. Young, G. A. Zangenberg, and M. A. Zoccoli.** 1996. Simplified hot start PCR. *Nature* **381:** 445–446.
21. **Blaser, M. J., G. I. Perez-Perez, H. Kleanthous, T. L. Cover, R. M. Peek, P. H. Chyou, G. N. Stemmermann, and A. Nomura.** 1995. Infection with *Helicobacter pylori* strains possessing cagA is associated with an increased

risk of developing adenocarcinoma of the stomach. *Cancer Res.* **55:**2111–2115.

22. **Blomqvist, G., L. Wesslen, C. Pahlson, E. Hjelm, B. Pettersson, T. Nikkila, U. Allard, O. Svensson, M. Uhlen, B. Morein, and G. Friman.** 1997. Phylogenetic placement and characterization of a new alpha-2 proteobacterium isolated from a patient with sepsis. *J. Clin. Microbiol.* **35:**1988–1995.
23. **Boddinghaus, B., T. Rogall, T. Flohr, H. Blocker, and E. C. Bottger.** 1990. Detection and identification of mycobacteria by amplification of rRNA. *J. Clin. Microbiol.* **28:**1751–1759.
24. **Boland, G. J., R. A. de Weger, M. G. Tilanus, C. Ververs, K. Bosboom-Kalsbeek, and G. C. de Gast.** 1992. Detection of cytomegalovirus (CMV) in granulocytes by polymerase chain reaction compared with the CMV antigen test. *J. Clin. Microbiol.* **30:**1763–1767.
25. **Boom, R., C. J. Sol, R. Heijtink, P. M. Wertheim-van Dillen, and J. van der Noordaa.** 1991. Rapid purification of hepatitis B virus DNA from serum. *J. Clin. Microbiol.* **29:**1804–1811.
26. **Boom, R., C. J. Sol, M. M. Salimans, C. L. Jansen, P. M. Wertheim-van Dillen, and J. van der Noordaa.** 1990. Rapid and simple method for purification of nucleic acids. *J. Clin. Microbiol.* **28:**495–503.
27. **Bottger, E. C., A. Teske, P. Kirschner, S. Bost, H. R. Chang, V. Beer, and B. Hirschel.** 1992. Disseminated "Mycobacterium genavense" infection in patients with AIDS. *Lancet* **340:**76–80.
28. **Brenner, D. J., S. P. O'Connor, D. G. Hollis, R. E. Weaver, and A. G. Steigerwalt.** 1991. Molecular characterization and proposal of a neotype strain for *Bartonella bacilliformis*. *J. Clin. Microbiol.* **29:**1299–1302.
29. **Brenner, D. J., S. P. O'Connor, H. H. Winkler, and A. G. Steigerwalt.** 1993. Proposals to unify the genera *Bartonella* and *Rochalimaea*, with descriptions of *Bartonella quintana* comb. nov., *Bartonella vinsonii* comb. nov., *Bartonella henselae* comb. nov., and *Bartonella elizabethae* comb. nov., and to remove the family *Bartonellaceae* from the order *Rickettsiales*. *Int. J. Syst. Bacteriol.* **43:**777–786.
30. **Brian, M. J., M. Frosolono, B. E. Murray, A. Miranda, E. L. Lopez, H. F. Gomez, and T. G. Cleary.** 1992. Polymerase chain reaction for diagnosis of enterohemorrhagic *Escherichia coli* infection and hemolytic-uremic syndrome. *J. Clin. Microbiol.* **30:**1801–1806.
31. **Brown, K. E., J. R. Hibbs, G. Gallinella, S. M. Anderson, E. D. Lehman, P. McCarthy, and N. S. Young.** 1994. Resistance to parvovirus B19 infection due to lack of virus receptor (erythrocyte P antigen). *N. Engl. J. Med.* **330:**1192–1196.
32. **Buck, G. E.** 1996. Detection of *Bordetella pertussis* by rapid-cycle PCR and colorimetric microwell hybridization. *J. Clin. Microbiol.* **34:**1355–1358.
33. **Buffone, G. J., G. J. Demmler, C. M. Schimbor, and J. Greer.** 1991. Improved amplification of cytomegalovirus DNA from urine after purification of DNA with glass beads. *Clin. Chem.* **37:**1945–1949.
34. **Busch, M. P., J. C. Wilber, P. Johnson, L. Tobler, and C. S. Evans.** 1992. Impact of specimen handling and storage on detection of hepatitis C virus RNA. *Transfusion* **32:**420–425.
35. **Caniza, M. A., D. L. Granger, K. H. Wilson, M. K. Washington, D. L. Kordick, D. P. Frush, and R. B. Blitchington.** 1995. Bartonella henselae: etiology of pulmonary nodules in a patient with depressed cell-mediated immunity. *Clin. Infect. Dis.* **20:**1505–1511.
36. **Cao, Y., L. Qin, L. Zhang, J. Safrit, and D. D. Ho.** 1995. Virologic and immunologic characterization of long-term survivors of human immunodeficiency virus type 1 infection. *N. Engl. J. Med.* **332:**201–208.
37. **Cardarelli-Leite, P., K. Blom, C. M. Patton, M. A. Nicholson, A. G. Steigerwalt, S. B. Hunter, D. J. Brenner, T. J. Barrett, and B. Swaminathan.** 1996. Rapid identification of *Campylobacter* species by restriction fragment length polymorphism analysis of a PCR-amplified fragment of the gene coding for 16S rRNA. *J. Clin. Microbiol.* **34:**62–67.
38. **Carmody, M. W., and C. P. Vary.** 1993. Inhibition of DNA hybridization following partial dUTP substitution. *BioTechniques* **15:**692–699.
39. **Carpentier, E., B. Drouillard, M. Dailloux, D. Moinard, E. Vallee, B. Dutilh, J. Maugein, E. Bergogne-Berezin, and B. Carbonnelle.** 1995. Diagnosis of tuberculosis by Amplicor *Mycobacterium tuberculosis* test: a multicenter study. *J. Clin. Microbiol.* **33:**3106–3110.
40. **Carroll, K. C., R. B. Leonard, P. L. Newcomb-Gayman, and D. R. Hillyard.** 1996. Rapid detection of the staphylococcal mecA gene from BACTEC blood culture bottles by the polymerase chain reaction. *Am. J. Clin. Pathol.* **106:**600–605.
41. **Caussy, D., W. Orr, A. D. Daya, P. Roth, W. Reeves, and W. Rawls.** 1988. Evaluation of methods for detecting human papillomavirus deoxyribonucleotide sequences in clinical specimens. *J. Clin. Microbiol.* **26:**236–243.
42. **Cembrowski, G. S.** 1990. The pursuit of quality in clinical laboratory analyses. *Clin. Chem.* **36:**1602–1604.
43. **Centers for Disease Control and Prevention.** 1993. Update: outbreak of hantavirus infection—southwestern United States, 1993. *Morbid. Mortal. Weekly Rep.* **42:**477–479.
44. **Chamberlain, J. S., R. A. Gibbs, J. E. Ranier, P. N. Nguyen, and C. T. Caskey.** 1988. Deletion screening of the Duchenne muscular dystrophy locus via multiplex DNA amplification. *Nucleic Acids Res.* **16:**11141–11156.
45. **Chen, S. M., J. S. Dumler, J. S. Bakken, and D. H. Walker.** 1994. Identification of a granulocytotropic *Ehrlichia* species as the etiologic agent of human disease. *J. Clin. Microbiol.* **32:**589–595.
46. **Chernesky, M. A., H. Lee, J. Schachter, J. D. Burczak, W. E. Stamm, W. M. McCormack, and T. C. Quinn.** 1994. Diagnosis of *Chlamydia trachomatis* urethral infection in symptomatic and asymptomatic men by testing first-void urine in a ligase chain reaction assay. *J. Infect. Dis.* **170:**1308–1311.
47. **Ching, S., H. Lee, E. W. Hook III, M. R. Jacobs, and J. Zenilman.** 1995. Ligase chain reaction for detection of *Neisseria gonorrhoeae* in urogenital swabs. *J. Clin. Microbiol.* **33:**3111–3114.
48. **Choo, Q. L., G. Kuo, A. J. Weiner, L. R. Overby, D. W. Bradley, and M. Houghton.** 1989. Isolation of a cDNA clone derived from a blood-borne non-A, non-B viral hepatitis genome. *Science* **244:**359–362.
49. **Choo, Q. L., K. H. Richman, J. H. Han, K. Berger, C. Lee, C. Dong, C. Gallegos, D. Coit, R. Medina-Selby, and P. J. Barr.** 1991. Genetic organization and diversity of the hepatitis C virus. *Proc. Natl. Acad. Sci. USA* **88:**2451–2455.
50. **Cimino, G. D., H. B. Gamper, S. T. Isaacs, and J. E. Hearst.** 1985. Psoralens as photoactive probes of nucleic acid structure and function: organic chemistry, photochemistry, and biochemistry. *Annu. Rev. Biochem.* **54:**1151–1193.
51. **Cimino, G. D., K. Metchette, S. T. Isaacs, and Y. S. Zhu.** 1990. More false-positive problems. *Nature* **345:**773–774. (Letter; comment.)
52. **Cimino, G. D., K. C. Metchette, J. W. Tessman, J. E. Hearst, and S. T. Isaacs.** 1991. Post-PCR sterilization: a

method to control carryover contamination for the polymerase chain reaction. *Nucleic Acids Res.* **19:**99–107.
53. **College of American Pathologists.** 1988. *Professional Relations Manual,* 9th ed. College of American Pathologists Press, Northfield, Ill.
54. **Collier, A. C., R. W. Coombs, D. A. Schoenfeld, R. L. Bassett, J. Timpone, A. Baruch, M. Jones, K. Facey, C. Whitacre, V. J. McAuliffe, H. M. Friedman, T. C. Merigan, R. C. Reichman, C. Hooper, and L. Corey.** 1996. Treatment of human immunodeficiency virus infection with saquinavir, zidovudine, and zalcitabine. *N. Engl. J. Med.* **334:**1011–1017.
55. **Collins, M. D., E. Falsen, J. Lemozy, E. Akervall, B. Sjoden, and P. A. Lawson.** 1997. Phenotypic and phylogenetic characterization of some *Globicatella*-like organisms from human sources: description of *Facklamia hominis* gen. nov., sp. nov. *Int. J. Syst. Bacteriol.* **47:**880–882.
56. **Compton, J.** 1991. Nucleic acid sequence-based amplification. *Nature* **350:**91–92.
57. **Conville, P. S., J. F. Keiser, and F. G. Witebsky.** 1989. Mycobacteremia caused by simultaneous infection with *Mycobacterium avium* and *Mycobacterium intracellulare* detected by analysis of a BACTEC 13A bottle with the Gen-Probe kit. *Diagn. Microbiol. Infect. Dis.* **12:**217–219.
58. **Conway, B., L. J. Bechtel, K. A. Adler, R. T. D'Aquila, J. C. Kaplan, and M. S. Hirsch.** 1992. Comparison of spot-blot and microtitre plate methods for the detection of HIV-1 PCR products. *Mol. Cell. Probes* **6:**245–249.
59. **Coombs, R. W., D. R. Henrard, W. F. Mehaffey, J. Gibson, E. Eggert, T. C. Quinn, and J. Phillips.** 1993. Cell-free plasma human immunodeficiency virus type 1 titer assessed by culture and immunocapture-reverse transcription-polymerase chain reaction. *J. Clin. Microbiol.* **31:**1980–1986.
60. **Cousins, D. V., S. D. Wilton, B. R. Francis, and B. L. Gow.** 1992. Use of polymerase chain reaction for rapid diagnosis of tuberculosis. *J. Clin. Microbiol.* **30:**255–258.
61. **Covacci, A., S. Censini, M. Bugnoli, R. Petracca, D. Burroni, G. Macchia, A. Massone, E. Papini, Z. Xiang, and N. Figura.** 1993. Molecular characterization of the 128-kDa immunodominant antigen of *Helicobacter pylori* associated with cytotoxicity and duodenal ulcer. *Proc. Natl. Acad. Sci. USA* **90:**5791–5795.
62. **Coyle, M. B., L. C. Carlson, C. K. Wallis, R. B. Leonard, V. A. Raisys, J. O. Kilburn, M. Samadpour, and E. C. Bottger.** 1992. Laboratory aspects of "*Mycobacterium genavense*," a proposed species isolated from AIDS patients. *J. Clin. Microbiol.* **30:**3206–3212.
63. **Crotty, P. L., R. A. Staggs, P. T. Porter, A. A. Killeen, and R. C. McGlennen.** 1994. Quantitative analysis in molecular diagnostics. *Hum. Pathol.* **25:**572–579.
64. **Dahl, M. L., and L. Bertilsson.** 1993. Genetically variable metabolism of antidepressants and neuroleptic drugs in man. *Pharmacogenetics* **3:**61–70.
65. **Dean, M., M. Carrington, C. Winkler, G. A. Huttley, M. W. Smith, R. Allikmets, J. J. Goedert, S. P. Buchbinder, E. Vittinghoff, E. Gomperts, S. Donfield, D. Vlahov, R. Kaslow, A. Saah, C. Rinaldo, R. Detels, and S. J. O'Brien.** 1996. Genetic restriction of HIV-1 infection and progression to AIDS by a deletion allele of the CKR5 structural gene. *Science* **273:**1856–1862.
66. **de Lamballerie, X., C. Zandotti, C. Vignoli, C. Bollet, and P. de Micco.** 1992. A one-step microbial DNA extraction method using "Chelex 100" suitable for gene amplification. *Res. Microbiol.* **143:**785–790.
67. **de Morais, S. M., G. R. Wilkinson, J. Blaisdell, K. Nakamura, U. A. Meyer, and J. A. Goldstein.** 1994. The major genetic defect responsible for the polymorphism of S-mephenytoin metabolism in humans. *J. Biol. Chem.* **269:**15419–15422.
68. **Denniston, K. J., B. H. Hoyer, A. Smedile, F. V. Wells, J. Nelson, and J. L. Gerin.** 1986. Cloned fragment of the hepatitis delta virus RNA genome: sequence and diagnostic application. *Science* **232:**873–875.
69. **Desjardin, L. E., M. D. Perkins, L. Teixeira, M. D. Cave, and K. D. Eisenach.** 1996. Alkaline decontamination of sputum specimens adversely affects stability of mycobacterial mRNA. *J. Clin. Microbiol.* **34:**2435–2439.
70. **Detmer, J., R. Lagier, J. Flynn, C. Zayati, J. Kolberg, M. Collins, M. Urdea, and R. Sanchez-Pescador.** 1996. Accurate quantification of hepatitis C virus (HCV) RNA from all HCV genotypes by using branched-DNA technology. *J. Clin. Microbiol.* **34:**901–907.
71. **Dewar, R. L., H. C. Highbarger, M. D. Sarmiento, J. A. Todd, M. B. Vasudevachari, R. T. Davey, Jr., J. A. Kovacs, N. P. Salzman, H. C. Lane, and M. S. Urdea.** 1994. Application of branched DNA signal amplification to monitor human immunodeficiency virus type 1 burden in human plasma. *J. Infect. Dis.* **170:**1172–1179.
72. **Dharakul, T., S. Songsivilai, S. Viriyachitra, V. Luangwedchakarn, B. Tassaneetritap, and W. Chaowagul.** 1996. Detection of *Burkholderia pseudomallei* DNA in patients with septicemic melioidosis. *J. Clin. Microbiol.* **34:** 609–614.
73. **DiDomenico, N., H. Link, R. Knobel, T. Caratsch, W. Weschler, Z. G. Loewy, and M. Rosenstraus.** 1996. COBAS AMPLICOR: fully automated RNA and DNA amplification and detection system for routine diagnostic PCR. *Clin. Chem.* **42:**1915–1923.
74. **Drake, T. A., J. A. Hindler, O. G. Berlin, and D. A. Bruckner.** 1987. Rapid identification of *Mycobacterium avium* complex in culture using DNA probes. *J. Clin. Microbiol.* **25:**1442–1445.
75. **Drancourt, M., J. Pelletier, A. A. Cherif, and D. Raoult.** 1997. *Gordona terrae* central nervous system infection in an immunocompetent patient. *J. Clin. Microbiol.* **35:** 379–382.
76. **Dumler, J. S., K. M. Asanovich, J. S. Bakken, P. Richter, R. Kimsey, and J. E. Madigan.** 1995. Serologic cross-reactions among *Ehrlichia equi, Ehrlichia phagocytophila,* and human granulocytic *Ehrlichia. J. Clin. Microbiol.* **33:** 1098–1103.
77. **Dumler, J. S., S. M. Chen, K. Asanovich, E. Trigiani, V. L. Popov, and D. H. Walker.** 1995. Isolation and characterization of a new strain of *Ehrlichia chaffeensis* from a patient with nearly fatal monocytic ehrlichiosis. *J. Clin. Microbiol.* **33:**1704–1711.
78. **Ehrlich, G. D., and S. J. Greenberg.** 1994. *PCR-Based Diagnostics in Infectious* Diseases. Blackwell Scientific Publications, Inc., Oxford, United Kingdom.
79. **Ehrlich, H. A.** 1991. Caveats of polymerase chain reaction. *Clin. Microbiol. Newsl.* **13:**149–151.
80. **Eisenstein, B. I.** 1990. The polymerase chain reaction. A new method of using molecular genetics for medical diagnosis. *N. Engl. J. Med.* **322:**178–183.
81. **Enroth, H., and L. Engstrand.** 1995. Immunomagnetic separation and PCR for detection of *Helicobacter pylori* in water and stool specimens. *J. Clin. Microbiol.* **33:** 2162–2165.
82. **Espy, M. J., R. Patel, C. V. Paya, and T. F. Smith.** 1995. Comparison of three methods for extraction of viral nucleic acids from blood cultures. *J. Clin. Microbiol.* **33:** 41–44.
83. **Espy, M. J., and T. F. Smith.** 1995. Comparison of SHARP signal system and Southern blot hybridization analysis for detection of cytomegalovirus in clinical specimens by PCR. *J. Clin. Microbiol.* **33:**3028–3030.

84. **Espy, M. J., T. F. Smith, and D. H. Persing.** 1993. Dependence of polymerase chain reaction product inactivation protocols on amplicon length and sequence composition. *J. Clin. Microbiol.* **31:**2361–2365.
85. **Fahrlander, P. D., and A. Klausner.** 1988. Amplifying DNA probe signals: a Christmas tree approach. *Bio/Technology* **6:**1165–1168.
86. **Falkow, S.** 1997. Perspectives series: host/pathogen interactions. Invasion and intracellular sorting of bacteria: searching for bacterial genes expressed during host/pathogen interactions. *J. Clin. Invest.* **100:**239–243.
87. **Fedorko, D. P., N. A. Nelson, and C. P. Cartwright.** 1995. Identification of microsporidia in stool specimens by using PCR and restriction endonucleases. *J. Clin. Microbiol.* **33:**1739–1741.
88. **Felmlee, T. A., Q. Liu, A. C. Whelen, D. Williams, S. S. Sommer, and D. H. Persing.** 1995. Genotypic detection of *Mycobacterium tuberculosis* rifampin resistance: comparison of single-strand conformation polymorphism and dideoxy fingerprinting. *J. Clin. Microbiol.* **33:** 1617–1623.
89. **Felmlee, T. A., R. P. Oda, D. A. Persing, and J. P. Landers.** 1995. Capillary electrophoresis of DNA potential utility for clinical diagnoses. *J. Chromatogr. A* **717:** 127–137.
90. **Figueroa, J. E., and P. Densen.** 1991. Infectious diseases associated with complement deficiencies. *Clin. Microbiol. Rev.* **4:**359–395.
91. **Findlay, J. B., S. M. Atwood, L. Bergmeyer, J. Chemelli, K. Christy, T. Cummins, W. Donish, T. Ekeze, J. Falvo, and D. Patterson.** 1993. Automated closed-vessel system for in vitro diagnostics based on polymerase chain reaction. *Clin. Chem.* **39:**1927–1933.
92. **Floyd, M. M., L. S. Guthertz, V. A. Silcox, P. S. Duffey, Y. Jang, E. P. Desmond, J. T. Crawford, and W. R. Butler.** 1996. Characterization of an SAV organism and proposal of *Mycobacterium triplex* sp. nov. *J. Clin. Microbiol.* **34:**2963–2967.
93. **Fodor, S. P., R. P. Rava, X. C. Huang, A. C. Pease, C. P. Holmes, and C. L. Adams.** 1993. Multiplexed biochemical assays with biological chips. *Nature* **364:** 555–556.
94. **Forghani, B., J. W. Hurst, and G. R. Shell.** 1991. Detection of the human immunodeficiency virus genome with a biotinylated DNA probe generated by polymerase chain reaction. *Mol. Cell. Probes* **5:**221–228.
95. **Frankel, G., L. Riley, J. A. Giron, J. Valmassoi, A. Friedmann, N. Strockbine, S. Falkow, and G. K. Schoolnik.** 1990. Detection of *Shigella* in feces using DNA amplification. *J. Infect. Dis.* **161:**1252–1256.
96. **Fredericks, D. N., and D. A. Relman.** 1996. Sequence-based identification of microbial pathogens: a reconsideration of Koch's postulates. *Clin. Microbiol. Rev.* **9:**18–33.
97. **Fuchs, P. G., F. Girardi, and H. Pfister.** 1988. Human papillomavirus DNA in normal, metaplastic, preneoplastic and neoplastic epithelia of the cervix uteri. *Int. J. Cancer* **41:**41–45.
98. **Funke, G., N. Alvarez, C. Pascual, E. Falsen, E. Akervall, L. Sabbe, L. Schouls, N. Weiss, and M. D. Collins.** 1997. *Actinomyces europaeus* sp. nov., isolated from human clinical specimens. *Int. J. Syst. Bacteriol.* **47:** 687–692.
99. **Furrer, B., U. Candrian, P. Wieland, and J. Luthy.** 1990. Improving PCR efficiency. *Nature* **346:**324. (Letter.)
100. **Geha, D. J., J. R. Uhl, C. A. Gustaferro, and D. H. Persing.** 1994. Multiplex PCR for identification of methicillin-resistant staphylococci in the clinical laboratory. *J. Clin. Microbiol.* **32:**1768–1772.
101. **Gerritsen, M. J., T. Olyhoek, M. A. Smits, and B. A. Bokhout.** 1991. Sample preparation method for polymerase chain reaction-based semiquantitative detection of *Leptospira interrogans* serovar hardjo subtype hardjobovis in bovine urine. *J. Clin. Microbiol.* **29:**2805–2808.
102. **Girotti, S., M. Musiani, E. Ferri, G. Gallinella, M. Zerbini, A. Roda, G. Gentilomi, and S. Venturoli.** 1996. Chemiluminescent immunoperoxidase assay for the dot blot hybridization detection of Parvovirus B19 DNA using a low light imaging device. *Anal. Biochem.* **236:**290–295.
103. **Granato, P. A., and M. R. Franz.** 1990. Use of the Gen-Probe PACE system for the detection of *Neisseria gonorrhoeae* in urogenital samples. *Diag. Microbiol. Infect. Dis.* **13:**217–221.
104. **Grattard, F., P. Berthelot, M. Reyrolle, A. Ros, J. Etienne, and B. Pozzetto.** 1996. Molecular typing of nosocomial strains of *Legionella pneumophila* by arbitrarily primed PCR. *J. Clin. Microbiol.* **34:**1595–1598.
105. **Greer, C. E., S. L. Peterson, N. B. Kiviat, and M. M. Manos.** 1991. PCR amplification from paraffin-embedded tissues. Effects of fixative and fixation time. *Am. J. Clin. Path.* **95:**117–124.
106. **Greisen, K., M. Loeffelholz, A. Purohit, and D. Leong.** 1994. PCR primers and probes for the 16S rRNA gene of most species of pathogenic bacteria, including bacteria found in cerebrospinal fluid. *J. Clin. Microbiol.* **32:** 335–351.
107. **Guatelli, J. C., K. M. Whitfield, D. Y. Kwoh, K. J. Barringer, D. D. Richman, and T. R. Gingeras.** 1990. Isothermal, in vitro amplification of nucleic acids by a multienzyme reaction modeled after retroviral replication. *Proc. Natl. Acad. Sci. USA* **87:**1874–1878.
108. **Haas, W. H., P. Kirschner, S. Ziesing, H. J. Bremer, and E. C. Bottger.** 1993. Cervical lymphadenitis in a child caused by a previously unknown mycobacterium. *J. Infect. Dis.* **167:**237–240.
109. **Hall, G. S., K. Pratt-Rippin, and J. A. Washington.** 1992. Evaluation of a chemiluminescent probe assay for identification of *Histoplasma capsulatum* isolates. *J. Clin. Microbiol.* **30:**3003–3004.
110. **Hamed, K. A., P. R. Dormitzer, C. K. Su, and D. A. Relman.** 1994. *Haemophilus parainfluenzae* endocarditis: application of a molecular approach for identification of pathogenic bacterial species. *Clin. Infect. Dis.* **19:** 677–683.
111. **Hammer, S. M., D. A. Katzenstein, M. D. Hughes, H. Gundacker, R. T. Schooley, R. H. Haubrich, W. K. Henry, M. M. Lederman, J. P. Phair, M. Niu, M. S. Hirsch, and T. C. Merigan.** 1996. A trial comparing nucleoside monotherapy with combination therapy in HIV-infected adults with CD4 cell counts from 200 to 500 per cubic millimeter. *N. Engl. J. Med.* **335:**1081–1090.
112. **Hankin, R. C.** 1992. In situ hybridization: principles and applications. *Lab. Med.* **23:**764–770.
113. **Haqqi, T. M., G. Sarkar, C. S. David, and S. S. Sommer.** 1988. Specific amplification with PCR of a refractory segment of genomic DNA. *Nucleic Acids Res.* **16:**11844.
114. **Hardman, W. J., G. M. Benian, T. Howard, J. E. McGowan, Jr., B. Metchock, and J. J. Murtagh.** 1996. Rapid detection of mycobacteria in inflammatory necrotizing granulomas from formalin-fixed, paraffin-embedded tissue by PCR in clinically high-risk patients with acid-fast stain and culture-negative tissue biopsies. *Am. J. Clin. Pathol.* **106:**384–389.
115. **Heim, M., and U. A. Meyer.** 1990. Genotyping of poor metabolisers of debrisoquine by allele-specific PCR amplification. *Lancet* **336:**529–532.
116. **Heller, R., B. Jaulhac, P. Charles, D. De Briel, V. Vincent, C. Bohner, Y. Piemont, and H. Monteil.** 1996. Identification of *Mycobacterium shimoidei* in a tubercu-

losis-like cavity by 16S ribosomal DNA direct sequencing. *Eur. J. Clin. Microbiol. Infect. Dis.* **15:**172–175.

117. **Hendricks, D. A., B. J. Stowe, B. S. Hoo, J. Kolberg, B. D. Irvine, P. D. Neuwald, M. S. Urdea, and R. P. Perrillo.** 1995. Quantitation of HBV DNA in human serum using a branched DNA (bDNA) signal amplification assay. *Am. J. Clin. Pathol.* **104:**537–546.
118. **Hermans, P. W., S. K. Saha, W. J. van Leeuwen, H. A. Verbrugh, A. van Belkum, and W. H. Goessens.** 1996. Molecular typing of *Salmonella typhi* strains from Dhaka (Bangladesh) and development of DNA probes identifying plasmid-encoded multidrug-resistant isolates. *J. Clin. Microbiol.* **34:**1373–1379.
119. **Herrmann, B., T. Nystrom, and H. Wessel.** 1996. Detection of *Neisseria gonorrhoeae* from air-dried genital samples by single-tube nested PCR. *J. Clin. Microbiol.* **34:** 2548–2551.
120. **Higgins, J. A., S. Radulovic, M. E. Schriefer, and A. F. Azad.** 1996. *Rickettsia felis*: a new species of pathogenic rickettsia isolated from cat fleas. *J. Clin. Microbiol.* **34:** 671–674.
121. **Hirschel, B., H. R. Chang, N. Mach, P. F. Piguet, J. Cox, J. D. Piguet, M. T. Silva, L. Larsson, P. R. Klatser, and J. E. Thole.** 1990. Fatal infection with a novel, unidentified mycobacterium in a man with the acquired immunodeficiency syndrome. *N. Engl. J. Med.* **323:** 109–113.
122. **Ho, S. A., J. A. Hoyle, F. A. Lewis, A. D. Secker, D. Cross, N. P. Mapstone, M. F. Dixon, J. I. Wyatt, D. S. Tompkins, and G. R. Taylor.** 1991. Direct polymerase chain reaction test for detection of *Helicobacter pylori* in humans and animals. *J. Clin. Microbiol.* **29:**2543–2549.
123. **Hunsaker, W. R., H. Badri, M. Lombardo, and M. L. Collins.** 1989. Nucleic acid hybridization assays employing dA-tailed capture probes. II. Advanced multiple capture methods. *Anal. Biochem.* **181:**360–370.
124. **Innis, M. A., D. H. Delfand, J. J. Sninsky, and T. J. White.** 1990. *PCR Protocols: A Guide to Methods and Applications*. Academic Press, Inc., San Diego, Calif.
125. **Innis, M. A., K. B. Myambo, D. H. Gelfand, and M. A. Brow.** 1988. DNA sequencing with *Thermus aquaticus* DNA polymerase and direct sequencing of polymerase chain reaction-amplified DNA. *Proc. Natl. Acad. Sci. USA* **85:**9436–9440.
126. **Isaacs, S. T., J. W. Tessman, K. C. Metchette, J. E. Hearst, and G. D. Cimino.** 1991. Post-PCR sterilization: development and application to an HIV-1 diagnostic assay. *Nucleic Acids Res.* **19:**109–116.
127. **Islam, D., and A. A. Lindberg.** 1992. Detection of *Shigella dysenteriae* type 1 and *Shigella flexneri* in feces by immunomagnetic isolation and polymerase chain reaction. *J. Clin. Microbiol.* **30:**2801–2806.
128. **Jacob, S., D. Baudy, E. Jones, L. Xu, A. Mason, F. Regenstein, and R. P. Perrillo.** 1997. Comparison of quantitative HCV RNA assays in chronic hepatitis C. *Am. J. Clin. Pathol.* **107:**362–367.
129. **Johansson, I., E. Lundqvist, L. Bertilsson, M. L. Dahl, F. Sjoqvist, and M. Ingelman-Sundberg.** 1993. Inherited amplification of an active gene in the cytochrome P450 CYP2D locus as a cause of ultrarapid metabolism of debrisoquine. *Proc. Natl. Acad. Sci. USA* **90:**11825–11829.
130. **Jou, N. T., R. B. Yoshimori, G. R. Mason, J. S. Louie, and M. R. Liebling.** 1997. Single-tube, nested, reverse transcriptase PCR for detection of viable *Mycobacterium tuberculosis*. *J. Clin. Microbiol.* **35:**1161–1165.
131. **Jouanguy, E., F. Altare, S. Lamhamedi, P. Revy, J. F. Emile, M. Newport, M. Levin, S. Blanche, E. Seboun, A. Fischer, and J. L. Casanova.** 1996. Interferon-gamma-receptor deficiency in an infant with fatal bacille Calmette-Guerin infection. *N. Engl. J. Med.* **335:** 1956–1961.
132. **Jungkind, D., S. Direnzo, K. G. Beavis, and N. S. Silverman.** 1996. Evaluation of automated COBAS AMPLICOR PCR system for detection of several infectious agents and its impact on laboratory management. *J. Clin. Microbiol.* **34:**2778–2783.
133. **Kain, K. C., A. E. Brown, H. K. Webster, R. A. Wirtz, J. S. Keystone, M. H. Rodriguez, J. Kinahan, M. Rowland, and D. E. Lanar.** 1992. Circumsporozoite genotyping of global isolates of *Plasmodium vivax* from dried blood specimens. *J. Clin. Microbiol.* **30:**1863–1866.
134. **Keene, W. E., E. Sazie, J. Kok, D. H. Rice, D. D. Hancock, V. K. Balan, T. Zhao, and M. P. Doyle.** 1997. An outbreak of *Escherichia coli* O157:H7 infections traced to jerky made from deer meat. *JAMA* **277:**1229–1231.
135. **Kellogg, J. A., J. W. Seiple, J. L. Klinedinst, E. S. Stroll, and S. H. Cavanaugh.** 1995. Improved PCR detection of *Chlamydia trachomatis* by using an altered method of specimen transport and high-quality endocervical specimens. *J. Clin. Microbiol.* **33:**2765–2767.
136. **Kenten, J. H., J. Casadei, J. Link, S. Lupold, J. Willey, M. Powell, A. Rees, and R. Massey.** 1991. Rapid electrochemiluminescence assays of polymerase chain reaction products. *Clin. Chem.* **37:**1626–1632.
137. **Kenzelmann, M., and K. Muhlemann.** 1997. Pitfalls of PCR: cross-reactivity with joyride *E. coli* nucleic acid. *BioTechniques* **23:**204–206.
138. **Kessler, H. H., B. Santner, H. Rabenau, A. Berger, A. Vince, C. Lewinski, B. Weber, K. Pierer, D. Stuenzner, E. Marth, and H. W. Doerr.** 1997. Rapid diagnosis of enterovirus infection by a new one-step reverse transcription-PCR assay. *J. Clin. Microbiol.* **35:**976–977.
139. **Kidd, A. H., M. Jonsson, D. Garwicz, A. E. Kajon, A. G. Wermenbol, M. W. Verweij, and J. C. De Jong.** 1996. Rapid subgenus identification of human adenovirus isolates by a general PCR. *J. Clin. Microbiol.* **34:**622–627.
140. **Kirschner, P., B. Springer, U. Vogel, A. Meier, A. Wrede, M. Kiekenbeck, F. C. Bange, and E. C. Bottger.** 1993. Genotypic identification of mycobacteria by nucleic acid sequence determination: report of a 2-year experience in a clinical laboratory. *J. Clin. Microbiol.* **31:** 2882–2889.
141. **Kitchin, P. A., Z. Szotyori, C. Fromholc, and N. Almond.** 1990. Avoidance of PCR false positives. *Nature* **344:**201. (Letter.)
142. **Kiviat, N. B., L. A. Koutsky, C. W. Critchlow, D. A. Galloway, D. A. Vernon, M. L. Peterson, P. E. McElhose, S. J. Pendras, C. E. Stevens, and K. K. Holmes.** 1990. Comparison of Southern transfer hybridization and dot filter hybridization for detection of cervical human papillomavirus infection with types 6, 11, 16, 18, 31, 33, and 35. *Am. J. Clin. Pathol.* **94:**561–565.
143. **Kolbert, C. P., E. S. Bruinsma, A. S. Abdulkarim, E. K. Hofmeister, R. B. Tompkins, S. R. Telford III, P. D. Mitchell, J. Adams-Stich, and D. H. Persing.** 1997. Characterization of an immunoreactive protein from the agent of human granulocytic ehrlichiosis. *J. Clin. Microbiol.* **35:**1172–1178.
144. **Kozal, M. J., N. Shah, N. Shen, R. Yang, R. Fucini, T. C. Merigan, D. D. Richman, D. Morris, E. Hubbell, M. Chee, and T. R. Gingeras.** 1996. Extensive polymorphisms observed in HIV-1 clade B protease gene using high-density oligonucleotide arrays. *Nature Med.* **2:** 753–759.
145. **Kramer, F. R., and P. M. Lizardi.** 1989. Replicatable RNA reporters. *Nature* **339:**401–402.
146. **Kreader, C. A.** 1996. Relief of amplification inhibition

in PCR with bovine serum albumin or T4 gene 32 protein. *Appl. Environ. Microbiol.* **62:**1102–1106.

147. **Kwoh, D. Y., G. R. Davis, K. M. Whitfield, H. L. Chappelle, L. J. DiMichele, and T. R. Gingeras.** 1989. Transcription-based amplification system and detection of amplified human immunodeficiency virus type 1 with a bead-based sandwich hybridization format. *Proc. Natl. Acad. Sci. USA* **86:**1173–1177.
148. **Kwok, S., and R. Higuchi.** 1989. Avoiding false positives with PCR. *Nature* **339:**237–238.
149. **Lage, A. P., A. Fauconnier, A. Burette, Y. Glupczynski, A. Bollen, and E. Godfroid.** 1996. Rapid colorimetric hybridization assay for detecting amplified *Helicobacter pylori* DNA in gastric biopsy specimens. *J. Clin. Microbiol.* **34:**530–533.
150. **Lanciotti, R. S., C. H. Calisher, D. J. Gubler, G. J. Chang, and A. V. Vorndam.** 1992. Rapid detection and typing of dengue viruses from clinical samples by using reverse transcriptase-polymerase chain reaction. *J. Clin. Microbiol.* **30:**545–551.
151. **La Rocco, M. T., A. Wanger, H. Ocera, and E. Macias.** 1994. Evaluation of a commercial rRNA amplification assay for direct detection of *Mycobacterium tuberculosis* in processed sputum. *Eur. J. Clin. Microbiol. Infect. Dis.* **13:**726–731.
152. **Laskus, T., J. Rakela, M. J. Nowicki, and D. H. Persing.** 1995. Hepatitis B virus core promoter sequence analysis in fulminant and chronic hepatitis B. *Gastroenterology* **109:** 1618–1623.
153. **Lawson, P. A., E. Falsen, E. Akervall, P. Vandamme, and M. D. Collins.** 1997. Characterization of some *Actinomyces*-like isolates from human clinical specimens: reclassification of *Actinomyces suis* (Soltys and Spratling) as *Actinobaculum suis* comb. nov. and description of *Actinobaculum schaalii* sp. nov. *Int. J. Sys. Bacteriol.* **47:** 899–903.
154. **Lebech, A. M., and K. Hansen.** 1992. Detection of *Borrelia burgdorferi* DNA in urine samples and cerebrospinal fluid samples from patients with early and late Lyme neuroborreliosis by polymerase chain reaction. *J. Clin. Microbiol.* **30:**1646–1653.
155. **Leibovitz, E., H. Pollack, T. Moore, J. Papellas, L. Gallo, K. Krasinski, and W. Borkowsky.** 1995. Comparison of PCR and standard cytological staining for detection of *Pneumocystis carinii* from respiratory specimens from patients with or at high risk for infection by human immunodeficiency virus. *J. Clin. Microbiol.* **33:**3004–3007.
156. **Lewis, J. S., O. Fakile, E. Foss, G. Legarza, A. Leskys, K. Lowe, and D. Powning.** 1993. Direct DNA probe assay for *Neisseria gonorrhoeae* in pharyngeal and rectal specimens. *J. Clin. Microbiol.* **31:**2783–2785.
157. **Liang, T. J., K. Hasegawa, N. Rimon, J. R. Wands, and E. Ben-Porath.** 1991. A hepatitis B virus mutant associated with an epidemic of fulminant hepatitis. *N. Engl. J. Med.* **324:**1705–1709.
158. **Lipshutz, R. J., D. Morris, M. Chee, E. Hubbell, M. J. Kozal, N. Shah, N. Shen, R. Yang, and S. P. Fodor.** 1995. Using oligonucleotide probe arrays to access genetic diversity. *BioTechniques* **19:**442–447.
159. **Liu, R., W. A. Paxton, S. Choe, D. Ceradini, S. R. Martin, R. Horuk, M. E. MacDonald, H. Stuhlmann, R. A. Koup, and N. R. Landau.** 1996. Homozygous defect in HIV-1 coreceptor accounts for resistance of some multiply-exposed individuals to HIV-1 infection. *Cell* **86:** 367–377.
160. **Loeffelholz, M. J., C. A. Lewinski, S. R. Silver, A. P. Purohit, S. A. Herman, D. A. Buonagurio, and E. A. Dragon.** 1992. Detection of *Chlamydia trachomatis* in endocervical specimens by polymerase chain reaction. *J. Clin. Microbiol.* **30:**2847–2851.
161. **Longo, M. C., M. S. Berninger, and J. L. Hartley.** 1990. Use of uracil DNA glycosylase to control carry-over contamination in polymerase chain reactions. *Gene* **93:** 125–128.
162. **Lorincz, A. T., M. H. Schiffman, W. J. Jaffurs, J. Marlow, A. P. Quinn, and G. F. Temple.** 1990. Temporal associations of human papillomavirus infection with cervical cytologic abnormalities. *Am. J. Obstet. Gynecol.* **162:**645–651.
163. **Lund, A., Y. Wasteson, and O. Olsvik.** 1991. Immunomagnetic separation and DNA hybridization for detection of enterotoxigenic *Escherichia coli* in a piglet model. *J. Clin. Microbiol.* **29:**2259–2262.
164. **MacGowan, A. P., K. O'Donaghue, S. Nicholls, J. McLauchlin, P. M. Bennett, and D. S. Reeves.** 1993. Typing of *Listeria* spp. by random amplified polymorphic DNA (RAPD) analysis. *J. Med. Microbiol.* **38:**322–327.
165. **Mahbubani, M. H., A. K. Bej, R. D. Miller, R. M. Atlas, J. L. DiCesare, and L. A. Haff.** 1991. Detection of bacterial mRNA using polymerase chain reaction. *BioTechniques* **10:**48–49.
166. **Mantero, G., A. Zonaro, A. Albertini, P. Bertolo, and D. Primi.** 1991. DNA enzyme immunoassay: general method for detecting products of polymerase chain reaction. *Clin. Chem.* **37:**422–429.
167. **Matthews, J. A., and L. J. Kricka.** 1988. Analytical strategies for the use of DNA probes. *Anal. Biochem.* **169:** 1–25.
168. **Maurin, M., V. Roux, A. Stein, F. Ferrier, R. Viraben, and D. Raoult.** 1994. Isolation and characterization by immunofluorescence, sodium dodecyl sulfate-polyacrylamide gel electrophoresis, Western blot, restriction fragment length polymorphism-PCR, 16S rRNA gene sequencing, and pulsed-field gel electrophoresis of *Rochalimaea quintana* from a patient with bacillary angiomatosis. *J. Clin. Microbiol.* **32:**1166–1171.
169. **McCaustland, K. A., S. Bi, M. A. Purdy, and D. W. Bradley.** 1991. Application of two RNA extraction methods prior to amplification of hepatitis E virus nucleic acid by the polymerase chain reaction. *J. Virol. Methods* **35:** 331–342.
170. **McHale, R. H., P. M. Stapleton, and P. L. Bergquist.** 1991. Rapid preparation of blood and tissue samples for polymerase chain reaction. *BioTechniques* **10:**20–23.
171. **McHugh, T. D., A. R. Ramsay, E. A. James, R. Mognie, and S. H. Gillespie.** 1995. Pitfalls of PCR: misdiagnosis of cerebral nocardia infection. *Lancet* **346:**1436. (Letter.)
172. **McOmish, F., P. L. Yap, B. C. Dow, E. A. Follett, C. Seed, A. J. Keller, T. J. Cobain, T. Krusius, E. Kolho, and R. Naukkarinen.** 1994. Geographical distribution of hepatitis C virus genotypes in blood donors: an international collaborative survey. *J. Clin. Microbiol.* **32:** 884–892.
173. **Mellors, J. W., L. A. Kingsley, C. R. Rinaldo, Jr., J. A. Todd, B. S. Hoo, R. P. Kokka, and P. Gupta.** 1995. Quantitation of HIV-1 RNA in plasma predicts outcome after seroconversion. *Ann. Intern. Med.* **122:**573–579.
174. **Mellors, J. W., C. R. Rinaldo, Jr., P. Gupta, R. M. White, J. A. Todd, and L. A. Kingsley.** 1996. Prognosis in HIV-1 infection predicted by the quantity of virus in plasma. *Science* **272:**1167–1170.
175. **Meyer, U. A.** 1994. Pharmacogenetics: the slow, the rapid, and the ultrarapid. *Proc. Natl. Acad. Sci. USA* **91:** 1983–1984.
176. **Miller, L. H., S. J. Mason, J. A. Dvorak, M. H. McGinniss, and I. K. Rothman.** 1975. Erythrocyte receptors for

(*Plasmodium knowlesi*) malaria: Duffy blood group determinants. *Science* **189:**561–563.

177. **Miller, N., S. G. Hernandez, and T. J. Cleary.** 1994. Evaluation of Gen-Probe Amplified Mycobacterium Tuberculosis Direct Test and PCR for direct detection of *Mycobacterium tuberculosis* in clinical specimens. *J. Clin. Microbiol.* **32:**393–397.
178. **Misrahi, M., J.-P. Teglas, M. N'Go, M. Burgard, M.-J. Mayaux, C. Rouzioux, J.-F. Delfraissy, and S. Blanche.** 1998. CCR5 chemokine receptor variant in HIV-1 mother-to-child transmission and disease progression in children. *JAMA* **279:**277–280.
179. **Mitchell, P. S., M. J. Espy, T. F. Smith, D. R. Toal, P. N. Rys, E. F. Berbari, D. R. Osmon, and D. H. Persing.** 1997. Laboratory diagnosis of central nervous system infections with herpes simplex virus by PCR performed with cerebrospinal fluid specimens. *J. Clin. Microbiol.* **35:** 2873–2877.
180. **Monstein, H. J., E. Kihlstrom, and A. Tiveljung.** 1996. Detection and identification of bacteria using in-house broad range 16S rDNA PCR amplification and genus-specific DNA hybridization probes, located within variable regions of 16S rRNA genes. *APMIS* **104:**451–458.
181. **Monteiro, L., D. Bonnemaison, A. Vekris, K. G. Petry, J. Bonnet, R. Vidal, J. Cabrita, and F. Megraud.** 1997. Complex polysaccharides as PCR inhibitors in feces: *Helicobacter pylori* model. *J. Clin. Microbiol.* **35:**995–998.
182. **Mori, J., and J. P. Clewley.** 1994. Polymerase chain reaction and sequencing for typing rhinovirus RNA. *J. Med. Virol.* **44:**323–329.
183. **Morrison, E. A., G. Y. Ho, S. H. Vermund, G. L. Goldberg, A. S. Kadish, K. F. Kelley, and R. D. Burk.** 1991. Human papillomavirus infection and other risk factors for cervical neoplasia: a case-control study. *Int. J. Cancer* **49:** 6–13.
184. **Mullis, K. B.** 1990. The unusual origin of the polymerase chain reaction. *Sci. Am.* **262:**56–65.
185. **Musser, J. M., V. Kapur, J. E. Peters, C. W. Hendrix, D. Drehner, G. D. Gackstetter, D. R. Skalka, P. L. Fort, J. T. Maffei, and L. L. Li.** 1994. Real-time molecular epidemiologic analysis of an outbreak of *Streptococcus pyogenes* invasive disease in US Air Force trainees. *Arch. Pathol. Lab. Med.* **118:**128–133.
186. **Myers, T. W., and D. H. Gelfand.** 1991. Reverse transcription and DNA amplification by a *Thermus thermophilus* DNA polymerase. *Biochemistry* **30:**7661–7666.
187. **Nakagiri, I., K. Ichihara, K. Ohmoto, M. Hirokawa, and N. Matsuda.** 1993. Analysis of discordant test results among five second-generation assays for anti-hepatitis C virus antibodies also tested by polymerase chain reaction-RNA assay and other laboratory and clinical tests for hepatitis. *J. Clin. Microbiol.* **31:**2974–2980.
188. **Neefs, J. M., Y. Van de Peer, P. De Rijk, S. Chapelle, and R. De Wachter.** 1993. Compilation of small ribosomal subunit RNA structures. *Nucleic Acids Res.* **21:** 3025–3049.
189. **Newport, M. J., C. M. Huxley, S. Huston, C. M. Hawrylowicz, B. A. Oostra, R. Williamson, and M. Levin.** 1996. A mutation in the interferon-gamma-receptor gene and susceptibility to mycobacterial infection. *N. Engl. J. Med.* **335:**1941–1949.
190. **Nichol, S. T., C. F. Spiropoulou, S. Morzunov, P. E. Rollin, T. G. Ksiazek, H. Feldman, A. Sanchez, J. Childs, S. Zaki, and C. J. Peters.** 1993. Genetic identification of a hantavirus associated with an outbreak of acute respiratory illness. *Science* **262:**914–917.
191. **Niederhauser, C., C. Hofelein, B. Wegmuller, J. Luthy, and U. Candrian.** 1994. Reliability of PCR decontamination systems. *PCR Methods Appl.* **4:**117–123.
192. **Nocton, J. J., F. Dressler, B. J. Rutledge, P. N. Rys, D. H. Persing, and A. C. Steere.** 1994. Detection of Borrelia burgdorferi DNA by polymerase chain reaction in synovial fluid from patients with Lyme arthritis. *N. Engl. J. Med.* **330:**229–234.
193. **Nowak, R.** 1995. Genome mappers have a hot time at Cold Spring Harbor. *Science* **268:**1134–1135.
194. **Orita, M., H. Iwahana, H. Kanazawa, K. Hayashi, and T. Sekiya.** 1989. Detection of polymorphisms of human DNA by gel electrophoresis as single-strand conformation polymorphisms. *Proc. Natl. Acad. Sci. USA* **86:** 2766–2770.
195. **Orle, K. A., C. A. Gates, D. H. Martin, B. A. Body, and J. B. Weiss.** 1996. Simultaneous PCR detection of *Haemophilus ducreyi*, *Treponema pallidum*, and herpes simplex virus types 1 and 2 from genital ulcers. *J. Clin. Microbiol.* **34:**49–54.
196. **Pachl, C., J. A. Todd, D. G. Kern, P. J. Sheridan, S. J. Fong, M. Stempien, B. Hoo, D. Besemer, T. Yeghiazarian, and B. Irvine.** 1995. Rapid and precise quantification of HIV-1 RNA in plasma using a branched DNA signal amplification assay. *J. Acquired Immune Defic. Synd. Hum. Retrovirol.* **8:**446–454.
197. **Panaccio, M., and A. Lew.** 1991. PCR based diagnosis in the presence of 8% (v/v) blood. *Nucleic Acids Res.* **19:** 1151.
198. **Pasternack, R., P. Vuorinen, A. Kuukankorpi, T. Pitkajarvi, and A. Miettinen.** 1996. Detection of *Chlamydia trachomatis* infections in women by Amplicor PCR: comparison of diagnostic performance with urine and cervical specimens. *J. Clin. Microbiol.* **34:**995–998.
199. **Paxton, W. A., S. R. Martin, D. Tse, T. R. O'Brien, J. Skurnick, N. L. VanDevanter, N. Padian, J. F. Braun, D. P. Kotler, S. M. Wolinsky, and R. A. Koup.** 1996. Relative resistance to HIV-1 infection of CD4 lymphocytes from persons who remain uninfected despite multiple high-risk sexual exposure. *Nature Med.* **2:**412–417.
200. **Pease, A. C., D. Solas, E. J. Sullivan, M. T. Cronin, C. P. Holmes, and S. P. Fodor.** 1994. Light-generated oligonucleotide arrays for rapid DNA sequence analysis. *Proc. Natl. Acad. Sci. USA* **91:**5022–5026.
201. **Perelson, A. S., P. Essunger, Y. Cao, M. Vesanen, A. Hurley, K. Saksela, M. Markowitz, and D. D. Ho.** 1997. Decay characteristics of HIV-1-infected compartments during combination therapy. *Nature* **387:**188–191.
202. **Perez, M., Y. Rikihisa, and B. Wen.** 1996. *Ehrlichia canis*-like agent isolated from a man in Venezuela: antigenic and genetic characterization. *J. Clin. Microbiol.* **34:** 2133–2139.
203. **Persing, D. H., T. F. Smith, F. C. Tenover, and T. J. White (ed.).** 1993. *Diagnostic Molecular Biology: Principles and Applications*. ASM Press, Washington, D.C.
204. **Persing, D. H.** 1996. *PCR Protocols for Emerging Infectious Diseases*. ASM Press, Washington, D.C.
205. **Persing, D. H.** 1991. Polymerase chain reaction: trenches to benches. *J. Clin. Microbiol.* **29:**1281–1285.
206. **Persing, D. H., B. L. Herwaldt, C. Glaser, R. S. Lane, J. W. Thomford, D. Mathiesen, P. J. Krause, D. F. Phillip, and P. A. Conrad.** 1995. Infection with a babesia-like organism in northern California. *N. Engl. J. Med.* **332:**298–303.
207. **Persing, D. H., D. Mathiesen, W. F. Marshall, S. R. Telford, A. Spielman, J. W. Thomford, and P. A. Conrad.** 1992. Detection of *Babesia microti* by polymerase chain reaction. *J. Clin. Microbiol.* **30:**2097–2103.
208. **Peterson, E. M., R. Lu, C. Floyd, A. Nakasone, G. Friedly, and L. M. de la Maza.** 1989. Direct identification of *Mycobacterium tuberculosis*, *Mycobacterium avium*, and *Mycobacterium intracellulare* from amplified primary cul-

tures in BACTEC media using DNA probes. *J. Clin. Microbiol.* **27**:1543–1547.

209. **Pfaller, M. A., and M. G. Cormican.** 1996. Role of the microbiology laboratory in monitoring and identifying resistance: use of molecular biology. *New Horizons* **4**: 361–369.
210. **Piatak, M., Jr., K. C. Luk, B. Williams, and J. D. Lifson.** 1993. Quantitative competitive polymerase chain reaction for accurate quantitation of HIV DNA and RNA species. *BioTechniques* **14**:70–81.
211. **Poljak, M., and K. Seme.** 1996. Rapid detection and typing of human papillomaviruses by consensus polymerase chain reaction and enzyme-linked immunosorbent assay. *J. Virol. Methods* **56**:231–238.
212. **Pollard-Knight, D., C. A. Read, M. J. Downes, L. A. Howard, M. R. Leadbetter, S. A. Pheby, E. McNaughton, A. Syms, and M. A. Brady.** 1990. Nonradioactive nucleic acid detection by enhanced chemiluminescence using probes directly labeled with horseradish peroxidase. *Anal. Biochem.* **185**:84–89.
213. **Popper, H. H., E. Winter, and G. Hofler.** 1994. DNA of *Mycobacterium tuberculosis* in formalin-fixed, paraffin-embedded tissue in tuberculosis and sarcoidosis detected by polymerase chain reaction. *Am. J. Clin. Pathol.* **101**: 738–741.
214. **Quinn, T. C., L. Welsh, A. Lentz, K. Crotchfelt, J. Zenilman, J. Newhall, and C. Gaydos.** 1996. Diagnosis by AMPLICOR PCR of *Chlamydia trachomatis* infection in urine samples from women and men attending sexually transmitted disease clinics. *J. Clin. Microbiol.* **34**: 1401–1406.
215. **Ramzan, N. N., E. Loftus, Jr., L. J. Burgart, M. Rooney, K. P. Batts, R. H. Wiesner, D. N. Fredricks, D. A. Relman, and D. H. Persing.** 1997. Diagnosis and monitoring of Whipple disease by polymerase chain reaction. *Ann. Intern. Med.* **126**:520–527.
216. **Reid, R., M. Greenberg, A. B. Jenson, M. Husain, J. Willett, Y. Daoud, G. Temple, C. R. Stanhope, A. I. Sherman, and G. D. Phibbs.** 1987. Sexually transmitted papillomaviral infections. I. The anatomic distribution and pathologic grade of neoplastic lesions associated with different viral types. *Am. J. Obstet. Gynecol.* **156**: 212–222.
217. **Reischl, U., and B. Kochanowski.** 1995. Quantitative PCR. A survey of the present technology. *Mol. Biotechnol.* **3**:55–71.
218. **Relman, D. A., J. S. Loutit, T. M. Schmidt, S. Falkow, and L. S. Tompkins.** 1990. The agent of bacillary angiomatosis. An approach to the identification of uncultured pathogens. *N. Engl. J. Med.* **323**:1573–1580.
219. **Relman, D. A., T. M. Schmidt, A. Gajadhar, M. Sogin, J. Cross, K. Yoder, O. Sethabutr, and P. Echeverria.** 1996. Molecular phylogenetic analysis of *Cyclospora*, the human intestinal pathogen, suggests that it is closely related to Eimeria species. *J. Infect. Dis.* **173**:440–445.
220. **Relman, D. A., T. M. Schmidt, R. P. MacDermott, and S. Falkow.** 1992. Identification of the uncultured bacillus of Whipple's disease. *N. Engl. J. Med.* **327**:293–301.
221. **Revets, H., D. Marissens, S. de Wit, P. Lacor, N. Clumeck, S. Lauwers, and G. Zissis.** 1996. Comparative evaluation of NASBA HIV-1 RNA QT, AMPLICOR-HIV monitor, and QUANTIPLEX HIV RNA assay, three methods for quantification of human immunodefiency virus type 1 RNA in plasma. *J. Clin. Microbiol.* **34**: 1058–1064.
222. **Reznicek, M., M. Bale, and M. Pfaller.** 1991. Application of DNA probes to antimicrobial susceptibility testing of Legionella pneumophila. *Diagn. Microbiol. Infect. Dis.* **14**:7–10.
223. **Rikihisa, Y., N. Zhi, G. P. Wormser, B. Wen, H. W. Horowitz, and K. E. Hechemy.** 1997. Ultrastructural and antigenic characterization of a granulocytic ehrlichiosis agent directly isolated and stably cultivated from a patient in New York state. *J. Infect. Dis.* **175**:210–213.
224. **Roberts, T. C., and G. A. Storch.** 1997. Multiplex PCR for diagnosis of AIDS-related central nervous system lymphoma and toxoplasmosis. *J. Clin. Microbiol.* **35**: 268–269.
225. **Romero, J. L., S. Descoteaux, S. Reed, E. Orozco, J. Santos, and J. Samuelson.** 1992. Use of polymerase chain reaction and nonradioactive DNA probes to diagnose *Entamoeba histolytica* in clinical samples. *Arch. Med. Res.* **23**:277–279.
226. **Rota, P. A., A. S. Khan, E. Durigon, T. Yuran, Y. S. Villamarzo, and W. J. Bellini.** 1995. Detection of measles virus RNA in urine specimens from vaccine recipients. *J. Clin. Microbiol.* **33**:2485–2488.
227. **Rys, P. N., and D. H. Persing.** 1993. Preventing false positives: quantitative evaluation of three protocols for inactivation of polymerase chain reaction amplification products. *J. Clin. Microbiol.* **31**:2356–2360.
228. **Saiki, R. K., D. H. Gelfand, S. Stoffel, S. J. Scharf, R. Higuchi, G. T. Horn, K. B. Mullis, and H. A. Erlich.** 1988. Primer-directed enzymatic amplification of DNA with a thermostable DNA polymerase. *Science* **239**: 487–491.
229. **Salomon, R. N.** 1995. Introduction to quantitative reverse transcription polymerase chain reaction. *Diagn. Mol. Pathol.* **4**:82–84.
230. **Samson, M., F. Libert, B. J. Doranz, J. Rucker, C. Liesnard, C. M. Farber, S. Saragosti, C. Lapoumeroulie, J. Cognaux, C. Forceille, G. Muyldermans, C. Verhofstede, G. Burtonboy, M. Georges, T. Imai, S. Rana, Y. Yi, R. J. Smyth, R. G. Collman, R. W. Doms, G. Vassart, and M. Parmentier.** 1996. Resistance to HIV-1 infection in Caucasian individuals bearing mutant alleles of the CCR-5 chemokine receptor gene. *Nature* **382**: 722–725.
231. **Sarkar, G., and S. Sommer.** 1990. More light on PCR contamination. *Nature* **347**:340–341. (Letter.)
232. **Sarrazin, C., G. Herrmann, W. K. Roth, J. H. Lee, S. Marx, and S. Zeuzem.** 1997. Prevalence and clinical and histological manifestation of hepatitis G/GBV-C infections in patients with elevated aminotransferases of unknown etiology. *J. Hepatol.* **27**:276–283.
233. **Saweljew, P., J. Kunkel, A. Feddersen, M. Baumert, J. Baehr, W. Ludwig, S. Bhakdi, and M. Husmann.** 1996. Case of fatal systemic infection with an *Aureobacterium* sp.: identification of isolate by 16S rRNA gene analysis. *J. Clin. Microbiol.* **34**:1540–1541.
234. **Schachter, J., W. E. Stamm, T. C. Quinn, W. W. Andrews, J. D. Burczak, and H. H. Lee.** 1994. Ligase chain reaction to detect *Chlamydia trachomatis* infection of the cervix. *J. Clin. Microbiol.* **32**:2540–2543.
235. **Schmidt, B., R. R. Muellegger, C. Stockenhuber, H. P. Soyer, S. Hoedl, A. Luger, and H. Kerl.** 1996. Detection of *Borrelia burgdorferi*-specific DNA in urine specimens from patients with erythema migrans before and after antibiotic therapy. *J. Clin. Microbiol.* **34**:1359–1363.
236. **Schriefer, M. E., J. B. Sacci, Jr., J. S. Dumler, M. G. Bullen, and A. F. Azad.** 1994. Identification of a novel rickettsial infection in a patient diagnosed with murine typhus. *J. Clin. Microbiol.* **32**:949–954.
237. **Schwab, K. J., R. De Leon, and M. D. Sobsey.** 1996. Immunoaffinity concentration and purification of waterborne enteric viruses for detection by reverse transcriptase PCR. *Appl. Environ. Microbiol.* **62**:2086–2094.
238. **Scotto, J., M. Hadchouel, C. Hery, J. Yvart, P. Tiollais,**

and C. Brechot. 1983. Detection of hepatitis B virus DNA in serum by a simple spot hybridization technique: comparison with results for other viral markers. *Hepatology* **3:**279–284.

239. **Secchiero, P., D. Zella, R. W. Crowley, R. C. Gallo, and P. Lusso.** 1995. Quantitative PCR for human herpesviruses 6 and 7. *J. Clin. Microbiol.* **33:**2124–2130.

240. **Shirai, H., M. Nishibuchi, T. Ramamurthy, S. K. Bhattacharya, S. C. Pal, and Y. Takeda.** 1991. Polymerase chain reaction for detection of the cholera enterotoxin operon of *Vibrio cholerae*. *J. Clin. Microbiol.* **29:**2517–2521.

241. **Shu, L. L., W. J. Bean, and R. G. Webster.** 1993. Analysis of the evolution and variation of the human influenza A virus nucleoprotein gene from 1933 to 1990. *J. Virol.* **67:**2723–2729.

242. **Slupphaug, G., I. Alseth, I. Eftedal, G. Volden, and H. E. Krokan.** 1993. Low incorporation of dUMP by some thermostable DNA polymerases may limit their use in PCR amplifications. *Anal. Biochem.* **211:**164–169.

243. **Smith, K. R., S. Ching, H. Lee, Y. Ohhashi, H. Y. Hu, H. C. Fisher III, and E. W. Hook III.** 1995. Evaluation of ligase chain reaction for use with urine for identification of *Neisseria gonorrhoeae* in females attending a sexually transmitted disease clinic. *J. Clin. Microbiol.* **33:**455–457.

244. **Smith, M. W., M. Dean, M. Carrington, C. Winkler, G. A. Huttley, D. A. Lomb, J. J. Goedert, T. R. O'Brien, L. P. Jacobson, R. Kaslow, S. Buchbinder, E. Vittinghoff, D. Vlahov, K. Hoots, M. W. Hilgartner, and S. J. O'Brien.** 1997. Contrasting genetic influence of *CCR2* and *CCR5* variants on HIV-1 infection and disease progression. *Science* **277:**959–965.

245. **Southern, E. M.** 1975. Detection of specific sequences among DNA fragments separated by gel electrophoresis. *J. Mol. Biol.* **98:**503–517.

246. **Sritharan, V., and R. H. Barker, Jr.** 1991. A simple method for diagnosing *M. tuberculosis* infection in clinical samples using PCR. *Mol. Cell. Probes* **5:**385–395.

247. **Stockman, L., K. A. Clark, J. M. Hunt, and G. D. Roberts.** 1993. Evaluation of commercially available acridinium ester-labeled chemiluminescent DNA probes for culture identification of *Blastomyces dermatitidis*, *Coccidioides immitis*, *Cryptococcus neoformans*, and *Histoplasma capsulatum*. *J. Clin. Microbiol.* **31:**845–850.

248. **Strickler, J. G., and C. M. Copenhaver.** 1990. In situ hybridization in hematopathology. *Am. J. Clin. Pathol.* **93:**S44–S48.

249. **Tang, Y. W., M. K. Hopkins, C. P. Kolbert, P. A. Hartley, P. J. Severance, and D. H. Persing.** 1998. Bordetella holmesii-like organisms associated with septicemia, endocarditis, and respiratory failure. *Clin. Infect. Dis.* **26:**389–392.

250. **Tang, Y. W., P. N. Rys, B. J. Rutledge, P. S. Mitchell, T. F. Smith, and D. H. Persing.** 1998. Comparative evaluation of colorimetric microtiter plate systems for detection of herpes simplex virus in cerebrospinal fluid. *J. Clin. Microbiol.* **36:**2714–2717.

251. **Tang, Y. W., N. M. Ellis, M. K. Hopkins, D. H. Smith, D. E. Dodge, and D. H. Persing.** 1998. Comparison of phenotypic and genotypic techniques for identification of unusual aerobic pathogenic gram-negative bacilli. *J. Clin. Microbiol.* **36:**3674–3679.

252. **Tang, Y. W., G. W. Procop, and D. H. Persing.** 1997. Molecular diagnosis of infectious diseases. *Clin. Chem.* **43:**2021–2038.

253. **Tang, Y. W., M. J. Espy, D. H. Persing, and T. F. Smith.** 1997. Molecular evidence and clinical significance of herpesvirus coinfection in central nervous system. *J. Clin. Microbiol.* **35:**2869–2872.

254. **Tang, Y. W., S. L. Ruo, X. Xu, A. Sanchez, S. P. Fisher-Hoch, J. B. McCormick, and Z. Y. Xu.** 1990. Hantavirus strains isolated from rodentia and insectivora in rural China differentiated by polymerase chain reaction assay. *Arch. Virol.* **115:**37–46.

255. **Tedder, D. G., R. Ashley, K. L. Tyler, and M. J. Levin.** 1994. Herpes simplex virus infection as a cause of benign recurrent lymphocytic meningitis. *Ann. Intern. Med.* **121:**334–338.

256. **Telenti, A., P. Imboden, F. Marchesi, T. Schmidheini, and T. Bodmer.** 1993. Direct, automated detection of rifampin-resistant *Mycobacterium tuberculosis* by polymerase chain reaction and single-strand conformation polymorphism analysis. *Antimicrob. Agents Chemother.* **37:**2054–2058.

257. **Tenover, F. C.** 1988. Diagnostic deoxyribonucleic acid probes for infectious diseases. *Clin. Microbiol. Rev.* **1:**82–101.

258. **Tenover, F. C., R. D. Arbeit, and R. V. Goering.** 1997. How to select and interpret molecular strain typing methods for epidemiological studies of bacterial infections: a review for healthcare epidemiologists. *Infect. Control Hosp. Epidemiol.* **18:**426–439.

259. **Thanos, M., G. Schonian, W. Meyer, C. Schweynoch, Y. Graser, T. G. Mitchell, W. Presber, and H. J. Tietz.** 1996. Rapid identification of *Candida* species by DNA fingerprinting with PCR. *J. Clin. Microbiol.* **34:**615–621.

260. **Thomas, D. L., Y. Nakatsuji, J. W. Shih, H. J. Alter, K. E. Nelson, J. A. Astemborski, C. M. Lyles, and D. Vlahov.** 1997. Persistence and clinical significance of hepatitis G virus infections in injecting drug users. *J. Infect. Dis.* **176:**586–592.

261. **Turkoglu, S., Y. Lazizi, H. Meng, A. Kordosi, P. Dubreuil, B. Crescenzo, S. Benjelloun, P. Nordmann, and J. Pillot.** 1996. Detection of hepatitis E virus RNA in stools and serum by reverse transcription-PCR. *J. Clin. Microbiol.* **34:**1568–1571.

262. **Urdea, M. S., T. Horn, T. J. Fultz, M. Anderson, J. A. Running, S. Hamren, D. Ahle, and C. A. Chang.** 1991. Branched DNA amplification multimers for the sensitive, direct detection of human hepatitis viruses. *Nucleic Acids Symp. Ser.* **24:**197–200.

263. **van Belkum, A., J. Kluytmans, W. van Leeuwen, R. Bax, W. Quint, E. Peters, A. Fluit, C. Vandenbroucke-Grauls, A. van den Brule, and H. Koeleman.** 1995. Multicenter evaluation of arbitrarily primed PCR for typing of *Staphylococcus aureus* strains. *J. Clin. Microbiol.* **33:**1537–1547.

264. **Vandamme, A. M., J. C. Schmit, S. Van Dooren, K. Van Laethem, E. Gobbers, W. Kok, P. Goubau, M. Witvrouw, W. Peetermans, E. De Clercq, and J. Desmyter.** 1996. Quantification of HIV-1 RNA in plasma: comparable results with the NASBA HIV-1 RNA QT and the AMPLICOR HIV monitor test. *J. Acquired Immune Defic. Syndr. Hum. Retrovirol.* **13:**127–139.

265. **VanDevanter, D. R., P. Warrener, L. Bennett, E. R. Schultz, S. Coulter, R. L. Garber, and T. M. Rose.** 1996. Detection and analysis of diverse herpesviral species by consensus primer PCR. *J. Clin. Microbiol.* **34:**1666–1671.

266. **van Embden, J. D., M. D. Cave, J. T. Crawford, J. W. Dale, K. D. Eisenach, B. Gicquel, P. Hermans, C. Martin, R. McAdam, and T. M. Shinnick.** 1993. Strain identification of *Mycobacterium tuberculosis* by DNA fingerprinting: recommendations for a standardized methodology. *J. Clin. Microbiol.* **31:**406–409.

267. **van Gemen, B., R. van Beuningen, A. Nabbe, D. van Strijp, S. Jurriaans, P. Lens, and T. Kievits.** 1994. A

one-tube quantitative HIV-1 RNA NASBA nucleic acid amplification assay using electrochemiluminescent (ECL) labelled probes. *J. Virol. Methods* **49:**157–167.

268. **Verweij, P. E., J. P. Latge, A. J. Rijs, W. J. Melchers, B. E. De Pauw, J. A. Hoogkamp-Korstanje, and J. F. Meis.** 1995. Comparison of antigen detection and PCR assay using bronchoalveolar lavage fluid for diagnosing invasive pulmonary aspergillosis in patients receiving treatment for hematological malignancies. *J. Clin. Microbiol.* **33:**3150–3153.
269. **von Herbay, A., H. J. Ditton, and M. Maiwald.** 1996. Diagnostic application of a polymerase chain reaction assay for the Whipple's disease bacterium to intestinal biopsies. *Gastroenterology* **110:**1735–1743.
270. **Vrielink, H., H. L. Zaaijer, H. T. Cuypers, C. L. van der Poel, M. Woerdeman, P. N. Lelie, C. Winkel, and H. W. Reesink.** 1997. Evaluation of a new HTLV-I/II polymerase chain reaction. *Vox Sang.* **72:**144–147.
271. **Wagar, E. A.** 1996. Direct hybridization and amplification applications for the diagnosis of infectious diseases. *J. Clin. Lab. Anal.* **10:**312–325.
272. **Wages, J. M., L. Dolenga, and A. F. Fowler.** 1993. Electrochemiluminescent detection and quantitation of PCR-amplified DNA. *Amplifications* **10:**1–6.
273. **Walder, R. Y., J. R. Hayes, and J. A. Walder.** 1993. Use of PCR primers containing a 3′-terminal ribose residue to prevent cross-contamination of amplified sequences. *Nucleic Acids Res.* **21:**4339–4343.
274. **Walker, G. T., M. S. Fraiser, J. L. Schram, M. C. Little, J. G. Nadeau, and D. P. Malinowski.** 1992. Strand displacement amplification—an isothermal, in vitro DNA amplification technique. *Nucleic Acids Res.* **20:** 1691–1696.
275. **Walker, G. T., M. C. Little, J. G. Nadeau, and D. D. Shank.** 1992. Isothermal in vitro amplification of DNA by a restriction enzyme/DNA polymerase system. *Proc. Natl. Acad. Sci. USA* **89:**392–396.
276. **Walsh, E. E., K. M. McConnochie, C. E. Long, and C. B. Hall.** 1997. Severity of respiratory syncytial virus infection is related to virus strain. *J. Infect. Dis.* **175:** 814–820.
277. **Wang, J. T., T. H. Wang, J. C. Sheu, S. M. Lin, J. T. Lin, and D. S. Chen.** 1992. Effects of anticoagulants and storage of blood samples on efficacy of the polymerase chain reaction assay for hepatitis C virus. *J. Clin. Microbiol.* **30:**750–753.
278. **Weitzman, I., and R. C. Summerbell.** 1995. The dermatophytes. *Clin. Microbiol. Rev.* **8:**240–259.
279. **Welsh, J., and M. McClelland.** 1990. Fingerprinting genomes using PCR with arbitrary primers. *Nucleic Acids Res.* **18:**7213–7218.
280. **Wetmur, J. G.** 1991. DNA probes: applications of the principles of nucleic acid hybridization. *Crit. Rev. Biochem. Mol. Biol.* **26:**227–259.
281. **Weyant, R. S., D. G. Hollis, R. E. Weaver, M. F. Amin, A. G. Steigerwalt, S. P. O'Connor, A. M. Whitney, M. I. Daneshvar, C. W. Moss, and D. J. Brenner.** 1995. *Bordetella holmesii* sp. nov., a new gram-negative species associated with septicemia. *J. Clin. Microbiol.* **33:**1–7.
282. **Whelen, A. C., T. A. Felmlee, J. M. Hunt, D. L. Williams, G. D. Roberts, L. Stockman, and D. H. Persing.** 1995. Direct genotypic detection of *Mycobacterium tuberculosis* rifampin resistance in clinical specimens by using single-tube heminested PCR. *J. Clin. Microbiol.* **33:** 556–561.
283. **White, T. J., R. Madej, and D. H. Persing.** 1992. The polymerase chain reaction: clinical applications. *Adv. Clin. Chem.* **29:**161–196.
284. **Wicher, K., G. T. Noordhoek, F. Abbruscato, and V. Wicher.** 1992. Detection of *Treponema pallidum* in early syphilis by DNA amplification. *J. Clin. Microbiol.* **30:** 497–500.
285. **Wiedbrauk, D. L.** 1992. Molecular methods for virus detection. *Lab. Med.* **23:**737–742.
286. **Wilke, W. W., R. N. Jones, and L. D. Sutton.** 1995. Automation of polymerase chain reaction tests. Reduction of human errors leading to contamination. *Diag. Microbiol. Infect. Dis.* **21:**181–185.
287. **Wobeser, W. L., M. Krajden, J. Conly, H. Simpson, B. Yim, M. D'Costa, M. Fuksa, C. Hian-Cheong, M. Patterson, A. Phillips, R. Bannatyne, A. Haddad, J. L. Brunton, and S. Krajden.** 1996. Evaluation of Roche Amplicor PCR assay for *Mycobacterium tuberculosis*. *J. Clin. Microbiol.* **34:**134–139.
288. **Woese, C. R.** 1987. Bacterial evolution. *Microbiol. Rev.* **51:**221–271.
289. **Woods, J. P., D. Kersulyte, R. W. Tolan, Jr., C. M. Berg, and D. E. Berg.** 1994. Use of arbitrarily primed polymerase chain reaction analysis to type disease and carrier strains of *Neisseria meningitidis* isolated during a university outbreak. *J. Infect. Dis.* **169:**1384–1389.
290. **Woolley, A. T., and R. A. Mathies.** 1995. Ultra-high-speed DNA sequencing using capillary electrophoresis chips. *Anal. Chem.* **67:**3676–3680.
291. **Wu, D. Y., and R. B. Wallace.** 1989. The ligation amplification reaction (LAR)—amplification of specific DNA sequences using sequential rounds of template-dependent ligation. *Genomics* **4:**560–569.
292. **Yamada, O., T. Matsumoto, M. Nakashima, S. Hagari, T. Kamahora, H. Ueyama, Y. Kishi, H. Uemura, and T. Kurimura.** 1990. A new method for extracting DNA or RNA for polymerase chain reaction. *J. Virol. Methods* **27:**203–209.
293. **Yang, L., J. H. Weis, E. Eichwald, C. P. Kolbert, D. H. Persing, and J. J. Weis.** 1994. Heritable susceptibility to severe *Borrelia burgdorferi*-induced arthritis is dominant and is associated with persistence of large numbers of spirochetes in tissues. *Infect. Immun.* **62:**492–500.
294. **Yerly, S., A. Gervaix, V. Simonet, M. Caflisch, L. Perrin, and W. Wunderli.** 1996. Rapid and sensitive detection of enteroviruses in specimens from patients with aseptic meningitis. *J. Clin. Microbiol.* **34:**199–201.
295. **Yoshioka, K., S. Kakumu, T. Wakita, T. Ishikawa, Y. Itoh, M. Takayanagi, Y. Higashi, M. Shibata, and T. Morishima.** 1992. Detection of hepatitis C virus by polymerase chain reaction and response to interferon-alpha therapy: relationship to genotypes of hepatitis C virus. *Hepatology* **16:**293–299.
296. **Young, K. K., R. M. Resnick, and T. W. Myers.** 1993. Detection of hepatitis C virus RNA by a combined reverse transcription-polymerase chain reaction assay. *J. Clin. Microbiol.* **31:**882–886.
297. **Zein, N. N., J. Rakela, E. L. Krawitt, K. R. Reddy, T. Tominaga, and D. H. Persing.** 1996. Hepatitis C virus genotypes in the United States: epidemiology, pathogenicity, and response to interferon therapy. *Ann. Intern. Med.* **125:**634–639.
298. **Zheng, H., T. C. Peret, V. B. Randolph, J. C. Crowley, and L. J. Anderson.** 1996. Strain-specific reverse transcriptase PCR assay: means to distinguish candidate vaccine from wild-type strains of respiratory syncytial virus. *J. Clin. Microbiol.* **34:**334–337.

BACTERIOLOGY

VOLUME EDITORS
ELLEN JO BARON AND PATRICK R. MURRAY

SECTION EDITORS
GARY V. DOERN, MARY JANE FERRARO, PETER H. GILLIGAN, J. MICHAEL JANDA, AND ALEXANDER VON GRAEVENITZ

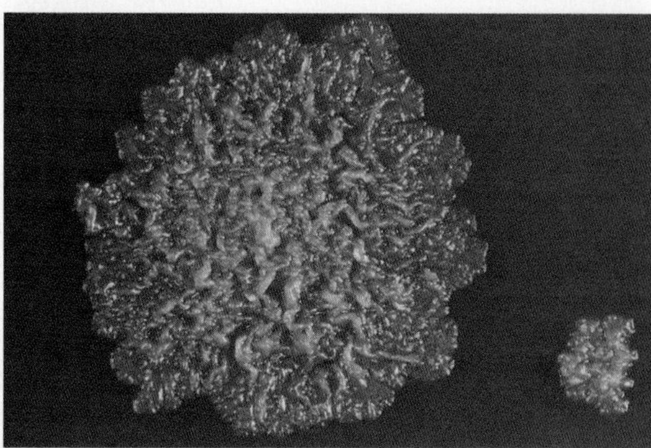

Tsukamurella tyrosinosolvens colony grown for 5 days on a heart infusion agar plate with 5% rabbit blood (*photograph by Jim Gathany, CDC*).

IV

GRAM-NEGATIVE BACTERIA

(continued)

Taxonomy and Classification of Bacteria*

PATRICK A. D. GRIMONT

14

Bacterial systematics or taxonomy originated from the need to distinguish pathogenic bacteria, especially those causing specific diseases such as typhoid, tuberculosis, syphilis, and anthrax, from commensal or saprophytic bacteria found in the same habitat. Before the antibiotic era, bacterial taxonomy was of interest primarily to medical microbiologists. Such interest declined when more emphasis was put on antimicrobial resistance and pathogenic mechanisms. However, for epidemiological studies and surveillance, precise identification is needed and species identification is a primary epidemiological marker. It is interesting that the tremendous development of biotechnology and subsequent interest in microbial diversity (which requires precise characterization of microorganisms) led to a renewed interest in bacterial taxonomy. Taxonomic methods evolving from the use of empirical biochemical tests to molecular characterization combined to meet the needs of industry and modern medicine.

DEFINITIONS

Systematics, the science of classification of living organisms, includes three parts: classification, nomenclature, and identification.

Classification

The aim of classification is to delineate groups of organisms about which one can generalize knowledge obtained from studying a few strains. Such a group is called a taxon (pl. taxa) irrespective of its hierarchic level. For example, if an organism belongs to the *Proteobacteria* phylogenetic branch, we can expect a gram-negative type of cell wall, the presence of endotoxin, and relative resistance to penicillin (61). If the taxon is *Escherichia coli*, we may assume that almost all the genetic and biochemical knowledge accumulated for strain K-12 is applicable to other strains of the same species. A search for pathogenic factors or antibiotic resistance mechanisms associated with a strain is much easier when the taxonomic position of the strain is known.

Bacterial classification is now phylogenetically based, and molecular methods are used to establish relationships. Multilocus enzyme electrophoresis (MLEE) and restriction fragment length polymorphism are often used to decide whether two isolates are derived from a single strain and thus belong to the same clone. A bacterial species can be seen as a set of clones sharing most of their DNA sequences. Such a genetic community relationship is characterized by quantitative total DNA hybridization. Delineation of clones and species is a major activity in practical taxonomic work. Taxonomic levels above the species, e.g., genus, family, order, and class, are especially useful in the process of communication in the scientific community and in the ability to generalize about a set of species without stating all the species names. The taxonomic hierarchy relies mostly on 16 or 23S rRNA sequence comparisons. Such a comparison is often displayed in the form of a phylogenetic tree, which shows species relationships but, unfortunately, no taxon boundaries. Enhancing a phylogenetic tree with phenotypic properties (morphological, physiological, biochemical, or chemotaxonomical properties) allows the grouping of species in genera, genera in families, families in orders, and orders in classes. The classification process is not complete unless molecular and phenotypic descriptions of the studied taxa are provided. Descriptive properties constitute a database from which a subset may be used for identification.

Nomenclature

Microbiologists from different countries use their own language to report clinical findings. Biological nomenclature is a universal vocabulary which can be used in any language. Names of organisms are treated as Latin names and indicated as such by using italics or by underlining. Since Linnaeus, organisms are given a double name; the first one is the genus name (written with the first letter capitalized), and the second one is the species epithet (no capital initial). The *International Code of Nomenclature of Bacteria* (81) includes rules on how to name bacteria and how to use the names. The aim is that a species in a given taxonomic position should have a single name. Any microbiologist may name a new species, provided that the proposal is supported by sufficient data and that the nomenclatural rules are followed. Each taxonomic name should be represented by a nomenclatural type. A species is represented by a type strain, which must be deposited in a recognized culture collection and thus made available to everybody. A genus is represented by a type species. In further studies, if a species (or a genus) is

* This chapter contains information presented in chapter 20 by Ellen Jo Baron, Alice S. Weissfeld, Pamela A. Fuselier, and Don J. Brenner in the sixth edition of this Manual.

subdivided into two species (or two genera), the name of the species (or the genus) will remain with the species (or the genus) which includes the nomenclatural type. If two species (or genera) are united, the name of the united taxon should be the older of the two species (genus) names. To avoid endless bibliographic searches, a list of approved bacterial names was published in 1980 (80). Names which were published before 1980 and which were not listed have lost standing in the nomenclature. Names given to newly described taxa have standing in the nomenclature once they are published or announced in the *International Journal of Systematic Bacteriology* (IJSB). Lists validating names published in other journals appear in all issues of IJSB. When nomenclatural rules are difficult to apply or in case of contested priority, the Judicial Commission of the International Committee on Bacterial Systematics (ICSB) issues an Opinion, which is published in IJSB. The validity of names or Opinions issued by the Judicial Commission is strictly limited to nomenclature as governed by the *Bacteriological Code* (81). The validity of a name has nothing to do with the scientific value of the taxonomic position implied by the name. Furthermore, the Judicial Commission and ICSB have no legal authority to decide whether a classification is correct. Science is not done by committees but by scientists. However, the Judicial Commission and ICSB will ensure that for a given taxonomic position, the proper nomenclature is used. A provisional nomenclature has been proposed for nonculturable bacteria (62).

Identification

Identification is a process whereby an organism is recognized as belonging to a known species and designated accordingly. Identification is based on the comparison between phenotypic characteristics of the isolate and those published for known families, genera, and species or on simplified molecular methods. Microbiologists faced with identifying many strains within a limited time frame and budget cannot (at present) determine full 16S rRNA sequences and quantitative DNA-DNA hybridization for all strains. If an isolate belongs to an undescribed species, identification is impossible until a complete taxonomic study is performed. Reference centers often have many unidentified strains awaiting taxonomic study. Such studies are usually started when several similar strains are collected. There is no rule governing the minimal number of strains which should support the description of a new species. Although emerging pathogens or bacterial species with unique properties have been described from the study of a single isolate, it is not reasonable to describe a species based on study of a single strain when its clinical, biotechnological, or environmental importance is limited or unknown.

CLASSIFICATION METHODS

For many years, bacterial taxonomy was empirical and subjective, with taxonomists arguing about which characteristics were most important for classification. The use of numerical taxonomy in 1959 was the first attempt at an objective classification scheme (82). This boosted taxonomic research. In 1969, the use of DNA-DNA hybridization (7) eventually led to the definition of a genomic species (90). After 1975, comparison of rRNA sequences, first by hybridization (18) and then by cataloging and sequencing (94), provided the means to arrange bacterial species into a phylogenetic tree. The use of different methods to arrive at taxonomic conclusions is called polyphasic taxonomy (12).

Phenotypic Characterization of Bacteria

Phenotype has always been an indicator of biodiversity. Computer comparison of phenotypic characters (numerical taxonomy [see below]) was the first objective method in bacterial taxonomy.

Morphology

The appearance of bacteria growing as colonies on agar media and as suspensions in broth media is often characteristic of a particular genus and, in some cases, species. The same is true of cellular morphology as viewed microscopically. The presence or absence of surface appendages such as flagella, pili, and capsular material can also be of taxonomic importance.

Physiology

The ability to grow in the presence of atmospheric oxygen is an important taxonomic determinant. The following method is of general application. An agar medium, devoid of nitrate, is melted and boiled in a long, thin screw-cap test tube and, when cooled near 45°C, is inoculated with a drop of a diluted culture. The contents of the tube are mixed gently to allow the bacterial cells to produce colonies at all depths of the medium. Strictly aerobic bacteria develop colonies at and up to a few millimeters below the surface. These bacteria are unable to ferment organic compounds. Strictly anaerobic bacteria develop colonies in the depth of the medium and not in the vicinity of the surface. Microaerophilic bacteria develop colonies at a point midway between the bottom and top of the tube. These are strictly aerobic bacteria that require oxygen at a partial pressure lower than that present in air. Bacteria growing at all depths are called facultatively anaerobic bacteria. This term includes bacteria which are capable of both aerobic and anaerobic metabolism and anaerobic bacteria which are oxygen tolerant. When nitrate, sulfate, or carbonate is added to the agar medium, some aerobic bacteria develop in the depth of the medium; these are capable of anaerobic respiration. An interesting case is that of *Haemophilus influenzae*, a facultative anaerobe which requires both hemin and NAD for growth. Without hemin, catalase and cytochromes cannot be synthesized in an active form and the bacterium appears strictly anaerobic.

A more complete study of relationships with oxygen would include the detection and identification of cytochromes, catalase, superoxide dismutase, and sensitivity to cyanide. In a cytochrome chain, the last enzyme is cytochrome oxidase, which reacts with oxygen. The oxidase test is typically positive only with bacteria which produce cytochrome *c*.

The range of temperatures allowing growth is often of taxonomic value. Minimum, optimum, and maximum temperatures for growth can be determined easily. Relationships with sodium ions allow the definition of nonhalophilic, moderately halophilic, hyperhalophilic, or halotolerant bacteria. Optimal pH and extreme pH values compatible with growth are also useful taxonomic characteristics.

Determination of growth factor requirements is essential before performing any nutritional study. A number of species are prototropic and can grow in a minimal medium containing an organic carbon source; ammonium ion as a source of nitrogen; calcium, magnesium, and iron salts; trace elements; and a phosphate buffer. Some species are auxotrophic for one or more growth factors (vitamins, amino acids, purines, pyrimidines, coenzymes, or hemin).

Biochemical Activities

Biochemical tests used in microbiology (conventional tests) are empirical tests which imperfectly reflect the metabolic activities of bacteria. In contrast to the tests used by biochemists (which are done quantitatively on cell extracts with known protein contents), tests used by microbiologists generally involve substrates in complex media and an undefined number of bacterial cells. Carbon source utilization tests are extremely useful in taxonomy (31, 83). They require a defined minimal medium and pure carbon sources and are valid only when the temperature, NaCl, $MgCl_2$, and growth factor requirements are met.

Antigenic Structure

Bacterial cells are composed of numerous different antigens, which may be distinguished by using either polyclonal or monoclonal antibodies in a variety of different immunoassays (see chapter 12 for details). From a practical point of view, surface antigens consisting of proteins, polysaccharides, and lipopolysaccharides are most often detected by the use of monospecific polyclonal antibodies in a whole-cell agglutination assay. Antigenic characteristics serve to categorize bacteria at a subspecies level into serotypes or serogroups. Two examples clearly illustrate this point. Currently, two species of *Salmonella* are genetically valid: *S. enterica* and *S. bongori*. Among these two species are more than 1,500 serotypes based on the presence or absence of polysaccharide (somatic), fimbrial, flagellar, and/or capsular antigens. *Streptococcus pneumoniae* can be distinguished into approximately 90 serotypes based on antigenically distinct capsular polysaccharides.

Chemical Composition

Whole-cell protein electrophoresis often yields species-specific patterns (88). However, the patterns are very complex, with overlapping bands, and pattern comparison requires a computer. Since patterns are compared as track intensity curves, standardization of electrophorectic conditions is essential. A few laboratories have constructed whole-cell protein electrophoresis databases for use in species identification, but between-laboratory comparisons are rare.

Enzyme electrophoresis has taxonomic value (79). In MLEE, several (10 to 20) enzymes, which are single-gene products, are subjected to electrophoresis. For each enzyme, an inventory of all observed electromorphs is obtained and the genetic distance between each pair of strains, which is the proportion of enzymes for which the strains show different electromorphs, is calculated. This approach has been used to define clones within a bacterial population. Different species are usually clearly differentiated by MLEE.

Chromatography of lipids, phospholipids, mycolic acids (in high-G+C-ratio gram-positive bacteria), fatty acids (91), isoprenoid quinones (11), and peptidoglycan hydrolysates (78) constitutes chemotaxonomy. These methods are essential for some bacterial groups. Gas-liquid chromatography of fatty acids has been standardized, and a system (65) for the characterization and identification of bacteria has been commercialized.

Numerical Taxonomy

Phenotypic data are often too numerous to be analyzed without the help of a computer. Historically, the application of numerical taxonomy principles, made possible with computers, brought objectivity to the field and boosted research in taxonomy (82). The essential principle of numerical taxonomy (Adansonian principle) is that, a priori, all phenotypic characters are given equal weight. Some physiologists and geneticists may be shocked by this principle, knowing that some characters are controlled by several genes whereas others are controlled by a single gene. However, the genetic basis of a phenotypic character is usually known for only a few strains. Numerical taxonomists reason that if some characters are taxonomically important, they will appear as classificatory (i.e., those describing taxa) when the results are analyzed. Originally, complex or quantitative characters were subdivided into unit characters, assigned values of 1, 0, or equivocal, and encoded to have additive or nonadditive effects. A data matrix is entered with one row per strain (operational taxonomic unit [OTU]) and one unit character per column.

A program then compares all pairs of strains, scoring characteristics which are positive for both strains ($S1$), negative for both strains ($S0$), negative for the first strain and positive for the second strain ($D0$), and the reverse case ($D1$). Two similarity coefficients are usually employed and differ in the way in which negative matches are considered. The Jaccard coefficient (S_J) ignores negative matches ($S0$): $S_J = S1/(S1 + D0 + D1)$. The simple-matching coefficient (S_{SM}) considers negative matches: $S_{SM} = (S0 + S1)/(S0 + S1 + D0 + D1)$. When the proportion of positive characters (vigor) varies widely in a collection of strains under study, these coefficients may yield quite different results.

Instead of similarity, one may prefer to determine distance coefficients. Distance (d) is the complement of similarity ($d = 1 - S_J$ or $d = 1 - S_{SM}$). However, distance may not respect genometric rules, and the sum distances AB and BC may be smaller than AC. To make these distances Euclidean, their square roots are used. A third coefficient is sometimes used and separates vigor and pattern components from distance coefficients (82). The pattern distance (DP) is calculated as $DP = \sqrt{(4 \times D0 \times D1)/(S0 + S1 + D0 + D1)}$. Thus, when all positive characteristics of organism A are included in the set of positive characteristics of organism B, the pattern distance is zero (even when B has many more positive characters). Vigor and pattern analysis was little used, probably because, for conventional tests, the significance of positive characteristics is not always obvious. Should antimicrobial susceptibility or antimicrobial resistance be scored positive? Is a positive indole test indicating the production of indole (which most bacteria should do) or the lack of indole catabolism? With the growing use of carbon source utilization tests, the concept of vigor and pattern becomes straightforward. Application of this concept to the *Enterobacteriaceae* shows *Shigella* to be a less vigorous subset of *Escherichia coli* (29a). The coefficients calculated as mentioned above constitute the similarity (or distance) matrix.

By using the similarity/distance matrix, a clustering algorithm builds a hierarchic classification and draws a taxonomic tree, called a dendrogram or phenogram, based on phenotypic characters. Two major clustering algorithms are commonly used. With single linkage, a strain joins a cluster at the distance level corresponding to the shortest distance between that strain and any strain in the cluster. Two clusters merge at the level of the shortest distance between a member of one cluster and a member of the other cluster. With the unweighted pair group method using averages (UPGMA), a strain joins a cluster at the distance level corresponding to the average distance between that strain and all strains in the cluster. The advantage of single linkage is that it is independent of the initial strain order. The disadvantage is chaining, causing clusters to merge too quickly in the distance scale. The advantage of UPGMA is that the relationships displayed in a dendrogram are less distorted than with other methods. Dendrograms are also more pleasant to look at than those of single linkage. The only disadvantage of UPGMA is that it is a pair group method; i.e., if two (or more) unclustered strains have a same average distance to a cluster, only one strain will join the cluster at that distance level (always the first or last considered). This action may increase the average distance of the other unclustered strain(s) to the now enlarged cluster. The final dendrogram may be different when the original strain order is different. The major clusters are likely to have the same composition, but the detailed branching differs. This feature is rarely taken into consideration in published papers. Clusters are called phenons when based on phenotypic characters; there are usually no clear phenon limits. One may use an arbitrary distance limit to delineate phenons or take into account the distinctness of phenons and have phenons formed at different distance levels in a single dendrogram.

The final step in numerical taxonomy is to extract classificatory characteristics, i.e., those which have played a role in the classification process because they were more or less correlated (positively or negatively). Test statistics are obtained for each phenon, and the best tests allowing phenon differentiation are delineated. These may be proposed for identification purposes.

The major problem with dendrograms is that species limits are not indicated. Furthermore, bacterial groups differ considerably in their metabolic versatility, and phenotypic differences may not parallel genomic differences. Nucleic acid methods are now used to delineate species. When confronting phenograms and DNA relatedness data, it is often possible to match phenons with genomic species provided that phenon limits are set to match DNA relatedness data. Numerical taxonomy is now used to delineate the phenotypic diversity of a strain collection and to select strains representative of such diversity. Selected strains can then be used in DNA relatedness studies or 16S rRNA sequencing.

Genotypic Classification of Bacteria

Useful Properties of Nucleic Acids

Most bacterial chromosomes consist of a single circular double-stranded DNA molecule. DNA from a strain is characterized by its nucleotide sequence, size, and G+C molar ratio. The G+C ratio determines the thermal denaturation midpoint (melting temperature, T_m) of a given DNA sample in a solution of a given ionic composition. The T_m of DNA sample A is higher than that of sample B when the G+C ratio of A is higher than that of B. For a given DNA sample, the T_m increases when the sodium molarity increases in the medium. The T_m decreases proportionally with the amount of formamide or dimethyl sulfoxide in the medium. The T_m also decreases when DNA is fragmented. When a DNA solution is heated well above the T_m (e.g., boiled) or when the medium is very alkaline (e.g., pH 10), the two strands separate (denaturation). If the denatured DNA solution is quickly placed in an ice bath, it remains denatured. If the denatured DNA solution is kept at a temperature between room temperature and T_m − 15°C, the strands reassociate (anneal). Reassociation is faster when the temperature is higher (but still below T_m − 15°C) or the sodium concentration is higher (marked increase between 0.0 and 0.4 M, smaller increase between 0.4 and 1.0 M) or the DNA concentration is higher. Reassociation is also faster when the DNA is fragmented. It is slower when the genome complexity is higher.

Some enzymes are known to react with DNA. Double-stranded DNA can be hydrolyzed by DNase I or nuclease P1. With very low concentrations of DNase I, breaks can be randomly made on either strand. Single-stranded (and not double-stranded) DNA can be selectively hydrolyzed by S1 nuclease under precise conditions (presence of sodium and zinc ions, precise pH, temperature above 45°C). Single-stranded RNA can be hydrolyzed by RNases. Restriction endonucleases recognize specific palindromic sequences 4 to 14 nucleotides long. For a given genome, restriction endonuclease cleavage yields a finite number of fragments corresponding to the number of cleavage sites.

Methods for Determining the G+C Ratio

When Lee et al. (50) showed the taxonomic usage of the DNA base composition, they used paper chromatography of bases obtained after hydrolysis of DNA with formic acid. After elution from paper, the base concentration was determined spectrophotometrically. This method lacked precision since some base decomposition occurred during hydrolysis. The following two methods, described in 1962, were reference methods for 30 years. (i) Buoyant density of DNA in CsCl is linearly correlated to the G+C ratio. The method (77) required analytical ultracentrifugation for 44 h, was very precise, and needed only small amounts of DNA. (ii) The thermal denaturation midpoint (T_m) of DNA in a given buffer is linearly correlated with the G+C ratio (54). T_m is interpolated from the evolution of the absorbance of the DNA solution in a cuvette when the temperature is increased. The absorbance at 260 nm of denatured DNA is higher than that of native (double-stranded) DNA.

The above techniques have now been replaced by high-performance liquid chromatography of nucleotides obtained after P1 nuclease digestion of DNA (58).

Methods for Labeling Nucleic Acids

To monitor a nucleic acid hybridization reaction, it is often necessary to label one of the reacting nucleic acids. Several methods are available, including nick translation (72), random priming, and direct labeling (49). Radioactive DNA can be quantified by liquid scintillation counting or gamma counting. Chemically labeled DNA can be detected specifically. Biotin reacts with avidin, and avidin can react with a biotinylated enzyme. Acetylaminofluorene is detected by a mouse monoclonal antibody, which is detected by an enzyme-linked anti-mouse antibody. The enzymes are detected by colorimetric reactions.

Methods for DNA-DNA Hybridization

Several methods are available for total-genome comparison by means of quantitative DNA-DNA hybridization (29). DeLey et al. (17) devised a DNA hybridization method that relies on renaturation rates measured optically with a recording spectrophotometer. The standard error is about 2 to 5% (2, 17, 37). Pure, high-molecular-weight DNA must be used. The advantage of the method is that radioisotopes are not required.

Following the discovery (63) that single-stranded DNA binds strongly to nitrocellulose, Denhardt (20) proposed a nitrocellulose filter hybridization method which has since been the basis of various procedures. In a typical procedure, single-stranded (heat-denatured or alkali-treated) unlabeled DNA is immobilized on a nitrocellulose filter. The filter is then treated so that it will not bind any more DNA (prehybridization step). Any radioactive single-stranded DNA incubated with this filter either will bind to the immobilized DNA and resist being washed off the filter or will be washed off. The amount of DNA reassociation is estimated by measuring the radioactivity of the filter. The results of heterologous reactions (i.e., reactions involving DNAs from different strains) are calculated relative to those of homologous reactions (i.e., reactions with labeled and unlabeled DNA from the same strain). This method, which is routinely used in molecular biology for qualitative or semiquantitative detection of hybridization, is not precise enough for taxonomy.

DNA relatedness can be more precisely measured by competition experiments. In this method, unlabeled DNA immobilized on filters and radioactive DNA are from the same reference strain. Hybridization is allowed to proceed in the presence of a large amount of unlabeled, sheared, denatured competitor DNA. An experiment without competitor DNA (0% competition) and an experiment with the homologous DNA used as competitor (100% competitions) serve as controls. The relatedness between competitor and reference DNAs is deduced from the reduction in filter-bound radioactivity due to the competitor and is compared with the 0 and 100% competition control experiments. Colorimetric methods derived from the filter method have been proposed (24, 39). Their reproducibility must be evaluated.

In the hydroxyapatite and the S1 nuclease methods, a small amount of sheared, radiolabeled, denatured DNA and a larger amount of sheared unlabeled, denatured DNA are mixed and allowed to reassociate under optimal conditions (0.4 M sodium ion) for the time necessary for complete reassociation. Then reassociated DNA fragments are separated from nonreassociated fragments by either hydroxyapatite chromatography (7) or selective digestion of single-stranded fragments by S1 nuclease (14).

A major advantage of the free-solution methods is the ability to study the thermal stability of reassociated DNA. After completion of hybridization at the optimal temperature, the temperature is raised by 5°C increments. At each temperature, a sample is taken for digestion by S1 nuclease. The temperature at which half of the reassociated DNA is denatured (T_m) is determined by interpolation. The value, called ΔT_m, or divergence, is the difference between the T_m of the homologous reaction and that of the heterologous reaction. The standard error in ΔT_m determination is between 0.7 and 1.7°C (32).

Different methods may give different percent reassociation values. A linear correlation exists between the percent reassociation obtained by the spectrophotometric method and that obtained by the nitrocellulose filter method for reassociation values above 20 to 30% (19, 37). Reassociation values below 30% are not reliable when obtained by the spectrophotometric method. Reassociation values above 80% are often similar irrespective of the method used. However, 50% reassociation in either the hydroxyapatite method or the filter method corresponds to about 25% reassociation in the S1 nuclease method. The difference occurs because the hydroxyapatite and filter methods retain fully or partly reassociated fragments, the radioactivity of which is counted as reassociated, whereas the S1 nuclease (an endonuclease) digests nonreassociated parts of reassociated fragments. Thus, the percent reassociation determined by the S1 nuclease method is often lower than that determined by other methods, especially when DNA fragments are partially reassociated. It should be noted that ΔT_m values determined by either the hydroxyapatite method or the S1 nuclease method are similar (32).

Interpretation of Quantitative DNA-DNA Hybridization Data

Since the earliest experiments with DNA-DNA hybridization, it was found that DNA from strains which were considered to belong to a single species showed generally high relatedness (above 70% percent reassociation) whereas DNA from different species generally showed much lower reassociation (less than 50%). It is not possible to assign a strict percent relatedness limit to delineate species, since different methods give different values and these values are affected by genome size differences. For example, if two DNA molecules, A and B, with B containing exactly sequence A plus 20% genome with no match in A are tested, the results will depend on which strand is labeled. When A is labeled, the percent relatedness between A and B should be 100%. When B is labeled, the percent relatedness should be 80%. In practice, interpretation problems occur in the 55 to 75% range. It is therefore important to determine ΔT_m values, since these values are robust and independent of genome size differences or methods. ΔT_m values of 0 to 2°C are not very different from 0°C and indicate a pair of strains belonging to a single subspecies in a single species. Values of 3 to 5°C are often observed for strains belonging to different subspecies within a single species. Values above 7°C always indicate different species (29).

An international committee has issued the following definition of a genomospecies: "The phylogenetic definition of a species generally would include strains with approximately 70% or greater DNA-DNA relatedness and with 5°C or less ΔT_m. Both values must be considered." (90). Most of the time, these criteria are fulfilled. As a result, some medically important organisms which have been split in the past appear to be single species whereas some environmental organisms which had been grouped previously are now being subdivided (6). Although a "good" genus contains species which are 30 to 55% related by DNA-DNA hybridization, many genera contain species which are less closely related. Thus, DNA-DNA hybridization is not a safe method for genus delineation.

Quantitative RNA-DNA Hybridization

All living cells contain rRNA. The rRNAs are currently designated by their sedimentation constant (Svedberg, S). Prokaryotes have 5S, 16S, and 23S rRNA. In most bacteria, rRNA genes are organized in the *rrn* operon with genes coding for 16S, 23S, and 5S in that order, with intergenic spacers between genes. These operons are present in 1 to 11 copies on the chromosome.

Purified rRNA is labeled in vivo or in vitro by direct labeling or by reverse transcription. Because of the variable number of gene copies, the rRNA relatedness cannot be determined reliably as percent reassociation and two approaches have been used: thermal denaturation midpoint [$T_m(e)$] determination of rRNA-DNA reassociated molecules (18) and a competition method (41).

rRNA-DNA hybridization was the first approach to bacterial phylogeny and has allowed the restructuring of a number of bacterial genera. However, rRNA-DNA relatedness has to be determined experimentally, and this requires large collections of reference DNAs and labeled rRNAs. As a result, this approach has been limited to a few laboratories.

rRNA Sequence Comparison

The greatest advantage of rRNA sequencing over rRNA-DNA hybridization is that each sequence which has been determined can be deposited in a database available to other workers (21). Therefore, to position a new organism in a phylogenetic tree, it is sufficient to determine its rRNA sequence and to compare the sequence to those available. If the sequence has been properly determined and verified, it should constitute "definitive" data. The most useful rRNA molecule for phylogenetic studies is 16S rRNA (or its gene), which contains about 1,500 nucleotides and can be sequenced in 1 day. More than 10,000 sequences are available in databases (64). 5S rRNA contains about 150 nucleotides (limited amount of information), and 23S rRNA contains about 3,000 nucleotides (limited number of sequences available).

It has been suggested that taxonomic conclusions based on sequence data found in databases may be incorrect because these sequences either are incomplete or contain errors. A critical selection of sequences from databases is therefore required.

Sequencing Methods

Earlier approaches (RNA cataloging) involved cleavage of rRNA by specific RNases and chemical sequencing of the oligonucleotides produced. This was labor-intensive and limited to a very few laboratories. Nonetheless, RNA cataloging allowed the first phylogenetic tree representing major bacterial groups to be drawn (94).

Currently used sequencing methods derive from that of Sanger et al. (76). An oligonucleotide primer binds to a complementary sequence on the single-stranded nucleic acid matrix (DNA or RNA) whose sequence is to be determined. An enzyme (DNA polymerase or reverse transcriptase) then polymerizes a complementary strand by adding nucleotides at the 3′ end of the primer. These nucleotides in the reaction mixture are deoxyribonucleotides (dA, dT, dG, and dC). If the reaction mixture also contains a dideoxyribonucleotide (ddA, ddT, ddG, or ddC), strand extension will stop as soon as the dideoxyribonucleotide is incorporated. By careful dosing of the dideoxyribonucleotide (e.g., ddT), its incorporation becomes a random event. Thus, the product of the reaction will be a set of polynucleotides extending from the primer to any position where ddT may have been incorporated. This corresponds to adenine nucleotide (A) on the matrix. The same type of reaction is done in parallel with each dideoxyribonucleotide. These polynucleotides are separated by polyacrylamide gel electrophoresis, with migration being dependent on the size (the smallest oligonucleotide migrates first). Since either the primer or dideoxyribonucleotides are labeled (radioactive or fluorescent labeling), it is easy to deduce the nucleotide on the matrix which corresponds to an observed band (oligo- or polynucleotide) on the gel (as seen on an autoradiogram or machine-capture fluorogram). Machines are now available to automatically read the sequence while fluorescent bands pass in front of a laser beam.

In rRNA sequencing, primers hybridizing conserved regions of 16S or 23S rRNA were used in association with reverse transcriptase and dideoxyribonucleotides (48). However, the rRNA matrix had to be pure and not fragmented, and incorporation errors were often caused by reverse transcriptase. The method became much easier when the 16S rRNA gene was amplified by PCR and either sequenced on both strands (4) or cloned in M13 phage single-stranded DNA and sequenced (75).

Sequence Comparison

Sequence alignment is helped by the presence of zones with various degrees of conservation (including some almost invariant zones). Problems arise with hypervariable zones, where deletions or insertions occurred during evolution, and when remotely related bacteria are being compared. Publicly available software (e.g., CLUSTAL) can align a number of sequences automatically. However, these alignments should be carefully inspected and when necessary corrected manually. Once sequences are aligned, they can be compared. Several methods based on different phylogenetic hypotheses and other assumptions about evolution are available. These include distance, parsimony, and maximum-likelihood methods.

Phylogenetic distance takes into account the probability of reverse mutations. For each sequence pair, a distance coefficient, K_{nuc}, is calculated from the proportion (P) of nucleotide positions where nucleotides are different (43). The distance matrix obtained is then subjected to cluster analysis. Although UPGMA as used in numerical taxonomy can be useful, methods yielding additive trees are often preferred. Additive trees allow the calculation of the approximate distance between two organisms, A and B, by summing all branch lengths linking A and B (except perpendicular links between branches which have no distance meaning). The most popular algorithm for this method is neighbor joining (74). Trees can be rooted (and the root selected at will) and will then appear like a dendrogram with uneven branch lengths, or they can be unrooted, with branches extending from an imaginary core. Interpretation of such trees should focus on branch lengths and not on tree aesthetics.

Parsimony methods select phylogenetic trees that minimize the number of nucleotide substitutions required to explain the data (94).

Maximum-likelihood methods consider the mutation probability at each nucleotide position. They evaluate the likelihood that a given evolutionary model will yield the observed sequences. The inferred phylogeny is that with the highest likelihood (94).

These methods have a number of variants depending on a priori decisions (independent evolution of sites or branches; constant or variable evolution speed among branches; weight of transitions, transversions, deletions, and insertions). Different methods often give different trees. A phylogenetic hypothesis is stronger when the three approaches (distance, parsimony, and maximum likelihood) converge to give trees with the same overall grouping. Some resampling methods, such as bootstrap testing for tree robustness, are available. The process begins with a set A of aligned sequences, with L sequences (lines) and N nucleotide positions (columns). The bootstrap method will build a set B with L lines by taking columns (nucleotide sites) at random N times. A phylogenetic tree is then built. Such bootstrap analysis is done 100 to 1,000 times, and a consensus tree is built which indicates, at each branching, the number (or percent) of trees which yielded such branching. A higher figure means more robust branching.

Interpretation

Even the most beautiful phylogenetic tree does not indicate the limits of a genus, family, or order. When a phylogenetic group (i.e., a branch of any level) has common phenotypic features, it is fairly easy to recognize it as constituting a taxon, and the level of such taxa is decided by comparison with the branching level of known taxa (genera, families, etc.). When members of a named taxon (e.g., a genus) are found to be spread across a phylogenetic tree, the arguments in favor of splitting such taxa into smaller phylogenetically homogeneous taxa are strong. The best example has been shown by the genus *Pseudomonas* sensu lato, which has been split into phylogenetically homogeneous genera (e.g., *Pseudomonas* sensu stricto, *Chryseomonas*, *Flavimonas*, *Burkholderia*, *Ralstonia*, *Comamonas*, *Acidovorax*, *Hydrogenophaga*, *Telluria*, *Stenotrophomonas*, *Brevundimonas*, *Aminobacter*, *Oligotropha*, *Zavarsinia*, *Sphingomonas*, and *Devosia* [44]). However, in many cases, the limits of a phylogenetic group are fuzzy: expanding the group causes less phenotypic characters to be shared, and reducing the group increases the phenotypic homogeneity. Should the genera *Legionella* and *Vibrio* be split into smaller genera? Should *Plesiomonas shigelloides* be included in the family *Enterobacteriaceae*? Should *Xanthomonas maltophilia* be placed in a separate genus, *Stenotrophomonas*? These questions cannot be answered by simply looking at a phylogenetic tree. There are currently no molecular definitions of a genus or a family.

The greatest practical application of sequence comparison has been the identification of specific sequences at any taxonomic level. Examination of aligned sequences often allows the observation of short (about 20-nucleotide) parts of the rRNA sequence which are invariant within a taxon and which differ from the corresponding sequence part of other taxa. Knowledge of these specific sequences is now used for identification.

IDENTIFICATION AND TYPING

Until recently, identification had two major limitations. A pure culture had to be available for study, and identification of a bacterium failed if the corresponding species had not been described. These limitations have been recently addressed by molecular methods. Growth and isolation of bacteria from a complex population generally selects some species which are able to grow under the chosen conditions. Therefore, since efforts to grow and describe pathogenic bacteria have been made for a century, identification of pathogens is much easier than identification of environmental bacteria.

Phenotypic Identification

There are two strategies for the detection and identification of bacteria depending on whether the studied specimen is likely to contain a single strain (or very few strains) or a complex flora. In the former case (a single strain in a normally sterile site), the strain is allowed to multiply in rich broth (under aerobic and anaerobic conditions) and streaked on rich, nonselective agar media to purify the strain from any contaminant. An essential step is to orient the identification toward some major bacterial group. This is done by careful examination of cultures, microscopic examination, and application of a few tests which can be done with part of a colony (e.g., catalase and oxidase). Identification consists of performing biochemical tests which are appropriate for the bacterial group involved. Most identification errors or delays can be traced back to the initial steps of the identification process. The results (coded or not) are compared with a printed or computerized database. Some identification systems include identification software, which uses a probabilistic identification algorithm. When the bacterial species corresponding to the isolate under study is not included in the database (new species or wrong database), identification fails.

In the latter case (a complex bacterial flora), the approach taken is dependent upon the objective. If the objective is to isolate a given species or bacterial group, selective conditions must be used (medium; temperature; aerobic, anaerobic, or microaerophilic conditions) to return to the former case. Often, more than one bacterial species may be sought. This requires the use of a number of selective conditions. Inadequate choice of selective conditions may cause the search for the etiologic agent to fail.

Another problem arose more recently. Most phenotypic identification schemes were devised to distinguish bacterial pathogens from phenotypically related bacteria. Molecular taxonomy delineates new species each year, some of which are opportunistic pathogens. Phenotypic identification of these new species is increasingly difficult with the currently available phenotypic tests.

Conventional Epidemiological Typing

Typing is a means of establishing subspecific relationships (or lack thereof) between different organisms of the same species. Such information may be of clinical or epidemiologic value.

Biotyping

An epidemic strain can sometimes be differentiated from other strains of the same species by biochemical tests. Generally, the larger the number of biochemical characteristics comprising the biotyping scheme, assuming roughly equal probabilities of a positive or negative reaction with each biochemical, the greater the utility of the system. Biotyping systems (often empirical systems) relying on one or a few reactions have limited discriminatory power. The minimal requirement of such systems is reproducibility.

Serotyping

Because of its ability to distinguish bacteria at the subspecific level, serotyping is often a useful epidemiologic tool. This technique, however, has two major limitations. First, bacteria from different species or strains within the same species often possess cross-reacting antigens. For instance, certain strains of *E. coli* cross-react antigenically with encapsulated type b *Haemophilus influenzae*. Second, it is clear that within a given clonal group, antigenic variation is often seen to occur in nature. An example of this is the "capsular antigen switching" that occurs within a single clone of *Streptococcus pneumoniae*.

Phage Typing

Phage typing is used to determine the sensitivity of bacteria to a set of selected bacteriophages. The surface of an agar plate is inoculated with a broth culture of a test bacterium. After the plate has dried, a small drop of each phage suspension (in a given order) is deposited on the agar surface and the plate is marked so that the position of each phage drop can easily be deduced. After a 5- to 18-h incubation at 30 to 37°C, the plate is examined for clearing or plaque formation at the drop positions. The set of reactions given by an isolate is compared to a chart showing the set of reactions for each known phage type. If a match is found, the phage type of the isolate is identified.

For certain organisms, e.g., *Salmonella* serotype Typhi, phage typing has great epidemiologic usefulness. For other organisms, such as *Pseudomonas aeruginosa* and *Serratia marcescens*, which commonly harbor several prophages and plasmids (some of which can be lost in subcultures), phage typing is of limited value. Phage typing, while cost-efficient, is technically demanding, labor-intensive, and tedious. In many cases, phage typing has been replaced by molecular methods.

Bacteriocin Typing

Bacteriocins are protein-containing substances produced by many gram-negative and gram-positive bacteria. Bacteriocins react with specific bacterial surface receptors and kill the bacteria. The activity spectrum of bacteriocins from gram-negative bacteria is often limited to a narrow taxonomic group; e.g., a bacteriocin produced by a strain of species A is active against some other strains of species A but rarely against strains of other species. However, bacteriocins of gram-positive bacteria often have a wider spectrum of activity. The word "bacteriocin" may be applied to very different structures. Two bacteriocin categories have been defined. The first consists of protein structures which can be ultracentrifuged, are trypsin resistant, and are dissociated at pH 2. Electron microscopy shows incomplete phage-like or phage tail structures. The second category includes proteins which cannot be easily ultracentrifuged, have no shape under the electron microscope, are hydrolyzed by trypsin, and are not dissociated at pH 2. Known colicins belong to this category. Genes encoding bacteriocins are found on plasmids or the bacterial chromosome.

Typing can be performed by testing susceptibility to or production of bacteriocins (25, 26). Drops of the different bacteriocins are deposited on an agar plate which has been surface inoculated with a test bacterium. After incubation, a clear zone at a drop position indicates susceptibility to the corresponding bacteriocin. The power of bacteriocin susceptibility testing depends on the diversity and choice of the set of bacteriocin-producing bacteria.

For bacteriocin production testing, a set of indicator strains known to exhibit different bacteriocin susceptibilities is used. Strains can be tested for bacteriocin production by spot inoculating on an agar plate, incubating the culture, killing by chloroform vapors, and overlaying with agar containing an indicator strain. Clear zones are observed above bacteriocin-producing cultures. In a second method, strains are grown in broth with mitomycin C induction and centrifuged. The presence of a bacteriocin in supernatants is tested by depositing drops of supernatants on agar plates which have been inoculated with indicator strains. After incubation, a clear zone at a drop position indicates that a bacteriocin has been produced by the corresponding culture. The power of bacteriocin production testing depends on the diversity and choice of the set of bacteriocin-susceptible (indicator) bacteria.

Phenotypic Methods with Universal Applications

The problem with conventional phenotypic tests is that a given test procedure is often applicable only to a restricted bacterial group. Tests with broader application include carbon source utilization (33), gas-liquid chromatography of end products or cellular fatty acids (23, 36, 65, 85), protein electrophoresis (13), and MLEE (79).

Application of Nucleic Acid Methods to Species Identification and Typing

There are two major strategies for nucleic acid-based identification. The first uses specific probes which react with sequences that are found only in the bacterial groups to be detected or identified. The result of such tests is often "yes" or "no." The second strategy uses universal probes to generate complex results (patterns or sequences) which lead to identification after comparison with a database. In specific systems, the reaction between a probe and the corresponding target sequence is the key to specificity.

Choice of the Target of a Nucleic Acid Probe or Amplification System

There are two major options for the target; one is the detection of a bacterium harboring a given gene (a gene coding for a given function), and the other is the detection of a taxonomic entity. There may be a few cases where a given gene is found in all strains of a given species and not in other species (e.g., the β-glucuronidase gene and *E. coli*). However, as more strains are studied, these cases become more unusual.

The best applications of specific probes or amplification systems are the detection of genes involved in pathogenicity, such as in *E. coli*. Thus, probes and amplification systems are available for genes coding for Shiga-like toxins produced by enterohemorrhagic *E. coli* (EHEC) or *Shigella dysenteriae* 1, thermostable and thermolabile enterotoxins produced by enterotoxic *E. coli* (ETEC), intimin (gene *eae*) associated with enteropathogenic *E. coli* (EPEC) and some EHEC strains, invasive properties of *Shigella* and enteroinvasive *E. coli* (EIEC), colonization factors and other adhesins, siderophores (aerobactin), and hemolysins (42, 47, 51, 60).

Genes encoding antimicrobial resistance can also be detected by the use of probes or amplification systems. It should be stressed that what is detected is a gene coding for a given resistance mechanism (67). Lack of detection of a given resistance gene does not mean that the strain is susceptible to an antimicrobial agent; it only means that the given gene is absent. Other resistance genes and mechanisms that have not been searched for may be present. Thus, nucleic acid probes targeted toward resistance genes are of great epidemiological interest, although they cannot replace antimicrobial susceptibility testing.

Only protein antigens (e.g., flagellin) are direct gene products. Restriction of amplified flagellin genes has been used for typing bacteria (45). Other antigens are produced through more or less complex metabolic pathways, involving several genes. Some of these genes may encode key enzymes, and their detection may, indirectly, indicate the presence of given antigens. This has been used for the detection of *S. typhi* Vi antigen (involving *viaA* and *viaB*) by use of a *viaB*-specific probe or amplification system (35). The detection is also positive for Vi-positive strains of serotypes Paratyphi C and Dublin and rare strains of *Citrobacter freundii*.

Genes coding for any enzyme can also be detected by probe or amplification systems. Examples of applications are the detection of *E. coli* β-glucuronidase or β-galactosidase (3) or *Staphylococcus aureus* thermonuclease (5). In all cases, the probe or amplification system specificity is, at best, that of the target gene. Some genes may be present in different species, and some functions or mechanisms (virulence or antibiotic resistance) may be encoded by different genes.

A Taxonomic Entity

Early attempts to make species-specific probes involved random cloning of chromosomal DNA and determination of the specificity of some clones. This approach often fails because of its lack of taxonomic basis. It has been shown that when total-DNA restriction fragments are deprived of fragments hybridizing with rRNA, the resulting mixture can be used as a species-specific probe (30). Thus, any DNA fragment which does not carry rRNA genes may show some specificity. Common random amplified polymorphic DNA (RAPD) fragments shared by patterns created from different strains have been extracted and used as probes (57). However, it remains to be demonstrated that selecting a common RAPD band gives a more specific probe than taking any band not carrying rRNA genes.

The use of oligonucleotide probes complementary to specific parts of rRNA sequences is the best taxonomic approach to identification at present. Probes can be designed to hybridize with rRNA from all bacteria or only eubacteria or a given phylogenetic branch down to the species level. A taxon-specific probe can be designed if the taxon represents a valid phylogenetic group. Therefore, there can be no probe for the genus *Pseudomonas* sensu lato (as known 20 years ago). However, there are probes for *Proteobacteria* branches, *Pseudomonas* sensu stricto, or *Pseudomonas aeruginosa* (1). Unfortunately, some closely related species cannot be distinguished by rRNA-based probes (27).

Detection of the Reaction

Early studies used filter hybridization. This method may still be used when it is necessary to screen colonies (colony blot) or a number of isolates (dot blot) for the presence of a given gene. Probes are easily digoxigenin labeled. After hybridization and washing, the filter is treated with alkaline phosphatase-conjugated anti-digoxigenin antibodies, 5-bromo-4-chloro-3-indolyphosphate, and nitroblue tetrazolium. A blue to purple color develops where the probe has bound.

Solution Hybridization

Some commercial kits have used solution hybridization with hydroxyapatite separation of free radioactive probe from bound probe (22).

Reverse Hybridization

Cloned or oligonucleotide probes can be bound to a surface (filter, microplate, or microchip). A number of different specific probes can thus be bound on a single surface. The target gene of an isolate is amplified, labeled, and allowed to react with the probe-bearing surface. After washing and visualization of the label, the surface is examined for evidence of binding to a probe, allowing identification. This approach allows multiple identifications when the amplification is carried out on specimens containing a mixture of microorganisms (73).

In Situ Hybridization

Bacterial cells collected on a filter (or a specially treated glass slide) can be fixed and permeabilized so as to maintain the cellular shapes. A fluorescent oligonucleotide probe can access rRNA and bind to the complementary sequence if present. This approach (fluorescent in situ hybridization) allows the visualization of hybridized cells, including their shape, grouping, and relationship with human cells. Probes with diverse specificities can be used to visualize all bacteria or a given phylogenetic branch, genus, or species (1). With a good choice of fluorescent chromophores (bound to different probes) and UV filters, multicolor reactions can be obtained. The method is fast (2 to 3 h) and less prone to artifacts than is PCR. However, it suffers from the relatively low sensitivity of microscopic observation. The present in situ technology is restricted to the use of rRNA as target. Other targets (rRNA or genes) require the amplification of either the target or the signal.

PCR—a Special Case of Probe Hybridization

As described in detail in chapter 13, PCR is a method whereby specific segments of either DNA or RNA are amplified into thousands of copies. These can be analyzed by agarose gel electrophoresis, where they appear as a band of the expected size (as deduced from the known sequence of the target DNA). Further proof of the presence of the target DNA can be obtained by hybridization with an oligonucleotide probe targeting a zone located in the amplified part of the target sequence (other than that reacting with the primers). The method is so sensitive that contamination of equipment and reagents with polynucleotides (DNA fragments) occasionally occurs. Extreme care should be taken to avoid contamination. Controls must be included in all experiments to detect possible contamination.

Although species-specific PCR systems have been proposed, the main application of PCR is in the detection of pathogenicity genes. When available, multiplex systems, using a mixture of primers to amplify DNA fragments of different sizes, are convenient.

Universal Approaches to the Identification of Any Bacterium

When no hypothesis on the identification of a microorganism is available, the use of specific probes is almost impossible (or too tedious). A universal approach is then needed.

Partial rRNA Sequencing

Knowledge of 16S rRNA (or *rrs* gene) sequences allows the selection of parts of the sequence which are sufficient for identification. Such gene segments can be amplified from clinical specimens by using universal primers. The amplified product is then sequenced, and the sequence is compared with databases. This approach has been particularly successful for the identification of *Bartonella henselae*, *B. quintana*, and *Tropheryma whippelii* in clinical samples (69–71). However, universal primers often amplify sequences matching those of the *Enterobacteriaceae* or *Pseudomonas* species. These may originate from dead bacteria in polymorphonuclear or monocytic cells or from production-contaminated *Taq* polymerase. For this reason, amplification with branch-specific primers may be preferred (16). Amplification of sequences corresponding to these bacteria and to gram-positive cocci (which are also widespread in nature) may be very difficult to interpret unless in situ hybridization shows bacterial forms associated with these sequences.

When an undescribed organism is isolated, sequencing of the 16S rRNA (or *rrs* gene) may be the only way to locate it in the taxonomic tree when phenotypic properties do not suggest a family or genus (15).

Ribotyping

When bacterial DNA is cleaved by a common restriction endonuclease, numerous fragments are generated. After agarose gel electrophoresis and transfer of the fragments to a membrane, the complexity of the fragment pattern can be reduced by visualization of a subset of fragments. By using 16S plus 23S rRNA as a probe, a simpler pattern is obtained (28). This method has been called rRNA gene restriction pattern determination (28) or ribotyping (84). The ability of ribotyping to uncover the taxonomic diversity of a collection of *Pseudomonas* isolates was recently demonstrated (8). The method has recently been improved by the use of a mixture of five digoxigenin-labeled oligonucleotides as the probe (68). Computer identification of ribotypes is feasible provided that the error associated with fragment length determination is known (53). The use of ribotyping for species identification relies on the availability of databases and logical identification algorithms that are able to give more weight to species-specific bands. A machine for fully automated ribotyping is available (66).

PCR Ribotyping

Amplification of the space between the *rrs* and *rrl* genes has been used in identification or typing (56); this method is called PCR ribotyping (46). However, the patterns obtained have different resolutions depending on the bacterial species studied.

ARDRA

Restriction of the amplified *rrs* gene cannot have the same resolution as the full 16S rRNA sequence and thus cannot be used as a general identification method (87). However, amplification of a 5-kb DNA segment comprising most of the *rrs* (16S) and *rrl* (23S) genes and the intergenic spacer followed by restriction by one to three endonucleases may be of general interest, allowing the differentiation of closely related species (38). In addition to ribotyping, many molecular typing methods have been proposed. However, only a few are widely used. This method is called amplified ribosomal DNA restriction analysis (ARDRA).

Restriction of Amplified DNA Fragment

Any gene can be amplified provided that two invariant (or quasi-invariant) regions to which primers can be directed occur in its sequence. The best example is flagellin genes, which have highly conserved sequences at both gene extremities and a highly variable central region. Restriction analysis of amplified flagellin genes correlates with antigenic diversity (45).

Pulsed-Field Gel Electrophoresis

Restriction endonucleases which recognize rare cleavage sites on the bacterial chromosome can be selected. Compared to common cleavage sites, rare cleavage sites either are more complex nucleotide combinations (the *Not*I site is about 12 nucleotides long) or have a less probable nucleotide composition (e.g., the *Dra*I site, which includes only nucleotides with A and T bases, is rare on high-G+C-ratio DNA, and the *Sma*I site, which includes only nucleotides with G and C bases, is rare on low-G+C-ratio DNA). Restriction fragments are so large that they do not migrate in agarose gel electrophoresis unless a special method is used to force the DNA threads through the agarose sieve (e.g., electric field rotation or field inversion). These special electrophoretic techniques are known as pulsed-field gel electrophoresis (PFGE) (10). PFGE is the most discriminative molecular typing method (55). The best results are obtained with rather expensive equipment, and the use of optimal conditions for PFGE is essential. Criteria have been proposed for the epidemiological interpretation of PFGE patterns (86).

Random Amplification with a Single Primer

A single oligonucleotide may serve as primer for amplification provided that it recognizes on both DNA strands complementary sequences which are close enough that the space between then can be amplified. This principle has been used in a family of techniques. Arbitrarily primed PCR (AP-PCR) uses oligonucleotides of about 20 bases with low-stringency annealing, incorporation of radioactive nucleotides, and visualization of amplified products by polyacrylamide gel electrophoresis (92). RAPD uses oligonucleotides of about 10 bases, stringent annealing, and visualization of amplified products by agarose gel electrophoresis (93). Because of its simplicity, RAPD is widely used in clinical microbiology. DNA-amplified fingerprinting uses very short oligonucleotides (5 bases) (9). The major problem with random amplification using a single primer is interlaboratory reproducibility. One study showed that different RAPD patterns were obtained when different thermocyclers or different *Taq* polymerase were used (59).

Amplification of Repetitive Elements

Several sequences which were found repeated on various bacterial chomosomes have been targets for PCR (52, 89).

Amplified Fragment Length Polymorphism

In the patented method called amplified fragment length polymorphism (AFLP), DNA is restricted by using two endonucleases. Short oligonucleotide adapters are ligated to fragment sticky ends. A selective amplification is performed with two primers complementary to a sequence comprising an adapter and part of the restriction site. The choice of primers allows the amplification of a subset of restriction fragments, resulting in a 30- to 40-fragment pattern (40). The method seems very promising.

The Future of Identification

There is no question that the future of identification is in the development of computerized databases. Since the natural environment is the reservoir of opportunistic pathogens, many new bacterial species (mostly environmental) are being described and many more are still to be discovered. Identification without the use of a database will be almost impossible. The major problem that can be envisioned is control of database quality. Companies that distribute kits or identification systems often provide the user with a database. In some instances, the database is of limited utility. A database should be built based on well-characterized strains identified by DNA hybridization or rRNA sequencing. Databases that are contributed to by anyone (e.g., major sequence databases) often contain wrong sequences, either because earlier methods were error-prone or because misidentified strains were used. These databases are still useful for research purposes, since experienced researchers can differentiate good from bad sequences. However, such databases cannot be used in clinical microbiology laboratories without refinement. The World Wide Web (Internet) will certainly be the place to access identification databases.

New technologies, such as fast sequencing on microchips, will probably bring sequencing closer to the clinical laboratory. Such developments should be sustained by taxonomic work to avoid the accumulation of meaningless sequences. In the meantime, the joint use of phenotypic tests and molecular methods based on DNA restriction suffices to meet the needs of clinical laboratories.

REFERENCES

1. **Amann, R. I., W. Ludwig, and K.-H Schleifer.** 1995. Phylogenetic identification and in situ detection of individual microbial cells without cultivation. *Microbiol. Rev.* **59:**143–169.
2. **Baess, I., and M. W. Bentzon.** 1978. Deoxyribonucleic acid hybridization between different species of mycobacteria. *Acta Pathol. Microbiol. Scand. Sect. B* **86:**71–76.

3. **Bej, A. K., J. L. Dicesare, L. Haff, and R. M. Atlas.** 1991. Detection of *Escherichia coli* and *Shigella* spp. in water by using the polymerase chain reaction and gene probes for *uid*. *Appl. Environ. Microbiol.* **57:**1013–1017.
4. **Böttger, E. C.** 1989. Rapid determination of bacterial ribosomal RNA sequences by direct sequencing of enzymatically amplified DNA. *FEMS Microbiol. Lett.* **65:** 171–176.
5. **Brakstad, O. G., and J. A. Maeland.** 1995. Direct identification of *Staphylococcus aureus* in blood cultures by detection of the gene encoding the thermostable nuclease or the gene product. *APMIS* **103:**209–218.
6. **Brenner, D. J., G. R. Fanning, G. V. Miklos, and A. G. Steigerwalt.** 1973. Polynucleotide sequence relatedness among *Shigella* species. *Int. J. Syst. Bacteriol.* **23:**1–7.
7. **Brenner, D. J., G. R. Fanning, A. V. Rake, and K. E. Johnson.** 1969. A batch procedure for thermal elution of DNA from hydroxyapatite. *Anal. Biochem.* **28:**447–459.
8. **Brosch, R., M. Lefevre, F. Grimont, and P. A. D. Grimont.** 1996. Taxonomic diversity of pseudomonads revealed by computer-interpretation of ribotyping data. *Syst. Appl. Microbiol.* **19:**541–555.
9. **Caetano-Anolles, G., B. J. Bassam, and P. M. Gresshoff.** 1991. DNA amplification fingerprinting using very short arbitrary oligonucleotide primers. *Bio/Technology* **9:** 553–556.
10. **Cantor, C. R., C. L. Smith, and M. K. Mathew.** 1988. Pulse-field gel electrophoresis of very large DNA molecules. *Annu. Rev. Biophys. Chem.* **17:**287–304.
11. **Collins, M. D., and D. Jones.** 1981. Distribution of isoprenoid quinone structural types in bacteria and their taxonomic implications. *Microbiol. Rev.* **45:**316–354.
12. **Colwell, R. R.** 1970. Polyphasic taxonomy of the genus *Vibrio*: numerical taxonomy of *Vibrio cholerae*, *Vibrio parahaemolyticus*, and related *Vibrio* species. *J. Bacteriol.* **104:** 410–433.
13. **Costas, M.** 1992. Classification, identification, and typing of bacteria by the analysis of their one–dimensional polyacrylamide gel electrophoretic protein patterns. *Adv. Electrophor.* **5:**351–408.
14. **Crosa, J. H., D. J. Brenner, and S. Falkow.** 1973. Use of a single-strand specific nuclease for analysis of bacterial and plasmid deoxyribonucleic acid homo- and heteroduplexes. *J. Bacteriol.* **115:**904–911.
15. **Dauga, C., M. Gillis, P. Vandamme, E. Ageron, F. Grimont, K. Kersters, D. DeMahenge, Y. Peloux, and P. A. D. Grimont.** 1993. *Balneatrix alpica* gen.nov., sp. nov., a bacterium associated with pneumonia and meningitis in a spa therapy centre. *Res. Microbiol.* **144:**35–46.
16. **Dauga, C., I. Miras, and P. A. D. Grimont.** 1997. Strategy for detection and identification of bacteria based on 16S rRNA genes in suspected cases of Whipple's disease. *J. Med. Microbiol.* **46:**1–8.
17. **DeLey, J., H. Cattoir, and A. Reynaerts.** 1970. The quantitative measurement of DNA hybridization from renaturation rates. *Eur. J. Biochem.* **12:**133–142.
18. **DeLey, J., and J. De Smedt.** 1975. Improvement of the membrane filter method for DNA-rRNA hybridization. *Antonie Leeuwenhoek J. Microbiol. Serol.* **41:**287–307.
19. **DeLey, J., and R. Tijtgat.** 1970. Evaluation of membrane filter methods for DNA-DNA hybridization. *Antonie Leeuwenhoek J. Microbiol. Serol.* **36:**461–474.
20. **Denhardt, D. T.** 1966. A membrane filter technique for the detection of complementary DNA. *Biochem. Biophys. Res. Commun.* **23:**641–646.
21. **DeRijk, P., J.-M. Neefs, Y. Van de Peer, and R. DeWachter.** 1992. Compilation of small ribosomal subunit RNA sequences. *Nucleic Acids Res.* **20:**2075–2089.
22. **Edelstein, P. H., R. N. Bryan, R. K. Enns, D. E. Kohne, and D. L. Kacian.** 1987. Retrospective study of Gen-Probe rapid diagnostic system for detection of legionellae in frozen clinical respiratory tract samples. *J. Clin. Microbiol.* **25:**1022–1026.
23. **Embley, T. M., and R. Wait.** 1994. Structural lipids of eubacteria, p. 121–163. *In* M. Goodfellow and A. G. O'Donnell (ed.), *Modern Microbial Methods. Chemical Methods in Prokaryotic Systematics.* John Wiley & Sons, Chichester, England.
24. **Ezaki, T., Y. Hashimoto, and E. Yabuuchi.** 1989. Fluorometric deoxyribonucleic acid-deoxyribonucleic acid hybridization in microdilution wells as an alternative to membrane filter hybridization in which radioisotopes are used to determine genetic relatedness among bacterial strains. *Int. J. Syst. Bacteriol.* **39:**224–229.
25. **Farmer, J. J., III.** 1972. Epidemiological differentiation of *Serratia marcescens*: typing by bacteriocin production. *Appl. Microbiol.* **23:**218–225.
26. **Farmer, J. J., III.** 1972. Epidemiological differentiation of *Serratia marcescens*: typing by bacteriocin sensitivity. *Appl. Microbiol.* **23:**226–231.
27. **Fox, G. E., J. D. Wisotzkey, and P. Jurtshuk.** 1992. How close is close: 16S rRNA sequence identity may not be sufficient to guarantee species identity. *Int. J. Syst. Bacteriol.* **42:**166–170.
28. **Grimont, F., and P. A. D. Grimont.** 1986. Ribosomal ribonucleic acid gene restriction patterns as possible taxonomic tools. *Ann. Inst. Pasteur Microbiol.* **137B:**165–175.
29. **Grimont, P. A. D.** 1988. Use of DNA reassociation in bacterial classification. *Can. J. Microbiol.* **34:**541–546.
29a.**Grimont, P. A. D.** Unpublished data.
30. **Grimont, P. A. D., F. Grimont, N. Desplaces, and P. Tchen.** 1985. DNA probe for *Legionella pneumophila*. *J. Clin. Microbiol.* **21:**431–437.
31. **Grimont, P. A. D., F. Grimont, H. L. C. Dulong de Rosnay, and P. H. A. Sneath.** 1977. Taxonomy of the genus *Serratia*. *J. Gen. Microbiol.* **98:**39–66.
32. **Grimont, P. A. D., M. Y. Popoff, F. Grimont, C. Coynault, and M. Lemelin.** 1980. Reproducibility and correlation study of three deoxyribonucleic acid hybridization procedures. *Curr. Microbiol.* **4:**325–330.
33. **Grimont, P. A. D., M. Vancanneyt, M. Lefevre, K. Vandemeulebroeke, L. Vauterin, R. Brosch, K. Kersters, and F. Grimont.** 1996. Ability of Biolog and Biotype-100 systems to reveal the taxonomic diversity of the pseudomonads. *Syst. Appl. Microbiol.* **19:**510–527.
34. **Gurtler, V., V. A. Wilson, and B. C. Mayall.** 1991. Classification of medically important clostridia using restriction endonuclease site differences of PCR-amplified 16S rDNA. *J. Gen. Microbiol.* **137:**2673–2679.
35. **Hashimoto, Y, Y. Itho, Y. Fujinaga, A. Q. Khan, F. Sultana, M. Miyake, K. Hirose, H. Yamamoto, and T. Ezaki.** 1995. Development of nested PCR based on the ViaB sequence to detect *Salmonella typhi*. *J. Clin. Microbiol.* **33:**775–777.
36. **Holdeman, L. V., and W. E. C. Moore.** 1977. *Anaerobe Laboratory Manual*, 4th ed. Virginia Polytechnic Institute and State University, Blacksburg.
37. **Huss, V. A. R., H. Festl, and K. H. Schleifer.** 1983. Studies on the spectrophotometric determination of DNA hybridization from renaturation rates. *Syst. Appl. Microbiol.* **4:**184–192.
38. **Ibrahim, A., P. Gerner-Smidt, and A. Sjostedt.** 1996. Amplification and restriction endonucelase digestion of a large fragment of genes coding for rRNA as a rapid method for discrimination of closely related pathogenic bacteria. *J. Clin. Microbiol.* **34:**2894–2896.
39. **Jahnke, K.-D.** 1994. A modified method of quantitative colorimetric DNA-DNA hybridization on membrane fil-

ters for bacterial identification. *J. Microbiol. Methods* **20:** 273–288.

40. **Janssen, P., R. Coopman, G. Huys, J. Swings, M. Bleeker, P. Vos, M. Zabeau, and K. Kersters.** 1996. Evaluation of the DNA fingerprinting method AFLP™ as a new tool in bacterial taxonomy. *Microbiology* **142:** 1881–1893.
41. **Johnson, J. L., and B. Harich.** 1983. Comparisons of procedures for determining ribosomal ribonucleic acid similarities. *Curr. Microbiol.* **9:**111–120.
42. **Johnson, J. R.** 1991. Virulence factors in *Escherichia coli* urinary tract infection. *Clin. Microbiol. Rev.* **4:**80–128.
43. **Jukes, T. H., and C. R. Cantor.** 1969. Evolution of protein molecules, p. 21–132. *In* H. N. Munro (ed.), *Mammalian Protein Metabolism*. Academic Press, Inc., New York, N.Y.
44. **Kersters, K., W. Ludwig, M. Vancanneyt, P. DeVos, M. Gillis, and K.-H. Schleifer.** 1996. Recent changes in the classification of the pseudomonads: an overview. *Syst. Appl. Microbiol.* **19:**465–477.
45. **Kilger, G., and P. A. D. Grimont.** 1993. Differentiation of *Salmonella* phase 1 flagellar antigen types by restriction of the amplified *fliC* gene. *J. Clin. Microbiol.* **31:** 1108–1110.
46. **Kostman, J. R., T. D. Edlin, J. L. Lipuma, and T. L. Stull.** 1992. Molecular epidemiology of *Pseudmonas cepacia* determined by polymerase chain reaction ribotyping. *J. Clin. Microbiol.* **30:**2084–2087.
47. **Kuhnert, P., J. Hacker, I. Muhldorfer, A. P. Burnens, J. Nicolet, and J. Frey.** 1997. Detection system for *Escherichia coli*-specific virulence genes: absence of virulence determinants in B and C strains. *Appl. Environ. Microbiol.* **63:**703–709.
48. **Lane, D. J., B. Pace, G. J. Olsen, D. A. Stahl, M. L. Sogin, and N. R. Pace.** 1985. Rapid determination of 16S ribosomal RNA sequences for phylogenetic analyses. *Proc. Natl. Acad. Sci. USA* **82:**6955–6959.
49. **Leary, J. J., and J. L. Ruth.** 1989. Nonradioactive labeling of nucleic acid probes, p. 33–57. *In* B. Swaminathan and G. Prakash (ed.), *Nucleic Acid and Monoclonal Antibody Probes—Applications in Diagnostic Microbiology*. Marcel Dekker, Inc., New York, N.Y.
50. **Lee, K. Y., R. Wahl, and E. Barbu.** 1956. Contenu en bases puriques et pyrimidiques des acides deoxyribonucleiques des bacteries. *Ann. Inst. Pasteur* **91:**212–224.
51. **Levine, M.** 1987. *Escherichia coli* that cause diarrhea: enterotoxigenic, enteropathogenic, enteroinvasive, enterohemorrhagic, and enteroadherent. *J. Infect. Dis.* **155:** 377–389.
52. **Lupski, J. R., and G. E. Weinstock.** 1992. Short, interspersed repetitive DNA sequences in prokaryotic genomes. *J. Bacteriol.* **174:**4525–4529.
53. **Machado, J., F. Grimont, and P. A. D. Grimont.** 1998. Computer identification of *Escherichia coli* rRNA gene restriction patterns. *Res. Microbiol* **149:**119–135.
54. **Marmur, J., and P. Doty.** 1962. Determination of the base composition of deoxyribonucleic acid from its thermal denaturation temperature. *J. Molec. Biol.* **5:**109–118.
55. **Maslow, J. N., M. E. Mulligan, and R. D. Arbeit.** 1993. Molecular epidemiology: application of contemporary techniques to the typing of microorganisms. *Clin. Infect. Dis.* **17:**153–164.
56. **McClelland, M., C. Petersen, and J. Welsh.** 1992. Length polymorphism in tRNA intergeneric spacers detected by using the polymerase chain reaction can distinguish streptococcal strains and species. *J. Clin. Microbiol.* **30:**1499–1504.
57. **Menard, C., P. Gosselin, J. F. Duhaime, and C. Mouton.** 1994. Polymerase chain reaction using arbitrary primer for the design and construction of a DNA probe specific for *Porphyromonas gingivalis*. *Res. Microbiol.* **145:** 595–602.
58. **Meshbah, M., U. Premachandran, and W. Whitman.** 1989. Precise measurement of the G+C content of deoxyribonucleic acid by high-performance liquid chromatography. *Int. J. Syst. Bacteriol.* **39:**159–167.
59. **Meunier, J.-R., and P. A. D. Grimont.** 1993. Factors affecting reproducibility of random amplified polymorphic DNA fingerprinting. *Res. Microbiol.* **144:**373–379.
60. **Muhldorfer, I., and J. Hacker.** 1994. Genetic aspects of *Escherichia coli* virulence. *Microb. Pathog.* **16:**171–181.
61. **Murray, R. G. E., D. J. Brenner, R. R. Colwell, P. DeVos, M. Goodfellow, P. A. D. Grimont, N. Pfennig, E. Stackebrandt, and G. A. Zavarsin.** 1990. Report of the ad hoc committee on approaches to taxonomy within the *Proteobacteria*. *Int. J. Syst. Bacteriol.* **40:**213–215.
62. **Murray, R. G. E., and K. H. Schleifer.** 1994. Taxonomic notes: a proposal for recording the properties of putative taxa of procaryotes. *Int. J. Syst. Bacteriol.* **44:**174–176.
63. **Nygaard, A. P., and B. D. Hall.** 1963. A method for the detection of RNA-DNA complexes. *Biochem. Biophys. Res. Commun.* **12:**98–104.
64. **Olsen, G. J., G. Larsen, and C. R. Woese.** 1991. The ribosomal RNA database project. *Nucleic Acids Res.* **19**(Suppl.)**:**2017–2021.
65. **Osterhout, G. J., V. H. Shull, and J. D. Dick.** 1991. Identification of clinical isolates of gram-negative nonfermentative bacteria by an automated cellular fatty acid identification system. *J. Clin. Microbiol.* **29:**1822–1830.
66. **Pfaller, M. A., C. Wendt, R. J. Holls, R. P. Wenzel, S. J. Fritschel, J. J. Neubauer, and L. A. Herwaldt.** 1996. Comparative evaluation of an automated ribotyping system versus pulse-field gel electrophoresis for epidemiological typing of clinical isolates of *Escherichia coli* and *Pseudomonas aeruginosa* from patients with recurrent Gram-negative bacteremia. *Diagn Microbiol. Infect. Dis.* **25:**1–8.
67. **Ploy, M. C., H. Giamarellou, P. Bourlioux, P. Courvalin, and T. Lambert.** 1994. Detection of aac(6′)-I genes in amikacin-resistant *Acinetobacter* spp. by PCR. *Antimicrob. Agents Chemother.* **38:**2925–2928.
68. **Regnault, B., F. Grimont, and P. A. D. Grimont.** 1997. Universal ribotyping method using a chemically labelled oligonucleotide probe mixture. *Res. Microbiol.* **148:** 649–659. (Erratum, **149:**73, 1998.)
69. **Relman, D. A.** 1993. The identification of uncultured microbial pathogens. *J. Infect. Dis.* **168:**1–8.
70. **Relman, D. A., J. S. Loutit, T. M. Schmidt, S. Falkow, and L. S. Tompkins.** 1990. The agent of bacillary angiomatosis—an approach to the identification of uncultured pathogens. *N. Engl. J. Med.* **323:**1573–1580.
71. **Relman, D. A., T. M. Schmidt, R. P. MacDermott, and S. Falkow.** 1992. Identification of the uncultured bacillus of Whipple's disease. *N. Engl. J. Med.* **327:**293–301.
72. **Rigby, P. W. J., M. Dieckmann, C. Rhodes, and P. Berg.** 1977. Labeling deoxyribonucleic acid to high specific activity in vitro by nick translation with DNA polymerase I. *J. Mol. Biol.* **113:**237–251.
73. **Rijpens, N. P., G. Jannes, M. VanAsbroeck, L. M. F. Herman, and R. Rossau.** 1995. Simultaneous detection of *Listeria* spp. and *Listeria monocytogenes* by reverse hybridization with 16S-23S rRNA spacer probes. *Mol. Cell. Probes* **9:**423–432.
74. **Saitou, N., and M. Nei.** 1987. The neighbor-joining method: a new method for reconstructing phylogenetic trees. *Mol. Biol. Evol.* **4:**406–425.
75. **Sambrook, J., E. F. Fritsch, and T. Maniatis.** 1989. *Molecular Cloning: a Laboratory Manual*, 2nd ed. Cold Spring Harbor Laboratory, Cold Spring Harbor, N.Y.

76. **Sanger, F., S. Nicklen, and A. R. Coulson.** 1977. DNA sequencing with chain-terminating inhibitors. *Proc. Natl. Acad. Sci. USA* **74:**5463–5467.
77. **Schildkraut, C. L., J. Marmur, and P. Doty.** 1962. Determination of the base composition of deoxyribonucleic acid from its buoyant density in CsCl. *J. Mol. Biol.* **4:** 430–442.
78. **Schleifer, K. H., and O. Kandler.** 1972. Peptidoglycan types of bacterial cell wall and their taxonomic implications. *Bacteriol. Rev.* **36:**407–477.
79. **Selander, R. K., D. A. Caugant, H. Ochman, J. M. Musser, M. N. Gilmour, and T. S. Whittam.** 1986. Methods of multilocus enzyme electrophoresis for bacterial population genetics and systematics. *Appl. Environ. Microbiol.* **51:**873–884.
80. **Skerman, V. B. D., V. McGowan, and P. H. A. Sneath.** 1980. Approved list of bacterial names. *Int. J. Syst. Bacteriol.* **30:**225–420.
81. **Sneath, P. H. A. (ed).** 1992. *International Code of Nomenclature of Bacteria: Bacteriological Code, 1990 Revision.* American Society for Microbiology, Washington, D.C.
82. **Sneath, P. H. A., and R. R. Sokal.** 1973. *Numerical Taxonomy.* W. H. Freeman & Co., San Francisco, Calif.
83. **Stanier, R. Y., N. J. Palleroni, and M. Doudoroff.** 1966. The aerobic pseudomonads: a taxonomic study. *J. Gen. Microbiol.* **43:**159–271.
84. **Stull, T., J. J. LiPuma, and T. D. Edlind.** 1988. A broad-spectrum probe for molecular epidemiology of bacteria: ribosomal RNA. *J. Infect. Dis.* **157:**280–286.
85. **Suzuki, K., M. Goodfellow, and A. G. O'Donnell.** 1993. Cell envelopes and classification, p. 195–250. *In* M. Goodfellow and A. G. O'Donnell (ed.), *Handbook of New Bacterial Systematics.* Academic Press, Ltd., London, England.
86. **Tenover, F. C., R. D. Arbeit, R. V. Doering, P. A. Mickelsen, B. E. Murray, D. H. Persing, and B. Swaminathan.** 1995. Interpreting chromosomal DNA restriction patterns produced by pulse-field gel electrophoresis: criteria for bacterial strain typing. *J. Clin. Microbiol.* **33:** 2233–2239.
87. **Vaneechoutte, M., R. Rossau, P. DeVos, M. Gillis, D. Janssens, N. Paepe, A. DeRouck, T. Fiers, G. Claeys, and K. Kersters.** 1992. Rapid identification of bacteria of the *Comamonadaceae* with amplified ribosomal DNA-restriction analysis (ARDRA). *FEMS Microbiol. Lett.* **93:** 227–234.
88. **Vauterin, L., J. Swings, and K. Kersters.** 1993. Protein electrophoresis and classification, p. 251–280. *In* M. Goodfellow and A. G. O'Donnell (ed.), *Handbook of New Bacterial Systematics.* Academic Press, Ltd., London, England.
89. **Versalovic, J., T. Kroeuth, and J. R. Lupski.** 1991. Distribution of repetitive DNA sequences in eubacteria and application to fingerprinting of bacterial genomes. *Nucleic Acids Res.* **19:**6823–6831.
90. **Wayne, L. G., D. J. Brenner, R. R. Colwell, P. A. D. Grimont, O. Kandler, M. I. Krichevsky, L. H. Moore, W. E. C. Moore, R. G. E. Murray, E. Stackebrandt, M. P. Starr, and H. G. Truper.** 1987. Report of the ad hoc committee on reconciliation of approaches to bacterial systematics. *Int. J. Syst. Bacteriol.* **37:**463–464.
91. **Welch, D. F.** 1991. Applications of cellular fatty acid analysis. *Clin. Microbiol. Rev.* **4:**422–438.
92. **Welsh, J., and M. McClelland.** 1990. Fingerprinting genomes using PCR with arbitrary primers. *Nucleic Acids Res.* **18:**7213–7219.
93. **Williams, J. G. K., A. R. Kubelic, K. J. Livak, J. A. Rafalski, and S. V. Tingey.** 1990. DNA polymorphisms amplified by arbitrary primers are useful as genetic markers. *Nucleic Acids Res.* **18:**6531–6535.
94. **Woese, C. R.** 1987. Bacterial evolution. *Microbiol. Rev.* **51:**221–271.

Algorithm for Identification of Aerobic Gram-Positive Cocci

KATHRYN L. RUOFF

15

Initial identification of gram-positive cocci recovered from cultures incubated in the presence of oxygen can be accomplished by the tests shown in Table 1. Most of the organisms in this category are "aerotolerant anaerobes," i.e., organisms that grow anaerobically or in the presence of oxygen but do not use oxygen metabolically. The remaining genera display different relationships to oxygen, ranging from facultative (*Staphylococcus* and *Stomatococcus*, which form larger colonies when cultured in the presence of oxygen) to microaerophilic (*Aerococcus*, which grows poorly if at all under anaerobic conditions) to obligately aerobic (*Micrococcus* and *Alloiococcus*).

The genera included in this group form colonies with different appearances on blood agar. While many of the organisms form non-beta-hemolytic colonies (alpha- or gamma-hemolytic), strains of streptococci, staphylococci, and enterococci may be beta-hemolytic. Depending on the organism, colonies can vary in size, pigmentation, and other aspects of gross appearance, and in one genus (*Abiotrophia*) colonies display "satelliting" behavior, growing adjacent to the colonies of other bacteria that excrete necessary growth factors into the surrounding medium.

Colony morphologies as well as other tests used for initial characterization of these organisms are described in various chapters of this Manual. Special care should be taken in the examination of Gram stains, since cellular morphology and arrangement is a key trait for accurate identification of the organisms in Table 1. As noted in chapter 19, Gram stains should be made with growth from broth cultures and examined for either a "streptococcal" morphology, consisting of gram-positive cocci or coccobacilli in pairs and chains, or a "staphylococcal" morphology, in which cells appear as cocci arranged in pairs, clusters, and tetrads. It should be remembered that unrelated genera may display similar cellular morphologies and that no taxonomic kinship is implied by division of these bacteria into two groups based on their appearance in the Gram stain.

While most of the organisms described in Table 1 are catalase negative, some genera produce strongly positive catalase reactions (*Micrococcus* and *Staphylococcus*) or reactions that can vary, depending on the strain, from negative or weakly positive to positive (*Alloiococcus*, *Stomatococcus*, and *Aerococcus*). Accurate catalase test results are observed when the test is performed with bacterial cells that have been cultured on media devoid of blood or other sources of heme groups, since organisms showing a negative result under these conditions may exhibit positive or weakly positive reactions when grown in the presence of heme compounds.

Although a few of the genera included in Table 1 contain some of the most virulent and important bacterial pathogens known (e.g., *Streptococcus pyogenes*, *Streptococcus pneumoniae*, and *Staphylococcus aureus*), many of the organisms in this group function as opportunistic pathogens whose clinical significance has been appreciated only recently. The list of genera of aerobic gram-positive cocci that have been recovered from human infections will no doubt continue to expand as more opportunists are recognized and as future taxonomic refinements of these bacteria occur.

TABLE 1 Differentiating features of gram-positive cocci that grow aerobically

Catalase[a]	Clusters[a]	Pairs, chains[a]	Obligate aerobe	Oxidase[a]	PYR[b]	Growth in NaCl[a]	LAP[a]	Esculin[b]	Vanco-mycin[a]	Micro-aerophilic	Satellite behavior[a]	Growth at: 10°C[a]	Growth at: 45°C[a]	Organism (chapter)
+	+		+	+		+[c]								*Micrococcus* (16)
				−		+[d]								*Alloiococcus* (19)
			−			+[c]								*Staphylococcus* (16)
						−[c]								*Stomatococcus* (19)
−	+				+		+	+						*Stomatococcus* (19)
								−						*Gemella* (19)
						+[d]	−			+				*Aerococcus viridans* (19)
										−				*Helcococcus* (19)
						−[d]	−	+						*Helcococcus* (19)
								−						*Gemella* (19)
					−	+[d]			S[e]					*Aerococcus urinae* (19)
						−[c]			S					*Stomatococcus* (19)
									R					*Pediococcus* (19)
	−	+			+		+		S		+			*Abiotrophia* (19)
											−	+	+	*Enterococcus* (18)
													−	*Lactococcus* (19)
					−		+		S			−	−/+	*Streptococcus* (17)
												+	−	*Lactococcus* (19)
							−		R					*Leuconostoc* (19)

[a] See chapter 19 for the method of performing this test.
[b] See chapter 17 for the method of performing this test.
[c] Growth in the presence of 5% sodium chloride (see chapter 19 for method).
[d] Growth in the presence of 6.5% sodium chloride (see chapter 19 for method).
[e] S, sensitive; R, resistant.

Staphylococcus and *Micrococcus*

WESLEY E. KLOOS AND TAMMY L. BANNERMAN

16

TAXONOMY

Members of the genera *Staphylococcus* and *Micrococcus* are catalase-positive, gram-positive cocci and were, up until recently, placed together with the genera *Stomatococcus* and *Planococcus* in the family *Micrococcaceae* (126). This family is not a phylogenetically coherent group, and the results of DNA base composition (135), DNA-rRNA hybridization (67), and comparative oligonucleotide cataloguing of 16S rRNA (98, 139) studies have indicated that staphylococci and micrococci are not closely related. The genus *Staphylococcus* is most closely related to the newly described genus *Macrococcus* (72), but it also has a relatively close relationship to the genera *Bacillus*, *Salinicoccus*, *Gamella*, *Listeria*, *Planococcus*, and *Brochothrix*. These genera are tentatively arranged together with staphylococci and several other genera in the family *Bacillaceae* (19) of the broad *Bacillus-Lactobacillus-Streptococcus* cluster (99, 138) or order *Bacillales* (19). On the other hand, the genus *Micrococcus* is most closely related to the genus *Arthrobacter* of the coryneform or actinomycete group (137, 139). The genus *Micrococcus* has recently been dissected into the six genera *Micrococcus* (containing the species *Micrococcus luteus* and *Micrococcus lylae*), *Kocuria* (containing the former species *Micrococcus roseus*, *Micrococcus varians*, and *Micrococcus kristinae*), *Kytococcus* (the former *Micrococcus sedentarius*), *Nesterenkonia* (the former *Micrococcus halobius*), *Dermacoccus* (the former *Micrococcus nishinomiyaensis*), and *Arthrobacter* (the former *Micrococcus agilis*, a member of the "*Arthrobacter globiformis-Arthrobacter citreus* group") (87, 136). The genus *Kocuria* is more closely related to the genera *Stomatococcus* and *Rothia* than to other actinomycetes, and the genus *Kytococcus* is most closely related to the genus *Dermacoccus* (136).

DESCRIPTION OF THE GENERA

Members of the genus *Staphylococcus* are gram-positive cocci (0.5 to 1.5 μm in diameter) that occur singly and in pairs, tetrads, short chains (three or four cells), and irregular grape-like clusters. Ogston (113) introduced the name "staphylococcus" (from *staphylé*, a bunch of grapes) for the group of micrococci causing inflammation and suppuration. Rosenbach (123) used the term in a taxonomic sense and provided the first description of the genus *Staphylococcus*. Staphylococci are nonmotile, non-spore forming, and usually catalase positive, and they are usually unencapsulated or have limited capsule formation. Most species are facultative anaerobes. Except for *Staphylococcus saccharolyticus* and *S. aureus* subsp. *anaerobius*, their growth is more rapid and abundant under aerobic conditions. These exceptional organisms are also catalase negative. Some uncommon strains of staphylococci may require the presence of CO_2 or other metabolites (hemin, menadione, etc.) or a hypertonic medium for growth. The genome size of staphylococci is in the range of 2,000 to 3,000 kb (47, 72, 120).

Members of the genus *Micrococcus* are gram-positive cocci (1 to 1.8 μm in diameter), occurring mostly in pairs, tetrads, and irregular clusters. Micrococci and staphylococci have been confused with one another for more than a century on the basis of their rather similar cell morphologies, Gram staining results, and positive catalase activities. Both genera are commonly found living on mammalian skin and may be present in various human and veterinary clinical specimens, although micrococci are found less frequently than staphylococci and are generally regarded as saprophytes rather than as opportunistic pathogens. Cohn (27) introduced the genus *Micrococcus* to represent small spherical bacteria such as staphylococci, micrococci, and streptococci as well as some other groups. Evans et al. (41) proposed separating staphylococci from micrococci on the basis of their relation to oxygen. The facultative cocci were placed in the genus *Staphylococcus*, and the obligate aerobes were placed in the genus *Micrococcus*. Although we now know that there are some exceptions to this proposal, it aided in placing staphylococcal and micrococcal systematics on a fruitful course. By the mid-1960s, a clear distinction could be made between staphylococci and micrococci on the basis of their DNA base compositions (135). Members of the genus *Staphylococcus* have a DNA G + C content of 30 to 39 mol%, whereas members of the genus *Micrococcus* have a G + C content within the range of 66 to 75 mol%. The cell wall of staphylococci contains peptidoglycan and teichoic acid (127). The diamino acid present in the peptidoglycan is L-lysine, and the interpeptide bridge of the peptidoglycan consists of oligoglycine peptides (susceptible to the action of lysostaphin). Depending on the species and relative amount of glycine present in the growth medium, some glycine residues may be substituted with L-serine or L-alanine. Cell wall teichoic acids of staphylococci may be poly(polyolphosphate), poly(glycerolphosphate-glycosylphosphate), or poly(glycosylphosphate), depending on the species. Glycerol or ribitol or both occur as typical components of poly(polyolphosphate) teichoic acids. Substituents of these teichoic acids may include *N*-acetylgalactosamine, glucose, and *N*-acetylglucosamine. Members of the genus *Micrococcus* have no glycine in the interpeptide bridge of the peptidoglycan and do not have teichoic acids. The respiratory chains of staphylococci and micrococci differ in cytochrome and menaquinone composition. Most staphylococci contain only *a*- and *b*-type cytochromes, whereas micrococci also have *c*- and *d*-type cytochromes. The exceptional species *S. lentus*, *S. sciuri*, and *S. vitulus* contain *a*-, *b*-, and *c*-type cytochromes. Staphylococci contain unsaturated polyisoprenoid side chains in their menaquinones, whereas micrococci have hydrogenated menaquinones. In the clinical laboratory, staphylococci can be easily distinguished from micrococci on the basis of the former's resistance to bacitracin and susceptibility to furazolidone (5).

Members of the genus *Macrococcus* (including the species *Macrococcus caseolyticus* [formerly *Staphylococcus caseolyticus*], *Macrococcus equipercicus*, *Macrococcus bovicus*, and *Macrococcus carouselicus*) can be distinguished from staphylococci on the basis of their generally higher G + C DNA contents (38 to 45 mol%), absence of cell wall teichoic acids (with the possible exception of *M. caseolyticus*), smaller genome size of approximately 1,500 to 1,800 kb, larger Gram-stained cell size of 1.3 to 2.5 μm in diameter, and unique ribotype and macrorestriction patterns (72). Macrococci can be distinguished from most species of staphylococci (except *S. sciuri*, *S. lentus*, and *S. vitulus*) by the former's oxidase activity. They are susceptible to a wide range of antibiotics and do not exhibit the antibiotic resistance profiles characteristic of many staphylococcal species. However, like staphylococci and salinicocci, macrococci have a cell wall peptidoglycan that has L-lysine as the diamino acid and that has an interpeptide bridge that is susceptible to the action of lysostaphin. Since macrococci have not yet been isolated and identified from clinical specimens and have a rather restricted host range on only cetaceans, artiodactyls, and/or perissodactyls, they will not be described further in this chapter. The main characteristics used to differentiate staphylococci from micrococci and other gram-positive cocci encountered in the clinical laboratory are listed in Table 1.

The genus *Staphylococcus* is currently composed of 32 species (44, 70, 71) and 15 subspecies (55, 70, 71, 73, 76), as depicted in Table 2. The genus *Micrococcus* is currently composed of the two species *M. luteus* and *M. lylae* (88, 136). *M. luteus* is the most common micrococcal species found in nature and in clinical specimens. The more distantly related species *Kocuria varians*, *Kocuria kristinae*, and *Kytococcus sedentarius* are occasionally found in clinical specimens and can be distinguished from micrococci on the basis of their cell wall peptidoglycan compositions, aliphatic hydrocarbon compositions, menaquinone compositions, and cellular fatty acid compositions and by several simple tests listed below in the section on the identification of *Micrococcus* species (88, 136).

NATURAL HABITATS

Staphylococci are widespread in nature, although they are mainly found living on the skin, skin glands, and mucous membranes of mammals and birds. They are sometimes found in the mouth, blood, mammary glands, and intestinal, genitourinary, and upper respiratory tracts of these hosts. Staphylococci generally have a benign or symbiotic relationship with their host; however, if the natural cutaneous barriers are damaged by trauma, inoculation by needles, or direct implantation of medical devices (foreign bodies), these organisms may gain entry into the host tissues or colonize foreign bodies and develop the lifestyle of a pathogen. Infected tissues of the host may support large populations of staphylococci, and in some situations, they may persist for long periods. The presence of enterotoxigenic strains of staphylococci (most notably, certain strains of *S. aureus*) in various food products is regarded as a public health hazard because of the ability of these strains to produce intoxication or food poisoning.

Staphylococci found on humans and other primates include *S. aureus*, *S. epidermidis*, *S. capitis*, *S. caprae*, *S. saccharolyticus*, *S. warneri*, *S. pasteuri*, *S. haemolyticus*, *S. hominis*, *S. lugdunensis*, *S. auricularis*, *S. saprophyticus*, *S. cohnii*, *S. xylosus*, and *S. simulans* (68, 70, 71, 81). Most of the species listed above produce resident populations on humans. However, *S. xylosus* and *S. simulans* are usually only transients on humans and are primarily acquired from domestic animals and their products. Some of the human staphylococcal species are temporary residents or transients on domestic animals. *S. aureus* is occasionally found on various mammals and on some host species may be represented by different ecovars (36, 104). *S. schleiferi*, *S. intermedius*, *S. simulans*, and *S. felis* are commonly found living on carnivora (71, 81). However, *S. schleiferi* may produce serious infections in humans (42, 61) and *S. intermedius* may produce infections in humans as a result of dog bites (142). *S. lutrae* has recently been isolated from the European otter, a carnivore (44). *S. xylosus*, *S. kloosii*, and *S. sciuri* are common residents on a variety of rodents (71). *S. hyicus*, *S. chromogenes*, *S. sciuri*, *S. lentus*, and *S. vitulus* are common residents of ungulates and, in addition, may be isolated from their food products (37, 73, 149). The last three species are also common residents of cetaceans, such as dolphins and whales (71).

Some *Staphylococcus* species and subspecies demonstrate habitat or niche preferences on their particular hosts (68). For example, *S. capitis* subsp. *capitis* is found as large populations on the adult human head, especially the scalp and forehead, where sebaceous glands are numerous and well developed. *S. capitis* subsp. *ureolyticus* is also found on the head, but it may produce relatively large populations in the axillae of some individuals (6). *S. auricularis* has a strong preference for the external auditory meatus. *S. hominis* and *S. haemolyticus* generally produce larger populations in areas of the skin where apocrine glands are numerous, such as the axillae and pubic areas. *S. aureus* prefers the anterior nares as a habitat, especially in the adult human.

Certain *Staphylococcus* species are found frequently as etiologic agents of a variety of human and animal infections. In this chapter, we will be concerned primarily with the identification of *S. aureus*, *S. epidermidis*, *S. haemolyticus*, *S. lugdunensis*, *S. warneri*, and *S. saprophyticus*, species most commonly associated with human infections, and *S. intermedius* and *S. hyicus*, species of special veterinary interest. *S. schleiferi* has been considered a significant pathogen in some European countries but has seldom been isolated from infections in the United States.

Micrococci are widespread in nature and are commonly found on the skin of humans and other mammals (77, 82, 88). They are generally believed to be temporary residents or transients and are most frequently found on the exposed skin of the face, arms, hands, and legs.

TABLE 1 Differentiation of members of the genus *Staphylococcus* from other gram-positive cocci[a]

Genus and exceptional species	Mol% G + C of DNA	Strict aerobe	Facultative anaerobe or microaerophile	Strict anaerobe	Tetrad cell arrangement	Strong adherence on agar	Motility	Growth on: 5% NaCl agar	6.5% NaCl agar	12% NaCl agar	P agar in 18 h[b]	Catalase[c]	Benzidine test[d]	Modified oxidase test[e]	Anaerobic acid from glucose[f]	Aerobic acid from glycerol	Growth on Schleifer-Kramer agar[g]	Resistance to: Lysostaphin (200 μg/ml)	Erythromycin (0.4 μg/ml)	Bacitracin (0.04 U)[h]	Furazolidone (100 μg)[i]
Staphylococcus	30–39	–	d	–	d	–[j]	–	+	+	d	+	+	+	–	d	+	+	–	+	+	–
S. aureus subsp. *anaerobius*		–	±	±	–	–	–	+	+	d	–	–	–	–	+	+	ND	–	+	ND	–
S. saccharolyticus		–	±	±	+	–	–	+	+	±	–	–	±	–	+	+	ND	–	+	ND	–
S. hominis		±[k]	±	–	+	–	–	+	+	±	+	+	+	–	+	+	+	–	+	+	–
S. auricularis		–	+	–	+	–	–	+	+	±	–	+	+	–	+	+	ND	–	+	+	–
S. saprophyticus, *S. cohnii*, *S. xylosus*		d	d	–	–	–	–	+	+	±	+	+	+	–	–	+	+	–	+	+	–
S. kloosii, *S. equorum*, *S. arlettae*		±	±	–	–	–	–	+	+	±	d	+	+	–	–	+	+	–	+	+	–
S. intermedius		–	+	–	–	–	–	+	+	+	+	+	+	–	+	+	±	–	+	+	–
S. sciuri, *S. lentus*, *S. vitulus*		±	±	–	d	–	–	+	+	d	d	+	+	+	–	+	+	–	+	+	–
Macrococcus[l]	38–45	±	±	–	d	–	–	+	+	±	d	+	+	+	–	d	ND	–	+	+	–
Enterococcus	34–42	–	+	–	–	–	d	+	+	(±)	±	–	–	–	+	d	(±)	+	+	+	–
Streptococcus	34–46	–	+	d	–	–	–	d	d	–	–	–	–	–	+	d	–	+	–	d	–
Aerococcus	35–40	–	+	–	+	–	–	+	+	+	–	–	–	–	(+)	ND	ND	+	ND	–	–
Planococcus	39–52	+	–	–	d	–	+	+	+	+	–	+	+	ND	–	–	ND	+	ND	ND	–
Stomatococcus	56–60	–	+	–	d	+	–	–	–	–	–	±	+	–	+	d	ND	+	ND	–	d
Micrococcus and related genera	66–75	+	–	–	+	–	–	+	+	d	–	+	+	+	–	–	–	+	–[m]	–	+
Kocuria kristinae	67	±	±	–	+	–	–	+	+	±	–	+	+	+	(+)	+	(±)	+	–	–	+

[a] Symbols and abbreviations: +, 90% or more species or strains positive; ±, 90% or more species or strains weakly positive; –, 90% or more species or strains negative; d, 11 to 89% of species or strains positive; ND, not determined; parentheses, a delayed reaction.

[b] Growth on P agar is under aerobic conditions and at 35 to 37°C. Positive growth is indicated for detectable colony formation of at least 1 mm in diameter; ± indicates detectable colony formation between 0.5 and 1 mm in diameter. Growth on sheep or bovine blood agar is slightly greater but less discriminative between staphylococci and other genera.

[c] Sometimes weak catalase or pseudocatalase reaction can be observed in certain strains of species designated catalase negative. In some species, catalase activity may be activated by hemin supplementation.

[d] Benzidine test detects the presence of cytochromes. Some strains of benzidine test-negative species can synthesize cytochromes on aerobic media supplemented with hemin.

[e] See reference 127.

[f] Standard oxidation-fermentation test (41, 127).

[g] Growth (KRAN agar supplemented with sodium azide, potassium thiocyanate, lithium chloride, and glycine) (128) is under aerobic conditions and at 35 to 37°C for 24 to 48 h. Positive growth is indicated for a number of CFU on selective medium comparable to that on plate count agar and a colony of 0.5 mm in diameter; ± indicates a significant reduction in the numbers of CFU on the selective medium compared to that on plate count agar, and parentheses indicate a colony of pinpoint size to 0.5 mm in diameter.

[h] Disk is used. Positive indicates resistance and no zone of inhibition. *Micrococcus*, *Kocuria*, *Kytococcus*, *Stomatococcus*, and *Aerococcus* spp. are susceptible and have inhibition zone sizes of 10 to 25 mm in diameter.

[i] Disk is used. Positive indicates resistance and from no zone of inhibition to 9 mm. Susceptible species have inhibition zone sizes of 15 to 35 mm in diameter.

[j] Some strains of *S. epidermidis* adhere tenaciously to the surface of agar, and this property is correlated with heavy slime production.

[k] *S. hominis* does not demonstrate growth in the anaerobic portion of a thioglycolate medium within 24 h and may produce only very poor growth in this portion following 3 to 5 days of incubation. However, it will grow and ferment glucose anaerobically (standard oxidation-fermentation test). Failure to grow anaerobically in thioglycolate may be due in part to inhibition by certain of the ingredients.

[l] *Macrococcus* species can also be differentiated from *Staphylococcus* species on the basis of their generally larger Gram-stained cell size (≥2 μm) and larger number of chromosome fragments produced by digestion with *Not*I (12 to 36 fragments) (72).

[m] A few *Micrococcus* strains demonstrate high-level (MIC, ≥50 μg/ml) erythromycin resistance.

CLINICAL SIGNIFICANCE

Staphylococcus

The coagulase-positive species *S. aureus* is well documented as a human opportunistic pathogen. Nosocomial infections caused by *S. aureus* have been a major cause of morbidity and mortality. *S. aureus* infections are often acute and pyogenic and, if untreated, may spread to surrounding tissue or via bacteremia to metastatic sites (involving other organs). Some of the most common infections caused by *S. aureus* involve the skin, and they include furuncles or boils, cellulitis, impetigo, and postoperative wound infections of various sites. Some of the more serious infections produced by *S. aureus* are bacteremia, pneumonia, osteomyelitis, acute endocarditis, myocarditis, pericarditis, cerebritis, meningitis, scalded skin syndrome, and abscesses of the muscle, urogenital tract, central nervous system, and various intra-abdominal organs. Food poisoning is often attributed to staphylococcal enterotoxin.

Toxic shock syndrome (TSS), a community-acquired disease, has also been attributed to infection or colonization with *S. aureus*. A single clone has been shown to cause the majority of the cases (110). TSS is prevalent in young, menstruating females who use certain types of highly absorbent tampons (145). TSS-associated nongenital *S. aureus* has also been described in men and nonmenstruating women. TSS is associated with strains that produce and secrete the exotoxin toxic shock syndrome toxin 1 (TSST-1) (129). TSST-1 production appears to be limited to the species *S. aureus* (128a). TSST-1 is a member of a superantigen family that has the ability to stimulate T cells (25) and induce tumor necrosis factor (114) and the cytokine interleukin-1 (115). Methods for recognizing TSST-1 production include radioimmunoassay, enzyme-linked immunosorbent assay, reversed passive latex agglutination (RPLA) (available from Oxoid, Ogdensburg, N.Y.), and PCR (62).

Methicillin-resistant *S. aureus* (MRSA) emerged in the 1980s as a major clinical and epidemiologic problem in hospitals. Presently, hospitals of all sizes are facing the MRSA problem. Recommendations for the management or control of the spread of MRSA have been made available (16, 17, 108). Nasal carriage of *S. aureus* or MRSA has been suggested as a risk factor for the development of infections. Strategies for eliminating the nasal carriage of this species, thus reducing the infection rate, have been proposed by Kluytmans and coworkers (83).

The coagulase-negative *Staphylococcus* (CoNS) species as a group constitute a major component of the normal microflora of humans. The role of CoNS species in causing nosocomial infections has been recognized and well documented over the last two decades, especially for the species *S. epidermidis*. The infection rate has been correlated with the increase in the use of prosthetic and indwelling devices and the growing number of immunocompromised patients in hospitals. The need exists for the accurate identification of CoNS, so that precise delineation of the clinical disease produced by this group of bacteria and the determination of the etiologic agent can be accomplished. A review of CoNS has summarized results that are helpful in identifying the etiologic agent (74). These results included (i) the isolation of a strain in pure culture from the infected site or body fluid (most contaminated clinical specimens produce mixed cultures of different strains and/or species; however, some infections may be the consequence of more than one strain or species) and (ii) the repeated isolation of the same strain or combination of strains over the course of the infection. *S. epidermidis* has been documented as a pathogen in numerous cases of bacteremia, and native and prosthetic valve endocarditis, in surgical wounds, and in urinary tract, cerebrospinal fluid, prosthetic joint, peritoneal dialysis-related, opthalmologic, and intravascular catheter-related infections (32, 124). *S. saprophyticus* is an important opportunistic pathogen in human urinary tract infections, especially in young, sexually active females (46). It has also been proposed as an agent of nongonococcal urethritis in males or a cause of other sexually transmitted diseases, prostatitis, wound infections, and septicemia. *S. haemolyticus*, the second most frequently encountered CoNS species associated with human infections, has been implicated in native valve endocarditis, septicemia, peritonitis, urinary tract infections, and wound, bone, and joint infections (74, 124). Other CoNS species have been implicated in a variety of infections. For example, *S. capitis*, *S. caprae*, *S. lugdunensis*, *S. saccharolyticus*, *S. simulans*, and *S. warneri* have been implicated in endocarditis; *S. capitis*, *S. hominis*, *S. schleiferi*, *S. simulans*, and *S. warneri* have been implicated in septicemia; *S. warneri* and *S. simulans* have been implicated in osteomyelitis; *S. cohnii* has been implicated in native valve endocarditis and pneumonia; *S. lugdunensis*, *S. cohnii*, *S. xylosus*, *S. schleiferi*, *S. hominis*, and *S. caprae* have been implicated in urinary tract infections; *S. cohnii* and *S. lugdunensis* have been implicated in arthritis; *S. schleiferi* has been implicated in wound and joint infections; *S. lugdunensis* has been implicated in endophthalmitis; and *S. capitis*, *S. lugdunensis*, *S. schleiferi*, and *S. warneri* have been implicated in catheter infections (74, 124). *S. hominis* subsp. *novobiosepticus*, a newly described and unusual novobiocin-resistant subspecies, has been isolated with increasing frequency during the 1990s from human blood cultures, and in many cases, it appears to be associated with clinically significant septicemia (76, 150). In many cases patients with infections caused by CoNS have predisposing or underlying diseases affecting the immune system and had also experienced surgery or intravascular manipulations. CoNS and *S. aureus* will continue to be infective agents in the future (8, 148).

The coagulase-positive species *S. intermedius* and the coagulase-variable species *S. hyicus* are of particular importance in veterinary infections. *S. aureus* and these two coagulase-positive species are serious opportunistic pathogens of animals. *S. intermedius* has been associated with a variety of canine infections including otitis externa, pyoderma, abscesses, reproductive tract infections, mastitis, and wound infections (38, 81). *S. intermedius* infections in humans are usually associated with animal bites. This species has been implicated in a food-poisoning outbreak involving butter-blend products (66). *S. hyicus* has been implicated in infectious exudative epidermitis and septic polyarthritis in pigs and mastitis in cows (38, 81).

CoNS are a major cause of foreign-body infections. Nonspecific and/or specific adhesion of bacteria to biomaterials may be the first step involved in foreign-body infections caused by CoNS species (51). This step is followed by the production of slime or glycocalyx (60, 118). Clinical isolates of CoNS species that display a polysaccharide-adhesion (PS-A) are generally more adherent to catheters in vitro and elaborate significant quantities of biofilm (107). Some clinical isolates display PS-A without producing measurable quantities of slime, yet they are adherent to polymers. Prevention of the formation of the biofilm may involve the use of special foreign-body polymers, modification of the polymer surface, or the addition of antiinfective materials

TABLE 2 Differentiation of *Staphylococcus* species

Species	Characteristics																
	Colony size (large)[b]	Colony pigment[c]	Anaerobic growth[d]	Aerobic growth[e]	Staphylocoagulase	Clumping factor[f]	Heat-stable nuclease	Hemolysins[g]	Catalase[h]	Oxidase[i]	Alkaline phosphatase	Arginine arylamidase	Pyrrolidonyl arylamidase[j]	Ornithine decarboxylase	Urease[j]	β-Glucosidase[j]	β-Glucuronidase[j]
S. aureus subsp. *aureus*	+	+	+	+	+	+	+	+	+	−	+	−	−	−	d	+	−
S. aureus subsp. *anaerobius*	−	−	(+)	(±)	+	−	+	+	−	−	+	ND	ND	ND	ND	−	−
S. epidermidis	−	−	+	+	−	−	−	(d)	+	−	+[m]	−	−	(d)	+	(d)	−
S. capitis subsp. *capitis*	−	−	(+)	+	−	−	−	(d)	+	−	−	−	−	−	−	−	−
S. capitis subsp. *ureolyticus*	−	(d)	(+)	+	−	−	−	(d)	+	−	−	−	(d)	−	+	−	−
S. caprae	d	−	(+)	+	−	−	−	(d)	+	−	(+)	−	d	−	+	−	−
S. saccharolyticus	−	−	+	(±)	−	−	−	−	−	−	d	−	ND	ND	ND	ND	ND
S. warneri	d	d	+	+	−	−	−	(d)	+	−	−	−	−	−	+	+	d
S. pasteuri[n]	d	d	+	+	−	−	−	(d)	+	−	−	−	−	−	+	+	+
S. haemolyticus	+	d	(+)	+	−	−	−	(+)	+	−	−	−	+	−	−	d	d
S. hominis subsp. *hominis*	−	d	−	+	−	−	−	−	+	−	−	−	−	−	+	−	−
S. hominis subsp. *novobiosepticus*[o]	d	−	−	+	−	−	−	−	+	−	−	−	−	−	+	−	−
S. lugdunensis	d	d	+	+	−	(+)	−	(+)	+	−	−	−	+	+	d	+	−
S. schleiferi subsp. *schleiferi*	−	−	+	+	−	+	+	(+)	+	−	+	−	+	−	−	−	−
S. schleiferi subsp. *coagulans*	d	−	+	+	+	−	+	(+)	+	−	+	−	ND	−	ND	ND	ND
S. muscae	−	−	+	+	−	−	−	(+)	+	−	+	−	ND	−	−	ND	ND
S. auricularis	−	−	(±)	(+)	−	−	−	−	+	−	−	+	d	−	−	−	−
S. saprophyticus subsp. *saprophyticus*	+	d	(+)	+	−	−	−	−	+	−	−	−	−	−	+	d	−
S. saprophyticus subsp. *bovis*	−	+	+	+	−	−	−	−	+	−	−	−	+	−	+	ND	−
S. cohnii subsp. *cohnii*	d	−	d	+	−	−	−	(d)	+	−	−	−	−	−	−	−	−
S. cohnii subsp. *urealyticum*	+	d	(+)	+	−	−	−	(d)	+	−	+	−	d	−	+	−	+
S. xylosus	+	d	d	+	−	−	−	−	+	−	d	−	d	−	+	+	+
S. kloosii	d	d	−	+	−	−	−	(d)	+	−	d	−	d	−	d	d	d
S. equorum	−	−	−	(+)	−	−	−	(d)	+	−	(+)	−	−	−	+	ND	+
S. arlettae	d	+	−	+	−	−	−	−	+	−	(+)	−	−	−	−	ND	+
S. gallinarum	+	d	(+)	+	−	−	−	(d)	+	−	(+)	−	−	−	+	+	d
S. simulans	+	−	+	+	−	−	−	(d)	+	−	(d)	−	+	−	+	−	d
S. carnosus	+	−	+	+	−	−	−	−	+	−	+	−	+	−	−	−	−
S. piscifermentans	+	−	+	+	−	−	−	−	+	−	+	−	ND	ND	+	+	−
S. felis	+	−	+	+	−	−	−	(d)	+	−	+	ND	ND	ND	+	−	−
S. lutrae	−	−	+	+	+	−	(±)	+	+	−	+	ND	ND	ND	+	ND	ND
S. intermedius	+	−	(+)	+	+	d	+	d	+	−	+	−	+	−	+	d	−
S. delphini	+	−	(+)	+	+	−	−	+	+	−	+	ND	ND	ND	+	ND	ND
S. hyicus	+	−	+	+	d	−	+	−	+	−	+	−	−	−	d	d	+
S. chromogenes	+	+	+	+	−	−	−	−	+	−	+	−	d	−	+	d	−
S. sciuri subsp. *sciuri*	+	d	(+)	+	−	−	−	(±)	+	+	+	−	−	−	−	+	−
S. sciuri subsp. *carnaticus*	−	d	(d)	+	−	d[p]	−	(±)	+	+	d	−	−	−	−	+	−
S. sciuri subsp. *rodentium*	d	d	(d)	+	−	+[p]	−	(±)	+	+	d	−	−	−	−	+	−
S. lentus	−	d	(±)	(+)	−	−	−	−	+	+	(±)	−	−	−	−	+	−
S. vitulus	−	+	−	(+)	−	−	−	−	+	+	−	ND	−	−	−	d	−

[a] Symbols and abbreviations (unless otherwise indicated): +, 90% or more strains positive; ±, 90% or more strains weakly positive; −, 90% or more strains negative; d, 11 to 89% of strains positive; ND, not determined. Parentheses indicate a delayed reaction.

[b] Positive is defined as a colony diameter of ≥6 mm after incubation on P agar at 34 to 35°C for 3 days and at room temperature (ca. 25°C) for an additional 2 days.

[c] Positive is defined as the visual detection of carotenoid pigments (e.g., yellow, yellow-orange, or orange) during colony development at normal incubation or room temperatures. Pigments may be enhanced by the addition of milk, fat, glycerol monoacetate, or soaps to P agar.

[d] In a semisolid thioglycolate medium. Symbols: +, moderate or heavy growth down the tube within 18 to 24 h; ±, heavier growth in the upper portion of the tube and weaker growth in the lower, anaerobic portion of the tube; −, no visible growth within 48 h, but very weak diffuse growth or a few scattered, small colonies may be observed in the lower portion of the tube by 72 to 96 h. Parentheses indicate delayed growth appearing within 24 to 72 h, sometimes noted as large discrete colonies in the lower portion of the tube.

[e] On P agar or bovine, sheep, or human blood agar at 34 to 37°C. *S. equorum* grows slowly at 35 to 37°C; its optimum growth temperature is 30°C. The anaerobic species *S. saccharolyticus* and *S. aureus* subsp. *anaerobius* grow very slowly in the presence of air. Aerobic growth may be increased slightly by subculture in the presence of air. *S. aureus* subsp. *anaerobius* requires the addition of blood, serum, or egg yolk for growth on primary isolation medium. *S. auricularis*, *S. lentus*, and *S. vitulus* produce just detectable colonies on P agar in 24 to 36 h, and these colonies remain very small (1 to 2 mm in diameter).

[f] Detected in rabbit or human plasma (slide coagulase test). Human plasma is preferred for the detection of clumping factor with *S. lugdunensis* and *S. schleiferi*. Latex agglutination is somewhat less reliable for detection of clumping factor of fibrinogen affinity factor in *S. lugdunensis*.

β-Galactosidase[j]	Arginine utilization[j]	Acetoin production	Nitrate reduction	Esculin hydrolysis	Novobiocin resistance[k]	Polymyxin B resistance[l]	Acid (aerobically) from: D-Trehalose	D-Mannitol	D-Mannose	D-Turanose	D-Xylose	D-Cellobiose	L-Arabinose	Maltose	α-Lactose	Sucrose	N-Acetylglucosamine	Raffinose
−	+	+	+	−	−	+	+	+	+	+	−	−	−	+	+	+	+	−
−	ND	−	−	−	−	ND	−	ND	−	ND	−	−	−	+	−	+	−	−
−	d	+	+	−	−	+	−	−	(+)	(d)	−	−	−	+	d	+	−	−
−	d	d	d	−	−	−	−	+	+	−	−	−	−	−	−	(+)	−	−
−	+	d	+	−	−	ND	−	+	+	−	−	−	−	+	(d)	+	−	−
−	+	+	+	−	−	−	(+)	d	+	−	−	−	−	(d)	+	−	−	−
ND	+	ND	+	ND	−	ND	−	−	(+)	ND	−	−	−	−	−	−	ND	−
−	d	+	d	−	−	−	+	d	−	(d)	−	−	−	(+)	d	+	−	−
−	d	d	d	−	−	ND	+	d	−	(d)	−	−	−	(d)	d	+	−	−
−	+	+	+	−	−	−	+	d	−	(d)	−	−	−	+	d	+	+	−
−	d	d	d	−	−	−	d	−	−	+	−	−	−	+	d	(+)	d	−
−	−	d	d	−	+	ND	−	−	−	ND	−	−	−	+	d	(+)	−	−
−	−	+	+	−	−	d	+	−	+	(d)	−	−	−	+	+	+	+	−
(+)	+	+	+	−	−	−	d	−	+	−	−	−	−	−	−	−	(+)	−
ND	+	+	+	−	−	ND	−	d	+	−	−	−	−	−	d	d	ND	−
−	−	−	+	−	−	ND	+	−	−	+	+	−	−	−	−	+	ND	−
(d)	d	−	(d)	−	−	−	(+)	−	−	(d)	−	−	−	(+)	−	d	−	−
+	−	+	−	−	+	−	+	d	−	+	−	−	−	+	d	+	d	−
d	−	d	+	−	+	ND	+	+	−	+	−	−	−	+	−	+	+	−
−	−	d	−	−	+	−	+	d	(d)	−	−	−	−	(d)	−	−	−	−
+	−	d	−	−	+	−	+	+	+	−	−	−	−	(+)	+	−	d	−
+	−	d	d	d	+	−	+	+	+	d	+	−	d	+	d	+	+	−
d	−	d	−	d	+	−	+	+	−	−	(d)	−	d	d	(d)	(±)	−	−
d	−	−	+	d	+	ND	+	+	+	d	+	(d)	+	d	d	+	d	−
d	−	−	−	−	+	ND	+	+	+	+	+	−	+	+	+	+	−	+
d	−	−	+	+	+	−	+	+	+	+	+	+	+	+	d	+	+	+
+	+	d	+	−	−	−	d	+	d	−	−	−	−	(±)	+	+	+	−
+	+	+	+	−	−	−	d	+	+	−	−	−	−	−	d	−	ND	−
(d)	+	−	+	d	−	ND	+	d	−	−	−	−	−	d	d	d	ND	−
+	+	−	+	ND	−	ND	+	+	+	ND	−	−	−	−	+	d	+	−
+	−	−	+	ND	−	ND	+	d	+	ND	+	ND	ND	+	+	ND	ND	ND
+	d	−	+	−	−	−	+	(d)	+	d	−	−	−	(±)	d	+	+	−
ND	+	−	+	ND	−	ND	−	(+)	+	ND	−	ND	−	+	+	+	ND	ND
−	+	−	+	−	−	+	+	−	+	−	−	−	−	−	+	+	+	−
−	+	−	+	−	−	+	+	d	+	d	−	−	−	d	+	+	d	−
−	−	−	+	+	+	−	+	+	(d)	(±)	(d)	+	d	(d)	(d)	+	−	−
−	−	−	+	+	+	−	+	+	(d)	ND	+	(d)	d	(d)	(d)	+	−	−
−	−	−	+	+	+	−	(+)	+	(+)	ND	(d)	d	(d)	(d)	−	+	−	−
−	−	−	+	+	+	−	+	+	(+)	(±)	(±)	+	d	d	d	+	d	+
−	−	−	+	d	+	ND	(d)	+	−	−	d	d	−	−	−	+	−	−

[g] Hemolysis on bovine blood agar. Symbols and abbreviations: +, wide zone of hemolysis within 24 to 36 h; (+), delayed moderate to wide zone of hemolysis within 48 to 72 h; (d), no or delayed hemolysis; −, no or only very narrow zone (≤1 mm) of hemolysis within 72 h. Some of the strains designated negative may produce a slight greening or browning of blood agar.

[h] Catalase and cytochrome synthesis cannot be induced in *S. aureus* subsp. *anaerobius* by the addition of H_2O_2 or hemin to the culture medium. Catalase can be induced in *S. saccharolyticus* by hemin supplementation. In this species, cytochromes *a* and *b* are present in small quantities.

[i] Determined by the modified oxidase test to detect the presence of cytochrome *c*.

[j] Determined primarily by commercial rapid identification tests.

[k] Positive is defined as an MIC of 1.6 μg/ml or a growth inhibition zone diameter of ≥16 mm with a 5-μg novobiocin disk.

[l] Positive is defined as a growth inhibition zone diameter of <10 mm with a 300-U polymyxin B disk.

[m] Alkaline phosphatase activity is negative for approximately 6 to 15% of strains of *S. epidermidis*, depending on the population sampled. A low but significant number of clinical isolates have been phosphatase negative.

[n] rRNA gene restriction site polymorphism with pBA2 as a probe can distinguish this species from other staphylococcal species, including *S. warneri* (24).

[o] All strains tested were also resistant to penicillin G, methicillin, oxacillin, gentamicin, and streptomycin.

[p] Positive reactions are by the Staph Latex agglutination test (Remel), which detects clumping factor and/or protein A.

to foreign bodies (122). Prevention of staphylococcal diseases in the future may also involve the use of vaccines by using the strategies discussed by Lee and Pier (97).

Micrococcus

Members of the genus *Micrococcus* and the related coccal genera *Kocuria* and *Kytococcus* are generally considered to be harmless saprophytes that inhabit or contaminate the skin, mucosa, and perhaps also the oropharynx; however, they can be opportunistic pathogens in certain immunocompromised patients. *M. luteus* has been implicated as the causative agent in some cases of intracranial abscesses, pneumonia, septic arthritis, and meningitis (75, 88). *K. sedentarius* has been associated with prosthetic valve endocarditis (102) and is often associated with pitted keratolysis (112). Other infections associated with micrococci and their relatives included bacteremia, continuous ambulatory peritoneal dialysis-related peritonitis, and infection of a cerebrospinal fluid shunt (101).

COLLECTION, TRANSPORT, AND STORAGE OF SPECIMENS

The general principles of collection, transport, and storage of specimens as described in chapter 4 of this Manual are applicable to staphylococci and micrococci. No special methods or precautions are usually required for these organisms because they are easily obtained from clinical material from most infection sites and are relatively resistant to drying and to moderate temperature changes. Some strains of staphylococci may require anaerobic conditions or CO_2 supplementation for satisfactory growth, but these survive transport and limited storage in air.

DIRECT EXAMINATION

The direct microscopic examination of normally sterile fluids such as cerebrospinal fluid and joint aspirates may be useful. Direct examination of certain nonsterile fluids may also be very useful if the microscopist carefully evaluates the specimen by noting the presence of inflammatory cells versus epithelial cells. Even if large numbers of gram-positive cocci are present, only a presumptive report of "gram-positive cocci resembling staphylococci (or micrococci)" should be made. This report must be confirmed by culture and appropriate identification techniques. It must also be emphasized that microscopy by itself cannot adequately differentiate various species of staphylococci or micrococci from one another or from planococci, some streptococci, aerococci, various anaerobic cocci, or other cocci related to micrococci.

ISOLATION PROCEDURES

Considering the widespread distribution of staphylococci and micrococci over the body surface, careful and thoughtful procedures should be used to isolate organisms from the focus or foci of infection without collecting surrounding normal flora (74). Distinguishing contaminants from the infecting staphylococci and micrococci continues to be a challenge for the clinical laboratory.

Several isolation procedures are currently available for the diagnosis of central venous catheter infections, although the best choice remains controversial. They include quantitative blood cultures taken from blood drawn from a peripheral catheter (39, 152) or quantitative catheter segment cultures (134), semiquantitative counts taken from a distal segment of the catheter (4), and differential positivity times of cultures of blood drawn simultaneously from a central venous catheter and peripheral sites without requiring removal of the catheter (13). With the use of anti-infective catheters, the addition of inhibitors to the sampling medium may be necessary to obtain correct colony counts (130).

Native and prosthetic valve endocarditis is often associated with staphylococcal bacteremia. The most convincing laboratory findings include the rapid isolation of staphylococci from more than one blood culture, a high intensity of bacteremia, and the presence of the same strain(s) in sequential isolations (2, 65). Generally, in patients with suspected bacterial endocarditis, three blood cultures are sufficient to isolate the etiologic agent. It is essential that blood for culture be collected aseptically and from separate venipuncture sites in the event that a contaminant is accidentally introduced at one of the sites.

For infections of prosthetic joints, aspiration of the joint space will commonly yield the infecting bacteria. Washing or ultrasonic oscillation of the prosthesis upon removal may be used to loosen adherent organisms embedded in a biofilm matrix (9, 146). Aspirates and washings should subsequently be Gram stained and cultured for identification of the infecting organism(s).

A freshly voided, midstream, clean-catch urine sample is usually satisfactory for making a determination of urinary tract infections (UTIs). Suprapubic aspiration may be indicated in patients who have a low bacterial count in clean-catch specimens, in neonates, and in young infants. Sometimes UTI due to *S. saprophyticus* may be accompanied by a bacteremia with the same organism (50). In most cases, other CoNS are not considered to be the etiologic agents of UTIs.

The basic procedures for culture and isolation described in chapter 5 of this Manual should be followed. Every specimen should be plated onto blood agar (preferably sheep blood agar) and other media as indicated. On blood agar, abundant growth of most staphylococcal species occurs within 18 to 24 h and abundant growth of micrococci occurs within 36 to 48 h. Since most species cannot be distinguished from one another during this time period, colonies should be picked at this time only for preliminary identification testing (e.g., when specimens are taken from patients with acute infections). Colonies should be allowed to grow for at least an additional 2 to 3 days before the primary isolation plate is confirmed for species or strain composition (79, 80). This growth period is particularly important if it is necessary to sample more than one colony to obtain sufficient inocula and for determining the predominant organism or presence of a pure culture. Failure to hold plates for 72 h can result in (i) selection of more than one species or strain if two or more colonies are sampled to produce an inoculum, (ii) selection of an organism(s) not producing the infection if the specimen contains two or more different species or strains, and (iii) incorrect labeling of a mixed culture as a pure culture. Colonies should be Gram stained, subcultured, and tested for genus, species, and strain properties. It should be noted that most staphylococci of major medical interest produce growth in the upper as well as the lower anaerobic portions of a thioglycolate broth or semisolid agar (80).

Specimens from heavily contaminated sources such as feces should also be streaked onto a selective medium such as Schleifer-Krämer agar (128), mannitol-salt agar, Columbia colistin-nalidixic acid agar, lipase-salt-mannitol agar (Remel, Lenexa, Kans.), or phenylethyl alcohol agar. These media inhibit the growth of gram-negative organisms but allow staphylococci and certain other gram-positive cocci to grow. On selective media, incubation should be extended to at least 48 to 72 h for discernible colony development.

IDENTIFICATION

Staphylococcus Species

Staphylococcus species can be identified on the basis of a variety of conventional phenotypic characters (71, 75, 81) (Table 2). The most clinically significant species can be identified on the basis of several key characteristics (Table 3). Species can also be identified on the basis of molecular phenotypic properties such as cellular fatty acids (91), multilocus enzymes (154), and whole-cell polypeptides (26) and genotypic properties such as chromosome restriction fragments (10), macrorestriction patterns (7, 47), and ribotypes (34, 149). Most of the molecular methods are currently confined to the reference or research laboratory.

Some laboratories may choose to restrict complete species identification of the CoNS to isolates from normally sterile sites such as blood (when considered to be clinically significant) or joint or cerebrospinal fluid and to distinguish routinely (i) *S. saprophyticus* from other CoNS isolated from urine, (ii) *S. epidermidis*, *S. lugdunensis*, and *S. schleiferi* isolated from colonized shunts, catheters, or prosthetic devices, and (iii) *S. epidermidis*, *S. lugdunensis*, *S. haemolyticus*, and *S. warneri* isolated from soft-tissue infections or endocarditis.

Colonial Appearance

On nonselective blood agar, nutrient agar, tryptic soy agar, brain heart infusion agar, or P agar, isolated colonies of most staphylococci are 1 to 3 mm in diameter within 24 h and 3 to 8 mm in diameter by 3 days of incubation in air at 34 to 37°C, depending on the species (81). The exceptional species *S. aureus* subsp. *anaerobius*, *S. saccharolyticus*, *S. auricularis*, *S. equorum*, *S. vitulus*, and *S. lentus* grow more slowly than other staphylococci and usually require 24 to 36 h for detectable colony development. Colony morphology can be a useful supplementary characteristic in the identification of species. Descriptions should be made for isolated colonies that have developed for several days at 34 to 37°C followed by 2 days of growth at room temperature. Comparisons should be made with type strains of recognized species.

Colonies of *S. aureus* are usually large (6 to 8 mm in diameter), smooth, entire, slightly raised, and translucent. On P agar, they become nearly transparent by 3 to 5 days of incubation. The colonies of most strains are pigmented, ranging from cream-yellow to orange. Some unusual strains of *S. aureus* produce dwarf colonies. Rare strains with relatively large capsules produce colonies that are smaller and more convex than those of unencapsulated strains and have a glistening, wet appearance. *S. epidermidis* colonies are relatively small and range from 2.5 to 6 mm in diameter, depending on the particular strain. Pigment is not usually detected. Some of the slime-producing strains are extremely sticky and adhere to the agar surface. Colonies of *S. haemolyticus* are usually larger than those of *S. epidermidis* and *S. hominis* and range from 5 to 9 mm in diameter. They are smooth, butyrous, and opaque, like those of the related species *S. hominis*, and may be unpigmented or cream to yellow-orange in color. Colonies of *S. lugdunensis* are usually 4 to 7 mm in diameter, are smooth and glossy, and may be unpigmented or cream to yellow-orange in color. The edge is entire and rather flat, while the center is slightly domed. They are sometimes confused with colonies of *S. warneri*. *S. schleiferi* colonies are usually 3 to 5 mm in diameter and unpigmented. They are smooth and glossy and are slightly convex with entire edges. Colonies of *S. saprophyticus* are large (5 to 8 mm in diameter), entire, very glossy, opaque, smooth, butyrous, and more convex than the colonies of the aforementioned species. Approximately one-half of the strains are pigmented, ranging from cream to yellow-orange. Colonies of *S. intermedius* and *S. hyicus* are relatively large, usually 5 to 8 mm in diameter. They are slightly convex, entire, smooth, glossy, and usually unpigmented. Colonies of *S. intermedius* are translucent. Those of *S. hyicus* are more opaque, becoming translucent with prolonged incubation.

Coagulase Production

The ability to clot plasma continues to be the most widely used and generally accepted criterion for the identification of pathogenic staphylococci often associated with acute infections, such as *S. aureus* in humans and animals and *S. intermedius* and *S. hyicus* in animals. Two different coagulase tests can be performed: a tube test for free coagulase and a slide test for bound coagulase or clumping factor (75). While the tube test is definitive, the slide test may be used as a rapid screening technique to identify *S. aureus*. A positive slide test may also aid in the identification of the newer species *S. lugdunensis* and *S. schleiferi* (Table 3). A variety of plasmas may be used for either test; however, dehydrated rabbit plasma containing EDTA is commercially available and most satisfactory with the exception that human plasma is somewhat more satisfactory for the identification of *S. lugdunensis* and *S. schleiferi*. Human plasma should not be used unless it has been carefully tested for a lack of infectious agents, clotting capability, and inhibitors.

The tube coagulase test is best performed by mixing 0.1 ml of an overnight culture in brain heart infusion broth with 0.5 ml of reconstituted plasma (preferably in a glass tube), incubating the mixture at 37°C in a water bath or heat block for 4 h, and observing the tube for clot formation by slowly tilting the tube 90° from the vertical. Alternatively, a large, well-isolated colony on a noninhibitory agar can be transferred into 0.5 ml of reconstituted plasma and incubated as described above. Any degree of clotting constitutes a positive test. However, a flocculent or fibrous precipitate is not a true clot and should be recorded as a negative result. Incubation of the test overnight has also been recommended for *S. aureus*, since a small number of strains may require longer than 4 h for clot formation. For veterinary clinical laboratories, it is important to note that some strains of *S. intermedius* and most coagulase-producing strains of *S. hyicus* require more than 4 h of incubation for a positive coagulase test. Clot formation by these species may require 12 to 24 h of incubation. If the incubation time exceeds 4 h, the following points must be considered: (i) staphylokinase produced by some strains may lyse the clot after prolonged incubation, yielding false-negative results; (ii) if the plasma used is not sterile (and some are not), either false-positive or false-negative results may occur; and (iii) an inoculum from an agar-grown colony may not be pure, and a contaminant may produce false-positive results after prolonged incubation. In this regard, plasma containing EDTA is superior to citrated plasma because citrate-utilizing organisms (e.g., some streptococci) may produce clot formation by consum-

TABLE 3 Key tests for identification of the most clinically significant *Staphylococcus* species

Species	Test[a]																			
	Colony pigment[b]	Staphylo-coagulase	Clumping factor[b]	Heat-stable nuclease	Alkaline phospha-tase	Pyrrol-idonyl arylami-dase[b]	Ornithine decarbox-ylase	Urease[b]	β-Galacto-sidase[b]	Acetoin produc-tion	Novo-biocin resist-ance[b]	Poly-myxin B resist-ance[b]	Acid (aerobically) from:							
													D-Trehal-ose	D-Man-nitol	D-Man-nose	D-Turan-ose	D-Xyl-ose	D-Cello-biose	Malt-ose	Su-crose
S. aureus subsp. *aureus*	+	+	+	+	+	−	−	d	−	+	−	+	+	+	+	+	−	−	+	+
S. epidermidis	−	−	−	−	+	−	(d)	+	−	+	−	+	−	−	(+)	(d)	−	−	+	+
S. haemolyticus	d	−	−	−	−	+	−	−	−	+	−	−	+	d	−	(d)	−	−	+	+
S. hyicus (veterinary)	−	d	−	+	+	−	−	d	−	−	−	+	+	−	+	−	−	−	−	+
S. intermedius (veterinary)	−	+	d	+	+	+	−	+	+	−	−	−	+	(d)	+	d	−	−	(±)	+
S. lugdunensis	d	−	(+)	−	−	+	+	d	−	+	−	d	+	−	+	(d)	−	−	+	+
S. saprophyticus subsp. *saprophyticus*	d	−	−	−	−	−	−	+	+	+	+	−	+	d	−	+	−	−	+	+
S. schleiferi subsp. *schleiferi*	−	−	+	+	+	+	−	−	(+)	+	−	−	d	−	+	−	−	−	−	−
S. warneri	d	−	−	−	−	−	−	+	−	+	−	−	+	d	−	(d)	−	−	(+)	+

[a] Symbols and abbreviations: +, 90% or more species or strains positive; ±, 90% or more species or strains weakly positive; −, 90% or more species or strains negative; d, 11 to 89% of species or strains positive; ND, not determined. Parentheses indicate a delayed reaction.

[b] Descriptions are the same as in Table 2.

ing the citrate. For those uncommon *S. aureus* strains requiring a longer clotting period, other characteristics (Table 3) should also be tested to confirm their identities. Additional characteristics are required to identify rare coagulase-negative mutants and some encapsulated strains.

The slide coagulase test is performed by making a heavy uniform suspension of growth in distilled water, stirring the mixture to a homogeneous composition so as not to confuse clumping with autoagglutination, adding 1 drop of plasma, and observing for clumping within 10 s. The slide test is very rapid and more economical of plasma than the tube test. However, 10 to 15% of *S. aureus* strains may yield a negative result, which requires that the isolates be reexamined by the tube test. Slide tests must be read quickly because false-positive results may appear with reaction times longer than 10 s. In addition, colonies for testing must not be picked from media containing high concentrations of salt (e.g., mannitol-salt agar) because autoagglutination and false-positive results may occur. Some uncommon strains of *S. intermedius* may give a positive slide test result. Alternative methods for the slide test include several commercial hemagglutination slide tests for clumping factor and latex agglutination tests that detect both clumping factor and protein A, although latex agglutination tests may not always yield the same reaction as the slide test. The latex agglutination tests often have a higher specificity and sensitivity than the conventional slide test for the identification of *S. aureus*, although they are generally less reliable for the identification of *S. lugdunensis*. Some members of the *S. saprophyticus* and *S. sciuri* species groups and *Macrococcus* species may produce positive results with latex agglutination tests, but they are usually negative for the slide test. A latex agglutination test that detects both serotype 5 and serotype 8 capsular polysaccharides of *S. aureus* is reliable for the identification of methicillin-susceptible *S. aureus* and MRSA strains (45). When the organism being tested is suspected of being *S. aureus*, negative slide tests should be confirmed by the tube coagulase test.

Heat-Stable Nuclease

A heat-stable staphylococcal nuclease (thermonuclease [TNase]) that has endo- and exonucleolytic properties and that can cleave DNA or RNA is produced by most strains of *S. aureus*, *S. schleiferi*, *S. intermedius*, and *S. hyicus*. Some strains of *S. epidermidis*, *S. simulans*, and *S. carnosus* demonstrate a weak TNase activity. TNase can be detected by using a metachromatic agar diffusion procedure and DNA-toluidine blue agar (95). A seroinhibition test has been developed to distinguish *S. aureus* TNase from those of other species (96). A commercial TNase test with toluidine blue agar is available (Remel), and the results can be interpreted in 4 h.

Phosphatase Activity

Phosphatase activity can be determined by using a modification of the technique of Pennock and Huddy (117), in which a 0.005 M solution of phenolphthalein diphosphate (sodium salt in 0.01 M citric acid-sodium citrate buffer [pH 5.8]) is used as the substrate. Color is developed by the addition of 4-aminoantipyrine and potassium ferricyanide. Phosphatase activity is indicated by the development of a deep red color. A newer, alternative method for determining phosphatase activity based on the hydrolysis of *p*-nitrophenylphosphate into P_i and *p*-nitrophenol by alkaline phosphatase has been incorporated into several of the commercial biochemical test systems for staphylococcal species identification. Phosphatase activity is indicated by the release of yellow *p*-nitrophenol from the colorless substrate. Key Scientific Company (Roundrock, Tex.) manufactures an alkaline phosphatase tablet that may detect activity in staphylococci, although it has not yet been widely accepted because it has a small database.

Strains of *S. aureus*, *S. schleiferi*, *S. intermedius*, and *S. hyicus* and most strains of *S. epidermidis* are alkaline phosphatase positive. Phosphatase-negative strains of *S. epidermidis* can be distinguished from the related species *S. hominis* on the basis of their strong anaerobic growth in thioglycolate within 18 to 24 h or resistance to polymyxin B (300-U disk).

Pyrrolidonyl Arylamidase Activity

Pyrrolidonyl arylamidase (pyrrolidonase) activity can be determined by the hydrolysis of pyroglutamyl-β-naphthylamide (L-pyrrolidonyl-β-naphthylamide [PYR]) into L-pyrrolidone and β-naphthylamine, which combines with a PYR reagent (*p*-dimethylaminocinnamaldehyde) to produce a red color. A commercial kit containing PYR broth and PYR reagent (Carr-Scarborough Microbiologicals, Inc., Stone Mountain, Ga.) is recommended for use in the identification of group A streptococci and enterococci and is also useful for distinguishing certain staphylococcal species (57). A slight modification of the standard procedure is required. A loopful of a 24-h agar slant culture or several well-isolated colonies are dispersed in the PYR broth (containing 0.01% PYR) to a turbidity of a McFarland no. 2 standard. The suspension is incubated at 35°C for 2 h. After incubation, 2 drops of PYR reagent is added to each tube without mixing. The development of a dark purple-red color within 2 min is indicative of a positive activity. A yellow, orange, or pink color is considered a negative result. Alternatively, the basic features of the test have been incorporated into several of the commercial biochemical test panels for the identification of staphylococcal species. *S. haemolyticus*, *S. lugdunensis*, *S. schleiferi*, and *S. intermedius* are usually pyrrolidonase positive.

Ornithine Decarboxylase Activity

A positive ornithine decarboxylase activity can identify the species *S. lugdunensis* with considerable accuracy. Ornithine decarboxylase activity can be determined by a slight modification of the test described by Moeller (105). Decarboxylase basal medium (Becton Dickinson Microbiology Systems, Sparks, Md.; Difco Laboratories, Detroit, Mich.; GIBCO Laboratories, Grand Island, N.Y.) is prepared according to the instructions of the manufacturer, 1% (wt/vol) L-ornithine dihydrochloride is added, and the final medium is adjusted to pH 6 with 1 N sodium hydroxide before sterilization. The medium is dispensed in 3- to 4-ml amounts in small (13- by 100-mm) screw-cap tubes and autoclaved at 121°C for 10 min. A loopful of an overnight agar slant culture or several well-isolated colonies are dispersed in the test broth, followed by overlaying of each tube with 4 to 5 mm of sterile mineral oil. Inoculated tubes should be incubated at 35 to 37°C for up to 24 h. They can be read initially as early as 8 h for the positive identification of most strains of *S. lugdunensis*; at this time, *S. epidermidis* will produce negative results. A positive reaction is indicated by alkalinization of the medium, with a change in the initial grayish color or slight yellowing (caused by the initial fermentation of glucose) to violet (caused by decarboxylation of L-ornithine). A yellow color at 24 h indicates a negative result.

Urease Activity

A conventional urease test broth (Urea R broth; Difco) with a reduced buffer capacity can be used to detect urease activity within 4 h in staphylococcal species. The test detects the release of ammonia from urea, resulting in an increase in pH, which is shown by a change in the phenol red indicator from yellow or orange to red or cerise. At present, comprehensive studies with this medium for the identification of staphylococcal species have not been reported. However, a miniaturization of this urease test has been incorporated into several of the commercial biochemical test systems for identification of staphylococcal species and is represented by a large database. *S. epidermidis*, *S. intermedius*, and most strains of *S. saprophyticus* are usually urease positive.

β-Galactosidase Activity

Detection of high levels of β-galactosidase activity for the differentiation of certain staphylococcal species can be accomplished by commercial biochemical test systems that use 2-naphthol-β-D-galactopyranoside as a substrate. Fast blue BB salt in 2-methoxyethanol is added to the test well after an appropriate incubation period to detect the free β-naphthol released by β-galactosidase. A positive activity is indicated by a plum purple color. By this assay, *S. intermedius* and most strains of *S. saprophyticus* are β-galactosidase positive; *S. schleiferi* is delayed or weakly positive.

Acetoin Production

Acetoin production from glucose or pyruvate is a useful alternative characteristic for distinguishing *S. aureus* (positive) from another coagulase-positive species, *S. intermedius* (negative), and coagulase-positive strains of *S. hycius* (negative). The rapid paper disk method of Davis and Hoyling (33) is recommended for this test. The accuracy of the disk test is comparable to that of conventional Voges-Proskauer tests requiring longer incubation times. Alternatively, acetoin production can be determined by a miniaturized Voges-Proskauer test incorporated into several of the commercial biochemical test systems for staphylococcal species identification.

Novobiocin Resistance

A simple disk diffusion test for estimating novobiocin susceptibility and distinguishing *S. saprophyticus* from other clinically important species can be performed by use of a 5-μg novobiocin disk on either P agar (80), Mueller-Hinton agar (1), or tryptic soy sheep blood agar (49). With an inoculum suspension equivalent in turbidity to a 0.5 McFarland opacity standard and incubation at 35 to 37°C for overnight to 24 h, novobiocin resistance is indicated by an inhibition zone diameter of ≤16 mm with any of these media. A rapid disk elution procedure with either manual or automated instrument interpretation has also been reported to predict novobiocin resistance after only 4 to 5 h of incubation (56). Novobiocin resistance is intrinsic to *S. saprophyticus* and several other species (Table 2), but it is uncommon in the other clinically important species.

Polymyxin B Resistance

A simple disk diffusion test for estimating polymyxin B susceptibility to distinguish several of the clinically important species can be done by using a 300-U polymyxin B disk (57). The test can be performed on any of the media mentioned above for estimation of novobiocin resistance. However, the largest database has been obtained with the use of tryptic soy sheep blood agar. Test conditions should be similar to those described above for novobiocin resistance. The 5-μg novobiocin disk and the 300-U polymyxin B disk can be tested on the same inoculated plate. Polymyxin B resistance is indicated by an inhibition zone diameter of <10 mm. *S. aureus*, *S. epidermidis*, *S. hyicus*, and *S. chromogenes* are usually resistant. Some strains of *S. lugdunensis* are also resistant.

Acid Production from Carbohydrates

Acid production from carbohydrates can be easily detected by using the agar plate method of Kloos and Schleifer (80). Carbohydrate reactions are also incorporated into several of the commercial biochemical test systems for staphylococcal species identification. These systems use a more acid-sensitive indicator than the bromcresol purple (pH ≤ 5.2) of the agar plate method. For this and other reasons, the results obtained by conventional carbohydrate tests (Tables 2 and 3) may be slightly different from those obtained with rapid commercial biochemical test systems.

S. epidermidis can be distinguished from other novobiocin-susceptible species by its production of acid from maltose and sucrose and the absence of acid production from trehalose and mannitol. Some uncommon strains of this species may produce acid from trehalose. These isolates can be distinguished from other species on the basis of phosphatase activity, anaerobic growth in thioglycolate, polymyxin B resistance, colony morphology, and absence of ornithine decarboxylase and pyrrolidonase activities. *S. lugdunensis* can be identified by its production of acid from trehalose, mannose, maltose, and sucrose and absence of acid production from mannitol. *S. schleiferi* produces acid from mannose and sometimes from trehalose but does not produce acid from mannitol, maltose, or sucrose. *S. saprophyticus* can be distinguished from other novobiocin-resistant species by its production of acid from sucrose and turanose and the absence of acid production from mannose, xylose, cellobiose, arabinose, and raffinose.

Identification of Species by Using Commercial Biochemical or Nucleic Acid Test Systems

Several manufacturers of commercial identification systems (see chapter 11 of this Manual) and automated instruments have released products that can identify a number of the *Staphylococcus* species with an accuracy of 70 to >90% with relative speed and simplicity (74, 119). Since their introduction, systems have been improved and expanded to include more species. Their reliability will continue to increase as the result of a growing database and the development of more discriminating tests. *S. aureus*, *S. epidermidis*, *S. capitis*, *S. haemolyticus*, *S. saprophyticus*, *S. simulans*, and *S. intermedius* can be identified reliably by most of the commercial systems now available. For some systems, reliability depends on additional testing, as suggested by the manufacturer. Additional testing might include determination of coagulase, clumping factor, or ornithine decarboxylase activity, anaerobic growth in thioglycolate, or novobiocin resistance. If one or more of these key tests are not included in the particular manufacturer's product, identification could be uncertain with respect to some species. Identification systems now available include the following: RAPIDEC Staph (identification of *S. aureus*, *S. epidermidis*, and *S. saprophyticus*) and API STAPH (bioMérieux Vitek, Inc., Hazelwood, Mo.); Vitek, a fully automated microbiology system that uses a Gram Positive Identification (GPI) Card (bioMérieux

Vitek); MicroScan Pos ID panel (read manually or on MicroScan instrumentation) and MicroScan Rapid Pos ID panel (read by the WalkAway systems) (in addition, the ID systems are available with antimicrobial agents for susceptibility testing) (Dade MicroScan, Inc., West Sacramento, Calif.); Crystal Gram-Positive Identification System, Crystal Rapid Gram-Positive Identification System, Sceptor *Staphylococcus* MIC/ID Panel, Sceptor Gram-Positive Breakpoint/ID Panel, and the frozen Pasco MIC/ID Gram-Positive Panel (Becton Dickinson Microbiology Systems); GP MicroPlate test panel (read manually, using Biolog computer software for interpretation, or automatically with the Biolog MicroStation) (Biolog, Hayward, Calif.); Microbial Identification System (MIS), which automates microbial identification by combining cellular fatty acid analysis with computerized high-resolution gas chromatography (MIDI, Newark, Del.); and the fully automated RiboPrinter Microbial Characterization System (Qualicon, Inc., Wilmington, Del.), based on ribotype pattern analysis (genetic fingerprinting).

Rapid detection of the species *S. aureus* can be done by the AccuProbe culture identification test for *S. aureus* (Gen-Probe, Inc., San Diego, Calif.). This test is a DNA probe assay directed against rRNA, and it is very accurate (100% specificity). Tube coagulase-negative and slide test-negative strains of *S. aureus* can be identified correctly by the AccuProbe test. *S. aureus* may be identified also by using the new immunoenzymatic assay (IEA) developed by Guardati and coworkers (52). The IEA is based on a monoclonal antibody (MAb), MAb C1-10/11, prepared against the *S. aureus* endo-β-*N*-acetylglucosaminidase (SaG). The 100% specificity of IEA depends on the unique chemical-physical properties of the SaG of *S. aureus*. Remel manufactures a variety of individual test media and reagents that aid in identifying the genus *Staphylococcus* and certain of its species. The products include Coagulase Plasma, Coagulase Mannitol broth, Baird Parker Agar, DNase Test Agar with Methyl Green, Staph Latex Kit, Thermonuclease Agar with Toluidine Blue, Mannitol Salt Agar, and Vogel-Johnson Agar to aid in the presumptive identification of *S. aureus*. The uncommon coagulase-negative subspecies *S. schleiferi* subsp. *schleiferi* and the veterinary species *S. intermedius* can also produce positive reactions with several of these test products. The Lysostaphin Test Kit differentiates staphylococci from micrococci and their relatives, and the Microdase Disk, a rapid oxidase test, differentiates micrococci from most staphylococci.

Micrococcus Species

Pigment production and colony morphology may be used as simple tests in the presumptive identification of *Micrococcus* species and other related gram-positive cocci (82, 88). Several other phenotypic characters can be used to identify micrococci in the clinical laboratory (88, 136). *M. lylae* can be distinguished from *M. luteus* by its cream-white and unpigmented colonies, lack of growth on inorganic nitrogen agar, and lysozyme resistance. However, a small percentage of *M. luteus* strains produce cream-white colonies. *Micrococcus* species can be distinguished from the genus *Kocuria* on the basis of their inability to produce acid, aerobically, from D-glucose and β-D-fructose. Furthermore, the species *K. varians* and *K. rosea* can be distinguished from micrococci by the former species' nitrate reduction and negative or only weak oxidase activity, and *K. kristinae* can be distinguished from micrococci by the former's production of acid, aerobically, from glycerol and D-mannose, production of acetoin, and hydrolysis of esculin. The orange-pigmented species *Dermacoccus nishinomiyaensis* can be distinguished from micrococci by the former's small pale orange colonies, nitrate reduction, and lack of growth on 7.5% NaCl agar. *K. sedentarius* differs from micrococci by being resistant to penicillin and methicillin and exhibiting arginine dihydrolase activity. Colonies of this species usually produce a water-soluble pigment and grow more slowly than those of micrococci. *Nesterenkonia halobia* can be easily separated from micrococci, because it requires at least 5% NaCl for growth.

Strain Identification

Members of a bacterial strain constitute a population of cells descended from a common ancestor at a relatively recent point in time. In the most recent examples, a strain represents a clonal population with each of its members being genetically identical (isogenic) and demonstrating identical phenotypic characteristics (69). It is also reasonable to consider a strain as representing a clonal population in which some of its members differ from one another only on the basis of one or a few mutations or the loss or acquisition of an extrachromosomal element (e.g., phage, plasmid, and transposon). Strain identification is very important in distinguishing contaminants from the etiologic agent. Multiple isolations of the same strain demonstrate a higher likelihood that the strain is clinically significant. Strain delineation is important in examining isolates from individual patients as well as those in outbreak situations. General considerations for epidemiologic typing of bacteria are discussed in chapter 7 of this Manual.

Strain typing may be accomplished by a variety of methods, including the examination of phenotypic and genotypic characters. Most tests require special media, techniques, and/or instrumentation and would be better performed in a reference laboratory. Nevertheless, some approaches to strain identification, such as the description of colony morphology and the development of biotype profiles and antibiograms, can be considered by the small clinical laboratory. Colony morphology is a character that can identify individual strains in many of the staphylococcal species. In general, strain colony recognition has little impact on patient care associated with the treatment of acute illness caused by *S. aureus*. However, strain colony recognition is useful when a coagulase-negative *Staphylococcus* species or *Micrococcus* species is suspected in situations involving chronic infections and treatment failure. Colonies should be allowed to develop on the primary isolation medium for 3 to 4 days at 35 to 37°C, followed by 2 days at room temperature for an initial screening. Colonies of the same strain generally exhibit similar features of size, consistency, edge, profile, lustre, and color on nonselective media commonly used for the culture of staphylococci or micrococci. Certain strains may exhibit variant morphotypes, and in these situations chromosomal analyses should help to clarify the relationship of each morphotype. At least one colony of each morphotype should be selected from the primary isolation plate for subsequent analyses. Members of the same strain usually have the same biotype profile. However, further differentiation may be necessary if the strain has a common biotype profile. Antibiograms are commonly determined in the laboratory, and highly standardized procedures have been established. A unique susceptibility pattern can serve as a valuable marker. The more common patterns will provide some support for identification if testing is confined to a small area or community. On occasion, a strain may demonstrate a variation in pattern due to the acquisition or loss of antibiotic resistance genes or their activity, making identification more difficult.

Most *Staphylococcus* species contain a variety of different plasmids (78, 100). Consequently, plasmid composition can serve as a valuable typing system for strain identification. In most staphylococcal species there is a relationship between the antibiotic resistance pattern and the presence of certain plasmids carrying resistance genes. In this regard, plasmid composition may not be entirely independent of the antibiogram. For plasmids of identical size, restriction endonuclease fragment analysis may provide additional information for making a determination of identity. Such plasmids are considered to be different if their fragment patterns are different. Unfortunately, some common plasmids are highly conserved (e.g., small tetracycline [*tetK*] resistance plasmids or small erythromycin [*ermC*] resistance plasmids) and often have identical fragment patterns irrespective of the strain or species carrying them. Some strains exhibit clonal variations in their plasmid profiles. This variation is most often represented by the addition or deletion of an entire plasmid or a restriction fragment within a plasmid, although occasionally different recombinant plasmids may be observed.

Cellular fatty acid profiling may be useful as a screening tool in epidemiologic studies, in addition to its use in the identification of *Staphylococcus* species and subspecies (12, 92). Electrophoretic analysis of multilocus enzymes has proved to be useful in distinguishing strains of *S. aureus* isolated from various sources (109, 111). Molecular typing techniques that examine the chromosome, such as field-inversion gel electrophoresis (FIGE) (48), pulsed-field gel electrophoresis (PFGE) of *SmaI*-digested genomic DNA (7, 47), and ribotyping (54, 144), have successfully delineated staphylococcal strains. Although we would expect that restriction fragment patterns are quite stable and similar among members of the same strain, some clonal variation has been observed with certain strains with respect to the size and number of fragments present. Such variation might be explained by the acquisition or loss of prophages, transposition events, and/or recombination events with resident extrachromosomal DNA. PCR is currently being investigated for its usefulness in the typing of staphylococcal strains. Target sequences include IS256 elements in MRSA strains (35), 16S-23S rRNA intergenic spacer sequences (53, 90, 94), and random amplified polymorphic DNA (11, 147).

ANTIBIOTIC SUSCEPTIBILITIES

Nosocomial infections caused by methicillin-resistant staphylococci pose a serious problem for health care institutions. The detection of resistance in these isolates has been hampered due to the variability in the standard techniques used to determine methicillin resistance. The resistant strains are often heteroresistant to β-lactam antibiotics in that two subpopulations (one susceptible and the other resistant) coexist within a culture (23). Each cell in the population may carry the genetic information for resistance, but only a small fraction (10^{-8} to 10^{-4}) can actually express the resistant phenotype under in vitro testing conditions. The resistant subpopulation usually grows much more slowly than the susceptible subpopulation and therefore may be missed when in vitro testing is performed. The successful detection of heteroresistant strains depends largely on promotion of the growth of the resistant subpopulations, which is favored by neutral pH, cooler temperatures (30 to 35°C), the presence of NaCl (2 to 4%), and possible prolonged incubation (up to 48 h) (30, 103). Detection of MRSA and methicillin-resistant *S. epidermidis* can be done by the methods recommended by the National Committee for Clinical Laboratory Standards as described in chapters 118 and 121 of this Manual. Rapid detection of the *mecA* gene by PCR (86, 125), DNA hybridization (89, 133), or a commercially available fluorescence test (59, 121) has been found to be accurate and provide results more quickly than standard susceptibility tests. Caution should be taken in the use of DNA probes in antibiotic susceptibility testing, since the probes only indicate gene sequences and the potential of the bacterium to demonstrate antibiotic resistance (143). They do not necessarily discriminate between functional and nonfunctional genes. Furthermore, the widespread animal staphylococcal species *S. sciuri* has a native *mecA* homolog that is different from the homolog found in MRSA and other methicillin-resistant staphylococci (31, 73, 76). The two *mecA* homologs share about 79 to 80% base pair similarity and appear to be rather similar by DNA hybridization; however, they can be distinguished by PCR conducted under different conditions of stringency and they are expressed differently. Typical *S. sciuri* strains carrying their native *mecA* homolog are susceptible or express uniform borderline resistance to methicillin, whereas staphylococci carrying the MRSA *mecA* homolog express heterogeneous resistance to methicillin. *S. sciuri* is rarely isolated from human infections; it is somewhat more frequently isolated from animal infections.

With the increase in methicillin resistance in *Staphylococcus* species, other antibiotics have been used in the treatment of serious infections caused by this group of bacteria. The glycopeptide vancomycin has been regarded as the drug of choice for the treatment of infections due to methicillin-resistant staphylococci. However, the appearance of vancomycin-intermediate isolates (MICs, 8 to 16 μg/ml) of *S. aureus* and other staphylococcal species and the potential for the development of resistance require the need for prudent use of the drug (21, 22, 93, 132, 151). Interim guidelines have been established to prevent and control staphylococcal infections associated with reduced susceptibility to vancomycin (20).

Recent reviews have summarized the antimicrobial susceptibilities of staphylococcal isolates to various drugs (3, 29, 71, 106, 116). Multidrug resistance is more frequent in *S. haemolyticus*, *S. epidermidis*, *S. hominis*, and *S. aureus* than in other staphylococcal species isolated in the clinical laboratory. Increased levels of resistance to alternative antimicrobial agents used for therapy including aminoglycosides, the glycopeptide teicoplanin, quinolones, tetracyclines, macrolides, lincosamides, and trimethroprim-sulfamethoxazole make the treatment of multidrug-resistant staphylococcal infections difficult. Attempts to eradicate nasal carriage of *S. aureus* by the use of mupirocin have met with some success. Mupirocin has been used to decrease the numbers of exit-site infections in dialysis patients (14, 84) and surgical site infections in cardiac patients (85), although resistance to mupirocin has been observed (18, 153). A variety of new compounds for effective therapy are under investigation, including the new fluoroquinolone trovafloxacin (15, 28), oxazolidinones (43, 63, 64), glycylcyclines (141), illudinic acid (40), and new glycopeptides (131).

Micrococci appear to be susceptible to most antibiotics. Successful treatment has occurred with the use of vancomycin, penicillin, gentamicin, clindamycin, or a combination of these antibiotics (101).

EVALUATION, INTERPRETATION, AND REPORTING OF RESULTS

Considering the widespread reputation of the species, it is prudent to consider *S. aureus* as the etiologic agent when it is isolated from a clinical specimen. The identities of suspected isolates should be confirmed on the basis of coagulase testing and also preferably on the basis of the biochemical profile with a commercial identification system. At a significant but reasonable initial cost, the AccuProbe culture identification test for *S. aureus* (Gen-Probe) may be used to accurately identify the uncommon tube coagulase-negative and slide test-negative strains of *S. aureus* and could be used for the routine identification of the species. Strains of *S. aureus* should be monitored in the advent of outbreaks and for the surveillance of nosocomial populations. Phage typing of *S. aureus* is being replaced by molecular typing methods in reference laboratories for the monitoring of strains.

It is a common practice to consider *S. epidermidis* as an etiologic agent when it is isolated from colonized shunts or catheters in association with bacteremia and from prosthetic devices in association with clinical and pathologic evidence and *S. saprophyticus* as the etiologic agent when it is isolated from patients with UTI, especially if the bacteria are present in large numbers or as the predominant organism. Although these assessments are not always accurate, they are based on the known pathogenic potential of these species. Traditionally, in UTIs colony counts of ≥100,000 CFU/ml in two or more cultures of midstream urine indicate a significant bacteriuria or UTI. Since staphylococci grow relatively slowly in urine, it has been suggested that lower colony counts of 100 to 10,000 CFU/ml should be considered an appropriate range for significant bacteriuria in the presence of pyuria (58, 140). Repeated isolation of a predominant strain or a strain in pure culture is quite convincing when attempting to determine the etiologic agent. For many of the other staphylococcal species and for micrococcal species, it is imperative that individual strains be identified and monitored, preferably over the course of the infection, before their etiology can be evaluated. In the small clinic or small community hospital laboratory, CoNS species are seldom identified, although isolates of interest are sometimes sent to private or other reference laboratories for identification to the species, subspecies, or strain level. When it is deemed necessary to identify the etiologic agent, e.g., as a result of treatment failure or during an outbreak, it is important that one or more aged (≥72 h) colonies of a particular morphotype be isolated from the primary isolation plate for each culture to be identified. The practice of pooling two or more younger (24- to 48-h) colonies in the preparation of an inoculum or culture carries with it the risk of producing a mixed culture resulting in an erroneous identification and erroneous accompanying antibiogram. Selecting only one young colony from a primary isolation plate carries with it the risk of missing the actual etiologic agent.

At many large community and teaching hospitals, state health departments, and the Centers for Disease Control and Prevention (CDC), both conventional and molecular methods are being performed for the complete identification of staphylococci. CoNS species and subspecies are usually identified on the basis of their phenotypic characters by commercial rapid identification systems and some supplemental conventional methods (discussed above). Any isolation of the species *S. aureus* should be considered suspect and processed for a confirmed identification together with an antibiogram. *S. aureus* strains isolated from patients with TSS may be tested for their ability to produce TSST-1 in the routine laboratory by the commercially available RPLA (Oxoid) or by using the services of the Microbiology Reference Laboratory (Cyprus, Calif.) and Toxin Technology (Sarasota, Fla.). In general, a combination of two or more conventional typing techniques is used for strain identification. Ribotyping, PFGE, and/or FIGE appear to be the most objective and discriminatory molecular techniques currently available. Initial guidelines for the interpretation of PFGE banding patterns from investigations in outbreaks of *S. aureus* are being established at CDC.

REFERENCES

1. **Almeida, R. J., and J. H. Jorgensen.** 1982. Use of Mueller-Hinton agar to determine novobiocin susceptibility of coagulase-negative staphylococci. *J. Clin. Microbiol.* **16:** 1155–1156.
2. **Archer, G. L.** 1985. Coagulase-negative staphylococci in blood cultures: a clinician's dilemma. *Infect. Control* **6:** 477–478.
3. **Archer, G. L., and M. W. Climo.** 1994. Antimicrobial susceptibility of coagulase-negative staphylococci. *Antimicrob. Agents Chemother.* **38:**2231–2237.
4. **Aufwerber, E., S. Ringertz, and U. Ransjö.** 1991. Routine semiquantitative cultures and central venous catheter-related bacteremia. *APMIS* **99:**627–630.
5. **Baker, J. S.** 1984. Comparison of various methods for differentiation of staphylococci and micrococci. *J. Clin. Microbiol.* **19:**875–879.
6. **Bannerman, T. L., and W. E. Kloos.** 1991. *Staphylococcus capitis* subsp. *urealyticus* subsp. nov. from human skin. *Int. J. Syst. Bacteriol.* **41:**144–147.
7. **Bannerman, T. L., G. A. Hancock, F. C. Tenover, and J. M. Miller.** 1995. Pulsed-field gel electrophoresis as a replacement for bacteriophage typing of *Staphylococcus aureus*. *J. Clin. Microbiol.* **33:**551–555.
8. **Bannerman, T. L., D. L. Rhoden, S. K. McAllister, J. M. Miller, and L. A. Wilson.** 1997. The source of coagulase-negative staphylococci in the endophthalmitis vitrectomy study: a comparison of eyelid and intraocular isolates using pulsed-field gel electrophoresis. *Arch. Ophthalmol.* **115:** 357–361.
9. **Bergamini, T. M., D. F. Bandyk, and D. Govostis.** 1989. Identification of *Staphylococcus epidermidis* vascular graft infections: a comparison of culture techniques. *J. Vasc. Surg.* **9:**665–670.
10. **Bialkowska-Hobrzanska, H., D. Jaskot, and O. Hammerberg.** 1990. Evaluation of restriction endonuclease fingerprinting of chromosomal DNA and plasmid profile analysis for characterization of multiresistant coagulase-negative staphylococci in bacteremic neonates. *J. Clin. Microbiol.* **28:**269–275.
11. **Bingen, E., M. C. Barc, N. Brahimi, E. Vilmer, and F. Beaufils.** 1995. Randomly amplified polymorphic DNA analysis provides rapid differentiation of methicillin-resistant coagulase-negative staphylococcus bacteremia isolates in pediatric hospital. *J. Clin. Microbiol.* **33:** 1657–1659.
12. **Birnbaum, D., L. Herwaldt, D. E. Low, M. Noble, M. Pfaller, R. Sherertz, and A. W. Chow.** 1994. Efficacy of microbial identification system for epidemiologic typing of coagulase-negative staphylococci. *J. Clin. Microbiol.* **32:**2113–2119.
13. **Blot, F., E. Schmidt, G. Nitenberg, C. Tancrède, B. Leclercq, A. Laplanche, and A. Andremont.** 1998. Earlier positivity of central-venous- versus peripheral-blood cultures is highly predictive of catheter-related sepsis. *J. Clin. Microbiol.* **36:**105–109.
14. **Boelaert, J. R., H. W. Van Landuyt, B. Z. Gordts,**

Y. A. De Baere, S. A. Messer, and L. A. Herwaldt. 1996. Nasal and cutaneous carriage of *Staphylococcus aureus* in hemodialysis patients: the effect of nasal mupirocin. *Infect. Control Hosp. Epidemiol.* **17:**809–811.
15. **Bonilla, H. F., L. T. Zarins, S. F. Bradley, and C. A. Kauffman.** 1996. Susceptibility of ciprofloxacin-resistant staphylococci and enterococci to trovafloxacin. *Diagn. Microbiol. Infect. Dis.* **26:**17–21.
16. **Boyce, J. M.** 1991. Should we vigorously try to contain and control methicillin-resistant *Staphylococcus aureus? Infect. Control Hosp. Epidemiol.* **12:**46–54.
17. **Boyce, J. M.** 1995. Strategies for controlling methicillin-resistant *Staphylococcus aureus* in hospitals. *J. Chemother.* **7**(Suppl. 3)**:**81–85.
18. **Bradley, S. F., M. A. Ramsey, T. M. Morton, and C. A. Kauffman.** 1995. Mupirocin resistance: clinical and molecular epidemiology. *Infect. Control Hosp. Epidemiol.* **16:**354–358.
19. **Cato, E. P., and E. Stackebrant.** 1989. Taxonomy and phylogeny, p. 1–26. *In* N. P. Minton and D. J. Clarke (ed.), *Clostridia.* Plenum Press, New York, N.Y.
20. **Centers for Disease Control and Prevention.** 1997. Interim guidelines for the prevention and control of staphylococcal infections associated with reduced susceptibility to vancomycin. *Morbid. Mortal. Weekly Rep.* **46:**626–628, 635–636.
21. **Centers for Disease Control and Prevention.** 1997. Reduced susceptibility of *Staphylococcus aureus* to vancomycin—Japan, 1996. *Morbid. Mortal. Weekly Rep.* **46:** 624–644.
22. **Centers for Disease Control and Prevention.** 1997. Update: *Staphylococcus aureus* with reduced susceptibility to vancomycin—United States, 1997. *Morbid. Mortal. Weekly Rep.* **46:**813–815.
23. **Chambers, H. F.** 1988. Methicillin-resistant staphylococci. *Clin. Microbiol. Rev.* **1:**173–186.
24. **Chesneau, O., A. Morvan, F. Grimont, H. Labischinski, and N. El Solh.** 1993. *Staphylococcus pasteuri* sp. nov., isolated from human, animal, and food specimens. *Int. J. Syst. Bacteriol.* **43:**237–244.
25. **Choi, Y., B. Kotzin, L. Herron, J. Callahan, P. Marrack, and J. Kappler.** 1989. Interaction of *Staphylococcus aureus* toxin "superantigens" with human T cells. *Proc. Natl. Acad. Sci. USA* **86:**8941–8945.
26. **Clink, J., and T. H. Pennington.** 1987. Staphylococcal whole-cell polypeptide analysis: evaluation as a taxonomic and typing tool. *J. Med. Microbiol.* **23:**41–44.
27. **Cohn, F.** 1872. Untersuchungen uber Bacterien. *Beitr. Biol. Pflanz. Bd. 1, Heft* **2:**127–224.
28. **Coque, T. M., K. V. Singh, and B. E. Murray.** 1996. Comparative in-vitro activity of the new fluoroquinolone trovafloxacin (CP-99, 219) against gram-positive cocci. *J. Antimicrob. Chemother.* **37:**1011–1016.
29. **Cormican, M. G., and R. N. Jones.** 1996. Emerging resistance to antimicrobial agents in gram-positive bacteria. Enterococci, staphylococci, and nonpneumococcal streptococci. *Drugs* **51**(Suppl. 1)**:**6–12.
30. **Coudron, P. E., D. L. Jones, H. P. Dalton, and G. L. Archer.** 1986. Evaluation of laboratory tests for detection of methicillin-resistant *Staphylococcus aureus* and *Staphylococcus epidermidis. J. Clin. Microbiol.* **24:**764–769.
31. **Couto, I., H. De Lencastre, E. Severina, W. E. Kloos, J. A. Webster, R. J. Hubner, I. Santos Sanches, and A. Tomasz.** 1996. Ubiquitous presence of a *mecA* homologue in natural isolates of *Staphylococcus sciuri. Microb. Drug Resist.* **2:**377–391.
32. **Crossley, K. B., and G. L. Archer (ed.).** 1997. *The Staphylococci in Human Disease.* Churchill Livingstone, New York, N.Y.
33. **Davis, G. H. G., and B. Hoyling.** 1973. Use of a rapid acetoin test in the identification of staphylococci and micrococci. *Int. J. Syst. Bacteriol.* **23:**281–282.
34. **DeBuyser, M.-L., A. Morvan, S. Aubert, F. Dilasser, and N. El Solh.** 1992. Evaluation of ribosomal RNA gene probe for the identification of species and subspecies within the genus *Staphylococcus. J. Gen. Microbiol.* **138:** 889–899.
35. **Deplano, A., M. Vaneechoutte, G. Verschraegen, and M. J. Struelens.** 1997. Typing of *Staphylococcus aureus* and *Staphylococcus epidermidis* strains by PCR analysis of inter-IS*256* spacer length polymorphisms. *J. Clin. Microbiol.* **35:**2580–2587.
36. **Devriese, L. A.** 1984. A simplified scheme for biotyping *Staphylococcus aureus* strains isolated from different animal species. *J. Appl. Bacteriol.* **56:**215–220.
37. **Devriese, L. A.** 1986. Coagulase-negative staphylococci in animals, p. 51–57. *In* P.-A. Mårdh and K. H. Schleifer (ed.), *Coagulase-Negative Staphylococci.* Almqvist & Wiksell International, Stockholm, Sweden.
38. **Devriese, L. A.** 1990. Staphylococci in healthy and disease animals. *J. Appl. Bacteriol. Symp. Suppl.* **69:**71S–80S.
39. **Douard, M. C., G. Arlet, G. Leverger, R. Paulien, C. Maintrop, E. Clemente, B. Eurin, and G. Scharson.** 1991. Quantitative blood cultures for diagnosis and management of catheter-related sepsis in pediatric hematology and oncology patients. *Intensive Care Med.* **17:**30–35.
40. **Dufresne, C., K. Young, F. Pelaez, A. Gonzalez del Val, D. Valentino, A. Graham, G. Platas, A. Bernard, and D. Zink.** 1997. Illudinic acid, a novel illudane sesquiterpene antibiotic. *J. Natural Products* **60:**188–190.
41. **Evans, J. B., W. L. Bradford, Jr., and C. F. Niven.** 1955. Comments concerning the taxonomy of the genera *Micrococcus* and *Staphylococcus. Int. Bull. Bacteriol. Nomencl. Taxon.* **5:**61–66.
42. **Fleurette, J., M. Bes, Y. Brun, J. Freney, F. Forey, M. Coulet, M. E. Reverdy, and J. Etienne.** 1989. Clinical isolates of *Staphylococcus lugdunensis* and *S. schleiferi*: bacteriological characteristics and susceptibility to antimicrobial agents. *Res. Microbiol.* **140:**107–118.
43. **Ford, C. W., J. C. Hamel, D. M. Wilson, J. K. Moerman, D. Stapert, R. J. Yancey, Jr., D. K. Hutchinson, M. R. Barbachyn, and S. J. Brickner.** 1996. In vivo activities of U-100592 and U-100766, novel oxazolidinone antimicrobial agents, against experimental bacterial infections. *Antimicrob. Agents Chemother.* **40:**1508–1513.
44. **Foster, G., H. M. Ross, R. A. Hutson, and M. D. Collins.** 1997. *Staphylococcus lutrae* sp. nov., a new coagulase-positive species isolated from otters. *Int. J. Syst. Bacteriol.* **47:**724–726.
45. **Fournier, J.-M., A. Bouvet, D. Mathieu, F. Nato, A. Boutonnier, R. Gerbal, P. Brunengo, C. Saulnier, N. Sagot, B. Slizewicz, and J.-C. Mazie.** 1993. New latex reagent using monoclonal antibodies to capsular polysaccharide for reliable identification of both oxacillin-susceptible and oxacillin-resistant *Staphylococcus aureus. J. Clin. Microbiol.* **31:**1342–1344.
46. **Gatterman, S. G., and K. B. Crossley.** 1997. Urinary tract infections, p. 493–508. *In* K. B. Crossley and G. L. Archer (ed.), *The Staphylococci in Human Disease.* Churchill Livingstone, New York, N.Y.
47. **George, C. G., and W. E. Kloos.** 1994. Comparison of the *Sma*I-digested chromosomes of *Staphylococcus epidermidis* and the closely related species *Staphylococcus capitis* and *Staphylococcus caprae. Int. J. Syst. Bacteriol.* **44:**404–409.
48. **Goering, R. V., and M. A. Winters.** 1992. Rapid method for epidemiological evaluation of gram-positive cocci by field inversion gel electrophoresis. *J. Clin. Microbiol.* **30:** 577–580.
49. **Goldstein, J., R. Schulman, E. Kelly, G. McKinley, and**

J. Fung. 1983. Effect of different media on determination of novobiocin resistance for differentiation of coagulase-negative staphylococci. *J. Clin. Microbiol.* **18:**592–595.

50. **Golledge, C. L.** 1988. *Staphylococcus saprophyticus* bacteremia. *J. Infect. Dis.* **157:**215.
51. **Gristina, A. G., G. Giridhar, B. Gabriel, A. Kreger, and Q. Myrvik.** 1994. The present status of biomaterial-associated infection, p. 313–333. *In* T. Wadström, I. A. Holder, and G. Kronvall (ed.), *Molecular Pathogenesis of Surgical Infections.* Gustav Fischer Verlag, New York, N.Y.
52. **Guardati, M. C., C. A. Guzmàn, G. Piatti, and C. Pruzzo.** 1993. Rapid methods for identification of *Staphylococcus aureus* when both human and animal staphylococci are tested: comparison with a new immunoenzymatic assay. *J. Clin. Microbiol.* **31:**1606–1608.
53. **Gurtler, V., and H. D. Barrie.** 1995. Typing of *Staphylococcus aureus* strains by PCR-amplification of variable-length 16S-23S rDNA spacer regions: characterization of spacer sequences. *Microbiology* **141:**1255–1265.
54. **Hadorn, K., W. Lenz, F. H. Kayser, I. Shalit, and C. Krasemann.** 1990. Use of a ribosomal RNA gene probe for epidemiological study of methicillin and ciprofloxacin resistant *Staphylococcus aureus*. *Eur. J. Clin. Microbiol. Infect. Dis.* **9:**649–653.
55. **Hájek, V., H. Meugnier, M. Bes, Y. Brun, F. Fiedler, Z. Chmela, Y. Lasne, J. Fleurette, and J. Freney.** 1996. *Staphylococcus saprophyticus* subsp. *bovis* subsp. nov. isolated from bovine nostrils. *Int. J. Syst. Bacteriol.* **46:** 792–796.
56. **Harrington, B. J., and J. M. Gaydos.** 1984. Five-hour novobiocin test for differentiation of coagulase-negative staphylococci. *J. Clin. Microbiol.* **19:**279–280.
57. **Hébert, G. A., C. G. Crowder, G. A. Hancock, W. R. Jarvis, and C. Thornsberry.** 1988. Characteristics of coagulase-negative staphylococci that help differentiate these species and other members of the family *Micrococcaceae*. *J. Clin. Microbiol.* **26:**1939–1949.
58. **Hovelius, B.** 1986. Epidemiological and clinical aspects of urinary tract infections caused by *Staphylococcus saprophyticus*, p. 195–202. *In* P.-A. Mårdh and K. H. Schleifer (ed.), *Coagulase-Negative Staphylococci.* Almqvist & Wiksell International, Stockholm, Sweden.
59. **Ieven, M., H. Jansens, D. Ursi, J. Verhoeven, and H. Goossens.** 1995. Rapid detection of methicillin resistance in coagulase-negative staphylococci by commercially available fluorescence test. *J. Clin. Microbiol.* **33:** 2183–2185.
60. **Jansen, B., F. Schumacher-Perdreau, G. Peters, and G. Pulverer.** 1989. New aspects in the pathogenesis and prevention of polymer-associated foreign-body infections caused by coagulase-negative staphylococci. *J. Invest. Surg.* **2:**361–380.
61. **Jean-Pierre, H., H. Darbas, A. Jean-Roussenq, and G. Boyer.** 1989. Pathogenicity in two cases of *Staphylococcus schleiferi*, a recently described species. *J. Clin. Microbiol.* **27:**2110–2111.
62. **Johnson, W. M., and S. D. Tyler.** 1993. PCR detection of genes for enterotoxins, exfoliative toxins, and toxic shock syndrome toxin-1 in *Staphylococcus aureus*, p. 294–299. *In* D. H. Persing, T. F. Smith, F. C. Tenover, and T. J. White (ed.), *Diagnostic Molecular Microbiology Principles and Applications.* American Society for Microbiology, Washington, D.C.
63. **Jorgensen, J. H., M. L. McElmeel, and C. W. Trippy.** 1997. In vitro activities of the oxazolidinone antibiotics U-100592 and U-100766 against *Staphylococcus aureus* and coagulase-negative *Staphylococcus* species. *Antimicrob. Agents Chemother.* **41:**465–467.
64. **Kaatz, G. W., and S. M. Seo.** 1996. In vitro activities of oxazolidinone compounds U100592 and U100766 against *Staphylococcus aureus* and *Staphylococcus epidermidis*. *Antimicrob. Agents Chemother.* **40:**799–801.
65. **Karchmer, A. W., and G. M. Caputo.** 1986. Endocarditis due to coagulase-negative staphylococci, p. 179–187. *In* P.-A. Maårdh and K. H. Schleifer (ed.), *Coagulase-Negative Staphylococci.* Almqvist & Wiksell International, Stockholm, Sweden.
66. **Khambaty, F. M., R. W. Bennett, and D. B. Shah.** 1994. Application of pulsed-field gel electrophoresis to the epidemiological characterization of *Staphylococcus intermedius* implicated in a food-related outbreak. *Epidemiol. Infect.* **113:**75–81.
67. **Kilpper, R., U. Buhl, and K. H. Schleifer.** 1980. Nucleic acid homology studies between *Peptococcus saccharolyticus* and various anaerobic and facultive anaerobic Gram-positive cocci. *FEMS Microbiol. Lett.* **8:**205–210.
68. **Kloos, W. E.** 1986. Ecology of human skin, p. 37–50. *In* P.-A. Maårdh and K. H. Schleifer (ed.), *Coagulase-Negative Staphylococci.* Almqvist & Wiksell International, Stockholm, Sweden.
69. **Kloos, W. E.** 1990. Systematics and the natural history of staphylococci. 1. *J. Appl. Bacteriol. Symp. Suppl.* **69:** 25S–37S.
70. **Kloos, W. E.** 1997. Taxonomy and systematics of staphylococci indigenous to humans, p. 113–137. *In* K. B. Crossley and G. L. Archer (ed.), *The Staphylococci in Human Disease.* Churchill Livingstone, New York, N.Y.
71. **Kloos, W. E.** 1998. *Staphylococcus*, p. 577–632. *In* L. Collier, A. Balows, and M. Sussman (ed.), *Topley & Wilson's Microbiology and Microbial Infections*, vol. 2, 9th ed. Edward Arnold, London, United Kingdom.
72. **Kloos, W. E., D. N. Ballard, C. G. George, J. A. Webster, R. J. Hubner, W. Ludwig, K. H. Schleifer, F. Fiedler, and K. Schubert.** 1998. Delimiting the genus *Staphylococcus* through description of *Macrococcus caseolyticus* gen. nov., comb. nov. and the new species *Macrococcus equipercicus* sp. nov., *Macrococcus bovicus* sp. nov., and *Macrococcus carouselicus* sp. nov. *Int. J. Syst. Bacteriol.* **48:**859–877.
73. **Kloos, W. E., D. N. Ballard, J. A. Webster, R. J. Hubner, A. Tomasz, I. Couto, G. L. Sloan, H. P. DeHart, F. Fiedler, K. Schubert, H. De Lencastre, I. Santos Sanches, H. E. Heath, P. A. LeBlanc, and Å. Ljungh.** 1997. Ribotype delineation and description of *Staphylococcus sciuri* subspecies and their potential as reservoirs of methicillin resistance and staphylolytic enzyme genes. *Int. J. Syst. Bacteriol.* **47:**313–323.
74. **Kloos, W. E., and T. L. Bannerman.** 1994. Update on clinical significance of coagulase-negative staphylococci. *Clin. Microbiol. Rev.* **7:**117–140.
75. **Kloos, W. E., and T. L. Bannerman.** 1995. *Staphylococcus* and *Micrococcus*, p. 282–298. *In* P. R. Murray, E. J. Baron, M. A. Pfaller, F. C. Tenover, and R. H. Yolken (ed.), *Manual of Clinical Microbiology*, 6th ed. American Society for Microbiology, Washington, D.C.
76. **Kloos, W. E., C. G. George, J. S. Olgiati, L. Van Pelt, M. L. McKinnon, B. L. Zimmer, E. Muller, M. P. Weinstein, and S. Mirrett.** 1998. *Staphylococcus hominis* subsp. *novobiosepticus* subsp. nov., a novel trehalose- and *N*-acetyl-D-glucosamine-negative, novobiocin- and multiple antibiotic-resistant subspecies isolated from human blood cultures. *Int. J. Syst. Bacteriol.* **48:**799–812.
77. **Kloos, W. E., and M. S. Musselwhite.** 1975. Distribution and persistence of *Staphylococcus* and *Micrococcus* species and other aerobic bacteria on human skin. *Appl. Microbiol.* **30:**381–395.
78. **Kloos, W. E., B. S. Orban, and D. D. Walker.** 1981. Plasmid composition of *Staphylococcus* species. *Can. J. Microbiol.* **27:**271–278.
79. **Kloos, W. E., and K. H. Schleifer.** 1975. Isolation and

characterization of staphylococci from human skin. II. Description of four new species: *Staphylococcus warneri*, *Staphylococcus capitis*, *Staphylococcus hominis*, and *Staphylococcus simulans*. *Int. J. Syst. Bacteriol.* **25:**62–79.

80. **Kloos, W. E., and K. H. Schleifer.** 1975. Simplified scheme for routine identification of human *Staphylococcus* species. *J. Clin. Microbiol.* **1:**82–88.
81. **Kloos, W. E., K. H. Schleifer, and F. Götz.** 1991. The genus *Staphylococcus*, p. 1369–1420. *In* A. Balows, H. G. Truper, M. Dworkin, W. Harder, and K. H. Schleifer (ed.), *The Prokaryotes*, 2nd ed. Springer-Verlag, New York, N.Y.
82. **Kloos, W. E., T. G. Tornabene, and K. H. Schleifer.** 1974. Isolation and characterization of micrococci from human skin, including two new species: *Micrococcus lylae* and *Micrococcus kristinae*. *Int. J. Syst. Bacteriol.* **24:** 79–101.
83. **Kluytmans, J., A. van Belkum, and H. Verbrugh.** 1997. Nasal carriage of *Staphylococcus aureus*: epidemiology, underlying mechanisms, and associated risks. *Clin. Microbiol. Rev.* **10:**505–520.
84. **Kluytmans, J. A., M. J. Manders, E. van Bommel, and H. Verbrugh.** 1996. Elimination of nasal carriage of *Staphylococcus aureus* in hemodialysis patients. *Infect. Control Hosp. Epidemiol.* **17:**793–797.
85. **Kluytmans, J. A., J. W. Mouton, M. F. VandenBergh, M. J. Manders, A. P. Maat, J. H. Wagenvoort, M. F. Michel, and H. A. Verbrugh.** 1996. Reduction of surgical-site infections in cardiothoracic surgery by elimination of nasal carriage of *Staphylococcus aureus*. *Infect. Control Hosp. Epidemiol.* **17:**780–785.
86. **Kobayashi, N., H. Wu, K. Kojima, K. Taniguchi, S. Urasawa, N. Uehara, Y. Omizu, Y. Kishi, A. Yagihashi, and I. Kurokawa.** 1994. Detection of *mecA*, *femA*, and *femB* genes in clinical strains of staphylococci using polymerase chain reaction. *Epidemiol. Infect.* **113:**259–266.
87. **Koch, C., and E. Stackebrandt.** 1995. Reclassification of *Micrococcus agilis* (Ali-Cohen 1889) to *Arthrobacter* as *Arthrobacter agilis* comb. nov. and emendation of the genus *Arthrobacter*. *Int. J. Syst. Bacteriol.* **45:**837–839.
88. **Kocur, M., W. E. Kloos, and K. H. Schleifer.** 1991. The genus *Micrococcus*, p. 1300–1311. *In* A. Balows, H. G. Truper, M. Dworkin, W. Harder, and K. H. Schleifer (ed.), *The Prokaryotes*, 2nd ed. Springer-Verlag, New York, N.Y.
89. **Kolbert, C. P., J. E. Connolly, M. J. Lee, and D. H. Persing.** 1995. Detection of staphylococcal *mecA* gene by chemiluminescent DNA hybridization. *J. Clin. Microbiol.* **33:**2179–2182.
90. **Kostman, J. R., M. B. Alden, M. Mair, T. D. Edlind, J. J. LiPuma, and T. L. Stull.** 1995. A universal approach to bacterial molecular epidemiology by polymerase chain reaction ribotyping. *J. Infect. Dis.* **171:**204–208.
91. **Kotilainen P., P. Huovinen, and E. Eerola.** 1991. Application of gas-liquid chromatographic analysis of cellular fatty acids for species identification and typing of coagulase-negative staphylococci. *J. Clin. Microbiol.* **29:** 315–322.
92. **Kotilainen, P., P. Huovinen, and E. Eerola.** 1995. Use of gas-liquid chromatography for subgrouping coagulase-negative staphylococci during a nosocomial sepsis outbreak. *Eur. J. Clin. Microbiol. Infect. Dis.* **14:**412–420.
93. **Krcmery, V., Jr., J. Trupl, L. Drgona, J. Lacka, E. Kukuckova, and E. Oravcova.** 1996. Nosocomial bacteremia due to vancomycin-resistant *Staphylococcus epidermidis* in four patients with cancer, neutropenia, and previous treatment with vancomycin. *Eur. J. Clin. Microbiol. Infect. Dis.* **15:**259–261.
94. **Kumari, D. N., V. Keer, P. M. Hawkey, P. Parnell, N. Joseph, J. F. Richardson, and B. Cookson.** 1997. Comparison and application of ribosome spacer DNA amplicon polymorphisms and pulsed-field gel electrophoresis for differentiation of methicillin-resistant *Staphylococcus aureus* strains. *J. Clin. Microbiol.* **35:**881–885.
95. **Lachica, R. V. F., P. D. Hoeprich, and C. Genigeorgis.** 1972. Metachromatic agar-diffusion microslide technique for detecting staphylococcal nuclease in foods. *Appl. Microbiol.* **23:**168–169.
96. **Lachica, R. V. F., S. S. Jang, and P. D. Hoeprich.** 1979. Thermonuclease seroinhibition test for distinguishing *Staphylococcus aureus* and other coagulase-positive staphylococci. *J. Clin. Microbiol.* **9:**141–143.
97. **Lee, J. C., and G. B. Pier.** 1997. Vaccine-based strategies for prevention of staphylococcal diseases, p. 631–654. *In* K. B. Crossley and G. L. Archer (ed.), *The Staphylococci in Human Disease*. Churchill Livingstone, New York, N.Y.
98. **Ludwig, W., K. H. Schleifer, G. E. Fox, E. Seewaldt, and E. Stackebrandt.** 1981. A phylogenetic analysis of staphylococci, *Peptococcus saccharolyticus* and *Micrococcus mucilaginosus*. *J. Gen. Microbiol.* **125:**357–366.
99. **Ludwig, W., E. Seewaldt, R. Kilpper-Bälz, K. H. Schleifer, L. Magrum, C. R. Woese, G. F. Fox, and E. Stackebrandt.** 1985. The phylogenetic position of *Streptococcus* and *Enterococcus*. *J. Gen. Microbiol.* **131:**543–551.
100. **Lyon, B. R., and R. Skurray.** 1987. Antimicrobial resistance of *Staphylococcus aureus*: genetic basis. *Microbiol. Rev.* **51:**88–134.
101. **Magee, J. T., I. A. Burnett, J. M. Hindmarch, and R. C. Spencer.** 1990. *Micrococcus* and *Stomatococcus* spp. from human infections. *J. Infect.* **16:**67–73.
102. **Manzell, J. P., J. A. Kellogg, and E. Q. Rogers.** 1989. *Micrococcus sedentarius* as a cause of prosthetic valve endocarditis, abstr. C-208, p. 428. *In Abstracts of the 89th Annual Meeting of the American Society for Microbiology 1989*. American Society for Microbiology, Washington, D.C.
103. **McDougal, L. K., and C. Thornsberry.** 1984. New recommendations for disk diffusion antimicrobial susceptibility tests for methicillin-resistant (heteroresistant) staphylococci. *J. Clin. Microbiol.* **19:**482–488.
104. **Meyer, W.** 1967. A proposal for subdividing the species *Staphylococcus aureus*. *Int. J. Syst. Bacteriol.* **17:**387–389.
105. **Moeller, V.** 1955. Simplified tests for some amino acid decarboxylases and for the arginine dihydrolase system. *Acta Pathol. Microbiol. Scand.* **36:**158–172.
106. **Moreira, B. M., and R. S. Daum.** 1995. Antimicrobial resistance in staphylococci. *Pediatr. Clin. N. Am.* **42:** 619–648.
107. **Muller, E., S. Takeda, H. Shiro, D. Goldmann, and G. B. Pier.** 1993. Occurrence of capsular polysaccharide/ adhesin among clinical isolates of coagulase-negative staphylococci. *J. Infect. Dis.* **168:**1211–1218.
108. **Mulligan, M. E., K. A. Murray-Leisure, B. S. Ribner, H. C. Standiford, J. F. John, J. A. Korvick, C. A. Kauffman, and V. L. Yu.** 1993. Methicillin-resistant *Staphylococcus aureus*: a consensus review of the microbiology, pathogenesis, and epidemiology with implications for prevention and management. *Am. J. Med.* **94:**313–328.
109. **Musser, J. M., and V. Kapur.** 1992. Clonal analysis of methicillin-resistant *Staphylococcus aureus* strains from intercontinental sources: association of the *mec* gene with divergent phylogenetic lineages implies dissemination by horizontal transfer and recombination. *J. Clin. Microbiol.* **30:**2058–2063.
110. **Musser, J. M., P. M. Schlievert, A. W. Chow, P. Ewan, B. N. Kreiswirth, V. T. Rosdahl, A. S. Naidu, W. White, and R. K. Selander.** 1990. A single clone of *Staphylococcus aureus* causes the majority of cases of toxic shock syndrome. *Proc. Natl. Acad. Sci. USA* **87:**225–229.
111. **Musser, J. M., and R. K. Selander.** 1990. Genetic analysis of natural populations of *Staphylococcus aureus*, p. 59–67.

In R. P. Novick (ed.), *Molecular Biology of the Staphylococci*. VCH Publishers, New York, N.Y.

112. **Nordstom, K. M., K. J. McGinley, J. M. Zechman, and J. J. Leyden.** 1987. Similarities between *Dermatophilus congolensis* and *Micrococcus sedentarius*: identity of the etiologic agent of pitted keratolysis, abstr. R-21, p. 244. *In Abstracts of the 87th Annual Meeting of the American Society for Microbiology 1987*. American Society for Microbiology, Washington, D.C.
113. **Ogston, A.** 1883. *Micrococcus* poisoning. *J. Anat. Physiol.* **17:**317–324.
114. **Parsonnet, J., and Z. A. Gillis.** 1988. Production of tumor necrosis factor by human monocytes in response to toxic shock syndrome toxin-1 *J. Infect. Dis.* **158:**1026–1033.
115. **Parsonnet, J., R. K. Hickman, D. D. Eardley, and G. B. Pier.** 1985. Induction of human interleukin-1 by toxic shock syndrome toxin-1. *J. Infect. Dis.* **151:**514–522.
116. **Paulsen, I. T., N. Firth, and R. A. Skurray.** 1997. Resistance to antimicrobial agents other than β-lactams, p. 175–212. *In* K. B. Crossley and G. L. Archer (ed.), *The Staphylococci in Human Disease*. Churchill Livingstone, New York, N.Y.
117. **Pennock, C. A., and R. B. Huddy.** 1967. Phosphatase reaction of coagulase-negative staphylococci and micrococci. *J. Pathol. Bacteriol.* **93:**685–688.
118. **Peters, G., F. Schumacher-Perdreau, B. Jansen, M. Bey, and G. Pulverer.** 1987. Biology of *S. epidermidis* extracellular slime, p. 15–32. *In* G. Pulverer, P. G. Quie, and G. Peters (ed.), *Pathogenicity and Clinical Significance of Coagulase-Negative Staphylococci*. Gustav Fischer Verlag, Stuttgart, Germany.
119. **Pfaller, M. A., and L. A. Herwaldt.** 1988. Laboratory, clinical, and epidemiological aspects of coagulase-negative staphylococci. *Clin. Microbiol. Rev.* **1:**281–299.
120. **Prevost, G., B. Jaulhac, and Y. Piemont.** 1992. DNA fingerprinting by pulsed-field gel electrophoresis is more effective than ribotyping in distinguishing among methicillin-resistant *Staphylococcus aureus* isolates. *J. Clin. Microbiol.* **30:**967–973.
121. **Qadri, S. M. H., Y. Ueno, H. Imambaccus, and E. Almodovar.** 1994. Rapid detection of methicillin-resistant *Staphylococcus aureus* by Crystal MRSA ID System. *J. Clin. Microbiol.* **32:**1830–1832.
122. **Raad, I., R. Hachem, A. Zermeno, M. Dumo, and G. P. Bodey.** 1996. In vitro antimicrobial efficacy of silver iontophoretic catheter. *Biomaterials* **17:**1055–1059.
123. **Rosenbach, F. J.** 1884. *Mikro-organismen bei den Wund-Infections-Krankheiten des Menschen*. J. F. Bergmann, Wiesbaden, Germany.
124. **Rupp, M. E., and G. L. Archer.** 1994. Coagulase-negative staphylococci: pathogens associated with medical progress. *Clin. Infect. Dis.* **19:**231–245.
125. **Salisbury, S. M., L. M. Sabatini, and C. A. Spiegel.** 1997. Identification of methicillin-resistant staphylococci by multiplex polymerase chain reaction assay. *Am. J. Clin. Pathol.* **107:**368–373.
126. **Schleifer, K. H.** 1986. Gram-positive cocci, p. 999–1002. *In* J. G. Holt, P. H. A. Sneath, N. S. Mair, and M. S. Sharpe (ed.), *Bergey's Manual of Systematic Bacteriology*, vol. 2. The Williams & Wilkins Co., Baltimore, Md.
127. **Schleifer, K. H.** 1986. Taxonomy of coagulase-negative staphylococci, p. 11–26. *In* P.-A. Mårdh and K. H. Schleifer (ed.), *Coagulase-Negative Staphylococci*. Almqvist & Wiksell International, Stockholm, Sweden.
128. **Schleifer, K. H., and E. Krämer.** 1980. Selective medium for isolating staphylococci. *Zentralbl. Bakteriol. Parasitenkd. Infektionskr. Hyg. Abt. 1 Orig. Reihe C* **1:**270–280.

128a. **Schlievert, P.** Personal communication.

129. **Schlievert, P. M., K. N. Shands, B. B. Dan, G. P. Schmid, and R. D. Nishimura.** 1981. Identification and characterization of an exotoxin from *Staphylococcus aureus* associated with toxic shock syndrome. *J. Infect. Dis.* **143:** 509–516.
130. **Schmitt, S. K., C. Knapp, G. S. Hall, D. L. Longworth, J. T. McMahon, and J. A. Washington.** 1996. Impact of chlorhexidine-silver sulfadiazine-impregnated central venous catheters on in vitro quantitation of catheter-associated bacteria. *J. Clin. Microbiol.* **34:**508–511.
131. **Schwalbe, R. S., A. C. McIntosh, S. Qaiyumi, J. A. Johnson, R. J. Johnson, K. M. Furness, W. J. Holloway, and L. Steele-Moore.** 1996. In vitro activity of LY333328, an investigational glycopeptide antibiotic, against enterococci and staphylococci. *Antimicrob. Agents Chemother.* **40:**2416–2419.
132. **Schwalbe, R. S., J. T. Stapleton, and P. H. Gilligan.** 1987. Emergence of vancomycin resistance in coagulase-negative staphylococci. *N. Engl. J. Med.* **316:**927–931.
133. **Shimaoka, M., M. Yoh, A. Segawa, Y. Takarada, and K. Yamamoto.** 1994. Development of enzyme-labeled oligonucleotide probe for detection of *mecA* gene in methicillin-resistant *Staphylococcus aureus*. *J. Clin. Microbiol.* **32:**1866–1869.
134. **Siegman-Igra, Y., M. Anglim, D. E. Shapiro, K. A. Adal, B. A. Strain, and B. M. Farr.** 1997. Diagnosis of vascular catheter-related bloodstream infection: a meta-analysis. *J. Clin. Microbiol.* **35:**928–936.
135. **Silvestri, L. G., and L. R. Hill.** 1965. Agreement between deoxyribonucleic acid base composition and taxonomic classification of gram-positive cocci. *J. Bacteriol.* **90:** 136–140.
136. **Stackebrandt, E., C. Koch, O. Gvozdiak, and P. Schumann.** 1995. Taxonomic dissection of the genus *Micrococcus: Kocuria*, gen. nov., *Nesterenkonia* gen. nov., *Kytococcus* gen. nov., *Dermacoccus* gen. nov., and *Micrococcus* Cohn 1872 gen. emend. *Int. J. Syst. Bacteriol.* **45:** 682–692.
137. **Stackebrandt, E., B. J. Lewis, and C. R. Woese.** 1980. The phylogenetic structure of the coryneform group of bacteria. *Zentralbl. Bakteriol. Parasitenkd. Infektionskr. Hyg. Abt. 1 Orig. Reihe C* **2:**137–149.
138. **Stackebrandt, E., and M. Teuber.** 1988. Molecular taxonomy and phylogenetic position of lactic acid bacteria. *Biochimie* **70:**317–324.
139. **Stackebrandt, E., and C. R. Woese.** 1979. A phylogenetic dissection of the family *Micrococcaceae*. *Curr. Microbiol.* **2:**317–322.
140. **Stamm, W. E.** 1988. Protocol for diagnosis of urinary tract infection: reconsidering the criterion for significant bacteriuria. *Urology* **32**(Suppl.):6–10.
141. **Sum, P. E., V. J. Lee, R. T. Testa, J. J. Hlavka, G. A. Ellestad, J. D. Bloom, Y. Gluzman, and F. P. Tally.** 1994. Glycylcyclines. 1. A new generation of potent antibacterial agents through modification of 9-aminotetracyclines. *J. Med. Chem.* **37:**184–188.
142. **Talan, D., D. Staatz, A. Staatz, E. J. Goldstein, K. Singer, and G. D. Overturf.** 1989. *Staphylococcus intermedius* in canine gingiva and canine-inflicted human wound infections: laboratory characterization of a newly recognized zoonotic pathogen. *J. Clin. Microbiol.* **27:**78–81.
143. **Tenover, F. C.** 1988. Diagnostic deoxyribonucleic acid probes for infectious diseases. *Clin. Microbiol. Rev.* **1:** 82–101.
144. **Thomson-Carter, F. M., P. E. Carter, and T. H. Pennington.** 1989. Differentiation of staphylococcal species and strains by ribosomal RNA gene restriction patterns. *J. Gen. Microbiol.* **135:**2093–2097.
145. **Tierno, P. M., Jr., and B. A. Hanna.** 1989. Ecology of toxic shock syndrome: amplification of toxic shock syn-

drome toxin 1 by materials of medical interest. *Rev. Infect. Dis.* **11**(Suppl. 1)**:**S182–S186.

146. **Tollefson, D. F., D. F. Bandyk, H. W. Kaebnick, G. R. Seabrook, and J. B. Towne.** 1987. Surface biofilm disruption-enhanced recovery of microorganisms from vascular prostheses. *Arch. Surg.* **122:**38–43.
147. **Van Belkum, A., J. Kluytmans, W. van Leeuwen, R. Bax, W. Quint, E. Peters, A. Fluit, C. Vandenbroucke-Grauls, A. van den Brule, H. Koeleman, W. Melchers, J. Meis, A. Elaichouni, M. Vaneechoutte, F. Moonens, N. Maes, M. Struelens, F. Tenover, and H. Verbrugh.** 1995. Multicenter evaluation of arbitrarily primed PCR for typing of *Staphylococcus aureus* strains. *J. Clin. Microbiol.* **33:**1537–1547.
148. **Viagappan, M., and M. C. Kelsey.** 1995. The origin of coagulase-negative staphylococci isolated from blood cultures. *J. Hosp. Infect.* **30:**217–223.
149. **Webster, J. A., T. L. Bannerman, R. Hubner, D. N. Ballard, E. Cole, J. Bruce, F. Fiedler, K. Schubert, and W. E. Kloos.** 1994. Identification of the *Staphylococcus sciuri* species group with *Eco*RI fragments containing rRNA sequences and description of *Staphylococcus vitulus* sp. nov. *Int. J. Syst. Bacteriol.* **44:**454–460.
150. **Weinstein, M. P., S. Mirrett, L. Van Pelt, M. McKinnon, B. L. Zimmer, W. E. Kloos, and L. B. Reller.** 1998. Clinical importance of identifying coagulase-negative staphylococci isolated from blood cultures: evaluation of MicroScan Rapid and Dried Overnight Gram-Positive Panels versus a conventional reference method. *J. Clin. Microbiol.* **36:**2089–2092.
151. **Weiss, K., D. Rouleau, and M. Laverdiere.** 1996. Cystitis due to vancomycin-intermediate *Staphylococcus saprophyticus*. *J. Antimicrob. Chemother.* **37:**1039–1040.
152. **Whimbey, E., B. Wong, T. E. Kiehn, and D. Armstrong.** 1984. Clinical correlations of serial quantitative blood cultures determined by lysis-centrifugation in patients with persistent septicemia. *J. Clin. Microbiol.* **19:** 766–771.
153. **Zakrzewska-Bode, A., H. L. Muytjens, and K. D. Liem.** 1995. Mupirocin resistance in coagulase-negative staphylococci, after topical prophylaxis for the reduction of colonization of central venous catheters. *J. Hosp. Infect.* **31:** 189–193.
154. **Zimmerman, R. J., and W. E. Kloos.** 1976. Comparative zone electrophoresis of esterases of *Staphylococcus* species isolated from mammalian skin. *Can. J. Microbiol.* **22:** 771–779.

Streptococcus

KATHRYN L. RUOFF, R. A. WHILEY, AND D. BEIGHTON

17

TAXONOMY

Broad changes in the classification of the streptococci have resulted from molecular taxonomic studies of the genus *Streptococcus*. The enterococci (previously considered group D streptococci) and the lactococci (previously considered group N streptococci) now reside in their own genera, *Enterococcus* and *Lactococcus*, respectively (70). Although traditional phenotypic criteria (hemolytic reactions, Lancefield serological groups) for classification of the streptococci are still useful in certain circumstances, the older classification schemes must be tempered by new taxonomic knowledge. For beta-hemolytic streptococci, we now know that unrelated species may produce identical Lancefield antigens and that strains genetically related at the species level may have heterogeneous Lancefield antigens.

In spite of these exceptions to the traditional rules of streptococcal taxonomy, hemolytic reactions and Lancefield serological tests can still be used to divide the streptococci into broad categories as a first step in identification of clinical isolates. Beta-hemolytic isolates with Lancefield group A, C, or G antigen can be subdivided into two groups: large-colony (>0.5 mm in diameter) and small-colony (<0.5 mm in diameter) formers. Large-colony-forming group A (*Streptococcus pyogenes*), C, and G strains are "pyogenic" streptococci replete with a variety of effective virulence mechanisms. The small-colony-forming beta-hemolytic strains with group A, C, or G Lancefield antigens are genetically different from the pyogenic strains and belong to the anginosus or "*Streptococcus milleri*" species group (which includes *S. anginosus*, *S. intermedius*, and *S. constellatus*). In spite of the existence of these groupable, beta-hemolytic strains, members of the anginosus species group are considered to be "viridans" streptococci, the majority of which display alpha-hemolytic or nonhemolytic reactions. Although the small-colony-forming strains may participate in infection (notably abscesses), they are also found as commensals whose pathogenic abilities appear to be much more subtle than those of the pyogenic streptococci. *Streptococcus agalactiae* is still identified reliably by its production of Lancefield group B antigen or other phenotypic traits.

Among non-beta-hemolytic streptococcal strains, alpha-reacting isolates can be separated into the species *Streptococcus pneumoniae* (optochin and bile susceptible) and the viridans division, composed of a number of species. It has been recently suggested (50) that organisms known as the nutritionally variant streptococci are not closely enough related to streptococci to be included in the genus *Streptococcus*. A new genus named *Abiotrophia* has been proposed to accommodate these bacteria, which are described in further detail in chapter 19. Streptococci with Lancefield's group D antigen include the nonhemolytic species *Streptococcus bovis*. Organisms previously thought to be anaerobic streptococci have been shown to be unrelated to members of the genus *Streptococcus* (59).

DESCRIPTION OF THE GENUS

Bergey's Manual of Systematic Bacteriology (42) describes streptococci as Gram-positive, catalase-negative facultatively anaerobic bacteria forming spherical or ovoid cells less than 2 μm in diameter. The reader is referred to Procedures for Initial Differentiation of Genera with Negative or Weak Catalase Reactions in chapter 19 for a description of the catalase test. Although the streptococci grow in the presence of oxygen, they are unable to synthesize heme compounds and are therefore incapable of respiratory metabolism. Some strains of *S. pneumoniae* and certain viridans species require elevated (5%) CO_2 levels for growth; the growth of many streptococcal isolates is stimulated in a CO_2-enriched atmosphere. Streptococci are nutritionally fastidious, with variable nutritional requirements, and growth on complex media is enhanced by the addition of blood or serum. Glucose and other carbohydrates are metabolized fermentatively, and lactic acid is produced as the major metabolic end product. Gas is not produced as a result of glucose metabolism. Isolates of streptococci produce the enzyme leucine aminopeptidase, but production of pyrrolidonyl arylamidase (PYR) is rare among streptococci, occurring only in isolates of *S. pyogenes* and some strains of pneumococci.

NATURAL HABITATS

Streptococci are usually found as parasites of humans and other animals. While some streptococci function as virulent pathogens, other strains live harmoniously with their hosts as normally avirulent commensals. Streptococci are transient colonizers of skin and resident colonizers of mucous membranes. They can be isolated as part of the normal flora of the alimentary, respiratory, and genital tracts.

CLINICAL SIGNIFICANCE

Group A Streptococci (*S. pyogenes*)

Beta-hemolytic, bacitracin-susceptible, PYR-positive, large-colony-forming streptococci with Lancefield's group A antigen are included in the species *S. pyogenes* and represent one of the most impressive human pathogens. The numerous virulence factors of *S. pyogenes* (M protein, lipoteichoic acid, enzymes, and toxins) allow it to cause a wide array of serious infections including pharyngitis, respiratory infection, skin (impetigo, erysipelas) and soft tissue infections, endocarditis, meningitis, puerperal sepsis, and arthritis. Infection with toxin-producing strains can result in scarlet fever or more serious toxic shock-like symptoms.

Group A streptococcal pharyngitis is characterized by pharyngeal pain, swelling, and erythema accompanied by fever and anterior cervical adenopathy. Suppurative sequelae of streptococcal pharyngitis may result from the spread of infection to contiguous tissue or from bacteremic dissemination. Nonsuppurative sequelae include rheumatic fever and acute glomerulonephritis. While either of these conditions may follow pharyngitis, only glomerulonephritis is linked with group A streptococcal infections of the skin.

In recent years, there has been an increase in the number of reports from North America and Europe of severe group A streptococcal infection associated with a toxic shock-like syndrome. Many of the streptococcal isolates from these patients produce M protein type 1 or 3, but current hypotheses suggest that streptococcal pyrogenic exotoxins are more directly involved in the production of severe infection with shock. The ability of pyrogenic exotoxins to act as superantigens, like the staphylococcal toxic shock toxin, is thought to contribute to the production of shock in these infections (73).

Group B Streptococci

Beta-hemolytic streptococci with Lancefield's group B antigen (*S. agalactiae*) are an important cause of serious neonatal infection characterized by sepsis and meningitis. Colonization of the maternal genital tract is associated with colonization of infants and risk of neonatal disease. Early-onset infection occurs within the first few days after delivery and often is associated with pneumonia, while late-onset disease usually appears after 1 week of age. Group B streptococci are also associated with postpartum infections. Conditions that predispose nonpregnant adults to group B streptococcal infection include diabetes mellitus, cancer, and human immunodeficiency virus infection. Group B infections of adults include bacteremia, endocarditis, skin and soft tissue infection, and osteomyelitis (82).

Other Beta-Hemolytic Streptococci

Human isolates of group C and G streptococci that form large colonies are pyogenic streptococci similar to *S. pyogenes* with respect to virulence traits; they cause a wide range of serious infections such as bacteremia, endocarditis, meningitis, septic arthritis, and infections of the respiratory tract and skin. The clinical symptoms of pharyngeal infection caused by these streptococci are similar to those of group A pharyngitis, except for the strong association of *S. pyogenes* with nonsuppurative sequelae. Poststreptococcal glomerulonephritis has, however, also occasionally been associated with outbreaks of group C pharyngitis (5, 27). Strains of large-colony-forming group C and G streptococci normally isolated from animals have also been noted infrequently as agents of human infection.

Small-colony-forming beta-hemolytic streptococcal strains may express Lancefield group A, C, F, or G antigen or may be nongroupable. These streptococci are usually identified as members of the anginosus or "*S. milleri*" group of species (see Viridans Streptococci, below). Although these organisms can be isolated from pyogenic infections (notably abscesses), they appear to reside in the pharynx as commensals and are not considered to be agents of pharyngitis (77).

Streptococcus pneumoniae

The pneumococcus is an important agent of community-acquired pneumonia that may be accompanied by bacteremia. Oropharyngeal carriage of pneumococci is common and contributes to the difficulty in interpreting the significance of pneumococci in cultures of expectorated sputum. Other pneumococcal infections include otitis media, sinusitis, meningitis, and endocarditis. Vaccines designed to protect against infection by pneumococci with predominant capsular polysaccharide types are now available.

Viridans Streptococci

Viridans streptococci are normal inhabitants of the oral cavity, gastrointestinal tract, and female genital tract, and they are often considered to be contaminants when isolated from blood cultures. However, their presence may be associated with subacute bacterial endocarditis, especially in patients with prosthetic valves; *S. sanguis, S. mitis, S. oralis*, and *S. gordonii* are frequently isolated (13, 23). *S. intermedius* is often isolated as a member of the polymicrobial flora of deep-seated abscesses, notably in the liver and brain (85). Other members of the anginosus or "*S. milleri*" group may be isolated from oral abscesses, with *S. anginosus* also being isolated from female genital infections. The viridans streptococci are playing an increasing role in infections in neutropenic patients (11). Complications associated with bacteremia in these patients include endocarditis, acute respiratory distress syndrome, and shock (12, 28). The major species causing infections in neutropenic patients are *S. oralis, S. mitis*, and *S. salivarius* (7, 48). The use of commercial kits to identify the viridans streptococci has meant that in many studies *S. oralis* is identified incorrectly as "*S. mitis*."

Streptococcus bovis

Bacteremia caused by *S. bovis* isolates, particularly biotype I, is associated with malignancies of the gastrointestinal tract (68). These organisms are also agents of endocarditis and have been isolated from patients with meningitis (66).

Other Streptococci Isolated Infrequently from Human Clinical Specimens

A few streptococcal species that appear to be pathogens primarily in animals have been documented as agents of human infection. *S. suis*, a pathogen of swine, has been noted as an agent of meningitis in humans (74). Some *S. suis* strains can produce a beta-hemolytic reaction on horse blood agar, but all are alpha-hemolytic on agars containing sheep blood. These organisms are serologically heterogeneous, with strains expressing Lancefield group R, S, or T antigen and a variety of capsular antigens (75). *S. porcinus*, also a pathogen of pigs, has been identified occasionally as an agent of human infection (29). Strains of this species are beta-hemolytic on sheep blood agar and may produce Lancefield group E, P, U, or V antigen; while positive for the production of PYR like *S. pyogenes*, *S. porcinus* is bacitracin resistant. *S. porcinus* strains produce a positive CAMP reaction but are differentiated from group B streptococci by virtue of their ability to produce PYR.

S. iniae, a fish pathogen, has been associated with cellulitis, bacteremia, endocarditis, and meningitis in humans who had a history of handling fish (often tilapia, a freshwater fish) while suffering from percutaneous injuries. Molecular typing evidence suggested that an invasive clone of the organism was responsible for causing observed cases of disease in humans as well as in fish. *S. iniae* strains form a narrow zone of beta-hemolysis surrounded by a larger alpha-hemolytic zone and are sometimes mistakenly characterized as alpha-hemolytic. Beta-hemolysis is reliably observed in anaerobically incubated cultures. *S. iniae* strains are PYR positive and Voges-Proskauer negative, and they show variable suceptibilities to bacitracin, making some isolates physiologically similar to *S. pyogenes*. They do not, however, react with Lancefield group A or other group antisera (79, 80).

COLLECTION, TRANSPORT, AND STORAGE OF SPECIMENS

Specimens suspected of harboring streptococci should be collected by methods outlined elsewhere in this manual. In general, a transport system need not be used if the transport time is under 2 h. Although some streptococci (e.g., *S. pyogenes*) can survive desiccation and refrigeration, other strains (e.g., pneumococci) are fairly fragile, and thus every effort should be made to process specimens as soon as possible.

Recommendations have recently been formulated by the Centers for Disease Control and Prevention for collection of specimens used to establish carriage of group B streptococci in pregnant women (16). Pregnant women should be cultured at 35 to 37 weeks' gestation. Rectal and vaginal swabs should be collected and placed into a nonnutritive moist swab transport system. The specimens may be held under refrigeration or at room temperature for up to 4 days before culture in a selective broth medium (see Special Procedures for Group B Streptococci, below).

ISOLATION PROCEDURES

General Procedures

Many commonly used nonselective laboratory media support the growth of streptococci; complex media enriched with blood are desirable because the hemolytic reaction of the streptococcal isolate may be determined early in the identification process. Hemolytic patterns may vary with the source of animal blood or type of basal medium used in blood agars. Media selective for gram-positive bacteria (e.g., phenylethyl alcohol or Columbia with colistin and nalidixic acid agars) will also support the growth of streptococci.

Cultures for isolation of streptococci should be incubated at 35 to 37°C. Ambient atmospheres are suitable for many streptococci, but since pneumococci and some viridans strains require elevated CO_2 concentrations, incubation in an atmosphere containing 5% CO_2 or in a candle jar will enhance the recovery of streptococcal isolates. Streptococci grow well in anaerobic atmospheres, but their facultative nature makes anaerobic incubation unnecessary for isolation.

Special Procedures for Throat Cultures

Complex media containing 5% sheep blood are usually recommended for the culture of throat specimens because NADase activity in sheep blood reduces the NAD content to levels insufficient for the growth of *Haemophilus haemolyticus*, a commensal that forms colonies that might be confused with those of beta-hemolytic streptococci. Throat swabs should be rolled firmly over one-sixth of the plate to deposit the specimen. A loop is used to carefully streak the inoculum over the surface of the plate. The loop is then used (without sterilization) to stab the agar several times in an area of the plate that has not been streaked, in an effort to deposit beta-hemolytic streptococci beneath the agar surface. Subsurface growth will display the most reliable hemolytic reactions, due to the activity of both oxygen-stable and oxygen-labile streptolysins. Other procedures involving overnight incubation of swabs in broth for enrichment of streptococci and a pour-streak plate method for culturing throat specimens have also been described (32).

In a coherent review of methods designed to improve recovery of beta-hemolytic streptococci from throat specimens, Kellogg (52) concluded that 90 to 95% of *S. pyogenes* isolates from symptomatic patients should be detected by any of the following protocols: sheep blood agar incubated anaerobically for 48 h, sheep blood agar incubated aerobically for 48 h without CO_2 supplementation (a coverglass may be placed over the primary inoculation area to reduce oxygen tension and enhance hemolysis), and sheep blood agar plus trimethoprim-sulfamethoxazole incubated anaerobically for 48 h. Cultures should be examined after 18 to 24 h of incubation and reincubated if negative, with a final examination at 48 h. Increased isolations of group A streptococci on sheep blood agar during the second 24 h of incubation have ranged from 2 to 46% in published studies. Incubation of throat culture plates in a CO_2-enriched atmosphere seems to encourage the recovery of non-group A beta-hemolytic streptococci. There is no consensus on whether a predominance of large-colony-forming group C or G streptococci should be reported. The reader is referred to Kellogg's review (52) and a study evaluating two commercially available selective media (81) for further details.

Special Procedures for Group B Streptococci

Detection of group B streptococci in the genital tracts of pregnant women can identify infants at risk for infection and guide intrapartum administration of antibiotics. As described above, vaginal and rectal swabs, or a single swab inserted into the vagina and then the rectum, should be collected at 35 to 37 weeks of gestation and inoculated into a selective broth medium. The Centers for Disease Control and Prevention recommend the use of Todd-Hewitt broth containing either 10 μg of colistin per ml and 15 μg of nalidixic acid per ml or 8 μg of gentamicin per ml and 15 μg of nalidixic acid per ml. Selective media are commercially available and should be incubated for 18 to 24 h before being subcultured to sheep blood agar. The blood agar subcultures should be examined for group B streptococci after 24 h of incubation and, if negative at the first observation, should be reexamined after a second 24-h incubation (16).

IDENTIFICATION

Direct Detection

Direct detection of streptococci by Gram stains is most useful when applied to specimens that are normally devoid of indigenous streptococcal flora. The Quellung test is a more specific method for microscopic detection of pneumococci in specimens and relies on the visual enhancement of the pneumococcal capsule after reaction of the streptococci with anticapsular antisera (32). Other specific microscopic methods for detecting group A and B streptococci have involved immunofluorescent staining (32).

Direct detection of streptococcal antigens has been used to identify group A streptococci in throat specimens. The sensitivities of these techniques depend not only on the method used but also on the numbers of streptococci present in the sample. In general, streptococci are transferred from the swab containing the specimen to a chemical (e.g., nitrous acid) or enzymatic (e.g., pronase) extraction solution. After a short incubation period, antigen in the suspension is detected by agglutination methods (36), enzyme immunoassay (26, 45), or other methods (37, 41). While antigen detection methods are rapid and specific, false-negative results may occur with specimens containing small numbers of streptococci. Since low streptococcal counts may be clinically significant, negative antigen detection tests should be followed up with culture (36).

Antigen detection techniques have also been used for the rapid identification of group B streptococci in urogenital specimens. Of the methods involving direct detection from specimens, latex agglutination assays (39), enzyme immunoassay methods (38, 88), and optical immunoassay methods (15) have not proven sensitive enough to detect low levels of colonization and are consequently not recommended for screening pregnant women for group B streptococcal carriage. These methods do, however, seem to be effective in identifying heavily colonized women. Older methods, involving incubation of specimens in a selective medium for 5 to 20 h before antigen testing via agglutination, will reveal even light colonization (58).

Normally sterile body fluids may also be tested directly for streptococcal antigens. Commercially available products that detect the Lancefield antigen of group B streptococci and the capsular polysaccharide antigen of penumococci may be used to determine the presence of these organisms in cerebrospinal fluid and in blood cultures. The clinical usefulness of these rapid bacterial antigen detection tests is, however, currently being debated (76).

A nucleic acid probe-based test for the direct detection of group A streptococci in throat swabs is commercially available (43). Additional evaluation of this or similar products is necessary before their true utility and cost-effectiveness can be established. The use of commercially available nucleic acid probe tests for the direct detection of *S. pneumoniae* and group B streptococci from positive blood cultures has also been described (20), along with probe-based detection of group B streptococci in genital specimens (56).

Hemolytic Reactions

Beta-hemolysis appears as complete clearing (lysis of erythrocytes) of the medium. This reaction may be obscured by the inhibition of streptolysin O by oxygen, or production of peroxide by streptococci growing in air or in the presence of increased CO_2 concentrations; thus, anaerobic incubation or observation of hemolysis in the area of stabs in the agar is optimal for accurate determination of beta-hemolytic reactions. In the alpha-hemolytic reaction, erythrocytes are not completely lysed but growth is surrounded by greenish discoloration of the agar due to streptococcal action on hemoglobin. Nonhemolytic or gamma-hemolytic streptococci have no effect on blood agar.

Description of Colonies

Streptococcal colonies vary in color from gray to whitish and usually glisten, although dry colonies are also observed. The beta-hemolytic pyogenic streptococci of groups A, C, and G form relatively large colonies (>0.5 mm in diameter after 24 h of incubation) compared with the pinpoint colonies of the small-colony-forming beta-hemolytic strains of the anginosus or "*S. milleri*" group. Strains of *S. pyogenes* occasionally form mucoid colonies.

Cultures of the small-colony-forming beta-hemolytic streptococci and other anginosus group strains may produce a distinct odor, which has been described as buttery or caramel-like and has been attributed to the production of diacetyl by these bacteria (17). Colonies of group B streptococci tend to be larger and have less pronounced zones of beta-hemolysis than do other beta-hemolytic strains; some group B strains are nonhemolytic.

Alpha-hemolytic colonies with depressions in their centers are characteristic of pneumococci, while colonies of viridans streptococci have a domed appearance. Pneumococci may also produce different amounts of capsular polysaccharide, contributing to a mucoid colonial appearance. Some viridans streptococcal strains, along with *S. bovis*, form nonhemolytic, grayish colonies.

Identification of Beta-Hemolytic Isolates: Serological Tests

Numerous products using rapid antigen extraction methods and agglutination techniques for antigen detection are available commercially for the Lancefield grouping of beta-hemolytic isolates. Descriptions of older antigen extraction methods and a protocol for precipitin testing can be found elsewhere (32). The presence of the group B antigen seems to correlate closely with a strain's identity as *S. agalactiae*, and most group F beta-hemolytic small-colony-forming strains appear to be members of the anginosus or "*S. milleri*" group of species. Lancefield antigens of groups A, C, and G, however, are not specific for a single streptococcal species. Organisms with these antigens can be differentiated by biochemical tests, as summarized in Table 1. When beta-hemolytic isolates that fail to react with Lancefield group A, B, C, F, or G antisera are encountered, physiological characterization may aid in identification.

Identification of Beta-Hemolytic Isolates: Physiological Tests

PYR Test

The PYR test determines the activity of PYR, also called pyrrolidonyl aminopeptidase, an enzyme produced by *S. pyogenes* but not by other beta-hemolytic streptococci except for the rarely encountered animal-associated species *S. porcinus* and *S. iniae* (see Other Streptococci Isolated Infrequently from Human Clinical Specimens, above). Products using rapid methods for performance of the PYR test are commercially available. Since other organisms that may be isolated along with *S. pyogenes* may also give a positive PYR reaction, only pure cultures or isolated colonies of beta-hemolytic streptococci should be tested. Beta-hemolytic strains of enterococci might be confused with *S. pyogenes*, since both organisms are PYR positive. Differences in colony size and morphology and other traits should allow for differentiation of these bacteria (see chapter 18).

TABLE 1 Differentiating characteristics of beta-hemolytic streptococci of human origin[a]

Lancefield group	Colony size	Species	PYR	VP[b]	CAMP	BGUR
A	Large	*S. pyogenes*	+	−	−	
A	Small	Anginosus group[c]	−	+	−	
B		*S. agalactiae*	−		+	
C	Large	*S. dysgalactiae* subsp. *equisimilis*[d]	−	−	−	+
C	Small	Anginosus group[c]	−	+	−	−
F	Small	Anginosus group[c]	−	+	−	
G	Large	*S. dysgalactiae* subsp. *equisimilis*[d]	−	−	−	+
G	Small	Anginosus group[c]	−	+	−	−
Nongroupable	Small	Anginosus group[c]	−	+	−	

[a] Abbreviations and symbols: +, positive; −, negative; CAMP, CAMP test for synergistic hemolysis.

[b] VP test results for group B streptococci (*S. agalactiae*) have been omitted from the table due to conflicting reports in the literature (32, 42), which may have resulted from the use of different test methods. The VP test result is not critical for the identification of group B streptococci.

[c] Also called the "*S. milleri*" group.

[d] Current data suggest that large-colony-forming group C and G beta-hemolytic strains of human origin are related at the species level. The name *S. dysgalactiae* subsp. *equisimilis* has been proposed for these streptococci (78). The ability to ferment trehalose and sorbitol was used in the past to differentiate group C beta-hemolytic streptococci into the species *S. equi*, *S. equisimilis*, and *S. zooepidemicus*. See the text and Table 2 for the current classification of group C and G streptococci.

Bacitracin Susceptibility

Although *S. pyogenes* can be identified rapidly by antigenic methods or the PYR test, a test for bacitracin susceptibility can be helpful in differentiating *S. pyogenes* from small-colony-forming group A strains or from other PYR-positive, beta-hemolytic species (see Other Streptococci Isolated Infrequently from Human Clinical Specimens, above). A 0.04-U bacitracin disk is applied to a sheep blood agar plate that has been heavily inoculated with three or four colonies of a pure culture of the streptococcus to be tested. After overnight incubation at 35°C, any zone of inhibition around the disk is interpreted as susceptibility (30).

VP Test

The Voges-Proskauer (VP) test for acetoin production will differentiate small-colony-forming beta-hemolytic anginosus ("*S. milleri*") group strains with Lancefield group A, C, or G antigens from large-colony-forming pyogenic strains with the same Lancefield antigens (Table 1). Facklam and Washington (32) described a version of this test for streptococci in which overnight growth from an entire agar plate culture is used to inoculate 2 ml of VP broth. After 6 h of incubation at 35°C, Coblentz reagents A and B are added, and the tube is shaken and incubated at room temperature for 30 min. A positive test is indicated by the development of a cherry red (or even slightly pink) color.

BGUR Test

The BGUR test assays for the action of β-D-glucuronidase (BGUR), an enzyme produced by human isolates of large-colony-forming beta-hemolytic group C and G streptococci but not by their small-colony-forming anginosus group ("*S. milleri*") counterparts (Table 1). Rapid methods for the BGUR test are commercially available. In addition, the use of methylumbelliferyl-β-D-glucuronide-containing MacConkey agar, normally used for the isolation and presumptive identification of *Escherichia coli*, in a rapid fluorogenic assay for BGUR in streptococcal strains has been described (55).

Differentiation of Large-Colony Group C and G Isolates by Carbohydrate Fermentation Tests

Traditionally, large-colony-forming group C isolates have been differentiated into species on the basis of their ability to ferment various carbohydrates. Studies of the genetic relatedness of group C and G streptococci have, however, shown that human isolates classified in the traditional group C species *S. equisimilis* are genetically similar enough to large-colony-forming group G human isolates to be classified in the same species, which was given the name *S. dysgalactiae*. Strains formerly classified as *S. zooepidemicus* were considered, on the basis of genetic data, to form a subspecies of *S. equi* (33). A subsequent study of these organisms proposed the division of *S. dysgalactiae* into two subspecies, *S. dysgalactiae* subsp. *equisimilis* to accommodate beta-hemolytic large-colony-forming group C and G strains isolated from humans and *S. dysgalactiae* subsp. *dysgalactiae* as the name for beta-, alpha-, and nonhemolytic animal strains with group C or L antigen (78). *S. canis*, an additional species composed of beta-hemolytic group G streptococci normally isolated from animals, has been noted as an infrequent cause of human infection (11).

Table 2 displays some differentiating features of the currently recognized species of large-colony-forming beta-hemolytic streptococci that may express Lancefield group C or G antigen. The table includes their reactions in trehalose and sorbitol fermentation broths, media that have traditionally been used to differentiate strains isolated from human clinical infections. Heart infusion broth containing 1.0% carbohydrate and bromcresol purple as an indicator (62) can be used for characterization of these bacteria if differentiation beyond the level of Lancefield serological characteristics is desired. Strains of group C and G streptococci that are normally isolated from domesticated animals are occasionally reported as agents of human infection.

CAMP Test

The majority of group B streptococci produce a diffusable extracellular protein (CAMP factor) that acts synergistically with staphylococcal beta lysin to lyse erythrocytes. Single straight streaks of the streptococcus to be tested and a beta lysin-producing *Staphylococcus aureus* strain are made perpendicular to each other and about 3 to 4 mm apart on the surface of a sheep blood agar plate. After overnight incubation in ambient atmosphere at 35°C, a positive test is characterized by an arrowhead-shaped zone of complete hemolysis in the area into which both staphylococcal beta lysin and CAMP factor have diffused (32). An alternative

TABLE 2 Differentiating features of human and animal strains of large-colony-forming beta-hemolytic streptococci with Lancefield's group C or G antigen[a]

Species	Lancefield antigen(s)	Hosts	Trehalose	Sorbitol
S. dysgalactiae subsp. *equisimilis*[b]	C, G	Humans	+	−
S. dysgalactiae subsp. *dysgalactiae*[b]	C, L	Animals	+	−[c]
S. equi subsp. *equi*	C	Animals	−	−
S. equi subsp. *zooepidemicus*	C		−	+
S. canis[d]	G	Animals	−	−[c]

[a] Symbols: +, positive; −, negative.

[b] *S. dysgalactiae* subsp. *equisimilis*, characteristically isolated from humans, exhibits proteolytic activity on human fibrin and streptokinase activity on human plasminogen. Both activities are lacking in *S. dysgalactiae* subsp. *dysgalactiae* strains, which are normally isolated from animals and may be alpha- or nonhemolytic as well as beta-hemolytic and may produce Lancefield group C or L antigen (78).

[c] Exceptions may occur.

[d] Most strains of *S. canis* are negative for the production of BGUR, in contrast to most other strains of large-colony-forming beta-hemolytic group C or G streptococci.

method, using beta lysin-containing disks, has also been described (87).

Hippurate Hydrolysis Test

The ability to hydrolyze hippurate is an alternate test for the presumptive identification of group B streptococci. A rapid version of this test involves incubating cells in a 1% aqueous sodium hippurate solution for 2 h and detecting glycine formed as an end product of hippurate hydrolysis with ninhydrin reagent (47).

Identification of Beta-Hemolytic Isolates: Nucleic Acid Probe Tests

Nucleic acid probes for identification of cultured isolates of group A and B streptococci are currently available (19, 43).

Identification of Non-Beta-Hemolytic Isolates: Serological Tests

Serological testing can be useful for revealing non-beta-hemolytic strains of group B streptococci. Testing for Lancefield's group D antigen may aid in the identification of *S. bovis*, but this antigen is not easily demonstrated in some strains. Moreover, the group D antigen is nonspecific; it is produced by certain streptococci and by members of the genera *Enterococcus* and *Pediococcus*. Physiological testing is more reliable for identifying non-beta-hemolytic isolates.

Identification of Non-Beta-Hemolytic Streptococci: Physiological Tests

Table 3 summarizes the physiological characteristics of non-beta-hemolytic (alpha- and nonhemolytic) streptococci. It should be remembered that non-beta-hemolytic strains of group B streptococci can be differentiated from the streptococci mentioned below by the CAMP test or serological testing. The optochin and bile solubility tests are used to differentiate pneumococci from viridans streptococci; viridans streptococci can be further characterized to the species or species group level by using physiological testing and identification kits [see Identification of Viridans and Group D Streptococci (*S. bovis*), below].

The nonhemolytic streptococci may belong to the species *S. bovis* or to various viridans species. The ability of *S. bovis* to hydrolyze the glycoside esculin in the presence of 40% bile distinguishes it from the majority of viridans strains. Complete characterization of *S. bovis* to the biotype level can be accomplished with commercially available products (69). The CAMP test may be of use for testing isolates suspected of being non-beta-hemolytic group B streptococci.

Optochin Test

Commercially available optochin disks are applied to a quarter of a blood agar plate that has been streaked with a few colonies of the organism to be tested. After overnight incubation at 35°C in either a candle jar or CO_2 incubator, inhibition zones are measured. Zones of >14 mm with a 6-mm disk or >16 mm with a 10-mm disk are indicative of inhibition and identify the isolate as *S. pneumoniae*. Isolates displaying smaller zones of inhibition should be subjected to an additional test for bile solubility to confirm their identity (32).

Bile Solubility Test

Aliquots containing 0.5 ml of a 0.5 to 1.0 McFarland saline suspension of the organisms to be tested are added to each of two small (13- by 100-mm) test tubes. An equal amount (0.5 ml) of 2% sodium deoxycholate (bile) is added to one tube, while 0.5 ml of saline is added to the second tube as a control. A positive bile solubility test (indicative of pneumococci) appears as clearing in the presence of deoxycholate but not in the control tube after incubation at 35°C for up to 2 h (32). In some reports, 10% sodium deoxycholate has been used in this procedure, resulting in a final deoxycholate concentration of 5% instead of 1% as in the method in reference 32.

In a plate method for testing bile solubility, a drop of a solution of 10% sodium deoxycholate is placed directly on a colony of the strain to be tested. The plate can be kept at room temperature or placed into an aerobic incubator at 35°C for approximately 15 min until the reagent dries but must be kept level to prevent the reagent from running over the plate and washing away the colony. Pneumococcal colonies will disappear or be flattened, while bile-resistant streptococcal colonies will be unaffected (6). The use of 2% sodium deoxycholate in this method has been documented in older reports in the literature.

TABLE 3 Differentiation of non-beta-hemolytic streptococci[a]

Streptococcus	Optochin susceptible	Bile soluble	Bile esculin
S. pneumoniae[b]	+	+	−
Viridans streptococci	−	−	−[c]
S. bovis	−	−	+

[a] Symbols: +, positive; −, negative. Strains of group B streptococci (*S. agalactiae*) may be non-beta-hemolytic; serological methods or the CAMP or hippurate hydrolysis test should be used to rule out possible group B strains.

[b] Some strains of *S. pneumoniae* may be PYR positive.

[c] Occasional strains of viridans streptococci produce weakly positive bile esculin reactions.

Bile Esculin Test

Bile esculin medium (available from commercial sources) in either plates or slants should be inoculated with one to three colonies of the organism to be tested and incubated at 35°C in an ambient atmosphere for up to 48 h. A definitive blackening of plated media or blackening of at least half of an agar slant is considered a positive test, indicative of *S. bovis* (32). A few viridans strains are positive in this test or display weakly positive reactions that are difficult to interpret (69). Isolates from patients with serious infections (e.g., endocarditis) should be more completely characterized (see below), as opposed to being identified as *S. bovis* on the basis of the bile esculin test alone.

Identification of Non-Beta-Hemolytic Isolates: Nucleic Acid Probe Tests

A nucleic acid probe test for identification of pneumococcal isolates is now commercially available (21).

Identification of Viridans and Group D Streptococci (*S. bovis*)

Viridans streptococci have traditionally been difficult to identify (71). The relatively limited usefulness of traditional methods such as possession of a Lancefield group antigen, the type of hemolysis produced on blood agar, and species delineation by phenotypic testing alone has often been made worse by nomenclatural differences (31, 44). Application of chemotaxonomic and genome-based techniques, particularly DNA-DNA reassociation, has led to a considerable increase in the number of species recognized, and in retrospect it is easy to appreciate how the taxonomic complexity of the viridans streptococci defied resolution for so long. However, improved identification schemes that provide a means by which the currently recognized viridans species may be identified have been developed (8, 54). Commercially available identification kits have also begun to adjust to this increase in the number of species by expanding their repertoire of tests (35). However, it should be noted that the nomenclature systems used among these products are not always uniform (44). In addition, it may be that not all recognized species are represented in the database and that identification "problem areas" may persist, requiring the use of additional tests before a confident identification can be made (35, 53).

In a study of the genus *Streptococcus* based on sequence comparisons of the small-subunit (16S) rRNA gene, a total of six species groups were demonstrated, five of which include the species considered in this section. These five were designated (i) the mitis group, (ii) the anginosus group, (iii) the mutans group, (iv) the salivarius group, and (v) the bovis group (51). Two alpha-hemolytic species, *S. acidominimus* and *S. suis* (the latter is beta-hemolytic on horse blood), remained ungrouped in this and also in a similar, previous study (10), while *S. ferus*, a candidate for inclusion in the mutans group of species, isolated from rats, has yet to be unequivocally classified. The members of these species groups commonly isolated from humans and their differential physiological traits are shown in Tables 4 to 6. Brief descriptions of these species are given below.

Mitis Group

The mitis group includes *S. mitis*, *S. sanguis*, *S. parasanguis*, *S. gordonii*, *S. crista*, and *S. oralis*, together with *S. pneumoniae*. This group of alpha-hemolytic streptococci includes several species that are of known clinical significance, together with others for which few or no clinical data have been collected. The classification and nomenclature of the members of this group have been a source of considerable confusion in the past. Current species descriptions for *S. sanguis*, *S. gordonii*, *S. oralis*, and *S. mitis*, all of which are found in mature dental plaque, are those of Kilian et al. (54), who provide a comprehensive review and discussion of the history of these species epithets and the taxa to which they have been applied. Both *S. parasanguis* and *S. crista* have been described more recently (40, 85). *S. sanguis* forms part of the normal dental plaque flora of humans and is among the most common species of viridans streptococci isolated from bacterial endocarditis when the strains isolated were identified according to modern species definitions (24). Strains produce extracellular polysaccharide (dextran) from sucrose to give hard, adherent, smooth colonies. The majority of strains react with Lancefield group H antiserum raised against strain Blackburn (British group H). Subdivision of *S. sanguis* on the basis of biochemical characteristics has been suggested, although it is difficult to equate the biovars of one study (54) with the biotypes of another (8); the clinical relevance of these is unknown. *S. gordonii* is also relatively common in patients with bacterial endocarditis, and the majority of strains produce colonies like those of *S. sanguis* on sucrose agar. Strains of this species frequently react with Lancefield group H antiserum raised against strain F90A (ATCC 12396) or against strain Blackburn. One point of confusion with these streptococci has been that the previous type strain of *S. mitis* prior to the emended description of this species by Kilian et al. (54) was strain NCTC 3165 but has since been replaced by a new type strain, NCTC 12261^T. NCTC 3165 was subsequently included within *S. gordonii*. *S. oralis* and *S. mitis* are both characterized by an unusual cell wall type, which contains ribitol teichoic acid and lacks significant amounts of rhamnose. *S. oralis* is relatively common in patients with endocarditis; *S. mitis* is found less frequently. Extracellular polysaccharide production is a variable characteristic of *S. oralis* and is negative in *S. mitis*. *S. parasanguis* and *S. crista* are the two most recent additions to the mitis group, and little clinical information about them is currently available. *S. parasanguis* has been isolated from clinical specimens (throats, blood, and urine), while *S. crista* strains originated from the mouth and upper respiratory tract (dental plaque, periodontal abscess, and throat). Both are alpha-hemolytic and hydrolyze arginine but not esculin. Extracellular polysaccharide production is negative for *S. parasanguis* and is a variable characteristic of *S. crista*. The latter species is also characterized by the presence of lateral tufts of fibrils on the cell surface. Differential characteristics of species in the mitis group are shown in Table 4.

Anginosus Group

The anginosus group includes *S. anginosus*, *S. constellatus*, and *S. intermedius*. A confused nomenclatural history surrounds this group, which now includes streptococci previously referred to as *Streptococcus*-MG, hemolytic and nonhemolytic streptococci possessing the type antigens of Lancefield group F, the minute-colony-forming streptococci of Lancefield groups F and G, *S. milleri*, the "*Streptococcus milleri* group," *S.* MG-*intermedius*, *S. anginosus-constellatus*, *S. anginosus*, *S. constellatus*, and *S. intermedius*. Currently the group is divided into three distinct, closely related species that have retained the names *S. anginosus*, *S. constellatus*, and *S. intermedius*, albeit with emended descriptions (84, 86). Together, these form part of the oral and genitouri-

TABLE 4 Differentiation of species in the mitis group[a]

Test	*S. sanguis* biotype 1[b]	*S. sanguis* biotype 2[b]	*S. sanguis* biotype 3[b]	*S. parasanguis*	*S. gordonii*	*S. crista*	*S. oralis*	*S. mitis*
Enzyme activity								
β-D-Fucosidase	−	+	+	V	−	−	−	−
β-*N*-Acetylgal[c]	−	−	−	+	V	+	+	−
Neuraminidase	−	−	−	−	−	−	+	V
α-L-Fucosidase	−	−	−	V	+	+	−	−
β-*N*-Acetylglu[d]	−	V	+	+	+	+	+	−
α-D-Glucosidase	−	−	−	+	V	−	+	+
β-D-Glucosidase	V	+	V	V	+	−	−	−
α-Arabinosidase	−	−	−	V	−	−	−	−
α-D-Galactosidase	V	+	−	+	−	−	V	V
β-D-Galactosidase	−	V	+	+	V	V	V	V
Acid from:								
Amygdalin	−	+	−	V	+	−	−	−
Inulin	V	V	V	−	+	−	−	−
Mannitol	−	−	−	−	−	−	−	−
N-Acetylglucosamine	+	+	+	+	+	+	+	+
Raffinose	+	+	−	V	−	−	V	+
Sorbitol	V	V	−	−	−	−	−	−
Arbutin	+	+	V	V	+	+	−	−
Lactose	+	+	+	+	+	V	+	V
Melibiose	+	V	−	V	−	−	V	+
Hydrolysis of:								
Arginine	+	+	+	+	+	V	−	−
Esculin	+	+	−	V	+	−	V	−
Production of:								
Acetoin (VP test)	−	−	−	−	−	−	−	−
Urease	−	−	−	−	−	−	−	−
Hyaluronidase	−	−	−	−	−	−	−	−

[a] Symbols: +, positive; −, negative; V, variable.
[b] Biotypes are those of Beighton et al. (8).
[c] β-*N*-Acetyl-gal, β-*N*-acetylgalactosaminidase.
[d] β-*N*-Acetylglu, β-*N*-acetylglucosaminidase.

nary flora and are isolated from the gastrointestinal tract. They are clinically significant, being associated with purulent infections at oral and nonoral sites. Strains may be non-, alpha-, or beta-hemolytic on blood agar, although a higher proportion of *S. intermedius* strains are nonhemolytic. Growth is frequently enhanced in the presence of 5% CO_2, with some strains requiring anaerobic conditions. No extracellular polysaccharide is produced. *S. anginosus* strains may possess Lancefield group A, C, F, or G antigens or be nongroupable. Mannitol-fermenting strains of this species are frequently isolated from the female genitourinary tract, although the role of these in infections is uncertain. *S. constellatus* strains are frequently beta-hemolytic and mainly possess Lancefield group F antigens or are nongroupable, although some strains may be of group A, C, or G. Strains of this species have been relatively frequently isolated from thoracic sites and from the respiratory tract, although anatomical associations in infections are less clear than for the other members of the group. *S. intermedius* seems to be less serologically diverse with respect to Lancefield group antigens than the other group members, with strains being either nongroupable or of group F. There is a strong association between this species and brain and liver abscesses. Differential characteristics of the species in the anginosus group are shown in Table 5.

Mutans Group

The mutans group includes *S. mutans*, *S. sobrinus*, *S. cricetus*, *S. rattus*, *S. downei*, and *S. macacae*. These species are associated with dental caries in humans and animals and are characterized by the production of water-soluble and -insoluble extracellular polysaccharides from sucrose and by the ability to produce acid from a relatively wide range of carbohydrates. *S. mutans* and *S. sobrinus* are the species most frequently isolated from dental plaque and carious lesions in humans, whereas *S. cricetus* and *S. rattus* are rarely recovered. *S. downei* and *S. macacae* are isolated from monkeys. *S. mutans* cells may form short rods on solid media or in broth culture under acidic conditions. On blood agar, colonies are often hard and adherent, usually alpha-hemolytic, with occasional strains giving beta-hemolysis. *S. sobrinus* strains are mostly nonhemolytic or occasionally alpha-hemolytic. On sucrose-containing agar, colonies are rough, heaped, and surrounded by liquid containing glucan. *S. rattus* colonies are rubbery on sucrose agar or, as with *S. cricetus*, may be rough and heaped with surrounding liquid glucan.

Differential characteristics of *S. mutans* and *S. sobrinus* are shown in Table 6.

Salivarius Group

The salivarius group includes *S. salivarius*, *S. vestibularis*, and *S. thermophilus*. *S. salivarius* and *S. vestibularis* both inhabit the human oral cavity, in contrast to the third member of the group, *S. thermophilus*, which is isolated from dairy sources. *S. salivarius* is isolated from most areas within the mouth, especially the tongue, mucosal surfaces, and saliva. *S. vestibularis* was initially isolated from the oral vestibule, although the full extent of its colonization of the oral surfaces has not been determined. Neither species is considered an important pathogen; however, *S. salivarius* occasionally causes septicemia in neutropenic patients. *S. salivarius* strains are usually non- or alpha-hemolytic on blood agar and form distinctive colonies on sucrose agar due to the production of extracellular polysaccharide, resulting in large, mucoid colonies (soluble fructan, levan) or large, hard colonies that may pit the agar (insoluble glucan, dextran). A high proportion of *S. salivarius* strains react with Lancefield group K antiserum. Urease production is a characteristic of approximately half (proportions vary among studies) of *S. salivarius* strains isolated. *S. vestibularis* is alpha-hemolytic and urease positive and does not produce extracellular polysaccharide from sucrose. Differential characteristics of *S. salivarius* and *S. vestibularis* are shown in Table 6.

TABLE 5 Differentiation of species in the anginosus group[a]

Test	*S. anginosus*	*S. constellatus*	*S. intermedius*
Enzyme activity			
β-D-Fucosidase	−	−	+
β-N-Acetyl-gal[b]	−	−	+
Neuraminidase	−	−	+
α-L-Fucosidase	−	−	−
β-N-Acetyl-glu[c]	−	−	+
α-D-Glucosidase	V	+	+
β-D-Glucosidase	+	−	V
α-Arabinosidase	V	−	−
α-D-Galactosidase	V	−	−
β-D-Galactosidase	V	V	+
Acid from:			
Amygdalin	+	V	V
Inulin	−	−	−
Mannitol	−	−	−
N-Acetylglucosamine	V	V	+
Raffinose	V	−	−
Sorbitol	−	−	−
Arbutin	+	+	+
Lactose	+	V	+
Melibiose	V	V	V
Hydrolysis of:			
Arginine	+	+	+
Esculin	+	V	+
Production of:			
Acetoin (VP test)	+	+	+
Urease	−	−	−
Hyaluronidase	−	+	+

[a] Symbols: +, positive; −, negative; V, variable.
[b] β-N-Acetyl-gal, β-N-acetylgalactosaminidase.
[c] β-N-Acetyl-glu, β-N-acetylglucosaminidase.

Bovis Group

The bovis group includes *S. bovis*, *S. alactolyticus*, and *S. equinus*. Despite the clinical significance of *S. bovis* in endocarditis and colon cancer, the confusing array of biotypes presented by human and bovine strains together has hindered the classification and identification of this group of streptococci. DNA-DNA reassociation studies have revealed considerable heterogeneity (18, 34, 63), with the most recent showing a clear separation of human strains of *S. bovis* from animal strains and the division of the latter into two distinct homology groups. *S. bovis* strains from humans are described as being typical (biotype I, able to ferment mannitol and produce copious amounts of extracellular polysaccharide, glucan, from sucrose) or variant (biotype II, unable to ferment mannitol or produce glucan). Commercial kits (Rapid ID STREP [bioMérieux, Marcy l'Etoile, France] or API 20Strep [BioMérieux Vitek, Hazelwood, Mo.]) subdivide biotype II strains into biotypes II/1 and II/2 on the basis of the production of both β-glucuronidase and β-galactosidase and the production of acid from trehalose but not from glycogen by the latter. *S. bovis* and *S. mutans* strains may resemble each other due to the production of glucan, fermentation of mannitol, and growth on bile esculin agar. However, *S. bovis* does not ferment sorbitol, is able to ferment starch or glycogen, and gives a Lancefield group D serological reaction. The differentiation of *S. bovis* from *S. salivarius* strains has been suggested on the basis of the Lancefield group D reaction; ability to grow on bile esculin agar; fermentation of mannitol, inulin, and starch; and urease production (68). *S. bovis* strains are virtually always β-galactosidase negative and α-galactosidase positive, in contrast to *S. salivarius* strains. In addition, β-glucuronidase production by *S. bovis* biotype II/2 may be a useful test. The biochemical characteristics of *S. bovis* are shown in Table 6.

As larger numbers of strains are examined, there is little doubt that the taxonomy of the viridans streptococci will continue to change with the addition of newly recognized species and emended descriptions of established ones. These streptococci will continue to present something of a challenge to those looking for a comprehensive identification scheme that is of use in the clinical laboratory.

Identification of Viridans Streptococci: Physiological Tests

Fluorogenic Substrates

4-Methylumbelliferyl linked substrates (Sigma Chemical Co.) are dissolved in a minimum volume of dimethyl sulfoxide and diluted in 50 mM Tris(hydroxymethyl)methyl-2-aminoethanesulfonic acid buffer (pH 7.5) (TES) to a final concentration of 100 μg/ml. Colonies from Columbia blood agar containing 5% (vol/vol) defibrinated horse blood are suspended in TES to approximately 10^8 organisms/ml (optical density at 620 nm of 0.1), and 50 μl of bacterial suspension is added to 20 μl of fluorogenic substrate solution in a flat-bottom microtiter tray well. After incubation at 37°C for 3 h, substrate degradation is visualized as bright blue fluorescence when viewed under UV light. This test format may be scored qualitatively on a UV transilluminator with a UV lamp or quantitatively in a UV plate reader. Standard-

TABLE 6 Biochemical characteristics of *S. mutans*, *S. sobrinus*, *S. salivarius*, *S. vestibularis*, and *S. bovis*[a]

Test	*S. mutans*	*S. sobrinus*	*S. salivarius*	*S. vestibularis*	*S. bovis*
Enzyme activity					
β-D-Fucosidase	−	−	V	−	NA
β-*N*-Acetyl-gal[b]	−	−	−	−	NA
Neuraminidase	−	−	−	−	NA
α-L-Fucosidase	−	−	−	−	NA
β-*N*-Acetyl-glu[c]	−	−	−	−	−
α-D-Glucosidase	+	+	V	V	NA
β-D-Glucosidase	+	−	V	−	+
α-Arabinosidase	−	−	+	+	NA
α-D-Galactosidase	V	−	−	−	V
β-D-Galactosidase	+	+	+	+	−^{V}[d]
Acid from:					
Amygdalin	+	−	V	V	V
Inulin	+	−	V	−	+
Mannitol	+	+	−	−	+$^{-}$[d]
N-Acetylglucosamine	+	−	V	V	+
Raffinose	+	−	V	−	+
Sorbitol	+	V	−	−	−
Arbutin	V	−	+	V	V
Lactose	+	+	+	V	+
Melibiose	+	−	−	−	+
Hydrolysis of:					
Arginine	−	−	−	−	−
Esculin	V	−	+	V	+
Production of:					
Acetoin (VP test)	+	+	+	−	+
Urease	−	−	V	+	−
Hyaluronidase	−	−	−	−	−

[a] Symbols: +, positive; −, negative; V, variable; NA, data not available.
[b] β-*N*-Acetyl-gal, β-*N*-acetylgalactosaminidase.
[c] β-*N*-Acetyl-glu, β-*N*-acetylglucosaminidase.
[d] Test scores in superscript are for "variant" strains (see the text). Variant strains are also variable (V) for glucuronidase and do not produce extracellular polysaccharide.

ized conditions for incubation should be applied to obtain consistent results with these substrates (1).

Carbohydrate Fermentation

Carbohydrate (1.0% [wt/vol]) is added to 24 g of thioglycolate broth medium per liter (without dextrose or indicator [Difco, Detroit, Mich.]) containing 16 g of purple broth base (Difco) per liter (57). Three drops of carbohydrate solution per well in a microtiter plate is inoculated with one drop of an overnight culture in Todd-Hewitt broth (Oxoid, Basingstoke, England). Incubation is carried out at 37°C for 24 h anaerobically. Acid production is indicated by the formation of a yellow color.

Arginine Hydrolysis

Arginine hydrolysis is a key reaction in the identification of viridans streptococci, and several test methods are described in the literature. Discrepancies can occur between them (83). Two commonly used methods are detailed here. (i) Moeller's decarboxylase broth containing arginine (commercially available) should be inoculated with the test organism, overlaid with mineral oil, and incubated at 35 to 37°C for up to 7 days. Degradation of arginine results in an increase in pH, indicated by the development of a purple color. Negative results are indicated by a yellow color, which is due to acid accumulation from metabolism of glucose only. (ii) Yeast extract (0.5%, wt/vol) (Difco), 0.5% (wt/vol) tryptone (Difco), 0.5% (wt/vol) glucose, 0.2% (wt/vol) K_2HPO_4, and 0.3% (wt/vol) L-arginine monohydrochloride are dissolved in water and sterilized by autoclaving, and three drops are added to a microtiter plate well. Cultures are incubated anaerobically for 24 h at 37°C. Production of ammonia is detected by the appearance of an orange color on addition of a drop of Nessler's reagent (9). Method ii was used to generate the data in Tables 4 to 6. The fact that results may vary with the method used should be taken into account when comparing arginine hydrolysis results from different laboratories.

Urea Hydrolysis Test

Christensen urea agar (available commercially) is inoculated and incubated at 35°C for up to 7 days. Development of a pink color indicates a positive reaction. An alternative format is to dispense Christensen's medium made up without agar into a microtiter tray well and, after inoculation, overlay it with oil prior to incubation.

VP Test

(i) For the Facklam and Washington (32) version of the VP test, see Identification of Beta-Hemolytic Isolates: Physiological Tests, above. (ii) A 1.5-ml volume of 0.5% (wt/vol) peptone, 0.5% (wt/vol) K_2HPO_4, and 0.5% (wt/vol) glucose (pH 7.5) is dispensed into bottles and autoclaved. After inoculation, incubation is carried out at 37°C for 2 to 4 days. After the addition of 0.6 ml of α-napthol dissolved in ethanol and 0.2 ml of 40% KOH, the bottles are shaken. A positive reaction is indicated by the formation of a cherry red color (weak reactions may result in a pink color).

Esculin Hydrolysis

(i) Esculin agar slants (available commercially) are inoculated and incubated for up to 1 week. A positive reaction appears as a blackening of the medium; no change in color indicates a negative esculin hydrolysis test. (ii) A broth version incorporates 1.0% (wt/vol) proteose peptone (Oxoid), 0.5% (wt/vol) yeast extract (Difco), 0.1% (vol/vol) Tween 80, 0.05% (wt/vol) ferric ammonium citrate, 1.0% (wt/vol) sodium acetate, 0.5% (wt/vol) esculin, 0.5% (vol/vol) each salt solution containing (a) 10% (wt/vol) K_2HPO_4 and 10% (wt/vol) KH_2PO_4 or (b) 11% (wt/vol) $MgSO_4.7H_2O$, 0.68% (wt/vol) $FeSO_4.7H_2O$, and 2.03% (wt/vol) $MgSO_4.4H_2O$ (final pH = 6.8).

Hyaluronidase Production

(i) Hyaluronidase activity can be detected on agar plates containing 400 μg of hyaluronic acid (sodium salt) from human umbilical cord (Sigma) per ml and 1% (wt/vol) bovine serum albumin (fraction V; Sigma) by the method of Smith and Willett (72). Strains are stabbed into the agar, and after overnight incubation at 37°C anaerobically, hyaluronidase activity is disclosed by flooding the plate with 2 M acetic acid. A positive test is revealed by the appearance of a clear zone around the stab. (ii) Homer et al. (46) have also described a quantitative method of determining hyaluronidase activity that is carried out in microtiter trays.

Production of Extracellular Polysaccharide

Strains are streaked out for single colonies on sucrose-containing agar. The two most commonly used media are (i) mitis-salivarius agar containing 0.001% (wt/vol) potassium tellurite (Difco) and (ii) tryptone yeast cystine agar (Lab M, Bury, England). Incubation should be carried out for up to 5 days at 37°C.

Two other tests found to be useful, particularly in helping to discriminate among the oralis group species, are production of immunoglobulin A protease (54) and amylase binding (25). However, these tests are unlikely to be used in routine clinical microbiology laboratories at present.

SEROLOGICAL TESTS

Serological tests are available to detect immune responses to both extracellular products (streptolysin O, hyaluronidase, DNase B, NADase, and streptokinase) and cellular components (M protein, group A antigen) of *S. pyogenes* in patient sera. These tests are useful in demonstrating antecedent streptococcal infection in patients who lack documentation of recent infection but who present with nonsuppurative sequelae (rheumatic fever, glomerulonephritis). Ayoub and Harden (3) provide a further discussion and describe methods for performing these tests.

ANTIBIOTIC SUSCEPTIBILITIES

In spite of reports of resistance in certain isolates, penicillin remains the drug of choice for treatment of infections caused by most streptococci, while narrow-spectrum cephalosporins, erythromycin, and vancomycin serve as alternative choices for treatment (14, 61). Although erythromycin resistance among group A streptococci is not common in North America, resistance has been observed in a number of locales worldwide (32). Susceptibility to tetracycline is variable among streptococcal strains. Although the streptococci are, as of this writing, considered to be susceptible to vancomycin, one recent report described the isolation of a vancomycin-resistant *S. bovis* strain during routine screening of stool specimens for vancomycin-resistant enterococci (65). This *S. bovis* isolate appears to have acquired enterococcal *vanB* vancomycin resistance genes, but to date no vancomycin-resistant streptococci have been isolated from sites of infection.

Penicillin treatment failures have been ascribed to tolerance, a situation in which bacterial growth is inhibited by penicillin but the bactericidal activity of the drug is greatly reduced. Tolerance has been described in vitro for beta-hemolytic and viridans streptococci, but testing for this trait is prone to technical problems. Other possible explanations for treatment failure, especially in pharyngitis, include the presence of beta-lactamase-producing bacteria at the site of infection (32) and poor patient compliance with dosing regimens. Concern about the efficacy of penicillin alone for effective treatment of life-threatening infections has led to the use of synergistic combinations of drugs (e.g., penicillin and gentamicin) for treatment of severe group B disease (32), and endocarditis due to viridans streptococci that are relatively resistant to penicillin (22).

The most notable trends in changing antimicrobial susceptibility patterns among the streptococci are penicillin resistance and multiple resistance in pneumococci and increasing frequencies of penicillin resistance in viridans streptococci. Among the viridans streptococci, penicillin resistance, both intermediate and high level, has been documented in the United States (23), the United Kingdom (60), Europe (67), and South Africa (64). *S. mitis* isolates are notable for displaying penicillin resistance, and South African workers have also observed high-level gentamicin resistance in *S. mitis* strains. No synergistic beta-lactam/aminoglycoside effect was observed in these high-level-gentamicin-resistant strains (64). It should be remembered that viridans strains identified as "*S. mitis*" will include a significant proportion of strains which would be identified as *S. oralis* if more discriminatory tests had been applied. While anginosus ("*S. milleri*") group isolates have been found to be generally penicillin susceptible by some workers (23, 49), there are also reports that suggest the impending emergence of penicillin resistance in these organisms (4).

Penicillin resistance in pneumococci has been reported in areas all over the world, and its incidence appears to be increasing. The reported frequencies of penicillin-resistant pneumococcal strains are variable, depending on the geographical location. Extended-spectrum cephalosporins (e.g., ceftriaxone or cefotaxime) have been used successfully to treat serious infections caused by penicillin-resistant pneumococci, but resistance to these agents also seems to be increasing. Pneumococcal strains displaying resistance to a variety of other antibiotics (erythromycin, tetracycline, chloramphenicol, or trimethoprim-sulfamethoxazole) have been encountered. Multiple resistance (resistance to three or more classes of antibiotics) may occur in the presence or absence of penicillin resistance (2).

EVALUATION, INTERPRETATION, AND REPORTING OF RESULTS

Beta-hemolytic streptococci and pneumococci are virulent pathogens, and consequently the detection and reporting of these organisms from all types of specimens have been emphasized in the clinical laboratory. Timely evaluation and reporting of throat specimens positive for *S. pyogenes* will allow for prompt antibiotic treatment, reducing the risk of nonsuppurative sequelae. While large-colony group C and G streptococci (*S. dysgalactiae* subsp. *equisimilis*) have been documented as agents of pharyngitis, evidence suggests that small-colony-forming beta-hemolytic streptococci (anginosus or "*S. milleri*" group) are constituents of the normal throat flora (77), although they may function as pathogens in infections other than pharyngitis.

The identification of viridans streptococci to the species or group level should be reserved for isolates from serious infections, particularly from endocarditis, abscesses, and infections in neutropenic patients. Since viridans streptococci are causative agents of shock, endocarditis, and pulmonary infections in neutropenic patients (13, 28), careful evaluation of the significance of these streptococci in blood cultures from members of this patient population is required. Viridans streptococci from blood cultures in neutropenic patients should be identified, since this may assist in the treatment of complications which may be common in these patients. It should be remembered that anginosus ("*S. milleri*") group organisms recovered from abscess or wound specimens, even when other organisms are present, are likely to be pathogens and not contaminants. As mentioned above, *S. bovis* biotyping may be useful because of a correlation between biotype I and endocarditis and gastrointestinal cancer.

REFERENCES

1. **Ahmet, Z., M. Warren, and E. T. Houang.** 1995. Species identification of members of the *Streptococcus milleri* group isolated from the vagina by ID 32 Strep system and differential phenotypic characteristics. *J. Clin. Microbiol.* **33:** 1592–1595.
2. **Applebaum, P. C.** 1996. Epidemiology and *in vitro* susceptibility of drug-resistant *Streptococcus pneumoniae*. *Pediatr. Infect. Dis. J.* **15:**932–939.
3. **Ayoub, E. M., and E. Harden.** 1997. Immune response to streptococcal antigens: diagnostic methods, p. 450–457. *In* N. R. Rose, E. Conway DeMarcario, J. D. Folds, H. C. Lane, and R. M. Nakamura (ed.), *Manual of Clinical Laboratory Immunology*, 5th ed. American Society for Microbiology, Washington, D.C.
4. **Bantar, C., L. Fernandez Canigia, S. Relloso, A. Lanza, H. Bianchini, and J. Smayevsky.** 1996. Species belonging to the "*Streptococcus milleri*" group: antimicrobial susceptibility and comparative prevalence in significant clinical specimens. *J. Clin. Microbiol.* **34:**2020–2022.
5. **Barnham, M., T. J. Thornton, and K. Lange.** 1983. Nephritis caused by *Streptococcus zooepidemicus* (Lancefield group C). *Lancet* **i:**945–948.
6. **Baron, E. J., L. R. Peterson, and S. M. Finegold.** 1994. Conventional and rapid microbiological methods for identification of bacteria and fungi, p. 97–122. *In* E. J. Baron, L. R. Peterson, and S. M. Finegold (ed.), *Bailey and Scott's Diagnostic Microbiology*, 9th ed. C. V. Mosby, St. Louis, Mo.
7. **Beighton, D., A. D. Carr, and B. A. Oppenheim.** 1994. Identification of viridans streptococci associated with bacteraemia in neutropaenic cancer patients. *J. Med. Microbiol.* **40:**202–204.
8. **Beighton, D., J. M. Hardie, and R. A. Whiley.** 1991. A scheme for the identification of viridans streptococci. *J. Med. Microbiol.* **35:**367–372.
9. **Beighton, D., R. R. B. Russell, and H. Hayday.** 1981. The isolation and characterization of *Streptococcus mutans* serotype h from dental plaque of monkeys (*Macacae fascicularis*). *J. Gen. Microbiol.* **124:**271–279.
10. **Bentley, R. W., J. A. Leigh, and M. D. Collins.** 1991. Intrageneric structure of *Streptococcus* based on comparative analysis of small subunit rRNA sequences. *Int. J. Syst. Bacteriol.* **41:**487–494.
11. **Bert, F., and N. Lambert-Zechovsky.** 1997. Septicemia caused by *Streptococcus canis* in a human. *J. Clin. Microbiol.* **35:**777–779.
12. **Bochud, P. Y., T. Calandra, and P. Francioli.** 1994. Bacteremia due to viridans streptococci in neutropenic patients: a review. *Am. J. Med.* **97:**256–264.
13. **Bochud, P. Y., P. Eggiman, T. Calandra, G. van Melle, L. Saghafi, and P. Francioli.** 1994. Bacteremia due to viridans streptococcus in neutropenic patients with cancer: clinical spectrum and risk factors. *Clin. Infect. Dis.* **20:**469–470.
14. **Bouvet, A., A. Durand, C. Devine, J. Etienne, C. Leport, and the Groupe d'Enquêsue l'Endocardite en France 1990–1991.** 1994. In vitro susceptibility to antibiotics of 200 strains of streptococci and enterococci isolated during infective endocarditis, p. 72–73. *In* A. Totalian (ed.), *Pathogenic Streptococci: Present and Future*. Lancer Publications, St. Petersburg, Russia.
15. **Carroll, K. C., D. Ballou, M. Varner, H. Chun, R. Traver, and J. Salyer.** 1996. Rapid detection of group B streptococcal colonization of the genital tract by a commercial optical immunoassay. *Eur. J. Clin. Microbiol. Infect. Dis.* **15:**206–210.
16. **Centers for Disease Control and Prevention.** 1996. Prevention of perinatal group B streptococcal disease: a public health perspective. *Morbid. Mortal. Weekly Rep.* **45**(RR-7)**:**1–24.
17. **Chew, T. A., and J. M. B. Smith.** 1992. Detection of diacetyl (caramel odor) in presumptive identification of the "*Streptococcus milleri*" group. *J. Clin. Microbiol.* **30:** 3028–3029.
18. **Coykendall, A. L., and K. B. Gustafson.** 1985. Deoxyribonucleic acid hybridizations among strains of *Streptococcus salivarius* and *Streptococcus bovis*. *Int. J. Syst. Bacteriol.* **35:** 274–280.
19. **Daly, J. A., N. L. Clifton, K. C. Seskin, and W. M. Gooch III.** 1991. Use of rapid, nonradioactive DNA probes in culture confirmation tests to detect *Streptococcus agalactiae*, *Haemophilus influenzae*, and *Enterococcus* spp. from pediatric patients with significant infections. *J. Clin. Microbiol.* **29:**80–82.
20. **Davis, T. E., and D. D. Fuller.** 1991. Direct identification of bacterial isolates in blood cultures by using a DNA probe. *J. Clin. Microbiol.* **29:**2192–2196.
21. **Denys, G. A., and R. B. Carey.** 1992. Identification of *Streptococcus pneumoniae* with a DNA probe. *J. Clin. Microbiol.* **30:**2725–2727.
22. **Dinubile, M. J.** 1990. Treatment of endocarditis caused by relatively resistant nonenterococcal streptococci: is penicillin enough? *Rev. Infect. Dis.* **12:**112–117.
23. **Doern, G. V., M. J. Ferraro, A. B. Brueggemann, and K. L. Ruoff.** 1996. Emergence of high rates of antimicrobial resistance among viridans group streptococci in the United States. *Antimicrob. Agents Chemother.* **40:**891–894.
24. **Douglas, C. W. I., J. Heath, K. K. Hampton, and F. E. Preston.** 1993. Identity of viridans streptococci isolated from cases of infective endocarditis. *J. Med. Microbiol.* **39:** 179–182.
25. **Douglas, C. W. I., A. A. Pease, and R. A. Whiley.** 1990.

Amylase-binding as a discriminator among oral streptococci. *FEMS Microbiol. Lett.* **66:**193–198.

26. **Drulak, M., W. Bartholomew, L. LaScolea, D. Amsterdam, N. Gunnersen, J. Yong, C. Fijalkowski, and S. Winston.** 1991. Evaluation of the modified Visuwell Strep-A enzyme immunoassay for detection of group-A *Streptococcus* from throat swabs. *Diagn. Microbiol. Infect. Dis.* **14:** 281–285.
27. **Duca, E., G. Teodorovici, C. Radu, A. Vita, P. Talasman-Niculescu, E. Bernescu, C. Feldi, and V. Rosca.** 1969. A new nephritogenic streptococcus. *J. Hyg. Camb.* **67:**691–698.
28. **Elting, L. S., G. P. Bodey, and B. H. Keefe.** 1992. Septicemia and shock syndrome due to viridans streptococci: a case-control study of predisposing factors. *Clin. Infect. Dis.* **14:**1201–1207.
29. **Facklam, R., J. Elliott, N. Pigott, and R. Franklin.** 1995. Identification of *Streptococcus porcinus* from human sources. *J. Clin. Microbiol.* **33:**385–388.
30. **Facklam, R. R.** 1980. Streptococci and aerococci, p. 88–110. *In* E. H. Lennette, A. Balows, W. J. Hausler, Jr., and J. P. Truant (ed.), *Manual of Clinical Microbiology*, 3rd ed. American Society for Microbiology, Washington, D.C.
31. **Facklam, R. R.** 1984. The major differences in the American and British Streptococcus taxonomy schemes with special reference to *Streptococcus milleri*. *Eur. J. Clin. Microbiol.* **3:**91–93.
32. **Facklam, R. R., and J. A. Washington II.** 1991. *Streptococcus* and related catalase-negative gram-positive cocci, p. 238–257. *In* A. Balows, W. J. Hausler, Jr., K. L. Herrmann, H. D. Isenberg, **and** H. J. Shadomy (ed.), *Manual of Clinical Microbiology*, 5th ed. American Society for Microbiology, Washington, D.C.
33. **Farrow, J. A. E., and M. D. Collins.** 1984. Taxonomic studies on streptococci of serological groups C, G and L and possibly related taxa. *Syst. Appl. Microbiol.* **5:**483–493.
34. **Farrow, J. A. E., J. Kruze, B. A. Phillips, A. J. Bramley, and M. D. Collins.** 1984. Taxonomic studies on *Streptococcus bovis* and *Streptococcus equinus*: description of *Streptococcus alactolyticus* sp. nov. and *Streptococcus saccharolyticus*. sp. nov. *Syst. Appl. Microbiol.* **5:**467–482.
35. **Freney, J., S. Bland, J. Etienne, M. Desmonceux, J. M. Boeufgras, and J. Fleurette.** 1992. Description and evaluation of the semiautomated 4-hour Rapid ID 32 Strep method for identification of streptococci and members of related genera. *J. Clin. Microbiol.* **30:**2657–2661.
36. **Gerber, M. A.** 1986. Diagnosis of group A beta-hemolytic streptococcal pharyngitis, use of antigen detection tests. *Diagn. Microbiol. Infect. Dis.* **4:**5S–15S.
37. **Gerber, M. A., M. F. Randolph, and K. K. DeMeo.** 1990. Liposome immunoassay for rapid identification of group A streptococci directly from throat swabs. *J. Clin. Microbiol.* **28:**1463–1464.
38. **Granato, P. A., and M. T. Petosa.** 1991. Evaluation of a rapid screening test for detecting group B streptococci in pregnant women. *J. Clin. Microbiol.* **29:**1536–1538.
39. **Green, M., B. Dashefsky, E. R. Wald, S. Laifer, J. Harger, and R. Guthrie.** 1993. Comparison of two antigen assays for rapid intrapartum detection of vaginal group B streptococcal colonization. *J. Clin. Microbiol.* **31:**78–82.
40. **Handley, P., A. Coykendall, D. Beighton, J. M. Hardie, and R. A. Whiley.** 1991. *Streptococcus crista* sp. nov., a viridans streptococcus with tufted fibrils, isolated from the human oral cavity and throat. *Int. J. Syst. Bacteriol.* **41:** 543–547.
41. **Harbeck, R. J., J. Teague, G. R. Crossen, D. M. Maul, and P. L. Childers.** 1993. Novel, rapid optical immunoassay technique for detection of group A streptococci from pharyngeal specimens: comparison with standard culture methods. *J. Clin. Microbiol.* **31:**839–844.
42. **Hardie, J. M.** 1986. Genus *Streptococcus* Rosenbach 1884, 22^{AL}, p. 1043–1071. *In* P. H. A. Sneath, N. S. Mair, M. E. Sharpe, and J. G. Holt (ed.), *Bergey's Manual of Systematic Bacteriology*, vol. 2. The Williams & Wilkins Co., Baltimore, Md.
43. **Heelan, J. S., S. Wilbur, G. Depetris, and C. Letourneau.** 1996. Rapid antigen testing for group A streptococcus by DNA probe. *Diagn. Microbiol. Infect. Dis.* **24:**65–69.
44. **Hinnebusch, C. J., D. M. Nikolai, and D. A. Bruckner.** 1991. Comparison of API Rapid STREP, Baxter Microscan Rapid Pos ID Panel, BBL Minitek Differential Identification System, IDS RapID STR System, and Vitek GPI to conventional biochemical tests for identification of viridans streptococci. *Am. J. Clin. Pathol.* **96:**459–463.
45. **Hoffman, S.** 1990. Detection of group A streptococcal antigen from throat swabs with five diagnostic kits in general practice. *Diagn. Microbiol. Infect. Dis.* **13:**209–215.
46. **Homer, K. A., L. Denbow, and R. A. Whiley.** 1993. Chondroitin sulfate depolymerase and hyaluronidase activities of viridans streptococci determined by a sensitive spectrophotometric assay. *J. Clin. Microbiol.* **31:** 1648–1651.
47. **Hwang, M. N., and G. M. Ederer.** 1975. Rapid hippurate hydrolysis method for presumptive identification of group B streptococci. *J. Clin. Microbiol.* **1:**114–115.
48. **Jacobs, J. A., H. C. Schouten, E. E. Stobberingh, and P. B. Soeters.** 1995. Viridans streptococci isolated from the bloodstream. Relevance of species identification. *Diagn. Microbiol. Infect. Dis.* **22:**267–273.
49. **Jacobs, J. A., and E. E. Stobberingh.** 1996. In-vitro antimicrobial susceptibility of the '*Streptococcus milleri*' group (*Streptococcus anginosus*, *Streptococcus constellatus* and *Streptococcus intermedius*). *J. Antimicrob. Chemother.* **37:** 371–375.
50. **Kawamura, Y., X. Hou, F. Sultana, S. Liu, H. Yamamoto, and T. Ezaki.** 1995. Transfer of *Streptococcus adjacens* and *Streptococcus defectivus* to *Abiotrophia* gen. nov. as *Abiotrophia adiacens* comb. nov. and *Abiotrophia defectiva* comb. nov., respectively. *Int. J. Syst. Bacteriol.* **45:**798–803.
51. **Kawamura, Y., X.-G. Hou, F. Sultana, H. Miura, and T. Ezaki.** 1995. Determination of 16S rRNA sequences of *Streptococcus mitis* and *Streptococcus gordonii* and phylogenetic relationships among members of the genus *Streptococcus*. *Int. J. Syst. Bacteriol.* **45:**406–408.
52. **Kellogg, J.** 1990. Suitability of throat culture procedures for detection of group A streptococci and as reference standards for evaluation of streptococcal antigen detection kits. *J. Clin. Microbiol.* **28:**165–169.
53. **Kikuchi, K., T. Enari, K.-I. Totsuka, and K. Shimizu.** 1995. Comparison of phenotypic characteristics, DNA-DNA hybridization results, and results with a commercial rapid biochemical and enzymatic reaction system for identification of viridans group streptococci. *J. Clin. Microbiol.* **33:**1215–1222.
54. **Kilian, M., L. Mikkelsen, and J. Henrichsen.** 1989. Taxonomic study of viridans streptococci: description of *Streptococcus gordonii* sp. nov. and emended descriptions of *Streptococcus sanguis* (White and Niven 1946), *Streptococcus oralis* (Bridge and Sneath 1982), and *Streptococcus mitis* (Andrewes and Horder 1906). *Int. J. Syst. Bacteriol.* **39:** 471–484.
55. **Kirby, R., and K. L. Ruoff.** 1995. Cost-effective, clinically relevant method for rapid identification of beta-hemolytic streptococci and enterococci. *J. Clin. Microbiol.* **33:** 1154–1157.
56. **Kircher, S. M., M. P. Meyer, and J. A. Jordan.** 1996. Comparison of a modified DNA hybridization assay with

standard culture enrichment for detecting group B streptococci in obstetric patients. *J. Clin. Microbiol.* **34:**342–344.

57. **Kral, T. A., and L. Daneo-Moore.** 1981. Biochemical differentiation of certain oral streptococci. *J. Dent. Res.* **60:** 1713–1718.
58. **Lim, D. V., W. J. Morales, and A. F. Walsh.** 1987. Lim group B strep broth and coagglutination for rapid identification of group B streptococci in preterm pregnant women. *J. Clin. Microbiol.* **25:**452–453.
59. **Ludwig, W., M. Weizenegger, R. Kilpper-Balz, and K. H. Schleiffer.** 1988. Phylogenetic relationships of anaerobic streptococci. *Int. J. Syst. Bacteriol.* **38:**15–18.
60. **McWhinney, P. H. M., S. Patel, R. A. Whiley, J. M. Hardie, S. H. Gillespie, and C. C. Kibbler.** 1993. Activities of potential therapeutic and prophylactic antibiotics against blood culture isolates of viridans group streptococci from neutropenic patients receiving ciprofloxacin. *Antimicrob. Agents Chemother.* **37:**2493–2495.
61. **Moellering, R. C., Jr.** 1995. Principles of anti-infective therapy, p. 199–212. *In* G. L. Mandell, J. E. Bennett, and R. Dolin (ed.), *Mandell, Douglas and Bennett's Principles and Practice of Infectious Diseases*, 4th ed. Churchill Livingstone, New York, N.Y.
62. **Nash, P., and M. M. Krenz.** 1991. Culture media, p. 1226–1288. *In* A. Balows, W. J. Hausler, Jr., K. L. Herrmann, H. D. Isenberg, and H. J. Shadomy (ed.), *Manual of Clinical Microbiology*, 5th ed. American Society for Microbiology, Washington, D.C.
63. **Nelms, L. F., D. A. Odelson, T. R. Whitehead, and R. B. Hespell.** 1995. Differentiation of ruminal and human *Streptococcus bovis* strains by DNA homology and 16S rRNA probes. *Curr. Microbiol.* **31:**294–300.
64. **Potgieter, E., M. Carmichael, H. J. Koornhof, and L. J. Chalkley.** 1992. In vitro antimicrobial susceptibility of viridans streptococci isolated from blood cultures. *Eur. J. Clin. Microbiol. Infect. Dis.* **11:**543–546.
65. **Poyart, C., C. Pierre, G. Quesne, B. Pron, P. Berche, and P. Trieu-Cuot.** 1997. Emergence of vancomycin resistance in the genus *Streptococcus*: characterization of a vanB transferable determinant in *Streptococcus bovis*. *Antimicrob. Agents Chemother.* **41:**24–29.
66. **Purdy, R. A., B. Cassidy, and T. J. Marrie.** 1990. *Streptococcus bovis* meningitis: report of 2 cases. *Neurology* **40:** 1782–1784.
67. **Renneberg, J., L. L. Niemann, and E. Gutschik.** 1997. Antimicrobial susceptibility of 278 streptococcal blood isolates to seven antimicrobial agents. *J. Antimicrob. Chemother.* **39:**135–140.
68. **Ruoff, K. L., M. J. Ferraro, J. Holden, and L. J. Kunz.** 1984. Identification of *Streptococcus bovis* and *Streptococcus salivarius* in the clinical laboratory. *J. Clin. Microbiol.* **20:** 223–226.
69. **Ruoff, K. L., S. I. Miller, C. V. Garner, M. J. Ferraro, and S. B. Calderwood.** 1989. Bacteremia with *Streptococcus bovis* and *Streptococcus salivarius*: clinical correlates of more accurate identification of isolates. *J. Clin. Microbiol.* **27:** 305–308.
70. **Schleifer, K. H., and R. Kilpper-Balz.** 1987. Molecular and chemotaxonomic approaches to the classification of streptococci, enterococci and lactococci: a review. *Syst. Appl. Microbiol.* **10:**1–19.
71. **Sherman, J. M.** 1937. The streptococci. *Bacteriol. Rev.* **1:** 3–97.
72. **Smith, R. F., and N. P. Willett.** 1968. Rapid plate method for screening hyaluronidase and chondroitin sulfatase-producing microorganisms. *Appl. Microbiol.* **16:**1434–1436.
73. **Stevens, D. L.** 1995. Streptococcal toxic-shock syndrome: spectrum of disease, pathogenesis, and new concepts in treatment. *Emerg. Infect. Dis.* **3:**69–78.
74. **Tambyah, P. A., G. Kumarasinghe, H. L. Chan, and K. O. Lee.** 1997. *Streptococcus suis* infection complicated by purpura fulminans and rhabdomyolysis: case report and review. *Clin. Infect. Dis.* **24:**710–712.
75. **Tarradas, C., A. Arenas, A. Maldonado, I. Luque, A. Miranda, and A. Perea.** 1994. Identification of *Streptococcus suis* isolated from swine: proposal for biochemical parameters. *J. Clin. Microbiol.* **32:**578–580.
76. **Thomas, J. G.** 1994. Routine CSF antigen detection for agents associated with bacterial meningitis: another point of view. *Clin. Microbiol. Newsl.* **16:**89–95.
77. **Turner, J. C., A. Fox, K. Fox, C. Addy, C. Z. Garrison, B. Herron, C. Brunson, and G. Betcher.** 1993. Role of group C beta-hemolytic streptococci in pharyngitis: epidemiologic study of clinical features associated with isolation of group C streptococci. *J. Clin. Microbiol.* **31:**808–811.
78. **Vandamme, P., B. Pot, E. Falsen, K. Kersters, and L. A. DeVries.** 1996. Taxonomic study of Lancefield streptococcal groups C, G, and L (*Streptococcus dysgalactiae*) and proposal of *S. dysgalactiae* subsp. *equisimilis* subsp. nov. *Int. J. Syst. Bacteriol.* **46:**774–781.
79. **Weinstein, M., D. E. Low, A. McGeer, B. Willey, D. Rose, M. Coulter, P. Wyper, A. Borczyk, and M. Lovgren.** 1996. Invasive infection with *Streptococcus iniae*-Ontario, 1995–1996. *Morbid. Mortal. Weekly Rep.* **45:** 650–653.
80. **Weinstein, M. R., M. Litt, D. A. Kertesz, P. Wyper, D. Rose, M. Coulter, A. McGeer, R. Facklam, C. Ostach, B. M. Willey, A. Borczyk, and D. E. Low.** 1997. Invasive infections due to a fish pathogen, *Streptococcus iniae*. *N. Engl. J. Med.* **337:**589–594.
81. **Welch, D. F., D. Hensel, D. Pickett, and S. Johnson.** 1991. Comparative evaluation of selective and nonselective culture techniques for isolation of group A beta-hemolytic streptococci. *Am. J. Clin. Pathol.* **95:**587–590.
82. **Wessels, M. R., and D. L. Kasper.** 1993. The changing spectrum of group B streptococcal disease. *N. Engl. J. Med.* **328:**1843–1844.
83. **West, P. W. J., H. A. Foster, Q. Electricwala, and A. Alex.** 1996. Comparison of five methods for the determination of arginine hydrolysis by viridans streptococci. *J. Med. Microbiol.* **45:**501–504.
84. **Whiley, R. A., and D. Beighton.** 1991. Emended descriptions and recognition of *Streptococcus constellatus*, *Streptococcus intermedius*, and *Streptococcus anginosus* as distinct species. *Int. J. Syst. Bacteriol.* **41:**1–5.
85. **Whiley, R. A., H. Y. Fraser, C. W. I. Douglas, J. M. Hardie, A. M. Williams, and M. D. Collins.** 1990. *Streptococcus parasanguis* sp. nov., an atypical viridans streptococcus from human clinical specimens. *FEMS Lett.* **68:** 115–122.
86. **Whiley, R. A., H. Fraser, J. M. Hardie, and D. Beighton.** 1990. Phenotypic differentiation of *Streptococcus intermedius*, *Streptococcus constellatus*, and *Streptococcus anginosus* strains within the "*Streptococcus milleri* group." *J. Clin. Microbiol.* **28:**1497–1501.
87. **Wilkinson, H. W.** 1977. CAMP-disk test for presumptive identification of group B streptococci. *J. Clin. Microbiol.* **6:**42–45.
88. **Wust, J., G. Hebisch, and K. Peters.** 1993. Evaluation of two enzyme immunoassays for rapid detection of group B streptococci in pregnant women. *Eur. J. Clin. Microbiol. Infect. Dis.* **12:**124–127.

Enterococcus

RICHARD R. FACKLAM, DANIEL F. SAHM, AND LÚCIA MARTINS TEIXEIRA

18

TAXONOMY

Genetic evidence that *Streptococcus faecalis* and *Streptococcus faecium* were sufficiently different from the other members of the genus *Streptococcus* to merit a separate genus, as originally proposed by Kalina (61), was provided by Schleifer and Kilpper-Balz in 1984 (101). It has been 15 years since this proposal, and it is generally accepted that the genus *Enterococcus* is valid. Since 1984, 17 other species have been proposed for inclusion in the genus *Enterococcus* (16–19, 25, 42, 66, 73, 94, 95, 116). Genetic evidence for these proposals has been provided by DNA-DNA and DNA-rRNA hybridization studies as well as by 16S rRNA sequencing.

Enterococcus solitarius (16) and *Enterococcus seriolicida* (66) belong in the genera *Tetragenococcus* and *Lactococcus* (29), respectively, based on 16S rRNA analysis (20, 35, 106, 117). These two species also fail to react with the AccuProbe *Enterococcus* probe manufactured by GenProbe Inc. (San Diego, Calif.). This probe is based on a DNA oligomer having a structure complementary to a segment of enterococcal rRNA (22, 37). All strains of known *Enterococcus* species, except the type strains of *Enterococcus cecorum*, *Enterococcus columbae*, and *Enterococcus saccharolyticus*, react positively with this probe.

DNA relatedness studies performed in our laboratory indicated that *Enterococcus flavescens* (94) and *Enterococcus casseliflavus* are closely related at the species level (104). *E. casseliflavus* should be retained as the species denomination.

DESCRIPTION OF THE GENUS

The enterococci are gram-positive cocci that occur singly, in pairs, and in short chains. The cells are sometimes coccobacillary when Gram stains are prepared from agar plate growth. They are more oval and are found in chains when Gram stains are prepared from thioglycolate broth. The enterococci are facultatively anaerobic, and optimum growth occurs at 35°C. Most strains grow at 10 and 45°C. All strains grow in broth containing 6.5% NaCl and hydrolyze esculin in the presence of 40% bile salts (bile-esculin medium). Motility is observed with some species. Most enterococci hydrolyze pyrrolidonyl-β-naphthylamide (PYR); the exceptions to this are *E. cecorum*, *E. columbae*, and *E. saccharolyticus*. All strains hydrolyze leucine-β-naphthylamide (LAP). Enterococci do not contain cytochrome enzymes, but on occasion the catalase test appears positive. A pseudocatalase is sometimes produced, and a weak effervescence is observed in the catalase test. This occurs when strains of *E. faecalis* are grown on blood-containing medium; it is not known if any other *Enterococcus* species behave in the same manner. Nearly all strains are homofermentative, gas is not produced, and lactic acid is the end product of glucose fermentation. Most strains produce a cell wall-associated glycerol teichoic acid antigen, which is identified as the streptococcal group D antigen. Detection of the group D antigen is sometimes difficult and depends upon the extraction procedure and the quality of the antiserum used (64, 110). The G+C content of the DNA ranges from 37 to 45 mol% (101).

Tests for differentiating the enterococci from other catalase-negative gram-positive cocci that are primarily arranged in chains are listed in Table 1.

The majority of other genera of catalase-negative gram-positive cocci are discussed in chapters 17 and 19. Note that because strains of *Lactococcus*, *Leuconostoc*, *Pediococcus*, and *Vagococcus* (15) have been isolated from human infections (40), the presumptive identification of enterococci on the basis of the bile-esculin reaction and growth in 6.5% NaCl broth can be erroneous (Table 1). Tetragenococci (20), which also have phenotypic characteristics similar to those of the enterococci, have been split from the genus *Pediococcus* and have not been isolated from human sources.

The most accurate presumptive identification of a catalase-negative gram-positive coccus as an *Enterococcus* strain can be accomplished by demonstrating that the unknown strain is PYR and LAP positive and grows in 6.5% NaCl and at 45°C. Demonstrating by extraction and serological reaction with group-specific antiserum that an unknown strain has group D antigen may be helpful in identification of some strains, but these reactions should be interpreted cautiously. Most of the pediococcus strains and about half of the leuconostoc strains isolated from human infections also have group D antigens (40, 41). Delayed or weak reactions with anti-group D serum can be observed with some vagococcal strains (103). Confirmation of a strain as an *Enterococcus* strain requires complete identification to the species level. Positive reactions with the AccuProbe *Enterococcus* test (GenProbe, Inc., San Diego, Calif.) can also be used to confirm an unknown strain as an *Enterococcus* strain (unpublished data). However, all *Vagococcus* strains we have

TABLE 1 Phenotypic characteristics of facultatively anaerobic, catalase-negative, gram-positive cocci in chains[a]

Genus	Van	Gas	PYR	LAP	BE	NaCl	Growth at: 10°C	Growth at: 45°C	Mot	Hem
Enterococcus	S[b]	−	+	+	+	+	+	+	v	α/β/n
Lactococcus	S	−	+	+	+	v	+	v	−	α/n
Vagococcus	S	−	+	+	+	+	+	v	+	α/n
Streptococcus	S	−	−[c]	+	−[d]	−[e]	−	v	−	α/β/n
Abiotrophia	S	−	+	+	−	−	v	−	−	α/n
Globicatella	S	−	+	−	−	+	−	−	−	α
Leuconostoc	R	+	−	−	v	v	+	v	−	α/n

[a] Abbreviations and symbols: Van, susceptibility to vancomycin (30-μg disk); Gas, gas produced from glucose in Mann, Rogosa, Sharpe *Lactobacillus* broth (MRS); PYR, production of PYR; LAP, production of LAP; BE, reaction on bile-esculin medium; NaCl, growth in broth containing 6.5% NaCl; Mot, motility; Hem, hemolysis on blood agar containing 5% sheep blood; α, alpha-hemolysis; β, beta-hemolysis; n, no hemolysis; S, susceptible; R, resistant; −, ≤5% positive reaction; +, ≥95% positive reaction; v, variable reaction.

[b] Some strains are vancomycin resistant but still show a small zone of inhibition around the disk; other strains grow right up to the disk and are vancomycin resistant under the defined screening test criteria.

[c] *Streptococcus pyogenes* (group A streptococci), *S. iniae*, and *S. porcinus* are PYR positive; all others are negative.

[d] Of viridans streptococci, 5 to 10% are bile-esculin positive.

[e] Some beta-hemolytic streptococci grow in 6.5% NaCl broth.

tested also have reacted with the AccuProbe *Enterococcus* genetic probe (103).

NATURAL HABITATS

The nature of these bacteria, which permits growth and survival in harsh environments, allows them to persist almost everywhere. Enterococci can be found in soil, food, water, plants, animals, birds, and insects (4, 27, 28, 32, 63, 81). In humans, as in other animals, the enterococci inhabit the gastrointestinal tract and the female genital tract. The prevalence of the different enterococcal species appears to vary according to the host and is also influenced by age, diet, and other factors that may be related to changes in the physiologic conditions (26). *E. faecalis* is one of the most common bacteria isolated from the gastrointestinal tracts of humans. It is likely that *E. faecium* is also commonly found in the gastrointestinal tracts of humans (36, 74). Because of changes in taxonomy, it is difficult to determine the distribution of other enterococcal species in humans as well as in other sources. The available limited information on the distribution of distinct enterococcal species in animal and environmental sources indicates that there are differences from the distribution in humans (25–28, 88).

CLINICAL SIGNIFICANCE

The ubiquitous nature of enterococci requires caution in establishing the clinical significance of a particular isolate so that unnecessary work and potentially misleading laboratory reports can be avoided whenever possible. This is especially important for in vitro susceptibility testing decisions (see Antimicrobial Susceptibilities, below).

Murray (82) has thoroughly reviewed and summarized the variety of infections in which enterococci are involved. Urinary tract infections are the most common. Enterococci are implicated in approximately 10% of all such infections (44) and in 16% of nosocomial urinary tract infections (100). Enterococcal bacteriuria usually occurs in patients with underlying structural abnormalities and/or in those who have undergone urologic manipulations (79). Intra-abdominal or pelvic wound infections are the next most commonly encountered infections. However, these wound cultures are frequently polymicrobial, and the role of enterococci in this setting remains controversial (87). Enterococci are being recovered from wound infections at an increasing rate, which probably results from increased antibiotic usage and emerging resistance among these organisms (79, 82, 100).

Bacteremia is the third most common type of infection, and enterococci are the third leading cause of nosocomial bacteremia (51, 54, 72, 79, 100). These infections occur most often in elderly patients who have serious underlying medical problems, and they also occur in other immunocompromised patients who have had prolonged hospitalization and have received antimicrobial therapy (1, 51). Although endocarditis is a serious enterococcal infection, it is less common than bacteremia. Enterococci are estimated to cause between 5 and 20% of cases of bacterial endocarditis (75, 114). Enterococcal endocarditis is more common in the elderly and in patients with degenerative valvular diseases or genitourinary conditions. *E. faecalis* is the most commonly encountered species in this setting, but various other species also have been implicated as causes of endocarditis (39).

Enterococcal infections of the respiratory tract or the central nervous system can occur but are rare (82). The significance of isolates from these sites should be carefully evaluated before any clinical decisions are made.

Although the spectrum of infections caused by enterococci has remained relatively unchanged since the review by Murray in 1990 (82), the prevalence of these organisms as nosocomial pathogens is clearly increasing. Enterococci are second only to *Escherichia coli* as agents of nosocomial urinary tract infections and third (behind *Staphylococcus aureus* and coagulase-negative staphylococci) as agents of nosocomial bacteremia (100). This trend is likely to continue as the overall population ages and more people are placed at risk of infection due to a generalized deterioration of health with increasing age (75).

COLLECTION, TRANSPORT, AND STORAGE OF SPECIMENS

The standard methods of collecting blood, urine, wound culture specimens, and other swab specimens should be adequate for the collection of enterococci (see chapters 4 and 5).

The transport of enterococci is simple and can take place with almost any transport media or with swabs that are kept dry. Like most clinical samples, the transported material should be cultured as soon as possible, preferably within 1 h.

Enterococci can be stored indefinitely when lyophilized. Cultures frozen at −70°C can be stored for several years. Most *Enterococcus* strains survive for several months at 4°C on ordinary agar slants.

ISOLATION PROCEDURES

Trypticase soy–5% sheep blood agar, brain heart infusion–5% sheep blood agar, or any blood agar base containing 5% animal blood supports the growth of enterococci. Some strains of *E. faecalis* are beta-hemolytic on agar bases containing rabbit, horse, or human blood but non-beta-hemolytic on the same base media containing sheep blood. Some cultures of *Enterococcus durans* are beta-hemolytic regardless of the type of blood used. All other species are usually alpha-hemolytic or nonhemolytic. All enterococci grow at 35 to 37°C, and they do not require an atmosphere containing increased levels of carbon dioxide, although some strains grow better in this atmosphere. If the clinical sample is likely to contain gram-negative bacteria, bile-esculin azide, Pfizer selective enterococcus, or some other commercially prepared medium containing azide is excellent as the primary isolation medium. Other media, such as Columbia colistin-nalidixic acid agar (CNA) or phenylethyl alcohol agar (PEA), have been used successfully to isolate enterococci. The advantage of CNA over PEA is that the hemolytic reaction can be read from CNA but not from PEA. The use of selective media for the isolation of enterococci has been previously reviewed (26, 38). Since then, several new media have been described, including those containing chromogenic substrates for the isolation of enterococci from urine (76, 118) and cephalexin-aztreonam-arabinose agar for the selective isolation of *E. faecium* from heavily contaminated sites (45).

The increasing incidence of vancomycin-resistant enterococci (VRE) has created a need for the development of vancomycin-containing selective media for the early detection of these bacteria from humans and animals (34, 36, 50, 68, 109, 112, 113). Although there is no uniformly accepted screening method for detecting colonization by VRE, Enterococcosel-vancomycin broth and brain heart infusion-vancomycin agar have both shown promising results as useful methods for the rapid and selective isolation of VRE from fecal specimens (68, 112, 113). Enterococcosel broth and brain heart infusion agar are commercially available, and vancomycin can easily be added to achieve the desired concentration (usually 6 μg/ml).

Because a laboratory report of VRE can initiate a cascade of infection control events that are time-consuming and costly (43), laboratories must be certain of the epidemiological importance of any suspected VRE isolate. The transferable and high-level VanA and VanB resistance associated with *E. faecalis* and *E. faecium* is the intended focus of infection control efforts. In contrast, the intrinsic low-level VanC resistance, which is not transferable and is not associated with wide dissemination of resistant strains, is much less likely to be important to the surveillance efforts of infection control personnel (46, 80, 99). Therefore, while the use of sensitive methods for isolating VRE from surveillance specimens such as stools and urine is important, the need to establish protocols to rapidly determine the identification to species or the likely underlying mechanism of resistance (i.e., VanA, VanB, or VanC [see chapter 121]) is equally important (99).

IDENTIFICATION OF *ENTEROCOCCUS* SPECIES

Once it is established that the unknown catalase-negative gram-positive coccus is *Enterococcus* or closely related genus (*Lactococcus* or *Vagococcus*), the tests listed in Table 2 can be used to identify the species. Because of the recognition of several different phenotypic variants of *E. faecium* (105), as well as variants of *E. faecalis*, *E. casseliflavus*, and *E. gallinarum* (104), and the decision to include *Lactococcus* and *Vagococcus*, it was necessary to expand the species identification table. It is best to separate the species into five groups based on acid formation in mannitol and sorbose broths and hydrolysis of arginine (Table 2).

The five species in group I form acid in both of the above-mentioned carbohydrate broths but do not hydrolyze arginine.

Group II comprises the enterococcal species that form acid in mannitol broth and hydrolyze arginine but fail to form acid from sorbose. There are atypical strains that fail to hydrolyze arginine or form acid in mannitol broth. *Lactococcus* strains are also included in group II because the phenotypic characteristics of the two *Lactococcus* species (*L. garvieae* and *L. lactis*) found in humans are similar to those of the *Enterococcus* species in this group.

Group III consists of *E. durans*, *E. hirae*, and *E. dispar*. These three species hydrolyze arginine but do not form acid in mannitol, sorbose, or sorbitol broth.

Group IV species do not form acid in mannitol or sorbose broth and fail to hydrolyze arginine.

Group V consists of *E. columbae* and *Vagococcus*. Similar to the *Lactococcus* situation above, *Vagococcus* is included here because of its phenotypic similarity to the species of *Enterococcus*, especially those in this group.

The species in each group are then identified by specific reactions (Table 2). The species in group I are identified by their reactions in arabinose broth and raffinose broth and utilization of pyruvate. *E. avium* and *E. raffinosus* form acid in arabinose. *E. raffinosus* forms acid in raffinose broth, whereas *E. avium* does not. *E. malodoratus* forms acid in raffinose broth but not arabinose broth. *E. raffinosus* forms acid in both, while *E. pseudoavium* forms acid in neither. *E. saccharolyticus* forms acid in raffinose broth but not in arabinose broth, similar to *E. malodoratus*. *E. saccharolyticus* does not utilize pyruvate, whereas *E. malodoratus* does.

E. faecalis is the only member of group II to tolerate tellurite and utilize pyruvate. *E. faecium* and *E. gallinarum* have similar characteristics but can be differentiated by the motility test, susceptibility to efrotomycin (EFRO), and acid formation in methyl α-D-glucopyranoside (MGP) (10). Preparation of EFRO disks is described in section IX, as they are not available commercially at this time. *E. gallinarum* is motile and resistant to EFRO and forms acid in MGP broth, but *E. faecium* is not motile, is susceptible to EFRO, and does not form acid in MGP broth. *E. casseliflavus* and *E. mundtii* are pigmented (yellow). *E. casseliflavus* is motile and resistant to EFRO and forms acid in MGP broth, but *E. mundtii* gives the opposite reactions.

The members of group III are easily identified by their reactions in the pyruvate, arabinose, raffinose, and sucrose tests. *E. durans* is negative in all four tests. *E. hirae* is positive

TABLE 2 Phenotypic characteristics used for the identification of *Enterococcus* species and related genera[a]

Species	MAN	SOR	ARG	ARA	SBL	RAF	TEL	MOT	PIG	SUC	PYU	MGP	EFRO
Group I													
E. avium	+	+	−	+	+	−	−	−	−	+	+	+	R
E. malodoratus	+	+	−	−	+	+	−	−	−	+	+	−	S
E. raffinosus	+	+	−	+	+	+	−	−	−	+	+	+	R
E. pseudoavium	+	+	−	−	+	−	−	−	−	+	+	+	R
E. saccharolyticus	+	+	−	−	+	+	−	−	−	+	−	+	R
Group II													
E. faecalis	+*	−	+*	−	+	−	+	−	−	+*	+	−[b]	R
Lactococcus spp.	+	−	+	−	−	−	−	−	−	v	−	−	S
E. faecium	+*	−	+	+	v	v	−	−	−	+*	−	−	S
E. casseliflavus	+	−	+*	+	v	+	−*	+*	+*	+	v	+	R
E. mundtii	+	−	+	+	v	+	−	−	+	+	−	−	S
E. gallinarum	+*	−	+*	+	−	+	−	+*	−	+	−	+	R
Group III													
E. durans	−	−	+	−	−	−	−	−	−	−	−	−	S
E. hirae	−	−	+	−	−	v	−	−	−	+	−	−	S
E. dispar	−	−	+	−	−	+	−	−	−	+	+	+	R
Group IV													
E. sulfureus	−	−	−	−	−	+	−	−	+	+	−	+	R
E. cecorum	−	−	−	−	+	+	−	−	−	+	+	−	R
Group V													
E. columbae	+	−	−	+	+	+	−	−	−	+	+	−	R
V. fluvialis	+	−	−	−	+	−	−	+	−	+	−	+	R

[a] Abbreviations and symbols: MAN, mannitol; SOR, sorbose; ARG, arginine; ARA, arabinose; SBL, sorbitol; RAF, raffinose; TEL, 0.04% tellurite; MOT, motility; PIG, pigment; SUC, sucrose; PYU, pyruvate; MGP, methyl-α-D-glucopyranoside; EFRO, efrotomycin disk (100 μg); +, >90%; −, <10% positive; v, variable; +* or −*, occasional exceptions (<3% of strains show aberrant reactions); R, resistant; S, sensitive.

[b] Some strains turn positive after a 2-week incubation.

in one or both of the raffinose and sucrose tests and negative in the tests for arabinose fermentation and utilization of pyruvate. *E. dispar* is positive in the test for utilization of pyruvate and production of acid from raffinose and sucrose but negative in the arabinose test.

The two species included in group IV, *E. sulfureus* and *E. cecorum*, can be differentiated by their opposite reactions in the tests involving acid production from sorbitol, pigmentation, utilization of pyruvate, and acid production from MGP broth.

The members of group V can be differentiated on the basis of their reactions in the arabinose, raffinose, pyruvate, MGP, and motility tests.

All the tests listed in Tables 1 and 2 are described in section IX as well as in references 39 to 41.

Commercially available kits and devices that claim to identify the *Enterococcus* species are not very useful and may in fact lead to erroneous identifications (102). These kits and devices generally identify *E. faecalis* quite accurately, but other species are not adequately identified.

Analysis of electrophoretic whole-cell protein profiles has been shown to be reliable for the differentiation and identification of typical and atypical *Enterococcus* strains (24, 77, 88, 103, 105). Species-specific rRNA probes have been used to identify *E. faecalis* and *E. faecium* (3). Restriction fragment length polymorphism (RFLP) of rDNA was used to identify four species of enterococci isolated from bovine sources (60). Donabedian et al. (31) tested contour-clamped homogeneous electric field electrophoresis (CHEF) for the identification of five enterococcal species. Tyrrell et al. (111) found that PCR amplification of the intergenic spacer region (ITS-PCR between the 16S and 23S rRNA genes) produced amplicon profiles characteristic of the several *Enterococcus* species examined. Other PCR-based techniques have been used to identify clinically relevant enterococcal isolates (24, 33). Of the molecular techniques used to identify the enterococcal species, only the whole-cell protein profile technique has been performed in more than one laboratory and appears to be practical for identification of all the *Enterococcus* species.

The majority of clinical isolates of enterococci (80 to 90%) are *E. faecalis*. *E. faecium* is found in 5 to 10% of enterococcal infections (8, 9, 49, 53, 97). In one recent study, the ratio of *E. faecalis* to *E. faecium* from clinical specimens was 4:1 (58). The other enterococcal species are identified less frequently. However, clusters of infections with *E. raffinosus* (12) and *E. casseliflavus* (86) have been reported. Therefore, the distribution of species varies with each clinical setting. *E. avium*, *E. gallinarum*, *E. mundtii*, *E. durans*, *E. hirae*, and *E. faecalis* variant strains have been isolated from human sources but only rarely (39). *E. malodoratus*, *E. pseudoavium*, *E. saccharolyticus*, *E. sulfureus*, *E. cecorum*, and *E. columbae* have not been isolated from human sources. All the *Vagococcus* strains isolated to date from humans have been *V. fluvialis* (103).

TYPING METHODS

Until a few years ago, enterococcal infections were traditionally considered to be acquired endogenously from the patient's own normal flora and their epidemiology had attracted little attention. Recently, increased interest has been focused on the epidemiology of enterococcal infections in part because of the documentation of *Enterococcus* as a nosocomial pathogen. Furthermore, the emergence and dissemination of multiple antimicrobial resistance traits among enterococcal strains and the evidence supporting the concept of exogenous acquisition of enterococcal infections have generated an additional need for typing the isolates as a means of assisting infection control and epidemiologic studies both within and among various medical institutions. Epidemiologic investigations of enterococcal infections have been limited by the lack of simple, highly reproducible, and sufficiently discriminatory typing systems.

Classic typing methods have included biotyping, antimicrobial resistance profiles, serologic characterization, bacteriocin typing, and bacteriophage typing (21, 70, 71). Although these approaches have occasionally yielded useful information, they generally are time-consuming and difficult to reproduce and/or interpret. These techniques frequently fail to adequately discriminate among strains, and for some, the reagents are not readily available; therefore, they have limited value in epidemiologic studies.

The advent of various molecular techniques has substantially enhanced our ability to differentiate enterococcal isolates and has provided critical insights into epidemiologic aspects of nosocomial enterococcal infections, especially in relation to outbreaks due to strains that exhibit clinically important antimicrobial resistance. As a result of the introduction of more discriminatory typing methods, it has been possible to demonstrate that strains can be exogenously acquired by direct and indirect contact among patients (23, 69, 91, 96, 115, 120, 121). Intrahospital transmission and interhospital spread, even among institutions located in different geographical areas, have also been documented for antimicrobially resistant enterococci (13, 98, 115).

The first molecular techniques developed for typing of enterococci were the analysis of plasmid profiles (6, 14, 30, 70, 90, 119) and the restriction enzyme analysis of genomic DNA by conventional electrophoresis (5, 55, 56, 62, 67). However, problems in interpretation were encountered with the use of these methods. The most useful methods of typing the enterococci include analysis of chromosomal DNA restriction endonuclease profiles by pulsed-field gel electrophoresis (PFGE) either by field inversion gel electrophoresis (FIGE) (7, 47) or, ideally, by CHEF (31, 48, 52, 84, 91–93). Multilocus enzyme electrophoresis (11, 110), ribotyping (48, 65, 93, 97, 119), and the PCR-based typing methods, such as the random amplified polymorphic DNA (RAPD-PCR) assay (2, 59), have also been used to type the enterococci. Comparative investigations involving more than one of these techniques indicate that analysis of *Sma*I restriction digests of genomic DNA by PFGE appears to be widely useful for studying enterococcal species exhibiting a variety of antimicrobial resistance patterns (11, 13, 14, 30, 78, 83, 85, 90–92, 107). In comparison with ribotyping (48, 93) and multilocus enzyme electrophoresis (11, 108), PFGE showed definite advantages in strain discrimination. Recent reports led to the conclusion that random amplification of polymorphic DNA (RAPD)-PCR and PFGE are comparable in efficiency for the investigation of VRE outbreaks (2, 36). Multiplex PCR-RFLP was also found to be a useful and convenient method for the rapid detection and discrimination of VRE genotypes (89). Although there is not a single definitive typing technique for enterococci, the most conclusive data indicate that PFGE is currently the single most useful and reliable method.

ANTIMICROBIAL SUSCEPTIBILITIES AND EVALUATION, INTERPRETATION, AND REPORTING OF RESULTS

The unpredictable nature of enterococcal susceptibility to antimicrobial agents dictates that in vitro testing be done; when and against which antimicrobial agents it is done depend on the site of infection and the significance of a particular isolate. Additionally, because acquired resistance to penicillins, vancomycin, and high levels of aminoglycosides has been described for a variety of enterococcal species, the decision to perform susceptibility testing should not be influenced by the species of the isolate. The methods that should be used for testing enterococci are discussed in detail in chapter 121.

Susceptibility testing for resistance to synergy should be done with any enterococcal isolate implicated in infections for which combination therapy is indicated, e.g., isolates from blood or cerebrospinal fluid. Enterococci are also frequently encountered in polymicrobial infections associated with the gastrointestinal tract or superficial wounds of hospitalized patients. Their pathogenic significance in such settings is uncertain, but susceptibility testing is warranted when predominant or heavy growth is observed (79).

Testing of enterococcal isolates from lower urinary tract infections is optional, since these infections usually respond to therapy with ampicillin. However, many hospital infection control programs require routine testing as a means of surveillance for VRE. Ciprofloxacin, levofloxacin, norfloxacin, nitrofurantoin, or tetracycline can also be used, but the prevalence of resistance to these agents is higher (83). In cases of treatment failure, testing is always warranted.

Occasionally, there is interest in the susceptibility of an enterococcal isolate to β-lactam antibiotics other than ampicillin (e.g., mezlocillin, piperacillin, azlocillin, amoxicillin-clavulanate, ampicillin-sulbactam, and imipenem). Although these antibiotics do not offer any significant advantages over ampicillin when they are used against enterococci, they may be of interest for use against polymicrobial infections involving enterococci and gram-negative bacilli. Ampicillin, along with a test for β-lactamase production, can be used to predict resistance to these other β-lactam antibiotics. Therefore, selection of these other drugs for testing is rarely needed. A positive test for β-lactamase production (see chapter 121) indicates resistance to ampicillin and the acylureidopenicillins (e.g., azlocillin, mezlocillin, and piperacillin). Resistance to ampicillin by disk diffusion or dilution methods would probably indicate penicillin-binding protein-mediated resistance to these agents, β-lactam–β-lactamase inhibitor combinations, and imipenem (57).

Although in vitro methods for detecting vancomycin resistance are thoroughly discussed (see chapter 121), issues regarding *van*C-containing species (i.e., *E. gallinarum* and *E. casseliflavus*) need to be emphasized. Disk diffusion will not detect the level of resistance usually associated with *van*C genotypes, but *van*C-containing strains usually produce growth on vancomycin agar screen tests (46). Because the clinical significance of the level of resistance expressed by VanC-containing strains is uncertain, the implications of these two in in vitro testing issues for patient management are uncertain. However, as discussed above, for therapeutic, infection control, and surveillance reasons, the need to differentiate VanA or VanB strains from VanC strains is quite evident. Because screening by growth on vancomycin agar fails to help with this important distinction, other criteria are needed. These criteria include species identification. VanC resistance has yet to be described in *E. faecalis* or *E. faecium*, so that growth on the screen by either of these species is probably due to VanA or VanB resistance. However, VanA resistance together with VanC resistance has been described in a single strain of *E. gallinarum*, so that identification of an organism to a species that usually harbors only VanC resistance does not completely rule out the presence of higher-level vancomycin resistance. In this regard, determining vancomycin MICs is useful because VanC resistance alone does not produce MICs of >16 μg/ml whereas VanA and VanB usually result in MICs of >32 μg/ml. Resistance to other agents such as ampicillin and aminoglycosides also is uncommon among VanC isolates.

Of importance is the observation that while enterococci are often discussed in terms of the multiple drug resistance they can express, two of the most problematic resistance profiles, ampicillin and vancomycin resistance, are by far most commonly associated with *E. faecium* (57). In terms of resistance surveillance, this is an important issue. Because ampicillin resistance and vancomycin resistance in *E. faecalis* are relatively uncommon compared to their resistance in *E. faecium*, widespread emergence and dissemination of these resistances in *E. faecalis* would significantly add to the current problem of multiply resistant enterococci. For the purposes of therapy and meaningful surveillance, enterococcal species identification is important.

Testing agents to which enterococci are intrinsically resistant is contraindicated. The results of such tests are superfluous and can be dangerously misleading. The drugs that should not be tested include aztreonam, any cephalosporin, clindamycin, methicillin (or oxacillin), trimethoprim-sulfamethoxazole, and aminoglycosides at standard concentrations. For instances when testing a urinary tract isolate is appropriate, ampicillin, ciprofloxacin, levofloxacin, nitrofurantoin, norfloxacin, or tetracycline could be selected (58).

REFERENCES

1. **Awada, A., P. Van der Auwera, F. Meunier, D. Daneau, and J. Klastersky.** 1992. Streptococcal and enterococcal bacteremia in patients with cancer. *Clin. Infect. Dis.* **15:** 33–48.
2. **Barbier, N., P. Sauinier, E. Chachaty, S. Dumontier, and A. Andremont.** 1996. Random amplified polymorphic DNA typing versus pulsed-field gel electrophoresis for epidemiologic typing of vancomycin-resistant enterococci. *J. Clin. Microbiol.* **34:**1096–1099.
3. **Beimfohr, D., A. Krause, R. Amann, W. Ludwig, and K. H. Schleifer.** 1993. *In situ* identification of lactococci, enterococci and streptococci. *Syst. Appl. Microbiol.* **16:** 450–456.
4. **Blaimont, B., J. Charlier, and G. Wauters.** 1995. Comparative distribution of *Enterococcus* species in faeces and clinical samples. *Microb. Ecol. Health Dis.* **8:**87–92.
5. **Bodnar, U. R., G. A. Noskin, T. Suriano, I. Cooper, B. E. Reisberg, and L. R. Peterson.** 1996. Use of in-house studies of molecular epidemiology and full species identification for controlling spread of vancomycin-resistant *Enterococcus faecalis* isolates. *J. Clin. Microbiol.* **34:** 2129–2132.
6. **Boyce, J. M., S. M. Opal, G. Potter-Bynoe, R. G. LaForge, M. J. Zervos, G. Furtado, G. Victor, and A. A. Medeiros.** 1992. Emergence and nosocomial transmission of ampicillin-resistant enterococci. *Antimicrob. Agents Chemother.* **36:**1032–1039.
7. **Boyle, J. F., S. A. Soumakis, A. Rendo, J. A. Herrington, D. G. Gianarkis, B. E. Thurberg, and B. G. Painter.** 1993. Epidemiologic analysis and genotypic characterization of nosocomial outbreak of vancomycin-resistant enterococci. *J. Clin. Microbiol.* **31:**1280–1285.
8. **Bryce, E. A., S. J. V. Zemcov, and A. M. Clarke.** 1991. Species identification and antibiotic resistance patterns of the enterococci. *Eur. J. Clin. Microbiol. Infect. Dis.* **10:** 745–747.
9. **Buschelman, B. J., B. J. Bale, and R. N. Jones.** 1993. Species identification and determination of high-level aminoglycoside resistance among enterococci. Comparison study of sterile body fluid isolates. *Diagn. Microbiol. Infect. Dis.* **16:**119–122.
10. **Carvalho, M. G. S., L. M. Teixeira, and R. R. Facklam.** 1998. Use of tests for acidification of methyl-α-D-glucopyranoside and susceptibility to efrotomycin for differentiation of strains of *Enterococcus* and some related genera. *J. Clin. Microbiol.* **36:**1584–1587.
11. **Carvalho, M. G. S., M. C. E. Vianni, J. A. Elliott, M. Reeves, R. R. Facklam, and L. M. Teixeira.** 1997. Molecular analysis of *Lactococcus garvieae* and *Enterococcus gallinarum* isolated from water buffalos with subclinical mastitis. *Adv. Exp. Med. Biol.* **418:**401–404.
12. **Chirurgi, V. A., S. E. Oster, A. A. Goldberg, M. J. Zervos, and R. E. McCabe.** 1991. Ampicillin-resistant *Enterococcus raffinosus* in an acute-care hospital: case-control study and antimicrobial susceptibilities. *J. Clin. Microbiol.* **29:**2663–2665.
13. **Chow, J. W., A. Kuritza, D. M. Shlaes, M. Green, D. F. Sahm, and M. J. Zervos.** 1993. Clonal spread of vancomycin-resistant *Enterococcus faecium* between patients in three hospitals in two states. *J. Clin. Microbiol.* **31:** 1609–1611.
14. **Clark, N. C., R. C. Cooksey, B. C. Hill, J. M. Swensen, and F. C. Tenover.** 1993. Characterization of glycopeptide-resistant enterococci from U.S. hospitals. *Antimicrob. Agents Chemother.* **37:**2311–2317.
15. **Collins, M. D., C. Ash, J. A. E. Farrow, S. Wallbanks, and A. M. Williams.** 1989. 16S ribosomal ribonucleic acid sequence analyses of lactococci and related taxa. Description of *Vagococcus fluvialis* gen. nov., sp. nov. *J. Appl. Bacteriol.* **67:**453–460.
16. **Collins, M. D., R. R. Facklam, J. A. E. Farrow, and R. Williamson.** 1989. *Enterococcus raffinosus* sp. nov., *Enterococcus solitarius* sp. nov. and *Enterococcus pseudoavium* sp. nov. *FEMS Microbiol. Lett.* **57:**283–288.
17. **Collins, M. D., J. A. E. Farrow, and D. Jones.** 1986. *Enterococcus mundtii* sp. nov. *Int. J. Syst. Bacteriol.* **36:** 8–12.
18. **Collins, M. D., D. Jones, J. A. E. Farrow, R. Kilpper-Balz, and K. H. Schleifer.** 1984. *Enterococcus avium* nom. rev., comb. nov.; *E. casseliflavus* nom. rev., comb. nov.; *E. durans* nom. rev., comb. nov.; *E. gallinarum* comb. nov.; and *E. malodoratus* sp. nov. *Int. J. Syst. Bacteriol.* **34:** 220–223.
19. **Collins, M. D., U. M. Rodrigues, N. E. Pigott, and R. R. Facklam.** 1991. *Enterococcus dispar* sp. nov. a new *Enterococcus* species from human sources. *Lett. Appl. Microbiol.* **12:**95–98.
20. **Collins, M. D., A. M. Williams, and S. Wallbanks.** 1990. The phylogeny of *Aerococcus* and *Pediococcus* as determined by 16S rRNA sequence analysis: description of *Tetragenococcus* gen. nov. *FEMS Microbiol. Lett.* **70:** 255–262.

21. **Coudron, P. E., C. G. Mayhall, R. R. Facklam, A. C. Spadora, V. A. Lamb, M. R. Lybrand, and H. P. Dalton.** 1984. *Streptococcus faecium* outbreak in a neonatal intensive care unit. *J. Clin. Microbiol.* **20:**1044–1048.
22. **Daly, J. A., N. L. Clifton, K. C. Seskin, and W. M. Gooch III.** 1991. Use of rapid, nonradioactive DNA probes in culture confirmation tests to detect *Streptococcus agalactiae*, *Haemophilus influenzae*, and *Enterococcus* spp. from pediatric patients with significant infections. *J. Clin. Microbiol.* **29:**80–82.
23. **Dembry, L. M., K. Uzoke, and M. J. Zervos.** 1996. Control of endemic glycopeptide-resistant enterococci. *Infect. Control Hosp. Epidemiol.* **17:**286–292.
24. **Descheemaeker, P., C. Lammens, B. Pot, P. Vandamme, and H. Goossens.** 1997. Evaluation of arbitrarily primed PCR analysis and pulsed-field gel electrophoresis of large genomic DNA fragments for identification of enterococci important in human medicine. *Int. J. Syst. Bacteriol.* **47:** 555–561.
25. **Devriese, L. A., K. Ceyssens, U. M. Rodrigues, and M. D. Collins.** 1990. *Enterococcus columbae*, a species from pigeon intestines. *FEMS Microbiol. Lett.* **71:**247–252.
26. **Devriese, L. A., M. D. Collins, and R. Wirth.** 1992. The genus *Enterococcus*, p. 1465–1481. *In* A. Balows, H. G. Truper, M. Dworkin, W. Harder, and K. H. Schleifer (ed.). *The Procaryotes. A Handbook on the Biology of Bacteria: Ecophysiology, Isolation, Identification, Applications*, 2nd ed. Springer-Verlag, New York, N.Y.
27. **Devriese, L. A., J. I. Cruz Cloque, P. DeHerdt, and F. Haesebrouck.** 1992. Identification and composition of the tonsilar and anal enterococci and streptococcal flora of dogs and cats. *J. Appl. Bacteriol.* **73:**421–425.
28. **Devriese, L. A., L. Laurier, P. DeHerdt, and F. Haesebrouck.** 1992. Enterococcal and streptococcal species isolated from faeces of calves, young cattle and dairy cows. *J. Appl. Bacteriol.* **72:**29–31.
29. **Domenech, A., J. Prieta, J. F. Fernandez-Garayzabal, M. D. Collins, D. Jones, and L. Dominquez.** 1993. Phenotypic and phylogenetic evidence for a close relationship between *Lactococcus garvieae* and *Enterococcus seriolicida*. *Microbiologia* **9:**63–68.
30. **Donabedian, S. M., J. W. Chow, J. M. Boyce, R. E. McCabe, S. M. Markowitz, P. E. Couldron, A. Kuritza, C. L. Pierson, and M. J. Zervos.** 1992. Molecular typing of ampicillin-resistant, non-β-lactamase-producing *Enterococcus faecium* isolates from diverse geographic areas. *J. Clin. Microbiol.* **30:**2757–2761.
31. **Donabedian, S. M., J. W. Chow, D. M. Shlaes, M. Green, and J. Zervos.** 1995. DNA hybridization and contour-clamped homogeneous electric field electrophoresis for identification of enterococci to the species level. *J. Clin. Microbiol.* **33:**141–145.
32. **Dutka, B. J., and K. K. Kwan.** 1978. Comparison of eight media-procedures for recovering faecal streptococci from water under winter conditions. *J. Appl. Bacteriol.* **45:** 333–340.
33. **Dutka-Malen, S., S. Evers, and P. Courvalin.** 1995. Detection of glycopeptide resistance genotypes and identification to the species level of clinically relevant enterococci by PCR. *J. Clin. Microbiol.* **33:**24–27.
34. **Edberg, S. C., C. J. Hardalo, C. Kontnick, and S. Campbell.** 1994. Rapid detection of vancomycin-resistant enterococci. *J. Clin. Microbiol.* **32:**2182–2184.
35. **Elliott, J. A., M. D. Collins, N. E. Pigott, and R. R. Facklam.** 1991. Differentiation of *Lactococcus lactis* and *Lactococcus garvieae* from humans by comparison of whole-cell protein patterns. *J. Clin. Microbiol.* **29:**2731–2734.
36. **Endtz, H. P., N. van den Braak, A. van Belkum, J. A. J. W. Kluytmans, J. G. M. Doeleman, L. Spanjaard, A. Voss, A. J. L. Weersink, C. J. E. Vanderbroucke-Grauls, A. G. M. Buiting, A. van Duin, and H. A. Verbrugh.** 1997. Fecal carriage of vancomycin-resistant enterococci in hospitalized patients and those living in the community in The Netherlands. *J. Clin. Microbiol.* **35:** 3026–3031.
37. **Enns, R. K.** 1988. DNA probes: an overview and comparison with current methods. *Lab. Med.* **19:**295–300.
38. **Facklam, R. R.** 1976. A review of the microbiological techniques for the isolation and identification of streptococci. *Crit. Rev. Clin. Lab. Sci.* **6:**287–317.
39. **Facklam, R. R., and M. D. Collins.** 1989. Identification of *Enterococcus* species isolated from human infections by a conventional test scheme. *J. Clin. Microbiol.* **27:** 731–734.
40. **Facklam, R. R., and J. A. Elliott.** 1995. Identification, classification, and clinical relevance of catalase-negative, gram-positive cocci, excluding the streptococci and enterococci. *Clin. Microbiol. Rev.* **8:**479–495.
41. **Facklam, R. R., D. Hollis, and M. D. Collins.** 1989. Identification of gram-positive coccal and coccobacillary vancomycin-resistant bacteria. *J. Clin. Microbiol.* **27:** 724–730.
42. **Farrow, J. A. E., and M. D. Collins.** 1985. *Enterococcus hirae*, a new species that includes amino acid assay strains causing NCDO 1258 and strains causing growth depression in young chickens. *Int. J. Syst. Bacteriol.* **35:**73–75.
43. **Federal Register.** 1994. Preventing the spread of vancomycin resistance—report from the hospital infection control practices advisory committee. *Fed. Regist.* **59**(v): 25758–25763.
44. **Felmingham, D., A. P. R. Wilson, A. I. Quintana, and R. N. Gruneberg.** 1992. *Enterococcus* species in urinary tract infection. *Clin. Infect. Dis.* **15:**295–301.
45. **Ford, M., J. D. Perry, and F. K. Gould.** 1994. Use of cephalexin-aztreonam-arabinose agar for selective isolation of *Enterococcus faecium*. *J. Clin. Microbiol.* **32:** 2999–3001.
46. **Free, L., and D. F. Sahm.** 1995. Investigation of the reformulated Remel Synergy Quad Plate for detection of high-level aminoglycoside and vancomycin resistance among enterococci. *J. Clin. Microbiol.* **33:**1643–1645.
47. **Goering, R. V., and M. A. Winters.** 1992. Rapid method for epidemiological evaluation of gram-positive cocci by field inversion gel electrophoresis. *J. Clin. Microbiol.* **30:** 577–580.
48. **Gordillo, M. E., K. V. Singh, and B. E. Murray.** 1993. Comparison of ribotyping and pulsed-field gel electrophoresis for subspecies differentiation of strains of *Enterococcus faecalis*. *J. Clin. Microbiol.* **31:**1570–1574.
49. **Gordon, S., J. M. Swenson, B. C. Hill, N. E. Pigott, R. R. Facklam, R. C. Cooksey, C. Thornsberry, Enterococcal Study Group, W. R. Jarvis, and F. C. Tenover.** 1992. Antimicrobial susceptibility patterns of common and unusual species of enterococci causing infections in the United States. *J. Clin. Microbiol.* **30:**2373–2378.
50. **Gordtz, B., H. Van Landuyt, M. Ieven, P. Vandamme, and H. Goossens.** 1995. Vancomycin-resistant enterococci colonizing the intestinal tracts of hospitalized patients. *J. Clin. Microbiol.* **33:**2842–2846.
51. **Graninger, W., and R. Ragette.** 1992. Nosocomial bacteremia due to *Enterococcus faecalis* without endocarditis. *Clin. Infect. Dis.* **15:**49–57.
52. **Green, M., K. Barbadora, S. Donabedian, and M. J. Zervos.** 1995. Comparison of field inversion gel electrophoresis with contour-clamped homogeneous electric field electrophoresis as a typing method for *Enterococcus faecium*. *J. Clin. Microbiol.* **33:**1554–1557.
53. **Guiney, M., and G. Urwin.** 1993. Frequency and antimicrobial susceptibility of clinical isolates of enterococci. *Eur. J. Clin. Microbiol. Infect. Dis.* **12:**362–366.
54. **Gullberg, R. M., S. R. Homann, and J. P. Phair.** 1989.

Enterococcal bacteremia: analysis of 75 episodes. *Rev. Infect. Dis.* **11:**74–85.

55. **Hall, L. M. C., B. Duke, M. Guiney, and R. Williams.** 1992. Typing of *Enterococcus* species by DNA restriction fragment analysis. *J. Clin. Microbiol.* **30:**915–919.
56. **Hall, L. M. C., B. Duke, G. Urwin, and M. Guiney.** 1992. Epidemiology of *Enterococcus faecalis* urinary tract infection in a teaching hospital in London, United Kingdom. *J. Clin. Microbiol.* **30:**1953–1957.
57. **Hindler, J. A., and D. F. Sahm.** 1992. Controversies and confusion regarding antimicrobial susceptibility testing of enterococci. *Antimicrob. Newsl.* **8:**65–74.
58. **Huycke, M. M., D. F. Sahm, and M. S. Gilmore.** 1998. Multiple-drug resistant enterococci: the nature of the problem and an agenda for the future. *Emerg. Infect. Dis.* **4:**239–249.
59. **Issack, M. J., E. G. M. Power, and G. L. French.** 1996. Investigation of an outbreak of vancomycin-resistant *Enterococcus faecium* by random amplified polymorphic DNA (RAPD) assay. *J. Hosp. Infect.* **33:**191–200.
60. **Jayarao, B. M., J. J. E. Dore, Jr., and S. P. Oliver.** 1992. Restriction fragment length polymorphism analysis of 16S ribosomal DNA of *Streptococcus* and *Enterococcus* species of bovine origin. *J. Clin. Microbiol.* **30:**2235–2240.
61. **Kalina, A. P.** 1970. The taxonomy and nomenclature of enterococci. *Int. J. Syst. Bacteriol.* **20:**185–189.
62. **Kaufhold, A., and P. Ferrieri.** 1993. Molecular investigation of clinical *Enterococcus faecium* isolates highly resistant to gentamicin. *Zentralbl. Bakteriol. Abt. 1 Orig. B* **278:**83–101.
63. **Kibbey, H. J., C. Hagedorn, and E. L. McCoy.** 1978. Use of fecal streptococci as indicators of pollution in soil. *Appl. Environ. Microbiol.* **35:**711–717.
64. **Knudtson, L. M., and P. A. Hartman.** 1993. Comparison of four latex agglutination kits to rapidly identify Lancefield group D enterococci and fecal streptococci. *J. Rapid Methods Autom. Microbiol.* **1:**301–304.
65. **Kuhn, I., L. G. Burman, S. Haeggman, K. Tullus, and B. E. Murray.** 1995. Biochemical fingerprinting compared with ribotyping and pulsed-field gel electrophoresis of DNA for epidemiological typing of enterococci. *J. Clin. Microbiol.* **33:**2812–2817.
66. **Kusuda, R., K. Kawai, F. Salati, C. R. Banner, and J. L. Fryer.** 1991. *Enterococcus seriolicida* sp. nov., a fish pathogen. *Int. J. Syst. Bacteriol.* **41:**406–409.
67. **Lacoux, P. A., J. Z. Jordens, C. M. Fentin, M. Guiney, and T. H. Pennington.** 1992. Characterization of enterococcal isolates by restriction enzyme analysis of genomic DNA. *Epidemiol. Infect.* **109:**69–80.
68. **Landman, D., J. M. Quale, E. Oydna, B. Willey, V. Ditore, M. Zaman, K. Patel, G. Saurina, and W. Huang.** 1996. Comparison of five selective media for identifying fecal carriage of vancomycin-resistant enterococci. *J. Clin. Microbiol.* **34:**751–752.
69. **Livornese, L. L., Jr., S. Dias, C. Samel, B. Romanowski, S. Taylor, P. May, P. Pitsakis, G. Woods, D. Kaye, M. E. Levison, and C. C. Johnson.** 1992. Hospital-acquired infection with vancomycin-resistant *Enterococcus faecium* transmitted by electronic thermometers. *Ann. Intern. Med.* **117:**112–116.
70. **Luginbuhl, L. M., H. A. Rotbart, R. R. Facklam, M. H. Roe, and J. A. Elliott.** 1987. Neonatal enterococcal sepsis: case-control study and description of an outbreak. *Pediatr. Infect. Dis. J.* **6:**1022–1030.
71. **Maekawa, S., M. Yoshioka, and Y. Kumamoto.** 1992. Proposal of a new scheme for the serological typing of *Enterococcus faecalis* strains. *Microbiol. Immunol.* **36:** 671–681.
72. **Maki, D. G., and W. A. Agger.** 1988. Enterococcal bacteremia: clinical features, the risk of endocarditis, and management. *Medicine (Baltimore)* **67:**248–269.
73. **Martinez-Murcia, A. J., and M. D. Collins.** 1991. *Enterococcus sulfureus*, a new yellow-pigmented *Enterococcus* species. *FEMS Microbiol. Lett.* **80:**69–74.
74. **Mead, G. C.** 1978. Streptococci in the intestinal flora of man and other non-ruminant animals, p. 245–261. *In* F. A. Skinner and L. B. Quesnel (ed.), *Streptococci.* Academic Press, Inc. (London) Ltd., London, United Kingdom.
75. **Megran, D. W.** 1992. Enterococcal endocarditis. *Clin. Infect. Dis.* **15:**63–71.
76. **Merlino, J., S. Siarakas, G. J. Robertson, G. R. Funnel, T. Gottlieb, and R. Bradbury.** 1996. Evaluation of CHROMagar orientation for differentiation and presumptive identification of gram-negative bacilli and *Enterococcus* species. *J. Clin. Microbiol.* **34:**1788–1793.
77. **Merquior, V. L. C., J. M. Peralta, R. R. Facklam, and L. M. Teixeira.** 1994. Analysis of electrophoretic whole-cell protein profiles as a tool for characterization of *Enterococcus* species. *Curr. Microbiol.* **28:**149–153.
78. **Miranda, A. G., K. V. Singh, and B. E. Murray.** 1991. DNA fingerprinting of *Enterococcus faecium* by pulsed-field gel electrophoresis may be a useful epidemiologic tool. *J. Clin. Microbiol.* **29:**2752–2757.
79. **Moellering, R. C., Jr.** 1992. Emergence of *Enterococcus* as a significant pathogen. *Clin. Infect. Dis.* **14:**1173–1178.
80. **Morris, J. G., D. K. Shay, J. N. Hebden, R. J. McCarter, B. E. Perdue, W. Jarvis, J. A. Johnston, T. C. Dowling, L. B. Polish, and R. S. Schwalbe.** 1995. Enterococci resistant to multiple antimicrobial agents, including vancomycin. *Ann. Intern. Med.* **123:**250–259.
81. **Mundt, J. O., W. F. Graham, and I. E. McCarty.** 1967. Spherical lactic acid-producing bacteria of Southern-grown raw and processed vegetables. *Appl. Environ. Microbiol.* **15:**1303–1308.
82. **Murray, B. E.** 1990. The life and times of the *Enterococcus. Clin. Microbiol. Rev.* **3:**46–65.
83. **Murray, B. E., H. A. Lopardo, E. A. Rubeglio, M. Frosolono, and K. V. Singh.** 1992. Intrahospital spread of a single gentamicin-resistant, β-lactamase-producing strain of *Enterococcus faecalis* in Argentina. *Antimicrob. Agents Chemother.* **36:**230–232.
84. **Murray, B. E., K. V. Singh, J. D. Heath, B. R. Skharma, and G. M. Weinstock.** 1990. Comparison of genomic DNAs of different enterococcal isolates using restriction endonucleases with infrequent recognition sites. *J. Clin. Microbiol.* **28:**2059–2063.
85. **Murray, B. E., K. V. Singh, S. M. Markowitz, H. A. Lopardo, J. E. Patterson, M. J. Zervos, E. Rubeglio, G. M. Eliopoulos, L. B. Rice, F. W. Goldstein, S. G. Jenkins, G. M. Caputo, R. Nasnas, L. S. Moore, E. S. Wong, and G. Weinstock.** 1991. Evidence for clonal spread of a single strain of β-lactamase-producing *Enterococcus (Streptococcus) faecalis* in six hospitals in five states. *J. Infect. Dis.* **163:**780–785.
86. **Nauschuetz, W. F., S. B. Trevino, L. S. Harrison, R. N. Longfield, L. Fletcher, and W. G. Wortham.** 1993. *Enterococcus casseliflavus* as an agent of nosocomial bloodstream infections. *Med. Microbiol. Lett.* **2:**102–108.
87. **Nichols, R. L., and A. C. Muzik.** 1992. Enterococcal infections in surgical patients: the mystery continues. *Clin. Infect. Dis.* **15:**72–76.
88. **Niemi, R. M., S. I. Niemela, D. H. Bamford, J. Hantula, T. Hyvarinen, T. Forsten, and A. Raateland.** 1993. Presumptive fecal streptococci in environmental samples characterized by one-dimensional sodium dodecyl sulfate-polyacrylamide gel electrophoresis. *Appl. Environ. Microbiol.* **59:**2190–2196.
89. **Patel, R., J. R. Uhl, P. Kohner, K. K. Hopkins, and F. R. Corkerill III.** 1997. Multiplex PCR detection of *vanA*, *vanB*, *vanC-1*, and *vanC-2/3* genes in enterococci. *J. Clin. Microbiol.* **35:**703–707.
90. **Patterson, J. E., K. V. Singh, and B. E. Murray.** 1991.

Epidemiology of an endemic strain of β-lactamase-producing *Enterococcus faecalis*. *J. Clin. Microbiol.* **29:** 2513–2516.

91. **Pegues, D. A., C. F. Pegues, P. L. Hibberd, D. S. Ford, and D. C. Hooper.** 1997. Emergence and dissemination of a highly vancomycin-resistant *vanA* strain of *Enterococcus faecium* at a large teaching hospital. *J. Clin. Microbiol.* **35:** 1565–1570.
92. **Perlada, D. E., A. G. Smulian, and M. T. Cushion.** 1997. Molecular epidemiology and antibiotic susceptibility of enterococci in Cincinnati, Ohio: a prospective citywide survey. *J. Clin. Microbiol.* **35:**2342–2347.
93. **Plessis, P., T. Lamy, P. Y. Donnio, F. Autuly, I. Grulois, P. Y. Le Prise, and J. L. Avril.** 1995. Epidemiologic analysis of glycopeptide-resistant *Enterococcus* strains in neutropenic patients receiving prolonged vancomycin administration. *Eur. J. Clin. Microbiol. Infect. Dis.* **14:** 959–963.
94. **Pompei, R., F. Berlutti, M. C. Thaller, A. Ingianni, G. Cortis, and B. Dainelli.** 1992. *Enterococcus flavescens* sp. nov., a new species of enterococci of clinical origin. *Int. J. Syst. Bacteriol.* **42:**365–369.
95. **Rodrigues, U., and M. D. Collins.** 1990. Phylogenetic analysis of *Streptococcus saccharolyticus* based on 16S rRNA sequencing. *FEMS Microbiol. Lett.* **71:**231–234.
96. **Rubin, L. G., V. Tucci, E. Cercenado, G. Eliopoulos, and H. D. Isenberg.** 1992. Vancomycin-resistant *Enterococcus faecium* in hospitalized children. *Infect. Control Hosp. Epidemiol.* **13:**700–705.
97. **Ruoff, K. L., L. de la Maza, M. J. Murtagh, J. D. Spargo, and M. J. Ferraro.** 1990. Species identities of enterococci isolated from clinical specimens. *J. Clin. Microbiol.* **28:** 435–437.
98. **Sader, H. S., M. A. Pfaller, F. C. Tenover, R. J. Hollis, and R. N. Jones.** 1994. Evaluation and characterization of multiresistant *Enterococcus faecium* from 12 U.S. medical centers. *J. Clin. Microbiol.* **32:**2840–2842.
99. **Sahm, D. F., L. Free, C. Smith, M. Eveland, and L. M. Mundy.** 1997. Rapid characterization schemes for surveillance isolates of vancomycin-resistant enterococci. *J. Clin. Microbiol.* **35:**2026–2030.
100. **Schaberg, D. R., D. H. Culver, and R. P. Gaynes.** 1991. Major trends in the microbial etiology of nosocomial infection. *Am. J. Med.* **91:**79S–82S.
101. **Schleifer, K. H., and R. Kilpper-Balz.** 1984. Transfer of *Streptococcus faecalis* and *Streptococcus faecium* to the genus *Enterococcus* nom. rev. as *Enterococcus faecalis* comb. nov. and *Enterococcus faecium* com. nov. *Int. J. Syst. Bacteriol.* **34:**31–34.
102. **Singer, D. A., E. M. Jochimsen, P. Gielerak, and W. R. Jarvis.** 1996. Pseudo-outbreak of *Enterococcus durans* infections and colonization associated with introduction of an automated identification system software update. *J. Clin. Microbiol.* **34:**2685–2687.
103. **Teixeira, L, M., M. G. S. Carvalho, V. L. C. Merquior, A. G. Steigerwalt, D. J. Brenner, and R. R. Facklam.** 1997. Phenotypic and genotypic characterization of *Vagococcus fluvialis*, including strains isolated from human sources. *J. Clin. Microbiol.* **35:**2778–2781.
104. **Teixeira, L. M., M. G. S. Carvalho, V. L. C. Merquior, A. G. Steigerwalt, M. G. M. Teixeira, D. J. Brenner, and R. R. Facklam.** 1997. Recent approaches on the taxonomy of the enterococci and some related microorganisms. *Adv. Exp. Med. Biol.* **418:**397–400.
105. **Teixeira, L. M., R. R. Facklam, A. G. Steigerwalt, N. E. Pigott, V. L. C. Merquior, and D. J. Brenner.** 1995. Correlation between phenotypic characteristics and DNA relatedness within *Enterococcus faecium* strains. *J. Clin. Microbiol.* **33:**1520–1523.
106. **Teixeira, L. M., V. L. C. Merquior, M. C. E. Vianni, M. G. S. Carvalho, S. E. L. Fracalanzza, A. G. Steigerwalt, D. J. Brenner, and R. R. Facklam.** 1996. Phenotypic and genotypic characterization of atypical *Lactococcus garvieae* strains isolated from water buffalos with subclinical mastitis and confirmation of *L. garvieae* as a senior subjective synonym of *Enterococcus seriolicida*. *Int. J. Syst. Bacteriol.* **46:**664–668.
107. **Thal, L. A., J. W. Chow, J. E. Patterson, M. B. Perri, S. Donabedian, D. B. Clewell, and M. J. Zervos.** 1993. Molecular characterization of highly gentamicin-resistant *Enterococcus faecalis* isolates lacking high-level streptomycin resistance. *Antimicrob. Agents Chemother.* **37:** 134–137.
108. **Tomayko, J. F., and B. E. Murray.** 1995. Analysis of *Enterococcus faecalis* isolates from intercontinental sources by multilocus enzyme electrophoresis and pulsed-field gel electrophoresis. *J. Clin. Microbiol.* **33:**2903–2907.
109. **Toye, B., J. Shymanski, M. Bobrowska, W. Woods, and K. Ramotar.** 1997. Clinical and epidemiological significance of enterococci intrinsically resistant to vancomycin (possessing the *vanC* genotype). *J. Clin. Microbiol.* **35:** 3166–3170.
110. **Truant, A. L., and V. Satishchandran.** 1993. Comparison of Streptex versus PathoDx for group D typing of vancomycin-resistant *Enterococcus*. *Diagn. Microbiol. Infect. Dis.* **16:**89–91.
111. **Tyrrell, G. J., R. N. Bethune, B. Willey, and D. E. Low.** 1997. Species identification of enterococci via intergenic ribosomal PCR. *J. Clin. Microbiol.* **35:**1054–1060.
112. **Van Horn, K. G., C. A. Gedris, and K. M. Rodney.** 1996. Selective isolation of vancomycin-resistant enterococci. *J. Clin. Microbiol.* **34:**924–927.
113. **Van Horn, K. G., C. A. Gedris, K. M. Rodney, and J. B. Mitchell.** 1996. Evaluation of commercial vancomycin agar screen plates for detection of vancomycin-resistant enterococci. *J. Clin. Microbiol.* **34:**2042–2044.
114. **Watanakunakorn, C., and T. Burkert.** 1993. Infective endocarditis at a large community teaching hospital, 1980–1990. *Medicine* **72:**90–102.
115. **Willey, B. M., A. J. McGree, M. A. Ostrowski, B. N. Kreiswirth, and D. E. Low.** 1994. The use of molecular typing techniques in the epidemiologic investigation of resistant enterococci. *Infect. Control Hosp. Epidemiol.* **15:** 548–556.
116. **Williams, A. M., J. A. E. Farrow, and M. D. Collins.** 1989. Reverse transcriptase sequencing of 16S ribosomal RNA from *Streptococcus cecorum*. *Lett. Appl. Microbiol.* **8:** 185–189.
117. **Williams, A. M., U. M. Rodrigues, and M. D. Collins.** 1991. Intrageneric relationships of *Enterococci* as determined by reverse transcriptase sequencing of small-subunit rRNA. *Res. Microbiol.* **142:**67–74.
118. **Willinger, B., and M. Manafi.** 1995. Evaluation of new chromogenic agar medium for the identification of urinary tract pathogens. *Lett. Appl. Microbiol.* **20:**300–302.
119. **Woodford, N., D. Morrison, B. Cookson, and R. C. George.** 1993. Comparison of high-level gentamicin-resistant *Enterococcus faecium* isolates from different continents. *Antimicrob. Agents Chemother.* **37:**681–684.
120. **Woodford, N., D. Morrison, A. P. Johnson, V. Briant, R. C. George, and B. Cookson.** 1993. Application of DNA probes for rRNA and *vanA* genes to investigation of a nosocomial cluster of vancomycin-resistant enterococci. *J. Clin. Microbiol.* **31:**653–658.
121. **Zervos, M. J., S. Dembinski, T. Mikesell, and D. R. Schaberg.** 1986. High-level resistance to gentamicin in *Streptococcus faecalis*: risk factors and evidence for exogenous acquisition of infection. *J. Infect. Dis.* **153:** 1075–1083.

Leuconostoc, Pediococcus, Stomatococcus, and Miscellaneous Gram-Positive Cocci That Grow Aerobically

KATHRYN L. RUOFF

19

TAXONOMY

The bacteria included in this chapter are taxonomically diverse gram-positive cocci. All, however, share the characteristic of being infrequent clinical isolates found as opportunistic agents of infection in hosts who are usually compromised. Many of the genera discussed here are members of the normal flora of the oral cavity, respiratory or alimentary tracts, or skin. Most of these organisms resemble other, more well known clinical isolates (i.e., streptococci, enterococci, and staphylococci) and consequently may be mistaken for members of those genera. These bacteria may have been misidentified or overlooked in clinical cultures in the past or may represent emerging pathogens in compromised patient populations. Table 1 lists the organisms included here along with some of their basic characteristics. The references listed in Table 1 should be consulted for detailed taxonomic information.

Most organisms listed in Table 1 exhibit fairly low G+C contents (30 to 45 mol%) and are not currently affiliated with taxa above the genus level. Although *Stomatococcus* (55 to 60 mol% G+C) and *Micrococcus* (64 to 75 mol% G+C) are both included along with staphylococci in the family *Micrococcaceae*, Stackebrandt (65) has noted that both of these genera probably belong (along with other non-staphylococcal organisms) in a yet-to-be described family. Stomatococci have been classified in the past as either micrococci or staphylococci. The genus *Planococcus*, traditionally classified in the family *Micrococcaceae*, is a motile coccus that is isolated from marine environments and that is now considered to be closely related to the genus *Bacillus* (18).

The genus *Lactococcus* is composed of organisms formerly classified as Lancefield group N streptococci (62). Motile *Lactococcus*-like organisms with the Lancefield group N antigen (a teichoic acid antigen) have been classified in the genus *Vagococcus* (20, 69). The vagococci also resemble the enterococci, and Facklam and Elliott (31) reported that *Vagococcus* isolates examined at the Centers for Disease Control and Prevention gave positive reactions in a commercially available nucleic acid-based probe test for enterococci.

The recently described genus *Abiotrophia* was proposed to accommodate organisms previously known as the nutritionally variant or satelliting streptococci (43). These bacteria were initially considered nutritional mutants of viridans group streptococcal strains, most notably of the species *Streptococcus mitis*. The work of Bouvet and colleagues (11) suggested that these organisms were really members of two novel streptococcal species given the names *Streptococcus defectivus* and *Streptococcus adjacens*. A comparative analysis of 16S rRNA sequences led Kawamura and coworkers (43) to propose the creation of a new genus, *Abiotrophia*, containing two species, *Abiotrophia defectiva* and *Abiotrophia adiacens*, to accommodate these bacteria. A third species, *Abiotrophia elegans*, was described in 1998 (58).

Members of the intrinsically vancomycin-resistant genus *Pediococcus* previously known as the species *Pediococcus halophilus* have been reclassified in the recently described genus *Tetragenococcus* (23). Tetragenococci have not, however, been isolated from human clinical specimens.

The organism now known as *Gemella morbillorum* was noted in 1917 by Tunicliff (67), who was searching for the etiologic agent of measles. The organism that she isolated from cultures of blood from numerous measles patients was originally named *Diplococcus rubeolae*. This bacterium has also been known as *Diplococcus morbillorum*, *Peptostreptococcus morbillorum*, and *Streptococcus morbillorum* until a proposal to include it in the genus *Gemella* was made in 1988 (46). *Gemella haemolysans* was originally classified as a *Neisseria*, due to its gram-variable or even gram-negative nature, and its cellular morphology (diplococci with flattened adjacent sides). The recently described genus *Dolosigranulum* shows phenotypic similarities with *Gemella*, although it is not closely related to *Gemella* strains (3).

Aerococcus urinae, a new species in the genus *Aerococcus*, is pyrrolidonyl arylamidase (PYR) negative and leucine aminopeptidase (LAP) positive, showing reactions opposite those of *Aerococcus viridans* in these important identification tests. Despite these phenotypic differences, molecular biology-based taxonomic studies suggest that *A. urinae* should remain in the *Aerococcus* genus. Organisms currently included in the *A. urinae* species are fairly heterogeneous and can probably be subdivided into at least two subspecies (17).

The sole species of the genus *Alloiococcus* was originally named *Alloiococcus otitis* (1), but von Graevenitz (68) recommended that it be renamed *Alloiococcus otitidis*, in keeping with the rules of the Bacteriological Code. Six of the 11 genera listed in Table 1 have been described since 1982 (*Stomatococcus*, *Lactococcus*, *Globicatella*, *Helcococcus*, *Alloiococcus*, *Abiotrophia*). The examination of gram-positive

TABLE 1 Some characteristics of infrequently isolated gram-positive cocci that grow aerobically[a,b]

Genus	Catalase	Relationship to oxygen	Appearance of Gram stain[c]	Reference
Streptococcus-like				
Abiotrophia	−	Facultative	c, cb, rods[d]	43
Globicatella	−	Facultative	cb, pr, ch	19
Lactococcus	−	Facultative	cb, pr, ch	62
Leuconostoc	−	Facultative	cb, pr, ch	37
Staphylococcus-like				
Aerococcus	− or w	Microaerophilic	c, pr, tet, cl	30
Alloiococcus	+[e]	Aerobic	cb, pr, tet	1
Gemella[f]	−	Aerobic or facultative[g]	c, pr, ch, cl[h]	56
Helcococcus	−	Facultative	c, pr, ch, cl	21
Micrococcus	+	Aerobic	c, cl, tet	61
Pediococcus	−	Facultative	c, pr, tet, cl	38
Stomatococcus	−, +, or w	Facultative	c, pr, cl	61

[a] Abbreviations and symbols: +, positive; −, negative; w, weak; cb, coccobacilli; pr, pairs; ch, chains; c, cocci; tet, tetrads; cl, clusters.

[b] Information on *Dolosigranulum, Vagococcus,* and *Facklamia* has been omitted from the table due to a lack of information on their characteristics and clinical significance. See text for information on these organisms.

[c] Morphology is most characteristic for organisms grown in broth.

[d] Cells are often pleomorphic; morphology varies with the medium on which cells have been grown.

[e] *Alloiococcus* strains may be negative by the catalase test, especially when they are grown on medium devoid of blood.

[f] G. *haemolysans* is easily decolorized and may appear gram variable or gram negative.

[g] G. *haemolysans* prefers an aerobic growth atmosphere, while G. *morbillorum* flourishes under anaerobic conditions.

[h] G. *haemolysans* cells usually occur as diplococci with adjacent sides flattened, while G. *morbillorum* cells are found in pairs, sometimes with cells of unequal sizes in a given pair, and chains.

cocci by molecular biology-based taxonomic methods has encouraged the delineation of these new groups of organisms and the refinement of a genetically based taxonomy for the gram-positive cocci.

DESCRIPTION OF THE GENERA

The organisms included in this chapter form gram-positive coccoid cells, but G. *haemolysans* may appear to be a gram-variable or gram-negative organism due to the ease with which its cells are decolorized. Cell shape and arrangement can aid in dividing these organisms into two broad groups, as listed in Table 1: those with a "streptococcal-like" Gram staining result (coccobacilli in pairs and chains) or those with a "staphylococcal-like" Gram staining result (more spherical cocci in pairs, tetrads, or clusters). Members of the genus *Abiotrophia* (formerly the nutritionally variant streptococci) may form coccobacilli arranged in pairs and chains, but these organisms also may appear pleomorphic, especially when they are grown under less than optimal nutritional conditions. The division of these diverse bacteria into two groups on the basis of cellular shape and arrangement serves only as an aid in identification; no relatedness of organisms is implied by this grouping. With the exception of the infrequently isolated vagococci, these organisms are nonmotile.

Most of the genera are facultative anaerobes, but *Micrococcus* and *Alloiococcus* are obligate aerobes. *Aerococcus* is classified as a microaerophile that grows poorly if at all under anaerobic conditions. The obligately aerobic genera are catalase positive, but strains of *Alloiococcus* have been described as being weakly catalase positive (31). Some strains of *Aerococcus* may exhibit weakly positive catalase reactions due to nonheme catalase activity, while *Stomatococcus* isolates, capable of heme synthesis, may evidence negative, weakly positive, or strongly positive reactions when tested with 3% hydrogen peroxide. None of the genera are beta-hemolytic on routinely used blood agars, but G. *haemolysans* is described as producing beta-hemolysis on agars supplemented with rabbit or horse blood (56).

NATURAL HABITATS

Some of the genera discussed here are members of the normal flora of the oral cavity or upper respiratory tract (*Stomatococcus, Gemella, Abiotrophia*) or colonize the skin (*Helcococcus*). Foods and vegetation are normal habitats for lactococci, pediococci, and leuconostocs; these genera may also be found as normal flora of the alimentary tract, but thorough data supporting this contention are lacking. Aerococci and micrococci are environmental isolates that can also be found on human skin. Although they have been isolated from human sources, the natural habitats of globicatellas, alloiococci, and some of the other organisms mentioned here are not well characterized.

CLINICAL SIGNIFICANCE

Although the organisms included in this chapter may be present as contaminants in clinical cultures, they are also isolated infrequently as opportunistic pathogens. These bacteria appear to be of low virulence and are normally pathogenic only in compromised hosts. Infection often occurs in previously damaged tissues (e.g., heart valves) or may be nosocomial and associated with prolonged hospitalization, antibiotic treatment, invasive procedures, and the presence of foreign bodies. Specimens likely to yield significant isolates of these bacteria are blood, cerebrospinal fluid, urine, and wound specimens.

Lactococcus

Difficulties in distinguishing lactococci from either streptococci or enterococci have probably led to the misidentification of clinical *Lactococcus* isolates in the past and may have contributed to the paucity of reports concerning the clinical role of these bacteria. Elliott and coworkers (27) studied the phenotypic characteristics of a number of lactococcal strains isolated from blood, patients with urinary tract infections, and an eye wound culture. The authors observed that three of the blood culture isolates were from patients diagnosed with prosthetic valve endocarditis. Other reports have noted cases of native-valve lactococcal endocarditis (48, 55). Due to the existence of very few isolates from human sources, not much is known about the clinical significance of members of the genus *Vagococcus*, motile organisms which, like lactococci, elaborate the Lancefield group N antigen (31).

Abiotrophia

Organisms formally known as nutritionally variant streptococci are normal residents of the oral cavity but have been identified as agents of endocarditis involving both native and prosthetic valves. These organisms have also been isolated from patients with ophthalmic infections (52).

Leuconostoc and *Pediococcus*

The vancomycin-resistant genera *Leuconostoc* and *Pediococcus* have been recognized in clinical specimens since the mid-1980s. Handwerger and colleagues (41) noted host defense impairment, invasive procedures breaching the integument, gastrointestinal symptoms, and prior antibiotic treatment as common features among adult patients infected with *Leuconostoc*. They also observed a predisposition to *Leuconostoc* bacteremia among neonates, suggesting that during delivery infants may become colonized with leuconostocs inhabiting the maternal genital tract. In addition to causing bacteremia, leuconostocs have also been isolated from cerebrospinal fluid, peritoneal dialysate fluid, and wounds.

The clinical significance of *Pediococcus* is less well documented. Mastro and coworkers (49) could find no clearly defined syndrome associated with the isolation of *Pediococcus acidilactici* from blood cultures in nine cases that they reviewed. They concluded that while this organism may be an opportunist in severely compromised patients, further data were needed to clarify its clinical significance. More recent reports have described *P. acidilactici* as an agent of septicemia and hepatic abscess (39, 63).

Gemella

G. haemolysans has been isolated as a pathogen from patients with endocarditis (15), meningitis (36), and a total knee arthroplasty (26). The other currently described member of this genus, *G. morbillorum*, has been isolated (when still classified as a streptococcus; see Taxonomy above) from cultures of blood, respiratory, genitourinary, wound, and abscess specimens (32), and from a patient with an infection in an arteriovenous shunt (5). Little is known about the clinical significance of *Dolosigranulum*, a genus that is phenotypically similar but not closely related to *Gemella*. The genus description is based on only two human clinical isolates (3).

Aerococcus

Although aerococci appear as contaminants in clinical cultures, occasional reports have noted a clinically significant role for these organisms in cases of endocarditis and bacteremia (24, 44, 53). A relatively new *Aerococcus* species, *A. urinae* (2), has been implicated as a urinary tract pathogen in patients predisposed to infection (16) and also as an agent of endocarditis (47, 64).

Globicatella

Globicatella sanguis, the sole species in the genus, has been isolated from patients with bacteremia, urinary tract infection, and meningitis (19). The recently described species *Facklamia hominis* (22) is closely related to but phenotypically and phylogenetically distinct from *Globicatella*. The six clinical isolates of *F. hominis* recognized to date have originated from genitourinary, blood, and wound specimens.

Helcococcus

Helcococcus kunzii, the only species in this recently described genus, has been isolated from intact skin of the lower extremities (40), as well as from wound cultures (notably foot ulcers) containing a mixture of bacteria (21). Consequently, the clinical significance of this organism is difficult to interpret, since it may be present merely as a colonizer of the wound site. The ability of this species to function as an opportunist was, however, suggested by its isolation in pure culture from an infected sebaceous cyst (54).

Stomatococcus

A 1978 report by Rubin and colleagues (59) of endocarditis caused by "*Micrococcus mucilaginosus incertae sedis*" represents the first well-documented account of disease caused by the organism currently called *Stomatococcus mucilaginosus*. Numerous reports of infection due to this organism began appearing in the middle to late 1980s. McWhinney and coworkers (50) and Ascher et al. (4) reviewed published descriptions of *Stomatococcus* infections (endocarditis, bacteremia, intravascular catheter infection, meningitis, peritonitis) and noted serious underlying disease, neutropenia, the presence of a foreign body, cardiac valve disease, or intravenous drug use as predisposing factors. Destruction of oral mucous membranes as a result of chemo- or radiotherapy was hypothesized to play a role in the dissemination of stomatococci from their normal habitat in the oral cavity.

Alloiococcus

Alloiococci have been isolated from the middle ear fluid of children with chronic otitis media. The observation of intracellular alloiococci and significant levels of inflammatory cells in middle ear fluids bearing this organism led Faden and Dryja (34) to suggest that *Alloiococcus* may play a pathogenic role in persistent otitis media.

Micrococcus

While micrococci appear as contaminants in cultures of clinical material, they may occasionally participate in infections like endocarditis (45).

COLLECTION, TRANSPORT, AND STORAGE OF SPECIMENS

The organisms described in this chapter have all been isolated from routine cultures of clinical specimens, and special requirements for the collection and processing of specimens have not been described. Since these bacteria are either facultative anaerobes, microaerophilic, or obligately aerobic, the aerobic collection, transport, and storage methods described in chapter 4 of this Manual should allow their isolation.

ISOLATION PROCEDURES

Generally, there are no special requirements for isolation of the group of bacteria discussed here; general recommenda-

TABLE 2 Differentiating features of gram-positive cocci with negative or weakly positive catalase reactions[a,b]

Genus	PYR	VAN	LAP	Gas[c]	Esculin hydrolysis	Growth in 6.5% NaCl
Streptococcus	V[d]	S	+	−	V	V[e]
Enterococcus	+	V[f]	+	−	+	+
Lactococcus	V	S	+	−	V[g]	V
Abiotrophia	+	S	+	−	V	−
Leuconostoc	−	R	−	+	V	V
Pediococcus	−	R	+	−	V[g]	V
Gemella	+	S	V	−	−	−
Aerococcus viridans	+	S	−	−	V	+
Aerococcus urinae	−	S	+	−	V	+
Helcococcus	+	S	−	−	+	V
Globicatella	+	S	−	−	+	+
Stomatococcus	+[g]	S	+	−	+	−

[a] Abbreviations and symbols: +, positive; −, negative; V, variable; S, susceptible; R, resistant; VAN, vancomycin.
[b] Information on *Dolosigranulum, Vagococcus,* and *Facklamia* has been omitted from the table due to a lack of information on their characteristics and clinical significance. See text for information on these organisms.
[c] Gas production from glucose in sealed MRS broth.
[d] *Streptococcus pyogenes* and some strains of pneumococci are PYR positive.
[e] Viridans group streptococci and group D streptococci are negative; group B streptococci may be positive.
[f] Vancomycin-resistant enterococcal strains have been described, but the majority of isolates are susceptible.
[g] Most strains are positive.

tions for the culture of blood, body fluids, and other specimens should be followed (see chapter 5). These organisms are likely to be isolated on rich, nonselective media (e.g., blood or chocolate agar or thioglycolate broth) since they are nutritionally fastidious. If selective isolation of the vancomycin-resistant genera *Leuconostoc* and *Pediococcus* is desired, Thayer-Martin medium may be used to inhibit normal flora or other contaminating microorganisms (60). Some of the genera (e.g., *Alloiococcus* and *Helcococcus*) grow slowly, forming tiny colonies that may not be visible unless extended incubation (48 to 72 h) is used.

Members of the genus *Abiotrophia* usually grow on chocolate agar, on brucella agar with 5% horse blood, and in thioglycolate broth but not on Trypticase soy agar with 5% sheep blood. These organisms can be cultured on nonsupportive media that have been appropriately supplemented (see Additional Procedures for Characterization of Genera with Negative or Weak Catalase Reactions, *Abiotrophia*, below).

IDENTIFICATION

The suggestions for identification presented in this section reflect currently available information on the infrequently isolated gram-positive cocci that grow aerobically. Additional taxonomic studies with and observations for clinical isolates may alter future protocols and introduce additional organisms into the identification schemes presented here. Although the Gram staining morphology is prone to subjective interpretation, it has been used as a major decision point in the identification protocols, with two general categories: Gram staining morphology resembling that of streptococci, meaning coccobacilli in pairs and chains, versus staphylococcal morphology, consisting of coccoid (usually more spherical) cells arranged in pairs, clusters, or tetrads. Broth-grown cells (thioglycolate broth is suitable) should be used to make morphological determinations. The flow diagrams in this section should not be used for definitive identification; in most cases additional procedures (Tables 2 and 3) are recommended before an identification to the genus level is made. Identifications of unfamiliar organisms from important specimens should be confirmed by a reference laboratory.

Procedures for Initial Differentiation of Genera with Negative or Weak Catalase Reactions

Initial testing of catalase-negative or weakly positive isolates with "streptococcal" (Fig. 1) or "staphylococcal" (Fig. 2) Gram staining morphologies is represented in the flow diagrams. Note that *Gemella* strains may display either type of cellular morphology, depending on the species (see Additional Procedures for Characterization of Genera with Negative or Weak Catalase Reactions below). Descriptions of tests for these organisms follow.

Catalase Test

If a positive catalase reaction is observed with growth from blood-containing medium, growth from a medium devoid of blood (e.g., brain heart infusion agar) should be used to repeat the catalase test. A loopful of growth is transferred to a microscope slide or an empty petri dish and is observed

TABLE 3 Characteristics differentiating catalase-positive or weakly positive gram-positive cocci[a]

Genus	Catalase	Obligately aerobic	Oxidase	Salt tolerance
Staphylococcus	+	−	−	+[b]
Stomatococcus	−, +, or w	−	−	−[b]
Micrococcus	+	+	+	+[b]
Alloiococcus	+ or w	+	−	+[c]

[a] Abbreviations and symbols: +, positive; −, negative; w, weak.
[b] Growth in the presence of 5% NaCl. This characteristic is tested on nutrient agar supplemented with 5% NaCl.
[c] Growth in the presence of 6.5% NaCl. This characteristic is tested by using salt tolerance medium for gram-positive cocci (see Growth in 6.5% NaCl in the text).

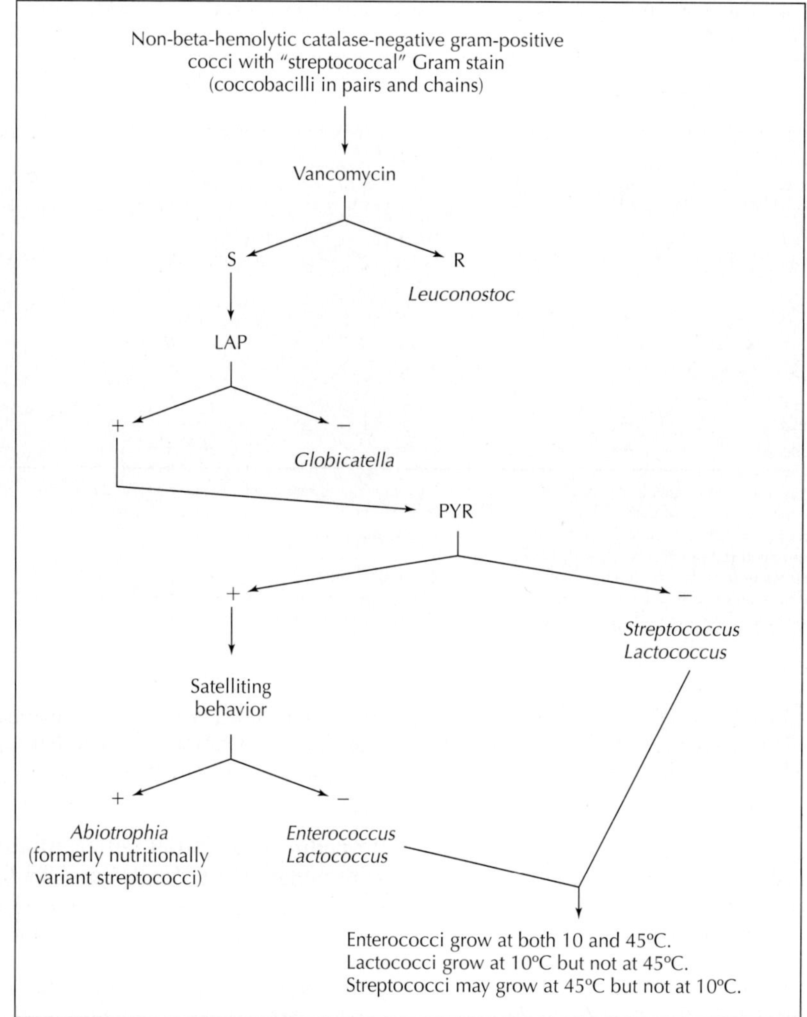

FIGURE 1 Identification of non-beta-hemolytic catalase-negative or weakly positive gram-positive cocci that grow aerobically. *Abiotrophia* stains may exhibit pleomorphic forms. S, susceptible; R, resistant; +, positive; −, negative. The genera *Vagococcus* and *Facklamia* have been omitted from the figure due to a lack of information on their characteristics and clinical significance. See the text for information on these organisms.

for the evolution of bubbles after the addition of a drop of 3% H_2O_2. It may be necessary to use a hand lens to detect weakly positive reactions.

Vancomycin Susceptibility Test

By the method of Facklam and Washington (33) a heavy inoculum (5 to 10 colonies) is spread with a loop over half of a plate containing Trypticase soy agar with 5% sheep blood. After placing a 30-μg vancomycin disk in the center of the inoculated area, the plate is incubated overnight in a CO_2-enriched atmosphere at 35°C. Any zone of inhibition indicates susceptibility, while resistant strains exhibit no inhibition zone.

LAP Test

The LAP test determines the presence of the enzyme leucine aminopeptidase. An assay for this enzyme is contained in some commercially available identification kits (e.g., the API Rapid Strep System [BioMerieux Vitek, Hazelwood, Mo.]), or a rapid disk test for LAP is also available commercially (Carr-Scarborough Microbiologicals, Inc., Stone Mountain, Ga.). Manufacturer's instructions should be followed when performing the test.

Growth in 6.5% NaCl

Salt-supplemented heart infusion broth with or without an acid-base indicator may be used for the detection of growth in 6.5% NaCl. According to the method of Facklam and Washington (33), salt-supplemented broth containing bromcresol purple is inoculated with two to three colonies of the organism to be tested and is incubated at 35°C for up to 72 h. Turbidity with or without a color change from purple to yellow (due to the production of acid) indicates growth.

PYR Test

See Identification of Beta-Hemolytic Isolates: Physiological Tests in chapter 17 for a description of the PYR test. Rapid disk tests are commercially available.

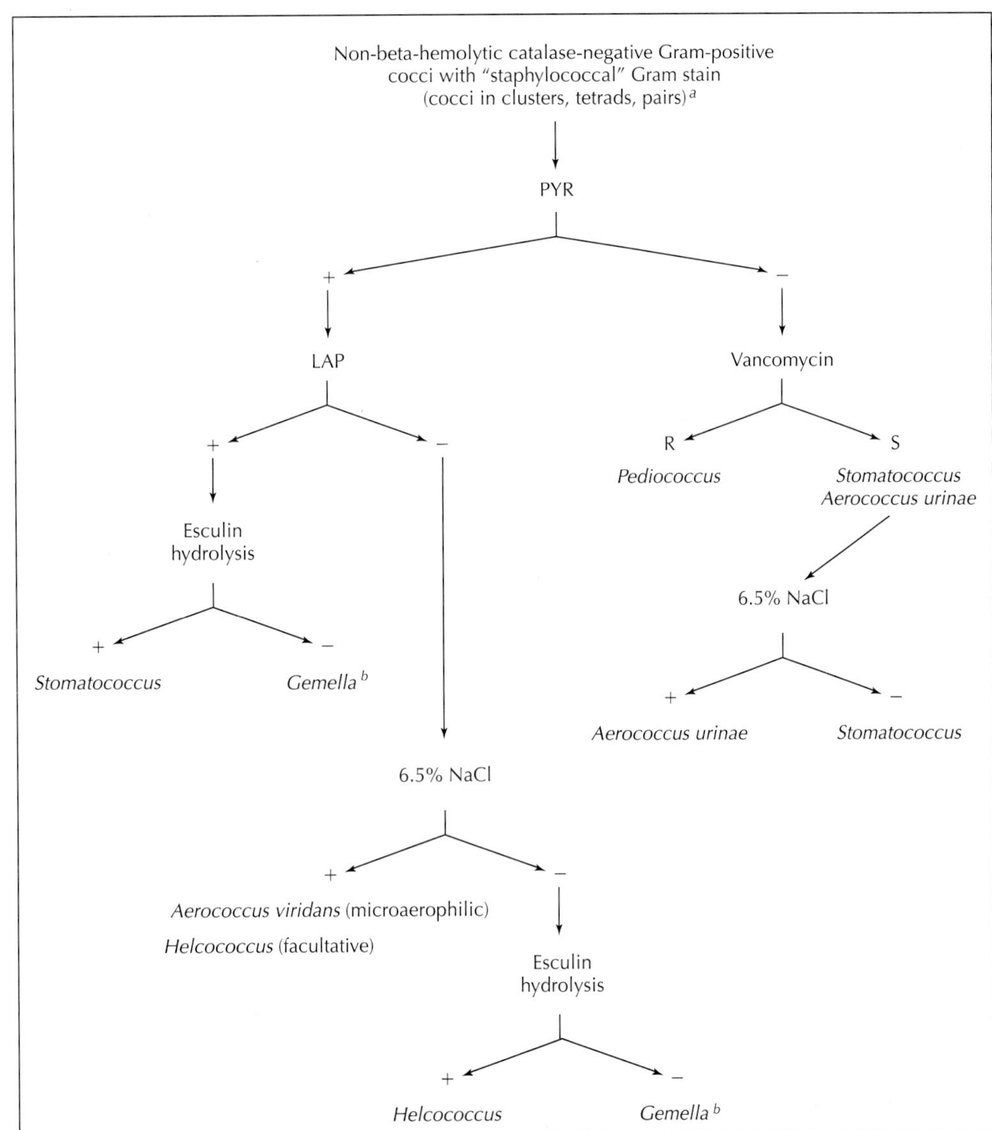

FIGURE 2 Identification of non-beta-hemolytic catalase-negative or weakly catalase-positive gram-positive cocci. S, susceptible; R, resistant; +, positive; −, negative. [a]Characteristics of *Micrococcus*, *Stomatococcus*, and *Alloiococcus*, organisms which tend to have positive catalase reactions, are displayed in Table 3. [b]Gram-stained cells of *G. morbillorum* may appear "streptococcal," but cells in a given pair are often of unequal sizes. *Dolosigranulum* is phenotypically similar but is not closely related to *Gemella*. It has been omitted from the figure due to a lack of information on its characteristics and clinical significance. See the text for information on this genus.

Esculin Hydrolysis Test

See Identification of Viridans Streptococci: Physiological Tests in chapter 17 for a description of the esculin hydrolysis test.

Additional Procedures for Characterization of Genera with Negative or Weak Catalase Reactions

Lactococcus

Facklam and Washington (33) recommended growth temperature tests for distinguishing lactococci from streptococci and enterococci. Consult Fig. 1 for the growth temperature characteristics of each genus. Broths are inoculated with a single colony or drop of a broth culture of the test strain and are incubated at 35°C for up to 7 days. A water bath is recommended for incubation of cultures at 45°C. Turbidity with or without a change in the broth's indicator to yellow indicates a positive test result.

If it is important to rule out enterococci, suspicious isolates can be tested with a commercially available nucleic acid probe test for the genus *Enterococcus*. *Lactococcus lactis* and *Lactococcus garvieae* are the species most commonly isolated from clinical specimens. Further information on the differentiation of *Lactococcus* isolates to the species level may be found elsewhere (27, 29, 62).

Abiotrophia

In a test for satelliting behavior, the strain to be examined is streaked for confluent growth on a medium that fails to support growth or that supports only weak growth. A single cross streak of *Staphylococcus aureus* (strain ATCC 25923 is suitable) is applied to the inoculated area. After incubation at 35°C in an atmosphere containing elevated levels of CO_2, strains of *Abiotrophia* will grow only in the vicinity of the staphylococcal growth. Alternatively, medium can be supplemented with pyridoxal, in the form of an aqueous stock solution of filter-sterilized 0.01% pyridoxal. This solution, which can be stored frozen, should be added to the medium to achieve a final concentration of 0.001%. Disks containing pyridoxal may also be used in the satelliting tests and are commercially available (Remel, Lenexa, Kans.) Compilations of additional phenotypic traits for *Abiotrophia* species, including their behavior on commercially available identification systems, can be found elsewhere (7, 12, 25, 58).

Leuconostoc and *Pediococcus*

Members of the genera *Leuconostoc* and *Pediococcus* produce on blood agar small, alpha-hemolytic or nonhemolytic colonies that can appear similar to those of viridans group streptococci. In addition to different cellular morphologies (Table 1), these vancomycin-resistant genera, along with vancomycin-resistant strains of lactobacilli that form short coccoid cells, may be separated by tests for gas production from glucose and arginine degradation. Leuconostocs produce gas and are always arginine negative. Lactobacilli are variable in both tests, but a positive arginine test result for a gas-producing strain would rule out the identity of the organism as a leuconostoc. Pediococci are gas production negative and show variable reactions in the arginine test, although *P. acidilactici* and *Pediococcus pentosaceus*, the two species commonly found in clinical material, are arginine hydrolysis positive.

Gas production is measured by inoculating MRS (lactobacillus deMan, Rogosa, and Sharpe) broth (commercially available) with the test organism, sealing the culture with melted petrolatum, and incubating the culture for up to 7 days at 35°C. Gas production is evidenced by displacement of the petrolatum plug (33). The arginine hydrolysis test can be performed with Moeller's decarboxylase broth containing arginine, as described in Identification of Viridans Streptococci: Physiological Tests in chapter 17. Lancefield group D antigen can be detected in pediococci (33). References 6, 28, 33, and 57 should be consulted for further information on the identification of *Leuconostoc* and *Pediococcus* to the species level.

The organism formerly known as *P. halophilus* was recently reclassified as *Tetragenococcus halophilus* (23). Although this organism shares some phenotypic characteristics with pediococci, it is vancomycin susceptible. Although there are no current reports of clinical isolates of *T. halophilus*, this species should be suspected if vancomycin-susceptible, *Pediococcus*-like strains are encountered.

Gemella

Facklam and Washington (33) state that all *Gemella* species are PYR positive but that *G. morbillorum* displays a weakly positive reaction in the PYR test. Earlier studies (8, 9) generally support these data, but they record some isolates of both species as being negative in the PYR test. Facklam and Washington (33) note that a large inoculum must be used when performing the PYR test with these bacteria in order to avoid false-negative results. LAP is usually absent from isolates of *G. haemolysans* but is present in strains of *G. morbillorum* (8, 9). On blood agar media, gemellas form small colonies that are similar in appearance to those of viridans group streptococci. The slow growth of some *Gemella* strains may lead to confusion of these organisms with *Abiotrophia* (formerly called nutritionally variant streptococci). A test for satelliting behavior will separate these two groups of bacteria (33).

Cells of *G. haemolysans* are easily decolorized and resemble those of neisserias, since they occur in pairs with the adjacent sides flattened. *G. haemolysans* prefers an aerobic growth atmosphere. *G. morbillorum* cells are gram positive and are arranged in pairs and short chains; individual cells in a given pair may be of unequal sizes. *G. morbillorum* is described as favoring anaerobic growth conditions.

Aerococcus

In addition to the traits listed in Table 2, aerococci are characterized by displaying weak or no growth when incubated in an anaerobic atmosphere (30). This trait can be tested by incubating one of a pair of duplicate blood agar plate cultures of the organism in question in an anaerobic atmosphere and incubating the other one in an aerobic atmosphere and comparing the growth after 24 to 48 h. When grown aerobically, *A. viridans* forms alpha-hemolytic colonies that, depending on the observer, could be confused with those of either viridans group streptococci or enterococci. *A. urinae* forms small (0.5 mm in diameter after 24 h of incubation) alpha-hemolytic, convex, shiny, transparent colonies on blood agar media. *A. urinae* is PYR negative and LAP positive, in contrast to *A. viridans* (2). Additional information on the identifying characteristics of *A. urinae* can be found elsewhere (16), and recognition of a second biotype (esculin hydrolysis-positive) of this species is described elsewhere (17).

Helcococcus

In addition to the characteristics listed in Table 2, most isolates of the slowly growing organism *Helcococcus* produce an API Rapid Strep (BioMereiux Vitek, Hazelwood, Mo.) profile of 4100413, corresponding to an identification of "doubtful" *A. viridans*. Colonial morphology (tiny gray, usually slightly alpha-hemolytic colonies), good growth under anaerobic conditions, and stimulation of growth by the addition of serum or Tween 80 to the medium differentiate *H. kunzii* from aerococci (21).

Globicatella

G. sanguis isolates resemble viridans group streptococci with respect to colonial and cellular morphology but differ from viridans group streptococci by displaying a positive PYR reaction, a negative LAP reaction, and salt tolerance. Although these physiological traits are identical to those of *A. viridans*, *Globicatella*'s streptococcal cellular morphology distinguishes it from aerococci (19). *F. hominis* is closely related to but is readily differentiated from *Globicatella*. The small number of *Facklamia* strains so far studied form weakly alpha-hemolytic colonies composed of cocci arranged in pairs or groups. Isolates display variable reactions in the PYR test, but they are uniformly positive for LAP and arginine hydrolysis. *Facklamia* strains fail to produce acid from glucose and many other carbohydrates and are negative for esculin hydrolysis, but they will, like *Globicatella* isolates, grow in the presence of elevated (5%) salt concentrations (22).

Stomatococcus

See Procedures for Differentiation of Genera with Positive or Weakly Positive Catalase Reactions below.

Procedures for Differentiation of Genera with Positive or Weakly Positive Catalase Reactions

Table 3 lists some distinguishing characteristics of micrococci, stomatococci, and alloiococci and compares them with those of staphylococci. On blood agar media, stomatococci form transparent to white, nonhemolytic colonies that are described as mucoid, sticky, or rubbery and that often adhere to the agar. *Stomatococcus* is distinguished from the other genera by its inability to grow in the presence of 5% NaCl. Nutrient agar that has been supplemented with 5% NaCl is suitable for determining salt tolerance in stomatococci, micrococci, and staphylococci. Studies with *Alloiococcus* have used 6.5% salt broth, as described above in Growth in 6.5% NaCl. The slowly growing (small alpha-hemolytic colonies form on blood agar after 48 h of incubation) *Alloiococcus* is differentiated from stomatococci and staphylococci by virtue of its obligately aerobic nature. A negative oxidase test distinguishes *Alloiococcus* from the other obligate aerobe in this group, *Micrococcus*.

Micrococci form colonies that are usually entire and smooth, but the colonies may be rough for some strains. Colonies may also be pigmented (yellow, orange, or pinkish). *Micrococcus* is the only oxidase-positive genus among the organisms grouped in Table 3. The modified oxidase test described by Faller and Schleifer (35) should be used when testing these organisms and is performed by smearing a colony from sheep blood agar onto a piece of filter paper. A modified oxidase reagent, consisting of 6% tetramethylphenylenediamine hydrochloride (available from Eastman Kodak, Rochester, N.Y.) in dimethyl sulfoxide (Sigma Chemical Co., St. Louis, Mo.), is dropped onto the bacterial growth. The development of a dark blue color within 2 min indicates a positive oxidase reaction. The test is also available in the form of a ready-to-use disk impregnated with the oxidase reagent (Remel, Lenexa, Kans.). The reader is referred to the references for further details concerning the characterization of *Stomatococcus* (4, 50, 51) and *Alloiococcus* (1, 34).

ANTIBIOTIC SUSCEPTIBILITIES

Limited information on the in vitro antimicrobial susceptibility of *Lactococcus lactis* and *Lactococcus garvieae* strains isolated from humans suggests that *L. garvieae* isolates are less susceptible to penicillin and cephalothin than are strains of *L. lactis*. The uniform resistance of *L. garvieae* versus the uniform susceptibility to clindamycin of the *L. lactis* strains examined by Elliott and Facklam (29) led them to propose a test for clindamycin susceptibility as an aid in the differentiation of these two species. In clinical practice, patients with lactococcal endocarditis have successfully been treated either with penicillin alone or with penicillin and gentamicin (48, 55).

The vancomycin-resistant genera *Leuconostoc* and *Pediococcus* are also resistant to teicoplanin. Although they are usually susceptible to imipenem, minocycline, chloramphenicol, and gentamicin, the penicillin MICs for these genera correspond to the moderately susceptible category (66).

The penicillin MICs for *Abiotrophia* isolates cover a range of values, with the majority of strains classified as either susceptible or relatively resistant. There is also variability in their susceptibilities to aminoglycosides, but no cases of high-level resistance have been reported. A synergistic effect between beta-lactam agents and aminoglycosides has been demonstrated for isolates of *Abiotrophia* (42).

A. viridans and *G. haemolysans* appear to be susceptible to penicillin and vancomycin and display a low level of resistance to aminoglycosides (13, 14). Buu-Hoi and colleagues (13) noted that while *A. viridans* seems to be naturally susceptible to macrolides, tetracyclines, and chloramphenicol, resistance to these agents has been observed. *A. urinae* has been described as susceptible to penicillin and vancomycin but resistant to sulfonamides and netilmicin (16). Buu-Hoi and coworkers (14) demonstrated a synergistic effect of penicillin and gentamicin against *G. haemolysans*.

Resistance to penicillin has been documented among some *Stomatococcus* strains, and the patterns of susceptibility to other commonly used antimicrobial agents seem to vary with the isolate (4, 50, 51). Stomatococci are uniformly susceptible to vancomycin. The observation that *Stomatococcus* exhibits poor or no growth on Mueller-Hinton agar and Mueller-Hinton agar with sheep blood may make susceptibility testing problematic (50, 51).

A reveiw of micrococcal endocarditis in patients who had undergone cardiac surgery noted that penicillin MICs ranged from 3.12 to 40.0 μg/ml and that vancomycin MICs spanned from 1.56 to 10.0 μg/ml. All of the *Micrococcus* isolates tested were susceptible to cephalothin (45). A study of 19 *A. otitidis* isolates revealed the absence of beta-lactamase but the presence of intermediate levels of resistance to beta-lactam agents and resistance to trimethoprim-sulfamethoxazole (10).

EVALUATION, INTERPRETATION, AND REPORTING OF RESULTS

Since the gram-positive cocci included in this chapter may appear in clinical cultures as contaminants or as part of the normal flora, efforts to identify them should be made only when isolates are considered to be clinically significant (i.e., isolated repeatedly, in pure culture, or from normally sterile sites). It should be remembered that these bacteria are opportunists; isolation from an immunocompetent patient may not have the same significance as isolation from a compromised host. Communication with clinicians should guide the microbiology laboratory in evaluating the significance of these infrequently isolated organisms.

Vancomycin susceptibility testing should be performed routinely for significant isolates. The documentation of resistance to this antibiotic not only will guide therapy but will also aid in the identification of the isolate. The method mentioned in this chapter, using a nonstandardized inoculum, seems to be fairly reliable for determining susceptibility to this drug for identification purposes. Since general standardized susceptibility test methods for these infrequently isolated gram-positive cocci do not exist, caution should be observed in interpretation of in vitro susceptibility test results. A reference laboratory should be consulted for identification or confirmation of the identities of unfamiliar organisms.

REFERENCES

1. **Aguirre, M., and M. D. Collins.** 1992. Phylogenetic analysis of *Alloiococcus otitis* gen. nov., sp. nov., an organism

from human middle ear fluid. *Int. J. Syst. Bacteriol.* **42:** 79–83.

2. **Aguirre, M., and M. D. Collins.** 1992. Phylogenetic analysis of some *Aerococcus*-like organisms from urinary tract infections: description of *Aerococcus urinae* sp. nov. *J. Gen. Microbiol.* **138:**401–405.
3. **Aguirre, M., D. Morrison, B. D. Cookson, F. W. Gay, and M. D. Collins.** 1993. Phenotypic and phylogenetic characterization of some *Gemella*-like organisms from human infections: description of *Dolosigranulum pigrum* gen. nov., sp. nov. *J. Appl. Bacteriol.* **75:**608–612.
4. **Ascher, D. P., C. Zbick, C. White, and G. W. Fischer.** 1991. Infections due to *Stomatococcus mucilaginosus*: 10 cases and review. *Rev. Infect. Dis.* **13:**1048–1052.
5. **Bannatyne, R. M., and I. W. Fong.** 1992. *Gemella morbillorum* infection in an arteriovenous shunt. *Clin. Microbiol. Newsl.* **14:**7–8.
6. **Barreau, C., and G. Wagener.** 1990. Characterization of *Leuconostoc lactis* strains from human sources. *J. Clin. Microbiol.* **28:**1728–1733.
7. **Beighton, D., K. A. Homer, A. Bouvet, and A. R. Storey.** 1995. Analysis of enzymatic activities for differentiation of two species of nutritionally variant streptococci, *Streptococcus defectivus* and *Streptococcus adjacens*. *J. Clin. Microbiol.* **33:**1584–1587.
8. **Berger, U.** 1985. Prevalence of *Gemella haemolysans* on the pharyngeal mucosa of man. *Med. Microbiol. Immunol.* **174:** 267–274.
9. **Berger, U., and A. Pervanidis.** 1986. Differentiation of *Gemella haemolysans* (Thjotta and Boe 1938) Berger 1960, from *Streptococcus morbillorum* (Prevot 1933) Holdeman and Moore 1974. *Zentbl. Bakteriol. Parasitenkd. Infektionskr. Hyg. Abt. 1 Orig. Reihe A* **261:**311–321.
10. **Bosley, G. S., A. M. Whitney, J. M. Pruckler, C. W. Moss, M. Daneshvar, T. Sih, and D. F. Talkington.** 1995. Characterization of ear fluid isolates of *Alloiococcus otitidis* from patients with recurrent otitis media. *J. Clin. Microbiol.* **33:**2876–2880.
11. **Bouvet, A., F. Grimont, and P. A. D. Grimont.** 1989. *Streptococcus defectivus* sp. nov. and *Streptococcus adjacens* sp. nov., nutritionally variant streptococci from human clinical specimens. *Int. J. Syst. Bacteriol.* **39:**290–294.
12. **Bouvet, A., F. Villeroy, F. Cheng, C. Lamesch, R. Williamson, and L. Gutmann.** 1985. Characterization of nutritionally variant streptococci by biochemical tests and penicillin-binding proteins. *J. Clin. Microbiol.* **22:**1030–1034.
13. **Buu-Hoi, A., C. LeBouguenec, and T. Horaud.** 1989. Genetic basis of antibiotic resistance in *Aerococcus viridans*. *Antimicrob. Agents Chemother.* **33:**529–534.
14. **Buu-Hoi, A., A. Sapoetra, C. Branger, and J. F. Acar.** 1982. Antimicrobial susceptibility of *Gemella haemolysans* isolated from patients with subacute endocarditis. *Eur. J. Clin. Microbiol.* **1:**102–106.
15. **Chatelain, R., J. Croize, P. Rouge, C. Massot, H. Dabernat, J. C. Auvergnat, A. Buu-Hoi, J. P. Stahl, and F. Bimet.** 1982. Isolment de *Gemella haemolysans* dans trois cas d'endocardites bacteriennes. *Med. Mal. Infect.* **12:** 25–30.
16. **Christensen, J. J., H. Vibits, J. Ursing, and B. Korner.** 1991. *Aerococcus*-like organism, a newly recognized potential urinary tract pathogen. *J. Clin. Microbiol.* **29:** 1049–1053.
17. **Christensen, J. J., A. M. Whitney, L. M. Teixeira, A. G. Steigerwalt, R. R. Facklam, B. Korner, and D. J. Brenner.** 1997. *Aerococcus urinae*: intraspecies genetic and phenotypic relatedness. *Int. J. Syst. Bacteriol.* **47:**28–32.
18. **Claus, D., D. Fritze, and M. Kocur.** 1992. Genera related to the genus *Bacillus*-*Sporolactobacillus*, *Sporosarcina*, *Planococcus*, *Filibacter*, and *Caryophanon*, p. 1769–1791. *In* A. Balows, H. G. Truper, M. Dworkin, W. Harder, and K.-H. Schleifer (ed.), *The Prokaryotes*, 2nd ed., vol. 2. Springer-Verlag, New York, N.Y.
19. **Collins, M. D., M. Aguirre, R. R. Facklam, J. Shallcross, and A. M. Williams.** 1992. *Globicatella sanguis* gen. nov., sp. nov., a new gram-positive catalase negative bacterium from human sources. *J. Appl. Bacteriol.* **73:**433–437.
20. **Collins, M. D., C. Ash, J. A. E. Farrow, S. Wallbanks, and A. M. Williams.** 1989. 16S ribosomal ribonucleic acid sequence analyses of lactococci and related taxa. Description of *Vagococcus fluvialis* gen. nov., sp. nov. *J. Appl. Bacteriol.* **67:**453–460.
21. **Collins, M. D., R. R. Facklam, U. M. Rodrigues, and K. L. Ruoff.** 1993. Phylogenetic analysis of some *Aerococcus*-like organisms from clinical sources: description of *Helcococcus kunzii* gen. nov., sp. nov. *Int. J. Syst. Bacteriol.* **43:** 425–429.
22. **Collins, M. D., E. Falsen, J. Lemozy, E. Åkervall, B. Sjödén, and P. A. Lawson.** 1997. Phenotypic and phylogenetic characterization of some *Globicatella*-like organisms from human sources: description of *Facklamia hominis* gen. nov., sp. nov. *Int. J. Syst. Bacteriol.* **47:**880–882.
23. **Collins, M. D., A. M. Williams, and S. Wallbanks.** 1990. The phylogeny of *Aerococcus* and *Pediococcus* as determined by 16S rRNA sequence analysis: description of *Tetragenococcus* gen. nov. *FEMS Microbiol. Lett.* **70:**255–262.
24. **Colman, G.** 1967. *Aerococcus*-like organisms isolated from human infections. *J. Clin. Pathol.* **20:**294–297.
25. **Davis, J. M., and M. M. Peel.** 1994. Identification of ten clinical isolates of nutritionally variant streptococci by commercial streptococcal identification systems. *Aust. J. Med. Sci.* **15:**52–55.
26. **Eggelmeijer, F., P. Petit, and B. A. C. Dijkmans.** 1992. Total knee arthroplasty infection due to *Gemella haemolysans*. *Br. J. Rheumatol.* **31:**67–69.
27. **Elliott, J. A., M. D. Collins, N. E. Pigott, and R. R. Facklam.** 1991. Differentiation of *Lactococcus lactis* and *Lactococcus garvieae* from humans by comparison of whole-cell protein patterns. *J. Clin. Microbiol.* **29:**2731–2734.
28. **Elliott, J. A., and R. R. Facklam.** 1993. Identification of *Leuconostoc* spp. by analysis of soluble whole-cell protein patterns. *J. Clin. Microbiol.* **31:**1030–1033.
29. **Elliott, J. A., and R. R. Facklam.** 1996. Antimicrobial susceptibilities of *Lactococcus lactis* and *Lactococcus garvieae* and a proposed method to discriminate between them. *J. Clin. Microbiol.* **34:**1296–1298.
30. **Evans, J. B.** 1986. Genus *Aerococcus* Williams, Hirch and Cowan 1953, 475^{AL}, p. 1080. *In* P. H. A. Sneath, N. S. Mair, M. E. Sharpe, and J. G. Holt (ed.), *Bergey's Manual of Systematic Bacteriology*, vol. 2. The Williams & Wilkins Co., Baltimore, Md.
31. **Facklam, R., and J. A. Elliott.** 1995. Identification, classification, and clinical relevance of catalase-negative, gram-positive cocci, excluding the streptococci and enterococci. *Clin. Microbiol. Rev.* **8:**479–495.
32. **Facklam, R. R.** 1977. Physiological differentiation of viridans streptococci. *J. Clin. Microbiol.* **5:**184–201.
33. **Facklam, R. R., and J. A. Washington II.** 1991. *Streptococcus* and related catalase-negative gram-positive cocci, p. 238–257. *In* A. Balows, W. J. Hausler, Jr., K. L. Herrmann, H. D. Isenberg, and H. J. Shadomy (ed.), *Manual of Clinical Microbiology*, 5th ed. American Society for Microbiology, Washington, D.C.
34. **Faden, H., and D. Dryja.** 1989. Recovery of a unique bacterial organism in human middle ear fluid and its possible role in chronic otitis media. *J. Clin. Microbiol.* **27:** 2488–2491.
35. **Faller, A., and K.-H. Schleifer.** 1981. Modified oxidase

and benzidine tests for separation of staphylococci from micrococci. *J. Clin. Microbiol.* **13:**1031–1035.

36. **Garcia-Marcos, J. A., M. Meseguer, and F. Baquero.** 1992. Meningitis due to *Gemella haemolysans*. *Clin. Microbiol. Newsl.* **14:**142–143.
37. **Garvie, E. I.** 1986. Genus *Leuconostoc* van Tieghem 1878, 198[AL] emend mut. char. Hucker and Pederson 1930, 66[AL], p. 1071–1075. *In* P. H. A. Sneath, N. S. Mair, M. E. Sharpe, and J. G. Holt (ed.), *Bergey's Manual of Systematic Bacteriology*, vol. 2. The Williams & Wilkins Co., Baltimore, Md.
38. **Garvie, E. I.** 1986. Genus *Pediococcus* Claussen 1903, 68[AL], p. 1075–1079. *In* P. H. A. Sneath, N. S. Mair, M. E. Sharpe, and J. G. Holt (ed.), *Bergey's Manual of Systematic Bacteriology*, vol. 2. The Williams & Wilkins Co., Baltimore, Md.
39. **Golledge, C. L., N. Stingemore, M. Aravena, and K. Joske.** 1990. Septicemia caused by vancomycin-resistant *Pediococcus acidilactici*. *J. Clin. Microbiol.* **28:**1678–1679.
40. **Haas, J., S. L. Jernick, R. J. Scardina, J. Teruya, A. M. Caliendo, and K. L. Ruoff.** 1997. Colonization of skin by *Helcococcus kunzii*. *J. Clin. Microbiol.* **35:**2759–2761.
41. **Handwerger, S., H. Horowitz, K. Coburn, A. Kolokathis, and G. P. Wormser.** 1990. Infection due to *Leuconostoc* species: six cases and review. *Rev. Infect. Dis.* **12:**602–610.
42. **Johnson, C. C., and A. R. Tunkel.** 1995. Viridans streptococci and groups C and G streptococci, p. 1845–1861. *In* G. L. Mandell, J. E. Bennett, and R. Dolin (ed.), *Mandell, Douglas and Bennett's Principles and Practice of Infectious Diseases*, 4th ed. Churchill Livingstone, New York, N.Y.
43. **Kawamura, Y., X. Hou, F. Sultana, S. Liu, H. Yamamoto, and T. Ezaki.** 1995. Transfer of *Streptococcus adjacens* and *Streptococcus defectivus* to *Abiotrophia* gen. nov. as *Abiotrophia adiacens* comb. nov. and *Abiotrophia defectiva* comb. nov., respectively. *Int. J. Syst. Bacteriol.* **45:**798–803.
44. **Kern, W., and E. Vanek.** 1987. *Aerococcus* bacteremia associated with granulocytopenia. *Eur. J. Clin. Microbiol.* **6:**670–673.
45. **Keys, T. F., and W. L. Hewitt.** 1973. Endocarditis due to micrococci and *Staphylococcus epidermidis*. *Arch. Intern. Med.* **132:**216–220.
46. **Kilpper-Balz, R., and K. H. Schleifer.** 1988. Transfer of *Streptococcus morbillorum* to the genus *Gemella* as *Gemella morbillorum* comb. nov. *Int. J. Syst. Bacteriol.* **38:**442–443.
47. **Kristensen, B., and G. Nielsen.** 1995. Endocarditis caused by *Aerococcus urinae*, a newly recognized pathogen. *Eur. J. Clin. Microbiol. Infect. Dis.* **14:**49–51.
48. **Mannion, P. T., and M. M. Rothburn.** 1990. Diagnosis of bacterial endocarditis caused by *Streptococcus lactis*. *J. Infect.* **21:**317–318.
49. **Mastro, T. D., J. S. Spika, P. Lozano, J. Appel, and R. R. Facklam.** 1990. Vancomycin-resistant *Pediococcus acidilactici*: nine cases of bacteremia. *J. Infect. Dis.* **161:** 956–960.
50. **McWhinney, P. H. M., C. C. Kibbler, S. H. Gillespie, S. Patel, D. Morrison, A. V. Hoffbrand, and H. G. Prentice.** 1992. *Stomatococcus mucilaginosus*: an emerging pathogen in neutropenic patients. *Clin. Infect. Dis.* **14:**641–646.
51. **Mitchell, P. S., B. J. Huston, R. N. Jones, L. Holcomb, and F. P. Koontz.** 1990. *Stomatococcus mucilaginosus* bacteremias; typical case presentations, simplified diagnostic criteria, and a literature review. *Diagn. Microbiol. Infect. Dis.* **13:**521–525.
52. **Ormerod, L. D., K. L. Ruoff, D. M. Meisler, P. J. Wasson, J. C. Kinter, S. P. Dunn, J. H. Lass, and I. Van de Rijn.** 1991. Infectious crystalline keratopathy. Role of nutritionally variant streptococci and other bacterial factors. *Ophthalmology* **98:**159–169.
53. **Parker, M. T., and L. C. Ball.** 1976. Streptococci and aerococci associated with systemic infection in man. *J. Med. Microbiol.* **9:**275–302.
54. **Peel, M. M., J. M. Davis, K. J. Griffin, and D. L. Freedman.** 1997. *Helcococcus kunzii* as sole isolate from an infected sebaceous cyst. *J. Clin. Microbiol.* **35:**328–329.
55. **Pellizzer, G., P. Benedetti, F. Biavasco, V. Manfrin, M. Franzetti, M. Scagnelli, C. Scarparo, and F. de Lalla.** 1996. Bacterial endocarditis due to *Lactococcus lactis* subsp. *cremoris*: case report. *Clin. Microbiol. Infect.* **2:**230–232.
56. **Reyn, A.** 1986. Genus *Gemella* Berger 1960, 253[AL], p. 1081–1082. *In* P. H. A. Sneath, N. S. Mair, M. E. Sharpe, and J. G. Holt (ed.), *Bergey's Manual of Systematic Bacteriology*, vol. 2. The Williams & Wilkins Co., Baltimore, Md.
57. **Riebel, W. J., and J. A. Washington.** 1990. Clinical and microbiologic characteristics of pediococci. *J. Clin. Microbiol.* **28:**1348–1355.
58. **Roggenkamp, A., M. Abele-Horn, K.-H. Trebesius, U. Tretter, I. B. Autenreith, and J. Heesemann.** 1998. *Abiotrophia elegans* sp. nov., a possible pathogen in patients with culture-negative endocarditis. *J. Clin. Microbiol.* **36:** 100–104.
59. **Rubin, S. J., R. W. Lyons, and A. J. Murcia.** 1978. Endocarditis associated with cardiac catheterization due to a gram-positive coccus designated *Micrococcus mucilaginosus incertae sedis*. *J. Clin. Microbiol.* **7:**546–549.
60. **Ruoff, K. L., D. R. Kuritzkes, J. S. Wolfson, and M. J. Ferraro.** 1988. Vancomycin-resistant gram-positive bacteria isolated from human sources. *J. Clin. Microbiol.* **26:** 2064–2068.
61. **Schleifer, K. H.** 1986. Family I. *Micrococcaceae* Prevot 1961, 31[AL], p. 1003–1035. *In* P. H. A. Sneath, N. S. Mair, M. E. Sharpe, and J. G. Holt (ed.), *Bergey's Manual of Systematic Bacteriology*, vol. 2. The Williams & Wilkins Co., Baltimore, Md.
62. **Schleifer, K. H., J. Kraus, C. Dvorak, R. Kilpper-Balz, M. D. Collins, and W. Fischer.** 1985. Transfer of *Streptococcus lactis* and related streptococci to the genus *Lactococcus* gen. nov. *Syst. Appl. Microbiol.* **6:**183–195.
63. **Sire, J. M., P. Y. Donnio, R. Mensard, P. Pouedras, and J. L. Avril.** 1992. Septicemia and hepatic abscess caused by *Pediococcus acidilactici*. *Eur. J. Clin. Microbiol. Infect. Dis.* **11:**623–625.
64. **Skov, R. L., M. Klarlund, and S. Thorsen.** 1995. Fatal endocarditis due to *Aerococcus urinae*. *Diagn. Microbiol. Infect. Dis.* **21:**219–221.
65. **Stackebrandt, E.** 1992. The genus *Stomatococcus*, p. 1320–1322. *In* A. Balows, H. G. Truper, M. Dworkin, W. Harder, and K. H. Schleifer (ed.), *The Prokaryotes*, vol. 2, 2nd ed. Springer-Verlag, New York, N.Y.
66. **Swenson, J. M., R. R. Facklam, and C. Thornsberry.** 1990. Antimicrobial susceptibility of vancomycin-resistant *Leuconostoc, Pediococcus,* and *Lactobacillus* species. *Antimicrob. Agents Chemother.* **34:**543–549.
67. **Tunicliff, R.** 1917. The cultivation of a micrococcus from blood in pre-eruptive and eruptive stages of measles. *JAMA* **68:**1028–1030.
68. **von Graevenitz, A.** 1993. Revised nomenclature of *Alloiococcus otitis*. *J. Clin. Microbiol.* **31:**472.
69. **Wallbanks, S., A. J. Martinez-Murcia, J. L. Fryer, B. A. Phillips, and M. D. Collins.** 1990. 16S rRNA sequence determination for members of the genus *Carnobacterium* and related lactic acid bacteria and description of *Vagococcus salmoninarum* sp. nov. *Int. J. Syst. Bacteriol.* **40:** 224–230.

Algorithm for Identification of Aerobic Gram-Positive Rods

GUIDO FUNKE

20

The aim of this algorithm for aerobic gram-positive rods is to guide the reader to the appropriate chapter for further information. This algorithm emphasizes that Gram stain (performed on 24- to 48-h-old colonies) and macroscopic morphologies are the initial key features for the differentiation of aerobic gram-positive rods. All strains of aerobic gram-positive rods (except the non-rapidly growing mycobacteria) are initially grown on blood agar plates.

Regular rods are organisms with cells whose longitudinal edges are usually not curved but are parallel. If spore formation is not observed initially, it can be tested on a nutritionally depleted medium. Catalase activity should be tested with media lacking heme groups. The type of metabolism can be checked in oxidative-fermentative media (OF) or in cystine Trypticase agar (CTA) medium. Irregular rods are organisms with cells whose longitudinal edges are curved and not parallel. Diagnostic end products of glucose metabolism can be detected by chromatographic methods only. Slight beta-hemolysis is best observed when cells are incubated in a CO_2-enriched atmosphere. Yellow- or orange-pigmented rods are always irregular rods. Some *Corynebacterium* spp., which are not medically relevant, as well as some *Brevibacterium* spp., may also exhibit a yellow pigment. Furthermore, some genera that stain partially acid-fast (e.g., *Gordona* and *Rhodococcus*) may also show a yellow-orange pigment. Rods exhibiting vegetative substrate filaments show branched hyphae, which either form spores or reproduce by fragmentation. It is obvious that vegetative substrate filaments might not be present initially (i.e., within 48 h), and so these organisms are prone to initial misidentification.

In particular, for the yellow-orange genera (e.g., *Microbacterium*/*Aureobacterium*, *Cellulomonas*, and "*Corynebacterium aquaticum*"), as well as the rods exhibiting vegetative substrate filaments, chemotaxonomic methods must be used for definitive identification to the genus level; for example, all partially acid-fast bacteria can be identified to the genus level by analysis of mycolic acids.

It is often not considered that genera which contain strict anaerobic gram-positive rods may also contain aerobically growing species. This is particularly true for the genus *Actinomyces* (as it is presently defined). *Clostridium tertium* (a strong gas producer) may also grow aerobically. Finally, it should be mentioned that some aerobic gram-positive cocci (e.g., *Leuconostoc* spp.) might initially be misidentified as gram-positive rods because of their initial Gram stain appearance. Likewise but less frequently, some gram-positive rods (e.g., *Rhodococcus* spp.) might be initially misidentified as gram-positive cocci because of their initial Gram stain appearance.

This algorithm should serve only as the basis of a very preliminary identification of an unknown aerobic gram-positive rod, and the reader is referred to the above-mentioned chapters for further information.

TABLE 1 Algorithm for identification of aerobic gram-positive rods (*Continued*)

Cellular morphology	Yellow-orange pigment	Vegetative substrate filaments	Spore formation	Catalase	Metabolism[a]	H_2S production in TSI	Other unusual Gram stain features	Diagnostic end product of glucose metabolism[b]	Slight β-hemolysis	Slow acid production	Acid-fast stain	Partially acid-fast stain	Aerial vegetative filaments	Motility	Growth at 50°C	Organism (chapter)
Regular			+													*Bacillus* incl. *Paeni-*, *Brevi-*, *Aneurini-*, and *Virgibacillus* (23)
			−	+	O											*Kurthia* (22)
					F											*Listeria* (22)
				−		+										*Erysipelothrix* (22)
						−										*Lactobacillus* (47)
Irregular	−			+			Club-shaped rods									*Corynebacterium* (21)
							Slim, long rods									*Turicella* (21)
							Very coccoid rods									*Dermabacter* (21)
							May show jointed rods									*Arthrobacter* (21)
							May show short rods									*Brevibacterium* (21)
							May show branching									*Actinomyces* (47), *Rothia* (21), *Propionibacterium* (47)
				−			Coccoid rods, Gram variable									*Gardnerella* (21)
								S	+ −							*Arcanobacterium* (21) *Actinomyces* (47)
								A								*Bifidobacterium* (47)

(*Continued on next page*)

TABLE 1 Algorithm for identification of aerobic gram-positive rods (*Continued*)

Cellular morphology	Yellow-orange pigment	Vegetative substrate filaments	Spore formation	Catalase	Metabolism[a]	H_2S production in TSI	Other unusual Gram stain features	Diagnostic end product of glucose metabolism[b]	Slight β-hemolysis	Slow acid production	Acid-fast stain	Partially acid-fast stain	Aerial vegetative filaments	Motility	Growth at 50°C	Organism (chapter)
								L								*Rothia* (21)
	+	+														*Oerskovia* (21)
		−		+	O					+						*Curtobacterium* (21)
										−						*Microbacterium/Aureobacterium* "*Corynebacterium aquaticum*" (both 21)
					F											*Microbacterium/Aureobacterium*, *Cellulomonas*, *Exiguobacterium* (all 21)
				−												*Microbacterium/Aureobacterium* (21)
	−	+									+					*Mycobacterium* (25)
											−	+	+			*Nocardia* (24)
													−			*Tsukamurella*, *Gordona*, *Rhodococcus*, *Dietzia* (all 24)
												−		+		*Dermatophilus* (24)
														−		*Micromonospora*, *Actinomadura* (both 24)
													+		+	*Saccharomonospora*, *Saccharopolyspora*, *Thermoactinomyces* (all 24)
															−	*Actinomadura*, *Amycolata*, *Amycolatopsis*, *Nocardiopsis*, *Streptomyces* (all 24)

[a] O, oxidative; F, fermentative.
[b] S, succinic acid; A, acetic acid; L, lactic acid.

Coryneform Gram-Positive Rods*

GUIDO FUNKE AND KATHRYN A. BERNARD

21

This chapter deals with aerobically growing, asporogenous, irregularly shaped, non-partially acid-fast, gram-positive rods generally called "coryneforms." The term "coryneform" is actually somehow misleading since only true *Corynebacterium* spp. exhibit a typical club-shaped ("*coryne*," meaning "club" in ancient Greek) morphology, whereas all the other bacteria discussed in this chapter show an irregular morphology. However, in our experience, the term "coryneforms" is a common and convenient expression used by many clinical microbiologists, and therefore, the term will be permanently applied in this chapter.

The coryneform bacteria which were, for didactical reasons, not included in this chapter comprise *Rhodococcus* spp. (chapter 24), *Actinomyces* spp. (in particular, the most frequently encountered species on aerobic plates, *A. europaeus*, *A. neuii*, *A. radingae*, and *A. turicensis*), *Propionibacterium* spp. (*P. acnes*, *P. avidum*, and *P. granulosum*), and *Propioniferax innocua* (see chapter 47), whereas *Arcanobacterium* spp. are included. *Gardnerella vaginalis* is included in this chapter but is discussed separately. Regularly shaped aerobically growing gram-positive rods (*Listeria*, *Erysipelothrix*, and *Kurthia*; *Bacillus*; *Clostridium tertium*; and *Lactobacillus*) are covered in chapters 22, 23, 46, and 47, respectively. Taxa which might be initially misdiagnosed as coryneform bacteria also include partially acid-fast bacteria and other nocardioform actinomycetes (see chapter 24) as well as rapidly growing mycobacteria (see chapter 25).

Within the last few years the field of coryneform bacteria has been evolving rapidly, particularly as far as the number of medically relevant taxa is concerned.

GENERAL TAXONOMY

All the genera described in this chapter except *Exiguobacterium* and *Gardnerella* belong to the lineage of the gram-positive bacteria with high guanine-plus-cytosine (G+C) content. They are most diverse and are differentiated by chemotaxonomic features (Table 1). Recent phylogenetic investigations, in particular, 16S rRNA gene sequencing, have, in general, confirmed the framework set by chemotaxonomic investigations. The 16S rRNA gene sequencing data demonstrate that the genera *Corynebacterium* and *Turicella* are more closely related to the partially acid-fast bacteria and to the genus *Mycobacterium* than to the other coryneform organisms covered in this chapter (62, 100, 124). The genus *Arthrobacter*, which contains rods, is phylogenetically intermixed with the genus *Micrococcus*, which contains cocci (45, 74). Other genera which are phylogenetically closely related include *Aureobacterium* and *Microbacterium* (109, 132), *Oerskovia* and *Cellulomonas* (55), as well as *Rothia*, *Arcanobacterium*, and *Actinomyces* (101). The genus *Dermabacter* is loosely associated with the genera *Arthrobacter* and *Micrococcus*, whereas the genus *Brevibacterium* forms a distinct line of descent (13).

DESCRIPTIONS OF THE GENERA

Genus *Corynebacterium*

The genus *Corynebacterium* is presently composed of 46 species (and two taxon groups), 31 of which are medically relevant. The species which are not known to be isolated from humans or to cause diseases in humans are *C. kutscheri*, *C. renale*, *C. cystitidis*, *C. pilosum*, *C. mycetoides*, *C. flavescens*, *C. vitaeruminis*, *C. glutamicum*, *C. callunae*, *C. bovis*, *C. variabilis*, *C. ammoniagenes*, *C. mastitidis*, *C. camporrealensis*, and *C. phocae*. Eighteen of the 31 medically important *Corynebacterium* species have been defined since 1995 (Table 2).

The cell wall of corynebacteria contains *meso*-diaminopimelic acid (*m*-DAP) as the diamino acid as well as short-chain mycolic acids with 22 to 36 carbon atoms (22, 24). *C. amycolatum* and *C. kroppenstedtii* are the only genuine *Corynebacterium* species which do not possess mycolic acids (21, 23). The corynebacterial cell wall also contains arabinose and galactose (22), but their detection is not recommended for the routine clinical laboratory. Palmitic ($C_{16:0}$), oleic ($C_{18:1\omega9c}$), and stearic ($C_{18:0}$) acids are the main cellular fatty acids (CFAs) in all corynebacteria, and tuberculostearic acid (TBSA) can also be found in some species like *C. urealyticum* and *C. confusum* (7, 53). The G+C content of *Corynebacterium* spp. varies from 46 mol% (in *C. kutscheri*) to 74 mol% (in *C. auris*) (63), indicating the enormous diversity within this genus. The phylogenetic relationships within the genus *Corynebacterium* were outlined in 1995 (100, 124), creating an extensive and reliable database for future comparative 16S rRNA gene studies, e.g., for the delineation of new species. These fundamental

*This chapter contains information presented in chapter 29 by Jill E. Clarridge and Carol A. Spiegel in the sixth edition of this Manual.

TABLE 1 Some chemotaxonomic features of coryneform bacteria

Genus	Major CFAs	Mycolic acids	Peptidoglycan diamino acid[a]	Acyl type
Corynebacterium	18:1ω9c, 16:0, 18:0	+[b]	*m*-DAP	Acetyl
Turicella	18:1ω9c, 16:0, 18:0	–	*m*-DAP	Glycolyl
Arthrobacter	15:0*ai*, 17:0*ai*, 15:0*i*	–	LYS	Acetyl
Brevibacterium	15:0*ai*, 17:0*ai*, 15:0*i*	–	*m*-DAP	Acetyl
Dermabacter	17:0*ai*, 15:0*ai*, 16:0*i*	–	*m*-DAP	ND[c]
Rothia	15:0*ai*, 17:0*ai*, 16:0*i*	–	LYS	ND
Exiguobacterium	17:0*ai*, 15:0*ai*, 16:0, 13:0*i*	–	LYS	ND
Oerskovia	15:0*ai*, 15:0*i*, 17:0*ai*	–	LYS	Acetyl
Cellulomonas	15:0*ai*, 16:0, 17:0*ai*	–	ORN	Acetyl
Microbacterium	15:0*ai*, 17:0*ai*, 16:0*i*	–	LYS	Glycolyl
Aureobacterium	15:0*ai*, 17:0*ai*, 16:0*i*	–	ORN	Glycolyl
Curtobacterium	15:0*ai*, 17:0*ai*, 16:0*i*	–	ORN	Acetyl
"*Corynebacterium aquaticum*"	17:0*ai*, 15:0*ai*, 16:0*i*	–	DAB	ND
Arcanobacterium	18:1ω9c, 16:0, 18:0	–	LYS	ND
Gardnerella	16:0, 18:1ω9c, 14:0	–	LYS	ND

[a] m-DAP, *meso*-diaminopimelic acid; LYS, lysine; ORN, ornithine; DAB, diaminobutyric acid.
[b] Exceptions: *C. amycolatum* and *C. kroppenstedtii*.
[c] ND, no data.

TABLE 2 Chronology of recently proposed or recognized medically relevant coryneform bacteria since publication of the previous edition of the *Manual of Clinical Microbiology*

Year of definition or recognition	Genus *Corynebacterium* (reference)	Other genera (reference)
1994	*C. jeikeium* (four genomospecies) (114)	*Aureobacterium* spp. (64)
1995	*C. macginleyi* (120) *C. ulcerans* (121) *C. argentoratense* (118) *C. glucuronolyticum* (39) *C. auris* (48)	*Microbacterium* spp. (42) *Cellulomonas* spp. (55)
1996		*Brevibacterium otitidis* (99) *Arthrobacter* spp., *Arthrobacter cumminsii* (45, 54)
1997	*C. coyleae* (56) *C. lipophiloflavum* (46) *C. imitans* (41) *C. mucifaciens* (49) *C. singulare* (122) *C. durum* (116)	*Arcanobacterium pyogenes* comb. nov. (101) *Arcanobacterium bernardiae* comb. nov. (101)
1998	*C. falsenii* (127) *C. riegelii* (50) *C. thomssenii* (151) *C. kroppenstedtii* (23) *C. confusum* (53) *C. sundsvallense* (20) *C. sanguinis* (44)	*Aureobacterium resistens* (51) *Rothia dentocariosa* genomospecies 2 (75) *Curtobacterium* spp. (38)

studies have confirmed that *C. amycolatum* is a true member of the genus *Corynebacterium*.

Gram staining of corynebacteria shows slightly curved, gram-positive rods with sides not parallel and sometimes slightly wider ends, giving some of the bacteria a typical club shape (Fig. 1a). Corynebacteria whose morphologies differ from this morphology include *C. durum*, *C. matruchotii*, and *C. sundsvallense* (see below under each species). Cells infrequently stain unevenly. If *Corynebacterium* cells are taken from fluid media, they are arranged as single cells, in pairs, in V forms, in palisades, or in clusters with a so-called Chinese letter appearance. It is again emphasized that the club-shaped form of the rods is observed only for true *Corynebacterium* spp. Corynebacteria are always catalase positive, and the medically relevant species are all nonmotile. The genus *Corynebacterium* includes both fermenting and nonfermenting species.

Genus *Turicella*

The genus *Turicella* is the sister genus of the genus *Corynebacterium* (100, 124) but contains *T. otitidis* as the only species. The cell wall contains *m*-DAP, but mycolic acids are not present (62). The main CFAs for *T. otitidis* are the same as those for *Corynebacterium* spp., but all *T. otitidis* strains also contain significant amounts of TBSA (2 to 10% of all CFAs) (62). *T. otitidis* is the only coryneform bacterium that has a polar lipid profile without glycolipids (113). The G+C content varies between 65 and 72 mol% (62).

Gram staining shows relatively long gram-positive rods which are not branched (Fig. 1b). *T. otitidis* is catalase positive and nonmotile and exhibits a respiratory metabolism.

Genus *Arthrobacter*

The genera *Arthrobacter* and *Micrococcus* are so closely related phylogenetically that it has been stated that micrococci are, in fact, arthrobacters which are unable to express rod forms (74). Presently, the genus *Arthrobacter* contains 19 species (45). Lysine is the diamino acid of the cell wall, and $C_{15:0ai}$ is the overall dominating CFA which represents more than 50% of all CFAs in most *Arthrobacter*

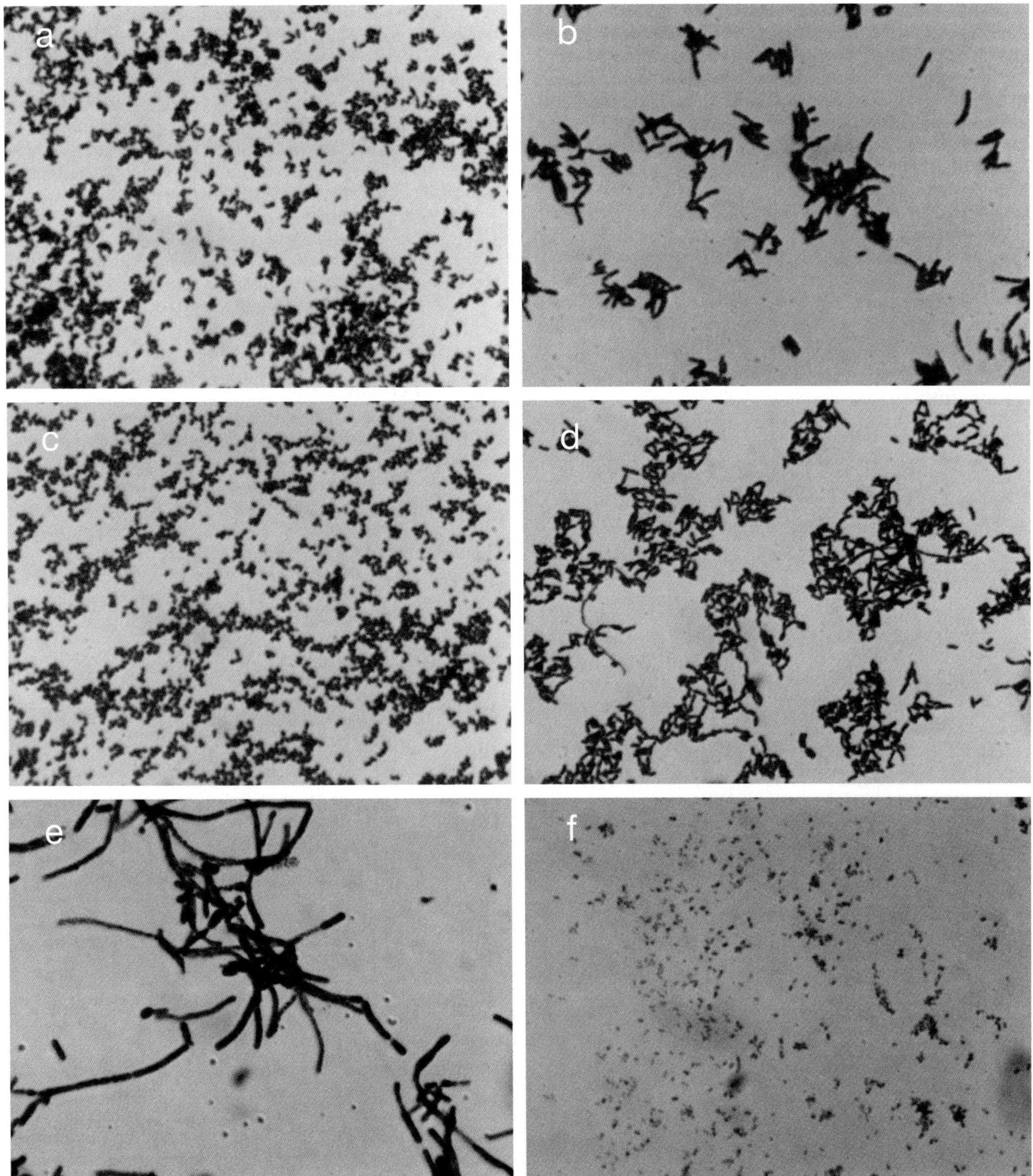

FIGURE 1 Gram stain morphologies of *Corynebacterium diphtheriae* ATCC 14779 after 48 h of incubation (a), *Turicella otitidis* DSM 8821 (48 h) (b), *Dermabacter hominis* ATCC 51325 (48 h) (c), *Corynebacterium durum* DMMZ 2544 (72 h) (d), *Corynebacterium matruchotii* ATCC 14266 (24 h) (e), and *Gardnerella vaginalis* ATCC 14018 (48 h) (f).

species. The G + C content varies between 59 and 70 mol%, indicating the diversity within the genus.

Gram staining may demonstrate a rod-coccus cycle (i.e., rod forms in younger cultures and cocci in older colonies) when cells are grown on rich media (e.g., Columbia base agar). Jointed rods (i.e., rods in a rectangular form) may also be observed in younger cultures (i.e., after 24 h) but may not be demonstrable for every species. Arthrobacters are catalase positive, motility is variable, and they always exhibit a respiratory metabolism.

Genus *Brevibacterium*

The genus *Brevibacterium* presently comprises six species, and some more species may be defined within the next few years. *m*-DAP is the diamino acid of the cell wall. $C_{15:0ai}$ and $C_{17:0ai}$ usually represent more than 75% of all CFAs (40). The G+C content varies between 60 and 67 mol%.

Gram staining demonstrates relatively short rods which may develop into cocci when cultures are getting older (rod-coccus cycle). Brevibacteria are catalase positive and nonmotile and have a respiratory metabolism.

Genus *Dermabacter*

The genus *Dermabacter* presently comprises only one species, *D. hominis*. *m*-DAP is the diamino acid of the cell wall, and $C_{15:0ai}$ and $C_{17:0ai}$ usually account for 40 to 60% of all CFAs. The G+C content range is between 60 and 62 mol% (73).

Gram staining shows very short rods (Fig. 1c) which are often initially misinterpreted as cocci. *D. hominis* strains are catalase positive and nonmotile and possess a fermentative metabolism.

Genus *Rothia*

The genera *Stomatococcus* and *Actinomyces* (discussed in chapters 19 and 47, respectively) are closely related to the genus *Rothia* (6, 101). This genus presently comprises only the species *R. dentocariosa*, but it is expected that further *Rothia* species will be defined in the near future (6, 75). Lysine is the diamino acid of the cell wall, and $C_{15:0ai}$ and $C_{17:0ai}$ usually represent 40 to 60% of all CFAs. The G+C content ranges between 47 and 53 mol%.

Rothia strains can be quite pleomorphic by Gram staining, showing coccoid and rod forms, but filamentous forms are normally not observed. They have variable catalase reactions, are nonmotile, and exhibit a fermentative metabolism.

Genus *Exiguobacterium*

The genus *Exiguobacterium* is phylogenetically related to the so-called group 2 bacilli (36). Presently, *E. aurantiacum* (25) and *E. acetylicum* (previously called *Brevibacterium acetylicum*) (36) are the only two species described for this genus, but *E. aurantiacum* has, except for one case (4a), not been isolated from human clinical material so far. Lysine is the diamino acid of the cell wall, and $C_{15:0ai}$ and $C_{17:0ai}$ comprise only about 30 to 40% of the total CFAs. *E. acetylicum* contains significant amounts of $C_{13:0}$ and $C_{13:0ai}$, which are not found in any other coryneform taxon (7). The G+C content is about 47 mol%.

Exiguobacteria present as relatively short rods in young cultures. Strains are catalase positive and motile and have a fermentative metabolism.

Genus *Oerskovia*

The correct phylogenetic placement of the genus *Oerskovia* has been debated for a long time (55). In older textbooks oerskoviae were assigned to the nocardioform group of organisms due to their morphological features. This includes extensive branching, vegetative hyphae, and penetration into agar, but they have no aerial hyphae. However, there is now abundant phylogenetic evidence that *Oerskovia* spp. are closely related to the genus *Cellulomonas* (55) but not to the mycolic acid-containing genera like *Nocardia*. Only two species, *O. turbata* and *O. xanthineolytica*, have been described. *Cellulomonas cellulans* is probably a synonym of *O. xanthineolytica*. Lysine is the diamino acid of the cell wall, and $C_{15:0ai}$ and $C_{15:0ai}$ are the main CFAs in oerskoviae, comprising about 40 to 60% of all CFAs. The G+C content is 70 to 75 mol%.

Gram staining shows coccoid to rod-shaped bacteria which originate from the breaking up of mycelia. *Oerskovia* spp. are catalase positive, motility is variable, and they are fermentative.

Genus *Cellulomonas*

The genus *Cellulomonas* presently comprises eight species, of which only *C. hominis* has been described as being isolated from humans (55). Some more *Cellulomonas* species derived from clinical material may be described in the near future. Ornithine is the diamino acid of the cell wall, and $C_{15:0ai}$ and $C_{16:0}$ are the main CFAs. The G+C content is 71 to 76 mol%.

Gram staining shows small, thin rods. All *Cellulomonas* spp. except *C. fermentans* are catalase positive, their motility is variable, all except *C. hominis* are cellulolytic (*C. hominis* did not hydrolyze cellulose in the test system used [55]), and they have a fermentative metabolism.

Genus *Microbacterium*

Microbacteria belong to the peptidoglycan type B (i.e., cross-linkage between positions 2 and 4 of the two peptide subunits) actinomycetes. There are presently six validated species (148), but proposals for additional species are expected in the near future. Lysine is the diamino acid of the cell wall, and $C_{15:0ai}$ and $C_{17:0ai}$ are the two main CFAs, usually representing more than 75% of the total CFAs (42). The G+C content of *Microbacterium* spp. is 69 to 75 mol%.

Microbacteria are short rods. Catalase activity and motility are variable, and almost all strains show a fermentative metabolism.

Genus *Aureobacterium*

Aureobacteria also belong to the peptidoglycan type B actinomycetes. Fourteen species are presently extant, with *A. resistens* being the only species primarily isolated from human clinical specimens (51, 147). It is expected that many more new *Aureobacterium* species, derived both from the environment and from patients, will appear in the literature soon. In contrast to microbacteria, *Aureobacterium* spp. possess ornithine as the diamino acid, and $C_{15:0ai}$ and $C_{17:0ai}$ usually do not represent more than 75% of all CFAs (64). The G+C contents span from 65 to 76 mol%, indicating the diversity within this genus.

Gram staining often shows thin rods with no branching. Catalase activity is variable, as is motility. Aureobacteria usually have an oxidative metabolism.

Genus *Curtobacterium*

Curtobacterium spp. also belong to the peptidoglycan type B actinomycetes. Presently, six species are validly described. As for *Aureobacterium* spp. ornithine is the diamino acid but the interpeptide bridge is composed of ornithine only, whereas it consists of (glycine)-ornithine in aureobacteria. Curtobacteria and aureobacteria also possess different menaquinones (MKs; MK-9 versus MK-11,12) and peptidoglycan acyl types (acetyl versus glycolyl) (Table 1). $C_{15:0ai}$ and $C_{17:0ai}$ represent more than 75% of all CFAs (38). The G+C contents range from 68 to 75 mol%.

Gram staining shows small and short rods with no branching. Catalase activity is positive, motility is observed in most strains, and all strains show a respiratory metabolism which proceeds slowly in oxidizing carbohydrates.

"Corynebacterium aquaticum"

"*C. aquaticum*" strains belong to the peptidoglycan B type actinomycetes and therefore cannot be true corynebacteria, which actually possess an A type of peptidoglycan (i.e., cross-linkage between positions 3 and 4 of the two peptide subunits). This taxon awaits assignment to its own genus (with an unknown number of species). Diaminobutyric acid is the diamino acid of the cell wall peptidoglycan (in contrast to *m*-DAP in true corynebacteria), and $C_{15:0ai}$ and $C_{17:0ai}$, as in aureobacteria, are the main CFAs but represent <75% of all CFAs (64). The G+C content is about 73 mol%.

Gram staining shows thin rods with no branching, as observed for aureobacteria. The strains are catalase positive and motile and have a respiratory metabolism.

Genus *Arcanobacterium*

The genus *Arcanobacterium* contains the type species *A. haemolyticum*, the recently from the genus *Actinomyces* reclassified species *A. pyogenes* and *A. bernardiae*, as well as *A. phocae* isolated from the common seal (101). Lysine is the diamino acid of the cell wall, whereas in *Actinomyces* spp. lysine or ornithine is found. Arcanobacteria contain menaquinones of the MK-9(H_4) type, whereas the *Actinomyces* spp. examined so far have the MK-10(H_4) type. The main CFAs of arcanobacteria are $C_{16:0}$, $C_{18:1\omega9c}$, and $C_{18:0}$ (as in *Corynebacterium* spp. and *T. otitidis*), but significant amounts of $C_{10:0}$, $C_{12:0}$, and $C_{14:0}$ may also be detected (7). The G+C content is 48 to 52 mol%.

Gram staining of arcanobacteria shows irregular gram-positive rods. All arcanobacteria except *A. phocae* are catalase negative, and they are nonmotile and fermentative.

NATURAL HABITAT

Many species of corynebacteria are part of the normal flora of the skin and mucous membranes in humans and mammals. The habitat for a minority of the species (e.g., *Corynebacterium callunae* and *C. ammoniagenes*) is the environment. It is noteworthy that not all corynebacteria are equally distributed over skin and mucous membranes but that many of them occupy a specific niche. *C. diphtheriae* can be isolated from the nasopharynx as well as from skin lesions, which actually represent a reservoir for the spread of diphtheria. Important opportunistic pathogens like *C. amycolatum*, *C. striatum*, and *D. hominis* are part of the normal human skin flora but have thus far not been recovered from throat swabs from healthy individuals (141). Coryneform bacteria prominent in the oropharynx include *C. durum* and *R. dentocariosa* (141). *C. auris* and *T. otitidis* seem to have an almost exclusive preference for the external auditory canal (52), and in nearly every instance that *C. macginleyi* has been isolated, it has been isolated from eye specimens (37a). Another *Corynebacterium* with a distinctive niche is *C. glucuronolyticum*, which is almost exclusively isolated from genitourinary specimens from males (39). *C. urealyticum*, another genitourinary pathogen, has, like *C. jeikeium*, also been cultured from the inanimate hospital environment (95).

The natural habitat of arcanobacteria is not fully understood, but *A. haemolyticum* is recovered from throat as well as from wound swabs (16, 80), whereas *A. bernardiae* has mainly been found in abscesses adjacent to skin (37a). It is unclear whether the two species are part of the normal skin and/or the gastrointestinal flora. *A. pyogenes* is found on mucous membranes of cattle, sheep, and swine. Brevibacteria can be found on dairy products (e.g., cheese) but are also inhabitants of the human skin (40, 65). Arthrobacters are some of the most frequently isolated bacteria when soil samples are cultured, but *Arthrobacter cumminsii* seems to be present on the human skin (54). Members of the genera *Exiguobacterium*, *Oerskovia*, *Cellulomonas*, *Microbacterium*, and *Aureobacterium* have their habitats in the inanimate environment (e.g., soil and activated sludge). *Microbacterium* spp. have also been recovered from hospital environments (42). Curtobacteria are plant pathogens (38), and "*C. aquaticum*" strains have been isolated mainly from water.

CLINICAL SIGNIFICANCE

Estimating the clinical significance of coryneform bacteria isolated from clinical specimens is often most confusing for clinical bacteriologists. This is in part due to the natural habitat of coryneform bacteria, which may lead to their recovery if specimens are not taken correctly. The reader is referred to the guidelines on minimal microbiological requirements in publications on disease associations of coryneform bacteria (63).

Coryneform bacteria should be identified to the species level if they are isolated (i) from normally sterile body sites, e.g., blood (except perhaps if only one of multiple specimens became positive), (ii) from adequately collected clinical material if they are the predominant organisms, and (iii) from urine specimens if they are the only bacteria encountered and the bacterial count is $>10^4$/ml or if they are the predominant organisms and the total bacterial count is $>10^5$/ml.

The clinical significance of coryneform bacteria is strengthened by the following findings: (i) multiple specimens are positive for coryneform bacteria, (ii) coryneform bacteria are present by direct Gram staining and a strong leukocyte reaction is also observed, and (iii) other organisms recovered from the same material are of low pathogenicity.

For a comprehensive summary of all case reports published on individual coryneform bacteria, the reader is referred to a recently published review article (63). The most frequently reported coryneforms as well as their established disease associations are listed in Table 3.

Historically, diphtheria caused by *C. diphtheriae* (or *C. ulcerans*) is the most important infectious disease for which coryneform bacteria are responsible. Therefore, special attention is given to that disease in this chapter. Due to immunization programs the disease has nearly disappeared in countries with high socioeconomic standards. However, the disease is still endemic in some subtropical and tropical countries as well as among individuals of certain ethnic groups (e.g., native or indigenous peoples in the Americas and Australia). Moreover, since the beginning of the 1990s, diphtheria has reemerged in the states of the former Soviet Union. This epidemic had its peak in 1994, when about 40,000 new cases were reported (107). Despite increased global travel activities, only a few imported cases have been reported by countries with well-developed health care systems.

The main manifestation of diphtheria is as an upper respiratory tract illness with a sore throat, dysphagia, lymphadenitis, low-grade fever, malaise, and headache. A nasopharyngeal adherent membrane which may occasionally lead to obstruction is characteristic. The severe systemic effects of diphtheria include myocarditis, neuritis, and kidney damage caused by the *C. diphtheriae* exotoxin, which is encoded by a bacteriophage carrying the *tox* gene. *C. diphtheriae* may also cause cutaneous diphtheria or endocarditis (with either toxin-positive or toxin-negative strains). Some people with poor hygienic standards (e.g., drug and alcohol abusers) are prone to colonization (on the skin more often than in the

TABLE 3 Most frequently reported disease associations of coryneform bacteria

Taxon	Disease or disease association	Reference(s)[a]
C. amycolatum	Wound infections, foreign body infections, bacteremia, urinary tract infections, respiratory tract infections	4, 47, 137
CDC group F-1	Urinary tract infections	
CDC group G	Catheter infections, bacteremia, endocarditis, wound infections, eye infections	
C. diphtheriae	Throat diphtheria, cutaneous diphtheria, endocarditis (mainly nontoxigenic strains), pharyngitis (nontoxigenic strains)	9, 103
C. glucuronolyticum	Genitourinary tract infections (males)	
C. jeikeium	Endocarditis, bacteremia, wound infections, foreign body infections	63, 105
C. macginleyi	Eye infections	
C. minutissimum	Wound infections, respiratory tract infections	152
C. pseudodiphtheriticum	Respiratory tract infections, endocarditis	1, 72, 81, 105
C. pseudotuberculosis	Lymphadenitis (occupational), ulcerative lymphangitis, abscess formation, abortion (animals)	104
C. riegelii	Urinary tract infections (females)	50
C. striatum	Wound infections, respiratory tract infections, foreign body infections	11, 78, 85, 137, 144
C. ulcerans	Respiratory diphtheria, mastitis in cattle	9
C. urealyticum	Urinary tract infections, endocarditis, bacteremia, wound infections	63, 128
Arthrobacter spp.	Bacteremia, foreign body infections, urinary tract infections	35, 45, 54
Brevibacterium spp.	Bacteremia, foreign body infections, malodorous feet	40, 65
D. hominis	Wound infections, bacteremia	5, 17, 61
R. dentocariosa	Endocarditis, bacteremia, respiratory tract infections	63
CDC group 4	Genitourinary tract infections (females)	68
Oerskovia spp.	Foreign body infections, bacteremia	66
Cellulomonas spp.	Bacteremia	55
Microbacterium spp.	Foreign body infections, bacteremia	42, 43
Aureobacterium spp.	Bacteremia	64, 96
A. bernardiae	Abscess formation (together with mixed anaerobic flora)	57
A. haemolyticum	Pharyngitis in older children, wound and soft tissue infections, osteomyelitis, endocarditis	16, 63, 80
A. pyogenes	Abscess formation, wound or soft tissue infections, bacteremia (both humans and animals)	63
G. vaginalis	Bacterial vaginosis, endometritis, postpartum sepsis	18

[a] References for taxa without references are the authors' observations.

pharynx) by *C. diphtheriae* strains, which are often nontoxigenic.

COLLECTION, TRANSPORT, AND STORAGE OF SPECIMENS

In general, coryneform bacteria do not need special handling when samples are collected.

C. diphtheriae

The diagnosis of diphtheria is primarily a clinical one. The physician should notify the receiving laboratory immediately of suspected diphtheria. In case of respiratory diphtheria, material for culture should be obtained on a swab (either a cotton- or a polyester-tipped swab) from the inflamed areas in the nasopharynx. Multisite sampling (nasopharynx) is thought to increase sensitivity. If membranes are present and can be removed (swabs from beneath the membrane are most valuable), they should also be sent to the microbiology laboratory (although *C. diphtheriae* might not be culturable from those in every instance). Nasopharyngeal swabs should be obtained from suspected carriers. It is preferable that the swabs are immediately transferred to the microbiology laboratory for culturing. If the swabs must be sent to the laboratory, semisolid transport media (e.g., Amies [see chapter 130]) ensure the maintenance of the bacteria. If the transport time exceeds 24 h, the use of silica gel transport media is recommended. All coryneform bacteria are relatively resistant to drying and moderate temperature changes. Material from patients with suspected cases of wound diphtheria can be obtained by swab or aspiration.

After the appropriate isolation media have been inoculated (see below under Isolation Procedures and Incubation), the swabs taken from diphtheritic membranes should be subject to Neisser or Loeffler methylene blue staining. However, it is noteworthy that the sensitivity of the microscopic examination is limited.

A PCR-based direct detection system for diphtheria toxin has been described by the Centers for Disease Control and Prevention (CDC) (91). Their system had the highest sensitivity when Dacron polyester-tipped swabs were used and when silica gel packages were stored at 4°C rather than at room temperature. CDC accepts swabs, pieces of diphtheria membranes, or biopsy tissue for this assay (9).

Long-term preservation in skim milk at −70°C is applicable to all coryneform bacteria. The same skim milk tubes except for those containing lipophilic corynebacteria can be thawed and put into the freezer again, and this can be done several times (37a). For nonlipophilic coryneforms good results were also observed with Microbank tubes (Pro-Lab Diagnostics, Austin, Tex.) (37a). The advantage of using these tubes is that individual pellets can be taken out of the tube. Coryneform bacteria can also be stored for decades when they are kept lyophilized in an appropriate medium (e.g., 0.9% NaCl containing 2% bovine serum albumin) (139).

ISOLATION PROCEDURES AND INCUBATION

Coryneform bacteria including *C. diphtheriae* can be readily isolated from a sheep blood agar (SBA)-based selective medium containing 100 μg of fosfomycin per ml (plus 12.5 μg of glucose-6-phosphate per ml) since nearly all coryneforms (except *Actinomyces* spp. and *D. hominis*) are highly resistant to this compound (134, 141). It is also possible to put disks containing 50 μg of fosfomycin (plus 50 μg of glucose-6-phosphate) (Becton Dickinson BBL, Cockeysville, Md.) on an SBA plate and then examining the colonies which grow around the disk. Selective media for coryneform bacteria containing furazolidone (Furoxone; 50 to 100 μg/ml) have also been described. If lipophilic corynebacteria like *C. jeikeium* or *C. urealyticum* are sought, then 0.1 to 1.0% Tween 80 (Merck, Darmstadt, Germany) should be added to an SBA plate. It is also possible to streak sterile filtered Tween 80 with a cotton swab onto SBA plates. Selective media for *C. jeikeium* and *C. urealyticum* have been described (139). Coryneform bacteria do not grow on MacConkey agar. If "coryneform" bacteria are recovered from this medium, they should be examined carefully to rule out rapidly growing mycobacteria (3, 63, 77).

With very few exceptions (some microbacteria, aureobacteria, and curtobacteria, which have optimal growth temperatures of between 30 and 35°C), the medically relevant coryneform bacteria all grow at 37°C. It is desirable to culture specimens for coryneform bacteria in a CO_2-enriched atmosphere since some taxa, e.g., *Rothia* and *Arcanobacterium* spp., grow much better under those conditions (37, 134). Nearly all medically relevant coryneform bacteria grow within 48 h, so primary culture plates should not be incubated longer than that. However, if liquid media are used (e.g., for specimens from normally sterile body sites), these should be checked after 5 days by Gram staining for the presence of coryneform bacteria (only if growth is observed with the naked eye) before they are discarded.

It is recommended that urine specimens be incubated for longer than 24 h to check for the presence of *C. urealyticum* but only when patients are symptomatic or have alkaline urine or struvite crystals in their urine sediment (128).

C. diphtheriae

The primary plating media for the cultivation of *C. diphtheriae* should be SBA plus one selective medium (Cystine-Tellurite blood agar [CTBA] or Tinsdale medium) (32). If silica gel is used as a transport medium, the desiccated swabs need to be additionally incubated overnight in broth (supplemented with either plasma or blood), which should then be streaked onto the primary plating medium. The plates are read after 18 to 24 h of incubation at 37°C, preferably in a 5% CO_2-enriched atmosphere. Tellurite inhibits the growth of many noncoryneform bacteria, but even a few *C. diphtheriae* strains are sensitive to potassium tellurite and will therefore not grow on CTBA but may grow on SBA (32). It is noteworthy that growth on CTBA and tellurite reduction are not specific for *C. diphtheriae* since many other coryneforms may also produce black (albeit smaller) colonies. The best medium for direct culturing of *C. diphtheriae* is probably Tinsdale medium, as recommended by the World Health Organization (WHO) Diphtheria Reference Laboratory (Public Health Laboratory Service, London, United Kingdom). However, the limitations of Tinsdale medium are its relatively short shelf life (<4 weeks) and the necessity to add horse serum to it. On Tinsdale plates both tellurite reductase activity (as shown by black colonies) and cystinase activity (as shown by a brown halo around the colonies) can be observed. If neither CTBA nor Tinsdale medium is available, colistin-nalidixic acid blood agar (CNA) plates are recommended for the isolation of *C. diphtheriae* or any other coryneform bacterium. It is necessary to pick multiple colonies from CNA plates to rule out *C. diphtheriae* (first Gram staining, then subculturing, and subsequent biochemical testing). Nonselective Loeffler serum slants are no longer recommended for the primary isolation of *C. diphtheriae* because of overgrowth by other bacteria (but *C. diphtheriae* cells with polar bodies are produced on Loeffler or Pai slants only).

IDENTIFICATION AND TYPING SYSTEMS

Basic tests available in every microbiology laboratory are of great value for the identification of coryneform bacteria. The Gram staining morphology of the cells can exclude the assignment to many genera and can even lead to the assignment to the correct genus (e.g., to the genus *Corynebacterium*, *Turicella*, or *Dermabacter*) (see Fig. 1a to c). Morphology, size, pigment, odor, and hemolysis of colonies are also valuable criteria in the differential diagnosis of coryneform bacteria.

von Graevenitz and Funke (138) have outlined a biochemical identification system for coryneform bacteria which was based on previous results from Hollis (68) and Hollis and Weaver (69). This system includes the following reactions: catalase; test for fermentation or oxidation (in our experience, this is best observed in semisolid cystine Trypticase agar [CTA] medium [rather than on triple sugar iron or oxidation-fermentation media], with fermentation indicated by acid or alkali production in the entire tube and oxidation found at the surface of the tube); motility; nitrate reduction; urea hydrolysis; esculin hydrolysis; acid production from glucose, maltose, sucrose, mannitol, and xylose; CAMP reaction with a β-hemolysin-producing strain of *Staphylococcus aureus* (e.g., strain ATCC 25923), i.e., positive reaction indicated by an augmentation of the effect of *S. aureus* β-hemolysin on erythrocytes, resulting in a complete hemolysis in an arrowhead configuration (Fig. 2); and a test for lipophilia, which is performed only for catalase-positive colonies <0.5 mm in diameter. For the test for lipophilia, colonies are subcultured onto ordinary SBA and onto a 0.1 to 1% Tween 80-containing SBA plate. Lipophilic corynebacteria develop colonies up to 2 mm in diameter after 24 h on the Tween-supplemented agar. It has also been suggested that growth in brain heart infusion broth with and without supplementation of 1% Tween 80 be compared, and strains which grow only in the supplemented broth can be called lipophilic. The identification protocols given in this chapter are, in principle, based on the identification system of von Graevenitz and Funke (138) mentioned above (see also Tables 4 and 5).

The presently available commercial identification systems include the API (RAPID) Coryne system (bioMérieux, Marcy l'Etoile, France), the Biolog GP plate (Biolog, Hayward, Calif.), the RapID CB Plus system (Remel, Norcross, Ga.), the MicroScan panel (Dade Microscan, Sacramento, Calif.), the BBL Crystal GP system (Becton-Dickinson),

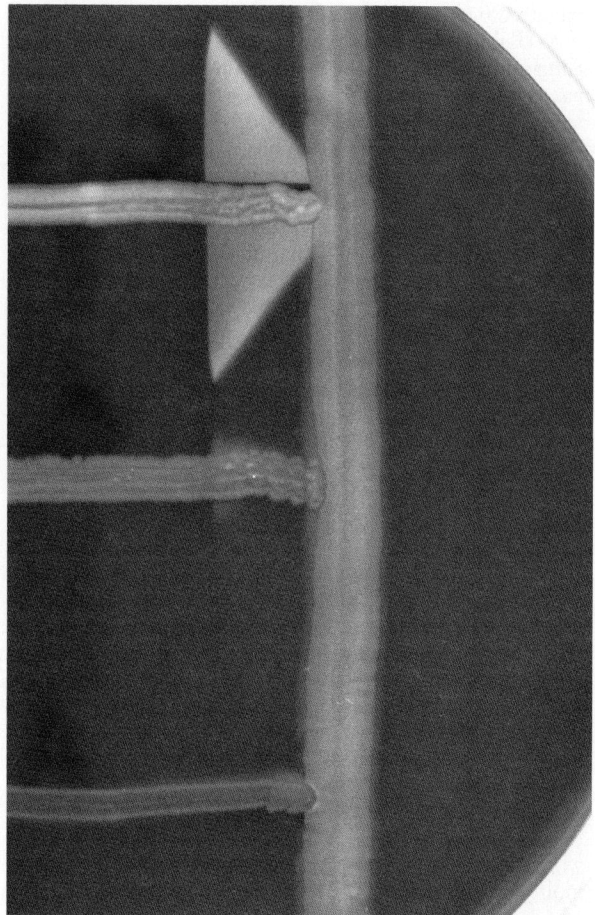

FIGURE 2 CAMP reactions of different coryneform bacteria after 24 h. (Top) *C. glucuronolyticum* DMMZ 891 (positive reaction). (Middle) *C. diphtheriae* ATCC 14779 (negative reaction). (Bottom) *A. haemolyticum* ATCC 9345 (reverse CAMP reaction). The vertical streak is *S. aureus* ATCC 25923.

and the MCN GP plate (Merlin Diagnostics, Bornheim-Hersel, Germany). So far, evaluations have been published only for the first three systems (58, 60, 71, 79). The API Coryne system contains 49 taxa in its present database (version 2.0). In a comprehensive multicenter study it was found that 90.5% of the strains belonging to the taxa included were correctly identified, with additional tests needed for correct identification for 55.1% of all strains tested (60). The results were highly reproducible if the manufacturer's recommendations for use were rigorously followed. It was concluded that the system is a useful tool for the identification of the diverse group of coryneform bacteria encountered in the routine clinical laboratory. In a stress test, the RapID CB Plus system correctly identified 80.9% of the strains to the genus and species levels and 12.2% to the genus level but with less accurate species designations; it was also concluded that this system may perform well under the conditions of a routine clinical laboratory (58). The Biolog GP plate system (database version 3.50) identified only about 60% of all strains tested to the correct genus level or to the correct species level (79). However, in the meantime the company has significantly improved both the technology and the database, but published evaluations of the revised system are still pending. The latter is also true for the three other commercial identification systems. The Vitek system (see chapter 11) has the disadvantage of a relatively limited database for coryneform bacteria. It is always important to question critically the identifications provided by any commercial identification system and to correlate the results with basic characteristics such as macroscopic morphology and Gram staining results.

For some identifications the use of the commercial API 50CH system (bioMérieux) has been found to be useful. For example, when applying the AUX medium (usually attached to the kit for gram-negative nonfermenters [bioMérieux]) to the API 50CH system, utilization reactions which allow the differentiation of *Brevibacterium* spp. can be observed (40).

A reference laboratory would also use chromatographic techniques for further characterization of coryneform bacteria. The presence of mycolic acids and their chain lengths can be detected by either thin-layer chromatography (TLC), gas chromatography and mass spectrometry, or high-performance liquid chromatography (24, 30). These methods can be useful for the differentiation of *Corynebacterium* spp. (mycolic acids of 22 to 36 carbon atoms) from the partially acid-fast bacteria (mycolic acids of 30 to 78 carbon atoms) but may also provide evidence that a coryneform bacterium is not a *Corynebacterium* (exceptions are *C. amycolatum* and *C. kroppenstedtii*) if mycolic acids are not detected. The detection of the diamino acid of the peptidoglycan by one-dimensional TLC is of certain value for determining the genus to which a particular strain belongs (Table 1). In some cases, partial hydrolysates of the peptidoglycan are separated by two-dimensional TLC to reveal the interpeptide bridge of the peptidoglycan in order to distinguish between genera having the same diamino acid in the peptide moiety. For example, the yellow-pigmented aureobacteria and curtobacteria both have ornithine as their diamino acids, but aureobacteria have (glycine)-ornithine as the interpeptide bridge, whereas curtobacteria possess ornithine only.

The analysis of CFAs by means of gas-liquid chromatography with the Sherlock system (MIDI Inc., Newark, Del.) is an extremely useful method for the identification of coryneform bacteria. This system is, in general, able to identify coryneform bacteria to the genus level, but identification to the species level is, in most cases, impossible, although the commercial database suggests that it is possible (140). This is due to the very closely related CFA profiles of coryneform bacteria belonging to the same genus (7) and because the quantitative profiles observed strongly depend on the incubation conditions. When a laboratory creates its individual database based on its own entries, species identification becomes possible in some cases (4a). The mycolic acids of some corynebacteria (e.g., *C. auris*) are cleaved at the temperature (300°C) produced in the injection port of the system, resulting in fatty acids which were identified as, e.g., $C_{17:1\omega6c}$ to $C_{\omega9c}$, by the Sherlock system (48).

Molecular genetic identification systems for coryneform bacteria are also recommended for reference laboratories only. A genus-specific probe for the genus *Corynebacterium* directed against positions 653 to 682 of the 16S rRNA gene has been described (70). Restriction fragment length polymorphism analysis of the partly amplified and digested 16S rRNA gene has been demonstrated to be of use for the identification of species within the genera *Corynebacterium* and *Brevibacterium* (14, 135). Some corynebacteria may also be identified to the species level by examination of the length of the 16S-23S rRNA intergenic spacer region (2). rRNA gene restriction fragment length polymorphism analysis (ribotyping) has recently been demonstrated to allow the identification of corynebacteria if three different restriction enzymes (*Bst*EII, *Sma*I, and *Sph*II) are used (10). In particular, potentially new corynebacterial species can be checked by this method for clustering with already established species. For molecular genetic investigations within genera which possess high levels of 16S rRNA gene homology (>97.5%), other essential genes (e.g., *gyrB* and *rpoC*) will become targets for future investigations. For pure taxonomic investigations of coryneform bacteria, full-length 16S rRNA gene sequencing, and, in selected cases, quantitative DNA-DNA hybridizations might be necessary but will be restricted to the reference laboratory.

It is emphasized that unidentifiable, clinically significant coryneform bacteria should be sent to an established reference laboratory experienced in corynebacterial identification.

DESCRIPTIONS OF GENERA AND SPECIES

Genus *Corynebacterium*

C. accolens

C. accolens (94) is mainly found in specimens from eyes, ears, nose, and the oropharynx. Colonies are, as for all other lipophilic corynebacteria, convex, smooth, and <0.5 mm in diameter on SBA. Initially, *C. accolens* strains had been described to exhibit satellitism in the vicinity of *S. aureus* strains, but this phenomenon simply indicated their lipophilism (this is not the recommended method for the testing of lipophilism [see above under Identification and Typing Systems]). *C. accolens* has a variable pyrazinamidase reaction but is negative for alkaline phosphatase, thus differentiating it from the morphologically and biochemically closely related CDC group G bacteria. The API Coryne and RapID CB Plus systems correctly identify *C. accolens* (58, 60). *C. accolens* strains are susceptible to a broad spectrum of antibiotics.

C. afermentans subsp. afermentans

C. afermentans subsp. *afermentans* (115) is part of the normal human skin flora and has so far been isolated mainly from blood cultures. Colonies are whitish, convex with regular edges, creamy, and about 1 to 1.5 mm in diameter after 24 h of incubation. *C. afermentans* subsp. *afermentans* has an oxidative metabolism. The API Coryne system provides the numerical code of 2100004 for this species. About 60% of all strains of this taxon are CAMP reaction positive. *C. afermentans* subsp. *afermentans* can be differentiated from *C. auris* and *T. otitidis* (both of which give the same API numerical code) by the consistency of its colonies (*C. auris* is slightly adherent to agar) and morphology on Gram staining (*T. otitidis* has longer cells). Further differential reactions include the carbohydrate utilization reaction tested with either the Biolog GP plate or the bioMérieux biotype 100 gallery (48, 113), but these techniques are not applicable in the routine clinical laboratory. *C. afermentans* subsp. *afermentans* is generally susceptible to β-lactam antibiotics.

C. afermentans subsp. lipophilum

Strains belonging to the species *C. afermentans* subsp. *lipophilum* (115) have mainly been isolated from blood cultures as well as from superficial wounds. Colonies are, typically for lipophilic corynebacteria, convex, smooth, and <0.5 mm in diameter after 24 h. *C. afermentans* subsp. *lipophilum* has an oxidative metabolism and does not produce acid from any of the carbohydrates usually tested (Table 4). It is the only species of lipophilic corynebacteria which may exhibit a positive CAMP reaction. *C. afermentans* subsp. *lipophilum* is not included in the API Coryne database, and the numerical profile observed for the species is 2100004. Strains are usually susceptible to β-lactam antibiotics.

C. amycolatum

C. amycolatum is part of the normal human skin flora but was not recovered from throat swabs from healthy persons (141). *C. amycolatum* is the most frequently encountered *Corynebacterium* species in human clinical material (63, 76). Colonies are very typically dry, waxy, and grayish white with irregular edges and are 1 to 2 mm in diameter after 24 h of incubation (Fig. 3a). *C. amycolatum* actually has a fermentative metabolism, but when CTA media are used for the observation of acid production from carbohydrates, *C. amycolatum* often appears to resemble an oxidizer (i.e., main acid production at the surface of the medium). Strains of *C. amycolatum* are remarkable for their variability in basic biochemical reactions (Table 4) and had been often misidentified in the past as the biochemically similar species *C. xerosis*, *C. striatum*, or *C. minutissimum* (26, 47, 142, 152). These four species can be differentiated by the following reactions: *C. amycolatum* and *C. minutissimum* do not grow at 20°C but *C. xerosis* and *C. striatum* do; in addition, *C. xerosis* does not ferment glucose at 42°C, whereas the other three species do, and *C. minutissimum* and *C. striatum* produce alkali from formate but *C. amycolatum* and *C. xerosis* do not (143). When tested on Mueller-Hinton agar supplemented with 5% sheep blood, nearly all *C. amycolatum* strains were resistant to the vibriocidal compound O/129 (150-μg disks) (Oxoid, Basingstoke, United Kingdom), as indicated by no zone of inhibition around the disk (47). In contrast, only 4% of all *C. amycolatum* strains were resistant to O/129 when tested on Mueller-Hinton agar with 5% horse blood (76). The API Coryne system identifies this species very well, but in every case additional reactions must be carried out in order to confirm the identification of *C. amycolatum* (60). All *C. amycolatum* strains produce propionic acid as the major end product of glucose metabolism (47, 142, 152). In contrast to many other corynebacteria, *C. amycolatum* exhibits only weak or no leucine arylamidase activity. The identification may also be suggested by the absence of mycolic acids (4). In addition, it may be shown that acyl phosphatidylglycerol is a major phospholipid in *C. amycolatum* in contrast to other *Corynebacterium* spp., in which other phospholipids are predominant (146). It is noteworthy that *C. amycolatum* strains are often multidrug resistant (59) and that *C. amycolatum* can be a serious opportunistic pathogen (47, 63, 76).

C. argentoratense

C. argentoratense (118) has almost exclusively been isolated from the human throat. Colonies are cream colored, nonhemolytic, slightly rough, and 2 mm in diameter after 48 h of incubation. Glucose fermentation by *C. argentoratense* is quite rapid, which differentiates it from the slowly fermenting species *C. coyleae*. *C. argentoratense* is the only medically relevant *Corynebacterium* species expressing α-chymotrypsin activity, which can be observed in the API ZYM (bioMérieux) system. Although *C. argentoratense* is phylogenetically closely related to *C. diphtheriae*, it does not harbor the *tox* gene coding for the diphtheria toxin.

TABLE 4 Identification of medically relevant *Corynebacterium* spp.[a]

Species	Fermentation/ oxidation	Lipophilism	Nitrate reduction	Urease	Esculin hydrolysis	Pyrazinamidase	Alkaline phosphatase	Acid production from: Glucose	Maltose	Sucrose	Mannitol	Xylose	CAMP reaction	Other traits
C. *accolens*	F	+	+	–	–	V	–	+	–	V	V	–	–	
C. *afermentans* subsp. *afermentans*	O	–	–	–	–	+	+	–	–	–	–	–	V	
C. *afermentans* subsp. *lipophilum*	O	+	–	–	–	+	+	–	–	–	–	–	V	
C. *amycolatum*	F	–	V	V	–	+	+	+	V	V	–	–	–	Most O/129 resistant
C. *argentoratense*	F	–	–	–	–	+	V	+	–	–	–	–	–	Chymotrypsin positive
C. *auris*	O	–	–	–	–	+	+	–	–	–	–	–	+	Slight adherence to agar, cleaved mycolics
C. *confusum*	F	–	+	–	–	+	+	(+)	–	–	–	–	–	Tyrosine negative
C. *coyleae*	F	–	–	–	–	+	+	(+)	–	–	–	–	+	
CDC group F-1	F	+	V	+	–	+	–	+	+	+	–	–	–	
CDC group G	F	+	V	–	–	+	+	+	V	V	–	–	–	Fructose positive, anaerobic growth positive
C. *diphtheriae* biotype *gravis*	F	–	+	–	–	–	–	+	+	–	–	–	–	Glycogen positive
C. *diphtheriae* biotype *intermedius*	F	+	+	–	–	–	–	+	+	–	–	–	–	
C. *diphtheriae* biotypes *mitis* and *belfanti*	F	–	+/–[b]	–	–	–	–	+	+	–	–	–	–	Glycogen negative
C. *durum*	F	–	+	(V)	(V)	+	–	+	+	+	V	–	–	Adherence to agar
C. *falsenii*	F	–	–	(+)	–	(+)	+	(+)	V	–	–	–	–	Yellowish
C. *glucuronolyticum*	F	–	V	V	V	+	V	+	V	+	–	V	+	β-Glucuronidase positive
C. *imitans*	F	–	–	–	–	(+)	+	+	+	(+)	–	–	+	Tyrosine negative, O/129 resistant

C. *jeikeium*	O	+	−	−	−	+	+	+	V	−	−	−	−	Fructose negative, anaerobic growth negative
C. *kroppenstedtii*	F	+	−	−	+	+	−	+	ND	+	−	−	−	Lacking mycolic acids
C. *lipophiloflavum*	O	+	−	−	−	+	+	−	−	−	−	−	−	Yellow
C. *macginleyi*	F	+	+	−	−	−	+	+	−	+	V	−	−	
C. *matruchotii*	F	−	+	−	V	+	−	+	+	+	−	−	−	"Whip handle" (upon Gram staining)
C. *minutissimum*	F	−	−	−	−	+	+	+	+	V	V	−	−	Tyrosine positive
C. *mucifaciens*	O	−	−	−	−	+	+	+	−	V	−	−	−	Very mucoid colonies
C. *propinquum*	O	−	+	−	−	V	V	−	−	−	−	−	−	Tyrosine positive
C. *pseudodiphtheriticum*	O	−	+	+	−	+	V	−	−	−	−	−	−	
C. *pseudotuberculosis*	F	−	V	+	−	−	V	+	+	V	−	−	REV	
C. *riegelii*	F	−	−	+	−	V	V	−	(+)	−	−	−	−	
C. *sanguinis*	F	−	−	−	−	+	+	(+)	−	−	−	−	−	Yellowish
C. *singulare*	F	−	−	+	−	+	+	+	+	+	−	−	−	Tyrosine positive
C. *striatum*	F	−	+	−	−	+	+	+	−	V	−	−	V	Tyrosine positive
C. *sundsvallense*	F	−	−	+	−	V	V	+	+	+	−	−	−	Sticky colonies
C. *thomssenii*	F	−	−	+	−	+	+	+	+	+	−	−	−	*N*-Acetyl-*β*-glucosaminidase positive, sticky colonies
C. *ulcerans*	F	−	−	+	−	−	+	+	+	−	−	−	REV	Glycogen positive
C. *urealyticum*	O	+	−	+	−	+	V	−	−	−	−	−	−	
C. *xerosis*	F	−	V	−	−	+	+	+	+	+	−	−	−	O/129 susceptible

[a] Abbreviations and symbols: V, variable; parentheses, delayed or weak reaction; ND, no data; REV, reverse CAMP reaction; F, fermentation; O, oxidation; +, positive reaction; −, negative reaction.
[b] C. *diphtheriae* biotype *mitis* is nitrate reductase positive, and C. *diphtheriae* biotype *belfanti* is nitrate reductase negative.

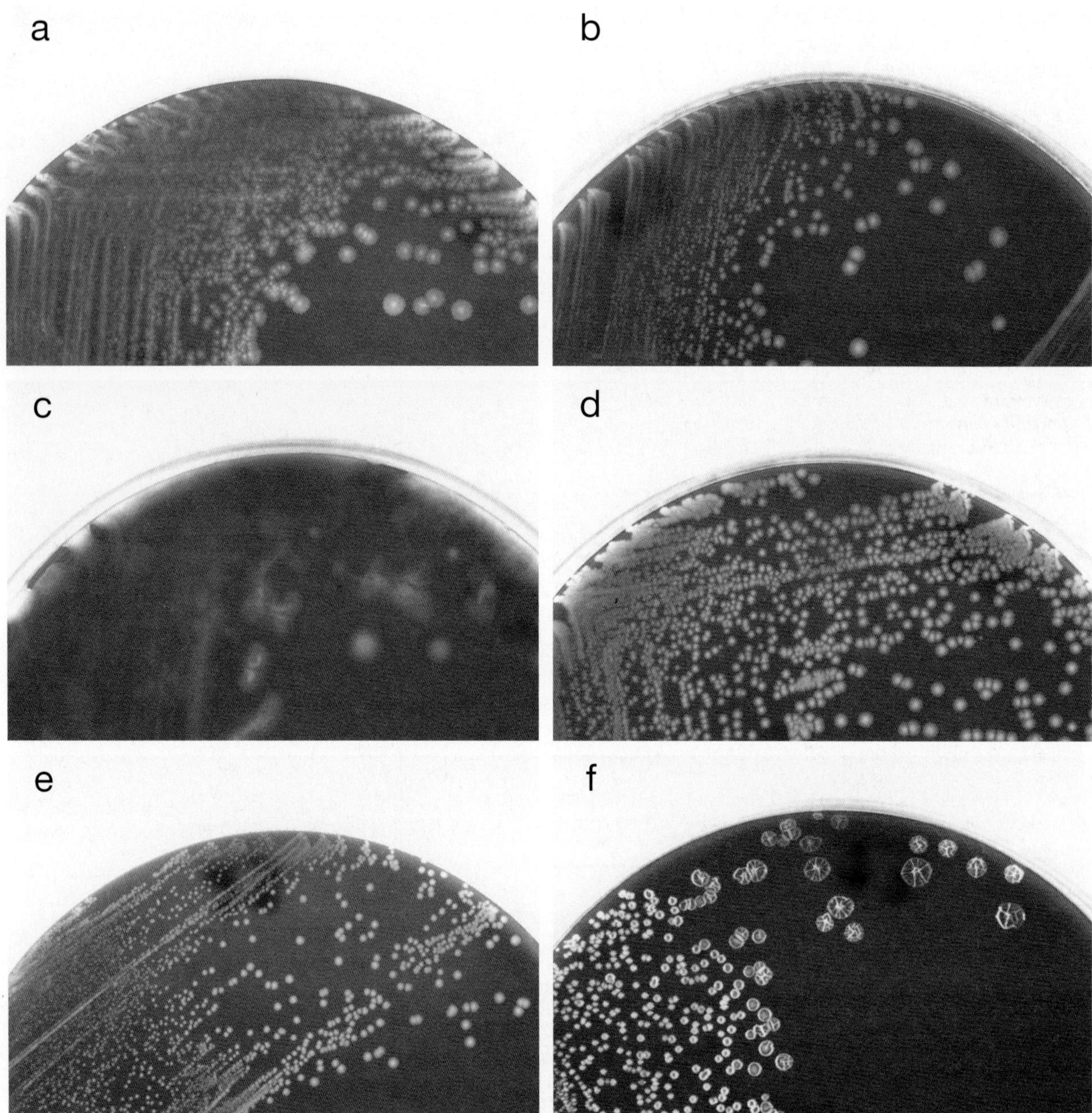

FIGURE 3 Colony morphologies of different coryneform bacteria after 48 h of incubation on SBA. (a) *C. amycolatum* LCDC 91-0077; (b) *C. diphtheriae* ATCC 14779; (c) *C. mucifaciens* LCDC 97-0202; (d) *C. striatum* ATCC 6940; (e) *D. hominis* ATCC 51325; and (f) *R. dentocariosa* LCDC 95-0154.

C. auris

C. auris (48) has almost exclusively been isolated from the ear region. Colonies are dryish, are slightly adherent to but do not penetrate agar, become slightly yellowish with time, and have diameters ranging from 1 to 2 mm after 48 h of incubation. *C. auris* does not produce acid from any of the carbohydrates usually tested. However, utilization reactions applying either the Biolog GP plate or the bioMérieux biotype 100 system may help in distinguishing *C. auris* from *C. afermentans* subsp. *afermentans* and *T. otitidis*, but in the clinical routine laboratory this can also be achieved by morphologic differentiation (see under *C. afermentans* subsp. *afermentans*). All *C. auris* strains are strongly CAMP test positive. The API Coryne system provides the numerical code 2100004 for this species. Abundant degradation products of mycolic acids are observed when CFA patterns are determined with the Sherlock system. It is noteworthy that the MICs of β-lactam antibiotics for *C. auris* strains are elevated, but the molecular mechanism for this is not known at present (59).

C. confusum

C. confusum (53) has been isolated from patients with foot infections as well as from a blood culture. Colonies are whitish, glistening, convex, creamy, and up to 1.5 mm in diameter after 48 h. Acid from glucose is produced only very weakly, becoming visible in the API Coryne or the API 50CH gallery only after 48 to 72 h. Weak growth under anaerobic conditions corresponds to slow fermentative acid production. It is advisable to incubate the API Coryne system after 24 h for another day in those cases in which the results for acid production are ambiguous (i.e., only a slight change in the color of the indicator). After 48 h of incubation the API Coryne system provides the numerical code 3100304 for this species. The species is correctly identified by the RapID CB Plus system (58). If glucose fermentation is judged to be negative, *C. confusum* strains can be misidentified as *C. propinquum*. However, in contrast to this species, *C. confusum* does not hydrolyze tyrosine and contains small amounts of TBSA (2 to 3%), whereas *C. propinquum* hydrolyzes tyrosine but does not contain TBSA. *C. confusum* is differentiated from *C. coyleae* and *C. argentoratense* by its ability to reduce nitrate.

C. coyleae

C. coyleae (56) has mainly been isolated from cultures of blood and other normally sterile body fluids, but it may also be recovered from genitourinary specimens (37a). Colonies are whitish and slightly glistening with entire edges and are about 1 mm in diameter after 24 h. The consistency of the colonies is either creamy or sticky. A slow fermentative acid production from glucose and a strongly positive CAMP reaction are the most significant phenotypic characteristics. *C. coyleae* is positive for cystine arylamidase, which is not observed for many other corynebacteria. The API Coryne numerical codes observed are 2100304 and 6100304, indicating that *C. coyleae* is consistently positive for ribose fermentation, whereas the biochemically similar species *C. argentoratense* is variable for this reaction. The API Coryne database lists only 6% glucose-fermenting *C. coyleae* strains, and therefore, when applying this commercial identification system, the clinical microbiologist may not receive a correct identification (60). However, the two numerical profiles given above combined with a positive CAMP reaction are highly indicative of *C. coyleae*. This species is correctly identified by the RapID CB Plus system (58).

CDC Group F-1 Bacteria

CDC group F-1 bacteria (120) have not been given a species name. Although genetically distinct, no distinguishing phenotypic markers which clearly allow their separation from other defined *Corynebacterium* spp. have been found. The characteristics of the CDC group F-1 bacteria are consistent with the definition of the genus *Corynebacterium* in all respects. The strains are lipophilic and are the only lipophilic fermentative *Corynebacterium* species able to hydrolyze urea. Of note is the negative alkaline phosphatase reaction (Table 4). CDC group F-1 strains are usually susceptible to penicillin but are often resistant to macrolides.

CDC Group G Bacteria

CDC group G bacteria (120) possess all chemotaxonomic features of true corynebacteria but cannot be given a species name since it has so far been impossible to find phenotypic traits allowing a unanimous definition (120). These lipophilic strains can be separated from *C. jeikeium* by anaerobic growth and fermentative acid production from fructose (114). Further biochemical features of CDC group G bacteria are given in Table 4. The API Coryne system correctly identifies CDC group G bacteria. They might be multidrug resistant, but the most frequently observed resistance is to macrolides and lincosamides.

C. diphtheriae

C. diphtheriae is commonly divided into four biotypes, biotypes *gravis*, *mitis*, *belfanti*, and *intermedius*; biotype differentiation is recommended by WHO (32) and CDC (9), although biotypes cannot be assigned separate subspecies status (121), nor is biotyping satisfactory for epidemiologic tracking. Initially, these biotypes were defined by differences in colony morphology and biochemical reactions (Table 4). However, only *C. diphtheriae* biotype *intermedius* can be diagnosed on the basis of colonial morphology (small, gray, or translucent lipophilic colonies) (28) as well as positive dextrin fermentation. Other *C. diphtheriae* biotypes produce larger (up to 2 mm after 24 h) white or opaque colonies (Fig. 3b) which are indistinguishable from each other. The lipophilic biotype *C. diphtheriae* biotype *intermedius* occurs only rarely in clinical infections, and *C. diphtheriae* biotype *belfanti* strains almost never harbor the diphtheria toxin gene.

Presumptive identification of *C. diphtheriae* (as well as of *C. pseudotuberculosis* and *C. ulcerans*) may be made by testing suspicious gram-positive rods for the presence of cystinase (as detected by using Tinsdale medium or diagnostic tablets [Rosco, Taastrup, Denmark]) and the absence of pyrazinamidase (diagnostic tablets are available from Key Scientific Products, Round Rock, Tex.). The API Coryne system identifies *C. diphtheriae* strains, with additional tests needed for the differentiation of *C. diphtheriae* biotype *mitis*-*C. diphtheriae* biotype *belfanti* and *C. diphtheriae* biotype *intermedius* (60). Large amounts of propionic acid are produced as the end product of glucose metabolism (37). *C. diphtheriae* strains are distinct from all other coryneform bacteria (except *C. pseudotuberculosis* and *C. ulcerans*) in their CFA patterns by the presence of a large volume of $C_{16:1\omega7c}$ (part of the so-called summed Feature 4, which also includes $C_{15iso2OH}$) (7).

Diphtheria Toxin Testing

It is recommended that at least 10 colonies of *C. diphtheriae* and related species be tested for diphtheria toxin by the Elek method in a laboratory with skill in performing the test and in interpreting the test results. The modified Elek method described by the WHO Diphtheria Reference Unit was initially used to characterize strains from the epidemic in Russia and Ukraine (34). This test was described as being faster than the original version (16 to 24 h compared with 48 h) and less technically problematic than the original version. The modification uses 3 ml of Elek medium (in which 0.5 ml of sterile newborn bovine serum was added to 2.5 ml of molten Elek base [ICN Biomedicals, Thame, United Kingdom] at 45°C) in 4.5-cm plates. The plates were inoculated with heavy inocula of test and control strains. An antitoxin disk (10 IU/disk) (antitoxin supplier, Swiss Serum and Vaccine Institute, Bern, Switzerland) is placed on the plate 9 mm away from the strains. The plates are incubated for up to 48 h at 37°C in air, but it was found that final readings of the precipitin lines can be done at 24 h (34) (Fig. 4). A similar modification of the Elek test which uses only 4.5 IU of diphtheria antitoxin in a central well on the agar plate and which can test up to 24 isolates on the same plate has recently been described (112). A 3-h enzyme-linked immunosorbent assay for the detection of diphtheria toxin from clinical isolates of *Corynebacterium*

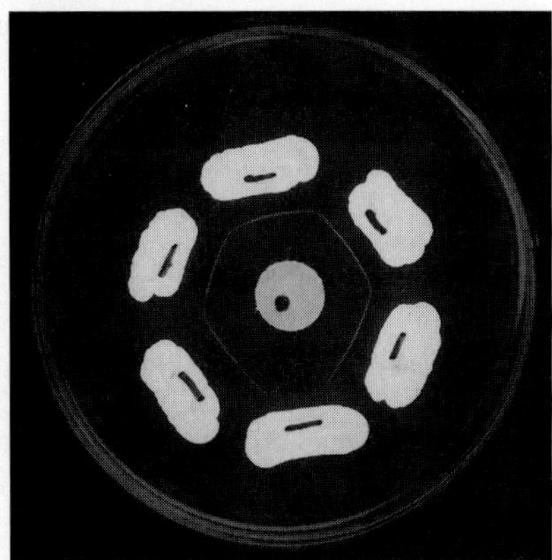

FIGURE 4 Modified Elek test (see text) with antitoxin disk in the center. Strains are (clockwise starting at noon) NCTC 3984 (weakly toxin-positive *C. diphtheriae* biotype *gravis*), NCTC 10648 (strongly toxin-positive *C. diphtheriae* biotype *gravis*), a test strain (which was found to be a toxin producer), NCTC 10356 (nontoxigenic *C. diphtheriae* biotype *belfanti*), another test strain (also a toxin producer), and, again, NCTC 10648. The photo was kindly supplied by K. H. Engler (WHO Diphtheria Reference Unit, Central Public Health Laboratory, London, United Kingdom).

spp. has recently been developed by the WHO Diphtheria Reference Unit (33).

PCR-based methods for the detection of the diphtheria toxin gene (*tox*) in grown bacteria have been described (67, 82, 89, 98). In addition, *tox* PCR assays applied directly to clinical specimens are encouraged by CDC (9), particularly because isolation is not always possible for patients already receiving antibiotics. However, a PCR-positive patient from whom bacteria are not isolated or without a histopathologic diagnosis and without an epidemiologic linkage to a patient with a laboratory-confirmed case of diphtheria should be classified as having a "probable case" of diphtheria, since to date there are insufficient data to conclude that a PCR-positive result always infers diphtheria. Also, detection of the toxin gene in samples by PCR cannot automatically be attributed to one species because *C. diphtheriae* as well as *C. ulcerans* and *C. pseudotuberculosis* may harbor the bacteriophage which carries the diphtheria toxin gene. Furthermore, *tox*-containing, nontoxigenic isolates have been described and characterized further (19). "Nontoxigenic" *C. diphtheriae* strains, i.e., those which do not express toxin in the Elek test or those which lack a detectable diphtheria toxin gene by PCR, have caused serious disease such as cases or outbreaks of skin disease or endocarditis among homeless people, alcoholics, and intravenous drug abusers (63).

Typing Methods

Outbreaks of *C. diphtheriae* in the states of the former Soviet Union and other outbreaks have been studied by whole-cell peptide analysis, whole genome restriction fragment length polymorphism analysis, ribotyping, pulsed-field gel electrophoresis, PCR–single-strand conformation polymorphism (PCR-SSCP) analysis of *tox* and *dtxR* (i.e., the regulatory element of the diphtheria toxin) as well as of the 16S-23S rRNA spacer region, and multilocus enzyme electrophoresis (31, 63, 92, 93, 103, 107). Sequencing studies with *C. diphtheriae* strains from the recent epidemic in the former Soviet Union have shown that point mutations within the *tox* gene were silent mutations, whereas multiple point mutations (which even led to amino acid substitutions) were observed for the *dtxR* gene, corresponding to the heterogeneity of outbreak strains as revealed by PCR-SSCP analysis (90).

C. diphtheriae strains are susceptible to β-lactam antibiotics. A minority of *C. diphtheriae* strains might be resistant to macrolides, and rifampin resistance has also been reported recently in a very few strains (27, 102).

C. durum

So far, *C. durum* (116) has been exclusively isolated from respiratory tract specimens. The majority of the strains described in the original paper on *C. durum* were primarily isolated after 2 to 3 days from nonselective charcoal-buffered yeast extract plates inoculated with sputa or bronchial washings (116). *C. durum* is the most frequent *Corynebacterium* isolated from throat swabs of healthy persons (141). Its pathogenic potential is unclear at present. *C. durum* is a peculiar nonlipophilic organism that forms colonies of only 0.5 to 1 mm in diameter after aerobic incubation for 72 h. They are beige and rough with convolutions, have an irregular margin, and strongly adhere to agar if they are grown under aerobic conditions. Gram staining of aerobic cultures shows long and filamentous rods which are highly unusual (except in *C. matruchotii*) for true corynebacteria (Fig. 1d). They are not observed when cells are grown in a 10% CO_2-enriched atmosphere (116). Strains grow only weakly under anaerobic conditions. They always reduce nitrate, and some exhibit weak and delayed urease and esculinase activities. The majority (but not all [141]) of *C. durum* strains ferment mannitol, which is another very unusual feature for true corynebacteria (Table 4). The API Coryne codes observed for *C. durum* include 3000135, 3001135, 3040135, 3400115, 3400135, 3400305, 3400325, and 3400335, indicating that all strains are negative for alkaline phosphatase. Only a small number of *C. durum* strains have been tested with the RapID system, and all were correctly identified (58). It is most likely that some strains identified as *C. matruchotii* in the past may actually have been *C. durum* strains. *C. matruchotii* and *C. durum* can easily be differentiated because the latter ferments galactose and very often mannitol, which is not observed for the *C. matruchotii* type strain; in contrast, the *C. matruchotii* type strain exhibits α-glucosidase activity, which is not observed in *C. durum* (110, 116). It has recently been shown that some *C. durum* strains also express β-galactosidase activity and ferment ribose (141).

C. falsenii

C. falsenii strains (127) have so far been isolated only from sterile body fluids. Colonies are whitish, glistening, and smooth with entire edges and are 1 to 2 mm in diameter after 24 h. After 72 h they exhibit a yellowish pigment which becomes even more intense after 120 h. This bright yellow pigment is not observed in any other nonlipophilic *Corynebacterium* encountered in clinical specimens except in the rarely isolated species *C. sanguinis* and the rarely found species *C. xerosis* (the colonies of the latter are dry in contrast to *C. falsenii* colonies). The most characteristic biochemical features of *C. falsenii* are a slow but fermentative acid production from glucose, a weak pyrazinamidase reaction, and a weak urease activity which becomes visible in either Christensen's urea broth or the API Coryne system after overnight incubation only. The API Coryne code observed for *C. falsenii* is 2101304.

C. glucuronolyticum

C. seminale (119) is a later synonym of *C. glucuronolyticum* (39). This species is probably part of the normal genitourinary flora of males, while its presence in females is uncertain. Colonies are whitish-yellowish, convex, and creamy, and colonies are 1 to 1.5 mm in diameter after 24 h. The fermentative species *C. glucuronolyticum* is remarkable for its variability in basic biochemical reactions (Table 4). It is the only medically relevant *Corynebacterium* exhibiting β-glucuronidase activity. When urease activity is present it is abundant in Christensen's urea broth, becoming positive after only 5 min of incubation at room temperature (39). *C. glucuronolyticum* is also one of the very few corynebacteria which are able to hydrolyze esculin. All *C. glucuronolyticum* strains are CAMP reaction positive (Fig. 2). With the exception of strains which are alkaline phosphatase positive, the API Coryne strip identifies *C. glucuronolyticum* well (60). Propionic acid is one of the major end products of glucose metabolism (39). *C. glucuronolyticum* strains are often tetracycline resistant and may also exhibit resistance to macrolides and lincosamides (59).

C. imitans

The only *C. imitans* strain described to date was isolated from a nasopharyngeal specimen of a child suspected of having throat diphtheria (41). The same strain was also isolated from three adult contacts. This was the first well-documented case of the person-to-person transmission of a *Corynebacterium* other than *C. diphtheriae* in a nonhospital setting. It is presently not known how many other people are carriers of *C. imitans*. Colonies are whitish-grayish, glistening with entire edges, creamy, and 1 to 2 mm in diameter. The strain did not produce a brown halo on Tinsdale medium but was tellurite reductase positive. Interestingly, Neisser staining was positive for polar bodies. Pyrazinamidase activity was weak only, as was fermentation of sucrose, which may lead to the initial misdiagnosis of an atypical *C. diphtheriae* strain. It is not unlikely that *C. imitans* may also have been misidentified as *C. minutissimum* in the past since the basic biochemical reactions of both taxa are quite similar (Table 4). However, *C. imitans* is CAMP reaction positive and does not hydrolyze tyrosine, whereas the opposite reactions are observed for *C. minutissimum*. The API Coryne system provided the numerical code 2100324 for *C. imitans*, indicating a negative α-glucosidase reaction, whereas all *C. diphtheriae* strains express this enzyme. It is also noteworthy that almost all toxin-harboring *C. diphtheriae* strains (except the less pathogenic biotype *C. diphtheriae* biotype *belfanti*) reduce nitrate, whereas *C. imitans* was negative for this reaction. Neither the diphtheria toxin gene nor its gene product could be detected in the *C. imitans* strain examined. *C. imitans* is resistant to O/129, while *C. diphtheriae* is not.

C. jeikeium

C. jeikeium is one of the most frequently encountered corynebacteria in clinical specimens (63, 117, 140). Nosocomial transmission has been described (63). It is often resistant to multiple antibiotics (including penicillin and gentamicin), but this cannot be used as a taxonomic characteristic because the phenotypically closely related CDC group G bacteria may also demonstrate multidrug resistance. By quantitative DNA-DNA hydridization experiments, it has also been shown that the presently defined species *C. jeikeium* includes two genomospecies for which penicillin and gentamicin MICs are low but which could otherwise not be differentiated phenotypically from the resistant *C. jeikeium* strains and which were therefore not proposed as independent species (114). Colonies of *C. jeikeium* are tiny, low, entire, and grayish white. *C. jeikeium* is a strict aerobe which may oxidatively produce acid from glucose and sometimes from maltose but not from fructose (CDC group G bacteria are positive for acid production from fructose). The RapID CB Plus system correctly identifies *C. jeikeium*, as does the API Coryne system if ancillary tests are used (58, 60). As for all other lipophilic corynebacteria, imperfectly cleaved mycolic acids coeluting with CFAs at or near equivalent chain lengths (ECLs) of 14.966 to 15.000 or ECLs of 16.7 to 16.8 have never been observed among *C. jeikeium* strains (4a, 7).

C. kroppenstedtii

C. kroppenstedtii (23) is a newly described species that is rarely found and that has been isolated from the sputum of a patient with pulmonary disease. Apart from *C. amycolatum*, it is the only *Corynebacterium* lacking mycolic acids. Colonies are grayish translucent, slightly dry, and less than 0.5 mm in diameter after 24 h of incubation at 37°C. *C. kroppenstedtii* is lipophilic and is one of the few medically relevant *Corynebacterium* species exhibiting esculinase activity. Other biochemical characteristics are given in Table 4. It can be separated from *C. durum*, *C. matruchotii*, and *C. glucuronolyticum* by its colony morphology and from *C. glucuronolyticum* also by its negative CAMP reaction.

C. lipophiloflavum

C. lipophiloflavum (46) is represented by only a single strain which has been isolated from a patient with bacterial vaginosis. It has the same biochemical screening pattern as *C. urealyticum* except that it exhibits a strong yellow pigment and weaker urease activity (Table 4). In contrast to most *C. urealyticum* strains (129), the *C. lipophiloflavum* strain observed was not multidrug resistant.

C. macginleyi

C. macginleyi (120) has almost exclusively been isolated from eye specimens. Colonies are typical for lipophilic corynebacteria (see above). When grown on Tween 80–SBA plates (better growth is usually found on plates supplemented with 0.1% Tween 80 than on those supplemented with 1.0% Tween 80), some *C. macginleyi* strains exhibit a rose pigment which is not seen for any other lipophilic *Corynebacterium* species. *C. macginleyi* is one of the very few *Corynebacterium* species not expressing pyrazinamidase activity (Table 4). Another peculiar feature is that most strains ferment mannitol, while the majority of other corynebacteria are unable to do so. The API Coryne system correctly identifies *C. macginleyi* (60). Strains belonging to this species are susceptible to a broad spectrum of antibiotics (37a).

C. matruchotii

C. matruchotii (110) is thought to be a natural inhabitant of the oral cavity, particularly on calculus and plaque deposits. It is a very rare human pathogen, primarily being cited as the subject of dental studies. Microcolonies appear flat, filamentous, and spider-like, but macrocolonies have a variable appearance. *C. matruchotii* demonstrates a very unusual appearance by Gram staining in that so-called whip handles (i.e., filamentous bacteria with a single short bacillus adjacent to the end of the filament creating the illusion of a whip) are observed (Fig. 1e). This microscopic presentation is consistent even when isolates which had been preserved for many years in a culture collection are stained. It has recently been demonstrated that heterogeneity exists among *C. matruchotii* strains obtained from international culture collections and that some strains represented were misidentified *C. durum* strains (110). *C. matruchotii* strains are consistently negative for galactose, whereas *C. durum* strains are positive. The API Coryne system database does not contain *C. matruchotii*; the numerical codes observed for *C. matruchotii* include 7000325, 7010325, and 7050325.

C. minutissimum

C. minutissimum is part of the normal human skin flora. Its association with erythrasma is highly questionable (152). Colonies of *C. minutissimum* are whitish-grayish, shiny and moist, convex, and circular, have entire edges, and are about 1 to 1.5 mm in diameter after 24 h. Most of the colonies are creamy, but some may also have a sticky consistency. *C. minutissimum* strains have a fermentative metabolism and produce acid from sucrose variably. Very few *C. minutissimum* strains are also able to produce acid from mannitol (152). The API Coryne system identifies *C. minutissimum*, with additional tests being necessary for most of the strains (60). Many *C. minutissimum* strains are pyrrolidonyl arylamidase positive. *C. minutissimum* strains exhibit DNase activity (152), and nearly all strains hydrolyze tyrosine, whereas only a very few strains exhibit a positive CAMP reaction. Lactic and succinic acids are the major end products of glucose metabolism (37, 152). Some isolates belong to the few fermentative *Corynebacterium* spp. which possess TBSA in their cell membranes. Nearly all *C. minutissimum* strains are susceptible to O/129 (150-μg disk); i.e., they exhibit an inhibition zone around the disk (usually between 20 and 35 mm).

C. mucifaciens

C. mucifaciens (49) has mainly been isolated from blood cultures and other sterile body fluids. Colonies are very distinct because they are slightly yellow and very mucoid (Fig. 3c). In fact, *C. mucifaciens* is the only presently known *Corynebacterium* species exhibiting those mucoid colonies; this characteristic strongly reminds the bacteriologist of *Rhodococcus equi* colonies. An extracellular substance (probably polysaccharides) causing connective filaments between the cells has been demonstrated as the ultrastructural correlate of the mucoid colonies. Colonies are about 1 to 1.5 mm after 24 h of incubation and have entire edges. They appear less mucoid after extended incubation for 96 h. *C. mucifaciens* has an oxidative metabolism. It consistently produces acid from glucose, but acid production from sucrose is variable. The API Coryne numerical codes 2100104, 2100105, 6100104, and 6100105 have been observed for *C. mucifaciens*. *C. mucifaciens* is enzymatically less active than *R. equi* which exhibits α- and β-glucosidase activities not observed for *C. mucifaciens*. In addition, *C. mucifaciens* produces acid from glycerol, fructose, and mannose, but acid production from these sugars is not seen in *R. equi* strains. Tuberculostearic acid can be detected in amounts of 1 to 2% of the total CFAs. β-Lactam antibiotics and aminoglycosides show very good activities against *C. mucifaciens*.

C. propinquum

C. propinquum is the closest phylogenetic relative of *C. pseudodiphtheriticum* (100, 124) and has the same niche (i.e., the oropharynx) as *C. pseudodiphtheriticum*. Colonies are whitish and matted with entire edges and are 1 to 2 mm in diameter after 24 h of incubation. This species reduces nitrate and hydrolyzes tyrosine but does not hydrolyze urea (Table 4). The API Coryne system and the RapID CB Plus system correctly identify *C. propinquum* strains (58, 60).

C. pseudodiphtheriticum

C. pseudodiphtheriticum is part of the normal oropharyngeal flora. Colonies are whitish, slightly dry with entire edges, and 1 to 2 mm in diameter after 48 h of incubation. This nonfermenting species reduces nitrate and hydrolyzes urea but does not produce acid from any of the commonly tested carbohydrates (Table 4). Some strains hydrolyze tyrosine. The API Coryne system and the RapID CB Plus system correctly identify *C. pseudodiphtheriticum* strains (58, 60). For this species, imperfectly cleaved mycolic acids coeluting with CFAs have been demonstrated (4a). *C. pseudodiphtheriticum* strains are susceptible to β-lactam antibiotics, but resistance to macrolides and lincosamides has been observed.

C. pseudotuberculosis

C. pseudotuberculosis is phylogenetically closely related to *C. diphtheriae* (100, 124), may also harbor the diphtheria toxin gene, and contains large amounts of $C_{16:1\omega7c}$ (7). Colonies are yellowish white, opaque, and convex with a matted surface and are about 1 mm in diameter after 24 h. Like *C. ulcerans*, *C. pseudotuberculosis* is positive for urease and the reverse CAMP test (complete inhibition of the effect of *S. aureus* β-hemolysin on sheep erythrocytes is achieved by streaking the presumed *C. pseudotuberculosis* strain in a right angle toward *S. aureus* and overnight incubation; a β-hemolysin inhibition zone in the form of a triangle is observed, as is the case for *A. haemolyticum* [Fig. 2]). *C. pseudotuberculosis* is variable for both nitrate reduction and sucrose fermentation. The API Coryne system and the RapID CB Plus panel correctly identify this species (58, 60).

C. riegelii

C. riegelii strains so far have been exclusively isolated from females with urinary tract infections (50). Colonies are whitish, glistening, and convex with entire margins and are of up to 1.5 mm in diameter after 48 h of incubation. Some colonies are of a creamy consistency, whereas others are sticky. *C. riegelii* strains exhibit a very strong urease activity with Christensen's urea broth, becoming positive within 5 min at room temperature after inoculation. A very peculiar characteristic of *C. riegelii* is the slow fermentation of maltose but not glucose. No other defined *Corynebacterium* exhibits this feature (Table 4). The weak anaerobic growth of *C. riegelii* corresponds to the weak fermentative metabolism. The API Coryne system codes observed for *C. riegelii* include 0101224, 2001224, and 2101224.

C. sanguinis

The presently known strains of *C. sanguinis* were isolated from blood cultures (44). Colonies are yellowish, smooth, slightly dryish, and up to 1.5 mm in diameter after 48 h of incubation. Slow fermentative acid production from glucose but not from maltose or sucrose and the presence of small amounts of TBSA (2 to 3%) are the most significant phenotypic features. *C. sanguinis* can be differentiated from *C. coyleae* by its negative CAMP reaction, from *C. falsenii* by its negative urease reaction, and from *C. confusum* by its yellow pigment and the inability to reduce nitrate. *C. argentoratense* produces acid from glucose more rapidly than *C. sanguinis* and also exhibits larger colonies after 24 h of incubation. The numerical API Coryne system code for *C. sanguinis* is 6100304.

C. singulare

Two strains of *C. singulare* have been described recently (122): one strain came from semen and the other came from a blood culture. Colonies are circular and slightly convex with entire margins and are of a creamy consistency, as observed for *C. minutissimum* and *C. striatum*. Key biochemical reactions are like those for *C. minutissimum*, except that urease activity can be observed (Table 4). The numerical API Coryne system profile is 6101125, indicating that pyrrolidonyl arylamidase activity is observed. Like *C. minutissimum* and *C. striatum*, *C. singulare* also hydrolyzes tyrosine. *C. singulare* can be differentiated from *C. minutissimum* by certain carbon source utilization tests (e.g., D-turanose and *N*-acetyl-D-glucosamine) performed by applying the bioMérieux biotype 100 gallery, but this is not advisable for the routine clinical laboratory. *C. singulare* does not produce propionic acid but does produce succinic acid as an end product of glucose metabolism, differentiating it from *C. amycolatum*.

C. striatum

C. striatum is part of the normal human skin flora. Nosocomial transmission of *C. striatum* has been well documented (11, 78). Colonies are convex, circular, shiny and moist, and creamy with entire edges and are about 1 to 1.5 mm in diameter after 24 h of incubation (Fig. 3d). Some investigators have described *C. striatum* colonies as somewhat like those of small coagulase-negative staphylococci (86). *C. striatum* has a fermentative metabolism, and acid production from sucrose is variable. The API Coryne system identifies *C. striatum*, but with additional tests needed in most of the cases (60). A few *C. striatum* strains might also be nitrate reductase negative (37a). All *C. striatum* strains hydrolyze tyrosine, and some strains are CAMP reaction positive; however, the CAMP reaction of *C. striatum* strains is usually not as strong as that of other CAMP test-positive species (e.g., *C. auris* or *C. glucuronolyticum*). Lactic and succinic acids are the major end products of glucose metabolism (37). All *C. striatum* strains are susceptible to O/129. Resistance to macrolides and lincosamides due to the presence of an rRNA methylase has been described (123). *C. striatum* may also be resistant to quinolones and tetracyclines (84).

C. sundsvallense

C. sundsvallense (20) is a newly described species that has been isolated from blood cultures, a vaginal swab, and a sinus drainage from an infected groin. Colonies of this nonlipophilic species are buff or slightly yellowish, are adherent to agar, and have a sticky consistency. Gram staining shows bulges or knobs at the ends of some rods, and these are not seen in any other corynebacteria. Fermentation of glucose, maltose, and sucrose is slow (Table 4). *C. sundsvallense* can be separated from *C. durum* by its positive α-glucosidase reaction and its inability to ferment galactose. It is further differentiated from *C. matruchotii* by expressing urease but not nitrate reductase activity and by not producing propionic acid as the major end product of glucose metabolism.

C. thomssenii

C. thomssenii (151) is a rarely found species and has been repeatedly isolated from a patient with pleural effusion. This species is fastidious and slowly growing, resulting in colonies of <0.5 mm after 48 h, but it is not lipophilic. After 96 h colonies are molar tooth-like, very sticky, and slightly adherent to agar. *C. thomssenii* is the only *Corynebacterium* species expressing *N*-acetyl-β-glucosaminidase activity, which can be observed either in the API Coryne system or in the API ZYM system. Acid is slowly and fermentatively produced from glucose, maltose, and sucrose, and the resulting API Coryne code for *C. thomssenii* is 2121125.

C. ulcerans

Phylogenetically, *C. ulcerans* (121) is, together with *C. pseudotuberculosis*, the closest relative of *C. diphtheriae* (100, 124), can also harbor the diphtheria toxin gene, and contains significant amounts of $C_{16:1\omega7c}$ (7). Colonies are somewhat dry and waxy and gray-white with light hemolysis and are 1 to 2 mm in diameter after 24 h. *C. ulcerans* may be differentiated from *C. diphtheriae* by urease activity and a reverse CAMP reaction (Table 4) (see also Fig. 2). Strains of *C. ulcerans* are positive for glycogen, starch, and trehalose fermentation. The API Coryne system and the RapID CB Plus identification strip correctly identify *C. ulcerans* (58, 60).

C. urealyticum

C. urealyticum is one of the more frequently isolated clinically significant corynebacteria in clinical specimens (63, 117). *C. urealyticum* is strongly associated with urinary tract infections. Recovery of this bacterium is often associated with urine with an alkaline pH, resulting in struvite crystals. As for all other lipophilic corynebacteria, colonies are pinpoint, convex, smooth, and whitish-grayish on regular SBA. *C. urealyticum* is a strict aerobe and has very strong urease activity (Table 4). Commercial identification systems correctly identify *C. urealyticum*. It is almost always multidrug resistant (63, 117, 129), but rare penicillin-susceptible strains have also been described (150).

C. xerosis

The natural habitat of *C. xerosis* (47) is unknown, although it has recently been isolated from vaginal swabs (37a). Colonies are dry, granular, and yellowish with irregular edges and are of 1 to 1.5 mm in diameter after 24 h. It is emphasized that nearly all "*C. xerosis*" strains which appeared in the literature before 1996 may have been misidentified *C. amycolatum* strains (47). *C. striatum* strains were also misidentified as *C. xerosis* in the past (26). *C. xerosis* has a fermentative metabolism, is variable for the presence of nitrate reductase, but always expresses α-glucosidase as well as leucine arylamidase activities. Because *C. xerosis* was thought to be rarely encountered in clinical specimens, it was not included in the API Coryne system version 2.0 database. The numerical profiles observed for *C. xerosis* strains include 2110325 and 3110325. The RapID CB Plus system correctly identifies *C. xerosis* (58). Lactic acid is the major end product of glucose metabolism, and strains are susceptible to O/129.

Biochemical Reactions for Other Genera

The key biochemical reactions for the genera other than *Corynebacterium* are given in Table 5.

Genus *Turicella*

T. otitidis is almost exclusively isolated from clinical specimens from the ear region, but it does not cause otitis media with effusion in children (52). Colonies are whitish, convex, and creamy with entire edges and are 1 to 1.5 mm in diameter after 48 h of incubation. Some young colonies show a greenish appearance when taken away from the plates with a swab. The distinctive Gram staining morphology of *T. otitidis* is given in Fig. 1b. Differentiation from *C. auris* and

TABLE 5 Identification of medically relevant coryneform bacteria other than *Corynebacterium* spp.[a]

Taxon	Catalase	Fermentation/ oxidation	Motility	Nitrate reduction	Urease	Esculin hydrolysis	Acid production from:					Other traits
							Glucose	Maltose	Sucrose	Mannitol	Xylose	
Turicella otitidis	+	O	−	−	−	−	−	−	−	−	−	CAMP reaction positive, long rods
Arthrobacter spp.	+	O	V	V	V	V	V	V	V	−	−	
Brevibacterium spp.	+	O	−	V	−	−	V	V	V	−	−	Odor
Dermabacter hominis	+	F	−	−	−	+	+	+	+	−	V	Small rods
Rothia dentocariosa	V	F	−	+	−	+	+	+	+	−	−	Adherence
Exiguobacterium acetylicum	+	F	+	V	−	+	+	+	+	+	−	
Oerskovia spp.	+	F	V	+	−	+	+	+	+	−	+	Agar penetration
Cellulomonas spp.	+	F	V	+	−	+	+	+	+	V	+	
Microbacterium spp.	V	F	V	V	−	+	+	+	+	+	V	
Aureobacterium spp.	V	O	V	V	V	V	+	+	V	V	V	
Curtobacterium spp.	+	O	V	−	−	+	+	V	V	V	+	
"*Corynebacterium aquaticum*"	+	O	+	V	−	V	+	V	V	+	+	
Arcanobacterium haemolyticum	−	F	−	−	−	−	+	+	V	−	−	Reverse CAMP reaction positive
Arcanobacterium pyogenes	−	F	−	−	−	V	+	V	V	V	+	
Arcanobacterium bernardiae	−	F	−	−	−	−	+	+	−	−	−	
Gardnerella vaginalis	−	F	−	−	−	−	+	+	V	−	−	

[a] Abbreviations and symbols: +, positive reaction; −, negative reaction; V, variable; O, oxidation; F, fermentation.

C. afermentans subsp. *afermentans* is readily achieved by morphologic features, but utilization reactions may also assist in the differentiation of these taxa (48, 113). All *T. otitidis* strains are strongly CAMP reaction positive and give the numerical code 2100004 in the API Coryne system. The MICs of β-lactam antibiotics for many strains are very low; some strains might be resistant to macrolides and clindamycin (59).

Genus *Arthrobacter*

Arthrobacter spp. have not been described as part of the normal human flora; however, there is now evidence that the recently described species *A. cumminsii* is a normal commensal organism. The latter species seems to be the most frequently isolated *Arthrobacter* species from clinical specimens (54). *Arthrobacter* colonies are usually whitish-grayish, slightly glistening, creamy, and 2 mm or greater in diameter after 24 h. *A. cumminsii* is slightly smaller than the other arthrobacters and may also exhibit a sticky consistency (54). *Arthrobacter* spp. usually do not oxidize any of the carbohydrates routinely tested and do not express a cheese-like smell, as is often found for the phenotypically closely related brevibacteria. Some arthrobacters are motile, whereas brevibacteria are always nonmotile. Like brevibacteria, *Arthrobacter* spp. express DNase and have gelatinase activity (45). The identification of arthrobacters might be achieved by carbohydrate utilization tests, but this should be performed only in reference laboratories. *A. cumminsii* has a distinctive CFA pattern, with $C_{14:0i}$ and $C_{14:0}$ each representing 2 to 4% of all CFAs (45). The penicillin MICs for most *Arthrobacter* strains are low (45). Aminoglycosides and quinolones show only very weak activities against *A. cumminsii* strains (54).

Genus *Brevibacterium*

Some *Brevibacterium* spp. are part of the normal human skin flora. Colonies are whitish-grayish, convex, creamy, and 2 mm or greater in diameter after 24 h. *B. mcbrellneri* colonies have a more granular appearance and are dryer than those of other brevibacteria (87). Some brevibacteria may develop a yellowish or greenish pigment after prolonged incubation. Many *Brevibacterium* strains isolated from human clinical material give off a distinctive cheese-like odor. Brevibacteria are nonmotile, are halotolerant (6.5% NaCl), and form methanethiol from methionine, but this test is specific for brevibacteria only when it is read within 2 h (40). Brevibacteria can be identified to the species level by carbohydrate utilization tests (40, 99). More than 95% of all clinical *Brevibacterium* isolates are *B. casei* (40). The MICs of β-lactam antibiotics for brevibacteria are often elevated (59).

Genus *Dermabacter*

D. hominis strains are part of the normal skin flora. Colonies are whitish, convex, of a creamy or sticky consistency, and 1 to 1.5 mm in diameter after 48 h (Fig. 3e) and have a characteristic pungent odor (5). *D. hominis* strains are sometimes mistaken for small-colony coagulase-negative staphylococci. The Gram staining result is distinctive, with coccobacillary or coccoidal forms (Fig. 1c). The key biochemical reactions are given in Table 5. *D. hominis* is one of the few coryneform bacteria with a variable reaction for xylose fermentation. It is the only catalase-positive coryneform bacterium (except *Actinomyces neuii* [37]) that is able to decarboxylate lysine and ornithine (5, 61, 68). The API Coryne system and the RapID CB Plus panel correctly identify this species (58, 60). *D. hominis* strains may be resistant to aminoglycosides (59, 61).

Genus *Rothia*

Colonies of *R. dentocariosa* are whitish, raised, and smooth or rough or have a "spoke-wheel" form (Fig. 3f), and they are up to 2 mm in diameter after 48 h. *Rothia* strains usually grow better in a CO_2-enriched atmosphere. The biochemical features of *R. dentocariosa* are given in Table 5. The API Coryne system correctly identifies *R. dentocariosa* (60). Its CFA composition is of the branched-chain type (7), which allows differentiation from the biochemically similar species *C. matruchotii*, *C. durum*, and *A. viscosus*, all of which also occupy the oropharynx. *R. dentocariosa* may also be confused with *D. hominis* and *Propionibacterium avidum*, both of which, in contrast, always exhibit smooth colonies.

Evidence which may provide additional precision to the description of *R. dentocariosa* and to documentation of the existence of additional species in this genus is accumulating. Heterogeneity among *R. dentocariosa* strains had been demonstrated by pyrolysis mass spectrometry (131). In a study of the pharyngeal bacterial flora of healthy adults, it was demonstrated that one-third of all *R. dentocariosa* strains isolated were catalase negative (141). Recent 16S rRNA gene sequencing data for *R. dentocariosa* (75) and *R. dentocariosa*-like strains (6) (identical to *R. dentocariosa* by colony morphology, phenotypic tests, and CFA composition but catalase negative and with a tendency toward being exclusively "coccoidal" by microscopic examination) suggested that there is heterogeneity in the genus. Unexpectedly, some *R. dentocariosa*-like strains examined were nearly identical to *Stomatococcus mucilaginosus* by 16S rRNA gene sequencing analysis; however, *S. mucilaginosus* has adherent mucoid yellowish colonies and a unique CFA pattern. The MICs of aminoglycosides for some *R. dentocariosa* strains are elevated (134).

CDC group 4 is a provisional name for bacteria which are phenotypically and by CFA composition closely related to *R. dentocariosa* except that they exhibit charcoal gray or black colonies (4a, 68). Not much is known about this taxon except that strains have primarily been recovered from the female genitourinary tract. Conclusive studies of the phylogenetic relationship of CDC group 4 bacteria to *R. dentocariosa* have not yet been published.

Genus *Exiguobacterium*

It is not known whether exiguobacteria are part of the indigenous bacterial flora of humans. Colonies of *E. acetylicum* are plain, golden-yellow to orange, and up to 2 mm in diameter after 24 h of incubation. Acid from carbohydrates is rapidly produced by fermentative metabolism. Exiguobacteria are motile and often oxidase positive. They might be confused with microbacteria, but CFA analysis provides a clear-cut distinction between the two genera (Table 1). The pathogenic potential of *E. acetylicum* seems to be rather low since it has been isolated from different sources (e.g., skin, wounds, and cerebrospinal fluid [69]), but case reports on infectious diseases due to *E. acetylicum* are not extant. Cases of pseudobacteremia due to *E. acetylicum* have been observed. By confirmatory 16S rRNA gene analysis, one *E. aurantiacum* strain from a blood culture has been identified recently (4a).

Genus *Oerskovia*

Oerskoviae are usually acquired from the environment (e.g., soil). Colonies are pale yellow to phosphorous yellow, convex, and creamy; they slightly penetrate into the agar; and they are approximately 1 to 2 mm in diameter after 24 h. *Oerskovia* spp. rapidly produce acid from sugars by fermentation. They also exhibit a very strong esculin reaction. Oerskoviae are well identified by the API Coryne system (60). Hydrolysis of either xanthine or hypoxanthine differentiates *O. xanthineolytica* (positive for both reactions) from *O. turbata* (negative for both reactions).

Genus *Cellulomonas*

Cellulomonas strains are usually acquired from the environment. Colonies are first whitish or pale or bright yellow, but after 7 days nearly all *Cellulomonas* strains are somewhat yellow. Colonies vary between 0.5 and 1.5 mm in diameter after 24 h, are convex and creamy, and have entire edges. *Cellulomonas* spp. are variable for the fermentation of mannitol. Other key biochemical reactions of *Cellulomonas* spp. are given in Table 5. The majority of *Cellulomonas* strains express cellulase activity, demonstrated by incubating a heavy bacterial suspension (McFarland no. 6 standard) with a piece of sterile copy paper in a 0.9% NaCl solution for 10 days, resulting in dissolution of the paper (55).

Genus *Microbacterium*

Microbacteria should always be considered when yellow- or yellow-orange-pigmented fermentative coryneform bacteria are isolated. Most of the strains are catalase positive, but catalase-negative strains have recently been observed (37a). Microbacteria grow relatively weakly under anaerobic conditions. Many *Microbacterium* strains are nitrate reductase negative, which separates them from the phenotypically closely related genus *Cellulomonas*, all of whose presently defined species are nitrate reductase positive (Table 5). Microbacteria may ferment mannitol but not xylose, whereas the lack of xylose fermentation has not been observed for the *Cellulomonas* strains described so far. A reference laboratory further differentiates microbacteria from *Cellulomonas* spp. by the chemotaxonomic features outlined in Table 1 (e.g., lysine versus ornithine as the diamino acid). Resistance to aminoglycosides was observed in some *Microbacterium* strains (42, 43).

Genus *Aureobacterium*

For many years, aureobacteria had been mistakenly identified as "*C. aquaticum*" (64). Aureobacteria comprise the largest group of yellow-pigmented oxidative coryneform bacteria isolated from human clinical specimens. All shades of yellow pigment are observed, ranging from pale to bright yellow. The pigment usually develops very rapidly, whereas in "*C. aquaticum*" strains pigment production is delayed (64). Most *Aureobacterium* strains show gelatinase activity and hydrolyze casein, neither of which is seen in "*C. aquaticum*" (64). For other biochemical reactions, see Table 5. Species identification is almost impossible since for many defined *Aureobacterium* species the type strain is the only representative, preventing the creation of a comprehensive database. Final identification to the species level is best achieved by chemotaxonomic (interpeptide bridges) and molecular genetic (16S rRNA gene sequencing) investigations, which are usually performed only in reference laboratories. The recently proposed species *A. resistens* is resistant to vancomycin but is susceptible to teicoplanin (51). Other aureobacteria are usually susceptible to vancomycin, but susceptibility to other antimicrobial agents is unpredictable (64), and therefore, every individual clinically significant strain must be tested.

Genus *Curtobacterium*

Curtobacteria are yellow- or yellow-orange-pigmented oxidative coryneform bacteria. In contrast to most aureobacteria, they produce acid from carbohydrates very slowly (within 4 to 7 days) (38). Curtobacteria are usually nitrate reductase negative but strongly hydrolyze esculin (Table 5). *C. pusillum* and related strains have a most unusual CFA composition which is not observed in any other coryneform bacteria, with feature 7 ($C_{18:1\omega9c/\omega12t/\omega7c}$) representing more than 50% of all CFAs (38). Again, the differentiation of curtobacteria is very difficult and should be performed in a reference laboratory. The MICs of macrolides and rifampin for curtobacteria are very low (38).

"*C. aquaticum*" and Other Yellow-Pigmented Bacteria

True "*C. aquaticum*" strains are very rarely encountered in clinical specimens. They are always motile, do not hydrolyze either gelatin or casein, and have stronger DNase activity than aureobacteria (64). Their yellow pigment develops relatively slowly within 3 to 4 days. The MICs of vancomycin for some "*C. aquaticum*" strains were shown to be elevated (8 μg/ml) (64), but the precise mechanism of this resistance is not known.

Other yellow-pigmented coryneform bacteria which contain diaminobutyric acid in their cell wall include *Clavibacter*, *Rathayibacter*, and *Agromyces*, which are mainly plant pathogens and which have not been isolated from humans so far.

Genus *Arcanobacterium*

The genus *Arcanobacterium* comprises four species, all of which exhibit beta-hemolysis on SBA. The three medically relevant species *A. haemolyticum*, *A. pyogenes*, and *A. bernardiae* are all catalase negative and show a fermentative glucose metabolism, with succinic and lactic acids as their major end products. All arcanobacteria grow and express beta-hemolysis best in a CO_2-enriched atmosphere.

The colonies of the type species, *A. haemolyticum*, are <0.5 mm in diameter after 48 h of incubation at 37°C, and two morphotypes have been described: one rough type isolated mainly from the respiratory tract and one smooth type isolated mainly from wounds (16). The biochemical reactions of *A. haemolyticum* are given in Table 5. Of major value for the identification of *A. haemolyticum* is the so-called reverse CAMP reaction (see the description of the reverse CAMP reaction in the section on *C. pseudotuberculosis*) (Fig. 2). The protein responsible for this phenomenon is a phospholipase D excreted by *A. haemolyticum*, and this protein is genetically and functionally similar to the ones expressed by *C. ulcerans* and *C. pseudotuberculosis* (29, 88). *A. haemolyticum* as well as the two other medically relevant arcanobacteria are correctly identified by the API Coryne system (60).

A. pyogenes colonies are the largest of all arcanobacteria colonies, with diameters of up to 1 mm after 48 h of incubation. Of all the arcanobacteria this species also shows the sharpest zone of beta-hemolysis on SBA. The protein responsible for hemolysis, named pyolysin, is also an important virulence factor in vivo (8). Gram stains may show some branching rods. *A. pyogenes* is the only *Arcanobacterium* species that expresses β-glucuronidase activity and that is capable of fermenting xylose.

A. bernardiae shows glassy, whitish colonies of <0.5 mm in diameter after 48 h. Some colonies have a creamy consistency, whereas others are sticky. Gram staining shows relatively short rods without branching. Most *A. bernardiae* strains belong to the very few coryneform bacteria that are able to ferment glycogen. Another peculiar feature of *A. bernardiae* strains is their ability to produce acid faster from maltose than from glucose.

The MICs of all β-lactams, rifampin, and tetracycline for arcanobacteria are very low, whereas aminoglycosides and quinolones have reduced activities against arcanobacteria (15, 134). A single *A. haemolyticum* strain carrying the *vanA* gene conferring resistance to vancomycin has been described (108). Macrolides also exhibit excellent activities against arcanobacteria and are an alternative to β-lactam antibiotics for the treatment of infections since treatment failures due to β-lactam antibiotics because of the inability of β-lactam antibiotics to act intracellularly have been reported.

ANTIMICROBIAL SUSCEPTIBILITIES

The susceptibility patterns for each taxon were given with the descriptions of each taxon (see above). Since the antimicrobial susceptibility of coryneform bacteria is not predictable in every case, susceptibility testing should always be performed with clinically significant isolates (see the section Clinical Significance). Due to the emergence of vancomycin-resistant gram-positive organisms, it has become inappropriate to recommend glycopeptides as first-line drugs for the treatment of infections caused by coryneform bacteria. It is also noteworthy that some coryneform bacteria (e.g., *A. resistens*) are intrinsically vancomycin resistant.

The National Committee for Clinical Laboratory Standards (NCCLS) has not explicitly published guidelines for the susceptibility testing of coryneform bacteria. However, clinical laboratories are often asked to carry out susceptibility testing with coryneform bacteria. A pragmatic approach includes disk diffusion testing on Mueller-Hinton agar supplemented with 5% sheep blood. Incubation is at 35°C in ambient air for 24 h, and for very few strains 48 h is required. Exceptions are lipophilic corynebacteria, *R. dentocariosa*, and arcanobacteria, which should be incubated in a 5% CO_2-enriched atmosphere. Interpretation criteria are those established for staphylococci, although other investigators have advocated the use of the criteria for streptococci when assessing the activity of penicillin against *Corynebacterium* spp. (145). The laboratory report should indicate which interpretive criteria have been used.

MICs can be determined by either the E-test or the agar dilution or broth microdilution method. The results of the E-test (AB Biodisk, Solna, Sweden) have been shown to correlate well with those of both the broth microdilution and the agar dilution methods for *Corynebacterium* spp. (83, 149). It should be carried out on Mueller-Hinton agar supplemented with 5% sheep blood. The same medium is used for the agar dilution method (59), but this method is not applicable in the routine laboratory and, rather, should be used in studies with individual antimicrobial agents. The commercial MCN broth microdilution system (Merlin Diagnostics, Bornheim-Hersel, Germany) has proved to be useful for the determination of the MICs for coryneform bacteria (41, 49, 134). However, this method has so far not been correlated with NCCLS methodologies. MICs should be reported without interpretive criteria, but if required by the clinician, the criteria applied should be mentioned and the report should indicate that there are presently no established standards for coryneform bacteria.

For some fastidious coryneform bacteria, e.g., the lipophilic corynebacteria, it might be necessary to supplement the agar with 0.01 to 0.1% Tween 80 in order to achieve optimal growth, but again, no comparative studies on this subject have been published so far.

EVALUATION, INTERPRETATION, AND REPORTING OF RESULTS

The guidelines related to when coryneform bacteria should be identified to the species level (see the section Clinical Significance) are also applicable for evaluating and interpreting culture results; i.e., whenever coryneform bacteria are identified to the species level, the results should be reported.

In the rare case of microscopically suspected *C. diphtheriae* (i.e., a positive Neisser staining result) the physician in charge of the patient should be notified immediately, although culture results and toxin testing results become available only later.

It is evident that repeated isolation of a predominant strain of a coryneform bacterium or a coryneform bacterium growing in pure culture suggests an etiological relationship to the patient's disease. If coryneform bacteria are present in blood cultures, the physician in charge should be notified immediately, and it should be emphasized when reporting that the clinical significance of the coryneform bacteria must be carefully examined by cooperation between the microbiology laboratory and the physician. In our experience, one positive blood culture out of two or three aerobically and anaerobically incubated pairs of blood cultures is hardly ever clinically significant (except in cases of treated endocarditis). Care must be taken in the interpretation of the results for those patients for whom half or more of the blood specimens taken for culture become positive for coryneform bacteria, in particular when lipophilic corynebacteria are cultured, since not all blood samples taken from patients with endocarditis due to lipophilic corynebacteria may eventually become positive (126).

On the other hand, coryneform bacteria should be reported as "normal flora" when they are grown in equal or smaller numbers from nonsterile sites together with other resident flora. It is suggested that the primary isolation plates be retained for at least 72 h before they are discarded in order to have the opportunity to assess the bacterial population retrospectively.

APPENDIX 1
Genus *Gardnerella*

The genus *Gardnerella* does not have a particular phylogenetic relation to any of the established genera described in this chapter. It is remotely related to the genus *Bifidobacterium*. *G. vaginalis* is the only species belonging to the genus *Gardnerella*. Studies on the ultrastructure of the cell wall of *G. vaginalis* have demonstrated that it has a cell wall similar to that of the gram-positive bacteria but that it is much thinner (i.e., there is a smaller peptidoglycan layer) than the cell walls of other gram-positive bacteria (125). Lysine is the diamino acid of the cell wall, and CFAs are similar to those detected in *Actinomyces* spp., *Arcanobacterium* spp., and *Corynebacterium* spp., with $C_{16:0}$ and $C_{18:1\omega9c}$ predominating. The G+C content of 42 to 44 mol% is lower than that of every other genus described in this chapter.

Gram stains show thin gram-variable rods or coccobacilli (Fig. 1f). Catalase is not produced, and cells are nonmotile and have a slow fermentative metabolism.

Natural habitat

G. vaginalis can be found in the anorectal flora of healthy adults of both sexes as well as in that of children (18). It is also part of the endogenous vaginal flora in women of reproductive age (133). The optimal pH for the growth of G. *vaginalis* is between 6 and 7. The organism can also be recovered from the urethras of the male partners of women with bacterial vaginosis (BV) (18).

Clinical significance

G. *vaginalis* is associated with BV and represents one but not the sole cause of this entity (130). Recurrent BV is due to reinfection rather than to relapse (i.e., overgrowth of the previously colonizing biotype) (12). In pregnant women, BV may lead to preterm birth, premature rupture of membranes, and chorioamnionitis (18). G. *vaginalis* may also be recovered from cultures of blood from patients with postpartum or postabortal fevers and may also cause infections in newborns (18). Although it might be recovered from the urethras of males, its disease association in males is questionable.

Collection, transport, and storage of specimens

Vaginal and extravaginal specimens can be collected with cotton-tipped swabs. It is best to take one swab for direct examination and to take another swab for culture if necessary, such as for epidemiologic studies. If culture media cannot be directly inoculated, then the swab should be placed in a transport medium (e.g., Amies) and culture should be done within 24 h.

It is noteworthy that G. *vaginalis* is susceptible to sodium polyanethol sulfonate (SPS), so an SPS-free medium (or an SPS medium supplemented with gelatin) should be used in order to achieve optimal recovery of G. *vaginalis* from blood culture systems whenever G. *vaginalis* is suspected (111).

Isolation and identification

The "gold standard" for the diagnosis of BV is direct examination of vaginal secretions and not the culture of G. *vaginalis* since G. *vaginalis* can also be recovered from healthy women. A bedside test for BV is examination of the vaginal discharge to detect the typical "fishy" trimethylamine odor which is enhanced after alkalinization with 10% KOH. The typical smear of vaginal discharge from BV patients shows "clue cells" (bacteria covering epithelial cell margins) together with mixed flora consisting of large numbers of small gram-negative (predominantly *Prevotella* and *Porphyromonas* spp.) and gram-variable (G. *vaginalis*) rods and coccobacilli, whereas lactobacilli are almost absent. It is recommended that a standardized Gram staining interpretative scheme be used in order to improve the reproducibility of this method (97).

Although not recommended for routine laboratory procedures, the isolation of G. *vaginalis* can support the diagnosis of BV. Vaginal swabs are cultured on Vaginalis agar (see chapter 130 for the preparation) or on human blood bilayer Tween agar (133) and should be semiquantitatively streaked out with a loop. Incubation is at 35 to 37°C in a 5% CO_2-enriched atmosphere or in a candle jar. Beta-hemolysis is observed on human or rabbit blood-containing media but not on SBA. Plates may be checked for the growth of diffuse beta-hemolytic colonies of $<$0.5 mm in diameter after 24 h, but very often G. *vaginalis* is best observed after 48 h. Gram staining of the suspected colonies confirms the diagnosis of G. *vaginalis*.

Eight G. *vaginalis* biotypes had been proposed on the basis of the reactions for lipase, β-galactosidase, and hippurate hydrolysis (106), with biotypes 1, 5, and 6 being the ones that are most commonly found (12). The diagnostic value of these biotypes is questionable since they have not been demonstrated to be associated with certain diseases or certain forms of disease. They may have some value for longitudinal studies, but molecular genetic typing methods are most likely to be superior to biotyping. G. *vaginalis* strains are consistently α-glucosidase and starch hydrolysis positive, but only 90% of all G. *vaginalis* strains hydrolyze hippurate. The API Coryne system identifies G. *vaginalis* well (60). Confirmation of the identification of G. *vaginalis* can also be achieved by antimicrobial agent disk inhibition tests with 50 μg of metronidazole (inhibition present), 5 μg of trimethoprim (inhibition present), and 1 mg of sulfonamide (inhibition absent).

Recently, G. *vaginalis*-like organisms recovered from patients with BV have been demonstrated to represent *Actinomyces turicensis* strains (136). G. *vaginalis* can be differentiated from these organisms in that it has acetic acid as the main end product of glucose fermentation and is unable to produce acid from xylose, whereas A. *turicensis* strains have succinic acid as the end product and produce acid from xylose.

Antimicrobial susceptibilities

Metronidazole is the drug of choice both for local therapy of BV and for systemic therapy of extravaginal infections caused by BV-associated flora. Systemic infections due to G. *vaginalis* alone can be treated with ampicillin or amoxicillin since β-lactamase-producing G. *vaginalis* strains have not been observed so far. Susceptibility testing for G. *vaginalis* is not recommended, and no specific NCCLS guidelines are extant.

REFERENCES

1. **Ahmed, K., K. Kawakami, K. Watanabe, H. Mitsushima, T. Nagatake, and K. Matsumoto.** 1995. *Corynebacterium pseudodiphtheriticum*: a respiratory tract pathogen. *Clin. Infect. Dis.* **20:**41–46.
2. **Aubel, D., F. N. R. Renaud, and J. Freney.** 1997. Genomic diversity of several *Corynebacterium* species identified by amplification of the 16S-23S rRNA gene spacer regions. *Int. J. Syst. Bacterol.* **47:**767–772.
3. **Barnass, S., K. Holland, and S. Tabaqchali.** 1991. Vancomycin-resistant *Corynebacterium* species causing prosthetic valve endocarditis successfully treated with imipenem and ciprofloxacin. *J. Infect.* **22:**161–169.
4. **Barreau, C., F. Bimet, M. Kiredjian, N. Rouillon, and C. Bizet.** 1993. Comparative chemotaxonomic studies of mycolic acid-free coryneform bacteria of human origin. *J. Clin. Microbiol.* **31:**2085–2090.

4a. **Bernard, K.** Unpublished observation.

5. **Bernard, K., M. Bellefeuille, D. G. Hollis, M. I. Daneshvar, and C. W. Moss.** 1994. Cellular fatty acid composition and phenotypic and cultural characterization of CDC fermentative coryneform groups 3 and 5. *J. Clin. Microbiol.* **32:**1217–1222.
6. **Bernard, K., J. Winstanley, C. Munro, and M. Coulthart.** 1997. Characterization of bacteria which closely resemble catalase-negative *Rothia dentocariosa*, isolated from clinical specimens, abstr. PS-14. *In Abstracts of the 65th Annual Conference of the Canadian Association of Clinical Microbiology and Infectious Diseases*. Canadian Association of Clinical Microbiology and Infectious Diseases, Vancouver, British Columbia, Canada.
7. **Bernard, K. A., M. Bellefeuille, and E. P. Ewan.** 1991. Cellular fatty acid composition as an adjunct to the identification of asporogenous, aerobic gram-positive rods. *J. Clin. Microbiol.* **29:**83–89.
8. **Billington, S. J., B. H. Jost, W. A. Cuevas, K. R. Bright, and J. G. Songer.** 1997. The *Arcanobacterium* (*Actinomyces*) *pyogenes* hemolysin, pyolysin, is a novel member of the thiol-activated cytolysin family. *J. Bacteriol.* **179:** 6100–6106.
9. **Bisgard, K. M., C. Vitek, A. Golaz, T. Popovic, and M. Wharton.** Diphtheria. Centers for Disease Control and Prevention, Atlanta, Ga. Available from http://www.cdc.gov/nip/manual/diphther/diphther.htm.
10. **Björkroth, J., H. Korkeala, and G. Funke.** rRNA gene restriction fragment length polymorphism as an identification tool for *Corynebacterium* spp. Submitted for publication.
11. **Brandenburg, A. H., A. van Belkum, C. van Pelt, H. A. Bruining, J. W. Mouton, and H. A. Verbrugh.** 1996. Patient-to-patient spread of a single strain of *Corynebacterium striatum* causing infections in a surgical intensive care unit. *J. Clin. Microbiol.* **34:**2089–2094.
12. **Briselden, A. M., and S. L. Hillier.** 1990. Longitudinal

study of the biotypes of *Gardnerella vaginalis*. *J. Clin. Microbiol.* **28:**2761–2764.

13. **Cai, J., and M. D. Collins.** 1994. Phylogenetic analysis of species of the *meso*-diaminopimelic acid-containing genera *Brevibacterium* and *Dermabacter*. *Int. J. Syst. Bacteriol.* **44:**583–585.
14. **Carlotti, A., and G. Funke.** 1994. Rapid distinction of *Brevibacterium* species by restriction analysis of rDNA generated by polymerase chain reaction. *Syst. Appl. Microbiol.* **17:**380–386.
15. **Carlson, P., S. Kontiainen, and O. V. Renkonen.** 1994. Antimicrobial susceptibility of *Arcanobacterium haemolyticum*. *Antimicrob. Agents Chemother.* **38:**142–143.
16. **Carlson, P., K. Lounatmaa, and S. Kontiainen.** 1994. Biotypes of *Arcanobacterium haemolyticum*. *J. Clin. Microbiol.* **32:**1654–1657.
17. **Cartuyvels, R., J. Verhaegen, W. E. Peetermans, and G. Wauters.** 1996. Report of a case of *Dermabacter hominis* bacteremia. *Med. Microbiol. Lett.* **5:**418–425.
18. **Catlin, B. W.** 1992. *Gardnerella vaginalis*: characteristics, clinical considerations, and controversies. *Clin. Microbiol. Rev.* **5:**213–237.
19. **Cianciotto, N. P., and N. B. Groman.** 1997. Characterization of bacteriophages from *tox*-containing, non-toxigenic isolates of *Corynebacterium diphtheriae*. *Microb. Pathog.* **22:**343–351.
20. **Collins, M. D., K. A. Bernard, R. A. Hutson, B. Sjödén, and E. Falsen.** *Corynebacterium sundsvallense* sp. nov., from human clinical specimens. Submitted for publication.
21. **Collins, M. D., R. A. Burton, and D. Jones.** 1988. *Corynebacterium amycolatum* sp. nov. a new mycolic acid-less *Corynebacterium* species from human skin. *FEMS Microbiol. Lett.* **49:**349–352.
22. **Collins, M. D., and C. S. Cummins.** 1986. Genus *Corynebacterium*, p. 1266–1276. *In* P. H. A. Sneath, N. S. Mair, M. E. Sharpe, and J. G. Holt (ed.), *Bergey's Manual of Systematic Bacteriology*, vol. 2. The Williams & Wilkins Co., Baltimore, Md.
23. **Collins, M. D., E. Falsen, E. Akervall, B. Sjödén, and N. Alvarez.** Characterization of novel non-mycolic acid-containing *Corynebacterium*: description of *Corynebacterium kroppenstedtii* sp. nov. *Int. J. Syst. Bacteriol.*, in press.
24. **Collins, M. D., M. Goodfellow, and D. E. Minnikin.** 1982. A survey of the structures of mycolic acids in *Corynebacterium* and related taxa. *J. Gen. Microbiol.* **128:** 129–149.
25. **Collins, M. D., B. M. Lund, J. A. E. Farrow, and K. H. Schleifer.** 1983. Chemotaxonomic study of an alkalophilic bacterium, *Exiguobacterium aurantiacum* gen. nov., sp. nov. *J. Gen. Microbiol.* **129:**2037–2042.
26. **Coyle, M. B., R. B. Leonard, D. J. Nowowiejski, A. Malekniazi, and D. J. Finn.** 1993. Evidence of multiple taxa within commercially available reference strains of *Corynebacterium xerosis*. *J. Clin. Microbiol.* **31:** 1788–1793.
27. **Coyle, M. B., B. H. Minshew, J. A. Bland, and P. C. Hsu.** 1979. Erythromycin and clindamycin resistance in *Corynebacterium diphtheriae* from skin lesions. *Antimicrob. Agents Chemother.* **16:**525–527.
28. **Coyle, M. B., D. J. Nowowiejski, J. Q. Russell, and N. B. Groman.** 1993. Laboratory review of reference strains of *Corynebacterium diphtheriae* indicated mistyped *intermedius* strains. *J. Clin. Microbiol.* **31:**3060–3062.
29. **Cuevas, W., and G. Songer.** 1993. *Arcanobacterium haemolyticum* phospholipase D is genetically and functionally similar to *Corynebacterium pseudotuberculosis* phospholipase D. *Infect. Immun.* **61:**4310–4316.
30. **de Briel, D., F. Couderc, P. Riegel, F. Jehl, and R. Minck.** 1992. High-performance liquid chromatography of corynomycolic acids as a tool in identification of *Corynebacterium* species and related organisms. *J. Clin. Microbiol.* **30:**1407–1417.
31. **De Zoysa, A., A. Efstratiou, R. C. George, M. Jahkala, J. Vuopio-Varkila, S. Deshevoi, G. Tseneva, and Y. Rikushin.** 1995. Molecular epidemiology of *Corynebacterium diphtheriae* from northwestern Russia and surrounding countries studied by using ribotyping and pulsed-field gel electrophoresis. *J. Clin. Microbiol.* **33:**1080–1083.
32. **Efstratiou, A., and P. A. C. Maple.** 1994. *Manual for the Laboratory Diagnosis of Diphtheria*. Document ICP/EPI 038 (C). The Expanded Programme on Immunization in the European Region of WHO, World Health Organization Europe, Copenhagen, Denmark.
33. **Engler, K., and A. Efstratiou.** 1997. A rapid ELISA for the confirmation of diphtheria caused by toxigenic *Corynebacterium* spp., poster 1522. *In 8th European Congress of Clinical Microbiology and Infectious Diseases*, Lausanne, Switzerland.
34. **Engler, K., T. Glushkevich, I. K. Mazurova, R. C. George, and A. Efstratiou.** 1997. A modified Elek test for detection of toxigenic corynebacteria in the diagnostic laboratory. *J. Clin. Microbiol.* **35:**495–498.
35. **Esteban, J., J. Bueno, J. Perez-Santonja, and F. Soriano.** 1996. Endophthalmitis involving an *Arthrobacter*-like organism following intraocular lens implantation. *Clin. Infect. Dis.* **23:**1180–1181.
36. **Farrow, J. A. E., S. Wallbanks, and M. D. Collins.** 1994. Phylogenetic interrelationships of round-spore-forming bacilli containing cell walls based on lysine and the non-spore-forming genera *Caryophanon*, *Exiguobacterium*, *Kurthia*, and *Planococcus*. *Int. J. Syst. Bacteriol.* **44:**74–82.
37. **Früh, M., A. von Graevenitz, and G. Funke.** 1998. Use of second-line biochemical and susceptibility tests for the differential diagnosis of coryneform bacteria. *Clin. Microbiol. Infect.* **4:**332–338.

37a. **Funke, G.** Unpublished observations and data.

38. **Funke, G., M. Aravena-Roman, N. Weiss, and P. A. Lawson.** Coryneform bacteria very rarely encountered in clinical specimens: description of *Curtobacterium* spp. isolated from human clinical material. Submitted for publication.
39. **Funke, G., K. A. Bernard, C. Bucher, G. E. Pfyffer, and M. D. Collins.** 1995. *Corynebacterium glucuronolyticum* sp. nov. isolated from male patients with genitourinary infections. *Med. Microbiol. Lett.* **4:**204–215.
40. **Funke, G., and A. Carlotti.** 1994. Differentiation of *Brevibacterium* spp. encountered in clinical specimens. *J. Clin. Microbiol.* **32:**1729–1732.
41. **Funke, G., A. Efstratiou, D. Kuklinska, R. A. Hutson, A. de Zoysa, K. H. Engler, and M. D. Collins.** 1997. *Corynebacterium imitans* sp. nov. isolated from patients with suspected diphtheria. *J. Clin. Microbiol.* **35:** 1978–1983.
42. **Funke, G., E. Falsen, and C. Barreau.** 1995. Primary identification of *Microbacterium* spp. encountered in clinical specimens as CDC coryneform group A-4 and A-5 bacteria. *J. Clin. Microbiol.* **33:**188–192.
43. **Funke, G., G. Haase, N. Schnitzler, N. Schrage, and R. R. Reinert.** 1997. Endophthalmitis due to *Microbacterium* species: case report and review of *Microbacterium* infections. *Clin. Infect. Dis.* **24:**713–716.
44. **Funke, G., L. Hoyle, and M. D. Collins.** *Corynebacterium sanguinis* sp. nov., isolated from human blood cultures. Submitted for publication.
45. **Funke, G., R. A. Hutson, K. A. Bernard, G. E. Pfyffer, G. Wauters, and M. D. Collins.** 1996. Isolation of *Arthrobacter* spp. from clinical specimens and description of

Arthrobacter cumminsii sp. nov. and *Arthrobacter woluwensis* sp. nov. *J. Clin. Microbiol.* **34:**2356–2363.

46. **Funke, G., R. A. Hutson, M. Hilleringmann, W. R. Heizmann, and M. D. Collins.** 1997. *Corynebacterium lipophiloflavum* sp. nov. isolated from a patient with bacterial vaginosis. *FEMS Microbiol. Lett.* **150:**219–224.
47. **Funke, G., P. A. Lawson, K. A. Bernard, and M. D. Collins.** 1996. Most *Corynebacterium xerosis* strains identified in the routine clinical laboratory correspond to *Corynebacterium amycolatum*. *J. Clin. Microbiol.* **34:** 1124–1128.
48. **Funke, G., P. A. Lawson, and M. D. Collins.** 1995. Heterogeneity within Centers for Disease Control and Prevention coryneform group ANF-1-like bacteria and description of *Corynebacterium auris* sp. nov. *Int. J. Syst. Bacteriol.* **45:**735–739.
49. **Funke, G., P. A. Lawson, and M. D. Collins.** 1997. *Corynebacterium mucifaciens* sp. nov., an unusual species from human clinical material. *Int. J. Syst. Bacteriol.* **47:** 952–957.
50. **Funke, G., P. A. Lawson, and M. D. Collins.** 1998. *Corynebacterium riegelii* sp. nov., an unusual species isolated from female patients with urinary tract infections. *J. Clin. Microbiol.* **36:**624–627.
51. **Funke, G., P. A. Lawson, F. S. Nolte, N. Weiss, and M. D. Collins.** 1998. *Aureobacterium resistens* sp. nov. exhibiting vancomycin resistance and teicoplanin susceptibility. *FEMS Microbiol. Lett.* **158:**89–93.
52. **Funke, G., T. Linder, D. Holzmann, and D. Nadal.** *Turicella otitidis* and *Corynebacterium auris* are not causing otitis media with effusion in children. Submitted for publication.
53. **Funke, G., C. R. Osorio, R. Frei, P. Riegel, and M. D. Collins.** *Corynebacterium confusum* sp. nov., isolated from human clinical specimens. *Int. J. Syst. Bacteriol.*, in press.
54. **Funke, G., M. Pagano-Niederer, B. Sjödén, and E. Falsen.** 1998. Characteristics of *Arthrobacter cumminsii*, the most frequently encountered *Arthrobacter* species in human clinical specimens. *J. Clin. Microbiol.* **36:** 1539–1543.
55. **Funke, G., C. Pascual Ramos, and M. D. Collins.** 1995. Identification of some clinical strains of CDC coryneform group A-3 and group A-4 bacteria as *Cellulomonas* species and proposal of *Cellulomonas hominis* sp. nov. for some group A-3 strains. *J. Clin. Microbiol.* **33:**2091–2097.
56. **Funke, G., C. Pascual Ramos, and M. D. Collins.** 1997. *Corynebacterium coyleae* sp. nov., isolated from human clinical specimens. *Int. J. Syst. Bacteriol.* **47:**92–96.
57. **Funke, G., C. Pascual Ramos, J. Fernandez-Garayzabal, N. Weiss, and M. D. Collins.** 1995. Description of human-derived Centers for Disease Control coryneform group 2 bacteria as *Actinomyces bernardiae* sp. nov. *Int. J. Syst. Bacteriol.* **45:**57–60.
58. **Funke, G., K. Peters, and M. Aravena-Roman.** 1998. Evaluation of the RapID CB Plus system for identification of coryneform bacteria and *Listeria* spp. *J. Clin. Microbiol.* **36:**2439–2442.
59. **Funke, G., V. Pünter, and A. von Graevenitz.** 1996. Antimicrobial susceptibility patterns of some recently established coryneform bacteria. *Antimicrob. Agents Chemother.* **40:**2874–2878.
60. **Funke, G., F. N. R. Renaud, J. Freney, and P. Riegel.** 1997. Multicenter evaluation of the updated and extended API (RAPID) Coryne database 2.0. *J. Clin. Microbiol.* **35:**3122–3126.
61. **Funke, G., S. Stubbs, G. E. Pfyffer, M. Marchiani, and M. D. Collins.** 1994. Characteristics of CDC group 3 and group 5 coryneform bacteria isolated from clinical specimens and assignment to the genus *Dermabacter*. *J. Clin. Microbiol.* **32:**1223–1228.
62. **Funke, G., S. Stubbs, G. E. Pfyffer, M. Marchiani, and M. D. Collins.** 1994. *Turicella otitidis* gen. nov., sp. nov., a coryneform bacterium isolated from patients with otitis media. *Int. J. Syst. Bacteriol.* **44:**270–273.
63. **Funke, G., A. von Graevenitz, J. E. Clarridge III, and K. A. Bernard.** 1997. Clinical microbiology of coryneform bacteria. *Clin. Microbiol. Rev.* **10:**125–159.
64. **Funke, G., A. von Graevenitz, and N. Weiss.** 1994. Primary identification of *Aureobacterium* spp. isolated from clinical specimens as "*Corynebacterium aquaticum*." *J. Clin. Microbiol.* **32:**2686–2691.
65. **Gruner, E., A. G. Steigerwalt, D. G. Hollis, R. S. Weyant, R. E. Weaver, C. W. Moss, M. Daneshvar, J. M. Brown, and D. J. Brenner.** 1994. Human infections caused by *Brevibacterium casei*, formerly CDC groups B-1 and B-3. *J. Clin. Microbiol.* **32:**1511–1518.
66. **Harrington, R. D., C. G. Lewis, J. Aslanzadeh, P. Stelmach, and A. E. Woolfrey.** 1996. *Oerskovia xanthineolytica* infection of a prosthetic joint: case report and review. *J. Clin. Microbiol.* **34:**1821–1824.
67. **Hauser, D., M. R. Popoff, M. Kiredjian, P. Boquet, and F. Bimet.** 1993. Polymerase chain assay for diagnosis of potentially toxinogenic *Corynebacterium diphtheriae* strains: correlation with ADP-ribosylation activity assay. *J. Clin. Microbiol.* **31:**2720–2723.
68. **Hollis, D. G.** 1992. Potential new CDC coryneform groups. Handout at the 92nd General Meeting of the American Society for Microbiology 1992. American Society for Microbiology, Washington, D.C.
69. **Hollis, D. G., and R. E. Weaver.** 1981. *Gram-Positive Organisms: A Guide to Identification*. Special Bacteriology Section, Centers for Disease Control, Atlanta, Ga.
70. **Hou, X. G., Y. Kawamura, F. Sultana, K. Hirose, M. Miyake, Y. Otsuka, S. Misawa, T. Oguri, H. Yamamoto, and T. Ezaki.** 1997. Genetic identification of members of the genus *Corynebacterium* at genus and species levels with 16S rDNA-targeted probes. *Microbiol. Immunol.* **41:** 453–460.
71. **Hudspeth, M. K., S. H. Gerardo, D. M. Citron, and E. J. C. Goldstein.** 1998. Evaluation of the RapID CB Plus system for identification of *Corynebacterium* species and other gram-positive rods. *J. Clin. Microbiol.* **36:**543–547.
72. **Izurieta, H. S., P. M. Strebel, T. Youngblood, D. G. Hollis, and T. Popovic.** 1997. Exudative pharyngitis possibly due to *Corynebacterium pseudodiphtheriticum*, a new challenge in the differential diagnosis of diphtheria. *Emerg. Infect. Dis.* **3:**65–68.
73. **Jones, D., and M. D. Collins.** 1988. Taxonomic studies on some human cutaneous coryneform bacteria: description of *Dermabacter hominis* gen. nov. sp. nov. *FEMS Microbiol. Lett.* **51:**51–56.
74. **Koch, C., F. A. Rainey, and E. Stackebrandt.** 1994. 16S rDNA studies on members of *Arthrobacter* and *Micrococcus*: an aid for their future taxonomic restructuring. *FEMS Microbiol. Lett.* **123:**167–172.
75. **Kronvall, G., M. Lannér-Sjöberg, L. V. von Stedingk, H. S. Hanson, B. Pettersson, and E. Falsen.** Whole-cell protein and partial 16S rRNA gene sequence analysis suggest the existence of a second *Rothia* species. *Clin. Microbiol. Infect.*, in press.
76. **Lagrou, K., J. Verhaegen, M. Janssens, G. Wauters, and L. Verbist.** 1998. Prospective study of catalase-positive coryneform organisms in clinical specimens: identification, clinical relevance, and antibiotic susceptibility. *Diagn. Microbiol. Infect. Dis.* **30:**7–15.
77. **Larkin, J. A., R. G. Shashy, and C. A. Gonzalez.** 1997. Difficulties in differentiating a rapidly growing *Mycobacte-*

rium species from diphtheroids in an immunocompromised patient. *Clin. Microbiol. Newsl.* **19:**109–111.

78. **Leonard, R. B., D. J. Nowowiejski, J. J. Warren, D. J. Finn, and M. B. Coyle.** 1994. Molecular evidence of person-to-person transmission of a pigmented strain of *Corynebacterium striatum* in intensive care units. *J. Clin. Microbiol.* **32:**164–169.
79. **Lindenmann, K., A. von Graevenitz, and G. Funke.** 1995. Evaluation of the Biolog system for the identification of asporogenous, aerobic gram-positive rods. *Med. Microbiol. Lett.* **4:**287–296.
80. **Mackenzie, A., L. A. Fuite, F. T. H. Chan, J. King, U. Allen, N. MacDonald, and F. Diaz-Mitoma.** 1995. Incidence and pathogenicity of *Arcanobacterium haemolyticum* during a 2-year study in Ottawa. *Clin. Infect. Dis.* **21:**177–181.
81. **Manzella, J. P., J. A. Kellogg, and K. S. Parsey.** 1995. *Corynebacterium pseudodiphtheriticum*: a respiratory tract pathogen in adults. *Clin. Infect. Dis.* **20:**37–40.
82. **Martinetti-Lucchini, G., E. Gruner, and M. Altwegg.** 1992. Rapid detection of diphtheria toxin by the polymerase chain reaction. *Med. Microbiol. Lett.* **1:**276–283.
83. **Martinez-Martinez, L., M. C. Ortega, and A. I. Suarez.** 1995. Comparison of E-test with broth microdilution and disk diffusion for susceptibility testing of coryneform bacteria. *J. Clin. Microbiol.* **33:**1318–1321.
84. **Martinez-Martinez, L., A. Pascual, K. Bernard, and A. I. Suarez.** 1996. Antimicrobial susceptibility pattern of *Corynebacterium striatum*. *Antimicrob. Agents Chemother.* **40:**2671–2672.
85. **Martinez-Martinez, L., A. I. Suarez, J. Rodriguez-Bano, K. Bernard, and M. A. Muniain.** 1997. Clinical significance of *Corynebacterium striatum* isolated from human samples. *Clin. Microbiol. Infect.* **6:**634–639.
86. **Martinez-Martinez, L., A. I. Suarez, J. Winstanley, M. C. Ortega, and K. Bernard.** 1995. Phenotypic characteristics of 31 strains of *Corynebacterium striatum* isolated from clinical samples. *J. Clin. Microbiol.* **33:**2458–2461.
87. **McBride, M. E., K. M. Ellner, H. S. Black, J. E. Clarridge, and J. E. Wolf.** 1993. A new *Brevibacterium* sp. isolated from infected genital hair of patients with white piedra. *J. Med. Microbiol.* **39:**255–261.
88. **McNamara, P. J., W. A. Cuevas, and J. G. Songer.** 1995. Toxic phospholipases D of *Corynebacterium pseudotuberculosis*, *C. ulcerans* and *Arcanobacterium haemolyticum*: cloning and sequence homology. *Gene* **156:**113–118.
89. **Mikhailovich, V. M., V. G. Melnikov, I. K. Mazurova, I. K. Wachsmuth, J. D. Wenger, M. Wharton, H. Nakao, and T. Popovic.** 1995. Application of PCR for detection of toxigenic *Corynebacterium diphtheriae* strains isolated during the Russian diphtheria epidemic, 1990 through 1994. *J. Clin. Microbiol.* **33:**3061–3063.
90. **Nakao, H., I. K. Mazurova, T. Glushkevich, and T. Popovic.** 1997. Analysis of heterogeneity of *Corynebacterium diphtheriae* toxin gene, *tox*, and its regulatory element, *dtxR*, by direct sequencing. *Res. Microbiol.* **148:**45–54.
91. **Nakao, H., and T. Popovic.** 1997. Development of a direct PCR assay for detection of the diphtheria toxin gene. *J. Clin. Microbiol.* **35:**1651–1655.
92. **Nakao, H., and T. Popovic.** 1998. Development of a rapid ribotyping method for *Corynebacterium diphtheriae* by using PCR single-strand conformation polymorphism: comparison with standard ribotyping. *J. Microbiol. Methods* **31:**127–134.
93. **Nakao, H., J. M. Pruckler, I. K. Mazurova, O. V. Narvskaia, T. Gluskhevich, V. F. Marijevski, A. N. Kravetz, B. S. Fields, I. K. Wachsmuth, and T. Popovic.** 1996. Heterogeneity of diphtheria toxin gene, *tox*, and its regulatory element, *dtxR*, in *Corynebacterium diphtheriae* strains causing epidemic diphtheria in Russia and Ukraine. *J. Clin. Microbiol.* **34:**1711–1716.
94. **Neubauer, M., J. Sourek, M. Ryc, J. Bohacek, M. Mara, and J. Mnukova.** 1991. *Corynebacterium accolens* sp. nov., a gram-positive rod exhibiting satellitism, from clinical material. *Syst. Appl. Microbiol.* **14:**46–51.
95. **Nieto, E., J. Zapardiel, and F. Soriano.** 1996. Environmental contamination by *Corynebacterium urealyticum* in a teaching hospital. *J. Hosp. Infect.* **32:**78–79.
96. **Nolte, F. S., K. E. Arnold, H. Sweat, E. F. Winton, and G. Funke.** 1996. Vancomycin-resistant *Aureobacterium* species cellulitis and bacteremia in a patient with acute myelogenous leukemia. *J. Clin. Microbiol.* **34:**1992–1994.
97. **Nugent, R. P., M. A. Krohn, and S. L. Hillier.** 1991. Reliability of diagnosing bacterial vaginosis is improved by a standardized method of Gram stain interpretation. *J. Clin. Microbiol.* **29:**297–301.
98. **Pallen, M. J.** 1991. Rapid screening for toxigenic *Corynebacterium diphtheriae* by polymerase chain reaction. *J. Clin. Pathol.* **44:**1025–1026.
99. **Pascual, C., M. D. Collins, G. Funke, and D. G. Pitcher.** 1996. Phenotypic and genotypic characterisation of two *Brevibacterium* strains from the human ear: description of *Brevibacterium otitidis* sp. nov. *Med. Microbiol. Lett.* **5:** 113–123.
100. **Pascual, C., P. A. Lawson, J. A. E. Farrow, M. Navarro Gimenez, and M. D. Collins.** 1995. Phylogenetic analysis of the genus *Corynebacterium* based on 16S rRNA gene sequences. *Int. J. Syst. Bacteriol.* **45:**724–728.
101. **Pascual Ramos, C., G. Foster, and M. D. Collins.** 1997. Phylogenetic analysis of the genus *Actinomyces* based on 16S rRNA gene sequences: description of *Arcanobacterium phocae* sp. nov., *Arcanobacterium bernardiae* comb. nov., and *Arcanobacterium pyogenes* comb. nov. *Int. J. Syst. Bacteriol.* **47:**46–53.
102. **Patey, O., F. Bimet, J. P. Emond, E. Estrangin, P. Riegel, B. Halioua, S. Dellion, and M. Kiredjian.** 1995. Antibiotic susceptibilities of 38 non-toxigenic strains of *Corynebacterium diphtheriae*. *J. Antimicrob. Chemother.* **36:** 1108–1110.
103. **Patey, O., F. Bimet, P. Riegel, B. Halioua, J. P. Emond, E. Estrangin, S. Dellion, J. M. Alonso, M. Kiredjian, A. Dublanchet, C. Lafaix, and the Coryne Study Group.** 1997. Clinical and molecular study of *Corynebacterium diphtheriae* systemic infections in France. *J. Clin. Microbiol.* **35:**441–445.
104. **Peel, M. M., G. G. Palmer, A. M. Stacpoole, and T. G. Kerr.** 1997. Human lymphadenitis due to *Corynebacterium pseudotuberculosis*: report of ten cases from Australia and review. *Clin. Infect. Dis.* **24:**185–191.
105. **Petit, P. L. C., J. W. Bok, J. Thompson, A. G. M. Buiting, and M. B. Coyle.** 1994. Native-valve endocarditis due to CDC coryneform group ANF-3: report of a case and review of corynebacterial endocarditis. *Clin. Infect. Dis.* **19:**897–901.
106. **Piot, P., E. van Dyck, M. Peeters, J. Hale, P. A. Totten, and K. K. Holmes.** 1984. Biotypes of *Gardnerella vaginalis*. *J. Clin. Microbiol.* **20:**677–679.
107. **Popovic, T., S. Y. Kombarova, M. W. Reeves, H. Nakao, I. K. Mazurova, M. Wharton, I. K. Wachsmuth, and J. D. Wenger.** 1996. Molecular epidemiology of diphtheria in Russia, 1985–1994. *J. Infect. Dis.* **174:** 1064–1072.
108. **Power, E. G. M., Y. H. Abdulla, H. G. Talsania, W. Spice, S. Aathithan, and G. L. French.** 1995. *van*A genes in vancomycin-resistant clinical isolates of *Oerskovia turbata* and *Arcanobacterium* (*Corynebacterium*) *haemolyticum*. *J. Antimicrob Chemother.* **36:**595–606.
109. **Rainey, F., N. Weiss, H. Prauser, and E. Stackebrandt.**

1994. Further evidence for the phylogenetic coherence of actinomycetes with group B-peptidoglycan and evidence for the phylogenetic intermixing of the genera *Microbacterium* and *Aureobacterium* as determined by 16S rDNA analysis. *FEMS Microbiol. Lett.* **118:**135–140.

110. **Rassoulian Barrett, S. L., L. C. Carlson, B. T. Cookson, K. A. Bernard, and M. B. Coyle.** Molecular evidence of diversity within reference strains of *Corynebacterium matruchotii*. Submitted for publication.
111. **Reimer, L. G., and L. B. Reller.** 1985. Effect of sodium polyanetholesulfonate and gelatin on the recovery of *Gardnerella vaginalis* from blood culture media. *J. Clin. Microbiol.* **21:**686–688.
112. **Reinhardt, D. J., A. Lee, and T. Popovic.** 1998. Antitoxin-in-membrane and antitoxin-in-well assays for detection of toxigenic *Corynebacterium diphtheriae*. *J. Clin. Microbiol.* **36:**207–210.
113. **Renaud, F. N. R., A. Grégory, C. Barreau, D. Aubel, and J. Freney.** 1996. Identification of *Turicella otitidis* isolated from a patient with otorrhea associated with surgery: differentiation from *Corynebacterium afermentans* and *Corynebacterium auris*. *J. Clin. Microbiol.* **34:**2625–2627.
114. **Riegel, P., D. de Briel, G. Prévost, F. Jehl, and H. Monteil.** 1994. Genomic diversity among *Corynebacterium jeikeium* strains and comparison with biochemical characteristics. *J. Clin. Microbiol.* **32:**1860–1865.
115. **Riegel, P., D. de Briel, G. Prévost, F. Jehl, H. Monteil, and R. Minck.** 1993. Taxonomic study of *Corynebacterium* group ANF-1 strains: proposal of *Corynebacterium afermentans* sp. nov. containing the subspecies *C. afermentans* subsp. *afermentans* subsp. nov. and *C. afermentans* subsp. *lipophilum* subsp. nov. *Int. J. Syst. Bacteriol.* **43:** 287–292.
116. **Riegel, P., R. Heller, G. Prevost, F. Jehl, and H. Monteil.** 1997. *Corynebacterium durum* sp. nov., from human clinical specimens. *Int. J. Syst. Bacteriol.* **47:** 1107–1111.
117. **Riegel, P., R. Ruimy, R. Christen, and H. Monteil.** 1996. Species identities and antimicrobial susceptibilities of corynebacteria isolated from various clinical sources. *Eur. J. Clin. Microbiol. Infect. Dis.* **15:**657–662.
118. **Riegel, P., R. Ruimy, D. de Briel, G. Prévost, F. Jehl, F. Bimet, R. Christen, and H. Monteil.** 1995. *Corynebacterium argentoratense* sp. nov., from human throat. *Int. J. Syst. Bacteriol.* **45:**533–537.
119. **Riegel, P., R. Ruimy, D. de Briel, G. Prévost, F. Jehl, F. Bimet, R. Christen, and H. Monteil.** 1995. *Corynebacterium seminale* sp. nov., a new species associated with genital infections in male patients. *J. Clin. Microbiol.* **33:** 2244–2249.
120. **Riegel, P., R. Ruimy, D. de Briel, G. Prévost, F. Jehl, R. Christen, and H. Monteil.** 1995. Genomic diversity and phylogenetic relationships among lipid-requiring diphtheroids from humans and characterization of *Corynebacterium macginleyi* sp. nov. *Int. J. Syst. Bacteriol.* **45:** 128–133.
121. **Riegel, P., R. Ruimy, D. de Briel, G. Prévost, F. Jehl, R. Christen, and H. Monteil.** 1995. Taxonomy of *Corynebacterium diphtheriae* and related taxa, with recognition of *Corynebacterium ulcerans* sp. nov., nom. rev. *FEMS Microbiol. Lett.* **126:**271–276.
122. **Riegel, P., R. Ruimy, F. N. R. Renaud, J. Freney, G. Prevost, F. Jehl, R. Christen, and H. Monteil.** 1997. *Corynebacterium singulare* sp. nov., a new species for urease-positive strains related to *Corynebacterium minutissimum*. *Int. J. Syst. Bacteriol.* **47:**1092–1096.
123. **Roberts, M. C., R. B. Leonard, R. Briselden, F. D. Schoenknecht, and M. B. Coyle.** 1992. Characterization of antibiotic resistant *Corynebacterium striatum* strains. *J. Antimicrob. Chemother.* **30:**463–474.
124. **Ruimy, R., P. Riegel, P. Boiron, H. Monteil, and R. Christen.** 1995. Phylogeny of the genus *Corynebacterium* deduced from analyses of small-subunit ribosomal DNA sequences. *Int. J. Syst. Bacteriol.* **45:**740–746.
125. **Sadhu, K., P. A. G. Domingue, A. W. Chow, J. Nelligan, N. Cheng, and J. W. Costerton.** 1989. *Gardnerella vaginalis* has a gram-positive cell-wall ultrastructure and lacks classical cell-wall lipopolysaccharide. *J. Med. Microbiol.* **29:**229–235.
126. **Sewell, D. L., M. B. Coyle, and G. Funke.** 1995. Prosthetic valve endocarditis caused by *Corynebacterium afermentans* subsp. *lipophilum* (CDC coryneform group ANF-1). *J. Clin. Microbiol.* **33:**759–761.
127. **Sjödén, B., G. Funke, A. Izquierdo, E. Akervall, and M. D. Collins.** 1998. Description of some coryneform bacteria isolated from human clinical specimens as *Corynebacterium falsenii* sp. nov. *Int. J. Syst. Bacteriol.* **48:** 69–74.
128. **Soriano, F., J. M. Aguado, C. Ponte, R. Fernandez-Roblas, and J. L. Rodriguez-Tudela.** 1990. Urinary tract infection caused by *Corynebacterium* group D2: report of 82 cases and review. *Rev. Infect. Dis.* **12:**1019–1034.
129. **Soriano, F., J. Zapardiel, and E. Nieto.** 1995. Antimicrobial susceptibilities of *Corynebacterium* species and other non-spore-forming gram-positive bacilli to 18 antimicrobial agents. *Antimicrob. Agents Chemother.* **39:**208–214.
130. **Spiegel, C. A.** 1991. Bacterial vaginosis. *Clin. Microbiol. Rev.* **4:**485–502.
131. **Sutcliffe, I. C., G. P. Manfio, K. P. Schaal, and M. Goodfellow.** 1997. An investigation of the intra-generic structure of *Rothia* by pyrolysis mass spectrometry. *Zentralbl. Bakteriol. Parasitenkd. Infektionskr. Hyg. Abt. 1 Orig.* **285:**204–211.
132. **Takeuchi, M., and A. Yokota.** 1994. Phylogenetic analysis of the genus *Microbacterium* based on 16S rRNA gene sequences. *FEMS Microbiol. Lett.* **124:**11–16.
133. **Totten, P. A., R. Amsel, J. Hale, P. Piot, and K. K. Holmes.** 1982. Selective differential human blood bilayer media for isolation of *Gardnerella* (*Haemophilus*) *vaginalis*. *J. Clin. Microbiol.* **15:**141–147.
134. **Troxler, R., A. von Graevenitz, and G. Funke.** Antimicrobial susceptibility patterns of infrequently isolated coryneform bacteria. Submitted for publication.
135. **Vaneechoutte, M., P. Riegel, D. de Briel, H. Monteil, G. Verschraegen, A. De Rouck, and G. Claeys.** 1995. Evaluation of the applicability of amplified rDNA-restriction analysis (ARDRA) to identification of species of the genus *Corynebacterium*. *Res. Microbiol.* **146:**633–641.
136. **van Esbroeck, M., P. Vandamme, E. Falsen, M. Vancanneyt, E. Moore, B. Pot, F. Gavini, K. Kersters, and H. Goossens.** 1996. Polyphasic approach to the classification and identification of *Gardnerella vaginalis* and unidentified *Gardnerella vaginalis*-like coryneforms present in bacterial vaginosis. *Int. J. Syst. Bacteriol.* **46:**675–682.
137. **von Graevenitz, A., L. Frommelt, V. Pünter-Streit, and G. Funke.** 1998. Diversity of coryneforms found in infections following prosthetic joint insertion and open fractures. *Infection* **26:**36–38.
138. **von Graevenitz, A., and G. Funke.** 1996. An identification scheme for rapidly and aerobically growing gram-positive rods. *Zentralbl. Bakteriol. Parasitenkd. Infektionskr. Hyg. Abt. 1 Orig.* **284:**246–254.
139. **von Graevenitz, A., and T. Krech.** 1992. The genus *Corynebacterium*—medical, p. 1172–1187. *In* A. Balows, H. G. Trüper, M. Dworkin, W. Harder, and K. H. Schleifer (ed.), *The Prokaryotes*, vol. 2. Springer-Verlag, New York, N.Y.

140. **von Graevenitz, A., V. Pünter, E. Gruner, G. E. Pfyffer, and G. Funke.** 1994. Identification of coryneform and other gram-positive rods with several methods. *APMIS* **102:**381–389.

141. **von Graevenitz, A., V. Pünter-Streit, P. Riegel, and G. Funke.** 1998. Coryneform bacteria in throat cultures of healthy individuals. *J. Clin. Microbiol.* **36:**2087–2088.

142. **Wauters, G., A. Driessen, E. Ageron, M. Janssens, and P. A. D. Grimont.** 1996. Propionic acid-producing strains previously designated as *Corynebacterium xerosis*, *C. minutissimum*, *C. striatum*, and CDC group I2 and group F2 coryneforms belong to the species *Corynebacterium amycolatum*. *Int. J. Syst. Bacteriol.* **46:**653–657.

143. **Wauters, G., B. van Bosterhaut, M. Janssens, and J. Verhaegen.** 1998. Identification of *Corynebacterium amycolatum* and other nonlipophilic fermentative corynebacteria of human origin. *J. Clin. Microbiol.* **36:**1430–1432.

144. **Weiss, K., A. C. Labbé, and M. Laverdière.** 1996. *Corynebacterium striatum* meningitis: case report and review of an increasingly important *Corynebacterium* species. *Clin. Infect. Dis.* **23:**1246–1248.

145. **Weiss, K., M. Laverdière, and R. Rivest.** 1996. Comparison of antimicrobial susceptibilities of *Corynebacterium* species by broth microdilution and disk diffusion methods. *Antimicrob. Agents Chemother.* **40:**930–933.

146. **Yagüe, G., M. Segovia, and P. L. Valero-Guillén.** 1997. Acyl phosphatidylglycerol: a major phospholipid of *Corynebacterium amycolatum*. *FEMS Microbiol. Lett.* **151:**125–130.

147. **Yokota, A., M. Takeuchi, T. Sakane, and N. Weiss.** 1993. Proposal of six new species in the genus *Aureobacterium* and transfer of *Flavobacterium esteraromaticum* Omelianski to the genus *Aureobacterium* as *Aureobacterium esteraromaticum* comb. nov. *Int. J. Syst. Bacteriol.* **43:**555–564.

148. **Yokota, A., M. Takeuchi, and N. Weiss.** 1993. Proposal of two new species in the genus *Microbacterium: Microbacterium dextranolyticum* sp. nov. and *Microbacterium aurum* sp. nov. *Int. J. Syst. Bacteriol.* **43:**549–554.

149. **Zapardiel, J., E. Nieto, M. I. Gegundez, I. Gadea, and F. Soriano.** 1994. Problems in minimum inhibitory concentration determinations in coryneform organisms—comparison of an agar dilution and the Etest. *Diagn. Microbiol. Infect. Dis.* **19:**171–173.

150. **Zapardiel, J., E. Nieto, and F. Soriano.** 1997. Urinary tract infections caused by beta-lactam-sensitive *Corynebacterium urealyticum*. *Eur. J. Clin. Microbiol. Infect. Dis.* **16:**174–176.

151. **Zimmermann, O., C. Spröer, R. M. Kroppenstedt, E. Fuchs, H. G. Köchel, and G. Funke.** 1998. *Corynebacterium thomssenii* sp. nov., a *Corynebacterium* with *N*-acetyl-β-glucosaminidase activity from human clinical specimens. *Int. J. Syst. Bacteriol.* **48:**489–494.

152. **Zinkernagel, A. S., A. von Graevenitz, and G. Funke.** 1996. Heterogeneity within *Corynebacterium minutissimum* strains is explained by misidentified *Corynebacterium amycolatum* strains. *Am. J. Clin. Pathol.* **106:**378–383.

Listeria, Erysipelothrix, and *Kurthia**

JACQUES BILLE, JOCELYNE ROCOURT, AND BALA SWAMINATHAN

22

LISTERIA

Taxonomy

The genus *Listeria* was first included in the broad group of coryneform bacteria in the 7th edition of *Bergey's Manual of Determinative Bacteriology* in 1957. In 1986, the use of 16S rRNA partial sequencing unambiguously located *Listeria* within the *Clostridium* subbranch, together with the genera *Staphylococcus, Streptococcus, Lactobacillus,* and *Brochothrix* (45). This phylogenetic position of *Listeria* is consistent with the low guanine-plus-cytosine (G+C) content of its DNA (36 to 38%), the presence of lipoteichoic acids, and the lack of mycolic acids (71).

Listeria monocytogenes remained the only recognized species in this genus during the two decades after its discovery until the description of *L. denitrificans* (now *Jonesia denitrificans* [62]) in 1948, *L. grayi* in 1966, and *L. murrayi* in 1971 (76). DNA-DNA homology and 16S rRNA sequencing results obtained during the last decade demonstrate that this genus comprises two lines of descent: one contains *L. monocytogenes* and genomically closely related species (*L. innocua, L. ivanovii* subsp. *ivanovii, L. ivanovii* subsp. *londoniensis, L. welshimeri,* and *L. seeligeri*), and the other contains *L. grayi* (now in one species with *L. murrayi*) (16, 21, 63). This structure of the genus *Listeria* is supported by classification based on multilocus enzyme electrophoresis results (15). Only *L. monocytogenes* causes infection in humans, while *L. ivanovii* is occasionally responsible for abortion in animals. The other species are nonpathogenic.

Description of the Genus

Members of the genus *Listeria* are asporogenous, nonbranching, regular, short (0.5 to 2 μm by 0.4 to 0.5 μm) gram-positive rods that occur singly or in short chains. Filaments 6 to 20 μm long may occur in older or rough cultures. The organisms are motile at 28°C by means of one to five peritrichous flagella. Colonies are small (1 to 2 mm after 1 or 2 days of incubation at 37°C), smooth, and blue-gray on nutrient agar when examined under obliquely transmitted light. The optimum growth temperature is between 30 and 37°C, but growth occurs at 4°C within a few days. *Listeria* spp. are facultatively anaerobic. Catalase is produced except in a few strains (23), and the oxidase test is negative. Acid is produced from D-glucose and other sugars. The Voges-Proskauer and methyl red tests are positive. Esculin is hydrolyzed in a few hours. Urea and gelatin are not hydrolyzed. Neither indole nor H_2S is produced. The cell wall contains a directly cross-linked peptidoglycan based on *meso*-diaminopimelic acid, as well as lipoteichoic acid, but no mycolic acid; the major menaquinone (MK-7) contains seven isoprene units. The G+C content of the DNA is 36 to 38% (71). The two predominant cellular fatty acids are a-$C_{15:0}$ and a-$C_{17:0}$ (branched-chain type) (7).

Natural Habitats

Listeria species are widely distributed in the environment. They have been isolated from soil, decaying vegetable matter, silage, sewage, water, animal feed, fresh and frozen poultry, fresh and processed meats, raw milk, cheese, slaughterhouse waste, and asymptomatic human and animal carriers (71). *L. monocytogenes* has been isolated from numerous species of mammals, birds, fish, crustaceans, and insects (24). Nevertheless, the primary habitats of *L. monocytogenes* are considered to be the soil and decaying vegetable matter, in which it survives and grows saprophytically. Because of its widespread occurrence, *L. monocytogenes* has many opportunities to enter food production and processing environments (24, 64).

Clinical Significance

In nonpregnant human adults, *L. monocytogenes* primarily causes meningitis, encephalitis, or septicemia (51, 69). Elderly patients or persons with predisposing conditions that lower cell-mediated immunity, such as transplants, lymphomas, and AIDS, are especially susceptible. On rare occasions, patients have no recognizable predisposing conditions. The tropism of *L. monocytogenes* for the central nervous system leads to severe disease, often with high mortality (20 to 50%) or with neurologic sequelae among survivors (19).

In pregnant women, *L. monocytogenes* often causes an influenza-like bacteremic illness that, if untreated, may lead to amnionitis and infection of the fetus, resulting in abortion, stillbirth, or premature birth. Early diagnosis can be made in some cases by detecting *L. monocytogenes* in maternal blood cultures; at birth, the diagnosis is made by detecting the organism in cerebrospinal fluid (CSF), blood, amni-

* This chapter contains information presented in chapter 29 by Jill E. Clarridge and Carol A. Spiegel in the sixth edition of this Manual.

otic fluid, respiratory secretions, placental or cutaneous swabs, gastric aspirates, or meconium of the neonate. Direct microscopic visualization of gram-positive rods in these specimens could be invaluable for early diagnosis of the disease.

Focal infections rarely occur after an episode of bacteremia. However, primary cutaneous listeriosis with or without bacteremia has been reported among veterinarians and abattoir workers, who acquire the illness through contact with infected animal tissues. Endocarditis, arthritis, osteomyelitis, intra-abdominal abscesses, endophthalmitis, and pleuropulmonary infections have been described infrequently (2).

The incubation period and infective dose have not been firmly established. Reported incubation times vary from a few days to 2 to 3 months. Gastrointestinal symptoms such as diarrhea have been observed in some individuals with systemic listeriosis but were not commonly associated with ingestion of contaminated food. A transient carrier state exists in 2 to 20% of animals and humans (24). Recently, one outbreak of gastroenteritis with fever but without progression to invasive disease was linked to the consumption of milk highly contaminated by *L. monocytogenes*, adding *Listeria* to the causes of food poisoning (22). Similar outbreaks of febrile gastroenteritis due to *L. monocytogenes* have been reported from Denmark and Italy (32, 65). Therefore, the possibility of infection with *L. monocytogenes* should be considered in investigations of gastroenteritis in which routine enteric pathogens have been ruled out. Cervicovaginal carriage in women (also pregnant ones) seems to be nonexistent.

Listeriosis can occur sporadically or epidemically; in both, contaminated foods are the primary vehicles of transmission. A few limited, non-food-related nosocomial outbreaks, mainly in nurseries, have been described. The number of sporadic cases of listeriosis in countries that report the illness is typically in the range of 0.5 to 0.8 cases per 100,000 persons; during outbreaks of food-borne disease, the incidence may rise to 5 cases per 100,000 persons (11). Foods implicated as vehicles of infection include coleslaw (cabbage), soft cheeses, paté, poultry, turkey frankfurters, mushrooms, milk, and pork tongue in jelly. Large numbers of organisms ($>10^3$ CFU/g) were detected in foods quantitatively assayed for the organism (24).

The pathogenesis of *L. monocytogenes* in human infections is unclear. However, after contaminated food has been ingested, the development of an invasive infection in some individuals depends on several factors: host susceptibility, gastric acidity, inoculum size, and virulence factors of the organism. After penetrating the epithelial barrier of the intestinal tract, *L. monocytogenes* can grow within hepatic and splenic macrophages, destroying them with listeriolysin, a hemolytic protein that binds to lipids of the host cell membrane. Immunity to listeriosis relies mainly on T-cell-mediated activation of macrophages by lymphokines; the role of humoral defenses is not fully understood (64).

Collection, Transportation, and Storage of Specimens

Laboratory Safety

The infectious dose for listeriosis has not been determined, and it may depend, in part, on the susceptibility of the host. Therefore, laboratorians working with *L. monocytogenes* should be made aware of this potential risk and advised to be particularly cautious when working with this organism (38).

Specimens

Clinical

L. monocytogenes is readily isolated from clinical specimens obtained from normally sterile sites (blood, CSF, amniotic fluid, placenta, or fetal tissue). These specimens should be immediately cultured or stored at 4°C for up to 48 h. Stool specimens are more productive than rectal swabs when epidemiologic studies of carriage rates are undertaken. A 1-g sample of stool can be inoculated into 100 ml of a selective enrichment broth (detailed below) and then shipped at room temperature by overnight mail. If this is not possible, the stools should be shipped frozen on dry ice by overnight mail. Other nonsterile-site specimens may be stored at 4°C for 24 to 48 h. To avoid overgrowth of *L. monocytogenes* by contaminating members of the microflora during longer periods of storage, freezing of specimens at −20°C is recommended.

Foods

Food samples must be collected aseptically in sterile containers. Whenever possible, foods packaged in the original containers should be collected. Attempts should be made to collect at least 100 g of a sample. Samples may be placed in sterile bags and shipped on ice by overnight mail. Ice cream and other frozen products are best transported in the frozen state in the original container and must not be thawed until immediately before analysis. Although *L. monocytogenes* is relatively resistant to freezing, repeated freezing and thawing may adversely affect its viability.

Isolates

Cultures of *Listeria* spp. may be shipped to a distant laboratory on a non-glucose-containing agar slant (such as heart infusion agar or tryptic soy agar) packaged to conform with the requirements for interstate shipment of etiologic agents (U.S. Code of Federal Regulations, 42CFR, part 72).

Isolation Procedures

Culture

Clinical specimens from normally sterile sites can be directly plated on tryptic soy agar containing 5% sheep, horse, or rabbit blood. Samples for blood culture can be inoculated into conventional blood culture broth. Clinical specimens obtained from nonsterile sites and foods and environmental specimens should be selectively enriched for *Listeria* spp. before being plated.

The U.S. Department of Agriculture (USDA) method and The Netherlands Government Food Inspection Service (NGFIS) method are used together at the Centers for Disease Control and Prevention to isolate *L. monocytogenes* from nonsterile-site clinical specimens and foods (31). Individually, the two methods are approximately 75% sensitive; in conjunction with each other, they are 90% sensitive. The USDA method involves enrichment of the specimen in University of Vermont (UVM) primary selective enrichment broth (1 part sample plus 9 parts broth) at 30°C. After 24 h, 0.1 ml of the enrichment culture is plated on lithium chloride-phenylethanol-moxalactam (LPM) agar and Oxford or modified Oxford agar (see section IX) (3). Another 0.1 ml of the enrichment culture is added to 10 ml of UVM secondary selective enrichment broth, which is incubated for an additional 24 h. The secondary enrichment culture is plated as described above. The plates are incubated at 35°C and examined after 24 and 48 h. All of the media named above are described in the compendium by Atlas and Parks (3) and in the fifth edition of this Manual (50). Also, they may be purchased commercially.

The NGFIS method involves enrichment of the specimen in liquid polymyxin-acriflavine-lithium chloride-ceftazidime-esculin-mannitol (PALCAM; see section IX)-egg yolk broth (74) at 30°C and plating of the enrichment culture on commercially available PALCAM agar at 24 and 48 h. The PALCAM agar is incubated at 30°C for 48 h under microaerobic conditions (5% oxygen, 7.5% carbon dioxide, 7.5% hydrogen, 80% nitrogen).

LPM agar (41) was developed as a highly selective but nondifferential medium for the isolation of *Listeria* species. Colonies on LPM agar are examined under a stereozoom microscope (magnification, ×15 to ×25) with oblique lighting directed to the microscope stage by a concave mirror positioned at a 45° angle to the incident light (Henry illumination). *Listeria* colonies appear blue, while colonies of other bacteria appear yellowish or orange.

Oxford and PALCAM agars contain selective differential chemicals that eliminate the need for examination under oblique lighting. On Oxford and modified Oxford agars, *Listeria* colonies appear black, are 1 to 3 mm in diameter, and are surrounded by a black halo after 24 to 48 h of incubation at 37°C. Color formation is due to the hydrolysis of esculin by *Listeria* spp. and the formation of black iron-phenol compounds in the medium. On PALCAM agar, *Listeria* colonies appear gray-green, are approximately 2 mm in diameter, and have black sunken centers; esculin, ferric iron, D-mannitol, and phenol red contribute to this color formation. Recently, an enhanced hemolysis agar (EHA) has been proposed as an alternative for PALCAM agar; EHA can differentiate *L. monocytogenes* from *L. innocua* on the basis of hemolysis (8).

Suspect colonies (3 to 10 colonies per plate) are transferred to tryptic soy agar with 5% sheep blood and incubated for 18 h at 35°C for further workup.

Rapid Detection

Commercially available tests for the rapid detection of *Listeria* species from food samples in selective enrichment broths are based on immunoassays that use monoclonal antibodies (Listeria-Tek [Organon-Teknika, Belgium], Listeria immunoenzymatic detection kit [Transia, France], Listeria visual immunoassay [Tecra, Australia], Vidas-Lis [bioMérieux, France], Listeria rapid test [Unipath/Oxoid Clearview, Basingstoke, United Kingdom], Vidas-LMO [bioMérieux]). These tests are genus specific. Lister test (VICAM, Watertown, Mass.), Vidas-LMO [bioMérieux], and a DNA-probe *L. monocytogenes* assay (Gene-Trak, Framingham, Mass.) are *L. monocytogenes* specific (9). These kits are not designed for the analysis of clinical specimens, for diagnosis, or for treatment.

L. monocytogenes DNA in CSF and tissue (fresh or in paraffin blocks) can be specifically detected by PCR-based tests (36, 68). The PCR assay, available only in specialized laboratories, is highly sensitive and specific and could be particularly useful when prior administration of antimicrobial agents compromises culture.

Identification

Genus Identification

A simplified identification is based on the following tests: Gram stain, observation of tumbling motility in a wet mount, positive catalase reaction, acid production from D-glucose, esculin hydrolysis, and positive Voges-Proskauer and methyl red reactions.

Species Identification

The scheme for identification of *Listeria* species is shown in Table 1. Identification of *Listeria* isolates to the species level is crucial, because all species can contaminate foods but only *L. monocytogenes* is of public health concern. Identification is based on a limited number of biochemical markers, among which hemolysis is essential to differentiating between *L. monocytogenes* and the most frequently isolated nonpathogenic *Listeria* species, *L. innocua*.

Hemolysis

Only three species, *L. monocytogenes*, *L. seeligeri*, and *L. ivanovii*, are hemolytic on sheep blood agar plates. Recent studies indicated hemolysin to be the major virulence factor of *L. monocytogenes*; however, hemolysis alone cannot be used as an indicator of the presence of a virulent species, because *L. seeligeri* is hemolytic but nonpathogenic. *L. monocytogenes* and *L. seeligeri* produce narrow zones of hemolysis that frequently do not extend much beyond the edge of the colonies, whereas *L. ivanovii* exhibits a wide zone of hemolysis (Fig. 1).

The CAMP test uses a β-lysin-producing *Staphylococcus aureus* or *Rhodococcus equi* strain streaked in one direction on a sheep blood agar plate and test cultures of *Listeria* spp. streaked at right angles to (but not touching) the *S. aureus* and *R. equi* lines. According to *Bergey's Manual of Systematic Bacteriology* (71), hemolysis of *L. monocytogenes* and *L. seeligeri* is enhanced in the vicinity of the *S. aureus* streak, and *L. ivanovii* hemolysis is enhanced in the vicinity of *R. equi* (typical picture of a shovel [Fig. 2]). However, because many investigators have reported observing a synergistic hemolysis reaction between *L. monocytogenes* and *R. equi*, this CAMP reaction must be interpreted with caution. A β-lysin disk (Remel, Lenexa, Kans.) could be used to observe hemolysis enhancement of *L. monocytogenes* with β-lysin from *S. aureus*.

Acid Production from Carbohydrates

L. monocytogenes is always D-xylose negative and α-methyl-D-mannoside positive. Rare atypical strains may be L-rhamnose negative.

Miniaturized Biochemical Tests

The API-Listeria test (bioMérieux Vitek, Inc., Hazelwood, Mo.) was specifically designed for the genus *Listeria* and includes 10 biochemical differentiation tests in a microtube format. It includes a patented "DIM" test, based on the absence or presence of arylamidase, which distinguishes between *L. monocytogenes* and *L. innocua* without the need for further tests for hemolytic activity (12). Another system based on 15 biochemical tests (Micro-ID Listeria [Organon-Teknika]) performs equally well but needs an additional test for hemolytic activity to differentiate *L. monocytogenes* from *L. innocua* (5).

DNA Probe Assay for Colony Confirmation

A 30-min chemiluminescence DNA probe assay is available (Gen-Probe, San Diego, Calif.) for the rapid confirmation of *L. monocytogenes* from colonies on primary isolation plates. This assay was highly specific for *L. monocytogenes* in two independent evaluations (52, 56).

TABLE 1 Biochemical differentiation of species in the genus *Listeria*[a]

Characteristic	*L. grayi*	*L. innocua*	*L. ivanovii*	*L. ivanovii* subsp. *londoniensis*	*L. monocytogenes*	*L. seeligeri*	*L. welshimeri*
β-Hemolysis	–	–	+ +[b]	+ +	+	+	–
CAMP test reaction							
S. aureus	–	–	–	–	+	+	–
R. equi	–	–	+	+	±	–	–
Acid production from:							
Mannitol	+	–	–	–	–	–	–
α-Methyl-D-mannoside	+	+	–	–	+	–	+
L-Rhamnose	V	V	–	–	+	–	V
Soluble starch	+	–	–	–	–	ND	ND
D-Xylose	–	–	+	+	–	+	+
Ribose	V	–	+	–	–	–	–
N-Acetyl-β-D-mannosamine			–	+			
Hippurate hydrolysis	–	+	+	+	+	ND	ND
Reduction of nitrate	±	–	–	–	–	ND	ND
Associated serovars	S	4ab, US, 6a, 6b	5	5	1/2a, 1/2b, 1/2c, 3a, 3b, 3c, 4a, 4ab, 4b, 4c, 4d, 4e, 7	1/2a, 1/2b, 1/2c, US, 4b, 4d, 6b	1/2b, 4c, 6a, 6b, US

[a] See references 16 and 71. Symbols and abbreviations: +, ≥90% of strains are positive; –, ≥90% of strains are negative; ND, not determined; V, variable; US, undesignated serotype; S, specific.
[b] + +, Usually a wide zone or multiple zones; ±, variable.

Differentiation of the Genus *Listeria* from Other Genera

Because they share some characteristics, *Listeria* spp. and some other gram-positive bacteria may be confused. *Streptococcus* spp. may be differentiated from *Listeria* spp. on the basis of Gram stain morphology, motility, and catalase activity. *Erysipelothrix* spp. differ from *Listeria* spp. in motility, catalase reaction, and ability to grow at 4°C (*Erysipelothrix* spp. do not grow at that temperature). Among the background microflora of foods, *Lactobacillus* spp. are usually nonmotile and catalase negative, *Brochothrix* spp. are unable to grow at 37°C, and *Kurthia* spp. are strictly aerobic and esculin negative.

Determination of Pathogenicity

Methods in which laboratory animals are used for evaluation of the virulence potential of *Listeria* isolates are available but are not used routinely, because most, if not all, wild

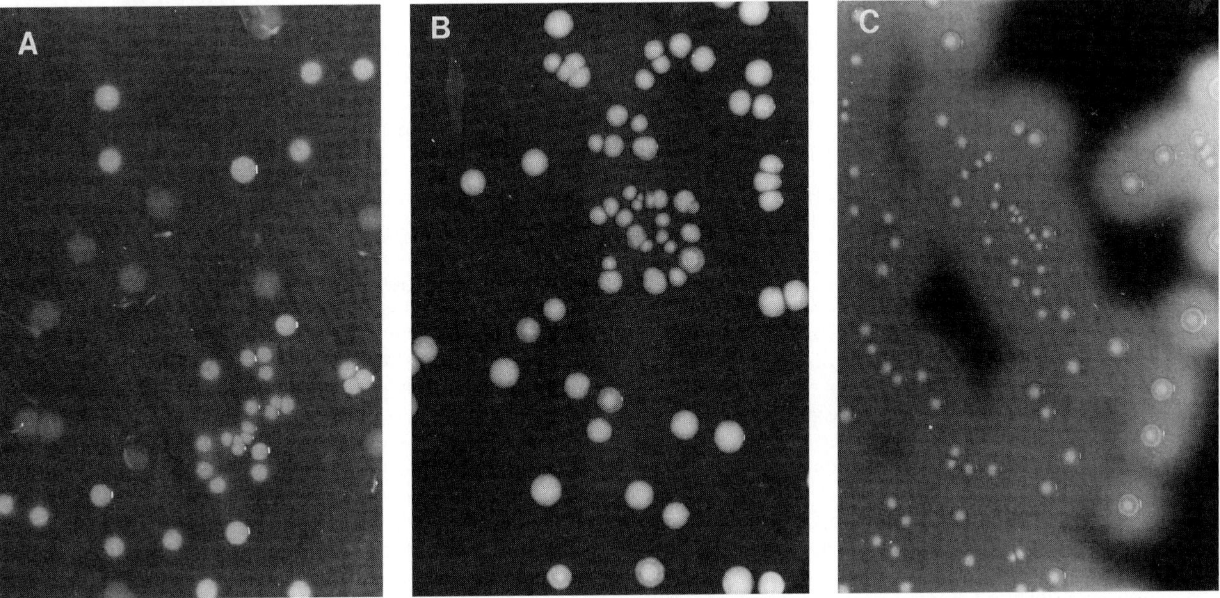

FIGURE 1 Macroscopic view of colonies on 5% human blood agar plates after 24 h of incubation. (A) *L. monocytogenes*: discrete zone of beta-hemolysis under the removed colonies. (B) *L. innocua*: no hemolysis. (C) *L. ivanovii*: wide zone of beta-hemolysis around the colonies.

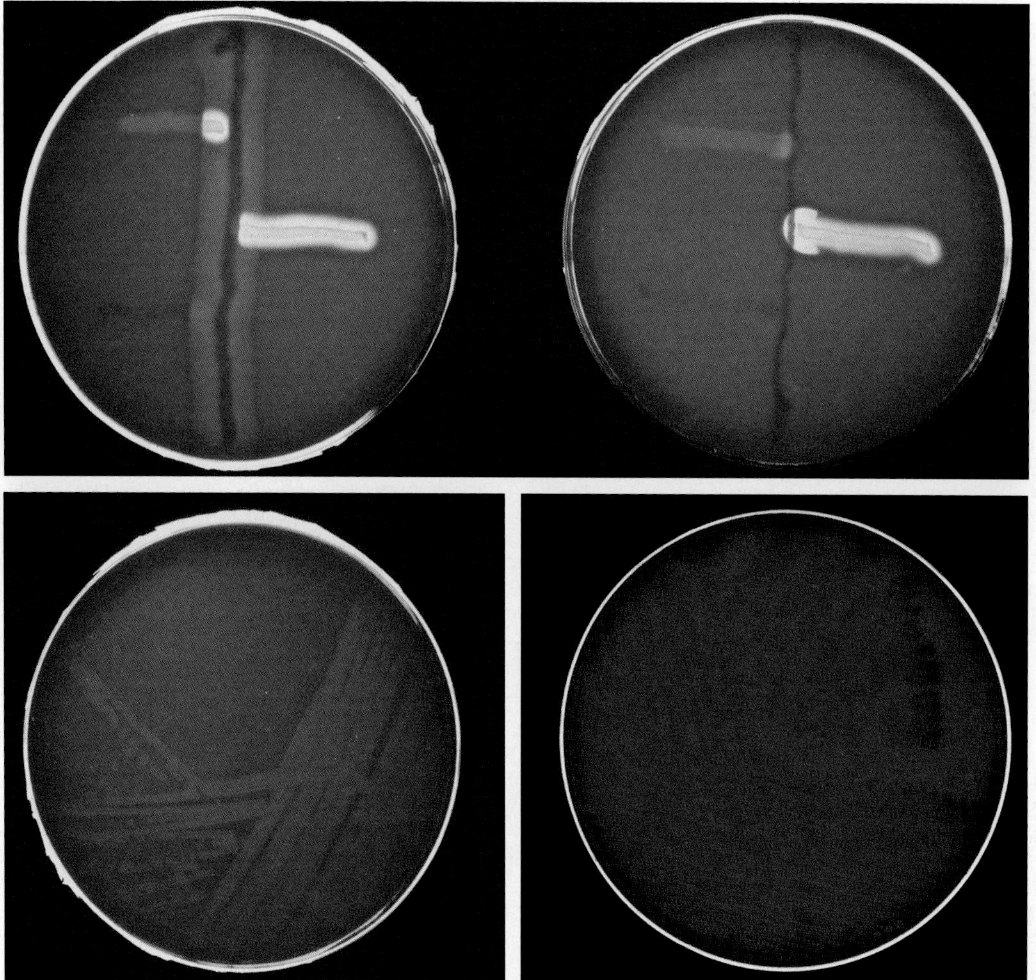

FIGURE 2 (top plates) CAMP test done with *R. equi* (left plate) and *S. aureus* (right plate). Upper left, *L. monocytogenes*; lower left, *L. innocua*; middle right, *L. ivanovii*.
FIGURE 3 (bottom plate, left) *E. rhusiopathiae* on sheep blood agar (48-h incubation at 37°C in 5% CO_2).
FIGURE 4 (bottom plate, right) *K. zopfii* on sheep blood agar (72-h incubation at room temperature).

isolates of *L. monocytogenes* are virulent. These tests include intraperitoneal inoculation of mice, inoculation of the chorioallantoic membranes of embryonated eggs, and inoculation of the conjunctivas of rabbits (Anton test). A sensitive immunocompromised-mouse model in which relatively small numbers of virulent listeriae cause the deaths of these immunosuppressed animals within 3 days has been developed (72). Also, cell culture cytotoxicity assays with the human intestinal epithelial line Caco-2 have been developed to determine the virulence potential of *Listeria* isolates in vitro (64). While the results generally agree with those of animal tests, cytotoxicity assays do not provide as quantitative a measure of virulence as do the animal tests (50% lethal dose determination). Also, some outbreak-associated *L. monocytogenes* isolates show very little cytotoxicity in the Caco-2 cell assays (58).

Typing Techniques

Serotyping

Listeria strains are divided into serotypes on the basis of somatic (O) and flagellar (H) antigens (70). Thirteen serotypes (1/2a, 1/2b, 1/2c, 3a, 3b, 3c, 4a, 4ab, 4b, 4c, 4d, 4e, and 7) of *L. monocytogenes* are known; 4bX, a variant of serotype 4b, was implicated in a listeriosis outbreak traced to contaminated paté in England (48). Serotyping antigens are shared among *L. monocytogenes*, *L. innocua*, *L. seeligeri*, and *L. welshimeri*. Most human disease is caused by serotypes 1/2a, 1/2b, and 4b; therefore, serotyping alone is not sufficiently discriminating for subtyping purposes. Nevertheless, serotyping serves a useful purpose as a first-level discriminator. Also, unlike other subtyping methods, serotype designations are universal. Determination of the serotype also facilitates the selection of appropriate controls for molecular subtyping methods. A recently introduced commercial kit for serotyping *Listeria* (Denka Seiken, Tokyo, Japan) is under evaluation.

Phage Typing

Because of the low discriminating ability of serotyping, phage typing was the only means of distinguishing between strains of the same serotype before the introduction of molecular methods. *Listeria* phages were isolated from lysogenic strains of all *Listeria* species and from sewage (44, 61). A multicenter study involving four laboratories was organized in 1981 to select an international set of phages among those isolated in France and Germany and to define a standardized method (58). Phage typing has been successfully used in clinical and epidemiologic evaluations involving recurrent infections in humans, nosocomial infections, and common-source outbreaks (11, 26, 42, 47, 67). The isolation of strains with the same phage type both from patients involved in epidemics and from the foods implicated by case-control studies confirmed the food-borne transmission of listeriosis. Despite its usefulness, phage typing is hampered by the non-typeability of some strains; the percentage of nontypeable strains may vary according to the origin of the strain (food and environmental isolates are frequently nontypeable). An improved method of reverse phage typing may represent an interesting alternative in this regard (43, 44).

Multilocus Enzyme Electrophoresis

Typically, 10 to 25 enzyme loci are examined by multilocus enzyme electrophoresis (MLEE) for each strain. Each unique mobility variant of an enzyme is given a unique numeric allele designation. Each strain is defined by a string of numerical values for the alleles examined (electrophoretic type). MLEE has been applied with great success to epidemiologic investigations of outbreaks and sporadic disease (10, 14, 57, 59, 69). Strains implicated in three food-borne outbreaks were determined by MLEE to be identical or highly related (57); this finding has caused some investigators to hypothesize that outbreaks are caused by a few clones that probably possess unique virulence factors. Nevertheless, MLEE alone may not be adequate to subtype serotype 4b, because large numbers of epidemiologically unrelated strains cluster in a few electrophoretic types (69). MLEE has also been very useful in taxonomic studies and in differentiating among *Listeria* species (15).

DNA Microrestriction Patterns

Characterization of chromosomal DNA by restriction endonuclease analysis or ribosomal DNA gene restriction patterns (ribotyping) has been used to differentiate *L. monocytogenes* strains in different serotypes and within a given serotype, in particular serotype 4b, which is most frequently involved in outbreaks. Microrestriction patterns generated by frequently cutting restriction enzymes (e.g., *Eco*RI) have proved useful in epidemiologic investigations (4, 54), although the complexity of patterns makes it difficult to compare the patterns of several strains. Ribotyping simplifies the microrestriction patterns by rendering visible only the DNA fragments containing part or all of the ribosomal genes, but its discriminating ability, particularly for serotype 4b, may not be adequate (4, 29, 34, 35, 53).

DNA Macrorestriction Patterns

Brosch et al. (18) evaluated the pulsed-field gel electrophoresis (PFGE) method for the World Health Organization (WHO) multicenter international typing study of *L. monocytogenes*. Four laboratories participated in using PFGE to analyze 80 coded strains. Two restriction endonucleases (*Apa*I and *Sma*I) were used by all laboratories; one laboratory used an additional restriction endonuclease (*Asc*I). Agreement of the typing data among the four laboratories ranged from 79 to 90%. A total of 69% of the strains were placed in exactly the same genomic group by all four laboratories; most of the epidemiologically related strains were correctly identified by all four laboratories. This study validated the previous claims that PFGE is a highly discriminating and reproducible method for subtyping *L. monocytogenes* and is particularly useful for subtyping serotype 4b isolates, which are not typed satisfactorily by most other typing methods.

Random Amplified Polymorphic DNA

Boerlin et al. (17) performed an extensive evaluation of random amplified polymorphic DNA (RAPD) by typing 100 *L. monocytogenes* isolates which had been characterized by serotyping, phage typing, MLEE analysis, restriction endonuclease analysis, and ribotyping. They found RAPD to be highly discriminating. O'Donoghue et al. (55) found RAPD to be useful for typing serogroup 1/2; also, they found that the method distinguished serotype 4bX strains involved in a paté-associated outbreak from other serotype 4b isolates. Wernars et al. (77) evaluated RAPD for the WHO collaborative study. Six laboratories participated in the study. By using three different 10-mer primers, the median reproducibility of the RAPD results obtained by the six participants was 86.5% (range, 0 to 100%). Failure in reproducibility was due mainly to results obtained with one particular primer. The participants concluded that RAPD analysis is a rapid and relatively simple technique for epidemiologic typing of *L. monocytogenes* isolates and that reproducible and useful results can be obtained. Despite the simplicity and high discriminating ability of RAPD, much more work is needed to make RAPD typing a standard technique for general and widespread use. Its primary drawback is the inconsistent reproducibility of patterns.

Present Status of Subtyping

The vast majority of *L. monocytogenes* strains causing sporadic infections or outbreaks belong to the three serotypes 1/2a, 1/2b, and 4b. Strains of serotype 1/2a are highly heterogeneous and thus are easily differentiated by any of the molecular methods and by phage typing when the strains are phage typeable. In contrast, strains of serotype 4b are more closely related and optimal differentiation probably necessitates the combined use of several methods. This has been confirmed by the first results of an international multicenter study aimed at evaluating the different subtyping methods for *L. monocytogenes* and at standardizing the most promising one (13).

Serologic Tests

Serologic responses to whole-cell antigens are not diagnostic, because of antigenic cross-reactivity between *L. monocytogenes* and other gram-positive bacteria such as staphylococci, enterococci, and *Bacillus* species. Furthermore, patients with culture-confirmed listeriosis have had undetectable antibody levels (69). Determination of antibody levels to listeriolysin O may be of value both for invasive listeriosis and for febrile gastroenteritis (6). A recent serologic method based on the detection of antibodies against recombinant truncated forms of listeriolysin O may be more specific, but additional studies must be performed before serologic tests can be recommended (27).

Antimicrobial Susceptibilities

The pattern of antimicrobial susceptibility and resistance of *L. monocytogenes* has been relatively stable for many years. In vitro, the organism is susceptible to penicillin, ampicillin, gentamicin, erythromycin, tetracycline, rifampin, and chloramphenicol (66, 78) but only moderately susceptible to quinolones (33). However, many of these antimicrobial agents are only bacteriostatic. Penicillin or ampicillin with or without an aminoglycoside is usually recommended for the treatment of listeriosis. Studies in vitro and in animal models have shown that an aminoglycoside enhances the antimicrobial (bactericidal) activity of penicillin against *L. monocytogenes* (49). Trimethoprim-sulfamethoxazole and aminoglycosides are among the few anti-infective agents that are bactericidal to *L. monocytogenes*; only trimethoprim-sulfamethoxazole has been used occasionally with success. Recently, resistance plasmids conferring resistance to chloramphenicol, macrolides, and tetracyclines have been found in several clinical isolates of *L. monocytogenes* and have raised concern for the future (30). Cephalosporins are ineffective in vitro and should never be administered when listeriosis is suspected.

Evaluation, Interpretation, and Reporting of Results

Colonies from blood, CSF, or other normally sterile-site specimens that show subdued beta-hemolysis on blood agar should be subjected to motility tests, Gram staining, and sugar fermentation tests to confirm the identification. They may resemble group B streptococcal colonies on blood agar plates. The CAMP test is not necessary on a routine basis, and the β-lysin test may be substituted for it. Use of the API-Listeria test may eliminate the need for enhanced hemolysis testing altogether.

If *L. monocytogenes* is present in small numbers in CSF, direct examination of Gram-stained clinical specimens may be of little or no value. Also, Gram-stained *Listeria* cells closely resemble other gram-positive bacteria such as streptococci, enterococci, or corynebacteria. If antimicrobial therapy was initiated before a CSF specimen was obtained, the culture results may be negative. In these instances, Gram staining may be useful, but additional confirmation by methods such as PCR (for laboratories that have the capability) may be needed.

Serologic responses to whole-cell antigens are unreliable, although in culture-negative cases, determination of the serologic response to listeriolysin O may be of diagnostic value retrospectively.

ERYSIPELOTHRIX

Taxonomy

Included at one time in the coryneform group, *Erysipelothrix* is now classified within the regular non-spore-forming gram-positive rods, a group that comprises the genera *Listeria* and *Lactobacillus*. The genus *Erysipelothrix* has two species, *E. rhusiopathiae* and *E. tonsillarum* (73). *E. rhusiopathiae*, which is widely distributed in nature and can be carried by a variety of animals, has been recognized for more than 100 years as the agent of swine erysipelas, and it occasionally causes erysipeloid, a human cutaneous infection usually localized to the hands and fingers (60).

Description of the Genus

Erysipelothrix organisms are mesophilic, facultatively anaerobic, non-spore-forming, non-acid-fast, gram-positive bacteria that appear microscopically as short rods (0.2 to 0.5 μm by 0.8 to 2.5 μm) with rounded ends and occur singly, in short chains, or in long nonbranching filaments (60 μm or more in length). They are nonmotile and grow in complex media at a wide range of temperatures (5 to 42°C; optimum, 30 to 37°C) and at alkaline pH (6.7 to 9.2; optimum, 7.2 to 7.6). Like *Listeria*, they can grow in the presence of high concentrations of sodium chloride (up to 8.5%). Metabolically, *Erysipelothrix* organisms are catalase negative and oxidase negative, do not hydrolyze esculin, and weakly ferment glucose without the production of gas. They are methyl red and Voges-Proskauer negative, and they do not produce indole or hydrolyze urea; however, they distinctively produce H_2S in triple sugar iron agar (37). Key fatty acids are $C_{16:0}$ and $C_{18:cis9}$ (7).

Natural Habitat

E. rhusiopathiae is widespread in nature and is remarkably persistent under environmental conditions such as low temperature, alkaline pH, and within organic matter favoring survival. The organism is parasitic on mammals, birds, and fish but is most frequently associated with pigs. Contamination of water and soil from the feces and urine of sick and asymptomatic animals often occurs.

E. tonsillarum has been recovered from water and from the tonsils of healthy swine.

Clinical Significance

Infection with *E. rhusiopathiae* is a zoonosis. Many animal species, especially turkeys and swine, carry the organism in their digestive tracts or tonsils. *E. rhusiopathiae* causes chronic or acute swine erysipelas. Other domestic and wild animals and birds also can be affected, in particular sheep, rabbits, cattle, and turkeys. Infection is most probably acquired by ingestion of contaminated matter (60).

In humans, *E. rhusiopathiae* mostly causes erysipeloid, a localized cellulitis developing within 2 to 7 days around the inoculation site. The disease is contracted through skin abrasion, injury, or a bite on the hands or arms of individuals handling animals or animal products. Erysipeloid is an occupational disease, occurring most frequently in veterinarians, butchers, and particularly fish handlers. The lesion usually is violaceous and painful, indurated with edema and inflammation but without suppuration, and clearly delineated at the border. Regional lymphangitis may be present, as well as an adjacent arthritis. Dissemination and endocarditis can occur, especially in immunocompromised patients; their prognosis is generally poor (28). Healing usually takes 2 to 4 weeks, sometimes months, and relapses are common. No apparent immunity develops after an episode of erysipeloid.

E. tonsillarum has not yet been recovered from humans.

Collection, Transport, and Storage of Specimens

Biopsy specimens from erysipeloid lesions are the best source of *E. rhusiopathiae*. Care should be taken to cleanse and disinfect the skin before sampling. The organisms typically are located deep in the subcutaneous layer of the leading edge of the lesion; hence, a biopsy of the entire thickness of the dermis at the periphery of the lesion should be taken for Gram stain and culture. Swabs from the surface of the skin are not useful. In patients with disseminated disease, the organism can be cultured from blood without special procedures.

Isolation Procedures

Microscopic Examination

Generally, direct examination of Gram-stained biopsy specimens is of little value. However, the presence of long, slender, gram-positive rods in tissue from an individual with a consonant history is suggestive of erysipeloid.

Culture

Biopsy specimens should be plated on blood agar or chocolate blood agar, placed in tryptic soy or Schaedler broth, and incubated at 35°C aerobically or in 5% CO_2 for 7 days. Blood from patients with septicemia or endocarditis can be plated directly onto blood agar plates for primary isolation or inoculated in commercial blood culture systems. *E. rhusiopathiae* colonies generally develop in 1 to 3 days, being pinpoint (<0.1 to 0.5 mm in diameter) on blood agar plates after 24 h of incubation. At 48 h, two distinct colony types can be observed (Fig. 3). The smaller, smooth colonies are 0.3 to 1.5 mm in diameter, transparent, convex, and circular with entire edges. Larger, rough colonies are flatter and more opaque and have a matte surface and an irregular, fimbriated edge. A zone of greenish discoloration frequently develops underneath the colonies on blood agar plates after 2 days of incubation (37).

Rapid Detection

A genus-specific PCR amplification system involving a DNA sequence coding for 16S rRNA has been used in pig samples (46).

Identification

Gram Stain of Colonies from a 24-h Blood Agar Plate

Cells stain gram positive but can decolorize and appear gram negative, with gram-positive granules giving a beaded effect. Cells from smooth colonies appear as rods or coccobacilli, sometimes in short chains. Cells from rough colonies appear as long filaments, often more than 60 μm in length.

Biochemical Identification of *E. rhusiopathiae*

E. rhusiopathiae is catalase negative; lactose and H_2S positive; and nitrate, urease, esculin, gelatin, xylose, mannose, maltose, and sucrose negative. *E. tonsillarum* differs biochemically from *E. rhusiopathiae* by being sucrose positive. Vitek automated systems, as well as API Coryne, usually identify *E. rhusiopathiae* correctly.

Differentiation of *Erysipelothix* from Related Genera

Genera that have morphologic and physiologic characteristics in common with *Erysipelothrix* include *Lactobacillus, Listeria, Brochothrix,* and *Kurthia*. All are regular nonpigmented, non-spore-forming, gram-positive rods (39). A major discriminatory test is that *E. rhusiopathiae* produces H_2S in triple sugar iron whereas species of the other genera do not. Furthermore, *Listeria, Brochothrix,* and *Kurthia* species are catalase positive. In addition, *Listeria* isolates are motile, are esculin positive, and are not alpha-hemolytic. *Brochothrix* isolates strongly ferment carbohydrates, are Voges-Proskauer positive, and do not grow above 30°C. *Kurthia* species are strict aerobes, motile, and nonhemolytic. Corynebacteria and streptococci also can be confused with *E. rhusiopathiae*, but careful examination of the cell morphology should facilitate the distinction.

The production of H_2S in triple sugar iron by a gram-positive bacterium is usually indicative of *E. rhusiopathiae*, because very few gram-positive bacteria of clinical origin produce H_2S. Exceptions include some *Bacillus* strains, but they are easily differentiated from *E. rhusiopathiae* by cellular morphology and spore formation. An additional trait highly characteristic of *E. rhusiopathiae* is its "pipe cleaner" pattern of growth in gelatin stab cultures incubated at 22°C (37, 75).

Typing Systems

Twenty-two serovars of *E. rhusiopathiae* have been identified on the basis of heat-stable somatic antigens. Although most isolates are serovar 1 or 2, no serotyping schemes are available for routine use in clinical laboratories (37). Both MLEE and ribotyping methods have been applied to *Erysipelothrix* strains and have shown an important genetic diversity (1, 20). In these studies, serotyping was unreliable for use as an epidemiologic tool.

Pathogenicity Testing

Most strains of *E. rhusiopathiae* are virulent for mice in a mouse protection test.

Serologic Tests

Since humans apparently do not develop immunity after an episode of erysipeloid, there are no serologic tests for routine use to demonstrate antibodies to *E. rhusiopathiae*. Active immunization of animals with a live attenuated vaccine protects against erysipelas (60); however, a natural infection of erysipeloid in humans does not prevent relapses or reinfection from occurring.

Antibiotic Susceptibility

E. rhusiopathiae isolates are generally susceptible to penicillin, cephalosporins, clindamycin, imipenem, tetracycline, chloramphenicol, erythromycin, and the fluoroquinolones; they are usually resistant to aminoglycosides, sulfonamides, and vancomycin. Penicillin is the treatment of choice for both localized and systemic infections (28).

KURTHIA

Once thought to be related to coryneform bacteria, *Kurthia* is now known to be closer to the genera *Bacillus, Staphylococcus, Streptococcus,* and *Lactobacillus* (40). On the basis of 16S rRNA sequence analysis, *Kurthia* clusters at the periphery of the second phylogenetic group of *Bacillus* genus and represents a distinct, somewhat distant line of descent from it (25).

Kurthia organisms are strictly aerobic, non-spore-forming, non-acid-fast, gram-positive bacteria that appear microscopically either as large bacilli in chains, often in parallel (0.8 to 1.2 μm in diameter by 2 to 4 μm in length), or as unbranched filaments. In older cultures, they tend to appear as coccoid cells to short rods. *Kurthia* cells are motile (peritrichous flagella) and grow at an optimum temperature of 25 to 30°C. Metabolically, *Kurthia* organisms are catalase positive and oxidase negative and are nonfermentative. Major cellular fatty acids are $C_{16:0}$, i-$C_{15:0}$, and a-$C_{15:0}$ (7).

Kurthia organisms are frequently isolated from the environment (soil, surface water, wood), from animals (chicken, pigs, dogs), and from meat and meat products.

A number of strains identified as *Kurthia* spp. have been isolated from various clinical samples, including those from patients with endocarditis; however, this has not occurred during the last 20 years, and the clinical evidence of the pathogenicity of *Kurthia* has never been confirmed (40).

Kurthia appears on blood agar plates as nonhemolytic, large, cream to yellow colonies. These colonies could be confused with *Bacillus* colonies (Fig. 4). On yeast nutrient gelatin agar slant, incubated at 25°C, *Kurthia* organisms produce a characteristic "bird's feather" growth.

Of the two species of *Kurthia* described, *K. zopfii* does not grow at 45°C and produces nonpigmented colonies, whereas *K. gibsonii* does grow at 45°C and produces yellow or cream colonies.

Serologic tests are not available for *Kurthia* spp., and their susceptibility to antibiotics has not been established.

REFERENCES

1. **Ahrné, S., I.-M. Stenström, N. E. Jensen, B. Pettersson, M. Uhlén, and G. Molin.** 1995. Classification of *Erysipelothrix* strains on the basis of restriction fragment length polymorphisms. *Int. J. Syst. Bacteriol.* **45:**382–385.
2. **Armstrong, D.** 1995. *Listeria monocytogenes*, p. 1880–1885. *In* G. L. Mandell, J. E. Bennett, and R. Dolin (ed.), *Principles and Practice of Infectious Diseases*, 4th ed. Churchill Livingstone, Inc., New York, N.Y.
3. **Atlas, R. M., and L. C. Parks (ed.).** 1993. *Handbook of Microbiological Media*. CRC Press, Inc., Boca Raton, Fla.
4. **Baloga, A. O., and S. K. Harlander.** 1991. Comparison of methods for discrimination between strains of *Listeria monocytogenes* from epidemiological surveys. *Appl. Environ. Microbiol.* **57:**2324–2331.
5. **Bannerman, E., M.-N. Yersin, and J. Bille.** 1992. Evaluation of the Organon-Teknika MICRO-ID LISTERIA System. *Appl. Environ. Microbiol.* **58:**2011–2015.
6. **Berche P., K. A. Reich, M. Bonnichon, J.-L. Beretti, C. Geoffroy, J. Raveneau, P. Cossart, J.-L. Gaillard, P. Geslin, H. Kreis, and M. Véron.** 1990. Detection of anti-listeriolysin O for serodiagnosis of human listeriosis. *Lancet* **ii:**624–627.
7. **Bernard, K. A., M. Bellefeuille, and E. P. Ewan.** 1991. Cellular fatty acid composition as an adjunct to the identification of asporogenous, aerobic gram-positive rods. *J. Clin. Microbiol.* **29:**83–89.
8. **Beumer, R. R., M. C. te Giffel, and L. J. Cox.** 1997. Optimization of hemolysis in enhanced hemolysis agar (EHA), a selective medium for the isolation of *Listeria monocytogenes*. *Lett. Appl. Microbiol.* **24:**421–425.
9. **Beumer, R. R., M. C. te Giffel, M. T. C. Kok, and F. M. Rombouts.** 1996. Confirmation and identification of *Listeria* spp. *Lett. Appl. Microbiol.* **22:**448–452.
10. **Bibb, W. F., B. G. Gellin, R. Weaver, B. Schwartz, B. D. Plikaytis, M. W. Reeves, R. W. Pinner, and C. V. Broome.** 1990. Analysis of clinical and food-borne isolates of *Listeria monocytogenes* in the United States by multilocus enzyme electrophoresis and application of the method to epidemiologic investigations. *Appl. Environ. Microbiol.* **56:** 2133–2141.
11. **Bille, J.** 1990. Epidemiology of human listeriosis in Europe, with special reference to the Swiss outbreak, p. 71–74. *In* A. J. Miller, J. L. Smith, and G. A. Somkuti (ed.), *Foodborne Listeriosis*. Elsevier, Amsterdam, The Netherlands.
12. **Bille, J., B. Catimel, E. Bannerman, C. Jacquet, M.-N. Yersin, I. Caniaux, D. Monget, and J. Rocourt.** 1992. API-Listeria, a new and promising one-day system to identify *Listeria* isolates. *Appl. Environ. Microbiol.* **58:** 1857–1860.
13. **Bille, J., and J. Rocourt.** 1996. WHO international multicenter *Listeria monocytogenes* subtyping study—rationale and set-up of the study. *Int. J. Food Microbiol.* **32:**251–262.
14. **Boerlin, P., and J.-C. Piffaretti.** 1991. Typing of human, animal, food, and environmental isolates of *Listeria monocytogenes* by multilocus enzyme electrophoresis. *Appl. Environ. Microbiol.* **57:**1624–1629.
15. **Boerlin, P., J. Rocourt, and J.-C. Piffaretti.** 1991. Taxonomy of the genus *Listeria* by using multilocus enzyme electrophoresis. *Int. J. Syst. Bacteriol.* **41:**59–64.
16. **Boerlin, P., J. Rocourt, F. Grimont, P. A. D. Grimont, C. Jacquet, and J.-C. Piffaretti.** 1992. *Listeria ivanovii* subsp. *londoniensis* subsp. nov. *Int. J. Syst. Bacteriol.* **42:**69–73.
17. **Boerlin, P., E. Bannerman, F. Ischer, J. Rocourt, and J. Bille.** 1995. Typing of *Listeria monocytogenes*: a comparison of random amplification of polymorphic DNA with 5 other methods. *Res. Microbiol.* **146:**35–49.
18. **Brosch, R., M. Brett, B. Catimel, J. B. Luchansky, B. Ojeniyi, and J. Rocourt.** 1996. Genomic fingerprinting of 80 strains from the WHO multicenter international typing study of *Listeria monocytogenes* via pulsed-field gel electrophoresis (PFGE). *Int. J. Food Microbiol.* **32:**343–355.
19. **Büla, C. J., J. Bille, and M. P. Glauser.** 1995. An epidemic of food-borne listeriosis in Western Switzerland: description of 57 cases involving adults. *Clin. Infect. Dis.* **20:** 66–72.
20. **Chooromoney, K. N., D. J. Hampson, G. J. Eamens, and M. J. Turner.** 1994. Analysis of *Erysipelothrix rhusiopathiae* and *Erysipelothrix tonsillarum* by multilocus enzyme electrophoresis. *J. Clin. Microbiol.* **32:**371–376.
21. **Collins, M. D., S. Wallbanks, D. J. Lane, J. Shah, R. Nietupski, J. Smida, M. Dorsch, and E. Stackebrandt.** 1991. Phylogenetic analysis of the genus *Listeria* based on reverse transcriptase sequencing of 16S rRNA. *Int. J. Syst. Bacteriol.* **41:**240–246.
22. **Dalton, C. B., C. C. Austin, J. Sobel, P. S. Hayes, W. F. Bibb, L. M. Graves, B. Swaminathan, M. E. Proctor, and P. M. Griffin.** 1997. An outbreak of gastroenteritis and fever due to *Listeria monocytogenes* in milk. *N. Engl. J. Med.* **336:**100–105.
23. **Elsner, H.-A., I. Sobottka, A. Bubert, H. Albrecht, R. Laufs, and D. Mack.** 1996. Catalase-negative *Listeria monocytogenes* causing lethal sepsis and meningitis in an adult hematologic patient. *Eur. J. Clin. Microbiol. Infect. Dis.* **15:**965–967.
24. **Farber, J. M., and P. I. Peterkin.** 1991. *Listeria monocytogenes*, a food-borne pathogen. *Microbiol. Rev.* **55:**476–511.
25. **Farrow, J. A. E., S. Wallbanks, and M. D. Collins.** 1994. Phylogenetic relationships of round spore-forming bacilli containing cell walls based on lysine and nonspore-forming *Caryophanon*, *Exiguobacterium*, *Kurthia*, and *Planococcus*. *Int. J. Syst. Bacteriol.* **44:**74–82.
26. **Fleming, D. W., S. L. Cochi, K. L. MacDonald, J. Brondum, P. S. Hayes, B. D. Plikaytis, M. B. Holmes, A. Audurier, C. V. Broome, and A. L. Reingold.** 1985. Pasteurized milk as a vehicle of infection in an outbreak of listeriosis. *N. Engl. J. Med.* **312:**404–407.
27. **Gholizadeh, Y., C. Poyart, M. Juvin, J.-L. Beretti, J. Croizé, P. Berche, and J.-L. Gaillard.** 1996. Serodiagnosis of listeriosis based upon detection of antibodies against recombinant truncated forms of listeriolysin O. *J. Clin. Microbiol.* **34:**1391–1395.
28. **Gorby, G. L., and J. E. Peacock, Jr.** 1988. *Erysipelothrix rhusiopathiae* endocarditis: microbiologic, epidemiologic, and clinical features of an occupational disease. *Rev. Infect. Dis.* **10:**317–325.
29. **Graves, L. M., B. Swaminathan, M. W. Reeves, and J. Wenger.** 1991. Ribosomal DNA fingerprinting of *Listeria monocytogenes* using a digoxigenin-labeled DNA probe. *Eur. J. Epidemiol.* **7:**77–82.
30. **Hadorn, K., H. Hächler, A. Schaffner, and F. H. Kayser.** 1993. Genetic characterization of plasmid-encoded multiple antibiotic resistance in a strain of *Listeria monocytogenes*

causing endocarditis. *Eur. J. Clin. Microbiol. Infect. Dis.* **12:**928–937.

31. **Hayes, P. S., L. M. Graves, B. Swaminathan, G. W. Ajello, G. B. Malcolm, R. E. Weaver, R. Ransom, K. Deaver, B. D. Plikaytis, A. Schuchat, J. D. Wenger, R. W. Pinner, C. V. Broome, and The Listeria Study Group.** 1992. Comparison of three selective enrichment methods for the isolation of *Listeria monocytogenes* from naturally contaminated foods. *J. Food Prot.* **55:**952–959.
32. **Heitmann M., P. Gerner-Smidt, and O. Heltberg.** 1997. Gastroenteritis caused by *Listeria monocytogenes* in a private day-care facility. *Pediatr. Infect. Dis. J.* **16:**827–828.
33. **Hof, H., T. Nichterlein, and M. Kretschmar.** 1997. Management of listeriosis. *Clin. Microbiol. Rev.* **10:**345–357.
34. **Jacquet, C., S. Aubert, N. El Sohl, and J. Rocourt.** 1992. Use of rRNA gene restriction patterns for the identification of *Listeria* species. *Syst. Appl. Microbiol.* **15:**42–46.
35. **Jacquet, C., J. Bille, and J. Rocourt.** 1992. Typing of *Listeria monocytogenes* by restriction fragment length polymorphism of the ribosomal ribonucleic acid gene region. *Zentralbl. Bakteriol. Mikrobiol. Hyg. Ser. A* **276:**356–365.
36. **Jaton, K., R. Sahli, and J. Bille.** 1992. Development of polymerase chain reaction assays for detection of *Listeria monocytogenes* in clinical cerebrospinal fluid samples. *J. Clin. Microbiol.* **30:**1931–1936.
37. **Jones, D.** 1986. Genus *Erysipelothrix* Rosenbach 1909, 367^{AL}, p. 1245–1249. *In* P. H. Sneath, N. S. Mair, M. E. Sharpe, and J. G. Holt (ed.), *Bergey's Manual of Systematic Bacteriology*, vol. 2. The Williams & Wilkins Co., Baltimore, Md.
38. **Jones, G. L. (ed.).** 1989. *Isolation and Identification of* Listeria monocytogenes. Centers for Disease Control, Atlanta, Ga.
39. **Kandler, O., and N. Weiss.** 1986. Regular, nonsporing Gram-positive rods, p. 1208–1209. *In* P. H. Sneath, N. S. Mair, M. E. Sharpe, and J. G. Holt (ed.), *Bergey's Manual of Systematic Bacteriology*, vol. 2. The Williams & Wilkins Co., Baltimore, Md.
40. **Keddie, R. M., and S. Shaw.** 1986. Genus *Kurthia* Trevisan 1885, 92^{AL}, p. 1255–1257. *In* P. H. Sneath, N. S. Mair, M. E. Sharpe, and J. G. Holt (ed.), *Bergey's Manual of Systematic Bacteriology*, vol. 2. The Williams & Wilkins Co., Baltimore, Md.
41. **Lee, W. H., and D. McClain.** 1986. Improved *Listeria monocytogenes* selective agar. *Appl. Environ. Microbiol.* **52:** 1215–1217.
42. **Linnan, M. J., L. Mascola, X. D. Lou, V. Goulet, S. May, C. Salminen, D. W. Hird, M. L. Yonekura, P. Hayes, R. Weaver, A. Audurier, B. D. Plikaytis, S. L. Fannin, A. Kleks, and C. V. Broome.** 1988. Epidemic listeriosis associated with Mexican-style cheese. *N. Engl. J. Med.* **319:** 823–828.
43. **Loessner, M. J.** 1991. Improved procedure for bacteriophage typing of *Listeria* strains and evaluation of new phages. *Appl. Environ. Microbiol.* **57:**882–884.
44. **Loessner, M. J., and M. Busse.** 1990. Bacteriophage typing of *Listeria* species. *Appl. Environ. Microbiol.* **56:**1912–1918.
45. **Ludwig, W., K.-H. Schleifer, and E. Stackebrandt.** 1984. 16S rRNA analysis of *Listeria monocytogenes* and *Brochothrix thermosphacta*. *FEMS Microbiol. Lett.* **25:**199–204.
46. **Makino, S.-L., Y. Okada, T. Maruyama, K. Ishikawa, T. Takahashi, M. Nakamura, T. Ezaki, and H. Morita.** 1994. Direct and rapid detection of *Erysipelothrix rhusiopathiae* DNA in animals by PCR. *J. Clin. Microbiol.* **32:** 1526–1531.
47. **McLauchlin, J., A. Audurier, and A. G. Taylor.** 1986. Aspects of the epidemiology of human *Listeria monocytogenes* infections in Britain 1967–1984; the use of serotyping and phage typing. *J. Med. Microbiol.* **22:**367–377.
48. **McLauchlin, J., S. M. Hall, S. K. Velani, and R. J. Gilbert.** 1991. Human listeriosis and paté: a possible association. *Br. Med. J.* **303:**773–775.
49. **Moellering, R. C., G. Medoff, I. Leech, C. Wennersten, and L. J. Kunz.** 1972. Antibiotic synergism against *Listeria monocytogenes*. *Antimicrob. Agents. Chemother.* **1:**30–34.
50. **Nash, P., and M. M. Krenz.** 1991. Culture media, p. 1226–1288. *In* A. Balows, W. J. Hausler, Jr., K. L. Herrmann, H. D. Isenberg, and H. J. Shadomy (ed.), *Manual of Clinical Microbiology*, 5th ed. American Society for Microbiology, Washington, D.C.
51. **Nieman, R. E., and B. Lorber.** 1980. Listeriosis in adults, a changing pattern: report of eight cases and a review of the literature, 1968–1978. *Rev. Infect. Dis.* **2:**207–227.
52. **Ninet, B., E. Bannerman, and J. Bille.** 1992. Assessment of the Accuprobe *Listeria monocytogenes* culture identification reagent kit for rapid colony confirmation and its application in various enrichment broths. *Appl. Environ. Microbiol.* **58:**4055–4059.
53. **Nocera, D., M. Altwegg, G. Martinetti Lucchini, E. Bannerman, F. Ischer, J. Rocourt, and J. Bille.** 1993. Characterization of *Listeria* strains from a foodborne listeriosis outbreak by rDNA gene restriction patterns compared to four other typing methods. *Eur. J. Clin. Microbiol. Infect. Dis.* **12:**162–169.
54. **Nocera, D., E. Bannerman, J. Rocourt, K. Jaton Ogay, and J. Bille.** 1990. Characterization by DNA restriction endonuclease analysis of *Listeria monocytogenes* strains related to the Swiss epidemic of listeriosis. *J. Clin. Microbiol.* **28:**2259–2263.
55. **O'Donoghue, K., K. Bowker, J. McLauchlin, D. S. Reeves, P. M. Bennett, and A. P. MacGowan.** 1995. Typing of *Listeria monocytogenes* by random amplified polymorphic DNA (RAPD) analysis. *Int. J. Food Microbiol.* **27:** 245–252.
56. **Okwumabua, O., B. Swaminathan, P. Edmonds, J. Wenger, J. Hogan, and M. Alden.** 1992. Evaluation of a chemiluminescent DNA probe assay for the rapid confirmation of *Listeria monocytogenes*. *Res. Microbiol.* **143:** 183–189.
57. **Piffaretti, J.-C., H. Kressebuch, M. Aeschbacher, J. Bille, E. Bannerman, J. M. Musser, R. K. Selander, and J. Rocourt.** 1989. Genetic characterization of clones of the bacterium *Listeria monocytogenes* causing epidemic disease. *Proc. Natl. Acad. Sci. USA* **86:**3818–3822.
58. **Pine, L., S. Kathariou, F. Quinn, V. George, J. D. Wenger, and R. E. Weaver.** 1991. Cytopathogenic effects in enterocytelike Caco-2 cells differentiate virulent from avirulent *Listeria* strains. *J. Clin. Microbiol.* **29:**990–996.
59. **Pinner, R. W., A. Schuchat, B. Swaminathan, P. S. Hayes, K. A. Deaver, R. E. Weaver, B. D. Plikaytis, M. Reeves, C. V. Broome, J. D. Wenger, and The Listeria Study Group.** 1992. Role of foods in sporadic listeriosis. II. A microbiologic and epidemiologic investigation. *JAMA* **267:**2046–2050.
60. **Reboli, A. C., and W. E. Farrar.** 1989. *Erysipelothrix rhusiopathiae*: an occupational pathogen. *Clin. Microbiol. Rev.* **2:** 354–359.
61. **Rocourt, J., A. Audurier, A. L. Courtieu, J. Durst, S. Ortel, A. Schrettenbrunner, and A. G. Taylor.** 1985. A multicenter study on the phage typing of *Listeria monocytogenes*. *Zentralbl. Bakteriol. Mikrobiol. Hyg. Ser. A* **259:** 489–497.
62. **Rocourt, J., U. Wehmeyer, and E. Stackebrandt.** 1987. Transfer of *Listeria denitrificans* to a new genus, *Jonesia denitrificans* comb. nov. *Int. J. Syst. Bacteriol.* **37:**266–270.
63. **Rocourt, J., P. Boerlin, F. Grimont, C. Jacquet, and J.-C. Piffaretti.** 1992. Assignment of *Listeria grayi* and *Listeria murrayi* to a single species, *Listeria grayi*, with a revised

description of *Listeria grayi*. *Int. J. Syst. Bacteriol.* **42:** 171–174.

64. **Rocourt, J., and P. Cossart.** 1997. *Listeria monocytogenes*, p. 337–352. *In* M. P. Doyle, L. R. Beuchat, and T. J. Montville (ed.), *Food Microbiology: Fundamentals and Frontiers*. ASM Press, Washington, D.C.
65. **Salamina, G., E. Dalle Donne, A. Niccolini, G. Poda, D. Cesaroni, M. Bucci, R. Fini, M. Maldini, A. Schuchat, B. Swaminathan, W. Bibb, J. Rocourt, N. Binkin, and S. Salmaso.** 1996. A foodborne outbreak of gastroenteritis involving *Listeria monocytogenes* in Northern Italy. *Epidemiol. Infect.* **117:**429–436.
66. **Scheld, W. M.** 1983. Evaluation of rifampin and other antibiotics against *Listeria monocytogenes* in vitro and in vivo. *Rev. Infect. Dis.* **5**(Suppl. 3)**:**S593–S599.
67. **Schlech, W. F., III, P. M. Lavigne, R. A. Bortolussi, A. C. Allen, E. V. Haldane, A. J. Wort, A. W. Hightower, S. E. Johnson, S. H. King, E. S. Nicholls, and C. V. Broome.** 1983. Epidemic listeriosis—evidence for transmission by food. *N. Engl. J. Med.* **308:**203–206.
68. **Schuchat, A., C. Lizano, C. V. Broome, B. Swaminathan, C. Kim, and K. Winn.** 1991. Outbreak of neonatal listeriosis associated with mineral oil. *Pediatr. Infect. Dis. J.* **10:** 183–189.
69. **Schuchat, A., B. Swaminathan, and C. V. Broome.** 1991. Epidemiology of human listeriosis. *Clin. Microbiol. Rev.* **4:** 169–183.
70. **Seeliger, H. P. R., and K. Hohne.** 1979. Serotyping of *Listeria monocytogenes* and related species. *Methods Microbiol.* **13:**31–49.
71. **Seeliger, H. P. R. and D. Jones.** 1986. Genus *Listeria* Pirie, 1940, 383[AL], p. 1235–1245. *In* P. H. Sneath, N. S. Mair, M. E. Sharp, and J. G. Holt (ed.), *Bergey's Manual of Systematic Bacteriology*, vol. 2. The Williams & Wilkins Co., Baltimore, Md.
72. **Stelma, G. N., A. L. Reyes, J. T. Peeler, D. W. Francis, J. M. Hunt, P. L. Spaulding, C. H. Johnson, and J. Lovett.** 1987. Pathogenicity test for *Listeria monocytogenes* using immunocompromised mice. *J. Clin. Microbiol.* **25:** 2085–2089.
73. **Takahashi, T., T. Fujisawa, Y. Tamura, S. Suzuki, M. Muramatsu, T. Sawada, Y. Benno, and T. Mitsuoka.** 1992. DNA relatedness among *Erysipelothrix rhusiopathiae* strains representing all twenty-three serovars and *Erysipelothrix tonsillarum*. *Int. J. Syst. Bacteriol.* **42:**469–473.
74. **van Netten, P., I. Perales, A. van de Moosdijk, G. D. W. Curtis, and D. A. A. Mossel.** 1989. Liquid and solid differential media for the detection and enumeration of *Listeria monocytogenes* and other *Listeria* spp. *Int. J. Food Microbiol.* **8:**299–316.
75. **Weaver, R. E.** 1985. *Erysipelothrix*, p. 209–210. *In* E. H. Lennette, A. Balows, W. J. Hausler, Jr., and H. J. Shadomy (ed.), *Manual of Clinical Microbiology*, 4th ed. American Society for Microbiology, Washington, D.C.
76. **Welshimer, H. J., and A. L. Meredith.** 1971. *Listeria murrayi*: a nitrate-reducing mannitol-fermenting *Listeria*. *Int. J. Syst. Bacteriol.* **21:**3–7.
77. **Wernars, K., P. Boerlin, A. Audurier, E. G. Russell, G. D. W. Curtis, L. Herman, and V. van der Mee-Marquet.** 1996. The WHO multicenter study on *Listeria monocytogenes* subtyping: random amplification of polymorphic DNA (RAPD). *Int. J. Food Microbiol.* **32:**325–341.
78. **Wiggins, G. L., W. L. Albritton, and J. C. Feeley.** 1978. Antibiotic susceptibility of clinical isolates of *Listeria monocytogenes*. *Antimicrob. Agents. Chemother.* **12:**854–860.

Bacillus and Recently Derived Genera*

NIALL A. LOGAN AND PETER C. B. TURNBULL

23

TAXONOMY

The family *Bacillaceae* accommodates a diversity of endospore-forming bacteria which range from obligate aerobes to strict anaerobes, from rods to cocci, from psychrophiles to thermophiles, and from alkaliphiles to acidophiles. The most familiar groups are *Bacillus* and *Clostridium*, but these genera, especially, encompass great diversity, and both have recently undergone subdivision.

The need for subdividing *Bacillus* has long been recognized from its DNA base composition range of 32 to 69 mol% G+C and the arrangements that have emerged from numerical taxonomies of phenotypic data (35). Studies with 16S rRNA have now allowed a start to be made on breaking the genus down into more manageable and better-defined groups (3, 45). So far, five new genera have been proposed: *Alicyclobacillus* (58), which contains three species of thermoacidophiles; *Paenibacillus* (4), containing 20 species and including organisms formerly called *Bacillus polymyxa*, *Bacillus macerans*, *Bacillus alvei*, and the honey bee pathogens *Bacillus larvae* and *Bacillus pulvifaciens* (now both subspecies of *Paenibacillus larvae* [23]); *Brevibacillus* (46), containing 10 species and including organisms formerly called *Bacillus brevis* and *Bacillus laterosporus; Aneurinibacillus* (46), with *Aneurinibacillus aneurinilyticus* and two other species; and *Virgibacillus* (25) with *Virgibacillus pantothenticus* and one other species. Further proposals are likely to include a genus to accommodate the thermophile *Bacillus stearothermophilus* and related species. The long-established genus *Sporosarcina* contains the motile, spore-forming coccus *Sporosarcina ureae*, which is closely related to *Bacillus sphaericus*. A more distantly related species, *Sporosarcina halophila*, has been placed in a new genus, *Halobacillus* (49), along with two new species of spore-forming halophilic rods. Another new genus, *Amphibacillus*, was proposed in 1990 for three strains of catalase-negative, facultatively anaerobic endospore formers (40).

Bacillus continues to accommodate the best-known species such as *Bacillus subtilis* (the type species), *Bacillus anthracis*, *Bacillus cereus*, *Bacillus licheniformis*, *Bacillus megaterium*, *Bacillus pumilus*, *B. sphaericus*, and *Bacillus thuringiensis*. With 50 valid species, it remains a large genus. Many of its species fall into several apparently distinct rRNA sequence groups such as the "*B. subtilis* group," the "*B. cereus* group," and the "*B. sphaericus* group," but although such divisions may also be phenotypically distinguishable, intermediate organisms may make satisfactory subdivision difficult. New species of aerobic endospore formers are regularly described (41 were described between 1993 and mid-1997, during which period only four proposals for merging species had been made), but often on the basis of information for very few strains.

DESCRIPTIONS OF THE GENERA

The production of resistant endospores in the presence of oxygen remains the defining feature for the genus *Bacillus*, and this character also applies to the new genera *Alicyclobacillus*, *Aneurinibacillus*, *Brevibacillus*, *Halobacillus*, *Paenibacillus*, and *Virgibacillus*. Sporangial morphology remains a valuable character in identification (see Fig. 2).

Members are gram-positive (in young cultures) but sometimes gram-variable or frankly gram-negative, rod-shaped, endospore-forming organisms which may be aerobic or facultatively anaerobic. They are mostly catalase positive and may be motile by means of peritrichous flagella. Most species are mesophilic, but *Bacillus* contains some thermophiles and psychrophiles, and *Paenibacillus* contains one psychrophilic species. Because *Alicyclobacillus* species are thermoacidophilic and *Halobacillus* strains are moderately halophilic, such organisms are unlikely to be isolated in a clinical laboratory, and so these two genera will not be considered further.

Unfortunately, taxonomic progress has not revealed readily determinable features characteristic of each genus. However, *Paenibacillus* species tend to produce swollen sporangia with ellipsoidal spores, and most *Aneurinibacillus* and *Brevibacillus* species produce acid from very few carbohydrates. *Bacillus* shows a wide range of sporangial morphologies and carbohydrate test patterns. A further difficulty is that many recently described species represent genomic groups disclosed by DNA-DNA pairing experiments, and routine phenotypic characters for distinguishing some of them are very few and of unproven value.

NATURAL HABITATS

Most *Bacillus*, *Aneurinibacillus*, *Brevibacillus*, *Paenibacillus*, and *Virgibacillus* species are saprophytes widely distributed

* This chapter contains information presented in chapter 28 by Peter C. B. Turnbull and John M. Kramer in the sixth edition of this Manual.

in the natural environment, but some species are opportunistic or obligate pathogens of animals, including humans, other mammals, and insects. The main habitats are soils of all kinds, ranging from acid to alkaline, hot to cold, and fertile to desert, and the water columns and bottom deposits of fresh and marine waters. Their spores readily survive distribution in soils, dusts, and aerosols from these natural environments to a wide variety of other habitats. Dried foods such as spices, milk powders, and farinaceous products are often quite heavily contaminated with spores. *B. anthracis* is, for all intents and purposes, an obligate pathogen of animals and humans; if it ever multiplies in the environment, it probably does so only rarely. Its close relative, *B. cereus*, is now well established as an opportunistic pathogen, and other aerobic endospore formers can also, from time to time, be opportunistic pathogens. Six organisms are important as insect pathogens: *B. thuringiensis* (another close relative of *B. anthracis*), *Bacillus popilliae*, *Bacillus lentimorbus*, *B. sphaericus*, and the two *P. larvae* subspecies.

CLINICAL SIGNIFICANCE

The majority of aerobic endospore formers apparently have little or no pathogenic potential and are rarely associated with disease in humans or other animals. The principal exceptions to this are *B. anthracis* and *B. cereus*, but other species, particularly those of the *B. subtilis* group, have been implicated in food poisoning and other human and animal infections. The resistance of the spores to heat, radiation, disinfectants, and desiccation also results in troublesome contaminations of operating rooms, surgical dressings, pharmaceutical products, and foods.

B. anthracis

Anthrax remains the best-known clinical condition caused by a *Bacillus* species. It is primarily a disease of herbivores, and before an effective vaccine became available in the 1930s, anthrax was one of the foremost causes of mortality in such animals worldwide. Humans contract anthrax directly or indirectly from animals. The development and application of veterinary and human vaccines, together with improvements in factory hygiene, sterilization procedures for imported animal products, and increased use of artificial alternatives to animal hides or hair, have resulted in marked declines in anthrax cases, but the disease continues to be endemic in countries that lack efficient vaccination policies. Because the spores survive in soil for many years, *B. anthracis* is exceedingly difficult to eradicate from areas where it is endemic, and regions where *B. anthracis* is not endemic must be alert for the arrival of the organism in imported animal products.

In comparison with herbivores, humans are moderately resistant to anthrax. Human anthrax is traditionally classified as either (i) nonindustrial, resulting from close contact with infected animals or their carcasses after death from the disease, or (ii) industrial, as acquired by those employed in the processing of wool, hair, hides, bones, or other animal products. Nonindustrial cases are usually cutaneous infections, but *B. anthracis* meningitis (32, 51) and intestinal anthrax are occasionally reported (33). Industrial anthrax is also usually cutaneous, but the pulmonary form can result from inhalation of spore-laden dust. A few reports of laboratory-acquired infections exist (43). Cutaneous cases account for 95 to 99% of human cases of anthrax worldwide. The disease is of the point-source type, and direct human-to-human transmission is exceedingly rare; direct animal-to-animal transmission within a species (i.e., excluding the case of carnivores feeding on meat from anthrax-infected carcasses) is likewise very rare. *B. anthracis* is always high on the list of potential agents in discussions of biological warfare. Unfortunately, this has attached an unjustified doomsday image to the natural disease, because nature cannot remotely emulate the overwhelmingly massive exposures that could be created artificially for human warfare.

Cutaneous infection occurs through a break in the skin, and so the lesions generally occur on exposed regions of the body. Fewer than 20% of untreated cases of cutaneous anthrax are fatal, and the rare fatalities seen today either follow obstruction of the airways by the extensive edema which may accompany face and neck lesions or are sequelae of secondary cellulitis or meningitis. The intestinal and pulmonary forms are more often fatal because they go unrecognized until it is beyond the time for effective therapy.

The incubation period for cutaneous anthrax is generally 2 to 3 days, with extremes of approximately 12 h to 2 weeks. Initially, a small pimple or papule appears; and over the next 24 h a ring of vesicles develops around it, and it ulcerates, dries, and blackens into the characteristic eschar. The eschar enlarges, becoming thick and adherent to underlying tissues over the ensuing week. The lesion is surrounded by edema which may be very extensive. Pus and pain are normally absent; their presence or the presence of marked lymphangitis and fever probably indicates secondary bacterial infection.

Intestinal anthrax is essentially cutaneous anthrax occurring on the intestinal mucosa, and it usually results from eating meat from an anthrax-infected carcass. Mild gastroenteritis symptoms may be followed by vomiting, fever, abdominal pain, hematemesis, bloody diarrhea, and massive ascites in the last hours of life. In pulmonary anthrax, the inhaled spores are carried from the lungs by macrophages to the lymphatic system, where they germinate and multiply, ultimately leading to fatal septicemia. Prior to the onset of the final, hyperacute phase, symptoms are insidious and nonspecific, lasting for 1 to a few days.

In any patients with fatal anthrax, generalized symptoms may be mild (fatigue, malaise, and slight fever) or absent prior to the sudden onset of acute illness; this is characterized by dyspnea, cyanosis, severe pyrexia, and disorientation followed by circulatory failure, shock, coma, and death, all within a few hours. Depending somewhat on the host species, there is a rapid buildup of the bacteria in the blood over the last few hours, with terminal levels of 10^7 to 10^9/ml in the most-susceptible species. Considerable progress is being made in elucidating the manner in which the toxin of *B. anthracis* produces the signs and symptoms of the disease (44).

Opportunistic Pathogens

Opportunistic infections with *Bacillus* species other than *B. anthracis* have been reported since the late 19th century. A common feature of such reports, right up to the present, has been emphasis on the importance of interpreting isolates of *Bacillus* in the light of any other species cultured and the clinical context, and the danger of dismissing them as mere contaminants. Case histories continue to warrant published reports because investigators feel that awareness needs to be improved. In the case of posttraumatic endophthalmitis, *Bacillus* species, particularly *B. cereus*, may be the second most commonly isolated organisms after *Staphylococcus epidermidis* (15). For reviews of reports, see references 8, 19, 33, and 41.

B. cereus Group

B. cereus is next in importance to *B. anthracis* as a pathogen of humans (and other animals), causing food-borne illness and opportunistic infections, and its ubiquity ensures that cases are not uncommon.

In relation to food-borne illness, *B. cereus* is the etiological agent of two distinct food-poisoning syndromes. (i) The diarrheal type, caused by a heat-labile enterotoxic complex and characterized by abdominal pain with diarrhea 8 to 16 h after ingestion of the contaminated food, is associated with a diversity of foods from meats and vegetable dishes to pastas, desserts, cakes, sauces, and milk (31). (ii) The emetic type, caused by a heat-stable enterotoxin, and characterized by nausea and vomiting 1 to 5 h after eating the offending food, is predominantly associated with Oriental rice dishes, although occasionally other foods such as pasteurized cream, milk pudding, pastas, and reconstituted formulas have been implicated (31). Fulminant liver failure associated with the emetic toxin has been reported (38). Both syndromes arise from *B. cereus* spores that have survived cooking and that have then germinated, producing vegetative cells that have multiplied during storage. Strains of *Bacillus mycoides* and *B. thuringiensis*, which are close relatives of *B. cereus*, may also produce the diarrheal toxin, and *B. thuringiensis* has indeed been implicated in cases of gastroenteritis (14).

The toxigenic basis of *B. cereus* food poisoning and other infections is beginning to be understood (6, 47), but no toxins or other virulence factors have yet been identified to account for symptoms periodically associated with other *Bacillus* species.

B. cereus is also a virulent and destructive ocular pathogen, and it is fortunate that cases are rare. Endophthalmitis is the most serious condition; it may follow penetrating trauma of the eye or hematogenous spread, and it evolves very rapidly. Its rarity means that prompt and appropriate treatment may be instituted too late, and loss both of vision and of the eye is usual (15). Other infections occur mainly in persons predisposed by neoplastic disease, immunosuppression, alcoholism or other drug abuse, or some other underlying condition, and they include bacteremia, septicemia, meningitis, brain hemorrhage, endocarditis, pneumonia, empyema, pleurisy, lung abscess, brain abscess, osteomyelitis, salpingitis, and primary cutaneous infections. Wound infections, mostly in otherwise healthy persons, have been reported following surgery, road traffic and other accidents, scalds, burns, and plaster fixation and in umbilical stumps; some became necrotic and gangrenous, and one burn infection was fatal (19). There have been reports of wound, burn, and ocular infections with *B. thuringiensis* (14).

Other Species

Reports of infections with non-*B. cereus* group species are comparatively rare, but the infections are very diverse (8, 19, 33, 41). *B. licheniformis* has been reported from ventriculitis following the removal of a meningioma, cerebral abscess after penetrating orbital injury, septicemia following arteriography, bacteremia during pregnancy with eclampsia and acute fibrinolysis, peritonitis with bacteremia in an immunologically normal person with volvulus and small-bowel perforation, and ophthalmitis and corneal ulcer after trauma. This organism has often been isolated in association with bovine and ovine abortion. There have also been reports of L-form organisms, phenotypically similar to *B. licheniformis*, occurring in human blood and other body fluids. There is strong circumstantial evidence that *B. licheniformis* can cause a food-borne diarrheal illness (8, 33).

The name *B. subtilis* was often used to mean any aerobic, endospore-forming organism, but since 1970 there have been reports of infection in which identification of this species appears to have been made accurately. They include cases associated with neoplastic disease (fatal pneumonia and bacteremia, a septicemia, and an infection of a necrotic axillary tumor in breast cancer patients), breast prosthesis and ventriculoatrial shunt infections, endocarditis in a drug abuser, and surgical wound-drainage sites. *B. subtilis* has also been implicated in food-borne illness and cases of bovine mastitis and ovine abortion (8, 33).

Organisms identified as *Bacillus circulans* have been isolated from patients with meningitis, a cerebrospinal fluid shunt infection, and endocarditis; a wound infection in a cancer patient; and a patient with a bite wound. *Bacillus coagulans* has been isolated from a corneal infection and a bacteremia and in association with a bovine abortion. *B. pumilus* has been found in cases of pustule and rectal fistula infection and in association with bovine mastitis. *B. sphaericus* has been implicated in a fatal lung pseudotumor and meningitis (8, 33).

B. brevis has been isolated from corneal infection and has been implicated in several incidents of food poisoning; since these reports, the species has been split (see the section Taxonomy above) and transferred to the new genus *Brevibacillus*. Strains of the new species, *Brevibacillus agri*, have been isolated in association with an outbreak of waterborne illness in Sweden, and other *Brevibacillus* species have been found in human blood and bronchoalveolar lavage specimens. *Brevibacillus laterosporus* has been reported in association with a severe case of endophthalmitis (8, 33).

Paenibacillus alvei has been isolated from patients with meningitis, a prosthetic hip infection in a patient with sickle cell anemia, and a wound infection, and in association with *Clostridium perfringens* from a patient with gas gangrene. *Paenibacillus macerans* has been isolated from a wound infection following removal of a malignant melanoma and in association with a bovine abortion, and *Paenibacillus polymyxa* has been isolated in association with an ovine abortion (33).

COLLECTION, TRANSPORT, AND STORAGE OF SPECIMENS

For the isolation of species other than *B. anthracis* from clinical specimens, no special precautions are needed, and the specimens can be collected, transported, and cultivated in the normal way. Aerobic endospore formers are quite hardy and usually survive transport to the laboratory either in freshly collected specimens or in a standard transport medium.

Safety Aspects in Relation to Anthrax

Despite its frightening reputation, anthrax is not highly contagious. Cutaneous anthrax is readily treated and is life-threatening only in exceptional cases; the infectious doses in the human pulmonary and intestinal forms (which are also treatable if they are recognized early) are generally very high (50% lethal dose, >10,000 spores). Precautions therefore need to be sensible, not extreme (see also chapter 9).

When collecting specimens related to suspected anthrax, disposable gloves, disposable apron or overalls, and disinfectable boots should be worn. If dusty samples suspected of harboring high numbers of anthrax spores are involved, the use of headgear and dust masks should be considered. Disposable items should be discarded in suitable containers for autoclaving followed by incineration. Nonautoclavable items should be immersed overnight in 10 to 30% formalin (4 to 12% formaldehyde solution, according to the perceived extent of spore contamination). Items that cannot be so immersed should be placed in bags for transfer to a formaldehyde fumigation facility. Formalin is also the best disinfectant for specimen spillages; when this is considered impractical, 10% hypochlorite solution can be used (55).

Human Anthrax

In all cases, specimens from possible sources of the infection (carcasses, hides, hair, bones, etc.) should be sought.

Cutaneous Anthrax

Swabs are appropriate for collecting the vesicular exudate found in early lesions. In the well-formed eschar where vesicular exudate is absent, the edge of the eschar should be lifted up with forceps and fluid should be obtained by application of a capillary tube under the edge. Adequate material should be submitted for both culture and a M'Fadyean-stained smear.

Intestinal Anthrax

Anthrax will be suspected only if an adequate history of the patient is known. If the patient is not severely ill, a fecal specimen may be collected. However, isolation of *B. anthracis* may not be successful. If the patient is severely ill, blood should also be cultured, although isolation of *B. anthracis* may not be possible after antimicrobial treatment. A M'Fadyean-stained blood smear may reveal the capsulate rods, or if treatment has been initiated, capsule "ghosts" may be visible. Postmortem blood collected by venipuncture (a characteristic of anthrax is nonclotting blood at death) should be examined by M'Fadyean-stained smear and culture. Any hemorrhagic fluid from the nose, mouth, or anus should be cultured. If these are positive, no further specimens are needed. If these are negative, specimens of peritoneal fluid, spleen, and/or mesenteric lymph nodes, aspirated by techniques that avoid the spillage of fluids, may be collected for smear and culture. Histology is optional and probably only of academic interest.

Pulmonary Anthrax

Again, anthrax will be suspected only if the history of the patient suggests it. Unless the patient is severely ill, immediate specimen collection is probably unnecessary and the person should be treated and simply observed; paired serum specimens (obtained when the patient is first seen and >10 days later) may be useful for confirmation of the diagnosis. The approach given for intestinal anthrax should be followed for blood specimens obtained from severely ill patients and those obtained postmortem.

Novel Tests

The M'Fadyean polychrome methylene blue staining method has proved to be a remarkably successful rapid diagnostic test since 1903. However, with the increasing rarity of the disease in developed countries, reliable stain is difficult to obtain. An excellent alternative, a rapid immunochromatographic, on-site test, has been developed at the Naval Medical Research Laboratory, Bethesda, Md. (10), but it is not yet commercially available. PCR methods are available in specialist laboratories for confirmation of virulent isolates, but as yet, procedures for direct diagnosis have not been fully developed.

Animal Anthrax

Anthrax should be considered the possible cause of death in herbivorous animals which have died suddenly and unexpectedly, particularly if hemorrhage from the nose, mouth, or anus has occurred and if death has taken place at a site with *any* history of anthrax.

Carcasses 1 to 2 Days Old

Due to the nonclotting nature of blood in anthrax victims, it is usually possible to aspirate a few drops of blood from a vein, with which (i) a M'Fadyean-stained smear and (ii) a direct plate culture on blood agar may be made.

When cervical edema is present, smears and cultures of fluid aspirated from the enlarged mandibular and suprapharyngeal lymph nodes should be made. In porcine intestinal anthrax, which may be obvious only at necropsy, organisms are usually visible in stained smears made from mesenteric lymph nodes, but they are usually not visible in blood smears.

Older Putrefying Carcasses

B. anthracis competes poorly with putrefactive organisms and may not be visible in smears after 2 to 3 days, and culture is necessary for confirmation of the diagnosis. Sections of tissue or any blood-stained material should be collected. If the animal has been opened, spleen or lymph node specimens should be taken. The best specimens may be soil samples taken from beneath the nose and anus, where they have been contaminated with the terminal hemorrhagic exudate.

Other Specimens

Tests for the presence of *B. anthracis* may be requested for a variety of specimens, such as animal products from regions of endemicity, soil or other materials from old burial or tannery sites, or other materials associated with outbreaks (e.g., sewage sludge). At present, culture by the selective agar techniques described below is the only available approach.

ISOLATION PROCEDURES

All the clinically significant isolates reported to date are of species that grow and often sporulate on routine laboratory media such as blood agar at 37°C. It seems unlikely that many clinically important but more fastidious strains are being missed for the want of special media or growth conditions. Maintenance is simple if spores can be obtained, but it is a mistake to assume that a primary culture or subculture on blood agar will automatically yield spores if it is stored on the bench or in the incubator. It is best to grow the organism on nutrient agar containing 5 mg of manganese sulfate per liter for a few days and refrigerate the culture when microscopy shows that most cells have sporulated. For most species, sporulated cultures on slants of this medium, sealed after incubation, can survive in a refrigerator for years. Alternatively, slopes can be frozen at −70°C or cultures can be lyophilized.

Normally Sterile Specimens

Aerobic endospore formers are usually easily recoverable on blood or nutrient agar after overnight incubation at 37°C.

Specimens with Mixed Microflora

In specimens submitted for food-poisoning investigations or for isolation of *B. anthracis* from old carcasses, animal products, or environmental specimens, the organisms will mostly be present as spores. Heating at 62.5°C for 15 min will both heat shock the spores and effectively destroy non-spore-forming contaminants (solid samples should first be emulsified in sterile, deionized water; 1:2 [wt/vol]). An alternative is to "alcohol shock" the spore by adding filter-sterilized 95 to 100% ethanol to a final concentration of 1:1 (vol/vol) and holding the spores for 30 to 60 min at room temperature. Direct plate cultures are made on blood, nutrient, or selective agar, as appropriate, by spreading up to 250-μl volumes of the undiluted treated sample and 10-, 100-, and 1,000-fold dilutions of the treated sample.

Enrichment procedures are generally inappropriate for isolations from clinical specimens; exceptions include searches for *B. anthracis* in old specimens or *B. cereus* in stool specimens more than 3 days after a food-poisoning episode. In these circumstances, enrichment may be carried out by adding nutrient or tryptic soy broth with polymyxin B (100,000 U/liter) to the heat-treated (not ethanol-treated) specimen.

The best selective medium for *B. anthracis* is polymyxin B-lysozyme EDTA-thallous acetate (PLET) agar (30, 41, 42). For environmental specimens, animal products, or specimens from old carcasses, spread 0.25-ml aliquots of the undiluted heat- or alcohol-treated suspension and 1:10, 1:100, and 1:1,000 dilutions of the heat- or alcohol-treated suspension of the specimen across PLET agar plates. These are best read after incubation at 37°C for 36 to 40 h. Roughly circular, creamy white colonies of 1 to 3 mm in diameter with a ground-glass texture are subcultured on (i) blood agar plates to test for gamma phage and penicillin susceptibility and for hemolysis and (ii) directly or subsequently in blood to look for capsule production.

Several selective agars have been designed for the isolation, identification, and enumeration of *B. cereus* (56). The essential ingredients of these are egg yolk, mannitol, and an indicator, exploiting the lecithin-hydrolyzing but mannitol-negative nature of *B. cereus*. Pyruvate and polymyxin may be included for further selectivity. Three satisfactory formulations are mannitol, egg yolk, and polymyxin B agar; polymyxin B, egg yolk, mannitol, and bromthymol blue agar; and *Bacillus cereus* medium (56). There are no selective media for other aerobic endospore formers, but spores can be selected for by heat or alcohol treatment. If a suspension of part of the specimen is held at 80°C for 10 min, the vegetative cells of both spore formers and non-spore formers will be killed, but the heat-resistant spores not only will survive but may be heat shocked into subsequent germination. The other part of the specimen is cultivated without heat treatment in case the endospore formers are present only in the vegetative phase or the spores are very heat sensitive (in the latter case, alcohol treatment may help). This approach is not appropriate for human specimens because spores may be sparse or absent.

IDENTIFICATION

Before attempting to identify an organism to the species level, it is important to establish that any suspect isolate really is an aerobic endospore former and that other kinds of inclusions are not being mistaken for spores. A Gram-stained smear showing gram-positive cells with unstained areas suggestive of spores can be stripped of oil with acetone-alcohol, washed, and then stained for spores. While the KOH (22) and L-alanine-4-nitroanilide (11) tests are valuable for rapid determination of the Gram reaction, microscopy is still necessary to confirm that the organism is a spore former. Phase-contrast microscopy (at a ×1,000 magnification) should be used if available, as it is greatly superior to and much more convenient than spore staining. Sporangial morphology should be observed at the same time, because it is most valuable in routine identification (see Fig. 2). Spores are larger, more phase bright, and more regular in shape, size, and position than other kinds of inclusions such as poly-β-hydroxybutyrate (PHB) granules (see Fig. 2d).

Members of the *B. cereus* group (*B. anthracis*, *B. cereus*, *B. mycoides*, and *B. thuringiensis*) and *B. megaterium* will produce large amounts of storage material when they are grown on carbohydrate media, but on routine media this vacuolate or foamy appearance is rarely sufficiently pronounced to cause confusion. Isolates of other organisms have occasionally been submitted to reference laboratories as *Bacillus* species because they were large, aerobic, gram-positive rods, even though sporulation had not been observed or because PHB granules or other storage inclusions had been mistaken for spores.

Bacillus contains facultative anaerobes as well as strict aerobes, and this can be a valuable characteristic in identification. For example, *B. licheniformis* and *B. subtilis*, which have very similar colonial (see Fig. 1j) and microscopic (see Fig. 2e) morphologies, are facultatively anaerobic and strictly aerobic, respectively; likewise, the two large-celled species *B. cereus* and *B. megaterium* (see Fig. 2b and d) are facultatively anaerobic and strictly aerobic, respectively. This may be tested for with anaerobically incubated plate cultures with aerobic controls.

In the most widely used diagnostic scheme for *Bacillus* species (21), 18 species were split into three groups according to their sporangial morphologies and were then further divided by biochemical and physiological tests. Although this approach was effective, identification was still complicated, owing to the need for special media and problems of between-strain variation, but much of the latter was a reflection of unsatisfactory taxonomy. Logan and Berkeley (36) addressed these problems with a large database for 38 clearly defined taxa using miniaturized tests in the API 20E and 50CHB systems (bioMérieux, Marcy l'Etoile, France), and this is in common use. bioMérieux also offers a *Bacillus* card for the Vitek automated identification system. However, because many new species have been proposed since these schemes were established and the phenotypic groupings that they used do not always correlate with the current, phylogenetically led classification, updated API and Vitek databases need to be prepared. Biolog (Biolog Inc., Hayward, Calif.) also offers a *Bacillus* database. The effectiveness of such kits can vary with the genera and species of aerobic endospore formers concerned, but they are improving with continuing development and increased databases. It should be stressed that their use should always be preceded by the appropriate basic characterization tests described below, principally spore and colony characteristics, motility, hemolysis, and the egg yolk reaction.

Other approaches include chemotaxonomic fingerprinting by fatty acid methyl ester (FAME) profiling, polyacrylamide gel electrophoresis analysis, pyrolysis mass spectrometry, and Fourier-transform infrared spectroscopy. All these approaches have been successfully applied either across the genera or to small groups. As with genotypic profiling methods, large databases of authentic strains are necessary; some of these are commercially available, such as the Microbial Identification System software (Microbial ID Inc., Newark, Del.) database for FAME analysis.

From the point of view of the routine diagnostic labora-

TABLE 1 Characters for differentiating reactive *Bacillus*, *Paenibacillus*, and *Virgibacillus* species[a]

Character[b]	*Bacillus*															*Paenibacillus*				
	B. subtilis group				*B. cereus* group					*B. circulans* group										
	B. subtilis	*B. amyloliquefaciens*	*B. licheniformis*	*B. pumilus*	*B. cereus*[c]	*B. anthracis*	*B. thuringiensis*	*B. mycoides*	*B. megaterium*	*B. circulans*	*B. firmus*	*B. lentus*	*B. coagulans*	*B. stearothermophilus*	*B. thermodenitrificans*	*P. polymyxa*	*P. alvei*	*P. macerans*	*P. validus*	*Virgibacillus pantothenticus*
Rod mean diameter (μm)	0.8	0.8	0.8	0.7	1.4	1.3	1.4	1.3	1.5	0.8	0.8	0.8	0.8	0.9	0.8	0.9	0.8	0.7	0.8	0.6
Chains of cells	(−)	(+)	(+)	−	+	+	+	+	+	−	−	(+)	v	−	v	−	(−)	−	−	+
Motility	+	+	+	+	+	−	+	−	+	+	+	+	+	+	−	+	+	+	+	+
Sporangia[d]																				
Spore shape	E	E	E(C)	C,E	E(C) [E]	E	E(C)	E	E,S	E	E	E	E	E	E	E	E(C)	E	E	E,S
Spore position	S,C	S,T	S,C	S,C	S,C	S	S	S(C)	S,C	S,T	S(C)	S,C	S,T	S,T	S	S,C	S,C	S,T	S,T	S,T
Sporangium swollen	−	−	−	−	−	−	−	−	−	+	v	v	+	+	−	+	+	+	+	+
Parasporal crystals	−	−	−	−	−	−	+	−	−	−	−	−	−	−	−	−	−	−	−	−
Parasporal bodies	−	−	−	−	−	−	−	−	−	−	−	−	−	−	−	−	−	−	−	−
Anaerobic growth	−	−	+	−	+	+	+	+	−	+	−	−	+	−	−	+	+	+	−	+
Growth at:																				
50°C	v	v	+	v	−	−	−	−	−	−	−	−	+	+	+	−	−	v	v	v
65°C	−	−	−	−	−	−	−	−	−	−	−	−	−	+	+	−	−	−	−	−
Egg yolk reaction	−	−	−	−	+	+	+	+	−	−	−	−	−	−	−	−	−	−	−	−
Casein hydrolysis	+	+	+	+	+	+	+	+	+	−	+	v	v	(+)	(−)	+	+	−	−	+
Starch hydrolysis	+	+	+	−	+	+	+	+	+	+	+	+	+	+	+	+	+	+	+	+
Arginine dihydrolase	−	−	+	−	v[(−)]	−	+	v	−	(−)	−	−	v	−	−	−	−	−	−	(−)
Indole production	−	−	−	−	−	−	−	−	−	−	−	−	−	−	−	−	+	−	−	−
Gelatin hydrolysis	+	+	+	+	+	(+)	+	+	+	−	v	v	−	+	+	+	+	v	−	+
Nitrate reduction	+	+	+	−	(+)[+]	+	+	(+)	−	v	(+)	(+)	(−)	v	(+)	v	−	−	v	v
Gas from carbohydrates	−	−	−	−	−	−	−	−	−	−	−	−	−	−	−	+	−	+	−	−
Acid from:																				
D-Arabinose	−	−	−	−	−	−	−	−	−	−	−	−	−	−	−	−	−	+	−	+
Glycerol	+	+	+	+	+[v]	−	+	+	+	v	−	v	+	(+)	v	+	+	+	+	+
Glycogen	+	+	+	−	+[−]	+	+	+	+	+	−	v	−	+	−	+	v	+	v	−
Inulin	(+)	−	v	−	−	−	−	−	+	(+)	−	(−)	−	−	−	+	−	+	v	−
Mannitol	+	+	+	+	−	−	−	−	+	+	v	(+)	v	−	v	+	−	+	+	−
Salicin	+	+	+	+	+[−]	−	(+)	(+)	+	+	−	+	+	(−)	v	+	v	+	−	+
D-Trehalose	+	+	+	+	+	+	+	+	+	+	v	(+)	+	+	+	+	v	+	+	+

[a] Symbols and abbreviations: +, >85% positive; (+), 75 to 84% positive; v, variable (26 to 74% positive); (−), 16 to 25% positive; −, 0 to 15% positive.

[b] Arginine dihydrolase, indole production, gelatin hydrolysis, and nitrate reduction reactions were determined by using the tests in the API 20E strip. Acid from carbohydrate reactions were determined by using the API 50CHB system.

[c] Reactions shown in brackets are for the biotype isolated particularly in connection with outbreaks of emetic-type food poisoning and for strains of serovars 1, 3, 5, and 8, which are commonly associated with such outbreaks.

[d] Spore shape: C, cylindrical; E, ellipsoidal; S, spherical. Spore position: C, central or paracentral; S, subterminal; T, terminal. The commonest shapes and positions are listed first, and those given in parentheses are infrequently observed.

tory, the aerobic endospore formers comprise two groups: the reactive ones that will give positive results in various routine biochemical tests (and which are therefore more amenable to identification) and the nonreactive ones that give few if any positive results in such tests. Nonreactive isolates tend to dominate the identification requests sent to reference laboratories. Tables 1 and 2, largely based upon data for strains proven to be authentic, show reactions for some species belonging to both of these groups. Either or both of the identification approaches of Gordon et al. (21) and the API system outlined above may be used in conjunction with the tables. Characters for identifying other species may be found in references 13, 24, 26, and 36.

B. cereus Group

Colonies of *B. cereus* and its relatives are very variable but are readily recognized (Fig. 1a to c). They are characteristically large (2 to 7 mm in diameter) and vary in shape from circular to irregular, with entire to undulate, crenate, or fimbriate edges; they have matte or granular textures. Smooth and moist colonies are not uncommon, however. The minimum temperature for growth is between 15 and 20°C, and the maximum temperature for growth is between 40 and 45°C, with the optimum being about 37°C. Although colonies of *B. anthracis* and *B. cereus* can be very similar in appearance, those of the former are generally smaller and nonhemolytic, may show more spiking or tailing along the lines of inoculation streaks, and are very tenacious compared with the usually more butyrous consistency of *B. cereus* colonies, so that they may be pulled into standing peaks with a loop. *B. mycoides* produces characteristic rhizoid or hairy-looking, adherent colonies which readily cover the whole agar surface.

It is generally easy to distinguish virulent *B. anthracis*

TABLE 2 Characters for differentiating nonreactive *Bacillus*, *Aneurinibacillus*, and *Brevibacillus* species[a]

Character[b]	*Bacillus*		*Aneurinibacillus aneurinilyticus*	*Brevibacillus*		
	B. sphaericus	*B. badius*		*B. brevis*	*B. agri*	*B. laterosporus*
Rod mean diameter (μm)	1.0	0.9	0.8	0.9	0.9	0.9
Chains of cells	−	+	−	−	−	−
Motility	+	+	+	+	+	+
Sporangia[c]						
Spore shape	S(E)	E	E	E	E	E
Spore position	S,T	S,C,T	S,C	S,C	S,C	S,C
Sporangium swollen	+	−	+	+	+	+
Parasporal crystals	−	−	−	−	−	−
Parasporal bodies	−	−	−	−	−	+
Anaerobic growth	−	−	−	−	−	+
Growth at:						
50°C	−	+	+	−	v	−
65°C	−	−	−	−	−	−
Casein hydrolysis	v	+	−	+	+	+
Gelatin hydrolysis	−	+	−	+	+	+
Nitrate reduction	−	−	+	+	−	+
Acid from:						
Glycerol	−	−	+	v	−	+
Mannitol	−	−	−	v	+	+
D-Trehalose	−	−	−	−	v	+
Assimilation of:						
D-Fructose	(−)	−	−	+	+	+
D-Gluconate	+	−	v	+	+	−
D-Glucosamine	(−)	−	−	+	−	−
Glutarate	(−)	+	+	−	−	−
DL-lactate	+	+	+	−	+	−
Putrescine	(−)	+	+	−	+	−
D-Trehalose	−	−	−	+	+	+

[a] Symbols and abbreviations: +, >85% positive; (+), 75 to 84% positive; v, variable (26 to 74% positive); (−), 16 to 25% positive; −, 0 to 15% positive.

[b] Gelatin hydrolysis and nitrate reduction reactions were determined by using the tests in the API 20E strip. Acid from carbohydrate reactions were determined by using the API 50CHB system, and assimilation reactions were determined by using the API Biotype 100 system; both kinds of reactions may also be investigated by using the media described in reference 34, along with appropriate reference strains.

[c] Spore shape: C, cylindrical; E, ellipsoidal; S, spherical. Spore position: C, central or paracentral; S, subterminal; T, terminal. The commonest shapes and positions are listed first, and those given in parentheses are infrequently observed.

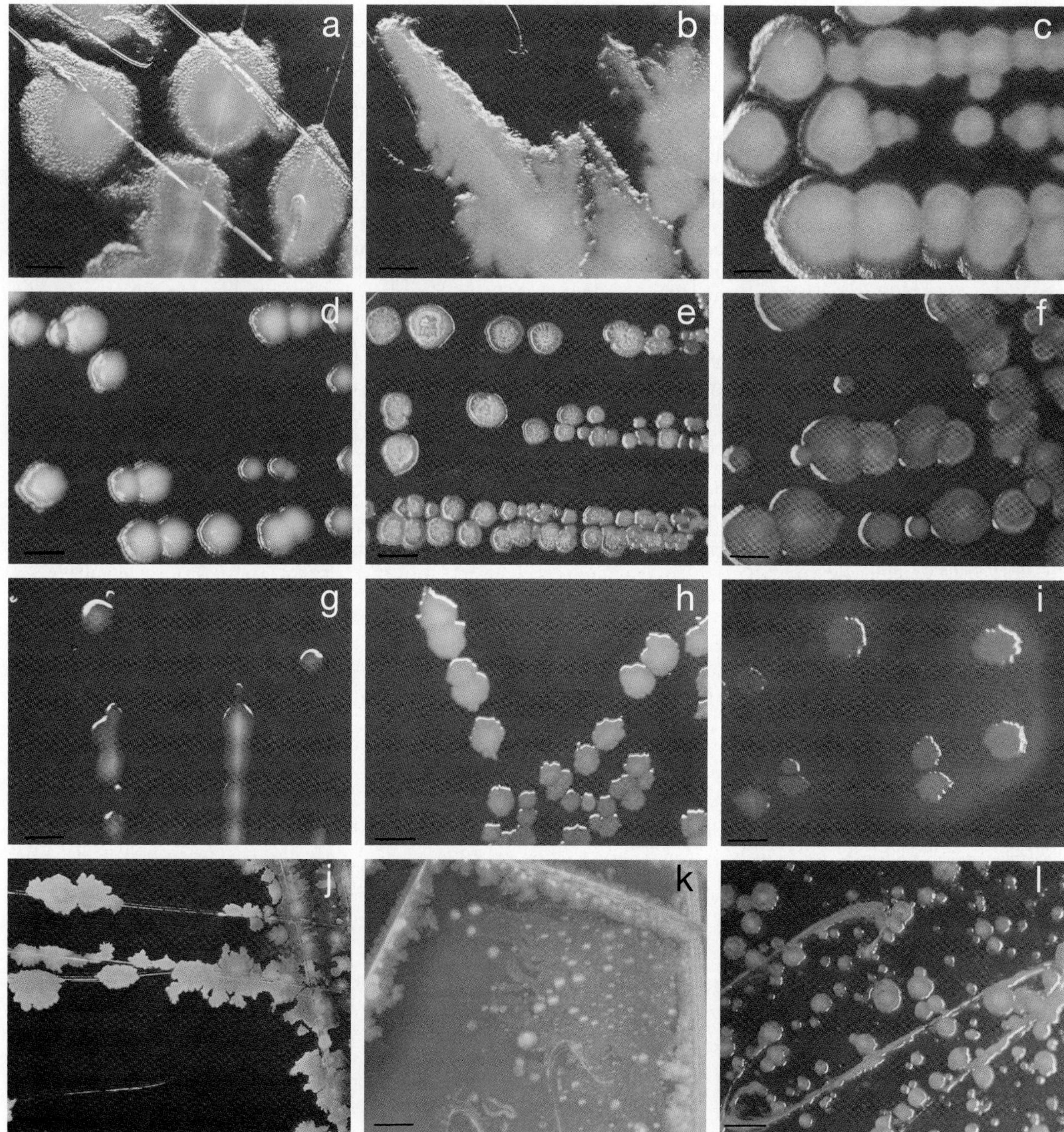

FIGURE 1 Colonies of endospore-forming bacteria on blood agar (a to i) and nutrient agar (j to l) after 24 to 36 h at 37°C. Bars, 2 mm. (a) *B. anthracis*; (b) *B. cereus*; (c) *B. thuringiensis*; (d) *B. megaterium*; (e) *B. pumilus*; (f) *B. sphaericus*; (g) *Brevibacillus brevis*; (h) *Brevibacillus laterosporus*; (i) *Paenibacillus polymyxa*; (j) *B. subtilis*; (k) *B. circulans*; (l) *P. alvei*.

from other members of the *B. cereus* group. An isolate that has the correct colonial morphology (Fig. 1a) and that is white or gray in color, nonhemolytic or only weakly hemolytic, nonmotile, susceptible to the diagnostic "gamma phage" (if available) and penicillin (42, 55), and able to produce the characteristic capsule (see Fig. 2a) is *B. anthracis*. An isolate that shows the characteristic phenotype but that is unable to produce capsules may be an avirulent form lacking either or both capsule or toxin genes (54) and should be referred to a specialist laboratory; such isolates are generally found in environmental samples and are frequently identified in routine laboratories as *B. cereus* and discarded. Primer sequences are now available for confirming the presence of the toxin and capsule genes and hence the virulence of an isolate. Molecular studies are giving valuable insights into genetic profiles among the *B. cereus* group (2, 28).

The capsule of virulent *B. anthracis* can be demonstrated on nutrient agar containing 0.7% sodium bicarbonate incubated overnight under 5 to 7% CO_2 (candle jars perform well). Colonies of the capsulate *B. anthracis* appear mucoid, and the capsule can be visualized by staining smears with M'Fadyean's polychrome methylene blue or India ink (55). Alternatively, and more simply, 2.5 ml of blood (defibrinated horse blood seems best; fetal calf serum is quite good) can be inoculated with a pinhead quantity of growth from the initial suspect colony, incubated statically for 6 to 18 h at 37°C, and M'Fadyean stained for capsules. Very rarely, doubt may persist and inoculation of a light suspension of the culture into a mouse or guinea pig (the latter is more susceptible) may be necessary to confirm the identity or at least its virulence. A M'Fadyean-stained blood smear made at death (about 48 h after inoculation) will reveal large numbers of the typical large, capsulate, square-ended rods mostly in chains (Fig. 2a).

The key characteristics for recognizing and distinguishing the *B. cereus* group are colonial morphology (Fig. 1a to c); the presence of large cells, often in chains, producing ellipsoidal spores not swelling the sporangia (Fig. 2b and c); the presence of facultative anaerobes; and egg yolk reaction (i.e., lecithinase) positive. Negative or very weak hemolysis and lack of motility distinguish *B. anthracis* and *B. mycoides* from *B. cereus* and *B. thuringiensis*. *B. cereus*, *B. mycoides*, *B. thuringiensis*, and, to a lesser extent, *B. anthracis* synthesize lecithinases, forming opaque zones of precipitation around colonies on egg yolk agar. Differentiation of *B. thuringiensis* from *B. cereus* is largely dependent on observation of the parasporal insecticidal toxin crystals of *B. thuringiensis* in sporulated cultures (after 2 to 5 days) by phase-contrast microscopy (Fig. 2c) or staining (42) and the demonstration of insecticidal activity (50).

Other Species

Other species show a very wide range of colonial morphologies both within and between species after 24 to 48 h (Fig. 1). They vary from moist and glossy (Fig. 1f to i) through granular to wrinkled (Fig. 1e); the shape varies from round to irregular (Fig. 1d to i), sometimes spreading (Fig. 1k and l), with entire through undulate or crenate to fimbriate edges (Fig. 1d to j); sizes range from 1 to 5 mm; color commonly ranges from buff or creamy gray to off-white, but some strains may produce orange pigment; hemolysis may be absent, slight, or marked, partial, or complete (Fig. 1h); elevations range from effuse through raised to convex; consistency is usually butyrous, but mucoid and dry, adherent colonies are not uncommon. Despite this diversity, *Bacillus* colonies are not generally difficult to recognize, and some species have characteristic yet seemingly infinitely variable colonial morphologies, as does the *B. cereus* group (Fig. 1a to c; for further illustrations, see reference 42).

B. subtilis and *B. licheniformis* produce similar colonies which are exceptionally variable in appearance and which often appear to be mixed cultures (Fig. 1j); colonies are irregular in shape and of moderate (2 to 4 mm) diameter and range from moist and butyrous or mucoid, with margins varying from undulate to fimbriate through membranous with an underlying mucoid matrix, with or without mucoid beading at the surface, to rough and crusty as they dry. The "licheniform" colonies of *B. licheniformis* tend to be quite adherent.

Rotating and migrating microcolonies, which may show spreading growth (Fig. 1k), have been observed macroscopically in about 13% of strains received as *Bacillus circulans* (37), but this very heterogeneous species continues to undergo radical taxonomic revision, with many spreading strains being assigned to other species. Motile, spreading microcolonies, which commonly have an unpleasant smell, are more typical of *P. alvei* (Fig. 1l).

Other species that have been encountered in the clinical laboratory include *Bacillus coagulans*, *B. megaterium*, *B. pumilus*, and *B. sphaericus*; *B. brevis* and *B. laterosporus* (now both *Brevibacillus*); and *B. macerans* and *B. polymyxa* (now both *Paenibacillus*); and they do not produce particularly distinctive growth (Fig. 1d to i). Further illustrations can be seen in reference 42, but it must be appreciated that only a few species have colonies sufficiently characteristic or invariant to allow tentative identification, even by the experienced worker.

Microscopic morphologies, particularly of sporangia (Fig. 2), are much more helpful than colonial characters for distinguishing between species. Vegetative cells are usually round ended, but those of *P. alvei* may be tapered (Fig. 2l). The large cells of *B. megaterium* may accumulate PHB (Fig. 2d) and appear vacuolate or foamy when grown on glucose nutrient agar. Overall, cell widths vary from about 0.5 to 1.5 μm, and lengths vary from 1.5 to 8 μm. Most strains of these species are motile. Spore shapes vary from cylindrical (Fig. 2f) through ellipsoidal (Fig. 2b, c to e, g, and i to l) to spherical (Fig. 2d and h); bean- or kidney-shaped, curved-cylindrical, and pear-shaped spores are also seen occasionally. Spores may be terminally (Fig. 2h), subterminally (Fig. 2b, c, f, g, and i), or centrally (Fig. 2e and j) positioned within sporangia and may distend them (Fig. 2g to k). Despite within-species and within-strain variation, sporangial morphologies tend to be characteristic of species and may allow tentative identification by the experienced worker. One species, *Brevibacillus laterosporus*, produces very distinctive ellipsoidal spores which have thickened rims on one side so that they appear to be laterally displaced in the sporangia (Fig. 2j).

All these species are mesophilic and will grow well at between 30 and 37°C. Minimum temperatures for growth lie mostly between 5 and 20°C, and maximum temperatures for growth mostly lie between 35 and 50°C. Strains of *B. coagulans* may be slightly thermophilic and grow at temperatures of up to 55 to 60°C.

SEROLOGICAL TESTS

Species and Strain Differentiation

Early attempts at developing simple serological differentiation systems for *Bacillus* species were always plagued by problems of cross-reacting antigens and, in the case of spores, hydrophobic surface properties leading to autoagglutination. Monoclonal antibody tests based on specific epitopes in the spore cortex or cell wall of *B. anthracis* that may reliably distinguish *B. anthracis* from other closely related *Bacillus* species are not yet available. Similarly, *B. anthracis* strain differentiation has long proved to be particularly challenging; up until about 5 years ago, the species largely defied investigators' attempts to devise methods for distinguishing isolates from each other for epidemiological or strategic purposes. Some success at overcoming the problems posed is being achieved by amplified fragment length polymorphism analysis (27, 28).

A strain differentiation system for *B. cereus* based on flagellar (H) antigens is available at the Food Hygiene Laboratory, Central Public Health Laboratory, Colindale, London, United Kingdom, for investigations of food-poisoning outbreaks or other *B. cereus*-associated clinical problems (31).

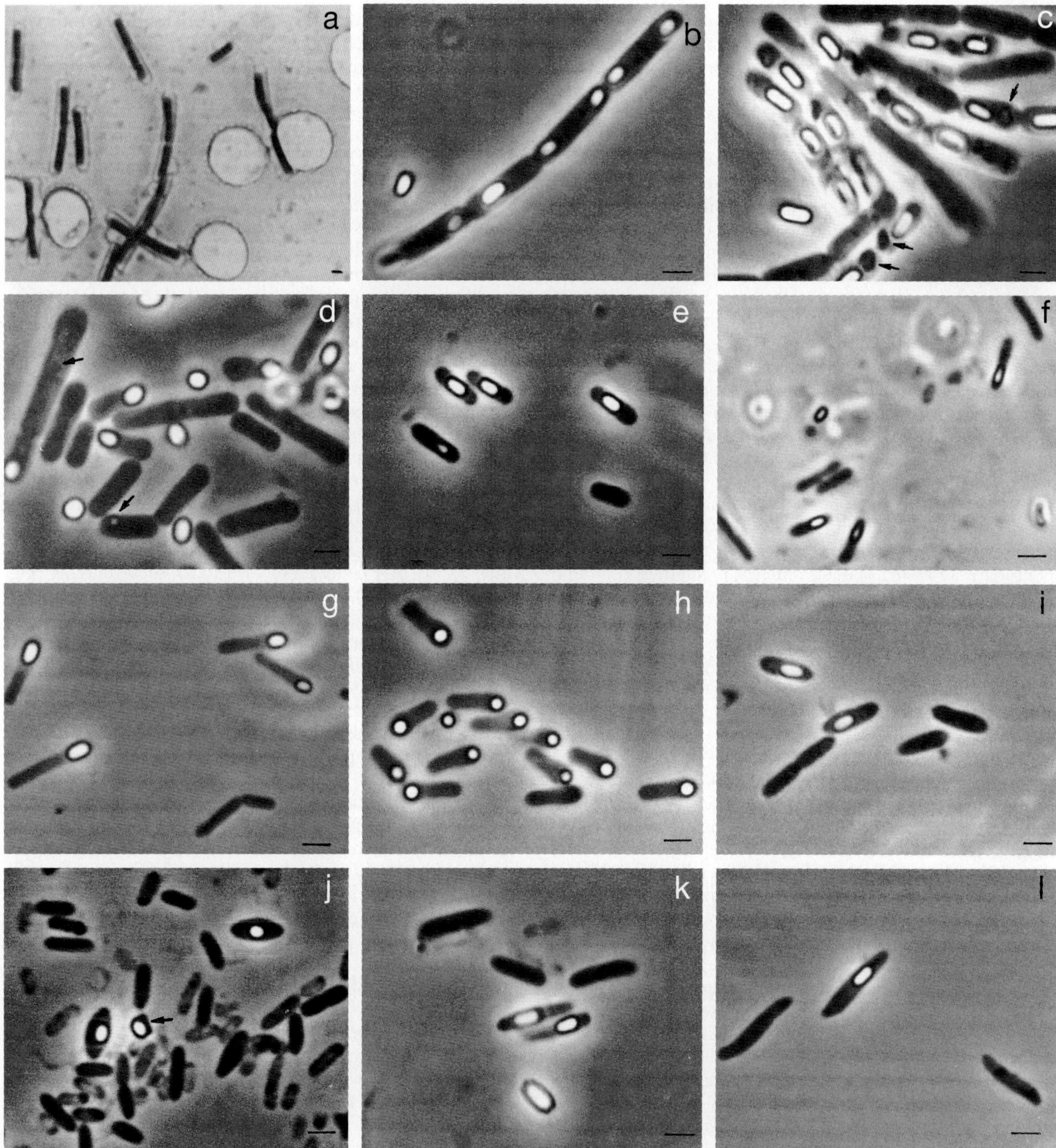

FIGURE 2 Photomicrographs of endospore-forming bacteria viewed by bright-field (a) and phase-contrast (b to l) microscopy. Bars, 2 μm. (a) *B. anthracis*, M'Fadyean stain showing capsulate rods in bovine blood smear; (b) *B. cereus*, broad cells with ellipsoidal, subterminal spores not swelling the sporangia; (c) *B. thuringiensis*, broad cells with ellipsoidal, subterminal spores not swelling the sporangia and showing parasporal crystals of insecticidal toxin (arrows); (d) *B. megaterium*, broad cells with ellipsoidal and spherical, subterminal, and terminal spores not swelling the sporangia and showing PHB inclusions (arrows); (e) *B. subtilis*, ellipsoidal, central, and subterminal spores not swelling the sporangia; (f) *B. pumilus*, slender cells with cylindrical, subterminal spores not swelling the sporangia; (g) *B. circulans*, ellipsoidal, subterminal spores swelling the sporangia; (h) *B. sphaericus*, spherical, terminal spores swelling the sporangia; (i) *Brevibacillus brevis*, ellipsoidal, subterminal spores, with one swelling its sporangium slightly; (j) *Brevibacillus laterosporus*, ellipsoidal, central spores with thickened rims on one side (arrow) swelling the sporangia; (k) *P. polymyxa*, ellipsoidal, paracentral to subterminal spores swelling the sporangia slightly; (l) *P. alvei*, cells with tapered ends, ellipsoidal, paracentral to subterminal spores not swelling the sporangium.

B. thuringiensis strains are classified on the basis of their flagellar antigens; 58 serovars based on H-antigenic subfactors are currently recognized (14, 17). This is done at the Pasteur Institute, Paris, France, and at Abbott Laboratories, North Chicago, Ill.

Toxin and Antitoxin Detection

The three protein components of anthrax toxin (protective antigen [PA], lethal factor [LF], and edema factor [EF]) and antibodies to them are usable in enzyme immunoassay systems. For routine confirmation of anthrax infection or for monitoring responses to anthrax vaccines, antibodies against protective antigen alone appear to be satisfactory; they have proved to be useful for epidemiological investigations with humans and animals. In human anthrax, however, early treatment sometimes prevents antibody development (53). Current human vaccines are either alum precipitates of cell-free products containing high levels of PA and little LF and EF or live spore suspensions from noncapsulating strains (48, 52); a new-generation anthrax vaccine might be based on recombinant PA used with an adjuvant (39).

In countries of the former USSR, a skin test with Anthraxin, a heat-stable extract from a noncapsulate strain of *B. anthracis* which has been licensed for human and animal use since 1962, is widely acclaimed for use in the retrospective diagnosis of anthrax (48). The delayed-type hypersensitivity is interpreted as indicating cell-mediated immunity to anthrax and can be used to diagnose anthrax retrospectively or to evaluate the vaccine-induced immune status after periods of several years. Anthraxin does not contain highly specific anthrax antigens and depends on the nature of anthrax rather than the specificity of the antigens involved. This is also true of the Ascoli test, which, dating from 1911, must be one of the oldest antigen detection tests in microbiology. It is a precipitin test that uses hyperimmune serum raised to *B. anthracis* whole-cell antigen to provide rapid retrospective evidence of anthrax infection in an animal from which the material being tested was derived. The test is still in use in eastern Europe and central Asia.

The enterotoxin complex responsible for the diarrheal type of *B. cereus* food poisoning has been increasingly well characterized. Two commercial kits are available for its detection in foods and feces: the Oxoid BCET-RPLA (product code TD950; Oxoid Ltd., Basingstoke, United Kingdom) and the TECRA VIA (product code BDEVIA48; TECRA Diagnostics, Roseville, New South Wales, Australia) (7). However, these kits detect different antigens, and there is some controversy about their reliabilities (7, 9, 16). Other assays, based on tissue culture, have also been developed (9, 12). Similarly, the emetic toxin of *B. cereus* has been identified as a dodecadepsipeptide (1), and a semiquantitative vacuolation response of cultured HEp-2 cells may be used for its assay in food extracts or culture filtrates.

ANTIMICROBIAL SUSCEPTIBILITIES

B. anthracis is almost invariably susceptible to penicillin; few published reports of resistant isolates appear to exist (32). It is also susceptible to gentamicin, erythromycin, and chloramphenicol, and tests with primates have shown infection to respond to ciprofloxacin and doxycycline (20). It is normally susceptible to streptomycin and to narrow-spectrum cephalosporins but is resistant to expanded-spectrum and broad-spectrum cephalosporins (18).

B. cereus and *B. thuringiensis* produce a broad-spectrum β-lactamase and are thus resistant to penicillin, ampicillin, and cephalosporins. They are also resistant to trimethoprim, but they are almost always susceptible to clindamycin, erythromycin, chloramphenicol, vancomycin, and the aminoglycosides and are usually sensitive to tetracycline and sulfonamides. Clindamycin with gentamicin, given early, appears to be the best treatment for ophthalmic infections caused by *B. cereus*. Oral ciprofloxacin has been used successfully in the treatment of *B. cereus* wound infections (29).

Information on the treatment of infections caused by other aerobic endospore formers is sparse, but an in vitro study showed that although there was much variation between species, many strains were sensitive to penicillins, semisynthetic penicillins, and cephalosporins (57). Gentamicin was effective in treating a case of *B. licheniformis* ophthalmitis, and a cephalosporin was effective against *B. licheniformis* bacteremia and septicemia. Metronidazole was the principal agent in the successful treatment of a brain abscess associated with penicillin- and chloramphenicol-resistant *B. licheniformis*. *B. subtilis* endocarditis in a drug abuser was successfully treated with a cephalosporin, and gentamicin was successful against a case of *B. subtilis* septicemia. Penicillin or its derivatives or cephalosporins are probably the best first choices for treatment of infections attributed to aerobic endospore formers other than members of the *B. cereus* group.

EVALUATION, INTERPRETATION, AND REPORTING OF RESULTS

Apart from *B. anthracis*, the majority of *Bacillus* species are common environmental contaminants. For this reason, the isolation of a *Bacillus* species from a single clinical specimen is generally not a sufficient basis for incriminating the organism as the etiological agent of the condition being investigated. However, many clinically significant isolates of *Bacillus* were certainly disregarded in the past, and the perceived difficulties of identification may have contributed to this. In the opinion of Barnham (5), however, moderate or heavy growth of *Bacillus* species from wounds is usually significant. *B. cereus* infections of the eye are emergencies, and isolations from this site should always be taken seriously and reported to the physician immediately.

From the point of view of the clinical laboratory, the most important questions to ask about an aerobic spore-forming isolate are the following: Was it isolated in pure culture or at least apparently dominating the flora? Was it isolated in large numbers? Was it isolated more than once? Is it a member of the *B. cereus* group? A repeatedly isolated aerobic endospore former found in large numbers in pure culture, particularly from blood cultures, is most unlikely to be a mere contaminant. Histopathology and specialist tests on the toxigenicity of the isolate may also help in making a decision about the relevance of the isolate.

Low-level contamination of foodstuffs by aerobic endospore formers is common, as is asymptomatic transient fecal carriage by human and animal populations. Therefore, in food-borne illness investigations, qualitative isolation tests are insufficient. The ideal criteria for proving that an aerobic endospore former is the etiological agent are the isolation of significant numbers ($>10^5$ CFU/g) of the organism from the epidemiologically incriminated food (and, in the case of suspected *B. cereus* food poisoning, detection of emetic toxin and/or enterotoxin) together with recovery of the same strain (biovar, serovar, phagovar, plasmid type, etc.)

in significant numbers from acute-phase specimens (feces or vomitus) from the patients.

In practice, it is rare that these ideal criteria can be met. A complete set of the appropriate food and clinical specimens is seldom available; and the epidemiological aspects of the outbreak, such as incubation times, clinical symptoms, the types of food implicated, and the time lapse and manner in which the food was stored between the episode and specimen collection, must all be considered along with the laboratory findings in forming conclusions as to the etiology.

B. anthracis continues to be generally regarded as an obligate pathogen. Its continued existence in the ecosystem appears to depend on a periodic multiplication phase within an animal host, and its environmental presence reflects contamination from an animal source at some time in the past rather than self-maintenance within the environment. Demonstration of capsulating *B. anthracis* from human and animal specimens, even in low numbers, confirms a clinical suspicion of anthrax, because the bacterium is rapidly destroyed by putrefactive processes after the host's death.

REFERENCES

1. **Agata, N., M. Mori, M. Ohta, S. Suwan, I. Ohtani, and M. Isobe.** 1994. A novel dodecadepsipeptide, cereulide, isolated from *Bacillus cereus* causes vacuole formation in HEp-2 cells. *FEMS Microbiol. Lett.* **121:**31–34.
2. **Andersen, G. L., J. M. Simchock, and K. H. Wilson.** 1996. Identification of a region of genetic variability among *Bacillus anthracis* strains and related species. *J. Bacteriol.* **178:**377–384.
3. **Ash, C., J. A. E. Farrow, S. Wallbanks, and M. D. Collins.** 1991. Phylogenetic heterogeneity of the genus *Bacillus* revealed by comparative analysis of small-subunit-ribosomal RNA sequences. *Lett. Appl. Microbiol.* **13:**202–206.
4. **Ash, C., F. G. Priest, and M. D. Collins.** 1993. Molecular identification of rRNA group 3 bacilli (Ash, Farrow, Wallbanks and Collins) using a PCR probe test. *Antonie Leeuwenhoek* **64:**253–260.
5. **Barnham, M.** 1980. *B. cereus* infections. *J. Clin. Pathol.* **33:**314.
6. **Beecher, D. J., and J. D. MacMillan.** 1990. A novel bicomponent hemolysin from *Bacillus cereus. Infect. Immun.* **58:** 2220–2227.
7. **Beecher, D. J., and A. C. Lee Wong.** 1994. Identification and analysis of the antigens detected by two commercial *Bacillus cereus* diarrheal enterotoxin immunoassay kits. *Appl. Environ. Microbiol.* **60:**4614–4616.
8. **Berkeley, R. C. W., and N. A. Logan.** 1997. *Bacillus, Alicyclobacillus* and *Paenibacillus*, p. 185–204. *In* A. M. Emmerson, P. M. Hawkey, and S. H. Gillespie (ed.), *Principles and Practice of Clinical Bacteriology*. John Wiley & Sons, Chichester, United Kingdom.
9. **Buchanan, R. L., and F. J. Schultz.** 1994. Comparison of the Tecra VIA kit, Oxoid BCET-RPLA kit and CHO cell culture assay for the detection of *Bacillus cereus* diarrhoeal enterotoxin. *Lett. Appl. Microbiol.* **19:**353–356.
10. **Burans, J., A. Keleher, T. O'Brien, J. Hager, A. Plummer, and C. Morgan.** 1996. Rapid method for the diagnosis of *Bacillus anthracis* infection in clinical samples using a hand-held assay. *Salisbury Med. Bull.* **87**(Special Suppl.): 36–37.
11. **Cerny, G.** 1978. Studies on the aminopeptidase test for the distinction of gram-negative from gram-positive bacteria. *Eur. J. Appl. Microbiol.* **5:**113–122.
12. **Christiansson, A., N. Satyanarayan, I. Nilsson, T. Wadström, and H.-E. Pettersson.** 1989. Toxin production by *Bacillus cereus* dairy isolates in milk at low temperatures. *Appl. Environ. Microbiol.* **55:**2595–2600.
13. **Claus, D., and R. C. W. Berkeley.** 1986. Genus *Bacillus* Cohn 1872, p. 1105–1139. *In* P. H. A. Sneath, N. S. Mair, M. E. Sharpe, and J. G. Holt (ed.), *Bergey's Manual of Systematic Bacteriology*, vol. 2. The Williams & Wilkins Co., Baltimore, Md.
14. **Damgaard, P. H., P. E. Granum, J. Bresciani, M. V. Torregrossa, J. Eilenberg, and L. Valentino.** 1997. Characterization of *Bacillus thuringiensis* isolated from infections in burn wounds. *FEMS Immunol. Med. Microbiol.* **18:**47–53.
15. **Davey, R. T., Jr., and W. B. Tauber.** 1987. Posttraumatic endophthalmitis: the emerging role of *Bacillus cereus* infection. *Rev. Infect. Dis.* **9:**110–123.
16. **Day, T. L., S. R. Tatani, S. Notermans, and R. W. Bennett.** 1994. A comparison of ELISA and RPLA for detection of *Bacillus cereus* diarrhoeal enterotoxin. *J. Appl. Bacteriol.* **77:**9–13.
17. **de Barjac, H., and E. Franchon.** 1990. Classification of *Bacillus thuringiensis. Entomophaga* **35:**233–240.
18. **Doganay, M., and N. Aydin.** 1991. Antimicrobial susceptibility of *Bacillus anthracis. Scand. J. Infect. Dis.* **23:** 333–335.
19. **Drobniewski, F. A.** 1993. *Bacillus cereus* and related species. *Clin. Microbiol. Rev.* **6:**324–338.
20. **Friedlander, A. M., S. L. Welkos, M. L. M. Pitt, J. W. Ezzell, P. W. Worsham, B. E. Ivins, J. R. Lowe, G. B. Howe, P. Mikesell, and W. B. Lawrence.** 1993. Postexposure prophylaxis against experimental inhalation anthrax. *J. Infect. Dis.* **167:**1239–1242.
21. **Gordon, R. E., W. C. Haynes, and C. H.-N. Pang.** 1973. *The Genus* Bacillus. *Agriculture Handbook No. 427*. U.S. Department of Agriculture, Washington, D.C.
22. **Gregersen, T.** 1978. Rapid method for distinction of gram-negative from gram-positive bacteria. *Eur. J. Appl. Microbiol.* **5:**123–127.
23. **Heyndrickx, M., K. Vandemeulebroecke, B. Hoste, P. Janssen, K. Kersters, P. De Vos, N. A. Logan, N. Ali, and R. C. W. Berkeley.** 1996. Reclassification of *Paenibacillus* (formerly *Bacillus*) *pulvifaciens* (Nakamura 1984) Ash et al. 1994, a later subjective synonym of *Paenibacillus* (formerly *Bacillus*) *larvae* (White 1906) Ash et al. 1994, as a subspecies of *P. larvae*, with emended description of *P. larvae* with *P. larvae* subsp. *larvae* and *P. larvae* subsp. *pulvifaciens. Int. J. Syst. Bacteriol.* **46:**270–279.
24. **Heyndrickx, M., K. Vandemeulebroecke, P. Scheldeman, K. Kersters, P. De Vos, N. A. Logan, A. M. Aziz, N. Ali, and R. C. W. Berkeley.** 1996. A polyphasic reassessment of the genus *Paenibacillus*, reclassification of *Bacillus lautus* (Nakamura 1984) as *Paenibacillus lautus* comb. nov. and of *Bacillus peoriae* (Montefusco et al. 1993) as *Paenibacillus peoriae* comb. nov., and emended descriptions of *P. lautus* and of *P. peoriae. Int. J. Syst. Bacteriol.* **46:**988–1003.
25. **Heyndrickx, M., L. Lebbe, M. Vancanneyt, K. Kersters, P. De Vos, G. Forsyth, and N. A. Logan.** 1998. *Virgibacillus*: a new genus to accommodate *Bacillus pantothenticus* (Proom and Knight 1950). Emended description of *Virgibacillus pantothenticus. Int. J. Syst. Bacteriol.* **48:**99–106.
26. **Heyndrickx, M., L. Lebbe, M. Vancanneyt, K. Kersters, P. De Vos, N. A. Logan, G. Forsyth, S. Nazli, N. Ali, and R. C. W. Berkeley.** 1997. A polyphasic reassessment of the genus *Aneurinibacillus*, reclassification of *Bacillus thermoaerophilus* (Meier-Stauffer et al. 1996) as *Aneurinibacillus thermoaerophilus* comb. nov., and emended descriptions of *A. aneurinolyticus*, of *A. migulanus*, and of *A. thermoaerophilus. Int. J. Syst. Bacteriol.* **47:**808–817.
27. **Jackson, P. J., E. A. Walthers, A. S. Kalif, K. L. Richmond, D. M. Adair, K. K. Hill, C. R. Kuske, G. L. Andersen, K. H. Wilson, M. E. Hugh-Jones, and P. Keim.** 1997.

Characterization of the variable-number tandem repeats in *vrrA* from different *Bacillus anthracis* isolates. *Appl. Environ. Microbiol.* **63:**1400–1405.
28. **Keim, P., A. Kalif, J. Schupp, K. Hill, S. E. Travis, K. Richmond, D. M. Adair, M. Hugh-Jones, C. R. Kuske, and P. J. Jackson.** 1997. Molecular evolution and diversity in *Bacillus anthracis* as detected by amplified fragment length polymorphism markers. *J. Bacteriol.* **179:**818–824.
29. **Kemmerly, S. A., and G. A. Pankey.** 1993. Oral ciprofloxacin therapy for *Bacillus cereus* wound infection and bacteremia. *Clin. Infect. Dis.* **16:**189.
30. **Knisely, R. F.** 1966. Selective medium for *Bacillus anthracis*. *J. Bacteriol.* **92:**784–786.
31. **Kramer, J. M., and R. J. Gilbert.** 1992. *Bacillus cereus* gastroenteritis, p. 119–153. *In* A. T. Tu (ed.), *Food Poisoning. Handbook of Natural Toxins*, vol. 7. Marcel Dekker, Inc., New York, N.Y.
32. **Lalitha, M. K., and M. K. Thomas.** 1997. Penicillin resistance in *Bacillus anthracis*. *Lancet* **349:**1522.
33. **Logan, N. A.** 1988. *Bacillus* species of medical and veterinary importance. *J. Med. Microbiol.* **25:**157–165.
34. **Logan, N. A.** 1989. Numerical taxonomy of violet-pigmented, gram-negative bacteria and description of *Iodobacter fluviatile* gen. nov., comb. nov. *Int. J. Syst. Bacteriol.* **40:**450–456.
35. **Logan, N. A.** 1994. *Bacterial Systematics*. Blackwell Scientific Publications, Oxford, United Kingdom.
36. **Logan, N. A., and R. C. W. Berkeley.** 1984. Identification of *Bacillus* strains using the API system. *J. Gen. Microbiol.* **130:**1871–1882.
37. **Logan, N. A., D. C. Old, and H. M. Dick.** 1985. Isolation of *Bacillus circulans* from a wound infection. *J. Clin. Pathol.* **38:**838–839.
38. **Mahler, H., A. Pasi, J. M. Kramer, P. Schulte, A. C. Scoging, W. Bär, and S. Krähenbühl.** 1997. Fulminant liver failure in association with the emetic toxin of *Bacillus cereus*. *N. Engl. J. Med.* **336:**1142–1148.
39. **Miller, J., B. W. McBride, R. J. Manchee, P. Moore, and L. W. J. Baillie.** 1998. Production and purification of recombinant protective antigen and protective efficacy against *Bacillus anthracis*. *Lett. Appl. Microbiol.* **26:**56–60.
40. **Niimura, Y., E. Koh, F. Yanagida, K.-I. Suzuki, K. Komagata, and M. Kozaki.** 1990. *Amphibacillus xylanus* gen. nov., sp. nov., a facultatively anaerobic sporeforming xylan-digesting bacterium which lacks cytochrome, quinone, and catalase. *Int. J. Syst. Bacteriol.* **40:**297–301.
41. **Norris, J. R., R. C. W. Berkeley, N. A. Logan, and A. G. O'Donnell.** 1981. The genera *Bacillus* and *Sporolactobacillus*, p. 1711–1742. *In* M. P. Starr, H. Stolp, H. G. Truper, A. Balows, and H. G. Schlegel (ed.), *The Prokaryotes: a Handbook on Habitats, Isolation and Identification of Bacteria*, vol. 2. Springer-Verlag, Berlin, Germany.
42. **Parry, J. M., P. C. B. Turnbull, and J. R. Gibson.** 1983. *A Colour Atlas of* Bacillus *Species*. Wolfe Medical Publications, London, United Kingdom.
43. **Pike, R. M., S. E. Sulkin, and M. L. Schulze.** 1965. Continuing importance of laboratory-acquired infections. *Am. J. Public Health* **55:**190–199.
44. **Quinn, C. P., and P. C. B. Turnbull.** 1997. Anthrax, p. 799–818. *In* L. H. Collier, A. Balows, M. Sussman, and W. J. Hausler (ed.), *Topley and Wilson's Microbiology and Microbial Infections*, vol. 3. Edward Arnold, London, United Kingdom.
45. **Rössler, D., W. Ludwig, K.-H. Schleifer, C. Lin, T. J. McGill, J. D. Wisoztskey, P. Jurtshuk, Jr., and G. E. Fox.** 1991. Phylogenetic diversity in the genus *Bacillus* as seen by 16S rRNA sequencing studies. *Syst. Appl. Microbiol.* **14:** 266–269.
46. **Shida, O., H. Takagi, K. Kadowaki, and K. Komagata.** 1996. Proposal for two new genera, *Brevibacillus* gen. nov. and *Aneurinibacillus* gen. nov. *Int. J. Syst. Bacteriol.* **46:** 939–946.
47. **Shinagawa, K., H. Konuma, H. Sekita, and S. Sugii.** 1995. Emesis of rhesus monkeys induced by intragastric administration with the HEp-2 vacuolation factor (cereulide) produced by *Bacillus cereus*. *FEMS Microbiol. Lett.* **130:**87–90.
48. **Shlyakhov, E., and E. Rubinstein.** 1994. Human live anthrax vaccine in the former USSR. *Vaccine* **12:**727–730.
49. **Spring, S., W. Ludwig, M. C. Marquez, A. Ventosa, and K.-H. Schleifer.** 1996. *Halobacillus* gen. nov., with descriptions of *Halobacillus litoralis* sp. nov. and *Halobacillus trueperi* sp. nov., and transfer of *Sporosarcina halophila* to *Halobacillus halophilus* comb. nov. *Int. J. Syst. Bacteriol.* **46:**492–496.
50. **Stahly, D. P., R. E. Andrews, and A. A. Yousten.** 1992. The genus *Bacillus*—insect pathogens, p. 1697–1745. *In* A. Balows, H. G. Trüper, M. Dworkin, W. Harder, and K. H. Schleifer (ed.) *The Prokaryotes: a Handbook on the Biology of Bacteria: Ecophysiology, Isolation, Identification, Applications*, 2nd ed., vol. 2. Springer-Verlag, New York, N.Y.
51. **Tabatabaie, P., and A. Syadati.** 1993. *Bacillus anthracis* as a cause of bacterial meningitis. *Pediatr. Infect. Dis. J.* **12:** 1035–1037.
52. **Turnbull, P. C. B.** 1991. Anthrax vaccines: past, present and future. *Vaccine* **9:**533–539.
53. **Turnbull, P. C. B., M. Doganay, P. M. Lindeque, B. Aygen, and J. McLaughlin.** 1992. Serology and anthrax in humans, livestock and Etosha National Park wildlife. *Epidemiol. Infect.* **108:**299–313.
54. **Turnbull, P. C. B., R. A. Hutson, M. J. Ward, M. N. Jones, C. P. Quinn, N. J. Finnie, C. J. Duggleby, J. M. Kramer, and J. Melling.** 1992. *Bacillus anthracis* but not always anthrax. *J. Appl. Bacteriol.* **72:**21–28.
55. **Turnbull, P. C. B., R. Böhm, H. G. B. Chizyuka, T. Fujikura, M. E. Hugh-Jones, and J. Melling.** 1993. *Guidelines for the Surveillance and Control of Anthrax in Humans and Animals*. WHO/Zoon./93.170. World Health Organization, Geneva, Switzerland.
56. **van Netten, P., and J. M. Kramer.** 1992. Media for the detection and enumeration of *Bacillus cereus* in foods: a review. *Int. J. Food Microbiol.* **17:**85–99.
57. **Weber, D. J., S. M. Saviteer, W. A. Rutala, and C. A. Thomann.** 1988. In vitro susceptibility of *Bacillus* spp. to selected antimicrobial agents. *Antimicrob. Agents Chemother.* **32:**642–645.
58. **Wisotzkey, J. D., P. Jurtshuk, Jr., G. E. Fox, G. Deinhard, and K. Poralla.** 1992. Comparative sequence analyses on the 16S rRNA (rDNA) of *Bacillus acidocaldarius*, *Bacillus acidoterrestris*, and *Bacillus cycloheptanicus* and proposal for creation of a new genus, *Alicyclobacillus* gen. nov. *Int. J. Syst. Bacteriol.* **42:**263–269.

Nocardia, Rhodococcus, Gordona, Actinomadura, Streptomyces, and Other Actinomycetes of Medical Importance*

JUNE M. BROWN, MICHAEL M. McNEIL, AND EDWARD P. DESMOND

24

TAXONOMY

The systematics of the aerobic actinomycetes began as a largely intuitive discipline based on microscopic morphology but has become increasingly objective with the introduction and application of modern taxonomic procedures, notably, chemosystematic, molecular systematic, and numerical taxonomic methods. Although the property of branched, filamentous hyphae that either form spores or reproduce by fragmentation remains central to the definition of an actinomycete, it is clear that many actinomycete genera are only distantly related phylogenetically (47, 121, 135). Although more than 40 genera are currently described as aerobic actinomycetes, only 18 genera appear to be relevant to human and veterinary medicine. The medically important genera include *Actinomadura, Corynebacterium, Dermatophilus, Gordona, Mycobacterium, Nocardia, Nocardiopsis, Oerskovia, Rhodococcus, Streptomyces, Saccharomonospora, Saccharopolyspora, Thermoactinomyces, Tsukamurella,* the putative, unculturable agent of Whipple's disease, *Tropheryma whippelii,* and, to a lesser extent, *Amycolata, Amycolatopsis,* and *Micromonospora.* The main characteristics used for the identification of the clinically important aerobic actinomycetes to the genus level are given in Table 1. The family *Nocardiaceae* includes the genera *Nocardia, Gordona, Rhodococcus,* and *Skermania.* Closely related to this taxon are the families *Mycobacteriaceae* (i.e., the genera *Mycobacterium* and *Tsukamurella*) and *Corynebacteriaceae* (i.e., the genera *Corynebacterium, Dietzia,* and *Turicella*). All of these families are collectively known as the mycolic acid-containing genera (formerly, the families *Corynebacteriaceae* [C], *Mycobacteriaceae* [M], and *Nocardiaceae* [N] were known as the CMN-taxon). Members of the CMN-taxon have a set of chemical markers in common (i.e., the cell wall components *meso*-diaminopimelic acid [*meso*-DAP], arabinose, and galactose and the mycolic acids) and a specific cellular fatty acid pattern. This combination of chemical markers is diagnostic for all members of the CMN-taxon except *Turicella,* which is not able to synthesize mycolic acids (47) (Table 2).

* This chapter contains information presented in chapter 30 by Blaine L. Beaman, Michael A. Saubolle, and Richard J. Wallace in the sixth edition of this Manual.

DESCRIPTION OF THE GENERA

Nocardia

The transfer of *Nocardia amarae* to the genus *Gordona* as *Gordona amarae* and the suggestion that *Nocardia pinensis* merits generic status within the family *Nocardiaceae* but not in the genus *Nocardia* leave the genus *Nocardia* as a relatively homogeneous taxon (38). The genus *Nocardia* is currently composed of 11 validly described species (30, 38, 59, 198). The characteristics used to differentiate the eight medically important *Nocardia* species are given in Table 3. Members of the reconstituted genus *Nocardia* form extensively branched hyphae that fragment into rod-shaped to coccoid, nonmotile elements and usually form aerial hyphae, which at times are visible only microscopically (59). Nocardiae are characterized by the presence of *meso*-DAP, arabinose, and galactose in their wall peptidoglycan (wall chemotype IV) (96), having muramic acid in the *N*-glycolated form; having diphosphatidylglycerol, phosphatidylethanolamine, phosphatidylinositol, and phosphatidylinositol mannosides as their major phospholipids; having major amounts of straight-chain, unsaturated, and tuberculostearic acids; having mycolic acids with 40 to 60 carbon atoms; and having DNAs that are rich in guanine-plus-cytosine content (64 to 72 mol%) (59).

Rhodococcus

Recent taxonomic revisions have reassigned certain members of the genus *Rhodococcus* to two genera: *Gordona* (84, 145) and *Mycobacterium* (27). These and other recent taxonomic reassignments have been summarized in Table 4. The members of the genus *Rhodococcus* consist of a diverse group of organisms that are quite variable in their morphology, biochemical characteristics, growth patterns, and capacity to cause disease. The differentiation of the genus *Rhodococcus* from related genera is given in Table 2. The differential characteristics within the genus *Rhodococcus* are given in Table 5.

Gordona

In 1988, Stackebrandt et al. (161) reintroduced the genus *Gordona* to accommodate microorganisms previously considered rhodococci on the basis of comparative analyses of genes coding for 16S rRNA. The species assigned to the genus *Gordona* include the former *Rhodococcus bronchialis, Rhodococcus rubropertinctus, Rhodococcus sputi,* and *Rhodo-*

TABLE 1 Tests used for the presumptive identification of the aerobic actinomycetes to the genus level[a]

Genus	Vegetative filaments		Conidia	Acid-fast nature	Presence of the following in whole cells[b]		Mycolic acids	Metabolism of glucose	Growth at 50°C	Arylsulfatase	Growth in lysozyme
	Substrate	Aerial			DAP isomer	Sugars					
Actinomadura	+	V	V	−	*meso*	Mad	−	O	−	−	−
Amycolata	+	+	V	−	*meso*	Arab, Gal	−	O	−	−	−
Amycolatopsis	+	+	V	−	*meso*	Arab, Gal	−	O	−	−	−
Corynebacterium	+	−	−	−	*meso*	Arab, Gal	+	O	−	−	−
Dermatophilus[c]	+	−	−	−	*meso*	Mad	−	F	−	−	NT
Gordona	+	−	−	W	*meso*	Arab, Gal	+	O	−	−	V
Micromonospora	+	−	+	−	*meso*	Arab, Xyl	−	O	−	−	−
Mycobacterium	+	−	−	+	*meso*	Arab, Gal	+	O	−	+	−
Nocardia	+	+	V	W	*meso*	Arab, Gal	+	O	−	−	+
Nocardiopsis	+	+	+	−	*meso*	None	−	O	−	−	−
Oerskovia[c]	+	−	−	−	None	Gal	−	F	−	−	+
Rhodococcus	+	−	−	−	*meso*	Arab, Gal	+	O	−	−	V
Saccharomonospora	+	+	+	−	*meso*	Arab, Gal	−	O	+	−	−
Saccharopolyspora	+	+	+	−	*meso*	Arab, Gal	−	O	+	−	V
Streptomyces	+	+	+	−	L	None	−	O	−	−	−
Thermoactinomyces	+	+	+	−	*meso*	Arab, Gal	−	O	+	−	+
Tsukamurella	+	−	−	W	*meso*	Arab, Gal	+	O	−	−	+

[a] Data adapted from McNeil and Brown (107). Abbreviations and symbols: +, 90% or more of strains are positive; −, 90% or more of the strains are negative; V, 11 to 89% of the strains are positive; O, oxidative; F, fermentative; NT, not tested; Mad, madurose; Arab, arabinose; Gal, galactose; Xyl, xylose; W, weakly or partially acid fast.

[b] As determined by the method of Becker et al. (15) for whole-cell DAP and sugars.

[c] Both genera are motile.

coccus terrae that have mycolic acids with between 48 and 66 carbon atoms and major amounts of dihydrogenated menaquinones with 9 isoprene units (72). Two other taxa, *Nocardia amarae* and *Rhodococcus aichiensis*, have been transferred to the genus *Gordona* as *Gordona amarae* and *Gordona aichiensis*, respectively (84). Other species that have recently been affiliated with the *Gordona* taxon, *Gordona hydrophobica* (16) and *Gordona hirsuta* (83), were isolated from biofilters for waste gas treatment (16). These taxa, along with *G. amarae*, have not been isolated from clinical specimens. Members of the genus *Gordona* are aerobic, gram-positive, slightly acid-fast, nonmotile short rods (0.5 to 0.2 μm in diameter) that have a rod-coccus growth cycle. The cells do not form spores or capsules and usually do not produce aerial hyphae. The differentiation of the genus *Gordona* from related genera is given in Table 2. The differential characteristics of the medically important members of the genus *Gordona* are given in Table 6.

Tsukamurella

The genus *Tsukamurella* was first described in humans in 1971 by Tsukamura (172) and was isolated from the sputum

TABLE 2 Differential characteristics of the mycolic acid-containing genera[a]

Genus	Acid-fast nature	Macroscopic aerial filaments	Arylsulfatase production in 14 days	Range of no. of carbon atoms in mycolic acids	Presence of: Tuberculostearic acid	Presence of: Phosphatidylethanolamine	Presence of: Phosphatidylinositol and phosphatidylinositol mannosides	Menaquinone(s)	N-Glycolyl in glycan moiety of wall	DNA G+C content (mol%)
Corynebacterium	−	−	−	22–36	−	—[b]	+	MK-8 (H_2), MK-9 (H_2)	−	51–67
Dietzia	−	−	−	34–38	+	+	−	MK-8 (H_2)	−	73
Gordona	W	−	−	48–66	+	+	+	MK-9 (H_2)	+	63–69
Mycobacterium	+	−	+	60–90	+	+	+	MK-9 (H_2)	+	70–72
Nocardia	W	+	−	44–60	+	+	+	MK-8 (H_4-ω-cycl)[c]	+	64–72
Rhodococcus	W	−	−	34–64	+	+	+	MK-8 (H_2)	+	63–73
Tsukamurella	W	−	−	64–78	+	+	+	MK-9	+	67–68

[a] Data are from McNeil and Brown (107) and Rainey et al. (136). Abbreviations and symbols: −, 90% or more of the strains are negative; +, 90% or more of the strains are positive; W, weakly or partially acid fast.

[b] —, some *Corynebacterium* species contain phosphatidylethanolamine (136).

[c] Data are from Rainey et al. (136).

TABLE 3 Characteristics differentiating the medically important species of the genus *Nocardia*[a]

Characteristics	*N. asteroides* sensu stricto		*N. brasiliensis*	*N. brevicatena* complex	*N. farcinica*	*N. nova*	*N. otitidiscaviarum*	*N. pseudobrasiliensis*	*N. transvalensis* complex			
	Type I	Type VI							*N. asteroides* type IV	Sensu stricto	New taxon I	New taxon II
Species isolated from humans	+	+	+	+	+	+	+	+	+	+	+	+
Species implicated in human infection	+	+	+	+	+	+	+	+	+	+	+	+
Decomposition of:												
Adenine	–	–	–	–	–	–	–	+	–	–	–	–
Casein	–	–	+	–	–	–	–	+	–	–	–	–
Hypoxanthine	–	–	+	–	–	–	+	+	+	+	+	+
Tyrosine	–	–	+	–	–	–	–	+	–	–	–	–
Xanthine	–	–	–	–	–	–	+	–	–	–	–	–
Utilization of the following as sole carbon source:												
Adonitol (ribitol)	–	–	–	–	–	–	–	–	–	+	+	+
L-Arabinose	–	–	–	–	–	–	V	–	–	–	–	–
Citrate	+	V	+	–	–	–	–	+	+	+	+	+
i-Erythritol	–	–	–	–	+	–	–	–	+	+	V	V
D-Galactose	–	V	+	–	–	–	–	+	–	+	+	V
D-Glucose	+	+	+	–	+	+	+	+	+	+	V	V
i-*myo*-Inositol	–	–	+	–	–	–	+	+	–	+	+	–
D-Mannitol	–	–	+	–	–	–	V	+	–	V	+	V
L-Rhamnose	–	V	–	V	+	–	–	–	–	–	–	–
D-Sorbitol (D-glucitol)	–	–	–	–	–	–	–	–	–	+	+	–
D-Trehalose	V	V	+	V	–	V	V	+	+	+	+	+
Growth at or in:												
45°C	V	V	–	V	+	–	V	–	NT	NT	NT	NT
Lysozyme broth	+	+	+	V	+	+	+	+	+	+	+	+

Hydrolysis of acetamide	–	V	–	–	+	–	–	+	–	–	–	–
Production of arylsulfatase	–	–	–	–	–	+	–	–	–	–	–	–
Resistance to[b]:												
Amikacin (MIC, >16 μg/ml)	–	–	–	–	–	–	–	–	+	+	V	V
Gentamicin (zone, ≤10 mm)	–	–	NT	±	+	±	NT	NT	+	+	+	+
Kanamycin (MIC, ≥16 μg/ml)	–	±	NT	–	+	±	NT	NT	+	+	+	+
Tobramycin (zone, <20 mm)	–	–	NT	+	+	±	NT	–	+	+	+	+
Ciprofloxacin (MIC, ≥4 μg/ml)	+	–	–	–	–	+	NT	–	NT	NT	NT	NT
Ampicillin (MIC, ≥4 μg/ml)	+	+	V	–	+	–	+	V	NT	NT	NT	NT
Amoxicillin-clavulanate (MIC, ≥64/32 μg/ml)	NT	NT	–	V	–	+	+	V	V	+	V	–
Cefamandole (zone, <20 mm)	–	–	V	V	+	–	NT	NT	NT	NT	NT	NT
Cefotaxime (MIC, ≥64 μg/ml)	–	–	V	–	+	–	V	NT	NT	NT	NT	NT
Ceftriaxone (MIC, ≥64 μg/ml)	–	–	V	–	+	–	V	NT	NT	NT	NT	NT
Erythromycin (zone, <30 mm)	+	+	–	+	+	–	+	–	+	+	+	+

[a] Data were reported previously (29, 147, 186, 187, 190, 191, 198). Abbreviations and symbols: –, 90% or more of the strains are negative; +, 90% or more of the strains are positive; V, 11 to 89% of the strains are positive; NT, not tested.

[b] Disk content (μg) was as follows: gentamicin, 10 μg; tobramycin, 10 μg; cefamandole, 30 μg; and erythromycin, 30 μg. Methodology adapted from Wallace and Steele (189). Briefly, the inoculum was adjusted to a turbidity equivalent to that of a 0.5 McFarland barium sulfate standard and was streaked onto a Mueller-Hinton agar plate, the plate was incubated at 35°C, and the zone of inhibition was read at 48 h.

TABLE 4 Recent taxonomic changes in the *Gordona-Rhodococcus* complex

Present or new (reference)	Previous (reference)
Dietzia maris (136)	*Rhodococcus maris* (Nesterenko et al. 1982) (76)
Gordona amarae (84)	*Nocardia amarae* (Lechevalier and Lechevalier 1974) (56)
Gordona aichiensis (84)	*Rhodococcus aichiensis* (Tsukamura 1982) (56)
Gordona bronchialis (161)	*Rhodococcus bronchialis* (Tsukumura 1974) (56)
Gordona hydrophobica (16)	
Gordona hirsuta (83)	
Gordona rubropertincta (161)	*Rhodococcus rubropertinctus* (Tsukamura 1974) (56)
Gordona sputi (145, 161)	*Rhodococcus sputi* (Tsukamura and Yano 1985), *Rhodococcus obuensis*, and *Rhodococcus chubiensis* (Tsukamura 1982) (56)
Gordona terrae (161)	*R. terrae* (Tsukamura 1974) (56)
Mycobacterium chlorophenolicus (27)	*R. chlorophenolicus* (Apajalahti et al. 1986) (56)
Rhodococcus equi (57)	*Corynebacterium equi* (Magnusson 1923)
Rhodococcus fascians (82)	*Rhodococcus luteus* (Nesterenko et al. 1982) (56)
Rhodococcus rhodochrous (135)	*Rhodococcus roseus* (Tsukamura 1991) (204)

of patients with tuberculosis. *Tsukamurella paurometabola* was referred to variously as *Rhodococcus aurantiacus* or *Gordona aurantiaca* (161, 174) until 16S rRNA gene sequence analysis comparison found it to be identical to *Corynebacterium paurometabolum* (40). Therefore, *R. aurantiacus* was removed from the genus *Rhodococcus*, renamed *T. paurometabola*, and assigned a new type strain (40). Recently, four additional species have been assigned to the genus *Tsukamurella: T. inchonensis*, *T. pulmonis*, *T. tyrosinosolvens*, and *T. wratislaviensis* (64, 204–206). Yassin et al. (204–206) have clearly shown that levels of 16S rRNA gene sequence similarity of >99% exist between *Tsukamurella* strains, but this high level of similarity does not indicate membership in the same species. The major chemotaxonomic characteristics that distinguish the genus *Tsukamurella* from other mycolic acid-containing taxa are summarized in Table 2 (206). The characteristics that differentiate the members within the genus *Tsukamurella* are given in Table 7.

Actinomadura

Actinomadura was first recognized in 1894 by Vincent (183), who named the organism "*Streptothrix madurae*" and described it as the causative agent of madura foot. Subsequently, the taxonomy of the genus has undergone numerous revisions on the basis of the application of chemical, numerical phenetic, and molecular systematic methods (78). The genus is now well defined and is composed of 26 validly described species (78). Before the recent polyphasic taxonomic study of Trujillo and Goodfellow (170) in 1997, only two species of *Actinomadura*, *A. madura* and *A. pelletieri*, were clinically significant. Those investigators examined 31 strains received either as *A. madurae* or *A. pelletieri* and assigned these strains to four clusters. Two clusters received as *A. pelletieri* were studied by using the results from pyrolysis mass spectrometric and PCR amplification fingerprinting analyses and were separated into two distinct cluster groups that were strongly supported by numerical phenetic analyses based on degradative, enzymatic, nutritional, and physiological results. The separation of the latter two cluster groups was also supported by chemotaxonomic and DNA relatedness data. Thus, Trujillo and Goodfellow (170) proposed that the cluster merited species status equivalent to *A. madurae* and *A. pelletieri* within the genus *Actinomadura* and were classified as *Actinomadura latina*. Members of the genus *Actinomadura* are gram-positive, nonfragmenting bacilli that have branched substrate and aerial hyphae that each carry up to 15 arthrospores. The major characteristics that separate this genus from other aerobic actinomycetes are given in Table 1.

Streptomyces

From 1940 through 1957, more than 1,000 *Streptomyces* species were described (131). By 1970, the total had increased to 3,100, although many had inadequate taxonomic descriptions or have been cited only in patent literature (169). Identification to the species level was based on a limited number of subjectively chosen features with a heavy emphasis on morphology and pigmentation. However, after exhaustive phenetic studies Williams et al. (194, 196) suggested that the heavy weighting given to morphologic characters in prior classifications was no longer justified. They suggested that there should be relatively few cluster groups (or species) within the genus and assigned more than 300 species of *Streptomyces* and *Streptoverticillium* to 41 minor cluster (2 to 5 strains in each cluster) and 22 single-member clusters and 20 major (6 to 71 strains) clusters that were provisionally considered species groups. These species or cluster groups were named after the earliest validly described species that they contained following the principle of priority; in most cases the other species within a cluster are listed as subjective synonyms of this name. For example, since *Streptomyces anulatus* has precedence over *Streptomyces griseus*, *S. anulatus* is the name of the species or cluster group containing *S. griseus* as a subjective synonym (196). Recently, Goodfellow et al. (58) studied representative strains studied by Williams et al. (196) to evaluate the original numerical classification and clarify the taxonomy of these species groups, in particular the *Streptomyces albidoflavus* species group. Those investigators used characters usually used for streptomycetes and newly applied rapid enzyme tests based on the fluorophores. From their studies, they concluded that, at present, this genus includes too few species and that *S. albidoflavus* encompasses at least three species, two of which, *S. albidoflavus* and *S. anulatus*, can be equated with genomic species. Since the numerical taxonomic studies (60–63, 194) that provided an invaluable framework for streptomycete taxonomy and identification, there have been several additional studies based on phylogenetic analyses with 16S rRNA sequence data and on the ribosomal AT-L30 proteins and N-terminal amino acid sequences (121, 122, 200), numerical phenetic studies with 329 miniaturized tests (79), sodium dodecyl sulfate-polyacrylamide gel electrophoresis (SDS-PAGE) (102), DNA-DNA relatedness studies (88–90), and restriction endonuclease fingerprinting of large DNA fragments from strains of *Streptomyces* by pulsed-field gel electrophoresis (20). Since the studies

TABLE 5 Differential characteristics of the genus *Rhodococcus*[a]

Characteristic	*R. coprophilus*	*R. equi*	*R. erythropolis*	*R. fascians*	*R. globerulus*	*R. marinonascens*	*R. rhodnii*	*R. rhodochrous*	*R. ruber*
Species isolated from humans	–	+	–	–	–	–	–	–	–
Species implicated as cause of human infections	–	+	–	–	–	–	–	–	–
Morphogenetic sequence	AH-R-C	R-C	RB-R-C	H-R-C	RB-R-C	H-R-C	RB-R-C	RB-R-C	H-R-C
Pigment	Orange	Pink	Orange to red	Yellow	Pink to red	Cream to pink	Red	Rose	Red
Decomposition of:									
Adenine	–	+	+	+	–	–	–	V	V
Tyrosine	–	–	V	+	–	V	V	V	+
Utilization of the following as sole carbon source:									
D-Galactose	–	+	V	+	–	NT	+	V	V
i-*myo*-Inositol	–	–	+	–	–	+	–	–	V
D-Mannitol	–	–	+	+	V	–	+	+	+
L-Rhamnose	–	V	–	–	–	–	–	–	V
D-Sorbitol	–	–	+	+	V	V	–	+	+
D-Sucrose	–	–	+	+	V	NT	–	V	V
Citrate	–	–	+	V	+	NT	–	V	V

[a] Data are adapted from references 56 and 82. Abbreviations and symbols: AH-R-C, aerial hypha-rod-coccus; R-C, rod-coccus; RB-R-C, rudimentary branching-rod-coccus; H-R-C, hypha-rod-coccus growth cycle; +, positive, –, negative; V, variable; NT, not tested.

TABLE 6 Differential physiological characteristics of the medically important *Gordona* species[a]

Characteristic	*G. aichiensis*	*G. bronchialis*	*G. rubropertincta*	*G. sputi*	*G. terrae*
Species isolated from humans	+	+	+	+	+
Species implicated as cause of human infections	ND	+	+	+	+
Presence of synnemata or rare microscopic hyphae	–	+	–	–	–
Utilization of the following as sole carbon source[b]:					
D-Galactose	+	–	+	+	+
i-*myo*-Inositol	–	+	–	–	–
D-Mannitol	–	–	+	+	+
Raffinose	–	–	–	+	+
L-Rhamnose	–	–	–	–	+
D-Sorbitol	–	–	+	+	+
Citrate	+	–	+	–	+

[a] Data are adapted from references 16, 56, 84, and 145. Abbreviations and symbols: +, ≥90% of the strains are positive; –, ≥90% of the strains are negative; ND, not determined.

[b] Concentration used to determine carbon source utilization was 1.0% except for growth on citrate, which was tested at 0.1%.

TABLE 7 Differential characteristics of the genus *Tsukamurella*[a]

Characteristic	*T. inchonensis*	*T. paurometabola*	*T. pulmonis*	*T. tyrosinosolvens*	*T. wratislaviensis*
Species isolated from humans	+	+	+	+	−
Species implicated as cause of human disease	+	+	+	+	−
Decomposition of:					
Hypoxanthine	+	−	−	+	+
Xanthine	−	−	−	+	+
Tyrosine	−	−	−	+	+
Utilization of the following as sole carbon source:					
Cellobiose	+	−	−	−	−
Maltose	+	−	−	+	+
i-*myo*-Inositol	+	−	−	+	+
D-Mannitol	+	−	+	+	+
D-Sorbitol	+	−	+	+	+
Citrate	+	+	−	V	−
Utilization of acetamide as sole carbon and nitrogen source:	+	−	+	+	−
Growth at 45°C	+	−	−	−	NT

[a] Data are adapted from references 164 and 204–206. Abbreviations and symbols: +, positive; −, negative; V, variable; NT, not tested.

based on rRNA found discrepancies between the results of phylogenetic studies and phenetic analyses, it was concluded that the presently used physiologic tests reflect too small a portion of the genome to be universally useful in streptomycete species characterization. Those investigators (20, 58, 79, 88–90, 102, 121, 122) also concluded that high levels of DNA-DNA relatedness (>90%) and high similarity values with low-frequency restriction fragment analysis will probably be valuable for the delineation of actinomycete species (20). The major characteristics that differentiate the genus *Streptomyces* from other related genera are given in Table 1.

Other Aerobic Actinomycetes

The genus *Nocardiopsis* was described by Meyer (113) for microorganisms previously designated "*Streptothrix dassonvillei*," "*Nocardia dassonvillei*," or "*Actinomadura dassonvillei*." Currently, the genus *Nocardiopsis* consists of seven validly described species in the family *Nocardiopsiaceae*: *Nocardiopsis alba* (207), *Nocardiopsis dassonvillei* (113), *Nocardiopsis halophila* (3), *Nocardiopsis listeri* (71), *Nocardiopsis lucentensis* (203), *Nocardiopsis prasina* (207), and *Nocardiopsis synnemataformans* (207). Members of the genus *Nocardiopsis* exhibit fragmentation of substrate and aerial hyphae into zigzag chains of arthrospores that are characteristic for this genus (113). These microorganisms contain *meso*-DAP but no diagnostically important carbohydrate (cell wall chemotype III) (96). Other features include a lack of mycolic acids, the presence of muramic acid of the acetyl type, and DNA G+C contents of between 64 and 69 mol% (137, 207). The current differentiation of the *Nocardiopsis* species is based on the color of the hyphae and physiological characteristics (Table 8).

Dermatophilosis was first recognized as an infectious disease in 1915 by Van Saceghem (180), who described the disease in cattle in the former Belgian Congo. The disease was first reported in the United States in 1961 (26). In 1995, Masters et al. (104) described a new species, *Dermatophilus chelonae*, from chelonids (two turtles and one tortoise). Members of the genus *Dermatophilus* are characterized by a unique life cycle, at the beginning and end of which they are motile zoospores of 0.5 μm in diameter. The characteristics that separate the genus *Dermatophilus* from other actinomycetes are given in Table 1.

The genus *Micromonospora* is known primarily as the microbiologic source of clinically significant antimicrobial agents, especially the aminoglycosides and macrolides. The characteristics that separate the genus *Micromonospora* from other actinomycetes are given in Table 1.

Three genera of thermophilic actinomycetes are considered of medical importance: *Saccharomonospora* spp., *Saccharopolyspora* spp. (or *Faenia* spp.), and *Thermoactinomyces* spp. Within these three genera, there is one important species of *Saccharomonospora* (*S. viridis*), one important species of *Saccharopolyspora* (*S. rectivirgula* ["*Faenia rectivirgula*"]), and three important species of *Thermoactinomyces* (*T. thalpophilus*, *T. sacchari*, and *T. vulgaris*). Thermotolerance to 50°C or above is a pathognomonic characteristic for all of the thermophilic species. In addition, all of these species form *meso*-DAP and lack mycolic acids in their cell walls. Although the first practical scheme for the identification of the thermophilic actinomycetes was developed in 1975 by Kurup and Fink (87) and has remained clinically useful, this group of microorganisms has undergone numerous taxonomic changes (178).

Amycolatopsis orientalis ("*Nocardia*" *orientalis*, "*Streptomyces orientalis*") is primarily known for the production of the antimicrobial agent vancomycin (129). Although these isolates had a cell wall composition similar to that of the true nocardiae (presence of *meso*-DAP, arabinose, and galactose), they do not contain mycolic acids.

TABLE 8 Differential characteristics of the genus *Nocardiopsis*[a]

Characteristic	*N. alba*	*N. dassonvillei*	*N. halophila*	*N. listeri*	*N. lucentensis*	*N. prasina*	*N. synnemataformans*
Species isolated from humans	−	+	−	−	−	−	+
Species implicated as cause of human disease	−	+	−	−	−	−	+
Color of substrate hyphae	Colorless	Yellow, orange to brown	Yellow to coral red	Colorless	Yellow to brown	Colorless	Deep pimiento
Decomposition of:							
Adenine	+	+	+	+	+	−	+
Casein	+	+	+	+	+	+	+
Hypoxanthine	+	+	+	+	+	−	+
Tyrosine	+	+	−	+	+	+	+
Xanthine	+	+	−	+	−	+	+
Utilization of the following as sole carbon source:							
Cellobiose	+	+	NT	−	+	−	+
D-Galactose	+	+	−	−	−	−	+
D-Glucose	+	+	−	−	+	−	+
i-*myo*-Inositol	−	−	+	−	+	−	+
Maltose	+	−	+	−	+	−	+
D-Mannitol	−	+	+	−	+	−	+
Raffinose	−	−	−	−	+	−	−
L-Rhamnose	+	w	+	−	+	−	+
Sucrose	−	+	−	−	+	−	−
Trehalose	+	+	NT	−	+	−	−
D-Xylose	−	+	+	−	−	−	+

[a] Data are from references 3, 71, 203, and 207. Abbreviations and symbols: +, positive; −, negative; w, weakly positive; NT, not tested.

Amycolata autotrophica is a rare human pathogen that has recently been removed from the genus *Nocardia*. The reclassification was based on the fact that these microorganisms lack mycolic acids; however, their cell wall compositions are remarkably similar to those of true nocardiae (98).

In 1992, Relman and colleagues (140) reported a technique in which oligonucleotide primers specific for Whipple's disease bacillus were used in a PCR to amplify sequences of bacterial 16S rRNA directly from infected tissues. Following a comparative 16S rRNA sequence analysis, they concluded that the disease is caused by an as yet uncultured and uncharacterized actinomycete, which they named *Tropheryma whippelii* (140).

NATURAL HABITATS

The aerobic actinomycetes are ubiquitous in the environment; they have been isolated worldwide from soil, freshwater, marine water, and organic matter (54). *Nocardia* spp. and related bacteria are considered saprophytic soil microorganisms that are primarily responsible for the decomposition of organic plant material (54, 123, 128). Although *N. asteroides* appears to be geographically widespread, most cases of *N. brasiliensis* infection in the United States have originated in the Southeast or Southwest (160). No environmental source for *N. transvalensis* has yet been identified. However, as has been found for *N. asteroides*, soil is a probable reservoir for this unusual actinomycete.

The species of the genus *Rhodococcus* are widely distributed in the environment: *R. coprophilus*, *R. equi*, *R. erythropolis*, *R. fascians*, *R. globerulus*, *R. rhodochrous*, and *R. ruber* have been isolated from soil; *R. coprophilus* and *R. equi* have been isolated from herbivore dung; *R. fascians* has been isolated from plants and the intestinal tracts of carp; *R. marinonascens* has been isolated from the uppermost layer of marine sediments; and *R. rhodnii* has been isolated from the intestine of the reduviid bug (56). In 1984, Barton and Hughes (11) detected *R. equi* in 54% of soil samples examined and from intestinal contents, feces from the rectum, and dung of all grazing herbivorous species examined. Those investigators found a 10,000-fold increase in the rate of isolation of *R. equi* in dung from horses 1 to 2 weeks after its deposition by using an enrichment broth. This multiplication of *R. equi* has implications for the study of disease caused by *R. equi* in foals. Severe lung infections of foals occur because crowded foaling paddocks may provide an environment conducive to massive challenge with *R. equi* microorganisms at a time when the foals lack antibody or a functioning cell-mediated immune system (11).

Members of the genus *Gordona* are widely distributed: *G. aichiensis* has been isolated from human sputum (56); *G. bronchialis*, *G. rubropertincta*, *G. sputi*, and *G. terrae* have been isolated from sputa and soil (56); *G. amarae* has been isolated from foam formed on the surface of aeration tanks in activated-sludge sewage treatment plants (59); and *G. hirsuta* and *G. hydrophobica* have been isolated from biofilters for waste gas treatment (16).

Members of the genus *Tsukamurella* are psychrophilic microorganisms that grow best at temperatures cooler than the human basal body temperature. They are found naturally in soil, sludge, and arthropods.

The natural habitat of the pathogenic actinomadurae is thought to be the environment; these agents are inhabitants of the surface layers of the soil and may be introduced by percutaneous trauma and most commonly cause mycetomatous involvement of the lower extremity, although other sites of the human body may also be affected. *A. madurae* seems to be widespread in soil, whereas to date *A. pelletieri* has been found only in clinical specimens.

Very little is known about the role of *Streptomyces* species in natural environments, although evidence for their occurrence is extensive. Streptomycetes are widely distributed in terrestrial and aquatic habitats. Most are strict saprophytes, but some form parasitic associations with plants and animals. *S. somaliensis*, a well-established causal agent of actinomycetoma, is rarely reported in the United States, but has been reported in Mexico as well in African countries (74).

The natural reservoir for *Dermatophilus congolensis* is unknown; however, contaminated soil is a likely source (97). These organisms have a worldwide distribution but are most prevalent in the tropics and subtropics (209).

Thermophilic microorganisms are ubiquitous and can be found in water, air, soil and compost piles, home and industrial air-conditioning systems, house dusts, hay, and bagasse (solid plant residue left after sugar cane has been crushed for the extraction of sugar).

PATHOGENESIS

Nocardia

In studies by Beaman and Beaman (13), the virulence of *Nocardia* strains for mice was correlated with resistance to killing within macrophages, and a virulent strain, GUH-2, inhibited phagosome-lysosome fusion. In addition, nocardial superoxide dismutase and catalase activities may contribute to the resistance of the nocardiae to the oxidative killing mechanisms of phagocytes. Cord factor (trehalose-6,6″-dimycolate) in the nocardial cell envelope is toxic, inhibits phagosome-lysosome fusion, and appears to be associated with nocardial virulence (13).

The ability of *R. equi* to persist in and eventually destroy macrophages is the basis of its pathogenicity. Electron microscopic examination of cultured equine macrophages showed that organisms evaded killing by preventing phagosome-lysosome fusion, thus multiplying in and eventually killing the phagocytes (130). A heat-stable surface component of *R. equi*, possibly a capsular polysaccharide, has been identified and has been shown to inhibit oxygen-dependent cytotoxic mechanisms of horse neutrophils (130). Mycolic acid-containing glycolipid is a major cell wall component of *Rhodococcus* species and may be involved in pathogenesis. Strains of *R. equi* with mycolic acids of longer carbon chain lengths are more lethal in mice and cause greater granuloma formation than isolates with mycolic acids of shorter carbon chain lengths (117).

In *D. congolensis* infections, minor trauma to the skin as a result of thorn injury or the bite of an insect or tick is often the initiating event (5). Organisms propagate in the epidermis, and thick scab formation often occurs. Proteolytic enzymes of *D. congolensis* may be related to its virulence (5, 168). These enzymes may cause a dysfunction in epidermal differentiation or desquamation.

CLINICAL SIGNIFICANCE

Nocardia

Nocardia infections are rare in humans, occurring most frequently in patients who are severely immunocompromised (107). *Nocardia* infection is usually acquired by inhalation, but rarely, direct skin inoculation may be implicated. Nocardiosis appears to have a slight predilection for males and usually affects adults in the third and fourth decades of life. Most clinical infections in temperate countries have been caused by *N. asteroides* complex, *N. brasiliensis*, and rarely, *N. otitidiscaviarum*. The *N. asteroides* complex (including *N. asteroides* sensu stricto, *N. farcinica*, and *N. nova*) has been considered to be responsible for the majority of serious invasive infections. *N. brasiliensis* has been associated particularly with subcutaneous infections and is predominant in tropical countries (160). The new taxon, *N. pseudobrasiliensis*, which was recently separated from *N. brasiliensis*, generally appears to be associated with noncutaneous (pulmonary, central nervous system, or systemic) nocardiosis (13, 14, 99, 186). Although nocardiosis is most often considered a late-presenting, community-acquired infection, nosocomial outbreaks of nocardiosis in immunocompromised patients attributed to airborne, patient-to-patient transmission have been reported (150). The clinical manifestations, severity, and prognosis of disease in the infected patient are extremely variable and may be determined by factors such as the route of infection and the presence or absence of a properly functioning immune system. In immunocompetent hosts, localized subcutaneous infection may result from inoculation of these microorganisms at the time of surgery or from traumatic percutaneous inoculation as a result of outdoor activities. Although other *Nocardia* species may cause primary cutaneous infections, *N. brasiliensis* is the predominant causative agent (160).

In severely immunocompromised patients, the principal predisposing factors for nocardiosis include immunosuppressive therapy, particularly steroid drugs, neoplastic diseases, solid organ and bone marrow transplantation, chronic bronchopulmonary diseases, and AIDS; and the most common clinical presentations are invasive pulmonary infection and disseminated disease (14, 107). However, invasive disease may also occur in nonimmunocompromised patients. In addition, underlying pulmonary disorders (e.g., malignancy and tuberculosis) may predispose an individual to respiratory tract colonization with *Nocardia*. *Nocardia* spp. have also rarely been implicated as causes of mild clinical infections in humans, including pharyngitis, bronchitis, and otitis media (99).

Cutaneous nocardiosis may be subdivided into four clinical types: mycetoma, lymphocutaneous infection, superficial skin infection (abscess or cellulitis), and secondary cutaneous involvement with disseminated disease. Localized cutaneous nocardial infections may also present as either a chronically draining ulcerative lesion or a slowly expanding nodule and, less commonly, as pustules, abscesses, cellulitis, or pyoderma. Frequently, there may be spread beyond the initial cutaneous focus to involve the regional lymphatic system, and the disease may progress to the formation of lymphatic abscesses. When regional lymph node involvement occurs, this form of the disease is referred to as the lymphocutaneous syndrome. Since skin manifestations may be complications of disseminated disease, the finding of a cutaneous lesion in a patient should not always be attributed to local inoculation. In North and South America, Mexico, and Australia, *N. brasiliensis* is the chief cause of actinomycetoma; however, in Africa, S. *somaliensis* predominates (99). These infections most commonly affect patients in rural areas in developing countries. Patients with these chronic infections may give a history of specific minor localized traumatic injury. The foot is the commonest site of involvement; however, the hand, face, and neck may also be affected (107). Walking barefooted may be the major mode of acquisition of this infection since this potentially results in the feet receiving repeated, soil-contaminated puncture wounds.

Rarely, ocular infections with *Nocardia* spp. have been reported to occur in both apparently immunocompetent and immunocompromised patients. This type of infection may occur secondary to a traumatic injury with exogenous inoculation with *Nocardia* spp. and may result in keratitis and ultimately endophthalmitis (107). Endogenous *Nocardia* ocular infection may also occur in immunocompromised patients following bloodstream dissemination from a distant pulmonary or other infective focus, and all patients who present with this ocular infection should therefore undergo a thorough evaluation to exclude underlying disseminated disease (85).

Pulmonary nocardiosis may be associated with nonspecific clinical findings; however, immunocompetent patients may have a chronic course, whereas severely immunocompromised patients may have progressive, disseminated, and life-threatening infections. The most frequent clinical presentation may be a subacute or chronic, often necrotizing pneumonia which is frequently associated with cavitation (53, 107). Other presentations may include a slowly enlarging pulmonary nodule or pneumonia with an associated empyema (107). Infected patients are usually systemically ill. The usual pathologic process involves the formation of multiple necrotizing pulmonary abscesses (107). Infection readily spreads to the pleural surface or to distant sites, predominantly the skin and the brain (107). The formation of tissue granulomata, especially in the lung (107), is another common pathologic finding. Indolent progressive fibrosis may result following treatment or successful containment without therapy (107). The appearance on chest radiographic examination for patients with pulmonary nocardiosis may be pleomorphic and nonspecific (10, 107). Abnormalities commonly observed include localized infiltrates and irregular nodules (both of which may show evidence of cavitation), pleural effusions, and hilar lymphadenopathy. Local complications of invasive *Nocardia* pulmonary infections include pleural effusion, empyema, pericarditis, mediastinitis, superior vena cava obstruction, and rarely, the development of local chest wall and neck abscesses. Metastatic infective foci may be present but unrecognized at the time of the patient's initial presentation with pulmonary nocardiosis, and infection at these sites may not become clinically evident until after the patient has begun to receive antimicrobial therapy. In severely immunocompromised patients, pulmonary nocardiosis may progress rapidly, and the diagnosis should be considered if these patients present with acute necrotizing pulmonary infections. However, pulmonary *Nocardia* infection may also have a gradually progressive indolent course.

Disseminated nocardiosis is often a late-presenting and potentially life-threatening infection. It is most frequently endogenous (i.e., secondary to bloodstream spread) from a primary pulmonary infection (107, 197). However, very rarely it may result from a primary nonpulmonary (cutaneous) infection site (160). In patients with primary pulmonary nocardiosis, the development of disseminated infection may result in brain and skin lesions and invariably has a significant adverse effect on the patient's prognosis. The rate of mortality from disseminated nocardiosis ranges from 7 to 44% (12, 107, 197). In severely immunocompromised patients the mortality rate may be greater than 85% (107). Disseminated infection in susceptible patients may be caused by any of the *Nocardia* spp. identified as causing invasive pulmonary and cutaneous infections. As seen with pulmonary nocardiosis, the patients at highest risk for the development of disseminated infections are severely immunocompromised patients (25). The brain is the most frequent nonpulmonary site involved in disseminated nocardiosis (50), and cerebral nocardiosis is an important cause of cerebral space-occupying lesions. However, the infection may also involve multiple other deep organs including the kidney, spleen, and liver and, rarely, bone, skin, and joints (107). In the brain and other organs, abscess formation is a particularly common pathologic manifestation of disseminated infection (107). Patients with cerebral nocardiosis may present with acute signs of sepsis and intracranial mass effects (107). However, severely immunocompromised patients with nocardial cerebral abscesses may frequently be asymptomatic, and a prolonged latency (up to 3 years) may occur before this type of clinical presentation is seen in patients infected following the commencement of immunosuppression (107, 134). There may be clinical evidence of pulmonary nocardial infection in about one-third of the patients (28), and cultures of blood from these patients may also be positive for *Nocardia* spp. (8, 146). Computed tomographic scanning is an extremely useful technique for making the diagnosis and may also be used to monitor the patient's response to treatment (192). However, a definitive diagnosis may be established in the patient only following the performance of a brain biopsy that yields clinical specimens which are positive for *Nocardia* spp. on microbiologic culture and/or which show morphologically compatible microorganisms on histopathologic examination. Specific investigations for the detection of cerebral involvement are recommended for all patients with pulmonary and invasive nocardiosis since a brain abscess may be a common serious complication in these patients, and early lesions may be asymptomatic (49).

N. *farcinica* may cause a variety of clinical presentations, including cerebral abscess, keratitis, bacteremia, and pulmonary, kidney, and cutaneous infections (46, 112, 151). There is a clear importance for differentiating between N. *farcinica* and other members of the N. *asteroides* complex. This is because N. *farcinica* has a high degree of resistance to various antibiotics, especially to broad-spectrum cephalosporins, which makes drug treatment of the infection difficult (151, 191). N. *farcinica* occurs more frequently than was previously recognized (191), and mouse pathogenicity studies have demonstrated that this may be a more virulent species than others in the N. *asteroides* complex (42).

The clinical diseases associated with N. *nova* isolates are similar to those previously described for diseases due to N. *farcinica* and N. *asteroides* complex microorganisms. The reasons for the identification of these microorganisms include their susceptibility to erythromycin and broad-spectrum cephalosporins and their resistance to amoxicillin-clavulanate (152). Also, as suggested for N. *farcinica* infections, infection with N. *nova* may be more common than is presently suspected; however, the successful detection of these newly recognized species of microorganisms is dependent upon the performance of appropriate isolation and characterization techniques (187).

Infections with *N. transvalensis* have recently been reviewed by McNeil et al. (108). Initially recognized as a cause of mycetoma, *N. transvalensis* infections have also recently been reported to cause life-threatening invasive pulmonary and disseminated infections in severely immunocompromised patients (9, 108, 110). Importantly, clinical isolates of this unusual species may demonstrate a high level of inherent resistance to amikacin and aminoglycosides in general. In addition, therapy with trimethoprim-sulfamethoxazole (TMP-SMX) may not always be effective in this infection (108, 198). In a recent study by Wilson et al. (198), the designated subgroups of the *N. transvalensis* complex isolates showed differences in their geographic distributions. No isolates of the previous *N. asteroides* complex type IV (now considered a member of the *N. transvalensis* complex) were identified among the clinical isolates identified in Queensland, Australia. However, the majority (75%) of *N. transvalensis* isolates of the new taxon (taxon I) were from that location (198).

Rhodococcus

R. equi is a rare opportunistic pathogen found in severely immunocompromised patients and, most commonly in recent years, in human immunodeficiency virus (HIV)-infected persons (100). Most often, patients have a slowly progressive granulomatous pneumonia with lobar infiltrates frequently progressing to cavitating lesions visible on a chest radiograph. Other sites of infection include the central nervous system, pelvis, subcutaneous tissue, and lymphadenitis, where abscesses are found (154). Cases of lung infection caused by inhalation and cutaneous lesions caused by wound contamination have been documented; the latter are almost the only *R. equi* infections reported in healthy persons, frequently children (181). Despite increased awareness of this organism as an opportunistic pathogen in humans, delays in the accurate diagnosis of *R. equi* infection are still common (107, 154). Factors responsible for this may include the insidious onset of disease; the clinical resemblance of the infection to mycobacterial, fungal, and actinomycotic infections; and the relatively unremarkable bacteriologic profile of *R. equi*. Morphology, partial acid fastness, and a distinctive histopathologic profile in bronchial specimens contribute to an accurate clinical diagnosis. Histopathologic examination may reveal polymorphonuclear leukocytes with intracellular pleomorphic gram-positive bacteria, microabscesses, pseudotumors, and malakoplakia (154, 181). Malakoplakia is a relatively rare granulomatous inflammation not typically associated with histology of lung infection and can be a marker for this infection (154, 166). However, a conclusive diagnosis and differentiation from similar pathogens require the isolation and identification of *R. equi* from clinical specimens including sputum, bronchoalveolar lavage, and open-lung biopsy specimens. Cultures of blood from severely immunocompromised patients with focal *R. equi* infection often contain the organism. Sixty-five percent of cultures of blood from patients with HIV infection may be positive for *R. equi* (181). AIDS patients with documented *R. equi* pneumonia can have a >50% rate of mortality from *R. equi* infection and a course of illness punctuated by multiple relapses, which are common even when successful treatment is ultimately achieved (44, 100).

Gordona

G. (*Rhodococcus*) *terrae* has been a cause of primary cutaneous infection in a 7-year-old nonimmunocompromised female with a granulomatous forearm skin lesion and axillary lymphadenopathy (103). *Gordona* spp. have also been described from sputum specimens of patients with pulmonary disease (cavitary pulmonary tuberculosis or bronchiectasis), specifically, G. *aichiensis*, G. *bronchialis*, and G. *rubropertincta* (171, 172). Although G. *sputi* was observed in the sputa of patients with chronic pulmonary disease in another study of Tsukamura (173), it was not considered pathogenic. Recently, Buchman et al. (31) reported on two patients with long-term indwelling central venous catheters in whom *Gordona* bacteremia complicated the receipt of total parenteral nutrition at home. In 1994, Drancourt et al. (45) presented the first description of a brain abscess caused by G. *terrae* in an immunocompromised child. This patient's infection complicated receipt of antineoplastic chemotherapy for a primary cerebral rhabdoid tumor (45).

Tsukamurella

The first description of *T. paurometabola* was in 1971 by Tsukamura and Mizuno (176). The organism was isolated from the sputa of patients with tuberculosis in Japan (176). This microorganism appears to be pathogenic only in specific circumstances, such as with immunosuppression, when an indwelling foreign body is present, or when a patient has a chronic infection such as tuberculosis. Rare infections caused by *Tsukamurella* have been described in humans, including chronic lung infections (175, 176), subcutaneous abscesses and necrotizing tenosynovitis (174), cutaneous lesions (69), meningitis in a patient with hairy cell leukemia (132), peritonitis (35), catheter-related bacteremia in patients with cancer (93, 156), and acute myelogenous leukemia (39). A *Tsukamurella* infection has also been described in a patient undergoing hemodialysis (76). In addition, this organism has been isolated from an HIV-infected patient; however, it was thought to represent colonization, not a true infection (141). Although it is clear that all of these isolates are species of *Tsukamurella*, most probably they are not *T. paurometabola*, as this species is presently taxonomically defined (40). *T. inchonensis* was isolated from multiple cultures of blood obtained from a patient who had ingested hydrochloric acid and from another patient's necrotic lung tissue (204); *T. pulmonis* was isolated from the sputum of a patient with mycobacterial lung infection (205); and *T. tyrosinosolvens* strains were isolated from cultures of blood from two patients, both of whom had cardiac pacemakers, and from a patient with chronic lung infection (206).

Actinomadura

A. madurae is a frequent cause of actinomycotic mycetomas. In mycetomas, the etiologic agents occur in the form of granules. The majority of the reports of infections caused by this species are from tropical and subtropical countries. However, the higher prevalence of such infections in warm climates may also only be a reflection of patients' increased tendency for exposure by walking barefoot. A review of the species of aerobic actinomycetes identified by the Actinomycete Laboratory of the Centers for Disease Control and Prevention (CDC) from October 1985 through February 1988 from clinical specimens found that *A. madurae* accounted for 42 (11.5%) of the total of 366 isolates referred to the laboratory and that this species was second in frequency only to *N. asteroides*, which accounted for 98 (26.8%) of these isolates (109). The majority of these isolates in this study were from sputum (24 isolates; 57.1%) and wounds (13 isolates; 31%). However, 1 (2.4%) of the 42 isolates was from blood, which suggests a potential role for *A. madurae* as a colonizing and/or infecting microorganism in some patients. The new clinically important species *A. latina* has been isolated only from a mycetoma (170). However, there are a few recent reports of nonmycetomic infections caused by this microorganism. *A. madurae* peritonitis developed in a patient who was undergoing long-term ambulatory peritoneal dialysis and who had no history of travel to tropical regions (202). Interestingly, this patient's infection responded to intraperitoneal therapy with amikacin. In addition, in 1992, the first case of pneumonia caused by *A. madurae* in an AIDS patient was reported (111).

Streptomyces

Because most of the members of the genus *Streptomyces* are saprophytes, it has been traditional to minimize their significance in clinical microbiology. One species, *S. somaliensis*, has been identified as one of the etiologic agents of actinomycotic mycetoma in many countries, including Algeria, India, Malaysia, Mexico, Niger, Nigeria, Saudi Arabia, Somalia, South Africa, Sudan, the United States, and Venezuela (74). In these countries, this species has been associated in particular with mycetomas affecting the head and neck. The only case of nonmycetomic *S. somaliensis* infection was reported in 1970 in a patient with a perforated peritoneum (70). Several recent reviews suggest that it is no longer acceptable to consider this species the only species of this genus that is pathogenic for humans. Non-*S. somaliensis Streptomyces* spp. have been identified from clinical specimens from humans and animals (17, 109, 114). Those researchers (17, 109, 114) considered all of these species to be of potential medical importance. In two of the studies (109, 114), the majority of the *Streptomyces* isolates (from sputum, wound, blood, and brain) were identified as *S. anulatus* (*S. griseus*). In those reports (109, 114), the assignment to a species was based only on phenotypic characteristics and chemotaxonomic cell wall studies and not on the newer molecular taxonomic methods. There is a discrepancy between the large number of *S. anulatus* strains identified in these clinical reference laboratories and the relatively small number of publications claiming a disease association. However, *Streptomyces* spp. were clearly identified in large numbers throughout histopathologic sections in a patient with chronic pericarditis (155) and from a traumatic wound infection (210). In a report of infections caused by members of the order *Actinomycetales* in AIDS patients, Holtz et al. (75) described a patient who developed dual *Streptomyces* and *Mycobacterium tuberculosis* lymphadenitis. A *Streptomyces* sp. has been reported as the causative agent of pneumonia in an HIV-infected patient and as the causative agent of pneumonia and septic arthritis in an AIDS patient (2, 34). In these two patients, *Streptomyces* was the only microorganism identified from a specimen obtained by bronchoscopy (2) and from sputum and knee fluid (34). In 1995, Mossad et al. (116) described the first case of prosthetic valve endocarditis due to a *Streptomyces* sp. Other reports of *Streptomyces* infections have included septicemia and primary lung involvement, panniculitis, and brain abscess (107).

Other Actinomycetes

Dermatophilosis may occur in both wild and domestic animals and is usually manifest as severe skin lesions. In addition to cattle, the disease has been reported mainly in horses, goats, and sheep. Less commonly, the disease has been described in humans. Acquisition of *D. congolensis* by humans is usually the result of contact with the tissues of infected animals or contaminated animal products (67). Occupational groups that have the greatest risk for acquiring the infection include abattoir workers, butchers, dairy farmers, hunters, and veterinarians (208). However, in two patients, a physician and a patient with "hairy" leukoplakia, no such contact could be established (32). One report also described the isolation of this microorganism from a patient's contact lens, but no association with ocular infection was established (18). Microorganisms indistinguishable from *D. congolensis* have been seen and isolated from patients with pitted keratolysis, which characteristically attacks the soles of the feet (201). In addition, such involvement of human keratinized tissue is not surprising since the microorganism is known to liberate significant amounts of keratinase when cultured on an appropriate medium (73).

The first isolation of *N. dassonvillei* from a clinical specimen was in 1911 and was from a patient with conjunctivitis as reviewed by Grund and Kroppenstedt (71). Although there have been infrequent reports of clinical disease caused by *Nocardiopsis* species, *N. dassonvillei* is a potential cause of human infections, including mycetomas (157), skin infections (127, 158), and extrinsic alveolitis (19). In 1997, Yassin et al. (207) described a new species, *N. synnemataformans*, which was isolated from the sputum of a kidney transplant patient.

The members of the genus *Micromonospora* have rarely been encountered in human clinical specimens. In a recent review of the clinical isolates received in the Actinomycete Laboratory at CDC during a 29-month study period, only 6 of 366 were identified as members of this genus (109). In addition, to our knowledge, no descriptions of *Micromonospora* infections in humans have been published.

Relatively few species of thermophilic actinomycetes have been recognized to cause human disease. Repeated inhalation of dust containing these microorganisms or their spores may result in hypersensitivity pneumonitis or extrinsic allergic alveolitis, a serious disabling, immunologically mediated pulmonary disease that may affect agricultural, office, and industrial workers. Various names have been given to different forms of hypersensitivity pneumonitis. These names indicate either the high-risk occupational group affected, the substrate that gives rise to the particular antigen, or a specific type of environmental exposure. The best-characterized form of the disease is farmer's lung, which was first described in 1932 in a group of farmers in the United Kingdom and was associated with exposure to the dust of moldy hay (33). In 1963, the predominant sensitin from this source was identified to be *S. rectivirgula* (126); however, another species, *T. vulgaris*, may also be present and may induce the disease. Other forms of the disease and their associated sensitins include mushroom worker's lung, induced by exposure to moldy compost (*S. rectivirgula* and *T. vulgaris*); bagassosis, induced by exposure to moldy sugar cane (*T. sacchari* and *T. vulgaris*); air-conditioner-associated lung disease, resulting from contaminated ventilation ducts (*S. viridis* and *T. vulgaris*); and humidification system-induced disease, caused by contamination of the system's reservoir (*T. vulgaris*). Importantly, in addition to dust containing the actinomycetes, hypersensitivity pneumonitis may also result from inhalation of dust containing various fungi, avian serum proteins, and other substances. All of these particulate allergens are characterized by a small particle size (1 to 5 μm) that facilitates their penetration to the lung alveoli, where they can impinge and persist for long periods (92). Despite the variety of settings and multiple possible etiologies, the similar presenting symptoms and signs for these patients and the typical findings on histopathologic examination of pulmonary tissues are consistent with a singular pathologic process or disease entity, which has been termed hypersensitivity pneumonitis. Criteria useful for making the diagnosis of hypersensitivity pneumonitis induced by the thermophilic actinomycetes include (i) history of exposure to a potential environmental source of antigen in the patient's home or work environment, which may require an environmental investigation, air sampling for further delineation, or both steps; (ii) characteristic clinical, radiographic, and lung function findings, whose onset may occur or which may worsen within hours following exposure to antigen; (iii) demonstration in the patient's serum of precipitating antibodies (precipitins) to the causal antigen; and (iv) pulmonary infiltrates compatible with hypersensitivity pneumonitis visible on chest radiographs (92).

Of the 21 isolates of *A. orientalis* studied by Gordon et al. (68) in 1978, most were isolated from soil and vegetable matter, and the site of isolation for two isolates was reported to be cerebrospinal fluid (CSF) and an unknown clinical source. Nothing more is known about the pathogenicity of this microorganism.

During the last 20 years, only one published report has suggested that *A. autotrophica* is a potential human pathogen (36). Those investigators reviewed the case histories for eight patients. No patient described in the review had histopathologic evidence of infection; however, there was strong evidence supporting the possibility that this actinomycete was a pathogen in one patient with purulent pericarditis and suggestive evidence that it was a pathogen in three other patients: one with meningitis, one with a leg wound, and one with sepsis associated with bone marrow hypoplasia. In the four remaining patients, *A. autotrophica* was judged to have probably not been a significant pathogen.

Whipple's disease, or intestinal lipodystrophy, is a systemic disorder first described by George Whipple in 1907 (193). The disease predominates in middle-aged white males and is characterized by arthralgia, diarrhea, abdominal pain, and weight loss. Lymphadenopathy, fever, and increased skin pigmentation may be additional findings. The diagnosis is made by histologic demonstration of "foamy" macrophages infiltrating the lamina propria of the small intestine, which contain periodic acid-Schiff-positive inclusions. These inclusions are gram-positive bacilli (Whipple's bacilli), which may also be found extracellularly. They possess a unique cell wall structure. Therapy with antimicrobial agents ultimately effectively eradicates the organism. Patients with Whipple's disease show evidence of impaired cell-mediated immunity before and after successful treatment. However, infection with this microorganism has yet to be documented in a patient with AIDS.

COLLECTION, TRANSPORT, AND STORAGE OF SPECIMENS

The general principles of collection, transport, and storage are applicable to most aerobic actinomycetes. However, if samples are suspected of containing nocardiae, they should not be refrigerated or placed on ice prior to being transported. Some strains of *Nocardia* lose their viability after exposure to near-freezing temperatures. Since the respiratory tract is the most common portal of entry of the nocardiae, most specimens from patients with suspected nocardiosis are sputum, bronchoalveolar lavage fluid, transtracheal aspirates, or lung biopsy tissue. Extrapulmonary sites may also be infected, and tissue specimens (e.g., subcutaneous and/or brain biopsy specimens) as well as body fluids (e.g., blood and CSF) may be submitted. Normally sterile fluids and tissues should be transported to the laboratory promptly, especially if their collection required an invasive procedure. The use of invasive procedures is usual for the retrieval of specimens from patients with brain infections, since the CSF is usually negative for nocardiae, even though the patient may have extensive brain lesions. CSF should be cultured for nocardiae only in circumstances in which meningitis due to these organisms is suspected clinically, and these cultures should be held for at least 4 weeks.

Depending on the clinical presentation, the specimens that may yield rhodococci, gordonae, or tsukamurellae include blood, lower respiratory tract secretions, and intravascular catheter tips. Collection and transport techniques should follow submission protocols commonly used for routine microbiologic isolation studies.

If actinomycotic mycetoma is suspected, aspirates, if possible, rather than swabs of sinus tracts should always be collected for the isolation of *Actinomadura* species, *N. brasiliensis*, and *Streptomyces* species. If granules are present in this drainage material, they should be washed repeatedly in sterile saline to remove contaminating bacteria or fungi before shipment to a reference laboratory for study. If drainage is absent or minimal, biopsy of deeper tissue is necessary, or alternatively, specimens may include scrapings or aspirates from draining lesions.

DIRECT EXAMINATION

For patients with suspected nocardial infection and a compatible clinical picture, a definitive diagnosis usually depends on the demonstration of the organisms in smears or sections examined microscopically together with isolation and identification by microbiologic culture. The importance of direct microscopic examination of stained preparations of clinical specimens in the diagnosis of aerobic actinomycotic infections cannot be overemphasized. The specimens most frequently received in the clinical microbiology laboratory for evaluation include sputum, bronchoalveolar lavage fluid, exudate, or CSF. If possible, the material should be spread out in a petri dish and observed for clumps of the microorganisms, which may resemble granules. If clumps or granules are present, they should be selectively removed and crushed between two glass microscope slides for microscopic examination. In addition, duplicate direct smears of the clinical material should be always be prepared for staining, and one smear should be stained with Gram stain and the other should be stained by the modified Kinyoun method. On Gram-stained smears, Gram stain-positive branched filamentous hyphae (Fig. 1) that are similar in appearance to nocardiae in cultures are seen (Fig. 2); they measure from 0.5 to 1 μm in diameter and as much as 20 μm in length. To be of diagnostic value the hyphae must branch at right angles. Although the hyphae of nocardiae may resemble those of *Actinomyces* species in width, they are usually much longer and are more widely scattered throughout purulent material and the walls of the abscesses. In mycetomas, compact granules that are similar to those observed for the anaerobic actinomycetes are formed. Very rarely, clubbing has been seen with *N. asteroides* (105), but often, granules with clubbing are seen with *N. brasiliensis* and *N. otitidiscaviarum* (159). The hematoxylin and eosin stain is very useful for staining the tissue and the granules but does not stain the individual filaments (37) (Fig. 3). A tissue Gram staining procedure such as the Brown and Brenn (37) procedure is recommended for demonstrating the gram-positive fila-

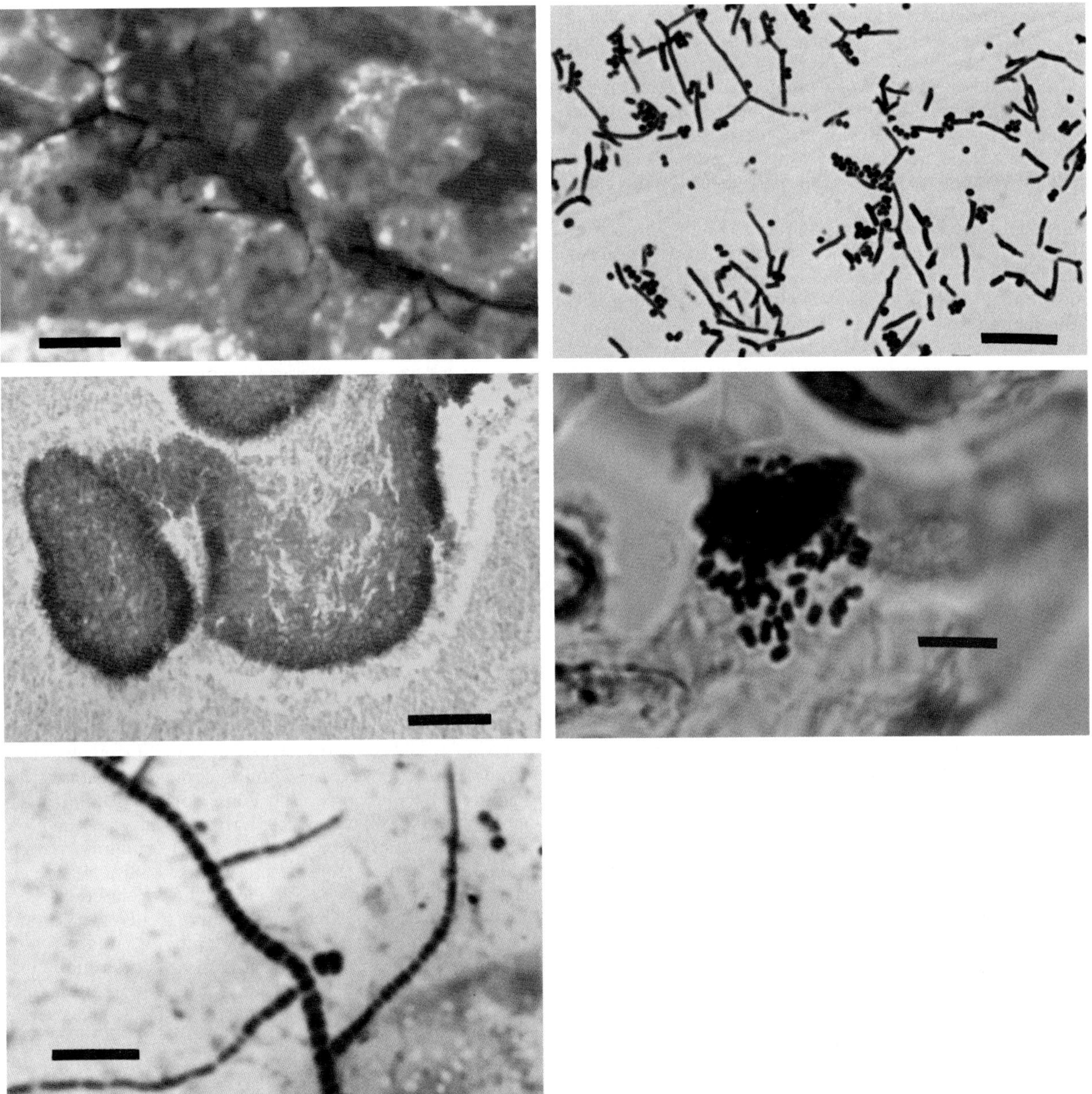

FIGURE 1 (Top left) *Nocardia asteroides*: branched, beady hyphae in a direct smear of sputum (Gram stain). Bar, 10 μm.
FIGURE 2 (Top right) *Nocardia farcinica*: branched hyphae, coccobacilli, and bacillary forms. A direct preparation from culture is shown (Gram stain). Bar, 10 μm.
FIGURE 3 (Middle left) *Nocardia brasiliensis*: granule in a section from a human mycetoma. No microorganisms are visible (hematoxylin and eosin stain). Bar, 40 μm.
FIGURE 4 (Middle right) *Rhodococcus equi*: coccobacillary forms in a section of human lung tissue (Brown and Brenn Gram stain). Bar, 10 μm.
FIGURE 5 (Bottom left) *Dermatophilus congolensis*: branched filaments divided in transverse and longitudinal planes with tapered fine hyphae. A direct preparation from infected subcutaneous tissue was used (Giemsa stain). Bar, 10 μm.

ments of nocardiae. The Gomori methenamine silver stain may also be useful. However, by both of these procedures, the filaments may not stain uniformly. Acid-fast stains are also of value in the histopathologic diagnosis of infections caused by *N. asteroides*, *N. brasiliensis*, and *N. otitidiscaviarum*. These species are frequently, but not always, acid fast in tissue sections stained by both the modified Kinyoun and the Fite-Faraco staining methods. *Actinomyces* and related species are usually not acid fast. These examinations may provide a rapid and presumptive diagnosis of the patient's infection, and the information that they yield may critically influence the clinician's choice of initial antimicrobial therapy.

In stained smears of clinical specimens, in particular, purulent material and tissue (obtained by biopsy, by surgery, and at autopsy), the coccoid or coccobacillary form of *R. equi* is usually seen intracellularly in macrophages and extracellularly (Fig. 4). However, bacillary *R. equi* forms have been reported in clinical specimens such as blood, bronchoalveolar lavage fluid, and sputum (43). In contrast, in all of the reported cases of non-*R. equi* rhodococcal infection, the direct smears prepared from clinical material have shown gram-positive coccobacilli, and in smears prepared from sputum, they were more filamentous than the level of filamentation reported for *R. equi* (124).

Although *D. congolensis* may be seen at any stage of development by direct examination of clinical materials, the appearance of branched filaments divided in their transverse and longitudinal planes is seen most frequently and is pathognomonic. These microorganisms may be seen in wet mounts or in smears of clinical material stained with methylene blue or by the Giemsa method (Fig. 5). A Gram-stained preparation is not likely to be helpful for visualizing these microorganisms because it is too dark and obscures crucial morphologic details.

ISOLATION

Since the aerobic actinomycetes are slowly growing microorganisms, their isolation from cultures of specimens obtained from normally sterile sites such as blood or CSF typically requires a prolonged incubation time (i.e., approximately 2 weeks). Isolation from tissue samples may take even longer (i.e., up to 3 weeks). These microorganisms grow satisfactorily on most of the nonselective media used for the isolation of bacteria, mycobacteria, and fungi. Blood specimens for culture may be inoculated into either conventional two-bottle broth blood culture systems, biphasic blood culture bottles, or automated radiometric or nonradiometric blood culture systems; each of these systems supports the growth of *Nocardia* microorganisms (146). However, satisfactory isolation of these microorganisms by these methods must still take into account factors such as maintaining the incubating cultures for up to 3 weeks and performing frequent and terminal subcultures (179). Blood specimens processed by lysis-centrifugation, exudates, joint fluid and CSF specimens, and homogenized tissue specimens are inoculated directly into media such as thioglycolate broth, Trypticase soy broth, or chopped-meat glucose broth. The thioglycolate broth medium, in addition to supporting the growth of aerobic actinomycetes, also supports the growth of anaerobic actinomycetes if these are present (149). Although the optimal blood culture method has not been defined, the use of the Isolator (Merck & Co., Inc., West Point, Pa.) system is probably best. All specimens from sterile sites may be inoculated directly onto a solid medium; however, the plates must be sealed in a manner that prevents dehydration.

The isolation of aerobic actinomycetes from the complex mixed flora of the soil and clinical specimens from sites that are normally nonsterile (e.g., samples from the respiratory tract and mycetomas) requires selective enrichment before these specimens are plated on selective isolation media. The isolation of *Nocardia* from soil and nonsterile sites may be difficult because its slow growth over 2 days to 3 weeks on routine culture media allows bacterial overgrowth to obscure the *Nocardia* colonies. Additionally, *Nocardia* is inhibited by the antibiotics in fungal culture media and often does not survive specimen digestive procedures used in mycobacterial culture techniques. The observation that some nocardial isolates may not survive in respiratory specimens has prompted studies of procedures that would facilitate the recovery of aerobic actinomycetes from these sources (107). In 1987, Murray et al. (119) demonstrated that digestion-decontamination of respiratory tract specimens with *N*-acetyl-L-cysteine, sodium hydroxide, and benzalkonium was toxic to *Nocardia*. Those same investigators studied Thayer-Martin medium containing colistin, nystatin, and vancomycin, a selective medium commonly used in clinical laboratories for the isolation of *Neisseria* species from contaminated specimens. Although this medium was not evaluated with clinical specimens, the successful results of this study with seeded sputum specimens encouraged further studies with this selective medium (179). Another promising medium is buffered-charcoal-yeast extract (BCYE) agar and selective BCYE agar that contained anisomycin, polymyxin, and vancomycin; these media are commonly used in clinical microbiology laboratories for the isolation of *Legionella* species from respiratory specimens (52, 182). However, one of the groups of investigators (182) found that pretreatment of the specimens with a low-pH (2.2) KCl-HCl solution for 4 min was necessary. No optimal method for isolating the aerobic actinomycetes from potentially contaminated specimens exists; however, the methods discussed above represent an improvement over the direct plating of these specimens directly on conventional media, such as Sabouraud dextrose agar (SDA), brain heart infusion agar, blood agar, or Lowenstein-Jensen medium.

After initial isolation, subcultures must be incubated at 25, 35, and 45°C to determine the optimal temperature for growth of the microorganisms. Most isolates of *N. asteroides* grow best at 35°C, while most isolates of *Streptomyces* grow best at 25°C. Any specimen suspected of containing a thermophilic actinomycete must also be incubated at 50°C since all thermophiles grow at this elevated temperature.

Isolation of *R. equi* requires selective media if the organisms are from soil or the feces of grazing herbivores. Recently, a new selective medium for *R. equi* containing ceftazidime (20 mg/liter) and novobiocin (25 mg/liter) in a Mueller-Hinton agar base was described (184). This selective medium proved to be less inhibitory for *R. equi* than the selective media devised in earlier studies and grew very few other nocardioforms.

Isolation of *D. congolensis* may be difficult. Clinical materials, preferably the underside of scabs, should be streaked onto a blood agar plate and incubated aerobically or in CO_2 at 35 to 37°C. Highly contaminated specimens may require passage in animals for successful isolation; crusts and scabs are ground and applied to the shaved and scarified skin of a rabbit (66). Cutaneous lesions develop in the animal within 2 to 7 days. Isolation of the microorganism in a pure culture of specimens from these infected sites may then be obtained.

IDENTIFICATION

Until recently, very little attention has been paid to the correct taxonomic assignment of clinically significant actinomycetes. The actinomycetes can be identified to the genus level on the basis of a variety of conventional phenotypic characteristics including microscopic (Gram and acid-fast staining) and macroscopic morphologies, growth requirements, metabolism of glucose, arylsulfatase production,

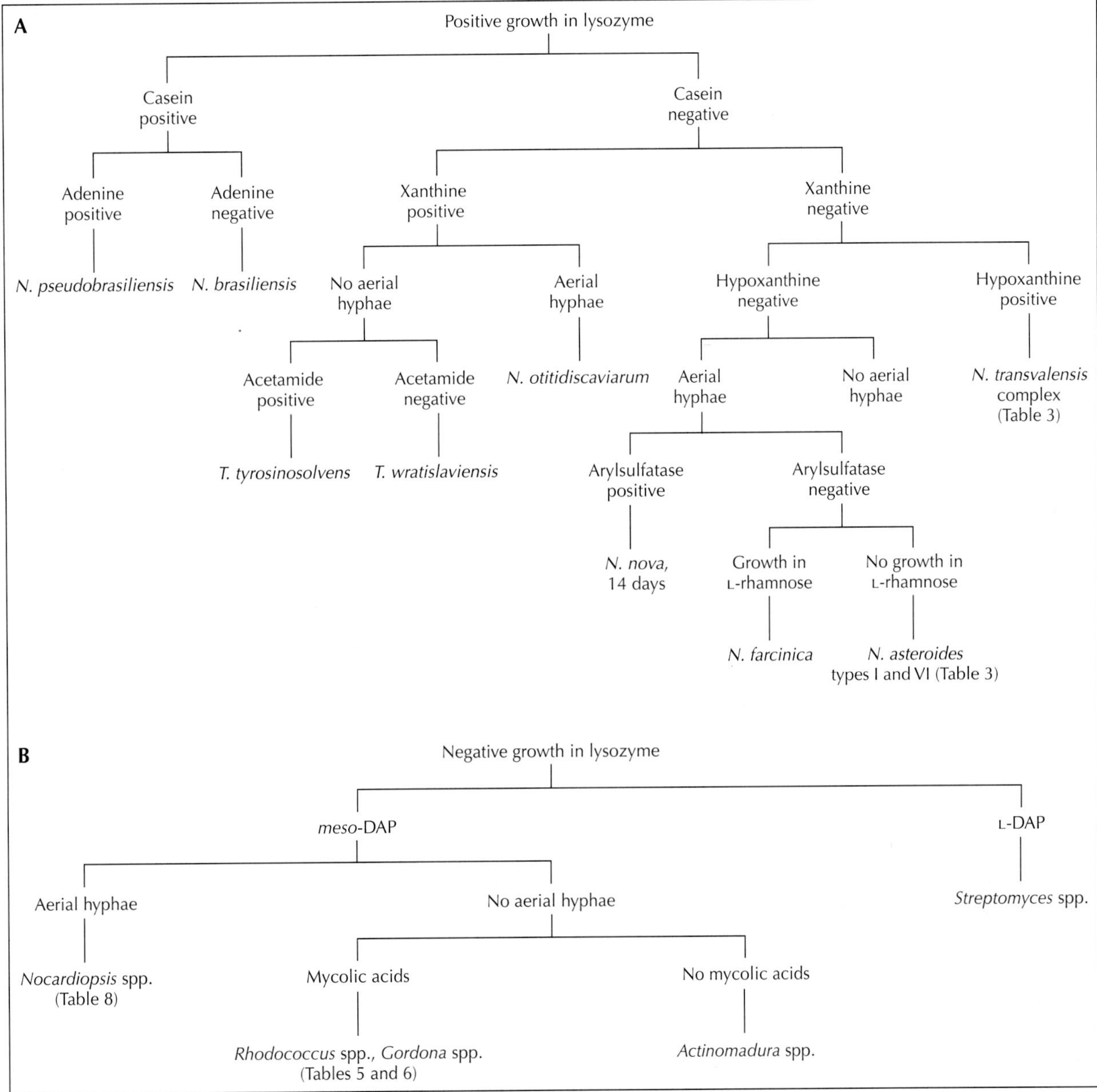

FIGURE 6 Schematic flow charts for the tentative identification of major medically important aerobic actinomycetes with positive (A) and negative (B) growth in lysozyme.

and growth in lysozyme and phenotypic molecular characteristics including the presence of whole-cell isomers of DAP and mycolic acid composition (Table 1). Some of these tests are beyond the capabilities of most clinical laboratories. However, both microscopic and macroscopic morphologies combined with a few physiologic tests can give a presumptive identification to the genus or species level. Schematic flowcharts for the tentative identification of medically important aerobic actinomycetes and related genera are given in Fig. 6A and B. Unfortunately, determination of the DAP isomer content is the only method of separating *Streptomyces* spp. from related genera. In addition to *Streptomyces* species, the definitive identification of the genera *Nocardiopsis* and *Actinomadura* requires referral of the isolate to a reference laboratory. As newer molecular techniques are applied to these organisms, many genera and species are being redefined. These genotypic methods include PCR-based methods, DNA hybridization, and sequencing of 16S rRNA. On primary isolation, typical colonial growth may be slow to appear. Cultures should be held for a week or more before being discarded as negative (107). Of importance, in some cases of pulmonary nocardiosis oft-repeated sputum cultures may not yield nocardial isolates; the retrieval of specimens by invasive procedures may be needed to make the diagnosis (107). The diagnostic yield of cultures of specimens obtained by invasive procedures such as transtracheal aspiration, bronchoscopic biopsy, and fine-needle aspiration has been reported to range between 85 and 90% (107). Therefore, particularly in the management of high-risk patients, clinicians must maintain a high degree of clinical suspicion for the diagnosis and, as indicated, perform invasive procedures for these patients. If necessary, clinicians should alert clinical microbiology and pathology laboratory personnel to use special methods to look for and identify microorganisms suspected of being *Nocardia* spp. (107).

Microscopic Morphology

The well-known acid fastness of *Nocardia* spp. is often more pronounced in clinical than in cultured material. By the modified Kinyoun technique, *Nocardia* spp. may be partially acid fast (showing both acid-fast and non-acid-fast bacilli and filaments). The presence of acid-fast branched filaments may be indicative of *Nocardia* spp.; however, in clinical material the result of acid-fast staining may be variable. Most isolates of *Nocardia* spp. in culture are weakly acid fast by the modified Kinyoun procedure when 1% sulfuric acid is used as a decolorizing agent (Fig. 7) (17). However, difficulties in the interpretation of the acid-fast staining result are frequently encountered. Variations in results may be dependent on the type of medium (medium containing high levels of lipid, such as Lowenstein-Jensen or Middlebrook 7H10, are best for demonstrating acid fastness). Of importance, isolates of *Streptomyces* spp. must be distinguished and may have acid-fast coccoid forms and non-acid-fast hyphae but are considered non-acid fast. The acid-fast staining procedure, long considered of primary importance in the identification of *Nocardia* spp., is a difficult test to standardize, and this may affect interpretation of its results. For example, if all of the acid-fast-stained smear appears bluish pink, the staining procedure must be repeated: there must be a contrast between the carbol fuchsin and the counterstain. Also, the demonstration of acid fastness by microorganisms grown in culture should be used only in conjunction with other tests as a supportive diagnostic test but not as an absolute diagnostic test (17). In cultures, these microorganisms' microscopic morphology is similar to that demonstrated in clinical material. They are gram positive with short to extensively branched vegetative hyphae of less than 1 μm in diameter. They may fragment into bacillary or coccoid, nonmotile forms. Short chains of conidia (two to three conidia) may be found on the aerial hyphae but are rarely seen on the substrate hyphae. The most satisfactory method for demonstrating the micromorphology of the nocardial culture is by direct in situ observation on a slide culture con-

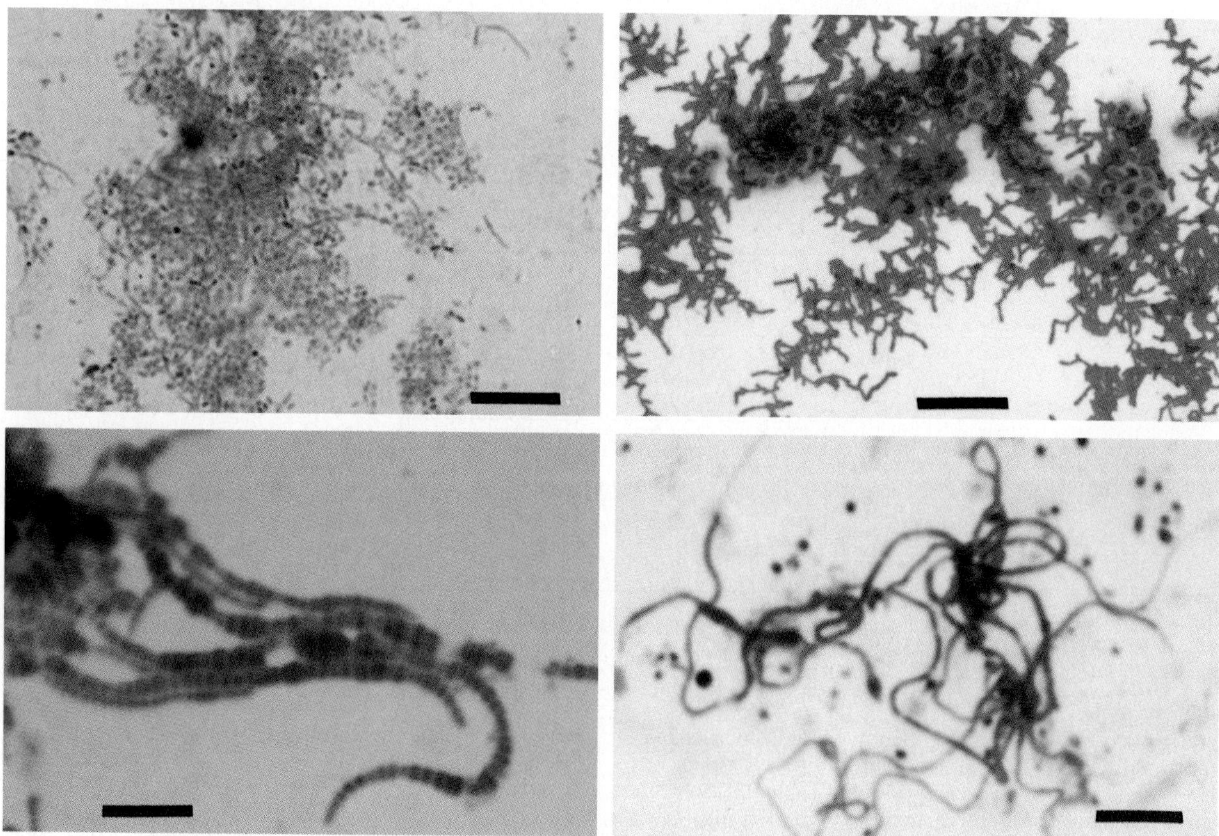

FIGURE 7 (Top left) *Nocardia farcinica*: rare acid-fast organisms from a smear of a Lowenstein-Jensen agar slant grown for 3 days (modified Kinyoun stain). Bar, 10 μm.
FIGURE 8 (Top right) *Rhodococcus rhodochrous*. The coccobacilli are arranged in a zigzag fashion. A slide culture preparation was grown on cornmeal agar without dextrose and was incubated for 1 week at 25°C (lactofuchsin stain). Bar, 10 μm.
FIGURE 9 (Bottom left) *Dermatophilus congolensis*. Branched filaments divided in transverse and longitudinal planes with tapered fine hyphae on a direct preparation from culture are shown (Giemsa stain). Bar, 10 μm.
FIGURE 10 (Bottom right) *Micromonospora* species. Fine branched hyphae with single spores on a direct preparation from culture are shown (Gram stain). Bar, 10 μm.

taining undisturbed colonies of the microorganism grown on a minimal medium such as tap water agar or cornmeal without dextrose (144). Culture preparations on these minimal media are incubated at 25°C and are examined periodically for 2 to 3 weeks. In examining slide cultures under the microscope, it is important to recognize a true branched substrate hypha, an aerial hypha, and sporulation. The substrate hyphae of *Nocardia* spp. appear as very fine, dichotomously branched filaments. Movement of the objective up and down through several planes will reveal aerial hyphae. The presence of aerial hyphae differentiates *Nocardia* spp. from other related genera such as *Corynebacterium*, *Gordona*, *Mycobacterium*, *Rhodococcus*, and *Tsukamurella*. The rapidly growing mycobacteria, which phenotypically resemble the nocardiae, have simple, relatively short substrate hyphae that branch at acute angles, in contrast to the complex hyphae of the nocardiae, which branch at right angles and which usually have secondary branches.

Rhodococci grow as coccobacilli arranged in a zigzag fashion (Fig. 8) on in situ slide cultures. The microscopic morphology of *R. equi* in culture is cyclic, varying from bacillary to coccoid depending on the incubation time and growth conditions. At 6 h on heart infusion agar (HIA) incubated at 35°C, these microorganisms are completely bacillary, but at 24 h they become completely coccoid. Gram-positive rudimentary branched filaments have reportedly been observed from cultures in liquid medium, especially from young cultures. The microscopic morphologies of the other *Rhodococcus* species are also cyclic, varying from a simple rod-coccus cycle in some species similar to *R. equi* to a more complex hypha-rod-coccus cycle in others (*R. coprophilus*, *R. fascians*, *R. marinonascens*, and *R. ruber*). *R. coprophilus*, *R. erythropolis*, *R. globerulus*, *R. rhodnii*, and *R. rhodochrous* are differentiated further into elementary branched hypha-rod-coccus cyclic forms (57). The branched hyphae may be rudimentary, highly transitory, or extensive. All of the rhodococci from clinical specimens are generally weakly acid fast when stained either by the modified Kinyoun method or by the Ziehl-Neelsen method.

Tsukamurellae are aerobic, gram-positive organisms and stain as slightly acid-fast bacilli with the modified Kinyoun stain (17). Most cells are long rods that fragment into three parts, which then separate and grow independently. The cells do not form spores or capsules or produce aerial hyphae.

The microscopic morphology of *D. congolensis* in culture is similar to that observed in clinical specimens. Depending on the age of the isolate and the type of medium used for culture, one may see completely coccal elements, many with flagellae or irregularly arranged cells in packets; germinating spores; or branched segmented or nonsegmented filaments (Fig. 9). Motility is usually evident in isolates from fresh cultures. If only cocci are seen and *D. congolensis* is suspected, younger cultures should be examined for hyphae.

The *Nocardiopsis* spp. produce hyphae that are long and branched and that fragment completely into zigzag chains of arthroconidia, which are characteristic of this species (113). The sporulation process was studied in detail by Williams et al. (195). They observed that the process is initiated by a single ingrowth of the hyphal wall, resulting in a cross wall. The first elements delimited are often long and are sometimes subdivided by further cross-wall formation. The process is completed by the disruption of the sheath between the spores. From these observations, it seems that the characteristic zigzag arrangement of developing spore chains is caused by lateral displacement of spores within the sheath (195).

The thermophilic actinomycetes are gram positive and non-acid fast. Individual thermophilic species are differentiated on the basis of their microscopic and macroscopic morphologies, in particular, the numbers of spores and the type of spore production. *S. rectivirgula* has short chains of spores that are on substrate and aerial hyphae, *S. viridis* has single spores only on aerial hyphae, and all three *Thermoactinomyces* species produce endospores. *T. vulgaris* has single endospores on sporophores on both aerial and substrate hyphae, *T. thalpophilus* has single endospores sessile on aerial and substrate hyphae, and *T. sacchari* has single endospores on sphorophores on both aerial and substrate hyphae.

Colonies of *Micromonospora* produce single spores on the substrate hyphae that are one of the well-defined characteristics of this genus (Fig. 10).

Microscopically, colonies of *A. orientalis* may produce aerial hyphae that form cylindrical, occasionally ovoid conidia in straight to flexuous chains. The substrate hyphae branch frequently and appear to zigzag at places.

Colonial Appearance

Aerial hyphae may be seen macroscopically in cultures, but in the early stages of growth they are seen only with the microscope. Macroscopic aerial hyphae may be lacking, sparse, or very abundant in *Nocardia* cultures; therefore, colonies may have a smooth appearance or, more commonly, a chalky white appearance reflecting the growth of aerial hyphae (Fig. 11). The gross morphology of the nocardiae is extremely variable and may differ depending on the medium or the incubation temperature used. The color of most colonies of *N. asteroides* complex varies from salmon pink to orange on SDA and HIA slants. The opacification of Middlebrook 7H10 agar with all isolates of *N. farcinica* studied is a useful adjunct for the identification of *N. farcinica* (51). *N. brasiliensis* colonies are usually orange-tan; in contrast, *N. otitidiscaviarum* colonies are usually pale tan in color. *N. transvalensis* colonies may vary in color from pale tan to violet.

The genus *Rhodococcus* consists of a diverse group of organisms that are quite variable in their colonial morphologies. These bacteria may produce rough, smooth, or mucoid and pigmented buff, coral, orange, or deep rose-colored colonies after several days of incubation. Growth occurs at 28 and 35°C but not at 45°C. *R. coprophilus* and *R. ruber* may demonstrate a few aerial hyphae, whereas none of the other *Rhodococcus* species form aerial hyphae. The colonial morphology of *R. equi* is diverse and consists of three major varieties. The classic colony type is pale pink and slimy in 2 to 4 days on HIA or on HIA containing 5% rabbit blood incubated aerobically at 35°C (Fig. 12). The second most frequent colony type is coral and nonslimy when the organism is grown on the same medium under similar incubation conditions. The third and least common colony type is pale yellow in color, nonslimy, and more opaque than the classic slimy type of colony and is identical to that of the *R. equi* type strain (ATCC 6939). Colorless colonial variants may also occur, particularly in *R. equi*.

Colonies of *G. sputi* are less pigmented than the other *Gordona* species; they are smooth, mucoid, and adherent to the media. *G. amarae* may produce feeble microscopically visible hyphae, and *G. bronchialis* may produce aerial synnemata consisting of unbranched filaments that coalesce and project upward and that may be confused with aerial hyphae. These bacteria produce dry, raised, beige colonies that become salmon colored after several days of culture (Fig. 13 and 14); however, the colonies of *G. amarae* and *G. hydro-*

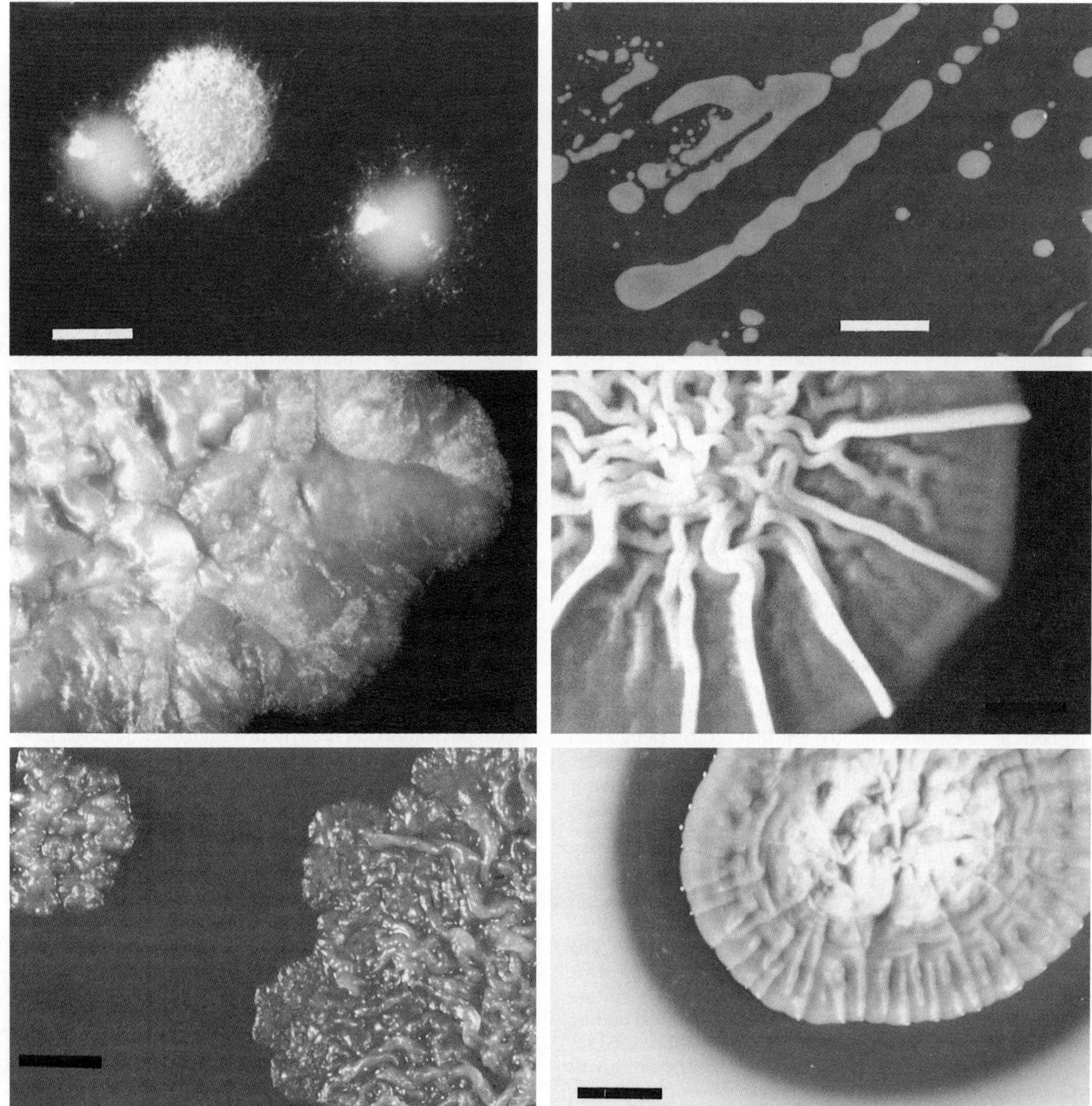

FIGURE 11 (Top left) *Nocardia farcinica* colonies with and without aerial hyphae grown for 5 days on heart infusion agar. Bar, 100 μm.

FIGURE 12 (Top right) Classic pink, slimy colonies of *Rhodococcus equi* grown for 5 days on an HIA plate with 5% rabbit blood. Bar, 100 μm.

FIGURE 13 (Middle left) *Gordona terrae* colony grown for 5 days on an HIA plate with 5% rabbit blood. Bar, 100 μm.

FIGURE 14 (Middle right) *Gordona bronchialis* colony grown for 5 days on an HIA plate with 5% rabbit blood. Bar, 100 μm.

FIGURE 15 (Bottom left) *Tsukamurella tyrosinosolvens* colony grown for 5 days on an HIA plate with 5% rabbit blood. Bar, 100 μm.

FIGURE 16 (Bottom right) *Streptomyces* colony grown for 10 days on a casein decomposition plate. Bar, 100 μm.

phobica remain beige. Growth occurs at 28 and 35°C but not at 45°C.

At 24 h on HIA containing 5% rabbit blood, colonies of the species *Tsukamurella* are usually 0.5 to 2.0 mm in diameter. These colonies are circular, usually have entire edges but may have rhizoid edges, are dry but easily emulsified, and are white to creamy to orange in color. Rough colonies are produced after prolonged incubation for up to 7 days. These colonies are characteristically cerebriform and do not produce aerial hyphae (Fig. 15). These colonies superficially resemble the rapidly growing mycobacteria, especially when they are cream in color. However, the mycobacteria can be differentiated from the genus *Tsukamurella* by arylsulfatase production within 14 days.

Colonies of *Actinomadura* species may be white to pink to red in color, are usually mucoid, and have a molar tooth appearance. Rare aerial hyphae are produced. *Actinomadura* species grow more slowly than other actinomycetes.

Colonies of *Streptomyces* species produce a wide variety of pigments that are responsible for coloration of the substrate and aerial hyphae; soluble pigments also may be produced (Fig. 16). Many strains of *Streptomyces* do not produce aerial hyphae.

D. congolensis has tiny (0.5 to 1.0 mm), round colonies at 24 h on HIA containing horse, sheep, or rabbit blood incubated at 35 to 37°C. The appearance of these colonies may vary, but they are usually gray-white and adherent, and they pit the medium. Later, in 2 to 5 days, they develop an orange pigment. Frequently, there is beta-hemolysis, which is improved with increased concentrations of carbon dioxide. This beta-hemolysis is also more prominent in areas of the medium where colonies are crowded. There is no growth on SDA.

The colonies of *N. dassonvillei* on organic media are abundant, coarsely wrinkled, and folded with a well-developed substrate mycelium and range in color from yellow to orange to brown; the colonies of *N. lucentesis* range from yellow to brown; the colonies of *N. synnemataformans* are deeply pimento colored; and the colonies of *N. alba*, *N. listeri*, and *N. prasina* are colorless (3, 71, 203, 207).

The color of the colonies of *Micromonospora* on agar media is initially pale yellow to light orange. With maturity, the colonies become progressively darker with the production of brown to black spores on some media, for example, SDA. Although some species have been reported to have maroon-purple and blue-green pigments, they have not been observed in the clinical laboratory.

The colonies of *S. rectivirgula* (*F. rectivirgula*) are usually yellow, and the colonies of *S. viridis* are blue-green. All of the colonies of *T. sacchari*, *T. thalpophilus*, and *T. vulgaris* are colorless to white.

The colonies of *A. orientalis* are cream or peach in color.

The colonies of *A. autotrophica* have cream-colored aerial hyphae and yellow to brown substrate hyphae.

Acid Production or Utilization of Carbohydrates

Two principal systems for testing the physiology of *Nocardia* spp. are the "Gordon" and "Goodfellow" methods. The former method, summarized by Berd (17) and Mishra et al. (114), has been found to be useful in differentiating the actinomycetes to the generic level on the basis of about 40 tests. However, Goodfellow and Lechevalier (59), using 140 characters, found that some of the taxa recognized by the Gordon method were heterogeneous, in particular, the *N. asteroides* complex. Acid production from carbohydrates is used in the Gordon method, and utilization of carbohydrates is used in the Goodfellow method for the differentiation of the actinomycetes. Tables 3, 5, 6, 7, and 8 use the utilization of carbohydrates to differentiate the medically important species within the genera *Nocardia*, *Rhodococcus*, *Gordona*, *Tsukamurella*, and *Nocardiopsis* (59, 64, 147, 187, 191, 198, 203, 206, 207). Usually, acid production from carbohydrates is comparable to carbohydrate utilization; however, early readings (<1 week) of acid production from some carbohydrates are important, since some carbohydrates (L-rhamnose and cellobiose) revert to negative reactions on prolonged incubation (191).

Isolates of *A. madurae* usually produce acid from adonitol, L-arabinose, cellobiose, i-erythritol, D-glucose, glycerol, D-mannitol, D-mannose, L-rhamnose, D-trehalose, and D-xylose. In contrast, the isolates of *A. pelletieri* are asaccharolytic; they produce acid only from D-glucose and D-trehalose (114). The carbohydrates utilized by isolates of the new taxon *A. latina* are similar to those utilized by *A. madurae* isolates except that *A. latina* does not utilize adonitol (170).

D. congolensis produces acid but not gas from glucose in fermentative basal medium in 48 h; however, it may produce acid transiently from galactose (acid in 48 h; negative in 2 weeks) (65). In addition, some strains produce acid from maltose in 1 to 2 weeks. No acid is produced from dulcitol, lactose, D-mannitol, salicin, D-sorbitol, sucrose, or D-xylose.

Decomposition of Substrates

The ability or inability of the aerobic actinomycetes to decompose adenine, casein, hypoxanthine, tyrosine, and xanthine continues to be a major and generally accepted criterion for the tentative identification of *N. brasiliensis*, *N. pseudobrasiliensis*, *N. otitidiscaviarum*, *N. transvalensis*, *Actinomadura* species, *Nocardiopsis* species, *Streptomyces* species, and *Tsukamurella* species. These tests are not useful for separating *N. asteroides* sensu stricto, *N. farcinica*, *N. nova*, and *N. brevicatena* from each other or from the related genera *Corynebacterium*, *Gordona*, *Mycobacterium*, and *Rhodococcus*. These tests are performed by inoculating growth onto the surfaces of quadrant plates containing adenine, hypoxanthine, tyrosine, or xanthine (0.4 g of each added to 100 ml of basal medium that contains 5 g of peptone, 3 g of beef extract, 15 g of agar, and 1,000 ml of distilled water) or casein plates (10 g of skim milk powder in 100 ml of distilled water and 2 g of agar in 100 ml are autoclaved separately, mixed, and poured into quadrant plates). The plates are incubated at 35°C (or 25°C if the isolate does not grow well at 35°C). Observe the casein plates at 7 and 14 days for clearing beneath and around the growth. Observe adenine, hypoxanthine, and tyrosine plates weekly for 4 weeks and xanthine plates weekly for 3 weeks for clearing of the crystals (17).

Isolates of *D. congolensis* may take up to 7 days to decompose casein. Hypoxanthine, tyrosine, and xanthine are not decomposed.

The thermophilic actinomycetes are separated by decomposition of the following substrates: adenine, casein, hypoxanthine, tyrosine, and xanthine (87, 91).

Most isolates of *Micromonospora* are strongly proteolytic; all isolates from human clinical specimens have decomposed casein and 75% have decomposed tyrosine (17). No isolates decompose hypoxanthine or xanthine.

Growth in Lysozyme

Growth in lysozyme is one of the most valuable tests for differentiating between nocardiae and other aerobic actinomycetes. The preparation of the lysozyme is as follows: 95

ml of sterile glycerol broth (peptone, 5 g; glycerol, 70 ml; and distilled water, 1,000 ml) is mixed with 5 ml of lysozyme solution (100 mg of lysozyme [Sigma Chemical Co., St. Louis, Mo.] in 100 ml of 0.01 N hydrochloric acid sterilized by filtration), and the mixture is dispensed into test tubes. These tubes and controls containing glycerol broth without lysozyme are inoculated with 1 drop of a culture suspension with a Pasteur pipette and are observed weekly for 4 weeks. The test is considered positive if good growth is noted in both tubes and negative if growth is good in the control tube but poor or absent in the tube containing the lysozyme (17). Except for 10 lysozyme-susceptible isolates of the *N. brevicatena* complex, all *Nocardia* species grow in the presence of lysozyme (29).

Arylsulfatase Production

Arylsulfatase production can be determined by a modification of the technique of Kubica and Ridgeon (86) in which a 0.008 M phenolphthalein disulfate solution in Middlebrook 7H9 broth is used as the substrate. Color is developed by the addition of 2 N sodium carbonate. Arylsulfatase activity is indicated by the development of a deep pink color (86). Strains of rapidly growing *Mycobacterium* are usually positive within 3 days; most strains of *N. nova* are positive within 14 days. These arylsulfatase-positive strains of *N. nova* can be distinguished from the *Mycobacterium* species by the presence of aerial hyphae.

Antibiogram

Wallace and colleagues (187, 190, 191) have shown that the determination of antimicrobial susceptibility results for amikacin, amoxicillin-clavulanate, ampicillin, cefotaxime, ciprofloxacin, erythromycin, and minocycline may be useful for species identification within the genus *Nocardia*, for example, *N. asteroides* sensu stricto (unnamed taxon group I, which is susceptible to amikacin, cefotaxime, ciprofloxacin, and minocycline, whose resistance to erythromycin is greater than its resistance to ampicillin, and which is resistant to amoxicillin-clavulanate; and unnamed taxon group VI, which is susceptible to amikacin, cefotaxime, ciprofloxacin, and minocycline, whose resistance to ampicillin is greater than its resistance to erythromycin, and which is resistant to amoxicillin-clavulanate); *N. farcinica* (which is susceptible to amikacin, amoxicillin-clavulanate, ciprofloxacin, and minocycline and resistant to ampicillin, cefotaxime, and erythromycin), and *N. nova* (which is susceptible to amikacin, ampicillin, erythromycin, and minocycline and resistant to amoxicillin-clavulanate and ciprofloxacin) (187, 190, 191).

Cell Wall Composition

Although the actinomycetous nature of an aerobic isolate is often immediately obvious, particularly if aerial hyphae are present, reliable differentiation of these aerobic actinomycetes to the genus level is usually possible only when chemotaxonomic techniques are used. These include examination of diagnostic cell wall components and testing for the presence or absence of mycolic acids, metabolism of glucose, and growth in lysozyme. The determination of certain diagnostic cell wall components provides especially useful data. In whole-microorganism hydrolysates, the presence or absence of 2,6-DAP and the differentiation of its isomers are of great diagnostic relevance. In addition, such hydrolysates may contain diagnostic sugars, which are also of value in the definitive identification of these microorganisms. The cell wall components that differentiate the major groups of the actinomycetes are given in Table 9. In routine work, the simplified techniques of Becker et al. (15), Lechevalier et al. (96), Berd (17), and Staneck and Roberts (162) are recommended for the detection of diagnostic amino acids and sugars. Before the analysis of whole-cell hydrolysates was introduced as a diagnostic tool, many isolates of *Micromonospora* spp. were likely discarded as unidentified actinomycetes. The application of this test, together with the characteristic formation of orange colonies that turn black and the production of single spores, may result in the more frequent identification of this rare species in the clinical laboratory (17).

Mycolic Acids

Qualitative evaluation of mycolic acid composition can be easily performed by thin-layer chromatography as recently described by Hamid et al. (72). The presence or absence of mycolic acid esters is one of the major tests used for the presumptive identification to the genus level (Table 2). McNabb et al. (106) studied an additional useful chemotaxonomic tool, fatty acid analysis, in a study of 568 type and reference strains of pathogenic aerobic actinomycetes by using the Microbial Identification System (Microbial Identification Inc., Newark, Del.). As further taxonomic revisions of the actinomycetes occur, fatty acid analysis may become one of the most practical methods for the rapid identification of this group of organisms.

TABLE 9 Major constituents of cell walls of actinomycetes[a]

Cell wall types	Major constituents	Whole-cell sugar pattern	
		Type	Diagnostic sugars
Streptomyces species or type I	L-DAP, glycine	None	None
Micromonospora species or type II	*meso*-DAP, glycine; hydroxy-DAP may also be present	D	Xylose, arabinose
Actinomadura species or type III	*meso*-DAP	B	Madurose[b]
Nocardiopsis species or type III	*meso*-DAP	C	None
Nocardia species or type IV, *Rhodococcus* species or type IV, *Gordona* species or type IV, *Tsukamurella* species or type IV	*meso*-DAP, arabinose, galactose	A	Arabinose, galactose

[a] All cell wall preparations contain major amounts of alanine, glutamic acid, glucosamine, and muramic acid.
[b] Madurose, 3-*O*-methyl-D-galactose.

Identification Using Commercial Biochemical or Miniaturized Test Systems

In contrast to the use of conventional, growth-dependent procedures for the identification of bacteria, the use of chromogenic enzyme substrates can rapidly detect constitutive enzymes produced by microorganisms.

Kilian (80) evaluated the API ZYM system (Societe Analytab Products Inc., La Balme Les Grottes, France) for its ability to rapidly identify members of the family *Actinomycetaceae* and related bacteria. In combination with the β-xylosidase test, catalase activity, and oxygen requirements, 12 of 19 enzymes screened proved to be of value for differentiating species of the family *Actinomycetaceae* and some related species within 4 h. In 1990, Boiron and Provost (24) further evaluated the API ZYM system for its ability to detect constitutive enzymes with chromogenic substrates.

A related application of rapid chromogenic substrate tests is the fluorogenic enzyme method described by Goodfellow and colleagues (55, 58) for studying the numerical taxonomy of both *Rhodococcus* and *Streptococcus* species. Other miniaturized studies include two Microscan (Dade MicroScan Inc., West Sacramento, Calif.) products, Rapid Anaerobe Identification and *Haemophilus-Neisseria* panels that test for preformed enzymes (21); the bioMerieux ID 32C Yeast Identification System (bioMerieux Vitek, Inc., Marcy l'Etoile, France) (118); and another system based on 273 phenotypic tests (79). However, the last approach with numerous tests is not applicable in the routine clinical laboratory and may be more suitable for specialized reference or research laboratories.

Identification Using Nucleic Acid Systems and Other Novel Methods

Recent advances in molecular techniques have shown promise as rapid and specific aids in the identification of many difficult-to-identify bacteria.

Recently, a PCR-restriction fragment length polymorphism identification schema has been used to identify all clinically significant species and taxa of aerobic actinomycetes, including *Actinomadura, Gordona, Nocardia, Rhodococcus, Streptomyces*, and *Tsukamurella* (163, 165, 198, 199). This methodology was as sensitive as, less time-consuming than (2 to 5 working days), and less labor-intensive than traditional methods (199). Although more time-consuming, ribotyping with a 16S rRNA gene probe was used for the identification of four different species within the *N. asteroides* complex (95) and isolates of the genera *Rhodococcus* and *Gordona* (94).

Diagnostic histopathology continues to be an essential counterpart of clinical microbiology. Application of in situ hybridization methods may be particularly beneficial when putative microorganisms are rare or have a nonspecific (coccoid) morphology, as seen with *R. equi* (30). An important and even more recent technological advance has been PCR analysis of 16S rRNA, which has further increased the sensitivity of detection of microorganisms that cannot be cultured on artificial media.

The original *T. whippelii* 16S rRNA gene PCR primers described by Relman et al. (140) in 1992 and subsequently modified have been successfully applied to small intestinal biopsy tissue, peripheral blood, pleural effusion cells, heart tissue, and vitreous fluid (41, 138–140, 143).

In 1995, Provost et al. (133) used the yeast killer system to separate species within the *N. asteroides* complex. Briefly, self-immune killer yeasts (*Pichia mrakii* K9 and *Pichia lynferdii* K76) secrete extracellular glycoproteins or killer toxins that produce different patterns of inhibition zones against three species of the *N. asteroides* complex. This method was relatively rapid (results were available after 5 days of incubation), economic, and feasible when it was compared to traditional methods that may take up to 3 weeks.

Comparative studies of the available phenetic and genetic methods that include well-characterized clinical and reference isolates are needed to determine which technique is best for the identification of each major pathogen.

Strain Identification

Typing systems based solely on phenotypic tests have limitations because the phenotypic traits of microorganisms may be inconsistently expressed. Therefore, additional stable phenotypic as well as genotypic assays are needed. In 1988, Morace et al. (115) described a biotyping method that has promise as a highly discriminatory epidemiologic tool. They found that 9 killer yeasts, grouped into triplets, selected from a panel of 44 yeasts belonging to the genera *Candida, Kluyveromyces, Pichia*, and *Saccharomyces* differentiated eight *Nocardia* test strains. However, this technique also has yet to be evaluated with a significant number of epidemiologically related *Nocardia* strains. Until such a study is performed, the usefulness of this method is unclear.

Molecular subtyping techniques have been successfully applied in the investigation of several nosocomial pseudo-outbreaks and nosocomial outbreaks as well as multiple, related isolates of the *N. asteroides* complex (101, 125) and *N. farcinica, N. brasiliensis, G. bronchialis*, and *T. paurometabola* (7, 23, 48, 112, 142, 164). The methods include *Pvu*II-, *Pst*I-, and *Sal*I-digested genomic DNA analysis (7, 112, 125, 142), pulsed-field gel electrophoresis (23, 101, 164), PCR analysis of randomly amplified polymorphic DNA (48, 101), ribotyping (7, 48, 94, 112, 142), and plasmid analysis (77, 142).

SEROLOGY

Most serologic tests for the actinomycetes have been hampered by a lack of specificity and sensitivity and are complicated further by the lack of antigenic homogeneity or the inability of some clinical isolates to secrete the antigen under study. A number of antigens have been proposed for serologic testing including the 26- and 24-kDa proteins (148), the 55-kDa protein (6); the 36-, 55-, and 62-kDa proteins (81); culture filtrates, cytoplasmic extracts, cord factor (trehalose dimycolate), and whole cells for the nocardiae (81); a soluble culture filtrate for *R. equi* (185); cell extracts for *Actinomadura* spp. (107); and culture extracts of the thermophilic actinomycetes (91). Serologic test methods included mostly enzyme-linked immunosorbent assay and Western blot techniques; however, immunodiffusion and indirect immunofluorescence methods have also been studied. Except for certain value in the diagnosis of hypersensitivity pneumonitis, most of these serologic tests are experimental but have some potential diagnostic value and may be useful as an indicator of response to therapy (148).

ANTIMICROBIAL THERAPY

Recent in vitro and in vivo studies, clinical observations, and taxonomic developments indicate that antimicrobial therapy must be adjusted to the particular species of *Nocardia* present, to the antimicrobial susceptibility patterns of individual strains, and to the site and type of infection (14, 99, 107). Sulfonamides (or the combination TMP-SMX) are the therapy of choice for nocardiosis. However, in patients with disease disseminated to the central nervous system or with depressed cell-mediated immunity, such as that which occurs in renal transplant recipients and HIV-infected patients, therapy may be complicated. The frequent use of TMP-SMX for the treatment of this infection may not be related as much to its properties of synergism or improved efficacy compared with that of sulfonamide treatment alone but may be related to its favorable pharmacokinetics (effective CSF penetration) and the general familiarity of clinicians with this drug combination. A problem not infrequently encountered in the therapy of HIV-infected patients is patient intolerance of TMP-SMX (167).

Antimicrobial therapy of pulmonary and/or systemic *R. equi* infections is problematic since the majority of patients have relapses, despite treatment, and the attributable mortality rate is high, especially among AIDS patients (100). Careful and repeated culture and susceptibility testing during treatment are essential for the detection of acquired resistance (120). One proposed regimen involves a parenteral glycopeptide plus imipenem for at least 3 weeks, followed by an oral combination of rifampin plus either macrolides or tetracycline (120).

The most appropriate drug treatment and duration of therapy for patients with infections due to other aerobic actinomycetes are unknown. Thus, performance of antimicrobial susceptibility tests with clinically significant isolates is needed and should preferably be performed at a specialized reference laboratory (1, 99).

Currently, no standards for antimicrobial susceptibility testing of the aerobic actinomycetes have been provided by the National Committee for Clinical Laboratory Standards. Over the years, a few studies have evaluated conventional methods of studying the susceptibilities of these microorganisms, including the disk diffusion (22, 188), broth dilution (22, 188, 189), and agar dilution (22, 153) methods. Recently, two newer methods, the epsilometer test (E-test [AB Biodisk, Solna, Sweden]) (22) and the radiometric broth method (153), have been evaluated. In 1997, Ambaye et al. (4) studied isolates of the members of the *N. asteroides* complex and compared the results of three conventional methods (the disk diffusion, broth dilution, and agar dilution methods) with those of the E-test and the radiometric methods for a panel of nine antimicrobial agents including amikacin, amoxicillin-clavulanate, ceftriaxone, ciprofloxacin, erythromycin, imipenem, minocycline, and TMP-SMX (4). Those workers determined that the radiometric broth method had the highest level of agreement when the results for all antimicrobial agents tested were combined; the agar dilution test method had the lowest level of agreement with the consensus interpretative results (4).

EVALUATION, INTERPRETATION, AND REPORTING OF RESULTS

The limited availability of laboratories with the appropriate capabilities for the identification of the actinomycetes is a problem. However, modern communications networks and the ability to rapidly ship specimens make the services of a few reference laboratories more widely available.

Determining whether a particular strain of *Streptomyces* is involved in a disease process can sometimes be difficult because most of these actinomycetes may be recovered from clinical specimens as contaminants. Many published case reports of disease associated with *Streptomyces* species are often cited, although they repeatedly provide minimal or erroneous laboratory data on the identification of the infecting organism. Therefore, to avoid these problems in future publications and to strengthen the establishment of a valid disease association, it is proposed that the following information be provided: (i) microscopic descriptions of the Gram staining result for the clinical material and the bacterial culture; (ii) macroscopic description of the size, pigment, odor, and hemolysis of colonies; (iii) descriptions of physiological reactions, including temperature requirements, decomposition of the substrates adenine, casein, hypoxanthine, tyrosine, and xanthine, and utilization of carbohydrates; (iv) results of chemotaxonomic investigations (e.g., cellular fatty acid analysis, presence or absence of mycolic acids, and cell wall analysis [the presence of L-DAP must be determined]); and (v) the results of molecular analysis (e.g., 16S rRNA gene sequence, G+C content, and DNA-DNA hybridization results) and pure culture or whether repeated isolation from a normally sterile site has been achieved.

REFERENCES

1. **Abu-Samra, M. T., S. E. Imbabi, and E. S. Mahgoub.** 1976. *Dermatophilus congolensis*. A bacteriological in vitro antibiotic sensitivity and histopathological study of natural infection in Sudanese cattle. *Br. Vet. J.* **132:**627–631.
2. **Ahmed, A. J.** 1996. *Streptomyces* infection in AIDS presenting with pneumonia and monarthritis. *Infect. Dis. Clin. Pract.* **5:**207–208.
3. **Al-tai, A. M., and J.-S. Ruan.** 1994. *Nocardiopsis halophila* sp. nov., a new halophilic actinomycete isolated from soil. *Int. J. Syst. Bacteriol.* **44:**474–478.
4. **Ambaye, A., P. C. Kohner, P. C. Wollan, K. L. Roberts, G. D. Roberts, and F. R. Cockerill III.** 1997. Comparison of agar dilution, broth microdilution, disk diffusion, E-test, and BACTEC radiometric methods for antimicrobial susceptibility testing of clinical isolates of the *Nocardia asteroides* complex. *J. Clin. Microbiol.* **35:**847–852.
5. **Ambrose, N. C.** 1996. The pathogenesis of dermatophilosis. *Trop. Anim. Health Prod.* **28:**29S–37S.
6. **Angeles, A. M., and A. M. Sugar.** 1987. Identification of a common immunodominant protein in culture filtrates of three *Nocardia* species and use in etiologic diagnosis of mycetoma. *J. Clin. Microbiol.* **25:**2278–2280.
7. **Auerbach, S. B., M. M. McNeil, J. M. Brown, B. A. Lasker, and W. R. Jarvis.** 1992. Outbreak of pseudoinfection with *Tsukamurella paurometabolum* traced to laboratory contamination: efficacy of a joint epidemiological and laboratory investigation. *Clin. Infect. Dis.* **14:**1015–1022.
8. **Avram, M. M., S. R. Nair, H. I. Lipner, and C. E. Cherubin.** 1978. Persistent nocardemia following renal transplantation. Association with pulmonary nocardiosis. *JAMA* **239:**2779–2780.
9. **Baghdadlian, H., S. Sorger, K. Knowles, M. McNeil, and J. Brown.** 1989. *Nocardia transvalensis* pneumonia in a child. *Pediatr. Infect. Dis. J.* **8:**470–471.
10. **Balikian, J. P., P. G. Herman, and S. Kopit.** 1978. Pulmonary nocardiosis. *Radiology* **126:**569–573.
11. **Barton, M. D., and K. L. Hughes.** 1984. Ecology of *Rhodococcus equi*. *Vet. Microbiol.* **9:**65–76.
12. **Beaman, B. L., J. Burnside, B. Edwards, and W. Causey.** 1976. Nocardial infections in the United States, 1972–1974. *J. Infect. Dis.* **134:**286–289.
13. **Beaman, B. L., and L. Beaman.** 1994. *Nocardia* species: host-parasite relationships. *Clin. Microbiol. Rev.* **7:**213–264.

14. **Beaman, B. L., P. Boiron, L. Beaman, G. H. Brownell, K. Schaal, and M. E. Gombert.** 1992. *Nocardia* and nocardiosis. *J. Med. Vet. Mycol.* **30:**317–331.
15. **Becker, B., M. P. Lechevalier, R. E. Gordon, and H. A. Lechevalier.** 1964. Rapid differentiation between *Nocardia* and *Streptomyces* by paper chromatography of whole-cell hydrolysates. *Appl. Microbiol.* **12:**421–423.
16. **Bendinger, B.** 1995. *Gordona hydrophobica* sp. nov., isolated from biofilters for waste gas treatment. *Int. J. Syst. Bacteriol.* **45:**544–548.
17. **Berd, D.** 1973. Laboratory identification of clinically important aerobic actinomycetes. *Appl. Microbiol.* **25:** 665–681.
18. **Berger, R. O., and B. W. Streeten.** 1981. Fungal growth in aphakic soft contact lenses. *Am. J. Ophthalmol.* **91:** 630–633.
19. **Bernatchez, H., and E. Lebreux.** 1991. *Nocardiopsis dassonvillei* recovered from a lung biopsy and a possible cause of extrinsic alveolitis. *Clin. Microbiol. Newsl.* **13:**174–175.
20. **Beyazova, M., and M. P. Lechevalier.** 1993. Taxonomic utility of restriction endonuclease fingerprinting of large DNA fragments from *Streptomyces* strains. *Int. J. Bacteriol.* **43:**674–682.
21. **Biehle, J. R., S. J. Cavalieri, T. Felland, and B. L. Zimmer.** 1996. Novel method for rapid identification of *Nocardia* species by detection of preformed enzymes. *J. Clin. Microbiol.* **34:**103–107.
22. **Biehle, J. R., S. J. Cavalieri, M. A. Saubolle, and L. J. Getsinger.** 1994. Comparative evaluation of the E test for susceptibility testing of *Nocardia* species. *Diagn. Microbiol. Infect. Dis.* **19:**101–110.
23. **Blumel, J., E. Blumel, A. F. Yassin, H. Schmidt-Rotte, and K. P. Schaal.** 1998. Typing of *Nocardia farcinica* by pulsed-field gel electrophoresis reveals an endemic strain as source of hospital infections. *J. Clin. Microbiol.* **36:** 118–122.
24. **Boiron, P., and F. Provost.** 1990. Enzymatic characterization of *Nocardia* spp. and related bacteria by API ZYM profile. *Mycopathologia* **110:**51–56.
25. **Braun, T. I., L. A. Kerson, and F. P. Eisenberg.** 1991. Nocardial brain abscesses in a pregnant woman. *Rev. Infect. Dis.* **13:**630–632.
26. **Bridges, C. H., and W. M. Romane.** 1961. Cutaneous streptothricosis in cattle. *J. Am. Vet. Med. Assoc.* **138:** 153–157.
27. **Briglia, M., R. I. Eggen, D. J. Van Elsas, and W. M. De Vos.** 1994. Phylogenetic evidence for transfer of pentachlorophenol-mineralizing *Rhodococcus chlorophenolicus* PCP-I(T) to the genus *Mycobacterium*. *Int. J. Syst. Bacteriol.* **44:**494–498.
28. **Bross, J. E., and G. Gordon.** 1991. Nocardial meningitis: case reports and review. *Rev. Infect. Dis.* **13:**160–165.
29. **Brown, B. A., R. W. Wilson, V. A. Steingrube, Z. Blacklock, and R. J. Wallace, Jr.** 1997. Characterization of a *Nocardia brevicatena* complex among clinical and reference isolates, abstr. C-65, p. 131. *In Abstracts of the 97th General Meeting of the American Society for Microbiology 1997*. American Society for Microbiology, Washington, D.C.
30. **Brown, J., M. McNeil, P. Greer, B. Lasker, R. Bluth, W. Schaffner, D. Oblack, J. Jahre, and S. Zaki.** 1991. Detection of *Rhodococcus equi* in tissues of HIV-infected patients by in situ hybridization using a biotinylated probe, abstr. D-26, p. 82. *In Abstracts of the 91st Annual Meeting of the American Society for Microbiology 1991*. American Society for Microbiology, Washington, D.C.
31. **Buchman, A. L., M. M. McNeil, J. M. Brown, B. A. Lasker, and M. E. Ament.** 1992. Central venous catheter sepsis caused by unusual *Gordona* (*Rhodococcus*) species: identification with a digoxigenin-labeled rDNA probe. *Clin. Infect. Dis.* **15:**694–697.
32. **Bunker, M. L., L. Chewning, S. E. Wang, and M. A. Gordon.** 1988. *Dermatophilus congolensis* and "hairy" leukoplakia. *J. Clin. Pathol.* **89:**683–687.
33. **Campbell, J. M.** 1932. Acute symptoms following work with hay. *Br. Med. J.* **2:**1143–1144.
34. **Caron, F., F. Borsa-Lebas, P. Boiron, E. Vasseur, C. Hennequin, M. Nouvellon, C. Dauga, J. F. Lemeland, and G. Humbert.** 1992. *Streptomyces* sp. as a cause of nodular pneumonia in an HIV infected patient? *Med. Microbiol. Lett.* **1:**297–303.
35. **Casella, P., A. Tommasi, and A. M. Tortorano.** 1987. Peritonite da *Gordona aurantiaca* (*Rhodococcus aurantiacus*) in dialisi peritoneale ambulatore continua. *Microbiologia* **2:** 47–48.
36. **Causey, W. A., and J. M. Brown.** 1974. Characteristics of isolates of *Nocardia autotrophica* (Takamiya and Tubaki) Hirsch recovered from clinical sources, p. 100–101. *In Proceedings of the 1st International Conference on the Biology of* Nocardia. McGowen Printing Co., Augusta, Ga.
37. **Chandler, F. W., W. Kaplan, and L. Ajello.** 1980. *A Color Atlas and Textbook of Histopathology of Mycotic Diseases*. Wolfe Medical Publications, London, United Kingdom.
38. **Chun, J., and M. Goodfellow.** 1995. A phylogenetic analysis of the genus *Nocardia* with 16S rRNA gene sequences. *Int. J. Syst. Bacteriol.* **45:**240–245.
39. **Clausen, C., and C. K. Wallis.** 1994. Bacteremia caused by *Tsukamurella* species. *Clin. Microbiol. Newsl.* **16:**6–8.
40. **Collins, M. D., J. Smida, M. Dorsch, and E. Stackebrandt.** 1988. *Tsukamurella* gen. nov., harboring *Corynebacterium paurometabolum* and *Rhodococcus aurantiacus*. *Int. J. Syst. Bacteriol.* **38:**385–391.
41. **Dauga, C., I. Miras, and P. A. Grimont.** 1997. Strategy for detection and identification of bacteria based on 16S rRNA genes in suspected cases of Whipple's disease. *J. Med. Microbiol.* **46:**340–347.
42. **Desmond, E. P., and M. Flores.** 1993. Mouse pathogenicity studies of *Nocardia asteroides* complex species and clinical correlations with human isolates. *FEMS Microbiol. Lett.* **110:**281–284.
43. **Doig, C., M. J. Gill, and D. L. Church.** 1991. *Rhodococcus equi*—an easily missed opportunistic pathogen. *Scand. J. Infect. Dis.* **23:**1–6.
44. **Donisi, A., M. G. Suardi, S. Casari, M. Longo, G. P. Cadeo, and G. Carosi.** 1996. *Rhodococcus equi* infection in HIV-infected patients. *AIDS* **10:**359–362.
45. **Drancourt, M., M. M. McNeil, J. M. Brown, B. A. Lasker, M. Maurin, M. Choux, and D. Raoult.** 1994. Brain abscess due to *Gordona terrae* in an immunocompromised child: case report and review of infections caused by *G. terrae*. *Clin. Infect. Dis.* **19:**258–262.
46. **Eggink, C. A., P. Wesseling, P. Boiron, and J. F. Meis.** 1997. Severe keratitis due to *Nocardia farcinica*. *J. Clin. Microbiol.* **35:**999–1001.
47. **Embley, T. M., and E. Stackebrandt.** 1994. The molecular phylogeny and systematics of the actinomycetes. *Annu. Rev. Microbiol.* **48:**257–289.
48. **Exmelin, L., B. Malbruny, M. Vergnaud, F. Prosvost, P. Boiron, and C. Morel.** 1996. Molecular study of nosocomial nocardiosis outbreak involving heart transplant recipients. *J. Clin. Microbiol.* **34:**1014–1016.
49. **Filice, G. A., and G. L. Simpson.** 1984. Management of *Nocardia* infections, p. 49–64. *In* J. S. Remington and M. N. Swartz (ed.), *Current Clinical Topics in Infectious Diseases*, vol. 5. McGraw-Hill Book Co., New York, N.Y.
50. **Findlay, J. C., B. M. Arafah, P. Silverman, and D. C. Aron.** 1992. Cushing's syndrome with cranial and pulmo-

nary lesions: necessity for tissue diagnosis. *South. Med. J.* **85:**204–206.

51. **Flores, M., and E. Desmond.** 1993. Opacification of Middlebrook agar as an aid in identification of *Nocardia farcinica*. *J. Clin. Microbiol.* **31:**3040–3041.
52. **Garratt, M. A., H. T. Holmes, and F. S. Nolte.** 1992. Selective buffered charcoal-yeast-extract medium for isolation of nocardiae from mixed cultures. *J. Clin. Microbiol.* **30:**1891–1892.
53. **Georghiou, P. R., and Z. M. Blacklock.** 1992. Infection with *Nocardia* species in Queensland. A review of 102 clinical isolates. *Med. J. Aust.* **156:**692–697.
54. **Goodfellow, M.** 1983. Ecology of actinomycetes. *Annu. Rev. Microbiol.* **37:**189–216.
55. **Goodfellow, M.** 1987. The taxonomic status of *Rhodococcus equi*. *Vet. Microbiol.* **14:**205–209.
56. **Goodfellow, M.** 1989. Genus *Rhodococcus* zopt 1891, p. 2362–2371. *In* S. T. Williams, M. E. Sharpe, and J. G. Holt (ed.), *Bergey's Manual of Systematic Bacteriology*, vol. 4. The Williams & Wilkins Co., Baltimore, Md.
57. **Goodfellow, M., and G. Alderson.** 1977. The actinomycete genus *Rhodococcus*. A home for the rhodochrous complex. *J. Gen. Microbiol.* **100:**99–122.
58. **Goodfellow, M., E. V. Ferguson, and J. J. Sanglier.** 1992. Numerical classification and identification of *Streptomyces* species. *Gene* **115:**225–233.
59. **Goodfellow, M., and M. P. Lechevalier.** 1989. Genus *Nocardia* Trevisan 1889, 9^{AL}, p. 2350–2361. *In* S. T. Williams, M. E. Sharpe, and J. G. Holt (ed.), *Bergey's Manual of Systematic Bacteriology*, vol. 4. The Williams & Wilkins Co., Baltimore, Md.
60. **Goodfellow, M., S. T. Williams, and G. Alderson.** 1986. Transfer of *Elytrosporangium brasiliense* Falcao de Morais et al., *Elytrosporangium carpinense* Falcao de Morais et al., *Elytrosporangium spirale* Falcao de Morais et al., *Microellobosporia* cinerea Cross et al., *Microellobosporia flavea* Cross et al., *Microellobosporia grisea* (Konev et al.) Pridham and *Microellobosporia violacea* (Tsyganov et al.) Pridham to the genus *Streptomyces* with amended descriptions of the species. *Syst. Appl. Microbiol.* **8:**48–54.
61. **Goodfellow, M., S. T. Williams, and G. Alderson.** 1986. Transfer of *Chainia* species to the genus *Streptomyces* with amended description of species. *Syst. Appl. Microbiol.* **8:** 55–60.
62. **Goodfellow, M., S. T. Williams, and G. Alderson.** 1986. Transfer of *Actinosporangium violaceum* Krasilnikov and Yuan, *Actinosporangium vitaminophilum* Shomura et al. and *Actinopycnidium caeruleum* Krasilikov to the genus *Streptomyces* with amended descriptions of the species. *Syst. Appl. Microbiol.* **8:**61–64.
63. **Goodfellow, M., S. T. Williams, and G. Alderson.** 1986. Transfer of *Kitasatoa purpurea* Matsumae and Hata to the genus *Streptomyces* as *Streptomyces purpureus* comb. nov. *Syst. Appl. Microbiol.* **8:**65–66.
64. **Goodfellow, M., J. Zakrzewska-Czerwinska, E. G. Thomas, M. Mordarski, A. C. Ward, and A. L. James.** 1991. Polyphasic taxonomic study of the genera *Gordona* and *Tsukamurella* including the description of *Tsukamurella wratislaviensis* sp. nov. *Zentralbl. Bakteriol. Parasitenkd. Infektionskr. Hyg. Abt. 1 Orig.* **275:**162–178.
65. **Gordon, M. A.** 1964. The genus *Dermatophilus*. *J. Bacteriol.* **88:**509–522.
66. **Gordon, M. A., and U. Perrin.** 1971. Pathogenicity of *Dermatophilus* and *Geodermatophilus*. *Infect. Immun.* **4:** 29–33.
67. **Gordon, M. A., I. F. Salkin, and W. B. Stone.** 1977. *Dermatophilus congolensis* enzootic in deer in New York State and vicinity. *J. Wildl. Dis.* **13:**184–190.
68. **Gordon, R. E., S. K. Mishra, and D. A. Barnett.** 1978. Some bits and pieces of the genus *Nocardia: N. carnea, N. vaccinii, N. transvalensis, N. orientalis* and *N. aerocoligenes*. *J. Gen. Microbiol.* **109:**69–78.
69. **Granel, F., A. Lozniewski, A. Barbaud, C. Lion, M. Dailloux, M. Weber, and J. L. Schmutz.** 1996. Cutaneous infection caused by *Tsukamurella paurometabolum*. *Clin. Infect. Dis.* **23:**839–840.
70. **Gruet, M., L. Maydat, and R. Ferro.** 1970. Peritonite a *Streptomyces somaliensis*. *Bull. Soc. Med. Afr. Noire* **15:** 609–610.
71. **Grund, E., and R. M. Kroppenstedt.** 1990. Chemotaxonomy and numerical taxonomy of the genus *Nocardiopsis*. *Int. J. Syst. Bacteriol.* **40:**5–11.
72. **Hamid, M. E., D. E. Minnikin, and M. Goodfellow.** 1993. A simple chemical test to distinguish mycobacteria from other mycolic-acid-containing actinomycetes. *J. Gen. Microbiol.* **139:**2203–2213.
73. **Hanel, H., J. Kalisch, M. Keil, W. C. Marsch, and M. Buslau.** 1991. Quantification of keratolytic activity from *Dermatophilus congolensis*. *Med. Microbiol. Immunol.* **180:** 45–51.
74. **Hay, R. J., E. S. Mahgoub, G. Leon, S. Al-Sogair, and O. Welsh.** 1992. Mycetoma. *J. Med. Vet. Mycol.* **30:**41–49.
75. **Holtz, H. A., D. P. Lavery, and R. Kapila.** 1992. *Actinomycetales* infection in the acquired immunodeficiency syndrome. *Ann. Intern. Med.* **102:**203–205.
76. **Jones, R. S., T. Fekete, A. L. Truant, and V. Satishchandran.** 1994. Persistent bacteremia due to *Tsukamurella paurometabolum* in a patient undergoing hemodialysis: case report and review. *Clin. Infect. Dis.* **18:**830–832. (Letter.)
77. **Jonsson, S., R. J. J. Wallace, S. I. Hull, and D. M. Musher.** 1986. Recurrent *Nocardia* pneumonia in an adult with chronic granulomatous disease. *Am. Rev. Respir. Dis.* **133:**932–934.
78. **Kampfer, P., W. Dott, and R. M. Kroppenstedt.** 1990. Numerical classification and identification of some nocardioform bacteria. *J. Gen. Appl. Microbiol.* **36:**309–331.
79. **Kampfer, P., R. M. Kroppenstedt, and W. Dott.** 1991. A numerical classification of the genera *Streptomyces* and *Streptoverticillium* using miniaturized physiological tests. *J. Gen. Microbiol.* **137:**1831–1891.
80. **Kilian, M.** 1978. Rapid identification of *Actinomycetaceae* and related bacteria. *J. Clin. Microbiol.* **8:**127–133.
81. **Kjelstrom, J. A., and B. L. Beaman.** 1993. Development of a serologic panel for the recognition of nocardial infections in a murine model. *Diagn. Microbiol. Infect. Dis.* **16:** 291–301.
82. **Klatte, S., K. Jahnke, R. M. Kroppenstedt, F. Rainey, and E. Stackebrandt.** 1994. *Rhodococcus luteus* is a later subjective synonym of *Rhodococcus fascians*. *Int. J. Syst. Bacteriol.* **44:**627–630.
83. **Klatte, S., R. M. Kroppenstedt, P. Schumann, K. Altendorf, and F. A. Rainey.** 1996. *Gordona hirsuta* sp. nov. *Int. J. Syst. Bacteriol.* **46:**876–880.
84. **Klatte, S., F. A. Rainey, and R. M. Kroppenstedt.** 1994. Transfer of *Rhodococcus aichiensis* Tsukamura 1982 and *Nocardia amarae* Lechevalier and Lechevalier 1974 to the genus *Gordona* as *Gordona aichiensis* comb. nov. and *Gordona amarae* comb. nov. *Int. J. Syst. Bacteriol.* **44:**769–773.
85. **Knouse, M. C., and B. Lorber.** 1990. Early diagnosis of *Nocardia asteroides* endophthalmitis by retinal biopsy: case report and review. *Rev. Infect. Dis.* **12:**393–398.
86. **Kubica, G. B., and A. L. Ridgeon.** 1961. The arylsulfatase activity of acid-fast bacilli. III. Preliminary investigation of rapidly growing acid-fast bacilli. *Am. Rev. Respir. Dis.* **83:**737–740.
87. **Kurup, V. P., and J. N. Fink.** 1975. A scheme for the identification of thermophilic actinomycetes associated

with hypersensitivity pneumonitis. *J. Clin. Microbiol.* **2:** 55–61.
88. **Labeda, D. P.** 1993. DNA related among strains of the *Streptomyces lavendulae* phenotypic cluster group. *Int. J. Syst. Bacteriol.* **43:**822–825.
89. **Labeda, D. P.** 1992. DNA-DNA hybridization in the systematics of *Streptomyces*. *Gene* **115:**249–253.
90. **Labeda, D. P., and A. J. Lyons.** 1991. Deoxyribonucleic acid relatedness among species of the "*Streptomyces cyaneus*" cluster. *Syst. Appl. Microbiol.* **14:**158–164.
91. **Lacey, J.** 1989. Genus *Faenia* Kurup and Agre 1983, 664[VP] (*Micropolyspora* Lechevalier, Soltorovsky and McDermont 1961, 11[AL]), p. 2387–2392. *In* S. T. Williams, M. E. Sharpe, and J. G. Holt (ed.), *Bergey's Manual of Systematic Bacteriology*, vol. 4. The Williams & Wilkins Co., Baltimore, Md.
92. **Lacey, J., J. Pepys, and T. Cross.** 1972. Actinomycetes and fungus spores in air as respiratory allergens, p. 151–184. *In* D. A. Shapton and R. G. Board (ed.), *Safety in Microbiology*. Academic Press, London, United Kingdom.
93. **Lai, K. K.** 1993. A cancer patient with central venous catheter-related sepsis caused by *Tsukamurella paurometabolum* (*Gordona aurantiaca*). *Clin. Infect. Dis.* **17:** 285–287.
94. **Lasker, B. A., J. M. Brown, and M. M. McNeil.** 1992. Identification and epidemiological typing of clinical and environmental isolates of the genus *Rhodococcus* with use of a digoxigenin-labeled rDNA gene probe. *Clin. Infect. Dis.* **15:**223–233.
95. **Laurent, F., A. Carlotti, P. Boiron, J. Villard, and J. Freney.** 1996. Ribotyping: a tool for taxonomy and identification of the *Nocardia asteroides* complex species. *J. Clin. Microbiol.* **34:**1079–1082.
96. **Lechevalier, H. A., M. P. Lechevalier, and B. Becker.** 1966. Comparison of the chemical composition of cell walls of nocardiae with that of other aerobic actinomycetes. *Int. J. Syst. Bacteriol.* **16:**151–166.
97. **Lechevalier, M. P.** 1989. Actinomycetes with multilocular sporangia, p. 2405–2417. *In* S. T. Williams, M. E. Sharpe, and J. G. Holt (ed.), *Bergey's Manual of Systematic Bacteriology*, vol. 4. The Williams & Wilkins Co., Baltimore, Md.
98. **Lechevalier, M. P., H. Prauser, D. P. Labeda, and J. S. Ruan.** 1986. Two new genera of nocardioform actinomycetes: *Amycolata* gen. nov. and *Amycolatopsis* gen. nov. *Int. J. Syst. Bacteriol.* **36:**29–37.
99. **Lerner, P. I.** 1996. Nocardiosis. *Clin. Infect. Dis.* **22:** 891–903.
100. **Linder, R.** 1997. *Rhodococcus equi* and *Arcanobacterium haemolyticum*: two "coryneform" bacteria increasingly recognized as agents of human infection. *Emerg. Infect. Dis.* **3:**145–153.
101. **Louie, L., M. Louie, and A. E. Simor.** 1997. Investigation of a pseudo-outbreak of *Nocardia asteroides* infection by pulsed-field gel electrophoresis and randomly amplified polymorphic DNA PCR. *J. Clin. Microbiol.* **35:** 1582–1584.
102. **Manchester, L., B. Pot, K. Kersters, and M. Goodfellow.** 1990. Classification of *Streptomyces* and *Streptoverticillium* species by numerical analysis of electrophoretic protein patterns. *Syst. Appl. Microbiol.* **13:**333–337.
103. **Martin, T., D. J. Hogan, F. Murphy, I. Natyshak, and E. P. Ewan.** 1991. *Rhodococcus* infection of the skin with lymphadenitis in a nonimmunocompromised girl. *J. Am. Acad. Dermatol.* **24:**328–332.
104. **Masters, A. M., T. M. Ellis, J. M. Carsons, S. S. Sutherland, and A. R. Gregory.** 1995. *Dermatophilus chelonae* sp. nov., isolated from chelonids in Australia. *Int. J. Syst. Bacteriol.* **45:**50–56.
105. **McClung, N. M.** 1960. Isolation of *Nocardia asteroides* from soils. *Mycologia* **52:**154–156.
106. **McNabb, A., R. Shuttleworth, R. Behme, and W. D. Colby.** 1997. Fatty acid characterization of rapidly growing pathogenic aerobic actinomycetes as a means of identification. *J. Clin. Microbiol.* **35:**1361–1368.
107. **McNeil, M. M., and J. M. Brown.** 1994. The medically important aerobic actinomycetes: epidemiology and microbiology. *Clin. Microbiol. Rev.* **7:**357–417.
108. **McNeil, M. M., J. M. Brown, P. R. Georghiou, A. M. Allworth, and Z. M. Blacklock.** 1992. Infections due to *Nocardia transvalensis*: clinical spectrum and antimicrobial therapy. *Clin. Infect. Dis.* **15:**453–463.
109. **McNeil, M. M., J. M. Brown, W. R. Jarvis, and L. Ajello.** 1990. Comparison of species distribution and antimicrobial susceptibility of aerobic actinomycetes from clinical specimens. *Rev. Infect. Dis.* **12:**778–783.
110. **McNeil, M. M., J. M. Brown, C. H. Magruder, K. T. Shearlock, R. A. Saul, D. P. Allred, and L. Ajello.** 1992. Disseminated *Nocardia transvalensis* infection: an unusual opportunistic pathogen in severely immunocompromised patients. *J. Infect. Dis.* **165:**175–178.
111. **McNeil, M. M., J. M. Brown, G. Scalise, and C. Piersimoni.** 1992. Nonmycetomic *Actinomadura madurae* infection in a patient with AIDS. *J. Clin. Microbiol.* **30:** 1008–1010.
112. **McNeil, M. M., S. Ray, P. E. Kozarsky, and J. M. Brown.** 1997. *Nocardia farcinica* pneumonia in a previously healthy woman: species characterization with use of a digoxigenin-labeled cDNA probe. *Clin. Infect. Dis.* **25:**933–934.
113. **Meyer, J.** 1976. *Nocardiopsis*, a new genus of the order actinomycetales. *Int. J. Syst. Bacteriol.* **26:**487–493.
114. **Mishra, S. K., R. E. Gordon, and D. A. Barnett.** 1980. Identification of nocardiae and streptomycetes of medical importance. *J. Clin. Microbiol.* **11:**728–736.
115. **Morace, G., G. Dettori, M. Sanguinetti, S. Manzara, and L. Polonelli.** 1988. Biotyping of aerobic actinomycetes by modified killer system. *Eur. J. Epidemiol.* **4:**99–103.
116. **Mossad, S. B., J. W. Tomford, R. Stewart, N. B. Ratliff, and G. S. Hall.** 1995. Case report of *Streptomyces* endocarditis of a prosthetic aortic valve. *J. Clin. Microbiol.* **33:** 3335–3337.
117. **Mosser, D. M., and M. K. Hondalus.** 1996. *Rhodococcus equi*: an emerging opportunistic pathogen. *Trends Microbiol.* **4:**29–33.
118. **Muir, D. B., and R. C. Pritchard.** 1997. Use of bioMerieux ID 32C yeast identification system for identification of aerobic actinomycetes of medical importance. *J. Clin. Microbiol.* **35:**3240–3243.
119. **Murray, P. R., R. L. Heeren, and A. C. Niles.** 1987. Effect of decontamination procedures on recovery of *Nocardia* spp. *J. Clin. Microbiol.* **25:**2010–2011.
120. **Nordmann, P.** 1995. Antimicrobial susceptibility of human isolates of *Rhodococcus equi*. *Med. Microbiol. Lett.* **4:**277–286.
121. **Ochi, K.** 1995. Phylogenetic analysis of mycolic acid-containing wall-chemotype IV actinomycetes and allied taxa by partial sequencing of ribosomal protein AT-L30. *Int. J. Syst. Bacteriol.* **45:**653–660.
122. **Ochi, K.** 1995. A taxonomic study of the genus *Streptomyces* by analysis of ribosomal protein AT-L30. *Int. J. Syst. Bacteriol.* **45:**507–514.
123. **Orchard, V. A., and M. Goodfellow.** 1980. Numerical classification of some named strains of *Nocardia asteroides* and related isolates from soil. *J. Gen. Microbiol.* **118:** 295–312.

124. **Osoagbaka, O. U.** 1989. Evidence for the pathogenic role of *Rhodococcus* species in pulmonary diseases. *J. Appl. Bacteriol.* **66:**497–506.

125. **Patterson, J. E., K. Chapin-Robertson, S. Waycott, P. Farrel, A. McGeer, M. M. McNeil, and S. C. Edberg.** 1992. Pseudoepidemic of *Nocardia asteroides* associated with a mycobacterial culture system. *J. Clin. Microbiol.* **30:**1357–1360.

126. **Pepys, J., P. A. Jenkins, G. N. Festenstein, P. H. Gregory, M. Lacey, and F. A. Skinner.** 1963. Thermophilic actinomycetes as a source of farmer's lung hay antigen. *Lancet* **ii:**607–611.

127. **Philip, A., and G. D. Roberts.** 1984. *Nocardiopsis dassonvillei* cellulitis of the arm. *Clin. Microbiol. Newsl.* **6:**14–15.

128. **Pier, A. C., and R. E. Fichtner.** 1981. Distribution of serotypes of *Nocardia asteroides* from animal, human, and environmental sources. *J. Clin. Microbiol.* **13:**548–553.

129. **Pittenger, R. C., and R. B. Brigham.** 1956. *Streptomyces orientalis* nov. sp., the source of vancomycin. *Antibiot. Chemother.* **6:**642–647.

130. **Prescott, J. F.** 1991. *Rhodococcus equi*: an animal and human pathogen. *Clin Microbiol. Rev.* **4:**20–34.

131. **Pridham, T. G., C. W. Hesseltine, and R. G. Benedict.** 1958. A guide for the classification of streptomycetes according to selected groups. *Appl. Microbiol.* **6:**52–79.

132. **Prinz, G., E. Ban, S. Fekete, and Z. Szabo.** 1985. Meningitis caused by *Gordona aurantiaca* (*Rhodococcus aurantiacus*). *J. Clin. Microbiol.* **22:**472–474.

133. **Provost, F., L. Polonelli, S. Conti, P. Fisicaro, M. Gerloni, and P. Boiron.** 1995. Use of yeast killer system to identify species of the *Nocardia asteroides* complex. *J. Clin. Microbiol.* **33:**8–10.

134. **Raby, N., G. Forbes, and R. Williams.** 1990. *Nocardia* infection in patients with liver transplants or chronic liver disease: radiologic findings. *Radiology* **174:**713–716.

135. **Rainey, F. A., J. Burghardt, R. M. Kroppenstedt, S. Klatte, and E. Stackebrandt.** 1995. Phylogenetic analysis of the genera *Rhodococcus* and *Nocardia* and evidence for the evolutionary origin of the genus *Nocardia* from within the radiation of *Rhodococcus* species. *Microbiology* **141:** 523–528.

136. **Rainey, F. A., S. Klatte, R. M. Kroppenstedt, and E. Stackebrandt.** 1995. *Dietzia*, a new genus including *Dietzia maris* comb. nov., formerly *Rhodococcus maris*. *Int. J. Syst. Bacteriol.* **45:**32–36.

137. **Rainey, F. A., N. Ward-Rainey, R. M. Kroppenstedt, and E. Stackebrandt.** 1996. The genus *Nocardiopsis* represents a phylogenetically coherent taxon and a distinct actinomycete lineage: proposal of *Nocardiopsaceae* fam. nov. *Int. J. Syst. Bacteriol.* **46:**1088–1092.

138. **Ramzan, N. N., E. Loftus, Jr., L. J. Burgart, M. Rooney, K. P. Batts, R. H. Wiesner, D. N. Fredricks, D. A. Relman, and D. H. Persing.** 1997. Diagnosis and monitoring of Whipple disease by polymerase chain reaction. *Ann. Intern. Med.* **126:**520–527.

139. **Relman, D. A.** 1997. Emerging infections and newly-recognised pathogens. *Neth. J. Med.* **50:**216–220.

140. **Relman, D. A., T. M. Schmidt, R. F. MacDermott, and S. Falkow.** 1992. Identification of the uncultured bacillus of Whipple's disease. *N. Engl. J. Med.* **327:**293–301.

141. **Rey, D., D. De Briel, R. Heller, P. Fraisse, M. Partisani, M. Leiva-Mena, and J. M. Lang.** 1995. *Tsukamurella* and HIV infection. *AIDS* **9:**1379.

142. **Richet, H. M., P. C. Craven, J. M. Brown, B. A. Lasker, C. Cox, M. M. McNeil, A. D. Tice, W. R. Jarvis, and O. C. Tablan.** 1991. A cluster of *Rhodococcus* (*Gordona*) *bronchialis* sternal-wound infections after coronary-artery bypass surgery. *N. Engl. J. Med.* **324:**104–109.

143. **Rickman, L. S., W. R. Freeman, W. R. Green, S. T. Feldman, J. Sullivan, V. Russack, and D. A. Relman.** 1995. Brief report: uveitis caused by *Tropheryma whippelii* (Whipple's bacillus). *N. Engl. J. Med.* **332:**363–366.

144. **Riddell, R. W.** 1950. Permanent stained mycological preparations obtained by slide culture. *Mycologia* **42:**265.

145. **Riegel, P., M. V. Kamne-Fotso, D. De Briel, G. Prévost, F. Jehl, Y. Piémont, and H. Monteil.** 1994. *Rhodococcus chubuensis* Tsukamura 1982 is a later subjective synonym of *Gordona sputi* (Tsukamura 1978) Stackebrandt 1989 comb. nov. *Int. J. Syst. Bacteriol.* **44:**764–768.

146. **Roberts, G. D., N. S. Brewer, and P. E. Hermans.** 1974. Diagnosis of nocardiosis by blood cultures. *Mayo Clinic Proc.* **49:**293–296.

147. **Ruimy, R., P. Riegel, A. Carlotti, P. Boiron, G. Bernardin, H. Monteil, R. J. Wallace, Jr., and R. Christen.** 1996. *Nocardia pseudobrasiliensis* sp. nov., a new species of *Nocardia* which groups bacterial strains previously identified as *Nocardia brasiliensis* and associated with invasive disease. *Int. J. Syst. Bacteriol.* **46:**259–264.

148. **Salinas-Carmona, M. C., O. Welsh, and S. M. Casillas.** 1993. Enzyme-linked immunosorbent assay for serological diagnosis of *Nocardia brasiliensis* and clinical correlation with mycetoma infections. *J. Clin. Microbiol.* **31:** 2901–2906.

149. **Schaal, K. P.** 1984. Laboratory diagnosis of actinomycete diseases, p. 441–456. *In* M. Goodfellow, M. Mordarski, and S. T. Williams (ed.), *The Biology of the Actinomycetes*. Academic Press, London, United Kingdom.

150. **Schaal, K. P.** 1991. Medical and microbiological problems arising from airborne infection in hospitals. *J. Hosp. Infect.* **18:**451–459.

151. **Schiff, T. A., M. M. McNeil, and J. M. Brown.** 1993. Cutaneous *Nocardia farcinica* infection in a nonimmunocompromised patient: case report and review. *Clin. Infect. Dis.* **16:**756–760.

152. **Schiff, T. A., M. Sanchez, J. Moy, D. Klirsfeld, M. M. McNeil, and J. M. Brown.** 1993. Cutaneous nocardiosis caused by *Nocardia nova* occurring in an HIV-infected individual: a case report and review of the literature. *J. Acquired Immune Defic. Syndr.* **6:**849–851.

153. **Scopetti, F., E. Iona, L. Fattorini, A. Goglio, N. Franceschini, G. Amicosante, and G. Orefici.** 1994. Activity of antimicrobial drugs evaluated by agar dilution and radiometric methods against strains of *Nocardia asteroides* isolated in Italy from immunocompromised patients. *J. Chemother.* **6:**29–34.

154. **Scott, M. A., B. S. Graham, R. Verrall, R. Dixon, W. Schaffner, and K. T. Tham.** 1995. *Rhodococcus equi*—an increasingly recognized opportunistic pathogen. Report of 12 cases and review of 65 cases in the literature. *Am. J. Clin. Pathol.* **103:**649–655.

155. **Shanley, J. D., K. Synder, and J. S. Child.** 1979. Chronic pericarditis due to *Streptomyces* species. *Am. J. Clin. Pathol.* **72:**107–110.

156. **Shapiro, C. L., R. F. Haft, N. M. Gantz, G. V. Doern, J. C. Christenson, R. O'Brien, J. C. Overall, B. A. Brown, and R. J. J. Wallace.** 1992. *Tsukamurella paurometabolum*: a novel pathogen causing catheter-related bacteremia in patients with cancer. *Clin. Infect. Dis.* **14:** 200–203.

157. **Sindhuphak, W., E. MacDonald, and E. Head.** 1985. Actinomycetoma caused by *Nocardiopsis dassonvillei*. *Arch. Dermatol.* **121:**1332–1334.

158. **Singh, S. M., J. Naidu, S. Mukerjee, and A. Malkani.** 1991. Cutaneous infections due to *Nocardiopsis dassonvillei* (Brocq-Rousseu) Meyer 1976, endemic in members of a family up to fifth degree relatives, abstr. PS1.91, p. 85. *In Program and Abstracts of the XI Congress of the International Society of Human and Animal Mycology*.

159. **Slack, J. M., and M. A. Gerencser.** 1975. Actinomyces, *Filamentous Bacteria*. Burgess Publishing Co., Minneapolis, Minn.
160. **Smego, R. A., Jr., and H. A. Gallis.** 1984. The clinical spectrum of *Nocardia brasiliensis* infection in the United States. *Rev. Infect. Dis.* **6:**164–180.
161. **Stackebrandt, E., J. Smida, and M. Collins.** 1988. Evidence of phylogenetic heterogeneity within the genus *Rhodococcus*: revival of the genus *Gordona* (Tsukamura). *J. Gen. Microbiol.* **35:**364–368.
162. **Staneck, J. L., and G. D. Roberts.** 1974. Simplified approach to identification of aerobic actinomycetes by thin-layer chromatography. *Appl. Microbiol.* **28:**226–231.
163. **Steingrube, V. A., B. A. Brown, J. L. Gibson, R. W. Wilson, J. Brown, Z. Blacklock, K. Jost, S. Locke, R. F. Ulrich, and R. J. Wallace, Jr.** 1995. DNA amplification and restriction endonuclease analysis for differentiation of 12 species and taxa of *Nocardia*, including recognition of four new taxa within the *Nocardia asteroides* complex. *J. Clin. Microbiol.* **33:**3096–3101.
164. **Steingrube, V. A., R. J. Wallace, Jr., B. A. Brown, Y. Pang, B. Zeluff, L. C. Steele, and Y. Zhang.** 1991. Acquired resistance of *Nocardia brasiliensis* to clavulanic acid related to a change in β-lactamase following therapy with amoxicillin-clavulanic acid. *Antimicrob. Agents Chemother.* **35:**524–528.
165. **Steingrube, V. A., R. W. Wilson, B. A. Brown, K. C. Jost, Jr., Z. Blacklock, J. L. Gibson, and R. J. Wallace, Jr.** 1997. Rapid identification of clinically significant species and taxa of aerobic actinomycetes, including *Actinomadura*, *Gordona*, *Nocardia*, *Rhodococcus*, *Streptomyces*, and *Tsukamurella* isolates, by DNA amplification and restriction endonuclease analysis. *J. Clin. Microbiol.* **35:** 817–822.
166. **Sutor, G. C., C. Fibich, P. Kirscher, M. Kuske, R. E. Schmidt, I. Schedel, and H. Deicher.** 1996. Poststenotic cavitating pneumonia due to *Rhodococcus dequi* in HIV infection. *AIDS* **10:**339–340.
167. **Telzak, E. E., J. Hii, B. Polsky, T. E. Kiehn, and D. Armstrong.** 1989. *Nocardia* infection in the acquired immunodeficiency syndrome. *Diagn. Microbiol. Infect. Dis.* **12:**517–519.
168. **Towersey, L., E. D. C. Martins, A. T. Londero, R. J. Hay, P. J. Soares Filho, C. M. Takiya, C. C. Martins, and O. F. Gompertz.** 1993. *Dermatophilus congolensis* human infection. *J. Am. Acad. Dermatol.* **29:**351–354.
169. **Treyo, W. O.** 1970. An evaluation of some concepts and criteria used in the speciation of streptomycetes. *Trans. N. Y. Acad. Sci.* **32:**989–997.
170. **Trujillo, M. E., and M. Goodfellow.** 1997. Polyphasic taxonomic study of clinically significant actinomadurae including the description of *Actinomadura latina* sp. nov. *Zentralb. Bakteriol. Parasitenkd. Infektionskr. Hyg. Abt. 1 Orig.* **285:**212–233.
171. **Tsukamura, M.** 1982. Differentiation between the genera *Rhodococcus* and *Nocardia* and between species of the genus *Mycobacterium* by susceptibility to bleomycin. *J. Gen. Microbiol.* **128:**2385–2388.
172. **Tsukamura, M.** 1971. Proposal of a new genus, *Gordona*, for slightly acid-fast organisms occurring in the sputa of patients with pulmonary disease and in soil. *J. Gen. Microbiol.* **68:**15–26.
173. **Tsukamura, M.** 1978. Numerical classification of *Rhodococcus* (formerly *Gordona*) organisms recently isolated from sputa of patients: description of *Rhodococcus sputi* Tsukamura sp. nov. *Int. J. Syst. Bacteriol.* **28:**169–181.
174. **Tsukamura, M., K. Hikosaka, K. Nishimura, and S. Hara.** 1988. Severe progressive subcutaneous abscesses and necrotizing tenosynovitis caused by *Rhodococcus aurantiacus*. *J. Clin. Microbiol.* **26:**201–205.
175. **Tsukamura, M., and K. Kawakami.** 1982. Lung infection caused by *Gordona aurantiaca* (*Rhodococcus aurantiacus*). *J. Clin. Microbiol.* **16:**604–607.
176. **Tsukamura, M., and S. Mizuno.** 1971. A new species *Gordona aurantiaca* occurring in sputa of patients with pulmonary disease. *Kekkaku* **46:**93–98.
177. **Tsukamura, M., and I. Yano.** 1985. *Rhodococcus sputi* sp. nov. nom. rev., and *Rhodococcus aurantiacus* sp. nov. nom. rev. *Int. J. Syst. Bacteriol.* **35:**364–368.
178. **Unsworth, B. A., and T. Cross.** 1980. Thermophilic actinomycetes implicated in farmer's lung; numerical taxonomy of *Thermoactinomyces* species, p. 389–390. *In* M. Goodfellow and R. G. Broad (ed.), *Microbiological Classification and Identification*. Academic Press, London, United Kingdom.
179. **Vannier, A. M., B. H. Ackerman, and L. F. Hutchins.** 1992. Disseminated *Nocardia asteroides* diagnosed by blood culture in a patient with disseminated histoplasmosis. *Arch. Pathol. Lab. Med.* **116:**537–539.
180. **Van Saceghem, R.** 1915. Dermatose contagieuse (impetigo contagieux). *Bull. Soc. Pathol. Exot. Filiales.* **8:** 354–359.
181. **Verville, T. D., M. M. Huycke, R. A. Greenfield, D. P. Fine, T. L. Kuhls, and L. N. Slater.** 1994. *Rhodococcus equi* infections of humans. 12 cases and a review of the literature. *Medicine (Baltimore)* **73:**119–132.
182. **Vickers, R. M., J. D. Rihs, and V. L. Yu.** 1992. Clinical demonstration of isolation of *Nocardia asteroides* on buffered charcoal-yeast extract media. *J. Clin. Microbiol.* **30:** 227–228.
183. **Vincent, M. H.** 1894. Etude sur le parasite du "pied de madura." *Ann. Inst. Pasteur* **8:**129–151.
184. **von Graevenitz, A., and V. Punter-Streit.** 1995. Development of a new selective plating medium for *Rhodococcus equi*. *Microbiol. Immunol.* **39:**283–284.
185. **Vullo, V., C. M. Mastroianni, M. Lichtner, F. Mengoni, E. Chiappini, C. D'Agostino, and S. Delia.** 1996. Serologic responses to *Rhodococcus equi* in individuals with and without human immunodeficiency virus infection. *Eur. J. Clin. Microbiol. Infect. Dis.* **15:**588–594.
186. **Wallace, R. J., Jr., B. A. Brown, Z. Blacklock, R. Ulrich, K. Jost, J. M. Brown, M. M. McNeil, G. Onyi, V. A. Steingrube, and J. Gibson.** 1995. New *Nocardia* taxon among isolates of *Nocardia brasiliensis* associated with invasive disease. *J. Clin. Microbiol.* **33:**1528–1533.
187. **Wallace, R. J., Jr., B. A. Brown, M. Tsukamura, J. M. Brown, and G. O. Onyi.** 1991. Clinical and laboratory features of *Nocardia nova*. *J. Clin. Microbiol.* **29:** 2407–2411.
188. **Wallace, R. J., Jr., E. J. Septimus, D. M. Musher, and R. R. Martin.** 1977. Disk diffusion susceptibility testing of *Nocardia* species. *J. Infect. Dis.* **35:**568–576.
189. **Wallace, R. J., Jr., and L. C. Steele.** 1988. Susceptibility testing of *Nocardia* species for the clinical laboratory. *Diagn. Microbiol. Infect. Dis.* **9:**155–166.
190. **Wallace, R. J., Jr., L. C. Steele, G. Sumter, and J. M. Smith.** 1988. Antimicrobial susceptibility patterns of *Nocardia asteroides*. *Antimicrob. Agents Chemother.* **32:** 1776–1779.
191. **Wallace, R. J., Jr., M. Tsukamura, B. A. Brown, J. Brown, V. A. Steingrube, Y. S. Zhang, and D. R. Nash.** 1990. Cefotaxime-resistant *Nocardia asteroides* strains are isolates of the controversial species *Nocardia farcinica*. *J. Clin. Microbiol.* **28:**2726–2732.
192. **Whelan, M. A., and K. Hilal Sadek.** 1986. Computer tomography as a guide in the diagnosis and follow up of brain abscess. *Radiology* **135:**663–671.

193. **Whipple, G. H.** 1907. A hitherto undescribed disease characterized anatomically by deposits of fat and fatty acids in the intestinal and mesenteric lymphatic tissues. *Johns Hopkins Hosp. Bull.* **18:**382–391.
194. **Williams, S. T., M. Goodfellow, G. Alderson, E. M. H. Wellington, P. H. A. Sneath, and M. J. Sachin.** 1983. Numerical classification of *Streptomyces* and related genera. *J. Gen. Microbiol.* **129:**1743–1813.
195. **Williams, S. T., G. P. Sharples, and R. M. Bradshaw.** 1974. Spore formation in *Actinomadura dassonvillei* (Brocq-Rousseau) Lechevalier and Lechevalier. *J. Gen. Microbiol.* **84:**415–419.
196. **Williams, S. T., E. M. H. Wellington, M. Goodfellow, G. Alderson, M. Sachin, and P. H. A. Sneath.** 1981. The genus *Streptomyces*—a taxonomic enigma. *Zentralbl. Bakteriol. Parasitenkd. Infektionskr. Hyg. Abt. 1 Orig. Suppl.* **11:**45–57.
197. **Wilson, J. P., H. R. Turner, K. A. Kirchner, and S. W. Chapman.** 1989. Nocardial infections in renal transplant recipients. *Medicine (Baltimore)* **68:**38–57.
198. **Wilson, R. W., V. A. Steingrube, B. A. Brown, Z. Blacklock, K. C. Jost, A. McNabb, W. D. Colby, J. R. Biehle, J. L. Gibson, and R. W. Wallace, Jr.** 1997. Recognition of a *Nocardia transvalensis* complex by resistance to aminoglycosides, including amikacin, and PCR-restriction fragment length polymorphism analysis. *J. Clin. Microbiol.* **35:**2235–2242.
199. **Wilson, R. W., V. A. Steingrube, B. A. Brown, and R. J. Wallace, Jr.** 1998. Clinical application of PCR-restriction enzyme pattern analysis for rapid identification of aerobic actinomycete isolates. *J. Clin. Microbiol.* **36:** 148–152.
200. **Witt, D., and E. Stackebrandt.** 1990. Unification of the genera *Streptoverticillium* and *Streptomyces*, and amendation of *Streptomyces* Waksman and Henrici 1943[AL] *Syst. Appl. Microbiol.* **13:**361–371.
201. **Woodger, A. J., M. Baxter, F. M. Rush-Munro, J. Brown, and W. Kaplan.** 1985. Isolation of *Dermatophilus congolensis* from two New Zealand cases of pitted keratolysis. *Aust. J. Dermatol.* **26:**29–35.
202. **Wust, J., H. Lanzendorfer, A. von Graevenitz, H. J. Gloor, and B. Schmid.** 1990. Peritonitis caused by *Actinomadura madurae* in a patient on CAPD. *Eur. J. Clin. Microbiol. Infect. Dis.* **9:**700–701.
203. **Yassin, A. F., E. A. Galinski, A. Wohlfarth, K. Jahnke, K. P. Schaal, and H. G. Truper.** 1993. A new actinomycete species, *Nocardiopsis lucentensis* sp. nov. *Int. J. Syst. Bacteriol.* **43:**266–271.
204. **Yassin, A. F., F. A. Rainey, H. Brzezinka, J. Burghardt, H. J. Lee, and K. P. Schaal.** 1995. *Tsukamurella inchonensis* sp. nov. *Int. J. Syst. Bacteriol.* **45:**522–527.
205. **Yassin, A. F., F. A. Rainey, H. Brzezinka, J. Burghardt, M. Rifai, P. Seifert, K. Feldmann, and K. P. Schaal.** 1996. *Tsukamurella pulmonis* sp. nov. *Int. J. Syst. Bacteriol.* **46:**429–436.
206. **Yassin, A. F., F. A. Rainey, J. Burghardt, H. Brzezinka, S. Schmitt, P. Seifert, O. Zimmermann, H. Mauch, D. Gierth, I. Lux, and K. P. Schaal.** 1997. *Tsukamurella tyrosinosolvens* sp. nov. *Int. J. Syst. Bacteriol.* **47:**607–614.
207. **Yassin, A. F., F. A. Rainey, J. Burghardt, D. Gierth, J. Ungerechts, I. Lux, P. Seifert, C. Bal, and K. P. Schaal.** 1997. Description of *Nocardiopsis synnemataformans* sp. nov., elevation of *Nocardiopsis alba* subsp. *prasina* to *Nocardiopsis prasina* comb. nov., and designation of *Nocardiopsis antarctica* and *Nocardiopsis alborubida* as later subjective synonyms of *Nocardiopsis dassonvillei*. *Int. J. Syst. Bacteriol.* **47:**983–988.
208. **Yeruham, I., A. Hadani, and D. Elad.** 1991. Human dermatophilosis (*Dermatophilus congolensis*) in dairymen in Israel. *Isr. J. Vet. Med.* **46:**114–116.
209. **Zaria, L. T.** 1993. *Dermatophilus congolensis* infection (Dermatophilosis) in animals and man. An update. *Comp. Immunol. Microbiol. Infect. Dis.* **16:**179–222.
210. **Zbinden, R., A. Zimmerman, and P. Boiron.** 1995. *Streptomyces* spp. as a cause of a wound infection. *Clin. Microbiol. Newsl.* **17:**167–168.

Mycobacterium

BEVERLY G. METCHOCK, FREDERICK S. NOLTE, AND RICHARD J. WALLACE, JR.

25

Tuberculosis remains a major global public health problem. The World Health Organization estimates that there are 8 million new cases and 3 million deaths directly attributable to the disease each year (70, 260). This makes tuberculosis the leading cause of death in many resource-poor and developing countries.

In the United States, tuberculosis steadily declined until 1985, when the downward trend was reversed. The number of cases of tuberculosis increased 18.4% between 1985 and 1991. The Centers for Disease Control and Prevention estimates that during that period 39,000 cases of tuberculosis occurred in excess of those expected if the pre-1985 downward trend had continued (39). A number of factors have facilitated the resurgence of tuberculosis in the United States. These include the advent of the AIDS epidemic, immigration from countries where the prevalence of tuberculosis is high, general deterioration of the health care infrastructure with concomitant incomplete tuberculosis therapy among homeless and noncompliant patients, transmission in high-risk environments, and the coincident increase in the number of cases of multidrug-resistant tuberculosis.

The number of cases of tuberculosis in the United States reported to the CDC peaked in 1992 (26,673 cases) (43). The substantial and consistent decline in the number of tuberculosis cases reported annually in the United States since 1992 reflects the effectiveness of prevention and control measures implemented during 1989 through 1993. These include the use of improved laboratory methods to allow prompt identification of *Mycobacterium tuberculosis*, broader use of antimicrobial susceptibility testing, expanded use of preventive therapy in high-risk groups, decreased transmission in congregative settings (e.g., hospitals and correctional facilities) as a result of implementation of infection control guidelines, improved follow-up of tuberculosis patients by health departments, and increased federal resources for assisting state and local tuberculosis control efforts. Although the overall number of new tuberculosis cases is decreasing nationally, there is still a significant increase in the number of cases within some population groups, particularly among persons born outside the United States and its territories (43).

There have also been major recent developments in the taxonomy and clinical conditions associated with nontuberculous mycobacteria (NTM), which are discussed later in this chapter. Currently, more than 80 species of NTM have been described.

Clinical mycobacteriology laboratories play an important role in the control of the spread of tuberculosis through the timely detection, isolation, identification, and drug susceptibility testing of *M. tuberculosis*. The methods described in this chapter enable laboratories to provide accurate results within a clinically relevant time frame. However, the level of service and the choice of methods used in an individual laboratory setting should be determined by the patient population served by the laboratory and the available resources.

TAXONOMY

The genus *Mycobacterium* is the only genus in the family *Mycobacteriaceae*. The high moles percent G+C content of the DNA of *Mycobacterium* species (62 to 70%) is similar to that of the other mycolic acid-producing bacteria, *Nocardia* (60 to 69%), *Rhodococcus* (59 to 69%), and *Corynebacterium* (51 to 59%).

A natural division occurs between slowly and relatively rapidly growing species of mycobacteria. Slow growers require more than 7 days to produce easily seen colonies on solid media from a dilute inoculum under ideal culture conditions. Rapid growers require less than 7 days under comparable conditions.

DESCRIPTION OF THE GENUS

The mycobacteria are slightly curved or straight bacilli, 0.2 to 0.6 by 1.0 to 10 μm in size, sometimes with branching. Filamentous or mycelium-like growth may occur but easily fragments into rods or coccoid elements. The organisms have cell walls with a high lipid content, including waxes having characteristic mycolic acids with long branched chains.

The high lipid content of the cell wall excludes the usual aniline dyes. Mycobacteria are not readily stained by Gram's method but are considered gram positive. Special staining procedures are used to promote the uptake of dye, and once stained, mycobacteria are not easily decolorized even with acid-alcohol. This resistance to decolorization by acid-alcohol is termed acid-fastness. Acid-fastness is partly or completely lost at some stage of growth by a proportion of the cells of some species.

The mycobacteria are aerobic, non-spore-forming, nonmotile bacilli. Colony morphology varies among the species, ranging from smooth to rough and from pigmented to nonpigmented. Diffusible pigment is rare, but colonies of some species are regularly or variably yellow, orange, or, rarely, pink. Some species require light to form pigment (photochromogens), and others form pigment in either the light or the dark (scotochromogens). Aerial filaments are rarely formed and are never visible without magnification.

Growth for mycobacteria is slow to very slow, with generation times ranging by species from 2 to more than 20 h. Easily visible colonies may be produced after 2 days to 8 weeks of incubation under optimal conditions depending upon the species. Optimal temperatures for growth vary widely among species, from 30 to almost 45°C. Most species adapt readily to growth on simple substrates, using ammonia or amino acids as nitrogen sources and glycerol as a carbon source in the presence of mineral salts. Some species require medium supplements such as hemin, mycobactins, or other iron transport compounds. *M. leprae* has not been cultured outside of living cells.

NATURAL HABITATS

The genus *Mycobacterium* includes obligate parasites, saprophytes, and opportunistic pathogens. Most species are free living in soil and water, but the major ecological niche for others such as *M. tuberculosis* complex and *M. leprae* is diseased tissue of humans and other warm-blooded animals.

Studies over the past 20 years have focused on piped water systems as a source of clinically important NTM. A number of species that have been rarely recovered from natural waters or soils are readily recovered from tap water in the same locale in the setting of clinical disease or frequent culture-positive specimens. The best examples of these are *M. kansasii*, *M. xenopi*, and *M. simiae* (3, 26, 148). Other species have been recovered from tap water and associated with nosocomial disease or pseudo-outbreaks. These include *M. avium* complex, *M. gordonae*, *M. fortuitum*, *M. peregrinum*, *M. abscessus*, and *M. mucogenicum* (3, 7, 84, 242).

A number of NTM species are presumed to be environmental but have yet to be recovered from soil or water. These include *M. ulcerans*, *M. haemophilum*, *M. asiaticum*, *M. shimoidei*, *M. szulgai*, and *M. genavense* (3). Failure to recover these organisms generally reflects their fastidious growth characteristics or lack of efforts to recover them. *M. genavense* was recently identified as the major pathogen causing mycobacteriosis in birds (174). The other listed species have not been shown to cause disease outside of humans.

CLINICAL SIGNIFICANCE

This section contains descriptions of the diseases associated with the clinically important species of *Mycobacterium*. Also included is a review of the diseases associated with the potentially pathogenic species.

M. tuberculosis Complex

Robert Koch was the first to establish the causal relationship of the tubercle bacillus to the disease tuberculosis. The organism was named *Mycobacterium tuberculosis* in 1886, presumably because the organism resembles the fungi in its slow growth and colony morphology.

Cases of tuberculosis are not evenly distributed throughout all segments of the U.S. population. Groups known to have a higher prevalence than the general population include medically underserved ethnic minorities, homeless persons, prison inmates, alcoholics, injecting drug users, the elderly, foreign-born persons from areas of high prevalence, and contacts of persons with active tuberculosis. Groups with a higher likelihood of progression from latent infection to active disease include persons with underlying medical conditions, persons who have been infected within the past 2 years, children of ≤4 years old, and persons with fibrotic lesions on chest radiographs. Human immunodeficiency virus (HIV) infection is the greatest known risk factor for the progression of latent infection to active tuberculosis. Combined HIV and tuberculosis infections, especially in association with drug resistance, have caused outbreaks with extremely high mortality rates (43).

M. tuberculosis is carried in airborne particles, known as droplet nuclei, that are generated when patients with pulmonary tuberculosis cough. These particles are 1 to 5 μm in size. Infection occurs when a susceptible person inhales the droplet nuclei, which then reach the terminal airways of the lungs. In the alveoli, the organisms are engulfed by the alveolar macrophages and may spread throughout the body. Usually, the host cell-mediated immune response limits the multiplication and spread of *M. tuberculosis*. However, some bacilli remain viable but dormant for many years after the initial infection. Patients latently infected with *M. tuberculosis* usually have a positive purified protein derivative (PPD) skin test but are asymptomatic and are not infectious. In general, persons with latent infections have a 10% risk during their lifetime for development of active tuberculosis. The risk is greatest within the first 2 years after infection. Patients with HIV have a 10 to 15% risk per year for progression of infection.

Pulmonary tuberculosis in adults is a slowly progressive inflammatory process characterized by intense chronic inflammation, necrosis, and caseation. The cavities that are formed in the lungs may rupture into bronchi, allowing large numbers of organisms to spread to other areas of the lungs and to be aerosolized by coughing, hence infecting other persons. The usual clinical features of pulmonary tuberculosis include cough, weight loss, low-grade fever, dyspnea, and chest pain. Tuberculosis in AIDS patients is much more rapidly progressive and often disseminates, sometimes without formation of typical granulomas. Other clinical manifestations of *M. tuberculosis* infection include cervical adenitis, skin infections, pericarditis, synovitis, and meningitis.

M. tuberculosis complex also includes the species *M. bovis*, *M. microti*, and *M. africanum*. *M. bovis* causes tuberculosis in cattle, humans and other primates, carnivores including dogs and cats, swine, parrots, and some birds of prey. The disease produced in humans is virtually indistinguishable from that caused by *M. tuberculosis* and is treated similarly. The bacillus of Calmette-Guérin (BCG), which is used as a vaccine against tuberculosis in many parts of the world, conforms to the properties described for *M. bovis* except that it is more attenuated in pathogenicity.

M. africanum is a cause of human tuberculosis in tropical Africa. It may represent an intermediate form between *M. tuberculosis* and *M. bovis*, and retention of *M. africanum* as a distinct species is probably not justified. *M. microti* causes naturally acquired generalized tuberculosis in voles and produces local lesions in guinea pigs, rabbits, and calves.

M. leprae

Leprosy (Hansen's disease) is a chronic, debilitating, granulomatous disease caused by *M. leprae*. The principal manifestations of the disease include anesthetic skin lesions and peripheral neuropathy with peripheral nerve thickening. Leprosy illustrates a continuous spectrum of disease from a localized, self-healing, granulomatous disease with very few demonstrable bacilli (tuberculoid leprosy) to a widespread, progressive form of the disease with massive numbers of M. *leprae* organisms due to the absence of cell-mediated immunity (lepromatous leprosy). The majority of leprosy patients have manifestations between these two polar forms and are clinically unstable. The medical complications of leprosy arise from nerve damage, immune reactions, and infiltration of the mycobacteria (25).

Recent estimates from the World Health Organization put the global prevalence of leprosy at 11 million persons, with the majority of cases occurring in South and Southeast Asia, Africa, and Latin America (143, 261). Although the disease has remained endemic in small pockets in the United States in Texas, Hawaii, California, and Louisiana (162), the majority of infections now seen in North America are acquired abroad. These imported cases of leprosy appear to present a negligible risk for transmission within the United States (143).

A patient with untreated lepromatous leprosy may discharge up to 8×10^8 acid-fast bacilli (AFB) in a single nose blow. Shedding from the nose, rather than from skin lesions, is important for transmission of the disease. Primary infection probably also occurs through the nose. Leprosy transmission is believed to result from prolonged and intimate contact with a person with multibacillary disease. It is recommended that all household contact of persons with leprosy be thoroughly evaluated for disease. The reservoir for M. *leprae* is not well established, but naturally occurring infections of the nine-banded armadillo have been documented in Texas and Louisiana.

M. *leprae* differs from all the other mycobacteria in that it cannot be cultured in vitro. The diagnosis of leprosy is essentially a clinical one, based on finding one or more signs of the disease supported by finding of AFB on slit skin smears or in skin biopsy specimens. In patients with lepromatous leprosy, nodules or plaques are the preferred sites for biopsies; specimens from these sites reveal numerous AFB. In patients with tuberculoid leprosy, the rims of lesions should be biopsied, but only a few or no AFB are found. The modified Fite stain (176) best reveals M. *leprae* in tissue. PCR assays for M. *leprae* are being evaluated (67, 116). Current chemotherapy, which should be initiated promptly following diagnosis, is highly effective for all forms of leprosy; infectiousness is generally lost within 3 days of treatment with multidrug regimens including rifampin (143).

M. avium Complex

M. *avium* complex (MAC) has traditionally consisted of 28 serotypes (referred to as serovars) of two distinct species, M. *avium* and M. *intracellulare*. Serovars 1 to 6, 8 to 11, and 21 are M. avium, while serovars 7, 12 to 20, and 22 to 28 are M. *intracellulare*. In the past M. *scofulaceum* (serovars 41 to 43) was often included in the group as M. *avium*-M. *intracellulare*-M. *scrofulaceum* (MAIS) complex. Inclusion of M. *scrofulaceum* with MAC is no longer appropriate, given recent advances in mycobacterial systematics (253) and the availability of better diagnostics (DNA probes and high-pressure liquid chromatography [HPLC]). M. *avium* and M. *intracellulare* are distinguishable by genetic methods that include DNA probes, 16S rRNA sequencing, and PCR-restriction fragment length polymorphism (RFLP) typing of the gene encoding the 65-kDa heat shock protein (HSP) (222). Three subspecies of M. *avium* have been proposed based on phenotypic characteristics and genetic studies: M. *avium* subspp. *avium*, *paratuberculosis*, and *silvaticum* (225). The International Working Group on Mycobacterial Taxonomy has suggested that there is taxonomic evidence for a third species within the MAC (252), which is generally referred to as the MAC-X strains. Isolates are recognized by the commercial DNA MAC probe but are negative with the M. *avium* or M. *intracellulare* probes.

MAC organisms are ubiquitous in nature and have been isolated from water, soil, plants, house dust, and other environmental sources. These are organisms of low pathogenicity, and single positive specimens with low numbers of organisms are not infrequently recovered from individuals without apparent disease. This complicates the interpretation of culture results, especially cultures of sputum and other respiratory tract specimens. The American Thoracic Society (ATS) has recently published revised diagnostic criteria to help with the interpretation of culture-positive respiratory specimens (3).

MAC infections have become increasingly common in North America and Europe, and MAC is the most common NTM cause of human disease. The greatest increase in MAC infections during the past decade has been in patients with AIDS.

Before the advent of AIDS, pulmonary disease was the most common presentation of MAC infection. Four clinical patterns of lung disease caused by MAC have been recognized: solitary nodules, nodular bronchiectasis, tuberculosis-like infiltrates, and diffuse infiltrates in immunocompromised patients (221). Tuberculosis-like disease (upper lobe fibrocavitary disease) due to MAC typically occurs in white men 45 to 60 years of age who are heavy smokers, many of whom abuse alcohol, and some of whom have preexisting lung disease. The clinical presentation is similar to tuberculosis, with productive cough, fatigue, fever, weight loss, and night sweats. Nodular bronchiectasis usually occurs in elderly nonsmoking women who have no predisposing disorders of the lungs or immune system other than associated bronchiectasis. These patients usually present with persistent cough (221). MAC organisms have been isolated from up to 20% of young adults with cystic fibrosis, particularly in the southeastern United States, but their contribution to the disease process is not yet established (127).

MAC is the leading cause of localized mycobacterial lymphadenitis in children. It typically occurs in children from 1 to 5 years of age. The disease is usually unilateral, involving nodes located in the submandibular, submaxillary, or preauricular areas. The route of infection is thought to be by way of the lymphatic vessels that drain the mouth and pharynx.

Disseminated MAC infections in patients without AIDS are extremely rare. They usually occur in patients with underlying malignancy or inherited or therapeutic immunodeficiency (107).

Patients with AIDS may present with focal or disseminated MAC infections. MAC is commonly isolated from sputum or stool cultures in patients with HIV infection. It is thought that MAC is acquired from the environment and colonizes either the respiratory or gastrointestinal tract before disseminating in HIV-infected patients (77, 106).

Focal infections commonly involve the lungs or gastrointestinal tract and occasionally involve peripheral lymph nodes (112). The clinical presentation of focal pulmonary disease due to MAC in AIDS patients is similar to that in other immunocompromised patients, but cavity formation is rare (<5%). There are few clinical or radiographic findings that distinguish MAC pulmonary disease from the pulmonary disease due to M. *tuberculosis* or the other opportunistic pulmonary pathogens that are of concern in this patient population. Peripheral lymphadenitis due to MAC occasionally occurs in HIV-infected individuals without disseminated disease (8).

Disseminated MAC infection in AIDS patients occurs usually 1 year or more after the diagnosis of AIDS is made, when the CD4 count is <100 cells/mm^3. Bacteremia occurs in almost all patients with disseminated MAC, and the organism is found almost exclusively in the circulating monocytes. With the frequent use of blood cultures, most patients are detected early, and the magnitude of mycobacteremia in most patients ranges from <1 to 10^2 CFU/ml. In disseminated disease, almost any organ system can be involved, with levels of mycobacteria in the tissues being as high as 10^{10} CFU/g of tissue.

AIDS patients are almost invariably infected with M. *avium* rather than M. *intracellulare* (3). In addition, relatively few serovars of M. *avium* account for the majority of the infections in AIDS patients, with serovars 1, 4, and 8 predominating in the United States.

M. fortuitum Complex

Because the two rapidly growing species, M. *fortuitum* and M. *chelonae* (formerly M. *chelonei*), shared a number of characteristics and were associated with similar types of infections, they were historically referred to collectively as the M. *fortuitum* complex. This taxonomic grouping has become less satisfactory with the recognition of additional species and taxa within the complex (e.g., M. *abscessus* and M. *mucogenicum*) (135, 196, 245), all of which differ in drug susceptibilities (219) and many of which differ in their type of clinical disease. For this reason, most of these species are discussed separately below. These taxa are different from slow-growing species in that they grow readily on blood agar or chocolate agar in 3 to 5 days (with the optimal incubation temperature).

M. abscessus

M. *abscessus* (formerly M. *chelonae* subsp. *abscessus*) is a nonpigmented, rapidly growing mycobacterium that is most closely related to M. *chelonae*. This species is responsible for almost 90% of the chronic lung disease due to rapidly growing species (94). It also is a common cause of post-traumatic wound infections (246), causes more than 90% of cases of post-tympanostomy tube otitis media (83), and produces disseminated cutaneous disease similar to that of M. *chelonae* in patients on chronic corticosteroids or other types of immune suppression. The organism is present in tap water and has been associated with a number of nosocomial outbreaks including sternal wound infections, mammaplasty wound infections, and bacteremia associated with contaminated hemodialysis equipment (84).

M. chelonae

M. *chelonae* (formerly M. *chelonae* subsp. *chelonae*) is the slowest-growing member of the complex and generally requires 28 to 30°C temperatures for primary isolation (196). It is most closely related to M. *abscessus* but can be separated from it by its ability to utilize citrate as the sole carbon source (196), by its drug susceptibility patterns (219), or by PCR-RFLP typing (222). NaCl tolerance is generally too unreliable to separate the two species.

This species of rapidly growing mycobacteria is the most likely to be encountered in immunosuppressed patients. The majority of clinical disease due to M. *chelonae* is a disseminated nodular skin disease in patients on steroids or other immunosuppression regimens (243). These patients usually present with multiple draining skin lesions but with minimal symptoms. Intravenous-catheter infections and posttraumatic wound infections also occur. The environmental reservoir for this species is unknown; it is relatively rare in tap water.

M. fortuitum Group

One group of four taxa that are closely related to (and include) M. *fortuitum* is dealt with collectively for reasons given below. These four taxa are known as the M. *fortuitum* group and include M. *fortuitum* (formerly M. *fortuitum* bv: fortuitum), M. *peregrinum* (formerly M. *fortuitum* bv: peregrinum), and M. *fortuitum* third biovariant complex sorbitol positive and M. *fortuitum* third biovariant complex sorbitol negative (135). These taxa have minimal differences in susceptibility to antimicrobial agents and produce similar clinical disease. The four taxa can be separated only by carbohydrate utilization (196), and this is done by few laboratories. Their separation is less important clinically than for M. *chelonae* and M. *abscessus*.

The M. *fortuitum* group is responsible for a number of different types of sporadic infections including osteomyelitis, cellulitis, surgical wound infections, posttraumatic wound infections, otitis media, and chronic pulmonary disease (246). More than 80% of sporadic cases due to the M. *fortuitum* group are due to M. *fortuitum* (246). In a large series of infections due to rapidly growing mycobacteria, the M. *fortuitum* group and M. *chelonae* occurred with equal frequency (246). M. *fortuitum* and M. *peregrinum* have been isolated from natural water and tap water, while M. *fortuitum* has also been isolated from soil and dust.

M. *fortuitum* has been the most common species associated with nosocomial outbreaks or pseudo-outbreaks due to rapidly growing mycobacteria along with M. *abscessus* (84).

M. mucogenicum

M. *mucogenicum* is a nonpigmented, rapidly growing mycobacterium. Biochemically similar to M. *chelonae* (7, 245), it was known as M. *chelonae*-like organism (MCLO) when first described in 1982 (7). It was given species status in 1995 based on 16S rRNA differences from other rapid growers (207). The organism is readily recovered from tap water samples, and its name reflects the finding that most strains are mucoid (245). It is most frequently recovered from a single sample of sputum, which is not clinically significant. It does produce clinical disease, most commonly catheter sepsis or posttraumatic wound infections (245).

M. genavense

M. *genavense* is a slow-growing NTM that was first isolated from the blood of an AIDS patients in Geneva, Switzerland (from which its name is derived); subsequent isolates were recovered from Austria, Germany, and the United States (19). It is the most common cause of mycobacterial disease in psittacine birds (parrots, parakeets, etc.) (174). Analysis of the 16S rRNA sequences indicates that these organisms are most closely related to M. *simiae*. Disseminated infections with M. *genavense* are clinically indistinguishable from those with MAC. The reservoir of the species is presumed to be environmental.

M. *genavense* was first isolated in BACTEC 13A medium only after extended incubation (6 to 8 weeks). It failed to grow on LJ, 7H11 agar, or other commonly used media for isolation of mycobacteria. Middlebrook 7H11 agar supplemented with mycobactin J consistently supported the growth of M. *genavense* (56). M. *genavense* almost certainly is an underrecognized cause of disseminated infections in AIDS patients and perhaps in other settings because of its failure to grow on solid media and its requirement for extended incubation even in BACTEC bottles, which precludes its detection in many mycobacteriology laboratories.

M. haemophilum

M. *haemophilum* was first isolated in 1978 from a subcutaneous lesion from a patient with Hodgkin's disease (179). The organism is unique among mycobacteria in its requirement for hemin or ferric ammonium citrate for growth. Approximately 50% of cases have been in patients with AIDS (216), with a relatively large number reported from New York City (37). The other 50% of cases have been in immunosuppressed individuals such as those with kidney or bone marrow transplantation or patients on chronic corticosteroid therapy (189). M. *haemophilum* has also been recovered from pediatric patients with localized cervical lymphadenopathy who have no underlying immunocompromising factors.

The clinical presentation is that of multiple skin nodules occurring in clusters or without a definite pattern, commonly involving the extremities. Abscesses, draining fistulaes, and osteomyelitis may be associated with the nodules. M. *haemophilum* infections may be underrecognized because of the nutritional requirements of the organism and its predilection for a low incubation temperature (30°C). The reservoir of this organism is presumed to be environmental, but the organism has yet to be recovered from an environmental site.

M. kansasii

M. *kansasii* is a photochromogenic species that was first characterized in 1953. Studies of the base sequences of the 16S rRNA suggest that M. *kansasii* is very closely phylogenetically related to the nonpathogenic, slowly growing, nonpigmented species, M. *gastri* (181). Recent studies have defined five genotypes of M. *kansasii*, most of which cause human disease (171).

A chronic pulmonary infection resembling classical tuberculosis is the usual disease produced by this organism (3). Most cases in the United States have been reported from California, Texas, Louisiana, Florida, Illinois, and Missouri. In the United States and many other countries, M. *kansasii* is second only to MAC as a cause of NTM lung disease (3, 90). M. *kansasii* has been cultured from tap water in municipalities around the world where clinical disease occurs, and tap water is believed to be the major reservoir associated with human disease (3).

Chronic pulmonary disease is the most common disease manifestation of M. *kansasii*; it classically involves the upper lobe, and there is evidence of cavities and scarring in most cases (3). Pleural effusions and hilar lymphadenopathy are rare. Pulmonary disease due to M. *kansasii* differs from that due to MAC in that fewer patients have underlying lung disease and the response to chemotherapy is much better (3).

Extrapulmonary infections are uncommon. They include cervical lymphadenitis in children (265), cutaneous and soft tissue infections (17), and musculoskeletal system involvement (66, 139, 250). M. *kansasii* rarely disseminates except in patients with severely impaired cellular immunity (e.g., those with organ transplants) and most recently in patients with AIDS (3, 192). This organism is the second most common opportunistic mycobacterial infection, after MAC, associated with AIDS.

M. malmoense

The species name M. *malmoense* is derived from Malmo, the city in Sweden from which the first case report originated in 1991 (179). Since its original description, disease due to this organism has been increasingly recognized in Northern Europe, including England, Scotland, Wales, Sweden, and France (3, 267). It remains rare in the United States and other areas of the world. M. *malmoense* infection may be more common than suspected, because it may require 8 to 12 weeks to isolate some strains, which is longer than many laboratories in the United States hold mycobacterial cultures.

Patients with M. *malmoense* infections are usually young children with cervical lymphadenitis or adults with chronic pulmonary disease (3). The latter are mostly middle-aged men with previously documented pneumoconiosis. In some regions of Northern Europe, M. *malmoense* is second only to MAC as a cause of these diseases. Extrapulmonary and disseminated infections have also been reported but only rarely. Recently, the species has been recovered from environmental cultures of soil and water (3).

M. marinum

M. *marinum* causes cutaneous infections as a result of trauma to the skin with subsequent exposure to contaminated freshwater fish tanks ("fish tank granuloma") or salt water. The disease occurs worldwide; in the United States, it is most common in southern coastal states. The skin lesions may be of two types. The more typical presentation is a single papulonodular lesion confined to one extremity, usually involving the elbow, knee, foot, toe, or finger. The lesion appears 2 to 3 weeks after inoculation and, with time, may become verrucous or ulcerated. A second variety resembles cutaneous sporotrichosis, in which the primary inoculation site is followed by secondary spread centrally along the lymphatics. More severe forms of the disease can occur, including tenosynovitis, arthritis, bursitis, and osteomyelitis. Disseminated infections and visceral involvement, including infections in patients with AIDS (71), have been reported but only rarely (88, 136).

M. simiae

As the name suggests, M. *simiae* was first isolated from monkeys. Clinical isolates generally come from a few geographic areas, including the southwestern United States (Texas, New Mexico, Arizona) (3, 57, 234), Israel (138), and the Caribbean including Cuba (3). The organism has been recovered from tap water in some of these areas, and most positive cultures are single positive specimens with low colony counts, suggesting that most represent environmental contamination. Clinical disease appears similar to that caused by MAC, and includes chronic pulmonary disease, osteomyelitis, and disseminated disease. Cases of M. *simiae* infection in AIDS patients have been reported (108).

M. szulgai

M. *szulgai* was first described as a distinct species in 1972. Although it is closely related to M. *malmoense* based on 16S rRNA sequences, phenotypic distinctions between the two species can be made easily (251). The distribution of this organism appears to be worldwide, but its natural reservoirs are unknown.

M. *szulgai* is an infrequent cause of human disease. In

one review, two-thirds of the 24 patients reported prior to 1987 presented with a chronic pulmonary disease that was indistinguishable from tuberculosis and occurred almost exclusively in middle-aged white men (142). The remaining presentations included olecranon bursitis, cervical adenitis, tenosynovitis, cutaneous infections, and osteomyelitis. Two cases of M. *szulgai* infection have been reported in AIDS patients (90).

M. ulcerans

M. *ulcerans* causes an ulcerating infection that usually involves the lower extremities and is limited to patients in localized geographic areas in the tropics, especially in Africa and Australia (3, 92). In Africa the disease is known as Buruli ulcer, and in Australia it is called Bairnsdale ulcer. The disease begins typically as a painless lump under the skin at the site of previous trauma. After a few weeks, a shallow ulcer develops at the site of the lump. The lesions may become necrotic and extend into the subcutaneous tissues. Satellite nodules may develop and ulcerate, but constitutional symptoms rarely occur unless the ulcers become superinfected. Severe limb deformities with contractures and scarring are common if the infection is untreated.

M. xenopi

M. *xenopi* was first isolated in 1957 from skin lesions on an African toad (*Xenopus laevis*), but it was not recognized as a human pathogen until 1965. By 1979, 50 cases of M. *xenopi* infections in humans had been reported, primarily from Great Britain, France, Denmark, Australia, and the United States (3). The optimal growth temperature for the species is 45°C, and it seems to frequent hot water systems (148, 203), including hot water storage tanks in hospitals. Nosocomial acquisition of infection and pseudoinfection has been described (55, 203). M. *xenopi* is being recovered with increasing frequency worldwide (including the United States), and in some areas such as Canada and southeast England, it is second only to MAC as an NTM clinical isolate (3, 267).

Pulmonary disease is the most common manifestation of infection (55, 197), usually occurring in patients with underlying lung disease such as chronic obstructive pulmonary disease or bronchiectasis. Pulmonary infections have been reported only in adults and occur in men more frequently than in women. The disease may be chronic, subacute, or acute. Clinically, the pulmonary infections in patients with M. *xenopi* resemble those in patients with M. *tuberculosis*, MAC, or M. *kansasii*. Extrapulmonary and disseminated infections have also been described in immunocompromised individuals, including renal transplant recipients, peritoneal dialysis patients, and patients with AIDS, but only rarely (5, 76).

Mycobacterium Species Rarely Recovered or Rarely Causing Human Disease

Several species of slowly growing mycobacteria, including M. *gordonae*, M. *scrofulaceum*, and M. *terrae* complex, are not infrequently recovered but are so rarely associated with human disease that they are best characterized as nonpathogens. Some of the case reports of infections attributable to these mycobacteria (especially in the era before molecular identification) lack sufficient documentation of the organism's identification or its disease association to confirm the validity of the cases. Other species (such as M. *asiaticum* or M. *shimoidei*) are pathogenic but are so rarely recovered that most laboratories will never see them. These two groups of species are described below.

M. asiaticum

M. *asiaticum* was first isolated from monkeys in 1965 but was not recognized as a distinct species until 1971. It is similar to M. *gordonae*, differing primarily in that M. *gordonae* is scotochromogenic whereas M. *asiaticum* is photochromogenic (253). The first published report of M. *asiaticum* human disease in 1983 described five patients in Australia with pulmonary disease (16). M. *asiaticum* has subsequently been isolated (infrequently) from patients with respiratory disease in the United States and elsewhere.

M. gastri

As opposed to M. *gordonae*, M. *gastri* is not frequently encountered in the clinical laboratory. Wayne and Sramek found only three reports of human infection attributed to M. *gastri* (253). None of the reports gave sufficient details of the properties of the organisms to conclusively identify them as M. *gastri*.

M. gordonae

M. *gordonae* is the most commonly encountered nonpathogenic species in clinical mycobacteriology laboratories. It is widely distributed in soil and water. In only 1 of the 38 published reports of M. *gordonae* infection was there convincing evidence that M. *gordonae* played a role in the patient's disease process (253). This sole clinically significant infection occurred in an AIDS patient with M. *gordonae* isolated from sputum and bone marrow.

M. scrofulaceum

The species name *scrofulaceum* was derived from scrofula, the historical term used to describe mycobacterial infections of the cervical lymph glands. Until the 1980s, M. *scrofulaceum* was the most common cause of mycobacterial cervical lymphadenitis in children (179). Since then, however, it has become a relatively infrequent cause of this disease, being replaced primarily by MAC. Other types of clinical disease are rare. They include pulmonary disease, disseminated disease, and rare cases of conjunctivitis, osteomyelitis, meningitis, and granulomatous hepatitis.

M. shimoidei

M. *shimoidei* was first described in 1988 in a Japanese patient in Japan with chronic cavitary lung disease (111). The organism is similar to M. *terrae* complex biochemically but can be identified by catalase and β-galactosidase tests. Only a few cases of clinical isolation or pulmonary disease have been reported since the first case description.

M. smegmatis

M. *smegmatis* is more commonly associated with human disease than are any of the other rapidly growing mycobacteria that do not belong to the M. *fortuitum* complex. It is similar to M. *fortuitum* by HPLC and by routine biochemical tests, except that M. *smegmatis* has a negative 3-day arylsulfatase test and clinical strains often have a late yellow-orange pigment at 7 to 10 days on 7H10 agar. An excellent review of the clinical conditions associated with M. *smegmatis* infection was published in 1988 (244). It has most often been associated with soft tissue lesions following trauma or surgery.

M. terrae Complex

M. terrae complex consists of three species, *M. terrae*, *M. nonchromogenicum*, and *M. triviale*. Separation of the members of the complex, especially *M. terrae* from *M. nonchromogenicum*, is difficult by all currently available methods. Clinical disease is generally limited to tenosynovitis of the hand following local trauma (144).

Chromogenic Rapidly Growing Mycobacteria

Other rapidly growing mycobacteria, some of which appear to be disease producing, have been recovered from clinical samples. They include *M. flavescens*, *M. neoaurum*, *M. thermoresistibile*, *M. mageritense*, *M. phlei*, *M. vaccae*, *M. aichiense*, *M. aurum*, *M. chubuense*, and *M. gadium*. In general, too few strains have been studied (especially in genetic studies) for us to be certain of the pathogenic potential of these species and their uniqueness.

New Species of Nontuberculous Mycobacteria

M. branderi

M. branderi was first described by Brander et al. in 1992 as 14 respiratory isolates collected in Finland (22). The strains had 2-week arylsulfatase activity, were nonpigmented, and were able to grow at 45°C. By 16S rRNA sequencing, the isolates were most closely related to *M. celatum*, *M. cookii*, and *M. xenopi* (131).

M. celatum

M. celatum is a slowly growing nonphotochromogenic species that was recently described by Butler et al. (32). *M. celatum* shares characteristics with MAC, *M. xenopi*, *M. malmoense*, and *M. shimoidei* but most closely resembles *M. xenopi*. Several subgroups have been identified, especially with the use of PCR-RFLP typing of the 65-kDa HSP-encoding gene (170). *M. celatum* can be differentiated from *M. xenopi* by its poor growth at 45°C, production of large colonies on 7H10 agar, and production of trace to 2% of the fatty acid 2-docosanol. A few strains have been misidentified as *M. tuberculosis* complex with a commercially available DNA probe test (Gen-Probe, San Diego, Calif.) (31).

Strains have been isolated from diverse geographic areas throughout the United States, Finland, and Somalia. Most strains have been isolated from respiratory tract specimens, but the organisms have been recovered from other sources including stool, spine, and blood. The clinical significance of these isolates was not defined. In one series, 32% of the patients from whom *M. celatum* was isolated were infected with HIV (32).

M. conspicuum

M. conspicuum was described in 1995 by Springer et al. (210), when they characterized isolates from two AIDS patients with disseminated disease. The organism was slow growing and produced dysgonic pale yellow colonies on solid media. An unusual feature is that the organisms did not grow at 37°C except in liquid media and produced good visible growth only at 22 to 31°C. They were able to grow in BACTEC medium at the higher temperatures, however. By 16S rRNA sequencing, the organism was shown to be most closely related to *M. asiaticum* and *M. gordonae* (210).

M. interjectum

M. interjectum was described by Springer et al. in 1993 based on two isolates recovered from the lymph node of a child with chronic lymphadenitis (208). The organism grows as dysgonic smooth scotochromogenic colonies which produce visible growth only within 21 to 28 days. Fatty-acid patterns by gas-liquid chromatography (GLC) were similar to those of *M. scrofulaceum*. By 16S rRNA sequencing, the organism was shown to be most closely related to *M. simiae*.

M. lentiflavum

M. lentiflavum was first reported in 1996 by Springer et al. (211), when they described a group of slowly growing pigmented organisms which had distinct HPLC and GLC patterns of mycolic acids. The majority of the isolates were from respiratory specimens. The organisms have a bright yellow pigment, do not grow at 45°C, and are generally resistant to the antituberculous agents (211).

M. triplex

M. triplex was characterized in 1996 by Floyd et al. (80), when they described an unusual group of slowly growing mycobacteria that resembled MAC. However, they were DNA probe negative for MAC. The majority of these isolates were from either lymph nodes or respiratory samples. By 16S rRNA sequencing, the organisms were shown to be most closely related to *M. genavense* and *M. simiae*. However, the organisms differ from *M. simiae* biochemically in that they do not produce any pigmentation, and their easy growth on solid media differentiates them from *M. genavense* (80).

COLLECTION, TRANSPORT, AND STORAGE OF SPECIMENS

Safety Procedures

Nosocomial transmission of *M. tuberculosis* from patients or specimens is of major concern to health care workers (34). Because of the low infective dose of *M. tuberculosis* for humans (50% infective dose, <10 bacilli), and in some laboratories a high rate of isolation of acid-fast organisms from clinical specimens (>10%), sputa and other clinical specimens from patients with suspected or known tuberculosis must be considered potentially infectious and handled with appropriate precautions (41). The control of aerosols and other forms of mycobacterial contamination in the laboratory is achieved by the use of properly functioning biologic safety cabinets (BSC), centrifuges with safety carriers, and meticulous processing techniques (see also chapter 9).

Classification of mycobacteriology laboratory practices should be based on risk assessment (i.e., volume of tests, prevalence of tuberculosis, rate of multidrug-resistant *M. tuberculosis*, types of testing). Biosafety Level 2 practices and facilities are required for laboratories assessed as low risk. Aerosol generating manipulations should be conducted in a Class I or II BSC. More rigorous Biosafety Level 3 practices and Level 2 facilities are required for laboratories assessed as being at higher risk. These laboratories process specimens for mycobacterial culture and propagate and manipulate cultures of *M. tuberculosis* (e.g., for identification and susceptibility testing). These practices require that laboratory access be restricted, that directional airflow be used to maintain the laboratory under negative pressure, and that workers wear special laboratory clothing and gloves when appropriate. Biosafety Level 3 practices and facilities are required for those laboratories growing *M. tuberculosis* to high volumes, working with large numbers of resistant isolates, or performing tests with unknown risk. A detailed description of safety requirements in the mycobacteriology laboratory is given in the CDC/NIH biosafety guide for laboratories (41).

All respiratory protective devices (respirators) used in the workplace should be certified by the National Institute for Occupational Safety and Health (NIOSH) (161). Respirators that contain a NIOSH-certified N-series filter with a 95% efficiency (N-95) rating are appropriate for use. These meet the recommendations from the CDC (42) for selection of respirators for protection against *M. tuberculosis*. The recommendations are as follows: (i) The unloaded filter must filter particles 0.3 μm in size with an efficiency of 95% at flow rates up to 50 liters/min. (ii) The respirator must have the ability to be qualitatively or quantitatively fit-tested to obtain a face-seal leakage rate of no more than 10%. (iii) It must have the ability to fit different facial sizes and characteristics, which is attained by making respirators available in at least three sizes. (iv) It must have the ability to check for face piece fit by the person wearing the respirator each time it is worn in accordance with OSHA standards. Surgical masks are not NIOSH-certified respirators and must not be used to provide respiratory protection.

The determination of when and if to use respiratory protective devices in the laboratory should be based on the risk assessment. A respirator program should be implemented by the laboratory and should include a written protocol describing when respirator use is necessary and procedures addressing (i) selection of the appropriate respirator, (ii) how to conduct fit-testing, and (iii) training of personnel in the use, fit-checking, and storage of the respirator.

All work involving specimens or cultures, such as making smears, inoculating media, adding reagents to biochemical tests, opening centrifuge cups, and sonication, must be performed in a BSC. The handling of all specimens suspected of containing mycobacteria (including specimens processed for other microorganisms), with the exception of centrifugation for concentration purposes, must be done within the BSC. Specimens that are to be taken out of the BSC should be covered before being transported. To further decrease aerosolization, paper towels soaked with a phenolic disinfectant can be used to cover work surfaces, to line discard pans, and to wipe the outside of culture tubes or containers. All work surfaces, including bench tops and the inside of the BSC, should be cleaned with an appropriate disinfectant before and after work. Effective disinfectants include Amphyl or other phenol-soap mixtures and 0.05 to 0.5% sodium hypochlorite (the concentration varies according to the nature of the contaminated surface). However, 5% phenol is no longer recommended as a surface disinfectant due to its documented toxicity to personnel. UV light is a useful adjunct for surface decontamination and may be applied to radiate the work area when it is not in use. Centrifuges should be used with aerosol-free safety carriers to contain debris in the event that tubes break. Use of electric incinerators rather than open flames is recommended. The excess inoculum from inoculating loops, wire, or spades may be removed by dipping the tool into a container of 95% ethanol in washed sand before placing it in an incinerator. The use of disposable inoculating loops is recommended. Syringes with permanently attached needles should be used if needles are required. An autoclave should be available in an easily accessible area and must be used to decontaminate infectious waste before it is removed to the disposal areas.

Personnel should be regularly monitored with the Mantoux PPD skin test (at least annually and more often if a conversion in the laboratory or the institution has been documented) (41, 122) to demonstrate conversions. Those with positive skin tests should be evaluated for active tuberculosis with a chest X-ray and clinical evaluation. Physical examinations should be performed when necessary. New converters should be referred to the Employee Health Department and the Infection Control Department for epidemiological evaluation. Laboratories should have written protocols describing procedures for handling laboratory accidents. In case of a laboratory accident with possible formation of aerosols, personnel should hold their breath, make sure BSCs are on and centrifuges are turned off, and then leave the room with the door closed for at least 30 min. (The length of time depends on the type of accident and the amount of risk.) With appropriate respiratory protection devices, personnel can return to the accident area to clean the spill. PPD-negative personnel should be skin tested 3 and 6 months after the accident. Persons who are immunocompromised should be discouraged from working in the mycobacteriology laboratory (41).

Specimen Collection and Submission

Most of the specimens submitted for mycobacterial culture are from the respiratory tract. Tissue, normally sterile body fluids, urine, and gastric aspirates are other commonly submitted specimens. Blood and stool specimens may be submitted from patients with AIDS.

Specimens should be collected and submitted in sterile, leakproof, disposable, appropriately labeled, laboratory-approved containers. Waxed containers must not be used, because they may result in false-positive smear results (122). Initial specimens should ideally be collected before the initiation of antimycobacterial chemotherapy. Specimens should be collected aseptically, or the collection method should bypass areas of contamination as much as possible, to minimize contamination with the indigenous flora. Contamination with tap water or other fluids that may contain either viable or nonviable environmental mycobacteria should be avoided, since saprophytic mycobacteria may result in false-positive culture and/or smear results (93, 242). In general, swabs are not recommended for the isolation of mycobacteria since they provide limited material and the hydrophobicity of the mycobacteria often compromises their isolation from swabs onto solid or broth media. Negative results from swab specimens are not reliable. No fixatives or preservatives should be used, and specimens should be transported to the laboratory in as short a time as practical to avoid overgrowth by contaminating bacteria and fungi. If transport to the laboratory is delayed more than 1 h, specimens except blood should be refrigerated. Once received in the laboratory, specimens should be refrigerated until processed. See chapter 4 for additional information on specimen collection.

Sputum

Sputum, both expectorated and induced, is the principal specimen obtained for the diagnosis of pulmonary tuberculosis. An early-morning specimen, preferably 5 to 10 ml, from a deep, productive cough should be collected on at least three, but usually not more than five or six consecutive days. Processing of additional specimens does not seem to improve recovery. Only two AFB smear-positive specimens are needed for the initial evaluation of pulmonary mycobacteriosis (215). For follow-up of smear-positive patients receiving therapy, specimens should be collected for smear examination at weekly intervals beginning 3 weeks after initiation of therapy. Repeat culture should be considered if the smears do not convert to negative. The requisition should include information about whether the specimen is induced or expectorated, to ensure proper handling, since induced sputa appear watery and much like saliva. The screening of sputum for upper respiratory tract contamination as done for bacteriologic workups is not performed for AFB cultures, but specimens should preferably be lower respiratory tract secretions. Any isolate of M. *tuberculosis*, even that in saliva, is considered significant. Pooled sputum specimens are unacceptable specimens for mycobacterial culture because of increased contamination and lower test sensitivity (122). Clinicians should consider the diagnosis of pulmonary mycobacterial disease in patients with or at risk for HIV infection even if the clinical presentation is unusual (105), and if tuberculosis is suspected, sputum samples should be collected even if results of chest X-ray examinations are negative.

Bronchoalveolar Lavage Fluids and Bronchial Washings

Invasive collection techniques may be necessary to diagnose pulmonary mycobacteriosis in some patients unable to produce sputum. Bronchial washings, bronchoalveolar lavage (BAL) fluid, transbronchial biopsy specimens, and brush biopsy specimens may all be collected during bronchoscopy. At least 5 ml of bronchial washing or BAL fluid should be collected in a sterile container. The bronchoscope must not become contaminated with tap water, which may contain saprophytic mycobacteria. The material obtained from bronchial brushings can be placed in a sterile tube containing approximately 10 ml of Middlebrook 7H9 broth supplemented with bovine serum albumin (final concentration, 1 to 2%) and Tween 80 (0.5%). Bronchial washings and BAL fluid can usually be sent directly to the laboratory in the containers in which they have been collected. Frequently, bronchoscopy causes the patient to produce sputum naturally for several days after the procedure, and specimens collected 1 or 2 days after bronchoscopy enhance the detection of mycobacteria. Transtracheal aspirates are not commonly submitted, but specimens collected by invasive techniques such as fine-needle aspiration and open-lung biopsy may be submitted in difficult cases.

Gastric Lavage Fluids

Aspiration of swallowed sputum from the stomach by gastric lavage may be necessary for infants, young children, and the obtunded. Samples of 5 to 10 ml should be collected on three consecutive days in a sterile container without a preservative. The fluid should be adjusted to neutral pH with 100 mg of sodium carbonate immediately after collection or within 4 h. If the specimen cannot be processed within 4 h, the laboratory should provide sterile disposable containers with 100 mg of sodium carbonate for collection. Unneutralized specimens are not acceptable, because acid is detrimental to mycobacteria. Fasting, early-morning specimens are recommended to obtain sputum swallowed during sleep. Saprophytic mycobacteria are frequently recovered from gastric lavage fluid and are often the cause of "false-positive" (i.e., not M. *tuberculosis*) smear results on these specimens.

Blood

Cultures for the isolation of mycobacteria from blood should be reserved for immunocompromised patients, particularly those with AIDS. The majority of disseminated mycobacterial infections are due to MAC. Positive MAC blood cultures are always associated with clinical evidence of disease (98). The Isolator lysis centrifugation system (Wampole Laboratories, Cranbury, N.J.) or the radiometric BACTEC 13A blood culture bottle (Becton-Dickinson Diagnostic Instrument Systems, Cockeysville, Md.) is recommended for mycobacterial blood cultures (2, 86, 124, 125, 256). Isolator tubes contain saponin, which lyses cells and releases intracellular mycobacteria. Sediment from the Isolator tube can be cultured onto egg-based or agar media. The use of Isolator blood sediments to inoculate BACTEC 12B medium is contraindicated because the sediments may be inhibitory to MAC (249). The BACTEC 13A bottle contains a lysing agent and is designed specifically for the recovery of mycobacteria from blood. The 13A medium can be directly inoculated with 5 ml of blood without the potential hazards associated with the lysis-centrifugation procedure. A potential disadvantage of using the BACTEC 13A medium is the inability to determine the number of CFU per volume of blood. However, the significance and necessity of obtaining quantitative data with each culture are unclear. The BACTEC blood culture system is discussed in more detail below. Direct inoculation of blood onto a solid medium is not recommended (2, 125).

The site should be disinfected as for routine blood culture. If blood has to be transported before inoculation of BACTEC media, sodium polyarethol sulfonate (SPS) or heparin is used as an anticoagulant; blood collected in EDTA or coagulated blood is not acceptable. MAC survives for prolonged periods in Isolator tubes, and so processing of Isolator tubes may be delayed for 24 h if absolutely necessary (99, 240).

Urine

The first morning specimen should be collected, either by catheterization or by midstream clean catch into a sterile container, on three consecutive days. Appropriate cleaning of genitalia should precede collection. Organisms accumulate in the bladder overnight, and the first morning void provides the best results. A minimum of 40 ml of urine is usually required for culture. For a suprapubic tap, as much as possible should be collected in a syringe with a Luer tip cap or other sterile container. Twenty-four-hour pooled specimens, catheter bag specimens, and small-volume (<40 ml, unless a larger volume is not obtainable) specimens are unacceptable.

Stools

Stool specimens (>1 g) should be collected in sterile, wax-free, disposable clean containers or transferred from a bedpan or plastic wrap stretched over the toilet bowl and sent directly to the laboratory. Stool specimens have been used for detection of MAC involvement of the gastrointestinal tracts of patients with AIDS, in conjunction with specimens from other sites.

Past recommendations have been that stool be cultured for mycobacteria only if the direct smear of unprocessed stool is positive for AFB. More recent studies showed the sensitivity of the smear to be only 32 to 34% (123, 155), suggesting that the fecal smear results should not determine whether a mycobacterium culture be performed. Routine screening cultures or smears are not effective ways to identify those patients at risk for developing disseminated MAC infection (99). Although detection of MAC in the gastrointestinal tract may be predictive of the development of disseminated infection (106), no data are available on the efficacy of antibiotic prophylaxis in patients with positive stool cultures and negative blood cultures. Therefore, routine screening of stool specimens for MAC is not recommended (47).

Body Fluids

Body fluids (e.g., cerebrospinal, pleural, peritoneal, and pericardial fluids) are aseptically collected by aspiration or surgical procedures. As much as possible should be collected in a sterile container or syringe with a Luer tip cap. Bloody specimens may be anticoagulated with SPS. Because certain body fluids (such as cerebrospinal fluid [CSF] and peritoneal dialysis effluent) may contain a small number of mycobacteria, larger specimen volumes increase culture yields. For CSF, at least 2 ml must be cultured. Small-volume specimens may be directly inoculated into broth.

Tissues (Lymph Node, Skin, Other Biopsy Material)

At least 1 g of tissue, if possible, should be aseptically collected into a sterile container without fixative or preservative. It must not be immersed in saline or other liquid or wrapped in gauze. For cutaneous ulcers, biopsy material should be collected from the periphery of the lesion. Specimens submitted in formalin are unacceptable.

Abscess Contents, Aspirated Fluid, Skin Lesions, and Wounds

As much material as possible should be aspirated into a syringe with Luer tip cap. The skin should be cleared with alcohol before the sample is collected. For cutaneous lesions, material is aspirated from under the margin of the lesion. The laboratory may provide 7H9 broth for the transport of small volumes of aspirates.

ISOLATION PROCEDURES

The laboratory diagnosis of mycobacterial diseases depends on the detection and recovery of AFB from clinical specimens. Microbiologists must be prepared to process and culture a variety of both respiratory and nonrespiratory specimens, some (but not all) of which are contaminated with the normal host flora. Because mycobacteria are slow growing and require long incubation times, a variety of nonmycobacterial organisms can overgrow cultures of specimens obtained from nonsterile sites. Appropriate digestion and decontamination procedures, culture media, and conditions of incubation must be selected to facilitate optimal recovery of mycobacteria (see also chapter 5).

Processing of Specimens

Normally Sterile Specimens

Tissues or body fluids collected aseptically usually do not require the digestion and decontamination procedures used with contaminated specimens. Decontamination of a specimen should be attempted only if the specimen is thought to be contaminated. If the need to decontaminate a specimen is not clear, the specimen may be refrigerated until the routine bacteriologic cultures are checked the next day. If routine cultures are not available, the specimen may be initially inoculated to blood or chocolate agar plates to check for sterility before being processed for mycobacteria (179).

Normally sterile tissues may be ground in sterile 0.85% saline or 0.2% bovine albumin and then inoculated directly to both solid and liquid media. Because body fluids commonly contain only small numbers of mycobacteria, they should be concentrated to maximize the yield of mycobacteria before inoculation of media. The fluids are centrifuged at $\geq$3,000 $\times$ g for 15 min, and the sediment is inoculated to liquid and solid media. When the volume of fluid submitted for culture is small, it may be added directly to liquid media such as Middlebrook 7H9 in a ratio of 1 part specimen to 5 parts broth, the BACTEC 12B vial, or another broth-based system. Specimens that would normally be inoculated directly may be decontaminated at some institutions due to problems with contamination specific to the institution.

Contaminated Specimens

Most specimens submitted for mycobacterial culture consist of a complex organic matrix contaminated with a variety of organisms that can rapidly outgrow the mycobacteria. Mucin may trap mycobacterial cells and protect contaminating bacteria from the action of decontaminating agents. Thus, mycobacteria are recovered optimally from clinical specimens through the use of procedures which reduce or eliminate contaminating bacteria while releasing mycobacteria trapped in mucin and cells. Liquefaction of certain specimens, particularly sputum, is often necessary. The mycobacteria are then concentrated to enhance detection in stained smears and by culture. No one method of digestion and decontamination is ideal for all clinical specimens, for all laboratories, and in all circumstances. The laboratorian must be aware of the inherent limitations of the various methods.

Digestion and Decontamination Methods

Sodium hydroxide, the most commonly used decontaminant, also serves as a mucolytic agent but must be used cautiously because it is only somewhat less harmful to tubercle bacilli than to the contaminating organisms. The stronger the alkali, the higher its temperature during the time it acts on the specimen, and the longer it is allowed to act, the greater will be the killing action on both contaminants and mycobacteria (133). Harsh decontamination can kill 20 to 90% of the mycobacteria in a clinical specimen (122, 132). Liquefaction is facilitated by vigorous mixing of a solution in a sealed container with a vortex-type mixer. To use the mixer properly and minimize aerosol production, the tube should be held on the vibrating base in such a way that churning, splashing, and foaming of the mixture are avoided. Homogenization should occur by centrifugal swirling, and this swirling should not be vigorous enough to allow material to rise to the cap. After agitation, there should be at least a 15-min delay before opening the tube to allow any fine aerosol droplets formed during the mixing to settle. All such procedures should be carried out in a BSC.

Most commonly, a combination liquefaction-decontamination mixture is used. *N*-Acetyl-L-cysteine (NALC), dithiothreitol, and several enzymes effectively liquefy sputum. These agents have no direct inhibitory effect on bacterial cells; however, their use permits treatment with lower concentrations of sodium hydroxide, thereby indirectly improving the recovery of mycobacteria. Addition of cetylpyridinium chloride (see Appendix 1) specimens mailed from remote collection stations to a central processing station has shown a good recovery of *M. tuberculosis* without overgrowth by contaminating bacteria (202).

Liquefaction and concentration of sputum for acid-fast staining may be conducted safely by first treating the specimens (in a class I or II BSC) with an equal volume of 5% sodium hypochlorite solution (undiluted household bleach) and waiting 15 min before centrifugation (122). Such a treated specimen cannot be cultured.

The type of procedures selected by the laboratory should reflect the number and types of specimens received and the time and staff required to process them. Even under the best of conditions, all currently available procedures are toxic for mycobacteria to some extent. Thus, the best yield of mycobacteria may be expected to result from the use of the mildest decontamination procedure that sufficiently controls contaminants. Strict adherence to specimen processing is mandatory to ensure survival of the maximal number of mycobacteria. Most laboratories process specimens in batches; current recommendations suggest that specimen batches should be processed daily (223). The most widely used digestion-decontamination method is the NALC–2% NaOH method. A variety of specimens can be processed by the NALC-NaOH method, and it is compatible with the BACTEC and other commercially available broth culture systems. Whatever method is used, great care must be taken to prevent laboratory cross-contamination of patient specimens during processing (198). A single positive culture for *M. tuberculosis* could be the basis of a diagnosis of tuberculosis, and thus a false-positive culture may have profound consequences for the clinical management of the patient, for epidemiologic investigations, and for public health control measures (see Quality Assurance, below).

Commonly used digestion-decontamination methods are described with step-by-step instructions in the guide by Kent and Kubica (122), the *Clinical Microbiology Procedures Handbook* (113), and Appendix 1 of this chapter. In general, the specimen is diluted with an equal volume of digestant and allowed to incubate for some time. A neutralizing buffer is added, and the specimen is centrifuged to sediment any AFB present. The centrifugation should be carried out at $\geq$3,000 $\times$ *g* for 15 min to get maximum recovery; some laboratorians recommend 3,800 $\times$ *g* (258, 259). The sediment is then inoculated onto the appropriate liquid and solid media.

Optimizing Decontamination Procedures

Excessive contamination is generally defined as a rate exceeding 5% of all digested and decontaminated specimens cultured. A high contamination rate (see Quality Assurance, below) suggests either too weak a decontaminant or incomplete digestion. One or a combination of several of the following measures may be used to help decrease the decontamination rate.

1. Cautiously increase the strength of the alkali treatment slightly; 4% NaOH will probably kill most tubercle bacilli.
2. Use a selective medium (one that contains antibiotics) in addition to a nonselective primary culture medium to inhibit the growth of bacterial and fungal contaminants. Selective 7H11 agar (Mitchison medium), Mycobactosel agar (BBL Microbiology Systems, Cockeysville, Md.), or the Gruft modification of Lowenstein-Jensen (L-J) medium should be considered. The most useful media for recovering MAC from stool specimens were Mitchison's selective 7H11 agar and Mycobactosel L-J medium (263).
3. Make sure specimens are completely digested; partially digested specimens may not be completely decontaminated. Increase the NALC concentration to digest thick, mucoid specimens.
4. Use an alternative digestion-decontamination procedure for problem specimen types. Respiratory secretions from patients with cystic fibrosis, often overgrown with pseudomonads, can successfully be decontaminated with NALC-NaOH followed by 5% oxalic acid treatment (255).

To determine the decontaminating capabilities of each new batch of reagents, the laboratory may wish to inoculate blood agar plates with four to six decontaminated sputum specimens in addition to inoculating mycobacterial media. Numbers of contaminants that grow after 48 h of incubation at 35°C should be minimal to none (122).

Acid-Fast Stain Procedures

Mycobacteria are difficult to stain. The large amount of lipids present in their cell walls renders them impermeable to the dyes used in the Gram stain, and the appearance of mycobacteria in a Gram-stained specimen may vary. Mycobacteria may be gram-invisible, they may appear as negatively stained images or "ghosts," or they may appear as beaded gram-positive rods (231). To an experienced microscopist, such an appearance may lead to the diagnosis of an unsuspected mycobacterial infection.

Mycobacteria are able to form stable complexes with certain arylmethane dyes such as fuchsin and auramine O. Although the exact nature of the acid-fast staining reaction is not completely understood, phenol in the primary stain allows penetration of the stain. The cell wall mycolic acid residues retain the primary stain even after exposure to acid-alcohol or strong mineral acids. This resistance to decolorization is required for an organism to be termed acid-fast. A counterstain is used to highlight the stained organisms for easier microscopic recognition. Information about specific staining procedures (carbol fuchsin and fluorochrome) is given in chapter 129.

Because acid-fast artifacts may be present in a smear, it is necessary to view the cell morphology carefully. AFB are approximately 1 to 10 μm long and typically are slender rods (0.2 to 0.6 μm wide) that may appear curved or bent. Individual bacilli may display heavily stained areas and areas of alternating stain, producing a beaded appearance. Some NTM species may appear pleomorphic, appearing as long filaments or coccoid forms, with uniform staining properties. *M. kansasii* organisms can often be suspected in stained sputum smears by their large size and cross-banding appearance. Cells of rapidly growing mycobacteria may be <10% acid-fast and may not stain with the fluorochrome stain (118). If the presence of a rapid grower is suspected and regular acid-fast stains are negative, it may be worthwhile staining over the smear with a carbol fuchsin stain in a weaker decolorizing process. Organisms that are truly acid fast are difficult to over-decolorize. Nonmycobacterial organisms with various degrees of acid fastness include *Rhodococcus* species, *Nocardia* species, *Legionella micdadei*, and the cysts of *Cryptosporidium*, *Isospora*, *Cyclospora*, and microsporidia.

Each slide made from a clinical specimen should be thoroughly examined for the presence of AFB. When a carbol fuchsin-stained smear is read, a minimum of 300 fields should be examined before the smear is reported as negative. Because the fluorochrome stain is read at a lower power than the carbol fuchsin stain, more material can be examined in a given period than could be examined on a fuchsin-stained smear. At the lower magnification, a minimum of 30 fields of view should be examined. This requires as little as 90 s. This ease of detection of AFB with the fluorochrome stain makes it the preferred staining method for clinical specimens, although to an inexperienced observer, fluorescent debris may be misinterpreted as bacilli. Positive fluorochrome smears can be restained by one of the carbol fuchsin methods to confirm the presence of AFB and to store slides for future reference (122).

All smears in which no AFB have been seen should be reported as negative. When acid-fast organisms are observed on a smear, the smear should be reported as positive and the staining method should be indicated. Information about

TABLE 1 Acid-fast smear evaluation and reporting[a]

Report	No. of AFB seen by staining method and magnification		
	Fuchsin stain	Fluorochrome stain	
	×1,000	×250	×450
No AFB seen	0	0	0
Doubtful; repeat	1–2/300 F[b] (3 sweeps)[c]	1–2/30 F (1 sweep)	1–2/70 F (1.5 sweeps)
1+	1–9/100 F (1 sweep)	1–9/10 F	2–18/50 F (1 sweep)
2+	1–9/10 F	1–9/F	4–36/10 F
3+	1–9/F	10–90/F	4–36/F
4+	>9/F	>90/F	>36/F

[a] Adapted from reference 122.
[b] F, microscope fields.
[c] In all cases, one full sweep refers to scanning the full length (2 cm) of a smear 1 cm wide by 2 cm long.

the quantity of AFB observed on the smear should be provided. The recommended interpretations and reporting of smear results are given in Table 1. If only one or two organisms are seen on an entire smear, this should be noted but not reported. Confirmation of this finding should be attempted by use of other smears from the same specimen or, if possible, smears prepared from a new specimen. Observations made with the fluorochrome smears should be converted to a format that equates these observations with those made with a 100× oil immersion objective.

The acid-fast stain, either direct and/or concentrated, should be used as an adjunct to culture. Definitive diagnosis of mycobacterial disease (except leprosy) requires growth of the microorganism. A minimum of 5×10^3 to 1×10^4 bacilli per ml of sputum is required for detection by smear, whereas culture detects as few as 10 to 100 viable organisms (122).

Although the sensitivity of the direct acid-fast smear examination for the diagnosis of mycobacterial infection is lower than that of culture methods, the acid-fast smear plays an important role in early diagnosis of mycobacterial infection because of the relatively long time required for mycobacteria to be detected by culture methods. It is important to detect the presence of mycobacterial disease as rapidly as possible for implementation of appropriate patient care and public health measures. Patients with positive smears are considered more likely to spread tuberculosis. The acid-fast stain also serves to confirm the acid-fast nature of organisms recovered from culture and to monitor the effectiveness of antimycobacterial therapy. Quantitation of a positive smear is also used as an aid in the determination of appropriate dilutions of a specimen for direct susceptibility testing.

The overall sensitivity of the direct smear has been reported to range from 22 to 80% (27, 141, 157). Factors influencing sensitivity include the types of specimens examined, centrifugation speed, the staining techniques, the experience of the reader, the culture methods used, and the patient population being evaluated. Respiratory specimens yield the highest smear positivity rate (141, 157). In practice, the fluorochrome stain is more sensitive than the carbol-fuchsin stain, probably because the fluorochrome stained smears are easier to read.

The specificity of the direct smear for the detection of mycobacteria is very high. Prolonged or too harsh specimen decontamination and short incubation of cultures may account for smear-positive, culture-negative results. Patients with pulmonary tuberculosis may have positive smears with negative cultures (for 2 to 10 weeks) during a course of appropriate treatment (128, 175). Cross contamination of slides during the staining process and the use of water contaminated with NTM during staining procedures are potential sources of false-positive results (69, 157, 242). Staining jars or dishes should not be used. Transfer of AFB in the oil used for microscopy may also occur. It is best to confirm positive smears by having them reviewed by another experienced reader.

Rapid and sensitive AFB stain results can be obtained by evaluation of sputum smears concentrated by cytocentrifugation (185). Sputa are liquefied and decontaminated by addition of an equal volume of 5% sodium hypochlorite prior to cytocentrifugation. The major limitation of this method is that a second specimen must be collected for culture.

The diagnostic yield of acid-fast stains of body fluids is less than for respiratory specimens because the concentration of mycobacteria is usually lower. A variety of techniques have been used to concentrate mycobacteria from CSF and other body fluids, but comparative data are lacking. Centrifugation is not an effective way to concentrate mycobacteria, since mycobacteria have a buoyant density of approximately 1 and, as a result, many organisms remain in the supernatant (130, 201). Sequential layering of several drops of uncentrifuged fluid on a slide or polycarbonate membrane filtration is probably the most effective means of concentrating mycobacteria for microscopy.

Culture Media

Many different media are available to use for the recovery of mycobacteria and include nonselective and selective medium, the latter containing one or more antibiotics to prevent overgrowth by contaminating bacteria or fungi. Broth medium is preferred for the initial isolation of mycobacteria. Solid media may be egg based or agar based; all contain malachite green, a dye which suppresses the growth of contaminating bacteria.

Egg-Based Media

Egg-based media contain whole eggs or egg yolks, potato flour, salts, and glycerol and are solidified by inspissation. These media have a long shelf life (several months when refrigerated) and support good growth of most mycobacteria. Also, materials in the inoculum and medium toxic to mycobacteria are neutralized. The disadvantages of these media include the difficulty in discerning colonies from debris and the inability to achieve accurate and consistent drug concentrations for susceptibility testing. When egg-based media become contaminated, the entire tube is involved and the media may completely liquefy.

Of the egg-based media, L-J medium is most commonly used in clinical laboratories. In general, L-J medium recovers *M. tuberculosis* well but is not as reliable for the recovery of other species. Petragnani medium contains about twice as much malachite green as does L-J medium and is most commonly used for recovery of mycobacteria from heavily contaminated specimens. American Trudeau Society medium contains a lower concentration of malachite green than L-J medium and is thus more easily overgrown by contaminants. The growth of mycobacteria on American Trudeau Society medium is less inhibited due to the low concentration of malachite green, resulting in the earlier growth of larger colonies.

Agar-Based Media

Agar-based media are transparent and provide a ready means for detecting early growth of microscopic colonies easily distinguished from inoculum debris. Colonies may be observed in 10 to 12 days, in contrast to 18 to 24 days with opaque egg-based media. Microscopic examination can be performed by simply turning the plate medium over and examining by focusing on the agar surface through the bottom of the plate and the agar at ×10 to ×100 magnification and may provide both earlier detection of growth than unaided visual examination and presumptive identification of the species of mycobacteria present. The use of thinly poured 7H11 agar plates (10 by 90 mm; Remel, Lenexa, Kans.) facilitates this process (254). Agar-based media can be used for susceptibility testing. They do not readily support the growth of contaminants (122); however, the plates are expensive to prepare and their shelf life is relatively short (1 month in the refrigerator). Care should be exercised in the preparation, incubation, and storage of the media, because excessive heat or light exposure may result in deterioration and in the release of formaldehyde, which is toxic to mycobacteria (150).

Middlebrook medium contains 2% glycerol, which enhances the growth of MAC. Additional supplements may be helpful for recovery of other mycobacteria and in certain situations. For example, the addition of 0.2% pyruvic acid is recommended if *M. bovis* is suspected (68), and 0.25% L-asparagine or 0.1% potassium aspartate must be added to 7H10 agar for maximal production of niacin (126). The addition of 0.1% enzymatic hydrolysate of casein to the Middlebrook 7H11 formulation (the only difference from 7H10) improves the recovery of isoniazid-resistant strains of *M. tuberculosis*.

Selective Media

The addition of antimicrobial agents to L-J, 7H10, or 7H11 medium may be helpful for eliminating the growth of contaminating organisms (147, 166). If selective medium is used for a particular specimen or specimen type, it should not be used alone but in conjunction with a nonselective agar- or egg-based medium. Egg-based selective media include L-J–Gruft with penicillin and nalidixic acid and Mycobactosel L-J medium with cycloheximide, lincomycin, and nalidixic acid. Mitchison selective 7H11 (7H11S) medium and its modifications contain carbenicillin (especially useful for inhibiting *Pseudomonas* spp.), polymyxin B, trimethoprim lactate, and amphotericin B.

Liquid Media

Middlebrook 7H9 and Dubos Tween albumin broths are commonly used for subculturing stock strains of mycobacteria and preparing the inoculum for drug susceptibility tests and other in vitro tests. 7H9 broth is used as the basal medium for several identification tests. Broth media also can be used for recovering organisms from specimens with low counts such as CSF. Tween 80 in liquid media acts as a surfactant and allows the dispersal of clumps of mycobacterial growth, resulting in more homogeneous growth.

BACTEC AFB System

The radiometric BACTEC AFB system (Becton Dickinson Diagnostic Instruments, Sparks, Md.) allows the detection of mycobacterial growth at a very early stage. The average detection time of positive cultures is decreased to <7 days for NTM and to 9–14 days for *M. tuberculosis*. An antimicrobial mixture/growth-promoting supplement containing polymixin B, amphotericin B, nalidixic acid, trimethoprim, and azlocillin (PANTA) and polyoxylene stearate is added to BACTEC 12B medium to suppress contaminants and enhance mycobacterial growth. Specimens processed by the Zephiran-trisodium phosphate, benzalkonium chloride, lauryl sulfate, or cetylpyridinium chloride method cannot be used with the BACTEC system, because the residual quantities of these substances in the inoculum inhibit mycobacterial growth. Highly cellular clinical specimens may give false-positive results soon after inoculation due to metabolic activity of the cells. BACTEC 13A medium is used for blood and bone marrow aspirate specimens. An enrichment fluid is added to a 13A vial before or after specimen inoculation.

The use of the BACTEC method has significantly improved the recovery rates and times of mycobacteria from respiratory secretions and other specimens (154, 178). This is particularly significant with smear-negative specimens and specimens from treated patients with chronic disease. Limitations of the BACTEC system include the inability to observe colony morphology, difficulty in recognizing mixed cultures, overgrowth by contaminants, cost, radioisotope disposal, and extensive use of needles.

The BACTEC TB system may be used for antimicrobial susceptibility testing (178) (see also chapter 124). Generally, the initial positive vial can be used directly for identification and drug susceptibility testing. It is good practice to subculture positive BACTEC vials onto solid media to obtain isolated colonies and abundant growth and to check for mixed cultures.

Biphasic Media

The Septi-Chek system (Becton Dickinson Microbiology Systems, Cockeysville, Md.) is a mycobacterial culture system consisting of a capped bottle containing 20 ml of modified 7H9 broth, under an enhanced (20%) CO_2 atmosphere, and a paddle containing three types of solid media, modified L-J, Middlebrook 7H11, and chocolate agars, encased in a plastic tube. Bacterial contamination is detected on the chocolate agar. The bottles and the paddles are supplied separately. Cultures are inoculated by removing the bottle cap, adding the processed specimen, and then attaching the paddle to the bottle. Solid media are inoculated after 24 h of incubation in an upright position by inverting the bottles. A supplement containing glucose, glycerin, oleic acid, pyridoxal HCl, catalase, albumin, azlocillin, nalidixic acid, trimethoprim, polymyxin B, and amphotericin B is added to the culture bottle before inoculation. During the incubation period, the bottles are periodically tipped to reinoculate the solid media as the cultures are being read. The sensitivity of this system is comparable to that of the BACTEC system

(114, 193). Although the average time to detection of growth is longer than with the BACTEC system, it is shorter than with conventional media. The system has not been evaluated for use with blood cultures.

Mycobacteria Growth Indicator Tube

The Mycobacteria Growth Indicator Tube (MGIT; Becton Dickinson Microbiology Systems) uses Middlebrook 7H9 broth and silicon rubber impregnated with a ruthenium metal complex as a fluorescence quenching-based oxygen sensor to detect growth of mycobacteria. The large amount of oxygen initially present in the medium quenches the fluorescence of the ruthenium complex, but growth of mycobacteria or other organisms in the broth depletes the oxygen, and the indicator fluoresces brightly when the tubes are illuminated with UV light at 365 nm. A Wood's lamp or a transilluminator can be used as the UV light source. The 7H9 broth is supplemented, prior to use, with oleic acid-albumin-dextrose to promote the growth of mycobacteria and the PANTA mixture of antimicrobial agents to suppress the growth of contaminants.

Overall, the sensitivity and time to growth detection of the MGIT system are similar to those of the BACTEC 460 system and superior to solid media in clinical evaluations (54, 168). However, the contamination rates for the MGIT system are higher than for the BACTEC 460 system, probably owing to the enrichments added to the MGIT broth, which enhance the growth of both mycobacteria and nonmycobacterial organisms.

The principal advantages of the MGIT system over the BACTEC 460 system include reduced opportunity for cross contamination of cultures, no need for needle inoculation, no radioisotopes, and no need for special instrumentation other than the UV light source. Its limitations include higher contamination rates, masking of fluorescence by blood or grossly bloody specimens, and possible lack of compatibility with some methods of digestion and decontamination of specimens (169). Susceptibility testing methods involving MGIT are in development, and an instrument that incubates, reads, and analyzes the data has recently been cleared by the Food and Drug Administration.

Automated, Continuously Monitored Systems

Three different automated, continuously monitored systems, initially designed for growth and detection of microorganisms in blood, have recently been adapted for myobacterial cultures. The BACTEC 9000 MB system (Becton Dickinson Diagnostic Instrument Systems) uses the same fluorescence quenching-based oxygen sensor used in the MGIT system to detect growth. The technology used in the ESP II system (AccuMed International, Westlake, Ohio) is based on detection of pressure changes in the headspace above the broth medium in a sealed bottle resulting from gas production or consumption due to growth of microorganisms. The MB/BacT system (Organon Teknika, Durham, N.C.) employs a colorimetric carbon dioxide sensor in each bottle to detect the growth of mycobacteria. Each of the systems includes a broth similar to 7H9 supplemented with various growth factors and antimicrobial agents.

The three systems have similar performance and operational characteristics. In clinical evaluations, all three systems had times to detection and recovery rates similar to those of the BACTEC 460 system and superior to those of conventional solid media (12, 167, 257, 268). The reported contamination rates have been higher with these systems than with the BACTEC 460 or solid media. All share the advantages over the radiometric broth system of having no cross contamination, being less labor-intensive, having continuous monitoring, using no radioisotopes, and having better data management. Since these systems are continuously monitored, the bottles must be incubated in the instruments for their entire life in the laboratory. As a result, these systems are both instrument and space intensive. The automated systems also lack the versatility of the BACTEC 460 system in that direct inoculation of blood and susceptibility testing applications are not yet available.

Heme-Containing Medium for *M. haemophilum*

M. haemophilum will grow on egg- or agar-based media only if they are supplemented with hemin, hemoglobin, or ferric ammonium citrate (64). Thus, specimens from skin lesions, joints, or bone should also be inoculated onto chocolate agar, Middlebrook 7H10 agar with hemolyzed sheep erythrocytes, hemin, or an X-factor disk, or L-J medium containing 1% ferric ammonium citrate to enhance the recovery of this organism (216). Broth media should be similarly supplemented.

Medium Selection

Medium selection for the isolation of mycobacteria and the culture reading schedule is usually based on personal preference and/or laboratory tradition. Both should be optimized for the most rapid detection of positive cultures and identification of mycobacterial isolates. The variety of media and methods available today is sufficient to permit laboratories to develop a system that is optimal for their patient population and administrative needs.

It is recommended that a broth-based system be used for primary mycobacterial isolation to favor rapid detection of positive cultures. For maximum recovery and to aid in the detection of mixed mycobacterial infections, one piece of conventional solid medium should be used in addition to the BACTEC 12B broth (212). Although clear agar medium permits earlier detection of mycobacteria, L-J medium often yields a greater number of positive cultures on prolonged incubation (133). The decision to use a broth system alone or with additional conventional medium should be made after reviewing each institution's own experience and requirements. All positive cultures, even if identified directly from the broth, must be subcultured to solid media to detect mixed cultures and to correlate direct identification results with colony morphology. The Septi-Chek system can be used as a stand-alone system. There is still insufficient data to determine whether the MGIT and the automated, continuously monitored systems could serve as stand-alone culture systems for mycobacteria.

Detection of colonies offers several advantages over detection of growth in broth, because colonial morphology can provide clues to identification and facilitate the selection of confirmatory tests including DNA probe tests. However, smears from BACTEC vials and other broth-based systems can provide important microscopic clues, such as cord formation, and it is possible to use the sediment from BACTEC vials for probe culture confirmation tests before the detection of growth on solid media (see below). The reliability of the criterion of cord formation for presumptive identification of *M. tuberculosis* should be determined within each laboratory (121, 156, 262).

Incubation

Temperature

The optimal incubation temperature for most specimens is 35 to 37°C. Exceptions to this include specimens obtained from skin and soft tissue suspected to contain *M. marinum*, *M. ulcerans*, *M. chelonae*, or *M. haemophilum*, since these organisms have a lower optimal growth temperature. For these specimens, a second set of media should be inoculated and incubated at 25 to 33°C. BACTEC vials should be incubated at 36 to 38°C because the optimal metabolism of the radiolabeled substrate occurs at 37 to 37.5°C for most species. Lower temperatures increase the detection time.

Atmosphere

An atmosphere of 5 to 10% CO_2 in air stimulates the growth of mycobacteria in primary isolation cultures performed with conventional media (9). Middlebrook agars require CO_2 atmosphere to ensure growth, while it is necessary to incubate egg media under CO_2 for only the first 7 to 10 days after inoculation (the log phase of growth); subsequently, L-J cultures can be removed to ambient-air incubators if space is limited. In the absence of CO_2 incubators, plates may be incubated in commercially available bags with CO_2-generating tablets. Candle extinction jars are unacceptable for use in the mycobacteriology laboratory because the oxygen tension is reduced below that required for growth of mycobacteria. BACTEC vials and the other commercially available broth systems do not require incubation at increased CO_2 concentrations.

Time

Mycobacterial cultures are generally held for 6 to 8 weeks before being discarded as negative. Specimens with positive smears that are culture negative should be held for an additional 4 weeks. Plates should be incubated medium side down until all the inoculum has been absorbed. Once the inoculum has been absorbed, plated media should be incubated inverted in CO_2-permeable polyethylene bags or sealed with CO_2-permeable shrink-seal or cellulose bands to prevent the media from drying out during the incubation period. Tubed media should be incubated in a slanted position with the screw caps loose for at least a week, until the sediment has been absorbed; they then can be incubated upright if space is needed. The caps on the tubes should be tightened at 2 to 3 weeks to prevent desiccation of the media. Specimens from skin lesions should be incubated for 8 to 12 weeks if *M. ulcerans* is suspected.

Reading Schedule

Mycobacteria are relatively slowly growing organisms, and thus cultures can be examined less frequently than examination of routine bacteriologic cultures. All solid media should be examined within 3 to 5 days after inoculation to permit early detection of rapidly growing mycobacteria and to enable prompt removal of contaminated cultures. Young cultures (up to 4 weeks of age) should be examined twice a week, whereas older cultures should be examined at weekly intervals. Use of a hand lens for opaque media and a microscope for agar media will facilitate the early detection of microcolonies. Conventional liquid media (7H9 or Dubos) used for primary isolation should be carefully examined weekly for particulate matter and stained and/or subcultured before being discarded as negative.

The reading schedule for BACTEC vials varies according to the laboratory workload. Low-volume laboratories may read cultures three times a week for the first 2 or 3 weeks and weekly thereafter for a total of 6 weeks, while high-volume laboratories may read cultures twice a week for the first 2 weeks and weekly thereafter. Some laboratories separate smear-positive specimens from smear-negative specimens and test the former more frequently, thus diminishing the workload. In addition, separation of "probable positive" cultures from negative ones will decrease the possibility of vial cross contamination by the instrument. With more frequent testing of all specimens, however, earlier detection of positive cultures is expected. Readings of negative cultures in 12B medium usually remain below a growth index of 10; a growth index of 10 or more is considered presumptively positive. At this point, the vials should be separated and tested daily. An acid-fast stain is performed when the growth index is >50 to determine whether the culture contains mycobacteria. The morphology of mycobacteria seen in smears from 12B medium may be used for presumptive identification of *M. tuberculosis* complex (262) or to decide how to progress with identification methods (121, 156). In addition, a smear of the broth from the vial may be Gram stained and/or the broth may be subcultured onto a sheep blood agar plate to determine whether contamination is present. When the growth index is 500 or more, BACTEC antimicrobial susceptibility testing can be performed (see below). Negative BACTEC 13A vials usually read 10 to 15. When the growth index reaches 20 or more, the culture is considered presumptively positive. A smear is prepared at this point and stained for AFB. If the smear is positive, the vial is incubated further or subcultured for subsequent testing. If the smear is negative, incubation and testing are continued.

The Septi-Chek and manual MGIT systems may be inspected for growth several times per week or daily for the first 1 to 2 weeks; Septi-Chek bottles should be inverted for reinoculation of the agar medium if growth is not observed. The systems are inspected weekly for growth thereafter.

IDENTIFICATION

Mycobacteria should always be identified to the species level if possible. According to traditional methods, mycobacteria are usually preliminarily identified by traits such as rate of growth and pigmentation (183). The preliminary grouping may provide presumptive identification of the organism and directs the selection of key biochemical tests to characterize the unknown mycobacteria (89, 122). Table 2 presents the characteristics of common species of mycobacteria recovered from clinical specimens. Many strains will have biochemical profiles and morphologic features compatible with the data in this table; however, variation occurs among strains and properties may deviate from those presented here. The traditional methods are well established, standardized, and relatively inexpensive but are slow in providing clinically relevant information and are limited in scope to the species for which a large number of strains have been studied. In many instances, it is necessary to identify the organisms based on a best-fit analysis. These methods may result in erroneous identifications (209).

Newer laboratory methods for mycobacterial identification include analysis of mycobacterial fatty acids by chromatography and genetic investigations through the use of nucleic acid probes, nucleic acid sequencing, and nucleic acid amplification. These new alternatives have limited the role of conventional identification methods. It is recommended that all laboratories perform initial identification of the *M. tuberculosis* complex by a rapid method (223). Although conventional methods are still widely used for the species of mycobacteria for which probe technology is not available, the use of rapid identification methods for all mycobacteria would allow prompt identification and reporting of results to physicians.

TABLE 2 Distinctive properties of cultivable mycobacteria encountered in clinical specimens[a]

Descriptive term	Species	Optimal temp (°C)	Usual colony morphology[b]	Pigmentation[c]	Niacin	Growth on T2H (10 μg/ml)	Nitrate reduction	Semi-quantitative catalase (mm of bubbles)	68°C catalase	Tween hydrolysis	Tellurite reduction	Tolerance to 5% NaCl	Iron uptake	Arylsulfatase, 3 day	MacConkey agar with crystal violet	Urease[d]	Pyrazinamidase, 4 day	Nucleic acid probes available
Slow growers																		
TB complex	*M. tuberculosis*	37	R	N (100)	+ (95)	+	+ (97)	<45 (89)	− (1)	± (68)	−/+ (36)	− (0)	−	− (0)	−	± 64	+	+[e]
	M. africanum	37	R	N	−	V	−	<45	−	−	−	−	−	−	−	+	−	+[e]
	M. bovis	37	Rt	N (100)	− (4)	−	− (9)	<45 (69)	− (2)	− (21)		− (0)	−	− (0)	−	± (50)	−	+[e]
	M. bovis BCG	37	R	N	−	−	−	<45	−	+/−		−	−	−		+	−	+[e]
Nonchromogens	MAC	37	St/R	N (87)	− (0)	+	− (4)	<45 (98)	± (60)	− (2)	+ (81)	− (0)	−	− (1)	−/+	− (2)	+	+
	M. xenopi	42	S	S (21)	− (0)	+	− (7)	>45 (85)	± (31)	− (12)	± (65)	− (0)	−	± (36)	−	− (0)	V	−
	M. haemophilum[f]	30	R	N		+	−	<45	−	−	−	−	−	−	−	−	+	−
	M. malmoense	37	S	N (88)	− (0)	+	− (1)	<45 (99)	−/+	+ (99)	+ (74)	− (0)	−	− (0)		− (9)	+	−
	M. shimoidei	37	R	N	−	+	−	<45	−	+		−	−	−	−	−	+	−
	M. genavense	37	St	N	−	+	−	>45	+	+			−	−		+	+	−
	M. celatum	37	S/St	N (100)	−	+	− (0)	<45 (100)	+ (100)	− (0)	+ (100)	− (0)	− (0)	+ (100)	− (0)	− (0)	+ (100)	−
	M. ulcerans	30	R	N	−	+	−	<45	+	−		−		−		V	−	−
	M. terrae complex	37	SR	N (93)	− (1)	+	± (67)	>45 (93)	+ (92)	+ (99)	−/+ (46)	− (2)	−	− (2)	V	− (13)	V	−
	M. triviale	37	R	N (100)	− (0)	+	+ (89)	>45 (100)	+ (100)	+ (100)	− (25)	+ (100)	−	± (56)	−	−/+ (33)	V	−
	M. gastri	30	S/SR/R	N (100)	− (0)	+	− (0)	<45 (100)	− (11)	+ (100)	± (50)	− (0)	−	− (0)		−/+ (44)	−	−
Chromogens	*M. kansasii*	37	SR/S	P (96)	− (4)	+	+ (99)	>45 (93)	+ (91)	+ (99)	−/+ (31)	− (0)	−	− (0)	−	−/+ (49)	−	+
	M. marinum	30	S/SR	P (100)	−/+ (21)	+	− (0)	<45	− (30)	+ (97)	−/+ (39)	− (0)	−	−/+ (41)[g]	−	+ (83)	+	−
	M. simiae	37	S	P (90)	± (63)	+	− (28)	>45 (93)	+ (95)	− (9)	+ (82)	− (0)	−	− (0)		± (69)	+	−
	M. asiaticum	37	S	P (86)	− (0)	+	− (5)	>45 (95)	+ (95)	+ (95)	− (20)	− (0)	−	− (0)		− (10)	−	−
	M. xenopi	42	S	N/S[c]	−	+	−	<45	+/−	−		−	−	+		−		−
	M. gordonae	37	S	S (99)	− (0)	+	− (1)	>45 (90)	+ (96)	+ (100)	− (29)	− (0)	−	V	−	V (31)	−/+	+
	M. scrofulaceum	37	S	S (97)	− (0)	+	− (5)	>45 (84)	+ (94)	− (2)	± (64)	− (0)	−	V	−	V (31)	±	−
	M. szulgai	37	S or R	S/P (93)	− (0)	+	+ (100)	>45 (98)	+ (93)	−/+ (49)	± (53)	− (0)	−	V	−	+ (72)	+	−
	M. flavescens	37	S	S (100)[h]	− (0)	+	+ (92)	>45 (94)	+ (100)	+ (100)	−/+ (44)	± (62)	−	− (0)	−	+ (72)	+	−
Rapid growers																		
Nonchromogens	*M. fortuitum* group[i]	28	R/S	N (100)	−	+	+ (100)	>45 (93)	+ (90)	−/+ (43)	+ (92)	+ (85)	+	+ (97)	+	+ (70)	+	−
	M. chelonae	28	S/R	N (100)	−/+	+	− (1)	>45 (92)	± (53)	−/+ (39)	+ (89)	V	−	+ (95)	+	+ (89)	+	−
	M. abscessus	28	S/R	N	−		−	>45		V		±	−	+	+	+		−
	M. mucogenicum	28	S	N	−		V	>45		+		−		+	+	+		−
	M. smegmatis	28	S/R	S (50)	−	+	+ (95)	<45 (82)	−	+	+	+	+ (100)	− (0)	+ (100)			−
Chromogens	*M. phlei*	28	R	S	−	+	+	>45	+	+	+	+	+	−	−			−
	M. vaccae	28	S	S	−	+	+	>45	+	+	+	V	+	−	−			−

[a] Modified from reference 179. Plus and minus signs indicate the presence and absence, respectively, of the feature; blank spaces indicate either that the information is not currently available or that the property is unimportant. V, Variable; ±, usually present; −/+, usually absent. The percentage of CDC-tested strains positive in each test is given in parentheses, and the test result is based on these percentages.

[b] R, rough; S, smooth; SR, intermediate in roughness; t, thin or transparent; f, filamentous extensions.

[c] P, photochromogenic; S, scotochromogenic; N, nonchromogenic (*M. szulgai* is scotochromogenic at 37°C and photochromogenic at 24°C).

[d] Urease test performed by the method of Steadham (213).

[e] Probe identifies *M. tuberculosis* complex.

[f] Requires hemin as growth factor.

[g] Arylsulfatase reaction at 14 days is positive.

[h] Young cultures may be nonchromogenic or possess only pale pigment that may intensify with age.

[i] Includes *M. fortuitum*, *M. perigrinum*, *M. fortuitum* third biovariant complex.

Growth Characteristics

Growth Rate and Preferred Growth Temperature

The growth rate refers to the length of time required to form mature colonies that are visible without magnification on solid media. Mycobacteria that form colonies clearly visible to the naked eye within 7 days on subculture are termed rapid growers, while those requiring longer periods are termed slow growers. The growth rate is determined as follows.

1. Dilute a 7-day broth culture or a saline suspension of the organism from a freshly grown slant or plate sufficiently to obtain isolated colonies.
2. Inoculate 0.1 ml of several 10-fold dilutions of the test organism onto either egg-based or agar-based medium and incubate at 35 to 37°C. Isolates suspected of being *M. ulcerans*, *M. marinum*, or *M. haemophilum* require incubation at 30 to 32°C.
3. Observe cultures at 5 to 7 days and weekly thereafter for visible colonies.

Growth in relation to temperature can usually be adequately determined by observing primary cultures or subcultures at 37 and 30°C. When more definitive identification is needed, isolates should be incubated at 24, 30, 35 to 37, and 42°C.

Pigmentation and Photoreactivity

Some mycobacteria produce carotenoid pigments without light. Others require photoactivation for pigment production. Mycobacteria are classified into three groups based on the production of pigments. Photochromogens produce nonpigmented colonies when grown in the dark and pigmented colonies only after exposure to light and reincubation. Scotochromogens produce deep yellow to orange colonies when grown in either the light or dark, and some strains may have an increased pigment production upon continuous exposure to light. Nonphotochromogens are nonpigmented in the light and dark or have only a pale yellow, buff, or tan pigment that does not intensify after light exposure. These responses to light exposure were originally delineated to aid in the identification of NTM; members of the *M. tuberculosis* complex, however, are considered nonphotochromogens, and pigmented mycobacteria can be reported as NTM in preliminary reports.

Pigment production should be studied for slow-growing isolates that are nonpigmented when grown in the dark and for pigmented isolates that have been exposed to light. Testing for pigment production should be done on young cultures and is usually more easily observed in cultures with isolated colonies (122). Three tubes of media are inoculated with a broth culture of the test organism diluted sufficiently to yield isolated colonies. Two tubes should be shielded from the light by being wrapped with aluminum foil, and the third should be uncovered so that it will be exposed to the ambient light in the incubator. When growth is first detected in the unshielded tube, the foil-wrapped tubes should be examined; and if growth is detected, one should be exposed to light (100-W tungsten bulb placed 20 to 25 cm from the culture, or fluorescent equivalent) for 3 to 5 h with its cap loosened. The loose cap allows induction of the soluble pigment, which is controlled by an oxygen-dependent, photoinducible enzyme. The tube should be reshielded and reincubated, and both shielded tubes should be reinspected after 24, 48, and 72 h for the development of pigment. Colonies in the light-exposed tube should be compared with those in the shielded tube. Interpretations of pigmentation patterns must be carefully evaluated, since variations within species occur. Most importantly, some MAC isolates can be pigmented. Scotochromogens should be tested for photochromogenicity at 25°C to detect *M. szulgai*, which is a scotochromogen at 37°C but a photochromogen at 25°C.

Colony Morphology

A tentative identification of the species of mycobacteria can be made by microscopically observing young (5- to 14-day-old) isolated colonies on plates inverted under the 10× power objective of a stereomicroscope with transmitted light, according to the scheme developed by Runyon (184). This is best accomplished with a clear agar medium like Middlebrook 7H10 or 7H11 agar so that colonies are easily visualized. Although grossly visible colonies may not yet be evident on the agar surface, they are commonly found by microscopic observation (254). Specific colony morphology features of commonly isolated mycobacteria are described in Table 3.

Conventional Biochemical Tests

After a mycobacterial isolate has been assigned to a preliminary subgroup based on growth characteristics (rate of growth, pigmentation, photoreactivity), it traditionally has been definitively identified to the species or complex level by conventional biochemical tests. Table 2 gives biochemical test profiles for the most commonly encountered species. The principles underlying these tests are described below. Detailed descriptions of methods, procedures and controls, and the primary references can be found in the *Clinical Microbiology Procedures Handbook* (113) and in the publication by Kent and Kubica (122). Basics of the procedures are given in Appendix 2 of this chapter. Many of the reagents and media are commercially available. Selected key tests, those useful for identifying the suspected species, are performed on the isolate based on the preliminary grouping. Preference is usually given to tests which will rule in an identification with a positive result rather than ruling out an identification by a negative test result. Suggested groupings of key biochemical tests for identification of mycobacteria are given in Table 4.

Arylsulfatase

Arylsulfatase hydrolyzes the bond between the sulfate group and the aromatic ring of tripotassium phenolphthalein disulfate incorporated into the growth medium, to form free phenolphthalein. The presence of phenolphthalein is indicated by a red color that develops when alkali is added. Most mycobacteria possess arylsulfatase activity, so the test conditions are varied to help identify various species. The 3-day test is used mainly to identify potentially clinically significant rapid growers. With few exceptions, only the *M. fortuitum* complex splits phenolphthalein from tripotassium phenolphthalein sulfate within 3 days. The 14-day test may be useful in the identification of slowly growing mycobacteria such as *M. marinum*, *M. asiaticum*, *M. szulgai*, *M. xenopi*, *M. triviale*, and *M. flavescens*. For the procedure, see Appendix 2.

Catalase

Catalase is an intracellular, soluble enzyme capable of degrading hydrogen peroxide (H_2O_2) to water and oxygen. The presence of the enzyme is detected by adding H_2O_2 to a culture of the test organisms and observing for the formation of oxygen bubbles in the reaction mixture. Virtually

TABLE 3 Growth characteristics of commonly isolated mycobacteria[a]

Organism	Growth rate (days)	Pigment production		Colony morphology on Middlebrook 7H10 agar
		Light	Dark	
M. abscessus	3–7	Buff	Buff	Rounded, smooth, matte, periphery entire or scalloped, no branching filaments; some colonies are rough and wrinkled
MAC	10–21	Buff to yellow	Buff to yellow	Thin, transparent, glistening or matte, smooth, entire, and rounded; some colonies rough and wrinkled
M. chelonae	3–7	Buff	Buff	Rounded, smooth, matte, periphery entire or scalloped, no branching filaments; some colonies are rough and wrinkled
M. fortuitum group	3–7	Buff	Buff	Circular, convex, wrinkled, or matte; branching filaments on periphery are obvious
M. gordonae	10–25	Yellow to orange	Yellow to orange	Round, smooth, convex, yellow to orange and glistening
M. kansasii	10–21	Yellow	Buff	Raised and smooth; some are rough and wrinkled; carotene crystals numerous after exposure to light
M. marinum	5–14	Yellow	Buff	Round, smooth; some may be wrinkled
M. mucogenicum	3–7	Buff	Buff	Round, smooth, highly mucoid
M. scrofulaceum	10–14	Yellow	Yellow	Smooth, moist, yellow, and round
M. simiae	7–14	Yellow	Buff	Smooth, domed, and slightly pigmented
M. terrae complex	10–21	Buff	Buff	Round, smooth, glistening, and sometimes colorless
M. tuberculosis complex	12–28	Buff	Buff	Flat, rough, spreading to irregular periphery
M. xenopi	28–42	Yellow	Buff	Small, domed, yellow, smooth or rough; at 45°C, resembles a miniature bird's nest

[a] Modified from reference 179.

all mycobacteria possess catalase enzymes, except for *M. gastri*, certain isoniazid-resistant mutants of *M. tuberculosis* and *M. bovis*, and some isoniazid-resistant strains of *M. kansasii*. Species of catalase-producing mycobacteria can be distinguished by quantitative differences in catalase activity demonstrated by intact cells in the semiquantitative catalase test and by the differences in heat stability detected by the 68°C catalase test (Appendix 2).

Growth on MacConkey Agar without Crystal Violet

Growth on MacConkey agar without crystal violet is used to distinguish the potentially pathogenic rapidly growing mycobacteria. Most isolates of the *M. fortuitum* complex usually grow on MacConkey agar without crystal violet, whereas isolates of the nonpathogenic (often pigmented) species of rapidly growing mycobacteria do not. *M. smegmatis* grows on this medium, but the 3-day arylsulfatase test distinguishes these species from organisms of the *M. fortuitum* complex. For the procedure, see Appendix 2.

Iron Uptake

The iron uptake test (Appendix 2) is used to detect rapid growers capable of converting ferric ammonium citrate to an iron oxide. The iron oxide is visible as a reddish brown "rust" color in the colonies. The medium shows a tan discoloration. Iron uptake is useful for distinguishing *M. chelonae* and *M. abscessus*, which are commonly negative, from *M. fortuitum* and most other rapid growers that are positive.

TABLE 4 Key tests for the identification of groups of mycobacteria

Nonphotochromogens	Photochromogens	Scotochromogens	Rapid growers
Niacin	Pigment	Nitrate reduction	Arylsulfatase (3 day)
Nitrate reduction	Growth rate (28°C)	Tween 80 hydrolysis	SQ catalase
SQ catalase	Niacin	SQ catalase	68°C catalase
Tween 80 hydrolysis	Nitrate reduction	Urease	MacConkey agar without CV
Urease	Tween 80 hydrolysis	Arylsulfatase (3 day) 42°C	NaCl tolerance (28°C)
T2H	Arylsulfatase (3 day) 28°C	NaCl tolerance	Iron uptake (28°C)
PZA	SQ catalase	Growth at 52°C	Nitrate reduction
NaCl tolerance		Photoactive pigment at 25°C	Utilization of sodium citrate, inositol, and mannitol
Arylsulfatase (3 day)			

Isolates of *M. mucogenicum* produce a less noticeable tan color (196). Slow growers are not capable of accumulating iron oxides.

Niacin Accumulation Test

Niacin (nicotinic acid) functions as a precursor in the biosynthesis of the coenzymes NAD and NADP. Although all mycobacteria produce nicotinic acid, comparative studies have shown that because of a blocked metabolic pathway for conversion of free niacin to nicotinic acid mononucleotide, *M. tuberculosis* accumulates niacin and excretes it into the culture medium from which it can be extracted. The niacin then is detected by its reaction with a cyanogen halide in the presence of a primary amine. Niacin-negative *M. tuberculosis* isolates are extremely rare. The niacin test (Appendix 2) should not be used alone to identify *M. tuberculosis*, however, because some strains of *M. simiae*, BCG, and other mycobacteria, although infrequently encountered, also accumulate niacin. The supportive tests of nitrate reduction and 68°C catalase are necessary to confirm the identification of *M. tuberculosis*. A paper strip version is available commercially (Difco Laboratories, Detroit, Mich.).

Nitrate Reduction

Mycobacteria differ quantitatively in their abilities to reduce nitrate to nitrite. The nitrate reduction test (Appendix 2) is valuable for the identification of some mycobacteria that possess similar characteristics of colony morphology, growth rate, and pigmentation. *M. tuberculosis*, *M. kansasii*, *M. szulgai*, some non-disease-associated strains of nonphotochromogens, *M. smegmatis*, and the *M. fortuitum* group are nitrate reductase positive. The test can be combined with the niacin paper strip test.

Pyrazinamidase

The enzyme pyrazinamidase hydrolyzes pyrazinamide (PZA) to pyrazinoic acid and ammonia. This acid is detected by the addition of ferrous ammonium sulfate to the culture medium. This test (Appendix 2) is most useful in separating *M. marinum* from *M. kansasii* and *M. bovis* from *M. tuberculosis*. *M. bovis* is negative even at 7 days, whereas *M. tuberculosis* is positive within 4 days. In addition, one mechanism for PZA resistance of *M. tuberculosis* appears to be the inability of the organism to produce pyrazinoic acid, which is assumed to be the active component of the drug PZA. A pyrazinamidase-negative *M. tuberculosis* isolate is assumed to be PZA resistant as well.

Sodium Chloride Tolerance

Few mycobacteria are able to grow in the presence of, or tolerate, 5% sodium chloride. *M. triviale* is the only slowly growing mycobacterium to do so. Pathogenic rapidly growing species, except *M. mucogenicum* and most isolates of *M. chelonae*, also grow in 5% NaCl. For the procedure, see Appendix 2.

Inhibition by Thiophene-2-Carboxylic Acid Hydrazide

Inhibition by thiophene-2-carboxylic acid hydrazide (T2H) is used to distinguish niacin-positive *M. bovis* from *M. tuberculosis* and other nonchromogenic, slowly growing mycobacteria. Most *M. bovis* isolates are susceptible to low concentrations of T2H (1 to 5 μg/ml), whereas *M. tuberculosis* and most other slowly growing mycobacteria are resistant. For the procedure, see Appendix 2.

Tellurite Reduction

Tellurite reductase reduces colorless potassium tellurite to a black metallic tellurium precipitate. *M. avium* complex has the ability to reduce tellurite within 3 to 4 days, whereas other mycobacteria require additional incubation. This distinctive property is used to separate MAC from most other nonphotochromogens. Some rapid growers can similarly reduce tellurite within this time frame. For the procedure, see Appendix 2.

Tween 80 Hydrolysis

Lipases produced by some mycobacterial species hydrolyze the detergent polyoxyethylene sorbitan monooleate (Tween 80) into oleic acid and polyoxyethylene sorbitol. Neutral red in the pH 7 test medium is bound by Tween 80 and is amber at a neutral pH. If Tween 80 is hydrolyzed, however, neutral red is no longer bound, and it reverts to its usual red color at pH 7. Of the nonphotochromogens, MAC and *M. xenopi* are usually negative, and of the scotochromogens, *M. scrofulaceum* is usually negative. For the procedure, see Appendix 2.

Urease

The ability of an isolate to hydrolyze urea to ammonia and CO_2 is useful in identifying both scotochromogens and nonphotochromogens. *M. scrofulaceum* is urease positive, whereas MAC organisms are urease negative. The urease test (Appendix 2) is helpful in the recognition of pigmented strains of MAC.

BACTEC P-Nitro-α-Acetylamino-β-Hydroxypropiophenone Test

Becton Dickinson offers the *p*-nitro-α-acetylamino-β-hydroxypropiophenone (NAP) test for identification of members of the *M. tuberculosis* complex directly from 12B medium. NAP is an intermediate compound in the synthesis of chloramphenicol and inhibits species in the *M. tuberculosis* complex (137, 153). Other mycobacterial species are inhibited only partially or not at all by this compound. If mycobacteria are inhibited, they are unable to metabolize in the presence of NAP and thus do not produce $^{14}CO_2$ in the BACTEC vial. Cultures of *M. tuberculosis* contaminated with bacteria or mixed with other mycobacteria may show resistance to NAP. Strains of *M. kansasii*, *M. gastri*, *M. szulgai*, *M. terrae*, and *M. triviale* are partially inhibited by NAP (137). Interpretation of the NAP test in the first 2 to 4 days may be misleading with these strains due to their longer lag phase. NAP may inhibit the growth of *M. marinum*, *M. chelonae*, and *M. xenopi* at 37°C, and thus the test may give "false-positive" results for these organisms when incubated at 37°C. However, incubation at temperatures other than 37°C is not routine and usually is performed only when problems are encountered. Isolates from wounds or skin should be incubated at both 30 and 37°C. NAP test results should always be confirmed by nucleic acid probe, chromatographic, or conventional methods of identification.

Chromatographic Analysis

Analysis of mycobacterial cell wall fatty acid composition by GLC and HPLC is recognized as a useful tool for the identification of mycobacteria (30, 227). Mycolic acids are high-molecular-weight fatty acids that are present in the cell walls of a restricted number of bacterial genera. The number of carbon atoms of mycolic acids is at a minimum

(22 to 38) in the genus *Corynebacterium* and increases in other genera with mycolic acids in the cell wall: *Rhodococcus* (34 to 52), *Nocardia* (44 to 60), *Gordona* (48 to 66), and *Tsukamurella* (64 to 78). The mycolic acid of the genus *Mycobacterium* contains the maximum number (60 to 90) of carbon atoms (103).

GLC

A GLC method for the analysis of short-chain fatty acids found in the cell wall of mycobacteria was developed in the 1970s (226, 227). The method used derivatives, usually the methyl esters, for the generation of characteristic fatty acid profiles. Organisms tested could be identified to the species level or placed into groups of two or three species that required a limited number of conventional biochemical tests for complete identification. A commercially available GLC identification system (MIDI, Newark, Del.) has hardware that consists of an autosampler, a gas chromatograph and detector, an integrator, and a computer. The software includes a library of fatty acid profiles of well-characterized mycobacteria and pattern recognition software that matches unknown profiles with those in the database. After several sample preparation steps, including saponification of bacterial cells, the extract is analyzed on a gas chromatograph with a fused-silica capillary column. A recent evaluation showed that the system correctly identified approximately 79% of the isolates tested when the first-rank choice was used, compared to traditional biochemical testing profiles (199). Optimal use of the system is derived by also considering colony morphology and selected biochemical tests (226). The current library is limited by the number of species included; the system can identify only mycobacteria for which fatty acid composition profiles have been entered into the database. A detailed procedure for the identification of mycobacteria by the MIDI system is included in the *Clinical Microbiology Procedures Handbook* (113).

HPLC

Reverse-phase HPLC of mycolic acid esters has also been shown to be a rapid, reproducible method for the identification of *Mycobacterium* species (30, 96, 224). Chromatographic profile analysis can be performed once visible growth is obtained on solid media. After several preparation steps, a gradient of methanol and dichloromethane (methylene chloride) is used to separate the mycolic acid esters, which are detected by UV spectrophotometry. Reproducible chromatographic patterns are used for the identification. Pattern recognition is performed by visual comparison of sample results with mycolic acid patterns from reference species of known mycobacteria. The mycolic acid patterns are consistent within various species of mycobacteria, and shared HPLC profiles between species are probably rare. CDC has recently published a standardized method for HPLC identification of mycobacteria (46). This manual is available from the CDC free of charge.

Correct HPLC pattern recognition requires training, and thus pattern recognition programs that match unknown samples with those in a database are necessary to simplify the ease of interpreting chromatograms. One computer-assisted pattern recognition technology has been evaluated with promising results (87), but inconsistencies have been reported among commercially available systems (177).

Although HPLC of mycolic acids is a rapid technique, it requires bacterial colonies grown in culture. Methods for assaying mycolic acids directly from BACTEC 12B media have been described (46). For identification of cultures grown in BACTEC culture media, the results should be compared with chromatograms for reference strains that were also grown in BACTEC culture media. Recently, HPLC with highly sensitive fluorescent detection (200-fold more sensitive than UV detection) has been used to detect *M. tuberculosis* and MAC directly in smear-positive sputum specimens (119).

Currently, HPLC methods are used for the identification of mycobacteria in research laboratories, large public health laboratories including the CDC, and referral laboratories. Both GLC and HPLC are technically complex, requiring expensive equipment and software; however, the costs of consumables are relatively low. These methods are rapid, providing definitive identification of an isolate in <2 h. Chromatographic analysis of lipids is an attractive alternative to conventional biochemical testing for large reference laboratories, and chromatography is finding increased use as the primary method for identification in those settings.

DNA Probes for Culture Confirmation

Beginning in 1987, DNA probes complementary to species-specific sequences of rRNA became commercially available for the identification of *M. tuberculosis* complex, *M. avium* complex, *M. avium*, *M. intracellulare*, *M. gordonae*, and *M. kansasii* (AccuProbe; Gen-Probe, San Diego, Calif.). These probes can be used to identify isolates that arise on solid culture medium or from broth culture. The tests can be performed with the growth from primary cultures, whereas conventional biochemical testing requires inoculation of subcultures and a subsequent delay in testing until adequate growth has occurred. The results of probe assays can be obtained in about 2 h. The original ^{125}I-labeled probes were both sensitive and specific (73, 158). The current acridinium ester-labeled AccuProbes are as sensitive and specific as the radioisotopically labeled probes (91, 140), have a long shelf life, and are associated with reduced biohazard, thus allowing more clinical laboratories access to the technology. See chapter 13 for principles of the AccuProbe method.

Probes can be combined with the BACTEC TB system to optimize rapid detection and identification of mycobacteria present in clinical samples (78, 165), but procedural modifications are required, especially with media containing blood (53, 79). No standard protocols are available for the combined use of the BACTEC vials and nucleic acid probes; generally, a portion of the broth culture (1.0 to 1.3 ml) is removed after a growth index of at least 100 is reached and placed into a 1.5-ml screw-cap microcentrifuge tube, and the bacilli are concentrated by centrifugation at 9,000 to 10,000 × *g* for at least 5 to 7 min. The microcentrifuge used should be equipped with aerosol-containing tube carriers or rotor. The supernatant is decanted, the pellet is resuspended in the detection reagents, and the testing proceeds as for testing colonies from solid media. Specimens containing blood are treated with 100 μl of 10% sodium dodecyl sulfate–50 mM EDTA (pH 7.2) before microcentrifugation to allow lysis of the erythrocytes and solubilization of the membranes. Pellets are washed with 1.0 to 1.5 ml of sterile water, centrifuged, and processed as above. These protocols are not FDA approved and therefore should be validated with appropriate control organisms by individual users. It has been recommended that a specimen blank be included with all probe assays from BACTEC blood cultures to help in evaluation of high nonspecific chemiluminescence seen with specimens containing blood (79). A positive and negative control specific for each probe should be run each time the assay is performed.

Users of the AccuProbe system should be aware of a problem with failure of the sonicating water baths that are used for lysis of the mycobacteria (247). Either transducer failure or mineral buildup in the sonicator tank can result in false-negative results, depending on the position of the sample in the water bath. If probe results do not correlate with clinical or culture observations, the test should be repeated or confirmed by an alternative method.

Although the number of probes commercially available is limited, their use can result in rapid identification of the vast majority of isolates found in clinical laboratories and eliminates the necessity for numerous biochemical tests for the identification process. The remaining isolates will require identification by biochemical reactions or chromatographic methods. Probes do not differentiate among M. *tuberculosis*, M. *bovis*, M. *bovis* BCG, M. *africanum*, and M. *microti*. Recent reports indicate that some isolates of M. *terrae* and M. *celatum* complex produce false-positive reactions with the M. *tuberculosis* complex probe (31, 190). The specificity of the M. *tuberculosis* complex probe has been increased by extending the length of the selection reagent step to 10 min (214).

DNA Sequencing

Genetic sequencing provides both identification and phylogenetic information. Although the method is highly accurate and rapid, it is expensive and labor-intensive, and its current use is restricted to a few research laboratories. These methods rely on the definition of species-specific nucleotide sequences, combined with a procedure for identifying these sequences. Hypervariable regions of 16S rRNA of mycobacteria have enough sequence variability to provide species differentiation, while sequence variability is generally conserved (180, 181). The nucleic acid is prepared by disruption of the mycobacterial cells, with subsequent PCR amplification of a portion of the 16S rRNA gene (129). One of the PCR primers is biotinylated to allow for single-strand solid-phase sequencing technology. The determined sequence of an unknown isolate is compared with known signature sequences, either manually or with the aid of a computer. Current instrumentation allows processing of a sample and final identification to be completed within one working day. 16S rRNA sequence determination has been used successfully for routine identification of mycobacterial isolates (129). Use of this technique has shown that the genus *Mycobacterium* is more complex than was previously believed and that it harbors new potentially pathogenic species such as M. *interjectum* (208), M. *conspicuum* (210), and yet to be characterized species (209). This diversity was not detected by conventional identification procedures, especially standard biochemical identification schemes (209). 16S rRNA gene sequence determination can also be used to identify extremely fastidious mycobacteria that, because of poor growth, are impossible to characterize biochemically (19).

Alternative approaches to DNA sequencing for the genetic characterization of mycobacteria involve PCR amplification of the 65-kDa heat shock protein-encoding gene followed by RFLP analysis (173, 222), PCR amplification of rRNA genes followed by RFLP (237), and PCR amplification of the 32-kDa protein-encoding gene (206).

Direct Detection and Identification by Nucleic Acid Amplification and Hybridization

The inherent limitations of culture-based diagnostic tests specific for M. *tuberculosis* and other mycobacterial species pose problems for both individual patient management and implementation of appropriate hospital infection control and public health control measures. An ideal diagnostic procedure would detect and identify mycobacteria directly from clinical specimens, thereby avoiding the relatively lengthy time required for culturing. Since specimens usually contain only a small number of tubercle bacilli, direct detection requires either an extremely sensitive and specific assay or a process by which a diagnostically useful component of the target organism can be "amplified" to a detectable level. Nucleic acid amplification (NAA) (also discussed in chapter 13) is one such process being actively developed and evaluated particularly for the diagnosis of tuberculosis and leprosy.

Many PCR assays (see also chapter 13) have been evaluated for their ability to offer a rapid diagnosis of tuberculosis. These in-house or "home brew" assays have recently been reviewed by several authors (81, 110, 188, 195), and the reader is referred to these reviews for the primary references. Most investigators studying the role of PCR in tuberculosis diagnosis have chosen the DNA insertion sequence IS*6110*, which reliably separates the M. *tuberculosis* complex organisms from all other mycobacteria (35). When applied to respiratory specimens for evaluations performed in clinical laboratories, the reported sensitivities of these assays generally range from 70 to 90% compared to culture and the specificities vary between 90 and 95%. The detection sensitivity of these assays is approximately 95% for smear-positive specimens but drops to as low as 50 to 60% for smear-negative specimens (a smear-positive specimen contains $>5 \times 10^3$/ml bacilli [see the section on the acid-fast stain procedure]).

The value of home brew PCR for the routine detection of M. *tuberculosis* in a clinical laboratory is unclear, but these assays are available through several commercial and research laboratories. None of these methods has been cleared by the FDA for use as an in vitro diagnostic product. Laboratories vary greatly on both the sensitivity and specificity of their assays (163), and the quality of testing may be personnel dependent.

Two commercial amplification assays have been cleared by the FDA for use as in vitro diagnostic products for detecting M. *tuberculosis* directly in AFB smear-positive respiratory specimens from untreated patients (not on antimycobacterial therapy or on antimycobacterial therapy for <7 days at the time of specimen collection). The Mycobacterium Tuberculosis Direct Test (MTD test) (GenProbe) was the first amplification assay for M. *tuberculosis* to be approved by the FDA for use in the United States. This test is based on transcription-mediated amplification of rRNA. The AMPLICOR MTB assay (Roche Molecular Systems, Branchburg, N.J.) is a PCR-based assay. Both are available in prepackaged kit form and give results comparable to those obtained with in-house PCR tests; the sensitivities for detecting M. *tuberculosis* from respiratory specimens vary between 70 and 100%, and the specificities are generally >98% (21, 51, 59, 109, 151, 241). The sensitivities for AFB smear-positive specimens are generally >95%, whereas sensitivities as low as 50% have been reported for smear-negative specimens. Limited data are available to guide the interpretation of the results of these tests for nonapproved indications (off-label uses), but initial reports of testing nonrespiratory specimens show promise (60, 75). The inability to distinguish live and dead organisms precludes DNA amplification from use in therapeutic monitoring (102).

Compared with amplification procedures, a significantly greater volume of specimen (up to 1 ml) is introduced into media for culture, thus favoring the latter process. However, culture may not be the best gold standard for comparison. The decontamination process can kill >90% of tubercle bacilli and thus produce false-negative culture results. Such dead bacilli may contain sufficient intact target nucleic acids to allow detection by an amplification procedure. Thus, additional analyses, such as a physician's clinical diagnosis of tuberculosis, may be necessary to determine the actual sensitivity and specificity of NAA tests for detecting a patient infected with *M. tuberculosis*. Occasionally, culture-positive specimens yield negative amplification results due to sampling variation and the presence of inhibitors of the amplification reactions. Specimens containing few bacilli may be subject to sampling variation, and simply repeating assays has been shown to increase sensitivity (117, 151). NAA tests allow the detection of *M. tuberculosis* in patient specimens within hours, compared with the 14 to 28 days usually required for culture. NAA on clinical specimens may also be useful when there is a need for rapid differentiation between *M. tuberculosis* complex infection and NTM infection, such as in AIDS patients. Additional clinical evaluations of NAA tests are necessary to reveal the ultimate utility of these tests for making patient management decisions.

The currently available NAA assays should be used only in conjunction with traditional culture isolation methods for maximum sensitivity of the laboratory diagnosis of tuberculosis. Each test result must be interpreted within the overall clinical setting in which it is used (4, 45). These tests may enhance diagnostic certainty but should be interpreted in a clinical context on the basis of local laboratory performance. Ideally, clinicians should provide patient information to the laboratory, and the laboratory should provide information about local test performance and interpretation both when the tests are ordered and when the results are reported (45), since the predictive values vary with the prevalence of tuberculosis and other mycobacterial disease.

Home brew assays and commercial assays have been used to identify *M. tuberculosis* from broth cultures (82, 104, 200). Since the lack of sensitivity is the main shortcoming of the NAA techniques and the specificity is more satisfactory, the tests can be used for organism identification. When culture in a liquid medium is combined with an amplification method, the time to diagnosis of *M. tuberculosis* can be shortened.

Other NAA assays based on a variety of different amplification strategies, as well as second-generation formats of the currently available assays, are being developed and/or are undergoing clinical evaluation by several manufacturers and will soon be available. These include ligase chain reaction (230), strand displacement amplification reaction (72), cycling probe technology (11), and nucleic acid sequence-based amplification (236). At present, NAA for *M. tuberculosis* cannot replace conventional diagnostic techniques, especially since strains should still be cultured for antimicrobial susceptibility testing.

STRAIN-TYPING SYSTEMS

Epidemiological studies of tuberculosis can be strengthened by the application of strain-typing systems (see also chapters 7 and 13). Historically, unusual drug susceptibility patterns and phage typing (205) have been used for this purpose, but they have significant limitations. DNA fingerprinting of *M. tuberculosis* has proven to be a powerful epidemiological tool (58, 74, 145). A standardized technique for RFLP analysis which exploits the variability in both the number and sites of chromosomal insertion of a 1,355-bp repetitive insertion sequence, IS*6110*, has been developed (238). The DNA of the vast majority of *M. tuberculosis* strains contains IS*6110*, whose number (0 to >25 copies) and location are unique to individual strains. The technique demonstrates relatedness among isolates due to the element's relative stability within a strain over time and the great variability in its number and position in the genomes among different strains (36, 145, 164). Changes in drug resistance profile do not alter a strain's fingerprint (36).

IS*6110* RFLP has become the most widely used technique for strain differentiation of *M. tuberculosis*. It involves growth of *M. tuberculosis*, extraction of DNA, restriction endonuclease digestion with *Pvu*II, Southern blotting, and probing for IS*6110*. The restriction enzyme cleaves the DNA at consistent sites within IS*6110*, resulting in DNA fragments with different molecular weights which can be separated electrophoretically on agarose gels. The sizes of the resulting IS*6110*-hybridizing fragments are determined by the use of molecular size markers, and the strain-specific patterns of isolates are compared. Two or more patients whose isolates demonstrate identical (or nearly identical) banding patterns are said to "cluster"—that is, to have the same strain of *M. tuberculosis*. RFLP patterns for *M. tuberculosis* have proven to be stable in outbreak situations. DNA fingerprinting of *M. tuberculosis* has been used as a tool during investigation of nosocomial outbreaks (10, 85), institutional outbreaks (58, 235), and community outbreaks (1, 220) of tuberculosis and for documentation of cross contamination in the laboratory (198). RFLP typing, which is both labor intensive and lengthy, is offered by seven regional laboratories in the United States through a program funded by CDC.

A secondary typing analysis may be required to further differentiate strains, especially when only a few bands (fewer than six) are revealed by RFLP (20, 28, 50). Secondary typing with the probe containing the polymorphic GC-rich repetitive sequences (PGRS) present in plasmid pTBN12 appears promising (20, 28, 50). Additional typing strategies have been developed, including quantification of nonrepetitive DNA spacers between direct-repeat (DR) sequences uniquely present in *M. tuberculosis* complex bacteria (65, 120). This typing technique, known as DR typing or spoligotyping (spacer oligotyping), is able to differentiate *M. bovis* from *M. tuberculosis*, a distinction which is often difficult to make by traditional methods (120).

IS*6110* RFLP provides results in several weeks. Haas et al. (97) developed a rapid, highly sensitive, and specific method for typing strains of *M. tuberculosis* that is based on the IS*6110* RFLP by PCR. The key feature of this method, termed mixed-linker PCR (ML-PCR), is the ability to amplify multiple restriction fragments containing IS*6110* sequences and variable sequences adjacent to the restriction site. ML-PCR requires small amounts of genomic DNA and does not rely on growing cultures or even viable cells, whereas traditional IS*6110* RFLP typing requires a 2- to 3-week-old subculture of the isolate or heavy growth on the original slant to provide enough DNA for analysis. Patterns generated by ML-PCR have shown a direct correlation to those obtained by the standard RFLP method, providing the same clustering of isolates (97). ML-PCR can also be applied directly to strongly smear-positive specimens (97), providing the opportunity for real-time epidemiology and early recognition of infection with known drug-resistant strains, long before the results of susceptibility tests are available.

Serovar distinctions with the MAC are based on a seroagglutination procedure originally developed by Schaefer (191). The serologic specificity of serovar antigens is conferred by oligosaccharide residues of the C-mycoside glycopeptidolipids (23). Strains are serotyped by a combination of thin-layer chromatography (232), enzyme-linked immunosorbent assay (ELISA) analysis of species and type-specific glycolipids (266), and the conventional seroagglutination procedure. Combined use of serotyping and species-specific DNA probes has shown that serovars 1 through 6 and 8 through 11 are M. *avium* while serovars 7, 12 through 17, 19, 20, and 25 are M. *intracellulare* (187). Serotyping is not currently available in the United States and is used primarily for research purposes.

Typing systems have also been used for strain comparison of NTM. Multilocus enzyme electrophoresis in combination with serotyping has been shown to be a potential epidemiologic tool for MAC (264).

Molecular methods allow the differentiation of M. *avium* from the other MAC species (225). More recently, molecular methods have been used to identify and track specific MAC strains. Digestion of MAC DNA with infrequently cutting restriction endonucleases and separation of the resultant DNA fragments by pulsed-field gel electrophoresis produce strain-specific, large-restriction-fragment patterns (146). RFLP assays with the M. *avium* insertion elements IS*1245* (95), IS*1311* (182), or both (172) have also been developed. Molecular characterization methods for other NTM, including M. *chelonae* and M. *abscessus* (84), M. *kansasii* (171), M. *xenopi* (203), and M. *celatum* (170), have been described. In addition to investigating strain relatedness and the epidemiology of NTM infections, these tools may be able to help define laboratory contamination.

IMMUNODIAGNOSTIC TESTS FOR TUBERCULOSIS

A variety of immunodiagnostic tests for tuberculosis based upon recognition of specific host responses to the infecting organism have been described. Historically, the first immunodiagnostic test was the tuberculin skin test. The shortcomings of this test include the inability to distinguish active disease from past sensitization and an unknown predictive accuracy (204). Various in vitro tests of cell-mediated immune response to mycobacterial antigens have been described, but they are expensive and technically demanding and provide no more diagnostic information than the tuberculin skin test does.

Much effort has been devoted to the development of serologic tests for tuberculosis, but no test has found widespread clinical use (18, 63). The specificity of serologic tests with crude antigen preparations is too low for clinical application. Specificity can be increased by using purified antigens but since not all patients respond to the same antigens, the increased specificity often results in decreased sensitivity (49, 63, 115). The sensitivity and specificity increase if ELISA results obtained with a set of purified antigens are combined. The antigens tested in serologic assays include the 38-kDa antigen (62, 115, 269), lipoarabinomannan (186), antigen 60 (52), and the antigen 85 complex (233).

The 38-kDa antigen was the first purified antigen to be extensively evaluated in a serologic test for tuberculosis. Most patients with tuberculosis produce antibody to it, and most healthy controls do not. A truncated form of the 38-kDa antigen has been cloned and expressed in *Escherichia coli*. This recombinant antigen is available from the World Health Organization.

Lipoarabinomannan, an antigenic lipopolysaccharide of mycobacteria, has been evaluated in serologic tests for tuberculosis. Antibody to this antigen is found in healthy controls, and the sensitivity and specificity of tests using this antigen are determined largely by choice of the cutoff titer. Antibody to lipoarabinomannan is measured in a commercially available serologic test for tuberculosis (DynaGen, Cambridge, Mass.).

Antigen 60 is a complex mixture of proteins, polysaccharides, and lipids obtained from BCG, which contains the major thermostable component of PPD. These antigens are shared by different mycobacterial species. Semipurified antigen 60 is used in a commercially available serodiagnostic test for tuberculosis (Anda Biologicals, Strasbourg, France). Antigen 85 complex-based serologic tests have also shown promise for serodiagnosis of tuberculosis, but none are commercially available yet.

A number of antigen capture assays based on ELISA, radioimmunoassay, or agglutination of antibody-coated latex particles have been described (61). The results reported for some assays have been promising for CSF, but the experience with sputum and other specimen types is limited. The sensitivities of immunoassays for detection of mycobacterial antigen in CSF ranged from 65.8 to 100% and the specificities ranged from 95 to 100% in six major studies (61). Another approach to detection of mycobacterial antigens is to apply an antigen detection test to a liquid culture after several days of incubation (217). The use of antigen tests cannot be recommended at this time.

ANTIMICROBIAL SUSCEPTIBILITY

The current approach to the treatment of tuberculosis is based on several principles that have evolved over the past 40 years (229). First, the relatively high rate of spontaneous mutations in M. *tuberculosis* that confer resistance to each antituberculosis drug preclude the use of a single drug for treatment. The treatment of tuberculosis should include at least two drugs to which the organism is susceptible, to prevent the emergence of drug-resistant strains. Second, to be successful, the treatment of smear-positive tuberculosis must continue well beyond the time when AFB are no longer present in the sputum. Third, although pretreatment susceptibility studies have minimal impact on the initial treatment of tuberculosis, such testing should be done because of the potential public health benefits. CDC recommends that initial isolates from all patients be tested for drug susceptibility to confirm the anticipated effectiveness of chemotherapy. Susceptibility testing should be repeated if the patient continues to produce culture-positive sputum after 3 months of treatment (223). The National Multidrug-Resistant TB Task Force recommends that drug susceptibility testing be performed on all initial and final M. *tuberculosis* isolates from each patient (38).

The first-line drugs in the treatment of tuberculosis are isoniazid (INH), rifampin, pyrazinamide, ethambutol, and streptomycin. Second-line drugs, *para*-aminosalicylic acid, ethionamide, cycloserine, capreomycin, kanamycin, amikacin, ciprofloxacin, ofloxacin, and rifabutin, should be used if resistance or toxicity occurs during administration of first-line drugs. Current recommendations for treatment of tuberculosis have been published by ATS and CDC (5, 44).

The emergence of strains of M. *tuberculosis* that are resistant to antimycobacterial agents is not a new problem but recently has become a serious concern. CDC conducted a nationwide survey of drug resistance among all patients with tuberculosis reported during the first quarter of 1991 (39). Overall, 14.9% of patients had isolates resistant to at least one antituberculosis drug and 3.3% had isolates resistant to both INH and rifampin. These findings showed an increase in drug resistance since a previous survey conducted from 1982 to 1986. The drug resistance is a much larger problem in certain cities, most notably New York City and Miami. Some organisms, such as the W family of M. *tuberculosis* (13), have been resistant to as many as seven drugs (INH, rifampin, kanamycin, ethambutol, ethionamide, streptomycin, and rifabutin). Recently, CDC reported the results of a follow-up nationwide survey of tuberculosis cases reported from 1993 to 1996 (152). INH resistance has remained relatively stable compared to the previous survey. In addition, the percentage of multidrug-resistant tuberculosis cases decreased to 2.2%, primarily due to a marked decrease among patients in New York City. The foreign-born and HIV-positive patients and those with prior tuberculosis have higher rates of drug resistance.

Strains of MAC are intrinsically resistant to antituberculosis drugs and many other antimicrobial agents due to the inability of these drugs to penetrate the lipid-rich cell wall. Recent studies have demonstrated the efficacy of rifabutin, clarithromycin, and azithromycin as single agents in the prophylaxis of disseminated MAC infection in patients with AIDS (3), and the use of one of these agents is recommended in all patients with CD4 counts of <75 cells (47). Antimycobacterial therapy appears to clear mycobacteremia in most patients (194) and to prolong the survival of patients with disseminated MAC infections. Current treatment recommendations have been published by the ATS (3).

In vitro susceptibility testing of MAC by using methods and interpretive criteria used for M. *tuberculosis* has no value in guiding the selection of drugs to treat MAC infection (3). There are no studies that have correlated in vitro susceptibility test results with clinical outcome, and there are no standardized methods for performing these tests. Until guidelines are established for performing and interpreting drug susceptibility tests for MAC, they should not be performed routinely (3). The one exception to this guideline is clarithromycin testing.

Clarithromycin has a low MIC (usually ≤ 8 μg/ml) for all pretreatment isolates of MAC. Following treatment failures or relapse, MAC isolates have been shown to have a point mutation at the 23S rRNA macrolide-binding site (149, 159) associated with a rise in the clarithromycin MIC to >32 μg/ml (101). Isolates resistant to clarithromycin are all cross-resistant to azithromycin (101), so testing of both drugs is not required.

Almost all strains of rapidly growing mycobacteria are resistant to the drugs used for tuberculosis. The antimicrobial agents used often depend upon the identification of the isolate and the results of drug susceptibility studies. Routine susceptibility testing of potentially active agents against clinically significant isolates is recommended. Agar disk elution and broth dilution methods for drug susceptibility testing of rapidly growing mycobacteria have been described previously (24, 218), and optimal methods are currently being assessed by an NCCLS subcommittee. Isolates of M. *chelonae* and M. *abscessus* tend to be much more resistant than the M. *fortuitum* group. Antimicrobial agents recommended for treatment of infections with rapidly growing mycobacteria and other mycobacterioses have been published by the ATS (3).

QUALITY ASSURANCE

Much of the information in this section was obtained from recent publications (6, 259). The reader should consult these publications for more information and access to the primary literature. In addition to the specific recommendations listed here, standard components of laboratory quality assurance, such as personnel competency, procedure manuals, proficiency testing, and quality control (QC) of media, tests, and reagents, should be in place (see chapter 2).

The Public Health Service introduced the levels-of-service concept for mycobacteriology laboratories in 1967. In this scheme, laboratories determine the level of service which best fits the needs of the patient population they serve, the experience of their personnel, their laboratory facilities, and the number of specimens they receive. The concept of levels of service is supported by the CDC and the ATS (100, 134). The College of American Pathologists (CAP) proposed extents of service for participation in mycobacterial interlaboratory comparison surveys. ATS levels I, II, and III correlate with CAP extents 2, 3, and 4. ATS makes no provision for laboratories in which no mycobacterial procedures are performed (CAP extent 1). Five types of mycobacteriology laboratories have been defined by the Clinical Laboratory Improvement Amendments (CLIA). These are modified from the extents described by CAP, but the definitions are awaiting consensus and may be modified in the future (259). All specimens submitted for mycobacterial examination should have cultures as well as smears performed. The ATS and the CDC recommend that laboratories examine a minimum of 10 to 15 AFB smears per week to maintain proficiency in performance and interpretation and process and culture 20 specimens per week to maintain proficiency in culture and the identification of M. *tuberculosis*. Recently, the Association of State and Territorial Public Health Laboratory Directors proposed that only two levels of service be designated: (i) specimen collection, specimen transport, and optional microscopy of at least 20 smears per week, and (ii) complete mycobacteriology service from microscopy to complete species identification and drug susceptibility testing (248).

Personnel working in the clinical mycobacteriology laboratory must have proper training and certification in the specific functions that they perform. Since many of the techniques used in mycobacteriology are not used elsewhere in the general bacteriology laboratory, personnel should be assigned to the mycobacteriology laboratory for extended periods if rotation through the other laboratory sections is necessary.

QC is vital for monitoring a laboratory's effectiveness in detecting and isolating mycobacteria because of the unique requirements involved, such as long incubating periods, special growth requirements, and the need for decontamination and digestion of specimens. The CLIA and accreditation programs represent the minimum acceptable standards of practice (259), and laboratories performing mycobacterial testing should follow QC recommendations in the scientific literature and in publications such as the *Clinical Microbiology Procedures Handbook* (113) and the ASTPHLD/CDC self-assessment document (6).

The laboratory must maintain a collection of well-characterized mycobacteria that are used for training, continuing education, and QC of test systems. These control organisms may be obtained from the American Type Culture Collection and proficiency testing programs. Frequently used stock cultures can be maintained on L-J slants or in 7H9 broth at 37°C or room temperature if they are subcultured monthly. Cultures on L-J slants may be held up to 1 year if stored at 4°C. Freezing of organisms suspended in skim milk or broth medium and storage at −20 to −70°C is the best option for long-term maintenance of stock cultures.

Routine QC tests are recommended with new lots of BACTEC 12B media and for media used with other commercial systems (113). Laboratories that prepare their own media must document the performance characteristics of each new lot. Many problems observed with mycobacterial culture media have been traced to the albumin-containing enrichments, and a turbidimetric test with *Bacillus subtilis* may be used to assess quality before culture media are prepared (33). The adequacy of mycobacterial growth can be assessed with stock cultures of *M. tuberculosis*, *M. kansasii*, *M. scrofulaceum*, *M. intracellulare*, and *M. fortuitum*. For media containing hemin or ferric ammonium citrate, *M. haemophilum* should be used. *E. coli* can be used to test the inhibitory capacity of selective media. Prolonged storage (>5 weeks) or exposure to light can result in the formation of formaldehyde in Middlebrook 7H10 and 7H11 agar, which is associated with poor growth of mycobacteria. To avoid this problem, new lots of media are put into use 1 week after inoculation of QC organisms. If the new lot fails QC testing, refrigerated aliquots of saved specimens can be reinoculated onto another lot or a different type of medium (179).

Ideally, positive control slides should be prepared from a concentrated sputum obtained from a patient with active tuberculosis. In practice, many laboratories use suspensions of stock cultures or seeded negative sputum as positive controls for acid-fast staining procedures. The *Clinical Microbiology Procedures Handbook* (113) describes a method for preparing control slides. Control slides are also commercially available. An increase in the percentage of smear-positive but culture-negative specimens of >2% (that cannot be attributed to response to antituberculosis therapy) or the presence of AFB in the negative controls suggests that the water or reagents used in the staining or the digestion procedures are contaminated with environmental mycobacteria (122). *M. gordonae* and *M. terrae* complex are most often involved. A procedure for detection of AFB in working solutions and reagents is described in the ASTPHLD/CDC document (6). AFB may also be carried over from one slide to another in the immersion oil used with the oil immersion lens. Oil should be removed from the lens after examining a positive slide. The sensitivity of the AFB smear is directly related to the relative centrifugal force (RCF) or g-force attained during centrifugation. Thus, laboratories should calculate the RCF of their centrifuge and periodically monitor and document that they are reaching sufficient RCF by checking the revolutions per minute with a tachometer. An RCF of at least 3,000 must be held for 15 min to achieve a 95% sedimentation rate and effective concentration of *M. tuberculosis* from sputum specimens (122).

Laboratories should monitor and document the contamination rates (percentage of specimens producing contaminating growth on culture media) for digested or decontaminated specimens. Contamination rates of 3 to 5% are generally considered acceptable. Rates below 3% may indicate that the decontamination procedure is too harsh and that the procedure should be modified to minimize the lethal effect on mycobacteria. Rates above 5% indicate too weak a decontamination procedure, which could compromise mycobacterial cultures due to overgrowth of contaminants (see Optimizing Decontamination Procedures, above).

The processes involved in culturing mycobacteria are naturally prone to errors because of the multiple steps involved in processing cultures, the viability of mycobacteria for long periods in the laboratory environment, and the large number of mycobacteria present in some specimens (29). In addition, some laboratories may batch specimens in volumes that exceed their capabilities (198). False-positive cultures may result from mislabeling, specimen switching during handling, specimen carryover (including proficiency testing specimens), contaminated reagents, or cross contamination between culture tubes or vials (29, 48, 74, 198). Inclusion of a "positive control" (e.g., a suspension of *M. tuberculosis*) in the processing of patient specimens is discouraged due to the risk of cross contamination. Cross contamination of culture vials in the BACTEC radiometric system, sometimes skipping several vials, due to inadequately sterilized sample needles has been documented (14, 239). False-positive cultures occur sporadically or as outbreaks, but sporadic false-positive cultures, and those due to NTM, may be more difficult to recognize. False-positive cultures may result in misdiagnosis, unnecessary and costly therapy and medical treatment, and unnecessary public health interventions. Timely recognition and investigation of false-positive cultures for *M. tuberculosis* require the cooperation of and communication between laboratories, clinicians, and health departments. Standardized laboratory procedures that minimize the potential for errors leading to false-positive cultures should be followed, and mechanisms should be in place to rapidly recognize their occurrence. Transfers or inoculation of cultures must be accomplished by using individual transfer pipettes, single-delivery diluent tubes, or disposable labware. The order in which specimens are processed and the media are inoculated should be recorded. Processing of a negative control specimen after patient specimens with the same digestion and decontamination solutions can be used as a method for detecting possible cross contamination by specimen contamination of the solutions (6). Alternatively, the processing solutions may be directly planted. Laboratories should prospectively track positivity rates and establish a threshold which, when exceeded, will prompt an investigation (198). The significance of an isolate may be determined by reviewing the order in which specimens were handled for all manipulations (e.g., initial processing, BACTEC readings, subculturing), the direct smear results, the time to positivity, and the clinical history. Cross contamination in the BACTEC system is probably rare if the manufacturer's recommendations for operation and maintenance are closely followed. Several recent reports document that the percentage of false-positive cultures ranges from 1.2 to 4% and that DNA fingerprinting provides a valuable tool for the study of false-positive results (29, 74, 85).

Laboratories should document the time required to report AFB smear results and to isolate, identify, and determine the antimicrobial susceptibility of *M. tuberculosis* to determine whether the results are available to the health care providers within a reasonable time. The CDC and others have recommended that AFB smear results be available and positive results be reported within 24 h of specimen receipt (6, 223). The time required for identification and susceptibility testing of *M. tuberculosis* should average 14 to 21 days and 15 to 30 days, respectively, from the time of specimen receipt (6, 38).

NAA-based assays require several levels of controls (e.g.,

to detect amplification inhibition and contamination between specimens) in addition to positive and negative controls (259). Laboratories may want to augment the manufacturer's recommendations with in-house controls. Used as approved by the FDA, NAA tests for M. *tuberculosis* diagnosis do not replace any previously recommended tests (45). Material from a clinical specimen should not be reserved for NAA testing if this compromises the ability to perform established tests. Laboratories testing patient specimens by research or home brew methods or by commercially available NAA assays for nonapproved or off-label indications and reporting results must validate the assay and establish its performance characteristics before putting it to diagnostic use. Available information is often insufficient to guide test interpretation. Approved guidelines for molecular diagnostic methods in clinical microbiology, in which the development, validation, quality assurance, and routine use of NAA assays are addressed in detail, are available from the National Committee for Clinical Laboratory Standards (160). However, basing the identification of M. *tuberculosis* on a sole positive home brew PCR result is not recommended because the results of these assays vary considerably (6, 40).

EVALUATION, INTERPRETATION, AND REPORTING OF RESULTS

Adequate funding and focused training are critical in maintaining state-of-the-art mycobacteriology laboratories (15, 228, 258). Laboratories play a pivotal role in the diagnosis and control of tuberculosis, and every effort should be made to implement sensitive and rapid methods for detection, identification, and susceptibility testing of M. *tuberculosis*. Specifically, these include (i) a fluorochrome stain for mycobacteria in smears; (ii) a broth-based or microcolony method for culture; (iii) NAP differentiation test, DNA probes, or chromatographic analysis for identification; and (iv) direct testing of smear-positive specimen concentrates by the radiometric or agar methods for susceptibility testing.

The 24-h turnaround time for AFB smear results presents a challenge to most laboratories. The daily processing of specimens required to meet this goal adds considerable expense to the laboratory budget. Whether these expenses would be offset by savings from outside the laboratory remains to be seen. In regions where tuberculosis is uncommon, less frequent processing is acceptable. Turnaround time goals for AFB smear results should be established for each institution after consultation with infection control practitioners and infectious-disease specialists.

NAA assays offer the promise of same-day detection and identification of M. *tuberculosis*. Implementation of this new technology presents several new challenges. Although the performance characteristics of many of these assays are quite good for smear-positive respiratory specimens, little information exists on their use for the diagnosis of paucibacillary pulmonary or extrapulmonary disease. Unfortunately, it is in the last two categories that these tests are likely to have the greatest clinical impact. The new technology will supplement rather than replace culture. Culture will still be required to obtain organisms for susceptibility testing and for detection of mycobacteria other than M. *tuberculosis*. The practicality, cost-effectiveness, and overall clinical utility of these NAA assays are not yet defined.

The significance of the isolation of NTM may be difficult to assess, since many species are opportunistic pathogens (3). The following criteria suggested by the ATS (3) are useful in establishing a role for NTM in a disease process: (i) repeated isolation of the same species from the same anatomical site or isolation of a large number of colonies on more than one occasion with positive AFB smears; (ii) clinical or radiographic evidence of disease; (iii) histopathologic evidence of the presence of granulomas and/or mycobacteria in tissues; (iv) increasing numbers of mycobacteria in sequential specimens; (v) isolation from a normally sterile site; (vi) predilection of the species to cause disease at that site; (vii) presence of predisposing conditions in the patient; and (viii) absence of other identifiable causes of disease. In addition to the above criteria, accurate identification of NTM will prevent rarely encountered pathogens from being mistaken for nonpathogenic species.

Accurate and timely reporting of results of AFB microscopy, culture, identification, and drug susceptibility tests is essential to effective management of individual patients and to appropriate implementation of public health and infection control measures. The use of the telephone or facsimile transmission for reporting avoids the inherent delays in preparing and mailing written reports (6). Laboratories should verbally report the first positive smear and subsequent positive smears if the quantitation increases after an initial decrease. Verbal reports should also be issued for the first positive culture and other information that may affect diagnosis or treatment, including preliminary identification and resistance of M. *tuberculosis* to antituberculosis drugs. All telephone reports should be documented in the laboratory. Written reports of the information reported verbally should be sent to the clinician caring for the patient, the infection control office, and the patient's medical record. To avoid duplication and delays in reporting, the procedures for notification need to be established in cooperation with primary care providers, infection control practitioners, infectious-disease specialists, respiratory medicine staff, public health officials, and other groups that may be responsible for the diagnosis and control of tuberculosis.

APPENDIX 1
Commonly Used Digestion-Decontamination Methods

Refer to references for detailed procedures and primary references (1, 2).

NALC-NaOH method

Reagents

Digestant: For each 100 ml, combine 50 ml of sterile 0.1 M (2.94%) trisodium citrate with 50 ml of 4% NaOH. The NaOH and citrate mixtures can be mixed, sterilized, and stored for future use. To this solution, add 0.5 g of powdered NALC just before use. Use within 24 h of addition of the NALC because the mucolytic action of NALC is inactivated on exposure to air.

Phosphate buffer: The buffer is 0.067 M and pH 6.8. Mix 50 ml of solution A (0.067 M Na_2HPO_4; 9.47 g of anhydrous Na_2HPO_4 in 1 liter of distilled water) and 50 ml of solution B (0.067 M KH_2PO_4; 9.07 g of KH_2PO_4 in 1 liter of distilled water). If the final buffer requires pH adjustment, add solution A to raise the pH or solution B to lower it.

BSA (optional): Use sterile 0.2% bovine serum albumin (BSA) fraction V (pH 6.8).

Procedure

1. Transfer up to 10 ml of specimen to a sterile, graduated, 50-ml plastic centrifuge tube labeled with appropriate identification. The tube should have a leakproof, aerosol-free screw cap.

Add an equal volume of the NALC-NaOH solution. The final concentration of NaOH in the tube is 1%.

2. Tighten the cap completely. Invert the tube so that the NALC-NaOH solution contacts all the inside surfaces of the tube and cap, and then mix the contents for approximately 20 s on a Vortex mixer. If liquefaction is not complete in this time, agitate the solution at intervals during the following decontamination period.

3. Allow the mixture to stand for 15 min at room temperature with occasional gentle shaking by hand. Avoid movement that causes aeration of the specimen. A small pinch of crystalline NALC may be added to viscous specimens for better liquefaction. Specimens should remain in contact with the decontaminating agent for only 15 min, since overprocessing results in reduced recovery of mycobacteria. If more active decontamination is needed, increase the concentration of NaOH.

4. Add phosphate buffer (pH 6.8), up to the 50-ml mark on the tube.

5. Centrifuge the solution for at least 15 min at ≥3,000 × *g*.

6. Decant the supernatant fluid into a splash-proof discard container containing a suitable disinfectant. Do not touch the lip of the tube to the discard container. Wipe the lip of each tube with disinfectant-soaked gauze (separate piece for each tube) to absorb drips, and recap.

7. Using a separate sterile pipette for each tube, add to the sediment 1 to 2 ml of sterile, 0.2% BSA fraction V (pH 6.8) or 1 to 2 ml of phosphate buffer (pH 6.8), and resuspend the sediment with the pipette or by shaking the tube gently by hand. BSA may have a buffering and detoxifying effect on the sediment and increases the adhesion of the specimen to solid media. However, BSA may lengthen BACTEC detection times.

8. Inoculate the specimens onto appropriate solid culture media and into broth media. Use a separate disposable capillary pipette for each specimen to deliver 3 drops to solid medium.

9. Prepare a smear for acid-fast staining. Use a sterile disposable pipette to place 1 drop of the sediment onto a clean, properly labeled microscope slide covering an area approximately 1 by 2 cm. Place the smears on an electric slide warmer at 65 to 75°C for 2 h to dry and fix them. Alternatively, air dry the smears and fix them by passing the slide three or four times through the blue cone of a flame. (Heat fixing does not always kill mycobacteria, and the slides are potentially infectious.)

10. Refrigerate the remaining sediment for later use if needed (direct susceptibility testing, further treatment if specimen is contaminated, etc.).

The NALC-NaOH method can be used to process gastric lavage specimens, tissues, stool, urine, and other body fluids. For neutralized gastric lavage specimens and other body fluids (≥10 ml), centrifuge at ≥3,000 × *g* for 30 min in sterile screw-cap 50-ml centrifuge tubes, decant the supernatants, resuspend the sediments in 2 to 5 ml of sterile distilled water, and proceed as for sputum. If a gastric lavage specimen is mucopurulent, add 50 mg of NALC powder per 50 ml of lavage fluid and vortex before centrifugation. Tissue that is not collected aseptically can be ground, placed in a tube, homogenized by vortexing, and processed as for sputum. For stool specimens, place approximately 1 g of a formed specimen or 1 to 5 ml of a liquid specimen in a total volume of 10 ml of 7H9 broth, sterile water, or sterile saline; vortex vigorously for 30 s; and then allow large particles to settle to the bottom of the tube for 15 min. Remove 7 to 8 ml of supernatant, place into a 50-ml centrifuge tube, and process as for sputum.

Sodium hydroxide method

Reagents

Digestant: NaOH solution (2 to 4%). Sterilize by autoclaving.

2 N HCl: Dilute 33 ml of concentrated HCl to 200 ml with water. Sterilize by autoclaving.

Phenol red indicator: Combine 20 ml of phenol red solution (0.4% in 4% NaOH) and 85 ml of concentrated HCl with distilled water to make 1,000 ml.

Phosphate buffer: The buffer is 0.067 M and pH 6.8. See the NALC-NaOH procedure for buffer preparation.

Procedure

Follow the steps described for the NALC-NaOH method, substituting 2% NaOH for the NALC-alkali digestant.

1. Transfer a maximum volume of 10 ml of specimen to a sterile 50-ml screw-cap plastic centrifuge tube. Add an equal volume of NaOH.

2. With the cap tightened, invert the tube and then agitate the mixture vigorously for 15 min on a mechanical mixer, or vortex vigorously and let stand for exactly 15 min. If it is necessary to reduce excessive contamination, the NaOH concentration can be increased to 3 or 4%.

3. Add phosphate buffer (pH 6.8) up to the 50-ml mark on the tube. Recap the tube, and swirl by hand to mix well.

4. Centrifuge the specimen at ≥3,000 × *g* for 15 min, decant the supernatant, and add a few drops of phenol red indicator to the sediment. Neutralize the sediment with HCl. Thoroughly mix the contents of the tube. Stop acid addition when the solution is persistently yellow.

5. Resuspend the sediment in 1 to 2 ml of phosphate buffer or sterile 0.1% BSA fraction V.

6. Inoculate the resuspended sediment to appropriate culture media, and prepare a smear.

Zephiran-trisodium phosphate method

Principle

This system can be used when the laboratory cannot monitor the exposure time to the decontaminating agent, since the timing of this digestion-decontamination process is not critical. Benzalkonium chloride (Zephiran), a quaternary ammonium compound, with trisodium phosphate selectively destroys many contaminants with little activity on tubercle bacilli. Zephiran is bacteriostatic to mycobacteria, and so the digested, centrifuged sediment must be neutralized with buffer before being inoculated onto agar medium. The phospholipids of egg medium neutralize this compound. It is incompatible with the BACTEC system.

Reagents

Zephiran-trisodium phosphate digestant: Dissolve 1 kg of trisodium phosphate ($Na_3PO_4 \cdot 12H_2O$) in 4 liters of hot distilled water. Add 7.5 ml of Zephiran concentrate (17% benzalkonium chloride [Winthrop Laboratories, New York, N.Y.]), and mix. Store at room temperature.

Neutralizing buffer: Neutralizing buffer is pH 6.6. Add 37.5 ml of 0.067 M disodium phosphate to 62.5 ml of 0.067 M monopotassium phosphate (for preparation of buffer solutions, see the NALC-NaOH procedure).

Procedure

1. Transfer a maximum volume of 10 ml of specimen to a sterile, 50-ml screw-cap plastic centrifuge tube. Add an equal volume of the Zephiran-trisodium phosphate digestant.

2. Tighten the cap, invert the tube, and then agitate the mixture vigorously for 30 min on a mechanical shaker. Permit the material to stand, without shaking, for an additional 30 min at room temperature.

3. Centrifuge the specimen at ≥3,000 × *g* for 15 min, decant the supernatant, and add 20 ml of neutralizing buffer. Vortex for 30 s to thoroughly suspend the sediment in the buffer. (The neutralizing buffer serves to inactivate traces of Zephiran in the sediment.)

4. Centrifuge the specimen again for 20 min.

5. Decant the supernatant, retaining some fluid to resuspend the sediment.

6. Inoculate egg-based medium, and make a smear. If the sediment is to be inoculated to agar-based medium, lecithin must be used as a neutralizer.

Oxalic acid method

Principle

The oxalic acid method is superior to alkali methods for processing specimens consistently contaminated with *Pseudomonas* species and certain other contaminants. Specimens processed by this method may be used with the BACTEC system. It can also be used to decontaminate a previously processed sediment when cultures are contaminated with *Pseudomonas*.

Reagents

5% oxalic acid
Physiologic saline (0.85%)
4% NaOH
Phenol red indicator or pH paper

Procedure

1. Add an equal volume of 5% oxalic acid to 10 ml of specimen in a 50-ml centrifuge tube.
2. Vortex the solution, and then allow it to stand at room temperature for 30 min with occasional shaking.
3. Add sterile physiologic saline to the 50-ml mark on the centrifuge tube. Recap the tube, and invert it several times to mix the contents.
4. Centrifuge for 15 min at ≥3,000 × *g*, decant the supernatant fluid, and add a few drops of phenol red indicator to the sediment. Alternatively, use pH paper.
5. Neutralize with 4% NaOH.
6. Resuspend the sediment, inoculate it to media, and make smear.

CPC method

Principle
Cetylpyridnium chloride (CPC), a quaternary ammonium compound, is used to decontaminate specimens, while sodium chloride effects liquefaction. CPC is bacteriostatic for mycobacteria inoculated onto agar-based media. This effect is not neutralized in the digestion process, and thus sediments from specimens treated with CPC should be inoculated only onto egg-based media.

This method is a means of digesting and decontaminating specimens in transit (>24 h). Mycobacteria remain viable for 8 days in the solution.

Reagents
CPC digestant-decontaminant: Dissolve 10 g of CPC and 20 g of NaCl in 1,000 ml of distilled water. The solution is self-sterilizing and remains stable if protected from light, extreme heat, and evaporation. Dissolve with gentle heat any crystals that might form in the working solution. Other ingredients include sterile water and sterile saline or 0.2% sterile BSA fraction V.

Procedure

1. Collect 10 ml or less of sputum in a 50-ml screw-cap centrifuge tube.
2. Inside a BSC, add an equal volume of CPC-NaCl, cap securely, and shake by hand until the specimen liquefies.
3. Package the specimen appropriately as specified by current postal regulations, and send it to a processing laboratory.
4. Upon receipt in the processing laboratory (allow at least 24 h for digestion-decontamination to be completed), dilute the digested-decontaminated specimen to the 50-ml mark with sterile distilled water and recap securely. Invert the tube several times to mix the contents.
5. Centrifuge at ≥3,000 × *g* for 15 min, decant the supernatant fluid, and suspend the sediment in 1 to 2 ml of sterile water, saline, or 0.2% BSA fraction V.
6. Inoculate the resuspended sediment onto egg medium, and make a smear.

Sulfuric acid method

Principle
The sulfuric acid method may be useful for urine and other body fluids that yield contaminated cultures when processed by one of the alkaline digestants.

Reagents

4% Sulfuric acid
4% Sodium hydroxide
Sterile distilled water
Phenol red indicator

Procedure

1. Centrifuge the entire specimen for 30 min at 3,000 × *g*. This may require several tubes.
2. Decant the supernatant fluids; pool the sediments if several tubes were used for a single specimen.
3. Add an equal volume of 4% sulfuric acid to the sediment.
4. Vortex, and let stand for 15 min at room temperature.
5. Fill the tube to the 50-ml mark with sterile water.
6. Centrifuge at ≥3,000 × *g* for 15 min and decant the supernatant.
7. Add 1 drop of phenol red indicator, and neutralize with 4% NaOH until a persistent pale pink color forms.
8. Inoculate the media, and make a smear.

References

1. **Isenberg, H. D.** 1993. *Clinical Microbiology Procedures Handbook*, vol. 1. American Society for Microbiology, Washington, D.C.
2. **Kent, P. T., and G. P. Kubica.** 1985. *Public Health Mycobacteriology: a Guide for the Level III Laboratory*. U.S. Department of Health and Human Services, Centers for Disease Control, Atlanta, Ga.

APPENDIX 2
Conventional Biochemical Tests

Refer to the references for detailed procedures, alternative procedures, and primary references (1, 2). Many of the reagents and media are available commercially.

Arylsulfatase test (3-day test)

Inoculum
Slightly turbid suspension.

Reagents
Substrate: Incorporate 1 ml of glycerol and 65 mg of tripotassium phenolphthalein disulfate (Nutritional Biochemicals Corp., Cleveland, Ohio) into 100 ml of melted Dubos oleic agar base (Wayne arylsulfatase agar). Dispense the mixture in 2-ml amounts into screw-cap vials (18 by 60 mm). Autoclave the vials, and permit the mixture to harden in an upright position.
Na_2CO_3, 1 M (10.6 g in water to make 100 ml).

Procedure
Inoculate the medium with 1 drop of the bacillary suspension. Incubate at 37°C for 3 days. Add 1 ml of Na_2CO_3 solution. A pink color indicates a positive test.

Controls
Use *M. fortuitum* and *M. avium* as positive and negative controls, respectively.

Semiquantitative catalase test

This test divides the mycobacteria into two groups, those producing a column of bubbles of <45 mm (low catalase) and those producing a column of bubbles of >45 mm (high catalase).

Inoculum
Use a 7-day broth culture or a cell suspension of comparable turbidity.

Reagents and medium
Freshly prepared 1:1 mixture of 10% Tween 80 and 30% H_2O_2
L-J deeps in screw-cap tubes (12 by 150 mm).

Procedure
Inoculate an L-J medium deep tube with 0.2 ml of the bacterial suspension. Incubate the medium for 2 weeks at 35°C with the cap loosened. Add 1 ml of the Tween-peroxide mixture, and measure the column of bubbles in millimeters after the tube has stood upright for 5 min at room temperature.

Controls
M. *tuberculosis* (produces a column of bubbles of <45 mm) and M. *kansasii* (>45 mm) as positive controls; uninoculated medium as negative control.

Heat-stable (68°C) catalase test

Inoculum
Well-developed, isolated colonies from egg-based media.

Reagents and medium
Freshly prepared mixture of 10% Tween 80 and 30% H_2O_2. Phosphate buffer (0.067 M, pH 6): 1.1 ml of 0.067 M Na_2HPO_4 (9.47 g of anhydrous Na_2HPO_4 in 1 liter of distilled water) and 38.9 ml of 0.067 M KH_2PO_4 (9.07 g of KH_2PO_4 in 1 liter of distilled water).

Procedure
Suspend several colonies in 0.5 ml of phosphate buffer in a screw-cap tube (16 by 125 mm). Place the tube in a 68°C water bath for 20 min. Cool to room temperature, and add 0.5 ml of the Tween-H_2O_2 mixture and observe bubbles (positive result). Hold for 20 min before discarding as negative.

Controls
M. *kansasii* and M. *tuberculosis* as positive and negative controls, respectively.

Growth on MacConkey agar without crystal violet

Inoculum
7- to 10-day broth culture.

Medium
MacConkey agar without crystal violet.

Procedure
Inoculate a plate of MacConkey agar without crystal violet with a 3-mm loopful of the broth culture, streaking for isolation. Incubate at 30°C. Examine for growth after 5 and 11 days.

Controls
M. *fortuitum* and M. *phlei* as positive and negative controls, respectively.

Iron uptake

Inoculum
Barely turbid aqueous suspension.

Reagent
Aqueous ferric ammonium citrate, 20%. Dispense and autoclave.

Procedure
Inoculate an L-J slant with 1 drop of a suspension of the strain. Incubate the L-J slant at 37°C until definite growth appears. Add about 1 drop of sterile citrate solution for each milliliter of the L-J medium. Incubate at 37°C for up to 21 days. A rusty brown color in the colonies and a tan discoloration of the medium indicate a positive result.

Controls
M. *fortuitum* and M. *chelonae* as positive and negative controls, respectively.

Niacin accumulation test (paper strip method)

Inoculum
Culture (>3 weeks old) on L-J medium showing heavy growth.

Reagent
Reagent-impregnated paper test strips are commercially available (Niacin Test Strips; Remel, Lenexa, Kans.).

Procedure
The directions supplied with the strips should be followed. Add 1.0 ml of sterile distilled water or saline to the L-J medium. Place the tube horizontally so that the fluid covers the entire surface. Allow ≥15 min for the extraction of niacin. Remove 0.6 ml of the extract to a 12- by 75-mm test tube. Insert the strip, and immediately seal the tube. Leave at room temperature for 15 min, with occasional agitation. Observe the color of the liquid in the tube against a white background. A yellow color in the liquid (not on the strip) is positive.

Controls
M. *tuberculosis* as positive control, and MAC and uninoculated medium as negative controls.

Nitrate reduction test (paper strip method)

Inoculum
Culture (>4 weeks old) on L-J medium showing heavy growth.

Reagent
Reagent-impregnated paper test strips are commercially available (Niacin Test Strips).

Procedure
The directions supplied with the strips should be followed. Add 1.0 ml of sterile distilled water or saline to a sterile 13- by 100-mm screw-cap test tube. Emulsify two 3-mm loopfuls of growth in the saline. Insert the strip; do not let the strip contact any fluid on the side of the tube. Cap the tube tightly, and incubate it in a vertical position at 37°C for 2 h. After 1 h, shake the tube gently without tilting it. After 2 h of incubation, tilt the tube six times to wet the entire strip, and allow the tube to remain slanted for 10 min with the liquid covering the strip. A blue color (light or dark) in the top portion of the strip indicates a positive reaction.

Controls
M. *tuberculosis* as positive control, and MAC and uninoculated medium as negative controls.

Pyrazinamidase

Inoculum
A 2- to 3-week-old culture.

Reagents
Dubos broth base containing 0.1 g of pyrazinamide, 2.0 g of pyruvic acid, and 15.0 g of agar per liter. Dispense in 15-ml amounts in screw-cap tubes. Autoclave and solidify agar in an upright position. Aqueous ferrous ammonium sulfate, freshly prepared.

Procedure
Heavily inoculate the agar with growth from the culture. The inoculum should be visible. Incubate at 37°C for 4 days. Add 1 ml of ferrous ammonium sulfate to the tubes, and place them in a refrigerator for 4 h. Examine then for a pink band in the agar (positive result).

Controls
MAC and uninoculated medium as positive and negative controls, respectively.

Sodium chloride tolerance

Inoculum
Barely turbid suspension.

Substrate
L-J medium containing 5% NaCl. L-J medium without salt should be used for a control.

Procedure
Inoculate the media (with and without NaCl) with 1 ml each of the bacterial suspension, and incubate at 37°C. Read for growth or no growth at 4 weeks.

Controls
M. *fortuitum* and M. *tuberculosis* as positive (growth) and negative (no growth) controls, respectively.

Inhibition by T2H

Inoculum
Barely turbid suspension in sterile water. Dilute 1 : 1,000 with sterile water.

Substrate
Middlebrook 7H11 medium. Incorporate 5 μg of T2H (Aldrich Chemical Co., Milwaukee, Wis.) per ml into the agar (cooled to 50°C in a water bath). Dispense in 5-ml amounts onto slants.

Procedure
Inoculate the T2H medium and control medium each with 3 drops of the 1 : 1,000 suspension, and incubate at 37°C. Record the time when growth is observed on the control medium. Maintain the T2H medium for an additional 3 weeks unless growth appears earlier. Record the organism as resistant if growth on the T2H medium is >1% of the growth on the control.

Controls
M. *tuberculosis* as positive (resistant) and M. *bovis* negative (inhibited) controls, respectively.

Tellurite reduction

Inoculum
Culture (7 days old) in 5 ml of 7H9 broth (fairly turbid).

Reagent
A 0.2% aqueous solution (0.1 g in 50 ml distilled water) of potassium tellurite. Dispense in 2- to 5-ml amounts, and autoclave.

Procedure
Add 2 drops of the tellurite solution to each culture, and return the cultures to the incubator. Examine the cultures daily for 4 days or more. A positive test is shown by a jet black precipitate.

Controls
MAC as positive control, and M. *kansasii* as negative control.

Tween 80 hydrolysis

Inoculum
Actively growing young culture on solid medium.

Reagents
100 ml of 0.067 M phosphate buffer (pH 7)
0.5 ml of Tween 80
0.1% Aqueous neutral red

Mix the three reagents in order. Dispense this substrate in 4-ml amounts in 16- by 125-mm screw-cap tubes, and autoclave at 121°C for 10 min. After autoclaving, the substrate should be straw or amber colored. Store in the dark at 4°C for no more than 2 weeks.

Procedure
Emulsify a 3-mm loopful of growth in a tube of substrate. Incubate at 37°C. Observe the tubes for a pink or red color after 1, 5, and 10 days. Do not shake the tubes. Record the number of days required for the first appearance of a pink or red color. A negative result is indicated by the substrate remaining amber-colored after 10 days.

Controls
M. *kansasii* and MAC as positive and negative controls, respectively.

Urease (Wayne method)

Inoculum
Actively growing colonies from solid medium.

Reagents
Mix 1 part of urea agar base concentrate with 9 parts of sterile distilled water. Do not add agar. Dispense 4-ml amounts into 16- by 125-mm screw-cap tubes, and store at 4°C.

Procedure
Emulsify a 3-mm loopful of growth in a tube of substrate. Incubate at 37°C for up to 3 days, and observe for a pink or red color (positive).

Controls
M. *scrofulaceum* and M. *gordonae* as positive and negative controls, respectively.

References

1. **Isenberg, H. D.** 1993. *Clinical Microbiology Procedures Handbook*, vol. 1. American Society for Microbiology, Washington, D.C.
2. **Kent, P. T., and G. P. Kubica.** 1985. *Public Health Mycobacteriology: a Guide for the Level III Laboratory*. U.S. Department of Health and Human Services, Centers for Disease Control, Atlanta, Ga.

REFERENCES

1. **Agerton, T., S. Valway, B. Gore, C. Pozsik, B. Plikaytis, C. Woodley, and I. Onorato.** 1997. Transmission of a highly drug-resistant strain (strain W1) of *Mycobacterium tuberculosis*. *JAMA* **278:**1073–1077.
2. **Agy, M. B., C. K. Wassis, J. J. Plorde, L. C. Carlson, and M. B. Coyle.** 1989. Evaluation of four mycobacterial blood culture media: BACTEC 13A, Isolator/BACTEC 12B, Isolator/Middlebrook Agar and a biphasic medium. *Diagn. Microbiol. Infect. Dis.* **12:**303–308.
3. **American Thoracic Society.** 1997. Diagnosis and treatment of disease caused by nontuberculous mycobacteria. *Am. J. Respir. Crit. Care Med. Suppl.* **156:**S1–S25.
4. **American Thoracic Society.** 1997. Rapid diagnostic tests for tuberculosis: what is the appropriate use? American Thoracic Society Workshop. *Am. J. Respir. Crit. Care Med.* **155:**1804–1814.
5. **American Thoracic Society/CDC.** 1994. Treatment of tuberculosis and tuberculosis infection in adults and children. *Am. J. Respir. Crit. Care Med.* **149:**1359–1374.
6. **Association of State and Territorial Public Health Laboratory Directors and U.S. Department of Health and Human Services, Public Health Service, Centers for Disease Control and Prevention.** 1995. Mycobacterium tuberculosis: *Assessing Your Laboratory*. Association of State and Territorial Public Health Laboratory Directors and Centers for Disease Control and Prevention, Atlanta, Ga.
7. **Band, J. D., J. I. Ward, D. W. Fraser, N. J. Peterson, V. A. Silcox, R. C. Good, P. R. Ostroy, and J. Kennedy.** 1982. Peritonitis due to a *Mycobacterium chelonei*-like organism associated with intermittent chronic peritoneal dialysis. *J. Infect. Dis.* **145:**9–17.
8. **Barbaro, D., V. Orcutt, and B. Coldiron.** 1989. *Mycobacterium avium-Mycobacterium intracellulare* infection limited to the skin and lymph nodes in patients with AIDS. *Rev. Infect. Dis.* **11:**625–628.
9. **Beam, E. R., and G. P. Kubica.** 1968. Stimulatory effects of carbon dioxide on the primary isolation of tubercle bacilli on agar containing medium. *Am. J. Clin. Pathol.* **50:**395–397.
10. **Beck-Sague, C., S. W. Dooley, M. D. Hutton, J. Otten, A. Breeden, J. T. Crawford, A. E. Pitchenik, C. Woodley, G. Cauthen, and W. R. Jarvis.** 1992. Hospital outbreak of multidrug-resistant *Mycobacterium tuberculosis* infections. Factors in transmission to staff and HIV-infected patients. *JAMA* **268:**1280–1286.
11. **Beggs, M. L., M. D. Cave, C. Marlowe, L. Cloney, P. Duck, and K. D. Eisenach.** 1996. Characterization of *Mycobacterium tuberculosis* complex direct repeat sequence for use in cycling probe reaction. *J. Clin. Microbiol.* **34:**2985–2989.

12. **Benjamin, W. H., Jr., A. Beverly, L. Gibbs, M. Waller, S. Nix, S. A. Moser, K. B. Waites, and M. Willert.** 1997. Comparison of the MB/BacT with a revised reconstitution fluid to the BACTEC 460 for detection of mycobacteria in clinical specimens, abstr. D-98. *In Program and Abstracts of the 37th Interscience Conference on Antimicrobial Agents and Chemotherapy*. American Society for Microbiology, Washington, D.C.
13. **Bifani, P. J., B. B. Plikaytis, V. Kapur, K. Stockbauer, X. Pan, M. L. Lutfey, S. Moghazeh, W. Eiser, T. M. Daniel, M. H. Kaplan, J. T. Crawford, J. M. Musser, and B. N. Kreiswirth.** 1996. Origin and interstate spread of a New York City multidrug-resistant *Mycobacterium tuberculosis* clone family. *JAMA* **275:**452–457.
14. **Bignardi, G. E., S. P. Barrett, R. Hinkins, P. A. Jenkins, and M. P. Rebec.** 1994. False positive *Mycobacterium avium-intracellulare* cultures with the BACTEC 460 TB system. *J. Hosp. Infect.* **26:**203–210.
15. **Bird, B. R., M. M. Denniston, R. E. Huebner, and R. C. Good.** 1996. Changing practices in mycobacteriology: a follow-up survey of state and territorial public health laboratories. *J. Clin. Microbiol.* **34:**554–559.
16. **Blacklock, Z., D. Dawson, D. Kane, and D. McEvoy.** 1983. *Mycobacterium asiaticum* as a potential pulmonary pathogen for humans. A clinical and bacteriologic review of five cases. *Am. Rev. Respir. Dis.* **127:**241–244.
17. **Bolivar, R., T. Satterwhite, and M. Floyd.** 1980. Cutaneous lesions due to *Mycobacterium kansasii*. *Arch. Dermatol.* **116:**207–208.
18. **Bothamley, G. H.** 1995. Serological diagnosis of tuberculosis. *Eur. Respir. J.* **8:**676S–688S.
19. **Böttger, E. C., A. Teske, P. Kirschner, S. Bost, H. R. Chang, V. Beer, and B. Hirschel.** 1991. Disseminated "*Mycobacterium genavense*" infection in patients with AIDS. *Lancet* **340:**76–80.
20. **Braden, C. R., G. L. Templeton, M. D. Cave, S. Valway, I. M. Onorato, K. G. Castro, D. Moers, Z. Yang, W. W. Stead, and J. H. Bates.** 1997. Interpretation of restriction fragment length polymorphism analysis of *Mycobacterium tuberculosis* isolates from a state with a large rural population. *J. Infect. Dis.* **175:**1446–1452.
21. **Bradley, S. P., S. L. Reed, and A. Catanzaro.** 1996. Clinical efficacy of the amplified *Mycobacterium tuberculosis* direct test for the diagnosis of pulmonary tuberculosis. *Am. J. Respir. Crit. Care Med.* **153:**1606–1610.
22. **Brander, E., E. Jantzen, R. Huttunen, A. Julkunen, and M. Katila.** 1992. Characterization of a distinct group of slowly growing mycobacteria by biochemical tests and lipid analysis. *J. Clin. Microbiol.* **30:**1972–1975.
23. **Brennan, P.** 1989. Structure of mycobacteria: recent developments in defining cell wall carbohydrates and proteins. *Rev. Infect. Dis.* **11:**S420–S430.
24. **Brown, B. A., J. M. Swenson, and R. J. Wallace, Jr.** 1991. Agar disk elution test for rapidly growing mycobacteria. p. 5.10.1–5.10.11 and 5.11.1–5.12.8. *In* H. D. Isenberg (ed.), *Clinical Microbiology Procedures Handbook*. American Society for Microbiology, Washington, D.C.
25. **Bryceson, A., and R. E. Pfaltzgraft.** 1990. *Leprosy*. Churchill-Livingstone, Edinburgh, United Kingdom.
26. **Bullin, C. H., and E. I. Tanner.** 1970. Isolation of *Mycobacterium xenopi* from water taps. *J. Hyg. Camb.* **68:** 97–100.
27. **Burdash, N. M., J. P. Manos, D. Ross, and E. R. Bannister.** 1976. Evaluation of the acid-fast smear. *J. Clin. Microbiol.* **4:**190–191.
28. **Burman, W. J., R. R. Reves, A. P. Hawkes, C. A. Rietmeijer, Z. Yang, H. El-Hajj, J. H. Bates, and M. D. Cave.** 1997. DNA fingerprinting with two probes decreases clustering of *Mycobacterium tuberculosis*. *Am. J. Respir. Crit. Care Med.* **155:**1140–1146.
29. **Burman, W. J., B. L. Stone, R. R. Reves, M. L. Wilson, Z. Yang, H. El-Hajj, J. H. Bates, and M. D. Cave.** 1997. The incidence of false-positive cultures for *Mycobacterium tuberculosis*. *Am. J. Respir. Crit. Care Med.* **155:**321–326.
30. **Butler, W. R., K. C. Jost, and J. O. Kilburn.** 1991. Identification of mycobacteria by high-performance liquid chromatography. *J. Clin. Microbiol.* **29:**2468–2472.
31. **Butler, W. R., S. P. O'Connor, M. A. Yakrus, and W. M. Gross.** 1994. Cross-reactivity of genetic probe for detection of *Mycobacterium tuberculosis* with newly described species *Mycobacterium celatum*. *J. Clin. Microbiol.* **32:** 536–538.
32. **Butler, W. R., S. P. O'Connor, M. A. Yakrus, R. W. Smithwick, B. B. Plikaytis, C. W. Moss, M. M. Floyd, C. L. Woodley, J. O. Kilburn, F. S. Vadney, and W. M. Gross.** 1993. *Mycobacterium celatum*. *Int. J. Syst. Bacteriol.* **43:**539–548.
33. **Butler, W. R., N. G. Warren, G. P. Kubica, and J. O. Kilburn.** 1990. Modified method for testing the quality of albumin-containing enrichments used in growth media for mycobacteria. *J. Clin. Microbiol.* **28:**1068–1070.
34. **Castro, K. G., and S. W. Dooley.** 1993. *Mycobacterium tuberculosis* transmission in healthcare settings: is it influenced by coinfection with human immunodeficiency virus? *Infect. Control Hosp. Epidemiol.* **14:**65.
35. **Cave, M. D., K. D. Eisenach, P. F. McDermott, J. H. Bates, and J. T. Crawford.** 1991. IS6110: conservation of sequence in the *Mycobacterium tuberculosis* complex and its utilization in DNA fingerprinting. *Mol. Cell. Probes* **5:**73–80.
36. **Cave, M. D., K. D. Eisenach, G. Templeton, M. Salfinger, G. Mazurek, J. H. Bates, and J. T. Crawford.** 1994. Stability of DNA fingerprint patterns produced with IS*6110* in strains of *Mycobacterium tuberculosis*. *J. Clin. Microbiol.* **32:**262–266.
37. **Centers for Disease Control.** 1991. *Mycobacterium haemophilum* infections—New York City Metropolitan Area, 1990–1991. *Morbid. Mortal. Weekly Rep.* **40:** 636–643.
38. **Centers for Disease Control.** 1992. National MDR-TB Task Force, National Action Plan to combat multidrug-resistant tuberculosis. *Morbid. Mortal. Weekly Rep.* **41**(RR-11)**:**1–71.
39. **Centers for Disease Control.** 1992. Tuberculosis morbidity—United States, 1991. *Morbid. Mortal. Weekly Rep.* **41:**240.
40. **Centers for Disease Control.** 1993. Diagnosis of tuberculosis by nucleic acid amplification methods applied to clinical specimens. *Morbid. Mortal. Weekly Rep.* **42:**686.
41. **Centers for Disease Control—National Institutes of Health.** 1993. *Biosafety in Microbiological and Biomedical Laboratories*, 3rd ed. HHS publication (CDC) 93-8395. U.S. Government Printing Office, Washington, D.C.
42. **Centers for Disease Control and Prevention.** 1994. Guidelines for preventing the transmission of *Mycobacterium tuberculosis* in health-care facilities. *Morbid. Mortal. Weekly Rep.* **43**(RR-13)**:**1–132.
43. **Centers for Disease Control and Prevention.** 1998. Tuberculosis morbidity—United States, 1997. *Morbid. Mortal. Weekly Rep.* **47:**253–257.
44. **Centers for Disease Control and Prevention.** 1996. Impact of HIV protease inhibitors on the treatment of HIV-infected tuberculosis patients with rifampin. *Morbid. Mortal. Weekly Rep.* **45:**921–925.
45. **Centers for Disease Control and Prevention.** 1996. Nucleic acid amplification tests for tuberculosis. *Morbid. Mortal. Weekly Rep.* **45:**950–952.

46. **Centers for Disease Control and Prevention.** 1996. *Standardized Method for HPLC Identification of Mycobacteria.* HHS publication. Centers for Disease Control and Prevention, Atlanta, Ga.
47. **Centers for Disease Control and Prevention.** 1997. USPHS/IDSA guidelines for the prevention of opportunistic infections in persons infected with human immunodeficiency virus. *Morbid. Mortal. Weekly Rep.* **46**(RR-12): 1–46.
48. **Centers for Disease Control and Prevention.** 1997. Multiple misdiagnoses of tuberculosis resulting from laboratory error—Wisconsin, 1996. *Morbid. Mortal. Weekly Rep.* **46:**797–801.
49. **Chan, S. L., Z. Reggiardo, T. M. Daniel, D. J. Girling, and D. A. Mitchison.** 1990. Serodiagnosis of tuberculosis using an ELISA with antigen 5 and a hemagglutination assay with glycolipid antigens. *Am. Rev. Respir. Dis.* **142:** 385–390.
50. **Chaves, F., Z. Yang, H. El Hajj, M. Alonso, W. J. Burman, K. D. Eisenach, F. Dronda, J. H. Bates, and M. D. Cave.** 1996. Usefulness of the secondary probe pTBN12 in DNA fingerprinting of *Mycobacterium tuberculosis*. *J. Clin. Microbiol.* **34:**1118–1123.
51. **Chin, D. P., D. M. Yajko, W. K. Hadley, C. A. Sanders, P. S. Nassos, J. J. Madej, and P. C. Hopewell.** 1995. Clinical utility of a commercial test based on the polymerase chain reaction for detecting *Mycobacterium tuberculosis* in respiratory specimens. *Am. J. Respir. Crit. Care Med.* **151:**1872–1877.
52. **Cocito, C. G.** 1991. Properties of the mycobacterial antigen complex A60 and its application to the diagnosis and prognosis of tuberculosis. *Chest* **100:**1687–1693.
53. **Conville, P. S., J. F. Keiser, and F. G. Witebsky.** 1989. Comparison of three techniques for concentrating positive BACTEC 13A bottles of mycobacterial DNA probe analysis. *Diagn. Microbiol. Infect. Dis.* **12:**309–313.
54. **Cornfield, D. B., K. G. Beavis, J. A. Greene, M. Bojac, and J. Bondi.** 1997. Mycobacterial growth and bacterial contamination in the mycobacteria growth indicator tube and BACTEC 460 culture systems. *J. Clin. Microbiol.* **35:** 2068–2071.
55. **Costrini, A. M., D. A. Mahler, W. M. Gross, J. E. Hawkins, R. Yesner, and N. D. D'Esopo.** 1981. Clinical and roentgenographic features of nosocomial pulmonary disease due to *Mycobacterium xenopi*. *Am. Rev. Respir. Dis.* **123:**104–109.
56. **Coyle, M. B., L. Carlson, C. Wallis, R. Leonard, V. Raisys, J. Kilburn, M. Samadpour, and E. Böttger.** 1992. Laboratory aspects of *Mycobacterium genavense*, a proposed species isolated from AIDS patients. *J. Clin. Microbiol.* **30:**3206–3212.
57. **Crossey, M. J., M. A. Yakrus, M. B. Cook, S. K. Rasmussen, T. M. McEntee, K. B. Oldewage, R. B. Ferguson, and J. C. McLaughlin.** 1994. Isolation of *Mycobacterium simiae* in a southwestern hospital and typing by multilocus enzyme electrophoresis, abstr. U38, p. 179. *In Abstracts of the 94th General Meeting of the American Society for Microbiology 1994*. American Society for Microbiology, Washington, D.C.
58. **Daley, C. L., P. M. Small, G. F. Schecter, G. K. Schoolnik, R. A. McAdam, R. Jacobs, Jr., and P. C. Hopewell.** 1992. An outbreak of tuberculosis with accelerated progression among persons infected with the human immunodeficiency virus: an analysis using restriction-fragment-length polymorphisms. *N. Engl. J. Med.* **326:**231–235.
59. **Daloviso, J. R., S. Montenegro-James, S. A. Kemmerly, C. F. Genre, R. Chambers, D. Greer, G. A. Pankey, D. M. Failla, K. G. Haydel, L. Hutchinson, M. F. Lindley, B. M. Nunez, A. Praba, K. D. Eisenach, and E. S. Cooper.** 1996. Comparison of the amplified *Mycobacterium tuberculosis* (MTB) direct test, Amplicor MTB PCR, and IS-6110-PCR for detection of MTB in respiratory specimens. *Clin. Infect. Dis.* **23:**1099–1106.
60. **D'Amato, R. F., L. H. Hochstein, P. M. Colaninno, M. Scardamaglia, K. Kim, A. J. Mastellone, R. C. Patel, S. Alkhuja, V. J. Tevere, and A. Miller.** 1996. Application of the Roche *Mycobacterium tuberculosis* (PCR) test to specimens other than respiratory secretions. *Diagn. Microbiol. Infect. Dis.* **24:**15–17.
61. **Daniel, T.** 1989. Rapid diagnosis of tuberculosis: laboratory techniques applicable in developing countries. *Rev. Infect. Dis.* **11:**S471–S478.
62. **Daniel, T., G. de Murillo, J. Sawyer, A. McLean Griffin, E. Pinto, S. Debanne, P. Espinosa, and E. Cespedes.** 1986. Field evaluation of enzyme-linked immunosorbent assay for the serodiagnosis of tuberculosis. *Am. Rev. Respir. Dis.* **134:**662–665.
63. **Daniel, T. M., and S. M. Debanne.** 1987. The serodiagnosis of tuberculosis and other mycobacterial diseases by enzyme-linked immunosorbent assay. *Am. Rev. Respir. Dis.* **158:**678–680.
64. **Dawson, D., and F. Jennis.** 1980. Mycobacteria with a growth requirement for ferric ammonium citrate identified as *Mycobacterium haemophilum*. *J. Clin. Microbiol.* **11:** 190–192.
65. **de la Salmoniére, Y.-O. G., H. M. Li, G. Torrea, A. Bunschoten, J. van Embden, and B. Gicquel.** 1997. Evaluation of spoligotyping in a study of the transmission of *Mycobacterium tuberculosis*. *J. Clin. Microbiol.* **35:**2210–2214.
66. **DeMerieux, P., E. Keystone, M. Hutcheon, and C. Laskin.** 1980. Polyarthritis due to *Mycobacterium kansasii* in a patient with rheumatoid arthritis. *Ann. Rheum. Dis.* **39:** 90–94.
67. **De Wit, M. Y. L., J. T. Douglas, J. McFadden, and P. R. Klaster.** 1993. Polymerase chain reaction for detection of *Mycobacterium leprae* in nasal swab specimens. *J. Clin. Microbiol.* **31:**502–506.
68. **Dixon, J. M. S., and E. H. Cuthbert.** 1967. Isolation of tubercle bacilli from uncentrifuged sputum on pyruvic acid medium. *Am. Rev. Respir. Dis.* **96:**119–122.
69. **Dizon, D., C. Mihailescu, and H. C. Bae.** 1976. Simple procedure for detection of *Mycobacterium gordonae* in water causing false-positive acid fast smears. *J. Clin. Microbiol.* **3:**211.
70. **Dolin, P. J., M. D. Raviglione, and A. Kochi.** 1993. Global tuberculosis incidence and mortality during 1990–2000. *Bull. W. H. O.* **72:**213–220.
71. **Dowell, M. E.** 1996. Disseminated *Mycobacterium marinum* in AIDS, p. 127. *In Program and Abstracts of the 34th Annual Meeting of the Infectious Disease Society of America*.
72. **Down, J. A., M. A. O'Connell, M. S. Dey, A. H. Walters, D. R. Howard, M. C. Little, W. E. Keating, P. Zwadyk, Jr., P. D. Haaland, D. A. McLauren III, and G. Cole.** 1996. Detection of *Mycobacterium tuberculosis* in respiratory specimens by strand displacement amplification of DNA. *J. Clin. Microbiol.* **34:**860–865.
73. **Drake, T. A., J. A. Hindler, O. G. W. Berlin, and D. Bruckner.** 1987. Rapid identification of *Mycobacterium avium* complex in culture using DNA probes. *J. Clin. Microbiol.* **25:**1442–1445.
74. **Dunlap, N. E., R. H. Harris, W. H. Benjamin, Jr., J. W. Harden, and D. Hafner.** 1995. Laboratory contamination of *Mycobacterium tuberculosis* cultures. *Am. J. Respir. Crit. Care Med.* **152:**1702–1704.
75. **Ehlers, S., R. Ignatius, T. Regnath, and H. Hahn.** 1996. Diagnosis of extrapulmonary tuberculosis by Gen-Probe

Amplified *Mycobacterium tuberculosis* Direct Test. *J. Clin. Microbiol.* **34:**2275–2279.

76. **El-Helou, P., A. Rachlis, I. Fong, S. Walmsley, A. Phillips, I. Salit, and A. E. Simor.** 1997. *Mycobacterium xenopi* infection in patients with human immunodeficiency virus infection. *Clin. Infect. Dis.* **25:**206–210.
77. **Ellner, J., M. Goldberger, and D. Parenti.** 1991. *Mycobacterium avium* infection and AIDS: a therapeutic dilemma in rapid evolution. *J. Infect. Dis.* **163:**1326–1335.
78. **Ellner, P. D., T. E. Kiehn, R. Cammarata, and M. Hosmer.** 1988. Rapid detection and identification of pathogenic mycobacteria by combining radiometric and nucleic acid probe methods. *J. Clin. Microbiol.* **26:** 1349–1352.
79. **Evans, K., A. Nakasone, P. Sutherland, L. de la Maza, and E. Peterson.** 1992. Identification of *Mycobacterium tuberculosis* and *Mycobacterium avium-M. intracellulare* directly from primary BACTEC cultures by using acridinium-ester-labeled DNA probes. *J. Clin. Microbiol.* **30:**2427–2431.
80. **Floyd, M. M., L. S. Guthertz, V. A. Silcox, P. S. Duffey, Y. Jang, E. P. Desmond, J. T. Crawford, and W. R. Butler.** 1996. Characterization of an SAV organism and proposal of *Mycobacterium triplex* sp. nov. *J. Clin. Microbiol.* **34:**2963–2967.
81. **Forbes, B. A.** 1997. Critical assessment of gene amplification approaches on the diagnosis of tuberculosis. *Immunol. Invest.* **26:**105–116.
82. **Forbes, B. A., and K. E. Hicks.** 1994. Ability of PCR assay to identify *Mycobacterium tuberculosis* in BACTEC 12B vials. *J. Clin. Microbiol.* **32:**1725–1728.
83. **Franklin, D. J., J. R. Starke, M. T. Brady, B. A. Brown, and R. J. Wallace, Jr.** 1994. Chronic otitis media after tympanostomy tube placement caused by *Mycobacterium abscessus*: a new clinical entity? *Am. J. Otol.* **15:**313–320.
84. **Fraser, V., and R. J. Wallace.** 1996. Nontuberculous mycobacteria, p. 1224–1237. *In* C. G. Mayhall (ed.), *Hospital Epidemiology and Infection Control*. The Williams & Wilkins, Co., Baltimore, Md.
85. **Frieden T. R., C. L. Woodley, J. T. Crawford, D. Lew, and S. M. Dooley.** 1996. The molecular epidemiology of tuberculosis in New York City: the importance of nosocomial transmission and laboratory error. *Tubercle Lung Dis.* **77:**407–413.
86. **Gill, V., and F. Stock.** 1987. Detection of *Mycobacterium avium-Mycobacterium intracellulare* in blood cultures using concentrated and unconcentrated blood in conjunction with radiometric detection systems. *Diagn. Microbiol. Infect. Dis.* **6:**119.
87. **Glickman, S. E., J. O. Kilburn, W. R. Butler, and L. S. Ramos.** 1994. Rapid identification of mycolic acid patterns of mycobacteria by high-performance liquid chromatography using pattern recognition software and a *Mycobacterium* library. *J. Clin. Microbiol.* **32:**740–745.
88. **Gombert, M., E. Goldstein, M. Corrado, A. Shin, and K. Butt.** 1981. Disseminated *Mycobacterium marinum* infection after renal transplantation. *Ann. Intern. Med.* **94:** 486–487.
89. **Good, R. C., V. A. Silcox, J. O. Kilburn, and B. D. Plikaytis.** 1985. Identification and drug susceptibility test results for *Mycobacterium* spp. *Clin. Microbiol. Newsl.* **7:** 133–135.
90. **Good, R. C., and D. E. Snider.** 1982. Isolation of nontuberculous mycobacteria in the United States 1980. *J. Infect. Dis.* **146:**829–833.
91. **Goto, M., S. Oka, K. Okuzumi, S. Kimur, and K. Shimada.** 1991. Evaluation of acridinium-ester labeled DNA probes for identification of *Mycobacterium tuberculosis* and *Mycobacterium avium-Mycobacterium intracellulare* complex in culture. *J. Clin. Microbiol.* **29:**2473–2476.
92. **Goutzamanis, J. J., and G. L. Gilbert.** 1995. *Mycobacterium ulcerans* infection in Australian children: report of eight cases and review. *Clin. Infect. Dis.* **21:**1186–1192.
93. **Graham, L., N. Warren, A. Tsang, and H. Dalton.** 1988. *Mycobacterium avium* complex pseudobacteruria from a hospital water supply. *J. Clin. Microbiol.* **26:** 1034–1036.
94. **Griffith, D. E., W. M. Girard, and R. J. Wallace, Jr.** 1993. Clinical features of pulmonary disease caused by rapidly growing mycobacteria: an analysis of 154 patients. *Am. Rev. Respir. Dis.* **147:**1271–1278.
95. **Guerrero, C., C. Permasconi, D. Burki, T. Bodmer, and A. Telenti.** 1994. A novel insertion element from *Mycobacterium avium*. IS*1245* is a specific marker for analysis of strain relatedness. *J. Clin. Microbiol.* **33:**304–307.
96. **Guthertz, L. S., S. D. Lim, Y. Yang, and P. S. Duffey.** 1993. Curvilinear-gradient high-performance liquid chromatography for identification of mycobacteria. *J. Clin. Microbiol.* **31:**1976–1881.
97. **Haas, W., W. R. Butler, C. Woodley, and J. Crawford.** 1993. Mixed-linker polymerase chain reaction: a new method for rapid fingerprinting of isolates of the *Mycobacterium tuberculosis* complex. *J. Clin. Microbiol.* **31:** 1293–1298.
98. **Havlik, J., C. Horsburgh, B. Metchock, P. William, S. Fan, and S. Thompson.** 1992. Disseminated *Mycobacterium avium* complex infection: clinical identification and epidemiologic trends. *J. Infect. Dis.* **165:**577–580.
99. **Havlik, J. A., B. Metchock, S. E. Thompson III, K. Barrett, D. Rimland, and C. R. Horsburgh Jr.** 1993. A prospective evaluation of *Mycobacterium avium* complex colonization of the respiratory and gastrointestinal tracts of persons with human immunodeficiency virus infection. *J. Infect. Dis.* **168:**1045–1048.
100. **Hawkins, J. E., R. C. Good, G. P. Kubica, P. R. J. Gangadharam, H. M. Gruft, K. D. Stottmeier, H. M. Sommers, and L. G. Wayne.** 1983. Levels of laboratory services for mycobacterial diseases: official statement of the American Thoracic Society. *Am. Rev. Respir. Dis.* **128:**213.
101. **Heifits, L., N. Mor, and J. Vanderkolk.** 1993. *Mycobacterium avium* strains resistant to clarithromycin and azithromycin. *Antimicrob. Agents Chemother.* **37:**2364–2370.
102. **Hellyer, T. J., T. W. Fletcher, J. H. Bates, W. W. Stead, G. L. Templeton, M. D. Cave, and K. D. Eisenach.** 1996. Strand displacement amplification and the polymerase chain reaction for monitoring response to treatment in patients with pulmonary tuberculosis. *J. Infect. Dis.* **173:** 934–941.
103. **Henrikson, H. P., and G. E. Pfyffer.** 1994. Mycobacterial mycolic acids. *Med. Microbiol. Lett.* **3:**49–57.
104. **Hernandez A., J. S. Bergmann, and G. L. Woods.** 1997. AMPLICOR MTB polymerase chain reaction test for identification of *Mycobacterium tuberculosis* in positive Difco ESP II broth cultures. *Diagn. Microbiol. Infect. Dis.* **27:**17–20.
105. **Holzman, R. S., P. C. Hopewell, A. E. Pitchenik, L. B. Reichman, and R. L. Stoneburner.** 1987. Diagnosis and management of mycobacterial infection and disease in persons with human immune deficiency virus infection. *Ann. Intern. Med.* **106:**254–256.
106. **Horsburgh, C., B. Metchock, J. McGowan, Jr., and S. Thompson.** 1992. Clinical implications of recovery of *Mycobacterium avium* complex from the stool or respiratory tract of HIV-infected individuals. *AIDS* **6:**512–514.
107. **Horsburgh, C. R., Jr., U. G. Mason III, D. C. Farhi, and M. D. Iseman.** 1985. Disseminated infection with *Mycobacterium avium-intracellulare*. A report of 13 cases and review of the literature. *Medicine* **64:**36–48.

108. **Huminer, D., S. Dux, Z. Samra, L. Kaufman, A. Lavy, C. S. Block, and S. D. Pitik.** 1993. *Mycobacterium simiae* infection in Israeli patients with AIDS. *Clin. Infect. Dis.* **17:**508–509.
109. **Ichiyama, S., Y. Iinuma, Y. Tawada, S. Yamori, Y. Hasegawa, H. Shimokata, and N. Nakashima.** 1996. Evaluation of GenProbe amplified *Mycobacterium tuberculosis* direct test and Roche-PCR microwell plate hybridization method (Amplicor Mycobacterium) for direct detection of mycobacteria. *J. Clin. Microbiol.* **34:**130–133.
110. **Ieven, M., and H. Goossens.** 1997. Relevance of nucleic acid amplification techniques for diagnosis of respiratory tract infections in the clinical laboratory. *Clin. Microbiol. Rev.* **10:**242–256.
111. **Imaeda, T., G. Broslawski, and S. Imaeda.** 1988. Genomic relatedness among mycobacterial species by nonisotopic blot hybridization. *Int. J. Syst. Bacteriol.* **38:** 151–156.
112. **Inderlied, C., C. Kempler, and L. Bermudez.** 1993. The *Mycobacterium avium* complex. *Clin. Microbiol. Rev.* **6:** 266–310.
113. **Isenberg, H. D. (ed.)** 1993. *Clinical Microbiology Procedures Handbook*, vol. 1. American Society for Microbiology, Washington, D.C.
114. **Isenberg, H. D., R. F. D'Amato, L. Heifets, P. R. Murray, M. Scardamaglia, M. C. Jacobs, P. Alperstein, and A. Niles.** 1991. Collaborative feasibility study of a biphasic system (Roche Septi-Check AFB) for rapid detection and isolation of mycobacteria. *J. Clin. Microbiol.* **29:** 1719–1722.
115. **Jackett, P. S., G. Bothamley, H. Batra, A. Mistry, D. Young, and J. Ivanyi.** 1988. Specificity of antibodies to immunodominant mycobacterial antigens in pulmonary tuberculosis. *J. Clin. Microbiol.* **26:**2313–2318.
116. **Job, C. K., J. Jayakumaaar, D. L. Williams, and T. P. Gillis.** 1997. Role of polymerase chain reaction in the diagnosis of early leprosy. *Int. J. Lepr. Other Mycobact. Dis.* **65:**461–464.
117. **Jonas, V., M. J. Alden, J. I. Curry, K. Kamisango, C. Knott, R. Lankford, J. Wolfe, and D. Moore.** 1993. Detection and identification of *Mycobacterium tuberculosis* directly from sputum sediments by amplification of rRNA. *J. Clin. Microbiol.* **31:**2410–2416.
118. **Joseph, S., E. Vaichulis, and V. Houk.** 1967. Lack of auramine-rhodamine fluorescence of Runyon group IV mycobacteria. *Am. Rev. Respir. Dis.* **95:**114.
119. **Jost, K., Jr., D. F. Dunbar, S. S. Barth, V. L. Headley, and L. B. Elliott.** 1995. Identification of *Mycobacterium tuberculosis* and *M. avium* complex directly from sputum and BACTEC 12B sputum cultures by high performance liquid chromatography with fluorescence detection and computer-driven pattern recognition models. *J. Clin. Microbiol.* **33:**1270–1277.
120. **Kamerbeek J., L. Schouls, A. Kolk, M. van Agterveld, D. van Soolingen, S. Kuijper, A. Bunschoten, H. Molhuizen, R. Shaw, M. Goyal, and J. van Embden.** 1997. Simultaneous detection and strain differentiation of *Mycobacterium tuberculosis* for diagnosis and epidemiology. *J. Clin. Microbiol.* **35:**907–914.
121. **Kaminski, D. A., and D. J. Hardy.** 1995. Selective utilization of DNA probes for identification of *Mycobacterium* species on the basis of cord formation in primary BACTEC 12B cultures. *J. Clin. Microbiol.* **33:**1548–1550.
122. **Kent, P. T., and G. P. Kubica.** 1985. *Public Health Mycobacteriology: a Guide for the Level III Laboratory*. U.S. Department of Health and Human Services, Centers for Disease Control, Atlanta, Ga.
123. **Kiehn, T. E., and R. Cammarata.** 1986. Laboratory diagnosis of mycobacterial infections in patients with acquired immunodeficiency syndrome. *J. Clin. Microbiol.* **24:** 708–711.
124. **Kiehn, T. E., and R. Cammarata.** 1988. Comparative recoveries of *Mycobacterium avium-M. intracellulare* from Isolator lysis-centrifugation and BACTEC 13A blood culture systems. *J. Clin. Microbiol.* **26:**760–761.
125. **Kiehn, T. E., F. F. Edwards, P. Brannon, A. Y. Tsang, M. Maio, J. W. M. Gold, E. Whimby, B. Wong, J. K. McClatchy, and D. Armstrong.** 1985. Infections caused by *Mycobacterium avium* complex in immunocompromised patients: diagnosis by blood culture and fecal examination, antimicrobial susceptibility tests, and morphological and seroagglutination characteristics. *J. Clin. Microbiol.* **21:**168–173.
126. **Kilburn, J. O., K. D. Stottmeier, and G. P. Kubica.** 1968. Aspartic acid as a precursor for niacin synthesis by tubercle bacilli grown on 7H10 agar medium. *Am. J. Clin. Pathol.* **50:**582–586.
127. **Kilby, J., P. Gilligan, J. Yankaskas, W. Highsmith, Jr., L. Edwards, and M. Knowled.** 1992. Nontuberculous mycobacteria in adult patients with cystic fibrosis. *Chest* **102:** 70–75.
128. **Kim, T. C., R. S. Blackman, K. M. Heatwole, T. Kim, and D. F. Rochester.** 1984. Acid fact bacilli in sputum smears of patients with pulmonary tuberculosis. Prevalence and significance of negative smears pretreatment and positive smears post-treatment. *Am. Rev. Respir. Dis.* **129:**264–268.
129. **Kirschner P., A. Meier, and E. C. Böttger.** 1993. Genotypic identification and detection of mycobacteria—facing novel and uncultured pathogens, p. 173–190. *In* D. H. Persing, T. F. Smith, F. C. Tenover, and T. J. White (ed.), *Diagnostic Molecular Microbiology*. American Society for Microbiology, Washington, D.C.
130. **Klein, G. C., M. M. Cummings, and C. H. Fish.** 1952. Efficiency of centrifugation as a method of concentrating tubercle bacilli. *Am. J. Clin. Pathol.* **22:**581–585.
131. **Koukila-Kähkölä, P., B. Springer, E. C. Böttger, L. Paulin, E. Jantzen, and M.-L. Katila.** 1995. *Mycobacterium branderi* sp. nov., a new potential human pathogen. *Int. J. Syst. Bacteriol.* **45:**549–553.
132. **Krasnow, I., and L. G. Wayne.** 1966. Sputum digestion. I. The mortality rate of tubercle bacilli in various digestion systems. *Am. J. Clin. Pathol.* **45:**352–355.
133. **Krasnow, I., and L. G. Wayne.** 1969. Comparison of methods for tuberculosis bacteriology. *Appl. Microbiol.* **18:**915–917.
134. **Kubica, G. P., W. M. Gross, J. E. Hawkins, H. M. Sommers, A. L. Vestal, and L. G. Wayne.** 1975. Laboratory services for mycobacterial diseases. *Am. Rev. Respir. Dis.* **112:**773–787.
135. **Kusunoki, S., and T. Ezaki.** 1992. Proposal of *Mycobacterium peregrinum* sp. nov., nom. rev., and elevation of *Mycobacterium chelonae* subsp. *abscessus* (Kubica et al.) to species status: *Mycobacterium abscessus* comb. nov. *Int. J. Syst. Bacteriol.* **42:**240–245.
136. **Lacaille, F., S. Blanche, C. Bodmer, C. Durand, Y. De Prost, and J. Gaillard.** 1990. Persistent *Mycobacterium marinum* infection in a child with probable visceral involvement. *Pediatr. Infect. Dis. J.* **9:**58–60.
137. **Laszlo, A., and S. H. Siddiqi.** 1984. Evaluation of a rapid radiometric differentiation test for the *Mycobacterium tuberculosis* complex by selective inhibition with *p*-nitro-a-acetylamino-b-hydroxypropiophenone. *J. Clin. Microbiol.* **19:**694–698.
138. **Lavy, A., and Y. Yoshpe-Purer.** 1982. Isolation of *Mycobacterium simiae* from clinical specimens in Israel. *Tubercle* **63:**279–285.

139. **Leader, M., P. Revell, and G. Clarke.** 1984. Synovial infection with *Mycobacterium kansasii*. *Ann. Rheum. Dis.* **43:**80–82.
140. **Lebrun, L., F. Espinasse, J. Povenda, and V. Vincent-Levy-Frebault.** 1992. Evaluation of nonradioactive DNA probes for identification of mycobacteria. *J. Clin. Microbiol.* **30:**2476–2478.
141. **Lipsky, B. J., J. Gates, F. C. Tenover, and J. J. Plorde.** 1984. Factors affecting the clinical value of microscopy for acid-fast bacilli. *Rev. Infect. Dis.* **6:**214–222.
142. **Maloney, J. M., C. R. Gregg, D. S. Stephens, F. A. Manian, and D. Rimland.** 1987. Infections caused by *Mycobacterium szulgai* in humans. *Rev. Infect. Dis.* **9:** 1120–1126.
143. **Mastro, T. D., S. C. Redd, and R. F. Breiman.** 1992. Imported leprosy in the United States, 1978 through 1988: an epidemic without secondary transmission. *Am. J. Public Health* **82:**1127–1130.
144. **May, D. C., J. E. Kutz, R. S. Howell, M. J. Raff, and J. C. Melo.** 1983. *Mycobacterium terrae* tenosynovitis: chronic infection in a previously healthy individual. *South. Med. J.* **76:**1445–1447.
145. **Mazurek, G., M. Cave, K. Eisenach, R. Wallace, J. Bates, and J. Crawford.** 1991. Chromosomal DNA fingerprint patterns produced with IS*6110* as strain-specific markers for epidemiologic study of tuberculosis. *J. Clin. Microbiol.* **29:**2030–2033.
146. **Mazurek, G. H., D. P. Chin, S. Hartman, V. Reddy, C. R. Horsburgh, Jr., T. A. Green, D. M. Yajko, P. C. Hopewell, A. L. Reingold, and J. T. Crawford.** 1997. Genetic similarity among *Mycobacterium avium* isolates from blood, stool, and sputum of persons with AIDS. *J. Infect. Dis.* **176:**976–983.
147. **McClatchy, J. K., R. F. Waggoner, W. Kanes, M. S. Cernick, and T. L. Bolton.** 1976. Isolation of mycobacteria from clinical specimens by use of selective 7H11 medium. *Am. J. Clin. Pathol.* **65:**412–416.
148. **McSwiggan, D. A., and C. H. Collins.** 1974. The isolation of *M. kansasii* and *M. xenopi* from water systems. *Tubercle* **55:**291–297.
149. **Meier, A., P. Kirschner, S. Burkhardt, V. A. Steingrube, B. A. Brown, R. J. Wallace, Jr., and E. C. Böttger.** 1994. Identification of mutations in 23S rRNA gene of clarithromycin-resistant *Mycobacterium intracellulare*. *Antimicrob. Agents Chemother.* **38:**381–384.
150. **Miliner, R. A., K. D. Stottmeier, and G. P. Kubica.** 1969. Formaldehyde: a photothermal activated toxic substance produced in Middlebrook 7H10 medium. *Am. Rev. Respir. Dis.* **99:**603–607.
151. **Miller, N., S. G. Hernandez, and T. J. Cleary.** 1994. Evaluation of Gen-Probe amplified Mycobacterium Tuberculosis direct test and PCR for direct detection of *Mycobacterium tuberculosis* in clinical specimens. *J. Clin. Microbiol.* **32:**393–397.
152. **Moore, M., I. M. Onorato, E. McCray, and K. G. Castro.** 1997. Trends in drug-resistant tuberculosis in the United States, 1993–1996. *JAMA* **278:**833–837.
153. **Morgan, M. A., K. A. Doerr, H. O. Hempel, N. L. Goodman, and G. D. Roberts.** 1985. Evaluation of the *p*-nitro-a-acetylamino-b-hydroxypropiophenone differential test for identification of *Mycobacterium tuberculosis* complex. *J. Clin. Microbiol.* **21:**634–635.
154. **Morgan, M. A., C. D. Horstmeier, D. R. DeYoung, and G. D. Roberts.** 1983. Comparison of radiometric method (BACTEC) and conventional culture media for recovery of mycobacteria from smear-negative specimens. *J. Clin. Microbiol.* **18:**384–388.
155. **Morris, A., L. B. Reller, M. Salfinger, K. Jackson, A. Sievers, and B. Dwyer.** 1993. Mycobacteria in stool specimens: the nonvalue of smears for predicting culture results. *J. Clin. Microbiol.* **31:**1385–1387.
156. **Morris, A. J., and L. B. Reller.** 1993. Reliability of cord formation in BACTEC media for presumptive identification of mycobacteria. *J. Clin. Microbiol.* **31:**2533–2534.
157. **Murray, P. R., C. Elmore, and D. J. Krogstad.** 1980. The acid-fast stain: a specific and predictive test for mycobacterial disease. *Ann. Intern. Med.* **92:**512–513.
158. **Musial, C. E., L. S. Tice, L. Stockman, and G. D. Roberts.** 1988. Identification of mycobacteria from culture by using the Gen-Probe rapid diagnostic system for *Mycobacterium avium* complex and *Mycobacterium tuberculosis* complex. *J. Clin. Microbiol.* **26:**2120–2123.
159. **Nash, K. A., and C. B. Inderlied.** 1995. Genetic basis of macrolide resistance in *Mycobacterium avium* isolated from patients with disseminated disease. *Antimicrob. Agents Chemother.* **39:**2625–2630.
160. **National Committee for Clinical Laboratory Standards.** 1994. Specifications for molecular microbiology methods for infectious diseases. NCCLS document MM-P. National Committee for Clinical Laboratory Standards, Villanova, Pa.
161. **National Institute of Occupational Safety and Health.** 1995. Respiratory protective devices: Final rules and notice. 42 CFR part 84. *Fed. Regist.* **60:**30335–30398.
162. **Neill, M. A., A. W. Hightower, and C. V. Broome.** 1985. Leprosy in the United States, 1971–1981. *J. Infect. Dis.* **152:**1064–1069.
163. **Noordhoek, G. T., J. D. A. van Embden, and A. H. J. Kolk.** 1996. Reliability of nucleic acid amplification for detection of *Mycobacterium tuberculosis:* an international collaborative quality control study. *J. Clin. Microbiol.* **34:** 2522–2525.
164. **Otal, I., C. Martín, V. Vincent-Lévy-Frebault, D. Thierry, and B. Giquel.** 1991. Restriction fragment length polymorphism analysis using IS*6110* as an epidemiologic marker in tuberculosis. *J. Clin. Microbiol.* **29:**1252–1254.
165. **Peterson, E. M., R. Lu, C. Floyd, A. Nakasone, G. Friledly, and L. M. DeLaMaza.** 1989. Direct identification of *Mycobacterium tuberculosis*, *Mycobacterium avium*, and *Mycobacterium intracellulare* from amplified primary cultures in BACTEC media using DNA probes. *J. Clin. Microbiol.* **27:**1543–1547.
166. **Petran, E. L., and H. D. Vera.** 1971. Media for selective isolation of mycobacteria. *Health Lab. Sci.* **8:**225–230.
167. **Pfyffer, G. E., C. Cieslak, H. M. Welscher, P. Kissling, and S. Rusch-Gerdes.** 1997. Rapid detection of mycobacteria in clinical specimen by using the automated BACTEC 9000 MB system and comparison with radiometric and solid-culture systems. *J. Clin. Microbiol.* **35:** 2229–2234.
168. **Pfyffer, G. E., H. M. Welscher, P. Kissling, C. Cieslak, M. J. Casal, J. Gutierrez, and S. Rusch-Gerdes.** 1997. Comparison of the mycobacteria growth indicator tube (MGIT) with radiometric and solid culture for recovery of acid-fast bacilli. *J. Clin. Microbiol.* **35:**364–368.
169. **Pfyffer, G. E., H. M. Welscher, and P. Kissling.** 1997. Pretreatment of clinical specimens with sodium dodecyl (lauryl) sulfate is not suitable for the mycobacteria growth indicator tube cultivation method. *J. Clin. Microbiol.* **35:** 2142–2144.
170. **Picardeau, M., T. J. Bull, G. Prod'Hom, A. L. Pozniak, D. C. Shanson, and V. Vincent.** 1997. Comparison of a new insertion element, IS*1407*, with established molecular markers for the characterization of *Mycobacterium celatum*. *Int. J. Syst. Bacteriol.* **47:**640–644.
171. **Picardeau, M., G. Prod'Hom, L. Raskine, M. P. LePennec, and V. Vincent.** 1997. Genotypic characterization

of five subspecies of *Mycobacterium kansasii*. *J. Clin. Microbiol.* **35:**25–32.

172. **Picardeau, M., and V. Vincent.** 1996. Typing of *Mycobacterium avium* isolates by PCR. *J. Clin. Microbiol.* **34:** 389–392.
173. **Plikaytis, B., B. Plikaytis, M. Yakrus, W. R. Butler, C. Woodley, V. A. Silcox, and T. M. Shinnick.** 1992. Differentiation of slowly growing *Mycobacterium* species, including *M. tuberculosis*, by gene amplification and restriction fragment length polymorphism analysis. *J. Clin. Microbiol.* **30:**1815–1822.
174. **Portaels, F., L. Realini, L. Bauwens, H. Hirschel, W. M. Meyers, and W. De Meurichy.** 1996. Mycobacteriosis caused by *Mycobacterium genavense* in birds kept in a zoo: 11-year survey. *J. Clin. Microbiol.* **34:**319–323.
175. **Rickman, T. W., and N. P. Moyer.** 1980. Increased sensitivity of acid-fast smears. *J. Clin. Microbiol.* **11:**618–620.
176. **Ridley, D. S., and C. K. Job.** 1985. The pathology of leprosy, p. 129. *In* R. C. Hastings (ed.), *Leprosy*. Churchill Livingstone, Inc., New York, N.Y.
177. **Roberts, G. D., E. C. Böttger, and L. Stockman.** 1996. Methods for the rapid identification of mycobacterial species. *Clin. Lab. Med.* **16:**603–615.
178. **Roberts, G. D., N. L. Goodman, L. Heifets, H. W. Larsh, T. H. Lindner, J. K. McClatchy, M. R. McGinnis, S. H. Siddiqi, and P. Wright.** 1983. Evaluation of the BACTEC radiometric method for recovery of mycobacteria and drug susceptibility testing of *Mycobacterium tuberculosis* from acid-fast smear-positive specimens. *J. Clin. Microbiol.* **18:**689–696.
179. **Roberts, G. D., E. W. Koneman, and Y. K. Kim.** 1991. *Mycobacterium*, p. 304–339. *In* A. Ballows, W. J. Hausler, Jr., K. L. Herrmann, H. D. Isenberg, and H. J. Shadomy (ed.), *Manual of Clinical Microbiology*, 5th ed. American Society for Microbiology, Washington, D.C.
180. **Rogall, T., T. Flohr, and E. C. Böttger.** 1990. Differentiation of *Mycobacterium* species by direct sequencing of amplified DNA. *J. Gen. Microbiol.* **136:**1915–1920.
181. **Rogall, T., J. Wolters, T. Flohr, and E. Böttger.** 1990. Towards a phylogeny and definition of species at the molecular level within the genus *Mycobacterium*. *Int. J. Syst. Bacteriol.* **40:**323–330.
182. **Roiz, M. P., E. Palenque, C. Guerrero, and M. J. Garcia.** 1995. Use of restriction fragment length polymorphism as a genetic marker for typing *Mycobacterium avium* strains. *J. Clin. Microbiol.* **33:**1389–1391.
183. **Runyon, E. H.** 1959. Anonymous mycobacteria in pulmonary disease. *Med. Clin. North Am.* **43:**273–290.
184. **Runyon, E. H.** 1970. Identification of mycobacterial pathogens using colony characteristics. *Am. J. Clin. Pathol.* **54:**578–586.
185. **Saceanu, C., N. Pfeiffer, and T. McLean.** 1993. Evaluation of sputum smears concentrated by cytocentrifugution for detection of acid-fast bacilli. *J. Clin. Microbiol.* **31:** 2371–2374.
186. **Sada, E., P. J. Brennan, T. Herrera, and M. Torres.** 1990. Evaluation of lipoarabinomannan for the serological diagnosis of tuberculosis. *J. Clin. Microbiol.* **28:** 2587–2590.
187. **Saito, H., H. Tomioka, K. Sato, H. Tasaka, and D. Dawson.** 1990. Identification of various serovar strains of *Mycobacterium avium* complex by using DNA probes specific for *Mycobacterium avium* and *Mycobacterium intracellulare*. *J. Clin. Microbiol.* **28:**1694–1697.
188. **Sandin, R. L.** 1996. Polymerase chain reaction and other amplification techniques in mycobacteriology. *Clin. Lab. Med.* **16:**617–639.
189. **Saubolle, M. A., T. E. Kiehn, M. H. White, M. F. Rudinsky, and D. Armstrong.** 1996. *Mycobacterium haemophilum*: microbiology and expanding clinical and geographic spectra of diseases in humans. *Clin. Microbiol. Rev.* **9:** 435–447.
190. **Saubolle, M. A., G. D. Roberts, N. L. Goodman, T. Davis, and V. Jonas.** 1993. Isolates of nontuberculous mycobacteria identified as members of tuberculosis complex, abstr. U-93. *In Abstracts of the 93rd General Meeting of the American Society for Microbiology* 1993. American Society for Microbiology, Washington, D.C.
191. **Schaefer, W.** 1979. Serological identification of atypical mycobacteria. *Methods Microbiol.* **13:**323–344.
192. **Scherer, R., R. Sable, M. Sonnenberg, S. Cooper, P. Spencer, S. Schwimmer, F. Kocka, P. Muthuswamy, and C. Kallick.** 1986. Disseminated infection with *Mycobacterium kansaii* in the acquired immunodeficiency syndrome. *Ann. Intern. Med.* **105:**710–712.
193. **Sewell, D., A. Rashad, W. Rourke, S. Poor, J. McCarthy, and M. Pfaller.** 1993. Comparison of the Septi-Chek AFB and BACTEC systems and conventional culture for recovery of mycobacteria. *J. Clin. Microbiol.* **31:** 2689–2691.
194. **Shafran, S. D., J. Singer, D. P. Zarowny, P. Phillips, I. Salit, S. L. Walmsley, I. W. Fong, M. J. Gill, A. R. Rachlis, R. G. Lalonde, M. M. Fanning, and C. M. Tsoukas.** 1996. A comparison of two regimens for the treatment of *Mycobacterium avium* complex bacteremia in AIDS: rifabutin, ethambutol, and clarithromycin versus rifampin, ethambutol, clofazimine, and ciprofloxacin. *N. Engl. J. Med.* **335:**377–383.
195. **Shinnick, T. M., and V. Jonas.** 1994. Molecular approaches to the diagnosis of tuberculosis, p. 517–530. *In* B. R. Bloom (ed.), *Tuberculosis*. American Society for Microbiology, Washington, D.C.
196. **Silcox, V. A., R. A. Good, and M. M. Floyd.** 1981. Identification of clinically significant *Mycobacterium fortuitum* complex isolates. *J. Clin. Microbiol.* **14:**686–691.
197. **Simor, A. E., I. E. Salit, and H. Vellend.** 1984. The role of *Mycobacterium xenopi* in human disease. *Am. Rev. Respir. Dis.* **129:**435–438.
198. **Small, P., N. McClenny, S. Sigh, G. Schoolnik, L. Tompkins, and P. Mickelsen.** 1993. Molecular strain typing of *Mycobacterium tuberculosis* to confirm cross-contamination in the mycobacteriology laboratory and modification of procedures to minimize occurrence of false-positive cultures. *J. Clin. Microbiol.* **31:**1677–1682.
199. **Smid, I., and M. Salfinger.** 1994. Mycobacterial identification by computer-aided gas-liquid chromatography. *Diagn. Microbiol. Infect. Dis.* **19:**81–88.
200. **Smith M. B., J. S. Bergmann, and G. L. Woods.** 1997. Detection of *Mycobacterium tuberculosis* in BACTEC 12B broth cultures by the Roche Amplicor PCR assay. *J. Clin. Microbiol.* **35:**900–902.
201. **Smithwick, R. W., and C. B. Stratigos.** 1981. Acid-fast microscopy on polycarbonate membrane filter sputum sediments. *J. Clin. Microbiol.* **13:**1109–1113.
202. **Smithwick, R. W., C. B. Stratigos, and H. L. David.** 1975. Use of cetylpyridinium chloride and sodium chloride for the decontamination of sputum specimens that are transported to the laboratory for the isolation of *Mycobacterium tuberculosis*. *J. Clin. Microbiol.* **1:**411–413.
203. **Sniadack, D. H., S. M. Ostroff, M. A. Karlix, R. W. Smithwick, B. Schwartz, M. A. Sprauer, V. A. Silcox, and R. C. Good.** 1993. A nosocomial pseudo-outbreak of *Mycobacterium xenopi* due to a contaminated potable water supply: lessons in prevention. *Infect. Control. Hosp. Epidemiol.* **14:**636–641.
204. **Snider, D.** 1982. The tuberculin skin test. *Am. Rev. Respir. Dis.* **125**(Suppl.)**:**108–118.

205. **Snider, D., W. Jones, and R. Good.** 1984. The usefulness of phage typing *Mycobacterium tuberculosis* isolates. *Am. Rev. Respir. Dis.* **130:**1095–1099.
206. **Soini, H., E. C. Böttger, and M. K. Viljanen.** 1994. Identification of mycobacteria by PCR-based sequence determination of the 32-kilodalton protein gene. *J. Clin. Microbiol.* **32:**2944–2947.
207. **Springer, B., E. C. Böttger, P. Kirschner, and R. J. Wallace, Jr.** 1995. Phylogeny of the *Mycobacterium chelonae*-like organism based on partial sequencing of the 16S rRNA gene and proposal of *Mycobacterium mucogenicum* sp. nov. *J. Clin. Microbiol.* **45:**262–267.
208. **Springer, B., P. Kirschner, G. Rost-Meyer, K.-H. Schroder, R. M. Kroppenstedt, and E. C. Böttger.** 1993. *Mycobacterium interjectum*, a new species isolated from a patient with chronic lymphadenitis. *J. Clin. Microbiol.* **31:**3083–3089.
209. **Springer, B., L. Stockman, K. Teschner, G. D. Roberts, and E. C. Böttger.** 1996. Two-laboratory collective study on identification of mycobacteria: molecular versus phenotypic methods. *J. Clin. Microbiol.* **34:**296–303.
210. **Springer, B., E. Tortoli, I. Richter, R. Grunewald, S. Rusch-Gerdes, K. Uschmann, F. Suter, M. D. Collins, R. M. Kroppenstedt, and E. C. Böttger.** 1995. *Mycobacterium conspicuum* sp. nov., a new species isolated from patients with disseminated infections. *J. Clin. Microbiol.* **33:** 2805–2811.
211. **Springer, B., W.-K. Wu, T. Bodmer, G. Haase, G. E. Pfyffer, R. M. Kroppenstedt, K.-H. Schroder, S. Emler, J. O. Kilburn, P. Kirschner, A. Telenti, M. B. Coyle, and E. C. Böttger.** 1996. Isolation and characterization of a unique group of slowly growing mycobacteria: description of *Mycobacterium lentiflavum* sp. nov. *J. Clin. Microbiol.* **34:**1100–1107.
212. **Stager, C., J. Libonati, S. Siddiqi, J. Davis, N. Hooper, J. Baker, and M. Carter.** 1991. Role of solid media when used in conjunction with the BACTEC system for mycobacterial isolation and identification. *J. Clin. Microbiol.* **29:**154–157.
213. **Steadman, J. E.** 1979. Reliable urease test for identification of mycobacteria. *J. Clin. Microbiol.* **10:**134–137.
214. **Stockman L., B. Springer, E. C. Böttger, and G. D. Roberts.** 1993. *Mycobacterium tuberculosis* nucleic acid probes for rapid diagnosis. *Lancet* **341:**1486.
215. **Stone, B. L., W. J. Burman, M. V. Hildred, E. A. Jarboe, R. R. Reves, and M. L. Wilson.** 1997. The diagnostic yield of acid-fast-bacillus smear-positive specimens. *J. Clin. Microbiol.* **35:**1030–1031.
216. **Straus, W. L., S. M. Ostroff, D. B. Jernigan, T. E. Kiehn, E. M. Sordillo, D. Armstrong, N. Boone, N. Schneider, J. O. Kilburn, V. A. Silcox, V. LaBombardi, and R. C. Good.** 1994. Clinical and epidemiologic characteristics of *Mycobacterium haemophilum*, an emerging pathogen in immunocompromised patients. *Ann. Intern. Med.* **120:**118–125.
217. **Strauss, E., N. Wu, M. A. H. Quraishi, and S. Levine.** 1981. Clinical application of the radioimmunoassay of secretory tuberculoprotein. *Proc. Natl. Acad. Sci. USA* **78:**3214–3217.
218. **Swenson, J. M., C. Thornsberry, and V. A. Silcox.** 1982. Rapidly growing mycobacteria: testing of susceptibility to 34 antimicrobial agents by broth microdilution. *Antimicrob. Agents Chemother.* **22:**186–192.
219. **Swenson, J. M., R. J. Wallace Jr., V. A. Silcox, and C. Thornsberry.** 1985. Antimicrobial susceptibility of *Mycobacterium fortuitum* and *Mycobacterium chelonae*. *Antimicrob. Agents Chemother.* **28:**807–811.
220. **Tabet, S. R., G. M. Goldbaum, T. M. Hooten, K. D. Eisenach, M. D. Cave, and C. M. Nolan.** 1994. Restriction fragment length polymorphism analysis detection of a community-based tuberculosis outbreak among persons infected with human immunodeficiency virus. *J. Infect. Dis.* **169:**189–192.
221. **Teirstein, A., B. Damsker, P. Kirschner, D. Krellenstein, R. Robinson, and M. Chuang.** 1990. Pulmonary infection with MAI: diagnosis, clinical patterns, treatment. *Mt. Sinai J. Med.* **57:**209–215.
222. **Telenti, A., F. Marchesi, M. Balz, F. Bally, E. C. Böttger, and T. Bodmer.** 1993. Rapid identification of mycobacteria to the species level by polymerase chain reaction and restriction enzyme analysis. *J. Clin. Microbiol.* **31:** 175–178.
223. **Tenover, F., J. Crawford, R. Huebner, L. Getter, C. R. Horsburgh, Jr., and R. C. Good.** 1993. The resurgence of tuberculosis: is your laboratory ready? *J. Clin. Microbiol.* **32:**767–770.
224. **Thibert, L., and S. Lapierre.** 1993. Routine application of high-performance liquid chromatography for identification of mycobacteria. *J. Clin. Microbiol.* **31:**1759–1763.
225. **Thorel, M.-F., M. Krichevsky, and V. Levy-Frebault.** 1990. Numerical taxonomy of mycobactin-dependent mycobacteria, emended description of *Mycobacterium avium*, and description of *Mycobacterium avium* subsp. avium subsp. nov., *Mycobacterium avium* subsp. *paratuberculosis* subsp. nov., and *Mycobacterium avium* subsp. *silvaticum* subsp. nov. *Int. J. Syst. Bacteriol.* **40:**254–260.
226. **Tisdall, P. A., D. R. DeYoung, G. D. Roberts, and J. P. Anhalt.** 1982. Identification of clinical isolates of mycobacteria with gas-liquid chromatography: a 10-month follow-up study. *J. Clin. Microbiol.* **16:**400–412.
227. **Tisdall, P. A., G. D. Roberts, and J. P. Anhalt.** 1979. Identification of clinical isolates of mycobacteria with gas-liquid chromatography alone. *J. Clin. Microbiol.* **10:** 506–514.
228. **Tokars, J. I., J. R. Rudnick, K. Kroc, L. Manangan, G. Pugliese, R. E. Huebner, J. Chan, and W. R. Jarvis.** 1996. U.S. hospital mycobacteriology laboratories: status and comparison with state public health department laboratories. *J. Clin. Microbiol.* **34:**680–685.
229. **Toosi, Z., and J. J. Ellner.** 1992. Tuberculosis, p. 1244–1245. *In* S. L. Gorbach, J. G. Bartlett, and N. R. Blacklow (ed.), *Infectious Diseases*. The W. B. Saunders Co., Philadelphia, Pa.
230. **Tortoli, E., F. Lavinia, and M. T. Simonetti.** 1997. Evaluation of a commercial ligase chain reaction kit (Abbott LCX) for direct detection of *Mycobacterium tuberculosis* in pulmonary and extrapulmonary specimens. *J. Clin. Microbiol.* **35:**2424–2426.
231. **Trifiro, S., A.-M. Bourgault, F. Lebel, and P. Rene.** 1990. Ghost mycobacteria on Gram stain. *J. Clin. Microbiol.* **28:**146.
232. **Tsang, A., I. Drupa, M. Goldberg, J. McClatchy, and P. Brennan.** 1983. Use of serology and thin-layer chromatography for the assembly of an authenticated collection of serovars within the *Mycobacterium avium-Mycobacterium intracellulare-Mycobacterium scrofulaceum* complex. *Int. J. Syst. Bacteriol.* **33:**285–292.
233. **Turner, M., J. P. van Vooren, J. deBruyn, E. Serruysl, P. Dierckz, and J. C. Yerhault.** 1988. Humoral immune response in human tuberculosis: immunoglobulins G, A, and M directed against the purified P32 protein antigen of *Mycobacterium bovis* bacillus Calmette-Guérin. *J. Clin. Microbiol.* **26:**1714–1719.
234. **Valero, G., J. Peters, J. H. Jorgensen, and J. R. Graybill.**

1995. Clinical isolates of *Mycobacterium simiae* in San Antonio, Texas. *Am. J. Respir. Crit. Care Med.* **152:** 1555–1557.

235. **Valway, S. E., R. B. Greifinger, M. Papania, J. O. Kilburn, C. Woodley, G. T. DiFerdinando, and S. W. Dooley.** 1994. Multidrug-resistant tuberculosis in the New York state prison system, 1990–1991. *J. Infect. Dis.* **170:**151–156.

236. **Vandervliet, G. M. E., R. A. F. Schukkink, B. Vangemen, P. Schepers, and P. R. Klaster.** 1993. Nucleic acid sequence-based amplification (NASBA) for the identification of mycobacteria. *J. Gen. Microbiol.* **139:** 2423–2429.

237. **Vaneechoutte, M., H. de Beenhouwer, G. Claeys, G. Verschraegen, A. de Rouck, N. Paepe, A. Elaichouni, and F. Portaels.** 1993. Identification of *Mycobacterium* species by using amplified ribosomal DNA restriction analysis. *J. Clin. Microbiol.* **31:**2061–2065.

238. **van Embden, J. D. A., M. D. Cave, J. T. Crawford, J. W. Dale, K. D. Eisenach, B. Gicquel, P. Hermans, C. Martin, R. McAdam, T. M. Shinnick, and P. M. Small.** 1993. Strain identification of *Mycobacterium tuberculosis* by DNA fingerprinting: recommendations for a standardized methodology. *J. Clin. Microbiol.* **31:** 406–409.

239. **Vannier, A., J. Tarrand, and P. Murray.** 1988. Mycobacterial cross contamination during radiometric culturing. *J. Clin. Microbiol.* **26:**1501–1505.

240. **von Reyn, C. F., S. Hennigan, S. Niemczyk, and N. J. Jacobs.** 1991. Effect of delays in processing on the survival of *Mycobacterium avium-M. intracellulare* in the isolator blood culture system. *J. Clin. Microbiol.* **29:** 1211–1214.

241. **Vuorinen, P., A. Miettinen, R. Vuento, and O. Hällström.** 1995. Direct detection of *Mycobacterium tuberculosis* complex in respiratory specimens by GenProbe amplified Mycobacterium Tuberculosis Direct Test and Roche Amplicor Mycobacterium Tuberculosis test. *J. Clin. Microbiol.* **33:**1856–1859.

242. **Wallace, R.** 1987. Nontuberculous mycobacteria and water: a love affair with increasing clinical importance. *Infect. Dis. Clin. North Am.* **1:**677–686.

243. **Wallace, R. J., Jr., B. A. Brown, and G. O. Onyi.** 1992. Skin, soft tissue, and bone infestions due to *Mycobacterium chelonae chelonae*: importance of prior corticosteroid therapy, frequency of disseminated infections, and resistance to oral antimicrobials other than clarithromycin. *J. Infect. Dis.* **166:**405–412.

244. **Wallace, R. J., Jr., D. R. Nash, M. Tsukamur, Z. M. Blacklock, and V. A. Silcox.** 1988. Human disease due to *Mycobacterium smegmatis*. *J. Infect. Dis.* **158:**52–59.

245. **Wallace, R. J., Jr., V. A. Silcox, M. Tsukamura, B. A. Brown, J. O. Kilburn, W. R. Butler, and G. O. Onyi.** 1993. Clinical significance, biochemical features, and susceptibility patterns of sporadic isolates of the *Mycobacterium chelonae*-like organism. *J. Clin. Microbiol.* **31:** 3231–3239.

246. **Wallace, R. J., Jr., J. M. Swenson, V. Silcox, R. Good, J. A. Tschen, and M. S. Stone.** 1983. Spectrum of disease due to rapidly growing mycobacteria. *Rev. Infect. Dis.* **5:** 657–679.

247. **Walton, D. T., and M. Valesco.** 1991. Identification of *Mycobacterium gordonae* from culture by the Gen-Probe rapid diagnostic system: evaluation of 218 isolates and potential sources of false-negative results. *J. Clin. Microbiol.* **29:**1850–1854.

248. **Warren, N. G., and J. R. Cordts.** 1996. Activities and recommendations by the Association of State and Territorial Public Health Laboratory Directors. *Clin. Lab. Med.* **16:**731–742.

249. **Wasilauskas, B., and R. Morrell, Jr.** 1994. Inhibitory effect of the isolator blood culture system on growth of *Mycobacterium avium-M. intracellulare* in BACTEC 12B bottles. *J. Clin. Microbiol.* **32:**654–657.

250. **Watanakunakorn, C., and A. Trott.** 1973. Vertebral osteomyelitis due to *Mycobacterium kansasii*. *Am. Rev. Respir. Dis.* **107:**846–850.

251. **Wayne, L.** 1985. The "atypical" mycobacteria: recognition and disease association. *Crit. Rev. Microbiol.* **12:** 185–222.

252. **Wayne, L., R. Good, M. Krichevsky, Z. Blacklock, H. David, D. Dawson, W. Gross, J. Hawkins, V. Levy-Frebault, C. McManus, F. Portaels, S. Rusch-Gerdes, K. Schroder, V. Silcox, M. Tsukamura, L. Van den Breen, and M. Yakrus.** 1991. Fourth report of the cooperative open-ended study of slowly growing mycobacteria of the International Working Group on Mycobacterial Taxonomy. *Int. J. Syst. Bacteriol.* **41:**463–472.

253. **Wayne, L., and H. Sramek.** 1992. Agents of newly recognized or infrequently encountered mycobacterial diseases. *Clin. Microbiol. Rev.* **5:**1–25.

254. **Welch, D., A. Guruswamy, S. Sides, C. Shaw, and M. Gilchrist.** 1993. Timely culture of mycobacteria which utilizes a microcolony method. *J. Clin. Microbiol.* **31:** 2178–2184.

255. **Whittier, S., K. Olivier, P. Gilligan, M. Knowles, P. Della-Latta, and The Nontuberculous Mycobacteria in Cystic Fibrosis Study Group.** 1997. Proficiency testing of clinical microbiology laboratories using modified decontamination procedures for detection of nontuberculous mycobacteria in sputum samples from cystic fibrosis patients. *J. Clin. Microbiol.* **35:**2706–2708.

256. **Witebsky, F. G., J. Keiser, P. Conville, R. Bryan, C. H. Park, R. Walker, and S. H. Siddiqi.** 1988. Comparison of BACTEC 13A medium and DuPont Isolator for detection of mycobacteria. *J. Clin. Microbiol.* **256:**1501–1505.

257. **Woods, G. L., G. Fish, M. Plaunt, and T. Murphy.** 1997. Clinical evaluation of Difco ESP culture system II for growth and detection of mycobacteria. *J. Clin. Microbiol.* **35:**121–124.

258. **Woods, G. L., T. A. Long, and F. G. Witebsky.** 1996. Mycobacterial testing in clinical laboratories that participate in the College of American Pathologists mycobacteriology surveys. Changes in practices based on responses to 1992, 1993, and 1995 questionnaires. *Arch. Pathol. Lab. Med.* **120:**429–435.

259. **Woods, G. L., and J. C. Ridderhof.** 1996. Quality assurance in the mycobacteriology laboratory. *Clin. Lab. Med.* **16:**657–675.

260. **World Health Organization.** 1994. TB epidemic outpaces new drug development.

261. **World Health Organization Study Group.** 1985. Epidemiology of leprosy in relation to control. World Health Organization technical report series 716. World Health Organization, Geneva, Switzerland.

262. **Yagupsky, P., D. Kaminski, K. Palmer, and F. Nolte.** 1990. Cord formation in BACTEC 7H12 medium for rapid, presumptive identification of *Mycobacterium tuberculosis* complex. *J. Clin. Microbiol.* **28:**1451–1453.

263. **Yajko, D. M., P. S. Nassos, C. A. Sanders, P. C. Gonzalez, A. L. Reingold, C. R. Horsburgh, P. Hopewell, D. P. Chin, and W. K. Hadley.** 1993. Comparison of four decontamination methods for recovery of *Mycobacterium avium* complex from stools. *J. Clin. Microbiol.* **31:** 302–306.

264. **Yakrus, M. A., M. W. Reeves, and S. B. Hunter.** 1992. Characterization of isolates of *Mycobacterium avium* sero-

types 4 and 8 from patients with AIDS by multilocus enzyme electrophoresis. *J. Clin. Microbiol.* **30:**1474–1478.

265. **Yamauchi, T., P. Ferrieri, and B. F. Anthony.** 1980. The aetiology of acute cervical adenitis in children: serological and bacteriological studies. *J. Med. Microbiol.* **13:**37–43.

266. **Yanagihara, D., V. Barr, C. Krisley, A. Tsang, J. McClatchy, and P. Brennan.** 1985. Enzyme-linked immunosorbent assay of glycolipid antigens for identification of mycobacteria. *J. Clin. Microbiol.* **21:**569–574.

267. **Yates, M. D., A. Pozniak, A. H. C. Uttley, R. Clarke, and J. M. Grange.** 1997. Isolation of environmental mycobacteria from clinical specimens in south-east England: 1973–1993. *Int. J. Tuberc. Lung Dis.* **1:**75–80.

268. **Zanetti, S., F. Ardito, L. Sechi, M. Sanguinetti, P. Molicotti, G. Delogu, M. P. Pinna, A. Nacci, and F. Fadda.** 1997. Evaluation of a nonradiometric system (BACTEC 9000MB) for detection of mycobacteria in human clinical samples. *J. Clin. Microbiol.* **35:**2072–2075.

269. **Zhou, A. T., W. L. Ma, P. Y. Zhang, and R. A. Cole.** 1996. Detection of pulmonary and extrapulmonary tuberculosis patients with the 38-kilodalton antigen from *Mycobacterium tuberculosis* in a rapid membrane-based assay. *Clin. Diagn. Lab. Immunol.* **3:**337–341.

Algorithms for Identification of Aerobic Gram-Negative Bacteria

PAUL C. SCHRECKENBERGER, J. MICHAEL JANDA, JANE D. WONG, AND ELLEN JO BARON

26

This algorithm is meant to assist in the identification of organisms that are not readily identified by methods in place in most clinical laboratories. Microbiologists planning to identify an unknown gram-negative rod begin with colonies on an agar plate. Our definition of "good growth on blood agar plate (BAP)" is the presence of distinct colonies (approximately 1 mm) on Trypticase soy agar–5% sheep blood after 24 h of incubation. Poor growth indicates that more than 24 h of incubation is necessary for the development of distinct colonies. If an organism fails to grow on BAP after 72 h, it is considered to show "no growth." Morphological and phenotypic criteria were chosen not only for their discriminatory value but also because the methods are available in most laboratories. Cellular morphology is determined by using a Gram stain from a young colony on a BAP. The description of "tiny coccobacilli" used for *Brucella* and *Francisella* implies almost indiscernible cells resembling grains of sand. For many organisms with pleomorphic morphologies, we chose to represent the dominant shape.

The urea test refers to conventional Christensen's urea reaction after 24 h of incubation, whereas the rapid urea result is read after 4 h. Glucose fermentation refers to an acid reaction in the butt of a Kligler iron agar (KIA) or triple sugar iron (TSI) tube. "Glucose oxidized" refers to acid production in the upper portion of oxidative-fermentative (OF) media. "BHI + serum" refers to BHI with 10% (vol/vol) serum added. The oxidase test refers to results obtained with the *N*,*N*,*N*,*N*-tetramethyl-*p*-phenylenediamine dihydrochloride reagent. Motility is best observed by preparing a wet preparation from a young colony on a BAP. Decarboxylase reactions are determined by using an extremely turbid inoculum in Moeller's media (heavier than usual inoculum). Polymyxin B sensitivity is indicated by any zone of inhibition surrounding a 300-U disk on a BAP. For difficult-to-identify organisms, Ehrlich's extraction method for indole detection is used (see chapter 35). "Esculin" refers to hydrolysis of esculin in medium without bile.

This algorithm is dichotomous, since many organisms may fall into more than one group due to phenotypic variability of a given trait. The presence of two or more atypical traits or a major variation from the ideal phenotype depicted in this algorithm, due to antibiotic use, auxotrophy, or other reasons, may limit the algorithm's utility. This algorithm is intended as a guide to a presumptive identification of an unknown isolate. The reference chapter describing that organism should be consulted to determine the definitive identification.

TABLE 1 Identification algorithm for gram-negative bacteria that grow well on blood agar

Cell morphology	Glucose fermented	Pigmented colonies	Oxidase	6% NaCl	Motility	Glucose oxidized	Rapid urea	Sucrose	Mannitol	Lysine decarboxylase or OF lactose	Lysine decarboxylase	OF maltose	Xylose or trehalose	Fluorescent pigment	Polymyxin B	Phenylalanine deaminase	H_2S in TSI	Indole	Esculin	Nitrate to gas	Organism group (chapter)
Rods	+	Purple																			*Chromobacterium* (36)
		Other	−	+																	*Vibrio metschnikovii* (31)
				−									+								*Enterobacteriaceae* (27–30)
													−			+					*Proteus*, *Morganella* (30)
																−	+				*Edwardsiella* (30)
																	−				*Pasteurella bettyae* (42)
			+	+																	*Vibrio* (31)
				−	−			+													*Pasteurella* (42)
								−													EF-4b (36)
					+																*Aeromonas*, *Plesiomonas* (32)
	−	Pink																			*Methylobacterium*, *Roseomonas* (35)
		Not pink	−		+	+			+	+											*Burkholderia cepacia* (34)
										Both negative		+									*Pseudomonas luteola*, *P. oryzihabitans* (33)
												−									*Burkholderia gladioli* (34)
									−		+										*Stenotrophomonas maltophilia* (34)
											−										*Sphingomonas paucimobilis* (35)
						−															*Bordetella trematum* (35, 40)

(Continued on next page)

TABLE 1 Identification algorithm for gram-negative bacteria that grow well on blood agar (*Continued*)

Cell morphology	Glucose fermented	Pigmented colonies	Oxidase	6% NaCl	Motility	Glucose oxidized	Rapid urea	Sucrose	Mannitol	Lysine decarboxylase or OF lactose	Lysine decarboxylase	OF maltose	Xylose or trehalose	Fluorescent pigment	Polymyxin B	Phenylalanine deaminase	H_2S in TSI	Indole	Esculin	Nitrate to gas	Organism group (chapter)
					–																*Acinetobacter*, *Bordetella*, NO-1, EO-5 (35), *Bordetella* (40)
			+		+	+								+							*Pseudomonas aeruginosa*, *P. fluorescens*, *P. putida* (33)
														–	R						*Burkholderia*, *Ralstonia* (34)
															S		+				*Shewanella* (35)
																	–	+			*Balneatrix* (35)
																		–	+		*S. paucimobilis*, *Ochrobactrum anthropi*, *Agrobacterium*, *Achromobacter* (35)
																			–		*O. anthropi* (35), *Pseudomonas* (33), *Acidovorax* (34)
						–	+														*Bordetella bronchiseptica* (40), *Oligella ureolytica*, IVc-2 (35)
							–												+		*Brevundimonas vesicularis* (34), O-1, O-2 (35)
																			–	+	*Pseudomonas* CDC grp. 1 (33), *Achromobacter xylosoxidans* subsp. denitrificans, WO-1 (35)
																				–	*Pseudomonas alcaligenes*, *P. pseudoalcaligenes* (33), *Brevundimonas diminuta* (34), various (35)
Diplococci			+																		*Neisseria*, *Moraxella catarrhalis* (38)
			–																		*Acinetobacter* (35)

TABLE 2 Identification algorithm for gram-negative bacteria with poor or no growth on blood agar

Growth on BAP	Growth only on:	Cellular morphology	Urea	Pigmented colonies	Oxidase	6% NaCl	H_2S in TSI	Cauliflower-like colony	O-shaped cells	Require X ± V	Organism group (chapter)
Poor growth on BAP		Tiny coccobacilli	+								*Brucella* (41)
			–		–						*Francisella* (44)
					+		+				*Francisella philomiragia* (44)
							–				*Bordetella* (40)
		Rods		Pink							*Methylobacterium*, *Roseomonas* (35)
				Other				+			*Bartonella* (43)
								–			*Haemophilus aphrophilus* (39), various (36)
		Diplococci							+		EO-2 (35)
									–		*Neisseria*, *Moraxella* (38)
No growth on BAP	Chocolate	Coccobacilli									*Neisseria* (38)
		Fusiform rods									*Capnocytophaga* (36)
		Rods						+			*Bartonella*, *Afipia* (43)
								–		+	*Haemophilus* (39)
										–	*Francisella* (44)
	BCYE[a]	Long gram-negative rods									*Legionella* (37)
		Regular rods			+						*Bordetella* (40)
					–						*Francisella* (44)
	BHI + serum	Pleomorphic, beaded filamentous rods									*Streptobacillus* (36)
		Small rods									*Bartonella*, *Afipia* (43)

[a] BCYE, buffered charcoal yeast extract agar.

Enterobacteriaceae: Introduction and Identification

J. J. FARMER III

27

INTRODUCTION

In the fifth edition of this Manual in 1991, Farmer and Kelly commented that it was becoming more difficult to cover the family *Enterobacteriaceae* in a single chapter. The family includes the plague bacillus *Yersinia pestis*; the typhoid bacillus *Salmonella* serotype Typhi (*Salmonella typhi*); four genera with species that often cause diarrhea and other intestinal infections; seven species that frequently cause nosocomial infections; many other organisms that occasionally cause human or animal infections; dozens of species that occasionally occur in human clinical specimens; and many other species that do not occur in human clinical specimens but can be confused with those that do. In the fifth edition, all these organisms were covered in a single chapter on *Enterobacteriaceae*, divided into six parts. In the sixth edition, the material on *Enterobacteriaceae* was divided among three chapters: an introduction to the family that described the overall plan for isolation and identification; a chapter that covered *Salmonella, Shigella, Escherichia coli*, and *Yersinia*, the four genera that comprise the enteric pathogens; and a chapter that covered the remaining genera and species in the family. In the current edition further subdivision has occurred and there are now four chapters on *Enterobacteriaceae*: chapters 27 through 30.

Because of space limitations, many topics in the present chapter are discussed briefly and only a few primary literature citations are given. Several books, reviews, and chapters are recommended for more detailed information (4, 12, 13, 22, 27, 33, 39, 71).

NOMENCLATURE AND CLASSIFICATION

The nomenclature and classification of the genera, species, subspecies, biogroups, and serotypes of the *Enterobacteriaceae* have always been topics for hot debate and differing opinions (12, 13, 22, 27, 33, 69, 71). Until recently, genera and species were defined by biochemical and antigenic analysis. Newer techniques such as nucleic acid hybridization and nucleic acid sequencing that measure evolutionary distance (see chapter 14) have made it possible to determine the evolutionary relationships of organisms in the family (13, 33). The use of DNA-DNA hybridization has led to the discovery of many new species and has resulted in the reclassification of some of the older ones (12, 13, 33).

This chapter includes the different names and classifications that clinical microbiologists are likely to encounter in the scientific literature and in material accompanying commercial products. The nomenclature and classification given in Table 1 are a compromise based on all available evidence and include most of the genera, species, subspecies, biogroups, and unnamed Enteric Groups included in the family. If two names are widely used for the same organism, both are given in this chapter with one in parentheses. Most of the "nonclinical" organisms in the family are also included because there is a possibility that they will be isolated from a human clinical specimen some day (33, 36).

Most of the newly described organisms in Table 1 are only very rarely found in clinical specimens (33); most clinically significant isolates belong to 20 to 25 species that have been well known for many years (27). This is illustrated by the lists of genera that most often cause bacteremia (Table 2), nosocomial infections (Table 3), and infections of the gastrointestinal tract (Table 4). The original citations for many of the newer genera (1, 9, 10, 35, 41, 43, 45, 46, 57–60, 63, 77, 88, 89) and species (2, 3, 7, 8, 14–19, 21, 23, 25, 28–31, 34, 36, 38, 40, 42, 44, 47–50, 52, 54–56, 61, 62, 64–66, 70, 73, 75, 77–79, 85, 90, 92) are given in the References section.

New Species

Several new species have been described since the sixth edition was published in 1995. These include *Buttiauxella ferragutiae* (77), *Buttiauxella gaviniae* (77), *Buttiauxella brennerae* (77), *Buttiauxella izardii* (77), *Buttiauxella noackiae** (77), *Buttiauxella warmboldiae* (77), *Citrobacter rodentium* (formerly *Citrobacter* species 9) (16), *Enterobacter kobei** (70), *Enterobacter pyrinus* (21), *Kluyvera cochleae* (77), and *Kluyvera georgiana** (77) (those found in human clinical specimens are indicated by an asterisk). These new species have been added to Table 1, except for *Enterobacter kobei* (reference strains have been unavailable). All newly described species of *Enterobacteriaceae* will eventually be studied and added.

The Expanding Number of *Enterobacteriaceae* Species

How many species of *Enterobacteriaceae* are there? There are probably many hundreds, if not thousands. This is becoming more apparent as methods such as DNA-DNA hybridization and 16S rRNA sequencing are being used routinely to study

TABLE 1 Biochemical reactions of the named species, biogroups, and Enteric Groups of the family *Enterobacteriaceae*[a]

Organism	Indole production	Methyl red	Voges-Proskauer	Citrate (Simmons)	Hydrogen sulfide (TSI)	Urea hydrolysis	Phenylalanine deaminase	Lysine decarboxylase	Arginine dihydrolase	Ornithine decarboxylase	Motility (36°C)	Gelatin hydrolysis (22°C)	Growth in KCN	Malonate utilization	D-Glucose, acid	D-Glucose, gas	Lactose fermentation	Sucrose fermentation	D-Mannitol fermentation	Dulcitol fermentation	Salicin fermentation	Adonitol fermentation	*myo*-Inositol fermentation	D-Sorbitol fermentation	L-Arabinose fermentation	Raffinose fermentation	L-Rhamnose fermentation	Maltose fermentation	D-Xylose fermentation	Trehalose fermentation	Cellobiose fermentation	alpha-Methyl-D-glucoside fermentation	Erythritol fermentation	Esculin hydrolysis	Melibiose fermentation	D-Arabitol fermentation	Glycerol fermentation	Mucate fermentation	Tartrate, Jordan's	Acetate utilization	Lipase (corn oil)	DNase at 25°C	Nitrate → Nitrite	Oxidase, Kovacs	ONPG test	Yellow pigment	D-Mannose fermentation
Budvicia																																															
B. aquatica[*] [b]	0	93	0	0	80	33	0	0	0	0	27	0	0	0	100	53	87	0	60	0	0	0	0	0	80	0	100	0	93	0	0	0	0	0	0	27	0	20	27	0	0	0	100	0	93	0	0
Buttiauxella																																															
B. agrestis	0	100	0	100	0	0	0	0	0	100	100	0	80	60	100	100	100	0	100	0	100	0	0	0	100	100	100	100	100	100	100	0	0	100	100	0	60	100	60	0	0	0	100	0	100	0	100
B. brennerae	0	100	0	0	0	0	0	0	0	33	100	0	100	100	100	100	67	0	100	0	100	67	0	0	100	100	33	100	100	100	100	0	0	100	100	67	67	67	0	0	0	0	100	0	100	0	100
B. ferragutiae	0	100	0	0	0	0	0	100	0	80	60	0	40	0	100	100	0	0	100	0	100	0	0	100	100	0	100	100	100	100	100	40	0	100	0	0	0	60	0	0	0	0	100	0	100	0	100
B. gaviniae	0	100	0	20	0	0	0	0	20	0	80	0	60	100	100	40	60	0	100	0	100	100	0	0	100	0	100	60	100	100	100	0	0	100	0	80	0	80	40	0	0	0	100	0	100	0	100
B. izardi	0	100	0	0	0	0	0	0	0	100	100	0	67	100	100	100	100	0	100	0	100	0	0	0	100	33	100	100	100	100	100	0	0	100	67	0	33	100	67	0	0	0	100	0	100	0	100
B. noackiae[*]	33	100	0	33	0	0	100	0	67	0	100	0	100	100	100	100	0	0	100	0	100	0	0	0	100	0	100	100	100	100	100	33	0	100	0	0	0	100	100	0	0	0	100	0	100	0	100
B. warmboldiae	0	100	0	33	0	0	100	0	0	0	100	0	33	100	100	100	0	0	100	0	100	0	67	0	100	0	100	100	100	100	100	0	0	100	0	0	0	0	0	0	0	0	100	0	100	0	100
Cedecea																																															
C. davisae[*]	0	100	50	95	0	0	0	0	50	95	95	0	86	91	100	70	19	100	100	0	99	0	0	0	0	10	0	100	100	100	100	5	0	45	0	100	0	0	0	0	91	0	100	0	90	0	100
C. lapagei[*]	0	40	80	99	0	0	0	0	80	0	80	0	100	99	100	100	60	0	100	0	100	0	0	0	0	0	0	100	0	100	100	0	0	100	0	100	0	0	0	60	100	0	100	0	99	0	100
C. neteri[*]	0	100	50	100	0	0	0	0	100	0	100	0	65	100	100	100	35	100	100	0	100	0	0	100	0	0	0	100	100	100	100	0	0	100	0	100	0	0	0	0	100	0	100	0	100	0	100
Cedecea species 3[*]	0	100	50	100	0	0	0	0	100	0	100	0	100	0	100	100	0	50	100	0	100	0	0	0	0	100	0	100	100	100	100	50	0	100	100	100	0	0	0	50	100	0	100	0	100	0	100
Cedecea species 5[*]	0	100	50	100	0	0	0	0	50	50	100	0	100	0	100	100	0	100	100	0	100	0	0	100	0	100	0	100	100	100	100	0	0	100	100	100	0	0	0	50	50	0	100	0	100	0	100
Citrobacter																																															
C. freundii[*]	33	100	0	78	78	44	0	0	67	0	89	0	89	11	100	89	78	89	100	11	0	0	0	100	100	44	100	100	89	100	44	11	0	0	100	0	100	100	100	44	0	0	100	0	89	0	100
C. diversus (koseri)[*]	99	100	0	99	0	75	0	0	80	99	95	0	0	95	100	98	50	40	99	40	15	99	0	99	99	0	99	100	100	100	99	40	0	1	0	98	99	95	90	75	0	0	100	0	99	0	100
C. amalonaticus[*]	100	100	0	95	5	85	0	0	85	95	95	0	99	1	100	97	35	9	100	1	30	0	0	99	99	5	100	99	99	100	100	2	0	5	0	0	60	96	96	86	0	0	99	0	97	0	100
C. farmeri[*]	100	100	0	10	0	59	0	0	85	100	97	0	93	0	100	96	15	100	100	2	9	0	0	98	100	100	100	100	100	100	100	75	0	0	100	0	65	100	93	80	0	0	100	0	100	0	100
C. youngae[*]	15	100	0	75	65	80	0	0	50	5	95	0	95	5	100	75	25	20	100	85	10	0	5	100	100	10	100	95	100	100	45	0	0	5	10	5	90	100	100	65	0	0	85	0	90	0	100
C. braakii[*]	33	100	0	87	60	47	0	0	67	93	87	0	100	0	100	93	80	7	100	33	0	0	0	100	100	7	100	100	100	100	73	33	0	0	80	0	87	100	93	53	0	0	100	0	80	0	100
C. werkmanii[*]	0	100	0	100	100	100	0	0	100	0	100	0	100	100	100	100	17	0	100	0	0	0	0	100	100	0	100	100	100	100	0	0	0	0	0	0	100	100	100	100	0	0	100	0	100	0	100
C. sedlakii[*]	83	100	0	83	0	100	0	0	100	100	100	0	100	100	100	100	100	0	100	100	17	0	0	100	100	0	100	100	100	100	100	0	0	17	100	0	83	100	100	83	0	0	100	0	100	0	100
C. rodentium[*]	0	100	0	0	0	100	0	0	0	100	0	0	0	100	100	100	100	0	100	0	0	0	0	100	100	0	100	100	100	100	100	0	0	0	0	0	0	100	100	0	0	0	100	0	100	0	100
Citrobacter species 10[*]	0	100	0	33	67	0	0	0	33	0	67	0	100	100	100	100	67	33	100	0	0	0	0	100	100	0	100	100	100	100	67	0	0	0	67	0	67	67	100	0	0	0	100	0	67	0	100
Citrobacter species 11[*]	100	100	0	100	67	67	0	0	67	0	100	0	100	0	100	100	67	33	100	100	33	0	0	100	100	33	100	100	100	100	100	0	0	0	33	0	100	100	100	33	0	0	100	0	100	0	100
Edwardsiella																																															
E. tarda[*]	99	100	0	1	100	0	0	100	0	100	98	0	0	0	100	100	0	0	0	0	0	0	0	0	9	0	0	100	0	0	0	0	0	0	0	0	30	0	25	0	0	0	100	0	0	0	100
E. tarda biogroup 1[*]	100	100	0	0	0	0	0	100	0	100	100	0	0	0	100	50	0	100	100	0	0	0	0	0	100	0	0	100	0	0	0	0	0	0	0	0	0	0	0	0	0	0	100	0	0	0	100
E. hoshinae[*]	50	100	0	0	0	0	0	100	0	95	100	0	0	100	100	35	0	100	100	0	50	0	0	0	13	0	0	100	0	100	0	0	0	0	0	0	65	0	0	0	0	0	100	0	0	0	100
E. ictaluri	0	0	0	0	0	0	0	100	0	65	0	0	0	0	100	50	0	0	0	0	0	0	0	0	0	0	0	100	0	0	0	0	0	0	0	0	0	0	0	0	0	0	100	0	0	0	100
Enterobacter																																															
E. aerogenes[*]	0	5	98	95	0	2	0	98	0	98	97	0	98	95	100	100	95	100	100	5	100	98	95	100	100	96	99	99	100	100	100	95	0	98	99	100	98	90	95	50	0	0	100	0	100	0	95
E. cloacae[*]	0	5	100	100	0	65	0	0	97	96	95	0	98	75	100	100	93	97	100	15	75	25	15	95	100	97	92	100	99	100	99	85	0	30	90	15	40	75	30	75	0	0	99	0	99	0	100
E. agglomerans group[*]	20	50	70	50	0	20	20	0	0	0	85	2	35	65	100	20	40	75	100	15	65	7	15	30	95	30	85	89	93	97	55	7	0	60	50	50	30	40	25	30	0	0	85	0	90	75	98
E. gergoviae[*]	0	5	100	99	0	93	0	90	0	100	90	0	0	96	100	98	55	98	99	0	99	0	0	0	99	97	99	100	99	100	99	2	0	97	97	97	100	2	97	93	0	0	99	0	97	0	100
E. sakazakii[*]	11	5	100	99	0	1	50	0	99	91	96	0	99	18	100	98	99	100	100	5	99	0	75	0	100	99	100	100	100	100	100	96	0	100	100	0	15	1	1	96	0	0	99	0	100	98	100
E. taylorae[*] *(cancerogenus)*	0	5	100	100	0	1	0	0	94	99	99	0	98	100	100	100	10	0	100	0	92	0	0	1	100	0	100	99	100	100	100	1	0	90	0	0	1	75	0	35	0	0	100	0	100	0	100
E. amnigenus biogroup 1[*]	0	7	100	70	0	0	0	0	9	55	92	0	100	91	100	100	70	100	100	0	91	0	0	9	100	100	100	100	100	100	100	55	0	91	100	0	0	35	9	0	0	0	100	0	91	0	100
E. amnigenus biogroup 2[*]	0	65	100	100	0	0	0	0	35	100	100	0	100	100	100	100	35	0	100	0	100	0	0	100	100	0	100	100	100	100	100	100	0	100	100	0	0	100	0	0	0	0	100	0	100	0	100
E. asburiae[*]	0	100	2	100	0	60	0	0	21	95	0	0	97	3	100	95	75	100	100	0	100	0	0	100	100	70	5	100	97	100	100	95	0	95	0	0	11	21	30	87	0	0	100	0	100	0	100

(continued on next page)

(Continued)

TABLE 1 Biochemical reactions of the named species, biogroups, and Enteric Groups of the family *Enterobacteriaceae*[a] (*Continued*)

Organism	Indole production	Methyl red	Voges-Proskauer	Citrate (Simmons)	Hydrogen sulfide (TSI)	Urea hydrolysis	Phenylalanine deaminase	Lysine decarboxylase	Arginine dihydrolase	Ornithine decarboxylase	Motility (36°C)	Gelatin hydrolysis (22°C)	Growth in KCN	Malonate utilization	D-Glucose, acid	D-Glucose, gas	Lactose fermentation	Sucrose fermentation	D-Mannitol fermentation	Dulcitol fermentation	Salicin fermentation	Adonitol fermentation	*myo*-Inositol fermentation	D-Sorbitol fermentation	L-Arabinose fermentation	Raffinose fermentation	L-Rhamnose fermentation	Maltose fermentation	D-Xylose fermentation	Trehalose fermentation	Cellobiose fermentation	alpha-Methyl-D-glucoside fermentation	Erythritol fermentation	Esculin hydrolysis	Melibiose fermentation	D-Arabitol fermentation	Glycerol fermentation	Mucate fermentation	Tartrate, Jordan's	Acetate utilization	Lipase (corn oil)	DNase at 25°C	Nitrate → Nitrite	Oxidase, Kovacs	ONPG test	Yellow pigment	D-Mannose fermentation
Enterobacter (continued)																																															
*E. hormaechei**	0	57	100	96	0	87	4	0	78	91	52	0	100	100	100	83	9	100	100	87	44	0	0	0	100	0	100	100	96	100	100	83	0	0	0	0	4	96	13	74	0	0	100	0	95	0	100
*E. intermedium**	0	100	100	65	0	0	0	0	0	89	89	0	65	100	100	100	100	65	100	100	100	0	0	100	100	100	100	100	100	100	100	100	0	100	100	0	100	100	100	0	0	0	100	0	100	0	100
E. cancerogenus	0	0	100	100	0	0	0	0	100	100	100	0	100	100	100	100	0	0	100	0	100	0	0	0	100	0	100	100	100	100	100	0	0	100	0	0	0	100	0	33	0	0	100	0	100	0	100
E. dissolvens	0	0	100	100	0	100	0	0	100	100	0	0	100	100	100	100	0	100	100	0	100	0	0	100	100	100	100	100	100	100	100	100	0	100	100	0	0	100	0	100	0	0	100	0	100	0	100
E. nimipressuralis	0	100	100	0	0	0	0	0	0	100	0	0	100	100	100	100	0	0	100	0	100	0	0	100	100	0	100	100	100	100	100	100	0	100	100	0	0	100	0	0	0	0	100	0	100	0	100
E. pyrinus	0	29	86	0	0	86	0	100	0	100	43	0	0	86	100	100	14	100	100	0	100	0	100	0	100	0	100	100	0	100	100	0	0	100	14	100	14	0	86	14	0	0	100	0	100	0	100
Escherichia																																															
*E. coli**	98	99	0	1	1	1	0	90	17	65	95	0	3	0	100	95	95	50	98	60	40	5	1	94	99	50	80	95	95	98	2	0	0	35	75	5	75	95	95	90	0	0	100	0	95	0	98
E. coli, inactive*	80	95	0	1	1	1	0	40	3	20	5	0	1	0	100	5	25	15	93	40	10	3	1	75	85	15	65	80	70	90	2	0	0	5	40	5	65	30	85	40	0	0	98	0	45	0	97
*E. fergusonii**	98	100	0	17	0	0	0	95	5	100	93	0	0	35	100	95	0	0	98	60	65	98	0	0	98	0	92	96	96	96	96	0	0	46	0	100	20	0	96	96	0	0	100	0	83	0	100
*E. hermannii**	99	100	0	1	0	0	0	6	0	100	99	0	94	0	100	97	45	45	100	19	40	0	0	0	100	40	97	100	100	100	97	0	0	40	0	8	3	97	35	78	0	0	100	0	98	98	100
*E. vulneris**	0	100	0	0	0	0	0	85	30	0	100	0	15	85	100	97	15	8	100	0	30	0	0	1	100	99	93	100	100	100	100	25	0	20	100	0	25	78	2	30	0	0	100	0	100	50	100
E. blattae	0	100	0	50	0	0	0	100	0	100	0	0	0	100	100	100	0	0	0	0	0	0	0	0	100	0	100	100	100	75	0	0	0	0	0	0	100	50	50	0	0	0	100	0	0	0	100
Shigella																																															
S. dysenteride (Group A)*	45	99	0	0	0	0	0	0	2	0	0	0	0	0	100	0	0	0	0	5	0	0	0	30	45	0	30	15	4	90	0	0	0	0	0	0	10	0	75	0	0	0	99	0	30	0	100
S. flexneri (Group B)*	50	100	0	0	0	0	0	0	5	0	0	0	0	0	100	3	1	1	95	1	0	0	0	29	60	40	5	30	2	65	0	0	0	0	55	1	10	0	30	8	0	0	99	0	1	0	100
S. boydii (Group C)*	25	100	0	0	0	0	0	0	18	2	0	0	0	0	100	0	1	0	97	5	0	0	0	43	94	0	1	20	11	85	0	0	0	0	15	0	50	0	50	0	0	0	100	0	10	0	100
S. sonnei (Group D)*	0	100	0	0	0	0	0	0	2	98	0	0	0	0	100	0	2	1	99	0	0	0	0	2	95	3	75	90	2	100	5	0	0	0	25	0	15	10	90	0	0	0	100	0	90	0	100
Ewingella																																															
*E. americana**	0	84	95	95	0	0	0	0	0	0	60	0	5	0	100	0	70	0	100	0	80	0	0	0	0	0	23	16	13	99	10	0	0	50	0	99	24	0	35	10	0	0	97	0	85	0	99
Hafnia																																															
*H. alvei**	0	40	85	10	0	4	0	100	6	98	85	0	95	50	100	98	5	10	99	0	13	0	0	0	95	2	97	100	98	95	15	0	0	7	0	0	95	0	70	15	0	0	100	0	90	0	100
H. alvei biogroup 1	0	85	70	0	0	0	0	100	0	45	0	0	0	45	100	0	0	0	55	0	55	0	0	0	0	0	0	0	0	70	0	0	0	0	0	0	0	0	30	0	0	0	100	0	30	0	100
Klebsiella																																															
*K. pneumoniae**	0	10	98	98	0	95	0	98	0	0	0	0	98	93	100	97	98	99	99	30	99	90	95	99	99	99	99	98	99	99	98	90	0	99	99	98	97	90	95	75	0	0	99	0	99	0	99
*K. oxytoca**	99	20	95	95	0	90	1	99	0	0	0	0	97	98	100	97	100	100	99	55	100	99	98	99	98	100	100	100	100	100	100	98	2	100	99	98	99	93	98	90	0	0	100	0	100	1	100
*K. ornithinolytica**	100	96	70	100	0	100	0	100	0	100	0	0	100	100	100	100	100	100	100	10	100	100	95	100	100	100	100	100	100	100	100	100	0	100	100	100	100	96	100	95	0	0	100	0	100	0	100
*K. planticola**	20	100	98	100	0	98	0	100	0	0	0	0	100	100	100	100	100	100	100	15	100	100	100	92	100	100	100	100	100	100	100	100	0	100	100	100	100	100	100	62	0	0	100	0	100	1	100
*K. ozaenae**	0	98	0	30	0	10	0	40	6	3	0	0	88	3	100	50	30	20	100	2	97	97	55	65	98	90	55	95	95	98	92	70	0	80	97	95	65	25	50	2	0	0	80	0	80	0	100
*K. rhinoscleromatis**	0	100	0	0	0	0	0	0	0	0	0	0	80	95	100	0	0	75	100	0	98	100	95	100	100	90	96	100	100	100	100	0	0	30	100	100	50	0	50	0	0	0	100	0	0	0	100
K. terrigena	0	60	100	40	0	0	0	100	0	20	0	0	100	100	100	80	100	100	100	20	100	100	80	100	100	100	100	100	100	100	100	100	0	100	100	100	100	100	100	20	0	0	100	0	100	0	100
Kluyvera																																															
*K. ascorbata**	92	100	0	96	0	0	0	97	0	100	98	0	92	96	100	93	98	98	100	25	100	0	0	40	100	98	100	100	99	100	100	98	0	99	99	0	40	90	35	50	0	0	100	0	100	0	100
*K. cryocrescens**	90	100	0	80	0	0	0	23	0	100	90	0	86	86	100	95	95	81	95	0	100	0	0	45	100	100	100	100	91	100	100	95	0	100	100	0	5	81	19	86	0	0	100	0	100	0	100
*K. georgiana**	100	100	0	100	0	0	0	100	0	100	100	0	83	50	100	17	83	100	100	33	100	0	0	0	100	100	83	100	100	100	100	100	0	100	100	0	33	83	50	83	0	0	100	0	100	0	100
K. cochleae	0	100	67	100	0	0	0	0	0	100	100	0	100	100	100	100	33	33	100	100	100	0	0	100	100	100	100	100	100	100	100	100	0	100	100	0	100	33	0	0	0	0	100	0	100	0	100
Leclercia																																															
*L. adecarboxylata**	100	100	0	0	0	48	0	0	0	0	79	0	97	93	100	97	93	66	100	86	100	93	0	0	100	66	100	100	100	100	100	0	0	100	100	96	3	93	83	28	0	0	100	0	100	37	100
Leminorella																																															
*L. grimontii**	0	100	0	100	100	0	0	0	0	0	0	0	0	0	100	33	0	0	0	83	0	0	0	0	100	0	0	0	83	0	0	0	0	0	0	0	17	100	100	0	0	0	100	0	0	0	0
*L. richardii**	0	0	0	0	100	0	0	0	0	0	0	0	0	0	100	0	0	0	0	0	0	0	0	0	100	0	0	0	100	0	0	0	0	0	0	0	0	50	100	0	0	0	100	0	0	0	0

(*Continued*)

TABLE 1 (*Continued*)

Organism	Indole production	Methyl red	Voges-Proskauer	Citrate (Simmons)	Hydrogen sulfide (TSI)	Urea hydrolysis	Phenylalanine deaminase	Lysine decarboxylase	Arginine dihydrolase	Ornithine decarboxylase	Motility (36°C)	Gelatin hydrolysis (22°C)	Growth in KCN	Malonate utilization	D-Glucose, acid	D-Glucose, gas	Lactose fermentation	Sucrose fermentation	D-Mannitol fermentation	Dulcitol fermentation	Salicin fermentation	Adonitol fermentation	*myo*-Inositol fermentation	D-Sorbitol fermentation
Moellerella																								
*M. wisconsensis**	0	100	0	80	0	0	0	0	0	0	0	0	70	0	100	0	100	100	60	0	0	100	0	0
Morganella																								
*M. morganii ss morganii**	95	95	0	0	20	95	95	1	0	95	95	0	98	1	99	90	1	0	0	0	0	0	0	0
M. morganii biogroup 1*	100	95	0	0	15	100	100	100	0	80	0	0	90	5	100	93	0	0	0	0	0	0	0	0
M. morganii ss sibonii 1*	50	86	0	0	7	100	93	29	0	64	79	0	79	0	100	86	0	7	0	0	0	0	0	0
Obesumbacterium																								
O. proteus biogroup 2	0	15	0	0	0	0	0	100	0	100	0	0	0	0	100	0	0	0	0	0	0	0	0	0
Pragia																								
P. fontium	0	100	0	89	89	0	22	0	0	0	100	0	0	0	100	0	0	0	0	0	78	0	0	0
Pantoea																								
P. dispersa	0	82	64	100	0	0	9	0	0	0	100	0	82	9	100	0	0	1	100	0	0	0	0	0
Photorhabdus																								
P. luminescens (25°C)	50	0	0	50	0	25	0	0	0	0	100	50	0	0	75	0	0	0	0	0	0	0	0	0
P. DNA group 5*	0	0	0	20	0	60	0	0	0	0	100	80	20	0	100	0	0	0	0	0	0	0	0	0
Proteus																								
*P. mirabilis**	2	97	50	65	98	98	98	0	0	99	95	90	98	2	100	96	2	15	0	0	0	0	0	0
*P. vulgaris**	98	95	0	15	95	95	99	0	0	0	95	91	99	0	100	85	2	97	0	0	50	0	0	0
*P. penneri**	0	100	0	0	30	100	99	0	0	0	85	50	99	0	100	45	1	100	0	0	0	0	0	0
P. myxofaciens	0	100	100	50	0	100	100	0	0	0	100	100	100	0	100	100	0	100	0	0	0	0	0	0
Providencia																								
*P. rettgeri**	99	93	0	95	0	98	98	0	0	0	94	0	97	0	100	10	5	15	100	0	50	100	90	1
*P. stuartii**	98	100	0	93	0	30	95	0	0	0	85	0	100	0	100	0	2	50	10	0	2	5	95	1
*P. alcalifaciens**	99	99	0	98	0	0	98	0	0	1	96	0	100	0	100	85	0	15	2	0	1	98	1	1
*P. rustigianii**	98	65	0	15	0	0	100	0	0	0	30	0	100	0	100	35	0	35	0	0	0	0	0	0
P. heimbachae	0	85	0	0	0	0	100	0	0	0	46	0	8	0	100	0	0	0	0	0	0	92	46	0
Rahnella																								
*R. aquatilis**	0	88	100	94	0	0	95	0	0	0	6	0	0	100	100	98	100	100	100	88	100	0	0	94
Salmonella																								
Group I[c] strains*																								
Most serotypes*	1	100	0	95	95	1	0	98	70	97	95	0	0	0	100	96	1	1	100	96	0	0	35	95
Serotype Typhi*	0	100	0	0	97	0	0	98	3	0	97	0	0	0	100	0	1	0	100	0	0	0	0	99
Serotype Choleraesuis*	0	100	0	25	50	0	0	95	55	100	95	0	0	0	100	95	0	0	98	5	0	0	0	90
Serotype Paratyphi A*	0	100	0	0	10	0	0	0	15	95	95	0	0	0	100	99	0	0	100	90	0	0	0	95
Serotype Gallinarum*	0	100	0	0	100	0	0	90	10	1	0	0	0	0	100	0	0	0	100	90	0	0	0	1
Serotype Pullorum*	0	90	0	0	90	0	0	100	10	95	0	0	0	0	100	90	0	0	100	0	0	0	0	10
Group II strains*	2	100	0	100	100	0	0	100	90	100	98	2	0	95	100	100	1	1	100	90	5	0	5	100
Group IIIa strains*	1	100	0	99	99	0	0	99	70	99	99	0	1	95	100	99	15	1	100	0	0	0	0	99
Group IIIb strains*	2	100	0	98	99	0	0	99	70	99	99	0	1	95	100	99	85	5	100	1	0	0	0	99
Group IV strains*	0	100	0	98	100	2	0	100	70	100	98	0	95	0	100	100	0	0	98	0	60	5	0	100
Group V strains*	0	100	0	94	100	0	0	100	94	100	100	0	100	0	100	94	0	0	100	94	0	0	0	100
Group VI strains*	0	100	0	89	100	0	0	100	67	100	100	0	0	0	100	100	22	0	100	67	0	0	0	0

Organism	L-Arabinose fermentation	Raffinose fermentation	L-Rhamnose fermentation	Maltose fermentation	D-Xylose fermentation	Trehalose fermentation	Cellobiose fermentation	alpha-Methyl-D-glucoside fermentation	Erythritol fermentation	Esculin hydrolysis	Melibiose fermentation	D-Arabitol fermentation	Glycerol fermentation	Mucate fermentation	Tartrate, Jordan's	Acetate utilization	Lipase (corn oil)	DNase at 25°C	Nitrate → Nitrite	Oxidase, Kovacs	ONPG test	Yellow pigment	D-Mannose fermentation
Moellerella																							
*M. wisconsensis**	0	100	0	30	0	0	0	0	0	0	100	75	10	0	30	10	0	0	90	0	90	0	100
Morganella																							
*M. morganii ss morganii**	0	0	0	0	0	0	0	0	0	0	0	0	5	0	95	0	0	0	90	0	10	0	98
M. morganii biogroup 1*	0	0	0	0	0	0	0	0	0	0	0	0	100	0	100	0	0	0	90	0	20	0	100
M. morganii ss sibonii 1*	0	0	0	0	0	100	0	0	0	0	0	0	7	7	100	0	0	0	100	0	0	0	100
Obesumbacterium																							
O. proteus biogroup 2	0	0	15	50	15	85	0	0	0	0	0	0	0	0	15	0	0	0	100	0	0	0	85
Pragia																							
P. fontium	0	0	0	0	0	0	0	0	0	78	0	0	0	0	0	0	0	0	100	0	0	0	0
Pantoea																							
P. dispersa	100	0	91	82	100	100	55	0	0	0	0	100	27	0	9	100	0	0	91	0	91	27	100
Photorhabdus																							
P. luminescens (25°C)	0	0	0	25	0	0	0	0	0	0	0	0	0	0	50	0	0	0	0	0	0	50	100
P. DNA group 5*	0	0	0	0	0	0	0	0	0	0	0	0	0	0	60	20	0	0	0	0	0	60	100
Proteus																							
*P. mirabilis**	0	1	1	0	98	98	1	0	0	0	0	0	70	0	87	20	92	50	95	0	0	0	0
*P. vulgaris**	0	1	5	97	95	30	0	60	1	50	0	0	60	0	80	25	80	80	98	0	1	0	0
*P. penneri**	0	1	0	100	100	55	0	80	0	0	0	0	55	0	85	5	45	40	90	0	1	0	0
P. myxofaciens	0	0	0	100	0	100	0	100	0	0	0	0	100	0	100	0	100	50	100	0	0	0	0
Providencia																							
*P. rettgeri**	0	5	70	2	10	0	3	2	75	35	5	100	60	0	95	60	0	0	100	0	5	0	100
*P. stuartii**	1	7	0	1	7	98	5	0	0	0	0	0	50	0	90	75	0	10	100	0	10	0	100
*P. alcalifaciens**	1	1	0	1	1	2	0	0	0	0	0	0	15	0	90	40	0	0	100	0	1	0	100
*P. rustigianii**	0	0	0	0	0	0	0	0	0	0	0	0	5	0	50	25	0	0	100	0	0	0	100
P. heimbachae	0	0	100	54	8	0	0	0	0	0	0	92	0	0	69	0	0	0	100	0	0	0	100
Rahnella																							
*R. aquatilis**	100	94	94	94	94	100	100	0	0	100	100	0	13	30	6	6	0	0	100	0	100	0	100
Salmonella																							
Group I[c] strains*																							
Most serotypes*	99	2	95	97	97	99	5	2	0	5	95	0	5	90	90	90	0	2	100	0	2	0	100
Serotype Typhi*	2	0	0	97	82	100	0	0	0	0	100	0	20	0	100	0	0	0	100	0	0	0	100
Serotype Choleraesuis*	0	1	100	95	98	0	0	0	1	0	45	1	0	0	85	1	0	0	98	0	0	0	95
Serotype Paratyphi A*	100	0	100	95	0	100	5	0	0	0	95	0	10	0	0	0	0	0	100	0	0	0	100
Serotype Gallinarum*	80	10	10	90	70	50	10	0	1	0	0	0	0	50	100	0	0	10	100	0	0	0	100
Serotype Pullorum*	100	1	100	5	90	90	5	0	0	0	0	0	0	0	0	0	0	0	100	0	0	0	100
Group II strains*	100	0	100	100	100	100	0	8	0	15	8	0	25	96	50	95	0	0	100	0	15	0	95
Group IIIa strains*	99	1	99	98	100	99	1	1	0	1	95	1	10	90	5	90	0	2	100	0	100	0	100
Group IIIb strains*	99	1	99	98	100	99	1	1	0	1	95	1	10	30	20	75	0	2	100	0	92	0	100
Group IV strains*	100	0	98	100	100	100	50	0	0	0	100	5	0	0	65	70	0	0	100	0	0	0	100
Group V strains*	94	0	88	100	100	100	0	0	0	0	94	0	0	88	0	100	0	0	100	0	94	0	100
Group VI strains*	100	0	100	100	100	100	0	0	0	0	89	0	33	89	100	89	0	0	100	0	44	0	100

(*Continued*)

TABLE 1 Biochemical reactions of the named species, biogroups, and Enteric Groups of the family *Enterobacteriaceae*[a] (*Continued*)

Organism	Indole production	Methyl red	Voges-Proskauer	Citrate (Simmons)	Hydrogen sulfide (TSI)	Urea hydrolysis	Phenylalanine deaminase	Lysine decarboxylase	Arginine dihydrolase	Ornithine decarboxylase	Motility (36°C)	Gelatin hydrolysis (22°C)	Growth in KCN	Malonate utilization	D-Glucose, acid	D-Glucose, gas	Lactose fermentation	Sucrose fermentation	D-Mannitol fermentation	Dulcitol fermentation	Salicin fermentation	Adonitol fermentation	*myo*-Inositol fermentation	D-Sorbitol fermentation	L-Arabinose fermentation	Raffinose fermentation	L-Rhamnose fermentation	Maltose fermentation	D-Xylose fermentation	Trehalose fermentation	Cellobiose fermentation	alpha-Methyl-D-glucoside fermentation	Erythritol fermentation	Esculin hydrolysis	Melibiose fermentation	D-Arabitol fermentation	Glycerol fermentation	Mucate fermentation	Tartrate, Jordan's	Acetate utilization	Lipase (corn oil)	DNase at 25°C	Nitrate → Nitrite	Oxidase, Kovacs	ONPG test	Yellow pigment	D-Mannose fermentation
Serratia																																															
*S. marcescens**	1	20	98	98	0	15	0	99	0	99	97	90	95	3	100	55	2	99	99	0	95	40	75	99	0	2	0	96	7	99	5	0	1	95	0	0	95	0	75	50	98	98	98	0	95	0	99
S. marcescens biogroup 1*	0	100	60	30	0	0	0	55	4	65	17	30	70	0	100	0	4	100	96	0	92	30	30	92	0	0	0	70	0	100	4	0	0	96	0	0	92	0	50	4	75	82	83	0	75	0	100
S. liquefaciens group*	1	93	93	90	0	3	0	95	0	95	95	90	90	2	100	75	10	98	100	0	97	5	60	95	98	85	15	98	100	100	5	5	0	97	75	0	95	0	75	40	85	85	100	0	93	0	100
*S. rubidaea**	0	20	100	95	0	2	0	55	0	0	85	90	25	94	100	30	100	99	100	0	99	99	20	1	100	99	1	99	99	100	94	1	0	94	99	85	20	0	70	80	99	99	100	0	100	0	100
S. odorifera biogroup 1*	60	100	50	100	0	5	0	100	0	100	100	95	60	0	100	0	70	100	100	0	98	50	100	100	100	100	95	100	100	100	100	0	0	95	100	0	40	5	100	60	35	100	100	0	100	0	100
S. odorifera biogroup 2*	50	60	100	97	0	0	0	94	0	0	100	94	19	0	100	13	97	0	97	0	45	55	100	100	100	7	94	100	100	100	100	0	7	40	96	0	50	0	100	65	65	100	100	0	100	0	100
*S. plymuthica**	0	94	80	75	0	0	0	0	0	0	50	60	30	0	100	40	80	100	100	0	94	0	50	65	100	94	0	94	94	100	88	70	0	81	93	0	50	0	100	55	70	100	100	0	70	0	100
*S. ficaria**	0	75	75	100	0	0	0	0	0	0	100	100	55	0	100	0	15	100	100	0	100	0	55	100	100	70	35	100	100	100	100	8	0	100	40	100	0	0	17	40	77	100	92	8	100	0	100
S. entomophila	0	20	100	100	0	0	0	0	0	0	100	100	100	0	100	0	0	100	100	0	100	0	0	0	0	0	0	100	40	100	0	0	0	100	0	60	0	0	100	80	20	100	100	0	100	0	100
"*Serratia*" *fonticola**	0	100	9	91	0	13	0	100	0	97	91	0	70	88	100	79	97	21	100	91	100	100	30	100	100	100	76	97	85	100	6	91	0	100	98	100	88	0	58	15	0	0	100	0	100	0	100
Tatumella																																															
*T. ptyseos**	0	0	5	2	0	0	90	0	0	0	0	0	0	0	100	0	0	98	0	0	55	0	0	0	0	11	0	0	9	93	0	0	0	0	25	0	7	0	0	0	0	0	98	0	0	0	100
Trabulsiella																																															
*T. guamensis**	40	100	0	88	100	0	0	100	50	100	100	0	100	0	100	100	0	0	100	0	13	0	0	100	100	0	100	100	100	100	100	0	0	40	0	0	0	100	50	88	0	0	100	0	100	0	100
Xenorhabdus																																															
X. nematophilus (25°C)	40	0	0	0	0	0	0	0	0	0	100	80	0	0	80	0	0	0	0	0	0	0	0	0	0	0	0	0	0	0	0	0	0	0	0	0	0	0	60	0	0	20	20	0	0	60	80
Yersinia																																															
*Y. enterocolitica**	50	97	2	0	0	75	0	0	0	95	2	0	2	0	100	5	5	95	98	0	20	0	30	99	98	5	1	75	70	98	75	0	0	25	1	40	90	0	85	15	55	5	98	0	95	0	100
*Y. frederiksenii**	100	100	0	15	0	70	0	0	0	95	5	0	0	0	100	40	40	100	100	0	92	0	20	100	100	30	99	100	100	100	100	0	0	85	0	100	85	5	55	15	55	0	100	0	100	0	100
*Y. intermedia**	100	100	5	5	0	80	0	0	0	100	5	0	10	5	100	18	35	100	100	0	100	0	15	100	100	45	100	100	100	100	96	77	0	100	80	45	60	6	88	18	12	0	94	0	90	0	100
*Y. kristensenii**	30	92	0	0	0	77	0	0	0	92	5	0	0	0	100	23	8	0	100	0	15	0	15	100	77	0	0	100	85	100	100	0	0	0	0	45	70	0	40	8	0	0	100	0	70	0	100
*Y. rohdei**	0	62	0	0	0	62	0	0	0	25	0	0	0	0	100	0	0	100	100	0	0	0	0	100	100	62	0	0	38	100	25	0	0	0	50	0	38	0	100	0	0	0	88	0	50	0	100
Y. aldovae	0	80	0	0	0	60	0	0	0	40	0	0	0	0	100	0	0	20	80	0	0	0	0	60	60	0	0	0	40	80	0	0	0	0	0	0	0	0	100	0	0	0	100	0	0	0	100
*Y. bercovieri**	0	100	0	0	0	60	0	0	0	80	0	0	0	0	100	0	20	100	100	0	20	0	0	100	100	0	0	100	100	100	100	0	0	20	0	0	0	0	100	0	0	0	100	0	80	0	100
*Y. mollaretii**	0	100	0	0	0	20	0	0	0	80	0	0	0	0	100	0	40	100	100	0	20	0	0	100	100	0	0	60	60	100	100	0	0	0	0	0	20	0	100	0	0	0	100	0	20	0	100
*Y. pestis**	0	80	0	0	0	5	0	0	0	0	0	0	0	0	100	0	0	0	97	0	70	0	0	50	100	0	1	80	90	100	0	0	0	50	20	0	50	0	0	0	0	0	85	0	50	0	100
*Y. pseudotuberculosis**	0	100	0	0	0	95	0	0	0	0	0	0	0	0	100	0	0	0	100	0	25	0	0	0	50	15	70	95	100	100	0	0	0	95	70	0	50	0	50	0	0	0	95	0	70	0	100
"*Yersinia*" *ruckeri**	0	97	10	0	0	0	0	50	5	100	0	30	15	0	100	5	0	0	100	0	0	0	0	50	5	5	0	95	0	95	5	0	0	0	0	0	30	0	30	0	30	0	75	0	50	0	100
Yokenella (Koserella)																																															
*Y. regensburgei**	0	100	0	92	0	0	0	100	8	100	100	0	92	0	100	100	0	0	100	0	8	0	0	0	100	25	100	100	100	100	100	0	0	67	92	0	0	0	0	25	0	0	100	0	100	0	100
Enteric Group 58*	0	100	0	85	0	70	0	100	0	85	100	0	100	85	100	85	30	0	100	85	100	0	0	100	100	0	100	100	100	100	100	55	0	0	0	0	30	0	60	45	0	0	100	0	100	0	100
Enteric Group 59*	10	100	0	100	0	0	30	0	60	0	100	0	80	90	100	100	80	0	100	0	100	0	0	0	100	0	100	100	100	100	100	10	0	100	0	10	10	60	50	50	0	0	100	0	100	25	100
Enteric Group 60*	0	100	0	0	0	50	0	0	0	100	75	0	0	100	100	100	0	0	50	0	0	0	0	0	25	0	75	0	0	100	0	0	0	0	0	0	75	0	75	0	0	0	100	0	100	0	100
Enteric Group 63	0	100	0	0	0	0	0	100	0	100	65	0	0	0	100	100	0	0	100	0	100	0	0	100	100	0	100	100	100	100	100	65	0	100	0	0	0	65	0	0	0	0	100	0	100	0	100
Enteric Group 64	0	100	0	50	0	0	0	0	50	0	100	0	100	100	100	50	100	0	100	0	100	100	0	0	100	0	100	100	100	100	100	0	0	100	0	100	0	100	50	0	0	0	100	0	100	0	100
Enteric Group 68*	0	100	50	0	0	0	0	0	0	0	0	0	100	0	100	0	0	100	100	0	50	0	0	0	0	0	0	50	0	100	0	0	0	0	0	0	50	0	0	0	0	100	100	0	0	0	100
Enteric Group 69	0	0	100	100	0	0	0	0	100	100	100	0	100	100	100	100	100	25	100	100	100	0	0	100	100	100	100	100	100	100	100	100	0	100	100	0	0	100	0	25	0	0	100	0	100	0	100

[a] Each number is the percentage of positive reactions after 2 days of incubation at 36°C (unless a different temperature is indicated). The vast majority of these positive reactions occur within 24 h. Reactions that become positive after 2 days are not considered. Abbreviations: TSI, triple sugar iron agar; ONPG, *o*-nitrophenyl-*β*-D-galactopyranoside.

[b] An "*" indicates that the organism occurs in human clinical specimens.

[c] The roman numerals refer to the seven *Salmonella* subgroups that are biochemically and genetically distinct.

TABLE 2 Distribution of *Enterobacteriaceae*, *Vibrionaceae*, and other organisms in patients with bacteremia[a]

Organism	No. of cases/yr[b] in England and Wales
Family *Enterobacteriaceae*	
Escherichia coli	9,680
Klebsiella species	2,075
Proteus species	1,516
Enterobacter species	1,316
Salmonella, all serotypes	413
Salmonella, serotypes Typhi and Paratyphi	140
Serratia species	368
Citrobacter species	326
Providencia species	55
Family *Vibrionaceae*	
Aeromonas species	40
Other organisms (for comparison)	
Staphyloccus aureus	9,016
Streptococcus pneumoniae	5,871
Enterococcus species	2,821
Pseudomonas aeruginosa	1,154
Neisseria meningitidis	1,096
Bacteroides species	907
Streptococcus species, group B	766
Pseudomonas species	765
Acinetobacter species	557
Clostridium species	380
Hemophilus influenzae	348
Bacillus species	255
Branhamella/Moraxella species	70
Listeria species	67
Campylobacter species	57
Mycobacterium avium-intracellulare	40

[a] Data are for bacteremia (blood, bone marrow, spleen, or heart) from published surveillance reports for England and Wales. Bacteremia is not a reportable disease in the United States.

[b] Data are adapted from the *CDR Weekly, Communicable Disease Report* (volume 8, no. 20, 15 May 1998). The tabulations for the first 19 weeks of the years 1997 and 1998 were averaged and then multiplied by 2.737 to extrapolate them to a full year.

strains isolated from human clinical specimens, plants, animals, and the environment. One example is the recent study of Müller et al. (77), who found six new species of *Buttiauxella* and one new species of *Kluyvera* in a large collection of strains isolated from snails. Clinical microbiologists should always be aware that most of the *Enterobacteriaceae* that they encounter every day will belong to just a few of the many species described. However, the expanding number of *Enterobacteriaceae* species is becoming a serious problem for reference laboratories and for commercial identification systems, whose identification methods are becoming inadequate for complete and accurate identification. Strains of *Enterobacteriaceae* isolated from plants, animals, and the environment can belong to any of the described species (Table 1), not just the species that were originally isolated from human clinical specimens. When a commercial identification gives an unusual organism for a final identification, there are several possibilities to consider: the identification is correct, just unusual; the identification is incorrect for a number of possible reasons; another aerobic or anaerobic organism is present and the biochemical profile is the result of all the metabolic activities of the mixture; or a handling or coding error was made somewhere along the way. Before a final report of an unusual organism is issued, it is advisable to do as much checking as possible. This could include repeating the biochemical tests in the same commercial system after confirming the absence of a contaminating aerobic or anaerobic organism; testing the isolate in another commercial identification system; and comparing the strain's antibiogram with known patterns reported for this organism. If these steps do not resolve the problem, the state health department can be contacted for advice, and the culture will often be accepted for further study. It is not uncommon for our reference laboratory to receive strains with a request such as: "Commercial identification system 1 called this species A, system 2 called it species B, and the state health department thinks it is neither of these but is species C. Please give us your opinion."

Changes in Classification

There is no designated international body that considers all proposed changes in classification and then issues a formal ruling on whether to accept them. For many years there has been a Subcommittee on *Enterobacteriaceae* of the International Committee on Systematic Bacteriology, whose responsibility is the nomenclature and classification of *Enterobacteriaceae*. This Subcommittee can make recommendations on these matters but has rarely done so in the past. Even if this Subcommittee studies a specific change in classification, it can only make a recommendation, which can then be accepted or rejected by the scientific community. It should be emphasized that changes in classification are decided by usage not by judicial action. Sometimes two classifications are widely used, and both can be "correct." Classifications are correct if they conform to all the nomenclatural rules in the *Bacteriological Code* (*International Code of Nomenclature of Bacteria*), but they can be useful or not useful.

Changes in Classification Incorporated in Table 1

Since the sixth edition of this Manual, some changes in classification have been proposed in the literature. Several of these appear to be clearly justified and have been incorporated in Table 1, but others have not been fully discussed or accepted by the scientific community. Table 1 gives the classification used by the Enteric Reference Laboratory, Foodborne and Diarrheal Diseases Laboratory Section, at the Centers for Disease Control and Prevention, which may differ from other classifications.

Xenorhabdus-Photorhabdus

Based on ecological, phenotypic, and molecular evidence, Boemare et al. (9) proposed to reclassify the organism *Xenorhabdus luminescens* in a new genus, *Photorhabdus* as *Photorhabdus luminescens*. This change seems very logical and prudent because it separates *Xenorhabdus* and *Photorhabdus*, two genera that are phenotypically distinct and distantly related by DNA-DNA hybridization. In Table 1, the organism formerly known (36) as *Xenorhabdus luminescens* DNA hybridization group 5 is now classified as *Photorhabdus* DNA hybridization group 5. Clinical microbiologists should be aware of this organism because it occasionally occurs in human clinical specimens and has caused a few cases of bacteremia and wound infection (36).

TABLE 3 Important causes of nosocomial infections in the United States[a]

Organism	No. (%) of isolates				
	Urinary tract infection	Wound or surgical site	Pneumonia	Blood	Total
Enterobacteriaceae					
Escherichia coli	20,218 (25.1)	3,600 (9.2)	1,607 (5.2)	1,511 (5.2)	27,871 (13.7)
Enterobacter, all species	4,232 (5.2)	2,850 (7.3)	3,257 (10.6)	1,316 (4.5)	12,757 (6.2)
Klebsiella pneumoniae	5,544 (6.9)	1,250 (3.2)	2,230 (7.2)	1,280 (4.4)	11,015 (5.4)
Proteus mirabilis	4,077 (5.1)	1,246 (3.2)	779 (2.5)	197 (0.7)	4,662 (2.3)
Citrobacter, all species	1,553 (1.9)	598 (1.5)	418 (1.4)	174 (0.6)	2,912 (1.4)
Serratia marcescens	688 (0.9)	548 (1.4)	1,112 (3.6)	351 (1.2)	3,010 (1.5)
Other organisms for comparison					
Enterococci	12,595 (15.6)	4,998 (12.8)	607 (2.0)	2,594 (9.0)	22,033 (10.8)
Pseudomonas aeruginosa	9,309 (11.5)	3,169 (8.1)	5,162 (16.8)	1,095 (3.8)	20,307 (9.9)
Staphylococcus aureus	1,569 (2.1)	7,371 (18.8)	5,352 (17.4)	4,625 (16.0)	23,187 (11.4)
Coagulase-negative staphylococci	3,035 (3.8)	5,147 (13.1)	637 (2.1)	8,481 (29.3)	20,465 (10.0)
Candida albicans	5,933 (7.4)	984 (2.5)	1,419 (4.6)	1,380 (4.8)	10,706 (5.2)
Streptococcus, all species	1,265 (1.6)	1,303 (3.3)	1,050 (3.4)	1,053 (3.6)	4,998 (2.4)
Candida, other species	1,763 (2.2)	229 (0.6)	245 (0.8)	879 (3.0)	3,370 (1.7)

[a] The first figure is the number of isolates; the number in parentheses is the percentage. Based on nosocomial infection surveillance of over 200,000 cases for the United States, 1986 to 1989 (86) and 1990 to 1996 (unpublished data).

Citrobacter diversus-Citrobacter koseri

The names *Citrobacter diversus* and *Citrobacter koseri* have both been used in the literature for some time, but the name *Citrobacter diversus* has been used much more frequently. Many workers recognized the phenotypic similarity of these two organisms and thought that they might be the same. The name *Citrobacter diversus* became the correct name for this organism on 1 January 1980, when the *Approved Lists of Bacterial Names* was issued, because under the laws of priority it was the older name. However, in 1993 the Judicial Commission of the International Committee on Systematic Bacteriology issued an Opinion (66) that the name *Citrobacter koseri* should be conserved over the name *Citrobacter diversus*, even though the name *Citrobacter diversus* was the older name, the correct name for the organism under the rules of the *Bacteriological Code*, and the name used most frequently in the literature. This "opinion" needs much more discussion by the scientific community, which is beyond the scope of this chapter; therefore, both names are included in Table 1.

Other Proposed Changes in Nomenclature and Classification

Enterobacter agglomerans Group-*Pantoea*

In 1972, Ewing and Fife (29) redefined the name *Enterobacter agglomerans* to include a wide variety of organisms known under many different names. These investigators also defined 11 different biogroups to recognize the phenotypic diversity of the many strains included in *Enterobacter agglomerans*. This name has become a useful one for clinical microbiologists and has been used extensively in the literature. Systematic analysis by Brenner and coworkers using DNA-DNA hybridization indicated that *Enterobacter agglomerans* is very heterogeneous, with at least 14 DNA hybridization groups (12). For this reason, the names "*Enterobacter agglomerans* complex" or "*Enterobacter agglomerans* group" (33) have been used to better indicate the heterogenicity of this "species." However, it has been very difficult to find simple tests to differentiate and identify all of the DNA hybridization groups (33). For this reason, workers have been reluctant to subdivide the *Enterobacter agglomerans* group until a definitive classification could be proposed (33). However, Gavini et al. (43) recently took the first step in a more logical classification for this complex group. They confirmed the close relatedness of a group of six strains that Brenner et al. had defined as "DNA hybridization group 13 of *Enterobacter agglomerans*" and proposed that this group be classified in a new genus, *Pantoea*. They also defined a new species in the genus, *Pantoea dispersa* (43), that corresponded to DNA hybridization group 3 of *Enterobacter agglomerans* of Brenner (12). The removal of these strains formerly classified in two DNA-DNA hybridization groups of *Enterobacter agglomerans* into a new genus, *Pantoea*, is a logical first attempt to reduce the heterogenicity of the genus *Enterobacter* and is based on sound scientific evidence.

However, this new classification has caused some problems. Some authors have broadened the original definition of Gavini et al. for *Pantoea agglomerans*. Gavini et al. were very careful to define *Pantoea agglomerans* to include only the strains that were closely related by DNA-DNA hybridization to strain ATCC 27155. Similarly, *Pantoea dispersa* was carefully defined to include only the strains that were highly related by DNA-DNA hybridization to the type strain of this new species, ATCC 14589. For the genus *Pantoea* and its species to remain homogeneous and well defined, these original species definitions must be adhered to very strictly. Since DNA-DNA hybridization is not routinely available and since simple tests are not available to definitively identify strains to the level of DNA hybridization group, it seems prudent to retain the vernacular name "*Enterobacter agglomerans* group" as a convenient name for clinical microbiologists for routine identification. This term is defined biochemically in Table 1, and it should be emphasized that it is used merely for convenience and because the name *Enterobacter agglomerans* is well understood and widely used in the literature. Eventually, this term will be replaced with a better classification. When definitive testing in a

TABLE 4 *Salmonella* and *Shigella* serotypes in the United States[a]

Rank and serotype	No. of isolates
Salmonella serotypes	
1 Enteritidis	9,566
2 Typhimurium	9,500
3 Heidelberg	1,998
4 Newport	1,985
5 Montevideo	1,227
6 Javiana	749
7 Oranienburg	689
8 Hadar	658
9 Agona	606
10 Munchen	595
11 Thompson	587
12 Saintpaul	562
13 Branderup	532
14 Infantis	503
15 Typhi	440
16 Poona	415
17 Paratyphi B	337
18 Anatum	270
19 Java	250
20 Mbandaka	223
Subtotal (20 most common serotypes)	31,692
Other important (invasive) serotypes:	
Paratyphi A	79
Paratyphi C	22
Choleraesuis	34
Other serotypes, or not typed	10,649
Total *Salmonella* isolates	34,520
Shigella serotypes	
1 *Shigella sonnei* (serogroup D)	11,094
2 *Shigella flexneri* (serogroup B)	4,015
3 *Shigella boydii* (serogroup C)	396
4 *Shigella dysenteriae* (serogroup A)	181
Shigella, not completely typed	1,573
Total *Shigella* isolates	17,259

[a] Data are from the latest published annual summaries from the Centers for Disease Control and Prevention. *Salmonella* Surveillance for 1996 and *Shigella* Surveillance for 1993 to 1995.

reference laboratory (usually including DNA hybridization) is done, more precise names can be used in reporting. Examples could include *Pantoea agglomerans* (DNA hybridization group 13), *Pantoea dispersa* (DNA hybridization group 3), *Enterobacter agglomerans* DNA hybridization group 1, *Enterobacter agglomerans* DNA hybridization group 2, *Enterobacter agglomerans* DNA hybridization group 12, etc. Precise identification to the level of DNA-DNA hybridization group is not available to the clinical microbiologist and will be limited to bacterial taxonomists and *Enterobacteriaceae* reference laboratories until simple identification methods become available.

Enterobacter taylorae-Enterobacter cancerogenus

Enterobacter taylorae and *Enterobacter cancerogenus* may be two names for the same organism (44). However, they have different type strains; therefore, they are not "objective synonyms" under the rules of the *Bacteriological Code*. Until the identity of these two organisms is confirmed by other laboratories, both names will be used (Table 1).

Nomenclature, Classification, and Reporting of the Genus *Salmonella*

After much study and discussion, there is now good agreement on most of the nomenclature and classification of the genus *Salmonella* (27, 37, 76, 81, 83). However, there are still several problem areas where different names or classifications are being used. These include the names *Salmonella choleraesuis* versus *Salmonella enterica*; the use of the terms "serotype" (sometimes abbreviated as ser.) versus "serovar"; the best way to write the names of the serotypes (serovars); the use of names versus antigenic formulas for some of the serotypes; and the argument whether some well-known serotype names should be eliminated and combined with other serotypes. Most of these points are discussed by McWhorter-Murlin and Hickman-Brenner (76), who summarize the differences between the nomenclature used at CDC (see chapter 28 for examples of this nomenclature and usage) and that used at the Institut Pasteur.

Historical Species Concept in the Genus *Salmonella*

Until the 1970s, the species concept in the genus *Salmonella* was based on epidemiology, host range, biochemical reactions, and antigenic structure (the O antigen, phases 1 and 2 of the H antigen, and the Vi antigen, if present), and strains that differed in one or all of these properties were given distinct names. Names such as *Salmonella typhi*, *Salmonella choleraesuis* (originally some names were written with a hyphen, which was eventually dropped), *Salmonella paratyphi* A, *Salmonella paratyphi* A var. *durazzo*, *Salmonella typhimurium*, *Salmonella typhimurium* var. *copenhagen*, *Salmonella enteritidis*, and *Salmonella newport* began to appear, and the list rapidly expanded to hundreds of names. Some workers believed that these names really represented biological species (69), but others thought they were antigenic and biochemical varieties with an uncertain evolutionary relationship. However, there was universal agreement that the names were an extremely useful way to communicate about the particular serotypes. Most authors wrote the serotype names in italics as a species in the genus *Salmonella*, for example, *Salmonella typhimurium* (37).

Basis for the Current Classification of the Genus *Salmonella*

In 1973, Crosa et al. (24) used DNA-DNA hybridization to show that *Salmonella* strains could be grouped into five main evolutionary groups. Two (possibly three) additional groups are now known (11, 81, 83). The vast majority of strains that cause infections in humans occurred in DNA hybridization group 1 (I). Strains isolated from animals and the environment clustered together into the four other groups, designated DNA groups 2 (II), 3a (IIIA), 3b (IIIB), and 4 (IV). Over the years, different authors have used different terms to refer to these evolutionary groups: DNA-DNA hybridization groups (24), multilocus enzyme electrophoresis clusters (11, 83), subgenera (69), species (see the *Approved Lists of Bacterial Names*), and subspecies (76, 81, 82).

A Single Species of *Salmonella*—*Salmonella choleraesuis*

Crosa et al. (24) showed that all five groups of *Salmonella* were very highly related. With the species definition usually used in DNA hybridization, these five groups could be considered as belonging to the same species. Under the rules of the *Bacteriological Code*, the name of this species is *Salmonella choleraesuis*. However, this species name can cause confusion, since *Salmonella choleraesuis* would have two totally different meanings, one as a species and one as a serotype.

A Single Species of *Salmonella—Salmonella enterica*

There has been support for making an exception to the rules of the *Bacteriological Code* and using a name that would not cause confusion. There was a formal proposal to coin a new name, *Salmonella enterica*, that would replace the name *Salmonella choleraesuis* as the species name to represent most of the serotypes of *Salmonella*. The main advantage of this proposal is that it would reduce confusion by using a new name that has never been used as a serotype name. However, the proposal to change the name from *Salmonella choleraesuis* to *Salmonella enterica* was denied by the Judicial Commission of the International Committee on Systematic Bacteriology; hence, the name *Salmonella choleraesuis* remains the correct name. A second proposal to the Judicial Commission is being prepared; if approved, it would change the status of *Salmonella enterica* from "without standing in nomenclature, thus illegitimate" to "with standing in nomenclature, and legitimate." The name *Salmonella enterica* is being used by the World Health Organization's International Center for *Salmonella* (81) and by some of the World Health Organization's National Centers for *Salmonella*, including the one in the United States (76). The name is also appearing in the literature.

Different Nomenclatures for Serotype Names

Another point of disagreement concerns the method of writing serotype names. For almost 100 years, serotype names have been written as species (the "serotype as species" nomenclature), and this method is still widely used. An example of this nomenclature: "*Salmonella enteritidis* is now the most common serotype in the United States and in many European countries."

Recently, the World Health Organization's International Center for *Salmonella*, a laboratory at the Institut Pasteur, Paris, France, introduced a different nomenclature in which the serotype name is capitalized and not written in italics. In this nomenclature, the name *Salmonella enteritidis* in the previous paragraph would be written in one of the following ways: "*Salmonella* serovar Enteriditis," "*Salmonella* ser. Enteritidis," or "*Salmonella* Enteritidis." The nomenclature described by McWhorter-Murlin and Hickman-Brenner (76) is similar, but they recommend using the term "serotype" instead of "serovar." The main advantage of these nomenclatures is that they do not artificially treat the serotypes as species. The main disadvantage is that they create a new nomenclature, which differs from one that has been widely accepted and used for many years, since there have been literally hundreds of thousands of uses of the "serotype as species" nomenclature in the literature. The International *Salmonella* Center's nomenclature is being used (often with modifications) by some of the National Centers for *Salmonella*, including the one at the Centers for Disease Control and Prevention (76). However, other National Centers for *Salmonella*, such as the one in England, continue to use the "serotype as species" nomenclature (for examples, see publications from the World Health Organization's National Center for *Salmonella* in England and epidemiological tabulations in the English epidemiological bulletin, *CDR Reports*). Since *Salmonella* names are being written differently by different authors and different National Centers for *Salmonella*, it is not surprising that the literature is beginning to reflect this variety of names. Recent examples of the way "serotype Typhimurium" is being written include *Salmonella* serotype Typhimurium, *Salmonella* ser. Typhimurium, *Salmonella typhimurium*, *Salmonella* Typhimurium, *Salmonella* typhimurium, *Salmonella* serovar Typhimurium, and *Salmonella* serovar typhimurium. When the above variations are combined with the four species/subspecies possibilities, i.e., *Salmonella choleraesuis*, *Salmonella choleraesuis* subspecies *choleraesuis*, *Salmonella enterica*, and *Salmonella enterica* subspecies *enterica*, the number of possible variations is multiplied considerably (one example of the over two dozen possible ones is *Salmonella enterica* subspecies *enterica* serovar Typhimurium).

Laboratory Reports for Isolates of *Salmonella*

Most clinical microbiology laboratories will identify a *Salmonella* isolate with a commercial identification system and then usually with *Salmonella* antisera. These two methods usually give definitive results, and a report can be issued such as "*Salmonella* serogroup B." Thus, fortunately, clinical microbiology laboratories are usually immune from the above problems in their reporting. A reference laboratory can do definitive serotyping and biochemical testing and can determine a complete serotype. A report such as "*Salmonella* serotype Typhimurium" can be issued. The advantage of this simple wording of reports is that it avoids the subgenus/species/subspecies concept entirely and concentrates on the actual laboratory results, which should be easily understood.

Nomenclature for Shiga Toxins/Verotoxins Produced by *E. coli* and *Shigella*

In a similar vein to the problems described for *Salmonella*, several different names are being used in the literature for the cytotoxins produced by *E. coli* and *Shigella*. This topic is critical because of the importance of *E. coli* O157 and other strains that produce these toxins (see chapter 28). Several different commercial assays for these toxins are being marketed; thus it is essential to read the package insert carefully to determine exactly which toxin(s) the kit is detecting, and to word laboratory reports accordingly.

For almost 100 years, it has been known that *Shigella dysenteriae* O1 produces a potent cytotoxin known as Shiga toxin. More recently, it has been shown that certain diarrheagenic strains of *E. coli* produced a similar toxin that was first detected because it was cytotoxic for Vero cells in tissue culture. A number of recent studies have defined these proteins from *Shigella dysenteriae* O1 and *E. coli*, and there is agreement that they comprise a family of toxins. They are being referred to in the literature as Shiga toxin, Shiga-like toxins, and verotoxins; and at least five different toxins are involved (20). The main disagreement in the literature is that some workers have referred to these cytotoxins produced by *E. coli* as "Shiga-like toxins," but others have used the term "verotoxins" (VT). Recently, Calderwood et al. summarized the data available and proposed a new nomenclature for the toxins and for their corresponding genes (20). They recommended that strains of *E. coli* that produce these toxins be called "Shiga toxin-producing" *E. coli*, which would replace the previous term, "Shiga-like toxin producing." They also recommended that the new toxin name be cross-referenced with the corresponding verotoxin name. With this nomenclature, a laboratory report for a stool culture might be worded, "positive for *E. coli* O157:H7, which produces Shiga toxins Stx1 (VT1) and Stx2 (VT2)." Hopefully the differences between the groups using the two different nomenclatures can be resolved, resulting in a single nomenclature in the literature.

DESCRIPTION OF THE FAMILY *ENTEROBACTERIACEAE*

Most organisms in the family *Enterobacteriaceae* share the following properties: they are gram negative and rod shaped; do not form spores; are motile by peritrichous flagella or nonmotile; grow on peptone or meat extract media without the addition of sodium chloride or other supplements; grow well on MacConkey agar; grow both aerobically and anaerobically; are active biochemically; ferment (rather than oxidize) D-glucose and other sugars, often with gas production; are catalase positive and oxidase negative; reduce nitrate to nitrite; contain the enterobacterial common antigen; and have a 39 to 59% guanine-plus-cytosine (G + C) content of DNA (4). Species in the family should also be more closely related (by techniques that measure evolutionary distance) to *Escherichia coli*, the type species of the type genus of the family, than they are to organisms in other families.

NATURAL HABITATS

Enterobacteriaceae are widely distributed on plants and in soil, water, and the intestines of humans and animals (4). Some species occupy very limited ecological niches. *Salmonella typhi* causes typhoid fever and is found only in humans (53). In contrast, strains of *Klebsiella pneumoniae* are distributed widely in the environment and contribute to biochemical and geochemical processes (71). However, strains of *K. pneumoniae* also cause human infections, ranging from asymptomatic colonization of the intestinal, urinary, and respiratory tracts to fatal pneumonia, septicemia, and meningitis.

CLINICAL SIGNIFICANCE

Strains of *Enterobacteriaceae* are associated with abscesses, pneumonia, meningitis, septicemia, and infections of wounds, the urinary tract, and the intestines. They are a major component of the normal intestinal flora of humans but are relatively uncommon at other body sites. Several species of *Enterobacteriaceae* are very important causes of nosocomial infections (Table 3). *Enterobacteriaceae* may account for 80% of clinically significant isolates of gram-negative bacilli and 50% of clinically significant bacteria in clinical microbiology laboratories. They account for nearly 50% of septicemia cases (Table 2), more than 70% of urinary tract infections, and a significant percentage of intestinal infections.

Human Extraintestinal Infections

Except for the species of *Shigella*, which rarely cause infections outside the gastrointestinal tract, many species of *Enterobacteriaceae* commonly cause extraintestinal infections. However, a small number of species, i.e., *E. coli*, *Klebsiella pneumoniae*, *K. oxytoca*, *Proteus mirabilis*, *Enterobacter aerogenes*, *Enterobacter cloacae*, and *Serratia marcescens*, account for most of these infections (Tables 2 and 3). Urinary tract infections, primarily cystitis, are the most common (86), followed by respiratory, wound, bloodstream, and central nervous system infections. Many of these infections, especially sepsis and meningitis, are life-threatening and are often hospital acquired. Because of the severity of these infections, prompt isolation, identification, and susceptibility testing of *Enterobacteriaceae* isolates are essential.

Human Intestinal Infections

Several organisms in the family *Enterobacteriaceae* are also important causes of intestinal infections of humans (Table 4) and animals worldwide. Although other species in the family have been associated with diarrhea (91) or even implicated as causes of diarrhea, only organisms in four genera, *Escherichia* (26, 32, 68, 93), *Salmonella* (24, 37, 53, 81), *Shigella* (27), and *Yersinia* (6, 67, 84), have been clearly documented as enteric pathogens. These four genera are discussed in chapters 28 and 30. Other *Enterobacteriaceae* such as *Citrobacter*, *Edwardsiella*, *Hafnia*, *Morganella*, *Proteus*, *Klebsiella*, *Enterobacter*, and *Serratia*, have occasionally been implicated (4, 91). Strains that produce biologically active compounds (these are often overstated as being "enterotoxin-producing strains") of these *Enterobacteriaceae* have been isolated from people with diarrhea (91), but the etiological roles of these strains are uncertain. Some laboratories issue reports for stool cultures such as, "*Klebsiella pneumoniae* isolated in essentially pure culture (10 of 10 colonies tested); please consult the laboratory to discuss possible significance," to reflect this drastic change in the stool flora. There is no evidence that strains of these other genera are important causes of diarrhea.

SPECIMEN COLLECTION, TRANSPORT, AND PROCESSING

Extraintestinal Specimens

Enterobacteriaceae are recovered from infections at many different body sites, and normal practices (see chapters 4 and 5) for collecting blood, respiratory, wound, urine, and other specimens should be followed.

Intestinal Specimens

Stool cultures are usually submitted to the laboratory with a request to isolate and identify the cause of a possible intestinal infection, usually manifested as diarrhea. The groups of *Enterobacteriaceae* usually associated with diarrhea in the United States are *Salmonella*, *Shigella*, and certain pathogenic strains of *E. coli* and *Yersinia enterocolitica*.

Stool specimens require special attention to both collection and transportation and should be obtained early in the course of illness, when the causative agent is likely to be present on primary plates in the largest numbers. At this stage, the use of enrichment broths should be unnecessary. Except for typhoid fever, the isolation rate for enteric pathogens declines as the patient recovers. Freshly passed stool is a better specimen than rectal swabs, since there is less chance for improper collection and since mucus and blood-stained portions can be selected for culture. Stool cultures should be plated within 2 h of collection, to recover fastidious pathogens such as *Shigella*. If rapid processing is not possible, a small portion of feces or a swab coated with feces should be placed in transport medium. Commonly used transport media include Stuart, Amies, Cary-Blair, and buffered glycerol saline. Cary-Blair is probably the best overall transport medium for diarrheal stools. Specimens held in transport media should be refrigerated until examined. In certain circumstances, such as with infants or during mass screening in outbreak investigations, rectal swabs may be useful. Mucosa within the rectal vault must be sampled for these specimens to be of optimum value. Many different procedures have been described for processing stool specimens. In cases of chronic or severe diarrhea, rare pathogens should also be considered. More information about the isolation, identification, typing, and virulence testing of isolates of *Salmonella*, *Shigella*, *E. coli*, and *Y. enterocolitica* is given in chapters 28 and 30.

Microscopic Examination

Stool specimens should be examined visually for the presence of blood or mucus, but microscopic examination should not be done routinely because of its lack of specificity (22, 26, 51, 80). Although identification by fluorescent-antibody staining is theoretically possible for all enteric pathogens, it has been of limited success because the method is difficult and there are many serological cross-reactions among the species of *Enterobacteriaceae* (27). This technique has been limited to detection of *Salmonella* strains (primarily by the food industry) and certain serogroups of *E. coli* and to outbreak investigations.

ISOLATION

Extraintestinal Specimens

Most strains of *Enterobacteriaceae* grow readily on the plating media commonly used in clinical microbiology laboratories. Specimens from body sites that are normally sterile are cultured on blood or chocolate agar. Urine, respiratory tract, and wound specimens, which are likely to contain mixtures of organisms, are almost always cultured on selective media to enhance the recovery of *Enterobacteriaceae*. MacConkey agar, generally interchangeable with eosin methylene blue (EMB) agar, is usually used, because it allows a preliminary grouping of enteric and other gram-negative bacteria. The most common isolates of *Enterobacteriaceae* have a characteristic appearance on blood agar and MacConkey agar that is useful for preliminary identification (Table 5). Broth enrichment can increase the isolation rate if small numbers of *Enterobacteriaceae* are present, but this step is not normally required.

Intestinal Specimens

Media that should be used routinely for intestinal specimens include a nonselective medium such as blood agar, a differential medium of low to moderate selectivity such as MacConkey agar, and a more selective differential medium such as xylose-lysine-deoxycholate (XLD) agar or Hektoen enteric (HE) agar. A broth enrichment such as selenite (or GN or tetrathionate) can be included, particularly if the specimen is not optimal. A highly selective medium such as brilliant green agar or bismuth sulfite agar can also be included for isolating strains of *Salmonella*. A plate of sorbitol-MacConkey (SMAC) agar can be added to enhance the isolation of Shiga toxin-producing strains of *E. coli* O157:H7. This medium should be used if the stool is frankly bloody or if the patient has a diagnosis of hemolytic-uremic syndrome (HUS), and it can be used for all fecal specimens if resources permit (see chapter 28). When *Y. enterocolitica* is suspected, a selective-differential medium, such as CIN (cefsulodin-irgasan-novobiocin) agar (also called *Yersinia* selective agar), can be added (see chapter 30). A complete stool culture procedure should also include media for isolation of *Campylobacter* and possibly *Vibrio* strains in areas where cholera and other *Vibrio* infections are common.

IDENTIFICATION

There are many different approaches to identifying strains of *Enterobacteriaceae* (33).

Conventional Biochemical Tests in Tubes

Tube testing was once used by all clinical microbiology laboratories, and it is still widely used in reference and public health laboratories (27, 33). Although many laboratories prepare their own media from commercial dehydrated powders, most of the common media are also available commercially in glass tubes that are ready to inoculate. Growth from a single colony is inoculated into each tube, and the tests are read at 24 h and usually also at 48 h. In the Enteric Reference Laboratory, most tests are read for 7 days. Unfortunately, the media and tests are not completely standardized, and few laboratories use exactly the same formulations or procedures. Even with these variables, this approach usually results in correct identifications of the common species of *Enterobacteriaceae*. Table 1 gives the results for *Enterobacteriaceae* in 47 tests (for the media and methods used to generate the data in this table, see references 31 and 53).

Computer Analysis To Assist in Identification

Two microcomputer programs have been developed in the Enteric Reference Laboratory to assist with the identifica-

TABLE 5 Colonial appearance of some of the most common *Enterobacteriaceae* on MacConkey agar and sheep blood agar[a]

Genus or species	Appearance and typical colony diameter on:	
	MacConkey agar	Sheep blood agar[b]
Salmonella and *Shigella*	Colorless, flat, 2–3 mm	Smooth, 2–3 mm
Yersinia enterocolitica	Colorless, <1 mm	Smooth, <1 mm
Escherichia coli (lactose positive)	Red, usually surrounded by precipitated bile, 2–3 mm	Smooth, 2–3 mm
Escherichia coli (lactose negative)	Colorless, 2–3 mm	Smooth, 2–3 mm
Klebsiella pneumoniae	Pink, mucoid, 3–4 mm	Mucoid, 3–4 mm
Enterobacter	Pink, not as mucoid as *Klebsiella*, 2–4 mm	Smooth, 3–4 mm
Proteus vulgaris and *Proteus mirabilis*	Colorless, flat, often swarm slightly, 2–3 mm	Swarm in waves to cover plate
Other *Proteus*, *Providencia*, and *Morganella* species	Colorless, flat, no swarming, 2–3 mm	Flat, 2–3 mm, no swarming

[a] Most strains appear this way, but there are exceptions.
[b] Unlike *Vibrionaceae*, most strains of *Enterobacteriaceae* are nonhemolytic. However, a few strains of *E. coli* are strongly hemolytic.

tion of *Enterobacteriaceae* cultures. "George" and "Strain matcher" were described in the 1985 review of the family (33). A detailed description and information for obtaining them is available by contacting the author and is being prepared for the Internet.

Screening Tests, Using All Information Available

Over the years, the *Enterobacteriaceae* reference laboratories have found that many genera, species, and serotypes can be tentatively identified by a minimum number of screening tests (Table 6). These tests may be more useful in a reference or research laboratory that does not have to deal with all of the regulatory aspects of testing human clinical specimens. More precise identification can be made by using more tests or commercial identification systems. For example, a blood isolate has the following properties: colonies on MacConkey agar are 2 to 3 mm in diameter, are bright red and nonmucoid, and have precipitated bile around them; they are indole positive and 4-methylumbelliferyl-β-D-glucuronidase (MUG) positive; they grow at 44.5°C; and they are antibiotic resistant. These results are completely compatible with *Escherichia coli*. Similarly, an isolate from the feces of a diarrhea patient has the following properties: colonies on MacConkey agar are 2 to 3 mm in diameter and colorless; colonies on XLD agar are 2 to 3 mm and black; the isolate agglutinates in *Salmonella* polyvalent serum and in O-group

TABLE 6 Screening tests for genera and species of *Enterobacteriaceae* often isolated from human clinical specimens[a]

Organism (genus, species, or serotype)	Test or property[b]
Citrobacter	Citrate$^+$, lysine decarboxylase$^-$, often grows on CIN agar, strong characteristic odor
Enterobacter	Variable biochemically, citrate$^+$, VP$^+$, resistant to cephalothin
Escherichia coli	Extremely variable biochemically, indole$^+$, MUG$^+$, grows at 44.5°C, sometimes antibiotic resistant, molecular test: PhoE^{+d}
Escherichia coli O157:H7	Colorless colonies on sorbitol-MacConkey agar, MUG$^-$, D-sorbitol$^-$ (or delayed), agglutinates in O157 serum and H7 serum
Hafnia	Lysed by *Hafnia* specific bacteriophage[c]; often more active biochemically at 25 than 36°C
Klebsiella	Mucoid colonies, encapsulated cells, nonmotile, lysine$^+$, very active biochemically, ferment most sugars, VP$^+$, malonate$^+$, resistant to carbenicillin and ampicillin
Proteus-Providencia-Morganella	Phenylalanine$^+$, tyrosine hydrolysis$^+$, often urea$^+$, resistant to colistin
Morganella	Very inactive biochemically, no swarming, citrate$^-$, H_2S^-, ornithine$^+$, gelatin$^-$, lipase$^-$, urea$^+$
Proteus	Swarms on blood agar, pungent odor, H_2S^+, gelatin$^+$, lipase$^+$
Proteus mirabilis	Urea$^+$, indole$^-$, ornithine$^+$, maltose$^-$
Proteus vulgaris	Urea$^+$, indole$^+$, ornithine$^-$, maltose$^+$
Providencia	No swarming, H_2S^-, ornithine$^-$, gelatin$^-$, lipase$^-$
Salmonella	Lactose$^-$, sucrose$^-$, H_2S^+, O1 phage^{+c}, MUCAP^{+d}, agglutinates in polyvalent serum[b], typical colonies on media selective or differential for *Salmonella* (brilliant green agar, SS agar, Rambach agar, etc.), lysed by *Salmonella*-specific bacteriophage,[c] often antibiotic resistant
Salmonella typhi	H_2S^+ (trace amount only), agglutinates in group D serum
Serratia	DNase$^+$, gelatinase$^+$, lipase$^+$, resistant to colistin and cephalothin
Serratia marcescens	L-Arabinose$^-$
Serratia, other species	L-Arabinose$^+$
Shigella	Nonmotile, lysine$^-$, gas$^-$, agglutinates in polyvalent serum, biochemically inactive, often antibiotic resistant, molecular test: PhoE^{+d}
Shigella boydii	Agglutinates in group C serum, D-mannitol$^+$
Shigella dysenteriae	Agglutinates in group A serum, D-mannitol$^-$
Shigella dysenteriae O1	Catalase$^-$, agglutinates in O1 serum, Shiga toxin$^+$
Shigella flexneri	Agglutinates in group B serum, D-mannitol$^+$
Shigella sonnei	Agglutinates in group D serum, D-mannitol$^+$, ornithine decarboxylase$^+$, lactose$^+$ (delayed), colony variation: smooth to rough
Yersinia	Grows on CIN agar, often more active biochemically at 25 than 36°C (motile at 25°C, nonmotile at 36°C), urea$^+$
Yersinia enterocolitica, pathogenic serotypes	CR-MOX$^+$, pyrazinamidase$^-$, salicin$^-$, esculin$^-$, agglutinates in O sera: 3; 4,32; 5,27; 8; 9; 13a,13b; 18; 20; or 21
Yersinia enterocolitica O3 (a pathogenic serotype)	D-Xylose$^-$, agglutinates in O3 serum, tiny colonies at 24 h on plating media
Yersinia enterocolitica, nonpathogenic serotypes	CR-MOX$^-$, pyrazinamidase$^+$, salicin$^+$, esculin$^+$, no agglutination in O sera: 3; 4,32; 5,27; 8; 09; 13a,13b; 18; 20; and 21

[a] This table gives only the general properties of the genera, species, serogroups, so there will be exceptions. See Table 1 and chapters 28 to 30 for more details and more precise data. The properties listed for a genus or group of genera generally apply for each of its species, and the properties listed for a species generally apply for each of its serotypes.

[b] Biochemical test results are given as percentages in Table 1. The serologic tests refer to slide agglutination in group or individual antisera for *Salmonella*, *Shigella*, *Yersinia*, or *E. coli*.

[c] These are two bacteriophage tests useful for identification.

[d] Abbreviations: CIN, cefsulodin-irgasan-novobiocin agar (a plating medium selective for *Yersinia*); CR-MOX, Congo red, magnesium oxalate agar (a differential medium useful for distinguishing pathogenic from nonpathogenic strains of *Yersinia*); MUCAP, 4-methylumbelliferyl caprylate (a genus-specific test for *Salmonella*); MUG, 4-methylumbelliferyl-β-D-glucuronidase; ONPG, *o*-nitrophenyl-β-D-galactopyranoside; PhoE, a test done by PCR that is sensitive and specific for *E. coli* and *Shigella* (see the text); VP, Voges-Proskauer.

B serum; the 4-methylumbelliferyl caprylate (MUCAP) test is positive; lysis by bacteriophage O1 is positive; and it is antibiotic resistant. All these results are compatible with *Salmonella* serogroup B.

"Kits" for Identification

A kit is defined as a series of miniaturized or standardized tests that are available commercially. The approach in using kits is similar to the conventional tube method, with the main differences being in the miniaturization, number of tests available, suspending medium, and method of reading and interpreting results (sometimes by machine). Kits are now used by most American laboratories; they are discussed in chapter 11. Kits usually give the correct identification for the most common species of *Enterobacteriaceae*, but they may not be as accurate for some of the new species. It is important to check the instruction manual to determine which organisms are included in the database and the number of strains that were used to define each organism. The main problem with kit-based identification is that the tests used (usually about 20 tests) are becoming inadequate to differentiate all of the current species of *Enterobacteriaceae* given in Table 1. This is also a problem with conventional tube tests when an inadequate number is used. Unusual identifications or "no identification" obtained with a kit should be checked by other methods.

Molecular Methods of Identification

Molecular methods have proved useful for identification to the level of family, genus, species, serotype, clone, and strain and for differentiation of pathogenic from nonpathogenic strains (see chapter 13). For example, a PCR test for the *phoE* gene appears to be a sensitive and specific test for determining if a culture belongs to *Escherichia-Shigella* (87). However, few if any of these molecular methods are commercially available. Commercial methods also must be approved by the Food and Drug Administration for use on human clinical specimens in the United States. These problems have greatly restricted the use of molecular methods for *Enterobacteriaceae* in clinical microbiology laboratories. However, they have proved extremely useful in a research setting. To conform with the CLIA (Clinical Laboratory Improvement Amendments of 1988, also called CLIA '88) regulations, it is necessary to report these research results with a disclaimer unless all the CLIA requirements have been met.

Problem Strains

Most strains of *Enterobacteriaceae* grow rapidly on plating media and on media used for biochemical identification, but occasionally a slow-growing or fastidious strain is encountered. Some strains grow poorly on blood agar but much better on chocolate agar incubated in a candle jar. This characteristic suggests a possible nutritional requirement or a mutation involving respiration. There are slow-growing strains of *E. coli*, *K. pneumoniae*, and *Serratia marcescens*, and typical biochemical reactions of these strains usually require extended incubation. Another type of problem organism is sometimes isolated from patients who are taking antimicrobial agents. Li et al. described such "pleiotropic" (having multiple phenotypic expression) mutants of *S. marcescens* (74) and *Salmonella* after exposure to gentamicin. These strains react atypically in many of the standard biochemical tests and are difficult to identify. A different type of pleiotropic mutant induced by chemical exposure was reported by Lannigan and Hussian (72). A *Salmonella* strain lost the ability to produce hydrogen sulfide, reduce nitrate to nitrite, and produce gas from glucose because of chlorate resistance acquired after exposure to Dakin's solution (a solution that contains chlorate and is found in hospitals). Some atypical and slow-growing strains become more typical and grow better when they are transferred several times. Laboratories occasionally isolate strains that grow rapidly but do not have biochemical reactions that fit any of the described species, biogroups, or Enteric Groups of *Enterobacteriaceae*. At present, this type of culture can only be reported as "unidentified." It may be an atypical strain of one of the organisms listed in Table 1, or it may belong to a new species that has not been described. Additional testing at a state, national, or international reference laboratory can often answer this question, and has in the past led to the discovery of new causes of human infections (12, 16, 33, 77).

ANTIBIOTIC SUSCEPTIBILITY

Several methods are available for testing the antibiotic susceptibility of *Enterobacteriaceae*, but the most popular are disk diffusion (5) and broth dilution (see chapter 118). In addition, the reader should consult a current textbook or review of infectious diseases for a description of antibiotic usage in clinical practice.

When antibiotics were first introduced, there was only slight resistance among the species of *Enterobacteriaceae*. Today, antibiotic resistance is much more common among strains isolated from humans and animals. Resistance patterns vary depending on the organism and its origin.

Intrinsic Resistance

Intrinsic resistance is a genetic property of most strains of a species and evolved long before the clinical use of antibiotics. This evolution can best be shown by studying strains isolated and stored before the antibiotic era or by studying strains from nature that presumably have had less exposure to antibiotics. For example, essentially all strains of *Serratia marcescens* have intrinsic resistance to penicillin G, colistin, and cephalothin. Table 7 lists some species of *Enterobacteriaceae* and their intrinsic resistance patterns.

The Antibiogram as a Marker in Epidemiological Studies

Antibiotic susceptibility testing is usually done on isolates that are clinically significant (see chapter 7) and provides an "antibiogram" that is useful for comparing isolates in epidemiologic studies. When the selective ecological pressure of antibiotics is changed, the resistance patterns of epidemic (or endemic) strains may also change. These changes have been documented in outbreaks that have lasted for several months or longer. Even with these limitations in stability, the antibiogram is probably the most useful and practical laboratory marker for comparing strains and can be extremely helpful in recognizing infection problems.

Use of Antibiograms for Identification

The antibiogram of a culture can be compared with those of known isolates (Table 7) to provide a different approach to identification. When the antibiogram and identification are incompatible (for example, a culture of *Klebsiella* that is susceptible to ampicillin and carbenicillin, or a culture of *Enterobacter* that is susceptible to cephalothin), the culture should be streaked and checked for purity. In addition, both the identification and the antibiogram may have to be repeated.

TABLE 7 Intrinsic antimicrobial resistance in some of the common *Enterobacteriaceae*

Genus or species	Most strains are resistant to:
Buttiauxella species	Cephalothin
Cedecea species	Polymyxins, ampicillin, cephalothin
Citrobacter amalonaticus	Ampicillin
Citrobacter freundii	Cephalothin
Citrobacter diversus	Cephalothin, carbenicillin
Edwardsiella tarda	Colistin
Enterobacter cloacae	Cephalothin
Enterobacter aerogenes	Cephalothin
Many other *Enterobacter* species	Cephalothin
Escherichia hermannii	Ampicillin, carbenicillin
Ewingella americana	Cephalothin
Hafnia alvei	Cephalothin
Klebsiella pneumoniae	Ampicillin, carbenicillin
Kluyvera ascorbata	Ampicillin
Kluyvera cryocrescens	Ampicillin
Proteus mirabilis	Polymyxins, tetracycline, nitrofurantoin
Proteus vulgaris	Polymyxins, ampicillin, nitrofurantoin, tetracycline
Morganella morganii	Polymyxins, ampicillin, cephalothin
Providencia rettgeri	Polymyxins, cephalothin, nitrofurantoin, tetracycline
Other *Providencia* species[a]	Polymyxins, nitrofurantoin
Serratia marcescens[b]	Polymyxins, cephalothin, nitrofurantoin
Serratia fonticola	Ampicillin, carbenicillin, cephalothin
Other *Serratia* species	Polymyxins,[c] cephalothin

[a] Most strains of *Providencia stuartii* are also resistant to cephalothin and tetracycline.

[b] *Serratia marcescens* can also be resistant to ampicillin, carbenicillin, streptomycin, and tetracycline.

[c] Resistance to polymyxins is common in *Serratia* species, but some strains have zones of 10 to 12 mm or larger.

Some of the material in this chapter was taken from or adapted from publications by authors from the Centers for Disease Control and Prevention, including other chapters and reviews of the family. I thank these authors for allowing me to use this material with a minimum of editing and rewriting. Thanks also to Robert Gaines, Hospital Infections Program, Centers for Disease Control and Prevention, for providing the unpublished data in Table 3 for 1992 to 1996 and to the many people who did biochemical testing of the cultures listed in Table 1.

REFERENCES

1. **Aldová, E., O. Hausner, D. J. Brenner, Z. Kocmoud, J. Schindler, B. Potužníková, and P. Petráš.** 1988. *Pragia fontium* gen. nov., sp. nov. of the family *Enterobacteriaceae*, isolated from water. *Int. J. Syst. Bacteriol.* **38:**183–189.
2. **Aleksić, S., A. G. Steigerwalt, J. Bockemühl, G. P. Huntley-Carter, and D. J. Brenner.** 1987. *Yersinia rohdei* sp. nov. isolated from human and dog feces and surface water. *Int. J. Syst. Bacteriol.* **37:**327–332.
3. **Bagley, S. T., R. J. Seidler, and D. J. Brenner.** 1981. *Klebsiella planticola* sp. nov.: a new species of *Enterobacteriaceae* found primarily in nonclinical environments. *Curr. Microbiol.* **6:**105–109.
4. **Balows, A., H. G. Trüper, M. Dworkin, W. Harder, and K.-H. Schleifer (ed.).** 1992. *The Prokaryotes*, 2nd ed, vol. 3, p. 2673–2937. Springer-Verlag KG, Berlin, Germany.
5. **Bauer, A. W., W. M. M. Kirby, J. C. Sherris, and M. Turck.** 1966. Antibiotic susceptibility testing by a standardized single disk method. *Am. J. Clin. Pathol.* **45:** 493–496.
6. **Bercovier, H., D. J. Brenner, J. Ursing, A. G. Steigerwalt, G. R. Fanning, J. M. Alonso, G. A. Carter, and H. H. Mollaret.** 1980. Characterization of *Yersinia enterocolitica sensu stricto*. *Curr. Microbiol.* **4:**201–206.
7. **Bercovier, H., A. G. Steigerwalt, A. Guiyoule, G. Huntley-Carter, and D. J. Brenner.** 1984. *Yersinia aldovae* (formerly *Yersinia enterocolitica*-like group X2): a new species of *Enterobacteriaceae* isolated from aquatic ecosystems. *Int. J. Syst. Bacteriol.* **34:**166–172.
8. **Bercovier, H., J. Ursing, D. J. Brenner, A. G. Steigerwalt, G. R. Fanning, G. P. Carter, and H. H. Mollaret.** 1980. *Yersinia kristensenii*: a new species of *Enterobacteriaceae* composed of sucrose-negative strains (formerly called *Yersinia enterocolitica* or *Yersinia enterocolitica*-like). *Curr. Microbiol.* **4:**219–224.
9. **Boemare, N. E., R. J. Akhurst, and R. G. Mourant.** 1993. DNA relatedness between *Xenorhabdus* spp. (*Enterobacteriaceae*), symbiotic bacteria of entomopathogenic nematodes, and a proposal to transfer *Xenorhabdus luminescens* to a new genus, *Photorhabdus* gen. nov. *Int. J. Syst. Bacteriol.* **43:**249–255.
10. **Bouvet, O. M. M., P. A. D. Grimont, C. Richard, E. Aldova, O. Hausner, and M. Gabrhelova.** 1985. *Budvicia aquatica* gen. nov., sp. nov.: a hydrogen sulfide-producing member of the *Enterobacteriaceae*. *Int. J. Syst. Bacteriol.* **35:** 60–64.
11. **Boyd, E. F., F.-S. Wang, T. S. Whittam, and R. K. Selander.** 1996. Molecular genetic relationships of the salmonellae. *Appl. Environ. Microbiol.* **62:**804–808.
12. **Brenner, D. J.** 1992. Additional genera of *Enterobacteriaceae*, p. 2922–2937. *In* A. Balows, H. G. Trüper, M. Dworkin, W. Harder, and K.-H. Schleifer (ed.), *The Prokaryotes*, 2nd ed. Springer-Verlag KG, Berlin, Germany.
13. **Brenner, D. J.** 1992. Introduction to the family *Enterobacteriaceae*, p. 2673–2695. *In* A. Balows, H. G. Trüper, M. Dworkin, W. Harder, and K.-H. Schleifer (ed.), *The Prokaryotes*, 2nd ed. Springer-Verlag KG, Berlin, Germany.
14. **Brenner, D. J., H. Bercovier, J. Ursing, J. M. Alonso, A. G. Steigerwalt, G. R. Fanning, G. P. Carter, and H. H. Mollaret.** 1980. *Yersinia intermedia*: a new species of *Enterobacteriaceae* composed of rhamnose-positive, melibiose-positive, raffinose-positive strains (formerly called atypical *Yersinia enterocolitica* or *Yersinia enterocolitica*-like). *Curr. Microbiol.* **4:**207–212.
15. **Brenner, D. J., B. R. Davis, A. G. Steigerwalt, C. F. Riddle, A. C. McWhorter, S. D. Allen, J. J. Farmer III, Y. Saitoh, and G. R. Fanning.** 1982. Atypical biogroups of *Escherichia coli* found in clinical specimens and description of *Escherichia hermannii* sp. nov. *J. Clin. Microbiol.* **15:** 703–713.
16. **Brenner, D. J., P. A. D. Grimont, A. G. Steigerwalt, G. R. Fanning, E. Ageron, and C. F. Riddle.** 1993. Classification of citrobacteria by DNA hybridization: designation of *Citrobacter farmeri* sp. nov., *Citrobacter youngae* sp. nov., *Citrobacter braakii* sp. nov., *Citrobacter werkmanii* sp. nov., *Citrobacter sedlakii* sp. nov., and three unnamed *Citrobacter* genomospecies. *Int. J. Syst. Bacteriol.* **43:**645–658.
17. **Brenner, D. J., A. C. McWhorter, A. Kai, A. G. Steigerwalt, and J. J. Farmer III.** 1986. *Enterobacter asburiae* sp. nov., a new species found in clinical specimens, and reassignment of *Erwinia dissolvens* and *Erwinia nimipressuralis* to the genus *Enterobacter* as *Enterobacter dissolvens* comb.

nov. and *Enterobacter nimipressuralis* comb. nov. *J. Clin. Microbiol.* **23:**1114–1120.

18. **Brenner, D. J., A. C. McWhorter, J. K. Leete Knutson, and A. G. Steigerwalt.** 1982. *Escherichia vulneris*: a new species of *Enterobacteriaceae* associated with human wounds. *J. Clin. Microbiol.* **15:**1133–1140.
19. **Brenner, D. J., C. Richard, A. G. Steigerwalt, M. A. Asbury, and M. Mandel.** 1980. *Enterobacter gergoviae* sp. nov.: a new species of *Enterobacteriaceae* found in clinical specimens and the environment. *Int. J. Syst. Bacteriol.* **30:** 1–6.
20. **Calderwood, S. B., D. W. K. Acheson, G. T. Keusch, T. J. Barrett, P. M. Griffin, N. A. Strockbine, B. Swaminathan, J. B. Kaper, M. M. Levine, B. S. Kaplan, H. Karch, A. D. O'Brien, T. G. Obrig, Y. Takeda, P. I. Tarr, and I. K. Wachsmuth.** 1996. Proposed new nomenclature for SLT (VT) family. *ASM News* **62:**118–119.
21. **Chung, Y. R., D. J. Brenner, A. G. Steigerwalt, B. S. Kim, H. T. Kim, and K. Y. Cho.** 1993. *Enterobacter pyrinus* sp. nov., an organism associated with brown leaf spot disease of pear trees. *Int. J. Syst. Bacteriol.* **43:**157–161.
22. **Collier, L., A. Balows, and M. Sussman (ed).** 1998. *Topley and Wilson's Microbiology and Microbial Infections*, 9th ed., vol. 2 and 3. Edward Arnold, London, England.
23. **Cosenza, B. J., and J. D. Podgwaite.** 1966. A new species of *Proteus* isolated from larvae of the gypsy moth *Porthetria dispar* (L.). *Antonie Leeuwenhoek J. Microbiol. Serol.* **32:** 187–191.
24. **Crosa, J. H., D. J. Brenner, W. H. Ewing, and S. Falkow.** 1973. Molecular relationships among the salmonelleae. *J. Bacteriol.* **115:**307–315.
25. **Dickey, R. S., and C. H. Zumoff.** 1988. Emended description of *Enterobacter cancerogenus* comb. nov. (formerly *Erwinia cancerogena*). *Int. J. Syst. Bacteriol.* **38:**371–374.
26. **DuPont, H. L., S. B. Formal, R. B. Hornick, M. J. Snyder, J. P. Libonati, D. G. Sheahan, E. H. LaBrec, and J. P. Kalas.** 1971. Pathogenesis of *Escherichia coli* diarrhea. *N. Engl. J. Med.* **285:**1–9.
27. **Ewing, W. H.** 1986. *Edwards and Ewing's Identification of Enterobacteriaceae*, 4th ed. Elsevier Science Publishing Co., New York, N.Y.
28. **Ewing, W. H., B. R. Davis, M. A. Fife, and E. F. Lessel.** 1973. Biochemical characterization of *Serratia liquefaciens* (Grimes and Hennerty) Bascomb et al. (formerly *Enterobacter liquefaciens*) and *Serratia rubidaea* comb. nov. and designation of type and neotype strains. *Int. J. Syst. Bacteriol.* **23:**217–225.
29. **Ewing, W. H., and M. A. Fife.** 1972. *Enterobacter agglomerans* (Beijerinck) comb. nov. (the *herbicola-lathyri* bacteria). *Int. J. Syst. Bacteriol.* **22:**4–11.
30. **Ewing, W. H., A. J. Ross, D. J. Brenner, and G. R. Fanning.** 1978. *Yersinia ruckerii* sp. nov., the redmouth (RM) bacterium. *Int. J. Syst. Bacteriol.* **28:**37–44.
31. **Farmer, J. J., III, M. A. Asbury, F. W. Hickman, D. J. Brenner, and The *Enterobacteriaceae* Study Group.** 1980. *Enterobacter sakazakii*: a new species of "*Enterobacteriaceae*" isolated from clinical specimens. *Int. J. Syst. Bacteriol.* **30:**569–584.
32. **Farmer, J. J., III, and B. R. Davis.** 1985. H7 antiserum-sorbitol fermentation medium: a single tube screening medium for detecting *Escherichia coli* O157:H7 associated with hemorrhagic colitis. *J. Clin. Microbiol.* **22:**620–625. (*Note:* This paper has a misprint in the formula for MacConkey sorbitol agar. The paper says to use 22.2 grams of MacConkey agar base; the correct amount is 40 grams, which is given in the instructions on the bottle.)
33. **Farmer, J. J., III, B. R. Davis, F. W. Hickman-Brenner, A. McWhorter, G. P. Huntley-Carter, M. A. Asbury, C. Riddle, H. G. Wathen, C. Elias, G. R. Fanning, A. G. Steigerwalt, C. M. O'Hara, G. K. Morris, P. B. Smith, and D. J. Brenner.** 1984. Biochemical identification of new species and biogroups of *Enterobacteriaceae* isolated from clinical specimens. *J. Clin. Microbiol.* **21:**46–76.
34. **Farmer, J. J., III, G. R. Fanning, B. R. Davis, C. M. O'Hara, C. Riddle, F. W. Hickman-Brenner, M. A. Asbury, V. Lowery, and D. J. Brenner.** 1984. *Escherichia fergusonii* and *Enterobacter taylorae*: two new species of *Enterobacteriaceae* isolated from clinical specimens. *J. Clin. Microbiol.* **21:**77–81.
35. **Farmer, J. J., III, G. R. Fanning, G. P. Huntley-Carter, B. Holmes, F. W. Hickman, C. Richard, and D. J. Brenner.** 1981. *Kluyvera*: a new (redefined) genus in the family *Enterobacteriaceae*: identification of *Kluyvera ascorbata* sp. nov. and *Kluyvera cryocrescens* sp. nov. in clinical specimens. *J. Clin. Microbiol.* **13:**919–933.
36. **Farmer, J. J., III, J. H. Jorgensen, P. A. D. Grimont, R. J. Akhurst, G. O. Poinar, Jr., E. Ageron, G. V. Pierce, J. A. Smith, G. P. Carter, K. L. Wilson, and F. W. Hickman-Brenner.** 1989. *Xenorhabdus luminescens* (DNA hybridization group 5) from human clinical specimens. *J. Clin. Microbiol.* **27:**1594–1600.
37. **Farmer, J. J., III, A. C. McWhorter, D. J. Brenner, and G. K. Morris.** 1984. The *Salmonella-Arizona* group of *Enterobacteriaceae*: nomenclature, classification and reporting. *Clin. Microbiol. Newsl.* **6:**63–66.
38. **Farmer, J. J., III, N. K. Sheth, J. A. Hudzinski, H. D. Rose, and M. F. Asbury.** 1982. Bacteremia due to *Cedecea neteri* sp. nov. *J. Clin. Microbiol.* **16:**775–778.
39. **Farmer, J. J., III, J. G. Wells, P. M. Griffin, and I. K. Wachsmuth.** 1987. *Enterobacteriaceae* infections, p. 233–296. *In* B. B. Wentworth (ed.), *Diagnostic Procedures for Bacterial Infections*, 7th ed. American Public Health Association, Washington, D.C.
40. **Ferragut, C., D. Izard, F. Gavini, K. Kersters, J. DeLey, and H. Leclerc.** 1983. *Klebsiella trevisanii*: a new species from water and soil. *Int. J. Syst. Bacteriol.* **33:**133–142.
41. **Ferragut, C., D. Izard, F. Gavini, B. Lefebre, and H. Leclerc.** 1981. *Buttiauxella*, a new genus of the family *Enterobacteriaceae*. *Zentralbl. Bakteriol. Parasitenkd. Infektionskr. Hyg. Abt. 1. Orig. Reihe C* **2:**33–44.
42. **Gavini, F., C. Ferragut, D. Izard, P. A. Trinel, H. Leclerc, B. Lefebvre, and D. A. A. Mossel.** 1979. *Serratia fonticola*, a new species from water. *Int. J. Syst. Bacteriol.* **29:**92–101.
43. **Gavini, F., J. Mergaert, A. Beji, C. Mielcarek, D. Izard, K. Kersters, and J. De Ley.** 1989. Transfer of *Enterobacter agglomerans* (Beijerinck 1888) Ewing and Fife 1972 to *Pantoea* gen. nov. as *Pantoea agglomerans* comb. nov. and description of *Pantoea dispersa* sp. nov. *Int. J. Syst. Bacteriol.* **39:**337–345.
44. **Grimont, P. A. D., and E. Ageron.** 1989. *Enterobacter cancerogenus* (Urosevic, 1966) Dickey and Zumoff 1988, a senior subjective synonym of *Enterobacter taylorae* Farmer et al. (1985). *Res. Microbiol.* **140:**459–465.
45. **Grimont, P. A. D., J. J. Farmer III, F. Grimont, M. A. Asbury, D. J. Brenner, and C. Deval.** 1983. *Ewingella americana* gen. nov., sp. nov., a new *Enterobacteriaceae* isolated from clinical specimens. *Ann. Microbiol. (Inst. Pasteur)* **134A:**39–52.
46. **Grimont, P. A. D., F. Grimont, J. J. Farmer III, and M. A. Asbury.** 1981. *Cedecea davisae* gen. nov., sp. nov., and *Cedecea lapagei* sp. nov., new *Enterobacteriaceae* from clinical specimens. *Int. J. Syst. Bacteriol.* **31:**317–326.
47. **Grimont, P. A. D., F. Grimont, C. Richard, B. R. Davis, A. G. Steigerwalt, and D. J. Brenner.** 1978. Deoxyribonucleic acid relatedness between *Serratia plymuthica* and other *Serratia* species, with a description of *Serratia odorifera* sp.

nov. (type strain: ICPB 3995). *Int. J. Syst. Bacteriol.* **28:** 453–463.

48. **Grimont, P. A. D., F. Grimont, C. Richard, and R. Sakazaki.** 1980. *Edwardsiella hoshinae*, a new species of *Enterobacteriaceae*. *Curr. Microbiol.* **4:**347–351.
49. **Grimont, P. A. D., F. Grimont, and M. P. Starr.** 1979. *Serratia ficaria* sp. nov., a bacterial species associated with smyrna figs and the fig wasp *Blastophaga psenes*. *Curr. Microbiol.* **2:**277–282.
50. **Grimont, P. A. D., T. A. Jackson, E. Ageron, and M. J. Noonan.** 1988. *Serratia entomophila* sp. nov. associated with amber disease in the New Zealand grass grub *Costelytra zealandica*. *Int. J. Syst. Bacteriol.* **38:**1–6.
51. **Harris, J. C., H. L. DuPont, and R. B. Hornick.** 1971. Fecal leukocytes in diarrheal illness. *Ann. Intern. Med.* **76:** 697–703.
52. **Hawke, J. P., A. C. McWhorter, A. G. Steigerwalt, and D. J. Brenner.** 1981. *Edwardsiella ictaluri* sp. nov., the causative agent of enteric septicemia of catfish. *Int. J. Syst. Bacteriol.* **31:**396–400.
53. **Hickman, F. W., and J. J. Farmer III.** 1978. *Salmonella typhi*: identification, antibiograms, serology, and bacteriophage typing. *Am. J. Med. Technol.* **44:**1149–1159.
54. **Hickman, F. W., J. J. Farmer III, A. G. Steigerwalt, and D. J. Brenner.** 1980. Unusual groups of *Morganella* ("*Proteus*") *morganii* isolated from clinical specimens: lysine-positive and ornithine-negative biogroups. *J. Clin. Microbiol.* **12:**88–94.
55. **Hickman, F. W., A. G. Steigerwalt, J. J. Farmer III, and D. J. Brenner.** 1982. Identification of *Proteus penneri* sp. nov., formerly known as *P. vulgaris* indole negative or as *Proteus vulgaris* biogroup 1. *J. Clin. Microbiol.* **15:** 1097–1102.
56. **Hickman-Brenner, F., J. J. Farmer III, A. G. Steigerwalt, and D. J. Brenner.** 1983. *Providencia rustigianii*: a new species in the family *Enterobacteriaceae* formerly known as *Providencia alcalifaciens* biogroup 3. *J. Clin. Microbiol.* **15:** 1057–1060.
57. **Hickman-Brenner, F. W., G. P. Huntley-Carter, G. R. Fanning, D. J. Brenner, and J. J. Farmer III.** 1985. *Koserella trabulsii*, a new genus and species of *Enterobacteriaceae* formerly known as Enteric Group 45. *J. Clin. Microbiol.* **21:**39–42.
58. **Hickman-Brenner F. W., G. P. Huntley-Carter, Y. Saitoh, A. G. Steigerwalt, J. J. Farmer III, and D. J. Brenner.** 1984. *Moellerella wisconsensis*, a new genus and species of *Enterobacteriaceae* found in human stool specimens. *J. Clin. Microbiol.* **19:**460–463.
59. **Hickman-Brenner, F. W., M. P. Vohra, G. P. Huntley-Carter, G. R. Fanning, V. A. Lowery III, D. J. Brenner, and J. J. Farmer III.** 1985. *Leminorella*, a new genus of *Enterobacteriaceae*: identification of *Leminorella grimontii* sp. nov. and *Leminorella richardii* sp. nov. found in clinical specimens. *J. Clin. Microbiol.* **21:**234–239.
60. **Hollis, D. G., F. W. Hickman, G. R. Fanning, J. J. Farmer III, R. E. Weaver, and D. J. Brenner.** 1981. *Tatumella ptyseos* gen. nov., sp. nov., a member of the family *Enterobacteriaceae* found in clinical specimens. *J. Clin. Microbiol.* **14:**79–88.
61. **Izard, D., C. Ferragut, F. Gavini, K. Kersters, J. DeLey, and H. Leclerc.** 1981. *Klebsiella terrigena*, a new species from soil and water. *Int. J. Syst. Bacteriol.* **31:**116–127.
62. **Izard, D., F. Gavini, and H. Leclerc.** 1980. Polynucleotide sequence relatedness and genome size among *Enterobacter intermedium sp. nov.* and the species *Enterobacter cloacae* and *Klebsiella pneumoniae*. *Zentralbl. Bakteriol. Parasitenkd. Infektionskr. Hyg. Abt. I Orig. Reihe C* **1:**51–60.
63. **Izard, D., F. Gavini, P. A. Trinel, and H. Leclerc.** 1979. *Rahnella aquatilis*, nouveau membre de la famille des *Enterobacteriaceae*. *Ann. Microbiol. (Inst. Pasteur)* **130A:** 163–177.
64. **Izard, D., F. Gavini, P. A. Trinel, and H. Leclerc.** 1981. Deoxyribonucleic acid relatedness between *Enterobacter cloacae* and *Enterobacter amnigenus* sp. nov. *Int. J. Syst. Bacteriol.* **31:**35–42.
65. **Jensen, K. T., W. Frederiksen, F. W. Hickman-Brenner, A. G. Steigerwalt, C. F. Riddle, and D. J. Brenner.** 1992. Recognition of *Morganella* subspecies, with proposal of *Morganella morganii* subspecies *morganii* subsp. nov. and *Morganella morganii* subspecies *sibonii* subsp. nov. *Int. J. Syst. Bacteriol.* **42:**613–620.
66. **Judicial Commission of the International Committee on Systematic Bacteriology.** 1993. Rejection of the name *Citrobacter diversus* Werkman and Gillen. *Int. J. Syst. Bacteriol.* **43:**392.
67. **Kandolo, K., and G. Wauters.** 1985. Pyrazinamidase activity in *Yersinia enterocolitica* and related organisms. *J. Clin. Microbiol.* **21:**980–982.
68. **Karmali, M. A.** 1989. Infection by verocytotoxin-producing *Escherichia coli*. *Clin. Microbiol. Rev.* **2:**15–38.
69. **Kauffmann, F.** 1966. *The Bacteriology of Enterobacteriaceae*. The Williams & Wilkins Co., Baltimore, Md.
70. **Kosako, Y., K. Tamura, R. Sakazaki, and K. Miki.** 1996. *Enterobacter kobei* sp. nov., a new species of *Enterobacteriaceae* resembling *Enterobacter cloacae*. *Curr. Microbiol.* **33:** 261–265.
71. **Krieg, N. R., and J. G. Holt (ed.).** 1984. *Bergey's Manual of Systematic Bacteriology*, vol. 1, p. 408–516. The Williams & Wilkins Co., Baltimore, Md.
72. **Lannigan, R., and Z. Hussian.** 1993. Wound isolate of *Salmonella typhimurium* that became chlorate resistant after exposure to Dakin's solution: concomitant loss of hydrogen sulfide production, gas production, and nitrate reduction. *J. Clin. Microbiol.* **31:**2497–2498.
73. **Le Minor, L., M. Y. Popoff, B. Laurent, and D. Hermant.** 1986. Individualisation d'une septième sous-espèce de *Salmonella: S. choleraesuis* subsp. *indica* subsp. nov. *Ann. Microbiol. (Inst. Pasteur)* **137B:**211–217.
74. **Li, K., J. J. Farmer III, and A. Coppola.** 1974. A novel type of resistant bacteria induced by gentamicin. *Trans. N. Y. Acad. Sci.* **36:**369–396.
75. **McWhorter, A. C., R. L. Haddock, F. A. Nocon, A. G. Steigerwalt, D. J. Brenner, S. Aleksic, J. Bockemuhl, and J. J. Farmer III.** 1991. *Trabulsiella guamensis*, a new genus and species of the family *Enterobacteriaceae* that resembles *Salmonella* subgroups 4 and 5. *J. Clin. Microbiol.* **29:** 1480–1485.
76. **McWhorter-Murlin, A. C., and F. W. Hickman-Brenner.** 1994. *Identification and Serotyping of* Salmonella *and an Update of the Kauffmann-White Scheme*; *Appendix A, Kauffmann-White Scheme, Alphabetical List of* Salmonella *Serotypes* (updated 1994); *Appendix B, Kauffmann-White Scheme, List of* Salmonella *Serotypes by O Group* (updated 1994). Foodborne and Diarrheal Diseases Laboratory Section, Centers for Disease Control and Prevention, Atlanta, Ga.
77. **Müller, H. E., D. J. Brenner, G. R. Fanning, P. A. D. Grimont, and P. Kämpfer.** 1996. Emended description of *Buttiauxella agrestis* with recognition of six new species of *Buttiauxella* and two new species of *Kluyvera: Buttiauxella ferragutiae* sp. nov., *Buttiauxella gaginiae* sp. nov., *Buttiauxella brennerae* sp. nov., *Buttiauxella izardii* sp. nov., *Buttiauxella noackiae* sp. nov., *Buttiauxella warmboldiae* sp. nov., *Kluyvera cochleae* sp. nov., and *Kluyvera georgiana* sp. nov. *Int. J. Syst. Bacteriol.* **46:**50–63.
78. **Müller, H. E., C. M. O'Hara, G. R. Fanning, F. W. Hickman-Brenner, J. M. Swenson, and D. J. Brenner.** 1986.

Providencia heimbachae, a new species of *Enterobacteriaceae* isolated from animals. *Int. J. Syst. Bacteriol.* **36:**252–256.

79. **O'Hara, C. M., A. G. Steigerwalt, B. C. Hill, J. J. Farmer III, G. R. Fanning, and D. J. Brenner.** 1989. *Enterobacter hormaechei*, a new species of the family *Enterobacteriaceae* formerly known as enteric group 75. *J. Clin. Microbiol.* **27:** 2046–2049.
80. **Pickering, L. K., H. L. DuPont, J. Olarte, R. Conklin, and C. Ericsson.** 1977. Fecal leucocytes in enteric infections. *Am. J. Clin. Pathol.* **68:**562–565.
81. **Popoff, M. Y., and L. Le Minor.** 1997. *Antigenic Formulas of the* Salmonella *Serovars*, 7th revision. WHO Collaborating Centre for Reference and Research on *Salmonella*. Institut Pasteur, Paris, France.
82. **Popoff, M. Y., and L. Le Minor.** 1997. *Guidelines for the Preparation of* Salmonella *Antisera.* WHO Collaborating Centre for Reference and Research on *Salmonella*. Institut Pasteur, Paris, France.
83. **Reeves, M. W., G. M. Evins, A. A. Heiba, B. D. Plikaytis, and J. J. Farmer III.** 1989. Clonal nature of *Salmonella typhi* and its genetic relatedness to other salmonellae as shown by multilocus enzyme electrophoresis, and proposal of *Salmonella bongori* comb. nov. *J. Clin. Microbiol.* **27:** 313–320.
84. **Riley, G., and S. Toma.** 1989. Detection of pathogenic *Yersinia enterocolitica* by using Congo red-magnesium oxalate agar medium. *J. Clin. Microbiol.* **27:**213–214.
85. **Sakazaki, R., K. Tamura, Y. Kosako, and E. Yoshizaki.** 1989. *Klebsiella ornithinolytica* sp. nov., formerly known as ornithine-positive *Klebsiella oxytoca*. *Curr. Microbiol.* **18:** 201–206.
86. **Schaberg, D. R.** 1991. Major trends in the microbial etiology of nosocomial infections. *Ann. Intern. Med.* **91**(Suppl. 3B)**:**72S–75S.
87. **Sprierings, G., C. Ockhuijsen, H. Hofstra, and J. Tommassen.** 1993. Polymerase chain reaction for the specific detection of *Escherichia coli/Shigella*. *Res. Microbiol.* **144:** 557–564.
88. **Tamura, K., R. Sakazaki, Y. Kosako, and E. Yoshizaki.** 1986. *Leclercia adecarboxylata* gen. nov., comb. nov., formerly known as *Escherichia adecarboxylata*. *Curr. Microbiol.* **13:**179–184.
89. **Thomas, G. M., and G. O. Poinar, Jr.** 1979. *Xenorhabdus* gen. nov., a genus of entomopathogenic nematophilic bacteria of the family *Enterobacteriaceae*. *Int. J. Syst. Bacteriol.* **29:**352–360.
90. **Ursing, J., D. J. Brenner, H. Bercovier, G. R. Fanning, A. G. Steigerwalt, J. Brault, and H. H. Mollaret.** 1980. *Yersinia frederiksenii*: a new species of *Enterobacteriaceae* composed of rhamnose-positive strains (formerly called atypical *Yersinia enterocolitica* or *Yersinia enterocolitica*-like). *Curr. Microbiol.* **4:**213–217.
91. **Wadstrom, T., A. Aust-Kettis, D. Habte, J. Holmgren, G. Meeuwisse, R. Mollby, and O. Soderlind.** 1976. Enterotoxin-producing bacteria and parasites in stool of Ethiopian children with diarrhoeal disease. *Arch. Dis. Child.* **51:**865–870.
92. **Wauters, G., M. Janssens, A. G. Steigerwalt, and D. J. Brenner.** 1988. *Yersinia mollaretii* sp. nov. and *Yersinia bercovieri* sp. nov., formerly called *Yersinia enterocolitica* biogroups 3A and 3B. *Int. J. Syst. Bacteriol.* **38:**424–429.
93. **Wells, J. G., B. R. Davis, I. K. Wachsmuth, L. W. Riley, R. S. Remis, R. Sokolow, and G. K. Morris.** 1983. Laboratory investigation of hemorrhagic colitis outbreaks associated with a rare *Escherichia coli* serotype. *J. Clin. Microbiol.* **18:**512–520.

Escherichia, Shigella, and *Salmonella**

CHERYL A. BOPP, FRANCES W. BRENNER, JOY G. WELLS, AND NANCY A. STROCKBINE

28

TAXONOMY

Escherichia, Shigella, and *Salmonella* are classified in the family *Enterobacteriaceae*, which is addressed in chapter 27 (37). Species in these three genera are gram-negative rods that grow well on MacConkey agar (MAC). When these organisms are motile, it is by peritrichous flagella; however, all strains of *Shigella* spp. and some strains of *Escherichia* and *Salmonella* are nonmotile. All ferment D-glucose; *Escherichia* and *Salmonella* strains usually produce gas. *Escherichia coli* and *Shigella* are phenotypically similar and, with the exception of *Shigella boydii* 13, would be considered the same species by DNA-DNA hybridization analysis (21).

NATURAL HABITATS

These three genera are most commonly isolated from the intestines of humans and animals. Because *E. coli* is ubiquitous in human and animal feces, the presence of this species in water is considered to be an indicator of fecal contamination. Some species or serotypes are isolated only from humans (e.g., *Salmonella* serotype Typhi and *Shigella dysenteriae* 1), while others (e.g., *Salmonella* serotype Gallinarum and *Salmonella* serotype Marina) are strongly associated with certain animal hosts. These genera can be isolated from fecally contaminated foods or water but probably do not occur as free-living organisms in the environment. *Salmonella* strains can, however, survive for long periods of time in the environment (perhaps years) (53).

COLLECTION, TRANSPORT, AND STORAGE OF FECAL SPECIMENS

Information on the collection, transport, and storage of specimens from extraintestinal sites is provided in chapter 4 of this Manual.

Fecal specimens can include whole stools, swabs prepared from whole stools, or rectal swabs with visible fecal staining. Ideally, stool specimens should be examined as soon as they are received in the laboratory. If whole stool specimens will not be processed immediately, they should be either refrigerated or frozen at −70°C as soon as possible after collection. All fecal specimens that cannot be examined within 1 to 2 h and all rectal swabs should be immediately placed in transport medium and refrigerated. The swab should be completely covered by the transport medium to keep it sufficiently moist for optimal recovery of the organisms. If specimens in transport medium will not be examined within 3 days, they should be frozen immediately, preferably at −70°C.

Many of the commercially available transport media (e.g., Cary-Blair, Stuart's, and Amies transport media) are satisfactory for these organisms. Although acceptable for the transport of *E. coli*, *Salmonella*, and *Shigella*, buffered glycerol saline should not be used for specimens that must also be tested for *Campylobacter* and *Vibrio*.

ESCHERICHIA

Description of the Genus

The genus *Escherichia* is composed of motile or nonmotile bacteria that conform to the definitions of the family *Enterobacteriaceae* (37). There are five species in this genus: *Escherichia blattae*, *E. coli*, *Escherichia fergusonnii*, *Escherichia hermannii*, and *Escherichia vulneris*. The type species is *E. coli*. Biochemical reactions typical of each *Escherichia* species are listed in chapter 27.

Clinical Significance

Of the five *Escherichia* species, *E. coli* is the species most commonly isolated from human specimens. It is part of the bowel flora of healthy individuals; however, certain strains may cause extraintestinal and intestinal infections in immunocompromised as well as healthy individuals. Urinary tract infections, bacteremia, meningitis, and diarrheal disease are the most common clinical syndromes caused primarily by a limited number of pathogenic clones of *E. coli* (see chapter 27). *E. hermannii* and *E. vulneris* are most frequently obtained from wound infections but have also been isolated from infections at other body sites (10). *E. fergusonnii* has been most frequently obtained from human feces. *E. blattae*, which is a commensal organism of cockroaches, is not isolated from human specimens.

Diarrheagenic *E. coli*

There are at least four categories of recognized diarrheagenic *E. coli*: Shiga toxin-producing *E. coli* (STEC) (also referred to as enterohemorrhagic *E. coli* [EHEC]), enterotoxigenic *E. coli* (ETEC), enteropathogenic *E. coli* (EPEC), and enter-

* This chapter contains information presented in chapter 33 by Larry D. Gray in the sixth edition of this Manual.

oinvasive *E. coli* (EIEC). The salient clinical features of infection and the pathogenic mechanisms of strains in these categories of diarrheagenic *E. coli* were recently reviewed by Nataro and Kaper (69). There are also several other groups of putative diarrheagenic *E. coli*, including enteroaggregative *E. coli* (EaggEC) and various toxin-producing *E. coli* strains, but the clinical significance of these organisms is unclear.

STEC: O157 and Other STEC Serogroups

We will refer to the STEC category of diarrheagenic *E. coli* according to the toxins that these organisms produce, e.g., STEC rather than EHEC, because the essential genetic features that define organisms capable of causing hemorrhagic colitis and hemolytic-uremic syndrome (HUS) are not clear. *E. coli* serotypes O157:H7 and O157:nonmotile (NM) (O157 STEC) produce one or more Shiga toxins, also called verocytotoxins, and are the most commonly identified diarrheagenic *E. coli* isolates in North America and Europe.

E. coli O157:H7 and other STEC serotypes cause a broad spectrum of illness that can present as mild nonbloody diarrhea, severe bloody diarrhea (hemorrhagic colitis), and HUS (43). Additional symptoms of *E. coli* O157:H7 infection include abdominal cramps and lack of fever. Of patients with O157 STEC diarrhea, approximately 6% develop HUS, a condition characterized by microangiopathic hemolytic anemia, thrombocytopenia, and acute renal failure.

O157 STEC is thought to cause at least 80% of cases of HUS in North America and is recognized as a common cause of bloody diarrhea in developed countries (43). In a recently published survey of 10 U.S. hospitals, the rates of isolation of O157 STEC from fecal specimens exceeded those of other common enteric pathogens, particularly *Shigella* (92), in some geographic areas and some age groups. Many U.S. clinical laboratories do not routinely culture stools for O157 STEC; as a result, many illnesses are not detected (19).

O157 STEC colonizes dairy and beef cattle, and not surprisingly, ground beef has caused more O157 STEC outbreaks than any other vehicle of transmission (43). Other known vehicles of transmission include raw milk, sausage, roast beef, unchlorinated municipal water, apple cider, raw vegetables, salads, and mayonnaise. O157 STEC spreads easily from person to person because the infectious dose is low; outbreaks associated with person-to-person spread have occurred in schools, long-term-care institutions, families, and day-care facilities (7).

At least 100 serotypes of non-O157 STEC have been isolated from persons with diarrhea or HUS (Table 1). In

TABLE 1 Serotypes of *E. coli* isolated from human diarrheal illness

ETEC	EPEC	EIEC	STEC			
O6:NM	O26:NM	O28ac:NM	O1:NM	O50:H7	O113:H21	O153:H25
O6:H16	O26:H11	O29:NM	O1:H1	O52:H25	O113:H53	O157:NM
O8:NM	O55:NM	O112ac:NM	O1:H7	O55:NM	O114:H4	O157:H7
O8:H9	O55:H6	O115:NM	O2:H1	O55:H7	O114:H48	O163:H19
O11:H27	O55:H7	O124:NM	O2:H5	O55:H10	O115:H10	O165:NM
O15:H11	O86:NM	O124:H7	O2:H6	O73:H34	O115:H18	O165:H10
O20:NM	O86:H2	O124:H30	O2:H7	O75:H5	O117:H4	O165:H19
O25:NM	O86:H34	O135:NM	O4:NM	O82:H8	O118:H12	O165:H25
O25:H42	O111ab:NM	O136:NM	O4:H10	O84:H2	O118:H30	O166:H12
O27:NM	O111ab:H2	O143:NM	O5:NM	O85:NM	O119:H5	O166:H15
O27:H7	O111ab:H12	O144:NM	O5:H16	O86:H10	O119:H6	OX3:H21
O27:H20	O111ab:H21	O152:NM	O6:NM	O88:NM	O120:H19	Orough:H20[a]
O49:NM	O114:NM	O164:NM	O6:H1	O91:NM	O121:NM	ONT:NM[b]
O63:H12	O114:H2	O167:NM	O6:H28	O91:H14	O121:H8	ONT:H1
O78:H11	O119:H6		O18:NM	O91:H21	O121:H19	ONT:H28
O78:H12	O125ac:H21		O18:H7	O100:H32	O125:NM	
O85:H7	O126:H27		O22:H8	O101:H19	O125:H8	
O114:H21	O127:NM		O22:H16	O103:H2	O126:NM	
O115:H21	O127:H6		O23:H7	O103:H6	O126:H8	
O126:H9	O127:H9		O23:H16	O104:NM	O126:H21	
O128ac:H12	O128ab:H2		O25:NM	O104:H21	O128:NM	
O128ac:H21	O142:H6		O26:NM	O105:H18	O128:H2	
O128ac:H27	O158:H23		O26:H2	O110:H19	O128:H8	
O148:H28			O26:H8	O111:NM	O128:H12	
O149:H4			O26:H11	O111:H2	O128:H25	
O153:H45			O26:H32	O111:H7	O132:NM	
O159:NM			O38:H21	O111:H8	O133:H53	
O159:H4			O39:H4	O111:H30	O141:NM	
O159:H20			O45:NM	O111:H34	O145:NM	
O166:H27			O45:H2	O111:HNT	O145:H25	
O167:H5			O48:H21	O112:H21	O146:NM	
O169:H41			O50:NM	O113:H2	O146:H21	
				O113:H7		

[a] Orough, O antigen rough and serotype not determined.
[b] NT, not typeable.

some geographic areas, non-O157 STEC strains, particularly *E. coli* serotypes O111:NM and O26:H11, are more commonly isolated than O157 STEC (1, 43, 101). In the United States, non-O157 STEC strains are less frequently encountered than O157 STEC strains, and outbreaks attributed to these strains are rare (6, 26, 43). Because most laboratory methods for the detection of O157 STEC do not detect non-O157 STEC, the numbers of documented infections with serotypes other than O157:H7 or O157:NM are probably underestimated.

ETEC

ETEC, which produces heat-labile *E. coli* enterotoxin (LT) or heat-stable *E. coli* enterotoxin (ST), or both LT and ST, is an important cause of diarrhea in developing countries, particularly among young children (69). ETEC also is a frequent cause of traveler's diarrhea. Although in the past ETEC was rarely implicated as a cause of epidemic illness in the United States and Japan, it has become an increasingly common etiologic agent of diarrheal outbreaks in both countries (68). Nine U.S. outbreaks were reported to the Centers for Disease Control and Prevention (CDC) from 1992 to 1997, while only four outbreaks occurred during the preceding 10 years (32, 112). ETEC is infrequently identified in the United States, but this is undoubtedly attributable, at least in part, to the fact that few laboratories are capable of identifying this pathogen. ETEC strains, particularly those associated with outbreaks, tend to cluster in a few serotypes (Table 1).

The most prominent symptoms of ETEC illness are diarrhea and abdominal cramps sometimes accompanied by nausea and headache, but usually with little vomiting or fever (32). Although ETEC is usually associated with relatively mild watery diarrhea, illness in recent ETEC outbreaks has been notable for its prolonged duration (25).

EPEC

In the past, EPEC strains were defined as certain *E. coli* serotypes that were epidemiologically associated with infantile diarrhea but that did not produce enterotoxins or Shiga toxins and that were not invasive. The traditional EPEC serotypes, as defined by the World Health Organization (WHO), are listed in Table 1; most of these serotypes show a distinct pattern of localized adherence to HeLa and HEp-2 cells. These serotypes usually also demonstrate actin aggregation in the fluorescent actin stain test, which correlates with the attaching-and-effacing lesion in vivo (69).

From the late 1940s to the early 1960s, serotypes of EPEC were associated with outbreaks of infantile diarrhea in hospital nurseries. The incidence of nursery outbreaks in developed countries has declined since the 1960s, but several outbreaks of EPEC diarrhea have occurred since then in day-care centers and nurseries in the United States (69). EPEC infections are rare in developed countries but are a common cause of infantile diarrhea in the developing world. Because of the lack of simple diagnostic methods for EPEC, few laboratories attempt to identify these organisms.

The symptoms of severe, prolonged, and nonbloody diarrhea, vomiting, and fever in infants or young toddlers are characteristic of EPEC illness (69). Infection with EPEC has been associated with chronic diarrhea; sequelae may include malabsorption, malnutrition, weight loss, and growth retardation.

EIEC

EIEC strains invade cells of the colon and produce a generally watery but occasionally bloody diarrhea by a pathogenic mechanism similar to that of *Shigella.* EIEC is very rare in the United States and is much less common than ETEC or EPEC in the developing world (69). EIEC strains, like ETEC and EPEC, are associated with a few characteristic serotypes (Table 1). Three large outbreaks of diarrhea caused by EIEC have been reported in the United States (69).

Putative Diarrheagenic *E. coli*

EAggEC, which exhibits a specific pattern of aggregative adherence to HEp-2 cells in culture, has been associated with diarrhea in children in Chile, persistent diarrhea in children in Mexico and Kenya, and bloody diarrhea in children in India (69). These organisms may also have a role in chronic diarrhea among human immunodeficiency virus-infected patients (80). EAggEC was isolated from children with diarrhea during an outbreak in Japan (46).

Diffusely adherent *E. coli* (DAEC) strains, which exhibit a diffuse pattern of adherence to HEp-2 cells in culture, have been implicated as causes of diarrhea in some studies but not others (69). Little is known about their associated clinical syndrome, epidemiology, and pathogenic mechanisms. In a retrospective case-control study, the majority of children infected with DAEC strains had watery diarrhea without blood or fecal leukocytes (79). In one study, an age-dependent susceptibility to DAEC was observed; DAEC infections were significantly associated with diarrhea among children 1 to 5 years of age but were not associated with illness among infants (57).

Cytotoxic necrotizing factor (CNF)-producing *E. coli* strains were first described by Caprioli et al. (23), who observed strains producing a toxin that induced morphological alterations (multinucleation) and death in tissue cultures. Two forms have been described: CNF1 and CNF2. CNF1-producing strains were originally detected in infants with enteritis (23) and later from humans with extraintestinal infections (17, 24). Most CNF1-producing strains are also hemolytic, although the toxin is distinct from hemolysin (24). CNF2-producing strains have been isolated from animals with diarrhea (33, 73, 94). The role of these strains in human diarrheal disease has not been definitively determined (69).

Johnson and Lior (48) first described cytolethal distending toxin (CLDT)-producing *E. coli* strains as strains that demonstrated a heat-labile factor which induced cytotonic and cytotoxic changes similar to those caused by LT in Chinese hamster ovary cells (48). This factor did not affect Y-1 cells. The results of one study in Bangladesh suggested that CLDT-producing *E. coli* is not associated with diarrhea, but other studies are needed to establish the status of these as etiologic agents (3, 69).

Isolation Procedures

Note that this chapter does not cover isolation procedures for extraintestinal infections. Refer to chapter 5 for more information.

Isolation Procedures for STEC

Laboratories should culture all stools for O157 STEC or, at a minimum, all stools from patients with bloody diarrhea. A recently published study showed that a history of bloody diarrhea was more predictive of infection with O157 STEC than visibly bloody stools; therefore, laboratorians should consider this information if it is available (92). Some laboratories limit culture for O157 STEC to stools from children, but many of these infections occur in adults (19, 92).

Stools from asymptomatic patients should not necessarily be discarded if a retrospective diagnosis of O157 STEC is sought. Although most patients infected with O157 STEC excrete the pathogen for only a few days, several studies have established that it may be fecally shed for up to 30 days or more after the onset of diarrhea (102).

Culture for non-O157 STEC should be considered for all patients with a history of bloody diarrhea without another identified cause or, at a minimum, all patients with severe diarrhea requiring hospitalization or patients with HUS whose stool cultures are negative for O157 STEC (1,104). Numerous strategies can be used to isolate STEC. The decision of how extensively to attempt to identify STEC infections is best guided by the prevalence of these organisms in the population served and in the availability of laboratory resources.

Enrichment

Although broth enrichment is widely used for the recovery of O157 STEC from foods, there is little evidence that it enhances isolation from human fecal specimens. However, immunomagnetic separation (IMS), a technique shown to increase the rate of isolation of O157 STEC from food specimens, has been adapted to culture of stools (29, 30, 49). IMS enhances the detection of O157 STEC from patients with HUS, patients presenting an extended period of time after the onset of illness, asymptomatic carriers, or specimens that have been stored or transported improperly (29, 30, 49). The O157-specific beads are available commercially (anti-*E. coli* O157 Dynabeads; Dynal, Inc., Lake Success, N.Y.) but are not approved by the U.S. Food and Drug Administration for use with clinical specimens. Laboratories seeking to isolate another serogroup of STEC can coat magnetic beads with the respective O-specific antibody (78).

Plating Media

Because O157 STEC strains ferment lactose, they are impossible to differentiate from other lactose-fermenting organisms on lactose-containing media. Most O157 STEC strains do not ferment the carbohydrate D-sorbitol overnight, in contrast to the approximately 80% of other *E. coli* strains that ferment sorbitol rapidly. For this reason, sorbitol was substituted for lactose in traditional MAC to create sorbitol MAC (SMAC) (63). Selective testing of sorbitol-nonfermenting colonies from SMAC simplifies the isolation of O157 STEC and conserves antisera because fewer colonies must be screened (63). In some areas of central Europe, sorbitol-fermenting O157 STEC strains are commonly isolated from patients with HUS (16); these organisms are very rare in North America (47, 98).

Tellurite and the antimicrobial cefixime have been added to SMAC to increase its selectivity (115). Rhamnose was also added to SMAC to enhance the discrimination of O157 STEC strains, which do not ferment rhamnose (115). Cefixime-tellurite SMAC (CT-SMAC) is mostly used for culture of animal and food specimens because of its selectivity, but it also is used for culture of human specimens (29, 49). However, it has been reported that a few O157:NM strains fail to grow on CT-SMAC (49). Cefixime-rhamnose SMAC is more expensive to prepare and therefore is not used as widely as CT-SMAC.

Plating media containing the substrate 4-methylumbelliferyl-β-D-glucuronide (MUG) have been used to isolate O157 STEC. Unlike other *E. coli* strains, most *E. coli* O157:H7 and O157:NM strains that produce Shiga toxins lack the β-glucuronidase enzyme and are MUG negative (89). These media are most useful for animal and food specimens but do not detect most non-O157 STEC strains because they are MUG positive. Several chromogenic media that have been designed for the isolation of both O157 and non-O157 STEC are available, but to our knowledge there are no published evaluations for human specimens.

Commercial Rapid Diagnostic Methods

An immunofluorescence assay that uses fluorescein-labeled O157-specific antibody (Kirkegaard & Perry Laboratories Inc., Gaithersburg, Md.) was developed for the rapid visualization of the organisms in stools by fluorescence microscopy (75). In addition, a commercial immunoassay (*E. coli* O157 Antigen Detection Kit; LMD Laboratories, Carlsbad, Calif.) is available for the detection of O157 strains in stool specimens (36, 76). Both of these assays can detect sorbitol-positive *E. coli* O157 strains, in contrast to culture in SMAC, which does not detect such strains, but additional testing is needed to distinguish nontoxigenic serogroup O157 strains from toxigenic strains. Because these two assays target the O157 antigen, they do not detect non-O157 STEC.

Another commercial enzyme immunoassay (EIA; Premier EHEC; Meridian Diagnostics, Inc., Cincinnati, Ohio) detects Shiga toxin in stool filtrates or broth cultures of stool specimens. In several published studies, this assay has been reported to be sensitive and specific, although it is not able to detect the Shiga toxin variant Stx2e and may produce false-positive reactions with *Pseudomonas aeruginosa* isolates (5, 14, 50, 74).

Because false-positive tests occur and because determination of the serotype responsible is important, isolation of STEC from fecal specimens that are positive by one of the rapid diagnostic methods described above should always be attempted. Ascertaining the serologic and molecular characteristics of a particular strain can be valuable for outbreak investigations.

Screening Procedures for STEC Strains

For the isolation of O157 STEC from SMAC, colorless (nonfermenting) colonies are selected and tested with O157 antiserum or latex reagent by the procedures recommended by the manufacturer (96). If the O157 latex reagent is used, it is important to test positive colonies with the latex control reagent because some sorbitol-nonfermenting organisms will react nonspecifically with latex. The manufacturers of these kits recommend that strains reacting with both the antigen-specific and control latex reagents be heated and retested. However, in a study that followed this procedure, none of the nonspecifically reacting strains were subsequently identified as O157 STEC (18).

Although the MUG reaction is most frequently used as a differential characteristic when culturing for O157 STEC from food or water, some laboratories find that this test, used in conjunction with sorbitol fermentation and O157 antiserum, is helpful for screening for these strains from human specimens (89). MUG-positive, urease-positive O157 STEC strains have been isolated in the United States but are still rare (44, 98).

Another marker that can be used for screening is production of a characteristic *E. coli* hemolysin, referred to as enterohemolysin, which is distinct from the α-hemolysin produced by other *E. coli* strains (13). Enterohemolysin is produced by virtually all O157 STEC strains and 60 to 80% of non-O157 STEC strains. A special medium, washed sheep blood agar supplemented with calcium (WSBA-Ca), is used as a differential medium for the detection of enterohemolytic activity (13). Enterohemolysin-producing colonies can be differentiated from α-hemolysin-producing colonies on WSBA-Ca because the latter are visible after 3 to 4 h of incubation. The WSBA-Ca plates are examined at 3 to 4 h, and colonies are marked for the appearance of α-hemolysin and are examined again after 18 to 24 h. No *E. coli* strains that produce both α-hemolysin and enterohemolysin have been reported; therefore, colonies that display hemolysis only after overnight incubation are selected for further testing. Because many non-O157 STEC strains do not demonstrate the enterohemolytic phenotype and because enterohemolytic nontoxigenic strains have been reported, additional screening methods should be used in conjunction with WSBA-Ca medium (11, 12, 88, 113). WSBA-Ca also can be used for the isolation of enterohemolytic strains, but to clearly discern the hemolysis reaction, well-isolated colonies must be obtained, which frequently entails spread-plating of serial dilutions of a broth enrichment culture (15).

Presumptive O157 STEC isolates that have been identified by the screening procedures described above should be sent to a reference laboratory for confirmation of the presence of the H7 antigen or the production of Shiga toxin (see Identification below). Presumptive non-O157 STEC strains should be tested for Shiga toxin, serotyped, and confirmed biochemically as *E. coli*.

Isolation Methods for ETEC, EPEC, EIEC, and the Putative Diarrheagenic *E. coli*

Methods for the identification of ETEC, EPEC, EIEC, and the putative diarrheagenic *E. coli* are generally available only in reference or research settings. Public health and reference laboratories usually examine specimens for these pathogens only when an outbreak is suspected.

ETEC should be considered a possible etiologic agent of watery diarrheal illness for which no pathogen has been identified by routine culture methods. EPEC should be considered a possible pathogen in outbreaks of severe nonbloody diarrhea occurring in infants or young toddlers, particularly in nursery or day-care settings. Specimens should have been examined and found to be negative for routine bacterial pathogens. EIEC should be considered a possible etiologic agent in outbreaks of diarrhea when other routine bacterial pathogens have been ruled out.

If isolation is to be attempted, fecal specimens should be plated on a differential medium of low selectivity (e.g., MAC). It is generally recommended that 5 to 20 colonies, mostly lactose fermenting but with a representative sample of nonfermenting colonies, be selected and inoculated to a nonselective agar slant. These colonies are then screened by techniques for the identification of virulence-associated characteristics appropriate to the pathogen being sought (see Virulence Testing below). Arrangements to send *E. coli* isolates from well-characterized outbreaks to CDC for testing can be made through local and state health departments.

Screening Procedures

Biochemical screening techniques are not useful for ETEC or EPEC because they cannot be distinguished from other *E. coli* strains by these methods. Many EIEC strains are nonmotile and fail to decarboxylate lysine, and these characteristics have been used for screening. However, the laboratorian should be aware that EIEC strains can be positive for either of these characteristics.

For many years, commercial companies produced antisera to the classical EPEC somatic (O) and capsular (K) antigens, and these were used by laboratorians to presumptively identify these organisms. Evidence indicates that this approach yields many false-positive results because many *E. coli* strains that are not classical EPEC strains agglutinate in the polyvalent sera. The classical EPEC strains were defined on the basis of both O and H (flagellar) antigens (Table 1); therefore, further testing in H antisera would reduce the number of false-positive reports. However, this type of testing is not practical for the average clinical microbiology laboratory.

Identification

Biochemical Identification

Generally, confirmation of diarrheagenic *E. coli* should include sufficient biochemical testing to confirm that the strain is an *E. coli* strain. Biochemical identification of presumptive O157 STEC isolates is one way of detecting other species which cross-react with O157 antiserum or latex reagents. These organisms include *Salmonella* O group N, *Yersinia enterocolitica* serotype O9, *Citrobacter freundii*, and *E. hermannii*. The laboratory's normal procedure for biochemical identification of *E. coli* should be suitable, whether it is a standard procedure with biochemicals in a tube or a commercial system known to be reliable for the identification of members of the family *Enterobacteriaceae*. Special biochemical tests (cellobiose fermentation, growth in the presence of KCN) may be necessary to differentiate *E. hermannii* from *E. coli*, but because *E. hermannii* is rarely detected in stool specimens, use of these tests is not cost-effective for most laboratories. Methods of biochemical identification and the specific biochemical reactions typical of *Escherichia* spp. and other members of the family *Enterobacteriaceae* are discussed in chapter 27. Manual and automated identification systems are covered in chapter 11.

Serotyping

The serologic classification of *E. coli* is generally based on two types of antigens: the O antigen (somatic) and the H antigen (flagellar) (10, 37). These antigens are most commonly identified by the tube agglutination test with antisera prepared against the different antigenic components. The O and H antigens of *E. coli* are stable and reliable strain characteristics, and although there are at least 170 O antigens and 50 H antigens, the actual number of serotype combinations associated with diarrheal disease is limited (Table 1).

Determination of the O and H serotypes of *E. coli* strains implicated in diarrheal disease is particularly useful in epidemiologic investigations as well as in the identification of certain classes of diarrheagenic *E. coli*. Complete serotyping is beyond the capacity of most reference laboratories because it is labor-intensive and would require the availability of a large number of specific antisera. If an outbreak for which common enteric pathogens have been ruled out as the cause has occurred, arrangements can be made through local and state health departments to send *E. coli* isolates to CDC for virulence testing and serotyping.

Serologic Confirmation of O157 STEC

Confirmation of *E. coli* O157:H7 requires identification of the H7 flagellar antigen. H7-specific antiserum is commercially available, but identification of the H7 flagellar antigen often requires multiple passages before the flagellar antigen is detected (96). Isolates that are nonmotile or that are negative for the H7 antigen should be tested for the production of Shiga toxins or the presence of genes encoding for Shiga toxins.

Approximately 85% of O157 isolates from humans received by CDC are serotype O157:H7, 12% are nonmotile, and 3% are H types other than H7 (98). *E. coli* O157:NM strains frequently produce Shiga toxin and are otherwise very similar to O157:H7, but no O157 strain from human illness with an H type other than H7 has been found to produce Shiga toxin (40, 98, 107).

Virulence Testing

STEC (primarily non-O157 STEC), ETEC, EPEC, EIEC, and EAggEC (and other putative diarrheagenic *E. coli*) are identified by the detection of their respective virulence-associated factors (characteristic toxins, adherence, or invasiveness). Techniques for virulence testing include bioassays (e.g., cell culture or in vivo testing), immunologic methods (e.g., immunoblotting or EIA), or the detection of gene sequences by DNA-based methods (e.g., PCR or colony blot hybridization). The laboratory's capability for performing the different types of assays will guide its selection of appropriate tests.

Most methods involve the screening of isolated colonies by one of the techniques discussed below in this Virulence Testing section. If PCR techniques are used, a sweep of confluent growth from a MAC plate rather than numerous individual colonies may be screened. If the PCR assay is positive, isolated colonies may then be picked and screened individually. This approach has worked well for some laboratories (9, 98, 112).

STEC

Two distinct Shiga toxins, Stx1 and Stx2, also referred to as verocytotoxins, have been described, and two variant forms of Stx2, Stx2c and Stx2e, have been described (22). All of these toxins are similar to the Shiga toxin expressed by *S. dysenteriae* 1, and the Stx1 toxins produced by O157 STEC and other STEC serotypes are virtually identical. STEC may produce either the Stx1 or the Stx2 toxin or both toxins.

In addition to the production of Shiga toxin, many STEC strains possess such virulence-associated characteristics as the production of intimin, a 60-MDa EHEC plasmid that also has a role in cell adherence, and enterohemolysin production, which was discussed earlier (69).

The production of Stx or the genes encoding Stx can be detected by a variety of biologic, immunologic, or nucleic acid-based assays (1, 69, 101). Protocols for performing several of these tests (e.g., cell culture, DNA probing, and PCR) are provided by Smith and Scotland (93) and Olsvik and Strockbine (72).

To our knowledge, studies evaluating commercial kits for the detection of Stx in broth culture have been published for only two of these assays, the Premier EHEC kit (described earlier in the section on commercial rapid diagnostics) and a latex agglutination test (VTEC-RPLA; Denka Seiken Co., Ltd., Tokyo, Japan) (15, 50, 74).

ETEC

The enterotoxins produced by ETEC, ST and LT, have been purified and sequenced and may be detected by a variety of biologic, immunologic, and nucleic acid-based assays (69). Two ST toxins that are structurally distinct but that show a high degree of homology have been identified. Most ETEC outbreaks in the United States have been caused by strains that produce ST only or ST in combination with LT.

At least two commercial immunoassays are available for the identification of ETEC strains from culture supernatants: one which detects ST and another which detects LT. One kit (ST EIA; Denka Seiken Co., Ltd.) is in the format of a competitive EIA for the detection of ST only (90, 97). A reversed passive latex agglutination assay (VET-RPLA; Oxoid, Ogdensburg, N.Y.) detects both cholera toxin and LT, which are highly related antigenically. The effectiveness of the VET-RPLA may be optimized by use of a culture medium designed for LT production rather than the medium recommended by the manufacturer (114).

EPEC

Laboratory identification of EPEC involves the identification of virulence-associated characteristics, particularly patterns of adherence to certain cells, by tissue culture methods, immunoassay, or nucleic acid-based methods.

No commercial kits are available for the detection of attachment-related virulence factors (e.g., intimin and the EPEC adherence factor [EAF], which is plasmid mediated) (69). An EIA has been described for the detection of EAF-positive *E. coli*, but the specific antibody is not commercially available.

To diagnose EPEC illness, a laboratory may find it convenient to set up one of the DNA-based assays with either oligonucleotide probes or primers that detect *eaeA* (intimin gene) or the EAF plasmid. Alternately, a laboratory with tissue culture facilities may set up cell culture adherence assays for the localized adherence pattern typically expressed by EAF-positive EPEC.

EIEC

EIEC can be identified by various in vivo assays, immunoassays, and nucleic acid-based assays for invasiveness. No commercial kits or reagents are available for the detection of EIEC. Laboratories wishing to diagnose these infections may set up a cell culture invasion assay or DNA-based assays for the *ipaC* or *ipaH* invasion-related factors (69, 91). A laboratory with the capability to perform plasmid DNA electrophoresis may find it useful to detect the large 120- to 140-MDa plasmid associated with invasiveness, but this plasmid is easily lost when the isolate is subcultured. Because of shared invasiveness-related characteristics, these assays will also detect *Shigella* strains.

Subtyping

Several methods of subtyping have been used for *E. coli* O157:H7 isolates. In particular, pulsed-field gel electrophoresis (PFGE) methods are useful (69, 101). Determination of the serotype and the antimicrobial susceptibility pattern is usually adequate for defining outbreak strains of ETEC, EPEC, and EIEC. Plasmid typing or PFGE methods may also be helpful for distinguishing between background isolates and outbreak strains, but neither method has been widely used for these groups of *E. coli*.

Serodiagnostic Tests

At the present time, serodiagnostic tests for diarrheagenic *E. coli* are primarily research methods useful only for seroepidemiology surveys and not for the diagnosis of sporadic infections. Assays that measure antibody response to lipopolysaccharide (LPS) have been used to diagnose STEC infection in HUS patients who are culture negative for these organisms (69).

Antimicrobial Susceptibilities

STEC

Antimicrobial therapy for O157 STEC infection has not been demonstrated to be efficacious and safe, except for cases of cystitis and pyelonephritis (43). Consequently, determination of the antimicrobial susceptibility pattern is usually meaningful only for epidemiologic purposes, as was the case in an outbreak linked to a municipal water supply in which all O157 STEC isolates were resistant to streptomycin, sulfisoxazole, and tetracycline (103).

Until recently, *E. coli* O157:H7 isolates were almost uniformly sensitive to antimicrobial agents. However, since the early 1990s, O157 and other STEC strains have demonstrated slowly increasing levels of resistance to certain antibiotics, particularly streptomycin, sulfonamides, and tetracycline (38, 51, 92).

ETEC, EPEC, EIEC, and Other Diarrheagenic *E. coli*

Treatment with an appropriate antibiotic can reduce the severity and duration of symptoms of ETEC infection (69, 87). Antimicrobial resistance, particularly to tetracycline, is common among ETEC strains isolated from outbreaks in the United States (32).

Antibiotic treatment also can be helpful for diarrhea caused by EPEC (69). Most strains associated with outbreaks are resistant to multiple antimicrobial agents (34). Little information about the efficacy of antimicrobial treatment or the prevalence of resistance is available for EIEC or other putative diarrheagenic *E. coli* (e.g., EAggEC). Determination of the antimicrobial susceptibility pattern may be helpful in establishing whether an isolate is associated with an outbreak.

Interpretation and Reporting of Results

STEC

A presumptive diagnosis of an O157 STEC (isolate positive for O157 antigen) or a non-O157 STEC (isolate positive for Shiga toxin) infection should be reported to the clinician as soon as the laboratory obtains this result. If the laboratory obtains positive results for a stool specimen by a commercial immunoassay, a preliminary report should be made to the physician with a note that these results are not considered final until they are confirmed by the isolation of STEC from the patient. It would be helpful to indicate on the report that some STEC strains cause diarrhea and HUS. Clusters and outbreaks of illness associated with STEC should be reported to public health authorities. Presumptive STEC isolates should be confirmed by demonstration of the H7 antigen or an assay for Shiga toxin and should be identified biochemically as *E. coli.*

ETEC, EPEC, and EIEC

Generally, the ETEC, EPEC, and EIEC classes of diarrheagenic *E. coli* are identified only during outbreak investigations. A laboratorian reporting these results, which usually will be a retrospective diagnosis obtained by a reference laboratory, should provide an explanation of the clinical significance of these organisms and should perhaps refer the clinician to the reference laboratory for further information. All suspected outbreaks should be reported to public health authorities.

SHIGELLA

Description of the Genus

The genus *Shigella* is composed of nonmotile bacteria that conform to the definition of the family *Enterobacteriaceae* (37). There are four serogroups of *Shigella* that historically have been treated as species: serogroup A as *S. dysenteriae,* serogroup B as *Shigella flexneri,* serogroup C as *Shigella boydii,* and serogroup D as *Shigella sonnei.* The type species is *S. dysenteriae.* With few exceptions, for example, certain strains of *S. flexneri* 6, *S. boydii* 13, and *S. boydii* 14, *Shigella* does not form gas from fermentable carbohydrates. Compared with *Escherichia, Shigella* strains are less active in their use of carbohydrates. *S. sonnei* strains ferment lactose on extended incubation, but other species generally do not use this substrate in conventional medium.

Clinical Significance

Members of the genus *Shigella* have been recognized since the late 19th century as causative agents of bacillary dysentery (2). *Shigella* causes bloody diarrhea (dysentery) and nonbloody diarrhea. Shigellosis often begins with watery diarrhea accompanied by fever and abdominal cramps but may progress to classic dysentery with scant stools containing blood, mucus, and pus. All four species of *Shigella* are capable of causing dysentery, but *S. dysenteriae* 1 has been associated with a particularly severe form of illness thought to be related to its production of Shiga toxin. Infection can also be asymptomatic, particularly infection with *S. sonnei* strains. Although these organisms are very important as causes of gastrointestinal infections, they rarely cause other types of infections. Complications of shigellosis include HUS, which is associated with *S. dysenteriae* 1 infection, and Reiter chronic arthritis syndrome, which is associated with *S. flexneri* infection (2). The identification of *Shigella* species is important for both clinical and epidemiologic purposes.

Humans and other large primates are the only natural reservoirs of *Shigella* bacteria. Most transmission is by person-to-person spread, but infection is also caused by ingestion of contaminated food or water. Shigellosis is most common in situations in which hygiene is limited (e.g., child-care centers and other institutional settings). In populations without running water and indoor plumbing, shigellosis can become an endemic problem. Sexual transmission of *Shigella* among homosexual men also occurs.

In the United States, approximately 20,000 cases of shigellosis are reported each year, but an estimated 400,000 infections are undetected. Up to 20% of all U.S. cases of shigellosis are related to international travel. Most infections in the United States and other developed countries are caused by *S. sonnei; S. flexneri* is the second most common serogroup.

In the developing world, the most prevalent serogroups are *S. flexneri* and *S. dysenteriae* 1, with the latter being the most frequent cause of epidemic dysentery. Since 1979, a prolonged *S. dysenteriae* 1 epidemic has affected southern Africa, and major epidemics have also occurred in other parts of Africa, in Asia, and in Central America. Infection with *S. dysenteriae* 1 is associated with high rates of morbidity and mortality in developing countries, particularly when antimicrobial resistance or its misdiagnosis as amoebiasis makes appropriate treatment problematic.

Isolation Procedures

Enrichment and Plating Media

There is no reliably effective enrichment medium for all serotypes of *Shigella,* but gram-negative (GN) broth and Se-

TABLE 2 Differentiation of *E. coli-Shigella*

Test	Reaction of the following species[a]:		
	Shigella	*E. coli* inactive	*E. coli*
Lysine decarboxylase	−	V	+
Motility	−	−	+
Gas from glucose	−	−	+
Acetate utilization	−	V	+
Christiansen's citrate	−	V	d
Mucate	−	V	+
Lactose	−	d	+

[a] Abbreviations: −, negative; +, positive; V, less than or equal to 50% positive; d, less than or equal to 25% positive.

lenite broth are frequently used. For the optimal isolation of *Shigella*, two different selective media should be used: a general-purpose plating medium of low selectivity (e.g., MAC) and a more selective agar medium (e.g., xylose lysine desoxycholate agar [XLD]). Desoxycholate citrate agar (DCA) and Hektoen Enteric agar (HE) are suitable alternatives to XLD as media with moderate to high selectivities. Salmonella-shigella agar (SS) should be used with caution because it inhibits the growth of some strains of *S. dysenteriae* 1.

Screening Procedures

Shigella strains appear as lactose- or xylose-nonfermenting colonies on the isolation media described above. *S. dysenteriae* 1 colonies may be smaller on all of these media, and these strains generally grow best on media with low selectivities (e.g., MAC). *S. dysenteriae* 1 colonies on XLD agar are frequently very tiny, unlike other *Shigella* species.

Suspect colonies may be screened biochemically or serologically. Some laboratories inoculate suspected *Shigella* isolates onto a single screening medium (e.g., Kligler iron agar [KIA] or triple sugar iron agar [TSI]) before biochemical and serologic testing. On KIA or TSI, *Shigella* species characteristically produce an alkaline slant and an acid butt (K/A) but do not produce gas or H_2S. A few strains of *S. flexneri* 6 and a very few strains of *S. boydii* produce gas in KIA or TSI. The motility test, the urea test (*Shigella* does not produce urease), or the lysine decarboxylase reaction can be used in conjunction with TSI or KIA to screen isolates before doing serologic testing (Table 2). Isolates that react typically with the screening biochemicals should be tested with grouping antisera or identified with a complete set of biochemical tests, with automated systems or self-contained commercial kits being satisfactory. Confirmation requires both biochemical and serologic identification, and laboratories that do not have the resources for both types of tests should send *Shigella* isolates to a reference laboratory.

Identification

Biochemical

Because the somatic antigens of most serotypes of *Shigella* are either identical to or related to those of *E. coli*, presumptive *Shigella*, as well as suspicious cultures that are serologically negative, should be tested further biochemically.

Shigella and inactive *E. coli* (anaerogenic or lactose nonfermenting) are frequently difficult to distinguish by routine biochemical tests. Table 2 lists certain reactions useful for discriminating between *Shigella* and *E. coli*. See Table 1 in chapter 27 for the biochemical reactions of *Shigella*.

Serotyping

Serologic testing is needed for the identification of *Shigella* isolates. In fact, the four species of *Shigella* are serologically defined anaerogenic biotypes of *E. coli*. Three of the four serogroups, *S. dysenteriae*, *S. flexneri*, and *S. boydii*, are made up of a number of serotypes. *S. sonnei* is made up of a single serotype and is the most common serotype in the United States, followed by *S. flexneri*. *S. dysenteriae* and *S. boydii* are rare. Although *S. dysenteriae* and *S. sonnei* are biochemically distinct, *S. flexneri* and *S. boydii* are often biochemically indistinguishable. Serologic grouping is essential for the separation of *S. flexneri* and *S. boydii* and is required for the confirmation of *S. dysenteriae* and *S. sonnei*.

Serologic identification is typically performed by slide agglutination with polyvalent somatic (O) antigen grouping sera, followed, in some cases, by testing with monovalent antisera for specific serotype identification. Monovalent antiserum to *S. dysenteriae* 1 is required to identify this serotype and is not widely available. Because of the potentially serious nature of illness associated with this serotype, isolates that agglutinate in serogroup A reagent should be sent to a reference laboratory immediately for further serotyping.

Biochemically typical *Shigella* isolates that agglutinate poorly or that do not agglutinate at all should be suspended in saline and heated in a water bath at 100°C for 15 to 30 min. After such treatment, the suspension is cooled and retested for agglutination on a slide.

Subtyping

A variety of methods have been used to subtype *Shigella*, including colicin typing (particularly for *S. sonnei*), plasmid profiling, restriction fragment length polymorphism analysis, PFGE, and ribotyping (4, 20, 39, 41, 60, 100). For an overview of the epidemiologic use of typing methods, refer to chapter 7 in this Manual.

Serodiagnostic Tests

Several groups have developed serodiagnostic assays based on several antigens possessed by *Shigella* (59, 99, 111). These assays are practical only in research settings for seroepidemiology surveys and are not currently used for the diagnosis of infection in individual patients who are acutely ill.

Antimicrobial Susceptibilities

Shigella infections are often treated with antimicrobial agents. Because of the widespread antimicrobial resistance among *Shigella* strains, all isolates should undergo susceptibility testing. Reporting of susceptibility results to the clinician is particularly important for *S. dysenteriae* 1 isolates. Infections caused by these strains are often acquired during international travel to areas where most strains are multidrug resistant (106). In certain areas of Africa and Asia, *S. dysenteriae* 1 strains are resistant to all locally available antimicrobial agents, including nalidixic acid. These resistant *S. dysenteriae* 1 strains are still susceptible to the fluoroquinolones, but use of these drugs in developing countries is usually precluded by their high cost (87).

Interpretation and Reporting of Results

A preliminary report of suspect *Shigella* infection may be issued if biochemical or serologic screening tests are positive. If serotyping results are available, these should also be reported, particularly if the isolate is *S. dysenteriae* 1. The isolate should be tested for its susceptibility to antimicrobial agents. Before issuing a final report, isolates should be confirmed by both serologic and biochemical methods. Isolates, particularly those from individuals with dysentery-like illness, that are biochemically identified as *Shigella* but that are serologically negative may be new serotypes of *Shigella* and should be sent to a reference laboratory for further characterization. Isolates from sites other than the gastrointestinal tract that resemble *Shigella* should be carefully scrutinized for gas production and other differentiating characteristics (Table 2) as well as sent for confirmation, because they are more likely to be anaerogenic *E. coli*, rough strains of which may even cross-react with *Shigella* antiserum.

SALMONELLA

Description of the Genus

The genus *Salmonella* is composed of motile bacteria that conform to the definition of the family *Enterobacteriaceae* (37). Two species are currently recognized in the genus *Salmonella: Salmonella enterica*, which is composed of six subspecies (*S. enterica* subsp. *enterica* [designated subspecies I], *S. enterica* subsp. *salamae* [subspecies II], *S. enterica* subsp. *arizonae* [subspecies IIIa], *S. enterica* subsp. *diarizonae* [subspecies IIIb], *S. enterica* subsp. *houtenae* [subspecies IV], *S. enterica* subsp. *indica* [subspecies VI]), and *Salmonella bongori* (formerly subspecies V) (82). The type species is *S. enterica* subsp. *enterica*. See the nomenclature section below and chapter 27 for a discussion of these six subspecies and *S. bongori*.

Subspecies I strains are usually isolated from humans and warm-blooded animals. Subspecies II, IIIa, IIIb, IV, and VI strains and *S. bongori* are usually isolated from cold-blooded animals and the environment (rarely from humans). The biochemical tests useful for subspecies differentiation and in the identification of *Salmonella* are given in Tables 3 and 4, respectively.

Nomenclature for *Salmonella* and Distribution of Serotypes

The WHO Collaborating Centre for Reference and Research on *Salmonella*, which is located at the Pasteur Institute in Paris, France, designates serotypes (serovars) belonging to *S. enterica* subsp. *enterica* or subspecies I with a name which is related to the geographical place where the serotype was first isolated (81). The serotype name is written in roman (not italicized) letters, and the first letter is a capital letter (for example, *Salmonella* serotype [ser.] Typhimurium or *Salmonella* Typhimurium). Serotypes belonging to other subspecies are designated by their antigenic formulae following the subspecies name (for example, *S. enterica* subsp. *salamae* ser. 50:z:e,n,x or *Salmonella* serotype II 50:z:e,n,x). The National *Salmonella* Reference Laboratory at CDC uses this nomenclature, with the minor deviation of using the term "serotype" instead of "serovar," and strongly encourages its use because it communicates the appropriate taxonomic relationship of the more than 2,400 antigenically distinct members of these two species.

Currently, there are 2,435 *Salmonella* serotypes. Most of these serotypes, including *Salmonella* serotype Typhi, belong to subspecies I (1,435 recognized serotypes) and are found in O groups A, B, C_1, C_2, D, E_1, E_2, E_3, and E_4. The two most commonly isolated serotypes in the United States are *Salmonella* serotypes Typhimurium and Enteritidis (28). Serotypes belonging to subspecies II (485 serotypes), IIIa (94 serotypes), IIIb (321 serotypes), IV (69 serotypes), VI (11 serotypes), and *S. bongori* (20 serotypes) are primarily found in O groups F (O11) through O67 (the higher O groups) (54–56, 84). The genus "*Arizona*" was incorporated into the genus *Salmonella* as subspecies IIIa (*S. enterica* subsp. *arizonae*) containing the monophasic strains and subspecies IIIb (*S. enterica* subsp. *diarizonae*) containing the diphasic strains (86).

TABLE 3 Biochemical reactions useful for differentiating *Salmonella* species and subspecies[a]

Test	Reaction of the following species or subspecies (no. of strains tested):						
	S. enterica					*S. bongori* V (16)	*S. enterica* VI (9)
	I (650)	II (146)	IIIa (120)	IIIb (155)	IV (120)		
Dulcitol	+	+	–	–	–	+	d[b]
Lactose	–	–	–[c]	+[d]	–	–	d[e]
ONPG (*o*-nitrophenyl-β-D-galactopyranoside)	–	–[f]	+	+	–	+	d[g]
Salicin	–	–	–	–	+[h]	–	–
Sorbitol	+	+	+	+	+	+	–
Galacturonate	–	+	–	+	+	+	+
Malonate	–	+	+	+	–	–	–
Mucate	+	+	+	–[i]	–	+	+
Growth in KCN	–	–	–	–	+	+	–
Gelatin	–	+	+	+	+	–	+
L-(+)-Tartrate (*d*-tartrate[j])	+	–	–	–	–	–	–

[a] See Table 4 for description of reactions.
[b] A total of 67% were positive.
[c] A total of 15% were positive.
[d] A total of 85% were positive.
[e] A total of 22% were positive.
[f] A total of 15% were positive.
[g] A total of 44% were positive.
[h] A total of 60% were positive.
[i] A total of 30% were positive.
[j] Sodium potassium tartrate (37).

TABLE 4 Biochemical tests useful in differentiating *Salmonella* from other members of the family *Enterobacteriaceae* and identifying *Salmonella* serotypes Typhi and Paratyphi A[a]

Test	Nontyphoidal *Salmonella* subsp. I reaction	*Salmonella* serotype Typhi reaction	*Salmonella* serotype Paratyphi A reaction
TSI	K/Ag	K/A	K/Ag
H_2S (TSI)	+	$+^{weak}$	− or $+^{weak}$
Indole	−	−	−
Citrate (Simmons)	+	−	−
Urea	−	−	−
Lysine decarboxylase	+	+	−
Arginine dihydrolase	+	d	(+)
Ornithine decarboxylase	+	−	+
Motility	+	+	+
Mucate	+	−	−
Malonate	−	−	−
L(+)-Tartrate (*d*-tartrate[b])	+	+	−
Growth in KCN	−	−	−
Glucose	Ag	A	Ag
Lactose	−	−	−
Salicin	−	−	−
Dulcitol	Ag	−	$Ag^{2\ days}$
Sorbitol	Ag	A	Ag
ONPG (*o*-nitrophenyl-β-D-galactopyranoside)	−	−	−
Galacturonate	−	−	−

[a] Reactions after incubation at 37°C. K, alkaline slant; A, acid; g, gas; +, 90% or more positive within 1 or 2 days; (+), positive reaction after 3 or more days; −, no reaction (90% or more) in 7 days; d, different reactions [+, (+), −]. Adapted from Ewing (37). See Table 3 for reactions of the other subspecies.
[b] Sodium potassium tartrate (37).

Clinical Significance

Strains of nontyphoidal *Salmonella* usually cause an intestinal infection (accompanied by diarrhea, fever, and abdominal cramps) that often lasts 1 week or longer. Persons of all ages are affected; the incidence is highest in infants. *Salmonella* is ubiquitous in animal populations, and human illness is usually linked to foods of animal origin. Salmonellosis also is transmitted by direct contact with animals, by nonanimal foods, by water, and occasionally, by human contact (67, 105). Each year, an estimated 1 million to 4 million cases of illness and 1,000 deaths are caused by nontyphoidal salmonellosis in the United States (105).

Typhoid fever is a serious bloodstream infection common in the developing world. However, it is rare in the United States, where approximately 400 cases are reported each year; >70% of U.S. cases are related to foreign travel (65). Typhoid fever typically presents with a sustained debilitating high fever and headache, without diarrhea. Illness is milder in young children (nonspecific fever) (65, 67). Humans are the only reservoir and may be healthy carriers. Typhoid fever typically has a low infectious dose ($<10^3$) and a long, highly variable incubation period (1 to 6 weeks). It is transmitted through person-to-person contact or fecally contaminated food and water. A syndrome similar to typhoid fever is caused by "paratyphoidal" strains of *Salmonella: Salmonella* serotypes Paratyphi A, Paratyphi B, and Paratyphi C. These serotypes are rare in the United States.

Disease caused by *Salmonella* serotype Enteritidis in the United States is part of an expanding global pandemic. The proportion of reported *Salmonella* isolates in the United States that were *Salmonella* serotype Enteritidis increased from 5% in 1976 to 26% in 1994, with the incidence of human infection highest in New England and the mid-Atlantic region (28). From 1985 to 1995, state and territorial health departments reported 582 *Salmonella* serotype Enteritidis outbreaks to CDC. In these outbreaks, the dominant location was a commercial venue (e.g., restaurants, delicatessens, and cafeterias). The dominant identified vehicles were foods containing raw or lightly cooked shell eggs. The WHO Collaborating Center for Enteric Phage Typing developed a phage typing system that is used internationally to monitor *Salmonella* serotype Enteritidis phage types (45). Although phage type 8 is currently the most common in the United States, an increase in *Salmonella* serotype Enteritidis infection in California and other western states that began during 1993 and 1994 is largely due to the introduction of phage type 4 (77, 95). Phage type 4 emerged in Europe, Russia, and Mexico during the 1980s and caused a striking increase in the reported numbers of cases of illness. In many countries, phage type 4 replaced all other phage types and spread rapidly through poultry and human populations (95).

A strain of *Salmonella* serotype Typhimurium phage type 104 resistant to ampicillin, chloramphenicol, streptomycin, sulfonamides, and tetracycline has emerged in the United Kingdom and the United States as the predominant strain of this serotype. This phage type is referred to by the WHO Center for Enteric Phage Typing as Definitive Type 104 (DT104). In 1997, the first outbreak of pentadrug-resistant DT104 infection in the United States was reported (27).

Isolation Procedures

Enrichment

Maximal recovery of *Salmonella* from fecal specimens is obtained by using an enrichment broth, although isolation from acutely ill persons is usually possible by direct plating of specimens. Enrichment broths for *Salmonella* are usually highly selective and will inhibit certain serotypes of *Salmonella*. The three selective enrichment media most widely used to isolate *Salmonella* from fecal specimens are tetrathionate broth, tetrathionate broth with brilliant green, and Selenite broth (SEL). SEL has the advantage in that it also can be used for the recovery of *Salmonella* serotype Typhi and *Shigella*, although its value as an enrichment for the latter has not been clearly established. Newer enrichment media (e.g., modified semisolid Rappaport-Vassiliadis) can also be helpful in selecting for *Salmonella* (35). Strains that may be inhibited by selective enrichment broths are best isolated by direct plating or enrichment in a nonselective broth (e.g., GN broth).

Plating Media

Many different plating media are used to isolate *Salmonella* from fecal specimens. These media are differential and vary from slightly selective to highly selective. Media of low selectivity include MAC and eosin methylene blue (EMB). Media of intermediate selectivity include XLD, DCA, SS, and HE. Highly selective media include bismuth sulfite agar (BS), which is the preferred medium for the isolation of *Salmonella* serotype Typhi, and brilliant green agar. New selective media include Rambach agar, xylose-lysine-Tergitol 4 (XLT4) agar, *Salmonella* detection and identification medium, and novobiocin-brilliant green-glycerol-lactose agar (35). BS, XLD, and HE all have H_2S indicator systems, which are necessary for the detection of lactose-positive *Salmonella*. Most laboratories today use HE or XLD because these media can also be used for the isolation of *Shigella*.

In the developing world, typhoid fever is frequently diagnosed solely on clinical grounds, but isolation of the causative organism is necessary for a definitive diagnosis. *Salmonella* serotype Typhi is more frequently isolated from blood cultures than from fecal specimens. Blood cultures are positive for 80% of typhoid patients during the first week of fever but show decreasing positive results thereafter.

Several commercial rapid diagnostic tests are available for the testing of foods, but to our knowledge, none has been evaluated in the literature for use with fecal specimens.

Screening Procedures

A latex agglutination kit has been described for screening for *Salmonella* from SEL enrichment broth (Wellcolex Color *Salmonella*; Murex Diagnostics, Inc., Norcross, Ga.) (66). This can also be used to screen individual colonies from primary plates.

Suspect colonies can be inoculated onto a screening medium such as KIA or TSI. On KIA or TSI, most *Salmonella* strains produce a K/Ag+ reaction, indicating that glucose is fermented with gas and H_2S production. On these media, *Salmonella* serotype Typhi isolates characteristically are K/A but do not produce gas and only a small amount of H_2S is visible at the site of the stab and in the stab line. Lysine iron agar is also a useful screening medium because most *Salmonella* isolates, even those which ferment lactose, decarboxylate lysine and produce H_2S. Alternately, isolates may be identified by a battery of biochemical tests or by slide agglutination with antisera for *Salmonella* O groups A, B, C_1, C_2, D, and E. Isolates suspected of being *Salmonella* serotype Typhi should be tested serologically with *Salmonella* Vi and O group D antisera (see discussion below).

If the biochemical reactions for a particular isolate are not characteristic but *Salmonella* antigens are found, the cultures should be plated on MAC or EMB to obtain a pure culture, tested biochemically by a complete set of tests, or forwarded to a reference laboratory.

Identification

Clinical laboratories may issue a preliminary report of *Salmonella* when an isolate is positive either with O group antisera or by biochemical identification methods. Clinical laboratories should consider that an isolate is confirmed as *Salmonella* when both determination of the O serogroup and biochemical identification have been completed. The methods described below for serotyping are intended primarily for reference laboratories.

Biochemical Identification

Suspect colonies from one of the differential plating media mentioned above can be identified biochemically as *Salmonella* spp. with traditional media in tubes or commercial biochemical systems. Methods of biochemical identification and specific commercial manual and automated identification systems are covered in chapter 11. The species and subspecies of *Salmonella* can be identified biochemically, as indicated in Tables 3 and 4. Table 4 lists the biochemical reactions of the tests that are helpful for distinguishing *Salmonella* serotypes Typhi and Paratyphi A from nontyphoidal *Salmonella*.

Serotyping

Salmonella spp. are serotyped according to their O (somatic) antigens, Vi (capsular) antigen, and H (flagellar) antigens (64). The antigenic formulae of *Salmonella* serotypes are listed in the Kauffman-White scheme and are expressed as follows: O antigen(s), Vi (when present): H antigen(s) (phase 1): H antigen(s) (phase 2, when present). Updating of the Kauffman-White scheme is the responsibility of the WHO Collaborating Centre for Reference and Research on *Salmonella*. The Kauffman-White scheme is updated annually with a listing of new serotypes (81), and the latest revision of the complete scheme is published every 5 years (82).

Determination of O Antigens

O (heat-stable somatic) antigens are identified by first testing the isolate in O grouping antisera, which react with one or several antigens in each group, and then in the appropriate O single-factor antisera, which react with individual antigens (64). The approach most commonly used for determining O antigens is to initially test the isolates by slide agglutination in antisera against O groups A to E_4 because 98 to 99% of *Salmonella* isolates belong to one of these O groups. If no agglutination occurs in antisera for the first nine O groups, the isolate is tested in pools containing the remaining *Salmonella* O antisera, O11 through O67.

Detection of the Vi Antigen and Identification of *Salmonella* Serotype Typhi (9,12,[Vi]:d:−)

The Vi antigen, a heat-labile capsular antigen, is commonly found in *Salmonella* serotype Typhi strains and is useful for the identification of this serotype. It is also occasionally detected in *Salmonella* serotype Dublin, *Salmonella* serotype Paratyphi C, and some *Citrobacter* strains. Vi antigen is identified by slide agglutination with a specific antiserum.

If *Salmonella* serotype Typhi is suspected, the culture is first tested live (unheated) in O group D antiserum (which contains antibodies to O antigens 9 and 12) and Vi antiserum on a slide. If only the Vi antiserum is positive, the bacterial suspension is heated in boiling water for 15 min, cooled, and tested again in the same antisera. After heating, *Salmonella* serotype Typhi isolates will be negative in the Vi antiserum but positive in the O group D antiserum. Expression of the Vi antigen by *Salmonella* serotype Typhi is variable but tends to occur more frequently in freshly isolated cultures than in cultures that have been subcultured. If the strain is typical for *Salmonella* serotype Typhi on TSI (see Screening Procedures above), is urease negative, and reacts in O group D or Vi antisera, a presumptive report is made. Before a final report is issued, the isolate's identity is confirmed with a set of biochemical tests (Table 4) and determination of the H (flagellar) antigen (see below). *Salmonella* serotype Typhi strains typically express only one flagellar antigen which is Hd.

Determination of H Antigens

H (flagellar) antigens are typically determined by tube agglutination tests with broth cultures as antigens and H typing and single-factor (absorbed) antisera. Isolates are initially tested with H typing antisera, which recognize individual or multiple antigens, and then with H single-factor antisera, which recognize individual antigens. Most *Salmonella* serotypes are either monophasic (express one type of H antigen) or diphasic (express two different types of H antigen). It is generally believed that in diphasic serotypes an individual cell expresses antigens from only one phase at a time, even though both phases may be detected in the whole culture.

In cultures that have a mixture of cells in different phases, it is possible to detect both phases of a diphasic strain in a single assay. When only one phase is detected (either phase 1 or phase 2), the strain should be inoculated into a semisolid medium to which sterile antiserum of the detected phase has aseptically been added. Growth of the strain in this semisolid agar immobilizes cells expressing the detected antigen(s) and allows the growth of bacteria expressing the antigen(s) in the other phase. After phase reversal, the strain is tested in appropriate H typing and single-factor antisera to complete the serotyping. A strain must be actively motile to ensure the good development of H antigens, and sometimes it must be passed through one or more tall tubes of semisolid agar before H antigens can be detected. When a *Salmonella* strain is nonmotile, it is identified biochemically (Table 4) and by the O antigens that it expresses.

Identification Problems

If a strain with a biochemical profile consistent with that of *Salmonella* cannot be typed with the first nine *Salmonella* O antisera (groups A to E) or in the higher *Salmonella* O antisera (groups 11 to 67), it may be due to one of the following:

1. The strain expresses the Vi capsular antigen, which can block the binding of antibodies against the O antigens.
2. The strain is rough, i.e., fails to make complete O antigens. Rough strains have a tendency to cross agglutinate in different antisera.
3. The strain is mucoid and will not agglutinate in antisera.

When O antigens are not recognized, a strain is confirmed as a *Salmonella* species by its H antigens and a set of biochemical tests (Tables 3 and 4).

Many laboratories are likely to miss *Salmonella* serotype Paratyphi A, because they do not screen with O group A antiserum and because it is H_2S negative and lysine negative (Table 4). *Salmonella* serotype Java is often misidentified as *Salmonella* serotype Paratyphi B because these two serotypes have identical antigenic formulas (4,5,12:b:[1,5]). However, disease caused by *Salmonella* serotype Paratyphi B is usually typhoid-like and rare in the United States, while *Salmonella* serotype Java infection is usually typical nontyphoidal salmonellosis. These strains can also be distinguished biochemically (serotype Java is tartrate positive, but serotype Paratyphi B is tartrate negative).

Because *Citrobacter* and *E. coli* strains may possess O, H, or Vi antigens that are related to those of *Salmonella*, biochemical identification may be necessary to confirm that an isolate is *Salmonella* (see Table 4 in this chapter and Table 1 in chapter 27).

Subtyping

For common serotypes (e.g., Typhimurium, Enteritidis, and Typhi) subtyping methods other than serotyping are frequently used. Various phenotypic methods (e.g., phage typing, antimicrobial susceptibility pattern determination, and biotyping) have been used to subtype *Salmonella* strains (108). More recently, genotyping methods (e.g., plasmid fingerprinting, multilocus enzyme electrophoresis, PFGE, IS*200* profiling, and random amplified polymorphic DNA analysis) have been developed for subtyping within serotypes of *Salmonella* (8, 58, 70, 71, 108). For an overview of the epidemiologic use of typing methods, refer to chapter 7 in this Manual.

Serodiagnostic Tests

The Widal test, which is the most commonly used method for the serodiagnosis of *Salmonella* enteric fever, measures agglutinating antibodies to the O and H antigens of *Salmonella* serotype Typhi (53). The Widal test, which is used when serotype Typhi cannot be isolated, may produce false-negative and false-positive reactions and does not provide a definitive diagnosis of individual cases of infection. Other serodiagnostic techniques have been developed for the detection of antibodies to various antigens (e.g., outer membrane proteins, lipopolysaccharide, flagellin protein, and Vi antigen). Vi assays are particularly helpful in situations in which samples for culture are unobtainable or are unlikely to be positive, such as retrospective epidemiologic investigations in which chronic carriers are being sought (61).

Antimicrobial Susceptibilities

Antimicrobial therapy is not recommended for uncomplicated *Salmonella* gastroenteritis. Therefore, routine susceptibility testing of these isolates is not warranted for the purposes of treatment. However, determination of antimicrobial resistance patterns is often valuable for surveillance purposes and may be performed periodically to monitor the development and spread of antimicrobial resistance among these strains.

In contrast to uncomplicated salmonellosis, treatment with the appropriate antimicrobial agent can be crucial for patients with invasive *Salmonella* and typhoidal infections (52), and the susceptibilities of these isolates should be tested as soon as possible. The untreated case mortality rate for typhoid fever is >10%; when patients with typhoid fever are treated with appropriate antibiotics, the rate should be <1%.

Since 1979 and 1980, CDC has conducted studies at 5-year intervals to monitor the antimicrobial resistance of nontyphoidal *Salmonella* strains causing infections in humans in the United States. These investigations found an increasing prevalence of antimicrobial resistance, from 16% during 1979 and 1980 to 29% during 1989 and 1990 (52, 62, 85). Data obtained in a 1996 survey of *Salmonella* isolates revealed that 37% were resistant to at least one antimicrobial agent (31). Recent reports from abroad have also noted an increasing level of resistance to one or more antimicrobial agents in *Salmonella* isolates, particularly in *Salmonella* serotype Typhi strains (83, 87, 110).

In contrast to the gradual increase in the overall level of resistance among all *Salmonella* serotypes is the recent emergence in both the United Kingdom and the United States of multidrug-resistant *Salmonella* serotype Typhimurium DT104. The incidence of DT104 has dramatically increased during the past 7 years in proportion to that of non-DT104 serotype Typhimurium strains (27). Currently, approximately 30% of all *Salmonella* serotype Typhimurium isolates in the United States possess this pentadrug resistance pattern, whereas the rates were 7% in 1990 and <1% in 1980 (42). In the United Kingdom, 6% of the DT104 isolates identified are also resistant to ciprofloxacin (109).

Interpretation and Reporting of Results

A preliminary report can be issued as soon as a presumptive identification of *Salmonella* is obtained. In most situations, a presumptive identification would be based on biochemical findings obtained either by traditional or commercial systems or by a serologic reaction in *Salmonella* O grouping antisera. A confirmed identification requires biochemical and serologic identification methods. Because the National *Salmonella* Surveillance System depends on the receipt of serotype information for *Salmonella* strains isolated in the United States for the tracking of outbreaks of infection, laboratories should follow the procedures recommended by their state health departments for submitting isolates for further characterization, including complete serotyping. The susceptibilities of typhoidal *Salmonella* strains and strains from normally sterile sites should be tested, and the strains should be forwarded to a reference or public health laboratory for complete biochemical and serologic characterization.

REFERENCES

1. **Abbott, S. L.** 1997. Laboratory aspects of non-O157 toxigenic *E. coli*. *Clin. Microbiol. Newsl.* **19:**105–108.
2. **Acheson, D. W. K., and G. T. Keusch.** 1995. *Shigella* and enteroinvasive *Escherichia coli.*, p. 763–784. *In* M. J. Blaser, J. I. Ravdin, H. B. Greenberg, and R. L. Guerrant (ed.), *Infections of the Gastrointestinal Tract.* Raven Press, New York, N.Y.
3. **Albert, M. J., S. M. Faruque, A. S. Faruque, K. A. Bettelheim, P. K. Neogi, N. A. Bhuiyan, and J. B. Kaper.** 1996. Controlled study of cytolethal distending toxin-producing *Escherichia coli* infections in Bangladeshi children. *J. Clin. Microbiol.* **34:**717–719.
4. **Albert, M. J., K. V. Singh, B. E. Murray, and J. Erlich.** 1990. Molecular epidemiology of *Shigella* infection in Central Australia. *Epidemiol. Infect.* **105:**51–57.
5. **Allerberger, F., D. Rossboth, M. P. Dierich, S. Aleksic, H. Schmidt, and H. Karch.** 1996. Prevalence and clinical manifestations of Shiga toxin-producing *Escherichia coli* infections in Austrian children. *Eur. J. Clin. Microbiol. Infect. Dis.* **15:**545–550.
6. **Banatvala, N., M. M. DeBeukelaer, P. M. Griffin, T. J. Barrett, K. D. Greene, J. H. Green, and J. G. Wells.** 1996. Shiga-like toxin-producing *Escherichia coli* O111 and associated hemolytic-uremic syndrome: a family outbreak. *Pediatr. Infect. Dis. J.* **15:**1008–1011.
7. **Belongia, E. A., M. T. Osterholm, J. T. Soler, D. A. Ammend, J. E. Braun, and K. L. MacDonald.** 1993. Transmission of *Escherichia coli* O157:H7 infection in Minnesota child day-care facilities. *JAMA* **269:**883–888.
8. **Beltran, P., J. M. Musser, R. Helmuth, J. J. Farmer III, W. M. Frerichs, I. K. Wachsmuth, K. Ferris, A. C. McWhorter, J. G. Wells, A. Cravioto, and R. K. Selander.** 1988. Toward a population genetic analysis of *Salmonella*: genetic diversity and relationships among strains of serotypes *S. choleraesuis, S. derby, S. dublin, S. enteritidis, S. heidelberg, S. infantis, S. newport,* and *S. typhimurium*. *Proc. Natl. Acad. Sci. USA* **85:**7753–7757.
9. **Besser-Wiek, J., D. Boxrud, J. Bender, M. Sullivan, L. Carroll, and F. Leano.** 1996. Selective media, broth enrichment, immunomagnetic separation, and PCR broth culture assay for detection of *E. coli* O157:H7 in fecal samples, abstr. C364, p. 65. *In Abstracts of the 96th General Meeting of the American Society for Microbiology 1996.* American Society for Microbiology, Washington, D.C.
10. **Bettelheim, K. A.** 1992. The genus *Escherichia*, p. 2696–2736. *In* A. Balows, H. G. Truper, M. Dworkin, W. Harder, and K.-H. Schleifer (ed.), *The Prokaryotes,* 2nd ed. Springer-Verlag KG, Berlin, Germany.
11. **Bettelheim, K. A.** 1995. Identification of enterohaemorrhagic *Escherichia coli* by means of their production of enterohaemolysin. *J. Appl. Bacteriol.* **79:**178–180.
12. **Beutin, L., S. Aleksic, S. Zimmerman, and K. Gleier.** 1994. Virulence factors and phenotypical traits of verotoxigenic strains of *Escherichia coli* isolated from human patients in Germany. *Med. Microbiol. Immunol.* **183:** 13–21.
13. **Beutin, L., M. A. Montenegro, I. Orskov, F. Orskov, J. Proada, S. Zimmerman, and R. Stephan.** 1989. Close association of verocytotoxin (Shiga-like toxin) production with enterohemolysin production in strains of *Escherichia coli*. *J. Clin. Microbiol.* **27:**2559–2564.
14. **Beutin, L., S. Zimmerman, and I. Gleier.** 1996. *Pseudomonas aeruginosa* can cause false-positive identification of verocytotoxin (Shiga-like toxin) production by a commercial enzyme immune assay system for the detection of Shiga-like toxins (SLTs). *Infection* **24:**267–268.
15. **Beutin, L., S. Zimmerman, and I. Gleier.** 1996. Rapid detection and isolation of Shiga-like toxin (verocytotoxin)-producing *Escherichia coli* by direct testing of individual enterohemolytic colonies from washed sheep blood agar plates in the VTEC-RPLA assay. *J. Clin. Microbiol.* **34:**2812–2814.
16. **Bitzan, M., K. Ludwig, M. Klemt, H. Konig, J. Buren, and D. E. Muller-Wiefel.** 1993. The role of *Escherichia coli* O157 infections in the classical (enteropathic) haemolytic uraemic syndrome: results of a Central European multicentre study. *Epidemiol. Infect.* **110:**183–196.
17. **Blanco, J. E., J. Blanco, M. Blanco, M. P. Alonso, and W. H. Jansen.** 1994. Serotypes of CNF1-producing *Escherichia coli* strains that cause extra intestinal infections in humans. *Eur. J. Epidemiol.* **10:**707–711.
18. **Borczyk, A. A., N. Harnett, M. Lombos, and H. Lior.** 1990. False-positive identification of *Escherichia coli* O157 by commercial latex agglutination tests. *Lancet* **336:** 946–947.
19. **Boyce, T. G., A. G. Pemberton, J. G. Wells, and P. M. Griffin.** 1995. Screening for *Escherichia coli* O157:H7: a nationwide survey of clinical laboratories. *J. Clin. Microbiol.* **33:**3275–3277.
20. **Bratoeva, M. P., J. F. Jopn, and N. L. Barg.** 1992. Molecular epidemiology of trimethoprim-resistant *Shigella boydii* serotype 2 strains from Bulgaria. *J. Clin. Microbiol.* **30:** 1428–1431.
21. **Brenner, D. J.** 1992. Introduction to the family *Enterobacteriaceae*, p. 2673–2695. *In* A. Balows, H. G. Truper, M. Dworkin, W. Harder, and K.-H. Schleifer (ed.), *The Prokaryotes,* 2nd ed. Springer-Verlag KG, Berlin, Germany.
22. **Calderwood, S. G., D. W. K. Acheson, G. T. Keusch, T. J. Barrett, P. M. Griffin, N. A. Strockbine, B. Swaminathan, J. B. Kaper, M. M. Levine, B. S. Kaplan, H. Karch, A. D. O'Brien, T. G. Obrig, Y. Takeda, P. I. Tarr, and I. K. Wachsmuth.** 1996. Proposed new nomenclature for SLT (VT) family. *ASM News* **62:**118–119.

23. **Caprioli, A., V. Falbo, L. G. Roda, F. M. Ruggeri, and C. Zona.** 1983. Partial purification and characterization of an *Escherichia coli* toxic factor that induces morphological cell alterations. *Infect. Immun.* **39:**1300–1306.
24. **Caprioli, A., V. Falbo, F. M. Ruggeri, L. Baldassarri, R. Bisicchia, G. Ippolito, E. Romoli, and G. Donelli.** 1987. Cytotoxic necrotizing factor production by hemolytic strains of *Escherichia coli* causing extra intestinal infections. *J. Clin. Microbiol.* **25:**146–149.
25. **Centers for Disease Control and Prevention.** 1994. Foodborne outbreaks of enterotoxigenic *Escherichia coli*—Rhode Island and New Hampshire, 1993. *Morbid. Mortal. Weekly Rep.* **43:**81–89.
26. **Centers for Disease Control and Prevention.** 1995. Outbreak of acute gastroenteritis attributable to *Escherichia coli* serotype O104:H21—Helena, Montana, 1994. *Morbid. Mortal. Weekly Rep.* **44:**501–503.
27. **Centers for Disease Control and Prevention.** 1997. Multidrug-resistant *Salmonella* serotype Typhimurium—United States, 1996. *Morbid. Mortal. Weekly Rep.* **46:** 308–310.
28. **Centers for Disease Control and Prevention.** 1997. *Salmonella Surveillance, 1996.* Centers for Disease Control and Prevention, Atlanta, Ga.
29. **Chapman, P. A., and C. A. Siddons.** 1996. A comparison of immunomagnetic separation and direct culture for the isolation of verocytotoxin-producing *Escherichia coli* O157 from cases of bloody diarrhoea, non-bloody diarrhoea and asymptomatic contacts. *J. Med. Microbiol.* **44:**267–271.
30. **Cubbon, M. D., J. E. Coia, M. F. Hanson, and F. M. Thomson-Carter.** 1996. A comparison of immunomagnetic separation, direct culture and polymerase chain reaction for the detection of verocytotoxin-producing *Escherichia coli* O157 in human faeces. *J. Med. Microbiol.* **44:** 219–222.
31. **Dabney, P., C. Bopp, F. Tenover, L. Tollefson, F. Angulo, and the NAMS Working Group.** 1997. National Antimicrobial Monitoring System: antimicrobial resistance in human isolates of *Salmonella* and *Escherichia coli* O157, abstr. C-136, p. 144. *In Abstracts of the 97th General Meeting of the American Society for Microbiology 1997.* American Society for Microbiology, Washington, D.C.
32. **Dalton, C. B., E. D. Mintz, R. V. Tauxe, and J. G. Wells.** 1995. Enterotoxigenic *E. coli* (ETEC) outbreaks in and around the United States, 1977–1994: a clinical and epidemiologic profile, abstr. K-148, p. 314. *In Program and Abstracts of the 35th Interscience Conference on Antimicrobial Agents and Chemotherapy.* American Society for Microbiology, Washington, D.C.
33. **De Rycke, J., J. F. Guillot, and R. Boivin.** 1987. Cytotoxins in nonenterotoxigenic strains of *Escherichia coli* isolated from feces of diarrheic calves. *Vet. Microbiol.* **15:** 137–150.
34. **Donnenberg, M. S.** 1995. Enteropathogenic *Escherichia coli*, p. 709–726. *In* M. J. Blaser, P. D. Smith, J. I. Ravdin, H. B. Greenberg, and R. L. Guerrant (ed.), *Infections of the Gastrointestinal Tract.* Raven Press, New York, N.Y.
35. **Dusch, H., and M. Altwegg.** 1995. Evaluation of five new plating media for isolation of *Salmonella* species. *J. Clin. Microbiol.* **33:**802–804.
36. **Dylla, B. L., E. A. Vetter, J. G. Hughes, and F. R. Cockerill III.** 1995. Evaluation of an immunoassay for direct detection of *Escherichia coli* O157 in stool specimens. *J. Clin. Microbiol.* **33:**222–224.
37. **Ewing, W. H.** 1986. *Edwards and Ewing's Identification of Enterobacteriaceae,* 4th ed. Elsevier Science Publishing Co. Inc., New York, N.Y.
38. **Farina, C., A. Goglio, G. Conedera, F. Minelli, and A. Capriolo.** 1996. Antimicrobial susceptibility of *Escherichia coli* O157 and other enterohemorrhagic *Escherichia coli* isolated in Italy. *Eur. J. Clin. Microbiol. Infect. Dis.* **15:** 351–353.
39. **Faruque, S. M., K. Haider, M. M. Rahman, A. R. M. A. Alim, Q. S. Ahmad, M. J. Albert, and R. B. Sack.** 1992. Differentiation of *Shigella flexneri* strains by rRNA gene restriction patterns. *J. Clin. Microbiol.* **30:** 2996–2999.
40. **Fields, P. I., K. Blom, H. J. Hughes, L. O. Helsel, P. Feng, and B. Swaminathan.** 1997. Molecular characterization of the gene encoding H antigen in *Escherichia coli* and development of a PCR-restriction fragment length polymorphism test for identification of *E. coli* O157:H7 and O157:NM. *J. Clin. Microbiol.* **35:**1066–1070.
41. **Gebre-Yohannes, A., and B. S. Drasar.** 1990. Plasmid profiles of *Shigella dysenteriae* type 1 isolates from Ethiopia with special reference to R-plasmids. *J. Med. Microbiol.* **33:**101–106.
42. **Glynn, M. K., C. Bopp, W. Dewitt, P. Dabney, M. Mokhtar, and F. J. Angulo.** 1998. Emergence of multidrug-resistant *Salmonella enterica* serotype Typhimurium DT104 infections in the United States. *N. Engl. J. Med.* **338:**1333–1338.
43. **Griffin, P. M.** 1995. *Escherichia coli* O157:H7 and other enterohemorrhagic *Escherichia coli*, p. 739–761. *In* M. J. Blaser, J. I. Ravdin, H. B. Greenberg, and R. L. Guerrant (ed.), *Infections of the Gastrointestinal Tract.* Raven Press, New York, N.Y.
44. **Hayes, P. S., K. Blom, P. Feng, J. Lewis, N. A. Strockbine, and B. Swaminathan.** 1995. Isolation and characterization of a β-glucuronidase-producing strain of *Escherichia coli* O157:H7 in the United States. *J. Clin. Microbiol.* **33:**3347–3348.
45. **Hickman-Brenner, F. W., A. D. Stubbs, and J. J. Farmer III.** 1991. Phage typing of *Salmonella enteritidis* in the United States. *J. Clin. Microbiol.* **29:**2817–2823.
46. **Itoh, Y., I. Nagano, M. Kunishima, and T. Ezaki.** 1997. Laboratory investigation of enteroaggregative *Escherichia coli* O untypable:H10 associated with a massive outbreak of gastrointestinal illness. *J. Clin. Microbiol.* **35:** 2546–2550.
47. **Johnson, W. M.** Personal communication.
48. **Johnson, W. M., and H. Lior.** 1988. A new heat-labile cytolethal distending toxin (CLDT) produced by *Escherichia coli* isolates from clinical material. *Microb. Pathog.* **4:**103–113.
49. **Karch, H., C. Janetzki-Mittman, S. Aleksic, and M. Datz.** 1996. Isolation of enterohemorrhagic *Escherichia coli* O157 strains from patients with hemolytic-uremic syndrome by using immunomagnetic separation, DNA-based methods, and direct culture. *J. Clin. Microbiol.* **34:** 516–519.
50. **Kehl, K. S., P. Havens, C. E. Behnke, and D. W. K. Acheson.** 1997. Evaluation of the Premier EHEC assay for detection of Shiga toxin-producing *Escherichia coli*. *J. Clin. Microbiol.* **35:**2051–2054.
51. **Kim, H. H., M. Samadpour, L. Grimm, C. R. Clausen, T. E. Besser, M. Baylor, J. M. Kobayashi, M. A. Neill, F. D. Schoenknecht, and P. I. Tarr.** 1994. Characteristics of antibiotic-resistant *Escherichia coli* O157:H7 in Washington State, 1984–1991. *J. Infect. Dis.* **170:**1606–1609.
52. **Lee, L. A., N. D. Puhr, E. K. Mahoney, N. H. Bean, and R. V. Tauxe.** 1994. Increase in antimicrobial-resistant *Salmonella* infections in the United States, 1989–1990. *J. Infect. Dis.* **170:**128–134.
53. **Le Minor, L.** 1992. The genus *Salmonella*, p. 2760–2774. *In* A. Balows, H. G. Truper, M. Dworkin, W. Harder, and K.-H. Schleifer (ed.), *The Prokaryotes,* 2nd ed. Springer-Verlag KG, Berlin, Germany.

54. **Le Minor, L., G. Chamoiseau, E. Barbe, C. Charie-Marsaines, and L. Egron.** 1969. Dix nouveau serotypes de *Salmonella* isoles au Tchad. *Ann. Inst. Pasteur (Paris)* **116:**775–780.
55. **Le Minor, L., M. Y. Popoff, B. Laurent, and D. Herman.** 1986. Individualization d'une septieme sous-espece de *Salmonella: S. choleraesuis* subsp. *Indica* subsp. nov. *Ann. Inst. Pasteur/Microbiol.* **137B:**211–217.
56. **Le Minor, L., M. Veron, and M. Y. Popoff.** 1982. Taxonomie des *Salmonella. Ann. Inst. Pasteur/Microbiol.* **133B:** 223–243.
57. **Levine, M. M., C. Ferreccio, V. Prado, M. Cayazzo, P. Abrego, J. Martinez, L. Maggi, M. M. Baldini, W. Martin, D. Maneval, B. Kay, L. Guers, H. Lior, S. S. Wasserman, and J. P. Nataro.** 1993. Epidemiologic studies of *Escherichia coli* diarrheal infections in a low socioeconomic level peri-urban community in Santiago, Chile. *Am. J. Epidemiol.* **138:**849–869.
58. **Lin, A. W., M. A. Usera, T. J. Barrett, and R. A. Goldsby.** 1996. Application of random amplified polymorphic DNA analysis to differentiate strains of *Salmonella enteritidis. J. Clin. Microbiol.* **34:**870–876.
59. **Lindberg, A. A., P. D. Cam, N. Chan, L. K. Phu, D. D. Trach, G. Lindberg, K. Karlsson, A. Karnell, and E. Ekwall.** 1991. Shigellosis in Vietnam: seroepidemiologic studies with use of lipopolysaccharide antigens in enzyme immunoassays. *Rev. Infect. Dis.* **13**(Suppl. 4):S213–S237.
60. **Litwin, C. M., A. L. Storm, S. Chipowsky, and K. J. Ryan.** 1991. Molecular epidemiology of *Shigella* infections: plasmid profiles, serotype correlation, and restriction endonuclease analysis. *J. Clin. Microbiol.* **29:** 104–108.
61. **Losonsky, G. A., and M. M. Levine.** 1997. Immunologic methods for diagnosis of infections caused by diarrheagenic members of the families *Enterobacteriaceae* and *Vibrionaceae*, p. 484–497. *In* N. R. Rose, E. Conway de Macario, J. D. Folds, H. C. Lane, and R. M. Nakamura (ed.), *Manual of Clinical Laboratory Immunology*, 5th ed. ASM Press, Washington, D.C.
62. **MacDonald, K. L., M. L. Cohen, N. T. Hargrett-Bean, J. G. Wells, N. D. Puhr, S. F. Collin, and P. A. Blake.** 1987. Changes in antimicrobial resistance of *Salmonella* isolated from humans in the United States. *JAMA* **258:** 1496–1499.
63. **March, S. B., and S. Ratnam.** 1986. Sorbitol-MacConkey medium for detection of *Escherichia coli* O157:H7 associated with hemorrhagic colitis. *J. Clin. Microbiol.* **23:** 869–872.
64. **McWhorter-Murlin, A. C., and F. W. Hickman-Brenner.** 1994. *Identification and Serotyping of* Salmonella *and an Update of the Kauffmann-White Scheme*. Centers for Disease Control and Prevention, Atlanta, Ga.
65. **Mermin, J. H., J. M. Townes, M. Gerber, N. Dolan, E. D. Mintz, and R. V. Tauxe.** 1998. Typhoid fever in the United States, 1985–1994: changing risks of international travel and increasing antimicrobial resistance. *Arch. Intern. Med.* **158:**633–638.
66. **Metzler, J., and I. Nachamkin.** 1988. Evaluation of a latex agglutination test for the detection of *Salmonella* and *Shigella* spp. by using broth enrichment. *J. Clin. Microbiol.* **26:**2501–2504.
67. **Miller, S. I., E. L. Hohmann, and D. A. Pegues.** 1995. *Salmonella* (including *Salmonella* Typhi), p. 2013–2033. *In* G. L. Mandell, J. E. Bennett, and R. Dolin (ed.), *Principles and Practice of Infectious Diseases*. Churchill Livingstone, New York, N.Y.
68. **Mitsuda, T., T. Muto, M. Yamada, N. Kobayashi, M. Toba, Y. Aihara, A. Ito, and S. Yokata.** 1998. Epidemiological study of a food-borne outbreak of enterotoxigenic *Escherichia coli* O25:NM by pulsed-field gel electrophoresis and randomly amplified polymorphic DNA analysis. *J. Clin. Microbiol.* **36:**652–656.
69. **Nataro, J. P., and J. B. Kaper.** 1998. Diarrheagenic *Escherichia coli. Clin. Microbiol. Rev.* **11:**142–201.
70. **Navaro, F., T. Llovett, M. A. Echeita, P. Coll, A. Aladueña, M. A. Usera, and G. Prats.** 1996. Molecular typing of *Salmonella enterica* serovar *Typhi. J. Clin. Microbiol.* **34:**2831–2834.
71. **Olsen, J. E., M. N. Skov, O. Angen, E. J. Threlfall, and M. Bisgaard.** 1997. Genomic relationships between selected phage types of *Salmonella enterica* subsp. *enterica* serotype *typhimurium* defined by ribotyping, IS200 typing, and PFGE. *Microbiology* **43:**1471–1479.
72. **Olsvik, O., and N. A. Strockbine.** 1993. PCR detection of heat-stable, heat-labile, and Shiga-like toxin genes in *Escherichia coli*, p. 271–276. *In* D. H. Persing, T. F. Smith, F. C. Tenover, and T. J. White (ed.), *Diagnostic Molecular Microbiology: Principles and Applications*. American Society for Microbiology, Washington, D.C.
73. **Oswald, E., J. DeRycke, J. F. Guillot, and R. Boivin.** 1989. Cytotoxic effect of multinucleation in HeLa cell cultures associated with the presence of Vir plasmid in *Escherichia coli* strains. *FEMS Microbiol. Lett.* **58:**95–100.
74. **Park, C. H., K. M. Gates, N. M. Vandel, and D. L. Hixon.** 1996. Isolation of Shiga-like toxin producing *Escherichia coli* (O157 and non-O157) in a community hospital. *Diagn. Microbiol. Infect. Dis.* **26:**69–72.
75. **Park, C. H., D. L. Hixon, W. L. Morrison, and C. B. Cook.** 1994. Rapid diagnosis of enterohemorrhagic *Escherichia coli* O157:H7 directly from fecal specimens using immunofluorescence stain. *Am. J. Clin. Pathol.* **101:** 91–94.
76. **Park, C. H., N. M. Vandel, and D. L. Hixon.** 1996. Rapid immunoassay for detection of *Escherichia coli* O157 directly from stool specimens. *J. Clin. Microbiol.* **34:** 988–990.
77. **Passaro, D. J., R. Reporter, L. Mascola, L. Kilman, G. B. Malcolm, H. Rolka, S. S. Werner, and D. J. Vugia.** 1996. Epidemic *Salmonella enteritidis* infection in Los Angeles County, California. The predominance of phage type 4. *West. J. Med.* **163**(3)**:**126–130.
78. **Paton, A. W., R. M. Ratcliff, R. M. Doyles, J. Seymour-Murray, D. Davos, J. A. Lanser, and J. C. Paton.** 1996. Molecular microbiological investigation of an outbreak of hemolytic-uremic syndrome caused by dry fermented sausage contaminated with Shiga-like toxin-producing *Escherichia coli. J. Clin. Microbiol.* **34:**1622–1627.
79. **Poitrineau, P., C. Forestier, M. Meyer, C. Jallat, C. Rich, G. Malpuech, and C. De Champs.** 1995. Retrospective case-control study of diffusely adhering *Escherichia coli* and clinical features in children with diarrhea. *J. Clin. Microbiol.* **33:**1961–1962.
80. **Polotsky, Y., J. P. Nataro, D. Kotler, T. J. Barrett, and J. M. Orenstein.** 1997. HEp-2 cell adherence patterns, serotyping, and DNA analysis of *Escherichia coli* isolates from eight patients with AIDS and chronic diarrhea. *J. Clin. Microbiol.* **35:**1952–1958.
81. **Popoff, M. Y., J. Bockemühl, and F. W. Hickman-Brenner.** 1997. Supplement 1996 (no. 40) to the Kauffmann-White scheme. *Res. Microbiol.* **148:**811–814.
82. **Popoff, M. Y., and L. Le Minor.** 1997. *Antigenic Formulas of the* Salmonella *Serovars*, 7th revision. WHO Collaborating Centre for Reference and Research on Salmonella, Pasteur Institute, Paris, France.
83. **Ramos, J. M., J. M. Ales, M. Cuenca-Estrella, R. Fernandez-Roblas, and F. Soriano.** 1996. Changes in susceptibility of *Salmonella enteritidis*, *Salmonella typhimurium*, and *Salmonella virchow* to six antimicrobial agents in a

Spanish hospital, 1980–1994. *Eur. J. Clin. Microbiol. Infect. Dis.* **15:**85–88.

84. **Reeves, M. W., G. M. Evins, A. A. Heiba, B. D. Plikaytis, and J. J. Farmer III.** 1989. Clonal nature of *Salmonella typhi* and its genetic relatedness to other salmonellae as shown by multilocus enzyme electrophoresis and proposal of *Salmonella bongori* comb. nov. *J. Clin. Microbiol.* **27:**313–320.
85. **Riley, L. W., M. L. Cohen, J. E. Seals, M. J. Blaser, K. A. Birkness, N. T. Hargrett, S. M. Martin, and R. A. Feldman.** 1984. Importance of host factors in human salmonellosis caused by multiresistant strains of *Salmonella. J. Infect. Dis.* **149:**878–883.
86. **Rohde, R.** 1979. Serological integration of all known *Arizona* species into the Kauffmann-White schema. *Zentbl. Bakteriol. Parasitenkd. Infektionskr. Hyg. I. Abt. Orig. Reihe* A **243:**148–176.
87. **Sack, R. B., M. Rahman, M. Yunus, and E. H. Khan.** 1997. Antimicrobial resistance in organisms causing diarrheal disease. *Clin. Infect. Dis.* **24**(Suppl. 1)**:**S102–S105.
88. **Schmidt, H., and H. Karch.** 1996. Enterohemolytic phenotypes and genotypes of Shiga toxin-producing *Escherichia coli* O111 strains from patients with diarrhea and hemolytic-uremic syndrome. *J. Clin. Microbiol.* **34:** 2364–2367.
89. **Scotland, S. M., T. Cheasty, A. Thomas, and B. Rowe.** 1991. Beta-glucuronidase activity of Vero cytotoxin-producing strains of *Escherichia coli*, including serogroup O157, isolated in the United Kingdom. *Lett. Appl. Microbiol.* **13:**42–44.
90. **Scotland, S. M., G. A. Willshaw, B. Said, H. R. Smith, and B. Rowe.** 1989. Identification of *Escherichia coli* that produce heat-stable enterotoxin ST_A by a commercially available enzyme-linked immunoassay and comparison of the assay with infant mouse and DNA probe tests. *J. Clin. Microbiol.* **27:**1697–1699.
91. **Sethabutr, O., P. Echeverria, C. W. Hoge, L. Bodhidatta, and C. Pitarangsi.** 1994. Detection of *Shigella* and enteroinvasive *Escherichia coli* by PCR in the stools of patients with dysentery in Thailand. *J. Diarrhoeal Dis. Res.* **12:**265–269.
92. **Slutsker, L., A. A. Ries, K. D. Greene, J. G. Wells, L. Hutwagner, and P. M. Griffin.** 1997. *Escherichia coli* O157:H7 diarrhea in the United States: clinical and epidemiologic features. *Ann. Intern. Med.* **126:**505–513.
93. **Smith, H. R., and S. M. Scotland.** 1993. Isolation and identification methods for *Escherichia coli* O157 and other Vero cytotoxin producing strains. *J. Clin. Pathol.* **46:** 10–17.
94. **Smith, H. W.** 1974. A search for transmissible pathogenic characters in invasive strains of *Escherichia coli*: the discovery of a plasmid-controlled toxin and a plasmid-controlled lethal character closely associated, or identical, with colicine V. *J. Gen. Microbiol.* **83:**95–111.
95. **Sobel, J., A. Hirshfeld, K. McTigue, C. Nichols, C. Burnette, S. Mottice, F. Brenner, G. Malcolm, and D. Swerdlow.** 1996. *Salmonella* Enteritidis phage type 4 pandemic reaches Utah, abstr. LB27. *In Program and Abstracts of the 36th Interscience Conference on Antimicrobial Agents and Chemotherapy*. American Society for Microbiology, Washington, D.C.
96. **Sowers, E. G., J. G. Wells, and N. A. Strockbine.** 1996. Evaluation of commercial latex reagents for identification of O157 and H7 antigens of *Escherichia coli*. *J. Clin. Microbiol.* **34:**1286–1289.
97. **Stavric, S., B. Buchanan, and J. Speirs.** 1992. Comparison of a competitive enzyme immunoassay kit and the infant mouse assay for detecting *Escherichia coli* heat-stable enterotoxin. *Lett. Appl. Microbiol.* **14:**47–50.
98. **Strockbine, N. A.** Unpublished data.
99. **Strockbine, N. A., S. V. Fernandez, B. Mahon, E. V. Oaks, W. Picking, and E. D. Mintz.** 1997. Serologic response to invasion plasmid antigens and lipopolysaccharide among individuals infected with *Shigella sonnei*, abstr. V-20, p. 577. *In Abstracts of the 97th General Meeting of the American Society for Microbiology 1997*. Washington, D.C.
100. **Strockbine, N. A., J. Parsonnet, K. Greene, J. A. Kiehlbauch, and I. K Wachsmuth.** 1991. Molecular epidemiologic techniques in analysis of epidemic and endemic *Shigella dysenteriae* type 1 strains. *J. Infect. Dis.* **163:**406–409.
101. **Strockbine, N. A., J. G. Wells, C. A. Bopp, and T. J. Barrett.** 1998. Overview of detection and subtyping methods, p. 331–356. *In* J. B. Kaper and A. D. O'Brien (ed.), Escherichia coli *O157:H7 and Other Shiga Toxin-Producing* E. coli *strains*. ASM Press, Washington, D.C.
102. **Swerdlow, D. L., and P. M. Griffin.** 1997. Duration of faecal shedding of *Escherichia coli* O157:H7 among children in day-care centres. *Lancet* **349:**745–746.
103. **Swerdlow, D. L., B. A. Woodruff, R. C. Brady, P. M. Griffin, S. Tippen, H. D. Donnell, E. Geldreich, B. J. Payne, A. Meyer, J. G. Wells, K. D. Greene, M. Bright, N. H. Bean, and P. A. Blake.** 1992. A waterborne outbreak in Missouri of *Escherichia coli* O157:H7 associated with bloody diarrhea and death. *Ann. Intern. Med.* **117:** 812–819.
104. **Tarr, P. I., and M. A. Neill.** 1996. Perspective: the problem of non-O157:H7 Shiga toxin (verocytotoxin)-producing *Escherichia coli*. *J. Infect. Dis.* **174:**1136–1139.
105. **Tauxe, R. V.** 1996. An update on *Salmonella*. *Health Environ. Digest* **10:**1–4.
106. **Tauxe, R. V., N. D. Puhr, J. G. Wells, N. Hargrett-Bean, and P. A. Blake.** 1990. Antimicrobial resistance of *Shigella* isolates in the USA: the importance of international travelers. *J. Infect. Dis.* **162:**1107–1111.
107. **Thomas, A., H. Chart, T. Cheasty, H. R. Smith, J. A. Frost, and B. Rowe.** 1993. Vero cytotoxin-producing *Escherichia coli*, particularly serogroup O157, associated with human infections in the United Kingdom: 1989–91. *Epidemiol. Infect.* **110:**591–600.
108. **Threlfall, E. J., and J. A. Frost.** 1990. The identification, typing, and fingerprinting of *Salmonella*: laboratory aspects and epidemiological applications. *J. Appl. Bacteriol.* **68:** 5–16.
109. **Threlfall, E. J., J. A. Frost, L. R. Ward, and B. Rowe.** 1996. Increasing spectrum of resistance in multiresistant *Salmonella typhimurium*. *Lancet* **347:**1053–1054.
110. **Threlfall, E. J., B. Rowe, and L. R. Ward.** 1993. A comparison of multiple drug resistance in salmonellas from humans and food animals in England and Wales, 1981 and 1990. *Epidemiol. Infect.* **111:**189–197.
111. **Verbrugh, H. A., D. R. Mekkes, R. P. Verkoyen, and J. E. Landbeer.** 1987. Widal type serology using live antigen for diagnosis of *Shigella flexneri* dysentery. *Eur. J. Clin. Microbiol. Infect. Dis.* **5:**540–542.
112. **Wells, J. G.** Unpublished data.
113. **Willshaw, G. A., S. M. Scotland, H. R. Smith, and B. Rowe.** 1992. Properties of Vero cytotoxin-producing *Escherichia coli* of human origin of O serogroups other than O157. *J. Infect. Dis.* **166:**797–802.
114. **Yam, W. C., M. L. Lung, and M. H. Ng.** 1992. Evaluation and optimization of a latex agglutination assay for detection of cholera toxin and *Escherichia coli* heat-labile toxin. *J. Clin. Microbiol.* **30:**2518–2520.
115. **Zadik, P. M., P. A. Chapman, and C. A. Siddons.** 1993. Use of tellurite for the selection of verocytotoxigenic *Escherichia coli* O157. *J. Med. Microbiol.* **39:**155–158.

Klebsiella, Enterobacter, Citrobacter, and *Serratia**

SHARON ABBOTT

29

TAXONOMY

Despite many nomenclatural changes over the last few years, the taxonomy within the genera *Klebsiella*, *Enterobacter*, *Citrobacter*, and *Serratia* remains unsettled. *Citrobacter* contains nine named species and two unnamed genomospecies (14). Five new species and the unnamed groups arose from DNA hybridization studies of the heterogeneous *Citrobacter freundii* complex (Table 1). Other changes include replacement of the name *Citrobacter diversus*, which was ruled a nomen dubium in 1994, with the name *Citrobacter koseri* (30), and elevation of *Citrobacter amalonaticus* biogroup 1 strains to species status as *Citrobacter farmeri* (2). The number of *Enterobacter* species has expanded to 14 with the transfer of three groups from *Erwinia* (14) (Table 1) and the addition of *Enterobacter hormaechei* (21) and *Enterobacter kobei* (16). The correct name for strains previously designated *Enterobacter taylorae* is *Enterobacter cancerogenus* (25). Besides these changes, both *Enterobacter cloacae* and *Enterobacter agglomerans* are known to be heterogeneous species containing at least 5 and 18 DNA groups, respectively (14). *E. agglomerans* was transferred to a new genus, *Pantoea*, in 1989. For more information on *Pantoea*, refer to chapter 27. Resolution of the genetic diversity within these nomenspecies in the future will undoubtedly reshape this genus by the addition of new members and changes to existing species. *Klebsiella* has remained relatively stable with seven species; the last addition to this genus, *Klebsiella ornithinolytica*, occurred in 1989 (14). It should be remembered that *Klebsiella ozaenae* and *Klebsiella rhinoscleromatis* are subspecies of *Klebsiella pneumoniae* but for convenience are referred to as if they were species. The number of species within *Serratia* is dependent upon whether *Serratia liquefaciens* is considered a "group" or as three distinct species (*S. liquefaciens* sensu stricto, *Serratia proteamaculans*, and *Serratia grimesii*). Since conventional biochemicals readily available to most clinical laboratories cannot separate these species, they will be referred to as the *S. liquefaciens*-group in this chapter. Although *Serratia* consists of eight species, both *Serratia marcescens* and *Serratia odorifera* contain biogroups.

* This chapter contains information presented in chapter 34 by Mary J. R. Gilchrist in the sixth edition of this Manual.

DESCRIPTION OF GENERA

All four genera belong to the family *Enterobacteriaceae* and are gram-negative, facultative anaerobic rods or coccobacilli ranging from 0.3 to 1.0 μm in width to 0.6 to 6.0 μm in length. Prototrophic strains grow readily on ordinary media. Among these genera, auxotrophic strains from clinical specimens are rare. However, cysteine-requiring urinary isolates of *K. pneumoniae*, which grow as pinpoint colonies on routine media, do occur. If encountered, these strains require supplementation of biochemical media or commercial identification systems with 0.63 mM cysteine for accurate identification. While some strains of *Serratia plymuthica* may not grow at 37°C, most other members of these genera grow well between 25 and 37°C. Essentially only *Klebsiella* spp. are encapsulated, but strains from all genera may grow as mucoid or rough colonies. Two genera produce pigment. Some strains of *S. marcescens* and most *Serratia rubidaea* and *S. plymuthica* strains produce a red pigment, prodigiosin, which may appear throughout a colony or as a red center or margin. *Enterobacter sakazakii* and some strains of *E. (Pantoea) agglomerans* form yellow-pigmented colonies which range from bright to pale yellow. Weak pigment producers may be detected only by observing growth placed on a swab or filter paper. Yellow pigment may be enhanced by incubation at 25°C. *S. odorifera* strains, true to their name, produce a distinctive pungent (potato-like) odor due to the production of alkyl-methoxypyrazines (11).

NATURAL HABITAT

Members of the genera *Klebsiella*, *Enterobacter*, *Citrobacter*, and *Serratia* are widespread throughout the environment (Table 1), although the citrobacters are primarily inhabitants of the intestinal tract. Their presence in the environment therefore may reflect fecal excretion by humans and animals; the natural habitat of some *Citrobacter* species is unknown.

All four genera are well-recognized nosocomial pathogens. Except for wounds, where *K. pneumoniae* ranks sixth, the National Nosocomial Infections Surveillance System lists *Enterobacter* species and *K. pneumoniae* as the fifth most common agents of nosocomial urinary tract (UT), wound, and bloodstream infections (24). They rank third and fourth, respectively, as causes of hospital-acquired pneumonia. Although less prevalent than other etiologic agents,

TABLE 1 Nomenclature, isolation source, and significance of the currently recognized members of the genera *Citrobacter*, *Enterobacter*, *Klebsiella*, and *Serratia*[a]

Current designation	Previous designation	Proposed or other designation	Clinical data: Frequency	Clinical data: Source	Clinical data: Significance	Enviromental data
Citrobacter						
C. amalonaticus			+ +	**Stool**, blood, Wd, UT, RT	2	Unk; one isolation from an animal
C. braakii	*C. freundii* complex		+ + +	**Stool**, UT, RT, Wd	2	Similar to *C. freundii*; some species have unknown reservoir
C. farmeri	*C. amalonaticus* biogroup 1		+ +	**Stool**, UT, Wd	2	Unk
C. freundii			+ + + +	All sites; stool most common	1	Water, soil, fish, animals, food
C. koseri	*C. diversus*		+ + +	All sites	1	Unk
C. rodentium	*C. freundii* complex genomospecies 9		–			Pathogenic for mice
C. sedlakii	*C. freundii* complex		+	Stool, blood, CSF	2	Same as for *C. braakii*
C. werkmanii	*C. freundii* complex		+ +	**Stool**, Wd	3	Same as for *C. braakii*
C. youngae	*C. freundii* complex		+ + + +	**Stool**, UT, blood, CSF	2	Same as for *C. braakii*
DNA group 10	*C. freundii* complex	*Citrobacter gillenii*	+	Stool	3	Food
DNA group 11	*C. freundii* complex	*Citrobacter murlinae*	+	Stool, blood	1	Same as for *C. braakii*
Enterobacter						
E. aerogenes			+ + + +	All sites	1	Water, soil, sewage, animal feces, dairy products
E. agglomerans		*Pantoea agglomerans*	+ + +	All sites	2	Plants, soil, water
E. amnigenus			+	RT, Wd, stool	3	Plants
Biogroup 1						
Biogroup 2						
E. asburiae			+ +	**UT**, RT, stool, Wd, blood	2	Water
E. cancerogenus	*E. taylorae*		+ +	**Wd**, RT, stool	2	Animals, water
E. cloacae			+ + + +	All sites	1	Water, soil, sewage, meat
E. dissolvens	*Erwinia dissolvens*		–			Diseased corn stalks
E. gergoviae			+ +	**RT**, UT, blood	2	Water, cosmetics
E. hormaechei	Enteric group 75		+	RT, Wd, blood	2	Unk; one isolation from a frog
E. intermedius	*E. intermedium*		+	Wd, blood, bile, stool	2	Water, soil

E. kobei	*E. cloacae* VP⁻		Unk	Unk	Unk	Food
E. nimipressuralis	*Erwinia nimipressuralis*		–			Diseased elm trees
E. pyrinus	*Erwinia pyrinus*		–			Diseased pear trees
E. sakazakii			+ +	**RT**, **Wd**, CSF	1	Unk
Klebsiella						
K. ornithinolytica	*Klebsiella* group 47		+	Wd, UT, blood	2	Food
K. oxytoca			+ + + +	Any site	1	Similar to *K. pneumoniae*
K. planticola[b]	*K. trevisanii*		Unk	Unk	3	Plants, water
K. pneumoniae			+ + + +	All sites; RT and UT most common	1	Plants, vegetables, animals, soil, water, wood and paper mills
K. pneumoniae subsp. *ozaenae*		*Klebsiella ozaenae*	+ +	**Nasal discharge** RT, UT, blood, eye	2	Unk
K. pneumoniae subsp. *rhinoscleromatis*		*Klebsiella rhinoscleromatis*	+ +	**Nasal discharge**	1	Unk
K. terrigena[b]			Unk	Unk	3	Soil, water
Serratia						
S. entomophila			–			New Zealand grass grub, water
S. ficaria			+	RT, wounds	3	Fig wasp, figs, plants
S. fonticola			+	**Wd**, RT	3	Water, birds
S. liquefaciens-group		*Serratia liquefaciens* sensu stricto, *Serratia proteamaculans*, *Serratia grimesii*	+ + +	RT, Wd	2	Plants, insects, small mammals, chickens, dairy products
S. marcescens			+	Any site; RT most common	1	Water, soil, plants, vegetables, insects, animals
S. marcescens biogroup 1			+	**UT**, RT	2	Unk
S. odorifera			+	**RT**, Wd, stool, blood, UT	2	Plants
Biogroup 1						
Biogroup 2						
S. plymuthica			+	RT	3	Water, plants, small mammals
S. rubidaea			+	RT, Wd, blood, UT, stool	2	Water, plants

[a] Symbols and abbreviations: + + + +, frequent; + + +, occasional; + +, rare; +, very rare; –, not yet isolated from humans; Wd, wounds or abscesses; UT, urinary tract; RT, respiratory tract; CSF, cerebrospinal fluid; Unk, unknown; 1, major pathogenic species of humans; 2, proven cause of disease in rare instances; 3, isolated from humans, significance unknown. Bold denotes most common source. Data are from references 2, 11, 12, 14, 16, 21, 25, and 30.

[b] May be misidentified as *K. pneumoniae*; cannot be separated from this species by routine biochemical tests.

Klebsiella and *Enterobacter* cause significant infections. For instance, in one study, when found intraoperatively, *Klebsiella* had a 68% probability and *Enterobacter* species had a 100% probability of causing a wound infection; probability rates for *Escherichia coli* or *Staphylococcus aureus*, which were isolated three times more often during surgery, were only 31 and 55%, respectively (27). While *K. pneumoniae* and *E. cloacae* cause sepsis four to five times less often than gram-positive organisms, they are two times more likely to cause patient mortality (28).

Klebsiella is commonly carried on human skin, in the nasopharynx, and in the bowel; of these, feces is probably the most significant source of patient infections (19). Approximately one-third of patients carry *Klebsiella* in their stools, but carriage rates may increase as much as threefold with hospitalization and antimicrobial usage in adults. Fecal carriage rates for children may be as high as 90 to 100% without antimicrobial therapy. Nosocomial *Enterobacter* colonization or infection is frequently associated with contaminated medical devices and instrumentation; however, *Enterobacter* species are commonly consumed in food, and an endogenous source should also be considered (14).

Citrobacter species and *S. marcescens* are the cause of 1 to 2% of nosocomial UT, wound, and bloodstream infections (24). *S. marcescens* causes 4% of hospital-acquired pneumonias, ranking as the sixth most common agent in this category (24). *Citrobacter* is most commonly isolated from the UT, where it is generally present in pure culture (60 to 75%) and is clinically significant (60 to 65%) (8, 18). Sepsis involving *Citrobacter* is often polymicrobic (14). Mortality rates as high as 48 to 50% have been reported; death is more often associated with polymicrobic than monomicrobic infections. *C. koseri* sepsis arising from endogenous sources typically originates from the genitourinary tract, while *C. freundii* bacteremia or septicemia arises from the UT, gallbladder, or gastrointestinal tract (5). *Citrobacter* meningitis is almost exclusively associated with *C. koseri* and involves children <2 months of age, with the highest onset rates noted in neonates with a mean age of 7 days (14). An exceedingly high number (>75%) of these infants develop brain abscesses, with those surviving generally afflicted with neurological defects. The most prominent risk factor is prior colonization; during outbreaks colonization rates of 27% have been noted (the normal rate is <1%) (17, 31). Person-to-person spread from personnel and less often from a mother to her offspring is the most likely source; sampling of inanimate or environmental reservoirs in hospitals usually fails to yield *Citrobacter*.

Serratia spp. are notorious nosocomial pathogens. The predominant mode of transmission is person to person, but various medical apparatuses, intravenous fluids, and other solutions have often been implicated as well (14). Patients with indwelling catheters, particularly for UT infections, serve as a primary reservoir for transmission via hospital personnel. In children the gastrointestinal tract is a common source of *Serratia* infections. Outbreaks transmitted by hand are often insidious and may occur over a long period of time, subsiding and peaking a number of times before recognition and infection control efforts can contain them.

The ability to trace the spread or involvement of these nosocomial pathogens in outbreaks has become a major responsibility and problem for the laboratory. Biotyping with commercially available identification systems is seldom suitably discriminatory unless an unusual marker or profile is present. Biotyping schemes that use carbon assimilation tests have been developed, particularly for *Serratia* (11). The typing of all four genera by traditional typing methods (serotyping, bacteriocin typing, and bacteriophage typing) would necessitate the use of multiple sets of reagents which are not readily available. Molecular techniques including plasmid analysis, ribotyping, pulsed-field gel electrophoresis (PFGE), and various PCR methods all appear to be satisfactorily discriminatory. However, since a single technique applicable to all strains is preferable, PFGE is currently the most universally accepted technique for epidemiological studies. The disadvantage of a long turnaround time (usually 4 days) has been partially overcome by a rapid PFGE protocol which is suitable for most enteric bacteria as well as other common clinical strains (10).

ISOLATION

For the most part none of the clinically relevant strains covered in this chapter present difficulties in isolation from sterile body sites. Cockerill et al. (4) did find, however, that when blood was cultured both *E. cloacae* and *S. marcescens* grew significantly better in aerobic culture than in nonvented or anaerobic culture; no difference was noted for other major species of these genera. *S. marcescens* was recovered significantly more often by the Isolator system than by the Septi-Check system (67 versus 38 isolations; $P = 0.006$). Isolation from nonsterile body or environmental

TABLE 2 Separation of members of the genus *Citrobacter*[a]

Species	Ind	ODC	Mal	Acid production from the following:			
				Sucrose	Dulcitol	Melibiose	Adonitol
C. amalonaticus	+	+	−	−	−	−	−
C. braakii	V	+	−	−	V	+	−
C. farmeri	+	+	−	+	−	+	−
C. freundii sensu stricto	V	−	V	V	V	+	−
C. rodentium	−	+	+	−	−	−	−
C. sedlakii	V	+	+	−	+	+	−
C. werkmanii	−	−	+	−	−	V	−
C. youngae	V	−	−	V	V	+	−
DNA genomospecies 10	−	−	+	V	−	V	−
DNA genomospecies 11	+	−	−	V	+	V	−

[a] Abbreviations and symbols: Ind, indole production; ODC, ornithine decarboxylase production; Mal, malonate utilization; +, ≥85% of strains; V, 15 to 85% of strains; −, ≤15% of strains.

TABLE 3 Differentiation of *Enterobacter* species[a]

Species	Production of the following:			VP reaction	Acid production from the following:							Yellow pigment
	LDC	ADH	ODC		Sucrose	Adonitol	Sorbitol	Rhamnose	α-Methyl-D-glucoside	Esculin	Melibiose	
Human species												
E. aerogenes	+	−	+	+	+	+	+	+	+	+	+	−
E. agglomerans	−	−	−	V	V	−	V	V	−	V	V	V
E. amnigenus biogroup I	−	−	V	+	+	−	−	+	V	+	+	−
E. asburiae	−	V	+	−	+	−	+	−	+	+	−	−
E. cancerogenus	−	+	+	+	−	−	−	+	−	+	−	−
E. cloacae	−	+	+	+	+	V	+	+	V	V	+	−
E. gergoviae	+	−	+	+	+	−	−	+	−	+	+	−
E. hormaechei	−	V	+	+	+	−	−	+	V	−	−	−
E. intermedius	−	−	V	+	V	−	+	+	+	+	+	−
E. kobei	−	+	+	−	+	−	+	+	+	V	+	−
E. sakazakii	−	+	+	+	+	−	−	+	+	+	+	+
Environmental species												
E. amnigenus biogroup II	−	V	+	+	−	−	+	+	+	+	+	−
E. dissolvens	−	+	+	+	+	−	+	+	+	+	+	−
E. nimipressuralis	−	−	+	+	−	−	+	+	+	+	+	−
E. pyrinus[b]	NA	NA	NA	+	+	−	−	+	−	+	+	−

[a] Abbreviations and symbols: LDC, lysine decarboxylase; ADH, arginine dihydrolase; ODC, ornithine decarboxylase; VP, Voges-Proskauer; +, ≥90% of strains; V, 10 to 90% of strains, −, ≤10% of strains; NA, not available.
[b] Separated from *E. gergoviae* by positive reactions in potassium cyanide broth and *myo*-inositol.

TABLE 4 Separation of some members of the genus *Klebsiella*[a]

Species	Ind	ODC	VP	Mal	ONPG
K. ornithinolytica	+	+	V	+	+
K. oxytoca	+	−	+	+	+
K. ozaenae	−	−	−	−	V
K. pneumoniae	−	−	+	+	+
K. rhinoscleromatis	−	−	−	+	−

[a] Abbreviations and symbols: Ind, indole production; ODC, ornithine decarboxylase production; VP, Voges-Proskauer reaction; Mal, malonate utilization; ONPG, *o*-nitrophenyl-*β*-D-galactopyranoside production; +, ≥90% of strains; V, 10 to 90% of strains; −, ≤10% of strains.

sites may require specialized media. Two media for *Serratia* include DNase-toluidine blue-cephalothin agar (7) and caprylate-thallous (CT) agar (26); neither will recover *Serratia fonticola* but are suitable for most other species. CT medium is not as effective for the isolation of *Serratia* from environmental specimens as it is for its isolation from nonsterile body sites. A 0.5% L-tyrosine medium can be used for *Citrobacter* isolation (20). Several media have been formulated for *Klebsiella*; a MacConkey-based agar substituting 1% inositol for lactose with 50 μg of carbenicillin per ml is probably simplest to make (11). Special media have not been developed for *Enterobacter*.

IDENTIFICATION

The biochemical tests most useful for separating the species within each genera are given in Tables 2 through 5. Full biochemical profiles for each species can be found in chapter 27. Identification problems arising from the use of commercial systems vary with each genus. *Serratia* species except for the *S. liquefaciens*-group are generally easily identified by commercial systems; separation of members within the *S. liquefaciens*-group requires carbon assimilation tests (14). These tests can be performed with a minimal agar to which neutralized carbon sources are added or a combination of the API 50CH, API 50 AO, and API 50 AA (carbohydrate, organic acid, and amino acid panels, respectively; bioMérieux, Hazelwood, Mo.) strips can be used (11). *Citrobacter* identification is hampered because few systems include newer species in their databases at this time. Automated systems appear to fare worse than manual systems, with <90% accuracy in identifying the *C. freundii* complex (14). Many strains require supplemental conventional biochemical tests, especially for the differentiation of *C. koseri* from *C. amalonaticus*. Most commonly used commercial systems have difficulties identifying *C. amalonaticus*, with incorrect identifications being obtained for 6 to 41% of strains tested (14). Of the *Klebsiella* species, *K. ozaenae* and *K. rhinoscleromatis* do the poorest in commercial systems, probably as a result of slow growth; these species can be difficult to separate with conventional biochemicals as well. Members of the genus *Enterobacter* appear to confound commercial systems more often than any of the other three genera. Six commonly used systems failed to identify one or more of several species (*E. cloacae*, *Enterobacter aerogenes*, *E.* [*Pantoea*] *agglomerans*, and *E. sakazakii*) with ≥90% accuracy a total of 14 times (14).

ANTIMICROBIAL SUSCEPTIBILITY

As with many bacteria, emerging antimicrobial resistance among members of these genera is becoming increasingly worrisome (1, 3, 13, 15, 22, 23). A 1994 study involving 43 medical centers across the United States found that 28.4% of *C. freundii* strains and 31% of *E. cloacae* strains were resistant to ceftazidime mediated by type I cephalosporinases and that 7.1% of *Klebsiella* spp. were resistant as a result of the presence of an extended-spectrum *β*-lactamase (ESBL) (15). Resistance was not restricted to a few institutions because 35 to 42 of the 43 facilities reported finding organisms resistant to these agents. Fluoroquinolone resistance (with the rate of resistance ranging from 6.3 to 14.4%)

TABLE 5 Biochemical characterization of members of the genus *Serratia*[a]

Species	Production of the following:		Mal utilization	Acid production from the following:								Red pigment	Odor
	LDC	ODC		Arabinose	Rham	Xyl	Suc	Adon	Sorb	Cello	Arabitol[b]		
S. entomophila[c]	−	−	−	−	−	V	+	−	−	−	V	−	−
S. ficaria	−	−	−	+	V	+	+	−	+	+	+	−	V
S. fonticola	+	+	V	+	V	V	V	+	+	−	+	−	−
S. liquefaciens-group	+	+	−	+	V	+	+	−	+	−	−	−	−
S. marcescens	+	+	−	−	−	−	+	V	+	−	−	V	−
S. marcescens biogroup 1	V	+	−	−	−	−	+	V	+	−	−	NA	−
S. odorifera biogroup 1	+	+	−	+	+	+	+	V	+	+	−	−	+
S. odorifera biogroup 2	+	−	−	+	+	+	−	V	+	+	−	−	+
S. plymuthica[d]	−	−	−	+	−	+	+	−	V	V	−	+	−
S. rubidaea	V	−	+	+	−	+	+	+	−	+	V	+	−

[a] Abbreviations and symbols: LDC, lysine decarboxylase; ODC, ornithine decarboxylase; Mal, malonate; Rham, rhamnose; Xyl, xylose; Suc, sucrose; Adon, adonitol; Sorb, sorbitol; Cello, cellobiose; +, ≥90% of strains; V, 10 to 90% of strains; −, ≤10% of strains; NA, information not available.

[b] Available in the API 50 CH system (bioMérieux).

[c] Growth at 37°C, but biochemical characterization is optimal at 30°C.

[d] May fail to grow at 37°C.

was found in all four genera. Approximately two-thirds of the study hospitals reported that *Enterobacter* and *Klebsiella* species were resistant to quinolones. While imipenem resistance was limited to two of the four genera, *Enterobacter* spp. and *S. marcescens* (4.0 and 5.2%, respectively), and was found in less than a third of the hospitals, its presence is disturbing. Because resistance, as demonstrated in this and other multicenter studies (1), varies both from hospital to hospital and regionally within any country, it is incumbent upon each institution to establish and monitor susceptibility profiles relevant for its patient population.

However, susceptibility data for some members of these genera are difficult to establish because they are infrequently isolated. Freney et al. (9) performed susceptibility testing with 120 isolates belonging to 13 of the more unusual species of *Klebsiella*, *Enterobacter*, and *Serratia*. Overall, they found that their susceptibilities were similar to those of conventional species within each genus (9).

While routine methods for testing the susceptibilities of these bacteria are well established, specialized techniques are required to determine the presence of ESBLs. A double-disk diffusion test is probably the most commonly used method, but other procedures including a three-dimensional test, the Vitek ESBL (Vitek; bioMérieux) test, and the Etest ESBL (AB Biodisk, Solna, Sweden) screen have also been examined (6, 23, 29). Specific methods can be found in section VIII of this Manual.

EVALUATION, INTERPRETATION, AND REPORTING OF RESULTS

When any of the species included in this chapter are identified with a high level of accuracy (>90% probability) by a commercial system, the identification is probably reliable. However, when an organism is isolated from a source where it may be considered significant, such as blood or cerebrospinal fluid, and the identification has a probability of <90%, the isolate should be identified in-house by conventional methods or sent to a reference laboratory and tested by conventional techniques. In the interim, the isolate may be reported to the physician with a presumptive identification. For those strains seen more commonly (i.e., *E. cloacae* and *S. marcescens*), the antimicrobial susceptibility profile may be a helpful adjunct for deciding if identifications with lower probabilities are reliable. Rare species that are identified with low probabilities should always be sent to a reference laboratory accompanied by a brief history.

REFERENCES

1. **ASCP Susceptibility Group.** 1996. United States geographic bacteria susceptibility patterns. *Am. J. Clin. Pathol.* **106:**275–281.
2. **Brenner, D. J., P. A. D. Grimont, A. G. Steigerwalt, G. R. Fanning, E. Ageron, and C. F. Riddle.** 1993. Classification of citrobacteria by DNA hybridization: designation of *Citrobacter farmeri* sp. nov., *Citrobacter youngae* sp. nov., *Citrobacter braakii* sp. nov., *Citrobacter werkmanii* sp. nov., *Citrobacter sedlakii* sp. nov., and three unnamed *Citrobacter* genomospecies. *Int. J. Syst. Bacteriol.* **43:**645–658.
3. **Chartrand, S. A., K. J. Thompson, and C. C. Sanders.** 1996. Antibiotic-resistant, gram-negative bacillary infections. *Semin. Pediatr. Infect. Dis.* **7:**187–203.
4. **Cockerill, F. R., III, J. G. Hughes, E. A. Vetter, R. A. Mueller, A. L. Weaver, D. M. Ilstrup, J. E. Rosenblatt, and W. R. Wilson.** 1997. Analysis of 281,797 consecutive blood cultures performed over an eight-year period: trends in microorganisms isolated and the value of anaerobic culture of blood. *Clin. Infect. Dis.* **24:**403–418.
5. **Drelichman, V., and J. D. Band.** 1985. Bacteremias due to *Citrobacter diversus* and *Citrobacter freundii*. *Arch. Intern. Med.* **145:**1808–1810.
6. **Emery, C. L., and L. A. Weymouth.** 1997. Detection and clinical significance of extended-spectrum β-lactamases in a tertiary-care medical center. *J. Clin. Microbiol.* **35:**2061–2067.
7. **Farmer, J. J., III, F. Silva, and D. R. Williams.** 1973. Isolation of *Serratia marcescens* on deoxyribonuclease-toluidine blue-cephalothin agar. *Appl. Microbiol.* **25:**151–152.
8. **Fields, B. N., M. M. Uwaydah, L. J. Kunz, and M. N. Swarz.** 1967. The so-called "paracolon" bacteria. *Am. J. Med.* **42:**89–106.
9. **Freney, J., M. O. Husson, F. Gavini, S. Madier, A. Martra, D. Izard, H. Leclerc, and J. Fleurette.** 1988. Susceptibilities to antibiotics and antiseptics of new species of the family *Enterobacteriaceae*. *Antimicrob. Agents Chemother.* **32:**873–876.
10. **Gautom, R. K.** 1997. Rapid pulsed-field gel electrophoresis protocol for typing of *Escherichia coli* O157:H7 and other gram-negative organisms in 1 day. *J. Clin. Microbiol.* **35:**2977–2980.
11. **Grimont, F., and P. A. D. Grimont.** 1981. The genus *Serratia*, p. 2822–2848. *In* M. P. Starr, H. Stolp, H. G. Trüper, and H. G. Schlegel (ed.), *The Prokaryotes: a Handbook on Habitats, Isolation, and Identification of Bacteria*. Springer-Verlag, Berlin, Germany.
12. **Grimont, F., P. A. D. Grimont, and C. Richard.** 1991. The genus *Klebsiella*, p. 2775–2796. *In* M. P. Starr, H. Stolp, H. G. Trüper, A. Balows, and H. G. Schlegel (ed.), *The Prokaryotes: a Handbook on the Biology of Bacteria: Ecophysiology, Isolation, Identification, Applications*. Springer-Verlag, Berlin, Germany.
13. **Jacoby, G. A., and A. A. Medeiros.** 1991. More extended-spectrum β-lactamases. *Antimicrob. Agents Chemother.* **35:**1697–1704.
14. **Janda, J. M., and S. L. Abbott.** 1998. *The Enterobacteria*. Lippincott-Raven, Philadelphia, Pa.
15. **Jones, R. N., E. N. Kehrberg, M. E. Erwin, S. C. Anderson, and the Fluoroquinolone Resistance Surveillance Group.** 1994. Prevalence of important pathogens and antimicrobial activity of parenteral drugs at numerous medical centers in the United States. I. Study on the threat of emerging resistances: real or perceived? *Diagn. Microbiol. Infect. Dis.* **19:**203–215.
16. **Kosako, Y., K. Tamura, R. Sakazaki, and K. Miki.** 1996. *Enterobacter kobei* sp. nov., a new species of the family *Enterobacteriaceae* resembling *Enterobacter cloacae*. *Curr. Microbiol.* **33:**261–265.
17. **Lin, F.-Y. C., W. F. Devoe, C. Morrison, J. Libonati, P. Powers, R. J. Gross, B. Rowe, E. Israel, and J. G. Morris.** 1987. Outbreak of neonatal *Citrobacter diversus* meningitis in a suburban hospital. *Pediatr. Infect. Dis. J.* **6:**50–55.
18. **Lipsky, B. A., E. W. Hook III, A. A. Smith, and J. J. Plorde.** 1980. *Citrobacter* infections in humans: experience at the Seattle Veterans Administration Medical Center and a review of the literature. *Rev. Infect. Dis.* **2:**746–760.
19. **Montgomerie, J. Z.** 1979. Epidemiology of *Klebsiella* and hospital-associated infections. *Rev. Infect. Dis.* **1:**736–753.
20. **Müller, H. E.** 1986. Occurrence and clinical significance of tyrosine clearing positive *Citrobacter freundii* in human faecal specimens. *Zentralbl. Bakteriol. Parasitenkd. Infektionskr. Hyg. Abt. 1 Orig. Reihe A* **262:**412–416.
21. **O'Hara, C. M., A. G. Steigerwalt, B. C. Hill, J. J. Farmer III, G. R. Fanning, and D. J. Brenner.** 1989. *Enterobacter hormaechei*, a new species of the family *Enterobacteriaceae*

formerly known as enteric group 75. *J. Clin. Microbiol.* **27:** 2046–2049.

22. **Rasmussen, B. A., and K. Bush.** 1997. Carbapenem-hydrolyzing β-lactamases. *Antimicrob. Agents Chemother.* **41:** 223–232.
23. **Sanders, C. C., A. L. Barry, J. A. Washington, C. Shubert, E. S. Moland, M. M. Traczewski, C. Knapp, and R. Mulder.** 1996. Detection of extended-spectrum β-lactamase-producing members of the family *Enterobacteriaceae* with the Vitek ESBL test. *J. Clin. Microbiol.* **34:** 2997–3001.
24. **Schaberg, D. R., D. H. Culver, and R. P. Gaynes.** 1991. Major trends in the microbial etiology of nosocomial infection. *Am. J. Med.* **91**(Suppl. 3B):72S–75S.
25. **Schønheyder, H. C., K. T. Jensen, and W. Frederiksen.** 1994. Taxonomic notes: synonymy of *Enterobacter cancerogenus* (Uroševič 1966) Dickey and Zumoff 1988 and *Enterobacter taylorae* Farmer et al. 1985 and resolution of an ambiguity in the biochemical profile. *Int. J. Syst. Bacteriol.* **44:** 586–587.
26. **Starr, M. P., P. A. D. Grimont, F. Grimont, and P. B. Starr.** 1976. Caprylate-thallous agar medium for selectively isolating *Serratia* and its utility in the clinical laboratory. *J. Clin. Microbiol.* **4:**270–276.
27. **Twum-Danso, K. C. Grant, S. A. Al-Suleiman, S. Abdel-Khader, M. S. Al-Awami, H. Al-Breiki, S. Taha. A.-A. Ashoor, and L. Wosornu.** 1992. Microbiology of postoperative wound infection: a prospective study of 1770 wounds. *J. Hosp. Infect.* **21:**29–37.
28. **Vallés, J., C. León, and F. Alvarez-Lerma.** 1997. Nosocomial bacteremia in critically ill patients: a multi-center study evaluating epidemiology and prognosis. *Clin. Infect. Dis.* **24:**387–395.
29. **Vercauteren, E., P. Descheemaeker, M. Ieven, C. C. Sanders, and H. Goossens.** 1997. Comparison of screening methods for detection of extended-spectrum β-lactamases and their prevalence among blood isolates of *Escherichia coli* and *Klebsiella* spp. in a Belgian teaching hospital. *J. Clin. Microbiol.* **35:**2191–2197.
30. **Wayne, L. G.** 1994. Actions of the Judicial Commission of the International Committee on Systematic Bacteriology on requests for opinions published between January 1985 and July 1993. *Int. J. Syst. Bacteriol.* **44:**177–178.
31. **Williams, W. W., J. Mariano, M. Spurrier, H. D. Donnell, Jr., R. L. Breckenridge, Jr., R. L. Anderson, I. K. Wachsmuth, C. Thornsberry, D. R. Graham, D. W. Thibeault, and J. R. Allen.** 1984. Nosocomial meningitis due to *Citrobacter diversus* in neonates: new aspects of epidemiology. *J. Infect. Dis.* **150:**229–235.

Yersinia and Other *Enterobacteriaceae**

STOJANKA ALEKSIC AND JOCHEN BOCKEMÜHL

30

YERSINIA SPECIES

Taxonomy

In 1944, Van Loghem proposed the transfer of *Pasteurella pestis* and *P. pseudotuberculosis* to his newly defined genus *Yersinia*, named after Alexandre Yersin, who had first isolated the plague bacillus in 1894. In 1964, Frederiksen further included *Pasteurella* X (syn. *Bacterium enterocoliticum*), which previously had been described by Schleifstein and Coleman.

Following intensive taxonomic studies in the 1980s, the genus *Yersinia* at present includes 10 established species: *Y. pestis*, *Y. pseudotuberculosis*, *Y. enterocolitica*, *Y. frederiksenii*, *Y. intermedia*, *Y. kristensenii*, *Y. bercovieri* (75), *Y. mollaretii* (75), *Y. rohdei*, and *Y. aldovae*. The taxonomic status of "Y." *ruckeri*, a fish pathogen, is still uncertain. *Y. pestis*, *Y. pseudotuberculosis*, and certain strains of *Y. enterocolitica* are of pathogenic importance for humans and certain warm-blooded animals, whereas the other species are of environmental origin and may, at best, act as opportunists. However, they are frequently isolated from clinical materials and therefore have to be identified to the species level.

Members of the genus *Yersinia* exhibit 10 to 32% relatedness to other members of the *Enterobacteriaceae* by DNA-DNA hybridization. The DNA G+C content of the genus is in the range of 46.0 to 48.5 mol%. Based on DNA-DNA hybridization, *Y. enterocolitica* sensu stricto exhibits 43 to 64% relatedness to *Y. pestis* and *Y. pseudotuberculosis* (22). However, *Y. pestis* and *Y. pseudotuberculosis* are so closely related that Bercovier et al. (4) suggested that *Y. pestis* should be classified as a subspecies of *Y. pseudotuberculosis*. Initially, the World Health Organization adopted this proposal; however, it was finally rejected following worldwide protest and nonacceptance (77).

Description of the Genus

Members of the genus *Yersinia* are non-spore-forming, gram-negative or gram-variable, rod-shaped or coccoid cells, 0.5 to 0.8 μm in width and 1 to 3 μm in length. Except for *Y. pestis*, which is nonmotile, the other species are motile at 22 to 30°C but not at 37°C; motile cells are peritrichously flagellated (41). Yersiniae grow under aerobic and anaerobic culture conditions between 0 and 45°C, with an optimum at 25 to 28°C, on nonselective and certain selective media. Only *Y. pestis* has special nutritional requirements for L-valine, L-methionine, L-phenylalanine, and glycine or L-threonine.

Glucose is fermentatively utilized, with the formation of acid; gas and hydrogen sulfide are not produced. There is no growth in the presence of KCN. Phenylalanine and tryptophan are not deaminated, gelatin is not liquefied, lysine is not decarboxylated, and arginine is not dehydrolyzed. Nitrate is reduced to nitrite, catalase is produced, but oxidase is absent. Acetoin (Voges-Proskauer reaction) is produced at 25 to 28°C (not at 37°C) by most strains of *Y. enterocolitica*, *Y. frederiksenii*, *Y. intermedia*, and *Y. aldovae* but not by the remaining *Yersinia* species. With the exception of *Y. pestis*, urease is produced at 25 to 28°C. Ornithine is decarboxylated by all the species but *Y. pestis* and *Y. pseudotuberculosis*.

Virulence Factors of Pathogenic *Yersinia*

Y. pestis, *Y. pseudotuberculosis*, and the pathogenic bioserotypes of *Y. enterocolitica* are similar insofar as they show preference for the lymphatic tissue and can be spread via the bloodstream. They seem to have the same basic virulence mechanism, although their routes of invasion as well as the clinical symptoms they cause are different. A majority of genes involved in pathogenicity are located on virulence plasmids, although some are chromosomally determined.

The three pathogenic species share a 70- to 75-kb plasmid carrying a number of genes, whose products may be classified into four main categories (64, 68): adhesin/invasin (YadA; not important in *Y. pestis*), excreted antiphagocytic proteins (YopE, YopH, and YopM in the three species; LcrV in *Y. pestis*; YpkA in *Y. pseudotuberculosis*), processing and excretion-related proteins for *Yersinia* outer proteins (Ysc), and regulatory proteins (Lcr). Loss of the plasmid results in decreased pathogenicity and inability to cause disseminated disease.

Chromosomally encoded virulence factors of *Y. enterocolitica* and *Y. pseudotuberculosis* include Inv (invasin) and Ail (attachment-invasion locus), which both contribute to invasion of the body. In *Y. pestis*, an important pathogenicity island termed the *pgm* locus carries the genes for a hemin storage system (Hms) and a siderophore named yersiniabactin (Ybt). These virulence factors are expressed at 25 and/or 37°C. The role of a thermostable enterotoxin produced by

* This chapter contains information presented in chapter 33 by Larry D. Gray and chapter 34 by Mary J. R. Gilchrist in the sixth edition of this Manual.

pathogenic strains of Y. *enterocolitica* is still under discussion, although a clinical association has been suggested (19).

Natural Habitats

Y. pestis

Rodents are the natural reservoir of the plague bacteria. Transmission in these populations occurs mainly via their fleas but occasionally also by direct contact and cannibalism. According to the density of the organisms in the infected host, fleas may acquire up to 300 bacteria during one blood meal (64). In the flea, the infection is restricted to the alimentary tract, including the salivary glands and stomach. Fleas possessing a pronounced proventriculus are especially capable of transmitting *Y. pestis* effectively. At 3 to 9 days after the infected blood meal, the organisms have multiplied to such an extent that the bacterial masses block the stomach and proventriculus and impede newly ingested blood from reaching the stomach. This causes the hungry flea to suck intensively and to regurgitate the mixture of bacteria and blood into the mammalian host, who thus may be infected with up to 20,000 organisms by one flea attack (3). Maintenance of natural plague depends on the cyclic transmission between fleas and mammals. Due to the ability to reduce its organic nutritional requirements, *Y. pestis* is able to survive for prolonged periods in the unique niche of its host, the stomach and proventriculus. Furthermore, it may express mechanisms for prolonged viability in soil and water (12, 65).

More than 200 mammalian species have been reported to be naturally infected with *Y. pestis*; however, rodents are of principal importance. Highly susceptible hosts include various species of mice, rats, voles, gerbils, ground squirrels, rabbits, and prairie dogs. If such susceptible populations migrate into areas occupied by infected species, this may be followed by dramatic increases in mortality and decimation of the invaders. Their fleas then search for new hosts, including humans, and transmit the disease. Such epizootic outbreaks have occurred in the past and were the cause of many of the large classical epidemics. Today, plague is more or less confined to endemic foci in Africa, the Americas, and Asia, where local epidemics or increased incidences may occur. In the United States, domestic cats repeatedly have been infected, and this mode of infection has caused 18 human cases since 1977 (28). However, of 286 cases for which the modes of transmission were determined during 1970 to 1995, 223 (78%) were caused by flea bites; therefore, the overall importance of cats is quite minor (14).

Plague Pandemics

Plague is one of the oldest recorded infectious diseases. Some historical and geographical data suggest the Himalayas to be the most likely birthplace (58). From there, the disease spread east toward China, south to the Indian subcontinent, and west toward the Middle East and Europe. More than 150 epidemics, most of them associated with three main pandemics, have been reported.

It has been hypothesized that the first (A.D. 541 to 544), second (A.D. 1330 to 1480), and third (A.D. 1855) pandemics were caused by three different but genetically constant biotypes of *Y. pestis*, i.e., Antiqua, Medievalis, and Orientalis, respectively (20). However, recent studies in Madagascar, using ribotyping for the clonal characterization of local isolates from various periods, have demonstrated the emergence of genetic variants in different areas of endemic infection (34).

Between 1981 and 1995, 25 countries reported a total of 21,087 cases to the World Health Organization, showing an increasing trend of morbidity with an average fatality rate of about 10% (80). Major epidemics and outbreaks in Tanzania (1991), Zaire (1992 to 1993), Peru (1993 to 1994), India (1994), and Madagascar (1995) with fatality rates of 4.6 to 22.3% have demonstrated that plague is far from being eradicated.

Enteropathogenic and Nonpathogenic *Yersinia* Species

Y. enterocolitica and *Y. pseudotuberculosis* are distributed worldwide but occur mainly in the moderate and subtropical climatic areas of the Americas; Europe; north, central, and east Asia; South Africa; and Australia. On the other hand, they are rare or lacking in the tropical regions of Africa and southeast Asia.

Y. pseudotuberculosis is found in numerous wild and domestic mammals as well as birds. Outbreaks occur mainly in captive rodent populations (fur farming and experimental animals), zoo animals, poultry farms (turkeys, ducks, and pigeons), and pet-bird breeding. The disease may vary from acute septicemia to a subacute or chronic course with fever, weakness, diarrhea, respiratory disorders, and paralysis. In wild, domestic, and pet animals, sporadic cases of pseudotuberculosis or asymptomatic infections prevail. The main reservoirs of *Y. pseudotuberculosis* are rodents (mice and rats), lagomorphs (hares and rabbits), and wild birds. The organisms survive for prolonged periods in soil and river water (26). About half of the strains examined in our laboratory originated from organs of deceased wild and domestic animals (hares, rabbits, wild ducks, birds, sheep, pigs, and cats). Strains of human origin have been isolated from stool specimens, intestinal specimens obtained at surgery (lymph nodes, ileum, appendix), and occasional blood cultures of leukemic patients.

Y. enterocolitica has a wide distribution and can be found in humans, in all warm-blooded wild, domestic, and pet animals, and occasionally in or on reptiles, fish, and shellfish. The organisms are also isolated from food, soil, and surface water. Pigs are important reservoirs for the human pathogenic serogroups O:3 and O:9; the organisms especially colonize the pigs' tonsils. Only certain serogroups are obligatory pathogens for animals; these include O:1,2a,3 (biotype 3) and O:2a,2b,3 (biotype 5) for chinchillas, hares, rabbits, cattle, sheep, and goats. These serogroups occasionally have also caused disease in humans. The remaining serotypes, including the human pathogens, usually cause asymptomatic infections in animals.

Whereas the nonpathogenic serotypes of *Y. enterocolitica* biotype 1A (see Table 2) apparently are able to propagate independently in the environment, this is less likely for the pathogenic serotypes; however, these may survive for prolonged periods outside their hosts. Thus, contaminated surface water, soil, and vegetation may become sources for infections of humans and animals.

Y. frederiksenii, *Y. kristensenii*, *Y. intermedia*, *Y. rohdei*, *Y. aldovae*, *Y. mollaretii*, and *Y. bercovieri* are primarily environmental organisms but occasionally colonize warm- and cold-blooded hosts in a transient manner. *Y. mollaretii*, *Y. intermedia*, *Y. bercovieri*, and *Y. kristensenii* seem to be especially adapted to the aquatic environment and frequently have been found to colonize filter systems of drinking water plants (2). "Y." *ruckeri* is a fish pathogen, which causes "red mouth disease."

Clinical Significance

Y. pestis (Plague)

The clinical course of plague in animals and humans is similar. Following infection by a flea or animal bite or via otherwise injured skin or mucous membrane, the organisms enter the bloodstream, where they are transported to the nearest lymph node. Ingested by macrophages, the *Y. pestis* organisms survive and proliferate there. An intense inflammatory response produces the characteristic swelling or "bubo" which gives the bubonic plague its name. Depending on the immunity of the host, bacteria leaking into the bloodstream may cause a secondary septicemia and be transported to various organs. This stage of the disease, septicemic plague, may be followed by meningitis or pneumonia when the organisms parasitize the alveolar macrophages. Patients suffering from pneumonic plague can transmit *Y. pestis* via aerosols to other persons. The resulting form of primary pneumonia is usually followed by a very acute course, since *Y. pestis* acquired from another human already expresses all the virulence factors required for the disease. Patients with plague often develop necrotic lesions in the peripheral blood vessels, giving the skin a blackish coloration which, in the past, led to the name "black death" (68).

Human plague can thus be classified into three general syndromes, i.e., bubonic plague, primary and secondary septicemic plague, and pneumonic plague (18, 64).

Highly susceptible animal species usually develop acute to subacute septicemic plague with necrosis or necrotic nodules in the lymph nodes, liver, and spleen; they succumb to the infection within approximately 6 days. Cats typically develop acute febrile illness followed by bacteremia, pneumonia, and buboes; they die within 6 to 20 days (28). More resistant animal species experience bubonic plague characterized by lymphadenopathy with purulent focal necrosis. Animals usually respond to symptomatic as well as asymptomatic infection by seroconversion.

Plague induces a long-lasting immunity, which, however, is not absolute (13). Two types of vaccine are available: one is derived from an attenuated, Pgm-deficient strain (live vaccine [Institut Pasteur, Paris, France]), and the other consists of a formalin-inactivated whole-cell preparation from a virulent strain of *Y. pestis* (available in the United States [57]). Although controlled field trials are lacking, the latter proved to have a certain effectiveness in soldiers exposed to virulent plague bacteria during the Vietnam war (57). Altogether, the protection is variable and particularly low against the pneumonic form. Vaccination is therefore limited to certain conditions such as staff working with virulent *Y. pestis* cultures or military personnel operating in areas of endemic infection.

Y. enterocolitica, Y. pseudotuberculosis, and Nonpathogenic Species

Infections due to *Y. enterocolitica* and *Y. pseudotuberculosis* may be acquired by ingestion of contaminated food or water or, rarely, by direct person-to-person transmission, e.g., in kindergartens, schools, or hospitals. *Y. enterocolitica* is a common cause of human infection, whereas *Y. pseudotuberculosis* is primarily an animal pathogen and infects humans only rarely. The incubation period varies between 4 and 7 days in *Y. enterocolitica* and is unknown for *Y. pseudotuberculosis* (13).

Both species have affinity for the lymphoid tissue and probably penetrate into the ileal mucosa via the M cells, which, together with B- and T-lymphoid cells and macrophages, form the follicles of Peyer's patches. From the underlying tissue, they enter the lymph nodes and multiply there (9). The inflammatory response causes pain in the lower abdominal region, which is a typical symptom and may be mistaken for appendicitis.

Intestinal yersiniosis may present in three clinical forms: enteritis, terminal ileitis or mesenteric lymphadenitis causing "pseudoappendicitis," and septicemia (10). Watery, sometimes bloody stools are characteristic of *Y. enterocolitica* but are rarely caused by *Y. pseudotuberculosis*. Bloody diarrhea is observed mainly in adults and less frequently in children, and it is often accompanied by fever, vomiting, and, typically, abdominal pain. Terminal ileitis, mesenteric lymphadenitis, and pseudoappendicitis are produced by both species and are the characteristic symptoms in *Y. pseudotuberculosis* infection, which is especially common in children older than 5 years and juveniles. Whereas adults usually overcome intestinal yersiniosis within 1 to 2 weeks, disease in children may last for up to 4 weeks.

Septicemia is a rare event, which occurs in adults mostly in association with severe underlying disease such as metabolic disorders (diabetes), liver disease (toxic and viral cirrhosis), immunodeficiency (AIDS), or neoplastic processes. Focal abscesses may be produced in various organs following the spread of the organisms in the bloodstream. A special case is septicemia in patients with iron overload due to hemolytic anemia (thalassemia, sickle cell disease, or aplastic anemia) or undergoing therapeutic application of iron compounds. Siderophore (yersiniabactin)-producing strains of *Y. enterocolitica* groups O:8, O:13a,13b, and O:20 have been isolated from patients with hemolytic anemia, whereas the non-siderophore-producing strains of serogroups O:3 and O:9 are associated with iron compound treatment (16, 38).

Since the mid-1970s, septicemia caused by transfusion of contaminated blood and blood products has been noted worldwide (15, 59). Amazingly, in all reported cases, only the non-siderophore-producing serogroups O:3, O:9, O:5,27, and O:1,2a,3 have been recovered from blood specimens. Serogroup O:8 has not been isolated from transfusion-related *Yersinia* septicemia; it was shown that O:8 more readily loses serum resistance at 4°C than do other pathogenic serogroups (11). Growth experiments with fresh whole blood have shown that after a lag phase of 4 days, counts of 5×10^6/ml *Y. enterocolitica* O:3 developed within 21 days at 4°C (70).

Following intestinal infection by both *Y. enterocolitica* and *Y. pseudotuberculosis*, extraintestinal disease develops in some patients, particularly those who display histocompatibility antigen HLA-B27. These sequelae include reactive arthritis, myocarditis, glomerulonephritis, thyroiditis, and erythema nodosum. It has been shown that certain *Yersinia* antigens have similarities to host antigens of the joints, to thyroid epithelial cells, and to HLA-B27, causing circulating antibodies to bacterial surface structures to cross-react with the host tissue even if the infection has already ceased (31, 71). These sequelae usually have a favorable prognosis, but they may last for years.

A special form of *Y. pseudotuberculosis* infection is the Far East scarlet fever-like disease, which hitherto has only been observed in eastern parts of the former USSR and in Japan. The disease is characterized by high fever, arthritis, and scarlet fever-like exanthema following an intestinal infection (69). Recently, it has been shown that strains causing this syndrome are significantly associated with the production of a novel superantigen designated *Y. pseudotuberculosis*-derived mitogen (YPM). The encoding gene, *ypm*, was detected in 95 to 100% of *Y. pseudotuberculosis* strains from the Far East, in contrast to only 17% in European clinical isolates (81).

Y. kristensenii, *Y. intermedia*, *Y. mollaretii*, *Y. bercovieri*, *Y. frederiksenii*, and *Y. rohdei* are frequently isolated from clinical materials, but a specific pathogenic potential in these organisms has not been established. Their role in opportunistic infections of immunocompromised hosts has yet to be elucidated.

Collection, Transport, and Storage of Specimens

Safety Procedures

Local and state health authorities must be immediately notified of suspected and presumptive cases of plague. Furthermore, plague is notifiable to the World Health Organization according to the International Health Regulations.

Y. pestis is a pathogen in biohazard risk group III and should be handled in a containment laboratory. Standard bacteriological practices of biosafety level 2 are usually sufficient for clinical laboratories, but special precautions must be used if aerosols are produced or deceased animals are handled. Such activities, as well as procedures with cultures of *Y. pestis*, should be performed in a class III biological safety cabinet. Laboratory staff must be protected against skin contact and inhalation of aerosols, e.g., by using gloves and a face mask (73).

If *Y. pestis* was not expected but is discovered in the course of examination, the activities must be stopped. The isolate should be preserved for further identification and susceptibility testing in a class III safety cabinet, and all remaining culture materials should be destroyed by autoclaving. The laboratory bench and equipment used for handling of the material must be disinfected. Laboratory personnel must be informed of possible clinical symptoms and are obligated to immediately report any signs of disease. If infection cannot be ruled out, prophylaxis with orally administered tetracycline may be considered.

Specimen Collection and Transport

In humans, *Y. pestis* can be isolated from blood (at least three samples taken within 24 h), by bubo aspiration (obtained by injection of 1 ml of sterile saline and immediate aspiration), from sputum, from throat swabs or throat washings, from skin swabs or scrapings, and from cerebrospinal fluid in patients with meningitis. At autopsy, blood and tissue specimens from the buboes, liver, spleen, and lungs should be collected.

Living or dead animals should be treated with an insecticide before specimens are collected; fleas are collected for bacteriological examination. Blood from the heart and tissue specimens from lymph nodes, liver, spleen, and other organs are collected; bone marrow and brain tissue are appropriate specimens from decaying cadavers. *Y. pestis* may even be isolated 1 to 2 months postmortem if the material is inoculated into mice, rats, or guinea pigs. Cary-Blair medium is a suitable transport medium for swabs.

Isolation of *Y. enterocolitica* and *Y. pseudotuberculosis* is attempted from stool specimens in patients with intestinal disease, from blood in patients with septicemia, from lymph nodes, intestinal tissue, or pus if abdominal surgery or biopsy has been performed, and in certain cases from nasopharyngeal swabs. Feces, mesenteric and pharyngeal lymphatic tissue, abscess material, or nodules in the liver and spleen are collected from animals. Examination of food and water may be useful for epidemiological reasons; local public health authorities should assist with such studies.

In the late stage of the disease (two or more weeks after onset), if antibiotics have been administered, or if appropriate material cannot be recovered for culture, serum specimens should be taken for detection of specific antibodies against the three pathogenic *Yersinia* species.

For transport and storage of suspected clinical specimens or cultures of *Yersinia* species, the general principles described in chapter 4 are applicable.

Isolation Procedures

Y. pestis

Microscopy after Giemsa, Wright, Wayson (see section IX), or methylene blue staining may be helpful; a typical stain is supportive but not confirmatory. *Y. pestis* organisms present in clinical material commonly display bipolarity resembling "safety pins" due to retention of stain by the cytoplasm (Fig. 1); this morphology is not displayed by Gram staining or in cultured organisms. *Y. pestis* is coccoid or rod shaped.

Direct microscopic detection of the capsular F1 antigen in clinical specimens can be attempted by use of a fluorescent antibody stain. Alternatively, the presence of F1 antigen can be tested for by enzyme-linked immunosorbent assay (ELISA). The antibody is available at the Centers for Disease Control and Prevention (CDC) or at national reference laboratories.

Capsular F1 antigen is expressed mainly at 37°C. Samples that have been refrigerated for more than 30 h, cells from cultures incubated below 35°C, or extracts from fleas will be negative (64). A positive fluorescent F1 antigen test may be taken as presumptive evidence of *Y. pestis* infection.

PCR (62) with primers derived from the *pla* (plasminogen activator protein) and *caf1* (capsular F1 antigen) genes, which are harbored by two different *Y. pestis* virulence

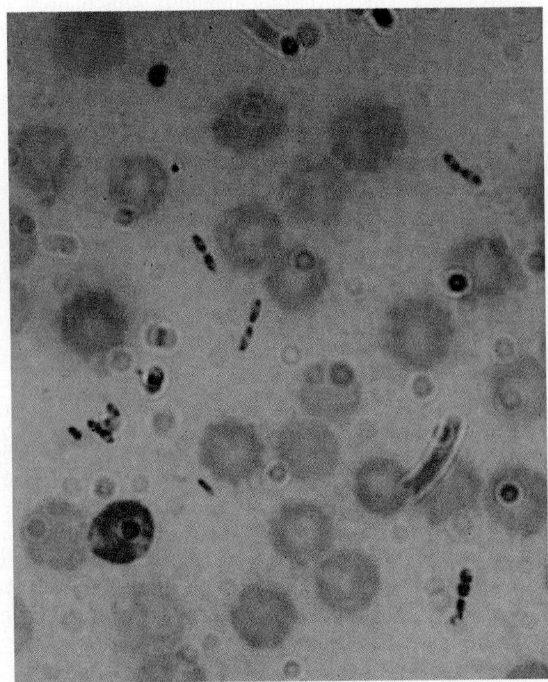

FIGURE 1 Methylene blue-stained blood smear of *Y. pestis* in mice.

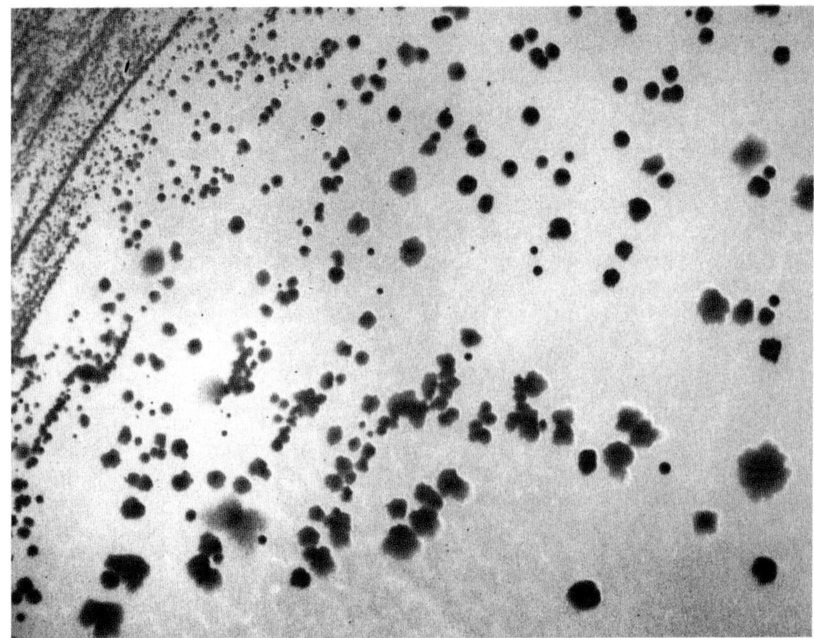

FIGURE 2 Growth of *Y. pestis* on CIN agar (cefsulodin content, 4 μg/ml) after 48 h at 28°C.

plasmids, is a rapid and sensitive method for the presumptive diagnosis of plague in clinical specimens or fleas. However, the method has not yet been sufficiently validated and should be performed only by a specialized laboratory.

Animal testing can be used if heavily contaminated specimens have to be examined. The samples are homogenized in sterile saline, of which 0.1 to 0.2 ml is subcutaneously or intraperitoneally inoculated into mice, rats, or guinea pigs. If virulent *Y. pestis* organisms are present, the animals die within 2 to 6 days and the organisms can be reisolated from the blood, liver, and spleen. Again, safety considerations restrict this procedure to specialized laboratories.

Isolation of the organisms in culture is the most certain etiological proof of *Y. pestis* infection. Nonselective media, such as 5% blood agar or brain heart infusion (BHI) agar, can be used for sterile materials such as blood, bubo aspirates, or biopsy specimens. Selective media such as MacConkey agar and cefsulodin-irgasan-novobiocin (CIN) (1b) agar with reduced cefsulodin content (4 μg/ml) are suitable for contaminated specimens such as sputum and swabs (throat, skin, and organs). Enrichment cultures of sterile specimens should be made in BHI broth. Blood specimens may be enriched in commercial blood culture media. For contaminated materials, MacConkey broth can be used. As a specific selective enrichment medium, CIN broth with 4 μg of cefsulodin per ml may be used (1b) (see section IX). Fluid and plate cultures are incubated at 35°C for 7 days before they are reported negative.

On all solid media, *Y. pestis* grows as pinpoint colonies after a 24-h incubation at 35°C. The morphology becomes more typical after 48 h, when the organisms are nonhemolytic on blood agar, smooth or mucoid on BHI agar, and lactose negative on MacConkey agar. Larger colonies have irregular edges (Fig. 2), demonstrating a "hammered-metal" appearance under a dissecting microscope. Upon further growth, the centers of the colonies are raised and older colonies often assume a "fried-egg" configuration.

Y. enterocolitica, Y. pseudotuberculosis, and Other *Yersinia* Species

Certain chromosomal and plasmid-located virulence genes, such as *inv, ail, yst, yadA,* and *virF*, have been used for the detection of pathogenic *Y. enterocolitica* and *Y. pseudotuberculosis* by PCR and DNA colony blot hybridization (36, 40, 51, 52). These methods, however, are not required in the clinical laboratory because isolation of *Y. enterocolitica* and *Y. pseudotuberculosis* usually is not problematic. Both species grow well on all nonselective or moderately selective media used for the isolation of *Enterobacteriaceae*.

Enrichment of stool specimens is usually not necessary for patients with diarrhea but is advised if solid stools are examined, e.g., for detection of healthy excreters or in cases of terminal ileitis or postinfectious arthritis. As a simple and efficient enrichment broth for intestinal *Yersinia* species, 0.15 M phosphate-buffered saline (pH 7.4) can be used. The cultures are kept at 4°C for up to 21 days with weekly subcultures. However, this method also propagates the nonpathogenic *Yersinia* species, which may overgrow the pathogens or render their identification difficult.

Except for cold-enrichment procedures, cultures for intestinal *Yersinia* species should preferably be incubated at 25 to 30°C, which yields better growth than incubation at 35°C. CIN agar is the best selective agar. This medium is commercially available with different cefsulodin concentrations, 4 and 8 μg/ml. We suggest the lower concentration, which produces better growth of *Y. enterocolitica* and *Y. pseudotuberculosis* and also allows for the isolation of *Y. pestis* and *Aeromonas* species. Suspected colonies of *Y. enterocolitica* (and *Aeromonas*) are approximately 2 mm in diameter after 48 h at 28 to 30°C. They are recognized by their red center surrounded by a translucent zone ("bulls-eye"), which is lacking in *Y. pseudotuberculosis*. MacConkey and salmonella-shigella agar may also be used for isolation of enteropathogenic yersiniae. The organisms grow as lactose-negative, pinpoint or flat colonies 1 mm in diameter after

TABLE 1 Biochemical differentiation of *Yersinia* species after incubation at 25°C for 48 h[a]

Species	Reaction[a]:										
	Motility	Voges-Proskauer	Indole	Citrate (Simmons)	Ornithine	Sucrose	Rhamnose	Cellobiose	Melibiose	Sorbose	Fucose
Y. pestis	−	−	−	−	−	−	−	−	d	−	−
Y. pseudotuberculosis	+	−	−	−	−	−	+	−	+	−	−
Y. enterocolitica	+	+	d	−	+	+	−	+	−	d	d
Y. intermedia	+	+	+	d	+	+	+	+	+	+	d
Y. frederiksenii	+	+	+	d	+	+	+	+	−	+	+
Y. kristensenii	+	−	d	−	+	−	−	+	−	+	d
Y. aldovae	+	+	−	d	+	−	+	−	−	+	d
Y. rohdei[b]	+	−	−	+	+	+	−	+	d	+	−
Y. mollaretii	+	−	−	−	+	+	−	+	−	+	−
Y. bercovieri	+	−	−	−	+	+	−	+	−	−	+

[a] +, ≥90% of strains positive; d, 11 to 89% of strains positive; −, ≥90% of strains negative.
[b] *Y. rohdei* biotype 1: melibiose +, raffinose +; biotype 2: melibiose −, raffinose −.

24 h at 25 to 30°C, depending on the selectivity of the media.

Identification

Yersiniae are metabolically more active at 25 to 30°C than at 35°C. Therefore, incubation at lower temperatures is indispensible for most biochemical tests and should be used for the reactions listed in Tables 1 and 2. Commercial bacteriological identification systems, on the other hand, are based on results obtained at 35°C. Biochemical reactions for yersiniae at 35°C can be found in chapter 27. At this temperature, the growth rate is lower and delayed or inconsistent biochemical reactions may occur. Furthermore, differential tests for *Yersinia* spp., as summarized in Table 1, are not included in most identification systems, leading to wrong or doubtful diagnoses, especially in the hands of inexperienced laboratory workers. This is especially true for metabolically inactive species, such as *Y. pestis*. Therefore, it is strongly advised to forward *Yersinia* isolates to a reference laboratory whenever the laboratory diagnosis does not agree with the clinical picture, when the material from which it had been isolated is unusual, or when the growth appearance in culture is atypical.

Y. pestis is identified by the biochemical reactions summarized in Table 1, in conjunction with Table 1 in chapter 27. After 2 to 5 days of incubation at 25 to 30°C, the organisms are nonmotile, ferment glucose without production of gas, and hydrolyze esculin but do not decarboxylate ornithine or hydrolyze urea. In fluid media, they show a stalagtitic growth, which sediments after slight shaking.

If *Y. pestis* is suspected, the isolate should be sent without delay to the CDC Plague Branch, Fort Collins, Colo., or to state reference centers.

Y. enterocolitica, *Y. pseudotuberculosis*, and the nonpathogenic *Yersinia* species are characterized by anaerogenic fermentation of glucose and other carbohydrates, urease production, motility below 30°C but not at 35°C, and lack of phenylalanine deaminase and lysine decarboxylase, respectively. However, *Y. enterocolitica* strains produce small gas bubbles of about 2 mm in diameter if tested in glucose broth with a Durham tube. Differentiation within the genus *Yersinia* is performed by the tests summarized in Table 1. For further differentiation of related genera, refer to Table 1 in chapter 27.

Strains of *Y. enterocolitica* should be further characterized by their biotypes, since strains of biotype 1A are mostly nonpathogenic (Table 2). Positive reactions with salicin and esculin are indicative of this biotype. On the other hand, pathogenic serotypes of *Y. enterocolitica* are associated with biotypes 1B, 2, 3, 4, and 5, respectively (Tables 2 and 3), which may be helpful if agglutinating sera are not available.

The presence of the 70-kb virulence plasmid and expression of YadA in strains of *Y. enterocolitica* and *Y. pseudotuberculosis* can reliably be determined by the autoagglutination test (54). If the test is positive, parallel cultures in tubes containing MR-VP medium (Difco) at room temperature and at 37°C show clearing of the medium with growth agglutinating at the bottom of the tube after 24 to 48 h at 37°C, in contrast to a uniform turbidity at room temperature. Virulence plasmid-negative strains, on the other hand, grow with uniform turbidity at both temperatures (Fig. 3).

The virulence plasmid is easily lost after subcultures at 35°C. Virulent strains grown on nutrient agar at 25 to 30°C frequently dissociate into small (plasmid-positive) and large (plasmid-negative) colonies. Less common phenotypic tests for recognizing virulent organisms are the uptake of Congo red at temperatures below 30°C (66) and calcium dependence at 37°C on magnesium oxalate agar (39).

Serotyping of isolates of *Y. enterocolitica* and *Y. pseudotu-*

TABLE 2 Biotypes of *Y. enterocolitica*[a] after incubation at 25°C for 48 h

Test	Reaction[b] for biotype:					
	1A	1B	2	3	4	5
Lipase (Tween esterase)	+	+	−	−	−	−
Esculin	+	−	−	−	−	−
Salicin	+	−	−	−	−	−
Indole	+	+	(+)	−	−	−
Xylose	+	+	+	+	−	d
Trehalose	+	+	+	+	+	−
$NO_3 \rightarrow NO_2$	+	+	+	+	+	−
DNase	−	−	−	−	+	+
Proline peptidase	d	−	−	−	−	−
β-D-Glucosidase	+	−	−	−	−	−
Pyrazinamidase[c]	+	−	−	−	−	−

[a] Modified from reference 76.
[b] +, ≥90% of strains positive; d, 11 to 89% of strains positive; −, ≥90% of strains negative; (+), weakly positive reaction.
[c] According to Kandolo and Wauters (50).

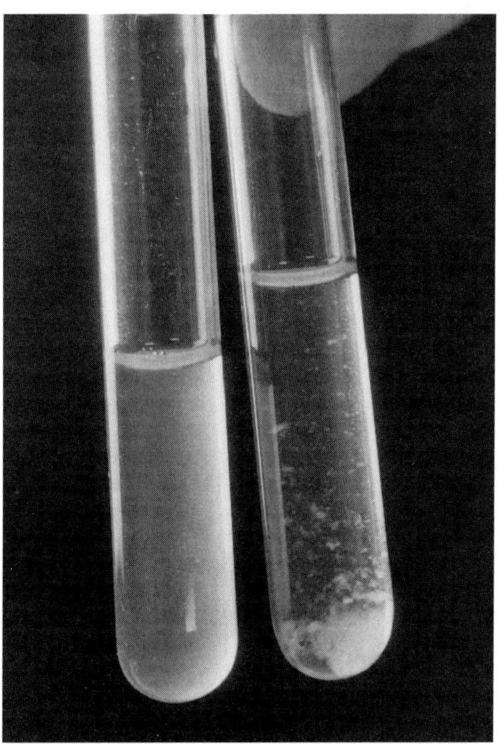

FIGURE 3 Autoagglutination test in MR-VP medium (Difco) after a 24-h incubation at 37°C and slight shaking. Left, virulence plasmid-negative strain of *Y. enterocolitica* O: 6,30 (biotype 1A); right, virulence plasmid-positive strain of *Y. enterocolitica* O:3 (biotype 4).

berculosis is appropriate for epidemiologic and diagnostic reasons. Enteropathogenic strains of *Y. enterocolitica* fall into a narrow scope of serotypes which are associated with distinct biotypes (Table 3) (1a), and characterization of isolates by their bioserotypes is advantageous since these traits are stable, in contrast to the virulence plasmid, which is easily lost. The pathogenic serogroups O:8, O:4,32, O:13a,13b, O:18, O:20, and O:21 are found nearly exclusively in the United States; they all belong to biotype 1B (American strains). Worldwide, serogroups O:3 (biotype 4), O:5,27 (biotypes 2 and 3), and O:9 (biotypes 2 and 3) prevail; the first two mentioned now are increasingly identified in the United States. Serogroups O:1,2a,3 (biotype 3) and O:2a,2b,3 (biotype 5) are pathogenic for animals and humans but are rarely isolated from patients.

Rarely, O antigens associated with pathogenic *Y. enterocolitica* are found in nonpathogenic yersiniae; however, these strains are serologically distinguished by their H antigens and by their biochemical reactions (1a). The typical H antigens, combined with O groups of pathogenic *Y. enterocolitica*, are listed in Table 3. Altogether, 297 serotypes associated with 76 O antigens and 44 H antigens have been identified so far in *Y. enterocolitica*, *Y. frederiksenii*, *Y. kristensenii*, *Y. intermedia*, *Y. bercovieri*, *Y. mollaretii*, and *Y. rohdei* (74). *Y. pseudotuberculosis* can be divided into 14 O and 5 H antigens on the basis of the diagnostic typing scheme of Tsubokura and Aleksic (72). These authors furthermore distinguished four biotypes on the basis of melibiose, raffinose, and citrate (Simmon's) utilization.

Serological Tests

The use of paired serum samples from the acute and convalescent phases of the disease or taken at 1- to 2-week intervals is preferable for serological tests. In plague, capsular F1 is the target antigen. The antibody response can be tested by a passive hemagglutination assay or ELISA. A titer of ≥1:10 directed against F1 antigen in a validated test system is presumptive and a fourfold rise or fall of the antibody titer is confirmatory of recent infection in persons who have not previously been infected or vaccinated; these tests are available at the CDC (64). It should be mentioned, however, that cases of clinical and even fatal plague in patients with reduced expression of F1 antigen and low antigenic response have been reported (42).

Antibodies directed against the pathogenic serogroups O:3, O:9, O:5,27, and O:8 of *Y. enterocolitica* can be detected by tube or microtiter agglutination with heated (1 h at 100°C) (O antigens) and formalin-killed whole-cell preparations (OH antigens) in parallel (79). Agglutination tests for *Y. pseudotuberculosis* are performed with formalin-killed cells (OH antigens). Reference sera with known titers must be tested in parallel since the antigens are not stable; this is especially true for OH antigens. O-antigen titers of ≥1:40 and OH-antigen titers of ≥1:160 or a fourfold rise of the titers in paired sera may be considered confirmatory. OH-antigen titers persist longer than do titers against O antigens and are used to assess the course of the infection in follow-up examinations. It is important to know that *Y. enterocolitica* O:9 and *Brucella* species cross-react with identical titers. Whole-cell antigens absorbed to microtiter wells can be used for separate detection of immunoglobulin G (IgG) and IgA antibodies by indirect enzyme immunoassay (32). When performed under standardized conditions, the above tests are reliable for the diagnosis of intestinal infections (terminal ileitis, lymphadenitis, and pseudoappendicitis). The tests are performed in specialized laboratories; test kits are commercially available in Europe but not in the United States (Sifin, Berlin, Germany; Sanofi Diagnostics Pasteur, Freiburg, Germany).

Reactive arthritis seems to be especially associated with the formation of IgA antibodies. These can be tested by either ELISA or immunoblotting with excreted protein antigens (Yops) (37). The latter method is preferred because it detects both *Y. enterocolitica* and *Y. pseudotuberculosis* infection and does not cross-react with *Brucella*. Test kits are commercially available (DPC Biermann GmbH, Bad Nauheim, Germany).

Treatment and Antibiotic Susceptibilities

Early treatment of plague with antibiotics is mandatory in view of the high mortality, which is over 50% in untreated patients (13, 64). Streptomycin is still the antibiotic of choice (13, 64). Most treated patients recover rapidly and become afebrile within 3 days. Vestibular and hearing functions should be monitored, especially in high-risk patients such as pregnant women, elderly persons, and patients with previous hearing problems. Alternatively, tetracycline may be given orally (13, 64). In patients with meningitis, chloramphenicol can be administered intravenously (64). Other antibiotics such as sulfonamides, trimethoprim-sulfamethoxazole, kanamycin, or ampicillin appear to be less effective than streptomycin (13).

Whereas antibiotic resistance in plague has never been a recognized problem, multidrug resistance mediated by a transferable plasmid has been recently identified in an isolate from a patient in Madagascar (27). The strain

TABLE 3 Pathogenic Y. *enterocolitica* O and H antigens, biotypes, origin, and distribution

O antigen	H antigen	Biotype	Origin	Distribution
1,2a,3	a,b,c	3	Chinchilla	Europe, United States
2a,2b,3	b,c	5	Hare, goat, rabbit, monkey	Europe
3	a,b,c	4	Human, dog, pig	Europe, Japan, North and South America, South Africa, Australia
	a,b,c,v		Dog, cat, rat	
	a,b		Human	
	a,c		Pig, pork	
	b,c		Human	
	c		Human, pig, chicken meat	
4,32	b,e,f,i	1B	Human, food	United States
5,27	a,b,c	2 or 3	Human, dog, pig, monkey	Europe, Japan, North America, Australia
	b,c		Dog, milk, water	
	b,c,v		Human	
8	b,e,f,i	1B	Human, milk, pig, drinking water	North America, Japan, Europe[a]
	b,e,f,i,v		Human, pig	
9	a,b	2 or 3	Human, pig	Europe, Japan, Canada, Australia
	a,b,c		Human, dog, cat, rat	
	a,b,v		Human	
13a,13b	a,b,i	1B	Human, monkey, milk	North America
18	b,e,f,i	1B	Human	United States
20	b,e,f,i	1B	Human, monkey, rat, milk	United States
21	b,e,f,i	1B	Human, rat flea (O: Tacoma)	North America

[a] Single isolates from Italy and The Netherlands.

was resistant to ampicillin, chloramphenicol, kanamycin, streptomycin, spectinomycin, sulfonamides, tetracycline, and minocycline. This observation is alarming and might become a new issue within the growing problem of emerging infectious diseases.

Intestinal infections with Y. *enterocolitica* and Y. *pseudotuberculosis* mostly are self-limited and need no specific antibiotic treatment. In immunocompromised patients, enteritis may be treated prophylactically and desferoxamine treatment (if applied) should be stopped. Oral doxycycline or trimethoprim-sulfamethoxazole has been recommended for such patients as well as for complicated gastrointestinal or focal extraintestinal infections in general (17).

In contrast to Y. *pseudotuberculosis*, Y. *enterocolitica* serogroups O:3 and O:9 produce two chromosomally determined β-lactamases (types A and B, respectively), whereas O:5,27 produces type B β-lactamase only. These account for resistance to ampicillin, cephalothin, and carbenicillin. Y. *enterocolitica* O:8 is susceptible to ampicillin but variably resistant to carbenicillin and cephalothin. β-Lactamase activity in O:8 strains is distinct from that in strains of serogroups O:3 and O:9 (9). In vitro antibacterial activity does not necessarily reflect in vivo efficacy. Clinically, administration of broad-spectrum cephalosporins, often in combination with aminoglycosides, has resulted in a successful outcome for most patients with extraintestinal infections, including septicemia (9). Fluoroquinolones, alone or in combination with aminoglycosides or extended-spectrum cephalosporins, have also proven efficacious (29).

Interpretation and Reporting of Results

Clinically, plague should be suspected if the patient has recently returned from, or lives in, an area of endemic infection; reported a history of contact with rodents, house cats, or flea bites; and presents with a severe febrile disease. The presence of painful swelling of inguinal, axillary, or cervical lymph nodes, septicemia, pneumonia, or meningitis is indicative. Detection of typical morphology in Wayson or methylene blue-stained smears of clinical material is supportive, and the diagnosis is confirmed by isolation of the organisms and identification by biochemical reactions and detection of specific virulence factors. At the earliest suspicion of plague, be it on clinical or bacteriological grounds, the case must immediately be reported to the local and state health administrations and further diagnostic steps should be performed by, or in close collaboration with, the CDC.

Enteropathogenic Y. *enterocolitica* and Y. *pseudotuberculosis* must be taken into consideration in patients with enteritis of unknown origin, in patients complaining of persistent abdominal pain (terminal enteritis, lymphadenitis, or pseudoappendicitis), and in patients with arthritis following intestinal illness. Detection of Y. *pseudotuberculosis* or pathogenic serogroups of Y. *enterocolitica* in stool specimens is confirmatory if no other enteropathogenic organisms are isolated. However, in patients with terminal ileitis and mesenteric lymphadenitis, as well as in those with reactive arthritis, isolation of the organisms from stool specimens is rare. Septicemic yersiniosis is not associated with specific clinical features; isolation of either *Yersinia* strain from blood cultures is confirmatory.

Determination of antibodies directed against the prevailing serogroups of *Y. pseudotuberculosis* and pathogenic *Y. enterocolitica* in a quantitative agglutination test (Widal reaction), by ELISA, or by immunoblotting is diagnostic for intestinal infections as well as extraintestinal complications (reactive arthritis and other conditions).

Isolates of *Y. enterocolitica* should always be tested according to their biotypes and serogroups, since all pathogenic strains are associated with defined bioserogroups (Table 3). Detection of the 70-kb virulence plasmid by either genotypic (PCR or DNA colony blot hybridization) or phenotypic (autoagglutination test) methods should be reported. Isolates of *Y. enterocolitica* biotype 1A generally lack virulence markers of classical invasive *Yersinia* strains and therefore are considered nonpathogenic. However, a novel mechanism of invading tissue culture cells has recently been identified in a number of such strains, and a role for them in the etiology of diarrhea was suggested (33). Until more facts are available, biotype 1A strains might tentatively be regarded as causative if they are isolated in large numbers from a patient with diarrhea, if no other enteropathogens are isolated, and if they disappear from the intestines after cessation of the symptoms.

Y. frederiksenii, *Y. kristensenii*, *Y. intermedia*, *Y. mollaretii*, *Y. bercovieri*, *Y. rohdei*, and *Y. aldovae* have no established pathogenic potential in immunocompetent patients. Their detection in stool specimens should be reported as "nonpathogenic yersiniae isolated."

PROTEUS, PROVIDENCIA, AND *MORGANELLA* SPECIES

The genera *Proteus* (named after a Greek polymorphic sea god), *Providencia*, and *Morganella* traditionally have been included in the tribe *Proteeae* of the family *Enterobacteriaceae*. Ten species (41) are attributed to these genera, i.e., *Proteus vulgaris*, *P. mirabilis*, *P. penneri*, and *P. myxofaciens*; *Providencia rettgeri*, *P. stuartii*, *P. alcalifaciens*, *P. rustigianii*, and *P. heimbachae*; and *Morganella morganii* subsp. *morganii* and *M. morganii* subsp. *sibonii* (46, 48). They have a number of diagnostic traits in common and therefore are treated together.

Proteeae are ubiquitous in the environment and reside in the intestines of healthy humans and animals. These organisms are especially associated with urinary tract infections. It has been assumed that alkalinization of the urine due to urea hydrolysis with production of ammonium hydroxide promotes stone formation (60). These deposits act as foreign bodies that obstruct the urinary flow and serve as a nidus for persistent infections. Thus, *Proteus and Providencia* urinary tract infections tend to become chronic and to destroy the renal parenchyma. Various factors in *P. mirabilis*, *P. vulgaris*, and *P. penneri*, such as flagellae, fimbriae, outer membrane proteins, cell wall and capsular lipopolysaccharides, urease, and hemolysins, have been suggested to promote virulence (67).

P. mirabilis is the clinically most important species within the *Proteeae*. Up to 10% of all uncomplicated urinary tract infections are caused by this species, which, however, may also cause wound infection and septicemia. Recently, a role for *P. mirabilis* as an etiological agent in rheumatoid arthritis has been suggested (78). Nevertheless, most nosocomial infections caused by members of the *Proteeae* are due to the indole-positive species rather than to *P. mirabilis*. These species are often isolated from infected wounds, respiratory tract specimens, and blood. For *M. morganii*, it was recently shown that the majority of clinical isolates belonged to subsp. *morganii* (46). *P. myxofaciens* and *P. heimbachae* seem to be without clinical importance.

Antibiotic treatment of infections caused by the *Proteeae* may be difficult due to the high frequency of aminoglycoside resistance among the indole-positive species. Newer cephalosporins or quinolones are usually effective, depending on the results of antibiotic susceptibility testing.

Proteus, *Providencia*, and *Morganella* grow well on all nonselective as well as moderately selective media designed for the isolation of *Enterobacteriaceae*. Apart from nonselective fluid media, *Proteus* spp. furthermore propagate in selenite and tetrathionate broth used for the enrichment of salmonellae, but they seem to be inhibited in Rappaport-Vassiliadis medium (section IX). On selective solid media, *Proteeae* grow with clear, lactose-negative colonies. *P. mirabilis* and *P. vulgaris* produce black, *Salmonella*-like colonies on salmonella-shigella or desoxycholate citrate agar. The latter species are furthermore recognized by their swarming growth on nonselective solid media.

Most *Proteeae* exhibit a characteristic smell (some have an odor resembling chocolate cake), which is indicative. They all produce phenylalanine deaminase and grow in the presence of potassium cyanide (except *P. heimbachae*), but they do not decarboxylate lysine. Urease is produced by *Proteus* spp., *M. morganii*, *P. rettgeri*, and occasionally *P. stuartii* but not by *P. alcalifaciens*, *P. rustigianii*, and *P. heimbachae*. *Proteus* spp., in contrast to *Providencia* spp. and *Morganella*, fail to ferment mannose. Strains of *P. mirabilis*, *P. penneri*, *P. myxofaciens*, and *P. heimbachae* are indole negative, whereas the other species in the tribe are positive. For a list of the biochemical reactions used to differentiate the *Proteeae* species, refer to Table 1 in chapter 27.

For epidemiologic purposes, biotyping may be helpful. On the basis of gas production from glucose and fermentation of adonitol and inositol, two biotypes may be distinguished in *P. alcalifaciens* and three may be distinguished in *P. stuartii* (22, 23). Results of utilization of salicin and rhamnose can detect four biotypes among *P. rettgeri* strains (22, 23). Seven biotypes have been defined in the two subspecies of *M. morganii*, i.e., subsp. *morganii* (trehalose negative) and subsp. *sibonii* (trehalose positive) (46, 48).

O antigens of the *Proteeae* cross-reacting with antibodies against O antigens of *Salmonella*, *Shigella*, or *Escherichia coli* may be misleading in the stool culture laboratory, where agglutinating antisera are used for primary identification of suspected isolates of enteropathogenic organisms.

OTHER *ENTEROBACTERIACEAE*

The following genera and species comprise organisms which are less frequently isolated in the clinical laboratory or which have been recognized and defined only recently. Clinically, they do not show a specific pathogenic potential and may instead act as opportunists. They meet the definitions of *Enterobacteriaceae*, but some possess particular traits which may be of diagnostic interest. In contrast to other *Enterobacteriaceae*, *Xenorhabdus* spp. are catalase negative. *Photorhabdus luminescens* can be recognized by its luminescence. Nitratase is absent in *Xenorhabdus* spp., *Photorhabdus* sp., *Erwinia* spp., and most *Pantoea* spp. Some species produce pigmented colonies at temperatures below 30°C; yellow colony coloration may occur in *Leclercia adecarboxylata, Pantoea* spp., *Erwinia* spp., and *Photorhabdus luminescens* (24, 30). Hydrogen sulfide production, which is a guiding reaction for *Salmonella, Proteus*, and *Citrobacter freundii*, is also found in *Leminorella* spp., *Budvicia aquatica, Edwardsiella tarda, Pragia fontium*, and *Trabulsiella guamensis*. Differentiation of these species by biochemical reactions is shown in Table 1 in chapter 27. Their inclusion in the database of commercially available identification systems has been evaluated by Gilchrist (30) and is summarized in chapter 5.

Budvicia sp.

Budvicia, with the single species *B. aquatica*, was first proposed by Aldová and coworkers and formally described by Bouvet et al. (10a). Most strains originate from water, but a few strains have been isolated from human feces. *B. aquatica* produces hydrogen sulfide.

Buttiauxella sp.

The taxonomic status of *Buttiauxella* has recently been emended, and seven species have been defined, i.e., *B. agrestis, B. ferragutiae* (formerly CDC enteric group 63), *B. gaviniae* (formerly CDC enteric group 64), *B. brennerae, B. izardii, B. noackiae* (formerly CDC enteric group 59), and *B. warmboldiae* (61). They are biochemically similar to *Kluyvera* spp. and have been isolated mainly from environmental specimens such as water, soil, and mollusks. A pathogenic potential has not been established.

Cedecea spp.

There are five species included in the genus *Cedecea*, of which only three have been named, i.e., *C. davisae, C. lapagei*, and *C. neteri*. The organisms are rarely isolated from clinical specimens of hospitalized patients. Most strains have been isolated from sputum, and rare cases of bacteremia due to *C. neteri* are cited in the literature (1). Strains of *C. neteri* resistant to extended-spectrum cephalosporins have been identified in hospitalized children (5). *Cedecea* spp. may be distinguished from similar *Serratia* strains by their lack of DNase activity.

Edwardsiella spp.

The genus *Edwardsiella* was established in 1965 and to date includes three species: *E. tarda* with two biogroups, i.e., "wild type" and biogroup 1, *E. hoshinae*, and *E. ictaluri*. Their principal habitat seems to be cold-blooded animals such as fish and reptiles and their environment. Of the three species, only *E. tarda* is associated with human disease. The predominant clinical picture is a *Salmonella*-like enteritis, which may occur in all age groups but has a special preference for young children and old people. The disease has been reported mainly in tropical and subtropical climates, e.g., Thailand (7), Panama (53), and the southern United States (44). Asymptomatic infections are not rare. Posttraumatic wound infections have been described in connection with water-associated and other environmental accidents. Occasional cases of septicemia, meningitis, or internal abscesses are related mostly to a severe underlying illness. Possible virulence factors for diarrheal disease include a plasmid-mediated heat-stable enterotoxin (6), penetration into HeLa and HEp-2 cells (47), and an iron-regulated hemolysin (45). *E. hoshinae* is uncommon in human clinical specimens and is isolated mainly from water, healthy birds, and reptiles. *E. ictaluri* is a fish pathogen without clinical importance for humans.

In stool cultures, *E. tarda* of the wild-type biogroup may be mistaken for *Salmonella* on media such as MacConkey, desoxycholate-citrate, salmonella-shigella, xylose-lysine-desoxycholate, Kligler iron, or TSI agar. The wild-type biogroup produces indole, hydrogen sulfide, and lysine decarboxylase but fails to ferment most carbohydrates and is not agglutinated by *Salmonella* antisera. A characteristic trait is its resistance to colistin, which may be incorporated into culture media (10 to 100 μg/ml) for selective isolation of the organisms. In contrast, *E. tarda* biogroup 1, which has been isolated only from freshwater and reptiles, is more active, producing acid from D-mannitol, L-arabinose, and sucrose but not producing hydrogen sulfide on Kligler or TSI agar. If antibiotic treatment of *E. tarda* infection is required, ampicillin, trimethoprim-sulfamethoxazole, and ciprofloxacin have all been effective.

Erwinia spp.

Erwinia spp. colonize plants, where they may be pathogens. They are a heterogeneous group of organisms, which need further taxonomic study. In the clinical microbiological laboratory, only one case of urinary tract infection due to *E. persicinus* has been described (63). These organisms are not included in the databases of commercially available identification systems, where they are likely to be misidentified as *Pantoea agglomerans*.

Ewingella sp.

Ewingella, with a single species, *E. americana*, has been isolated rarely from respiratory infections, blood cultures, and wound infections of hospitalized patients. Biochemically, it is similar to the genus *Cedecea*. In our laboratory, we have received single isolates which had been misidentified as *Y. pestis* by inexperienced laboratory personnel using commercial identification systems.

Hafnia sp.

The genus *Hafnia* is composed of a single species, *H. alvei*, which for many years had been a member of the genus *Enterobacter*. The natural habitats are the gastrointestinal tracts of humans and other warm-blooded animals (particularly birds) as well as the environment (surface water, sewage, food, and dairy products). In general, *Hafnia* strains may contribute to opportunistic infections in the hospital, where they are associated with respiratory and urinary tract infections, bacteremia, meningitis, or mixed infections in wounds and abscesses (35). Recently, a potential role for causing diarrheal illness has been suggested following community and hospital-associated outbreaks (25); virulence factors similar to the attaching-effacing phenotype of *E. coli* have been described (43). These strains, however, possess unusual biochemical properties, atypical of the genus as a whole. Nevertheless, these observations merit further attention.

Hafnia strains grow on all nonspecific and most moderately selective media used for the isolation of *Enterobacteriaceae*, where they produce flat, colorless (lactose and sucrose-negative) colonies. Most strains are inhibited in selenite and tetrathionate broth. The organisms produce lysine and ornithine decarboxylases and ferment glucose, with the formation of gas. Indole and urease are not produced. The Voges-Proskauer reaction and the citrate utilization (Simmon's) test are generally positive at 22°C but not consistently positive at 35°C. Hydrogen sulfide may be weakly positive on SIM but not on Kligler iron or TSI agar. The organisms grow in the presence of potassium cyanide. *Hafnia* strains are usually susceptible to piperacillin, imipenem, quinolones, and the newer cephalosporins.

Kluyvera spp.

Four species, i.e., *K. ascorbata*, *K. georgiana*, *K. cryocrescens*, and *K. cochleae*, are now included in the genus *Kluyvera* (61). The organisms are of environmental origin and are occasionally associated with opportunistic infections in the hospital. Primary infections such as single cases of pyelonephritis and soft tissue infection have been described.

Leclercia sp.

The single species, *L. adecarboxylata*, was previously included in the genus *Escherichia*. The organisms are occasionally isolated from clinical specimens (including blood and sputum) and from the environment.

Leminorella spp.

The genus *Leminorella* includes two species, *L. grimontii* and *L. richardii*. Both produce hydrogen sulfide on media used for the isolation of *Salmonella*, but they are otherwise biochemically inactive. Most strains have been isolated from feces and occasionally from urine. A specific role in causing disease has not been established.

Moellerella sp.

The genus *Moellerella* contains a single species, *M. wisconsensis*. Most isolates have been obtained from stool specimens or water, but they seem to be without special clinical importance. *M. wisconsensis* is a biochemically inactive species.

Pantoea spp.

The genus *Pantoea* was established in 1989 to include strains of the former *Erwinia herbicola-Enterobacter agglomerans* complex. Today, the genus has seven species, i.e., *P. agglomerans*, *P. dispersa*, *P. punctata*, *P. citrea*, *P. terrea*, *P. ananas*, and *P. stewartii* subsp. *stewartii* and subsp. *indologenes* (49, 56). The organisms reside on plants and in the environment. *P. agglomerans* is an occasional opportunist in wounds, urine, and blood specimens.

Photorhabdus sp.

The genus *Photorhabdus* was proposed in 1993 to include the single species *P. luminescens*, which previously was a member of the genus *Xenorhabdus* (8). The natural habitat is the intestinal lumen of entomogenous nematodes, but the organisms have also been isolated from human blood, wound, and abdominal infections (24). At 35°C, they grow on MacConkey agar, produce yellow pigment, and are bioluminescent and catalase positive, but they do not reduce nitrate to nitrate (8, 24).

Pragia sp.

The single species included in the genus *Pragia*, *P. fontium*, has its habitat in surface water. Clinical importance has not been established, but the organisms produce hydrogen sulfide and therefore may cause confusion in the clinical microbiological laboratory.

Rahnella sp.

Rahnella aquatilis, the only species, has been isolated mostly from water specimens, but occasional nosocomial infections in immunocompromised patients have been reported. In Germany, 20 patients developed bacteremia following transfusion of contaminated blood (1b). Recently, a possible importance as an aeroallergen in sawmill workers has been suggested (21).

Tatumella sp.

Tatumella is composed of a single species, *T. ptyseos*. The organisms have been isolated occasionally from sputum and rarely from urine and blood cultures. *Tatumella* strains are unusual insofar as they produce lateral flagella at 22°C but are nonmotile at 35°C. Furthermore, the organisms are biochemically more active at temperatures below 30°C.

Trabulsiella sp.

Described in 1991, the genus *Trabulsiella* includes a single species, *T. guamensis* (55). Only a few strains have been isolated from environmental sources and stool specimens, but a pathogenic role has not yet been attributed to them. Biochemically, they are very similar to *Salmonella* subspp. 4 and 5, but they are not agglutinated by *Salmonella* O and H antisera.

Xenorhabdus spp.

The genus *Xenorhabdus* consists almost entirely of symbionts of entomopathogenic nematodes (8). To date, four species have been recognized, i.e., *X. nematophilus*, *X. bovienii*, *X. poinarii*, and *X. beddingii* (8). The organisms best grow at temperatures below 30°C and are not bioluminescent. A pathogenic potential for human infections has not been established.

Yokenella sp.

The only species of the genus *Yokenella* is *Y. regensburgei*. An identical species, *Koserella trabulsii* (formerly CDC enteric group 45), had been independently published shortly after *Y. regensburgei*, and the name of the latter has priority over *K. trabulsii* (55). The organisms have occasionally been isolated from the respiratory tract, wounds, urine, and feces of humans, but primarily they seem to belong to the bacterial flora of insects.

REFERENCES

1. **Aguilera, A., J. Pascual, E. Loza, J. Lopez, G. Garcia, F. Liano, C. Quereda, and J. Ortuno.** 1995. Bacteriaemia with *Cedecea neteri* in a patient with systemic lupus erythematosus. *Postgrad. Med. J.* **71:**179–180.

1a. **Aleksic, S.** 1995. Occurrence of *Y. enterocolitica* O:3, O:9 and O:8 in different species. Their corresponding H antigens and origin. *Contrib. Microbiol. Immunol.* **13:**89–92.

1b. **Aleksic, S.** Unpublished data.

2. **Aleksic, S., and J. Bockemühl.** 1988. Serological and biochemical characteristics of 416 *Yersinia* strains from well water and drinking water plants in the Federal Republic of Germany: lack of evidence that these strains are of public health importance. *Zentralbl. Bakteriol. Parasitenkd. Hyg. Abt. 1 Orig. Reihe B* **185:**527–533.

3. **Barnes, A. M., and T. J. Quan.** 1992. Plague, p. 1285–1291. *In* S. L. Gorbach, J. G. Bartlett, and N. R. Blacklow (ed.), *Infectious Diseases*. The W. B. Saunders Co., Philadelphia, Pa.

4. **Bercovier, H., H. H. Mollaret, J. M. Alonso, J. Brault, G. R. Fanning, A. G. Steigerwalt, and D. J. Brenner.** 1980. Intra- and interspecies relatedness of *Yersinia pestis* by DNA hybridization and its relationship to *Yersinia pseudotuberculosis*. *Curr. Microbiol.* **4:**225–229.

5. **Berkowitz, F. E., and B. Metchock.** 1995. Third generation cephalosporin-resistant gram-negative bacilli in the

feces of hospitalized children. *Pediatr. Infect. Dis. J.* **14:** 97–100.

6. **Bockemühl, J., V. Aleksic, R. Wokatsch, and S. Aleksic.** 1983. Pathogenicity tests with strains of *Edwardsiella tarda*: detection of a heat-stable enterotoxin. *Zentralbl. Bakteriol. Parasitenkd. Hyg. Abt. 1 Orig. Reihe A* **255:**464–471.
7. **Bockemühl, J., R. Pan-Urai, and F. Burkhardt.** 1971. *Edwardsiella tarda* associated with human disease. *Pathol. Microbiol.* **37:**393–401.
8. **Boemare, N. E., R. J. Akhurst, and R. G. Mourant.** 1993. DNA relatedness between *Xenorhabdus* spp. (*Enterobacteriaceae*), symbiotic bacteria of entomopathogenic nematodes, and a proposal to transfer *Xenorhabdus luminescens* to a new genus, *Photorhabdus* gen. nov. *Int. J. Syst. Bacteriol.* **43:**249–255.
9. **Bottone, E. J.** 1997. *Yersinia enterocolitica*: the charisma continues. *Clin. Microbiol. Rev.* **10:**257–276.
10. **Bottone, E. J., C. R. Gullans, and M. F. Sierra.** 1987. Disease spectrum of *Yersinia enterocolitica* serogroup O:3, the predominant cause of human infection in New York City. *Contrib. Microbiol. Immunol.* **9:**56–90.

10a. **Bouvet, O. M. M., P. A. D. Grimont, C. Richard, E. Aldová, O. Hausner, and M. Gabrhelova.** 1985. *Budvicia aquatica* gen. nov., sp. nov.: a hydrogen sulfide-producing member of the *Enterobacteriaceae*. *Int. J. Syst. Bacteriol.* **35:** 60–64.

11. **Buchholz, D. H., J. P. AuBuchon, E. L. Snyder, R. Kandler, S. Edberg, V. Piscitelli, C. Pickard, and P. Napychank.** 1992. Removal of *Yersinia enterocolitica* from AS-1 red cells. *Transfusion* **32:**667–672.
12. **Butler, T.** 1989. The black death past and present. 1. Plague in the 1980s. *Trans. R. Soc. Trop. Med. Hyg.* **83:** 458–460.
13. **Butler, T.** 1994. *Yersinia* infections: centennial of the discovery of the plague bacillus. *Clin. Infect. Dis.* **19:**655–661.
14. **Centers for Disease Control and Prevention.** 1997. Summary of notifiable diseases, United States 1996. *Morbid. Mortal. Weekly Rep.* **45:**vii–ix.
15. **Centers for Disease Control and Prevention.** 1997. Red blood cell transfusions contaminated with *Yersinia enterocolitica*—United States, 1991–1996, and initiation of a national study of detecting bacteria-associated transfusion reactions. *Morbid. Mortal. Weekly Rep.* **46:**553–555.
16. **Chin, H. Y., D. M. Flynn, A. V. Hoffrand, and D. Politis.** 1986. Infection with *Yersinia enterocolitica* in patients with iron overload. *Br. Med. J.* **292:**97.
17. **Cover, T. L., and R. C. Aber.** 1989. *Yersinia enterocolitica*. *N. Engl. J. Med.* **321:**16–24.
18. **Crook, L. D., and B. Tempest.** 1992. Plague, a clinical review of 27 cases. *Arch. Intern. Med.* **152:**1253–1256.
19. **Delor, I., and G. R. Cornelis.** 1992. Role of *Yersinia enterocolitica* Yst toxin in experimental infection of young rabbits. *Infect. Immun.* **60:**4269–4277.
20. **Devignat, R.** 1951. Variétés de l'espèce *Pasteurella pestis*. Nouvelle hypothèse. *Bull. W. H. O.* **4:**247–263.
21. **Dutkiewicz, J., E. T. Krysinska-Traczyk, C. Skorska, J. Milanowski, J. Sitkowska, E. Dutkiewicz, A. Matuszyk, and B. Fafrowicz.** 1997. Microflora of the air in sawmills as a potential occupational hazard: concentration and composition of microflora and immunologic reactivity of workers to microbiological aeroallergens. *Pneumonol. Alergol. Pol.* **64**(Suppl. 1):25–31. (In Polish.)
22. **Ewing, W. H.** 1986. Identification of *Enterobacteriaceae*, 4th ed. Elsevier Science Publishing, Inc., New York, N.Y.
23. **Farmer, J. J., III.** 1995. *Enterobacteriaceae*: introduction and identification, p. 438–449. *In* P. R. Murray, E. J. Baron, M. A. Pfaller, F. C. Tenover, and R. H. Yolken (ed.), *Manual of Clinical Microbiology*, 6th ed. American Society for Microbiology, Washington, D.C.
24. **Farmer, J. J., III, J. H. Jorgensen, P. A. D. Grimont, R. J. Akhurst, G. O. Poinar, E. Ageron, G. V. Pierce, J. A. Smith, G. P. Carter, K. L. Wilson, and F. W. Hickman-Brenner.** 1989. *Xenorhabdus luminescens* (DNA hybridization group 5) from human clinical specimens. *J. Clin. Microbiol.* **27:**1594–1600.
25. **Fazal, B. A., I. E. Justman, G. S. Tutatt, and E. E. Telzak.** 1997. Community acquired *Hafnia alvei* infection. *Clin. Infect. Dis.* **24:**527–528.
26. **Fukushima, H., M. Gomyoda, K. Shiozawa, S. Kaneko, and M. Tsubokura.** 1988. *Yersinia pseudotuberculosis* infection contracted through water contaminated by a wild animal. *J. Clin. Microbiol.* **26:**584–585.
27. **Galimand, M., A. Guiyoule, G. Gerbaud, B. Rasoamanana, S. Chanteau, E. Carniel, and P. Courvalin.** 1997. Multidrug resistance in *Yersinia pestis* mediated by a transferable plasmid. *N. Engl. J. Med.* **337:**677–680.
28. **Gasper, P. W., A. M. Barnes, T. J. Quan, J. P. Benziger, L. G. Carter, M. L. Beard, and G. O. Maupin.** 1993. Plague (*Yersinia pestis*) in cats: description of experimentally induced disease. *J. Med. Entomol.* **30:**20–26.
29. **Gayraud, M., M. R. Scavizzi, H. H. Mollaret, L. Guillevine, and M. J. Hornstein.** 1993. Antibiotic treatment of *Yersinia enterocolitica* septicemia: a retrospective review of 43 cases. *Clin. Infect. Dis.* **17:**405–410.
30. **Gilchrist, M. J. R.** 1995. *Enterobacteriaceae*: opportunistic pathogens and other genera, p. 457–464. *In* P. R. Murray, E. J. Baron, M. A. Pfaller, F. C. Tenover, and R. H. Yolken (ed.), *Manual of Clinical Microbiology*, 6th ed. American Society for Microbiology, Washington, D.C.
31. **Granfors, K., S. Jalkannen, R. R. von Essen, R. Lahesmaa-Rantala, O. Isomäki, K. Pekkola-Haino, and A. Toivanen.** 1989. *Yersinia* antigens in synovial-fluid cells from patients with reactive arthritis. *N. Engl. J. Med.* **320:** 216–221.
32. **Granfors, K., M. K. Viljanen, and A. Toivanen.** 1981. Measurement of immunoglobulin M, immunoglobulin G, and immunoglobulin A antibodies against *Yersinia enterocolitica* by enzyme-linked immunosorbent assay. Comparison of lipopolysaccharide and whole bacterium as antigen. *J. Clin. Microbiol.* **14:**6–14.
33. **Grant, T., V. Bennet-Wood, and R. M. Robins-Browne.** 1998. Identification of virulence-associated characteristics in clinical isolates of *Yersinia enterocolitica* lacking classical virulence markers. *Infect. Immun.* **66:**1113–1120.
34. **Guiyoule, A., B. Rasoamanana, C. Buchrieser, P. Michel, S. Chanteau, and E. Carniel.** 1997. Recent emergence of new variants of *Yersinia pestis* in Madagascar. *J. Clin. Microbiol.* **35:**2826–2833.
35. **Gunthard, H., and A. Pennekamp.** 1997. Clinical significance of extraintestinal *Hafnia alvei* isolates from 61 patients and review of the literature. *Clin. Infect. Dis.* **22:** 1040–1045.
36. **Harnett, N., J. P. Lin, and C. Krishnan.** 1996. Detection of pathogenic *Yersinia enterocolitica* using the multiplex polymerase chain reaction. *Epidemiol. Infect.* **117:**59–67.
37. **Heesemann, J., C. Eggers, and J. Schröder.** 1987. Serological diagnosis of yersiniosis by immunoblot technique using virulence-associated antigen of enteropathogenic yersiniae. *Contrib. Microbiol. Immunol.* **9:**285–289.
38. **Heesemann, J., K. Hantke, T. Vocke, E. Saken, A. Rakin, I. Stojiljkovic, and R. Berner.** 1993. Virulence of *Yersinia enterocolitica* is closely associated with siderophore production, expression of an iron-repressible outer membrane polypeptide of 65.000 Da and pesticin sensitivity. *Mol. Microbiol.* **8:**397–408.
39. **Higuchi, K., and J. I. Smith.** 1961. Studies on the nutrition and physiology of *Pasteurella pestis*. VI. A differential plat-

ing medium for the estimation of mutation rate to avirulence. *J. Bacteriol.* **81:**605–608.

40. **Hill, W. E., A. R. Datta, P. Feng, K. A. Lampel, and W. L. Payne.** 1995. Identification of foodborne bacterial pathogens by gene probes, p. 24.01–24.33. *In* U.S. Food and Drug Administration (ed.), *Bacteriological Analytical Manual*, 8th ed. AOAC International, Gaithersburg, Md.
41. **Holt, J. G., N. R. Krieg, P. H. A. Sneath, J. T. Staley, and S. T. Williams.** 1994. *Bergey's Manual of Determinative Bacteriology*, p. 175–190, 203–222. The Williams & Wilkins Co., Baltimore, Md.
42. **Isaäcson, M., D. Levy, B. J. Te, W. N. Pienaar, H. D. Bubb, J. A. Louw, and D. K. Genis.** 1973. Unusual cases of human plague in Southern Africa. *S. Afr. Med. J.* **47:** 2109–2113.
43. **Ismaili, A., B. Bouske, I. C. de Azavedo, S. Ratnam, M. A. Karmali, and P. M. Sherman.** 1997. Heterogeneity in phenotypic and genotypic characteristics among strains of *Hafnia alvei*. *J. Clin. Microbiol.* **34:**2973–2979.
44. **Janda, J. M., and S. L. Abbott.** 1993. Infections associated with the genus *Edwardsiella*: the role of *E. tarda* in human disease. *Clin. Infect. Dis.* **17:**742–748.
45. **Janda, J. M., and S. L. Abbott.** 1993. Expression of an iron-regulated hemolysin from *Edwardsiella tarda*. *FEMS Microbiol. Lett.* **111:**275–280.
46. **Janda, M., S. L. Abbott, S. Kashe, and T. Robin.** 1996. Biochemical investigation of biogroups and subspecies of *Morganella morganii*. *J. Clin. Microbiol.* **34:**108–113.
47. **Janda, J. M., S. L. Abbott, and L. S. Oshiro.** 1991. Penetration and replication of *Edwardsiella tarda* in HEp-2 cells. *Infect. Immun.* **59:**154–161.
48. **Jensen, K. T., W. Frederiksen, F. W. Hickman-Brenner, A. G. Steigerwalt, C. F. Riddle, and D. J. Brenner.** 1992. Recognition of *Morganella morganii* subspecies with proposal of *M. morganii* subsp. *morganii* and *M. morganii* subsp. *sibonii*. *Int. J. Syst. Bacteriol.* **42:**613–620.
49. **Kageyama, B., M. Nakae, S. Yagi, and T. Sonoyama.** 1992. *Pantoea punctata* sp. nov., *Pantoea citrea* sp. nov., and *Pantoea terrea* sp. nov. isolated from fruit and soil samples. *Int. J. Syst. Bacteriol.* **42:**203–210.
50. **Kandolo, K., and G. Wauters.** 1985. Pyrazinamidase activity in *Yersinia enterocolitica* and related organisms. *J. Clin. Microbiol.* **21:**980–982.
51. **Kapperud, G., K. Dommarsness, M. Skurnik, and E. Hornes.** 1990. A synthetic oligonucleotide probe based on the *yopA* gene for detection and enumeration of virulent *Yersinia enterocolitica*. *Appl. Environ. Microbiol.* **56:** 17–23.
52. **Kapperud, G., T. Vardund, E. Skjerve, E. Hornes, and T. E. Michaelsen.** 1993. Detection of pathogenic *Yersinia enterocolitica* in foods and water by immunomagnetic separation, nested polymerase chain reaction, and colorimetric detection of amplified DNA. *Appl. Environ. Microbiol.* **59:**2938–2944.
53. **Kourany, M., M. A. Vasquez, and R. Saenz.** 1977. Edwardsiellosis in man and animals in Panama: clinical and epidemiological characteristics. *Am. J. Trop. Med. Hyg.* **26:**1183–1190.
54. **Laird, W. J., and D. C. Cavanaugh.** 1980. Correlation of autoagglutination and virulence of yersiniae. *J. Clin. Microbiol.* **11:**430–432.
55. **McWhorter, A. C., R. L. Haddock, F. A. Nocon, A. G. Steigerwalt, D. J. Brenner, S. Aleksic, J. Bockemühl, and J. J. Farmer III.** 1991. *Trabulsiella guamensis*, a new genus and species of the family *Enterobacteriaceae* that resembles *Salmonella* subgroups 4 and 5. *J. Clin. Microbiol.* **29:** 1480–1485.
56. **Mergaert, J., L. Verdonck, and K. Kersters.** 1993. Transfer of *Erwinia ananas* (synonym, *Erwinia uredovora*) and *Erwinia stewartii* to the genus *Pantoea* emend. as *Pantoea ananas* (Serrano 1928) comb. nov. and *Pantoea stewartii* (Smith 1898) comb. nov., respectively, and description of *Pantoea stewartii* subsp. *indologenes* subsp. nov. *Int. J. Syst. Bacteriol.* **43:**162–173.
57. **Meyer, K. F.** 1970. Effectiveness of live or killed plague vaccines in man. *Bull. W. H. O.* **42:**653–666.
58. **Mollaret, H. H.** 1995. Fifteen centuries of yersiniosis. *Contrib. Microbiol. Immunol.* **13:**1–4.
59. **Mollaret, H. H., P. Wallet, A. Gilton, E. Carniel, and N. Duedari.** 1989. Le choc septique transfusionnel du à *Yersinia enterocolitica*. A propos de 19 cas. *Med. Malad. Infect.* **19:**186–192.
60. **Mosher, D. M., D. P. Griffith, D. Yawa, and R. D. Rossen.** 1975. Role of urease in pyelonephritis resulting from urinary tract infection with *Proteus*. *J. Infect. Dis.* **131:** 177–181.
61. **Müller, H. E., D. J. Brenner, G. R. Fanning, P. A. D. Grimont, and P. Kämpfer.** 1996. Emended description of *Buttiauxella agrestis* with recognition of six new species of *Buttiauxella* and two new species of *Kluyvera*: *Buttiauxella ferragutiae* sp. nov., *Buttiauxella gaviniae* sp. nov., *Buttiauxella brennerae* sp. nov., *Buttiauxella izardii* sp. nov., *Buttiauxella noackiae* sp. nov., *Buttiauxella warmboldiae* sp. nov., *Kluyvera cochleae* sp. nov., and *Kluyvera georgiana* sp. nov. *Int. J. Syst. Bacteriol.* **46:**50–63.
62. **Norkina, O. V., A. N. Kulichenko, A. L. Gintsburg, I. V. Tuchkov, Y. A. Popov, M. U. Aksenov, and I. G. Drosdov.** 1994. Development of a diagnostic test for *Yersinia pestis* by the polymerase chain reaction. *J. Appl. Bacteriol.* **76:**240–245.
63. **O'Hara, C. M., A. G. Steigerwalt, B. C. Hill, J. M. Miller, and D. J. Brenner.** 1998. First report of a human isolate of *Erwinia persicinus*. *J. Clin. Microbiol.* **36:**248–250.
64. **Perry, R. D., and J. D. Fetherston.** 1997. *Yersinia pestis*—etiologic agent of plague. *Clin. Microbiol. Rev.* **10:** 35–66.
65. **Poland, J. D., T. J. Quan, and A. M. Barnes.** 1994. Plague, p. 93–112. *In* G. W. Beran (ed.), *Handbook of Zoonoses*, Sect. A. *Bacterial, Rickettsial, Chlamydial, and Mycotic Diseases*, 2nd ed. CRC Press, Inc., Ann Arbor, Mich.
66. **Prpic, K., R. M. Robins-Browne, and B. Davey.** 1983. Determination between virulent and avirulent *Yersinia enterocolitica* isolates by using Congo red agar. *J. Clin. Microbiol.* **18:**486–489.
67. **Rozalzki, A., Z. Sidoreczyk, and K. Kotelko.** 1997. Potential virulence factors of *Proteus* bacilli. *Microbiol. Mol. Biol. Rev.* **61:**65–89.
68. **Salyers, A. A., and D. D. Whitt.** 1994. *Bacterial Pathogenesis*, p. 213–228. American Society for Microbiology, Washington, D.C.
69. **Sato, K.** 1987. *Yersinia pseudotuberculosis* infection in children. Manifestations and epidemiology. *Contrib. Microbiol. Immunol.* **9:**111–116.
70. **Stenhouse, M. A. E., and L. V. Milner.** 1982. *Yersinia enterocolitica*: a hazard in blood transfusion. *Transfusion* **22:** 396–398.
71. **Toivanen, P., and A. Toivanen.** 1994. Does *Yersinia* induce autoimmunity? *Int. Arch. Allergy Immunol.* **104:** 107–111.
72. **Tsubokura, M., and S. Aleksic.** 1995. A simplified antigenic scheme for serotyping of *Yersinia pseudotuberculosis*. Phenotypic characterization of reference strains and preparation of O and H factor sera. *Contrib. Microbiol. Immunol.* **13:**99–105.
73. **U.S. Department of Health and Human Services.** 1988. *Biosafety in Microbiological and Biomedical Laboratories*. HHS publication no. CDC 88-8395. U.S. Department of Health and Human Services, Washington, D.C.

74. **Wauters, G., S. Aleksic, J. Charlier, and G. Schulze.** 1991. Somatic and flagellar antigens of *Yersinia enterocolitica* and related species. *Contrib. Microbiol. Immunol.* **12:** 239–243.
75. **Wauters, G., M. Janssens, A. G. Steigerwalt, and D. J. Brenner.** 1988. *Yersinia mollaretii* sp. nov. and *Yersinia bercovieri* sp. nov. formerly called *Yersinia enterocolitica* biogroups 3A and 3B. *Int. J. Syst. Bacteriol.* **38:**424–429.
76. **Wauters, G., K. Kandolo, and M. Janssens.** 1987. Revised biogrouping scheme of *Yersinia enterocolitica*. *Contrib. Microbiol. Immunol.* **9:**14–21.
77. **Williams, J.** 1983. Warning on a new potential for laboratory-acquired infections as a result of the new nomenclature for the plague bacillus. *Bull. W. H. O.* **61:**545–546.
78. **Wilson, C., A. Thakore, D. Isenberg, and A. Ebringer.** 1997. Correlation between anti-*Proteus* antibodies and isolation rates of *P. mirabilis* in rheumatoid arthritis. *Rheumatol. Infect.* **16:**187–189.
79. **Winblad, S.** 1969. Erythema nodosum associated with infection with *Yersinia enterocolitica*. *Scand. J. Infect. Dis.* **1:** 11–16.
80. **World Health Organization.** 1997. Human plague in 1995. *Weekly Epidemiol. Rec.* **72:**344–347.
81. **Yoshino, K. I., T. Ramamurthy, G. B. Nair, H. Fukushima, Y. Ohtomo, N. Takeda, S. Kaneko, and T. Takeda.** 1995. Geographical heterogeneity between Far East and Europe in prevalence of *ypm* gene encoding the novel superantigen among *Yersinia pseudotuberculosis* strains. *J. Clin. Microbiol.* **33:**3356–3358.

*Vibrio**

DAVID L. TISON

31

TAXONOMY

The genus *Vibrio* is classified in the family *Vibrionaceae* (7). Detailed information on the family *Vibrionaceae* can be found in reference texts (22, 36). Descriptions of the clinical and epidemiologic features of the pathogenic *Vibrio* species can be found in review articles (35, 75).

DESCRIPTION OF THE GENUS

Species in the genus *Vibrio* are facultatively anaerobic, gram-negative, curved or straight rods measuring about 0.5 to 0.8 μm in diameter and 1.4 to 2.4 μm in length. Most pathogenic *Vibrio* spp. are motile by means of a single, sheathed polar flagellum. Species which swarm on agar media have unsheathed, peritrichous flagella. Glucose is fermented by all *Vibrio* species, usually without the production of gas. Indophenol oxidase is produced and nitrate is reduced by all pathogenic *Vibrio* species except *V. metschnikovii*. Sodium is required or stimulates the growth of all pathogenic *Vibrio* spp.

About one-third of the more than 35 species in the genus *Vibrio* are pathogenic for humans. Nearly half of the species in the genus *Vibrio* have been described in the past 20 years. *V. cholerae* Pacini 1854 is the type species of the genus (7).

NATURAL HABITATS

Pathogenic *Vibrio* species are found as part of the autochthonous microbial community in brackish and marine environments in temperate or tropical regions throughout the world. *V. cholerae* and *V. mimicus* have been isolated from freshwater lakes and rivers and from birds and herbivores in areas geographically removed from marine and coastal waters (12, 55, 61, 62). The incidence and density of pathogenic *Vibrio* spp. decrease significantly as water temperatures fall below 20°C. *Vibrio* spp. can be found in the water column and surface sediment and are associated with mollusks and crustaceans. Human disease results from ingestion of water containing pathogenic *Vibrio* spp., the consumption of contaminated food, or exposure of wounds to water in environments where pathogenic *Vibrio* spp. are present. The pathogenic *Vibrio* species and the most common types of infections that they cause are listed in Table 1.

CLINICAL SIGNIFICANCE

V. cholerae O1

V. cholerae serogroup O1 is the etiologic agent of epidemic cholera. The organism was described by Pacini in 1854, the same year that John Snow identified the link between drinking water and cholera in Soho, London, with his historic Broad Street pump study (11). The bacterial etiology of cholera was confirmed by Robert Koch in 1883 when he isolated the cholera bacillus from pond water during a cholera outbreak in Egypt (42).

Documentation of the disease in the modern medical literature began in 1817, at the beginning of the first cholera pandemic (an epidemic affecting many countries) (58). The current cholera pandemic, pandemic seven, began in 1961. *V. cholerae* O1 has two biogroups, classical and El Tor. The classical biogroup was historically isolated during cholera epidemics on the Indian subcontinent. This changed with the seventh pandemic, which has predominantly been caused by the El Tor biogroup (38). The history of pandemic cholera has been extensively reviewed (11, 38, 58).

The severity of disease resulting from *V. cholerae* O1 infection ranges from asymptomatic or inapparent to the most severe form, referred to as "cholera gravis" (38). The severity of disease caused by the classical and El Tor biogroups of *V. cholerae* O1 varies (38). About 75% of infections with the El Tor biogroup and about 60% of infections with the classical biogroup are asymptomatic (38). Infection with the classical biogroup results in mild or moderate disease in 30% of infected individuals and severe disease in 11% of infected individuals. In contrast, El Tor strains produce mild or moderate disease in 23% of infected individuals and severe disease in only 2% of infected individuals (38).

The incubation period of cholera ranges from several hours to 5 days, depending on the inoculum size (38). The buffering effect of food on gastric acidity reduces the infective dose of *V. cholerae* O1 to about 10^6 vibrios, whereas it is about 10^{11} CFU at normal gastric acidity (38).

Cholera symptoms result from the action of cholera toxin (CT), which is a chromosomally mediated, heat-labile en-

* This chapter contains information presented in chapter 35 by James C. McLaughlin in the sixth edition of this Manual.

TABLE 1 Clinical syndromes associated with *Vibrio* species

Species	Disease presentation[a]	Clinical significance[b]	Relative frequency[c]	Major clinical sources
V. cholerae O1	Cholera	1	+	Feces
V. cholerae O139	Cholera	1	0	Feces
V. cholerae non-O1	Gastroenteritis	1	+ + +	Feces, blood
V. parahaemolyticus	Gastroenteritis	1	+ + +	Feces, wound
V. vulnificus	Bacteremia, wound infections	1	+ + +	Blood, wound
V. hollisae	Gastroenteritis	2	+ +	Feces
V. alginolyticus	Wound infections	2	+ +	Ear, wound
V. mimicus	Gastroenteritis	2	+ +	Feces
V. damsela	Wound infections	2	+	Wound
V. fluvialis	Gastroenteritis	3	+ +	Feces
V. metschnikovii	Gastroenteritis	3	+	Feces
V. furnissii	Gastroenteritis	3	0	
V. cincinnatiensis	Bacteremia, meningitis	3	0	
V. carchariae	Wound infection	3	0	

[a] Primary clinical presentation.

[b] 1, major pathogen; 2, causes sporadic infections; 3, rare or pathogenicity unproven, on the basis of data from references 31 and 45.

[c] Relative recovery rate in the United States on the basis of the rate of recovery of all pathogenic *Vibrio* spp.; + + +, common, + +, occasional, +, rare, 0, not isolated during major surveys of *Vibrio* infections in the United States.

terotoxin. CT has a high level of similarity to the plasmid-mediated, heat-labile enterotoxin (LT) of *Escherichia coli* (38). CT is an oligomeric protein composed of an A subunit and five B subunits. The B subunits bind to ganglioside GM_1 receptors on the membranes of intestinal epithelial cells, while the A subunit activates adenylate cyclase, producing increased levels of cyclic AMP and resulting in the hypersecretion of water and electrolytes. The outpouring of water and electrolytes into the lumen of the intestine causes copious purging, resulting in the severe dehydration associated with the classical clinical presentation of cholera (9, 38).

The initial symptoms of cholera are an increase in peristalsis followed by loose stools, which rapidly progress to the watery, mucus-flecked, "rice-water" stools characteristic of cholera. In cholera gravis, the rate of fluid loss quickly reaches 500 to 1,000 ml/h (38). Vomiting often occurs in the early stages of cholera. There is little abdominal pain, although muscle cramping may result from dehydration and electrolyte imbalance. Dehydration, hypovolemic shock, hypoglycemia, and metabolic acidosis must all be managed to prevent death in patients with cholera (9, 38).

Rehydration and electrolyte replacement therapy is the primary means of cholera treatment and is described in detail by Bennish (9) and Kaper et al. (38). Patients with mild and moderate cases of cholera can usually be managed with oral rehydration therapy (ORT) and do not require hospitalization. Fluids for ORT whose electrolyte, base, and glucose compositions vary from those recommended by the World Health Organization (WHO) should not be used. Vomiting is not a contraindication for ORT.

Cholera gravis requires immediate medical care to manage the symptoms described above. WHO recommends intravenous rehydration with Ringer's lactate to which potassium chloride (10 meq/liter) has been added. Hypoglycemia requires the addition of intravenous glucose. If isotonic saline is used to correct hypovolemia, it must be supplemented with potassium, base, and glucose. Intravenous rehydration should be given to infuse 2 liters in the first 30 min for adults. If this improves the patient's clinical condition, the infusion rate can be slowed to deliver 100 ml/kg of body weight within the first 4 h of therapy. Children should receive 30 ml/kg in the first hour and additional 40 ml/kg in the next 2 h (9, 38, 71).

Antimicrobial therapy may reduce the duration of diarrhea and the period of excretion of *V. cholerae* (38). Treatment should begin after the patient is clinically stabilized and vomiting has subsided. Tetracyclines are the antimicrobial agents of choice (71). The incidence of tetracycline-resistant strains of *V. cholerae* O1 is increasing (74), and infections with such strains require regimens of treatment with alternative agents such as erythromycin, trimethoprim-sulfamethoxazole, or furazolidone. Although efficacy data are limited, the in vitro activities of quinolones suggest that these agents may prove to be effective against *V. cholerae* O1 strains which are resistant to other antimicrobial agents (38).

V. cholerae O139 Bengal

The ability to produce CT and epidemic cholera was limited to the O1 serogroup of *V. cholerae* until a new serogroup emerged in October 1992, when an epidemic of cholera-like disease broke out in Madras, India (3). This new serogroup of *V. cholerae* was given the designation O139 Bengal to distinguish it from the 138 somatic antigen groups of *V. cholerae* which had previously been characterized. The onset of this epidemic of cholera caused by *V. cholerae* O139 Bengal has been suggested to be the beginning of the eighth cholera pandemic (72). By 1994, *V. cholerae* O139 had spread to more than a half dozen Asian countries and it had been imported to the United Kingdom and the United States (3). *V. cholerae* O139 was rapidly replaced with a new clone of *V. cholerae* O1 El Tor in 1994 (23). This was followed by the reemergence of *V. cholerae* O139 as the cause of the epidemic in the spring of 1996 (65).

V. cholerae O139 produces CT and shares several characteristics with *V. cholerae* O1 biotype El Tor, from which it probably developed by genetic recombination (10). Unlike the O1 serovar, O139 strains produce a capsule, as do other non-O1 *V. cholerae* serovars (79). *V. cholerae* O1 and O139 both must now be considered during outbreaks of epidemic cholera. Clinically, the disease caused by these organisms is the same. However, this poses new challenges for laboratory diagnosis and the epidemiologic investigations of cholera epidemics, which were limited to the O1 serovar in the past.

V. cholerae non-O1/O139

Other *V. cholerae* serogroups have been collectively referred to as non-O1, nonagglutinating (NAG) vibrios, or noncholera vibrios. Non-O1/O139 *V. cholerae* strains do not produce CT, with rare exceptions, and they do not cause epidemic disease (51). Several other toxins have been identified from non-O1/O139 *V. cholerae* strains. These include a hemolysin similar to that produced by El Tor *V. cholerae* O1; a heat-stable enterotoxin very similar to that produced by *E. coli*, referred to as NAG-ST; and a hemolysin termed NAG-rTDH, which is related to the thermostable direct hemolysin (TDH) of *V. parahaemolyticus* (32).

Non-O1/O139 *V. cholerae* strains are the etiologic agents of self-limiting gastroenteritis and may also cause wound infections and bacteremia (31, 35, 51). The capsule produced by non-O1/O139 *V. cholerae* strains is a factor in the ability of these organisms to cause bacteremia, probably by blocking the bactericidal activity of serum (38, 51). Preexisting liver disease was identified as a significant risk factor and predictor of fatality from septicemia caused by non-O1/O139 *V. cholerae*, *V. parahaemolyticus*, and *V. vulnificus* (31). An outbreak of diarrhea caused by non-O1/O139 *V. cholerae*, predominantly serovars O10 and O12, was recently reported in Peru (17). Morris (50) presented a review of the epidemiology of non-O1 *V. cholerae* disease.

V. mimicus

V. mimicus was classified as sucrose-negative *V. cholerae* until nucleic acid homology studies showed that these strains constituted a new species (20). *V. mimicus* has a spectrum of disease and characteristics similar to those of non-O1 *V. cholerae*, including O antigens in common with those of several non-O1 *V. cholerae* serogroups. A survey of *Vibrio* infections in Florida over a 13-year period identified *V. mimicus* predominantly as an agent of gastroenteritis, with the occurrence of rare cases of bacteremia and wound infection (31). An outbreak of diarrheal disease caused by *V. mimicus* after the consumption of raw turtle eggs has also been reported (15). Rare strains which produce CT have been found, but epidemic disease is not produced. The production of TDH appears to be associated with the production of disease by *V. mimicus*, as is the case for *V. parahaemolyticus* (78).

V. parahaemolyticus

V. parahaemolyticus was first identified as a cause of human disease after an outbreak of gastroenteritis in Japan in 1950 (37). Food-borne outbreaks and isolated cases occur throughout the world and are commonly the result of consumption of contaminated seafood (37). Crabs, prawns, scallops, oysters, and clams have been identified as sources of *V. parahaemolyticus* disease (37). The characteristics of *V. parahaemolyticus* gastroenteritis include nausea, vomiting, abdominal cramps, low-grade fever, and chills. The diarrhea is watery and occasionally bloody. Cases are usually self-limiting after 2 to 3 days' duration; however, severe and rare fatal cases have occurred. Wound, eye, and ear infections may occasionally result from exposure to marine environments where *V. parahaemolyticus* is present. *V. parahaemolyticus* can be found in temperate and tropical coastal waters worldwide, as are other pathogenic *Vibrio* spp. *V. parahaemolyticus* is the pathogenic *Vibrio* species most frequently isolated from clinical specimens in the United States (31, 45).

The virulence of *V. parahaemolyticus* is associated with the production of a TDH. This hemolysin is detected by the lysis of human erythrocytes on Wagatsuma medium and is known as the Kanagawa phenomenon (64). Strains which produce hemolysin are referred to as Kanagawa positive. This characteristic has been used epidemiologically as an indicator of the pathogenic potential of environmental isolates of *V. parahaemolyticus*. An increase in the numbers of urease-producing *V. parahaemolyticus* strains has been noted by clinical laboratories (40). A recently published study has documented the link between urease production and the TDH-related hemolysin (*trh*) gene (70). It appears that urease production, which can be reliably detected by routine laboratory methods, might be used as an indicator of the virulence of *V. parahaemolyticus* isolates.

V. vulnificus

Among the pathogenic *Vibrio* species, *V. vulnificus* causes the most severe disease. The septicemia and wound infections caused by this organism progress rapidly and are frequently fatal. Wounds and bullous lesions resulting from the hematogenous spread of *V. vulnificus* require extensive debridement. The consumption of raw oysters is the predominant source of systemic infection with *V. vulnificus* (73). This is in contrast to the case for other *Vibrio* spp. for which a variety of other mollusks and crustaceans serve as vehicles of transmission. This type of infection occurs most commonly in individuals with preexisting hepatic disease (31). The increased iron availability caused by liver disease has been shown to be a factor placing an individual at high risk of acquiring *V. vulnificus* infection (31).

Biogroup 2 of *V. vulnificus* (76), which was originally isolated from diseased eels, has recently been identified as an agent of human wound infections (5). The environmental distribution of *V. vulnificus* is similar to those of other pathogenic *Vibrio* species. The early literature documenting disease caused by *V. vulnificus* has referred to this organism as *Beneckia vulnifica*, Centers for Disease Control and Prevention (CDC) group EF-3, or the "lactose-positive" (Lac$^+$ or L$^+$) vibrio (75).

V. alginolyticus

V. alginolyticus is most commonly isolated from patients with external ear infections (otitis externa) acquired by swimming in seawater (22). It may also infect wounds which have been exposed to marine waters. *V. alginolyticus* was the third most frequent *Vibrio* species isolated from wound infections in Florida over a 13-year period (31). The older literature refers to *V. alginolyticus* as biotype 2 of *V. parahaemolyticus* (22). *V. alginolyticus* is the most halophilic of the pathogenic *Vibrio* species, with nearly 70% of strains growing in the presence of NaCl at concentrations as high as 10% (22).

V. fluvialis

V. fluvialis was originally isolated from patients with diarrhea in Bangladesh, and it has subsequently been reported as a cause of diarrhea in patients with sporadic cases of diarrhea throughout the world (22). This organism was referred to as group F vibrios and CDC group EF-6 (33) before it was named a new *Vibrio* species in 1981 (44). Rare fatal cases of gastroenteritis caused by *V. fluvialis* have been reported (41). This organism has the same environmental distribution as other *Vibrio* species.

V. furnissii

The aerogenic biogroup 2 of *V. fluvialis* was found to be a genetically distinct species and was named *V. furnissii* in 1983 (14). The pathogenicity of *V. furnissii*, which on rare occasions is isolated from feces, is questionable (22). A recent report of *V. furnissii* isolated from patients with diarrheal disease suggests that this organism may have clinical significance (19). *V. furnissii* is found in the same marine environments as other pathogenic *Vibrio* species.

V. hollisae

V. hollisae has been isolated from the feces of individuals with gastroenteritis and on rare occasions from patients with wound infections and bacteremia (1, 49). Seafood consumption and exposure to marine waters are the sources of infection with *V. hollisae*, as they are for the other pathogenic *Vibrio* species. This organism was referred to as CDC group EF-13 or Enteric Group 42 prior to its designation as a new *Vibrio* species in 1982 (30). A TDH gene is common to all *V. hollisae* strains (54). This gene is distantly related to the TDH gene which is found in a minority of *V. parahaemolyticus*, *V. cholerae* non-O1, and *V. mimicus* strains (54).

V. damsela

V. damsela was named a new *Vibrio* species in 1981 after it was isolated from ulcers on damselfish (47). The same organism had been isolated from a number of humans with wound infections resulting from exposure to seawater. These isolates had been submitted to CDC for identification, where they were given the preliminary designation CDC group EF-5 (22). *V. damsela* was rarely isolated during two surveys of *Vibrio* disease in the United States (31). *V. damsela* has been reported from patients with fatal cases of bacteremia resulting from wound infections (24, 57, 69).

Other *Vibrio* Species

V. metschnikovii was originally reported from a single patient with bacteremia and cholecystitis. Three additional cases of *V. metschnikovii* bacteremia have been reported (25, 26). Five cases of diarrheal disease in infants attributed to *V. metschnikovii* have also been reported (18). However, these patients were not screened for any other bacterial or viral enteric pathogens. An additional six clinical isolates were reported by Farmer and Hickman-Brenner (22) among strains submitted to CDC for identification. This organism has been isolated from marine environments as well as from shellfish, birds, river water, and sewage (43). *V. metschnikovii* requires only trace amounts of Na^+ for growth, suggesting that it may have an environmental distribution similar to that of non-O1 *V. cholerae*.

V. cincinnatiensis was first reported from a single patient with bacteremia and meningitis (13). In addition, five clinical isolates have been reported from the CDC Enteric Reference laboratory collection (22).

V. carchariae was described from a single patient with a wound infection following a shark bite (56). *V. carchariae* and *V. harveyii* are very similar, if not identical, phenotypically, as indicated by the data presented by Farmer and Hickman-Brenner (22). Since *V. harveyii* has taxonomic precedence over *V. carchariae*, further work is needed to clarify the validity of *V. carchariae* as a separate species.

COLLECTION, TRANSPORT, AND STORAGE OF SPECIMENS

Specimens should be collected as early in the clinical course as possible and before the initiation of antimicrobial therapy. Fecal specimens for culture of *V. cholerae*, *V. parahaemolyticus*, and the other less common *Vibrio* species which cause gastroenteritis should be placed in Cary-Blair transport medium and stored at room temperature (39). Buffered glycerol saline transport media are not adequate for maintaining the viability of pathogenic *Vibrio* species (21). Rectal swab specimens or vomitus for culture may also be collected from patients with suspected cholera. In epidemic situations, specimens from cholera patients may be inoculated into alkaline-peptone water or a few drops of specimen may be placed onto filter paper, gauze, or cotton which is then sealed in a plastic bag containing a few drops of sterile saline to prevent drying (34). Maintaining the moisture content of the specimen is the most important factor in maintaining the viability of vibrios.

Specimens from extraintestinal sources, such as wounds and blood, should be collected by standard procedures (40, 77).

DIRECT DETECTION

Dark-field and phase-contrast microscopy have been used to screen liquid or rice-water fecal specimens for *V. cholerae* (8, 39). Liquid stool or enrichment broth is examined for the presence of organisms with a darting or "shooting star" motility. If the addition of *V. cholerae* O1 antiserum results in the cessation of motility, a presumptive identification of *V. cholerae* can be made. In nonepidemic settings microscopy should not be used to rule out *Vibrio* infections. The pleomorphic microscopic morphology of the vibrios renders microscopy unreliable except for determining the Gram stain reaction of this group of organisms.

Direct fluorescent-antibody staining of smears from liquid stools has also been used to identify *V. cholerae* O1 (27). A coagglutination test with monoclonal antibodies against the O1 antigen (16) is commercially available (Cholera-Screen; New Horizons Diagnostics Corp., Columbia, Md.). A colloidal gold-based colorimetric immunoassay (28) is also available for the direct detection of *V. cholerae* O1 in fecal specimens (Cholera SMART; New Horizons Diagnostics Corp.).

Kits for the direct detection of *V. cholerae* O139 Bengal have also been developed (29, 59).

Detection of CT

Animal and cell culture assays have been used in the past to detect CT (52). Modifications of an enzyme-linked immunosorbent assay (ELISA) with purified GM_1 ganglioside receptor as the capture molecule (63) are now commonly used to detect CT. A latex agglutination kit for the detection of CT (VET-RPLA; Oxoid Limited, Basingstoke, Hampshire, England) has been shown to have excellent sensitivity and specificity (4).

A number of nucleic acid-based probes and PCR assays have been developed for use on a research basis for the detection of the *ctx* gene and are discussed in detail by Kaper et al. (38).

ISOLATION PROCEDURES

It is very important that any history of travel to an area where vibrios are endemic or a history of consumption of seafood or exposure to seawater be communicated to the diagnostic microbiology laboratory at the time that a specimen is submitted. This information may affect how the specimen is inoculated for culture. It will also aid the microbiologist during the examination of culture plates and help determine which microbial identification procedures are used.

Pathogenic *Vibrio* species grow on several types of culture media routinely used in the clinical laboratory. Trypticase soy agar, with or without blood, supports the growth of the pathogenic *Vibrio* species, since it contains 0.5% NaCl, as do most culture media used in the clinical laboratory. Pathogenic *Vibrio* species may be alpha-, beta-, or nonhemolytic on blood agar. Most pathogenic *Vibrio* species will also grow on moderately selective enteric media, such as MacConkey agar containing lactose or sorbitol. *Vibrio* species will appear as nonfermenters on MacConkey agars after overnight incubation, with rare exceptions. Colonies from nonselective media or nonfermenting colonies from MacConkey agar should be tested for oxidase activity to avoid false-negative reactions. Spot oxidase testing of individual colonies is recommended since it is more sensitive than dropping the oxidase reagent onto the plate and picking positive colonies (39). Oxidase-positive colonies should be subcultured for identification. Use of these media for fecal and wound specimens in conjunction with oxidase screening is sufficient for the routine isolation of the pathogenic *Vibrio* species (39, 77).

In outbreak situations or in areas where vibrios are endemic during summer months, it may be helpful to use a medium selective for vibrios such as thiosulfate-citrate-bile salts-sucrose (TCBS) agar. Sucrose-fermenting colonies, such as *V. cholerae* and *V. alginolyticus* colonies, will be yellow and sucrose-nonfermenting colonies, such as *V. parahaemolyticus*, *V. vulnificus*, and *V. mimicus* colonies, will be green on TCBS agar plates after overnight incubation. This medium was originally developed for the isolation of *V. cholerae* from patients during a cholera epidemic. Other pathogenic *Vibrio* species may grow poorly or not at all on TCBS agar due to lot-to-lot variations in commercial TCBS agar. The selective nature of the medium may be inhibitory to some organisms such as *V. hollisae*, *V. damsela*, *V. metschnikovii*, and *V. cincinnatiensis* (48). Variations in TCBS agar formulations among manufacturers also affect the variety of organisms isolated. The formulation produced by Eiken (Tokyo, Japan) is more selective than those produced by Oxoid (Basingstoke, Hampshire, England) and Difco (Detroit, Mich.). Those produced by the last two companies may support the growth of a variety of *Vibrio* spp., *Aeromonas* spp., and *Plesiomonas* spp. (22). Enrichment of fecal specimens in alkaline peptone water with subculture of a sample from the surface of the broth after 5 to 8 h of incubation to TCBS agar may also be used in epidemic situations. Taurocholate-tellurite-gelatin agar may also be used as a selective and differential medium for the isolation of *V. cholerae* from fecal specimens (39).

IDENTIFICATION

The genus *Vibrio* is oxidase positive and ferments glucose. The former phenotype differentiates *Vibrio* spp. from the members of the family *Enterobacteriaceae* and the latter from the pseudomonads and other nonfermenting gram-negative rods. Inoculation of a triple sugar iron (TSI) agar or a Kligler iron agar (KIA) slant is useful for identifying the fermentative phenotype of *Vibrio*. Once an organism has been found to be fermentative and oxidase positive, differentiation among the genera *Vibrio*, *Aeromonas*, and *Plesiomonas* must be done. The distinguishing characteristics of these pathogens are given in Table 2.

All *Vibrio* species grow to higher densities in nutrient broth or on nutrient agar when NaCl is added. Most culture media used in diagnostic microbiology laboratories contain at least 0.5% NaCl; therefore, nutrient broth or agar which does not contain NaCl (Difco) is useful for determining the requirement for NaCl. Since most diagnostic microbiology laboratories do not stock prepared nutrient broth, it may be useful to keep dehydrated nutrient broth powder on hand. The powder can be reconstituted and filter sterilized in small volumes sufficient for the testing of the occasional isolate. Nutrient broth can be prepared with distilled water and a 6% NaCl solution.

TABLE 2 Characteristics differentiating the species pathogenic for humans in the genera *Vibrio*, *Aeromonas*, and *Plesiomonas*[a]

Characteristic	*V. cholerae*, *V. mimicus*	Other *Vibrio* spp.	*Aeromonas*	*Plesiomonas*
Growth in nutrient broth or on nutrient agar (Difco)				
0% NaCl	+	−	+	+
6% NaCl	+	+	−	−
Susceptibility to O/129				
10 μg	+[b]	+/−	−	+/−
150 μg	+[b]	+	−	+/−
Ampicillin (10 μg) susceptibility	+/−	+[c]	−	−
Gas from glucose	−	−[d]	+/−	−
String test	+	+[c]	−	−
Fermentation of:				
m-Inositol	−	−[e]	−	+
L-Arabinose	−	−/+	+/−	−

[a] Adapted from reference 36. +, >90% positive; −, >90% negative; +/−, variable, >50% positive; −/+, variable, <50% positive.
[b] Most strains of *V. cholerae* isolated in India are now resistant.
[c] Except for some strains of *V. parahaemolyticus*.
[d] Except *V. furnissii*.
[e] Except *V. cincinnatiensis* and some strains of *V. metschnikovii*.

TABLE 3 Characteristics of pathogenic *Vibrio* species[a]

Test	Test reaction[b]											
	V. cholerae	*V. mimicus*	*V. parahaemolyticus*	*V. alginolyticus*	*V. vulnificus*	*V. damsela*	*V. fluvialis*	*V. furnissii*	*V. hollisae*	*V. metschnikovii*	*V. cincinnatiensis*	*V. carchariae*
Oxidase	+	+	+	+	+	+	+	+	+	−	+	+
Indole	+	+	+	+/−	+	−	−/+	−/+	+	−/+	−	+
Voges-Proskauer	+/−	−	−	+	−	+	−	−	−	+	−	+/−
Citrate, Simmons	+	+	−	−	+/−	−	+	+	−	+/−	−/+	−
ONPG[c]	+	+	−	−	+/−	−	−/+	−/+	−	+/−	+/−	−
Urea hydrolysis	−	−	+/−	−	−	−	−	−	−	−	−	−
Gelatin hydrolysis	+	+/−	+	+	+/−	−	+/−	+/−	−	+/−	−	−
Motility	+	+	+	+	+	−/+	+/−	+/−	−	+/−	+/−	−
Polymyxin B inhibition	−/+	+	+/−	+/−	−	+/−	+	+/−	+	+	+	+
Arginine, Moeller	−	−	−	−	−	+	+	+	−	+/−	−	−
Lysine, Moeller	+	+	+	+	+	+/−	−	−	−	−/+	+/−	+
Ornithine, Moeller	+	+	+	+/−	+/−	−	−	−	−	−	−	−
Acid production from:												
D-Glucose	+	+	+	+	+	+	+	+	+	+	+	+/−
L-Arabinose	−	−	+/−	−	−	−	+	+	+	−	+	−
D-Arabitol	−	−	−	−	−	−	+/−	+/−	−	−	−	−
Cellobiose	−	−	−	−	+	−	−/+	−/+	−	−	+	+/−
Lactose	−	−/+	−	−	+/−	−	−	−	−	+/−	−	−
Maltose	+	+	+	+	+	+	+	+	−	+	+	+
D-Mannitol	+	+	+	+	−/+	−	+	+	−	+	+	+/−
Salicin	−	−	−	−	+	−	−	−	−	−	+	−
Sucrose	+	−	−	+	−/+	−	+	+	−	+	+	+/−

[a] Adapted from reference 22.
[b] +, >90% positive; +/−, variable; >50% positive; −/+, variable; <50% positive; −, <10% positive.
[c] ONPG, *o*-nitrophenyl-β-D-galactopyranoside.

Growth in nutrient broth or on nutrient agar with and without salt will allow the differentiation among *Vibrio*, *Aeromonas*, and *Plesiomonas* (Table 2). *Aeromonas* spp. and *Plesiomonas* spp. will grow in nutrient broth without added salt. *V. cholerae* and *V. mimicus* will also grow in nutrient broth or agar without added NaCl. These *Vibrio* species, which are arginine dehydrogenase (ADH) negative and lysine decarboxyl (LDC) and ornithine decarboxylase (ODC) positive, can be differentiated from most *Aeromonas* spp. and *Plesiomonas* spp., which are ADH positive. The LDC, ODC, and ADH set of reactions is also useful for distinguishing between phenotypic groups of *Vibrio* spp. (Table 3).

The vibriostatic compound 2,4-diamino-6,7-diisopropylpteridine (O/129) has been used on disks at concentrations of 10 and 150 μg/ml as a means of identifying *Vibrio* species. Testing is done by the methods for standardized disk antimicrobial susceptibility testing, with any zone of inhibition around an O/129 disk regarded as positive. Many *V. cholerae* strains isolated from recent epidemics have been found to be resistant to O/129 as well as other antimicrobial agents (60). Non-O1 *V. cholerae* resistance to O/129 has also been reported. Although this test may be useful for the identification of *Vibrio* spp. isolated outside of epidemic situations, the results should be interpreted with caution and should be used in conjunction with the results of the salt requirement test for the reliable identification of pathogenic *Vibrio* species.

Another test which may be useful for the presumptive identification of *Vibrio* spp. is the string test. Growth from a suspect colony is taken with a loop and stirred in 0.5% sodium deoxycholate on a glass slide. Most diagnostic microbiology laboratories will have 10% sodium deoxycholate on hand for bile solubility testing for the identification of *Streptococcus pneumoniae*. This reagent can be diluted to a final concentration of 0.5% for use in the string test. *Vibrio* spp. will lyse and produce a viscous suspension, which is seen when the loop is pulled from the slide and a string of viscous material is pulled up from the slide (39). *Aeromonas* and *Plesiomonas* are not lysed, so they do not produce a viscous string and are therefore string test negative.

V. cholerae O1 is divided into the classical and El Tor biogroups or biotypes for epidemiologic purposes. The classical biogroup of *V. cholerae* O1 is negative by the Voges-Proskauer test and is negative for the hemolysis of sheep erythrocytes and agglutination of chicken erythrocytes. The El Tor biogroup has historically been positive by these tests. The El Tor strains isolated since the early 1960s have been nonhemolytic (6, 38). The classical biogroup is inhibited by polymyxin B (50 U), whereas the El Tor biogroup is not. Several bacteriophages are also biogroup specific. Biogrouping of *V. cholerae* O1 is a valuable epidemiologic tool but is not of use for diagnostic purposes in the clinical microbiology laboratory.

Many of the commercial identification systems currently used in diagnostic microbiology laboratories use substrates or tests which have not been used in the past for the identification of pathogenic *Vibrio* species. The number of strains of individual species in the manufacturers' databases may be limited, so the results obtained with these systems, especially for the uncommon *Vibrio* species, should be interpreted with caution. Misidentification of *Aeromonas veronii* biovar veronii as *V. cholerae* and *A. caviae* as *V. fluvialis* has been documented (2).

Some of the older kit identification systems which use conventional biochemical tests may be useful for identifying pathogenic *Vibrio* species. Increasing the NaCl concentration of the inoculation solution to 1% may give results which are more reliably compared to those from reference laboratories such as CDC (22, 40). However, misidentification of an *Aeromonas* sp. as a *Vibrio* sp. may also occur with these kit systems (2).

TABLE 4 Unique phenotypic characteristics useful for identifying some of the pathogenic *Vibrio* spp.

Species	Phenotype	Reaction
V. parahaemolyticus	Urea	+[a]
V. hollisae	LDC/ODC/ADH	−/−/−
V. metschnikovii	Oxidase/nitrate	−/−
V. furnissii	Gas from glucose	+
V. cincinnatiensis	*m*-Inositol	+

[a] Not all strains of *V. parahaemolyticus* are urease positive.

Individual tests which are key for the identification of the pathogenic *Vibrio* species include the LDC, ODC, ADH tests, as mentioned above. *V. cholerae*, *V. mimicus*, *V. parahaemolyticus*, *V. alginolyticus*, and *V. vulnificus* are LDC positive, ODC positive, and ADH negative. *V. cholerae* and *V. mimicus* grow in nutrient broth or on nutrient agar without NaCl, while the other species in this group do not. Many *V. parahaemolyticus* strains isolated from clinical specimens are urease positive, which distinguishes this species. It is important for laboratories which use TSI agar reactions and urease activity for the screening of isolates from stool specimens to include an oxidase test to avoid discarding *V. parahaemolyticus* strains which would have an alkaline slant over an acid butt on TSI agar and are urease positive. Distinguishing features for *V. alginolyticus* are growth in 10% NaCl and swarming on agar media. The serious nature of the infection is often a clue as to the possible identification of *V. vulnificus*. This organism will also ferment lactose after 24 to 48 h of incubation.

V. fluvialis, *V. furnissii*, and *V. damsela* are ADH positive and LDC and ODC negative. *V. furnissii* produces gas, which may be seen in the butt of TSI agar or KIA slants. *V. damsela* is LDC, ODC, and ADH negative, which distinguishes it from the other pathogenic *Vibrio* species. *V. metschnikovii* is oxidase negative, so it may be difficult to differentiate from the members of the family *Enterobacteriaceae*, although it is nitrate negative, which distinguishes this organism from the members of the family *Enterobacteriaceae* and other pathogenic *Vibrio* species. *V. cincinnatiensis* and *V. carchariae* are very rare clinical isolates which are best identified by a reference laboratory. Unique phenotypic characteristics which are useful in identifying some of the pathogenic *Vibrio* spp. are listed in Table 4.

Most diagnostic microbiology laboratories isolate *Vibrio* spp. infrequently and may not have the expertise or supplemental media necessary to definitively identify pathogenic *Vibrio* species. Any organism which is isolated from feces and which is suspected of being *V. cholerae* should be sent to a state reference laboratory as soon as possible. Any other *Vibrio* species isolated in the clinical laboratory should also be referred to a reference laboratory for confirmation of the identification unless that laboratory has significant experience and expertise in the identification of these organisms.

SEROLOGIC TESTS

V. cholerae has 155 somatic (O) antigens, and these have been characterized (68). The different somatic antigen groups are referred to as serogroups or serovars (38). A flagellar (H) antigen is also produced; however, it is of limited usefulness since common epitopes exist among all the *Vibrio* species (38).

V. cholerae can be serotyped or subtyped further on the basis of minor O antigens, referred to as O factors A, B, and C. *V. cholerae* strains which produce both A and B O factors are referred to as subgroup O1 Ogawa, those which produce O factors A and C are subgroup O1 Inaba, and those which produce O factors A, B, and C are subgroup Hikojima. The Hikojima subgroup is rare and unstable (38) and is not recognized by some authorities, who report only the Ogawa and Inaba subgroups (40). Serologic subgrouping should be done by centralized or reference laboratories in areas where *V. cholerae* is epidemic.

Antibody detection may be useful for the retrospective diagnosis of *V. cholerae* disease. Antibody tests are particularly useful for the diagnosis of suspected cases of *V. cholerae* disease which were not confirmed by culture. The two main serologic tests for these purposes are assays for the vibriocidal antibody and the cholera antitoxin antibody (38). The procedures for these assays have been described by Losonsky and Levine (46). Most individuals develop both vibriocidal and antitoxin immune responses within 10 days postexposure (38). In areas where *V. cholerae* disease is not endemic, vibriocidal titers return to the baseline within 1 to 6 months, while antitoxin titers decline over a 1- to 2-year period but do not return to the baseline (38).

A serotyping scheme for *V. parahaemolyticus* has been used for epidemiologic purposes but is not useful for assessing clinical significance (37). *V. parahaemolyticus* has 13 thermostable O-antigen groups and more than 60 heat-labile capsular (K) antigens. Antibodies for *V. parahaemolyticus* serotyping are commercially available (Accurate Chemical and Scientific, Westbury, N.Y.). A scheme for serotyping of *V. vulnificus* has also been described (66). *V. vulnificus* has seven O-antigen serovars which are identified with heat-killed strains. Heating is required to remove the heat-labile masking antigen of most live strains of *V. vulnificus*. A combined serotyping scheme composed of 35 O-antigen groups is used for *V. fluvialis* and *V. furnissii* (67).

ANTIMICROBIAL SUSCEPTIBILITY TESTING

The pathogenic *Vibrio* species grow well on Mueller-Hinton agar without added salt. Testing can be done by the disk diffusion or the broth microdilution method by standardized procedures for antimicrobial susceptibility testing. Interpretive standards for *V. cholerae* tested with ampicillin, tetracycline, trimethoprim-sulfamethoxazole, chloramphenicol, and sulfonamides are published in document M100-S8 of the National Committee for Clinical Laboratory Standards (53). Standardized breakpoints for other *Vibrio* sp. have not been published. Extensive data for antimicrobial susceptibility testing of *Vibrio* spp. are presented by Farmer and Hickman-Brenner (22). Reports of increasing resistance among *V. cholerae* strains isolated during epidemics indicate that antimicrobial susceptibilities may need to be closely monitored in the future (60).

INTERPRETATION AND REPORTING OF RESULTS

The isolation of a pathogenic *Vibrio* species from a clinical specimen should be considered a significant finding. Positive results should be telephoned to the physician who submitted the specimen for testing, especially if *V. cholerae* is isolated from feces or if *V. vulnificus* is isolated from any clinical specimen. Reporting of antimicrobial susceptibility test results is probably not warranted for the clinical management of self-limited diarrheal disease, but these data may be useful in the laboratory for identification purposes. Antimicrobial susceptibility test results should be reported for extraintestinal isolates since this information may help direct the management of a patient's infection. It should be noted in any report of antimicrobial susceptibility test results that the data have been interpreted by using standards which have not been validated for the pathogenic *Vibrio* species other than *V. cholerae*.

REFERENCES

1. **Abbott, S. L., and J. M. Janda.** 1994. Severe gastroenteritis associated with *Vibrio hollisae* infection: report of two cases and review. *Clin. Infect. Dis.* **18:**310–312.
2. **Abbott, S. L., L. S. Seli, M. Catino, Jr., M. A. Hartley, and J. M. Janda.** 1998. Misidentification of unusual *Aeromonas* species as members of the genus *Vibrio*: a continuing problem. *J. Clin. Microbiol.* **36:**1103–1104.
3. **Albert, M. J.** 1994. *Vibrio cholerae* O139 Bengal. *J. Clin. Microbiol.* **32:**2345–2349.
4. **Almeida, M. J., F. W. Hickman-Brenner, E. G. Sowers, N. D. Puhr, J. J. Farmer III, and I. K. Wachsmuth.** 1990. Comparison of a latex agglutination assay and an enzyme-linked immunosorbent assay for detecting cholera toxin. *J. Clin. Microbiol.* **28:**128–130.
5. **Amaro, C., and E. G. Biosca.** 1996. *Vibrio vulnificus* biotype 2, pathogenic for eels, is also an opportunistic pathogen for humans. *Appl. Environ. Microbiol.* **62:**1454–1457.
6. **Barrett, T. J., and P. A. Blake.** 1981. Epidemiological usefulness of changes in hemolytic activity of *Vibrio cholerae* El Tor during the seventh pandemic. *J. Clin. Microbiol.* **13:**126–129.
7. **Baumann, P., A. L. Furniss, and J. V. Lee.** 1984. Genus I. *Vibrio* Pacini 1854, 411[AL], p. 518–538. *In* N. R. Krieg and J. G. Holt (ed.), *Bergey's Manual of Systematic Bacteriology*, vol. 1. The Williams & Wilkins Co. Baltimore, Md.
8. **Benenson, A. S., M. R. Islam, and W. B. Greenough III.** 1964. Rapid identification of *Vibrio cholerae* by darkfield microscopy. *Bull. W. H. O.* **30:**827–831.
9. **Bennish, M. L.** 1994. Cholera: pathophysiology, clinical features, and treatment, p. 229–255. *In* I. K. Wachsmuth, P. A. Blake, and O. Olsvik (ed.), Vibrio cholerae *and Cholera: Molecular to Global Perspectives*. ASM Press, Washington, D.C.
10. **Bik, E. M., A. E. Bunschoten, R. D. Gouw, and F. R. Mooi.** 1995. Genesis of the novel epidemic *Vibrio cholerae* O139 Bengal: evidence for horizontal transfer of genes involved in polysaccharide synthesis. *EMBO J.* **14:**209–216.
11. **Blake, P. A.** 1994. Historical perspectives on pandemic cholera, p. 293–295. *In* I. K. Wachsmuth, P. A. Blake, and O. Olsvik (ed.), Vibrio cholerae *and Cholera: Molecular to Global Perspectives*. ASM Press, Washington, D.C.
12. **Bockemuhl, J., K. Roch, B. Wohlers, V. Aleksic, S. Aleksic, and R. Wokatsch.** 1986. Seasonal distribution of facultatively enteropathogenic vibrios (*Vibrio cholerae, Vibrio mimicus, Vibrio parahaemolyticus*) in the freshwater of the Elbe River in Hamburg. *J. Appl. Bacteriol.* **60:**435–442.
13. **Brayton, P. R., R. B. Bode, R. R. Colwell, M. T. MacDonell, H. L. Hall, D. J. Grimes, P. A. West, and T. N. Bryant.** 1986. *Vibrio cincinnatiensis* sp. nov., a new human pathogen. *J. Clin. Microbiol.* **23:**104–108.
14. **Brenner, D. J., F. W. Hickman-Brenner, J. V. Lee, A. G. Steigerwalt, G. R. Fanning, D. G. Hollis, J. J. Farmer III, R. E. Weaver, and R. J. Seidler.** 1983. *Vibrio furnissii*

(formerly aerogenic biogroup of *Vibrio fluvialis*), a new species isolated from human feces and the environment. *J. Clin. Microbiol.* **18:**816–824.

15. **Campos, E., H. Bolanos, M. T. Acuna, G. Diaz, M. C. Matamoros, H. Raventos, L. M. Sanchez, O. Sanchez, and C. Barquero.** 1996. *Vibrio mimicus* diarrhea following ingestion of raw turtle eggs. *Appl. Environ. Microbiol.* **62:** 1141–1144.
16. **Colwell, R. R., J. A. K. Hasan, A. Huq, L. Loomis, R. J. Siebeling, M. Torres, S. Galvez, S. Islam, M. Tamplin, and D. Bernstein.** 1992. Development and evaluation of a rapid, simple, sensitive monoclonal antibody-based coagglutination test for direct detection of *Vibrio cholerae* O1. *FEMS Immunol. Med. Microbiol.* **8:**293–298.
17. **Dalsgaard, A., M. J. Albert, D. N. Taylor, T. Shimada, R. Meza, O. Serichantalergs, and P. Echeverria.** 1995. Characterization of *Vibrio cholerae* non-O1 serogroups obtained from an outbreak of diarrhea in Lima, Peru. *J. Clin. Microbiol.* **33:**2715–2722.
18. **Dalsgaard, A., A. Alarcon, C. F. Lanata, T. Jensen, H. J. Hansen, F. Delgado, A. I. Gil, M. E. Penny, and D. Taylor.** 1996. Clinical manifestations and molecular epidemiology of five cases of diarrhoea in children associated with *Vibrio metschnikovii* in Arequipa, Peru. *J. Med. Microbiol.* **45:**494–500.
19. **Dalsgaard, A., P. Glerup, L. L. Hoybye, A. M. Paarup, R. Meza, M. Bernal, T. Shimada, and D. N. Taylor.** 1997. *Vibrio furnissii* isolated from humans in Peru: a possible human pathogen? *Epidemiol. Infect.* **119:**143–149.
20. **Davis, B. R., G. R. Fanning, J. M. Madden, A. G. Steigerwalt, H. B. Bradford, Jr., H. L. Smith, Jr., and D. J. Brenner.** 1981. Characterization of biochemically atypical *Vibrio cholerae* strains and designation of a new pathogenic species, *Vibrio mimicus*. *J. Clin. Microbiol.* **14:**631–639.
21. **DeWitt, W. E., E. J. Gangarosa, I. Huq, and A. Zarifi.** 1971. Holding media for the transport of *Vibrio cholerae* from field to laboratory. *Am. J. Trop. Med. Hyg.* **20:** 685–688.
22. **Farmer, J. J., III, and F. Hickman-Brenner.** 1992. The genera *Vibrio* & *Photobacterium*, p. 2952–3011. *In* A. Balows, H. G. Tüper, and K. H. Schleifer (ed.), *The Prokaryotes: a Handbook on the Biology of Bacteria. Ecophysiology, Isolation, Identification, Applications*, vol. 3. Springer-Verlag, New York, N.Y.
23. **Faruque, S. M., K. M. Ahmed, A. R. M. Abdul Alim, F. Qadri, A. K. Siddique, and M. J. Albert.** 1997. Emergence of a new clone of toxigenic *Vibrio cholerae* O1 biotype El Tor displacing *V. cholerae* O139 Bengal in Bangladesh. *J. Clin. Microbiol.* **35:**624–630.
24. **Fraser, S. L., B. K. Purcell, B. Delgado, Jr., A. E. Baker, and A. C. Whelen.** 1997. Rapidly fatal infection due to *Photobacterium* (*Vibrio*) *damsela*. *Clin. Infect. Dis.* **25:** 935–936.
25. **Hansen, W., J. Freney, H. Benyagoub, M.-N. Letouzey, J. Gigi, and G. Wauters.** 1993. Severe human infections caused by *Vibrio metschnikovii*. *J. Clin. Microbiol.* **31:** 2529–2530.
26. **Hardardittir, H., K. Vikenes, A. Digranes, J. Lassen, and A. Halstensen.** 1994. Mixed bacteremia with *Vibrio metschnikovii* in an 83-year-old female patient. *Scand. J. Infect. Dis.* **26:**493–494.
27. **Hasan, J. A. K., D. Bernstein, A. Huq, L. Loomis, M. L. Tamplin, and R. R. Colwell.** 1994. Cholera DFA: an improved direct fluorescent-monoclonal antibody staining kit for rapid detection and enumeration of *Vibrio cholerae* O1. *FEMS Microbiol. Lett.* **120:**143–148. (Erratum, **122:** 201.)
28. **Hasan, J. A. K., A. Huq, M. L. Tamplin, R. J. Siebeling, and R. R. Colwell.** 1994. A novel kit for rapid detection of *Vibrio cholerae* O1. *J. Clin. Microbiol.* **32:**249–252.
29. **Hasan, J. A. K., A. Huq, G. B. Nair, S. Garg, A. K. Mukhopadhyay, L. Loomis, D. Bernstein, and R. R. Colwell.** 1995. Development and testing of monoclonal antibody-based rapid immunodiagnostic kits for direct detection of *V. cholerae* O139 synonym Bengal. *J. Clin. Microbiol.* **33:**2935–2939.
30. **Hickman-Brenner, F. W., J. J. Farmer III, D. G. Hollis, G. R. Fanning, A. G. Steigerwalt, R. E. Weaver, and D. J. Brenner.** 1982. Identification of *Vibrio hollisae* sp. nov. from patients with diarrhea. *J. Clin. Microbiol.* **15:** 395–401.
31. **Hlady, W. G., and K. C. Klontz.** 1996. The epidemiology of *Vibrio* infections in Florida, 1981–1993. *J. Infect. Dis.* **173:**1176–1183.
32. **Honda, T., M. Arita, T. Takeda, M. Yoh, and T. Miwatani.** 1985. Non-O1 *Vibrio cholerae* produces two newly identified toxins related to *Vibrio parahaemolyticus* hemolysin and *Escherichia coli* heat-stable enterotoxin. *Lancet* **ii:** 163–164.
33. **Huq, M. I., A. K. M. J. Alam, D. J. Brenner, and G. K. Morris.** 1980. Isolation of *Vibrio*-like group EF-6 from patients with diarrhea. *J. Clin. Microbiol.* **11:**621–624.
34. **Huq, M. I., and M. M. Rahaman.** 1983. Blotting paper strip for the transport of stool specimens for laboratory diagnosis of cholera. *Indian J. Med. Res.* **78:**765–768.
35. **Janda, J. M., C. Powers, R. G. Bryant, and S. L. Abbott.** 1988. Current perspectives on the epidemiology and pathogenesis of clinically significant *Vibrio* spp. *Clin. Microbiol. Rev.* **1:**245–267.
36. **Janda, J. M.** 1998. *Vibrio, Aeromonas & Plesiomonas*, p. 1065–1089. *In* L. Collier (ed.), *Topley & Wilson's Microbiology & Microbial Infections*, 9th ed. Oxford University Press, New York, N.Y.
37. **Joseph, S. W., R. R. Colwell, and J. B. Kaper.** 1982. *Vibrio parahaemolyticus* and related halophilic vibrios. *Crit. Rev. Microbiol.* **10:**77–124.
38. **Kaper, J. B., J. G. Morris, Jr., and M. M. Levine.** 1995. Cholera. *Clin. Microbiol. Rev.* **8:**48–86.
39. **Kay, B. A., C. A. Bopp, and J. G. Wells.** 1994. Isolation and identification of *Vibrio cholerae* O1 from fecal specimens, p. 3–25. *In* I. K. Wachsmuth, P. A. Blake, and O. Olsvik (ed.), Vibrio cholerae *and Cholera: Molecular to Global Perspectives*. ASM Press, Washington, D.C.
40. **Kelly, M. T., F. W. Hickman-Brenner, and J. J. Farmer III.** 1992. *Vibrio*, p. 384–395. *In* A. Balows, W. J. Hausler, Jr., K. L. Hermann, H. D. Isenberg, and H. J. Shadomy (ed.), *Manual of Clinical Microbiology*, 5th ed. American Society for Microbiology, Washington, D.C.
41. **Klontz, K. C., D. E. Cover, F. N. Hyman, and R. C. Mullen.** 1994. Fatal gastroenteritis due to *Vibrio fluvialis* and nonfatal bacteremia due to *Vibrio mimicus*: unusual vibrio infections in two patients. *Clin. Infect. Dis.* **19:** 541–542.
42. **Koch, R.** 1884. An address on cholera and its bacillus. *Br. Med. J.* **2:**403–407, 453–459.
43. **Lee, J. V., T. J. Donovan, and A. L. Furniss.** 1978. Characterization, taxonomy, and emended description of *Vibrio metschnikovii*. *Int. J. Syst. Bacteriol.* **28:**99–111.
44. **Lee, J. V., P. Shread, L. Furniss, and T. N. Bryant.** 1981. Taxonomy and description of *Vibrio fluvialis* sp. nov. (synonym group F vibrios, group EF-6). *J. Appl. Bacteriol.* **50:** 73–94.
45. **Levine, W. C., P. M. Griffin, and the Gulf Coast *Vibrio* Working Group.** 1993. *Vibrio* infections on the Gulf Coast: results of the first year of regional surveillance. *J. Infect. Dis.* **167:**479–483.

46. **Losonsky, G. A., and M. M. Levine.** 1997. Immunologic methods for diagnosis of infections caused by diarrheagenic members of the families *Enterobacteriaceae* and *Vibrionaceae*, p. 484–497. *In* N. R. Rose, E. C. de Macario, J. D. Folds, H. C. Lane, and R. M. Nakamura (ed.), *Manual of Clinical Immunology*, 5th ed. ASM Press, Washington, D.C.

47. **Love, M. D., D. Teebken-Fisher, J. E. Hose, J. J. Farmer III, F. W. Hickman-Brenner, and G. R. Fanning.** 1981. *Vibrio damsela*, a marine bacterium, causes skin ulcers on the damselfish *Chromis punctipinnis*. *Science* **214:**1139–1140.

48. **McLaughlin, J. C.** 1994. *Vibrio*, p. 465–476. *In* P. R. Murray, E. J. Baron, M. A. Pfaller, F. C. Tenover, and R. H. Yolken (ed.), *Manual of Clinical Microbiology*, 6th ed. American Society for Microbiology, Washington, D.C.

49. **Morris, J. G., Jr., R. Wilson, D. G. Hollis, R. E. Weaver, H. G. Miller, C. O. Tacket, R. W. Hickman, and P. A. Blake.** 1982. Illness caused by *Vibrio damsela* and *Vibrio hollisae*. *Lancet* **i:**1294–1297.

50. **Morris, J. G., Jr.** 1990. Non-O group 1 *Vibrio cholerae*: a look at the epidemiology of an occasional pathogen. *Epidemiol. Rev.* **12:**179–191.

51. **Morris, J. G., Jr.** 1994. Non-O group 1 *Vibrio cholerae* strains not associated with epidemic disease, p. 103–115. *In* I. K. Wachsmuth, P. A. Blake, and O. Ølsvik (ed.), Vibrio cholerae *and Cholera: Molecular to Global Perspectives*. ASM Press, Washington, D.C.

52. **Nair, G. B., and Y. Takeda.** 1994. Detection of toxins of *Vibrio cholerae* O1 and non-O1, p. 53–67. *In* I. K. Wachsmuth, P. A. Blake, and O. Ølsvik (ed.), Vibrio cholerae *and Cholera: Molecular to Global Perspectives*. ASM Press, Washington, D.C.

53. **National Committee for Clinical Laboratory Standards.** 1998. *Performance Standards for Antimicrobial Susceptibility Testing*. Eighth Informational Supplement. NCCLS document M100-S8. National Committee for Clinical Laboratory Standards, Wayne, Pa.

54. **Nishibuchi, M., J. M. Janda, and T. Ezaki.** 1996. The thermostable direct hemolysin gene (*tdh*) of *Vibrio hollisae* is dissimilar in prevalence to and phylogenetically distant from the *tdh* genes of other vibrios: implications in the horizontal transfer of the *tdh* gene. *Microbiol. Immunol.* **40:** 59–65.

55. **Ogg, J. E., R. A. Ryder, and H. L. Smith, Jr.** 1989. Isolation of *Vibrio cholerae* from aquatic birds in Colorado and Utah. *Appl. Environ. Microbiol.* **55:**95–99.

56. **Pavia, A. T., J. A. Bryan, K. L. Maher, T. R. Hester, Jr., and J. J. Farmer III.** 1989. *Vibrio carchariae* infection after a shark bite. *Ann. Intern. Med.* **111:**85–86.

57. **Perez-Tirse, J., J. F. Levine, and M. Mecca.** 1993. *Vibrio damsela*: a cause of fulminant septicemia. *Arch. Intern. Med.* **153:**1838–1840.

58. **Pollitzer, R.** 1959. *Cholera*. World Health Organization, Geneva, Switzerland.

59. **Qadri, F., J. A. K. Hasan, J. Hossain, A. Chowdhury, Y. A. Begum, T. Azim, L. Loomis, R. B. Sack, and M. J. Albert.** 1995. Evaluation of the monoclonal antibody-based kit Bengal SMART for rapid detection of *Vibrio cholerae* O139 synonym Bengal in stool specimens. *J. Clin. Microbiol.* **33:**732–734.

60. **Ramamurthy, T., A. Pal, S. C. Pal, and G. B. Nair.** 1992. Taxonomic implications of the emergence of high frequency of occurrence of 2,4-diamino-6,7-diisopropylpteridine-resistant strains of *Vibrio cholerae* from clinical cases of cholera in Calcutta, India. *J. Clin. Microbiol.* **30:**742–743.

61. **Rhodes, J. B., D. Schweitzer, and J. E. Ogg.** 1985. Isolation of non-O1 *Vibrio cholerae* associated with enteric disease of herbivores in western Colorado. *J. Clin. Microbiol.* **22:**572–575.

62. **Rhodes, J. B., H. L. Smith, Jr., and J. E. Ogg.** 1986. Isolation of non-O1 *Vibrio cholerae* serovars from surface waters in western Colorado. *Appl. Environ. Microbiol.* **51:** 1216–1219.

63. **Sack, D. A., S. Huda, P. K. B. Neogi, R. R. Daniel, and W. M. Spira.** 1980. Microtiter ganglioside enzyme-linked immunosorbent assay for *Vibrio* and *Escherichia coli* heat-labile enterotoxins and antitoxin. *J. Clin. Microbiol.* **11:** 35–40.

64. **Sakazaki, R., K. Tamura, T. Kato, Y. Obara, S. Yamai, and K. Hobo.** 1968. Studies on the enteropathogenic, facultatively halophilic bacteria, *Vibrio parahaemolyticus* III: enteropathogenicity. *Jpn. J. Med. Sci. Biol.* **21:**325–331.

65. **Sharma, C., S. Maiti, A. K. Mukhopadhyay, A. Basu, I. Basu, G. B. Nair, R. Mukhopadhyay, B. Das, S. Kar, R. K. Ghosh, and A. Ghosh.** 1997. Unique organization of the CTX genetic element in *Vibrio cholerae* O139 strains which reemerged in Calcutta, India, in September 1996. *J. Clin. Microbiol.* **35:**3348–3350.

66. **Shimada, T., and R. Sakazaki.** 1984. On the serology of *Vibrio vulnificus*. *Jpn. J. Med. Sci. Biol.* **37:**241–246.

67. **Shimada, T., Y. Kosako, K. Inoue, M. Ohtomo, S. Matsushita, S. Yamada, and Y. Kudoh.** 1991. *Vibrio fluvialis* and *Vibrio furnissii* serotyping scheme for international use. *Curr. Microbiol.* **22:**335–337.

68. **Shimada, T., E. Arakawa, K. Itoh, T. Okitsu, A. Matsushima, Y. Asai, S. Yamai, T. Nakazato, G. B. Nair, M. J. Albert, and Y. Takeda.** 1994. Extended serotyping scheme for *Vibrio cholerae*. *Curr. Microbiol.* **28:**175–178.

69. **Shin, J. H., M. G. Shin, S. P. Suh, D. W. Ryang, J. S. Rew, and F. S. Nolte.** 1996. Primary *Vibrio damsela* septicemia. *Clin. Infect. Dis.* **22:**856–857.

70. **Suthienkul, O., M. Ishibashi, T. Iida, N. Nettip, S. Supavej, B. Eampokalap, M. Mankino, and T. Honda.** 1996. Urease production correlates with the possession of the TRH gene in *Vibrio parahaemolyticus* strains isolated in Thailand. *J. Infect. Dis.* **172:**1405–1408.

71. **Swerdlow, D., and A. A. Reis.** 1992. Cholera in the Americas: guidelines for the clinician. *JAMA* **267:**1495–1499.

72. **Swerdlow, D., and A. A. Reis.** 1993. *Vibrio cholerae* non-O1—the eighth pandemic? *Lancet* **342:**382–383.

73. **Tacket, C. O., F. Hickman-Brenner, and P. A. Blake.** 1984. Clinical features and an epidemiological study of *Vibrio vulnificus* infections. *J. Infect. Dis.* **149:**558–561.

74. **Takeda, Y., T. Takeda, S. C. Pal, and G. B. Nair.** 1992. Serovar, biotype, phage type, toxigenicity, and antibiotic susceptibility patterns of *Vibrio cholerae* isolated during two consecutive cholera seasons (1989–90) in Calcutta. *Indian J. Med. Res. Sect. A* **95:**125–129.

75. **Tison, D. L., and M. T. Kelly.** 1982. *Vibrio* species of medical importance. *Diagn. Microbiol. Infect. Dis.* **2:** 263–276.

76. **Tison, D. L., M. Nishibuchi, J. D. Greenwood, and R. J. Seidler.** 1982. *Vibrio vulnificus* biogroup 2: new biogroup pathogenic for eels. *Appl. Environ. Microbiol.* **44:**640–646.

77. **Tison, D. L.** 1987. *Vibrio* infections, p. 599–611. *In* B. B. Wentworth (ed.), *Diagnostic Procedures for Bacterial, Mycotic and Parasitic Infections*, 7th ed. American Public Health Association, Washington, D.C.

78. **Uchimura, M., K. Koiwai, Y. Tsuruoka, and H. Tanaka.** 1993. High prevalence of thermostable direct hemolysis (TDH)-like toxin in *Vibrio mimicus* strains isolated from diarrhoeal patients. *Epidemiol. Infect.* **111:**49–53.

79. **Weintraub, A., G. Widmalm, P.-E. Jansson, M. Jansson, K. Hultenby, and M. J. Albert.** 1994. *Vibrio cholerae* O139 Bengal possesses a capsular polysaccharide which confers increased virulence. *Microb. Pathog.* **16:**235–241.

Aeromonas and *Plesiomonas**

MARTIN ALTWEGG

32

TAXONOMY

Members of the genera *Aeromonas* and *Plesiomonas* are oxidase-positive, gram-negative rods with mainly polar flagellation and both respiratory and fermentative metabolism (facultative anaerobes) (95, 104). On the basis of these characteristics, they were listed as belonging to the family *Vibrionaceae* in the first edition of *Bergey's Manual of Systematic Bacteriology* (18). More recently, mainly on the basis of molecular genetic evidence, it has been proposed that aeromonads should be classified in a separate family, *Aeromonadaceae* (32, 79), whereas *Plesiomonas* seems most closely related to the genus *Proteus* in the family *Enterobacteriaceae* (79).

While the genus *Plesiomonas* still includes only a single species, *Plesiomonas shigelloides* (63, 104), four phenotypically separable *Aeromonas* species, *A. hydrophila*, *A. caviae*, *A. sobria*, and *A. salmonicida*, with the last one having three subspecies (*A. salmonicida* subsp. *salmonicida*, *A. salmonicida* subsp. *masoucida*, and *A. salmonicida* subsp. *achromogenes*), were recognized in 1984 (95). Thereafter, several new phenotypic species and DNA hybridization groups (HGs) have been described, some of which are not yet named (Table 1). The following new *Aeromonas* species and subspecies have not been mentioned in the 6th edition of the *Manual of Clinical Microbiology* (63) or have been newly described or named since then: *A. ichthiosmia* (107), *A. enteropelogenes* (106), *A. encheleia* (38), *A. bestiarum* (4), *A. popoffii* (57), and *A. salmonicida* subsp. *smithia* (16). Despite this progress, the taxonomy of aeromonads is still very confusing due to inconsistencies in the relevant literature resulting in reclassifications or extended descriptions of existing taxa. The following issues warrant special attention. (i) Strains originally assigned to HG8 and HG10 have later been shown to belong to a single species, *A. veronii* (HG8/10), consisting of two biovars, *A. veronii* biovar veronii (esculin hydrolysis and ornithine decarboxylase positive) and *A. veronii* biovar sobria (esculin hydrolysis and ornithine decarboxylase negative) (21). Clinical isolates previously identified as *A. sobria* are actually *A. veronii* biovar sobria. Strains of the genomic species *A. sobria* (*A. sobria* sensu stricto: HG7) have not yet been found in clinical specimens. (ii) *A. enteropelogenes* and *A. ichthiosmia* have now been shown to be most probably identical to the earlier proposed species *A. trota* and *A. veronii* biovar sobria, respectively (31). The former names should therefore not be used until the issue has been resolved by the Taxonomic Working Group on *Aeromonas* that has been established within the *Vibrionaceae* Subcommittee of the International Committee on Systemic Bacteriology (21). (iii) Very recently, it has been shown by a polyphasic approach that the strains originally described as *A. eucrenophila* (105) do not represent a homogeneous species but, rather, represent two subgroups, subgroups I and II (55). While only subgroup I (including five of the original strains) is now regarded as *A. eucrenophila*, subgroup II could not be differentiated from members of *A. encheleia* and HG11 strains. This has led to the emended description of the two species *A. eucrenophila* and *A. encheleia* (58).

DESCRIPTION OF THE GENERA

Members of the genus *Aeromonas* (21, 63, 95, 115) are gram-negative, straight, rod-shaped to coccoid cells with rounded ends. They are 1.0 to 3.5 μm long and 0.3 to 1.0 μm wide, and most possess polar, usually monotrichous flagella with a wavelength of 1.7 μm. Peritrichous flagella may be formed in young cultures on solid medium. Nonmotile species are *A. salmonicida* and *A. media*, but strains of the other species may occasionally lack flagella as well. Aeromonads are oxidase and catalase positive, reduce nitrate to nitrite, and ferment D-glucose (as well as many other carbohydrates) to acid or to acid and gas. Many exoenzymes, i.e., amylase, DNase, esterases, peptidases, arylamidases, and other hydrolytic enzymes, are produced (22, 115). Their main cellular fatty acids are hexadecanoic acid (16:0), hexadecenoic acid (16:1), and octadecenoic acid (18:1) (56, 75), and the guanine-plus-cytosine content of their DNA is in the range of between 57 and 63% (57, 58, 95). They grow over a wide temperature range (0 to 45°C); human (mesophilic) strains grow at between 10 and 42°C (46), whereas the nonmotile, psychrophilic species have a maximum growth temperature of 37°C (*A. media*) or lower (*A. salmonicida*) (5, 63). Some mesophilic strains are biochemically more active at 22°C than at 37°C. In brain heart infusion medium at 28°C, growth occurs at between pH 4.5 and 9.0 and in the presence of NaCl concentrations of between 0 and 4% (90). *Aeromonas* spp. are resistant to the vibriostatic

* This chapter contains information presented in chapter 36 by J. Michael Janda, Sharon L. Abbott, and Amy M. Carnahan in the sixth edition of this Manual.

TABLE 1 Currently recognized genomic and phenotypic species in the genus *Aeromonas* and their occurrence in clinical specimens

DNA HG	Genospecies	Phenospecies	Occurrence in clinical specimens[a]	Remarks
1	*A. hydrophila*	*A. hydrophila*	+ +	
2	*A. bestiarum*	*A. hydrophila*	+	
3	Nonmotile, psychrophilic			
	A. salmonicida subsp. *salmonicida*	*A. salmonicida*	−	
	A. salmonicida subsp. *achromogenes*		−	
	A. salmonicida subsp. *masoucida*		−	
	A. salmonicida subsp. *smithia*		−	
	Motile, mesophilic			
	Unnamed	*A. hydrophila*	+	
4	*A. caviae*	*A. caviae*	+ +	
5A	(*A. media*) Unnamed	*A. caviae*	+	HGs 5A and 5B may constitute two subspecies, with HG 5B consisting of two biovars
5B	*A. media*	*A. media*	−	
		A. caviae	+	
6	*A. eucrenophila*	*A. eucrenophila*	−[b]	Extended description (55, 58); some of the original *A. eucrenophila* strains have been reclassified as *A. encheleia.*
7	*A. sobria*	*A. sobria*	−	
8	*A. veronii* biovar sobria	*A. sobria*	+ +	Includes *A. ichthiosmia* strains (31, 107)
10	*A. veronii* biovar *veronii*	*A. veronii*	+	
9	*A. jandaei*	*A. jandaei*	+	
11	*A. encheleia*	*A. encheleia*	−	Extended description (55, 58); includes *A. encheleia*, HG 11 strains, and some of the previous *A. eucrenophila* strains
12	*A. schubertii*	*A. schubertii*	+	
13	Unnamed	*Aeromonas* group 501	+[c]	Indole positive, lysine decarboxylase negative
14	*A. trota*	*A. trota*	+	Includes *A. enteropelogenes* strains (31, 106)
15	*A. allosaccharophila*	*A. allosaccharophila*	−[d]	
16	*A. popoffii*	*A. popoffii*	−	

[a] + +, common; +, rare; −, not isolated to date.
[b] One strain of unknown significance was isolated from the wound of a human in Switzerland (58).
[c] Only two strains are known; these are related to *A. schubertii* (48).
[d] One strain was isolated from a diarrheic stool specimen in the United States (78).

compound 2,4-diamino-6,7-diisopropylpteridine (O/129), but rare O/129-susceptible strains have been reported (23).

Members of the species *P. shigelloides* (formerly known as C27 or *A. shigelloides*), the only species of the genus *Plesiomonas* (104), are straight, gram-negative rods with rounded ends. They are about 3.0 μm long and 0.8 to 1.0 μm wide, and they are usually motile, with two to five lophotrichous flagella with wavelengths of 3.5 to 4.0 μm in stained preparations. Nonmotile flagellated and nonmotile atrichous strains may occur. In very young cultures (2 to 4 h old) lateral flagella with shorter wavelengths (less than 1.7 μm) have been observed in addition to polar flagella. *Plesiomonas* is oxidase and catalase positive, reduces nitrate to nitrite, and ferments D-glucose (as well as a few other carbohydrates) without the production of gas. The main cellular fatty acids are hexadecanoic acid (16:0), hexadecenoic acid (16:1), octadecanoic acid (18:0), and octadecenoic acid (18:1) (26). The percentage ratios of 16:1 to 16:0 fatty acids and of 18:1 to 18:0 fatty acids can be used to differentiate *P. shigelloides* (ratios of 0.8 and 1.5, respectively) from aeromonads (ratios of 1.2 and 6.0, respectively). *Plesiomonas* DNA has a guanine-plus-cytosine content of 51% and can grow over a wide temperature range (8 to 45°C). *Plesiomonas* strains tolerate NaCl concentrations of from 0 to 5% and a pH of from 4.0 to 8.0 (81). Most strains are susceptible to O/129.

NATURAL HABITATS

Aeromonads are mainly found in aquatic ecosystems worldwide, with densities ranging from <1 to about 1,000 cells per ml of groundwater, drinking water at treatment plants and in water distribution systems, clean rivers, lakes, and storage reservoirs. Higher densities, i.e., up to $>10^8$ cells per ml, are found in wastewater, treated sewage, crude sewage, and domestic sewage sludge (50). Occasionally, *Aero-*

monas may also be found in marine environments, although these organisms seem to prefer salt waters interfacing with fresh waters. Especially for low-nutrient waters, these numbers may be an underestimate considering the fact that *Aeromonas*, like many other gram-negative bacteria, may enter a viable but noncultivable state (50, 94). Although environmental strains may express a number of putative virulence factors, there is now increasing evidence that strains associated with clinical infections are usually, but not always, from genomic species different from those isolated from drinking water and environmental sources (86, 110). Various *Aeromonas* species occur widely and in very high numbers in both fresh and processed foods, where they can grow or at least survive even when the food is held at adequate refrigeration temperatures, i.e., at approximately 4°C (91). However, a direct link between food and disease has been documented only very rarely (14, 19). *Aeromonas* species are associated with a wide variety of diseases in warm- and cold-blooded vertebrates, including frogs, fish, reptiles, snakes, birds, and humans (39). Certain genomic species (HGs 1, 4, and 8) seem to predominate in clinical specimens (10, 73), while others are mainly considered environmental (Table 1) (4, 38, 57, 63).

The aquatic distribution of *P. shigelloides* is limited by its minimum growth temperature of 8°C and its lack of halophilism. It may be found in fresh and estuarine water rather than in a marine environment, primarily in tropical countries (15, 20, 111). However, it has also been shown to occur in surface water in Middle Europe (103). Its animal host range is wider than that of *Aeromonas* (freshwater fish, shellfish, oysters, toads, snakes, monkeys, dogs, cats, goats, pigs, poultry, and cattle) (20, 115).

CLINICAL SIGNIFICANCE

Aeromonas

There are two major disease categories associated with *Aeromonas* spp.: intestinal infections and extraintestinal infections (septicemia and wound, ocular, bone and joint, intra-abdominal, and other infections) (12, 60, 114). Not all species are found at identical frequencies in the various syndromes; e.g., *A. caviae*, a quite common cause of milder, self-limiting gastroenteritis, is rarely, if ever, seen as a cause of extraintestinal infections, especially septicemia (61). Extraintestinal infections are usually either secondary to gastroenteritis (e.g., septicemia) or due to traumatic injury and subsequent contact with contaminated water.

Diarrheal Disease

Definitive experimental evidence for the causative role of *Aeromonas* spp. in gastrointestinal disorders is still lacking. Studies with volunteers have failed, although strains possessing various putative virulence factors were used (83). However, most epidemiological studies have shown that the presence of these organisms in stools is significantly more often associated with diarrhea than with the carrier state (12, 65), and several recent studies have documented a direct link between food contaminated with *Aeromonas* species and the development of gastrointestinal disease, thus supporting the clinical significance of these organisms. A case of moderate diarrhea was reported after consumption of a ready-to-eat shrimp cocktail, with *A. hydrophila* being isolated both from the incriminated food and from the stool of the patient. Both isolates had identical ribotypes (14). Similarly, investigators described a patient who developed severe *Aeromonas* infection after shucking shellfish (41). Furthermore, a small outbreak involving 22 of 27 people at a Swedish *landgang* (smorgasbord) was recently described (72). Patients developed within 20 to 34 h typical signs of acute diarrheal illness of short duration. High numbers of *A. hydrophila* were isolated from all the meat samples tested.

Aeromonas-associated gastroenteritis may affect both children and adults (42, 101), with the highest seasonal incidence occurring during the summer months (higher temperatures presumably result in higher numbers of organisms in both contaminated food and water (44, 85). In developed countries two populations, children and travelers, seem to be primarily affected (12, 65, 97). This may be explained by the following observations (12): (i) different species are predominant at different geographical locations; e.g., *A. hydrophila* and *A. veronii* biovar sobria (formerly called *A. sobria*) were the main isolates from clinical as well as from environmental specimens in Australia and Thailand, whereas European and American studies revealed a majority of *A. caviae* isolates; (ii) the predominant species are associated with childhood diarrhea; i.e., the frequencies of isolation of the various *Aeromonas* species from children were highest for *A. veronii* biovar sobria and *A. hydrophila* in Australia, whereas *A. caviae* was most often found in Europe and in the United States, with the highest incidence being in children younger than 5 years of age. In contrast, species other than *A. caviae* were significantly more often isolated from Swiss adults than from children. It has been speculated that mild gastrointestinal infections are caused by *A. caviae* in children, leading to some type of immunity against this particular species but not against the other species to which individuals would remain susceptible when coming into contact with them later during their lives (e.g., as travelers). This has been nicely illustrated in a study performed in Thailand in which *Aeromonas* species were significantly more often isolated from diarrheic Peace Corps volunteers than from controls, whereas the isolation frequencies from symptomatic and asymptomatic Thais were about equally high (93).

As is the case for most enteropathogenic organisms, clinical symptoms do not allow a presumptive diagnosis of the etiological agent. *Aeromonas*-associated gastrointestinal infections tend to be generally mild, self-limiting diseases with watery diarrhea. However, rare reports have described seriously ill patients with bloody stools and numerous fecal leukocytes, very much resembling the bacillary dysentery caused by *Shigella*. There seems to be a tendency toward acute illness in developing countries and in children in industrialized countries, whereas *Aeromonas* infection appears to be a rather chronic disease in adults in developed regions (12). It is likely that these differences in clinical presentation are somehow related to the species involved. A clue to this may be that putative virulence factors (hemolysins and other products) are more frequently found in *A. hydrophila* and *A. veronii* biovar sobria than in *A. caviae* (52, 113).

Wound Infections

Skin and soft tissue (60, 61) are the second most common sites after the gastrointestinal tract from which *Aeromonas* spp. are isolated. Most skin and soft tissue *Aeromonas* infections are due to *A. hydrophila* or *A. veronii*, occur after traumatic exposure to contaminated water or soil, and predominantly involve the lower extremities. Manifestations include acute inflammation of subcutaneous tissues with induration which can be treated successfully by surgical debridement and adequate antimicrobial chemotherapy. However, in compromised patients (patients with diabetes, cirrhosis, agranulocytopenia, etc.) more severe and even fatal infections including myonecrosis and ecthyma gangrenosum may occur. Astonishing and as yet unexplained observations are the facts that about 75% of *Aeromonas*-associated wound infections have been observed in males and that more than 90% of them have been recorded in adults, although traumas are more frequently encountered in children than in adults. Soft tissue infections ranging from purulent discharge to necrosis have been reported after the use of medicinal leeches (*Hirudo medicinalis*) to relieve venous congestion after reconstructive surgery (76, 109). Leeches are known to harbor aeromonads in their gut, from which they can reach the wound during attachment.

Septicemia

Although there are rare patients with no known predisposing condition (43), *Aeromonas* septicemia is usually seen in association with hepatitis, biliary or pancreatic disease, or malignancy, particularly acute leukemia, aplastic anemia, and solid tumors (61, 115). The overall incidence appears to be very low (<1% of all episodes of sepsis) in the United States, while the numbers in Southeast Asia are considerably higher (70). *Aeromonas* bacteremia is most often seen in adult males with classic signs of sepsis (fever in >90% of the patients and chills in >70% of the patients). *A. hydrophila* and *A. veronii* (both biotypes) cause more than 90% of all reported episodes of *Aeromonas* bacteremia (61). As with gastroenteritis, the majority of cases of septicemia are observed during the warmer months of the year. The fatality rate is in the range of between 30 and 70% (60, 70).

Ocular Infections

Eye infections caused by *Aeromonas* are rare. They range from mild conjunctivitis to corneal ulcer and endophthalmitis (60, 68) and are usually associated with contact lenses or penetrating injuries. Asymptomatic conjunctival colonization has been described (108). A double infection with *A. hydrophila* and *P. shigelloides* was observed in an 8-year-old boy who sustained a corneal laceration following an injury caused by a fishhook. He rapidly developed endophthalmitis, and both organisms were cultured from the anterior chamber after enucleation (30).

Respiratory Tract Infections

Although aeromonads are often cultured from respiratory tract specimens such as throat swabs, sputum, and tracheal secretions, most isolates represent transient colonization rather than true infection. Bona fide *Aeromonas*-associated pneumonia has adequately been documented in a number of patients, with the responsible organisms being isolated both from the respiratory tract and from the blood (61). Most of these infections were associated with an underlying disease or with water contact (swimming, near drowning) and had fatal outcomes (37). Very recently, a case of *A. hydrophila* lung abscess was described in a previously healthy individual (54).

Miscellaneous Infections

Aeromonas spp. may be found in patients with various other infections. However, it is difficult to evaluate the clinical significance of all these isolates unless the organisms are found in pure culture. Infections that have been attributed to aeromonads include meningitis (117), osteomyelitis (35, 68), septic arthritis (25), peritonitis (87), endocarditis (89), cholecystitis (92), and urinary tract infections (68, 116).

Plesiomonas

As with *Aeromonas* spp., *P. shigelloides* has been implicated as the causative agent of gastroenteritis as well as of extraintestinal infections, primarily septicemia (20). Although feeding experiments with humans did result in the excretion of the organism from about one-third of the volunteers but not in diarrhea (47), several epidemiological studies suggest that *Plesiomonas* is a possible agent in gastrointestinal disease (115). In addition, well-investigated outbreaks of diarrheal disease, mainly in Japan, have been attributed to this organism (51, 112). Human carriers are very rare except in areas where the organism is endemic (e.g., up to 24% in Thailand) (93). Infections have been associated with travel to or residence in tropical and subtropical countries, with the consumption of raw seafood, or with exposure to amphibians or reptiles (20, 100). Similar to *Aeromonas* spp., the peak season of *Plesiomonas*-associated diarrheal disease appears to be the summer months. The spectrum of illness ranges from short-lived episodes of watery stools to several days of dysentery-like diarrhea (49, 80) and has not been reported to affect particular age groups more often than others.

Extraintestinal infections due to *P. shigelloides*, primarily septicemia and meningitis, are very rare but are severe and have been associated with a high mortality rate (20). Occasionally, this organism has been isolated from anatomic sources other than feces, blood, and cerebrospinal fluid of both immunocompromised patients and patients with no known underlying disease (34, 40, 59, 88).

COLLECTION, TRANSPORT, AND STORAGE OF SPECIMENS

Both *Aeromonas* and *Plesiomonas* are nonfastidious organisms that survive under a wide variety of conditions; e.g., aeromonads survive for up to 5 days after inoculation in glycerol-buffered saline (82). Although systematic investigations are essentially lacking, special precautions do not seem to be necessary for this group of organisms. Hence, multipurpose transport media are recommended for swabs, whereas Cary-Blair transport medium is certainly appropriate for fecal specimens. However, stool samples are preferable to rectal swabs for the recovery of either agent (63).

ISOLATION PROCEDURES

Aeromonas and *Plesiomonas* grow on most common, routinely used media (e.g., blood or chocolate agar and most enteric differential agars) (36). Their isolation from clinical specimens other than feces therefore does not pose any problems. With stool and environmental specimens, a wide variety of specially designed differential and/or selective media have been used mainly for the isolation of *Aeromonas* spp. (66).

Aeromonas

For stool specimens, blood agar (with or without ampicillin) and cefsulodin-irgasan-novobiocin (CIN) agar have proven useful. Both have advantages and disadvantages: CIN agar can be used for the simultaneous recovery of *Yersinia* spp. and is quite selective, but direct oxidase testing from CIN agar is not recommended because mannitol can be fermented, resulting in a low pH and a possibly false-negative oxidase test result (7, 53). In addition, CIN agar containing 4 rather than 15 μg of cefsulodin per ml should be used due to inhibition of many *Aeromonas* strains by higher concentrations of this selective agent (6, 7). Blood agar with 10 μg of ampicillin per ml allows direct oxidase testing but is not very selective and nonhemolytic strains (e.g., *A. caviae*) may be missed. In addition, susceptibility to ampicillin has been reported for *Aeromonas* spp. and is a key feature of *A. trota* (24, 69). For reasons of cost-effectiveness, many laboratories look for *Aeromonas* spp. on MacConkey, Hektoen enteric, or other agars used for the isolation of *Salmonella* and *Shigella*. Since many aeromonads are sucrose or lactose positive, some strains may easily be missed. Thiosulfate-citrate-bile salts-sucrose agar (TCBS) is often inhibitory to *Aeromonas* strains and therefore should not be used (115). Alkaline peptone water is the most effective enrichment broth for aeromonads; however, the clinical significance of additional isolates has been questioned.

Plesiomonas

The low incidence of *P. shigelloides* in the United States and Europe may preclude the use of a separate medium such as inositol-bile salts-brilliant green (IBG) agar. When present in large numbers, such strains can be isolated on regular enteric medium (115). If IBG agar is used, direct oxidase testing is to be avoided because a fermentable sugar is present in the medium. Because a considerable number of *Plesiomonas* strains are susceptible to ampicillin, media containing this antibiotic should not be used (99). The use of alkaline peptone water as enrichment is controversial, and bile peptone broth, also effective as enrichment for other members of the *Vibrionaceae*, has been shown to be superior.

IDENTIFICATION

A presumptive identification of the genera *Vibrio*, *Aeromonas*, and *Plesiomonas* can be made for oxidase-positive strains that grow on MacConkey agar and ferment D-glucose (115). Considering the multitude of *Vibrio* and *Aeromonas* species, an assignment to one of these two genera is not always without problems and essentially includes testing for resistance to the vibriostatic compound O/129, for growth in 6% NaCl, and for the presence of ornithine decarboxylase. However, it should be borne in mind that increasing resistance to O/129 has been observed in *Vibrio cholerae*. In contrast, identification of *P. shigelloides* is usually straightforward on the basis of its unique biochemical properties (lysine decarboxylase, ornithine decarboxylase, and arginine dihydrolase positive, a combination not found in any *Aeromonas* or *Vibrio* species).

Commercially available identification kits are not very reliable for the identification of members of the family *Vibrionaceae*. The three main problems are as follows. (i) Aeromonads are at best identified to the level of the three phenospecies that most often occur in clinical specimens, i.e., *A. hydrophila*, *A. caviae*, and *A. veronii* (66). Often, the name *A. sobria* is still used as a synonym for the now correct designation *A. veronii* biovar sobria. The other species are usually not included in the databases due to the lack of reliable tests for the separation of the species (98). Conventional biochemical tests that allow the identification of *P. shigelloides* and the various phenotypic *Aeromonas* species are listed in Table 2. Tests useful for differentiation within phenotypic *A. hydrophila* strains (e.g., HGs 1 to 3) and within phenotypic *A. caviae* strains (e.g., HGs 4, 5A, and 5B) are given in Tables 3 and 4, respectively. It is noteworthy that some biochemical tests are temperature and/or medium dependent; e.g., Fay and Barry's medium detects lysine decarboxylase faster and more sensitively than either Møller's or Falkow's medium (11). (ii) *A. caviae* is frequently misidentified as *Vibrio fluvialis*. However, these two species can easily be differentiated by using the basic tests mentioned above (e.g., salt tolerance) and esculin hydrolysis (positive for *A. caviae* and negative for *V. fluvialis*) (115). (iii) *A. veronii* biovar veronii may be confused with *V. cholerae* since both are ornithine decarboxylase positive. In addition, resistance to O/129 is now rather common for *V. cholerae*.

Almost any method available for the subtyping of *Aeromonas* has also been evaluated as a tool for the identification of unknown strains and as an approach to addressing taxonomic problems (9, 21). These methods, however, are not applicable in a routine setting. Among the methods that have yielded useful results are multilocus enzyme electrophoresis, ribotyping, cellular fatty acid analysis, amplified fragment length polymorphism analysis, and 16S rRNA sequence analysis. Other methods like bacteriophage typing, protein fingerprinting, and serotyping have little or no taxonomic value but still may be valuable tools for epidemiological investigations.

SEROLOGIC TESTS

As is the case for many other intestinal pathogens, the demonstration of an immune response to *Aeromonas* spp. is not a reliable diagnostic test. However, a fourfold or greater rise in antibody titers between acute- and convalescent-phase sera has been demonstrated in certain patients. In other studies no differences in titers were found between sera from patients and controls (65). Several techniques (tube agglutination, immunoblotting, and enzyme-linked immunosorbent assay) with various antigens have been used, but none has received general acceptance due to low sensitivity and limited specificity (74). Intestinal secretory immunoglobulin A (IgA) against the homologous strains were found in patients shedding *A. hydrophila* or *A. veronii* biovar sobria but not in those excreting *A. caviae*. This was considered an indicator for the increased enteropathogenicity of the former two species (64). In addition, IgG antibody responses to *Aeromonas* isolates have been described in the sera of divers. Repeated exposure was considered necessary for the generation of a specific systemic immune response (77). The presence of serum O agglutinins against the patient's own isolates has also been described for *P. shigelloides* gastroenteritis (33) and cholecystitis (28), but no major studies on the diagnostic value of measuring the immune response in patients have been published.

Serotyping of *Aeromonas* strains can be done in very few laboratories. Serotyping has revealed that genomospecies are serologically heterogeneous, i.e., most serogroups can be found in more than one species, and that serogroups O:11, O:34, and O:16 seem to be of special importance in human infections (62). Serologic cross-reactions between *A. trota* and *V. cholerae* O:139 Bengal have been described (3), but these seem to be the exception rather than the rule (62). Two serotyping schemes have been published for *Plesiomonas*. Cross-reactions have particularly been observed with *Shigella* (*S. sonnei* and *S. dysenteriae*) (20) and have sometimes led, when serotyping was available, to the initial misidentification of *P. shigelloides* as *Shigella* (1).

TABLE 2 Relevant biochemical properties of *P. shigelloides* and the various phenotypic *Aeromonas* spp. to be expected in clinical specimens[a]

Characteristic	Response							
	A. hydrophila	*A. caviae*	*A. veronii* biovar sobria	*A. veronii* biovar veronii	*A. jandaei*	*A. schubertii*	*A. trota*	*P. shigelloides*
DNase	+	+	+	+	ND	+	ND	−
Urea hydrolysis	−	−	−	−	−	−	ND	−
Growth in KCN medium	+	+	v	v	ND	−	ND	−
Indole	+	+	+	+	+	−	+	+
Gas from glucose	+	−	+	+	+	−	+	−
Arginine dihydrolase	+	+	+	−	+	+	+	+
Lysine decarboxylase	+	−	+	+	+	+	+	+
Ornithine decarboxylase	−	−	−	+	−	−	−	+
Voges-Proskauer	+	−	+	+	+	−[b]	−	−
Acid from:								
L-Arabinose	+	+	−	−	−	−	−	−
Lactose	−	+	−	−	ND	−	ND	−
Sucrose	+	+	+	+	−	−	−	−
m-Inositol	−	−	−	−	−	−	−	+
D-Mannitol	+	+	+	+	+	−	+	−
Salicin	+	+	−	+	−	−	−	v
Cellobiose	v	+	v	v	−	−	+	−
Esculin hydrolysis	+	+	−	+	−	−	−	−
β-hemolysis on sheep blood agar	+	−	+	+	+	V	V	−
Susceptibility to:								
Cephalothin	−	−	+	+	−	+	−	+
Ampicillin	−	−	−	−	−	−	+	+
O/129, 10 μg/150 μg	−/−	−/−	−/−	−/−	−/−	−/−	−/−	+/+

[a] +, positive; −, negative; V, variable (20 to 80% positive); ND, no data available.
[b] Depending on the method used (58).

TABLE 3 Identification of genomic species within phenotypic *A. hydrophila*[a]

Characteristic	HG1, *A. hydrophila*		HG2, *A. bestiarum*		HG3, unnamed (*A. salmonicida*)	
	25°C	35°C	25°C	35°C	25°C	35°C
Acid from:						
Phenylpyruvic acid	+	V	+	V	+	+
D-Rhamnose	−	−	+	+	−	−
D-Sorbitol	−	−	−	−	+	+
Lactose		−		−		+
Salicin		+		−		+
Utilization of:						
DL-Lactate	V	V	−	−	−	−
Urocanic acid	−	−	+	+	+	+
Elastase	+	V	+	−	+	V
Gluconate oxidation		V		−		−
Lysine decarboxylase	+	+	+	−	+	V

[a] Results for some tests may vary in relation to incubation temperature. Data are from previous reports (2, 4). −, <25% of strains positive; V, 25 to 75% of strains positive; +, >75% of strains positive.

TABLE 4 Identification of genomic species within the *A. caviae* complex[a]

Characteristic	HG4, *A. caviae*	HG5A, unnamed (*A. media*)	HG5B, *A. media*
Acid from:			
Lactose	V	+	+
Cellobiose	V	+	+
Utilization of:			
DL-Lactate	+	−	+
Citrate	+	−	−

[a] The incubation temperature was 30°C. Data are from previous reports (10, 45) −, <25% of strains positive; V, 25 to 75% of strains positive; +, >75% of strains positive.

ANTIBIOTIC SUSCEPTIBILITIES

Most *Aeromonas* spp. are resistant to penicillin, ampicillin, carbenicillin, and ticarcillin but susceptible to expanded- and broad-spectrum cephalosporins, aminoglycosides, carbapenems, chloramphenicol, tetracyclines, trimethoprim-sulfamethoxazole, and the quinolones (63). Most aeromonads produce inducible β-lactamases (84). Rapid commercial systems should be used with caution because very major errors have been observed with β-lactam antibiotics (102). Susceptibility to cephalothin is correlated to the species; i.e., most *A. veronii* biovar sobria strains are susceptible, whereas *A. hydrophila* and *A. caviae* strains are resistant. *A. trota* is peculiar in its uniform susceptibility to ampicillin. The use of ampicillin in selective medium may consequently lead to an underestimation of the prevalence of this species. Recently, *Aeromonas* strains from Taiwan have been shown to be more resistant to tetracycline, trimethoprim-sulfamethoxazole, some cephalosporins, and aminoglycosides than strains from the United States and Australia (71).

P. shigelloides seems to be susceptible to most major classes of antibiotics including trimethoprim (alone or in combination with sulfamethoxazole), cephalosporins, chloramphenicol, and quinolones (67). Most strains produce a β-lactamase(s) that can be detected by the nitrocefin method and are therefore resistant to penicillins unless these are combined with a β-lactamase inhibitor (29). Many strains may also be resistant to the aminoglycosides (except netilmicin) and to the tetracyclines (67).

INTERPRETATION AND REPORTING OF RESULTS

While the clinical significance of *Aeromonas* isolates from extraintestinal sources is often quite obvious, especially if they are recovered in pure cultures, their causative role in patients with gastrointestinal diseases is usually difficult to assess. In the absence of other enteric pathogens (including rotaviruses in children), a significance may be assumed for most isolates in patients younger than about the age of 10 years. In adults (mainly those with a history of recent travel to a tropical country), only phenotypic *A. hydrophila* and *A. veronii* (both biovars) seem to be significant. Consequently, it seems reasonable to differentiate and report at least these species in a routine diagnostic setting. For research purposes, however, it is mandatory to determine genomic species in order to facilitate the definition of a species-associated disease spectrum in the future. The determination of an immune response may be helpful as well, but no tests have been standardized, nor have their sensitivities and specificities been adequately determined. The use of molecular biology-based techniques like PCR for the detection of *Aeromonas* or *Plesiomonas* directly in clinical specimens or for the detection of putative virulence factors in isolates (17) is not appropriate for a diagnostic laboratory as long as no clear associations either between clinical syndromes and particular species or between clinical syndromes and the presence of particular virulence factors have been established.

REFERENCES

1. **Abbott, S. L., R. P. Kokka, and J. M. Janda.** 1991. Laboratory investigations on the low pathogenic potential of *Plesiomonas shigelloides*. *J. Clin. Microbiol.* **29:**148–153.
2. **Abbott, S. L., W. K. W. Cheung, S. Kroske-Bystrom, T. Malekzadeh, and J. M. Janda.** 1992. Identification of *Aeromonas* strains to the genospecies level in the clinical laboratory. *J. Clin. Microbiol.* **30:**1262–1266.
3. **Albert, M. J., M. Ansaruzzaman, T. Shimada, A. Rahman, N. A. Bhuiyan, S. Nahar, F. Qadri, and M. S. Islam.** 1995. Characterization of *Aeromonas trota* strains that cross-react with *Vibrio cholerae* O139 Bengal. *J. Clin. Microbiol.* **33:**3119–3123.
4. **Ali, A., A. Carnahan, M. Altwegg, J. Lüthy-Hottenstein, and S. Joseph.** 1996. *Aeromonas bestiarum* sp. nov. (formerly genomospecies DNA group 2 *A. hydrophila*), a new species isolated from non-human sources. *Med. Microbiol. Lett.* **5:**156–165.
5. **Allen, D. A., B. Austin, and R. R. Colwell.** 1993. *Aeromonas media*, a new species isolated from river water. *Int. J. Syst. Bacteriol.* **33:**599–604.
6. **Alonso, J. L., I. Amoros, and M. A. Alonso.** 1996. Differential susceptibility of aeromonads and coliforms to cefsulodin. *Appl. Environ. Microbiol.* **62:**1885–1888.
7. **Altorfer, R., M. Altwegg, J. Zollinger-Iten, and A. von Graevenitz.** 1985. Growth of *Aeromonas* spp. on cefsulodin-irgasan-novobiocin agar selective for *Yersinia enterocolitica*. *J. Clin. Microbiol.* **22:**478–480.
8. **Altwegg, M.** 1985. *Aeromonas caviae*: an enteric pathogen? *Infection* **13:**228–230.
9. **Altwegg, M.** 1996. Subtyping methods for *Aeromonas* species, p. 109–125. *In* B. Austin, M. Altwegg, P. J. Gosling, and S. Joseph (ed.), *The Genus* Aeromonas. John Wiley & Sons Ltd., Chichester, England.
10. **Altwegg, M., A. G. Steigerwalt, R. Altwegg-Bissig, J. Lüthy-Hottenstein, and D. J. Brenner.** 1990. Biochemical identification of *Aeromonas* genospecies isolated from humans. *J. Clin. Microbiol.* **28:**258–264.
11. **Altwegg, M., A. von Graevenitz, and J. Zollinger-Iten.** 1987. Medium and temperature dependence of decarboxylase reactions in *Aeromonas* spp. *Curr. Microbiol.* **14:** 1–4.
12. **Altwegg, M., and H. K. Geiss.** 1989. *Aeromonas* as a human pathogen. *Crit. Rev. Microbiol.* **16:**253–286.
13. **Altwegg, M., and M. Jöhl.** 1987. Isolation frequency of *Aeromonas* species in relation to patient age. *Eur. J. Clin. Microbiol.* **6:**55–56.
14. **Altwegg, M., G. Martinetti Lucchini, J. Lüthy-Hottenstein, and M. Rohrbach.** 1991. *Aeromonas*-associated gastroenteritis after consumption of contaminated shrimp. *Eur. J. Clin. Microbiol. Infect. Dis.* **10:**44–45.
15. **Arai, T., N. Ikejima, T. Itoh, S. Sakai, T. Shimada, and R. Sakazaki.** 1980. A survey of *Plesiomonas shigelloides* from aquatic environments, domestic animals, pets and humans. *J. Hyg. Camb.* **84:**203–211.
16. **Austin, D. A., D. McIntosh, and B. Austin.** 1989. Taxonomy of fish associated *Aeromonas* spp., with the descrip-

tion of *Aeromonas salmonicida* subsp. *smithia* subsp. nova. *Syst. Appl. Microbiol.* **11:**277–290.

17. **Baloda, S. B., K. Krovacek, L. Eriksson, T. Linne, and I. Mansson.** 1995. Detection of aerolysin gene in *Aeromonas* strains isolated from drinking water, fish and foods by the polymerase chain reaction. *Comp. Immunol. Microbiol. Infect. Dis.* **18:**17–26.
18. **Baumann, P., and R. H. W. Schubert.** 1984. Family II. *Vibrionaceae* Véron, 1965, 5245, p. 516–617. *In* N. R. Krieg and J. G. Holt (ed.), *Bergey's Manual of Systematic Bacteriology*, vol. 1. The Williams & Wilkins Co., Baltimore, Md.
19. **Bernadeschi, P., I. Bonnechi, and G. Cavallini.** 1988. *Aeromonas hydrophila* infection after cockles ingestion. *Haematologia* **73:**545.
20. **Brenden, R. A., M. A. Miller, and J. M. Janda.** 1988. Clinical disease spectrum and pathogenic factors associated with *Plesiomonas shigelloides* infections in humans. *Rev. Infect. Dis.* **10:**303–316.
21. **Carnahan, A., and M. Altwegg.** 1996. Taxonomy, p. 1–38. *In* B. Austin, M. Altwegg, P. J. Gosling, and S. Joseph (ed.), *The Genus* Aeromonas. John Wiley & Sons Ltd., Chichester, England.
22. **Carnahan, A. M., M. O'Brien, S. W. Joseph, and R. R. Colwell.** 1988. Enzymatic characterization of three *Aeromonas* species using API peptidase, API 'osidase', and API esterase test kits. *Diagn. Microbiol. Infect. Dis.* **10:** 195–203.
23. **Carnahan, A. M., and S. W. Joseph.** 1993. Systematic assessment of geographically and clinically diverse aeromonads. *Syst. Appl. Microbiol.* **16:**72–84.
24. **Carnahan, A. M., T. Chakraborty, G. R. Fanning, D. Verma, A. Ali, J. M. Janda, and S. W. Joseph.** 1991. *Aeromonas trota*, sp. nov., an ampicillin-susceptible species isolated from clinical specimens. *J. Clin. Microbiol.* **29:**1206–1210.
25. **Chmel, H., and D. Armstrong.** 1976. Acute arthritis caused by *Aeromonas hydrophila*: clinical and therapeutic aspects. *Arthritis Rheum.* **19:**169–172.
26. **Chou, S., E. Aldova, and S. Kasatiya.** 1991. Cellular fatty acid composition of *Plesiomonas shigelloides*. *J. Clin. Microbiol.* **29:**1072–1074.
27. **Chowdhury, M. A. R., H. Yamanaka, S. Miyoshi, and S. Shinoda.** 1990. Ecology of mesophilic *Aeromonas* spp. in aquatic environment of a temperate region and relationship with some biotic and abiotic environmental parameters. *Zentralbl. Bakteriol. Parasitenkd. Infektionskr. Hyg. Abt. 1 Orig.* **190:**344–356.
28. **Claesson, B. E. B., D. E. W. Holmlund, C. A. Lindhagen, and T. W. Mätzsch.** 1984. *Plesiomonas shigelloides* in acute cholecystitis: a case report. *J. Clin. Microbiol.* **20:** 985–987.
29. **Clark, R. B., P. D. Lister, L. Arneson-Rotert, and J. M. Janda.** 1990. In vitro susceptibilities of *Plesiomonas shigelloides* to 24 antibiotics and antibiotic-β-lactamase-inhibitor combinations. *Antimicrob. Agents Chemother.* **34:**159–160.
30. **Cohen, K. L., P. R. Holyk, L. R. McCarthy, and R. L. Peiffer.** 1983. *Aeromonas hydrophila* and *Plesiomonas shigelloides* endophthalmitis. *Am. J. Ophthalmol.* **96:** 403–404.
31. **Collins, M. D., A. J. Martinez-Murcia, and J. Cai.** 1994. *Aeromonas enteropelogenes* and *Aeromonas ichthiosmia* are identical to *Aeromonas trota* and *Aeromonas veronii*, respectively, as revealed by small-subunit rRNA sequence analysis. *Int. J. Syst. Bacteriol.* **43:**855–856.
32. **Colwell, R. R., M. R. MacDonell, and J. DeLey.** 1986. Proposal to recognize the family *Aeromonadaceae* fam. nov. *Int. J. Syst. Bacteriol.* **36:**473–477.
33. **Cooper, R. G., and G. W. Brown.** 1968. *Plesiomonas shigelloides* in South Australia. *J. Clin. Pathol.* **21:** 715–718.
34. **Curti, A. J., J. H. Lin, and K. Szabo.** 1985. Overwhelming post-splenectomy infection with *Plesiomonas shigelloides* in a patient cured of Hodgkin's disease. *Am. J. Clin. Pathol.* **83:**522–524.
35. **Deghrar, A., P. Nenormandie, J. M. Feron, J. F. Signoret, and A. Patel.** 1997. *Aeromonas hydrophila* bone infection. *Presse Med.* **26:**415.
36. **Desmond, E., and J. M. Janda.** 1986. Growth of *Aeromonas* species on enteric agars. *J. Clin. Microbiol.* **23:** 1065–1067.
37. **Ender, P. T., M. J. Dolan, D. Dolan, J. C. Farmer, and G. P. Melcher.** 1996. Near-drowning-associated *Aeromonas* pneumonia. *J. Emerg. Med.* **14:**737–741.
38. **Esteve, C., M. C. Gutierrez, and A. Ventosa.** 1995. *Aeromonas encheleia* sp. nov., isolated from European eels. *Int. J. Syst. Bacteriol.* **45:**462–466.
39. **Farmer, J. J., III, M. J. Arduino, and F. W. Hickman-Brenner.** 1992. The genera *Aeromonas* and *Plesiomonas*, p. 3012–3028. *In* A. Balows, H. G. Trüper, M. Dworkin, W. Harder, and K. H. Schleifer (ed.), *The Prokaryotes*, 2nd ed. Springer-Verlag, New York, N.Y.
40. **Fischer, K., T. Chakraborty, H. Hof, R. Kirchner, and O. Wamsler.** 1988. Pseudoappendicitis caused by *Plesiomonas shigelloides*. *J. Clin. Microbiol.* **26:**2675–2677.
41. **Flynn, T. J., and I. G. Knipp.** 1987. Seafood shucking as an etiology for *Aeromonas hydrophila* infection. *Arch. Intern. Med.* **147:**1816–1817.
42. **George, W. L., M. M. Nakata, J. Thompson, and M. L. White.** 1985. *Aeromonas* related diarrhea in adults. *Arch. Intern. Med.* **145:**2207–2211.
43. **Golik, A., Y. Leonov, F. Schlaeffer, I. Gluskin, and G. Lewinsohn.** 1990. *Aeromonas* species bacteremia in nonimmunocompromised hosts: two case reports and a review of the literature. *Isr. J. Med. Sci.* **26:**87–90.
44. **Gomez Campdera, J., P. Munoz, F. Lopez Prieto, R. Rodriguez Fernandez, M. Robles, M. Rodriguez Creixems, and E. Bouza Santiago.** 1996. Gastroenteritis due to *Aeromonas* in pediatrics. *An. Esp. Pediatr.* **44:** 548–552.
45. **Hänninen, M. L., and A. Siitonen.** 1995. Distribution of *Aeromonas* phenospecies and genospecies among strains isolated from water, foods or from human clinical samples. *Epidemiol. Infect.* **115:**39–50.
46. **Hänninen, M.-L.** 1994. Phenotypic characteristics of the three hybridization groups of *Aeromonas hydrophila* complex isolated from different sources. *J. Appl. Bacteriol.* **76:** 455–462.
47. **Herrington, D. A., S. Tzipori, R. M. Robins-Browne, B. D. Tall, and M. M. Levine.** 1987. In vitro and in vivo pathogenicity of *Plesiomonas shigelloides*. *Infect. Immun.* **55:**979–985.
48. **Hickman-Brenner, F. W., G. R. Fanning, M. J. Arduino, D. J. Brenner, and J. J. Farmer III.** 1988. *Aeromonas schubertii*, a new mannitol-negative species found in human clinical specimens. *J. Clin. Microbiol.* **26:** 1561–1564.
49. **Holmberg, S. D., I. K. Wachsmuth, F. W. Hickman-Brenner, P. A. Blake, and J. J. Farmer.** 1986. *Plesiomonas* enteric infections in the United States. *Ann. Intern. Med.* **105:**690–694.
50. **Holmes, P., L. M. Niccolls, and D. P. Sartory.** 1996. The ecology of mesophilic *Aeromonas* in the aquatic environment, p. 127–150. *In* B. Austin, M. Altwegg, P. J. Gosling, and S. Joseph (ed.), *The Genus* Aeromonas. John Wiley & Sons Ltd., Chichester, England.
51. **Hori, M., K. Hayashi, K. Maeshima, M. Kigawa, T.**

Miyasoto, Y. Yoneda, and Y. Hagihara. 1966. Food poisoning caused by *Aeromonas shigelloides* with an antigen common to *Shigella dysenteriae* 7. *J. Jpn. Assoc. Infect. Dis.* **39:**433–441.

52. **Howard, S. P., S. MacIntyre, and J. T. Buckley.** 1996. Toxins, p. 267–286. *In* B. Austin, M. Altwegg, P. J. Gosling, and S. Joseph (ed.), *The Genus* Aeromonas. John Wiley & Sons Ltd., Chichester, England.
53. **Hunt, L. K., T. L. Overman, and R. B. Otero.** 1981. Role of pH in oxidase variability of *Aeromonas hydrophila*. *J. Clin. Microbiol.* **13:**1054–1059.
54. **Hur, T., K. C. Cheng, and J. M. Hsieh.** 1995. *Aeromonas hydrophila* lung abscess in a previously healthy man. *Scand. J. Infect. Dis.* **27:**295.
55. **Huys, G., M. Altwegg, M.-L. Hänninen, M. Vancanneyt, L. Vauterin, R. Coopman, U. Torck, J. Lüthy-Hottenstein, P. Janssen, and K. Kersters.** 1996. Genotypic and chemotaxonomic description of two subgroups in the species *Aeromonas eucrenophila* and their affiliation to *A. encheleia* and *Aeromonas* DNA hybridization group 11. *Syst. Appl. Microbiol.* **19:**616–623.
56. **Huys, G., M. Vancanneyt, R. Coopman, P. Janssen, E. Falsen, M. Altwegg, and K. Kersters.** 1994. Cellular fatty acid composition as a chemotaxonomic marker for the differentiation of phenospecies and hybridization groups in the genus *Aeromonas*. *Int. J. Syst. Bacteriol.* **44:**651–658.
57. **Huys, G., P. Kämpfer, M. Altwegg, I. Kersters, A. Lamb, R. Coopman, J. Lüthy-Hottenstein, M. Vancanneyt, P. Janssen, and K. Kersters.** 1997. *Aeromonas popoffii* sp. nov., a mesophilic bacterium isolated from drinking water production plants and reservoirs. *Int. J. Syst. Bacteriol.* **47:**1165–1171.
58. **Huys, G., P. Kämpfer, M. Altwegg, R. Coopman, P. Janssen, M. Gillis, and K. Kersters.** 1997. Inclusion of *Aeromonas* DNA hybridization group 11 in *Aeromonas encheleia* and extended description of the species *Aeromonas eucrenophila* and *A. encheleia*. *Inst. J. Syst. Bacteriol.* **47:**1157–1164.
59. **Ingram, C. W., A. J. Morrison, Jr., and R. E. Levitz.** 1987. Gastroenteritis, sepsis, and osteomyelitis caused by *Plesiomonas shigelloides* in an immunocompetent host: case report and review of the literature. *J. Clin. Microbiol.* **25:**1791–1793.
60. **Janda, J. M., and P. S. Duffey.** 1988. Mesophilic aeromonads in human disease: current taxonomy, laboratory identification, and infectious disease spectrum. *Rev. Infect. Dis.* **10:**980–997.
61. **Janda, J. M., and S. L. Abbott.** 1996. Human pathogens, p. 151–173. *In* B. Austin, M. Altwegg, P. J. Gosling, and S. Joseph (ed.), *The Genus* Aeromonas. John Wiley & Sons Ltd., Chichester, England.
62. **Janda, J. M., S. L. Abbott, S. Khashe, G. H. Kellogg, and T. Shimada.** 1996. Further studies on biochemical characteristics and serologic properties of the genus *Aeromonas*. *J. Clin. Microbiol.* **34:**1930–1933.
63. **Janda, J. M., S. L. Abbott, and A. M. Carnahan.** 1995. *Aeromonas* and *Plesiomonas*, p. 477–482. *In* P. R. Murray, E. J. Baron, M. A. Pfaller, F. C. Tenover, and R. H. Yolken (ed.), *Manual of Clinical Microbiology*, 6th ed. American Society for Microbiology, Washington, D.C.
64. **Jiang, Z. D., A. C. Nelson, J. J. Mathewson, C. D. Ericsson, and H. L. DuPont.** 1991. Intestinal secretory immune response to infection with *Aeromonas* species and *Plesiomonas shigelloides* among students from the United States in Mexico. *J. Infect. Dis.* **164:**979–982.
65. **Joseph, S. W.** 1996. *Aeromonas* gastrointestinal disease: a case study in causation, p. 311–335. *In* B. Austin, M. Altwegg, P. J. Gosling, and S. Joseph (ed.), *The Genus* Aeromonas. John Wiley & Sons Ltd., Chichester, England.
66. **Joseph, S. W., and A. Carnahan.** 1994. The isolation, identification, and systematics of the motile *Aeromonas* species. *Annu. Rev. Fish Dis.* **4:**315–343.
67. **Kain, K. C., and M. T. Kelly.** 1989. Antimicrobial susceptibility of *Plesiomonas shigelloides* from patients with diarrhea. *Antimicrob. Agents Chemother.* **33:**1609–1610.
68. **Khardori, N., and V. Fainstein.** 1988. *Aeromonas* and *Plesiomonas* as etiological agents. *Annu. Rev. Microbiol.* **42:**395–419.
69. **Kilpatrick, M. E., J. Escarmilla, A. L. Bourgeois, J. J. Adkins, and R. C. Rockhill.** 1987. Overview of four U.S. Navy overseas research studies on *Aeromonas*. *Experientia* **43:**365–366.
70. **Ko, W. C., and Y. C. Chuang.** 1995. *Aeromonas* bacteremia: review of 59 episodes. *Clin. Infect. Dis.* **20:**1298–1304.
71. **Ko, W. C., K. W. Yu, C. Y. Liu, C. T. Huang, H. S. Leu, and Y. C. Chuang.** 1996. Increasing antibiotic resistance in clinical isolates of *Aeromonas* strains in Taiwan. *Antimicrob. Agents Chemother.* **40:**1260–1262.
72. **Krovacek, K., S. Dumontet, E. Ericksson, and S. B. Balada.** 1995. Isolation and virulence profiles of *Aeromonas hydrophila* implicated in an outbreak of food poisoning in Sweden. *Microbiol. Immunol.* **39:**655–661.
73. **Kuijper, E. J., A. G. Steigerwalt, B. S. C. I. M. Schoenmakers, M. F. Peeters, H. C. Zanen, and D. J. Brenner.** 1989. Phenotypic characterization and DNA relatedness in human fecal isolates of *Aeromonas* spp. *J. Clin. Microbiol.* **27:**132–138.
74. **Kuijper, E. J., I. van Alphen, M. F. Peeters, and D. J. Brenner.** 1990. Human serum antibody response to the presence of *Aeromonas* spp. in the intestinal tract. *J. Clin. Microbiol.* **28:**584–590.
75. **Lambert, M. A., F. W. Hickman-Brenner, J. J. Farmer III, and C. W. Moss.** 1983. Differentiation of *Vibrionaceae* species by their cellular fatty acid composition. *Int. J. Syst. Bacteriol.* **33:**777–792.
76. **Lineaweaver, W. C., M. K. Hill, G. M. Buncke, S. Follansbee, H. J. Bunck, R. K. M. Wong, E. K. Manders, J. C. Grotting, J. Anthony, and S. J. Mathes.** 1992. *Aeromonas hydrophila* infections following use of medicinal leeches in replantation and flap surgery. *Ann. Plast. Surg.* **29:**238–244.
77. **Losonsky, G. A., J. A. Hasan, A. Huq, S. Kaintuck, and R. R. Colwell.** 1994. Serum antibody responses of divers to waterborne pathogens. *Clin. Diagn. Lab. Immunol.* **1:**182–185.
78. **Martinez-Murcia, A. J., C. Esteve, E. Garay, and M. D. Collins.** 1992. *Aeromonas allosaccharophila* sp. nov., a new mesophilic member of the genus *Aeromonas*. *FEMS Microbiol. Lett.* **91:**199–206.
79. **Martinez-Murcia, A. J., S. Benlloch, and M. D. Collins.** 1992. Phylogenetic interrelationships of members of the genera *Aeromonas* and *Plesiomonas* as determined by 16S ribosomal DNA sequencing: lack of congruence with results of DNA-DNA hybridizations. *Int. J. Syst. Bacteriol.* **42:**412–421.
80. **McNeeley, D., P. Ivy, J. C. Craft, and I. Cohen.** 1984. *Plesiomonas*: biology of the organism and diseases in children. *Pediatr. Infect. Dis.* **3:**176–181.
81. **Miller, M. L., and J. A. Koburger.** 1986. Tolerance of *Plesiomonas shigelloides* to pH, sodium chloride and temperature. *J. Food Prot.* **49:**877–879.
82. **Morgan, D. R., P. C. Johnson, A. H. West, L. V. Wood, C. D. Ericsson, and H. L. DuPont.** 1984. Isolation of enteric pathogens from patients with travelers' diarrhea

using fecal transport media. *FEMS Microbiol. Lett.* **23:** 59–63.

83. **Morgan, D. R., P. C. Johnson, H. L. Dupont, T. K. Satterwhite, and L. V. Wood.** 1985. Lack of correlation between known virulence properties of *Aeromonas hydrophila* and enteropathogenicity for humans. *Infect. Immun.* **50:**62–65.
84. **Morita, K., N. Watanabe, S. Kurata, and M. Kanamori.** 1994. β-Lactam resistance of motile *Aeromonas* isolates from clinical and environmental sources. *Antimicrob. Agents Chemother.* **38:**253–255.
85. **Moyer, N. P.** 1987. Clinical significance of *Aeromonas* species isolated from patients with diarrhea. *J. Clin. Microbiol.* **25:**2044–2048.
86. **Moyer, N. P., G. Martinetti Lucchini, L. A. Holcomb, N. H. Hall, and M. Altwegg.** 1992. Application of ribotyping for differentiating aeromonads isolated from clinical and environmental sources. *Appl. Environ. Microbiol.* **58:**1940–1944.
87. **Munoz, P., V. Fernandez-Baca, T. Palaez, R. Sanchez, M. Rodriguez-Creixems, and E. Bouza.** 1994. *Aeromonas* peritonitis. *Clin. Infect. Dis.* **18:**32–37.
88. **Nolte, F. S., R. M. Poole, G. W. Murphy, C. Clark, and B. J. Panner.** 1988. Proctitis and fatal septicemia caused by *Plesiomonas shigelloides* in a bisexual man. *J. Clin. Microbiol.* **26:**388–391.
89. **Ong, K. R., E. Sordilli, and E. Frankel.** 1991. Unusual case of *Aeromonas hydrophila* endocarditis. *J. Clin. Microbiol.* **29:**1056–1057.
90. **Palumbo, S. A., D. R. Morgan, and R. L. Buchanan.** 1985. Influence of temperature, NaCl, and pH on the growth of *Aeromonas hydrophila. J. Food Sci.* **50:** 1417–1421.
91. **Palumbo, S. A.** 1996. The *Aeromonas hydrophila* group in food, p. 287–310. *In* B. Austin, M. Altwegg, P. J. Gosling, and S. Joseph (ed.), *The Genus* Aeromonas. John Wiley & Sons Ltd., Chichester, England.
92. **Parsons, W. J.** 1985. Acute cholecystitis due to *Aeromonas hydrophila. N. Y. State J. Med.* **85:**564–565.
93. **Pitarangsi, C., P. Echeverria, R. Whitmire, C. Tirapat, S. Formal, G. J. Dammin, and M. Tingtalapong.** 1982. Enteropathogenicity of *Aeromonas hydrophila* and *Plesiomonas shigelloides*: prevalence among individuals with and without diarrhea in Thailand. *Infect. Immun.* **35:** 666–673.
94. **Poffe, R., and E. Op de Beeck.** 1991. Enumeration of *Aeromonas hydrophila* from domestic wastewater treatment plants and surface waters. *J. Appl. Bacteriol.* **71:**366–370.
95. **Popoff, M.** 1984. Genus III. *Aeromonas* Kluyver and van Niel 1936, 398, p. 545–548. *In* N. R. Krieg and J. G. Holt (ed.), *Bergey's Manual of Systematic Bacteriology*, vol. 1. The Williams & Wilkins Co., Baltimore, Md.
96. **Rahim, Z., and B. A. Kay.** 1988. Enrichment for *Plesiomonas shigelloides* from stools. *J. Clin. Microbiol.* **26:** 789–790.
97. **Rautelin, H., A. Sivonen, A. Kuikka, O. V. Renkonen, V. Valtonen, H. Lehti, A. Kahanpaa, and T. U. Kosunen.** 1995. Role of *Aeromonas* isolated from feces of Finnish patients. *Scand. J. Infect. Dis.* **27:**207–210.
98. **Reina, J., and A. Lopez.** 1996. Gastroenteritis caused by *Aeromonas trota* in a child. *J. Clin. Pathol.* **49:**173–175.
99. **Reinhardt, J. F., and W. L. George.** 1985. Comparative in vitro activities of selected antimicrobial agents against *Aeromonas* species and *Plesiomonas shigelloides. Antimicrob. Agents Chemother.* **27:**643–645.
100. **Rutala, W. A., F. A. Sarubbi, C. S. Finch, J. N. MacCormack, and G. E. Steinkraus.** 1982. Oyster-associated outbreak of diarrhoeal disease possibly caused by *Plesiomonas shigelloides. Lancet* **i:**739.
101. **San Joaquin, V. H., and D. A. Pickett.** 1988. *Aeromonas*-associated gastroenteritis in children. *Pediatr. Infect. Dis. J.* **7:**53–57.
102. **Shadow, K. H., D. K. Giger, and C. C. Sanders.** 1993. Failure of the Vitek system to detect beta-lactam resistance in *Aeromonas* species. *Am. J. Clin. Pathol.* **100:** 308–310.
103. **Schubert, R. H. W.** 1981. On the ecology of *Plesiomonas shigelloides. Zentralbl. Bakteriol. Parasitenkd. Infektionskr. Hyg. Abt. 1 Orig. Reihe B* **172:**528–533.
104. **Schubert, R. H. W.** 1984. Genus IV. *Plesiomonas* Habs and Schubert 1962, 324, p. 548–550. *In* N. R. Krieg and J. G. Holt (ed.), *Bergey's Manual of Systematic Bacteriology*, vol. 1. The Williams & Wilkins Co., Baltimore, Md.
105. **Schubert, R. H. W., and M. Hegazi.** 1988. *Aeromonas eucrenophila* species nova *Aeromonas caviae*, a later and illegitimate synonym of *Aeromonas punctata. Zentralbl. Bakteriol. Parasitenkd. Infektionskr. Hyg. Abt. 1 Orig. Reihe A* **268:**34–39.
106. **Schubert, R. H. W., M. Hegazi, and W. Wahlig.** 1990. *Aeromonas enteropelogenes* species nova. *Hyg. Med.* **15:** 471–472.
107. **Schubert, R. H. W., M. Hegazi, and W. Wahlig.** 1990. *Aeromonas ichthiosmia* species nova. *Hyg. Med.* **15:** 477–479.
108. **Smith, J. A.** 1980. Ocular *Aeromonas hydrophila. Am. J. Ophthalmol.* **89:**449–451.
109. **Snower, D. P., C. Ruef, A. P. Kuritza, and S. C. Edberg.** 1989. *Aeromonas hydrophila* infection associated with the use of medicinal leeches. *J. Clin. Microbiol.* **28:**980–984.
110. **Tonolla, M., A. Demarta, and R. Peduzzi.** 1991. Multilocus genetic relationships between clinical and environmental *Aeromonas* strains. *FEMS Microbiol. Lett.* **81:** 193–200.
111. **Tsukamoto, T., Y. Kinoshita, T. Shimada, and R. Sakazaki.** 1978. Two epidemics of diarrheal disease possibly caused by *Plesiomonas shigelloides. J. Hyg.* **80:**275–280.
112. **Tsukamoto, T., Y. Kinoshita, T. Shimada, and R. Sakazaki.** 1978. Two epidemics of diarrhoeal disease possibly caused by *Plesiomonas shigelloides. J. Hyg. Camb.* **80:** 275–280.
113. **Turnbull, P. C. B., J. V. Lee, M. D. Miliotis, S. van de Walle, H. J. Koornhof, L. Jeffrey, and T. N. Bryant.** 1984. Enterotoxin production in relation to taxonomic grouping and source of isolation of *Aeromonas* species. *J. Clin. Microbiol.* **19:**175–180.
114. **von Graevenitz, A., and A. H. Mensch.** 1968. The genus *Aeromonas* in human bacteriology. Report of 30 cases and review of the literature. *N. Engl. J. Med.* **278:**245–249.
115. **von Graevenitz, A., and M. Altwegg.** 1991. *Aeromonas* and *Plesiomonas*, p. 396–401. *In* A. Balows, W. J. Hausler, Jr., K. L. Herrmann, H. D. Isenberg, and H. J. Shadomy (ed.), *Manual of Clinical Microbiology*, 5th ed. American Society for Microbiology, Washington, D.C.
116. **Washington, J. A.** 1972. *Aeromonas hydrophila* in clinical bacteriologic specimens. *Ann. Intern. Med.* **76:**611–614.
117. **Yadava, R., R. A. Seeler, M. Kalelkar, and J. E. Royal.** 1979. Fatal *Aeromonas hydrophila* sepsis and meningitis in a child with sickle cell anemia. *Am. J. Dis. Child.* **133:** 753–754.

Pseudomonas

DEANNA L. KISKA AND PETER H. GILLIGAN

33

TAXONOMY

The original classification of the genus *Pseudomonas* into five rRNA homology groups (53) has undergone extensive revision, resulting in the reclassification of four of the five homology groups into separate genera. The genus *Pseudomonas* sensu stricto is limited to homology group I and includes the type species, *P. aeruginosa*, as well as the *Pseudomonas* spp. listed in Table 1. The members of the other homology groups have been placed into separate genera, which include *Burkholderia*, *Stenotrophomonas*, *Comamonas*, *Shewanella*, *Ralstonia*, *Methylobacterium*, *Sphingomonas*, *Acidovorax*, and *Brevundimonas* (29). The genus *Pseudomonas* can be distinguished from other related genera on the basis of cellular fatty acid composition. Characteristic fatty acids include C16:0, C16:1 *cis* 9, and C18:1 *cis* 11 (67).

Among members of the genus *Pseudomonas*, there is marked heterogeneity at the nucleic acid and protein levels. The moles % G+C content for the genus ranges from 58 to 70% (53). Genetic variation occurs even at the species level. For example, *P. stutzeri* can be divided into seven "genomovars" based on 16S rRNA gene sequence analysis and DNA hybridization studies (61). Genomovar 6 is sufficiently different from the type strain that a new species name, *P. balearica* sp. nov., has been proposed (8). Likewise, *P. fluorescens* and *P. putida* can be divided into several genotypes based on 16S rRNA sequence analysis (36). Further studies with 16S rRNA data and ribosomal protein analysis may eventually demonstrate that some of these strains are equivalent to separate species (52). *Pseudomonas* CDC group 1 strains are of uncertain RNA homology but appear to be phenotypically similar to *P. alcaligenes*. *P. luteola* and *P. oryzihabitans*, formerly members of the genera *Chryseomonas* and *Flavimonas*, respectively, have been returned to the genus *Pseudomonas* based on 16S rRNA sequence analysis (3).

GENERAL DESCRIPTION

Pseudomonas spp. are aerobic, non-spore-forming, gram-negative rods which are straight or slightly curved (27). They are 1.5 to 5 μm long and 0.5 to 1.0 μm wide and possess a strictly respiratory metabolism with oxygen as the terminal electron acceptor. Some isolates can grow under anaerobic conditions by using nitrate or arginine as terminal electron acceptors. *Pseudomonas* spp. are motile due to the presence of one or more polar flagella. Clinical isolates are oxidase positive (with the exception of *P. luteola* and *P. oryzihabitans*) and catalase positive and grow on MacConkey agar, appearing as lactose nonfermenters. Most species degrade glucose oxidatively and convert nitrate to either nitrite or nitrogen gas. Certain species have distinctive colony morphologies or pigmentation. They are nutritionally quite versatile, with different species being able to utilize a variety of simple and complex carbohydrates, alcohols, and amino acids as carbon sources. Certain species can multiply at 4°C, but most are mesophilic, with optimal growth temperatures between 30 and 37°C.

NATURAL HABITATS

Pseudomonas spp. have a worldwide distribution with a predilection for moist environments (27). They are found in water and soil and on plants, including fruits and vegetables. Some *Pseudomonas* species are well recognized as phytopathogens, and many species were first described in that context. Because of their ability to survive in aqueous environments, these organisms, particularly *P. aeruginosa*, have become problematic in the hospital environment. *P. aeruginosa* has been found in a variety of aqueous solutions including disinfectants, ointments, soaps, irrigation fluids, eye drops, and dialysis fluids and equipment (49). *P. aeruginosa* is frequently found in the aerators and traps of sinks; in baby, whirlpool, and hydrotherapy baths; in respiratory therapy equipment; and on showerheads. It is also found on the surface of many types of raw fruits and vegetables; therefore, profoundly immunosuppressed individuals should not consume these foods because subsequent gastrointestinal colonization by *P. aeruginosa* may lead to bacteremia. In addition to its nosocomial sources, *P. aeruginosa* may be found in swimming pools, hot tubs, contact lens solutions, cosmetics, illicit injectable drugs, and the inner soles of sneakers. All have been sources of infection.

P. aeruginosa is found infrequently as part of the microbial flora of healthy individuals. In these persons, the gastrointestinal tract is the most frequent site of colonization, but other moist body sites, including the throat, nasal mucosa, and moist skin surfaces such as the axillae and perineum, may become colonized. Rates of colonization increase in hospitalized patients, particularly in those who have been hospitalized for extended periods and/or have received broad-spectrum antimicrobial therapy or chemotherapy.

TABLE 1 Characteristics of *Pseudomonas* spp. found in clinical specimens[a]

Test	*P. aeruginosa* (n = 201)	*P. fluorescens* (n = 155)	*P. putida* (n = 16)	*P. stutzeri* (n = 28)	*P. mendocina* (n = 4)	*P. pseudoalcaligenes* (n = 34)	*P. alcaligenes* (n = 26)	*Pseudomonas* sp. CDC group 1[6] (n = 31)	*P. luteola* (n = 34)	*P. oryzihabitans* (n = 36)
Oxidase	99	97	100	100	100	100	96	100	0	0
Growth										
MacConkey	100	100	100	100	100	100	96	97	100	100
Cetrimide	94	89	81 (6)	4	75 (25)	56 (18)	15	13 (6)	0	25 (28)
6.5% NaCl	65	43	100	80 (16)	100	62 (6)	41	14	74	62
42°C	100	0	0	69	100	94	0	48	94	33
Nitrate reduction	98	19	0	100	100	100	54	100	62	6
Gas from nitrate	93	3	0	100	100	0	0	100	0	0
Pyoverdin	65	96	93	0	0	0	0	0	0	0
Arginine dihydrolase	100	97	100	0	100	78	12	33	100	14
Lysine decarboxylase	0	0	0	0	0	0	0	0	0	7
Ornithine decarboxylase	0	0	0	0	0	0	0	0	0	3

Indole	0	0	0	0	0	0	0	0	0	0
Litmus milk	89 pep[b]	95 pep	62 k[b]	57 k	25 (75) k	38 k	46 k	39 k	44 k	57 k
Hydrolysis										
Urea	48 (9)	21 (31)	13 (44)	33 (22)	50	3 (6)	0	3 (7)	26 (38)	77
Gelatin	82	100	0	0	0	0	0	4	61	17
Acetamide	100	6 (12)	0	0	0	ND	ND	ND	ND	ND
Esculin	0	0	0	0	0	0	0	0	100	0
Acid from[c]:										
Glucose	97	100	100	96	100	9	0	0	100	100
Fructose	ND[d]	ND	ND	ND	ND	79 (21)	0	ND	ND	ND
Starch	ND	ND	ND	100	0	ND	ND	ND	ND	ND
Xylose	90	100	100	93 (7)	75 (25)	18 (12)	0	0	100	100
Lactose	<1	24	25 (13)	0	0	0	0	0	3 (24)	14 (22)
Sucrose	0	48	0	0	0	0	0	0	12	25
Maltose	<1	2	31	100	0	0	0	0	100	97
Mannitol	70	53	25	89	0	0	0	0	76 (18)	100
Simmons citrate	95	93	94 (6)	82 (14)	100	26 (9)	57 (8)	42 (6)	100	97
No. of flagella	1	>1	>1	1	1	1	1	1	>1	1

[a] Percentage of strains positive; percentage in parentheses represents strains with delayed reactions. Data from reference 69.
[b] Type of reaction on litmus milk; pep, peptonization; k, alkaline.
[c] Oxidative-fermentation basal medium with 1% carbohydrate.
[d] ND, no data.

The colonization sites in these patients are similar to those in healthy persons but also include the lower respiratory tract, especially in intubated patients (54).

The distribution of other *Pseudomonas* spp. in the environment is similar to that of *P. aeruginosa*. Contamination of aqueous solutions, such as distilled water, soaps, disinfectants, and injectable medicines, with these organisms has led to pseudoinfections, most commonly pseudobacteremia, as well as true bacteremia and other infections (11, 30, 40, 51, 66).

P. pseudoalcaligenes has a highly unusual habitat. It has been found at concentrations of $>10^8$ organisms/ml in metal-working fluid, a mixture of water and petroleum products. Metalworkers are exposed to aerosols containing 10^5 organisms per m^3 with no apparent ill effects (45).

CLINICAL SIGNIFICANCE

P. aeruginosa

P. aeruginosa is the most important human pathogen in the genus *Pseudomonas* with respect to both the numbers and types of infections caused and their associated morbidity and mortality (54). The spectrum of diseases caused by this agent ranges from superficial skin infections to fulminant sepsis.

Community-acquired *P. aeruginosa* infections in nonimmunocompromised individuals tend to be localized and frequently associated with contaminated water or solutions. Probably the most superficial infection associated with this organism is folliculitis, acquired in swimming pools, water slides, whirlpools, or hot tubs or by using contaminated sponges (11, 42).

Superficial *P. aeruginosa* infections of the ear canal frequently develop in persons, such as competitive swimmers, involved in aquatic sports. This condition is aptly named "swimmer's ear." It should not be confused with a much more severe ear infection called malignant otitis externa. In the latter infection, seen primarily in diabetics and the elderly, *P. aeruginosa* can invade the underlying tissues, damaging cranial nerves and causing a temporal bone and basilar skull osteomyelitis. Meningitis may result (62). Successful treatment of this infection requires surgical debridement and antimicrobial therapy.

P. aeruginosa infection of the eye usually follows minor trauma to the cornea. These infections are frequently associated with contact lens use. Contaminated contact lens solution and the use of tap water during lens care have been implicated as sources of infection (26). *P. aeruginosa* infection of the eye can cause corneal ulcers, which may progress to loss of ocular function if not promptly treated.

P. aeruginosa is a common cause of osteomyelitis of the calcaneus in children (15). A puncture wound, usually caused by a nail penetrating a sneaker, occurs within the month preceding the development of this infection. The inner pad of the sneaker is the source of *P. aeruginosa* (17).

The most severe community-acquired infection caused by *P. aeruginosa* is endocarditis in intravenous-drug users, resulting from the use of contaminated injectable drugs. Replacement of the infected valve is usually necessary (34). These individuals may also develop osteomyelitis of a variety of bones.

P. aeruginosa is a major cause of nosocomial infection. It is the leading cause of nosocomial respiratory tract infection and can be especially serious in the intubated patient in the intensive care unit, with a mortality of 40 to 50% (58). *P. aeruginosa* also causes nosocomial urinary tract infections, wound infections, peritonitis in patients on chronic ambulatory peritoneal dialysis, and bacteremia (2, 9). Wound infections due to *P. aeruginosa* are particularly troublesome in burn patients. Although the incidence of such infections has declined in these patients, the high rate of sepsis following wound infections is responsible for significant mortality rates (50).

Several years ago, *P. aeruginosa* was recognized as an important cause of morbidity and mortality among both pediatric and adult AIDS patients (16, 18, 65). AIDS patients who develop *P. aeruginosa* infections typically have CD4 counts of $< 50/\mu l$. Infections commonly seen in this patient population include bacteremia whose source is usually either soft tissue infections or central venous catheters, respiratory tract infections, and malignant otitis media. Infections are more frequently community acquired than nosocomial, and recurrences are common. Whether these infections will continue to pose a problem in this patient population is uncertain, given the potency of new antiretroviral regimens and the decreasing number of patients with very low CD4 counts.

An unusual "mucoid" phenotype of *P. aeruginosa* chronically infects approximately 70 to 80% of adolescents and adults with cystic fibrosis (CF) (20). Once infected, CF patients rarely, if ever, clear this organism. Overproduction of alginate, a polysaccharide polymer, is responsible for the wet, "mucoid" appearance typical of colonies of the mucoid phenotype. The events which surround the establishment of the mucoid phenotype in the lungs of CF patients are not well understood despite being the focus of intense study (23). It is speculated that following infection with a nonmucoid isolate, emergence of the mucoid phenotype is due to random mutation in the gene cluster that controls alginate synthesis. Growth of mucoid *P. aeruginosa* as "microcolonies," which are small clusters of organisms surrounded by large amounts of alginate, is central to the development of chronic infection in the airway of CF patients. This form of growth is believed to inhibit phagocytosis and to induce a significant immune response in the lungs of CF patients via the action of neutrophil-derived elastase. High levels of elastase damage the lungs and have a cumulative, deleterious effect on pulmonary function over a period of years or even decades, eventually resulting in death (23). Bacteremia is rare, probably due to the high level of circulating antibodies to various *P. aeruginosa* virulence factors in these patients (33). Mucoid *P. aeruginosa* occasionally is seen causing pulmonary infections in individuals with other chronic lung diseases or urinary tract infections secondary to indwelling catheters (46).

Other *Pseudomonas* Species

Pseudomonas species other than *P. aeruginosa* infrequently cause infection. Because of their low virulence, infections due to these species are often iatrogenic and are associated with the administration of contaminated solutions, medicines, and blood products or the presence of indwelling catheters (22, 40, 41, 57, 63).

P. fluorescens can be isolated from the skin of a small proportion of blood donors (56, 63), resulting in occasional transfusion-associated septicemia. *P. putida* has been reported as the agent of catheter-related bacteremia in cancer patients (1). Both *P. fluorescens* and *P. stutzeri* have been implicated in outbreaks of pseudobacteremia (30, 66). Contamination of bone marrow transplants by *Pseudomonas* spp.

during processing (39) may become more common as the numbers of these procedures increase.

P. stutzeri is an unusual cause of human infection, but it has been reported to cause bacteremia in the immunosuppressed (55) and pneumonia in alcoholics (13). It has also caused bacteremia in patients undergoing hemodialysis with contaminated dialysis fluid (22). *P. stutzeri* has also been recovered from wounds, the respiratory tracts of intubated patients, and the urinary tract; however, its pathogenic role in those settings is unclear (51).

P. oryzihabitans increasingly is being recognized as a cause of bacteremia in immunocompromised patients with central venous access devices. Because of the low virulence of *P. oryzihabitans*, patients bacteremic with this organism can be successfully treated with parenteral antimicrobial agents and do not require removal of their foreign bodies (41). This organism has also been reported to cause peritonitis in patients undergoing chronic ambulatory peritoneal dialysis. Cellulitis, abscesses, wound infections, and meningitis following neurosurgical procedures have also been reported (40).

P. luteola is a rare cause of infections in humans. There have been case reports of a variety of different infections including osteomyelitis, peritonitis, endocarditis, and meningitis in patients following a neurosurgical procedure. Bacteremia is the most frequently reported infection with this organism (57).

Other *Pseudomonas* species are found even less frequently in human infection. *P. alcaligenes* was the cause of catheter-related endocarditis in a bone marrow transplant recipient (44). *P. mendocina* has also been isolated from a patient with endocarditis (5).

COLLECTION, TRANSPORT, AND STORAGE

Pseudomonas spp. can survive in a variety of hostile environments and at temperatures found in clinical settings. Therefore, standard collection, transport, and storage techniques as outlined in chapter 4 are sufficient to ensure the recovery of these organisms from clinical specimens.

DIRECT EXAMINATION

Pseudomonas spp. have similar Gram stain morphologies and are not easily distinguished from other glucose-nonfermenting gram-negative bacilli. Mucoid *P. aeruginosa* can be seen as microcolonies in the sputum of CF patients. They appear as clusters of thin gram-negative rods surrounded by more darkly staining amorphous gram-negative material. Multiplex PCR for the direct detection of *P. aeruginosa* and related fluorescent pseudomonads has been reported, but little clinical experience with this technique is currently available (14). Because of the rapid growth and ease of identification of *P. aeruginosa* and the need to perform susceptibility testing on clinically significant isolates, rapid molecular methods for detecting this organism currently have little practical value. Serological diagnosis of pseudomonad infections is not typically done.

CULTURE AND ISOLATION

Pseudomonas spp. grow well on standard laboratory media such as 5% sheep blood or chocolate agar. These media can be used to recover the organisms from clinical specimens such as cerebrospinal fluid, joint fluid, or peritoneal dialysis fluid, where a mixed flora is not anticipated. All members of the genus *Pseudomonas* grow in broth blood culture systems; therefore, special blood culture techniques such as the Isolator system are not required. Isolation of these organisms from specimens with a mixed flora is facilitated by the use of selective media. MacConkey agar is a useful selective medium for the isolation of most *Pseudomonas* spp., including mucoid strains of *P. aeruginosa* from CF patients. Selective agents such as cetrimide, acetamide, nitrofurantoin, and 9-chloro-9-[4-(diethylamino)phenyl]-9,10-dihydro-10-phenylacridine hydrochloride (C390) may be used to isolate *P. aeruginosa* from clinical and environmental samples (12, 25, 35, 37).

IDENTIFICATION

P. aeruginosa, P. fluorescens, and *P. putida*

P. aeruginosa isolates are easily recognized on primary isolation media on the basis of their characteristic colony morphology, production of diffusible pigments if present, and a grape-like or corn taco-like odor. Colonies are usually spreading and flat, have serrated edges, and have a metallic sheen which is often associated with autolysis of the colonies (70). Other colony variants exist, including smooth, coliform, gelatinous, dwarf, and mucoid forms. Mucoid colony variants are particularly prevalent in respiratory tract specimens from CF patients (20). *P. aeruginosa* produces a number of water-soluble pigments including the yellow-green or yellow-brown fluorescent pigment pyoverdin (also produced by *P. fluorescens* and *P. putida*). When pyoverdin combines with the blue, water-soluble, phenazine pigment, pyocyanin, the bright green color characteristic of *P. aeruginosa* is created. This organism may also produce one of two other water-soluble pigments: pyorubrin (red) or pyomelanin (brown to brown-black). *P. aeruginosa* can be confidently identified on the basis of a positive oxidase test, a triple sugar iron (TSI) agar reaction of alkaline over no change, growth at 42°C, and production of bright blue to blue-green, red, or brown diffusible pigments on Mueller-Hinton or other non-dye-containing agars.

Occasional *P. aeruginosa* strains produce only pyoverdin, which would not differentiate them from *P. fluorescens* or *P. putida*. The ability of *P. aeruginosa* to grow at 42°C distinguishes it from these two species (Table 1). Nonpigmented *P. aeruginosa* strains may also occur; frequently, they are highly mucoid strains recovered from the respiratory secretions of CF patients. In practice, the finding of a highly mucoid, glucose-nonfermenting, gram-negative rod in respiratory specimens from CF patients is sufficient to identify the organism as *P. aeruginosa*. However, when a nonpigmented isolate is recovered in a clinical setting other than this, key biochemical characteristics of *P. aeruginosa* besides those already mentioned include oxidation of glucose but not disaccharides, hydrolysis of acetamide, and reduction of nitrates to nitrogen gas. Additional characteristics include resistance to the combination of C390 and phenanthroline, the presence of the exotoxin A gene (~95% of strains), and the presence of the C19:0cyc11–12 fatty acid (12, 67, 68).

P. fluorescens and *P. putida* are the other members of the fluorescent pseudomonad group (pyoverdin producers) which are recovered from clinical specimens. Unlike *P. aeruginosa*, they do not possess a distinctive colony morphology or odor. In most clinical settings, there is little need to differentiate these organisms since they are of low virulence and usually not of clinical significance. However, because of the well-known association between *P. fluorescens* and contaminated blood products, accurate identification of isolates from patients who recently received blood products and developed bacteremia may be important. *P. fluorescens* can be differentiated from *P. putida* based on its ability to grow at 4°C and its ability to degrade gelatin; *P. putida* can do neither. A significant number of *P. fluorescens* isolates require 4 to 7 days of incubation for accurate detection of gelatin degradation.

Other fluorescent pseudomonads are rarely encountered in clinical specimens, since most are phytopathogens. Identification as "*Pseudomonas* species not *aeruginosa*" and susceptibility testing of the isolates, when appropriate, will be sufficient in most circumstances. When necessary, these isolates can be referred to reference laboratories, where more extensive biochemical batteries and cell wall fatty acid analysis can be used to establish a definitive identification. Recently, PCR amplification of 16S rDNA followed by restriction fragment length polymorphism analysis was used to successfully identify and characterize members of the fluorescent pseudomonad group (36).

P. stutzeri Group

The *P. stutzeri* group consists of three organisms: *P. stutzeri*, CDC group Vb-3, and *P. mendocina*. Because of their biochemical and morphologic similarities, CDC group Vb-3 should be considered a biovar of *P. stutzeri*. Of this group, *P. stutzeri* is most frequently encountered in clinical specimens. Most *P. stutzeri* isolates are easily recognized on primary isolation media by their distinctive dry, wrinkled colony morphology, which is similar to the morphology of *Burkholderia pseudomallei*. *P. stutzeri* colonies can pit or adhere to the agar and are buff to brown. The adherence can make removal of colonies from agar medium difficult. Because of the difficulty in making suspensions of specific turbidity, commercial identification and susceptibility systems may not work well with this organism. Not all isolates of *P. stutzeri* produce wrinkled colonies, and such strains are not readily distinguishable from other pseudomonads. *P. mendocina* is rarely recovered as a human pathogen (5). It is occasionally recovered from environmental cultures since it can be found, like other pseudomonads, in water and soil. The colonies are smooth and flat, producing a brownish yellow pigment; they are not readily distinguished from other pseudomonads.

Key biochemical characteristics of the *P. stutzeri* group are the ability to reduce nitrates to nitrogen gas, the ability to oxidize glucose but not lactose, and growth in 6.5% NaCl. Both *P. mendocina* and CDC group Vb-3 demonstrate arginine dihydrolase activity, whereas *P. stutzeri* does not. Otherwise, *P. stutzeri* and CDC group Vb-3 are indistinguishable by commonly used biochemical tests. Most strains of *P. stutzeri* and CDC group Vb-3 oxidize maltose and mannitol, whereas *P. mendocina* cannot metabolize these sugars.

P. alcaligenes, P. pseudoalcaligenes, and *Pseudomonas* sp. CDC Group 1

P. alcaligenes, *P. pseudoalcaligenes*, and *Pseudomonas* sp. CDC group 1 are encountered rarely in clinical and environmental samples (44). They do not have a distinctive colony morphology, nor do they produce pigments. Compared to other pseudomonads, they are biochemically inert. Characteristics that distinguish them from other biochemically inert gram-negative rods are a positive oxidase reaction, motility due to a polar flagellum, and growth on MacConkey agar. Most strains of *P. pseudoalcaligenes* and some strains of *P. alcaligenes* reduce nitrates to nitrites. CDC group 1 can be distinguished from these two species by its ability to reduce nitrates to nitrogen gas. *P. alcaligenes* is distinguished from *P. pseudoalcaligenes* by its inability to oxidize sugars while *P. pseudoalcaligenes* will weakly oxidize fructose. Isolates of these organisms are difficult to identify, and many laboratories, especially those using commercial systems, may appropriately call these isolates "*Pseudomonas* sp. not *aeruginosa*." If the clinical situation dictates that a definitive identification is required, assistance from reference laboratories should be sought.

P. luteola and *P. oryzihabitans*

P. luteola and *P. oryzihabitans* can be distinguished from other pseudomonads by their negative oxidase reaction and production of an intracellular, nondiffusible yellow pigment. Both organisms typically exhibit rough, wrinkled, adherent colonies or, more rarely, smooth colonies. *P. luteola* can be differentiated from *P. oryzihabitans* on the basis of its ability to hydrolyze *o*-nitrophenyl-β-D-galactopyranoside (ONPG) and esculin.

Use of Commercial Systems for Identification of *Pseudomonas* spp.

Many laboratories use commercial systems rather than conventional biochemical tests to identify *Pseudomonas* spp. Commercial systems developed for the identification of glucose-nonfermenting gram-negative rods include the N/F system (Remel Laboratories, Lenexa, Kans.), Vitek AutoMicrobic System gram-negative identification (GNI) card and API 20NE (bioMerieux Vitek, Hazelwood, Mo.), RapID NF Plus (Innovative Diagnostics Systems, Inc., Atlanta, Ga.), MicroScan W/A Neg Combo panels (Dade MicroScan, Inc., West Sacramento, Calif.), Crystal E/NF (Becton Dickinson, Cockeysville, Md.), and Cobas Micro ID-E/NF (Becton Dickinson Diagnostic Instrument Systems, Sparks, Md.). It may take from 4 to 48 h to obtain an identification with these systems depending on whether the system identifies the organism on the basis of preformed enzymes (rapid) or substrate utilization.

The accuracy of these commercial systems for identifying pigmented *P. aeruginosa* ranges from 70 to 100% but, on average, is greater than 90% (4, 19, 32, 59, 60). However, the use of an expensive commercial system for identification of *P. aeruginosa* is unwarranted when a few simple tests will suffice. When the commercial systems are challenged with nonpigmented, atypical *P. aeruginosa* strains, many of them perform inadequately (31). The most accurate system in this regard appears to be RapID NF Plus, which does not rely on pigment production as a key characteristic for identification (31).

Although the *Pseudomonas* spp. listed in Table 1 are in most of the commercial system databases, published evaluations of these systems often include very few, if any, *Pseudomonas* spp. other than *P. aeruginosa* (19, 59, 60). However, certain statements can be made concerning the value of commercial systems in identifying some *Pseudomonas* spp. RapID NF Plus and API 20NE appear to accurately identify *P. fluorescens* and *P. putida*, although the former system does not distinguish between these two species (4, 32). Differentiating these organisms is clinically relevant if a patient develops bacteremia with a blood transfusion as a potential source. These systems also appear to perform well with *P. stutzeri* (4, 32). However, if other *Pseudomonas* spp. are encountered or if other commercial systems are used, identification should be confirmed by alternative methods if clinically indicated.

TYPING SYSTEMS

Because of the importance of *P. aeruginosa* as a cause of nosocomial outbreaks and its role in lung disease in CF patients, there has been great interest in developing typing systems to study the clonal relationship among *P. aeruginosa* isolates. Before the development of molecular typing methods, serotyping based on the smooth lipopolysaccharide of *P. aeruginosa* was considered the most practical, discriminatory, and reproducible typing technique compared with antibiograms, phage typing, bacteriocin typing, and biotyping (28). One of the major shortcomings of this technique was that it could not type mucoid strains of *P. aeruginosa* which have rough lipopolysaccharide. Mucoid strains either agglutinated with multiple antisera, autoagglutinated, or failed to agglutinate at all.

Molecular methods have the advantage over serotyping of being able to type essentially all strains, and studies have shown them to discriminate among *P. aeruginosa* strains of the same serotype (38). Ribotyping, pulsed-field gel electrophoresis (PFGE), and a variety of PCR-based techniques have been used to type *P. aeruginosa*. PFGE has been reported to be the most discriminatory and reproducible of these methods (24). In most circumstances, ribotyping is sufficiently discriminatory to be useful in studying the molecular epidemiology of *P. aeruginosa*. In addition, this technique is much more rapid and less labor-intensive than PFGE.

ANTIMICROBIAL SUSCEPTIBILITY

Community-acquired isolates of *P. aeruginosa* are usually susceptible to the antipseudomonal penicillins (ticarcillin and piperacillin), the aminoglycosides (gentamicin, tobramycin, and amikacin), ciprofloxacin, cefoperazone, ceftazidime, meropenem, and imipenem. Susceptibility is less predictable for other broad-spectrum cephalosporins (ceftriaxone and cefotaxime), and the monobactam, aztreonam. The organism is uniformly resistant to antistaphylococcal penicillins, ampicillin, amoxicillin-clavulanic acid, ampicillin-sulbactam, tetracyclines, macrolides, rifampin, chloramphenicol, trimethoprim/sulfamethoxazole, narrow- and extended-spectrum cephalosporins, and oral broad-spectrum cephalosporins (cefixime and cefpodoxime).

Nosocomially acquired *P. aeruginosa* isolates tend to be more resistant to antimicrobial agents than are community-acquired strains, frequently displaying resistance to multiple classes of antimicrobial agents. Development of resistance during monotherapy with either cell wall-active agents (antipseudomonal penicillins, cefoperazone, and ceftazidime) or ciprofloxacin occurs frequently (7, 64).

Susceptibility testing of *P. aeruginosa* isolates recovered from respiratory secretions of CF patients presents a special challenge to the clinical microbiologist for two reasons. First, several different morphotypes are often present in sputa from these patients. Although frequently clonally related (10), these individual morphotypes may have significantly different antibiograms. Testing individual morphotypes is labor-intensive and expensive. Studies done to compare testing of individual morphotypes with testing of mixtures of those morphotypes have shown that mixed-morphotype testing does not detect resistance as accurately as individual-morphotype testing does (47). Second, the accuracy of commercially available susceptibility testing for the mucoid morphotype has been evaluated only with the E-test (AB BioDisk North America Inc., Piscataway, N.J.). Although this technique showed good correlation with a reference MIC method, it is too expensive for routine testing (43). Until evaluations of commercial susceptibility test systems are available, the U.S. Cystic Fibrosis Foundation is recommending that disc diffusion testing be performed on *P. aeruginosa* isolates recovered from CF patients (21).

In the final stages of chronic CF lung infection, *P. aeruginosa* may be resistant to all available antimicrobial agents. In these patients, high-dose aerosolized tobramycin may be of value. It should be noted that by using this treatment strategy, the achievable tobramycin concentration in the airways is in a range of 100 to 200 μg/ml of secretion. Therefore, laboratories involved in the care of these patients should be able to offer testing either by MIC or E-test to determine the tobramycin MIC of these pan-resistant organisms, especially at ranges up to 200 μg/ml (21).

INTERPRETATION OF RESULTS

P. aeruginosa is considered a true pathogen when isolated from any sterile site. Recovery of this organism from sites which harbor an indigenous microflora is significant when it is associated with a typical clinical syndrome, such as folliculitis or otitis externa. Colonization of the upper airways and endotracheal tubes can occur in intubated patients and must be distinguished from true infection in this setting (6), because patients with pneumonia have a high mortality rate and require aggressive antimicrobial therapy. Gram stains of secretions obtained by endotracheal suction which reveal large quantities of gram-negative rods and polymorphonuclear leukocytes are supportive of the diagnosis of nosocomial pneumonia (6). The absence of gram-negative rods and the presence of squamous epithelial cells indicate that the specimen is not useful for determining if the patient has pneumonia and should be rejected (48).

The presence of *P. aeruginosa*, especially isolates with a mucoid phenotype, in the respiratory tract of a young child may indicate that the individual has CF. Testing for the presence of chloride in the sweat should then be initiated to determine if the child has this disease. In cultures from patients with CF, the different colony morphotypes of *P. aeruginosa* (smooth, rough, or mucoid) should be reported. The presence of mucoid colonies suggests chronic infection in these patients.

The recovery of multiple *P. aeruginosa* isolates with the same, unusual antibiogram or phenotypic characteristic(s) in a nosocomial setting should alert laboratory and infection control personnel to the possibility of nosocomial outbreaks or, occasionally, pseudoepidemics due to *P. aeruginosa*.

Although other pseudomonads are isolated infrequently from clinical specimens, they have been associated with infections, particularly bacteremias. Recovery of these organisms from blood, sterile fluids, or blood unit bags should be considered significant until proven otherwise. The hospital infection control unit should be notified if an unusual pseudomonad is isolated from more than one patient, since contaminated hospital equipment or injectables may be involved (22, 57, 63). In these situations, consideration should be given to sending the isolates to a reference laboratory for definitive identification. The clinical significance of these organisms in specimens from contaminated sites is often unclear. These organisms may cause wound infections, cellulitis, abscesses, and pneumonia, although only rarely. In these instances, the specimen Gram stain, the predominance of the organism in culture, and the absence of more common pathogens should be used to guide judgment of whether the organism is significant.

REFERENCES

1. **Anaissie, E., V. Fainstein, P. Miller, K. Hassamali, S. Pitlik, G. P. Bodey, and K. Rolston.** 1987. *Pseudomonas putida*: newly recognized pathogen in patients with cancer. *Am. J. Med.* **82:**1191–1194.
2. **Anonymous.** 1997. National Nosocomial Surveillance (NNIS) report, data summary from October 1986–April 1997, issued May 1997. A report from NNIS System. *Am. J. Infect. Control* **25:**477–487.
3. **Anzai, Y., Y. Kudo, and H. Oyaizu.** 1997. The phylogeny of the genera *Chryseomonas*, *Flavimonas*, and *Pseudomonas* supports synonymy of these three genera. *Int. J. Syst. Bacteriol.* **47:**249–251.
4. **Appelbaum, P. C., and D. J. Leathers.** 1984. Evaluation of the Rapid NFT system for identification of gram-negative, nonfermenting rods. *J. Clin. Microbiol.* **20:**730–734.
5. **Aragone, M. R., D. M. Maurizi, and L. O. Clara.** 1992. *Pseudomonas mendocina*, an environmental bacterium isolated from a patient with human infective endocarditis. *J. Clin. Microbiol.* **30:**1583–1584.
6. **Baselski, V.** 1993. Microbiologic diagnosis of ventilator-associated pneumonia. *Infect. Dis. Clin. North Am.* **7:** 331–357.
7. **Bell, S. M., J. N. Pham, and J. Y. M. Lanzarone.** 1985. Mutation of *Pseudomonas aeruginosa* to piperacillin resistance mediated by β-lactamase production. *J. Antimicrob. Chemother.* **15:**665–670.
8. **Bennasar, A., R. Rossello-Mora, J. Lalucat, and E. R. B. Moore.** 1996. 16S rRNA gene sequence analysis relative to genomovars of *Pseudomonas stutzeri* and proposal of *Pseudomonas balearica* sp. nov. *Int. J. Syst. Bacteriol.* **46:** 200–205.
9. **Bernardini, J., B. Piraino, and M. Sorkin.** 1987. Analysis of continuous ambulatory peritoneal dialysis-related *Pseudomonas aeruginosa* infections. *Am. J. Med.* **83:**829–832.
10. **Bingen, E., E. Denamur, B. Picard, P. Goullet, N. Lambert-Zechovsky, P. Foucaud, J. Navarro, and J. Elion.** 1992. Molecular epidemiological analysis of *Pseudomonas aeruginosa* strains causing failure of antibiotic therapy in cystic fibrosis patients. *Eur. J. Clin. Microbiol. Infect. Dis.* **11:**432–437.
11. **Bottone, E. J., and A. A. Perez, Jr.** 1993. *Pseudomonas aeruginosa* folliculitis acquired through use of a contaminated loofah sponge: an unrecognized potential public health problem. *J. Clin. Microbiol.* **31:**480–483.
12. **Campbell, M. E., S. W. Farmer, and D. P. Speert.** 1988. New selective medium for *Pseudomonas aeruginosa* with phenanthroline and 9-chloro-9-[4-(diethylamino)phenyl]-9,10-dihydro-10-phenylacridine hydrochloride. *J. Clin. Microbiol.* **26:**1910–1912.
13. **Carratala, J., A. Salazar, J. Mascaro, and M. Santin.** 1992. Community-acquired pneumonia due to *Pseudomonas stutzeri*. *Clin. Infect. Dis.* **14:**792.
14. **De Vos, D., A. Lim, Jr., J.-P. Pirnay, M. Struelens, C. Vandenvelde, L. Duinslaeger, A. Vanderkelen, and P. Cornelis.** 1997. Direct detection and identification of *Pseudomonas aeruginosa* in clinical samples such as skin biopsy specimens and expectorations by multiplex PCR based on two outer membrane lipoprotein genes, *oprI* and *oprL*. *J. Clin. Microbiol.* **35:**1295–1299.
15. **Faden, H., and M. Grossi.** 1991. Acute osteomyelitis in children: reassessment of etiologic agents and their clinical characteristics. *Am. J. Dis. Child.* **145:**65–69.
16. **Fichtenbaum, C. J., K. Woeltje, and W. G. Powderly.** 1994. Serious *Pseudomonas aeruginosa* infections in patients infected with human immunodeficiency virus: a case-control study. *Clin. Infect. Dis.* **19:**417–422.
17. **Fisher, M. C., J. F. Goldsmith, and P. H. Gilligan.** 1985. Sneakers as a source of *Pseudomonas aeruginosa* in children with osteomyelitis following puncture wounds. *J. Pediatr.* **106:**607–609.
18. **Flores, G., J. J. Stavola, and G. J. Noel.** 1993. Bacteremia due to *Pseudomonas aeruginosa* in children with AIDS. *Clin. Infect. Dis.* **16:**706–708.
19. **Geiss, H. K., and M. Geiss.** 1992. Evaluation of a new commercial system for the identification of Enterobacteriaceae and non-fermentative bacteria. *Eur. J. Clin. Microbiol. Infect. Dis.* **11:**610–616.
20. **Gilligan, P. H.** 1991. Microbiology of airway disease in patients with cystic fibrosis. *Clin. Microbiol. Rev.* **4:**35–51.
21. **Gilligan, P. H.** 1996. Report on the consensus document for microbiology and infectious diseases in cystic fibrosis. *Clin. Microbiol. Newsl.* **18:**83–87.
22. **Goetz, A., V. L. Yu, J. E. Hanchett, and J. D. Rihs.** 1983. *Pseudomonas stutzeri* bacteremia associated with hemodialysis. *Arch. Intern. Med.* **143:**1909–1912.
23. **Govan, J. R. W., and V. Deretic.** 1996. Microbial pathogenesis in cystic fibrosis: mucoid *Pseudomonas aeruginosa* and *Burkholderia cepacia*. *Microbiol. Rev.* **60:**539–574.
24. **Grundman, H., C. Schneider, D. Hartung, F. D. Daschner, and T. L. Pitt.** 1995. Discriminatory power of three DNA-based typing techniques for *Pseudomonas aeruginosa*. *J. Clin. Microbiol.* **33:**528–534.
25. **Hedberg, M.** 1969. Acetamide agar medium selective for *Pseudomonas aeruginosa*. *Appl. Microbiol.* **17:**481.
26. **Holland, S. P., J. S. Pulido, T. K. Shires, and J. W. Costerton.** 1993. *Pseudomonas aeruginosa* ocular infections, p. 159–176. *In* R. B. Fick, Jr. (ed.), Pseudomonas aeruginosa: *the Opportunist*. CRC Press, Inc., Boca Raton, Fla.
27. **Holt, J. G., N. R. Kreig, P. H. A. Sneath, J. T. Staley, and S. T. Williams.** 1994. Genus *Pseudomonas*, p. 93–94 and 151–168. *In Bergey's Manual of Determinative Bacteriology*, 9th ed. The Williams & Wilkins Co., Baltimore, Md.
28. **International *Pseudomonas aeruginosa* Typing Study Group.** 1994. A multicenter comparison of methods for typing strains of *Pseudomonas aeruginosa* predominantly from patients with cystic fibrosis. *J. Infect. Dis.* **169:** 134–142.
29. **Kersters, K., W. Ludwig, M. Vancanneyt, P. DeVos, M. Gillis, and K.-H. Schleifer.** 1996. Recent changes in the classification of the pseudomonads: an overview. *Syst. Appl. Microbiol.* **19:**465–477.
30. **Keys, T. F., L. J. Melton III, M. D. Maker, and D. M. Ilstrup.** 1983. A suspected hospital outbreak of pseudobacteremia due to *Pseudomonas stutzeri*. *J. Infect. Dis.* **147:** 489–493.
31. **Kiska, D. L., A. Kerr, M. C. Jones, J. A. Caracciolo, B. Eskridge, M. Jordan, S. Miller, D. Hughes, N. King, and P. H. Gilligan.** 1996. Accuracy of four commercial systems for identification of *Burkholderia cepacia* and other gram-negative nonfermenting bacilli recovered from patients with cystic fibrosis. *J. Clin. Microbiol.* **34:**886–891.
32. **Kitch, T. T., M. R. Jacobs, and P. C. Appelbaum.** 1992. Evaluation of the 4-hour RapID NF Plus method for identification of 345 gram-negative nonfermentative rods. *J. Clin. Microbiol.* **30:**1267–1270.
33. **Klinger, J. D., D. C. Straus, C. B. Hilton, and J. A. Bass.** 1978. Antibodies to proteases and exotoxin A of *Pseudomonas aeruginosa* in patients with cystic fibrosis: demonstration by radioimmunoassay. *J. Infect. Dis.* **138:** 49–58.
34. **Komshian, S. V., O. C. Tablan, W. Palutke, and M. P. Reyes.** 1990. Characteristics of left-sided endocarditis due to *Pseudomonas aeruginosa* in the Detroit Medical Center. *Rev. Infect. Dis.* **12:**693–702.
35. **Krueger, C. L., and W. Sheikh.** 1987. A new selective medium for isolating *Pseudomonas* spp. from water. *Appl. Environ. Microbiol.* **53:**895–897.

36. **Laguerre, G., L. Rigottier-Gois, and P. Lamanceau.** 1994. Fluorescent *Pseudomonas* species categorized by using polymerase chain reaction (PCR)/restriction fragment analysis of 16S rDNA. *Mol. Ecol.* **3:**479–487.
37. **Lambe, D. W., and P. Stewart.** 1972. Evaluation of Pseudosel agar as an aid in the identification of *Pseudomonas aeruginosa*. *Appl. Microbiol.* **23:**377–381.
38. **Lau, Y. J., P. Y. F. Liu, B. S. Hu, J. M. Shyr, Z. Y. Shi, W. S. Tsai, Y. H. Lin, and C. Y. Tseng.** 1995. DNA fingerprinting of *Pseudomonas aeruginosa* serotype 011 by enterobacterial repetitive intergenic consensus-polymerase chain reaction and pulsed-field gel electrophoresis. *J. Hosp. Infect.* **31:**61–66.
39. **Lazarus, H. M., M. Magalhaes-Silverman, R. M. Fox, R. J. Creger, and M. Jacobs.** 1991. Contamination during in vitro processing of bone marrow for transplantation: clinical significance. *Bone Marrow Transplant.* **7:**241–246.
40. **Lin, R.-D., P.-R. Hsueh, J.-C. Chang, L.-J. Teng, S.-C. Chang, S.-W. Ho, W.-C. Hsieh, and K.-T. Luh.** 1996. *Flavimonas oryzihabitans* bacteremia: clinical features and microbiological characteristics of isolates. *Clin. Infect. Dis.* **24:**867–873.
41. **Lucas, K. G., T. E. Kiehn, K. A. Sobeck, D. Armstrong, and A. E. Brown.** 1994. Sepsis caused by *Flavimonas oryzihabitans*. *Medicine* **73:**209–214.
42. **Maniatis, A. N., C. Karkavitsas, N. A. Maniatis, E. Tsiftsakis, V. Genimata, and N. J. Legakis.** 1995. *Pseudomonas aeruginosa* folliculitis due to non-0:11 serogroups: acquisition through use of contaminated synthetic sponges. *Clin. Infect. Dis.* **21:**437–439.
43. **Marley, E. F., C. Mohla, and J. M. Campos.** 1995. Evaluation of E-test for determination of antimicrobial MICs for *Pseudomonas aeruginosa* isolates from cystic fibrosis patients. *J. Clin. Microbiol.* **33:**3191–3193.
44. **Martino, P., A. Micozzi, M. Venditti, G. Gentile, C. Girmenia, R. Raccah, S. Santilli, N. Alessandri, and F. Mandelli.** 1990. Catheter-related right-sided endocarditis in bone marrow transplant recipients. *Rev. Infect. Dis.* **12:** 250–257.
45. **Mattsby-Baltzer, I., L. Edebo, B. Järvholm, B. Lavenius, and T. Soderstrom.** 1990. Subclass distribution of IgG and IgA antibody response to *Pseudomonas pseudoalcaligenes* in humans exposed to metal-working fluid. *J. Allergy Clin. Immunol.* **6:**231–238.
46. **McAvoy, M. J., V. Newton, A. Paull, J. Morgan, P. Gacesa, and N. J. Russell.** 1989. Isolation of mucoid *Pseudomonas aeruginosa* from non-CF patients and characterization of the structure of secreted alginate. *J. Med. Microbiol.* **28:**1831–1839.
47. **Morlin, G. L., D. L. Hedges, A. L. Smith, and J. L. Burns.** 1994. Accuracy and cost of antibiotic susceptibility testing of mixed morphotypes of *Pseudomonas aeruginosa*. *J. Clin. Microbiol.* **32:**1027–1030.
48. **Morris, A. J., D. C. Tanner, and L. B. Reller.** 1993. Rejection criteria for endotracheal aspirates from adults. *J. Clin. Microbiol.* **31:**1027–1029.
49. **Morrison, A. J., Jr., and R. P. Wenzel.** 1984. Epidemiology of infections due to *Pseudomonas aeruginosa*. *Rev. Infect. Dis.* **6**(Suppl. 3)**:**S627–S642.
50. **Mousa, H. A.** 1997. Aerobic, anaerobic and fungal burn wound infections. *J. Hosp. Infect.* **37:**317–323.
51. **Noble, R. C., and S. B. Overman.** 1994. *Pseudomonas stutzeri* infection. A review of hospital isolates and a review of the literature. *Diagn. Microbiol. Infect. Dis.* **19:**51–56.
52. **Ochi, K.** 1995. Comparative ribosomal protein sequence analyses of a phylogenetically defined genus, *Pseudomonas*, and its relatives. *Int. J. Syst. Bacteriol.* **45:**268–273.
53. **Palleroni, N. J., R. Kunisawa, R. Contopoulou, and M. Doudoroff.** 1973. Nucleic acid homologies in the genus *Pseudomonas*. *Int. J. Syst. Bacteriol.* **23:**333–339.
54. **Pollack, M.** 1994. *Pseudomonas aeruginosa*, p. 1980–2003. *In* G. L. Mandell, J. E. Bennett, and R. Dolin (ed.), *Principles and Practice of Infectious Diseases*, 4th ed. Churchill Livingstone, Inc., New York, N.Y.
55. **Potvliege, C., J. Jonckheer, C. Lenclud, and W. Hansen.** 1987. *Pseudomonas stutzeri* pneumonia and septicemia in a patient with multiple myeloma. *J. Clin. Microbiol.* **25:** 458–459.
56. **Puckett, A., G. Davison, C. C. Entwistle, and J. A. J. Barbara.** 1992. Post-transfusion septicaemia 1980–1989: importance of donor arm cleansing. *J. Clin. Pathol.* **45:** 155–157.
57. **Rahav, G., A. Simhon, Y. Mattan, A. E. Moses, and T. Sacks.** 1995. Infections with *Chryseomonas luteola* (CDC Group Ve-1) and *Flavimonas oryzihabitans* (CDC Group Ve-2). *Medicine* **74:**83–88.
58. **Rello, J., P. Jubert, J. Valles, A. Artigas, M. Rue, and M. S. Niederman.** 1996. Evaluation of outcome for intubated patients with pneumonia due to *Pseudomonas aeruginosa*. *Clin. Infect. Dis.* **23:**973–978.
59. **Rhoads, S., L. Marinelli, C. A. Imperatrice, and I. Nachamkin.** 1995. Comparison of the MicroScan Walkaway system and Vitek system for identification of gram-negative bacteria. *J. Clin. Microbiol.* **33:**3044–3046.
60. **Robinson, A., Y. S. McCarter, and J. Tetreault.** 1995. Comparison of Crystal enteric/nonfermenter system, API 20E system, and Vitek Automicrobic system for identification of gram-negative bacilli. *J. Clin. Microbiol.* **33:** 364–370.
61. **Rossello, R., E. Garcia-Valdes, J. Lalucat, and J. Ursing.** 1991. Genotypic and phenotypic diversity of *Pseudomonas stutzeri*. *Syst. Appl. Microbiol.* **14:**150–157.
62. **Rubin, J., and V. L. Yu.** 1990. Malignant external otitis: insights into pathogenesis, clinical manifestations, diagnosis, and therapy. *Am. J. Med.* **85:**391–398.
63. **Scott, J., F. E. Boulton, J. R. W. Govan, R. S. Miles, D. B. L. McClelland, and C. V. Prowse.** 1988. A fatal transfusion reaction associated with blood contaminated with *Pseudomonas fluorescens*. *Vox Sang.* **54:**201–204.
64. **Scully, B. E., M. F. Parry, H. C. Neu, and W. Mandell.** 1986. Oral ciprofloxacin therapy of infections due to *Pseudomonas aeruginosa*. *Lancet* **i:**819–822.
65. **Shepp, D. H., I. T.-L. Tang, M. B. Ramundo, and M. H. Kaplan.** 1994. Serious *Pseudomonas aeruginosa* infection in AIDS. *J. Acquired Immune Defic. Syndr.* **7:**823–831.
66. **Simor, A. E., J. Ricci, A. Lau, R. M. Bannatyne, and L. Ford-Jones.** 1985. Pseudobacteremia due to *Pseudomonas fluorescens*. *Pediatr. Infect. Dis. J.* **4:**508–512.
67. **Stead, D. E.** 1992. Grouping of plant-pathogenic and some other *Pseudomonas* spp. by using cellular fatty acid profiles. *Int. J. Syst. Bacteriol.* **42:**281–295.
68. **Vasil, M. L., C. Chamberlain, and C. C. R. Grant.** 1986. Molecular studies of *Pseudomonas* exotoxin A gene. *Infect. Immun.* **52:**538–548.
69. **Weyant, R. S., C. W. Moss, R. E. Weaver, D. G. Hollis, J. G. Jordan, E. C. Cook, and M. I. Daneshvar.** 1995. Identification of unusual pathogenic gram-negative aerobic and facultatively anaerobic bacteria, p. 318–319, 340–341, and 470–503. The Williams & Wilkins Co. Baltimore, Md.
70. **Zierdt, C. H.** 1971. Autolytic nature of iridescent lysis in *Pseudomonas aeruginosa*. *Antonie Leeuwenhoek* **37:** 319–337.

Burkholderia, Stenotrophomonas, Ralstonia, Brevundimonas, Comamonas, and *Acidovorax*

PETER H. GILLIGAN AND SUSAN WHITTIER

34

TAXONOMY

The original description of the genus *Pseudomonas* included a wide variety of aerobic gram-negative rods. Subsequently, the genus was divided into five groups on the basis of RNA homology (83). Recent studies have led to either the reclassification or the general acceptance of new genus designations for four of these five groups. The use of DNA-rRNA hybridization, DNA-DNA hybridization, and 16S rRNA sequencing techniques has played an important role in the reclassification of these four rRNA homology groups (Table 1).

On the basis of DNA-DNA and DNA-rRNA homology studies, organisms in homology group II are sufficiently different from organisms in homology group I (*Pseudomonas aeruginosa* and related organisms) to belong to the genus *Burkholderia*. Four species recognized as human or animal pathogens (*Burkholderia cepacia, Burkholderia mallei, Burkholderia pseudomallei,* and *Burkholderia gladioli*) formerly called *Pseudomonas* have been assigned to the genus *Burkholderia* (141). Recent taxonomic studies by polyacrylamide gel electrophoresis whole-cell protein analysis and DNA-rRNA hybridization studies have shown that *B. cepacia* can be subdivided into four genomovars, genomovars I to IV (120). It has been proposed that one of these genomovars, type II, be designated *Burkholderia multivorans* because it can be phenotypically differentiated from the other genomovars of *B. cepacia*. Another species, *Burkholderia vietnamiensis*, which is closely related to *B. cepacia*, has recently been found in rice paddies in Vietnam. Human infections have not been associated with this organism (39). Other species of *Burkholderia* including *Burkholderia cocovenenans, Burkholderia andropogonis, Burkholderia glumae, Burkholderia caryophylli, Burkholderia vandii,* and *Burkholderia plantarii* are plant pathogens and will not be discussed further here (39, 109).

Two *Burkholderia* species and an *Alicaligenes* species have been reclassified as members of the new genus *Ralstonia* on the basis of DNA homology, cellular lipid composition, and 16S rRNA analysis. *Burkholderia pickettii* (a human pathogen), *Burkholderia solanacearum*, and *Alcaligenes eutropha* (both plant pathogens) have all been reclassified as members of the genus *Ralstonia* (142).

Organisms in group III are now classified in a new family, the *Comamonadaceae*, which includes the genera *Comamonas* and *Acidovorax* (136). The genus *Comamonas* was originally created in 1985 and included a single species, *Comamonas terrigena*. Two years later *Pseudomonas acidovorans* and *Pseudomonas testosteroni* were reclassified as members of the genus *Comamonas* (115). Originally, *Acidovorax facilis* was classified as *Hydrogenomonas facilis* on the basis of its ability to oxidize hydrogen (98). Poly-β-hydroxybutyrate metabolism studies resulted in the transfer of this species to the genus *Pseudomonas*, along with a new species called *Pseudomonas delafieldii* (23). Recent studies of DNA-rRNA hybridization led to the proposal of a new genus, *Acidovorax*, which includes three species, *Acidovorax facilis, Acidovorax delafieldii,* and *Acidovorax temperans*, all of which are members of homology group III (137).

Brevundimonas diminuta and *Brevundimonas vesicularis* were originally classified as members of homology group IV and were referred to as *Pseudomonas* species (5). Phenotypically, this categorization seemed appropriate. However, on the basis of DNA-rRNA hybridization studies, 16S rRNA cataloging, and 16S rRNA sequencing, the reclassification as *Brevundimonas* constituting homology group IV was proposed (99). This genus includes the organisms *B. diminuta* and *B. vesicularis*.

The genomic classification of *Stenotrophomonas maltophilia* has been a circuitous one. In 1961, the organism was designated *Pseudomonas maltophilia* on the basis of flagellar characteristics (51). Although significant rRNA homology differences were demonstrated between *P. maltophilia* and the other pseudomonads, this genus designation remained until the early 1980s. In 1983, the transfer of this bacteria to the genus *Xanthomonas* was proposed (112). This proposal was based on genotypic and phenotypic characteristics including DNA-rRNA hybridizations, cellular fatty acid (CFA) composition, and growth parameters. However, many differences were also noted, including flagellum number, nitrate reduction, fimbriation, and plant pathogenicity. Therefore, a new genus designation of *Stenotrophomonas*, homology group V, consisting of the species *S. maltophilia* and *Stenotrophomonas africana* has been proposed (27, 82).

GENERAL DESCRIPTION

Burkholderia, Ralstonia, Brevundimonas, Acidovorax, and *Comamonas* spp. are aerobic, non-spore-forming, gram-negative rods which are straight or slightly curved. They are 1 to 5 μm in length and 0.5 to 1.0 μm in width (49).

TABLE 1 Current classification of selected *Pseudomonas* homology group II to V organisms which have been recovered from humans

Pseudomonas homology group	Former species designation	Current species designation
II	*Pseudomonas cepacia*	*Burkholderia cepacia*
	Pseudomonas gladioli	*Burkholderia gladioli*
	Pseudomonas mallei	*Burkholderia mallei*
	Pseudomonas (*Burkholderia*) *pickettii*	*Ralstonia pickettii*
	Pseudomonas pseudomallei	*Burkholderia pseudomallei*
III	*Pseudomonas acidovorans*	*Comamonas acidovorans*
	Pseudomonas testosteroni	*Comamonas testosteroni*
	Pseudomonas delafieldii	*Acidovorax delafieldii*
	Hydrogenomonas facilis	*Acidovorax facilis*
IV	*Pseudomonas diminuta*	*Brevundimonas diminuta*
	Pseudomonas vesicularis	*Brevundimonas vesicularis*
V	*Pseudomonas* (*Xanthomonas*) *maltophilia*	*Stenotrophomonas maltophilia*
		Stenotrophomonas africana

Stenotrophomonas spp. are straight bacilli and tend to be slightly smaller (0.4 to 0.7 μm wide by 0.7 to 1.8 μm long) (49). With the exception of *B. mallei*, these organisms are motile due to the presence of one or more polar flagella (81). These bacteria are catalase positive, and most are oxidase positive. With the exception of certain strains of *B. vesicularis*, they grow on MacConkey agar and appear as nonfermenters. The majority of species degrade glucose oxidatively, and most degrade nitrate to either nitrite or nitrogen gas. Certain species have distinctive colony morphologies or pigmentation. They are nutritionally quite versatile, with different species being able to utilize a variety of simple and complex carbohydrates, alcohols, and amino acids as carbon sources. Certain species can multiply at 4°C, but most are mesophilic, with optimal growth temperatures of between 30 and 37°C (81).

NATURAL HABITATS

Burkholderia, *Stenotrophomonas*, *Ralstonia*, *Brevundimonas*, *Comamonas*, and *Acidovorax* spp. are environmental organisms found in water, in soil, and on plants including fruits and vegetables. They have a worldwide distribution. Members of these genera are well recognized as phytopathogens, and many species were first described in that context. Because of their ability to survive in aqueous environments, these organisms have become particularly problematic in the hospital environment.

The natural distribution of *B. cepacia* is being intensively studied because of interest in its use as a biologic control agent in the bioremediation of soils contaminated with toxic wastes and its pathogenicity in patients with cystic fibrosis (CF) (44). Studies have shown that unlike *P. aeruginosa*, *B. cepacia* is infrequently recovered from environmental sites such as sinks, swimming pools, pond water, showers, and salad bars (44, 70). These data suggest that the acquisition of *B. cepacia* from natural environments by CF patients may be more difficult than the acquisition of *P. aeruginosa*.

B. pseudomallei is found primarily in tropical and subtropical areas; the highest prevalence of disease (melioidosis) is found in northern Australia and Southeast Asia. The disease is particularly prevalent in the rice-growing regions of northern Thailand because of high concentrations of the organism in rice paddy surface water (21, 64).

CLINICAL SIGNIFICANCE

Burkholderia spp.

The genus *Burkholderia* contains two organisms frequently encountered as human pathogens, *B. pseudomallei* and *B. cepacia*.

B. pseudomallei is the etiologic agent of melioidosis. The organism is acquired either by inhalation or by contact of cut or abraded skin with contaminated soil or water (21, 64). There appears to be a broad spectrum of disease ranging from asymptomatic infection (as judged by serologic surveys) to chronic infection to fulminant sepsis (58, 64). Mortality in patients with fulminant sepsis approaches 90%, with high-grade bacteremia as evidenced by >100 CFU/ml of blood or a positive blood culture within 24 h being poor prognostic signs (116, 128). The organism frequently produces abscesses in organs of the reticuloendothelial system such as the lungs, liver, spleen, and lymph nodes. Abscesses can also occur in skin, soft tissue, joints, and bones. Multiple rather than single lesions are common. Chronic infections with this organism can mimic those of *Mycobacterium tuberculosis*. Like *M. tuberculosis*, this organism can survive within phagocytes (55), produce nodular lesions visible on chest radiograph, and granulomatous lesions in a variety of tissues and can lie dormant for years and then reactivate (64). Infections of the central nervous system are unusual. When it occurs, encephalitis with peripheral neuropathy is more characteristic than a pyogenic meningitis (139). Relapse following appropriate antimicrobial therapy occurs in 5% of patients (25). Molecular genotyping indicates that relapse rather than reinfection usually occurs in these patients (25).

Melioidosis is most prevalent in Southeast Asia and northern Australia but occurs in tropical and subtropical regions throughout the world. Concern exists that a significant number of Vietnam War veterans are latently infected with the organism that causes this disease, *B. pseudomallei*; reactivation may become increasingly common as that population ages (61). As travel to Southeast Asia has become more frequent for individuals living in industrialized countries, reports of infection in travelers returning to Europe and the United States are becoming more common (10, 135). This organism should be considered in the differential diagnosis of any individual with a fever of unknown origin or a tuberculosis-like disease who has a travel history to a region of endemicity, even if travel preceded the illness by decades (10, 61).

B. cepacia is well recognized as a nosocomial pathogen, causing infections associated with contaminated equipment, medications, and disinfectants including povidone-iodine and benzalkonium chloride (107). These infections include bacteremia, particularly in patients with indwelling catheters, urinary tract infection, septic arthritis, peritonitis, and respiratory tract infection (80, 87). Nosocomial outbreaks of *B. cepacia* respiratory tract infections in ventilated patients have been attributed to contamination of nebulizers or medication such as albuterol given by nebulizers (86, 93). Because *B. cepacia* is of low virulence, morbidity and mortality associated with these infections are low. *B. cepacia* pseudobacteremia due to contaminated disinfectants has been described (20, 80). Isolation of *B. cepacia* from the blood of multiple patients over a short period of time should be investigated for possible pseudobacteremia.

B. cepacia is emerging as an important pathogen in two patient populations with genetic diseases, CF and chronic granulomatous disease (37, 78). In the United States, approximately 6 to 7% of adult CF patients are infected with this organism (33). CF patients chronically infected with *B. cepacia* have decreased survival rates compared to the rates for those who are uninfected. Approximately 20 to 30% of CF patients who become infected with *B. cepacia* develop the "cepacia syndrome." These patients frequently have mild lung disease prior to *B. cepacia* infection but show a rapid decline in lung function, frequent bacteremia (an unusual occurrence in CF patients), and death due to lung failure. Autopsy results have revealed multiple lung abscesses containing *B. cepacia*, a pathologic finding similar to that seen in fulminant *B. pseudomallei* disease (37). Interestingly, host factors appear to play an important role in who develops the cepacia syndrome since molecular typing studies have shown a wide spectrum of disease in CF patients infected with the same clone (43, 44).

Molecular typing techniques have played an important role in our understanding of the epidemiology of *B. cepacia* in CF patients. A clone of this bacterium which has a highly unusual adhesin called cable pilin (42) has been shown to have been spread from a CF center in Canada to other Canadian centers as well as centers in England and Scotland and then on to CF centers in continental Europe (101, 111). Studies suggest that transmission occurs primarily via close personal contact, with kissing being implicated as one transmission mode (43). However, more conventional modes of transmission such as inhalation of aerosols from infected patients may also be involved. Studies with powerful air sampling systems show that *B. cepacia* can be found in the air of rooms following chest physiotherapy of infected CF patients, a daily practice in this patient population (30). These studies have resulted in the segregation of *B. cepacia*-infected patients, a practice which is traumatic for the patients and their families. Making this problem even more complex is the observation in some CF centers that all *B. cepacia*-infected patients are colonized with genetically unique strains, suggesting environmental rather than person-to-person or common-source acquisition (52, 100, 110).

Because of their profound immunosuppression, CF patients who have received lung transplants are particularly vulnerable to infection with *B. cepacia*. In addition, nosocomial *B. cepacia* infections have occurred in this patient population, with a mortality rate of 80% (105). Conversely, genotype analysis in one CF center showed that the CF patients infected with *B. cepacia* posttransplantation harbored the same organism prior to transplantation (110). The decision to perform lung transplants on *B. cepacia*-infected CF patients remains controversial (1a).

B. gladioli has also been isolated from the respiratory secretions of CF patients. This organism was first recognized due to its ability to grow on a selective medium used to isolate *B. cepacia* (19). Several reports have implicated this organism as the cause of pulmonary exacerbation in CF patients (7, 56, 138). Like *B. cepacia*, it has also caused infections in patients with chronic granulomatous disease and has also been seen in other immunocompromised patients (96, 117).

B. mallei is the etiologic agent of glanders, a disease of livestock, particularly horses, mules, and donkeys. Human disease due to this organism has not been reported in the United States in more than 50 years (97).

Stenotrophomonas

S. maltophilia has become a significant nosocomial pathogen, and in fact, the vast majority of all clinical infections caused by this organism are hospital acquired. *S. maltophilia* can be a colonizer in certain patient populations, including immunosuppressed patients (34) and those with CF (41, 127). However, in many hospitalized patients who are immunocompromised, infection is becoming more frequent and has been associated with substantial morbidity and mortality. Risk factors for colonization or infection include mechanical ventilation (107), broad-spectrum antibiotic prophylaxis (107), chemotherapeutic regimens (4, 68, 71), catheterization (28, 125), and neutropenia (107, 125). Infections caused by *S. maltophilia* are numerous and include bacteremia (68, 71, 107), meningitis (40, 75), urinary tract infection (125), mastoiditis (107), epididymitis (107), conjunctivitis (88), endocarditis (46), continuous ambulatory peritoneal dialysis-associated peritonitis (113), bursitis (84), keratitis (108), endophthalmitis (57), cholangitis (85), and a wide range of mucocutaneous and soft-tissue infections that may mimic disseminated fungal infections (124). Pneumonia is an uncommon occurrence, and isolation from the respiratory tract is usually indicative of colonization (54).

Recently, a new species of *Stenotrophomonas* has been proposed, *S. africana* (27). This organism was isolated from the spinal fluid of a human immunodeficiency virus-positive Rwandan refugee with primary meningoencephalitis. Analysis of the 16S rRNA gene sequence demonstrated significant homology with *S. maltophilia*.

Other Genera

In general, *Acidovorax* spp., *Brevundimonas* spp., *Comamonas* spp., and *Ralstonia* spp. are infrequently isolated from clinical specimens. *Acidovorax* spp. have been isolated from a variety of clinical sources; however, their role as true pathogens has not been established (137). *B. vesicularis* bacteremia was reported in a hemodialysis patient, a patient with sickle cell anemia, and an immunosuppressed individual (77, 90, 121). It has been isolated from peritoneal dialysis fluid, an oral abscess, and a scalp wound (15, 60). It has also been recognized in cervical specimens because of its ability to produce bright orange colonies on Thayer-Martin agar (79). *B. diminuta* has been associated with a limited number of bacteremias (60).

Although typically regarded as nonpathogenic (115), *Comamonas* spp. have been recovered from a variety of environmental and clinical sites and have been linked to certain disease states. One report described 10 adult cases of *Comamonas testosteroni* infections, with the most common site of isolation being the peritoneal cavity (6). The majority of these infections were polymicrobic. *Comamonas acidovorans* has also been reported to cause infection. It has been identified as the etiologic agent of bacteremia (17, 29, 131), intravenous drug use-associated endocarditis (50), indwelling central venous catheter-associated bacteremia (17), ocular infections (12), and acute suppurative otitis (94).

Ralstonia pickettii has been recovered from a variety of clinical specimens (95) and is an infrequent cause of bacteremia (26, 35, 62), meningitis (31), endocarditis (45), and osteomyelitis (133). It has been identified in several nosocomial outbreaks due to contamination of intravenous products (32), "sterile" water (67), saline (18), chlorhexidine solutions (133), respiratory therapy solutions (69), and intravenous catheters (92). It has also been associated with pseudobacteremias (126) and asymptomatic colonization (69). *R. pickettii* may be recovered from the respiratory tracts of CF patients. Because of biochemical similarities, *R. pickettii* may be confused with *B. cepacia*. *R. pickettii* does not appear to cause pulmonary disease exacerbations in CF patients.

COLLECTION, TRANSPORT, AND STORAGE

Members of all of the genera described in this chapter can survive in a variety of hostile environments and at temperatures found in clinical settings. Therefore, standard collection, transport, and storage techniques as outlined in chapter 4 are sufficient to ensure the recovery of these organisms from clinical specimens.

DIRECT EXAMINATION

The genera described in this chapter have similar morphologies and are not easily distinguished from each other on the basis of Gram staining results. Direct Gram stains of clinical specimens for the detection of *B. pseudomallei* are generally negative (53). Because septicemia with *B. pseudomallei* is frequently fatal, several rapid, direct detection methods have been developed in research laboratories including urinary antigen detection by latex agglutination (LA) and enzyme immunosorbent assay (EIA), direct fluorescent-antibody (DFA) staining, and PCR (24, 47, 103, 129). The EIA for detection of urinary antigen is more sensitive than LA, with an overall sensitivity of 70% and an even higher sensitivity (84%) for septicemic patients. Cross-reactions with other urinary tract pathogens including *Klebsiella pneumoniae* and *Escherichia coli* have been reported with EIA but not LA, so EIA results must be interpreted cautiously (24, 103).

Antibody raised against heat-killed, whole cells of *B. pseudomallei* have been used to prepare a reagent for DFA staining. When this DFA reagent was used to stain clinical specimens from patients with suspected melioidosis, it showed a sensitivity (73%) similar to those of other bacterial DFA stains. The reagent apparently does not cross-react with other organisms, although the number of isolates tested for cross-reaction was small (129).

Preliminary reports on the use of PCR for the direct detection of *B. pseudomallei* in clinical specimens indicate that the currently used primer sets and assay conditions are sensitive but lack specificity (47). PCR techniques for the detection of *B. cepacia* have also been described. Studies of the direct detection of *B. cepacia* in respiratory secretions of CF patients by PCR are currently inconclusive, but this technique has been very helpful in the identification of isolates of this organism (16, 66).

CULTURE AND ISOLATION

Organisms of the genera described in this chapter have been recovered from a variety of clinical specimens. These organisms grow well on standard laboratory media such as 5% sheep blood or chocolate agar. Such media can be used to recover the organisms from clinical specimens such as cerebrospinal fluid, joint fluid, or peritoneal dialysis fluid when a mixed flora is not anticipated. All members of these genera which have been reported to be recovered from blood, including *B. pseudomallei* (116), will grow in broth blood culture systems within the standard 5-day incubation period so special blood culture techniques such as lysis-centrifugation or extended incubation periods are not required.

Isolation of these organisms from specimens with mixed flora is facilitated by the use of selective media. With the exception of *B. vesicularis*, MacConkey agar is a useful selective medium for the isolation of most species of these genera.

Burkholderia species will grow on MacConkey agar, but the use of specific selective media with the ability to inhibit *P. aeruginosa* is preferred for the isolation of *B. cepacia* and *B. pseudomallei*. Three media, PC (*Pseudomonas cepacia*) agar (38), OFPBL (oxidative-fermentative base, polymyxin B, bacitracin, lactose) agar (132), and BCSA (*B. cepacia* selective agar) (48), are useful for the recovery of *B. cepacia* from respiratory secretions of CF patients. All three media contain antimicrobials that inhibit the growth of *P. aeruginosa*, which will grow on these media infrequently. Each medium has distinct disadvantages. BCSA has not been evaluated with clinical specimens. *B. gladioli* isolates may be confused with *B. cepacia* isolates because *B. gladioli* produces an intense yellow pigment on OFPBL agar. PC agar may be too selective, not allowing the growth of a small percentage of *B. cepacia* isolates (14). However, proficiency surveys indicate that PC and OFPBL media are more effective than MacConkey agar for the isolation of *B. cepacia* (114).

Ashdown medium is effective for the isolation of *B. pseudomallei*; crystal violet and gentamicin act as selective agents. It has been shown to be superior to MacConkey agar or MacConkey agar supplemented with colistin for the recovery of *B. pseudomallei* from clinical specimens containing mixed bacterial flora such as throat, rectal, and sputum specimens (3, 140). An enrichment broth consisting of Ashdown medium supplemented with 50 mg of colistin per liter allowed the recovery of 25% more *B. pseudomallei* isolates compared with the amount recovered by direct plating of clinical specimens on Ashdown agar (130).

The isolation of *Acidovorax* species on media routinely used in the clinical laboratory has not been described.

IDENTIFICATION

Burkholderia spp.

Burkholderia spp. can be recovered on most aerobically incubated primary isolation media used in the clinical laboratory to isolate enteric gram-negative bacilli. Some members of the *Burkholderia* genus have distinctive characteristics. *B. pseudomallei* colonies vary from smooth and mucoid to dry and wrinkled. The dry, wrinkled colonial morphotype will allow this organism to be recognized in specimens with a mixed bacterial flora. This wrinkled colonial morphotype is similar to that of *Pseudomonas stutzeri*, and because of the clinical significance of *B. pseudomallei*, it is important to distinguish the two. In addition to its distinctive colonial morphology, *B. pseudomallei* has a pungent, earthy odor. On Ashdown medium, the colonies are typically dry, wrinkled, and violet-purple. These characteristics are sufficiently distinct to make a presumptive identification of *B. pseudomallei* (140).

B. cepacia, especially when recovered from the respiratory tracts of CF patients, may require 3 days of incubation before colonies are seen on selective media. On MacConkey agar, these colonies may be punctate and tenacious, while on blood agar or selective medium such as PC or OFPBL agar the colonies will be smooth and slightly raised; occasional isolates will be mucoid. On MacConkey agar, colonies of *B. cepacia* will frequently become dark pink to red due to the oxidation of lactose after extended incubation (4 to 7 days). Most clinical isolates are nonpigmented, but on iron-containing media such as a triple sugar iron (TSI) slant, many strains will produce a bright yellow pigment. *B. cepacia* has a characteristic dirt-like odor.

B. mallei is the most easily identified member of this genus because it is nonmotile (Table 2). Other characteristics helpful in identifying *B. mallei* are the reduction of nitrate to nitrite, arginine dihydrolase activity, and oxidation of glucose. It fails to oxidize sucrose or maltose (134).

Because of the importance of *B. pseudomallei* and *B. cepacia* as human pathogens, accurate identification of these or-

TABLE 2 Characteristics of *Burkholderia* spp. and *Ralstonia pickettii* from clinical specimens[a]

Test	% Positive strains						
	B. pseudomallei (n = 70)	*B. mallei* (n = 8)	*B. cepacia* (n = 159)	*B. gladioli* (n = 58)	*R. pickettii* Biovar 1 (n = 70)	*R. pickettii* Biovar 2 (n = 54)	*R. pickettii* Biovar 3 (n = 31)[b]
Oxidase	100	25	86	47	100	100	100
Growth							
MacConkey	100	88	100	97	99	100	100
Cetrimide	0	0	44	3	1	0	0
42°C	100	0	83	9	83	3	84
Nitrate reduction	100	100	57	43	100	100	13
Gas from nitrate	100	0	0	0	86	100	0
Arginine dihydrolase	100	100	0	2	6	0	3
Lysine decarboxylase	0	0	80	0	0	0	0
Ornithine decarboxylase	0	0	48	0	0	0	0
Hemolysis	0	0	0	0	0	0	0
Hydrolysis:							
Urea	13	12	60	30	100	100	81
Citrate	77	0	94	93	99	100	100
Gelatin	79	0	20	12	12	38	30
Esculin	59	0	63	0	0	0	0
Acid from:							
Glucose[c]	100	100	100	98	100	100	100
Xylose	86	12	100	98	100	100	100
Lactose	99	12	99	9	100	0	100
Sucrose	66	0	86	0	0	0	0
Maltose	99	0	99	0	100	0	100
Mannitol	94	62	100	91	0	0	100
Motile	100	0	100	100	100	100	100
No. of flagella	>2	0	>2	>2	1–2	1–2	1–2

[a] Data are from reference 134.
[b] Also referred to as *Pseudomonas thomasii* in reference 134.
[c] Oxidation-fermentation basal medium with 1% carbohydrates.

ganisms is important. Key characteristics of *B. pseudomallei* include a positive oxidase reaction, production of gas from nitrate, multitrichous polar flagella, arginine dihydrolase and gelatinase activities, and oxidation of a wide variety of carbohydrates. An acid slant on TSI results from oxidation of both lactose and sucrose. *B. pseudomallei* has a characteristic CFA profile with large amounts (>20%) of hexadecanoic acid ($C_{16:0}$) and the cyclopropane acid *cis*-11,12-methylene octadecanoic acid ($C_{19:0\ cyclo\ 11-12}$) and significant amounts (>10%) of *cis*-9,10-methylene hexadecanoic acid ($C_{17:0\ cyclo}$) and *cis*-11-octadecenoic acid ($C_{18:1\ cis\ 11}$) (123, 134). The other *Burkholderia* spp. pathogenic for humans, *B. cepacia*, *B. mallei*, and *B. gladioli*, have CFA patterns very similar to that for *B. pseudomallei* (72, 109, 134). CFA analysis is useful only when differentiating these organisms from other genera.

Recent studies have suggested that there are two different biotypes of *B. pseudomallei* on the basis of the ability of isolates to assimilate arabinose. Isolates capable of assimilating arabinose are usually environmental and of low virulence in animal models; clinical isolates are unable to assimilate arabinose and are highly virulent in animal models (11, 102). Partial sequence analysis of 16S rRNA suggests that the arabinose-assimilating, environmental isolates may actually represent a new species of *Burkholderia*, but no new name has been proposed (11).

B. pseudomallei can be distinguished from *P. stutzeri* by arginine dihydrolase and gelatinase activities, lactose oxidation, and numbers of flagella (Table 2). The NFT (BioMerieux-Vitek, Hazelwood, Mo.) is the only commercial identification system that has been adequately evaluated for accuracy in identifying *B. pseudomallei*. One study with 400 isolates showed an overall accuracy of >99% (22). The identification of a clinical isolate as *B. pseudomallei* by any other kit system requires confirmation, preferably with conventional biochemicals. Because of the clinical importance and highly virulent nature of this organism in at least some patients, clinicians should be notified as soon as possible if this organism is suspected.

Because of its role in CF lung disease and the resulting segregation of infected CF patients, both the taxonomy and modes of identification of *B. cepacia* have been the objects of intense research over the past few years. Key biochemical characteristics of *B. cepacia* include a positive oxidase reaction in 86% of the isolates, lysine decarboxylase activity by 80% of the isolates, multitrichous polar flagella, and utilization of a wide variety of mono- and disaccharides including lactose.

The two major genomovars encountered clinically, genomovars II and III, can be differentiated as follows: genomovar II is lysine decarboxylase and sucrose negative and genomovar III is positive for both of these biochemicals (120). Differentiating certain isolates of *B. cepacia* from isolates of *R. pickettii* and *B. gladioli* can be very difficult biochemically, especially for genomovar II strains (120). Reduction of nitrate to gas is a characteristic of many but not all *R. pickettii* strains. *B. cepacia* isolates are typically unable to reduce nitrates to nitrites, and no strain can reduce nitrites to nitrogen gas. *R. pickettii* isolates, specifically biovar 3 isolates (also referred to as *Pseudomonas thomasii*), that fail to reduce nitrate to nitrogen gas can be very difficult to distinguish from *B. cepacia* isolates that can reduce nitrates to nitrites. CFA analysis may be helpful in distinguishing between these two species (142). *B. gladioli* isolates are unable to oxidize lactose, maltose, and sucrose and can usually be differentiated from *B. cepacia* on the basis of these phenotypic characteristics. However, isolates which have selected phenotypic characteristics consistent with both *B. gladioli* and *B. cepacia* have been recovered from CF patients, making differentiation between the two species extremely difficult, especially since these isolates have the same CFA profiles (8, 72, 109).

Many laboratories use commercial kit systems rather than conventional biochemical tests to identify *Burkholderia* spp. and phenotypically related organisms. These include the N/F system (Remel Laboratories, Lenexa, Kans.), the AutoMicrobic System Gram-negative identification (GNI) card and Rapid NFT (bioMerieux Vitek), the RapID NF plus system (Innovative Diagnostics Systems, Inc., Atlanta, Ga.), and the autoSCAN W/A Rapid Neg Combo (RNC) 1 panel (Baxter MicroScan, West Sacramento, Calif.). The general principles of these kits are described in chapter 11.

A recent evaluation of four of these kits for the identification of isolates of *Burkholderia* and related organisms recovered from CF patients showed relatively poor accuracy in the identification of *B. cepacia*, *B. gladioli*, and *R. pickettii*. One commercial system did not even have *B. gladioli* in its database. *B. cepacia* isolates were misidentified as other species, and other species were misidentified as *B. cepacia* (59). In most clinical settings, this would be of minimal importance. However, for CF patients, accuracy as close to 100% as possible is essential because CF patients infected or colonized with *B. cepacia* often become medical and social outcasts due to concern over the spread of the organism to other individuals with CF (44). When *B. cepacia*, *B. gladioli*, or *R. pickettii* is identified by a commercial system from a CF patient, the identity of the isolate should be confirmed by conventional biochemical testing (134) and, if necessary, CFA analysis or molecular techniques. To aid clinical microbiologists in the United States, the U.S. Cystic Fibrosis Foundation has established a *B. cepacia* Reference Laboratory which uses a combination of phenotypic and genotypic methods to confirm the identities of suspected *B. cepacia* isolates (66).

Of the *Ralstonia* species, only *R. pickettii* has been isolated from clinical specimens. The three species can be differentiated on the basis of motility and flagellation. *R. pickettii* has a polar monotrichous flagellum, while *Ralstonia eutropha* has peritrichous flagella. *Ralstonia solanacearum* is nonmotile (134, 142).

S. maltophilia

Key features for identifying *S. maltophilia* include a negative oxidase reaction, oxidation of glucose and maltose with a more intense reaction with the latter, a tuft of polar flagella, and a positive DNase reaction. Detection of extracellular DNase activity by *S. maltophilia* is a key to differentiating this species from most other glucose-oxidizing, gram-negative bacilli. It can be detected on tube or plate DNase medium with a methyl green indicator. DNase-positive organisms produce a zone of clearing around the colonies on this medium (see chapter 130). Care must be taken when interpreting the DNase reaction, because one report documented the misidentification of *S. maltophilia* as *B. cepacia* partially on the basis of false-negative DNase reactions that were finalized within 48 h of incubation rather than 72 h (13). Selected isolates of *Flavobacterium* spp. and *Shewanella* spp. may also be DNase positive (see chapter 35). On sheep blood agar, colonies appear rough and lavender-green and have an ammonia odor. *S. maltophilia* has a characteristic CFA profile with large amounts (>30%) of 13-methyl tetradecanoic acid ($C_{15:0\ iso}$) and lesser amounts (>10%) of 12-

methyl tetradecanoic acid ($C_{15:0\ anteiso}$) and *cis*-9-hexadecenoic acid ($C_{16:1\ cis\ 9}$) (134).

Acidovorax species, rarely encountered in clinical and environmental samples, are straight to slightly curved gram-negative bacilli which occur either singly or in short chains. They are oxidase positive, may be pigmented, and have one to two polar flagella (Table 3). Urease activity varies among strains (134, 137).

B. diminuta and *B. vesicularis* are infrequently encountered in clinical and environmental samples and have growth requirements for specific vitamins, including pantothenate, biotin, and cyanocobalamin. An additional growth requirement for *B. diminuta* is cysteine. All strains of *B. diminuta* will grow on MacConkey agar, while 43% of *B. vesicularis* strains will grow on this medium (Table 3). On primary isolation media, *B. diminuta* colonies are tan, while many strains of *B. vesicularis* are characterized by a yellow-orange intracellular pigment. These organisms are oxidase

TABLE 3 Characteristics of *Acidovorax*, *Brevundimonas*, *Comamonas*, and *Stenotrophomonas* spp. found in clinical specimens[a]

Test	% Strains positive							
	A. delafieldii (n = 2)	*A. facilis* (n = 2)	*A. temperans* (n = 2)	*B. diminuta* (n = 68)	*B. vesicularis* (n = 94)	*C. acidovorans* (n = 69)	*C. testosteroni* (n = 1)	*S. maltophilia* (n = 228)
Oxidase	100	100	100	100	98	100	100	0
Growth								
MacConkey	100	0	100	100	43	100	100	100
Cetrimide	0	0	0	0	0	4	0	2
6.0% NaCl	0	0	0	21	23	6	0	22
42°C	50	0	100	38	19	29	100	48
Nitrate reduction	100	100	100	3	5	99	100	39
Gas from nitrate	0	0	100	0	0	0	0	0
Pigment	Yellow; soluble	None	Yellow; soluble	Brown-tan; soluble	52%; yellow-orange; insoluble	26%; fluorescent	Tan; soluble	Brown-tan; soluble
Arginine dihydrolase	100	100	0	0	0	0	0	0
Lysine decarboxylase	0	0	0	0	0	0	0	93
Ornithine decarboxylase	0	0	0	0	0	0	0	0
Indole	0	0	0	0	0	0	0	0
Hemolysis	0	0	0	0	0	0	0	1
Hydrolysis								
Urea	100	100	50	13	2	0	0	3
Citrate	100	0	0	1	1	94	100	34
Gelatin	0	100	0	68	25	11	0	93
Esculin	0	0	0	5	88	0	0	39
Acid from								
Glucose[b]	100	100	100	21	87	0	0	85
Xylose	85	100	0	0	27	0	0	35
Lactose	0	0	0	0	0	0	0	60
Sucrose	0	0	0	0	0	0	0	63
Maltose	0	0	0	0	94	0	0	100
Mannitol	50	100	50	0	0	100	0	0
H_2S[c]	100	100	100	34	49	57	0	95
Motility	100	100	100	100	100	100	100	100
No. of flagella	1–2	1–2	1–2	1–2	1–2	>2	>2	>2

[a] Data are from reference 134.
[b] Oxidation-fermentation basal medium with 1% carbohydrate.
[c] Lead acetate paper.

positive, have one to two polar flagella, and weakly oxidize glucose (*B. vesicularis* more so than *B. diminuta*). The vast majority fail to reduce nitrate to nitrite. The most reliable method for differentiating these two species is the test for esculin hydrolysis. Almost all strains of *B. vesicularis* (88%) are reported to hydrolyze this substrate, while *B. diminuta* strains rarely do (5%) (134).

Comamonas spp. are straight to slightly curved gram-negative bacilli which occur singly or in pairs. The organisms are catalase and oxidase positive and have a single tuft of polar flagella. All *Comamonas* species reduce nitrate to nitrite, and *C. acidovorans* oxidizes fructose and mannitol and may produce a soluble yellow to tan pigment (134, 136).

TYPING SYSTEMS

Several molecular methodologies for assessing strain relatedness in nosocomial outbreak investigations are available. These methods have proven to be much more discriminatory and reproducible than phenotypically based systems (9, 18, 91, 110, 119). Pulsed-field gel electrophoresis (PFGE) and ribotyping are the most accurate, albeit technically challenging, typing methods. They have been used to study outbreaks and more global epidemiologic questions for *B. cepacia* (86, 110, 111), *B. pseudomallei* (118), *R. pickettii* (18, 26), and *S. maltophilia* (9, 63, 119). Restriction endonuclease *Xba*I or *Spe*I, frequently used for chromosomal digestion in PFGE, usually yields 20 to 30 fragments for analysis. This is not surprising since *B. cepacia* strains have been shown to have as many as four chromosomes and a very large genome size of 5 to 9 Mb (65).

Typing methods have not been reported for *Brevundimonas*, *Comamonas*, or *Acidovorax* spp.

SEROLOGIC TESTS

Of the organisms discussed in this chapter, serologic tests have been used clinically to diagnose only *B. pseudomallei* infections. The indirect hemagglutination assay (IHA) is the most widely used test in regions of endemicity. Because of high antibody background levels in healthy individuals (1), cross-reactions with other organisms including *B. cepacia* (1), and the rapid onset of septicemic disease, IHA is of limited clinical value. Even individual titers with high relative values lack both sensitivity and specificity. Fourfold changes in IHA titers between acute- and convalescent-phase sera may be of use in patients with subacute or chronic infection (76). EIAs with a variety of different antigens have also been described. Although more sensitive and specific than IHA, these EIAs have been used only in research settings. False-positive results also occur with these tests due to cross-reactions or subclinical infections (122).

ANTIMICROBIAL SUSCEPTIBILITY

B. pseudomallei is usually susceptible to the antipseudomonal penicillins, cefoperazone, ceftazidime, ampicillin-sulbactam, amoxicillin-clavulanic acid, chloramphenicol, and tetracyclines. Susceptibility to the fluoroquinolones is variable. Most isolates are resistant to the aminoglycosides and trimethoprim-sulfamethoxazole (TMP-SMX) (104, 106, 143). The organism is uniformly resistant to antistaphylococcal penicillins, ampicillin, rifampin, and the narrow- and expanded-spectrum cephalosporins. Antimicrobial resistance has been reported to emerge during therapy with chloramphenicol. These resistant isolates may show cross-resistance to tetracyclines, TMP-SMX, and quinolones (22a).

B. cepacia is one of the most antimicrobial agent-resistant organisms encountered in the clinical laboratory. The organism is usually susceptible only to piperacillin, azlocillin, cefoperazone, ceftazidime, chloramphenicol, and TMP-SMX. Susceptibility to imipenem and meropenem is variable, and a small percentage of isolates may be susceptible to kanamycin (89). Strains recovered from CF patients who have received repeated antimicrobial courses will frequently be resistant to all known antimicrobial agents (37).

S. maltophilia is inherently resistant to many antibiotics. In addition, the slow growth rate and increased mutation rate often result in discordance between in vitro susceptibility results and clinical outcome (36). Resistance develops quickly and against several classes of antimicrobial agents. Resistance to beta-lactam agents is mediated by the production of at least two β-lactamases, one of which is resistant to β-lactamase inhibitors and degrades imipenem. Aminoglycoside and quinolone resistance is the result of mutations in outer membrane proteins. TMP-SMX is the drug of choice, and in vitro data suggest that the combination of aztreonam and clavulanic acid may be effective (35a), although in vivo validation is necessary. There is no standardized susceptibility testing method specific for this genus. Although difficulties have been reported with all methods, the broth microdilution method, the E test (144), or the agar dilution method is preferred over the disk susceptibility method because of interpretation inconsistencies associated with disk susceptibility testing (2).

In general, the *Comamonas* species are susceptible to expanded- and broad-spectrum cephalosporins, carbapenems, quinolones, and TMP-SMX (6). *C. acidovorans* isolates are frequently resistant to the aminoglycosides.

Interpretative standards for *P. aeruginosa* are applicable to the susceptibility testing of *Burkholderia*, *Stenotrophomonas*, *Acidovorax*, *Brevundimonas*, *Comamonas*, and *Ralstonia* spp. The disk diffusion method is not recommended (73, 74).

REFERENCES

1. **Anuntunagool, N., P. Rugdech, and S. Sirisinha.** 1993. Identification of specific antigens of *Pseudomonas pseudomallei* and evaluation of their efficacies for diagnosis of melioidosis. *J. Clin. Microbiol.* **31:**1232–1236.

1a. **Aris, R. M., P. H. Gilligan, I. P. Neuringer, K. K. Gott, J. Rea, and J. R. Yankaskas.** 1997. The effect of panresistant bacteria in cystic fibrosis on lung transplant outcome. *Am. J. Respir. Crit. Care Med.* **155:**1699–1704.

2. **Arpi, M., M. A. Victor, I. Mortenson, A. Gottschau, and B. Bruun.** 1996. In vitro susceptibility of 124 *Xanthomonas maltophilia* isolates: comparison of the agar dilution method with the E test and two agar diffusion methods. *APMIS* **104:**108–114.

3. **Ashdown, L. R.** 1979. An improved screening technique for isolation of *Pseudomonas pseudomallei* from clinical specimens. *Pathology* **11:**293–297.

4. **Balaz, M., A. Demitrovicova, S. Spanik, L. Drgona, I. Krupova, S. Grausova, K. Kralovicova, J. Trupl, A. Kunova, and V. Krcmery.** 1996. Etiology of bacteremia in patients with various malignancies: is there an association between certain antineoplastic drugs and microorganisms? *Bratislavske Lekarske Listy* **97:**675–679.

5. **Ballard, R. W., M. Doudoroff, and R. Y. Stanier.** 1968. Taxonomy of the aerobic pseudomonads: *Pseudomonas diminuta* and *Pseudomonas vesicularis*. *J. Gen. Microbiol.* **53:** 349–361.

6. **Barbaro, D. J., and P. A. Mackowiak.** 1987. *Pseudomonas testosteroni* infections: eighteen recent cases and review of the literature. *Rev. Infect. Dis.* **9:**124–129.
7. **Barker, P. M., R. E. Wood, and P. H. Gilligan.** 1997. Lung infection with *Burkholderia gladioli* in a child with cystic fibrosis: acute clinical and spirometric deterioration. *Pediatr. Pulmon.* **24:**123–125.
8. **Baxter, I. A., P. A. Lambert, and I. N. Simpson.** 1997. Isolation from clinical sources of *Burkholderia cepacia* possessing characteristics of *Burkholderia gladioli*. *J. Antimicrob. Chemother.* **39:**169–175.
9. **Bingen E. D., K. Denamur, and J. Elion.** 1994. Use of ribotyping in epidemiological surveillance of nosocomial outbreaks. *Clin. Microbiol. Rev.* **7:**311–327.
10. **Bouvy, J. J., J. E. Degener, C. Stijnen, M. P. W. Gallee, and B. van der Berg.** 1986. Septic melioidosis after a visit to Southeast Asia. *Eur. J. Clin. Microbiol.* **5:**655–656.
11. **Brett, P. J., D. Deshazer, and D. E. Woods.** 1997. Characterization of *Burkholderia pseudomallei* and *Burkholderia pseudomallei*-like strains. *Epidemiol. Infect.* **118:**137–148.
12. **Brinser, J. H., and E. Torczynski.** 1977. Unusual *Pseudomonas* corneal ulcers. *Am. J. Ophthalmol.* **84:**462–466.
13. **Burdge, D. R., M. A. Noble, M. E. Campbell, V. L. Krell, and D. P. Speert.** 1995. *Xanthomonas maltophilia* misidentified as *Pseudomonas cepacia* in cultures of sputum from patients with cystic fibrosis: a diagnostic pitfall with major clinical implications. *Clin. Infect. Dis.* **20:**445–448.
14. **Burns, J. L., D. K. Clark, and G. L. Morlin.** 1993. Effect of specimen storage temperature on the ability to recover *Pseudomonas cepacia* from sputum. *Pediatr. Pulmon. Suppl.* **9:**256–257.
15. **Calegari, L., K. Gezuele, E. Torres, and C. Carmona.** 1996. Botryomycosis caused by *Pseudomonas vesicularis*. *Int. J. Dermatol.* **35:**817–818.
16. **Campbell, P. W., III, J. A. Phillips III, G. L. Heidecker, M. R. S. Krishnamani, R. Zahorchak, and T. L. Stull.** 1995. Detection of *Pseudomonas (Burkholderia) cepacia* using PCR. *Pediatr. Pulmon.* **20:**44–49.
17. **Castagnola, E., L. Tasso, M. Conte, M. Nantron, A. Barretta, and R. Giacchino.** 1994. Central venous catheter-related infection due to *Comamonas acidovorans* in a child with non-Hodgkin's lymphoma. *Clin. Infect. Dis.* **19:**559–560.
18. **Chetoui, H., P. Melin, M. J. Struelens, E. Delhalle, M. Mutro Nigo, R. De Ryck, and P. De Mol.** 1997. Comparison of biotyping, ribotyping, and pulsed-field gel electrophoresis for investigation of a common-source outbreak of *Burkholderia pickettii* bacteremia. *J. Clin. Microbiol.* **35:**1398–1403.
19. **Christenson, J. C., D. F. Welch, G. Mukwaya, M. J. Muszynski, R. E. Weaver, and D. J. Brenner.** 1989. Recovery of *Pseudomonas gladioli* from respiratory tract specimens of patients with cystic fibrosis. *J. Clin. Microbiol.* **27:**270–273.
20. **Craven, D. E., B. Moody, M. G. Connolly, N. R. Kollisch, K. D. Stottmeier, and W. R. McCabe.** 1981. Pseudobacteremia caused by povidone-iodine solution contaminated with *Pseudomonas cepacia*. *N. Engl. J. Med.* **305:**621–623.
21. **Dance, D. A. B.** 1991. Melioidosis: the tip of the iceberg? *Clin. Microbiol. Rev.* **4:**52–60.
22. **Dance, D. A. B., V. Wuthiekanun, P. Naigowit, and N. J. White.** 1989. Identification of *Pseudomonas pseudomallei* in clinical practice: use of simple screening tests and API 20NE. *J. Clin. Pathol.* **42:**645–648.

22a. **Dance, D. A. B., V. Wuthiekanun, W. Chaowagul, and N. J. White.** 1989. The antimicrobial susceptibility of *Pseudomonas pseudomallei*. Emergence of resistance *in vitro* and during treatment. *J. Antimicrob. Chemother.* **24:**295–309.

23. **Davis, D. H., R. Y. Stanier, M. Doudoroff, and M. Mandel.** 1970. Taxonomic studies on some gram negative polarly flagellated "hydrogen bacteria" and related species. *Arch. Mikrobiol.* **70:**1–13.
24. **Desakorn, V., M. D. Smith, V. Wuthiekanun, D. A. B. Dance, H. Aucken, P. Suntharasamai, A. Rajchanuwong, and N. J. White.** 1994. Detection of *Pseudomonas pseudomallei* antigen in urine for diagnosis of melioidosis. *Am. J. Trop. Med. Hyg.* **51:**627–633.
25. **Desmarchelier, P. M., D. A. B. Dance, W. Chaowagul, Y. Suputtamongkol, N. J. White, and T. L. Pitt.** 1993. Relationships among *Pseudomonas pseudomallei* isolates from patients with recurrent melioidosis. *J. Clin. Microbiol.* **31:**1592–1596.
26. **Dimech, W. J., A. G. Hellyar, M. Kotiw, D. Marcon, S. Ellis, and M. Carson.** 1993. Typing of strains from a single-source outbreak of *Pseudomonas pickettii*. *J. Clin. Microbiol.* **31:**3001–3006.
27. **Drancourt, M., C. Bollet, and D. Raoult.** 1997. *Stenotrophomonas africana* sp. nov., an opportunistic human pathogen in Africa. *Int. J. Syst. Bacteriol.* **47:**160–163.
28. **Elting, L. S., S. Khadori, G. Bodey, and G. P. Fainstein.** 1990. Nosocomial infections caused by *Xanthomonas maltophilia*: a case-control study of predisposing factors. *Infect. Control Hosp. Epidemiol.* **11:**134–138.
29. **Ender, T. E., D. P. Dooley, and R. H. Moore.** 1996. Vascular catheter-related *Comamonas acidovorans* bacteremia managed with preservation of the catheter. *Pediatr. Infect. Dis. J.* **15:**918–920.
30. **Ensor, E., H. Humphrey, D. Peckham, C. Webster, and A. J. Knox.** 1996. Is *Burkholderia* (*Pseudomonas*) *cepacia* disseminated from cystic fibrosis patients during physiotherapy? *J. Hosp. Infect.* **32:**9–15.
31. **Fass, R. J., and J. Barnishan.** 1976. Acute meningitis due to a *Pseudomonas*-like group Va-1 bacillus. *Ann. Intern. Med.* **84:**51–52.
32. **Fernandez, C., I. Wilhelm, E. Andradas, C. Gaspar, J. Gomez, J. Romera, J. Mariano, O. Corral, M. Rubio, J. Elviro, and J. Fereres.** 1996. Nosocomial outbreak of *Burkholderia pickettii* infection due to a manufactured intravenous product used in three hospitals. *Clin. Infect. Dis.* **22:**1092–1095.
33. **Fitzsimmons, S. C.** 1993. The changing epidemiology of cystic fibrosis. *J. Pediatr.* **122:**1–9.
34. **Fujita, J., I. Yamadori, G. Xu, S. Hojo, K. Negayama, H. Miyawaki, Y. Yamaji, and J. Takahara.** 1996. Clinical features of *Stenotrophomonas maltophilia* in immunocompromised patients. *Respir. Med.* **90:**35–38.
35. **Fujita, S., T. Yoshida, and F. Matsubara.** 1981. *Pseudomonas pickettii* bacteremia. *J. Clin. Microbiol.* **13:**781–782.

35a. **Garcia-Rodriguez, J. A., J. E. Garcia Sanchez, M. I. Garcia Garcia, E. Garcia Sanchez, and J. L. Munoz Bellido.** 1991. Antibiotic susceptibility profile of *Xanthamonas maltophilia*: In vitro activity of beta-lactam/beta-lactamase inhibitor combinations. *Diagn. Microbiol. Infect. Dis.* **14:**239–243.

36. **Garrison, M. W., D. E. Anderson, D. M. Campbell, K. C. Carroll, C. L. Malone, and J. D. Anderson.** 1996. *Stenotrophomonas maltophilia*: emergence of multidrug resistant strains during therapy and in an in vitro pharmodynamic chamber model. *Antimicrob. Agents Chemother.* **40:**2859–2864.
37. **Gilligan, P. H.** 1991. Microbiology of airway disease in patients with cystic fibrosis. *Clin. Microbiol. Rev.* **4:**35–51.
38. **Gilligan, P. H., P. A. Gage, L. M. Bradshaw, D. V. Schidlow, and B. T. DeCicco.** 1985. Isolation medium for the recovery of *Pseudomonas cepacia* from respiratory secretions of patients with cystic fibrosis. *J. Clin. Microbiol.* **22:**5–8.
39. **Gillis, M., T. V. Van, R. Hardin, M. Goor, P. Hebbar,**

A. Willems, P. Segers, K. Kersters, T. Heulin, and M. P. Fernandez. 1995. Polyphasic taxonomy in the genus *Burkholderia* leading to an emended description of the genus and proposition of *Burkholderia vietnamiensis* sp. nov. for the N_2-fixing isolates from rice in Vietnam. *Int. J. Syst. Bacteriol.* **45:**274–289.

40. **Girijaratnakumari, T., A. Raja, R. Ramani, B. Antony, and P. G. Shivananda.** 1993. Meningitis due to *Xanthomonas maltophilia*. *J. Postgrad. Med.* **39:**153–155.
41. **Gladman G., P. J. Connor, R. F. Williams, and T. J. David.** 1992. Controlled study of *Pseudomonas cepacia* and *Pseudomonas maltophilia* in cystic fibrosis. *Arch. Dis. Child.* **67:**192–195.
42. **Goldstein, R., L. Sun, R.-Z. Jiang, U. Sajjan, J. F. Forstner, and C. Campanelli.** 1995. Structurally variant classes of pilus appendage fibers coexpressed from *Burkholderia* (*Pseudomonas*) *cepacia*. *J. Bacteriol.* **177:**1039–1052.
43. **Govan, J. R. W., P. H. Brown, J. Maddison, C. J. Doherty, J. W. Nelson, M. Dodd, A. P. Greening, and A. K. Webb.** 1993. Evidence for transmission of *Pseudomonas cepacia* by social contact in cystic fibrosis. *Lancet* **342:** 15–19.
44. **Govan, J. R. W., J. E. Hughes, and P. Vandamme.** 1996. *Burkholderia cepacia*: medical, taxonomic, and ecological issues. *J. Med. Microbiol.* **45:**395–407.
45. **Graber, C. D., L. Jervey, W. E. Ostrander, A. H. Sally, and R. E. Weaver.** 1968. Endocarditis due to a lanthanic, unclassified gram-negative bacterium (group IVd). *Am. J. Clin. Pathol.* **49:**220–223.
46. **Gutierrez, R. F., M. M. Masia, J. Cortes, V. Ortez de la Tabla, V. Mainar, and A. Vilar.** 1996. Endocarditis caused by *Stenotrophomonas maltophilia*: case report and review. *Clin. Infect. Dis.* **23:**1261–1265.
47. **Haase, A., M. Brennan, S. Barrett, Y. Woods, S. Huffam, D. O'Brien, and B. Currie.** 1998. Evaluation of PCR for diagnosis of melioidosis. *J. Clin. Microbiol.* **36:**1039–1041.
48. **Henry, D. A., M. E. Campbell, J. J. LiPuma, and D. P. Speert.** 1997. Identification of *Burkholderia cepacia* isolates from patients with cystic fibrosis and use of a simple selective medium. *J. Clin. Microbiol.* **35:**614–619.
49. **Holt, J. G., N. R. Krieg, P. H. A. Sneath, J. T. Staley, and S. T. Williams (ed.).** 1994. *Bergey's Manual of Determinative Bacteriology*, 9th ed., p. 73, 80, 93, and 100. The Williams & Wilkins Co., Baltimore, Md.
50. **Horowitz, H., S. Gilroy, S. Feinstein, and G. Gilardi.** 1990. Endocarditis associated with *Comamonas acidovorans*. *J. Clin. Microbiol.* **28:**143–145.
51. **Hugh, R., and E. Ryschenkow.** 1961. *Pseudomonas maltophilia*, an *Alcaligenes*-like organism. *J. Gen. Microbiol.* **26:** 123–132.
52. **Hutchinson, G. R., S. Parker, J. A. Pryor, F. Duncan-Skingle, P. N. Hoffman, M. E. Hodson, M. E. Kauffman, and T. L. Pitt.** 1996. Home-use nebulizers: a potential primary source of *Burkholderia cepacia* and other colisitin-resistant, gram-negative bacteria in patients with cystic fibrosis. *J. Clin. Microbiol.* **43:**584–587.
53. **Ip, M., L. G. Osterberg, P. Y. Chau, and T. A. Raffin.** 1995. Pulmonary melioidosis. *Chest* **108:**1420–1424.
54. **Irifune, K., T. Ishida, K. Shimoguchi, J. Ohtake, T. Tanaka, N. Morikawa, M. Kaku, H. Koga, S. Kohno, and K. Hara.** 1994. Pneumonia caused by *Stenotrophomonas maltophilia* with a mucoid phenotype. *J. Clin. Microbiol.* **32:** 2856–2857.
55. **Jones, A. L., T. J. Beveridge, and D. E. Woods.** 1996. Intracellular survival of *Burkholderia pseudomallei*. *Infect. Immun.* **64:**782–790.
56. **Kahyaoglu, O., B. Nolan, and A. Kumar.** 1995. Empyema and bloodstream infection caused by *Burkholderia gladioli* in a patient with cystic fibrosis after lung transplantation. *Pediatr. Infect. Dis. J.* **15:**637–638.
57. **Kaiser, G. M. P. C. Tso, R. Morris, and D. McCurdy.** 1997. *Xanthomonas maltophilia* endophthalmitis after cataract extraction. *Am. J. Ophthalmol.* **123:**410–411.
58. **Kanaphun, P., N. Thirawattanasuk, Y. Suputtamongkol, P. Naigowit, D. A. B. Dance, M. D. Smith, and N. J. White.** 1993. Serology and carriage of *Pseudomonas pseudomallei*: a prospective study in 1000 hospitalized children in northeast Thailand. *J. Infect. Dis.* **167:**230–233.
59. **Kiska, D. L., A. Kerr, M. C. Jones, J. A. Caraccioli, B. Eskridge, M. Jordan, S. Miller, D. Hughes, N. King, and P. H. Gilligan.** 1996. Accuracy of four commercial systems for the identification of *Burkholderia cepacia* and other gram-negative nonfermenting bacilli recovered from patients with cystic fibrosis. *J. Clin. Microbiol.* **34:**886–891.
60. **Koneman, E. W., S. D. Allen, W. M. Janda, P. C. Schreckenberger, and W. C. Winn, Jr.** 1992. The nonfermentative gram negative bacilli, p. 185–242. *In Color Atlas and Textbook of Diagnostic Microbiology*, 4th ed. J. B. Lippincott Co., Philadelphia, Pa.
61. **Koponen, M. A., D. Zlock, D. L. Palmer, and T. L. Merlin.** 1991. Melioidosis: forgotten, not gone! *Arch. Intern. Med.* **151:**605–608.
62. **Lacey, S., and S. V. Want.** 1991. *Pseudomonas pickettii* infections in a pediatric oncology unit. *J. Hosp. Infect.* **17:** 45–51.
63. **Laing, F. P., K. Ramotar, R. R. Reed, N. Alfieri, A. Kureishi, E. A. Henderson, and T. O. Louie.** 1995. Molecular epidemiology of *Xanthomonas maltophilia* colonization and infection in the hospital environment. *J. Clin. Microbiol.* **33:**513–518.
64. **Leelarasamee, A., and S. Bovornkitti.** 1989. Melioidosis: review and update. *Rev. Infect. Dis.* **11:**413–425.
65. **Lessie, T. G., W. Hendrickson, B. D. Manning, and R. Devereux.** 1996. Genomic complexity and plasticity of *Burkholderia cepacia*. *FEMS Microbiol. Lett.* **144:**117–128.
66. **LiPuma, J. J.** 1997. Is it *Burkholderia cepacia*? Does it matter? *Pediatr. Pulmon. Suppl.* **14:**88–89.
67. **Maki, D. G., B. S. Klein, R. D. McCormick, C. J. Alvarado, M. A. Zilz, S. M. Stolz, C. A. Hassemer, J. Gould, and A. R. Liegel.** 1991. Nosocomial *Pseudomonas pickettii* bacteremias traced to narcotic tampering: a case for selective drug screening of health care personnel. *JAMA* **265:** 981–986.
68. **Martino, R., C. Martinez, R. Pericas, R. Salazar, C. Sola, S. Brunet, A. Sureda, and A. Domingo-Albos.** 1996. Bacteremia due to glucose non-fermenting gram-negative bacilli in patients with hematological neoplasias and solid tumors. *Eur. J. Clin. Microbiol. Infect. Dis.* **15:**610–615.
69. **McNeil, M. M., S. L. Solomon, R. L. Anderson, B. J. Davis, R. F. Spengler, R. E. Reisberg, C. Thornsberry, and W. J. Martone.** 1985. Nosocomial *Pseudomonas pickettii* colonization associated with a contaminated respiratory therapy solution in a special care nursery. *J. Clin. Microbiol.* **22:**903–907.
70. **Mortensen, J. E., M. C. Fisher, and J. J. LiPuma.** 1995. Recovery of *Pseudomaonas cepacia* and other *Pseudomonas* species from the environment. *Infect. Control Hosp. Epidemiol.* **16:**30–32.
71. **Muder, R. R., A. P. Harris, S. Muller, M. Edmond, J. W. Chow, K. Papadakis, M. W. Wagener, G. P. Bodey, and J. M. Steckelberg.** 1996. Bacteremia due to *Stenotrophomonas maltophilia*: a prospective multicenter study of 91 episodes. *Clin. Infect. Dis.* **22:**508–512.
72. **Mukwaya, G. M., and D. F. Welch.** 1989. Subgrouping of *Pseudomonas cepacia* by cellular fatty acid composition. *J. Clin. Microbiol.* **27:**2640–2646.
73. **National Committee for Clinical Laboratory Standards.**

1995. *Methods for Dilution Antimicrobial Susceptibility Tests for Bacteria That Grow Aerobically*. Approved standard M7-A4. National Committee for Clinical Laboratory Standards, Wayne, Pa.

74. **National Committee for Clinical Laboratory Standards.** 1998. *Performance Standards for Antimicrobial Susceptibility Testing*. Eighth Information Supplement. Approved standard M100-S8. National Committee for Clinical Laboratory Standards, Wayne, Pa.
75. **Nguyen, M. H., and R. R. Muder.** 1994. Meningitis due to *Xanthomonas maltophilia*: case report and review. *Clin. Infect. Dis.* **19:**325–326.
76. **Norzah, A., M. Y. Rohani, P. T. Chang, and A. G. M. Kamel.** 1996. Indirect hemagglutination antibodies against *Burkholderia pseudomallei* in normal blood donors and suspected cases of melioidosis in Malaysia. *Southeast Asian J. Trop. Med. Public Health* **27:**263–266.
77. **Oberhelman, R. A., J. R. Humbert, and F. W. Santorelli.** 1994. *Pseudomonas vesicularis* causing bacteremia in a child with sickle cell anemia. *South. Med. J.* **87:**821–822.
78. **O'Neil, K. M., J. H. Herman, J. F. Modlin, E. R. Moxon, and J. A. Winkelstein.** 1986. *Pseudomonas cepacia*: an emerging pathogen in chronic granulomatous disease. *J. Pediatr.* **108:**940–942.
79. **Otto, L. A., B. S. Deboo, E. L. Capers, and M. J. Pickett.** 1978. *Pseudomonas vesicularis* from cervical specimens. *J. Clin. Microbiol.* **7:**341–345.
80. **Pallent, L. J., W. B. Hugo, D. J. W. Grant, and A. Davies.** 1983. *Pseudomonas cepacia* as contaminant and infective agent. *J. Hosp. Infect.* **4:**9–13.
81. **Palleroni, N. J.** 1984. Genus I. *Pseudomonas* Migula 1894, 237^{AL}, p. 141–199. *In* N. R. Krieg and J. G. Holt (ed.), *Bergey's Manual of Systematic Bacteriology*, vol. 1. The Williams & Wilkins Co., Baltimore, Md.
82. **Palleroni, N. J., and J. F. Bradbury.** 1993. *Stenotrophomonas*, a new bacterial genus for *Xanthomonas maltophilia* (Hugh 1980) Swings et al. *Int. J. Syst. Bacteriol.* **43:** 606–609.
83. **Palleroni, N. J., R. Kunisawa, R. Contopoulou, and M. Doudoroff.** 1973. Nucleic acid homologies in the genus *Pseudomonas*. *Int. J. Syst. Bacteriol.* **23:**333–339.
84. **Papadakis, K. A., S. E. Vartivarian, M. E. Vassilaki, and E. J. Anaissie.** 1996. Septic prepatellar bursitis caused by *Stenotrophomonas maltophilia*. *Clin. Infect. Dis.* **22:** 388–389.
85. **Papadakis, K. A., S. E. Vartivarian, M. E. Vassilaki, and E. J. Anaissie.** 1995. *Stenotrophomonas maltophilia*: an unusual cause of biliary sepsis. *Clin. Infect. Dis.* **21:**1032–1034.
86. **Pegues, C. F., D. F. Pegues, D. S. Ford, P. L. Hibberd, L. A. Carson, C. M. Raine, and D. C. Hooper.** 1996. *Burkholderia cepacia* respiratory acquisition: epidemiology and molecular characterization of a large nosocomial outbreak. *Epidemiol. Infect.* **116:**309–317.
87. **Pegues, D. A., L. A. Carson, R. L. Anderson, M. J. Norgard, T. A. Agent, W. R. Jarvis, and C. H. Woernle.** 1993. Outbreak of *Pseudomonas cepacia* bacteremia in oncology patients. *Clin. Infect. Dis.* **16:**407–411.
88. **Penland, R. L., and K. R. Wilhelmus.** 1996. *Stenotrophomonas* ocular infections. *Arch. Ophthalmol.* **114:**433–436.
89. **Pitkin, D. H., W. Sheikh, and H. L. Nadler.** 1997. Comparative in vitro activity of meropenem versus other extended-spectrum antimicrobials against randomly chosen and selected resistant clinical isolates tested in 26 North American centers. *Clin. Infect. Dis.* **24**(Suppl. 2): S238–S248.
90. **Planes, M., A. Ramirez, F. Fernandez, J. A. Capdevila, and C. Tolosa.** 1992. *Pseudomonas vesicularis* bacteremia. *Infection* **20:**367–368.
91. **Rabkin, C. S., W. R. Jarvis, R. L. Anderson, J. Govan, J. Kliger, J. LiPuma, W. Jarvis, W. J. Martone, H. Monteil, C. Richard, S. Shigeta, A. Sosa, T. Stull, J. Swenson, and D. Woods.** 1989. *Pseudomonas cepacia* typing systems: collaborative study to assess their potential in epidemiologic investigations. *Rev. Infect. Dis.* **11:** 600–607.
92. **Raveh, D., A. Simhon, Z. Gimmon, T. Sacks, and M. Shapiro.** 1993. Infections caused by *Pseudomonas pickettii* in association with permanent indwelling intravenous devices: four cases and a review. *Clin. Infect. Dis.* **17:** 877–880.
93. **Reboli, A. C., R. Koshinski, K. Arias, K. Marks-Austin, D. Stiertz, and T. L. Stull.** 1996. An outbreak of *Burkholderia cepacia* lower respiratory tract infection associated with contaminated albuterol nebulization solution. *Infect. Control Hosp. Epidemiol.* **17:**741–743.
94. **Reina, J., I. Llompart, and P. Alomar.** 1991. Acute suppurative otitis caused by *Comamonas acidovorans*. *Clin. Microbiol. Newsl.* **13:**38–39.
95. **Riley, P. S., and R. E. Weaver.** 1975. Recognition of *Pseudomonas pickettii* in the clinical laboratory: biochemical characterization of 62 strains. *J. Clin. Microbiol.* **1:** 61–64.
96. **Ross, J. P., S. M. Holland, V. J. Gill, E. S. DeCarlo, and J. I. Gallin.** 1995. Severe *Burkholderia* (*Pseudomonas*) *gladioli* infection in chronic granulomatous disease: report of two successfully treated cases. *Clin. Infect. Dis.* **21:** 1291–1293.
97. **Sanford, J. P.** 1995. *Pseudomonas* species including melioidosis and glanders, p. 2003–2009. *In* G. L. Mandell, J. E. Bennett, and R. Dolin (ed.), *Principles and Practice of Infectious Diseases*, 4th ed. Churchill-Livingstone, New York, N.Y.
98. **Schatz, A., and C. Bovell, Jr.** 1952. Growth and hydrogenase activity of a new bacterium, *Hydrogenomonas facilis*. *J. Bacteriol.* **63:**87–98.
99. **Segers, P., M. Vancanneyt, B. Pot, U. Torck, B. Hoste, D. Dewettinck, E. Falsen, K. Kersters, and P. De Vos.** 1994. Classification of *Pseudomonas diminuta* Leifson and Hugh 1954 and *Pseudomonas vesicularis* Busing, Doll, and Freytag 1953 in *Brevundimonas* gen. nov. as *Brevundimonas diminuta* comb. nov. and *Brevundimonas vesicularis* comb. nov., respectively. *Int. J. Syst. Bacteriol.* **44:**499–510.
100. **Segonds, C., E. Bingen, G. Couetdic, S. Mathy, N. Brahimi, N. Marty, P. Plesiat, Y. Michel-Briand, and G. Chabanon.** 1997. Genotypic analysis of *Burkholderia cepacia* isolates from 13 French cystic fibrosis centers. *J. Clin. Microbiol.* **35:**2055–2060.
101. **Smith, D. L., L. B. Gumery, E. G. Smith, D. E. Stableforth, M. E. Kaufmann, and T. L. Pitt.** 1993. Epidemic of *Pseudomonas cepacia* in an adult cystic fibrosis unit: evidence of person-to-person transmission. *J. Clin. Microbiol.* **31:**3017–3022.
102. **Smith, M. D., B. J. Angus, V. Wuthiekanun, and N. J. White.** 1997. Arabinose assimilation defines a nonvirulent biotype of *Burkholderia pseudomallei*. *J. Clin. Microbiol.* **65:**4319–4321.
103. **Smith, M. D., V. Wuthiekunan, A. L. Walsh, N. Teerawattanasook, V. Desakorn, Y. Suputtamongkol, T. L. Pitt, and N. J. White.** 1995. Latex agglutination for rapid detection of *Pseudomonas pseudomallei* antigen in urine of patients with melioidosis. *J. Clin. Pathol.* **48:**174–176.
104. **Smith, M. D., V. Wuthiekunan, A. L. Walsh, and N. J. White.** 1994. Susceptibility of *Pseudomonas pseudomallei* to some newer beta-lactam antibiotics and antibiotic combinations using time-kill studies. *J. Antimicrob. Chemother.* **33:**145–149.
105. **Snell, G. I., A. de Hoyos, M. Krajden, T. Winton, and J.**

R. Maurer. 1993. *Pseudomonas cepacia* in lung transplant recipients with cystic fibrosis. *Chest* **103:**466–471.
106. **Sookpranee, T., M. Sookpranee, M. A. Mellencamp, and L. C. Preheim.** 1991. *Pseudomonas pseudomallei*, a common pathogen in Thailand that is resistant to the bactericidal effects of many antibiotics. *Antimicrob. Agents Chemother.* **35:**484–489.
107. **Spencer, R. C.** 1995. The emergence of epidemic, multiple-antibiotic resistant *Stenotrophomonas maltophilia* and *Burkholderia cepacia*. *J. Hosp. Infect.* **30**(Suppl.)**:**453–464.
108. **Spraul, C. W., G. E. Lang, and G. K. Lang.** 1996. *Xanthomonas maltophilia* keratitis associated with contact lenses. *CLAO J. (Contact Lens Assoc. Ophthalmol.)* **22:**158.
109. **Stead, D. E.** 1992. Grouping of plant-pathogenic and some other *Pseudomonas* spp. by using cellular fatty acid profiles. *Int. J. Syst. Bacteriol.* **42:**281–285.
110. **Steinbach, S., L. Sun, R.-Z. Jiang, P. Gilligan, P. Flume, T. M. Egan, and R. Goldstein.** 1994. Transmissibility of *Pseudomonas cepacia* infection in clinic patients and lung-transplant recipients with cystic fibrosis. *N. Engl. J. Med.* **331:**981–987.
111. **Sun, L., R.-Z. Jiang, S. Steinbach, A. Holmes, C. Campanelli, J. Forstner, U. Sajjan, Y. Tan, M. Riley, and R. Goldstein.** 1995. The emergence of a highly transmissible lineage of *cbl*$^+$ *Pseudomonas* (*Burkholderia*) *cepacia* causing CF centre epidemics in North America and Britain. *Nat. Med.* **1:**661–666.
112. **Swing, J., P. de Vos, M. van den Mooter, and J. de Ley.** 1983. Transfer of *Pseudomonas maltophilia* Hugh 1981 to the genus *Xanthomonas* as *Xanthomonas maltophilia* (Hugh 1981) comb. nov. *Int. J. Syst. Bacteriol.* **33:**409–413.
113. **Szeto, C. C., P. K. Li, C. B. Leung, A. W. Yu, S. F. Lui, and K. N. Lai.** 1997. *Xanthomonas maltophilia* peritonitis in uremic patients receiving continuous ambulatory peritoneal dialysis. *Am. J. Kidney Dis.* **29:**91–95.
114. **Tablan, O. C., L. A. Carson, L. B. Cusick, L. A. Bland, W. J. Martone, and W. R. Jarvis.** 1987. Laboratory proficiency test results on use of selective media for isolating *Pseudomonas cepacia* from simulated sputum specimens of patients with cystic fibrosis. *J. Clin. Microbiol.* **25:** 485–487.
115. **Tamaoka, J., D. M. Ha, and K. Komagata.** 1987. Reclassification of *Pseudomonas acidovorans* den Dooren de Jong 1926 and *Pseudomonas testosteroni* Marcus and Talalay 1956 as *Comamonas acidovorans* comb. nov. and *Comamonas testosteroni* comb. nov., with an emended description of the genus *Comamonas*. *Int. J. Syst. Bacteriol.* **37:**52–59.
116. **Tiangitayakorn, C., S. Songsivilai, N. Piyasangthong, and T. Dharakul.** 1997. Speed of detection of *Burkholderia pseudomallei* in blood cultures and its correlation with clinical outcome. *Am. J. Trop. Med.* **57:**96–99.
117. **Trotter, J. A., T. L. Kuhis, D. A. Pickett, S. Reyes de la Rocha, and D. F. Welch.** 1990. Pneumonia caused by a newly recognized pseudomonad in a child with chronic granulomatous disease. *J. Clin. Microbiol.* **28:**1120–1124.
118. **Vadivelu, J., S. D. Puthucheary, A. Mifsud, B. S. Drasar, D. A. B. Dance, and T. L. Pitt.** 1997. Ribotyping and DNA macrorestriction analysis of isolates of *Burkholderia pseudomallei* from cases of melioidosis in Malaysia. *Trans. R. Soc. Trop. Med. Hyg.* **91:**358–460.
119. **Van Couwenberghe, C., and S. Cohen.** 1994. Analysis of epidemic and endemic isolates of *Xanthomonas maltophilia* by contour clamped homogeneous electric field gel electrophoresis. *Infect. Control Hosp. Epidemiol.* **15:** 691–696.
120. **Vandamme, P., B. Holmes, M. Vancanneyt, T. Coenye, B. Hoste, R. Coopman, H. Revets, S. Lauwers, M. Gillis, K. Kersters, and J. R. W. Govan.** 1997. Occurrence of multiple genomovars of *Burkholderia cepacia* in cystic fibrosis patients and proposal of *Burkholderia multivorans* sp. nov. *Int. J. Syst. Bacteriol.* **47:**1188–1200.
121. **Vanholder, R., E. Vanhaecke, and S. Ringoir.** 1992. *Pseudomonas* septicemia due to deficient disinfectant mixing during reuse. *Int. J. Artif. Organs* **15:**19–24.
122. **Van Phung, L., Y. Han, S. Oka, H. Hotta, M. D. Smith, P. Theerparakun, E. Yabuuchi, and I. Yano.** 1995. Enzyme-linked immunosorbent assay (ELISA) using a glycolipid antigen for serodiagnosis of melioidosis. *FEMS Microbiol. Lett.* **12:**259–264.
123. **Van Phung, L. M., T. Thi Bich Chi, H. Hotta, E. Yabuuchi, and I. Yano.** 1995. Cellular lipid and fatty acid composition of *Burkholderia pseudomallei* strains from human and environment in Viet Nam. *Microbiol. Immunol.* **39:**105–116.
124. **Vartivarian, S. E., K. A. Papadakis, J. A. Palacios, J. T. Manning, and E. J. Anaissie.** 1994. Mucocutaneous and soft tissue infections caused by *Xanthomonas maltophilia*. A new spectrum. *Ann. Intern. Med.* **121:**969–973.
125. **Vartivarian, S. E., K. A. Papadakis, and E. J. Anaissie.** 1996. *Stenotrophomonas maltophilia* urinary tract infection. A disease that is usually severe and complicated. *Arch. Intern. Med.* **156:**433–435.
126. **Verschraegen, G., G. Claeys, G. Meeus, and M. Delanghe.** 1985. *Pseudomonas pickettii* as a cause of pseudobacteremia. *J. Clin. Microbiol.* **21:**278–279.
127. **Vu-Thien, H., D. Moissenet, M. Valcin, C. Dulot, G. Tournier, and A. Garbarg-Chenon.** 1996. Molecular epidemiology of *Burkholderia cepacia*, *Stenotrophomonas maltophilia* and *Alcaligenes xylosoxidans* in a cystic fibrosis center. *Eur. J. Clin. Microbiol. Infect. Dis.* **15:**876–879.
128. **Walsh, A. L., M. D. Smith, V. Wuthiekanun, Y. Suputtamongkol, W. Chaowagul, D. A. B. Dance, B. Angus, and N. J. White.** 1995. Prognostic significance of quantitative bacteremia in septicemic melioidosis. *Clin. Infect. Dis.* **21:**1498–1500.
129. **Walsh, A. L., M. D. Smith, V. Wuthiekanun, Y. Suputtamongkol, V. Desakorn, W. Chaowagul, and N. J. White.** 1994. Immunofluorescence microscopy for the rapid diagnosis of melioidosis. *J. Clin. Pathol.* **47:** 377–379.
130. **Walsh, A. L., V. Wuthiekanun, M. D. Smith, Y. Suputtamongkol, and N. J. White.** 1995. Selective broth for the isolation of *Pseudomonas pseudomallei* from clinical samples. *Trans. R. Soc. Trop. Med. Hyg.* **89:**124.
131. **Weinstein, R. A., W. E. Stamm, L. Kramer, and L. Corey.** 1976. Pressure monitoring devices: an overlooked source of nosocomial infection. *JAMA* **236:**936–938.
132. **Welch, D. F., M. J. Muszynski, C. H. Pai, M. J. Marcon, M. M. Hribar, P. H. Gilligan, J. M. Matsen, P. A. Ahlin, B. C. Hilman, and S. A. Chartrand.** 1987. Selective and differential medium for recovery of *Pseudomonas cepacia* from the respiratory tracts of patients with cystic fibrosis. *J. Clin. Microbiol.* **25:**1730–1734.
133. **Wertheim, W. A., and D. M. Markovitz.** 1992. Osteomyelitis and intervertebral discitis caused by *Pseudomonas pickettii*. *J. Clin. Microbiol.* **30:**2506–2508.
134. **Weyant, R. S., C. W. Moss, R. E. Weaver, D. G. Hollis, J. G. Jordan, E. C. Cook, and M. I. Daneshvar.** 1996. *Identification of Unusual Pathogenic Gram-Negative Aerobic and Facultatively Anaerobic Bacteria*, 2nd ed. The Williams & Wilkins Co., Baltimore, Md.
135. **Wilks, D., S. K. Jacobson, A. M. L. Lever, and M. Farrington.** 1994. Fatal melioidosis in a tourist returning from Thailand. *J. Infect.* **29:**87–90.
136. **Willems, A., J. De Ley, M. Gillis, and K. Kersters.** 1991. *Comamonadaceae*, a new family encompassing the acidovorans rRNA complex, including *Variovorax paradoxus*

gen. nov., comb nov., for *Alcaligenes paradoxus* (Davis 1969). *Int. J. Syst. Bacteriol.* **41:**445–450.

137. **Willems, A., E. Falsen, B. Pot, B. Hoste, P. Vandamme, M. Gillis, K. Kersters, and J. De Ley.** 1990. *Acidovorax*, a new genus for *Pseudomonas facilis*, *Pseudomonas delafieldii*, E. Falsen (EF) Group 13, EF Group 16 and several clinical isolates with the species *Acidovorax* comb. nov., *Acidovorax delafieldii* comb. nov., and *Acidovorax temperans* sp. nov. *Int. J. Syst. Bacteriol.* **40:**384–398.
138. **Wilsher, M. L., J. Kolbe, A. J. Morris, and D. F. Welch.** 1997. Nosocomial acquisition of *Burkholderia gladioli* in patients with cystic fibrosis. *Am. J. Respir. Crit. Care Med.* **155:**1436–1438.
139. **Woods, M. L., II, B. J. Currie, D. M. Howard, A. Tierney, A. Watson, N. M. Anstey, J. Philpott, V. Asche, and K. Withnall.** 1992. Neurological melioidosis: seven cases from the Northern Territory of Australia. *Clin. Infect. Dis.* **15:**163–169.
140. **Wuthiekanun, V., D. A. B. Dance, Y. Wattanagoon, Y. Supputtamongkol, W. Chaowagul, and N. J. White.** 1990. The use of selective media for the isolation of *Pseudomonas pseudomallei* in clinical practice. *J. Med. Microbiol.* **33:**121–126.
141. **Yabuuchi, E., Y. Kosako, H. Oyaizu, I. Yano, H. Hotta, Y. Hashimoto, T. Ezaki, and M. Arakawa.** 1992. Proposal of *Burkholderia* gen. nov. and transfer of seven species of the genus *Pseudomonas* homology group II to the new genus, with the type species *Burkholderia cepacia* (Palleroni and Holmes 1981) comb. nov. *Microbiol. Immunol.* **36:**1251–1275.
142. **Yabuuchi, E., Y. Kosako, I. Yano, H. Hotta, and Y. Nishiuchi.** 1995. Transfer of two *Burkholderia* and an *Alcaligenes* species to *Ralstonia* gen. nov.: proposal of *Ralstonia pickettii* (Ralston, Palleroni and Doudoroff 1973) comb. nov., *Ralstonia solanacearum* (Smith 1896) comb. nov. and *Ralstonia eutropha* (Davis 1969) comb. nov. *Microbiol. Immunol.* **39:**897–904.
143. **Yamamoto, T., P. Naigowit, S. Dejsirilert, D. Chiewsilp, E. Kondo, T. Yokota, and K. Kanai.** 1990. In vitro susceptibilities of *Psuedomonas pseudomallei* to 27 antimicrobial agents. *Antimicrob. Agents Chemother.* **34:** 2027–2029.
144. **Yao, J. D., M. Louie, L. Louie, J. Goodfellow, and A. E. Simor.** 1995. Comparison of E test and agar dilution for antimicrobial susceptibility testing of *Stenotrophomonas maltophilia*. *J. Clin. Microbiol.* **33:**1428–1430.

Acinetobacter, Achromobacter, Alcaligenes, Moraxella, Methylobacterium, and Other Nonfermentative Gram-Negative Rods

PAUL C. SCHRECKENBERGER AND ALEXANDER VON GRAEVENITZ

35

The organisms covered in this chapter belong to a group of taxonomically diverse nonfermentative gram-negative bacilli. They all share the common phenotypic features of failing to acidify the butt of Kligler or triple sugar iron agar or of oxidative-fermentative media, and they grow significantly better under aerobic conditions than under anaerobic conditions; many strains fail to grow anaerobically. Most of the organisms covered in this chapter are either nonmotile or motile with peritrichous flagella, the oxidase reaction is variable, and with the exception of *Neisseria elongata*, all are catalase positive.

Methods used to grow and identify this group are those used for *Pseudomonas* spp. (see chapter 33). Initial incubation should be at 35 to 37°C, although many pink-pigmented strains grow only at ≤30°C and can be detected only on plates left at room temperature after the initial readings. Note that many of these organisms display better growth at 30°C. In such cases, all identification tests should be carried out at that temperature. In fact, some of the commercial kits, such as the API 20NE, are designed to be incubated at 30°C. Growth on certain selective primary media (e.g., MacConkey or salmonella-shigella agar) is variable; there can be significant lot-to-lot variations in the media. Nonfermenters that grow on MacConkey agar generally form colorless colonies.

Although certain nonfermenting bacilli (NFBs) can on occasion be frank pathogens, e.g., *Pseudomonas aeruginosa, Burkholderia pseudomallei,* and *Chryseobacterium meningosepticum*, NFBs are generally considered to be of low virulence and often occur in mixed cultures, making it difficult to determine when to work up cultures and when to perform susceptibility studies. Decisions regarding the significance of NFBs in a clinical specimen must take into account the clinical condition of the patient and the source of the specimen submitted for culture. In general, the recovery of an NFB in pure culture from a normally sterile site warrants identification and susceptibility testing, whereas predominant growth of an NFB from a culture of an endotracheal specimen from a patient with no clinical signs or symptoms of pneumonia would not be worked up further. Because many NFBs exhibit resistance to multiple antibiotics, patients who are on multiple-antibiotic regimens often become colonized with NFBs, which for them is part of their normal colonizing flora. NFB species isolated in mixed cultures can usually be reported as a descriptive identification, e.g., "growth of *P. aeruginosa* and two varieties of nonfermenting gram-negative bacilli not further identified." Often, a Gram stain made from the clinical material can provide a clue as to the significance of organisms that may grow in culture and aid in the laboratory decision on how far to work up the specimen.

Decisions about performing susceptibility testing are further complicated by the fact that there are no National Committee for Clinical Laboratory Standards interpretive breakpoints for the organisms included in this chapter except for *Acinetobacter* species. Furthermore, the results obtained with certain organisms (e.g., *Chryseobacterium* species) by the disk diffusion and E-test methods do not correlate with the results obtained by conventional MIC methods (see discussion later in this chapter). In general, laboratories should be guarded in performing susceptibility testing with the organisms included in this chapter. When clinical necessity dictates that susceptibility testing be performed, an MIC method is recommended, and a disclaimer should be amended to the report indicating that the method performed has not been validated for the organism tested and that MIC interpretive breakpoints are not currently available.

When laboratory identification of this group of organisms is deemed necessary, a simplified approach is recommended, whereby unknown isolates are initially characterized and placed into one of eight groups on the basis of microscopic morphology, oxidase reaction, motility, acidification of carbohydrates, H_2S production, indole production, and production of pink-pigmented colonies (Fig. 1). Further characterization is made on the basis of the biochemical reactions given in Tables 1 to 9. Additional differential tests can be found in other publications (54, 110, 181). Carbon assimilation is determined in mineral basal medium as described by Gilardi (54) and Nash and Krenz (124) (see section IX in this Manual). In the authors' experience indole production is best demonstrated by inoculation of heart infusion broth and incubation at 35 to 37°C, followed by extraction with xylene and the addition of Ehrlich's reagent. The oxidase test is performed with *N,N,N,N*-tetramethyl-*p*-phenylenediamine dihydrochloride (1%). Motility is easily determined by preparing a wet mount preparation of a young colony from a blood agar plate. For some strains, motility can best be demonstrated after incubation of cultures at room temperature.

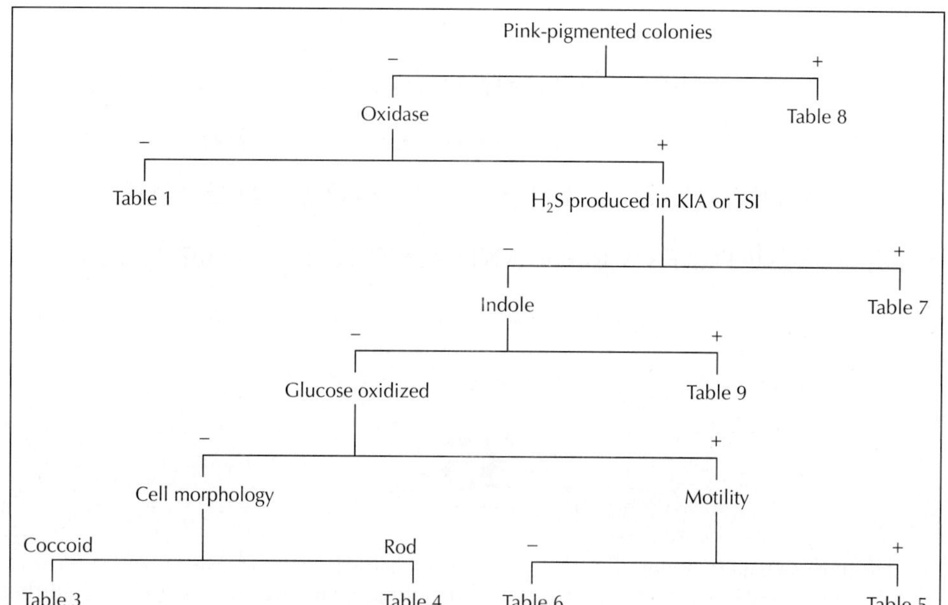

FIGURE 1 Identification of miscellaneous gram-negative nonfermenters. KIA, Kligler iron agar; TSI, triple sugar iron agar.

Traditional diagnostic systems, e.g., those based on oxidative-fermentative media, aerobic low-peptone media, or buffered single substrates (61), have now been replaced in many laboratories by commercial kits. The ability of commercial kits to identify this group of nonfermenters is variable and often results in an identification only to the genus or group level (12, 107). If such kits are used, the laboratory must be familiar with the extent of the database; organisms not included will, of course, not be identified correctly. Because assimilation test results often depend on the basal medium used, most of those results are not included in the tables presented here. Identification of nonfermenters by automated fatty acid analysis has also been attempted (172). In view of the difficulties inherent in this approach (128), it is recommended that fatty acid profiles be used only in conjunction with traditional or commercial diagnostic systems. The fatty acid profiles for the most common species of nonfermenting bacilli have been published by Weyant and colleagues (181).

OXIDASE-NEGATIVE GROUP

See Table 1.

Acinetobacter spp.

The genus *Acinetobacter* consists of strictly aerobic, gram-negative coccobacillary rods that are oxidase negative, nonmotile, nitrate negative, and nonfermentative. Individual cells are 1 to 1.5 by 1.5 to 2.5 μm in size, sometimes difficult to decolorize, and frequently arranged in pairs. In the stationary growth phase and on nonselective agars, coccobacillary forms predominate, while early growth in fluid media and growth on plates containing cell wall-active antimicrobial agents yield mostly rods. Colonies are smooth, opaque, and slightly smaller than those of members of the family *Enterobacteriaceae*. Many strains grow on MacConkey agar as either colorless or slightly pinkish colonies. Some strains are fastidious, showing punctate colonies on blood agar, and fail to grow in nutrient broth (181). Certain glucose-oxidizing acinetobacters may also cause a unique brown discoloration of blood agar into which glucose is incorporated (154). Differential and selective media have been used to isolate *Acinetobacter* spp. (82, 94).

The genus was originally placed within the family *Neisseriaceae* but was more recently moved to the family *Moraxellaceae* (147). Studies based on DNA-DNA hybridization have resulted in the description of 21 DNA homology groups (also called genomospecies) within the genus *Acinetobacter* (15, 17, 51, 92, 125, 162); 16 of these DNA homology groups can be differentiated by means of biochemical and growth tests (Table 2), although only seven species have been named (15, 125). Genomospecies 1, 2, 3, and 13 of Tjernberg and Ursing (162) may be difficult to separate in the clinical laboratory and have been referred to as the *Acinetobacter calcoaceticus-Acinetobacter baumannii* complex (52). Most glucose-oxidizing nonhemolytic clinical strains are *A. baumannii*, most glucose-negative nonhemolytic ones are *Acinetobacter lwoffii*, and most hemolytic ones are *Acinetobacter haemolyticus*. A transformation assay that can be used for the genus-level identification of *Acinetobacter* has been described (98, 181). This is a research technique that involves the mixing of crude DNA extracts of test strains with the cellular mass of an amino acid auxotroph. Genetically related test strains will convert the auxotroph to prototrophy. This conversion is evidenced by the subsequent growth of colonies from the auxotroph-crude DNA test mixture on a basal mineral salts medium (181).

Acinetobacter species are widely distributed in nature and in the hospital environment, are the second most commonly isolated nonfermenters in human specimens (*P. aeruginosa* is the most common), are able to survive on moist and dry surfaces (53), and may be present on healthy human skin (151). The species most frequently isolated is *A. baumannii* (with 19 biotypes identified by assimilation tests [16] and 34 serovars [163]), followed by *A. lwoffii*, *A. haemolyticus*, *Acinetobacter johnsonii*, genomospecies 3 (with 26 serovars

TABLE 1 Oxidase-negative, coccoid, or rod-shaped nonfermenters[a]

Test	*Acinetobacter* spp.	Group EO-5	Group NO-1	*Bordetella holmesii* (NO-2)	*Bordetella parapertussis*	*Bordetella trematum*	*Pseudomonas* (*Chryseomonas*) *luteola*	*Pseudomonas* (*Flavimonas*) *oryzihabitans*	*Stenotrophomonas maltophilia*
Motility	–	–	–	–	–	+	+	+	+
Pigmentation	–	Pale yellow[b]	–	Brown soluble pigment[c]	–	–	Yellow	Yellow	Greenish tan
Growth on MacConkey agar	V	–	V	+	+	+	+	+	+
Growth at 42°C	V	–	V	–	–	+	V	V	V
Nitrate to nitrite	–	–	+	–	–	V	V	–	V
Esculin hydrolysis	–	–	–	–	–	–	+	–	+
Gelatin hydrolysis	V	–	–	–	–	–	V	–	+
Urease (Christensen)	V	+[d]	–	–	+	–	V	V	–
Arginine dihydrolase	–	–	–	–	–	–	V	–	–
DNase	–	ND	ND	ND	ND	ND	–	–	+
ONPG	–	ND	–	–	–	–	+	–	+
Starch hydrolysis	–	ND	ND	ND	–	–	V	V	–
Acid from:									
Glucose	V	+	–	–	–	–	+	+	+
Maltose	V	–	–	–	–	–	+	+	+
Sucrose	–	–	–	–	–	–	–	V	V
Mannitol	–	–	–	–	–	–	+	+	–
Xylose	V	+	–	–	–	–	+	+	V
CFAs	16:0[e], 16:1ω7c, 18:1ω9c	16:0, 18:1ω7c	16:0, 16:1ω7c, 18:1ω7c	16:0, 17:0cyc	16:0, 17:0cyc	16:0, 17:0cyc	16:0, 16:1ω7c, 18:1ω7c	16:0, 16:1ω7c, 18:ω7c	i-15:0, a-15:0

[a] Data are from references 38, 65, 109, 169, 180, and 181. *P. luteola* and *P. oryzihabitans* are covered in chapter 33, *S. maltophilia* is covered in chapter 34, and *Bordetella* species are covered in chapter 40. Symbols and abbreviations: +, ≥90% of strains positive; –, ≥90% of strains negative; ND, no data available; V, variable; ONPG, *o*-nitrophenyl-β-D-galactopyranoside; CFAs, main cellular fatty acids.

[b] Insoluble pale yellow pigment produced by some strains.

[c] Brown soluble pigment produced on heart infusion-tyrosine agar.

[d] Reaction may be weak or delayed in some strains.

[e] Cannot distinguish *Acinetobacter* species by cellular fatty acid composition (181).

TABLE 2 Phenotypic characteristics of 17 *Acinetobacter* genomospecies

Test	% Positive strains in the following genomospecies[a]:															
	1 (8)	2 (121)	3 (15)	4 (23)	5 (17)	6 (3)	7 (23)	8/9 (34)	10 (4)	11 (4)	12 (3)	13 (9)	14 (3)	15 (2)	16 (4)	17 (2)
Growth at:																
37°C	100	100	100	100	100	100	0	100	100	100	100	89	100	100	100	75
41°C	0	100	100	0	90	0	0	0	0	0	0	0	0	0	0	0
44°C	0	100	0	0	0	0	0	0	0	0	0	0	0	0	0	0
Gelatin hydrolysis[b]	0	0	0	96	0	100	0	0	0	0	0	100	100	100	100	100
Acid from glucose[b]	100	95	100	52	0	66	0	6	100	0	33	100	100	0	0	0
Hemolysis on SBA	0	0	0	100	0	100	0	0	0	0	0	100	100	100	100	100
Utilization of[b]:																
trans-Aconitate	100	99	100	52	0	0	0	0	0	0	0	11	67	0	0	50
β-Alanine	100	95	94	0	0	0	0	0	100	100	0	0	100	0	75	100
DL-4-Aminobutyrate	100	100	100	100	88	0	35	40	100	100	100	11	100	0	25	100
L-Arginine	100	98	100	96	95	100	35	0	0	0	100	100	100	50	100	100
Azelate	100	90	100	0	0	0	0	100	50	25	100	0	100	0	0	0
Citrate	100	100	100	91	82	100	100	0	100	100	0	100	100	100	100	100
Glutarate	100	100	100	0	0	0	0	0	100	100	100	0	100	0	0	100
L-Histidine	100	98	94	96	100	100	0	0	100	100	0	100	100	100	100	100
DL-Lactate	100	100	100	0	100	0	100	100	100	100	100	100	100	100	100	100
D-Malate	0	98	100	96	100	66	22	76	100	100	0	100	66	50	100	100
Malonate	100	98	87	0	0	0	13	0	0	0	100	11	100	0	50	50

[a] Data are from Bouvet and Grimont (15) for genomospecies 1 to 12 and from Bouvet and Jeanjean (17) for genomospecies 13 to 17. See those papers for methodology. *Acinetobacter* genomospecies: 1, *A. calcoaceticus*; 2, *A. baumannii*; 3, unnamed; 4, *A. haemolyticus*; 5, *A. junii*; 6, unnamed; 7, *A. johnsonii*; 8 and 9 (phenotypically inseparable), *A. lwoffii*; 10 and 11, unnamed; 12, *A. radioresistens*; 13 to 17, unnamed. Genomospecies 13 and 15 of Tjernberg and Ursing (162) do not correspond to genomospecies 13 and 15 of Bouvet and Jeanjean (17), while genomospecies 14 of the former authors corresponds to genomospecies 13 of the latter authors (100). Numbers in parentheses after genomospecies numbers indicate numbers of strains.

[b] Incubation at 30°C. This table lists only 11 utilization tests, while Gerner-Smidt et al. (52) recommend 14 tests for diagnostic purposes.

[163]), and genomospecies 6 (18, 100, 151, 162). *Acinetobacter* spp. are generally considered to be nonpathogenic to healthy individuals but may cause infections in debilitated individuals. The ability of this microorganism to acquire resistance to multiple antimicrobial agents and its high capacity for survival on most environmental surfaces have led to an increased concern regarding hospital-acquired infections due to this organism. Corbella and colleagues (35) have shown that the digestive tracts of patients in intensive care units are important epidemiologic reservoirs for multidrug-resistant *A. baumannii* infections in hospital outbreaks, and they suggest that a fecal surveillance program might be considered for early implementation of patient isolation precautions in an outbreak setting. Hospital-acquired infections are most likely to involve the respiratory tract (most often related to endotracheal tubes or tracheostomies), urinary tract, and wounds (including catheter sites) and may progress to septicemia (9, 11, 33, 152). Sporadic cases of continuous ambulatory peritoneal dialysis-related peritonitis, endocarditis, meningitis, osteomyelitis, and arthritis have also been reported (9, 96). There is an increasing number of reports of *Acinetobacter* species as agents of nosocomial pneumonia, particularly ventilator-associated pneumonia in patients confined to hospital intensive care units (9). Risk factors are antibiotic treatment and/or surgery, instrumentation, and stay in intensive care units; clinical isolates, however, are more often colonizers than infecting agents (9, 33). Hospital outbreaks have been investigated by various typing methods (11, 62, 114). Community-acquired *Acinetobacter* pneumonias in which a fatal outcome was strongly associated with inappropriate initial antibiotic therapy have also been reported (5). Cephalothin is ineffective, while trimethoprim-sulfamethoxazole, imipenem, ampicillin-sulbactam, ticarcillin-clavulanate, piperacillin-tazobactam, amoxicillin-clavulanate, doxycycline, and quinolones are effective against most strains (9, 33, 150, 173), but susceptibility testing is required for each clinically significant strain. Multidrug-resistant strains occur mostly among members of the *A. calcoaceticus*-*A. baumannii* complex and strains of *A. haemolyticus* (150, 183).

CDC Group EO-5

CDC group EO (eugonic oxidizer) 5 (38) consists of glucose-oxidizing gram-negative rods that have a biochemical profile similar to that of *A. baumannii*. They are nonmotile and oxidase negative, but unlike *Acinetobacter* species, they fail to grow on MacConkey agar. Other characteristics are given in Table 1. Isolates have been recovered from blood, peritoneal fluid, transtracheal aspirates, gallbladders, and an arm wound (38).

CDC Group NO-1

CDC group NO-1 bacteria (65) are oxidase negative, asaccharolytic, nonmotile, coccoid to medium-sized gram-negative rods that form small colonies on sheep blood agar (SBA). Other differential features are listed in Table 1. Nitrate, but not nitrite, is reduced; however, since approximately 3% of asaccharolytic *Acinetobacter* spp. reduce nitrate, the definitive differential test between the two groups is the transformation assay (98, 181), which is negative with group NO-1. Most strains have been isolated from human wounds resulting from dog or cat bites. They are susceptible to antibiotics used to treat infections caused by gram-negative organisms, including aminoglycosides, beta-lactam antibiotics, tetracyclines, quinolones, and sulfonamides (65).

Bordetella spp.

The *Bordetella* species are discussed in detail in chapter 40 of this Manual. There are six *Bordetella* spp. that are nonfastidious and that will grow on ordinary culture media (i.e., SBA and MacConkey agar), and they biochemically resemble either *Acinetobacter* spp. or *Alcaligenes* spp. Three species (*Bordetella holmesii*, *Bordetella parapertussis*, *Bordetella trematum*) are oxidase negative (see Table 1), and three species (*Bordetella avium*, *Bordetella bronchiseptica*, *Bordetella hinzii*) are oxidase positive (see Table 4). *Bordetella holmesii* (formerly CDC group NO-2) is nitrate negative (differentiating it from NO-1 strains) and produces a brown soluble pigment on heart infusion-tyrosine agar. Other differential tests are given in Table 1. *B. bronchiseptica* is rapid urease positive and must be differentiated from CDC group IVc-2 and *Oligella ureolytica* (see Table 4).

Flavimonas and *Chryseomonas*

The species *Flavimonas oryzihabitans* and *Chryseomonas luteola* have recently been reclassified as species in the genus *Pseudomonas* (6, 109) and as such are covered in chapter 33 of this Manual. They are included in Table 1 in this chapter to aid in the laboratory identification of oxidase-negative nonfermenting rods.

OXIDASE-POSITIVE, INDOLE-NEGATIVE, ASACCHAROLYTIC, COCCOID-SHAPED NONFERMENTERS

See Table 3.

Moraxella spp.

The classification of species belonging to the family *Moraxellaceae* is still evolving and has been recently reviewed by Pettersson and colleagues (133). Members of the genus *Moraxella* are oxidase-positive, nonmotile, asaccharolytic coccobacilli that are often plump, occur predominantly in pairs and sometimes in short chains, and have a tendency to resist Gram stain decolorization.

Moraxellae are parasitic on human skin and mucous membranes. The most frequently isolated species is *Moraxella nonliquefaciens*, which forms smooth, translucent to semiopaque colonies 0.1 to 0.5 mm in diameter after 24 h and 1 mm in diameter after 48 h of growth on SBA plates. Occasionally, these colonies spread and pit the agar. The colonial morphologies of *Moraxella lincolnii* (168), *Moraxella osloensis*, and *Psychrobacter phenylpyruvicus* (formerly *Moraxella phenylpyruvica* [20]) are similar, but pitting is rare. On the other hand, pitting is common for *Moraxella lacunata*, whose colonies are smaller and form dark haloes on chocolate agar. Colonies of *Moraxella atlantae* are small (usually 0.5 mm in diameter) and show pitting and spreading (19). Most *Moraxella canis* colonies resemble those of members of the family *Enterobacteriaceae* (large, smooth colonies) and may produce a brown pigment when grown on starch-containing Mueller-Hinton agar (93). Some strains may also produce very slimy colonies resembling colonies of *Klebsiella pneumoniae* (93). Microscopically, *M. canis* resembles *Moraxella catarrhalis* (*Branhamella catarrhalis*), which is discussed in chapter 38 of this Manual. Animal species include *Moraxella bovis*, which is isolated from healthy cattle and other animals, including horses, *Moraxella boevrei*, *Moraxella caprae*, *Moraxella caviae*, *Moraxella cuniculi*, and *Moraxella ovis*.

Biochemical reactions for the human isolates are listed in Table 3. Most laboratories do not determine the species

TABLE 3 Oxidase-positive, indole-negative, asaccharolytic, coccoid-shaped nonfermenters[a]

Test	*Moraxella lacunata*	*Moraxella nonliquefaciens*	*Moraxella canis*	*Moraxella catarrhalis*	*Moraxella lincolnii*	*Moraxella osloensis*	*Moraxella atlantae*	*Psychrobacter phenylpyruvicus*[b]	*Oligella urethralis*	*Oligella ureolytica*
Motility	–	–	–	–	–	–	–	–	–	+[c]
Catalase	+	+	+	+	+	+	+	+	+	+
Hemolysis (SBA)	α/–	–	–	–	–	–	–	slβ/–	slβ/–	slβ/–
Growth on										
MacConkey agar	–	–	+	–	–	V	+	+	+	V
At 42°C	–	V	ND	V	–	–	V	V	+	V
Urease	–	–	–	–	–	–	–	+	–	++
Phenylalanine deaminase	D	–	–	V	ND	V	–	+	+	+
Gelatin hydrolysis	+[c]	–	–	–	–	–	–	–	–	–
Nitrate to nitrite	+	+	+	+	–	V	–	V	–	+
Nitrite reduction	–	–	V	+	V	–	–	–	+	+
DNase	–	–	+	+	–	–	–	–	–	–
Penicillin[d]	S	S	S	R/S[e]	S	S	S	V	S	S
CFAs	16:0, 16:1ω7c, 18:1ω9c	18:1ω9c, 16:1ω7c, 16:0	18:1ω9c	16:1ω7c, 17:1ω8c, 18:1ω9c	16:0, 16:1ω7c, 18:1ω9c	16:1ω7c, 18:1ω9c	16:0, 18:2, 18:1ω9c, 18:0	16:0, 16:1ω7c, 18:1ω9c, 18:2	16:0, 18:1ω7c	16:0, 18:1ω7c

[a] Data are from references 19, 54, 93, 121, 146, 168, and 181. For truest microscopic morphology, perform Gram staining with a sample from enrichment broth culture incubated for 2 h at 35°C. For abbreviations, see Table 1, footnote *a*. Other abbreviations: α, alpha-hemolysis; slβ, diffuse beta-hemolysis underneath colonies on SBA; D, different data reported in literature; S, susceptible; R, resistant; + +, strong positive reaction.

[b] *Brucella* species may be misidentified as *Psychrobacter* (*Moraxella*) *phenylpyruvicus* in some commercial identification systems; see comments in text. *Brucella* species are covered in detail in chapter 41 of this Manual.

[c] May be delayed or difficult to demonstrate.

[d] Test performed by directly inoculating surface of SBA in a manner that will produce a uniform lawn of growth, immediately placing a 10-U penicillin disc on the agar surface, and incubating in room atmosphere at 35°C for 18 to 24 h. Any strain with a zone of inhibited growth around the penicillin disc is interpreted as susceptible for identification purposes.

[e] Some strains, particularly those in Europe, may be beta-lactamase negative and therefore penicillin susceptible.

of moraxellae because of the similarity in pathogenic significance of the species and because many strains are somewhat fastidious and biochemical reactions are often negative or equivocal. A separation between M. *lacunata* and nonspreading M. *nonliquefaciens* may prove difficult, because gelatin hydrolysis (by any method) and liquefaction of Loeffler slants may take more than 1 week. In some instances, fatty acid analysis may help determine the species (181); in other cases, quantitative transformation of a high-level streptomycin resistance marker can be used (99). The differential diagnosis of P. *phenylpyruvicus* and *Brucella* spp. is of great practical importance and requires microscopy (*Brucella* spp. are tiny coccobacilli) and tests for phenylalanine deaminase and acid formation from xylose. The former is positive for P. *phenylpyruvicus* and the latter is positive for *Brucella* spp. Microbiologists should be aware that *Brucella* species that are unwittingly inoculated into certain commercial identification systems will be misidentified as M. *phenylpyruvica* (now called P. *phenylpyruvicus*) (7, 8, 131). The tributyrin test may be positive for several *Moraxella* spp. and therefore cannot be used to separate them from M. *catarrhalis* (132). Likewise, γ-glutamyl aminopeptidase occurs not only in M. *canis* but also in some strains of other moraxellae (93).

M. *osloensis*, M. *nonliquefaciens*, and M. *lincolnii* are part of the normal flora of the human respiratory tract, while most M. *canis* strains have been found in the upper respiratory tracts of dogs and cats. These and other moraxellae are rare agents of infections (conjunctivitis, keratitis, meningitis, septicemia, endocarditis, arthritis, and otolaryngologic infections) (56, 97). Most strains are susceptible to penicillin and its derivatives, cephalosporins, tetracyclines, quinolones, and aminoglycosides (47, 54, 145, 157). Production of beta-lactamase has been only rarely reported in *Moraxella* species other than M. *catarrhalis* (97, 145).

Oligella spp.

The genus *Oligella* consists of two species: *Oligella urethralis* (formerly *Moraxella urethralis* and CDC group M-4) and *Oligella ureolytica* (formerly CDC group IVe) (146). O. *urethralis* is nonmotile, while most strains of O. *ureolytica* are motile by peritrichous flagella. Biochemical features which help differentiate *Oligella* spp. from *Moraxella* spp. are shown in Table 3. O. *urethralis* is similar to *Moraxella* spp. in that isolates are coccobacillary, oxidase positive, and nonmotile. Colonies are smaller than those of M. *osloensis* and are opaque to whitish. O. *urethralis* and M. *osloensis* share additional biochemical similarities, e.g., accumulation of poly-β-hydroxybutyric acid and failure to hydrolyze urea, but can be differentiated on the basis of nitrite reduction, growth at 42°C, and alkalinization of formate, itaconate, proline, and threonine (positive for all O. *urethralis* strains and negative for all M. *osloensis* strains) (135).

Colonies of O. *ureolytica* grow slowly on blood agar, producing pinpoint colonies after 24 h but large colonies after 3 days of incubation. Colonies are white, opaque, entire, and nonhemolytic. O. *ureolytica* strains are both phenylalanine deaminase and rapid urease positive, with the urease reaction often turning positive within minutes after inoculation. In this regard, O. *ureolytica* is similar to B. *bronchiseptica* and CDC group IVc-2 from which it must be differentiated. Both *Oligella* spp. have been isolated chiefly from the human urinary tract, and both have been reported to cause urosepsis (137, 144). A case of septic arthritis due to O. *urethralis* has also been reported (117). O. *urethralis* is generally susceptible to most antibiotics, including penicillin, while O. *ureolytica* exhibits variable susceptibility patterns (47, 54).

OXIDASE-POSITIVE, INDOLE-NEGATIVE, ASACCHAROLYTIC, ROD-SHAPED NONFERMENTERS

See Table 4.

Alcaligenes and *Achromobacter* spp.

Members of these genera are rods (0.5 by 1 to 0.5 by 2.6 μm) with peritrichous flagella. Both phylogenetically and biochemically, they are closely related to members of the genus *Bordetella* (see chapter 40 in this Manual). They occur mainly in the environment and show limited action on carbohydrates. Colonies are nonpigmented and similar in size to those of *Acinetobacter* spp. Medically important species are divided into the asaccharolytic species (Table 4) including *Alcaligenes faecalis*, *Achromobacter piechaudii*, and *Achromobacter xylosoxidans* subsp. *denitrificans* (formerly *Alcaligenes xylosoxidans* subsp. *denitrificans* [169, 184a]), and the saccharolytic species (Table 5) *Achromobacter xylosoxidans* subsp. *xylosoxidans* (formerly *Alcaligenes xylosoxidans* subsp. *xylosoxidans* [169, 184a]). A. *faecalis* is the most frequently isolated species and characteristically produces colonies with a thin, spreading, irregular edge. Some strains (previously named "*Alcaligenes odorans*") produce a characteristic fruity odor (sometimes described as the odor of green apples) and cause a greenish discoloration of blood agar medium. A key biochemical feature of this species is its ability to reduce nitrite but not nitrate. The asaccharolytic species are rarely observed as human pathogens (106, 175), but A. *xylosoxidans* subsp. *xylosoxidans* is a relatively frequent agent of infection, particularly as a cause of septicemia in nosocomial settings (31, 43, 175). A. *xylosoxidans* subsp. *xylosoxidans* has also been found to colonize the respiratory tracts of intubated children and patients with cystic fibrosis, leading to exacerbation of pulmonary symptoms (44). Methods for epidemiologic typing of A. *xylosoxidans* subsp. *xylosoxidans* have been described previously (31, 112). Susceptibilities are unpredictable except for susceptibility to piperacillin and ticarcillin-clavulanic acid (13, 54, 157, 175).

Myroides

Vancanneyt and colleagues (166) determined that the organism formerly classified as *Flavobacterium odoratum* consisted of a heterogeneous group which comprised two distinct species for which they proposed the names *Myroides odoratus* and *Myroides odoratimimus*. Cells of both species stain as gram-negative rods 0.5 μm in diameter and 1 to 2 μm long. Various colony types may occur, but most colonies are yellow pigmented and form effuse, spreading colonies that may be confused with the colony morphology of a *Bacillus* species. A characteristic fruity odor (similar to the odor of A. *faecalis*) is produced by most strains. *Myroides* spp. grow on most media including MacConkey agar. Growth occurs at 18 to 37°C but not at 42°C. They are asaccharolytic but are oxidase, catalase, urease, and gelatinase positive. Indole is not produced, and nitrite (but not nitrate) is reduced (Table 4). There are no routine phenotypic tests for differentiating the two *Myroides* species, with determination of their differences being confined to assimilation tests and cellular fatty acid analyses ($C_{13:0}$ and $C_{15:0}$) (166). Organisms identified as M. *odoratus* have been reported mostly from urine but have also been found in wound, sputum, blood, and ear specimens. Clinical infection with *Myroides* spp. is exceedingly rare; however, a case of rapidly

TABLE 4 Oxidase-positive, indole-negative, asaccharolytic, rod-shaped nonfermenters[a]

Test	*Alcaligenes faecalis*	*Achromobacter xylosoxidans* subsp. *denitrificans*	*Achromobacter piechaudii*	*Bordetella avium*	*Bordetella bronchiseptica*	*Bordetella hinzii*	*Myroides odoratus*-*Myroides odoratimimus*	*Neisseria weaveri*	*Neisseria elongata* subsp. *nitroreducens*[b]	CDC group IVc-2	Gilardi Rod Group 1
Motility	+	+	+	+	+	+	–	–	–	+	–
Catalase	+	+	+	+	+	+	+	+	–	+	+
Growth on MacConkey agar	+	+	+	+	+	+	V	V	V	+	+
Nitrate to nitrite	–	+	+	–	+	–	–	–	+	–	–
Nitrite reduced	+	+	–	–	–	–	V	+	+	–	–
Urease	–	D	–	–	++	V	+	–	–	++	–
Phenylalanine deaminase	–	–	–	–	V	V	V	w+	–	–	++
Acetamide hydrolysis	+	V	–	+	–	+	–	–	–	–	–
Malonate utilization	+	+	+	–	+	+	ND	ND	ND	ND	ND
DNase	–	–	–	–	–	–	+	–	–	–	–
Penicillin[c]	V	V	V	S	R	V	V	S	S	R/S	S
CFAs	3-OH-14:0, 16:0, 16:1ω7c, 17:0cyc	16:0, 16:1ω7c, 17:0cyc	16:0, 16:1ω7c, 17:0cyc	16:0, 17:0cyc	16:0, 16:1ω7c, 17:0cyc	16:0, 17:0cyc	i-15:0	16:0, 16:1ω7c, 18:1ω7c	16:0, 16:1ω7c, 18:1ω7c	16:0, 16:1ω7c, 17:0cyc, 18:1ω7c	14:0, 16:0, 18:1ω7c, 19:0cyc

[a] Data are from references 41, 54, 106, 120, 170, and 181. For truest microscopic morphology perform Gram staining with samples from enrichment broth culture incubated for 2 h at 35°C. Also consider *Brucella* (chapter 41), *Comamonas*, *Acidovorax*, and *Brevundimonas* (chapter 34), and the alkaline *Pseudomonas* species (chapter 33). For abbreviations, see Table 1, footnote *a*, and Table 3, footnote a. Other abbreviations: w, weak.

[b] *N. elongata* subsp. *elongata* has the same biochemical and CFA profile as *N. elongata* subsp. *nitroreducens* except that nitrate is not reduced. *Neisseria elongata* subsp. *glycolytica* can be differentiated on the basis of a positive catalase reaction, a negative nitrate reaction, and production of weak acid from glucose (181).

[c] Test performed by directly inoculating surface of SBA in a manner that will produce a uniform lawn of growth, immediately placing a 10-U penicillin disc on the agar surface, and incubating in room atmosphere at 35°C for 18 to 24 h. Any strain with a zone of inhibited growth around the penicillin disc is interpreted as susceptible for identification purposes.

progressive necrotizing fasciitis and bacteremia has been reported (88). Most strains are resistant to penicillins, cephalosporins, aminoglycosides, aztreonam, and carbapenems (78).

Neisseria weaveri and *Neisseria elongata* subsp. *nitroreducens*

The previously unnamed *Moraxella*-like species, CDC groups M-5 and M-6, have now been placed in the genus *Neisseria* as *N. weaveri* (CDC group M-5) (3, 68) and *N. elongata* subsp. *nitroreducens* (CDC group M-6) (58). *N. weaveri* is found as part of the normal oral flora of dogs and is associated with human wound infections and septicemia resulting from dog bites (3, 26, 68). *N. elongata* subsp. *nitroreducens* has been reported to cause bacteremia, endocarditis, and osteomyelitis (182). The *Neisseria* species are covered in detail in chapter 38.

CDC Group IVc-2

The unnamed species CDC group IVc-2 is a short to medium-sized gram-negative rod that is asaccharolytic and motile by peritrichous flagella. Cells may stain irregularly. It is rapid urease positive and can be differentiated from the phenotypically similar organisms *B. bronchiseptica* and *O. ureolytica* by a negative nitrate reduction test. It has been isolated from a variety of human sources and has been reported to cause septicemia and peritonitis (4, 122, 138). A procedure for molecular typing of strains in epidemiologic investigations has been reported (118). It is often resistant to ampicillin, cephalothin, and aminoglycosides (47, 54).

Gilardi Rod Group 1

Gilardi rod group 1 consists of oval to medium-length asaccharolytic gram-negative rods that resemble *N. weaveri* in many respects except that Gilardi rod group 1 isolates grow on MacConkey agar, do not reduce nitrite, and are strongly phenylalanine deaminase positive, producing a dark green slant after the addition of $FeCl_3$ (10%), while *N. weaveri*, when positive, produces a weak to moderate reaction (Table 4). Isolates of Gilardi rod group 1 have been recovered from a variety of human sources including leg, arm, and foot wounds, an oral lesion, urine, and blood; however, their pathogenic potential has yet to be determined (120). They are susceptible to many antimicrobial agents including various penicillins, cephalothin, and chloramphenicol (54, 120).

OXIDASE-POSITIVE, INDOLE-NEGATIVE, SACCHAROLYTIC, MOTILE, ROD-SHAPED NONFERMENTERS

See Table 5.

Agrobacterium radiobacter

The genus *Agrobacterium* contains several species of plant pathogens occurring worldwide in soils. Four distinct species of *Agrobacterium* are recognized: *Agrobacterium radiobacter* (formerly *Agrobacterium tumefaciens* and CDC group Vd-3), *Agrobacterium rhizogenes* (subsequently transferred to the genus *Sphingomonas* as *Sphingomonas rosa*), *Agrobacterium vitis*, and *Agrobacterium rubi* (149). The separation of the phenotypically indistinguishable species *A. tumefaciens* and *Agrobacterium radiobacter* was based on the presence of a plant tumor-inducing plasmid that was present in *A. tumefaciens* but absent from *A. radiobacter*. Genetic studies have now shown that these two species are the same and a proposal has been made to reject the name *A. tumefaciens* and to designate *A. radiobacter* as the type species for the genus *Agrobacterium* (149). Cells are 0.6 to 1.0 by 1.5 to 3.0 μm long and occur singly and in pairs. Colonies of *A. radiobacter* grow optimally at 25 to 28°C but will grow at 35°C as well. They appear circular, convex, smooth, and nonpigmented to light beige on SBA with a diameter of 2 mm at 48 h. Colonies may appear wet and become extremely mucoid and pink on MacConkey agar with prolonged incubation. *A. radiobacter* has most frequently been isolated from blood, followed by peritoneal dialysate, urine, and ascitic fluid (45, 91). The majority of cases of *A. radiobacter* infection have occurred in patients with transcutaneous catheters or implanted biomedical prostheses, and effective treatment often requires removal of the device (46). Most strains are susceptible to broad-spectrum cephalosporins, carbapenems, tetracyclines, and gentamicin but not to tobramycin (54, 175). Testing of individual isolates is recommended for clinically significant cases.

Agrobacterium Yellow Group

Organisms in the *Agrobacterium* yellow group are represented by slender, medium to long gram-negative rods that produce a yellow insoluble growth pigment and that most closely resemble *Sphingomonas paucimobilis* and CDC group O organisms. Growth on MacConkey agar is variable, motility occurs via a single polar flagellum, tests for oxidase and catalase are positive, and glucose, xylose, lactose, sucrose, and maltose but not mannitol are oxidized (Table 5). Isolates have been recovered from blood and peritoneal fluid (160, 181).

Ochrobactrum anthropi and "*Achromobacter*" Groups B, E, and F

O. anthropi is the name given to the urease-positive "*Achromobacter*" species formerly designated CDC group Vd (biotypes 1 and 2) (77) and is also identical to "*Achromobacter*" groups A, C, and D of Holmes et al. (76). It is a medium-length rod with peritrichous flagella, but an individual cell may have only a single flagellum. Colonies on SBA resemble those of members of the family *Enterobacteriaceae* except that those of *Ochrobactrum* are smaller. Colonies measure about 1 mm in diameter and appear circular, low convex, smooth, shining, and entire. *O. anthropi* has been isolated from various environmental and human sources, predominantly from patients with catheter-related bacteremias (32, 57, 77, 102), and from one patient with meningitis (28). Pulsed-field gel electrophoresis and PCR genome fingerprinting based on repetitive chromosomal sequences have both been used successfully for epidemiologic typing of outbreak strains (171). *O. anthropi* is susceptible to aminoglycosides, carbenicillin, fluoroquinolones, imipenem, tetracycline, and trimethoprim-sulfamethoxazole but is resistant to other antimicrobial agents (54, 102, 175).

"*Achromobacter*" groups B and E constitute biotypes of a single new species that has yet to be named (69, 70, 72). "*Achromobacter*" group F is genetically distinct from groups B and E (69, 70). Biovars A, C, and D are biovars of *O. anthropi* (181). "*Achromobacter*" group B has been isolated from patients with septicemia (71, 95). Isolates of "*Achromobacter*" groups E and F have also been recovered from blood (69, 70). Susceptibility to chloramphenicol, ciprofloxacin, gentamicin, imipenem, tobramycin, and trimethoprim-sul-

TABLE 5 Oxidase-positive, indole-negative, saccharolytic, motile, rod-shaped nonfermenters[a]

Test	*Agrobacterium radiobacter*	"*Agrobacterium* yellow group"	*Achromobacter xylosoxidans* subsp. *xylosoxidans*	*Ochrobactrum anthropi*	*Achromobacter* group B	*Achromobacter* group E	*Achromobacter* group F	OFBA-1	CDC group O-1	CDC group O-2	CDC group O-3	*Sphingomonas paucimobilis*[b]	*Pseudomonas*-like group 2	CDC group WO-1
Motility	+	+[c]	+	+	+	+	+	+	+	+	+	+	+	+
Growth on MacConkey agar	+	V	+	+	+	+	−	+	V	V	−	V	+	V
Pigment	−	y	−	−	−	−	−	−	y	y	−	y	ND	y/−
DNase	−	ND	−	−	−	−	−	−	ND	ND	ND	−	−	ND
ONPG	+	−	−	−	+	+	−	−	ND	ND	ND	+	+	ND
Arginine dihydrolase	−	−	V	V	−	+	−	+	−	V	−	−	−	−
Nitrate to nitrite	V	−	+	+	+	+	+	+	−	V	V	−	−	+
Nitrate to gas	−	−	V	+	+	−	−	+	−	−	−	−	−	V
Urease	+	−[d]	−	+	+	+	+	−	−	V	−	−	+	V
Phenylalanine deaminase	+	−	−	+	ND	ND	ND	+	ND	ND	ND	V	+	ND
Esculin hydrolysis	+	+	−	V	+	+	+	−	+	V	+	+	−	−
Acid from:														
Glucose	+	+	+	+	+	+	+	+	+[e]	V	+	+	+	+[e]
Maltose	+	+	−	V	+	+	+	−	−	+[e]	+	+	−	−
Sucrose	+	+	−	V	+	+	+	ND	−	+[e]	+	+	−	−
Mannitol	+	−	−	V	+	−	+	−	−	−	−	−	+	+[e]
Xylose	+	+	+	+	+	+	+	ND	−	−	+	+	+	−
Polymyxin B[f]	S	ND	S	S	ND	ND	ND	S	ND	ND	ND	S	V	ND
CFAs	16:0, 18:1ω7c, 19:0cyc11–12	ND	16:0, 16:1ω7c, 17:0cyc	18:0, 18:1ω7c, 19:0cyc	18:1ω7c	18:1ω7c	ND	16:0, 17:0cyc, 19:0cyc11–12	ND	ND	16:0, 16:1ω7c, 18:1ω7c	16:0, 18:1ω7c	16:0, 16:1ω7c, 18:1ω7c	16:0, 16:1ω7c, 18:1ω7c

[a] Data are from references 37, 54, 67, 76, 77, 160, 177, and 181. Also consider *Pseudomonas* species (chapter 33) and *Burkholderia* and *Ralstonia* species (chapter 34). For abbreviations, see Table 1, footnote *a*, and Table 3, footnote *a*. Other abbreviations: y, yellow.

[b] Approximately 6% of strains are oxidase negative (54).

[c] Motile at room temperature, nonmotile at 37°C (160).

[d] Swann et al. (160) report a negative urease test result; Weyant et al. (181) report a delayed positive urease test result.

[e] Reaction may be weak or delayed.

[f] Test performed by directly inoculating the surface of SBA in a manner that will produce a uniform lawn of growth, immediately placing a 300-U polymyxin B disc on the agar surface, and incubating in room atmosphere at 35°C for 18 to 24 h. Any strain with a zone of inhibited growth around the polymyxin B disc is interpreted as susceptible for identification purposes.

famethoxazole has been reported for isolates of "*Achromobacter*" group B recovered from blood (71, 95).

OFBA-1

OFBA-1 is an unclassified medium to long gram-negative, motile rod with one to two polar flagella that has the unusual property of producing acid in oxidative-fermentative base medium without carbohydrate, thus the acronym "OFBA." The organism most closely resembles *P. aeruginosa* biochemically due to beta-hemolysis, growth at 42°C, the presence of arginine dihydrolase, nitrate reduction to gas, and utilization of most carbohydrates (177, 181). Unlike *P. aeruginosa*, it is negative for pyocyanin and pyoverdin production and acetamide hydrolysis. Isolates have been recovered from blood, a leg ulcer, an abdominal wound, a bronchial wash, and a catheter tunnel infection in a patient on continuous ambulatory peritoneal dialysis (177, 181).

CDC Groups O-1, O-2, and O-3

CDC groups O-1, O-2, and O-3 are phenotypically similar, motile, usually oxidase-positive, gram-negative rods. Groups O-1 and O-2 are yellow pigmented and most closely resemble *Agrobacterium* yellow group and *Sphingomonas* species. These organisms grow poorly or not at all on MacConkey agar, usually hydrolyze esculin, but are otherwise inactive. All are motile, although motility may be difficult to demonstrate. Group O-1 cells appear as uniformly short gram-negative rods; group O-2 cells appear as slightly pleomorphic rods, with some cells appearing thin in the central portion with thickened ends; and group O-3 cells appear as thin, medium to slightly long, curved rods with tapered ends (sickle-like) (37, 181). Group O-3 is the only group in which yellow growth pigment is not produced and the only group of predominantly curved rods. Most isolates of O-3 grow well on CAMPY CVA (campylobacter agar with cefoperazone, vancomycin, and amphotericin B) plates under microaerophilic conditions, thus creating the potential for misidentification of O-3 organisms as *Campylobacter* (37). Isolates of all three O groups have come from a variety of clinical sources; however, the pathogenic potential of these organisms is unknown.

Sphingomonas spp.

On the basis of its 16S rRNA sequence and the presence of unique sphingoglycolipid and ubiquinone types, the new genus *Sphingomonas* was created for the organism formerly known as *Pseudomonas paucimobilis* and CDC group IIk-1 (185). The genus *Sphingomonas* presently contains 16 species, but only *S. paucimobilis*, which is designated the type species, is important clinically. It is characterized by medium to long motile rods with a polar flagellum. However, few cells are actively motile in broth culture, thus making motility a difficult characteristic to demonstrate. Motility occurs at 18 to 22°C but not at 37°C. The oxidase reaction is positive, although Gilardi (54) has reported that only 94% of the strains are oxidase positive. Colonies grown on blood agar medium are yellow pigmented and slowly growing, with only small colonies observed after 24 h of incubation. Growth occurs at 37°C but not at 42°C, with optimum growth occurring at 30°C (130). *S. paucimobilis* is widely distributed in the environment, including water, and has been isolated from a variety of clinical specimens, including blood, cerebrospinal fluid, peritoneal fluid, urine, wounds, vagina, and cervix and from the hospital environment (73, 86, 119, 139). Most strains are susceptible to tetracycline, chloramphenicol, trimethoprim-sulfamethoxazole, aminoglycosides, and fluoroquinolones; susceptibility to other antimicrobial agents varies (47, 54).

Pseudomonas-Like Group 2

The organisms in *Pseudomonas*-like group 2 were previously included in a heterogeneous group of organisms designated CDC group IVd (105). Strains are oxidase positive and motile with polar tufts of flagella and are both phenylalanine deaminase and urease positive (54). Other characteristics are given in Table 5. Colonies tend to stick to the agar. Human clinical isolates have been obtained from the respiratory tract, blood, spinal fluid, feces, urine, and dialysate (55, 105, 108). They are susceptible to most antibiotics used against gram-negative rods except polymyxin B (54).

CDC Group WO-1

Members of CDC group WO-1 (weak oxidizer) are oxidase positive and motile with one or two polar flagella. Motility may be difficult to detect in motility media and is best detected by wet preparation. Some strains produce soluble pigments (yellow, tan, amber, olive green, or brown) and weakly oxidize glucose and mannitol, often requiring 3 to 7 days of incubation (67). Other characteristics are listed in Table 5. Human isolates have come from blood, urine, cerebrospinal fluid, and other sources (67). No genetic or susceptibility data have been published.

OXIDASE-POSITIVE, INDOLE-NEGATIVE, SACCHAROLYTIC, NONMOTILE, COCCOID OR ROD-SHAPED NONFERMENTERS

See Table 6.

Sphingobacterium and *Pedobacter*

Sphingobacterium spp. are yellow-pigmented, oxidase-positive, indole-negative, gram-negative rods. They have no flagella but may exhibit sliding motility. They are nonproteolytic and produce acid from carbohydrates. The currently described species of *Sphingobacterium* are *Sphingobacterium multivorum* (formerly *Flavobacterium multivorum*, CDC group IIk-2), *Sphingobacterium spiritivorum* (includes species formerly designated *Flavobacterium spiritivorum*, *Flavobacterium yabuuchiae*, and CDC group IIK-3), *Sphingobacterium mizutae*, *Sphingobacterium thalpophilum*, *Sphingobacterium faecium*, *Sphingobacterium antarcticus*, and unnamed species *Sphingobacterium* genomospecies 1 and 2 (161, 184). The former *Sphingobacterium* species *Sphingobacterium heparinum* and *Sphingobacterium piscium* have been placed in a new genus *Pedobacter* as *Pedobacter heparinus* and *Pedobacter piscium*, respectively (158). The genus *Pedobacter* contains several species of heparinase-producing bacteria found in soil, activated sludge, or fish and has strong similarities to the genus *Sphingobacterium* and the misclassified species *Flexibacter canadensis*. Steyn and colleagues (158) have shown that all these organisms constitute a separate rRNA branch in the rRNA superfamily V, for which they have proposed a new family called the *Sphingobacteriaceae* (158). *S. multivorum* and *S. spiritivorum* are the two species that have been most frequently recovered from human clinical specimens. They can be distinguished from the similar organism *S. paucimobilis* (formerly IIk-1) by lack of motility, urease production, and resistance to polymyxin B (*S. paucimobilis* is usually motile, urease negative, and usually susceptible to polymyxin B) (Table 5). *S. multivorum* has been isolated from various clinical specimens but has only rarely been associ-

TABLE 6 Oxidase-positive, indole-negative, saccharolytic, nonmotile, coccoid or rod-shaped nonfermenters[a]

Test	*Sphingobacterium mizutae*	*Sphingobacterium multivorum*	*Sphingobacterium spiritivorum*	*Sphingobacterium thalpophilum*	CDC group EO-2[b]	CDC group EO-3	*Psychrobacter immobilis*[c]	CDC group EF-4b[d]
Motility	–	–	–	–	–	–	–	–
Growth on MacConkey agar	–	+	V	+	V	+	+	V
Pigment	sl y	sl y	sl y	sl y	y/–	y	–	–
DNase	–	V	+	+	–	ND	–	ND
ONPG	+	+	+	+	V	ND	–	ND
Arginine dihydrolase	V	–	V	–	–	–	–	–
Nitrate to nitrite	–	–	–	+	V	–	V	+
Nitrate to gas	–	–	–	–	–	–	–	–
Urease	–	+	+	+	V	+	V	–
Phenylalanine deaminase	+	V	+	–	–	ND	ND	ND
Esculin hydrolysis	+	+	+	+	–	–	–	–
Acid from:								
Glucose	+	+	+	+	+	+	V	+
Maltose	+	+	+	+	V	V	–	–
Sucrose	+	+	+	+	–	–	–	–
Mannitol	–	–	+	–	V	w+	–	–
Xylose	+	+	+	+	+	+	V	–
Polymyxin B[e]	R	R	R	R	S	ND	ND	S
CFAs	i-15:0, i-2-OH-15:0, 16:1ω7c	i-15:0, i-2-OH-15:0, 16:1ω7c	i-15:0, i-2-OH-15:0	i-15:0, i-2-OH-15:0, 16:1ω7c	ND	ND	16:1ω7c, 18:1ω9c	16:1ω7c, 16:0, 18:1ω7c

[a] Data are from references 40, 54, 90, 121, and 181. For abbreviations, see Table 1, footnote *a*, and Table 3, footnote *a*. Other abbreviations: sl, slightly; y, yellow; w, weak.
[b] O-shaped cells seen on Gram staining.
[c] Rose-like odor noted from agar cultures.
[d] Popcorn-like odor noted from agar cultures.
[e] Test performed by directly inoculating the surface of SBA in a manner that will produce a uniform lawn of growth, immediately placing a 300-U polymyxin B disc on the agar surface, and incubating in room atmosphere at 35°C for 18 to 24 h. Any strain with a zone of inhibited growth around the polymyxin B disc is interpreted as susceptible for identification purposes.

ated with serious infections (peritonitis and two patients with sepsis) (50, 75). Blood and urine have been the most common sources for the isolation of *S. spiritivorum* (74). *Sphingobacterium* species are generally resistant to aminoglycosides and polymyxin B, while they are susceptible in vitro to the quinolones and trimethoprim-sulfamethoxazole (54, 157). Susceptibility to beta-lactam antibiotics is variable, requiring testing of individual isolates (54).

CDC Group EF-4b

CDC group EF-4b along with EF-4a were originally designated eugonic fermenter group 4 (EF-4). However, CDC group EF-4b strains do not ferment glucose, do not hydrolyze arginine, and do not produce gas from nitrate, which separate them from the glucose-fermenting strains now designated EF-4a (see chapter 36). EF-4b strains are coccoid to short rods that are nonmotile and oxidase and catalase positive. Colonies on culture plates are nonpigmented and are reported to smell like popcorn. Most isolates have been recovered from human infections following dog and cat bites (181).

CDC Groups EO-2 and EO-3 and *Psychrobacter immobilis*

The classification of eugonic oxidizer groups EO-2 and EO-3 and *P. immobilis* is incomplete. All are strongly oxidase positive, nonmotile, saccharolytic coccobacilli and grow, sometimes poorly, on MacConkey agar. In contrast to the two EO groups, *P. immobilis* grows best at 20°C and only occasionally at 37°C. Cultures of EO-2 have an odor resembling that of phenylethyl alcohol agar (roses), while EO-3 strains have a yellow, nondiffusible pigment that is not observed with either EO-2 or *P. immobilis* (121). Microscopically, EO-2 is characterized by distinctive O-shaped cells upon Gram stain examination due to the presence of vacuolated or peripherally stained cells, and *P. immobilis* is characterized by paired organisms. *P. immobilis* can be confirmed by transformation studies (121). These three groups have all been isolated from clinical specimens; *P. immobilis* has also been isolated from food (90, 121). There are no reports of clinical infections due to EO-2 and EO-3 and only rare reports of disease due to *P. immobilis* (115).

Genus *Shewanella*

See Table 7.

The organism formerly called *Pseudomonas putrefaciens*, *Alteromonas putrefaciens*, *Achromobacter putrefaciens*, and CDC group Ib has now been placed in the genus *Shewanella* (116). Colonies on SBA are convex, circular, smooth, and occasionally mucoid, produce a brown-to-tan soluble pigment, and cause green discoloration of the medium. Cells are long, short, or filamentous. Motility is due to a single polar flagellum. Ornithine decarboxylase, nitrate reductase, and DNase are always produced, and with few exceptions, H_2S is produced in Kligler and triple sugar iron agars (they are the only nonfermenters that produce H_2S in these media). Three biovars have been described by Gilardi (54). Biovar 1 is primarily found in foodstuffs and the environment, while biovars 2 and 3 are found mainly in clinical samples. The Centers for Disease Control and Prevention (CDC) recognizes two biotypes based upon the requirement of NaCl for growth, oxidation of sucrose and maltose, and the ability to grow on salmonella-shigella agar (181). Owen et al. (129) have shown that organisms identified as *Shewanella putrefaciens* comprise at least four clearly separated genomic groups (groups I to IV). Ziemke et al. (186) have

TABLE 7 *Shewanella* spp.[a]

Test	*S. putrefaciens*	*S. alga*
Oxidase	+	+
H_2S in KIA	+	+
DNase	+	+
Ornithine decarboxylase	+	+
Acid from:		
Sucrose	+[b]	−
Maltose	+[b]	−
Glucose	V	−
Ribose	−	V
Growth in 6.5% NaCl	−[c]	+
Growth at 42°C	−[c]	+[c]
Source	Dairy, fish	Human
CFAs	i-15:0, 16:1ω7c, 17:1ω8c	i-15:0, 16:1ω7c, 17:1ω8c

[a] Data are from references 54, 103, and 181. For abbreviations, see Table 1, footnote *a*. Other abbreviations: KIA, Kligler iron agar.

[b] Variable results were reported by Khashe and Janda (103).

[c] Variable results were reported by Weyant et al. (181).

proposed the new species *Shewanella baltica*, for strains belonging to genomic group II of Owen et al. (129), which have been isolated mostly from the Baltic Sea and which grow at 4°C but not at 37°C (186). Based upon the taxonomic proposals of Nozue and colleagues (127) and Simidu et al. (156), strains belonging to genomic group IV of Owen et al. (129) (synonymous with Gilardi biovar 2 and CDC biotype 2) should be identified as *Shewanella alga* (see Table 7). Khashe and Janda (103) have reported that *S. alga* is the predominant human clinical isolate (77%), while *S. putrefaciens* (Gilardi biovar 1, CDC biotype 1) represents the majority of nonhuman isolates (89%). Although an infrequent isolate in the clinical laboratory, *S. putrefaciens-S. alga* has been recovered from a wide variety of clinical specimens and has been associated with a broad range of human infections including cellulitis, otitis media, ocular infection, abscesses, osteomyelitis, peritonitis, and septicemia (22, 25, 30, 36, 81, 104). Many of these infections were probably caused by the biovar now named *S. alga*. They are generally susceptible to most antimicrobial agents effective against gram-negative rods except penicillin and cephalothin (47, 54, 175). Recent investigations have noted that the mean MICs of penicillin, ampicillin, and tetracycline for *S. alga* were higher than the corresponding MICs for *S. putrefaciens* (103, 174).

PINK-PIGMENTED NONFERMENTERS

See Table 8.

Methylobacterium spp.

Members of the genus *Methylobacterium* are pink-pigmented bacteria that are able to utilize methanol as a sole source of carbon and energy, although this characteristic may be lost on subculture. They occur mostly on vegetation but may also be found in the hospital environment. Nine named species (*Methylobacterium extorquens*, *Methylobacterium organophilum*, *Methylobacterium rhodinum*, *Methylobacterium rhodesianum*, *Methylobacterium zatmanii*, *Methylobacterium aminovorans*, *Methylobacterium radiotolerans*, *Methylobacterium mesophilicum*, and *Methylobacterium fujisawaense*) and

TABLE 8 *Methylobacterium* and *Roseomonas* spp.[a]

Test	*Methylobacterium* spp.	*Roseomonas* spp.
Oxidase	+	+
Oxidation of methanol	+	−
Growth on MacConkey agar	−	+
Growth at 42°C	−	+
Urease	+	+
Starch hydrolysis	+	+
MBM + acetate	+	−
Colonies appear dark when exposed to long-wave UV light	+	−
Colony morphology	Dry, coral	Mucoid, pink
Gram staining morphology	Vacuolated rods	Coccoid rods
CFAs	18:1ω7c	*R. gilardii*: 16:0, 18:1ω7c, 2-OH-19:0cyc, and 19:0cyc$^{11-12}$; *other Roseomonas spp*.: 16:0 and 18:1ω7c

[a] Data are from references 54, 143, 178, and 181. For abbreviations, see Table 1, footnote *a*. Other abbreviations: MBM, mineral base medium.

additional unassigned biovars are recognized on the basis of carbon assimilation type, electrophoretic type, and DNA-DNA homology grouping (59, 60, 164). Most human strains belong to the species *Methylobacterium mesophilicum* (formerly *Pseudomonas mesophilica*, *Pseudomonas extorquens*, and *Vibrio extorquens*). This species is oxidase positive and motile by one polar or lateral flagellum, although motility is often difficult to demonstrate. Isolates are slowly growing on ordinary media, producing 1-mm-diameter colonies in 4 to 5 days on SBA, modified Thayer-Martin, Sabouraud, buffered charcoal-yeast extract, and Middlebrook 7H11 agars, with the best growth occurring on Sabouraud agar and usually no growth occurring on MacConkey agar. Optimum growth occurs from 25 to 30°C. Colonies are dry and appear pink or coral in incandescent light. Under UV light, *Methylobacterium* species appear dark due to absorption of UV light (143). On Gram staining the cells appear as large, vacuolated, pleomorphic rods that stain poorly and that may resist decolorization. Oxidation of sugars (xylose and sometimes glucose) is weak; urea and starch are hydrolyzed. *Methylobacterium* species have been reported to cause septicemia, continuous ambulatory peritoneal dialysis-related peritonitis, skin ulcers, synovitis, and other infections as well as pseudoinfections (48, 101, 113). Drugs active against *Methylobacterium* species include aminoglycosides and trimethoprim-sulfamethoxazole, whereas beta-lactam drugs show variable patterns of activity (24, 54). They are best tested for susceptibility by the agar or broth dilution method at 30°C for 48 h (24).

Roseomonas spp.

Members of the new genus *Roseomonas* (143) are also pink pigmented but differ in morphologic and biochemical characteristics from *Methylobacterium* spp. (Table 8). They are nonvacuolated and rather plump and coccoid and form mostly pairs and short chains. They grow on SBA, modified Thayer-Martin agar, and, usually, MacConkey agar at 37°C, but the best growth is observed on Sabouraud agar. Colonies are mucoid and runny. They are separated from *Methylobacterium* by their inability to oxidize methanol and to assimilate acetamide and by a lack of absorption of long-wave UV light (143). All strains are weakly oxidase positive (often after 30 s) or oxidase negative, catalase positive, and urease positive. The genus includes three named species (*Roseomonas gilardii*, *Roseomonas cervicalis*, and *Roseomonas fauriae*) and three unnamed genomospecies (143). Clinical isolates have been recovered from blood, wounds, exudates, abscesses, genitourinary sites, continuous ambulatory peritoneal dialysis fluid, and bone (2, 111, 123, 142, 143, 148, 159). In a review of the laboratory, clinical, and epidemiologic data for 35 patients from whom *Roseomonas* was isolated, Struthers and colleagues (159) reported that *Roseomonas* spp. appear to have a low pathogenic potential for humans but that some species, particularly *R. gilardii*, may be significant pathogens in persons with underlying medical complications. *Roseomonas* species are susceptible to aminoglycosides, tetracycline, and imipenem (143); however, in patients with catheter-related infections, eradication of the organism has proven difficult unless the infected catheter is removed (2, 142).

OXIDASE-POSITIVE, INDOLE-POSITIVE, NONMOTILE OR MOTILE, YELLOW-PIGMENTED NONFERMENTERS

See Table 9.

Family *Flavobacteriaceae* and CDC Groups IIc, IIe, IIg, IIh, and IIi

The taxonomy of organisms belonging to the genus *Flavobacterium* and other closely aligned genera has undergone extensive revision resulting in an emended description of the family *Flavobacteriaceae* and an emended classification and description of the genus *Flavobacterium* (10, 166, 167). These changes are summarized below.

1. *Flavobacterium balustinum*, *Flavobacterium gleum*, *Flavobacterium indologenes*, *Flavobacterium indoltheticum*, *Flavobacterium meningosepticum*, and *Flavobacterium scophthalmum* have been moved to a new genus, *Chryseobacterium*, with *Chryseobacterium gleum* being the type species (167).
2. *Flavobacterium breve* represents a distinct genetic taxon and has been reclassified as *Empedobacter brevis* (167).
3. *Flavobacterium odoratum* has been placed in a new genus, *Myroides*, as *Myroides odoratus* and *M. odoratimimus* (166) (see above).
4. The emended genus of *Flavobacterium* contains the following species: *Flavobacterium aquatile*, *Flavobacterium branchiophilum*, *Flavobacterium columnare*, *Flavobacterium flevense*, *Flavobacterium hydatis*, *Flavobacterium johnsoniae*, *Flavobacterium pectinovorum*, *Flavobacterium psychrophilum*, *Flavobacterium saccharophilum*, and *Flavobacterium succin-*

TABLE 9 Oxidase-positive, indole-positive, nonfermentative gram-negative rods[a]

Test	*Chryseobacterium meningosepticum*	*Chryseobacterium indologenes-Chryseobacterium gleum*	CDC group					*Weeksella virosa*	*Bergeyella zoohelcum*	*Empedobacter brevis*	*Balneatrix alpica*
			IIc	IIe	IIg	IIh	IIi				
Yellow pigment	sl	Bright	–	Pale	Pale	Pale	Pale	Pale	–	Pale	Pale
Flexirubin pigment (insoluble)	–	+	–	–	–	–	–	–	–	+	ND
Other pigments (soluble)	V[b]	V[c]	+[b]	V[c]	–	+[b]	V[c]	+[b]	+[c]	+[b]	+[c]
Motility	–	–	–	–	–	–	–	–	–	–	+
Nitrate to nitrite	–	V	–	–	–	–	–	–	–	–	+
Growth on MacConkey agar	V	V	–	–	+	–	–	–	–	D	–
Growth at 42°C	V	V	–	–	V	–	D	V	–	–	+
ONPG	+	V	ND	ND	ND	–	+	–	–	–	–
Starch hydrolysis[d]	–	+	ND	+	ND	+	V	–	–	V	–
Urease[d]	–	–	–	–	–	–	–	–	+ +	–	–
DNase[d]	+	–	ND	D	–	V	–	–	–	+	–
Esculin hydrolysis	+	+	+	–	–	+	+	–	–	–	–
Gelatin hydrolysis	+	+	V	–	–	D	–	+	+	+	–
Acid from:											
Glucose	+	+	+	+	–	+	+	–	–	V	+
Maltose	+	+	+	+	–	+	+	–	–	+	+
Sucrose	–	V	+	–	–	–	+	–	–	–	–
Mannitol	+	–	–	–	–	–	–	–	–	–	+
Xylose	–	V	–	–	–	–	+	–	–	–	–
Penicillin[e]	R	R	ND	S	ND	V	V	S	S	R	S
Polymyxin B[f]	R	R	ND	S	S	V	R	S	R	R	ND
CFAs	i-15:0, i-2-OH-15:0, i-3-OH-17:0	i-15:0, i-2-OH-15:0, i-3-OH-17:0, i-17:1ω8c	i-15:0, i-2-OH-15:0, i-3-OH-17:0, i-17:1ω8c	i-15:0, a-15:0, i-2-OH-15:0, i-17:1ω8c	16:0, 16:1ω7c, 18:1ω7c	i-15:0, a-15:0, i-2-OH-15:0, i-3-OH-17:0	ND	i-15:0, i-2-OH-15:0	i-15:0	i-15:0, 16:1ω7c	16:1ω7c, 16:0, 18:1ω7c

[a] Data are from references 41, 64, 66, 79, 80, and 181. For abbreviations, see Table 1, footnote *a*, and Table 3, footnote *a*. Other abbreviations: sl, slight.

[b] Tan to brown (late).

[c] Tan to yellow.

[d] Results are dependent on the choice of medium, reagents, and length of incubation. Variations with different lots of starch have been reported, indole positivity may be stronger with tryptophan than with tryptone or heart infusion broth, higher concentrations of urea (2%) may cause inhibition of growth, and DNase agar with methyl green is less satisfactory than either a dye-free medium or one with toluidine blue. For an in-depth review, see Pickett (134).

[e] Test performed by directly inoculating surface of SBA in a manner that will produce a uniform lawn of growth, immediately placing a 10-U penicillin disc on the agar surface, and incubating in room atmosphere at 35°C for 18 to 24 h. Any strain with a zone of inhibited growth around the penicillin disc is interpreted as susceptible for identification purposes.

[f] Test performed by directly inoculating surface of SBA in a manner that will produce a uniform lawn of growth, immediately placing a 300-U polymyxin B disc on the agar surface, incubating in room atmosphere at 35°C for 18 to 24 h. Any strain with a zone of inhibited growth around the polymyxin B disc is interpreted as susceptible for identification purposes.

icans (10). These remaining species of *Flavobacterium* are all indole negative and are not found in human clinical specimens.

5. *Weeksella zoohelcum* has been reclassified as *Bergeyella zoohelcum* (167). *Weeksella virosa* remains the type species and only species in the genus *Weeksella*.

Chryseobacterium, Empedobacter, and Unnamed CDC Groups

The natural habitats of *Chryseobacterium*, *Empedobacter*, and unnamed CDC groups are soil, plants, foodstuff, and water sources, including those in hospitals. Species in these genera are oxidase positive, indole positive, and nonmotile. The indole reaction is often weak and difficult to demonstrate; therefore, the more sensitive Ehrlich method should be used. Pigment formation with these organisms is variable. Colonies of *Chryseobacterium meningosepticum* are smooth and fairly large (1 to 2 mm in diameter after 24 h) but show only weak (if any) production of yellow pigment. In contrast, colonies of *Chryseobacterium indologenes* are deep yellow due to the production of the water-insoluble pigment flexirubin (134). Colonies of *Empedobacter brevis* are pale yellow. Microscopically, cells of *C. meningosepticum*, *C. indologenes*, and groups IIe, IIh, and IIi are thinner in their central portions than in their peripheral portions and include filamentous forms; IIh cells are significantly smaller than those of other species. It should be emphasized that test results (e.g., tests for DNase, indole, urea, and starch hydrolysis) are dependent on the choice of medium, reagents, and length of incubation (134). Phenotypic separation between *C. indologenes* and *C. gleum* has been difficult; however, acid production from xylose and growth at 41°C are consistently positive for DNA groups clustering around the type strain of *C. gleum* (165).

C. indologenes is the most frequent human isolate, although it rarely has clinical significance (175). *C. indologenes* has been documented to cause bacteremia in hospitalized patients with severe underlying disease, although the mortality rate is relatively low even among patients who were administered antibiotics without activity against *C. indologenes* (84). Nosocomial infections due to *C. indologenes* have been linked to the use of indwelling devices during the hospital stay (85, 87). *C. meningosepticum* is the species most often associated with significant disease in humans, causing neonatal meningitis, nosocomial miniepidemics (155) that are verifiable by ribotyping (34), and, rarely, adult pneumonia and septicemia (14, 153, 175). A case of respiratory colonization and infection following aerosolized polymyxin B treatment has also been described (23). *E. brevis* and unnamed CDC groups IIc, IIe, IIg, IIh, and IIi are rarely recovered from clinical material, and little is known about their involvement in clinical disease. One case of meningitis caused by CDC group IIe has been reported (179), and the phenotypic characteristics of several clinical isolates of CDC groups IIc and IIg have also been recently described (64, 66). The appropriate choice of effective antimicrobial agents for treatment of chryseobacteria infections is difficult. *Chryseobacterium* spp. are inherently resistant to many antimicrobial agents commonly used to treat infections caused by gram-negative bacteria (aminoglycosides, beta-lactam antibiotics, tetracylines, chloramphenicol) but are often susceptible to agents generally used to treat infections caused by gram-positive bacteria (rifampin, clindamycin, erythromycin, sparfloxacin, trimethoprim-sulfamethoxazole, vancomycin) (47, 54, 157, 175). While early investigators recommended vancomycin for the treatment of serious *C. meningosepticum* infections (63, 136), recent studies have shown that minocycline, rifampin, trimethoprim-sulfamethoxazole, and quinolones have greater in vitro activities (14, 49, 157). Among the quinolones, sparfloxacin and levofloxacin are more active than ciprofloxacin and ofloxacin (157). Di Pentima and colleagues (42) have provided evidence to suggest that the combination of intravenous vancomycin and rifampin is an appropriate regimen for initial empirical therapy of *C. meningosepticum* meningitis in newborns. *C. indologenes* is reported to be uniformly resistant to cephalothin, cefotaxime, ceftriaxone, aztreonam, aminoglycosides, erythromycin, clindamycin, vancomycin, and teicoplanin, while *C. indologenes* susceptibility to piperacillin, cefoperazone, ceftazidime, imipenem, quinolones, minocycline, and trimethoprim-sulfamethoxazole is variable, requiring testing of individual isolates (84, 85, 157, 176). Further complicating the choice of appropriate antimicrobial therapy is the fact that MIC breakpoints for resistance and susceptibility of chryseobacteria have not been established by the National Committee for Clinical Laboratory Standards, and the results of disk diffusion testing have been shown to be unreliable in predicting the antimicrobial susceptibilities of *Chryseobacterium* (*Flavobacterium*) species (1, 29, 49, 176). The E-test has been shown to be a possible alternative to the standard agar dilution method for testing susceptibility to cefotaxime, ceftazidime, amikacin, minocycline, ofloxacin, and ciprofloxacin but not piperacillin (83). Definitive therapy for clinically significant isolates should be guided by individual susceptibility patterns determined by an MIC method.

Weeksella and *Bergeyella*

Vandamme and colleagues (167) have shown that *Weeksella virosa* (formerly CDC group IIf) (79) and *Weeksella zoohelcum* (formerly CDC group IIj) (80) represent separate genetic taxa and thus have proposed the reclassification of one of these species, *Weeksella zoohelcum*, as *Bergeyella zoohelcum*. These organisms are 0.6 to 2 to 3 μm long, with parallel sides and rounded ends. Both species are oxidase positive, are indole positive, fail to grow on MacConkey agar, are nonpigmented, and are nonsaccharolytic. Both species have the unusual feature of being susceptible to penicillin, a feature that allows them to be easily differentiated from the related genera *Flavobacterium* and *Sphingobacterium*. *W. virosa* colonies are mucoid and adherent to the agar and develop tan to brown pigmentation; *B. zoohelcum* colonies are sticky and tan to yellow. *W. virosa* is urease negative and polymyxin B susceptible; *B. zoohelcum* is rapid urease test positive and polymyxin B resistant. *W. virosa* occurs mainly in urine and vaginal samples (79, 141), whereas *B. zoohelcum* is isolated mainly from wounds caused by animal bites (mostly dog bites) (80, 140). Reports of meningitis or septicemia due to *B. zoohelcum* have occurred in patients either bitten by a dog (21) or with continuous contact with cats (126). Both organisms are susceptible to most antibiotics (54); however, at present no specific antibiotic treatment is recommended. Therefore, antibiotic susceptibility testing should be performed for significant clinical isolates.

Balneatrix

The genus *Balneatrix* contains a single species, *Balneatrix alpica* (39), which was first isolated in 1987 during an outbreak of pneumonia and meningitis among persons who attended a hot spring (37°C) spa in southern France (27, 39, 89). Isolates were recovered from blood, cerebrospinal fluid, and sputum of eight patients, and one isolate was recovered from water. The bacterium is described as a gram-negative straight or curved rod, it is motile by a single polar flagellum, and it is strictly aerobic. Growth occurs at 20 to 46°C, and it produces colonies that are 2 to 3 mm in diameter, convex, and smooth. The center of the colonies is pale yellow after 2 to 3 days and pale brown after 4 days. Growth occurs on chocolate and tryptic soy agars but not on MacConkey agar. It is oxidase positive and nonfermentative, but it oxidizes glucose, mannose, fructose, maltose, sorbitol, mannitol, glycerol, and inositol. Indole is produced and nitrate is reduced to nitrite (Table 9). Gelatin is weakly hydrolyzed, and it is positive for lecithinase. *B. alpica* is reported to be susceptible to penicillin G and all other beta-lactam antibiotics and to all aminoglycosides, chloramphenicol, tetracycline, erythromycin, sulfonamides, trimethoprim, ofloxacin, and nalidixic acid. It is resistant to clindamycin and vancomycin (27).

REFERENCES

1. **Aber, R. C., C. Wennersten, and R. C. Moellering, Jr.** 1978. Antimicrobial susceptibility of flavobacteria. *Antimicrob. Agents Chemother.* **14:**483–487.
2. **Alcala, L., F. J. Vasallo, E. Cercenado, F. Garcia-Garrote, M. Rodriquez-Creixems, and E. Bouza.** 1997. Catheter-related bacteremia due to *Roseomonas gilardii* sp. nov. *J. Clin. Microbiol.* **35:**2712. (Letter.)
3. **Andersen, B. M., A. G. Steigerwalt, S. P. O'Connor, D. G. Hollis, R. S. Weyant, R. E. Weaver, and D. J. Brenner.** 1993. *Neisseria weaveri* sp. nov., formerly CDC group M-5, a gram-negative bacterium associated with dog bite wounds. *J. Clin. Microbiol.* **31:**2456–2466.
4. **Anderson, R. R., P. Warnick, and P. C. Schreckenberger.** 1997. Recurrent CDC group IVc-2 bacteremia in a human with AIDS. *J. Clin. Microbiol.* **35:**780–782.
5. **Anstey, N. M., B. J. Currie, and K. M. Withnall.** 1992. Community-acquired *Acinetobacter* pneumonia in the Northern Territory of Australia. *Clin. Infect. Dis.* **14:** 83–91.
6. **Anzai, Y., Y. Kudo, and H. Oyaizu.** 1997. The phylogeny of the genera *Chryseomonas*, *Flavimonas*, and *Pseudomonas* supports synonymy of these three genera. *Int. J. Syst. Bacteriol.* **47:**249–251.
7. **Barham, W. B., P. Church, J. E. Brown, and S. Paparello.** 1993. Misidentification of *Brucella* species with use of rapid bacterial identification systems. *Clin. Infect. Dis.* **17:**1068–1069.
8. **Batchelor, B. I., R. J. Brindle, G. F. Gilks, and J. B. Selkon.** 1992. Biochemical misidentification of *Brucella melitensis* and subsequent laboratory-acquired infections. *J. Hosp. Infect.* **22:**159–162.
9. **Bergogne-Berezin, E., and K. J. Towner.** 1996. *Acinetobacter* spp. as nosocomial pathogens: microbiological, clinical, and epidemiological features. *Clin. Microbiol. Rev.* **9:**148–165.
10. **Bernardet, J.-F., P. Segers, M. Vancanneyt, F. Berthe, K. Kersters, and P. Vandamme.** 1996. Cutting a Gordian knot: emended classification and description of the genus *Flavobacterium*, emended description of the family *Flavobacteriaceae*, and proposal of *Flavobacterium hydatis*, nom. nov. (basonym, *Cytophaga aquatilis* Strohl and Tait 1978). *Int. J. Syst. Bacteriol.* **46:**128–148.
11. **Bernards, A. T., A. J. de Beaufort, L. Dijkshoorn, and C. P. A. van Boven.** 1997. Outbreak of septicaemia in neonates caused by *Acinetobacter junii* investigated by amplified ribosomal DNA restriction analysis (ARDRA) and four typing methods. *J. Hosp. Infect.* **35:**129–140.
12. **Bernards, A. T., J. van der Toorn, C. P. A. van Boven, and L. Dijkshoorn.** 1996. Evaluation of the ability of a commercial system to identify *Acinetobacter* genomic species. *Eur. J. Clin. Microbiol. Infect. Dis.* **15:**303–308.
13. **Bizet, C., F. Tekaia, and A. Philippon.** 1993. In-vitro susceptibility of *Alcaligenes faecalis* compared with those of other *Alcaligenes* spp. to antimicrobial agents including seven β-lactams. *J. Antimicrob. Chemother.* **32:**907–910.
14. **Bloch, K. C., R. Nadarajah, and R. Jacobs.** 1997. *Chryseobacterium meningosepticum*: an emerging pathogen among immunocompromised adults. *Medicine (Baltimore)* **76:**30–40.
15. **Bouvet, P. J. M., and P. A. D. Grimont.** 1986. Taxonomy of the genus *Acinetobacter* with the recognition of *Acinetobacter baumannii* sp. nov., *Acinetobacter haemolyticus* sp. nov., *Acinetobacter johnsonii* sp. nov., and *Acinetobacter junii* sp. nov. and emended descriptions of *Acinetobacter calcoaceticus* and *Acinetobacter lwoffii*. *Int. J. Syst. Bacteriol.* **36:**228–240.
16. **Bouvet, P. J. M., and P. A. D. Grimont.** 1987. Identification and biotyping of clinical isolates of *Acinetobacter*. *Ann. Inst. Pasteur/Microbiol.* **138:**569–578.
17. **Bouvet, P. J. M., and S. Jeanjean.** 1989. Delineation of new proteolytic genomic species in the genus *Acinetobacter*. *Res. Microbiol.* **140:**291–299.
18. **Bouvet, P. J. M., S. Jeanjean, J. F. Vieu, and L. Dijkshoorn.** 1990. Species, biotype, and bacteriophage type determinations compared with cell envelope protein profiles for typing *Acinetobacter* strains. *J. Clin. Microbiol.* **28:** 170–176.
19. **Bovre, K., J. E. Fuglesang, N. Hagen, E. Jantzen, and L. O. Froholm.** 1976. *Moraxella atlantae* sp. nov. and its distinction from *Moraxella phenylpyruvica*. *Int. J. Syst. Bacteriol.* **26:**511–521.
20. **Bowman, J. P., J. Cavanagh, J. J. Austin, and K. Sanderson.** 1996. Novel *Psychrobacter* species from antarctic ornithogenic soils. *Int. J. Syst. Bacteriol.* **46:**841–848.
21. **Bracis, R., K. Seibers, and R. M. Julien.** 1979. Meningitis caused by group IIj following a dog bite. *West. J. Med.* **131:**438–440.
22. **Brink, A. J., A. van Straten, and A. J. van Rensburg.** 1995. *Shewanella* (*Pseudomonas*) *putrefaciens* bacteremia. *Clin. Infect. Dis.* **20:**1327–1332.
23. **Brown, R. B., D. Phillips, M. J. Barker, R. Pieczarka, M. Sands, and D. Teres.** 1989. Outbreak of nosocomial *Flavobacterium meningosepticum* respiratory infections associated with use of aerosolized polymyxin B. *Am. J. Infect. Control* **17:**121–125.
24. **Brown, W. J., R. L. Sautter, and A. E. Crist, Jr.** 1992. Susceptibility testing of clinical isolates of *Methylobacterium* species. *Antimicrob. Agents Chemother.* **36:** 1635–1638.
25. **Butt, A. A., J. Figueroa, and D. H. Martin.** 1997. Ocular infection caused by three unusual marine organisms. *Clin. Infect. Dis.* **24:**740.
26. **Carlson, P., S. Kontiainen, P. Anttila, and E. Eerola.** 1997. Septicemia caused by *Neisseria weaveri*. *Clin. Infect. Dis.* **24:**739.
27. **Casalta, J. P., Y. Peloux, D. Raoult, P. Brunet, and H. Gallais.** 1989. Pneumonia and meningitis caused by a new nonfermentative unknown gram-negative bacterium. *J. Clin. Microbiol.* **27:**1446–1448.
28. **Centers for Disease Control and Prevention.** 1996. *Ochrobactrum anthropi* meningitis associated with cadaveric pericardial tissue processed with a contaminated solution—Utah, 1994. *Morbid. Mortal. Weekly Rep.* **45:** 671–673.
29. **Chang, J.-C., P.-R. Hsueh, J.-J. Wu, S.-W. Ho, W.-C. Hsieh, and K.-T. Luh.** 1997. Antimicrobial susceptibility of flavobacteria as determined by agar dilution and disk diffusion methods. *Antimicrob. Agents Chemother.* **41:** 1301–1306.

30. **Chen, Y.-S., Y.-C. Liu, M.-Y. Yen, J.-H. Wang, J.-H. Wang, S.-R. Wann, and D.-L. Cheng.** 1997. Skin and soft-tissue manifestations of *Shewanella putrefaciens* infection. *Clin. Infect. Dis.* **25:**225–229.
31. **Cheron, M., E. Abachin, E. Guerot, M. El-Bez, and M. Simonet.** 1994. Investigation of hospital-acquired infections due to *Alcaligenes denitrificans* subsp. *xylosoxidans* by DNA restriction fragment length polymorphism. *J. Clin. Microbiol.* **32:**1023–1026.
32. **Cieslak, T. J., M. L. Robb, C. J. Drabick, and G. W. Fischer.** 1992. Catheter-associated sepsis caused by *Ochrobactrum anthropi*: report of a case and review of related nonfermentative bacteria. *Clin. Infect. Dis.* **14:**902–907.
33. **Cisneros, J. M., M. J. Reyes, J. Pachon, B. Becerril, F. J. Caballero, J. L. Garcia-Garmendia, C. Ortiz, and A. R. Cobacho.** 1996. Bacteremia due to *Acinetobacter baumannii*: epidemiology, clinical findings, and prognostic features. *Clin. Infect. Dis.* **22:**1026–1032.
34. **Colding, H., J. Bangsborg, N.-E. Fiehn, T. Bennekov, and B. Bruun.** 1994. Ribotyping for differentiating *Flavobacterium meningosepticum* isolates from clinical and environmental sources. *J. Clin. Microbiol.* **32:**501–505.
35. **Corbella, X., M. Pujol, J. Ayats, M. Sendra, C. Ardanuy, M. A. Dominguez, J. Linares, J. Ariza, and F. Gudiol.** 1996. Relevance of digestive tract colonization in the epidemiology of nosocomial infections due to multiresistant *Acinetobacter baumannii*. *Clin. Infect. Dis.* **23:** 329–334.
36. **Dan, M., R. Gutman, and A. Biro.** 1992. Peritonitis caused by *Pseudomonas putrefaciens* in patients undergoing continuous ambulatory peritoneal dialysis. *Clin. Infect. Dis.* **14:**359–360.
37. **Daneshvar, M. I., B. Hill, D. G. Hollis, C. W. Moss, J. G. Jordan, J. P. MacGregor, F. Tenover, and R. S. Weyant.** 1998. CDC group O-3: phenotypic characteristics, fatty acid composition, isoprenoid quinone content, and in vitro antimicrobic susceptibilities of an unusual gram-negative bacterium isolated from clinical specimens. *J. Clin. Microbiol.* **36:**1674–1678.
38. **Daneshvar, M. I., D. G. Hollis, C. W. Moss, J. G. Jordan, J. P. MacGregor, and R. S. Weyant.** 1998. Eugonic oxidizer group 5: an unusual gram-negative nonfermenter isolated from clinical specimens, abstr. C-204, p. 165. *In Abstracts of the 98th General Meeting of the American Society for Microbiology 1998*. American Society for Microbiology, Washington, D.C.
39. **Dauga, C., M. Gillis, P. Vandamme, E. Ageron, F. Grimont, K. Kersters, C. de Mahenge, Y. Peloux, and P. A. D. Grimont.** 1993. *Balneatrix alpica* gen. nov., sp. nov., a bacterium associated with pneumonia and meningitis in a spa therapy centre. *Res. Microbiol.* **144:**35–46.
40. **Dees, S. B., G. M. Carlone, D. Hollis, and C. W. Moss.** 1985. Chemical and phenotypic characteristics of *Flavobacterium thalpophilum* compared with those of other *Flavobacterium* and *Sphingobacterium* species. *Int. J. Syst. Bacteriol.* **35:**16–22.
41. **Dees, S. B., C. W. Moss, D. G. Hollis, and R. E. Weaver.** 1986. Chemical characterization of *Flavobacterium odoratum*, *Flavobacterium breve*, and *Flavobacterium*-like groups IIe, IIh, and IIf. *J. Clin. Microbiol.* **23:**267–273.
42. **Di Pentima, M. C. E. O. Mason, Jr., and S. L. Kaplan.** 1998. In vitro antibiotic synergy against *Flavobacterium meningosepticum*: implications for therapeutic options. *Clin. Infect. Dis.* **26:**1169–1176.
43. **Duggan, J. M., S. J. Goldstein, C. E. Chenoweth, C. A. Kauffman, and S. F. Bradley.** 1996. *Achromobacter xylosoxidans* bacteremia: report of four cases and review of the literature. *Clin. Infect. Dis.* **23:**569–576.
44. **Dunne, W. M., Jr., and S. Maisch.** 1995. Epidemiological investigation of infections due to *Alcaligenes* species in children and patients with cystic fibrosis: use of repetitive-element-sequence polymerase chain reaction. *Clin. Infect. Dis.* **20:**836–841.
45. **Dunne, W. M., Jr., J. Tillman, and J. C. Murray.** 1993. Recovery of a strain of *Agrobacterium radiobacter* with a mucoid phenotype from an immunocompromised child with bacteremia. *J. Clin. Microbiol.* **31:**2541–2543.
46. **Edmond, M. B., S. A. Riddler, C. M. Baxter, B. M. Wicklund, and A. W. Pasculle.** 1993. *Agrobacterium radiobacter*: a recently recognized opportunistic pathogen. *Clin. Infect. Dis.* **16:**388–391.
47. **Fass, R. J., and J. Barnishan.** 1980. In vitro susceptibility of nonfermentative gram-negative bacilli other than *Pseudomonas aeruginosa* to 32 antimicrobial agents. *Rev. Infect. Dis.* **2:**841–853.
48. **Flournoy, D. J., R. L. Petrone, and D. W. Voth.** 1992. A pseudo-outbreak of *Methylobacterium mesophilica* isolated from patients undergoing bronchoscopy. *Eur. J. Clin. Microbiol. Infect. Dis.* **11:**240–243.
49. **Fraser, S. L., and J. H. Jorgensen.** 1997. Reappraisal of the antimicrobial susceptibilities of *Chryseobacterium* and *Flavobacterium* species and methods for reliable susceptibility testing. *Antimicrob. Agents Chemother.* **41:** 2738–2741.
50. **Freney, J., W. Hansen, C. Ploton, H. Meugnier, S. Madier, N. Bornstein, and J. Fleurette.** 1987. Septicemia caused by *Sphingobacterium multivorum*. *J. Clin. Microbiol.* **25:**1126–1128.
51. **Gerner-Smidt, P., and I. Tjernberg.** 1993. *Acinetobacter* in Denmark. II. Molecular studies of the *Acinetobacter calcoaceticus-Acinetobacter baumannii* complex. *APMIS* **101:**826–832.
52. **Gerner-Smidt, P., I. Tjernberg, and J. Ursing.** 1991. Reliability of phenotypic tests for identification of *Acinetobacter* species. *J. Clin. Microbiol.* **29:**277–282.
53. **Getchell-White, S. I., L. G. Donowitz, and D. H. M. Gröschel.** 1989. The inanimate environment of an intensive care unit as a potential source of nosocomial bacteria: evidence for long survival of *Acinetobacter calcoaceticus*. *Infect. Control Hosp. Epidemiol.* **10:**402–407.
54. **Gilardi, G. L.** 1990. *Identification of Glucose-Nonfermenting Gram-Negative Rods*. North General Hospital, New York, N.Y.
55. **Graber, C. D., L. P. Jervey, W. E. Ostrander, L. H. Salley, and R. E. Weaver.** 1968. Endocarditis due to a lanthanic, unclassified gram-negative bacterium (group IVd). *Am. J. Clin. Pathol.* **49:**220–223.
56. **Graham, D. R., J. D. Band, C. Thornsberry, D. G. Hollis, and R. E. Weaver.** 1990. Infections caused by *Moraxella*, *Moraxella urethralis*, *Moraxella*-like groups M-5 and M-6, and *Kingella kingae* in the United States, 1953–1980. *Rev. Infect. Dis.* **12:**423–431.
57. **Gransden, W. R., and S. J. Eykyn.** 1992. Seven cases of bacteremia due to *Ochrobactrum anthropi*. *Clin. Infect. Dis.* **15:**1068–1069.
58. **Grant, P. E., D. J. Brenner, A. G. Steigerwalt, D. G. Hollis, and R. E. Weaver.** 1990. *Neisseria elongata* subsp. *nitroreducens* subsp. nov., formerly CDC group M-6, a gram-negative bacterium associated with endocarditis. *J. Clin. Microbiol.* **28:**2591–2596.
59. **Green, P. N., and I. J. Bousfield.** 1983. Emendation of *Methylobacterium* Patt, Cole, and Hanson 1976; *Methylobacterium rhodinum* (Heumann 1962) comb. nov. corrig.; *Methylobacterium radiotolerans* (Ito and Iizuka 1971) comb. nov. corrig.; and *Methylobacterium mesophilicum* (Austin and Goodfellow 1979) comb. nov. *Int. J. Syst. Bacteriol.* **33:**875–877.
60. **Green, P. N., I. J. Bousfield, and D. Hood.** 1988. Three new *Methylobacterium* species: *M. rhodesianum* sp. nov.,

M. *zatmanii* sp. nov., and M. *fujisawaense* sp. nov. *Int. J. Syst. Bacteriol.* **38:**124–127.

61. **Greenwood, J. R.** 1985. Methods of isolation and identification of glucose-nonfermenting gram-negative rods, p. 1–16. *In* G. L. Gilardi (ed.), *Nonfermentative Gram-Negative Rods: Laboratory Identification and Clinical Aspects.* Marcel Dekker, Inc., New York, N.Y.
62. **Grundmann, H. J., K. J. Towner, L. Dijkshoorn, P. Gerner-Smidt, M. Maher, H. Seifert, and M. Vaneechoutte.** 1997. Multicenter study using standardized protocols and reagents for evaluation of reproducibility of PCR-based fingerprinting of *Acinetobacter* spp. *J. Clin. Microbiol.* **35:**3071–3077.
63. **Hawley, H. B., and D. W. Gump.** 1973. Vancomycin therapy of bacterial meningitis. *Am. J. Dis. Child.* **126:** 261–264.
64. **Hollis, D. G., M. I. Daneshvar, C. W. Moss, and C. N. Baker.** 1995. Phenotypic characteristics, fatty acid composition, and isoprenoid quinone content of CDC group IIg bacteria. *J. Clin. Microbiol.* **33:**762–764.
65. **Hollis, D. G., C. W. Moss, M. I. Daneshvar, L. Meadows, J. Jordan, and B. Hill.** 1993. Characterization of Centers for Disease Control group NO-1, a fastidious, nonoxidative, gram-negative organism associated with dog and cat bites. *J. Clin. Microbiol.* **31:**746–748.
66. **Hollis, D. G., C. W. Moss, M. I. Daneshvar, and P. L. Wallace-Shewmaker.** 1996. CDC group IIc: phenotypic characteristics, fatty acid composition, and isoprenoid quinone content. *J. Clin. Microbiol.* **34:**2322–2324.
67. **Hollis, D. G., R. E. Weaver, C. W. Moss, M. I. Daneshvar, and P. L. Wallace.** 1992. Chemical and cultural characterization of CDC group WO-1, a weakly oxidative gram-negative group of organisms isolated from clinical sources. *J. Clin. Microbiol.* **30:**291–295.
68. **Holmes, B., M. Costas, S. L. W. On, P. Vandamme, E. Falsen, and K. Kersters.** 1993. *Neisseria weaveri* sp. nov. (formerly CDC group M-5), from dog bite wounds of humans. *Int. J. Syst. Bacteriol.* **43:**687–693.
69. **Holmes, B., M. Costas, A. C. Wood, and K. Kersters.** 1990. Numerical analysis of electrophoretic protein patterns of "*Achromobacter*" group B, E and F strains from human blood. *J. Appl. Bacteriol.* **68:**495–504.
70. **Holmes, B., M. Costas, A. C. Wood, R. J. Owen, and D. D. Morgan.** 1990. Differentiation of *Achromobacter*-like strains from human blood by DNA restriction endonuclease digest and ribosomal RNA gene probe patterns. *Epidemiol. Infect.* **105:**541–551.
71. **Holmes, B., R. Lewis, and A. Trevett.** 1992. Septicaemia due to *Achromobacter* group B: a report of two cases. *Med. Microbiol. Lett.* **1:**177–184.
72. **Holmes, B., C. W. Moss, and M. I. Daneshvar.** 1993. Cellular fatty acid compositions of "*Achromobacter* groups B and E." *J. Clin. Microbiol.* **31:**1007–1008.
73. **Holmes, B., R. J. Owen, A. Evans, H. Malnick, and W. R. Willcox.** 1977. *Pseudomonas paucimobilis*, a new species isolated from human clinical specimens, the hospital environment, and other sources. *Int. J. Syst. Bacteriol.* **27:** 133–146.
74. **Holmes, B., R. J. Owen, and D. G. Hollis.** 1982. *Flavobacterium spiritivorum*, a new species isolated from human clinical specimens. *Int. J. Syst. Bacteriol.* **32:**157–165.
75. **Holmes, B., R. J. Owen, and R. E. Weaver.** 1981. *Flavobacterium multivorum*, a new species isolated from human clinical specimens and previously known as group IIK, biotype 2. *Int. J. Syst. Bacteriol.* **31:**21–34.
76. **Holmes, B., C. A. Pinning, and C. A. Dawson.** 1986. A probability matrix for the identification of gram-negative, aerobic, non-fermentative bacteria that grow on nutrient agar. *J. Gen. Microbiol.* **132:**1827–1842.
77. **Holmes, B., M. Popoff, M. Kiredjian, and K. Kersters.** 1988. *Ochrobactrum anthropi* gen. nov., sp. nov. from human clinical specimens and previously known as group Vd. *Int. J. Syst. Bacteriol.* **38:**406–416.
78. **Holmes, B., J. J. S. Snell, and S. P. Lapage.** 1979. *Flavobacterium odoratum*: a species resistant to a wide range of antimicrobial agents. *J. Clin. Pathol.* **32:**73–77.
79. **Holmes, B., A. G. Steigerwalt, R. E. Weaver, and D. J. Brenner.** 1986. *Weeksella virosa* gen. nov., sp. nov. (formerly group IIf), found in human clinical specimens. *Syst. Appl. Microbiol.* **8:**185–190.
80. **Holmes, B., A. G. Steigerwalt, R. E. Weaver, and D. J. Brenner.** 1986. *Weeksella zoohelcum* sp. nov. (formerly group IIj), from human clinical specimens. *Syst. Appl. Microbiol.* **8:**191–196.
81. **Holt, H. M., P. Sogaard, and B. Gahrn-Hansen.** 1997. Ear infections with *Shewanella alga*: a bacteriologic, clinical and epidemiologic study of 67 cases. *Clin. Microbiol. Infect.* **3:**329–334.
82. **Holton, J.** 1983. A note on the preparation and use of a selective and differential medium for the isolation of the *Acinetobacter* spp. from clinical sources. *J. Appl. Bacteriol.* **66:**24–26.
83. **Hsueh, P.-R., J.-C. Chang, L.-J. Teng, P.-C. Yang, S.-W. Ho, W.-C. Hsieh, and K.-T. Luh.** 1997. Comparison of Etest and agar dilution method for antimicrobial susceptibility testing of *Flavobacterium* isolates. *J. Clin. Microbiol.* **35:**1021–1023.
84. **Hsueh, P.-R., T.-R. Hsiue, J.-J. Wu, L.-J. Teng, S.-W. Ho, W.-C. Hsieh, and K.-T. Luh.** 1996. *Flavobacterium indologenes* bacteremia: clinical and microbiological characteristics. *Clin. Infect. Dis.* **23:**550–555.
85. **Hsueh, P.-R., L.-J. Teng, S.-W. Ho, W.-C. Hsieh, and K.-T. Luh.** 1996. Clinical and microbiological characteristics of *Flavobacterium indologenes* infections associated with indwelling devices. *J. Clin. Microbiol.* **34:** 1908–1913.
86. **Hsueh, P.-R., L.-J. Teng, P.-C. Yang, Y.-C. Chen, H.-J. Pan, S.-W. Ho, and K.-T. Luh.** 1998. Nosocomial infections caused by *Sphingomonas paucimobilis*: clinical features and microbiological characteristics. *Clin. Infect. Dis.* **26:**676–681.
87. **Hsueh, P.-R., L.-J. Teng, P.-C. Yang, S.-W. Ho, W.-C. Hsieh, and K.-T. Luh.** 1997. Increasing incidence of nosocomial *Chryseobacterium indologenes* infections in Taiwan. *Eur. J. Clin. Microbiol. Infect. Dis.* **16:**568–574.
88. **Hsueh, P.-R., J.-J. Wu, T.-R. Hsiue, and W.-C. Hsieh.** 1995. Bacteremic necrotizing fasciitis due to *Flavobacterium odoratum*. *Clin. Infect. Dis.* **21:**1337–1338.
89. **Hubert, B., A. de Mahenge, F. Grimont, C. Richard, Y. Peloux, C. de Mahenge, J. Fleurette, and P. A. D. Grimont.** 1991. An outbreak of pneumonia and meningitis caused by a previously undescribed gram-negative bacterium in a hot spring spa. *Epidemiol. Infect.* **107:** 373–381.
90. **Hudson, M. J., D. G. Hollis, R. E. Weaver, and C. G. Galvis.** 1987. Relationship of CDC group EO-2 and *Psychrobacter immobilis*. *J. Clin. Microbiol.* **25:**1907–1910.
91. **Hulse, M., S. Johnson, and P. Ferrieri.** 1993. *Agrobacterium* infections in humans: experience at one hospital and review. *Clin. Infect. Dis.* **16:**112–117.
92. **Ibrahim, A., P. Gerner-Smidt, and W. Liesack.** 1997. Phylogenetic relationship of the twenty-one DNA groups of the genus *Acinetobacter* as revealed by 16S ribosomal DNA sequence analysis. *Int. J. Syst. Bacteriol.* **47:** 837–841.
93. **Jannes, G., M. Vaneechoutte, M. Lannoo, M. Gillis, M. Vancanneyt, P. Vandamme, G. Verschraegen, H. van Heuverswyn, and R. Rossau.** 1993. Polyphasic taxonomy leading to the proposal of *Moraxella canis* sp. nov. for *Moraxella catarrhalis*-like strains. *Int. J. Syst. Bacteriol.* **43:**438–449.

94. **Jawad, A., P. M. Hawkey, J. Heritage, and A. M. Snelling.** 1994. Description of Leeds *Acinetobacter* Medium, a new selective and differential medium for isolation of clinically important *Acinetobacter* spp., and comparison with Herellea agar and Holton's agar. *J. Clin. Microbiol.* **32:**2353–2358.

95. **Jenks, P. J., and E. J. Shaw.** 1997. Recurrent septicaemia due to "*Achromobacter* group B." *J. Infect.* **34:**143–145.

96. **Jimenez-Mejias, M. E., J. Pachon, B. Becerril, J. Palomino-Nicas, A. Rodriguez-Cobacho, and M. Revuelta.** 1997. Treatment of multidrug-resistant *Acinetobacter baumannii* meningitis with ampicillin/sulbactam. *Clin. Infect. Dis.* **24:**932–935.

97. **Johnson, D. W., G. Lum, G. Nimmo, and C. M. Hawley.** 1995. *Moraxella nonliquefaciens* septic arthritis in a patient undergoing hemodialysis. *Clin. Infect. Dis.* **21:** 1039–1040.

98. **Juni, E.** 1972. Interspecies transformation of *Acinetobacter*: genetic evidence for a ubiquitous genus. *J. Bacteriol.* **112:**917–931.

99. **Juni, E., G. A. Heym, M. J. Maurer, and M. L. Miller.** 1987. Combined genetic transformation and nutritional assay for identification of *Moraxella nonliquefaciens*. *J. Clin. Microbiol.* **25:**1691–1694.

100. **Kämpfer, P.** 1993. Grouping of *Acinetobacter* genomic species by cellular fatty acid composition. Med. *Microbiol. Lett.* **2:**394–400.

101. **Kaye, K. M., A. Macone, and P. H. Kazanjian.** 1992. Catheter infection caused by *Methylobacterium* in immunocompromised hosts: report of three cases and review of the literature. *Clin. Infect. Dis.* **14:**1010–1014.

102. **Kern, W. V., M. Oethinger, A. Kaufhold, E. Rozdzinski, and R. Marre.** 1993. *Ochrobactrum anthropi* bacteremia: report of four cases and short review. *Infection* **21:** 306–310.

103. **Khashe, S., and J. M. Janda.** 1998. Biochemical and pathogenic properties of *Shewanella alga* and *Shewanella putrefaciens*. *J. Clin. Microbiol.* **36:**783–787.

104. **Kim, J. H., R. A. Cooper, K. E. Welty-Wolf, L. J. Harrell, P. Zwadyk, and M. E. Klotman.** 1989. *Pseudomonas putrefaciens* bacteremia. *Rev. Infect. Dis.* **11:**97–104.

105. **King, A., B. Holmes, I. Phillips, and S. P. Lapage.** 1979. A taxonomic study of clinical isolates of *Pseudomonas pickettii*, "*P. thomasii*" and "group IVd" bacteria. *J. Gen. Microbiol.* **114:**137–147.

106. **Kiredjian, M., B. Holmes, K. Kersters, I. Guilvout, and J. de Ley.** 1986. *Alcaligenes piechaudii*, a new species from human clinical specimens and the environment. *Int. J. Syst. Bacteriol.* **36:**282–287.

107. **Kiska, D. L., A. Kerr, M. C. Jones, J. A. Caracciolo, B. Eskridge, M. Jordan, S. Miller, D. Hughes, N. King, and P. H. Gilligan.** 1996. Accuracy of four commercial systems for identification of *Burkholderia cepacia* and other gram-negative nonfermenting bacilli recovered from patients with cystic fibrosis. *J. Clin. Microbiol.* **34:**886–891.

108. **Knuth, B. D., M. R. Owen, and R. Latorraca.** 1969. Occurrence of an unclassified organism group IVd. *Am. J. Med. Technol.* **35:**227–232.

109. **Kodama, K., N. Kimura, and K. Komagata.** 1985. Two new species of *Pseudomonas: P. oryzihabitans* isolated from rice paddy and clinical specimens and *P. luteola* isolated from clinical specimens. *Int. J. Syst. Bacteriol.* **35:** 467–474.

110. **Koneman, E. W., S. D. Allen, W. M. Janda, P. C. Schreckenberger, and W. C. Winn, Jr.** 1997. *Color Atlas and Textbook of Diagnostic Microbiology*, 5th ed., p. 253–320. J. B. Lippincott Co., Philadelphia, Pa.

111. **Lewis, L., F. Stock, D. Williams, S. Weir, and V. J. Gill.** 1997. Infections with *Roseomonas gilardii* and review of characteristics used for biochemical identification and molecular typing. *Am. J. Clin. Pathol.* **108:**210–216.

112. **Lin, Y.-H., P. Y.-F. Liu, Z.-Y. Shi, Y.-J. Lau, and B.-S. Hu.** 1997. Comparison of polymerase chain reaction and pulsed-field gel electrophoresis for the epidemiological typing of *Alcaligenes xylosoxidans* subsp. *xylosoxidans* in a burn unit. *Diagn. Microbiol. Infect. Dis.* **28:**173–178.

113. **Liu, J.-W., J.-J. Wu, H.-M. Chen, A.-H. Huang, W.-C. Ko, and Y.-C. Chuang.** 1997. *Methylobacterium mesophilicum* synovitis in an alcoholic. *Clin. Infect. Dis.* **24:** 1008–1009.

114. **Liu, P. Y.-F., and W.-L. Wu.** 1997. Use of different PCR-based DNA fingerprinting techniques and pulsed-field gel electrophoresis to investigate the epidemiology of *Acinetobacter calcoaceticus-Acinetobacter baumannii* complex. *Diagn. Microbiol. Infect. Dis.* **28:**19–28.

115. **Lloyd-Puryear, M., D. Wallace, T. Baldwin, and D. G. Hollis.** 1991. Meningitis caused by *Psychrobacter immobilis* in an infant. *J. Clin. Microbiol.* **29:**2041–2042.

116. **MacDonell, M. T., and R. R. Colwell.** 1985. Phylogeny of the Vibrionaceae, and recommendation for two new genera, *Listonella* and *Shewanella*. *Syst. Appl. Microbiol.* **6:** 171–182.

117. **Mesnard, R., J. M. Sire, P. Y. Donnio, J. Y. Riou, and J. L. Avril.** 1992. Septic arthritis due to *Oligella urethralis*. *Eur. J. Clin. Microbiol. Infect. Dis.* **11:**195–196.

118. **Moissenet, D., M.-D. Tabone, J.-P. Girardet, G. Leverger, A. Garbarg-Chenon, and H. Vu-Thien.** 1996. Nosocomial CDC group IV c-2 bacteremia: epidemiological investigation by randomly amplified polymorphic DNA analysis. *J. Clin. Microbiol.* **34:**1264–1266.

119. **Morrison, A. J., and J. A. Shulman.** 1986. Community-acquired bloodstream infection caused by *Pseudomonas paucimobilis*: case report and review of literature. *J. Clin. Microbiol.* **24:**853–855.

120. **Moss, C. W., M. I. Daneshvar, and D. G. Hollis.** 1993. Biochemical characteristics and fatty acid composition of Gilardi rod group 1 bacteria. *J. Clin. Microbiol.* **31:** 689–691.

121. **Moss, C. W., P. L. Wallace, D. G. Hollis, and R. E. Weaver.** 1988. Cultural and chemical characterization of CDC groups EO-2, M-5, and M-6, *Moraxella* (*Moraxella*) species, *Oligella urethralis*, *Acinetobacter* species, and *Psychrobacter immobilis*. *J. Clin. Microbiol.* **26:**484–492.

122. **Musso, D., M. Drancourt, J. Bardot, and R. Legre.** 1994. Human infection due to the CDC group IVc-2 bacterium: case report and review. *Clin. Infect. Dis.* **18:**482–484. (Letter.)

123. **Nahass, R. G., R. Wisneski, D. J. Herman, E. Hirsh, and K. Goldblatt.** 1995. Vertebral osteomyelitis due to *Roseomonas* species: case report and review of the evaluation of vertebral osteomyelitis. *Clin. Infect. Dis.* **21:** 1474–1476.

124. **Nash, P., and M. M. Krenz.** 1991. Culture media, p. 1226–1288. *In* A. Balows, W. J. Hausler, Jr., K. L. Herrmann, H. D. Isenberg, and H. J. Shadomy (ed.), *Manual of Clinical Microbiology*, 5th ed. American Society for Microbiology, Washington, D.C.

125. **Nishimura, Y., T. Ino, and H. Hzuka.** 1988. *Acinetobacter radioresistens* sp. nov. isolated from cotton and soil. *Int. J. Syst. Bacteriol.* **38:**209–211.

126. **Noell, F., M. F. Gorce, C. Garde, and C. Bizet.** 1989. Isolation of *Weeksella zoohelcum* in septicaemia. *Lancet* **ii:** 332. (Letter.)

127. **Nozue, H., T. Hayashi, Y. Hashimoto, T. Ezaki, K. Hamasaki, K. Ohwada, and Y. Terawaki.** 1992. Isolation and characterization of *Shewanella alga* from human clinical specimens and emendation of the description of *S.*

alga Simidu et al., 1990, 335. *Int. J. Syst. Bacteriol.* **42:** 628–634.

128. **Osterhout, G. J., V. H. Shull, and J. D. Dick.** 1991. Identification of clinical isolates of gram-negative nonfermentative bacteria by an automated cellular fatty acid identification system. *J. Clin. Microbiol.* **29:**1822–1830.
129. **Owen, R. J., R. M. Legros, and S. P. Lapage.** 1978. Base composition, size and sequence similarities of genome deoxyribonucleic acids from clinical isolates of *Pseudomonas putrefaciens*. *J. Gen. Microbiol.* **104:**127–138.
130. **Palleroni, N. J.** 1984. Family I. Pseudomonadaceae, p. 141–219. *In* N. R. Krieg and J. G. Holt (ed.), *Bergey's Manual of Systematic Bacteriology*, vol. 1. The Williams & Wilkins Co., Baltimore, Md.
131. **Peiris, V., S. Fraser, M. Fairhurst, D. Weston, and E. Kaczmarski.** 1992. Laboratory diagnosis of brucella infection: some pitfalls. *Lancet* **339:**1415–1416.
132. **Perez, J. L., A. Pulido, F. Pantozzi, and R. Martin.** 1990. Butyrate esterase (Tributyrin) spot test, a simple method for immediate identification of *Moraxella* (*Branhamella*) *catarrhalis*. *J. Clin. Microbiol.* **28:**2347–2348.
133. **Pettersson, B., A. Kodjo, M. Ronaghi, M. Uhlen, and T. Tonjum.** 1998. Phylogeny of the family *Moraxellaceae* by 16S rRNA sequence analysis, with special emphasis on differentiation of *Moraxella* species. *Int. J. Syst. Bacteriol.* **48:**75–89.
134. **Pickett, M. J.** 1989. Methods for identification of flavobacteria. *J. Clin. Microbiol.* **27:**2309–2315.
135. **Pickett, M. J., A. von Graevenitz, G. E. Pfyffer, V. Punter, and M. Altwegg.** 1996. Phenotypic features distinguishing *Oligella urethralis* from *Moraxella osloensis*. *Med. Microbiol. Lett.* **5:**265–270.
136. **Plotkin, S. A., and J. C. McKitrick.** 1966. Nosocomial meningitis of the newborn caused by a *Flavobacterium*. *JAMA* **198:**194–196.
137. **Pugliese, A., B. Pacris, P. E. Schoch, and B. A. Cunha.** 1993. *Oligella urethralis* urosepsis. *Clin. Infect. Dis.* **17:** 1069–1070.
138. **Ramos, J. M., F. Soriano, M. Bernacer, J. Esteban, and J. Zapardiel.** 1993. Infection caused by the nonfermentative gram-negative bacillus CDC group IV c-2: case report and literature review. *Eur. J. Clin. Microbiol. Infect. Dis.* **12:** 456–458.
139. **Reina, J., A. Bassa, I. Llompart, D. Portela, and N. Borrell.** 1991. Infections with *Pseudomonas paucimobilis*: report of four cases and review. *Rev. Infect. Dis.* **13: 1072–1076.**
140. **Reina, J., and N. Borrell.** 1992. Leg abscess caused by *Weeksella zoohelcum* following a dog bite. *Clin. Infect. Dis.* **14:**1162–1163. (Letter.)
141. **Reina, J., J. Gil, F. Salva, J. Gomez, and P. Alomar.** 1990. Microbiological characteristics of *Weeksella virosa* (formerly CDC group IIf) isolated from the human genitourinary tract. *J. Clin. Microbiol.* **28:**2357–2359.
142. **Richardson, J. D.** 1997. Failure to clear a *Roseomonas* line infection with antibiotic therapy. *Clin. Infect. Dis.* **25:**155.
143. **Rihs, J. D., D. J. Brenner, R. E. Weaver, A. G. Steigerwalt, D. G. Hollis, and V. L. Yu.** 1993. *Roseomonas*, a new genus associated with bacteremia and other human infections. *J. Clin. Microbiol.* **31:**3275–3283.
144. **Rockhill, R. C., and L. I. Lutwick.** 1978. Group IVe-like gram-negative bacillemia in a patient with obstructive uropathy. *J. Clin. Microbiol.* **8:**108–109.
145. **Rosenthal, S. L., L. F. Freundlich, G. L. Gilardi, and F. Y. Clodomar.** 1978. In vitro antibiotic sensitivity of *Moraxella* species. *Chemotherapy (Basel)* **24:**360–363.
146. **Rossau, R., K. Kersters, E. Falsen, E. Jantzen, P. Segers, A. Union, L. Nehls, and J. de Ley.** 1987. *Oligella*, a new genus including *Oligella urethralis* comb. nov. (formerly *Moraxella urethralis*) and *Oligella ureolytica* sp. nov. (formerly CDC group IVe): relationship to *Taylorella equigenitalis* and related taxa. *Int. J. Syst. Bacteriol.* **37:**198–210.
147. **Rossau, R., A. Van Landschoot, M. Gillis, and J. de Ley.** 1991. Taxonomy of *Moraxellaceae* fam. nov., a new bacterial family to accommodate the genera *Moraxella*, *Acinetobacter*, and *Psychrobacter* and related organisms. *Int. J. Syst. Bacteriol.* **41:**310–319.
148. **Sandoe, J. A. T., H. Malnick, and K. W. Loudon.** 1997. A case of peritonitis caused by *Roseomonas gilardii* in a patient undergoing continuous ambulatory peritoneal dialysis. *J. Clin. Microbiol.* **35:**2150–2152.
149. **Sawada, H., H. Ieki, H. Oyaizu, and S. Matsumoto.** 1993. Proposal for rejection of *Agrobacterium tumefaciens* and revised descriptions for the genus *Agrobacterium* and for *Agrobacterium radiobacter* and *Agrobacterium rhizogenes*. *Int. J. Syst. Bacteriol.* **43:**694–702.
150. **Seifert, H., R. Baginski, A. Schulze, and G. Pulverer.** 1993. Antimicrobial susceptibility of *Acinetobacter* species. *Antimicrob. Agents Chemother.* **37:**750–753.
151. **Seifert, H., L. Dijkshoorn, P. Gerner-Smidt, N. Pelzer, I. Tjernberg, and M. Vaneechoutte.** 1997. Distribution of *Acinetobacter* species on human skin: comparison of phenotypic and genotypic identification methods. *J. Clin. Microbiol.* **35:**2819–2825.
152. **Seifert, H., A. Strate, and G. Pulverer.** 1995. Nosocomial bacteremia due to *Acinetobacter baumannii*: clinical features, epidemiology and predictors of mortality. *Medicine (Baltimore)* **74:**340–349.
153. **Sheridan, R. I., C. M. Ryan, M. S. Pasternack, J. M. Weber, and R. G. Tompkins.** 1993. Flavobacterial sepsis in massively burned pediatric patients. *Clin. Infect. Dis.* **17:**185–187.
154. **Siau, H., K.-Y. Yuen, P.-L. Ho, W. K. Luk, S. S. Y. Wong, P. C. Y. Woo, R. A. Lee, and W.-T. Hui.** 1998. Identification of acinetobacters on blood agar in presence of D-glucose by unique browning effect. *J. Clin. Microbiol.* **36:**1404–1407.
155. **Siegman-Igra, Y., D. Schwartz, G. Soferman, and N. Konforti.** 1987. *Flavobacterium* group IIb bacteremia: report of a case and review of *Flavobacterium* infections. *Med. Microbiol. Immunol.* **176:**103–111.
156. **Simidu, U., K. Kita-Tsukamoto, T. Yasumoto, and M. Yotsu.** 1990. Taxonomy of four marine bacterial strains that produce tetrodotoxin. *Int. J. Syst. Bacteriol.* **40:** 331–336.
157. **Spangler, S. K., M. A. Visalli, M. R. Jacobs, and P. C. Appelbaum.** 1996. Susceptibilities of non-*Pseudomonas aeruginosa* gram-negative nonfermentative rods to ciprofloxacin, ofloxacin, levofloxacin, D-ofloxacin, sparfloxacin, ceftazidime, piperacillin, piperacillin-tazobactam, trimethoprim-sulfamethoxazole, and imipenem. *Antimicrob. Agents Chemother.* **40:**772–775.
158. **Steyn, P. L., P. Segers, M. Vancanneyt, P. Sandra, K. Kersters, and J. J. Joubert.** 1998. Classification of heparinolytic bacteria into a new genus, *Pedobacter*, comprising four species: *Pedobacter heparinus* comb. nov., *Pedobacter piscium* comb. nov., *Pedobacter africansus* sp. nov. and *Pedobacter saltans* sp. nov.: proposal of the family *Sphingobacteriaceae* fam. nov. *Int. J. Syst. Bacteriol.* **48:**165–177.
159. **Struthers, M., J. Wong, and J. M. Janda.** 1996. An initial appraisal of the clinical significance of *Roseomonas* species associated with human infections. *Clin. Infect. Dis.* **23:** 729–733.
160. **Swann, R. A., S. J. Foulkes, B. Holmes, J. B. Young, R. G. Mitchell, and S. T. Reeders.** 1985. "*Agrobacterium* yellow group" and *Pseudomonas paucimobilis* causing peri-

tonitis in patients receiving continuous ambulatory peritoneal dialysis. *J. Clin. Pathol.* **38:**1293–1299.

161. **Takeuchi, M., and A. Yokota.** 1992. Proposals of *Sphingobacterium faecium* sp. nov., *Sphingobacterium piscium* sp. nov., *Sphingobacterium heparinum* comb. nov., *Sphingobacterium thalpophilum* comb. nov. and two genospecies of the genus *Sphingobacterium*, and synonymy of *Flavobacterium yabuuchiae* and *Sphingobacterium spiritivorum*. *J. Gen. Appl. Microbiol.* **38:**465–482.
162. **Tjernberg, I., and J. Ursing.** 1989. Clinical strains of *Acinetobacter* classified by DNA-DNA hybridization. *APMIS* **97:**595–605.
163. **Traub, W. H., and B. Leonhard.** 1994. Serotyping of *Acinetobacter baumannii* and genospecies 3: an update. *Med. Microbiol. Lett.* **3:**120–127.
164. **Urakami, T., H. Araki, K.-I. Suzuki, and K. Komagata.** 1993. Further studies of the genus *Methylobacterium* and description of *Methylobacterium aminovorans* sp. nov. *Int. J. Syst. Bacteriol.* **43:**504–513.
165. **Ursing, J., and B. Bruun.** 1991. Genotypic heterogeneity of *Flavobacterium* group IIb and *Flavobacterium breve*, demonstrated by DNA-DNA hybridization. *APMIS* **99:** 780–786.
166. **Vancanneyt, M., P. Segers, U. Torck, B. Hoste, J.-F. Bernardet, P. Vandamme, and K. Kersters.** 1996. Reclassification of *Flavobacterium odoratum* (Stutzer 1929) strains to a new genus, *Myroides*, as *Myroides odoratus* comb. nov. and *Myroides odoratimimus* sp. nov. *Int. J. Syst. Bacteriol.* **46:**926–932.
167. **Vandamme, P., J.-F. Bernardet, P. Segers, K. Kersters, and B. Holmes.** 1994. New perspectives in the classification of the flavobacteria: description of *Chryseobacterium* gen. nov., *Bergeyella* gen. nov., and *Empedobacter* nom. rev. *Int. J. Syst. Bacteriol.* **44:**827–831.
168. **Vandamme, P., M. Gillis, M. Vancanneyt, B. Hoste, K. Kerster, and E. Falsen.** 1993. *Moraxella lincolnii* sp. nov., isolated from the human respiratory tract, and reevaluation of the taxonomic position of *Moraxella osloensis*. *Int. J. Syst. Bacteriol.* **43:**474–481.
169. **Vandamme, P., M. Heyndrickx, M. Vancanneyt, B. Hoste, P. De Vos, E. Falsen, K. Kersters, and K.-H. Hinz.** 1996. *Bordetella trematum* sp. nov., isolated from wounds and ear infections in humans, and reassessment of *Alcaligenes denitrificans* Ruger and Tan 1983. *Int. J. Syst. Bacteriol.* **46:**849–858.
170. **Vandamme, P., J. Hommez, M. Vancanneyt, M. Monsieurs, B. Hoste, B. Cookson, C. H. Wirsing Von Konig, K. Kersters, and P. J. Blackall.** 1995. *Bordetella hinzii* sp. nov., isolated from poultry and humans. *Int. J. Syst. Bacteriol.* **45:**37–45.
171. **Van Dijck, P., M. Delmee, H. Ezzedine, A. Deplano, and M. J. Struelens.** 1995. Evaluation of pulsed-field gel electrophoresis and rep-PCR for the epidemiological analysis of *Ochrobactrum anthropi* strains. *Eur. J. Clin. Microbiol. Infect. Dis.* **14:**1099–1102.
172. **Veys, A., W. Callewaert, E. Waelkens, and K. van den Abbeele.** 1989. Application of gas-liquid chromatography to the routine identification of nonfermenting gram-negative bacteria in clinical specimens. *J. Clin. Microbiol.* **27:** 1538–1542.
173. **Visalli, M. A., M. R. Jacobs, T. D. Moore, F. A. Renzi, and P. C. Appelbaum.** 1997. Activities of β-lactams against *Acinetobacter* genospecies as determined by agar dilution and E-test MIC methods. *Antimicrob. Agents Chemother.* **41:**767–770.
174. **Vogel, B. F., K. Jørgensen, H. Christensen, J. E. Olsen, and L. Gram.** 1997. Differentiation of *Shewanella putrefaciens* and *Shewanella alga* on the basis of whole-cell protein profiles, ribotyping, phenotypic characterization, and 16S rRNA gene sequence analysis. *Appl. Environ. Microbiol.* **63:**2189–2199.
175. **von Graevenitz, A.** 1985. Ecology, clinical significance, and antimicrobial susceptibility of infrequently encountered glucose-nonfermenting gram-negative rods, p. 181–232. *In* G. L. Gilardi (ed.), *Nonfermentative Gram-Negative Rods: Laboratory Identification and Clinical Aspects.* Marcel Dekker, Inc., New York, N.Y.
176. **von Graevenitz, A., and M. Grehn.** 1977. Susceptibility studies on *Flavobacterium* II-b. *FEMS Microbiol. Lett.* **2:** 289–292.
177. **von Graevenitz, A., G. E. Pfyffer, M. J. Pickett, R. E. Weaver, and J. Wust.** 1993. Isolation of an unclassified non-fermentative gram-negative rod from a patient on continuous ambulatory peritoneal dialysis. *Eur. J. Clin. Microbiol. Infect. Dis.* **12:**568–570.
178. **Wallace, P. L., D. G. Hollis, R. E. Weaver, and C. W. Moss.** 1990. Biochemical and chemical characterization of pink-pigmented oxidative bacteria. *J. Clin. Microbiol.* **28:**689–693.
179. **Watson, K. C., and I. Muscat.** 1983. Meningitis caused by a *Flavobacterium*-like organism (CDC IIe strain). *J. Infect.* **7:**278–279.
180. **Weyant, R. S., D. G. Hollis, R. E. Weaver, M. F. M. Amin, A. G. Steigerwalt, S. P. O'Connor, A. M. Whitney, M. I. Daneshvar, C. W. Moss, and D. J. Brenner.** 1995. *Bordetella holmesii* sp. nov., a new gram-negative species associated with septicemia. *J. Clin. Microbiol.* **33:** 1–7.
181. **Weyant, R. S., C. W. Moss, R. E. Weaver, D. G. Hollis, J. G. Jordan, E. C. Cook, and M. I. Daneshvar.** 1996. *Identification of Unusual Pathogenic Gram-Negative Aerobic and Facultatively Anaerobic Bacteria*, 2nd ed. The Williams & Wilkins Co., Baltimore, Md.
182. **Wong, J. D., and J. M. Janda.** 1992. Association of an important *Neisseria* species, *Neisseria elongata* subsp. *nitroreducens*, with bacteremia, endocarditis, and osteomyelitis. *J. Clin. Microbiol.* **30:**719–720.
183. **Wood, C. A., and A. C. Reboli.** 1993. Infections caused by imipenem-resistant *Acinetobacter calcoaceticus* biotype *anitratus*. *J. Infect. Dis.* **168:**1602–1603.
184. **Yabuuchi, E., T. Kaneko, I. Yano, C. W. Moss, and N. Miyoshi.** 1983. *Sphingobacterium* gen. nov., *Sphingobacterium spiritivorum* comb. nov., *Sphingobacterium multivorum* com. nov., *Sphingobacterium mizutae* sp. nov., and *Flavobacterium indologenes* sp. nov.: glucose-nonfermenting gram-negative rods in CDC groups IIk-2 and IIb. *Int. J. Syst. Bacteriol.* **33:**580–598.

184a. **Yabuuchi, E., Y. Kawamura, Y. Kosako, and T. Ezaki.** 1998. Emendation of genus *Achromobacter* and *Achromobacter xylosoxidans* (Yabuuchi and Yano) and proposal of *Achromobacter ruhlandii* (Packer and Vishniac) comb. nov., *Achromobacter piechaudii* (Kiredjian et al.) comb. nov., and *Achromobacter xylosoxidans* subsp. *denitrificans* (Ruger and Tan) comb. nov. *Microbiol. Immunol.* **42:** 429–438.

185. **Yabuuchi, E., I. Yano, H. Oyaizu, Y. Hashimoto, T. Ezaki, and H. Yamamoto.** 1990. Proposals of *Sphingomonas paucimobilis* gen. nov. and comb. nov., *Sphingomonas parapaucimobilis* sp. nov., *Sphingomonas yanoikuyae* sp. nov., *Sphingomonas adhaesiva* sp. nov., *Sphingomonas capsulata* comb. nov., and two genospecies of the genus *Sphingomonas*. *Microbiol. Immunol.* **34:**99–119.
186. **Ziemke, F., M. G. Hofle, J. Lalucat, and R. Rossello-Mora.** 1998. Reclassification of *Shewanella putrefaciens* Owen's genomic group II as *Shewanella baltica* sp. nov. *Int. J. Syst. Bacteriol.* **48:**179–186.

Actinobacillus, Capnocytophaga, Eikenella, Kingella, and Other Fastidious or Rarely Encountered Gram-Negative Rods*

REINIER MUTTERS

36

DESCRIPTION OF THE GROUP

The term "fastidious bacteria" has traditionally been applied to organisms that grow poorly or not at all on conventional culture media (e.g., blood agar, chocolate agar, or MacConkey agar), require a capnophilic or microaerophilic atmosphere, and may require prolonged incubation before growth is detected. The specialized growth requirements can also complicate biochemical identification of these isolates. Thus, the fact that the organisms are uncommon pathogens may in part reflect the difficulties encountered in their isolation and identification.

With the exception of their fastidious growth properties, the gram-negative bacteria described in this chapter are heterogeneous. The organisms can vary in size from very short, small coccobacilli (e.g., *Kingella*) to organisms that are fusiform and that have curved shapes (e.g., *Capnocytophaga*) or very long filaments (e.g., *Streptobacillus*). Likewise, the colonial morphology can range from small, dry, pitting colonies (e.g., *Eikenella*) to colonies that can spread ("glide") over the agar surface (e.g., *Capnocytophaga*).

TAXONOMY

Actinobacillus is classified with *Pasteurella* and *Haemophilus* in the family *Pasteurellaceae* (19, 54). The precise taxonomic placement of species in the genus *Actinobacillus* is currently unresolved. On the basis of DNA hybridization and analysis of the 16S rRNA gene sequences, *Actinobacillus* consists of six species: *Actinobacillus equuli*, *Actinobacillus ureae*, *Actinobacillus hominis*, *Actinobacillus lignieresii*, *Actinobacillus suis*, and the V factor-dependent species *Actinobacillus pleuropneumoniae*. Four other species are candidates for this genus: Bisgaard's unnamed taxon 11, an avian hemolytic *Actinobacillus*-like species (53), *Actinobacillus capsulatus*, and a newly described species, *Actinobacillus minor* (43). *Actinobacillus actinomycetemcomitans* has been classified in the genus *Actinobacillus*; however, DNA homology and 16S rRNA sequencing studies have demonstrated a close relationship to *Haemophilus aphrophilus* and *Haemophilus segnis*. None of these three species belongs in the genus *Actinobacillus* or *Haemophilus* and will likely be classified in a new genus in the future. However, for practical purposes, *A. actinomycetemcomitans* will be discussed in this chapter, and the other two species will be discussed in chapter 39. Other species that should be reclassified in a different genus include *Actinobacillus muris*, *Actinobacillus delphinicola*, "*Actinobacillus seminis*," and the heterogeneous *Actinobacillus salpingitidis* group. The taxonomic positions of *Actinobacillus porcinus* and *Actinobacillus indolicus* also remain unclear, although they are closely related to *Haemophilus parasuis* (43). The taxonomic relationships among these organisms need to be clarified, and one or more new genera will likely be formed in the family *Pasteurellaceae*.

Most of the *Actinobacillus* species are animal pathogens with a narrow host spectrum. The species of medical relevance for humans are *A. ureae*, *A. hominis*, *A. lignieresii*, and *A. actinomycetemcomitans* (29, 62). *A. muris*, *A. suis*, *A. pleuropneumoniae*, and *A. minor* may also be uncommon causes of human disease.

The genus *Capnocytophaga* was proposed in 1979 (42) and consisted of three species: *Capnocytophaga ochracea* (the former CDC group DF-1 organisms), *Capnocytophaga sputigena*, and *Capnocytophaga gingivalis* (70, 79). The genus was then expanded to include *Capnocytophaga canimorsus* (former CDC group DF-2) and *Capnocytophaga cynodegmi* (CDC group DF-2-like organisms) (5). In contrast to the first three species, which are part of the indigenous flora of humans, the last two species are isolated from dog mouths and are associated with human infections after dog bites. Finally, the genus was expanded to include *Capnocytophaga haemolytica* and *Capnocytophaga granulosa*, which are isolated from the human oral cavity (82). On the basis of 16S rRNA sequencing, the genus can be divided into three clusters: (i) *C. ochracea*, *C. sputigena*, and *C. haemolytica*; (ii) *C. gingivalis* and *C. granulosa*; and (iii) *C. canimorsus* and *C. cynodegmi*. Although most isolates within these species have homogeneous DNA banding patterns, *C. ochracea* and *C. cynodegmi* are more heterogeneous and may be subdivided in the future (76).

Eikenella was initially classified as *Bacteroides corrodens* because the organism's characteristic growth into the agar ("pitting") was mistaken for anaerobic growth. Later these organisms were reclassified as *Bacteroides ureolyticus* (formerly *B. corrodens*) (strict anaerobic strains) and *Eikenella corrodens* (microaerophilic strains). DNA hybridization studies and analysis of 16S rRNA sequences grouped all

* This chapter contains information presented in chapter 39 by Barry Holmes, M. John Pickett, and Dannie G. Hollis in the sixth edition of this Manual.

initial isolates of *Eikenella* into a single species, *E. corrodens*, and placed the genus in the family *Neisseriaceae* (16, 32, 60). Organisms originally classified as HB-1 were also demonstrated to be identical to *E. corrodens* and were reclassified in this species. Recent studies have suggested that one or more new species of *Eikenella* may exist. Phenotypically aberrant strains have been recovered from animals, and genomic analysis has demonstrated that a human isolate is distantly related to *E. corrodens* (9). Two subspecies of *E. corrodens* have also been characterized on the basis of differences in cellular carbohydrates (34).

The three species of *Kingella* (*Kingella kingae*, *Kingella denitrificans*, and the newly described *Kingella oralis*) and the unnamed CDC eugonic fermenters (groups EF-4a and EF-4b) were placed in the family *Neisseriaceae* on the basis of the results of nucleic acid hybridization and 16S rRNA sequencing (16, 18, 60). Both *Kingella* and group EF-4 belong to DeLey's rRNA superfamily III.

The family *Cardiobacteriaceae* consists of three genera: *Cardiobacterium*, *Dichelobacter*, and *Suttonella*. *Cardiobacterium* consists of a single species, *Cardiobacterium hominis; Bacteroides nodosus*, a pathogen of sheep, goats, and cattle, was reclassified in the new genus *Dichelobacter* (*Dichelobacter nodosus*); and *Suttonella indologenes* (formerly *Kingella indologenes*) was removed from the genus *Kingella* and was reclassified in the new, monospecific genus *Suttonella*. The new family *Cardiobacteriaceae* is placed in the gamma division of the class *Proteobacteria* (17).

CDC dysgonic fermenters (group DF-3 and DF-3-like organisms) share several biochemical properties with *Capnocytophaga* species but are genetically unrelated to this genus. Group DF-3 is most closely related to the anaerobic gram-negative bacilli *Bacteroides forsythus* and *Bacteroides distasonis*, but the definitive phylogenetic affiliation is unresolved.

The genus *Chromobacterium* consists of two species, *Chromobacterium violaceum* and *Chromobacterium fluviatile*. On the basis of 16S rRNA sequence data and the results of nucleic acid hybridization analysis, *Chromobacterium* is related to the genera *Eikenella* and *Kingella* and belongs in the emended family *Neisseriaceae*. *Chromobacterium* forms a deep branch in the beta group of the class *Proteobacteria* (16, 60).

The taxonomic position of *Streptobacillus* with the sole species *Streptobacillus moniliformis* remains unclear. This genus may be related to members of the order *Mycoplasmatales*, which would be consistent with the observation that *S. moniliformis* has a low G+C content (24 to 25%) and can spontaneously change into L forms.

ACTINOBACILLUS

Actinobacillus species are gram-negative, non-spore-forming rods with a mean size of 0.4 by 1.0 μm. Coccobacillary and short rods are observed from colonies growing on solid media, while long, narrow rods can be seen in glucose-containing broth media. Actinobacilli grow both aerobically and anaerobically at 36°C, with growth enhanced in a humid 5 to 10% carbon dioxide atmosphere. Colonies on chocolate or sheep blood agar are small, with a diameter of 1 to 2 mm, and may be sticky upon primary isolation.

Natural Habitat and Clinical Significance

Actinobacilli are frequent residents of the mucous membranes of the respiratory tracts and genitourinary tracts of healthy individuals and animals. The bacteria produce disease when they are introduced into healthy tissues (e.g., periodontal tissue) through trauma or localized injury, and disease is more common in individuals with compromised immune defenses, in elderly people, and following viral infections.

Human disease is primarily associated with three species which exclusively colonize humans: *A. actinomycemcomitans*, *A. ureae*, and *A. hominis*. Other species of *Actinobacillus* colonize animals such as cattle, pigs, or hares, which can serve as reservoirs for opportunistic infections in humans.

A. actinomycetemcomitans is a microaerophilic species that was first isolated from actinomycotic lesions. However, the species has greater medical importance as a common cause of periodontitis and systemic infections such as endocarditis and abscess formation, particularly in the brain. Of the approximately 350 anaerobic or microaerophilic species associated with human periodontal disease, *A. actinomycetemcomitans* is the most common cause of juvenile periodontitis and is commonly isolated from diseased tissues from adults (45, 46, 66, 74). Potential virulence factors include the production of leukotoxin (83) and collagenase (57). As a complication in advanced periodontal lesions, *A. actinomycetemcomitans* and other fastidious gram-negative bacteria such as *Capnocytophaga* and *E. corrodens* have been isolated from the inflamed tissues surrounding unsuccessful bone implants (2). Periodontal disease is also a predisposing factor for the development of infective endocarditis caused by *A. actinomycetemcomitans*, as well as by *C. hominis*, *E. corrodens*, and *Kingella* spp. (23).

A. ureae and *A. hominis* are opportunistic pathogens that are primarily isolated from sputum and tracheal secretions from patients with chronic respiratory tract diseases and pneumonia. Systemic infections (i.e., bacteremia and meningitis) have also been reported (77). Although no definitive studies have demonstrated that these organisms are part of the normal indigenous flora, it is assumed that they colonize the upper respiratory tracts of healthy individuals. Earlier reports that *A. ureae* (formerly *Pasteurella ureae*) was isolated from laboratory mice are inconclusive because definitive identification tests were not performed (49).

A number of human infections caused by *A. lignieresii* and *A. equuli* have been described. Most infections involved animal bites, with the organisms isolated from cultures of wound or blood specimens. Although the identifications of many isolates appear in doubt, the etiologies of some infections are well documented. For example, the recovery of *A. lignieresii* from a subcutaneous abscess was confirmed by DNA-DNA hybridization (20, 62), and the identification of *A. equuli* from a horse bite wound was also documented conclusively (51).

Human infections caused by other *Actinobacillus* species have not been described. However, contact with colonized animals may result in human infections. Thus, identification tests for the species most commonly isolated from animals (i.e., *A. minor*, *A. muris*, *A. pleuropneumoniae*, and *A. suis*) are discussed below.

Culture and Isolation

Specimens submitted for the isolation of *Actinobacillus* species include tracheal secretions, bronchial washings and lavages, wound aspirates, and cerebrospinal fluid, tissue biopsy, and blood specimens. Isolation of the bacteria requires the use of weakly alkaline, enriched growth media such as blood agar with 5 to 8% sheep blood or chocolate agar supplemented with vitamins and either hemoglobin or lysed blood (sheep or horse blood). Blood agar will need to be

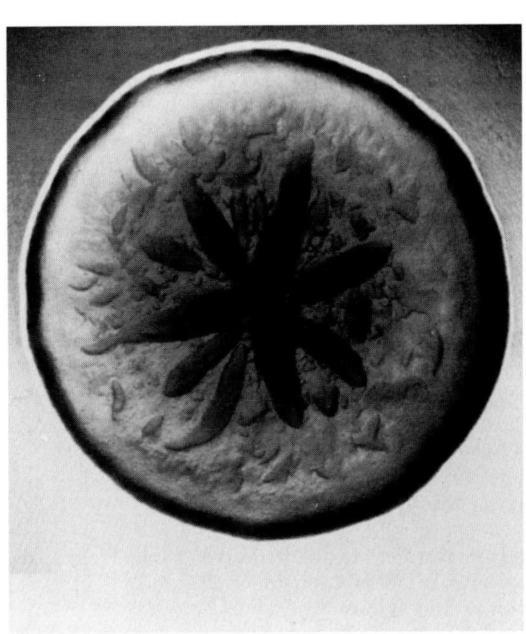
 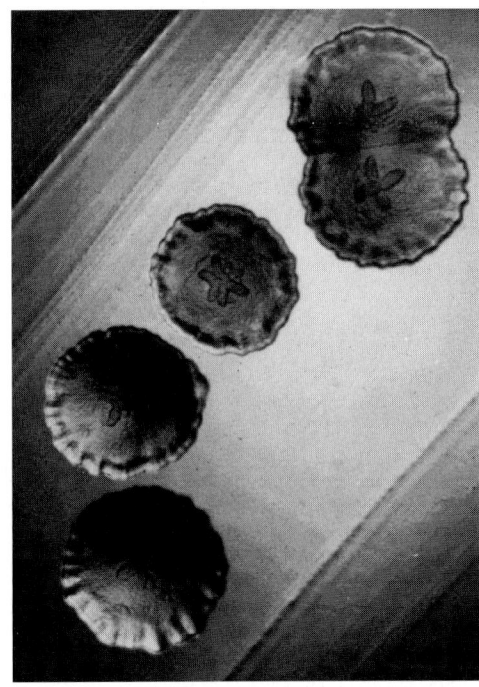

FIGURE 1 Star-shaped colonies of *A. actinomycetemcomitans*.

supplemented with NAD for the isolation of V factor-dependent species (i.e., *A. pleuropneumoniae* and *A. minor*). Agar media should be incubated in a humid atmosphere of 5% CO_2 or anaerobically for 24 to 72 h.

A. actinomycetemcomitans will appear as 1- to 3-mm-diameter colonies after incubation for 2 to 3 days. Colonies are round, smooth, and grayish white with central wrinkling and are strongly adherent to the agar surface. Older colonies on serum-containing agar will develop star-like inner structures that are visible by microscopy (Fig. 1). Gram-stained cells reveal small, oval, coccobacillary rods. Colonies of *A. ureae* on blood or chocolate agar are 0.5 to 1 mm in diameter, smooth, convex, and nonhemolytic, with slight blackening of the agar under the colonies being observed. *A. hominis* produces 1- to 2-mm-diameter colonies after 24 h. The colonies are initially transparent but change to grayish white after 48 h. Adherent, rough, 1- to 2-mm-diameter colonies of *A. equuli* are observed on primary isolation, whereas smooth, buttery colonies develop after several subcultures. *A. lignieresii* colonies are also adherent on primary isolation, appearing grayish white on chocolate or blood agar. *A. suis* produces hemolytic, adherent colonies on blood agar, with a white to ivory-colored center and transparent edges. *A. minor* has characteristically small, smooth, gray colonies (<1 mm in diameter) on chocolate agar after 48 h of incubation.

A. actinomycetemcomitans is a significant cause of human periodontal disease; however, recovery of this organism in culture is difficult because it may be overgrown by the multiple species of other bacteria present in diseased tissues. For that reason, molecular techniques such as PCR and culture hybridization have been developed for the detection and identification of *A. actinomycetemcomitans* (26, 56, 63, 66).

Identification

The phenotypic properties used to differentiate the fastidious gram-negative rods discussed in this chapter are summarized in Table 1. All *Actinobacillus* species are positive by either the oxidase or the alkaline phosphatase reaction, with most strains being positive by both reactions. Nitrates are reduced to nitrite but not gas, no growth is observed on Simmons citrate medium, the arginine dihydrolase reaction is negative, and no acid is produced from adonitol and sorbose. The phenotypic characteristics used to separate members of the family *Pasteurellaceae* are listed in Table 2. Additional reactions that are useful for characterizing *Actinobacillus* spp. include positive urease test, acid production from mannitol but not from *meso*-inositol and *d*-sorbitol, negative reactions by the methyl red test, and negative reactions for indole production, ornithine decarboxylase, and ONPF (α-fucosidase). NAD (V-factor) dependency is characteristic of *Haemophilus* species; however, DNA-DNA hybridization studies have shown that this requirement is not unique to *Haemophilus* (48, 55). *A. pleuropneumoniae* and *A. minor* both require V factor for growth. Additionally, the lack of V-factor dependency does not exclude *Haemophilus* because it has been described previously that strains of *H. parainfluenzae* grow in the absence of V factor (81). Heme (X-factor) dependency has never been observed in *Actinobacillus*.

The differential characteristics of *Actinobacillus* species are summarized in Table 3. *A. actinomycetemcomitans* is strongly catalase positive; ferments fructose, galactose, and maltose; and fails to ferment inositol, salicin, sorbitol, sucrose, and trehalose. Most strains ferment mannose and xylose. Negative reactions are observed for urease activity, indole production, ornithine decarboxylase, esculin hydrolysis, and the *o*-nitrophenyl-β-D-galactopyranoside (ONPG) test.

A. equuli forms H_2S on lead acetate paper, is ONPG positive, and produces acid from fructose, lactose, maltose, mannitol, melibiose (some strains have delayed reactions), raffinose, sucrose, trehalose (delayed reactions), and xylose.

TABLE 1 Phenotypic properties used to differentiate fastidious or unusual gram-negative rods[a]

Reaction	*Actinobacillus*	*Capnocytophaga*	*Eikenella*	*Kingella*	EF-4a	EF-4b	*Cardiobacterium*	*Suttonella*	CDC group DF-3	*Streptobacillus*	*Chromobacterium*
Oxidase	+	V	+	+	+	+	+	+	−	−	V
Catalase	V	V	−	−	+	+	−	V	V	−	+
Growth on MacConkey agar	V	−	−	−	V	V	−	V	−	−	+
Simmons citrate	−	−	−	−	−	V	−	−	−	−	V
Nitrate reductase	+	−	+	V	+	+	−	−	−	−	+
Arginine dihydrolase	−	V	−	−	V	−	−	−	−	−	+
Urease	V	−	−	−	−	−	−	−	−	−	V
Indole production	−	−	−	−	−	−	+	+	V	−	V
Acid from:											
Mannitol	V	−	−	−	−	−	+	−	−	−	−
Glucose	+	+	−	+	F	O	+	+	+	+	+

[a] Symbols and abbreviations: +, positive reaction; −, negative reaction; V, variable reaction; F, ferments glucose; O, oxidizes glucose. Most data are from Dewhirst et al. (17, 18) and Weyant et al. (78).

No acid is produced from inositol, salicin, and sorbitol, and esculin hydrolysis and ornithine decarboxylase are negative. The G+C content of *A. equuli* DNA is 40.0 to 41.8 mol%.

A. ureae strains form acid from fructose, maltose, mannitol (delayed), and sucrose but not from galactose, inositol, lactose, sorbitol, trehalose, or xylose. The strains are also negative by the ONPG test, for the ornithine decarboxylase reaction, and for indole production. *A. hominis* can be distinguished from *A. ureae* by acid production from galactose, trehalose, and xylose; most strains acidify mannitol; some strains produce acid from lactose; and some strains hydrolyze esculin. *A. hominis* has positive urease and ONPG reactions, has variable production of acid from salicin, and is negative or weakly positive for catalase. The G+C content of the DNA is 41.2 to 43.7 mol%.

A. lignieresii is oxidase and alkaline phosphatase positive and produces acid from fructose, maltose, mannitol, mannose, sucrose, and xylose (the reaction can be delayed). Negative reactions are observed for ONPG, ornithine decarboxylase, indole production, and gelative liquefaction; and acid is typically not produced from galactose, inositol, salicin, sorbitol, or trehalose. The G+C content of the DNA is 41.8 to 42.6 mol%.

A. muris and *A. pleuropneumoniae* resemble *A. ureae*. *A. muris* is distinguished from *A. ureae* by the ability to hydrolyze esculin and produce acid from salicin. *A. pleuropneumoniae* is dependent on V factor for growth, has a positive ONPG reaction (delayed), and produces acid from lactose and xylose.

TABLE 2 Phenotypic characteristics separating the genera in the family *Pasteurellaceae*[a]

Reaction	*Actinobacillus* sensu stricto	*Pasteurella* sensu stricto	*Haemophilus* sensu stricto
Hemolysis	V	−	V
Urease	+	V	V
X-factor dependence	−	−	+
Acid from:			
Mannitol	+	V	−
Mannose	V	+	V

[a] Symbols and abbreviations: +, positive reaction; −, negative reaction; V, variable reaction.

A. suis hydrolyzes esculin, has positive ONPG and urease reactions, and produces acid from arabinose, galactose, lactose, maltose, mannose, melibiose, salicin, sucrose, trehalose, and xylose. The G+C content of the DNA is 40.5 mol%.

The newly described species, *A. minor*, is V-factor dependent and ONPG positive and produces acid from lactose, maltose, mannose, raffinose, and sucrose. Indole is not produced, the ornithine decarboxylase reaction is negative, and no acid is produced from arabinose, esculin, inositol, inulin, or sorbitol. The G+C content of the DNA is 38.2 mol%. The major cellular fatty acids of *Actinobacillus* include 14:0, 16:1ω7c, and 16:0.

Antimicrobial Susceptibilities

Actinobacilli are generally susceptible to many antibiotics. Although *A. actinomycetemcomitans* is resistant to penicillin, the other *Actinobacillus* species are susceptible to many beta-lactam antibiotics. The cephalosporins, carbapenems, and combinations of penicillins with β-lactamase inhibitors have good activities against *Actinobacillus* species. Aminoglycosides are active but should be combined with a beta-lactam antibiotic. Fluoroquinolones, such as ciprofloxacin, ofloxacin, and levofloxacin, also have good activity against actinobacilli. Tetracycline and metronidazole treatment combined with subgingival debridement has been effective in treating periodontitis caused by *A. actinomycetemcomitans* (11, 50).

CAPNOCYTOPHAGA

Capnocytophaga spp. are thin, spindle-shaped, gram-negative rods, are 1 to 3 mm in length, and are morphologically similar to fusobacteria. Curved filaments and coccoid forms can also be seen. Movement of the organisms in the microscopic field has been described as "gliding motility." *Capnocytophaga* spp. grow aerobically in 5 to 10% CO_2, as well as anaerobically. Nonhemolytic colonies are very small on blood agar after 1 day of incubation and reach a size of 2 to 3 mm in diameter only after 2 to 4 days. The colonies are convex or flat with irregular edges, with spreading

TABLE 3 Differential characteristics of *Actinobacillus*[a]

Reaction	*A. actinomycetemcomitans*	*A. equuli*	*A. ureae*	*A. hominis*	*A. lignieresii*	*A. muris*	*A. pleuropneumoniae*	*A. suis*	*A. minor*
V-factor dependence	−	−	−	−	−	−	+	−	+
Alkaline phosphatase	+	+	+	+	+	−	+	+	ND
Ornithine decarboxylase	−	−	−	−	−	−	+	−	−
Esculin hydrolysis	−	−	−	(V)	−	+	−	+	−
Urease	−	+	+	+	+	+	+	+	+
ONPG	−	+	−	+	−	−	(+)	+	+
Acid from:									
Arabinose	−	V	−	−	V	−	−	+	−
Cellobiose	−	−	−	−	−	−	−	+	ND
Galactose	+	V	−	+	V	−	V	V	ND
Lactose	−	+	−	(V)	V	−	(+)	(+)	+
Maltose	+	+	+	+	+	+	V	+	+
Mannitol	(+)	+	(+)	+	+	+	+	−	−
Mannose	V	+	V	−	+	+	+	+	+
Melibiose	−	+	−	(+)	−	−	V	+	ND
Raffinose	−	+	−	+	V	−	V	+	+
Salicin	−	−	−	V	−	+	−	+	ND
Sorbitol	−	−	−	−	−	−	−	−	−
Sucrose	−	+	+	+	+	+	+	+	+
Trehalose	−	(+)	−	+	−	−	−	+	ND
Xylose	+	+	−	+	(+)	−	+	+	ND

[a] Symbols and abbreviations: +, positive reaction; parentheses, delayed reaction; −, negative reaction; V, variable reaction; ND, not determined. Data are from Møller et al. (43), Mutters et al. (47), and Weyant et al. (78).

growth and pitting of the agar observed. *C. haemolytica* may be weakly hemolytic, but this property is lost after a few subcultures. *C. ochracea* colonies may have a bitter almond odor.

Natural Habitat and Clinical Significance

C. gingivalis, *C. granulosa*, *C. haemolytica*, *C. ochracea*, and *C. sputigena* are members of the human oral flora, while *C. canimorsus* and *C. cynodegmi* colonize the oral cavities of cats and dogs. The species that colonize humans are opportunistic pathogens and have been implicated in periodontal disease as well as systemic infections. *C. gingivalis* and *C. ochracea* are associated with juvenile periodontitis (14), *C. sputigena* is associated with adult periodontitis, and *C. granulosa* and *C. haemolytica* are isolated from supragingival dental plaque from adults. Localized infections (e.g., abscess formation, keratitis, and endophthalmitis) and systemic infections (e.g., septicemia, peritonitis, endocarditis, and osteomyelitis) are observed in both immunocompetent and immunocompromised patients (3, 7, 24, 25, 28, 61, 64). *C. canimorsus* and *C. cynodegmi* are responsible for infectious complications of animal bites. *C. cynodegmi* causes localized wound infections, while *C. canimorsus* has been associated with septicemia and other severe infections (5, 22, 44, 52).

Culture and Isolation

Capnocytophaga spp. have been recovered from subgingival plaque, dental pockets, tracheal secretions, bronchoscopy specimens, aspirates of wounds and abscesses, and blood. The organisms grow best at 35 to 37°C in an aerobic atmosphere with 5 to 10% CO_2 or in an anaerobic atmosphere and on Columbia agar with 5% sheep blood, heart infusion agar with 5% rabbit serum, or standard chocolate agar. The organisms do not grow on MacConkey agar.

Identification

With relatively few exceptions, all *Capnocytophaga* spp. are negative for indole production, lysine and ornithine decarboxylase, and motility. Fermentation of carbohydrates is difficult to measure and should be performed in serum-enriched medium with a large inoculum of organisms (5). Acid production from glucose, mannose, and maltose but not mannitol or xylose is observed with all species. The characteristics that are used to identify individual species are summarized in Table 4.

Phenotypic differentiation among *C. gingivalis*, *C. ochracea*, and *C. sputigena* is difficult. All three species are negative for oxidase and catalase activity, as well as arginine dihydrolase. *C. ochracea* can be distinguished from *C. sputigena* by acid production from galactose and glycogen and by a negative reaction for nitrate reductase. *C. gingivalis* can be differentiated from the other two species by negative or variable reactions for esculin hydrolysis and lactose and raffinose acidification. The other two species of *Capnocytophaga* that colonize humans, *C. granulosa* and *C. haemolytica*, are separated by positive reactions for nitrate reductase, esculin hydrolysis, and acidification of glycogen and inulin for *C. haemolytica*. *Capnocytophaga* species isolated from animals (i.e., *C. canimorsus* and *C. cynodegmi*) are differentiated from the species isolated from humans by positive oxidase, catalase, and arginine dihydrolase reactions. Negative tests for acid production from inulin, raffinose, and sucrose differentiate *C. canimorsus* from *C. cynodegmi*.

Alternative techniques for the detection and identification of *Capnocytophaga* spp. have been developed. Although these tests are not commercially available at this time, the seven species can be identified by DNA homology analyses (70, 79), restriction fragment length polymorphism analysis of 16S rRNA (80), and the profiles of its cellular proteins (40). Most species yield a 15:0 major cellular fatty acid.

TABLE 4 Differential characteristics of *Capnocytophaga*[a]

Reactions	*C. gingivalis*	*C. granulosa*	*C. haemolytica*	*C. ochracea*	*C. sputigena*	*C. canimorsus*	*C. cynodegmi*
Oxidase	−	−	−	−	−	+	+
Catalase	−	−	−	−	−	+	+
Nitrate reductase	−	−	+	−	+	−	−
Arginine dihydrolase	−	−	−	−	−	+	+
Esculin hydrolysis	V	−	+	+	+	V	+
Acid from:							
Galactose	−	ND	ND	+	−	+	V
Glycogen	+	−	+	+	−	+	V
Inulin	+	−	V	+	+	−	V
Lactose	−	ND	ND	+	V	+	+
Mannose	+	+	+	+	+	+	(+)
Raffinose	−	ND	ND	V	V	−	V
Sucrose	+	+	+	+	+	−	+

[a] Symbols and abbreviations: +, positive reaction; parentheses, delayed reaction; −, negative reaction; V, variable reaction; ND, not determined. Data are from Brenner et al. (5), Conrads et al. (13), Weyant et al. (78), and Yamamoto et al. (82).

Antimicrobial Susceptibilities

Capnocytophaga spp. are usually susceptible to extended-spectrum cephalosporins, carbapenems, fluoroquinolones, chloramphenicol, clindamycin, and erythromycin and are resistant to aztreonam, aminoglycosides, trimethoprim, and metronidazole (31, 33, 65). Most strains are susceptible to penicillin, although β-lactamase production has been described (59).

EIKENELLA

Cells of *E. corrodens* are slender, straight, and 1.5 to 4 μm in length with rounded ends. *E. corrodens* is nonmotile, but twitching movements may be observed in colonies removed from some agar media. After 2 days of incubation on chocolate or blood agar, colonies of less than 1 mm in diameter will appear. Most strains pit or corrode the agar by splitting polygalacturonic acid. This is not observed for all isolates, and corroding and noncorroding strains can be observed on the same culture plate. Upon initial isolation, colonies are transparent and gray but can develop a slight yellow color with prolonged incubation. A distinct odor similar to that of *Haemophilus* may be noticed.

Natural Habitat and Clinical Significance

E. corrodens is a commensal organism of the human oral cavity and is responsible for both oral and extraoral infections. It is a prevalent pathogen in subgingival plaques from adults with periodontitis (68) and has been recovered from patients with a variety of other infections and conditions including pleuropulmonary infections, postsurgical wound infections, soft-tissue abscesses, arthritis, meningitis, endocarditis, and septicemia (15, 27, 38, 39, 71).

Culture and Isolation

E. corrodens has been recovered from a variety of specimens or sites including dental plaque, dental pockets, periodontal tissues, lower respiratory tract specimens, aspirates from wounds and abscesses, and blood and other normally sterile fluids. Growth on agar medium is slow, with 2 to 4 days being required before well-developed colonies are observed. *E. corrodens* is facultatively anaerobic, but growth is best in 5% CO_2 at 36°C. Heme is required for aerobic growth, so colonies will develop on blood and chocolate agars but not on MacConkey agar.

Identification

E. corrodens is positive for oxidase, nitrate reductase, and ornithine decarboxylase. Negative reactions are observed for catalase, lysine decarboxylase, arginine dihydrolase, esculin hydrolysis, urease, indole production, and acidification of carbohydrates (Table 5). The G+C content of *E. corrodens* DNA is 56 to 58 mol%. Recently, a catalase-positive strain of *E. corrodens* was described. This probably represents a new species within the genus (18). The heterogeneity of *E. corrodens* isolates has also been demonstrated by analysis of cellular carbohydrates (34) and outer membrane proteins and lipopolysaccharides (8).

Antimicrobial Susceptibilities

E. corrodens is susceptible to penicillin, ampicillin, amoxicillin-clavulanic acid, expanded- and broad-spectrum cephalosporins, carbapenems, quinolones, and tetracycline. Strains are resistant to narrow-spectrum cephalosporins, clindamycin, and metronidazole.

KINGELLA AND CDC GROUP EF-4

Kingella and CDC group EF-4 organisms are nonmotile, non-spore-forming, gram-negative rods in the family *Neisseriaceae*. *Kingella* spp. are coccobacillary, 0.6 to 1 μm in diameter, and 2 to 3 μm in length. They occur in pairs and short chains and can be confused with *Neisseria* spp. EF-4 organisms are also coccobacillary but occur singly.

Natural Habitat and Clinical Significance

Kingella spp. are part of the normal bacterial flora on mucous membranes of the human respiratory tract. *K. kingae* is an opportunistic pathogen responsible for endocarditis, osteomyelitis, and septicemia (1, 10). *K. oralis* has been isolated from dental plaque, but its role in periodontal disease is unknown. *K. denitrificans* is not commonly isolated but has

TABLE 5 Phenotypic characteristics of *E. corrodens*, *Kingella*, and CDC group EF-4[a]

Reaction	*E. corrodens*	*K. denitrificans*	*K. kingae*	*K. oralis*	EF-4a	EF-4b
Oxidase	+	+	+	+	+	+
Catalase	−	−	−	−	+	+
Nitrate reductase	+	+	−	−	+	+
Arginine dihydrolase	−	−	−	ND	+	−
Lysine decarboxylase	V	−	−	−	−	−
Ornithine decarboxylase	+	−	−	−	−	−
Esculin hydrolysis	−	−	−	−	−	−
Acid from:						
Glucose	−	(+)	(+)	W	+	(+)
Maltose	−	−	(+)	−	−	−
Sucrose	−	−	−	−	−	−
Major cellular fatty acids	16:1ω7c, 16:0, 18:1ω7c	12:0, 14:0, 16:0, 18:2, 18:1ω9c	14:0, 16:1ω7c, 16:0	NA	16:1ω5, 16:0, 18:1ω7c	16:1ω7c, 16:0, 18:1ω7c

[a] Symbols and abbreviations: +, positive reaction; parentheses, delayed reaction; −, negative reaction; V, variable reaction; W, weak reaction; ND, not determined; NA, not available. Data are from Møller et al. (43), Mutters et al. (47), and Weyant et al. (78).

been associated with endocarditis (73). EF-4 strains are part of the normal oral flora of dogs and cats and produce disease in humans following animal bites, scratches, or contamination of a preexisting wound. EF-4a is more commonly associated with dogs, while EF-4b is more commonly associated with cats (35, 78).

Culture and Isolation

Kingella spp. and EF-4 have been isolated from blood, wound, and abscess specimens, dental plaque, and periodontal tissues. *Kingella* and EF-4 strains grow aerobically at 36°C on blood and chocolate agars incubated for 2 or more days. Growth is enhanced in a 5% CO_2 atmosphere. *K. kingae* colonies but not the other species are beta-hemolytic on blood agar. Colonies of *Kingella* are smooth and convex, although spreading, corroding colonies with twitching cellular motility can be seen. Some strains of EF-4 are weakly pigmented, with tan to pale yellow colonies observed.

Identification

The phenotypic characteristics of *Kingella* and EF-4 are summarized in Table 5. *Kingella* and EF-4 are oxidase positive, do not produce indole, and generally fail to acidify carbohydrates with the exception of glucose. EF-4 is catalase positive, and *Kingella* (with the exception of some strains of *K. oralis*) is catalase negative. *K. kingae* is differentiated from the other *Kingella* spp. by acidification of maltose (delayed reaction). The G+C content of DNA is 47.3 mol%. *K. denitrificans* is the only species of *Kingella* with nitrate reductase activity. The G+C contents of *K. denitrificans* and *K. oralis* are 54.1 to 54.8 and 56 to 58 mol%, respectively. EF-4 is differentiated from *Kingella* by a positive catalase reaction and the ability of many strains to grow on MacConkey agar. EF-4a usually digests gelatin and exhibits arginine dihydrolase activity. Colonies can have a popcorn-like smell. The G+C content of EF-4 ranges from 49.3 to 50.9 mol%.

Antibiotic Susceptibilities

Kingella and EF-4 are susceptible to penicillin and most other antibiotics including erythromycin, tetracycline, chloramphenicol, and sulfonamides.

CARDIOBACTERIUM AND *SUTTONELLA*

Cells of *C. hominis* are gram-negative rods and are 1.0 to 3.0 μm long. They can appear pleomorphic with bulbous ends and arranged in rosette clusters, but this property is lost on media enriched with yeast extract. Cells of *S. indologenes* appear as gram-negative rods 3 μm in length. As with *Kingella* and *Cardiobacterium* spp., *S. indologenes* resists decolorization.

The members of the family *Cardiobacteriaceae* are residents of the human respiratory tract and, occasionally, the urogenital tract. As the name implies, *C. hominis* is associated with endocarditis (6, 58), with 4.8% of cases of gram-negative endocarditis being caused by this organism (12). *C. hominis*-like strains have been isolated from human dental plaque and from patients with periodontitis. *S. indologenes* has been implicated in endocarditis (37) and human eye infections (72, 75).

Isolates of *Cardiobacterium* and *Suttonella* have been recovered from blood, corneal scrapings, and periodontal specimens. They grow on blood agar and chocolate agar but not on MacConkey agar. Small (diameter, 1 mm), circular, flat colonies are seen after 2 days of incubation in a microaerophilic atmosphere at 36°C. *Cardiobacterium* colonies are yellowish to white, and *Suttonella* colonies are gray and translucent. Both genera exhibit twitching motility, and the edges of the colonies tend to spread.

Differential characteristics useful for the identification of *Cardiobacterium* and *Suttonella* are summarized in Table 6. Both genera are positive for oxidase and indole production and acid production from glucose, fructose, mannose, and sucrose and are negative for nitrate reduction, urease production, and esculin hydrolysis. *C. hominis* can be separated from *S. indologenes* by its negative alkaline phosphatase reaction and acid production from maltose, sorbitol, or mannitol. Some strains of *S. indologenes* acidify maltose weakly. Only the indole-negative *C. hominis*-like strains acidify trehalose.

Cardiobacterium and *Suttonella* are susceptible to most antibiotics, including penicillin, all cephalosporins, carbapenems, aminoglycosides, chloramphenicol, and tetracyclines. Clindamycin resistance has been reported for *C. hominis*, but no strains have been found to produce β-lactamases.

CDC GROUP DF-3 AND DF-3-LIKE ORGANISMS

DF-3 organisms are fastidious, nonmotile, coccobacillary rods. DF-3 strains have been isolated from blood, wounds,

TABLE 6 Phenotypic characteristics of *Cardiobacterium*, *Suttonella*, CDC group DF-3, *Chromobacterium*, and *Streptobacillus*[a]

Reaction	*C. hominis*	*S. indologenes*	DF-3	DF-3-like	*C. violaceum*	*S. moniliformis*
Oxidase	+	+	−	−	V	−
Catalase	−	−	−	V	+	−
Nitrate reductase	−	−	−	−	+	−
Arginine dihydrolase	−	−	−	−	+	+
Alkaline phosphatase	−	+	ND	ND	ND	ND
Esculin hydrolysis	−	−	+	V	−	V
Urease	−	−	−	−	V	−
Indole production	+	+	V	+	V	−
Acid from:						
Glucose	+	+	(+)	(+)	+	(W)
Lactose	−	−	(+)	(+)	−	−
Maltose	+	V	(+)	(+)	−	(W)
Mannitol	V	−	−	−	−	−
Sucrose	+	+	+	−	V	−
Xylose	−	−	+	−	−	−
Major cellular fatty acids	14:0, 16:0, 18:1ω7c	15:0, 16:1ω7c, 16:0, 18:1ω7c	15:0-*i*, 15:0-*a*, 16:0, 18:2,	15:0-*i*, 15:0-*a*, 16:0, 18:2, 3-OH-17:0-*i*	16:1ω7c, 16:0, 18:1ω7c	NA

[a] Symbols and abbreviations: +, positive reaction; W, weak reaction; parentheses, delayed reaction; V, variable reaction; −, negative reaction; ND, not determined; NA, not available. Data are from Weyant et al. (78).

stool, peritoneal fluid, urine, and abscesses (78). The role of DF-3 as a cause of diarrhea in immunocompromised patients has not been determined (4). DF-3-like organisms have been recovered from finger, foot, and hand wounds and from blood specimens (78). DF-3 is a capnophilic, facultative anaerobe that grows slowly on blood and chocolate agars but not on MacConkey agar. DF-3-like strains can be distinguished from DF-3 strains by their weak beta-hemolytic activities.

Both groups of organisms are negative for oxidase activity, nitrate reduction, and urease activity (Table 6). Most strains produce indole and hydrolyze esculin. DF-3 strains are negative for catalase, while DF-3-like strains have variable catalase activity. Carbohydrate fermentation tests should be supplemented with two drops of rabbit or horse serum. Delayed glucose, lactose, and maltose activities are observed. Acid production in xylose differentiates DF-3 strains from DF-3-like strains and DF-3 strains from *C. hominis* and *S. indologenes* strains.

CHROMOBACTERIUM

Of the two species of *Chromobacterium*, only *C. violaceum* has been implicated in human disease. These facultatively anaerobic, gram-negative rods are 1.5 to 3.5 μm in length, are straight or slightly curved with rounded ends, and are arranged singly, in pairs, or in short chains. Convex, smooth, violet colonies are formed on simple peptone medium. Unpigmented variants may occur with the violet colonies.

C. violaceum is found in the soil and water of tropical and subtropical areas. Human infections rarely occur and generally follow contamination of cutaneous lesions with soil or water. Localized wound infections or septicemic infections with abscesses in multiple internal organs have been reported, as have diarrhea and urinary tract infections (30, 67, 69). The mortality rate is high for patients with disseminated infections.

C. violaceum grows on simple peptone agar and on MacConkey agar. Some strains are slightly hemolytic on blood agar. Preliminary identification of this organism is aided by the violet pigmentation and positive reactions for catalase and nitrate reduction. Variable reactions are observed for oxidase, urease, and indole production. Acid is produced from glucose, usually without gas formation, but not from maltose, mannitol, or xylose. Acidification of sucrose is variable. The arginine dihydrolase test is positive, but lysine and ornithine decarboxylation reactions are negative. The G+C content of the type strain is 67.2 mol%.

C. violaceum is susceptible to aminoglycosides, chloramphenicol, and tretracyclines but is resistant to penicillins and cephalosporins (36).

STREPTOBACILLUS

S. moniliformis is highly pleomorphic, 0.3 to 0.5 μm in width, and 1 to 5 μm in length; however, extremely long (100 to 150 μm), unbranched filaments can be seen. Young cultures appear homogeneous, while older cultures can have long chains with moniliaceous swellings resembling a string of pearls which later break into coccobacillary forms. Spontaneous reversion to L forms also occurs.

S. moniliformis occurs naturally in the nasopharynges and oropharynges of wild and laboratory rats. Human infections result either from rodent bites (rat bite fever) or through the consumption of contaminated milk or other foods (Haverhill fever). Clinical symptoms of infection with *S. moniliformis* develop after an incubation period of 10 or more days. Onset is characterized by the abrupt onset of high fever, chills, intense headache, vomiting, and severe migratory arthralgias. The site of the bite is generally healed at this stage, and lymphadenitis is rare. A petechial or measles-like rash develops, particularly over the extremities, including the palms and soles. Complications can include arthritis, cardiac involvement (endocarditis, myocarditis, pericarditis), abscess formation, pneumonia, hepatitis, nephritis, and meningitis. Haverhill fever differs from rat bite fever by more severe vomiting and a high incidence of pharyngitis. Without adequate therapy, the illness may persist over a period of months, with the mortality rate being as high as 10%.

More commonly, the fever falls spontaneously after 3 to 5 days of illness, and full recovery occurs within 2 weeks.

S. moniliformis is recovered from blood, synovial fluid, and aspirates from abscesses. The specimens should be mixed with an equal volume of 2.5% sodium citrate to prevent clotting before the specimens can be examined microscopically. Fluid specimens should be concentrated by centrifugation, with 0.1 ml of the sediment inoculated onto heart infusion agar or into broth supplemented with 10% horse serum (or 15% rabbit blood or ascitic fluid) and 10% yeast extract. The sodium polyanetholesulfonate present in most blood culture broths is inhibitory to *S. moniliformis*. A portion of the sediment should also be examined microscopically by either Gram or Giemsa staining. Within 3 days, round, smooth, butyrous, gray colonies 1 to 2 mm in diameter will appear on serum agar incubated at 36°C in a humid atmosphere with 10% CO_2. Mycoplasma-like colonies with a characteristic fried egg appearance may appear with the colonies. Broth cultures should be examined after 2 to 3 days for the presence of downy, bread crumb-like, whitish granules ("puff balls"). They are observed mainly on the surfaces of the erythrocytes and at the bottom of the culture. Broth cultures with growth should be subcultured immediately to both solid and liquid media because *S. moniliformis* will die rapidly when the pH of the broth decreases.

S. moniliformis is relatively inert. Negative reactions are observed for catalase, oxidase, nitrate reduction, and indole production; arginine but not urea is hydrolyzed; and glucose and maltose are acidified weakly (Table 6). The phenotypic properties may be determined in cysteine tryptic agar base (41).

Penicillin G is the treatment of choice (21). Although penicillin is active against the bacillary forms, an aminoglycoside must be added to eliminate the L forms. Penicillin can also be combined with chloramphenicol or with erythromycin. Tetracyclines can be used to eliminate the L forms.

REFERENCES

1. **Adachi, R., O. Hammerberg, and H. Richardson.** 1983. Infective endocarditis caused by *Kingella kingae*. *Can. Med. Assoc. J.* **128:**1087–1089.
2. **Augthun, M., and G. Conrads.** 1997. Microbial findings of deep peri-implant bone defects. *Int. J. Oral Maxillofac. Implant.* **12:**106–112.
3. **Baranda, M. M., V. A. Arrieta, J. H. Almaraz, M. P. Rodriguez, M. A. Oraeta, and C. A. Errasti.** 1984. Two cases of *Capnocytophaga* bacteremia, one with endocarditis. *Can. Med. Assoc. J.* **130:**1420. (Letter.)
4. **Blum, R. N., C. D. Berry, M. G. Phillips, D. L. Hamlos, and E. W. Koneman.** 1992. Clinical illness associated with isolation of dysgonic fermenter 3 from stool samples. *J. Clin. Microbiol.* **30:**396–400.
5. **Brenner, D. J., D. G. Hollis, G. R. Fanning, and R. E. Weaver.** 1989. *Capnocytophaga canimorsus* sp. nov. (formerly CDC group DF-2), a cause of septicemia following dog bite, and *C. cynodegmi* sp. nov., a cause of localized wound infection following dog bite. *J. Clin. Microbiol.* **27:** 231–235.
6. **Bruun, B., J. Buch, E. Kirkegaard, and P. Bjaeldager.** 1983. Endocarditis caused by *Cardiobacterium hominis*. Two case reports. *Acta Pathol. Microbiol. Immunol. Scand. Sect. B* **91:**325–328.
7. **Buu-Hol, A. Y., S. Joundy, and J. F. Acar.** 1988. Endocarditis caused by *Capnocytophaga ochracea*. *J. Clin. Microbiol.* **26:**1061–1062.
8. **Chen, C.-K. C., G. J. Sunday, J. J. Zambon, and M. E. Wilson.** 1990. Outer membrane protein and lipopolysaccharide heterogeneity among *Eikenella corrodens* isolates. *J. Infect. Dis.* **162:**664–671.
9. **Chen, C.-K. C., T. V. Potts, and M. E. Wilson.** 1990. DNA homologies shared among *E. corrodens* isolates and other corroding bacilli from the oral cavity. *J. Periodontal Res.* **25:**106–112.
10. **Chinh, T. L.** 1983. *Kingella* (*Moraxella*) *kingae* infections. *Am. J. Dis. Child.* **137:**1212–1213.
11. **Christersson, L. A., and J. J. Zambon.** 1993. Suppression of subgingival *Actinobacillus actinomycetemcomitans* in localized juvenile periodontitis by systemic tetracycline. *J. Clin. Periodontol.* **20:**395–401.
12. **Cohen, P. S., J. H. Maguire, and L. Weinstein.** 1980. Infective endocarditis caused by gram-negative bacteria: a review of the literature, 1945–1977. *Prog. Cardiovasc. Dis.* **22:**205–242.
13. **Conrads, G., R. Mutters, I. Seyfarth, and K. Pelz.** 1998. DNA-probes for the differentiation of *Capnocytophaga* species. *Mol. Probes* **11:**323–328.
14. **Conrads, G., R. Mutters, J. Fischer, A. Brauner, R. Lütticken, and F. Lampert.** 1996. PCR reaction and dot-blot hybridization to monitor the distribution of oral pathogens within plaque sample of periodontally healthy individuals. *J. Periodontol.* **67:**994–1003.
15. **Decker, M. D., B. S. Graham, E. B. Hunter, and S. M. Liebowitz.** 1986. Endocarditis and infections of intravascular devices due to *Eikenella corrodens*. *Am. J. Med. Sci.* **292:** 209–212.
16. **Dewhirst, F. E., B. J. Paster, and P. L. Bright.** 1989. *Chromobacterium*, *Eikenella*, *Kingella*, *Neisseria*, *Simonsiella*, and *Vitreoscilla* species comprise a major branch of the beta group Proteobacteria by 16S ribosomal ribonucleic acid sequence comparison: transfer of *Eikenella* and *Simonsiella* to the family *Neisseriaceae* (emend.). *Int. J. Syst. Bacteriol.* **39:**258–266.
17. **Dewhirst, F. E., B. J. Paster, S. la Fontaine, and J. I. Rood.** 1990. Transfer of *Kingella indologenes* (Snell and Lapage 1976) to the genus *Suttonella* gen. nov. as *Suttonella indologenes* comb. nov.; transfer of *Bacteroides nodosus* (Beveridge 1941) to the genus *Dichelobacter* gen. nov. as *Dichelobacter nodosus* comb. nov.; and assignment of the genera *Cardiobacterium*, *Dichelobacter*, and *Suttonella* to *Cardiobacteriaceae* fam. nov. in the gamma division of *Proteobacteria* on the basis of 16S rRNA sequence comparisons. *Int. J. Syst. Bacteriol.* **40:**426–433.
18. **Dewhirst, F. E., C.-K. C. Chen, B. Paster, and J. J. Zambon.** 1993. Phylogeny of species in the family *Neisseriaceae* isolated from human dental plaque and description of *Kingella orale* sp. nov. *Int. J. Syst. Bacteriol.* **43:**490–499.
19. **Dewhirst, F. E., B. J. Paster, I. Olsen, and G. J. Fraser.** 1993. Phylogeny of the *Pasteurellaceae* determined by comparison of 16S ribosomal ribonucleic acid sequences. *Zentbl. Bakteriol. Parasitenkd. Infektionskr. Hyg. Abt. 1 Orig.* **279:**35–44.
20. **Eckert, F., A. Stenzel, R. Mutters, W. Frederiksen, and W. Mannheim.** 1991. Some unusual members of the family *Pasteurellaceae* isolated from human sources—phenotypic features and genomic relationships. *Zentralbl. Bakteriol. Parasitenkd. Infektionskr. Hyg. Abt. 1 Orig.* **275:**143–155.
21. **Edwards, R., and R. G. Finch.** 1986. Characterisation and antibiotic susceptibilities of *Streptobacillus moniliformis*. *J. Med. Microbiol.* **21:**39–42.
22. **Ehrbar, H.-U., J. Gubler, S. Harbarth, and B. Hirschel.** 1996. *Capnocytophaga canimorsus* sepsis complicated by myocardial infarction in two patients with normal coronary arteries. *Clin. Infect. Dis.* **23:**335–336.
23. **El Khizzi, N., S. A. Lasab, and A. O. Osoba.** 1997. HACEK group endocarditis at the Riyadh Armed Forces Hospital. *J. Infect.* **34:**69–74.

24. **Elster, A. D., A. B. Macone, and J. R. Kasser.** 1983. Osteomyelitis caused by *Capnocytophaga ochracea*. *J. Pediatr. Orthop.* **3:**613–615.
25. **Esteban, J., M. Albalate, C. Caramelo, A. Reyero, A. Carriazo, J. Hernandez, A. Ortiz, and F. Soriano.** 1995. Peritonitis involving a *Capnocytophaga* sp. in a patient undergoing continuous ambulatory peritoneal dialysis. *J. Clin. Microbiol.* **33:**2471–2472.
26. **Flemmig, T. F., S. Rüdiger, U. Hofmann, H. Schmidt, B. Plaschke, A. Strätz, B. Klaiber, and H. Karch.** 1995. Identification of *Actinobacillus actinomycetemcomitans* in subgingival plaque by PCR. *J. Clin. Microbiol.* **33:** 3102–3105.
27. **Flesher, S. A., and E. J. Bottone.** 1989. *Eikenella corrodens* cellulitis and arthritis of the knee. *J. Clin. Microbiol.* **27:** 2606–2608.
28. **Font, R., V. Jay, R. Misra, D. Jones, and K. Wilhelmus.** 1994. *Capnocytophaga* keratitis: a clinicopathologic study of three patients, including electron microscopic observations. *Ophthalmology* **101:**1929–1934.
29. **Frederiksen, W.** 1993. Ecology and significance of Pasteurellaceae in man—an update. *Zentralbl. Bakteriol. Parasitenkd. Infektionskr. Hyg. Abt. 1 Orig.* **279:**27–34.
30. **Georghiou, P. R., G. M. O'Kane, S. Siu, and R. J. Kemp.** 1989. Near-fatal septicemia with *Chromobacterium violaceum*. *Med. J. Aust.* **150:**720–721.
31. **Gomez-Garces, J., J. Alos, J. Sanchez, and R. Gogollos.** 1994. Bacteremia by multidrug-resistant *Capnocytophaga sputigena*. *Clin. Microbiol. Rev.* **32:**1067–1069.
32. **Göthe, E., R. Mutters, and W. Mannheim.** 1989. Deoxyribonucleic acid relatedness and phenotypic variation among human isolates of *Eikenella corrodens*. *Zentralbl. Bakteriol. Parasitenkd. Infektionskr. Hyg. Abt. 1 Orig.* **271:**61–69.
33. **Hawkey, P. M., S. D. Smith, J. Haynes, H. Malnick, and S. W. Forlenza.** 1987. In vitro susceptibility of *Capnocytophaga* species to antimicrobial agents. *Antimicrob. Agents Chemother.* **31:**331–332.
34. **Heiske, A., and R. Mutters.** 1996. Cytochemical subtypes of *Eikenella corrodens* demonstrated by cellular carbohydrate patterns. *Med. Microbiol. Lett.* **5:**204–215.
35. **Holmes, B., and M. S. Ahmed.** 1981. Group EF-4: a *Pasteurella*-like organism, p. 161–174. *In* M. Kilian, W. Frederiksen, and E. L. Biberstein (ed.), *Haemophilus, Pasteurella, and Actinobacillus*. Academic Press, London, United Kingdom.
36. **Holmes, B., M. J. Pickett, and D. G. Hollis.** 1995. Unusual gram-negative bacteria, including *Capnocytophaga, Eikenella, Pasteurella,* and *Streptobacillus*, p. 499–508. *In* P. R. Murray, E. J. Baron, M. A. Pfaller, F. C. Tenover, and R. H. Yolken (ed.) *Manual of Clinical Microbiology*, 6th ed. American Society for Microbiology, Washington, D.C.
37. **Jenny, D. B., P. W. Letendre, and G. Iverson.** 1987. Endocarditis caused by *Kingella indologenes*. *Rev. Infect. Dis.* **9:**787–789.
38. **Joshi, N., T. O'Bryan, and P. C. Apppelbaum.** 1991. Pleuropulmonary infections caused by *Eikenella corrodens*. *Rev. Infect. Dis.* **13:**1207–1212.
39. **Kentos, A., P. de Vuyst, M. J. Struelens, F. Jacobs, P. de Franquen, B. Delaere, P. Demaeyer, and J. P. Thys.** 1995. Lung abscess due to *Eikenella corrodens:* three cases and review. *Eur. J. Clin. Microbiol. Infect. Dis.* **14:** 146–148.
40. **Kwhaja, K. J., P. Parish, M. J. Aldred, and W. G. Wade.** 1990. Protein profiles of *Capnocytophaga* species. *J. Appl. Bacteriol.* **68:**385–390.
41. **Lambe, D. W. Jr., A. W. McPhedran, J. A. Mertz, and P. Stewart.** 1973. *Streptobacillus moniliformis* isolated from a case of Haverhill fever: biochemical characterization and inhibitory effect of sodium polyethanol sulfonate. *Am. J. Clin. Pathol.* **60:**854–860.
42. **Leadbetter, E. R., S. C. Holt, and S. S. Sokransky.** 1979. *Capnocytophaga*: new genus of gram-negative gliding bacteria. I. General characteristics, taxonomic considerations and significance. *Arch. Microbiol.* **122:**9–16.
43. **Møller, K., V. Fussing, P. A. D. Grimont, B. J. Paster, F. E. Dewhirst, and M. Kilian.** 1996. *Actinobacillus minor* sp. nov., *Actinobacillus porcinus* sp. nov., and *Actinobacillus indolicus* sp. nov., three new V factor-dependent species from the respiratory tract of pigs. *Int. J. Syst. Bacteriol.* **46:** 951–956.
44. **Mossad, S. B., A. E. Lichtin, G. S. Hall, and S. M. Gordon.** 1997. Diagnosis: *Capnocytophaga canimorsus* septicemia. *Clin. Infect. Dis.* **24:**123.
45. **Mueller, H. P., T. Eger, D. Lobinsky, S. Hoffmann, and L. Zoeller.** 1997. A longitudinal study of *Actinobacillus actinomycetemcomitans* in army recruits. *J. Periodontal Res.* **32**(1 Pt. 1):69–78.
46. **Müller, H. P., and L. Flores-de-Jacoby.** 1985. The composition of the subgingival microflora of young adults suffering from juvenile periodontitis. *J. Clin. Periodontol.* **12:** 113–123.
47. **Mutters, R., K. Piechulla, and W. Mannheim.** 1984. Phenotypic differentiation of *Pasteurella sensu stricto* and the *Actinobacillus* group. *Eur. J. Clin. Microbiol.* **3:**225–229.
48. **Mutters, R., K. Piechulla, K.-H. Hinz, and W. Mannheim.** 1985. *Pasteurella avium* (Hinz and Kunjara 1977) comb. nov. and *Pasteurella volantium* sp. nov. *Int. J. Syst. Bacteriol.* **35:**5–9.
49. **Mutters, R., W. Frederiksen, and W. Mannheim.** 1984. Lack of evidence for the occurrence of *Pasteurella ureae* in rodents. *Vet. Microbiol.* **9:**83–93.
50. **Noyan, U., S. Yilmaz, B. Kuru, T. Kadir, O. Acar, and E. Bueget.** 1997. A clinical and microbiological evaluation of systemic and local metronidazole delivery in adult periodontitis patients. *J. Clin. Periodontol.* **24:**158–165.
51. **Peel, M. M., K. A. Hornidge, M. Luppino, A. M. Stacpoole, and R. E. Weaver.** 1991. *Actinobacillus* spp. and related bacteria in infected wounds of humans bitten by horses and sheep. *J. Clin. Microbiol.* **29:**2535–2538.
52. **Pers, C., B. Gahrn-Hansen, and W. Frederiksen.** 1996. *Capnocytophaga canimorsus* septicemia in Denmark, 1982–1995: a review of 39 cases. *Clin. Infect. Dis.* **23:** 71–75.
53. **Piechulla, K., M. Bisgaard, H. Gerlach, and W. Mannheim.** 1985. Taxonomy of some recently described *Pasteurella/Actinobacillus*-like organisms as indicated by deoxyribonucleic acid relatedness. *Avian Pathol.* **14:** 281–311.
54. **Pohl, S.** 1981. Validation of new names and new combinations previously effectively published outside the IJSB. List no. 7. *Int. J. Syst. Bacteriol.* **31:**382–383.
55. **Pohl, S., H. U. Bertschinger, W. Frederiksen, and W. Mannheim.** 1983. Transfer of *Haemophilus pleuropneumoniae* and the *Pasteurella haemolytica*-like organism causing porcine necrotic pleuropneumonia to the genus *Actinobacillus* (*Actinobacillus pleuropneumoniae* comb. nov.) on the basis of phenotypic and deoxyribonucleic acid relatedness. *Int. J. Syst. Bacteriol.* **33:**510–514.
56. **Riggio, M. P., and A. Lennon.** 1997. Rapid identification of *Actinobacillus actinomycetemcomitans, Haemophilus aphrophilus,* and *Haemophilus paraphrophilus* by restriction enzyme analysis of PCR-amplified 16S rRNA genes. *J. Clin. Microbiol.* **35:**1630–1632.
57. **Robertson, P. B., M. Lantz, P. T. Marucha, K. S. Kornman, C. L. Trummel, and S. C. Holt.** 1982. Collagenolytic activity associated with *Bacteroides* species and *Actinobacillus actinomycetemcomitans*. *J. Periodontal Res.* **17:**275–283.

58. **Robinson, W. J. and A. S. Vitelli.** 1985. Infectious endocarditis caused by *Cardiobacterium hominis*. *South. Med. J.* **78:**1020–1021.
59. **Roscoe, D. L., S. J. V. Zemcov, D. Thornber, R. Wise, and A. M. Clarke.** 1992. Antimicrobial susceptibilities and β-lactamase characterization of *Capnocytophaga* species. *Antimicrob. Agents Chemother.* **36:**2197–2200.
60. **Rossau, R., G. Vandenbusche, S. Thielemans, P. Seegers, H. Grosch, E. Göthe, W. Mannheim, and J. De Ley.** 1989. Ribosomal ribonucleic acid similarities and deoxyribonucleic acid homologies of *Neisseria, Kingella, Eikenella, Simonsiella, Alysiella*, and Centers for Disease Control groups EF-4 and M-5 in the emended family *Neisseriaceae*. *Int. J. Syst. Bacteriol.* **39:**185–198.
61. **Rubsamen, P. E., W. M. McLeish, S. Pflugfelder, and D. Miller.** 1993. *Capnocytophaga* endophthalmitis. *Ophthalmology* **100:**456–459.
62. **Sakazaki, R., E. Yoshizaki, K. Tamura, and S. Kuramochi.** 1984. Increased frequency of isolation of *Pasteurella* and *Actinobacillus* species and related organisms. *Eur. J. Clin. Microbiol.* **3:**244–248.
63. **Savitt, E. D., M. N. Strzemko, K. K. Vaccaro, W. J. Peros, and C. K. French.** 1988. Comparison of cultural methods and DNA probe analysis for the detection of *Actinobacillus actinomycetemcomitans, Bacteroides gingivalis*, and *Bacteroides intermedius* in subgingival plaque samples. *J. Periodontol.* **59:**431–438.
64. **Seger, R., J. Kloeti, A. von Graevenitz, J. Wüst, J. Briner, U. Willi, and H. Siegrist.** 1982. Cervical abscess due to *Capnocytophaga ochracea*. *Pediatr. Infect. Dis.* **1:**170–172.
65. **Singh, N., K. Anderegg, and V. Yu.** 1993. Resistance of *Capnocytophaga* species to beta-lactam antibiotics. *Clin. Infect. Dis.* **17:**284–285.
66. **Slots, J., D. Feik, and T. E. Rams.** 1990. *Actinobacillus actinomycetemcomitans* and *Bacteroides intermedius* in human periodontitis. *J. Clin. Periodontol.* **17:**659–662.
67. **Sneath, P. H. A.** 1960. A study of the bacterial genus *Chromobacterium*. *Iowa St. J. Sci.* **34:**243–500.
68. **Soder, P. O., L. J. Jin, and B. Soder.** 1993. DNA probe detection of periodontopathogens in advanced periodontitis. *Scand. J. Dent. Res.* **101:**363–370.
69. **Sorensen, R. U., M. R. Jacobs, and S. B. Shurin.** 1985. *Chromobacterium violaceum* adenitis acquired in the northern United States as a complication of chronic granulomatous disease. *Pediatr. Infect. Dis.* **4:**701–702.
70. **Speck, H., R. M. Kroppenstedt, and W. Mannheim.** 1987. Genomic relationships and species differentiation in the genus *Capnocytophaga*. *Zentralbl. Bakteriol. Parasitenkd. Infektionskr. Hyg. Abt. 1 Orig. Reihe A* **266:**390–402.
71. **Stoloff, A. L., and M. L. Gillies.** 1986. Infections with *Eikenella corrodens* in a general hospital: a report of 33 cases. *Rev. Infect. Dis.* **8:**50–53.
72. **Sutton, R. G. A., M. F. O'Keeffe, M. A. Bundock, J. Jeboult, and M. P. Tester.** 1972. Isolation of a new *Moraxella* from corneal abscess. *J. Med. Microbiol.* **5:**148–150.
73. **Swann, R. A., and B. Holmes.** 1984. Infective endocarditis caused by *Kingella denitrificans*. *J. Clin. Pathol.* **37:** 1384–1387.
74. **Tinoco, E. M., M. I. Beldi, C. A. Loureiro, M. Lana, F. Camedelli, N. M. Tinoco, P. Gjermo, and H. R. Preus.** 1997. Localized juvenile periodontitis and *Actinobacillus actinomycetemcomitans* in a Brazilian population. *Eur. J. Oral Sci.* **105:**9–14.
75. **Van Bijsterveld, O. P.** 1970. New *Moraxella* strain isolated from angular conjunctivitis. *Appl. Microbiol.* **20:**405–408.
76. **Vandamme, P., M. Vancanneyt, A. van Belkum, P. Segers, W. G. V. Quint, K. Kersters, B. J. Paster, and F. E. Dewhirst.** 1996. Polyphasic analysis of strains of the genus *Capnocytophaga* and Centers for Disease Control group DF-3. *Int. J. Syst. Bacteriol.* **46:**782–791.
77. **Verhaegen, J., H. Verbraeken, A. Cabuy, J. Vandeven, and J. Vandepitte.** 1988. *Actinobacillus* (formerly *Pasteurella*) *ureae* meningitis and bacteraemia: report of a case and review of the literature. *J. Infect.* **17:**249–253.
78. **Weyant, R. S., C. W. Moss, R. E. Weaver, D. G. Hollis, J. J. Jordan, E. C. Cook, and M. I. Daneshvar.** 1996. *Identification of Unusual Pathogenic Gram-Negative Aerobic and Facultatively Anaerobic Bacteria*, 2nd ed. The Williams & Wilkins Co., Baltimore, Md.
79. **Williams, B. L., and B. F. Hammond.** 1979. *Capnocytophaga*: new genus of gram-negative gliding bacteria. IV. DNA base composition and sequence homology. *Arch. Microbiol.* **122:**29–33.
80. **Wilson, M. J., W. G. Wade, and A. J. Weightman.** 1995. Restriction fragment length polymorphism analysis of PCR-amplified 16S ribosomal DNA of human *Capnocytophaga*. *J. Appl. Bacteriol.* **78:**394–401.
81. **Windsor, H. M., R. C. Gromokova, and H. J. Koornhof.** 1991. Plasmid-mediated NAD independence in *Haemophilus parainfluenzae*. *J. Gen. Bacteriol.* **137:**2415–2421.
82. **Yamamoto, T., S. Kajiura, Y. Hirai, and T. Watanabe.** 1994. *Capnocytophaga haemolytica* sp. nov. and *Capnocytophaga granulosa* sp. nov., from human dental plaque. *Int. J. Syst. Bacteriol.* **44:**324–329.
83. **Zambon J. J., C. DeLuca, J. Slots, and R. J. Genco.** 1983. Studies of leukotoxin from *Actinobacillus actinomycetemcomitans* using the promyelotic HL-60 cell line. *Infect. Immun.* **40:**205–212.

Legionella

WASHINGTON C. WINN, JR.

37

The medical significance of the genus *Legionella* was first recognized after an epidemic of pneumonia among members of the Pennsylvania American Legion during the United States bicentennial celebration (1976) in Philadelphia (35, 81). In fact, members of the genus had been isolated by inoculation of guinea pigs and characterized as "rickettsia-like organisms" as long ago as 1943 (48, 80). A combination of epidemic disease, media attention, and the resultant marshalling of full scientific resources caused a rapid transformation of these bacterial curiosities into established pathogens.

TAXONOMY

In many respects, *Legionella* spp. and legionellosis are children of the technology age. Technology has facilitated many of the epidemics, by producing either the means for efficient transmission of bacteria or medical advances that reduce the resistance of patients to infection. Similarly, the taxonomy has been based from the outset on genetic analysis, tempered by recognition of phenotypic characteristics and practical considerations. The newly isolated bacterium from Philadelphia was unrelated to previously described pathogens. For that reason, a new family (*Legionellaceae*), a new genus (*Legionella*), and a new species (*pneumophila*) were established (12). This new family is a part of the gamma subgroup of the class *Proteobacteria* (37). Subsequently, a burgeoning number of additional species have been defined, primarily on the basis of genetic and serologic analysis (Table 1). Some of the newly recognized species have been isolated from both human and environmental sources; others have been isolated only from the environment to date. With increasingly sophisticated analysis becoming available, genetic diversity in a single serogroup (38) and phenotypic variation among genetically homogeneous strains (43, 44) have been recognized. Serological cross-reactions between genetically disparate species have also been described. The implications of this dichotomy between phenotypic and genotypic characteristics are exciting for epidemiologic studies and potentially significant for diagnostic microbiologists, but taxonomists have only begun to address the issue. Brenner and colleagues have suggested the creation within the species *Legionella pneumophila* of three subspecies, based on genomic relationship and with crossing of serological groups (11). Recently, the name "*L. lytica*" has been proposed for strains that have been isolated only from amoebae; these strains were previously designated "*Legionella*-like amoebal pathogens" or *Sarcobium lyticum* (8).

DESCRIPTION OF THE GENUS

The genus *Legionella* consists of thin, faintly staining gram-negative non-spore-forming bacilli (Fig. 1A) that generally measure 0.3 to 0.9 μm by 1.5 to 5 μm in clinical specimens but may become filamentous in culture. *Legionella* spp. require L-cysteine for growth on initial isolation from clinical and environmental sources, and growth is enhanced by inclusion of iron salts in the medium. The members of the genus are aerobic (stimulated by 5% CO_2), nonsaccharolytic, and relatively inert biochemically. Most species are weakly oxidase and catalase positive, gelatinase positive, and motile by means of one or more polar or subpolar flagella. The expression of flagella is inconstant, however, and may be temperature dependent (89). The fatty acid composition, isoprenoid quinone content, carbohydrate characterization, and peptide analysis of *Legionella* spp. can be used to identify individual isolates and to group related species if these tools are available in the laboratory (27, 34, 51, 64). *L. micdadei* is weakly acid fast in tissues and clinical specimens (Fig. 1B), but this characteristic is lost after isolation on agar media (86). The characteristics of the genus *Legionella* are summarized in Table 2.

NATURAL HABITATS

Legionella spp. are widespread in the environment and are associated almost exclusively with surface and potable waters or moist environments. The potable sources may be easily recognized as drinking facilities, such as taps and faucets, or less obvious distribution sites, such as showerheads and public fountains. A variety of *Legionella* spp., including *L. pneumophila*, *L. micdadei*, and, most prominently, *L. longbeachae* serogroup 1, have been isolated from potting soil stored at room temperature for 7 months but not from soils that had thoroughly dried out (101). Isolation of *L. micdadei* from water sources has been considerably more difficult to accomplish than isolation of *L. pneumophila*.

It is clear that environmental microbes are important for the survival and growth of legionellae in nature, because inclusion of the complex microbiota found in tap water is

TABLE 1 Selected characteristics of *Legionella* species[a]

Legionella sp.	Serogroup	Isolated from: Humans	Isolated from: Environment	Autofluorescence	Gelatin liquefaction	Motility, flagellum	Brown pigment	Hippurate hydrolysis	Major cellular fatty acids[d]
L. pneumophila[b] subsp. *pneumophila* subsp. *fraseri* subsp. *pascullei*	15	Yes	Yes	–	+	+	+[c]	+	15:0*a*, 16:0*i*, 16:1ω7*c*
L. micdadei[b]	1	Yes	Yes	–	–	+	–	–	15:0*a*, 16:1B, 16:0*i*, 17:0*a*
L. bozemanii	2	Yes	Yes	BW	+	+	+	–	15:0*a*, 16:0*i*, 16:0, 17:0*a*, 17:0cyc
L. dumoffii	1	Yes	Yes	BW	+	+	+[c]	–	15:0*a*, 16:0*i*, 17:0*a*, 17:0cyc
L. feeleii[b]	2	Yes	Yes	–	–	+	+[c]	±	15:0*a*, 16:1A*i*, 16:0*i*, 16:1ω7c, 16:0
L. gormanii	1	Yes	Yes	BW	+	+	+	–	15:0*a*, 16:0*i*, 16:1ω7*c*, 16:0, 17:0*a*, 17:0cyc
L. hackeliae	2	Yes	No	–	+	+	+	–	15:0*a*, 16:0*i*, 16:1ω7*c*, 17:0*a*
L. israelensis	1	Yes	Yes	–	+[c]	+	–	–	15:0*a*, 16:0*i*, 17:0*a*
L. jordanis	1	Yes	Yes	–	+	+	+	–	15:0*a*, 16:0*i*, 17:0*a*
L. sainthelensi	2	Yes	Yes	–	+	+	+[c]	–	15:0*a*, 16:0*i*, 16:1ω7*c*, 17:0*a*
L. longbeachae	2	Yes	Yes	–	+	+	+	–	15:0*a*, 16:0*i*, 16:1ω7*c*
L. maceachernii	1	Yes	Yes	–	+	+	+	–	15:0*a*, 16:0*i*, 16:1ω7*c*, 17:0*a*
L. oakridgensis	1	Yes	Yes	–	+	–	+	–	16:0*i*, 16:1ω7*c*, 16:0, 17:0cyc, 18:0*i*
L. wadsworthii	1	Yes	No	YG	+	+	–	–	15:0*a*, 16:0*i*, 17:0*a*
L. birminghamensis	1	Yes	No	YG	+	+	–	–	NA
L. cincinnatiensis	1	Yes	No	–	+	+	+	–	NA
L. anisa[b]	1	Yes	Yes	BW[c]	+	+	+	–	15:0*a*, 16:0*i*
L. tucsonensis	1	Yes	No	BW	+	+	–	–	NA
L. lansingensis	1	Yes	No	–	–	+	–	–	NA
L. cherrii	1	No	Yes	BW	+	+	+	–	15:0*a*, 16:0*i*, 17:0*a*
L. erythra	2	No	Yes	R (c)	+	+	+	–	15:0*a*, 16:0*i*, 16:1ω7*c*, 16:0, 17:0*a*
L. jamestownensis	1	No	Yes	–	+	+	+	–	15:0*a*, 16:0*i*, 17:0*a*
L. parisiensis	1	No	Yes	BW	+	+	+	–	15:0*a*, 16:0*i*, 17:0cyc
L. shakespearei	1	No	Yes	–	+	+	–	–	NA
L. santicrucis	1	No	Yes	–	+	+	+	–	15:0*a*, 16:0*i*, 16:1ω7*c*, 16:0

(Continued on next page)

TABLE 1 Selected characteristics of *Legionella* species[a] (*Continued*)

Legionella sp.	Serogroup	Isolated from: Humans	Isolated from: Environment	Autofluorescence	Gelatin liquefaction	Motility, flagellum	Brown pigment	Hippurate hydrolysis	Major cellular fatty acids[d]
L. steigerwaltii	1	No	Yes	BW	+	+	+	–	15:0*a*, 16:0*i*, 16:0, 17:0cyc
L. adelaidensis	1	No	Yes	–	+	+	–	–	NA
L. fairfieldensis	1	No	Yes	–	–	–	–	–	NA
L. brunensis	1	No	Yes	–	+	+	+[c]	–	NA
L. moravica	1	No	Yes	–	+	+	+[c]	–	NA
L. quinlivanii	2	No	Yes	–	±	+	+	–	NA
L. gratiana	1	No	Yes	–	+	+	–	–	NA
L. quateirensis	1	No	Yes	–	+	+	+	–	NA
L. nautarum	1	No	Yes	–	–	–	–	–	NA
L. worsleiensis	1	No	Yes	–	+	+	+	–	NA
L. londiniensis	1	No	Yes	–	+	–	+	±[c]	NA
L. geestiana	1	No	Yes	–	+	+	+[c]	+[c]	NA
L. rubrilucens	1	No	Yes	R[c]	+	+	+	–	15:0*a*, 16:0*i*, 16:1ω7*c*, 16:0
L. spiritensis	2	No	Yes	–	+	+	+	+[c]	15:0*a*, 16:0*i*, 16:1ω7*c*, 17:0*a*
L. waltersii	1	No	Yes	–	+	+	–	+	NA
"*L. lytica*" (amoebal pathogens)	1	No	Yes	NA	NA	NA	NA	NA	NA
Unnamed species and genomospecies	≥1	NA	NA	NA	NA	NA	NA	NA	NA

[a] Characteristics derived from multiple references. +, ≥90% positive; –, ≥90% negative; ±, most strains positive; V, variable; YG, yellow-green fluorescence; BW, blue-white fluorescence; R, red fluorescence; ND, not done; NA not available.
[b] Associated with outbreaks of Pontiac fever.
[c] Rare strains are negative or weakly positive only.
[d] From reference 64.

necessary for the growth of *L. pneumophila* in water suspensions in vitro (117). An increasing body of evidence suggests that environmental protozoa are the most important factor for the survival and growth of legionellae in nature (94). A variety of free-living amoebae and ciliated protozoa have been isolated along with *Legionella* spp. from environmental water sites suspected as sources of *Legionella* infection (5). *Legionella* spp. multiply intracellularly within the amoebae, much as they do within human monocytes and macrophages (5, 94). In fact, on occasion, environmental strains of *Legionella* spp. are successfully isolated on agar media only after cocultivation of water samples with amoebae (31) or preincubation of water samples that contain amoebae before subculture onto agar (98). Additionally, some nonculturable strains in environmental samples may be detected only by the use of amplification techniques, either directly (82) or after coincubation with amoebae (45). Wadowsky and colleagues demonstrated that the growth-promoting activity of

FIGURE 1 (A) Gram's stain of *L. pneumophila* serogroup 1 from scraping of formalin-fixed lung tissue. Numerous thin gram-negative bacilli of various lengths are clearly demonstrated. Intracellular bacteria are evident in polymorphonuclear neutrophils. The counterstain is safranin with 0.05% basic fuchsin. Although *Legionella* spp. are not usually demonstrated in sputum, they may be seen with Gram's stain if sufficient numbers are present. Magnification, ×2,500. (B) Acid-fastness of *L. micdadei* in tissue; Ziehl-Neelsen stain. The bacteria are not acid-fast when isolated on agar. Magnification, ×1,250. (C) Growth of *L. pneumophila* serogroup 1 on BCYEα agar with (left) and without (right) antibiotics. Heavy growth of this isolate from sputum was obtained on both plates. Colonies on the nonselective medium are small, presumably inhibited by the normal flora including yeasts. (D) *L. pneumophila* serogroup 1. The faceted, cut-glass appearance of the colonies under reflected light is evident with the use of a dissecting microscope. (E) *L. pneumophila* serogroup 1 on BCYEα agar. The "sticky" appearance of the colonies is evident. (F) Autofluorescence of some *Legionella* spp. The blue-white fluorescence of *L. bozemanii* under long-wavelength UV light is apparent. *L. pneumophila* and *L. micdadei* do not fluoresce. (G) Direct immunofluorescence of *L. pneumophila* serogroup 1. Fluorescein-isothiocyanate conjugate polyclonal antiserum was used. Magnification, ×400.

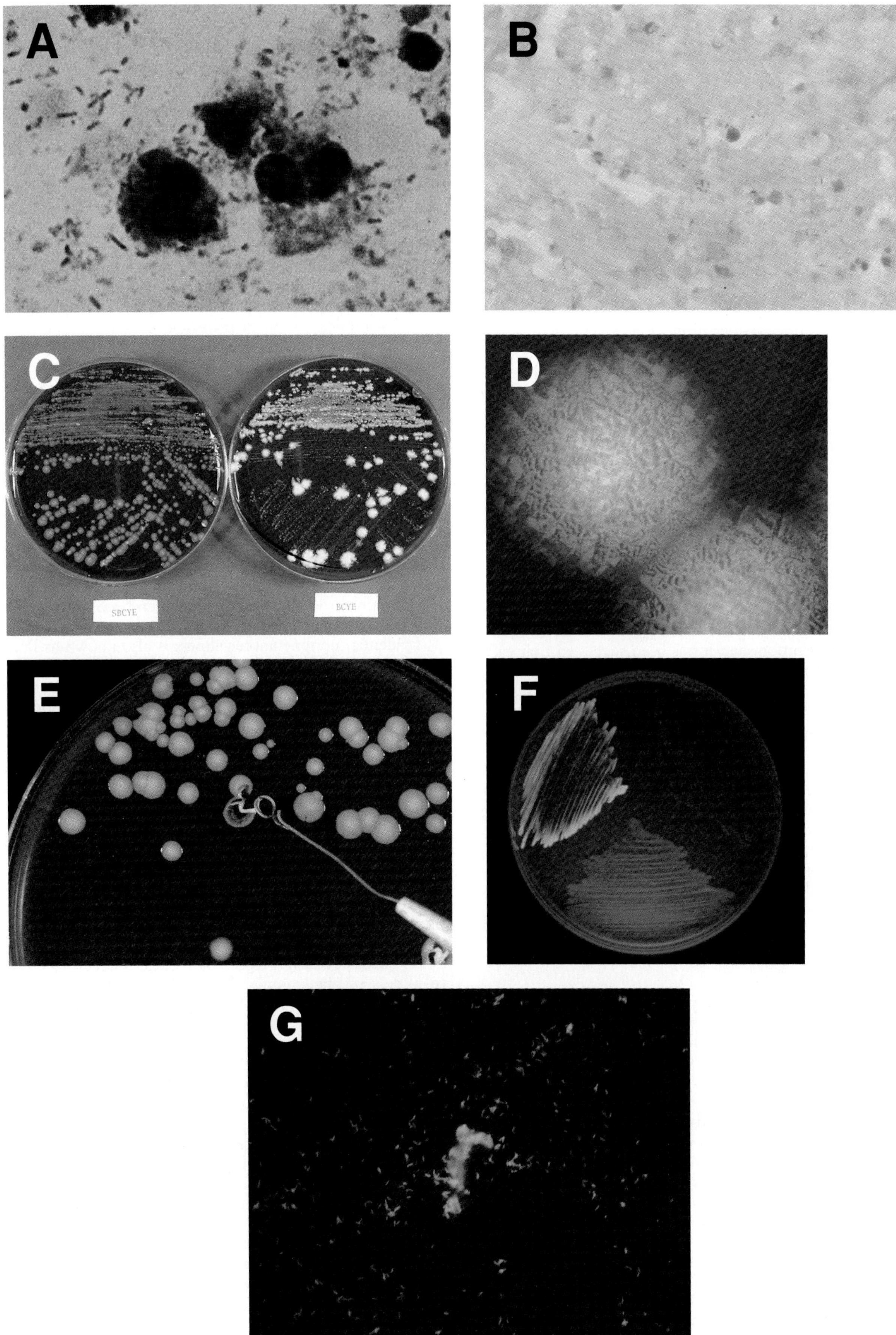
A
B
C
D
SBCYE
BCYE
E
F
G

TABLE 2 Characteristics of the genus *Legionella*

Faintly staining, thin, gram-negative, non-spore-forming bacilli
Requirement for L-cysteine on primary isolation
Mottled, cut-glass colonies on BCYEα agar under low magnification (dissecting microscope)
Growth stimulation by iron compounds
Utilization of amino acids for growth
Nonutilization of carbohydrates for growth
High concentrations of branched-chain fatty acids
Isoprenoid quinones (ubiquinones) with >10 isoprene units in side chain

tap water was eliminated by filtration through a 1 μm-pore-size membrane filter, a procedure that removed amoebae, but not heterotrophic bacteria from the system (110).

The environmental niches in which *Legionella* spp. are found may also have practical implications for attempts at eradication and control. *Legionella* spp. in tap water (62) and adherent to plumbing surfaces (116) may be more resistant to chlorine and other biocides than are *Legionella* spp. cultured in vitro.

Although *Legionella* spp. are widespread in the environment, colonization of natural and artificial water sources depends heavily on the local environment. In one study, the percentage of water samples positive for *Legionella* spp. over a 6-month period ranged from 0 to 72%; there were no institutional factors that could be associated with positive cultures (76). The same strain of *Legionella* tends to persist in a given institution, and it has been suggested that each water outlet serves as a microecologic unit (76). It is likely that one or more of the environmental cofactors discussed above is operative in the microenvironments. Colonization of peripheral water outlets in homes (1) and in hospitals (2) has been correlated with reduced hot-water temperature, which is presumably insufficient to kill the bacteria. Protection of legionellae within the intracellular milieu of free-living, environmental, heat-tolerant amoebae may be one of the reasons for the difficulty in eradicating *Legionella* spp. from potable and surface waters.

Animals may possess antibodies to *Legionella* spp., but there is no evidence that human infection results from contact with animals. Colonization of humans with *Legionella* spp. occurs rarely, if ever. Isolation of this genus from clinical specimens is usually associated with overt clinical disease.

CLINICAL SIGNIFICANCE

Legionella infections can be classified into four categories: (i) subclinical infection, (ii) nonpneumonic disease, (iii) pneumonia, and (iv) extrapulmonary inflammatory disease. The 1976 Philadelphia epidemic was referred to as Legionnaires' disease. A more general term is legionellosis or *Legionella* infection of a specific type, such as pneumonia. Cases in each category may occur as part of an epidemic, may occur sporadically or nosocomially, or may be community acquired. Nosocomial *Legionella* pneumonia and community-acquired pneumonia that require hospitalization have been estimated to represent 1 to 4% of all pneumonias in each category. Extrapolations from a recent study of sporadic *Legionella* pneumonia acquired in the community yield an estimate of 17,000 to 23,000 cases per year nationally (78). Failure to utilize available diagnostic tools may result in the mistaken impression that *Legionella* infections are not occurring in a hospital or a community (104). For *Legionella* infections in particular, national extrapolations are potentially misleading because of the critical importance of the local microenvironment. Even a demonstration that *Legionella* spp. contaminate natural or potable water systems does not predict the subsequent occurrence of human disease.

Although the number of species within the genus *Legionella* continues to increase, the vast majority of human infections are caused by *L. pneumophila*, particularly serogroups 1 and 6, or by *L. micdadei* (78, 92). Most of the clinical information therefore comes from experience with these two species. It is very likely, however, that any species is capable of causing serious human disease, particularly if the patient is sufficiently immunosuppressed. As judged by case reports, the epidemiology, clinical presentation, and pathology of infections caused by other *Legionella* spp. are similar to those caused by *L. pneumophila* and *L. micdadei.*

Subclinical infection can be inferred from the frequent occurrence worldwide of antibodies to *Legionella* spp. (up to 30%; commonly 5 to 10%) in the absence of recognized episodes of pneumonia (7, 88, 102). Although some surveys have documented higher titers in some groups with potentially higher risk than in the general population, there are no consistent correlations with potential occupational or recreational exposure. Even if a portion of the positive serological tests represent cross-reactions, the magnitude and reproducibility of the prevalence of antibodies cannot be dismissed. Although most subclinical infections occur in healthy hosts, the phenomenon has even been described in transplant patients (19, 50).

Epidemic, nonpneumonic illness is also known as Pontiac fever, named after the location of the first recognized episode. The infection is characterized by a very high attack rate (>95%) among those exposed, a short incubation period (hours to several days), a self-limited illness, and the absence of pulmonary infiltrates on chest radiographs. Prominent symptoms include fever, malaise, myalgias, and cough, a nonspecific flu-like syndrome. The initial episode was caused by *L. pneumophila* serogroup 1 (40). Subsequently, outbreaks have been attributed to *L. feeleii, L. anisa,* and *L. micdadei.* Nosocomial outbreaks of Pontiac fever have not been described. Pontiac fever is by definition an epidemic disease. Patients have contracted pneumonia and a nonpneumonic, Pontiac fever-like illness after exposure to the same environmental source (39). Sporadic cases of nonpneumonic illness, which are indistinguishable clinically from Pontiac fever, may represent a bridge between subclinical illness and pneumonia.

Pneumonia is the most frequent manifestation of *Legionella* infection. The onset is usually abrupt with high fever, malaise, myalgias, headache, and a nonproductive cough (32, 59). When sputum is produced, it often contains some polymorphonuclear neutrophils, but bacteria that are morphologically compatible with *Legionella* spp. are not usually demonstrated by Gram's stain. The inflammatory response in human lungs consists of macrophages, polymorphonuclear neutrophils, or, most commonly, a mixture of the two cell types (115). The intense inflammatory exudate results in necrotizing infection and macroscopically visible abscesses in approximately 20% of patients. It is ironic that this often intense cellular exudate in the airspaces is so poorly mobilized into expectorated sputum. For this reason, sputum sent for detection of *Legionella* should not undergo the standard screening (49) and rejection process based on squamous epithelial cells. Extrapulmonary manifestations, particularly confusion and diarrhea, are frequently prominent, but investigators have not been able to differentiate *Legionella* infection from other bacterial pneumonias in multiple prospective studies. The nonproductive cough suggests atypical pneumonia, to be differentiated especially from *Mycoplasma pneumoniae* and *Chlamydia pneumoniae* infections in outpatients. A rapid progression of pulmonary infiltrates and the frequent extension to other lobes and to the contralateral lung suggest infection with other gram-negative bacilli, particularly if colonizing enteric bacilli contaminate sputum specimens. Failure of the pneumonia to respond to therapy with expanded-spectrum cephalosporins and aminoglycosides suggests that *Legionella* should be included in the differential diagnosis of severe pneumonia, including nosocomial infections. Abscesses are commonly documented pathologically in fatal cases (115) and are recognized radiographically in a small minority of patients (30). Convalescence is often prolonged, and radiographic resolution may be protracted. Chronic residua with scarring have been described in rare cases (16).

Dissemination of bacteria through the bloodstream occurs frequently in severe *Legionella* pneumonia. In a prospective study of *Legionella* infection, 6 (38%) of 16 patients with culture-proved infection had positive blood cultures (93). The frequency of bacteremia in mild disease is unclear. Occasionally, a secondary focus of metastatic infection will occur after direct extension from the infected lung or after bacteremic spread. Pleural empyema, pericarditis, myocarditis, endocarditis, pancreatitis, pyelonephritis, peritonitis, cellulitis, hepatic abscess, abscesses related to the gastrointestinal tract, and infections of intravascular prosthetic devices have been described (70, 114). The list can be expected to expand as clinical experience grows, but it is important to document the microbial etiology of unusual occurrences rigorously. In addition, noninfectious complications, including skin rashes, encephalitis, arthritis, acute renal failure, and myoglobinuria, have been associated with *Legionella* infection.

Although most extrapulmonary lesions develop concurrently with or shortly after the episode of pneumonia, occasional infections have been described in the absence of obvious pulmonary infection (70). Most dramatically, an outbreak of primary sternal wound infections was traced to direct introduction of bacteria into the wounds during bathing (69).

Legionella infections are a result of interactions among the traditional triad of factors: bacterium, environment, and human host. Cell-mediated immunity plays a critical role in *Legionella* infections, as might be expected for a facultative intracellular pathogen. The role of humoral immunity is not clear. Activation of monocyte/macrophages is the critical operational step, and polymorphonuclear neutrophils may also be important for limiting bacterial growth. The preponderance of certain species and serotypes in human infection suggests the presence of virulence factors, which have not yet been clearly defined.

Although *Legionella* spp. may cause serious disease in apparently healthy individuals, severe infection and death occur most commonly in patients with diminished host defenses. The most commonly documented risk factors have been cigarette smoking and chronic obstructive lung disease, chronic cardiovascular disease, renal failure, and immunosuppression caused by underlying disease or by therapy (28, 78). Transplantation of organs and therapy with high doses of steroids have been implicated as risk factors with particular frequency. More recently, infection with human immunodeficiency virus has been recognized as an additional risk factor (9, 78). Neutropenia has been notably absent from the list of prominent risk factors.

The link between virulent bacteria in the environment and an immunosuppressed patient is often difficult to establish. The best-documented route for transmission of infection is the generation of an infective aerosol from a *Legionella*-contaminated water source. The most direct documentation of cooling-tower water as a source of infectious aerosol occurred when two maintenance workers entered an operating cooling tower to do repairs (39). Although questioned by some authorities (83), the epidemiologic evidence is convincing that water drift from evaporative condensers and cooling towers is responsible for epidemics of *Legionella* infection. Other open-water sources that have been implicated as sources of infectious aerosols include whirlpool spas and public water fountains.

Most sporadic *Legionella* infections and some epidemics are caused by contaminated potable water that has been aerosolized by vehicles such as humidifiers, nebulizers, misters, and showerheads. This association has been documented for infections acquired in the home as well as in the hospital (105). In addition to inhalation of aerosols, aspiration of contaminated potable water is a probable mechanism for infection of the lower respiratory tract (109). Entry through the gastrointestinal tract has been suggested to explain abdominal infections, although this portal of entry has not been proved. As described above, direct entry of bacteria into a fresh wound may cause nosocomial *Legionella* infection (69, 70).

The only recognized source of *Legionella* infection is colonized water, especially when aerosols are produced. There has been no evidence of human-to-human transmission or of documented laboratory infections. The usual laboratory safety precautions are adequate for *Legionella* spp. unless a procedure is likely to produce significant aerosols.

COLLECTION, TRANSPORT, AND STORAGE OF SPECIMENS

Specimens should be obtained from the site of infection, (see chapter 4) if localized disease is present. Lower respiratory tract secretions should be collected by usual methods and submitted to the laboratory as soon as possible. There are no data to suggest the appropriate number or timing of sputum specimens. If clinical suspicion is high, several sputum samples should be submitted, because small numbers of organisms may be present. Careful induction of sputum by nebulization has the potential for increasing the yield from expectorated sputum, but there are no clinical trials on the subject. Although suspensions of NaCl reduce the recovery of *Legionella* spp., there is little alternative to procedures such as bronchoscopy or sputum induction, which require the use of nebulized saline. Delayed specimens should not be rejected, because *Legionella* has been recovered after storage of specimens for several days at room temperature. Microscopic screening protocols, commonly used when bacterial pneumonia is suspected, should not be used for selecting samples to be cultured, because the cellular composition of sputum does not predict the recovery of *L. pneumophila* (49). If the presence of urinary antigen is to be tested for, a clean-catch sample should be obtained.

Blood cultures should be collected from seriously ill, hospitalized patients with documented pneumonia, because a positive culture is definitive evidence of infection. Dissemination of bacteria through the bloodstream is common in very ill, often terminally ill patients, as judged by positive blood cultures (93) and by demonstration of legionellae in peripheral organs (29). Among the major blood culture systems, only the BACTEC instrument has been evaluated in a prospective study (93). *L. pneumophila* has been isolated from both aerobic and anaerobic bottles, but blind subculture onto buffered charcoal yeast extract agar supplemented with α-ketoglutarate (BCYEα) medium is required (93). Lysis-centrifugation has been used to isolate *L. pneumophila* from seeded blood (18), but clinical experience has been limited (107a). If lysis-centrifugation is used in the laboratory for other purposes, it is convenient to adapt the method for recovery of *Legionella*. The laboratory should be notified that *Legionella* spp. are suspected, because special handling is required. There is often a considerable delay before the diagnosis of Legionnaires' disease is considered, well after routine blood cultures have been collected. In this situation, diagnosis may be expedited by staining fluid from conventional bottles with acridine orange and/or subculturing an aliquot onto BCYE α agar.

Serum for antibody studies should be collected as soon as possible. A convalescent-phase specimen should be obtained at least 6 weeks after the onset of infection. When infection is undifferentiated, as in Pontiac fever, documentation of the etiology must depend on serological studies and detection of urinary antigen (36).

Environmental water samples should be taken from all potential sources in clean screw-cap containers. For documentation of low levels of *Legionella* colonization, volumes of at least 1 liter should be collected. Sampling of potable-water systems should include sediment from hot-water tanks and swab samples of faucets and showerheads. If the water has recently been chlorinated, 0.5 ml of 0.1 N sodium thiosulfate should be added to each liter of water (15). Faucets and showers should be sampled with a wooden shaft swab after removal of the aerator or showerhead. The swab is then placed in 3 to 5 ml of water from the same fixture. Careful epidemiologic investigation is essential in documenting the significance of any colonized environmental sites.

DIRECT DETECTION

Investigators have attempted to develop procedures for early diagnosis by detection of antigens or nucleic acids in clinical specimens (Table 3). The initial approach, direct immunofluorescence of respiratory secretions, has a reported sensitivity of 25 to 70% for *L. pneumophila* serogroup 1(14, 24). The specificity of the test is greater than 95%. False-positive results occur both because of cross-reactions with other bacteria and because of contamination with environmental *Legionella* spp. A monoclonal fluorescein-conjugated antibody to a species-specific outer membrane protein antigen of *L. pneumophila* produces cleaner staining and fewer cross-reactions (106). In areas of low disease prevalence, the positive predictive value of direct immunofluorescence is unacceptably low. The combination of low sensitivity and false-positive tests in a low-prevalence environment indicates that this test should not be performed in most clinical situations.

Detection of *Legionella* antigen in urine and other body fluids has also been used successfully to diagnose *Legionella* infections expeditiously by radioimmunoassay, enzyme immunoassay, or latex agglutination (99). An enzyme immunoassay for serogroup 1 *L. pneumophila* antigen that has a sensitivity of 70% or greater and a very high specificity is commercially available (Binax, Portland, Maine) (56, 91). Cross-reactions have been demonstrated between urinary antigens of several *L. pneumophila* serogroups (60). Antigen may be excreted for months; therefore, a positive urinary assay does not equate precisely with acute infection (61).

L. pneumophila nucleic acid has been successfully detected in clinical specimens by using various "home brew" reagents and a commercially available amplification assay, which has, however, been approved only for environmental samples (52, 55, 58, 68, 79). The sensitivity of the amplification methods has been equivalent or superior to that of culture techniques, but clinical experience is limited. Inhibitors of amplification have been documented when legionellae are suspended in homogenized lung tissue (100). Positive amplification tests have been recorded in patients without other laboratory evidence of Legionnaires' disease; some of these appeared to be false-positive reactions (52, 73). It is not clear whether the discrepancies represent greater sensitivity of the amplification system, specificity or contamination problems with the molecular techniques, the presence of noncultivable legionellae (as has been suggested for environmental specimens [45]) or a combination of these factors.

ISOLATION

The classic triad of diagnostic approaches is available for the diagnosis of *Legionella* infections; isolation of the bacter-

TABLE 3 Diagnostic tests for *Legionella* infection

Test	Commercially available	Specimen type	Sensitivity (%)	Specificity (%)	Comments
Culture	Yes	Lower respiratory tract, wound, blood, tissue	70	100	Preferred method; detects all species and serogroups
Direct immunofluorescence	Yes	Lower respiratory tract, wound, tissue	25–70	>95	Not recommended for routine use; reagents for limited species and serogroups available
Radioimmunoassay	No	Urine	70–90	>99	*L. pneumophila* serogroup 1 only
Enzyme immunoassay (EIA)	Yes	Urine	70–90	>99	*L. pneumophila* serogroup 1 only
Latex agglutination	Yes	Urine	55–90	85–99	*L. pneumophila* serogroup 1 only; commercial products perform at low end
Serology (indirect immunofluorescence)	Yes	Serum	70–80	>95	Reagents available for limited species and serogroups; ancillary to culture

ium in culture, direct detection of bacterial antigens or nucleic acids in clinical specimens, and documentation of a serological response to the bacterium. The overwhelmingly preferred diagnostic method is culture (120). The sensitivity of culture is comparable to that of other methods, and the specificity is 100%, a significant advantage when the prevalence of disease in the test population is low. The widespread distribution of *Legionella* spp. in water systems even produced a false-positive culture result when a postmortem sample was apparently contaminated with water from the autopsy room (67). Although the results of culture are not available immediately, most isolates are recovered within 72 h, a clinically relevant time frame for assessment of therapy and clinical response.

The standard for isolation of *Legionella* spp. from clinical specimens is BCYEα agar, a medium that was developed from the pioneering efforts of the late James Feeley (33) (see chapter 130). Yeast extract is included as a rich source of nutrients; L-cysteine, iron compounds, and α-ketoglutarate are added to stimulate growth. Activated charcoal serves as a scavenger of a variety of toxic compounds, such as superoxide radicals and peroxides, that are produced in the medium, especially after exposure to light. Other methods that have been used to minimize the effects of inhibitory substances include washing the yeast extract agar and adding albumin, either as a substitute for charcoal or as a second protective measure. ACES [*N*-(2-acetamido)-2-aminoethanesulfonic acid] buffer, incorporated in BCYEα agar, provides an optimal pH for *Legionella* growth without causing inhibitory effects. Although BCYEα agar is the standard, it is worth noting that *L. pneumophila* has been isolated on commercially prepared chocolate agar.

When specimens from nonsterile sources are cultured, selective media or treatments should be used to inhibit other bacteria (Fig. 1C). The most commonly used selective medium consists of BCYEα agar supplemented with polymyxin B, anisomycin, and either cefamandole or vancomycin. It is essential that a noninhibitory medium be inoculated also, because some strains, particularly of species other than *L. pneumophila*, are inhibited by the antibiotics, with the cephalosporin mixtures being more inhibitory than those containing vancomycin (66). Brief treatment of sputum specimens with heat (26) or with acid (14) may enhance the recovery of *Legionella* spp. from clinical specimens, but the techniques have not been widely used. A 10% solution of sputum is made in 0.2 M HCl-KCl (pH 2.2), after which the mixture is vortexed until it is homogeneous. Aliquots are plated onto agar after a total contact time of 5 min. Alternatively, the sputum is heated to 60°C for 2 min. Pretreatment of water specimens is essential for the recovery of legionellae from the mixture of diverse environmental microorganisms. Selective media are efficient at suppressing the indigenous upper respiratory flora in outpatients, so the additional pretreatment is most likely to be efficacious in patients who are colonized with nosocomial bacteria, such as *Pseudomonas* spp., that are resistant to the antibiotics incorporated into the selective agars. Acid treatment provided little additional yield from specimens that originated in the lower respiratory tract, such as those in bronchoalveolar lavage fluids (14). Treatment of seeded water specimens with acid reduced the quantity of *L. pneumophila* recovered by approximately 30% (10). In some clinical studies, heat treatment of sputum reduced the number of isolates (84). Heat or acid treatment also imposes a workload burden on the laboratory; therefore, the decision to use these techniques must be made in each laboratory. They cannot substitute for using both nonselective and selective agar media.

When environmental samples are cultured, it is useful to add glycine to the basic BCYEα medium in addition to the vancomycin-polymyxin B-anisomycin mixture (15). With the addition of bromothymol blue and bromocresol purple for differential coloration of some *Legionella* spp., the agar becomes modified Wadowsky-Yee medium (see chapter 130). Acidification of the sample for 15 min at pH 2.0 to 2.2 by addition of acid buffer (0.2 M HCl, 0.2 M KCl) followed by neutralization to pH 7.0 with 0.1 N KOH is also useful for environmental samples. Potable-water specimens should be concentrated by filtration through a 0.22-μm-pore-size filter (15). Boulanger and Edelstein reported that filtration was superior to centrifugation at 8,150 $\times$ *g* for 15 min for the recovery of seeded legionellae in water samples. Flat polycarbonate filters (Nucleopore type) were more efficient than cast filters (Millipore type) (10). After concentration, the sediment is resuspended or the filters are vortexed in 10 to 20 ml of the original water. Swab specimens are expressed into their water suspending medium before inoculation.

Preincubation of water samples at 35°C may increase the yield from lightly contaminated samples, putatively by allowing the multiplication of bacteria within environmental amoebae (98). The relationship between *Legionella* spp. and free-living amoebae has been exploited for the diagnosis of both human infection and environmental colonization. Isolation of *Legionella*-like bacteria from sputum specimens and of *L. micdadei* from water samples only after incubation of the samples with amoebae has been reported (31, 95). These enrichment techniques may be appropriate for use by specialized reference laboratories. Procedures for processing water samples are available from several sources (13, 15).

Commercially available media are of variable quality (57, 66), but several manufacturers have maintained the production of high-quality media. If the media are made in-house, it is important to be aware of variable performance of the agar bases (21). Cost-effective alternatives for the buffering agent are described elsewhere (23). Quality control should be performed with bacterial strains that have been passaged minimally on agar. Laboratory-adapted strains, including some available from the American Type Culture Collection, will grow well on some media that do not support the growth of fresh clinical isolates (57). If commercial quality control data are used, documentation of the procedures can be requested.

Inoculated plates should be streaked for isolation, incubated for a minimum of 5 days in a humid atmosphere, and observed daily for growth. CO_2 at 2 to 5% may stimulate the growth of some species, but higher concentrations of CO_2 may be inhibitory. Young colonies can be detected perhaps 12 to 24 h earlier if a dissecting microscope is used for examination.

IDENTIFICATION

Colonies of BCYEα or selective BCYEα agar should be selected for Gram staining if they are not represented on other enriched medium, such as sheep blood agar or chocolate agar, or if they have a characteristic macroscopic appearance. Viewed through a dissecting microscope (Fig. 1D), the colonies have a "mottled" surface, an iridescent red-blue-green sheen, or a faceted "cut-glass" appearance. Although the colonies themselves are round and entire, the play of light on the surface produces an appearance of irregularity or complex internal structure. As colony growth continues, the iridescence can be appreciated with the naked eye, particularly where growth is confluent. Another clue is the sticky consistency that colonies of *L. pneumophila* often have when manipulated with a bacteriologic loop (Fig. 1E).

Legionella spp. stain very poorly with the usual safranin counterstain. The staining time for the safranin counterstain should be prolonged. Alternatively, 0.05% basic fuchsin can be used alone or added to the safranin stain to increase the intensity of the staining. If a Gram stain of the suspect colonies reveals thin, pale-staining gram-negative bacilli, the colonies should be subcultured for demonstration of cysteine dependence. The most rigorous test of dependence is to subculture the isolate to two agar media that differ only in the presence of l-cysteine (see chapter 130). For laboratories in which *Legionella* spp. are infrequently isolated, it may be inconvenient and costly to stock the additional cysteine-deficient media. An acceptable alternative is subculture of the isolate onto BCYEα agar and sheep blood agar in parallel. Microbiologic judgment must be used, because dichotomous growth on blood agar and BCYEα agar could result from differences in nutrient composition. Similarly, bacteria other than *Legionella* spp., including thermophilic spore-forming bacilli (107), *Francisella tularensis* (96), and *Bordetella pertussis* (87), are dependent on L-cysteine for growth or on charcoal for removal of inhibitory substances. In the case of *Bordetella* and *Francisella*, the problem is complicated by similar morphology in Gram stains, cross-reactions with some *Legionella* antisera (6, 87, 96), and potential clinical presentation as lower respiratory tract infection. Careful analysis of colony morphology may suggest the correct identification, which can be confirmed by application of appropriate serological or genetic analysis.

Biochemical tests are of little use in the differentiation of *Legionella* spp. from other genera or in the differentiation of species within the genus. The genus is asaccharolytic, and other reactions are weak, variable, or temperature dependent. The accompanying table of reactions, used judiciously and with caution, may provide confirmatory information (Table 1). The hippurate hydrolysis test is useful for biochemical confirmation of the most common pathogenic species, *L. pneumophila* (47); however, the diagnostic utility of this test has been diminished by the variability of more recently isolated species. Although autofluorescence of colonies under long-wavelength UV light (Wood's lamp) distinguishes certain *Legionella* spp. (Fig. 1F), the infrequency of occurrence of the fluorescent species in human disease compromises the clinical utility of the test. Browning of tyrosine-containing media is more variable, and rare isolates of *L. pneumophila* do not produce the expected result. Catalase and oxidase reactions and bacterial motility may be weak and difficult to detect.

For practical purposes, serological typing of putative *Legionella* isolates is the simplest approach and is sufficient for characterization of most isolates in clinical laboratories. The power of serological analysis has been eroded by cross-reactions among *Legionella* species and serogroups and between *Legionella* spp. and other genera; these cross-reactions are being reported with increasing frequency. The positive predictive value is probably acceptably high if the isolate is identified as a commonly isolated pathogen, such as *L. pneumophila* serogroup 1 or 6, *L. micdadei*, or *L. dumoffii*, and if other microbiologic criteria for *Legionella* spp. are fulfilled.

Although agglutinating antisera are commercially available, the most common procedure has been direct immunofluorescence with polyclonal or monoclonal antibodies (Fig. 1G). Commercially available polyclonal antibodies (Meridian Diagnostics, Cincinnati, Ohio) are directed at serogroup-specific antigens, probably lipopolysaccharide, and must be used for serotyping (22). Bacterial suspensions should be sparse to minimize quenching of fluorescence by the antigenic mass, which may produce a weakly positive reaction. The polyclonal reagents cross-react with some environmental organisms and human pathogens, in particular *Pseudomonas fluorescens*, *P. aeruginosa*, *Bacteroides fragilis*, *F. tularensis*, *Capnocytophaga* sp., and *Bordetella pertussis* (see also Serological Tests below). A monoclonal fluoresceinated antiserum against a species-specific outer membrane protein antigen of *L. pneumophila* (Genetic Systems, Redmond, Wash.) produces a cleaner background and does not cross-react with the common non-*Legionella* pathogens (20, 106).

Definitive identification of isolates requires genetic analysis by techniques that are beyond the reach of most clinical laboratories. Characterization of fatty acid, isoprenoid quinone, carbohydrate, and peptide composition have also been used to identify *Legionella* spp. (27, 34, 51, 64), but these techniques are also restricted to highly specialized laboratories. Isolates should be sent to a reference laboratory for definitive identification if (i) serological analysis indicates an infrequently isolated species or serotype, (ii) phenotypic characteristics suggest *Legionella* sp. but available antisera do not react with the isolate, (iii) the isolate reacts with antisera to more than one serogroup or species, and/or (iv) the phenotypic characteristics are atypical.

SEROLOGICAL TESTS

Serological tests are useful for epidemiologic studies of prevalence and for diagnosis of suspected cases in which the patient does not have pneumonia or is not able to produce adequate lower respiratory secretions. Such tests are an adjunct to microbiologic diagnosis and should not be used as a substitute for it. The disadvantages of serological tests are that the diagnosis is usually retrospective and that cross-reactions among *Legionella* spp. and with other bacteria make the result presumptive.

A variety of methods, including microagglutination, enzyme immunoassay, and counterimmunoelectrophoresis, have been developed to measure the serological response. The most frequently used test is indirect immunofluorescence, which is commercially available from a variety of sources and has been extensively evaluated (24, 113, 119). The immunologic response includes antibodies of the immunoglobulin G (IgG), IgM, and, to a lesser extent, IgA classes (113). It is important to use an antiglobulin reagent that detects all classes. IgM antibody can be measured to provide an early provisional serological diagnosis with a single serum specimen. However, this antibody class can persist for many months in some patients (119).

The sensitivity of serological diagnosis is approximately 80% (24, 112). Seroconversion occurs in most patients within 3 weeks, but patients should be monitored for at least 6 weeks. At least 15% of patients seroconvert later than 6 weeks (24). The most common criterion for seroconversion is an increase in the antibody titer of at least fourfold to 1: 128 (113). A single titer cannot be used to diagnose individual infections and is only presumptive in studies of epidemic disease (91).

The specificity of serological diagnosis has been estimated to be 96 to 99% (112, 113). In areas where there is a moderate incidence of infection, demonstration of seroconversion results in an acceptable predictive value for *Legionella* infection. Where disease is rare (1% of patients tested or less), the predictive value is considerably lower, resulting in a more presumptive diagnosis. Serological cross-reactions have been demonstrated with *P. aeruginosa*, *P. fluorescens*, *Burkholderia pseudomallei*, *P. alcaligenes*, *Stenotrophomonas* spp., *Flavobacterium* spp., *Bacillus cereus* spores, *Bacteroides fragilis*, *Bordetella pertussis*, *F. tularensis*, *Campylobacter jejuni*, and members of the *Enterobacteriaceae* such as *Citrobacter freundii*. Heat-killed and formalin-inactivated bacteria have been most frequently used in indirect immunofluorescence tests, with the former producing higher titers (111). The immunologic response is directed against lipopolysaccharide and protein antigens. The genus-specific 60-kDa protein antigen, for instance, has epitopes that are shared with 39 non-*Legionella* bacterial species (90). Some patients respond with antibodies that react with a single serogroup; others develop a more diverse response (113). To detect the spectrum of *Legionella* infections, therefore, it is important to test multiple antigens, but the precise identity of the infecting species cannot be determined with certainty. Absorption of patient sera with cross-reacting antigens provides greater specificity but makes the assay more complicated and decreases sensitivity (90, 112).

ANTIMICROBIAL SUSCEPTIBILITIES

In vitro antimicrobial susceptibility results do not correlate well with the clinical response; therefore, routine testing is not appropriate. It has been suggested that the intracellular location of legionellae in phagocytes is responsible for the dichotomy. In addition, some antibiotics are bound by the activated charcoal in media that are typically used for susceptibility testing of *Legionella* spp. The standard therapy for *Legionella* infection is erythromycin, although no prospective, randomized clinical trials have ever been performed. Increased mortality has been correlated with increasing delay in the initiation of erythromycin chemotherapy (46). Rifampin is often added to treat severe, life-threatening disease. Natural resistance to these antibiotics has not yet occurred. Trimethoprim-sulfamethoxazole, several quinolone antibiotics, and new macrolides such as clarithromycin and azithromycin have been used successfully, but clinical experience is limited. Failures of quinolone therapy have been recorded (63, 97).

EVALUATION, INTERPRETATION, AND REPORTING OF RESULTS

Respiratory secretions or other clinically indicated sites should be cultured. Urine should be tested for *L. pneumophila* serogroup 1 antigen if feasible. Blood cultures should be collected from hospitalized patients for *Legionella* culture. Positive results should be called to the caregiver and to the epidemiologist. An acute-phase serum sample for serological analysis should be collected and stored; if a specific diagnosis is not made during the acute infection, convalescent-phase sera should be obtained 3 weeks later and again at 6 weeks if seroconversion has not occurred. An increase in antibody titer of at least fourfold to 1:128 or greater is presumptive evidence of acute infection.

The clinical microbiologist may also be called upon to participate in investigations of epidemic disease and in decisions about control of *Legionella* infection. A variety of molecular techniques are now available for characterizing isolated strains and matching isolates from clinical and environmental sources (4). In addition to monoclonal antibody typing (41, 103, 108), investigators have used plasmid analysis (41, 103), multilocus alloenzyme electrophoresis (25, 71, 75, 108), restriction enzyme digestion with conventional agarose electrophoresis (108), macrorestriction analysis of genomic DNA with pulsed-field gel electrophoresis (53, 72), restriction fragment length polymorphism of rRNA genes (ribotyping) (3, 41), and arbitrarily primed PCR (41, 42, 65). All the approaches have successfully characterized environmental and clinical isolates from single-patient exposures or epidemics. Plasmid analysis has the disadvantage that it cannot be used for strains that lack a plasmid. Multiple approaches may be necessary to provide the most reliable characterization of isolates (74); it is no longer adequate to employ serological characterization alone.

It is potentially possible, although not easy, to prevent *Legionella* infections by controlling exposure to bacteria in the aquatic environment. There are several schools of thought on the proper approach to monitoring for the presence of *Legionella* spp. and *Legionella* infections (17, 54, 118). It is clear that attention should be concentrated on the individuals at highest risk, particularly immunosuppressed patients in hospitals. In addition, commonsense measures should be instituted. Only sterile water should be used in situations in which aerosols will be generated or when direct contact with sick patients will ensue. Attention should be paid to the proximity of air intake vents to potential generators of aerosols. Environmental- and potable-water systems should be maintained according to established protocols and manufacturer instructions.

Monitoring of clinical disease can be focused most efficiently on high-risk patients by using culture of respiratory secretions (77). Microbiologic characterization of fatal cases of pneumonia from the autopsy room represents another approach to the surveillance of *Legionella* infection. Routine microbiologic surveillance of the environment in the absence of documented human infection is controversial. Once clinical infection has been documented, several methods of environmental control are available (85). Each has advantages and drawbacks, and none is permanent; therefore, continued environmental surveillance is required.

REFERENCES

1. **Alary, M., and J. R. Joly.** 1991. Risk factors for contamination of domestic hot water systems by legionellae. *Appl. Environ. Microbiol.* **57:**2360–2367.
2. **Alary, M., and J. R. Joly.** 1992. Factors contributing to the contamination of hospital water distribution systems by legionellae. *J. Infect. Dis.* **165:**565–569.
3. **Bangsborg, J. M., P. Gerner-Smidt, H. Colding, N. E. Fiehn, B. Bruun, and N. Hoiby.** 1995. Restriction fragment length polymorphism of rRNA genes for molecular typing of members of the family *Legionellaceae*. *J. Clin. Microbiol.* **33:**402–406.
4. **Barbaree, J. M.** 1993. Selecting a subtyping technique for use in investigations of legionellosis epidemics, p. 169–172. *In* J. M. Barbaree, R. F. Breiman, and A. P. Dufour (ed.), *Legionella: Current Status and Emerging Perspectives*. American Society for Microbiology, Washington, D.C.
5. **Barbaree, J. M., B. S. Fields, J. C. Feeley, G. W. Gorman, and W. T. Martin.** 1986. Isolation of protozoa from water associated with a legionellosis outbreak and demonstration of intracellular multiplication of *Legionella pneumophila*. *Appl. Environ. Microbiol.* **51:**422–424.

6. **Benson, R. F., W. L. Thacker, B. B. Plikaytis, and H. W. Wilkinson.** 1987. Cross-reactions in *Legionella* antisera with *Bordetella pertussis* strains. *J. Clin. Microbiol.* **25:** 594–596.
7. **Bettelheim, K. A., R. V. Metcalfe, and H. Sillars.** 1982. Levels of antibody against *Legionella pneumophila* serotype 1 in healthy populations in five areas in New Zealand. *J. Clin. Microbiol.* **16:**555–557.
8. **Birtles, R. J., T. J. Rowbotham, D. Raoult, and T. G. Harrison.** 1996. Phylogenetic diversity of intra-amoebal legionellae as revealed by 16S rRNA gene sequence comparison. *Microbiology* **142:**3525–3530.
9. **Blatt, S. P., M. J. Dolan, C. W. Hendrix, and G. P. Melcher.** 1994. Legionnaires' disease in human immunodeficiency virus-infected patients: eight cases and review. *Clin. Infect. Dis.* **18:**227–232.
10. **Boulanger, C. A., and P. H. Edelstein.** 1995. Precision and accuracy of recovery of *Legionella pneumophila* from seeded tap water by filtration and centrifugation. *Appl. Environ. Microbiol.* **61:**1805–1809.
11. **Brenner, D. J., A. G. Steigerwalt, P. Epple, W. F. Bibb, R. M. McKinney, R. W. Starnes, J. M. Colville, R. K. Selander, P. H. Edelstein, and C. W. Moss.** 1988. *Legionella pneumophila* serogroup Lansing 3 isolated from a patient with fatal pneumonia, and descriptions of *L. pneumophila* subsp *pneumophila* subsp. nov., *L. pneumophila* subsp. *fraseri* subsp. nov., and *L. pneumophila* subsp. *pascullei* subsp. nov. *J. Clin. Microbiol.* **26:**1695–1703.
12. **Brenner, D. J., A. G. Steigerwalt, and J. E. McDade.** 1979. Classification of the legionnaires' disease bacterium: *Legionella pneumophila,* genus novum, species nova, of the family Legionellaceae, familia nova. *Ann. Intern. Med.* **90:** 656–658.
13. **Brindle, R. J., P. J. Stannett, and R. N. Cunliffe.** 1987. *Legionella pneumophila*: comparison of isolation from water specimens by centrifugation and filtration. *Epidemiol. Infect.* **99:**241–247.
14. **Buesching, W. J., R. A. Brust, and L. W. Ayers.** 1983. Enhanced primary isolation of *Legionella pneumophila* from clinical specimens by low-pH treatment. *J. Clin. Microbiol.* **17:**1153–1155.
15. **Centers for Disease Control and Prevention.** 1992. *Procedures for the Recovery of Legionella from the Environment.* U.S. Department of Health and Human Services, Atlanta, Ga.
16. **Chastre, J., G. Raghu, P. Soler, P. Brun, F. Basset, and C. Gibert.** 1987. Pulmonary fibrosis following pneumonia due to acute Legionnaires' disease. Clinical, ultrastructural, and immunofluorescent study. *Chest* **91:**57–62.
17. **Dennis, P. J.** 1990. Reducing the risk of Legionnaires' disease. *Ann. Occup. Hyg.* **34:**189–193.
18. **Dorn, G. L., and W. R. Barnes.** 1979. Rapid isolation of *Legionella pneumophila* from seeded donor blood. *J. Clin. Microbiol.* **10:**114–115.
19. **Dowling, J. N., A. W. Pasculle, F. N. Frola, M. K. Zaphyr, and R. B. Yee.** 1984. Infections caused by *Legionella micdadei* and *Legionella pneumophila* among renal transplant recipients. *J. Infect. Dis.* **149:**703–713.
20. **Edelstein, P. H., K. B. Beer, J. C. Sturge, A. J. Watson, and L. C. Goldstein.** 1985. Clinical utility of a monoclonal direct fluorescent reagent specific for *Legionella pneumophila*: comparative study with other reagents. *J. Clin. Microbiol.* **22:**419–421.
21. **Edelstein, P. H., and M. A. Edelstein.** 1991. Comparison of different agars used in the formulation of buffered charcoal yeast extract medium. *J. Clin. Microbiol.* **29:**190–191.
22. **Edelstein, P. H., and M. A. C. Edelstein.** 1989. Evaluation of the Merifluor-*Legionella* immunofluorescent reagent for identifying and detecting 21 *Legionella* species. *J. Clin. Microbiol.* **27:**2455–2458.
23. **Edelstein, P. H., and M. A. C. Edelstein.** 1993. Comparison of three buffers used in the formulation of buffered charcoal yeast extract medium. *J. Clin. Microbiol.* **31:** 3329–3330.
24. **Edelstein, P. H., R. D. Meyer, and S. M. Finegold.** 1980. Laboratory diagnosis of Legionnaires' disease. *Am. Rev. Respir. Dis.* **121:**317–327.
25. **Edelstein, P. H., C. Nakahama, J. O. Tobin, K. Calarco, K. B. Beer, J. R. Joly, and R. K. Selander.** 1986. Paleoepidemiologic investigation of legionnaires' disease at Wadsworth Veterans Administration Hospital by using three typing methods for comparison of legionellae from clinical and environmental sources. *J. Clin. Microbiol.* **23:** 1121–1126.
26. **Edelstein, P. H., J. B. Snitzer, and J. A. Bridge.** 1982. Enhancement of recovery of *Legionella pneumophila* from contaminated respiratory tract specimens by heat. *J. Clin. Microbiol.* **16:**1061–1065.
27. **Ehret, W., K. Jacob, and G. Ruckdeschel.** 1987. Identification of clinical and environmental isolates of *Legionella pneumophila* by analysis of outer-membrane proteins, ubiquinones and fatty acids. *Zentralbl. Bakteriol. Mikrobiol. Hyg. Ser. A* **266:**261–275.
28. **England, A. C., III, D. W. Fraser, B. D. Plikaytis, T. F. Tsai, G. Storch, and C. V. Broome.** 1981. Sporadic legionellosis in the United States: the first thousand cases. *Ann. Intern. Med.* **94:**164–170.
29. **Evans, C. P., and W. C. Winn, Jr.** 1981. Extrathoracic localization of *Legionella pneumophila* in Legionnaires' pneumonia. *Am. J. Clin. Pathol.* **76:**813–815.
30. **Fairbank, J. T., A. C. Mamourian, P. A. Dietrich, and J. C. Girod.** 1983. The chest radiograph in Legionnaires' disease. Further observations. *Radiology* **147:**33–34.
31. **Fallon, R. J., and T. J. Rowbotham.** 1990. Microbiological investigations into an outbreak of Pontiac fever due to *Legionella micdadei* associated with use of a whirlpool. *J. Clin. Pathol.* **43:**479–483.
32. **Fang, G. D., V. L. Yu, and R. M. Vickers.** 1989. Disease due to the *Legionellaceae* (other than *Legionella pneumophila*). Historical, microbiological, clinical, and epidemiological review. *Medicine (Baltimore)* **68:**116–132.
33. **Feeley, J. C., R. J. Gibson, G. W. Gorman, N. C. Langford, J. K. Rasheed, D. C. Mackel, and W. B. Baine.** 1979. Charcoal-yeast extract agar: primary isolation medium for *Legionella pneumophila. J. Clin. Microbiol.* **10:**437–441.
34. **Fox, A., P. Y. Lau, A. Brown, S. L. Morgan, Z. T. Zhu, M. Lema, and M. D. Walla.** 1984. Capillary gas chromatographic analysis of carbohydrates of *Legionella pneumophila* and other members of the family *Legionellaceae. J. Clin. Microbiol.* **19:**326–332.
35. **Fraser, D. W., T. R. Tsai, W. Orenstein, W. E. Parkin, H. J. Beecham, R. G. Sharrar, J. Harris, G. F. Mallison, S. M. Martin, J. E. McDade, C. C. Shepard, and P. S. Brachman.** 1977. Legionnaires' disease: description of an epidemic of pneumonia. *N. Engl. J. Med.* **297:**1189–1197.
36. **Friedman, S., K. Spitalny, J. Barbaree, Y. Faur, and R. McKinney.** 1987. Pontiac fever outbreak associated with a cooling tower. *Am. J. Public Health* **77:**568–572.
37. **Fry, N. K., S. Warwick, N. A. Saunders, and T. M. Embley.** 1991. The use of 16S ribosomal RNA analyses to investigate the phylogeny of the family *Legionellaceae. J. Gen. Microbiol.* **137:**1215–1222.
38. **Garrity, G. M., E. M. Elder, B. Davis, R. M. Vickers, and A. Brown.** 1982. Serological and genotypic diversity among serogroup 5-reacting environmental *Legionella* isolates. *J. Clin. Microbiol.* **15:**646–653.
39. **Girod, J. C., R. C. Reichman, W. C. Winn, Jr., D. N.**

Klaucke, R. L. Vogt, and R. Dolin. 1982. Pneumonic and nonpneumonic forms of legionellosis. The result of a common-source exposure to *Legionella pneumophila*. *Arch. Intern. Med.* **142:**545–547.

40. **Glick, T. H., M. B. Gregg, B. Berman, G. Mallison, W. W. Rhodes, Jr., and I. Kassanoff.** 1978. Pontiac fever. An epidemic of unknown etiology in a health department. I. Clinical and epidemiologic aspects. *Am. J. Epidemiol.* **107:** 149–160.
41. **Gomez-Lus, P., B. S. Fields, R. F. Benson, W. T. Martin, S. P. O'Connor, and C. M. Black.** 1993. Comparison of arbitrarily primed polymerase chain reaction, ribotyping, and monoclonal antibody analysis for subtyping *Legionella pneumophila* serogroup 1. *J. Clin. Microbiol.* **31:**1940–1942.
42. **Grattard, F., P. Berthelot, M. Reyrolle, A. Ros, J. Etienne, and B. Pozzetto.** 1996. Molecular typing of nosocomial strains of *Legionella pneumophila* by arbitrarily primed PCR. *J. Clin. Microbiol.* **34:**1595–1598.
43. **Harrison, T. G., N. A. Saunders, A. Haththotuwa, N. Doshi, and A. G. Taylor.** 1992. Further evidence that genotypically closely related strains of *Legionella pneumophila* can express different serogroup specific antigens. *J. Gen. Microbiol.* **37:**155–161.
44. **Harrison, T. G., N. A. Saunders, A. Haththotuwa, G. Hallas, R. J. Birtles, and A. G. Taylor.** 1990. Phenotypic variation amongst genotypically homogeneous *Legionella pneumophila* serogroup 1 isolates: implications for the investigation of outbreaks of Legionnaires' disease. *Epidemiol. Infect.* **104:**171–180.
45. **Hay, J., D. V. Seal, B. Billcliffe, and J. H. Freer.** 1995. Non-culturable *Legionella pneumophila* associated with *Acanthamoeba castellanii*: detection of the bacterium using DNA amplification and hybridization. *J. Appl. Bacteriol.* **78:**61–65.
46. **Heath, C. H., D. I. Grove, and D. F. Looke.** 1996. Delay in appropriate therapy of *Legionella* pneumonia associated with increased mortality. *Eur. J. Clin. Microbiol. Infect. Dis.* **15:**286–290.
47. **Hebert, G. A.** 1981. Hippurate hydrolysis by *Legionella pneumophila*. *J. Clin. Microbiol.* **13:**240–242.
48. **Hebert, G. A., C. W. Moss, L. K. McDougal, F. M. Bozeman, R. M. McKinney, and D. J. Brenner.** 1980. The rickettsia-like organisms TATLOCK (1943) and HEBA (1959): bacteria phenotypically similar to but genetically distinct from *Legionella pneumophila* and the WIGA bacterium. *Ann. Intern. Med.* **92:**45–52.
49. **Ingram, J. G., and J. F. Plouffe.** 1994. Danger of sputum purulence screens in culture of *Legionella* species. *J. Clin. Microbiol.* **32:**209–210.
50. **Jacobs, F., C. Liesnard, J. P. Goldstein, M. J. Struelens, G. Primo, J. L. Leclerc, and J. P. Thys.** 1990. Asymptomatic *Legionella pneumophila* infections in heart transplant recipients. *Transplantation* **50:**174–175.
51. **Jantzen, E., A. Sonesson, T. Tangen, and J. Eng.** 1993. Hydroxy-fatty acid profiles of *Legionella* species: diagnostic usefulness assessed by principal component analysis. *J. Clin. Microbiol.* **31:**1413–1419.
52. **Jaulhac, B., M. Nowicki, N. Bornstein, O. Meunier, G. Prevost, Y. Piemont, J. Fleurette, and H. Monteil.** 1992. Detection of *Legionella* spp. in bronchoalveolar lavage fluids by DNA amplification. *J. Clin. Microbiol.* **30:** 920–924.
53. **Johnson, W. M., K. Bernard, T. J. Marrie, and S. D. Tyler.** 1994. Discriminatory genomic fingerprinting of *Legionella pneumophila* by pulsed-field electrophoresis. *J. Clin. Microbiol.* **32:**2620–2621.
54. **Joly, J. R.** 1993. Monitoring for the presence of *Legionella*: where, when, and how? p. 211–216. *In* J. M. Barbaree, R. F. Breiman, and A. P. Dufour (ed.), *Legionella: Current Status and Emerging Perspectives*. American Society for Microbiology, Washington, D.C.
55. **Jonas, D., A. Rosenbaum, S. Weyrich, and S. Bhakdi.** 1995. Enzyme-linked immunoassay for detection of PCR-amplified DNA of legionellae in bronchoalveolar fluid. *J. Clin. Microbiol.* **33:**1247–1252.
56. **Kazandjian, D., R. Chiew, and G. L. Gilbert.** 1997. Rapid diagnosis of *Legionella pneumophila* serogroup 1 infection with the Binax enzyme immunoassay urinary antigen test. *J. Clin. Microbiol.* **35:**954–956.
57. **Keathley, J. D., and W. C. Winn, Jr.** 1985. Comparison of media for recovery of clinical isolates of *Legionella pneumophila*. *Am. J. Clin. Pathol.* **83:**498–499.
58. **Kessler, H. H., F. F. Reinthaler, A. Pschaid, K. Pierer, B. Kleinhappl, E. Eber, and E. Marth.** 1993. Rapid detection of *Legionella* species in bronchoalveolar lavage fluids with the EnviroAmp Legionella PCR amplification and detection kit. *J. Clin. Microbiol.* **31:**3325–3328.
59. **Kirby, B. D., K. M. Snyder, R. D. Meyer, and S. M. Finegold.** 1980. Legionnaires' disease: report of sixty-five nosocomially acquired cases and review of the literature. *Medicine (Baltimore)* **59:**188–205.
60. **Kohler, R. B., L. J. Wheat, M. L. French, P. L. Meenhorst, W. C. Winn, Jr., and P. H. Edelstein.** 1985. Cross-reactive urinary antigens among patients infected with *Legionella pneumophila* serogroups 1 and 4 and the Leiden 1 strain. *J. Infect. Dis.* **152:**1007–1012.
61. **Kohler, R. B., W. C. Winn, Jr., and L. J. Wheat.** 1984. Onset and duration of urinary antigen excretion in Legionnaires disease. *J. Clin. Microbiol.* **20:**605–607.
62. **Kuchta, J. M., S. J. States, J. E. McGlaughlin, J. H. Overmeyer, R. M. Wadowsky, A. M. McNamara, R. S. Wolford, and R. B. Yee.** 1985. Enhanced chlorine resistance of tap water-adapted *Legionella pneumophila* as compared with agar medium-passaged strains. *Appl. Environ. Microbiol.* **50:**21–26.
63. **Kurz, R. W., W. Graninger, T. P. Egger, H. Pichler, and K. H. Tragl.** 1988. Failure of treatment of *Legionella* pneumonia with ciprofloxacin. *J. Antimicrob. Chemother.* **22:**389–391.
64. **Lambert, M. A., and C. W. Moss.** 1989. Cellular fatty acid compositions and isoprenoid quinone contents of 23 *Legionella* species. *J. Clin. Microbiol.* **27:**465–473.
65. **Ledesma, E., M. L. Camaro, E. Carbonell, T. Sacristan, A. Marti, S. Pellicer, J. Llorca, P. Herrero, and M. A. Dasi.** 1995. Subtyping of *Legionella pneumophila* isolates by arbitrarily primed polymerase chain reaction. *Can. J. Microbiol.* **41:**846–848.
66. **Lee, T. C., R. M. Vickers, V. L. Yu, and M. M. Wagener.** 1993. Growth of 28 *Legionella* species on selective culture media: a comparative study. *J. Clin. Microbiol.* **31:** 2764–2768.
67. **Lightfoot, N. F., I. R. Richardson, J. Shrimanker, and D. J. Farrell.** 1991. Post-mortem isolation of *Legionella* due to contamination. *Lancet* **337:**376.
68. **Lisby, G., and R. Dessau.** 1994. Construction of a DNA amplification assay for detection of *Legionella* species in clinical samples. *Eur. J. Clin. Microbiol. Infect. Dis.* **13:** 225–231.
69. **Lowry, P. W., R. J. Blankenship, W. Gridley, N. J. Troup, and L. S. Tompkins.** 1991. A cluster of *Legionella* sternal-wound infections due to postoperative topical exposure to contaminated tap water. *N. Engl. J. Med.* **324:** 109–113.
70. **Lowry, P. W., and L. S. Tompkins.** 1993. Nosocomial legionellosis: a review of pulmonary and extrapulmonary syndromes. *Am. J. Infect. Control* **21:**21–27.
71. **Luck, P. C., E. Dinger, J. H. Helbig, V. Thurm, H. Keuchel, C. Presch, and M. Ott.** 1994. Analysis of *Legionella*

pneumophila strains associated with nosocomial pneumonia in a neonatal intensive care unit. *Eur. J. Clin. Microbiol. Infect. Dis.* **13**:565–571.

72. **Luck, P. C., J. H. Helbig, H. J. Hagedorn, and W. Ehret.** 1995. DNA fingerprinting by pulsed-field gel electrophoresis to investigate a nosocomial pneumonia caused by *Legionella bozemanii* serogroup 1. *Appl. Environ. Microbiol.* **61**: 2759–2761.
73. **Maiwald, M., M. Schill, C. Stockinger, J. H. Helbig, P. C. Luck, W. Witzleb, and H. G. Sonntag.** 1995. Detection of *Legionella* DNA in human and guinea pig urine samples by the polymerase chain reaction. *Eur. J. Clin. Microbiol. Infect. Dis.* **14**:25–33.
74. **Mamolen, M., R. F. Breiman, J. M. Barbaree, R. A. Gunn, K. M. Stone, J. S. Spika, D. T. Dennis, S. H. Mao, and R. L. Vogt.** 1993. Use of multiple molecular subtyping techniques to investigate a Legionnaires' disease outbreak due to identical strains at two tourist lodges. *J. Clin. Microbiol.* **31**:2584–2588.
75. **Marques, M. T., N. Bornstein, and J. Fleurette.** 1995. Combined monoclonal antibody typing, multilocus enzyme electrophoresis, soluble protein profiles and plasmid analysis of clinical and environmental *Legionella pneumophila* serogroup 1 isolated in a Portuguese hospital. *J. Hosp. Infect.* **30**:103–110.
76. **Marrie, T. J., D. Haldane, G. Bezanson, and R. Peppard.** 1992. Each water outlet is a unique ecological niche for *Legionella pneumophila*. *Epidemiol. Infect.* **108**:261–270.
77. **Marrie, T. J., S. Macdonald, K. Clarke, and D. Haldane.** 1991. Nosocomial legionnaires' disease: lessons from a four-year prospective study. *Am. J. Infect. Control* **19**:79–85.
78. **Marston, B. J., H. B. Lipman, and R. F. Breiman.** 1994. Surveillance for Legionnaires' disease. Risk factors for morbidity and mortality. *Arch. Intern. Med.* **154**:2417–2422.
79. **Matsiota-Bernard, P., E. Pitsouni, N. Legakis, and C. Nauciel.** 1994. Evaluation of commercial amplification kit for detection of *Legionella pneumophila* in clinical specimens. *J. Clin. Microbiol.* **32**:1503–1505.
80. **McDade, J. E., D. J. Brenner, and F. M. Bozeman.** 1979. Legionnaires' disease bacterium isolated in 1947. *Ann. Intern. Med.* **90**:659–661.
81. **McDade, J. E., C. C. Shepard, D. W. Fraser, T. R. Tsai, M. A. Redus, and W. R. Dowdle.** 1977. Legionnaires' disease: isolation of a bacterium and demonstration of its role in other respiratory disease. *N. Engl. J. Med.* **297**: 1197–1203.
82. **Miller, L. A., J. L. Beebe, J. C. Butler, W. Martin, R. Benson, R. E. Hoffman, and B. S. Fields.** 1993. Use of polymerase chain reaction in an epidemiologic investigation of Pontiac fever. *J. Infect. Dis.* **168**:769–772.
83. **Muder, R. R., V. L. Yu, and A. H. Woo.** 1986. Mode of transmission of *Legionella pneumophila*. A critical review. *Arch. Intern. Med.* **146**:1607–1612.
84. **Munro, R., S. Neville, D. Daley, and J. Mercer.** 1994. Microbiological aspects of an outbreak of Legionnaires' disease in south western Sydney. *Pathology* **26**:48–51.
85. **Muraca, P. W., V. L. Yu, and A. Goetz.** 1990. Disinfection of water distribution systems for *Legionella*: a review of application procedures and methodologies. *Infect. Control Hosp. Epidemiol.* **11**:79–88.
86. **Myerowitz, R. L., A. W. Pasculle, J. N. Dowling, G. J. Pazin, M. Puerzer, R. B. Yee, C. R. Rinaldo, Jr., and T. R. Hakala.** 1979. Opportunistic lung infection due to "Pittsburgh Pneumonia Agent." *N. Engl. J. Med.* **301**: 953–958.
87. **Ng, V. L., M. York, and W. K. Hadley.** 1989. Unexpected isolation of *Bordetella pertussis* from patients with acquired immunodeficiency syndrome. *J. Clin. Microbiol.* **27**: 337–338.
88. **Nichol, K. L., C. M. Parenti, and J. E. Johnson.** 1991. High prevalence of positive antibodies to *Legionella pneumophila* among outpatients. *Chest* **100**:663–666.
89. **Ott, M., P. Messner, J. Heesemann, R. Marre, and J. Hacker.** 1991. Temperature-dependent expression of flagella in *Legionella*. *J. Gen. Microbiol.* **137**:1955–1961.
90. **Plikaytis, B. B., G. M. Carlone, C. P. Pau, and H. W. Wilkinson.** 1987. Purified 60-kilodalton *Legionella* protein antigen with *Legionella*-specific and nonspecific epitopes. *J. Clin. Microbiol.* **25**:2080–2084.
91. **Plouffe, J. F., T. M. File, Jr., R. F. Breiman, B. A. Hackman, S. J. Salstrom, B. J. Marston, and B. S. Fields.** 1995. Reevaluation of the definition of Legionnaires' disease: use of the urinary antigen assay. Community Based Pneumonia Incidence Study Group. *Clin. Infect. Dis.* **20**: 1286–1291.
92. **Reingold, A. L., B. M. Thomason, B. J. Brake, L. Thacker, H. W. Wilkinson, and J. N. Kuritsky.** 1984. *Legionella* pneumonia in the United States: the distribution of serogroups and species causing human illness. *J. Infect. Dis.* **149**:819.
93. **Rihs, J. D., V. L. Yu, J. J. Zuravleff, A. Goetz, and R. R. Muder.** 1985. Isolation of *Legionella pneumophila* from blood with the BACTEC system: a prospective study yielding positive results. *J. Clin. Microbiol.* **22**:422–424.
94. **Rowbotham, T. J.** 1980. Preliminary report on the pathogenicity of *Legionella pneumophila* for freshwater and soil amoebae. *J. Clin. Pathol.* **33**:1179–1183.
95. **Rowbotham, T. J.** 1983. Isolation of *Legionella pneumophila* from clinical specimens via amoebae, and the interaction of those and other isolates with amoebae. *J. Clin. Pathol.* **36**:978–986.
96. **Roy, T. M., D. Fleming, and W. H. Anderson.** 1989. Tularemic pneumonia mimicking Legionnaires' disease with false-positive direct fluorescent antibody stains for *Legionella*. *South. Med. J.* **82**:1429–1431.
97. **Salord, J. M., P. Matsiota-Bernard, F. Staikowsky, M. Kirstetter, J. Frottier, and C. Nauciel.** 1993. Unsuccessful treatment of *Legionella pneumophila* infection with a fluoroquinolone. *Clin. Infect. Dis.* **17**:518–519.
98. **Sanden, G. N., W. E. Morrill, B. S. Fields, R. F. Breiman, and J. M. Barbaree.** 1992. Incubation of water samples containing amoebae improves detection of legionellae by the culture method. *Appl. Environ. Microbiol.* **58**: 2001–2004.
99. **Sathapatayavongs, B., R. B. Kohler, L. J. Wheat, A. White, and W. C. Winn, Jr.** 1983. Rapid diagnosis of Legionnaires' disease by latex agglutination. *Am. Rev. Respir. Dis.* **127**:559–562.
100. **Schlenk, R., A. Wildfeuer, and O. Haferkamp.** 1993. Identification of *Legionella pneumophila* in various specimens by the polymerase chain reaction. *Arzneim-Forsch.* **43**:1249–1252.
101. **Steele, T. W., C. V. Moore, and N. Sangster.** 1990. Distribution of *Legionella longbeachae* serogroup 1 and other legionellae in potting soils in Australia. *Appl. Environ. Microbiol.* **56**:2984–2988.
102. **Storch, G., P. S. Hayes, D. L. Hill, and W. B. Baine.** 1979. Prevalence of antibody to *Legionella pneumophila* in middle- aged and elderly Americans. *J. Infect. Dis.* **140**: 784–788.
103. **Stout, J. E., J. Joly, M. Para, J. Plouffe, C. Ciesielski, M. J. Blaser, and V. L. Yu.** 1988. Comparison of molecular methods for subtyping patients and epidemiologically linked environmental isolates of *Legionella pneumophila*. *J. Infect. Dis.* **157**:486–495.
104. **Stout, J. E., and V. L. Yu.** 1997. Current concepts: legionellosis. *N. Engl. J. Med.* **337**:682–687.
105. **Stout, J. E., V. L. Yu, P. Muraca, J. Joly, N. Troup,**

and L. S. Tompkins. 1992. Potable water as a cause of sporadic cases of community-acquired legionnaires' disease. *N. Engl. J. Med.* **326:**151–155.

106. **Tenover, F. C., P. H. Edelstein, L. C. Goldstein, J. C. Sturge, and J. J. Plorde.** 1986. Comparison of cross-staining reactions by *Pseudomonas* spp. and fluorescein-labeled polyclonal and monoclonal antibodies directed against *Legionella pneumophila. J. Clin. Microbiol.* **23:**647–649.

107. **Thacker, L., R. M. McKinney, C. W. Moss, H. M. Sommers, M. L. Spivack, and T. F. O'Brien.** 1981. Thermophilic sporeforming bacilli that mimic fastidious growth characteristics and colonial morphology of *Legionella. J. Clin. Microbiol.* **13:**794–797.

107a. **Tompkins, L. S., B. J. Roessler, S. C. Redd., L. E. Markowitz, and M. L. Cohen.** 1988. *Legionella* prosthetic-valve endocarditis. *N. Engl. J. Med.* **318:**530–535.

108. **Tompkins, L. S., N. J. Troup, T. Woods, W. Bibb, and R. M. McKinney.** 1987. Molecular epidemiology of *Legionella* species by restriction endonuclease and alloenzyme analysis. *J. Clin. Microbiol.* **25:**1875–1880.

109. **Venezia, R. A., M. D. Agresta, E. M. Hanley, K. Urquhart, and D. Schoonmaker.** 1994. Nosocomial legionellosis associated with aspiration of nasogastric feedings diluted in tap water. *Infect. Control Hosp. Epidemiol.* **15:** 529–533.

110. **Wadowsky, R. M., L. J. Butler, M. K. Cook, S. M. Verma, M. A. Paul, B. S. Fields, G. Keleti, J. L. Sykora, and R. B. Yee.** 1988. Growth-supporting activity for *Legionella pneumophila* in tap water cultures and implication of hartmannellid amoebae as growth factors. *Appl. Environ. Microbiol.* **54:**2677–2682.

111. **Wilkinson, H. W., and B. J. Brake.** 1982. Formalin-killed versus heat-killed *Legionella pneumophila* serogroup 1 antigen in the indirect immunofluorescence assay for legionellosis. *J. Clin. Microbiol.* **16:**979–981.

112. **Wilkinson, H. W., D. D. Cruce, and C. V. Broome.** 1981. Validation of *Legionella pneumophila* indirect immunofluorescence assay with epidemic sera. *J. Clin. Microbiol.* **13:**139–146.

113. **Wilkinson, H. W., A. L. Reingold, B. J. Brake, D. L. McGiboney, G. W. Gorman, and C. V. Broome.** 1983. Reactivity of serum from patients with suspected legionellosis against 29 antigens of Legionellaceae and *Legionella*-like organisms by indirect immunofluorescence assay. *J. Infect. Dis.* **147:**23–31.

114. **Winn, W. C., Jr.** 1988. Legionnaires disease: historical perspective. *Clin. Microbiol. Rev.* **1:**60–81.

115. **Winn, W. C., Jr., and R. L. Myerowitz.** 1981. The pathology of the *Legionella* pneumonias. A review of 74 cases and the literature. *Hum. Pathol.* **12:**401–422.

116. **Wright, J. B., I. Ruseska, and J. W. Costerton.** 1991. Decreased biocide susceptibility of adherent *Legionella pneumophila. J. Appl. Bacteriol.* **71:**531–538.

117. **Yee, R. B. and R. M. Wadowsky.** 1982. Multiplication of *Legionella pneumophila* in unsterilized tap water. *Appl. Environ. Microbiol.* **43:**1330–1334.

118. **Yu, V. L., T. R. J. Beam, R. M. Lumish, R. M. Vickers, J. Fleming, C. McDermott, and J. Romano.** 1987. Routine culturing for *Legionella* in the hospital environment may be a good idea: a three-hospital prospective study. *Am. J. Med. Sci.* **294:**97–99.

119. **Zimmerman, S. E., M. L. French, S. D. Allen, E. Wilson, and R. B. Kohler.** 1982. Immunoglobulin M antibody titers in the diagnosis of Legionnaires' disease. *J. Clin. Microbiol.* **16:**1007–1011.

120. **Zuravleff, J. J., V. L. Yu, J. W. Shonnard, B. K. Davis, and J. D. Rihs.** 1983. Diagnosis of Legionnaires' disease. An update of laboratory methods with new emphasis on isolation by culture. *JAMA* **250:**1981–1985.

Neisseria and *Branhamella**

JOAN S. KNAPP AND EMILY H. KOUMANS

38

TAXONOMY

Neisseria species and *Branhamella catarrhalis* are classified with the genera *Moraxella, Kingella,* and *Acinetobacter* in the family *Neisseriaceae* (10). The genus *Neisseria* contains species isolated from humans and animals. The taxonomic positions of some *Neisseria* species (*Neisseria caviae, N. ovis,* and *N. cuniculi*) and *B. catarrhalis* are currently uncertain. Two proposals have been made with regard to the taxonomic position of the species *B. catarrhalis*: that the species be assigned to the genus *Moraxella* (*Moraxella catarrhalis*) in the family *Moraxellaceae* or to its own genus, *Branhamella,* in the family *Branhamaceae* (14, 80). Although the name *Moraxella* is used widely, neither name has yet taken precedence; the name *B. catarrhalis* will be used throughout this chapter because the cardinal characteristics used to identify isolates—cell morphology and positive oxidase reaction—are more similar to those used to identify *Neisseria* spp. than to those used to identify *Moraxella* spp. The genera *Eikenella, Simonsiella,* and *Alysiella*; CDC groups EF-4 and M-5 (*N. weaverii* sp. nov.); and *N. macacae, N. polysaccharea,* and *N. iguanae* have also been assigned to the family *Neisseriaceae* (6, 10, 43, 77, 92). Descriptions of species in this chapter will be limited to those of human origin. Information relating to species of animal origin will be limited to a table of differential characteristics that should be consulted when a gram-negative diplococcus which is not readily identifiable as a human *Neisseria* species, e.g., an isolate from a wound inflicted by an animal bite, is isolated.

An extensive discussion of the genetic relatedness among *Neisseria* and related species is beyond the scope of this chapter. However, elegant studies of the genetic relatedness between species have been published (27, 81). The relatedness between species can be summarized as follows: (i) *N. gonorrhoeae* and *N. meningitidis* (and *N. kochii*) are very closely related; (ii) *N. lactamica, N. polysaccharea, N. cinerea,* and *N. flavescens* are related to *N. gonorrhoeae* and each other more distantly; and (iii) strains of the "saccharolytic" *Neisseria* species (*N. subflava* bv. subflava, *N. subflava* bv. flava, and *N. subflava* bv. perflava, *N. sicca,* and *N. mucosa*) are distantly related to the first two groups. As anticipated, *B. catarrhalis* and *Kingella denitrificans* are still more distantly related, as are the species of animal origin.

DESCRIPTION OF THE GENUS

Neisseria species (except *N. elongata*) and *B. catarrhalis* are gram-negative diplococci with adjacent sides flattened to give a characteristic kidney or coffee bean appearance observed in stained smears (91). Cells divide in two planes at right angles to each other, resulting in tetrads. Cells range in size from 0.6 to 1.5 μm, depending on the species, source of the isolate, and age of the culture. Occasionally, giant cells may be observed in some cultures. *N. elongata* and *K. denitrificans* are gram-negative coccobacilli which may form diplobacilli; the diplobacilli of *K. denitrificans* isolates may resemble diplococci and thus may be confused with *N. gonorrhoeae*. Cells are nonmotile and do not produce endospores. The cells of some species are encapsulated, and some species produce a yellow-green carotinoid pigment. Cells of some species, most notably *N. gonorrhoeae*, may autolyze in culture after approximately 24 h of incubation.

Most *Neisseria, Branhamella,* and *Kingella* strains have complex growth requirements; some strains may be exquisitely sensitive to fatty acids, necessitating the incorporation of soluble starch in growth media. All species are aerobic and have an optimal growth temperature of 35 to 37°C; *B. catarrhalis* strains are tolerant of lower temperatures and may grow well at 28°C. The growth of many *Neisseria* species is enhanced by humidity and CO_2, and strains of some species, notably *N. gonorrhoeae*, require CO_2. All species are oxidase positive and, with the exception of *N. elongata* and *K. denitrificans*, are catalase positive. Species have limited metabolic activities and are differentiated by their abilities to produce catalase, produce acid from a few carbohydrates, produce polysaccharide from sucrose, produce DNase, reduce nitrate and nitrite, oxidize fatty acids such as tributyrin, and produce certain enzymes.

Neisseria species are oxidative, not fermentative; i.e., they produce acid from carbohydrates by oxidation, not fermentation. Because these species are oxidative and produce less acid from carbohydrates than do fermentative organisms and because they also produce ammonia from peptones, which may neutralize any acid produced from carbohydrates, acid production must be determined in a medium with a low

* This chapter contains information presented in chapter 26 by Joan S. Knapp and Roselyn J. Rice in the sixth edition of this Manual.

protein/carbohydrate ratio and a sensitive indicator such as phenol red (56). The terms carbohydrate utilization and carbohydrate degradation should not be used to describe the results obtained in acid production tests. Some species, e.g., *N. cinerea*, may use glucose but rapidly overoxidize acid to carbon dioxide, with the result that acid does not accumulate in the reaction tube, even though the carbohydrate has been used (56). Thus, the term acid production is the most accurate term to describe the reaction observed in laboratory diagnostic tests.

NATURAL HABITAT

Most *Neisseria* species are nonpathogenic and are normal inhabitants only of the oro- and nasopharyngeal mucous membranes of humans (58). On rare occasions, nonpathogenic species may be isolated from other mucous membranes, but these sites should be considered to be opportunistic sites of colonization rather than normal habitats. Among *Neisseria* species, only strains of *N. meningitidis* and *N. gonorrhoeae* are considered pathogens. Strains of *N. gonorrhoeae* are always considered pathogenic and may infect exposed anogenital and oropharyngeal mucous membranes. Strains of *N. meningitidis* may colonize the oro- and nasopharynges as nonpathogens in a "carrier" state and may colonize exposed anogenital mucosal membranes, particularly of homosexual men (49); some strains may cause epidemic and acute meningitis.

The normal patterns of oro- and nasopharyngeal colonization by *Neisseria* species were studied extensively in the early 1900s, but many species were misidentified owing to the use of inappropriate differential tests and media (56). Recent studies have demonstrated that both adults and children may be colonized simultaneously by several *Neisseria* species or by multiple strains of the *N. subflava* biovar perflava-*N. sicca* group (55, 58). Patterns of colonization appear to be stable, persisting for several months in adults (58). Similarly, colonization by strains of *N. meningitidis* may persist for many months. *N. lactamica* is isolated more frequently from children and young adolescents than from adults; the isolation of *N. polysaccharea* may vary geographically (7, 8, 38). *B. catarrhalis* is rarely isolated from the oropharynx of a healthy adult but may be carried more frequently in children and older adults (58, 90). The frequency and persistence of colonization by *K. denitrificans* appear to vary geographically (50, 58, 59).

CLINICAL SIGNIFICANCE

N. gonorrhoeae

Gonorrhea is second only to *Chlamydia trachomatis* infections in the number of cases reported to the Centers for Disease Control and Prevention (CDC); it is estimated, however, that only one-half of cases are reported (18). The number of reported cases of gonorrhea increased steadily from 1964 to 1977, fluctuated through the early 1980s, and then increased until 1987, and since 1987 the number has decreased annually (18). The incidence of gonorrhea is highest in high-density urban areas among persons under 24 years of age who have multiple sexual partners and engage in unprotected sexual intercourse. Recently, increases in gonorrhea prevalence have been noted among men who have sex with men (19). The decline in gonorrhea prevalence may be attributed to recommendations, in the United States, for the routine use of highly effective antimicrobial agents to treat gonorrhea (15, 20). Factors that may contribute to the persistence and spread of gonorrhea are the occurrence of asymptomatic infections (particularly in women), which may be transmitted unknowingly between sexual partners, and the high-frequency spread of infections by persons with multiple sexual partners, including those who exchange sex for money or drugs.

N. gonorrhoeae is highly susceptible to adverse environmental conditions, including extreme temperatures and drying; the organism does not survive long outside its host. Gonorrhea is transmitted by direct, close, usually sexual contact between individuals. Infections are transmitted more efficiently from an infected man to a woman (in 50 to 60% of instances of one sexual exposure) than from an infected woman to a man (in 35% of instances of one sexual exposure). Transmission of gonorrhea to neonates usually occurs during birth. Transmission of gonorrhea to older infants is often associated with allegations of sexual abuse by an adult or older adolescent. Nonsexual human (skin-skin or skin-mucous membrane inoculation or autoinoculation) or fomite transmission (excluding laboratory accidents) has not been documented.

Uncomplicated Gonorrhea

The majority of gonococcal infections are uncomplicated lower genital tract infections caused by direct infection of the columnar epithelium of mucosal membranes. In men, acute urethritis with symptoms including a scant clear to a copious purulent discharge, burning during urination, and an increase in urination frequency usually occurs within 7 days after infection. Asymptomatic infections are estimated to occur in 10 to 50% of infected men. If untreated, men may develop epididymitis, prostatitis, and urethral stricture. In women, the primary site of infection is usually the endocervix; symptomatic uncomplicated infections are characterized by a vaginal discharge, dysuria, and an erythematous, friable cervical os. Asymptomatic infections in women often manifest as low-grade or no endocervical inflammation or discharge. In prepubertal girls, gonococcal infections may present as vulvovaginitis. Local complications may include urethral vestibular abscesses, salpingitis, tubo-ovarian abscesses, and pelvic inflammatory disease (PID).

Oropharyngeal and Anorectal Infections

Persons practicing receptive oral or anal intercourse may acquire oral or anorectal gonococcal infections. However, women who do not engage in anal intercourse may acquire anorectal infections by contamination from cervical secretions. Anorectal infections may be asymptomatic. Symptoms of anorectal infections may include a copious purulent discharge, burning or stinging pain, tenesmus, and blood in stools. Symptomatic oropharyngeal infections may manifest as a mild pharyngitis. Oropharyngeal and anorectal infections may also be asymptomatic.

Conjunctivitis

Ocular infections, which are most frequently diagnosed in newborns exposed to infected secretions during birth (ophthalmia neonatorum) but which are also occasionally seen in adults, must be treated promptly to prevent blindness. Conjunctival infections involve tearing and edema associated with a purulent exudate. If the infection is not treated, scarring or perforation of the cornea may occur. In industrial countries, neonatal blindness due to gonococcal infections has largely been eliminated by the routine application of prophylactic agents such as silver nitrate drops or erythromycin or tetracycline ointment to the eyes of newborns.

PID

If left untreated, endocervical infections may ascend locally to cause PID manifested as endometritis, salpingitis, pelvic peritonitis, or tubo-ovarian abscesses. It is estimated that 8 to 10% of women with endocervical gonococcal infections may develop PID, the most serious complication of which is permanent damage to the reproductive system. Although other organisms, including *C. trachomatis* and anaerobes, are associated with the development of PID, gonococci have been isolated from 10 to 70% of patients with PID and are believed to play a major role in initial episodes of this syndrome. Anaerobic vaginal and gut flora have been associated more frequently with subsequent episodes of PID. The inflammatory response to infections may result in scarring and blockage of the fallopian tubes and, subsequently, infertility and ectopic pregnancies. Fitz-Hugh-Curtis syndrome (perihepatitis) may be associated with gonococcal PID, as with chlamydial PID. A diagnosis of PID must be considered for women with lower abdominal pain and adnexal tenderness. Although laparoscopy is the best method for diagnosing PID if the inflammation has reached the fallopian tubes and the pelvic peritoneum, this procedure is rarely performed, and endocervical specimens for *N. gonorrhoeae* and *C. trachomatis* must be taken. PID should be treated empirically with recommended antimicrobial regimens with broad-spectrum activity against not only *N. gonorrhoeae* but also *C. trachomatis* and anaerobes (20).

DGI

Approximately 1 to 3% of persons with gonorrhea may develop disseminated gonococcal infection (DGI), which often has been associated with untreated asymptomatic infections, although persons deficient in complement components C7, C8, or C9 are more likely to develop DGI. Gonococci may be isolated from blood from fewer than 50% of patients. Patients may develop "dermatitis-arthritis" syndrome, with fever, chills, skin lesions, and diffuse arthralgias in the hands, feet, ankles, and elbows. Skin lesions, which occur most frequently on the extensor surfaces of the hands and feet, may be macular, pustular, hemorrhagic lesions with central necrosis. A small number of patients develop septic arthritis, usually monoarticular arthritis, and gonococci may be isolated from approximately 50% of patients. A few patients may also develop endocarditis or meningitis. A diagnosis of DGI may be based on the identification of gonococci from synovial fluid, blood, or cerebrospinal fluid (CSF). However, DGI must be differentiated from meningococcemia.

Because gonococci are rarely observed in clinical specimens and the organism cannot be isolated from many patients, a presumptive diagnosis of DGI may be based on the isolation of gonococci from a mucosal site in the patient or the patient's sexual partner, the observation of skin lesions on the extremities, or the resolution of symptoms when the patient is treated with an appropriate antimicrobial agent. Cases of DGI have been associated with highly penicillin-susceptible organisms. However, due to recent case reports of antibiotic-resistant strains causing DGI, persons with suspected or confirmed DGI should be treated with appropriate extended-spectrum antimicrobial regimens.

N. meningitidis

Meningococci are isolated most frequently from the oro- or nasopharynges of asymptomatic carriers. Meningococcal colonization may persist for several weeks to several months and may occur in as many as 5 to 15% of individuals; higher carriage rates may occur in confined populations such as military recruits. Because meningococci do not survive well outside their human host and have no alternate host, transmission of meningococcal strains usually occurs by direct contact with contaminated respiratory secretions or airborne droplets. Sexual transmission of meningococcal strains may cause lower genital tract infections in women (37) and homosexual men, resulting in anogenital carriage in addition to oro- and nasopharyngeal carriage (37, 46). Because meningococci may be isolated from anogenital sites infected by gonococci, for medicolegal purposes, it is necessary to identify to the species level neisserial isolates from these sites by confirmatory tests.

Meningococci may disseminate from the nasopharynx to cause meningococcemia and/or meningitis. The incidence of meningococcemia is highest in school-age children, adolescents, and young adults. In some individuals, the disease progresses rapidly, resulting in the fulminant death of a previously healthy person within hours of the onset of symptoms (death rates are as high as 3% in patients with meningococcal meningitis and in 17% of patients with meningococcemia) (85). Close contacts of persons with meningococcemia are at highest risk for acquiring the disease and must receive immediate prophylaxis.

Meningococcemia is usually characterized by profound vascular effects including a petechial or purpuric skin rash that occurs in about 75% of patients. In fulminating infections (Waterhouse-Friderichsen syndrome), fulminant sepsis and disseminated intravascular coagulation occur, resulting in shock and, usually, death.

Meningococci have also caused arthritis—a relatively frequent complication of meningococcemia—and, rarely, purulent conjunctivitis, sinusitis, endocarditis, and primary pneumonia. Persons with inherited deficiencies in their complement systems are at greater risk for acquiring systemic meningococcal infections and may experience repeated episodes. On rare occasions, endocervical meningococcal infections have been associated with PID.

B. catarrhalis

Although *B. catarrhalis* has been recognized as a cause of human infections since the early 1900s, the variety of infections caused by this species has been documented only in the past 10 to 15 years (30). *B. catarrhalis* causes infections ranging from acute, localized infections such as otitis media, sinusitis, and bronchopneumonia to life-threatening, systemic diseases including endocarditis and meningitis. *B. catarrhalis* causes 10 to 15% of cases of otitis media (36) and a similar proportion of cases of sinusitis (53). In addition, this organism causes a large proportion of cases of lower respiratory tract infections in elderly patients with chronic obstructive pulmonary diseases and is only exceeded by *Haemophilus influenzae* and *Streptococcus pneumoniae* as a causative agent of acute purulent exacerbations of chronic bronchitis (30). *B. catarrhalis* is also associated with frank pneumonia. Infections of the maxillary sinuses, middle ear, or bronchi may occur through contiguous spread of organisms from their normal habitat.

The status of *B. catarrhalis* as a member of the oropharyngeal flora deserves reevaluation. Descriptions, in the early 1900s, of *N. catarrhalis* in the normal oropharyngeal flora were probably incorrect; for many years, strains of *N. cinerea* were misidentified as *N. catarrhalis* (56). *B. catarrhalis* is not frequently isolated from the oropharynges of healthy adults (53, 58, 90). The species was, however, isolated from some individuals with signs of respiratory infections but only for the duration of those symptoms (55). Although the species may be part of the normal flora in the nasopharynx or upper respiratory tract rather than in the oropharynx, it is possible that *B. catarrhalis* colonizes in a carrier state, similar to *N. meningitidis*. Additional longitudinal studies of the colonization, by *B. catarrhalis*, of the respiratory tract of healthy children and adults are required to answer this question. From a practical perspective, *B. catarrhalis* must be distinguished from *Neisseria* species in the clinical laboratory.

Other *Neisseria* Species

Most *Neisseria* species isolated from humans are considered commensal inhabitants of the oro- and nasopharynges of healthy persons. *N. flavescens* has been isolated only once in association with an outbreak of meningitis. Most species have been implicated as an etiologic agent in one or more of the following infections: meningitis, bacteremia, endocarditis, empyema, pericarditis, and pneumonia (42). *N. lactamica* has been isolated from the urogenital tract (51). When isolated from normally sterile sites, *N. gonorrhoeae* and *N. meningitidis* must be identified and distinguished from commensal *Neisseria* species. *N. cinerea*, which has been isolated on gonococcal selective media from patients with endocervical and rectal infections, from neonates with conjunctivitis, and from patients with lymphadenitis, has been misidentified repeatedly as *N. gonorrhoeae* (23, 26, 31, 61). *N. lactamica* and *N. polysaccharea*, both of which are isolated on selective media, must be differentiated from *N. meningitidis*. *N. kochii*, considered a subspecies of *N. gonorrhoeae*, has been isolated in Egypt from patients with conjunctivitis and urethritis (56). Strains of *N. kochii* have colonial morphologic characteristics of *N. meningitidis* and biochemical characteristics of *N. gonorrhoeae*. This species has not been described in the United States, but depending on the diagnostic tests used for identification, isolates would be described as *N. gonorrhoeae* or a nontypeable, maltose-negative *N. meningitidis*. Under normal conditions, strains of *N. subflava* biovars and *N. elongata* are part of the normal flora of the oro- or nasopharnyx, and their isolation from these sites should be considered normal. The isolation of *N. subflava* biovars and *N. elongata* from other sites should be considered noteworthy; their identification as etiologic agents of infections, however, should be evaluated in the context of the other organisms isolated from the specimen, where they may occur as secondary colonizers of infections. Occasionally, *Neisseria* species of animal origin may be isolated from bite wounds inflicted by cats or dogs (40, 43). Thus, it is important to keep animal species in mind when the characteristics of a gram-negative, oxidase-positive diplococcus are not those of a described human species.

COLLECTION, TRANSPORT, AND STORAGE OF SPECIMENS FOR CULTURE

N. gonorrhoeae

Specimens for the isolation of *N. gonorrhoeae* may be obtained from the genital tract, urine, anal area, oropharynx, conjunctiva, Bartholin's gland, fallopian tubes, endometrium, blood, joint fluid, skin lesions, or gastric contents of neonates as described in *Cumitech 4A* (33), *Cumitech 17A* (5), and chapter 4 of this Manual (Table 1). A few special precautions and procedures mentioned here may facilitate isolation of the organism. Although endocervical specimens are appropriate for sexually active girls and women, prepubescent females may be infected in the vaginal mucosa. A Dacron or Rayon swab may be rubbed against the posterior vaginal wall for 10 to 15 s to absorb secretions, or if the hymen is intact, the specimen may be collected from the vaginal orifice. Cotton swabs may be used if cotton is treated to neutralize toxicity; cotton swabs should not be used if there is any doubt that the cotton has been treated. Urethral specimens should be collected at least 1 h after the patient has urinated. Clean-catch, midstream urine specimens (5 to 10 ml) should be centrifuged and the sediment should be inoculated onto a selective medium for the isolation of *N. gonorrhoeae*. Anorectal swabs that are contaminated with fecal material should be discarded, and a second specimen should be obtained. Blood cultures may have a low yield because sodium polyanetholsulfonate (SPS), which is found

TABLE 1 Body sites or specimens and culture media for the isolation of *N. gonorrhoeae*, *N. meningitidis*, and *B. catarrhalis*

Species	Syndrome	Gender[a]	Site(s) or specimen(s)	Media
N. gonorrhoeae	Uncomplicated	Female	Endocervix (Bartholin's gland), rectum,[b] urethra, pharynx[b]	Selective
		Male		
		Heterosexual	Urethra	Selective
		Homosexual	Urethra, rectum,[b] pharynx[b]	Selective
	PID	Female	Endocervix, endometrium,[c] fallopian tubes[c]	Selective, nonselective
	DGI		Endocervix (female), urethra (male), skin lesions	Selective, nonselective
			Joint fluid	Nonselective, selective
			Blood	Blood culture medium
	Ophthalmia		Conjunctiva	Nonselective
N. meningitidis	Meningitis		CSF, skin lesions	Nonselective
			Blood	Blood culture medium
			Nasopharynx	Selective, nonselective
B. catarrhalis	Pneumonia		Sputum (transtracheal aspirates)	Nonselective
	Otitis media		Tympanocentesis[d]	Nonselective
	Sinus		Sinus biopsy[d]	Nonselective

[a] Only if samples from different sites of males and females are cultured.
[b] If there is a history of oral-genital or anal-genital exposure.
[c] If a laparoscopic examination is performed.
[d] Not routinely performed.

in most commercial blood culture broths, is toxic for *N. gonorrhoeae*. The toxicity of SPS may be circumvented by using a gelatin-containing medium or collecting the specimen in an Isolator system tube (Wampole, Cranbury, N.Y.) and immediately inoculating the specimen on an SPS-free culture medium. Skin lesion specimens should be kept moist and ground or minced before inoculation of the culture medium. Gonococci are more likely to be isolated from a punch biopsy specimen of skin than from an aspirate; nonselective and selective media should be inoculated.

N. meningitidis

Specimens for the isolation of meningococci should be immediately transported to the laboratory under ambient conditions. These organisms are highly susceptible to temperature extremes and desiccation. Specimens may include CSF, blood, petechial aspirates, biopsy samples, joint fluid, conjunctival swabs, sputum or transtracheal aspirates, and nasopharyngeal swabs. Because there is some evidence that SPS is toxic to *N. meningitidis*, tubes containing this component should not be used for blood specimens when meningococcemia is suspected. Nasopharyngeal swabs produce a higher yield than oropharyngeal specimens.

B. catarrhalis

Tympanocentesis fluid and sinus aspirates are the ideal specimens from which to isolate the causative agents of otitis media and sinusitis, respectively. These specimens are rarely collected because the procedures used to retrieve them are costly and invasive and cause much discomfort to the patient. Thus, these infections are usually treated empirically. On the basis of a comparison of Gram staining and culture results for sputum and transtracheal aspirates, sputum is a satisfactory specimen for the isolation of *B. catarrhalis* from patients with lower respiratory infections (2).

Specimen Transport

The best method for preserving viable organisms is the inoculation of specimens directly onto a nutritive medium and incubation at 35 to 37°C in a CO_2-enriched atmosphere immediately after collection. Specimens from sites with normal flora should be inoculated onto a selective medium such as modified Thayer-Martin (MTM), Martin-Lewis (ML), or New York City (NYC) medium. Nasopharyngeal specimens for *N. meningitidis* may be inoculated onto chocolate and blood agar media. Joint fluid, conjunctival specimens, or specimens from sterile sites may also be inoculated onto a nonselective medium such as chocolate medium supplemented with IsoVitaleX (or an equivalent supplement). Specimens for the isolation of meningococci may be inoculated onto a blood agar medium. If specimens must be transported to a local laboratory and it is not possible to immediately incubate the inoculated media before transport, it is more important to place the inoculated plates in a CO_2-enriched atmosphere than to incubate them at 35 to 37°C. Inoculated media may be held at room temperature in a CO_2-enriched atmosphere in either candle extinction jars or commercial CO_2-generating systems such as JEMBEC plates (65) for up to 5 h without an appreciable loss of viability. If inoculated specimens must be transported between locations in very hot or very cold weather, it is recommended that containers be placed in an insulated Styrofoam container. If specimens must be transported to a distant town, the inoculated media should be incubated for 18 to 24 h before being transported, and the specimen should arrive within 48 h.

Before the development of the nutritive transport systems, specimens for the isolation of gonococci were shipped to laboratories in buffered, nonnutritive transport media. Although gonococci survive in these media for 6 to 12 h, their viability decreases rapidly after 6 to 12 h, so that they may not be recovered after 24 h. In addition, the specimen is diluted, thus reducing the probability of isolating organisms. With the development of commercial zipper-locked, CO_2-generating systems, semisolid transport media such as Stuart's or Amies medium are no longer recommended for the transport of gonococcal specimens.

Media, Specimen Inoculation, and Incubation Conditions

Procedures for the transport of specimens for the isolation, identification, and storage of organisms apply not only to *N. gonorrhoeae* and *N. meningitidis* but also to *B. catarrhalis* and the commensal *Neisseria* and related species which may occasionally be associated with these infections.

Selective Media

Selective media for *N. gonorrhoeae* and *N. meningitidis*, such as MTM and ML media, contain four antimicrobial agents: vancomycin (MTM, 3 μg/ml; ML, 4 μg/ml) to inhibit gram-positive bacteria; colistin (7.5 μg/ml) to inhibit gram-negative bacteria including the commensal *Neisseria* species; trimethoprim lactate (5 μg/ml) to inhibit swarming *Proteus* species; and an antifungal agent (MTM, 13.5 μg of nystatin per ml; ML, 20 μg of anisomycin per ml) (64, 66). NYC medium is a clear medium in which hemolyzed horse erythrocytes, horse plasma, and yeast dialysate are substituted for the hemoglobin and supplements contained in the chocolate agar-based media (34). NYC medium contains the following antimicrobial agents: vancomycin, 2 μg/ml; colistin, 5.5 μg/ml; amphotericin B, 1.2 μ/ml; and trimethoprim lactate, 3 μg/ml. When prepared properly and used while fresh, these media all permit the selective isolation of *N. gonorrhoeae* and *N. meningitidis* while inhibiting the growth of most commensal *Neisseria* species. It should be noted, however, that strains of the commensal species *N. lactamica* and *K. denitrificans* are also routinely isolated on selective media; occasionally, some strains of *N. subflava* bv. perflava, *N. cinerea*, *N. polysaccharea*, and *B. catarrhalis* are also isolated on selective media (3). NYC medium also permits the growth of large-colony mycoplasmas and *Ureaplasma urealyticum* (T-cell mycoplasmas).

Some gonococcal strains, especially AHU strains (so named because they require arginine, hypoxanthine, and uracil for growth on chemically defined media), are susceptible to the concentrations of vancomycin used in selective media. Although AHU isolates accounted for more than 50% of isolates in some geographic regions in the United States in the mid-1970s, they are now rare (83). Still other gonococci may be susceptible to trimethoprim. It is advisable for laboratorians to consider periodic assessment of the adequacy of isolation of potentially more fastidious strains of *N. gonorrhoeae* through a quality assessment program that compares isolation rates on selective and nonselective isolation media.

Nonselective Media

Ideally, specimens from sterile sites such as joint fluids, skin lesions, and conjunctiva should be inoculated onto both nonselective and selective media. A disadvantage of transporting specimens on nonselective media is that any contaminating organism may overgrow a pathogenic species.

Contaminating organisms may be introduced into the specimen during the collection process, during handling of the specimen and its container, or in the condensation that develops during the incubation process. Specimens received on nonselective medium are incubated as described above for specimens received on selective media.

Specimens for the isolation of *B. catarrhalis* and nasopharyngeal specimens for the isolation of *N. meningitidis* may be inoculated onto 5% sheep blood agar in addition to or in place of chocolate agar. Since gonococcal strains may not grow on blood agar, specimens should be inoculated onto chocolate agar if there is a possibility that gonococci will be isolated from the specimen.

Blood Culture Media

Most blood culture media (tryptic soy, Columbia, and brain heart infusion media) support the growth of gonococci and meningococci, provided the inoculated medium is vented and incubated in a CO_2-enriched atmosphere. However, avoid blood culture media that contain SPS, which may be toxic for some strains of *N. gonorrhoeae* and *N. meningitidis*. Media that contain gelatin (Carr Scarborough Microbiological, Decatur, Ga.) neutralize the effect of SPS (32). Lysed blood also neutralizes the toxicity of SPS; thus, cell lysis in the Isolator system (Wampole, Cranbury, N.Y.) overcomes the toxicity of SPS (86).

Incubation Conditions

Gonococci are the most fastidious of the *Neisseria* species, require complex growth media, and are highly susceptible to toxic substances such as fatty acids. In addition, although some gonococci require CO_2 for growth, the growth of all species is enhanced by a CO_2-enriched atmosphere. Thus, cultures for the isolation of *N. gonorrhoeae* or *N. meningitidis* species are always incubated at 35 to 37°C in a CO_2-enriched, humid atmosphere.

CO_2-Enriched Atmosphere

CO_2 incubators are desirable if large numbers of specimens must be processed. Alternate methods for providing a CO_2-enriched atmosphere (candle extinction jars or commercial CO_2-generating systems) may be used when specimens must be transported to a laboratory or when only small numbers of specimens are processed. A candle extinction jar produces a CO_2 concentration of 3 to 5%. It is important (i) to use a nonscented candle (the vapor from scented candles may be toxic) and (ii) to relight the candle if the jar is opened to add more plates.

Humidity

Both gonococci and meningococci require increased humidity for good growth. The humidity in incubation chambers may be increased in several ways: placing a pan of water on the bottom shelf of a CO_2 incubator; placing moistened but not dripping paper towels on the bottom of the candle extinction jar (these should be replaced frequently); or placing a few drops of sterile saline or culture broth onto the surface of the culture medium, allowing it to soak in before inoculation, and sealing the plates in a zipper-locked bag with a CO_2-generating tablet. It is not necessary to replace the moistened towels each time that the jar is opened; however, it is advisable to replace the towels at least once a week to ensure that they do not become a source of contamination, particularly with fungi.

Storage

Cultures

An isolate will usually survive for no longer than 48 h in culture, although some isolates may survive for 72 to 96 h. Isolates should be subcultured every 18 to 24 h to maintain maximum viability. An 18- to 24-h culture should be used for inoculation in any diagnostic test that requires viable organisms and antimicrobial susceptibility tests. Similarly, isolates that are stored by freezing or lyophilization should also be subcultured at least once after the initial recovery culture before being used in a diagnostic test.

Frozen Storage

Long-term storage of gonococcal isolates is achieved with a −70°C freezer, in liquid nitrogen (−196°C), or by lyophilization (freeze drying). To store frozen isolates, dense suspensions of 18- to 24-h pure cultures are prepared in tryptic soy broth containing 20% glycerin. As many as 99% of the cells in a suspension may be destroyed during the freezing and the thawing of the preparations due to physical destruction (shearing) of cells by crystals of the suspending medium that form during the freezing process. For this reason, frozen preparations of gonococcal isolates should not be repeatedly thawed and refrozen. The loss of cells during freezing may be minimized by "flash" freezing the specimen in an acetone or alcohol bath containing dry ice. Some isolates may survive storage at −20°C for up to 2 weeks. The use of freezing media containing glycerin results in a "softer" product from which a sample may be taken with a sterile bacterial loop without thawing the preparation.

Lyophilization

Some laboratories may have access to lyophilization (freeze-drying) facilities. To prepare lyophilates, 18- to 24-h cultures of isolates are suspended in special lyophilization media and are distributed in small aliquots (usually 0.25 to 0.5 ml) in lyophilization ampoules. As with frozen storage, ca. 99% of the organisms are killed during the freezing process. Skim milk is not recommended as a suspending medium for the lyophilization of *Neisseria* species because fatty acids in the milk may be toxic for some organisms and it is impossible to determine the density of the suspension. The suspensions are frozen at −70°C or in an ethanol-dry ice bath and are dried in a vacuum for 18 to 24 h until the moisture has evaporated. The dried preparation should be powdery; if the preparation is syrupy, the vial should be discarded. One ampoule should also be opened immediately to ascertain that the preparation is viable and pure and to verify the identity of the organism and important characteristics, e.g., antimicrobial susceptibilities. Ampoules are best stored at 4 to 10°C or −20°C; storage at room temperature is not recommended. Oxygen may diffuse slowly into the ampoule through the thin seal, particularly with thin-walled ampoules. Thus, one ampoule should be opened every 1 to 2 years to confirm that the preparation is viable. If the preparation is not viable after 48 h of incubation, new ampoules must be prepared.

ISOLATION PROCEDURES

Inoculated Agar Media

Incubate inoculated specimens on selective or nonselective media for up to 72 h, examining plates at 24-h intervals. If no growth is observed after 72 h, the culture should be reported as "no growth." Colonies of *N. gonorrhoeae* vary in diameter from 0.5 to 1.0 mm owing to the formation of different colony types (11). When examining cultures for *N. gonorrhoeae*, remember that AHU strains may produce atypically small colonies (ca. 0.25 mm in diameter) compared with those of most gonococcal strains (0.5 to 1 mm in diameter). In contrast, after incubation for 18 to 24 h, colonies of *N. meningitidis* are usually larger (1 to 2 mm in diameter) and flatter than those of *N. gonorrhoeae*. Colonies of encapsulated serogroup A and C strains may be mucoid. Among the *Neisseria* and related species, colonies of *N. lactamica, N. cinerea, N. polysaccharea, N. kochii*, and *K. denitrificans* are similar in size, appearance, and consistency to those of *N. gonorrhoeae* and *N. meningitidis*. Colonies of *B. catarrhalis* and the saccharolytic species *N. subflava, N. sicca*, and *N. mucosa* are usually 1 to 3 mm in diameter and opaque, and they vary in color from grayish pink (*B. catarrhalis*) to yellow (*N. subflava*). Colonies vary in consistency. The pinkish brown colonies of *B. catarrhalis* have a friable, "hockey puck" consistency and may be moved intact over the surface of the medium with a bacteriologic loop; colonies disintegrate in chunks when broken with a loop. Colonies of *N. subflava* bv. perflava and *N. mucosa* are convex, glistening, and butyrous; colonies of *N. subflava* bv. subflava and *N. subflava* bv. flava are low convex to flat with a matte surface and a slightly friable consistency. Colonies of *N. sicca* may adhere to the agar surface and become wrinkled with prolonged incubation.

Blood Agar

Although many gonococcal strains do not grow on sheep blood agar, the more robust strains may grow quite luxuriantly on this medium. The colonial morphologic characteristics of *Neisseria* species and *B. catarrhalis* on sheep blood agar are similar to those on chocolate agar except for the pigmentation. Like the colonies of *N. lactamica, N. cinerea, N. polysaccharea*, and *N. kochii*, colonies of *N. gonorrhoeae* and *N. meningitidis* on blood agar are grayish to white and more opaque than on chocolate media. Similarly, the pigmentation and opacity of colonies of the other species are more pronounced on blood agar than on chocolate agar.

IDENTIFICATION

Gram Stain

A Gram stain may be performed immediately after the specimen is collected. If smears are too thick, the decolorization process may not adequately decolorize diplococci in clumps or the smear may be overdecolorized, with the result that some gram-positive organisms may appear to be gram negative. If a Gram stain cannot be performed on-site, a smear should be prepared and transported to a laboratory for staining and interpretation.

Gram-stained smears of urethral discharge from men with symptomatic gonococcal urethritis usually contain two or more intracellular, gram-negative diplococci in occasional polymorphonuclear leukocytes (PMNs); many PMNs contain no diplococci (Fig. 1). Other bacteria are rarely seen in these smears. Gram-negative, intracellular diplococci may not be observed in smears from men with early symptomatic infections, although many extracellular diplococci may be observed in stringy, mucoid material.

Gram-stained smears from endocervical and anorectal specimens must be interpreted carefully, with attention being paid to the quality of the smear. If endocervical specimens have been collected properly and are not diluted with cervical mucus or contaminated with vaginal secretions, a reliable observation of gram-negative diplococci may be made. Similarly, mucopurulent material from rectal specimens collected through an anoscope may provide an acceptable specimen for a Gram stain (Fig. 2). However, because both vaginal and anorectal mucosa are colonized with gram-negative coccobacilli and bipolarly staining enteric bacteria, there is a danger of overinterpreting these smears, and results should be considered presumptive until confirmed by culture. Report the Gram stain characteristics, the cell morphology, and the number of all organisms present in the smear together with the types of cells (PMNs, squamous epithelial cells). Note whether intracellular, gram-negative diplococci are observed in PMNs and quantify the number either by the terms few, moderate, or many or by scoring from 1+ to 4+.

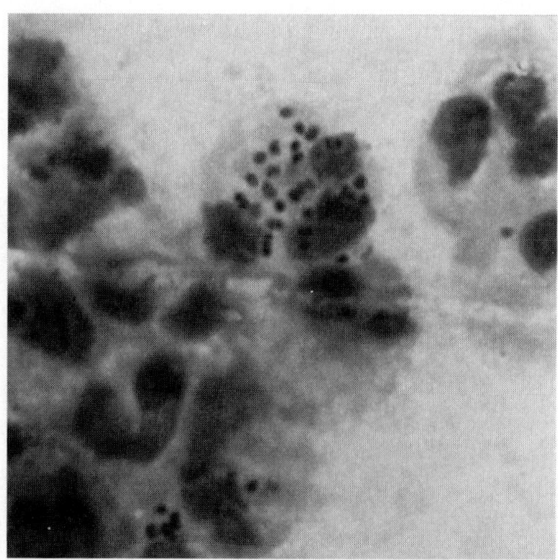

FIGURE 1 Gram stain of male urethral exudate. Some PMNs contain many diplococci; others contain none. Magnification, ×1,500.

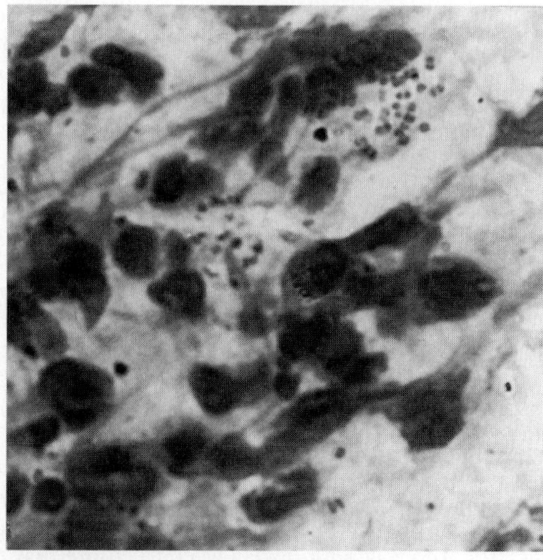

FIGURE 2 Gram stain of mucopurulent rectal exudate showing many diplococci inside PMNs. Magnification, ×1,500.

Antigen Detection, Nucleic Acid Probe Tests, and Nucleic Acid Amplification Tests for *N. gonorrhoeae*

Direct nonculture tests are available for detecting *N. gonorrhoeae* in patient specimens. These tests are useful for screening specimens from patients in geographically isolated locations where culture facilities are not available and specimens for culture confirmation cannot be transported to a laboratory within 48 h of collection. In addition, the development of combination nucleic acid probe tests and nucleic acid amplification tests permits the simultaneous detection of *C. trachomatis* and *N. gonorrhoeae*.

An enzyme-linked immunosorbent assay (Gonozyme; Abbott Laboratories, North Chicago, Ill.) detects gonococcal antigen. This test has been reported to be as sensitive and specific as the Gram stain for detecting gonococci in male urethral specimens and first-void urine specimens (79) but is less sensitive for detecting gonococci in endocervical specimens (84). Because the antigen detection test may cross-react with commensal *Neisseria* and related species (56), this test can be used only to make a presumptive diagnosis of a gonococcal infection.

A direct, nonculture nucleic acid probe test (PACE II [probe assay chemiluminescence enhanced]; GenProbe, San Diego, Calif.) has been used to detect *N. gonorrhoeae* in specimens from patients from populations at high risk for gonorrhea (39, 62, 73). This test detects gonococcal nucleic acid directly in patient specimens in 2 h. This test is highly sensitive and specific for detecting *N. gonorrhoeae* in urogenital and endocervical specimens but is less sensitive for detecting gonococci in pharyngeal and rectal specimens from patients at high risk for gonorrhea (39, 62, 73). There have been small numbers of false-negative (probe-negative, culture-positive) and false-positive (probe-positive, culture-negative) results with this test. A probe competition assay may clarify the result obtained by the initial probe test, especially if the initial result falls in the "gray zone." Because the PACE II test does not allow isolation and confirmed identification of an etiologic agent, culture and definitive identification procedures must be used to identify isolates from nongenital specimens, isolates from sexual abuse or assault victims, and isolates collected to monitor antimicrobial resistance. In addition, the PACE II test should be combined with culture when patients with asymptomatic infections are screened.

Recently, a nucleic acid amplification test, the ligase chain reaction (Abbott Laboratories), has been cleared by the Food and Drug Administration for the detection of *N. gonorrhoeae* in endocervical, urine, and vaginal specimens (12, 44, 87). Additional tests, a PCR (Roche Diagnostic Systems, Branchburg, N.J.) and a transcription-mediated amplification (TMA; GenProbe) test, are being developed for the detection of *N. gonorrhoeae* infections. These tests may also permit the concurrent detection of *C. trachomatis*. Nucleic acid amplification tests do not appreciably increase the number of cases of gonorrhea detected compared with the numbers detected with a proficient specimen transport and culture system. These tests do, however, permit the detection of *N. gonorrhoeae* in urine, thus avoiding the necessity for endocervical examinations and the retrieval of urethral swabs specimens. In addition to technical issues related to these tests, test results must be interpreted with care in the context of a clinical diagnosis. For example, since gonococcal DNA may still be present in specimens for up to 3 weeks after successful treatment of an infection, amplification tests should not be used to assess test of cure. The results of nucleic acid amplification tests may be used only to make a presumptive diagnosis of a gonococcal infection and are inadmissible evidence in medicolegal cases.

Latex Agglutination and Coagglutination Tests for *N. meningitidis*

Currently, there are no immunologic tests that permit the presumptive laboratory identification of gonorrhea by the detection of gonococcal antigens in patient sera. Commercial latex agglutination tests (Becton Dickinson Microbiology Systems, Cockeysville, Md.; Wellcome Diagnostics, Research Triangle Park, N.C.) and coagglutination tests (Pharmacia, Rahway, N.J.) are used to detect meningococcal antigens in body fluids. These kits contain a polyvalent antibody reagent for serogroups A, C, Y, and W135 and a separate reagent for serogroup B that also detects the cross-reacting *Escherichia coli* K1 antigen. Antigen detection tests should always be run in conjunction with Gram stain and culture. Positive results provide a rapid, presumptive diagnosis that permits early administration of appropriate therapy. Negative results do not, however, exclude a diagnosis of meningococcemia. A PCR test has also been developed for the detection of meningococci; however, this test is not commercially available (71).

Multiplex PCR for *B. catarrhalis*

A recent study has indicated that multiplex PCR tests with middle ear effusion specimens may provide a direct method for the presumptive identification of *B. catarrhalis* as an etiologic agent of chronic otitis media (41). This test also offers the advantage that other pathogens, such as *S. pneumoniae*, *H. influenzae*, and *Alloiococcus otitidis*, may also be detected.

IDENTIFICATION

Presumptive Identification

Identification of *Neisseria* and related species may be made at two levels, presumptive and confirmed. A presumptive identification of a neisserial infection may be made with a Gram stain and oxidase test and simply indicates that a gram-negative, oxidase-positive diplococcus has been isolated from a specimen; a laboratory diagnosis of *N. gonorrhoeae* cannot be made on the basis of these tests alone. Although antimicrobial therapy may be initiated on the basis of a presumptive test result, additional tests must be performed to identify (confirm) an isolate.

To perform a Gram stain, a thin smear should be prepared by emulsifying one suspect colony in a drop of water. Care must also be taken to distinguish gram-negative coccobacilli from gram-negative diplococci. Cells of some *K. denitrificans* may appear to be diplococci but can be identified as bacilli by a cell elongation test (Fig. 3) (13). The suspect organism is inoculated onto a chocolate agar plate, and a 10-IU penicillin disk is placed on the inoculated area. After incubation for 18 to 24 h, growth is harvested from the edge of the zone of inhibition and stained with crystal violet or safranin. In subinhibitory concentrations of penicillin, bacilli form long bacillary forms due to their inability to divide. In contrast, true diplococci will retain their characteristic cell morphology.

An oxidase test should also be performed on suspect colonies (remember, however, that oxidase reagents are toxic for gonococci; thus, if oxidase reagent is placed on colonies that must be isolated, they must be subcultured immedi-

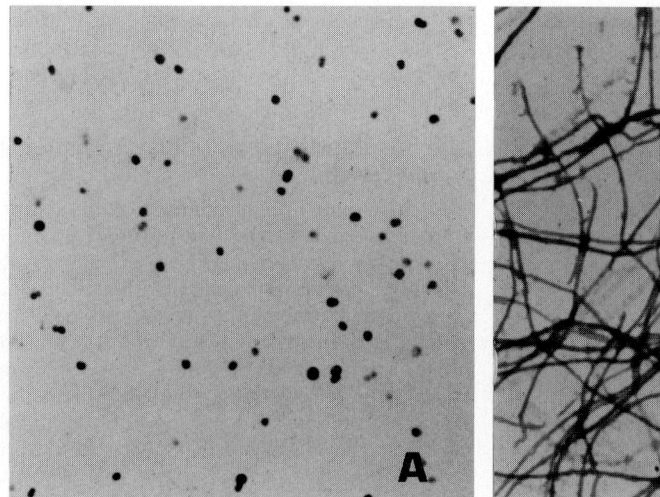
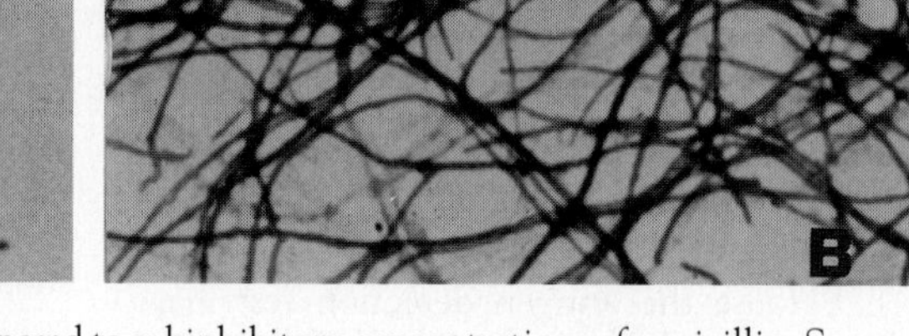

FIGURE 3 Cocci (A) and bacilli (B) exposed to subinhibitory concentrations of penicillin. Some cocci are swollen but still coccoid; bacilli form long strings. Magnification, ×1,000.

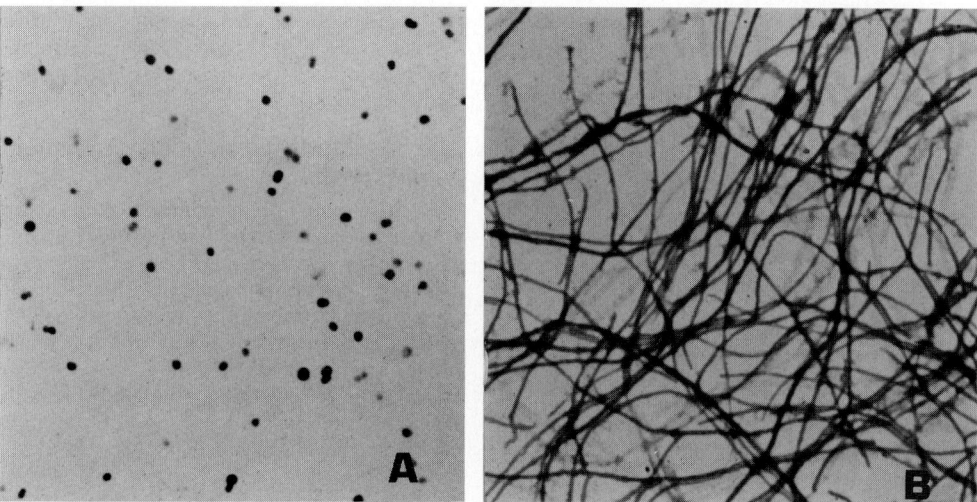

ately). It is preferable not to perform the oxidase test on the plate (particularly when few colonies are present) but to perform the test by Kovac's modification by harvesting growth with a sterile platinum (not nichrome) loop and placing it onto a filter paper freshly impregnated with oxidase reagent. Alternately, dispense a drop of oxidase reagent onto the growth from a suspect colony harvested on a sterile swab; oxidase-positive cells will immediately turn purple. In some instances, only one suspect colony is present on a plate. Because, occasionally, a subculture from this colony may not grow, restreak and reincubate the primary culture plate after preparing a Gram stain, subculturing the colony, and performing an oxidase test by one of the alternative methods; dispersed cells will usually grow luxuriantly and permit isolation of the organism. A presumptive identification of a *Neisseria* species or *B. catarrhalis* may be made when colonies of gram-negative, oxidase-positive diplococci are detected in the culture.

Confirmatory Identification

Members of three genera (*Neisseria, Branhamella,* and *Kingella*) must be considered when *Neisseria* species of clinical importance are being identified; characteristics that differentiate between these genera and the genus *Moraxella* are given in Table 2. Because *N. meningitidis*, commensal *Neisseria* species, and *B. catarrhalis* may occasionally be isolated from infections traditionally associated with *N. gonorrhoeae* and vice versa, tests must be performed to differentiate among these species. Characteristics that differentiate among these and other *Neisseria* spp. are given in Table 3. A variety of commercial tests are available for the identification of *Neisseria* and related species. Tests range from those that measure one parameter of the organism, e.g., detection of acid or enzymes, to tests that measure several parameters, e.g., acid production, enzymes, and nitrate reduction. Most tests are designed to differentiate among species isolated on selective media; thus, when organisms are isolated on nonselective media, it is important to determine if they can grow on selective media, i.e., if they are colistin resistant, before using such tests to identify an isolate. Some tests require inoculation with growth from pure subcultures of suspect colonies on a nonselective medium (chocolate or blood agar), whereas other tests may be inoculated with growth from primary culture plates. In addition, because problems have been identified with most rapid tests, it is important to conduct internal evaluations of any test that will be routinely used to identify organisms. A panel of named strains of *Neisseria* and related species should be used to assess the performance characteristics of the test and to select additional tests that must be performed to identify isolates accurately.

Considering the social and medicolegal implications of misidentifying a gram-negative, oxidase-positive diplococcus, the clinical laboratorian must be skilled in knowing on what specimens tests may be performed, how the tests must be performed, the limitations of the tests chosen to identify an isolate, and additional tests that must be performed to confirm the identity of an isolate. The number of tests that must be performed will depend on the level of identification required. For example, if a specimen has been collected specifically to confirm a clinical diagnosis of gonorrhea or meningococcal infection, tests may be performed specifically to distinguish *N. gonorrhoeae* or *N. meningitidis* from other species. In contrast, if the etiology of an infection is unknown, it will be necessary to identify the organism to the species level. In addition, if specimens have been collected as a result of allegations of sexual abuse or assault, it is also necessary to identify an isolate to the species level; in this instance, the identification must be made with two tests

TABLE 2 Differential characteristics for genera of the family *Neisseriaceae*

Genus	Cell morphology	Oxidase	Catalase	Acid from glucose
Neisseria	Diplococcus/rod	+	+[a]	V[b]
Branhamella	Diplococcus	+	+	−
Kingella	Coccobacillus[c]	+	−	+
Moraxella	Rod	+	+	−

[a] Strains of *N. elongata* may be catalase negative.
[b] Acid from glucose is species dependent.
[c] Cells may appear as diplococci.

TABLE 3 Characteristics of *Neisseria* and related species of human origin[a]

Species	Colony morphology on chocolate medium	Growth on: MTM, ML, and NYC media	Growth on: Chocolate or blood agar (22°C)	Growth on: Nutrient agar (35°C)	Acid from: GLU	Acid from: MAL	Acid from: LAC	Acid from: SUC	Acid from: FRU	Reduction of NO_3	Polysaccharide from SUC	DNase
N. gonorrhoeae[b]	Beige to gray-brown, translucent, smooth, 0.5–1 mm in diam	+	0	0	+	0	0	0	0	0	0	0
N. meningitidis	Beige to gray-brown, translucent, smooth, 1–3 mm in diam, encapsulated, mucoid	+	0	V	+	+	0	0	0	0	0	0
N. lactamica	Beige to gray-brown, translucent, smooth, 1–2 mm in diam	+	V	+	+	+	+	0	0	0	0	0
N. cinerea[c]	Beige to gray-brown to yellowish, translucent, smooth, 1–2 mm in diam	V	0	+	0	0	0	0	0	0	0	0
N. polysaccharea	Beige to gray-brown, translucent, smooth, 1–2 mm in diam	V	+	+	+	+	0	0	0	0	0	0
N. subflava[d]	Greenish yellow, opaque, 1–3 mm in diam, smooth to rough, sometimes adherent	V	+	+	+	+	0	V	V	0	V	0
N. sicca	White, opaque, 1–3 mm in diam, dry, adherent, wrinkled with age	0	+	+	+	+	0	+	+	0	+	0
N. mucosa	Greenish yellow, opaque, 1–3 mm in diam	0	+	+	+	+	0	+	+	+	+	0
N. flavescens	Yellow, opaque, 1–2 mm in diam, smooth	0	+	+	0	0	0	0	0	0	+	0
N. elongata[e]	Gray-brown, translucent, smooth, 1–2 mm in diam, glistening, dry, claylike consistency	0	+	+	0	0	0	0	0	0	0	0
B. catarrhalis	Pinkish-brown, opaque, 1–3 mm in diam, dry, "hockey puck" consistency	V	+	+	0	0	0	0	0	+	0	+
K. denitrificans	Beige to gray-brown, translucent, smooth, 1–2 mm in diam	+	NT	+	+	0	0	0	0	+	0	0

[a] Symbols and abbreviations: +, strains typically positive but genetic mutants may be negative; V, strain dependent; NT, not tested; GLU, glucose; MAL, maltose; LAC, lactose; SUC, sucrose; FRU, fructose.

[b] *N. kochii* is considered to be a subspecies of *N. gonorrhoeae*; isolates of *N. kochii* exhibit characteristics of both *N. gonorrhoeae* and *N. meningitidis* but will be identified as *N. gonorrhoeae*, by tests routinely used for the identification of *Neisseria* spp.

[c] Some strains grow on selective media.

[d] Includes biovars subflava, flava, and perflava. *N. subflava* bv. perflava strains produce acid from sucrose and fructose and produce polysaccharide from sucrose; *N. subflava* bv. flava strains produce acid from fructose; *N. subflava* bv. flava and *N. subflava* bv. subflava do not produce polysaccharide.

[e] Rod-shaped organism. Catalase test is weakly positive or negative compared with those of other *Neisseria* spp. (catalase positive). Results in the table are for *N. elongata* subsp. *elongata*. Strains of *N. elongata* subsp. *glycolytica* may produce a weak acid reaction from D-glucose, are catalase positive, do not reduce nitrate, but reduce nitrite. Strains of *N. elongata* subsp. *nitroreducans*, formerly CDC group M-6, may produce a weak acid reaction from D-glucose, are catalase negative, and reduce nitrate and nitrite.

that measure different parameters, e.g., acid production and biochemical tests or serologic or probe confirmation tests.

Colistin susceptibility is particularly useful for differentiating between the colistin-susceptible, commensal *Neisseria* species and colistin-resistant species, particularly when a specimen has been inoculated only on a nonselective medium. Colistin resistance may be determined either by inoculating the isolate on MTM or ML medium or by placing a 10-μg colistin disk onto an inoculated chocolate agar plate. Strains that grow luxuriantly on selective media or show no inhibition zone in the disk test may be interpreted as being colistin resistant. Strains of *N. gonorrhoeae*, *N. meningitidis*, *N. lactamica*, some strains of *N. polysaccharea*, and *K. denitrificans* are colistin resistant and will grow luxuriantly on colistin-containing media. However, remember also that some strains of *N. cinerea*, *N. subflava* bv. perflava, and *B. catarrhalis* may also be isolated on selective media and may grow when they are subcultured on these media. The performance of a colistin susceptibility test will indicate the appropriateness of the use of confirmatory tests that are designed to differentiate between organisms isolated on selective media.

Biochemical Tests

Acid Production from Carbohydrates

Neisseria and related species may be differentiated by their patterns of acid production from glucose, maltose, lactose, sucrose, and fructose, although acid production from fructose is not routinely determined (Table 3). The advantage of acid production tests is that they provide a reaction profile that permits immediate differentiation among several groups of *Neisseria* species and that their use is not limited to the testing of strains isolated on selective media. Although acid production from carbohydrates by *Neisseria* species has traditionally been determined in CTA (cystine Trypticase agar) Medium containing 1% carbohydrate, this medium is no longer recommended, because it is designed to detect acid production by fermentative organisms and is relatively insensitive for the detection of acid produced by the oxidative *Neisseria* species (56). Rapid methods, e.g., QuadFERM+ (bio-Mérieux Vitek, Hazelwood, Mo.), permit the detection of acid from neisseriae within several hours. The patterns of acid production by strains permit immediate confirmed identification of *N. lactamica* (the only species which produces acid from lactose) and elimination of some other species (*N. subflava* bv. perflava, *N. sicca*, and *N. mucosa*) from further consideration unless species identification is required. Without additional tests, strains of commensal *Neisseria* spp. may be misidentified as *N. gonorrhoeae*, *N. meningitidis*, or *B. catarrhalis* (21). *N. polysaccharea*, *N. subflava* bv. flava, and *N. subflava* bv. subflava, which produce acid from glucose and maltose, may be misidentified as *N. meningitidis* (21). *K. denitrificans*, which produces acid from glucose, may be misidentified as *N. gonorrhoeae* (21). *N. cinerea* may be misidentified as *B. catarrhalis* in some tests if additional differential tests are not performed (21). In addition to confusion between species with identical acid production patterns, false-positive and false-negative acid reactions have resulted in misidentification of some isolates. Specifically, some gonococcal isolates, particularly AHU isolates, have been described as glucose negative because they failed to produce detectable acid in some tests. Conversely, some strains of *N. cinerea*, which are considered glucose negative, may produce weak acid reactions from glucose in some tests (28, 56).

Chromogenic Enzyme Substrate Tests

Enzyme substrate tests (Gonochek II [bio-Mérieux Vitek], Identicult-Neisseria [Adams Scientific, West Warwick, R.I.]) permit rapid differentiation among species isolated on gonococcal selective media; differentiation is limited, however, to *N. gonorrhoeae*, *N. meningitidis*, *N. lactamica*, and *B. catarrhalis*. *N. lactamica* produces β-galactosidase, *N. meningitidis* produces γ-glutamylaminopeptidase, and *N. gonorrhoeae* produces hydroxyprolylaminopeptidase; *B. catarrhalis* produces none of these enzymes (24). The major problem associated with enzyme substrate tests is that strains of *N. cinerea*, *N. polysaccharea*, *N. sicca*, *N. mucosa*, the *N. subflava* biovars, and *K. denitrificans* are hydroxyprolylaminopeptidase positive and may be misidentified as *N. gonorrhoeae* if tested only by an enzyme substrate test (21). In spite of these problems, enzyme substrate tests permit differentiation between *N. meningitidis* (γ-glutamylaminopeptidase-positive) and *N. polysaccharea* and *N. subflava* biovars (hydroxyprolylaminopeptidase positive, γ-glutamylaminopeptidase negative) and maltose-negative variants of *N. meningitidis* (γ-glutamylaminopeptidase positive) which may be misidentified in acid production tests (82).

Multitest Identification Systems

Some commercial tests include not only acid production tests but also other biochemical tests, including tests for enzyme substrates, DNase, nitrate reduction, and β-lactamase production; some of these tests are intended for the concurrent identification of *Haemophilus* and *Neisseria* and related species. These systems identify *N. gonorrhoeae*, *N. meningitidis*, and *B. catarrhalis*, although additional tests may be required to identify some isolates (47, 48, 78). The QuadFERM+ test is a multitest system in which a DNase test (which differentiates between *N. cinerea* [DNase negative] and *B. catarrhalis* [DNase positive]) is included with acid production tests and a β-lactamase test. No problems have been reported with the acid production component of this test; *N. cinerea* does not produce detectable acid, and AHU gonococcal isolates produce clearly positive acid reactions from glucose. Some problems have been encountered with the β-lactamase test, which is an acidometric test in this product.

Serologic Tests for Identification of *N. gonorrhoeae*

Fluorescent-Antibody Tests

A monoclonal fluorescent-antibody test (*Neisseria gonorrhoeae* Culture Confirmation Test; Syva Co., Palo Alto, Calif.) is available for the culture confirmation of *N. gonorrhoeae*. Although this test is sensitive and specific (56), some gonococcal strains do not react with this reagent (56), and nonspecific Fc binding with nongonococcal isolates may occur if mixed cultures are used. The advantage of this test is that it can be performed with growth from a single colony of a gram-negative organism on a primary isolation plate even if the culture is not pure.

Coagglutination Tests for *N. gonorrhoeae*

Two coagglutination tests are available: these are the Phadebact GC Monoclonal Antibody test (Karo Bio Diagnostics AB, Huddinge, Sweden), which permits subgrouping of gonococcal isolates into WI (protein IA) and WII/WIII (protein IB) groups, and the GonoGen I (New Horizons Diagnostics, Columbia, Md.). Tests are performed in a similar manner; test and control reagents are reacted with a

TABLE 4 Characteristics of *Neisseria* species of animal origin[a]

Species	Cell morphology	Acid from:				Reduction of:		Polysaccharide from SUC	Tributyrin hydrolysis
		GLU	MAL	LAC	SUC	NO_3	NO_2		
N. canis	Diplococcus	0	0	0	0	+	0	0	0
N. caviae	Diplococcus	0	0	0	0	+	+	NT	+
N. cuniculi	Diplococcus	0	0	0	0	0	0	NT	+
N. macacae	Diplococcus	+	+	+	+	−	+	+	−
N. iguanae	Diplococcus	V	0	NT	0	+	V	+	NT
N. ovis	Diplococcus	0	0	0	0	+	0	NT	+
N. weaveri	Rod	0	0	0	0	0	+	NT	NT

[a] Data are from previous reports (6, 43, 91, 92). Symbols and abbreviations: +, strains typically positive but genetic mutants may be negative (−); V, strain dependent; NT, not tested; GLU, glucose; MAL, maltose; LAC, lactose; SUC, sucrose.

drop of a boiled suspension of suspect organisms. A positive reaction is recorded if an agglutinin is formed with the test reagent but not with the control reagent. Because coagglutination tests can be performed with growth from primary culture plates, an identification of *N. gonorrhoeae* may be obtained some 24 h earlier than is possible with tests that require a pure culture for inoculation. However, some gonococcal strains have not reacted in these tests, and cross-reactions have been noted with strains of *N. meningitidis*, *N. lactamica*, *N. cinerea*, and *K. denitrificans* in tests performed in accordance with the manufacturer's directions (56). Thus, an alternative test should be used to confirm an identification of *N. gonorrhoeae* when (i) isolates suspected of being gonococci fail to react or give equivocal reactions with a reagent, (ii) positive reactions are obtained with isolates from extragenital sites in patients at low risk for gonorrhea, and (iii) positive reactions are obtained with isolates from genital or extragenital sites from children, whether or not sexual abuse is suspected.

Gonogen II

Gonogen II is a serologic test in which monoclonal antibodies have been conjugated to colloidal gold. Colonies of suspect organisms are suspended in a lysing solution, a drop of which is mixed with the monoclonal antibody-gold conjugate. After mixing for 2 to 10 min, the mixture is passed through a microfilter that retains the antigen-antibody complex. When *N. gonorrhoeae* is present, a red color is seen on the filter; with nongonococcal isolates, the filter remains white or becomes pale pink.

Nucleic Acid Probe Culture Confirmation Tests

A DNA probe test (AccuProbe; Gen-Probe) is a culture confirmation test for *N. gonorrhoeae* (63). The test format is similar to that of the PACE II nonculture test for the direct detection of *N. gonorrhoeae* in specimens. This test is highly sensitive and specific for the identification of *N. gonorrhoeae* compared with rapid acid production and coagglutination tests (97).

Additional Tests

Nitrate and Nitrite Reduction Tests

The nitrate reduction test is useful for differentiating between strains of *N. gonorrhoeae* (nitrate negative) and *K. denitrificans* or *B. catarrhalis* (nitrate positive). The nitrate test is performed in a standard nitrate broth which is inoculated heavily to give a dense suspension of organisms. The nitrite reduction test is performed in a similar base medium containing nitrite (0.1%, 0.01%, and 0.001%). Although the nitrite reduction test is not useful for differentiating between human *Neisseria* spp., both the nitrate and nitrite reduction tests are important for differentiating between neisserial species of animal origin (Table 4).

Superoxol Test

The superoxol test is analogous to the catalase test, but it is performed with a 30% hydrogen peroxide solution and has been recommended for differentiating between *N. gonorrhoeae* and other *Neisseria* and related species (4). Reagent is dropped onto growth on a chocolate (not blood) agar plate, and the degree of bubbling is observed. Gonococci typically give an immediate, explosive (++++) reaction. Reevaluation of this test shows that most *Neisseria* spp. give weak reactions (++) with the superoxol reagent, although some strains of *N. meningitidis* and *B. catarrhalis* may give ++++ reactions in this test (96). This test may be most useful for differentiating between *N. gonorrhoeae* strains (++++ reaction) and *N. cinerea* strains (++ reaction) and *K. denitrificans* (superoxol negative) (96).

Polysaccharide from Sucrose

The polysaccharide test is not commercially available but is particularly useful for differentiating between *N. polysaccharea* (polysaccharide positive) and *N. meningitidis* (polysaccharide negative). Strains of *N. flavescens* are polysaccharide positive, as are strains of *N. subflava* bv. perflava, *N. sicca*, and *N. mucosa*; strains of *N. subflava* bv. flava and *N. subflava* bv. subflava are polysaccharide negative. The test is performed on a starch-free base medium that supports growth of the organism and to which 1% sucrose is added. The traditional medium with 5% sucrose is inhibitory for many strains (58). Inoculated media are incubated at 35 to 37°C for 24 to 48 h. A drop of Gram's iodine is added to isolated colonies; if polysaccharide has been produced, the growth will immediately turn dark brown to purple. The reaction will fade with time but can be redeveloped by adding more iodine solution. The inoculated medium should be tested for no longer than the 48 h of incubation, since polysaccharide-producing organisms will metabolize the polysaccharide on prolonged incubation, resulting in the possibility of a false-negative reaction. It should also be noted that some commercially prepared Gram's iodine solutions will not produce a positive reaction with polysaccharide-positive *Neisseria* spp.

Tributyrin Hydrolysis

B. catarrhalis strains hydrolyze tributyrin, whereas other human *Neisseria* species do not metabolize this substrate. Several tests have been developed to detect this activity and provide a rapid method for confirming this species (74).

STRAIN TYPING SYSTEMS

N. gonorrhoeae

Typing systems used to differentiate between strains of *N. gonorrhoeae* include auxotyping (a nutritional typing system) and serotyping with monoclonal antibodies in coagglutination tests (60, 83). A dual auxotype-serovar classification system provides greater discrimination among strains than is possible with either typing system alone (83). Auxotyping involves determination of the requirement of strains for individual metabolites for growth on a chemically defined medium. For example, if a strain fails to grow on a medium from which arginine has been omitted, the strain is recorded as arginine requiring. Thus, strains with single or multiple growth requirements may be identified. Serotyping is performed with a panel of monoclonal antibody coagglutination reagents; monoclonal antibodies are directed against epitopes on the protein I molecule in the gonococcal outer membrane (83). Strains are divided into two major serogroups, serogroups IA and IB, on the basis of the protein I species expressed by the strain; further subdivision into serovars is made according to patterns of reaction with a panel of six protein IA- and protein IB-specific antibody reagents. Typing systems are not used for the identification of isolates as *N. gonorrhoeae*. Rather, they are used to compare isolates for molecular epidemiologic investigations, which may range from studies of the dynamics of gonococcal strains in communities and the geographic spread of antimicrobial-resistant strains to comparison between strains for medicolegal investigations (60, 83).

Gonococcal isolates may also be characterized by their plasmid content. At least six different β-lactamase plasmids have been described in *N. gonorrhoeae*; these as well as two conjugative plasmids (one possessing a TetM determinant) have also been used to study the distribution of gonococcal strains (83). Strains possessing the TetM determinant may, with PCR-based tests, be assigned to one of two types: American or Dutch (45). Mutations in the *gyrA* and *parC* genes in strains exhibiting decreased susceptibilities to fluoroquinolones may also be characterized (25). In addition, molecular typing methods such as pulsed-field gel electrophoretic techniques, which allow characterization of strains with no distinct antimicrobial resistance patterns, have been used to study gonococcal strains that do not exhibit distinct antimicrobial resistance patterns (95).

N. meningitidis

Meningococci are subgrouped into serological groups on the basis of the presence of capsular polysaccharide or outer membrane protein antigens. Although 13 serogroups are currently recognized (A, B, C, D, 29E, H, I, K, L, W135, X, Y, and Z), strains belonging to groups A, B, C, Y, and W135 are most frequently implicated in systemic disease (98). Classically, group A and C strains cause epidemic meningococcal disease; group B strains are usually associated with sporadic infections during interepidemic periods, although they have been implicated in localized outbreaks. In recent years, group Y strains have increasingly been reported from patients with meningococcal pneumonia (22). During epidemics, carriers tend to be colonized with the prevailing serogroup. Other serogroups associated with conditions of crowding (military recruits) and social disruption (refugees) are isolated sporadically from both carriers and patients with disease. In sub-Saharan Africa and certain Scandinavian countries, outbreaks of meningococcal group A and C disease are common. In North America, groups B and C are commonly associated with sporadic cases of septicemia and/or meningitis and, occasionally, with regionally contained outbreaks. The utility of other methods for molecular epidemiologic typing, including antigenic analyses of outer membrane proteins, multilocus enzyme electrophoresis, ribotyping, PCR, and pulsed-field gel electrophoresis, is being investigated (1, 54, 88, 94).

ANTIBIOTIC SUSCEPTIBILITIES

Antimicrobial resistance is now widespread among strains of *N. gonorrhoeae* and occurs as both chromosomally mediated resistance to a variety of agents and plasmid-mediated resistance to penicillins (penicillinase [β-lactamase] producing) and to tetracycline (tetracycline-resistant *N. gonorrhoeae*) (52, 75). Owing to the increased frequency of penicillin- and tetracycline-resistant strains of *N. gonorrhoeae* (Fig. 4), CDC has recommended that selected extended-spectrum cephalosporins and newer fluoroquinolones be used as primary therapy against uncomplicated gonococcal infections (20). Although tetracycline is no longer recommended for the treatment of gonorrhea, dual therapy including tetracycline or azithromycin is recommended for the empiric treatment of concurrent chlamydial infections. Although CDC no longer recommends test-of-cure cultures, if symptoms persist after treatment with one of the recommended thera-

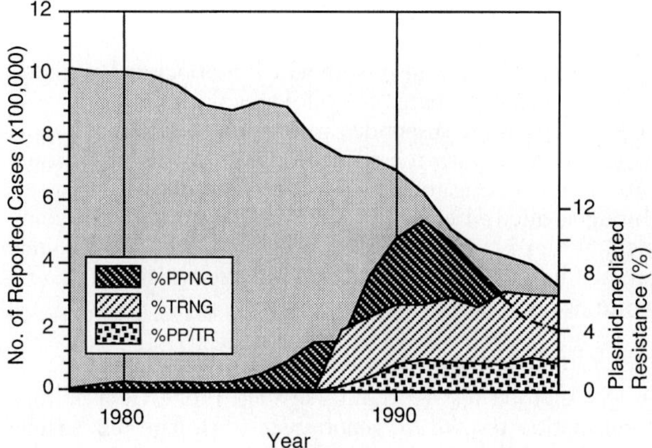

FIGURE 4 Percentage of cases of gonorrhea and frequency of gonorrhea caused by strains of *N. gonorrhoeae* with plasmid-mediated resistance to penicillin (PPNG), tetracycline (TRNG), and both penicillin and tetracycline (PP/TR) in the United States, 1978 to 1996, compared with the total number of reported cases. The number of cases of infection with strains with plasmid-mediated resistance to penicillin are based on a combination of passive surveillance of strains with plasmid-mediated resistance to penicillin (1978 to 1987) and data provided by active surveillance in the Gonococcal Isolate Surveillance Project. Data for *N. gonorrhoeae* strains resistant to tetracycline and to both penicillin and tetracycline are provided by the Gonococcal Isolate Surveillance Project.

pies, patients should be reevaluated for *N. gonorrhoeae* infection and the susceptibilities of any resulting gonococcal isolate should be determined (20). Although resistance to extended-spectrum cephalosporins has not been documented, failure of infections to respond to treatment with CDC-recommended doses of fluoroquinolones (MIC of ciprofloxacin, $\geq$1.0 μg/ml; MIC of ofloxacin, $\geq$2.0 μg/ml) has been documented (17, 76, 89); strains with clinically significant resistance to fluoroquinolones are now widespread in the Far East (57). Strains exhibiting decreased susceptibility to fluoroquinolones are endemic in Ohio (35).

The susceptibilities of gonococcal isolates are determined by an agar dilution method or by a disk diffusion method recommended by the National Committee for Clinical Laboratory Standards (68–70). β-Lactamase production may be determined by a highly sensitive nitrocefin test (72). Ideally, susceptibilities to penicillin, tetracycline, spectinomycin, an extended-spectrum cephalosporin, and a fluoroquinolone should be determined. At a minimum, susceptibilities to the agents routinely used to treat gonorrhea should be determined; in clinical settings where PID is treated, susceptibility to antigonococcal agents (cefoxitin or cefotetan) recommended for the treatment of PID, should be tested. Because more isolates have remained susceptible to extended-spectrum cephalosporins, resistance to both penicillin and tetracycline may serve as an indicator of decreased susceptibility to the extended-spectrum cephalosporins (93). Determination of spectinomycin susceptibilities is recommended if this agent is used as an alternative therapy for uncomplicated gonococcal infections.

Because resistance to fluoroquinolones has emerged and resistance to extended-spectrum cephalosporins may emerge, it is important to determine the susceptibilities of gonococcal isolates from patients whose symptoms persist after treatment. Isolates that exhibit resistance or decreased susceptibility to the agent (zone inhibition diameter less than the criterion for susceptibility) should be submitted to a reference laboratory for confirmation. If possible, laboratories should implement a routine surveillance program to monitor the susceptibilities of gonococcal isolates in order to detect changes that may indicate the emergence of clinically significant resistance to therapeutic agents that may compromise treatment outcomes.

N. meningitidis

Although penicillin G has remained effective for the treatment of meningococcal infections including meningitis, meningococci exhibiting chromosomally mediated and plasmid-mediated resistance to penicillin and tetracycline have been reported (29, 67). Chloramphenicol is still recommended as an alternative for treating meningococcal infections in patients allergic to penicillin. Because of the development of resistance over the years, sulfonamides are no longer recommended for the treatment of meningococcal infections.

The narrow-spectrum cephalosporins are not recommended for therapy of meningococcal disease. In vitro susceptibility studies of newer extended-spectrum cephalosporins, e.g., cefotaxime, ceftriaxone, cefoperazone, and ceftizoxime, have demonstrated the excellent activities of these agents against meningococcal isolates.

Chemoprophylaxis is recommended to reduce nasopharyngeal meningococcal carriage, particularly in contacts of patients with meningococcal infection and in potential contacts in families, military installations, schools, and closed populations, to prevent further transmission and disease. Rifampin, minocycline, and more recently, some of the newer fluoroquinolones, e.g., ciprofloxacin, reduce the meningococcal carrier state.

B. catarrhalis

In the early antibiotic era, *B. catarrhalis* was highly susceptible to penicillins, but currently an estimated 85% of strains produce β-lactamase. Recent in vitro susceptibility testing of *B. catarrhalis* has shown that the majority of clinical isolates remain susceptible to cephamycins, cephalosporins, β-lactamase-stable penicillins (e.g., amoxicillin-clavulanate), tetracyclines, and trimethoprim-sulfamethoxazole. Limited experience with quinolones suggests that these agents are active against β-lactamase-positive and -negative strains.

Other *Neisseria* Species

Comprehensive in vitro susceptibility data are not available for commensal *Neisseria* species. Occasional reports of clinical disease caused by other *Neisseria* species such as endocarditis, meningitis, empyema, pneumonia, and ocular infections should prompt clinicians to administer antimicrobial therapy guided by in vitro susceptibility testing. Generally, commensal *Neisseria* species have been reported to be susceptible at least in vitro to penicillin, ampicillin, and tetracyclines, although some strains may possess the Tet M determinant. Strains of *N. cinerea*, however, appear to exhibit uniformly decreased susceptibility or resistance to erythromycin (MICs, 4 to 16 μg/ml) when tested by procedures for *N. gonorrhoeae* (55). This is of some concern because ocular infections with *N. cinerea* in newborns may not respond to prophylaxis with erythromycin ointment (9). Thus, in vitro susceptibility testing is recommended for any gram-negative, oxidase-positive diplococcus isolated from ocular and other clinically relevant specimens.

EVALUATION, INTERPRETATION, AND REPORTING OF RESULTS

The level of testing and the format for reporting of laboratory results should be directed by the sociodemographic characteristics, e.g., age and gender of the patient clientele served, and a working knowledge of the incidence and prevalence of clinically significant disease caused by *Neisseria* species, e.g., gonorrhea or meningococcal meningitis, in that population. When specimens are collected from patients at high risk for gonorrhea and there are no sociologic or medicolegal implications of a diagnosis of gonorrhea, a presumptive identification of *N. gonorrhoeae* may be sufficient if the diagnosis is intended to facilitate prompt and effective treatment of infections. However, when specimens are collected to confirm a clinical diagnosis in patients, e.g., women and children at low risk for gonorrhea, special concerns apply to the laboratory processing and retention of specimens because of the medicolegal consequences that may ensue if an organism is identified as *N. gonorrhoeae*. Laboratorians and clinicians must know the patient population that they serve and decide to what levels of specificity identifications of *Neisseria* and related species must be made.

Special protocols should be developed for processing specimens from alleged victims of sexual abuse and assault. In these instances, organism identifications must be confirmed by at least two confirmatory tests that detect different characteristics of the organism. It must be emphasized also that accurate communication between the clinician and laboratory is essential to ensure that specimens of potential medicolegal importance are processed according to these criteria. In too many instances, because a specimen has not been clearly marked as being from a child, an organism has been identified with only one confirmatory test and discarded according to a routine protocol.

In general, however, with the exception of high-risk patients for whom presumptive identifications may suffice, similar principles apply to the identification of all gram-negative, oxidase-positive diplococci. Many tests are available for the confirmation of the identities of gram-negative, oxidase-positive diplococcal isolates from clinical specimens. Although many tests for the identification of *Neisseria* and related species are marketed as confirmatory tests, most do not provide sufficient information to accurately identify an isolate to the species level without the performance of additional tests. As noted earlier in the chapter, several species may give identical reactions in some tests; e.g., maltose-negative *N. meningitidis* and *K. denitrificans* may give reactions identical to those of *N. gonorrhoeae* in some acid production tests. In addition, problems have been identified with most tests for the identification of *N. gonorrhoeae* and related species, e.g., false-negative acid production reactions from glucose with *N. gonorrhoeae* or false-positive reactions from glucose with *N. cinerea.*

Culture confirmation tests are preferred for the identification of *Neisseria* and related species because they require the isolation of an organism which can be examined by multiple tests if the results of the primary tests are equivocal. In general, multitest systems provide the most information about several biochemical characteristics that may, in some cases, allow identification of an isolate. These tests are most useful if identification to the species level is required and may help characterize isolates in rare instances when hybrid organisms may be isolated (56). Rapid identification tests, including serologic and nucleic acid probe or amplification tests, that provide a yes-no answer, i.e., an isolate either is or is not *N. gonorrhoeae*, may be adequate if it is necessary only to eliminate *N. gonorrhoeae* as the causative agent; these tests are of limited usefulness when identification to the species level is required.

Reporting

Because of the serious social and medicolegal consequences of misdiagnosing gonorrhea or misidentifying strains of *N. gonorrhoeae*, CDC has recommended criteria for reporting diagnoses of gonorrhea (16). Three levels of diagnosis are defined: these are suggestive, which is defined on the basis of clinical findings; presumptive; and definitive, with the last two levels including the results of laboratory diagnostic tests.

A suggestive diagnosis is defined by the presence of (i) a mucopurulent endocervical or urethral exudate on physical examination and (ii) sexual exposure to a person infected with *N. gonorrhoeae*. A presumptive diagnosis of gonorrhea is made on the basis of two of the following three criteria: (i) typical gram-negative intracellular diplococci on microscopic examination of a smear of urethral exudate (men) or endocervical secretions (women); (ii) growth of *N. gonorrhoeae* from the urethra (men) or endocervix (women) on culture medium and demonstration of typical colonial morphology, positive oxidase reaction, and typical gram-negative morphology; and/or (iii) detection of *N. gonorrhoeae* by nonculture laboratory tests (e.g., antigen detection, nucleic acid probe tests, or nucleic acid amplification tests). A definitive diagnosis requires (i) isolation of *N. gonorrhoeae* from sites of exposure (e.g., urethra, endocervix, throat, or rectum) by culture (usually on a selective medium) and demonstration of typical colonial morphology, positive oxidase reaction, and typical gram-negative morphology and (ii) confirmation of isolates by biochemical, enzymatic, serologic, or nucleic acid tests, e.g., carbohydrate utilization, rapid enzyme substrate tests, serologic methods such as coagglutination or fluorescent-antibody tests, or DNA probe confirmation test.

For reporting purposes, the laboratory should perform species-level identification and confirmation with appropriate tests in order to report a definitive result of "*N. gonorrhoeae* confirmed" for the clinician unless otherwise requested. If an organism suspected to be *N. gonorrhoeae* is tested by rapid tests but not by additional confirmatory tests that compensate for problems associated with the primary test and is reported as "presumptive *N. gonorrhoeae*," it is important that a clinician receiving this report understands that additional tests may be required to confirm this identification. Ideally, to avoid confusion, an organism should be reported only as "gram-negative, oxidase-positive diplococcus isolated" unless it has been identified to the species level with sufficient tests to ensure the accuracy of the identification.

REFERENCES

1. **Achtman, M., B. A. Crowe, A. Olyhoek, W. Strittmatter, and G. Morelli.** 1988. Recent results on epidemic meningococcal meningitis. *J. Med. Microbiol.* **26:**172–177.
2. **Ainsworth, S. M., S. B. Nagy, L. A. Morgan, G. R. Miller, and J. L. Perry.** 1990. Interpretation of Gram-stained sputa containing *Moraxella (Branhamella) catarrhalis. J. Clin. Microbiol.* **28:**2559–2560.
3. **Anand, C. M., F. Ashton, H. Shaw, and R. Gordon.** 1991. Variability in growth of *Neisseria polysaccharea* on colistin-containing selective media for *Neisseria* spp. *J. Clin. Microbiol.* **29:**2434–2437.
4. **Arko, R. J., and T. Odugbemi.** 1984. Superoxol and amylase inhibition tests for distinguishing gonococcal and nongonococcal cultures growing on selective media. *J. Clin. Microbiol.* **20:**1–4.
5. **Baron, E. J., G. H. Cassell, L. B. Duffy, D. A. Eschenbach, J. R. Greenwood, S. M. Harvey, N. E. Madinger, E. M. Peterson, and K. B. Waites.** 1993. *Cumitech 17A: Laboratory Diagnosis of Female Genital Tract Infections.* Coordinating ed., E. J. Baron. American Society for Microbiology, Washington, D.C.
6. **Barrett, S. J., L. K. Slater, R. J. Montall, and P. H. A. Sneath.** 1994. A new species of *Neisseria* from iguanid lizards, *Neisseria iguanae* sp. nov. *Lett. Appl. Microbiol.* **18:** 200–202.
7. **Blakebrough, I. S., V. M. Greenwood, H. C. Whittle, A. K. Bradley, and H. M. Gilles.** 1982. Epidemiology of infections due to *Neisseria meningitidis* and *Neisseria lactamica* in a northern Nigerian community. *J. Infect. Dis.* **146:** 626–637.
8. **Boquete, M. T., C. Marcos, and J. A. Saez-Niéto.** 1986. Characterization of *Neisseria polysacchareae* sp. nov. (Riou, 1983) in previously unidentified noncapsular strains of *Neisseria meningitidis. J. Clin. Microbiol.* **24:**973–975.
9. **Bourbeau, P., V. Holla, and S. Piemontese.** 1990. Ophthalmia neonatorum caused by *Neisseria cinerea. J. Clin. Microbiol.* **28:**1640–1641.
10. **Bøvre, K.** 1984. Family VIII. *Neisseriaceae* Prévot, p. 288–309. *In* N. R. Krieg (ed.), *Manual of Systematic Bacteriology*, vol. 1. The Williams & Wilkins Co., Baltimore, Md.
11. **Brown, W. J., and S. J. Kraus.** 1974. Gonococcal colony types. *JAMA* **228:**862–863.
12. **Buimer, M., G. J. J. van Doornum, S. Ching, P. G. H.**

Peerbooms, P. K. Plier, D. Ram, and H. H. Lee. 1996. Detection of *Chlamydia trachomatis* and *Neisseria gonorrhoeae* by ligase chain reaction-based assays with clinical specimens from various sites: implications for diagnostic testing and screening. *J. Clin. Microbiol.* **34:**2395–2400.

13. **Catlin, B. W.** 1975. Cellular elongation under the influence of antibacterial agents: way to differentiate coccobacilli from cocci. *J. Clin. Microbiol.* **1:**102–105.
14. **Catlin, B. W.** 1991. *Branhamaceae* fam. nov., a proposed family to accommodate the genera *Branhamella* and *Moraxella*. *Int. J. Syst. Bacteriol.* **41:**320–323.
15. **Centers for Disease Control.** 1987. Antibiotic-resistant strains of *Neisseria gonorrhoeae*: policy guidelines for detection, management, and control. *Morbid. Mortal. Weekly Rep.* **36**(Suppl. 5S)**:**1S–18S.
16. **Centers for Disease Control.** 1991. *Sexually Transmitted Diseases Clinical Practice Guidelines*. Centers for Disease Control, Atlanta, Ga.
17. **Centers for Disease Control and Prevention.** 1995. Fluoroquinolone resistance in *Neisseria gonorrhoeae*—Colorado and Washington, 1995. *Morbid. Mortal. Weekly Rep.* **44:** 761–764.
18. **Centers for Disease Control and Prevention.** 1997. *Sexually Transmitted Diseases Surveillance 1996*. Centers for Disease Control and Prevention, Atlanta, Ga.
19. **Centers for Disease Control and Prevention.** 1997. Gonorrhea among men who have sex with men—selected sexually transmitted diseases clinics, 1993–1996. *Morbid. Mortal. Weekly Rep.* **4:**889–902.
20. **Centers for Disease Control and Prevention.** 1998. 1998 Sexually transmitted diseases treatment guidelines. *Morbid. Mortal. Weekly Rep.* **47:**59–63.
21. **Centers for Disease Control and Prevention.** 1998. *Identification of* Neisseria *and Related Species*. Electronic publication (http://www.cdc.gov/ncidod/dastlr/gcdir/NeIdent/Index.html). Centers for Disease Control and Prevention, Atlanta, Ga.
22. **Centers for Disease Control and Prevention.** 1996. Serogroup Y meningococcal disease—Illinois, Connecticut, and selected areas, United States, 1989–1996. *Morbid. Mortal. Weekly Rep.* **45:**1010–1013.
23. **Clausen, C. R., J. S. Knapp, and P. A. Totten.** 1984. Lymphadenitis due to *Neisseria cinerea*. *Lancet* **i:**908.
24. **D'Amato, R. F., L. A. Eriquez, K. M. Tomfohrde, and E. Singerman.** 1978. Rapid identification of *Neisseria gonorrhoeae* and *Neisseria meningitidis* by using enzyme profiles. *J. Clin. Microbiol.* **7:**77–81.
25. **Deguchi, T., M. Yasuda, M. Nakano, S. Ozeki, T. Ezaki, I. Saito, and Y. Kawada.** 1996. Quinolone-resistant *Neisseria gonorrhoeae*: correlations of alterations in the GyrA subunit of DNA gyrase and the ParC subunit of topoisomerase IV with antimicrobial susceptibility profiles. *Antimicrob. Agents Chemother.* **40:**1020–1023.
26. **Denison, M. R., S. Perlman, and R. D. Anderson.** 1988. Misidentification of *Neisseria* species in a neonate with conjunctivitis. *Pediatrics* **81:**877–878.
27. **Dewhirst, F. E., B. H. Paster, and P. L. Bright.** 1989. *Chromobacterium*, *Eikenella*, *Kingella*, *Neisseria*, *Simonsiella*, and *Vitreoscilla* species comprise a major branch of the beta group proteobacteria by 16S ribosomal ribonucleic acid sequence comparison: transfer of *Eikenella* and *Simonsiella* to the family *Neisseriaceae* (emend.). *Int. J. Syst. Bacteriol.* **39:**258–266.
28. **Dillon, J. R., M. Carballo, and M. Pauze.** 1988. Evaluation of eight methods for identification of pathogenic *Neisseria* species: *Neisseria* Kwik, RIM-N, Gonobio-Test, Minitek, Gonochek II, GonoGen, Phadebact Monoclonal GC OMNI test, and Syva Micro Trak test. *J. Clin. Microbiol.* **26:**493–497.
29. **Dillon, J. R., M. Pauzé, and K.-H. Yeung.** 1983. Spread of penicillinase-producing and transfer plasmids from the gonococcus to *Neisseria meningitidis*. *Lancet* **i:**779–781.
30. **Doern, G. V.** 1986. *Branhamella catarrhalis*—an emerging human pathogen. *Diagn. Microbiol. Infect. Dis.* **4:**191–201.
31. **Dossett, J. H., P. C. Appelbaum, J. S. Knapp, and P. A. Totten.** 1985. Proctitis associated with *Neisseria cinerea* misidentified as *Neisseria gonorrhoeae* in a child. *J. Clin. Microbiol.* **21:**575–577.
32. **Eng, J., and E. Holten.** 1977. Gelatin neutralization of the inhibitory effect of sodium polyanethol sulfonate on *Neisseria meningitidis* in blood culture. *J. Clin. Microbiol.* **6:** 1–3.
33. **Evangelista, A. T., and H. R. Beilstein.** 1993. *Cumitech 4A: Laboratory Diagnosis of Gonorrhea*. Coordinating ed., C. Abramson. American Society for Microbiology, Washington, D.C.
34. **Faur, Y. C., M. H. Weisburd, M. E. Wilson, and P. S. May.** 1973. A new medium for the isolation of pathogenic Neisseria (NYC medium). 1. Formulation and comparisons with standard media. *Health Lab. Sci.* **10:**44–52.
35. **Fox, K. K., J. S. Knapp, K. K. Holmes, E. W. Hook III, F. N. Judson, S. E. Thompson, J. A. Washington, and W. L. Whittington.** 1997. Antimicrobial resistance in *Neisseria gonorrhoeae* in the United States, 1988–1994: the emergence of decreased susceptibility to the fluoroquinolones. *J. Infect. Dis.* **157:**1396–1403.
36. **Giebink, G. S.** 1989. The microbiology of otitis media. *Pediatr. Infect. Dis. J.* **8:**518–520.
37. **Given, K. F., B. W. Thomas, and A. G. Johnston.** 1977. Isolation of *Neisseria meningitidis* from the urethra, cervix, and anal canal: further observations. *Br. J. Vener. Dis.* **53:** 109–112.
38. **Gold, R., I. Goldschneider, M. L. Lepow, T. F. Draper, and M. Randolph.** 1978. Carriage of *Neisseria meningitidis* and *Neisseria lactamica* in infants and children. *J. Infect. Dis.* **137:**112–121.
39. **Granato, P. A., and M. R. Franz.** 1990. Use of the Gen-Probe PACE system for the detection of *Neisseria gonorrhoeae* in urogenital samples. *Diagn. Microbiol. Infect. Dis.* **13:**217–221.
40. **Guibourdenche, M., T. Lambert, and J.-Y. Riou.** 1989. Isolation of *Neisseria canis* in mixed culture for a patient after a cat bite. *J. Clin. Microbiol.* **27:**1673–1674.
41. **Hendolin, P. H., A. Markkanen, Y. Ylikoski, and J. J. Wahlfors.** 1997. Use of multiplex PCR for simultaneous detection of four bacterial species in middle ear effusions. *J. Clin. Microbiol.* **35:**2854–2858.
42. **Herbert, D. A., and J. Ruskin.** 1981. Are the "nonpathogenic" neisseriae pathogenic? *Am. J. Clin. Pathol.* **75:** 739–742.
43. **Holmes, B., M. Costas, S. L. W. On, P. VanDamme, E. Falsen, and K. Kersters.** 1993. *Neisseria weaveri* sp. nov. (formerly CDC group M-5), from dog bite wounds of humans. *Int. J. Syst. Bacteriol.* **43:**687–693.
44. **Hook, E. W., S. F. Ching, J. Stephens, K. F. Hardy, K. R. Smith, and H. H. Lee.** 1997. Diagnosis of *Neisseria gonorrhoeae* infections in women by using the ligase chain reaction on patient-obtained vaginal swabs. *J. Clin. Microbiol.* **35:**2129–2132.
45. **Ison, C. A., N. Tekki, and M. J. Gill.** 1993. Detection of the tetM determinant in *Neisseria gonorrhoeae*. *Sex. Transm. Dis.* **20:**329–333.
46. **Janda, W. M., M. Bohnhoff, J. A. Morello, and S. A. Lerner.** 1980. Prevalence and site pathogen studies of *Neisseria meningitidis* and *N. gonorrhoeae* in homosexual men. *JAMA* **244:**2060–2064.
47. **Janda, W. M., J. J. Bradna, and P. Ruther.** 1989. Identification of *Neisseria* spp., *Haemophilus* spp., and other fastidi-

ous gram-negative bacteria with the MicroScan *Haemophilus-Neisseria* identification panel. *J. Clin. Microbiol.* **27:** 869–873.

48. **Janda, W. M., P. J. Malloy, and P. C. Schreckenberger.** 1987. Clinical evaluation of the Vitek *Neisseria-Haemophilus* identification card. *J. Clin. Microbiol.* **25:**37–41.
49. **Janda, W. M., J. A. Morello, S. A. Lerner, and M. Bohnhoff.** 1983. Characteristics of pathogenic *Neisseria* spp. isolated from homosexual men. *J. Clin. Microbiol.* **17:**85–91.
50. **Janda, W. M., J. G. Ulanday, M. Bohnhoff, and L. J. LeBeau.** 1985. Evaluation of the RIM N, Gonochek II, and Phadebact systems for the identification of pathogenic *Neisseria* spp. and *Branhamella catarrhalis*. *J. Clin. Microbiol.* **21:**734–737.
51. **Jephcott, A. E., and R. S. Morton.** 1982. Isolation of *Neisseria lactamica* from a genital site. *Lancet* **ii:**739–740.
52. **Johnson, S. R., and S. A. Morse.** 1988. Antibiotic resistance in *Neisseria gonorrhoeae*: genetics and mechanisms of resistance. *Sex. Transm. Dis.* **15:**217–224.
53. **Jourismies-Somer, H. R., S. Savolainen, and J. S. Ylikoski.** 1989. Comparison of the nasal bacterial floras in two groups of healthy subjects and in patients with acute maxillary sinusitis. *J. Clin. Microbiol.* **27:**2736–2743.
54. **Kertesz, D. A., S. K. Byrne, and A. W. Chow.** 1993. Characterization of *Neisseria meningitidis* by polymerase chain reaction and restriction endonuclease digestion of the porA gene. *J. Clin. Microbiol.* **31:**2594–2598.
55. **Knapp, J. S.** Unpublished observations.
56. **Knapp, J. S.** 1988. Historical perspectives and identification of *Neisseria* and related species. *Clin. Microbiol. Rev.* **1:**415–431.
57. **Knapp, J. S., K. K. Fox, D. L. Trees, and W. L. Whittington.** 1997. Fluoroquinolone resistance in *Neisseria gonorrhoeae*. *Emerg. Infect. Dis.* **24:**142–148.
58. **Knapp, J. S., and E. W. Hook III.** 1988. Prevalence and persistence of *Neisseria cinerea* and other *Neisseria* spp. in adults. *J. Clin. Microbiol.* **26:**896–900.
59. **Knapp, J. S., S. R. Johnson, J. M. Zenilman, M. C. Roberts, and S. A. Morse.** 1989. High-level tetracycline resistance resulting from TetM in strains of *Neisseria* spp., *Kingella denitrificans*, and *Eikenella corrodens*. *Antimicrob. Agents Chemother.* **32:**765–757.
60. **Knapp, J. S., M. R. Tam, R. C. Nowinski, K. K. Holmes, and E. G. Sandström.** 1984. Serological classification of *Neisseria gonorrhoeae* using monoclonal antibodies directed against gonococcal outer membrane protein I. *J. Infect. Dis.* **150:**44–48.
61. **Knapp, J. S., P. A. Totten, M. H. Mulks, and B. H. Minshew.** 1984. Characterization of *Neisseria cinerea*, a nonpathogenic species isolated on Martin-Lewis medium selective for pathogenic *Neisseria* species. *J. Clin. Microbiol.* **19:**63–67.
62. **Lewis, J. S., O. Fakile, E. Foss, G. Legarza, A. Leskys, K. Lowe, and D. Powning.** 1993. Direct DNA probe assay for *Neisseria gonorrhoeae* in pharyngeal and rectal specimens. *J. Clin. Microbiol.* **31:**2783–2785.
63. **Lewis, J. S., D. Kranig-Brown, and D. A. Trainor.** 1990. DNA probe confirmatory test for *Neisseria gonorrhoeae*. *J. Clin. Microbiol.* **28:**2349–2350.
64. **Martin, J. E., J. H. Armstrong, and P. B. Smith.** 1974. New system for cultivation of *Neisseria gonorrhoeae*. *Appl. Microbiol.* **27:**802–805.
65. **Martin, J. E., Jr., and R. L. Jackson.** 1975. A biological environment chamber for the culture of *Neisseria gonorrhoeae*. *J. Am. Vener. Dis. Assoc.* **2:**28–30.
66. **Martin, J. E., and J. S. Lewis.** 1977. Anisomycin: improved antimycotic activity in modified Thayer-Martin medium. *Public Health Lab.* **35:**53–62.
67. **Mendelman, P. M., J. Campos, D. O. Chaffin, D. A. Serfass, A. L. Smith, and J. A. Saez Nieto.** 1988. Relative penicillin G resistance in *Neisseria meningitidis* and reduced affinity of penicillin-binding protein 3. *Antimicrob. Agents Chemother.* **32:**706–709.
68. **National Committee for Clinical Laboratory Standards.** 1993. *Methods for Dilution Antimicrobial Susceptibility Tests for Bacteria That Grow Aerobically*. Approved standard M7-A3. National Committee for Clinical Laboratory Standards, Villanova, Pa.
69. **National Committee for Clinical Laboratory Standards.** 1993. *Performance Standards for Antimicrobial Disk Susceptibility Tests*, 5th ed. Approved standard M2-A5. National Committee for Clinical Laboratory Standards, Villanova, Pa.
70. **National Committee for Clinical Laboratory Standards.** 1998. *Performance Standards for Antimicrobial Susceptibility Testing*. M100-S8. National Committee for Clinical Laboratory Standards, Wayne, Pa.
71. **Ni, H., A. I. Knight, K. Cartwright, W. H. Palmer, and J. McFadden.** 1992. Polymerase chain reaction for diagnosis of meningococcal meningitis. *Lancet* **340:**1432–1434.
72. **O'Callaghan, C. H., A. Morris, S. M. Kirby, and A. H. Shingler.** 1972. Novel method for detection of beta-lactamases by using a chromogenic cephalosporin substrate. *Antimicrob. Agents Chemother.* **1:**283–288.
73. **Panke, E. S., L. I. Yang, P. A. Leist, P. Magevny, R. J. Fry, and R. F. Lee.** 1991. Comparison of Gen-Probe DNA probe test and culture for the detection of *Neisseria gonorrhoeae* in endocervical specimens. *J. Clin. Microbiol.* **29:** 883–888.
74. **Pérez, J. L., A. Pulido, F. Pantozzi, and R. Martin.** 1990. Butyrate esterase (tributyrin) spot test, a simple method for immediate identification of *Moraxella (Branhamella) catarrhalis*. *J. Clin. Microbiol.* **28:**2347–2348.
75. **Rice, R. J., and J. S. Knapp.** 1994. Comparative in vitro activities of penicillin G, amoxicillin-clavulanic acid, selected cephalosporins, and quinolone antimicrobial agents against representative resistance phenotypes of *Neisseria gonorrhoeae*. *Antimicrob. Agents Chemother.* **38:**155–158.
76. **Ringuette, L., T. Trudeau, T. Turcotte, K. Yeung, R. Rémes, L. Perron, and I. Le Corre.** 1996. Emergence of *Neisseria gonorrhoeae* strains with decreased susceptibility to ciprofloxacin—Quebec, 1994–1995. *Can. Commun. Dis. Rep.* **22:**121–125.
77. **Riou, J.-Y., and M. Guibourdenche.** 1987. *Neisseria polysaccharea* sp. nov. *Int. J. Syst. Bacteriol.* **37:**163–165.
78. **Robinson, M. J., and T. R. Oberdorfer.** 1983. Identification of pathogenic *Neisseria* species with RapID NH system. *J. Clin. Microbiol.* **17:**400–404.
79. **Roongpisuthipong, A., J. S. Lewis, S. J. Kraus, and S. A. Morse.** 1988. Gonococcal urethritis diagnosed from enzyme immunoassay of urine sediment. *Sex. Transm. Dis.* **15:**192–195.
80. **Rossau, R. G., A. van Landschoot, M. Gillis, and J. de Ley.** 1991. Taxonomy of *Moraxellaeae* fam. nov., a new bacterial family to accommodate the genera *Moraxella*, *Acinetobacter*, and *Psychrobacter* and related organisms. *Int. J. Syst. Bacteriol.* **41:**310–319.
81. **Rossau, R., G. Vandenbussche, S. Thielemans, P. Segers, H. Grosch, E. Göthe, W. Mannheim, and J. E. DeLey.** 1989. Ribosomal ribonucleic acid cistron similarities and deoxyribonucleic acid homologies of *Neisseria*, *Kingella*, *Eikenella*, *Simonsiella*, *Alysiella*, and Centers for Disease Control groups EF-4 and M-5 in the emended family *Neisseriaceae*. *Int. J. Syst. Bacteriol.* **39:**185–198.
82. **Saez-Nieto, J. A., A. Fenoll, J. Bazquez, and J. Casal.** 1982. Prevalence of maltose-negative *Neisseria meningitidis* variants during an epidemic period in Spain. *J. Clin. Microbiol.* **15:**78–81.

83. **Sarafian, S. K., and J. S. Knapp.** 1989. Molecular epidemiology of gonorrhea. *Clin. Microbiol. Rev.* **2:**S49–S55.

84. **Schachter, J., W. M. McCormick, R. F. Smith, R. M. Parks, R. Bailey, and A. C. Ohlin.** 1984. Enzyme immunoassay for diagnosis of gonorrhea. *J. Clin. Microbiol.* **19:** 57–59.

85. **Schuchart, A., K. Robinson, J. E. Wenger, L. H. Harrison, M. Farley, A. L. Reingold, L. Lefkowitz, and B. A. Perkins.** 1997. Bacterial meningitis in the United States in 1995. *N. Engl. J. Med.* **14:**970–976.

86. **Scribner, R. K., and D. F. Welch.** 1984. Neutralization of the inhibitory effect of sodium polyanetholsulfonate on *Neisseria meningitidis* in blood cultures processed with the Du Pont Isolator system. *J. Clin. Microbiol.* **20:**40–42.

87. **Smith, K. R., S. Ching, H. Lee, Y. Ohhashi, H. Y. Yu, H. C. Fisher III, and E. W. Hook III.** 1995. Evaluation of ligase chain reaction for use with urine for identification of *Neisseria gonorrhoeae* in females attending a sexually transmitted disease clinic. *J. Clin. Microbiol.* **33:**455–457.

88. **Strathdee, C. A., S. D. Tyler, A. Ryan, W. M. Johnson, and F. E. Ashton.** 1993. Genomic fingerprinting of *Neisseria meningitidis* associated with group C meningococcal disease in Canada. *J. Clin. Microbiol.* **31:**2506–2508.

89. **Tapsall, J. W., R. R. Schultz, R. Lovett, and R. Munro.** 1992. Failure of 500 mg ciprofloxacin therapy in male urethral gonorrhoea. *Med. J. Aust.* **156:**143.

90. **Vaneechoutte, M., G. Verschraegen, G. Claeys, B. Weise, and A. M. van den Abeele.** 1990. Respiratory tract carrier rates of *Moraxella (Branhamella) catarrhalis* in adults and children and interpretation of the isolation of *M. catarrhalis* from sputum. *J. Clin. Microbiol.* **28:**2647–2680.

91. **Vedros, N. A.** 1984. Genus I. *Neisseria* Trevisan 1885, 105AL, p. 290–296. *In* N. R. Krieg (ed.), *Bergey's Manual of Systematic Bacteriology*, vol. 1. The Williams & Wilkins Co., Baltimore, Md.

92. **Vedros, N. A., C. Hoke, and P. Chun.** 1983. *Neisseria macacae* sp. nov., a new *Neisseria* species isolated from the oropharynges of rhesus monkeys (*Macaca mulatta*). *Int. J. Syst. Bacteriol.* **33:**515–520.

93. **Whittington, W. L., and J. S. Knapp.** 1988. Trends in antimicrobial resistance in *Neisseria gonorrhoeae* in the United States. *Sex. Transm. Dis.* **15:**202–210.

94. **Woods, T. C., L. O. Helsel, B. Swaminathan, W. F. Bibb, R. W. Pinner, B. G. Gellin, S. F. Collin, S. H. Waterman, M. W. Reeves, D. J. Brenner, and C. V. Broome.** 1992. Characterization of *Neisseria meningitidis* serogroup C by multilocus enzyme electrophoresis and ribosomal DNA restriction profiles (ribotyping). *J. Clin. Microbiol.* **30:** 132–137.

95. **Xia, M., M. C. Roberts, W. L. Whittington, K. K. Holmes, J. S. Knapp, J. R. Dillon, and T. Wi.** 1996. *Neisseria gonorrhoeae* with decreased susceptibility to ciprofloxacin: pulsed-field gel electrophoresis typing of strains from North America, Hawaii, and the Philippines. *Antimicrob. Agents Chemother.* **40:**2439–2440.

96. **Young, H., A. B. Harris, and J. W. Tapsall.** 1984. Differentiation of gonococcal and nongonococcal neisseriae by the superoxol test. *Br. J. Vener. Dis.* **60:**87–89.

97. **Young, H., and A. Moyes.** 1993. Comparative evaluation of AccuProbe culture identification test for *Neisseria gonorrhoeae* and other rapid methods. *J. Clin. Microbiol.* **31:** 1996–1999.

98. **Zollinger, W. D., B. L. Brandt, and E. C. Tramont.** 1986. Immune response to *Neisseria meningitidis*, p. 346–352. *In* N. R. Rose, H. Driedman, and J. L. Fahey (ed.), *Manual of Clinical Laboratory Immunology*, 3rd ed. American Society for Microbiology, Washington, D.C.

Haemophilus

JOSEPH M. CAMPOS

39

TAXONOMY

Haemophilus species remain the cause of a wide spectrum of human infections, despite the dramatic reduction in the incidence of *Haemophilus influenzae* type b infections over the past 10 years (5). The *Haemophilus* species encountered clinically include *H. influenzae*, *H. parainfluenzae*, *H. ducreyi*, *H. aphrophilus*, *H. paraphrophilus*, *H. haemolyticus*, *H. parahaemolyticus*, and *H. segnis*. Available evidence, however, suggests that *H. ducreyi* is only distantly related to the other members of the genus and should be reassigned to another genus (26). *H. aphrophilus* appears to be closely related genetically and physiologically to *Actinobacillus actinomycetemcomitans*, and perhaps the two will be placed in the same genus in the future.

The organism we know today as *H. influenzae* was described initially by Pfeiffer in 1892, who recovered it from the sputa of several patients suffering from influenza virus infections. The genus name, however, was not proposed officially for the organism until 1920 (100). Pittman (73) described the six capsular serotypes of *H. influenzae* in 1931 and recognized that members of serotype b were the most likely to cause invasive infection.

DESCRIPTION OF THE GENUS

Haemophilus species are oxidase positive, pleomorphic, gram-negative bacilli. Their catalase reaction is variable, and they are facultatively anaerobic. Growth is optimal for most species when cultures are incubated in a humid environment containing 5 to 7% CO_2 at 33 to 37°C.

Most species exhibit fastidious nutritional requirements and grow in the laboratory only when provided with complex, nutrient-rich media. Some isolates are found when satellite colonies are noticed around colonies of other microorganisms excreting essential nutrients into the medium. The unique growth requirements of the individual species of *Haemophilus* are discussed later in the chapter.

NATURAL HABITATS

Most *Haemophilus* species are normal residents of the upper respiratory tracts of humans and other animals. Some species are found as colonizers of the gastrointestinal and urogenital tracts.

CLINICAL SIGNIFICANCE

Many types of *Haemophilus* infection occur in humans, ranging from those which are uncomplicated and easily managed (e.g., conjunctivitis, sinusitis, and otitis media) to those which are invasive and life-threatening (e.g., meningitis, pericarditis, and endocarditis) (93). Species of *Haemophilus* implicated as human pathogens are *H. influenzae* (including biogroup aegyptius), *H. parainfluenzae*, *H. ducreyi*, and *H. aphrophilus*. The species *H. haemolyticus*, *H. parahaemolyticus*, *H. segnis*, and *H. paraphrophilus* are highly unusual causes of infection and will be discussed only briefly.

H. influenzae

The major virulence factor of *H. influenzae* strains causing invasive infection is the polysaccharide capsule. Encapsulated strains belong to one of six serotypes (serotypes a to f) and are known as the "typeable strains." Unencapsulated strains are referred to as the "nontypeable strains."

Before the widespread use of effective vaccines, serotype b strains caused the vast majority of invasive *Haemophilus* infections in the United States. Approximately 0.5% of children in the United States below the age of 5 years suffered from serious infections caused by *H. influenzae* type b (17). The peak incidence of infection was 6 to 7 months of age. *H. influenzae* type b was the leading cause of bacterial meningitis and epiglottitis in children less than 5 years of age (18, 38). It was also a major cause of pericarditis, pneumonia, septic arthritis, osteomyelitis, and facial cellulitis in the same age group. Attendance of preschool-age children at day-care centers was a significant risk factor for the development of primary *H. influenzae* disease (71).

A sharp reduction in the incidence of serotype b infection began in the mid-1980s and was likely due to vaccine administration, rifampin prophylaxis of disease contacts, and the availability of more efficacious therapeutic agents (61). From 1987 through 1994, the incidence of invasive infection among U.S. children less than 5 years of age declined by 95% (13). The Immunization Practices Advisory Committee of the Centers for Disease Control and Prevention currently recommends administration of a licensed *H. influenzae* type b conjugate vaccine to all children beginning at the age of 2 months (11).

In the years leading up to the vaccine era, most of the typeable strains recovered from bacteremic patients were serotype b. Serotype f strains have constituted the large majority of the non-type b encapsulated strains (82). In a study conducted in Georgia, the proportion of serotype f isolates responsible for invasive *H. influenzae* disease rose from 1% in 1989 to 17% in 1994. Approximately 75% of cases occurred in adults, with an overall mortality rate of 30% (95).

Person-to-person spread of *H. influenzae* occurs by inhalation of aerosolized respiratory droplets. Upper respiratory tract colonization rates in humans may be as high as 50%. Colonization with type b strains, however, is unusual in healthy infants (0.7%) and children (3 to 5%) and is very rare in adults (62).

Unencapsulated (nontypeable) strains may also cause infection, but such infections usually occur at sites contiguous with the upper respiratory tract. They typically are not spread to other sites via the bloodstream. Molecular analysis suggests that the nontypeable strains of *H. influenzae* were derived from encapsulated ancestors (84).

Nontypeable strains of *H. influenzae* cause a variety of infections in adults and in older children (85). Lower respiratory tract infections (febrile tracheobronchitis and pneumonia), often with bacteremia, are reported most often. Approximately 25% of all cases of invasive *H. influenzae* infection presently occur in adults (32). The majority of these patients have underlying medical problems that predispose them to infection. These problems include malignancy, chronic obstructive pulmonary disease, alcoholism, human immunodeficiency virus type 1 (HIV-1) infection, and pregnancy. Approximately 80% of invasive isolates have been nontypeable (49).

Unencapsulated strains of *H. influenzae* cause noninvasive respiratory tract infection in young children, community-acquired pneumonia and exacerbation of chronic bronchitis in adults, and occasional invasive infections in healthy and immunocompromised patients of all ages (35, 48, 65). Approximately 19% of children with cystic fibrosis yield growth of nontypeable *H. influenzae* from respiratory tract specimens (33). In young children, these organisms are the second leading cause of otitis media (after *Streptococcus pneumoniae*) (6). A subgroup of these organisms (formerly referred to as *H. aegyptius* or the Koch-Weeks bacillus) is the leading cause of purulent bacterial conjunctivitis (92, 98). During the spring of 1984, an outbreak of severe childhood illness characterized by high fever, abdominal pain and vomiting, hemorrhagic skin lesions, vascular collapse, and death occurred in São Paulo State, Brazil (7). Laboratory investigation revealed that strains belonging to a single clone of *H. influenzae* biogroup aegyptius were the cause of the epidemic, later referred to as Brazilian purpuric fever (BPF) (8). Conventional laboratory testing is unable to differentiate the BPF clone of *H. influenzae* biogroup aegyptius from *H. influenzae* biogroup III (88). The outer membrane protein profiles of the two biogroups are different, however, and can be used to distinguish the biogroups (10).

H. ducreyi

H. ducreyi causes chancroid, a sexually transmitted disease characterized by shallow genital ulceration that may be accompanied by inguinal lymphadenopathy. Most cases occur among the lower socioeconomic groups in the tropical climates of Africa, Asia, and Latin America. In recent years, however, miniepidemics of chancroid have occurred at sites far removed from the tropics. More than 4,000 cases were reported in the United States each year from 1987 through 1990. During the 20-year period between 1965 and 1984, an average of only 925 cases per year was reported. Since 1990, the number of annual cases had declined to fewer than 400 in 1996 (12).

The lesion begins as a tender papule that becomes pustular and then ulcerated over the course of 2 days. Individual lesions may coalesce to form larger ulcers. The lesions in most patients are painful and thus are easily distinguished from syphilitic chancres. Tender unilateral inguinal lymphadenitis (bubo formation) is found in 50% of cases. Recent data suggest that the existence of genital ulceration, such as those of chancroid, increases the risk of HIV-1 infection during homosexual or heterosexual contact (83, 94).

See the recent review by Trees and Morse (91) for in-depth information regarding *H. ducreyi* and chancroid.

H. parainfluenzae

H. parainfluenzae is considered part of the commensal flora of the upper respiratory tract. There are situations (*H. parainfluenzae* endocarditis is an example) in which this organism behaves as a life-threatening pathogen (22). Detection of this organism in blood cultures can be difficult because of the fastidious nature of the organism (16). The organism is also an occasional cause of secondary bacteremia and urethritis in adults (69, 86).

H. aphrophilus

H. aphrophilus is another upper respiratory tract inhabitant that can be the cause of serious infections. Endocarditis and brain abscess are the most common presentations, with pneumonia, meningitis, and secondary bacteremia occurring less frequently (4). The species name *aphrophilus* originates from the wine-making term "aphros," referring to the froth formed during the fermentation of grape juice. The name is an indirect reference to the organism's requirement for CO_2 during incubation.

Other Species

An unnamed genospecies of *Haemophilus* genetically related to *H. influenzae* and *H. haemolyticus* has been described in patients with serious urogenital, neonatal, and maternal-infant infections (75, 76). Characterization of these isolates by currently used criteria has identified them as nontypeable *H. influenzae* belonging to biotypes I to IV. They preferentially colonize the urogenital tract. They are known to cause chorioamnionitis and bacteremia during pregnancy and infections in neonates during premature labor and rupture of the membranes (34). Quite likely, these organisms will be assigned to a distinct, thus far unnamed species.

Other species of *Haemophilus*, e.g., *H. paraphrophilus*, *H. haemolyticus*, and *H. segnis*, are part of the human upper respiratory tract flora and very rarely cause infection.

COLLECTION, TRANSPORT, AND STORAGE OF SPECIMENS

Specimens containing *Haemophilus* spp. should be as free as possible of other microorganisms because of the likelihood that colonies of other microorganisms will obscure the presence of *Haemophilus* spp. Careful selection and disinfection (where appropriate) of specimen collection sites cannot be overemphasized.

Blood

The majority of cases of *H. influenzae* type b bacteremia in young children are of a high magnitude (>100 CFU per ml), obviating the need to collect as large a quantity of blood as is collected from adults (3). However, approximately one-quarter of young patients exhibit organism counts of <10 CFU/ml (9), and 10 to 20% of low-magnitude cases of bacteremia in children are caused by *H. influenzae* (40). Ideally, a minimum of 0.5 ml of blood and preferably several milliliters of blood should be collected for culture. The recommendations published in *Cumitech 1B* (30) for adults should be followed for patients older than 7 years of age.

Body Fluids

For laboratories that use conventional centrifugation to concentrate cerebrospinal fluid (CSF) specimens before Gram staining and culture, at least 1 ml of CSF should be submitted to make the centrifugation worthwhile. CSF collected from patients partially treated with antimicrobial agents should be of sufficient volume to permit microbial antigen detection tests (discussed below) as well as Gram staining and culture. Other body fluids likely to contain *Haemophilus* spp. (e.g., synovial fluid, pericardial fluid, and pleural fluid) should be collected in amounts that make both Gram staining and culture possible.

Ocular Specimens

Patients with conjunctivitis caused by *H. influenzae* usually present with copious amounts of purulent discharge. Pus should be collected on the tips of calcium alginate flexible-shaft swabs. Swabs should be placed in modified Stuart's transport medium during delivery to the laboratory.

Respiratory Specimens

The major difficulty with proving that a *Haemophilus* sp. is causing a lower respiratory tract infection is avoiding interference from commensal upper respiratory tract flora. Specimen collection techniques that bypass the upper respiratory tract or that protect lower respiratory tract specimens from contamination with flora in the upper respiratory tract are recommended. Collection of secretions from patients with epiglottitis should not be attempted unless emergency airway maintenance procedures can be initiated rapidly. Such patients are at extreme risk of life-threatening laryngospasm.

The utility of cultures of nasopharyngeal specimens for identification of the etiology of otitis media has been controversial for several years. Most recently, these cultures were shown to have minimal positive predictive value (71%) for nontypeable *H. influenzae* disease and very little positive predictive value for *S. pneumoniae* and *Moraxella catarrhalis* infections (31). Schwartz et al. (80) found the positive predictive value of culture to be highest when 2+ or more growth of a single pathogen was recovered.

Genital Specimens

The specimen of choice for the laboratory diagnosis of chancroid is material collected from the exposed base or margin of the lesion. Needle aspirates of pus from buboes of patients manifesting inguinal lymphadenitis augment, but should not replace, lesional smears and cultures.

Recovery of nonchancroid isolates from the urogenital tract can be accomplished by collecting urethral specimens with a flexible-shaft minitip swab (preferred) or by obtaining clean-catch midstream urine specimens that are immediately inoculated onto an appropriate culture medium.

DIRECT EXAMINATION

Microscopic Examination

Observation of *Haemophilus* under the microscope is hampered by the relatively small size of these organisms. Biological stains such as the Gram and acridine orange (AO) stains facilitate their detection by enhancing the contrast between the bacteria and the background. Methanol fixation of smears, a standard step during AO staining, also enhances the appearance of *Haemophilus* in Gram stains compared to its appearance after heat fixation (see chapter 20). The Quellung reaction, usually associated with identification and serotyping of *S. pneumoniae*, may also be used for recognition of encapsulated strains of *H. influenzae*.

Gram Stain

Microscopic examination of Gram-stained body fluid smears can enable the early detection of life-threatening *H. influenzae* infection. Although definitive identification of *H. influenzae* cannot be made microscopically, presumptive identification by an experienced microscopist is reliable.

The primary limitation of the Gram stain, as is the case with other microscopic assays, is its lack of sensitivity (~10^4 CFU/ml). Approximately 85% of cases of culture-proven *H. influenzae* meningitis yield positive Gram-stained CSF smears (36). Conventional centrifugation and preparation of smears from resuspended sediments increase the sensitivity 5- to 10-fold, provided there is a sufficient quantity of the specimen (≥1.0 ml) to make centrifugation worthwhile. Use of cytocentrifugation increases the sensitivity of the Gram stain by as much as 100-fold compared to that with the use of uncentrifuged or conventionally centrifuged Gram-stained CSF smears (81).

Gram stain has also been advocated for use in the presumptive diagnosis of chancroid. *H. ducreyi* organisms typically exhibit the "school of fish" arrangement, although this is more often seen with smears prepared from broth culture suspensions than lymph node aspirates. Published studies have reported the sensitivity of Gram staining to be less than 50% (67).

Wayson Stain

Another limitation of the Gram stain is the lack of contrast between stained microorganisms and specimen artifacts. The tiny gram-negative bacilli of *H. influenzae* can be camouflaged effectively by the gram-negative proteinaceous strands frequently found in infected body fluids. Wayson-stained smears yield dark blue bacteria, light blue proteinaceous strands, and light blue or purple inflammatory cells (20). These smears cannot be restained with Gram reagents, however, and new smears are necessary to demonstrate the Gram stain reactions of organisms.

AO Stain

The AO stain enables the detection of 10-fold fewer *Haemophilus* spp. than the Gram stain (51). However, the better sensitivity of the AO stain is at least partially negated when specimens contain large numbers of inflammatory cells that can interfere with the detection of tiny fluorescent bacteria. AO stain-positive smears can be restained with Gram reagents to determine the Gram stain reactions of the bacteria that are present (59).

Antigen Detection Assays

Many laboratories today have discontinued body fluid and urine antigen detection for *H. influenzae* type b and the other agents of bacterial meningitis. The reasons are that (i) testing is expensive, (ii) the results have little if any impact on patient management, and (iii) some positive results (especially those from urine) are falsely positive.

Laboratories that continue to offer body fluid antigen

detection use particle agglutination assays that are available from several commercial sources.

Particle Agglutination

Commercially available particle agglutination assays for *H. influenzae* type b antigen are of two types: those based upon the agglutination of immunoglobulin G (IgG)-sensitized latex particles (LPA) and those based upon staphylococcal protein A-mediated coagglutination (SPAMC) of IgG-coated staphylococcal cells. Both assays furnish results in less than 10 min and require no specialized equipment, although use of a mechanical rotator makes both assays more convenient to perform. More importantly, both assay types are 10- to 100-fold more sensitive than their predecessor, counterimmunoelectrophoresis (24, 52). Direct comparison of LPA and SPAMC found them to be equivalent at detecting *H. influenzae* type b antigen in CSF (56). However, LPA was superior to SPAMC when body fluids from patients with culture-proven nonmeningeal *H. influenzae* type b infections were tested. Neither assay is sufficiently sensitive to replace culture.

LPA detection of *H. influenzae* type b antigen in CSF (23) and urine (41) has been reported as long as 21 days after immunization with *H. influenzae* type b vaccine. Laboratory personnel should alert clinicians of this possibility when unexpectedly positive test results are obtained for children of vaccine age.

Other Methods

Immunofluorescence (44) and enzyme immunoassays (78) have been described for the detection of *H. ducreyi* antigen. Evaluation of the immunofluorescence assay versus culture yielded sensitivities of 93% for ulcer specimens and 89% for bubo specimens; however, the specificities were only 63 and 56%, respectively. The poor specificities were thought to reflect the insensitivity of the culture method used. The enzyme immunoassay demonstrated a sensitivity and a specificity of 100% each during a limited evaluation of 30 patients.

DNA Probe Assays

PCR-based DNA probe assays have been developed in research settings for the noncultural detection of *H. ducreyi* in genital ulcer specimens (15, 70, 99). One assay used broad-specificity primers that amplified rRNA from a wide variety of bacteria followed by the use of specific probes labeled with [^{32}P]ATP for recognition of amplified *H. ducreyi* rRNA sequences. Comparison of PCR assay performance with that of culture during testing of clinical specimens revealed a sensitivity as high as 98% but a specificity of only 51%. Most of the "falsely" positive PCR results were attributed to truly infected patients who yielded falsely negative cultures.

CULTURE AND ISOLATION

Attempts to grow *Haemophilus* spp. in culture must take into account the nutritionally fastidious properties of these microorganisms. All species, with the exception of laboratory-adapted strains of *H. aphrophilus*, require either exogenous hemin (X factor) or NAD (V factor), or both. Strains of some species (e.g., *H. influenzae* biogroup aegyptius and *H. ducreyi*) exhibit requirements for other nutrients which, when met, facilitate their growth in culture. Most species grow well on conventional chocolate agar but do not grow at all on standard 5% sheep blood agar. The latter medium may have adequate amounts of X factor, but metabolically useful V factor is found only within intact erythrocytes. The original recipe for chocolate agar included a heating step during which sheep erythrocytes were lysed and NADase, the V factor-destroying enzyme, was inactivated. Most commercial chocolate agar available today is prepared by adding hemoglobin and vitamin supplements to a nutritional agar base. Rennie et al. (77), following a comparison of six medium bases and seven growth supplements, reported that a medium comprising gonococcal agar base plus 5% chocolatized sheep blood and 1% yeast autolysate promoted the best growth of *H. influenzae*, *H. parainfluenzae*, and other less commonly encountered species of *Haemophilus* (excluding *H. ducreyi*).

Growth of *Haemophilus* spp. can be achieved on 5% sheep blood agar by cross streaking the medium with a *Staphylococcus* sp. *Haemophilus* spp. form satellite colonies along the length of the staphylococcal growth streak because of the excess X factor released during erythrocyte lysis and the excess V factor excreted by staphylococci during growth. Growth of *Haemophilus* spp. on a nutrient-rich, nonselective medium lacking X and V factors (e.g., Mueller-Hinton agar) can be obtained by applying commercially available filter paper disks or strips saturated with X, V, or X+V factors to the surface of the medium. This technique is used by some laboratories during the identification of *Haemophilus* isolates to the species level. Colonies of *Haemophilus* spp. tend to be small and translucent after overnight incubation on chocolate agar. Their presence among the mixed flora of respiratory tract specimens is easily overlooked. This problem is particularly vexing when culturing sputa from cystic fibrosis patients, whose sputa usually yield large numbers of spreading, mucoid *Pseudomonas aeruginosa* colonies on culture. Since nontypeable *H. influenzae* is a significant pulmonary pathogen in these patients, its detection is highly desirable. Inoculation and anaerobic incubation of chocolate agar supplemented with 300 μg of bacitracin per ml has been successful. Similar success with the use of NAG medium (blood agar base, *N*-acetyl-D-glucosamine, hemin, NAD, and bacitracin) has also been reported (63).

Body fluid and bronchoscopically obtained specimens from which growth of *Haemophilus* spp. is a possibility should be inoculated onto 5% sheep blood agar and chocolate agar. Inoculation of other agar media or an enrichment broth (e.g., modified eugonic broth, enriched thioglycolate broth, or Fildes broth) is not warranted in most situations. Agar media should be incubated at 35 to 37°C for 48 to 72 h in an aerobic atmosphere containing 5 to 10% CO_2. *Haemophilus* colonies tend to be small and translucent and exude a mouse nest odor owing to their production of indole from tryptophan. Encapsulated strains of *H. influenzae* form glistening colonies that are somewhat larger after overnight incubation than nonencapsulated strains.

Conjunctival swabs for the detection of nontypeable *H. influenzae* and members of biogroup aegyptius should be inoculated onto 5% sheep blood agar and chocolate agar (or, preferably, enriched chocolate agar [chocolate agar plus 1% IsoVitaleX], if available). Cultures should be incubated at 35 to 37°C for 72 h in an aerobic atmosphere containing 5 to 10% CO_2.

Lymph node aspirates from patients with suspected chancroid should be inoculated onto selective nutritionally rich media such as Hammond gonococcal medium (gonococcal agar base containing 5% fetal calf serum, 1% bovine hemoglobin, 1% cofactors-vitamins-amino acids [CVA] enrichment, and 3 μg of vancomycin per ml), Fildes-enriched gonococcal medium (gonococcal agar base containing 5% Fildes reagent, 5% horse blood, and 3 μg of vancomycin per ml), or enriched Mueller-Hinton agar ((Mueller-Hinton agar base containing 5% chocolatized horse blood, 1% CVA enrichment, and 3 μg of vancomycin per ml) (21, 54). Vancomycin is present in these media to suppress the growth of contaminating gram-positive cutaneous flora. Use of two different media has been shown to augment the recovery of *H. ducreyi* over that from a single medium (64). Cultures should be incubated at 33 to 35°C for 72 h in an aerobic atmosphere containing 5 to 10% CO_2. There is evidence that recovery rates are as much as 21% greater when cultures are incubated at 33°C instead of 35°C (79).

IDENTIFICATION

X- and V-Factor Requirements

The standard procedure for identifying an isolate which exhibits microscopic and colonial properties suggestive of *Haemophilus* is to determine its X- and V-factor requirements.

A long-standing, still popular method for determining an isolate's X- and V-factor requirements uses factor-impregnated filter paper strips. A McFarland 0.5 standardized suspension of the isolate is prepared in sterile normal saline. The suspension is swabbed to the surface of a 150-mm Mueller-Hinton agar plate, and then the X, V, and X+V filter paper strips are applied to the medium surface. Care must be taken not to prepare too heavy a suspension and thus experience X- or V-factor carryover from the primary growth medium. The strips should not be placed too close to one another to avoid obtaining confusing results. The plate is examined after overnight incubation to determine which of the growth factor strips promoted satelliting growth.

Inzana et al. (39) described a broth medium alternative to the agar-based X- and V-factor strip test. The broth system consists of three tubes of brain heart infusion broth supplemented with X factor, V factor, or X+V factors. Tubes are inoculated from an organism suspension prepared in sterile normal saline and are incubated with aeration at 37°C. In most instances, the tubes can be read for turbidity after 4 to 5 h of incubation. Some V-factor-dependent strains require overnight incubation.

Perhaps the most convenient method for ascertaining X- and V-factor growth requirements is the commercially available quadrant plate approach. Laboratories may purchase prepoured plates in which each quadrant of the 100-mm plate contains Mueller-Hinton agar supplemented with either X factor, V factor, X+V factor, or X+V factor and horse erythrocytes (for determination of hemolytic properties). An organism suspension in sterile normal saline is prepared and is lightly inoculated onto each of the four quadrants. As mentioned earlier, heavy suspensions should be avoided to eliminate X- and V-factor carryover from the primary growth medium. After overnight incubation, the plate is examined to determine the isolate's X- and V-factor requirements as well as its horse erythrocyte hemolytic capability.

Porphyrin Test

The porphyrin test determines an isolate's X-factor requirement while avoiding the potential problem of X-factor carryover from primary culture media or X-factor contamination of test media (47). *Haemophilus* species which require X factor do not excrete porphobilinogen and porphyrins during growth because of enzymatic deficiencies in the hemin biosynthetic pathway. To perform the test, heavy suspensions of isolates are prepared in 0.5-ml quantities of 2 mM δ-aminolevulinic acid and 0.8 mM $MgSO_4$ in 0.1 M phosphate buffer (pH 6.9). Suspensions are incubated for 4 h at 37°C. The suspensions are illuminated with UV light (~360 nm) and are examined for red fluorescence. Fluorescence indicates enzymatic conversion of the δ-aminolevulinic acid substrate to porphyrins and, thus, X-factor independence. Lund and Blazevic (53) found the porphyrin test to be more rapid and more accurate than the X-factor satellitism test.

Biochemical Tests

In addition to determining growth requirements for X and/or V factors, biochemical tests can be performed to identify isolates to the species level (Table 1). The isolate's ability to hemolyze horse erythrocytes is useful for distinguishing *H. influenzae* from *H. haemolyticus* and *H. parainfluenzae* from *H. parahaemolyticus*. Fermentation of 1% glucose, sucrose, lactose, and/or mannose in phenol red broth base supplemented with X and V factors is useful for confirming the identification of all *Haemophilus* species. Biotyping of *H. influenzae* and *H. parainfluenzae* (37), as well as identification of *H. segnis* and the aegyptius biogroup of *H. influenzae*, can be achieved with growth-independent rapid assays

TABLE 1 Differential characteristics of *Haemophilus* species

Organism	X factor required[a]	V factor required	Hemolysis of horse blood	Glucose fermentation	Sucrose fermentation	Lactose fermentation	Mannose fermentation	Catalase	CO_2 enhancement of growth
H. influenzae[b]	+	+	−	+	−	−	−	+	+
H. haemolyticus	+	+	+	+	−	−	−	+	−
H. ducreyi	+	−	−	−	−	−	−	−	−
H. parainfluenzae	−	+	−	+	+	−	+	D[c]	D
H. parahaemolyticus	−	+	+	+	+	−	−	+	−
H. segnis	−	+	−	W[d]	W	−	−	D	−
H. paraphrophilus	−	+	−	+	+	+	+	−	+
H. aphrophilus	−	−	−	+	+	+	+	−	+

[a] As determined by the porphyrin test.
[b] Includes biogroup aegyptius.
[c] D, differences encountered.
[d] W, weak fermentation reaction.

TABLE 2 Differentiation of the biotypes of *H. influenzae* and *H. parainfluenzae*

Species and biotype	Indole	Urease	Ornithine decarboxylase
H. influenzae			
Biotype I	+	+	+
Biotype II	+	+	−
Biotype III[a]	−	+	−
Biotype IV	−	+	+
Biotype V	+	−	+
Biotype VI	−	−	+
Biotype VII	+	−	−
Biotype VIII	−	−	−
H. parainfluenzae[b]			
Biotype I	−	−	+
Biotype II	−	+	+
Biotype III	−	+	−
Biotype IV	+	+	+
Biotype VI	+	−	+
Biotype VII	+	+	−
Biotype VIII	+	−	−

[a] *H. influenzae* biotype III and *H. influenzae* biogroup aegyptius can be differentiated by analysis of outer membrane protein profiles.

[b] V-factor-dependent strains showing negative reactions in all three tests used for biotyping have been referred to as *H. parainfluenzae* biotype V (87). However, it is yet unclear whether such strains are *H. parainfluenzae* or are strains of *H. segnis* or *H. paraphrophilus*.

for indole, urease, and ornithine decarboxylase production (Table 2).

Several commercially available kits identify and biotype *Haemophilus* species as well. Evaluations have been published for the API 10E and API 20E systems (bioMérieux Vitek, St. Louis, Mo.), HNID System (Dade Behring, West Sacramento, Calif.), the RIM-H 1/RIM-H 2 system (Ortho Diagnostic Systems, Raritan, N.J.), and the API NH system (bioMérieux Vitek) (2, 72, 74). All were reported to be acceptably accurate compared to conventional biochemical test systems.

DNA Probes

A commercially available DNA probe for the identification of *H. influenzae* culture isolates is marketed under the Accuprobe product name (Gen-Probe, San Diego, Calif.). The principle of the method is hybridization of a chemiluminescent acridinium ester-labeled single-stranded DNA probe with complementary *H. influenzae* rRNA. A published assessment of the product found it to be extremely accurate compared to conventional test methods (19).

SEROLOGIC TESTS

Serotyping Methods

Within the *Haemophilus* genus, serotyping is appropriate only for the encapsulated strains of *H. influenzae*. Agglutination of organisms in type-specific antisera has been practiced for many years, but it requires sufficient cell mass to produce visible clumping of bacterial cells. An equally rapid method that requires fewer organisms and that produces easily interpreted results is the commercially available Phadebact Haemophilus Test (Boule Diagnostics AB, Huddinge, Sweden) staphylococcal coagglutination kit. The limitation of this kit is that it identifies type b strains only; non-type b encapsulated isolates are referred to collectively as types a and c to f. The traditional agglutination method described above must be used for the specific identification of these serotypes.

Detection of Antibodies to *Haemophilus* spp.

Chancroid is the only *Haemophilus* infection for which detection of antibodies for diagnostic and epidemiologic purposes has been used, although its level of accuracy has been less than impressive. Enzyme immunoassays for *H. ducreyi* IgG antibodies and IgM antibodies (25, 66) have been described. An evaluation of two enzyme immunoassays (adsorption and lipooligosaccharide enzyme immunoassays) for *H. ducreyi* IgG antibodies revealed sensitivities of 53 and 48%, respectively, and specificities of 71 and 89%, respectively (14).

Documentation of a satisfactory immunologic response to the *H. influenzae* type b vaccines can also be performed serologically. Assays in use include radioimmunoassay and enzyme immunoassay (97).

ANTIMICROBIAL SUSCEPTIBILITIES

As recently as 25 years ago, *Haemophilus* infections responded uniformly to treatment with ampicillin. Since then, ampicillin and penicillin resistance has become commonplace. Chloramphenicol resistance is no longer unusual in areas of the world where it is administered frequently. Doern et al. (28) reported that 36.4% of 1,537 U.S. isolates of *H. influenzae* isolates produced β-lactamase during a study reported in 1997. They also found rates of resistance to trimethoprim-sulfamethoxazole, tetracycline, and rifampin of 9.0, 1.3, and 0.3%, respectively. In comparison, a 1997 study of 816 *H. influenzae* isolates from Europe revealed 24% β-lactamase positivity, 7% trimethoprim-sulfamethoxazole resistance, and 1.2% tetracycline resistance (55).

Resistance of *H. influenzae* to ampicillin was first reported in Europe in 1972 (58) and in the United States in 1974 (46, 90). The mechanism of resistance was later found to be production of a plasmid-mediated β-lactamase (68, 89). Ampicillin resistance in *H. influenzae* caused by a mechanism other than the production of a β-lactamase was reported in 1980 (57). The mechanism appears to be structural alterations of penicillin-binding proteins that result in elevated MICs for all β-lactam agents including the cephalosporins (60).

Resistance of *H. influenzae* to chloramphenicol was first recognized in 1977. The cause was production of an inactivating enzyme, chloramphenicol acetyltransferase (1, 29, 96). Shortly thereafter, *H. influenzae* strains resistant to both ampicillin and chloramphenicol were reported (45).

Antimicrobial susceptibility testing of *H. ducreyi* is complicated by its fastidious nature. National Committee for Clinical Laboratory Standards standardized methods used for testing other species of *Haemophilus* (see below) fail to work with *H. ducreyi* because of its requirement for complex growth media. Moreover, the autoagglutination of *H. ducreyi* cells in suspension makes standardization of the inoculum density nearly impossible. The E-test method (AB Biodisk, Solna, Sweden) (see below) has shown promise as a test method suitable for *H. ducreyi* (50).

The fastidious growth requirements of *Haemophilus* spp. require special methods for antimicrobial agent susceptibility testing (27, 42, 43). Descriptions of these methods are presented in chapters 119 and 121.

EVALUATION, INTERPRETATION, AND REPORTING OF RESULTS

Laboratory diagnosis of *Haemophilus* infections can be approached from several directions. Culture is the mainstay for the diagnosis of serious infections, and that situation is likely to continue for at least the next several years. Rapid methods such as microscopy, antigen detection, and probing for nucleic acid sequences are important adjuncts but are neither sensitive nor specific enough today to replace culture. Serologic tests for *Haemophilus* infection are handicapped by their lack of sensitivity and specificity and by the time which must pass before antibodies reach detectable titers.

Culture results are extremely reliable, provided that the laboratory is using acceptable techniques for the recovery and identification of isolates. Cultures for the growth of *H. influenzae* should always include a chocolate agar plate or other medium containing both X and V factors. Even more enriched media are necessary for the growth of *H. ducreyi* from genital ulcer sites. Selective media are helpful for the recovery of *Haemophilus* from sites harboring other microorganisms, especially respiratory tract specimens from cystic fibrosis patients.

Isolation of *Haemophilus* spp. from sites not contiguous with the upper respiratory, gastrointestinal, or genitourinary tracts is usually clinically significant. Of greatest concern in young children are the typeable (encapsulated) *H. influenzae* strains, especially those belonging to serotype b. Fortunately, routine immunization of children in many countries of the world has sharply reduced the incidence of serotype b infections. *H. influenzae* (both typeable and nontypeable), *H. parainfluenzae*, and *H. aphrophilus* can be causes of life-threatening infection in older children and adults. Biotyping of *H. influenzae* and *H. parainfluenzae* isolates from such patients can be performed for epidemiologic or research purposes, but it is of little value for patient management. Detection of *H. ducreyi* in genital ulcers and lymph node aspirates is always clinically important.

Microscopic assays inherently lack sensitivity, requiring 10^3 CFU or more bacteria per ml to yield positive results. With the exception of the rarely used Quellung reaction, one is unable to identify *Haemophilus* definitively by microscopic observation. Accordingly, microscopic techniques should be limited to determining the presence or absence of microorganisms and help guide the selection of initial antimicrobial therapy.

Antigen detection immunoassays for *H. influenzae* type b also have restricted utility. The present-day practice of prescribing ampicillin and a broad-spectrum cephalosporin (e.g., cefotaxime or ceftriaxone) as empiric therapy for childhood bacterial meningitis has eliminated much of the urgency of identifying the infectious etiology. Clinicians are comfortable today with leaving meningitis patients on empiric therapy until culture and antimicrobial susceptibility results are available from the laboratory. The clinical value of antigen detection for patients with bacterial meningitis is so little that many laboratories perform this test only under extraordinary circumstances.

The most commonly encountered situation in which bacterial antigen detection has retained its clinical value is in the management of patients who present with partially treated meningitis. Gram-stained smears and cultures of samples from such patients are likely to be negative. A positive antigen detection test may be the only indication of the etiologic agent. Knowledge of the etiologic agent, especially in the case of *H. influenzae* type b and *Neisseria meningitidis* meningitis, is necessary for institution of correct prophylaxis measures.

Direct testing of genital specimens for *H. ducreyi* antigen or nucleic acid polymers holds much promise in that cultures for this microorganism are difficult and insensitive. Standardization and commercial availability of such assays are lacking, however, at the present time.

REFERENCES

1. **Azemun, P., T. Stull, M. Roberts, and A. L. Smith.** 1981. Rapid detection of chloramphenicol resistance in *Haemophilus influenzae*. *Antimicrob. Agents Chemother.* **20:** 168–170.
2. **Barbé, G., M. Babolat, J. M. Boeufgras, D. Monget, and J. Freney.** 1994. Evaluation of API NH, a new 2-hour system for identification of *Neisseria* and *Haemophilus* species and *Moraxella catarrhalis* in a routine clinical laboratory. *J. Clin. Microbiol.* **32:**187–189.
3. **Bell, L. M., G. Alpert, J. M. Campos, and S. A. Plotkin.** 1985. Routine quantitative blood cultures in children with *Haemophilus influenzae* or *Streptococcus pneumoniae* bacteremia. *Pediatrics* **76:**901–904.
4. **Bieger, R. C., N. S. Brewer, and J. A. Washington II.** 1978. *Haemophilus aphrophilus*: a microbiologic and clinical review and report of 42 cases. *Medicine* **57:**345–355.
5. **Bisgard, K. M., A. Kao, J. Leake, P. M. Strebel, B. A. Perkins, and M. Wharton.** 1998. *Haemophilus influenzae* invasive disease in the United States, 1994–1995: near disappearance of a vaccine-preventable childhood disease. *Emerg. Infect. Dis.* **4:**229–237.
6. **Bluestone, C. D., and J. O. Klein.** 1990. Otitis media—atelectasis and eustachian tube dysfunction, p. 320–486. *In* C. D. Bluestone and S. E. Stool (ed.), *Pediatric Otolaryngology*, 2nd ed. The W. B. Saunders Co., Philadelphia, Pa.
7. **Brazilian Purpuric Fever Study Group.** 1987. Brazilian purpuric fever: epidemic purpura fulminans associated with antecedent purulent conjunctivitis. *Lancet* **ii:**761–763.
8. **Brenner, D. J., L. W. Mayer, G. M. Carlone, L. H. Harrison, W. F. Bibb, M. C. de Cunto Brandileone, F. O. Sottnek, K. Irino, M. W. Reeves, J. M. Swenson, K. A. Birkness, R. S. Weyant, S. F. Berkley, T. C. Woods, A. G. Steigerwalt, P. A. D. Grimont, R. M. McKinney, D. W. Fleming, L. L. Gheesling, R. C. Cooksey, R. J. Arko, C. V. Broome, and the Brazilian Purpuric Fever Study Group.** 1988. Biochemical, genetic, and epidemiologic characterization of *Haemophilus influenzae* biogroup aegyptius (*Haemophilus aegyptius*) strains associated with Brazilian purpuric fever. *J. Clin. Microbiol.* **26:**1524–1534.
9. **Campos, J. M., and J. R. Spainhour.** 1985. Comparison of the Isolator 1.5 Microbial Tube with a conventional blood culture broth system for detection of bacteremia in children. *Diagn. Microbiol. Infect. Dis.* **3:**167–174.
10. **Carlone, G. M., F. O. Sottnek, and B. D. Plikaytis.** 1985. Comparison of outer membrane protein and biochemical profiles of *Haemophilus aegyptius* and *Haemophilus influenzae* biotype III. *J. Clin. Microbiol.* **22:**708–713.
11. **Centers for Disease Control.** 1991. Haemophilus b conjugate vaccines for prevention of *Haemophilus influenzae* type b disease among infants and children two months of age and older: recommendations of the Immunization Practices Advisory Committee (ACIP). *Morbid. Mortal. Weekly Rep.* **40**(No. RR-1)**:**1–7.
12. **Centers for Disease Control and Prevention.** 1996. *Sexually Transmitted Disease Surveillance, 1996*. U.S. Department of Health and Human Services, Atlanta, Ga.
13. **Centers for Disease Control and Prevention.** 1996.

Progress toward elimination of *Haemophilus influenzae* type b disease among infants and children—United States, 1987–1995. *Morbid. Mortal. Weekly Rep.* **45**(No. 42): 901–906.

14. **Chen, C. Y., K. J. Mertz, S. M. Spinola, and S. A. Morse.** 1997. Comparison of enzyme immunoassays for antibodies to *Haemophilus ducreyi* in a community outbreak of chancroid in the United States. *J. Infect. Dis.* **175:**1390–1395.
15. **Chui, L., W. Albritton, B. Paster, I. Maclean, and R. Marusyk.** 1993. Development of the polymerase chain reaction for diagnosis of chancroid. *J. Clin. Microbiol.* **31:** 659–664.
16. **Chunn, C. J., S. R. Jones, J. A. McCutchan, E. J. Young, and D. N. Gilbert.** 1977. *Haemophilus parainfluenzae* infective endocarditis. *Medicine* **56:**99–113.
17. **Cochi, S. L., C. V. Broome, and A. W. Hightower.** 1985. Immunization of US children with *Haemophilus influenzae* type b polysaccharide vaccine: a cost effectiveness model of strategy assessment. *JAMA* **253:**521–529.
18. **Dajani, A. S., B. I. Asmar, and M. C. Thirumoorthi.** 1979. Systemic *Haemophilus influenzae* disease: an overview. *J. Pediatr.* **94:**355–364.
19. **Daly, J. A., N. L. Clifton, K. C. Seskin, and W. M. Gooch III.** 1991. Use of rapid, nonradioactive DNA probes in culture confirmation tests to detect *Streptococcus agalactiae*, *Haemophilus influenzae*, and *Enterococcus* spp. from pediatric patients with significant infections. *J. Clin. Microbiol.* **29:**80–82.
20. **Daly, J. A., W. M. Gooch III, and J. M. Matsen.** 1985. Evaluation of the Wayson variation of a methylene blue staining procedure for the detection of microorganisms in cerebrospinal fluid. *J. Clin. Microbiol.* **21:**919–921.
21. **Dangor, Y., S. D. Miller, H. J. Koornhof, and R. C. Ballard.** 1992. A simple medium for the primary isolation of *Haemophilus ducreyi*. *Eur. J. Clin. Microbiol. Infect. Dis.* **11:** 930–934.
22. **Darras-Joly, C., O. Lortholary, J. L. Mainardi, J. Etienne, L. Guillevin, and J. Acar.** 1997. *Haemophilus* endocarditis: report of 42 cases in adults and review. *Clin. Infect. Dis.* **24:**1087–1094.
23. **Darville, T., R. F. Jacobs, R. A. Lucas, and B. Caldwell.** 1992. Detection of *Haemophilus influenzae* type b antigen in cerebrospinal fluid after immunization. *Pediatr. Infect. Dis. J.* **11:**243–244.
24. **Daum, R. S., G. R. Siber, J. S. Kamon, and R. R. Russell.** 1982. Evaluation of a commercial latex particle agglutination test for rapid diagnosis of *Haemophilus influenzae* type b infection. *Pediatrics* **69:**466–471.
25. **Desjardins, M., C. E. Thompson, L. G. Filion, J. O. Ndinya-Achola, F. A. Plummer, A. R. Ronald, P. Piot, and D. W. Cameron.** 1992. Standardization of an enzyme immunoassay for human antibody to *Haemophilus ducreyi*. *J. Clin. Microbiol.* **30:**2019–2024.
26. **Dewhirst, F. E., B. J. Paster, I. Olsen, and G. J. Fraser.** 1992. Phylogeny of 54 representative strains of species in the family *Pasteurellaceae* as determined by comparison of 16S rRNA sequences. *J. Bacteriol.* **174:**2002–2013.
27. **Doern, G. V.** 1992. In vitro susceptibility testing of *Haemophilus influenzae*: review of new National Committee for Clinical Laboratory Standards recommendations. *J. Clin. Microbiol.* **30:**3035–3038.
28. **Doern, G. V., A. B. Brueggemann, G. Pierce, H. P. Holley, Jr., and A. Rauch.** 1997. Antibiotic resistance among clinical isolates of *Haemophilus influenzae* in the United States in 1994 and 1995 and detection of β-lactamase-positive strains resistant to amoxicillin-clavulanate: results of a national multicenter surveillance study. *Antimicrob. Agents Chemother.* **41:**292–297.
29. **Doern, G. V., G. S. Daum, and T. A. Tubert.** 1987. In vitro chloramphenicol susceptibility testing of *Haemophilus influenzae*: disk diffusion procedures and assays for chloramphenicol acetyltransferase. *J. Clin. Microbiol.* **25:** 1453–1455.
30. **Dunne, W. M., Jr., F. S. Nolte, and M. L. Wilson.** 1997. *Cumitech 1B, Blood Cultures III*. Coordinating ed., J. A. Hindler. American Society for Microbiology, Washington, D.C.
31. **Faden, H., J. Stanievich, L. Brodsky, J. Bernstein, and P. L. Ogra.** 1990. Changes in nasopharyngeal flora during otitis media of childhood. *Pediatr. Infect. Dis. J.* **9:** 623–626.
32. **Farley, M. M., D. S. Stephens, P. S. Brachman Jr., C. Harvey, J. D. Smith, J. D. Wenger, and CDC Meningitis Surveillance Group.** 1992. Invasive *Haemophilus influenzae* disease in adults: a prospective, population-based surveillance. *Ann. Intern. Med.* **116:**806–812.
33. **Fitzsimmons, S.** 1997. *Cystic Fibrosis Foundation Patient Registry—1996 Annual Report*. Cystic Fibrosis Foundation, Bethesda, Md.
34. **Gill, M. V., P. E. Schoch, J. M. Musser, and B. A. Cunha.** 1995. Bacteremia and chorioamnionitis due to cryptic genospecies of *Haemophilus influenzae* biotype I. *Eur. J. Clin. Microbiol. Infect. Dis.* **14:**1088–1090.
35. **Gilsdorf, J. R.** 1987. *Haemophilus influenzae* non-type b infections in children. *Am. J. Dis. Child.* **141:**1063–1065.
36. **Greenlee, J. L.** 1990. Approach to diagnosis of meningitis. Cerebrospinal fluid evaluation. *Infect. Dis. Clin. N. Am.* **4:**583–597.
37. **Harper, J. J., and M. H. Tilse.** 1991. Biotypes of *Haemophilus influenzae* that are associated with noninvasive infections. *J. Clin. Microbiol.* **29:**2539–2542.
38. **Hickerson, S. L., R. S. Kirby, J. G. Wheeler, and G. E. Schutze.** 1996. Epiglottitis: a 9-year case review. *South. Med. J.* **89:**487–490.
39. **Inzana, T. J., J. Clarridge, and R. P. Williams.** 1987. Rapid determination of X/V growth requirements of *Haemophilus* species in broth. *Diagn. Microbiol. Infect. Dis.* **6:**93–100.
40. **Jaffe, D. M.** 1994. Occult bacteremia in children. *Adv. Pediatr. Infect. Dis.* **9:**237–258.
41. **Jones, R. G., J. W. Bass, M. E. Weisse, and J. M. Vincent.** 1991. Antigenuria after immunization with *Haemophilus influenzae* oligosaccharide CRM197 conjugate (HbOC) vaccine. *Pediatr. Infect. Dis. J.* **10:**557–559.
42. **Jorgensen, J. H., A. W. Howell, and L. A. Maher.** 1990. Antimicrobial susceptibility testing of less commonly isolated *Haemophilus* species using *Haemophilus* test medium. *J. Clin. Microbiol.* **28:**985–988.
43. **Jorgensen, J. H., A. W. Howell, and L. A. Maher.** 1991. Quantitative antimicrobial susceptibility testing of *Haemophilus influenzae* and *Streptococcus pneumoniae* by using the E-test. *J. Clin. Microbiol.* **29:**109–114.
44. **Karim, Q. N., G. Finn, C. S. F. Easmon, Y. Dangor, D. A. B. Dance, Y. F. Ngeow, and R. C. Ballard.** 1989. Rapid detection of *Haemophilus ducreyi* in clinical and experimental infections using monoclonal antibody: a preliminary evaluation. *Genitourin. Med.* **65:**361–365.
45. **Kenny, J. F., G. D. Isburg, and R. H. Michaels.** 1980. Meningitis due to *Haemophilus influenzae* type b resistant to both ampicillin and chloramphenicol. *Pediatrics* **66:**14–16.
46. **Khan, W., S. Ross, W. Rodriguez, G. Controni, and A. K. Saz.** 1974. *Haemophilus influenzae* type B resistant to ampicillin: a report of two cases. *JAMA* **229:**298–301.
47. **Kilian, M.** 1976. A taxonomic study of the genus *Haemophilus*, with the proposal of a new species. *J. Gen. Microbiol.* **93:**9–62.
48. **Klein, J. O.** 1997. Role of nontypeable *Haemophilus influen-*

zae in pediatric respiratory tract infections. *Pediatr. Infect. Dis. J.* **16:**S5–S8.

49. **Kostman, J. R., B. L. Sherry, C. L. Fligner, S. Egaas, P. Sheeran, L. Baken, J. E. Bauwens, C. Clausen, D. M. Sherer, J. J. Plorde, T. L. Stull, and P. M. Mendelman.** 1993. Invasive *Haemophilus influenzae* infections in older children and adults in Seattle. *Clin. Infect. Dis.* **17:** 389–396.
50. **Lagergard, T., A. Frisk, and B. Trollfors.** 1996. Comparison of the E-test with agar dilution for antimicrobial susceptibility testing of *Haemophilus ducreyi. J. Antimicrob. Chemother.* **38:**849–852.
51. **Lauer, B. A., L. B. Reller, and S. Mirrett.** 1981. Comparison of acridine orange and Gram stains for detection of microorganisms in cerebrospinal fluid and other clinical specimens. *J. Clin. Microbiol.* **14:**201–205.
52. **Leinonen, M., and H. Käyhty.** 1978. Comparison of counter-current immunoelectrophoresis, latex agglutination, and radioimmunoassay in detection of soluble capsular polysaccharide antigens of *Haemophilus influenzae* type b and *Neisseria meningitidis* of groups A or C. *J. Clin. Pathol.* **31:**1172–1176.
53. **Lund, M. E., and D. J. Blazevic.** 1977. Rapid speciation of *Haemophilus* with the porphyrin production test versus the satellite test for X. *J. Clin. Microbiol.* **5:**142–144.
54. **MacDonald, K., D. W. Cameron, G. Irungu, L. J. D'Costa, F. A. Plummer, L. A. Slaney, J. O. Ndinya-Achola, and A. R. Ronald.** 1989. Comparison of Sheffield media with standard media for the isolation of *Haemophilus ducreyi. Sex. Transm. Dis.* **16:**88–90.
55. **Manninen, R., P. Huovinen, and A. Nissinen.** 1997. Increasing antimicrobial resistance in *Streptococcus pneumoniae, Haemophilus influenzae,* and *Moraxella catarrhalis* in Finland. *J. Antimicrob. Chemother.* **40:**387–392.
56. **Marcon, M. J., A. C. Hamoudi, and H. J. Cannon.** 1984. Comparative laboratory evaluation of three antigen detection methods for diagnosis of *Haemophilus influenzae* type b disease. *J. Clin. Microbiol.* **19:**333–337.
57. **Markowitz, S. M.** 1980. Isolation of an ampicillin-resistant, non-β-lactamase-producing strain of *Haemophilus influenzae. Antimicrob. Agents Chemother.* **17:**80–83.
58. **Mathies, A. W., Jr.** 1972. Penicillins in the treatment of bacterial meningitis. *J. R. Coll. Physicians London* **6:** 139–146.
59. **McCarthy, L. R., and J. E. Senne.** 1980. Evaluation of acridine orange stain for detection of microorganisms in blood cultures. *J. Clin. Microbiol.* **11:**281–285.
60. **Mendelman, P. M., D. O. Chaffin, T. L. Stull, C. E. Rubens, K. D. Mack, and A. L. Smith.** 1984. Characterization of non-β-lactamase-mediated ampicillin resistance in *Haemophilus influenzae. Antimicrob. Agents Chemother.* **26:**235–244.
61. **Michaels, R. H., and O. Ali.** 1993. A decline in *Haemophilus influenzae* type b meningitis. *J. Pediatr.* **122:**407–409.
62. **Michaels, R. H., C. S. Poziviak, F. E. Stonebraker, and C. W. Norder.** 1976. Factors affecting pharyngeal *Haemophilus influenzae* type b colonization rates in children. *J. Clin. Microbiol.* **4:**413–417.
63. **Möller, L. V. M., G. J. Ruijs, H. G. M. Heijerman, J. Dankert, and L. van Alphen.** 1992. *Haemophilus influenzae* is frequently detected with monoclonal antibody 8BD9 in sputum samples from patients with cystic fibrosis. *J. Clin. Microbiol.* **30:**2495–2497.
64. **Morse, S. A.** 1989. Chancroid and *Haemophilus ducreyi. Clin. Microbiol. Rev.* **2:**137–157.
65. **Murphy, T. F., and M. A. Apicella.** 1987. Nontypable *Haemophilus influenzae*: a review of clinical aspects, surface antigens, and the human immune response to infection. *Rev. Infect. Dis.* **9:**1–15.
66. **Museyi, K., E. Van Dyck, T. Vervoot, D. Taylor, C. Hoge, and P. Piot.** 1988. Use of an enzyme immunoassay to detect serum IgG antibodies to *Haemophilus ducreyi. J. Infect. Dis.* **157:**1039–1043.
67. **Nsanze, H., M. V. Fast, L. J. D'Costa, P. Tukei, J. Curran, and A. R. Ronald.** 1981. Genital ulcers in Kenya: a clinical and laboratory study. *Br. J. Vener. Dis.* **59:** 378–381.
68. **O'Callaghan, C. H., A. Morris, S. M. Kirby, and A. H. Shingler.** 1972. Novel method for detection of β-lactamases by using a chromogenic cephalosporin substrate. *Antimicrob. Agents Chemother.* **1:**283–288.
69. **Oill, P. A., A. W. Chow, and L. B. Guze.** 1979. Adult bacteremic *Haemophilus parainfluenzae* infections. *Arch. Intern. Med.* **139:**985–988.
70. **Orle, K. A., C. A. Gates, D. H. Martin, B. A. Body, and J. B. Weiss.** 1996. Simultaneous PCR detection of *Haemophilus ducreyi, Treponema pallidum,* and herpes simplex virus types 1 and 2 from genital ulcers. *J. Clin. Microbiol.* **34:**49–54.
71. **Osterholm, M. T.** 1990. Invasive bacterial diseases and child day care. *Semin. Pediatr. Infect. Dis.* **1:**222–233.
72. **Palladino, S., B. J. Leahy, and T. L. Newall.** 1990. Comparison of the RIM-H rapid identification kit with conventional tests for the identification of *Haemophilus* spp. *J. Clin. Microbiol.* **28:**1862–1863.
73. **Pittman, M.** 1931. Variation and type specificity in the bacterial species *Hemophilus influenzae. J. Exp. Med.* **53:** 471–495.
74. **Quentin, R., I. Dubarry, C. Martin, B. Cattier, and A. Goudeau.** 1992. Evaluation of four commercial methods for identification and biotyping of genital and neonatal strains of *Haemophilus* species. *Eur. J. Clin. Microbiol. Infect. Dis.* **11:**546–549.
75. **Quentin, R., C. Martin, J. M. Musser, N. Pasquier-Picard, and A. Goudeau.** 1993. Genetic characterization of a cryptic genospecies of *Haemophilus* causing urogenital and neonatal infections. *J. Clin. Microbiol.* **31:**1111–1116.
76. **Quentin, R. A., A. Goudeau, R. J. Wallace, Jr., A. L. Smith, R. K. Selander, and J. M. Musser.** 1990. Urogenital, maternal and neonatal isolates of *Haemophilus influenzae*: identification of unusually virulent serologically nontypable clone families and evidence for a new *Haemophilus* species. *J. Gen. Microbiol.* **136:**1203–1209.
77. **Rennie, R., T. Gordon, Y. Yaschuk, P. Tomlin, P. Kibsey, and W. Albritton.** 1992. Laboratory and clinical evaluations of media for the primary isolation of *Haemophilus* species. *J. Clin. Microbiol.* **30:**1917–1921.
78. **Roggen, E. L., R. Pansaerts, E. Van Dyck, and P. Piot.** 1993. Antigen detection and immunological typing of *Haemophilus ducreyi* with a specific rabbit polyclonal serum. *J. Clin. Microbiol.* **31:**1820–1825.
79. **Schmid, G. P., Y. C. Faur, J. A. Valu, S. A. Sikandar, and M. M. McLaughlin.** 1995. Enhanced recovery of *Haemophilus ducreyi* from clinical specimens by incubation at 33 versus 35°C. *J. Clin. Microbiol.* **33:**3257–3259.
80. **Schwartz, R., W. J. Rodriguez, R. Mann, W. Khan, and S. Ross.** 1979. The nasopharyngeal culture in acute otitis media. *JAMA* **241:**2170–2173.
81. **Shanholtzer, C. J., P. J. Schaper, and L. R. Peterson.** 1982. Concentrated Gram-stained smears prepared with a cytospin centrifuge. *J. Clin. Microbiol.* **16:**1052–1056.
82. **Slater, L. N., J. Guarnaccia, S. Makintubee, and G. R. Istre.** 1990. Bacteremic disease due to *Haemophilus influenzae* capsular type f in adults: report of five cases and review. *Rev. Infect. Dis.* **12:**628–635.
83. **Stamm, W. E., H. H. Handsfield, A. M. Rompalo, R. L. Ashley, P. L. Roberts, and L. Corey.** 1988. The associa-

tion between genital ulcer disease and acquisition of HIV infection in homosexual men. *JAMA* **260:**1429–1433.

84. **St. Geme, J. W., III, A. Takala, E. Esko, and S. Falkow.** 1994. Evidence for capsule gene sequences among pharyngeal isolates of nontypeable *Haemophilus influenzae*. *J. Infect. Dis.* **169:**337–342.
85. **Strausbaugh, L. J.** 1997. *Haemophilus influenzae* infections in adults: a pathogen in search of respect. *Postgrad. Med.* **101:**191–192.
86. **Sturm, A. W.** 1986. *Haemophilus influenzae* and *Haemophilus parainfluenzae* in nongonococcal urethritis. *J. Infect. Dis.* **153:**165–167.
87. **Sturm, A. W.** 1986. Isolation of *Haemophilus influenzae* and *Haemophilus parainfluenzae* from genital-tract specimens with a selective medium. *J. Med. Microbiol.* **21:** 349–352.
88. **Swaminathan, B., L. W. Mayer, W. F. Bibb, G. W. Ajello, K. Irino, K. A. Birkness, C. F. Garon, M. W. Reeves, M. Cristina de Cunto Brandileone, F. O. Sottnek, D. J. Brenner, A. G. Steigerwalt, and the Brazilian Purpuric Fever Study Group.** 1989. Microbiology of Brazilian purpuric fever and diagnostic tests. *J. Clin. Microbiol.* **27:** 605–608.
89. **Sykes, R. B., M. Matthew, and C. H. O'Callaghan.** 1975. R-factor mediated beta-lactamase production by *Haemophilus influenzae*. *J. Med. Microbiol.* **8:**437–441.
90. **Tomeh, M. O., S. E. Starr, J. E. McGowan, Jr., P. M. Terry, and A. J. Nahmias.** 1974. Ampicillin-resistant *Haemophilus influenzae* type b infection. *JAMA* **229:** 295–297.
91. **Trees, D. L., and S. A. Morse.** 1995. Chancroid and *Haemophilus ducreyi*: an update. *Clin. Microbiol. Rev.* **8:** 357–375.
92. **Trottier, S., K. Stenberg, I. A. Von Rosen, and C. Svanborg.** 1991. *Haemophilus influenzae* causing conjunctivitis in day-care children. *Pediatr. Infect. Dis. J.* **10:**578–584.
93. **Turk, D. C.** 1984. The pathogenicity of *Haemophilus influenzae*. *J. Med. Microbiol.* **18:**1–16.
94. **Tyndall, M. S., A. R. Ronald, E. Agoki, W. Malisa, J. J. Bwayo, J. O. Ndinya-Achola, S. Moses, and F. A. Plummer.** 1996. Increased risk of infection with human immunodeficiency virus type 1 among uncircumcised men presenting with genital ulcer disease in Kenya. *Clin. Infect. Dis.* **23:**449–453.
95. **Urwin, G., J. A. Krohn, K. Deaver-Robinson, J. D. Wenger, and M. M. Farley.** 1996. Invasive disease due to *Haemophilus influenzae* serotype f: clinical and epidemiologic characteristics in the *H. influenzae* serotype b vaccine era. *Clin. Infect. Dis.* **22:**1069–1076.
96. **van Klingeren, B., J. D. A. van Embden, and M. Dessens-Kroon.** 1977. Plasmid-mediated chloramphenicol resistance in *Haemophilus influenzae*. *Antimicrob. Agents Chemother.* **11:**383–387.
97. **Vella, P. P., J. M. Staub, J. Armstrong, K. T. Dolan, C. M. Rusk, S. Szymanski, W. E. Greer, S. Marburg, P. J. Kniskern, T. L. Schofield, R. L. Tolman, F. Hartner, S. Pan, R. J. Gerety, and R. W. Ellis.** 1990. Immunogenicity of a new *Haemophilus influenzae* type b conjugate vaccine (meningococcal protein conjugate) (PedvaxHIB). *Pediatrics* **85**(Suppl.)**:**668–675.
98. **Wald, E. R.** 1997. Conjunctivitis in infants and children. *Pediatr. Infect. Dis. J.* **16:**S17–S20.
99. **West, B., S. M. Wilson, J. Changalucha, S. Patel, P. Mayaud, R. C. Ballard, and D. Mabey.** 1995. Simplified PCR for detection of *Haemophilus ducreyi* and diagnosis of chancroid. *J. Clin. Microbiol.* **33:**787–790.
100. **Winslow, C. E., J. Broadhurst, and R. E. Buchanan.** 1920. The families and genera of the bacteria: final report of the committee of the Society of American Bacteriologists on characterization and classification of bacterial types. *J. Bacteriol.* **5:**191–229.

*Bordetella**

JÖRG E. HOPPE

40

TAXONOMY

In the 9th edition of *Bergey's Manual of Determinative Bacteriology* of 1994, four species of the genus *Bordetella* are listed: *Bordetella pertussis*, *B. parapertussis*, *B. bronchiseptica*, and *B. avium* (32). *B. pertussis*, *B. parapertussis*, and *B. bronchiseptica* are closely related (99). They can be considered subtypes or subspecies of a single genospecies; however, this is controversial (63). Strains referred to as "*B. avium*-like" have now been assigned to a new species, *B. hinzii* (94). *B. holmesii* previously had the vernacular name "CDC nonoxidizer group 2" (101). Another recently described species has been named *B. trematum* (95).

DESCRIPTION OF THE GENUS

Bordetellae are small gram-negative coccobacilli (Fig. 1) (76). Some species are motile (Table 1). All are catalase-positive, strict aerobes and have only simple nutritional requirements including nicotinamide, organic sulfur (e.g., cysteine), and organic nitrogen (amino acids). Most bordetellae do not use carbohydrates as an energy source (99). *B. pertussis* is the most fastidious species within the genus. It does not grow on simple media (Table 1); however, Mueller-Hinton agar supplemented with 5% horse blood supports its growth (43). *B. pertussis* is inhibited by medium constituents such as unsaturated fatty acids, metal ions, colloidal sulfur, and peroxides. Starch, charcoal, albumin, blood, cyclodextrin, or other protective substances must be added to isolation media (for a review, see reference 85). *B. pertussis* grows slowly (mean generation time, 2.3 to 5 h [85]). It is susceptible to cold (70) and desiccation (1, 58). The other *Bordetella* species are less fastidious. *B. parapertussis* and *B. holmesii* are relatively slowly growing species as well.

Bordetellae produce a number of toxins and virulence factors (Table 2) (31, 80) which are involved in adherence and clinical disease. Pertussis toxin (PT) is produced only by *B. pertussis*; *B. parapertussis* and *B. bronchiseptica* possess but do not express the complete toxin operon (5). PT is a protein consisting of six subunits; it transfers ADP ribose to G proteins to inhibit their coupling of receptors to intracellular signal transduction pathways (31, 80). PT has a multitude of biological effects (for reviews, see references 31, 80, and 100). Adenylate cyclase toxin (ACT) inhibits host cells including immune effector cells by leading to high levels of intracellular cyclic adenosine 3′, 5′-phosphate. Tracheal cytotoxin (TCT) plays a major role in the initial pathology of pertussis by causing ciliostasis, inhibition of DNA synthesis, and cell death (31). The role of dermonecrotic toxin (heat-labile toxin) is still ill defined. In addition to the toxins, bordetellae produce adhesion molecules including filamentous hemagglutinin (FHA), pertactin (formerly known as the 69-kDa outer membrane protein), and fimbriae (also termed pili). Two virulence factors whose roles are still unclear have recently been described: serum resistance factor (termed BrkA) and tracheal colonization factor (74). The production of most virulence factors is regulated by a two-component signaling system, termed *bvg*, which is also responsible for the regulatory phenomena of phase variation and phenotypic modulation (100).

The pathogenesis of pertussis involves initial fimbria-mediated attachment of the organisms to epithelial and immune effector cells. Attachment is stabilized by FHA, pertactin, and PT. While PT and ACT help to counteract the host's immune system, TCT damages the respiratory epithelium (for a review, see reference 31). The hypothesis that pertussis is a monotoxin disease solely caused by PT (75) is increasingly being challenged by the concept that it is a multifactorial disease (31). However, mechanisms of immunity remain incompletely understood. While antibody plays a role in preventing colonization and combating toxin-mediated disease, complete bacterial clearance requires cellular immune responses (69).

NATURAL HABITATS

In the past, bordetellae were considered noninvasive parasites of the respiratory tracts of warm-blooded animals and humans with a tropism for the respiratory ciliated epithelium (99). However, *B. pertussis*, *B. parapertussis*, and *B. bronchiseptica* have mechanisms for attachment to, invasion of, and survival in epithelial cells and phagocytes (18). The significance of this is not yet clear, but it may be important in the protracted course of *Bordetella* infections or in the establishment of a quiescent or a chronic stage (74). *B. pertussis* has been isolated from the blood of an immunocompromised patient (51). It is a uniquely human pathogen,

* This chapter contains information presented in chapter 46 by Mario J. Marcon in the sixth edition of this Manual.

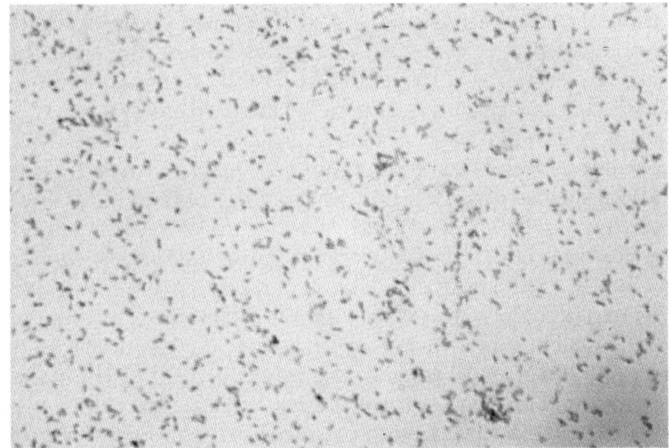

FIGURE 1 Tiny gram-negative coccobacilli typical of *B. pertussis* smear made from a colony.

whereas *B. parapertussis* is found both in humans and in lambs (74). *B. bronchiseptica* causes kennel cough in dogs and atrophic rhinitis in swine. It is rarely found in humans, in whom it causes pertussis-like symptoms in immunocompetent hosts (91) and various infections in immunocompromised patients (106). Coryza in turkey poults is the main disease due to *B. avium* (53); *B. avium* infections have not been observed in humans. *B. hinzii* has been isolated from the respiratory tracts of birds, in which it appears to be apathogenic (94); few isolates have so far been reported from humans. *B. holmesii* has been isolated from cultures of blood from immunocompromised patients (101); *B. trematum* has been isolated from wounds and ear infections (95).

CLINICAL SIGNIFICANCE

B. pertussis is the predominant cause of pertussis (whooping cough). The disease has an incubation period of 6 to 20 days (mean, 7 to 10 days). Classical pertussis is an illness of three stages (the catarrhal, paroxysmal, and convalescent stages). It starts like a viral upper respiratory tract infection with coryza and mild cough (catarrhal stage; duration, 1 to 2 weeks). Cough becomes more prominent with staccato attacks, posttussive whooping, and vomiting (paroxysmal stage; duration, 2 to 6 weeks). Fever, pharyngitis, and signs and symptoms of systemic illness are usually absent. During the convalescent stage (duration, several weeks) the cough gradually decreases in frequency and severity (13). Complications are mainly due to the effects of the paroxysms and include anoxia, cyanosis, atelectasis, and bronchiectasis. Secondary infections due to *Haemophilus influenzae*, *Streptococcus pneumoniae*, *Streptococcus pyogenes*, or *Staphylococcus aureus* manifest as pneumonia or otitis media. Encephalopathy is the most serious form of central nervous system complications (13).

Typical pertussis occurs mainly during primary infection in unimmunized children, but 25 to 30% of such children present with mild or atypical clinical pictures (50); they are thus not suspected of suffering from pertussis but spread the disease (12). Adults play an important role in transmission as well. Their disease may take the typical form; more often they suffer from long-standing cough without whooping

TABLE 1 Differential phenotypic characteristics of *Bordetella* spp.[a]

Characteristic	Response[b]						
	B. pertussis	*B. parapertussis*	*B. bronchiseptica*	*B. avium*	*B. hinzii*	*B. holmesii*	*B. trematum*
Growth on:							
Blood agar	−	+	+	+	+	+	+
MacConkey agar	−	±	+	+	+	+	+
Oxidase	+	−	+	+	+	−	−
Nitrate reduction	−	−	+	−	−	−	±
Urease production	−	+ (24 h)	+ (4 h)	−	±	−	−
Motility, 37°C	−	−	+	+	+	−	+

[a] Modified from references 32, 63, 94, 95, and 101.
[b] Responses: +, activity or growth present; −, not present; ±, may or may not be present.

TABLE 2 Virulence factors of *Bordetella* spp.[a]

Virulence factor	*B. pertussis*	*B. parapertussis*	*B. bronchiseptica*	*B. avium*	Probable role in pathogenicity
PT	+	−	−	−	Adhesion, invasion, interference with immune effector cells
FHA	+	+	+	−	Adhesion, invasion
ACT	+	+	+	+	Interference with immune effector cells
Pertactin	+	+	+	NK[b]	Adhesion, invasion
Tracheal cytotoxin	+	+	+	+	Ciliostasis, cytotoxicity
Heat-labile toxin	+	+	+	+	Local inflammation, cytotoxicity
Fimbriae	+	+	+	+	Adhesion, invasion

[a] Modified from reference 74.
[b] NK, not known.

which is frequently misdiagnosed (78, 87). Vaccine-induced immunity in pertussis is relatively short-lived, and naturally acquired immunity also wanes with time (12, 78, 104). Thus, neither vaccination nor pertussis in childhood can prevent adult pertussis with certainty. Neonates are susceptible to pertussis with potentially fatal consequences (7). Whooping and even cough may be absent; apnea is the hallmark of pertussis in neonates and young infants.

Typical pertussis can be recognized clinically during the paroxysmal stage, but organisms other than *B. pertussis* can cause pertussis-like disease. These include *B. parapertussis*, *B. bronchiseptica*, *Chlamydia trachomatis* (in young infants), and certain viruses (adenoviruses and respiratory syncytial virus).

Pertussis remains a disease with significant morbidity and mortality. There are more than 350,000 deaths annually worldwide, with the majority occurring in young infants (12). Pertussis is a highly communicable disease; >90% of susceptible household contacts may contract it (9). Immunized contacts can become transiently colonized and remain asymptomatic (29), but a long-lasting carrier state has not been observed. In populations with low immunization rates, pertussis is epidemic. It remains endemic in populations with high vaccination rates such as in the United States. Vaccinated persons, especially adults whose immunity has waned, can circulate *B. pertussis* within the population via colonization and subclinical infection (9, 12). In both types of populations, epidemic cycles of pertussis occur every 2 to 5 years. In nonvaccinating countries, most pertussis cases are seen in children 2 to 5 years of age (50); in the United States, 40 to 50% of reported cases occur in young infants and 30% occur in adults (9).

Traditional pertussis vaccines consist of killed and partially detoxified whole *B. pertussis* organisms; they are 80 to 90% efficacious but are associated with a high rate of minor adverse events (13). Therefore, acellular vaccines consisting of one to five components of *B. pertussis* (PT, FHA, pertactin, agglutinogens) have been developed, and these are better tolerated. Their strong efficacy even in young infants has been shown in recent clinical trials (for an overview, see reference 77).

Infections caused by *B. parapertussis* are not rare. Approximately 40% of them remain asymptomatic; another 40% result in nonspecific "bronchitis." Fewer than 20% of infected individuals, mainly young children, suffer from a pertussis-like disease (61). Conversely, fewer than 5% of pertussis cases are caused by *B. parapertussis* (58, 61). In these patients, the clinical picture is indistinguishable from that of pertussis but tends to be less severe (30). Lymphocytosis is seen less frequently in parapertussis than in pertussis. Since *B. parapertussis* does not produce PT but can cause a clinical picture similar to that of pertussis, it is unlikely that PT is the main cause of the typical cough of pertussis (30, 102). Dual infections with *B. pertussis* and *B. parapertussis* occur (83); infection with one species does not protect a person from subsequent infection with the other (61).

COLLECTION, TRANSPORT, AND STORAGE OF SPECIMENS

Respiratory secretions are the obvious specimen used for direct bacteriological diagnosis of pertussis. Patients usually are not sick enough to justify invasive diagnostic measures such as bronchoalveolar lavage. Exceptions include AIDS patients (73) and other immunocompromised patients. Specimens are usually obtained from the upper respiratory tract. The use of nasopharyngeal (NP), i.e., pernasal, swabs results in higher rates of isolation of *B. pertussis* than the use of cough plates (57). The use of NP aspirates obtained with flexible catheters and by suction with a syringe (27) leads to even higher *Bordetella* isolation rates than those obtained by the use of NP swabs (24), and NP aspirates are also preferred for PCR (66), since more material is obtained and several diagnostic methods can be performed in parallel. Unfortunately, NP swabs are still the standard specimen used in most countries. The technique of obtaining NP swabs is simple; a thin swab with a flexible wire is introduced flat and is pushed forward with gentle downward pressure on the lower nasal floor to the posterior wall of the nasopharynx. The swab is rotated for a few seconds before it is gently withdrawn. Leaving the swab in the nasopharynx for a longer period has not been shown to increase the yield. Thick swabs such as those used for throat cultures are unsuitable for NP swabbing. Anterior nasal swabs are inadequate. The cultural yield from throat swabs is lower than that from NP swabs for two reasons (8, 64). One, the throat does not contain ciliated respiratory epithelium, and two, the diversity of the throat flora exceeds that of the nasopharynx, resulting in higher contamination rates (20, 58). With regard to PCR, large comparative studies of NP and throat swabs are lacking.

The swab material is of importance. Cotton is least suitable for bordetellae (46) since some fibers contain inhibitors (58). Calcium alginate swabs (CalgiFybr; PurFybr, Inc., Munster, Ind.) are best for the isolation of bordetellae since they lack toxicity and enable better release of organisms because of the partial dissolution of the fibers (34, 46). Dacron fibers are slightly inferior to alginate fibers for culture but are preferred for PCR since both alginate fibers and the aluminum components of their shafts were inhibitory in some PCR assays (98).

For culture, direct plating of NP swabs or aspirates at the bedside or in the office is the method of choice (1, 40, 79). When this is not possible, NP aspirates collected in 1% Casamino Acids (Difco Laboratories, Detroit, Mich.) in phosphate-buffered saline (pH 7.4) may be stored at 4°C for several days (27). A transport medium must be used for NP swabs. It is less satisfactory than direct plating, since the latter enables a more rapid diagnosis and yields a significantly higher number of *Bordetella* isolates (40). NP swabs should never be transported dry. The choice of medium depends on the delay between collection and plating (63, 88): If a transport time of <2 h is expected, Casamino Acids broth may be used (11) and specimens can be transported at room temperature. If the delay is longer but <24 h, Amies medium with charcoal transported at room temperature is satisfactory (105). If a longer transport time is anticipated, a medium containing nutrients and selective agents that inhibit the commensal NP flora is preferable (48). The semisolid transport medium of Regan and Lowe (81) fulfills these requirements; it is in fact an enrichment medium. It contains charcoal agar base (Oxoid Inc., Ogdersburg, N.Y.) at a concentration half of that used in the agar plates (see below) but with the same supplements, i.e., 10% horse blood and 40 mg of cephalexin per liter. Regan-Lowe transport medium has a shelf-life of 4 to 8 weeks. It may be prepared as slants; the swab specimen is streaked onto the agar surface and is then submerged into the agar and the swab shaft is cut off (63).

If transport systems (combinations of swabs and media) are mailed, they will be exposed to ambient temperatures during transport. Bordetellae survive this exposure significantly better if transport systems are incubated at 36°C for 1 to 2 days prior to mailing (34, 46, 48). During this preincubation the organisms start multiplying again and the medium thus contains greater numbers of bacteria, making survival during transport more likely. On the other hand, preincubation delays final diagnosis and also increases overgrowth of the more rapidly growing cephalexin-resistant commensal flora. If transport systems are transported at 4°C, overgrowth is suppressed but *B. pertussis* colony numbers decrease by >75% (70). Thus, the higher contamination rate after preincubation must be weighed against the substantial loss of bordetellae during refrigeration, which may render the isolation of small inocula impossible. Leaving swabs in transport media at room temperature is the worst solution. Bordetellae will not multiply significantly, but overgrowth will occur (27). The ambient temperature in a given locale should also be taken into account (92). In the author's experience in Germany, preincubation is preferable, and transport by mail at ambient temperatures is of course much more practical than transport under refrigeration. Once bordetellae have grown on agar, plates or slants may be mailed without a loss of viability even if the transport lasts for several days (33).

NP swabs for PCR should be mailed dry or suspended in saline (71). Transport conditions for NP aspirates for PCR have not been studied systematically. In the laboratory, NP aspirates are treated with a mucolytic agent and are then centrifuged to pellet the bacteria. After removal of the supernatant, the pellet is resuspended in water and boiled. Whichever methods are selected for the collection and transport of NP specimens in a particular clinical setting, it is imperative that detailed instructions and appropriate collection materials be readily available (63, 92). The "*B. pertussis* collection kit" which contains an agar plate, a transport medium, and a swab (20) is a good example, and helpful details may also be found in the *Clinical Microbiology Procedures Handbook* (14, 88).

DIRECT EXAMINATION

DFA Test

The direct fluorescent-antibody (DFA) test uses commercially available (Difco) polyclonal, fluorescein-labeled, species-specific antibodies against *B. pertussis* and *B. parapertussis* for the direct detection of the organisms in NP specimens. Organism viability is not a prerequisite. Unlike culture and PCR, DFA testing does not incorporate multiplication of the bacteria or their genetic material. Like PCR but unlike culture, DFA testing provides rapid results; this explains the continuing attractiveness of this time-honored method. A number of studies have documented the lack of sensitivity and specificity of DFA testing (17, 26). Sensitivity is limited by the number of organisms present in the secretions and by the lack of multiplication. Cross-reaction with organisms of the NP flora makes the results of DFA tests technically difficult to interpret, resulting in rates of false positivity as high as 88.4% (17). Much depends on the technical skill and experience of the technicians who perform the test and read the test results. Preparation of reagents, quality control, test performance, and subjectivity of interpretation of the DFA test present some challenges even to good laboratories (63). Laboratories proficient in both DFA testing and culture for bordetellae should obtain a DFA test sensitivity of at least 60% and a specificity of at least 90% in comparison with the results of culture (20). DFA testing should be performed only with simultaneous culturing (20, 63, 71). Slides should be dried, heat fixed, and stained on the day of receipt. They should be prepared with a coverslip and fluorescent-antibody mounting fluid (Difco) and should be viewed under oil immersion at a magnification of between ×600 and ×1,000. The organisms appear as small coccobacillary rods with strong peripheral apple green fluorescence and dark centers. The *B. parapertussis* conjugate may be used as a negative staining control for *B. pertussis* and vice versa (20, 63, 88).

Recently, a monoclonal antibody (termed BL-5) which recognizes the lipooligosaccharide of *B. pertussis* has been developed. Compared with culture, the sensitivity and specificity of fluorescein-conjugated BL-5 in DFA smears were 65.1 and 99.6%, respectively (65). This monoclonal antibody in combination with one specific for *B. parapertussis* is now commercially available as a dual fluorochrome DFA reagent (Biotex Laboratories, Edmonton, Alberta, Canada). It is likely that in the long run DFA testing will be replaced by PCR since the latter method combines rapidity with a much higher sensitivity (71).

Nucleic Acid Detection

Detection of *Bordetella*-specific nucleic acids in NP specimens by DNA amplification methods such as PCR shows tremendous diagnostic potential (for reviews, see references 66 and 71 and chapter 13 of this Manual). Primers derived from four chromosomal regions have been used, including a PT promoter region (23, 82), a region upstream of the porin gene (60), the repetitive insertion sequences IS*481* of *B. pertussis* and IS*1001* of *B. parapertussis* (97), and the ACT gene (15). With the exception of the ACT gene, these primers are species specific. Some PCR assays are specific for *B. pertussis* (23); others allow the detection of *B. pertussis* and *B. parapertussis* (60, 97) or, in addition, *B. bronchiseptica* (82). The sensitivities of the assays with the various primers appear to be similar (66, 71). Nested primer systems (6, 83) and multiplex assays that simultaneously amplify two separate DNA targets may offer advantages regarding sensitivity and specificity.

Steps are necessary to prevent false-negative and false-positive PCR results. Factors that may lead to false-negative results include an insufficient number of bacteria in the nasopharynx (very early or late stage of disease) or in the specimen (inadequate sampling technique), the presence of an inhibitor in the sample, the loss or damage of bacteria or DNA during processing or storage, a prozone-like effect when very large amounts of DNA are present in the test tube (86), technical problems with the assay, and the low sensitivity of the detection system (66, 71). False-positive results may be caused by samples containing other organisms with DNA sequences homologous to those of the bordetellae, sample contamination with DNA or bacteria from laboratory *Bordetella* strains, and contamination of samples with DNA from previous amplifications (product carryover). Therefore, rigorous internal and external quality control systems are indispensable (66, 71).

Studies comparing PCR with culture have in general found good concordance. PCR-negative, culture-positive results have been observed for up to 26% of specimens (96); often, culture showed only a few colonies in such cases (29). PCR-positive, culture-negative results occur more frequently; in some studies the number of pertussis patients identified by PCR was severalfold higher than the number detected by culture (29, 86, 96). Unlike culture, PCR cannot distinguish between dead and viable bacteria. PCR is rapid, sensitive, and specific, but it is expensive, requires sophisticated equipment, and is at present insufficiently standardized (23, 71). It should be performed only in parallel with culture (86).

CULTURE AND ISOLATION

B. pertussis was originally isolated by Bordet and Gengou (10) on potato infusion agar supplemented with 4% glycerol and 50% rabbit blood. Modifications of this Bordet-Gengou (BG) agar containing 10% glycerol and 20% blood are still used (88). One of the disadvantages of BG agar is its short shelf-life. Plates more than 5 days old give inferior results (58). Ideally, BG agar plates should be made fresh with each use. Tubes of base medium can, however, be stored at 4°C for several weeks (88). Another disadvantage of BG agar is that suspensions of *B. pertussis* from this medium tend to be autoagglutinable (1, 58). Some commercial BG agar preparations support the growth of bordetellae only inadequately (105). In 1965 the Oxoid company marketed a charcoal agar base to be supplemented with 10% whole defibrinated horse blood (charcoal-horse blood [CHB] agar). Several studies have demonstrated the superiority of CHB agar to BG agar for the isolation of *B. pertussis* from clinical specimens (45, 56, 70, 79, 81, 93). CHB agar has also been shown to be superior to blood-free Oxoid and other charcoal agars (41), which stresses the importance of blood in *Bordetella* media. Plates of CHB agar supplemented with cephalexin (40 mg/liter) possess a shelf-life of 4 to 8 weeks. Some commercially prepared plated charcoal-blood agar media may not adequately support the growth of bordetellae (20, 33). A study comparing sheep blood with horse blood in charcoal agar noted more abundant and rapid growth and a more typical colony morphology of bordetellae on horse blood agar (39). Cyclodextrin solid medium (3), a synthetic blood-free medium resembling Stainer-Scholte broth (89), is superior to BG agar (3) but is inferior to CHB agar (70). Higher *Bordetella* isolation rates by combined use of BG and CHB media have been reported. It remains unclear if this was due just to the quantitative effect of inoculating two plates in parallel.

It has been shown with regard to streptococci that swabs release <10% of the initial inoculum when they are streaked onto solid media, while elution in a liquid medium enables the recovery of 50% of the initial inoculum (84). Since this is likely to apply also to bordetellae, it appears logical to use a liquid enrichment medium for NP swabs. The semisolid Regan-Lowe medium (81) may be used; it increased the *Bordetella* isolation rate by 6 to 14% in two studies (25, 105). Heptakis-supplemented Stainer-Scholte broth allowed the isolation of an additional 12% of isolates (105). Stainer-Scholte broth, which is mainly used for vaccine production, has a complicated composition and is not commercially available. Mueller-Hinton broth with 5% horse blood (43) has not been studied with clinical material. From a practical standpoint, the procedure suggested by Regan and Lowe (81) may be followed: if swabs have been plated directly or have been transported in Amies medium, they should be placed into Regan-Lowe medium and subcultured after 48 h of incubation. If swabs have been transported in Regan-Lowe medium and have been preincubated prior to transport, use of an enrichment medium is probably not necessary. Large studies evaluating this approach are lacking, as are studies on the use of NP aspirates and enrichment procedures.

Since bordetellae grow more slowly than most constituents of the normal NP flora, a selective antimicrobial agent is incorporated into *Bordetella* media to prevent overgrowth. At present, cephalexin (93) is the agent of choice. It is superior to penicillin, methicillin, lincomycin, and cefsulodin (103), but overgrowth by cephalexin-resistant flora (mainly *H. influenzae*, enterococci, and pseudomonads [33]) is not uncommon. Candidate agents with a broader inhibitory spectrum such as ceftibuten or cefetamet have yet to be studied. Growth of *B. pertussis* is slightly retarded on cephalexin-containing media (81). Some strains of *B. pertussis* are said to be inhibited by cephalexin; therefore, the use of both selective and nonselective media has been advocated (14). However, a large study found none of 233 isolates to be susceptible to 40 μg of cephalexin per ml (103). Therefore, the additional use of nonselective media is not warranted. If problems with contaminating fungi are often encountered, amphotericin B (50 mg/liter) (81) or anisomycin (20 mg/liter) (56) may be added to the agar.

The optimum temperature of incubation for bordetellae is 35 to 36°C (1, 58, 79). Adequate humidity is essential; therefore, plates must be poured thick (1). For the prevention of desiccation, simple plastic boxes with tightly closing lids (34) or candle jars with an unlit candle (20) may be used, or plates may be wrapped with a sealing tape that allows air exchange (63). Incubation should take place in ambient air without added carbon dioxide (39).

Plates are inspected for growth of contaminants or *B. bronchiseptica* after 24 h of incubation. Mature colonies of *B. parapertussis* usually become visible after 2 to 3 days of incubation, and colonies of *B. pertussis* usually become visible after 3 to 4 days of incubation. Plates must be incubated for at least 7 days before being discarded as negative. A recent study reported the additional recovery of 18% of isolates by extending the incubation to 12 days (52). Prolonged incubation seems to be particularly warranted when patients receive effective antimicrobial therapy or when their DFA test result has been positive (63). Occasionally, plates will be overgrown with contaminants, thus being uninterpretable; final reports should stress that the presence of bordetellae could not be excluded (63).

IDENTIFICATION

Fresh clinical isolates of *B. pertussis* have a typical colony morphology on CHB agar. They are small, smooth, and round and have a characteristic anthracite color, a shiny surface with a high convex shape (mercury droplet-like appearance), and a butyrous consistency. The color turns into a whitish grey as the colonies age. Subcultures of *B. pertussis* have grey colonies from the beginning. Young colonies of *B. bronchiseptica* are indistinguishable from those of *B. pertussis*, while young colonies of *B. parapertussis* are duller, slightly larger, and more grey than anthracite and assume a slight brownish green tint when aging (1, 33, 58). The morphology of *Bordetella* colonies on BG agar is similar; all three species produce zones of hemolysis (58).

Colonies of typical morphology are Gram stained; the safranin counterstain should be applied for 1 to 2 min to enhance the intensity of staining (58, 63). Bordetellae appear as gram-negative coccobacilli or short slender rods. Typical colonies are subjected to the oxidase reaction. *B. pertussis* and *B. bronchiseptica* are oxidase positive; *B. parapertussis* is oxidase negative. If the oxidase reaction is positive, identification is performed with *B. pertussis* antiserum, and *B. parapertussis* antiserum is used if the oxidase reaction is negative. It is not advisable to use both antisera on the same isolate because weak cross-reactions may occur (1, 33). Both fluorescent polyclonal antisera (Difco) and agglutinating polyclonal antisera (Difco; Murex Diagnostics, Inc., Norcross, Ga.; Denka Seiken, Tokyo, Japan) for *B. pertussis* and *B. parapertussis* are commercially available. For slide agglutination, a suspension of the organism approximately equivalent to a no. 3 McFarland standard is prepared in saline (14). Bordetellae do not always emulsify readily in saline. Clumping of bacteria is more often seen with older and/or dry colonies, which tend to produce ambiguous agglutination results. One may try to break up the clumps by forcing the suspension through a pipette (63, 79); however, it is better to subculture the isolate (preferably on antibiotic-free CHB agar), which leads to unequivocal agglutination results (33). Specific agglutination occurs rapidly, and only immediate reactions should be considered positive (58). Agglutination is often only of medium strength (approximately 2+ on a 1+ to 4+ scale) and is not as marked as that in latex-enhanced tests (34). The fluorescein-labeled antisera are the same as those used for the DFA test. A very dilute suspension of the organisms is prepared in phosphate-buffered saline; testing of suspensions that are too heavy may lead to false-negative results due to the dulling of fluorescence. False-positive reactions may occur due to cross-reactions with other small gram-negative bacilli, e.g., *Haemophilus* spp. (20).

If testing with antisera supplies clear-cut results, no additional steps are needed. If not, other methods of identification must be used (Table 1), including subcultures on sheep blood and MacConkey agar and biochemical identification. PCR may help to distinguish between *B. pertussis* and *B. parapertussis* (90). *B. bronchiseptica* may easily be confused with *B. pertussis*. The colony morphology of *B. bronchiseptica* is identical to that of *B. pertussis*; *B. bronchiseptica* is also oxidase positive and may agglutinate both *B. pertussis* and *B. parapertussis* antisera (33, 91). Unlike *B. pertussis*, it develops mature colonies after only 24 h of incubation (33, 58). Subcultures show that *B. bronchiseptica* grows on sheep blood and MacConkey agar. It can reliably be identified by commercial kits, e.g., API-NFT (BioMérieux Vitek, Inc., Hazelwood, Mo.) (33).

Quality control of media and identification procedures is essential. Stock strains of *B. pertussis* ATCC 9797 and *B. parapertussis* ATCC 15311 are adequate positive controls (14). In addition, fresh clinical isolates may be used (20), and these should be frozen as soon as possible. Long-term preservation is possible by lyophilization or by storage at −70°C in whole sheep blood (20) or in pure glycerol (33), while storage at −20°C preserves viability for several months and storage at 4°C preserves viability for 4 weeks (33, 34). Since stock cultures rapidly lose viability, they must be replaced fairly often. Both commercial and in-house-prepared media must undergo rigorous quality control. The control strains mentioned above are seeded in duplicate onto newly prepared and previously quality-controlled medium. With regard to colony count and size, the new medium must display a plating efficiency of at least 50% compared with that of the previously controlled medium (63).

SEROLOGIC TESTS

After infection with *B. pertussis*, specific antibodies of all isotypes are produced. Immune reactions against PT and FHA can be detected in >90% of infected patients and against pertactin, lipooligosaccharide, and fimbriae in 30 to 60% of infected patients (67). PT is the only antigen specific for *B. pertussis*. Nonencapsulated *H. influenzae* possesses antigens that cross-react with FHA and that may affect the specificity of pertussis serology (49). Low levels of antibody to all antigens may be found in healthy persons; therefore, quantitative assessment is essential (49, 108). Erythromycin therapy of pertussis does not significantly interfere with antibody production (21). The response to vaccination (mainly immunoglobulin M [IgM] and IgG) is directed against the antigens of the vaccine when an acellular vaccine is used and is directed against various antigens (mainly outer membrane and fimbrial antigens) when whole-cell vaccine is used (71). For the serodiagnosis of pertussis in patients, assessments of IgG and IgA antibodies to PT and FHA are the most useful assays (67). IgG against these antigens is produced in >80% of infected individuals, and IgA is produced in 40 to 60% of infected individuals. IgA occurs mainly after infection in both unvaccinated and vaccinated individuals (22) and rarely occurs as a response to vaccination and is thus valuable when it is present (72); however, young infants are often unable to produce IgA (96). On the other hand, specific IgA may persist in healthy populations as a result of subclinical infections (72, 108). It can also be detected in NP secretions and saliva (71). The value of measuring the levels of IgM antibodies to PT and FHA in serum is controversial. Some researchers found it helpful (28), while others saw little diagnostic value (22, 67). IgM levels are generally not elevated in infected, previously vaccinated individuals (67). IgA and IgM decline to low levels 3 to 5 months after the onset of the disease, while IgG levels remain elevated for a much longer period of time (19) (Fig. 2).

Many methods have been used to assess specific antibodies in serum including agglutination, complement fixation, immunoblotting, indirect hemagglutination, toxin neutralization, and enzyme-linked immunosorbent assays (ELISAs) (for reviews, see references 67 and 71 and chapter 12 of this Manual). The traditional method of agglutination has been converted to a micromethod (62). Agglutinating antibodies are mainly IgG directed against fimbrial antigens, pertactin, and/or lipooligosaccharide. Agglutination tests do not differentiate between antibody isotypes and are less sensitive than ELISAs (67). Recently, a particle agglutination test with improved sensitivity has been reported (2). ELISAs have become the method of choice in recent years (67, 71),

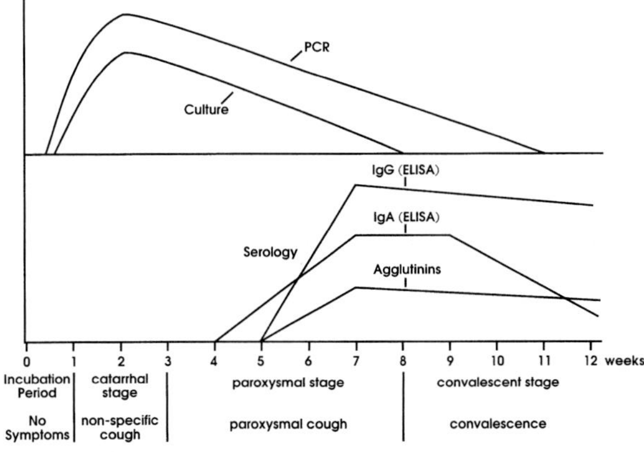

FIGURE 2 Schematic diagram of stages and symptoms of pertussis and value of culture, PCR, and serology in relation to duration of disease.

with solid-phase assays with microtiter plates being the most widely used. To improve standardization, most laboratories use reference sera from the Laboratory of Pertussis, Center for Biologics Evaluation and Research, Food and Drug Administration, Bethesda, Md. As antigen for the ELISA, whole or sonicated cells of *B. pertussis* have been used, but a significantly higher sensitivity was found when purified individual antigens (PT and FHA) were used in pooled form or, preferably, when individual antigens were used in combination (28).

EVALUATION AND INTERPRETATION OF RESULTS

No available method can detect 100% of pertussis cases. This refers also to the clinical picture, which is equivocal in patients with atypical or mild cases and is only of limited value as a reference standard for laboratory methods. Defining a case of pertussis is difficult and controversial (92). Due to its specificity of 100%, a positive culture is considered the "gold standard" for the diagnosis of pertussis. However, data on the sensitivity of culture vary from very low to >80% (12). Many factors affect this sensitivity, including time between disease onset and sampling (the highest isolation rate is during the catarrhal stage but decreases thereafter [Fig. 2] [57, 92]); age of the patient (higher isolation rate in infants [57]); immunization status (lower rate in vaccinated individuals [57, 92]); preceding effective antimicrobial therapy (57, 92); and maybe most importantly, experience with the collection, transport, and culturing of specimens. The sensitivity of PCR is superior to that of culture when only a few organisms are present in the nasopharynx or when their viability is reduced by antimicrobial therapy (16, 60, 86). In well-vaccinated communities, where patients often harbor only a few bordetellae, PCR is superior to culture (29, 96). It is as yet unknown if PCR is significantly superior to well-performed culture for untreated nonimmunized patients who present early, i.e., at the peak of infectivity (a situation common in nonvaccinating countries). Both PCR and culture depend on the presence of bordetellae in the nasopharynx and are negative for patients with advanced stages of pertussis (Fig. 2).

In nonvaccinating countries, serology for the first serum sample drawn early during the disease is often negative due to slow antibody production, and antibody does not become measurable before 1 or 2 weeks after the onset of the typical cough (19) (Fig. 2). A second serum sample drawn several weeks later will often confirm the diagnosis but is not helpful for the initial management of the patient. Demonstration of significant titer changes is the most reliable approach to the serodiagnosis of pertussis (67, 108). In well-vaccinated communities, however, the serology for the first sample may already be diagnostic due to a rapid anamnestic response of the immune system (22) and due to the fact that the diagnosis of "pertussis" is considered only at an advanced stage of the illness; therefore, the first serum is drawn late and shows a high titer. Accordingly, an initial high titer which may already have reached a plateau will be found; therefore, a significant titer rise cannot be expected. Even in this situation, however, a second serum sample may be needed to establish the diagnosis (26). If only one serum sample is available, pertussis can be considered likely if a patient has a test result more than 3 standard deviations above the control group mean in one assay or more than 2 standard deviations above the mean in two or more tests (67). On the other hand, false-negative results of serology sometimes occur even when several serum samples are collected (22); thus, the sensitivity of this method is not 100%. For adults with pertussis, serology is the most important diagnostic tool, since these patients often present late in the disease. Serology also plays an important role in epidemiological studies and in assessing the immunogenicities of pertussis vaccines (67, 71). In conclusion, both the choice of diagnostic methods and the interpretation of test results depend on the levels of vaccine use and disease activity in the community and the vaccination status of the individual patient. This information must be available to the laboratory performing diagnostic tests for pertussis.

ANTIMICROBIAL SUSCEPTIBILITY

Antimicrobial susceptibility testing of the fastidious slowly growing bordetellae is not standardized; widely divergent methods have been used (37). Indirect evidence with trimethoprim-sulfamethoxazole (TMP-SMX) suggests that the agar dilution method may be more relevant to the in vivo situation than the broth dilution method: low MICs were found by the agar dilution method but very high MICs were found by the broth dilution method (107); in vivo, TMP-SMX reliably eradicates *B. pertussis* (47). Mueller-Hinton agar with 5% horse blood seems to be the most suitable medium for use with the agar dilution method (43). MICs obtained by the E test (AB Biodisk, Piscataway, N.J., and Solna, Sweden) (see also chapter 118 of this Manual) correlate well with agar dilution test results for *B. parapertussis* (44). When the E test is used for *B. pertussis*, scanty growth of some isolates may pose problems (33). Disk diffusion methods are not standardized for the slowly growing bordetellae.

Routine susceptibility testing of *B. pertussis* and *B. parapertussis* is not necessary. *B. pertussis* in general continues to be susceptible to erythromycin. MICs mostly range from ≤0.008 to 0.5 μg/ml (35, 55). Recently, however, two highly erythromycin-resistant isolates of *B. pertussis* were found in Arizona (59) and Utah (54); the mechanism of resistance has not yet been elucidated.

Erythromycin is the agent of choice both for the treatment and for the chemoprophylaxis of pertussis (36). Treatment during the catarrhal stage shortens and ameliorates the disease, and the onset of therapy even during the early paroxysmal stage still has positive effects (36). In addition, erythromycin therapy terminates infectivity. Both the estolate and the ethylsuccinate forms of erythromycin reliably eradicate *B. pertussis* when the dosage of the agent is sufficiently high to achieve concentrations in the respiratory secretions well above the agent's MICs. The in vitro activities of the new macrolides against *B. pertussis* are similar to that of erythromycin (35). In vivo efficacy is likely, but clinical data are scanty (4). TMP-SMX is the agent of choice if erythromycin cannot be administered (47). Therapy with amoxicillin frequently leads to treatment failures (38). Several of the newer fluoroquinolones show good in vitro activity against bordetellae (42) and achieve high concentrations in respiratory secretions, but clinical experience is lacking. Oral cephalosporins are inactive against bordetellae.

B. parapertussis in general is more resistant than *B. pertussis* to antimicrobial agents (35, 55). Clinical studies on the antimicrobial therapy of parapertussis are lacking. Anecdotal experience suggests that TMP-SMX may be more effective in vivo than erythromycin (68). *B. bronchiseptica* is susceptible in vitro to some aminoglycosides (gentamicin, tobramycin, and amikacin), some penicillins (azlocillin, mezlocillin, and ticarcillin), some cephalosporins (cefoperazone and ceftazidime), chloramphenicol, and the tetracyclines, but it is resistant to erythromycin (106).

REFERENCES

1. **Abbott, J. D., M. E. Macaulay, and N. W. Preston.** 1982. *Bacteriological Diagnosis of Whooping Cough.* Broadsheet 105. Association of Clinical Pathologists, London, United Kingdom.
2. **Aoyama, T., T. Kato, Y. Takeuchi, K. Kato, K. Morokuma, and T. Hirai.** 1997. Simple, speedy, sensitive, and specific serodiagnosis of pertussis by using a particle agglutination test. *J. Clin. Microbiol.* **35:**1859–1861.
3. **Aoyama, T., Y. Murase, T. Iwata, A. Imaizumi, Y. Suzuki, and Y. Sato.** 1986. Comparison of blood-free medium (cyclodextrin solid medium) with Bordet-Gengou medium for clinical isolation of *Bordetella pertussis. J. Clin. Microbiol.* **23:**1046–1048.
4. **Aoyama, T., K. Sunakawa, S. Iwata, Y. Takeuchi, and R. Fujii.** 1996. Efficacy of short-term treatment of pertussis with clarithromycin and azithromycin. *J. Pediatr.* **129:** 761–764.
5. **Aricò, B., and R. Rappuoli.** 1987. *Bordetella parapertussis* and *Bordetella bronchiseptica* contain transcriptionally silent pertussis toxin genes. *J. Bacteriol.* **169:**2847–2853.
6. **Bäckman, A., B. Johansson, and P. Olcén.** 1994. Nested PCR for detection of *Bordetella pertussis* in clinical nasopharyngeal samples. *J. Clin. Microbiol.* **32:**2544–2548.
7. **Beiter, A., K. Lewis, E. F. Pineda, and J. D. Cherry.** 1993. Unrecognized maternal peripartum pertussis with subsequent fatal neonatal pertussis. *Obstet. Gynecol.* **82:** 691–693.
8. **Bejuk, D., J. Begovac, A. Bace, N. Kuzmanovic-Sterk, and B. Aleraj.** 1995. Culture of *Bordetella pertussis* from three upper respiratory tract specimens. *Pediatr. Infect. Dis. J.* **14:**64–65.
9. **Black, S.** 1997. Epidemiology of pertussis. *Pediatr. Infect. Dis. J.* **16:**S85–S89.
10. **Bordet, J., and O. Gengou.** 1906. Le microbe de la coqueluche. *Ann. Inst. Pasteur* **20:**731–741.
11. **Cassiday, P. K., G. N. Sanden, C. Toure Kane, S. M'Boup, and J. M. Barbaree.** 1994. Viability of *Bordetella pertussis* in four suspending solutions at three temperatures. *J. Clin. Microbiol.* **32:**1550–1553.
12. **Cherry, J. D.** 1996. Historical review of pertussis and the classical vaccine. *J. Infect. Dis.* **174**(Suppl. 3):S259–S263.
13. **Cherry, J. D., P. A. Brunell, G. S. Golden, and D. T. Karzon.** 1988. Report of the task force on pertussis and pertussis immunization—1988. *Pediatrics* **81:**939–984.
14. **Daughterty, M. P., J. Dolter, G. C. Evans, M. E. Griffith, B. A. Hummert, D. Linquist, M. M. Struthers, and J. D. Wong.** 1992. Processing of specimens for isolation of unusual organisms, p. 1.18.13–1.18.17. *In* H. Isenberg (ed.), *Clinical Microbiology Procedures Handbook,* vol. 1. American Society for Microbiology, Washington, D.C.
15. **Douglas, E., J. G. Coote, R. Parton, and W. McPheat.** 1993. Identification of *Bordetella pertussis* in nasopharyngeal swabs by PCR amplification of a region of the adenylate cyclase gene. *J. Med. Microbiol.* **38:**140–144.
16. **Edelman, K., S. Nikkari, O. Ruuskanen, Q. He, M. Viljanen, and J. Mertsola.** 1996. Detection of *Bordetella pertussis* by polymerase chain reaction and culture in the nasopharynx of erythromycin-treated infants with pertussis. *Pediatr. Infect. Dis. J.* **15:**54–57.
17. **Ewanowich, C. A., L. W. L. Chui, M. G. Paranchych, M. S. Peppler, R. G. Marusyk, and W. L. Albritton.** 1993. Major outbreak of pertussis in northern Alberta, Canada: analysis of discrepant direct fluorescent-antibody and culture results by using polymerase chain reaction methodology. *J. Clin. Microbiol.* **31:**1715–1725.
18. **Ewanowich, C. A., A. R. Melton, A. A. Weiss, R. K. Sherburne, and M. S. Peppler.** 1989. Invasion of HeLa 229 cells by virulent *Bordetella pertussis. Infect. Immun.* **57:** 2698–2704.
19. **Finger, H., and C. H. Wirsing von König.** 1985. Serological diagnosis of whooping cough. *Dev. Biol. Stand.* **61:** 331–335.
20. **Gilchrist, M. J. R.** 1991. *Bordetella,* p. 471–477. *In* A. Balows, W. J. Hausler, Jr., K. L. Herrmann, H. D. Isenberg, and H. J. Shadomy (ed.), *Manual of Clinical Microbiology,* 5th ed. American Society for Microbiology, Washington, D.C.
21. **Granström, G., and M. Granström.** 1994. Effect of erythromycin treatment on antibody responses in pertussis. *Scand. J. Infect. Dis.* **26:**453–457.
22. **Granström, G., B. Wretlind, C. R. Salenstedt, and M. Granström.** 1988. Evaluation of serologic assays for diagnosis of whooping cough. *J. Clin. Microbiol.* **26:**1818–1823.
23. **Grimprel, E., P. Bégué, I. Anjak, F. Betsou, and N. Guiso.** 1993. Comparison of polymerase chain reaction, culture, and Western immunoblot serology for diagnosis of *Bordetella pertussis* infection. *J. Clin. Microbiol.* **31:** 2745–2750.
24. **Hallander, H. O., E. Reizenstein, B. Renemar, G. Rasmuson, L. Mardin, and P. Olin.** 1993. Comparison of nasopharyngeal aspirates with swabs for culture of *Bordetella pertussis. J. Clin. Microbiol.* **31:**50–52.
25. **Hallander, H. O., J. Storsaeter, and R. Möllby.** 1991. Evaluation of serology and nasopharyngeal cultures for diagnosis of pertussis. *J. Infect. Dis.* **163:**1046–1054.
26. **Halperin, S. A., R. Bortolussi, and A. J. Wort.** 1989. Evaluation of culture, immunofluorescence, and serology for the diagnosis of pertussis. *J. Clin. Microbiol.* **27:** 752–757.
27. **Halperin, S. A., A. Kasina, and M. Swift.** 1992. Prolonged survival of *Bordetella pertussis* in a simple buffer after nasopharyngeal secretion aspiration. *Can. J. Microbiol.* **38:** 1210–1213.
28. **He, Q., J. Mertsola, J. P. Himanen, O. Ruuskanen, and M. K. Viljanen.** 1993. Evaluation of pooled and individual components of *Bordetella pertussis* as antigens in an enzyme immunoassay for diagnosis of pertussis. *Eur. J. Clin. Microbiol. Infect. Dis.* **12:**690–695.
29. **He, Q., G. Schmidt-Schläpfer, M. Just, H. C. Matter, S. Nikkari, M. K. Viljanen, and J. Mertsola.** 1996. Impact of polymerase chain reaction on clinical pertussis research: Finnish and Swiss experiences. *J. Infect. Dis.* **174:** 1288–1295.
30. **Heininger, U., K. Stehr, S. Schmitt-Grohé, C. Lorenz, R. Rost, P. D. Christenson, M. Überall, and J. D. Cherry.** 1994. Clinical characteristics of illness caused by *Bordetella parapertussis* compared with illness caused by *Bordetella pertussis. Pediatr. Infect. Dis. J.* **13:**306–309.
31. **Hewlett, E. L.** 1997. Pertussis: current concepts of pathogenesis and prevention. *Pediatr. Infect. Dis. J.* **16:**S78–S84.
32. **Holt, J. G., N. R. Krieg, P. H. A. Sneath, J. T. Staley, and S. T. Williams (ed.).** 1994. Differential characteristics of the species of the genus *Bordetella,* p. 136. *Bergey's Manual of Determinative Bacteriology,* 9th ed. The Williams & Wilkins Co., Baltimore, Md.
33. **Hoppe, J. E.** Unpublished data and observations.
34. **Hoppe, J. E.** 1988. Methods for isolation of *Bordetella pertussis* from patients with whooping cough. *Eur. J. Clin. Microbiol. Infect. Dis.* **7:**616–620.
35. **Hoppe, J. E., and A. Eichhorn.** 1989. Activity of new

macrolides against *Bordetella pertussis* and *Bordetella parapertussis*. *Eur. J. Clin. Microbiol.* **8:**653–654.

36. **Hoppe, J. E., and the Erythromycin Study Group.** 1992. Comparison of erythromycin estolate and erythromycin ethylsuccinate for treatment of pertussis. *Pediatr. Infect. Dis. J.* **11:**189–193.
37. **Hoppe, J. E., and A. Haug.** 1988. Antimicrobial susceptibility of *Bordetella pertussis*. *Infection* **16:**126–130.
38. **Hoppe, J. E., and A. Haug.** 1988. Treatment and prevention of pertussis by antimicrobial agents. *Infection* **16:** 148–152.
39. **Hoppe, J. E., and M. Schlagenhauf.** 1989. Comparison of three kinds of blood and two incubation atmospheres for cultivation of *Bordetella pertussis* on charcoal agar. *J. Clin. Microbiol.* **27:**2115–2117.
40. **Hoppe, J. E., and J. Schwaderer.** 1989. Direct plating versus use of transport medium for detection of *Bordetella* species from nasopharyngeal swabs. *Eur. J. Clin. Microbiol. Infect. Dis.* **8:**264–265.
41. **Hoppe, J. E., and J. Schwaderer.** 1989. Comparison of four charcoal media for the isolation of *Bordetella pertussis*. *J. Clin. Microbiol.* **27:**1097–1098.
42. **Hoppe, J. E., and C. G. Simon.** 1990. In vitro susceptibilities of *Bordetella pertussis* and *Bordetella parapertussis* to seven fluoroquinolones. *Antimicrob. Agents Chemother.* **34:** 2287–2288.
43. **Hoppe, J. E., and T. Tschirner.** 1995. Comparison of media for agar dilution susceptibility testing of *Bordetella pertussis* and *Bordetella parapertussis*. *Eur. J. Clin. Microbiol. Infect. Dis.* **14:**775–779.
44. **Hoppe, J. E., and T. Tschirner.** 1997. Comparison of E test and agar dilution for testing the activity of three macrolides against *Bordetella parapertussis*. *Diagn. Microbiol. Infect. Dis.* **28:**49–51.
45. **Hoppe, J. E., and R. Vogl.** 1986. Comparison of three media for culture of *Bordetella pertussis*. *Eur. J. Clin. Microbiol.* **5:**361–362.
46. **Hoppe, J. E., and A. Weiss.** 1987. Recovery of *Bordetella pertussis* from four kinds of swabs. *Eur. J. Clin. Microbiol.* **6:**203–205.
47. **Hoppe, J. E., U. Halm, H. J. Hagedorn, and A. Kraminer-Hagedorn.** 1989. Comparison of erythromycin ethylsuccinate and co-trimoxazole for treatment of pertussis. *Infection* **17:**227–231.
48. **Hoppe, J. E., S. Wörz, and K. Botzenhart.** 1986. Comparison of specimen transport systems for *Bordetella pertussis*. *Eur. J. Clin. Microbiol.* **5:**671–673.
49. **Isacson, J., B. Trollfors, J. Taranger, and T. Lagergard.** 1995. Acquisition of IgG serum antibodies against two *Bordetella* antigens (filamentous hemagglutinin and pertactin) in children with no symptoms of pertussis. *Pediatr. Infect. Dis. J.* **14:**517–521.
50. **Isacson, J., B. Trollfors, J. Taranger, G. Zackrisson, and T. Lagergard.** 1993. How common is whooping cough in a nonvaccinating country? *Pediatr. Infect. Dis. J.* **12:** 284–288.
51. **Janda, W. M., E. Santos, J. Stevens, D. Celig, L. Terrile, and P. C. Schreckenberger.** 1994. Unexpected isolation of *Bordetella pertussis* from a blood culture. *J. Clin. Microbiol.* **32:**2851–2853.
52. **Katzko, G., M. Hofmeister, and D. Church.** 1996. Extended incubation of culture plates improves recovery of *Bordetella* spp. *J. Clin. Microbiol.* **34:**1563–1564.
53. **Kersters, K., K. H. Hinz, A. Hertle, P. Segers, A. Lievens, O. Siegmann, and J. de Ley.** 1984. *Bordetella avium* sp. nov., isolated from the respiratory tracts of turkeys and other birds. *Int. J. Syst. Bacteriol.* **34:**56–70.
54. **Korgenski, E. K., and J. A. Daly.** 1997. Surveillance and detection of erythromycin resistance in *Bordetella pertussis* isolates recovered from a pediatric population in the Intermountain West region of the United States. *J. Clin. Microbiol.* **35:**2989–2991.
55. **Kurzynski, T. A., D. M. Boehm, J. A. Rott-Petri, R. F. Schell, and P. E. Allison.** 1988. Antimicrobial susceptibilities of *Bordetella* species isolated in a multicenter pertussis surveillance project. *Antimicrob. Agents Chemother.* **32:** 137–140.
56. **Kurzynski, T. A., D. M. Boehm, J. A. Rott-Petri, R. F. Schell, and P. E. Allison.** 1988. Comparison of modified Bordet-Gengou and modified Regan-Lowe media for the isolation of *Bordetella pertussis* and *Bordetella parapertussis*. *J. Clin. Microbiol.* **26:**2661–2663.
57. **Kwantes, W., D. H. M. Johnson, and W. O. Williams.** 1983. *Bordetella pertussis* isolation in general practice: 1977–79 whooping cough epidemic in West Glamorgan. *J. Hyg.* **90:**149–158.
58. **Lautrop, H.** 1960. Laboratory diagnosis of whooping cough or *Bordetella* infections. *Bull. W. H. O.* **23:**15–35.
59. **Lewis, K., M. A. Saubolle, F. C. Tenover, M. F. Rudinsky, S. D. Barbour, and J. D. Cherry.** 1995. Pertussis caused by an erythromycin-resistant strain of *Bordetella pertussis*. *Pediatr. Infect. Dis. J.* **14:**388–391.
60. **Li, Z., D. L. Jansen, T. M. Finn, S. A. Halperin, A. Kasina, S. P. O'Connor, T. Aoyama, C. R. Manclark, and M. J. Brennan.** 1994. Identification of *Bordetella pertussis* infection by shared-primer PCR. *J. Clin. Microbiol.* **32:** 783–789.
61. **Linnemann, C. C., Jr., and E. B. Perry.** 1977. *Bordetella parapertussis*. *Am. J. Dis. Child.* **131:**560–563.
62. **Manclark, C. R., B. D. Meade, and D. G. Burstyn.** 1986. Serological response to *Bordetella pertussis*, p. 388–394. *In* N. R. Rose, H. Friedman, and J. L. Fahey (ed.), *Manual of Clinical Laboratory Immunology*, 3rd ed. American Society for Microbiology, Washington, D.C.
63. **Marcon, M. J.** 1995. *Bordetella*, p. 566–573. *In* P. R. Murray, E. J. Baron, M. A. Pfaller, F. C. Tenover, and R. H. Yolken (ed.), *Manual of Clinical Microbiology*, 6th ed. American Society for Microbiology, Washington, D.C.
64. **Marcon, M. J., A. C. Hamoudi, H. J. Cannon, and M. M. Hribar.** 1987. Comparison of throat and nasopharyngeal swab specimens for culture diagnosis of *Bordetella pertussis* infection. *J. Clin. Microbiol.* **25:**1109–1110.
65. **McNicol, P., S. M. Giercke, M. Gray, D. Martin, B. Brodeur, M. S. Peppler, T. Williams, and G. Hammond.** 1995. Evaluation and validation of a monoclonal immunofluorescent reagent for direct detection of *Bordetella pertussis*. *J. Clin. Microbiol.* **33:**2868–2871.
66. **Meade, B. D., and A. Bollen.** 1994. Recommendations for use of the polymerase chain reaction in the diagnosis of *Bordetella pertussis* infections. *J. Med. Microbiol.* **41:**51–55.
67. **Meade, B. D., C. M. Mink, and C. R. Manclark.** 1990. Serodiagnosis of pertussis, p. 322–329. *In* C. R. Manclark (ed.), *Proceedings of the Sixth International Symposium on Pertussis*. DHHS publication no. (FDA) 90–1164. Food and Drug Administration, Bethesda, Md.
68. **Mertsola, J.** 1985. Mixed outbreak of *Bordetella pertussis* and *Bordetella parapertussis* infection in Finland. *Eur. J. Clin. Microbiol.* **4:**123–128.
69. **Mills, K. H. G., and K. Redhead.** 1993. Cellular immunity in pertussis. *J. Med. Microbiol.* **39:**163–164. (Editorial.)
70. **Morrill, W. E., J. M. Barbaree, B. S. Fields, G. N. Sanden, and W. T. Martin.** 1988. Effects of transport temperature and medium on recovery of *Bordetella pertussis* from nasopharyngeal swabs. *J. Clin. Microbiol.* **26:**1814–1817.
71. **Müller, F. M., J. E. Hoppe, and C. H. Wirsing von König.**

1997. Laboratory diagnosis of pertussis: state of the art in 1997. *J. Clin. Microbiol.* **35:**2435–2443.

72. **Nagel, J., and E. J. Poot-Scholtens.** 1983. Serum IgA antibody to *Bordetella pertussis* as an indicator of infection. *J. Med. Microbiol.* **16:**417–426.
73. **Ng, V. L., M. York, and W. K. Hadley.** 1989. Unexpected isolation of *Bordetella pertussis* from patients with acquired immunodeficiency syndrome. *J. Clin. Microbiol.* **27:** 337–338.
74. **Parton, R.** 1996. New perspectives on *Bordetella* pathogenicity. *J. Med. Microbiol.* **44:**233–235. (Editorial.)
75. **Pittman, M.** 1979. Pertussis toxin: the cause of the harmful effects and prolonged immunity of whooping cough. A hypothesis. *Rev. Infect. Dis.* **1:**401–412.
76. **Pittman, M.** 1984. Genus *Bordetella* Moreno-López 1952, 178, p. 388–393. *In* N. R. Krieg and J. G. Holt (ed.), *Bergey's Manual of Systematic Bacteriology*, vol. 1. The Williams & Wilkins Co., Baltimore, Md.
77. **Plotkin, S. A., and M. Cadoz.** 1997. The acellular pertussis vaccine trials: an interpretation. *Pediatr. Infect. Dis. J.* **16:** 508–517.
78. **Postels-Multani, S., H. J. Schmitt, C. H. Wirsing von König, H. L. Bock, and H. Bogaerts.** 1995. Symptoms and complications of pertussis in adults. *Infection* **23:** 139–142.
79. **Preston, N. W.** 1970. Technical problems in the laboratory diagnosis and prevention of whooping cough. *Lab. Pract.* **19:**482–486.
80. **Rappuoli, R.** 1994. Pathogenicity mechanisms of *Bordetella*. *Curr. Top. Microbiol. Immunol.* **192:**319–336.
81. **Regan, J., and F. Lowe.** 1977. Enrichment medium for the isolation of *Bordetella*. *J. Clin. Microbiol.* **6:**303–309.
82. **Reizenstein, E., B. Johansson, L. Mardin, J. Abens, R. Möllby, and H. O. Hallander.** 1993. Diagnostic evaluation of polymerase chain reaction discriminative for *Bordetella pertussis*, *B. parapertussi*, and *B. bronchiseptica*. *Diagn. Microbiol. Infect. Dis.* **17:**185–191.
83. **Reizenstein, E., L. Lindberg, R. Möllby, and H. O. Hallander.** 1996. Validation of nested *Bordetella* PCR in a pertussis vaccine trial. *J. Clin. Microbiol.* **34:**810–815.
84. **Ross, P. W.** 1977. The isolation of *Streptococcus pyogenes* from throat swabs. *J. Med. Microbiol.* **10:**69–76.
85. **Rowatt, E.** 1957. The growth of *Bordetella pertussis*: a review. *J. Gen. Microbiol.* **17:**297–326.
86. **Schläpfer, G., J. D. Cherry, U. Heininger, M. Überall, S. Schmitt-Grohé, S. Laussucq, M. Just, and K. Stehr.** 1995. Polymerase chain reaction identification of *Bordetella pertussis* infections in vaccinees and family members in a pertussis vaccine efficacy trial in Germany. *Pediatr. Infect. Dis. J.* **14:**209–214.
87. **Schmitt-Grohé, S., J. D. Cherry, U. Heininger, M. A. Überall, E. Pineda, and K. Stehr.** 1995. Pertussis in German adults. *Clin. Infect. Dis.* **21:**860–866.
88. **Sneed, J. O.** 1992. Laboratory diagnosis of pertussis, p. 1.14.9–1.14.13. *In* H. D. Isenberg (ed.), *Clinical Microbiology Procedures Handbook*, vol. 1. American Society for Microbiology, Washington, D.C.
89. **Stainer, D. W., and M. J. Scholte.** 1971. A simple chemically defined medium for the production of phase I *Bordetella pertussis*. *J. Gen. Microbiol.* **63:**211–220.
90. **Stefanelli, P., M. Giuliano, M. Bottone, P. Spigaglia, and P. Mastrantonio.** 1996. Polymerase chain reaction for the identification of *Bordetella pertussis* and *Bordetella parapertussis*. *Diagn. Microbiol. Infect. Dis.* **24:**197–200.
91. **Stefanelli, P., P. Mastrantonio, S. Z. Hausman, M. Giuliano, and D. L. Burns.** 1997. Molecular characterization of two *Bordetella bronchiseptica* strains isolated from children with coughs. *J. Clin. Microbiol.* **35:**1550–1555.
92. **Strebel, P. M., S. L. Cochi, K. M. Farizo, B. J. Payne, S. D. Hanauer, and A. L. Baughman.** 1993. Pertussis in Missouri: evaluation of nasopharyngeal culture, direct fluorescent antibody testing, and clinical case definitions in the diagnosis of pertussis. *Clin. Infect. Dis.* **16:**276–285.
93. **Sutcliffe, E. M., and J. D. Abbott.** 1972. Selective medium for the isolation of *Bordetella pertussis* and *parapertussis*. *J. Clin. Pathol.* **25:**732–733.
94. **Vandamme, P., J. Hommez, M. Vancanneyt, M. Monsieurs, B. Hoste, B. Cookson, C. H. Wirsing von König, K. Kersters, and P. J. Blackall.** 1995. *Bordetella hinzii* sp. nov., isolated from poultry and humans. *Int. J. Syst. Bacteriol.* **45:**37–45.
95. **Vandamme, P., M. Heyndrickx, M. Vancanneyt, B. Hoste, P. de Vos, E. Falsen, K. Kersters, and K. H. Hinz.** 1996. *Bordetella trematum* sp. nov., isolated from wounds and ear infections in humans, and reassessment of *Alcaligenes denitrificans* Rüger and Tan 1983. *Int. J. Syst. Bacteriol.* **46:**849–858.
96. **van der Zee, A., C. Agterberg, M. Peeters, F. Mooi, and J. Schellekens.** 1996. A clinical validation of *Bordetella pertussis* and *Bordetella parapertussis* polymerase chain reaction: comparison with culture and serology using samples from patients with suspected whooping cough from a highly immunized population. *J. Infect. Dis.* **174:**89–96.
97. **van der Zee, A., C. Agterberg, M. Peeters, J. Schellekens, and F. R. Mooi.** 1993. Polymerase chain reaction assay for pertussis: simultaneous detection and discrimination of *Bordetella pertussis* and *Bordetella parapertussis*. *J. Clin. Microbiol.* **31:**2134–2140.
98. **Wadowsky, R. M., S. Laus, T. Libert, S. J. States, and G. D. Ehrlich.** 1994. Inhibition of PCR-based assay for *Bordetella pertussis* by using calcium alginate fiber and aluminum shaft components of a nasopharyngeal swab. *J. Clin. Microbiol.* **32:**1054–1057.
99. **Weiss, A. A.** 1992. The genus *Bordetella*, vol. 3, p. 2530–2543. *In* A. Balows, H. G. Trüper, M. Dworkin, W. Harder, and K. H. Schleifer (ed.), *The Prokaryotes: a Handbook on the Biology of Bacteria: Ecophysiology, Isolation, Identification, Applications*, 2nd ed. Springer-Verlag, Berlin, Germany.
100. **Weiss, A. A., and E. L. Hewlett.** 1986. Virulence factors of *Bordetella pertussis*. *Annu. Rev. Microbiol.* **40:** 661–686.
101. **Weyant, R. S., D. G. Hollis, R. E. Weaver, M. F. M. Amin, A. G. Steigerwalt, S. P. O'Connor, A. M. Whitney, M. I. Daneshvar, C. W. Moss, and D. J. Brenner.** 1995. *Bordetella holmesii* sp. nov., a new gram-negative species associated with septicemia. *J. Clin. Microbiol.* **33:** 1–7.
102. **Wirsing von König, C. H., and H. Finger.** 1994. Role of pertussis toxin in causing symptoms of *Bordetella parapertussis* infection. *Eur. J. Clin. Microbiol. Infect. Dis.* **13:** 455–458.
103. **Wirsing von König, C. H., J. E. Hoppe, A. Tacken, and H. Finger.** 1990. Detection of *Bordetella pertussis* in clinical specimens, p. 315–320. *In* C. Manclark (ed.), *Proceedings of the Sixth International Symposium on Pertussis*, DHHS publication no. (FDA) 90-1164. Food and Administration, Bethesda, Md.
104. **Wirsing von König, C. H., S. Postels-Multani, H. L. Bock, and H. J. Schmitt.** 1995. Pertussis in adults: frequency of transmission after household exposure. *Lancet* **346:**1326–1329.
105. **Wirsing von König, C. H., A. Tacken, and H. Finger.** 1988. Use of supplemented Stainer-Scholte medium for the isolation of *Bordetella pertussis* from clinical material. *J. Clin. Microbiol.* **26:**2558–2560.
106. **Woolfrey, B. F., and J. A. Moody.** 1991. Human infec-

tions associated with *Bordetella bronchiseptica*. *Clin. Microbiol. Rev.* **4**:243–255.

107. **Zackrisson, G., J. E. Brorson, and B. Trollfors.** 1984. Influence of culture medium and inoculum size on susceptibility of *Bordetella pertussis* to antibacterial agents in vitro. *Eur. J. Clin. Microbiol.* **3**:566–567.

108. **Zackrisson, G., I. Krantz, T. Lagergard, P. Larsson, R. Sekura, N. Sigurs, J. Taranger, and B. Trollfors.** 1988. Antibody response to pertussis toxin in patients with clinical pertussis measured by enzyme-linked immunosorbent assay. *Eur. J. Clin. Microbiol. Infect. Dis.* **7**:149–154.

*Brucella**

DANIEL S. SHAPIRO AND JANE D. WONG

41

TAXONOMY

Brucella spp. were first described in 1887 by Surgeon David Bruce (15) while working as a British military doctor on the island of Malta. He named the organism *Micrococcus melitensis*. Zammitt demonstrated that the organism was shed in goat milk, which led to the prohibition of the consumption of goat milk products by British government personnel in 1906. By 1907, the attack rate in the Army and Navy was markedly reduced (76). Meanwhile, in Denmark, Bang (9) described *Bacillus abortus*, an organism which he found to be the agent of infectious abortion in cattle. Alice Evans (30) was the first to recognize the similarity between these two organisms, which were later placed in the same genus, *Brucella*, by Meyer and Shaw (55). Huddleson and Abell (44) later studied the production of H_2S by these strains, as well as their sensitivity to the dyes thionine and basic fuchsin. Huddleson (41) proposed that *Brucella* be divided into three species: *B. abortus*, *B. suis*, and *B. melitensis*. Further refinements to identification such as CO_2 requirements and rate of hydrolysis of urea have been made, and further species, *B. canis* (18, 47), *B. neotomae* (78), *B. ovis* (17), and a probable new species, *B. maris* (31), have been identified.

On the basis of DNA-DNA hybridization studies (82) on strains representing all recognized species and biovars of *Brucella*, it has been proposed that the genus *Brucella* comprises a single species, *Brucella melitensis*. Chromosomal restriction endonuclease analysis with *Eco*RI or *Hin*dIII demonstrate only minor differences between *Brucella* strains, supporting this proposal. However, chromosomal DNA analysis by pulsed-field gel electrophoresis with *Xba*I or *Not*I reveals genomic differences between the species (2). This confirms that at the DNA level the use of the natural host as a phenotypic characteristic is valid for classifying the genus *Brucella*. The International Committee on Systematic Bacteriology (24) stated that the existing vernacular names for the nomenspecies *Brucella abortus*, *Brucella suis*, *Brucella melitensis*, and the others can be retained for nontaxonomic purposes to avoid confusion. This approach will be followed here.

DESCRIPTION OF THE GENUS

Brucella species are gram-negative cocci or short rods, 0.5 to 0.7 by 0.6 by 1.5 μm, arranged singly or, less frequently, in pairs, short chains, or small groups. Capsules and spores are not produced. The cells are nonmotile and do not produce flagella. The organisms are aerobic, possessing a respiratory type of metabolism and having a cytochrome-based electron transport system with oxygen or nitrate as the terminal electron acceptor. They are chemoorganotrophic, and most strains require complex media containing several amino acids, thiamine, nicotinamide, and magnesium ions. Some strains may be induced to grow on minimal media containing an ammonium salt as the sole nitrogen source. Growth is improved by serum or blood, but hemin (X factor) and NAD (V factor) are not essential. The organisms are catalase positive, nitrate positive, and usually oxidase positive. Many strains require supplementary CO_2 for growth, especially on primary isolation. Colonies on serum dextrose agar or other clear media are transparent, raised, and convex, with an entire edge and smooth, shiny surface. They appear a pale honey color by transmitted light. Nonsmooth variants of the smooth species occur, but there are also stable nonsmooth species such as *B. canis* and *B. ovis*, with a distinctive host range. The optimum temperature is 37°C, but growth occurs between 20 and 40°C. They are intracellular parasites, transmissible to a wide range of animal species, including humans (23).

NATURAL HABITATS

Brucellosis is a zoonotic disease, and domestic animals serve as the reservoir. The members of the genus *Brucella* are important veterinary pathogens (80). The host range for *Brucella* spp. is extensive, but preferred hosts exist for each species. In addition to mammals, insects and ticks have been found to have *Brucella* infections and reptiles and amphibians have been experimentally infected with this organism (67). *Brucella abortus*, which most commonly infects cattle, has also been isolated from affected horses, American bison, buffalo, and yaks. *Brucella melitensis*, a more virulent species, naturally infects not only goats and sheep but also alpacas and camels. *Brucella suis* most commonly infects swine (including feral swine). In Brazil and Colombia, however, *B. suis* biovar 1 has become established in cattle. Cattle have, in some areas, become a more important source of *B. suis*

* This chapter contains information presented in chapter 44 by Nelson P. Moyer and Larry A. Holcomb in the sixth edition of this Manual.

infection than swine in human infections (25). In addition, *B. suis* has been isolated from caribou, reindeer, the European hare, and rodents. *Brucella canis*, which was isolated initially as a cause of abortions in kennel-bred dogs, is an uncommon but well-described cause of human brucellosis (52, 69, 70, 85). The organism has also been isolated from coyotes and foxes. *Brucella ovis*, isolated from sheep, and *Brucella neotomae*, found in rodents, appear to be nonpathogenic for humans. Recently described but not yet officially named, a new species likely to be included within the genus *Brucella* (unofficially *Brucella maris*) has been isolated from marine mammals but not humans (31, 68).

Transmission of brucellosis can be the result of ingestion, direct contact via skin abrasions and mucous membranes (including the conjunctiva), and inhalation (in abattoirs and laboratories). Risk factors for infection include the handling of infected animals, ingestion of contaminated animal products such as unpasteurized milk and milk products (including cow, goat, and camel milk) and meat, and the handling of cultures of *Brucella* spp. in laboratories. A common risk factor in the United States in individuals who are diagnosed with brucellosis is the consumption of imported cheese made from unpasteurized goat milk. Other people who have been infected include hunters who have acquired *B. suis* from feral swine. Because of aggressive vaccination campaigns in cattle, many countries are now essentially free of bovine brucellosis (25). This has significantly decreased the risk of this infection in individuals who historically have been at increased risk, including veterinarians, farmers, meat inspectors, and abattoir workers (16). Accidents with the live, attenuated *B. abortus* 19 vaccine resulting in infection continue to put veterinarians at risk (71).

CLINICAL SIGNIFICANCE

The number of cases of brucellosis peaked at more than 300 in the United States in 1975. Since then, the number has declined and has remained relatively stable at about 100 cases per year for the past 10 years (21).

Clinically, brucellosis may present acutely, subacutely, or as localized disease. When brucellosis presents subacutely, it may be confused with tuberculosis. This is not surprising because, like *Mycobacterium tuberculosis*, *Brucella* spp. are facultative intracellular organisms, and the immune system response to infection often results in the formation of granulomata. In an analysis of the 1,288 cases of brucellosis in the United States reported to the Center for Disease Control (CDC) from 1968 to 1974, seven symptoms were reported by more than half of the patients: fever (89%), chills (69%), weakness and malaise (64%), body aches and sweating (61%), and headache (51%). In addition, weight loss was reported in 41% of patients and anorexia was reported in 39%. Fever was more commonly intermittent (83%) than constant (17%). Of 2,047 patients with cases reported to the CDC from 1965 to 1974, 5 died (0.2%) but brucellosis was considered to be the primary cause of death in only 2 of these (33). Death due to brucellosis is uncommon and has been nearly universally associated with endocarditis (62).

In addition to presenting as a systemic illness, brucellosis may include involvement of the liver (hepatosplenomegaly and granulomas) (22), hematologic system, bones and joints (including arthritis, spondylitis, and osteomyelitis) (3, 7, 35, 53, 57), genitourinary tract of men (epididymo-orchitis) and women (abortion) (45, 49), central nervous system (meningitis, encephalitis, myelitis, radiculitis, cerebellar syndromes, psychiatric manifestations) (13, 72), eyes (73), skin (most frequently as papulonodular lesions) (8, 12), lung (miliary lesions or hilar adenopathy) (37, 38, 61), and, uncommonly but most seriously, of the heart (endocarditis) (1, 32, 36, 46, 62, 65).

COLLECTION, TRANSPORT, AND STORAGE OF SPECIMENS

The diagnosis of brucellosis may be definitively established by culture of the organism. Specimens should be cultured as soon as possible after collection or, if this is not possible, refrigerated. *Brucella* organisms are most frequently recovered from blood and bone marrow. They are occasionally recovered from biopsy specimens of spleen and liver and from abscesses. They are rarely recovered from specimens with a competing microflora. For serologic diagnosis of brucellosis, acute-phase serum should be collected at presentation of the patient as close to the onset of illness as possible and convalescent-phase serum should be collected 14 to 21 days later.

DIRECT EXAMINATION

Direct Gram stains are of little value in establishing the diagnosis of brucellosis, in large part due to the clinical material from which they are most typically recovered, i.e., blood and bone marrow. The use of PCR with peripheral-blood specimens and genus-specific primers, while experimental in the diagnosis of brucellosis, shows promise (66). In addition, PCR has been used to determine the species of *Brucella* isolates (14) and has shown 100% agreement with identifications made by conventional methods.

CULTURE AND ISOLATION

Blood and bone marrow aspirates are the clinical specimens from which *Brucella* is most commonly isolated. Culture of blood for *Brucella* has historically been performed by broth-based methods and has required prolonged incubation and the use of blind subcultures. Culture has also been performed with biphasic Castaneda medium. Currently available methods that have been advocated include both lysis-centrifugation (Isolator) blood cultures and the use of automated, continuous-monitoring blood culture instrumentation. In a large study from Saudi Arabia, 92.7% of 97 patient isolates of *Brucella* spp. (85 *B. melitensis* and 12 *B. abortus*) were detected within 5 days of incubation (10) with the BACTEC 9240 system. In a pediatric study (84) comparing the BACTEC 9240 system, using Peds Plus medium bottles, with the Isolator 1.5 microbial tubes, the BACTEC system detected all 28 positive cultures and the Isolator system detected 22 of 28 positive cultures (79%). In a single study, the older BACTEC NR system had a longer mean time to recovery than did lysis-centrifugation (Isolator) blood cultures (59). In another study (19), the BacT/Alert system often required blind subculture to detect *Brucella* spp. The ESP system has also been shown to recover *Brucella* spp., although there has been no published comparison with other methods involving clinical specimens. In studies with seeded blood culture bottles, the ESP system was essentially equivalent to the BACTEC 9240 and faster than the BACTEC NR 660 in the detection of *B. melitensis* (74). In laboratory practice, the ESP system has isolated *B. melitensis*, *B.*

abortus, and *B. canis* in 96 h or less (79). Although there are sufficient published data on the use of the BACTEC 9240 to suggest that blood cultures for *Brucella* do not require subculture when this system is used, there are insufficient data on other automated blood culture systems (ESP and BacT/Alert) to allow the same conclusion. It would therefore seem prudent to perform both early and terminal subcultures from the bottles in the ESP and BacT Alert systems when brucellosis is suspected clinically and to hold these bottles for a minimum of 21 days.

It is worthy of note that the culture of bone marrow aspirate was shown in one study (34) to be superior to that of blood cultures (Castaneda bottles). Of particular importance, bone marrow cultures remained positive in patients with subacute disease (9 to 10 patients) whereas blood cultures were less reliable (4 of 10 patients). In addition, for 10 patients who had received prior antibiotic therapy, bone marrow cultures were positive in 9 while blood cultures were positive in only 5. The time to detection was shorter in bone marrow cultures than in blood cultures. Since bone marrow aspirate is a somewhat invasive procedure and since positive cultures of blood or a diagnosis on the basis of serologic testing can often be established, it is not clear when the aspiration of bone marrow is an appropriate test. Although culture of other tissue such as lymph nodes and liver has been suggested, there are no controlled studies to assess the diagnostic utility of this procedure (34).

Brucella spp. grow on most standard laboratory media, e.g., brucella agar, blood agar, chocolate agar, and Trypticase soy agar (TSA), when incubated at 35°C in 5 to 10% CO_2. Some strains grow on MacConkey agar. It grows slowly, and 48 h of incubation may be needed for visible colonies to appear. The organism grows on selective media designed for *Neisseria gonorrhoeae* isolation, such as Martin Lewis medium or Thayer-Martin medium. This is useful in isolating the organism from a site likely to have an indigenous microflora, such as a surface wound or the lungs.

HANDLING *BRUCELLA* CULTURES IN THE MICROBIOLOGY LABORATORY

Brucellosis is one of the most commonly reported bacterial infections acquired in laboratories (27, 43). Over 100 laboratory infections with *Brucella* spp. have been well documented (40, 43, 54, 77, 81). *B. abortus*, *B. melitensis*, *B. suis*, and *B. canis* have all been known to cause illness in laboratory workers (25, 48). Of the 186 *Brucella* isolates processed by the California State Health Department Laboratory during the period from 1988 through 1997, 6% were from documented laboratory infections.

Within the laboratory, aerosolization is the primary mechanism of transmission (60). As a result, the appropriate handling of *Brucella* cultures requires biological safety level 3 precautions. Most laboratory infections of brucellosis do not follow a known accident or breach in technique. Laboratory infections can occur when microbiologists work on the laboratory bench with unknown cultures which in fact are *Brucella*. Suspicious colonies should be examined in a biological safety cabinet. The following characteristics can alert the microbiologist to the possibility that the culture is *Brucella*:

1. Gram stain characteristics: *Brucella* spp. are very small gram-negative coccobacilli, which may not take up the counterstain safranin very well and appear faintly staining. They have been described as appearing like "fine sand" (Fig. 1).

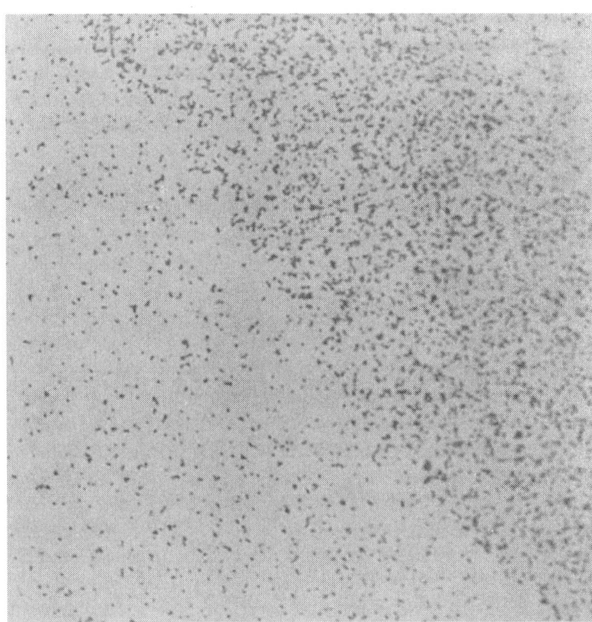

FIGURE 1 Gram stain of a *Brucella* sp. demonstrating the faintly staining, "fine sand" appearance. Photograph courtesy of David Lindquist.

2. Urea hydrolysis (performed in a biological safety cabinet): Most *Brucella* strains regardless of species, will appear urea positive on heavily inoculated Christensen's urea agar within 1 h (due to preformed enzyme).

Organisms with these characteristics require manipulation in a biological safety cabinet even if only to prepare a culture to send to a reference laboratory for identification.

IDENTIFICATION

Brucella spp. can be differentiated from similar organisms by the reactions in Table 1. Identification to the genus level is sufficient for treatment of the patient. Identification to the species and/or biovar level can be helpful for epidemiologic studies, although it is not very discriminating in the United States since the majority of the isolates are either *B. melitensis* or *B. abortus*. Confirmation of cultures as *Brucella* species can be achieved serologically by a tube agglutination test with the *Brucella* antiserum (Difco Laboratories, Detroit, Mich.) used as the positive control for the febrile agglutination test and a formalinized saline suspension (treatment for 24 h will ensure killing) of the suspected organism as the antigen. This test will confirm the culture as *Brucella* but will not discriminate among the species. Cross-reactions with other organisms such as *Afipia clevelandenesis*, *Francisella tularensis*, *Vibrio cholerae*, and *Yersinia enterocolitica* O:9 have been reported (11, 28, 29, 50). Cross-reactions are only of concern with *F. tularensis*, which has Gram stain characteristics similar to *Brucella* spp. Urease testing and growth characteristics will differentiate the two.

Identification to species level (Table 2) should be performed by a reference laboratory with appropriate class III facilities by experienced personnel. Tests necessary for species identification are CO_2 requirement, H_2S production, urea hydrolysis, dye sensitivities, and phage sensitivity.

TABLE 1 Differentiation of *Brucella* spp. from other fastidious, gram-negative coccobacilli[a]

Test	*Brucella* sp.	*Bordetella bronchiseptica*	*Acinetobacter* sp.	*Moraxella phenylpyruvica*	*Oligella ureolytica*	*Haemophilus influenzae*
Agglutination in *Brucella* antiserum	+[b]	−	−	−	−	−
Oxidase	+[b]	+	−	+	+	+
Motility	−	+	−	−	+/−	−
Urea	+	+	+/−	+	+	+/−
Nitrate reduction	+	+	−/+	+	+	NA[c]
Growth on blood agar	+	+	+	+	+	−
Gram stain morphology	Tiny ccb[c] stain faintly	Small rods and ccb, stain brightly	Large ccb, stain brightly	ccb, stain brightly	Tiny ccb	Small ccb

[a] Compiled from references 23 and 83.
[b] *B. canis* is oxidase variable and does not agglutinate in *Brucella* antiserum.
[c] ccb, coccobacilli; NA, not applicable.

CO_2 Requirement

The CO_2 test is done by streaking two agar plates (heart infusion agar, TSA, or sheep blood agar) with the suspected organism. Both plates are incubated at 35°C, one in 5% CO_2 and the other in ambient air. Enhancement of growth by 5% CO_2 is a characteristic of *B. abortus* but not the other commonly encountered *Brucella* spp., especially after primary isolation.

H_2S Production

To determine H_2S production, a milky suspension of the organism is inoculated onto a brucella agar slant. A lead acetate paper strip (Key Scientific Products, Round Rock, Tex.) is inserted into the tube so that it hangs down over the agar slant but does not touch it. The tube should be incubated at 35°C in 5% CO_2 for a total of 6 days. These tubes are read daily to determine the presence or absence of blackening of the lead acetate paper. The paper strip should be changed daily. *B. abortus* will produce a moderate amount of H_2S, with blackening of the strip on days 2 to 5. *B. melitensis* produces little if any H_2S detectable by this method. *B. suis* produces the most H_2S, with blackening of the strip occurring on days 1 to 6 (41).

Urea Hydrolysis

Urea hydrolysis has been reported to be a variable characteristic for *Brucella* spp., but in our experience almost all isolates of *Brucella* hydrolyze urea. The rate of urea hydrolysis varies with the species and is highest in *B. suis* (64). The suspension used for H_2S production is also used in this assay. Equal volumes of the organism suspension are mixed with Rustigian-Stuart urea broth (64) and incubated at room temperature. The tubes are observed for the development of a fuchsia color at 15-min intervals for the first 2 h. After this, they are read at approximately 6, 24, and 48 h. The development of a fuchsia color indicates urea hydrolysis. Rapid urea hydrolysis, as indicated by the development of a fuchsia color within 15 min, is indicative of *B. suis*. *B. abortus* and *B. melitensis* take at least 2 h to show any urea hydrolysis and may take more than 24 h to do so (64).

Dye Sensitivities

Dye sensitivity tests are based on the principle that certain dyes, when introduced into a medium which supports the growth of *Brucella*, have a bacteriostatic effect on *Brucella* which varies with the species (26, 39, 42). Only a microbiologist experienced at performing and interpreting dye sensitivity tests should perform them. There are two methods for performing dye sensitivity tests: (i) sensitivity to thionine and basic fuchsin at 20 and 40 μg and (ii) sensitivity to basic fuchsin, azure A, crystal violet, safranin, pyronin, and thionine dyes incorporated in dye tablets (Key Scientific Products) (56, 63).

To perform the test for sensitivity to thionine and basic fuchsin at 20 and 40 μg, sterile 0.1% solutions of thionine and basic fuchsin are added to brucella agar (without blood) to prepare four plates containing the following dye concentrations: 20 and 40 μg/ml of basic fuschin and thionine per plate. A control plate which contains no dyes is also used. A swab dipped in a turbid suspension of the test and control organisms (*B. abortus* 19, *B. melitensis* 16M [ATCC 23456], and *B. suis* 1330 [ATCC 23444]) is used to inoculate each plate. Up to six organisms can be tested on each plate as long as the streaks do not touch each other. The plates are

TABLE 2 Key characteristics of selected *Brucella* isolates[a]

Test	*B. abortus*	*B. melitensis*	*B. suis*	*B. canis*
Dye sensitivity				
Basic fuchsin	R[b]	R	S	S
Thionine	S	R	R	R
Urea hydrolysis	>90 min	>90 min	<90 min	<90 min
H_2S production	2–5 days	None	1–6 days	None
Lysis by Tb phage	+	−	−	−
Requirement for CO_2	+/−	−	−	−

[a] Reference 4.
[b] R, resistant; S, sensitive.

incubated in 5 to 10% CO_2 at 35°C and read for growth at 48 h or when growth appears. *B. abortus* 19 grows in the presence of basic fuschin but not thionine; *B. melitensis* 16M grows in the presence of both dyes; and *B. suis* 1330 grows in the presence of thionine but not basic fuschin (26, 42).

To perform the test for sensitivity to dyes incorporated into dye tablets, a single sweep across the brucella agar plate is made with a sterile cotton swab containing turbid suspension of the organism. Three streaks can be made on each plate. One tablet of each dye is placed on each line of inoculum. The plates are held at 4°C for 14 to 16 h to permit the dyes to diffuse into the medium before growth of the organism and then incubated at 35°C for 48 h in 5% CO_2 (63). The width of the zone of inhibition around the dye tablet is read in terms of millimeters from the edge of the tablet to the beginning of growth. A zone of 4 mm or greater is recorded as sensitive. No zone is recorded as resistant. *B. melitensis* is resistant to all six dyes; *B. suis* is sensitive to all of these dyes except thionine; and *B. abortus* is sensitive to thionine and azure A but resistant to basic fuchsin, crystal violet, pyronin, and safranin.

B. abortus Phage Sensitivity

A no. 3 McFarland standard (9 × 10^8 organisms/ml) suspension of the test and control (*B. abortus* 19) organisms is prepared, and one loopful of each organism is placed onto each of two nickel-sized areas of a fresh, dry brucella agar plate. The inoculated areas are allowed to dry. One loopful of Tbilisi (Tb) phage at routine test dilution (RTD) is placed onto the center of one spot of inoculum. To the other spot is added Tb phage at 10^4 × RTD. The plates are allowed to dry thoroughly, inverted, incubated in 5% CO_2 at 35°C, and examined for lysis at 24 and 48 h. The plates should not be read after 48 h, since resistant organisms may appear. *B. abortus* is lysed at both RTD and 10^4 × RTD. *B. melitensis* and *B. suis* are not lysed by Tb phage at either dilution. It has been reported that sometimes *B. suis* appears to be partially lysed by the phage at 10^4 × RTD (4).

SEROLOGIC TESTS

Serodiagnosis of brucellosis is most commonly made on the basis of the tube agglutination test (TAT). This assay, the most widely used in the literature, uses antigen from *B. abortus*. Other assays, including the rose Bengal test and the anti-*Brucella* Coombs' test, have been used as well. An advantage of the rose Bengal test is that the results may be obtained rapidly. The TAT assay does not detect *B. canis* antibodies (*B. canis* antibody testing is available from some veterinary laboratories) but will detect antibodies to the three major *Brucella* species pathogenic for humans (86). A single titer of ≥160 or a fourfold rise in titer is considered significant. In a modification of the assay, the use of 2-mercaptoethanol in the assay disrupts the disulfide bonds in immunoglobulin M (IgM), allowing measurement of only IgG. IgG antibody typically appears within weeks of infection and, in the absence of infection, usually persists (86). After cure, the IgG may be present for as long as 1 year (86). A slide agglutination test has been evaluated and reported to have a sensitivity of 97 to 100% and a specificity of 88 to 89% compared with the TAT (58).

Other serologic tests for *Brucella* antibodies have been developed, most notably enzyme-linked immunosorbent assays (ELISAs). The ELISA is more sensitive than the TAT in the diagnosis of brucellosis (86), including neurobrucellosis (6). Unfortunately, the ELISA is not commercially available and is less standardized from laboratory to laboratory than is the TAT.

ANTIMICROBIAL SUSCEPTIBILITY AND THERAPY

Susceptibility testing of *Brucella* species is not generally recommended. Most treatment failures in brucellosis are not due to drug resistance (75). Treatment of brucellosis requires combination antibiotic therapy for a prolonged period. Tetracyclines, aminoglycosides, rifampin, and trimethoprim-sulfamethoxazole have all been used with success in the treatment of brucellosis (75). Therapy usually consists of doxycycline for 45 days and streptomycin intramuscularly for the first 14 days. For young children, there is no clear consensus on recommendations (5) and suggested regimens include, for example, treatment with trimethoprim-sulfamethoxazole alone, in combination with rifampin, or in combination with gentamicin. Doxycycline and other tetracyclines are typically not recommended for use in this age group. In patients with endocarditis, surgery (including valve replacement) may be required in addition to antibiotic therapy. In those with central nervous system disease, the addition of rifampin may be considered (75). The quinolones have been associated with an unacceptably high relapse rate when used alone in the treatment of brucellosis (51).

EVALUATION AND INTERPRETATION OF TEST RESULTS

The isolation of any *Brucella* species from clinical material is always clinically significant, and physicians caring for the patients and appropriate public health agencies should always be notified. Unfortunately, cultures are only infrequently positive in patients with brucellosis; the diagnosis is more commonly established serologically. With the TAT, a single titer of ≥160 in an individual with a compatible clinical presentation or a fourfold rise in titer is considered clinically significant (20). However, individuals living in regions with endemic *Brucella* infection may have titers of ≥160 (86). Therefore, to establish a definitive serologic diagnosis in those individuals, acute- and convalescent-phase serum samples should be obtained and a fourfold rise in titer should be documented. Other caveats (86) when interpreting *Brucella* antibody titers include the following: (i) titers may be increased after subclinical infection; (ii) dilutions should be used to eliminate the prozone effect; and (iii) cross-reactions occur with some non-*Brucella* species including *Afipia clevelandensis* (28), *Francisella tularensis* (11), *Vibrio cholerae*, especially in individuals receiving the cholera vaccine (29), and *Yersinia enterocolitica* serotype O:9 (28, 50).

REFERENCES

1. **al-Kasab, S., M. R. al-Fagih, S. al-Yousef, M. A. Ali Khan, P. A. Ribeiro, S. Nazzal, and M. al-Zaibag.** 1988. Brucella infective endocarditis, successful combined medical and surgical therapy. *J. Thorac. Cardiovasc. Surg.* **95:**862–867.
2. **Allardet-Servent, A., G. Bourg, M. Ramuz, M. Pages, M. Bellis, and G. Roizes.** 1988. DNA polymorphism in strains of the genus *Brucella*. *J. Bacteriol.* **170:**4603–4607.
3. **al-Rawi, T. I., A. J. Thewaini, A. R. Shawket, and G. M. Ahmed.** 1989. Skeletal brucellosis in Iraqi patients. *Ann. Rheum. Dis.* **48:**77–79.
4. **Alton, G. G., L. M. Jones, R. D. Angus, and J. M. Verger.** 1988. *Techniques for the Brucellosis Laboratory*, p. 44. Institut National de la Recherche Agronomique, Paris.

5. **American Academy of Pediatrics.** 1997. Brucellosis, p. 157–159. *In* G. Peters (ed). *Red Book: Report of the Committee on Infectious Diseases.* American Academy of Pediatrics, Elk Grove Village, Ill.
6. **Araj, G. F., A. R. Lulu, M. A. Saadah, A. M. Mousa, I.-L. Strannegard, and R. A. Shakir.** 1986. Rapid diagnosis of central nervous system brucellosis by ELISA. *J. Neuroimmunol.* **12:**73–82.
7. **Ariza, J., F. Gudiol, J. Valverde, R. Pallares, P. Fernandez-Viladrich, G. Rufi, L. Espadaler, and F. Fernandez-Nogues.** 1985. Brucellar spondylitis: a detailed analysis based on current findings. *Rev. Infect. Dis.* **7:**656–664.
8. **Ariza, J., O. Servitje, R. Pallares, P. Fernandez Viladrich, G. Rufi, J. Peyri, and F. Gudiol.** 1989. Characteristic cutaneous lesions in patients with brucellosis. *Arch. Dermatol.* **125:**380–383.
9. **Bang, B.** 1897. The etiology of epizootic abortion. *J. Comp. Pathol. Ther.* **10:**125–149.
10. **Bannatyne, R. M., M. C. Jackson, and Z. Memish.** 1997. Rapid diagnosis of *Brucella* bacteremia by using the BACTEC 9240 system. *J. Clin. Microbiol.* **35:**2673–2674.
11. **Behan, K. A., and G. C. Klein.** 1982. Reduction of *Brucella* species and *Francisella tularensis* cross-reacting agglutinins by dithiothreitol. *J. Clin. Microbiol.* **16:**756–757.
12. **Berger, T. G., M. A. Guill, and D. K. Goette.** 1981. Cutaneous lesions in brucellosis. *Arch. Dermatol.* **117:**40–42.
13. **Bouza, E., M. Garcia de la Torre, F. Parras, A. Guerrero, M. Rodriguez-Creixems, and J. Gobernado.** 1987. Brucellar meningitis. *Rev. Infect. Dis.* **9:**810–822.
14. **Bricker, B. J., and S. M. Halling.** 1994. Differentiation of *Brucella abortus* bv. 1, 2, and 4, *Brucella melitensis, Brucella ovis*, and *Brucella suis* bv. 1 by PCR. *J. Clin. Microbiol.* **32:**2660–2666.
15. **Bruce, D.** 1887. Note on the discovery of a microorganism in Malta Fever. *Practitioner* **36:**161–170.
16. **Buchanan, T. M., L. C. Faber, and R. A. Feldman.** 1974. Brucellosis in the United States, 1960–1972, an abattoir-associated disease, part I. *Medicine* **53:**403–413.
17. **Buddle, M. B.** 1956. Studies on *Brucella ovis* (n. sp.), a cause of genital disease of sheep in New Zealand and Australia. *J. Hyg. Camb.* **54:**351–364.
18. **Carmichael, L. E., and D. W. Bruner.** 1968. Characteristics of a newly-recognized species of *Brucella* responsible for infectious canine abortions. *Cornell Vet.* **58:**579–592.
19. **Casas, J., Y. Partal, J. Llosa, J. Leiva, J. M. Navarro, and M. de la Rosa.** 1994. Detection of *Brucella* with an automatic hemoculture system: Bact/Alert. *Enferm. Infecc. Microbiol. Clin.* **12:**497–500. (In Spanish.)
20. **Centers for Disease Control and Prevention.** 1994. Brucellosis outbreak at a pork processing plant—North Carolina, 1992. *Morbid. Mortal. Weekly Rep.* **43:**113–116.
21. **Centers for Disease Control and Prevention.** 1997. Summary of notifiable diseases, United States, 1996. *Morbid. Mortal. Weekly Rep.* **53:**39.
22. **Cervantes, F., M. Bruguera, J. Carbonell, L. Force, and S. Webb.** 1982. Liver disease in brucellosis. A clinical and pathological study of 40 cases. *Postgrad. Med. J.* **58:**346–350.
23. **Corbel, M. J., and W. J. Brinley-Morgan.** 1984. Genus *Brucella*, p. 377–388. *In* N. R. Krieg and J. G. Holt (ed.), *Bergey's Manual of Systematic Bacteriology*, vol. 1. The Williams & Wilkins Co., Baltimore, Md.
24. **Corbel, M. J.** 1988. International Committee on Systematic Bacteriology subcommittee on the taxonomy of *Brucella*. *Int. J. Syst. Bacteriol.* **38:**450–452.
25. **Corbel, M. J.** 1997. Brucellosis: an overview. *Emerging Infect. Dis.* **3:**213–221.
26. **Cruickshank, J. C.** 1948. A simple method for testing dye sensitivity of *Brucella* species. *J. Pathol. Bacteriol.* **60:**328–329.
27. **Department of Health and Human Services, Public Health Service.** 1993. *Biosafety in Microbiological and Biomedical Laboratories*, 3rd ed. Department of Health and Human Services, Washington, D.C.
28. **Drancourt, M., P. Brouqui, and D. Raoult.** 1997. *Afipia clevelandensis* antibodies and cross-reactivity with *Brucella* spp. and *Yersinia enterocolitica* O:9. *Clin. Diagn. Lab. Immunol.* **4:**748–752.
29. **Eisele, C. W., N. B. McCullough, and G. A. Beal.** 1948. Brucella antibodies following cholera vaccination. *Ann. Intern. Med.* **28:**833–837.
30. **Evans, A. C.** 1918. Further studies on *Bacterium abortus* and related bacteria. II. A comparison of *Bacterium abortus* with *Bacterium bronchosepticus* and with the organism which causes Malta fever. *J. Infect. Dis.* **22:**580–593.
31. **Ewalt, D. R., J. B. Payeur, B. M. Martin, D. R. Cummins, and W. G. Miller.** 1994. Characteristics of a *Brucella* species from a bottlenose dolphin (*Tursiops truncatus*). *J. Vet. Diagn. Invest.* **6:**448–452.
32. **Fernandez-Guerrero, M. L., J. Martinell, J. M. Aguado, M. C. Ponte, J. Fraile, and G. de Rabago.** 1987. Prosthetic valve endocarditis caused by *Brucella melitensis*. A report of four cases successfully treated with tetracycline, streptomycin, and sulfamethoxazole and trimethoprim plus valve replacement. *Arch. Intern. Med.* **147:**1141–1143.
33. **Fox, M. D., and A. F. Kaufmann.** 1977. Brucellosis in the United States, 1965–1974. *J. Infect. Dis.* **136:**312–316.
34. **Gotuzzo, E., C. Carrillo, J. Guerra, and L. Llosa.** 1986. An evaluation of diagnostic methods for brucellosis—the value of bone marrow culture. *J. Infect. Dis.* **153:**122–125.
35. **Gotuzzo, E., C. Seas, J. G. Guerra, C. Carrillo, T. S. Bocanegra, A. Calvo, O. Castaneda, and G. S. Alarcon.** 1987. Brucellar arthritis: a study of 39 Peruvian families. *Ann. Rheum. Dis.* **46:**506–509.
36. **Grant, G. H., and C. L. Stote.** 1953. Rupture of the heart as a result of *Brucella abortus* endocarditis. *Br. Med. J.* **1:**914–916.
37. **Haden, R. L., and E. R. Kyger.** 1946. Pulmonary manifestations of brucellosis. *Clevel. Clin. Q.* **13:**220–227.
38. **Harvey, W. A.** 1948. Pulmonary brucellosis. *Ann. Intern. Med.* **28:**768–781.
39. **Hollis, D.** 1990. Personal communication.
40. **Howe, C., E. S. Miller, E. H. Kelly, H. L. Bookwalter, and H. V. Ellingson.** 1947. Acute brucellosis among laboratory workers. *N. Engl. J. Med.* **236:**741–747.
41. **Huddleson, I. F.** 1929. The differentiation of the species of the genus *Brucella*. *Mich. Agric. Exp. Stn. Tech. Bull.* **100:**1–16.
42. **Huddleson, I. F.** 1931. Differentiation of the species of the genus *Brucella*. *Am. J. Public Health* **21:**491–498.
43. **Huddleson, I. F., and M. Munger.** 1940. A study of an epidemic of brucellosis due to *Brucella melitensis*. *Am. J. Public Health* **30:**944–954.
44. **Huddleson, I. F., and E. Abell.** 1927. A biochemical method of differentiating *Brucella abortus* from *Brucella melitensis-paramelitensis*. *J. Bacteriol.* **13:**13.
45. **Ibrahim, A. I., R. Awad, S. D. Shetty, M. Saad, and N. E. Bilal.** 1988. Genito-urinary complications of brucellosis. *Br. J. Urol.* **61:**294–298.
46. **Jeroudi, M. O., M. A. Halim, E. J. Harder, M. B. Al-Siba'i, G. Ziady, and E. N. Mercer.** 1987. *Brucella* endocarditis. *Br. Heart J.* **58:**279–283.
47. **Jones, L. M., M. Zanardi, D. Leong, and J. B. Wilson.** 1968. Taxonomic position in the genus *Brucella* of the causative agent of canine abortion. *J. Bacteriol.* **95:**625–630.
48. **Kaufman, A. F., and J. M. Boyce.** 1995. Transmission of bacterial and rickettsial zoonoses in the laboratory, p.

93–104. *In* D. O. Fleming, J. H. Richardson, J. J. Tulis, and D. Vesley (ed.), *Laboratory Safety*, 2nd ed. ASM Press, Washington, D.C.

49. **Khan, M. S., M. S. Humayoon, and M. S. Al Manee.** 1989. Epididymo-orchitis and brucellosis. *Br. J. Urol.* **63:** 87–89.
50. **Kittelberger, R., P. G. Bundesen, A. Cloeckaert, I. Greiser Wilke, and J. J. Letesson.** 1998. Serological cross-reactivity between *Brucella abortus* and *Yersinia enterocolitica* O:9. IV. Evaluation of the M- and C-epitope antibody response for the specific detection of *B. abortus* infections. *Vet. Microbiol.* **60:**45–57.
51. **Lang, R., and E. Rubinstein.** 1992. Quinolones for the treatment of brucellosis. *Antimicrob. Agents Chemother.* **29:** 357–360.
52. **Lum, M. K., F. D. Pien, and D. M. Sasaki.** 1985. Human *Brucella canis* infection in Hawaii. *Hawaii Med. J.* **44:** 66–68.
53. **Madkour, M. M., H. S. Sharif, M. Y. Abed, and M. A. Al-Fayez.** 1988. Osteoarticular brucellosis: results of bone scintigraphy in 140 patients. *Am. J. Roentgenol.* **150:** 1101–1105.
54. **Martin-Mazuelos, E., M. C. Nogales, C. Florez, J. M. Gomez-Mateos, F. Lozano, and A. Sanchez.** 1994. Outbreak of *Brucella melitensis* among laboratory workers. *J. Clin. Microbiol.* **32:**2035–2036.
55. **Meyer, K. F., and E. B. Shaw.** 1920. A comparison of the morphologic, culture and biochemical characteristics of *B. abortus* and *B. melitensis*: studies on the genus *Brucella* nov. gen. I. *J. Infect. Dis.* **27:**173–184.
56. **Moriera-Jacob, M.** 1963. Safranine O: reliable selective dye for characterization of *Brucella suis*. *J. Bacteriol.* **86:** 599–600.
57. **Mousa, A. R., K. M. Elhag, M. Khogali, and A. A. Marafie.** 1988. The nature of human brucellosis in Kuwait: study of 379 cases. *Rev. Infect. Dis.* **10:**211–217.
58. **Moyer, N. P., G. M. Evins, N. E. Pigott, J. D. Hudson, C. E. Farshy, J. C. Feeley, and W. J. Hausler, Jr.** 1987. Comparison of serologic screening tests for brucellosis. *J. Clin. Microbiol.* **25:**1969–1972.
59. **Navas, E., A. Guerrero, J. Cobo, and E. Loza.** 1993. Faster isolation of *Brucella* spp. from blood by Isolator compared with BACTEC NR. *Diagn. Microbiol. Infect. Dis.* **16:** 79–81.
60. **Olle-Goig, J. D., and J. Canela-Soler.** 1987. An outbreak of *Brucella melitensis* infection by airborne transmission among laboratory workers. *Am. J. Public Health* **77:** 335–338.
61. **Patel, P. J., H. Al-Suhaibani, A. K. Al-Aska, T. M. Kolawole, and F. A. Al-Kasssimi.** 1988. The chest radiograph in brucellosis. *Clin. Radiol.* **39:**39–41.
62. **Peery, T. M., and L. F. Belter.** 1960. Brucellosis and heart disease. II. Fatal brucellosis: a review of the literature and report of new cases. *Am. J. Pathol.* **36:**673–697.
63. **Pickett, M. J., E. L. Nelson, R. E. Hoyt, and B. E. Eisenstein.** 1952. Speciation within the genus *Brucella*. I. Dye sensitivity of smooth brucellae. *J. Lab. Clin. Med.* **40:** 200–205.
64. **Pickett, M. J., E. L. Nelson, and J. D. Liberman.** 1953. Speciation within the genus *Brucella*. II. Evaluation of differential dye, biochemical, and serological tests. *J. Bacteriol.* **66:**210–219.
65. **Pratt, D. S., J. H. Tenney, C. M. Bjork, and L. B. Reller.** 1978. Successful treatment of *Brucella melitensis* endocarditis. *Am. J. Med.* **64:**897–900.
66. **Queipo-Ortuno, M. I., P. Morata, P. Ocon, P. Manchado, and J. D. Colmenero.** 1997. Rapid diagnosis of human brucellosis by peripheral-blood PCR assay. *J. Clin. Microbiol.* **35:**2927–2930.
67. **Ray, W. C.** 1979. Brucellosis (due to *Brucella abortus* and *B. suis*), p. 99–183. *In* J. H. Steele (ed.), *CRC Handbook Series in Zoonoses*, sect. A, vol. 1. CRC Press, Inc., Boca Raton, Fla.
68. **Ross, H. M., G. Foster, R. J. Reid, K. L. Jabans, and A. P. MacMillan.** 1994. *Brucella* species infection in sea mammals. *Vet. Rec.* **134:**359.
69. **Rousseau, P.** 1985. *Brucella canis* infection in a woman with fever of unknown origin. *Postgrad. Med.* **78:**249, 253–254, 257.
70. **Rumley, R. L., and S. W. Chapman.** 1986. *Brucella canis*: an infectious cause of prolonged fever of undetermined origin. *South. Med. J.* **79:**626–628.
71. **Schnurrenberger, P. R., J. F. Walker, and R. J. Martin.** 1975. *Brucella* infections in Illinois veterinarians. *J. Am. Vet. Med. Assoc.* **167:**1084–1088.
72. **Shakir, R. A., A. S. Al-Din, G. F. Araj, A. R. Lulu, A. R. Mousa, and M. A. Saadah.** 1987. Clinical categories of neurobrucellosis, a report on 19 cases. *Brain* **110**(Part I)**:**213–223.
73. **Solanes, M. P., J. Heatley, F. Arenas, and G. G. Ibarra.** 1953. Ocular complications in brucellosis. *Am. J. Ophthalmol.* **36:**675–689.
74. **Soler, P., P. Fraile, E. Golvano, and P. Peña.** 1993. Comparison of ESP128 (Difco Laboratories), Bactec 9240 and Bactec NR 660 for rapid diagnosis of fastidious aerobic microorganisms, abstr. 674. *In Abstracts of the 6th European Congress of Clinical Microbiology and Infectious Diseases*.
75. **Solera, J., E. Martinez-Alfaro, and A. Espinosa.** 1997. Recognition and optimum treatment of brucellosis. *Drugs* **53:**245–256.
76. **Spink, W. W.** 1956. *Brucellosis*, p. 9. The University of Minnesota Press, Minneapolis.
77. **Staszkiewicz, J., C. M. Lewis, J. Colville, M. Zervos, and J. Band.** 1991. Outbreak of *Brucella melitensis* among microbiology laboratory workers in a community hospital. *J. Clin. Microbiol.* **29:**287–290.
78. **Stoenner, H. G., and D. B. Lackman.** 1957. A new species of *Brucella* isolated from the desert woodrat *Neotoma lepida* Thomas. *Am. J. Vet. Res.* **18:**947–951.
79. **Sullivan, N.** 1997. Personal communication.
80. **Timoney, J. F., J. H. Gillespie, F. W. Scott, and J. E. Barlough.** 1988. The genus *Brucella*, p. 135–152. *In Hagan and Bruner's Microbiology and Infectious Diseases of Domestic Animals*, 8th ed. Comstock Publishing Associates, Cornell University Press, Ithaca, N.Y.
81. **Trevor, R. W., L. E. Cluff, R. N. Peeler, and I. L. Bennett.** 1959. Brucellosis. I. Laboratory-acquired acute infection. *Arch. Intern. Med.* **103:**381–397.
82. **Verger, J. M., F. Grimont, P. A. D. Grimont, and M. Grayon.** 1985. *Brucella*, a monospecific genus as shown by deoxyribonucleic acid hybridization. *Int. J. Syst. Bacteriol.* **35:**292–295.
83. **Weyant, R. S., C. W. Moss, R. E. Weaver, D. G. Hollis, J. G. Jordan, E. C. Cook, and M. I. Daneshaver.** 1996. *Identification of Unusual Pathogenic Gram-Negative Aerobic and Facultatively Anaerobic Bacteria*, 2nd ed. The Williams & Wilkins Co., Baltimore, Md.
84. **Yagupsky, P., N. Peled, J. Press, O. Abramson, and M. Abu-Rashid.** 1997. Comparison of Bactec 9240 Peds Plus medium and Isolator 1.5 microbial tube for detection of *Brucella melitensis* from blood cultures. *J. Clin. Microbiol.* **35:**1382–1384.
85. **Young, E. J.** 1983. Human brucellosis. *Rev. Infect. Dis.* **5:** 821–842.
86. **Young, E. J.** 1991. Serologic diagnosis of human brucellosis: analysis of 214 cases by agglutination tests and review of the literature. *Rev. Infect. Dis.* **13:**359–372.

Pasteurella

BARRY HOLMES, M. JOHN PICKETT, AND DANNIE G. HOLLIS

42

TAXONOMY

Perroncito, in 1878, was apparently the first to isolate and describe the organism known as the bacillus of fowl cholera (18). According to Gay (15), Huelle, in 1886, first noted that certain apparently separate but distinctive diseases of wild animals, cattle, swine, and rabbits, as well as fowl cholera, were not simply septicemias but septicemias of a distinctive sort, as shown by their tendency to produce capillary submucous hemorrhage and by the presence in each instance of a short, bipolar-staining bacterium. The following year, Trevisan suggested the generic name *Pasteurella* for these organisms. Subsequently, different species names were assigned to isolates according to the animal of origin, e.g., "*Pasteurella aviseptica*" from fowl and "*Pasteurella boviseptica*" from cattle. For a long time, the genus was recognized as containing three main species, *P. haemolytica*, *P. multocida*, and *P.* (now *Actinobacillus*) *ureae* (18).

Currently, some 20 species are included in the genus *Pasteurella*, although several of these, indicated by [*P.*], are not true members of the genus (see below). These 20 species are *P. multocida* (the type species of the genus), [*P.*] *aerogenes*, *P. bettyae*, *P. canis*, *P. dagmatis*, [*P.*] *haemolytica*, [*P.*] *pneumotropica*, *P. stomatis*, and [*Pasteurella*] "SP" group, all of which have so far been recovered from human specimens or associated with human disease, and the following which have yet to be isolated either at all or with any regularity from human clinical material: *P. anatis*, *P. avium*, *P. caballi*, *P. gallinarum*, *P. granulomatis*, *P. langaa*, *P. lymphangitidis*, *P. mairi*, *P. testudinis*, *P. trehalosi*, and *P. volantium* (7, 26, 29, 31, 32).

The genera *Actinobacillus* and *Pasteurella* are similar with respect to the moles percent G+C of their chromosomal DNA (ca. 40 to 45% in *Pasteurella* [7] and 40 to 43% in *Actinobacillus*) and their phenotypic features (notably fermentation of glucose, reduction of nitrate, and lack of motility) and in terms of animals being reservoirs for human disease. No single phenotypic feature definitively distinguishes the two genera (26), but an unknown organism can usually be identified based on the features of individual species.

DNA-DNA hybridization studies (26) have shown that several taxa previously assigned to the genus *Pasteurella* (*P. aerogenes*, *P. haemolytica*, and *P. pneumotropica*) are more closely related to members of the genus *Actinobacillus*. Comparisons of 16S rRNA sequences (8) confirm that these three species are not closely related to each other or to *Pasteurella* spp. Two biotypes of [*P.*] *haemolytica* were long recognized within the species: biotype A was xylose positive, esculin negative, and usually mannose negative, while biotype T was mannose positive, xylose negative, and usually esculin positive. However, these biotypes were found to exhibit only low levels of DNA-DNA hybridization to each other (2), and they have now each been accorded species status: biotype A is [*P.*] *haemolytica*, and biotype T (from sheep) is now *P. trehalosi* (32). Hybridization (26) and subsequent (32) numerical analysis of phenotypic characters detected more than 13 taxa in the genus *Pasteurella*.

NATURAL HABITATS AND CLINICAL SIGNIFICANCE

Pasteurella species have been recovered from lesions in many parts of the human body, especially animal bite wounds; there is a higher incidence of one or more pathogenic strains in gingival scrapings of cats than of dogs (14), and this could explain why *Pasteurella* infections in humans occur less often after dog bites than after cat bites. The occurrence of *Pasteurella* and related species in human infections has been reviewed by Escande and Lion (9) and by Frederiksen (12). In animals, they cause fowl cholera, hemorrhagic septicemia, mastitis, septic pleuropneumonia, snuffles, and other focal infections. Both healthy and diseased wild and domestic animals are the reservoirs for most human infections.

P. multocida is apparently a commensal in the upper respiratory tracts of fowl and mammals and possibly also of humans. In humans, it is associated with focal infections following animal bites, with chronic pulmonary disease, and with systemic disease including meningitis. A cytotoxin can be found in cell extracts of certain strains, particularly strains of capsular type D; for a fuller discussion of toxin production and pathogenicity of *P. multocida*, particularly in animals other than humans, see reference 18.

[*P.*] *aerogenes* has been recovered from aborted fetuses of swine and from animal bites, urine, and peritoneal fluid in humans. Ribotyping (together with phenotypic characterization) has been applied (22) to strains of this species from various animal and geographic origins, but the strains examined proved to constitute a well-defined group that could not be subdivided according to origin. Another organism that may resemble pasteurellae is the so-called [*Pasteurella*]

"SP" group, which is aerogenic like [*P.*] *aerogenes* and also is not a true member of the genus. It is usually isolated from guinea pigs and rabbits. Five cases of human infection have been reported, including a severe infection following a guinea pig bite (24).

P. bettyae (32), formerly CDC group HB-5 (37), was initially described with the grammatically incorrect name *P. bettii*, but the epithet was subsequently corrected (18, 19). The reservoir for this organism is currently unknown, but *P. bettyae* has been recovered from amniotic fluid, blood (usually of newborn babies), finger lesions, leg abscesses, placenta, rectal sites, surgical incisions, and urogenital specimens (particularly those of females), including exudates of genital ulcers, especially Bartholin gland abscesses (1, 37).

The oral cavity of dogs (*P. canis*) or of cats and dogs (*P. dagmatis*) is the reservoir for several species associated with bite wounds in humans. A second biotype of *P. canis* is found in cattle. The name *P. dagmatis* was proposed (26) for a group of pasteurellae originally referred to by the Centers for Disease Control and Prevention (CDC) as *Pasteurella* sp. "new species 1" (*Pasteurella* "gas") (37). Many of the 129 strains characterized by the CDC were recovered from localized wounds in humans following animal contact, particularly cat and dog bites. This species has also been implicated in infective endocarditis (33) and as a cause of septicemia in a diabetic patient following septicemia caused by *P. multocida* (11). [*P.*] *haemolytica* is relatively common as a cause of septicemia and mastitis in domestic animals but rarely causes disease in humans (40).

[*P.*] *pneumotropica* was initially associated with pulmonary infections in laboratory mice, and most of the strains processed at the CDC were recovered from mice and rats (37). It appears to be less common than other species of pasteurellae as an agent of either animal or human disease. Strains from humans reported in the past as belonging to this species are now more likely to have been strains of *P. dagmatis*. Strains of *P. stomatis* were recovered from the respiratory tracts of cats and dogs (26); the organism has been reported to cause human infection following cat or dog bites (20, 28).

A strain of *P. caballi*, found in the oral cavity of horses, has been isolated from an infected wound on a veterinary surgeon (3), as well as from a horse bite wound (10). Similarly, although most strains of *P. volantium* were recovered from fowl, one strain was isolated from a human tongue (26); all 10 strains that have been isolated required V factor (NAD) for growth.

Pasteurellae are not commonly recovered from clinical specimens. Between June 1996 and May 1997, the Clinical Microbiology Laboratories of the University of California Los Angeles Medical Center recovered 8 such isolates compared with 6,219 isolates of nonfastidious gram-negative rods (e.g., *Acinetobacter* spp., members of the *Enterobacteriaceae*, and *Pseudomonas aeruginosa* [unpublished data]).

SPECIMEN COLLECTION, TRANSPORT, AND PROCESSING

Specimens from infected bite wounds should be obtained surgically and transported and processed to facilitate the recovery of both aerobic and anaerobic bacteria (see chapter 4). Swabs should be avoided; aspirates or curettings are preferred. Pasteurellae usually grow well, and so routine procedures used with other types of specimens, including sputum and blood cultures, should be sufficient (37). Commercial 5% sheep blood agar (BA) plates should be used for isolation and propagation; these plates may be slightly less sensitive to bacterial hemolysins than is 5% rabbit blood agar prepared with heart infusion agar. Primary isolation may be best accomplished if the BA plates are incubated for up to 72 h in a humidified atmosphere of 3 to 5% CO_2, since some pasteurellae are capnophilic. Growth on MacConkey agar varies among species.

IDENTIFICATION

Pasteurella species are coccobacilli or rods, 1 to 2 μm long. They are nonmotile, facultatively anaerobic, and saccharolytic. Most strains recovered from clinical specimens are catalase, oxidase, indole, and sucrose positive; most decarboxylate ornithine; some are encapsulated. Oxidase tests should be performed on cultures grown on BA or chocolate agar medium; negative results may be obtained with other growth media (16). The oxidase test should be performed with the tetramethyl, not the dimethyl, reagent, because the former is more sensitive. For tests of indole production, tryptone medium should be incubated for 2 days and then Ehrlich reagent should be added after extraction with xylene.

A 10-U penicillin disk may be used as an aid to identification. *Pasteurella* species are typically penicillin susceptible, yielding a zone of inhibition of ≥15 mm when tested with a McFarland 0.5 inoculum suspension on a Mueller-Hinton agar plate.

Pasteurella species resemble several other moderately fastidious gram-negative rods (Table 1), in particular, *Actinobacillus* species. The differential phenotypic characteristics of species of *Pasteurella* that occur in human clinical specimens are shown in Table 2. The characteristics of species found exclusively in veterinary material are described elsewhere (26, 32); workers in this field must also consider a number of as yet unnamed taxa when identifying these organisms (see, for example, reference 6).

P. multocida colonies on 24-h BA plates are 1 to 2 mm in diameter and nonhemolytic. Like other pasteurellae and actinobacilli, *P. multocida* acidifies both the slant and butt of a triple sugar iron agar slant. Occasionally, a strain gives a weak or even negative result in the oxidase test; however, tests with the tetramethyl reagent only rarely give negative results. Tests for indole production, ornithine decarboxylase, and acidification of maltose and sucrose form the basis for definitive identification of this species (Table 2). Tests for acidification of dulcitol and sorbitol delineate three subspecies, subspp. *gallicida*, *multocida*, and *septica* (26).

Colonies of [*P.*] *aerogenes* on 1-day BA plates are 0.5 to 1 mm in diameter, convex, smooth, translucent, and nonhemolytic. This species grows well on MacConkey agar. Like several other species, [*P.*] *aerogenes* is urease positive and, as the name suggests, produces gas from glucose.

The capnophilic *P. bettyae* appears as coccobacilli and rods. Growth on BA plates for 24 h yields colonies that are 0.5 to 1.0 mm in diameter, convex, and smooth. All strains are weakly aerogenic. Of the usual battery of six sugars used by the CDC (i.e., D-glucose, lactose, maltose, D-mannitol, sucrose, and D-xylose), only glucose is acidified. Although *P. bettyae* and HB-5 are considered the same organism, their synonymy does not appear to have been confirmed by DNA-DNA homology studies; different proportions of strains giving positive reactions have been noted for them by different authors for catalase and oxidase production and maltose fermentation, and a major disparity in indole formation has been reported (32, 37).

TABLE 1 Salient features of *Pasteurella* species and similar bacteria[a]

Organism	No. of strains	Capnophilic	% of strains positive			
			Catalase	Oxidase	TSIA,[b] acid	
					Slant	Butt
Actinobacillus actinomycetemcomitans	120	+	99	19[c]	100	100
Actinobacillus equuli	19	−	73	100	100	100
Actinobacillus lignieresii	30	−	89	100	100	100
Actinobacillus suis	33	−	85	100	100	100
Actinobacillus (Pasteurella) ureae	97	−	63	99	100	99
Cardiobacterium hominis (IId)	65	+	1	100	93	84
DF-3	21	+	0	0	95	100
DF-3-like	7	+	29	0	29	29
EF-4a	97	−	100	100	3	73
EF-4b	34	−	100	100	0	6
Eikenella corrodens (HB-1)	506	+	8	100	0	0
Kingella denitrificans (TM-1)	60	−	10	100	2	0
Kingella kingae	137	−	0	100	21	11
Kingella oralis	11	−	9	100	ND[e]	ND
[*Pasteurella*] *aerogenes*	16	−	100	100	94	100
Pasteurella bettyae (HB-5)	88	+	1	61	100	100
Pasteurella canis	31	−	96	92	96	96
Pasteurella dagmatis[d]	129	−	99	98	100	100
[*Pasteurella*] *haemolytica*	30	−	96	96	100	100
Pasteurella multocida	225	−	98	96	99	92
[*Pasteurella*] *pneumotropica*	107	−	100	99	100	97
Pasteurella stomatis	8	−	100	100	100	100
Pasteurella sp. Bisgaard's taxon 16	30	−	100	100	100	100

[a] Data for this table are adapted from reference 37, except for data on *K. oralis*, which are from reference 19.
[b] TSIA, triple sugar iron agar.
[c] Of the strains tested, 95% were either oxidase negative or only weakly positive.
[d] *Pasteurella* "new species 1"; similar to *Pasteurella* sp. Bisgaard's taxon 16.
[e] ND, no data.

Biotype 1 strains of *P. canis* (26) are indole positive; biotype 2 strains from cattle are indole negative. The principal test for differentiating between *P. canis* and *P. multocida* is acidification of mannitol (Table 2).

After a 24-h incubation on BA plates, *P. dagmatis* colonies are 1 to 2 mm in diameter and nonhemolytic. Differential tests are for acidification of maltose and xylose, production of indole, decarboxylation of ornithine, and hydrolysis of urea (Table 2). Similar strains that are urea negative are probably *Pasteurella* sp. Taxon 16 (37).

[*P.*] *haemolytica* is indole and urease negative (Table 2). Freshly isolated strains are hemolytic but may lose this feature upon subculture. On 24-h BA plates, *P. pneumotropica* colonies are 0.5 to 1.5 mm in diameter, low convex, and nonhemolytic. Salient tests for identification include ornithine decarboxylase, hydrolysis of urea, and production of gas from glucose (Table 2).

Important differential tests for *P. stomatitis* include acidification of maltose and mannitol, production of indole, and decarboxylation of ornithine (Table 2).

Although not described in detail because little association with human disease has so far been reported, the following species deserve some consideration. *P. caballi* (29) differs from most other pasteurellae in being catalase negative. All of the 29 strains of *P. caballi* recovered from horses were aerogenic, did not grow on MacConkey agar, acidified neither L-arabinose nor trehalose, and were both urease and indole negative.

SEROLOGIC TYPING AND MOLECULAR METHODS

Typing methods used for *P. multocida* for epidemiological purposes include use of the API ZYM system (17), bacteriophages (27), and various DNA fingerprinting techniques (4, 30, 38, 39) as well as serologic testing. There are several somatic groups, and four capsular serotypes, A, B, D, and E, are recognized, with most human strains belonging to type A and the remainder belonging mostly to type D (the antigenic structure is described in detail by Holmes [18]). Serologic tests are not used for other species.

PCR analysis for the direct detection of toxigenic strains of *P. multocida* has been developed (23). A PCR method based on 16S rDNA and specific for [*P.*] *pneumotropica* has also been described (35).

TABLE 2 Differential features of *Pasteurella* species occurring in clinical specimens[a]

Feature	[P.] *aerogenes*	*P. bettyae* (HB-5)	*P. canis*	*P. dagmatis*[b]	[P.] *haemolytica*	*P. multocida*[c]	[P.] *pneumotropica*	*P. stomatis*
Acidified								
L-Arabinose	(+)	−	−	−	+	d	(−)	−
D-Galactose	+	−	+	+	+	+	+	+
Lactose	(−)	−	−	−	d	−	d	−
Maltose	+	d[d]	−	+	+	(−)	d	−
D-Mannitol	d	−	−	−	+	(+)	−	−
D-Mannose	+	d	+	+	(−)	+	+	+
Melibiose	d	−	−	−	−[e]	(−)	d	−
Raffinose	d	−	−	+,w	d	−	d	−
Sorbitol	(−)	−	−	−	+	d	−	−
Sucrose	+	−	+	+	+	+	+	+
D-Trehalose	−	−	d	+	−	d	(+)	+
D-Xylose	+	−	(−)	−	+	d	d	−
Beta-hemolysis (sheep cells)	−	−	−	−	(+)	−	−	−
Catalase	+	d	+	+	+	+	+	+
Esculin hydrolysis	−	−	−	−	d	−	−	−
Gas from D-glucose[f]	(+)	d,w	−	+,w	−	−	d	−
Growth on MacConkey agar	+	d	−	−	+	d	d	−
Indole production	(−)	−[g]	d,w	+	−	(+)	+	+,w
ONPG reaction[h]	d	−	−	−	d	−	+	−
Ornithine decarboxylase	d	−	+	−	−	d	+	−
Oxidase	d	−	+	+	+	+	+	+
Urease	+	−	−	+	−	−	+	−

[a] This table is adapted from reference 19, which includes data from 20 additional references and also includes *P. trehalosi* and *P. volantium*. Symbols and abbreviations: +, ≥90% of the strains are positive; (+), 80 to 89% of the strains are positive; d, 21 to 79% of the strains are positive; (−), 11 to 20% of the strains are positive; −, ≤10% of the strains are positive; w, weak reaction.

[b] Strains that are similar except for failing to produce urease are probably *Pasteurella* sp. Bisgaard's taxon 16 (37).

[c] Three subspecies: *P. multocida* subsp. *gallicida* is dulcitol and sorbitol positive; *P. multocida* subsp. *multocida* is dulcitol negative and sorbitol positive; *P. multocida* subsp. *septica* is dulcitol and sorbitol negative.

[d] Negative according to reference 37.

[e] Positive according to reference 7 and negative according to references 21 and 32.

[f] In Hugh-Leifson medium containing glucose, with incubation for 48 h at 37°C.

[g] Positive according to reference 37.

[h] Hydrolysis of *o*-nitrophenyl-β-D-galactopyranoside.

ANTIBIOTIC SUSCEPTIBILITY

Although numerous strains of bovine and porcine origin have been reported to be resistant to many antibiotics, resistance is rare among human isolates. Most isolates are susceptible to penicillin and tetracyclines (20, 36), with the latter, especially minocycline, being the usual drugs of choice for the treatment of local pasteurellosis in humans. Although macrolides have been proposed as a therapeutic alternative where tetracyclines are contraindicated (13), macrolide resistance has been reported (25); some strains are resistant to chloramphenicol (34). Fluoroquinolones appear to be effective in treating systemic pasteurellosis (13). *P. bettyae* is usually susceptible to many antimicrobial agents, including penicillin, but some strains produce β-lactamases (5).

INTERPRETATION AND REPORTING OF RESULTS

The main points to bear in mind are that *Pasteurella* species are associated predominantly with animals other than humans. Isolates are therefore rarely encountered in clinical laboratories but should be considered in the setting of animal bite wounds and lung infections, particularly where a pet is involved. For this reason, clinicians need to include clinical information with specimens from patients suspected of having *Pasteurella* infections. Most strains of this genus isolated in clinical laboratories will be catalase, oxidase, indole, ornithine, and sucrose positive and susceptible to penicillin (10-U disk).

REFERENCES

1. **Baddour, L. M., M. S. Gelfand, R. E. Weaver, T. C. Woods, M. Altwegg, L. W. Mayer, R. A. Kelley, and D. J. Brenner.** 1989. CDC group HB-5 as a cause of genitourinary infections in adults. *J. Clin. Microbiol.* **27:** 801–805.
2. **Bingham, D. P., R. Moore, and A. B. Richards.** 1990. Comparison of DNA:DNA homology and enzymatic activity between *Pasteurella haemolytica* and related species. *Am. J. Vet. Res.* **51:**1161–1166.
3. **Bisgaard, M., O. Heltberg, and W. Frederiksen.** 1991. Isolation of *Pasteurella caballi* from an infected wound on a veterinary surgeon. *APMIS* **99:**291–294.
4. **Blackwood, R. A., C. K. Rode, J. S. Read, I. H. Law, and C. A. Bloch.** 1996. Genomic fingerprinting by pulsed field gel electrophoresis to identify the source of *Pasteurella multocida* sepsis. *Pediatr. Infect. Dis. J.* **15:**831–833.
5. **Bogaerts, J., J. Verhaegen, W. M. Tello, S. Allen, L. Verbist, E. Van Dyck, and P. Piot.** 1990. Characterization, in vitro susceptibility, and clinical significance of CDC group HB-5 from Rwanda. *J. Clin. Microbiol.* **28:** 2196–2199.
6. **Boot, R., and M. Bisgaard.** 1995. Reclassification of 30 *Pasteurellaceae* strains isolated from rodents. *Lab. Anim.* **29:** 314–319.
7. **Carter, G. R.** 1984. Genus I. *Pasteurella* Trevisan 1887, 94[AL], Nom. cons. Opin. 13, Jud. Comm. 1954, 153, p. 552–557. *In* N. R. Krieg and J. G. Holt (ed.), *Bergey's Manual of Systematic Bacteriology*, vol. 1. The Williams & Wilkins Co., Baltimore, Md.
8. **Dewhirst, F. E., B. J. Paster, I. Olsen, and G. J. Fraser.** 1992. Phylogeny of 54 representative strains of species in the family *Pasteurellaceae* as determined by comparison of 16S rRNA sequences. *J. Bacteriol.* **174:**2002–2013.
9. **Escande, F., and C. Lion.** 1993. Epidemiology of human infections by *Pasteurella* and related groups in France. *Int. J. Med. Microbiol. Virol. Parasitol. Infect. Dis.* **279:** 131–139.
10. **Escande, F., E. Vallee, and F. Aubart.** 1997. *Pasteurella caballi* infection following a horse bite. *Zentralbl. Bakteriol.* **285:**440–444.
11. **Fajfar-Whetstone, C. J. T., L. Coleman, D. R. Biggs, and B. C. Fox.** 1995. *Pasteurella multocida* septicemia and subsequent *Pasteurella dagmatis* septicemia in a diabetic patient. *J. Clin. Microbiol.* **33:**202–204.
12. **Frederiksen, W.** 1993. Ecology and significance of *Pasteurellaceae* in man—an update. *Int. J. Med. Microbiol. Virol. Parasitol. Infect. Dis.* **279:**27–34.
13. **Gaillot, O., L. Guilbert, C. Maruejouls, F. Escande, and M. Simonet.** 1995. In-vitro susceptibility to thirteen antibiotics of *Pasteurella* spp. and related bacteria isolated from humans. *J. Antimicrob. Chemother.* **36:**878–880.
14. **Ganiere, J. P., F. Escande, G. Andre, and M. Larrat.** 1993. Characterization of *Pasteurella* from gingival scrapings of dogs and cats. *Comp. Immunol. Microbiol. Infect. Dis.* **16:** 77–85.
15. **Gay, F. P.** 1935. *Agents of Disease and Host Resistance.* Charles C Thomas, Baltimore, Md.
16. **Grehn, M., and F. Müller.** 1989. The oxidase reaction of *Pasteurella multocida* strains cultured on Mueller-Hinton medium. *J. Microbiol. Methods* **9:**333–336.
17. **Grehn, M., F. Müller, and R. Hugelshofer.** 1991. The API ZYM system as a tool for typing of *Pasteurella multocida* strains from humans. *J. Microbiol. Methods* **13:**201–206.
18. **Holmes, B.** 1998. *Actinobacillus, Pasteurella* and *Eikenella*, p. 1191–1215. *In* A. Balows and B. I. Duerden (ed.), *Topley & Wilson's Microbiology and Microbial Infections*, 9th ed., vol. 2. Edward Arnold, London, England.
19. **Holmes, B., M. J. Pickett, and D. G. Hollis.** 1995. Unusual gram-negative bacteria, including *Capnocytophaga, Eikenella, Pasteurella*, and *Streptobacillus*, p. 499–508. *In* P. R. Murray, E. J. Baron, M. A. Pfaller, F. C. Tenover, and R. H. Yolken (ed.), *Manual of Clinical Microbiology*, 6th ed. American Society for Microbiology, Washington, D.C.
20. **Holst, E., J. Rollof, L. Larsson, and J. P. Nielsen.** 1992. Characterization and distribution of *Pasteurella* species recovered from infected humans. *J. Clin. Microbiol.* **30:** 2984–2987.
21. **Kilian, M., and W. Frederiksen.** 1981. Identification tables for the *Haemophilus-Pasteurella-Actinobacillus* group, p. 281–290. *In* M. Kilian, W. Frederiksen, and E. L. Biberstein (ed.), Haemophilus, Pasteurella *and* Actinobacillus. Academic Press, Inc. (London), Ltd., London, England.
22. **Lester, A., P. Gerner-Smidt, B. Gahrn-Hansen, P. Sogaard, J. Schmidt, and W. Frederiksen.** 1993. Phenotypical characters and ribotyping of *Pasteurella aerogenes* from different sources. *Int. J. Med. Microbiol. Virol. Parasitol. Infect. Dis.* **279:**75–82.
23. **Lichtensteiger, C. A., S. M. Steenbergen, R. M. Lee, D. D. Polson, and E. R. Vimr.** 1996. Direct PCR analysis for toxigenic *Pasteurella multocida*. *J. Clin. Microbiol.* **34:** 3035–3039.
24. **Lion, C., M. C. Conroy, M. L. Dupuy, and F. Escande.** 1995. *Pasteurella* "SP" group infection after a guinea pig bite. *Lancet* **346:**901–902.
25. **McFarland, J. W., C. M. Berger, S. A. Froshauer, S. F. Hayashi, S. J. Hecker, B. H. Jaynes, M. R. Jefson, B. J. Kamicker, C. A. Lapinski, K. M. Lundy, et al.** 1997. Quantitative structure-activity relationships among macrolide antibacterial agents: in vitro and in vivo potency against *Pasteurella multocida*. *J. Med. Chem.* **40:** 1340–1346.
26. **Mutters, R., P. Ihm, S. Pohl, W. Frederiksen, and W. Mannheim.** 1985. Reclassification of the genus *Pasteurella* Trevisan 1887 on the basis of deoxyribonucleic acid homology, with proposals for the new species *Pasteurella dagmatis, Pasteurella canis, Pasteurella stomatis, Pasteurella anatis*, and *Pasteurella langaa*. *Int. J. Syst. Bacteriol.* **35:**309–322.
27. **Nielsen, J. P., and V. T. Rosdahl.** 1990. Development and epidemiological applications of a bacteriophage typing system for typing *Pasteurella multocida*. *J. Clin. Microbiol.* **28:**103–107.
28. **Pouëdras, P., P. Y. Donnio, Y. Le Tulzo, and J. L. Avril.** 1993. *Pasteurella stomatis* infection following a dog bite. *Eur. J. Clin. Microbiol. Infect. Dis.* **12:**65.
29. **Schlater, L. K., D. J. Brenner, A. G. Steigerwalt, C. W. Moss, M. A. Lambert, and R. A. Packer.** 1989. *Pasteurella caballi*, a new species from equine clinical specimens. *J. Clin. Microbiol.* **27:**2169–2174.
30. **Schuur, P. M., A. J. Haring, A. van Belkum, J. M. Draaisma, and A. G. Buiting.** 1997. Use of random amplification of polymorphic DNA in a case of *Pasteurella multocida* meningitis that occurred following a cat scratch on the head. *Clin. Infect. Dis.* **24:**1004–1006.
31. **Sneath, P. H. A., and M. Stevens.** 1985. A numerical taxonomic study of *Actinobacillus, Pasteurella* and *Yersinia*. *J. Gen. Microbiol.* **131:**2711–2738.
32. **Sneath, P. H. A., and M. Stevens.** 1990. *Actinobacillus rossii* sp. nov., *Actinobacillus seminis* sp. nov., nom. rev., *Pasteurella bettii* sp. nov., *Pasteurella lymphangitidis* sp. nov.,

Pasteurella mairi sp. nov., and *Pasteurella trehalosi* sp. nov. *Int. J. Syst. Bacteriol.* **40:**148–153.

33. **Sorbello, A. F., J. O'Donnell, J. Kaiser-Smith, J. Fitzharris, J. Shinkarow, and S. Doneson.** 1994. Infective endocarditis due to *Pasteurella dagmatis*: case report and review. *Clin. Infect. Dis.* **18:**336–338.
34. **Vassort-Bruneau, C., M. C. Lesage-Descauses, J.-L. Martel, J.-P. Lafont, and E. Chaslu-Dancla.** 1996. CAT III chloramphenicol resistance in *Pasteurella haemolytica* and *Pasteurella multocida* isolated from calves. *J. Antimicrob. Chemother.* **38:**205–213.
35. **Wang, R.-F., W. Campbell, W.-W. Cao, C. Summage, R. S. Steele, and C. E. Cerniglia.** 1996. Detection of *Pasteurella pneumotropica* in laboratory mice and rats by polymerase chain reaction. *Lab. Anim. Sci.* **46:**81–85.
36. **Weaver, R. E., D. G. Hollis, and E. J. Bottone.** 1985. Gram-negative fermentative bacteria and *Francisella tularensis*, p. 309–329. *In* E. H. Lennette, A. Balows, W. J. Hausler, Jr., and H. J. Shadomy (ed.), *Manual of Clinical Microbiology*, 4th ed. American Society for Microbiology, Washington, D.C.
37. **Weyant, R. S., C. Wayne Moss, R. E. Weaver, D. G. Hollis, J. G. Jordan, E. C. Cook, and M. I. Daneshvar.** 1995. *Identification of Unusual Pathogenic Gram-negative Aerobic and Facultatively Anaerobic Bacteria.* The Williams & Wilkins Co., Baltimore, Md.
38. **Wilson, M. A., R. M. Duncan, G. E. Nordholm, and B. M. Berlowski.** 1995. *Pasteurella multocida* isolated from wild birds of North America: a serotype and DNA fingerprint study of isolates from 1978 to 1993. *Avian Dis.* **39:**587–593.
39. **Wilson, M. A., M. J. Morgan, and G. E. Barger.** 1993. Comparison of DNA fingerprinting and serotyping for identification of avian *Pasteurella multocida* isolates. *J. Clin. Microbiol.* **31:**255–259.
40. **Yaneza, A. L., H. Jivan, P. Kumari, and M. S. Togoo.** 1991. *Pasteurella haemolytica* endocarditis. *J. Infect.* **23:**65–67.

Bartonella and *Afipia*

DAVID F. WELCH AND LEONARD N. SLATER

43

TAXONOMY

The genus *Bartonella* is named for A. L. Barton, who described the intraerythrocytic bacterium *Bartonella bacilliformis* in 1909. The genus *Afipia* is named for the Armed Forces Institute of Pathology, Washington, D.C., where *Afipia felis* was first described as an agent of cat scratch disease. *Bartonella* and *Afipia* are members of the α_2 subgroup of the *Proteobacteria* (32). The species formerly within *Rochalimaea* and *Grahamella* are now included in the genus *Bartonella* (4, 6), and in addition there is a newly recognized species (*B. clarridgeiae*) (10) and subspecies of *B. vinsonni* (subsp. *berkhoffii*) (26). Closely related genera, on the basis of 16S rRNA similarity, are *Brucella* and *Agrobacterium*, while members of the family *Rickettsiaceae* are more distantly related (6). All of the species classified within the genera *Bartonella* and *Afipia* have been genotypically analyzed by 16S rRNA sequencing and by DNA hybridization and found to satisfy currently accepted taxonomic guidelines.

DESCRIPTION OF THE GENERA

Bartonella spp. are small (0.6- by 1.0-μm) gram-negative rods that are often slightly curved. They are oxidase negative, aerobic, and highly fastidious. They do not produce acid from carbohydrates. All members of the genus can be cultured on enriched (blood-containing) bacteriologic culture medium in the presence of air or 5% CO_2. For the species documented to be commonly pathogenic for humans, the optimal growth temperature varies from 25–30°C (*B. bacilliformis*) to 35–37°C (*B. henselae*, *B. quintana*, and *B. elizabethae*). *B. clarridgeiae*, *B. vinsonii*, and *B. vinsonii* subsp. *berkhoffii* are potentially pathogenic, and they are variable with respect to optimal growth temperatures. The species derived from the genus *Grahamella* (*B. talpae*, *B. peromysci*, *B. grahamii*, *B. taylorii*, and *B. doshiae*) are found in erythrocytes of small rodents, birds, fish, and other animals; since they have not been documented as human pathogens, they are discussed no further in this chapter. Some members of the genus are motile. *B. bacilliformis* and *B. clarridgeiae* have flagella. Electron microscopy of *B. henselae* and *B. quintana* does not reveal flagella, but these organisms typically display twitching motility in wet mounts due to the presence of pili. The pili are also associated with marked cytoadherence and may mediate specific interaction with host endothelial cells and erythrocytes, leading to intracellular localization.

The genus *Afipia* consists of *A. felis*, *A. broomeae*, *A. clevelandensis*, and three unnamed *Afipia* genospecies (5). They differ from *Bartonella* spp. in that they are urease and oxidase positive. Most *Afipia* strains produce acid from D-xylose. Their generation time is usually shorter, and they are less fastidious nutritionally than *Bartonella* spp. *A. felis* is also a facultatively intracellular pathogen.

NATURAL HABITATS

Limited to the Andes mountain region of South America, *B. bacilliformis* had received little attention outside its zone of endemicity in recent years until related bacteria of the genus formerly named *Rochalimaea* were found to be pathogens in patients with AIDS. The strictly regional occurrence of *B. bacilliformis* is due to the limited distribution of its sand fly (*Lutzomyia verrucarum*) vector. *B. quintana* is globally distributed. Outbreaks of trench fever (also known as Volhynia fever, Meuse fever, His-Werner disease, shinbone fever, shank fever, and quintan or 5-day fever) have been focal and widely separated, often associated with conditions of poor sanitation and personal hygiene which may predispose to exposure to *Pediculus humanus*, the only known vector of *B. quintana*. Nonhuman vertebrate reservoirs have not been identified for *B. bacilliformis* or *B. quintana*.

B. henselae infection is globally endemic; serologic studies indicate that infection of domestic cats is worldwide, with the prevalence of antibodies in cats being higher in warm, humid climates, where cat fleas are abundant (8, 21, 47). Rates of bacteremia in cats can vary, even between geographically close locales, but generally tend to be higher among feral animals in any given locale. *B. henselae* bacteremia has been found in healthy domestic cats which have been specifically associated with bacillary angiomatosis (BA) or typical cat scratch disease (CSD) in their human contacts. Transmission of *B. henselae* to humans has been linked to cats by numerous studies. The major arthropod vector of *B. henselae* is the cat flea, *Ctenocephalides felis* (9). Fleas appear to serve primarily as vectors for cat-to-cat transmission; their contribution to human infection is not defined. *B. clarridgeiae* is also now recognized to be an agent of feline asymptomatic infection (10, 17, 18), which, like *A. felis* infection, appears occasionally to be transmitted to humans (25). As yet, much less is known about the full geographic distribution or potential vectors of these organisms. *A. felis* is apparently not a common zoonotic agent among cats or dogs. Although dogs have been linked epidemiologically to CSD, a recent study failed to implicate them in the epidemiology of CSD (14).

CLINICAL SIGNIFICANCE

Oroya Fever and Verruga Peruana: *B. bacilliformis*

The link between Oroya fever and verruga peruana was revealed tragically in 1885 by Daniel Carrión, a medical student who had himself injected with material from a verruga and subsequently died of Oroya fever. The eponym "Carrión's disease" has since denoted the full spectrum of *B. bacilliformis* infection. After a typical incubation period of about 3 weeks, acute *B. bacilliformis* infection results in bacteremic illness (Oroya fever) with often severe extravascular hemolysis and anemia. The illness may be insidious or abrupt in onset. Fever, chills, diaphoresis, headache, and mental status changes can be severe and are often associated with a rapid and profound anemia. During this stage, there can be associated lymphadenopathy and thrombocytopenia, severe myalgias and arthralgias, and complications of tissue hypoxia such as delirium, coma, dyspnea, or angina. For survivors, convalescence is associated with a decline of fever and a disappearance of erythrocyte-associated bacteria, but there is an apparent increased susceptibility to opportunistic infection. Without antimicrobial therapy, there can be a high fatality rate among persons lacking endemic exposure. Usually within months after acute infection, but sometimes longer, the late-stage manifestation of verruga peruana may become evident. In addition to nodular skin lesions of a variety of shapes and hues, mucosal and internal lesions can occur (35). Histologically, they reveal neovascular proliferation, with bacteria being evident in the affected tissue. Such lesions may develop at one site while receding at another, persist for months to years, and eventually become fibrotic with involution. At this stage, the prognosis for these patients is good.

Bacteremic Illness, Endocarditis: Primarily *B. quintana* and *B. henselae*

Mortality due to bacteremia with *B. quintana and B. henselae*, even when persistent, is apparently uncommon. In recent years, *B. quintana* bacteremic infection (trench fever) not associated with human immunodeficiency virus (HIV) infection has been identified sporadically, mainly in homeless persons in North America and Europe (20). Trench fever is characterized by a spectrum of self-limited clinical patterns. The incubation period may span 3 to 38 days before the sudden onset of chills and fevers. In the shortest form, a single bout of fever lasts 4 to 5 days. In the more typical periodic form, there are three to five and sometimes up to eight febrile paroxysms, each lasting about 5 days. The continuous form is manifested by 2 to 6 weeks of uninterrupted fever. Afebrile infection is the least common form. The illness may be accompanied by other nonspecific symptoms.

B. quintana or *B. henselae* bacteremia in HIV-infected persons is often characterized by insidious development of malaise, body aches, fatigue, weight loss, progressively higher and longer recurring fevers, and sometimes headache. Hepatomegaly may occur, but localizing symptoms or physical findings are often lacking. By way of contrast, *B. henselae* bacteremia in persons who are not infected with HIV more often presents with abrupt onset of fever, which may persist or become relapsing. Localized symptoms or physical findings remain unusual (39, 40, 45). Aseptic meningitis, other than in association with CSD, concurrent with bacteremia has been documented at least once in an immunocompetent host (28). *B. henselae* bacteremia can evolve into long-term asymptomatic persistence. *B. elizabethae*, *B. quintana*, and *B. henselae* have also been reported to cause endocarditis, commonly "blood-culture negative." *Bartonella* spp. may well represent important pathogens in this syndrome and should be added to the list of fastidious gram-negative organisms which have been similarly implicated, i.e., the HACEK group, comprising *Haemophilus*, *Actinobacillus*, *Cardiobacterium*, *Eikenella*, and *Kingella*.

Bacillary Angiomatosis and Peliosis: *B. quintana* and *B. henselae*

BA (also referred to as epithelioid angiomatosis or bacillary epithelioid angiomatosis) is a disorder of neovascular proliferation that was originally described as involving the skin and regional lymph nodes of HIV-infected persons (11, 24, 42). It has since been demonstrated to be able to involve a variety of internal organs including the liver, spleen, bone, brain, lungs, and bowel and to occur in other immunocompromised as well as immunocompetent hosts. In bacillary peliosis, which involves the liver and/or the spleen in HIV-infected and other immunosuppressed persons, the affected tissues contain numerous blood-filled, partially endothelial cell-lined cystic structures and fibromyxoid stroma with a mixture of inflammatory cells, dilated capillaries, and clumps of bacilli identified by Warthin-Starry staining. Either species can cause cutaneous lesions, but subcutaneous and osseous lesions are more often associated with *B. quintana* and hepatosplenic lesions are associated only with *B. henselae* (23). Cutaneous lesions of BA often arise in crops, but both the temporal pattern and the morphologic characteristics can vary. These lesions can be remarkably similar in gross and microscopic appearance to the lesions of verruga peruana, but the major differential diagnoses clinically are Kaposi's sarcoma and pyogenic granuloma. The histologic distinction from vascular tumors, including the presence in BA lesions of Warthin-Starry-staining bacilli, has been clearly defined. Inflammatory reactions to *B. henselae* infection without associated BA or peliosis but involving the liver, spleen, lymph nodes, heart, and bone marrow may occur. These granulomatous reactions are characterized by nodular collections of histiocytes, lymphocytes, and aggregates of neutrophils and karyorrhexic debris suggestive of microscopic abscess formation, and they resemble the lymph node lesions of CSD (27).

Cat Scratch Disease: *B. henselae, B. clarridgeiae,* and *Afipia felis*

The various manifestations comprising CSD have been recognized over the past 100 years, but "la maladie des griffes du chat" was not defined as a syndrome until 1950 (13). CSD remained an infection in search of an agent for more than 40 years after that. Hence, most cases have been identified by clinical and pathologic criteria, supplemented by reactions to nonstandardized skin test antigens in some cases. It is reasonable to ascribe the majority of CSD cases to *B. henselae* based on the numerous lines of evidence developed in recent years. However, it remains likely that occasional CSD cases can be caused by other agents, such as has been reported with *A. felis* (1, 5) and with *B. clarridgeiae* (25). Other *Afipia* spp. have been isolated from only skeletal and/or pleuropulmonary sites of one patient each and not in the setting of CSD; their roles as pathogens remain speculative.

CSD is the most commonly recognized manifestation of human infection with *Bartonella*. In the United States, the number of CSD cases is estimated to approach 25,000 annually (19). In typical CSD (about 89% of cases), a cutaneous papule or pustule develops at the site of inoculation (usually a scratch or bite) within a week after the contact (most commonly with a kitten). Regional lymphadenopathy develops in 1 to 7 weeks. About one-third of patients have fever, and about one-sixth develop lymph node suppuration. The histopathologic findings of the nodes include a mixture of inflammatory reactions such as granulomata and stellate necrosis.

Atypical CSD (about 11%) includes Parinaud's oculoglandular syndrome (self-limited granulomatous conjunctivitis and ipsilateral, usually preauricular, lymphadenitis) and various other presentations (29), such as self-limited granulomatous hepatitis/splenitis, retinitis, and encephalitis. The importance of accurate history regarding animal exposure cannot be overemphasized when evaluating a patient with findings consistent with one of these syndromes. Fortunately, in most cases of CSD, whether typical or atypical, spontaneous resolution occurs in 2 to 4 months.

HIV-Associated Neurologic Syndromes

B. henselae and *B. quintana* have been implicated in a small proportion of cases of HIV-associated brain lesions, meningoencephalitis, encephalopathy, or neuropsychiatric disease which cannot be ascribed to other causes. Intracerebral BA was first recognized in 1990 (41). *B. henselae* has also been identified by immunofluorescent staining and PCR amplification postmortem in the brains of AIDS patients with dementia and by the presence of elevated indices of *B. henselae*-reactive antibody in cerebrospinal fluid and serum (33). At least 4% of new cases of HIV-associated dementia or neuropsychological decline are estimated to result from *Bartonella* infections and therefore to be potentially treatable with antibiotics.

COLLECTION, TRANSPORT, AND STORAGE OF SPECIMENS

The specimen used to obtain most isolates of *Bartonella* and *Afipia* spp. is blood or tissue. The approaches typically used for recovery of other pathogens from these sites are generally suitable, although the fastidious nature of these organisms requires that precautions be taken to minimize the interval from collection to processing. If specimens must be stored, they should be kept frozen. A controlled study of the effects of blood collection and handling methods has shown that blood specimens which were collected from *B. henselae*-infected cats into both EDTA and Isolator (Wampole, Cranbury, N.J.) blood lysis tubes yielded good recovery and that blood collected into tubes containing EDTA can be plated after 26 days at −65°C with no loss of sensitivity (7). *Bartonella* spp. are broadly susceptible to antimicrobial agents in vitro and so specimens should be collected before antimicrobial therapy, especially with the tetracyclines and macrolides. *B. henselae* is also inhibited by concentrations of sodium polyanethol sulfonate (SPS) that are relevant to blood culture systems. Adding agents that neutralize SPS toxicity or the use of resin-containing media (primarily to lyse erythrocytes) is another precaution that should be taken if blood is cultured in commercially designed blood culture systems. Lytic blood culture systems (e.g., Isolator) combine the protective effect of free hemoglobin against SPS toxicity with the release of intracellular organisms.

DETECTION AND ISOLATION PROCEDURES

Direct Examination

Although stained blood films have been used to detect intraerythrocytic *B. bacilliformis* in patients with Oroya fever, the level of bacteremia associated with the other species is usually too low for this technique to be practical. Other means of direct examination that may prove useful include Warthin-Starry silver staining of fixed tissue sections and detection of organisms in tissue by an immunocytochemical labeling technique (34); however, reagents for immunocytochemical labeling are not widely available. Bacilli may be demonstrable by Warthin-Starry staining during the early stages of lymphadenopathy in patients with CSD, but they are typically not found during the later, granulomatous stage of inflammation. Successful staining of organisms in tissue by the Warthin-Starry method also depends on careful attention to the details of the procedure. Critical steps include washing glassware in potassium dichromate-sulfuric acid solution, making the developer from solutions heated separately at 54 to 56°C (and maintained at this temperature after they are mixed) for 30 min, and using the developer as soon as it is mixed.

Bartonella spp. can also be detected directly by amplification of DNA from tissue, pus, or skin lesions. A gene fragment specific for either citrate synthase or a heat shock protein of *B. henselae* is demonstrable by PCR in most patients with CSD (1, 38). Amplification of rRNA with universal primers followed by direct nucleotide sequence analysis of the amplification product or hybridization with a specific probe is another, more sensitive but more laborious approach. These tests are performed by a few reference laboratories or academic centers (e.g., MRL Reference Laboratory, Cypress, Calif.).

Culture

Since most isolates require more than 7 days of incubation before they can be detected, routine bacterial culture methods usually do not allow *Bartonella* spp. to be detected. Attempts to isolate *Bartonella* spp. may be driven by the clinical picture, but throughout the spectrum of manifestations, many symptoms are not distinctive enough to guide the diagnosis and thus to inform the laboratory that special cultures are needed. If clinically directed culturing is relied upon to detect *Bartonella* spp., it is indicated in the settings of atypical CSD (cultures are not recommended for diagnosis of most cases of CSD); fever of unknown origin with history of cat exposure; fever, lymphadenitis, or encephalitis of unknown origin in the immunocompromised patient; and BA and peliosis. Culture protocols designed to yield other slowly growing organisms (for example, *Histoplasma capsulatum* or *Mycobacterium avium* complex on noninhibitory media) can also result in the recovery of *Bartonella* spp. *A. felis* and *Bartonella* spp. also have been isolated (from lymph node biopsy samples or aspirates) by using various cell lines. HeLa cell or primary cell cultures of human monocytes support the growth of *A. felis*, and *B. henselae* and *B. quintana* grow in endothelial cell cultures. In both systems, elongated pleomorphic organisms become visible in Gimenez-stained preparations 72 h after inoculation of the cell cultures. A defined cell-free medium which permits the recovery of both *Afipia* and *Bartonella* spp. has also been described (46).

Therefore, in general any method designed to recover *Bartonella* spp. would also be adequate for the recovery of *Afipia* spp. since the latter are less fastidious.

Blood

The two fundamentally different blood culture practices of direct plating and using broth-based systems can be adapted for the detection of *Bartonella* spp. Isolator-processed blood should be plated on enriched (chocolate- or blood-containing) medium incubated at 35 to 37°C under conditions of 5 to 10% CO_2 and >40% humidity. For optimal growth, the medium should be as fresh as possible. Plates can be sealed with Parafilm or Shrink Seal after the first 24 h of incubation to preserve the moisture content of the medium. These plates usually can be incubated for up to 30 days without noticeable deterioration. Considering that the length of time required for the detection of *Bartonella* spp. allows other slowly growing pathogens, including *Mycobacterium tuberculosis*, to grow on the same plates, appropriate safety precautions should be taken with positive cultures.

Alternative approaches to the use of the Isolator include the use of a broth-based or biphasic culture system. Improved growth has been obtained in brucella both supplemented with hemin (250 μg/ml) and peptic digest of blood (8% Fildes reagent), but this technique has been applied primarily to propagation rather than primary isolation (37). Similarly, isolates can be propagated on buffered charcoal yeast extract medium, but this is not recommended for primary isolation of *Bartonella* spp. whereas it may be a practical approach for the recovery of *Afipia* spp. *B. henselae* has been isolated in the biphasic Septi-Chek system (Roche Diagnostics, Nutley, N.J.) after prolonged incubation (more than 40 days). Evidence of growth, if any, in the broth phase is provided by the presence of a pellicle or adherent film on the glass surface. Biphasic media reportedly serve to isolate *A. felis* (16), but experience to date is so limited that methods of choice, with the possible exception of the tissue culture protocol of Birkness et al. (3), cannot be stated with certainty.

Bartonella spp. usually grow best on solid or semisolid media. In broth, they often do not produce turbidity or convert enough oxidizable substrate to CO_2 for CO_2 detection-based blood culture systems to indicate growth. However, several isolates have been initially detected by using BACTEC and resin-containing media combined with acridine orange staining at the termination of a 7-day incubation period, with recovery subsequently being achieved by subculture to solid media. The optimal treatment of blood for recovery of *Bartonella* spp. probably involves the use of the Isolator in conjunction with freshly prepared rabbit heart infusion agar plates.

Tissue

B. henselae and *B. quintana* have been isolated from the liver, spleen, lymph nodes, and skin after homogenization either by direct plating or by cocultivation with an endothelial cell line (22). Although the cocultivation method may be more successful in recovering organisms from specimens such as tissue, it is not practical for most microbiology laboratories. Freshly prepared heart infusion agar containing 5 or 10% defibrinated rabbit or horse blood supports better growth of most strains than do other media such as chocolate or 5% sheep blood, although the last two have been used successfully. Other necessary conditions include a humid atmosphere and incubation for 3 to 4 weeks at 35 to 37°C. *B. bacilliformis* and *Afipia* spp. have a lower (25 to 30°C) optimal temperature for growth. Selective culture techniques have not been developed, and so recovery of isolates from certain specimens such as skin may be impossible if indigenous or contaminating organisms are present. The medium (modified RPMI 1640) described by Wong et al. (46) may also be useful for the recovery of *B. henselae* from both tissue and blood.

IDENTIFICATION

Bartonella spp.

Morphology

Colonies of *Bartonella* spp. are of two morphologic types: (i) irregular, raised, whitish, rough ("cauliflower" or "molar tooth" or "verrucous"), and dry in appearance or (ii) smaller, circular, tan, and moist in appearance, tending to pit and adhere to the agar. Both types are usually present in the same culture (Fig. 1). The degree of colony heterogeneity varies by species and by strain, with *B. henselae* typically being characterized by a greater proportion of rough colonies than *B. quintana*, which may even appear as uniformly smooth in primary cultures. Repeated subcultures of *B. henselae* tend to have increasing proportions of smooth colonies. Cultures of *B. henselae* on blood agar produce an odor similar to the caramel odor (diacetyl) produced by *Streptococcus milleri*. The Gram stain of a colony reveals small, gram-negative, slightly curved rods resembling *Campylobacter*, *Helicobacter*, or *Haemophilus*. Cells, especially of *B. henselae*, are very autoadherent, as can be demonstrated by attempting to scrape the colonies off of a culture plate with a loop. In a wet mount, there is twitching motility of cells. These features, plus a lengthy (>7-day) incubation before the appearance of colonies and negative catalase and oxidase reactions, are sufficient for presumptive identification of *B. henselae* or *B. quintana*. Additional methods may be used to confirm the identity of isolates, or isolates may be referred to a laboratory experienced with *Bartonella* spp. for confirmatory identification. Although not widely available, a reliable means of identification is immunofluorescence with antisera monospecific for each of these two species. Characterization with conventional tests produces results that identify the *Bartonella* spp. and distinguish them from *A. felis* (Table 1).

Motility

The isolates most likely to be encountered, i.e., *B. henselae* or *B. quintana*, do not possess flagella but do produce a twitching motion when suspended in saline and examined microscopically under a coverslip. This motility is presumably related to adherence, with both features being mediated by fine fimbriae (pili) that are visible in negatively stained preparations under the electron microscope.

Cellular Fatty Acid Composition

Determination of the cellular fatty acid composition by gas-liquid chromatography is outlined in chapter 11. Fatty acid methyl esters are prepared from cells harvested after 7 days of incubation at 35°C in 5% CO_2 on plates containing 5% rabbit blood heart infusion agar. This approach is useful for identifying and distinguishing *Bartonella* spp., since they have relatively simple gas-liquid chromatography profiles consisting mainly of $C_{18:1}$, $C_{18:0}$, and $C_{16:0}$ acids. *B. elizabethae* contains a larger amount of $C_{17:0}$ than do the other species. An unusual branched-chain fatty acid (11-methyloctadec-12-enoic acid) is found in *Afipia* spp. (5) but not in *Bartonella* spp.

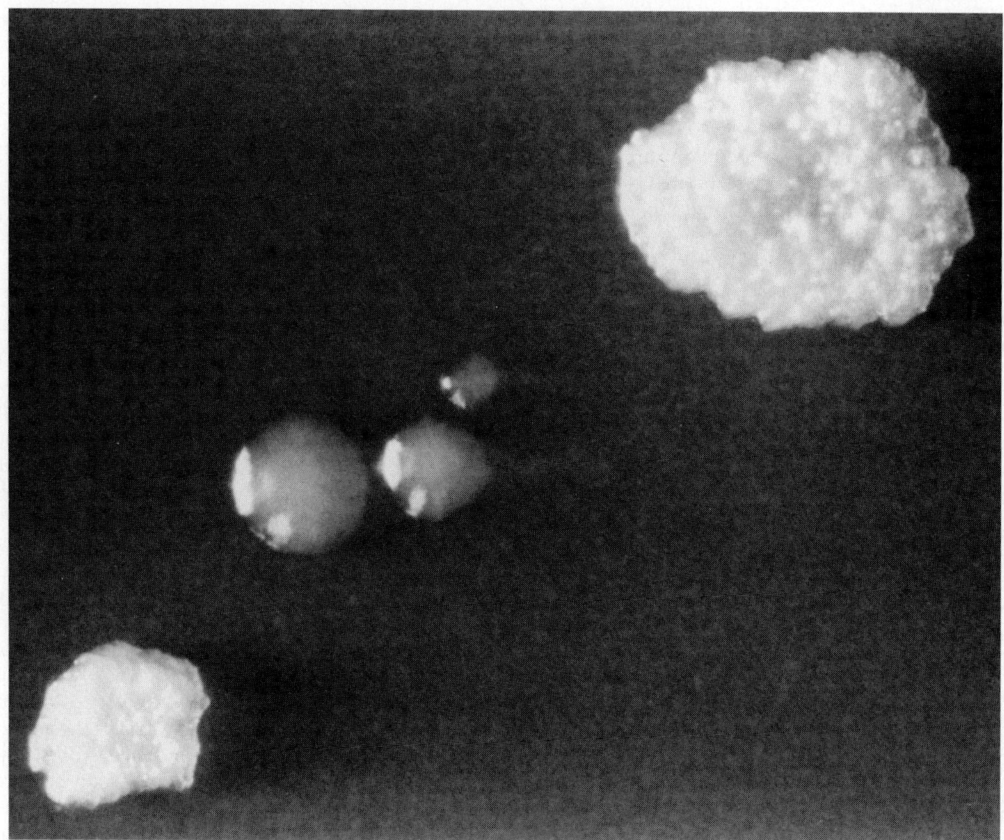

FIGURE 1 *B. henselae* after 7 days of incubation, showing heterogeneity of colonies. Magnification, ×40.

TABLE 1 Differential characteristics of commonly pathogenic *Bartonella* species and *A. felis*[a]

Characteristic	*B. bacilliformis*	*B. quintana*	*B. henselae*	*B. elizabethae*	*B. clarridgeiae*	*A. felis*
Gram reaction	–	–	–	–	–	–
Catalase	+	–	±	–	–	–
Oxidase	–	±	–	–	–	+
Nitrate reduction	–	–	–	–	–	+
Indole	–	–	–	–	–	–
Urease	–	–	–	–	–	+
Acid from carbohydrates[b]	–	–	–	–	–	–
Optimal growth temp (°C)	25–30	35–37	35–37	35–37	35–37	25–30
Growth in nutrient broth	–	–	–	–	–	+
Hemolysis	–	–	–	–	–	–
Flagella	+	–[c]	–[c]	–	+	+
Cellular fatty acids constituting >90% of total	$C_{18:1\omega7C}$, $C_{16:0}$, $C_{16:1\omega7C}$	$C_{18:1\omega7C}$, $C_{16:0}$, $C_{18:0}$	$C_{18:1\omega7C}$, $C_{18:0}$, $C_{16:0}$	$C_{18:1\omega7C}$, $C_{17:0}$, $C_{16:0}$	$C_{18:1\omega7C}$, $C_{18:0}$, $C_{16:0}$	$C_{18:1\omega7C}$, $C_{BR19:1}$, $C_{19:0cyc}$

[a] +, positive reaction; –, negative reaction; ±, negative or weakly positive.
[b] Glucose, lactose, maltose, mannitol, and sucrose.
[c] May demonstrate twitching motility in wet mounts.

Identification Kits

Although none of the various commercially available identification systems contain *Bartonella* spp. in their databases, the RapID ANA II, Rapid ID 32 A, and MicroScan rapid anaerobe systems have been used as aids to identification. With the MicroScan rapid anaerobe panel and careful adjustment of inoculum size, it is possible to distinguish *B. henselae* and *B. quintana* on the basis of biotype codes derived from the reactions in this panel (44). If the inoculum size used in performing the MicroScan tests is equivalent to a McFarland no. 3 standard, the biotype codes usually obtained are 10077640 (*B. henselae*), 10073640 (*B. quintana*), and 10077240 (*B. bacilliformis*). Difficulty in separating *B. quintana* from *B. henselae* is encountered when heavier inocula are used in these panels. In other systems, the biochemical reactivity of *B. quintana* and *B. henselae* has been enhanced by the addition of hemin to test media (15).

Afipia Species

Afipia spp. can be identified on the basis of conventional phenotypic tests. Due to weaker growth at 35 than 30°C, incubations should be carried out at the latter temperature. Colonies develop by 72 h on blood agar or on buffered charcoal yeast extract agar. They are greyish white, glistening, convex, and opaque. Delayed, weak growth of *A. clevelandensis* may occur on MacConkey agar. Biochemical characteristics useful in differentiation among the *Afipia* and *Bartonella* spp. are shown in Table 1.

Strain Identification

A PCR-based restriction fragment length polymorphism method has been applied by Matar et al. (30) to subtyping of isolates. Genomic DNA making up the spacer region between the 16S and 23S rRNA genes plus a portion of the 23S rRNA gene are amplified and then subjected to restriction endonuclease analysis. Different patterns are seen among the *Bartonella* spp., and at least seven subtypes within *B. henselae* have been determined, but no studies to date have made any epidemiologic correlations. Variants of *B. henselae* have also been found among bacteremic isolates from cats by using enterobacterial repetitive intergenic consensus PCR and sodium dodecyl sulfate-polyacrylamide gel electrophoresis (36). This genomic fingerprinting technique of the *B. henselae* isolates yielded two different patterns based on three distinct bands.

SEROLOGIC TESTS

Serologic testing is becoming a mainstay of diagnosis, particularly for the part of the clinical spectrum of diseases occupied by CSD and central nervous system infection. Since culturing of *Bartonella* spp. is difficult and time-consuming, these alternative means of identifying the infectious agents are important. However, serologic cross-reactions, most notably with *Coxiella burnetii* and *Chlamydia* spp., can occur. Human antibody responses to *Bartonella* species have been measured by a variety of techniques. The tests are performed commercially by most reference laboratories, and kits are available in Europe but not in the United States.

B. bacilliformis

Enzyme immunoassay (EIA) is the most sensitive test for detecting immunoglobulin G (IgG) antibodies among persons from regions of endemic infection. IgM antibodies can be detected by immunofluorescence in persons with active Oroya fever as well as in some persons without blood smear evidence of acute bacteremic infection.

B. quintana and *B. henselae*

EIA and radioimmunoprecipitation have proven to be comparable, and both are superior to hemagglutination or immunofluorescence assays in sensitivity. When the same EIA was used, all the patients in a small series of patients with acute primary or relapsed trench fever had measurable, although often low, levels of anti-*B. quintana* antibodies. Human antibody responses often have been substantially cross-reactive between *B. quintana* and *B. henselae* in tests in which whole organisms were used as the antigen. The differential magnitude of antibody reactions to either species in EIAs with component antigens may allow an inference about which species may be responsible for a particular infection. This would be especially important when the species cause overlapping syndromes such as fever with bacteremia or BA but is less important in CSD, where *B. quintana* is not implicated. The tests for *B. henselae* reported to date have undergone different degrees of scrutiny and corroboration, but most appear to have high sensitivity (85 to 90%) and specificity (>95%) (1, 38, 43). Persons with CSD develop IgM antibodies that can be measured early in the course of disease and IgG antibodies whose levels rise somewhat later and then decline over time. In general, the results of the immunofluorescence test and EIA for *B. henselae* antibodies have demonstrated reasonable correlation with each other and with the results of CSD skin testing. Since the skin test antigen for CSD is not commercially available or standardized and since it carries the potential risk of transmitting infection, serologic testing should replace skin testing in the diagnosis of CSD.

Afipia felis

The indirect fluorescent-antibody test and EIA for antibodies to *B. henselae* and *B. quintana*, both of which use bacterial whole-cell antigens, have been compared with one another, with an EIA for antibodies to *A. felis*, and with the findings of CSD antigen skin testing in evaluating patients with a clinical diagnosis of CSD (12, 43). Sera from CSD patients had no higher levels of antibodies to *A. felis* than did normal control sera, while most CSD patients had evidence of elevated anti-*Bartonella* antibodies by IFA and of anti-*Bartonella* IgM by EIA compared with controls. Therefore, there would appear to be limited, if any, roles for serologic testing to diagnose *Afipia* infections.

ANTIMICROBIAL SUSCEPTIBILITY

Antimicrobial susceptibility testing can be performed by incorporation of antimicrobial agents into either blood or chocolate agar or into *Haemophilus* test medium by using a broth microdilution technique. Testing of isolates is problematic for strains displaying the most fastidious growth characteristics. The E test (AB Biodisk, Solna, Sweden) can also be used to assess susceptibility. Generally, isolates of *Bartonella* spp. are susceptible in vitro to most antibacterial agents tested, including β-lactams, tetracyclines, macrolides, aminoglycosides, fluoroquinolones, vancomycin, rifampin, chloramphenicol, and trimethoprim-sulfamethoxazole but resistant to nalidixic acid. In vitro resistance to penicillin and ampicillin, tetracycline, or vancomycin has been noted. *B. quintana* is similar in its in vitro susceptibility pattern except for resistance to aminoglycosides. Moreover, the in vitro susceptibility of *B. henselae* and *B. quintana* does not predict the in vivo response to therapy. BA can develop and organisms can be recovered in the face of therapy with trimethoprim-sulfamethoxazole, β-lactam antibiotics, and fluoroquinolone antibiotics (23, 24). In contrast, therapy with rifampin, tetracyclines, or macrolides dramatically reduces culture recovery from BA and peliosis lesions and macrolide administration appears to protect against BA. The routine use of rifabutin, clarithromycin, and azithromycin for the prevention of *Mycobacterium avium* complex infections in persons with advanced HIV disease will probably also reduce the incidence of *Bartonella* infections in that population. There have been anecdotal reports of the utility of various agents in the treatment of CSD. However, only azithromycin has been demonstrated to accelerate the resolution of the lymphadenopathy of typical CSD in a placebo-controlled double-blinded study (2). Although the value of antibiotic therapy of CSD remains subject to debate, azithromycin should be considered the agent of choice if antimicrobial administration is contemplated. For BA and peliosis, bacteremia, endocarditis, and other manifestations of either *B. quintana* or *B. henselae* infection, erythromycin or doxycycline are the agents of choice based on their efficacy, low cost, and ease of administration. Despite in vitro findings suggesting likely susceptibility, treatment with a variety of β-lactams appears largely ineffective. Responses to trimethoprim-sulfamethoxazole and fluoroquinolones in other manifestations of *Bartonella* infections have been inconsistent. The standard treatment for *B. bacilliformis* infection is oral chloramphenicol.

Afipia spp. are more resistant than *Bartonella* spp. In axenic medium, *A. felis* displays susceptibility to imipenem, aminoglycosides, and rifampin by either the broth or the agar dilution technique. When grown in HeLa cells, *A. felis* is susceptible to amikacin and tobramycin but appears resistant to other compounds (31). It is generally nonsusceptible to penicillins, cephalosporins, and quinolones. Documented cases of infection due to *Afipia* are too few to draw conclusions about in vivo correlation.

EVALUATION, INTERPRETATION, AND REPORTING OF RESULTS

Serologic data provide the most cost-effective diagnosis of typical CSD. The sensitivity of serologic testing is 85 to 90% based on IgG detection and probably higher if IgM testing is included. The specificity of serologic testing is around 95% according to screening in other populations presumed to be uninfected and for other diseases. An optimized PCR assay would be expected to approach 100% sensitivity. Atypical CSD and other manifestations of *Bartonella* infection are usually best approached by serologic testing combined with culture or PCR. Serologic testing with antigens more specific than whole-cell antigens may also play a role in corroborating these entities. PCR amplification may enable the identification of *B. henselae* in clinical material such as cerebrospinal fluid or brain tissue in the absence of positive cultures. While the value of culturing for *Bartonella* spp. is limited in certain cases by practicality issues of fresh-medium availability, length of incubation, and unknown efficiency, the use of cultures in conjunction with serologic testing is justified in selected cases. In addition to blood, *B. henselae* and *B. quintana* have been cultured from a variety of tissue sources, albeit infrequently.

REFERENCES

1. **Avidor, B., Y. Kletter, S. Abulafia, Y. Golan, M. Ephros, and M. Giladi.** 1997. Molecular diagnosis of cat scratch disease: a two-step approach. *J. Clin. Microbiol.* **35:** 1924–1930.
2. **Bass, J. W., B. C. Freitas, A. D. Freitas, C. L. Sisler, D. S. Chan, J. M. Vincent, D. A. Person, J. R. Claybaugh, R. R. Wittler, M. E. Weisse, R. L. Regnery, and L. N. Slater.** 1998. Prospective randomized double-blind placebo-controlled evaluation of azithromycin for treatment of cat scratch disease. *Pediatr. Infect. Dis. J.* **17:**447–452.
3. **Birkness, K. A., V. G. George, E. H. White, D. S. Stephens, and F. D. Quinn.** 1992. Intracellular growth of *Afipia felis*, a putative etiologic agent of cat scratch disease. *Infect. Immun.* **60:**2280–2287.
4. **Birtles, R. J., T. G. Harrison, N. A. Saunders, and D. H. Molyneux.** 1995. Proposals to unify the genera *Grahamella* and *Bartonella*, with descriptions of *Bartonella talpae* comb. nov., *Bartonella peromysci* sp. nov., *Bartonella taylorii* sp. nov., and *Bartonella doshiae* sp. nov. *Int. J. Syst. Bacteriol.* **45:**1–8.
5. **Brenner, D. J., D. G. Hollis, C. W. Moss, C. K. English, G. S. Hall, V. Judy, J. Radosevic, K. A. Birkness, W. F. Bibb, F. D. Quinn, B. Swaminathan, R. E. Weaver, M. W. Reeves, S. P. O'Connor, P. S. Hayes, F. C. Tenover, A. G. Steigerwalt, B. A. Perkins, M. I. Daneshvar, B. C. Hill, J. A. Washington, T. C. Woods, S. B. Hunter, T. L. Hadfield, G. W. Ajelio, A. F. Kaufman, D. J. Wear, and J. D. Wenger.** 1991. Proposal of *Afipia* gen. nov., with *Afipia felis* sp. nov. (formerly the cat scratch disease bacillus), *Afipia clevelandensis* sp. nov. (formerly the Cleveland Clinic Foundation strain), *Afipia broomeae* sp. nov., and three unnamed genospecies. *J. Clin. Microbiol.* **29:** 2450–2460.
6. **Brenner, D. J., S. P. O'Connor, H. H. Winkler, and A. G. Steigerwalt.** 1993. Proposals to unify the genera *Bartonella* and *Rochalimaea*, with descriptions of *Bartonella quintana* comb. nov., *Bartonella vinsonii* comb. nov., *Bartonella henselae* comb. nov., and *Bartonella elizabethae* comb. nov., and to remove the family *Bartonellaceae* from the order *Rickettsiales*. *Int. J. Syst. Bacteriol.* **43:**777–786.
7. **Brenner, S. A., J. A. Rooney, P. Manzewitsch, and R. L. Regnery.** 1997. Isolation of *Bartonella (Rochalimaea) henselae*—effects of methods of blood collection and handling. *J. Clin. Microbiol.* **35:**544–547.
8. **Chomel, B. B., R. C. Abbott, R. W. Kasten, K. A. Floyd-Hawkins, P. H. Kass, C. A. Glaser, N. Pedersen, and J. E. Koehler.** 1995. *Bartonella henselae* prevalence in domestic cats in California: risk factors and association between bacteremia and antibody titers. *J. Clin. Microbiol.* **33:** 2445–2450.
9. **Chomel, B. B., R. W. Kasten, K. Floyd-Hawkins, B. Chi, K. Yamamoto, J. Roberts-Wilson, A. N. Gurfield, R. C. Abbott, N. Pederson, and J. E. Koehler.** 1996. Experimental transmission of *Bartonella henselae* by the cat flea. *J. Clin. Microbiol.* **34:**1952–1956.
10. **Clarridge, J. E., III, T. J. Raich, D. Pirwani, B. Simon, L. Tsai, M. C. Rodriguez-Barradas, R. Regnery, A. Zollo, D. C. Jones, and C. Rambo.** 1995. Strategy to detect and identify *Bartonella* species in a routine clinical laboratory yields *Bartonella henselae* from human immunodeficiency virus-infected patient and a unique *Bartonella* strain from his cat. *J. Clin. Microbiol.* **33:**2107–2113.
11. **Cockerell, C. J., G. F. Webster, M. A. Whitlow, and A. E. Friedman-Kien.** 1987. Epithelioid angiomatosis: a distinct vascular disorder in patients with the acquired immunodeficiency syndrome or AIDS-related complex. *Lancet* **ii:**6544–6546.
12. **Dalton, M. J., L. E. Robinson, J. Cooper, R. L. Regnery, J. G. Olson, and J. E. Childs.** 1995. Use of *Bartonella* antigens for the serologic diagnosis of cat-scratch disease

at a national referral center. *Arch. Intern. Med.* **155:** 1670–1676.

13. **Debré, R., M. Lamy, M. L. Jammet, L. Costil, and P. Mozziconacci.** 1950. La maladie des griffes de chat. *Semin. Hop. Paris.* **26:**1895–1904.
14. **Demers, D. M., J. W. Bass, J. M. Vincent, D. A. Person, D. K. Noyes, C. M. Staege, C. P. Samlaska, N. H. Lockwood, R. L. Regnery, and B. E. Anderson.** 1995. Cat-scratch disease in Hawaii: etiology and seroepidemiology. *J. Pediatr.* **127:**23–26.
15. **Drancourt, M., and D. Raoult.** 1993. Proposed tests for the routine identification of *Rochalimaea* species. *Eur. J. Clin. Microbiol.* **4:**112–114.
16. **English, C. K., D. J. Wear, A. M. Margileth, C. R. Lissner, and G. P. Walsh.** 1988. Cat-scratch disease. Isolation and culture of the bacterial agent. *JAMA* **269:**1347–1354.
17. **Gurfield, A. N., H.-J. Boulouis, B. B. Chomel, R. Heller, R. W. Kasten, K. Yamamoto, and Y. Piemont.** 1997. Coinfection with *Bartonelle clarridgeiae* and *Bartonella henselae* and with different *Bartonella henselae* strains in domestic cats. *J. Clin. Microbiol.* **35:**2120–2123.
18. **Heller, R., M. Artois, V. Xemar, D. De Briel, H. Gehin, B. Jaulhac, H. Monteil, and Y. Piemont.** 1997. Prevalence of *Bartonella henselae* and *Bartonella clarridgeiae* in stray cats. *J. Clin. Microbiol.* **35:**1327–1331.
19. **Jackson, L. A., B. A. Perkins, and J. D. Wenger.** 1993. Cat scratch disease in the United States: an analysis of three national databases. *Am. J. Public Health* **83:** 1707–1711.
20. **Jackson, L. A., and D. H. Spach.** 1996. Emergence of *Bartonella quintana* infection among homeless persons. *Emerging Infect. Dis.* **2:**141–144.
21. **Jameson, P., C. Greene, R. Regnery, M. Dryden, A. Marks, J. Brown, J. Cooper, B. Glaus, and R. Greene.** 1995. Prevalence of *Bartonella henselae* antibodies in pet cats throughout regions of North America. *J. Infect. Dis.* **172:**1145–1149.
22. **Koehler, J. E., F. D. Quinn, T. G. Berger, P. E. LeBoit, and J. W. Tappero.** 1992. Isolation of *Rochalimaea* species from cutaneous osseous lesions of bacillary angiomatosis. *N. Engl. J. Med.* **327:**1625–1632.
23. **Koehler, J. E., M. A. Sanchez, C. S. Garrido, M. J. Whitfield, F. M. Chen, T. G. Berger, M. C. Rodriguez-Barradas, P. E. LeBoit, and J. W. Tappero.** 1997. Molecular epidemiology of *Bartonella* infections in patients with bacillary angiomatosis-peliosis. *N. Engl. J. Med.* **337:** 1876–1883.
24. **Koehler, J. E., and J. W. Tappero.** 1993. Bacillary angiomatosis and bacillary peliosis in patients infected with human immunodeficiency virus. *Clin. Infect. Dis.* **17:** 612–624.
25. **Kordick, D. L., E. J. Hilyard, T. L. Hadfield, K. H. Wilson, A. G. Steigerwalt, D. J. Brenner, and E. B. Breitschwerdt.** 1997. *Bartonella clarridgeiae*, a newly recognized zoonotic pathogen causing inoculation papules, fever and lymphadenopathy (cat scratch disease). *J. Clin. Microbiol.* **35:**1813–1818.
26. **Kordick, D. L., B. Swaminathan, C. E. Greene, K. H. Wilson, A. M. Whitney, O. C. Steve, D. G. Hollis, G. M. Matar, A. G. Steigerwalt, G. B. Malcolm, P. S. Hayes, T. L. Hadfield, E. B. Breitschwerdt, and D. J. Brenner.** 1996. *Bartonella vinsonii* subsp. *berkhoffii* subsp. nov., isolated from dogs; *Bartonella vinsonii* subsp. *vinsonii*; and emended description of *Bartonella vinsonii*. *Int. J. Syst. Bacteriol.* **46:**704–709.
27. **Liston, T. E., and J. E. Koehler.** 1996. Granulatomous hepatitis and necrotizing splenitis due to *Bartonella henselae* in a patient with cancer: case report and review of hepatosplenic manifestations of *Bartonella* infection. *Clin. Infect. Dis.* **22:**951–957.
28. **Lucey, D., M. J. Dolan, C. W. Moss, M. Garcia, D. G. Hollis, S. Wegner, G. Morgan, R. Almeida, D. Leong, K. S. Greisen, D. F. Welch, and L. N. Slater.** 1992. Relapsing illness due to *Rochalimaea henselae* in normal hosts: implication for therapy and new epidemiologic associations. *Clin. Infect. Dis.* **14:**683–688.
29. **Margileth, A. M., D. J. Wear, and C. K. English.** 1987. Systemic cat scratch disease: report of 23 patients with prolonged or recurrent severe bacterial infection. *J. Infect. Dis.* **155:**390–402.
30. **Matar, G. M., B. Swaminathan, S. B. Hunter, L. N. Slater, and D. F. Welch.** 1993. Polymerase chain reaction-based restriction fragment length polymorphism analysis of a fragment of the ribosomal operon from *Rochalimaea* species for subtyping. *J. Clin. Microbiol.* **31:** 1730–1734.
31. **Maurin M., H. Lepocher, D. Mallet, and D. Raoult.** 1993. Antibiotic susceptibilities of *Afipia felis* in axenic medium and in cells. *Antimicrob. Agents Chemother.* **37:**1410–1413.
32. **O'Connor, S. P., M. Dorsch, A. G. Steigerwalt, D. J. Brenner, and E. Stackebrandt.** 1991. 16S rRNA sequences of *Bartonella bacilliformis* and cat scratch disease bacillus reveal phylogenetic relationships with the alpha-2 subgroup of the class *Proteobacteria*. *J. Clin. Microbiol.* **29:** 2144–2150.
33. **Patnaik, M., W. A. Schwartzman, and J. B. Peter.** 1995. *Bartonella henselae*: detection in brain tissue of patients with AIDS-associated neurological disease. *J. Invest. Med.* **43:** 368A.
34. **Reed, J., D. J. Brigati, S. D. Flynn, N. S. McNutt, K. W. Min, D. F. Welch, and L. N. Slater.** 1992. Immunocytochemical identification of *Rochalimaea henselae* in bacillary (epithelioid) angiomatosis, parenchymal bacillary peliosis, and persistent fever with bacteremia. *Am. J. Surg. Pathol.* **16:**650–657.
35. **Ricketts, W. E.** 1949. Clinical manifestations of Carrion's disease. *Arch. Intern. Med.* **84:**751–781.
36. **Sander, A., C. Buhler, K. Pelz, E. Voncramm, and W. Bredt.** 1997. Detection and identification of two *Bartonella henselae* variants in domestic cats in Germany. *J. Clin. Microbiol.* **35:**584–587.
37. **Schwartzman, W. A., C. A. Nesbit, and E. J. Baron.** 1993. Development and evaluation of a blood-free medium for determining growth curves and optimizing growth of *Rochalimaea henselae*. *J. Clin. Microbiol.* **31:**1882–1885.
38. **Scott, M. A., T. L. McCurley, C. L. Vnencakjones, C. Hager, J. A. McCoy, B. Anderson, R. D. Collins, and K. M. Edwards.** 1996. Cat scratch disease—detection of *Bartonella henselae* DNA in archival biopsies from patients with clinically, serologically, and histologically defined disease. *Am. J. Pathol.* **149:**2161–2167.
39. **Slater, L. N., D. F. Welch, D. Hensel, and D. W. Coody.** 1990. A newly recognized fastidious Gram-negative pathogen as a cause of fever and bacteremia. *N. Engl. J. Med.* **323:**1587–1593.
40. **Slater, L. N., D. F. Welch, and K. W. Min.** 1992. *Rochalimaea henselae* causes bacillary angiomatosis and peliosis hepatis. *Arch. Intern. Med.* **152:**602–606.
41. **Spach, D. H., L. A. Panther, D. R. Thorning, J. E. Dunn, J. J. Plorde, and R. A. Miller.** 1992. Intracerebral bacillary angiomatosis in a patient infected with the human immunodeficiency virus. *Ann. Intern. Med.* **116:**740–742.
42. **Stoler, M. H., T. A. Bonfiglio, R. T. Steigbigel, and M. Pereira.** 1983. An atypical subcutaneous infection associated with acquired immune deficiency syndrome. *Am. J. Clin. Pathol.* **80:**714–718.

43. **Szelc-Kelly, C. M., S. Goral, G. I. Perez-Perez, B. A. Perkins, R. L. Regnery, and K. M. Edwards.** 1995. Serologic responses to *Bartonella* and *Afipia* antigens in patients with cat scratch disease. *Pediatrics* **96:**1137–1142.
44. **Welch, D. F., D. M. Hensel, D. A. Pickett, V. H. San Joaquin, A. Robinson, and L. N. Slater.** 1993. Bacteremia in a child due to *Rochalimaea henselae*: a practical identification of isolates in the clinical laboratory. *J. Clin. Microbiol.* **31:**2381–2386.
45. **Welch, D. F., D. A. Pickett, L. N. Slater, A. G. Steigerwalt, and D. J. Brenner.** 1992. *Rochalimaea henselae* sp. nov., a cause of septicemia, bacillary angiomatosis, and parenchymal bacillary peliosis. *J. Clin. Microbiol.* **30:**275–280.
46. **Wong, M. T., D. C. Thornton, R. C. Kennedy, and M. J. Dolan.** 1995. A chemically defined liquid medium that supports primary isolation of *Rochalimaea* (*Bartonella*) *henselae* from blood and tissue specimens. *J. Clin. Microbiol.* **33:**742–744.
47. **Zangwill, K. M., D. H. Hamilton, B. A. Perkins, R. L. Regnery, B. D. Plikaytis, J. L. Hadler, M. L. Cartter, and J. D. Wenger.** 1993. Cat scratch disease in Connecticut. Epidemiology, risk factors, and evaluation of a new diagnostic test. *N. Engl. J. Med.* **329:**8–13.

*Francisella**

JANE D. WONG AND DANIEL S. SHAPIRO

44

TAXONOMY

First described in humans in 1907 and later in rodents (19), the causative agent of tularemia was called *Bacterium tularensis*. Beginning his work in 1920, Edward Francis dedicated his career to describing the clinical manifestations, diagnosis, and histopathology of tularemia (13). In 1974, the causative agent was renamed *Francisella tularensis* in recognition of his contributions. Early colloquial names, such as rabbit fever and deerfly fever in the United States, hare fever in Japan, and trappers' ailment in Europe and Asia, attest to the long-recognized association of tularemia with wild animals. *F. tularensis* biovar tularensis (type A), present in North America, is highly virulent for most mammals. Its reservoir appears to be the cottontail rabbit, and it is frequently transmitted by ticks (23). *F. tularensis* biovar palaearctica (type B) is found in Europe, Asia, and North America. It causes epizootics in beavers, voles, and muskrats. It is not considered to be as virulent as type A (23). Humans of any age, sex, or race are universally susceptible to infection with *F. tularensis*. The annual incidence of tularemia in humans in the United States has declined from several thousand in the 1930s to a few hundred in the 1990s, in concert with the disappearance of market hunting and trapping.

Other *Francisella* species have been described. *F. philomiragia*, originally *Yersinia philomiragia* (17), was first isolated from a dying muskrat found in a marshy area in Utah. This organism is associated with human illness, particularly in patients with underlying disease such as chronic granulomatous disease or myeloproliferative disorders or with a recent history of near drowning (15). Eighty-seven percent (13 of 15) of affected patients lived within 50 mi of a saltwater coastline or had intimate contact with brackish water (22, 32). *F. novicida* has been shown to be similar to *F. tularensis* in its genetic and pathogenicity characteristics and is now considered to be a third biovar of *F. tularensis*, *F. tularensis* biovar novicida (15).

DESCRIPTION OF THE GENUS

The organism is a small, gram-negative, pleomorphic, nonmotile, non-spore-forming coccobacillus measuring 0.2 by 0.2 to 0.7 μm. It is a strict aerobe, is nonpiliated, and possesses a thin capsule composed predominantly of lipid. Its cellular fatty acid profile is characterized by the presence of long-chain saturated and monosaturated C_{18} to C_{26} fatty acids, relatively large amounts of even-chain saturated acids ($C_{10:0}$, $C_{14:0}$, and $C_{16:0}$), and two long-chain hydroxy acids (3-OH $C_{16:0}$ and 3-OH $C_{18:0}$). This profile is unique to the genus *Francisella* (15, 16). In nature, the organism is rather hardy, persisting for many weeks in mud, water, and decaying animal carcasses. *F. tularensis* has been known to survive and proliferate within amoebae, as do *Legionella* species, a characteristic which may help it to survive in environments such as water and mud (2). The organism is extremely infectious. Biosafety level 2 is recommended for clinical laboratory work with suspected material, and biosafety level 3 is required for culturing the organism in large quantities (30).

NATURAL HABITATS

F. tularensis is widely distributed in nature and has been isolated from hundreds of animals, including numerous mammalian and avian species, arthropods, and domesticated animals, as well as water, mud, and animal feces (12).

The most frequent sources of human infection are wild rabbits of the genus *Sylvilagus*, which includes cottontail rabbits, marsh rabbits, and swamp rabbits. Jackrabbits and snowshoe hares are susceptible but have rarely been the source of human infection. The domestic rabbit has not been documented as a source of human infection (6). In the United States, tularemia has been most frequently reported from Missouri, Arkansas, and Oklahoma.

Other common sources of human infection are bloodsucking arthropod vectors, including ticks, deerflies, and mosquitoes. Less frequently, human cases have been reported to be transmitted by cats (5). Sheep, beavers, and muskrats have also been responsible for epidemics.

CLINICAL SIGNIFICANCE

The number of reported cases of tularemia in the United States in the 1980s and 1990s has been approximately 100 to 200 cases annually, with from one to four deaths. The number of reported cases has dropped dramatically since the 1940s, when the number of reported cases averaged

* This chapter contains information presented in chapter 43 by Scott J. Stewart in the sixth edition of this Manual.

1,180/year. Tularemia was deleted from the nationally notifiable disease list in 1995 (7).

Tularemia can be contracted by direct cutaneous inoculation, including contact with infected animals or a tick or deerfly bite, conjunctival inoculation, inhalation (28), and ingestion of infected undercooked animals and contaminated water. It has been speculated that *F. tularensis* can actually penetrate intact skin. Many cases of tularemia occur in individuals who hunt and skin animals.

Tularemia often begins abruptly with nonspecific symptoms including fever, chills, headache, and generalized aches. Cough and abdominal symptoms may also occur. The Centers for Disease Control and Prevention (CDC) case definitions of 1997 (8) define tularemia as an illness characterized by several distinct forms, including the following:

- Ulceroglandular (cutaneous ulcer with regional lymphadenopathy)
- Glandular (regional lymphadenopathy with no ulcer)
- Oculoglandular (conjunctivitis with preauricular lymphadenopathy)
- Oropharyngeal (stomatitis, pharyngitis, or tonsillitis and cervical lymphadenopathy)
- Intestinal (intestinal pain, vomiting, and diarrhea)
- Pneumonic (primary pleuropulmonary disease)
- Typhoidal (febrile illness without early localizing signs and symptoms)

The most common manifestation of *F. tularensis* in the United States is the ulceroglandular form, typically due to tick bites and contact with infected animals. A red papule develops and undergoes necrosis to form a tender ulcer at the site of cutaneous inoculation, and lymphatic spread results in regional lymphadenopathy. Bacteremia may subsequently occur. Ulcers present on the upper extremities are usually the result of direct inoculation from an infected mammal, such as a rabbit. Ulcers on the lower extremities, head, and back are usually the result of a bite of an arthropod vector.

Other clinical manifestations of tularemia are more unusual. The oculoglandular form results from conjunctival inoculation, either by aerosol inoculation or by autoinoculation with fingers. In addition to conjunctivitis, yellow conjunctival ulcers may be present. Regional lymphadenopathy involving the preauricular, submandibular, and cervical nodes may occur (20). The oropharyngeal form is often due to the ingestion of contaminated food and is characterized by the presence of stomatitis or painful pharyngitis or tonsillitis and cervical lymphadenopathy. The intestinal form is due to the ingestion of contaminated food or water and is associated with intestinal pain, vomiting, and diarrhea. The dose of organisms required to cause illness via ingestion, 10^8, is many orders of magnitude larger than the infective dose via the cutaneous or respiratory route (20). Pneumonic tularemia, due either to inhalation of organisms or to hematogenous dissemination to the lungs, may be seen as a community-acquired pneumonia in an individual who has had aerosol exposure (usually occupational exposure) to organisms. In addition to pneumonia, the patient may have an exudative pleural effusion. In typhoidal tularemia, the patient appears to be septic and lacks both the lymphadenopathy and the ulcers that are present in other forms of tularemia. This form of tularemia is more likely to be rapidly fatal and more difficult to diagnose than are forms associated with lymphadenopathy and/or ulcers.

TRANSPORT AND STORAGE OF SPECIMENS

As *F. tularensis* is an infection that is easily acquired within the laboratory, particular care should be taken to ensure that the specimens are collected, processed, and manipulated with strict attention to biosafety level 2 precautions. It is important that physicians notify laboratories when this organism is considered in the differential diagnosis because of its danger to laboratory personnel. Colonies resembling *F. tularensis* should be examined in a biological safety cabinet. Specimens from which *F. tularensis* can be isolated include infected ulcer scrapings, lymph node aspirates, gastric washings, sputum, and blood. If a specimen needs to be shipped to a laboratory for processing, it should be kept cold but not frozen. No transport medium is necessary.

DIRECT EXAMINATION

Gram staining of biopsy material is of little value, as the small, weakly staining organism cannot readily be distinguished from the background. A direct fluorescent-antibody (DFA) test is available at some state health department laboratories and at the CDC. Although a positive DFA test is a presumptive test when used on tissue specimens, this reagent is not known to cross-react with other organisms.

CULTURE AND ISOLATION

Bacterial isolation can be difficult because *F. tularensis* has specific growth requirements, grows slowly, and can be overgrown by contaminating organisms. In a study of over 1,000 human cases, 84% of which were laboratory confirmed by serologic evaluation, the organism was isolated in only slightly more than 10% of the cases (29). This finding suggests that it is necessary to examine cultures carefully for *Francisella* species in order to detect this relatively slowly growing organism, especially in specimens such as sputum or ulcer scrapings, in which competing flora may be present.

Direct isolation can be achieved from infected ulcer scrapings, lymph node aspirates, gastric washings, and sputum. The historical medium of choice is cystine-glucose-blood agar (27); however, good growth has been achieved with chocolate agar supplemented with IsoVitaleX and modified charcoal-yeast extract agar (33, 34). Although *F. tularensis* has a reputation for fastidious growth requirements, especially for cystine, not all strains are so exacting (25). Some strains can also grow on Columbia blood agar (3) and Trypticase soy agar (9). A heavy inoculum on an appropriate medium will yield a growth mass in 18 h, while individual colonies may require 2 to 4 days of incubation to reach 2 mm in size. Overgrowth by contaminating organisms can be reduced by incorporating 100 to 500 U of penicillin per ml into the medium. Selective media designed for the isolation of *Neisseria gonorrhoeae*, such as modified Thayer-Martin or modified Martin-Lewis medium, can also be used for contaminated material, such as ulcer specimens (26, 27, 34).

The Septi-Chek blood culture technique (10) has been shown to be successful in isolating *F. tularensis* from blood. Alternatively, lysis centrifugation with extended incubation in a medium such as chocolate agar or cystine-glucose-blood agar or a broth-based system with blind subculturing may also be useful in recovering this organism from blood.

TABLE 1 Presumptive identification of *F. philomiragia*, *F. tularensis* biovar novicida, *F. tularensis* biovar tularensis, and *F. tularensis* biovar palaearctica (15, 34)

Test or substrate	Result[a] for:			
	F. philomiragia (*n* = 16)	*F. tularensis* biovar novicida (*n* = 3)	*F. tularensis* biovar tularensis (type A)[b] (*n* = 69)	*F. tularensis* biovar palaearctica (type B)[b] (*n* = 43)
Small, gram-negative coccoid forms	100	100	100	100
Aerobic growth	100	100	100	100
Growth on MacConkey agar	14 (14)	(66)	6	0
Oxidase (Kovács) reaction	100	0	0	0
Triple sugar iron agar				
Acid slant	0	0	0	0
Acid butt	0	0	0	0
H_2S (slant or butt)	64 (36)	0	0	0
Growth in:				
Nutrient broth with 0% NaCl	0	0	10	0
Nutrient broth with 6% NaCl	86	66	0	0
Urease	0	0	0	0
Nitrate reduction	0	0	0	0
Acid from[c]:				
D-Glucose	57 (43)	(100)	92 (7)	79 (21)
Sucrose	57 (43)	100	0	0
Maltose	57 (43)	66	NT	NT
Glycerol	0	NT	71 (29)	0
Motility	0	0	0	0
Gelatin hydrolysis	75	0	0	0

[a] Test results are given as percent positive after 24 to 48 h (reaction delayed 3 to 7 days); NT, not tested.
[b] Cysteine or cystine is usually required for growth.
[c] Difco oxidation-fermentation basal medium is used for assaying acid production from carbohydrates for *F. philomiragia* and *F. tularensis* biovar novicida, and cysteine agar (carbohydrate base) (34) is used for *F. tularensis* biovar tularensis and *F. tularensis* biovar palaearctica.

IDENTIFICATION

Colonies are blue-gray, round, smooth, and slightly mucoid on cystine-glucose-blood agar and white, smooth, and moist on chocolate agar, modified Thayer-Martin medium, or modified Martin-Lewis medium. On medium containing blood, a small zone of alpha-hemolysis usually surrounds the colony. A slide agglutination test with a commercially available antiserum (2240-56-9; Difco, Detroit, Mich.) and a positive control antigen can be performed on a formalinized culture suspension for identification. The DFA test can also be used for culture confirmation. Biochemical reactions to determine biovars of *F. tularensis* (Table 1) are of no particular value and do not justify the additional risk to the microbiologist. Fermentation of glycerol or evidence of citrulline ureidase production serves to differentiate type A from type B (26). PCR has been used to demonstrate the infection experimentally (14, 18, 35) and has detected *F. tularensis* DNA in samples of skin lesions from humans with tularemia (23). PCR is a promising new technology for the detection of *F. tularensis* but is not yet routinely available.

SEROLOGY AND DIAGNOSIS

The clinical diagnosis of tularemia is often made in the absence of a positive culture for *F. tularensis* and relies upon serologic evidence of infection. The diagnosis is supported by evidence or history of a tick or deerfly bite, exposure to tissues of a mammalian host of *F. tularensis*, or exposure to potentially contaminated water. The CDC case definitions of 1997 (8) define the laboratory criteria for diagnosis and the case classification as follows:

Presumptive: elevated serum antibody titer to *F. tularensis* antigen (without documented fourfold or greater change) in a patient with no history of tularemia vaccination or detection of *F. tularensis* in a clinical specimen by the DFA test.

Confirmatory: isolation of *F. tularensis* in a clinical specimen or a fourfold or greater change in serum antibody titer to *F. tularensis* antigen.

Case classification: probable—a clinically compatible case with laboratory results indicative of presumptive infection; confirmed—a clinically compatible case with confirmatory laboratory results.

A number of serologic methods have been developed for the serologic evaluation of patients suspected of having tularemia; these include the standard tube agglutination assay, microagglutination test, enzyme-linked immunosorbent assay, and hemagglutination.

The most commonly used assay, the standard tube agglutination assay, which measures both immunoglobulin G and immunoglobulin M antibodies, can be performed with commercially available antigens (4087 [BBL Microbiology Systems, Cockeysville, Md.]; 2240-56-5 [Difco]). A titer of less than 1:20 is not diagnostic, due to nonspecific cross-reactions. A fourfold or greater change in serum antibody titer to *F. tularensis* antigen is diagnostic, and a single titer of 1:160 or greater is presumptive evidence of infection. The titers are usually negative in the first week of illness, are positive by the end of 2 weeks, and peak after 4 to 5 weeks (20). Titers of 1:20 to 1:80 can persist for years following infection (24). The microagglutination test (4), which is not routinely available, is more sensitive than the standard tube agglutination assay (21).

F. philomiragia and *F. tularensis* biovar novicida have caused human infections and cross-react with *F. tularensis*. Since these organisms are so closely related and cause similar diseases, these cross-reactions are not clinically significant (15). Cross-reactions with *Brucella* species and *Proteus vulgaris* OX19 may also complicate the interpretation of *F. tularensis* serology. In patients with fever of unknown orgin and in whom tularemia is suspected, agglutination tests for *F. tularensis*, *Brucella* species, and *P. vulgaris* OX19 should be done in parallel to determine if positive serologic responses are a result of infection or cross-reaction with another pathogen (24).

ANTIMICROBIAL SUSCEPTIBILITIES

Standardized antimicrobial susceptibility testing cannot be performed for isolates of *F. tularensis* unless modified Mueller-Hinton broth (supplemented with Ca^{2+} and Mg^{2+}, 2% IsoVitaleX, 0.1% glucose, and 0.025% ferric pyrophosphate) is used (1). The drug of choice for the treatment of tularemia has historically been streptomycin, which recently became available in the United States. This situation prompted a review of the use of alternative therapy for tularemia (11). In this review, the cure rate with streptomycin therapy (97%) exceeded that with gentamicin (86%), tetracycline (88%), chloramphenicol (77%), and tobramycin (50%). The relapse rate was also lower with streptomycin than with these alternative agents. There are limited, although positive, data on the use of imipenem-cilastatin and the quinolones ciprofloxacin and norfloxacin. Ceftriaxone was found to be ineffective.

An investigational, live attenuated vaccine has been developed by the U.S. Army Medical Research and Development Command at Fort Detrick, Md. This vaccine has been shown to stimulate both humoral immunity and cell-mediated immunity in volunteers. The duration of this immunity is currently unknown (31).

REFERENCES

1. **Baker, C. N., D. G. Hollis, and C. Thornsberry.** 1985. Antimicrobial susceptibility testing of *Francisella tularensis* with a modified Mueller-Hinton broth. *J. Clin. Microbiol.* **22:**212–215.
2. **Berdal, B. P., R. Mehl, N. K. Meidell, A.-M. Lorentzen-Styr, and O. Scheel.** 1996. Field investigations of tularemia in Norway. *FEMS Immunol. Med. Microbiol.* **13:**191–195.
3. **Bernard, K., S. Tessier, J. Winstanley, D. Chang, and A. Borczyk.** 1994. Early recognition of atypical *Francisella tularensis* strains lacking a cysteine requirement. *J. Clin. Microbiol.* **32:**551–553.
4. **Brown, S. L., F. T. McKinney, G. C. Klein, and W. Jones.** 1980. Evaluation of a safranin-O-stained antigen microagglutination test for *Francisella tularensis* antibodies. *J. Clin. Microbiol.* **11:**146–148.
5. **Capellan, J., and I. W. Fong.** 1993. Tularemia from a cat: case report and review of feline-associated tularemia. *Clin. Infect. Dis.* **16:**472–475.
6. **Centers for Disease Control.** 1986. Tularemia—New Jersey. *Morbid. Mortal. Weekly Rep.* **35:**747–753.
7. **Centers for Disease Control and Prevention.** 1994. Summary of notifiable diseases, United States. *Morbid. Mortal. Weekly Rep.* **43:**53.
8. **Centers for Disease Control and Prevention.** 1997. Case definitions for infectious conditions under public health surveillance. *Morbid. Mortal. Weekly Rep.* **46** (No. RR-10)**:** 53–54.
9. **Clarridge, J. E., T. J. Raich, A. Sjösted, G. Sandström, R. O. Darouiche, R. M. Shawar, P. R. Georghiou, C. Osting, and L. Vo.** 1996. Characterization of two unusual clinically significant *Francisella* strains. *J. Clin. Microbiol.* **34:**1995–2000.
10. **Doern, G. V., R. Davaro, M. George, and P. Campognone.** 1996. Lack of requirement for prolonged incubation of Septi-Check blood culture bottles in patients with bacteremia due to fastidious bacteria. *Diagn. Microbiol. Infect. Dis.* **24:**141–143.
11. **Enderlin, G., L. Morales, R. F. Jacobs, and I. T. Cross.** 1994. Streptomycin and alternative agents for the treatment of tularemia: review of the literature. *Clin. Infect. Dis.* **19:**42–47.
12. **Evans, M. E., D. W. Gregory, W. Schaffner, and Z. A. McGee.** 1985. Tularemia: a 30-year experience with 88 cases. *Medicine* (Baltimore) **64:**251–269.
13. **Francis, E.** 1925. Tularemia. *JAMA* **84:**1243–1250.
14. **Fulop, M., D. Leslie, and R. Titball.** 1996. A rapid, highly sensitive method for the detection of *Francisella tularensis* in clinical samples using the polymerase chain reaction. *Am. J. Trop. Med. Hyg.* **54:**364–366.
15. **Hollis, D. G., R. E. Weaver, A. G. Steigerwalt, J. D. Wenger, C. W. Moss, and D. J. Brenner.** 1989. *Francisella philomiragia* comb. nov (formerly *Yersinia philomiragia*) and *Francisella tularensis* biogroup novicida (formerly *Francisella novicida*) associated with human disease. *J. Clin. Microbiol.* **27:**1601–1608.
16. **Jantzen, E., B. P. Berdal, and T. Omland.** 1979. Cellular fatty acid composition of *Francisella tularensis*. *J. Clin. Microbiol.* **10:**928–930.
17. **Jensen W. I., C. R. Owen, and W. L. Jellison.** 1969. *Yersinia philomiragia* sp. nov., a new member of the *Pasteurella* group of bacteria, naturally pathogenic for the muskrat (*Ondatra zibethica*). *J. Bacteriol.* **100:**1237–1241.
18. **Long, G. W., J. J. Oprandy, R. B. Narayanan, A. H. Fortier, K. R. Porter, and C. A. Nacy.** 1993. Detection of *Francisella tularensis* in blood by polymerase chain reaction. *J. Clin. Microbiol.* **31:**152–154.
19. **McCoy, G. W., and C. W. Chapin.** 1912. Further observations on a plague-like disease of rodents with a preliminary note on the causative agent, Bacterium tularense. *J. Infect. Dis.* **10:**61–72.
20. **Penn, R. L.** 1995. *Francisella tularensis* (tularemia), p. 2060–2068. *In* G. L. Mandell, J. E. Bennett, and R. Dolin (ed.), *Mandell, Douglas and Bennett's Principles and Practice of Infectious Diseases*, 4th ed. Churchill Livingstone Inc., New York, N.Y.
21. **Sato, T., H. Fujita, Y. Ohara, and M. Homma.** 1990. Microagglutination test for early and specific serodiagnosis of tularemia. *J. Clin. Microbiol.* **28:**2372–2374.
22. **Sicherer, S. H., E. J. Asturias, J. A. Winkelstein, J. D. Dick, and R. E. Willoughby.** 1997. *Francisella philomiragia* sepsis in chronic granulomatous diseases. *Pediatr. Infect. Dis. J.* **16:**420–422.
23. **Sjöstedt, A., A. Tärnvik, and G. Sandström.** 1996. *Francisella tularensis*: host-parasite interaction. *FEMS Immunol. Med. Microbiol.* **13:**181–184.
24. **Snyder, M. J.** 1986. Immune response to *Francisella tularensis*, p. 377–378. *In* N. R. Rose, H. Friedman, and J. L. Fahey (ed.), *Manual of Clinical Immunology*, 3rd ed. American Society for Microbiology, Washington, D.C.
25. **Spach, D. H., W. C. Liles, G. L. Campbell, R. E. Quick, D. E. Anderson, and T. R. Fritsche.** 1993. Tick-borne diseases in the United States. *N. Engl. J. Med.* **329:** 936–947.
26. **Stewart, S. J.** 1988. Tularemia, p. 519–524. *In* A. Balows,

W. J. Hausler, Jr., M. Ohashi, and A. Turano (ed.), *Laboratory Diagnosis of Infectious Diseases: Principles and Practice*. Springer Verlag, New York, N.Y.

27. **Stewart, S. J.** 1981. Tularemia, p. 705–714. *In* A. Balows and W. J. Hausler, Jr. (ed.), *Diagnostic Procedures for Bacterial, Mycotic and Parasitic Infections*, 6th ed. American Public Health Association, Washington, D.C.
28. **Syrjälä, H., P. Kujala, V. Myllylä, and A. Salminen.** 1985. Airborne transmission of tularemia in farmers. *Scand. J. Infect. Dis.* **17:**371–375.
29. **Taylor, J. P., G. R. Istre, T. C. McChesney, F. T. Satalowich, R. L. Parker, and L. M. McFarland.** 1991. Epidemiologic characteristics of human tularemia in the southwest-central states, 1981–1987. *Am. J. Epidemiol.* **133:** 1032–1038.
30. **U.S. Department of Health and Human Services.** 1993. *Biosafety in Microbiological and Biomedical Laboratories*, 3rd ed., p. 91. U.S. Government Printing Office, Washington, D.C.
31. **Waag, D. M., G. Sandstrom, M. J. England, and J. C. Williams.** 1996. Immunogenicity of a new lot of *Francisella tularensis* live vaccine strain in human volunteers. *FEMS Immunol. Med. Microbiol.* **13:**205–209.
32. **Wenger, J. D., D. G. Hollis, R. E. Weaver, C. N. Baker, G. R. Brown, D. J. Brenner, and C. V. Broome.** 1989. Infection caused by *Francisella philomiragia* (formerly *Yersinia philomiragia*). *Ann. Intern. Med.* **110:**888–892.
33. **Westerman, E. L., and J. McDonald.** 1983. Tularemia pneumonia mimicking Legionnaires' disease: isolation of organism on CYE agar and successful treatment with erythromycin. *South. Med. J.* **76:**1169–1170.
34. **Weyant, R. S., C. W. Moss, R. E. Weaver, D. G. Hollis, J. G. Jordan, E. C. Cook, and M. I. Daneshvar.** 1996. *Identification of Unusual Pathogenic Gram-Negative Aerobic and Facultatively Anaerobic Bacteria*, 2nd ed., p. 362–365. The Williams & Wilkins Co., Baltimore, Md.
35. **Zhai, J., R. Yang, J. Lu, S. Zhang, M. Chen, F. Che, and H. Cui.** 1996. Detection of *Francisella tularensis* by the polymerase chain reaction. *J. Med. Microbiol.* **45:**477–482.

Algorithm for Identification of Anaerobic Bacteria

ELLEN JO BARON AND DIANE M. CITRON

45

Anaerobic bacteria are defined for purposes of this algorithm as organisms displaying better growth when incubated in an anaerobic atmosphere than when incubated in any atmosphere containing oxygen. These include some *Actinomyces* and *Propionibacterium* species and clostridia that grow poorly under aerobic conditions. Gram stain and colony morphologies are determined after a minimum of 48 h of incubation on a blood-containing agar medium supplemented with vitamin K and hemin. Fluorescence is determined in a dark room by holding the colonies close to the light from a Woods lamp (long-wave UV light, 366 nm) for as long as 60 s and observing them for colored fluorescence. In some cases, pigment is best observed by spreading some colony material onto a white cotton swab for contrast. Vancomycin sensitivity is defined as yielding a ≥10-mm zone of inhibition around a 5-μg vancomycin disc on anaerobic blood agar. The catalase test for anaerobes uses 10 to 15% H_2O_2 instead of the 3% used for testing aerobic bacteria. Although in most cases it will be easy to characterize an isolate as gram positive or gram negative, several species of clostridia usually stain gram negative or gram variable. Vancomycin sensitivity cannot differentiate them all, since *Porphyromonas* species (gram-negative coccobacilli) are vancomycin sensitive and some *Clostridium innocuum* (gram-variable rods) are sometimes vancomycin resistant, hence the dichotomous nature of this algorithm.

TABLE 1 Algorithm for identification of bacteria that grow better anaerobically than aerobically

Cellular morphology	Gram reaction	Spores seen on Gram stain	Black or tan colony or fluoresces red in UV light	Catalase	Spreading, irregular, peaked, or large colony	Large boxcar-shaped cells; double zone of beta-hemolysis	Vancomycin sensitive	Long, thin rods	Organism (chapter)
Rods or coccobacilli	+	+							*Clostridium* (46)
		−		+					*Actinomyces* or *Propionibacterum* (47)
				−	−	−			*Actinomyces*, *Lactobacillus*, or *Propionibacterum* (47)
						+			*Clostridium perfringens* (46)
					+	−			*Clostridium* (46)
	− or variable	+							*Clostridium* (46)
		−	+				+	−	*Porphyromonas* (48)
								+	C. *ramosum* (46)
			−				+		C. *clostridioforme* or C. *innocuum* (46)
							−		Gram-negative rods (48), C. *innocuum*[a] (46)
Cocci	+								*Peptostreptococcus* species (47)
	−								*Veillonella*, *Acidaminococcus*, or *Megasphaera* (48)

[a] Some C. *innocuum* strains are vancomycin resistant.

*Clostridium**

STEPHEN D. ALLEN, CHRISTOPHER L. EMERY, AND JEAN A. SIDERS

46

TAXONOMY

Originally described in 1880 by Prazmowski (105), the genus *Clostridium* differed from the genus *Bacillus* by including obligately anaerobic rods with central or subterminal heat-resistant spores that swell the cells (29). Currently, the genus *Clostridium* includes obligately anaerobic or aerotolerant spore-forming rods that do not form spores in the presence of air, are usually gram positive (at least in early stages of growth), and do not carry out a dissimilatory sulfate reduction (29, 31). Probably as a result of this simple definition, as Collins et al. suggested, the genus *Clostridium* has become one of the largest and most diverse genera of bacteria and "is clearly in need of revision (31)." Although significant genetic diversity within the genus has long been known (68), recent studies by Collins et al. (31), using 16S rRNA gene sequences determined by PCR direct sequencing and the construction of phylogenetic trees, revealed that the genus *Clostridium* is extremely heterogeneous and could be divided into several phylogenetic clusters. The type species, *Clostridium butyricum*, and most of the medically important *Clostridium* species were placed in cluster I, which was equivalent to rRNA group 1 of Johnson and Francis (68). Collins et al. named five new genera of spore-forming rods: *Caloramator*, *Filifactor*, *Moorella*, *Oxobacter*, and *Oxalophagus* (31). They also proposed 11 new species combinations. None of these new generic and species designations was of medical significance; however, changes in the nomenclature of some medically important clostridia will probably occur in the future. Currently, based upon the number of species validly published, there were 130 "official" species of *Clostridium* with standing in nomenclature as of 1 January 1998 (96, 116). Fortunately for the clinical microbiologist, the number of species commonly encountered as agents of infection in properly collected clinical specimens from humans is relatively small (Table 1).

DESCRIPTION OF THE GENUS

The vegetative cells of most species are rod shaped and straight or curved, but cells vary from short coccoid rods to long filamentous forms. The rod-shaped cells may be rounded, tapered, or blunt ended. Cells may occur singly, in pairs, or in chains of various lengths. In certain species (e.g., *C. cocleatum* and *C. spiroforme*), many rods may be joined to form tight coils or spiral configurations (28). Most species stain gram positive during the early stage of growth; however, some, such as *C. ramosum* and *C. clostridioforme*, almost always appear gram negative after overnight culture. Several species (e.g., *C. tetani*) appear gram negative by the time spores have formed. All but a few species are motile by means of peritrichous flagella. Nonmotile species isolated from clinical specimens include *C. perfringens*, *C. ramosum*, and *C. innocuum*. The spores of clostridia are ovoid to spherical and distend the vegetative cells. Certain species, e.g., *C. perfringens*, produce spores only under special culture conditions. Although the majority of *Clostridium* species are obligate anaerobes, there is considerable species variation with respect to oxygen toxicity; some species (e.g., *C. haemolyticum* and *C. novyi* type B) are strict obligate anaerobes and will not grow when exposed to even trace amounts of oxygen. A few aerotolerant species (*C. tertium*, *C. carnis*, *C. histolyticum*, and occasional strains of *C. perfringens*) show scant growth on solid media incubated in a 5 to 10% CO_2 incubator in air or in a candle jar.

Since aerotolerant clostridia may grow on the surface of fresh agar media under aerobic conditions, it is possible to confuse them with certain facultatively anaerobic *Bacillus* species. However, members of the genus *Clostridium* usually form spores only under anaerobic conditions and almost never produce catalase. Also, aerotolerant clostridia show much better growth (i.e., they form larger colonies) under anaerobic conditions than in air, whereas *Bacillus* species often form larger colonies on aerobically than anaerobically incubated media.

Catalase is not produced except in rare instances. If it is produced, the reaction is only weakly positive. In addition, clostridia lack a cytochrome system and thus react negatively in the cytochrome oxidase test. They do not have a mechanism for phosphorylation via an electron transport system. Energy is obtained via ATP by substrate level phosphorylation (28). Clostridia are usually fermentative, proteolytic, or both, but some are asaccharolytic and nonproteolytic. Many clostridia produce a range of short-chain fatty acids (e.g., acetate and butyrate) when grown in peptone-yeast extract-glucose or chopped-meat–carbohydrate medium, and many produce a variety of other fermentation products (e.g., acetone, butanol, and other alcohols).

* This chapter contains information presented in chapter 47 by Andrew B. Onderdonk and Stephen D. Allen in the sixth edition of this Manual.

TABLE 1 The *Clostridium* species most frequently encountered in clinical specimens at IUMC Anaerobe Laboratory in 1989 through 1997[a]

Species	Isolates	
	No.	% of total
C. perfringens	366	20
C. clostridioforme	304	17
C. innocuum	289	16
C. ramosum	234	13
C. difficile	202	11
C. butyricum	75	4
C. cadaveris	72	4
C. sporogenes	40	2
C. bifermentans	35	2
C. glycolicum	35	2
C. tertium	33	2
C. septicum	30	2
C. sordellii	21	1
C. paraputrificum	20	1
C. symbiosum	20	1
C. subterminale	14	1
C. baratii	13	1
Other recognized species[b]	24	1

[a] S. D. Allen and J. A. Siders, unpublished data. The total of 1,827 isolates does not include 171 isolates (9% of 1,998 isolates) that did not belong to a recognized species. All of the isolates were from properly collected specimens and did not include fecal samples for *C. difficile* testing.

[b] Includes one to six isolates of each of the following: *C. beijerinckii*, *C. botulinum type* A, *C. carnis*, *C. celatum*, *C. coccoides*, *C. cocleatum*, *C. ghoni*, *C. hastiforme*, *C. limosum*, *C. malenominatum*, *C. novyi type* A, *C. putrificum*, and *C. sphenoides*.

NATURAL HABITATS

Although *Clostridium* species are ubiquitous in nature, their principal habitats are the soil and the intestinal tracts of many animals including humans (120). The species most frequently isolated from soil are *C. subterminale*, *C. sordellii*, *C. sporogenes*, *C. indolis*, *C. bifermentans*, *C. mangenotii*, and *C. perfringens* (117). Others regularly found in soil samples, but somewhat less frequently, are *C. botulinum* and *C. tetani* (118). The widespread occurrence of *C. perfringens*, including its spores, in soil samples almost guarantees the frequent presence of this organism on surfaces exposed to dust contamination, including many food items (120). However, the average daily intake of *C. perfringens* on foods consumed by humans is probably small (e.g., $<5 \times 10^2$ organisms per day) (120).

Clostridia were recovered frequently from the feces of infants studied during the first week of life (125). However, breast-fed infants 1 month of age were less likely to be colonized by clostridia than formula-fed infants were. As reviewed elsewhere (120), the feces of infants 6 to 20 months old tend to contain about the same numbers of *C. perfringens* (essentially all toxin type A) as is the case for adults (e.g., $\sim 10^3$ to 10^8 CFU per g). The feces of infants commonly contain *C. difficile*, but it is seen less frequently in healthy adults (44, 129). Several additional *Clostridium* species reside in the lower intestinal tracts of humans as part of the normal flora. Examples of those commonly found include *C. innocuum*, *C. ramosum*, *C. paraputrificum*, *C. putrificum*, *C. sporogenes*, *C. tertium*, *C. bifermentans*, and *C. butyricum*. With certain notable exceptions, most species occur as harmless saprophytes.

Exogenous diseases, caused by clostridia from an external source (e.g., food-borne botulism, tetanus, and myonecrosis), are well known historically and are clinically important. Although usually acquired from the patient's own gastrointestinal tract, *C. difficile* may be spread exogenously from person to person during outbreaks of hospital-acquired diarrhea or colitis (73, 98). Endogenous infections involving clostridia that are a part of the host's own microflora are much more common, however. As is true for other endogenous infections involving anaerobes (endocarditis, brain abscess, aspiration pneumonia, intra-abdominal abscess, etc.), the development of clostridial disease is usually associated with special circumstances. Common predisposing factors include trauma, operative procedures, vascular stasis, obstruction, treatment of cancer patients with immunosuppressive agents or chemotherapeutic agents, prior treatment with antimicrobial agents (as in pseudomembranous colitis), and underlying illness such as leukemia, carcinoma, or diabetes mellitus. Under the right conditions, clostridia can invade and multiply in essentially any tissue of the body.

CLINICAL SIGNIFICANCE

C. perfringens and Associated Conditions

C. perfringens is the species most commonly isolated from human clinical specimens excluding feces. It is encountered in a wide variety of clinical settings ranging from simple contamination of wounds to traumatic or nontraumatic myonecrosis, clostridial cellulitis, intra-abdominal sepsis, gangrenous cholecystitis, postabortion infection with devastating septicemia, intravascular hemolysis, bacteremia in various clinical settings, aspiration pneumonia, necrotizing pneumonia, thoracic empyema, subdural empyema, and brain abscess (42, 54).

C. perfringens, also called *C. welchii* by some investigators, is commonly considered to be one of a group of organisms referred to as the histotoxic or tissue-destroying clostridia, the most common form of tissue destruction being gas gangrene. The histotoxic clostridia most commonly involved in gas gangrene (myonecrosis) are *C. perfringens* (80%), *C. novyi*, and *C. septicum*, followed by *C. histolyticum* and *C. bifermentans*. Other species such as *C. sordellii*, *C. fallax*, *C. sporogenes*, and *C. tertium* have been encountered in patients with myonecrosis, but their pathogenic significance is not certain.

Clostridial myonecrosis (gas gangrene) is a toxin-mediated breakdown of muscle tissue associated with growth of the organism. It is a rapidly progressive, life-threatening condition with liquefactive necrosis of muscle, gas (primarily insoluble hydrogen and nitrogen) formation, and associated clinical signs of toxemia. Blood cultures are positive in about 15% of patients (127).

In addition to the habitats mentioned above, *C. perfringens* has been isolated from the vaginal vaults or cervices of approximately 1 to 9% of healthy pregnant and nonpregnant women (33). Gas gangrene of the uterus, which is now rare in the United States, has occurred most frequently as a consequence of illegal or self-induced abortions. It has also followed spontaneous abortion or vaginal delivery in which the postabortal or puerperal uterus contained blood clots and fragments of necrotic placenta or fetal tissue along with a minimum number of clostridia that could proliferate within the endometrium and subsequently invade the uterine wall. Clostridial myonecrosis of the uterus is associated with fulminant and overwhelming septicemia, marked intravascular hemolysis with profound anemia, jaundice, hemoglobinuria, and excretion of urine that is burgundy wine colored. Patients become hypotensive and often experience cardiovascular collapse, cardiac failure, pulmonary edema, renal failure, and coma; they may die within hours after onset of the infection (131). A dirty, red-brown, foul-smelling vaginal discharge containing gas bubbles and a Gram-stained smear showing numerous gram-positive bacilli should suggest clostridial myonecrosis of the uterus.

The presence of gas at an infected site does not always signal clostridial myonecrosis. Various gas-producing bacteria may form gas in tissue without causing myonecrosis; those that do so most frequently, particularly after laceration-type wounds involving soft tissue other than muscle, are the clostridia, especially C. *perfringens* (7, 55). Crepitant cellulitis caused by clostridia, also called anaerobic cellulitis, characteristically involves subcutaneous tissues or retroperitoneal tissues and can progress to fulminant systemic disease (7, 8). In contrast to clostridial myonecrosis, the muscle is usually not involved to a significant extent and remains viable during crepitant cellulitis. Although both gas gangrene and crepitant cellulitis are serious, the outlook for patients who have clostridial infections confined to subcutaneous tissues is usually not as ominous as that for patients with myonecrosis, provided that the correct diagnosis and treatment are initiated early in the course of illness. Pertinent findings in crepitant cellulitis include abundant gas in the tissue, often more than in myonecrosis; tissue swelling without much discoloration of the overlying skin; minimal pain; and a thin, sweet-smelling or sometimes foul-smelling exudate that may contain numerous polymorphonuclear leukocytes and bacteria (7, 85). On occasion, however, polymorphonuclear leukocytes are absent because of the activity of the leukolytic toxins of the clostridia. The presence of boxcar-shaped, gram-variable rods and no leukocytes in a Gram-stained preparation of infected tissue should lead one to suspect clostridial infection. These infections may involve only clostridia but are frequently polymicrobial (7, 100).

Clostridium species are commonly encountered in a variety of polymicrobial infections involving the abdomen, including peritonitis, intra-abdominal abscesses, and septicemia in patients with obstructive or perforating lesions of the terminal ileum or large bowel (56). C. *perfringens* and C. *septicum* have been documented in patients with overwhelming sepsis and gangrenous necrosis of the small intestine or large bowel. C. *septicum* has been associated with carcinoma of the colon or other malignancy. Although it is clear that clostridia play a major pathogenic role in some life-threatening necrotizing infections of the intestinal tract, the role of clostridia during intra-abdominal infections must be assessed on an individual patient basis (78).

C. *perfringens* produces a variety of biologically active proteins, or toxins, that play an important role in pathogenicity (62, 86). On the basis of mouse lethality assays and specific neutralization of four toxins produced in culture fluids, five toxin types of C. *perfringens* have been identified (types A through E) (61) (Table 2). Clostridia of all five types that produce lethal toxins will produce a potent phospholipase, or alpha-toxin, which plays a major role in the pathogenesis of myonecrosis caused by C. *perfringens* (27, 101). Also referred to as a phospholipase C, the alpha-toxin has several additional properties (128). It produces the opaque zone of lecithin hydrolysis products that surrounds colonies of C. *perfringens* growing on egg yolk agar plates. It is also a hemolysin. It gives rise to an outer zone of partial hemolysis that encircles a smaller zone of complete hemolysis produced by theta-toxin (a heat-labile, oxygen-labile hemolysin easily detected around colonies of C. *perfringens* growing on sheep blood agar). The alpha-toxin is also active against the membranes of muscle cells, leukocytes, and platelets, and it has necrotizing activity that leads to the death of a variety of host cells and tissues. These effects are probably related to its interaction with eukaryotic cell membranes and hydrolysis of sphingomyelin and phosphatidylcholine, resulting in lysis of the affected cells (128). In addition to producing alpha-toxin, type B strains of C. *perfringens* produce lethal beta- and epsilon-toxins, type D strains produce lethal epsilon-toxin, and type E strains uniquely produce an iota-toxin as well as alpha-toxin (Table 2).

A variety of apparently less important bioactive proteins, or minor toxins, which may or may not serve as virulence factors, are produced by C. *perfringens* (108, 119). These include lambda-toxin (a protease), kappa-toxin (a collagenase), mu-toxin (a hyaluronidase), a neuraminidase, and a DNase (120, 131).

C. perfringens and Food Poisoning

C. *perfringens* is one of the most common bacterial causes of food-borne illness in the United States (113). During 1990 to 1992, it was second only to *Salmonella* spp. in the number of food-borne disease outbreaks caused by a known bacterial agent (20). Almost all U.S. outbreaks and cases of C. *perfringens* food-borne gastroenteritis appear to be due to type A strains (113). In C. *perfringens* type A food-borne disease, the food vehicle is almost always an improperly cooked meat or a meat product, such as gravy, that has cooled slowly after cooking or may have been inadequately reheated. Spores surviving the initial cooking germinate, and vegetative cells proliferate during slow cooling or insufficient reheating. C. *perfringens* type A food-borne illness should be suspected when there is an outbreak of diarrhea with crampy abdominal pain within about 7 to 15 h after the consumption of a suspected food (113). However, the incubation period may range up to 30 h. Most patients are afebrile; nausea and vomiting occur in less than one-third of patients, and the stools are frequently foamy and foul smelling. Illness results from the ingestion of food with about 10^8 viable vegetative cells, which, in the alkaline environment of the small intestine, undergo sporulation, producing an enterotoxin in the process (113). The enterotoxin, a single polypeptide with a molecular weight of about 35,000, accumulates within C. *perfringens* cells when they sporulate and is released into the intestine when the sporulating cells undergo lysis and release their spores (76). After it is released into the small intestine, the enterotoxin apparently binds to receptors on the surface of intestinal epithelial cells and causes cytotoxic damage to cell membranes and permeability alterations leading to diarrhea and cramping abdominal symptoms (76). Animal model studies have revealed that C. *perfringens* enterotoxin causes significant histopathological damage to the small intestine, including necrosis of villus cells (115). In humans, the illness is usually mild, and most patients recover within 2 to 3 days after onset. The diagnosis is problematic, and the disease undoubtedly is underdiagnosed. Laboratory confirmation has traditionally been performed by the culture from epidemiologically implicated food of at least 10^5 organisms per g and by the demonstration, using a quantitative spore selection technique, of median spore counts of at least 10^6 C. *perfringens* spores per g of feces collected within 24 h after the onset of illness (10,

TABLE 2 Distribution of major toxins among types of *C. perfringens*

Toxin type	Occurrence and country where originally found	Alpha-toxin		Beta-toxin		Epsilon-toxin		Iota-toxin	
		Presence or absence	Characteristics	Presence or absence	Characteristics	Presence or absence	Characteristics	Presence or absence	Characteristics
A[a]	Gas gangrene of humans and animals Intestinal flora of humans and animals Putrefactive processes in soil, etc. (United States) Food poisoning (United Kingdom)	+	Lethal, lecithinase, hemolytic, necrotizing	−	Lethal, necrotizing	−	Lethal, permease	−	Lethal, dermonecrotic, ADP-ribosylating
B	Lamb dysentery Enterotoxemia of foals (United Kingdom) Enterotoxemia of sheep and goats (Iran)	+		+		+		−	
C	Enterotoxemia of sheep (struck) (United Kingdom) Enteritis necroticans of humans (pig-bel) (Papua New Guinea)	+		+		−		−	
D	Enterotoxemia of sheep, lambs, goats, cattle, possibly humans (Australia)	+		−		+		−	
E	Sheep and cattle, pathogenicity doubted (United Kingdom)	+		−		−		+	

[a] Also called phospholipase C.

113). Assays that have been used to detect the enterotoxin include Vero cell toxin neutralization, Western immunoblotting (77), reverse passive latex agglutination (Oxoid USA, Columbia, Md.), and commercial enzyme-linked immunosorbent assay kits (TechLab, Blacksburg, Va.). Although PCR assays and digoxigenin-labeled probe assays (to detect all or part of the *C. perfringens* enterotoxin gene) (77) can indicate the potential of a *C. perfringens* isolate to produce enterotoxin in vitro without a requirement for sporulation, gene probe assays do not indicate whether an isolate can sporulate and produce enterotoxin within the intestinal tract of a patient (62). Laboratory testing for *C. perfringens* food-borne illness is a public health laboratory function that should be performed concomitantly with provision of epidemiologic support. Ideally, isolates of the same serotype can be cultured from epidemiologically incriminated food and ill persons but not from control subjects. Unfortunately, the experience with serotyping of *C. perfringens* at the Centers for Disease Control and Prevention (CDC) has not been highly successful (77).

C. perfringens may produce a severe necrotizing disease of the small bowel known as enteritis necroticans, which can occur sporadically or in an epidemic form. The syndrome has been called Darmbrand in Germany and pig-bel in Papua New Guinea (3). In this condition, seen mostly in children, there is evidence to suggest that *C. perfringens* type C, which either is present as part of the normal intestinal flora or is ingested with contaminated pork or other meat during a feast, proliferates in the small intestine and produces beta-toxin. Toxin production probably leads to focal paralysis, inflammation, hemorrhage, and segmental gangrenous necrosis of the intestine, particularly the jejunum. Among the factors likely to be involved in the pathogenesis of enteritis necroticans are (i) overeating, which might distend the bowel and cause partial obstruction; (ii) poor nutrition, which leads to low levels of production of the pancreatic proteases (particularly trypsin, which ordinarily destroys beta-toxins); and (iii) a diet rich in trypsin inhibitors (such as the semicooked sweet potatoes often eaten at pig feasts) (32, 84).

C. difficile and Antibiotic Colitis

C. *difficile*, the major cause of antibiotic-associated diarrhea and pseudomembranous colitis, is also the most frequently identified cause of hospital-acquired diarrhea (47, 69, 72, 94). The organism has been isolated from diverse natural habitats, including soil, hay, sand, dung from various large mammals (cows, donkeys, and horses), and the feces of dogs, cats, rodents, and humans (88). C. *difficile* is carried asymptomatically as part of the gastrointestinal flora of as many as half of all healthy neonates during the first year of life; the carriage rate decreases to the adult carrier rate of 3% or less in children older than 2 years (129). Carriage rates of C. *difficile* in asymptomatic adult populations have varied from 1.9% in Sweden to 15.4% of young adults in Japan (14, 99). As reviewed by Gerding et al., hospitalized patients frequently become colonized with this organism (47). McFarland et al. reported that 21% of 399 patients with negative cultures on admission to a hospital with a high prevalence of C. *difficile*-associated diarrhea acquired C. *difficile* during hospitalization (94). Of these patients, 63% remained asymptomatic while 37% developed diarrhea. Antimicrobial agents of all classes and several anticancer chemotherapeutic agents have been implicated in the development of C. *difficile*-associated diarrhea or pseudomembranous colitis (43, 51, 53). The most commonly reported agents are ampicillin, clindamycin, and cephalosporins (47, 52).

C. *difficile* produces at least three potential virulence factors: a 308-kDa enterotoxin (toxin A) that induces a positive fluid response in the rabbit ligated ileal loop model, a 270-kDa cytotoxin (toxin B) that induces cytopathic effects in numerous tissue culture cell lines (95), and a substance that inhibits bowel motility (71). Toxin A also produces cytopathic effects in cell cultures but is less potent than toxin B in most cell culture lines (95). Most strains tested for toxin in vitro produce either both toxins or no detectable toxin, although there are reports of one toxin being present without the other (25, 87); it is thought that toxins A and B are both important in the pathogenesis of C. *difficile*-associated disease. Both toxins interfere with the actin cytoskeletons of intestinal epithelial cells, thereby rendering the cells nonfunctional. As reviewed elsewhere, the mechanism through which toxins A and B disrupt the cytoskeleton involves modification of Rho family proteins by UDP-glucose-dependent glycosylation (95).

Although C. *difficile* is by far the major cause of antibiotic-associated diarrhea, there are reports suggesting that C. *perfringens* is another, less frequently identified, cause of antibiotic-associated diarrhea in the United Kingdom (24). Historically, *Staphylococcus aureus* was believed to cause antibiotic-associated colitis. However, supporting evidence for this has been lacking in recent years (19).

C. *difficile* is now one of the most commonly detected enteric pathogens in hospitalized patients and also is an important cause of enteric infections in nursing home residents (49, 73, 97). Despite the common perception that colitis caused by C. *difficile* is a problem only when antibiotics are used, patients with bowel stasis, those who have had bowel surgery, and those with no known risk factors can also develop C. *difficile*-induced gastrointestinal disease, although this form of the disease is less common than that associated with antibiotic use. Clinical symptoms range from mild diarrhea to toxic megacolon (46). In the most severe form, the disease may include bowel perforation and death, although these events are unlikely to occur in appropriately treated patients.

C. septicum and Bacteremia

C. *septicum* is isolated only rarely from the feces of healthy individuals and is not recovered often from cultures of blood from otherwise healthy individuals. Increasingly, the isolation of this organism from blood cultures has been associated with other underlying disease processes (discussed below). The finding of this swarming organism on blood agar plates incubated anaerobically after subculture from an anaerobic blood culture bottle is often a precursor to the diagnosis of a serious neoplastic disease. The portal of entry for C. *septicum* into the bloodstream is believed to be the ileocecal region of the bowel. Whether C. *septicum* is part of the indigenous microflora of this site, at least in low concentrations, has not been established. C. *septicum* has, however, been found in the lumens of 10 to 68% of normal appendixes and in 0 of 30 nonlumen appendiceal tissue samples from gangrenous or perforated appendices (21, 44).

Of particular interest has been the association of C. *septicum* bacteremia with malignancies, especially leukemia and lymphoma or carcinoma of the large bowel. As many as 70 to 85% of patients whose blood cultures are positive for this organism have some underlying malignancy (23, 75). Another clinically important association has been observed between C. *septicum* bacteremia, neutropenia, and enterocolitis involving the terminal ileum or cecum (22, 74, 82). The neutropenia has been related both to chemotherapy for leukemia or other neoplastic diseases and to cyclic neutropenia and drug-induced agranulocytosis.

Not all patients with C. *septicum* bacteremia have malignancy or neutropenic enterocolitis. Patients with diabetes mellitus, severe atherosclerotic cardiovascular disease, or gas gangrene may also develop C. *septicum* bacteremia (80). The clinical importance of recognizing C. *septicum* bacteremia and starting appropriate treatment without delay cannot be overemphasized. Patients with this condition are usually acutely and gravely ill, frequently have high temperatures, and often show metastatic spread of myonecrosis to distant anatomic sites. Mortality rates are significant (68% or greater). Although appropriate antibiotic therapy with β-lactam antibiotics and aggressive surgical intervention early in the course of the illness have both been recommended to aid in avoiding a devastating outcome (80, 81), some survivors have received antibiotics and supportive care alone (70).

C. botulinum and Botulism

C. *botulinum*, perhaps most often thought of as the cause of a rare but life-threatening food-borne illness, is widely distributed in soil and aquatic habitats throughout the world. Microorganisms designated C. *botulinum*, along with unique strains of C. *butyricum*, C. *baratii*, and C. *argentinense*, have the ability to produce the most lethal poison known, namely, botulinum neurotoxin (BoNT). There are seven antigenic toxin types of BoNT (A through G), determined by serologic toxin neutralization tests, and they serve as useful clinical and epidemiologic markers (11). Types A, B, E, and F are the principal causes of botulism in humans; and types C and D are associated primarily with botulism in birds and mammals (60). Type C can be subdivided into two toxin types, C1 and C2; C1 is a neurotoxin, and C2 is not a neurotoxin but produces vascular permeability and has enterotoxic activity. Bacteria that produce type G BoNT, now called C. *argentinense* (126), have been isolated from soil in Argentina and from autopsy materials from five individuals who died suddenly, but *C. argentinense* has not been clearly implicated in cases of botulism (60, 121). Regardless of serologic type, each BoNT is synthesized during growth of the organism as a single inactive protein (~150 kDa) that is released during lysis of the bacterial cells (86). Activation of the molecule requires proteolytic cleaveage into two disulfide-linked polypeptide chains. Thus, the active form of BoNT is a dichain neurotoxin containing a 50-kDa light chain and a 100-kDa heavy chain (111).

Botulism is currently classified into four categories: (i) classical food-borne botulism, an intoxication caused by the ingestion of preformed botulinal toxin in contaminated food; (ii) wound botulism, which results from elaboration of botulinal toxin in vivo after growth of *C. botulinum* in an infected wound; (iii) infant botulism, in which botulinal toxin is elaborated in vivo in the intestinal tract of an infant who has been colonized with *C. botulinum*; and (iv) botulism due to intestinal colonization in children older than infants and in adults (62). Regardless of the category of botulism, the toxin enters the bloodstream from the site where it was produced or absorbed and binds irreversibly at the neuromuscular junctions of motor neurons. The chemical identity of the receptor site(s) on the presynaptic membranes has not been determined. A portion of the toxin molecule probably penetrates the plasma membrane, possibly by receptor-mediated endocytosis, and thus is internalized into the nerve cell. The neurotoxin molecule acts within the nerve terminal at the neuromuscular junction to prevent the release of acetylcholine (111). The characteristic clinical hallmark of botulism is an acute flaccid paralysis, which begins with bilateral cranial nerve impairment involving muscles of the face, head, and pharynx and then descends symmetrically to involve muscles of the thorax and extremities. Death may result from respiratory failure caused by paralysis of the tongue or muscles of the pharynx that occlude the upper airway or from paralysis of the diaphragm and intercostal muscles. Patients diagnosed with food-borne or wound botulism should immediately receive trivalent (type ABE) antitoxin and intensive respiratory care.

C. botulinum and Infant Botulism

In the United States, infant botulism is the most frequently recognized form of botulism. Although it has been documented in at least 13 other countries, it is rare outside the United States (60). Of the 1,290 cases reported in the United States between 1976 and 1994, almost half were in California (11). Across the United States, the geographical distribution of toxin types in infant botulism cases has paralleled the distribution of *C. botulinum* toxin types in soil sampled from different locations (118). Type A has been the most frequent BoNT type in cases of infant botulism in states west of the Mississippi River, whereas type B cases have predominated east of the Mississippi (12). Interestingly, one infant from Hawaii had two different strains of *C. botulinum*; one strain was type A, and the other was type B (59). Two other cases were caused by a strain(s) of *C. botulinum* that produced toxins that required both type B antitoxin and type F antitoxin for neutralization (59). In another interesting case, type F infant botulism was caused by an organism that most closely resembled *C. baratii* in its culture and biochemical characteristics (58). Type E botulism, caused by toxigenic strains of *C. butyricum*, was confirmed in two infants from Italy (60). Although most infected infants are 3 weeks to 6 months old, the age range is 6 to 363 days (11). Preformed toxin has not been detected in any food or liquid ingested by these infants. To date, the only clearly defined risk factors have been breast-feeding and exposure to honey, which is a potential source of spores. The CDC has recommended that honey not be fed to infants less than 1 year old (123). Another concern is that spores have also been found in a limited number of samples of corn syrup, which is often given to infants for treatment of decreased frequency of bowel movement (123). However, there has been no demonstration of *C. botulinum* spores in corn syrup actually consumed by an infant with botulism. Whatever the sources of the spores, the ingested spores of *C. botulinum* germinate within the intestinal tract, and the vegetative cells multiply and produce the neurotoxin, which is then absorbed into the bloodstream. Decreased frequency of bowel movements, which may also be a sign of decreased intestinal motility, may be an additional risk factor for infant botulism (123). The decreased motility could lead to the spread of *C. botulinum* or its toxin from the colon to the small intestine, where the toxin is probably absorbed (123). The first sign of illness is invariably constipation, which is often overlooked. Infants who are ultimately hospitalized usually develop lethargy and mild weakness with feeding difficulties, pooled oral secretions, and an altered cry. They eventually become floppy, lose head control, and may go on to develop ophthalmoplegia, ptosis, flaccid facial expression, dysphagia, other signs of cranial nerve deficits, and generalized muscular weakness. Respiratory insuffiency necessitating respiratory therapy also may occur, as in other forms of botulism (12). There is a spectrum of clinical features in infant botulism, ranging from mild illness not requiring hospitalization to sudden death, and this syndrome accounts for a small percentage of cases of sudden infant death syndrome (13). The differential diagnosis of infant botulism includes sepsis, myasthenia gravis, failure to thrive, benign congenital hypotonia, and a variety of other conditions.

C. tetani and Tetanus

The strictly toxigenic disease caused by *C. tetani* is often associated with puncture wounds that do not appear to be serious infections, particularly in animals. The organism and its spores can be isolated from a variety of sources, including soil and the intestinal contents of numerous animal species. Toxin is elaborated at the site of apparent minor trauma and rapidly binds to neural tissue, provoking a characteristic paralysis and spasms (see below). Tetanus is largely a disease of nonimmunized animals and humans, since an effective toxoid has been in use for many years.

The clinical syndrome known as tetanus is an extremely dramatic illness produced by the action of a potent neurotoxin, tetanospasmin, which is elaborated by *C. tetani*. Spasticity is characteristic of tetanus, whereas flaccid paralysis is characteristic of botulism (35). These opposite clinical findings in tetanus and botulism result from the activity of the two toxins in different locations within the nervous system. Tetanospasmin acts within the central nervous system, wheras the activity of BoNT is confined to the peripheral nervous system. Tetanospasmin is synthesized as a single, inactive, polypeptide chain (150 kDa). Upon lysis of *C. tetani*, the toxin is cleaved by an intrinsic protease to produce a dichain, consisting of a heavy chain (100 kDa) and a light chain (50 kDa) linked by a disulfide bond (111). The heavy chain is the part of the molecule that binds to neuronal cells. The light chain, a zinc endopeptidase, binds to protein components of the neuroexocytotic apparatus and thus inhibits the exocytosis of the neurotransmitter (γ-aminobutyric acid in this case) at synapses within the central nervous system (111). Thus, inhibitory impulses to the motor neurons are blocked; uninhibited firing of motor nerve transmissions continues, resulting in prolonged muscle spasms of both flexor and extensor muscles that can persist for weeks. In the United States tetanus is reported most frequently in California, Michigan, Texas, Florida, and other areas of the rural South (67). While most cases involve persons aged ≥60 years, injection of drugs (i.e., "skin popping") has recently become an important risk factor in younger persons (67). It would be unusual for the clinical laboratory to be requested to isolate C. *tetani* from a wound, since tetanus usually presents few diagnostic problems for the clinician.

OTHER CLOSTRIDIAL DISEASES

Clostridium spp. and Bacteremia

At the Indiana University Medical Center (IUMC), where anaerobic blood cultures have remained a standard part of a high-volume blood culture system for many years, approximately 10% of all blood cultures have yielded clinically significant bacteria. Clostridia have usually accounted for about 0.5 to 2% of the significant isolates (4). The species encountered most frequently in positive blood cultures is C. *perfringens*, which usually represents 20 to ≥50% of the *Clostridium* isolates. Other *Clostridium* species found less frequently in positive blood cultures include C. *septicum*, C. *ramosum*, C. *clostridioforme*, C. *difficile*, C. *bifermentans*, C. *sordellii*, C. *tertium*, C. *paraputrificum*, C. *innocuum*, C. *butyricum*, C. *cadaveris*, and C. *sporogenes* (4, 26, 56). Underlying conditions commonly associated with clostridial bacteremia have included chronic alcoholism, sepsis following intra-abdominal surgery, necrosis of the small intestine and large bowel, genitourinary tract disorders (including septic abortions), cardiovascular disease, pulmonary diseases, underlying malignancy, diabetes, and decubitus ulcers (26, 54, 56). Bacteremia involving C. *perfringens* and certain other clostridia is not always associated with a serious underlying illness (54). Isolates are sometimes of doubtful significance or may even represent contaminants. Clostridia of the intestinal flora deposited transiently in the perianal area could be spread to a venipuncture site; alternatively, blood culture isolates could reflect transient bacteremia of no clinical significance.

Additional Clostridial Species of Interest

Numerous other clostridial species are occasionally associated with disease. Species such as C. *novyi*, C. *histolyticum*, C. *bifermentans*, C. *sordellii*, C. *fallax*, C. *sporogenes*, and C. *tertium* have all been associated with histotoxic clostridial disease (see the discussion of C. *perfringens*, above) (42, 120, 131). C. *sordellii* has also been cited as producing a cytotoxin similar to that of C. *difficile* (see the discussion of C. *difficile* above).

COLLECTION, TRANSPORT, AND STORAGE OF CLINICAL SPECIMENS

As with other anaerobic bacteria, the proper selection, collection, and transport of clinical specimens are extremely important for the laboratory diagnosis of clostridial infections. For recommended collection and transport procedures in general, refer to chapter 4. Several tissue specimens should be taken from the active site of infections when gas gangrene is suspected, because clostridia are often not distributed uniformly in pathological lesions. In addition to standard aspirates and tissues, selected clostridial illnesses require special specimens.

Specimens for Confirmation of *C. perfringens* Food-Borne Illness

For a laboratory confirmation of C. *perfringens* food-borne illness, most clinical laboratories need to use the services of a reference laboratory (e.g., local or state public health laboratory [see chapter 10]).

Specimens for *C. difficile* Culture and Toxin Assay

A single, freshly passed fecal specimen (ideally 10 to 20 ml of watery stool; minimum of 5.0 ml or 5 g) is the preferred specimen for C. *difficile* culture and toxin assay (45). To lessen the chance of obtaining positive culture results from patients merely colonized with the organism, we recommend that only liquid or unformed stool specimens be processed. Results of testing solid, formed stools are not likely to contribute to the diagnosis of C. *difficile*-associated disease. An exception could be made for epidemiologic surveys in which the objective is to determine the degree of C. *difficile* carriage in a population. Swab specimens are inadequate for the toxin assay because the volume of sample obtained is too small, although swabs have been used successfully to detect carriers during epidemiologic investigations (93). Other appropriate specimens include lumen contents and surgical or autopsy samples of the large bowel. Specimens should be transported in tightly sealed, leakproof plastic or glass containers. For optimal recovery, stool specimens should be cultured within 2 h of collection; although spores will survive in refrigerated stool for several days, there will probably be a large decrease in the number of viable vegetative cells of C. *difficile* in refrigerated specimens. Stools may be placed in an anaerobic environment (anaerobic transport vial or swab) if culture must be performed after storage. Adequate recovery of C. *difficile* may be expected from stools stored at 5°C for up to 2 days. Specimens for toxin assay may be stored at 5°C for up to 3 days and should be frozen at −70°C if a longer delay before the assay is performed is anticipated. Freezing at −20°C results in a dramatic loss of cytotoxin activity (4, 102).

Specimens for Suspected Neutropenic Enterocolitis Involving *C. septicum*

The specimens of choice for suspected neutropenic enterocolitis involving C. *septicum* are three blood cultures collected from three different venipuncture sites, stool (at least 25 g, or 25 ml if liquid), and lumen contents or tissue from the involved ileocecal area collected at surgery or autopsy and transported in tightly sealed leakproof containers. In addition, a biopsy sample of muscle (or an aspirate of fluid from the involved area, taken with a needle and syringe) should be collected if the patient is also suspected of having myonecrosis.

Specimens for *C. botulinum* Culture and Toxin Assay

The clinical diagnosis of food-borne botulism can be confirmed by the demonstration of BoNT in serum, feces, gastric contents, or vomitus or by the recovery of C. *botulinum* from the feces of the patient. The organism has been isolated only rarely from asymptomatic individuals during food-borne outbreaks (9). The demonstration of botulinal toxin and C. *botulinum* in suspected foods aids in determining the food item responsible for an outbreak, but it provides only indirect evidence to support a clinical diagnosis of botulism. Ideally, 15 to 20 ml of serum (not whole blood), 25 to 50 g of stool, and the suspect food(s) should be collected. Specimens from patients with suspected wound botulism include serum, feces, tissue, exudate, or swab samples from the wound. When infant botulism is suspected, serum (2 ml) and as much stool as possible should be collected. In most instances, the diagnosis of infant botulism has been confirmed by the detection of the toxin or *C. botulinum* or both in feces. Toxin has been detected in serum only infrequently in infants with this diagnosis.

Most hospital laboratories are not properly equipped to process specimens from patients suspected of having botulism. Attending physicians should notify their State Health Department or the CDC immediately when there is a suspected case of botulism so that appropriate action can be taken to establish the diagnosis, initiate treatment, and investigate the potential outbreak. The CDC provides epidemiologic aid and emergency laboratory services 24 h a day every day of the week. The appropriate CDC telephone number (24 h a day) for enteric disease epidemiologic aid is (404) 639-3753.

DIRECT EXAMINATION

The direct microscopic examination of clinical materials can provide extremely useful information for the physician in the diagnosis and treatment of clostridial infections. Gas gangrene is an extremely urgent situation, requiring a rapid clinical diagnosis. The direct examination of a Gram-stained smear of the wound may be of special aid to the clinician in establishing the diagnosis. Characteristic findings are the absence of inflammatory cells and other cellular outlines and the presence of clostridia in smears prepared from the central areas of the lesion. In contrast, nonclostridial anaerobic cellulitis may involve anaerobic cocci, facultatively anaerobic cocci, *Bacteroides* spp., *Fusobacterium* spp., and/or other microbial species. Cell outlines of striated muscle cells and granulocytes remain intact in the latter condition.

The usual Gram stain is satisfactory for the direct examination of a specimen. Special note should be made of gram-positive rods with or without spores, because sporulation in tissue is not common for the two most frequently encountered species in wound and abscess materials, *C. perfringens* and *C. ramosum*. *C. perfringens* usually appears as large, relatively short, fat, gram-positive rods in tissue smears; the cells of *C. ramosum* are more slender and longer (78). *C. perfringens* may or may not be encapsulated in smears from wounds; capsules usually are present in smears of endometrial specimens from postabortion *C. perfringens* infections. Special spore stains offer no advantage over Gram stains for the demonstration of spores. Examination with a phase microscope may be helpful if the spores are close to maturity. If spores are present, their shapes (spherical or oval) and positions (terminal, subterminal, or central) in the cells should be noted. An excellent medium for the demonstration of spores is a chopped-meat agar slant. The culture should be incubated anaerobically at 5 to 7°C below the optimum temperature for growth of clostridia. For most species, 30°C is satisfactory, but 37°C is better for inducing sporulation of *C. perfringens*. If spores are not visible, their presence may he deduced by subjecting a suspension of the isolate to heat (80°C) or ethanol treatment (described below).

CULTURE AND ISOLATION OF CLOSTRIDIA OTHER THAN *C. DIFFICILE*

A summary of useful procedures for culture and isolation of clostridia is provided below. For more detailed information on the topic, the *Clinical Microbiology Procedures Handbook* for anaerobic bacteriology (66), the manual by Summanen et al. (127), and the text by Koneman et al. (78) provide detailed procedures that should be applicable to most clinical situations. Clostridia usually produce good growth on commercially available CDC anaerobe blood agar and phenylethyl alcohol blood agar (PEA) after 1 to 2 days of incubation. Brucella 5% sheep blood agar, Columbia agar, or brain heart infusion agar supplemented with yeast extract, vitamin K, and hemin may also be used as the nonselective blood agar medium; colony characteristics vary on these different media. A few species, such as *C. perfringens*, form colonies after overnight incubation. When clostridia are suspected in wound or abscess specimens (e.g., from gas gangrene), it is recommended that egg yolk agar (modified McClung-Toabe formula) or neomycin egg yolk (NEY) agar be inoculated in addition to blood agar and PEA. Neomycin is added to inhibit some of the facultatively anaerobic gram-negative bacilli; thus, NEY medium is moderately selective.

After incubation, the blood agar and PEA cultures should be examined under a dissecting microscope, with particular note being made of the hemolysis pattern, colony structure, and any evidence of swarming or of motile colonies. Egg yolk agar should be examined for evidence of lecithinase or lipase production. Lecithinase activity is indicated in either medium by the development of an insoluble, opaque, whitish precipitate within the agar. An iridescent sheen or oil-on-water appearance (pearly layer) on the surface growth indicates lipase activity. Proteolysis, the third reaction that can be seen on egg yolk agar, is indicated by a zone of translucent clearing in the medium around the colonies. In addition to the modified McClung-Toabe egg yolk agar formulation, the same reactions can be visualized on the hemin-supplemented egg yolk agar formulation recommended by Summanen et al. (127) or on Lombard-Dowell egg yolk agar (78).

If swarming growth, such as that associated with swarming *Proteus* species, has covered the surface of the agar medium, another blood agar plate should be inoculated and incubated anaerobically for only 18 to 24 h. A subculture from the colonies should be performed as soon as the plates are taken from the anaerobe jar. If swarming is again observed, the isolate should be subcultured to a PEA plate to inhibit swarming. Alternatively, anaerobic blood agar made up with 4% (or higher-concentration) agar may be useful. This mixture is known as stiff blood agar (36). When isolated colonies can be picked, they should be subcultured to chopped-meat medium, and the culture should be incubated overnight and used for the inoculation of differential media. In addition, chopped-meat-carbohydrate broth (65) should be inoculated for gas-liquid chromatography.

Spore Selection Techniques

The treatment of specimens with heat (80°C) or ethanol aids in isolating clostridia from highly contaminated specimens (79). These procedures are commonly used in public health laboratories for the selective isolation of *C. botulinum* and *C. perfringens* from feces and foods (36, 62). In hospital microbiology laboratories, these techniques can aid in the isolation of *C. difficile* from feces and are less costly than cycloserine-cefoxitin-fructose agar (CCFA) medium (91).

They can also save time in isolation of clostridia from other kinds of specimens containing a mixture of microorganisms (e.g., wounds and abscesses) (78). Ethanol may be more effective than heat if the specimen contains relatively heat-sensitive clostridia (e.g., *C. botulinum* type E and some strains of *C. perfringens* involved in food-borne outbreaks) (79). Heat treatment may be more effective than alcohol if homogenization is incomplete and the specimen contains particulate matter that is not penetrated adequately by the alcohol. For any spore selection technique, an untreated control subculture should be prepared.

Alcohol Treatment

To a 1-ml sample of a fecal suspension, homogenate of a wound or exudate, etc., in a sterile screw-cap tube is added an equal volume of absolute (or 95%) ethanol (79). The specimen is mixed gently at room temperature (22 to 25°C for 1 h). An Ames aliquot mixer (Miles Laboratories, Inc., Elkhart, Ind.) is a convenient way to provide continuous mixing. The treated material is subcultured and used to inoculate chopped-meat–glucose (or chopped-meat–glucose–starch) medium, anaerobe blood agar, or egg yolk agar. The culture is incubated and inspected for growth. For stool specimens, it is often advantageous to perform the alcohol treatment with separate 1-ml samples from a series of 1:10 dilutions. This treatment helps the alcohol penetrate solid particles.

Heat Treatment

For heat treatment (36), a tube of chopped-meat–glucose–starch medium is preheated in an 80°C water bath for 5 min and 1 ml of sample suspension is added. The culture is heated for 10 min, and the tube is removed and cooled in cold water. The treated sample suspension is subcultured into an unheated tube of chopped-meat–glucose–starch medium and onto an anaerobe blood agar and egg yolk agar plate. The culture is incubated anaerobically and examined for growth.

Tests (Including Culture) for Diagnosis of *C. difficile* Disease

There are multiple methods for the detection of *C. difficile* and its toxins (Table 3). Controversy exists about which detection method or combination of methods is optimal. Toxin detection and neutralization by a tissue culture cytotoxin assay is often considered the "gold standard" when new detection methods are evaluated. Toxigenic culture, however, tests *C. difficile* isolates for toxin production and has higher sensitivity and equivalent specificity compared to the cytotoxicity assay (39, 104, 114, 124). In studies designed to evaluate the diagnostic utility of detection methods, a confirmed diagnosis of *C. difficile*-associated diarrhea (CDAD) on the basis of both clinical and laboratory criteria probably represents the ultimate gold standard.

Toxigenic culture, although it can require 3 to 4 days, may be the most reliable test for the diagnosis of CDAD (39, 103, 104, 114). Direct stool cytotoxin neutralization assays have not detected toxin in as many as 15 to 38% of patients with confirmed CDAD (39, 124). Unfortunately, some patients, without positive direct stool cytotoxin assay results, have progressed to pseudomembranous colitis and some of these have died (39, 83).

It is important to note that culture alone (without subsequent testing of all *C. difficile* isolates for toxin production) leads to lower specificity and misdiagnosis of CDAD when high background rates of asymptomatic *C. difficile* carriage exist. This situation has led some investigators to conclude that cytotoxicity assays are more specific than culture and that culture should not be used as a means of detecting *C. difficile* in patients with CDAD (57). However, for properly performed toxigenic culture, this conclusion does not hold.

To perform a toxigenic culture, a stool specimen or fecal swab should be inoculated directly onto CCFA (containing 500 μg of cycloserine) with horse blood (91). Commercially available CCFA with the recommended horse blood formulation (Remel, Lenexa, Kans.) has performed satisfactorily in our laboratory. The plates should be incubated anaerobically at 35 to 37°C for 18 to 24 h before observation. Following incubation, the use of a dissecting microscope is strongly recommended to select colonies of *C. difficile* for toxin analysis (78, 91, 104). Colonies of *C. difficile* are yellowish to white, circular to irregular, and flat, with a rhizoid or erose edge and a ground-glass appearance. The colonies have a distinctive odor like *p*-cresol (or horse manure). By using the dissecting microscope, four to six colonies with characteristics of *C. difficile* should be subcultured to chopped-meat carbohydrate or brain heart infusion broth and incubated anaerobically at 35 to 37°C for 24 h. Isolates are tested for in vitro toxin production by performing a cytotoxin assay on filtered 24-h broths. Because *C. difficile* recovery rates vary significantly when media from different manufacturers are used (91), the importance of appropriate quality control of commercially prepared CCFA cannot be overemphasized.

In addition to the use of CCFA medium, *C. difficile* from fecal samples can be isolated by using an alcohol or heat shock spore selection technique, as described above. If a spore selection technique is used, the alcohol- or heat-treated sample is inoculated onto anaerobe blood agar after treatment. After 18 to 24 h of incubation, colonies on anaerobe blood agar are nonhemolytic, 2 to 4 mm in diameter, creamy yellow to grey-white, and irregular, have a coarsely mottled to mosaic internal structure and a matte or dull surface, and are slightly raised when viewed under a dissecting microscope. The odor remains distinctive. Gram stain of *C. difficile* reveals gram-positive to gram-variable rods that are thin, even sided, and 0.5 μm wide by 3 to 5 μm long. If spores are present, they are subterminal. As described above (for CCFA), isolates obtained by a spore selection technique should also be tested for in vitro toxin production.

Presumptive identification of *C. difficile* can be made by demonstrating typical colonies, Gram stain morphology, and characteristic odor. Definitive identification depends on demonstration of the unique pattern of short-chain fatty acid metabolic products by gas-liquid chromatography (Table 4) and by biochemical characterization of isolates (38, 65, 78, 127).

Commercially available cytotoxin neutralization assays, including the *Clostridium difficile* TOX-B test (TechLab, Blacksburg, Va.) and the Bartels cytotoxicity assay (Bartels, Inc., Issaquah, Wash.), are designed to detect toxin B (2). Toxin neutralization assays are highly specific because parallel tests of a patient's stool sample are run with specific antisera, which neutralizes any toxin-mediated cytotoxic effect. No standards or National Committee for Clinical Laboratory Standards (NCCLS) guidelines exist for performing the cytotoxin neutralization assay (57). An accurate cytotoxin neutralization assay result, and hence an accurate comparison to other detection methods such as toxigenic culture, depends on multiple factors including specimen centrifugation, cell line, and the subjective interpretation of cytopathic effect (112). Submitting two additional stool specimens from patients suspected of having CDAD in-

TABLE 3 Methods and tests for the detection of *C. difficile* and its toxins

Method	Entity detected	Advantages	Limitations	Available tests and sources
Toxigenic culture	Organism	Most sensitive, specific	Efficiency varies from lab to lab, use of stereomicroscope recommended	CCFA with horse blood preferred; 500 μg of cycloserine and prereduction of medium increases the isolation rate of *C. difficile* (Remel, Lenexa, Kans.)
Latex agglutination	Glutamate dehydrogenase	Rapid, simple	Not extremely sensitive, does not distinguish between toxigenic and nontoxigenic strains of *C. difficile*	CDT (Becton Dickinson Microbiology Systems, Sparks, Md.) Meritec *C. difficile* (Meridian Diagnostics, Inc., Cincinnati, Ohio)
EIA	Glutamate dehydrogenase	Rapid, simple	More sensitive than latex agglutination, does not distinguish between toxigenic and nontoxigenic strains of *C. difficile*	ImmunoCard *C. difficile* (Meridian Diagnostics, Inc., Cincinnati, Ohio) Triage *C. difficile* panel (Biosite Diagnostics, Inc., San Diego, Calif.)
Tissue culture	Toxin B	Sensitive, specific	Most assays require 24–48 h to complete; Toxin B can be inactivated, resulting in false-negative results	*C. difficile* Tox-B Test (TechLab, Inc., Blacksburg, Va.) *C. difficile* Tox-B Test (Biowhittaker, Inc., Walkersville, Md.) *C. difficile* Toxititer (Bartels, Inc., Issaguah, Wash.) Cytoxi (Advanced Clinical Diagnostics, Toledo, Ohio)
EIA	Toxin A	Rapid, simple, specific	Some kits have higher sensitivity than others, some kits may yield indeterminant readings	*C. difficile* Toxin A (Oxoid, Inc., Ogdensburg, N.Y.) CD-Tox (Porton, Cambridge, England) Difco Cube Test (Difco, Detroit, Mich.) Premier (Meridian Diagnostics, Inc., Cincinnati, Ohio) Prospect II *C. difficile* Toxin A microplate (Alexon-Trend, Sunnyvale, Calif.) Tox A (Biowhittaker, Inc., Walkersville, Md.) Tox-A Test (TechLab, Inc., Blacksburg, Va.) Toxin A EIA (Bartels, Inc., Issaguah, Wash.) Toxin CD Test (Becton Dickinson Microbiology Systems, Sparks, Md.) Triage *C. difficile* panel (Biosite Diagnostics, Inc., San Diego, Calif.) VIDAS-CDA (bioMerieux Vitek, Hazelwood, Mo.)
EIA	Toxins A and B	Rapid, simple, specific		*C. difficile* Tox-A/B Test (TechLab, Inc., Blacksburg, Va.) Cd Toxin A + B (Rohm Pharma, Darmstadt, Germany) Premier Cytoclone (Meridian Diagnostics, Inc., Cincinnati, Ohio)

TABLE 4 Differential characteristics of commonly encountered clostridia[a]

Species	Spores	Egg yolk agar		Growth on aerobic blood agar	Gelatin hydrolysis	Milk digestion	Indole production	Carbohydrate fermentation						Principal metabolic products on PYG or CMC	Other	Cellular fatty acids[b]
		LEC	LIP					Glucose	Maltose	Lactose	Sucrose	Salicin	Manitol			
C. bifermentans	OS	+	–	–	+	+	+	+	w/–	–	–	–	–	A, (p), (ib), (b), (iv), (ic)	Urease negative	16:0, 18:1*cis* 9, 19cyc9, 10/:1
C. botulinum[c]																
Group I[d]	OS	–	+	–	+	+	–	+	–/w	–	–	–	–	A, (p), ib, B, IV, (v), (ic)		14:0, 16:0, 18:1*cis* 9, 18:1*cis* 9dma
Group II[d]	OS	–/+	+	–	+	+	–/+	+	V	–	–	–	–	A, P, B, (v)		14:0, 16:0, 18:1*cis* 9
Group III[d]	OS	–	+	–	+	–	–	+	+/w	–	+/w	–	–	A, B		14:0, 16:0, 18:1*cis* 9
C. butyricum	OS	–	–	–	–	–	–	+	+	+	+	+	–/+	A, B		16:0, 18:1*cis* 9
C. cadaveris	OT	–	–	–	+	+	+	+	–	–	–	–	–	A, (p), B (from PY = A, p, ib, v, iv)		14:0, 16:0, 18:1*cis* 9
C. chauvoei[e]	OS	–	–	–	+	–	–	+	+/w	+/w	+/w	–	–	A, B		14:0, 16:0, 18:1*cis* 9
C. clostridioforme	OS	–	–	–	–	–	–/+	+	+/w	+/–	–	+/–	–	A	Spores seldom observed; usually gram negative	16:0, 18:1*cis* 11dma
C. difficile	OS	–	–	–	+	–	–	+	–	–	–	–/w	+/–	A, (p), ib, B, iv, (v), ic		16:0, 16:0dma, 18:1*cis* 9, 19cyc 9, 10/:1
C. histolyticum	OS	–	–	V	+	+	–	–	–	–	–	–	–	A	Aerotolerant	14:0, 16:0, 18:1*cis* 9, 18:1cis 9dma
C. innocuum[f]	OT	–	–	–	–	–	–	+	–	–	+	+	+	A, B		16:0, 18:1*cis* 9
C. limosum	OS	+	–	–	+	+	–	–	–	–	–	–	–	A		12:0, 18:1*cis* 9, 18:1*cis* 9dma

C. *novyi* A	OS	+	+	−	+	−	−	+	V	−	−	−/+	−	A, P, B		14:0, 18:1*cis* 9, 18:1*cis* 9dma
C. *novyi* B	OS	+	−	−	+	+	+/−	+	V	−	−	−	−	A, P, B		14:0, 15:0, 16:0, 18:1*cis* 9
C. *paraputrificum*	OT	−	−	−	−	−	−	+	+	+	+	+	−	A, B		16:0, 18:1*cis* 9, 18:1*cis* 9dma
C. *perfringens*[f]	OS	+	−	−	+	+	−	+	+	+	+	−	−	A, (p), B	Spores seldom observed; double zone of hemolysis	12:0, 14:0
C. *ramosum*[f]	R/OT	−	−	−	−	−	−	+	+	+	+	+	+/−	A	Spores seldom observed; Frequently gram negative	16:0, 16:0dma, 18:1*cis* 9
C. *septicum*	OS	−	−	−	+	+	−	+	+	+	−	V	−	A, (p), B	Spreading colony	14:0, 16:0, 18:1*cis* 9
C. *sordellii*	OS	+	−	−	+	+	+	+	w/+	−	−	−	−	A, (p), (ib), (iv), (ic)	Usually urease positive	18:1*cis* 9, 19cyc 9, 10/:1
C. *sphenoides*	RS/T	−	−	−	−	−	−	+	+	w/+	w/−	w/+	w/+	A	Usually gram negative	16:0, 18:1*cis* 11dma
C. *sporogenes*	OS	−	+	−	+	+	−	+	−/w	−	−	−	−	A, (p), ib, B, iv, (v), (ic)		14:0, 16:0, 18:1*cis* 9
C. *subterminale*	OS	−/+	−	−	+	+	−	−	−	−	−	−	−	A, (p), ib, B, IV, (ic)		16:0, 18:1cis 9, 18:1*cis* 9dma
C. *tertium*	OT	−	−	+	−	−	−	+	+	+	+	+	+/w	A, B	Aerotolerant	14:0, 16:0, 18:1*cis* 9
C. *tetani*	RT	−	−	−	+	+/−	V	−	−	−	−	−	−	A, p, B		14:0, 18:1*cis* 9, 18:1*cis* 9dma

[a] Based on the use of PRAS media as described by Holdeman et al. (65). Key: +, positive reaction; −, negative reaction; V, variable reaction; w, weak reaction; /, either/or; O, oval; R, round; S, subterminal; T, terminal; LEC, lecithinase production; LIP, lipase production. Fermentation products: A, acetate; B, butyrate; F, formate; IB, isobutyrate; IC, isocaproate; IV, isovalerate; P, propionate; V, valerate. Parentheses indicate may or may not be present. Capital letters indicate major peaks; lowercase letters indicate minor peaks. PYG, peptone-yeast extract-glucose medium; CMC, chopped-meat–carbohydrate medium.

[b] Major fatty acid methyl esters (FAME) are listed. Data derived from the Moore database Version 3.9, September 1995, Sherlock, Microbial Identification System, MIDI, Inc., Newark, DE 19713.

[c] Group I contains proteolytic strains (A,B, and F); group II contains types C and D; and group III contains saccharolytic strains (B,E, and F).

[d] Toxin neutralization test required for identification.

[e] Pathogenic for herbivores.

[f] C. *innocuum*, C. *perfringens*, and C. *ramosum* are nonmotile.

creases toxin detection by only 10% (15). Because of the lower sensitivity of the cytotoxin neutralization assays, toxigenic culture should remain an option for the diagnostic evaluation of some patients with CDAD (39, 47, 104, 114).

Multiple enzyme immunoassays (EIAs) have been introduced by various manufacturers for detection of toxin A and/or toxin B in stool. Despite extensive testing, relatively few studies have compared EIAs to toxigenic culture in patients with confirmed CDAD. A review of the literature which summarized comparative studies for eight commercial EIA kits reported that the sensitivity and specificity ranged from 34 to 100% and 88 to 100%, respectively (57).

An EIA that detects glutamate dehydrogenase has been developed as a screening test for detecting *C. difficile* in stool specimens from patients with CDAD (124). The test exhibited a sensitivity and specificity of 74 to 88% and 95 to 100%, respectively, for patients meeting certain criteria for CDAD (17, 107, 124). When compared to the cytotoxicity assay alone (107, 124) or in combination with other toxin-specific EIAs (50), the sensitivity and specificity were 84 to 92% and 96 to 100%, respectively. The test is rapid to perform (15 to 20 min) and approaches the accuracy of cytotoxin neutralization assays and toxin-specific EIAs. A latex agglutination assay for glutamate dehydrogenase has also been developed, but it lacks sensitivity compared to the EIA for this enzyme (57).

PCR can detect the presence of *C. difficile* and differentiate between toxigenic and nontoxigenic strains, but lack of commercial kits and equipment has limited its use (45, 47). A single step assay which combines toxin gene detection and molecular typing has been developed (110).

Laboratory Investigation of *C. perfringens* Food-Borne Illness

Methods for the enumeration of *C. perfringens* in foods and *C. perfringens* spores in feces with egg yolk-free tryptose-sulfite-cycloserine agar are described in detail by Hauschild (63). Although methods for the detection of *C. perfringens* enterotoxin in feces have been described previously and are of considerable interest, these assays are still considered experimental and are generally not used in clinical laboratories, except in research settings (90, 113).

IDENTIFICATION OF CLOSTRIDIA OTHER THAN *C. DIFFICILE*

A number of strategies are available for the phenotypic characterization and identification of clostridia (36, 38, 65, 78, 127). One of the traditional methods has included the use of prereduced anaerobically sterilized (PRAS) media for the determination of fermentation profiles and other characteristics. To identify clostridia by this method, tubes of the PRAS media (available commercially, as listed in Table 4), prepared as described by Holdeman et al. (65), are inoculated. Although the CHO-based media of Dowell and Hawkins provide an excellent system for characterizing clostridia and can be used, Table 4 is based on results obtained with PRAS media, and a few of the reactions differ. Thus, if CHO-based media are used, the CDC publications on anaerobic bacteriology should be consulted (36). The cultures are incubated for 24 to 72 h at 35 to 37°C; overnight incubation is often sufficient for most clostridia because they grow rapidly. Gram stains of the chopped-meat culture are examined to determine the presence, positions, and shapes of the spores. If spores are not found, a tube of chopped-meat medium is inoculated, the culture is heated at 70°C for 10 min, and the tube is incubated. Growth in this heated tube usually indicates the presence of spores, although none may be apparent microscopically. Alternatively, an alcohol spore selection technique may be helpful for clostridia with heat-sensitive spores (79).

The presence of carbohydrate fermentation can be determined by measuring the pH (65). The metabolic products from chopped-meat–carbohydrate broth culture are determined by gas liquid chromatography (see chapter 11 of this Manual and reference 127 or 78). The results will not be identical if peptone-yeast extract-glucose is the culture medium (36, 65). In addition, analyses of cellular fatty acids are practical, accurate, and sensitive methods for characterization of isolates that simplify the identification of clostridia (Table 4) (6). The identification of *Clostridium* species can be made without the analyses of either metabolic products or cellular fatty acids, but such identification usually involves more time. The information listed in Table 4 will serve to identify most of the *Clostridium* species commonly isolated from clinical specimens. Information on additional tests and descriptions of differential characteristics of additional species can be found elsewhere (28, 36, 38, 62, 65, 78, 120, 127). In the current era of managed competition and ever-increasing budget tightening, there has been increasing interest in finding less costly alternatives to conventional identification procedures.

A number of commercial packaged kits have been marketed for the rapid identification of anaerobes; these are described in detail in the *Clinical Microbiology Procedures Handbook* (66). In general, Gram reaction, cellular morphology, colony characteristics, and aerotolerance of isolates should always be determined in conjunction with these packaged microsystems. When the kits are used to identify the clostridia, the results are incorrect relatively frequently (5, 18). Two of the more commonly encountered clostridia, *C. perfringens* and *C. ramosum*, were accurately identified with the RapID-ANA II (Innovative Diagnostic Systems, Inc., Atlanta, Ga.), but identifications were less likely to be correct for other common species (e.g., *C. difficile*, *C. innocuum*, and *C. clostridioforme*) (92). Similarly, the BBL Crystal anaerobe identification system (Becton Dickinson, Cockeysville, Md.) correctly identified 76.7% of *Clostridium* strains but did not identify any of the strains of *C. innocuum*, *C. sporogenes*, or *C. tetani* that were tested; in addition, some strains of *C. septicum* and *C. difficile* required retesting to achieve correct identifications (30). Another kit, the AN-Ident (bioMérieux Vitek, Hazelwood, Mo.), identified 98% of 53 *C. perfringens* and 100% of 20 *C. difficile* isolates correctly, but data were lacking with regard to the accuracy of this product for many other species that were not tested, including *C. septicum*, *C. clostridioforme*, and *C. innocuum* (106). Commercial packaged kits are not without significant costs, especially if clostridia other than *C. perfringens* are to be identified (18).

Presumptive Identification of Commonly Encountered Clostridia

Simplified flowcharts for presumptive identification of anaerobes by using minimal resources were devised recently by Baron and Citron (18). Somewhat different approaches and schema for the relatively low-cost presumptive identification of anaerobes have been described elsewhere (78, 127). The first 12 species listed in Table 1 represent 95% of all the *Clostridium* organisms isolated at the IUMC Anaerobe Lab. Some key characteristics that aid in the presumptive identification of these most common species, without the use of gas-liquid chromatography, commercial packaged kits, or other costly resources, are listed below. Based on their ability to hydrolyze gelatin, these 12 species can be divided into two groups: proteolytic (gelatin hydrolysis positive) and nonproteolytic (gelatin hydrolysis negative).

Proteolytic Group

- *C. perfringens*—double zone of hemolysis, boxcar-shaped rods, spores rare, lecithinase positive. *C. baratii* mimics these characteristics but does not hydrolyze gelatin.
- *C. difficile*—creamy-yellow to grey-white, irregular, coarse mottled to mosaic internal structure, matte or dull surface; subterminal to free spores or spores infrequent, gelatin hydrolysis can be slow for half the strains, mannitol positive.
- *C. cadaveris*—white-grey, entire to slightly irregular, raised to slightly convex; oval terminal spores, spot indole positive, DNase positive.
- *C. sporogenes*—medusa-head colonies, possible swarmer; subterminal and many free spores, lipase positive.
- *C. bifermentans*—grey-white, irregular, scalloped edge; many free spores often chaining, urease negative, indole and lecithinase positive. *C. sordellii* is similar but is urease positive.
- *C. septicum*—swarms, subterminal spores often "citron" forms, DNase positive, sucrose negative.

Nonproteolytic Group

- *C. clostridioforme*—colonies resemble *Bacteroides fragilis* but usually have a slightly irregular edge, gram negative, football shaped; spores are rare.
- *C. innocuum*—grey-white to brilliant greenish, coarsely mottled to mosaic internal structure; terminal spores may be difficult to find, nonmotile, mannitol positive, lactose and maltose negative.
- *C. ramosum*—colonies resemble *Bacteroides fragilis* but usually have a slight irregular edge; gram-variable, palisading, slender rods, nonmotile, mannitol positive.
- *C. butyricum*—very large irregular, mottled to mosaic internal structure, subterminal spores, ferments many carbohydrates.
- *C. tertium*—aerotolerant, terminal spores from anaerobically incubated media only.
- *C. glycolicum*—grey-white, entire to scalloped edge, convex; subterminal and free spores, DNase positive.

Toxin tests are necessary for the identification of a few species (36, 62, 120). *C. sporogenes* cannot be differentiated with certainty from the proteolytic group I strains of *C. botulinum* unless toxin tests are used. A few strains of group III *C. botulinum* produce lecithinase as well as lipase and are difficult to distinguish from *C. novyi* type A except by toxin tests or by the use of a *C. novyi* fluorescent-antibody conjugate (120). To test for toxin, the following procedure is used. Two tubes of chopped-meat–glucose medium are inoculated. One tube is incubated at 37°C overnight, and the other tube is incubated at 37°C for 3 days. If no toxin is found in the overnight culture, the 3-day culture is tested. The culture is centrifuged, and 1.2-ml volumes of the supernatant are placed in several tubes. Appropriate antiserum (0.3 ml) is added per tube for the various species suspected. The well-mixed suspensions are allowed to stand for 30 min at room temperature or at 37°C, and then 0.5-ml portions of control supernatant (without antiserum) and antiserum mixtures are injected intraperitoneally into each of two mice. The mice are observed for 3 days, and any deaths are recorded. Only specific sera for laboratory testing should be used for toxin identification; therapeutic sera are often unsatisfactory because they may contain antibodies to toxins of species other than those listed on the label. An excellent source of diagnostic clostridial antisera is TechLab. The analysis of cellular fatty acids provides a supplement to the methods described above, since the various types of *C. botulinum* can be presumptively identified on the basis of differences in their cellular fatty acid profiles (Table 4) (6, 48).

SUSCEPTIBILITY TO ANTIMICROBIAL AGENTS

Penicillin G shows excellent activity against most but not all strains of *C. perfringens* and has traditionally been considered the antibiotic of choice for the clostridia in general (109). However, resistance among *C. perfringens* isolates is increasing to the extent that alternative antimicrobial agents may have to be considered (78). β-Lactamase has not been demonstrated in *C. perfringens*. Resistance to penicillin in *C. perfringens* involves a decreased affinity of penicillin-binding protein I for penicillin (64). Resistance to penicillin is especially common in *C. ramosum*, *C. clostridioforme*, and *C. butyricum* (41, 109); these species produce β-lactamases that are induced by β-lactam antibiotics (64). *C. tertium* is also resistant to β-lactam antibiotics and is a bit unusual among the clostridia in that it also is resistant to metronidazole and clindamycin (54, 122).

Although clindamycin is still highly active against many species of commonly encountered anaerobic bacteria in the United States, a number of clostridial species are frequently resistant to it. Resistance to this antibiotic occurs in some strains of *C. ramosum*, *C. difficile*, *C. tertium*, *C. subterminale*, *C. innocuum*, *C. sporogenes*, and *C. perfringens* (130).

Chloramphenicol, piperacillin, metronidazole, imipenem, and combinations of β-lactam drugs with β-lactam inhibitors (e.g., ampicillin-sulbactam) are active against nearly all of the clostridia, with only a few exceptions (54, 78). The clostridia have shown variable resistance to the cephalosporins and tetracyclines, and they are usually resistant to the aminoglycosides. Many clostridia other than *C. perfringens* are resistant to cefoxitin, cefotaxime, ceftazidime, ceftizoxime, cefoperazone, and other broad-spectrum β-lactam drugs (41, 78, 109). In general, anaerobes are considered to be resistant to the quinolone agents, and the quinolones have not been recommended for treatment of mixed infections involving anaerobes, including those involving the clostridia. However, trovafloxacin, a new trifluoronaphthyridone agent introduced recently, is much more active than ciprofloxacin against a number of anaerobes (1). Although trovafloxacin appears promising, further data are needed relative to its activity against the clostridia.

Severe *C. difficile*-associated intestinal disease is usually treated with oral vancomycin or metronidazole, although most strains of *C. difficile* are susceptible to a number of antimicrobial agents in vitro (including penicillins, tetracycline, and quinolones). For patients unable to tolerate oral antibiotics but requiring therapy, parenteral vancomycin or metronidazole has been recommended (43). Antibiotic therapy often results in relapse of disease, so that discontinuation of the offending agent or change to an agent less likely to cause diarrhea should be considered the primary intervention of choice (43). A current concern about the use of vancomycin is the emergence of vancomycin-resistant enterococci (VRE) (112), coupled with the demonstration that VRE can transfer resistance into clostridia via plasmids (104). Thus, the use of oral vancomycin is being restricted in most hospitals because of concerns about VRE.

INTERPRETATION OF RESULTS

In decision-making about whether to implement *C. difficile* EIA toxin testing in the laboratory, the laboratory director is faced with the need to evaluate the merits of each EIA kit on an individual basis. EIAs provide same-day test results and acceptable specificity, but slightly lower sensitivities are commonly reported compared to those of toxigenic culture or cytotoxicity assays (16, 34, 47, 57). EIAs should not be relied upon as the sole laboratory test for *C. difficile* toxin. However, an EIA which detects both toxin A and toxin B may be optimal since *C. difficile* producing only toxin B has been isolated from a patient whose clinical history was consistent with CDAD (89). Such isolates would be missed by EIAs which test for toxin A only. Currently, the detection either of toxigenic *C. difficile* or of toxin(s) A and/or B in feces of patients with appropriate clinical findings is needed for the diagnosis of CDAD (47, 104). Reliable and timely results can be provided by culturing for the organism and performing a rapid EIA directly on the stool. If *C. difficile* is isolated but the toxin assay performed directly on feces is negative, *C. difficile* could be tested for toxin if warranted clinically.

The decision about which of the various test strategies available for the detection of *C. difficile* and its toxins should be chosen for an individual laboratory is the responsibility of the laboratory director. The Shea Position Paper provides an excellent review of the advantages and disadvantages of the different diagnostic procedures (47). For smaller laboratories without anaerobic chambers, incubation of the recommended formulation of prereduced CCFA in anaerobic jars, bags, and pouches provides acceptable recovery (40). New and easy-to-use anaerobic incubation systems which do not require the addition of water or a catalyst have recently been introduced (37). As described above, quality control of media and use of a stereomicroscope are essential for accurate isolation and identification of *C. difficile*. EIAs can be performed on isolates to detect toxin production and provide same-day results. Commercially available cytotoxin neutralization assays may provide a low-cost alternative to the more expensive EIAs, but they have a longer turnaround time and require experienced personnel for interpretation. Screening tests for glutamate dehydrogenase produced by *C. difficile* may allow rapid preliminary identification in nosocomial outbreaks and epidemiological investigations.

REFERENCES

1. **Aldridge, K. E., D. Ashcraft, and K. A. Bowman.** 1997. Comparative in vitro activities of trovafloxacin (CP 99, 219) and other antimicrobials against clinically significant anaerobes. *Antimicrob. Agents Chemother.* **41:**484–487.
2. **Allen, S., J. Siders, M. Riddell, J. Fill, and Y. Grant.** 1994. Comparison of the TechLab TOX-B Test for the detection of *Clostridium difficile* toxin with the Bartels Cytotoxicity Assay and culture for toxigenic *C. difficile*, abstr. C-6, p. 491. *In Abstracts of the 94th General Meeting of the American Society for Microbiology 1994*. American Society for Microbiology, Washington, D.C.
3. **Allen, S. D.** 1997. Pig-bel and other necrotizing disorders of the gut involving *Clostridium perfringens*, p. 717–724. *In* D. H. Connor, F. W. Chandler, D. A. Schwartz, H. J. Manz, and E. E. Lack (ed.), *Pathology of Infectious Diseases*. Appleton & Lange, Norwalk, Conn.
4. **Allen, S. D., and J. A. Siders.** 1998. Unpublished data.
5. **Allen, S. D., J. A. Siders, and L. M. Marler.** 1995. Current issues and problems in dealing with anaerobes in the clinical laboratory. *Clin. Lab. Med.* **15:**333–364.
6. **Allen, S. D., J. A. Siders, M. J. Riddell, J. A. Fill, and W. S. Wegener.** 1995. Cellular fatty acid analysis in the differentiation of *Clostridium* in the clinical microbiology laboratory. *Clin. Infect. Dis.* **20:**S198–S201.
7. **Altemeier, W. A., and W. R. Culbertson.** 1948. Acute non-clostridial crepitant cellulitis. *Surg. Gynecol. Obstet.* **87:**206–212.
8. **Altemeier, W. A., and W. L. Furste.** 1947. Gas gangrene. *Surg. Gynecol. Obstet.* **84:**507–523.
9. **Anonymous.** 1979. *Botulism in the United States, 1899–1977. Handbook for Epidemiologists, Clinicians and Laboratory Workers*. Center for Disease Control, Atlanta, Ga.
10. **Anonymous.** 1983. *Foodborne Disease Outbreaks Annual Summary—1980*. Centers for Disease Control, Atlanta, Ga.
11. **Arnon, S. S.** 1997. Human tetanus and human botulism, p. 95–115. *In* J. I. Rood, B. A. McClane, J. G. Songer, and R. W. Titball (ed.), *The Clostridia: Molecular Biology and Pathogenesis*. Academic Press, Inc., New York, N.Y.
12. **Arnon, S. S.** 1989. Infant botulism, p. 601–609. *In* S. M. Finegold and W. L. George (ed.), *Anaerobic Infections in Humans*. Academic Press, Inc., New York, N.Y.
13. **Arnon, S. S., K. Damus, and J. Chin.** 1981. Infant botulism: epidemiology and relation to sudden infant death syndrome. *Epidemiol. Rev.* **3:**45–66.
14. **Aronsson, B., R. Mollby, and C. E. Nord.** 1985. Antimicrobial agents and *Clostridium difficile* in acute enteric disease: epidemiological data from Sweden, 1980–1982. *J. Infect. Dis.* **151:**476–481.
15. **Aronsson, B., R. Mollby, and C. E. Nord.** 1984. Diagnosis and epidemiology of *Clostridium difficile* enterocolitis in Sweden. *J. Antimicrob. Chemother.* **14:**85–95.
16. **Barbut, F., C. Kajzer, N. Planas, and J.-C. Petit.** 1993. Comparison of three enzyme immunoassays, a cytotoxicity assay, and toxigenic culture for diagnosis of *Clostridium difficile*-associated diarrhea. *J. Clin. Microbiol.* **31:**963–967.
17. **Barbut, F., M. Mace, V. Lalande, P. Tilleul, and J.-C. Petit.** 1997. Clinical evaluation of the ImmunoCard Toxin A for the rapid diagnosis of *Clostridium difficile*-associated diarrhea, abstr. C-261, p. 166. *In Abstracts of the 97th General Meeting of the American Society for Microbiology 1997*. American Society for Microbiology, Washington, D.C.
18. **Baron, E. J., and D. M. Citron.** 1997. Anaerobic identification flowchart using minimal laboratory resources. *Clin. Infect. Dis.* **25:**S143–S146.
19. **Bartlett, J. G.** 1994. *Clostridium difficile:* history of its role as an enteric pathogen and the current state of knowledge about the organism. *Clin. Infect. Dis.* **18:**S265–S272.
20. **Bean, N. H., J. S. Goulding, C. Lao, and F. J. Angulo.** 1996. Surveillance for foodborne-disease outbreaks—United States, 1988–1992. *Morbid. Mortal. Weekly Rep. CDC Surveill. Summ.* **45:**1–66.
21. **Bennion, R. S., E. J. Baron, J. E. Thompson, Jr., J. Downes, P. Summanen, D. A. Talan, and S. M. Finegold.** 1990. The bacteriology of gangrenous and perforated appendicitis—revisited. *Ann. Surg.* **211:**165–171.
22. **Bignold, L. P., and H. P. Harvey.** 1979. Necrotising enterocolitis associated with invasion by *Clostridium septicum* complicating cyclic neutropaenia. *Aust. N. Z. J. Med.* **9:** 426–429.
23. **Bodey, G. P., S. Rodriguez, V. Fainstein, and L. S. Elting.**

1991. Clostridial bacteremia in cancer patients. A 12-year experience. *Cancer* **67:**1928–1942.

24. **Borriello, S. P., F. E. Barclay, A. R. Welch, M. F. Stringer, G. N. Watson, R. K. Williams, D. V. Seal, and K. Sullens.** 1985. Epidemiology of diarrhoea caused by enterotoxigenic *Clostridium perfringens*. *J. Med. Microbiol.* **20:** 363–372.
25. **Borriello, S. P., B. W. Wren, S. Hyde, S. V. Seddon, P. Sibbons, M. M. Krishna, S. Tabaqchali, S. Manek, and A. B. Price.** 1992. Molecular, immunological, and biological characterization of a toxin A-negative, toxin B-positive strain of *Clostridium difficile*. *Infect. Immun.* **60:**4192–4199.
26. **Brook, I.** 1989. Anaerobic bacterial bacteremia: 12-year experience in two military hospitals. *J. Infect. Dis.* **160:** 1071–1075.
27. **Bryant, A. E., and D. L. Stevens.** 1997. The pathogenesis of gas gangrene, p. 185–196. *In* J. I. Rood, B. A. McClane, J. G. Songer, and R. W. Titball (ed.), *The Clostridia: Molecular Biology and Pathogenesis*. Academic Press, Inc., New York, N.Y.
28. **Cato, E. P., W. L. George, and S. M. Finegold.** 1986. Genus *Clostridium* Prazmowski 1880, 23^{AL}, p. 1141–1200. *In* P. H. A. Sneath, N. S. Mair, M. E. Sharpe, and J. G. Holt (ed.), *Bergey's Manual of Systematic Bacteriology*, vol. 2. The Williams & Wilkins Co., Baltimore, Md.
29. **Cato, E. P., and E. Stackebrandt.** 1989. Taxonomy and phylogeny, p. 1–26. *In* N. P. Minton and D. J. Clark (ed.), *Clostridia*. Plenum Press, New York, N.Y.
30. **Cavallaro, J. J., L. S. Wiggs, and J. M. Miller.** 1997. Evaluation of the BBL Crystal Anaerobe identification system. *J. Clin. Microbiol.* **35:**3186–3191.
31. **Collins, M. D., P. A. Lawson, A. Willems, J. J. Cordoba, J. Fernandez-Garayzabal, P. Garcia, J. Cai, H. Hippe, and J. A. Farrow.** 1994. The phylogeny of the genus *Clostridium*: proposal of five new genera and eleven new species combinations. *Int. J. Syst. Bacteriol.* **44:**812–826.
32. **Cooke, R. M.** 1979. Pig bel. *Perspect. Pediatr. Pathol.* **5:** 137–152.
33. **Decker, W. H., and W. Hall.** 1966. Treatment of abortions infected with *Clostridium welchii*. *Am. J. Obstet. Gynecol.* **95:**395–399.
34. **Delmee, M., T. Mackey, and A. Hamitou.** 1992. Evaluation of a new commercial *Clostridium difficile* toxin A enzyme immunoassay using diarrhoeal stools. *Eur. J. Clin. Microbiol. Infect. Dis.* **11:**246–249.
35. **Dowell, V. R., Jr.** 1984. Botulism and tetanus: selected epidemiologic and microbiologic aspects. *Rev. Infect. Dis.* **6:**S202–S207.
36. **Dowell, V. R., Jr., and T. M. Hawkins.** 1977. *Laboratory Methods in Anaerobic Bacteriology*. CDC laboratory manual. DHEW publication (CDC) 78-8272. Centers for Disease Control, Atlanta, Ga.
37. **Emery, C. L., and S. D. Allen.** 1997. Evaluation of the AnaeroPack System® for broth microdilution susceptibility testing of clinically significant *Bacteroides* species, abstr. D-11, p. 85. *In Program and Abstracts of the 37th Interscience Conference on Antimicrobial Agents and Chemotherapy*. American Society for Microbiology, Washington, D.C.
38. **Engelkirk, P. G., J. Duben-Engelkirk, and V. R. Dowell, Jr.** 1992. *Principles and Practice of Clinical Anaerobic Bacteriology*. Star Publishing, Belmont, Calif.
39. **Fang, F. C., D. N. Gerding, and L. R. Peterson.** 1996. Diagnosis of *Clostridium difficile* colitis. *Ann. Intern. Med.* **125:**515–516. (Letter.)
40. **Fekety, R.** 1997. Guidelines for the diagnosis and management of *Clostridium difficile*-associated diarrhea and colitis. American College of Gastroenterology, Practice Parameters Committee. *Am. J. Gastroenterol.* **92:**739–750.
41. **Finegold, S. M.** 1989. Therapy of anaerobic infections, p. 793–818. *In* S. M. Finegold and W. L. George (ed.), *Anaerobic Infections in Humans*. Academic Press, Inc., New York, N.Y.
42. **Finegold, S. M., and W. L. George (ed.).** 1989. *Anaerobic Infections in Humans*. Academic Press, Inc., San Diego, Calif.
43. **George, W. L.** 1989. Antimicrobial agent-associated diarrhea and colitis, p. 661–678. *In* S. M. Finegold and W. L. George (ed.), *Anaerobic Infections in Humans*. Academic Press, Inc., New York, N.Y.
44. **George, W. L., and S. M. Finegold.** 1985. Clostridia in the human gastrointestinal flora, p. 1–37. *In* S. P. Borriello (ed.), *Clostridia in Gastrointestinal Disease*. CRC Press, Inc., Boca Raton, Fla.
45. **Gerding, D. N., and J. S. Brazier.** 1993. Optimal methods for identifying *Clostridium difficile* infections. *Clin. Infect. Dis.* **16:**S439–S442.
46. **Gerding, D. N., R. L. Gebhard, H. W. Sumner, and L. R. Peterson.** 1988. Pathology and diagnosis of *Clostridium difficile* disease, p. 259–286. *In* R. D. Rolfe and S. M. Finegold (ed.), *Clostridium difficile: Its Role in Intestinal Disease*. Academic Press, Inc., New York, N.Y.
47. **Gerding, D. N., S. Johnson, L. R. Peterson, M. E. Mulligan, and J. Silva, Jr.** 1995. *Clostridium difficile*-associated diarrhea and colitis. *Infect. Control Hosp. Epidemiol.* **16:** 459–477.
48. **Ghanem, F. M., A. C. Ridpath, W. E. Moore, and L. V. Moore.** 1991. Identification of *Clostridium botulinum*, *Clostridium argentinense*, and related organisms by cellular fatty acid analysis. *J. Clin. Microbiol.* **29:**1114–1124.
49. **Gilligan, P. H., L. R. McCarthy, and V. M. Genta.** 1981. Relative frequency of *Clostridium difficile* in patients with diarrheal disease. *J. Clin. Microbiol.* **14:**26–31.
50. **Gleaves, C., R. J. Dworkin, L. Olson, and M. Campbell.** 1997. Evaluation of the ImmunoCard Toxin A Test as compared to the cytotoxin method for detection of *Clostridium difficile* toxin in clinical specimens, abstr. C-266, p. 167. *In Abstracts of the 97th General Meeting of the American Society for Microbiology 1997*. American Society for Microbiology, Washington, D.C.
51. **Golledge, C. L., C. F. Carson, G. L. O'Neill, R. A. Bowman, and T. V. Riley.** 1992. Ciprofloxacin and *Clostridium difficile*-associated diarrhoea. *J. Antimicrob. Chemother.* **30:** 141–147.
52. **Golledge, C. L., T. McKenzie, and T. V. Riley.** 1989. Extended spectrum cephalosporins and *Clostridium difficile*. *J. Antimicrob. Chemother.* **23:**929–931.
53. **Golledge, C. L., and T. V. Riley.** 1995. *Clostridium difficile*-associated diarrhoea after doxycycline malaria prophylaxis. *Lancet* **345:**1377–1378. (Letter.)
54. **Gorbach, S. L.** 1998. *Clostridium perfringens* and other clostridia, p. 1925–1933. *In* S. L. Gorbach, J. G. Bartlett, and N. R. Blacklow (ed.), *Infectious Diseases*, 2nd ed. The W. B. Saunders Co., Philadelphia, Pa.
55. **Gorbach, S. L.** 1998. Gas gangrene and other clostridial skin and soft tissue infections, p. 915–922. *In* S. L. Gorbach, J. G. Barlett, and N. R. Blacklow (ed.), *Infectious Diseases*, 2nd ed. The W. B. Saunders Co., Philadephia, Pa.
56. **Gorbach, S. L., and H. Thadepalli.** 1975. Isolation of *Clostridium* in human infections: evaluation of 114 cases. *J. Infect. Dis.* **131:**S81–S85.
57. **Groschel, D. H.** 1996. *Clostridium difficile* infection. *Crit. Rev. Clin. Lab. Sci.* **33:**203–245.
58. **Hall, J. D., L. M. McCroskey, B. J. Pincomb, and C. L. Hatheway.** 1985. Isolation of an organism resembling *Clostridium barati* which produces type F botulinal toxin from an infant with botulism. *J. Clin. Microbiol.* **21:** 654–655.

59. **Hatheway, C. L.** 1988. Botulism, p. 111–133. *In* A. Balows, W. J. Hausler, Jr., M. Ohashi, and A. Turano (ed.), *Laboratory Diagnosis of Infectious Diseases: Principles and Practice*, vol. 1. Springer-Verlag, New York, N.Y.
60. **Hatheway, C. L.** 1998. *Clostridium botulinum*, p. 1919–1925. *In* S. L. Gorbach, J. G. Bartlett, and N. R. Blacklow (ed.), *Infectious Diseases*, 2nd ed. The W. B. Saunders Co., Philadelphia, Pa.
61. **Hatheway, C. L.** 1990. Toxigenic clostridia. *Clin. Microbiol. Rev.* **3:**66–98.
62. **Hatheway, C. L., and E. A. Johnson.** 1998. *Clostridium*: the spore-bearing anaerobes, p. 731–782. *In* A. Balows and B. I. Duerden (ed.), *Systematic Bacteriology*, 9th ed., vol. 2. Edward Arnold Publisher, London, United Kingdom.
63. **Hauschild, A. H.** 1975. Criteria and procedures for implicating *Clostridium perfringens* in food-borne outbreaks. *Can. J. Public Health* **66:**388–392.
64. **Hecht, D. W., M. H. Malamy, and F. P. Tally.** 1989. Mechanisms of resistance and resistance transfer in anaerobic bacteria, p. 755–769. *In* S. M. Finegold and W. L. George (ed.), *Anaerobic Infections in Humans*. Academic Press, Inc., New York, N.Y.
65. **Holdeman, L. V., E. P. Cato, and W. E. C. Moore.** 1977. *Anaerobe Laboratory Manual.* Virginia Polytechnic Institute and State University, Blacksburg.
66. **Isenberg, H. D.** 1992. *Clinical Microbiology Procedures Handbook*, vol. 1. American Society for Microbiology, Washington, D.C.
67. **Izurieta, H. S., R. W. Sutter, P. M. Strebel, B. Bardenheier, D. R. Prevots, M. Wharton, and S. C. Hadler.** 1997. Tetanus surveillance—United States, 1991–1994. CDC Surveillance Summaries. *Morbid. Mortal. Weekly Rep.* **46**(no. SS-2)**:**15–25.
68. **Johnson, J. L., and B. S. Francis.** 1975. Taxonomy of the clostridia: ribosomal ribonucleic acid homologies among the species. *J. Gen. Microbiol.* **88:**229–244.
69. **Johnson, S., C. R. Clabots, F. V. Linn, M. M. Olson, L. R. Peterson, and D. N. Gerding.** 1990. Nosocomial *Clostridium difficile* colonisation and disease. *Lancet* **336:** 97–100.
70. **Johnson, S., M. R. Driks, R. K. Tweten, J. Ballard, D. L. Stevens, D. J. Anderson, and E. N. Janoff.** 1994. Clinical courses of seven survivors of *Clostridium septicum* infection and their immunologic responses to alpha toxin. *Clin. Infect. Dis.* **19:**761–764.
71. **Justus, P. G., J. L. Martin, D. A. Goldberg, N. S. Taylor, J. G. Bartlett, R. W. Alexander, and J. R. Mathias.** 1982. Myoelectric effects of *Clostridium difficile*: motility-altering factors distinct from its cytotoxin and enterotoxin in rabbits. *Gastroenterology* **83:**836–843.
72. **Kelly, C. P., C. Pothoulakis, and J. T. LaMont.** 1994. *Clostridium difficile* colitis. *N. Engl. J. Med.* **330:**257–262.
73. **Kim, K. H., R. Fekety, D. H. Batts, D. Brown, M. Cudmore, J. Silva, Jr., and D. Waters.** 1981. Isolation of *Clostridium difficile* from the environment and contacts of patients with antibiotic-associated colitis. *J. Infect. Dis.* **143:** 42–50.
74. **King, A., A. Rampling, D. G. Wright, and R. E. Warren.** 1984. Neutropenic enterocolitis due to *Clostridium septicum* infection. *J. Clin. Pathol.* **37:**335–343.
75. **Kirchner, J. T.** 1991. *Clostridium septicum* infection. Beware of associated cancer. *Postgrad. Med.* **90:**157–160.
76. **Kokai-Kun, J. F., and B. A. McClane.** 1997. The *Clostridium perfringens* enterotoxin, p. 325–357. *In* J. I. Rood, B. A. McClane, J. G. Songer, and R. W. Titball (ed.), *The Clostridia: Molecular Biology and Pathogenesis*. Academic Press, Inc., New York, N.Y.
77. **Kokai-Kun, J. F., J. G. Songer, J. R. Czeczulin, F. Chen, and B. A. McClane.** 1994. Comparison of Western immunoblots and gene detection assays for identification of potentially enterotoxigenic isolates of *Clostridium perfringens*. *J. Clin. Microbiol.* **32:**2533–2539.
78. **Koneman, E. W., S. D. Allen, W. M. Janda, P. C. Schreckenberger, and W. C. Winn, Jr.** 1997. *Color Atlas and Textbook of Diagnostic Microbiology*, 5th ed. Lippincott-Raven Publishers, Philadelphia, Pa.
79. **Koransky, J. R., S. D. Allen, and V. R. Dowell, Jr.** 1978. Use of ethanol for selective isolation of sporeforming microorganisms. *Appl. Environ. Microbiol.* **35:**762–765.
80. **Koransky, J. R., M. D. Stargel, and V. R. Dowell, Jr.** 1979. *Clostridium septicum* bacteremia. Its clinical significance. *Am. J. Med.* **66:**63–66.
81. **Kornbluth, A. A., J. B. Danzig, and L. H. Bernstein.** 1989. *Clostridium septicum* infection and associated malignancy. Report of 2 cases and review of the literature. *Medicine* **68:**30–37.
82. **Kudsk, K. A.** 1992. Occult gastrointestinal malignancies producing metastatic *Clostridium septicum* infections in diabetic patients. *Surgery* **112:**765–772.
83. **Lashner, B. A., J. Todorczuk, D. F. Sahm, and S. B. Hanauer.** 1986. *Clostridium difficile* culture-positive toxin-negative diarrhea. *Am. J. Gastroenterol.* **81:**940–943.
84. **Lawrence, G., and R. Cooke.** 1980. Experimental pigbel: the production and pathology of necrotizing enteritis due to *Clostridium welchii* type C in the guinea-pig. *Br. J. Exp. Pathol.* **61:**261–271.
85. **Lorber, B.** 1995. Gas gangrene and other clostridium-associated diseases, p. 2182–2195. *In* G. L. Mandell, J. E. Bennett, and R. Dolin (ed.), *Mandell, Douglas and Bennett's Principles and Practice of Infectious Diseases*, 4th ed., vol. 2. Churchill Livingstone, Inc., New York, N.Y.
86. **Lyerly, D. M., and S. D. Allen.** 1997. The clostridia, p. 559–623. *In* A. M. Emmerson, P. Hawkey, and S. Gillespie (ed.), *Principles and Practice of Clinical Bacteriology*. John Wiley & Sons, Inc., New York, N.Y.
87. **Lyerly, D. M., L. A. Barroso, T. D. Wilkins, C. Depitre, and G. Corthier.** 1992. Characterization of a toxin A-negative, toxin B-positive strain of *Clostridium difficile*. *Infect. Immun.* **60:**4633–4639.
88. **Lyerly, D. M., H. C. Krivan, and T. D. Wilkins.** 1988. *Clostridium difficile*: its disease and toxins. *Clin. Microbiol. Rev.* **1:**1–18.
89. **Lyerly, D. M., L. M. Neville, D. T. Evans, J. Fill, S. Allen, W. Greene, R. Sautter, P. Hnatuck, D. J. Torpey, and R. Schwalbe.** 1998. Multicenter evaluation of the *Clostridium difficile* TOX A/B TEST. *J. Clin. Microbiol.* **36:** 184–190.
90. **Mahony, D. E., E. Gilliatt, S. Dawson, E. Stockdale, and S. H. Lee.** 1989. Vero cell assay for rapid detection of *Clostridium perfringens* enterotoxin. *Appl. Environ. Microbiol.* **55:**2141–2143.
91. **Marler, L. M., J. A. Siders, L. C. Wolters, Y. Pettigrew, B. L. Skitt, and S. D. Allen.** 1992. Comparison of five cultural procedures for isolation of *Clostridium difficile* from stools. *J. Clin. Microbiol.* **30:**514–516.
92. **Marler, L. M., J. A. Siders, L. C. Wolters, Y. Pettigrew, B. L. Skitt, and S. D. Allen.** 1991. Evaluation of the new RapID-ANA II system for the identification of clinical anaerobic isolates. *J. Clin. Microbiol.* **29:**874–878.
93. **McFarland, L. V., M. B. Coyle, W. H. Kremer, and W. E. Stamm.** 1987. Rectal swab cultures for *Clostridium difficile* surveillance studies. *J. Clin. Microbiol.* **25:**2241–2242.
94. **McFarland, L. V., M. E. Mulligan, R. Y. Kwok, and W. E. Stamm.** 1989. Nosocomial acquisition of *Clostridium difficile* infection. *N. Engl. J. Med.* **320:**204–210.
95. **Moncrief, J. S., D. M. Lyerly, and T. D. Wilkins.** 1997. Molecular biology of the *Clostridium difficile* toxins, p. 369–392. *In* J. I. Rood, B. A. McClane, J. G. Songer, and R. W. Titball (ed.), *The Clostridia: Molecular Biology and Pathogenesis*. Academic Press, Inc., New York, N.Y.

96. **Moore, W. E. C., and L. V. H. Moore.** 1992. *Index of the Bacterial and Yeast Nomenclatural Changes*. American Society for Microbiology, Washington, D.C.
97. **Mulligan, M. E.** 1984. Epidemiology of *Clostridium difficile*-induced intestinal disease. *Rev. Infect. Dis.* **6:** S222–S228.
98. **Mulligan, M. E., L. R. Peterson, R. Y. Kwok, C. R. Clabots, and D. N. Gerding.** 1988. Immunoblots and plasmid fingerprints compared with serotyping and polyacrylamide gel electrophoresis for typing *Clostridium difficile*. *J. Clin. Microbiol.* **26:**41–46.
99. **Nakamura, S., M. Mikawa, S. Nakashio, M. Takabatake, I. Okado, K. Yamakawa, T. Serikawa, S. Okumura, and S. Nishida.** 1981. Isolation of *Clostridium difficile* from the feces and the antibody in sera of young and elderly adults. *Microbiol. Immunol.* **25:**345–351.
100. **Nichols, R. L., and J. W. Smith.** 1975. Gas in the wound; what does it mean? *Surg. Clin. North Am.* **55:**1289–1296.
101. **Okabe, A., T. Shimizu, and H. Hayashi.** 1989. Cloning and sequencing of a phospholipase C gene of *Clostridium perfringens*. *Biochem. Biophys. Res. Commun.* **160:**33–39.
102. **Peterson, L. R., J. J. Holter, C. J. Shanholtzer, C. R. Garrett, and D. N. Gerding.** 1986. Detection of *Clostridium difficile* toxins A (enterotoxin) and B (cytotoxin) in clinical specimens. Evaluation of a latex agglutination test. *Am. J. Clin. Pathol.* **86:**208–211.
103. **Peterson, L. R., and P. J. Kelly.** 1993. The role of the clinical microbiology laboratory in the management of *Clostridium difficile*-associated diarrhea. *Infect. Dis. Clin. North Am.* **7:**277–293.
104. **Peterson, L. R., P. J. Kelly, and H. A. Nordbrock.** 1996. Role of culture and toxin detection in laboratory testing for diagnosis of *Clostridium difficile*-associated diarrhea. *Eur. J. Clin. Microbiol. Infect. Dis.* **15:**330–336.
105. **Prazmowski, A.** 1880. *Untersuchung über die entwicklungsgeschichte und fermentwirkung einiger Bakterien, Arten*. Hugo Voigt, Leipzig, Germany.
106. **Quentin, C., M. A. Desailly-Chanson, and C. Bebear.** 1991. Evaluation of AN-Ident. *J. Clin. Microbiol.* **29:** 231–235.
107. **Riddell, S., P. Gilligan, and L. McMillon.** 1997. Evaluation of the ImmunoCard Toxin A Membrane EIA for *Clostridium difficile* toxin A, abstr. C-254, p. 165. *In Abstracts of the 97th General Meeting of the American Society for Microbiology 1997*. American Society for Microbiology, Washington, D.C.
108. **Rood, J. I., B. A. McClane, J. G. Songer, and R. W. Titball (ed.).** 1997. *The Clostridia: Molecular Biology and Pathogenesis*. Academic Press, Inc., New York, N.Y.
109. **Rosenblatt, J. E.** 1989. Susceptibility testing of anaerobic bacteria. *Clin. Lab. Med.* **9:**239–254.
110. **Saulnier, P., E. Chachaty, F. Hilali, and A. Andremont.** 1997. Single-step polymerase chain reaction for combined gene detection and epidemiological typing in three bacterial models. *FEMS Microbiol. Lett.* **150:**311–316.
111. **Schiavo, G., and C. Montecucco.** 1997. The structure and mode of action of botulinum and tetanus toxins, p. 295–322. *In* J. I. Rood, B. A. McClane, J. G. Songer, and R. W. Titball (ed.), *The Clostridia: Molecular Biology and Pathogenesis*. Academic Press, Inc., New York, N.Y.
112. **Schleupner, M. A., D. C. Garner, K. M. Sosnowski, C. J. Schleupner, L. J. Barrett, E. Silva, D. Hirsch, and R. L. Guerrant.** 1995. Concurrence of *Clostridium difficile* toxin A enzyme-linked immunosorbent assay, fecal lactoferrin assay, and clinical criteria with *C. difficile* cytotoxin titer in two patient cohorts. *J. Clin. Microbiol.* **33:** 1755–1759.
113. **Shandera, W. X., C. O. Tacket, and P. A. Blake.** 1983. Food poisoning due to *Clostridium perfringens* in the United States. *J. Infect. Dis.* **147:**167–170.
114. **Shanholtzer, C. J., K. E. Willard, J. J. Holter, M. M. Olson, D. N. Gerding, and L. R. Peterson.** 1992. Comparison of the VIDAS *Clostridium difficile* toxin A immunoassay with *C. difficile* culture and cytotoxin and latex tests. *J. Clin. Microbiol.* **30:**1837–1840.
115. **Sherman, S., E. Klein, and B. A. McClane.** 1994. *Clostridium perfringens* type A enterotoxin induces tissue damage and fluid accumulation in rabbit ileum. *J. Diarrhoeal Dis. Res.* **12:**200–207.
116. **Skerman, V. B. D., V. McGowan, and P. H. A. Sneath.** 1989. *Approved Lists of Bacterial Names*, amended ed. American Society for Microbiology, Washington, D.C.
117. **Smith, L. D.** 1975. Common mesophilic anaerobes, including *Clostridium botulinum* and *Clostridium tetani*, in 21 soil specimens. *Appl. Microbiol.* **29:**590–594.
118. **Smith, L. D.** 1978. The occurrence of *Clostridium botulinum* and *Clostridium tetani* in the soil of the United States. *Health Lab. Sci.* **15:**74–80.
119. **Smith, L. D.** 1979. Virulence factors of *Clostridium perfringens*. *Rev. Infect. Dis.* **1:**254–262.
120. **Smith, L. D. S., and B. L. Williams.** 1984. *The Pathogenic Anaerobic Bacteria*, 3rd ed. Charles C Thomas, Springfield, Ill.
121. **Sonnabend, O., W. Sonnabend, R. Heinzle, T. Sigrist, R. Dirnhofer, and U. Krech.** 1981. Isolation of *Clostridium botulinum* type G and identification of type G botulinal toxin in humans: report of five sudden unexpected deaths. *J. Infect. Dis.* **143:**22–27.
122. **Speirs, G., R. E. Warren, and A. Rampling.** 1988. *Clostridium tertium* septicemia in patients with neutropenia. *J. Infect. Dis.* **158:**1336–1340.
123. **Spika, J. S., N. Shaffer, N. Hargrett-Bean, S. Collin, K. L. MacDonald, and P. A. Blake.** 1989. Risk factors for infant botulism in the United States. *Am. J. Dis. Child.* **143:**828–832.
124. **Staneck, J. L., L. S. Weckbach, S. D. Allen, J. A. Siders, P. H. Gilligan, G. Coppitt, J. A. Kraft, and D. H. Willis.** 1996. Multicenter evaluation of four methods for *Clostridium difficile* detection: ImmunoCard *C. difficile*, cytotoxin assay, culture, and latex agglutination. *J. Clin. Microbiol.* **34:**2718–2721.
125. **Stark, P. L., and A. Lee.** 1982. The microbial ecology of the large bowel of breast-fed and formula-fed infants during the first year of life. *J. Med. Microbiol.* **15:**189–203.
126. **Suen, J. C., C. L. Hatheway, A. G. Steigerwalt, and D. J. Brenner.** 1988. *Clostridium argentinense*, sp. nov.: a genetically homogenous group composed of all strains of *Clostridium botulinum* toxin type G and some nontoxigenic strains previously identified as *Clostridium subterminale* or *Clostridium hastiforme*. *Int. J. Syst. Bacteriol.* **38:** 375–381.
127. **Summanen, P., E. J. Baron, D. M. Citron, C. A. Strong, H. M. Wexler, and S. M. Finegold.** 1993. *Wadsworth Anaerobic Bacteriology Manual*, 5th ed. Star Publishing, Belmont, Calif.
128. **Titball, R. W.** 1993. Bacterial phospholipases C. *Microbiol. Rev.* **57:**347–366.
129. **Viscidi, R., S. Willey, and J. G. Bartlett.** 1981. Isolation rates and toxigenic potential of *Clostridium difficile* isolates from various patient populations. *Gastroenterology* **81:** 5–9.
130. **Wilkins, T. D., and T. Thiel.** 1973. Resistance of some species of *Clostridium* to clindamycin. *Antimicrob. Agents Chemother.* **3:**136–137.
131. **Willis, A. T.** 1969. *Clostridia of Wound Infection*. Butterworths, London, United Kingdom.

Peptostreptococcus, Propionibacterium, Lactobacillus, Actinomyces, and Other Non-Spore-Forming Anaerobic Gram-Positive Bacteria

ARNE C. RODLOFF, SHARON L. HILLIER, AND BERNARD J. MONCLA

47

The anaerobic gram-positive cocci and non-spore-forming rods constitute a genetically and phenotypically diverse group of bacteria. These organisms are, for the most part, components of the normal flora of the skin or mucosal surfaces of humans. As with many other anaerobes, they may become opportunistic pathogens when they are allowed to leave their normal habitat and gain access to normally sterile body tissue. Hence, infections are normally endogenous and require predisposing factors such as disruption of mucous membranes. Recovery of anaerobic gram-positive rods from clinical specimens is summarized in Table 1. They are most likely to be found in mixed infections together with anaerobic gram-negative rods or facultatively anaerobic organisms. These infective associations may cause wound infections, abscesses, or systemic infections such as peritonitis.

In cultures of clinical specimens, gram-positive cocci and non-spore-forming rods often go undetected or unrecognized by many clinical laboratories. Many of the species discussed in this chapter require extended anaerobic incubation for growth and/or complex growth media. For example, specimen-handling procedures and growth conditions that may be adequate for the recovery of *Bacteroides fragilis* or *Clostridium* species will not necessarily be suitable for the recovery of *Peptostreptococcus anaerobius* or *Mobiluncus curtisii*. Specimens from oral or pelvic abscesses will in all likelihood be negative for most anaerobes after 48 h of incubation, and extended anaerobic incubation is required to accurately define the etiologic agents of these infections. Extra attention to extended, uninterrupted anaerobic incubation on suitable media will provide an opportunity to detect these organisms.

After their recovery and isolation, members of this group of microorganisms are difficult to identify accurately. Most of the commercial rapid identification systems that identify many of the fast-growing anaerobic gram-negative rods correctly are woefully inadequate for identification of the organisms discussed in this chapter. However, correct identification at least to the genus level may provide useful information for the clinician. Thus, recovery of *Lactobacillus* species from the blood is suggestive of a genital or rectal source of the infection whereas recovery of a *Propionibacterium* species may suggest a skin source.

ANAEROBIC GRAM-POSITIVE COCCI

Description of the Genera

The genera *Peptostreptococcus* and *Peptococcus* include gram-positive obligately anaerobic non-spore-forming cocci. Cells may occur in pairs, tetrads, irregular masses, or chains. These species are chemoorganotrophs that metabolize peptones and amino acids to acetic acid and often produce isobutyric, butyric, isovaleric, or isocaproic acid. Obligately anaerobic cocci belonging to the genus *Streptoccus* produce lactic acid as the major product of glucose metabolism. The genera *Coprococcus* and *Ruminococcus* differ from the other genera in requiring a fermentable carbohydrate for growth.

Taxonomy

Major revisions in the taxonomy of gram-positive cocci occurred around 1983, when many species formerly in the genus *Peptococcus* were transferred to the genus *Peptostreptococcus* because of the similarities in the G+C contents of their DNAs (31, 32). They seem to be closely related to *Clostridium* spp. Since 1990, a number of new species of human origin have been described for the genus *Peptostreptococcus*. These include *P. hydrogenalis*, *P. vaginalis*, *P. lacrimalis*, *P. lactolyticus*, *P. harei*, *P. ivorii*, and *P. octavius* (30, 61, 72). *P. barnesae*, an obligately purine-utilizing species, has been found exclusively in chicken feces (94). The genus *Peptococcus* contains only one species, *Peptococcus niger* (119).

The genus *Streptococcus* currently includes three strictly anaerobic species, *S. hansenii*, *S. pleomorphus*, and *S. parvulus*. They are rarely found in clinical specimens. The taxonomic positions of these species remain unclear. Analyses of the 16S RNA, DNA base composition, and peptidoglycan type suggest that *S. hansenii* is related to *Clostridium coccoides* (120) and *Clostridium amniovalericum* whereas *S. pleomorphus* appears to be closely related to *Clostridium innocuum* (63). *S. parvulus*, which can be recovered from the gingival crevice, is more closely related to *Peptostreptococcus* species (17). *Gemella morbillorum* (formerly *Streptococcus morbillorum*) is occasionally isolated from clinical specimens but is considered microaerophilic and therefore is covered in chapter 19.

Anaerobic gram-positive cocci of other genera, including *Ruminococcus* and *Coprococcus*, can be isolated from the rumens of animals and the stomachs and bowels of human

TABLE 1 Recovery of anaerobic gram-positive rods and cocci from various specimen types[a]

Site	% of patients yielding isolates of:				
	Peptostreptococcus	*Actinomyces*	*Eubacterium*	*Lactobacillus*[b]	*Propionibacterium*
Appendix	23	11	34	21	6
Kidney abscess	83	0	17	0	17
Bladder abscess	100	0	50	0	0
Periurethral abscess	71	0	0	0	0
Bartholin gland abscess	42	0	8	4	0
Penile abscess	86	0	0	0	0
Scrotal or testicular abscess	48	5	5	0	0
Periapical abscess	68	14	9	23	0
Orofacial infection	33	0	13	33	0
Penile wound	66	0	0	0	0
Periodontal pockets[c]	60	75	43	NA[d]	15
Breast abscess	51	0	2	0	27
Peritonsillar abscess	36	0	0	2	10
Blood	11	0	2	0.2	36
Nostril (normal)	16	0	0	0	75
Vagina	87	7	3	14	22

[a] Data from references 4, 8, 9, 10, 11, 33, 46, and 121.
[b] Obligately anaerobic strains only.
[c] Moncla, unpublished data from University of Washington Periodontal Clinic, 1984 through 1989.
[d] NA, no attempts were made to recover *Lactobacillus* spp. in these studies.

beings. However, their isolation from clinical specimens is exceedingly rare.

Natural Habitat

The anaerobic gram-positive cocci are widely distributed as members of the normal flora in humans and animals. They can be recovered routinely from the skin, oropharynx, upper respiratory tract, gut, and urogenital tract (74); in particular, they are recovered from the vagina of 90% of pregnant women, with *P. prevotii*, *P. tetradius*, *P. magnus*, and *P. asaccharolyticus* being the most common species (46). Likewise, these organisms can be recovered from 60% of periodontal pocket specimens but are relatively uncommon in saliva. *Peptococcus niger* is present in the vaginas of 20 to 30% of pregnant women but has been only infrequently recovered from clinical specimens (46).

Clinical Significance

The role of "anaerobic streptococci" in human infections has been recognized since the early 1900s. Schwarz and Dieckmann published a report in 1926 on postpartum endometritis in 165 women (98). They recovered bacteria resembling *P. anaerobius* from blood and endometrial cultures from 28% of the patients and found another 13% "anaerobic streptococci" in the same cultures. The importance of anaerobic gram-positive cocci in the etiology of postpartum endometritis has since been confirmed in many studies. One more recent report (46) listed a wide variety of species recovered from the endometria of women with postpartum fever, including *P. magnus* (41%), *P. tetradius* (26%), *P. asaccharolyticus* (20%), *P. anaerobius* (19%), *P. prevotii* (15%), and, less frequently, *Peptococcus niger* (4%). These organisms are also frequently recovered from tubo-ovarian abscesses, the fallopian tubes or endometria of women with pelvic inflammatory disease, septic abortions, and patients with amnionitis and infection of the placental membranes (chorioamnionitis) (Table 1) (45). The isolation of *Peptostreptococcus* species from placental membranes is associated with preterm birth (45). In patients with pelvic inflamatory disease, these organisms are often part of a mixed infection in association with *Prevotella* and *Porphyromonas* species or facultatively anaerobic bacteria such as *Escherichia coli* (47).

Anaerobic gram-positive cocci are isolated from patients with a wide variety of head and neck infections, including periodontitis, chronic otitis media, chronic sinusitis, purulent nasopharyngitis, and brain abscess (9, 10, 12, 13). The source of anaerobic cocci in brain abscess is probably related to the presence of these bacteria in otitis and sinusitis and their subsequent spread into the central nervous system. Also, anaerobic gram-positive cocci present in the gingiva can spread hematogenously following dental manipulations or extractions to cause endocarditis or brain abscess. The organisms can also spread by aspiration from the oral cavity to cause pulmonary disease, such as pneumonitis, lung abscess, empyema, or necrotizing pneumonia. Again, these infections are usually polymicrobic.

Spillage of fecal contents into the peritoneum following appendicitis, diverticulitis, surgery, penetrating trauma, or cancer can lead to intra-abdominal mixed infections involving anaerobic gram-positive cocci, *Bacteroides* species, *Clostridium* species, and facultatively anaerobic bacteria such as members of the *Enterobacteriaceae* and enterococci. Intestinal perforation or cancer may also lead to liver abscess, which involves obligate anaerobes in at least half of all cases (5). In one recent study, *Peptostreptococcus* species were isolated in one of four specimens from patients with perforated appendicitis and peritonitis (4).

Bacteremia due to anaerobic gram-positive cocci most commonly follows obstetric or gynecologic infections, including postpartum endometritis and amnionitis. Over a 6-year period in Turku, Finland, *Peptostreptococcus* species were recovered from 7 of 57 patients who developed clinically significant bacteremias (91). Although none of these infections were lethal, they were considered to be clinically significant. An additional 24 patients developed clinically insignificant bacteremias, and 3 of these cases were due to *Peptostreptococcus* species. Thus, the recovery of *Peptostreptococcus* from the blood is not as frequently associated with fatal infection as is bacteremias due to *Bacteroides* species, but *Peptostreptococcus* spp. cannot be routinely interpreted as clinically insignificant. The most common isolates include *P. magnus*, *P. asaccharolyticus*, and *P. anaerobius* (8, 10). Infection of bone, joints, and grafts may also occur, with *P. magnus* being of major importance in these processes (6).

Peptococcus niger has been associated with sheep foot rot (81).

Collection and Transport of Specimens

The appropriate specimen collection and transport methods for anaerobic gram-positive cocci depend on the specimen site to be sampled. In general, aspirates or biopsy specimens are considered the optimal samples for culture of obligate anaerobic bacteria. Such specimens are less likely to be contaminated with microorganisms of the normal flora and are also less likely to be exposed to the detrimental effects of oxygen and desiccation. Appropriate samples should be transported to the laboratory within 30 min. Swab specimens should be discouraged. If the culture site does not yield sufficient amounts of aspirate, swab specimens may be accepted after consultation. In all cases, it is imperative to use an anaerobic transport system, since anaerobic cocci are quickly rendered nonviable when exposed to O_2. Anaerobic transport media that have been evaluated for use with anaerobic cocci include the B-D Port-a-Cul anaerobic transport tube (Becton-Dickinson Microbiology Products, Cockeysville, Md.) and the Anaerobic Specimen Collector (Becton-Dickinson Vacutainer Systems, Rutherford, N.J.). It has been demonstrated that *Peptostreptococcus* species had 100% viability after 24 h at room temperature in the Port-a-Cul but less than 60% viability after 24 h in the Anaerobic Specimen Collector (7). Additionally, since the vacutainer tube is specifically designed for swabs, its use cannot be recommended. A modified Stuart transport medium has also been reported to provide adequate protection for *P. magnus* and *P. anaerobius* for up to 48 h (7, 79, 110). Finally, an Amies medium without charcoal (Venturi Transystem; Copan Diagnostics, Corona, Calif.) was shown to be equivalent to Port-a-Cul in protecting *P. anaerobius*, and other anaerobes (51). However, in another study comparing the survival of *P. anaerobius* for 24 to 48 h in Port-a-Cul vials, Culturette EZ (Becton-Dickinson), and the Venturi Transystem Amies gel, none of the transport systems maintained more than 1% of the viable counts for 48 h (79). These data suggest that rapid transportation to the laboratory is essential irrespective of the transport system chosen if preservation of *Peptostreptococcus* species is desired. It should be noted that *P. anaerobius* is susceptible to sodium polyanethol sulfonate (Liquoid), and this characteristic has even been used for identification purposes (118). However, this also suggests that blood culture systems containing Liquoid as an additive are inadequate for the recovery of this species.

As pointed out above, specimens for culture of anaerobic cocci should always be transported to the laboratory as soon as possible. However, transport times of up to 24 h may be tolerated if an appropriate specimen (not swab) and anaerobic transport medium are used. The optimal temperature for transport is somewhat controversial. A report by Tvede and Hoiby indicates that transportation at either 4 or 22°C did not influence survival of anaerobic bacteria; however, our experience suggests better recovery when the specimens are held at 18 to 22°C (110).

Direct Examination

Although direct examination of clinical specimens with a Gram stain is imperative, little information about anaerobic cocci is gathered. Microscopically, facultatively anaerobic and obligately anaerobic cocci cannot be distinguished. Moreover, anaerobic cocci may display a rod shape, and, finally, cocci with a gram-negative cell wall structure (*Megasphaera*) may show a gram-positive appearance on initial microscopic examination.

Isolation Procedures

The anaerobic cocci grow well on most nonselective plating media suitable for anaerobic isolation. Brucella, Columbia, or Schaedler agar base supplemented with 5% sheep blood, vitamin K, and hemin generally yields good growth within 48 to 72 h. One report has suggested that Centers for Disease Control and Prevention (CDC) agar base gives better recovery of *P. tetradius*, *P. anaerobius*, and *P. asaccharolyticus* than does brucella blood agar (100).

There is no single selective medium for growing anaerobic gram-positive cocci. The addition of nalidixic acid and Tween 80 (125) or oxolinic acid (80) may enhance the recovery of anaerobes in mixed infections. Columbia CNA agar supplemented with glutathione and lead acetate can be used as a differential medium for *P. micros*. Unlike other cocci, *P. micros* rapidly utilizes the reduced form of glutathione to form hydrogen sulfide, which reacts with lead acetate to form a black precipitate under the colony in the medium (109).

Acceptable broth media include peptone yeast-extract glucose, chopped meat-glucose, and thioglycolate supplemented with hemin, vitamin K, and rabbit serum (5%). Supplementation with Tween (final concentration, 0.02%) may stimulate growth in broth media. Many laboratories no longer inoculate broth enrichment media for routine testing, including for isolation of anaerobes.

For recovery of *Peptostreptococcus* species from the blood, anaerobic tryptic or Trypticase soy broth incubated for a minimum of 5 days has been reported to be effective (20). By comparison, aerobic blood culture bottles never yield *Peptostreptococcus* species from the blood, and short-term incubation of blood culture bottles similarly failed to detect these organisms.

Identification Procedures

Anaerobic gram-positive cocci do not always stain as gram-positive cocci. For instance, *P. productus* and *P. anaerobius* may be elongated and resemble gram-positive coccobacilli. Any of the gram-positive cocci may lose gram positivity rapidly with age. To add to the confusion, anaerobic gram-negative cocci, including *Veillonella* and *Megasphaera* spp., appear at times to be gram positive. Preparation of Gram stains from a variety of media, both broth and solid, and examination of subcultures at different ages may help in assessing the correct cellular morphology and Gram stain reaction. Gram-positive cocci that resemble rods while on agar medium will assume a more coccoid appearance when grown in broth. Vancomycin susceptibility (5-μg disk on brucella blood agar) is useful for establishing that a microorganism is gram positive in instances in which gram-variable or gram-negative staining is observed (106).

Assignment of an anaerobic gram-positive coccus to a specific genus can be somewhat difficult, especially if gas chromatography is not available. Any identification of anaerobic gram-positive cocci that is made without the aid of chromatographic analysis of metabolic fatty acids must be considered presumptive. Even though the rapid identification systems can readily identify many species of anaerobic gram-positive cocci, the accuracy of the identification is directly related to the knowledge and experience of the individual reading the test (2, 15, 54, 73). For example, the reported accuracy of the RapID-ANA II for members of the genus *Peptostreptococcus* ranges from 15% for *P. prevotii* to 100% for *P. micros* (18, 66). In an evaluation of the rapid ID32A kit (bioMérieux Vitek, Inc., Hazelwood, Mo.), the system correctly identified only 1 of 12 *P. prevotii* isolates (75). The authors noted that *P. prevotii* is heterogeneous according to preformed enzyme profiles, and that the correct taxonomy may require further clarification. By contrast, *P. asaccharolyticus* is identified by most commercial systems. The difficulty in correctly identifying these organisms may be due in part to our lack of understanding of the true taxonomic status of some *Peptostreptococcus* species. The capabilities of several commercial systems to identify gram-positive anaerobic cocci are summarized in Table 2. Tables 3 and 4 can be used to further distinguish the genera and species.

The three species of *Peptostreptococcus* most commonly seen in clinical specimens are *P. magnus*, *P. anaerobius*, and *P. asaccharolyticus*. Colonies of *P. magnus* are minute to 0.5 mm in diameter, raised, dull, smooth, and nonhemolytic. The cells are 0.7 to 1.2 μm in diameter and appear in a tightly packed arrangement. *P. micros* colonies are minute to 1 mm, convex, and dull. The cells are smaller than those of *P. magnus*, being 0.3 to 0.7 μm in diameter. However, strain variability under different growth conditions makes differentiation of these two species on the basis of cellular morphology subjective. While most colonies of *P. micros* are smooth, a rough variant from periodontitis patients has also been described (112). The colonies of *P. anaerobius* are usually somewhat larger (1 mm in diameter) and nonhemolytic, while the individual cells are smaller (0.5 to 0.6 μm in diameter) than those of *P. magnus*. Very young cultures of *P. anaerobius* may have elongated cells in chains. The colonies of *P. anaerobius* may have a pungently sweet odor. *P. asaccharolyticus* colonies are minute to 2 mm in diameter and may have a slightly yellow pigment on blood agar. The individual cells are 0.5 to 1.5 μm in diameter and are arranged in pairs, tetrads, or irregular clumps.

The three newly described species of *Peptostreptococcus* are related to *P. prevotii*. These species, *P. vaginalis*, *P. lacrimalis*, and *P. lactolyticus*, appear as short chains or in masses. *P. hydrogenalis* cells are 0.7 to 1.8 μm in diameter and occur in short chains or masses.

Peptococcus niger is rarely recovered from clinical specimens, although it is likely that this isolate has gone unnoticed within mixed anaerobic cultures from clinical specimens. On initial isolation, the colonies are black to olive green. The pigment may not be visible to the naked eye but is evident under a dissecting microscope. It fades quickly upon exposure to oxygen. After subculture or in older cultures, the colony can take on a mustard yellow pigment. Colonies are convex and circular with a shiny, smooth appearance. They are weakly catalase positive. *Peptococcus niger* strains are indole, urease, and coagulase negative; nitrate is not reduced; and esculin and starch are not hydrolyzed. Hydrogen sulfide (in sulfide-indole-motility medium) and ammonia are produced. The only definitive means of differentiating *Peptococcus* from *Peptostreptococcus* spp. is by analyzing G+C ratios or by genetic sequencing. Unfortunately, this is not practical, and the peptococci must be presumptively identified on the basis of pigment production and the catalase reaction.

Antimicrobial Susceptibility

Most *Peptostreptococcus* isolates (96%) are susceptible to β-lactam antibiotics (Table 5). However, MICs as high as 64 μg/ml have been reported for ticarcillin and cefotaxime. Clindamycin and metronidazole are slightly less active: 84 and 88% of isolates, respectively, are susceptible. However, there is evidence of inducible macrolide-lincosamide resistance, with *P. asaccharolyticus* being the most resistant to erythromycin (87). Some strains that are clindamycin susceptible and erythromycin resistant have inducible clindamycin resistance. While most quinolones have limited activity against *Peptostreptococcus* species, the trifluoro-

TABLE 2 Identification of anaerobic gram-positive cocci by commercial systems[a]

Organism	No (%) of isolates			
	RapID-ANA II		AN-Ident	
	Tested	Identified to species level	Tested	Identified to species level
Peptostreptococcus spp.				
P. asaccharolyticus	53	49 (92)	4	4
P. magnus	40	39 (98)	5	5
P. anaerobius	31	22 (71)	5	4
P. micros	26	26 (100)	1	1
P. tetradius	4	3 (75)	9	5
P. prevotii	27	4 (15)	3	3
Peptococcus niger	0	Na[b]	1	0

[a] Data from references 2, 15, 18, 54, and 66
[b] NA, not applicable.

TABLE 3 Differential characteristics of *Peptostreptococcus* and *Peptococcus* spp.[a]

Species (no of strains examined)	Terminal VFA[b]	Indole	Production of[b]:			Carbohydrate fermentation reaction					Production of saccharolytic and proteolytic enzymes[b]										
			Urease	ALP	ADH	Glucose	Lactose	Raffinose	Ribose	Mannose	αGAL	βGAL	αGLU	βGUR	ArgA	ProA	PheA	LeuA	PyrA	TyrA	HisA
P. magnus (116)	A	–	–	d	d	–/w	–	–	–	–	–	–	–	–	+	–	–	+	+	–/w	–/w
P. micros (31)	A	–	–	+	–	–	–	–	–	–	–	–	–	–	+	+	+	+	+	+	+
P. heliotrinreducens (6)	A	–	–	–	+	–	–	–	–	–	–	–	–	–	d	+	+	+	–	w	w
P. productus (1)	A	–	–	–	–	+	+	+	d	d	+	–	+	–	–	–	–	–	–	–	–
P. bamesae (1)	A(B)	w	–	–	–	–	–	–	–	–	–	–	–	–	–	–	–	–	–	–	–
P. asaccharolyticus (52)	B	d	–	–	–	–	–	–	–	–	–	–	–	–	+	–	–	d	–	d	w
P. indolicus (6)	B	+	–	+		–	–	–	–	–	–	–	–	–	+	–	+	+	–	w	+
P. harei (13)	B	d	–	–	–	–	–	–	–	–	–	–	–	–	+	–	–	–/w	–	w	+
P. lacrimalis (1)	B	–	–	–	–	–	–	–	–	–	–	–	–	–	+	–	+	+	–	d	+
"*trisimilis*" group (4)[c]	B	+	–	d	–	+	w	–/w	–/w	+	–	d	–	–	–	–	–	–	+	–	–
P. hydrogenais (14)	B	+	d	–/w	–	+	+	+	–	+	–	–	d	–	–	–	–	–	–	–	–
P. prevotii (type strain)	B	–	+	–	–	–	–	+	+	+	+	–	+	+	+	–	–	–	+	w	+
P. tetradius (type strain)	B	–	+	–	–	–	–	–	–	+	–	–	+	+	+	–	w	+	w	w	w
prevotii/tetradius group (34)	B	–	?d	–	–	d	–	d	d	d	d	d	+	+	+	–	d	d	d	d	d
P. lactolyticus (1)	B	–	+	–	–	+	+	–	–	+	–	+	–	–	+	–	–	–	–	–	–
P. vaginalis (29)	B	?d	–	–/w	+	+	–	–	–	d	–	–	–	–	+	–	–	+	–	–	+
"β-GAL" group (24)[c]	B	–	·	w	d	+	+	–	+	+	–	w/+	–/w	–	+	–	–	+	w	–	–
P. ivorii (4)	IV	–	–	–	–	–	–	–	–	–	–	–	–	–	–	+	–	–	–	–	–
P. anaerobius (63)	IC(IV)	–	–	–	–	+	–	–	–	w	–	+	–	–	–	+	–	–	–	–	–
P. octavius (6)	C	–	–	–	–	+	–	–	+	+	–	–	–	–	–	+	–	–	w	–	–
P. niger (1)	C	–	–	–	–	–	–	–	–	–	–	–	–	–	–	–	–				

[a] Taken from reference 71.

[b] VFA, volatile fatty acids; A, acetate; B, butyrate; IV; isovalerate; IC, isocarborate; C, *n*-caproate; ALP, alkaline phosphatase; ADH, arginine dihydrolase; αGAL, α-galactosidase; βGAL, β-galactosidase; αGLU, α-glucosidase; βGUR, β-glucoronidase; ArgA, arginine arylamidase (AMD); ProA, proline AMD; PheA, phenylalanine AMD; LeuA, leucine AMD; PyrA, pyroglutamyl AMD; TyrA, tyrosine AMD, HisA, histidine AMD. –, >90% negative; w, weakly positive; +, >90% positive; d, different reactions.

[c] Undescribed strains that cluster in whole-cell composition as assessed by pyrolysis mass spectrometry.

TABLE 4 Biochemical characteristics of the anaerobic streptococci and *Gemella morbillorum*[a]

Characteristic	*G. morbillorum*	*S. hansenii*	*S. pleomorphus*	*S. parvulus*
Aerotolerance	+	−	−	−
Acid from:				
Cellobiose	−	−	−	+
Fructose	−	−	+	+
Galactose	−	+	−	+
Inulin	−	−	NT	+
Lactose	−	+	−	+
Maltose	w	+	−	+
Mannose	w	−	d	+
Salicin	−	−	−	+
Sucrose	w	−	−	+
Raffinose	−	+	NT	−
Production of H_2S	−	+	w	−
Esculin hydrolysis	−	d	NT	+

[a] +, positive; −, negative; w, weak; d, differs among strains; NT, not tested. All species produce lactic acid from carbohydrate fermentation and fail to ferment mannitol, sorbitol, and starch. Adapted from reference 102.

naphthyridone trovafloxacin had an MIC_{50} of 0.06 μg/ml and an MIC_{90} of 0.5 μg/ml against 14 *Peptostreptococcus* isolates. Ciprofloxacin was less active, having an MIC_{90} of 2 μg/ml against *Peptostreptococcus* isolates (1).

Evaluation, Interpretation, and Reporting of Results

The significance of finding anaerobic gram-positive cocci in clinical specimens depends on the specimen and the likelihood that it was contaminated by the physiologic flora of the skin or mucous membranes. Hence, interpretation of the culture result is dependent on the nature and quality of the specimen submitted to the laboratory. When anaerobic cocci are the only isolates in a clinical specimen, one still should keep in mind that they most often occur in mixed infection. This might have implications in selecting an appropriate antimicrobial therapy.

TABLE 5 Antimicrobic susceptibilities of *Peptostreptococcus* spp. and *Peptococcus niger*[a]

Antimicrobial agent	Breakpoint (mg/liter)	*Peptostreptococcus* species[b]: No. of strains tested	MIC_{50}[c] (mg/liter)	MIC_{90}[c] (mg/liter)	MIC range (mg/liter)	*Peptococcus niger*: No. of strains tested	MIC_{50} (mg/liter)	MIC range (mg/liter)
Penicillin G	2	60	0.2	8	≤0.06–128	4	0.1	0.1–0.5
Ampicillin	2	98	2	32	≤0.06–128	4	0.1	≤0.06–2
Piperacillin	128	35	0.5	8	≤0.06–32	4	0.2	≤0.06–0.5
Mezlocillin	128	35	0.5	16	≤0.06–128	4	0.2	0.2–1
Cefuroxime	16	35	0.5	16	≤0.06–≥256	4	0.2	≤0.06–1
Cefpodoxime		63	1	32	≤0.12–264	0		
Cefixime		63	8	≥64	0.5–≥64	0		
Cefoxitin	64	123	1	8	≤0.06–64	4	0.5	0.2–4
Cefoperazone	64	60	0.5	4	≤0.06–64	4	0.2	≤0.06–8
Cefotaxime	64	35	2	8	≤0.06–16	4	1	≤0.06–2
Imipenem	16	60	1	16	≤0.06–≥256	4	1	0.5–8
Clindamycin	4	88	2	16	≤0.06–128	0		
Linocomycin	4	35	4	≥256	≤0.06–≥256	4	8	0.5–32
Ofloxacin	4	83	2	16	≤0.06–32	0		
Norfloxacin	4	39	4	32	≤0.06–128	4	1	0.5–8
Ciprofloxacin	4	139	2	4	≤0.06–32	0		
Trovafloxacin	8	14	0.06	0.5	0.015–0.5	NA[d]	NA	NA
Tinidazole	32	35	2	32	≤0.06–≥256	4	1	1–16
Metronidazole	32	147	2	64	≤0.06–≥256	4	1	0.5–8
Tetracycline	16	35	2	16	≤0.06–32	4	1	0.2–8
Doxycycline		63	4	16	≤0.06–32	0	NA	NA

[a] Includes data compiled from references 1, 41, 64, 81, 115, and 116.
[b] Includes *P. anaerobius*, *P. prevotii*, *P. asaccharolyticus*, and *P. micros*.
[c] MIC_{50} and MIC_{90}, MICs at which 50% and 90% of strains, respectively, are inhibited.
[d] NA, not applicable.

ANAEROBIC NON-SPORE-FORMING GRAM-POSITIVE RODS

Description of the Genera

Members of the group of anaerobic non-spore-forming gram-positive rods are gram-positive asporogenous rods, obligately anaerobic or facultatively anaerobic, motile or nonmotile, chemoorganotrophs, and saccharolytic or asaccharolytic.

Taxonomy

The group of anaerobic non-spore-forming gram-positive rods includes the genera *Propionibacterium*, *Eubacterium*, *Bifidobacterium*, *Lactobacillus*, *Actinomyces*, and *Mobiluncus*. These genera are taxonomically quite diverse but share many phenotypic characteristics. In the past, bacterial taxonomy has relied heavily on descriptive aspects of these organisms, which has resulted in the grouping of genera into families that were probably not appropriate genetically; hence, numerous revisions are to be expected.

The gram-positive anaerobic bacteria may be separated on the basis of moles percent G+C into two major subdivisions, which appear to represent separate phylogenetic lines. The low-G+C subdivision represents a more ancient line and includes the genera *Lactobacillus*, *Clostridium*, *Eubacterium*, *Peptostreptococcus*, and *Peptococcus*. The high-G+C subdivision includes the genera *Bifidobacterium*, *Actinomyces*, *Propionibacterium*, and *Mobiluncus* (24, 60, 93, 124).

The genera fall into discrete units based on the amino acid content of the cell wall, the major end products of glucose fermentation, and the moles percent G+C (93, 95, 96, 102). *Actinomyces* cell walls contain lysine, aspartic acid, and ornithine, similar to *Bifidobacterium* cell walls. *Propionibacterium* cell walls may contain *meso*-DAP, LL-DAP, or lysine in place of diaminopimelic acid (DAP), and *Propionibacterium propionicum* (formerly *Actinomyces propionicus*, then *Arachnia propionica*) has LL-DAP or lysine in place of DAP (19, 25). There is some overlap in the moles percent G+C of all of these organisms (Table 6).

Several species of *Actinomyces* have been described more recently: *A. georgiae* (previously designated *Actinomyces* strain D08); *A. gerencseriae* (*A. israelii* serotype II); *A. neuii* (CDC group 1-like coryneform bacterium), with two subspecies, *neuii* and *anitratus*; and *A. bernardiae*, *A. hyovaginalis*, *A. radingae*, *A. turicensis*, *A. graevenitzii*, and *A. europaeus* (22, 35, 36, 37, 53, 84, 126). Recent studies on 16S rRNA sequences suggest that *A. pyogenes* and *A. bernardiae* should be assigned to the genus *Arcanobacterium* as *Arcanobacterium pyogenes* and *Arcanobacterium bernardiae*, respectively (85). The same group reported that 16S rRNA sequence data from *Actinomyces*, *Mobiluncus*, *Rothia*, and *Arcanobacterium* indicate that these genera are phylogenetically intermixed with *Actinomyces* species and that the genus *Actinomyces* clearly represents at least seven different distinct genera. See chapter 21 for a complete discussion of the actinomycetes that grow aerobically.

Addenda to the *Lactobacillus* species include *L. rimae* and *L. uli* (76). At least 34 species are currently recognized, and at least 19 other distinct groups of unnamed species are known, but only a few are encountered in the clinical laboratory.

Mobiluncus spp. (motile anaerobic curved rods) were first recovered in 1913 from the uterine discharge of a woman with postpartum endometritis. While other workers reported the recovery of similar anaerobic rods from vaginal specimens, this group of microorganisms was not recognized formally and given the name *Mobiluncus* until 1984 (104). The genus *Mobiluncus* is composed of obligately anaerobic, gram-variable or gram-negative, curved, non-spore-forming rods with tapered ends. The rods occur singly or in pairs and may have a gull-wing appearance. They are motile by multiple subpolar flagella. Even though single organisms stain gram negative to gram variable, they possess a multilayered gram-positive type of cell wall lacking the lipopolysaccharide 2-keto-3-deoxyoctulonic acid and hydroxylated fatty acids typically found in the cell walls of gram-negative organisms (16). These organisms are susceptible to vanco-

TABLE 6 Differentiation of anaerobic gram-positive rods[a,b]

Characteristic	*Actinomyces* spp.	*Propionibacterium propionicum*	*Bifidobacterium* spp.	*Lactobacillus* spp.	*Propionibacterium* spp.	*Eubacterium* spp.	*Mobiluncus* spp.
Strictly anaerobic	v	−	+	v	v	+	+
Motility	−	−	−	−	−	v	+
Catalase production	±[c]	−	−	−	v	−	−
VFA[d]	S, L, a	A, P, (I), (s)[e]	A, L[f]	L, (a), (s)	A, P, (iv), (s), (I)	A, B[g]	S, L, A
Indole production	−	−	−	−	v	−	−
Nitrate reduction	v	+	−	−	v	v	v
Mol% G+C of DNA	55–68	63–75	57–64	35–53	59–66	30–40	49–52

[a] Data compiled from references 24, 37, 70, 92, 95, 96, 101, 102, and 104.

[b] +, Most strains positive; −, most strains negative; v, variable results occur for different species of the same genus; VFA, volatile fatty acids; A, acetic acid; S, succinic acid; B, butyric acid; L, lactic acid; P, propionic acid; IV, isovaleric acid; () variable or, if produced, usually present only in trace amounts; lowercase letters represent products usually produced in small amounts.

[c] *A. viscosus* is the only member of the genus that produces catalase.

[d] Determined in peptone-yeast extract-glucose broth cultures.

[e] Under anaerobic conditions, *P. propionicum* ferments glucose to CO_2, acetic acid, propionic acid, and small amounts of lactic and succinic acids. In air, glucose is converted to CO_2 and acetic acid.

[f] Acetic and lactic acids are produced in a molar ratio of 3:2.

[g] Metabolic products formed by *Eubacterium* species vary (see Table 8).

mycin and resistant to colistin, which is consistent with the susceptibility patterns of other gram-positive organisms. The genus *Mobiluncus* does not conform to other families of anaerobic bacteria. Because the family *Bacteroidaceae* includes other genera of curved, anaerobic, rod-shaped bacteria that produce succinic acid, the genus *Mobiluncus* was tentatively placed into the family *Bacteroidaceae* in 1984. Partial reverse transcriptase sequencing of the 16S rRNA has demonstrated that the genus *Mobiluncus* is more closely related to the genus *Actinomyces* than to the *Bacteroidaceae* (60).

Natural Habitat

With the exception of *A. humiferus*, which is found exclusively in soil, the natural habitat of *Actinomyces* spp. appears to be the mucous membranes of humans and animals. *A. bovis*, *A. denticolens*, *A. howellii*, *A. hordeovulneris*, *A. hyovaginalis*, *A. slackii*, and *A. suis* have not been isolated from humans.

Bifidobacterium species are found in the intestines of humans and animals and in sewage. *Eubacterium* species are also found in the intestines and in the oral cavities (periodontia) of humans and other animals and in various plant products. *Propionibacterium* species can be isolated from skin and the oral cavity. Although most isolates of *Lactobacillus* species are facultative anaerobes, approximately 20% of the human isolates are obligately anaerobic. *Lactobacillus* species are found in the mouth (in both saliva and plaque), intestinal tract, and vagina of humans and other mammals. They are also found in a variety of food products.

The natural habitat of *Mobiluncus* spp. is the reproductive tract and rectum of humans and other primates. *Mobiluncus* species have been found in 50 to 65% of vaginal specimens from women with bacterial vaginosis (*Gardnerella vaginalis* vaginitis, nonspecific vaginitis) (50). However, they are recovered from fewer than 10% of specimens from women with normal, *Lactobacillus*-predominant flora. They may be recovered together with other bacteria associated with bacterial vaginosis from the vaginas of children with no history of sexual abuse. *Mobiluncus* spp. have been cultured from rectal swabs from women with bacterial vaginosis and from rectal and urethral specimens from male sex partners of women with bacterial vaginosis.

Clinical Significance in Actinomycosis

Information on the occurrence of anaerobic gram-positive rods in clinical materials is difficult to obtain, since many data on anaerobic infections are not reliable. Both methodologic and taxonomic problems contribute to our inability to obtain such data. However, results from individual laboratories specializing in anaerobes indicate that the prevalence of these anaerobes in various infections is much greater than is reflected by their isolation frequencies in many other clinical laboratories. For example, Finegold determined that *Actinomyces* spp. were isolated in his laboratory from 14% of the infections involving anaerobes, while other workers reported a much lower incidence (33).

Actinomycosis is the most frequently encountered disease entity involving *Actinomyces* spp. The incidence of actinomycosis in the United States is difficult to determine, since this disease is not reportable. While there are few recent reports on this subject, Slack and Gerencser concluded that "actinomycosis occurs throughout the world and is neither a rare nor a common disease" (101). Actinomycosis is observed twice as frequently in men as in women, and the anatomical distribution is about 60% cervicofacial, 15% thoracic, 20% abdominal, and 5% other types. Clinically, actinomycosis other than the cervicofacial type is often misdiagnosed as a malignant tumor.

Actinomycosis is characterized as a chronic granulomatous lesion that becomes suppurative and forms abscesses and draining sinuses (88). A purulent actinomycotic discharge, usually containing macroscopic sulfur granules that appear as whitish, yellow, or brown granular bodies, may be present. *A. israelii* is the most common cause of actinomycosis in humans, but other *Actinomyces* spp. (i.e., *A. naeslundii*, *A. odontolyticus*, and *A. viscosus*), as well as *Propionibacterium propionicum*, may also be etiologic agents. These infections are usually polymicrobic. Frequently, *Fusobacterium* spp., *Eikenella corrodens*, *Capnocytophaga* spp., *Actinobacillus actinomycetemcomitans*, black-pigmented *Prevotella* spp., *Porphyromonas asaccharolytica*, *Porphyromonas gingivalis*, and streptococci are also found in various combinations. It is believed that these associated microorganisms contribute significantly to the pathogenesis of actinomycosis.

Among animals, the incidence of actinomycosis is greatest in cattle, although infections have also been reported in dogs, sheep, goats, horses, cats, deer, moose, and antelope (101). Bovine actinomycosis (lumpy jaw) occurs when *A. bovis* gains entrance to the mandibular tissue following traumatic injury, after ingestion of rough plant material such as straw or silage, or via a broken tooth. *A. hordeovulneris* is of veterinary importance because it is an agent of actinomycosis (thoracic or abdominal) of dogs (14). In many cases, *A. viscosus* is isolated with *A. hordeovulneris*, suggesting that the natural habitat of the organism is the canine oral cavity. *A. suis* is believed to be involved in swine mammary gland actinomycosis. The pathogenic properties of. *A. denticolens*, *A. howellii*, and *A. slackii* are unknown.

Clinical Significance in Other Infections

A. israelii, *A. naeslundii*, *A. viscosus*, *A. odontolyticus*, *A. meyeri*, *A turicensis*, *A. radingae*, *A. neuii*, and *Arcanobacterium pyogenes* (see chapter 21) were found as causative agents in various diseases in humans and must be considered opportunistic pathogens (27). All except *A. pyogenes* and *A. meyeri* are found in large numbers in saliva and subgingival plaques. *A. viscosus* and *A. naeslundii* have been studied extensively and are believed to play significant roles in dental caries and periodontal disease (69). *Actinomyces* species may also be involved in pelvic inflammatory disease associated with intrauterine contraceptive devices (34, 108, 127). Evans estimated that between 1.6 and 11.6% of intrauterine device users have *A. israelii* infection (29). *Actinomyces* species are also reported to cause pyogenic liver abscess, with the majority of cases occurring in patients without preexisting oral disease or intra-abdominal infections (68).

Propionibacteria have been recovered from mixed infections of the skin (12, 28). The role of *Propionibacterium acnes* in acne vulgaris is widely accepted. Induction of proinflammatory cytokines (113) and/or specific cell-mediated immunity (55) by *Propionibacterium* antigens may play a role in the pathogenesis. Often, propionibacterial infections have been linked to surgical procedures or foreign bodies (52). *Propionibacterium* is the predominant member of the anaerobic flora from conjunctival cultures of adults and children and has been reported to cause uveitis and endophthalmitis. The organism has also proven to be pathogenic in infections of bone, joints, and the central nervous system (28). It may cause endocarditis especially after prosthetic valve implantation (42). *Propionibacterium* has been associated with the SAPHO syndrome (synovitis, acne, pustulosis, hyperostosis, and osteomyelitis) (59). Thus, although *Propionibacterium* species often originate from the normal flora, they can act as primary pathogens and should not be immediately dismissed as contaminants. However, in a recent study, recovery of *Propionibacterium* species from the blood accounted for only 5% of clinically significant bacteremias and 50% of clinically insignificant bacteremias, suggesting that this group of microorganisms is a more frequent cause of insignificant anaerobic bacteremias (91).

Finally, the ability of *Propionibacterium* spp. to modulate the immune response to unrelated antigens has been well documented (83, 90).

Propionibacterium propionicum is a recognized agent of lacrimal canaliculitis and produces abscesses in animals when injected.

Eubacterium species are not frequently encountered in clinical specimens, probably because of the difficulty in recognizing them. Eubacteria are usually isolated in mixed culture from abscesses and wounds and very rarely from blood cultures. *E. lentum* is the species most frequently observed. Several species have been associated with periodontal disease: *E. nodatum*, *E. timidum*, and *E. brachy* (48, 70, 114). A study by Hill et al. suggests that these species are involved in numerous infections at other sites such as head and neck, thorax, bones, skin, and pelvis (44).

Bifidobacterium species are infrequently encountered in clinical materials. *B. dentium* (formerly *Actinomyces eriksonii* and later *B. eriksonii*) appears to be the only *Bifidobacterium* species with pathogenic potential. It has been isolated from dental caries and from various clinical materials such as lower respiratory tract specimens. *B. longum* and *B. breve* are found only rarely in human clinical materials. Recent reports claim that administration of *B. breve* to preterm infants improved weight gain and reduced abnormal abdominal signs (56).

Most *Lactobacillus* species recovered from clinical specimens are microaerophilic, but obligately anaerobic isolates can also be recovered. They are rarely pathogenic and might even be beneficial in the treatment of bacterial vaginosis (78) and diarrhea (77, 86, 123). However, lactobacilli have been reported to cause endocarditis, neonatal meningitis, chorioamnionitis, pleuropulmonary infections, and bacteremia (3, 23, 26, 62). Lactobacilli may play a role in dental caries (89). Identification of anaerobic lactobacilli to the species level is extremely difficult and, given the low pathogenicity of the organisms, is rarely indicated. The difficulty in identifying lactobacilli can lead to confusion about the probable source of some infections due to *Lactobacillus* species. For example, a case of peritonitis associated with a vancomycin-resistant *Lactobacillus rhamnosus* in a continuous peritoneal dialysis patient was initially identified as being due to *L. acidophilus* (57). Superinfection from *Lactobacillus* spp. may be possible only in an immunocompromised host, and identification of this organism to the species level is often inaccurate because of the poor reproducibility of current methods.

The pathogenic potential of *Mobiluncus* spp. is not well understood. However, it is unclear whether the rare isolation of *Mobiluncus* spp. from clinical specimens is due to the inability of many laboratories to isolate and identify this fastidious microorganism or to its low pathogenicity. While *Mobiluncus* spp. are present in the vaginas of many women with bacterial vaginosis, their role in the etiology of this syndrome is not known. However, bacterial vaginosis in pregnant women is associated with premature rupture of membranes and preterm birth (67). The pathogenic potential of *Mobiluncus* spp. has been supported by its isolation from breast abscesses, umbilical discharge, and blood cultures (40, 105). *Mobiluncus* spp. can also be recovered from the endometrial aspirates of women with pelvic inflammatory disease and from the chorioamnion of the placenta from preterm deliveries. While they have been recovered in pure cultures from some sterile-site specimens, they are most often found in association with *Prevotella* and *Peptostreptococcus* species.

Collection and Transport of Specimens

This group includes microorganisms that are anaerobic, aerotolerant, or facultatively anaerobic. Therefore, samples should be treated as anaerobic and handled as outlined above for anaerobic cocci.

Direct Examination

Direct microscopic examination of clinical materials is an excellent presumptive method for detection of anaerobic gram-positive rods and should be used whenever possible. In oral pathology laboratories, specimens are sectioned, stained with Brown-Brenn stain, and examined for sulfur granules, which are considered diagnostic for actinomycosis (Fig. 1).

A variety of materials are suitable for examination for the presence of sulfur granules: surgically removed tissues, autopsy tissues, bronchial washes, body fluids, purulent exudates, intrauterine devices, Papanicolau smears, and gauze from draining wounds. Sulfur granules are irregular in shape and size (ranging from 0.1 to 5 mm), hard, and usually yellowish. They may be large enough to be seen with the unaided eye; granules from patients with oral actinomycosis sometimes resemble popcorn husks. If sulfur granules are observed, one granule should be removed with an inoculating needle, loop, or sterile forceps; placed in a drop of water on a microscope slide; and then gently crushed with a second slide. A wet mount should be examined under low power (×100). The granules have distinctly irregular edges. Upon reduction of the light intensity, the peripheries of the granules give the appearance of numerous club-shaped masses of filaments radiating from the granule, which is usually difficult to distinguish. The clubs should become very distinct at higher magnification (×1,000). They should be

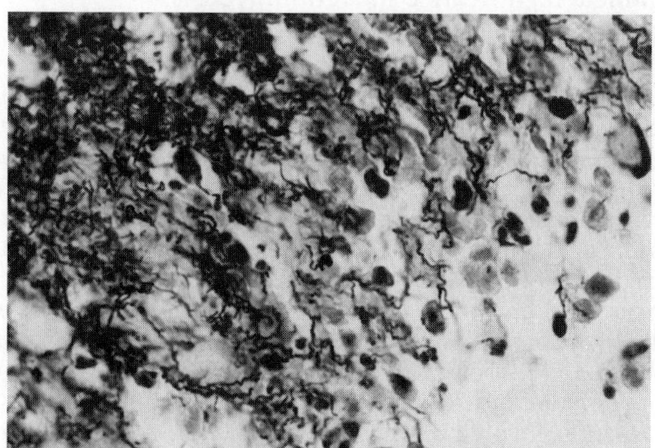

FIGURE 1 Microscopic morphology of *Actinomyces* species in a sulfur granule taken from an oral soft tissue section stained with the Brown-Brenn modification of the Gram stain. Note the characteristic appearance of the club-shaped filaments and the numerous polymorphonuclear leukocytes. Magnification, ×100. (Courtesy of Dolphine Oda, Department of Oral Biology, University of Washington, Seattle.)

refractile, and their appearance has been described as hyaline. Having made these initial observations, one must confirm the presence of filaments. The coverslip is removed, and the specimen is dried, heat fixed, and Gram stained. Gram-positive branched and unbranched filaments should be easily discernible.

However, it is usually necessary to fix, section, and stain tissue specimens to demonstrate sulfur granules. If the specimen is stained with hematoxylin-eosin, the eosinophilic clubs should be visible at the peripheries of the granules. Diphtheroidal cells and filaments should be apparent at the bases of the clubs. Visualization of the filaments in the granules is easier with a modified Gram stain such as MacCallum-Goodpasture or Brown-Brenn. Fixed and sectioned tissues can also be stained with fluorescent-antibody reagents, which are available in some public health laboratories. Other organisms that may produce granules with clubs are *Nocardia*, *Streptomyces*, and *Staphylococcus* species. The presence of *Staphylococcus* species can be ruled out by morphology and Gram reaction. To distinguish *Actinomyces* from *Nocardia* isolates, granules should be stained for acid-fastness by the modified acid fast stain (see section IX) (101).

Curved rods resembling *Mobiluncus* spp. can easily be identified in Gram-stained vaginal smears from women with bacterial vaginosis, which is the laboratory test of choice for diagnosis of this syndrome. Routine vaginal cultures for isolation of *Mobiluncus* spp. are never indicated.

Isolation Procedures

Clinicians should indicate clearly which specimens are to be cultured for the presence of non-spore-forming anaerobic gram-positive rods, particularly *Actinomyces* spp., since additional steps are required for proper setup and since the incubation should be extended. Routinely used anaerobic plate media, anaerobic blood culture media, enriched thioglycolate medium, and chopped-meat–glucose medium will support the growth of these microorganisms.

The usual procedures for anaerobes should be followed. Many of these organisms require a high moisture content for optimal growth, and so fresh medium should be used. Laboratories unable to prepare their own media may wish to consider the use of commercially prepared prereduced anaerobically sterilized blood agar available from Anaerobe Systems (San Jose, Calif.). These media have an extended shelf life of up to 6 months and yield results comparable to those obtained with fresh media (65).

Sulfur granules, if present, should be placed in a sterile petri dish and rinsed with thioglycolate broth. They should then be transferred with a sterile Pasteur pipette to a sterile tube or preferably a Ten Broeck grinder (available from various sources) with approximately 0.5 ml of thioglycolate broth. The granules should be crushed with the tip of a sterile glass rod and immediately inoculated on anaerobic blood agar and phenylethylalcohol blood agar plates (1 drop of inoculum each). The plates should be streaked to achieve well-isolated colonies. Thioglycolate broth medium should be inoculated with 2 drops of inoculum near the bottom of the tube; the screw caps should be left loose to allow exchange of gases. Media should be incubated in an anaerobic jar or anaerobic chamber at 35 to 37°C. The cultures should be examined for growth after 48 h and then reincubated for 5 to 7 days. It may be necessary to hold the plates for as long as 2 to 4 weeks. Plate media incubated in anaerobic glove boxes should be protected from desiccation.

Actinomyces species may grow on many common bacteriological media; however, isolation from specimens rich in microflora may be particularly troublesome. Therefore, the use of CC medium (see section IX) (43), which promotes the growth of actinomycetes and also allows the development of typical colonies, has been recommended.

Cervical swabs obtained via a catheter-protected device or intrauterine devices may present a considerable problem, since the number of organisms may be quite large and many different species are present. Traynor et al. described a method in which swabs are soaked in 5 ml of thioglycolate broth, the samples are diluted 10-fold in the same medium (10^{-1} to 10^{-4} dilutions), and the dilutions are plated on Columbia blood agar with and without 2.5 mg of metronidazole per liter (108). Although this method would not inhibit many organisms such as streptococci and lactobacilli, it appears to give results comparable to the visual results obtained by using fluorescent antibodies in a direct microscopic examination.

The importance of *Actinomyces* species in periodontal diseases and caries has spurred workers in the dental research field to develop selective media for recovery of these species from dental plaque (58). However, the usefulness of these media with other clinical materials has yet to be tested.

Identification Procedures

Traditionally, inclusion in a group of microorganisms was based primarily on morphologic and biochemical criteria. Although considerable progress has been made in understanding the taxonomy of anaerobic non-spore-forming gram-positive rods, reliable, accessible, and consistent tests for identification of many of these species are still not available. At least part of the problem stems from the difficulty in obtaining a uniform inoculum. As a result, identification in the clinical laboratory may be difficult.

Colony and cell morphologies are a means of presumptively separating anaerobic gram-positive rods into genera; however, these characteristics can be both variable and diverse. For example, *Actinomyces* species on blood agar yield numerous colony types, ranging from "smooth" to "molar tooth." Moreover, the colony appearance and micromorphology of *Actinomyces* and *Propionibacterium* species may vary with different culture medium used and the ages and conditions of culture. Excellent photographs and drawings may be found in references 49, 101, and 102.

The key for the presumptive genus identification of anaerobic gram-positive rods is depicted in Table 6. As shown, gas chromatography of metabolic products is an important tool in identifying gram-positive anaerobes. Some other genera may be eliminated from consideration by relatively simple means. The presence of bacterial endospores indicates *Bacillus* or *Clostridium* species. Some organisms appear more rod-like or diphtheroidal on solid medium than in broth culture. *Streptococcus mutans*, *Streptococcus intermedius*, *Gemella morbillorum*, and others form elongated cells on solid media more rapidly than in broth culture and may on initial inspection be mistaken for rods. *Nocardia*, *Rothia*, *Corynebacterium*, *Erysipelothrix*, and *Listeria* species may be ruled out as anaerobic gram-positive non-spore-forming bacilli by testing aerobic growth. The observation of rods with clubs or bifurcated ends should suggest a species of *Bifidobacterium*, but this morphology may also be observed in other genera. Non-partial-acid-fast branched filaments are good indicators of *Actinomyces* species.

Actinomyces species are facultatively anaerobic, except for *A. bovis* and *A. meyeri*, which are strict anaerobes or very rarely microaerophilic. All species grow best in primary cultures under anaerobic conditions. It may be difficult to obtain isolates in pure culture; therefore, several subcultures are recommended to ensure purity before biochemical tests are carried out.

Differentiation of several *Actinomyces* species may be difficult. *A. naeslundii* and *A. viscosus* are very similar phenotypically but differ in catalase production, with *A. viscosus* being positive. *A. israelii* and *Propionibacterium propionicum* both produce acetic and lactic acids as end products of carbohydrate metabolism; however, *Propionibacterium propionicum* produces propionic acid whereas *A. israelii* produces succinic acid. Differential characteristics for species of *Actinomyces*, *A. pyogenes*, and *Propionibacterium propionicum* are summarized in Table 7. Phenotypically, *A. israelii* and other *Actinomyces* species are very similar to *Eubacterium nodatum*, but the production of butyric acid by some *Eubacterium* species is a differential characteristic (44, 49). Some *Actinomyces* spp. actually require CO_2 before they can produce succinate.

Eubacterium spp. (Tables 8 and 9) are easily confused with other anaerobic gram-positive rods; however, gas-liquid chromatographic analysis of metabolic end products is very useful for differentiation (44, 49, 70) (Table 6). Cells may be either uniform or pleomorphic on Gram stain, and growth is obligately anaerobic. They are chemoorganotrophs and may or may not be saccharolytic. The moles percent G+C for the species ranges from 30 to 55%, demonstrating that the genus is a heterogeneous group. This conclusion is supported by the fact that the metabolic end products fall into three groups: (i) butyric acid plus other short-chain fatty acids and alcohols; (ii) a combination of lactic, acetic, and formic acids with H_2; and (iii) few or no detectable acids.

The cellular and colonial morphologic characteristics of *Rothia dentocariosa* (39) (see chapter 21) closely resemble those of *Actinomyces* spp. and to some extent those of *Nocardia* spp. Biochemically, *R. dentocariosa* is fermentative whereas *Nocardia* spp. are not; fermentation of glucose by *R. dentocariosa* does not produce succinic acid, whereas fermentation by *Actinomyces* spp. does.

The key characteristic (Table 10) of *Bifidobacterium* spp. is the production of acetate and lactate at a molar ratio of 2:3, which distinguishes these organisms from other lactic acid- and acetic acid-producing gram-positive anaerobic rods.

Lactobacillus spp. can usually be identified on the basis of long, parallel-sided, thin gram-positive rods on Gram stain; a negative catalase test; and a major lactic acid peak from glucose in gas chromatography.

There are currently two recognized species of *Mobiluncus*: *M. curtisii* and *M. mulieris*. They are oxidase, catalase, and indole negative, and H_2S is not produced. Both species of *Mobiluncus* are positive for proline aminopeptidase and α-D-glucosidase and negative for phosphatases and β-D-glucosidase. They are weakly saccharolytic, and they produce succinic and acetic acids during fermentation, with or without lactic acid. Growth is not stimulated by formate and fumarate. The strains are motile by multiple subterminal flagella. Colonies are colorless, translucent, smooth, and convex and may have a watery appearance, especially on very moist or fresh media. Colonies have a maximum diameter of 2 to 3 mm after 5 days of uninterrupted anaerobic incubation. They may be less than 1 mm in diameter after 2 days of incubation.

Although cells of both species are curved and slightly pointed rods, *M. curtisii* can be differentiated from *M. mulieris* most easily by its length and its gram-variable rather than gram-negative staining. *M. curtissi* is shorter (mean length, 1.7 μm) than *M. mulieris* (mean length, 2.9 μm). Typical strains of *M. curtisii* hydrolyze hippurate, but up to 73% of atypical *M. curtisii* isolates (*M. curtisii* group SLH 29) identified by DNA homology lack this ability (99). Gas-chromatographic analysis of peptone yeast broth supplemented with starch and 2% serum is of some use in distinguishing the two species. *M. curtisii* produces a major succinate and a minor acetate peak, while *M. mulieris* generally produces major succinate and acetate peaks with or without a minor lactate peak. Typical strains of *M. curtisii* are positive for α-D-galactosidase and arginine dihydrolase, while *M. mulieris* is negative for these two enzymes (Table 11).

Several commercial systems for the identification of anaerobic bacteria have been evaluated for gram-positive rods. While the number of isolates evaluated in each study is relatively small, the overall accuracy of these systems is low (Table 12). More recent reports suggest that molecular methods like PCR-restriction fragment length polymorphism may be helpful in permitting a definite identification of anaerobic gram-positive rods (99, 122).

As with aerobic gram-positive organisms, analysis of cellular fatty acids may aid in the identification of anaerobic bacteria (38). However, this technique does not lend itself to nonspecialist laboratories.

Antimicrobial Susceptibility

New information on the antimicrobial susceptibilities of anaerobic gram-positive rods is sparse compared with the information available on other anaerobic species. Many reports fail to give results for specific species, opting instead to combine data for the group. However, it is generally accepted that the anaerobic gram-positive non-spore-forming rods are susceptible to penicillin G, carbenicillin, and chloramphenicol (115, 117). Other antimicrobial agents, particularly metronidazole, have been reported to have various efficiencies. Clindamycin, erythromycin, and tetracycline were active against 94, 88, and 60% of isolates tested, respectively (107, 115, 116). *Mobiluncus curtisii* is uniformly resistant to metronidazole, but the clinical significance of this fact is doubtful (103). Women with bacterial vaginosis who are treated with oral or intravaginal metronidazole rarely have persistent *M. curtisii* immediately after therapy.

Eradication of some of these organisms from the sites of infection may be difficult, particularly in actinomycotic or actinomycosis-like infections, since blood supplies to the infected site(s) may be inadequate, multiple abscesses may be present, and surrounding granulation tissue may impede the penetration of antimicrobial agents. Therefore, in these cases surgical intervention and prolonged therapy is usually recommended (8, 33, 88).

Evaluation, Interpretation, and Reporting of Results

As with the anaerobic gram-positive cocci, interpretation of culture results may require additional clinical information about how the specimen was obtained. Specimens yielding anaerobic gram-positive rods will often yield two or three other organisms as well; therefore, one should not automatically dismiss mixed cultures as contaminated. On the other hand, since these microorganisms are members of the endogenous flora of the skin, oral cavity, genital tract, and gut, contamination by the normal flora during specimen acquisition is often a problem. Therefore, communication with the physician submitting the specimen for culture is essential.

TABLE 7 Characteristics of members of the genus *Actinomyces* and *Propionibacterium propionicum*[a, b]

Characteristic	*P. propionicum*	*A. viscosus*	*A. neuii*	*A. naeslundii*	*A. odontolyticus*	*A. gerencseriae*	*A. georgiae*	*A. graevenitzii*	*A. israelii*	*A. meyeri*	*A. turicensis*	*A. radingae*	*A. bernardiae*	*A. europaeus*	*A. pyogenes*	*A. hyovaginalis*
Catalase	−	+	+	−	−	−	−	−	−	−	−	−	−	−	−	−
Nitrate reduction	+	d	d	+	+	−	−	−	d	−	−	−	−	−	−	+
Gelatin hydrolysis	d	−	−	−	−	−	d		−	−		−			+	−
H_2S production	d	+	−	+	+		d		+	−					−	
Esculin hydrolysis	−	d		+	d	+	+	−	+	−	−	+	d	d	−	+
Pink pigment on blood agar	−	−		−	+[c]	−	−	−	−	−					−	
Urease	−	d	−	+	−	−	−	−	−	d	−	−	−	−	−	−
Acid from:																
meso-Inositol	d	d		+	−	d	d	+	+	−	+				d	d
Glycerol	d[d]		+	d	d	−	d	+	−	d	+				−	
Xylose		+	+	d	d	+	+	−	+	+	+	+	−	−	+	+
Raffinose	+	+	+	+	−	+	−		+	−				−	−	−
Trehalose	+	d	+	+	−	+	+	−	−	−	−				d	−
Mannitol	d	−	+	−	−	+	−	−	+	−	−	d	−	−	−	
Glycogen		d	−	d	d	−	+		−	d	−	−	+	d	+	
Beta-hemolysis on sheep blood agar	+	−	−	−	−	−	−		−	−	−/w	−/w	d	d	+	−
Mol% G + C	63–65	59–69	55–58	63–68	62	70–71	65–69		57–65	64–67			63–66	61–63	56–58	63

[a] Data adapted from references 22, 24, 39, 84, 93, 95, 101, and 102.
[b] +, positive reactions for 90 to 100% of strains tested; −, negative reactions for 90 to 100% of strains tested; d, variable reactions, no result, not available; w, weak.
[c] Pigmentation of A. *odontolyticus* may be variable and may take 7 to 10 days to develop. Exposure to oxygen may enhance pigmentation.
[d] Serovar 1, variable reaction; serovar 2 usually negative.

TABLE 8 Characteristics of nonsaccharolytic species of *Eubacterium*[a]

Species	Cellular characteristics	Colony morphology	Fatty acid production[b]	Utilization of pyruvate	Nitrate reduced	Gelatin hydrolyzed	Esculin hydrolyzed	Hydrogen produced
E. nodatum	Branched, filamentous, or club-shaped cells; nonmotile; 0.5–0.9 by 2.0–12 mm in PY[c]	Molar tooth, heaped, or raspberry; 0.5–1.0 mm in diameter		+	–	–	–	–
D-6 group[d]	Regular, variable length, occasional chaining, beading, or diphtheroidal	Circular, entire, convex	a, B, paa, (f), (l), (s), (hc)	–	–	–	–	+
E. brachy	Short or coccoidal, chaining, 0.4–0.8 by 0.1–3.0 mm in PY	Circular, entire, low convex, occasionally rough	ib, iv, ic (a), (f), (l), (s), (hc)	–, (+)	–	–	–	+
E. timidum	Short, regular to diphtheroidal, occasional clumps, 0.8–1.6 by 1.6–3.1 mm in PY	Circular, entire, low convex	paa (a), (f), (l), (s)	–	–	–	–	–
E. lentum	Short or coccoidal, occasional chains, 0.2–0.4 by 0.2–2.0 mm in PY	Circular, entire, low convex	(a), (f), (l), (s)	–	+	–	–	–
E. dolichum	Thin rods in long chains, slightly tapered, 0.4–0.6 by 1.6–6.0 mm in PYG[c]	Fails to grow on blood agar plate	b (l), (a)	–	–	w	–	–
E. combesii	Singles, pairs, short chains, and palisade arrangements; motile; 0.6–0.8 by 3.0–10 mm in PYG	Circular, entire to irregular convex, semiopaque, whitish yellow, shiny, smooth	A, B, iv, l, ib, (p), (f)	+	–	+	d	+
E. yurii	Straight rods with slightly rounded edges, form unique three-dimensional brushlike aggregates	Colonies spread on blood agar, measuring about 10 mm in 48 h; pale yellow pigment may be evident	B, A, p			–	–	
E. infirmum	Short rods (0.5 by 2.0 μm). cells occur as singles	Colonies are approximately 1 mm, circular, convex, and translucent	a, B					
E. tardum	Short rods (0.5 by 1.0–3.0 μm), cells may occur in singles and in diphtheroidal arrangements		B					
E. minutum	Short rods (0.5 by 1.0–1.5 μm), in singles, pairs, and clumps	Colonies on BHI-blood agar are 0.3–0.5 mm, circular, convex, entire, translucent	B or b	–	–	–	–	
E. saphenum[e]	Short rods	After 7 days, colonies are 0.3–0.5 mm, circular, convex, and translucent	a, b	–	–	–	–	

[a] Data compiled from references 21, 44, 48, 82, and 111.
[b] ic, isocaproate, iv, isovalerate; ib, isobutyrate; a, acetate; b, butyrate; l, lactate; s, succinate; f, formate; p, propionate; v, valerate; paa, phenylacetate; hc, hydrocinnamate. Capital letters represent ≥1 meq of product per 100 ml of culture; lowercase letters represent <1 meq of product per 100 ml of culture; products in parantheses are not produced uniformly. +, most strains positive; –, most strains negative; (+), usually positive but some strains give negative reaction; w, reaction weak; d, reaction variable.
[c] PY, peptone-yeast extract; PYG, peptone-yeast extract-glucose.
[d] An undescribed *Eubacterium* species that appears to be of clinical significance.
[e] Resembles *E. nodatum* except for lack of production of ammonia from arginine

TABLE 9 Flowchart for identification of selected *Eubacterium* spp.[a]

I. Butyric acid produced
- A. Caproic acid produced: *E. alactolyticus*
- B. Caproic acid not produced, acid from glucose
  - 1. Indole produced: *E. saburreum*
  - 2. Indole not produced
    - a. Nitrate reduced
      - i. Esculin hydrolyzed: *E. multiforme*
      - ii. Esculin not hydrolyzed: *E. monoforme*
    - b. Nitrate not reduced
      - i. Major lactic acid from glucose: *E. rectale*
      - ii. No major lactic acid from glucose
        - aa. Acid from glucose and esculin hydrolyzed: *E. limosum*
        - bb. No acid from glucose or maltose, gelatin hydrolyzed: *E. combesii*
        - cc. Weak acid from glucose and maltose, gelatin not hydrolyzed: *E. nodatum*

II. Butyric acid not produced
- A. Acid from glucose
  - 1. Indole produced: *E. tenue*
  - 2. Indole not produced
    - a. Major lactic acid from glucose: *E. aerofaciens*
    - b. No lactic acid from glucose: *E. contortum*
- B. No acid from glucose: *E. lentum*, *E. brachy*, *E. timidum*, *E. yurii*

[a] Modified from reference 70.

TABLE 10 Characteristics of *Bifidobacterium* spp.[a]

Species	Arabinose	Cellobiose	Fermentation of glycogen	Melezitose	Sucrose	Occurrence in human material			
						Clinical	Mouth	Feces	Vagina
B. dentium	+	+	+	+	+	+	+	+	+
B. bifidum	−	−	−	−	−	+		+	+
B. infantis	−	$-^{+}$	−	−	+			+	+
B. globosum	+	v	+	−	+			+	
B. breve	−	+	+	v	+	+		+	+
B. longum	+	$-^{+}$	−	$+^{w}$	+	+		+	
B. catenulatum	v	+	v	−	+			+	+
B. adolescentis	v	+	+	−	+			+	

[a] +, pH below 5.5, or positive; w, pH 5.5 to 5.9 or weak; −, pH above 5.9, or negative; v, variable; superscript, reaction of some strains of a species. Fermentation patterns of *Bifidobacterium* species overlap considerably; polyacrylamide gel electrophoresis or DNA-DNA homology or both are required for the definitive identification of some species. All *Bifidobacterium* species produce acid from glucose.

TABLE 11 Characteristics of *Mobiluncus* spp.[a]

Characteristic	*M. mulieris*[b]	*M. curtisii*	*M. curtisii* group SLH-29
Length (μm)	2.9	1.7	1.3–1.7
Gram reaction	−	v	−
Hippurate hydrolyzed	−	+	v (27%)
α-D-Galactosidase	−	+	v (7%)
Arginine dihydrolase	−	+	+
Proline aminopeptidase	+	+	+
α-D-Glucosidase	+	+	+
β-D-Glucosidase	−	−	−

[a] Adapted from references 99 and 104.
[b] v, variable; −, negative; +, positive.

TABLE 12 Identification of anaerobic gram-positive rods by commercial systems[a]

Organism	% Correctly identified to genus and species level (no. of isolates tested) by:				
	API 20A	Vitek ANI	PRAS II	RapID-ANA	AN-Ident
Actinomyces spp.	14 (7)	50 (6)	NT[b]	40 (5)	86 (7)
Propionibacterium spp.	90 (10)	89 (18)	66 (6)	NT	63 (16)
P. acnes	NT	NT	NT	96 (25)	NT
P. granulosum	NT	NT	NT	100 (2)	NT
E. lentum	100 (4)	33 (6)	100 (2)	69 (13)	100 (6)
E. limosum	NT	NT	NT	33 (3)	NT
Lactobacillus spp.	0 (1)	25 (4)	100 (1)	NT	100 (2)
Bifidobacterium spp.	0 (1)	75 (4)	NT	66 (3)	0 (1)

[a] Data compiled from references 2, 15, 54, 73, and 97.
[b] NT, not tested.

REFERENCES

1. **Aldridge, K. E., D. Ashcroft, and K. A. Bowman.** 1997. Comparative in vitro activities of trovafloxacin (CP 99,219) and other antimicrobials against clinically significant anaerobes. *Antimicrob. Agents Chemother.* **41:** 484–487.
2. **Appelbaum, P. C., C. S. Kaufmann, and J. W. Depenbusch.** 1985. Accuracy and reproducibility of a four-hour method for anaerobe identification. *J. Clin. Microbiol.* **21:** 894–898.
3. **Bayer, A. S., A. W. Chow, D. Betts, and L. B. Guze.** 1978. Lactobacillemia—report of nine cases. Important clinical and therapeutic considerations. *Am. J. Med.* **64:** 808–813.
4. **Bennion, R. S., J. E. Thompson, E. J. Baron, and S. M. Finegold.** 1990. Gangrenous and perforated appendicitis with peritonitis: treatment and bacteriology. *Clin. Ther.* **12:**31–44.
5. **Bjornson, H. S.** 1989. Biliary tract and hepatic infections, p. 333–347. *In* S. M. Finegold and W. L. George (ed.), *Anaerobic Infections in Humans*. Academic Press, Inc., San Diego, Calif.
6. **Bourgault, A. M., J. E. Rosenblatt, and R. H. Fitzgerald.** 1980. *Peptococcus magnus:* a significant human pathogen. *Ann. Intern. Med.* **93:**244–248.
7. **Brook, I.** 1987. Comparison of two transport systems for recovery of aerobic and anaerobic bacteria from abscesses. *J. Clin. Microbiol.* **24:**2020–2022.
8. **Brook, I.** 1988. Anaerobic bacteria in suppurative genitourinary infections. *J. Urol.* **141:**889–893.
9. **Brook, I.** 1988. Aerobic and anaerobic bacteriology of purulent nasopharyngitis in children. *J. Clin. Microbiol.* **26:** 592–594.
10. **Brook, I.** 1988. Recovery of anaerobic bacteria from clinical specimens in 12 years at two military hospitals. *J. Clin. Microbiol.* **26:**1181–1188.
11. **Brook, I.** 1988. Microbiology of non-puerperal breast abscesses. *J. Infect. Dis.* **157:**377–379.
12. **Brook, I., and E. H. Frazier.** 1993. Significant recovery of nonsporulating anaerobic rods from clinical specimens. *Clin. Infect. Dis.* **16:**476–480.
13. **Brook, I., R. B. Kiehlich, and S. Grimm.** 1981. Bacteriology of acute periapical abscess in children. *J. Endodontol.* **7:**378–380.
14. **Buchanan, A. M., J. L. Scott, M. A. Gerencser, B. L. Beaman, S. Jang, and L. Biberstein.** 1984. *Actinomyces hordeovulneris* sp. nov., an agent of canine actinomycosis. *Int. J. Syst. Bacteriol.* **34:**439–443.
15. **Burlage, R. S., and P. D. Ellner.** 1985. Comparison of the PRAS II, AN-Ident, and RapID ANA systems for identification of anaerobic bacteria. *J. Clin. Microbiol.* **22:**32–35.
16. **Carlone, G. M., M. L. Thomas, R. J. Arko, G. O. Guerrant, C. W. Moss, J. M. Swenson, and S. A. Morse.** 1986. Cell wall characteristics of *Mobiluncus* species. *Int. J. Syst. Bacteriol.* **36:**288–296.
17. **Cato, E. P.** 1983. Transfer of *Peptostreptococcus parvulus* (Weinberg, Nativelle, and Prevot 1937), Smith 1957 to the genus *Streptococcus: Streptococcus parvulus* (Weinberg, Nativelle, and Prevot 1937) comb. nov., nom. rev., emend. *Inst. J. Syst. Bacteriol.* **33:**82–84.
18. **Celig, D. M., and P. C. Schreckenberger.** 1991. Clinical evaluation of the RapID ANA II panel for identification of anaerobic bacteria. *J. Clin. Microbiol.* **29:**457–462.
19. **Charfreitag, O., M. O. Collins, and E. Stackebrandt.** 1988. Reclassification of *Arachnia propionica* as *Propionibacterium propionicus* comb. nov. *Int. J. Syst. Bacteriol.* **38:** 354–375.
20. **Cheeseman, S. L., S. J. Hiom, A. J. Weightman, and W. G. Wade.** 1996. Phylogeny of oral asaccharolytic *Eubacterium* species determined by 16S ribosomal DNA sequence comparison and proposal of *Eubacterium infirmum* sp. nov. and *Eubacterium tardum* sp. nov. *Int. J. Syst Bacteriol.* **46:** 957–959.
21. **Cockerill, F. R., J. G. Hughes, E. A. Vetter, R. A. Mueller, A. L. Weaver, D. M. Ilstrup, J. E. Rosenblatt, and W. R. Wilson.** 1997. Analysis of 281,797 consecutive blood cultures performed over an eight-year period: trends in microorganisms isolated and the value of anaerobic culture of blood. *Clin. Infect. Dis.* **24:**403–418.
22. **Collins, M. S., S. Stubbs, J. Hommez, and L. A. Devriese.** 1993. Molecular taxonomic studies of *Actinomyces*-like bacteria isolated from purulent lesions in pigs and description of *Actinomyces hyovaginalis* sp. nov. *Int. J. Syst. Bacteriol.* **43:**471–473.
23. **Cox, S. M., L. E. Phillips, L. J. Mercer, C. E. Stager, S. Waller, and S. Faro.** 1986. Lactobacillemia of amniotic fluid origin. *Obstet. Gynecol.* **68:**134–135.
24. **Cummins, C. S., and J. S. Johnson.** 1986. Genus I. *Propionibacterium* Orla Jensen 1909, 337[AL], p. 1346–1363. *In* P. H. A. Sneath, N. S. Mair, M. E. Sharpe, and J. G. Holt (ed.), *Bergey's Manual of Systematic Bacteriology*, vol. 2. The Williams & Wilkins Co., Baltimore, Md.
25. **Cummins, C. S., and C. W. Moss.** 1990. Fatty acid composition of *Propionibacterium propionicus* (*Arachnia propionica*). *J. Clin. Microbiol.* **40:**307–308.
26. **Davis, A. J., P. A. James, and P. M. Hawkey.** 1986. *Lactobacillus* endocarditis. *J. Infect.* **12:**169–174.
27. **Drancourt, M., O. Oules, V. Bouche, and Y. Peloux.**

1993. Two cases of *Actinomyces pyogenes* infection in humans. *Eur. J. Clin. Microbiol. Infect. Dis.* **12:**55–57.

28. **Edmiston, C. E.** 1991. *Arachnia* and *Propionibacterium*: casual commensals or opportunistic diphtheroids. *Clin. Microbiol. Newsl.* **13:**57–59.
29. **Evans, D. T. P.** 1993. *Actinomyces israelii* in the female genital tract: a review. *Genitourin. Med.* **69:**54–59.
30. **Ezaki, T., S. L. Liu, Y. Hashimoto, and E. Yabuchi.** 1990. *Peptostreptococcus hydrogenalis* sp. nov. from human fecal and vaginal flora. *Int. J. Syst. Bacteriol.* **40:**305–306.
31. **Ezaki, T., and E. Yabuuchi.** 1986. Transfer of *Peptococcus heliotrinreducens* corrig. to the genus *Peptostreptococcus*: *Peptostreptococcus heliotrinreducens* 1983a comb. nov. *Int. J. Syst. Bacteriol.* **36:**107–108.
32. **Ezaki, T., N. Yamamoto, K. Ninomiya, S. Suzuki, and E. Yabuuchi.** 1983. Transfer of *Peptococcus indolicus*, *Peptococcus asaccharolyticus*, *Peptococcus prevotii*, and *Peptococcus magnus* to the genus *Peptostreptococcus* and proposal of *Peptostreptococcus tetradius* sp. nov. *Int. J. Syst. Bacteriol.* **33:** 683–698.
33. **Finegold, S. M.** 1989. General aspects of anaerobic infection, p. 135–153. *In* S. M. Finegold and W. L. George (ed.), *Anaerobic Infections in Humans*. Academic Press, Inc., San Diego, Calif.
34. **Fiorino, A.-S.** 1996. Intrauterine contraceptive device-associated actinomycotic abscess and *Actinomyces* detection on cervical smear. *Obstet. Gynecol.* **87:**142–149.
35. **Funke, G., S. Stubbs, A. von Graevenitz, and M. O. Collins.** 1994. Assignment of human-derived CDC group 1 coryneform bacteria and CDC group 1-like bacteria to the genus *Actinomyces* as *Actinomyces neuii* subsp. neuii sp. nov. subsp. nov., and *Actinomyces neuii* subsp. *anitratus* subsp. nov. *Int. J. Syst. Bacteriol.* **44:**167–171.
36. **Funke, G., C. P. Ramos, J. F. Fernandez-Garayzabal, N. Weiss, and M. D. Collins.** 1995. Description of a human-derived Centers for Disease Control coryneform group 2 bacteria as *Actinomyces bernardiae* sp. nov. *Int. J. Syst. Bacteriol.* **45:**57–60.
37. **Funke, G., N. Alvarez, C. P. Ramos, E. Falsen, E. Akervall, L. Sabbe, L. Schouls, N. Weiss, and M. D. Collins.** 1997. *Actinomyces europaeus* sp. nov., isolated from human clinical specimens. *Int. J. Syst. Bacteriol.* **47:**687–692.
38. **Funke, G. N., A. von Graevenitz, J. E. Clarridge III, and K. A. Bernard.** 1997. Clinical microbiology of coryneform bacteria. *Clin. Microbiol. Rev.* **10:**125–159.
39. **Gerencser, M. A., and G. H. Bowden.** 1986. Genus *Rothia* Georg and Brown 1967, 68[AL], p. 1342–1346. *In* P. H. A. Sneath, N. S. Mair, M. E. Sharpe, and J. G. Holt (ed), *Bergey's Manual of Systematic Bacteriology*, vol. 2. The Williams & Wilkins Co., Baltimore, Md.
40. **Glupczynski, Y., M. Labbe, F. Crockaert, F. Pepersack, P. Van Der Auwera, and E. Yourassowsky.** 1984. Isolation of *Mobiluncus* in four cases of extragenital infections in adult women. *Eur. J. Clin. Microbiol.* **3:**433–435.
41. **Goldstein, E. J. C., and D. M. Citron.** 1991. Susceptibility of anaerobic bacteria isolated from intra-abdominal infections to ofloxacin and interaction of ofloxacin with metronidazole. *Antimicrob. Agents Chemother.* **35:**2447–2449.
42. **Günthard, H., A. Hany, M. Turina, and J. Wüst.** 1994. *Propionibacterium acnes* as a cause of aggressive aortic valve endocarditis and importance of tissue grinding: case report and review. *J. Clin. Microbiol.* **32:**3043–3045.
43. **Heinrich, S., and H. Korth.** 1967. Zur Nährbodenfrage in der Routinediagnostik der Aktinomykose: Ersatz unsicherer biologischer Substrate durch ein standardisiertes Medium, p. 16–20. *In* J.–H. Heite (ed.), *Krankheiten durch Aktinomyzeten und verwandte Erreger*. Springer-Verlag, Berlin, Hannover, Germany.
44. **Hill, G. B., O. M. Ayers, and A. P. Kohan.** 1987. Characterization and sites of infection of *Eubacterium nodatum*, *Eubacterium timidum*, *Eubacterium brachy*, and other asaccharolytic eubacteria. *J. Clin. Microbiol.* **25:**1540–1545.
45. **Hillier, S. L., M. A. Krohn, N. B. Kiviat, D. H. Watts, and D. A. Eschenbach.** 1991. Microbiologic causes and neonatal outcomes associated with chorioamnion infection. *Am. J. Obstet. Gynecol.* **165:**955–961.
46. **Hillier, S. L., M. A. Krohn, L. K. Rabe, S. J. Klebanoff, and D. A. Eschenbach.** 1993. Normal vaginal flora, H_2O_2-producing lactobacilli and bacterial vaginosis in pregnant women. *Clin. Infect. Dis.* **16**(Suppl. 4)**:**S273–S281.
47. **Hillier, S. L., D. H. Watts, M. F. Lee, and D. A. Eschenbach.** 1990. Etiology and treatment of post cesarean section endometritis after cephalosporin prophylaxis. *J. Reprod. Med.* **35:**322–328.
48. **Holdeman, L. V., E. P. Cato, J. A. Burmeister, and W. E. C. Moore.** 1980. Descriptions of *Eubacterium timidum* sp. nov., *Eubacterium brachy* sp. nov., and *Eubacterium nodatum* sp. nov. isolated from human periodontitis. *Int. J. Syst. Bacteriol.* **30:**163–169.
49. **Holdeman, L. V., E. P. Cato, and W. E. C. Moore (ed.).** 1977. *Anaerobe Laboratory Manual*, 4th ed. Virginia Polytechnic Institute and State University, Blacksburg.
50. **Holst, E., B. Wathne, B. Hovelius, and P.-A. Mårdh.** 1987. Bacterial vaginosis: microbiological and clinical findings. *Eur. J. Clin. Microbiol.* **6:**536–541.
51. **Hudspeth, M. K., D. M. Citron, and E. J. C. Goldstein.** 1997. Evaluation of a novel specimen transport system (Venturi Transystem) for anaerobic bacteria. *Clin. Infect. Dis.* **25:**132–133.
52. **Jakab, E., R. Zbinden, J. Gubler, C. Ruef, A. von Graevenitz, and M. Krause.** 1998. Severe infections caused by *Propionibacterium acnes*: an underestimated pathogen in late postoperative infections. *Yale J. Biol. Med.* **69:** 477–482.
53. **Johnson, J. L., L. V. H. Moore, B. Kaneko, and W. E. C. Moore.** 1990. *Actinomyces georgiae* sp. nov., *Actinomyces gerencseriae* sp. nov., designation of two genospecies of *Actinomyces naeslundii*, and inclusion of *A. naeslundii* serotypes II and III and *Actinomyces viscosus* serotype II in *A. naeslundii* genospecies 2. *Int. J. Syst. Bacteriol.* **40:**273–286.
54. **Karachewski, N. O., E. L. Busch, and C. L. Wells.** 1985. Comparison of PRAS II, RapID ANA, and API 20A systems for identification of anaerobic bacteria. *J. Clin. Microbiol.* **21:**122–126.
55. **Karvonen, S. L., L. Rasanen, W. J. Cunliffe, K. T. Holland, J. Karvonen, and T. Reunala.** 1994. Delayed hypersensitivity to *Propionibacterium acnes* in patients with severe nodular acne and acne fulminans. *Dermatology* **189:** 344–349.
56. **Kitajima, H., Y. Sumida, R. Tanaka, N. Yuki, H. Takayama, and M. Fujimura.** 1997. Early administration of *Bifidobacterium breve* to preterm infants: randomised controlled trial. *Arch. Dis. Child. Fetal Neonatal Med.* **76:**F101–F107.
57. **Klein, G., E. Zill, R. Schindler, and J. Louwers.** 1998. Peritonitis associated with vancomycin-resistant *Lactobacillus rhamnosus* in a continuous ambulatory peritoneal dialysis patient: organism identification, antibiotic therapy, and case report. *J. Clin. Microbiol.* **36:**1781–1783.
58. **Kornman, K. S., and W. J. Loesche.** 1978. New medium for isolation of *Actinomyces viscosus* and *Actinomyces naeslundii* from dental plaque. *J. Clin. Microbiol.* **7:**514–518.
59. **Kotilainen, P., R. Merilahti-Palo, O. P. Lehtonen, I. Manner, I. Helander, T. Mottonen, and E. Rintala.** 1996. *Propionibacterium acnes* isolated from sternal osteitis in a patient with SAPHO syndrome. *J. Rheumatol.* **23:** 1302–1304.
60. **Lassnig, C., M. Dorsch, J. Wolters, E. Schaber, G. Stöffler, and E. Stackebrandt.** 1989. Phylogenetic evidence

for the relationship between the genera *Mobiluncus* and *Actinomyces*. *FEMS Microbiol. Lett.* **65:**17–22.

61. **Li, N., Y. Hashimoto, S. Adnan, H. Miura, H. Yamamoto, and T. Ezaki.** 1992. Three new species of the genus *Peptostreptococcus* isolated from humans: *Peptostreptococcus vaginalis* sp. nov., *Peptostreptococcus lacrimalis* sp. nov., and *Peptostreptococcus lactolyticus* sp. nov. *Int. J. Syst. Bacteriol.* **42:**602–605.
62. **Lorenz, R. P., P. C. Appelbaum, R. M. Ward, and J. J. Botti.** 1982. Chorioamnionitis and possible neonatal infection associated with *Lactobacillus* species. *J. Clin. Microbiol.* **16:**558–561.
63. **Ludwig, W., R. Weizenegger, R. Kilpper-Bälz, and K. H. Schleifer.** 1988. Phylogenetic relationships of anaerobic streptococci. *Int. J. Syst. Bacteriol.* **38:**15–18.
64. **Madinger, N. E., J. A. McGregor, P. J. McKinney, S. T. Dembeck, C. S. Haskell, and Z. Johnson.** 1993. Comparative antibiotic susceptibilities of anaerobes associated with infection of the female reproductive tract. *Clin. Infect. Dis.* **16**(Suppl. 4)**:**S349–S352.
65. **Mangels, J. I., and B. P. Douglas.** 1989. Comparison of four commercial brucella agar media for growth of anaerobic organisms. *J. Clin. Microbiol.* **27:**2268–2271.
66. **Marler, L. M., J. A. Siders, L. C. Wolters, Y. Pettigrew, B. L. Skitt, and S. D. Allen.** 1991. Evaluation of the new RapID-ANA II system for the identification of clinical anaerobic isolates. *J. Clin. Microbiol.* **29:**874–878.
67. **McGregor, J. A., J. I. French, W. Jones, K. Milligan, P. J. McKinney. E. Patterson, and R. Parker.** 1994. Bacterial vaginosis is associated with prematurity and vaginal fluid mucinase and sialidase: results of a controlled trial of topical clindamycin cream. *Am. J. Obstet. Gynecol.* **170:** 1048–1060.
68. **Miyamoto, M. I., and F. C. Fang.** 1993. Pyogenic liver abscess involving *Actinomyces:* case report and review. *Clin. Infect. Dis.* **16:**303–309.
69. **Moore, L. V. H., W. E. C. Moore, E. P. Cato, R. M. Smibert, J. A. Burmeister, and A. M. Best.** 1987. Bacteriology of human gingivitis. *J. Dent. Res.* **6:**989–995.
70. **Moore, W. E. C., and L. V. H. Moore.** 1986. Genus *Eubacterium* Prevot 1938, 294[AL], p. 1353–1373. *In* P. H. A. Sneath, N. S. Mair, M. E. Sharpe, and J. G. Holt (ed.), *Bergey's Manual of Systematic Bacteriology*, vol. 2. The Williams & Wilkins Co., Baltimore, Md.
71. **Murdoch, D. A.** 1998. Gram-positive anaerobic cocci. *Clin. Microbiol. Rev.* **11:**81–120.
72. **Murdoch, D. A., M. D. Collins, A. Willems, J. M. Hardie, K. A. Young, and T. J. Magee.** 1997. Description of three new species of the genus *Peptostreptococcus* from human clinical specimens: *Peptostreptococcus harei* sp. nov., *Peptostreptococcus ivorii* sp. nov., and *Peptostreptococcus octavius* sp. nov. *Int. J. Syst. Bacteriol.* **47:**781–787.
73. **Murray, P. R., C. J. Weber, and A. C. Niles.** 1985. Comparative evaluation of three identification systems for anaerobes. *J. Clin. Microbiol.* **22:**52–55.
74. **Neut, C., V. Lesieur, C. Romond, and H. Beerens.** 1985. Analysis of gram-positive anaerobic cocci in oral, fecal and vaginal flora. *Eur. J. Clin. Microbiol.* **4:**435–437.
75. **Ng, J., L.-K. Ng, A. W. Chow, and J. R. Dillon.** 1994. Identification of five *Peptostreptococcus* species isolated predominantly from the female genital tract by using the rapid ID32A system. *J. Clin. Microbiol.* **32:**1302–1307.
76. **Olsen, I., J. L. Johnson, L. V. Moore, and W. E. Moore.** 1991. *Lactobacillus uli* sp. nov. and *Lactobacillus rimae* sp. nov. from the human gingival crevice and emended descriptions of *Lactobacillus minutus* and *Streptococcus parvulus*. *Int. J. Syst. Bacteriol.* **41:**261–266.
77. **Pant, A. R., S. M. Graham, S. J. Allen, S. Harikul, A. Sabchareon, L. Cuevas, and C. A. Hart.** 1996. *Lactobacillus* GG and acute diarrhoea in young children in the tropics. *J. Trop. Pediatr.* **42:**162–165.
78. **Parent, D., M. Bossens, D. Bayot, C. Kirkpatrick, F. Graf, F. E. Wilkinson, and R. R. Kaiser.** 1996. Therapy of bacterial vaginosis using exogenously-applied *Lactobacilli acidophili* and a low dose of estriol: a placebo-controlled multicentric clinical trial. *Arzneimittelforschung* **46:**68–73.
79. **Perry, J. L.** 1997. Assessment of swab transport systems for aerobic and anaerobic organism recovery. *J. Clin. Microbiol.* **35:**1269–1271.
80. **Petts, D. N., W. Champion, and G. Raymond.** 1988. Oxolinic acid as a selective agent for the isolation of nonsporing anaerobes from clinical material. *Lett. Appl. Microbiol.* **6:** 65–67.
81. **Piriz, S., R. Cuenca, J. Valle, and S. Vadillo.** 1992. Susceptibilities of anaerobic bacteria isolated from animals with ovine foot rot to 28 antimicrobial agents. *Antimicrob. Agents Chemother.* **36:**198–201.
82. **Poco, S. E., F. Nakazawa, M. Sato, and E. Hoshino.** 1996. *Eubacterium minutum* sp. nov., isolated from human periodontal pockets. *Int. J. Syst Bacteriol.* **46:**31–34.
83. **Pulverer G., J. Beuth, W. Roszkowski, H. Burrichter, K. Roszkowski, A. Yassin, H. L. Ko, and J. Jeljaszewicz.** 1990. Bacteria of human physiological microflora liberate immunomodulating peptides. *Zentralbl. Bakteriol.* **272:** 467–476.
84. **Ramos, C. P., E. Falsen, N. Alvarez, E. Åkervall, B. Sjöden, and M. D. Collins.** 1997. *Actinomyces graevenitzii* sp. nov., isolated from human clinical specimens. *Int. J. Syst. Bacteriol.* **47:**885–888.
85. **Ramos, C. P., G. Foster, and M. D. Collins.** 1997. Phylogenetic analysis of the genus *Actinomyces* based on 16S rRNA gene sequences: description of *Arcanobacterium phocae* sp. nov., *Arcanobacterium bernardiae* comb. nov., and *Arcanobacterium pyogenes* comb. nov. *Int. J. Syst. Bacteriol.* **47:**46–53.
86. **Raza, S., S. M. Graham, S. J. Allen, S. Sultana, L. Cuevas, and C. A. Hart.** 1995. *Lactobacillus* GG promotes recovery from acute nonbloody diarrhea in Pakistan. *Pediatr. Infect. Dis.* **14:**107–111.
87. **Reig, M., A. Moreno, and F. Baquero.** 1992. Resistance of *Peptostreptococcus* spp. to macrolides and lincosamides: inducible and constitutive phenotypes. *Antimicrob. Agents Chemother.* **36:**662–664.
88. **Reiner, S. L., J. M. Harrelson, S. E. Miller, G. B. Hill, and H. A. Gallis.** 1987. Primary actinomycosis of an extremity: a case report and review. *Rev. Infect. Dis.* **9:** 581–589.
89. **Roeters, F. J., J. S. van der Hoeven, R. C. Burgersdijk, and M. J. Schaeken.** 1995. Lactobacilli, mutant streptococci and dental caries: a longitudinal study in 2-year-old children up to the age of 5 years. *Caries Res.* **29:**272–279.
90. **Roszkowski, W., K. Roszkowski, H. L. Ko, J. Beuth, and J. Jeljaszewicz.** 1990. Immunomodulation by propionibacteria. *Zentralbl. Bakteriol.* **274:**289–298.
91. **Salonen, J. H., E. Erola, and O. Meurman.** 1998. Clinical significance and outcome of anaerobic bactermia. *Clin. Infect. Dis.* **26:**1413–1417.
92. **Schaal, K. P.** 1986. Genus *Actinomyces* Harz 1877, 133[AL], p. 1383–1418. *In* P. H. A. Sneath, N. S. Mair, M. E. Sharpe, and J. G. Holt (ed.), *Bergey's Manual of Systematic Bacteriology*, vol. 2. The Williams & Wilkins Co., Baltimore, Md.
93. **Schaal, K. P., G. M. Schofield, and G. Pulverer.** 1980. Taxonomy and clinical significance of *Actinomycetaceae* and *Propionibacteriaceae*. *Infection* **8**(Suppl. 2)**:**S122–S130.
94. **Schiefer-Ullrich, H., and J. R. Andreesen.** 1985. *Peptostreptococcus barnesae* sp. nov., a gram-positive, anaerobic, obligately partial purine utilizing coccus from chicken feces. *Arch. Microbiol.* **143:**26–31.

95. **Schofield, G. M., and K. P. Schaal.** 1980. Carbohydrate fermentation patterns of facultatively anaerobic actinomycetes using micromethods. *FEMS Microbiol. Lett.* **8:** 67–69.
96. **Schofield, G. M., and K. P. Schaal.** 1981. A numerical taxonomic study of members of the *Actinomycetaceae* and related taxa. *J. Gen. Microbiol.* **127:**237–259.
97. **Schreckenberger, P. C., D. M. Celig, and W. M. Janda.** 1988. Clinical evaluation of the Vitek ANI card for identification of anaerobic bacteria. *J. Clin. Microbiol.* **26:** 225–232.
98. **Schwarz, D., and W. J. Dieckmann.** 1926. Anaerobic streptococci: their role in puerperal infection. *South. Med. J.* **19:**470–479.
99. **Schwebke, J. R., S. A. Lukehart, M. C. Roberts, and S. L. Hillier.** 1991. Identification of two new antigenic subgroups within the genus *Mobiluncus*. *J. Clin. Microbiol.* **29:**2204–2208.
100. **Sheppard, A., C. Cammarata, and D. H. Martin.** 1990. Comparison of different medium basis for the semiquantitative isolation of anaerobes from vaginal secretions. *J. Clin. Microbiol.* **28:**455–457.
101. **Slack, J. M., and M. A. Gerencser.** 1975. *Actinomyces, Filamentous Bacteria: Biology and Pathogenicity*. Burgess Publishing Co., Minneapolis, Minn.
102. **Sneath, P. H. A., N. S. Mair, M. E. Sharpe, and J. G. Holt (ed.).** 1986. *Bergey's Manual of Systematic Bacteriology*, vol. 2. The Williams & Wilkins Co., Baltimore, Md.
103. **Spiegel, C. A.** 1987. Susceptibility of *Mobiluncus* species to 23 antimicrobial agents and 15 other compounds. *Antimicrob. Agents Chemother.* **31:**249–252.
104. **Spiegel, C. A., and M. Roberts.** 1984. *Mobiluncus* gen. nov., *Mobiluncus curtisii* subsp. *curtisii* sp. nov., *Mobiluncus curtisii* subsp. *holmesii* subsp. nov., and *Mobiluncus mulieris* sp. nov., curved rods from the human vagina. *Int. J. Syst. Bacteriol.* **34:**177–184.
105. **Sturm, A. W.** 1989. *Mobiluncus* species and other anaerobic bacteria in nonpuerperal breast abscess. *Eur. J. Clin. Microbiol.* **8:**789–792.
106. **Summanen, P., E. J. Baron, D. M. Citron, C. A. Strong, H. M. Wexler, and S. M. Finegold.** 1993. *Wadsworth Anaerobic Bacteriology Manual*, 5th ed. Star Publishing, Belmont, Calif.
107. **Sutter, V. L., and S. M. Finegold.** 1976. Susceptibility of anaerobic bacteria to 23 antimicrobial agents. *Antimicrob. Agents Chemother.* **10:**736–752.
108. **Traynor, R. M., D. Pavatt, H. L. D. Duguid, and I. D. Duncan.** 1981. Isolation of actinomycetes from cervical specimens. *J. Clin. Pathol.* **34:**914–916.
109. **Turng, B. F., J. M. Guthmiller, G. E. Minah, and W. A. Falkler, Jr.** 1996. Development and evaluation of a selective and differential medium for the primary isolation of *Peptostreptococcus micros*. *Oral Microbiol. Immunol.* **11:** 356–361.
110. **Tvede, M., and N. Hoiby.** 1992. Experimental studies of survival of anaerobic bacteria at 4°C and 22°C in two different transport systems. *APMIS* **100:**1048–1052.
111. **Uematsu, H., F. Nakazawa, T. Ikeda, and E. Hoshino.** 1993. *Eubacterium saphenus* sp. nov., isolated from human periodontal pockets. *Int. J. Syst Bacteriol.* **43:**302–304.
112. **van Dalen, P. J., T. J. M. van Steenbergen, M. M. Cowan, H. J. Busscher, and J. de Graaff.** 1993. Description of two morphotypes of *Peptostreptococcus micros*. *Int. J. Syst. Bacteriol.* **3:**787–798.
113. **Vowels, B. R., S. Yang, and J. J. Leyden.** 1995. Induction of proinflammatory cytokines by a soluble factor of *Propionibacterium acnes*: implications for chronic inflammatory acne. *Infect. Immun.* **63:**3158–3165.
114. **Wade, W. G.** 1996. The role of *Eubacterium* species in periodontal disease and other oral infections. *Microb. Ecol. Health Dis.* **9:**367–370.
115. **Wexler, H. M., and S. M. Finegold.** 1988. In vitro activity of cefotetan compared with that of other antimicrobial agents against anaerobic bacteria. *Antimicrob. Agents Chemother.* **32:**601–604.
116. **Wexler, H. M., and S. M. Finegold.** 1988. In vitro activity of cefoperazone plus sulbactam compared with that of other antimicrobial agents against anaerobic bacteria. *Antimicob. Agents Chemother.* **32:**403–406.
117. **Whiting, J. L., N. Cheng, and A. W. Chow.** 1987. Interactions of ciprofloxacin with clindamycin, metronidazole, cefoxitin, cefotaxime, and mezlocillin against gram-positive and gram-negative anaerobic bacteria. *Antimicrob. Agents Chemother.* **31:**1379–1382.
118. **Wideman, P. A., V. L. Vargo, D. Citronbaum, and S. M. Finegold.** 1976. Evaluation of the sodium polyanethol sulfonate disk test for the identification of *Peptostreptococcus anaerobius*. *J. Clin. Microbiol.* **4:**330–333.
119. **Wilkins, T. D., W. E. C. Moore, S. E. H. West, and L. V. Holdeman.** 1975. *Peptococcus niger* (Hall) Kluyver and van Niel 1936: emendation of description and designation of neotype strain. *Int. J. Syst. Bacteriol.* **25:**47–49.
120. **Willems, A., and M. D. Collins.** 1995. Phylogenetic analysis of *Ruminococcus flavefaciens*, the type species of the genus *Ruminococcus*, does not support the reclassification of *Streptococcus hansenii* and *Peptostreptococcus productus* as ruminococci. *Int. J. Syst. Bacteriol.* **45:**572–575.
121. **Williams, B. L., G. F. McCann, and F. D. Schoenknecht.** 1983. Bacteriology of dental abscesses of endodontic origin. *J. Clin. Microbiol.* **18:**770–774.
122. **Wilson, K. H., R. B. Blitchington, and R. C. Green.** 1990. Amplification of bacterial 16S ribosomal DNA with polymerase chain reaction. *J. Clin. Microbiol.* **28:** 1942–1946.
123. **Witsell, D. L., C. G. Garrett, W. G. Yarbrough, S. P. Dorrestein, A. F. Drake, and M. C. Weissler.** 1995. Effect of *Lactobacillus acidophilus* on antibiotic-associated gastrointestinal morbidity: a prospective randomized trial. *J. Otolaryngol.* **24:**230–233.
124. **Woese, C. R.** 1987. Bacterial evolution. *Microbiol. Rev.* **51:**221–271.
125. **Wren, M. W.** 1980. Multiple selective media for the isolation of anaerobic bacteria from clinical specimens. *J. Clin. Pathol.* **33:**61–65.
126. **Wüst, J., N. Weiss, G. Funke, and M. D. Collins.** 1995. Assignment of *Actinomyces pyogenes*-like (CDC coryneform group E) bacteria to the genus *Actinomyces* as *Actinomyces radingae* sp. nov. and *Actinomyces turicensis* sp. nov. *Lett. Appl. Microbiol.* **20:**76–81.
127. **Yoonessi, M., K. Crickard, I. S. Cellino, S. K. Satchidanand, and W. Fett.** 1985. Association of *Actinomyces* and intrauterine contraceptive devices. *J. Reprod. Med.* **30:** 48–52.

Bacteroides, Porphyromonas, Prevotella, Fusobacterium, and Other Anaerobic Gram-Negative Rods and Cocci

HANNELE R. JOUSIMIES-SOMER, PAULA H. SUMMANEN, AND SYDNEY M. FINEGOLD

48

TAXONOMY

The anaerobic gram-negative bacteria are part of the normal flora of the mouth, upper respiratory tract, intestinal tract, and urogenital tract of humans and animals. Anaerobic spirochetes are covered in chapter 54, and *Campylobacter* spp. other than *Campylobacter rectus*, *Campylobacter curvus* (formerly *Wolinella recta* and *Wolinella curva*), *Campylobacter gracilis* (formerly *Bacteroides gracilis*), and *Campylobacter showae* are discussed in chapter 50; the rest are discussed here. The initial differentiation of these genera is based on cellular morphology, motility, flagellar arrangement, and an analysis of metabolic end products by gas-liquid chromatography (GLC) (Table 1) (41, 86, 93). Species definition is based on biochemical characteristics, nucleic acid base composition, and homology (see chapter 14). *Acidaminococcus*, *Megasphaera*, and *Veillonella* are the genera of anaerobic, gram-negative cocci (Table 1). In the majority of clinical specimens, only organisms of the genera *Bacteroides*, *Porphyromonas*, *Prevotella*, *Fusobacterium*, *Campylobacter*, *Sutterella*, *Bilophila*, and *Veillonella* are encountered.

Bacteroides spp., *Porphyromonas* spp., *Prevotella* spp., *Fusobacterium* spp., *Campylobacter* spp., *Sutterella* sp., and *Bilophila* sp. may be presumptively characterized on the basis of colony and cellular morphology, pigment production, fluorescence under long-wave UV light, atmospheric growth characteristics, susceptibility to special-potency antibiotic disks, and certain rapidly determined biochemical characteristics. A definitive species-level identification requires a battery of biochemical tests, cellular fatty acid profiling, and occasionally molecular methods (see chapter 13). Definitive identification is not feasible for all anaerobic isolates because of financial constraints and is not ordinarily important for clinical purposes. Generally, for clinical purposes (especially for initiating empirical therapy), it is sufficient to know the broad groupings of isolates and their usual pattern of susceptibility to antimicrobial agents. However, all laboratories performing anaerobic cultures should be able to isolate different anaerobes, store them, and forward them to a reference laboratory for further testing if clinically indicated.

In recent years, the taxonomy of anaerobic bacteria, especially that of the gram-negative bacilli, has been in a state of great change, and this trend will continue. New species have been found, and old species have been renamed. The methods used for taxonomic studies have been based mainly on nucleic acid analyses such as DNA-DNA hybridization and 16S rRNA sequencing. The latter classification approach, based on phylogenetic relatedness, does not necessarily correlate with phenotypic characteristics, such as Gram-staining properties, morphology, atmospheric growth requirements, and sporulation—concepts that were earlier considered cornerstones in the classification of anaerobes (46). In fact, several species currently included in anaerobic gram-negative rods and all gram-negative cocci (*Butyrivibrio* spp., *Catonella morbi*, *Dialister pneumosintes*, *Fusobacterium* spp., *Leptotrichia* spp., *Johnsonella ignava*, *Tissierella* spp., *Mitsuokella multiacida*, *Selenomonas* spp., *Centipeda periodontii*, *Acidaminococcus fermentans*, *Megasphaera elsdenii*, and *Veillonella* spp.) cluster within the *Clostridium* subphylum of the gram-positive bacteria (Table 2) (17, 46, 97).

The genus *Bacteroides* now includes bile-resistant species that were formerly described as the "*Bacteroides fragilis*" group (including *B. eggerthii*) (86). However, *B. distasonis* seems to cluster close to *Porphyromonas* by 16S rRNA sequencing and will probably be relocated accordingly (80). Similarly, *Bacteroides splanchnicus* falls far outside the group and probably represents a new genus (80). On the other hand, *Prevotella heparinolytica* and *Prevotella zoogleoformans* are classified in the *B. fragilis* group, although they are sensitive to bile (80). Inclusion of these species warrants redefinition of the *B. fragilis* group. The taxonomic positions of other species still included in the genus *Bacteroides* remain uncertain, but all of these species will ultimately be transferred to other genera. The genera *Prevotella* (pigmented or nonpigmented saccharolytic organisms) and *Porphyromonas* (pigmented or nonpigmented asaccharolytic or weakly saccharolytic organisms) were previously included in the genus *Bacteroides*. The recently described *Oribaculum catoniae* (75), now is reclassified as *Porphyromonas catoniae* and is the only nonpigmented taxon among *Porphyromonas* (106). Similarly, *Hallella seregens* (75) was found to be identical to *Mitsuokella dentalis*, and they were combined to form a new species, *Prevotella dentalis*, within the genus *Prevotella* (107). *Prevotella ruminicola* (formerly *Bacteroides ruminicola*), from the rumen of cattle, is currently segregated into four species: *Prevotella ruminicola*, *Prevotella brevis*, *Prevotella bryantii*, and *Prevotella albensis* (4). Several other new species have recently been included in these genera, and new candidates await inclusion shortly (Table 2) (45, 46). Preliminary 16S rRNA sequencing results have identified at least two closely related pigmented, bile-resistant, saccharolytic, gram-nega-

TABLE 1 Differentiation of genera of gram-negative anaerobic bacteria

Characteristic	Genus
Rod-shaped cells or coccobacilli	
I. Nonmotile or peritrichous flagella	
A. Produce butyric acid (without isobutyric and isovaleric acids) ..	*Fusobacterium*
B. Produce major lactic acid	*Leptotrichia*
C. Produce acetic acid and hydrogen sulfide; reduce sulfate	*Desulfomonas*
D. Not as above (A, B, or C)	*Anaerorhabdus*
	Bacteroides
	Bilophila
	Campylobacter (gracilis)
	Catonella
	Dialister
	Dichelobacter
	Fibrobacter
	Johnsonella
	Megamonas
	Mitsuokella
	Porphyromonas
	Prevotella
	Rikenella
	Ruminobacter
	Sebaldella
	Sutterella
	Tissierella
II. Polar flagella	
A. Fermentative	
1. Produce butyric acid	*Butyrivibrio*
2. Produce succinic acid	
a. Spiral-shaped cells	*Succinivibrio*
b. Ovoid cells	*Succinimonas*
3. Produce propionic and acetic acids	*Anaerovibrio*
B. Nonfermentative	
1. Produce succinic acid from fumarate	*Campylobacter (Wolinella)*
2. Produce hydrogen sulfide; reduce sulfate	*Desulfovibrio*
III. Tufts of flagella on concave side of curved cells; fermentative	*Selenomonas*
IV. Flagella in a spiral arrangement along cell body; fermentative	*Centipeda*
V. Bipolar tufts of flagella	*Anaerobiospirillum*
Spherical or kidney bean-shaped cells	
I. Produce propionic and acetic acids	*Veillonella*
II. Produce butyric and acetic acids	*Acidaminococcus*
III. Produce isobutyric, butyric, isovaleric, valeric, and caproic acids	*Megasphaera*

tive "species" possibly conforming to a new genus (83). The asaccharolytic, formate- and fumarate-requiring gram-negative rods *Bacteroides ureolyticus*, *Campylobacter gracilis*, *C. curvus*, *C. rectus*, and *Sutterella wadsworthensis* are microaerophiles instead of true anaerobic bacteria (36, 103). *Wolinella recta* and *Wolinella curva* were transferred to the genus *Campylobacter* as *C. rectus* and *C. curvus*, respectively (101). *Wolinella succinogenes*, isolated from the bovine rumen, is currently the only species remaining in the genus *Wolinella*. Organisms formerly included in *Bacteroides gracilis* were a heterogeneous group in terms of bile resistance, composition of cellular fatty acids, atmospheric growth requirements, and antimicrobial susceptibility profiles, and they were placed in two different genera, *Campylobacter* and a new genus, *Sutterella* (100, 103). The taxonomic position of *B. ureolyticus* has remained uncertain; additional studies are required to determine whether these organisms should be transferred to *Campylobacter* or if they represent a new genus (100). New species have also been included in the other microaerophilic genera *Capnocytophaga* (see chapter 36) and *Leptotrichia* (37, 48, 110).

The anaerobic, gram-negative cocci are identified presumptively on the basis of colony and cellular morphology, fluorescence under long-wave UV light, susceptibility to special-potency antibiotic disks, and some rapidly determined biochemical characteristics. A definite identification relies on carbohydrate fermentation test results and fatty acid profiles of metabolic end products determined by GLC.

For recent taxonomic changes, see Table 2 and references 46 and 48.

DESCRIPTION OF THE GROUP

The anaerobic gram-negative bacteria are differentiated from the facultatively anaerobic bacteria by their inability

TABLE 2 Recent taxonomic changes and trends (since the sixth edition of *Manual of Clinical Microbiology*)

Current name	Synonym, taxonomic position	Reference
Acidaminococcus fermentans	Related to *Sporomusa* branch of *Clostridium* subphylum, cluster IX	97
Anaerobiospirillum thomasii	New species	62
Bacteroides distasonis	Related to *Porphyromonas* cluster	80
Bacteroides forsythus	Related to *Porphyromonas* cluster	80
Bacteroides furcosus	Related to *Porphyromonas* cluster	80
Bacteroides putredinis	Possibly related to *Rikenella*	80
Bacteroides pyogenes[a]	*Bacteroides tectum* homology group II (some strains)	32
Bacteroides splanchnicus	Possibly represents a new genus	80
Bacteroides tectum[a]	Related to *Bacteroides fragilis*	
Butyrivibrio species	Related to *Clostridium* subphylum, cluster XIVa	104
Campylobacter gracilis	*Bacteroides gracilis* (some strains)	100
Campylobacter showae	New species	24
Capnocytophaga granulosa	New species	110
Capnocytophaga haemolytica	New species	110
Catonella morbi	Related to *Clostridium* subphylum, cluster XIVa	75, 108
Centipeda periodontii	Related to *Selenomonas* species	97
Dialister pneumosintes	*Bacteroides pneumosintes;* related to *Sporomusa* branch of *Clostridium* subphylum, cluster IX	75, 105
Fusobacterium varium	*Fusobacterium pseudonecrophorum*	5
Johnsonella ignava	Related to *Clostridium* subphylum, cluster XIVa	75, 108
Leptotrichia sanguinegens	New species	37
Megasphaera elsdenii	Related to *Sporomusa* branch of *Clostridium* subphylum, cluster IX	97
Mitsuokella multiacida	Related to *Sporomusa* branch of *Clostridium* subphylum, cluster IX	97
Porphyromonas cangingivalis[a]	New species	18
Porphyromonas cansulci[a]	New species	18
Porphyromonas catoniae	*Oribaculum catoniae*	75, 106
Porphyromonas crevioricanis[a]	New species	39
Porphyromonas gingivicanis[a]	New species	39
Porphyromonas levii[a]	*Bacteroides levii*	87
Porphyromonas macacae[a]	*Bacteroides macacae, Porphyromonas salivosa*	58
Prevotella albensis[a]	*Bacteroides ruminicola* subsp. *ruminicola* biovar 7, *Prevotella ruminicola* (some strains)	4
Prevotella brevis[a]	*Bacteroides ruminicola* subsp. *brevis* biovars 1 and 2, *Prevotella ruminicola* (some strains)	4
Prevotella bryantii[a]	*B. ruminicola* subsp. *brevis* biovar 3, *Prevotella ruminicola* (some strains)	4
Prevotella dentalis	*Mitsuokella dentalis, Hallella seregens*	75, 107
Prevotella ruminicola[a]	*B. ruminicola* subsp. *ruminicola* biovar 1	4
Prevotella enoeca	New species	74
Prevotella heparinolytica	Related to *Bacteroides fragilis* group	80
Prevotella pallens	New species	53
Prevotella tannerae	New species	74
Prevotella zoogleoformans	Related to *Bacteroides fragilis* group	80
Selenomonas species	Related to *Sporomusa* branch of *Clostridium* subphylum, cluster IX	97
Sutterella wadsworthensis	New genus and species, *Bacteroides gracilis* (some strains)	103
Tissierella praeacuta	Related to *Clostridium* subphylum, cluster XII	25
Veillonella species	Related to *Sporomusa* branch of *Clostridium* subphylum, cluster IX	97

[a] Of animal origin.

to grow in the presence of oxygen and their susceptibility to metronidazole. Metronidazole resistance among anaerobes is extremely rare if proper anaerobic testing conditions are used; any unusual finding in this setting should trigger further testing. Some of the species included here are indeed microaerophiles and are often resistant to metronidazole; the appropriate atmospheric requirements should be determined for all isolates.

NATURAL HABITATS AND CLINICAL SIGNIFICANCE

Gram-negative anaerobic bacilli are the anaerobes most commonly encountered in clinical infections; they are found in more than half of the specimens yielding anaerobes (26, 27, 29, 93). The bile-resistant *B. fragilis* group is the most commonly encountered of the anaerobes in clinical specimens and is more resistant to antimicrobial agents than are most other anaerobes. *B. fragilis* and *Bacteroides thetaiotaomicron* are of the greatest clinical significance. They are recovered from most intra-abdominal infections and may occur in infections at other sites. Members of the *B. fragilis* group are major constituents of the normal colonic flora and are also found in smaller numbers in the female genital tract but are not common in the mouth or upper respiratory tract (27). *B. fragilis* strains producing a potent zinc-dependent metalloprotease or enterotoxin with a variety of pathological effects on intestinal mucosal cells have been recently identified (78). Enterotoxin-producing *B. fragilis* strains have been isolated from the intestinal tracts of young farm animals and small children with diarrhea and in cases of extra-abdominal infections including bacteremia, but they have also been isolated from fecal samples from healthy children and adults and from vaginal samples from pregnant women (51, 57, 79). Further epidemiological surveys are indicated to clarify the clinical significance of enterotoxin-producing *B. fragilis* findings in different settings. *Bacteroides splanchnicus*, formerly included in the *B. fragilis* group, is frequently isolated from patients with intra-abdominal infections.

The pigmented anaerobic gram-negative bacilli are composed of saccharolytic and asaccharolytic species of the genera *Prevotella* and *Porphyromonas* and a group of organisms probably representing a new genus and species (for an update, see references 45, 46, 48, and 83). Several species of these genera are found in human clinical specimens. *Prevotella corporis*, *P. denticola*, *P. intermedia*, *P. loescheii*, *P. melaninogenica*, *P. nigrescens*, *P. pallens* (a new species [53, 54]), *P. tannerae* (a new species [74]) *Porphyromonas endodontalis*, and *P. gingivalis* are found in the human oral cavity. Likewise, the nonpigmenting *Porphyromonas catoniae* (former *Oribaculum catoniae*) and nonpigmented variants of *P. endodontalis* are encountered mainly in the oral cavity (56, 96). Some are important pathogens in oral, dental, and bite infections and may produce infections of the head, neck, and lower respiratory tract. Some of the above-named pigmented organisms plus *Porphyromonas asaccharolytica* are also prevalent in the urogenital and intestinal tracts and are important in infections arising from these sources. In addition to the recently described *Porphyromonas endodontalis*-like organisms and the pigmented bile-resistant organisms mentioned above, *P. gingivalis* has been isolated from extraoral sources, especially from patients with appendicitis (30, 67, 83, 99). Nine *Porphyromonas* spp. of animal origin (*P. cangingivalis*, *P. canoris*, *P. cansulci*, *P. circumdentaria*, *P. crevioricanis*, *P. gingivalis* [catalase positive], *P. gingivicanis*, *P. levii*, and *P. macacae* [currently includes the former *P. salivosa*]) have been described (18, 39, 59, 87). *Porphyromonas* spp. of animal origin have been recently encountered in humans with animal bite infections (15, 30) Strains phenotypically similar to but genotypically different from *Porphyromonas levii* have been isolated from various types of human clinical infections including pleuropulmonary, skin, and soft tissue infections and bacterial vaginosis (38, 49).

The bile-sensitive, nonpigmented, saccharolytic *Prevotella* isolates from human samples presently include 12 species. They are found in the same settings as the pigmented gram-negative rods (30). *Prevotella bivia* and *P. disiens* are found in female patients with genital tract infections and less frequently in patients with oral infections; these strains are often resistant to the *β*-lactam antibiotics, including penicillin, aminopenicillins and cephalosporins. *Prevotella oris* and *P. buccae* are found in a variety of oral, pleuropulmonary (16), and other infections. The *P. oralis* group, which is relatively infrequently encountered in samples from humans, is now represented by *P. oralis*, *P. veroralis*, *P. buccalis*, and *P. oulorum*. The clinical significance of the recently described *Prevotella enoeca* from oral samples is poorly defined (74).

P. zoogleoformans (indole negative) is rarely isolated from human clinical specimens, whereas *P. heparinolytica* (indole positive) is often found in the oral cavity and in association with oral infections. As mentioned above, these bile-sensitive species cluster in the *Bacteroides fragilis* group and thus will probably be reclassified in the future. *Prevotella dentalis* (former *Mitsuokella dentalis* and *Hallella seregens*) (107) is a common isolate from infected root canals and from periodontal pockets. We have also encountered this organism in mandibular and gum abscesses and in sialadenitis (95). *Mitsuokella multiacida*, a nonmotile gram-negative anaerobic rod, sometimes isolated from the intestinal tract, is not related to *Prevotella dentalis* but is most closely related genetically to *Selenomonas* species, which in turn seem to belong to cluster IX of the *Clostridium* subphylum of the gram-positive bacteria (17). The nonpigmented, saccharolytic *Megamonas hypermegas* has not to our knowledge been isolated from human clinical specimens.

The nonpigmented, asaccharolytic or weakly fermentative species *Anaerorhabdus furcosus*, *Bacteroides capillosus*, *Bacteroides coagulans*, *Dialister pneumosintes* (formerly *B. pneumosintes*), *Bacteroides putredinis*, *Desulfomonas pigra*, *Desulfovibrio* spp., and *Tissierella praeacuta* inhabit the intestinal tract and have occasionally been recovered from miscellaneous infections (44). *Bacteroides forsythus*, a fusiform gram-negative rod, is a putative pathogen recovered from subgingival sites in patients with periodontitis and is often isolated together with *C. rectus* and *Fusobacterium nucleatum*. Phylogenetically, *B. forsythus* and *Bacteroides distasonis* (the latter currently a member of the *B. fragilis* group) are related to each other and most closely related to *Porphyromonas* species, but their final designations are still unsettled (80). Our group and others have encountered *Bacteroides tectum*, a member of the feline and canine oral flora and found in associated infections, in humans who have sustained animal bites (3, 30, 32). This organism and the phenotypically similar *Bacteroides pyogenes* have been isolated from subgingival sites in dogs with periodontitis (32). *Bilophila wadsworthia*, a bile-resistant organism, has been recovered from patients with acute appendicitis, gangrenous and perforated appendicitis, and related abscesses. It has also been isolated from various other clinical specimens including blood, brain abscess, liver abscess, pericardial fluid, joint fluid, and pleural fluid, as well as from human feces and vaginal and oral secretions (7, 8, 30, 50). *B. wadsworthia* is easily overlooked in cultures owing to its fastidious growth.

Members of the formate-fumarate-requiring *B. ureolyticus*-like group, including *B. ureolyticus*, *C. gracilis*, *C. curvus*, *C. rectus*, and the newly described *Sutterella wadsworthensis*, have been isolated from various types of infections. *B. ureolyticus* has been recovered from pulmonary, head and neck, intra-abdominal, urogenital, bone, and soft tissue infections. *B. gracilis* has been recognized as an important pathogen in serious visceral or head and neck infections and, in general, in infections above the diaphragm, and *Sutterella wadsworthensis* is an important pathogen in infections below the diaphragm, especially abdominal infections (69, 103). As noted above, *Sutterella wadsworthensis* is more resistant to antimicrobial agents such as metronidazole and some *β*-lactam drugs than is *Campylobacter gracilis* (69, 103). *Campylobacter* (formerly *Wolinella*) spp., *Campylobacter concisus*, and the recently described *Campylobacter showae* are primarily oral isolates found in patients with oral infections and periodontitis; *C. rectus* has been implicated as a putative pathogen at sites of active periodontal breakdown (22, 97).

Fusobacterium nucleatum is the *Fusobacterium* sp. most commonly encountered in clinical infections (10, 93). This organism is found in the mouth, genital, gastrointestinal, and upper respiratory tracts. It is often involved in the same types of infections as the pigmented *Prevotella* and *Porphyromonas* spp. Currently, *F. nucleatum* of human origin is divided into four different subspecies (10, 21, 33, 34). *Fusobacterium necrophorum* is a very virulent anaerobe that may cause severe infection, usually in children or young adults, originating from pharyngotonsillitis, sometimes in association with infectious mononucleosis (66). It was the most common anaerobe isolated from peritonsillar abscesses in young adults (47). In addition to peritonsillar abscesses, local complications include neck space infections and jugular vein septic thrombophlebitis. There may also be pleural effusion with empyema and multiple metastatic abscesses (most frequently in the lungs, pleural space, liver, and large joints) related to bacteremia (postanginal sepsis syndrome or Lemierre's disease) (66, 77). *F. necrophorum* is encountered much less often in serious infections now than in the era before antimicrobial agents, but this makes it more treacherous, because many clinicians may not be familiar with the problems. Erythromycin and the newer extended-spectrum macrolides, commonly used in upper respiratory tract infections such as tonsillitis, otitis media, and maxillary sinusitis, are not active against fusobacteria. *F. necrophorum* has been separated into two subspecies; *F. necrophorum* subsp. *necrophorum* contains the lipase-positive, hemagglutinin-producing biovar A, and *F. necrophorum* subsp. *funduliforme* contains the lipase-negative, non-hemagglutinin-producing biovar B (90). Furthermore, *F. pseudonecrophorum* was proposed to include strains belonging to biovar C; however, a subsequent study suggested that *F. pseudonecrophorum* is a synonym for *Fusobacterium varium* (5). *F. mortiferum* and *F. varium* are encountered mainly in patients with intra-abdominal infections. *F. alocis*, *F. sulci*, and *F. periodonticum* are isolated primarily from subgingival sites in patients with gingivitis and periodontitis (97). *F. russii* has been implicated in animal bite infections (30). *F. ulcerans* is found in tropical ulcer (1). *F. prausnitzii*, which is not a real fusobacterium but, rather, is related to some *Eubacterium* spp. and *Clostridium* spp. (102), is one of the major components of the fecal anaerobic flora, but little is known about its pathogenic potential.

Capnocytophaga spp. of human origin include two new species, *C. granulosa* and *C. haemolytica* (see chapter 36), in addition to *C. ochraceae*, *C. sputigena*, and *C. gingivalis* (110). These species are often isolated only in anaerobic culture, and they are common in the oral cavity and have been involved in bacteremia in immunocompromised patients with oral mucositis and other oral lesions (6, 9). *Leptotrichia buccalis* is a common oral organism and may also be found in the vagina and intestinal tract. It has been isolated from blood cultures in immunocompromised patients with similar oral conditions to patients with *Capnocytophaga* infections (6, 9) (see chapter 36). The newly proposed species *Leptotrichia sanguinegens* has been isolated from blood cultures of pregnant and elderly women and neonates (37). *Leptotrichia* spp. as well as *Capnocytophaga* spp. are sometimes β-lactamase producers and are resistant to aminoglycosides and vancomycin; *Leptotrichia* spp. are resistant to erythromycin as well (9, 30).

Selenomonas sputigena, *Selenomonas artemidis*, *Selenomonas dianae*, *Selenomonas flueggei*, *Selenomonas infelix*, and *Selenomonas noxia* are all oral organisms, as is *Centipeda periodontii*, which closely resembles and phylogenetically clusters with *Selenomonas* in the *Clostridium* subphylum of the gram-positive bacteria (17, 97); these organisms are found in subgingival sites in patients with periodontitis (76, 97).

The motile *Succinivibrio dextrinosolvens*, *Butyrivibrio fibrisolvens*, and *Desulfovibrio* spp. and the nonmotile, phylogenetically closely related *Desulfomonas pigra* are found as members of the normal colonic flora but are occasionally encountered in patients with clinical infections, such as appendicitis (8, 44). A new species of *Desulfovibrio*, provisionally named *Desulfovibrio fairfieldensis*, which has been recovered in a culture of blood from an immunocompromised patient and from a pyogenic liver abscess in another patient, was recently characterized and phylogenetically confirmed by 16S rRNA sequencing (68, 98). The sites of normal carriage of *Anaerobiospirillum succiniciproducens* and the newly described *Anaerobiospirillum thomasii* in humans are unknown, but *Anaerobiospirillum* species are common in the fecal flora of cats and dogs (62). Strains of *Anaerobiospirillum* have been isolated from blood cultures in immunocompromised patients and from fecal specimens of patients with diarrhea (61, 62). In the latter case, a zoonotic role for *Anaerobiospirillum* spp. has been proposed.

Acidaminococcus fermentans, *Megasphaera elsdenii*, and *Veillonella parvula* are part of the normal human fecal flora, and *V. parvula*, as well as *V. atypica* and *V. dispar*, is part of the normal oral flora. Anaerobic gram-negative cocci are rarely pathogenic. *Veillonella* spp. are isolated more frequently from clinical specimens than are *Megasphaera* or *Acidaminococcus* spp. *Veillonella* spp. have been encountered in patients with oral, bite-wound, head and neck, and miscellaneous soft tissue infections (93).

COLLECTION, TRANSPORT, AND STORAGE OF SPECIMENS

General guidelines for collection, transport, and storage of specimens are discussed in chapter 4. Sites normally harboring a rich indigenous flora, such as the intestinal tract or vagina, should not be sampled and cultured for anaerobes except under special circumstances and by using special methods (e.g., quantitative study of upper small bowel flora in patients with the blind-loop syndrome). Lower respiratory tract specimens and endometrial samples are especially difficult to obtain without contaminating the sample with indigenous flora. Double-lumen-catheter bronchial brushings and bronchoalveolar lavage fluid transported immediately to the laboratory under anaerobic condition and cultured quantitatively, as well as pleural fluid, represent good respiratory tract specimens. An endometrial suction curette (Pipelle; Unimar, Wilton, Conn.) biopsy provides a good sample from the endometrium (31). Instructions for collection of specimens from different body sites and by various methods are given in more detail elsewhere (28, 31, 42, 93).

Ulcers should be carefully debrided, and proper samples should be collected from the base or progressive edge, where bacteria actively multiply, rather than from unremoved crust or surface pus, which are often contaminated by other bacteria not reflecting the true infecting flora.

Pus, when present, is best aspirated into a syringe through a needle and injected into an anaerobic transport vial containing an oxidation-reduction indicator. Syringes used for aspiration should not be used as transporters because of the potential danger of needlestick injuries or accidental expulsion and because oxygen diffuses through plastic syringes. Pieces of infected tissue obtained by excision or biopsy are always preferable to pus, which is, in turn, preferable to a specimen obtained with a swab. Tissue samples are best transported in loosely capped containers with an anaerobic atmosphere in gas-impermeable bags. For small tissue and biopsy specimens and for subgingival and root canal samples, a semisolid anaerobic transport medium in which the specimen can be submerged may be used. The dental specimens can be collected with a curette or with the use of paper points after careful removal of supragingival plaque. The material from curettes or the paper points is transported in a transport medium, such as the VMGA III containing glass beads, to facilitate dispersion of aggregates in plaque (70). Swabs are prone to drying and may carry too small a volume of sample to be cultured on several media or quantitatively. More detailed information on transport systems can be found elsewhere (28, 31, 42, 93).

The conditions and time of transport should not affect the viability or relative proportions of bacteria present in the specimen if appropriate transport systems are used (6a). Fast transport is important when Gram stain and culture results are needed early for guidance of therapy. Specimens should not be refrigerated, because oxygen diffuses better at lower temperatures.

DIRECT DETECTION

The following methods of direct examination may be useful for the detection of gram-negative, non-spore-forming anaerobic bacteria: macroscopic examination, Gram stain, dark-field or phase-contrast microscopy, and GLC.

The gross appearance (purulence, necrotic tissue), fluorescence under long-wave (366-nm) UV light, and the odor of the specimen can give the laboratory valuable clues to the presence of anaerobes. A fetid or putrid odor due to volatile short-chain fatty acids and amines is always associated with the presence of anaerobes in the sample. Black, necrotic tissue and/or red fluorescence of the sample may be indicative of the presence of pigmented gram-negative rods.

Molecular methods such as nucleic acid probes used in the direct demonstration of some anaerobic oral (19, 92) and nonoral (82) gram-negative bacilli, as well as amplification and direct demonstration of nucleic acid sequences of anaerobes by 16S rRNA sequencing from clinical specimens, are not yet standardized and produced for commercial distribution or commonly used in clinical laboratories. In due time, they undoubtedly will offer a potential option when accurate identification and rapid diagnosis are indicated in laboratories supplied with appropriate equipment, competence, and funding (see chapter 13).

Of the conventional methods, the Gram stain is by far the simplest and the most likely to yield significant information. Gram-stained smears should be prepared from all specimens accepted for anaerobic culture. The morphotypes and relative quantities of both the host and bacterial cells present in the preparation will give clues to the presence of particular bacterial species and suggest the need for special selective media. Furthermore, the Gram stain information also provides quality control for specimen transport and isolation efficiency (31). It is recommended that direct smears be fixed in methanol for 30 s to preserve the host and bacterial cell morphologies (63). Standard Gram stain procedures and reagents are used, except that 0.5% basic fuchsin, which enhances the staining of gram-negative anaerobes, is used instead of safranin as the counterstain (93). In thick films from exudates and bloody fluids, recognition of organisms may be facilitated by staining with acridine orange. Dark-field and phase-contrast microscopy may be helpful in the detection of small, poorly staining organisms (*Dialister pneumosintes*), for the direct observation of motility (*Campylobacter* spp.), for noting spores (*Clostridium* spp.), and for the recognition of morphotypes not cultivable on ordinary media (spirochetes).

Direct gas-chromatographic analysis of specimens other than blood cultures does not add relevant information to what is obtainable from Gram-stained smears.

ISOLATION PROCEDURES AND MEDIA

The use of selective media along with nonselective media will increase the yield and save time in terms of recognition and isolation of colonies. Fresh or prereduced media (commercially available from Anaerobe Systems, Morgan Hill, Calif.) are recommended because they considerably increase the isolation efficiency (64, 81). Nonselective media made from different basal media differ in their abilities to support the growth of certain groups of anaerobes; brucella base is superior to Trypticase soy (CDC base agar) and Schaedler base for isolation of gram-negative bacilli, but CDC base better supports the growth of anaerobic gram-positive cocci. Brain heart infusion base is superior to Trypticase soy in isolation efficiency for *Eubacterium* species but inferior for pigmented gram-negative rods from subgingival and other samples (76, 89). Fastidious anaerobe agar (Lab M, Bury, England) produces luxuriant growth of fusobacteria and some formate-fumarate-requiring species and can be used as a base medium with or without selective agents. In academic centers performing large-scale anaerobic bacteriology, it would be ideal to use two different basal media to maximize the isolation efficiency (31).

Isolation methods have been published elsewhere (12, 84). The minimum medium setup includes (i) a nonselective, enriched, brucella base sheep blood agar plate supplemented with vitamin K_1 and hemin (BAP); (ii) a kanamycin-vancomycin laked sheep blood agar (KVLB) for the selection of *Bacteroides* and *Prevotella* spp. (KVLB allows the growth and rapid pigmentation of most *Prevotella* spp., but the concentration of vancomycin [7.5 μg/ml] in the medium will inhibit the growth of most *Porphyromonas* spp.; for the isolation of *Porphyromonas* spp., KVLB medium with a reduced vancomycin concentration (2 μg/ml) may be prepared [93]); and (iii) a *Bacteroides* bile-esculin agar plate (BBE) for specimens below the diaphragm for the selection and presumptive identification of the *B. fragilis* group and *Bilophila* sp. BBE and KVLB are also available as biplates. When indicated, a phenylethyl alcohol-sheep blood agar plate to prevent overgrowth by aerobic gram-negative rods and swarming of some clostridia may be inoculated. When fusobacteria are clinically suspected as the cause of infection, *Fusobacterium* neomycin-vancomycin agar or *Fusobacterium* selective agar may be used (93). Also, a selective medium for culturing *Anaerobiospirillum* spp. from fecal specimens has been described (61). After inoculation, the anaerobic plates should immediately be placed in an anaerobic environment. After incubation for 48 h at 35 to 37°C, the plates are examined. In routine clinical microbiology, a total incubation period of at least 7 days for primary plates is recommended. In our experience with shorter incubation times, some anaerobic species, such as *Porphyromonas* spp., may not be detected.

IDENTIFICATION

Different colony types are subcultured to a brucella BAP to which special-potency antibiotic disks (colistin, 10 μg; kanamycin, 1,000 μg; and vancomycin, 5 μg) are added (a nitrate disk may also be added) (Fig. 1) to a chocolate agar

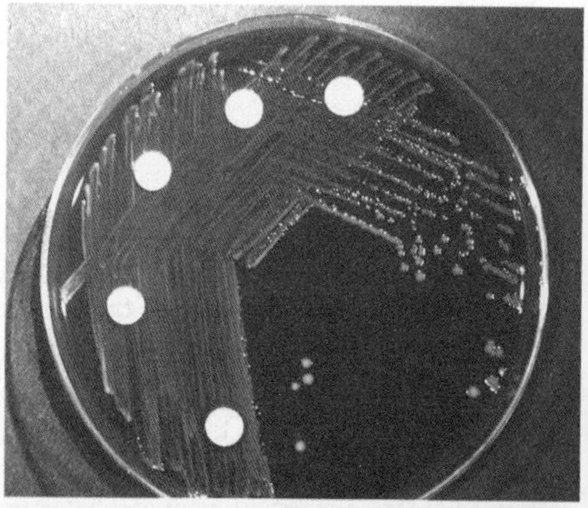

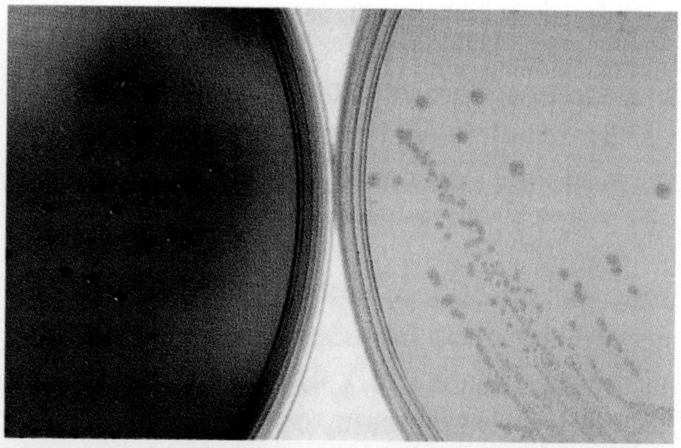

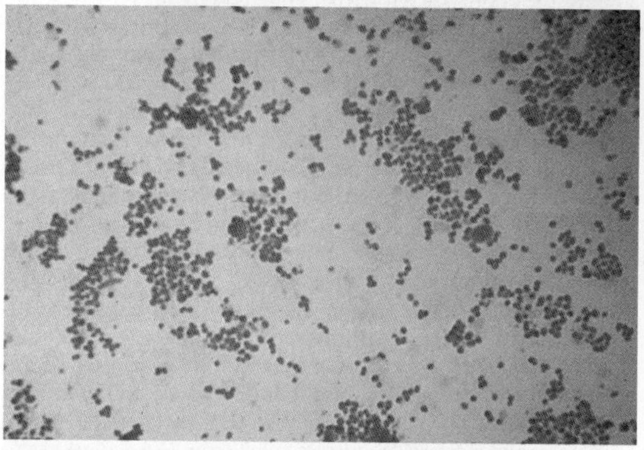

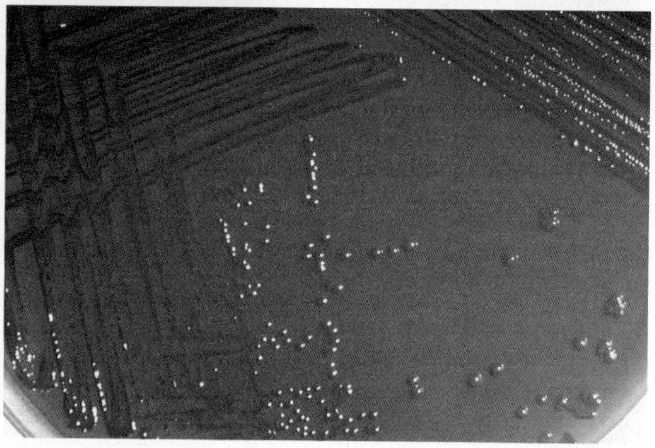

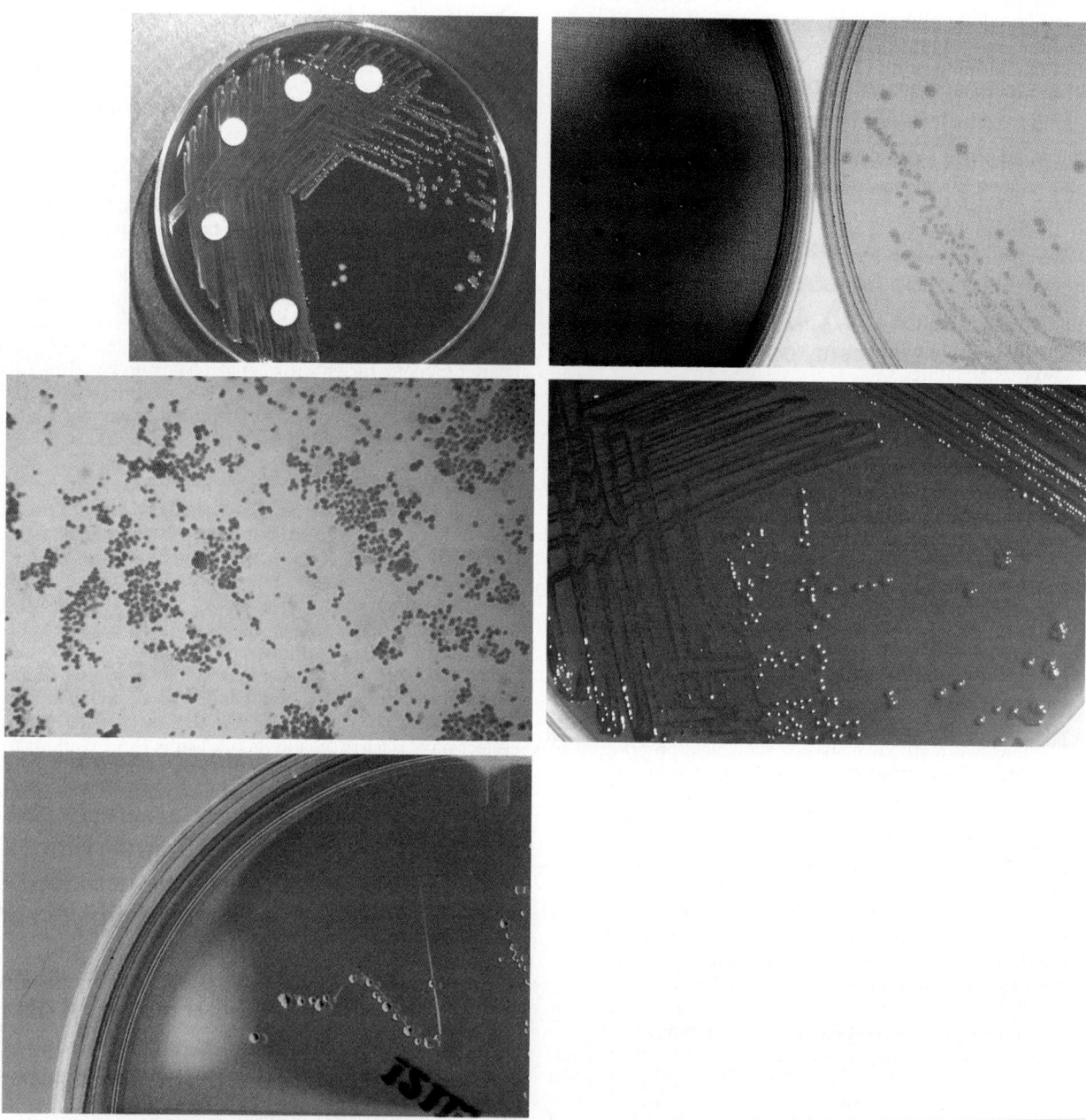

FIGURE 1 (top left) Placement of special-potency antibiotic disks. A blank disk for indole testing may be added (usually after growth has occurred).

FIGURE 2 (top right) Colonies of *Bacteroides fragilis* (left) and *Bacteroides vulgatus* (right) on BBE agar. Note the blackening of the agar and colonies due to esculin hydrolysis and bile precipitation.

FIGURE 3 (middle left) Coccobacillary cells of *Prevotella melaninogenica*.

FIGURE 4 (middle right) Pigmented colonies of *Porphyromonas* sp.

FIGURE 5 (bottom) Colonial morphology of *Bilophila wadsworthia* on BBE agar. Note the black centers.

plate that is incubated in 5–10% CO_2, and to blood agar which is incubated in air (for aerotolerance testing). Laked blood agar plates (LBA) for the rapid demonstration of pigment production (laked rabbit blood agar is the most reliable and effective medium) (45) and egg yolk agar plates (EYA) for the demonstration of lipase and proteolytic activity may also be inoculated at this point. The primary plates are reincubated along with the purity and test plates.

Preliminary Examination of Isolates

The characteristics that are noted and the tests that are made with colonies from the BAP are detailed Gram stain and colony morphology, pigment, fluorescence (long-wave UV-light) (the last two tests are also recorded from LBA), hemolysis, greening, pitting, spot indole reaction (*para*-dimethylaminocinnamaldehyde reagent), nitrate-nitrite reduction, special-potency antibiotic disk susceptibility, catalase (15% H_2O_2, preferably testing colonies from EYA), and motility from broth culture or plate (hanging drop/wet mount). Motile isolates are studied further as indicated in Table 1; most often, these are *Campylobacter* spp. Another approach is the use of Lombard-Dowell Presumpto plates (Presumpto I, II, and III; Carr Scarborough, Stone Mountain, Ga.; Remel Laboratories, Lenexa, Kans.) developed at the Centers for Disease Control and Prevention; these may give additional important information about the presumptive identification of the anaerobic gram-negative bacilli (23). Good growth is necessary for the proper interpretation of test results on this medium.

The primary plates are reinspected after 4 days or more to detect slow growers, new morphotypes, or late pigmenters. In oral microbiology, two rapid in situ tests have been used. The rapid differentiation of lactose-fermenting from lactose-nonfermenting species is performed by applying 4-methylumbelliferyl-D-galactoside reagent (Sigma Chemical Co., St. Louis, Mo.; catalog no. M-1633) to the colonies and screening for fluorescent (lactose-positive) colonies under long-wave UV light (MUG test) (2). The carboxy-L-arginine-7-amino-4-methylcoumarin amide HCl (CAAM) test demonstrates trypsin-like activity of suspected colonies of *Porphyromonas gingivalis*; the CAAM reagent (Sigma; catalog no. C-9396) is applied to the colonies, which are then screened for blue-white fluorescence under long-wave UV light (91).

Presumptive Identification of Species

Most of the clinically significant gram-negative rods can be placed into broad groups on the basis of relatively few tests, and some can be presumptively identified with ease (Table 3). The special-potency antibiotic disk pattern can be used to separate the gram-negative rods into several groups. A zone size equal to or greater than 10 mm is considered to indicate a susceptible isolate (93).

Most of the *Bacteroides* and *Prevotella* spp. are resistant to vancomycin and kanamycin and variable in susceptibility to colistin; *Porphyromonas* spp. are generally susceptible to vancomycin and resistant to colistin. The *B. fragilis* group can be identified presumptively by their special-potency antibiotic disk pattern (resistant to all three disks) and by growth equal to or greater than control growth in 20% bile determined by a tube test, by a bile disk test (93), or on a BBE agar plate (Fig. 2). Coccobacillary organisms that fluoresce red or produce black colonies are in the pigmented *Prevotella-Porphyromonas* spp. group (Fig. 3 and 4).

Fusobacterium spp., the *B. ureolyticus*-like group including *Campylobacter* spp., *Bilophila* sp., *Sutterella* sp., and *Leptotrichia* spp. are resistant to vancomycin but susceptible to both colistin and kanamycin. *B. ureolyticus*, *Campylobacter*, *Bilophila*, and *Sutterella* colonies are usually much smaller and more translucent than those of fusobacteria; *Leptotrichia* colonies are large and gray and have a convoluted ("brain surface") texture. Furthermore, the most commonly encountered fusobacteria, *F. nucleatum* and *F. necrophorum*, are indole positive and nitrate negative. Fusobacteria cells usually are bigger on microscopic inspection than are the other bacteria with the same identification disk profile, excluding the huge tapered cells of *Leptotrichia*. An anaerobic, gram-negative, catalase-negative rod that requires formate and fumarate for growth in broth culture or that pits agar may be presumptively identified as a *B. ureolyticus*-like organism. To document the formate-fumarate requirement, two tubes of peptone yeast (or thioglycolate) broth medium, with one containing the additive and the other not containing it (control), are inoculated and the intensity of growth is compared (Table 3, footnote *b*). A strongly catalase-positive, (often urease-positive) gram-negative rod (Fig. 5), stimulated by bile, can be presumptively identified as *Bilophila* sp. Microaerophilic, catalase- and urease-negative but bile-resistant organisms growing in a *Campylobacter* atmosphere most probably are *Sutterella wadsworthensis*.

Desulfomonas pigra (nonmotile), *Desulfovibrio* spp. (motile), and the capnophilic, often yellow-pigment-producing *Capnocytophaga* spp. are resistant to vancomycin and colistin but susceptible to kanamycin. *Desulfovibrio* cells are curved or spiral; *Capnocytophaga* cells resemble fusobacteria with tapered ends. *Selenomonas* spp. may have the the same special potency disk pattern, but we have also encountered strains that are susceptible to colistin. *Selenomonas* cells are curved and motile as are those of *Centipeda periodontii*, a closely related species that forms swarming colonies.

Most organisms not fitting the above-described groupings are *Bacteroides* spp. or *Prevotella* spp., but occasionally they are representatives of the other genera listed in Table 1.

Gram-negative cocci are sensitive to colistin and usually to kanamycin but resistant to vancomycin. Small, gram-negative cocci reducing nitrate or nitrite and growing as small, grayish-white, translucent colonies that may fluoresce red under UV light can be presumptively identified as *Veillonella* spp.

Rapid Identification

The anaerobic gram-negative rods that can be rapidly identified are shown in Table 3. Identification of the most commonly encountered bile-resistant members of the *Bacteroides fragilis* group is based on the special potency disk profile, and a few rapidly performed tests including catalase, indole, esculin and α-fucosidase (see Table 4, footnote *b*). On these grounds, the members of this group can be reported as *B. fragilis* group, most closely related to *B. fragilis*, or other organisms in this group according to the reactions obtained (Table 3 and 4). Further tests are performed when indicated. *Porphyromonas* spp. are easily identified, even to the species level, with the aid of a special-potency antibiotic disk profile; a few tests including indole, catalase, lipase, and some rapid enzyme tests (Table 3; also see Table 7) (20, 45). An indole- and lipase-positive coccobacillus that forms black-pigmented colonies or fluoresces red may be identified as *P. intermedia*/*P. nigrescens* group; a newly described species,

TABLE 3 Grouping of anaerobic gram-negative rods[a]

Species	Kanamycin (1,000 μg)	Vancomycin (5 μg)	Colistin (10 μg)	Growth in 20% bile	Catalase	Indole
B. fragilis group	R	R	R	+	V	V
Other *Bacteroides* spp.	R	R	V	$-^{+}$	$-^{+}$	V
Pigmented species	R	V	V	–	$-^{+}$	V
Porphyromonas spp.	R	S	R	–	V	$+^{-}$
Prevotella spp.	R^{s}	R	V	–	–	V
P. intermedia- P. nigrescens- P. pallens	R^{s}	R	S	–	–	+
P. loescheii	R	R	V	–	–	–
Other *Prevotella* spp.	R	R	V	–	$-^{+}$	$-^{+}$
B. ureolyticus-like group[f]	S	R	S	–	–	–
B. ureolyticus	S	R	S	–	–	–
Campylobacter spp.[g]	S	R	S	–	–	–
C. gracilis	S	R	S	–	–	–
Bilophila sp.[h]	S	R	S	+	+	–
Sutterella sp.	S	R	S	+	–	–
Desulfomonas pigra[i]	S	R	R	V	–	–
Desulfovibrio spp.[i]	S	R	R	V	–	–
Fusobacterium spp.	S	R	S	V	–	V
F. nucleatum	S	R	S	–	–	+
F. necrophorum	S	R	S	$-^{+}$	–	+
F. varium/F. mortiferum	S	R	S	+	–	V

[a] R, Resistant; S, susceptible; R^{s}, most strains resistant, some strains susceptible; V, variable; +, positive reaction for majority of strains; –, negative reaction; $+^{-}$, most strains positive; $-^{+}$, most strains negative, some strains positive.

[b] Compare the growth of the organism in an unsupplemented thioglycolate broth with growth in a broth supplemented with formate and fumarate additive: dissolve 3 g of sodium formate, 3 g of fumaric acid, and 20 pellets of sodium hydroxide in 50 ml of distilled water; adjust the pH to 7; and filter sterilize. Add 0.5 ml additive to 10 ml of culture broth (40, 93).

[c] Use the spot nitrate disk test (92a, 93).

[d] Make a heavy suspension of the organism in 0.5 ml of sterile urea broth (Difco Laboratories, Detroit, Mich.) or in sterile water, and insert a urea tablet (Rosco or WEE-Tabs). Incubate the tubes aerobically for up to 24 h. A bright pink or red is positive; this color usually appears within 15 to 30 min.

Prevotella pallens, resembles the former two but has lighter pigment and is lipase negative (53, 54). We have also encountered a few *P. asaccharolytica* strains that are lipase positive. A rapid enzyme test for α-glucosidase (Rosco, Taastrup, Denmark, or WEE-Tabs, Round Rock, Tex.) is helpful; *P. intermedia/P. nigrescens* and *P. pallens* are positive, and *P. asaccharolytica* is negative. Any indole-negative strains must be identified further by other biochemical tests. A lipase-positive, indole-negative pigmented gram-negative rod may be identified as *P. loescheii* or as Virginia Polytechnic Institute "*Prevotella* DIC-20" genospecies (109).

B. ureolyticus, *C. gracilis* and other "anaerobic" *Campylobacter* spp., and *Sutterella* sp. are thin gram-negative rods with rounded ends that produce the *Fusobacterium* disk pattern. The colonies are small and translucent or transparent and may produce greening of the agar. Three colony morphotypes exist: smooth and convex, pitting (Fig. 6), and spreading. All colony types can occur in the same culture. These organisms are asaccharolytic and nitrate or nitrite reducing, and they require supplementation of broth media with formate and fumarate for growth (Table 3, footnote *b*). *Campylobacter rectus*, *C. curvus*, *C. concisus*, and *C. showae* are motile and oxidase positive; unlike the first three, *C. showae* is catalase positive (24). *C. gracilis* is nonmotile and urease negative and thus can be differentiated from urease-positive *B. ureolyticus*. (Table 3, footnotes *d*, *e*, and *f*). *Bilophila* sp., which phenotypically resembles *B. ureolyticus*, is distinguished from the above-mentioned species by its resistance to bile and its strong catalase reaction. *Sutterella* sp. is also resistant to bile but is urease and catalase negative, characteristics that differentiate it from *Bilophila* (103).

F. nucleatum is a thin rod with tapering ends (Fig. 7) and is indole positive. The needle-shaped morphology is shared with the microaerophilic, indole-negative *Capnocytophaga* spp. and *Leptotrichia* spp., as discussed above. *F. nucleatum* fluoresces chartreuse under UV light and often produces greening of the agar after exposure to air. At least three different colony morphotypes of *F. nucleatum* exist. Due to considerable phenotypic and genotypic heterogeneity and uncertainty of the valid criteria to separate the *Fusobacterium nucleatum* subspecies, it is hard to judge whether the reported colony morphologies consistently coincide with the subspecies designations. *F. nucleatum* subsp. *nucleatum* colonies may be small, grayish white, and smooth; *F. nucleatum* subsp. *fusiforme* colonies may also be small (<0.5 to 1 mm), granular, and irregular (bread crumb shaped) (Fig. 8); and *F. nucleatum* subsp. *polymorphum* colonies often are large, speckled, smooth, translucent, and butyrous (34). *F. necrophorum* subsp. *necrophorum* is lipase positive and usually bile sensitive. It is a pleomorphic long rod with round ends and often has bizarre forms. It produces indole, fluoresces chartreuse, produces greening of the agar, and often demonstrates beta-hemolysis around the grayish to yellow dull, umbonate colonies (Fig. 9). Lipase-negative strains require further biochemical testing. *Fusobacterium mortiferum* is indole negative and extremely pleomorphic; it has filaments containing swollen areas with large, round bodies and exhibiting

Lipase	Slender cells with pointed ends	Growth stimulated by formate-fumarate[b]	Nitrate reduction[c]	Urease[d]	Motility[e]	Pitting of agar	Pigment	Brick red fluorescence
−								−
−								
V							+	$+^-$
$-^+$							+	$+^-$
V							+	+
$+^-$							+	+
V							+	+
$-^+$							−	−
−		+	+	V	V	V		
−		+	+	+	−	V		
−		+	+	−	$+^-$	V		
−		+	+	−	−	V		
−		−	+	$+^-$	−	−		
−		+	+	−	−	V		
−		−	V	V	−	−		
−		−	V	V	+	−		
V	V							
−	+		−					
$+^-$	−		−					
−	−							

[e] Check motility with a young broth culture supplemented with formate and fumarate.
[f] Formate and fumarate should be added to broth media for this group of organisms.
[g] *Campylobacter rectus*, *C. curvus*, and *C. showae*.
[h] Growth stimulated by 1% pyruvate (final concentration).
[i] Desulfoviridin positive. Inoculate a tube of liquid medium supplemented with 1% pyruvate and 0.25% magnesium sulfate. Incubate until turbidity indicates good growth. Centrifuge the tube to obtain a pellet. Pipette a heavy drop of the pellet onto a slide. Add a drop of 2 N NaOH to the pellet, and immediately observe under long-wave (366 nm) UV light. Positive, red fluorescence; negative, no fluorescence.

irregular staining (Fig. 10). *F. necrophorum* may have similar morphology but usually has fewer round bodies. A bile-resistant fusobacterium isolated from BBE agar may be identified presumptively as *F. mortiferum* or *F. varium*; however, other fusobacteria (e.g., *F. necrophorum* and *F. ulcerans*) may grow in 20% bile. Therefore, further testing is required to confirm the presumptive identification.

Small, gram-negative cocci, which have colonies fluorescing red under UV light and which reduce nitrate or nitrite, are probably *Veillonella* spp. *Megasphaera* cells are large (diameter, >1.5 μm). *Megasphaera* and *Acidaminococcus* colonies do not fluoresce.

Definitive Identification

A definitive identification of an anaerobic isolate should be obtained for all blood and visceral-space isolates; when the patient is gravely ill and not responding to treatment; and when a prolonged and expensive treatment is indicated. Definitive identification is also indicated in unusual case presentations, when a nosocomial infection is suspected, and in teaching-hospital settings.

The definite identification of most species requires certain additional biochemical tests, metabolic end product analysis, and/or whole-cell fatty acid profiling by GLC (93). Even in good research or reference laboratories, a percentage of strains will not be identified definitively. If such strains are isolated from blood or closed-space infections, molecular methods such as 16S rRNA sequencing may prove helpful if available or provided by the local reference center. Curved rods that are not *Campylobacter* spp. should be checked for motility and identified as set out in Table 1. Organisms with small, translucent, spreading colonies that are not *B. ureolyticus*-like should also be checked for motility. Very large fusiform rods that are isolated from the mouth or urogenital tract and have one pointed end, one blunt end, and grey, relatively large, sometimes spreading, convoluted colonies (often growing on neomycin-vancomycin agar on primary isolation) are suggestive of *Leptotrichia* spp. The characteristic GLC pattern shows major amounts of lactic acid. Tables 5 to 9 are based on reactions in prereduced, anaerobically sterilized (PRAS) liquid media (40, 93). A shortened and simplified scheme (arabinose, trehalose, rhamnose, and xylan) for the identification of the *B. fragilis* group by utilizing commercial PRAS biochemicals and 24-h postincubation addition of bromthymol blue has been described (14). **Do not interpret the results from other systems with the tables given here.** Gas-chromatographic analysis may be performed on broth that shows good growth of the organism (40, 93). Each lot of uninoculated broth must be assayed in parallel with samples to determine the background amounts of acetic and succinic acids, and if chopped-meat broth is used, an uninoculated broth is assayed for lactic acid. Fermentation end products vary depending on the substrate available to the organism. This may lead to misinterpretation of the GLC pattern and misidentification of the organism. For instance, saccharolytic organisms produce greater amounts of isoacids in the absence of a fermentable carbohy-

TABLE 4 Characteristics of the *B. fragilis* group[a]

Species	Growth in 20% bile	Indole	Catalase	Esculin hydrolysis	Arabinose	Cellobiose	Rhamnose	Salicin	Sucrose	Trehalose	Xylan	α-Fucosidase[b]	Fatty acids from PYG[c]
B. caccae	+	−	$-^{+}$	+	+	$+^{-}$	$+^{-}$	$-^{+}$	+	+	−	+	A, p, S (iv)
B. distasonis	+	−	$+^{-}$	+	$-^{+}$	+	V	+	+	+	−	−	A, p, S (pa,ib,iv,l)
B. eggerthii	+	+	−	+	+	$-^{+}$	$+^{-}$	−	−	−	+	−	A, p, S (ib,iv,l)
B. fragilis	+	−	+	+	−	$+^{-}$	−	−	+	−	−	+	A, p, S, pa (ib,iv,l)
B. merdae	+	−	$-^{+}$	+	$-^{+}$	V	+	+	+	+	−	−	A, p, S (ib,iv)
B. ovatus	+	+	$+^{-}$	+	+	+	+	+	+	+	+	+	A, p, S, pa (ib,iv,l)
B. stercoris	+	+	−	$+^{-}$	$-^{+}$	$-^{+}$	+	$-^{+}$	+	−	V	V	A, p, S, (ib,iv)
B. thetaiotaomicron	+	+	+	+	+	$+^{-}$	+	$-^{+}$	+	+	−	+	A, p, S, pa (ib,iv,l)
B. uniformis	W^{+}	+	$-^{+}$	+	+	+	$-^{+}$	$+^{-}$	+	$-^{w}$	V	+	a, p, l, S (ib,iv)
B. vulgatus	+	−	$-^{+}$	$-^{+}$	+	−	+	−	+	−	$-^{+}$	+	A, p, S

[a] +, Positive reaction for the majority of strains; −, negative reaction; V, variable reaction; W, weak reaction; $+^{-}$, most strains positive; $-^{+}$, most strains negative, some strains positive; $-^{w}$, most strains negative, some strains weakly positive. Sugars: +, pH < 5.5; W, pH 5.5 to 5.8; −, pH > 5.8.

[b] Make a heavy suspension (heavier than a McFarland no. 2 standard) of the organism in 0.25 ml of sterile saline. Insert a tablet of substrate (Rosco or WEE-Tab). Incubate for 4 h (or overnight). Yellow color, positive; colorless, negative.

[c] Capital letters indicate major metabolic products from peptone-yeast-glucose (PYG), lowercase letters indicate minor products, and parentheses indicate a variable reaction for the following fatty acids: A, acetic; P, propionic; IB, isobutyric; B, butyric; IV, isovaleric; V, valeric; L, lactic; S, succinic; PA, phenylacetic. Note that isoacids are primarily from carbohydrate-free media (e.g., peptone-yeast extract) for saccharolytic organisms.

drate, and a fermentable carbohydrate is required for the detection of lactic acid.

Colonies of the *B. fragilis* group on brucella BAP are 2 to 3 mm in diameter, circular, entire, convex, and gray to white. The cells may be uniform, bipolarly stained, or pleomorphic (some with vacuoles) (Fig. 11); this difference is medium and age dependent. The presence of ovoid cells suggests *B. ovatus*. Good growth in or stimulation by 20% bile (2% oxgall) is characteristic of the *B. fragilis* group; the exception to this rule is the poor growth of *B. uniformis* in bile. Some organisms not belonging to the *B. fragilis* group (non-*B. fragilis* group) are bile resistant. These include *B. splanchnicus*, *B. tectum*, *B. pyogenes*, *Mitsuokella multiacida*, *Bilophila* sp., *Sutterella* sp., the newly described pigmented organism (83), and some fusobacteria. Not all of these, however, grow on BBE agar. Morphologic characteristics, special-potency identification disks, and some biochemical reactions differentiate these species. Most of the *B. fragilis* group organisms blacken BBE agar (esculin hydrolyzed), although *B. vulgatus* may not hydrolyze esculin. Table 4 is a key for the differentiation of members of the bile-resistant *B. fragilis* group.

Members of the non-*B. fragilis* group, nonpigmented anaerobic gram-negative bacilli, form three major subgroups: (i) saccharolytic, (ii) saccharolytic and proteolytic, and (iii) asaccharolytic. Tables 5 and 6 list the more commonly encountered or clinically important species in this group.

The saccharolytic organisms fall into two categories, i.e., pentose fermenters and nonfermenters (arabinose and xylose are usually tested). Pentose fermentation may be difficult to demonstrate owing to suboptimal growth in the test medium; therefore, a screening test for the presence of the preformed enzyme β-xylosidase is recommended (for the procedure, see Table 4, footnote *b*). *P. oris* and *P. buccae* are pentose fermenters (Table 5). They are phenotypically very similar but can be differentiated by the α-fucosidase and *N*-acetyl-β-glucosaminidase tests (Table 4, footnote *b*) (20); furthermore, *P. buccae* is usually sensitive to the special-potency colistin disk whereas *P. oris* is not. *P. zoogleoformans* and *P. heparinolytica* may also ferment pentoses. Both produce viscous material in broth cultures, and the colonies often adhere to the agar on solid media. The positive indole reaction of *P. heparinolytica* differentiates these two species. The indole production is sometimes very difficult to demonstrate and should be tested from a pure culture on an EYA plate and/or from an "old" culture (>5 days old), because it tends to be a weak reaction. Other pentose fermenters include bile-resistant *M. multiacida* and *B. splanchnicus* and bile-susceptible *Prevotella dentalis*. Unlike most *Prevotella* and *Bacteroides* species, *Mitsuokella multiacida* is both nitrate and inositol positive. *Prevotella dentalis* forms characteristic, "water-drop," viscous colonies on blood agar. A positive *N*-acetyl-β-glucosaminidase reaction differentiates it from *Prevotella buccae*, and a negative α-fucosidase reaction differentiates it from *Prevotella oris*. The far better growth of *P. dentalis* on CDC blood agar than on brucella blood agar is an additional feature that facilitates the identification of the species. The species differentiation of the pentose fermenters of animal origin, *Prevotella ruminicola*, *P. brevis*, *P. bryantii*, and *P. albensis*, is based on the demonstration of extracellular enzyme activities, such as carboxymethyl cellulase, xylanase, and DNase (4).

Salicin, cellobiose, xylan, and sucrose are the key sugars in the differentiation of *Prevotella oralis*, *P. buccalis*, *P. veror-*

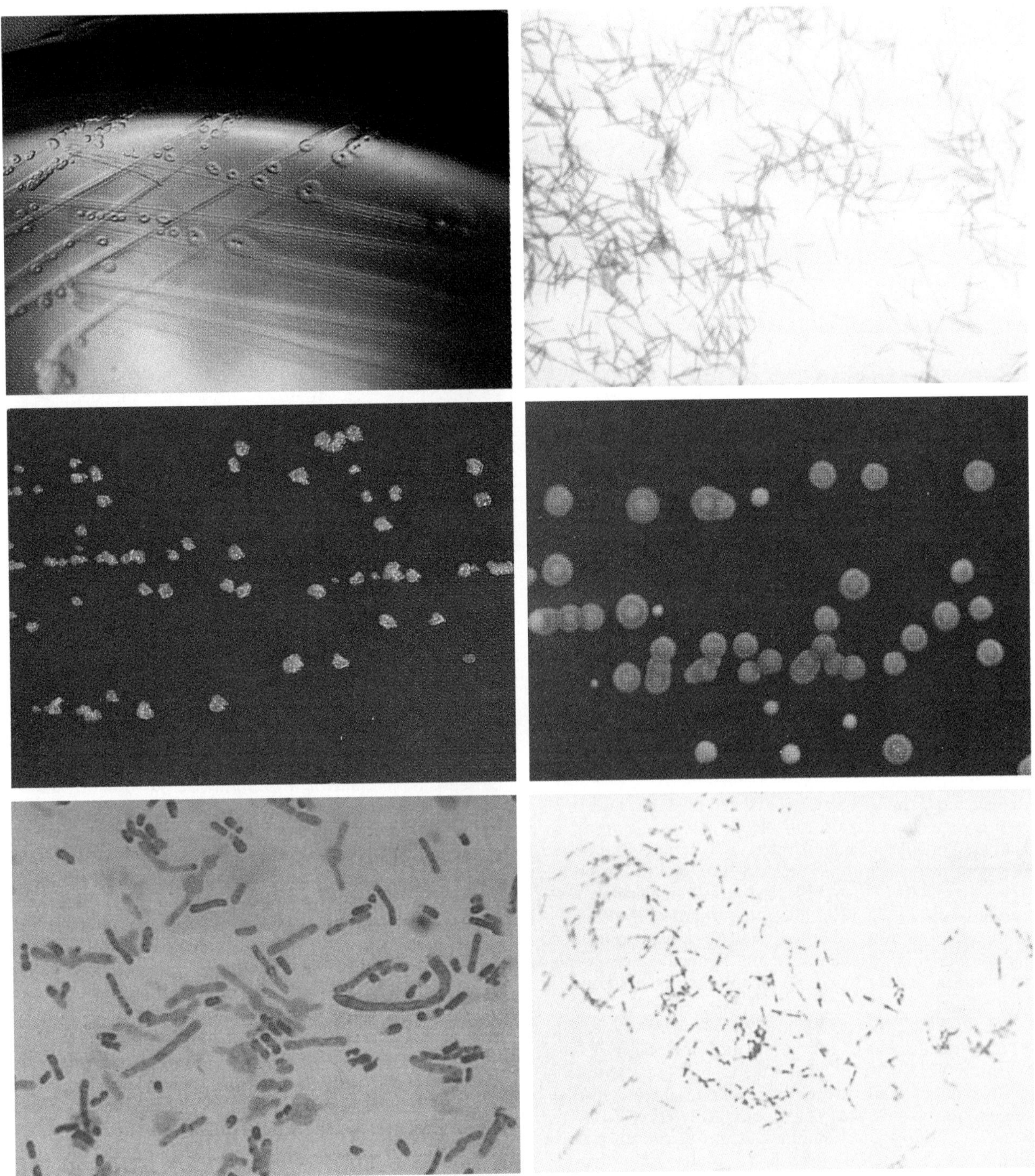

FIGURE 6 (top left) Pitting colonies of *Bacteroides ureolyticus.*

FIGURE 7 (top right) Cells of *Fusobacterium nucleatum.* Note the slender shape with pointed ends.

FIGURE 8 (middle left) Bread crumb-shaped colonies of *Fusobacterium nucleatum.* Note greening of the agar.

FIGURE 9 (middle right) Umbonate colonies of *Fusobacterium necrophorum.*

FIGURE 10 (bottom left) Microscopic morphology of *Fusobacterium mortiferum.* There is marked pleomorphism and irregularity of staining. Note the filaments with swellings along their course.

FIGURE 11 (bottom right) Pleomorphic, bipolar staining of *Bacteroides fragilis.*

TABLE 5 Characteristics of nonpigmented saccharolytic *Bacteroides* spp., *Mitsuokella* sp., and *Prevotella* spp.[a]

Subgroup and species	Growth in 20% bile	Indole	Esculin hydrolysis	Arabinose	Cellobiose	Glucose	Lactose	Salicin	Sucrose
Pentose fermenters									
B. splanchnicus	+	+	+	+	−	+	+	−	−
M. multiacida	+	−	+	+	+	+	+	+	+
P. buccae	−	−	+	+	+	+	+	+	+
P. dentalis	−	−	V	+	+	+	+	−	W
P. heparinolytica[e]	−	+	+	+	+	+	+	+	+
P. oris	−	−	+	+[−]	+	+	+	+	+
P. zoogleoformans[e]	−	−	+	V	+	+	+	V	+
Not pentose fermenters									
P. buccalis	−	−	+	−	+	+	+	−	+
P. enoeca	−	−	V	−	−	+	+	−	−
P. oralis	−	−	+	−	+	+	+	+	+
P. oulorum[g]	−	−	+	−	−	+	+	−	+
P. veroralis	−	−	+	−	+	+	+	−	+
Proteolytic									
P. bivia	−	−	−	−	−	+	+	−	−
P. disiens	−	−	−	−	−	+	−	−	−

[a] See Table 4, footnote *a*.
[b] See Table 4, footnote *b*.
[c] ONPG, *o*-nitrophenyl-*β*-D-galactopyranoside.
[d] See Table 4, footnote *c*.

alis, P. oulorum, and *P. enoeca* (Table 5). Furthermore, *P. oulorum* produces catalase and is lipase positive (73). Certain strains of the saccharolytic pigmented *Prevotella* spp. require more than 21 days to develop pigment, and these strains (especially *P. loescheii*) closely resemble *P. veroralis*. Darker, more opaque colonies and the salicin and cellobiose reactions may aid in differentiating the strains. According to recent reports (72, 74, 109), *P. loescheii, P. tannerae*, "*Prevotella* sp. strain DIC-20," and some strains of *P. melaninogenica, P. denticola, P. enoeca*, and *P. veroralis* cannot be differentiated by conventional biochemical tests; cellular fatty acid analysis was the only reliable method of separating these species.

P. bivia and *P. disiens* are both saccharolytic and strongly proteolytic (Table 5). Gelatin and milk are usually digested within 2 to 3 days (milk may take longer). Differentiation is based on lactose fermentation; *P. bivia* is lactose positive, and *P. disiens* is lactose negative. Furthermore, *P. bivia* is both *N*-acetyl-*β*-glucosaminidase and *α*-fucosidase positive but *P. disiens* is negative for both. Under long-wave UV light, *P. bivia* and *P. disiens* colonies may fluoresce light orange to pink (coral) and *P. disiens* also may produce a brown pigment on LBA that makes differentiation from the phenotypically similar *P. corporis* difficult. *P. bivia* and *P. enoeca* have the same phenotypic characteristics, but *P. enoeca* is gelatin negative; it is usually isolated from oral or orally associated sources, whereas *P. bivia* is more often found from nonoral samples.

Asaccharolytic, nonpigmented (Table 6) *Anaerorhabdus* spp., *Bacteroides* spp., and *Tissierella* spp. are infrequently isolated from clinical specimens. *B. capillosus* coagulates milk and may grow better with Tween 80-supplemented media. *Dialister pneumosintes* (formerly *Bacteroides pneumosintes*) is a very tiny rod best seen by dark-field microscopy (it closely resembles *Veillonella* spp. in the Gram stain), and it forms minute colonies that may require magnification to be seen. *B. forsythus* is a fusiform bacillus that exhibits a wide variety of enzyme activities including trypsin-like activity, *N*-acetyl-*β*-glucosaminidase, *α*-fucosidase, and *β*-glucuronidase. However, its growth is minimal in broth media, and it requires *N*-acetylmuramic acid; therefore, it is often seen as satellite colonies around other organisms, especially fusobacteria. *Desulfomonas* spp. are sulfate-reducing bacteria, and their presence can be confirmed by the desulfoviridin test (Table 3, footnote *i*); they can be differentiated from *Desulfovibrio* spp. by lack of motility. Despite the difference in motility, these two species are genetically closely related and both produce copious amounts of H_2S.

The pigmented *Prevotella* spp. and *Porphyromonas* spp. (Table 7) vary greatly in the degree and rapidity of pigment production, depending primarily on the type of blood and the composition of the base medium used in the agar. A period of 2 to 21 days may be required even on LRBA to detect pigmentation, which ranges from buff to tan to black. The identity of strains not showing pigmentation within 21 days must be established by other biochemical tests to avoid confusion with the *P. oralis* group organisms. The pigmented *Prevotella* and *Porphyromonas* spp. fluoresce pink, orange, or brick red under UV light. Fluorescence is best demonstrated in young cultures; in older cultures, especially on LBA, the fluorescence is more or less masked depending on the intensity of pigment production (45).

The indole-positive *Prevotella intermedia* and *P. nigrescens* produce dark pigment; *P. pallens* pigment is lighter. The use of oligonucleotide probes or determination of arbitrarily primed PCR and enzyme electrophoretic mobility profiles is needed in species differentiation. (54, 67, 88). The unusual

Xylose	Xylan	α-Fucosidase[b]	ONPG[c] (β-galactosidase)[b]	N-Acetyl-β-glucosaminidase[b]	β-Xylosidase[b]	Fatty acids from PYG[d]
–	–	+	+	+	–	A, P, S, ib, b, iv (I)
+		+	+	+	+	A, L, S
+		–	+	–	+	A, S (p,ib,b,iv,I)
V		–	+	+	V	A, S
+		+	+	+	+	A, p, S (iv)
+		+	+	+	+	A, S (p,ib,iv)
V		+	+	+	+	A, P, S (ib,iv)
–	–	+	+	+	–	a, iv, S
–		+	+	+	–	a, S
–	–	+	+	+	–[f]	A, S (I)
–	–	–	+	+	–	A, S
–	+	+	+	+	–	a, S
–		+	+	+	–	A, iv, S (ib)
–		–	–	–	–	A, S (p,ib,iv)

[e] Produces viscous sediment in broth, and colonies usually adhere to agar.
[f] Positive by 4-methylumbelliferyl substrates (60).
[g] Catalase positive.

special-potency antibiotic disk pattern (susceptible to vancomycin), in addition to asaccharolytic properties, separate most *Porphyromonas* spp. from the other pigment producers. *P. asaccharolytica*, *P. endodontalis*, and *P. gingivalis* are all asaccharolytic and phenotypically very similar. The key differential tests include phenylacetic acid production, trypsin-like activity, and *N*-acetyl-β-glucosaminidase and α-fucosidase activities (Table 7). Unlike most *Porphyromonas* spp., *P. catoniae*, *P. levii*, and *P. levii*-like organisms (frequently isolated from human clinical specimens) are indole negative and weakly saccharolytic; the latter characteristic is also shared with *P. macacae*. Most of the *Porphyromonas* spp. of animal origin are differentiated from the human strains by a positive catalase reaction, except for *P. crevioricanis*, which is catalase negative (45).

Table 8 characterizes the more commonly isolated fusobacteria. The conversion of threonine and lactate to propionic acid is important in the differentiation of these species. Bizarre pleomorphic rods with very large, round bodies are suggestive of *Fusobacterium mortiferum* (Fig. 10). This organism may grow on BBE agar and turn the agar black. *F. ulcerans*, isolated from tropical ulcers, closely resembles *F. mortiferum* but is esculin negative. *F. periodonticum*, an oral isolate, is indole positive and bile sensitive and converts threonine but not lactate to propionate. Contrary to earlier reports, we have failed to demonstrate glucose, fructose, or galactose fermentation by the type strain. In fact, this bacterium has been found to be phylogenetically related to *F. nucleatum*. *F. alocis*, *F. sulci*, and *F. russii* are indole negative and do not convert lactate or threonine to propionate; *F. russii* forms larger colonies. Preliminary phylogenetic studies suggest that *F. alocis* and *F. sulci* are not true fusobacteria but are related to gram-positive rods.

Veillonella spp. are nonfermentative and produce acetic and propionic acids (Table 9). *Acidaminococcus fermentans* produces acetic and butyric acids. *Megasphaera elsdenii* ferments glucose and produces multiple fatty acids, including caproic acid.

Other Approaches to Identification

Several microsystems for the identification of anaerobes are currently available. The API 20A (bio-Mérieux Vitek, Hazelwood, Mo.) and Minitek (BD Micro Systems, Cockeysville, Md.) are microtube biochemical systems that produce results in 24 to 48 h and have computerized databases. API 20A and Minitek are best suited for identification of saccharolytic, fast-growing organisms such as the *B. fragilis* group and many clostridia. Most asaccharolytic organisms cannot be identified by these systems, and some fastidious organisms (e.g., some *Prevotella* spp.) fail to grow in them. Even for many saccharolytic organisms, supplemental tests, including GLC, are often required for definitive identification. The color reactions in both of these systems are not always clear-cut, as shades of brown or no color (API 20A) and yellow-orange (Minitek) can make interpretation of the test results difficult.

The rapid (2-4-h) identification systems based on the detection of preformed (constitutive) enzymes by the use of chomogenic or fluorogenic substrates or a combination of the two include RapID ANA II (Innovative Diagnostic Systems, Inc., Atlanta, Ga.), Rapid ID 32A (bioMérieux, Marcy l'Etoile, France), ANI Card (bio-Mérieux Vitek Systems), AN-IDent and API ZYM (bioMérieux Vitek), MicroScan (Dade MicroScan, Sacramento, Calif.), and BBLCrystal Anaerobe (ANR) Identification (ID) system, (BD Micro Systems) as mentioned in chapter 11. The overall performance of these systems has varied from moderate to good; 60 to 90% of the isolates are identified to the species

TABLE 6 Characteristics of nonpigmented weakly saccharolytic or nonsaccharolytic gram-negative bacilli[a]

Species	Growth in 20% bile	Glucose	Catalase	Indole	Nitrate	Motility
Anaerorhabdus furcosus	$+^{-}$	W	−	−	−	−
Bilophila wadsworthia[f]	+	−	+	−	+	−
Bacteroides capillosus	$-^{+}$	W^{-}	−	−	−	−
B. coagulans	+	−	−	+	−	−
B. forsythus	−	−	−	−	−	−
B. putredinis	$+^{-}$	−	$+^{-}$	+	−	−
B. pyogenes[g]	+	W	−	−	−	−
B. tectum[g]	+	W	−	−	−	−
B. ureolyticus	−	−	$-^{+}$	−	+	−
Campylobacter spp.	−	−	−	−	+	$+^{-}$
C. gracilis	−	−	−	−	+	−
Desulfomonas pigra	V	−	−	−	V	−
Desulfovibrio spp.	V	−	−	−	V	+
Dialister pneumosintes	−	−	−	−	−	−
Sutterella wadsworthensis	+	−	−	−	+	−
Tissierella praeacuta	+	−	−	−	V	+

[a] See Table 4, footnote *a*.
[b] See Table 3, footnote *b*.
[c] See Table 3, footnote *i*.
[d] See Table 3, footnote *d*.
[e] See Table 4, footnote *c*.

TABLE 7 Characteristics of pigmented *Porphyromonas* spp. and *Prevotella* spp.[a]

Species	Indole	Lipase	Catalase	Fermentation of: Glucose	Cellobiose	Lactose	Sucrose	Esculin hydrolysis
Porphyromonas: asaccharolytic or weakly saccharolytic								
P. asaccharolytica	+	−	−	−	−	−	−	−
P. canoris[d]	+	−	+	−	−	−	−	−
P. cangingivalis	+	−	+	−	−	−	−	−
P. cansulci[d]	+	−	$+^{W}$	−	−	−	−	−
P. catoniae[e]	−	−	−	W	−	W	−	−
P. circumdentaria[d]	+	−	+	−	−	−	−	−
P. crevioricanis[d]	+	NA	−	−	−	−	−	−
P. endodontalis	+	−	−	−	−	−	−	−
P. gingivalis[f]	+	−	−	−	−	−	−	−
P. gingivicanis[d]	+	NA	+	−	−	−	−	−
P. levii[f]	−	−	−	W	−	W	−	−
P. macacae[d]	+	+	+	W	−	W	−	−
Prevotella: saccharolytic								
P. corporis	−	−	−	+	−	−	−	−
P. denticola	−	−	−	+	$-^{+}$	+	+	$+^{-}$
P. intermedia	+	$+^{-}$	−	+	−	−	$+^{-}$	−
P. loescheii	−	V	−	+	+	+	+	$+^{-}$
P. melaninogenica	−	−	−	+	$-^{+}$	+	+	$-^{+}$
P. nigrescens[h]	+	$+^{-}$	−	+	−	−	+	−
P. pallens	+	−	−	+	−	−	+	−
P. tannerae	−	−	−	+	−	+	V	−

[a] See Table 4, footnote *a*.
[b] Reaction by API ZYM System or Rosco Diagnostic tablets (see Table 4, footnote *b*).
[c] See Table 4, footnote *c*.
[d] Animal origin; may be isolated from bite infections; *P. macacae* presently includes the former *P. salivosa*; NA, information not available.

F/F Required[b]	Desulfoviridin[c]	Urease[d]	Esculin hydrolysis	Gelatin hydrolysis	Fatty acids from PYG[e]
−	−	−	+	$-^{w}$	a, l (s)
−	W^{-}	$+^{-}$	−	−	A (s)
−	−	−	+	$-^{W}$	a, s (p,l)
−	−	−	−	+	a (p,l,s)
−	−	−	+	+	A, S, pa
−	−	−	−	+	a, P, ib, b, IV, S (l), pa
−	−	−	+	+	a, P, ib, b, IV, S (l)
−	−	−	+	+	A, p, iv, S, pa
+	−	+	−	−	A, S
+	−	−	−	−	a, S
+	−	−	−	−	a, S
−	+	V	−	−	A
−	+	V	−	−	A
−	−	−	−	$-^{W}$	a (l,s)
+	−	−	−	−	a, S
−	−	−	−	+	A, p, ib, B, IV, s (l)

[f] Pyruvate (1%) stimulates growth. Dissolve 20 g of pyruvic acid in 100 ml of distilled water. Sterilize by filtration or autoclave at 121°C for 15 min. Add 0.5 ml of additive to 10 ml of culture medium.

[g] Animal origin, also isolated from bite infections in humans. Quantitative differences between some cellular fatty acids may help in differentiation of these species (32).

α-Fucosidase[b]	α-Galactosidase[b]	β-Galactosidase[b]	N-Acetyl-β-glucosaminidase[b]	Trypsin[b]	Chymotrypsin[b]	Fatty acids from PYG[c]
+	−	−	−	−	−	A, P, ib, B, IV, s
−	−	+	+	−	+	A, P, ib, b, IV, s
−	−	−	−	−	+	A, p, ib, B, IV
−	−	−	−	−	−	A, P, ib, B, IV, S, pa
+	$-^{+}$	+	+	$-^{+}$	$+^{-}$	a, P, iv, l, S
−	−	−	−	−	−	A, P, ib, b, IV, s, pa
−	NA	NA	−	−	NA	A, P, ib, b, IV, s, pa
−	−	−	−	−	−	A, P, ib, B, IV, s
−	−	$-^{g}$	+	+	−	A, P, ib, B, IV, s, pa
−	NA	NA	−	−	NA	A, p, ib, B, IV, s
−	−	+	+	−	+	A, P, ib, B, IV, s
−	+	$-^{g}$	+	+	+	A, P, ib, B, IV, s, pa
−	−	−	−	−	$+^{-}$	A, ib, iv, S (b)
+	+	+	+	−	−	A, S (ib,iv,l)
+	−	−	−	−	−	A, iv, S (p,ib)
+	+	+	+	−	−	a, S (l)
+	+	+	+	−	−	A, S (ib,iv,l)
+	−	−	−	−	−	A, iv, S (p,ib)
+	−	−	−	−	−	A, S (p,ib)
+	−	+	+	−	−	A, iv, S (ib)

[e] Nonpigmented.

[f] *P. gingivalis* does not show fluorescence; *P. levii*-like may show weak or no fluorescence.

[g] Negative by the API ZYM System; positive with the Rosco *o*-nitrophenyl-β-D-galactopyranoside test.

[h] *P. intermedia* has the same characteristics. Differentiation based on enzyme electrophoresis, oligonucleotide probe, or arbitrarily primed PCR (67, 88).

TABLE 8 Characteristics of *Fusobacterium* species[a]

Species	Distinctive cellular morphology	Indole	Growth in 20% bile	Lipase	Gas in glucose agar[b]	Fermentation of: Glucose	Fructose	Mannose	Esculin hydrolysis	Lactate converted to propionate	Threonine converted to propionate	Fatty acids from PYG[c]
F. gonidiaformans	Gonidial forms	+	−	−	4^{2}	−	−	−	−	−	+	A, p, B (l,s)
F. mortiferum[d]	Bizarre; round bodies	−	+	−	4	$+^{W}$	$+^{W}$	$+^{W}$	+	−	+	a, p, B (v,l,s)
F. naviforme	Boat shape	+	−	−	$-^{2}$	W^{-}	−	−	−	−	−	a, B, L (p,s)
F. necrophorum	Large, pleomorphic	+	$-^{+}$	$+^{-e}$	4^{2}	$-^{W}$	$-^{W}$	−	−	+	+	a, p, B (l,s)
F. nucleatum[f]	Slender, pointed ends	+	−	−	$-^{2}$	$-^{W}$	$-^{W}$	−	−	−	+	a, p, B (L,s)
F. russii[g]		−	−	−	2^{-}	−	−	−	−	−	−	a, B, L
F. varium		$+^{-}$	+	−	4	W^{+}	W^{+}	$+^{W}$	−	−	+	a, p, B, L (s)
F. ulcerans	Pointed ends, some with central round swellings	−	+	−	2	+	−	$+^{-}$	−	−	+	a, p, B, l (s)

[a] See Table 4, footnote *a*. $+^{W}$, Most strains positive, some strains weakly positive; $-^{W}$, most strains negative, some strains weakly positive; W^{-}, most strains weakly positive, some strains negative; W^{+}, most strains weakly positive, some strains positive.

[b] Gas in PYG agar deep: −, no gas detected; 2, splits agar horizontally; 4, agar is displaced to top of tube.

[c] See Table 4, footnote *c*.

[d] *o*-Nitrophenyl-β-D-galactopyranoside positive (see Table 4, footnote *b*).

[e] Lipase-positive strains *F. necrophorum* subsp. *necrophorum* and lipase-negative strains of *F. necrophorum* subsp. *funduliforme*.

[f] *F. periodonticum* has the same characteristics.

[g] *F. alocis* and *F. sulci* have the same characteristics; *F. russii* colonies are larger.

level (11, 13, 52, 85, 94). The rapid identification systems are indicated when an identification is not achieved by using tests described in "Rapid Identification", before more time-consuming tests, such as fermentation tests and GLC, are used. These systems are also suited for the identification of slow-gowing, fastidious gram-negative rods and cocci, since no growth in the test medium is required. When using rapid identification systems, all the information available on the organism should be considered. The performance of all these systems is, of course, affected by the source and nature of the isolates; the accuracy can be further increased by certain simple supplemental tests and by GLC. The API ZYM system, which allows the determination of 19 preformed enzymes in 4 h, does not have a database; only compiled data from different publications is available, but it is a useful supplement for the identification of clinically encountered anaerobic bacteria, especially the *Porphyromonas* spp. (Table 7) (20, 35, 99).

Individually available single, dual, or triple enzyme substrates containing tablets (Rosco Diagnostic Tablets [Rosco, Taastrup, Denmark]; WEE-TAB system [Key Scientific Products, Round Rock, Tex.]) are much cheaper than commercial kits; they can be applied in a number of situations and allow flexibility in tailoring the set to best suit special needs (20, 43). The use of 4-methylumbelliferone derivatives of many substrates (Sigma) permits rapid and inexpensive spot tests based on fluorescence (60, 65, 71, 82). It should be noted, however, that reactions obtained by fluorogenic and the different chromogenic test applications may not completely coincide, owing to divergent substrate concentrations, affinities, and buffering conditions in the differ ent systems. Therefore, it is important to report the system used in context when reporting enzyme reactions.

A recently developed method for the identification of anaerobes is based on the analysis of whole-cell fatty acids by capillary column GLC. An extensive database for anaerobes has been compiled, largely by the Virginia Polytechnic Institute Anaerobe Laboratory, and it is updated frequently (MIDI, Inc., Newark, Del.). An option for creating a cumulative database is also available. Nucleic acid probes are not yet standardized and are not commercially available for the identification of clinically important anaerobes. A number of oral microbiology laboratories and commercial concerns, however, have sets of probes designed for the identification of indicator bacteria of periodontal disease (19, 92). Determination of AP-PCR and enzyme electrophoretic mobility profiles may be useful in the differentiation of certain species such as *Prevotella intermedia* and *P. nigrescens* (67, 88). Identification of unusual isolates by 16S rRNA sequencing is being gradually adopted by reference laboratories and is also commercially available (see chapter 13).

SEROLOGICAL TESTS

Serological procedures are not practical for the identification of anaerobic bacteria from colonies. Furthermore, there are no standardized tests available for antibody or antigen detection in clinical specimens that would be useful for this group of organisms.

ANTIBIOTIC SUSCEPTIBILITIES

Susceptibility testing of anaerobes is discussed in chapter 120. Susceptibility patterns obtained in the Wadsworth Anaerobic Bacteriology Laboratory for the most commonly encountered gram-negative rods of clinical significance and

TABLE 9 Characteristics of gram-negative cocci[a]

Organism	Nitrate reduction	Catalase	Glucose	Fatty acids from PYG[b]
Veillonella spp.	+	V	−	A, p
Acidaminococcus fermentans	−	−	−	A, B
Megasphaera elsdenii	−	−	+	a, ib, b, iv, v, C

[a] +, Positive reaction for most strains; −, negative reaction for most strains; V, variable reaction.
[b] See Table 4, footnote c.

for *Veillonella* spp. are noted in Table 10. Resistance is increasingly common among anaerobic gram-negative bacilli. This is particularly true for the *Bacteroides fragilis* group, whose members are not uncommonly resistant to expanded- and broad-spectrum cephalosporins (including β-lactamase-resistant drugs such as cefoxitin) and clindamycin. Strains of the *B. fragilis* group with resistance to imipenem and metronidazole are also encountered. The previously reported resistance to several antimicrobial agents in the group containing both *Bacteroides gracilis* and *Sutterella wadsworthensis* was found to be due partly to a technical artifact (lack of formate-fumarate additive in susceptibility testing media). The true resistance, independent of the artifact, including resistance to metronidazole, seems to be confined to *Sutterella* (69).

β-Lactamase production (nitrocefin test positivity) is common among the *B. fragilis* group and in *Bilophila wadsworthia*; almost all strains are β-lactamase-positive. Approximately 30 to 50% of *Prevotella* spp. are also β-lactamase producers, and even higher proportions have been reported among certain species when several isolates per sample were tested (46, 55). Occasional strains of *Campylobacter gracilis*, *Bacteroides coagulans*, *B. splanchnicus*, *Desulfomonas pigra*, *Fusobacterium mortiferum*, *F. nucleatum*, *F. varium*, *Megamonas hypermegas*, *Mitsuokella multiacida*, and *Porphyromonas* spp. (especially those of animal origin) may produce β-lactamase.

Mechanisms of resistance other than β-lactamase (including high-level metalloenzyme) production include changes in penicillin-binding proteins and in outer membrane porin channels. Plasmids conferring resistance are also encountered.

EVALUATION, INTERPRETATION, AND REPORTING OF RESULTS

Because anaerobic bacteriology is time-consuming, several interim reports are desirable. The initial report can give Gram stain results. Bacterial and host cell morphologies, and their relative quantities seen in the smear, will give a good overall impression of the specimen quality, nature of polymicrobial infection, and even morphologies suggestive of certain anaerobes. Furthermore, Gram stain results will guide the laboratory in choosing media for optimal recovery of predicted organisms. At 24 h, preliminary information on the aerobic and facultatively anaerobic flora is available, and at 48 h, more definite information on the nonanaerobes and preliminary but clinically useful information on the anaerobes can be given (31).

Interpretation of results of a mixed culture containing multiple isolates is difficult. In general, bacterial isolates that are most predominant, empirically most virulent, and most resistant to antimicrobial agents should be given the most attention. Rough quantitation of different isolates recovered, together with Gram stain results (provided that the specimen was properly obtained and transported), is helpful because bacteria present in pure culture or in large numbers most probably are of major importance, as are organisms recovered on repeat culture and organisms isolated from normally sterile sites. The nature of the bacteria found also can give clues to their importance in the infectious process. Certain taxa are much more important clinically in terms of frequency of occurrence, severity of infection produced, and antimicrobial resistance. Organisms of the *Bacteroides fragilis* group, especially *B. fragilis* and *B. thetaiotaomicron*, are more virulent and/or resistant to antimicrobial drugs than are many other anaerobes. *Fusobacterium necrophorum* is an exceptionally virulent organism, producing serious infections such as postanginal sepsis syndrome. *F. nucleatum* may be found as the sole infecting agent in pleuropulmonary infections (16). *Bilophila wadsworthia* is present in small numbers in the bowel flora of healthy persons, yet it is the third most common anaerobe recovered from gangrenous or perforated appendices and is a common constituent of the microbiota in other intra-abdominal infections. Furthermore, the majority of the strains are β-lactamase producers. *Campylobacter gracilis* is often associated with severe infection occurring above the diaphragm. *Sutterella wadsworthensis* is associated with infections occurring below the diaphragm and has a high degree of resistance to certain antimicrobial agents, including metronidazole (69). *Porphyromonas gingivalis* is the putative key pathogen in aggressive forms of adult periodontitis and, together with *P. endodontalis*, is often involved in root canal infections and complications of these infections such as odontogenic sinusitis. Isolation of *Capnocytophaga* spp. or *Leptotrichia* spp. from blood cultures is often linked to patients with hematological malignancies and is a direct clue to oral mucosal lesions in the patient (6, 9, 30).

Bacteroides tectum, *B. pyogenes*, catalase-positive *Porphyromonas* spp., and *Fusobacterium russii* are often associated with the canine or feline oral flora and are thus prevalent in bite wound infections of humans (3, 30, 32, 43). Furthermore, the animal-derived *Porphyromonas* spp. are more often β-lactamase producers than are those isolated from humans (45).

Microbiologists must be professionally competent and willing to consult with clinicians on interpretation of the relevance of the findings. The laboratory should provide the clinician with a gradual introduction to new taxonomy by reporting both the new and old names in parallel for at least 1 to 2 years. Reports must be readily available for phone or direct contact. Statements of specimen quality and possible limitations of methods used serve as most important feedback to the clinician. Dialogue between the clinician and the microbiologist should be frequent.

TABLE 10 Activity of various drugs against anaerobic gram-negative bacteria (Wadsworth Agar Dilution Procedure)[a]

Drug	NCCLS breakpoint (μg/ml)	% Susceptible at breakpoint[b]							
		B. fragilis	*B. fragilis* group[c]	*Prevotella* spp.	*Porphyromonas* spp.	*Fusobacterium* spp.	*Sutterella* spp.[d]	*Bilophila* sp.[e]	*Veillonella* spp.
Cefoperazone	32	50–69	50–69	>95	>95	85–95		<50	
Cefotaxime	32	50–69	<50	>95	>95	85–95		70–84	
Cefotetan	32	85–95	50–69			85–95		>95	
Cefoxitin	32	>95	85–95	>95	>95	>95	>95	>95	
Ceftizoxime	64/32[f]	85–95	85–95	>95	>95	85–95	70–84	>95	
Ceftriaxone	32		<50	85–95	>95	85–95	>95		
Chloramphenicol	16	>95	>95	>95	>95	>95	>95	>95	>95
Clindamycin	4	85–95	70–84	>95	>95	>95	50–69	85–95	>95
Imipenem	8	>95	>95	>95	>95	>95	>95	>95	>95
Meropenem	8	>95	>95	>95	>95	>95	>95	>95	>95
Metronidazole	16	>95	>95	>95	>95	>95	70–84	>95	>95
Penicillin G[g]	1	<50	<50	<70	85–95	85–95		<50	70–90
Amoxicillin/clavulanate	8/4	85–95	85–95	>95	>95	85–95	>95	>95	
Piperacillin	64	>95	85–95	>95	>95	>95	85–95	>95	
Piperacillin/tazobactam	64/4	>95	>95	>95	>95	>95	85–95	>95	
Ticarcillin	64			>95	>95			>95	>95
Ticarcillin/Clavulanate	64/2	>95	>95	>95	>95	>95	>95	>95	>95
Trovafloxacin[h]	4	>95	>95	>95	>95	>95	85–95	>95	

[a] National Committee for Clinical Laboratory Standards (NCCLS M11-A4) approved method; data from Wadsworth Anaerobic Bacteriology Laboratory.
[b] According to the NCCLS-approved breakpoints (M11-A4), using the intermediate category as susceptible.
[c] Includes the species *B. fragilis*.
[d] The use of formate-fumarate additive is presently recommended (Table 3, footnote *b*).
[e] Addition of 1% pyruvate in the test medium recommended (Table 6, footnote *f*).
[f] 32 μg/ml is the breakpoint for broth microdilution test.
[g] Strains producing β-lactamase should be considered resistant.
[h] DU 6859A and clinafloxacin have equivalent activity.

REFERENCES

1. **Adriaans, B., and H. Shah.** 1988. *Fusobacterium ulcerans* sp. nov. from tropical ulcers. *Int. J. Syst. Bacteriol.* **38:** 447–448.
2. **Alcoforado, G. A., T. L. McKay, and J. Slots.** 1987. Rapid method for detection of lactose fermenting oral microorganisms. *Oral Microbiol. Immunol.* **2:**35–38.
3. **Alexander, C. J., D. M. Citron, S. Hunt Gerardo, M. C. Claros, D. Talan, and E. J. C. Goldstein.** 1997. Characterization of saccharolytic *Bacteroides* and *Prevotella* isolates from infected dog and cat bite wounds in humans. *J. Clin. Microbiol.* **35:**406–411.
4. **Avgustin, G., R. J. Wallace, and H. J. Flint.** 1997. Phenotypic diversity among ruminal isolates of *Prevotella ruminicola*: proposal of *Prevotella brevis* sp. nov., *Prevotella bryantii* sp. nov., and *Prevotella albensis* sp. nov. and redefinition of *Prevotella ruminicola*. *Int. J. Syst. Bacteriol.* **47:**284–288.
5. **Bailey, G. D., and D. N. Love.** 1993. *Fusobacterium pseudonecrophorum* is a synonym for *Fusobacterium varium*. *Int. J. Syst. Bacteriol.* **43:**819–821.
6. **Baquero, F., J. Fernández, F. Dionda, A. Erice, J. Pérez de Oteiza, J. A. Reguera, and M. Reig.** 1990. Capnophilic and anaerobic bacteremia in neutropenic patients: an oral source. *Rev. Infect. Dis.* **2**(Suppl. 12):S157–S160.

6a. **Baron, E. J., C. A. Strong, M. McTeague, M.-L. Väisänen, and S. M. Finegold.** 1995. Survival of anaerobes in original specimens transported by overnight mail services. *Clin. Infect. Dis.* **20**(Suppl. 2):S174–S177.

7. **Baron, E. J., M. Curren, G. Henderson, H. Jousimies-Somer, K. Lee, K. Lechowitz, C. A. Strong, P. Summanen, K. Tuner, and S. M. Finegold.** 1992. *Bilophila wadsworthia* isolates from clinical specimens. *J. Clin. Microbiol.* **30:**1882–1884.
8. **Baron, E. J., R. Bennion, J. Thompson, C. Strong, P. Summanen, M. McTeague, and S. M. Finegold.** 1992. A microbial comparison between acute and complicated appendicitis. *Clin. Infect. Dis.* **14:**227–231.
9. **Beebe, J. L., and E. W. Koneman.** 1995. Recovery of uncommon bacteria from blood: association with neoplastic disease. *Clin. Microbiol. Rev.* **8:**336–356.
10. **Bolstad, A. I., H. B. Jensen, and V. Bakken.** 1996. Taxonomy, biology, and periodontal aspects of *Fusobacterium nucleatum*. *Clin. Microbiol. Rev.* **9:**55–71.
11. **Burlage, R. S., and P. D. Ellner.** 1985. Comparison of the PRAS II, AN-Ident, and RapID ANA systems for identification of anaerobic bacteria. *J. Clin. Microbiol.* **22:**32–35.
12. **Byrd, L.** 1992. Examination of primary culture plates for anaerobic bacteria, p. 2.4.1–2.4.6. *In* H. D. Isenberg (ed.), *Clinical Microbiology Procedures Handbook*. American Society for Microbiology, Washington, D.C.
13. **Cavallaro, J. J., L. S. Wiggs, and J. M. Miller.** 1997. Evaluation of the BBL crystal anaerobe identification system. *J. Clin. Microbiol.* **35:**3186–3191.
14. **Citron, D. M., E. J. Baron, S. M. Finegold, and E. J. C. Goldstein.** 1990. Short prereduced anaerobically sterilized (PRAS) biochemical scheme for identification of clinical isolates of bile-resistant *Bacteroides* species. *J. Clin. Microbiol.* **28:**2220–2223.
15. **Citron, D. M., S. Hunt Gerardo, M.-C. Claros, F. Abrahamian, D. Talan, and E. J. C. Goldstein.** 1996. Incidence and characterization of *Porphyromonas* species isolated from infected dog and cat bite wounds in humans by biochemical and PCR fingerprinting. *Clin. Infect. Dis.* **23**(Suppl. 1): S78–S82.
16. **Civen, R., H. Jousimies-Somer, M. Marina, L. Borenstein, H. Shah, and S. M. Finegold.** 1995. A retrospective review of cases of anaerobic empyema and update of bacteriology. *Clin. Infect. Dis.* **20**(Suppl. 2):S224–S229.
17. **Collins, M. D., P. A. Lawson, and A. Willems.** 1994. The phylogeny of the genus *Clostridium*: proposal of five new genera and eleven new species combinations. *Int. J. Syst. Bacteriol.* **44:**812–826.
18. **Collins, M. D., D. N. Love, J. Karjalainen, A. Kanervo, B. Forsblom, A. Willems, S. Stubbs, E. Sarkiala, G. D. Bailey, D. I. Wigney, and H. Jousimies-Somer.** 1994. Phylogenetic analysis of members of the genus *Porphyromonas* and description of *Porphyromonas cangingivalis* sp. nov., and *Porphyromonas cansulci* sp. nov. *Int. J. Syst. Bacteriol.* **44:** 674–679.
19. **Dix, K., S. M. Watanabe, S. McArdle, D. I. Lee, C. Randolph, B. Moncla, and D. E. Schwartz.** 1990. Species specific oligonucleotide probes for the identification of periodontal bacteria. *J. Clin. Microbiol.* **28:**319–323.
20. **Durmaz, B., H. R. Jousimies-Somer, and S. M. Finegold.** 1995. Enzymatic profiles of *Prevotella*, *Porphyromonas*, and *Bacteroides* species obtained with the API ZYM system and Rosco diagnostic tablets. *Clin. Infect. Dis.* **20**(Suppl 2): S192–S194.
21. **Dzink, J. L., M. T. Sheenan, and S. S. Socransky.** 1990. Proposal of three subspecies of *Fusobacterium nucleatum* Knorr 1922: *Fusobacterium nucleatum* subsp. *nucleatum* subsp. nov.; *Fusobacterium nucleatum* subsp. *polymorphum* subsp. nov., nov. rev., comb. nov.; *Fusobacterium nucleatum* subsp. *vincentii* subsp. nov., nov. rev., comb. nov. *Int. J. Syst. Bacteriol.* **40:**74–78.
22. **Dzink, J. L., S. S. Socransky, and A. D. Haffajee.** 1988. The predominant cultivable microbiota of active and inactive lesions of destructive periodontal diseases. *J. Clin. Periodontol.* **15:**316–323.
23. **Engelkirk, P. G., J. Duben-Engelkirk, and V. R. Dowell, Jr.** 1992. *Principles and Practice of Clinical Anaerobic Bacteriology*. Star Publishing Co., Belmont, Calif.
24. **Etoh, Y., F. E. Dewhirst, B. J. Paster, A. Yamamoto, and N. Goto.** 1993. *Campylobacter showae* sp. nov., isolated from the human oral cavity. *Int. J. Syst. Bacteriol.* **3:43:** 631–639.
25. **Farrow, J. A. E., P. A. Lawson, H. Hippe, U. Gauglitz, and M. D. Collins.** 1995. Phylogenetic evidence that the gram-negative nonsporulating bacterium *Tissierella praeacuta* is a member of the *Clostridium* subphylum of the gram-positive bacteria and description of *Tissierella creatinini* sp. nov. *Int. J. Syst. Bacteriol.* **45:**436–440.
26. **Finegold, S. M.** 1995. Anaerobic infections in humans: an overview. *Anaerobe* **1:**3–9.
27. **Finegold, S. M.** 1995. Overview of clinically important anaerobes. *Clin. Infect. Dis.* **20:**S205–S207.
28. **Finegold, S. M., E. J. Baron, and H. M. Wexler.** 1991. *A Clinical Guide to Anaerobic Infections*. Star Publishing Co., Belmont, Calif.
29. **Finegold, S. M., and W. L. George (ed.).** 1989. *Anaerobic Infections in Humans*. Academic Press, Inc., San Diego, Calif.
30. **Finegold, S. M., and H. Jousimies-Somer.** 1997. Recently described anaerobic bacteria: medical aspects. *Clin. Infect. Dis.* **25**(Suppl. 2):S88–S93.
31. **Finegold S. M., H. R. Jousimies-Somer, and H. M. Wexler.** 1993. Current perspectives on anaerobic infections: diagnostic approaches. *Infect. Dis. Clin. North Am.* **7:** 257–275.
32. **Forsblom, B., D. N. Love, and H. R. Jousimies-Somer.** 1997. Characterization of anaerobic, gram-negative, nonpigmented saccharolytic rods from subgingival sites of dogs. *Clin. Infect. Dis.* **25** (Suppl. 2):S100–S106.
33. **Gharbia, S. E., and H. N. Shah.** 1992. *Fusobacterium nucleatum* subsp. *fusiforme* subsp. nov. and *Fusobacterium nucleatum* subsp. *animalis* subsp. nov. as additional subspecies within *Fusobacterium nucleatum*. *Int. J. Syst. Bacteriol.* **42:**296–298.
34. **Gharbia, S. E., H. N. Shah, P. A. Lawson, and M. Haapasalo.** 1990. The distribution and frequency of *Fusobacterium nucleatum* subspecies in the human oral cavity. *Oral Microbiol. Immunol.* **5:**324–327.
35. **Gruner, E., A. von Graevenitz, and M. Altwegg.** 1992. The API ZYM system: tabulated review from 1977 to date. *J. Microbiol. Methods* **16:**101–118.
36. **Han, Y.-H., R. M. Smibert, and N. R. Krieg.** 1991. *Wolinella recta*, *Wolinella curva*, *Bacteroides ureolyticus*, and *Bacteroides gracilis* are microaerophiles, not anaerobes. *Int. J. Syst. Bacteriol.* **41:**218–222.
37. **Hanff, P. A., J.-A. Rosol-Donoghue, C. A. Spiegel, K. H. Wilson, and L. H. Moore.** 1995. *Leptotrichia sanguinegens* sp. nov., a new agent of postpartum and neonatal bacteremia. *Clin. Infect. Dis.* **20**(Suppl. 2):S237–S239.

38. **Hillier, S. H., M. A. Krohn, L. K. Rabe, S. J. Klebanoff, and D. A. Eschenbach.** 1993. The normal vaginal flora, H_2O_2-producing lactobacilli, and bacterial vaginosis in pregnant women. *Clin. Infect. Dis.* **16**(Suppl. 4)**:**S273–S281.
39. **Hirasawa, M., and K. Takada.** 1994. *Porphyromonas gingivicanis* sp. nov. and *Porphyromonas crevioricanis* sp. nov., isolated from beagles. *Int. J. Syst. Bacteriol.* **44:**637–640.
40. **Holdeman, L. V., E. P. Cato, and W. E. C. Moore (ed.).** 1977. *Anaerobe Laboratory Manual*, 4th ed. Virginia Polytechnic Institute and State University, Blacksburg.
41. **Holdeman, L. V., R. W. Kelley, and W. E. C. Moore.** 1984. Anaerobic gram-negative straight, curved and helical rods. Family I. *Bacteroidaceae* Pribram 1933, 10^{AL}, p. 602–662. *In* N. R. Krieg and J. G. Holt (ed.), *Bergey's Manual of Systematic Bacteriology*, vol. 1. The Williams & Wilkins Co., Baltimore, Md.
42. **Holden, J.** 1992. Collection and transport of clinical specimens for anaerobic culture, p. 2.2.1–2.2.7. *In* H. D. Isenberg (ed.), *Clinical Microbiology Procedures Handbook*. American Society for Microbiology. Washington, D.C.
43. **Hudspeth, M. K., S. Hunt Gerardo, D. M. Citron, and E. J. C. Goldstein.** 1997. Growth characteristics and a novel method for identification (the WEE-TAB System) of *Porphyromonas* species isolated from infected dog and cat bite wounds in humans. *J. Clin. Microbiol.* **35:**2450–2453.
44. **Johnson, C. C., and S. M. Finegold.** 1987. Uncommonly encountered, motile, anaerobic gram-negative bacilli associated with infection. *Rev. Infect. Dis.* **9:**1150–1162.
45. **Jousimies-Somer, H. R.** 1995. Update on the taxonomy and the clinical and laboratory characteristics of pigmented anaerobic gram-negative rods. *Clin. Infect. Dis.* **20**(Suppl. 2)**:**S187–S191.
46. **Jousimies-Somer, H.** 1997. Recently described clinically important anaerobic bacteria: taxonomic aspects and update. *Clin. Infect. Dis.* **25**(Suppl. 2)**:**S78–S87.
47. **Jousimies-Somer, H., S. Savolainen, A. Mäkitie, and J. Ylikoski.** 1993. Bacteriologic findings in peritonsillar abscesses in young adults. *Clin. Infect. Dis.* **16**(Suppl. 4)**:** 292–298.
48. **Jousimies-Somer, H., and P. Summanen.** 1997. Microbiology terminology update: clinically significant anaerobic gram-positive and gram-negative bacteria (excluding spirochetes). *Clin. Infect. Dis.* **25:**11–14.
49. **Jousimies-Somer, H. R., P. Summanen, and S. M. Finegold.** 1995. *Bacteroides levii*-like organisms isolated from clinical specimens. *Clin. Infect. Dis.* **20**(Suppl. 2)**:** S208–S209.
50. **Kasten, M. J., J. E. Rosenblatt, and D. R. Gustafson.** 1992. *Bilophila wadsworthia* bacteremia in two patients with hepatic abscess. *J. Clin. Microbiol.* **30:**2502–2503.
51. **Kato, N. H., H. Kato, K. Watanabe, and K. Ueno.** 1996. Association of enterotoxigenic *Bacteroides fragilis* with bacteremia. *Clin. Infect. Dis.* **23:**S83–S86.
52. **Kitch, T. T., and P. C. Appelbaum.** 1989. Accuracy and reproducibility of the 4-hour ATB 32A method for anaerobe identification. *J. Clin. Microbiol.* **27:**2509–2513.
53. **Könönen, E., E. Eerola, E. V. G. Frandsen, J. Jalava, J. Mättö, S. Salmenlinna, and H. R. Jousimies-Somer.** 1998. Phylogenetic characterization and proposal of a new pigmented species to the genus *Prevotella: Prevotella pallens* sp. nov. *Int. J. Syst. Bacteriol.* **48:**47–51.
54. **Könönen, E., J. Mättö, M.-L. Väisänen-Tunkelrott, E. V. G. Frandsen, I. Helander, S. M. Finegold, and H. R. Jousimies-Somer.** 1998. Biochemical and genetic characterization of a *Prevotella intermedia/Prevotella nigrescens*-like organism. *Int. J. Syst Bacteriol.* **48:**39–46.
55. **Könönen, E., S. Nyfors, J. Mättö, S. Asikainen, and H. R. Jousimies-Somer.** 1997. β-Lactamase production among oral pigmented *Prevotella* species in young children. *Clin. Infect. Dis.* **25**(Suppl. 2)**:**S272–S274.
56. **Könönen, E., M.-L. Väisänen, S. M. Finegold, R. Heine, and H. Jousimies-Somer.** 1996. Cellular fatty acid analysis of *Porphyromonas catoniae*—a frequent colonizer of the oral cavity in children. *Anaerobe* **2:**329–335.
57. **Leszczynski, P., A. van Belkum, H. Pituch, H. Verbrugh, and F. Meisel-Mikolajczyk.** 1997. Vaginal carriage of enterotoxigenic *Bacteroides fragilis* in pregnant women. *J. Clin. Microbiol.* **35:**2899–2903.
58. **Love, D. N.** 1995. *Porphyromonas macacae* comb. nov., a consequence of *Bacteroides macacae* being a senior synonym of *Porphyromonas salivosa*. *Int. J. Syst. Bacteriol.* **45:**90–92.
59. **Love, D. N., J. Karjalainen, A. Kanervo, B. Forsblom, E. Sarkiala, G. D. Bailey, D. Wigney, and H. Jousimies-Somer.** 1994. *Porphyromonas canoris* sp. nov., an asaccharolytic, black pigmented species from periodontal pockets of dogs. *Int. J. Syst. Bacteriol.* **44:**204–208.
60. **Maiden, M. F. J., A. Tanner, and P. J. Macuch.** 1996. Rapid characterization of periodontal bacterial isolates by using fluorogenic substrate tests. *J. Clin. Microbiol.* **34:** 376–384.
61. **Malnick, H., K. Williams, J. Phil-Ebosie, and A. S. Levy.** 1990. Description of a medium for isolating *Anaerobiospirillum* spp., a possible cause for zoonotic disease, from diarrheal feces and blood of humans and use of the medium in a survey of human, canine, and feline feces. *J. Clin. Microbiol.* **28:**1380–1384.
62. **Malnick, H.** 1997. *Anaerobiospirillum thomasii* sp. nov., an anaerobic spiral bacterium isolated from the faeces of cats and dogs and from diarrheal feces of humans, and emendation of the genus *Anaerobiospirillum*. *Int. J. Syst. Bacteriol.* **47:**381–384.
63. **Mangels, J. I., M. Cox, and L. H. Lindberg.** 1984. Methanol fixation: an alternative to heat fixation of smears before staining. *Diagn. Microbiol. Infect. Dis.* **2:**129–137.
64. **Mangels, J. I., and B. P. Douglas.** 1989. Comparison of four commercial brucella agar media for growth of anaerobic organisms. *J. Clin. Microbiol.* **27:**2268–2271.
65. **Mangels, J. I., I. Edvalson, and M. Cox.** 1993. Rapid presumptive identification of *Bacteriodes fragilis* group organisms with use of 4-methylumbelliferone-derivative substrates. *Clin. Infect. Dis.* **16**(Suppl. 4)**:**S319–S321.
66. **Mann, K. A.** 1994. Lemierre's syndrome following infectious mononucleosis. *Clin. Microbiol. Newsl.* **16:**158–159.
67. **Mättö J., S. Asikainen, M.-L. Väisänen, M. Saarela, P. Summanen, S. M. Finegold, and H. R. Jousimies-Somer.** 1997. *Porphyromonas gingivalis, Prevotella intermedia* and *Prevotella nigrescens* in extraoral and some odontogenic infections. *Clin. Infect. Dis.* **25**(Suppl. 2)**:**S194–S198.
68. **McDougall, R., J. Robson, D. Paterson, and W. Tee.** 1997. Bacteremia caused by a recently described novel *Desulfovibrio* species. *J. Clin. Microbiol.* **35:**1805–1808.
69. **Molitoris, E., H. M. Wexler, and S. M. Finegold.** 1997. Sources and antimicrobial susceptibilities of *Campylobacter gracilis* and *Sutterella wadsworthensis*. *Clin. Infect. Dis.* **25**(Suppl. 2)**:**S264–S265.
70. **Möller, A. J. R.** 1966. Microbiological examination of root canals and periapical tissues of human teeth. *Odontol. Tidskr.* **74:**1–38.
71. **Moncla, B. J., P. Braham, L. K. Rabe, and S. L. Hillier.** 1991. Rapid presumptive identification of black-pigmented gram-negative anaerobic bacteria by using 4-methylumbelliferone derivatives. *J. Clin. Microbiol.* **29:**1955–1958.
72. **Moore, L. V. H., D. M. Bourne, and W. E. C. Moore.** 1994. Comparative distribution and taxonomic value of cellular fatty acids in thirty-three genera of anaerobic gram-negative bacilli. *Int. J. Syst. Bacteriol.* **44:**338–347.
73. **Moore, L. V. H., E. P. Cato, and W. E. C. Moore.** 1991. *Anaerobe Laboratory Manual Update: a Supplement to the VPI Anaerobe Laboratory Manual*, 4th ed. Virginia Polytechnic Institute and State University, Blacksburg.
74. **Moore, L. V. H., J. L. Johnson, and W. E. C. Moore.** 1994. Description of *Prevotella tannerae* sp. nov. and *Prevotella enoeca* sp. nov. from human gingival crevice and emendation of the description of *Prevotella zoogleoformans*. *Int. J. Syst. Bacteriol.* **44:**599–602.
75. **Moore, L. V. H., and W. E. C. Moore.** 1994. *Oribaculum catoniae* gen. nov., sp. nov.; *Catonella morbi* gen. nov., sp. nov.; *Hallella seregens* gen. nov., sp. nov.; *Johnsonella ignava* gen. nov., sp. nov.; and *Dialister pneumosintes* gen. nov., comb. nov., nom. rev., anaerobic gram-negative bacilli from the human gingival crevice. *Int. J. Syst. Bacteriol.* **44:** 187–192.

76. **Moore, W. E. C.** 1987. Microbiology of periodontal disease. *J. Periodont. Res.* **22:**335–341.
77. **Moreno, S., J. G. Altozano, B. Pinilla, J. C. Lopez, B. de Quiros, A. Ortega, and E. Bouza.** 1989. Lemierre's disease: postanginal bacteremia and pulmonary involvement caused by *Fusobacterium necrophorum*. *Rev. Infect. Dis.* **11:** 319–324.
78. **Obiso, R. J., D. M. Lyerly, R. L. Van Tassell, and T. D. Wilkins.** 1995. Proteolytic activity of the *Bacteroides fragilis* enterotoxin causes fluid secretion and intestinal damages in vivo. *Infect. Immun.* **63:**3820–3826.
79. **Pantosti, A., M. Malpeli, M. Wilks, M. G. Menozzi, and B. D'Ambrosio.** 1997. Detection of enterotoxigenic *Bacteroides fragilis* by PCR. *J. Clin. Microbiol.* **35:**2482–2486.
80. **Paster, B. J., F. E. Dewhirst, I. Olsen, and G. I. J. Fraser.** 1994. Phylogeny of *Bacteroides*, *Prevotella*, and *Porphyromonas* spp. and related bacteria. *J. Bacteriol.* **176:**725–732.
81. **Peterson, L. R.** 1997. Effect of media on transport and recovery of anaerobic bacteria. *Clin. Infect. Dis.* **25**(Suppl. 2)**:**S134–S136.
82. **Rabe, L. K., D. Sheiness, and S. L. Hillier.** 1995. Comparison of the use of oligonucleotide probes, 4-methylumbelliferyl derivatives, and conventional methods for identifying *Prevotella bivia*. *Clin. Infect. Dis.* **20**(Suppl. 2)**:**S195–S197.
83. **Rautio, M., H. Saxén, M. Lönnroth, M.-L. Väisänen, R. Nikku, and H. R. Jousimies-Somer.** 1997. Characteristics of an unusual anaerobic pigmented gram-negative rod isolated from normal and inflamed appendices. *Clin. Infect. Dis.* **25**(Suppl. 2)**:**S107–S110.
84. **Reichelsderfer, C., and J. I. Mangels.** 1992. Culture media for anaerobes, p. 2.3.1–2.3.8. *In* H. D. Isenberg (ed.), *Clinical Microbiology Procedures Handbook*. American Society for Microbiology, Washington, D.C.
85. **Schreckenberger, P. C., D. M. Celig, and W. M. Janda.** 1988. Clinical evaluation of the Vitek ANI card for identification of anaerobic bacteria. *J. Clin. Microbiol.* **26:** 225–230.
86. **Shah, H. N., and M. D. Collins.** 1989. Proposal to restrict the genus *Bacteroides* (Castellani and Chalmers) to *Bacteroides fragilis* and closely related species. *Int. J. Syst. Bacteriol.* **39:**85–87.
87. **Shah, H., M. D. Collins, I. Olsen, B. J. Paster, and F. E. Dewhirst.** 1995. Reclassification of *Bacteroides levii* (Holdeman, Cato, and Moore) in the genus *Porphyromonas* as *Porphyromonas levii* comb. nov. *Int. J. Syst. Bacteriol.* **45:** 586–588.
88. **Shah, H. N., and S. E. Gharbia.** 1992. Biochemical and chemical studies on strains designated *Prevotella intermedia* and proposal of a new pigmented species, *Prevotella nigrescens* sp. nov. *Int. J. Syst. Bacteriol.* **42:**542–546.
89. **Sheppard, A., C. Cammarata, and D. H. Martin.** 1990. Comparison of different bases for the semiquantitative isolation of anaerobes from vaginal secretions. *J. Clin. Microbiol.* **28:**455–457.
90. **Shinjo, T., T. Fujisawa, and T. Mitsuoka.** 1991. Proposal of two subspecies of *Fusobacterium necrophorum* (Flugge) Moore and Holdeman: *Fusobacterium necrophorum* subsp. *necrophorum* subsp. nov., nom. rev. (ex Flugge 1886), *Fusobacterium necrophorum* subsp. *funduliforme* subsp. nov., rev. (ex Halle 1898). *Int. J. Syst. Bacteriol.* **41:**395–397.
91. **Slots, J.** 1987. Detection of colonies of *Bacteroides gingivalis* by a rapid fluorescence assay for trypsin-like activity. *Oral Microbiol. Immunol.* **2:**139–141.
92. **Sockransky, S. S., S. Smith, L. Martin, B. J. Paster, F. E. Dewhirst, and A. E. Levin.** 1994. "Checkerboard" DNA-DNA hybridization. *BioTechniques* **17:**788–793.

92a. **Summanen, P.** 1992. Rapid disk and spot test for the identification of anaerobes. p 2.5.1.–2.5.10. *In* H. D. Isenberg (ed.), *Clinical Microbiology Procedures Handbook*. American Society for Microbiology, Washington, D.C.

93. **Summanen, P., E. J. Baron, D. M. Citron, C. Strong, H. M. Wexler, and S. M. Finegold.** 1993. *Wadsworth Anaerobic Bacteriology Manual*, 5th ed. Star Publishing Co., Belmont, Calif.
94. **Summanen, P., and H. Jousimies-Somer.** 1988. Comparative evaluation of Rap ID ANA and API 20A for identification of anaerobic bacteria. *Eur. J. Clin. Microbiol. Infect. Dis.* **7:**771–775.
95. **Summanen, P. H., P. J. Hancher, M. J. Flynn, and J. Slots.** 1996. Obstructive sialadenitis secondary to parotic sialolithiasis: a case report. *Anaerobe* **2:**81–84.
96. **Suzuki, K., T. Ikeda, H. Nakamura, and F. Yoshimura.** 1997. Isolation and characterization of a nonpigmented variant of *Porphyromonas endodontalis*. *Oral Microbiol. Immunol.* **12:**155–161.
97. **Tanner, A., M. F. J. Maiden, B. J. Paster, and F. E. Dewhirst.** 1994. The impact of 16S ribosomal RNA-based phylogeny on the taxonomy of oral bacteria. *Periodontology 2000* **5:**26–51.
98. **Tee, W., M. Dyall-Smith, W. Woods, and D. Eisen.** 1996. Probable new species of *Desulfovibrio* isolated from a pyogenic liver abscess. *J. Clin. Microbiol.* **34:**1760–1764.
99. **Väisänen, M.-L., M. Kiviranta, P. Summanen, S. M. Finegold, and H. R. Jousimies-Somer.** 1997. *Porphyromonas endodontalis*-like organisms isolated from extraoral sources. *Clin. Infect. Dis.* **23**(Suppl. 2)**:**S191–S193.
100. **Vandamme, P., M. I. Daneshvar, F. E. Dewhirst, B. J. Paster, K. Kersters, H. Goossens, and C. W. Moss.** 1995. Chemotaxonomic analyses of *Bacteroides gracilis* and *Bacteroides ureolyticus* and reclassification of *B. gracilis* as *Campylobacter gracilis* comb. nov. *Int. J. Syst. Bacteriol.* **45:**145–152.
101. **Vandamme, P., E. Falsen, R. Rossau, B. Hoste, P. Segers, R. Tytgat, and J. De Ley.** 1991. Revision of *Campylobacter*, *Helicobacter*, and *Wolinella* taxonomy: emendation of generic descriptions and proposal of *Arcobacter* gen. nov. *Int. J. Syst. Bacteriol.* **41:**88–103.
102. **Wang, R.-F., W.-W. Cao, and C. E. Gerniglia.** 1996. Phylogenetic analysis of *Fusobacterium prausnitzii* based on 16S rRNA gene sequence and PCR confirmation. *Int. J. Syst. Bacteriol.* **46:**341–343.
103. **Wexler, H. M., D. Reeves, P. H. Summanen, E. Molitoris, M. McTeague, J. Duncan, K. Wilson, and S. M. Finegold.** 1996. *Sutterella wadsworthensis* gen. nov., sp. nov., bile-resistant microaerophilic *Campylobacter gracilis*-like clinical isolates. *Int. J. Syst. Bacteriol.* **46:**252–258.
104. **Willems, A., M. Amat-Marco, and M. D. Collins.** 1996. Phylogenetic analysis of *Butyrivibrio* strains reveals three distinct groups of species within the *Clostridium* subphylum of the gram-positive bacteria. *Int. J. Syst. Bacteriol.* **46:**195–199.
105. **Willems, A., and M. D. Collins.** 1995. Phylogenetic placement of *Dialister pneumosintes* (formerly *Bacteroides pneumosintes*) within the *Sporomusa* subbranch of the *Clostridium* subphylum of the gram-positive bacteria. *Int. J. Syst. Bacteriol.* **45:**403–405.
106. **Willems, A., and M. D. Collins.** 1995. Reclassification of *Oribaculum catoniae* (Moore and Moore 1994) as *Porphyromonas catoniae* comb. nov. and emendation of the genus *Porphyromonas*. *Int. J. Syst. Bacteriol.* **45:**578–581.
107. **Willems, A., and M. D. Collins.** 1995. 16S rRNA gene sequences indicate that *Hallella seregens* (Moore and Moore) and *Mitsuokella dentalis* (Haapasalo et al.) are genotypically highly related and are members of the genus *Prevotella:* Emended description of the genus *Prevotella* (Shah and Collins) and description of *Prevotella dentalis* comb. nov. *Int. J. Syst. Bacteriol.* **45:**832–836.
108. **Willems, A., and M. D. Collins.** 1995. Evidence for the placement of the gram-negative *Catonella morbi* (Moore and Moore) and *Johnsonella ignava* (Moore and Moore) within the *Clostridium* subphylum of the gram-positive bacteria on the basis of 16S rRNA sequences. *Int. J. Syst. Bacteriol.* **45:**855–857.
109. **Wu, C.-C., J. L. Johnson, W. E. C Moore, and L. V. H. Moore.** 1992. Emended descriptions of *Prevotella denticola*, *Prevotella loescheii*, *Prevotella veroralis*, and *Prevotella melaninogenica*. *Int. J. Syst. Bacteriol.* **42:**536–541.
110. **Yamamoto, T., S. Kajiura, and T. Watanabe.** 1994. *Capnocytophaga haemolytica* sp. nov. and *Capnocytophaga granulosa* sp. nov. from human dental plaque. *Int. J. Syst. Bacteriol.* **44:**324–329.

Algorithms for Identification of Curved and Spiral-Shaped Gram-Negative Rods

PATRICK R. MURRAY

49

In contrast to the bacteria discussed in chapters 15 through 48, the microbes discussed in the next five chapters do not share phenotypic or genotypic properties. The only feature in common for the organisms presented in the following subsection is their microscopic appearance. They all are curved or spiral-shaped rods. Although this morphology is distinct for some genera (e.g., *Leptospira*), most of these bacteria cannot be identified simply by their size and shape. Additionally, microscopy is relatively insensitive for the detection of these bacteria in specific infections. For that reason, their detection requires a combination of tests including microscopy, antigen tests, molecular diagnostic tests, in vitro culture, and serologic tests. The following summarizes the epidemiology of infections caused by the bacteria discussed in chapters 50 to 54 (Table 1) and the diagnostic tests used for their detection (Table 2).

TABLE 1 Epidemiology of infections with *Arcobacter*, *Borrelia*, *Campylobacter*, *Helicobacter*, *Leptospira*, and *Treponema*

Organism	Disease	Reservoir	Vector or mode of transmission
Arcobacter butzleri	Bacteremia, endocarditis, peritonitis, gastroenteritis	Poultry, humans, other animals	Ingestion of contaminated food or water; fecal-oral
Arcobacter cryaerophilus	Bacteremia, gastroenteritis	Cattle, horses, domestic animals, humans	Ingestion of contaminated food or water; fecal-oral
Borrelia afzelii	Lyme disease	Rodents	Ixodes (hard ticks)
Borrelia burgdorferi	Lyme disease	Rodents	Ixodes (hard ticks)
Borrelia garinii	Lyme disease	Rodents	Ixodes (hard ticks)
Borrelia recurrentis	Epidemic relapsing fever	Humans	*Pediculus humanus* (human body louse)
Borrelia species (many)	Endemic relapsing fever	Rodents, chipmunks, squirrels, humans	*Ornithodoros* (soft ticks)
Campylobacter coli	Gastroenteritis	Contaminated foods (e.g., poultry), milk, water	Ingestion of contaminated food, milk, or water
Campylobacter fetus	Bacteremia, extraintestinal infections	Humans	Fecal-oral
Campylobacter jejuni	Gastroenteritis	Contaminated foods (e.g., poultry), milk, water	Ingestion of contaminated food, milk, or water
Campylobacter lari	Bacteremia, gastroenteritis, urinary tract infection	Gulls, other birds, dogs, cats, chickens	Fecal-oral
Campylobacter upsaliensis	Bacteremia, gastroenteritis	Humans	Fecal-oral
Helicobacter canis	Gastroenteritis	Dogs	Contact with infected dogs
Helicobacter cinaedi	Gastroenteritis, bacteremia, cellulitis, arthritis, meningitis	Humans, hamsters	Fecal-oral

(*Continued on next page*)

TABLE 1 (*Continued*)

Organism	Disease	Reservoir	Vector or mode of transmission
Helicobacter fennelliae	Gastroenteritis, bacteremia	Humans	Fecal-oral
Helicobacter pylori	Gastritis, peptic ulcer disease, gastric cancer	Humans, macaques, cats	Fecal-oral, oral-oral
Helicobacter pullorum	Gastroenteritis	Chickens	Ingestion of poultry
Helicobacter westmeadii	Febrile bacteremias	Humans	Fecal-oral
Leptospira species (many)	Leptospirosis (mild, self-limiting febrile illness to fulminant hepatorenal failure and death [Weil's disease])	Dogs, cattle, swine, mice, rats	Exposure to urine from infected animals, e.g., in contaminated water or food; contact with contaminated tissues
Treponema pallidum subsp. *pallidum*	Venereal syphilis	Humans	Sexual contact; transplacental
Treponema pallidum subsp. *endemicum*	Endemic syphilis (bejel)	Humans	Contact with infected mucous membranes
Treponema pallidum subsp. *pertenue*	Yaws	Humans	Skin contact
Treponema carateum	Pinta	Humans	Skin contact

TABLE 2 Diagnostic tests for *Arcobacter*, *Borrelia*, *Campylobacter*, *Helicobacter*, *Leptospira*, and *Treponema*

Organism	Diagnostic test[a]
Arcobacter spp.	**Microscopy:** Gram-negative, curved or helical rods; test sensitivity and specificity undefined **Antigen tests:** None described **Molecular tests:** PCR (research tool currently) **Culture:** Growth at 15, 25, and 30°C; variable growth at 37°C; generally no growth at 42°C; microaerophilic; can grow on selective media, e.g., Campy-CVA **Serologic tests:** Not available
Borrelia burgdorferi, *B. afzelii*, *B. garinii* (Lyme disease)	**Microscopy:** Spirochetes detected in skin biopsy specimens collected outside the periphery of an erythema migrans lesion or tissues; stain with Warthin-Starry silver stain or fluorescein-labeled antibodies; not detected in blood **Antigen tests:** Not available **Molecular tests:** May rapidly become the diagnostic test of choice; probes specific but insensitive; PCR highly sensitive and specific **Culture:** Spirochetes grow in BSK II medium in a microaerophilic atmosphere at 30–37°C; incubation for 6 weeks **Serologic tests:** Used to confirm clinical disease; IFA and ELISA most commonly used; poor specificity and test reproducibility but use of species-specific antigens rather than whole organism should improve this; titer of ≥ 1:256 considered positive; low titers in patients from areas without endemic infection should be confirmed by Western blotting; false-positive reactions with tick-borne relapsing fever, syphilis, leptospirosis, or periodontal disease
Borrelia spp. (louse- and tick-borne relapsing fever)	**Microscopy:** Test of choice; spirochetes detected with Romanowsky stains (e.g., Giemsa, Wright) in blood collected during febrile episodes **Antigen tests:** Not available **Molecular tests:** Not available **Culture:** Spirochetes grow in BSK II medium in a microaerophilic atmosphere at 30–37°C; incubation for 6 weeks **Serologic tests:** Use if negative blood smears; relapsing-fever specific antigen now available for serologic test, so specificity has improved

(*Continued on next page*)

TABLE 2 Diagnostic tests for *Arcobacter*, *Borrelia*, *Campylobacter*, *Helicobacter*, *Leptospira*, and *Treponema* (*Continued*)

Organism	Diagnostic test[a]
Campylobacter coli, *C. jejuni*	**Microscopy:** Thin, curved, poorly staining gram-negative rods; variable sensitivity **Antigen tests:** Genus-specific latex agglutination tests for culture confirmation only **Molecular tests:** Genus-specific probe for culture confirmation only; PCR (research only) developed but problems with specimen preparation to eliminate inhibitors in stool **Culture:** Test of choice; growth at 37 and 42°C on selective media (e.g., CCDA, CSM, SSM, Skirrow, Campy-CVA); microaerobic atmosphere **Serologic tests:** Not recommended for diagnosis; infected patients may have false-positive *Legionella* serologic reactions
Campylobacter fetus	**Microscopy:** Thin, curved, poorly staining gram-negative rods; not observed in blood specimens **Antigen tests:** Not available **Molecular tests:** Genus-specific probe for culture confirmation only **Culture:** Test of choice; growth at 37 but not 42°C; blood specimens should be inoculated onto nonselective blood agar and incubated in microaerobic atmosphere **Serologic tests:** Not recommended for diagnosis; infected patients may have false-positive *Legionella* serologic reactions
Campylobacter, other spp.	**Microscopy:** Thin, curved, poorly staining gram-negative rods; not observed in blood specimens **Antigen tests:** Not available **Molecular tests:** Genus-specific probe for culture confirmation only; PCR (research only) developed, but problems with specimen preparation to eliminate inhibitors in stool **Culture:** Test of choice; growth at 37 and 42°C in microaerobic atmosphere; selective media with cephalothin should not be used **Serologic tests:** Not recommended for diagnosis; infected patients may have false-positive *Legionella* serologic reactions
Helicobacter pylori	**Microscopy:** Organisms detected in gastric biopsy specimens with H&E, Giemsa, or Warthin-Starry silver stains; not in areas of intestinal metaplasia, gastric adenocarcinoma, or gastric MALT lymphomas **Antigen tests:** Test measuring urease production by the bacteria is useful for screening patients; gastric biopsy specimens should be tested (invasive) or the urea breath test should be used (noninvasive); both tests have sensitivity and specificity exceeding 90–95% **Molecular tests:** Species-specific PCR available (research test) but requires specimens collected by endoscopy and may not be cost-effective compared with the urease test or histopathologic tests **Culture:** Growth on selective and nonselective media in microaerobic atmosphere; incubation at 37°C for 5–7 days **Serologic tests:** IgG antibodies correlate with active infection; serum better than whole blood; EIA better than IFA or CF tests; asymptomatic or dyspeptic patients screened for anti-*H. pylori* IgG antibodies, with the urease test used to confirm negative serologic test result; urease or histopathologic test used for symptomatic patients
Helicobacter, other spp.	**Microscopy:** No value in direct fecal smears **Antigen tests:** No tests available (usually urease negative) **Molecular tests:** Species-specific PCR available (research test) **Culture:** Growth on selective media (e.g., Columbia or Skirrow's base with horse blood and antibiotics); incubation in microaerobic atmosphere at 37°C for 3–5 days **Serologic tests:** No commercial serology for enteric helicobacters
Leptospira spp.	**Microscopy:** Leptospires detected in blood, CSF, and tissues by either dark-field microscopy or DFA assay; dark-field microscopy is insensitive, and interpretation is subjective; DFA is more sensitive and specific **Antigen tests:** Not available **Molecular tests:** PCR is more sensitive than culture in first 10–14 days after onset; specimens include serum, urine, aqueous humor, and CSF; necessary to monitor for assay inhibitors **Culture:** Leptospires isolated in blood and CSF during first 10 days of disease; isolated from urine after 1 week; blood collected in heparin or sodium oxalate (avoid citrate); acidic urine avoided; selective Fletcher's or Ellinghausen's medium is used; incubation at room temperatures for up to 4 months (usually detected within first 2 weeks) **Serologic tests:** Most commonly used test; antibodies detected after 1 week of symptoms with peak at 3–4 weeks; MAT and ELISA highly sensitive and specific; titer of 1:200 is suggestive and ≥1:800 is strong evidence of disease; cross-reactions are seen with syphilis, relapsing fever, Lyme disease, and legionellosis

(*Continued on next page*)

TABLE 2 (*Continued*)

Organism	Diagnostic test[a]
Treponema pallidum subsp. *pallidum*	**Microscopy:** Spirochetes observed in lesions by dark-field microscopy or DFA; most sensitive test in primary syphilis, reliably positive in congenital and secondary syphilis, not sensitive in latent syphilis or neurosyphilis; DFA used for oral or perirectal lesions **Antigen tests:** Not available **Molecular tests:** PCR tests (research only) available; would be most useful for disease with only a few organisms (late manifestations) **Culture:** Not available **Serologic tests:** Nontreponemal (VDRL, RPR, USR, TRUST) and treponemal (FTA-ABS, FTA-ABS[DS], MHA-TP) tests available; nontreponemal tests are insensitive in primary and late syphilis; treponemal tests are insensive in primary syphilis, but positive reactions persist for life; both test types with false-positive reactions for patients with autoimmune disease, pregnancy, viral infections, malignancy, leprosy; neurosyphilis diagnosed with reactive serum treponemal test and a reactive VDRL in CSF; congenital syphilis supported by reactive IgM treponemal test and reactive VDRL in CSF
Treponema, other pathogenic spp.	**Microscopy:** Spirochetes observed in lesions by dark-field microscopy or DFA **Antigen tests:** Not available **Molecular tests:** PCR reactive with these organisms **Culture:** Not available **Serologic tests:** Reactive in syphilis tests

[a] BSK II, Barbour-Stoenner-Kelly II medium; Campy-CVA, Campy medium with cefoperazone, vancomycin, and amphotericin; CCDA, charcoal, cefoperazone, deoxycholate agar; CF, complement fixation; CSF, cerebrospinal fluid; CSM, charcoal-based selective medium; DFA, direct fluorescent antibody; EIA, enzyme immunoassay; ELISA, enzyme-linked immunosorbent assay; FTA-ABS, fluorescent treponemal antibody absorption; FTA-ABS [DS], FTA-ABS [double staining]; H&E, hematoxylin and eosin; IFA, indirect fluorescent antibodies; IgG, immunoglobulin G; MALT, mucosa-associated lymphoid tissue lymphoma; MAT, macroscopic agglutination test; MHA-TP, microhemagglutionation assay for antibodies to *T. pallidum*; RPR, rapid plasma reagin; SSM, semisolid blood-free motility medium; TRUST, toluidine red unheated-serum test; USR, unheated serum reagin; VDRL, Venereal Disease Research Laboratory test.

Campylobacter and *Arcobacter*

IRVING NACHAMKIN

50

DESCRIPTION OF THE GENUS

Two closely related genera, *Campylobacter* and *Arcobacter*, are included in the family *Campylobacteraceae* (119, 121). The family *Campylobacteraceae* includes 18 species and subspecies within the genus *Campylobacter* and four species in the genus *Arcobacter* (Table 1). Two species that were formerly classified in the genus *Wolinella* (*Wolinella curva* and *W. recta*) were reclassified as *Campylobacter* (121). Several species that were formerly classified as *Campylobacter* were reclassified in the genus *Arcobacter* and include *Arcobacter cryaerophilus* and *A. butzleri* (121, 122). The former *Campylobacter cinaedi* and *C. fennelliae* were reclassified in the genus *Helicobacter* (121) and are described in chapter 51 of this Manual. *C. hyoilei*, associated with porcine proliferative enteritis and previously thought to be a distinct species (2), is now considered to be identical to *C. coli* (123). *Bacteroides gracilis* was reclassified as *C. gracilis* (118), and *B. ureolyticus* is thought to be closely related to the genus *Campylobacter*; however, this classification is still uncertain. Some phenotypically unusual isolates of *C. gracilis* were recently reclassified into a new genus and species, *Sutterella wadsworthensis* (132).

Campylobacters are curved, S-shaped, or spiral rods that are 0.2 to 0.9 μm wide and 0.5 to 5.0 μm long. Campylobacters are gram-negative, non-spore-forming rods that may form spherical or coccoid bodies in old cultures or cultures exposed to air for prolonged periods. The organisms are motile by means of a single polar unsheathed flagellum at one or both ends. The species are generally microaerobic by means of a respiratory type of metabolism; however, some strains grow aerobically or anaerobically. An atmosphere containing increased hydrogen may be required by some species for microaerobic growth (119).

Arcobacters are gram-negative, slightly curved, curved, S-shaped, or helical non-spore-forming rods that are 0.2 to 0.9 μm wide and 1 to 3 μm long. The organisms are motile by means of a single polar unsheathed flagellum. Arcobacters grow at 15, 25, and 30°C but show variable growth at 37 and 42°C. The organisms are microaerobic and do not require an increased hydrogen concentration for growth. Arcobacters may grow aerobically at 30°C and anaerobically at 35 to 37°C. Most strains are nonhemolytic. *A. skirrowii* may be alpha-hemolytic. Most *Arcobacter* strains are susceptible to nalidixic acid but show a variable response to cephalothin (122).

CLINICAL SIGNIFICANCE

C. jejuni and *C. coli*

C. jejuni subsp. *jejuni* (referred to as *C. jejuni* throughout this chapter) and *C. coli* have been recognized since the late 1970s as agents of gastrointestinal infection. Many clinical and epidemiologic investigations have established *C. jejuni* as one of the most common causes of sporadic bacterial enteritis in the United States. Studies by the Centers for Disease Control and Prevention suggest that the overall infection rate is 1,000 per 100,000 population, determined by limited surveillance of *Campylobacter* infection in addition to estimates based on outbreak- and hospital-based studies in the United States. Over 2 million cases are estimated to occur annually, an incidence of infection similar to that in the United Kingdom and other developed nations (106). *C. jejuni* continues to be the most common enteric pathogen isolated from patients with diarrhea, as suggested by a preliminary study of the Food-borne Diseases Active Surveillance Network, FoodNet (96). *Campylobacter* infections are usually sporadic, occurring in the summer and early fall, and usually follow ingestion of improperly handled or improperly cooked food, primarily poultry products. The incidence of infection follows a bimodal age distribution, with the highest incidence occurring in infants and young children, followed by a second peak in young adults 20 to 40 years old. Outbreaks usually occur in the spring and fall and have been associated with ingestion of contaminated milk and water (106, 134).

The incidence of *Campylobacter* infection in developing countries such as Mexico and Thailand may be orders of magnitude higher than that in the United States (108). In developing countries, *Campylobacter* is frequently isolated from individuals who may or may not have diarrheal disease. Most symptomatic infections occur in infancy and early childhood, and incidence decreases with age. Travelers to developing countries are at risk for developing *Campylobacter* infection, with isolation rates of 0 to 39% having been reported in different studies (106, 108).

C. jejuni and *C. coli* are the most common *Campylobacter* species associated with diarrheal illness and are clinically indistinguishable. Most laboratories do not routinely distinguish these organisms. Approximately 5 to 10% of cases reported as being due to *C. jejuni* in the United States are

TABLE 1 Phenotypic properties of *Campylobacter* species[a]

Organism	Catalase	Nitrate reduction	Nitrite reduction	H_2 required	Urease	H_2S (TSI)	Hippurate hydrolysis	Indoxyl acetate hydrolysis	Growth at: 15°C	Growth at: 25°C	Growth at: 42°C	Growth in or on: 3.5% NaCl	Growth in or on: 1% Glycine	Growth in or on: MacConkey agar	Susceptibility to: Nalidixic acid	Susceptibility to: Cephalothin
C. *jejuni*	+	+	−	−	−	−	+	+	−	−	+	−	+	+	V	R
C. *jejuni* subsp. *doylei*	V	−	−	−	−	−	V	+	−	−	−	−	+	−	S	S
C. *coli*	+	+	−	−	−	−	−	+	−	−	+	−	+	+	S	R
C. *fetus*	+	+	−	−	−	−	−	−	−	+	−	−	+	+	V	S
C. *fetus* subsp. *venerealis*	+	+	−	−	−	−	−	−	−	+	−	−	−	+	R	S
C. *lari*	+	+	−	−	V	−	−	−	−	−	+	−	+	+	R	R
C. *upsaliensis*	W	+	−	−	−	−	−	+	−	−	+	−	V	−	S	S
C. *hyointestinalis*	+	+	−	V	−	+	−	−	−	+	+	−	+	+	R	S
C. *sputorum* biovar sputorum	−	+	+	−	−	+	−	−	−	−	+	−	+	+	S	S
C. *sputorum* biovar bubulus	−	+	+	−	−	+	−	−	−	−	+	+	+	−	R	S
C. *sputorum* biovar fecalis	+	+	+	−	−	+	−	−	−	−	+	−	+	+	R	S
C. *helveticus*	−	+	ND	−	ND	−	−	+	−	−	+	V	V	ND	S	S
C. *mucosalis*	−	+	+	+	−	+	−	−	−	−	+	−	+	+	R	S
C. *concisus*	−	+	+	+	−	+	−	−	−	−	+	−	+	+	R	R
C. *curvus*	−	+	+	+	−	+	−	+	−	−	+	−	+	ND	S	ND
C. *rectus*	−	+	+	+	−	+	−	+	−	−	W	−	+	ND	S	ND
C. *showae*	+	+	ND	+	−	+	−	+	−	−	+	−	V	ND	R	S
A. *cryaerophilus* group 1A	+	V	−	−	−	−	−	+	+	+	−	−	−	−	V	R
A. *cryaerophilus* group 1B	+	V	ND	−	−	−	−	+	+	+	−	−	−	+	S	V
A. *butzleri*	W	+	−	−	−	−	−	+	+	+	V	V	+	+	S	R
A. *nitrofigilis*	+	+	−	−	−	−	−	−	+	+	−	+	−	−	S	S
A. *skirrowii*	+	+	ND	−	−	−	−	+	+	+	V	V	V	−	S	S

[a] TSI, triple sugar iron; W, weak reaction; V, variable reaction; ND, not determined; S, susceptible; R, resistant. Adapted from references 27, 53, 87, 103, 119, and 122.

probably due to C. *coli*; this percentage may be higher in other parts of the world (108).

A spectrum of illness is seen during C. *jejuni* or C. *coli* infection; patients may be asymptomatic to severely ill. Symptoms and signs usually include fever, abdominal cramping, and diarrhea (with or without blood or fecal leukocytes) that lasts for several days to more than 1 week. Symptomatic infections are usually self-limited, but relapses may occur in 5 to 10% of untreated patients (10). *Campylobacter* infection may mimic acute appendicitis and result in unnecessary surgery. Extraintestinal infection and chronic sequelae of infection do occur and include bacteremia, reactive arthritis, bursitis, urinary tract infection, meningitis, endocarditis, peritonitis, erythema nodosum, pancreatitis, abortion, and neonatal sepsis (10). Bacteremia has been reported to occur at a rate of 1.5 per 1,000 intestinal infections, with the highest rate occurring in the elderly (101). Persistent diarrheal illness and bacteremia may occur in immunocompromised hosts, such as patients with human immunodeficiency virus infection (85), and may be difficult to treat. Deaths attributable to C. *jejuni* infection are uncommon but do occur (30, 106).

C. *jejuni* is now the most recognized antecedent cause of Guillain-Barré syndrome (GBS), an acute paralytic disease of the peripheral nervous system. Certain O serotypes, such as O:19, appear to be overrepresented in some GBS cases (55); other, more common serotypes are frequently reported as well (68, 75). The pathogenesis of *Campylobacter*-induced GBS is not completely understood but in part involves ganglioside-like epitopes in the *Campylobacter* lipopolysaccharide (71) that cross-react with reactive targets in peripheral nerve tissue as well as host susceptibility factors (42).

Little is known about the pathogenesis of *Campylobacter* infection. The infective dose of *Campylobacter* is not clearly defined; as few as 1,000 organisms may be capable of causing illness (9). The signs and symptoms of infection suggest an invasive mechanism of disease. In vitro and in vivo studies suggest that *Campylobacter* first colonizes the intestinal mucus layer by means of motility and then invades and/or translocates through the epithelial surface to the underlying tissue, where other putative virulence factors are then elaborated (135). C. *jejuni* has been reported to produce a cholera-like enterotoxin; however, other studies have refuted the significance of this finding. A *Campylobacter* toxin review was recently published (129).

C. fetus

C. *fetus* subsp. *fetus* (referred to as C. *fetus* throughout this chapter) is primarily associated with bacteremia and extraintestinal infection in patients with underlying diseases, which may lead to a poor outcome in some patients (10). C. *fetus* is also associated with septic abortions, septic arthritis, abscesses, meningitis, endocarditis, mycotic aneurysm, thrombophlebitis, peritonitis, and salpingitis (10). Gastroenteritis does occur with this species, but the incidence is probably underestimated because the organism does not grow well at 42°C and is usually susceptible to cephalothin, an antimicrobial agent used in some common selective media for stool cultures (23). C. *fetus* produces a surface protein capsule composed of a high-molecular-weight surface array protein that is essential for the virulence of the organism. This high-molecular-weight protein confers resistance to serum-mediated killing and phagocytosis and may explain why C. *fetus* is able to cause systemic infection (12). C. *fetus* subsp. *venerealis* is not associated with human infection.

C. upsaliensis

C. *upsaliensis* is a thermotolerant species that appears to be an important cause of diarrhea and bacteremia (35, 60). C. *upsaliensis* is susceptible to many antimicrobial agents present in C. *jejuni*-selective media; thus, most C. *upsaliensis* isolates are recovered by a filtration method (35). C. *upsaliensis* isolates occasionally may be recovered on some selective media.

C. lari

C. *lari* is a thermophilic species first isolated from gulls (of the genus *Larus*) and from other avian species, dogs, cats, and chickens. C. *lari* has been infrequently reported from humans with bacteremia and gastrointestinal and urinary tract infections. A waterborne outbreak of infection that occurred in 1985 affected over 100 individuals (107).

Other Species

Other *Campylobacter* species have been isolated from clinical specimens of patients with a variety of diseases, but their pathogenic role has not been determined. C. *jejuni* subsp. *doylei* is a nitrate-negative organism rarely recovered from patients with upper-gastrointestinal-tract infections and gastroenteritis (35, 104). C. *hyointestinalis* has been occasionally associated with proctitis and diarrhea in human infection (24). C. *concisus* has been associated primarily with periodontal disease but has also been isolated from patients with bacteremia, foot ulcer, and upper- and lower-gastrointestinal-tract infections (50, 120). The role of C. *concisus* as a cause of diarrheal disease has not been established, and one recent study suggests that the organism is not inherently pathogenic (125). C. *sputorum* biovar sputorum and C. *sputorum* biovar bubulus have been associated with lung, axillary, scrotal, and groin abscesses (69). C. *mucosalis* has been isolated from two children with enteritis (29). C. *helveticus* (103) has been recovered from domestic cats and dogs and has not been reported from human sources. C. *rectus* has been isolated primarily from patients with active periodontal infections (90) but has also been isolated from a patient with a pulmonary infection (102). C. *showae* has been isolated from the human gingival crevice (27). S. *wadsworthensis* (formerly C. *gracilis*) has been isolated from gingival crevices and from visceral, head, and neck infections in humans (118).

Arcobacter

Arcobacters are aerotolerant, *Campylobacter*-like organisms frequently isolated from bovine and porcine products of abortion and feces of animals with enteritis (131). Two of the four *Arcobacter* species have been associated with human infection. *A. butzleri* has been isolated from patients with bacteremia, endocarditis, peritonitis, and diarrhea (53, 79, 111, 122). *A. cryaerophilus* group 1B has been isolated from patients with bacteremia and diarrhea (44, 53, 122). *A. nitrofigilis* is a nitrogen-fixing bacterium found on the roots of a small marsh plant in Nova Scotia and has not been associated with human disease (66).

COLLECTION, TRANSPORT, AND STORAGE OF SPECIMENS

Fecal Samples

Fecal specimens are the preferred sample for isolating *Campylobacter* species from patients with gastrointestinal infections; however, rectal swabs are acceptable for cultures. For hospitalized patients, the "3-day" rule (rejection of specimens collected >72 h after admission) should be used as a criterion for the acceptability of routine cultures (41). For routine purposes, a single stool sample has high sensitivity for common enteric pathogens, but two samples may be desirable, depending upon clinical circumstances or delay in transport of the first sample, which could affect recovery (117). A transport medium should be used for transport of fecal specimens to the laboratory if a delay of more than 2 h is anticipated and for transport of rectal swabs. Cary-Blair medium containing a reduced agar concentration (1.6 g/liter) appears to be the most suitable transport medium for *Campylobacter* as well as other enteric pathogens (128). Specimens received in Cary-Blair medium should be stored at 4°C if processing is not performed immediately.

Blood

Campylobacter species, primarily *C. fetus*, *C. jejuni*, and *C. upsaliensis*, have been isolated from blood; however, in only a few studies have optimal conditions for isolating *Campylobacter* species from blood culture systems been evaluated. Both the BACTEC system (aerobic bottles) and the Septi-Chek system appear to support the growth of the common *Campylobacter* species (52, 58, 127). Other systems, such as anaerobic broth or lysis-centrifugation, may not be as sensitive (52).

DIRECT EXAMINATION

Campylobacters are not easily visualized with the safranin counterstain commonly used in the Gram stain procedure; carbolfuchsin or 0.1% aqueous basic fuchsin should be used as the counterstain for smears of stools or pure cultures (82, 95). Because of their characteristic microscopic morphology, campylobacters may be detected by direct Gram stain examination of stools obtained from patients with acute enteritis at a sensitivity ranging from 66 to 94% and at a very high specificity (82, 95).

Fecal leukocytes may be present during *Campylobacter* infection and have been reported in as few as 25% to as many as 80% of culture-proven cases (28, 33). Some authors have suggested that a test for the presence of leukocytes in stools be used for selective culturing to improve the cost-effectiveness of diagnosis (37). While the likelihood of *Campylobacter* or other enteroinvasive pathogens may be higher in the presence of fecal leukocytes, the absence of fecal leukocytes does not rule out disease (117). Thus, examination of stool samples for fecal leukocytes is not recommended as a test for predicting bacterial infection or for selective culturing for *Campylobacter* or other stool pathogens (28).

ISOLATION PROCEDURES

Most *Campylobacter* species require a microaerobic atmosphere containing approximately 5% O_2, 10% CO_2, and 85% N_2 for optimal recovery. Several manufacturers produce microaerobic gas generator packs that are suitable for routine use. A tri-gas incubator (115) or evacuation of an anaerobic incubator and replacement with the approximate gas mixture may also be used for routine cultures (73). The concentration of oxygen generated in candle jars is suboptimal for the isolation of *Campylobacter* and should not be used for routine laboratory isolation procedures (63). Some *Campylobacter* species, such as *C. sputorum*, *C. concisus*, *C. mucosalis*, *C. curvus*, *C. rectus*, and *C. hyointestinalis*, may require hydrogen for primary isolation and growth. These species may not be recovered under conventional microaerobic conditions since the amount of hydrogen generated in properly used commercial gas generator packs is <2% (74). A gas mixture of 10% CO_2, 6% H_2, and balanced N_2 used in an evacuation-replacement jar is sufficient for isolating hydrogen-requiring species (74).

Primary plating on selective media in combination with a filtration method (described below) is the optimal method for recovering a variety of *Campylobacter* species from clinical samples. A number of selective media are recommended for isolating *C. jejuni* and *C. coli*; these include blood-free media, such as charcoal-cefoperazone-deoxycholate agar (CCDA) (47), charcoal-based selective medium (CSM) (51), and semisolid blood-free motility medium (36), and blood-containing media, such as Skirrow medium (100) and Campy-CVA medium (93). A charcoal-based medium containing cefoperazone, amphotericin, and teicoplanin seems to be a very promising selective medium for the primary isolation of *C. upsaliensis* (5). To achieve the highest yield of *Campylobacter* organisms from stool samples, a combination of media including either CCDA or CSM as one of the media appears to be optimal (26, 38) and may increase the recovery of *Campylobacter* organisms by as much as 10 to 15% over the use of a single medium. If only a single medium can be used because of budget constraints, our laboratory has had very good experience with the Campy-CVA formulation, but a charcoal-based medium such as CCDA would work just as well.

Most of these selective media contain one or more antimicrobial agents, mainly cefoperazone, as the primary inhibitor of enteric bacterial flora. The antimicrobial agents, such as cephalothin, colistin, and polymyxin B, that are present in some selective medium formulations may be inhibitory to some strains of *C. jejuni* and *C. coli* (34, 77) and are inhibitory to *C. fetus*. *C. jejuni* subsp. *doylei*, *C. upsaliensis*, and *A. butzleri* generally do not grow on cephalothin-containing media. When choosing selective media for the primary isolation of *Campylobacter* from fecal samples, laboratories should use cefoperazone-containing media and discontinue using cephalothin-containing formulations.

If *Campylobacter* infection is suspected when blood specimens are drawn, broth media should be subcultured after 24 to 48 h on a nonselective blood agar plate incubated under microaerobic conditions at 37°C. This procedure will allow for the isolation of thermophilic and nonthermophilic species. Similarly, blood drawn in Isolator (Wampole Laboratories, Cranbury, N.J.) tubes for bacterial cultures should be incubated on a nonselective blood agar plate under microaerobic conditions at 37°C if *Campylobacter* infection is suspected. If a curved, gram-negative rod is observed upon Gram stain examination of a positive blood culture bottle, an aliquot should be cultured on a nonselective blood agar plate and incubated under microaerobic conditions at 37°C. An alternative staining method, such as acridine orange staining, may also be useful for detecting campylobacters in blood culture bottles if the Gram stain results are negative.

Optimal conditions for the recovery of *Arcobacter* species from clinical specimens have not been determined. *Arcobacter* species were first isolated on semisolid media designed to isolate *Leptospira* species (122, 131). *Arcobacter* species are aerotolerant and have been recovered on certain selective media, such as Campy-CVA medium (4), incubated under microaerobic conditions at 37°C and on nonselective media used with the filtration method. Several other media have been reported to recover *Arcobacter* species but have not been studied in clinical settings (4, 14, 21, 122).

Enrichment Cultures

A number of enrichment broths have been formulated to enhance the recovery of *Campylobacter* from stool samples; these include Preston enrichment (13), Campy-thio (11), *Campylobacter* enrichment broth (65), and other formulations (1, 20, 54, 98). Enrichment cultures may be beneficial when low numbers of organisms are expected because of delayed transport to the laboratory or because the acute stage of disease has passed (75, 110). The use of enrichment cultures as part of a routine stool culture setup has not been studied adequately and is probably not necessary.

Filtration

Various investigators have cultured stools by using a filtration method with a nonselective medium to isolate antibiotic-susceptible. *C. jejuni* and *C. coli* as well as *Campylobacter* species (34, 35) and *Arcobacter* species (53) that are susceptible to antibiotics present in most selective media. The method is based on the principle that campylobacters can pass through membrane filters (pore size, 0.45 μm to 0.65 μm) with relative ease (because of their motility), while other stool flora are retained during the short processing time. Cellulose acetate membrane filters with a 0.65-μm pore size are recommended for routine use (130). The filtration technique is performed by placing a sterile 0.65-μm cellulose acetate filter onto the surface of an agar medium such as antibiotic-free CCDA, CSM, or blood-containing medium. Ten to 15 drops of fecal suspension are placed on the filter, and the plate is incubated at 37°C for 1 h. The filter is removed and the plate is incubated at 37°C under microaerobic conditions, preferably in an atmosphere containing increased hydrogen (for the hydrogen-requiring species). Stool samples containing ~10^5 CFU of campylobacters per ml will be detected with this method; thus, the filtration method is not as sensitive as primary culturing with selective media (35). Therefore, filtration should be used to complement direct culturing on selective plating media and not as a replacement.

Species within the genera *Campylobacter* and *Arcobacter* have different optimal temperatures for growth. The choice of incubation temperature for routine stool cultures therefore is critical in determining the spectrum of species that will be isolated. By convention, most laboratories use 42°C as the primary incubation temperature for *Campylobacter*. This temperature allows the growth of *C. jejuni* and *C. coli* on selective media. *C. upsaliensis* also grows well at 42°C but usually is not recovered on selective media. *C. fetus* grows poorly at this temperature and generally is not recovered. *Arcobacter* species are not thermophilic and generally are not recovered at 42°C.

In contrast, most *Campylobacter* and *Arcobacter* species grow well at 37°C. Several selective media, such as Skirrow medium and semisolid blood-free motility medium, were devised for use at 42°C and have poor selective properties at 37°C, whereas CCDA and CSM have good selective properties at 37°C (26). Plates should be incubated for 72 h before being reported as negative.

Because of the expense of including several types of media and filtration in the initial workup for campylobacters, a practical approach is to use a single medium, such as Campy-CVA medium or CCDA (or equivalent) incubated at 42°C, for the isolation of thermophilic campylobacters in the workup of acute bacterial gastroenteritis. If the primary culture workup is unrevealing and, based on clinical consultation, additional testing is required, additional stool samples should be plated on multiple selective media, processed by the filtration method, and incubated at 37°C under microaerobic conditions.

IDENTIFICATION

Depending on the medium used, *Campylobacter* colonies may have different appearances. In general, *Campylobacter* spp. produce gray, flat, irregular, spreading colonies, particularly on freshly prepared media; spreading along the streak line is commonly seen. As the moisture content decreases, colonies may become round, convex, and glistening, with little spreading. Hemolysis on blood agar is not observed. *Arcobacter* spp. are morphologically similar to *Campylobacter* spp. (122).

For initial analysis, a Gram stain examination and an oxidase test should be performed. Oxidase-positive colonies exhibiting a characteristic Gram stain appearance (e.g., gram-negative, curved to S-shaped rods) on selective media incubated at 42°C under microaerobic conditions can be reliably reported as *Campylobacter* spp. until other biochemical tests are performed. Primary isolates should first be tested for hippurate hydrolysis (hippuricase activity), and positive isolates with the above characteristics should be reported as *C. jejuni* without further phenotypic tests. The Gram stain appearance of *Arcobacter* colonies may differ from that of typical *Campylobacter* colonies. *A. butzleri* is only slightly curved, and *A. cryaerophilus* tends to be much more helical.

Phenotypic assays still remain the most useful methods for the routine differentiation of common *Campylobacter* species. Because many *Campylobacter* and *Arcobacter* species are difficult to identify, however, molecular methods have been developed to differentiate a number of species. The most common species, *C. jejuni*, is relatively easy to identify phenotypically; however, hippurate-negative strains may be more difficult to identify. *C. coli* is similar biochemically to *C. jejuni*, except for the lack of hippuricase activity; molecular methods are needed to identify *C. coli*. *C. jejuni* and *C. coli* have been reported to be reliably differentiated based on polymorphisms in the *ceuE* gene (32), a GTPase gene (124), the 16S ribosomal DNA gene (19, 61), and the 23S ribosomal DNA gene (46) by PCR and/or PCR-restriction fragment length polymorphism analysis.

Several phenotypic tests have been described for identifying *Campylobacter* spp. The most routinely useful tests for initial identification include growth temperature studies (e.g., growth at 25, 37, and 42°C), catalase production, hippurate hydrolysis, indoxyl acetate hydrolysis, nitrate reduction, production of H_2S, and antibiotic susceptibility determined by the disk method (7). Methods for the routinely useful tests have been published elsewhere (7, 49, 73). To obtain consistent and reproducible results, a standardized suspension and inoculum should be used for performing phenotypic tests. For growth temperature and oxygen tolerance studies, a suspension of the organism in heart infusion broth or tryptic soy broth at a turbidity of a McFarland no. 1 standard should be used. A fiber-tipped swab dipped in the broth suspension should be used to make a single streak across a plate (Mueller-Hinton agar with 5% sheep blood is a suitable medium), and the plates should be incubated at the desired temperature and/or under the desired atmospheric conditions (7, 73).

Hydrolysis of sodium hippurate is the major test for distinguishing *C. jejuni* (and *C. jejuni* subsp. *doylei*) from other *Campylobacter* species. Strains that are isolated on selective media at 42°C, are oxidase positive, show characteristic microscopic morphology, and have a positive result for hippurate hydrolysis should be reported as *C. jejuni*; for routine clinical purposes, no other tests need to be performed. Methods for this test are described elsewhere (64, 89). Commercially available disk methods for rapid hippurate hydrolysis testing compare favorably with the tube method (18). A large inoculum (i.e., a full loop) should be used for this test. Occasional strains of *C. jejuni* may be hippurate hydrolysis negative (72, 116). Gas-liquid chromatography for detecting benzoic acid (liberated from the hydrolysis of sodium hippurate) is the most sensitive assay for hippurate hydrolysis (72) and can be used for more definitive determination. Molecular detection of the *hipO* (hippuricase) gene by PCR may be useful for identifying phenotypically negative isolates (39).

Inhibition (susceptibility) or resistance of *Campylobacter* spp. to nalidixic acid and cephalothin has routinely been used as an aid for species identification. Tests can be performed by standard disk diffusion techniques with any nonselective medium that supports the growth of the *Campylobacter* strain; 30-μg nalidixic acid and 30-μg cephalothin disks should be incubated at 37°C for nonthermophilic campylobacters and at 42°C for thermophilic strains for 1 to 2 days. Any zone of inhibition indicates susceptibility. Some variability does exist with this test, and even with *C. jejuni* and *C. coli*, some strains may not give the expected results. Some strains of *C. jejuni* and *C. coli* occasionally may be cephalothin susceptible. Nalidixic acid-resistant *C. jejuni* and *C. coli* strains have been noted by a number of investigators; in Europe, increasing resistance to fluoroquinolones has been noted (25, 91). Since there is cross-resistance between the fluoroquinolones and nalidixic acid, the finding of nalidixic acid resistance does not exclude the identification of *C. jejuni* or *C. coli*. Hippurate hydrolysis-positive strains should be reported as *C. jejuni*, regardless of the nalidixic acid disk results. Detection of a nalidixic acid-resistant strain of *C. jejuni* should also alert the laboratory and suggest to the physician that the strain may be resistant to fluoroquinolones, and further susceptibility testing may be warranted if antimicrobial therapy with this class of drugs is planned.

Indoxyl acetate hydrolysis (67, 87) is useful for differentiating some thermophilic *Campylobacter* species. The disk method is rapid (5 to 30 min) and easy to perform. Disks are prepared by making a 20% solution of indoxyl acetate in acetone and adding 25 μl to a blank paper disk (0.6 cm). The disk is dried at room temperature and stored at 4°C in a brown tube with desiccant. Disks are also available from commercial sources. A large loopful of growth from a plate is placed on the disk, and a drop of sterile distilled water is added. Hydrolysis of indoxyl acetate is indicated by the appearance of a dark blue or blue-green color. Weakly positive strains show a pale blue color in 10 to 30 min. No color change is indicative of a negative reaction.

Additional tests can be performed to aid in the identification of *Campylobacter* spp. (Table 1). The H_2S reaction on triple sugar iron medium works best if the medium is freshly prepared. The nitrate reduction test is performed with nitrate broth medium (73) as described by Barrett et al. (7). Nitrate broth medium is inoculated with 0.1 ml of bacterial suspension. Strains that do not grow in nitrate broth medium can be inoculated into semisolid Mueller-Hinton broth with 0.3% agar and 0.2% potassium nitrate by stabbing the agar several times with bacterial growth from an agar plate. Development of a red reaction after the addition of reagents indicates the reduction of nitrate.

Commercial systems for the identification of *Campylobacter* species have not been found to be more accurate than conventional tests (48). Molecular approaches with PCR-restriction fragment length polymorphism analysis appear to be promising as alternatives for distinguishing among various *Campylobacter* species (19, 46). Unfortunately, *Campylobacter* species are difficult to differentiate from *Arcobacter* species based on phenotypic tests. However, an aerotolerant species (i.e., growth under aerobic conditions) that grows on MacConkey agar (under microaerobic conditions) could be presumptively identified as an *Arcobacter* species. The failure to grow on MacConkey agar, however, does not rule out an *Arcobacter* species. PCR-based assays may ultimately be the most useful approach for accurately identifying *Arcobacter* species; some of these assays have been described recently (8, 40, 46).

NONCULTURE METHODS

A number of commercial systems have been developed as an aid to identifying *Campylobacter* spp. to the genus level. Two immunologic assays that use isolated colonies (ID Campy [Integrated Diagnostics, Baltimore, Md.]; Campyslide [BBL Microbiology Systems, Cockeysville, Md.]) (43, 76) can identify *C. jejuni* and *C. coli* but cannot differentiate the two. At the time of evaluation, the ID Campy (formerly Meritec Campy jcl; Meridian Diagnostics, Cincinnati, Ohio) assay could not reliably identify *C. lari* (76). A DNA probe (Accuprobe; Gen-Probe Inc., San Diego, Calif.) directed against *Campylobacter* RNA sequences can identify *C. jejuni*, *C. jejuni* subsp. *doylei*, *C. coli*, and *C. lari* and was 100% sensitive for all isolates tested (88, 114); however, the probe also hybridized with 2 of 17 *C. hyointestinalis* isolates (88). Thus, these methods may be useful for confirming *Campylobacter* if other tests are not conclusive.

Although a specific test for the detection of *Campylobacter* in fecal samples is not commercially available, several investigators have evaluated the PCR for directly detecting *Campylobacter* in stool samples (59, 61, 80, 81, 105, 126). The major obstacle in the development of a PCR assay for stools for use in the clinical laboratory is the lack of a simple and practical DNA extraction procedure for stools that eliminates PCR inhibitors.

EPIDEMIOLOGIC TYPING SYSTEMS

Many typing systems have been devised to study the epidemiology of *Campylobacter* infections; they vary in complexity and ability to discriminate between strains. These methods include serotyping, biotyping, bacteriocin sensitivity testing, detection of preformed enzymes, auxotyping, lectin binding, phage typing, multilocus enzyme electrophoresis, and molecular methods such as restriction endonuclease analysis, ribotyping, and PCR (83). The most frequently used system is serotyping. Two major serotyping schemes are used worldwide and detect heat-labile (HL) (62) and O (84) antigens. The HL serotyping scheme originally described by Lior et al. (62) can detect over 100 serotypes of *C. jejuni*, *C. coli*, and *C. lari*. Uncharacterized bacterial surface antigens and, in some serotypes, flagellar antigens are the serodeterminants for this serotyping scheme (3). The O serotyping scheme of Penner and Hennessy (84) detects 60 types of *C. jejuni* and *C. coli* (83) and is based on the detection of lipopolysaccharide antigens. Serotyping is performed only in a few reference laboratories because of the time and expense needed to maintain quality antisera. Commercially available HL serotyping reagents are generally of very poor quality (78). A combination of serotyping and molecular methods should be used for studying the epidemiology of *Campylobacter* infection.

SEROLOGIC TESTS

Serum immunoglobulin G (IgG), IgM, and IgA levels rise in response to infection, but serum and fecal IgA levels appear during the first few weeks of infection and then fall rapidly (10). Serum antibody assays vary in both sensitivity and specificity for detecting *Campylobacter* infection, and test performance appears to be population dependent. Patients with *Campylobacter* infection may have false-positive *Legionella* antibody tests (15). Serologic testing appears to be useful for epidemiologic investigations and is not recommended for routine diagnosis.

ANTIMICROBIAL SUSCEPTIBILITY

C. jejuni and *C. coli* show variable susceptibilities to a variety of antimicrobial agents, including macrolides, fluoroquinolones, aminoglycosides, chloramphenicol, nitrofurantoin, and tetracycline (10). Most isolates are not susceptible to cephalosporins and penicillins (10). Erythromycin has been the drug of choice for treating *C. jejuni* gastrointestinal infection, and ciprofloxacin (or equivalent) has been used as an alternative drug (10). Early therapy of *Campylobacter* infection with erythromycin or ciprofloxacin is effective in eliminating the organism from stools and may also reduce the duration of symptoms associated with infection (22, 33, 86, 94).

C. jejuni is generally susceptible to erythromycin, with resistance rates of less than 5% (92, 97). Rates of erythromycin resistance in *C. coli* vary considerably, with up to 80% of strains showing resistance in some studies (45, 57, 92, 109). Although ciprofloxacin has been effective in treating *Campylobacter* infection, the emergence of ciprofloxacin resistance during therapy has been reported (17, 33, 86, 112, 136). Several in vitro studies have suggested that resistance to fluoroquinolones is increasing (16, 25, 31, 91, 99, 133); thus, the effectiveness of this class of drugs may be diminished in the future. *C. jejuni* and *C. coli* may also produce a β-lactamase that appears to be active against amoxicillin, ampicillin, and ticarcillin; this enzyme has been reported to be inhibited by clavulanic acid but not by sulbactam or tazobactam (56).

Parenteral therapy is used to treat *C. fetus* systemic infection; drugs used include erythromycin, ampicillin, aminoglycosides, and chloramphenicol, depending upon the type of infection (10). *S. wadsworthensis* (formerly *C. gracilis*) is susceptible to a variety of antimicrobial agents (70) (see chapter 48).

Susceptibility tests for *Campylobacter* are not standardized; consequently, the literature contains some variability in the susceptibility data reported. Recommendations for agar dilution methods include the use of Mueller-Hinton agar supplemented with 5% horse or sheep blood and incubated for 24 to 48 h at 37°C under microaerobic conditions (6, 113). The E-test (PDM Epsilometer; AB Biodisk, Solna, Sweden), in which Mueller-Hinton agar supplemented with 5% sheep blood is incubated for 24 to 48 h at 37°C or for 20 to 24 h at 42°C, has been found to compare favorably with agar dilution methods (6, 45).

INTERPRETATION AND REPORTING OF RESULTS

Campylobacter species, including the common thermophilic species *C. jejuni* and *C. coli*, should be sought in all diarrheic stools submitted to the laboratory for routine stool culturing. The initial workup may also include a Gram stain of the stools to look specifically for *Campylobacter*; the presence of gull-shaped, curved gram-negative bacilli may be presumptively reported as *Campylobacter* species.

Isolation of *Campylobacter* from a patient with acute diarrhea is usually significant, since the carrier rate in developed countries is quite low; however, in developing countries, the significance may be more difficult to interpret, especially in the presence of other enteric pathogens. In acute infection, there is usually a high number of organisms in the stool; however, the quantity of organisms is neither related to the severity of infection nor indicative of a carrier state. Other species, such as *C. fetus* and *C. upsaliensis*, that may be important causes of diarrhea may not be isolated on routine selective media, and special methods and alternative incubation techniques would be required as described above. Isolation of oxidase-positive, catalase-positive, curved gram-negative rods that are hippurate hydrolysis positive can be identified as *C. jejuni* without further workup. Nalidixic acid disk identification test results may be misleading because of the increasing occurrence of fluoroquinoline resistance in *Campylobacter*. Thus, the isolation of a hippurate hydrolysis-positive strain that is resistant to nalidixic acid should still be reported as *C. jejuni*.

The importance of identifying other *Campylobacter* species depends upon the clinical circumstances, but identification should always be performed on isolates from blood or other sterile sites, since the results could influence antimicrobial therapy decisions. Given that fluoroquinolone resistance is increasing in *C. jejuni*, nonstandardized susceptibility testing may need to be performed on isolates from patients who fail to respond to initial empiric therapy or on isolates from patients with serious infection (i.e., bacteremia).

REFERENCES

1. **Agulla, A., F. J. Merino, P. A. Villasante, J. V. Saz, A. Diaz, and A. C. Velasco.** 1987. Evaluation of four enrichment media for isolation of *Campylobacter jejuni*. *J. Clin. Microbiol.* **25:**174–175.
2. **Alderton, M. R., V. Korolik, P. J. Coloe, F. E. Dewhirst, and B. J. Paster.** 1995. *Campylobacter hyoilei* sp. nov., associated with porcine proliferative enteritis. *Int. J. Syst. Bacteriol.* **45:**61–66.
3. **Alm, R. A., P. Guerry, M. E. Power, H. Lior, and T. J. Trust.** 1991. Analysis of the role of flagella in the heat-labile Lior serotyping scheme of thermophilic campylobacters by mutant allele exchange. *J. Clin. Microbiol.* **29:** 2438–2445.
4. **Anderson, K. F., J. A. Kiehlbauch, D. C. Anderson, H. M. McClure, and I. K. Wachsmuth.** 1993. *Arcobacter (Campylobacter) butzleri*-associated diarrheal illness in a nonhuman primate. *Infect. Immun.* **61:**2220–2223.
5. **Aspinall, S. T., D. R. A. Wareing, P. G. Hayward, and D. N. Hutchinson.** 1996. A comparison of a new campylobacter selective medium (CAT) with membrane filtration for the isolation of thermophilic campylobacters including *Campylobacter upsaliensis*. *J. Appl. Bacteriol.* **80:** 645–650.
6. **Baker, C. N.** 1992. The E-test and *Campylobacter jejuni*. *Diagn. Microbiol. Infect. Dis.* **15:**469–472.
7. **Barrett, T. J., C. M. Patton, and G. K. Morris.** 1988. Differentiation of *Campylobacter* species using phenotypic characterization. *Lab. Med.* **19:**96–102.
8. **Bastyns, K., D. Cartuyvels, S. Chapelle, P. Vandamme, H. Goossens, and R. De Wachter.** 1995. A variable 23S rDNA region is a useful discriminating target for genus-

specific and species-specific PCR amplification in *Arcobacter* species. *Syst. Appl. Microbiol.* **18:**353–356.

9. **Black, R. E., M. M. Levine, M. L. Clements, T. P. Hughs, and M. J. Blaser.** 1988. Experimental *Campylobacter jejuni* infections in humans. *J. Infect. Dis.* **157:** 472–480.
10. **Blaser, M. J.** 1995. *Campylobacter* and related species, p. 1948–1956. *In* G. L. Mandell, J. E. Bennett, and R. Dolin (ed.), *Principles and Practice of Infectious Diseases*. Churchill Livingstone, New York, N.Y.
11. **Blaser, M. J., I. D. Berkowitz, F. M. LaForce, J. Craven, L. B. Reller, and W. L. Wang.** 1979. *Campylobacter* enteritis: clinical and epidemiologic features. *Ann. Intern. Med.* **91:**179–185.
12. **Blaser, M. J., and Z. Pei.** 1993. Pathogenesis of *Campylobacter fetus* infections: critical role of high-molecular weight S-layer proteins in virulence. *J. Infect. Dis.* **167:** 372–377.
13. **Bolton, F. J., and L. Robertson.** 1982. A selective medium for isolating *Campylobacter jejuni/coli*. *J. Clin. Pathol.* **35:**462–467.
14. **Borczyk, A., S. D. Rosa, and H. Lior.** 1991. Enhanced recognition of *Campylobacter cryaerophila* in clinical and environmental specimens. abstr. C-267, p. 386. *In Abstracts of the 91st Annual Meeting of the American Society for Microbiology 1991*. American Society for Microbiology, Washington, D.C.
15. **Boswell, T. C. J., and G. Kudesia.** 1992. Serological cross-reactions between *Legionella pneumophila* and *Campylobacter* in the indirect fluorescent antibody test. *Epidemiol. Infect.* **109:**291–295.
16. **Bowler, I. C. J. W., M. Connor, M. P. A. Lessing, and D. Day.** 1996. Quinolone resistance and *Campylobacter* species. *J. Antimicrob. Chemother.* **38:**315.
17. **Burnens, A. P., M. Heitz, I. Brodard, and J. Nicolet.** 1996. Sequential development of resistance to fluoroquinolones and erythromycin in an isolate of *Campylobacter jejuni*. *Zentbl. Bakteriol. Parasitenkd. Infektionskr.* **283:** 314–321.
18. **Cacho, J. B., P. M. Aguirre, A. Hernanz, and A. C. Velasco.** 1989. Evaluation of a disk method for detection of hippurate hydrolysis by *Campylobacter* spp. *J. Clin. Microbiol.* **27:**359–360.
19. **Cardarelli-Leite, P., K. Blom, C. M. Patton, M. A. Nicholson, A. G. Steigerwalt, S. B. Hunter, D. J. Brenner, T. J. Barrett, and B. Swaminathan.** 1996. Rapid identification of *Campylobacter* species by restriction fragment length polymorphism analysis of a PCR-amplified fragment of the gene coding for 16S rRNA. *J. Clin. Microbiol.* **34:**62–67.
20. **Chan, F. T. H., and A. M. R. Mackenzie.** 1984. Advantage of using enrichment-culture techniques to isolate *Campylobacter jejuni* from stools. *J. Infect. Dis.* **149:** 481–482.
21. **de Boer, E., J. J. H. C. Tilburg, D. L. Woodward, H. Lior, and W. M. Johnson.** 1996. A selective medium for the isolation of *Arcobacter* from meats. *Lett. Appl. Microbiol.* **23:**64–66.
22. **Dryden, M. S., R. J. E. Gabb, and S. K. Wright.** 1996. Empirical treatment of severe acute community-acquired gastroenteritis with ciprofloxacin. *Clin. Infect. Dis.* **22:** 1019–1025.
23. **Edmonds, P., C. M. Patton, T. J. Barrett, G. K. Morris, A. G. Steigerwalt, and D. J. Brenner.** 1985. Biochemical and genetic characteristics of atypical *Campylobacter fetus* subsp. *fetus* isolated from humans in the United States. *J. Clin. Microbiol.* **21:**936–940.
24. **Edmonds, P., C. M. Patton, P. M. Griffin, T. J. Barrett, G. P. Schmid, C. N. Baker, M. A. Lambert, and D. J. Brenner.** 1987. *Campylobacter hyointestinalis* associated with human gastrointestinal disease in the United States. *J. Clin. Microbiol.* **25:**685–691.
25. **Endtz, H. P., G. J. Ruijs, B. van Klingeren, W. H. Jansen, T. van der Reyden, and R. P. Mouton.** 1991. Quinolone resistance in campylobacter isolated from man and poultry following the introduction of fluoroquinolones in veterinary medicine. *J. Antimicrob. Chemother.* **27:** 199–208.
26. **Endtz, H. P., G. J. Ruijs, A. H. Zwinderman, T. van der Reijden, M. Biever, and R. P. Mouton.** 1991. Comparison of six media, including a semisolid agar, for the isolation of various *Campylobacter* species from stool specimens. *J. Clin. Microbiol.* **29:**1007–1010.
27. **Etoh, Y., F. E. Dewhirst, B. J. Paster, A. Yamamoto, and N. Goto.** 1993. *Campylobacter showae* sp. nov., isolated from the human oral cavity. *Int. J. Syst. Bacteriol.* **43:**631–639.
28. **Fan, K., A. J. Morris, and L. B. Reller.** 1993. Application of rejection criteria for stool cultures for bacterial enteric pathogens. *J. Clin. Microbiol.* **31:**2233–2235.
29. **Figura, N., P. Guglielmetti, A. Zanchi, N. Partini, D. Armellini, P. F. Bayeli, M. Bugnoli, and S. Verdiani.** 1993. Two cases of *Campylobacter mucosalis* enteritis in children. *J. Clin. Microbiol.* **31:**727–728.
30. **Font, C., A. Cruceta, A. Moreno, O. Miro, B. Coll-Vinent, M. Almela, and J. Mensa.** 1997. Estudio de 30 pacientes con bacteremia por *Campylobacter* spp. *Med. Clin.* (Barcelona) **108:**336–340.
31. **Gaunt, P. N., and L. J. V. Piddock.** 1996. Ciprofloxacin resistant *Campylobacter* spp. in humans: an epidemiological and laboratory study. *J. Antimicrob. Chemother.* **37:** 747–757.
32. **Gonzalez, I., K. A. Grant, P. T. Richardson, S. F. Park, and M. D. Collins.** 1997. Specific identification of the enteropathogens *Campylobacter jejuni* and *Campylobacter coli* by using a PCR test based on the *ceuE* gene encoding a putative virulence determinant. *J. Clin. Microbiol.* **35:** 759–763.
33. **Goodman, L. J., G. M. Trenholme, R. L. Kaplan, J. Segreti, D. Hines, R. Petrak, J. A. Nelson, K. W. Mayer, W. Landau, and G. W. Parkhurst.** 1990. Empiric antimicrobial therapy of domestically acquired acute diarrhea in urban adults. *Arch. Intern. Med.* **150:**541–546.
34. **Goossens, H., M. De Boeck, H. Coignau, L. Vlaes, C. Van den Borre, and J.-P. Butzler.** 1986. Modified selective medium for isolation of *Campylobacter* spp. from feces: comparison with Preston medium, a blood-free medium, and a filtration system. *J. Clin. Microbiol.* **24:**840–843.
35. **Goossens, H., L. Vlaes, M. De Boeck, B. Pot, K. Kersters, J. Levy, P. de Mol, J. P. Butzler, and P. Vandamme.** 1990. Is "*Campylobacter upsaliensis*" an unrecognised cause of human diarrhoea? *Lancet* **335:**584–586.
36. **Goossens, H., L. Vlaes, I. Galand, C. Van den Borre, and J. P. Butzler.** 1989. Semisolid blood-free selective-motility medium for the isolation of campylobacters from stool specimens. *J. Clin. Microbiol.* **27:**1077–1080.
37. **Guerrant, R. L., and D. A. Bobak.** 1991. Bacterial and protozoal gastroenteritis. *N. Engl. J. Med.* **325:**327–340.
38. **Gun-Monro, J., R. P. Rennie, J. H. Thornley, H. L. Richardson, D. Hodge, and J. Lynch.** 1987. Laboratory and clinical evaluation of isolation media for *Campylobacter jejuni*. *J. Clin. Microbiol.* **25:**2274–2277.
39. **Hani, E., and V. L. Chan.** 1995. Expression and characterization of *Campylobacter jejuni* benzoylglycine amidohydrolase (hippuricase) gene in *Escherichia coli*. *J. Bacteriol.* **177:**2396–2402.
40. **Harmon, K. M., and I. V. Wesley.** 1996. Identification

of *Arcobacter* isolates by PCR. *Lett. Appl. Microbiol.* **23:** 241–244.

41. **Hines, J., and I. Nachamkin.** 1996. Effective use of the clinical microbiology laboratory for diagnosing diarrheal diseases. *Clin. Infect. Dis.* **23:**1292–1301.
42. **Ho, T. W., G. M. McKhann, and J. W. Griffin.** Human autoimmune neuropathies. *Annu. Rev. Neurosci.*, in press.
43. **Hodinka, R. L., and P. H. Gilligan.** 1988. Evaluation of the Campyslide agglutination test for confirmatory identification of selected *Campylobacter* species. *J. Clin. Microbiol.* **26:**47–49.
44. **Hsueh, P.-R., L.-J. Teng, P.-C. Yang, S.-K. Wang, S.-C. Chang, S.-W. Ho, W.-C. Hsieh, and K.-T. Luh.** 1997. Bacteremia caused by *Arcobacter cryaerophilus* 1B. *J. Clin. Microbiol.* **35:**489–491.
45. **Huang, M. B., C. N. Baker, S. Banerjee, and F. C. Tenover.** 1992. Accuracy of the E test for determining antimicrobial susceptibilities of staphylococci, enterococci, *Campylobacter jejuni*, and gram-negative bacteria resistant to antimicrobial agents. *J. Clin. Microbiol.* **30:**3243–3248.
46. **Hurtado, A., and R. J. Owen.** 1997. A molecular scheme based on 23S rRNA gene polymorphisms for rapid identification of *Campylobacter* and *Arcobacter* species. *J. Clin. Microbiol.* **35:**2401–2404.
47. **Hutchinson, D. N., and F. J. Bolton.** 1984. Improved blood free selective medium for the isolation of *Campylobacter jejuni* from faecal specimens. *J. Clin. Pathol.* **37:** 956–957.
48. **Huysmans, M. B., J. D. Turnidge, and J. H. Williams.** 1995. Evaluation of API Campy in comparison with conventional methods for identification of thermophilic campylobacters. *J. Clin. Microbiol.* **33:**3345–3346.
49. **Isenberg, H. (ed.).** 1992. *Clinical Microbiology Procedures Handbook*. American Society for Microbiology, Washington, D.C.
50. **Johnson, C. C., and S. M. Finegold.** 1987. Uncommonly encountered motile, anaerobic gram-negative bacilli associated with infection. *Rev. Infect. Dis.* **9:**1150–1162.
51. **Karmali, M. A., A. E. Simor, M. Roscoe, P. C. Flemming, S. S. Smith, and J. Lane.** 1986. Evaluation of a blood-free, charcoal-based, selective medium for the isolation of *Campylobacter* organisms from feces. *J. Clin. Microbiol.* **23:**456–459.
52. **Kasten, M. J., F. Allerberger, and J. P. Anhalt.** 1991. *Campylobacter* bacteremia: clinical experience with three different blood culture systems at Mayo Clinic 1984–1990. *Infection* **19:**88–90.
53. **Kiehlbauch, J. A., D. J. Brenner, M. A. Nicholson, C. N. Baker, C. M. Patton, A. G. Steigerwalt, and I. K. Wachsmuth.** 1991. *Campylobacter butzleri* sp. nov. isolated from humans and animals with diarrheal illness. *J. Clin. Microbiol.* **29:**376–385.
54. **Korhonen, L. K., and P. J. Martikainen.** 1990. Comparison of some enrichment broths and growth media for the isolation of thermophilic campylobacters from surface water samples. *J. Appl. Bacteriol.* **68:**593–599.
55. **Kuroki, S., T. Saida, M. Nukina, T. Haruta, M. Yoshioka, Y. Kobayashi, and H. Nakanishi.** 1993. *Campylobacter jejuni* strains from patients with Guillain-Barre syndrome belong mostly to Penner serogroup 19 and contain β-N-acetylglucosamine residues. *Ann. Neurol.* **33:** 243–247.
56. **Lachance, N., C. Gaudreau, F. Lamothe, and L. A. Larivière.** 1991. Role of the β-lactamase of *Campylobacter jejuni* in resistance to β-lactam agents. *Antimicrob. Agents Chemother.* **35:**813–818.
57. **Lachance, N., C. Gaudreau, F. Lamothe, and F. Turgeion.** 1993. Susceptibilities of β-lactamase-positive and -negative strains of *Campylobacter coli* to β-lactam agents. *Antimicrob. Agents Chemother.* **37:**1174–1176.
58. **Lastovica, A. J., E. Le Roux, and J. L. Penner.** 1989. "*Campylobacter upsaliensis*" isolated from blood cultures of pediatric patients. *J. Clin. Microbiol.* **27:**657–659.
59. **Lawson, A. J., D. Linton, J. Stanley, and R. J. Owen.** 1997. Polymerase chain reaction and speciation of *Campylobacter upsaliensis* and *C. helveticus* in human faeces and comparison with culture techniques. *J. Appl. Microbiol.* **83:**375–380.
60. **Lindblom, G.-B., E. Sjogren, J. Hansson-Westerberg, and B. Kaijser.** 1995. *Campylobacter upsaliensis*, *C. sputorum sputorum* and *C. concisus* as common causes of diarrhea in Swedish children. *Scand. J. Infect. Dis.* **27:** 187–188.
61. **Linton, D., A. J. Lawson, R. J. Owen, and J. Stanley.** 1997. PCR detection, identification to species level, and fingerprinting of *Campylobacter jejuni* and *Campylobacter coli* directly from diarrheic samples. *J. Clin. Microbiol.* **35:** 2568–2572.
62. **Lior, H., D. L. Woodward, J. A. Edgar, L. J. Laroche, and P. Gill.** 1982. Serotyping of *Campylobacter jejuni* by slide agglutination based on heat-labile antigenic factors. *J. Clin. Microbiol.* **15:**761–768.
63. **Luechtefeld, N. W., L. B. Reller, M. J. Blaser, and W.-L. L. Wang.** 1982. Comparison of atmospheres of incubation for primary isolation of *Campylobacter fetus* subsp. *jejuni* from animal specimens: 5% oxygen versus candle jar. *J. Clin. Microbiol.* **15:**53–57.
64. **MacFaddin, J. F.** 1980. Hippurate hydrolysis test, p. 141–162. *In* J. F. MacFaddin (ed.), *Biochemical Tests for Identification of Medical Bacteria*. The Williams & Wilkins Co., Baltimore, Md.
65. **Martin, W. T., C. M. Patton, G. K. Morris, M. E. Potter, and N. D. Puhr.** 1983. Selective enrichment broth for isolation of *Campylobacter jejuni*. *J. Clin. Microbiol.* **17:** 853–855.
66. **McClung, C. R., D. G. Patriquin, and R. E. Davis.** 1983. *Campylobacter nitrofigilis* sp. nov., a nitrogen-fixing bacterium associated with roots of *Spartina alterniflora* Loisel. *Int. J. Syst. Bacteriol.* **33:**605–612.
67. **Mills, C. K., and R. L. Cherna.** 1987. Indoxyl acetate hydrolysis. *J. Clin. Microbiol.* **25:**1560–1561.
68. **Mishu, B., and M. J. Blaser.** 1993. Role of infection due to *Campylobacter jejuni* in the initiation of Guillain-Barre syndrome. *Clin. Infect. Dis.* **17:**104–108.
69. **Mishu, B., C. M. Patton, and R. V. Tauxe.** 1992. Clinical and epidemiological features of non-jejuni, non-coli *Campylobacter* species, p. 31–41. *In* I. Nachamkin, M. J. Blaser, and L. S. Tompkins (ed.), Campylobacter jejuni: *Current Status and Future Trends*. American Society for Microbiology, Washington, D.C.
70. **Molitoris, E., H. M. Wexler, and S. M. Finegold.** 1997. Sources and antimicrobial susceptibilities of *Campylobacter gracilis* and *Sutterella wadsworthensis*. *Clin. Infect. Dis.* **25**(Suppl. 2):S264–S265.
71. **Moran, A. P., B. J. Appelmelk, and G. O. Aspinall.** 1996. Molecular mimicry of host structures by lipopolysaccharides of *Campylobacter* and *Helicobacter* spp.: implications in pathogenesis. *J. Endotoxin Res.* **3:**521–531.
72. **Morris, G. K., M. R. El Sherbeeny, C. M. Patton, H. Kodaka, G. L. Lombard, P. Edmonds, D. G. Hollis, and D. J. Brenner.** 1985. Comparison of four hippurate hydrolysis methods for identification of thermophilic *Campylobacter* spp. *J. Clin. Microbiol.* **22:**714–718.
73. **Morris, G. K., and C. M. Patton.** 1985. *Campylobacter*, p. 302–308. *In* E. Lennette, A. Balows, W. J. Hausler, Jr., and H. J. Shadomy (ed.), *Manual of Clinical Microbiology*. American Society for Microbiology, Washington, D.C.

74. **Nachamkin, I.** 1995. *Campylobacter* and *Arcobacter*, p. 483–491. *In* P. R. Murray, E. J. Baron, M. A. Pfaller, F. C. Tenover, and R. H. Yolken (ed.), *Manual of Clinical Microbiology*, 6th ed. ASM Press, Washington, D.C.
75. **Nachamkin, I.** 1997. Microbiologic approaches for studying *Campylobacter* in patients with Guillain-Barre syndrome. *Clin. Infect. Dis.* **176** (Suppl. 2):S106–S114.
76. **Nachamkin, I., and S. Barbagallo.** 1990. Culture confirmation of *Campylobacter* spp. by latex agglutination. *J. Clin. Microbiol.* **28:**817–818.
77. **Ng, L.-K., D. E. Taylor, and M. E. Stiles.** 1988. Characterization of freshly isolated *Campylobacter coli* strains and suitability of selective media for their growth. *J. Clin. Microbiol.* **26:**518–523.
78. **Nicholson, M. A., and C. M. Patton.** 1993. Evaluation of commercial antisera for serotyping heat-labile antigens of *Campylobacter jejuni* and *Campylobacter coli*. *J. Clin. Microbiol.* **31:**900–903.
79. **On, S. L. W., A. Stacey, and J. Smyth.** 1995. Isolation of *Arcobacter butzleri* from a neonate with bacteremia. *J. Infect.* **31:**225–227.
80. **Oyofo, B. A., Z. S. Mohran, S. El-Etr, M. O. Wasfy, and L. F. Peruski.** 1996. Detection of enterotoxigenic *Escherichia coli*, *Shigella*, and *Campylobacter* spp. by multiplex PCR assay. *J. Diarrhoeal Dis. Res.* **14:**207–210.
81. **Oyofo, B. A., S. A. Thornton, D. H. Burr, T. J. Trust, O. R. Pavlovskis, and P. Guerry.** 1992. Specific detection of *Campylobacter jejuni* and *Campylobacter coli* by using polymerase chain reaction. *J. Clin. Microbiol.* **30:** 2613–2619.
82. **Park, C. H., D. L. Hixon, A. S. Polhemus, C. B. Ferguson, S. L. Hall, C. C. Risheim, and C. B. Cook.** 1983. A rapid diagnosis of campylobacter enteritis by direct smear examination. *Am. J. Clin. Pathol.* **80:**388–390.
83. **Patton, C. M., and I. K. Wachsmuth.** 1992. Typing schemes: are current methods useful? p. 110–128. *In* I. Nachamkin, M. J. Blaser, and L. S. Tompkins (ed.), Campylobacter jejuni: *Current Status and Future Trends*. American Society for Microbiology, Washington, D.C.
84. **Penner, J. L., and J. N. Hennessy.** 1980. Passive hemagglutination technique for serotyping *Campylobacter fetus* subsp. *jejuni* on the basis of soluble heat-stable antigens. *J. Clin. Microbiol.* **12:**732–737.
85. **Perlman, D. M., N. M. Ampel, R. B. Schifman, D. L. Cohn, C. M. Patton, M. L. Aguirre, W.-L. L. Wang, and M. J. Blaser.** 1988. Persistent *Campylobacter jejuni* infections in patients infected with human immunodeficiency virus (HIV). *Ann. Intern. Med.* **108:**540–546.
86. **Petruccelli, B. P., G. S. Murphy, J. L. Sanchez, S. Walz, R. DeFraites, J. Gelnett, R. L. Haberberger, P. Echeverria, and D. N. Taylor.** 1992. Treatment of traveler's diarrhea with ciprofloxacin and loperamide. *J. Infect. Dis.* **165:**557–560.
87. **Popovic-Uroic, T., C. M. Patton, M. A. Nicholson, and J. A. Kiehlbauch.** 1990. Evaluation of the indoxyl acetate hydrolysis test for rapid differentiation of *Campylobacter*, *Helicobacter*, and *Wolinella* species. *J. Clin. Microbiol.* **28:** 2335–2339.
88. **Popovic-Uroic, T., C. M. Patton, I. K. Wachsmuth, and P. Roeder.** 1991. Evaluation of an oligonucleotide probe for identification of *Campylobacter* species. *Lab. Med.* **22:** 533–539.
89. **Pratt-Ripplin, K., and M. Pezzlo.** 1992. Identification of commonly isolated aerobic gram-positive bacteria, p. 1.20.21–1.20.22. *In* H. D. Isenberg (ed.), *Clinical Microbiology Procedures Handbook*. American Society for Microbiology, Washington, D.C.
90. **Rams, T. E., D. Feik, and J. Slots.** 1993. *Campylobacter rectus* in human periodontitis. *Oral Microbiol. Immunol.* **8:**230–235.
91. **Rautelin, H., O. V. Renkonen, and T. U. Kosunen.** 1991. Emergence of fluoroquinolone resistance in *Campylobacter jejuni* and *Campylobacter coli* in subjects from Finland. *Antimicrob. Agents Chemother.* **35:**2065–2069.
92. **Reina, J., N. Borrell, and A. Serra.** 1992. Emergence of resistance to erythromycin and fluoroquinolones in thermotolerant *Campylobacter* strains isolated from feces 1987–1991. *Eur. J. Clin. Microbiol. Infect. Dis.* **11:** 1163–1166.
93. **Reller, L. B., S. Mirrett, and L. G. Reimer.** 1983. Controlled evaluation of an improved selective medium for isolation of *Campylobacter jejuni*, abstr. C-274, p. 357. *In Abstracts of the 83rd Annual Meeting of the American Society for Microbiology 1983*. American Society for Microbiology, Washington, D.C.
94. **Salazar-Lindo, E., R. B. Sack, E. Chea-Woo, B. A. Kay, I. Piscoya, and R. Y. Leon-Barua.** 1986. Early treatment with erythromycin of *Campylobacter jejuni* associated dysentery in children. *J. Pediatr.* **109:**3555–3560.
95. **Sazie, E. S. M., and A. E. Titus.** 1982. Rapid diagnosis of *Campylobacter* enteritis. *Ann. Intern. Med.* **96:**62–63.
96. **Shallow, S., P. Daily, G. Rothrock, A. Reingold, D. Vugia, S. Waterman, T. Fiorentino, R. Marcus, R. Ryder, P. Mshar, J. L. Hadler, W. Vaughman, J. Koehler, P. Blake, K. E. Toomey, J. Hogan, V. Deneen, C. Hedberg, M. T. Osterholm, M. Cassidy, J. Townes, B. Shiferaw, P. Cieslak, K. Hedberg, and D. Fleming.** 1997. Foodborne Diseases Active Surveillance Network, 1996. *Morbid. Mortal. Weekly Rep.* **46:**258–261.
97. **Sjogren, E., B. Kaijser, and M. Werner.** 1992. Antimicrobial susceptibilities of *Campylobacter jejuni* and *Campylobacter coli* isolated in Sweden: a 10-year follow-up report. *Antimicrob. Agents Chemother.* **36:**2847–2849.
98. **Sjogren, E., G. B. Lindblom, and B. Kaijser.** 1987. Comparison of different procedures, transport media, and enrichment media for isolation of *Campylobacter* species from healthy laying hens and humans with diarrhea. *J. Clin. Microbiol.* **25:**1966–1968.
99. **Sjogren, E., G. B. Lindblom, and B. Kaijser.** 1997. Norfloxacin resistance in *Campylobacter jejuni* and *Campylobacter coli* isolates from Swedish patients. *J. Antimicrob. Chemother.* **40:**257–261.
100. **Skirrow, M. B.** 1977. *Campylobacter* enteritis: a "new" disease. *Br. Med. J.* **ii:**9–11.
101. **Skirrow, M. B., D. M. Jones, E. Sutcliffe, and J. Benjamin.** 1993. *Campylobacter* bacteremia in England and Wales, 1981–1991. *Epidemiol. Infect.* **110:**567–573.
102. **Spiegel, C. A., and G. Telford.** 1984. Isolation of *Wolinella recta* and *Actinomyces viscosus* from an actinomycotic chest wall mass. *J. Clin. Microbiol.* **20:**1187–1189.
103. **Stanley, J., A. P. Burnens, D. Linton, S. L. W. On, M. Costas, and R. J. Owen.** 1992. *Campylobacter helveticus* sp. nov., a new thermophilic species from domestic animals: characterization, and cloning of a species-specific DNA probe. *J. Gen. Microbiol.* **138:**2293–2303.
104. **Steele, T. W., and R. J. Owen.** 1988. *Campylobacter jejuni* subspecies *doylei* (subsp. nov.), a subspecies of nitrate-negative campylobacters isolated from human clinical specimens. *Int. J. Syst. Bacteriol.* **38:**316–318.
105. **Takeshi, K., T. Ikeda, A. Kubo, Y. Fujinaga, S. Makino, K. Oguma, E. Isogai, S. Yoshida, H. Sunagawa, T. Ohyama, and H. Kimura.** 1997. Direct detection by PCR of *Escherichia coli* O157 and enteropathogens in patients with bloody diarrhea. *Microbiol. Immunol.* **41:**819–822.
106. **Tauxe, R. V.** 1992. Epidemiology of *Campylobacter jejuni* infections in the United States and other industrialized nations, p. 9–19. *In* I. Nachamkin, M. J. Blaser, and L.

S. Tompkins (ed.), Campylobacter jejuni: *Current Status and Future Trends*. American Society for Microbiology, Washington, D.C.

107. **Tauxe, R. V., C. M. Patton, P. Edmonds, T. J. Barrett, D. J. Brenner, and P. A. Blake.** 1985. Illness associated with *Campylobacter laridis*, a newly recognized *Campylobacter* species. *J. Clin. Microbiol.* **21:**222–225.
108. **Taylor, D. N.** 1992. *Campylobacter* infections in developing countries, p. 20–30. *In* I. Nachamkin, M. J. Blaser, and L. S. Tompkins (ed.), Campylobacter jejuni: *Current Status and Future Trends*. American Society for Microbiology, Washington, D.C.
109. **Taylor, D. N., M. J. Blaser, P. Echeverria, C. Pitarangsi, L. Bodhidatta, and W.-L. Wang.** 1987. Erythromycin-resistant *Campylobacter* infections in Thailand. *Antimicrob. Agents Chemother.* **31:**438–442.
110. **Taylor, D. N., P. Echeverria, C. Pitarangsi, J. Seriwatana, L. Bodhidatta, and M. J. Blaser.** 1988. Influence of strain characteristics and immunity on the epidemiology of *Campylobacter* infections in Thailand. *J. Clin. Microbiol.* **26:**863–868.
111. **Taylor, D. N., J. H. Kiehlbauch, W. Tee, C. Pitarangsi, and P. Echeverria.** 1991. Isolation of group 2 aerotolerant *Campylobacter* species from Thai children with diarrhea. *J. Infect. Dis.* **163:**1062–1067.
112. **Tee, W., A. Mijch, E. Wright, and A. Yung.** 1995. Emergence of multidrug resistance in *Campylobacter jejuni* isolates from three patients infected with human immunodeficiency virus. *Clin. Infect. Dis.* **21:**634–638.
113. **Tenover, F. C., C. N. Baker, C. L. Fennell, and C. A. Ryan.** 1992. Antimicrobial resistance in *Campylobacter* species, p. 66–73. *In* I. Nachamkin, M. J. Blaser, and L. S. Tompkins (ed.), Campylobacter jejuni: *Current Status and Future Trends*. American Society for Microbiology, Washington, D.C.
114. **Tenover, F. C., L. Carlson, S. Barbagallo, and I. Nachamkin.** 1990. DNA probe culture confirmation assay for identification of thermophilic *Campylobacter* species. *J. Clin. Microbiol.* **28:**1284–1287.
115. **Thompson, J. S., D. S. Hodge, D. E. Smith, and Y. A. Yong.** 1990. Use of tri-gas incubator for routine culture of *Campylobacter* species from fecal specimens. *J. Clin. Microbiol.* **28:**2802–2803.
116. **Totten, P. A., C. M. Patton, F. C. Tenover, T. J. Barrett, W. E. Stamm, A. G. Steigerwalt, J. Y. Lin, K. K. Holmes, and D. J. Brenner.** 1987. Prevalence and characterization of hippurate-negative *Campylobacter jejuni* in King County, Washington. *J. Clin. Microbiol.* **25:**1747–1752.
117. **Valenstein, P., M. Pfaller, and M. Yungbluth.** 1996. The use and abuse of routine stool microbiology: a College of American Pathologists Q-probes study of 601 institutions. *Arch. Pathol. Lab. Med.* **120:**206–211.
118. **Vandamme, P., M. I. Daneshvar, F. E. Dewhirst, B. J. Paster, K. Kersters, H. Goossens, and C. W. Moss.** 1995. Chemotaxonomic analyses of *Bacteroides gracilis* and *Bacteroides ureolyticus* and reclassification of *B. gracilis* as *Campylobacter gracilis* comb. nov. *Int. J. Syst. Bacteriol.* **45:**145–152.
119. **Vandamme, P., and J. De Ley.** 1991. Proposal for a new family, *Campylobacteraceae*. *Int. J. Syst. Bacteriol.* **41:**451–455.
120. **Vandamme, P., E. Falsen, B. Pot, B. Hoste, K. Kersters, and J. De Ley.** 1989. Identification of EF group 22 campylobacters from gastroenteritis cases as *Campylobacter concisus*. *J. Clin. Microbiol.* **27:**1775–1781.
121. **Vandamme, P., E. Falsen, R. Rossau, B. Hoste, P. Segers, R. Tytgat, and J. De Ley.** 1991. Revision of *Campylobacter*, *Helicobacter*, and *Wolinella* taxonomy: emendation of generic descriptions and proposal of *Arcobacter* gen. nov. *Int. J. Syst. Bacteriol.* **41:**81–103.
122. **Vandamme, P., M. Vancanneyt, B. Pot, L. Mels, B. Hoste, D. Dewettinck, L. Vlaes, C. Van den Borre, R. Higgins, and J. Hommez.** 1992. Polyphasic taxonomic study of the emended genus *Arcobacter* with *Arcobacter butzleri* comb. nov. and *Arcobacter skirrowii* sp. nov., an aerotolerant bacterium isolated from veterinary specimens. *Int. J. Syst. Bacteriol.* **42:**344–356.
123. **Vandamme, P., L. J. VanDoorn, S. T. Alrashid, W. G. V. Quint, J. VanderPlas, V. L. Chan, and S. L. W. On.** 1997. *Campylobacter hyoilei* Alderton et al. 1995 and *Campylobacter coli* Veron and Chatelain 1973 are subjective synonyms. *Int. J. Syst. Bacteriol.* **47:**1055–1060.
124. **VanDoorn, L. J., B. A. J. Giesendorf, R. Bax, B. A. M. Van Der Zeijst, P. Vandamme, and W. G. V. Quint.** 1997. Molecular discrimination between *Campylobacter jejuni*, *Campylobacter coli*, *Campylobacter lari* and *Campylobacter upsaliensis* by polymerase chain reaction based on a novel putative GTPase gene. *Mol. Cell. Probes* **11:**175–185.
125. **Van Etterijck, R., J. Breynaert, H. Revets, T. Devreker, Y. Vandenplas, P. Vandamme, and S. Lauwers.** 1996. Isolation of *Campylobacter concisus* from feces of children with and without diarrhea. *J. Clin. Microbiol.* **34:**2304–2306.
126. **Waegel, A., and I. Nachamkin.** 1996. Detection and molecular typing of *Campylobacter jejuni* in fecal samples by polymerase chain reaction. *Mol. Cell. Probes* **10:**75–80.
127. **Wang, W.-L. L., and M. J. Blaser.** 1986. Detection of pathogenic *Campylobacter* species in blood culture systems. *J. Clin. Microbiol.* **23:**709–714.
128. **Wang, W.-L. L., L. B. Reller, B. Smallwood, N. W. Luechtefeld, and M. J. Blaser.** 1983. Evaluation of transport media for *Campylobacter jejuni* in human fecal specimens. *J. Clin. Microbiol.* **18:**803–807.
129. **Wassenaar, T. M.** 1997. Toxin production by *Campylobacter* spp. *Clin. Microbiol. Rev.* **10:**466–476.
130. **Wells, J. G., N. D. Puhr, C. M. Patton, M. A. Nicholson, M. A. Lambert, and R. C. Jerris.** 1989. Comparison of selective media and filtration for the isolation of *Campylobacter* from feces, abstr. C-231, p. 432. *In Abstracts of the 89th Annual Meeting of the American Society for Microbiology 1989*. American Society for Microbiology, Washington, D.C.
131. **Wesley, I. V.** 1994. *Arcobacter* infections, p. 181–190. *In* G. W. Beran (ed.), *CRC Handbook of Zoonosis*. CRC Press, Inc., Boca Raton, Fla.
132. **Wexler, H. M., D. Reeves, P. H. Summanen, E. Molitoris, M. McTeague, J. Duncan, K. H. Wilson, and S. M. Finegold.** 1996. *Sutterella wadsworthensis* gen. nov., sp. nov., bile-resistant microaerophilic *Campylobacter gracilis*-like clinical isolates. *Int. J. Syst. Bacteriol.* **46:**252–258.
133. **Wistrom, J., M. Jertborn, E. Ekwall, K. Norlin, B. Soderquist, A. Stromberg, R. Lundholm, H. Hogevik, L. Lagergren, G. Englund, and S. R. Norrby.** 1992. Empiric treatment of acute diarrheal disease with norfloxacin. *Ann. Intern. Med.* **117:**202–208.
134. **Wood, R. C., K. L. MacDonald, and M. T. Osterholm.** 1992. Campylobacter enteritis outbreaks associated with drinking raw milk during youth activities. A 10-year review of outbreaks in the United States. *JAMA* **268:**3228–3230.
135. **Wooldridge, K. G., and J. M. Ketley.** 1997. *Campylobacter* host cell interactions. *Trends Microbiol.* **5:**96–102.
136. **Wretlind, B., A. Stromberg, L. Ostlund, E. Sjogren, and B. Kaijser.** 1992. Rapid emergence of quinolone resistance in *Campylobacter jejuni* in patients treated with norfloxacin. *Scand. J. Infect. Dis.* **24:**685–686.

*Helicobacter**

JAMES VERSALOVIC AND JAMES G. FOX

51

TAXONOMY

Gastric spiral-shaped bacteria have been observed in animals and humans for more than 100 years. The first recorded observations of gastric spiral-shaped bacteria in animals were made by Rappin in 1881 and Bizzozero in 1893. In 1898, Salomon noted spiral bacteria in the stomachs of dogs, cats, and Norway rats (100). In 1982, *Campylobacter pyloridis* (later known as *Helicobacter pylori*) was successfully cultured from stomach biopsies of human patients with gastritis (118). Subsequently other spiral gram-negative bacteria were observed and isolated from the gastrointestinal tracts of mammals such as cats, dogs, ferrets, and rodents (23).

Initially, many spiral gram-negative bacteria isolated from the mammalian gastrointestinal tract were grouped as campylobacters. This classification was based on similar microscopic Gram stain morphologies, common microaerobic growth requirements, and a similar ecologic niche (Table 1). Ultrastructural differences such as the presence of sheathed flagella in helicobacter organisms provided clues that distinguished helicobacters from campylobacters. However, partial sequencing of 16S rRNA genes yielded evidence that *Campylobacter pylori* belonged in a different genus (97). The genus *Helicobacter* was formally distinguished from other gram-negative curved rods (e.g., *Campylobacter*) following extensive analysis of enzymatic activities, fatty acid profiles, growth characteristics, nucleic acid hybridization profiles, and 16S rRNA sequence analysis (31, 89, 114).

DESCRIPTION OF THE GENUS

The genus *Helicobacter* (which contains 19 formally named species as of September 1998) includes spiral or curved bacilli ranging from 0.3 to 1.0 μm in width and 1.5 to 10.0 μm in length. Helicobacters are gram-negative, non-spore-forming rods that may form spheroid or coccoid bodies with prolonged culture. These bacteria are motile and usually possess multiple bipolar sheathed flagella (Table 1). *H. pylori* isolates, in contrast to other *Helicobacter* species, have multiple monopolar sheathed flagella. Only two known helicobacters, *Helicobacter pullorum* and *Helicobacter rodentium*, have unsheathed flagella resembling the campylobacters. The canine gastric helicobacters, *Helicobacter bizzozeronii*, *Helicobacter felis*, and *H. salomonis*, as well as the human gastric pathogen "*Helicobacter heilmannii*" (formerly *Gastrospirillum hominis*), have distinctive tightly spiraled cytomorphologies under light and transmission electron microscopy (Fig. 1C). Notably, further biochemical and genetic analyses may establish an identity between "*H. heilmannii*" and *H. bizzozeronii*.

These organisms are microaerobic and possess a respiratory type of metabolism. Successful cultivation of helicobacters requires a humid atmosphere at 37°C with reduced levels of oxygen (5 to 10%) and increased levels of carbon dioxide (5 to 12%). Atmospheric hydrogen (as much as 5 to 10%) either is required or stimulates the growth of these organisms. Most *Helicobacter* species grow poorly, if at all, in routine aerobic or anaerobic atmospheres. A notable exception is the newly described *Helicobacter westmeadii* (113), which requires anaerobic conditions to be successfully cultivated on solid media. Several helicobacters, including *H. felis* (59), *Helicobacter hepaticus* (20), and *H. rodentium* (101), can grow both microaerobically and anaerobically.

Several biochemical and genetic criteria distinguish this genus, although significant intragenus variation exists with respect to each trait (Table 1). All helicobacters are oxidase positive and do not appear to ferment or oxidize carbohydrates by conventional biochemical tests. However, nuclear magnetic resonance spectroscopy studies have revealed the existence of carbohydrate catabolic activities in *H. pylori* (44). Members of the genus *Helicobacter* have G+C contents ranging from 30 to 48 mol% (23), similar to those of the campylobacters, which range from 29 to 45 mol% (114).

NATURAL HABITATS

Helicobacter species have been isolated from the gastrointestinal tracts of mammals and birds (Table 1). In this chapter, we will refer to gastric (stomach) and enteric (intestinal) helicobacters. The gastric helicobacters primarily inhabit the stomach either within or beneath the mucous gel layer adjacent to the epithelium and rarely invade the bloodstream (in contrast to the enteric helicobacters). *H. pylori* colonizes the cordia, corpus (body), and antrum (distal portion) of the human stomach (27a). These organisms may also be found transiently in saliva, feces, and areas of gastric metaplasia of the proximal small intestine (duodenum).

Both fecal-oral and oral-oral modes of interhuman trans-

* This chapter contains information presented in chapter 38 by Robert C. Jerris in the sixth edition of this Manual.

TABLE 1 Habitats and phenotypic characteristics of *Helicobacter* species[a]

Helicobacter taxon	Source(s)	Primary site	Catalase production	Nitrate reduction	Alkaline phosphatase	Urease	Indoxyl acetate hydrolysis	γ-Glutamyl transferase	Growth: At 42°C	Growth: With 1% glycine	Resistance to[b]: Nalidixic acid	Resistance to[b]: Cephalothin	Flagella
Human													
H. bizzozeronii[c]	Human, dog	Stomach	+	+	+	+	+	+	+	–	R	S	Bipolar
H. canis	Human, dog	Intestine	–	–	+	–	+	ND[d]	+	ND	S	I	Bipolar
H. cinaedi	Human, hamster	Intestine	+	+	–	–	–	–	–	+	S	I	Bipolar
H. fennelliae	Human	Intestine	+	–	+	–	+	–	–	+	S	S	Bipolar
H. pullorum	Human, chicken	Intestine	+	+	–	–	–	ND	+	ND	R	S	Monopolar
H. pylori	Human, macaque, cat	Stomach	+	–	+	+	–	+	–	–	R	S	Monopolar
H. westmeadii	Human	Unknown	+	+	+	–	ND	ND	–	ND	S	R	Monopolar
Nonhuman													
H. acinonyx	Cheetah	Stomach	+	–	+	+	–	+	–	–	R	S	Bipolar
H. bilis	Mouse, dog	Intestine	+	+	ND	+	–	ND	+	+	R	R	Bipolar
H. cholecystus	Hamster	Liver	+	+	+	–	–	–	+	+	I	R	Bipolar
H. felis	Cat, dog	Stomach	+	+	+	+	–	+	+	–	R	S	Bipolar
H. hepaticus	Mouse	Intestine	+	+	ND	+	+	ND	–	+	R	R	Bipolar
H. muridarum	Mouse, rat	Intestine	+	–	+	+	+	+	–	–	R	R	Bipolar
H. mustelae	Ferret, mink	Stomach	+	+	+	+	+	+	+	–	S	R	Peritrichous
H. nemestrinae	Macaque	Stomach	+	–	+	+	–	ND	+	–	R	S	Bipolar
H. pametensis	Birds, swine	Intestine	+	+	+	–	–	–	+	+	S	S	Bipolar
H. rodentium	Mouse	Intestine	+	+	–	–	–	–	+	+	R	R	Bipolar
H. salomonis	Dog	Stomach	+	+	+	+	+	+	–	ND	R	S	Bipolar
H. trogontum	Rat	Intestine	+	+	–	+	ND	+	+	ND	R	R	Bipolar
"*H. rappini*"[e]	Human, dog, sheep, mouse	Intestine	+	–	–	+	ND	+	+	–	R	R	Bipolar

[a] Data are from references 23, 50, and 113. All *Helicobacter* species are oxidase positive and lack the ability to oxidize or ferment carbohydrates in routine reactions.

[b] Resistance is determined by disk diffusion. Isolates are incubated for several days at 37°C on blood-containing medium containing 30-μg antibiotic disks. Microaerobic conditions are typically used, and exact incubation times vary between organisms. Resistance (R) is defined as the complete absence of an inhibition zone, whereas intermediate (I; inhibition zone usually <15 mm in diameter) and susceptible (S; inhibition zone usually >20 mm in diameter) isolates have visible inhibition zones of various sizes.

[c] Likely the same as "*H. heilmannii*." "*H. heilmannii*" (formerly *Gastrospirillum hominis*) has the same phenotype as listed here for *H. bizzozeronii*. Only a single "*H. heilmannii*" strain and a single example of *Helicobacter* sp. strain Mainz have been isolated by culture, and thus they have not been included in the table.

[d] ND, not determined.

[e] Formerly regarded as "*Flexispira rappini*."

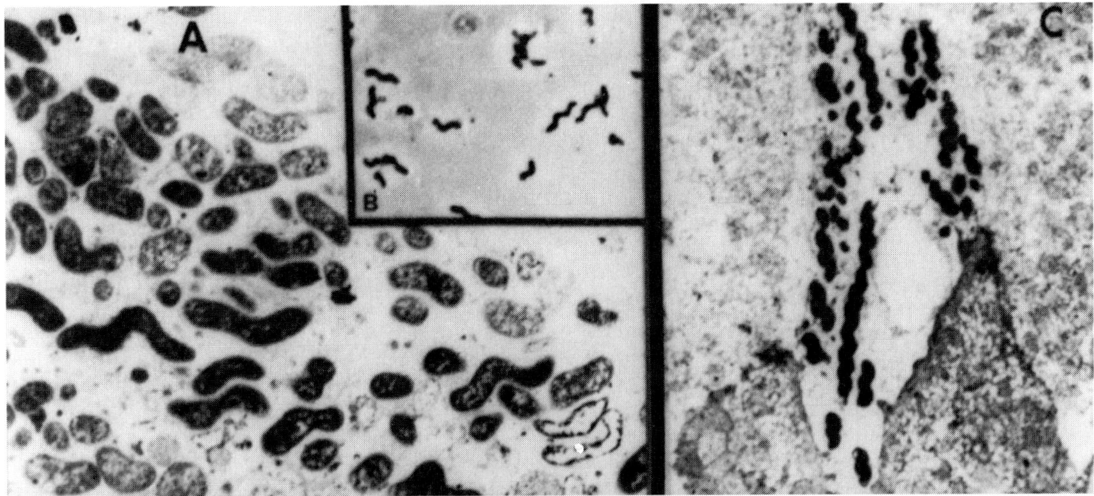

FIGURE 1 Microscopic morphology of *H. pylori* and "*H. heilmannii.*" (A) Transmission electron micrograph of a gastric biopsy specimen from an *H. pylori*-infected individual. (B) Phase-contrast micrograph of *H. pylori.* (C) Transmission electron micrograph of bacteria resembling "*H. heilmannii*" in the gastric pits of an infected cat. Adapted from reference 23 with permission.

mission are likely to represent the principal routes of dissemination of *H. pylori*. Crowded living conditions and the lack of hot running water have been associated with an increased likelihood of *H. pylori* infection (68, 74). Though *Helicobacter* organisms have never been cultured from environmental sources, *H. pylori* DNA was detected by PCR in Peruvian municipal water supplies (47) and raised the possibility of fecal-oral transmission via contaminated municipal water sources. Epidemiologic analyses of intrafamilial *H. pylori* infection support direct person-to-person spread, chiefly occurring in early childhood, as a primary mode of transmission (117, 119). Spouses of *H. pylori*-infected individuals may be at increased risk of infection (85), and a common *H. pylori* strain may colonize both marital partners (28).

H. pylori naturally infects other mammals such as cats (18) and nonhuman primates (39) and has caused experimental infections of laboratory mice (64). The presence of *H. pylori* in the saliva and feces of naturally infected cats has raised the possibility of zoonotic transmission from cats to humans (25). Some authors have suggested vector modes of transmission, since houseflies (*Musca domestica*) can harbor viable *H. pylori* on their bodies and within their excreta (35). Like *H. pylori*, "*H. heilmannii*" resides in the human stomach (45, 46). Evidence of canine-to-human transmission of "*H. heilmannii*" organisms has been reported (112), consistent with the increased prevalence of this infection in individuals with significant farm and pet animal exposure (107). *H. felis*, which is distinguished from "*H. heilmannii*" by periplasmic fibers, has also been implicated (though not confirmed by culture or sequencing) in zoonotic spread from an infected cat to a human caretaker (58).

In contrast to the gastric helicobacters, the enteric helicobacters inhabit the lower gastrointestinal tract (small intestine, colon, rectum, and hepatobiliary tract) of mammals and birds. In humans, enteric helicobacters (*Helicobacter canis*, *Helicobacter cinaedi*, *Helicobacter fennelliae*, *H. pullorum*, and "*Helicobacter rappini*") have been isolated from rectal swabs and feces (2, 7, 34, 57, 94, 98, 105, 106). *H. cinaedi* comprises part of the normal intestinal flora of hamsters (27), and evidence of hamster-to-human transmission has been reported (84). *H. canis* has been cultured from the bile, intestines, and feces of diarrheic dogs (106). Since *H. canis* has been cultured from the feces of both dogs and humans with gastroenteritis (7, 106), this organism, like "*H. heilmannii*," may be transmitted zoonotically from canines to humans. One avian helicobacter, *H. pullorum*, has been cultured from the intestines and feces of asymptomatic chickens, hens with hepatitis, and humans with gastroenteritis (6, 23, 105). It may be transmitted to humans by ingestion of contaminated poultry.

CLINICAL SIGNIFICANCE

Gastric Helicobacters

H. pylori has been associated with peptic ulcer disease and cancers of the human gastrointestinal tract. Warren and Marshall (118) first proposed the association of *Helicobacter pylori* with peptic ulcer disease and gastric cancer. In February 1994, the U.S. National Institutes of Health Consensus Development Conference concluded that *H. pylori* infection represents the major cause of peptic ulcer disease and stated that all patients with confirmed peptic ulcer disease associated with *H. pylori* infection should receive antimicrobial treatment (81). In June 1994, the International Agency for Research on Cancer Working Group of the World Health Organization identified *H. pylori* as a group I, or definite, human carcinogen. Approximately 50% of the world's population is estimated to be infected with *H. pylori*. Seroprevalence of *H. pylori* varies from 20% in young adults in developed countries to more than 50% (sometimes over 90%) in developing countries (65).

Persons infected with *H. pylori* may develop acute gastritis (abdominal pain, nausea, and vomiting) within 2 weeks following infection. *H. pylori* establishes a chronic infection, represented by an antrally predominant chronic active gastritis, in the majority of infected individuals. Many patients infected with *H. pylori* have recurrent abdominal symptoms (nonulcer dyspepsia) without ulcer disease (69). Inflammation of the duodenum (duodenitis) often occurs with *H. pylori* infection, and duodenal ulcers develop in as many as

16% of infected individuals. *H. pylori* infection has been associated with more than 90% of duodenal ulcers and the majority of gastric ulcers (65). In patients with long-standing *H. pylori* infection, persistent inflammation can lead to chronic atrophic gastritis. Chronic atrophic gastritis is a recognized precursor state for gastric ulcer disease and gastric adenocarcinoma (40). *H. pylori* infection represents an independent risk factor for the development of atrophic gastritis (52), gastric ulcer disease (109), gastric adenocarcinomas (82, 86), and gastric mucosa-associated lymphoid tissue (MALT) lymphomas (87, 122).

"*H. heilmannii*" has been observed in human gastric biopsy specimens (46, 104) and cultured from human stomach tissue (1). The species name has not been formally recognized, since significant nucleic acid sequence variation was found among various human isolates. Infection with "*H. heilmannii*" has been associated with peptic ulcer disease in swine (93) and abdominal pain, gastritis, and peptic ulcer disease in humans (45, 46). "*H. heilmannii*" was relatively uncommon, being present in only 0.5% of human esophagogastroduodenal (EGD) endoscopy specimens, in contrast to *H. pylori*, which was present in 59% of such specimens (46).

Helicobacter species have been observed in and isolated from the stomach tissue of other mammals, including cats, dogs, ferrets, rodents, and nonhuman primates (Table 1). Two nonhuman gastric helicobacters, *H. felis* and *Helicobacter mustelae*, represent important models for diseases associated with human helicobacter infections. *H. felis* was isolated from the stomachs of cats (59) and associated with chronic gastritis in cats and experimentally infected mice (60). *H. mustelae* was originally isolated from a duodenal ulcer in a ferret (19, 22) and has been associated with chronic active gastritis and peptic ulcer disease in ferrets from diverse geographic regions (23). More recently, *H. mustelae* has been implicated in the development of gastric adenocarcinomas (23) and gastric MALT lymphomas (14) in naturally infected ferrets.

Enteric Helicobacters

H. cinaedi and *H. fennelliae* have been implicated as causes of human gastroenteritis, particularly in immunocompromised individuals (34, 57, 94). Cases of human gastroenteritis have also been associated with infection by *H. canis* (106) and *H. pullorum* (23, 105). "*H. rappini*" (formerly "*Flexispira rappini*") is a helicobacter by 16S rRNA analysis (89) and has been implicated in cases of human gastroenteritis (2, 98). In contrast to *H. pylori*, *H. cinaedi* was identified from the blood of multiple patients with febrile bacteremia and was associated with multifocal cellulitis and monoarticular arthritis in a subset of infected individuals (5, 53). A neonate presumably contracted *H. cinaedi* bacteremia and meningitis from her mother during pregnancy (84). *H. fennelliae* has occasionally been isolated from human blood (80), and a closely related isolate, named *Helicobacter* sp. strain Mainz, was cultured from the blood and joint fluid of a human immunodeficiency virus-positive male with septic arthritis and recurrent fevers (49). Recently, *H. westmeadii* has been isolated from the blood of bacteremic human immunodeficiency virus-positive patients with persistent fevers (113). Presumably, these bacteremia-associated helicobacters invaded the bloodstream via colonization of the human gastrointestinal tract.

Several other enteric helicobacters have not been isolated to date from human specimens, even though they cause significant diseases in other mammals (Table 1). In addition to the stomach and intestine, *Helicobacter* organisms colonize and cause inflammation in the mammalian hepatobiliary tract. *H. hepaticus* infection was associated with multifocal necrotic hepatitis in several strains of barrier-maintained mice and was implicated in the development of hepatic adenomas and hepatocellular carcinomas in A/JCr mice and more recently in $B_6C_3F_1$ mice (20, 24). *Helicobacter bilis* was isolated from the bile, livers, and lower intestines of aged inbred mice with multifocal chronic hepatitis (26). Both *H. hepaticus* and *H. bilis* are capable of inducing proliferative colitis and typhlitis in *scid* mice (8, 102). Interestingly, *H. canis* has been isolated from the liver of a dog with necrotizing hepatitis (21).

COLLECTION, TRANSPORT, AND STORAGE OF SPECIMENS

Blood Specimens

Given that *H. pylori* specifically colonizes gastric mucosal epithelium and causes noninvasive gastric infections, it has rarely been isolated from blood. A single documented blood isolate of *H. pylori* in a lymphoma patient was of undetermined significance (79). However, enteric helicobacters, such as *H. cinaedi* (5, 53, 80, 84, 111), *H. fennelliae* (80), *Helicobacter* sp. strain Mainz (49), and *H. westmeadii* (113), have been isolated from human blood specimens. Blood culture isolates have been detected by using routine media with prolonged incubation (≥5 days) in automated instruments such as the BACTEC (Becton Dickinson, Franklin Lakes, N.J.) (5) and BacT/Alert (Organon Teknika, Durham, N.C.) systems (84). The instruments signal positive blood cultures with these organisms, and blind terminal subcultures are not required.

Feces

In contrast to the campylobacters and enteric helicobacters, the gastric helicobacters, *H. pylori* and "*H. heilmannii*," are not routinely isolated from human fecal specimens. The enteric helicobacters *H. canis* (7), *H. cinaedi* (34), *H. fennelliae* (54), *H. pullorum* (6), and "*H. rappini*" (2, 98) have been isolated on selective media from fresh fecal specimens of human patients with gastroenteritis, though little information is available regarding transport and storage of these specimens. Enteric helicobacters (e.g., *H. cinaedi* and *H. hepaticus*) are isolated from fresh rodent feces following homogenization by vortexing in phosphate-buffered saline. Homogenized samples are plated directly onto selective (horse or sheep) blood agar or following filtration (0.45-μm-pore-size filter) onto nonselective blood agar.

Gastric Biopsies

Gastric biopsy specimens are necessary for direct tissue diagnosis of *H. pylori* or "*H. heilmannii*" by the rapid urease test or histopathology. Furthermore, the proper collection, storage, and transport of gastric biopsy specimens are important for bacteriologic culture of *H. pylori*. Culture of *H. pylori* may be necessary for antimicrobial susceptibility testing, diagnostic confirmation, or epidemiologic studies. Importantly, "*H. heilmannii*"-like organisms have been rarely cultured from human tissue (1). Since *H. pylori* rapidly loses viability at room temperature, biopsy specimens that must be maintained at ambient temperature should be plated within 2 h. *H. pylori* is sensitive to desiccation and the ambient atmosphere, so appropriate transport media should be used. Recommended transport media include brucella broth with 20% glycerol, cysteine-Albimi broth with 20%

glycerol, isotonic saline with 4% glucose, and Stuart's transport medium (Difco, Detroit, Mich.) (38).

In contrast to Stuart's transport medium and physiological saline, glycerol-containing media may serve as both transport and storage media for biopsy specimens. Storage time, temperature, and media are important variables. Isolates from 81% of biopsy specimens stored at 4°C in glycerol-containing media for 1 week remained viable, whereas isolates from only 19% of biopsy specimens stored at 4°C for 2 weeks were cultivable (38). In contrast, 100% of biopsy specimens stored at −20°C in glycerol-containing media for 4 weeks remained culturable for *H. pylori*. Only cysteine-Albimi medium with 20% glycerol was evaluated for long-term storage, and 14 of 16 gastric biopsy specimens stored at least 5 years at −70°C yielded *H. pylori* (38). For prolonged transport (exceeding 4 days) of cultures by air mail, chocolate agar slants preincubated in a microaerobic atmosphere proved to be a better transport medium for the recovery of *H. pylori* than chocolate agar plates in Campy Pouches (BBL Microbiology Systems, Cockeysville, Md.) (123).

DIRECT EXAMINATION AND DETECTION

Antigen Detection

Though the published literature (63a) remains sparse, direct fecal antigen detection for the presence of *H. pylori* appears promising as a diagnostic alternative, especially for pediatric and dyspeptic patients. Meridian Diagnostics (Cincinnati, Ohio) has a commercial kit (Premier Platinum HpSA) currently available for the rapid, noninvasive detection of *H. pylori* antigens by enzyme immunoassay. *H. pylori* antigens from fresh human fecal specimens are detected by polyclonal antibodies adsorbed to microwells. This test was approved by the U.S. Food and Drug Administration in May 1998 for the diagnosis of *H. pylori* infection in symptomatic individuals. Questions remain regarding utility during follow-up after treatment and the assay's specificity with respect to the enteric helicobacters and campylobacters.

Biopsy and Histology

In patients with possible peptic ulcer disease, *H. pylori* infection is often diagnosed by direct detection of organisms in tissue collected at EGD endoscopy. In cases of duodenal ulcer disease, biopsy samples are taken from the gastric antrum and corpus. Adequate sampling is the primary issue affecting the sensitivity of histology, since *H. pylori* infection may be patchy. At least two, and preferably four, biopsy specimens (from the antrum and corpus) should be obtained. Following fixation in formalin, routine hematoxylin-and-eosin (H&E) staining and special stains (e.g., Giemsa stain) are performed for histopathology and organism detection, respectively. With H&E staining, an antrally predominant chronic active gastritis is observed in most *H. pylori*-infected individuals with duodenal ulcers. If gastric ulcers are found, biopsy specimens are taken from the region surrounding the ulcer in the stomach. In contrast to duodenal ulcer disease, chronic atrophic gastritis is often found in association with gastric ulcers. Patients with atrophic gastritis often lack prominent inflammation, and the sensitivity of histology for organism detection diminishes with increasing severity of glandular atrophy. *H. pylori* and "*H. heilmannii*" must be distinguished by organism morphology in gastric biopsy specimens (Fig. 1), since "*H. heilmannii*" also produces urease and is rarely cultivable. Importantly, organisms do not colonize areas of intestinal metaplasia, foci of gastric adenocarcinoma, or areas of advanced gastric MALT lymphomas.

DNA Amplification

Since rapid urease testing and histologic examination yield excellent sensitivities and specificities for the diagnosis of *H. pylori* infection, PCR amplification of gastric biopsy specimens may not be cost-effective. However, recent developments such as colorimetric hybridization of PCR products have increased the sensitivity of PCR detection 100-fold and may enable ultrasensitive detection of *H. pylori* in biopsy specimens (76). Species-specific PCR assays have been developed for other helicobacters such as *H. pullorum* (105) and *H. hepaticus* (96). PCR applications may facilitate the diagnosis of enteric helicobacter infection if biochemical identification or culture is problematic.

Currently, nucleic acid detection of *H. pylori* is available only in research settings because DNA probes and PCR amplification kits are not commercially available. Commercial reference laboratories are not currently offering DNA hybridization- or PCR-based testing for *H. pylori*, since nucleic acid detection requires endoscopic biopsy and offers no obvious advantages over noninvasive or other invasive diagnostic approaches.

Smear Evaluation

Imprint cytology specimens do not require overnight formalin fixation and provide a rapid adjunct to histopathologic examination of antral biopsy specimens. After biopsy specimens are collected with forceps, imprints are made by pressing a needle against the tissue on a glass slide or by simply rubbing the tissue over the slide. Cytology specimens may be prepared immediately after biopsy by staining the imprints with a rapid Giemsa or Gram stain, and *H. pylori* or "*H. heilmannii*" organisms may be directly visualized. Such an approach has been demonstrated to match or outperform conventional histology in multiple studies (12, 75, 88). When imprint smears were used, 30 of 32 biopsy specimens with positive cultures yielded visible organisms by Gram stain (88). "*H. heilmannii*" organisms were detected in 11 of 100 patients with dyspepsia by imprint cytology, and imprint cytology may be more sensitive than histology for detection of this organism (12). Direct fecal smears, like fecal cultures, have lacked utility for the diagnosis of *H. pylori*.

Urease Testing

H. pylori produces large amounts of extracellular urease which can be detected within hours following placement of gastric biopsy tissue in a urea-containing medium (43, 67). At least one fresh biopsy specimen from the gastric angle or antrum should be submitted for rapid urease testing, and biopsy specimens should be stored at 4°C. The sensitivity of rapid urease testing is maximized if specimens are obtained from the gastric angle (121) and multiple specimens are obtained (71).

Biopsy tissue can be placed in an agar gel in the CLOtest (Ballard Medical Products, Draper, Utah), an agar gel in the hp*fast* assay (GI Supply, Camp Hill, Pa.), or a reagent strip (PyloriTek; Serim Research Corp., Elkhart, Ind.). A pH indicator in the strip or gel causes a color change if urease is present and enables the diagnosis of *H. pylori* infection within 1 h for the strip test and at most 24 h (usually 3 h) for the agar gel tests (92, 124, 125). Since the sensitivity and specificity of the agar gel rapid urease tests approach or exceed 90% in multiple studies, agar gel-based rapid urease tests represent cost-effective methods to screen biopsy tissue for *H. pylori* infection.

Noninvasive urease testing by sampling human breath specimens has enabled the direct detection of *H. pylori* infection without endoscopy (32, 55, 66, 103). In 1996 and 1997, the U.S. Food and Drug Administration approved both ^{13}C-based (Meretek Diagnostics, Nashville, Tenn.) and ^{14}C-based (PY test, Ballard Medical Products, Draper, Utah) urea breath tests (UBT) for the diagnosis of *H. pylori*. In the UBT (61), a solution containing isotopically labeled urea is consumed by the patient. Isotopically labeled carbon dioxide formed by *H. pylori* urease activity in the stomach is absorbed into the bloodstream and exhaled in the breath sample collected 30 min after ingestion of labeled urea. The ^{13}C-labeled carbon dioxide must be detected by gas isotope ratio mass spectrometry, whereas the ^{14}C-labeled carbon dioxide may be analyzed by scintillation particle counting. The UBT has excellent sensitivity and specificity, with both exceeding 95% for the initial diagnosis of active infection in untreated patients (3, 65) and for treatment follow-up at 6 weeks after therapy (55, 103).

CULTURE AND ISOLATION PROCEDURES

Gastric Helicobacters

Unlike the campylobacters, *H. pylori* is usually diagnosed by nonculture methods such as histology, serology, or urease testing. However, the increasing prevalence of nitroimidazole and macrolide resistance (29) has revitalized efforts to culture organisms for antimicrobial susceptibility testing from patients with recurrent dyspepsia or ulcer disease. *H. pylori* may be routinely isolated by culture from human gastric biopsy samples.

H. pylori organisms, like most helicobacters, are microaerobes, requiring reduced oxygen concentrations and elevated levels of carbon dioxide. Helicobacters typically grow best in freshly prepared, moist media incubated in a warm (37°C) atmosphere with 5 to 10% carbon dioxide, 80 to 90% nitrogen, and 5 to 10% oxygen. Humid atmospheres enriched in hydrogen content (5 to 8%) improve the yield of *H. pylori*. Primary isolation of *H. pylori* from gastric biopsy specimens requires 5 to 7 days in a microaerobic atmosphere created by a variable atmosphere incubator, partially evacuated anaerobic jars with defined gas mixtures, or commercial gas-generating sachets (CampyPak Plus [BBL Microbiology Systems] and others). A dedicated CO_2 incubator (10 to 12% CO_2) is useful for subculturing *H. pylori* but is not reliable for primary isolation.

Selective and nonselective media (one plate each) enriched with blood or serum are recommended for the cultivation of *H. pylori* from gastric biopsy specimens. Such a strategy maximizes the sensitivity of culture. Various agar media, including brain heart infusion, brucella, Columbia, and Skirrow's supplemented with horse blood, horse serum, or sheep blood, have been used to cultivate *H. pylori* (42). We recommend commercially available brucella agar plates with 5% horse blood (BBL Microbiology Systems or Remel, Lenexa, Kans.) or brain heart infusion broth supplemented with 7% horse blood as a nonselective medium. One study documented the superiority of brain heart infusion agar supplemented with 7% fresh, whole defibrinated horse blood (96% recovery) over commercial Trypticase soy agar with 5% sheep blood (78% recovery) and Columbia blood agar with cyclodextrin (32% recovery) for the isolation of *H. pylori* (36). Three antibiotic supplements (10 mg of vancomycin per liter, 10 mg of amphotericin B per liter, and 5 mg of cefsulodin or trimethoprim per liter) are recommended for selective media to facilitate primary isolation. In the single report of "*H. heilmannii*" culture from human gastric biopsy samples (1), specimens were cultivated for up to 7 days on nonselective media containing 7% lysed horse blood (Statens Seruminstitut, Copenhagen, Denmark) in an atmosphere of 5% oxygen and 10% carbon dioxide.

Enteric Helicobacters

Selective, enriched media and a microaerobic atmosphere are essential for the cultivation of helicobacters from feces and rectal swabs. *H. canis*, *H. cinaedi*, *H. fennelliae*, *H. pullorum*, and "*H. rappini*" have been isolated from fecal specimens of humans with gastroenteritis. When *H. cinaedi* or *H. fennelliae* is cultured from feces or rectal swabs, specimens should be plated directly onto a selective medium and incubated for 3 to 7 days at 37°C. We recommend selective CVA medium (Columbia base with 5% sheep blood and cefoperazone, vancomycin, and amphotericin B; Remel) and a defined microaerobic atmosphere in partially evacuated anaerobic jars (10% carbon dioxide, 5% hydrogen, 5 to 10% oxygen) for the successful isolation of enteric helicobacters (6, 7) from human feces. Commercial gas-generating sachets (e.g., CampyPak Plus) have been used to isolate enteric helicobacters, but because of increased atmospheric hydrogen requirements, the amount of hydrogen may be inadequate in such systems.

Detection of enteric helicobacters in positive blood cultures may require special stains to detect organisms such as *H. cinaedi* and *H. westmeadii*. The authors of a multicenter study that included 22 *H. cinaedi* blood isolates noted that these thin, gull-winged organisms were generally not visible on Gram stains and required acridine orange staining, dark-field microscopy, or Giemsa staining for visualization (53). In the cases of *H. westmeadii* infection (113), dark-field microscopy revealed motile spiral bacilli in spite of negative Gram stains. Instrument-positive blood cultures should be stained with acridine orange or Giemsa stain if Gram stains are negative. Isolated cases of *H. pullorum* and *H. canis* were diagnosed by fecal culture, but no reports of direct detection of these organisms in blood or feces have been documented.

Nonselective media are preferred for the isolation of helicobacters from primary blood culture media and sterile body fluids. *H. cinaedi* from positive blood cultures has been subcultured in nonselective blood media (e.g., brucella or Columbia base with horse or sheep blood) in a microaerobic atmosphere (e.g., CampyPak Plus) (5). *H. westmeadii* (113) was subcultured from positive blood culture bottles and, in contrast to *H. cinaedi*, required strictly anaerobic conditions for 4 days on nonselective tryptic soy agar supplemented with 5% defibrinated horse blood. The only documented examples of *Helicobacter* cultivation from sterile body fluids other than blood are the isolation of *H. cinaedi* from cerebrospinal fluid in nonselective Trypticase soy broth (84) and the culture of *Helicobacter* sp. strain Mainz from joint fluid on nonselective blood agar (49).

IDENTIFICATION

Helicobacters reveal various colony phenotypes on blood agar ranging from the small, gray, translucent colonies of *H. pylori* to the diffuse, spreading growth of *H. felis*. Helicobacters have a characteristic morphology by light microscopy that resembles that of other gram-negative spiral or curved bacteria (Fig. 1). Most helicobacter isolates are motile if observed by phase-contrast microscopy. Helicobacters are routinely tested for cytochrome oxidase, catalase, and urease activities (72) (Table 1). All helicobacters are oxidase positive. Every *Helicobacter* species described to date except *H. canis* is catalase positive. Many, though not all, *Helicobacter* species, including *H. pylori*, are urease positive (Table 1).

Gastric Helicobacters

The morphology of helicobacters observed in gastric biopsies may differ markedly from that observed in a Gram-stained preparation of cultured organisms. For example, *H. pylori* usually appears as a slightly curved or straight rod in culture, whereas stained tissue biopsy specimens usually reveal a helical or more curved appearance. "*H. heilmannii*" is usually distinguished from *H. pylori* by its larger size and more pronounced helical morphology in gastric biopsy specimens (Fig. 1) (46). *H. felis* has been putatively identified in human gastric biopsy specimens (58) and cannot be distinguished from "*H. heilmannii*" by light microscopy.

H. pylori infection is presumptively diagnosed by microscopic morphology (Gram stain or biopsy) and the presence of catalase, oxidase, and urease activities. *Campylobacter jejuni*, a relative of *H. pylori*, has been identified in a gastric biopsy specimen from a patient with a gastric ulcer (99). That report highlights the need to perform biopsy-based rapid urease testing or the urea breath test with patients who are refractory to therapy and have spiral or curved gram-negative bacteria visible in gastric biopsy specimens. The rapid urease, indoxyl acetate hydrolysis, and hippurate hydrolysis tests distinguish *H. pylori* and *C. jejuni* (chapter 50) (83, 91). Commercial tests for urease (Christensen's agar slant; Remel), indoxyl acetate (Remel), and hippurate hydrolysis (Remel) are available and convenient for rapid identification of cultured specimens. In a study of 400 clinical isolates, all *H. pylori* isolates were positive for cytochrome oxidase, catalase, and urease activities (Table 1) (70). In contrast to *C. jejuni*, *H. pylori* is urease positive and lacks the ability to hydrolyze hippurate or indoxyl acetate.

Enteric Helicobacters

The enteric helicobacters possess several distinguishing biochemical characteristics. Several enteric helicobacters isolated from humans, such as *H. cinaedi*, *H. fennelliae*, *H. pullorum*, and *H. westmeadii*, lack urease activity. Distinguishing these catalase-positive, urease-negative helicobacters from campylobacters (e.g., *C. jejuni*) may be especially challenging. Unlike *C. jejuni* and *Campylobacter coli*, *H. cinaedi* and *H. fennelliae* do not survive at 42°C and *H. cinaedi* does not hydrolyze indoxyl acetate (Table 1) (91). Indoxyl acetate hydrolysis distinguishes *C. jejuni* and *C. coli* from *H. pullorum* (Table 1). *H. pullorum* is distinguished from *Campylobacter lari* only by its resistance to nalidixic acid. A nalidixic acid-resistant *C. lari* isolate would require species-specific PCR (105) for differentiation from *H. pullorum*. Unlike other helicobacters, *H. canis* is catalase and urease negative. To distinguish *H. canis* from catalase-negative campylobacters, the nitrate reduction and indoxyl acetate hydrolysis tests may be useful (Table 1).

SEROLOGIC TESTS

Serologic tests are being used extensively to screen dyspeptic patients for active *H. pylori* infection. Infection with *H. pylori* results in a vigorous local and systemic humoral response (90, 95). In contrast to serum immunoglobulin M (IgM), serum IgA and IgG levels persist for months or years and correlate with active infection (4, 77, 90). Only a minority (2%) of individuals did not show evidence of systemic seroconversion following infection (71). Anti-*H. pylori* serum IgG levels are more consistently elevated than serum IgA levels. Consequently, serum IgG immunoassays yield superior sensitivities and specificities in comparative studies with serum IgA assays (56, 63).

Commercial enzyme immunoassays detecting anti-*H. pylori* serum IgG are the tests of choice (reviewed in reference 56a) for primary screening of patients with uncomplicated infections. Anti-*H. pylori* serum IgG assays from various commercial sources have variable sensitivities (86 to 100%) and specificities (76 to 98%) (73, 120). Importantly, positive (95 to 100%) and negative (84 to 89%) predictive values for serology were comparable to those of histology, rapid urease testing, and UBT (10). Patients infected with "*H. heilmannii*" were usually negative by anti-*H. pylori* IgG assays (46). Serum IgA immunoassays may be used as second-line tests for assessing equivocal or possibly false-negative anti-*H. pylori* serum IgG results. In one study (51), over 7% of patients with a negative serum IgG test were found to have detectable anti-*H. pylori* serum IgA and symptoms consistent with *H. pylori* infection. With sensitivities of 39 to 82%, serum IgA assays lack the requisite sensitivity to serve as primary screening tests but may be useful in cases when infection is strongly suspected and the serum IgG result is negative or equivocal.

Though serum IgG assays remain the tests of choice for screening patient sera, whole-blood immunoassays are being used with increasing frequency in physicians' offices. Qualitative point-of-care immunoassays produce rapid results (4 to 10 min) with heparinized whole blood or capillary blood specimens. Rapid whole-blood immunoassays had lower sensitivities (usually 80 to 90%) than serum enzyme immunoassays, and concerns regarding interoffice variability with whole-blood assays were raised (15).

Sustained immunoglobulin responses to multiple antigens of *H. cinaedi* and *H. fennelliae* have been documented (17). Little is known about the nature of immunoglobulin class and subclass responses following infection by *H. cinaedi* and *H. fennelliae*. No commercial serologic assays have been developed to monitor infection with *H. cinaedi* or other enteric helicobacters.

ANTIBIOTIC SUSCEPTIBILITIES

Multidrug regimens are required to attain successful cure rates (exceeding 90%) for *H. pylori* infection (48). Either a nitroimidazole (e.g., metronidazole) or a macrolide (e.g., clarithromycin) must be included as part of the multidrug regimen to attain a high cure rate. "Antiacid" medications such as proton pump inhibitors (e.g., omeprazole) or H_2 antagonists (e.g., ranitidine) are usually added to reduce acid output and accelerate ulcer healing. The most successful treatment regimens include metronidazole-omeprazole-clarithromycin for 7 to 14 days, triple metronidazole-based therapy (tetracycline-metronidazole-bismuth) for 14 days, and triple clarithromycin-based therapy (tetracycline- or amoxicillin-clarithromycin-bismuth) for 14 days. The prevalence of *H. pylori* strains resistant to either metronidazole or clarithromycin has been reportedly increasing in various geographic regions (29, 62, 113a). Infections with *H. pylori* strains resistant to clarithromycin or metronidazole have been associated with a greater incidence of treatment failures than infections with susceptible strains (29, 113a).

Various susceptibility testing methods such as broth microdilution, disk diffusion, the E test, and agar dilution have been used to assess antimicrobial resistance in *H. pylori* (13, 37, 41). The National Committee for Clinical Laboratory Standards (NCCLS) has recently recommended an agar dilution standard for *H. pylori* susceptibility testing (78). Mueller-Hinton agar base with 5% sheep blood was selected by NCCLS for susceptibility testing by agar dilution. Resistance in vitro to clarithromycin by *H. pylori* appears to be clinically relevant, and an MIC breakpoint of 2 μg per ml has been proposed (37). Point mutations in the 23S rRNA gene confer stable macrolide resistance (116), and either of two predominant mutations (11, 116) may be detected by PCR amplification and restriction digestion (110, 115, 116) or oligonucleotide ligation (108). Multiple mutations in the NADPH nitroreductase gene (*rdxA*) appear to explain the molecular basis for metronidazole resistance in *H. pylori* (30a). In contrast to those of clarithromycin resistance, atmospheric conditions may significantly affect the MICs of metronidazole (37). Generally, metronidazole susceptibility in vitro means that treatment is likely to be successful, but metronidazole resistance does not necessarily correlate with treatment failure.

Eradication of "*H. heilmannii*" by antimicrobial therapy resulted in the resolution of gastritis and peptic ulcer disease (30, 45, 46). Since "*H. heilmannii*" has been rarely cultured, antibiotic susceptibility testing for only a single isolate has been reported (1). This isolate was susceptible to amoxicillin, metronidazole, and tetracycline. "*H. heilmannii*" infections have been successfully treated with bismuth alone and with combination therapies that included metronidazole or amoxicillin (1, 45, 46).

Effective therapy for *H. cinaedi* infection has included ciprofloxacin, gentamicin, or tetracycline for at least 2 to 3 weeks (5, 53, 84). In vitro susceptibility testing of *H. cinaedi* (16, 53, 54) appears to be meaningful, and resistance in vitro has been correlated with failures in patients treated with erythromycin (5) or ciprofloxacin (53). Relatively limited therapeutic experience is available for *H. fennelliae* infections. Gentamicin has been used successfully to treat bacteremia caused by *H. fennelliae* (80). One of two patients with *H. westmeadii* bacteremia was treated successfully with a combination β-lactam—aminoglycoside regimen (113). Neither in vitro susceptibility testing data nor treatment recommendations have been reported for cases of gastroenteritis caused by *H. canis* or *H. pullorum*. NCCLS recommendations are not available for antimicrobial susceptibility testing of organisms other than *H. pylori*.

INTERPRETATION AND REPORTING OF RESULTS

For the diagnosis of *H. pylori* infection, the patient's clinical status will dictate whether noninvasive or invasive approaches are used (9). Asymptomatic patients or patients with nonulcer dyspepsia who do not possess "alarm" features (33) should be screened initially by examining anti-*H. pylori* IgG levels in whole blood or serum. Positive rapid whole-blood immunoassays should be confirmed by IgG serologies. If serum IgG is negative or equivocal and clinical suspicion remains, the UBT is recommended as the method of choice to establish or exclude *H. pylori* infection without endoscopy. If arranging a separate breath collection is problematic for the patient, the same serum specimen could be used to determine serum IgA levels. A promising secondary test is fecal antigen detection to confirm a diagnosis of *H. pylori* infection. In the case of a symptomatic patient who must be assessed for active infection, the UBT should be utilized instead of serologic evaluation of anti-*H. pylori* IgG antibodies. As early as 6 weeks following therapy, the UBT can establish successful eradication or treatment failure.

Patients with "alarm" features (33) such as old age, weight loss, or gastrointestinal bleeding should undergo EGD endoscopy. Rapid urease testing of gastric biopsy specimens can be used to assess *H. pylori* infection status. If results are positive, results can be reported as "positive and consistent with *H. pylori* infection." Gastric biopsies may be interpreted by the histopathologist. Routine H&E staining indicates the nature of gastritis or the presence of gastric adenocarcinoma or gastric MALT lymphoma. *H. pylori* organisms may be visible with the Gram stain, the H&E stain, and special silver or Giemsa stains. "*H. heilmannii*" infection must be diagnosed by bacterial morphology in the gastric biopsy specimen, since this organism is rarely cultured.

In order to perform antimicrobial susceptibility testing, bacteriologic culture of *H. pylori* from gastric biopsies is recommended in the setting of apparent treatment failures. Successful culture of *H. pylori* from biopsies may be reported if organisms have the typical gram-negative morphology and cytochrome oxidase, catalase, and urease activity. Primary biopsy cultures should be incubated at least 7 to 10 days prior to a negative report. Susceptibility testing should be performed by the NCCLS reference method (78) or a substantially equivalent method.

The enteric helicobacters such as *H. cinaedi* and *H. fennelliae* must be isolated by microbiologic culture of blood or feces for a definitive diagnosis. If the Gram stain is negative, microscopic morphology may be assessed by a Giemsa stain, an acridine orange stain, or dark-field microscopy. Appropriate biochemical tests must be performed (Table 1). The enteric helicobacters are typically urease negative and may be easily confused with the campylobacters. Even with supplemental tests, the distinctions can be difficult without a genotypic test such as species-specific PCR amplification or DNA hybridization.

REFERENCES

1. **Andersen, L. P., A. Norgaard, S. Holck, J. Blom, and L. Elsborg.** 1996. Isolation of a "*Helicobacter heilmannii*"-like organism from the human stomach. *Eur. J. Clin. Microbiol. Infect. Dis.* **15:**95–96.
2. **Archer, J. R., S. Romero, A. E. Ritchie, M. E. Hamacher, B. M. Steiner, J. H. Bryner, and R. F. Schell.** 1988. Characterization of an unclassified microaerophilic bacterium associated with gastroenteritis. *J. Clin. Microbiol.* **26:**101–105.
3. **Bazzoli, F., M. Zagari, S. Fossi, P. Pozzaro, L. Ricciardiello, C. Mwangemi, A. Roda, and E. Roda.** 1997. Urea breath tests for the detection of *Helicobacter pylori* infection. *Helicobacter* **2:**S34–S37.
4. **Blecker, U., S. Lanciers, B. Hauser, D. Menta, and Y. Vandenplas.** 1995. Serology as a valid screening test for *Helicobacter pylori* infection. *Arch. Pathol. Lab. Med.* **119:**30–32.
5. **Burman, W. J., D. L. Cohn, R. R. Reves, and M. L. Wilson.** 1995. Multifocal cellulitis and monoarticular arthritis as manifestations of *Helicobacter cinaedi* bacteremia. *Clin. Infect. Dis.* **20:**564–570.
6. **Burnens, A. P., J. Stanley, R. Morgenstern, and J. Nicolet.** 1994. Gastroenteritis associated with *Helicobacter pullorum*. *Lancet* **344:**1569–1570.
7. **Burnens, A. P., J. Stanley, U. B. Schaad, and J. Nicolet.** 1993. Novel *Campylobacter*-like organism resembling *Heli-*

cobacter fennelliae isolated from a boy with gastroenteritis and from dogs. *J. Clin. Microbiol.* **31:**1916–1917.

8. **Cahill, R. J., C. J. Foltz, J. G. Fox, C. A. Dangler, F. Powrie, and D. B. Schauer.** 1997. Inflammatory bowel disease: an immunity-mediated condition triggered by bacterial infection with *Helicobacter hepaticus*. *Infect. Immun.* **65:**3126–3131.
9. **Cutler, A. F.** 1996. Testing for *Helicobacter pylori* in clinical practice. *Am J. Med.* **100:**5A-35S–5A-41S.
10. **Cutler, A. F., S. Havstad, C. Ma, M. Blaser, G. Perez-Perez, and T. Shubert.** 1995. Accuracy of invasive and noninvasive tests to diagnose *Helicobacter pylori* infection. *Gastroenterology* **109:**136–141.
11. **Debets-Ossenkopp, Y. J., M. Sparrius, J. G. Kusters, J. J. Kolkman, and C. M. J. E. Vandenbroucke-Grauls.** 1996. Mechanism of clarithromycin resistance in clinical isolates of *Helicobacter pylori*. *FEMS Microbiol. Lett.* **142:**37–42.
12. **Debongnie, J. C., J. Mairesse, M. Donnay, and X. Dekoninck.** 1994. Touch cytology: a quick, simple, screening test in the diagnosis of infections of the gastrointestinal mucosa. *Arch. Pathol. Lab. Med.* **118:**1115–1118.
13. **DeCross, A. J., B. J. Marshall, R. W. McCallum, S. R. Hoffman, L. J. Barrett, and R. L. Guerrant.** 1993. Metronidazole susceptibility testing for *Helicobacter pylori*: comparison of disk, broth, and agar dilution methods and their clinical relevance. *J. Clin. Microbiol.* **31:**1971–1974.
14. **Erdman, S. E., P. Correa, L. A. Coleman, M. D. Schrenzel, X. Li, and J. G. Fox.** 1997. *Helicobacter mustelae*-associated gastric MALT lymphoma in ferrets. *Am. J. Pathol.* **151:**273–280.
15. **The European *Helicobacter pylori* Study Group.** 1997. Current European concepts in the management of *Helicobacter pylori* infection. The Maastricht consensus report. *Gut* **41:**8–13.
16. **Flores, B. M., C. L. Fennell, K. K. Holmes, and W. E. Stamm.** 1985. In vitro susceptibilities of *Campylobacter*-like organisms to twenty antimicrobial agents. *Antimicrob. Agents Chemother.* **28:**188–191.
17. **Flores, B. M., C. L. Fennell, and W. E. Stamm.** 1989. Characterization of *Campylobacter cinaedi* and *C. fennelliae* antigens and analysis of the human immune response. *J. Infect. Dis.* **159:**635–640.
18. **Fox, J. G., M. Batchelder, B. Marini, L. Yan, L. Handt, X. Li, B. Shames, A. Hayward, J. Campbell, and J. C. Murphy.** 1995. *Helicobacter pylori*-induced gastritis in the domestic cat. *Infect. Immun.* **63:**2674–2681.
19. **Fox, J. G., T. Chilvers, C. S. Goodwin, N. S. Taylor, P. Edmonds, L. I. Sly, and D. J. Brenner.** 1989. *Campylobacter mustelae*, a new species resulting from the elevation of *Campylobacter pylori* subsp. *mustelae* to species status. *Int. J. Syst. Bacteriol.* **39:**301–303.
20. **Fox, J. G., F. E. Dewhirst, J. G. Tully, B. J. Paster, L. L. Yan, N. S. Taylor, M. J. Collins, P. L. Gorelick, and J. M. Ward.** 1994. *Helicobacter hepaticus* sp. nov., a microaerophilic bacterium isolated from livers and intestinal mucosal scrapings from mice. *J. Clin. Microbiol.* **32:** 1238–1245.
21. **Fox, J. G., R. Drolet, R. Higgins, S. Messier, L. Yan, B. E. Coleman, B. J. Paster, and F. E. Dewhirst.** 1996. *Helicobacter canis* isolated from a dog liver with multifocal necrotizing hepatitis. *J. Clin. Microbiol.* **34:**2479–2482.
22. **Fox, J. G., B. M. Edrise, and E. Cabot.** 1986. *Campylobacter*-like organisms isolated from gastric mucosa of ferrets. *Am. J. Vet. Res.* **47:**236–239.
23. **Fox, J. G., and A. Lee.** 1997. The role of *Helicobacter* species in newly recognized gastrointestinal tract diseases of animals. *Lab. Anim. Sci.* **47:**222–255.
24. **Fox, J. G., J. A. MacGregor, Z. Shen, X. Li, R. Lewis, and C. A. Dangler.** 1998. Comparison of methods of identifying *Helicobacter hepaticus* in $B_6C_3F_1$ mice used in a carcinogenesis bioassay. *J. Clin. Microbiol.* **36:**1382–1387.
25. **Fox, J. G., S. Perkins, L. Yan, Z. Shen, L. Attardo, and J. Pappo.** 1996. Local immune response in *Helicobacter pylori*-infected cats and identification of *H. pylori* in saliva, gastric fluid, and feces. *Immunology* **88:**400–406.
26. **Fox, J. G., L. L. Yan, F. E. Dewhirst, B. J. Paster, B. Shames, J. C. Murphy, A. Hayward, J. C. Belcher, and E. N. Mendes.** 1995. *Helicobacter bilis* sp. nov., a novel *Helicobacter* species isolated from bile, livers, and intestines of aged, inbred mice. *J. Clin. Microbiol.* **33:**445–454.
27. **Gebhart, C. J., C. L. Fennell, M. P. Murtaugh, and W. E. Stamm.** 1989. *Campylobacter cinaedi* is normal intestinal flora in hamsters. *J. Clin. Microbiol.* **27:**1692–1694.

27a. **Genta, R. M., R. M. Huberman, and D. Y. Graham.** 1994. The gastric cardia in *Helicobacter pylori* infection. *Hum. Pathol.* **25:**915–919.

28. **Georgopoulos, S. D., A. F. Mentis, C. A. Spiliadis, L. S. Tzouvelekis, E. Tzelepi, A. Moshopoulos, and N. Skandalis.** 1996. *Helicobacter pylori* infection in spouses of patients with duodenal ulcers and comparison of ribosomal RNA gene patterns. *Gut* **39:**634–638.
29. **Goddard, A. F., and R. P. H. Logan.** 1996. Antimicrobial resistance and *Helicobacter pylori*. *J. Antimicrob. Chemother.* **37:** 639–643.
30. **Goddard, A. F., R. P. H. Logan, J. C. Atherton, D. Jenkins, and R. C. Spiller.** 1997. Healing of duodenal ulcer after eradication of *Helicobacter heilmannii*. *Lancet* **349:** 1815–1816.

30a. **Goodwin, A., D. Kersulyte, G. Sisson, S. J. Veldhuyzen van Zanten, D. E. Berg, and P. S. Hoffman.** 1998. Metronidazole resistance in *Helicobacter pylori* is due to null mutations in a gene (*rdxA*) that encodes an oxygen-insensitive NADPH nitroreductase. *Mol. Microbiol.* **28:**383–393.

31. **Goodwin, C. S., J. A. Armstrong, T. Chilvers, M. Peters, M. D. Collins, L. Sly, W. McConnell, and W. E. S. Harper.** 1989. Transfer of *Campylobacter pylori* and *Campylobacter mustelae* to *Helicobacter* gen. nov. as *Helicobacter pylori* comb. nov. and *Helicobacter mustelae* comb. nov., respectively. *Int. J. Syst. Bacteriol.* **39:**397–405.
32. **Graham, D. Y., P. D. Klein, D. J. Evans, D. G. Evans, L. Alpert, A. R. Opekun, and T. W. Boutton.** 1987. *Campylobacter pylori* detected noninvasively by the ^{13}C-urea breath test. *Lancet* **i:**1174–1177.
33. **Graham, D. Y., and L. Rabeneck.** 1996. Patients, payers, and paradigm shifts: what to do about *Helicobacter pylori*. *Am. J. Gastroenterol.* **91:**188–190.
34. **Grayson, M. L., W. Tee, and B. Dwyer.** 1989. Gastroenteritis associated with *Campylobacter cinaedi*. *Med. J. Aust.* **150:**214–215.
35. **Grubel, P., J. S. Hoffman, F. K. Chong, N. A. Burstein, C. Mepani, and D. R. Cave.** 1997. Vector potential of houseflies (*Musca domestica*) for *Helicobacter pylori*. *J. Clin. Microbiol.* **35:**1300–1303.
36. **Hachem, C. Y., J. E. Clarridge, D. G. Evans, and D. Y. Graham.** 1995. Comparison of agar based media for primary isolation of *Helicobacter pylori*. *J. Clin. Pathol.* **48:** 714–716.
37. **Hachem, C. Y., J. E. Clarridge, R. Reddy, R. Flamm, D. G. Evans, S. K. Tanaka, and D. Y. Graham.** 1996. Antimicrobial susceptibility testing of *Helicobacter pylori*. *Diagn. Microbiol. Infect. Dis.* **24:**37–41.
38. **Han, S. W., R. Flamm, C. Y. Hachem, H. Y. Kim, J. E. Clarridge, D. G. Evans, J. Beyer, J. Drnec, and D. Y. Graham.** 1995. Transport and storage of *Helicobacter pylori* from gastric mucosal biopsies and clinical isolates. *Eur. J. Clin. Microbiol. Infect. Dis.* **14:**349–352.
39. **Handt, L. K., J. G. Fox, L. L. Yan, Z. Shen, W. J. Pouch, D. Ngai, S. L. Motzel, T. E. Nolan, and H. J. Klein.** 1997.

Diagnosis of *Helicobacter pylori* infection in a colony of rhesus monkeys (*Macaca mulatta*). *J. Clin. Microbiol.* **35:** 165–168.

40. **Hansson, L. E., O. Nyren, A. W. Hsing, R. Bergstrom, S. Josefsson, W. H. Chow, J. F. Fraumeni, Jr., and H. O. Adami.** 1996. The risk of stomach cancer in patients with gastric or duodenal ulcer disease. *N. Engl. J. Med.* **335:**242–249.
41. **Hardy, D. J., C. W. Hanson, D. M. Hensey, J. M. Beyer, and P. B. Fernandes.** 1988. Susceptibility of *Campylobacter pylori* to macrolides and fluoroquinolones. *J. Antimicrob. Chemother.* **22:**631–636.
42. **Hazell, S. L.** 1993. Cultural techniques for the growth and isolation of *Helicobacter pylori*, p. 273–283. *In* C. S. Goodwin and B. W. Worsley (ed.), Helicobacter pylori: *Biology and Clinical Practice.* CRC Press, Boca Raton, Fla.
43. **Hazell, S. L., T. J. Borody, A. Gal, and A. Lee.** 1987. *Campylobacter pyloridis* gastritis I: detection of urease as a marker of bacterial colonization and gastritis. *Am. J. Gastroenterol.* **82:**292–296.
44. **Hazell, S. L., and G. L. Mendz.** 1997. How *Helicobacter pylori* works: an overview of the metabolism of *Helicobacter pylori. Helicobacter* **2:**1–12.
45. **Heilmann, K. L., and F. Borchard.** 1991. Gastritis due to spiral shaped bacteria other than *Helicobacter pylori:* clinical, histological, and ultrastructural findings. *Gut* **32:** 137–140.
46. **Hilzenrat, N., E. Lamoureux, I. Weintrub, E. Alpert, M. Lichter, and L. Alpert.** 1995. *Helicobacter heilmannii*-like spiral bacteria in gastric mucosal biopsies. *Arch. Pathol. Lab. Med.* **119:**1149–1153.
47. **Hulten, K., S. W. Han, H. Enroth, P. D. Klein, A. R. Opekun, R. H. Gilman, D. G. Evans, L. Engstrand, D. Y. Graham, and F. A. K. El-Zaatari.** 1996. *Helicobacter pylori* in the drinking water in Peru. *Gastroenterology* **110:** 1031–1035.
48. **Hunt, R. H.** 1997. Peptic ulcer disease: defining the treatment strategies in the era of *Helicobacter pylori. Am. J. Gastroenterol.* **92:**36S–40S.
49. **Husmann, M., C. Gries, P. Jehnichen, T. Woelfel, G. Gerken, W. Ludwig, and S. Bhakdi.** 1994. *Helicobacter* sp. strain *Mainz* isolated from an AIDS patient with septic arthritis: case report and nonradioactive analysis of 16S rRNA sequence. *J. Clin. Microbiol.* **32:**3037–3039.
50. **Jalava, K., M. Kaartinen, M. Utriainen, I. Happonen, and M.-L. Hänninen.** 1997. *Helicobacter salomonis* sp. nov., a canine gastric *Helicobacter* sp. related to *Helicobacter felis* and *Helicobacter bizzozeronii. Int. J. Syst. Bacteriol.* **47:** 975–982.
51. **Jaskowski, T. D., T. B. Martins, H. R. Hill, and C. M. Litwin.** 1997. Immunoglobulin A antibodies to *Helicobacter pylori. J. Clin. Microbiol.* **35:**2999–3000.
52. **Kawaguchi, H., K. Haruma, K. Komoto, M. Yoshihara, K. Sumii, and G. Kajiyama.** 1996. *Helicobacter pylori* infection is the major risk factor for atrophic gastritis. *Am. J. Gastroenterol.* **91:**959–962.
53. **Kiehlbauch, J., R. V. Tauxe, C. N. Baker, and I. K. Wachsmuth.** 1994. *Helicobacter cinaedi*-associated bacteremia and cellulitis in immunocompromised patients. *Ann. Intern. Med.* **121:**90–93.
54. **Kiehlbauch, J. A., D. J. Brenner, D. N. Cameron, A. G. Steigerwalt, J. M. Makowski, C. N. Baker, C. M. Patton, and I. K. Wachsmuth.** 1995. Genotypic and phenotypic characterization of *Helicobacter cinaedi* and *Helicobacter fennelliae* strains isolated from humans and animals. *J. Clin. Microbiol.* **33:**2940–2947.
55. **Klein, P. D., H. M. Malaty, R. F. Martin, K. S. Graham, R. M. Genta, and D. Y. Graham.** 1996. Noninvasive detection of *Helicobacter pylori* infection in clinical practice: the ^{13}C urea breath test. *Am. J. Gastroenterol.* **91:**690–694.
56. **Kosunen, T. U., K. Seppala, S. Sarna, and P. Sipponen.** 1992. Diagnostic value of decreasing IgG, IgA, and IgM antibody titres after eradication of *Helicobacter pylori. Lancet* **339:**893–895.

56a. **Laheij, R. J. F., H. Straatman, J. B. M. J. Jansen, and A. L. M. Verbeek.** 1998. Evaluation of commercially available *Helicobacter pylori* serology kits: a review. *J. Clin. Microbiol.* **36:**2803–2809.

57. **Laughon, B. E., A. A. Vernon, D. A. Druckman, R. Fox, T. C. Quinn, F. Polk, and J. G. Bartlett.** 1988. Recovery of *Campylobacter* species from homosexual men. *J. Infect. Dis.* **158:**464–467.
58. **Lavelle, J. P., S. Landas, F. A. Mitros, and J. L. Conklin.** 1994. Acute gastritis associated with spiral organisms from cats. *Dig. Dis. Sci.* **39:**744–750.
59. **Lee, A., S. L. Hazell, J. O'Rourke, and S. Kouprach.** 1988. Isolation of a spiral-shaped bacterium from the cat stomach. *Infect. Immun.* **56:**2843–2850.
60. **Lee, A., and J. O'Rourke.** 1993. Gastric bacteria other than *Helicobacter pylori. Gastroenterol. Clin. N. Am.* **22:** 21–42.
61. **Logan, R. P. H.** 1993. Breath tests to detect *Helicobacter pylori*, p. 307–326. *In* C. S. Goodwin and B. W. Worsley (ed.), Helicobacter pylori: *Biology and Clinical Practice.* CRC Press, Boca Raton, Fla.
62. **Lopez-Brea, M., D. Domingo, I. Sanchez, and T. Alarcon.** 1997. Evolution of resistance to metronidazole and clarithromycin in *Helicobacter pylori* clinical isolates from Spain. *J. Antimicrob. Chemother.* **40:**279–281.
63. **Luzza, F., M. Maletta, M. Imeneo, A. Marcheggiano, C. Iannoni, L. Biancone, and F. Pallone.** 1995. Salivary-specific immunoglobulin G in the diagnosis of *Helicobacter pylori* infection in dyspeptic patients. *Am. J. Gastroenterol.* **90:**1820–1823.

63a. **Makristathis, A., E. Pasching, K. Schutze, M. Wimmer, M. L. Rotter, and A. M. Hirschl.** 1988. Detection of *Helicobacter pylori* in stool specimens by PCR and antigen enzyme immunoassay. *J. Clin. Microbiol.* **36:**2772–2774.

64. **Marchetti, M., B. Arico, D. Burroni, N. Figura, R. Rappuoli, and P. Ghiara.** 1995. Development of a mouse model of *Helicobacter pylori* infection that mimics human disease. *Science* **267:**1655–1658.
65. **Marshall, B. J.** 1994. *Helicobacter pylori. Am. J. Gastroenterol.* **89:**S116–S128.
66. **Marshall, B. J., and I. Surveyor.** 1988. Carbon-14 urea breath test for the diagnosis of *Campylobacter pylori* associated gastritis. *J. Nucl. Med.* **29:**11–16.
67. **Marshall, B. J., J. R. Warren, G. J. Francis, S. R. Langton, C. S. Goodwin, and E. D. Blincow.** 1987. Rapid urease test in the management of *Campylobacter pyloridis*-associated gastritis. *Am. J. Gastroenterol.* **82:**200–210.
68. **McCallion, W. A., L. J. Murray, A. G. Bailie, A. M. Dalzell, D. P. J. O'Reilly, and K. B. Bamford.** 1996. *Helicobacter pylori* infection in children: relation with current household living conditions. *Gut* **39:**18–21.
69. **McCarthy, C., S. Patchett, R. M. Collins, S. Beattie, C. Keane, and C. O'Morain.** 1995. Long-term prospective study of *Helicobacter pylori* in nonulcer dyspepsia. *Dig. Dis. Sci.* **40:**114–119.
70. **McNulty, C. A. M., and J. C. Dent.** 1987. Rapid identification of *Campylobacter pylori* (*C. pyloridis*) by preformed enzymes. *J. Clin. Microbiol.* **25:**1683–1686.
71. **Megraud, F.** 1996. Advantages and disadvantages of current diagnostic tests for the detection of *Helicobacter pylori. Scand. J. Gastroenterol.* **31:**57–62.
72. **Megraud, F., F. Bonnet, M. Garnier, and H. Lamouliatte.** 1985. Characterization of "*Campylobacter pyloridis*" by cul-

ture, enzymatic profile, and protein content. *J. Clin. Microbiol.* **22:**1007–1010.

73. **Meijer, B. C., J. C. Thijs, J. H. Kleibeuker, A. A. van Zwet, and R. J. P. Berrelkamp.** 1997. Evaluation of eight enzyme immunoassays for detection of immunoglobulin G against *Helicobacter pylori*. *J. Clin. Microbiol.* **35:**292–294.
74. **Mendall, M., P. M. Goggin, N. Molineaux, J. Levy, T. Toosy, D. Strachan, and T. C. Northfield.** 1992. Childhood living conditions and *Helicobacter pylori* seropositivity in adult life. *Lancet* **339:**896–897.
75. **Misra, S. P., M. Dwivedi, V. Misra, and S. C. Gupta.** 1993. Imprint cytology—a cheap, rapid and effective method for diagnosing *Helicobacter pylori*. *Postgrad. Med. J.* **69:**291–295.
76. **Monteiro, L., J. Cabrita, and F. Megraud.** 1997. Evaluation of performances of three DNA enzyme immunoassays for detection of *Helicobacter pylori* PCR products from biopsy specimens. *J. Clin. Microbiol.* **35:**2931–2936.
77. **Morris, A. J., M. R. Ali, G. I. Nicholson, G. I. Perez-Perez, and M. J. Blaser.** 1991. Long-term followup of voluntary ingestion of *Helicobacter pylori*. *Ann. Intern. Med.* **114:**662–663.
78. **National Committee for Clinical Laboratory Standards.** 1999. *Performance Standards for Antimicrobial Susceptibility Testing: Ninth Informational Supplement*. NCCLS document M100-S9. National Committee for Clinical Laboratory Standards, Villanova, Pa.
79. **Ndawula, E. M., R. J. Owen, G. Mihr, P. Borman, and A. Hurtado.** 1994. *Helicobacter pylori* bacteremia. *Eur. J. Clin. Microbiol. Infect. Dis.* **13:**621.
80. **Ng, V. L., W. K. Hadley, C. L. Fennell, B. M. Flores, and W. E. Stamm.** 1987. Successive bacteremias with "*Campylobacter cinaedi*" and "*Campylobacter fennelliae*" in a bisexual male. *J. Clin. Microbiol.* **25:**2008–2009.
81. **NIH Consensus Development Panel.** 1994. *Helicobacter pylori* in peptic ulcer disease. *JAMA* **272:**65–69.
82. **Nomura, A., G. N. Stemmerman, P.-H. Chyou, I. Kato, G. I. Perez-Perez, and M. J. Blaser.** 1991. *Helicobacter pylori* infection and gastric carcinoma among Japanese Americans in Hawaii. *N. Engl. J. Med.* **325:**1132–1136.
83. **On, S. L. W., and B. Holmes.** 1992. Assessment of enzyme detection tests useful in identification of campylobacteria. *J. Clin. Microbiol.* **30:**746–749.
84. **Orlicek, S. L., D. F. Welch, and T. L. Kuhls.** 1993. Septicemia and meningitis caused by *Helicobacter cinaedi* in a neonate. *J. Clin. Microbiol.* **31:**569–571.
85. **Parente, F., G. Maconi, O. Sangaletti, M. Minguzzi, L. Vago, E. Rossi, and G. Bianchi Porro.** 1996. Prevalence of *Helicobacter pylori* infection and related gastroduodenal lesions in spouses of *Helicobacter pylori* positive patients with duodenal ulcer. *Gut* **39:**629–633.
86. **Parsonnet, J., G. D. Friedman, D. P. Vanderstein, Y. Chang, J. H. Vogelman, N. Orentreich, and R. K. Sibley.** 1991. *Helicobacter pylori* infection and the risk of gastric carcinoma. *N. Engl. J. Med.* **325:**1127–1131.
87. **Parsonnet, J., S. Hansen, L. Rodriguez, A. B. Gelb, R. A. Warnke, E. Jellum, N. Orentreich, J. H. Vogelman, and G. D. Friedman.** 1994. *Helicobacter pylori* infection and gastric lymphoma. *N. Engl. J. Med.* **330:**1267–1271.
88. **Parsonnet, J., K. Welch, C. Compton, R. Strauss, T. Wang, P. Kelsey, and M. J. Ferraro.** 1988. Simple microbiologic detection of *Campylobacter pylori*. *J. Clin. Microbiol.* **26:**948–949.
89. **Paster, B. J., A. Lee, J. G. Fox, F. E. Dewhirst, L. A. Tordoff, G. J. Fraser, J. L. O'Rourke, N. S. Taylor, and R. Ferrero.** 1991. Phylogeny of *Helicobacter felis* sp. nov., *Helicobacter mustelae*, and related bacteria. *Int. J. Syst. Bacteriol.* **41:**31–38.
90. **Perez-Perez, G. I., B. M. Dworkin, J. E. Chodos, and M. J. Blaser.** 1988. *Campylobacter pylori* antibodies in humans. *Ann. Intern. Med.* **109:**11–17.
91. **Popovic-Uroic, T., C. M. Patton, M. A. Nicholson, and J. A. Kiehlbauch.** 1990. Evaluation of the indoxyl acetate hydrolysis test for rapid differentiation of *Campylobacter*, *Helicobacter*, and *Wolinella* species. *J. Clin. Microbiol.* **28:**2335–2339.
92. **Puetz, T., N. Vakil, S. Phadnis, B. Dunn, and J. Robinson.** 1997. The Pyloritek test and the CLOtest: accuracy and incremental cost analysis. *Am. J. Gastroenterol.* **92:**254–257.
93. **Queiroz, D. M. M., G. A. Rocha, E. N. Mendes, S. B. de Moura, A. M. R. Oliveira, and D. Miranda.** 1996. Association between *Helicobacter* and gastric ulcer disease of the pars esophagea in swine. *Gastroenterology* **111:**19–27.
94. **Quinn, T. C., S. E. Goodell, C. L. Fennell, S.-P. Wang, M. D. Schuffler, K. K. Holmes, and W. E. Stamm.** 1984. Infections with *Campylobacter jejuni* and *Campylobacter*-like organisms in homosexual men. *Ann. Intern. Med.* **101:**187–192.
95. **Rathbone, B. J., J. I. Wyatt, B. W. Worsley, S. E. Shires, L. K. Trejdosiewicz, R. V. Heatley, and M. S. Losowsky.** 1986. Systemic and local antibody responses to gastric *Campylobacter pyloridis* in non-ulcer dyspepsia. *Gut* **27:**642–647.
96. **Riley, L. K., C. L. Franklin, R. R. Hook, Jr., and C. Besch-Williford.** 1996. Identification of murine helicobacters by PCR and restriction enzyme analyses. *J. Clin. Microbiol.* **34:**942–946.
97. **Romaniuk, P. J., B. Zoltowska, T. J. Trust, D. J. Lane, G. J. Olsen, N. R. Pace, and D. A. Stahl.** 1987. *Campylobacter pylori*, the spiral bacterium associated with human gastritis, is not a true *Campylobacter* sp. *J. Bacteriol.* **169:**2137–2141.
98. **Romero, S., J. R. Archer, M. E. Hamacher, S. M. Bologna, and R. F. Schell.** 1988. Case report of an unclassified microaerophilic bacterium associated with gastroenteritis. *J. Clin. Microbiol.* **26:**142–143.
99. **Sahay, P., A. P. West, D. Birkenhead, and P. M. Hawkey.** 1995. *Campylobacter jejuni* in the stomach. *J. Med. Microbiol.* **43:**75–77.
100. **Salomon, H.** 1898. Über das Spirillum des Säugetiermagens und sein Verhalten zu den Belegzellen. *Zentbl. Bakteriol. Parasitenkd. Infektionskr. Hyg. Abt.* **19:**422–441.
101. **Shen, Z., J. G. Fox, F. E. Dewhirst, B. J. Paster, C. J. Foltz, L. Yan, B. Shames, and L. Perry.** 1997. *Helicobacter rodentium* sp. nov., a urease-negative *Helicobacter* species isolated from laboratory mice. *Int. J. Syst. Bacteriol.* **47:**627–634.
102. **Shomer, N. H., C. A. Dangler, M. D. Schrenzel, and J. G. Fox.** 1997. *Helicobacter bilis*-induced inflammatory bowel disease in *scid* mice with defined flora. *Infect. Immun.* **65:**4858–4864.
103. **Slomianski, A., T. Schubert, and A. F. Cutler.** 1995. [^{13}C] urea breath test to confirm eradication of *Helicobacter pylori*. *Am. J. Gastroenterol.* **90:**224–226.
104. **Solnick, J. V., J. O'Rourke, A. Lee, B. J. Paster, F. E. Dewhirst, and L. S. Tompkins.** 1993. An uncultured gastric spiral organism is a newly identified *Helicobacter* in humans. *J. Infect. Dis.* **168:**379–385.
105. **Stanley, J., D. Linton, A. P. Burnens, F. E. Dewhirst, S. L. W. On, A. Porter, R. J. Owen, and M. Costas.** 1994. *Helicobacter pullorum* sp. nov.—genotype and phenotype of a new species isolated from poultry and from human patients with gastroenteritis. *Microbiology* **140:**3441–3449.
106. **Stanley, J., D. Linton, A. P. Burnens, F. E. Dewhirst, R. J. Owen, A. Porter, S. L. W. On, and M. Costas.** 1993. *Helicobacter canis* sp. nov., a new species from dogs:

an integrated study of phenotype and genotype. *J. Gen. Microbiol.* **139:**2495–2504.

107. **Stolte, M., E. Wellens, B. Bethke, M. Ritter, and H. Eidt.** 1994. *Helicobacter heilmannii* (formerly *Gastrospirillum hominis*) gastritis: an infection transmitted by animals? *Scand. J. Gastroenterol.* **29:**1061–1064.
108. **Stone, G. G., D. Shortridge, J. Versalovic, J. Beyer, R. K. Flamm, D. Y. Graham, A. T. Ghoneim, and S. K. Tanaka.** 1997. A PCR-oligonucleotide ligation assay to determine the prevalence of 23S rRNA gene mutations in clarithromycin-resistant *Helicobacter pylori. Antimicrob. Agents Chemother.* **41:**712–714.
109. **Sung, J. J. Y., S. C. S. Chung, T. K. W. Ling, M. Y. Yung, V. K. S. Leung, E. K. W. Ng, M. K. K. Li, A. F. B. Cheng, and A. K. C. Li.** 1995. Antibacterial treatment of gastric ulcers associated with *Helicobacter pylori. N. Engl. J. Med.* **332:**139–142.
110. **Szczebara, F., L. Dhaenens, and M. O. Husson.** 1997. Evaluation of rapid molecular methods for detection of clarithromycin resistance in *Helicobacter pylori. Eur. J. Clin. Microbiol. Infect. Dis.* **16:**162–164.
111. **Tee, W., A. C. Street, D. Spelman, W. Munckhof, and A. Mijch.** 1996. *Helicobacter cinaedi* bacteraemia: varied clinical manifestations in three homosexual males. *Scand. J. Infect. Dis.* **28:**199–203.
112. **Thomson, M. A., P. Storey, R. Greer, and G. J. Cleghorn.** 1994. Canine-human transmission of *Gastrospirillum hominis. Lancet* **343:**1605–1607.
113. **Trivett-Moore, N. L., W. D. Rawlinson, M. Yuen, and G. L. Gilbert.** 1997. *Helicobacter westmeadii* sp. nov., a new species isolated from blood cultures of two AIDS patients. *J. Clin. Microbiol.* **35:**1144–1150.

113a. **Vakil, N., B. Hahn, and D. McSorley.** 1998. Clarithromycin-resistant *Helicobacter pylori* in patients with duodenal ulcer in the United States. *Am. J. Gastroenterol.* **93:**1432–1435.

114. **Vandamme, P., E. Falsen, R. Rossau, B. Hoste, P. Segers, R. Tytgat, and J. de Ley.** 1991. Revision of *Campylobacter, Helicobacter,* and *Wolinella* taxonomy: emendation of generic descriptions and proposal of *Arcobacter* gen. nov. *Int. J. Syst. Bacteriol.* **41:**88–103.
115. **Versalovic, J., M. S. Osato, K. Spakosky, M. P. Dore, R. Reddy, G. G. Stone, D. Shortridge, R. K. Flamm, S. K. Tanaka, and D. Y. Graham.** 1997. Point mutations in the 23S rRNA gene of *Helicobacter pylori* associated with different levels of clarithromycin resistance. *J. Antimicrob. Chemother.* **40:**283–286.
116. **Versalovic, J., D. Shortridge, K. Kibler, M. V. Griffy, J. Beyer, R. K. Flamm, S. K. Tanaka, D. Y. Graham, and M. F. Go.** 1996. Mutations in 23S rRNA are associated with clarithromycin resistance in *Helicobacter pylori. Antimicrob. Agents Chemother.* **40:**477–480.
117. **Vincent, P., F. Gottrand, P. Pernes, M. O. Husson, M. Lecomte-Houcke, D. Turck, and H. Leclerc.** 1994. High prevalence of *Helicobacter pylori* infection in cohabiting children. Epidemiology of a cluster, with special emphasis on molecular typing. *Gut* **35:**313–316.
118. **Warren, J. R., and B. Marshall.** 1983. Unidentified curved bacilli on gastric epithelium in active chronic gastritis. *Lancet* **i:**1273–1275.
119. **Webb, P. M., T. Knight, S. Greaves, A. Wilson, D. G. Newell, J. Elder, and D. Forman.** 1994. Relation between infection with *Helicobacter pylori* and living conditions in childhood: evidence for person to person transmission in early life. *Br. Med. J.* **308:**750–753.
120. **Wilcox, M. H., T. H. S. Dent, J. O. Hunter, J. J. Gray, D. F. J. Brown, D. G. D. Wight, and E. P. Wraight.** 1996. Accuracy of serology for the diagnosis of *Helicobacter pylori* infection—a comparison of eight kits. *J. Clin. Pathol.* **49:**373–376.
121. **Woo, J. S., H. M. T. El-Zimaity, R. M. Genta, M. M. Yousfi, and D. Y. Graham.** 1996. The best gastric site for obtaining a positive rapid urease test. *Helicobacter* **1:**256–259.
122. **Wotherspoon, A. C., C. Ortiz-Hidalgo, M. R. Falzon, and P. G. Isaacson.** 1991. *Helicobacter pylori*-associated gastritis and primary B-cell gastric lymphoma. *Lancet* **338:**1175–1176.
123. **Xia, H.-X., C. T. Keane, J. Chen, J. Zhang, E. J. Walsh, A. P. Moran, J.-S. Hua, F. Megraud, and C. A. O'Morain.** 1994. Transportation of *Helicobacter pylori* cultures by optimal systems. *J. Clin. Microbiol.* **32:**3075–3077.
124. **Yousfi, M. M., H. M. T. El-Zimaity, R. A. Cole, R. M. Genta, and D. Y. Graham.** 1996. Detection of *Helicobacter pylori* by rapid urease tests: is biopsy size a critical variable? *Gastrointest. Endosc.* **43:**222–224.
125. **Yousfi, M. M., H. M. T. El-Zimaity, R. A. Cole, R. M. Genta, and D. Y. Graham.** 1997. Comparison of agar gel (CLOtest) or reagent strip (PyloriTek) rapid urease tests for detection of *Helicobacter pylori* infection. *Am. J. Gastroenterol.* **92:**997–999.

Leptospira and *Leptonema*

ROBBIN S. WEYANT, SANDRA L. BRAGG, AND ARNOLD F. KAUFMANN

52

TAXONOMY

The family *Leptospiraceae* was first described in 1979 and consists of spiral-shaped bacteria with hooked ends in the order *Spirochaetales* (Fig. 1) (16). These organisms are the causative agents of leptospirosis, a zoonosis with a worldwide distribution. Two taxonomic systems, one based on serology and the other based on DNA-DNA hybridization, are currently recognized.

In the traditional serologic system the basic taxon is the serovar, and pathogenicity is the key criterion for differentiating between species (19, 42). Pathogenic serovars are assigned to the species *Leptospira interrogans*, and free-living nonpathogenic serovars comprise the species *Leptospira biflexa*. More than 218 *L. interrogans* serovars and at least 60 *L. biflexa* serovars are recognized (21). The serovars of each species are organized into serogroups on the basis of shared major antigens. Serogroup designation has no official taxonomic status and is intended primarily for laboratory use. For an example of the nomenclature of the classical taxonomic system, consider strain Ictero #1, the type strain of *L. interrogans*. This strain is in the serovar icterohaemorrhagiae of the serogroup Icterohaemorrhagiae of *L. interrogans*.

Molecular taxonomic studies of the family *Leptospiraceae* have shown a high degree of genetic heterogeneity within *L. interrogans* and *L. biflexa* (2, 3, 17, 30, 45). On the basis of this foundation, a phylogenetic taxonomic system was developed. In this system, serovars formerly considered to be *L. interrogans* have been assigned to seven named and five unnamed species: *L. interrogans*, *Leptospira noguchii*, *Leptospira weilii*, *Leptospira santarosai*, *Leptospira borgpetersenii*, *Leptospira kirschneri*, *Leptospira inadai*, and *Leptospira* genomospecies 1, 2, 3, 4, and 5. *L. biflexa* serovars have been assigned to one of five species in two genera: *L. biflexa*, *Leptospira meyeri*, *Leptospira wolbachii*, *Leptospira parva*, and *Leptonema illini*. The new genus name, *Turneria*, suggested for *L. parva* at the September 1990 meeting of the International Committee on Systematic Bacteriology Subcommittee on the Taxonomy of *Leptospira* (24), has not yet been validly published.

Table 1 presents the identification of some type and reference strains obtained with both systems (2, 3, 30, 45). With the exception of serogroup Ballum, the only serovar of which that has been studied thus far is *L. borgpetersenii*, all other serogroups show molecular heterogeneity. This heterogeneity has also been demonstrated among strains of the same serovar (Table 1). Therefore, the serologic identification of an isolate cannot be used to predict its molecular identification.

DESCRIPTION OF THE FAMILY

Members of the family *Leptospiraceae* are flexible helical rods of 0.1 μm in diameter and from 6 to greater than 12 μm in length (Fig. 1). The helical conformation is right-handed with more than 18 coils per cell. Usually, one or both ends of the cells are hooked. Individual cells stain faintly negative upon Gram staining, but they are best viewed by dark-field or phase-contrast microscopy. Members of the family *Leptospiraceae* are motile with two subterminal periplasmic flagella and are able to pass through 0.2-μm-pore-size filters. Their metabolism is aerobic, with long-chain fatty acids or long-chain alcohols used as primary energy and carbon sources.

NATURAL HABITAT

Leptospires have a worldwide distribution. These organisms may be free-living or may live in association with human or animal hosts. The organisms are excreted in the urine of infected animals and may survive for days to months in freshwater, soil, or mud. Humans are dead-end hosts in the chain of transmission, with possible incidents of person-to-person transmission rarely being reported. Pathogenic leptospires do not survive well in salt water or in environments with low pH or low humidity.

The distribution of *Leptospira* serovars varies by region and host species. Some commonly recognized associations between serovars and their hosts include canicola with dogs, pomona with cattle or swine, ballum with mice, and icterohaemorrhagiae with rats. A knowledge of the predominant serovars in the geographic region of interest is important for the development of effective methods for the diagnosis of leptospirosis.

CLINICAL SIGNIFICANCE

Infection usually results from direct or indirect exposure to the urine of infected animals (11). Indirect exposure through contaminated water and soil accounts for most spo-

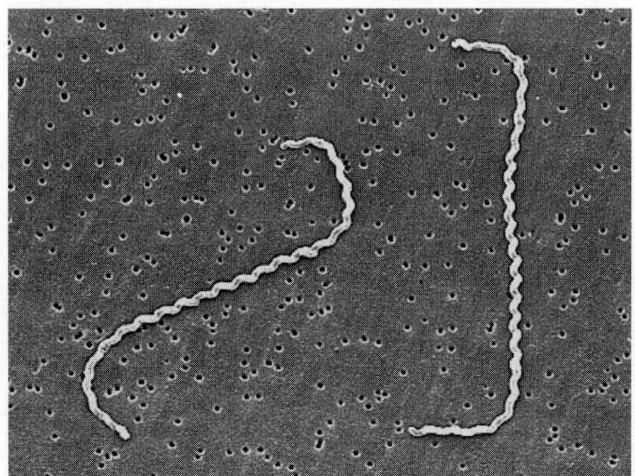

FIGURE 1 Scanning electron micrograph of leptospiral cells bound to a 0.2-μm filter. Magnification, approximately ×3,500.

radic cases, common-source outbreaks in swimmers, and cases in occupational groups such as rice farmers, sugarcane workers, sewer workers, and military personnel. Direct exposure occurs in pet owners, veterinarians, and persons working with livestock. Other modes of infection, such as animal bites, handling of infected animal tissues, and ingestion of contaminated food and water, are of less importance. Recent outbreaks involving large numbers of individuals have occurred after periods of heavier than normal rainfall and flooding in remote areas (7, 33, 46).

Leptospirosis exhibits a great variety of clinical manifestations, ranging from a mild self-limiting febrile illness (most patients) to a fulminating fatal illness associated with hepatorenal failure (Weil's disease). The incubation period is usually 7 to 14 days, but it can range from 2 to 21 days (11). Mild cases of disease are characterized by the sudden onset of low-grade fever, headache, and muscle pain which may last between 1 day and 2 weeks. Conjunctival infection, pharyngitis, hepatomegaly, and skin rash may also occur in the first several days of illness. Due to the nonspecificity of these symptoms, mild cases of leptospirosis may be confused with viral syndromes.

Leptospirosis is typically a biphasic illness (11, 20). The initial or septicemic phase lasts for 4 to 7 days. Leptospires disseminate widely throughout the body during this stage, and blood cultures are most productive for establishing the diagnosis. Following a 1- to 3-day quiescent period that is thought to reflect the initial onset of an immune response, the second phase, or the immune phase, begins. In anicteric leptospirosis, the less severe form of the disease, the immune phase is generally of a shorter duration and of lesser severity than the septicemic phase, and its most important features are meningitis (up to 40% of patients) and leptospiruria (>95% of patients). Urine cultures and serology are recommended for laboratory diagnosis during and after this phase of the illness. About 10% of patients develop icteric leptospirosis. The hallmarks of icteric leptospirosis (jaundice and azotemia) begin late in the septicemic phase and tend to obscure the biphasic nature of the disease. Icteric leptospirosis can be clinically severe, with a mortality rate of about 10%.

COLLECTION, TRANSPORT, AND STORAGE OF SPECIMENS

Blood, cerebrospinal fluid (CSF), and urine are the specimens of choice for the recovery of leptospires from patients with leptospirosis. The most appropriate specimens for culture during the first 10 days of illness are blood and CSF.

TABLE 1 Serologic and molecular identification of selected leptospiral strains

Strain	Serologic identification		Molecular identification
	Serogroup	Serovar	
Akiyami A	Autumnalis	autumnalis	*L. interrogans*
Fort Bragg	Autumnalis	fortbragg	*L. noguchii*
Butembo	Autumnalis	butembo	*L. kirschneri*
Sponslee	Sejroe	hardjo	*L. borgpetersenii*
Hardjoprajitno	Sejroe	hardjo	*L. interrogans*
Went 5	Sejroe	hardjo	*L. meyeri*
RGA^T	Icterohaemorrhagiae	icterohaemorrhagiae	*L. interrogans*
CZ 214K^T	Panama	panama	*L. noguchii*
Veldrat Batavia 46^T	Javanica	javanica	*L. borgpetersenii*
Celledoni^T	Celledoni	celledoni	*L. weilii*
LT 821^T	Shermani	shermani	*L. santarosai*
3522 C^T	Cynopteri	cynopteri	*L. kirschneri*
10^T	Lyme	lyme	*L. inadai*
Iowa City Frog^T	Ranarum	ranarum	*L. meyeri*
Patoc I^T	Semaranga	patoc	*L. biflexa*
H^T	Turneria	parva	*L. parva*
3055^T	Leptonema	illini	*Leptospira* illini
80–412	Ranarum	pinchang	*Leptospira* genomospecies 1
L 60^T	Manhao	manhao 3	*Leptospira* genomospecies 2
Waz Holland	Undesignated	holland	*Leptospira* genomospecies 3
LT 11–33	Icterohaemorrhagiae	hualin	*Leptospira* genomospecies 4
Sao Paulo	Semaranga	saopaulo	*Leptospira* genomospecies 5

These specimens should be collected prior to antibiotic treatment and while the patient is febrile. If culture media are not immediately available, blood should be collected in tubes containing heparin or sodium oxalate for transport. Tubes containing citrate solutions should be avoided, because citrate may be inhibitory (42). Specimens should be stored and transported under conditions that avoid freezing or excessive heat and should be inoculated into culture media within 1 week of collection.

After the first week of illness, the optimal source for isolation of leptospires is the urine. Extreme care should be taken to collect an uncontaminated specimen because most urine contaminants will overgrow leptospires in culture. Cultures should be inoculated as soon as possible, especially if the pH of the urine is acidic. Leptospires survive for only a few hours in acidic urine. If culture media are not immediately available, the urine can be diluted 1:10 in 1% bovine serum albumin and stored for a few days at 5 to 20°C.

For patients with fatal cases of leptospirosis, viable leptospires can be isolated from multiple tissues, particularly the liver, kidney, and brain (8). Samples should be collected and processed within 4 h of death because leptospires will not survive in autolytic tissues.

For epidemiologic investigations, freshwater ponds represent potential sources of pathogenic leptospires. Water should be collected in sterile containers and transported at room temperature to the laboratory within 72 h of collection (18).

Serologic procedures should always be included in the diagnostic workup for patients with leptospirosis. In most cases antibodies can be detected approximately 1 week after the onset of symptoms, and titers peak at 3 to 4 weeks postonset. A fourfold rise in titer between acute- and convalescent-phase serum samples is the most reliable indication of current infection, so the testing of paired serum specimens drawn at least 1 week apart is recommended. Acute-phase serum specimens should be collected within 14 days of the onset of disease, and convalescent-phase serum specimens should be collected at least 21 days postonset. If acute-phase sera are to be screened for the presence of immunoglobulin M (IgM) antibodies, these specimens should be collected at least 5 days postonset.

DIRECT DETECTION OF LEPTOSPIRES

A presumptive identification of leptospires can be made by direct microscopic methods. Blood, CSF, and tissues may be screened microscopically for the presence of leptospires by either dark-field microscopy or direct fluorescent-antibody assay. Blood is prepared for analysis by mixing 5 ml of freshly drawn whole blood with either 0.5 ml of 1% sodium oxalate or 1.0 ml of 1% heparin. The mixture is centrifuged at 500 × *g* for 15 min, and the supernatant is then transferred to another tube and centrifuged at 1,500 × *g* for 30 min. The supernatant is discarded, and a wet mount is prepared from the sediment. For urine or CSF, the sample is centrifuged at 1,500 × *g* for 30 min, the supernatant is discarded, and a wet mount is prepared from the sediment.

Tissues may be prepared for analysis by disruption in a sterile Ten Broeck tissue grinder or with a mortar and pestle and suspension in 9 parts sterile phosphate-buffered saline (PBS; pH 7.2 to 7.8). The resulting suspension is centrifuged at 500 × *g* for 15 min. The sediment is discarded, and the supernatant is poured into another tube and centrifuged at 1,500 × *g* for 30 min. The supernatant is discarded, and a wet mount is prepared from the sediment.

Dark-field microscopic examination of specimens processed as indicated above can be useful in establishing a rapid presumptive diagnosis but should not be relied upon as the sole diagnostic criterion. For specimens in which the number of leptospires is small, it may be difficult to find the organisms even after centrifugation. Experience and skill are required to differentiate leptospires from artifacts, such as fibrils or cellular extrusions. On a freshly prepared slide, the characteristic hooked ends of the leptospiral cells will usually be apparent, whereas the ends of artifacts are usually straight.

Numerous silver staining techniques, including the Warthin-Starry and Van Orden methods, have been described for visualizing leptospires in tissues (36). As with other microscopic techniques, sensitivity is poor for samples in which the number of leptospires is small.

A slightly more sensitive technique for visualizing leptospires in specimens is staining with fluorescein-conjugated antibodies for detection by UV microscopy. The National Veterinary Service Laboratory, Animal and Plant Health Inspection Service (APHIS), U.S. Department of Agriculture, Ames, Iowa, produces multivalent conjugates for the veterinary profession. These conjugates are available through local APHIS representatives.

For fluorescence microscopy, urine or CSF sediment is placed on a slide, air dried, and fixed in absolute alcohol for 10 min. The fixed specimen is reacted with the leptospiral conjugate for 2 h at 37°C. After washing the slide with PBS or saline, a coverslip is mounted with 10% PBS in glycerol (pH 7.5). A fluorescence microscope with a filter combination that is usually recommended for bacterial identification, such as a BG 12 exciter and an OG1 ocular filter, is recommended for examination of the slide (36).

Immunohistochemistry has proven useful for the sensitive and specific detection of leptospires in recent outbreak investigations (46). Although this technique has not been directly compared with direct immunofluorescence, it represents a promising non-fluorescence-based alternative.

In recent years PCR-based methods have been developed for the rapid detection of *Leptospira* DNA in human specimens (14, 27, 34, 39). Two of these methods have been evaluated in comparison to culture and serology with specimens from leptospirosis patients, and both appear to be more sensitive than culture for patients with serologically confirmed disease (6, 27). PCR analysis is most useful within the first 10 to 14 days after the onset of disease, when leptospiral DNA may be detected prior to the development of the humoral immune response. Specimens in which leptospiral DNA has been detected by PCR include serum, urine, aqueous humor, and CSF. When testing serum, care must be taken to avoid the erythrocyte fraction, which contains PCR inhibitors.

ISOLATION PROCEDURES

By using aseptic techniques, inoculate the specimens (see below) within 24 h into tubes containing 5 ml of a serum-containing semisolid medium, such as Fletcher's, Stuart's, Ellinghausen's (EMJH), or PLM-5 (see section IX of the Manual for formulations) (11, 36). Culture media can be made selective for leptospiral growth by the addition of neomycin (one 30-μg antimicrobial susceptibility disc per 5 ml) or 5-fluorouracil (5-FU) (200 μg/ml) (36). Media containing 5-FU tend to be more selective than neomycin-supplemented media; however, 5-FU may also slow the growth of leptospires. As soon as leptospiral growth is detected in selective media, either by sight or by dark-field microscopic examination, the culture should be transferred to nonselective media.

The inoculum volume for blood should be kept to a minimum due to the presence of inhibitory substances. Only 1 or 2 drops (approximately 50 μl per drop) should be added to 5 ml of medium. Inoculate three to five tubes per specimen, because the bacteremia tends to be of low titer. For CSF, as much as 0.5 ml of undiluted specimen per 5 ml of medium can be used.

To minimize problems with bacterial overgrowth, the following urine culture technique is recommended (36). Draw about 1 ml of urine from the specimen container into a sterile 2-ml syringe with an attached 2.5-cm, 20-gauge needle. Inoculate two tubes, each containing 5 ml of semisolid medium, with 1 drop of the undiluted urine from the syringe. One tube of each pair should contain a selective agent. Expel all but 0.1 ml of the urine and then draw 0.9 ml of sterile PBS into the syringe. Expel a few drops of the diluted urine before inoculating 1 drop of the 1 : 10 dilution into each of two tubes of semisolid medium. Repeat the dilution procedure two more times; the result will be a set of four pairs of tubes containing inoculated medium.

To culture tissues, use aseptic technique to remove a small piece of the organ and place this piece in the barrel of a sterile 5-ml syringe. Insert the plunger, and crush the specimen through the tip of the syringe into a tube of semisolid culture medium. The inoculum should be roughly the size of a pea (5 mm in diameter). Two tubes of medium, one selective and the other nonselective, should be inoculated per specimen.

To culture pond water, laboratory animal inoculation is used as a first step to overcome problems posed by overgrowth by saprophytic leptospires and other bacteria. Inject 3 ml of the water sample intraperitoneally into a weanling guinea pig. Obtain a heart blood specimen 4 h after inoculation for culture and a baseline serum sample. After 4 weeks euthanize the animal and obtain blood, kidney, and brain for serologic tests and culture.

Hold all leptospiral culture specimens at room temperature (20 to 30°C). Examine a drop of the culture medium by dark-field microscopy once a week for 5 weeks and then twice a month for 4 months before calling a culture negative. Although leptospires are usually detectable in positive cultures within 1 to 2 weeks, holding negative cultures for up to 4 months ensures that the patient's diagnosis is accurate for prognostic purposes.

In semisolid cultures leptospiral growth will initially appear as a diffuse zone near the top of the tube. As the culture matures, the leptospires will condense into a well-differentiated ring located at the level of the tube corresponding to the optimum oxygen tension for the organism (Dinger's ring). In general, the saprophytic serovars form rings closer to the top of the tube than the pathogenic serovars do. Leptospiral growth can be confirmed by examining a sample of the growth ring by dark-field microscopy.

Cultures in semisolid media should remain viable for at least 8 weeks at room temperature. For longer-term storage, cell suspensions containing 10% glycerol can be kept in liquid nitrogen.

IDENTIFICATION

Although significant progress has been made in recent years, the final identification of leptospiral isolates to the species or serovar level requires the use of techniques and reagents that are usually limited to reference laboratories. Once a positive culture is detected in the clinical laboratory, it should be shipped to a reference laboratory for further identification. Cultures in tubed semisolid media should be packaged in biohazard shipping containers and should be shipped at room temperature.

There are two general approaches to the identification of leptospires: serologic and molecular. The serologic approach can identify leptospires to the serogroup level by the microscopic agglutination test (MAT) with reference rabbit antisera raised against the type serovars of all recognized serogroups (36). MAT is performed with isolates that have been passaged at least three times in liquid medium, such as PLM-5 liquid. This effectively dilutes out agar granules that might produce agglutination artifacts and reduces nonspecific agglutination. The test is performed in a flat-bottom 96-well tissue culture plate. Reference sera are diluted with PBS in twofold steps from 1 : 25 through 1 : 3,200. Then, 50 μl of each serum dilution is mixed with 50 μl of an antigen suspension standardized at 100 to 200 organisms per high-power (magnification, ×450) field (an antigen density equivalent to a McFarland 0.5 or a Roessler 20 turbidity standard). The antigen-antiserum mixtures are incubated at room temperature for 1.5 to 4 h, and then the reactions are read by dark-field microscopy. The titer is defined as the highest antiserum dilution at which at least 50% of the leptospires are agglutinated (2+ agglutination). The final identification of an isolate to the serovar level requires the use of the agglutinin adsorption technique (36). This technique involves raising isolate-specific hyperimmune rabbit antiserum and requires the maintenance of many reference serovar strains and antisera. This technique is usually limited to reference laboratories.

An alternative method based on the use of a set of monoclonal antibodies is available for serovar identification. The reagents and procedures for this method are available from the World Health Organization (WHO)/Food and Agriculture Organization (FAO) Collaborative Center for Reference and Research on Leptospirosis, Royal Tropical Institute, Amsterdam, The Netherlands.

The genetic diversity of the member of the family *Leptospiraceae* has led to the investigation of molecular approaches for identification. Whole-chromosome restriction endonuclease patterns and ribotyping are used for serovar identification in some reference laboratories (25), and PCR-restriction fragment length polymorphism methods which differentiate between *L. illini* and *Leptospira* species (43) and between *L. interrogans* and *L. biflexa* (44) have been described. Randomly amplified polymorphic DNA fingerprinting and arbitrarily primed PCR represent two extremely promising approaches. Within the past 4 years investigators, using primarily reference strains, have successfully applied these methods to the identification of serovars (5, 10, 12, 29, 31). As these methods are applied to more clinical isolates, the utilities of these approaches will become more apparent.

SEROLOGIC TESTS

MAT with live antigen is the standard reference laboratory procedure for the detection of leptospiral antibodies (9, 36). Both highly sensitive and specific, MAT is the standard against which other serodiagnostic test procedures must be measured. This test, however, is time-consuming, difficult to standardize, and hazardous to perform. Some laboratories use formalin-killed antigens because they are less hazardous and are stable for about 2 weeks. Although the titers are somewhat lower and cross-reactivity is greater, the results obtained with killed antigens generally compare favorably with those obtained with live antigens (13).

The extensive antigenic diversity of leptospiral serovars and the partially serovar-specific nature of MAT necessitate the use of a battery of antigens. Because at the Centers for Disease Control and Prevention (CDC), Atlanta, Ga., we receive sera from sources worldwide, we use a panel of 23 antigens representing 21 serovars and 17 serogroups and supplement these with additional serovars as needed. Laboratories that serve a more localized geographic area may not require a panel this large. Knowledge of the serovars commonly isolated in the area is critical to the development of an appropriate panel.

Antigens for MAT are live 4- to 7-day-old cultures in PLM-5 broth adjusted to a turbidity equivalent to that of a McFarland 0.5 standard. MAT is performed in 96-well flat-bottom tissue culture plates, starting at a serum dilution of 1:50 (1:100 after the addition of antigen). Serial twofold dilutions of serum in PBS (50 μl/well) are mixed with an equal volume of antigen. As a positive control for each antigen, homologous rabbit antiserum is run in parallel with the patient's serum specimens. After incubation at room temperature for 1.5 to 4 h, the reactions are read at a magnification of $\times$ 100 on a dark-field microscope. The end point is the highest dilution that agglutinates 50% or more of the leptospires relative to the dilution for the buffer control.

Although MAT is considered the "gold standard" method for leptospirosis serology, its complexity limits its use to reference laboratories. A commercially produced indirect hemagglutination assay that uses a genus-specific antigen from serovar andamana (MRL Diagnostics, Cypress, Calif.) represents a U.S. Food and Drug Administration (FDA)-cleared alternative to MAT for diagnostic use in the United States. When this method was evaluated by CDC in 1975, it was found to be 92% sensitive and 95% specific compared to the results of MAT (37). A more recent evaluation of this assay performed by the Leptospira Laboratory, University of the West Indies, reports a positive predictive value of 95% and a negative predictive value of 100% for the detection of acute leptospirosis (22).

In recent years other alternatives to MAT which use either enzyme-linked immunosorbent assay (ELISA) or dipstick formats have been developed (15, 32, 35, 41). Initial evaluations suggest that these assays are highly sensitive and specific compared with MAT. A commercially available IgM ELISA (PanBio, Ltd., Brisbane, Australia) was recently evaluated with MAT-tested sera and was found to be 100% sensitive in detecting MAT-positive samples. Specificity values of 98% were found with specimens from asymptomatic donors, and specificity values of 93% were found with specimens from patients infected with other agents (41). Two dipstick methods (LEPTO Dipstick [Royal Tropical Institute, Amsterdam, The Netherlands] and Leptospira Dip-S-Ticks [Integrated Diagnostics, Baltimore, Md.]) have also recently been evaluated. In a study reported by Gussenhoven et al. [15], the LEPTO Dipstick detected antibodies in 76.4% of 284 serum specimens from leptospirosis patients (versus 81.3% for MAT) and was positive for 7.2% of 274 negative control serum specimens (versus 0.7% for MAT). An evaluation of the Dip-S-Ticks method by Levett et al. (23), which included sera from 23 leptospirosis patients and 26 controls, reported a positive predictive value of 79% and a predictive value of 100% for a negative test. Although neither the ELISA nor the dipstick methods have yet been cleared by FDA for diagnostic use, these methods, particularly the dipstick methods, have a tremendous potential for use in field studies. A recent study performed in our laboratory supported the usefulness of the LEPTO Dipstick assay for the detection of an outbreak of leptospirosis in Puerto Rico (33).

ANTIBIOTIC SUSCEPTIBILITIES

Standardized procedures have not been developed for antimicrobial susceptibility testing of leptospires. However, clinical experience, studies with experimental animals, and in vitro susceptibility testing have generally correlated (1, 20, 26, 28, 38, 40). The results of controlled clinical trials support the therapeutic efficacies of doxycycline and penicillin (26, 40), although in vitro testing has demonstrated strain variability in susceptibility to penicillins and tetracyclines (4, 28). In a hamster model ampicillin, bacampicillin, cyclacillin, piperacillin, mezlocillin, doxycycline, chlortetracycline, cefotaxime, and moxalactam were effective in preventing the death of infected animals (1). Further methodologic development and evaluation will be necessary before in vitro susceptibility testing can be recommended as a method for choosing therapeutic protocols.

EVALUATION, INTERPRETATION, AND REPORTING OF RESULTS

The first step in the diagnosis of leptospirosis involves the evaluation of serologic findings, supplemented with clinical and epidemiologic information. If the appropriate serovars are used, clinically significant MAT titers to *Leptospira* antigens can confirm a diagnosis of leptospirosis. A serologically confirmed case of leptospirosis is defined by a fourfold rise in the MAT titer to one or more serovars between acute- and convalescent-phase serum specimens run in parallel. A titer of at least 1:200 for a single serum specimen obtained after the onset of symptoms or a titer of at least 1:100 for consecutive specimens is suggestive but not diagnostic of leptospirosis. A titer of at least 1:800 in the presence of compatible symptoms is strong evidence of recent or current leptospirosis (11, 20), and in some recent outbreak investigations, a titer of 1:400 has been used to separate patients with leptospirosis from patients without the disease (33). Delayed seroconversions are common. We estimate that up to 10% of patients will not seroconvert within 30 days of clinical onset. We have observed cross-reactive antibody, sometimes with significant seroconversion, associated with syphilis, relapsing fever, Lyme disease, and legionellosis.

Negative results by direct examinations of specimens for leptospires or tests for leptospiral DNA for patients with elevated MAT titers do not necessarily rule out acute disease because MAT serology is more sensitive than microscopic or molecular tests. The isolation of leptospires in culture or the demonstration of leptospiral DNA by molecular methods confirms the diagnosis and differentiates between current infection and past exposure, which may not be clearly differentiated by serology.

Despite significant advances in the areas of molecular detection and characterization of leptospires and in the development of serologic tests for use in the field, there are still only a few laboratories throughout the world with the appropriate capabilities for *Leptospira* diagnostics. The reference laboratory for human leptospirosis for the United States is the WHO/FAO Collaborating Center for Reference and Research on Leptospirosis at CDC. Some other international reference laboratories for leptospirosis include the WHO/FAO Collaborating Centers in Amsterdam, The Netherlands, and Brisbane, Australia. Additional information regarding leptospirosis is available on the World Wide Web at the International Leptospirosis Society web site (http://www.monash.edu.au/informatics/micro/department/ilspage.htm). With the development of modern communications and transportation networks, the ability to rapidly ship specimens from even the remotest areas makes the services of these laboratories much more widely available than they were just a few years ago.

REFERENCES

1. **Alexander, A. D., and P. L. Rule.** 1986. Penicillins, cephalosporins, and tetracyclines in treatment of hamsters with fatal leptospirosis. *Antimicrob. Agents Chemother.* **30:** 835–839.
2. **Brendle, J. J., M. Rogul, and A. D. Alexander.** 1974. Deoxyribonucleic acid hybridization among selected leptospiral serotypes. *Int. J. Syst. Bacteriol.* **24:**205–214.
3. **Brenner, D. J., A. F. Kaufmann, K. R. Sulzer, A. G. Steigerwalt, F. C. Rogers, and R. S. Weyant.** Further determination of deoxyribonucleic acid relatedness between serogroups and serovars in the family *Leptospiraceae* with a proposal for *Leptospira alexanderi* sp. nov. and four new *Leptospira* genomospecies. Submitted for publication.
4. **Broughton, E. S., and L. E. Flack.** 1986. The susceptibility of a strain of *Leptospira interrogans* serogroup Icterohaemorrhagiae to amoxicillin, erythromycin, lincomycin, tetracycline, oxytetracycline, and minocycline. *Zentrbl. Bakteriol. Parasitenkd. Infectionskr. Hyg. Abt. 1 Orig. Reihe A* **261:** 425–431.
5. **Brown, P. D., and P. N. Levett.** 1997. Differentiation of *Leptospira* species and serovars by PCR-restriction endonuclease analysis, arbitrarily primed PCR and low-stringency PCR. *J. Med. Microbiol.* **46:**173–181.
6. **Brown, P. D., C. Gravecamp, D. G., Carrington, H. van de Kemp, R. A. Hartskeerl, C. N. Edwards, C. O. Everard, W. J. Terpstra, and P. N. Levett.** 1995. Evaluation of the polymerase chain reaction for early diagnosis of leptospirosis. *J. Med. Microbiol.* **43:**110–114.
7. **Centers for Disease Control and Prevention.** 1997. Outbreak of leptospirosis among white-water rafters—Costa Rica, 1996. *Morbid. Mortal. Weekly Rep.* **46:**577–579.
8. **Cole, J. R.** 1990. Spirochetes, p. 41–60. *In* G. R. Carter and J. R. Cole (ed.), *Diagnostic Procedures in Veterinary Bacteriology and Mycology*, 5th ed. Academic Press, Inc., New York, N.Y.
9. **Cole, J. R., C. R. Sulzer, and A. R. Pursell.** 1973. Improved microtechnique for the leptospiral microscopic agglutination test. *Appl. Microbiol.* **25:** 976–980.
10. **Corney, B. G., J. Colley, S. P. Djordjevic, R. Whittington, and G. C. Graham.** 1993. Rapid identification of some *Leptospira* isolates from cattle by random amplified polymorphic DNA fingerprinting. *J. Clin. Microbiol.* **31:** 2927–2932.
11. **Faine, S. (ed).** 1982. *Guidelines for the Control of Leptospirosis.* WHO offset publication no. 67. World Health Organization, Geneva, Switzerland.
12. **Gerritsen, M. A., M. A. Smits, and T. Olyhoek.** 1995. Random amplified polymorphic DNA fingerprinting for rapid identification of leptospiras of serogroup Sejroe. *J. Med. Microbiol.* **42:**336–339.
13. **Gochenour, W. S., C. A. Gleiser, and M. K. Ward.** 1958. Laboratory diagnosis of leptospirosis. *Ann. N. Y. Acad. Sci.* **70:**421–426.
14. **Gravekamp, C., H. Van de Kemp, M. Franzen, D. Carrington, G. J. Schoone, G. J. Van Eys, C. O. Everard, R. A. Hartskeerl, and W. J. Terpstra.** 1993. Detection of seven species of pathogenic leptospiras by PCR using two sets of primers. *J. Gen. Microbiol.* **139:**1691–1700.
15. **Gussenhoven, G. C., M. A. van der Hoorn, M. G. Goris, W. J. Terpstra, R. A. Hartskeerl, B. W. Mol, C. W. van Ingen, and H. L. Smits.** 1997. LEPTO dipstick, a dipstick assay for detection of *Leptospira*-specific immunoglobulin M antibodies in human sera. *J. Clin. Microbiol.* **35:**92–97.
16. **Hovind-Hougen, K.** 1979. *Leptospiraceae*, a new family to include *Leptospira* Noguchi 1917 and *Leptonema* gen. nov. *Int. J. Syst. Bacteriol.* **29:**245–251.
17. **Hovind-Hougen, K., W. A. Ellis, and A. Birch-Andersen.** 1981. *Leptospira parva* sp. nov.: some morphological and biological characters. *Zentrbl. Bakteriol. Parasitenkd. Infektionskr. Hyg. Abt. 1 Orig. Reihe A* **250:**343–354.
18. **Jackson, L. A., A. F. Kaufmann, W. G. Adams, M. B. Phelps, C. Andreasen, C. W. Langkop, B. J. Francis, and J. D. Wenger.** 1993. Outbreak of leptospirosis associated with swimming. *Pediatr. Infect. Dis. J.* **12:**48–54.
19. **Johnson, R. C., and S. Faine.** 1984. Family II *Leptospiraceae* Hovind-Hougen 1979, 245AL, p. 62–67. *In* N. R. Kreig and J. G. Holt (ed.), *Bergey's Manual of Systematic Bacteriology*, vol. 1. The Williams & Wilkins Co., Baltimore, Md.
20. **Kelley, P. W.** 1992. Leptospirosis, p. 1295–1301 *In* S. L. Gorbach, J. G. Bartlett, and N. R. Blacklow (ed.), *Infectious Diseases*. The W. B. Saunders Co., Philadelphia, Pa.
21. **Kmety, E., and H. Dikken.** 1993. *Classification of the Species* Leptospira interrogans *and History of Its Serovars.* University Press, Groningen, The Netherlands.
22. **Levett, P. N., and C. U. Worthington.** 1998. Evaluation of the indirect hemagglutination assay for diagnosis of acute leptospirosis. *J. Clin. Microbiol.* **36:**11–14.
23. **Levett, P. N., S. L. Branch, and H. Paxton.** 1997. Prospective evaluation of Dot-ELISA method for detection of acute leptospirosis, abstr. D-4, p. 83. *In Program and Abstracts of the 37th Interscience Conference on Antimicrobial Agents and Chemotherapy.* American Society for Microbiology, Washington, D.C.
24. **Marshall, R.** 1992. International Committee on Systematic Bacteriology, Subcommittee on the Taxonomy of *Leptospira*, minutes of the meetings, 13 and 15 September 1990, Osaka, Japan. *Int. J. Syst. Bacteriol.* **42:**330–334.
25. **Marshall, R. B., B. E. Wilton, and A. J. Robinson.** 1981. Identification of leptospiral serovars by restriction endonuclease analysis. *J. Med. Microbiol.* **14:**163–166.
26. **McClain, J. B. L., W. R. Ballou, S. M. Harrison, and D. L. Steinweg.** 1984. Doxycycline therapy for leptospirosis. *Ann. Intern. Med.* **100:**696–698.
27. **Merien, F., P. Amouriax, P. Perolat, G. Baranton, and I. St. Girons.** 1992. Polymerase chain reaction detection of *Leptospira* spp. in clinical samples. *J. Clin. Microbiol.* **30:** 2219–2224.
28. **Oie, S., K. Hironaga, A. Koshiro, H. Konishi, and Z. Yoshii.** 1983. In vitro susceptibilities of five *Leptospira* strains to 16 antimicrobial agents. *Antimicrob. Agents Chemother.* **24:**905–908.
29. **Ralph, D., M. McClelland, J. Welsh, G. Baranton, and P. Perolat.** 1993. *Leptospira* species categorized by arbitrarily primed polymerase chain reaction (PCR) and by mapped restriction polymorphisms in PCR-amplified rRNA genes. *J. Bacteriol.* **175:**973–981.
30. **Ramadass, P., B. D. W. Jarvis, R. J. Corner, D. Penny, and R. B. Marshall.** 1992. Genetic characterization of pathogenic *Leptospira* species by DNA hybridization. *Int. J. Syst. Bacteriol.* **42:**215–219.
31. **Ramadass, P., S. Meeranani, M. D. Venkatesha, A. Senthikumar, and K. Nachimuthu.** 1997. Characterization

of leptospiral serovars by randomly amplified polymorphic DNA fingerprinting. *Int. J. Syst. Bacteriol.* **47:**575–576.

32. **Ribiero, M. A., C. C. Souza, and S. H. Almeida.** 1995. Dot-ELISA for human leptospirosis employing immunodominant antigen. *J. Trop. Med. Hyg.* **98:**452–456.
33. **Sanders, E. J., J. G. Rigau-Perez, H. Smits, C. Deseda, T. Aye, S. Bragg, R. Speigel, and R. Weyant.** 1997. Hurricane-related leptospirosis in dengue-negative patients, Puerto Rico, abstr. 303. *In Abstracts of the 35th Annual Meeting of the Infectious Diseases Society of America.* Infectious Diseases Society of America, Alexandria, Va.
34. **Savio, M. L., C. Rossi, P. Fusi, S. Tagliabue, and M. L. Pacciarini.** 1994. Detection and identification of *Leptospira interrogans* serovars by PCR coupled with restriction endonuclease analysis of amplified DNA. *J. Clin. Microbiol.* **32:** 935–941.
35. **Silva, M. V., P. M. Nakamura, E. D. Camargo, L. Batista, A. J. Vaz, E. C. Romero, and A. P. Brandao.** 1997. Immunodiagnosis of human leptospirosis by dot-ELISA for the detection of IgM, IgG, and IgA antibodies. *Am. J. Trop. Med. Hyg.* **56:**650–655.
36. **Sulzer, C. R., and W. L. Jones.** 1978. Leptospirosis. *In Methods in Laboratory Diagnosis* (revised edition). Publication no. (CDC) 78-8275. U.S. Department of Health, Education, and Welfare, Washington, D.C.
37. **Sulzer, C. R., J. W. Glosser, F. Rogers, W. L. Jones, and M. Frix.** 1975. Evaluation of an indirect hemagglutination test for the diagnosis of human leptospirosis. *J. Clin. Microbiol.* **2:**218–221.
38. **Takafuji, E. T., J. W. Kirkpatrick, R. N. Miller, J. J. Karwacki, P. W. Kelley, M. W. Gray, K. M. McNeill, H. L. Timboe, R. E. Kane, and J. L. Sanchez.** 1984. An efficacy trial of doxycycline chemoprophylaxis against leptospirosis. *N. Engl. J. Med.* **310:**497–500.
39. **Van Eyes, G. J. J. M., C. Gravekamp, M. J. Gerritsen, W. Quint, M. T. E. Cornelissen, J. Ter Schegget, and W. J. Terpstra.** 1989. Detection of leptospires in urine by polymerase chain reaction. *J. Clin. Microbiol.* **27:** 2258–2262.
40. **Watt, G., L. P. Padre, M. L. Tuazon, C. Calubaquib, E. Santiago, C. P. Ranoa, and L. W. Laughlin.** 1988. Placebo-controlled trial of intravenous penicillin for severe and late leptospirosis. *Lancet* **i:**433–435.
41. **Winslow, W. E., D. J. Merry, M. L. Pirc, and P. L. Devine.** 1997. Evaluation of a commercial enzyme-linked immunosorbent assay for detection of immunoglobulin M antibody in diagnosis of human leptospiral infection. *J. Clin. Microbiol.* **35:**1938–1942.
42. **Wolff, J. W.** 1954. *The Laboratory Diagnosis of Leptospirosis.* Charles C Thomas, Publisher, Springfield, Ill.
43. **Woo, T. H., L. D. Smythe, M. L. Symonds, M. A. Norris, M. F. Dohnt, and B. K. Patel.** 1996. Rapid distinction between *Leptonema* and *Leptospira* by PCR amplification of 16S-23S ribosomal DNA spacer. *FEMS Microbiol. Lett.* **142:**85–90.
44. **Woo, T. H., L. D. Smythe, M. L. Symonds, M. A. Norris, M. F. Dohnt, and B. K. Patel.** 1997. Rapid distinction between *Leptospira interrogans* and *Leptospira biflexa* by PCR amplification of 23S ribosomal DNA. *FEMS Microbiol. Lett.* **150:**9–18.
45. **Yasuda, P. H., A. G. Steigerwalt, K. R. Sulzer, A. F. Kaufmann, F. Rogers, and D. J. Brenner.** 1987. Deoxyribonucleic acid relatedness between serogroups and serovars in the family *Leptospiraceae* with proposals for seven new *Leptospira* species. *Int. J. Syst. Bacteriol.* **37:**407–415.
46. **Zaki, S. R., W.-J. Shieh, and the Epidemic Working Group.** 1996. Leptospirosis associated with outbreak of acute febrile illness and pulmonary haemorrhage, Nicaragua, 1995. *Lancet* **347:**535–536.
47. **Zuerner, R. L., and C. A. Bolin.** 1990. Nucleic acid probe characterizes *Leptospira interrogans* serovars by restriction fragment length polymorphisms. *Vet. Microbiol.* **24:** 355–356.

Borrelia

TOM G. SCHWAN, WILLY BURGDORFER, AND PATRICIA A. ROSA

53

TAXONOMY

Bacteria of the genus *Borrelia* belong to one of two separate lineages of spirochetes (order *Spirochaetales*) that are taxonomically distinguished at the family level (140). The type species is *Borrelia anserina* (Sakharoff 1891). Species of this genus form a tight phylogenetic group within the family *Spirochaetaceae*. Other genera in this family include *Treponema, Spirochaeta, Serpulina, Cristispira* (97), and *Brevinema* (40). The second family of spirochetes is *Leptospiraceae*, which encompasses the genera *Leptospira* and *Leptonema*. Four additional genera of spirochetes have been named in GenBank submissions (*Ancona, Canela, Jequitaia,* and *Brachyspira*) but are not yet published. Spirochetes are one of the few major bacterial groups for which classical morphologic criteria and 16S rRNA sequence analyses agree in predicting the phylogenetic relationships among members of the group and their position as a distinct entity within the eubacterial kingdom (140). They are neither gram-positive nor gram-negative organisms.

DESCRIPTION OF THE GENUS

Borreliae are highly motile organisms that are 5 to 25 μm long and 0.2 to 0.5 μm wide (14). An outer membrane encloses the periplasmic flagella and the protoplasmic cylinder (61). The flagella (7 to 20 per terminus) are found beneath the outer membrane, attached subterminally to opposite ends of the protoplasmic cylinder, and they mediate both the motility and the shape of borreliae (53, 58).

The protoplasmic cylinder consists of the cell wall and the cytoplasmic membrane enclosing the protoplasmic contents of the cell. Microtubules have not been detected in the cytoplasm of borreliae, a trait that, along with unsheathed flagella, serves to distinguish them morphologically from the treponemes (14).

It is currently accepted that borreliae are microaerophilic (8), but evidence indicates that they can grow anaerobically (105). Borreliae require long-chain fatty acids for growth, and they produce lactic acid through glucose fermentation.

GENOME

Components

Borreliae have a unique genomic structure and organization composed of a linear chromosome (16, 30, 38, 49) and both linear and circular plasmids (9, 59, 126). Relapsing fever and Lyme disease borreliae have a linear chromosome of approximately 950 kb (30, 38, 49). Although a linear chromosome is presumed to be a borrelial trait, it has not been directly demonstrated for all members of the genus. Where analyzed, the chromosomal gene order is highly conserved, indicating that chromosomal recombination and rearrangements are rare (31). Most Lyme disease spirochetes contain a single 16S rRNA gene and two copies each of the 23S and 5S rRNA genes, clustered near the center of the chromosome (122). There is a putative origin of replication near the middle of the chromosome (51, 93), but the mechanisms of chromosome and plasmid replication and segregation in borreliae are undefined. Linear plasmids were first described in the relapsing fever spirochete *Borrelia hermsii* (104) and subsequently found in Lyme disease spirochetes (13). The linear plasmids and chromosome have covalently closed ends (13, 32, 51). Telomeric sequences of the chromosome and a subset of plasmids have been determined (32, 51, 57); similarity among all the sequences is limited to the terminal 25 bp, which constitute an inverted repeat. An extended region of the right chromosomal telomere is similar to linear plasmid sequences, suggesting that exchange with plasmid telomeres has occurred (32, 51).

The large gene family encoding the outer surface variable major proteins of the relapsing fever spirochete *B. hermsii* is located on linear plasmids (103). A gene conversion-like mechanism among these sequences results in antigenic variation and immune system evasion (87, 103). The linear plasmids of the Lyme disease spirochetes also contain genes encoding outer surface proteins (20, 141), including a highly variable locus that may result in antigenic variation similar to that in the relapsing fever spirochetes (87, 103). Circular plasmids in the Lyme disease spirochete contain a number of loci whose products may facilitate transmission of the spirochete from the tick to the mammal (83). A particularly attractive candidate is a plasmid gene encoding a major outer surface protein that is specifically induced during tick feeding (85, 110, 118).

Different isolates of Lyme disease and relapsing fever spirochetes exhibit nonidentical arrays of plasmids (9, 56, 116, 125). Relatedness among plasmids cannot be assigned strictly on the basis of size or structure. An interesting set of plasmids has been described in the Lyme disease spirochete; at least six separate but related 32-kbp circular plasmids can exist within a single spirochete (134). These 32-kbp plasmids contain extended regions of near identity interrupted by highly divergent loci (33). A related set of plasmids may exist in *B. hermsii* (116). The biological significance of this family of plasmids is unknown, but the variable regions encode antigenic proteins that are expressed in the mammalian environment (3, 104, 133, 136, 139).

Sequence

Borrelial DNA has a G+C content of approximately 30% (59). The complete nucleotide sequences of the chromosome and 11 plasmids from a Lyme disease spirochete have recently been determined (51). A total of 93% of the chromosome represents predicted coding sequences (open reading frames [ORFs]), in contrast to 71% of the plasmid DNA. Another distinction between plasmid and chromosomal sequences is the relative proportion of coding sequences that are similar to identified sequences in the database: 59% of the chromosomal ORFs are homologous to known sequences, whereas only 16% of the plasmid ORFs are homologous. Plasmid coding sequences exhibit a high degree of redundancy, with more than one-third of the ORFs belonging to paralogous gene families. These differences suggest that the chromosome and plasmids are not necessarily equivalent components of a segmented genome and may reflect different evolutionary histories and constraints.

The complete genomic sequence indicates that *B. burgdorferi* contains genes encoding a basic set of proteins for DNA replication, transcription, translation, and energy metabolism but is lacking most cellular biosynthetic pathways (51). This limited metabolic capacity presumably necessitates the acquisition of many essential components from the environment; consistent with this hypothesis, homologs of 16 different membrane transporters have been identified in the *B. burgdorferi* genome. Whereas genes encoding all of the enzymes of the glycolytic pathway were identified, none of the genes encoding proteins of the tricarboxylic acid cycle or oxidative phosphorylation were identified. The *B. burgdorferi* genome contains few genes that are recognizable as virulence determinants in other bacteria. A significant challenge to researchers interested in the pathogenesis of Lyme disease will be to identify the functions of a large number of gene products in order to define the molecular bases of particular phenotypes. This will require the ability to manipulate *B. burgdorferi* by a standard set of genetic techniques.

SPECIES DIVERSITY

All borreliae are transmitted by blood-feeding arthropods. Individual species of *Borrelia* differ in the arthropod vectors by which they are transmitted, their reservoir hosts, the diversity of species that they can infect, and the diseases they cause. All known species of *Borrelia* are transmitted by ticks, with only one exception, *B. recurrentis*, which is transmitted by the human body louse. These bacteria can be pathogenic for humans, domestic animals, rodents, and birds (48).

Recent studies have divided the Lyme disease spirochetes, *B. burgdorferi* sensu lato, into three separate species, *B. burgdorferi* sensu stricto, *B. garinii*, and *B. afzelii* (7). It is unclear whether they cause separate or identical diseases; however, preliminary results demonstrate that in Europe, different clinical manifestations may be associated with the three currently recognized species (138). Genetic analysis of the 16S rRNA gene of new isolates of *Borrelia* has led to the recent description and naming of many new species from ixodid ticks, although the public health significance of these spirochetes is unknown. Currently there are 36 recognized species of *Borrelia*, although 2 remain unnamed (4, 23) (Table 1). Many of the species associated with *Ornithodoros* ticks or relapsing fever cases that were established in the older literature, however, have not been isolated in pure culture or examined by the newer molecular techniques to compare their relatedness to well-characterized species.

NATURAL HABITATS

Except for *B. recurrentis* and *B. duttonii*, all species of *Borrelia* are maintained in nature by cycling through wild animals and the ticks that feed upon them. *B. recurrentis* and *B. duttonii* do not have a wild-animal reservoir (48). These two species of spirochetes infect only humans and the human body louse or *Ornithodoros moubata* ticks that feed on human blood. The ecological components that maintain *Borrelia* spp. in nature are quite diverse and widespread throughout the world (Table 1).

About two-thirds of the currently recognized species of *Borrelia* are transmitted by "soft" ticks of the family Argasidae (48). This group includes (i) the borreliae that cause tick-borne relapsing fever, which are transmitted by soft ticks of the genus *Ornithodoros* (Fig. 1A); (ii) *Borrelia coriaceae*, the putative agent of epidemic bovine abortion of cattle, which may be transmitted by *Ornithodoros coriaceus*; and (iii) *B. anserina*, the agent of fowl spirochetosis, which is transmitted by several species of soft ticks of another genus, *Argas* (Fig. 1B) (41). *B. recurrentis* also causes relapsing fever in humans but is unique among all the borreliae by not being transmitted by a tick. The sole vector of this spirochete is the human body louse, *Pediculus humanus humanus*. Although *B. recurrentis* infects mice and monkeys in the laboratory, the strict host preference of the human body louse for only humans is probably a primary factor restricting the distribution of this spirochete in nature. A recent analysis of isolates of *B. recurrentis* established from Ethiopian patients with louse-borne relapsing fever showed these spirochetes to be very closely related to the tick-borne *B. duttonii* (36, 37).

The remaining known species of *Borrelia* are transmitted by various species of "hard" ticks of the family Ixodidae. *B. burgdorferi* sensu stricto, *B. garinii*, and *B. afzelii*, the causative agents of Lyme disease and related disorders, are transmitted by numerous species of ticks in the genus *Ixodes* (Fig. 1C) (6, 73) and possibly by ticks in other genera as well (112).

Diverse vertebrate hosts are infected with borreliae in nature. With only a few exceptions, however, various species of rodents are the natural vertebrate hosts, and these rodent hosts, along with ticks, maintain most of the species of *Borrelia* in foci throughout many parts of the world (48). Except for *B. duttonii*, for which humans remain the only natural vertebrate hosts, tick-borne relapsing fever spirochetes all naturally infect small rodents. In western North America, *B. hermsii*, *B. turicatae*, and *B. parkeri* all naturally infect small rodents, primarily in the squirrel family. These three species appear to be maintained and transmitted only by their specific tick vectors, *Ornithodoros hermsi*, *Ornithodoros turicata*, and *Ornithodoros parkeri*, respectively. The unique ecological requirements of each of these species of tick therefore also influence the distribution of borreliae, the mammalian hosts infected, and the probability of humans entering the maintenance cycle and becoming infected. In

TABLE 1 Characteristics and distribution of arthropod-borne borreliae

Borrelia sp.	Arthropod vector	Animal reservoir	Distribution	Disease
B. recurrentis	*P. humanus humanus*	Humans	Worldwide	Louse-borne (epidemic) relapsing fever
B. duttonii	*O. moubata*	Humans	Central, Eastern, and Southern Africa	Tick-borne (endemic) relapsing fever
B. hispanica	*O. erraticus* (large variety)	Rodents	Spain, Portugal, Morocco, Algeria, Tunisia	Tick-borne relapsing fever
B. crocidurae, *B. merionesi*, *B. microti*, *B. dipodilli*	*O. erraticus* (small variety)	Rodents	Morocco, Libya, Egypt, Iran, Turkey, Senegal, Kenya	Tick-borne relapsing fever
B. persica	*O. tholozani* (syn. *O. papillipes*, *O. crossi?*)	Rodents	From West China and Kashmir to Iraq and Egypt, USSR, India	Tick-borne relapsing fever
B. caucasica	*O. verrucosus*	Rodents	Caucasus to Iraq	Tick-borne relapsing fever
B. latyschewii	*O. tartakowskyi*	Rodents	Iran, Central Asia	Tick-borne relapsing fever
B. hermsii	*O. hermsi*	Rodents, chipmunks, tree squirrels	Western United States	Tick-borne relapsing fever
B. turicatae	*O. turicata*	Rodents	Southwestern United States	Tick-borne relapsing fever
B. parkeri	*O. parkeri*	Rodents	Western United States	Tick-borne relapsing fever
B. mazzottii	*O. talaje* (*O. dugesi?*)	Rodents	Southern United States, Mexico, Central and South America	American tick-borne relapsing fever
B. venezuelensis	*O. rudis* (syn. *O. venezuelensis*)	Rodents	Central and South America	Tick-borne relapsing fever
B. brasiliensis	*O. brasiliensis*	?	South America (Brazil)	?
B. graingeri	*O. graingeri*	?	East Africa (Kenya)	One laboratory case
B. tillae	*O. zumpti*	Rodents	South Africa	?
B. queenslandica	*O. gurneyi*	Rodents	Australia	?
B. armenica	*O. alactagalis*	Rodents	Armenia	?
Borrelia sp. nov.	*Ornithodoros* sp. (?)	?	United States (Florida)	Canine borreliosis
Borrelia sp. nov.	*Ornithordoros* sp. (?)	?	Spain	Tick-borne relapsing fever
B. coriaceae	*O. coriaceus*	Deer (?) Cattle (?)	Western United States	Epizootic bovine abortion (?)
B. anserina	*Argas* spp.	Fowl	Worldwide	Avian borreliosis
B. burgdorferi	*I. scapularis*	Rodents	Eastern and Midwestern United States	Lyme disease
	I. pacificus	Rodents	Western United States	Lyme disease
	I. ricinus	Rodents	Europe	Lyme disease
B. garinii	*I. ricinus*	Rodents	Europe	Lyme disease
	I. uriae	Seabirds	Bipolar	?
B. afzelii	*I. persulcatus*	Rodents	Asian countries	Lyme disease
B. japonica	*I. ovatus*	Rodents	Japan	?
B. andersonii	*I. dentatus*	Rabbits	United States	?
B. miyamoti	*I. persulcatus*	Rodents	Japan	?
B. tanukii	*I. tanukii*, *I. ovatus*	Rodents	Japan	?
B. turdae	*I. turdus*	?	Japan	?
B. valaisiana	*I. ricinus*	?	The Netherlands, England, Switzerland	?
B. lusitaniae	*I. ricinus*	?	Portugal, Belorussia, Czech Republic	?
B. lonestari	*Amblyomma americanum*	?	United States	?
B. theileri	*Rhipicephalus* spp., probably other ixodid ticks	Cattle, horses, sheep	South Africa, Australia, North America, Europe	Tick spirochetosis

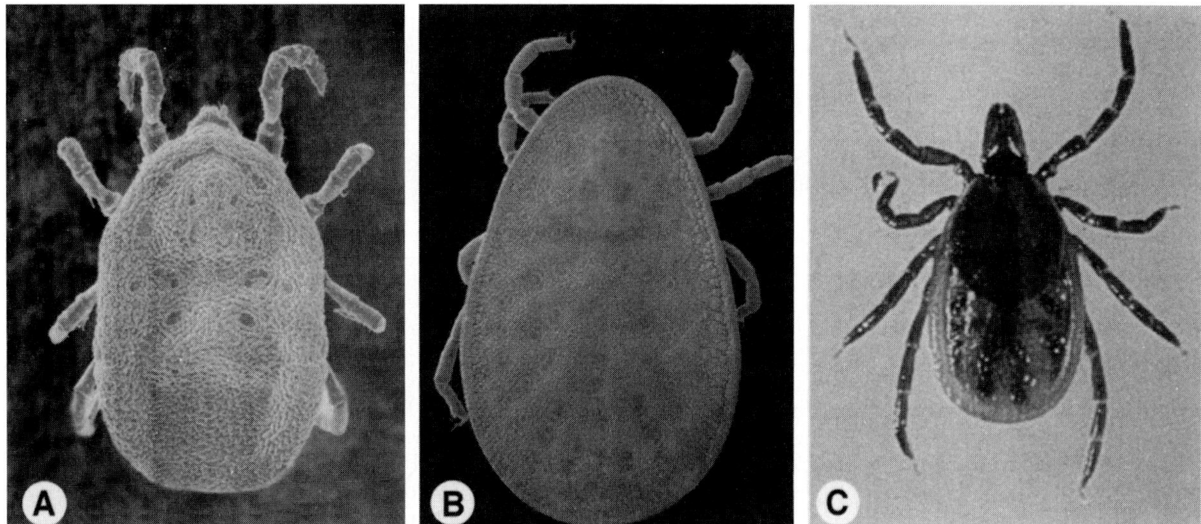

FIGURE 1 Three genera of ticks that are vectors of *Borrelia*. (A) *Ornithodoros*; (B) *Argas*; (C) *Ixodes*.

Florida, a "relapsing fever-like" *Borrelia* was isolated from a dog; however, the vector and natural reservoir for this unnamed spirochete are not known (23).

The diversity of vertebrate hosts that are naturally infected with Lyme disease spirochetes (*B. burgdorferi* sensu lato) is far greater than the types of hosts infected by any one species of relapsing fever spirochete (5, 6, 73). This diversity is probably influenced not so much by the species of mammals that the spirochetes are able to colonize but, rather, by the very different life cycles and behaviors displayed by the *Ornithodoros* and *Ixodes* ticks. *Ornithodoros* ticks (Fig. 1A) spend their entire lives in protected microhabitats closely associated with the nest or resting places of their host and source of blood. These ticks feed rapidly, usually in 10 to 45 min and usually at night, and for the rest of the time remain away from their hosts. All stages of these ticks, including larvae, multiple nymphs, and adults, most probably feed on the same species of mammal and are unlikely to be dispersed widely by the movements of their hosts.

The *Ixodes* ticks (Fig. 1C) that transmit Lyme disease spirochetes have life cycles and behaviors very different from those of the relapsing fever ticks. The specificity displayed by many of the relapsing fever borreliae for a single species of tick is not true for the Lyme disease spirochetes. *Ixodes* ticks are called "three-host" ticks, since each of the three stages in the life cycle (larva, single nymph, and adult) feeds on a different host (129). For the *Ixodes* species associated with Lyme disease, the larvae and nymphs feed primarily on small rodents. Many species of mammals as well as birds may be hosts for these ticks, and adult ticks feed primarily on a variety of mammal species, including deer, raccoons, domestic and wild carnivores, and larger domestic mammals such as horses. These *Ixodes* ticks all feed for prolonged periods, thus contributing significantly to their own dispersal in association with the movement of their host. They thereby encounter a greater diversity of hosts to subsequently feed upon. As a result, many species of small to large mammals play a role both in maintaining Lyme disease spirochetes in nature and in serving as hosts for the ticks that transmit these bacteria. The recent findings of Lyme disease spirochetes associated with seabirds and the seabird tick, *Ixodes uriae*, in the higher latitudes of both hemispheres add to an increasingly complex natural cycle for these spirochetes (94, 95).

All vectors become infected by ingesting spirochetes while feeding on the blood of an infected mammal or bird. Some species of ticks may also pass spirochetes to the next generation via eggs, a phenomenon referred to as vertical or transovarial transmission. This type of transmission has the potential to maintain spirochetal infections in ticks without the necessity for the ticks to feed on infectious vertebrate hosts. Although transovarial transmission of *B. burgdorferi* has been reported (71, 101), it is rare and has no importance in maintaining the spirochetes in nature.

The transmission of spirochetes from the arthropod vector to susceptible vertebrate hosts varies somewhat among the three types of vectors and is influenced by the type of infection established in the arthropod. *B. recurrentis*, the etiologic agent of louse-borne relapsing fever, is unique both in its vector, the human body louse, and in the way in which the spirochete is transmitted by this insect (28). In the louse, the spirochetes establish an infection restricted to the hemolymph and are absent from the salivary glands; hence, they are not transmitted by bite via saliva. Humans become infected only when body lice carrying the spirochetes are crushed, rupturing the outer skeleton and releasing the spirochetes onto the skin, where they will enter the body through either broken or intact skin (28).

The soft ticks that transmit the relapsing fever spirochetes do so primarily by bite via infected saliva. After ingestion by a soft tick, the borreliae penetrate the gut wall and disseminate to several organs, including the ovaries, synganglion (central ganglion), salivary glands, and sometimes also the coxal glands. Although *Ornithodoros* and *Argas* ticks (Fig. 1A and B) feed rapidly, transmission results either from the direct inoculation of infected saliva or from contamination of the bite wound with infected coxal fluid, which is excreted from pores near the base of each front leg of the tick (hard ticks do not have coxal glands).

In *Ixodes* ticks infected with *B. burgdorferi*, the spirochetes are usually restricted to the midgut during periods

TABLE 2 Human borrelioses, the arthropod vectors, and modes of spirochetal transmission

Disease	Vector		
	Arthropod species	Life stages	Mode of transmission
Louse-borne relapsing fever	Human body louse (*Pediculus humanus humanus*)	Nymphs and adults	Contamination with infected hemolymph
Tick-borne relapsing fever	Soft ticks (*Ornithodoros* spp.)	Nymphs and adults	Saliva and coxal fluid
Lyme disease	Hard ticks (*Ixodes* spp.)	Nymphs and adults	Saliva

when the ticks are off their hosts (25). However, during tick engorgement, spirochetes multiply and penetrate the midgut to invade the hemolymph and spread to the salivary glands, from which they may be transmitted via saliva that is secreted during the later stages of tick feeding (102, 142). The arthropod vectors and modes of spirochetal transmission associated with the human borrelioses are summarized in Table 2.

Several studies have demonstrated that transmission of *B. burgdorferi* seldom occurs during the first 24 to 48 h of tick feeding (102), although a recent laboratory study in Germany demonstrated that infected nymphal *I. ricinus* ticks transmitted spirochetes to approximately 50% of gerbils after only 16 h of attachment (66). As ticks feed for longer periods, however, the frequency with which *Ixodes* ticks infect mammalian hosts increases dramatically (102).

CLINICAL SIGNIFICANCE

Relapsing Fever in Humans

Relapsing fever in humans is a febrile, septicemic disease with sudden onset after an incubation period of 2 to 15 days. Fever persists for 3 to 7 days and is followed by an afebrile interval of several days to several weeks. Thereafter, as many as 13 relapses may occur, especially in untreated patients, as a result of antigenic variations in the causative borreliae. Detailed clinical descriptions of relapsing fever in humans have been presented elsewhere (24, 45, 130). During the acute, febrile episodes, patients may also experience shaking chills, severe headache, myalgias, arthralgias, nausea, and vomiting. A skin rash that is quite variable in form and may resemble the erythema migrans lesion associated with Lyme disease has also been reported for 28% of relapsing fever patients. Pregnant women who contract relapsing fever may abort their fetus or give birth to an infant infected via transplacental transmission (65). Long-term or chronic clinical manifestations may involve the respiratory and cardiovascular systems as well as the central nervous system (29). Such chronic cases of relapsing fever may resemble and be confused with chronic Lyme disease (74).

According to medical history, more than 50 million persons contracted louse-borne relapsing fever during the first half of this century, with epidemics occurring throughout Europe, Africa, Asia, and South America. Since 1967, however, louse-borne relapsing fever has been reported primarily from African countries, with the highest incidence occurring regularly in the highlands of Ethiopia.

Because of the sporadic occurrence of tick-borne relapsing fevers, extremely little is known about their incidence worldwide. In the United States during the period 1964 to 1993, 512 cases of tick-borne relapsing fever were recognized. Most occurred within the distributional area of *O. hermsi*, and a few occurred also within that of *O. turicata*. Outbreaks usually are sporadic and rarely involve more than two persons. Outbreaks involving a larger number have been recorded occasionally, with reports from the Pacific Northwest (137) as well as the Southwest, including the Grand Canyon (22). A recent retrospective analysis of patient histories within the Pacific Northwest identified 182 cases from 1980 to 1995, with the area of highest incidence occurring in northern Idaho and eastern Washington (45). Tick-borne relapsing fever is underreported in the United States because it is seldom recognized. Most patients are unaware of a tick bite, and unless a history of wilderness exposure, camping, or spending nights in old, rodent-infested cabins is given, the disease is rarely suspected during the initial period of fever (50).

Lyme Disease in Humans

Lyme disease is an endemic inflammatory disorder that usually begins in summer with the distinctive skin lesion erythema migrans, which occurs in 60 to 80% of patients and is often accompanied by headache, stiff neck, myalgias, arthralgias, malaise, fatigue, or swelling of the lymph nodes (131). Weeks to months later, some patients develop meningoencephalitis, myocarditis, or migrating musculoskeletal pain. Still later, patients may develop intermittent attacks of oligoarticular arthritis or chronic arthritis in the large joints, particularly the knees. First described after an outbreak among children in Lyme, Conn., in 1975 (132), the disease appears to be more severe than erythema chronicum migrans, a tick-borne associated syndrome observed as early as 1908 in Europe (2). The etiologic agent, *B. burgdorferi*, remained obscure until 1981, when it was discovered in *Ixodes scapularis* (= *Ixodes dammini*) in New York (26) and later in the European tick vector *Ixodes ricinus*. Other clinical syndromes in Europe that appear to be related to the same agent include lymphocytoma (lymphadenosis benigna cutis), acrodermatitis chronica atrophicans, tick-borne meningoradiculitis (Garin-Bujadoux-Bannwarth syndrome), and myositis (2, 106, 138).

While human cases of Lyme disease have been reported from most of the 48 contiguous United States, most cases have been from three geographical areas: the Northeast and Midwest, where *I. scapularis* is the principal vector; and the West, where *I. pacificus* carries the spirochete. Between 1975 and 1979, a total of 512 cases of Lyme disease were diagnosed. Of these, 503 occurred in northeastern, 5 in midwestern, and 4 in western states. In 1980, 226 cases of Lyme disease came to the attention of the Centers for Disease Control in Atlanta. In 1982, after the discovery of the causative agent, Lyme disease became a reportable disease and surveillance was intensified. Since then, the number of reported cases in the United States has increased, and nearly 98,000 human cases were reported from 1982 through 1996, with the highest incidence in Connecticut, New York, Rhode Island, and New Jersey.

Borrelioses in Animals

Borrelioses in rodents and lagomorphs may be similar to the diseases observed in humans. There may be one or more relapses accompanied by spirochetemias of various degrees. Not all animals are equally susceptible to the various *Borrelia* species, and even differences in susceptibility to various isolates of a single species of spirochete may be seen. Young animals are generally more susceptible and may die of the disease.

Avian borreliosis, caused by *B. anserina*, affects geese, ducks, turkeys, and chickens throughout the world and has been economically important in certain countries because it has caused severe losses to the poultry industry. Clinically, the disease begins with a high fever after an incubation period of about 4 days. The birds become cyanotic and have yellowish green diarrhea. During the early stages of the febrile reaction, spirochetes can be readily detected in the blood, and young birds can demonstrate incredibly high spirochetemias before death. Surviving birds recover after about 2 weeks and have long-lasting immunity. This disease of domestic birds is much less of a problem today because of the improved husbandry practices associated with commercial rearing of chickens and turkeys.

Tick spirochetosis caused by *B. theileri* in cattle, horses, and sheep in South Africa and recently also in Australia is a benign disease characterized by one to two attacks of fever, inappetence, weight loss, weakness, and anemia.

The Lyme disease spirochete, *B. burgdorferi*, does not adversely affect wild animals. However, it has been reported to cause arthritic manifestations with lameness, stiffness, and swollen joints in dogs, cows, and horses (27, 79, 80). White-footed mice (*Peromyscus leucopus*), once infected, probably remain so for their entire lives, although there are fluctuations in the percentage of ticks that become infected while feeding upon them (25, 76).

A *Borrelia* spirochete has also been isolated from *O. coriaceus*, the soft tick implicated as a vector of epizootic bovine abortion, which is a major disease of rangeland cattle in the western United States (72). Genetic and phenotypic characteristics revealed that this spirochete is a new species, named *B. coriaceae* (62). As yet, there is only circumstantial evidence that this organism is causally related to epizootic abortion, and as of 1998, no additional isolates of this spirochete have been described.

ANIMAL MODELS

Rabbits, hamsters, gerbils, mice, rats, dogs, and nonhuman primates are susceptible to *B. burgdorferi* infection and have been useful in studies related to the pathogenicity of this agent, pathogenesis of the disease and various clinical manifestations, treatment, and efficacy of vaccines (17, 34, 64, 88, 89, 99, 123).

COLLECTION, TRANSPORT, AND STORAGE OF SPECIMENS

Relapsing fever spirochetes can be isolated from infected ticks or lice, from human blood of patients with acute disease, or from the appropriate wild mammalian reservoir. Given the difficulty of collecting *Ornithodoros* ticks and the short time when wild mammals have spirochetes circulating in their peripheral blood, human patients acutely ill with relapsing fever are often the best sources for acquiring new isolates of these spirochetes.

The Lyme disease spirochetes *B. burgdorferi* sensu stricto, *B. garinii*, and *B. afzelii* can all be acquired from infected *Ixodes* ticks, various infected tissues of mammalian reservoirs, or human patients. Because this group of *Borrelia* spp. does not frequently produce detectable spirochetemias in mammals, blood does not yield spirochetes as often as other tissues such as the skin, urinary bladder, heart, and spleen (64, 115, 128). Although these spirochetes have been isolated from human blood, skin biopsy samples taken just outside the periphery of an erythema migrans lesion have been the best sources. For this procedure, the surface of the skin is disinfected with povidone-iodine (Betadine solution) and the 2-mm skin biopsy specimen is collected, placed directly into Barbour-Stoenner-Kelly (BSK) medium, and incubated at 33 to 35°C. If the specimen requires transportation to another location for culture, it should be sent in BSK or brain heart infusion medium on ice packs by overnight courier and then transferred to fresh BSK medium for incubation. Lyme disease spirochetes have also been isolated from human cerebrospinal fluid and only rarely from other tissues and fluids.

The maintenance of infectious spirochetes requires the use of laboratory animals such as rats or mice or live colonies of infected ticks. Relapsing fever spirochetes can be kept alive for several months in clotted whole blood collected from the infected mammal and held at 4°C. Repeated reinoculation of mice and subsequent storage of frozen blood can be used to maintain spirochetes in the laboratory for long periods. Vector ticks infected with their associated spirochetes (by feeding on infective mice) can be held for either one generation (*Ixodes* ticks) or months to several years (*Ornithodoros* ticks), thus maintaining infections of these bacteria that can then be passed into mice by inoculation or tick feeding. Lyme disease spirochetes can also be inoculated into laboratory mice, hamsters, or white-footed mice, which will probably remain infected for their entire lives and can be the source of *B. burgdorferi* through culture of their infected tissues.

DETECTION AND ISOLATION PROCEDURES

Detection

Diagnosis of clinical cases of relapsing fever and avian spirochetosis is based primarily on the detection of spirochetes in the peripheral blood of febrile persons and animals. During acute phases of relapsing fever, large numbers of spirochetes may circulate in the blood and can be detected by light or dark-field microscopy of wet preparations made from a drop of whole blood. Leishman, Giemsa, May-Grunwald, Wright, and other combinations of Romanowsky stains are used to stain thin- and thick-drop films for examination by conventional light microscopy (Fig. 2). Because microscopic detection of spirochetes requires that at least 10^4 to 10^5 organisms per ml of blood be present, spirochetes in the blood of mildly infected persons may be more readily detected by a microhematocrit concentration technique (52). For this technique, approximately three-fourths of a microhematocrit capillary tube is filled with citrated blood and centrifuged in a microhematocrit centrifuge for 2 min, and then the region of the tube containing the buffy coat is examined directly under a microscope at ×400 to ×1,000. Lyme disease spirochetes usually do not produce a microscopically detectable spirochetemia in humans or wild animals.

B. burgdorferi can be detected in tissue sections by light

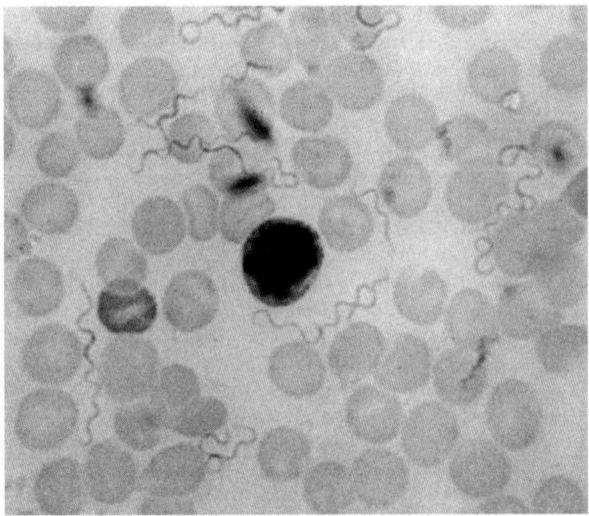

FIGURE 2 *B. hermsii* in a thin smear of rodent blood. Giemsa stain. Magnification, ×1,000.

microscopy involving various staining methods. The Warthin-Starry silver stain has been used often (19), as have immunologic stains that use fluoresceinated polyclonal antiserum. Staining indirectly with species-specific monoclonal antibodies followed by a secondary fluoresceinated antibody has the potential to both detect and identify spirochetes in clinical samples (15, 21, 96, 117). Such an approach, however, is costly and labor-intensive, preventing the use of this method in diagnostic laboratories.

Another strategy for the detection of *Borrelia* spp. has been to demonstrate the presence of DNA specific for certain species of spirochete. Hybridization probes were developed first to specifically identify the purified DNAs of *B. burgdorferi* and *B. hermsii* as well as whole spirochetes (121, 125). Although the probes were highly specific, their sensitivities were unsatisfactory, requiring a minimum of 2,800 to 10,000 spirochetes for detection. Subsequently, PCR-based assays specific for *B. burgdorferi* were developed. These assays are capable of detecting only one to five spirochetes (109), of classifying or typing spirochetes (86, 108), and of identifying the three currently recognized species, *B. burgdorferi*, *B. garinii*, and *B. afzelii* (84). Other workers have further developed PCR assays, amplifying other regions of the spirochete genome to identify *B. burgdorferi* DNA (82, 91) and to detect the spirochete in ticks (98) or in the urine or cerebrospinal fluid of human patients with Lyme disease (54, 92). Currently, the Mayo Clinic in Rochester, Minn., offers PCR for the laboratory confirmation of Lyme disease. The utility and sensitivity of PCR for detecting spirochetes in patients with chronic Lyme disease require further evaluation. The assay is hindered by the paucity of organisms in infected tissues and by potential contamination in the laboratory setting.

Isolation

In vitro cultivation of borreliae in liquid medium was first demonstrated by Kelly in 1971 (68). The medium currently used by most workers to isolate and maintain many species of *Borrelia* in the laboratory is BSK II medium (8, 12). A commercial preparation of the complete medium, BSK-H, is available from Sigma Chemical Co., St. Louis, Mo. The spirochetes are cultured most successfully when the medium has a neutral pH and is incubated in a microaerophilic environment at 30 to 37°C. The culture medium is monitored for spirochetes by dark-field microscopy for 4 to 6 weeks; cultures may be positive in less than a week or may require many months if the medium lacks gelatin and rabbit serum and is incubated at temperatures lower than 30°C (77). Once isolated in the medium, the spirochetes may be identified by reactivity with species-specific monoclonal antibodies, although hybridization with specific DNA probes or amplification of specific DNA by PCR can be done. Cultures of borreliae can be stored for several years at −70°C by adding a cryopreservative such as glycerol (10 to 20% final concentration) to the medium.

Various modifications of BSK medium have also been used successfully for the cultivation of borreliae from ticks as well as from human and other animal tissues. Borreliae are resistant to rifampin and phosphomycin, and these antibiotics can be added to the BSK-II medium (50 and 100 μg/ml, respectively) to reduce contamination of cultures by other bacteria. Amphotericin B (10 μg/ml) is also useful for reducing fungal contamination, especially when one is attempting to isolate borreliae from triturates of entire ticks. Various solidified media have been used to successfully grow *B. burgdorferi* (105), with recipes based on PMR (Preac-Mursic) and BSK media providing the greatest efficacy. Solid plating and serial dilution in liquid medium have been used to establish cultures of clonal populations of these spirochetes (69, 107, 120). Continuous serial passage for even short periods, however, may effect many biological changes in the spirochetes, thereby altering their phenotypic and genotypic characteristics (113, 114). However, cocultivation of *B. burgdorferi* with tick cells was shown to prolong spirochetal infectivity (70).

Animal Inoculation

Before the development of a successful culture medium, inoculation of susceptible laboratory animals for recovery of spirochetes was the only method available. Today, animal inoculation is not necessary to isolate Lyme disease spirochetes, since the BSK-II medium performs well for growth of these spirochetes from primary clinical, mammal, and tick sources. However, relapsing fever spirochetes are difficult to establish in culture when one is attempting to isolate them directly from infected human blood. Often, amplification of these spirochetes in laboratory mice followed by inoculation of fresh, infected mouse blood into BSK-II medium is required.

IDENTIFICATION

Historically, taxonomic identification of borreliae, particularly the relapsing fever spirochetes, has depended heavily on their geographical distribution and the natural arthropod vectors (39). This assumed specificity, however, does not always hold true. Thus, for most cases of tick-borne relapsing fevers, taxonomic identification of the etiologic agent is presumptive and is based on a history of exposure to a particular vector.

Morphologic criteria are not sufficient to distinguish among the species of *Borrelia*. Comparisons of total DNA by hybridization studies discriminate between the relapsing fever and Lyme disease spirochetes but may be of limited utility in distinguishing among the various species of relapsing fever spirochetes (59, 63). The development of methods that permit the identification of different relapsing fever species is hindered by the paucity of such isolates from clinical or natural sources. One monoclonal antibody that distinguishes *B. hermsii* from other species of *Borrelia* has been described (117), and such reagents for the specific identification of other relapsing fever spirochetes would be desirable.

Several molecular procedures to identify *B. burgdorferi* and to differentiate it from other pathogenic spirochetes are available (59, 121, 125), although as more species become named, their precise identification becomes more cumbersome. *B. burgdorferi* can be directly identified in tick midguts by fluorescent staining with species-specific monoclonal antibodies that recognize spirochetal outer surface proteins. It is also possible to identify *B. burgdorferi* in ticks by using PCR with specific primers. Direct identification of *B. burgdorferi* in clinical material by PCR is possible but is currently performed in only a few diagnostic laboratories. Methods to distinguish between *B. burgdorferi* and other borreliae include DNA probes and PCR assays based on sequences encoding flagellin (100), 16S rRNA (98), outer surface proteins (98), or other targets (54), as well as on the reactivity of bacterial isolates on immunoblots with species-specific monoclonal antibodies.

SEROLOGIC TESTS

Serologic confirmation of borrelioses is based on a diagnostic change in the titer of antibodies specific to the agent when sequential sera from a patient are compared. In the absence of an acute-phase serum sample, a single convalescent-phase serum sample with an antibody titer of 1:128 to 1:256 or above may be acceptable for confirmation of the diagnosis. However, many species of relapsing fever spirochetes have not yet been successfully isolated and maintained in artificial culture and are therefore not available for use as antigens in serologic tests. When a clinical history suggests an infection with borreliae not yet isolated, other available species can be useful as the test antigen due to considerable shared antigenicity among borrelial proteins. Promising results have been obtained by the indirect immunofluorescence assay (IFA) with cultured spirochetes as antigens, although specificity in such assays is lacking.

Lyme disease spirochetes are difficult to detect in human patients, and serologic tests are therefore the most practical and readily available methods for confirming the infection. Numerous types of serologic tests for Lyme disease have been described in the scientific literature, and new test kits have quickly inundated an increasingly competitive commercial market. Numerous reviews and editorials that describe some of these tests, their potential problems, and the lack of standardization have been published (10, 11, 44, 46).

The IFA uses Lyme disease spirochetes as a substrate fixed onto a glass microscope slide. While this test is easy to perform, there are problems with its specificity, reproducibility, and usefulness when large numbers of samples have to be tested, as well as in its subjective interpretation and lack of quantification. Owing to the presence of nonspecific antibodies in some normal serum samples, most workers require that a positive sample be reactive when diluted 1:256 or more, although not everyone adheres to this threshold for a positive result. Unfortunately, a titer of 256 or higher may occur if the patient has been exposed to other species of spirochetes or to even more distantly related bacteria that share antigens with the Lyme disease spirochete (10). Therefore, a patient who has not been exposed to *B. burgdorferi* but who has had tick-borne relapsing fever, syphilis, leptospirosis, or periodontal disease may have antibodies that react positively in a Lyme test (81). Visual determination of the titer end point is also somewhat subjective.

The enzyme-linked immunosorbent assay (ELISA), or enzyme immunoassay, is probably the most widely used serologic test for confirming Lyme disease in laboratories where large numbers of samples are routinely tested (10, 18, 78). The advantages of this type of assay over the IFA are the ability to quickly test many samples and the use of a spectrophotometric determination that is quantifiable and subject to statistical analysis. The assay in its simplest form uses microtiter plates in which wells are coated with either intact spirochetes or a suspension of spirochetal antigens produced by disrupting the bacteria by sonication. While this method is fast, efficient for testing many samples, and quantifiable with less subjective error, it has the same weaknesses of specificity as the IFA (81) and has become even less standardized than the IFA. As mentioned above, sera from patients exposed to some other pathogenic bacteria may give false-positive reactions. Also, there is considerable variation in how the ELISA is done and how the results are reported.

Because of the poor specificity of both the IFA and the ELISA, the Western immunoblot technique, considered by some investigators to be the "gold standard," can be more beneficial than these assays, especially in the diagnosis of patients with atypical clinical manifestations who live in areas where the disease is currently considered nonendemic. If the test is done properly, a negative serum sample can be identified with a high degree of confidence, although "seronegative Lyme disease" remains controversial for some clinicians and patient advocacy groups. Variation in banding patterns resulting from antibodies binding to one or more of the antigens raises the concern of what is really positive. Considerable differences in the reagents and methods used subject this procedure to the same types of interlaboratory variation that exist for the ELISA. However, several recent studies have addressed the use of Western blotting for the serodiagnosis of Lyme disease and have established criteria for defining positive reactivities in such tests (42, 43, 47, 60).

The potential lack of specificity for the IFA and ELISA described above has led investigators to search for components of the bacterium that can be used as diagnostic antigens to improve the specificities and sensitivities of serologic tests. Specific antigens have been obtained either by lysing the spirochetes and then selectively purifying the target antigen (35, 55, 67) or by using recombinant DNA techniques to clone genes, thereby expressing a specific spirochetal antigen in a foreign bacterial cell such as *Escherichia coli* (75, 124, 127). One such antigen, GlpQ of *B. hermsii*, is conserved among relapsing fever spirochetes but is absent in Lyme disease spirochetes and is highly immunogenic during infection in humans and other animals (119). This antigen has the potential to retrospectively identify true cases of relapsing fever, regardless of the infecting species, and to distinguish such cases from cases of Lyme disease. This antigen is not yet commercially available but is being developed into the ELISA format at the Rocky Mountain Laboratories for diagnostic use.

ANTIBIOTIC SUSCEPTIBILITIES

Many antibiotics are available to successfully treat borrelial infections; however, the choice of antibiotic, dosage, and duration and route of treatment are controversial, especially for Lyme disease. Tetracyclines are the drugs of choice in treating relapsing fever (48). They reduce the relapse rate and rid the central nervous system of spirochetes. However, the rapid destruction of organisms may provoke a severe Jarisch-Herxheimer reaction, and some antibiotics appear to promote a more severe reaction than others. Good results have been obtained with 0.5 g of tetracycline given orally every 6 h for 4 to 5 days or with a single oral dose of 100 mg of doxycycline. To avoid the Jarisch-Herxheimer reaction, a combined penicillin-tetracycline therapeutic regimen is recommended. It consists of 400,000 U of procaine penicillin administered intramuscularly followed the next day by 500 mg of tetracycline given orally every 6 h for 7 days (111).

Although all stages of Lyme disease may respond to antibiotic therapy, treatment regimens depend on the nature and severity of clinical manifestations (1, 90, 131). Antibiotics given early in the disease shorten the duration of the rash and prevent later illness, although some patients with severe early disease develop manifestations later despite recommended courses of antibiotics. Men, nonpregnant women, and children with early disease, mild neurological symptoms, and/or minor cardiac involvement have been treated orally with doxycycline (100 mg twice daily) or tetracycline HCl (250 to 500 mg three times daily) given for 10 to 30 days. Amoxicillin (250 to 500 mg three times daily, or 20 to 40 mg/kg of body weight per day for children) given for 10 to 30 days is also effective and is preferred for children under 8 years of age and for pregnant and lactating women. For patients who cannot take tetracycline and are allergic to penicillin, erythromycin at 250 mg four times daily (or 30 mg/kg/day for children) is recommended.

Patients with late neurological (focal central nervous system involvement) complications, severe Lyme arthritis, or severe cardiac involvement may require intravenous application of penicillin G or ceftriaxone. Whether "treatment failure" of some cases of late-stage Lyme disease actually reflects "true failure" or results instead from an initial misdiagnosis of Lyme disease is difficult to assess. A recent study examining Lyme disease in experimentally infected dogs suggests that treatment failure following high doses of amoxicillin or doxycycline may occur (135).

Borreliae are resistant to rifampin, phosphomycin, sulfonamides, and 5-fluorouracil (14). The molecular basis for these resistances is unknown; however, as discussed above, they have been useful when isolating borreliae from samples contaminated with other bacteria.

PREVENTION

Currently the most effective means of protection from Lyme disease is to reduce the exposure of humans to infected ixodid ticks. This is done by reducing one's activity in tick-infested areas, wearing protective clothing, using repellents, and performing frequent checks while in tick-infested areas to prevent ticks from attaching and feeding. Immunization with Bacterin, a whole-cell vaccine of inactivated *B. burgdorferi*, has been used in a commercial vaccine for dogs. Recombinant vaccines prepared from the spirochete's outer surface protein A (OspA) have now been tested in monkeys (99) and humans and are awaiting evaluation and approval by the U.S. Food and Drug Administration.

Tick-borne relapsing fever is most often acquired at night, when humans are asleep and fed upon by the infective, fast-feeding *Ornithodoros* ticks. Tick and rodent control in areas of endemic infection may help reduce the risk of infection but is practical only in small, restricted areas such as cabins and established campgrounds. No vaccines have been developed for relapsing fever.

EVALUATION, INTERPRETATION, AND REPORTING OF RESULTS

Tick-borne relapsing fever in the United States is not a reportable disease except in California, Idaho, Washington, Utah, and Texas. Therefore, the disease is certainly underrecognized, both in the United States and in other regions of the world where it is endemic. A presumptive diagnosis of human cases is based primarily on recurrent febrile episodes following exposure to habitats where infected *Ornithodoros* ticks (or infected human body lice) are known to occur. Cases are confirmed by demonstrating spirochetes in a smear made with blood collected during a febrile episode. Retrospective serologic confirmation of relapsing fever is now possible with the use of the recently identified GlpQ antigen (119).

Lyme disease is now reportable throughout the United States. Case recognition and reporting rely heavily on positive serologic test results (in lieu of detection or isolation of spirochetes) and clinical manifestations involving organ systems that are considered consistent for this disease. Therefore, unlike procedures for relapsing fever, serologic testing, evaluation, and reporting for Lyme disease have placed heavy demands on diagnostic laboratories. Because of the lack of standardization of the commonly used serologic tests (IFA and ELISA) and the significantly high frequency of false-positive results due to cross-reactive antibodies to other bacteria, the interpretation of a positive Lyme disease titer is very difficult without the patient's history. Thus, for many clinicians in areas where the disease is endemic, the diagnosis of Lyme disease is often based solely on clinical presentation with a possible exposure to or known history of *Ixodes* tick bite. A greater problem arises in regions where Lyme disease spirochetes and a proven vector are not yet known to occur. In such areas, caution must be taken not to place too much significance on a borderline or moderately positive titer to *B. burgdorferi* in the sera of patients who present with clinical manifestations similar to one of the many conditions described for Lyme disease. In such circumstances, second-step testing by Western blotting is required. Serologic tests that use single or multiple recombinant antigens with much greater specificities than tests with entire spirochetes as antigens are becoming available. With the emphasis on Western blotting and the use of recombinant antigens, these tests will become much more reliable and will either confirm or rule out a presumptive diagnosis of Lyme disease.

REFERENCES

1. **Abramowicz, M.** 1989. Treatment of Lyme disease. *Med. Lett.* **31:**57–59.
2. **Afzelius, A.** 1921. Erythema chronicum migrans. *Acta Dermatol. Venereol.* **2:**120–125.
3. **Akins, D. R., S. F. Porcella, T. Popova, D. Shevchenko, S. Baker, M. Li, M. V. Norgard, and J. D. Radolf.** 1995. Evidence for in vivo but not in vitro expression of a *Borrelia burgdorferi* outer surface protein F (OspF) homologue. *Mol. Microbiol.* **18:**507–520.
4. **Anda, P., W. Sanchez-Yebra, M. Del Mar Vitutia, E. P. Pastrana, I. Rodríguez, N. S. Miller, P. B. Backenson, and J. L. Benach.** 1996. A new *Borrelia* species isolated from patients with relapsing fever in Spain. *Lancet* **348:** 162–165.

5. **Anderson, J. F.** 1988. Mammalian and avian reservoirs of *Borrelia burgdorferi*. *Ann. N. Y. Acad. Sci.* **539:**180–191.
6. **Anderson, J. F.** 1989. Epizootiology of *Borrelia* in *Ixodes* tick vectors and reservoir hosts. *Rev. Infect. Dis.* **11:** 1451–1459.
7. **Baranton, G., D. Postic, I. Saint-Girons P. Boerlin, J. C. Piffaretti, M. Assous, and P. A. D. Grimont.** 1992. Delineation of *Borrelia burgdorferi* sensu stricto, *Borrelia garinii* sp. nov., and group VS461 associated with Lyme borreliosis. *Int. J. Syst. Bacteriol.* **42:**378–383.
8. **Barbour, A. G.** 1984. Isolation and cultivation of Lyme disease spirochetes. *Yale J. Biol. Med.* **57:**521–525.
9. **Barbour, A. G.** 1988. Plasmid analysis of *Borrelia burgdorferi*, the Lyme disease agent. *J. Clin. Microbiol.* **26:**475–478.
10. **Barbour, A. G.** 1988. Laboratory aspects of Lyme borreliosis. *Clin. Microbiol. Rev.* **1:**399–414.
11. **Barbour, A. G.** 1989. The diagnosis of Lyme disease: rewards and perils. *Ann. Intern. Med.* **110:**501–502.
12. **Barbour, A. G., W. Burgdorfer, S. F. Hayes, O. Peter, and A. Aeschlimann.** 1983. Isolation of a cultivable spirochete from Ixodes ricinus ticks of Switzerland. *Curr. Microbiol.* **8:**123–126.
13. **Barbour, A. G., and C. F. Garon.** 1987. Linear plasmids of the bacterium *Borrelia burgdorferi* have covalently closed ends. *Science* **237:**409–411.
14. **Barbour, A. G., and S. F. Hayes.** 1986. Biology of *Borrelia* species. *Microbiol. Rev.* **50:**381–400.
15. **Barbour, A. G., S. F. Hayes, R. A. Heiland, M. E. Schrumpf, and S. L. Tessier.** 1986. A Borrelia-specific monoclonal antibody binds to a flagellar epitope. *Infect. Immun.* **52:**549–554.
16. **Baril, C., C. Richaud, G. Baranton, and I. Saint Girons.** 1989. Linear chromosomes of *Borrelia burgdorferi*. *Res. Microbiol.* **140:**507–516.
17. **Barthold, S. W.** 1996. Lyme borreliosis in the laboratory mouse. *J. Spirochetal Tick-Borne Dis.* **3:**22–44.
18. **Berardi, V. P., K. E. Weeks, and A. C. Steere.** 1988. Serodiagnosis of early Lyme disease: analysis of IgM and IgG antibody responses by using an antibody-capture enzyme immunoassay. *J. Infect. Dis.* **158:**754–760.
19. **Berger, B. W.** 1989. Dermatologic manifestations of Lyme disease. *Rev. Infect. Dis.* **11:**S1475–S1481.
20. **Bergström, S., V. Bundoc, and A. G. Barbour.** 1989. Molecular analysis of linear plasmid-encoded major surface proteins, OspA and OspB, of the Lyme disease spirochete *Borrelia burgdorferi*. *Mol. Microbiol.* **3:**479–486.
21. **Blanchard-Channell, M., and J. L. Stott.** 1991. Characterization of *Borrelia coriaceae* antigens with monoclonal antibodies. *Infect. Immun.* **59:**2790–2798.
22. **Boyer, K. M., R. S. Munford, G. O. Maupin, C. P. Pattison, M. D. Fox, A. M. Barnes, W. L. Jones, and J. E. Maynard.** 1977. Tick-borne relapsing fever: an interstate outbreak originating at Grand Canyon National Park. *Am. J. Epidemol.* **105:**469–479.
23. **Breitschwerdt, E. B., W. L. Nicholson, A. R. Kiehl, C. Steers, D. J. Meuten, and J. F. Levine.** 1994. Natural infections with *Borrelia* spirochetes in two dogs from Florida. *J. Clin. Microbiol.* **32:**352–357.
24. **Bryceson, A. D. E., E. H. O. Parry, P. L. Perine, D. A. Warrell, D. Vukotich, and C. S. Leithead.** 1970. Louse-borne relapsing fever. A clinical and laboratory study of 62 cases in Ethiopia and a reconsideration of the literature. *J. Med.* **39:**129–170.
25. **Burgdorfer, W.** 1989. Vector/host relationships of the Lyme disease spirochete, *Borrelia burgdorferi*. *Rheum. Dis. Clin. North Am.* **15:**775–787.
26. **Burgdorfer, W., A. G. Barbour, S. F. Hayes, J. L. Benach, E. Grunwaldt, and J. P. Davis.** 1982. Lyme disease—a tick-borne spirochetosis? *Science* **216:**1317–1319.
27. **Burgess, E. C.** 1988. *Borrelia burgdorferi* infection in Wisconsin horses and cows. *Ann. N. Y. Acad. Sci.* **539:** 235–243.
28. **Buxton, P. A.** 1946. *The Louse: an Account of the Lice Which Infest Man. Their Medical Importance and Control*, p. 1–164. The Williams & Wilkins Co., Baltimore, Md.
29. **Cadavid, D., and A. G. Barbour.** 1998. Neuroborreliosis during relapsing fever: review of the clinical manifestations, pathology, and treatment of infections of humans and experimental animals. *Clin. Infect. Dis.* **26:**151–164.
30. **Casjens, S., and W. M. Huang.** 1993. Linear chromosomal physical and genetic map of *Borrelia burgdorferi*, the Lyme disease agent. *Mol. Microbiol.* **8:**967–980.
31. **Casjens, S., H. Ley, M. DeLange, P. Rosa, and W. Huang.** 1995. Linear chromosomes of Lyme disease agent spirochetes: genetic diversity and conservation of gene order. *J. Bacteriol.* **177:**2769–2780.
32. **Casjens, S., M. Murphy, M. DeLange, L. Sampson, R. van Vugt, and W. M. Huang.** 1997. Telomeres of the linear chromosome of Lyme disease spirochaetes: nucleotide sequence and possible exchange with linear plasmid telomeres. *Mol. Microbiol.* **26:**581–596.
33. **Casjens, S., R. van Vugt, K. Tilly, P. Rosa, and B. Stevenson.** 1997. Homology throughout the multiple 32-kilobase circular plasmids present in Lyme disease spirochetes. *J. Bacteriol.* **179:**217–227.
34. **Chang, Y.-F., R. K. Straubinger, R. H. Jacobson, J. B. Kim, T. J. Kim, D. Kim, S. J. Shin, and M. J. G. Appel.** 1996. Dissemination of *Borrelia burgdorferi* after experimental infection in dogs. *J. Spirochetal Tick-Borne Dis.* **3:**80–86.
35. **Coleman, J. L., and J. L. Benach.** 1987. Isolation of antigenic components from the Lyme disease spirochete: their role in early diagnosis. *J. Infect. Dis.* **155:**756–765.
36. **Cutler, S. J., D. Fekade, K. Hussein, K. A. Knox, A. Melka, K. Cann, A. R. Emilianus, D. A. Warrell, and D. J. M. Wright.** 1997. Successful in-vitro cultivation of *Borrelia recurrentis*. *Lancet* **343:**242. (Letter.)
37. **Cutler, S. J., J. Moss, M. Fukunaga, D. J. M. Wright, D. Fekade, and D. Warrell.** 1997. *Borrelia recurrentis* characterization and comparison with relapsing-fever, Lyme-associated, and other *Borrelia* spp. *Int. J. Syst. Bacteriol.* **47:** 958–968.
38. **Davidson, B., J. MacDougall, and I. Saint Girons.** 1992. Physical map of the linear chromosome of the bacterium *Borrelia burgdorferi* 212, a causative agent of Lyme disease, and localization of the rRNA genes. *J. Bacteriol.* **174:** 3766–3774.
39. **Davis, G. E.** 1956. The identification of spirochetes from human cases of relapsing fever by xenodiagnosis with comments on local specificity of tick vectors. *Exp. Parasitol.* **5:** 271–275.
40. **Defosse, D. L., R. C. Johnson, B. J. Paster, F. E. Dewhirst, and G. J. Fraser.** 1995. *Brevinema andersonii* gen. nov., sp. nov., an infectious spirochete isolated from the short-tailed shrew (*Blarina brevicauda*) and the white-footed mouse (*Peromyscus leucopus*). *Int. J. Syst. Bacteriol.* **45:**78–84.
41. **Diab, F. M., and Z. R. Soliman.** 1977. An experimental study of *Borrelia anserina* in four species of *Argas* ticks. Spirochete localization and densities. *Z. Parasitenkd.* **53:** 201–212.
42. **Dressler, F., R. Ackermann, and A. C. Steere.** 1994. Antibody responses to the three genomic groups of *Borrelia burgdorferi* in European Lyme borreliosis. *J. Infect. Dis.* **169:** 313–318.
43. **Dressler, F., J. A. Whalen, B. N. Reinhardt, and A. C. Steere.** 1993. Western blotting in the serodiagnosis of Lyme disease. *J. Infect. Dis.* **167:**392–400.
44. **Duffy, J., I. E. Mertz, G. H. Wobig, and J. A. Katzmann.**

1988. Diagnosing Lyme disease: the contribution of serologic testing. *Mayo Clin. Proc.* **63:**1116–1121.

45. **Dworkin, M. S., D. E. Anderson Jr., T. G. Schwan, P. C. Shoemaker, S. N. Banerjee, B. O. Kassen, and W. Burgdorfer.** 1998. Tick-borne relapsing fever in the northwestern United States and southwestern Canada. *Clin. Infect. Dis.* **26:**122–131.
46. **Eichenfield, A. H., and B. H. Athreya.** 1989. Lyme disease: of ticks and titers. *J. Pediatr.* **114:**328–332.
47. **Engstrom, S. M., E. Shoop, and R. C. Johnson.** 1995. Immunoblot interpretation criteria for serodiagnosis of early Lyme disease. *J. Clin. Microbiol.* **33:**419–427.
48. **Felsenfeld, O.** 1971. Borrelia. *Strains, Vectors, Human and Animal Borrelosis*, p. 180. Warren H. Green, Inc., St. Louis, Mo.
49. **Ferdows, M. S., and A. G. Barbour.** 1989. Megabase-sized linear DNA in the bacterium *Borrelia burgdorferi*, the Lyme disease agent. *Proc. Natl. Acad. Sci. USA* **86:**5969–5973.
50. **Fihn, S., and E. B. Larson.** 1980. Tick-borne relapsing fever in the Pacific Northwest: an underdiagnosed illness? *West. J. Med.* **133:**203–209.
51. **Fraser, C., et al.** 1997. Genomic sequence of a Lyme disease spirochete, *Borrelia burgdorferi*. *Nature* **390:**580–586.
52. **Goldschmid, J. M., and K. Mahomed.** 1972. The use of the microhematocrit technic for the recovery of *Borrelia duttonii* from the blood. *Am. J. Clin. Pathol.* **58:**165–169.
53. **Goldstein, S. F., N. W. Charon, and J. A. Kreiling.** 1994. *Borrelia burgdorferi* swims with a planar waveform similar to that of eukaryotic flagella. *Proc. Natl. Acad. Sci. USA* **91:**3433–3437.
54. **Goodman, J. L., P. Jurkovich, J. M. Kramber, and R. C. Johnson.** 1991. Molecular detection of persistent *Borrelia burgdorferi* in the urine of patients with active Lyme disease. *Infect. Immun.* **59:**269–278.
55. **Hansen, K., K. Pii, and A.-M. Lebech.** 1991. Improved immunoglobulin M serodiagnosis in Lyme borreliosis by using a 1L-capture enzyme-linked immunosorbent assay with biotinylated *Borrelia burgdorferi* flagella. *J. Clin. Microbiol.* **29:**166–173.
56. **Hinnebusch, B. J., A. G. Barbour, B. I. Restrepo, and T. G. Schwan.** 1998. Population structure of the relapsing fever spirochete *Borrelia hermsii* as indicated by polymorphism of two multigene families that encode immunogenic outer surface lipoproteins. *Infect. Immun.* **66:**432–440.
57. **Hinnebusch, B. J., S. Bergström, and A. G. Barbour.** 1990. Cloning and sequence analysis of linear plasmid telomeres of the bacterium *Borrelia burgdorferi*. *Mol. Microbiol.* **4:**811–820.
58. **Holt, S. C.** 1978. Anatomy and chemistry of spirochetes. *Microbiol. Rev.* **42:**114–160.
59. **Hyde, F. W., and R. C. Johnson.** 1984. Genetic relationship of Lyme disease spirochetes to *Borrelia, Treponema*, and *Leptospira* spp. *J. Clin. Microbiol.* **20:**151–154.
60. **Johnson, B. J. B., K. E. Robbins, R. E. Bailey, B.-L. Cao, S. L. Sviat, R. B. Craven, L. W. Mayer, and D. T. Dennis.** 1996. Serodiagnosis of Lyme disease: accuracy of a two-step approach using a flagella-based ELISA and immunoblotting. *J. Infect. Dis.* **174:**346–353.
61. **Johnson, R. C.** 1977. The spirochetes. *Annu. Rev. Microbiol.* **31:**89–106.
62. **Johnson, R. C., W. Burgdorfer, R. S. Lane, A. G. Barbour, S. F. Hayes, and F. W. Hyde.** 1987. *Borrelia coriaceae* sp. nov.: putative agent of epizootic bovine abortion. *Int. J. Syst. Bacteriol.* **328:**454–456.
63. **Johnson, R. C., F. W. Hyde, and C. M. Rumpel.** 1984. Taxonomy of the Lyme disease spirochete. *Yale J. Biol. Med.* **57:**529–537.
64. **Johnson, R. C., N. Marek, and C. Kodner.** 1984. Infection of Syrian hamsters with Lyme disease spirochetes. *J. Clin. Microbiol.* **20:**1099–1101.
65. **Jongen, V. H. W. M., J. Van Roosmalen, J. Tiems, J. Van Holten, and J. C. F. M. Wetsteyn.** 1997. Tick-borne relapsing fever and pregnancy outcome in rural Tanzania. *Acta Obstet. Gynecol. Scand.* **76:**834–838.
66. **Kahl, O., C. Janetzki-Mittmann, J. S. Gray, R. Jonas, J. Stein, and R. De Boer.** 1998. Risk of infection with *Borrelia burgdorferi* sensu lato for a host in relation to the duration of nymphal *Ixodes ricinus* feeding and the method of tick removal. *Zentrallol. Bakteriol.* **287:**41–52.
67. **Karlsson, M., G. Stiemstedt, M. Granstrom, E. Asbrink, and B. Wrettind.** 1990. Comparison of flagellum and sonicate antigens for serological diagnosis of Lyme borreliosis. *Eur. J. Clin. Microbiol. Infect. Dis.* **9:**169–177.
68. **Kelly, R.** 1971. Cultivation of *Borrelia hermsi*. *Science* **173:**443–444.
69. **Kurtti, T. J., U. G. Munderloh, R. C. Johnson, and G. G. Ahlstrand.** 1987. Colony formation and morphology in *Borrelia burgdorferi*. *J. Clin. Microbiol.* **25:**2054–2058.
70. **Kurtti, T. J., U. G. Munderloh, D. E. Krueger, R. C. Johnson, and T. G. Schwan.** 1993. Adhesion to and invasion of cultured tick (Acarina: Ixodidae) cells by *Borrelia burgdorferi* (Spirochaetales: Spirochaetaceae) and maintenance of infection. *J. Med. Entomol.* **30:**586–596.
71. **Lane, R. S., and W. Burgdorfer.** 1987. Transovarial and transstadial passage of *Borrelia burgdorferi* in the western black legged tick, *Ixodes pacificus*. *Am. J. Trop. Med. Hyg.* **37:**188–192.
72. **Lane, R. S., W. Burgdorfer, S. F. Hayes, and A. G. Barbour.** 1985. Isolation of a spirochete from the soft tick, *Ornithodoros coriaceus*: a possible agent of epizooric bovine abortion. *Science* **230:**85–87.
73. **Lane, R. S., J. Piesman, and W. Burgdorfer.** 1991. Lyme borreliosis: relation of its causative agent to its vectors and hosts in North America and Europe. *Annu. Rev. Entomol.* **36:**587–609.
74. **Lange, W. R., T. G. Schwan, and J. D. Frame.** 1991. Can protracted relapsing fever resemble Lyme disease? *Med. Hypotheses* **35:**77–79.
75. **LeFebvre, R. B., G.-C. Perng, and R. C. Johnson.** 1990. The 83-kilodalton antigen of *Borrelia burgdorferi* which stimulates immunoglobulin M (IgM) and IgG responses in infected hosts is expressed by a chromosomal gene. *J. Clin. Microbiol.* **28:**1673–1675.
76. **Levine, J. F., M. L. Wilson, and A. Spielman.** 1985. Mice as reserviors of the Lyme disease spirochete. *Am. J. Trop. Med. Hyg.* **34:**355–360.
77. **MacDonald, A. B., B. W. Berger, and T. G. Schwan.** 1990. Clinical implications of delayed growth of *Borrelia burgdorferi*. *Acta Trop.* **48:**89–94.
78. **Magnarelli, L. A., and J. F. Anderson.** 1988. Enzyme-linked immunosorbent assays for the detection of class-specific immunoglobulins to *Borrelia burgdorferi*. *Am. J. Epidemiol.* **127:**818–825.
79. **Magnarelli, L. A., J. F. Anderson, A. B. Schreier, and C. M. Ficke.** 1987. Clinical and serologic studies of canine borreliosis. *J. Am. Vet. Med. Assoc.* **191:**1089–1094.
80. **Magnarelli, L. A., J. F. Anderson, E. Shaw, J. E. Post, and P. C. Palka.** 1988. Borreliosis in equids in northeastern United States. *Am. J. Vet. Res.* **49:**359–362.
81. **Magnarelli, L. A., J. N. Miller, J. F. Anderson, and G. R. Riviere.** 1990. Cross-reactivity of nonspecific treponemal antibody in serologic tests for Lyme disease. *J. Clin. Microbiol.* **28:**1276–1279.
82. **Malloy, D. C., R. Y. Nauman, and H. Paxton.** 1990. Detection of *Borrelia burgdorferi* using the polymerase chain reaction. *J. Clin. Microbiol.* **28:**1089–1093.
83. **Margolis, N., D. Hogan, K. Tilly, and P. Rosa.** 1994.

Plasmid location of *Borrelia* purine biosynthesis gene homologs. *J. Bacteriol.* **176:**6427–6432.

84. **Marconi, R. T., and C. F. Garon.** 1992. Development of polymerase chain reaction primer sets for diagnosis of Lyme disease and for species-specific identification of Lyme disease isolates by 16S rRNA signature nucleotide analysis. *J. Clin. Microbiol.* **30:**2830–2834.
85. **Marconi, R. T., D. S. Samuels, and C. F. Garon.** 1993. Transcriptional analyses and mapping of the *ospC* gene in Lyme disease spirochetes. *J. Bacteriol.* **175:**926–932.
86. **Mathiesen, D. A., J. H. Oliver, Jr., C. P. Kolbert, E. D. Tullson, B. J. Johnson, G. L. Campbell, P. D. Mitchell, K. D. Reed, S. R. Telford III, R. S. Lane, and D. H. Persing.** 1997. Genetic heterogeneity of *Borrelia burgdorferi* in the United States. *J. Infect. Dis.* **175:**98–107.
87. **Meier, J., M. Simon, and A. G. Barbour.** 1985. Antigenic variation is associated with DNA rearrangements in a relapsing fever *Borrelia*. *Cell* **41:**403–409.
88. **Miller, J. N., D. M. Foley, J. T. Skare, C. I. Champion, E. S. Shang, D. R. Blanco, and M. A. Lovett.** 1996. The rabbit as a model for the study of Lyme disease pathogenesis and immunity. *J. Spirochetal Tick-Borne Dis.* **3:**6–14.
89. **Munson, E. L., B. K. DuChateau, D. A. Jobe, M. L. Padilla, S. D. Lovrich, J. R. Jensen, L. C. L. Lim, J. L. Schmitz, S. M. Callister, and R. F. Schell.** 1996. Hamster model of Lyme borreliosis. *J. Spirochetal Tick-Borne Dis.* **3:** 15–21.
90. **Nawakowski, J., and G. P. Wormser.** 1993. Treatment of early Lyme disease: infection associated with erythema migrans, p. 149–162. *In* P. K. Coyle (ed.), *Lyme Disease*. Mosby—Year Book, St. Louis, Mo.
91. **Nielsent, S. L., K. K. Y. Young, and A. G. Barbour.** 1990. Detection of *Borrelia burgdorferi* DNA by the polymerase chain reaction. *Mol. Cell. Probes* **4:**73–79.
92. **Nocton, J. J., B. J. Bloom, B. J. Rutledge, D. H. Persing, E. L. Logigian, C. H. Schmid, and A. C. Steere.** 1996. Detection of *Borrelia burgdorferi* DNA by polymerase chain reaction in cerebrospinal fluid in Lyme neuroborreliosis. *J. Infect. Dis.* **174:**623–627.
93. **Old, I., J. MacDougall, I. Saint Girons, and B. Davidson.** 1992. Mapping of genes on the linear chromosome of the bacterium *Borrelia burgdorferi*: possible locations for its origin of replication. *FEMS Microbiol. Lett.* **99:**245–250.
94. **Olsén, B., D. C. Duffy, T. G. T. Jaenson, A. Gylfe, J. Bonnedahl, and S. Bergström.** 1995. Transhemispheric exchange of Lyme disease spirochetes by seabirds. *J. Clin. Microbiol.* **33:**3270–3274.
95. **Olsén, B., T. G. T. Jaenson, L. Noppa, J. Bunikis, and S. Bergström.** 1993. A Lyme borreliosis cycle in seabirds and *Ixodes uriae* ticks. *Nature* **362:**340–342.
96. **Park, H. K., B. E. Jones, and A. G. Barbour.** 1986. Erythema chronicum migrans of Lyme disease: diagnosis by monoclonal antibodies. *J. Am. Acad. Dermatol.* **15:** 406–410.
97. **Paster, B. J., D. A. Pelletier, F. E. Dewhirst, W. G. Weisburg, V. Fussing, L. K. Poulsen, S. Dannenberg, and I. Schroeder.** 1996. Phylogenetic position of the spirochetal genus *Cristispira*. *Appl. Environ. Microbiol.* **62:**942–946.
98. **Persing, D. H., S. R. Telford III, A. Spielman, and S. W. Barthold.** 1990. Detection of *Borrelia burgdorferi* infection in *Ixodes dammini* ticks with the polymerase chain reaction. *J. Clin. Microbiol.* **28:**566–572.
99. **Philipp, M. T., Y. Lobet, R. P. Bohm, Jr., E. D. Roberts, V. A. Dennis, Y, Gu, R. C. Lowrie, Jr., P. Desmons, P. H. Duray, J. D. England, P. Hauser, J. Piesman, and K. Xu.** 1997. The outer surface protein A (OspA) vaccine against Lyme disease: efficacy in the rhesus monkey. *Vaccine* **15:**1872–1887.
100. **Picken, R. N.** 1992. Polymerase chain reaction primers and probes derived from flagellin gene sequences for specific detection of Lyme disease and North American relapsing fever. *J. Clin. Microbiol.* **30:**99–114.
101. **Piesman, J., J. G. Donahue, T. N. Mather, and A. Spielman.** 1986. Transovarially acquired Lyme disease spirochetes (*Borrelia burgdorferi*) in field-collected larval *Ixodes dammini* (Acari: Ixodidae). *J. Med. Entomol.* **23:**219.
102. **Piesman, J., T. N. Mather, R. J. Sinsky, and A. Spielman.** 1987. Duration of tick attachment and *Borrelia burgdorferi* transmission. *J. Clin. Microbiol.* **25:**557–558.
103. **Plasterk, R., M. Simon, and A. G. Barbour.** 1985. Transposition of structural genes to an expression sequence on a linear plasmid causes antigenic variation in *Borrelia hermsii*. *Nature* **318:**257–263.
104. **Porcella, S., T. Popova, D. Akins, M. Li, J. Radolf, and M. Norgard.** 1996. *Borrelia burgdorferi* supercoiled plasmids encode multi-copy tandem open reading frames and a lipoprotein gene family. *J. Bacteriol.* **178:** 3293–3307.
105. **Preac-Mursic, V., B. Wilske, and S. Reinhardt.** 1991. Culture of *Borrelia burgdorferi* on six solid media. *Eur. J. Clin. Microbiol. Infect. Dis.* **10:**1076–1079.
106. **Reimers, C. D., D. E. Pongratz, U. Neubert, A. Pilz, G. Hubner, M. Naegele, B. Wilske, P. H. Duray, and J. de Koning.** 1989. Myositis caused by *Borrelia burgdorferi*: report of four cases. *J. Neurol. Sci.* **91:**215–226.
107. **Rosa, P. A., and D. M. Hogan.** 1992. Colony formation by *Borrelia burgdorferi* in solid medium: clonal analysis of *osp* locus variants, p. 95–103. *In* U. G. Munderloh and T. J. Kurtii (ed.), *Proceedings of the First International Conference on Tick-Borne Pathogens at the Host-Vector Interface: an Agenda for Research*. University of Minnesota College of Agriculture, St. Paul, Minn.
108. **Rosa, P. A., D. Hogan, and T. G. Schwan.** 1991. Polymerase chain reaction analyses identify two distinct classes of *Borrelia burgdorferi*. *J. Clin. Microbiol.* **29:** 524–532.
109. **Rosa, P. A., and T. G. Schwan.** 1989. A specific and sensitive assay for the Lyme disease spirochete, *Borrelia burgdorferi*, using the polymerase chain reaction. *J. Infect. Dis.* **160:**1018–1029.
110. **Sadziene, A., B. Wilske, M. Ferdows, and A. G. Barbour.** 1993. The cryptic *ospC* gene of *Borrelia burgdorferi* B31 is located on a circular plasmid. *Infect. Immun.* **61:** 2192–2195.
111. **Salih, S. Y., and D. Mustafa.** 1977. Louse-borne relapsing fever. II. Combined penicillin and tetracycline therapy in 160 Sudanese patients. *Trans. R. Soc. Trop. Med. Hyg.* **71:**49–51.
112. **Schulze, T. L., G. S. Bowlen, E. M. Bosler, M. F. Lake, W. E. Parkin, R. Altman, B. G. Ormiston, and J. K. Shisler.** 1984. *Amblyomma americanum*: a potential vector of Lyme disease in New Jersey. *Science* **224:**601–603.
113. **Schwan, T. G., and W. Burgdorfer.** 1987. Antigenic changes of *Borrelia burgdorferi* as a result of in vitro cultivation. *J. Infect. Dis.* **156:**852–853.
114. **Schwan, T. G., W. Burgdorfer, and C. F. Garon.** 1988. Changes in infectivity and plasmid profile of the Lyme disease spirochete, *Borrelia burgdorferi*, as a result of in vitro cultivation. *Infect. Immun.* **56:**1831–1836.
115. **Schwan, T. G., W. Burgdorfer, M. E. Schrumpf, and R. H. Karstens.** 1988. The urinary bladder, a consistent source of *Borrelia burgdorferi* in experimentally infected white-footed mice (*Peromyscus leucopus*). *J. Clin. Microbiol.* **26:**893–895.
116. **Schwan, T. G., K. L. Gage, and J. Hinnebusch.** 1995. Analysis of relapsing fever spirochetes from the western United States. *J. Spirochetal Tick-Borne Dis.* **2:**3–8.

117. **Schwan, T. G., K. L. Gage, R. H. Karstens, M. E. Schrumpf, S. F. Hayes, and A. G. Barbour.** 1992. Identification of the tick-borne relapsing fever spirochete, *Borrelia hermsii*, with a species-specific monoclonal antibody. *J. Clin. Microbiol.* **30:**790–795.
118. **Schwan, T. G., J. Piesman, W. T. Golde, M. C. Dolan, and P. A. Rosa.** 1995. Induction of an outer surface protein on *Borrelia burgdorferi* during tick feeding. *Proc. Natl. Acad. Sci. USA* **92:**2909–2913.
119. **Schwan, T. G., M. E. Schrumpf, B. J. Hinnebusch, D. E. Anderson, and M. E. Konkel.** 1996. GlpQ: an antigen for serological discrimination between relapsing fever and Lyme borreliosis. *J. Clin. Microbiol.* **34:**2483–2492.
120. **Schwan, T. G., M. E. Schrumpf, and R. H. Karstens.** 1992. Rapid identification of small supercoiled plasmids in cloned populations of *Borrelia burgdorferi*, p. 89–94. *In* U. G. Munderloh and T. J. Kurtii (ed.), *Proceedings of the First International Conference on Tick-Borne Pathogens at the Host-Vector Interface: an Agenda for Research.* University of Minnesota College of Agriculture, St. Paul, Minn.
121. **Schwan, T. G., W. J. Simpson, M. E. Schrumpf, and R. H. Karstens.** 1989. Identification of *Borrelia burgdorferi* and *Borrelia hermsii* using DNA hybridization probes. *J. Clin. Microbiol.* **27:**1734–1738.
122. **Schwartz, J., A. Gazumyan, and I. Schwartz.** 1992. rRNA gene organization in the Lyme disease spirochete *Borrelia burgdorferi*. *J. Bacteriol.* **174:**3757–3765.
123. **Simon, M. M., R. Wallich, and M. D. Kramer.** 1996. *Borrelia burgdorferi* infection of inbred strains of mice provides insights into cellular and molecular parameters of pathogenesis and protection of Lyme disease: a viewpoint. *J. Spirochetal Tick-Borne Dis.* **3:**45–52.
124. **Simpson, W. J., W. Burgdorfer, M. E. Schrumpf, R. H. Karstens, and T. G. Schwan.** 1991. Antibody to a 39-kilodalton *Borrelia burgdorferi* antigen (P39) as a marker for infection in experimentally and naturally inoculated animals. *J. Clin. Microbiol.* **29:**236–243.
125. **Simpson, W. J., C. F. Garon, and T. G. Schwan.** 1990. *Borrelia burgdorferi* contains repeated DNA sequences that are species specific and plasmid associated. *Infect. Immun.* **58:**847–853.
126. **Simpson, W. J., C. F. Garon, and T. G. Schwan.** 1990. Analysis of supercoiled circular plasmids in infectious and non-infectious *Borrelia burgdorferi*. *Microb. Pathog.* **8:** 109–118.
127. **Simpson, W. J., M. E. Schrumpf, and T. G. Schwan.** 1990. Reactivity of human Lyme borreliosis sera with a 39-kilodalton antigen specific to *Borrelia burgdorferi*. *J. Clin. Microbiol.* **28:**1329–1337.
128. **Sinsky, R. J., and J. Piesman.** 1989. Ear punch biopsy method for detection and isolation of *Borrelia burgdorferi* from rodents. *J. Clin. Microbiol.* **27:**1723–1727.
129. **Sonenshine, D. E.** 1991. *Biology of Ticks*. Oxford University Press, New York, N.Y.
130. **Southern, P. M., and J. P. Sanford.** 1969. Relapsing fever: a clinical and microbiological review. *Medicine* **48:** 129–149.
131. **Steere, A. C.** 1989. Lyme disease. *N Engl. J. Med.* **321:** 586–596.
132. **Steere, A. C., S. E. Malawista, J. A. Hardin, S. Ruddy, P. W. Askenase, and W. A. Andiman.** 1977. Erythema chronicum migrans and Lyme arthritis: the enlarging clinical spectrum. *Ann. Intern. Med.* **86:**685–698.
133. **Stevenson, B. L., T. G. Schwan, and P. A. Rosa.** 1995. Temperature-related differential expression of antigens in the Lyme disease spirochete *Borrelia burgdorferi*. *Infect. Immun.* **63:**4535–4539.
134. **Stevenson, B., K. Tilly, and P. Rosa.** 1996. A family of genes located on four separate 32-kilobase circular plasmids in *Borrelia burgdorferi* B31. *J. Bacteriol.* **178:** 3508–3516.
135. **Straubinger, R. K., B. A. Summers, Y.-F. Chang, and M. J. G. Appel.** 1997. Persistence of *Borrelia burgdorferi* in experimentally infected dogs after antibiotic treatment. *J. Clin. Microbiol.* **35:**111–116.
136. **Suk, K., S. Das, W. Sun, B. Jwang, S. Barthold, R. Flavell, and E. Fikrig.** 1995. *Borrelia burgdorferi* genes selectively expressed in the infected host. *Proc. Natl. Acad. Sci. USA* **92:**4269–4273.
137. **Thompson, R. S., W. Burgdorfer, R. Russell, and B. J. Francis.** 1969. Outbreak of tick-borne relapsing fever in Spokane County, Washington. *JAMA* **210:**1045–1050.
138. **vanDam, A. P., H. Kuiper, K. Vos, A. Widjojokusumo, B. M. deJongh, L. Spanjaard, A. C. P. Ramselaar, M. D. Kramer, and J. Dankert.** 1993. Different genospecies of *Borrelia burgdorferi* are associated with distinct clinical manifestations of Lyme borreliosis. *Clin. Infect. Dis.* **17:** 708–717.
139. **Wallich, R., C. Brenner, M. Kramer, and M. Simon.** 1995. Molecular cloning and immunological characterization of a novel linear plasmid-encoded gene, *pG*, of *Borrelia burgdorferi* expressed only in vivo. *Infect. Immun.* **63:** 3327–3335.
140. **Woese, C. R.** 1987. Bacterial evolution. *Microbiol. Rev.* **51:**221–271.
141. **Zhang, J.-R., J. M. Hardham, A. G. Barbour, and S. J. Norris.** 1997. Antigenic variation in Lyme disease *Borrelia* by promiscuous recombination of VMP-like sequence cassettes. *Cell* **89:**275–285.
142. **Zung, J. L., S. Lewengrub, M. A. Rudzinska, A. Spielman, S. R. Telford, and J. Piesman.** 1989. Fine structural evidence for the penetration of the Lyme disease spirochete *Borrelia burgdorferi* through the gut and salivary tissues of *Ixodes dammini*. *Can. J. Zool.* **67:**1737–1748.

Treponema and Other Host-Associated Spirochetes

SANDRA A. LARSEN, STEVEN J. NORRIS, AND VICTORIA POPE

54

GENERAL TAXONOMY

The genus *Treponema* (order *Spirochaetales*, family *Spirochaetaceae*) includes four human pathogens (Table 1) and at least six human nonpathogens. In volume 1 of *Bergey's Manual of Systematic Bacteriology* (95), the nomenclature was restructured so that the species *Treponema pallidum* includes three of the human pathogens: *T. pallidum* subsp. *pallidum* (venereal syphilis), *T. pallidum* subsp. *endemicum* (endemic syphilis), and *T. pallidum* subsp. *pertenue* (yaws). *T. carateum* (pinta) remains a separate species owing to the lack of genetic information. The pathogenic treponemes in this group are very closely related, to the extent that they are distinguished primarily by their patterns of pathogenesis in humans and experimentally infected animals. They are morphologically indistinguishable and, where examined, have ≥95% DNA homology by hybridization (23), a high degree of sequence identity of known genes (65–67), nearly identical protein profiles (see reference 72 for a review), and shared reactivity with monoclonal antibodies (64). Recent data indicate that there may be some subspecies differences, as well as differences between *T. pallidum* and *T. paraluiscuniculi*, a rabbit pathogen, in the flanking-region sequences of the 15.5-kDa lipoprotein gene (14). According to structure, host dependence, and protein content, *T. paraluiscuniculi* appears to be closely related to the human pathogens; however, it causes venereal spirochetosis of rabbits and is not known to cause human disease.

In contrast to the close relationship among the human pathogens, *T. pallidum* subsp. *pallidum* has ≤5% DNA homology with other nonpathogenic spirochetes such as *T. phagedenis*, *T. refringens*, and *Serpulina* (formerly *Treponema*) *hyodysenteriae* (23, 98, 100). However, rRNA sequence similarities (74) indicated an evolutionary relationship between *T. pallidum*, *T. phagedenis*, *T. denticola*, and other treponemes. The sequence of the 1.13×10^6-bp *T. pallidum* subsp. *pallidum* Nichols genome was published in 1998 (28), and sequencing of the 3.0×10^6-bp *T. denticola* genome was begun in 1998. The resulting information will be of value in characterizing the similarities and differences of these organisms. Because of the distinctive nature of treponemes pathogenic to humans and other host-associated spirochetes, these two groups will be discussed separately below.

SPIROCHETES ASSOCIATED WITH HUMAN TREPONEMATOSES

Description of the Genus

T. pallidum is a spirochete ~0.18 μm in diameter and ranging in length from 6 to 20 μm (Fig. 1). Suspensions of *T. pallidum* are best visualized by dark-field microscopy, although the bacterium can also be seen by phase-contrast microscopy. Unstained organisms are not visible by standard bright-field microscopy because of the small cell diameter.

Morphologically, *T. pallidum* has regular helices (6 to 14 per cell) with a wavelength of 1.1 μm and an amplitude of ~0.3 μm. The ends are pointed and lack the hook shape characteristic of some commensal human spirochetes. Fresh preparations of the organism exhibit rapid rotation about the axis (the characteristic corkscrew motility) due to the action of flagella inserted in both ends and extending down the cell body within the periplasmic space (Fig. 1). Flexing and reversal of rotation can occur also, but translational motion is not observed unless *T. pallidum* is in a viscous medium.

Habitat and Distribution

The *T. pallidum* subspecies and *T. carateum* are obligate parasites of humans and are not known to have any animal or environmental reservoirs. Venereal syphilis has a worldwide distribution, with the incidence varying widely according to geographic location and socioeconomic groups (Table 1). Endemic syphilis is restricted to desert and temperate regions of North Africa and the Middle East. Yaws occurs most commonly in tropical or desert regions of Africa, South America, and Indonesia. Pinta is found primarily in tropical areas of Central and South America.

Clinical Significance

Syphilis is still a common sexually transmitted disease in many areas of the world, despite the availability of effective therapy. In 1995, the World Health Organization estimated that the worldwide incidence of sexually acquired syphilis was 0.4% (12 million cases) and that the prevalence was 1% (28 million cases) (112). In the United States, 52,995 cases were reported in 1996, including 11,387 cases of primary and secondary syphilis and 1,181 cases of congenital syphilis (10), a dramatic decrease from the 134,255 total

TABLE 1 Characteristics of the human treponematoses[a]

Organism	Disease	Distribution	Predominant age of onset	Transmission	Congenital infection
T. pallidum subsp. *pallidum*	Venereal syphilis	Worldwide	Adolescents, adults	Sexual contact	Yes
T. pallidum subsp. *pertenue*	Yaws (frambesia, pian)	Tropical areas, Africa, South America, Caribbean, Indonesia	Children	Skin contact	No
T. pallidum subsp. *endemicum*	Endemic syphilis (bejel, dichuchwa)	Arid areas, North Africa, Middle East	Children to adults	Mucous membrane	Rarely
T. carateum	Pinta (carate, cute)	Semiarid, warm areas, Central and South America	Children, adolescents	Skin contact	No

[a] See references 21, 22, 76, 77, and 110.

reported cases at the peak of a syphilis epidemic in 1990 (10).

Transmission of the treponematoses occurs through direct contact with active lesions. In venereal syphilis, the primary and secondary lesions are infectious and contain large numbers of organisms until the healing stage; for epidemiologic purposes, early latent cases (duration, ≤1 year) are also considered potentially infectious. *T. pallidum* and related organisms apparently penetrate mucous membranes and abrasions in the epidermis, establish a local infection in the dermis, and disseminate rapidly from the primary site.

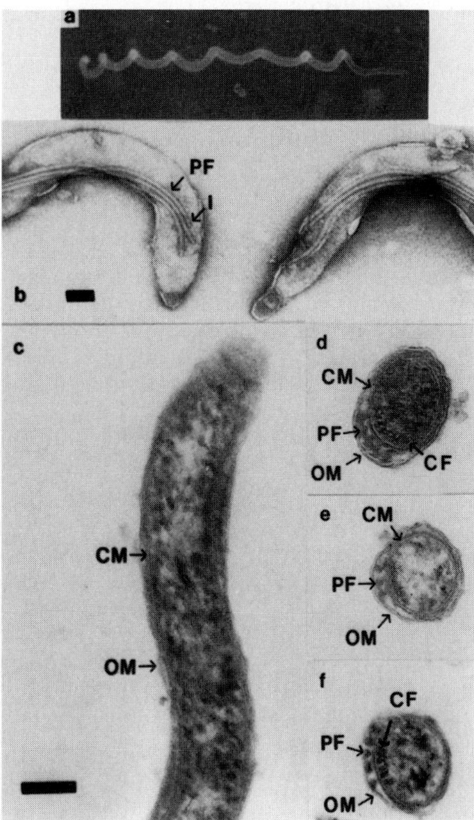

FIGURE 1 Morphology of *T. pallidum*. (A) Scanning electron micrograph showing spiral shape. (B) Negatively stained view of the tips of two organisms. Note the insertion points (I) of periplasmic flagella (PF) near the ends. (C to F) Electron micrographs of ultrathin sections, showing the outer membrane (OM), the cytoplasmic membrane (CM), periplasmic flagella (PF), and the location of the cytoplasmic filaments (CF). Bars, 0.1 μm. Reprinted with permission from reference 72.

Venereal syphilis exhibits a wide variety of clinical manifestations (Table 2). Early syphilis consists of the primary, secondary, and early latent stages. The primary stage is characterized by the chancre, a firm, indurated lesion with an ulcerated or crusted surface ranging in size from a few millimeters to 1 to 2 cm. Although disseminated infection occurs in virtually all infected individuals regardless of stage, multiple lesions arise in ~25% of patients with secondary syphilis. Numerous treponemes are often present in exudates from primary or secondary syphilitic lesions, and detection of organisms with the characteristic morphology and motility is still considered the only definitive means of diagnosis (see below).

About two-thirds of the syphilis cases reported in the United States are diagnosed at the latent (asymptomatic) stage, in which diagnosis is based solely on serologic reactivity and history. Longitudinal observations of untreated syphilis patients at the beginning of the 20th century indicated that approximately one-third remain latently infected for life, one-third undergo "biological cure" (i.e., lose serologic reactivity), and the remaining one-third develop tertiary manifestations (30). Tertiary syphilis, consisting of neurologic, cardiovascular, and gummatous forms, can develop decades after the initial infection (110). The cardiovascular and gummatous forms of syphilis are now rarely encountered, apparently because of effective therapy of early syphilis and antimicrobial therapy administered for other infections. Recent studies have shown that viable *T. pallidum* is present in the cerebrospinal fluid (CSF) of patients with the primary and secondary stages of syphilis, indicating that central nervous system infection occurs very early in the course of disease (53). Neurologic manifestations, including syphilitic meningitis, may occur as early as 3 months postinfection; thus, neurosyphilis should not be considered solely a late manifestation of the disease (38).

Congenital syphilis results from the transmission of *T. pallidum* across the placenta during pregnancy. Early congenital syphilis tends to occur when the mothers are afflicted with early syphilis during the course of pregnancy, resulting in stillbirth or fulminant infection of the newborn (Table 2). Late manifestations of congenital syphilis are the outcome of chronic untreated infection and can result in multiple

TABLE 2 Common manifestations of treponematoses

Venereal syphilis (*T. pallidum* subsp. *pallidum*)
- Primary (local): 10 to 90 days postinfection (avg, 21 days)
  - Chancre (single or multiple, skin or mucous membranes)
  - Regional lymphadenopathy
- Secondary (disseminated): 6 weeks to 6 months postinfection
  - Multiple secondary lesions (skin or mucous membranes)
  - Generalized lymphadenopathy, fever, malaise
  - Condylomata lata
  - Alopecia
  - Asymptomatic or symptomatic CNS[a] involvement (meningitis)
- Latent (early, ≤1-yr duration; late, >1-yr duration)
  - Reactive serologic tests for syphilis
  - Asymptomatic
- Tertiary (late, chronic): months to years postinfection
  - Gummatous (monocytic infiltrates, tissue destruction, any organ)
  - Cardiovascular (aortic aneurysm)
  - Neurosyphilis (paresis, tabes dorsalis, meningovascular syphilis)
- Congenital
  - Early (onset, <2 yr): fulminant, disseminated infection, mucocutaneous lesions, osteochondritis, anemia, hepatosplenomegaly, CNS involvement
  - Late (persistence, >2 yr): interstitial keratitis, bone and tooth deformities, eighth-nerve deafness, neurosyphilis, other tertiary manifestations

Yaws (*T. pallidum* subsp. *pertenue*)
- Early: onset 9 to 90 days postinfection (avg, 21 days)
  - Primary lesion (mother yaw): papular, nontender, often pruritic, crusted, or ulcerated
  - Disseminated lesions (daughter yaws): often resemble primary lesion or appearance may vary
  - Malaise, fever, lymphadenopathy
  - Osteitis, periostitis, other bone and joint manifestations
- Latent: positive serologic tests, no other signs of infection
- Late: 10% of patients
  - Destructive lesions of bone and cartilage (e.g., ulcerative rhinopharyngitis)
  - Hyperkeratotic skin lesions

Endemic syphilis (*T. pallidum* subsp. *endemicum*)
- Early
  - Primary lesion not usually detected
  - Secondary: multiple oropharyngeal, cutaneous lesions
  - Generalized lymphadenopathy
  - Periostitis
- Latent: positive serologic tests, no other signs of infection
- Late: destructive skin, bone, and cartilage lesions

Pinta (*T. carateum*): restricted to skin
- Early
  - Initial lesion: hyperkeratotic, pigmented papule or plaque
  - Disseminated skin lesions (pintids)
  - Regional lymphadenopathy
- Late: pigmentary changes in skin (hyper- and hypopigmentation)

[a] CNS, central nervous system.

stigmata (Table 2) that are often not obvious until the second decade of life.

Yaws, endemic syphilis, and pinta were common infections in areas of endemicity prior to the World Health Organization's eradication program beginning in 1948; in the early 1950s, it was estimated that 200 million people were exposed to yaws during their lifetimes (21, 22, 76, 77). Now, areas where the diseases are endemic are more restricted, but decreased surveillance has led to a recrudescence of incidence in many areas (58). Transmission of endemic treponematoses occurs through direct contact with early lesions or with contaminated fingers or drinking or eating utensils. Yaws and endemic syphilis commonly are transmitted among children (2 to 10 years of age), whereas pinta usually has a later onset (ages 15 to 30 years). Many of the manifestations of yaws and endemic syphilis are similar to those of venereal syphilis (Table 2); the lesions of pinta appear to be restricted to the skin. Congenital transmission of the endemic treponematoses is rare.

Diagnostic Parameters and Interpretation of Laboratory Tests

The following is a brief discussion of the parameters involved in the diagnosis of syphilis and other treponematoses. Procedures for the direct detection of *T. pallidum* and the serologic diagnosis of syphilis are described in detail in *A Manual of Tests for Syphilis* (48).

Diagnostic Criteria for Venereal Syphilis

For the laboratory diagnosis of syphilis, each stage has a particular testing requirement (Table 3) (9). Because *T. pallidum* cannot be readily cultured (18, 24, 70), other laboratory methods for the identification of infection have been developed. The current tests for syphilis fall into three categories: direct microscopic examination, used when lesions are present; nontreponemal tests, used for screening; and treponemal tests that are confirmatory. In the United States, the routine testing scheme is direct microscopic examination of lesion exudates, followed by a nontreponemal test which, if reactive, is confirmed by a treponemal test (Fig. 2).

During the primary stage, because serous fluids from the lesion contain numerous treponemes and development of humoral antibodies takes several weeks, dark-field microscopy or the direct fluorescent-antibody (DFA) test for *T. pallidum* (DFA-TP) (48) are the methods of choice for definitive identification. Humoral antibodies, as detected by the standard nontreponemal and treponemal serologic tests for syphilis, usually do not appear until 1 to 4 weeks after the chancre(s) has formed. By the secondary stage of syphilis the organism has invaded every organ of the body and virtually all body fluids. At this stage, with few if any exceptions, all serologic tests for syphilis are reactive; plus, treponemes may be found in lesions. The titer obtained by serologic tests may be higher among patients with secondary syphilis with coexistent human immunodeficiency virus (HIV) infection, but the choice of tests and the interpretation of test results for the diagnosis of secondary syphilis are the same for HIV-infected and uninfected patients (62). The relationship between the detection of treponemes in the CSF from patients with early syphilis and the development of late neurosyphilis and the potential for reducing any such increased risk of developing neurosyphilis through enhanced therapy has not been established (62). Nontreponemal and treponemal serologic tests are consistently reactive in the early latent stage, but the patient is asymptomatic. In the latent stage, the titers of reactive nontreponemal tests may be higher among patients with coexistent HIV and *T. pallidum* infections (7, 31, 44, 87) except for patients with advanced immunodeficiency, who may become falsely seronegative (32, 36). Even though possible false-negative serologic tests for syphilis in advanced AIDS should be con-

TABLE 3 Criteria for diagnosis of syphilis

Early syphilis
- Primary
  - Confirmed
    1. One or more chancres (ulcers)
    2. Direct microscopic identification of *T. pallidum* in clinical specimens
  - Probable (requires 1 *and* either 2 or 3)
    1. A clinically compatible case with one or more chancres
    2. Reactive nontreponemal test and no history of syphilis
    3. For persons with a history of syphilis, a fourfold increase in titer on a quantitative nontreponemal test when results of past tests are compared with the most recent test results
- Secondary
  - Confirmed
    - Direct microscopic identification of *T. pallidum* in clinical specimens
  - Probable (requires 1 *and* either 2 or 3)
    1. Skin or mucous membrane lesions typical of secondary syphilis
       a. Macular, papular, follicular, papulosquamous, or pustular
       b. Condylomata lata (anogenital region or mouth)
       c. Mucous patches (oropharynx or cervix)
    2. Reactive nontreponemal test titer of >1:4 and no previous history of syphilis
    3. For persons with a history of syphilis, a fourfold increase in the most recent nontreponemal test titer when compared with previous test results
- Early latent
  - Probable (requires 1, 2, 3, *and* 4 or 5)
    1. Absence of signs and symptoms of syphilis
    2. Reactive nontreponemal and treponemal test results
    3. A history of sexual exposure to a partner with confirmed or probable early syphilis (documented independently as duration <1 yr)
    4. A history of a nonreactive nontreponemal test the previous 12 mo
    5. A past history of syphilis therapy and a current fourfold increase in nontreponemal test titer compared with the previous test results
- Late latent
  - Probable (requires 1, 2, *and* 3 or 4)
    1. No evidence of having acquired the disease within the preceding 12 mo
    2. Absence of signs and symptoms
    3. Reactive nontreponemal and treponemal test results
    4. A past history of syphilis therapy and a current fourfold increase in nontreponemal test titer compared with the previous test results
- Latent of unknown duration
  - Probable (requires 1, 2, *and* 3 or 4)
    1. No evidence of having acquired the disease within the preceding 12 mo
    2. Absence of signs and symptoms
    3. Patient is aged 13–35 yr and has a nontreponemal titer of >1:32
    4. Patient is aged 13–35 yr and has a past history of syphilis therapy and a current fourfold increase in nontreponemal test titer compared with the previous test results

Late syphilis
- Benign and cardiovascular
  - Confirmed
    1. Clinically compatible case
    2. Observation by direct microscopic examination of treponemes in tissue sections by DFAT-TP or equivalent methods (PCR)
  - Probable
    1. Clinically compatible case
    2. A reactive treponemal test
    3. No known history of treatment for syphilis
  - Comment: Patients with any form of late syphilis should be evaluated for neurosyphilis
- Neurosyphilis
  - Confirmed (requires 1, 2, *and* 3 or 4)
    1. Clinical signs consistent with neurosyphilis
    2. A reactive serum treponemal test
    3. A reactive VDRL-CSF test
    4. Identification of *T. pallidum* in CSF or tissue by microscopic examination or equivalent methods
  - Probable
    1. Clinical signs consistent with neurosyphilis
    2. A reactive serum treponemal test
    3. Elevated CSF protein or leukocyte count in the absence of other known causes

Neonatal congenital syphilis
- Confirmed
  1. Clinically compatible case
  2. Demonstration of *T. pallidum* by direct microscopic examination of umbilical cord, placenta, nasal discharge, or skin lesion material
- Probable (requires 1, 2, and 3)
  1. An infant born to a mother who had untreated or inadequately[a] treated syphilis at delivery regardless of findings in the infant
  2. An infant with a reactive treponemal test result
  3. One of the following additional criteria:
     a. Clinical sign or symptom of congenital syphilis on physical examination
     b. Abnormal CSF finding without other cause
     c. Reactive VDRL-CSF test result
     d. Reactive IgM antibody test specific for syphilis
- Syphilitic stillbirth
  1. A fetal death that occurs after a 20-wk gestation or in which the fetus weighs >500 g
  2. Mother had untreated or inadequately[a] treated syphilis at delivery

[a] Nonpenicillin therapy or penicillin given less than 30 days before delivery.

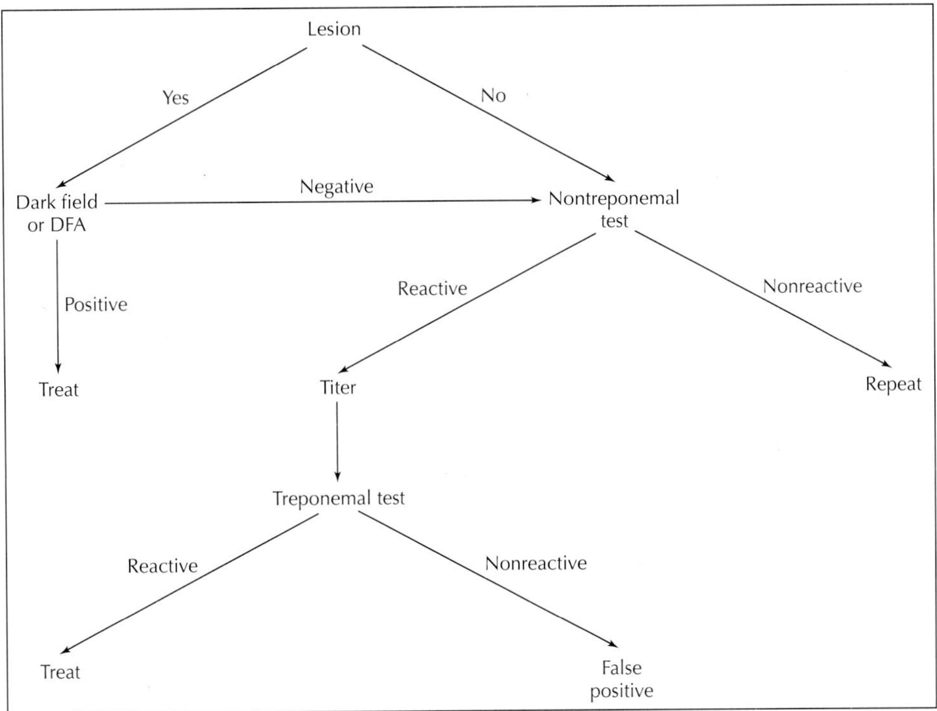

FIGURE 2 Routine screening scheme for early syphilis in the United States.

sidered, the approach to the detection of early latent syphilis is the same for HIV-infected and uninfected individuals (87). Routine CSF examination for the detection of neurosyphilis is probably indicated for the patient with coexistent latent syphilis and HIV infection (87), whereas the need for lumbar puncture in the HIV-uninfected patient with latent syphilis is controversial (8). During the late latent stage (duration of >1 year), the proportion of patients exhibiting reactive nontreponemal tests and the reactive titers of the nontreponemal tests decrease.

Symptoms of late or tertiary syphilis may occur 10 to 20 years after the initial infection. Although rare, earlier onset of late or tertiary syphilis has been reported for individuals coinfected with HIV (43). Approximately 71% of patients with late-stage syphilis have reactive nontreponemal tests; however, treponemal tests are almost always reactive and may be the only basis for diagnosis (Table 3). Diagnosis of cardiovascular syphilis is made on the basis of symptoms that indicate aortic insufficiency or aneurysm, reactive treponemal test results, and no known history of treatment for syphilis. Neurologic forms of syphilis (e.g., syphilitic meningitis) may develop during the secondary stage. Neurosyphilis as a complication of late syphilis may occur as early as 2 years after initial infection. Neurosyphilis may take many forms, yet symptoms consistent with neurosyphilis may not always be present (38). CSF examinations, such as the Venereal Disease Research Laboratory (VDRL)-CSF slide test or total protein and leukocyte counts, should be performed with the spinal fluid of patients with late latent syphilis and the spinal fluid of those with clinical symptoms and signs consistent with neurosyphilis (38). Diagnosis of neurosyphilis is based on a combination of these criteria (Table 3).

Diagnostic Criteria for Congenital Syphilis

A primary stage does not occur in congenital syphilis, because the organisms directly infect the fetal circulation (115). Treponemes or the effects thereof are detectable in almost every tissue of the infant. The standard serologic tests for syphilis, based on the measurement of immunoglobulin G (IgG), reflect antibodies passively transferred from the mother to the infant rather than IgM antibodies produced during gestation. Currently, the diagnosis of neonatal congenital syphilis depends on a combination of results from physical, radiographic, serologic, and direct microscopic examinations (Table 3). Clinical signs of congenital syphilis include hepatosplenomegaly, cutaneous lesions, osteochondritis, and snuffles (45, 110). Although some clinical manifestations may be present at birth, they are more often seen at 3 weeks to 6 months. At birth, up to 50% of the infants with congenital syphilis are asymptomatic; other stigmata that may develop later include tooth and bone malformations, deafness, blindness, and learning disabilities.

Diagnostic Criteria for Other Treponematoses

To date, no routine laboratory method has been devised to distinguish the other pathogenic treponematoses from each other or from syphilis. The standard serologic tests for syphilis are uniformly reactive with yaws, pinta, and nonvenereal endemic syphilis (bejel) (3). Western blotting (immunoblotting) assays do not differentiate the antibodies formed in syphilis from those formed in yaws or pinta (29, 65). Most molecular approaches, such as DNA sequencing, DNA probes analyses, and PCR techniques, have also failed to individualize the pathogenic treponemes (12, 65). Therefore, the clinical appearance of the lesions formed by *T. pallidum* subsp. *pertenue*, *T. pallidum* subsp. *pallidum*, *T. pallidum* subsp. *endemicum*, and *T. carateum*; the anatomical location of the lesion; the mode of transmission; and the age of the individual are the only criteria that can be used to diagnose these infections as separate entities (3) (Table 1).

Because yaws, pinta, and nonvenereal syphilis are often

childhood diseases, the nontreponemal test titers for adults from geographic regions in which endemic treponematoses were virtually eliminated by mass campaigns in the 1950s and 1960s are expected to be ≤1:8 (1). Therefore, any titer of >1:8 for adults from these regions is probably indicative of venereal syphilis. Likewise, titers of ≥1:8 for children indicate a possible resurgence of yaws in the populations of these areas (77).

Detection and Identification of *T. pallidum* in Tissue and Tissue Exudates

General Principles

In addition to being difficult to culture, treponemes are not readily detectable with common laboratory stains but can be visualized with silver stains (103). Therefore, when lesions are present, the most specific and easiest means of diagnosing syphilis is by direct detection of the organism. Currently, dark-field microscopy and DFA (DFA-TP) tests are commonly used to detect *T. pallidum*. A positive result on microscopic examination is definitive for syphilis if infection with other pathogenic treponemes can be excluded. When dark-field microscopy is used, the presence of morphologically similar parasitic spirochetes within and near the genitalia requires that *T. pallidum* be viewed in its "living state" in order to observe its characteristic morphology and motility. Samples for DFA-TP are air dried onto slides and therefore do not require cell viability or immediate examination. Labeled monoclonal antibodies are available from the Biological Products Branch of the Centers for Disease Control and Prevention (CDC). The DFA-TP test can also be performed by the Bacterial STD Branch of CDC.

The newest technique for the direct detection of *T. pallidum* is PCR (6, 11, 13, 33, 67, 68, 90, 111). PCR as a tool for detecting *T. pallidum* is used by only a few laboratories, and as of this writing a commercial test based on PCR is not available. However, the PCR test is available at CDC for patients with indications for neurosyphilis (i.e., reactive serum serology, abnormal CSF or neurologic systems, and a history of syphilis).

The oldest method of detection of infection with *T. pallidum* is animal infectivity testing. This technique probably offers the most sensitive method for detecting infectious treponemes and is used as the "gold standard" for measuring the sensitivities of detection methods, such as PCR (33, 90). However, use of animal infectivity is limited to research settings.

Specimen Collection

When collecting, preparing, and examining specimens, observe universal precautions (48). Specimens collected from the epidermal and mucosal lesions of primary, secondary, and early congenital syphilis are most useful, because these specimens may be obtained without using invasive procedures, and the lesions tend to contain large concentrations of treponemes. Briefly, a specimen for dark-field microscopy should consist of serous fluid free of erythrocytes, other organisms, and tissue debris. The lesion should be cleansed only if it is encrusted or obviously contaminated, and only tap water or physiologic saline (without antibacterial additives) should be used. Gentle abrasion of the lesion surface may be necessary to yield a clear serous fluid, which is then collected on a glass slide and covered with a coverslip. Because even the experienced observer may find it difficult or impossible to differentiate *T. pallidum* from other parasitic spirochetes of the mouth, dark-field microscopy should not be used for the examination of samples from oral lesions. It is essential that exudates be examined as soon as possible (ideally within 20 min) to ensure retention of motility of the organism. *T. pallidum* is very sensitive to exposure to oxygen, heat, nonphysiologic pH, and desiccation.

Lesion samples for direct fluorescence examination are collected in the manner described above for dark-field microscopy, except the samples are air dried. Motility of the organism is not required in the DFA-TP test. Because the conjugates used are specific for pathogenic strains of *Treponema*, the DFA-TP test is applicable to samples collected from both oral and rectal lesions. The use of the DFA-TP test has been extended to include the staining of tissue sections (DFAT-TP) (42, 48). Any tissue can be used, but most frequently, tissue for paraffin-embedded sections is collected from the brain, gastrointestinal tract, placenta, umbilical cord (Fig. 3), or skin. Often, DFAT-TP is used to diagnose late-stage or congenital syphilis, although organism concentrations are often low in late adult syphilis, in congenital syphilis, and in resolving lesions of early syphilis (93).

The sample source for PCR is controversial (69). For example, one study found whole blood and lesion material, both exudate and tissue, to be satisfactory samples for PCR, whereas the appropriateness of serum and CSF as sample sources for PCR is still under consideration (69, 111). Contamination of the samples collected for PCR with extraneous DNA from other specimens can be a major problem and may account for some of the variable results noted by some researchers.

Any specimen source can be used for rabbit infectivity testing as long as the material is less than 1 h old or was flash frozen immediately after collection and was maintained in liquid nitrogen or at temperatures of −78°C or below; 10% glycerol or 5% (vol/vol) dimethyl sulfoxide may be added to liquid specimens immediately prior to freezing.

Dark-Field Microscopy

Because of their narrow width, treponemes cannot be observed with the ordinary light microscope. Microscopes equipped with a double-reflecting or a single-reflecting dark-field condenser, a ×40 to ×45 objective, and a ×90 to ×100 objective with a funnel stop are needed to perform the dark-field examination (48). The slide is first scanned with the ×40 to ×45 objective. Once an organism is located, a small drop of immersion oil is placed on the coverslip, the objective is switched to the ×90 to ×100 objec-

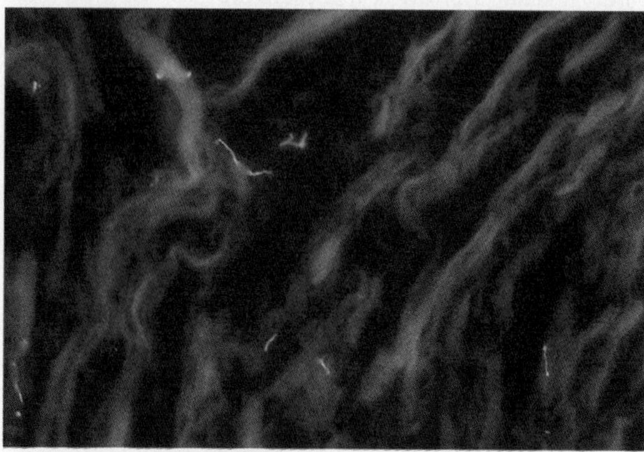

FIGURE 3 DFAT-TP of an umbilical cord section from a baby with congenital syphilis.

tive, and the organism is brought into focus. *T. pallidum* is distinguished from other spiral organisms by the tightness and regularity of the spirals and by the characteristic corkscrew movement. Positive findings on dark-field microscopic examination are reported as "organisms that have the characteristic morphology and motility of *T. pallidum* were found" and allow a specific and immediate diagnosis of syphilis. Also, primary syphilis can be diagnosed by dark-field microscopy before the appearance of reactive serologic tests. However, a negative dark-field microscopy finding does not exclude the diagnosis of syphilis, since the organisms may be too few to be demonstrated if the lesion is in the healing stage or if the infection has been altered by systemic or topical treatment. Adequate training and experience are necessary to make an accurate diagnosis by dark-field microscopy. The untrained observer may be deceived by artifacts such as cotton fibers and Brownian motion. When the direct microscopic examination results are negative, other sexually transmitted diseases that cause lesions, such as herpes and chancroid, should be considered.

DFA-TP Test

The easier to perform and more specific DFA-TP method has been used to detect the presence of *T. pallidum* subspecies in tissues, body fluids, secretions, and lesion exudates (48). A UV fluorescence microscope equipped with a dark-field condenser or epifluorescence illumination and the standard set of filters is required. The test detects pathogenic treponemes and differentiates them from nonpathogenic treponemes by an antigen-antibody reaction. For this reason, use of nonspecific fluorescent stains such as acridine orange is not recommended because nonpathogenic treponemes or artifacts may be confused with *T. pallidum*. Initially, samples are air dried, and immediately before staining, smears are fixed with either acetone for 10 min or 100% methanol for 10 s or slides are gently heat fixed. Smears are stained with fluorescein isothiocyanate (FITC)-labeled anti-*T. pallidum* globulins obtained from the sera of humans or rabbits with syphilis; these globulins have been absorbed with Reiter treponemes to remove cross-reacting antibodies. More recently, a mouse monoclonal antibody to *T. pallidum* has been used in the DFA-TP test (42). When fluorescing treponemes displaying typical morphology are seen by microscopic examination, results are reported as "treponemes immunologically specific for *T. pallidum* were observed by direct immunofluorescence." Negative results are reported as "treponemes were not observed by direct immunofluorescence." As with all tests for syphilis, the use of proper controls for the technique and for the reagents used in these methods is mandatory if the results are to be meaningful.

DFAT-TP Test

A combination of the DFAT-TP test and histological stains may be used to examine biopsy and autopsy material for the presence of pathogenic *Treponema* spp. (48). To perform the DFAT-TP test, tissue specimens obtained by punch biopsy or surgical excision are initially fixed for 24 h in 10% neutral-buffered formalin and are then embedded in paraffin blocks. Sections (2 μm) are attached to microscope slides and are then deparaffinized and pretreated with either NH_4OH or trypsin. Next, the slides are stained with a monoclonal antibody conjugate as for the DFA-TP test. A *T. pallidum*-infected rabbit testicular tissue section is used as the control. Results are reported as for the DFA-TP test.

PCR

The methods used for PCR have not been standardized, but one group of investigators (33, 90) has successfully used alkaline lysis extraction of the treponemal DNA in the sample. The primers and probe for detection of *T. pallidum* are prepared from the 47-kDa gene. After a 40-cycle series of denaturation, annealing, and extension, the PCR products are visualized by electrophoresis or dot blotting followed by hybridization with a ^{32}P-labeled probe and autoradiography. Nonradioactive probes may also be used. Although a commercial PCR for detection of *T. pallidum* in genital ulcers was under evaluation in 1995 and 1996 (61, 73), the manufacturer recently postponed further development until a later date.

Isolation Procedures

The *T. pallidum* subspecies and *T. carateum* cannot be cultivated in vitro by standard bacteriologic techniques. The pathogenic treponemes (except for *T. carateum*) can be propagated by inoculation of appropriate laboratory animals (108). This technique is capable of detecting one or two infectious treponemes under optimal conditions (55). Most recently, rabbit inoculation was used to demonstrate the presence of viable *T. pallidum* in the CSF of patients with early syphilis (53, 87). This method is not practical for routine diagnostic use because of the expense and technical difficulty.

Limited multiplication of *T. pallidum* subsp. *pallidum* has been obtained over a 10- to 20-day period in a complex tissue culture system, but continuous in vitro culture has not been achieved (18, 24, 70). The growth rate both in vivo and in vitro is very slow, with an estimated doubling time in vivo of 30 to 33 h. Recent evidence indicates that *T. pallidum* subsp. *pallidum* is a microaerophile rather than an anaerobe (17, 18). *T. pallidum* requires molecular oxygen for energy production through an oxidative phosphorylation mechanism, but it is extremely sensitive to oxygen radicals and will become nonviable within minutes to hours of exposure to atmospheric levels of oxygen. Therefore, survival is best in an atmosphere containing 1 to 5% O_2 and in media containing reducing agents. Glucose appears to provide the principal energy source, and serum is required for survival and growth.

Serologic Tests

General Principles

Humoral antibodies produced in response to *T. pallidum* infection become detectable in the primary stage and increase in concentration during the secondary stage. Antibody detection tests supplement the antigen detection methods used for the diagnosis of primary and secondary syphilis and are the only practical methods of diagnosis during early latent and late syphilis. As mentioned earlier, the serologic tests fall into one of two categories, nontreponemal or treponemal. Four nontreponemal tests and three treponemal tests are currently considered standard tests (Table 4).

Nontreponemal tests used for screening have the advantage of being widely available, inexpensive, convenient to perform with large numbers of specimens, and useful for determining the efficacy of treatment. Limitations of the nontreponemal serologic tests include their lack of sensitivity in early dark-field microscopy-positive primary syphilis and in late syphilis and the possibilities of a prozone reaction or of false-positive results. Treponemal tests use *T. pallidum* subsp. *pallidum* as the antigen and detect specific treponemal

TABLE 4 Standard status tests for syphilis

Type of test	Test name
Nontreponemal tests	VDRL slide Unheated serum reagin RPR 18-mm circle card TRUST
Treponemal tests	FTA-ABS test FTA-ABS double staining MHA-TP

antibodies that are usually related only to treponemal infections. Treponemal tests are primarily used to verify reactivity in the nontreponemal tests. The treponemal test may also be used to confirm a clinical impression of syphilis when the nontreponemal test is nonreactive but there is evidence of syphilis, such as might occur in late syphilis. Unfortunately, treponemal tests are technically more difficult and costly to perform than nontreponemal tests and cannot be used to monitor treatment. For 85% of persons successfully treated, test results remain reactive for years, if not a lifetime.

Specimen Collection

When collecting, preparing, and examining specimens, observe universal safety precautions (48). Serum is the specimen of choice for both nontreponemal and treponemal tests. However, the rapid plasma reagin (RPR) card test and toluidine red unheated serum test (TRUST) may also be performed with plasma samples. The technician must check the product insert to be sure that the plasma sample has not been stored for longer than the recommended storage time and that the blood was collected in the specified anticoagulant. Plasma cannot be used in the VDRL test, since the sample must be heated before testing, and plasma cannot be used in the treponemal tests for syphilis. The VDRL test is the only test that should be used for the testing of CSF. The CSF is not heated before the test is performed.

When screening for congenital syphilis, CDC recommends the testing of the mother's serum rather than cord blood. Recent studies compared the reactivities of the mother's serum, cord blood, and infant's serum and found that the maternal sample is the best indicator of infection, followed by neonatal serum, with cord blood being the least reactive (15, 79). Infant's serum is the specimen of choice for the IgM-specific tests.

Nontreponemal Tests

All available nontreponemal tests are based on an antigen composed of an alcoholic solution containing measured amounts of cardiolipin, cholesterol, and sufficient purified lecithin to produce standard reactivity (49). The nontreponemal (reagin) tests measure IgM and IgG antibodies to lipoidal material released from damaged host cells as well as antibodies to lipoprotein-like material and possibly cardiolipin released from the treponemes (2, 56). The antilipoidal antibodies are antibodies that can be produced not only as a consequence of syphilis and the other treponemal diseases but also in response to autoimmune diseases, pregnancy, nontreponemal diseases of an acute and chronic nature in which tissue damage occurs, and other conditions (see below).

The standard nontreponemal tests use flocculation of lipoidal particles to indicate reactivity. The test antigen is mixed with the patient's serum on a solid matrix and rotated for a specified number of minutes before reading of the results. Because of the lipid nature of the antigen, the lipid particles formed are barely visible. Likewise, the antigen-antibody complex that occurs with serum from individuals with syphilis remains suspended, and flocculation rather than agglutination or precipitation occurs. The VDRL and unheated serum reagin (USR) tests are flocculation tests requiring microscopic examination, whereas reactions in the RPR test and TRUST, because of the addition of colored particles, can be read without magnification. Each of the standard status nontreponemal tests can be performed as a quantitative test by preparing serial dilutions of the patient's serum to reach an endpoint titer. As qualitative tests, the nontreponemal tests are used to screen for syphilis. Quantitative tests are more informative than qualitative tests alone. Quantitative tests establish a baseline of reactivity from which change can be measured; this baseline allows evaluation of recent infection by demonstrating a fourfold rise in titer and helps to detect reinfection or relapse among persons with a persistently reactive (serofast) test for syphilis. All of the nontreponemal tests have approximately the same sensitivity and specificity (Table 5), but their reactivity levels may differ as a result of the variation in antigen preparation. The different levels of reactivity are reflected in the different endpoint titers obtained when the same serum sample is tested in the four tests. Because success or failure of treatment is based on just a fourfold decrease in titer, the serum sample used as the baseline should be drawn on the day that treatment is begun. Also, because of the variation in reactivity levels among the tests, the same test used in the initial testing should be used to monitor treatment.

Qualitative test results for the microscopic tests (the VDRL test and the USR test) are reported as reactive, weakly reactive, or nonreactive. Qualitative test results for the macroscopic tests (the RPR card test and TRUST) are reported as reactive (regardless of the size of the flocculant) or nonreactive. Quantitative results may be reported as the reciprocal of the dilution, for example, 4 dils or a titer of 4 rather than a 1:4 dilution. The endpoint reported is the last dilution giving a fully reactive, not weakly reactive, result. This variation in the reporting of quantitative test results between the microscopic and macroscopic tests partially accounts for the lower titers often reported for microscopic tests.

The interpretation of the results also depends on the population being tested. When the nontreponemal tests are used as a screening test in a low-risk population, all reactive results should be confirmed with a treponemal test. In low-risk populations, false-positive reactions may outnumber true-positive reactions. Nontreponemal test results must also be interpreted according to the stage of syphilis suspected. Approximately 30% of those with early primary syphilis have nonreactive nontreponemal test results on the initial visit. The nontreponemal test usually becomes reactive 1 to 4 weeks after the chancre appears. In secondary syphilis, nearly all patients will have nontreponemal test endpoint titers of $\geq$1:8. For patients with atypical lesions and/or nontreponemal test titers of $<$1:8, the nontreponemal tests should be repeated and a confirmatory treponemal test should be performed. Patients with late latent syphilis, i.e., with reactive nontreponemal and treponemal tests, no clinical or historical findings, and an unknown history of treatment or nonreactive serologic results, should be evaluated for potential asymptomatic neurosyphilis. Even without

TABLE 5 Percent sensitivity and specificity of serologic tests for syphilis

Test	Sensitivity (%)				Specificity (%) (nonsyphilis)
	Primary	Secondary	Latent	Late	
Nontreponemal tests					
VDRL	78 (74–87)[a]	100	95 (88–100)	71 (37–94)	98 (96–99)
RPR card	86 (77–100)	100	98 (95–100)	73	98 (93–99)
USR[b]	80 (72–88)	100	95 (88–100)		99
TRUST	85 (77–86)	100	98 (95–100)		99 (98–99)
Treponemal tests					
FTA-ABS test	84 (70–100)	100	100	96	97 (94–100)
MHA-TP	76 (69–90)	100	97 (97–100)	94	99 (98–100)
FTA-ABS DS[c]	80 (69–90)	100	100		98 (97–100)

[a] Range in CDC studies.
[b] USR, unheated serum reagin.
[c] DS, double staining.

treatment the nontreponemal test may be weakly reactive or even nonreactive in the late stages of syphilis.

Neurosyphilis should be suspected in patients with neurologic symptoms, reactive serum nontreponemal or treponemal tests, and a history indicating a lack of previous treatment. Diagnosis may be confirmed by a reactive VDRL test with CSF or demonstration of *T. pallidum* in CSF or tissue by microscopy, PCR, or rabbit infectivity assay. Neurosyphilis is usually accompanied by a predominantly mononuclear leukocytosis and elevated protein levels in the CSF, but these are nonspecific findings. When a patient is treated for neurosyphilis, the CSF cell count usually returns to normal first; this is followed by a return to normal of the CSF protein concentration and, finally, the nontreponemal serologic test result (49). However, the response of the quantitative VDRL test with CSF to treatment is less predictable; it may take many years for the nontreponemal test with CSF to become nonreactive, although the titer should drop progressively.

Congenital syphilis can be controlled by treating pregnant women. False-positive nontreponemal test results for samples from pregnant women have been reported, and reactive results should be confirmed by a treponemal test. Nontreponemal titers remaining from previous treatment for syphilis tend to increase nonspecifically during pregnancy. This increase in titer may be confused with the diagnosis of reinfection or relapse. An increase in titer may be considered nonspecific if previous treatment can be documented and if dark-field microscopy-positive lesions, a fourfold increase in titer, and a history of recent sexual exposure to a person with infectious syphilis are absent. Previously, the difference between the mother's nontreponemal test titer and the infant's titer at delivery was thought to be a means of distinguishing infected from uninfected infants. If the infant's titer was higher than that of the mother's, then the infant had congenital syphilis. However, the converse is not true. A lower titer in the infant's serum than in the mother's serum does not rule out congenital syphilis. Examination of serum sample pairs from mothers and infants for congenital syphilis indicated that only 22% of the infants had a titer higher than that of the mother (102).

In any form of syphilis, patients should be monitored to ensure that treatment was effective, i.e., that signs and symptoms have resolved and that the titer has declined. A fall in antibody titer following treatment establishes cure (26–28, 92), whereas a rise in titer following treatment indicates treatment failure or reinfection. To monitor the efficacy of treatment, quantitative nontreponemal tests should be performed with the patient's serum samples, which are drawn at 3- to 4-month intervals for at least 1 year. Following adequate therapy for initial episodes of primary and secondary syphilis, there should be at least a fourfold decline in the VDRL test titer by the third or fourth month and an eightfold decline in titer by the sixth to eighth month (48). When the RPR card test is used to monitor treatment, the initial fourfold decline in titer may not be observed until the sixth or eighth month after treatment (49). For most patients treated during the early stage of syphilis, the titers decline until little or no reaction is detected after 3 years (26, 28, 48, 49, 88). Patients who are treated in the latent or late stages or patients who have had multiple episodes of syphilis may show a more gradual decline in titer (25, 28, 87). A low titer will persist in approximately 50% of these patients after 2 years (25). As far as can be determined, this persistent seropositivity does not signify treatment failure or reinfection, and these patients are likely to remain serofast even if they are retreated (25). Recent studies indicate that HIV infection may delay the decline in antibody titer detected by nontreponemal tests for syphilis in patients with primary or secondary syphilis (87). The prognostic significance of this finding is unknown, since these patients did not experience clinical treatment failure during the 1-year posttreatment observation period. A delayed decline in antibody titer was not associated with detection of *T. pallidum* in CSF, and enhanced therapy did not appear to prevent the delay (87).

Prozone reactions occur in 1 to 2% of patients with secondary syphilis. Undiluted serum samples exhibiting a weakly reactive, an atypical, or, on rare occasions, a "rough negative" reaction should be diluted as in the quantitative assay, in which case the reactivity will increase and then decrease as the endpoint titer is approached. Dilution of the antibody to 1:16 is usually adequate to obtain the proper optimal concentration and a readily detectable reaction.

False-positive reactions can occur either acutely (<6 months' duration) as an outcome of viral infections, immunizations, or pregnancy or chronically (>6 months' duration) as a result of multisystem autoimmune diseases such as systemic lupus erythematosus or other conditions including narcotic addiction, aging, malignancy, or leprosy. False-positive reactions are generally low in titer (<1:8), but high-titer false-positive nontreponemal test results can be obtained for up to 10% of intravenous drug abusers.

Treponemal Tests

Three tests are considered standard treponemal tests (Table 4); all use *T. pallidum* as the antigen and are based on the detection of antibodies directed against cellular components (48). The treponemal tests are not intended for routine use as screening procedures. Their greatest value is in distinguishing positive nontreponemal test results from false-positive results and in establishing the diagnosis of late latent or late syphilis. Problems arise when these tests are used as screening procedures, because about 1% of the general population will have false-positive results. However, a reactive treponemal test result for a sample that is also reactive by a nontreponemal test is highly specific.

If used appropriately as confirmatory tests, the treponemal tests have few limitations; their greatest limitation is cost. Treponemal tests vary in their sensitivity for the detection of early primary syphilis (Table 5); this is related to the time of serum collection after lesion development. With primary syphilis, the microhemagglutination assay for antibodies to *T. pallidum* (MHA-TP) is less sensitive than the fluorescent treponemal antibody absorption (FTA-ABS) test and is probably less sensitive than the nontreponemal tests.

In the secondary stage of syphilis, the sensitivity of MHA-TP is equal to that of the nontreponemal and FTA-ABS tests. In the secondary and latent stages all of the treponemal tests are 100% reactive. Because the sensitivities of the nontreponemal tests decline to approximately 70% in the late stages of syphilis (Table 5), treponemal test results should be obtained if syphilis in these stages is suspected and the nontreponemal tests are nonreactive. The laboratory should be informed that late syphilis is suspected; otherwise, according to laboratory policy, a treponemal test may not be performed when the nontreponemal test result is nonreactive. Again, these findings should be interpreted in the light of treatment history, in that treponemal tests usually remain reactive following effective therapy.

As with the nontreponemal tests, all standard treponemal tests are reactive for congenital syphilis. Passively transferred treponemal antibodies should be catabolized and undetectable among noninfected infants between the ages of 12 and 18 months.

Although false-positive results by the treponemal tests are often transient and their cause is unknown, a definite association has been made between false-positive FTA-ABS test results and the diagnosis of systemic, discoid, and drug-induced varieties of lupus erythematosus (49). Patients with systemic lupus erythematosus can give false-positive FTA-ABS test results that exhibit an "atypical beading" fluorescence pattern. Patients whose serum specimens exhibit this type of reaction should be screened for autoimmune disease, including a test for serum anti-DNA antibodies. Unexplained reactive serologic results may also occur, particularly in elderly patients. Some false-positive reactions may be due to the failure of the sorbent used in the tests to remove all cross-reacting antibodies against group-, genus-, or family-specific antigens, e.g., antibodies to the organism that causes Lyme disease (40, 54). In these instances, the hemagglutination test or absorption with *T. phagedenis* Reiter may be the only means of differentiating between syphilis and a false-positive reaction.

Of the three treponemal test methods currently in use, MHA-TP gives fewer false-positive results. In general, the occurrence of false-positive hemagglutination test results is rare in healthy persons (<1%). Inconclusive hemagglutination test results have been reported for patients with infectious mononucleosis, especially in the presence of high heterophile antibody levels. Presumably, false-positive hemagglutination test results also occur with samples from drug addicts, patients with collagen disease, patients with leprosy, and patients with other miscellaneous conditions. In some cases, it is difficult to assess whether syphilis actually coexists with these other infections. If both the FTA-ABS test and MHA-TP are reactive, the sample is most likely (95%) from a person who has or has had syphilis (81). However, the final decision rests with clinical judgment.

FTA-ABS Tests

The FTA-ABS test is an indirect fluorescent-antibody technique (48). By this procedure, the antigen used is *T. pallidum* subsp. *pallidum* Nichols. The patient's serum is first diluted 1:5 in sorbent (an extract from cultures of the nonpathogenic Reiter treponeme) to remove group-specific treponemal antibodies that are produced in some persons in response to nonpathogenic treponemes. Next, the serum is layered on a microscope slide to which *T. pallidum* has been fixed. If the patient's serum contains *T. pallidum*-specific antibody, the antibody binds to the treponeme. FITC-labeled anti-human immunoglobulin is added, and it combines with the adherent patient antibodies, resulting in FITC-stained spirochetes that are visible when examined by fluorescence microscopy.

A modification of the standard FTA-ABS test is the FTA-ABS double staining test (Fig. 4). The FTA-ABS double staining technique uses a tetramethylrhodamine isothiocyanate-labeled, anti-human IgG globulin (Fig. 4B) and a counterstain with FITC-labeled anti-*T. pallidum* conjugate (Fig. 4A). The counterstain was developed for use with microscopes with incident illumination to eliminate the need to locate the treponemes by dark-field microscopy when the patient's serum does not contain antibodies to *T. pallidum*. Counterstaining of the organism ensures that the nonreactive result is due to the absence of antibodies and not to the absence of treponemes on the slide.

Results of both FTA-ABS tests are reported as reactive, reactive minimal, or nonreactive or as the observation of atypical fluorescence. Specimens initially read as 1+ (reactive minimal) should always be retested. If the results are again read as 1+, they should be reported as such with the statement that "in the absence of historical or clinical evidence of treponemal infection, this test result should be considered equivocal." A second specimen should be obtained 1 to 2 weeks after the initial specimen and submitted to the laboratory for serologic testing. Beaded fluorescence (e.g., atypical staining) should be reported to alert the physician to possible autoimmune diseases.

The sources for errors are numerous with the FTA-ABS tests, because they are multicomponent tests and each component must be matched with the other ones. Conjugates must be properly titrated, and controls for reactive, reactive minimal, and nonreactive samples and for nonspecific staining and sorbent must be included. Slides must be evaluated to ensure that the antigen is adhering. In addition, the microscope must be in proper operating condition with the appropriate filters in place.

MHA-TP

Passive hemagglutination of erythrocytes sensitized with antigen is an extremely simple method for the detection of

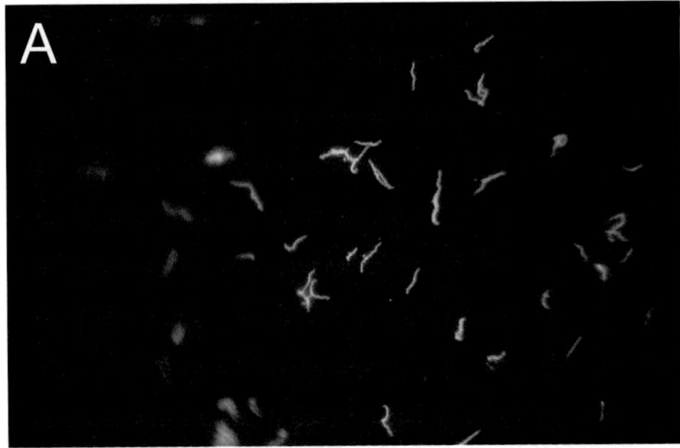

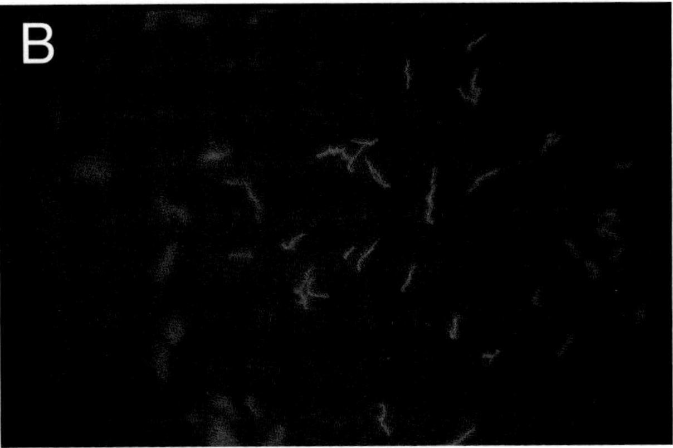

FIGURE 4 Fluorescent treponemal antibody-absorption double-staining test. (A) FITC-labeled anti-*T. pallidum* conjugate; (B) tetramethyl rhodamine isothiocyanate-labeled anti-human IgG.

antibody (48). The antigen used in the procedure is formalinized, tanned sheep erythrocytes sensitized with ultrasonicated material from *T. pallidum* Nichols. The patient's serum is first mixed with absorbing diluent made from nonpathogenic Reiter treponemes and other absorbents and stabilizers. The serum is then placed in a microtiter plate and sensitized sheep erythrocytes are added. Serum containing antibodies reacts with these cells to form a smooth mat of agglutinated cells in the microtiter plate. Unsensitized cells are used as a control for nonspecific reactivity.

Results are reported as reactive, nonreactive, or inconclusive. Reactive results are reported for a range of agglutination patterns, from a smooth mat of agglutinated cells surrounded by a smaller red circle of unagglutinated cells with hemagglutination outside the circle (1+) to a smooth mat of agglutinated cells covering the entire bottom of the well (4+). With highly reactive serum samples the edges of the mat are sometimes folded. Nonreactive results are reported when a definite compact button with or without a very small hole in its center forms in the center of the well. A button of unagglutinated cells having a small hole in the center is initially read as "±," and the test should be repeated. If the same pattern is again observed, then the report should be "nonreactive." If agglutination is observed with the unsensitized cells, then the test is repeated as follows. Twofold dilutions of the absorbed serum are prepared in absorbing diluent in two rows of the microtiter plate wells. Sensitized cells are added to each well in one row, and unsensitized cells are added to each well in the other row. A reactive result is reported, without reference to titer, if (i) the hemagglutination with sensitized cells is at least 2 doubling dilutions (four times greater) than that with unsensitized cells and (ii) the first dilution showing no hemagglutination with unsensitized cells has a 3+ or 4+ reaction with sensitized cells. Otherwise, the test results are reported as inconclusive.

Because the test is based on agglutination, quantitation of treponemal antibody is possible but has not proven to be worthwhile. Most studies demonstrate no practical relationship between the titer and either the progression of the disease or the clinical stage of syphilis diagnosed, and unlike the quantitative nontreponemal tests, the quantitative MHA-TP does not seem to be useful in posttreatment evaluations (49). The sources for error with MHA-TP are usually associated with the use of dusty or improper plates, pipetting errors, or vibrations in the laboratory.

Newer Serologic Tests for Syphilis

Several tests that use the enzyme immunoassay (EIA) format have been developed for the diagnosis of syphilis (41, 48, 51, 63, 75, 114). In the nontreponemal SpiroTek Reagin II test (Organon Teknika, Durham, N.C.), a VDRL antigen coats the wells of the microtiter plate. Anticardiolipin antibodies in the patient's serum adhere to the antigen in the wells, and this antibody reaction is detected by an anti-human IgG antibody labeled with peroxidase as the enzyme. For untreated syphilis, the test has a sensitivity of 97% and, in an uninfected population, a specificity of 97% (75). Like the other nontreponemal tests, the reactivity of the Reagin II test declines with treatment of the patients, but the test is not a quantitative technique.

Because infected infants can produce IgM in utero after 3 months of gestation and because the fetus can be infected with *T. pallidum* at any time during gestation, an EIA measuring IgM would appear to be appropriate. One such test, the Syphilis-M (Sanofi Diagnostics Pasteur, Chaska, Minn., and Trinity Biotech, Jamestown, N.Y.), is available commercially. This test is based on the use of anti-human IgM antibody to capture IgM in the patient's serum, followed by the use of a purified *T. pallidum* antigen to detect those IgM antibodies in the patient's serum directed toward *T. pallidum* (41). Next, a horseradish peroxidase-conjugated monoclonal antibody to *T. pallidum* is used to detect the antigen-patient antibody reaction through the enzyme's reaction with a substrate. One study found that the IgM capture EIA was more sensitive than the FTA-ABS 19S IgM test in detecting probable cases of congenital syphilis (102); however, another study found the test to be equal in sensitivity to the IgM Western blot for the detection of neonatal congenital syphilis but less sensitive than the Western blot for the detection of delayed-onset congenital syphilis (5).

Of the commercial IgG EIA (Spirotek Syphilis [Organon Teknika]; Syphilis-G [Sanofi Diagnostics Pasteur and Trinity Biotech]) designed to replace the FTA-ABS tests and MHA-TP as confirmatory tests for syphilis, initial evaluations have found all to have sensitivities and specificities similar to those of the other treponemal tests (51, 63, 114).

Another test format frequently used in the research laboratory is the Western blot for *T. pallidum*. This test is not commercially available but is performed in the Syphilis Diagnostic Immunology Activity Laboratory at CDC. The test uses IgG conjugate and appears to be at least as sensitive and specific as the FTA-ABS tests, and efforts have been made to standardize the procedure (7, 29). To date many investigators agree that the detection of antibodies to the immunodeterminants with molecular masses of 15.5, 17, 44.5, and 47 kDa appears to be diagnostic for acquired syphilis (72). The Western blot for *T. pallidum* has its greatest value as a diagnostic test for congenital syphilis when an IgM-specific conjugate is used (5, 19, 52, 90, 91). The IgM Western blot for congenital syphilis appears to have a greater specificity and sensitivity than the FTA-ABS 19S IgM test and IgM EIA. Unfortunately, the Western blot test is not yet commercially available.

Treatment and Antimicrobial Susceptibilities

The syphilis treatment guidelines recommended by CDC in 1998 are provided in Table 6 (8). Penicillin and its derivatives are the preferred antimicrobial agents for the treatment of syphilis and the other treponematoses. Early syphilis in immunologically normal patients can be treated effectively with a single dose of benzathine penicillin G. Neurosyphilis should be treated with either aqueous crystalline penicillin G or procaine penicillin, because benzathine penicillin does not achieve treponemacidal concentrations in the central nervous system. In one study, viable *T. pallidum* was present in the CSF of 12 of 40 untreated primary and secondary syphilis patients (53). Central nervous system infection persisted in some patients following benzathine penicillin therapy, regardless of HIV status (53, 87). In immunologically normal patients, the host apparently clears the remaining organisms, because the incidence of relapse is low in benzathine penicillin-treated patients. However, HIV-infected individuals may be susceptible to neurologic or ocular complications of syphilis following benzathine penicillin treatment (4). Therefore, some investigators have recommended that therapy appropriate for neurosyphilis be used for all patients coinfected with *T. pallidum* and HIV and that HIV-positive patients be examined carefully for clinical signs of neurologic involvement (e.g., CSF examination) prior to and after therapy (4, 37). However, Rolfs et al. (87) failed to show any benefit in treating primary or secondary syphilis in HIV-infected patients with an "enhanced" regimen (benzathine penicillin G plus amoxicillin plus probenecid). Late latent syphilis patients with evidence of neurosyphilis or other forms of active syphilis should have a CSF examination; if neurologic involvement is indicated, prolonged treatment with benzathine penicillin is recommended (Table 6).

Effective therapy of early syphilis may result in a Jarisch-Herxheimer reaction, consisting of fever and local intensification of lesions. This reaction, thought to result from the rapid release of treponemal antigens, occurs within the first 12 h of the initiation of therapy and usually resolves within 24 h.

Doxycycline and tetracycline can be used as alternative therapies for the treatment of penicillin-allergic individuals. Erythromycin is no longer recommended because of the occurrence of treatment failures and the possible existence of erythromycin-resistant strains (101), and the macrolides are contraindicated in pregnant women. For the pregnant patient with syphilis, the treatment guidelines suggest that penicillin allergy be documented by thorough questioning regarding the patient's history and by skin testing. If necessary, the patient may be desensitized to permit the use of penicillin therapy (8). A Jarisch-Herxheimer reaction occurring in pregnant women may cause premature labor, fetal distress, or (rarely) stillbirth. However, the high probability of fetal damage resulting from syphilitic infection in the absence of adequate therapy outweighs this risk.

Antimicrobial susceptibility testing is not straightforward, owing to the lack of a method for continuous culture of *T. pallidum*. A number of approaches have been used to determine the susceptibilities of representative strains (e.g., the Nichols strain) to antimicrobial agents, including in vitro loss of motility or infectivity, treatment of experimental animal infections, human trials, and examination of the susceptibilities of nonpathogenic, cultivable treponemes (80). Inhibition of protein synthesis and of in vitro multipli-

TABLE 6 Recommended treatment for syphilis[a]

Stage	Treatment[b]
Primary, secondary, or early latent disease (<1-yr duration)	Benzathine penicillin G, 2.4 U IM in one dose For patients allergic to penicillin (nonpregnant): doxycycline, 100 mg orally b.i.d. for 14 days, or tetracycline, 500 mg orally q.i.d. for 14 days
Late latent syphilis (>1-yr duration) or syphilis of unknown duration	Benzathine penicillin G, 7.2 $\times$ 10^6 U total, 2.4 $\times$ 10^6 U per wk for 3 consecutive wk; for patients allergic to penicillin (nonpregnant): doxycycline, 100 mg orally b.i.d. for 28 days, or tetracycline, 500 mg orally q.i.d. for 28 days[c]
Tertiary disease, excluding neurosyphilis	As for late latent disease, with appropriate management of complications
Neurosyphilis	Aqueous crystalline penicillin G, 18 $\times$ 10^6 to 24 $\times$ 10^6 U per day i.v. (3 $\times$ 10^6 to 4 $\times$ 10^6 U every 4 h) for 10 to 14 days, or procaine penicillin, 2.4 $\times$ 10^6 U per day i.m., plus probenecid, 500 mg orally q.i.d., both for 10 to 14 days
Syphilis during pregnancy	Penicillin regimen appropriate for the woman's stage of syphilis. Tetracycline, doxycycline, and erythromycin are contraindicated.[d] Insufficient data to recommend azithromycin or ceftriaxone.
Congenital syphilis	Aqueous crystalline penicillin G, 100,000 to 150,000 U per kg per day i.v. (50,000 U/kg i.v. every 12 h) for the first 7 days of life and every 8 h on days 8 to 10

[a] Adapted from references 8, 37, and 116; refer to these resources for further information.

[b] b.i.d., twice a day; q.i.d., four times a day; i.m., intramuscularly; i.v., intravenously.

[c] Patients treated for syphilis with regimens that do not include penicillin may be at increased risk for treatment failure. Assurance of compliance with therapy and follow-up are recommended for such patients.

[d] Women treated in the second half of pregnancy are at risk for premature labor and/or fetal stress due to a Jarisch-Herxheimer reaction. Tetracycline and doxycycline are contraindicated due to possible fetal bone and tooth damage, and erythromycin poses a high risk of treatment failure.

cation in a tissue culture system has been shown to be an effective means of determining susceptibility (71, 101). The MICs (in micrograms per milliliter) determined by the in vitro culture method were 0.0005 for penicillin G, 0.2 for tetracycline, 0.0007 for ceftriaxone, 0.04 for cefetamet, 0.004 for cefteram, and 0.007 for ceftazidime. Like other spirochetes, *T. pallidum* was relatively insensitive to seven quinolones tested (MIC range, 1 to 10 μg/ml) and to rifampin (MIC, 44 μg/ml). The minimal bactericidal concentration, as determined by loss of infectivity during in vitro culture, were one- to fivefold higher than the MICs (71).

T. pallidum strains appear to be uniformly susceptible to penicillin and other β-lactams. There is no evidence for the development of resistance to penicillin, as has occurred with *Neisseria gonorrhoeae* and other pathogens. Penicillin G provides greater inhibitory activity than cephalosporins and the other β-lactams tested. Ceftriaxone, amoxicillin, and ampicillin are active against *T. pallidum* in vitro and also appear to be effective in the treatment of early syphilis. Amoxicillin and ampicillin offer no theoretical advantage over benzathine penicillin G. Ceftriaxone has a long serum half-life and reaches high levels in the central nervous system. However, the cost is high, multiple doses are required, and there is a 3 to 7% risk of adverse reactions in penicillin-allergic individuals; in addition, the data on efficacy in patients are limited. Therefore, ceftriaxone is not currently recommended as an alternative therapy for early syphilis.

OTHER HUMAN HOST-ASSOCIATED SPIROCHETES

In addition to *T. pallidum* and related pathogens, a number of anaerobic treponemes and other spirochetes are parasites of humans. These include separate groups of spirochetes found in the oral cavity (particularly the gingival crevices), in sebaceous secretions in the genital region, and in the colon and rectum (Table 7). In general, these spirochetes are considered commensal organisms. However, there is evidence that spirochetes are involved in gingivitis and periodontal disease and that overgrowth of intestinal spirochetes may correlate with the occurrence of diarrhea or other bowel disorders.

Oral Spirochetes

A variety of spirochetes inhabit supragingival and subgingival plaques in humans; only a small proportion of these have been cultured in vitro and characterized (16). Those that have been cultivated and identified to the species level are within the genus *Treponema* (Table 7). They are spiral-shaped organisms ranging from 0.15 to 0.30 μm in diameter and from 5 to 16 μm in length (with lengths being variable within each species). Although the species differ from one another slightly in terms of cell diameter and helical configuration, it is generally not possible to identify them on morphologic grounds; genotypic characteristics and biochemical parameters such as growth requirements, carbohydrate fermentation, and enzymatic activities are used to identify species (95).

The oral spirochetes listed in Table 7 are difficult to isolate from healthy gingiva, but they increase both in prevalence and in number of organisms present in patients with gingivitis or periodontal disease. Treponemes are detected in the subgingival plaque of 88 to 97% of patients with periodontal disease (60). *T. socranskii* is the most common isolate in patients without periodontal disease, followed by *T. denticola* and *T. pectinovorum*. These organisms are isolated from a greater proportion of patients with periodontal disease than patients without the disease (60, 96, 97).

The procedures for isolation and characterization of oral spirochetes have been described previously (59, 60, 95–98). Briefly, treponemes may be cultured from samples of supragingival or subgingival material removed with a sterile dental scaler having a detachable tip or paper points. Samples should be examined by dark-field microscopy for the presence and morphologic characteristics of spirochetes. The plaque material is placed into tubes with sterile anaerobic dilution broth and small glass beads and is dispersed by vortexing for a few seconds. Tenfold dilutions are made and inoculated onto agar plates containing oral treponeme isolation medium, a complex peptone-yeast extract medium containing clarified rumen fluid and serum as sources of short- and long-chain fatty acids, respectively (59, 96). Alternatively, M10 medium or a modification thereof (47) may be used. Selection of treponemes can be achieved by addition of rifampin (2 μg/ml) and polymyxin B (800 U/ml) to the medium or by use of a membrane filter technique. By the latter technique, a sterile 45-μm-pore-size nitrocellulose filter with an average pore diameter of 0.15 to 0.3 μm is placed on the surface of agar isolation medium. A sterile O ring is sealed onto the filter with 3% molten agarose, and a few drops of the diluted sample are placed in the resulting

TABLE 7 Other human host-associated spirochetes

Type	Habitat	Species and groups	Reference(s)
Oral spirochetes	Dental plaque in gingival crevices	*Treponema denticola*	59, 60, 82, 95
		Treponema socranskii	60, 82, 97
		Treponema vincentii	59, 95
		Treponema pectinovorum	96
		Treponema skoliodontum	59, 95
		Treponema maltophilum	113
		Treponema medium	109
		Pathogen-related oral spirochetes	82–86, 94
Skin-associated spirochetes	Sebaceous secretions in genital region	*Treponema phagedenis*	59, 95
		Treponema refringens	
		Treponema minutum	
Intestinal spirochetes	Colon, rectum, feces	*Serpulina pilosicoli*	50, 105–107
		Brachyspira aalborgii	39

well. Treponemes are capable of translocating through the filter into the underlying medium, whereas other bacteria are trapped on the surface. Growth is indicated by a white, hazy appearance of the medium when the filter is removed after 1 to 2 weeks of incubation at 37°C. Subculture and single-colony isolation can be achieved by removing a plug from the area of growth and placing it in broth or semisolid medium and by streaking plates with 2- to 3-day cultures. At all stages, care should be taken to minimize exposure to air and to maintain strict anaerobic conditions during culture through the use of prereduced medium and an anaerobic chamber or anaerobic jars gassed with nitrogen with 5% carbon dioxide. Anaerobic jars with platinum catalyst may be evacuated and refilled three times with a nitrogen-hydrogen-carbon dioxide gas mixture; alternatively, a GasPak envelope (BBL, Baltimore, Md.) may be used.

Pathogen-related oral spirochetes (PROS) were found in plaque samples from a high proportion of patients with necrotizing ulcerative gingivitis or periodontitis but were absent from healthy subjects (82–86, 94). However, PROS and other spirochetes could be found in healthy gingival regions but could not be detected in most sites of periodontitis (82, 83), bringing into question the strength of the association of these organisms with periodontal disease. PROS have not been cultured in vitro and are identified by their reactivity with monoclonal antibodies specific for *T. pallidum* antigens, including the 37-kDa flagellar sheath protein (FlaA) and a major, 47-kDa lipoprotein. Gingivitis and periodontitis patients also expressed IgG antibodies reactive with 47-, 37-, 14-, and 12-kDa *T. pallidum* subsp. *pallidum* antigens, whereas a smaller proportion of healthy subjects had detectable antibodies against only the 47- and 37-kDa antigens (80). PROS were found in the periodontal tissue of ulcerative gingivitis patients (84, 86) and were capable of migrating through a mouse abdomen wall barrier, an invasive property shared with *T. pallidum* but not the cultivable oral treponemes (85). Oral spirochetes reactive with the anti-*T. pallidum* monoclonal antibodies were also detected in gorillas and dogs (94). Further studies are in progress to establish the taxonomic relationship between PROS and other spirochetes and to determine whether PROS represent frank pathogens.

NONPATHOGENIC SPIROCHETES OF THE GENITAL REGION

T. phagedenis, *T. refringens*, and *T. minutum* are treponemal species that inhabit the smegma (sebaceous secretions and desquamated epithelial cells) found beneath the prepuce and in other epithelial folds of the genital region. *T. phagedenis* and *T. refringens* are 0.20 to 0.25 μm in diameter, whereas *T. minutum* tends to be smaller in diameter (0.15 to 0.20 μm). Although *T. phagedenis* and *T. refringens* have been shown to have $\leq$5% homology with *T. pallidum* by DNA-DNA hybridization (23), comparison of 16S rRNA sequences indicates that they are related to the pathogenic treponemes. These harmless normal flora could potentially be misidentified as *T. pallidum* in dark-field microscopy preparations from skin sites. Careful cleansing of the site as described in the Specimen Collection section under Detection and Identification of *T. pallidum* in Tissue and Tissue Exudates obviates this possibility. The skin-associated treponemes may be collected with sterile moistened swabs and placed in anaerobic transport medium or directly into selective medium. They are readily cultured in peptone-yeast extract-glucose medium or in thioglycolate medium with 10% heat-inactivated rabbit serum under anaerobic conditions at 37°C (59).

INTESTINAL SPIROCHETES

The presence of spirochetes in the colon, rectum, and feces of humans has been recognized for more than a hundred years (89). Since the description of "human intestinal spirochetosis" in 1967 (35), there has been a resurgence in interest in the possible involvement of intestinal spirochetes in diarrhea and other gastrointestinal diseases (34), as well as in the apparently high prevalence of these organisms in homosexual males and HIV-infected individuals (89).

Morphologically, most human intestinal spirochetes are relatively short (3 to 6 μm on average) and are 0.2 to 0.4 μm in diameter with one to two helices per cell. Longer cells may also be present. They have pointed ends and four to six periplasmic flagella attached subterminally in a single row at each end of the cell. The human intestinal spirochetes identified thus far fall into two species: *Serpulina pilosicoli* and *Brachyspira aalborgii*. *S. pilosicoli* (106, 107) is related to the *Serpulina* species *S. hyodysenteriae*, *S. innocens*, *S. intermedia*, and *S. murdochii* (99). Thus far, *S. pilosicoli* is the only *Serpulina* species isolated from humans (50, 105–107). *S. pilosicoli* has a broad range of natural hosts, including swine, mice, rats, dogs, and chickens (20, 57, 78, 104, 106, 107). *B. aalborgii* (39) is genetically and phenotypically distinct from *S. pilosicoli* (46, 106). *S. pilosicoli* represents the vast majority of human intestinal spirochetes that have been isolated.

When observed in association with rectal or colonic tissue, these organisms are typically attached by the tip to the apical surface of the columnar epithelial cells. Although the spirochetes can form a dense layer visible by light microscopy (using silver staining or other staining techniques), signs of tissue damage or inflammation are usually absent.

A clear association between intestinal spirochetes and disease has not been established (89). Spirochetes can be present in healthy individuals as well as those with diarrhea or other gastrointestinal symptoms. In the early 1900s, several studies examined the presence of spirochetes in human stool specimens by light microscopy. In those studies with more than 100 patients, the proportion of subjects with spirochetes ranged from 3.3 to 61%. Recent examinations of rectal biopsy specimens from heterosexual patients by light and electron microscopy or culture have indicated the presence of spirochetes in 1.9 to 6.9% of subjects, and helical organisms were also found to be associated with normal and inflamed appendixes. Higher proportions of homosexual males have been reported to have intestinal spirochetes. At present, there is no clear evidence for an association between intestinal spirochetosis and HIV infection.

S. pilosicoli was isolated from routine anaerobic cultures of blood from seven critically ill patients, including those with stroke, ethylene glycol intoxication, severe arteriopathy, peritonitis, and myeloma (105). The clinical significance and cause-and-effect relationship of *S. pilosicoli* bacteremia and life-threatening illness remain to be determined.

For isolation, fresh stool specimens or rectal swabs should be examined by dark-field microscopy for the presence of spirochetes. Rectal biopsy samples can also serve as a source of material for culture or for histologic examination for spirochetes (89). Positive samples can be cultured under anaerobic conditions at 37°C by streaking them onto Trypticase soy agar medium with 5 to 10% defibrinated horse or calf blood and 400 μg of spectinomycin per ml (with or without 5 μg of polymyxin B per ml) to inhibit the growth of other bacteria. After 5 to 14 days of incubation, growth will appear as a thin film or as discrete, pinpoint colonies. Weak beta-hemolysis is typically observed. In the isolation of *S. pilosicoli* from anaerobic blood cultures, no growth signals were detected by automated culture systems, but the organisms could be observed by dark-field microscopy (105). No serologic procedures for detection of intestinal spirochetosis are available, and no data on antimicrobial susceptibility or treatment have been reported. Clearly, more information is needed to establish the potential medical importance of these organisms.

REFERENCES

1. **Antal, G. M., and G. Causse.** 1985. The control of endemic treponematoses. *Rev. Infect. Dis.* **7**(Suppl. 2)**:** S220–S226.
2. **Belisle, J. T., M. E. Brandt, J. D. Radolf, and M. V. Norgard.** 1994. Fatty acids of *Treponema pallidum* and *Borrelia burgdorferi* lipoproteins. *J. Bacteriol.* **176:**2151–2157.
3. **Benenson, A. S. (ed.).** 1990. Pinta, p. 323–324; Nonvenereal endemic syphilis, p. 425–426; and Yaws, p. 483–486. *In Control of Communicable Diseases in Man*, 15th ed. American Public Health Association, Washington, D.C.
4. **Berry, C. D., T. M. Hooten, A. C. Collier, and S. A. Lukehart.** 1987. Neurologic relapse after benzathine penicillin therapy for secondary syphilis in a patient with HIV infection. *N. Engl. J. Med.* **316:**1587–1589.
5. **Bromberg, K., S. Rawstron, and G. Tannis.** 1993. Diagnosis of congenital syphilis by combining *Treponema pallidum*-specific IgM detection with immunofluorescent antigen detection for *T. pallidum*. J. Infect. Dis. **168:**238–242.
6. **Burstain, J. M., E. Grimprel, S. A. Lukehart, M. V. Norgard, and J. D. Radolf.** 1991. Sensitive detection of *Treponema pallidum* by using the polymerase chain reaction. *J. Clin. Microbiol.* **29:**62–69.
7. **Byrne, R. E., S. Laske, M. Bell, D. Larson, J. Phillips, and J. Todd.** 1992. Evaluation of a *Treponema pallidum* Western immunoblot assay as a confirmatory test for syphilis. *J. Clin Microbiol.* **30:**115–122.
8. **Centers for Disease Control and Prevention.** 1998. 1998 Sexually transmitted diseases treatment guidelines. *Morbid. Mortal. Weekly Rep.* **47**(No. RR-1)**:**28–49.
9. **Centers for Disease Control and Prevention.** 1997. Conditions under public health surveillance. *Morbid. Mortal. Weekly Rep.* **46**(No. RR-10)**:**34–37.
10. **Centers for Disease Control and Prevention.** 1997. *Sexually Transmitted Disease Surveillance, 1996*, p. 83–104. U.S. Department of Health and Human Services, Atlanta, Ga.
11. **Centurion-Lara, A., C. Castro, J. M. Shaffer, W. C. Van Voorhis, C. M. Marra, and S. A. Lukehart.** 1997. Detection of *Treponema pallidum* by a sensitive reverse transcriptase PCR. *J. Clin. Microbiol.* **35:**1348–1352.
12. **Centurion-Lara, A., C. Castro, W. C. van Voorhis, and S. A. Lukehart.** 1996. Two 16S-23S ribosomal DNA intergenic regions in different *Treponema pallidum* subspecies contain tRNA genes. *FEMS Microbiol. Lett.* **143:**235–240.
13. **Centurion-Lara, A., T. Arroll, R. Castillo, J. M. Shaffer, C. Castro, W. C. Van Voorhis, and S. A. Lukehart.** 1997. Conservation of the 15-kilodalton lipoprotein among *Treponema pallidum* subspecies and strains and other pathogenic treponemes: genetic and antigenic analyses. *Infect. Immun.* **65:**1440–1444.
14. **Centurion-Lara, A., C. Castro, R. Castillo, J. M. Shaffer, W. C. van Voorhis, and S. A. Lukehart.** 1998. The flanking region sequences of the 15 kD lipoprotein gene differentiate pathogenic treponemes. *J. Infect. Dis.* **117:** 1036–1040.
15. **Chhabra, R. S., L. P. Brion, M. Castro, L. Freundlich, and J. H. Glaser.** 1993. Comparison of maternal sera, cord blood and neonatal sera for detection of presumptive congenital syphilis: relationship with maternal treatment. *Pediatrics* **91:**88–91.
16. **Choi, B. K., B. J. Paster, F. E. Dewhirst, and U. B. Göbel.** 1994. Diversity of cultivable and uncultivable oral spirochetes from a patient with severe destructive periodontitis. *Infect. Immun.* **62:**1889–1895.
17. **Cox, C. D.** 1983. Metabolic activities, p. 57–70. *In* R. F. Schell and D. M. Musher (ed.), *Pathogenesis and Immunology of Treponemal Infection*. Marcel Dekker, Inc., New York, N.Y.
18. **Cox, D. L., B. Riley, P. Chang, S. Sayahtaheri, S. Tassell, and J. Hevelone.** 1990. Effects of molecular oxygen, oxidation-reduction potential, and antioxidants upon in vitro replication of *Treponema pallidum* subsp. *pallidum*. *Appl. Environ. Microbiol.* **56:**3063–3072.
19. **Dobson, S. R. M., L. H. Taber, and R. E. Baughn.** 1988. Recognition of *Treponema pallidum* antigens by IgM and IgG antibodies in congenitally infected newborns and their mothers. *J. Infect. Dis.* **157:**903–910.
20. **Duhamel, G. E., N. Muniappa, M. R. Mathiesen, J. L. Johnson, J. Toth, R. O. Elder, and A. R. Doster.** 1995. Certain canine weakly beta-hemolytic intestinal spirochetes are phenotypically and genotypically related to spirochetes associated with human and porcine intestinal spirochetosis. *J. Clin. Microbiol.* **33:**2212–2215.
21. **Engelkens, H. J. H., J. Judanarso, A. P. Oranje, V. D. Vuzevski, P. L. A. Niemel, J. J. van der Sluis, and E. Stolz.** 1991. Endemic treponematoses. Part I. Yaws. *Int. J. Dermatol.* **30:**77–83.
22. **Engelkens, H. J. H., P. L. A. Niemel, J. J. van der Sluis, A. Meheus, and E. Stolz.** 1991. Endemic treponematoses. Part II. Pinta and endemic syphilis. *Int. J. Dermatol.* **30:** 231–238.
23. **Fieldsteel, A. H.** 1983. Genetics, p. 39–54. *In* R. F. Schell and D. M. Musher (ed.), *Pathogenesis and Immunology of Treponemal Infection*. Marcel Dekker, Inc., New York, N.Y.
24. **Fieldsteel, A. H., D. L. Cox, and R. A. Moeckli.** 1981. Cultivation of virulent *Treponema pallidum* in tissue culture. *Infect. Immun.* **32:**908–915.
25. **Fiumara, N. J.** 1979. Serologic responses to treatment of 128 patients with late latent syphilis. *Sex. Transm. Dis.* **6:** 243–246.
26. **Fiumara, N. J.** 1978. Treatment of early latent syphilis of less than one year's duration. *Sex. Transm. Dis.* **5:**85–88.
27. **Fiumara, N. J.** 1980. Treatment of primary and secondary syphilis; serological response. *JAMA* **243:**2500–2502.
28. **Fraser, C. M., et al.** 1998. Complete genome sequence of *Treponema pallidum*, the syphilis spirochete. *Science* **281:** 324–325.
29. **George, R. W., V. Pope, and S. A. Larsen.** 1991. Use of the Western blot for the diagnosis of syphilis. *Clin. Immunol. Newsl.* **8:**124–128.
30. **Gjestland, T.** 1955. The Oslo study of untreated syphilis: an epidemiologic investigation of the natural course of syphilis infection based upon a re-study of the Boeck-Bruusgaard material. *Acta Dermato.-Vener.* **35**(Suppl. 34)**:** 1–368.
31. **Gourevitch M. N., P. A. Selwyn, D. Davenny, D. Buono, E. E. Schoenbaum, R. S. Klein, and F. H. Friedland.** 1993. Effects of HIV infection on the serologic manifestation and response to treatment of syphilis in intravenous drug users. *Ann. Intern. Med.* **118:**350–355.
32. **Gregory, N., M. Sanchez, and M. R. Buchness.** 1990. The spectrum of syphilis in patients with human immunodeficiency virus infection. *J. Am. Acad. Dermatol.* **22:** 1061–1067.

33. **Grimprel, E., P. J. Sanchez, G. D. Wendel, J. M. Burstain, G. H. McCracken, J. D. Radolf, and M. V. Norgard.** 1991. Use of polymerase chain reaction and rabbit infectivity testing to detect *Treponema pallidum* in amniotic fluid. *J. Clin. Microbiol.* **29:**1711–1718.
34. **Hampson, D. J., and T. B. Stanton (ed.).** 1996. *Intestinal Spirochetes in Domestic Animals and Humans*. CAB International, Wallingford, Oxon, United Kingdom.
35. **Harland, W. A., and F. D. Lee.** 1967. Intestinal spirochaetosis. *Br. Med. J.* **3:**718–719.
36. **Hicks, C. B., P. M. Benson, G. P. Lupton, and E. C. Tramont.** 1987. Seronegative secondary syphilis in a patient infected with the human immunodeficiency virus (HIV) with Kaposi sarcoma. *Ann. Intern. Med.* **107:** 492–495.
37. **Hook, E. W., III.** 1989. Treatment of syphilis: current recommendations, alternatives, and continuing problems. *Rev. Infect. Dis.* **11**(Suppl. 6):S1511–S1517.
38. **Hook, E. W., III, and C. M. Marra.** 1992. Acquired syphilis in adults. *N. Engl. J. Med.* **326:**1060–1069.
39. **Hovind-Hougen, K., A. Birch-Andersen, R. Henrik-Nielsen, M. Orholm, J. O. Pedersen, P. S. Teglbjærg, and E. H. Thaysen.** 1982. Intestinal spirochetosis: morphological characterization and cultivation of the spirochete *Brachyspira aalborgii* gen. nov., sp. nov. *J. Clin. Microbiol.* **16:**1127–1136.
40. **Hunter, E. F., H. Russell, C. E. Farshy, J. S. Sampson, and S. A. Larsen.** 1986. Evaluation of sera from patients with Lyme disease in the fluorescent treponemal antibody-absorption tests for syphilis. *Sex. Transm. Dis.* **13:**232–236.
41. **Ijsselmuiden, O. E., J. J. van der Sluis, A. Mulder, E. Stolz, K. P. Bolton, and R. V. W. van Eijk.** 1989. An IgM capture enzyme-linked immunosorbent assay to detect IgM antibodies to treponemes in patients with syphilis. *Genitourin. Med.* **65:**79–83.
42. **Ito, F., R. W. George, E. F. Hunter, S. A. Larsen, and V. Pope.** 1992. Specific immunofluorescent staining of pathogenic treponemes with a monoclonal antibody. *J. Clin. Microbiol.* **30:**831–838.
43. **Johns, D. R., M. Tierney, and D. Felsenstein.** 1987. Alteration in the natural history of neurosyphilis by concurrent infection with the human immunodeficiency virus. *N. Engl. J. Med.* **316:**1569–1572.
44. **Jurado, R. L., J. Campbell, and P. D. Martin.** 1993. Prozone phenomenon in secondary syphilis: has its time arrived? *Arch. Intern. Med.* **153:**2496–2498.
45. **Kaufman, R. E., O. G. Jones, J. H. Blount, and P. J. Wiesner.** 1977. Questionnaire survey of reported early congenital syphilis, problems in diagnosis, prevention and treatment. *Sex. Transm. Dis.* **4:**135–139.
46. **Koopman, M. B. H., A. Käsbohrer, G. Beckmann, B. A. M. van der Zeijst, and J. G. Kusters.** 1993. Genetic similarity of intestinal spirochetes from humans and various animal species. *J. Clin. Microbiol.* **31:**711–716.
47. **Koseki, T., Y. Benno, Y. J. Zhang-Koseki, M. Umeda, and I. Ishikawa.** 1996. Detection frequencies and the colony-forming unit recovery of oral treponemes by different cultivation methods. *Oral Microbiol. Immunol.* **11:** 203–208.
48. **Larsen, S. A., E. F. Hunter, and S. J. Kraus (ed.).** 1990. *A Manual of Tests for Syphilis*, 8th ed., p. 1–165. American Public Health Association, Washington, D.C.
49. **Larsen, S. A., and B. M. Steiner.** 1995. Laboratory diagnosis and interpretation of tests for syphilis. *Clin. Microbiol. Rev.* **8:**1–21.
50. **Lee, J. I., A. J. McLaren, A. J. Lymbery, and D. J. Hampson.** 1993. Human intestinal spirochetes are distinct from *Serpulina hyodysenteriae*. *J. Clin. Microbiol.* **31:**16–21.
51. **Lefèvre, J. C., M. A. Bertrand, and R. Bauriaud.** 1990. Evaluation of the Captia enzyme immunoassays for detection of immunoglobulins G and M to *Treponema pallidum* in syphilis. *J. Clin. Microbiol.* **28:**1704–1707.
52. **Lewis, L. L., L. H. Taber, and R. E. Baughn.** 1990. Evaluation of immunoglobulin M Western blot analysis in the diagnosis of congenital syphilis. *J. Clin. Microbiol.* **28:** 296–302.
53. **Lukehart, S. A., E. W. Hook III, S. A. Baker-Zander, A. C. Collier, C. W. Critchlow, and H. H. Handsfield.** 1988. Invasion of the central nervous system by *Treponema pallidum*: implications for diagnosis and treatment. *Ann. Intern. Med.* **109:**855–862.
54. **Magnarelli, L. A., J. N. Miller, J. F. Anderson, and G. R. Riviere.** 1990. Cross-reactivity of nonspecific treponemal antibody in serologic tests for Lyme disease. *J. Clin. Microbiol.* **28:**1276–1279.
55. **Magnuson, H. J., H. Eagle, and R. Fleischman.** 1948. The minimal infectious inoculum of *Spirochaeta pallida* (Nichols strain) and a consideration of its rate of multiplication in vivo. *Am. J. Syph.* **32:**1–18.
56. **Matthews, H. M., T. K. Yang, and H. M. Jenkin.** 1979. Unique lipid composition of *Treponema pallidum* (Nichols virulent strain). *Infect. Immun.* **24:**713–719.
57. **McLaren, A. J., D. J. Trott, D. E. Swayne, S. L. Oxberry, and D. J. Hampson.** 1997. Genetic and phenotypic characterization of intestinal spirochetes colonizing chickens and allocation of known pathogenic isolates to three distinct genetic groups. *J. Clin. Microbiol.* **35:**412–417.
58. **Meheus, A., and G. M. Antal.** 1992. The endemic treponematoses: not yet eradicated. *World Health Stat. Q.* **45:** 228–237.
59. **Miller, J. N., R. M. Smibert, and S. J. Norris.** 1990. The genus *Treponema*. *In* A. Balows, H. G. Trüper, M. Dworkin, W. Harder, and K.-H. Schliefer (ed.), *The Prokaryotes. A Handbook on the Biology of Bacteria, Ecophysiology, Isolation, Identifications, and Applications*, 2nd ed. Springer Verlag, Inc., New York, N.Y.
60. **Moore, L. V. H., W. E. C. Moore, E. P. Cato, R. M. Smibert, J. A. Burmeister, A. M. Best, and R. R. Ranney.** 1987. Bacteriology of human gingivitis. *J. Dent. Res.* **66:** 989–995.
61. **Morse, S. A., D. L. Trees, Y. Htun, F. Radevbe, K. Orle, Y. Dangor, C. M. Beck-Sague, S. Schmid, G. Fehler, J. B. Weiss, and R. C. Ballard.** 1997. Comparison of clinical diagnosis and standard laboratory and molecular methods for the diagnosis of genital ulcer disease in Lesotho: association with human immunodeficiency virus infection. *J. Infect. Dis.* **175:**583–589.
62. **Musher, D. M.** 1991. Syphilis, neurosyphilis, penicillin and AIDS. *J. Infect. Dis.* **163:**1201–1206.
63. **Nayar, R., and J. M. Campos.** 1993. Evaluation of the DCL Syphilis-G enzyme immunoassay test kit for the serologic diagnosis of syphilis. *Am. J. Clin. Pathol.* **99:**282–285.
64. **Noordhoek, G. T., A. Cockayne, L. M. Schouls, R. H. Meloen, E. Stolz, and J. D. A. van Embden.** 1990. A new attempt to distinguish serologically the subspecies of *Treponema pallidum* causing syphilis and yaws. *J. Clin. Microbiol.* **28:**1600–1607. (Erratum, **28:**2853.)
65. **Noordhoek, G. T., H. J. H. Engelkens, J. Judanarso, J. van der Stek, G. N. M. Aelbers, J. J. van der Sluis, J. D. A. van Embden, and E. Stolz.** 1991. Yaws in West Sumatra, Indonesia: clinical manifestations, serological findings, and characterization of new treponema isolates by DNA probes. *Eur. J. Clin. Microbiol. Infect. Dis.* **10:**12–19.
66. **Noordhoek, G. T., P. W. M. Hermans, A. N. Paul, L. M. Schouls, J. J. van der Sluis, and J. D. A. van Embden.** 1989. *Treponema pallidum* subspecies *pallidum* (Nichols) and *Treponema pallidum* subspecies *pertenue* (CDC 2575)

differ in at least one nucleotide: comparison of two homologous antigens. *Microb. Pathog.* **6:**29–42.
67. **Noordhoek, G. T., B. Wieles, J. J. van der Sluis, and J. D. A. van Embden.** 1990. Polymerase chain reaction and synthetic DNA probes—a means of distinguishing the causative agents of syphilis and yaws? *Infect. Immun.* **58:** 2011–2013.
68. **Noordhoek, G. T., E. C. Wolters, M. E. J. De Jonge, and J. D. A. van Embden.** 1991. Detection by polymerase chain reaction of *Treponema pallidum* DNA in cerebrospinal fluid from neurosyphilis patients before and after antibiotic treatment. *J. Clin. Microbiol.* **29:**1976–1984.
69. **Norgard, M. V.** 1993. Clinical and diagnostic issues of acquired and congenital syphilis encompassed in the current syphilis epidemic. *Curr. Opin. Infect. Dis.* **6:**9–16.
70. **Norris, S. J., and D. G. Edmondson.** 1987. Factors affecting the multiplication and subculture of *Treponema pallidum* subsp. *pallidum* in a tissue culture system. *Infect. Immun.* **53:**534–539.
71. **Norris, S. J., and D. G. Edmondson.** 1988. In vitro culture system to determine the MICs and MBCs of antimicrobial agents against *Treponema pallidum* subsp. *pallidum* (Nichols strain). *Antimicrob. Agents Chemother.* **32:**68–74.
72. **Norris, S. J., and the *Treponema pallidum* Polypeptide Research Group.** 1993. Polypeptides of *Treponema pallidum*: progress toward understanding their structural, functional and immunologic roles. *Microbiol. Rev.* **57:**750–779.
73. **Orle, K. A., C. A. Gates, D. H. Marten, B. A., Body, and J. B. Weiss.** 1996. Simultaneous PCR detection of *Haemophilius ducreyi*, *Treponema pallidum*, and herpes simplex virus types 1 and 2 from genital ulcers. *J. Clin. Microbiol.* **34:**49–54.
74. **Paster, B. J., F. E. Dewhirst, and W. G. Weisburg.** 1991. Phylogenetic analysis of the spirochetes. *J. Bacteriol.* **173:** 6101–6109.
75. **Pedersen, N. S., O. Orum, and S. Mouritsen.** 1987. Enzyme-linked immunosorbent assay for detection of antibodies to venereal disease research laboratory (VDRL) antigen in syphilis. *J. Clin. Microbiol.* **25:**1711–1716.
76. **Perine, P. L., D. R. Hopkins, P. L. A. Niemel, R. K. St. John, G. Causse, and G. M. Antal.** 1984. *Handbook of Endemic Treponematoses: Yaws, Endemic Syphilis, and Pinta.* World Health Organization, Geneva, Switzerland.
77. **Perine, P. L., J. W. Nelson, J. O. Lewis, S. Liska, E. F. Hunter, S. A. Larsen, V. K. Agadzi, F. Kofi, J. A. K. Ofori, M. R. Tam, and M. A. Lovett.** 1985. New technologies for use in the surveillance and control of yaws. *Rev. Infect. Dis.* **7**(Suppl. 2)**:**S295–S299.
78. **Ramanathan, M., G. E. Duhamel, M. R. Mathiesen, and S. Messier.** 1993. Identification and partial characterization of a group of weakly beta-hemolytic intestinal spirochetes of swine distinct from *Serpulina innocens* isolate B256. *Vet. Microbiol.* **37**(1–2)**:**53–64.
79. **Rawstron, S. A., and K. Romberg.** 1991. Comparison of maternal and newborn serologic tests for syphilis. *Am. J. Dis. Child.* **145:**1383–1388.
80. **Rein, M. F.** 1976. Biopharmacology of syphilotherapy. *J. Am. Vener. Dis. Assoc.* **3:**109–127.
81. **Rein, M. F., G. W. Banks, L. C. Logan, S. A. Larsen, J. C. Feeley, D. S. Kellogg, and P. J. Wiesner.** 1980. Failure of the *Treponema pallidum* immobilization test to provide additional diagnostic information about contemporary problem sera. *Sex. Transm. Dis.* **7:**101–105.
82. **Riviere, G. R., K. S. Smith, N. Carranza, Jr., E. Tzagaroulaki, S. L. Kay, and M. Dock.** 1995. Subgingival distribution of *Treponema denticola*, *Treponema socranskii*, and pathogen-related oral spirochetes: prevalence and relationship to periodontal status of sampled sites. *J. Periodontol.* **66:**829–837.
83. **Riviere, G. R., K. S. Smith, E. Tzagaroulaki, S. L. Kay, X. Zhu, T. A. DeRouen, and D. F. Adams.** 1996. Periodontal status and detection frequency of bacteria at sites of periodontal health and gingivitis. *J. Periodontol.* **67:**109–115.
84. **Riviere, G. R., M. A. Wagoner, S. A. Baker-Zander, K. S. Weisz, D. F. Adams, L. Simonson, and S. A. Lukehart.** 1991. Identification of spirochetes related to *Treponema pallidum* in necrotizing ulcerative gingivitis and chronic periodontitis. *N. Engl. J. Med.* **325:**539–543.
85. **Riviere, G. R., K. S. Weisz, D. F. Adams, and D. D. Thomas.** 1991. Pathogen-related oral spirochetes from dental plaque are invasive. *Infect. Immun.* **59:**3377–3380.
86. **Riviere, G. R., K. S. Weisz, L. G. Simonson, and S. A. Lukehart.** 1991. Pathogen-related spirochetes identified within gingival tissue from patients with acute necrotizing ulcerative gingivitis. *Infect. Immun.* **59:**2653–2657.
87. **Rolfs, R. T., M. R. Joesoef, E. F. Hindershot, A. M. Rompalo, M. H. Augenbraun, M. Chiu, G. Bolan, S. C. Johnson, P. French, E. Steen, J. D. Radolf, and S. A. Larsen for the Syphilis & HIV Study Group.** 1997. A randomized trial of enhanced therapy for early syphilis in patients with and without human immunodeficiency virus infection. *N. Engl. J. Med.* **337:**307–314.
88. **Romanowski, B., R. Sutherland, F. H. Fick, D. Mooney, and E. J. Love.** 1991. Serologic response to treatment of infectious syphilis. *Ann. Intern. Med.* **114:**1005–1009.
89. **Ruane, P. J., M. M. Nakata, J. F. Reinhardt, and W. Lance George.** 1989. Spirochete-like organisms in the human gastrointestinal tract. *Rev. Infect. Dis.* **11:**184–196.
90. **Sanchez, P. J., G. D. Wendel, E. Grimprel, M. Goldberg, M. Hall, O. Arencibia-Mireles, J. D. Radolf, and M. V. Norgard.** 1993. Evaluation of molecular methodologies and rabbit infectivity testing for the diagnosis of congenital syphilis and neonatal central nervous system invasion by *Treponema pallidum*. *J. Infect. Dis.* **167:**148–157.
91. **Sanchez, P. J., G. H. McCracken, G. D. Wendel, K. Olsen, N. Threlkeld, and M. V. Norgard.** 1989. Molecular analysis of the fetal IgM response to *Treponema pallidum* antigen: implications for improved serodiagnosis of congenital syphilis. *J. Infect. Dis.* **159:**508–517.
92. **Schroeter, A. L., J. B. Lucas, E. V. Price, and V. H. Falcone.** 1973. Treatment of early syphilis and reactivity of serologic tests. *JAMA* **221:**471–476.
93. **Schwartz, D. A., S. A. Larsen, R. J. Rice, M. Fears, and C. Beck-Sague.** 1995. Pathology of the umbilical cord in congenital syphilis. *Hum. Pathol.* **26:**784–791.
94. **Simonson, L., L. Braswell, W. Falkler, A. Laws, D. Lloyd, S. Lukehart, and G. Riviere.** 1993. Human oral spirochete antigens in certain animal populations, abstr. D-133, p. 118. *In Abstracts of the 93rd General Meeting of the American Society for Microbiology 1993*. American Society for Microbiology, Washington, D.C.
95. **Smibert, R. M.** 1984. Genus III *Treponema* Schaudinn 1905, 1728^{AL}, p. 49–57. *In* N. R. Krieg and J. G. Holt (ed.), *Bergey's Manual of Systematic Bacteriology*, vol. 1. The Williams & Wilkins, Co., Baltimore, Md.
96. **Smibert, R. M., and J. A. Burmeister.** 1983. *Treponema pectinovorum* sp. nov. isolated from humans with periodontitis. *Int. J. Syst. Bacteriol.* **33:**852–856.
97. **Smibert, R. M., J. L. Johnson, and R. R. Ranney.** 1984. *Treponema socranskii* sp. nov., *Treponema socranskii* subsp. *socranskii* subsp. nov., *Treponema socranskii* subsp. *buccale* subsp. nov., and *Treponema socranskii* subsp. *paredis* subsp. nov. isolated from the human periodontia. *Int. J. Syst. Bacteriol.* **34:**457–462.
98. **Stanton, T. B.** 1992. Proposal to change the genus designation *Serpula* to *Serpulina* gen. nov. containing the species *Serpulina hyodysenteriae* comb. nov. and *Serpulina innocens* comb. nov. *Int. J. Syst. Bacteriol.* **42:**189–190.

99. **Stanton, T. B., E. Fournie-Amazouz, D. Postic, D. J. Trott, P. A. Grimont, G. Baranton, D. J. Hampson, and I. S. Girons.** 1997. Recognition of two new species of intestinal spirochetes: *Serpulina intermedia* sp. nov. and *Serpulina murdochii* sp. nov. *Int. J. Syst. Bacteriol.* **47:** 1007–1012.
100. **Stanton, T. B., N. S. Jensen, T. A. Casey, L. A. Tordoff, F. E. Dewhirst, and B. J. Paster.** 1991. Reclassification of *Treponema hyodysenteriae* and *Treponema innocens* in a new genus, *Serpula,* gen. nov., as *Serpula hyodysenteriae* comb. nov. and *Serpula innocens* comb. nov. *Int. J. Syst. Bacteriol.* **41:**50–58.
101. **Stapleton, J. T., L. V. Stamm, and P. J. Bassford, Jr.** 1985. Potential for development of antibiotic resistance in pathogenic treponemes. *Rev. Infect. Dis.* **7:**S314–S317.
102. **Stoll, B. J., F. K. Lee, S. A. Larsen, E. Hale, D. Schwartz, R. J. Rice, R. Ashby, R. Holmes, and A. J. Nahmias.** 1993. Improved serodiagnosis of congenital syphilis with combined assay approach. *J. Infect. Dis.* **167:** 1093–1099.
103. **Swisher, B. L.** 1987. Modified Steiner procedure for microwave staining of spirochetes and nonfilamentous bacteria. *J. Histotechnol.* **10:**241–243.
104. **Trott, D. J., R. F. Atyeo, J. I. Lee, D. A. Swayne, J. W. Stoutenburg, and D. J. Hampson.** 1996. Genetic relatedness amongst intestinal spirochaetes isolated from rats and birds. *Lett. Appl. Microbiol.* **23:**431–436.
105. **Trott, D. J., N. S. Jensen, I. Saint Girons, S. L. Oxberry, T. B. Stanton, D. Lindquist, and D. J. Hampson.** 1997. Identification and characterization of *Serpulina pilosicoli* isolates recovered from the blood of critically ill patients. *J. Clin. Microbiol.* **35:**482–485.
106. **Trott, D. J., T. B. Stanton, N. S. Jensen, G. E. Duhamel, J. L. Johnson, and D. J. Hampson.** 1996. *Serpulina pilosicoli* sp. nov., the agent of porcine intestinal spirochetosis. *Int. J. Syst. Bacteriol.* **46:**206–215.
107. **Trott, D. J., T. B. Stanton, N. S. Jensen, and D. J. Hampson.** 1996. Phenotypic characteristics of *Serpulina pilosicoli* the agent of intestinal spirochaetosis. *FEMS Microbiol. Lett.* **142:**209–214.
108. **Turner, T. B., and D. H. Hollander.** 1957. *Biology of the Treponematoses.* World Health Organization, Geneva, Switzerland.
109. **Umemoto, T., F. Nakazawa, E. Hoshino, K. Okada, M. Fukunaga, and I. Namikawa.** 1997. *Treponema medium* sp. nov., isolated from human subgingival dental plaque. *Int. J. Syst. Bacteriol.* **47:**67–72.
110. **U.S. Public Health Service.** 1968. *Syphilis: a Synopsis.* U.S. Public Health Service publication no. 1660. U.S. Government Printing Office, Washington, D.C.
111. **Wicher K., G. T. Noordhoek, F. Abbruscato, and V. Wicher.** 1992. Detection of *Treponema pallidum* in early syphilis by DNA amplification. *J. Clin. Microbiol.* **30:** 497–500.
112. **World Health Organization.** 1995. *Global Prevalence and Incidence of Selected Curable Sexually Transmitted Diseases: Overview and Estimates.* World Health Organization, New York, N.Y.
113. **Wyss, C., B. K. Choi, P. Schupbach, B. Guggenheim, and U. B. Gobel.** 1996. *Treponema maltophilum* sp. nov., a small oral spirochete isolated from human periodontal lesions. *Int. J. Syst. Bacteriol.* **46:**745–752.
114. **Young, H., A. Moyes, A. McMillan, and J. Patterson.** 1992. Enzyme immunoassay for antitreponemal IgG: screening or confirmatory test? *J. Clin. Pathol.* **45:**37–41.
115. **Zenker, P. N., and S. M. Berman.** 1990. Congenital syphilis: reporting and reality. *Am. J. Public Health* **80:** 271–272.
116. **Zenker, P. N., and R. T. Rolfs.** 1990. Treatment of syphilis, 1989. *Rev. Infect. Dis.* **12**(Suppl. 6)**:**S590–S608.

Algorithms for Identification of Mycoplasmas, Ureaplasma, and Obligate Intracellular Bacteria

PATRICK R. MURRAY

55

The bacteria discussed in chapters 56 to 60 differ from the bacteria described in the previous chapters by the lack of staining with the Gram stain and, with the exception of *Mycoplasma* and *Ureaplasma*, the requirement for intracellular growth. Thus, the two microbiology tests used most commonly, Gram stain and culture on artificial media, would not detect these organisms in clinical specimens. Diagnosis of these bacteria has traditionally been accomplished by staining clinical specimens with Romanowsky stains (e.g., Giemsa or Wright stain) or detecting an antibody response to infection by a variety of serological methods. More recently, our diagnostic yields have been improved considerably through refinements in culture procedures and the use of molecular diagnostic tools. The following tables summarize the epidemiology of infections caused by these bacteria (Table 1) and the diagnostic tests used for their detection (Table 2).

TABLE 1 Epidemiology of infections with *Chlamydia, Coxiella, Ehrlichia, Mycoplasma, Rickettsia,* and *Ureaplasma*

Organism	Disease	Reservoir	Vector and mode of transmission
Chlamydia pneumoniae	Pneumonia, bronchitis, sinusitis, pharyngitis, cardiovascular disease (?)	Humans	Inhalation of infectious aerosols
Chlamydia psittaci	Psittacosis (pneumonia), systemic infections (e.g., endocarditis)	Birds, domestic mammals	Inhalation of infectious aerosols
Chlamydia trachomatis	Endemic trachoma, inclusion conjunctivitis, lymphogranuloma venereum, urethritis, epididymitis, cervicitis, salpingitis, perihepatitis, pneumonia	Humans	Sexual contact, hand-eye contact, passage through infected birth canal
Coxiella burnetii	Acute or chronic Q fever: self-limited febrile illness, pneumonia, hepatitis, endocarditis, variety of systemic illnesses	Primarily cattle, sheep, goats, and parturient cats and dogs; less commonly many animal species and arthropods (e.g., ticks)	Inhalation of infectious aerosols, ingestion of contaminated milk, percutaneous
Ehrlichia chaffeensis	Human monocytotropic ehrlichiosis: high fever, headache, malaise, myalgia, gastrointestinal symptoms, arthralgia, central nervous system involvement	White-tailed deer, domestic dogs	Tick bite (*Amblyomma*)
Ehrlichia equi/ phagocytophila group	Human granulocytotropic ehrlichiosis: high fever, myalgias, headache, malaise, and gastrointestinal, respiratory, musculoskeletal, or central nervous system involvement	White-footed mouse, chipmunks, voles, and other small mammals; deer, sheep, cattle, and goats	Tick bite (*Ixodes, Dermacentor,* others [?])
Ehrlichia sennetsu	Sennetsu ehrlichiosis (mononucleosis-like glandular fever): rare self-limited febrile illness with chills, headache, malaise, sore throat, anorexia, and generalized lymphadenopathy	Unknown	Consumption of raw fish (?)
Mycoplasma hominis	Acute pyelonephritis, genital infections (?), systemic infections (?)	Humans	Sexual contact, vertical spread from mother to infant in utero or at birth
Mycoplasma pneumoniae	Pneumonia, tracheobronchitis, pharyngitis, and extrarespiratory complications	Humans	Contact with infectious aerosols or fomites
Orientia tsutsugamushi	Scrub typhus	Rats and other small mammals, marsupials, mites	Contamination of skin or mucous membranes with infected larval mites (chiggers), inhalation of infectious aerosols
Rickettsia akari	Rickettsialpox	Mice, voles, mites	Mite bite
Rickettsia prowazekii	Louse-borne typhus, Brill-Zinsser (recrudescent) disease	Humans, flying squirrels, lice	Contamination of skin or mucous membranes with louse or flea feces, inhalation of infectious aerosols
Rickettsia rickettsii	Rocky Mountain spotted fever	Rodents and other small mammals, ticks	Tick bite (*Dermacentor, Amblyomma*)
Rickettsia typhi	Murine typhus	Rats, opossums, fleas	Direct contact or inhalation of flea feces
Ureaplasma urealyticum	Urethritis, epididymo-orchitis, urinary calculi, spontaneous abortion, premature birth	Humans	Sexual contact, vertical spread from mother to infant in utero or at birth

TABLE 2 Diagnostic tests for *Chlamydia*, *Coxiella*, *Ehrlichia*, *Mycoplasma*, *Rickettsia*, and *Ureaplasma*

Organism	Diagnostic test[a]
Chlamydia pneumoniae	**Microscopy**: Organisms can be detected with the Giemsa stain and DFA test directed against LPS. Both tests are relatively insensitive. **Antigen tests**: Available EIA directed against LPS should detect all *Chlamydia* spp. but are licensed only for *C. trachomatis*. **Molecular tests**: Not commercially available. **Culture**: Grow best in HL cells and Hep-2 cells. **Serologic tests**: Genus-specific CF test is available, but the species-specific micro-IF test is the most sensitive and preferred test (diagnostic test of choice). Diagnosis confirmed by a fourfold or greater increase in titer, IgM titer of ≥1:16, or IgG titer of ≥1:512.
Chlamydia psittaci	**Microscopy**: Organisms can be detected with the Giemsa stain and DFA test directed against LPS. Both tests are relatively insensitive. **Antigen tests**: Available EIA directed against LPS should detect all *Chlamydia* spp. but are licensed only for *C. trachomatis*. **Molecular tests**: Not commercially available. **Culture**: Grow in a variety of cell lines including HeLa, McCoy, and monkey kidney cells. **Serologic tests**: Genus-specific CF test is useful for *C. psittaci*, although seroconversion occurs in only 50% of infections and may be delayed. Micro-IF is more sensitive and preferred (test of choice).
Chlamydia trachomatis	**Microscopy**: Organisms can be detected with the Giemsa stain and DFA test. Although the DFA is more sensitive than the Giemsa stain, neither test should be used alone. **Antigen tests**: Commercial EIA are available but are less sensitive than culture. Specificity is good, but the tests should not be used to screen low-prevalence populations. **Molecular tests**: Commercial probes and amplification assay (PCR, ligase chain reaction, transcription-mediated amplification) are available. The amplification assays are the most sensitive tests available (test of choice). **Culture**: Organisms can be cultured in a variety of cell lines (e.g., HeLa, McCoy, monkey kidney). Test sensitivity is dependent upon the quality of the submitted specimen (must contain infected cells). **Serologic tests**: Lymphogranuloma venereum can be diagnosed with a CF titer of >1:64 and compatible clinical picture. Micro-IF can also be used for lymphogranuloma venereum if the titer is rising, IgM titer is >1:32, or IgG titer is ≥1:2,000. The CF and Micro-IF tests cannot be reliably used to diagnose trachoma, inclusion conjunctivitis, or genital infections. Micro-IF used to confirm neonatal pneumonia (IgM titer, >1:32, IgG titer not useful).
Coxiella burnetii	**Microscopy**: DFA tests are available but are not used commonly because the sensitivity is poor. **Antigen tests**: Not commercially available. **Molecular tests**: PCR tests are available in research laboratories only. **Culture**: Organism can be cultured in cell lines (monkey kidney, Vero, human embryonic fibroblasts), egg yolk sacs, or laboratory animals. These tests are not performed commonly. **Serologic tests**: Diagnostic test of choice. The IFA test is the recommended test. A fourfold rise in titer or a phase II antibody titer of ≥1:256 is diagnostic of acute infection. Phase I antibody titers are generally much higher than phase II titers in chronic infections. A phase I IgG titer of ≥1:800 is considered diagnostic for endocarditis.
Ehrlichia chaffeensis	**Microscopy**: Giemsa or Wright stain of peripheral blood or buffy coat leukocytes is insensitive (positive in only about 1% of patients). **Antigen tests**: Not available. **Molecular tests**: EDTA-anticoagulated blood collected during the acute phase of illness is used for PCR amplification. Species- and genus-specific tests available. Likely to become the diagnostic test of choice. **Culture**: Peripheral blood (preferred) or CSF is inoculated onto specific cell lines for the isolation of *Ehrlichia*. Cultures are not commonly performed because they are rarely positive and can require 1 month or longer. **Serologic tests**: IFA is the most commonly used test. A fourfold or greater rise in titer or a peak titer of ≥1:64 is diagnostic. Partial cross-reactivity occurs with other *Ehrlichia* spp., and false-positive reactions are observed in some patients with Rocky Mountain spotted fever, Q fever, brucellosis, Lyme disease, or Epstein-Barr virus infections. Test sensitivity is believed to be high.
Ehrlichia equi/phagocytophila group	**Microscopy**: Giemsa or Wright stain of peripheral blood or buffy coat leukocytes is positive in 20 to 80% of patients. **Antigen tests**: Not available.

(Continued on next page)

TABLE 2 Diagnostic tests for *Chlamydia*, *Coxiella*, *Ehrlichia*, *Mycoplasma*, *Rickettsia*, and *Ureaplasma* (*Continued*)

Organism	Diagnostic test[a]
	Molecular tests: EDTA-anticoagulated blood collected during the acute phase of illness is used for PCR amplification. Species- and genus-specific tests available. Likely to become the diagnostic test of choice. **Culture**: Peripheral blood (preferred) or CSF is inoculated onto specific cell lines for the isolation of *Ehrlichia*. Positive cultures are more common than with the other ehrlichiae and are detected between 5 and 10 days. However, molecular tests are still preferred. **Serologic tests**: IFA is the most commonly used test. A fourfold or greater rise in titer or a peak titer of ≥1:80 is diagnostic. Positive titers are observed in asymptomatic patients in areas of endemic infection. The test sensitivity is believed to be high. False-positive reactions occur in patients with other rickettsial and ehrlichial infections, Q fever, or Epstein-Barr virus infections.
Ehrlichia sennetsu	**Microscopy**: Peripheral blood or buffy coat leukocytes can be stained with Giemsa or Wright stain. Test sensitivity is unknown. **Antigen tests**: Not available. **Molecular tests**: EDTA-anticoagulated blood collected during the acute phase of illness is used for PCR amplification. Species- and genus-specific tests are available. **Culture**: This *Ehrlichia* species is easily propagated in murine macrophage cell lines. **Serologic tests**: Not commercially available.
Mycoplasma hominis	**Microscopy**: Not useful. **Antigen tests**: Not commercially available. **Molecular tests**: PCR amplification tests have been developed but are less useful than culture. **Culture**: Organisms are isolated from a variety of specimens. The use of cotton swabs should be avoided. Mycoplasmas are extremely labile, and appropriate transport media must be used. Can be recovered on SP4 glucose broth and agar supplemented with arginine. Cultures are positive in 2–5 days. **Serologic tests**: Not useful.
Mycoplasma pneumoniae	**Microscopy**: Not useful. **Antigen tests**: A variety of tests (e.g., DFA, counterimmunoelectrophoresis, EIA, immunoblotting) have been developed but are insensitive and nonspecific. **Molecular tests**: Probe tests have been developed but are insensitive. They have been replaced by PCR amplification tests. The test sensitivity is high, but the specificity is unknown. Standardization is required, but this is likely to become the diagnostic test of choice. **Culture**: Organisms are isolated from a variety of specimens. The use of cotton swabs should be avoided. Mycoplasmas are extremely labile, and appropriate transport media must be used. Can be recovered on SP4 glucose broth and agar. Cultures are positive in 3 weeks or more. This test is insensitive. **Serologic tests**: CF has been used traditionally to measure seroconversion; however, it is insensitive and nonspecific. EIA are more sensitive and specific than CF, and IgM-specific tests are commercially available.
Orientia tsutsugamushi	**Microscopy**: Not useful. **Antigen tests**: Not available. **Molecular tests**: PCR amplification tests are performed with EDTA- or sodium citrate-anticoagulated blood collected during acute infection. **Culture**: Isolation is performed by intraperitoneal inoculation of mice. Not commonly performed. **Serologic tests**: The IFA test is the most sensitive and specific test. A titer of ≥1:64 for patients from areas without endemic infection is diagnostic. The indirect immunoperoxidase test has similar sensitivity and specificity to the IFA test at an IgG titer of ≥1:128 or IgM titer of ≥1:32. EIA have been developed but are not available in the United States.
Rickettsia akari	**Microscopy**: Heparinized blood collected during the acute febrile illness or a biopsy specimen of the skin rash or the margin of an eschar can be used for immunohistologic detection of rickettsiae. This is a sensitive, specific, and rapid test. Species- and group-specific tests are available. **Antigen tests**: Not available. **Molecular tests**: Not available. **Culture**: Heparin-anticoagulated plasma or buffy coat cells are inoculated into cell lines (e.g., Vero, L-929, HEL, MRC5). Infected cells are detected after 2–3 days by immunofluorescent staining of the monolayer cells. The test has poor sensitivity and is rarely performed. **Serologic tests**: The IFA test is the most sensitive and specific test. A titer of ≥1:64 for patients from areas without endemic infection is diagnostic. The indirect immunoperoxidase test has similar sensitivity and specificity to the IFA test at an IgG titer of ≥1:128 or IgM titer of ≥1:32.

(*Continued on next page*)

TABLE 2 *(Continued)*

Organism	Diagnostic test[a]
Rickettsia prowazekii	**Microscopy:** A biopsy specimen of the skin rash or the margin of an eschar can be used for immunohistologic detection of rickettsiae. This is a sensitive, specific, and rapid test. Species- and group-specific tests are available. **Antigen tests:** Not available. **Molecular tests:** PCR amplification tests are performed with EDTA- or sodium citrate-anticoagulated blood collected during acute infection. **Culture:** Heparin-anticoagulated plasma or buffy coat cells are inoculated into cell lines (e.g., Vero, L-929, HEL, MRC5). Infected cells are detected after 2–3 days by immunofluorescent staining of the monolayer cells. The test has poor sensitivity and is rarely performed. **Serologic tests:** The IFA test is the most sensitive and specific test. A titer of ≥1:64 for patients from areas without endemic infection is diagnostic. The indirect immunoperoxidase test has similar sensitivity and specificity to the IFA test at an IgG titer of ≥1:128 or IgM titer of ≥1:32.
Rickettsia rickettsii	**Microscopy:** Heparinized blood collected during the acute febrile illness or a biopsy specimen of the skin rash or the margin of an eschar can be used for immunohistologic detection of rickettsiae. Detection of rickettsiae in biopsy specimens has a sensitivity of 70% and a specificity of 100%. Species- and group-specific tests are available. **Antigen tests:** Not available. **Molecular tests:** PCR amplification tests are performed with EDTA- or sodium citrate-anticoagulated blood collected during acute infection. **Culture:** Heparin-anticoagulated plasma or buffy coat cells are inoculated into cell lines (e.g., Vero, L-929, HEL, MRC5). Infected cells are detected after 2–3 days by immunofluorescent staining of the monolayer cells. The test has poor sensitivity and is rarely performed. **Serologic tests:** The IFA test is the most sensitive and specific test. A titer of ≥1:64 for patients from areas without endemic infection is diagnostic. The indirect immunoperoxidase test has similar sensitivity and specificity to the IFA test at an IgG titer of ≥1:128 or IgM titer of ≥1:32. A latex agglutination test is available commercially. A diagnostic titer is >1:128. EIA are commercially available but are less sensitive and specific than the IFA test.
Rickettsia typhi	**Microscopy:** A biopsy specimen of the skin rash or the margin of an eschar can be used for immunohistologic detection of rickettsiae. This is a sensitive, specific, and rapid test. Species- and group-specific tests are available. **Antigen tests:** Not available. **Molecular tests:** PCR amplification tests are performed with EDTA- or sodium citrate-anticoagulated blood collected during acute infection. **Culture:** Heparin-anticoagulated plasma or buffy coat cells are inoculated into cell lines (e.g., Vero, L-929, HEL, MRC5). Infected cells are detected after 2–3 days by immunofluorescent staining of the monolayer cells. The test has poor sensitivity and is rarely performed. **Serologic tests:** The IFA test is the most sensitive and specific test. A titer of ≥1:64 for patients from areas without endemic infection is diagnostic. The indirect immunoperoxidase test has similar sensitivity and specificity to the IFA test at an IgG titer of ≥1:128 or IgM titer of ≥1:32. EIA are commercially available but are less sensitive and specific than the IFA test.
Ureaplasma urealyticum	**Microscopy:** Not useful. **Antigen tests:** Not commercially available. **Molecular tests:** PCR amplification tests have been developed but are considered less useful than culture. **Culture:** Ureaplasmas are isolated from a variety of specimens. The use of cotton swabs should be avoided. Organisms are extremely labile, and so appropriate transport media must be used. The organisms can be recovered on Shepard's 10B urea broth and 8A urea agar. Cultures are positive in 1–2 days. **Serologic tests:** Not useful.

[a] Abbreviations: CF, complement fixation; CSF, cerebrospinal fluid; DFA, direct fluorescent antibody; EIA, enzyme immunoassay; IFA, indirect immunofluorescent antibody; Ig, immunoglobulin; micro-IF, microimmunofluorescence.

Mycoplasma and *Ureaplasma*

KEN B. WAITES AND DAVID TAYLOR-ROBINSON

56

TAXONOMY AND NOMENCLATURE

Bacteria commonly referred to as mycoplasmas ("fungus form") are included within the class *Mollicutes* ("soft skin"), which comprises four orders, five families, eight genera, and more than 150 known species, as listed in Table 1. Table 2 lists 16 species isolated from humans, excluding occasional mycoplasmas that are usually isolated from animals but that have been detected in humans from time to time, usually in immunosuppressed hosts, and that are generally considered transient colonizers. Mollicutes are eubacteria which have evolved from clostridialike gram-positive cells by gene deletion. The recent availability of species-specific PCR technology is ameliorating difficulties of both culture and identification of fastidious mollicutes. Therefore, additional noncultivable, and thus presently unknown, species will likely be discovered.

DESCRIPTION OF *MOLLICUTES*

Mollicutes are smaller than conventional bacteria both in cellular dimensions and in genome size, making them the smallest free-living organisms known. Mycoplasmas associated with humans range from coccoid cells of about 0.2 to 0.3 μm in diameter, as in the case of *Ureaplasma urealyticum* and *Mycoplasma hominis* (48), to tapered rods of up to 2 μm in length, as in the case of *M. pneumoniae* and *M. penetrans* (76). Mollicutes are contained by a trilayered cell membrane and do not possess a cell wall. The permanent lack of a cell wall barrier makes the mollicutes unique among prokaryotes and differentiates them from bacterial L forms, for which the lack of the cell wall is but a temporary reflection of environmental conditions. The lack of a cell wall also renders these organisms insensitive to the activities of β-lactam antimicrobial agents, prevents them from staining by the Gram technique, and is largely responsible for their pleomorphic form. The extremely small genome (<600 kbp in the case of *M. genitalium*) and limited biosynthetic capabilities explain the parasitic or saprophytic existence for these organisms, their sensitivity to environmental conditions, and their fastidious growth requirements, which can complicate detection by culture. Mollicutes require enriched growth medium supplemented with nucleic acid precursors. Except for acholeplasmas, asteroleplasmas, and mesoplasmas, mollicutes require sterols in their growth media, and these are supplied by the addition of serum. Growth rates in culture medium vary among individual species, with generation times of approximately 1 h for *U. urealyticum*, 6 h for *M. pneumoniae*, and 16 h for *M. genitalium* (33).

Typical mycoplasmal colonies vary in diameter from 15 to ≥300 μm. Colonies of some species, such as *M. hominis*, often exhibit a "fried-egg" appearance owing to the contrast in deeper growth in the center of the colony with more shallow growth at the periphery (Fig. 1), while others, such as *M. pneumoniae*, produce spherical colonies. Whereas colonies of mycoplasmal species may be observed with the naked eye, those produced by *U. urealyticum* (referred to trivially as ureaplasmas) are typically much smaller (15 to 60 μm in diameter) and require low-power microscopic magnification (Fig. 2).

Mycoplasmas of human origin can be classified according to whether they ferment glucose, utilize arginine, or hydrolyze urea (Table 2). Except for the hydrolysis of urea, which is unique for ureaplasmas, these biochemical features are not sufficient for species distinction. Anaeroplasmas and asteroleplasmas, which occur in ruminants, are strictly anaerobic and oxygen sensitive, while most other mollicutes are facultative anaerobes.

Attachment of *M. pneumoniae* to host cells is a prerequisite for colonization and infection. Cytadherence, mediated by the P1 adhesin protein, is followed by induction of ciliostasis. *M. pneumoniae* stimulates B and T lymphocytes and induces the formation of autoantibodies which react with a variety of host tissues and the I antigen on erythrocytes and which are responsible for the production of cold agglutinins. *M. genitalium* also possesses a terminal structure, the MgPa adhesin, which facilitates its attachment to epithelial cells. The factors involved with *U. urealyticum* and *M. hominis* attachment have not been well characterized, but *U. urealyticum* is known to produce immunoglobulin A (IgA) protease, which may be associated with disease production. The production of hydrogen peroxides and the release of ammonia have also been implicated in the development of disease following infection by various mollicute species.

NATURAL HABITATS

Mollicutes are common in practically all mammalian species, as well as many other vertebrates in which they have been sought. Although most mollicutes have species-specific host-organism associations, some mycoplasmas and

TABLE 1 Classification and some distinguishing features of mycoplasmas (class *Mollicutes*)

Classification of class *Mollicutes*	Distinguishing features			
	Sterol required	Genome size (kbp)	Mol% G+C of DNA	Other
Order I: *Mycoplasmatales*				
Family I: *Mycoplasmataceae*				
Genus I: *Mycoplasma* (~100 species)	Yes	580–1,380	23–41	
Genus II: *Ureaplasma* (6 species)[a]	Yes	730–1,160	27–30	Urea metabolized
Order II: *Entomoplasmatales*				
Family I: *Entomoplasmataceae*				
Genus I: *Entomoplasma* (5 species)	Yes	790–1,140	27–29	
Genus II: *Mesoplasma* (12 species)	No	870–1,100	27–30	Requires 0.04% Tween 80
Family II: *Spiroplasmataceae*				
Genus I: *Spiroplasma* (33 species)	Yes	940–2,200	25–31	Helical structure
Order III: *Acholeplasmatales*[b]				
Family I: *Acholeplasmataceae*				
Genus I: *Acholeplasma* (13 species)	No	1,500–1,690	27–36	
Order IV: *Anaeroplasmatales*				
Family I: *Anaeroplasmataceae*				Obligate anaerobes
Genus I: *Anaeroplasma* (4 species)	Yes	~1,600	29–33	
Genus II: *Asteroleplasma* (1 species)	No	~1,600	40	

[a] *U. urealyticum* is the only species of human origin. It has at least 14 serovars which can be separated into two distinct biovars.
[b] Phytoplasmas are uncultivable mollicutes of plants and insects genetically related to the *Acholeplasmatales*, but they have not been assigned individual genus and species designations.

acholeplasmas of animal origin occur in a wide variety of different animal hosts. Mollicutes can also be isolated from insects (entomoplasmas) and plants (spiroplasmas).

In humans, mycoplasmas and ureaplasmas are mucosally associated, residing predominantly in the respiratory and urogenital tracts and rarely penetrating the submucosa, except in cases of immunosuppression or instrumentation, when they may invade the bloodstream and disseminate to many different organs and tissues throughout the body. Many mollicutes exist as commensal organisms in the oropharynx (*M. salivarium*, *M. orale*, *M. buccale*, *M. faucium*, *M. lipophilum*, and *Acholeplasma laidlawii*). *M. fermentans* has been detected by means of a PCR assay in the urogenital tract, the throat, and other body sites, including joints (34), but its primary site of colonization and true disease potential are incompletely understood. Oral commensal mycoplasmas may occasionally spread to the lower respiratory tract and can cause diagnostic confusion with *M. pneumoniae*.

The frequent occurrence of pathogenic species such as *M. hominis* and *U. urealyticum* in the lower urogenital tracts of healthy men and women has complicated complete understanding of their disease-producing capabilities. Organ-

TABLE 2 Primary sites of colonization, metabolism, and pathogenicity of mollicutes of human origin

Species	Primary site of colonization		Metabolism of:		Pathogenicity
	Oropharynx	Genitourinary tract	Glucose	Arginine	
M. salivarium	+	−	−	+	−
M. orale	+	−	−	+	−
M. buccale	+	−	−	+	−
M. faucium	+	−	−	+	−
M. lipophilum	+	−	−	+	−
M. pneumoniae	+	−	+	−	+
M. hominis	+	+	−	+	+
M. genitalium	?+	+	+	−	+
M. fermentans	+	+	+	+	+
M. primatum	−	+	−	+	−
M. spermatophilum	−	+	−	+	−
M. pirum	?	?	+	+	−
M. penetrans	−	+	+	+	?
U. urealyticum[a]	+	+	−	−	+
A. laidlawii	+	−	+	−	−
A. oculi	?	?	+	−	−

[a] Metabolizes urea.

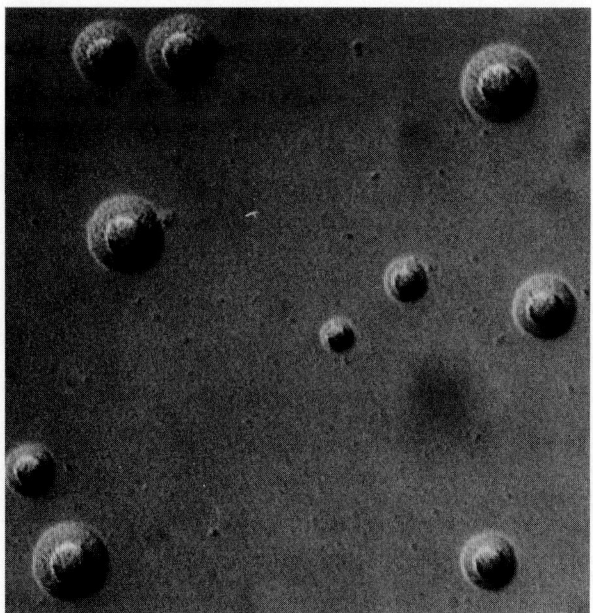

FIGURE 1 Fried-egg-type colonies of *M. hominis* up to 110 μm in diameter. Magnification, ×132.

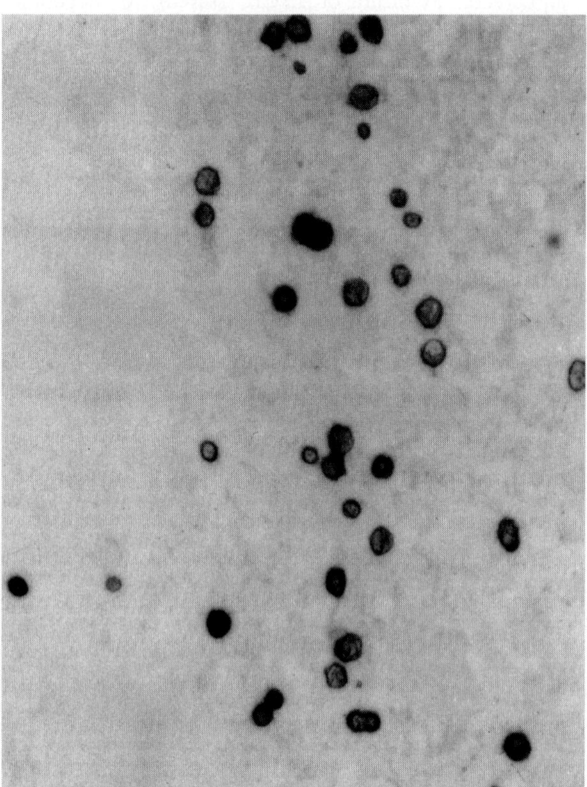

FIGURE 2 Granular brown colonies of *U. urealyticum* from a vaginal specimen growing on A 8 agar. Magnification, ×100.

isms such as *M. hominis*, although most commonly isolated from the urogenital tract, can also disseminate to other body sites, particularly if host defenses are impaired. Species such as *M. primatum*, *M. spermatophilum*, and *Acholeplasma oculi* have been detected in the urogenital tract but are not associated with disease. Recent studies in which PCR assays have been used have demonstrated the frequent occurrence of *M. genitalium* in the urogenital tract and of *M. penetrans* in the urine of homosexual males with human immunodeficiency virus (HIV)-associated disease (40, 73, 74). Although mycoplasmas are generally considered to be extracellular organisms, intracellular localization is now appreciated for *M. fermentans*, *M. penetrans*, *M. genitalium*, and possibly, *M. pneumoniae*. Intracellular localization may be responsible for protecting the organism from antibodies and antibiotics, as well as contributing to disease chronicity and difficulty in cultivation. Variations in the surface antigens of *M. hominis* and *U. urealyticum* may be related to the persistence of these organisms at invasive sites. In humans, mycoplasmas and ureaplasmas may be transmitted by direct contact between hosts, i.e., by venereal transmission through genital-genital or oral-genital contact, by vertical transmission from mother to offspring either at birth or in utero, by respiratory aerosols or fomites in the case of *M. pneumoniae*, or even by nosocomial acquisition through transplanted tissues.

CLINICAL SIGNIFICANCE

Respiratory Infections

M. pneumoniae was first identified and described in the early 1960s. It causes approximately 20% of all community-acquired pneumonias in the general population and up to 50% of pneumonias in certain confined groups (22, 59). Although *M. pneumoniae* has long been associated with pneumonias in school-age children, adolescents, and young adults, in recent years this organism has also been shown to occur endemically and occasionally epidemically in older persons, as well as children under 5 years of age (22, 59). The most typical clinical syndrome is tracheobronchitis, often accompanied by upper respiratory tract manifestations. Acute pharyngitis is uncommon. Pneumonia develops in about one-third of persons who are infected. The incubation period is generally 2 to 3 weeks, and spread throughout households is common. The organism may persist in the respiratory tract for several months after initial infection and sometimes for years in hypogammaglobulinemic patients (22, 65). The disease tends not to be seasonal, subclinical infections are common, and the disease is ordinarily mild. However, severe infections requiring hospitalization are known to occur, especially in middle-aged and elderly individuals. Extrapulmonary complications including meningoencephalitis, ascending paralysis, transverse myelitis, pericarditis, hemolytic anemia, arthritis, and mucocutaneous lesions occur in some patients. Other nonspecific manifestations include nausea, vomiting, and diarrhea. An autoimmune response is thought to play a role in extrapulmonary complications, but since *M. pneumoniae* has been isolated directly from cerebrospinal, pericardial, and synovial fluids, as well as from other extrapulmonary sites, direct invasion by this organism must be considered. Clinical manifestations are not sufficiently unique to allow differentiation from infections caused by other common bacteria, particularly *Chlamydia pneumoniae*.

M. fermentans has been recovered from the throats of children with pneumonia, in some of whom no other etiologic agent was identified, but the frequency of its occurrence in healthy children is not known (59). *M. fermentans* has been detected in adults with an acute influenza-like illness (39) and in bronchoalveolar lavage specimens from patients with AIDS and pneumonia (1). It is apparent that respiratory infection with *M. fermentans* is not necessarily linked with immunodeficiency, but it may also behave as an opportunistic respiratory pathogen.

Genitourinary Infections

Following puberty, *U. urealyticum* and *M. hominis* can be isolated from the lower genital tracts of the majority of sexually active adults, with *U. urealyticum* being the more common species detected. Difficulty in accepting *M. hominis* and *U. urealyticum* as causes of disease has arisen either because samples cannot be easily obtained from the affected site (for example, the fallopian tube) or because the organisms are recovered from asymptomatic individuals. Nevertheless, there is evidence that these species play etiologic roles in some genital tract diseases of both men and women. However, the organisms reach the upper genital tract and cause disease only in a subpopulation of individuals who are colonized in the lower tract.

Results of human and animal inoculation studies and observations of immunocompromised patients are supportive of the fact that ureaplasmas are a cause of nonchlamydial, nongonococcal urethritis (NGU) in men, with further evidence supplied by therapeutic and serologic studies (56, 61). There is no evidence to indicate that *M. hominis* is a cause of male urethritis (56). *M. genitalium* has been detected by PCR technology significantly more often in urethral specimens from men with acute NGU than from those without urethritis (30, 32). Antibody responses have been detected in some men with acute disease, and this mycoplasma has also produced urethritis in nonhuman primates (59). *M. fermentans*, *M. penetrans*, and *M. pirum* were not detected in the urethras of men with urethritis by PCR assays, suggesting that these organisms are unlikely to have a pathogenic role in individuals with this condition (17). In women, there is no evidence that *M. hominis* is a cause of the urethral syndrome, but *U. urealyticum* may be involved (53).

M. hominis and *U. urealyticum* have not been detected by culture of prostatic biopsy samples from patients with chronic abacterial prostatitis (18), nor has *M. genitalium* been found by PCR assay. In contrast, ureaplasmas have been recovered from an epididymal aspirate from a patient suffering from nonchlamydial, nongonococcal acute epididymo-orchiditis accompanied by a specific antibody response (31) and may be an infrequent cause of the disease. *U. urealyticum* produces urease and induces crystallization of struvite and calcium phosphates in urine in vitro (29) and calculi in animal models (66). In addition, ureaplasmas have been found more frequently in urinary calculi of patients with infection-type stones than in those of patients with metabolic-type stones, suggesting a possible causal association (29). *M. hominis* has been isolated from the upper urinary tracts only of patients with symptoms of acute pyelonephritis, often with an antibody response (68), and causes possibly about 5% of cases of such disease. Obstruction or instrumentation of the urinary tract may be a predisposing factor. *U. urealyticum* has not been associated with acute pyelonephritis in the same way.

Mollicutes do not cause vaginitis, but they are among the various microorganisms that proliferate in patients with bacterial vaginosis and may contribute to the condition (64). Bacterial vaginosis may lead to pelvic inflammatory disease (PID), and *M. hominis* has been isolated from the endometrium and fallopian tubes of about 10% of women with salpingitis diagnosed by laparoscopy and its presence is typically accompanied by a specific antibody response (64). However, assessment of the significance of this mycoplasma in an individual patient is difficult when several microorganisms are present. *U. urealyticum* has been isolated directly from affected fallopian tubes, but not in pure culture. This, together with the negative results of serologic tests and of tests in which nonhuman primates as well as fallopian tube organ cultures are inoculated (64), does not support a causal relationship for ureaplasmas in PID. *M. genitalium*, however, may play a role, as suggested by serologic data (42) and the results of nonhuman primate inoculation studies (64). It is unknown if mycoplasmas cause infertility in women. That *U. urealyticum* might cause involuntary infertility remains speculative (58), as does the possibility that ureaplasmas could affect sperm (27, 57).

Ureaplasmas have been isolated from the internal organs of spontaneously aborted fetuses and from stillborn and premature infants more often than from tissues from induced abortions or healthy full-term infants (63). The results from some serologic and therapeutic studies (27) have also supported a role for these organisms in fetal morbidity. Bacterial vaginosis is a possible confounding factor which must be considered in the association between ureaplasmas in the chorioamnion and low birth weight. Ureaplasmas in the chorioamnion are directly associated with inflammation (20) and may invade the amniotic sac early in pregnancy in the presence of intact fetal membranes, causing persistent infection and an adverse pregnancy outcome (9).

The notion that *M. hominis* organisms cause fever in some women after abortion or after a normal delivery is based on their isolation from the blood of about 10% of such women but not from afebrile women who have had abortions or from healthy pregnant women (27, 63). In addition, antibody responses have been detected in about half of febrile aborting women but in few of those who remain afebrile (27, 63). Similar observations have been made for the isolation of *U. urealyticum* (19). Case reports suggest that, at least in some individuals, *U. urealyticum* alone may play a causal role in spontaneous abortion and premature birth (12).

Neonatal Infections

Colonization of infants by genital mycoplasmas may occur by ascension of the mycoplasma from the lower genital tract of the mother at the time of delivery or in utero, earlier in gestation, and may be transient and without sequelae. The rate of vertical transmission may be 18 to 55% among infants born to colonized mothers (12). *U. urealyticum* and *M. hominis* may be isolated from neonates born to mothers with intact membranes and delivered by cesarean section, indicative of transplacental in utero transmission (12). Congenital pneumonia, bacteremia, progression to chronic lung disease of prematurity, and even death have occurred in very low birth weight infants (birth weight, <1,000 g) due to ureaplasmal infection of the lower respiratory tract (11). Both *M. hominis* and *U. urealyticum* have been isolated from maternal and umbilical cord blood, as well as from the blood of neonates. Both species can also invade the cerebrospinal fluid of neonates (70). Either mild, subclinical meningitis without sequelae or neurologic damage with permanent handicaps may ensue (70). Colonization of healthy full-term infants declines after 3 months of age, and fewer than 10% of older children and sexually inexperienced adults are colonized with genital mycoplasmas (12). While *M. fermentans* has been detected in pure culture from placenta and amniotic fluid in the presence of inflammation, no prospective studies have been performed to date to determine its occurrence and significance, if any, in neonates.

Routine screening of neonates for genital mycoplasmas is not clinically justified. However, if there is clinical, radiological, or laboratory evidence of pneumonia, meningitis, or overall instability, particularly in preterm neonates in whom there are no obvious alternative etiologies, infection with *M. hominis* or *U. urealyticum* should be considered.

Systemic Infections and Immunosuppressed Hosts

Extrapulmonary and extragenital mycoplasmal infections probably occur more often than is currently recognized. In many instances, these organisms are considered only after other likely etiologic agents have been excluded and/or if there is no improvement following treatment with antimicrobial agents inactive against mycoplasmas. *M. hominis* is alone among the pathogenic mycoplasmas of human origin which may occasionally be detected in routine bacteriologic cultures, so that many cases have been discovered accidentally, when mycoplasmas were not specifically sought. There is considerable evidence that mollicutes can cause invasive disease of the joints and respiratory tract with bacteremic dissemination in immunosuppressed persons, especially individuals with hypogammaglobulinemia (12, 25, 41, 61, 62, 65). Mycoplasmas are probably the most common etiologic agents of septic arthritis in the setting of congenital antibody deficiency states and should always be considered early when attempting to diagnose these conditions (12, 25, 41, 61, 62, 65). In some patients, the arthritis responds to antibiotic therapy, whereas in others, disease and organisms persist for many months, despite treatment with antimicrobial and anti-inflammatory agents and gamma globulin replacement. In some patients arthritis due to *U. urealyticum* has been associated with subcutaneous abscesses and chronic urethrocystitis (62, 65). *M. hominis* bacteremia has been demonstrated after renal transplantation, trauma, and genitourinary manipulations and has also been found in wound infections, brain abscesses, and osteomyelitis lesions (41). Numerous mycoplasmal species, including *M. fermentans*, *U. urealyticum*, *M. salivarium*, and *M. orale*, can be detected by culture and/or PCR in the synovial fluid of persons with rheumatoid arthritis, although the precise contribution of these organisms to this disease condition is still speculative (49). The significance of *M. fermentans* (34, 75), *M. penetrans* (40, 73, 74), and other mycoplasmas in persons infected with HIV, with or without AIDS, has received a great deal of attention and is currently a matter of debate. *M. hominis* has been isolated on numerous occasions from the sternal wounds of recipients of heart or lung transplants (59).

TYPE, COLLECTION, TRANSPORT, AND STORAGE OF SPECIMENS

Specimen Type and Collection

Body fluids appropriate for mycoplasmal culture include blood, synovial fluid, amniotic fluid, cerebrospinal fluid, urine, prostatic secretions, semen, wound aspirates, sputum, pleural fluid, bronchoalveolar lavage specimens, or other tracheobronchial secretions, depending on the clinical condition. Swabs from the nasopharynx, cervix or vagina, wounds, and urethra are also acceptable. Tissue specimens obtained by biopsy or at autopsy, including placenta, bone chips, and urinary calculi, can also be cultured. When swabs are obtained, care must be taken to sample the desired site vigorously to obtain as many cells as possible since mycoplasmas are cell associated. If determination of the localization of mycoplasmas in the genitourinary tract is desired, urine specimens can be obtained at various stages during urination or after prostatic massage. Care should be taken to avoid collection of specimens which are contaminated with lubricants or antiseptics commonly used in gynecologic practice. Calcium alginate, Dacron, or polyester swabs with aluminum or plastic shafts are preferred. Cotton swabs with wooden shafts should be avoided because of potential inhibitory effects. Swabs should always be removed from specimens before transportation to the laboratory.

Successful isolation of mycoplasmas from blood can be achieved by inoculating blood, free of anticoagulant, into liquid growth medium at the bedside at a 1:10 ratio, using as much blood as possible (at least 10 ml for adults). Mycoplasmas are inhibited by sodium polyanethol sulfonate, the anticoagulant used in most commercial blood culture media, but the inhibitory effect can be overcome by the addition of gelatin (1%; wt/vol) (44). Use of commercial blood culture media with or without automated blood culture instruments is not recommended for the detection of mycoplasmas.

Transport and Storage

Mycoplasmas are extremely sensitive to adverse environmental conditions, particularly drying and heat. Specimens should be inoculated at the bedside whenever possible, and an appropriate transport and/or culture medium should be used. Specific mycoplasma media such as SP 4 or 10 B broths (49, 68), 2 SP (10% heat-inactivated fetal calf serum with 0.2 M sucrose in 0.02 M phosphate buffer [pH 7.2]), and Trypticase soy broth with 0.5% bovine serum albumin are all acceptable transport media. 2 SP can also be used for sample preparation for PCR assays. Other media available commercially for transport and storage of specimens are Stuart's medium and Mycotrans (Irvine Scientific, Irvine, Calif.). A3B broth (Remel, Inc., Lenexa, Kans.) is available as a transport medium, whereas the Arginine Broth and 10 B and SP 4 transport broths of Remel also serve as growth media. Liquid specimens do not require a special transport medium if cultures can be inoculated within 1 h, provided that the specimens are protected from drying. Tissues can be placed in a sterile container which can be tightly closed and delivered to the laboratory immediately. Otherwise, tissue specimens should be placed in a transport medium if delay in culture inoculation is anticipated. Specimens should be refrigerated if immediate transportation to the laboratory is not possible. If specimens must be shipped and/or if the storage time is likely to exceed 24 h prior to processing, the specimen in transport medium should be frozen at −70°C to prevent the loss of viability and to minimize bacterial overgrowth if the specimen is from a nonsterile site. Mollicutes can be stored for long periods in appropriate growth or transport medium at −70°C or in liquid nitrogen (24). Frozen specimens can be shipped with dry ice to a reference laboratory if necessary. When specimens are to be examined, they should be thawed rapidly in a 37°C water bath.

NONCULTURAL DETECTION

Although culture is well adapted to species which can be isolated easily and rapidly from clinical specimens, such as *M. hominis* and *U. urealyticum*, it is not ideal for the detection of fastidious and/or extremely slowly growing organisms such as M. *genitalium* and, to a considerable degree, M. *pneumoniae*. The same types of specimens used for culture can also be used for the noncultural detection of mycoplasmas, but transportation conditions do not have to maintain organism viability. A number of different methods for the direct or amplified detection of mycoplasmas in clinical specimens have been described.

Antigen Detection Techniques

Rapid methods developed for the antigenic detection of M. *pneumoniae* have included direct immunofluorescence, counterimmunoelectrophoresis, immunoblotting, and antigen-capture enzyme immunoassay (EIA) (26, 37, 58). The utility and general acceptance of these techniques have been reduced by their low sensitivities and cross-reactivities with other mycoplasmas found in the respiratory tract. Use of optimum antibody mixtures can increase the sensitivity of detection within the range of 10^3 to 10^4 CFU/100 μl of specimen. Considering that the concentration of M. *pneumoniae* cells typically found in the sputum of patients is approximately 10^2 to 10^6 CFU/ml, this technique is at the limit of sensitivity for detection.

DNA Probes

DNA hybridization techniques for the diagnosis of M. *pneumoniae* infection were developed in the early 1980s (45). 16S rRNA genes have been widely used as targets, as have probes consisting of rDNA. Because probes are relatively insensitive, the more recently available amplified techniques such as PCR have largely supplanted them.

PCR

PCR systems based on 16S rRNA genes have been developed for a number of mycoplasma species (45). Other repetitive sequences which have been used are the insertion-like elements of M. *fermentans* (75), the P1 adhesin of M. *pneumoniae* (16), and the MgPa adhesin gene of M. *genitalium* (16, 32). Urease genes have been used for U. *urealyticum* (5). PCR assays have been used to detect M. *hominis* and U. *urealyticum* in the urogenital tract as well as at other body sites, including the respiratory tracts of neonates (4, 15, 28, 49). For slowly growing organisms such as M. *pneumoniae*, and especially for extremely fastidious species for which optimum cultivation techniques are not established, such as M. *genitalium* and M. *fermentans*, the use of PCR assays may be the only practical means of detecting their presence in clinical material. The sensitivity of PCR is very high, corresponding to a single organism when purified DNA is used. However, comparison of the PCR technique with culture and/or serology, in the case of M. *pneumoniae*, has yielded varied results, and large-scale experience with this procedure is still limited for any mollicute species. Positive PCR results for M. *pneumoniae* in culture-negative persons without evidence of respiratory disease suggest inadequate specificity or persistence of the organism after infection or its existence in asymptomatic carriers. Quantitative studies may be useful in drawing conclusions. PCR is also a very good tool for the identification of an unknown mycoplasma previously obtained by culture. It can be used for the characterization of strains within a species and for the detection of a specific feature, such as the presence of an antibiotic resistance determinant. PCR technology appears to be less valuable for routine diagnostic purposes in the case of the more rapidly growing and easily cultivable organisms, such as M. *hominis* and U. *urealyticum*. Presently, PCR detection of mycoplasmas and most other microorganisms of clinical significance is still too expensive and complex to be carried out routinely in most clinical microbiology laboratories. Some drawbacks must still be corrected, such as the problem of contamination and the presence of inhibitors. Multiplex PCR tests, which detect several mycoplasmas or even combinations of mycoplasmas and other agents of community-acquired pneumonia, such as C. *pneumoniae* and *Legionella pneumophila*, may eventually prove to be useful for screening purposes. The possible development of commercial PCR kits in the future should bring about better standardization of the technique, and if available at a reasonable cost, PCR could become a major method for the diagnosis of mycoplasmal infections. Detailed information concerning PCR methodology and controls has been described elsewhere (44).

ISOLATION PROCEDURES

Growth Media and Inoculation

Growth of mycoplasmas pathogenic for humans requires the presence of serum, growth factors such as yeast extract, and a metabolic substrate. No single formulation is ideal for all pertinent species due to the different properties, optimum pH, and substrate requirements of the different mycoplasmas. SP 4 glucose broth and agar (pH 7.5) (69) are the best media overall and can be used for both M. *pneumoniae* and M. *hominis*, provided that arginine is added for the latter organism. Shepard's (50) 10 B urea broth (pH 6.0) can be used for M. *hominis* and U. *urealyticum*, with A 8 (51) used as the corresponding solid medium. The compositions of these media are included in section IX of this Manual. Penicillin G or a broad-spectrum semisynthetic penicillin should be added to minimize bacterial overgrowth, especially for specimens from nonsterile sites. The addition of a pH indicator, such as phenol red, is important for the detection of growth because mycoplasmas usually do not produce turbidity in broth culture owing to their small cell size.

The lack of commercially prepared media in the past has effectively prevented many laboratories, except those in institutions with especially high volumes or specific research interests in mycoplasmal diseases, from offering on-site mycoplasma detection. For self-prepared media, quality control is crucial for each of the main components. These controls consist of the quantitative growth of a mycoplasma strain(s) in two media that differ only in the component to be tested. New lots or batches of broth are considered satisfactory if the numbers of organisms that grow are within 10- to 100-fold of the numbers that grow in the reference batch. Agar plates should support the growth of at least 90% of the colonies that are supported by the reference media. The sterility of commercially purchased medium components, such as horse serum, must be confirmed prior to their use. If a reference laboratory is to be used for mycoplasma testing, inquiry should be made of whether the medium used is self-prepared or purchased from a manufacturer, and there should also be verification of the type of quality control procedures performed. Quality control test organisms should include type strains, low-passage clinical isolates, and all 14 serotypes of U. *urealyticum* from frozen stocks. Type strains of M. *pneumoniae*, M. *hominis*, and U. *urealyticum* designated by the American Type Culture Collection are available commercially for quality control testing. Testing of the inhibitory properties of media against the growth of various other organisms likely present in specimens from nonsterile sites may also be worthwhile to prevent the loss of mycoplasmas due to overgrowth of contaminating organisms.

Specimens should always be mixed well before inoculation of the culture media, and fluids should be centrifuged (600 × *g* for 15 min) and the pellet should be inoculated. Urine should be filtered through a 0.45-μm-pore-size filter if bacterial contamination is suspected. Furthermore, it is wise to mince, not grind, tissues in broth prior to dilution. Serial dilution of specimens in broth to at least 10^{-3} with subculture of each dilution onto agar is an extremely important step in the cultivation process since it will help overcome possible interference by antibiotics, antibodies, and other inhibitors, including bacteria, that may be present in clinical specimens (58). Omission of this critical dilution step can be one reason why some laboratories have difficulty in recovering the organisms. Dilution also helps to overcome the problem of rapid decline in culture viability, which is particularly common with ureaplasmas, and it also provides information about the number of organisms present in the specimen. A DNA fluorochrome stain such as Hoechst 33258 may be useful when applied to body fluids such as amniotic fluid after cytocentrifugation, but it is not specific for mycoplasmas.

Incubation Conditions and Subcultures

Broths should be incubated at 37°C under atmospheric conditions. Agar plates are incubated in an atmosphere of room air supplemented with 5 to 10% CO_2 or 95% N_2 plus CO_2. Colonies of genital mycoplasmas may develop best under the latter conditions. The relatively rapid growth rates of *M. hominis* and *U. urealyticum* make identification of most positive cultures possible within 2 to 5 days, whereas *M. pneumoniae* requires 21 days or more. Several mycoplasmal species of human origin can produce similar biochemical reactions, and identification can be accomplished only by specific tests with the organisms once they are isolated. All broths which have changed color should be subcultured into a fresh tube of the corresponding broth (0.1 ml into 0.9 ml) and onto agar (0.02 ml). Subcultures must be performed soon after the color change occurs, particularly if the organism is *U. urealyticum*, because the culture can lose viability within a few hours. Subculture also increases the diagnostic yield since some strains from the original specimen inoculated initially onto solid medium may not grow sufficiently. Periodic blind subculture during incubation may improve the yield of *M. pneumoniae* and other mycoplasmas since a color change may not always be evident, even if growth occurs. Cultures should be incubated for at least 7 days before being designated negative for genital mycoplasmas and 4 weeks before being designated negative for *M. pneumoniae*. The growth rate of *M. fermentans* is similar to that of *M. pneumoniae*. However, for *M. fermentans*, *M. genitalium*, and mycoplasmas of human origin other than *M. pneumoniae*, *M. hominis*, or *U. urealyticum*, cultivation conditions are not well established. Due to the advent of PCR assays for use in research and reference laboratories, the need to refine culture techniques for these slowly growing and fastidious organisms is less critical than it was previously.

Development of Colonies

Broth cultures for *U. urealyticum* should be examined twice daily for up to 7 days for a color change resulting from the hydrolysis of urea because of the steep death phase of this organism in culture. This is less critical for *Mycoplasma* spp., for which once-daily inspection of broth cultures is sufficient. Agar plates should be examined with a stereomicroscope at ×20 to ×60 magnification daily for *U. urealyticum*, at 1- to 3-day intervals for *M. hominis*, and every 3 to 5 days for *M. pneumoniae* and other slower-growing species. Mycoplasmal colonies must be distinguished from artifacts such as air bubbles, water or lipid droplets, or other debris with which it can be confused. Colonies of *U. urealyticum* can be identified on A 8 agar by urease production in the presence of a $CaCl_2$ indicator. In this circumstance, the colonies are 15 to 30 μm in diameter and appear as brownish granular clumps on the agar surface (Fig. 2). *M. hominis* colonies are approximately 200 to 300 μm in diameter, are urease negative, and often have the typical fried-egg appearance (Fig. 1). Other species, such as *M. pneumoniae* and *M. genitalium*, will produce much smaller spherical colonies which may not demonstrate the fried-egg appearance (Fig. 1). The Dienes methylene blue stain applied directly to the agar plate can be very useful if there is uncertainty about whether or not mycoplasmal colonies are present. With this reagent, mycoplasmal colonies will stain blue. *M. hominis* is the only pathogenic mycoplasma of humans cultivable on bacteriologic media such as chocolate agar or blood agar, but the pinpoint translucent colonies are easily overlooked, and routine bacterial cultures may be discarded sooner than the time needed for *M. hominis* colonies to develop. The occurrence of suspicious colonies warrants subculture to a medium appropriate for the growth of mycoplasmas.

Commercial Media and Culture Kits

In response to the growing desires of many independent or hospital-based clinical laboratories to offer mycoplasmal cultures on-site, numerous companies have developed various transport and growth medium systems patterned after the original formulations developed by researchers in the field of mycoplasmology several years ago. Products available for use vary from one country to another.

A triphasic flask system containing broth and agar in a single flask is available for the isolation and identification of *U. urealyticum* and *M. hominis* (Mycotrim; Irvine Scientific, Irvine, Calif.). With this kit, growth in the broth medium as indicated by a color change can be verified by the observation of colonies. A comparable system, adapted to *M. pneumoniae* detection, is also available for respiratory specimens. Remel, Inc., has developed several formulations of transport and growth media, including 10 B broth, A 7 and A 8 agars, and SP 4 broth and agar. A comparison of Remel A 7 and A 8 agars showed that the latter is more sensitive than the Mycotrim system for the detection of genital mycoplasmas (6). Systems adapted to the quantitative detection and identification of *U. urealyticum* and *M. hominis* from urogenital specimens are available from commercial suppliers in Europe but not in North America at this time.

Problems with some of the commercially prepared products have included contamination of serum with mycoplasmas of animal origin and inadequate quality control. If commercially prepared media are to be used, it is advisable that laboratories perform internal quality control tests. Some kits and other commercial products have been evaluated to a limited degree (6, 43, 77), but no rigorous large-scale comparisons of commercially prepared media with reference media and techniques for the isolation of mycoplasmas have been reported. Commercial products and kits may be of particular value if the need to detect mycoplasmas arises infrequently in laboratories which do not specialize in mycoplasma detection, but users should be aware of the potential limitations of existing products.

IDENTIFICATION

Because of their cellular dimensions, mycoplasmas cannot be clearly visualized by routine light microscopy. The lack of a cell wall precludes visualization of mycoplasmas by Gram staining, but this procedure may prove useful for excluding the possibility that contaminating bacteria are present. *M. hominis* may occasionally appear as pinpoint colonies on bacteriologic media, and the lack of a Gram staining reaction by these colonies gives a clue as to their possible mycoplasmal identity, warranting further, more specific evaluation and subculture to a medium appropriate for the growth of mycoplasmas. Giemsa stains may be used, but the results can be difficult to interpret because of the presence of debris and artifacts in clinical specimens which can be confused with mycoplasmas due to their small size. Even though the numerous large-colony mycoplasmal species which may be isolated from humans cannot be identified on the basis of their colonial morphology or a particular biochemical profile, the body site of origin and the rate of growth, in conjunction with biochemical features, give some clues. For example, a slowly growing glycolytic organism from the respiratory tract which produces spherical colonies on SP 4 agar and which exhibits hemolytic activity and hemadsorption when colonies on agar are overlaid with guinea pig erythrocytes is likely to be *M. pneumoniae*. An alkaline color change which occurs after overnight incubation without turbidity in 10 B broth containing urea is almost certainly due to *U. urealyticum*, whereas a genital specimen that produces an alkaline reaction within 24 to 72 h in medium supplemented with arginine is likely to contain *M. hominis*.

In order to identify an organism completely to the species level, a number of different techniques are available, although they are more appropriately within the province of a reference laboratory rather than a hospital microbiology laboratory because of their complexity and the lack of widespread availability of the serologic reagents required. Agar growth inhibition with species-specific antisera impregnated in filter paper disks and applied to agar plates onto which the unknown organism is inoculated is one method, but several antisera may be required to encompass multiple strains within a given species. Because of possible cross-reactions between related species, such as *M. pneumoniae* and *M. genitalium*, rigorous proof of the specificity of the method must be documented by testing multiple isolates of the same species as controls. Epi-immunofluorescence or immunoperoxidase techniques enable colonies on agar to be identified directly so that mixtures of different species can be readily discerned. Immunoblotting with monoclonal antibodies, metabolism inhibition tests, mycoplasmacidal tests, and PCR assays have also been used to identify mycoplasmas to the species level (12, 55, 60). *U. urealyticum* serotypes have been identified by PCR, metabolism inhibition, mycoplasmacidal, agar growth inhibition, and epi-immunofluorescence tests (51, 54).

SEROLOGIC TESTS

M. pneumoniae Respiratory Disease

Historically, serology has been the most common laboratory means for the diagnosis of respiratory tract infections caused by *M. pneumoniae*. Although culture and, more recently, PCR are also used to detect the presence of *M. pneumoniae* in respiratory specimens, the persistence of the organism for variable lengths of time following acute infection makes it difficult to assess the significance of a positive test result without additional confirmatory tests such as tests for seroconversion. *M. pneumoniae* has both lipid and protein antigens which elicit antibody responses in patients with clinical infections, allowing several different serologic assays based on different antigens and technologies. However, some are impractical for routine diagnostic use, have not been developed sufficiently for use in clinical laboratories, and do not merit in-depth discussion here.

Complement fixation (CF) with the chloroform-methanol-extractable lipid antigen has often been the reference method for serologic testing for *M. pneumoniae* (21, 35). Although CF measures mainly the early IgM response, the test does not differentiate among antibody classes, which is desirable for the differentiation of acute from remote infection. Therefore, seroconversion in paired serum specimens collected 2 to 4 weeks apart provides optimum diagnostic accuracy by CF, particularly for adults over 40 years of age, in whom an IgM response may be minimal or absent, presumably because of reinfection (10). When present, the duration of detectable IgM may be variable (52). Antibody production may also be delayed in some patients with infections or even absent if the patient is immunosuppressed.

CF is far from being a "gold standard" for diagnosis. It suffers from low sensitivity because the glycolipid antigen mixture used is not specific for *M. pneumoniae* and may be found in other microorganisms, as well as human tissues and even plants. CF has reduced specificity due to cross-reactions with other organisms, most notably *M. genitalium* (38, 67) and may provide false-positive results due to the presence of cross-reactive autoantibodies induced by acute inflammation from other unrelated causes. Confirmation of positive CF results by Western blotting can overcome the problem with cross-reactivity but adds further to the time and expense of testing (10, 35).

Other serologic tests include an IgM-specific immunofluorescent-antibody (IFA) assay, direct hemagglutination, indirect hemagglutination with IgM capture, and particle agglutination (2, 3, 14). The last two tests tend to be more sensitive than CF, but specificities remain a problem. Performance of the IFA assay is technically simple, but interpretation of its results is subjective, and the presence of *M. pneumoniae*-specific IgG may interfere with the results (2). Microimmunofluorescence for IgM is more specific but is less sensitive than CF (52).

EIAs were developed in the 1970s and are marketed commercially by several companies. Various assays may require the use of washed whole organisms, sonicated whole-cell antigen preparations, detergent-lysed organisms, or other formulations. Thus, not all of the assays can be considered equivalent. EIAs are more sensitive than CF or culture, have good specificity, and are less technically demanding. For these reasons, EIA has replaced CF in many diagnostic laboratories (2, 10, 67). Like CF tests, early-generation EIAs sold commercially do not allow differentiation among antibody classes. The need for acute- and convalescent-phase sera collected 2 to 4 weeks apart and tested simultaneously for the accurate detection of acute *M. pneumoniae* infection by EIAs remains an obvious limitation to prompt diagnosis (21, 67). More recently, immunoglobulin class-specific EIA reagents have become available (2, 13). An EIA specific for IgM, the ImmunoCard (Meridian Diagnostics, Cincinnati, Ohio), has been developed for the rapid detection of an acute *M. pneumoniae* infection with a single serum specimen (2). The ImmunoCard has the advantages of being technically much simpler and quicker (10 min) in terms of assay performance than other types of assays. Its potential disadvantage is a lack of sensitivity for the detection of some *M. pneumoniae* infections in some adults, in whom the IgM response may be minimal. There remains a need for improved serologic reagents for the detection of acute *M. pneumoniae* infection. Purified P1 adhesin protein as the antigenic basis of such tests may eventually prove to be useful.

Cold agglutinins, detected by agglutination of type O Rh-negative erythrocytes at 4°C, occur in association with *M. pneumoniae* infection in about 50% of patients (10). Titers of 64 to 128 or a fourfold or greater rise in titer suggests a recent *M. pneumoniae* infection, but the test is nonspecific, and cold agglutinins may be induced by a wide variety of viral infections as well as noninfectious conditions such as collagen-vascular diseases.

Infections Due to Genital Mycoplasmas

The ubiquity of most genital mycoplasmas in humans makes interpretation of antibody titers difficult, and the mere existence of antibodies alone cannot be considered significant. However, when invasive extragenital disease occurs, elevation of antibody titers is often apparent. The unique susceptibility of hypogammaglobulinemic persons to invasive infections due to *U. urealyticum* testifies to the importance of the humoral immune response in providing protection against disease due to this organism (12). Although it has been suggested that increases in the titers of type-specific antibodies against certain ureaplasmal serovars occur in women with pregnancy wastage and in infants with respiratory disease compared to the titers in control patients, more comparative data from well-characterized and carefully matched control populations are needed to fully appreciate the value of antibody titer determinations in these settings (12). Patients with invasive infection caused by *M. hominis* almost without exception seroconvert or have a significant rise in existing antibody titer (27, 63, 64, 68).

No single serologic test has proved to be satisfactory for identifying genital mycoplasma infections. Serologic tests for *M. hominis* and *U. urealyticum* by the techniques of microimmunofluorescence, metabolism inhibition, and EIA have been described (7, 8, 54, 55, 60). A microimmunofluorescence assay for *M. genitalium* has also been developed (23) and has been shown to detect antibody responses in men with NGU (58) and women with salpingitis (42). This method is rapid, reproducible, and quite sensitive and specific, with there being less cross-reactivity with *M. pneumoniae* than is seen with other methods. CF has not been shown to be sufficiently sensitive or specific for use in identifying genital mycoplasmal infections. No serologic tests for genital mycoplasmas have been standardized and made commercially available, and they cannot be recommended for routine diagnostic purposes at present.

ANTIBIOTIC SUSCEPTIBILITIES

Methods Used

Several methods of susceptibility testing used for conventional bacteria have been used for the susceptibility testing of mycoplasmas. Agar dilution has been used extensively as a reference method (4, 36, 71). It has the advantages of a relatively stable endpoint over time, the inoculum size does not have a great effect, and it allows detection of mixed cultures readily. However, this technique is not practical for the testing of small numbers of strains or occasional isolates which may be encountered in diagnostic laboratories. Agar disk diffusion is not acceptable for the testing of mycoplasmas. Broth microdilution for the determination of MICs is probably the most practical and widely used method. It is economical, allows several antimicrobial agents to be tested in the same microtiter plate, but has numerous disadvantages in that preparation of dilutions of antimicrobial agents is labor-intensive and the endpoint tends to shift over time. Limited comparisons of the agar dilution versus the broth microdilution methods indicate that similar results may be obtained for erythromycin and tetracycline when they have been tested against *U. urealyticum* (71).

Preliminary studies with the Etest (AB BIODISK, Solna, Sweden) for the detection of tetracycline resistance in *M. hominis* yielded results comparable to those obtained by the broth microdilution method (72). Whether this technique will be suitable for *U. urealyticum* or slower-growing organisms, such as *M. pneumoniae*, has not been determined. The Etest has the advantages of the simplicity of agar-based testing, it has an endpoint which does not shift over time, it does not have a large inoculum effect, and it can easily be adapted for the testing of single isolates. The Etest is most cost-effective only if testing of a small number of drugs is of interest, such as screening for tetracycline resistance, due to the relatively high cost of individual antibiotic-containing Etest strips.

Irrespective of the test method, there are no universally accepted standards for pH, media, incubation conditions, or duration of incubation for performing mycoplasmal or ureaplasmal susceptibility tests. No MIC breakpoints specific for these organisms are endorsed by any regulatory agency. The lack of specific guidelines for susceptibility testing by the National Committee for Clinical Laboratory Standards has led to diverse and often inconsistent susceptibility profiles for mollicutes.

A control strain for which the MICs of the drugs being tested are reproducible must be included with each assay for validation purposes. This can be a commercially purchased type strain or a well-studied clinical isolate for which MICs are reproducible. An inoculum of 10^4 to 10^5 CFU/ml has been recommended as the optimum inoculum for broth-based testing (4). Nonstandardized conditions at low pH (6.0) can affect MICs, especially those of macrolides, making them appear less active in vitro, but such conditions may be required to achieve adequate growth of organisms such as *U. urealyticum* (36).

Bactericidal activity can be tested directly from the wells in broth microdilution MIC assays by removing the mixture of organisms and antibiotic, diluting the mixture so that it contains subinhibitory concentrations in fresh medium, and observing the diluted mixture for a color change as evidence of growth. Detailed descriptions of procedures for susceptibility testing techniques are available in reference texts (4).

Although some reference laboratories have adopted MIC breakpoints for other bacteria for use in the interpretation of MICs when testing mycoplasmas, this practice should be used with caution, and it may be preferable to merely report MICs and allow clinicians to draw their own conclusions about the suitability of a particular agent for use in the treatment of a specific infection. For most antimicrobial agents of potential use against mollicutes, organisms for which MICs are ≤ 1 μg/ml should be considered likely to be effectively treated. Tetracycline-resistant *M. hominis* and *U. urealyticum* can readily be distinguished by broth- or agar-based methods since the MICs for resistant strains are generally ≥ 8 μg/ml, whereas MICs for susceptible strains are consistently ≤2 μg/ml, with no overlap between the MICs for the two distinct populations (71, 72). Since susceptibility testing of mycoplasmas should be performed only under special circumstances, the most practical approach for laboratories which offer this service might be to test drugs on a case-by-case basis according to specific physician and patient needs, including only those agents being considered for actual treatment.

Commercial MIC panels in kits have been used in Europe. They consist of microwells containing dried antimicrobial agents, generally in two concentrations corresponding to the threshold proposed for conventional bacteria to classify a strain as susceptible, intermediate, or resistant. These kits give results comparable to those obtained by established means of making MIC determinations (4, 46).

Susceptibility Profiles and Antimicrobial Resistance

A great deal of conflicting information concerning the relative activities of various antimicrobial agents against mycoplasmas has arisen over the past few years. In addition to the lack of standardized techniques, the small sample sizes in studies described in published reports, the use of samples collected in a nonrandom manner without respect to drug exposure, the use of vague endpoints subject to fluctuation, and changes in resistance over time have further confounded the issue. Information on in vitro susceptibilities is greatest for M. *pneumoniae*, M. *hominis*, and U. *urealyticum*, but in some recent studies the activities of numerous antimicrobial agents against M. *fermentans* and M. *genitalium* have been evaluated. Although incompletely studied, M. *genitalium* has susceptibilities generally similar to those of M. *pneumoniae*, while M. *fermentans* has susceptibilities generally similar to those of M. *hominis*, with some exceptions. A comparison of the MICs of several antimicrobial agents tested against these mollicutes is presented in Table 3.

Due to the lack of a cell wall, mollicutes are innately resistant to all β-lactams. Sulfonamides, trimethoprim, and rifampin are also inactive. Resistance to macrolides and lincosamides is variable according to species, with M. *hominis* being resistant to erythromycin but susceptible to clindamycin. For U. *urealyticum*, the reverse is true. Newer macrolides and azalides have shown in vitro activity comparable to that of erythromycin against M. *pneumoniae* and U. *urealyticum*.

M. *pneumoniae* has remained predictably susceptible to tetracyclines and macrolides so that susceptibility testing is not indicated except for the in vitro evaluation of new and previously untested agents. Tetracycline resistance has been well documented in recent years in both M. *hominis* and U. *urealyticum*, to variable degrees, mediated by the *tet*M transposon which codes for a protein that binds to the ribosomes, protecting them from the actions of these drugs (47). The extent to which tetracycline resistance occurs in genital mycoplasmas varies geographically and according to prior antimicrobial exposure in different populations, but it may approach 40% for M. *hominis* in some groups. Other agents active at the bacterial ribosome such as streptogramins, aminoglycosides, and chloramphenicol may show in vitro inhibitory activity against some mollicute species.

Extragenital infections, often in immunocompromised hosts, may be caused by multidrug-resistant mycoplasmas, making guidance of chemotherapy by the results of in vitro susceptibility tests important in this clinical setting. Eradication of infection under these circumstances can be extremely difficult, requiring prolonged therapy, even when the organisms are susceptible to the expected agents. This difficulty highlights the facts that mollicutes are inhibited but not killed by most commonly used bacteriostatic antimicrobial agents at concentrations achievable in vivo and that a functioning immune system plays an integral part in their eradication. The need for bactericidal agents for the treatment of systemic infections in immunocompromised hosts has led to considerable interest in the fluoroquinolones. New quinolones such as trovafloxacin and sparfloxacin tend to have greater in vitro activity against mollicutes than older agents such as ciprofloxacin and ofloxacin.

TABLE 3 Ranges of MICs of various antimicrobial agents for M. *pneumoniae*, M. *hominis*, M. *fermentans*, M. *genitalium*, and U. *urealyticum*[a]

Antimicrobial agent	MIC range (μg/ml)				
	M. *pneumoniae*	M. *hominis*	M. *genitalium*	M. *fermentans*	U. *urealyticum*
Tetracycline	0.63–0.25	0.2–2[b]	ND[c]	0.1–1	0.05–2[b]
Doxycycline	0.02–0.5	0.1–2[b]	≤0.01–0.3	0.05–1	0.02–1[b]
Erythromycin	≤0.004–0.06	32–>1,000	≤0.01	0.5–64	0.02–4
Clarithromycin	≤0.004–0.125	16–>256	≤0.01	1–64	≤0.004–2
Azithromycin	≤0.004–0.01	4–64	≤0.01	≤0.003–0.05	0.5–4
Clindamycin	≤0.008–2	≤0.008–2	0.2–1	0.01–0.25	0.2–64
Chloramphenicol	2	4–25	ND	0.5–10	0.4–8
Gentamicin	4	2–16	ND	0.25–>500	0.1–13
Ciprofloxacin	0.5–2	0.1–4	2	0.02–>64	0.1–16
Ofloxacin	0.05–2	0.1–64	1–2	0.02–25	0.2–25
Levofloxacin	0.5–1	0.1–0.5	0.5–1	0.05	0.2–1
Sparfloxacin	≤0.008–0.5	<0.008–0.1	0.05–0.1	≤0.01–0.05	0.003–1
Trovafloxacin	0.12–0.5	0.03–0.06	ND	ND	0.06–0.5
Rifampin	ND	>1,000	ND	25–>50	>1,000
Quinupristin-dalfopristin	0.008–0.06	0.25–8	ND	ND	0.12–0.5
Nitrofurantoin	ND	6–500	ND	0.1–2.5	13–>1,000

[a] Data were compiled from multiple published studies in which different methods and often different antimicrobial concentrations were used.

[b] Tetracycline-susceptible strains only.

[c] ND, no data.

EVALUATION, INTERPRETATION, AND REPORTING OF RESULTS

Tests offered through diagnostic microbiology laboratories should focus on the species known to cause human disease and for which cultivation techniques are best defined. Unusual organisms or those for which cultivation conditions are not established may be detectable by PCR technology offered through a few specialized research or reference laboratories. Such organisms should be sought only after consultation with clinicians and personnel from the reference laboratory. Except for *U. urealyticum*, which can be identified by its urease production and distinct colonial morphology until species identification can be confirmed, a preliminary report of "large-colony *Mycoplasma* species" is appropriate. In many instances, as in the culturing of specimens from the lower genital tract, this may be sufficient. Isolates from normally sterile sites and/or from immunosuppressed persons should be identified to the species level if possible.

M. pneumoniae

Detection of *M. pneumoniae* in culture is time-consuming and not overly sensitive. However, isolation of the organism from respiratory tract specimens is clinically significant in most instances and should be correlated with the presence of clinical respiratory disease since a small proportion of asymptomatic carriers may exist. Detection by PCR technology is becoming more widely available through reference laboratories, but a positive result must still be correlated with clinical events. Reliable serology is critical for the accurate diagnosis of *M. pneumoniae* respiratory disease, and EIA for the detection of antibody is the method of choice. EIA is widely available, is more sensitive than culture, and has sensitivity for the detection of infection comparable to that of PCR. A fourfold rise in antibody titer in acute- and convalescent-phase sera is considered diagnostic. In children, adolescents, and young adults, a single positive IgM result with appropriate immunoglobulin class-specific reagents may be considered diagnostic in many cases.

M. hominis

M. hominis can be detected in culture within a few days. It may occasionally be discovered in routine bacteriologic media from appropriate clinical material, but this should not be relied upon for its detection. Its isolation in any quantity from normally sterile body fluids or tissues is significantly associated with disease, but quantitation of the organisms present may be of value in other circumstances. When mycoplasmas are detected at nonsterile sites such as the female lower genital tract in numbers of $\geq 10^5$ organisms, they are most likely to be associated with bacterial vaginosis.

U. urealyticum

U. urealyticum can be detected in culture within 24 to 48 h, and its characteristic colonial morphology and urease production are sufficient for its identification. Isolation in any quantity from normally sterile body fluids or tissues is significantly associated with disease. Fewer than 10^4 organisms in the male urethra is unlikely to be significant (27).

Identification of specific biovars or serovars of *U. urealyticum* is not practical or necessary for diagnostic purposes on the basis of presently available information. Whether there is a difference in the pathogenicity among the two biovars of this organism has been the subject of several evaluations, with inconclusive results. This issue is now being investigated more extensively owing to the advent of PCR technology, which allows isolates to be classified more readily.

Other Mycoplasmas

Optimum culture techniques for the detection of species other than *M. pneumoniae*, *M. hominis*, and *U. urealyticum* in clinical specimens are less well defined. However, detection of *M. genitalium* by a PCR assay without quantitation is likely to be significant.

REFERENCES

1. **Ainsworth, J. G., S. Hourshid, J. Clarke, D. Mitchell, J. N. Weber, and D. Taylor-Robinson.** 1994. Detection of *Mycoplasma fermentans* in HIV-positive individuals undergoing bronchoscopy. *IOM Lett.* **3:**319–320.
2. **Alexander, T. S., L. D. Gray, J. A. Kraft, D. S. Leland, M. T. Nikaido, and D. H. Willis.** 1996. Performance of Meridian ImmunoCard *Mycoplasma* test in a multicenter clinical trial. *J. Clin. Microbiol.* **34:**1180–1183.
3. **Barker, C. E., M. Sillis, and T. G. Wreghitt.** 1990. Evaluation of Serodia Myco II particle agglutination test for detecting *Mycoplasma pneumoniae* antibody: comparison with μ-capture ELISA and indirect immunofluorescence. *J. Clin. Pathol.* **43:**163–165.
4. **Bebear, C., and J. A. Robertson.** 1996. Determination of minimal inhibitory concentration, p. 189–197. *In* J. G. Tully and S. Razin (ed.), *Molecular and Diagnostic Procedures in Mycoplasmology*. Academic Press, Inc., New York, N.Y.
5. **Blanchard, A., J. Hentschel, L. Duffy, K. Baldus, and G. H. Cassell.** 1993. Detection of *Ureaplasma urealyticum* by polymerase chain reaction in the urogenital tract of adults, in amniotic fluid and in the respiratory tract of newborns. *Clin. Infect. Dis.* **17**(Suppl. 1):S83–S89.
6. **Broitman, N. L., C. M. Floyd, C. A. Johnson, L. M. de la Maza, and E. Peterson.** 1992. Comparison of commercially available media for detection and isolation of *Ureaplasma urealyticum* and *Mycoplasma hominis*. *J. Clin. Microbiol.* **30:** 1335–1337.
7. **Brown, M. B., G. H. Cassell, D. Taylor-Robinson, and M. C. Shepard.** 1983. Measurement of antibody to *Ureaplasma urealyticum* by an enzyme-linked immunosorbent assay and detection of antibody responses in patients with nongonococcal urethritis. *J. Clin. Microbiol.* **17:**288–295.
8. **Brown, M. B., G. H. Cassell, W. M. McCormack, and J. K. Davis.** 1987. Measurement of antibody to *Mycoplasma hominis* by an enzyme-linked immunosorbent assay and detection of antibody responses in women with postpartum fever. *Am. J. Obstet. Gynecol.* **156:**701–708.
9. **Cassell, G. H., R. O. Davis, K. B. Waites, P. A. Marriott, M. B. Brown, and J. K. Davis.** 1983. Isolation of *Mycoplasma hominis* and *Ureaplasma urealyticum* from amniotic fluid at 16–20 weeks of gestation: potential effect on outcome of pregnancy. *Sex. Transm. Dis.* **10(Suppl.):** 294–302.
10. **Cassell, G. H., G. Gambill, and L. Duffy.** 1996. ELISA in respiratory infections of humans, p. 123–136. *In* J. G. Tully and S. Razin (ed.), *Molecular and Diagnostic Procedures in Mycoplasmology*. Academic Press, Inc. New York, N.Y.
11. **Cassell, G. H., K. B. Waites, D. T. Crouse, P. T. Rudd, K. C. Canupp, S. Stagno, and G. R. Cutter.** 1988. Association of *Ureaplasma urealyticum* infection of the lower respiratory tract with chronic lung disease and death in very-low-birth-weight infants. *Lancet* **ii:**240–244.
12. **Cassell, G. H., K. B. Waites, and D. T. Crouse.** 1994. Mycoplasmal infections, p. 619–656. *In* J. S. Remington

and J. O. Klein (ed.), *Infectious Diseases of the Fetus and Newborn Infant*, 4th ed. The W. B. Saunders Co., Philadelphia, Pa.

13. **Cimolai, N., and A. C. H. Cheong.** 1996. An assessment of a new diagnostic indirect enzyme immunoassay for the detection of anti-*Mycoplasma pneumoniae* IgM. *Clin. Microbiol. Infect. Dis.* **105:**205–209.
14. **Coombs, R. R. A., G. Easter, P. Matejtschuk, and T. G. Wreghitt.** 1988. Red-cell IgM-antibody capture assay for the detection of *Mycoplasma pneumoniae*-specific IgM. *Epidemiol. Infect.* **100:**101–109.
15. **Cunliffe, N. A., S. Fergusson, F. Davidson, A. Lyon, and P. W. Ross.** 1996. Comparison of culture with the polymerase chain reaction for detection of *Ureaplasma urealyticum* in endotracheal aspirates of preterm infants. *J. Med. Microbiol.* **45:**27–30.
16. **de Barbeyrac, B., C. Berner-Poggi, F. Febrer, H. Renaudin, M. Dupon, and C. Bebear.** 1993. Detection of *Mycoplasma pneumoniae* and *Mycoplasma genitalium* in clinical samples by polymerase chain reaction. *Clin. Infect. Dis.* **17**(Suppl. 1)**:**83–89.
17. **Deguchi, T., C. B. Gilroy, and D. Taylor-Robinson.** 1996. Failure to detect *Mycoplasma fermentans*, *Mycoplasma penetrans*, or *Mycoplasma pirum* in the urethra of patients with acute nongonococcal urethritis. *Eur. J. Clin. Microbiol. Infect. Dis.* **15:**169–171.
18. **Doble, A., B. J. Thomas, P. M. Furr, M. M. Walker, J. R. W. Harris, R. O. Witherow, and D. Taylor-Robinson.** 1989. A search for infectious agents in chronic abacterial prostatitis utilizing ultrasound guided biopsy. *Br. J. Urol.* **64:**297–301.
19. **Eschenbach, D. A.** 1986. *Ureaplasma urealyticum* as a cause of post-partum fever. *Pediatr. Infect. Dis.* **5**(Suppl)**:** 258–261.
20. **Eschenbach, D. A.** 1993. *Ureaplasma urealyticum* and premature birth. *Clin. Infect. Dis.* **17**(Suppl. 1)**:**100–106.
21. **Fedorko, D. P., D. D. Emery, S. M. Franklin, and D. D. Congdon.** 1995. Evaluation of a rapid enzyme immunoassay system for serologic diagnosis of *Mycoplasma pneumoniae* infection. *Diagn. Microbiol. Infect. Dis.* **23:**85–88.
22. **Foy, H. M.** 1993. Infections caused by *Mycoplasma pneumoniae* and possible carrier state in different populations of patients. *Clin. Infect. Dis.* **17**(Suppl. 1)**:**37–46.
23. **Furr, P. M., and D. Taylor-Robinson.** 1984. Microimmunofluorescence technique for detection of antibody to *Mycoplasma genitalium*. *J. Clin. Pathol.* **37:**1072–1074.
24. **Furr, P. M., and D. Taylor-Robinson.** 1990. Long-term viability of stored mycoplasmas and ureaplasmas. *J. Med. Microbiol.* **31:**203–206.
25. **Furr, P. M., D. Taylor-Robinson, and A. D. B. Webster.** 1994. Mycoplasmas and ureaplasmas in patients with hypogammagobulinaemia and their role in arthritis: microbiological observations over 20 years. *Ann. Rheum. Dis.* **53:** 183–187.
26. **Gerstenecker, B., and E. Jacobs.** 1993. Development of a capture-ELISA for the specific detection of *Mycoplasma pneumoniae* in patient's material, p. 195–205. *In* I. Kahane and A. Adoni (ed.), *Rapid Diagnosis of Mycoplasmas*. Plenum Press, New York, N.Y.
27. **Glatt, A. E., W. M. McCormack, and D. Taylor-Robinson.** 1989. Genital mycoplasmas, p. 279–293. *In* K. K. Holmes, P. A. Mardh, P. F. Sparling, P. J. Wiesner, W. Cates, S. M. Lemon, and W. E. Stamm (ed.), *Sexually Transmitted Diseases*, 2nd ed. McGraw-Hill Book Co., New York, N.Y.
28. **Grau, O., R. Kovacic, R. Griffais, V. Launay, and L. Montagnier.** 1994. Development of PCR-based assays for the detection of two human mollicute species, *Mycoplasma penetrans* and *M. hominis*. *Mol. Cell. Probes* **8:**139–148.
29. **Grenabo, L., H. Hedelin, and S. Pettersson.** 1988. Urinary infection stones caused by *Ureaplasma urealyticum*: a review. *Scand. J. Infect. Dis.* **53**(Suppl.)**:**46–49.
30. **Horner, P. J., C. B. Gilroy, B. J. Thomas, R. O. M. Naidoo, and D. Taylor-Robinson.** 1993. Association of *Mycoplasma genitalium* with acute non-gonococcal urethritis. *Lancet* **342:**582–585.
31. **Jalil, N., A. Doble, C. Gilchrist, and D. Taylor-Robinson.** 1988. Infection of the epididymis by *Ureaplasma urealyticum*. *Genitourin. Med.* **64:**367–368.
32. **Jensen, J. S., S. A. Uldum, J. Sondergard-Anderson, J. Vuust, and K. Lind.** 1991. Polymerase chain reaction for detection of *Mycoplasma genitalium* in clinical samples. *J. Clin. Microbiol.* **29:**46–50.
33. **Jensen, J. S., H. T. Hansen, and K. Lind.** 1996. Isolation of *Mycoplasma genitalium* strains from the male urethra. *J. Clin. Microbiol.* **34:**286–291.
34. **Katseni, V. L., C. B. Gilroy, B. K. Ryait, K. Ariyoshi, P. D. Bieniasz, J. N. Weber, and D. Taylor-Robinson.** 1993. *Mycoplasma fermentans* in individuals seropositive and seronegative for HIV-1. *Lancet* **341:**271–273.
35. **Kenny, G. E.** 1992. Serodiagnosis, p. 505–512. *In* J. Maniloff, R. N. McElhaney, L. R. Finch, and J. B. Baseman (ed.), *Mycoplasmas: Molecular Biology and Pathogenesis*. American Society for Microbiology, Washington, D.C.
36. **Kenny, G. E., and F. D. Cartwright.** 1993. Effect of pH, inoculum size, and incubation time on the susceptibility of *Ureaplasma urealyticum* to erythromycin *in vitro*. *Clin. Infect. Dis.* **17**(Suppl. 1)**:**215–218.
37. **Kok, T. W., G. Varkanis, B. P. Marmion, J. Martin, and A. Esterman.** 1988. Laboratory diagnosis of *Mycoplasma pneumoniae* infection. I. Direct detection of antigen to respiratory exudates by enzyme immunoassay. *Epidemiol. Infect.* **101:**669–684.
38. **Lind, K.** 1982. Serological cross-reaction between *Mycoplasma genitalium* and *M. pneumoniae*. *Lancet* **ii:**1158–1159.
39. **Lo, S. C., D. J. Wear, S. L. Green, P. G. Jones, and J. F. Legler.** 1993. Adult respiratory distress syndrome with or without systemic disease associated with infections due to *Mycoplasma fermentans*. *Clin. Infect. Dis.* **17**(Suppl. 1)**:** 259–263.
40. **Lo, S. C., M. M. Hayes, J. G. Tully, R. Y. Wang, H. Kotani, P. F. Pierce, D. L. Rose, and J. W. K. Shih.** 1992. *Mycoplasma penetrans* sp. nov., from the urogenital trait of patients with AIDS. *Int. J. Syst. Bacteriol.* **42:**357–364.
41. **Meyer, R. D., and W. Clough.** 1993. Extragenital *Mycoplasma hominis* infections in adults: emphasis on immunosuppression. *Clin. Infect. Dis.* **17**(Suppl. 1)**:**243–249.
42. **Møller, B. R., D. Taylor-Robinson, and P. M. Furr.** 1984. Serologic evidence implicating *Mycoplasma genitalium* in pelvic inflammatory disease. *Lancet* **i:**1102–1103.
43. **Phillips, L. E., K. H. Goodrich, R. M. Turner, and S. Faro.** 1986. Isolation of *Mycoplasma* species and *Ureaplasma urealyticum* from obstetrical and gynecological patients by using commercially available medium formulations. *J. Clin. Microbiol.* **24:**377–379.
44. **Pratt, B.** 1990. Automatic blood culture systems: detection of *Mycoplasma hominis* in SPS-containing media, p. 778–781. *In* G. Staneck, G. H. Cassell, J. G. Tully, and R. F. Whitcomb (ed.), *Recent Advances in Mycoplasmology*. Gustav Fischer Verlag, Stuttgart, Germany.
45. **Razin, S.** 1994. DNA probes and PCR in diagnosis of mycoplasma infections. *Mol. Cell. Probes* **8:**497–511.
46. **Renaudin, H., and C. Bebear.** 1990. Evaluation des systemes *Mycoplasma* PLUS et SIR *Mycoplasma* pour la detection quantitative et l'etude de la sensibilite aux antibiotiques des mycoplasmes genitaux. *Pathol. Biol.* **38:** 431–435.
47. **Roberts, M. C.** 1992. Antibiotic resistance, p. 513–523.

In J. Maniloff, R. N. McElhaney, L. R. Finch, and J. B. Baseman (ed.), *Mycoplasmas: Molecular Biology and Pathogenesis*. American Society for Microbiology, Washington, D.C.

48. **Robertson, J. A., M. Alfa, and E. S. Boatman.** 1983. The morphology of the cells and colonies of *Mycoplasma hominis*. *Sex. Transm. Dis.* **10**(Suppl.)**:**232–239.
49. **Schaeverbeke, T., H. Renaudin, M. Clerc, L. Lequen, J. P. Vernhes, B. de Barbeyrac, B. Bannwarth, C. Bebear, and J. Dehais.** 1997. Systematic detection of mycoplasmas by culture and polymerase chain reaction (PCR) procedures in 209 synovial fluid samples. *Br. J. Rheum.* **36:**310–314.
50. **Shepard, M. C.** 1983. Culture media for ureaplasmas, p. 137–146. *In* S. Razin and J. G. Tully (ed.), *Methods in Mycoplasmology*, vol. 1. Academic Press, Inc., New York, N.Y.
51. **Shepard, M. C., and C. D. Lunceford.** 1978. Serological typing of *Ureaplasma urealyticum* isolates from urethritis patients by an agar growth inhibition method. *J. Clin. Microbiol.* **8:**566–574.
52. **Sillis, M.** 1990. The limitation of IgM assays in the serological diagnosis of *Mycoplasma pneumoniae* infection. *J. Med. Microbiol.* **33:**253–258.
53. **Stamm, W. E., K. Running, J. Hale, and K. K. Holmes.** 1983. Etiologic role of *Mycoplasma hominis* and *Ureaplasma urealyticum* in women with the acute urethral syndrome. *Sex. Transm. Dis.* **10**(Suppl.)**:**318–322.
54. **Taylor-Robinson, D.** 1983. Serological identification of ureaplasmas from humans, p. 57–63. *In* J. G. Tully and S. Razin (ed.), *Methods in Mycoplasmology*, vol. 2. Academic Press, Inc., New York, N.Y.
55. **Taylor-Robinson, D.** 1983. Metabolism inhibition test, p. 411–417. *In* J. G. Tully and S. Razin (ed.), *Methods in Mycoplasmology*, vol. 1. Academic Press, Inc., New York, N.Y.
56. **Taylor-Robinson, D.** 1985. Mycoplasmal and mixed infections of the human male urogenital tract and their possible complications, p. 27–63. *In* S. Razin and M. F. Barile (ed.), *The Mycoplasmas*, vol. 4. Academic Press, Inc., New York, N.Y.
57. **Taylor-Robinson, D.** 1986. Evaluation of the role of *Ureaplasma urealyticum* in infertility. *Pediatr. Infect. Dis.* **5**(Suppl.)**:**262–265.
58. **Taylor-Robinson, D.** 1989. Genital mycoplasma infections. *Clin. Lab. Med.* **9:**501–523.
59. **Taylor-Robinson, D.** 1996. Infections due to species of *Mycoplasma* and *Ureaplasma*: an update. *Clin. Infect. Dis.* **23:**671–684.
60. **Taylor-Robinson, D., and G. W. Csonka.** 1981. Laboratory and clinical aspects of mycoplasmal infections of the human genitourinary tract, p. 151–186. *In* J. W. Harris (ed.), *Recent Advances in Sexually Transmitted Diseases*, no. 2. Churchill Livingstone, Ltd., Edinburgh, United Kingdom.
61. **Taylor-Robinson, D., P. M. Furr, and A. D. B. Webster.** 1985. *Ureaplasma urealyticum* causing persistent urethritis in a patient with hypogammaglobulinaemia. *Genitourin. Med.* **61:**404–408.
62. **Taylor-Robinson, D., P. M. Furr, and A. D. B. Webster.** 1986. *Ureaplasma urealyticum* in the immunocompromised host. *Pediatr. Infect. Dis.* **5**(Suppl.)**:**236–238.
63. **Taylor-Robinson, D., and W. M. McCormack.** 1979. Mycoplasmas in human genitourinary infections, p. 307–366. *In* J. G. Tully and R. F. Whitcomb (ed.), *The Mycoplasmas*, vol. 2. Academic Press, Inc., New York, N.Y.
64. **Taylor-Robinson, D., and P. E. Munday.** 1988. Mycoplasmal infection of the female genital tract and its complications, p. 228–247. *In* M. J. Hare (ed.), *Genital Tract Infection in Women*. Churchill Livingstone, Ltd., Edinburgh, United Kingdom.
65. **Taylor-Robinson, D., A. D. B. Webster, P. M. Furr, and G. L. Asherson.** 1980. Prolonged persistence of *Mycoplasma pneumoniae* in a patient with hypogammaglobulinaemia. *J. Infect.* **2:**171–175.
66. **Texier-Maugein, J., M. Clerc, A. Vekris, and C. Bebear.** 1987. *Ureaplasma urealyticum*-induced bladder stones in rats and their prevention by flurofamide and doxycycline. *Isr. J. Med. Sci.* **23:**565–567.
67. **Thacker, W. L., and D. F. Talkington.** 1995. Comparison of two rapid commercial tests with complement fixation for serologic diagnosis of *Mycoplasma pneumoniae* infections. *J. Clin. Microbiol.* **33:**1212–1214.
68. **Thomsen, A. C.** 1978. Mycoplasmas in human pyelonephritis: demonstration of antibodies in serum and urine. *J. Clin. Microbiol.* **8:**197–202.
69. **Tully, J. G., D. L. Rose, R. F. Whitcomb, and R. P. Wenzel.** 1979. Enhanced isolation of *Mycoplasma pneumoniae* from throat washings with a newly modified culture medium. *J. Infect. Dis.* **139:**478–482.
70. **Waites, K. B., P. T. Rudd, D. T. Crouse. K. C. Canupp, K. G. Nelson, C. Ramsey, and G. H. Cassell.** 1988. Chronic *Ureaplasma urealyticum* and *Mycoplasma hominis* infections of central nervous system in preterm infants. *Lancet* **i:**17–21.
71. **Waites, K. B., T. A. Figarola, T. Schmid, D. M. Crabb, L. B. Duffy, and J. W. Simecka.** 1991. Comparison of agar versus broth dilution techniques for determining antibiotic susceptibilities of *Ureaplasma urealyticum*. *Diagn. Microbiol. Infect. Dis.* **14:**265–271.
72. **Waites, K. B., D. M. Crabb, L. B. Duffy, and G. H. Cassell.** 1997. Evaluation of the Etest for detection of tetracycline resistance in *Mycoplasma hominis*. *Diagn. Microbiol. Infect. Dis.* **27:**117–122.
73. **Wang, R. Y. H., J. W. K. Shih, T. Grandinetti, P. F. Pierce, M. M. Hayes, D. J. Wear, H. J. Alter, and S. C. Lo.** 1992. High frequency of antibodies to *Mycoplasma penetrans* in HIV-infected patients. *Lancet* **340:**1312–1316.
74. **Wang, R. Y. H., J. W. K. Shih, S. H. Weiss, T. Grandinetti, P. F. Pierce, M. Lange, H. J. Alter, D. J. Wear, C. L. Davies, R. K. Mayur, and S. C. Lo.** 1993. *Mycoplasma penetrans* infection in male homosexuals with AIDS: high seroprevalence and association with Kaposi's sarcoma. *Clin. Infect. Dis.* **17:**724–729.
75. **Wang, R. Y. H., W. S. Wu, M. S. Dawson, J. W. H. Shih, and S. C. Lo.** 1992. Selective detection of *Mycoplasma fermentans* by polymerase chain reaction and by using a nucleotide sequence within the insertion sequence-like element. *J. Clin. Microbiol.* **30:**245–248.
76. **Wilson, M. H., and A. M. Collier.** 1976. Ultrastructural study of *Mycoplasma pneumoniae* in organ culture. *J. Bacteriol.* **125:**332–339.
77. **Wood, J. C., R. M. Lu, E. M. Peterson, and L. M. de la Maza.** 1985. Evaluation of Mycotrim-GU for isolation of *Mycoplasma* species and *Ureaplasma urealyticum*. *J. Clin. Microbiol.* **22:**789–792.

Chlamydia

JULIUS SCHACHTER AND WALTER E. STAMM

57

The chlamydiae are among the more common pathogens throughout the animal kingdom (33). They are nonmotile, gram-negative, obligate intracellular bacteria. Their unique developmental cycle differentiates them from all other microorganisms (37). They replicate within the cytoplasm of host cells, forming characteristic intracellular inclusions that can be seen by light microscopy. They differ from the viruses by possessing both RNA and DNA and have cell walls quite similar in structure to those of gram-negative bacteria. They are susceptible to many broad-spectrum antibiotics, possess a number of enzymes, and have a restricted metabolic capacity. None of these metabolic reactions results in the production of energy. Hence, they have been considered energy parasites that use the ATP produced by the host cell for their own requirements.

TAXONOMY

Chlamydiae are presently placed in their own order, the *Chlamydiales*, family *Chlamydiaceae*, with one genus, *Chlamydia* (19, 37, 45). There are four species: *Chlamydia trachomatis*, *C. psittaci*, *C. pecorum*, and *C. pneumoniae*. *C. trachomatis* includes the organisms causing trachoma, inclusion conjunctivitis, lymphogranuloma venereum (LGV), and genital tract diseases. *C. trachomatis* also causes pneumonia in infants and occasionally in immunocompromised hosts, and it is associated with oligoarthritis (Reiter's syndrome). The three biovars within the species are trachoma, LGV, and murine. Similar organisms have been isolated from ferrets and swine, and while they appear to be *C. trachomatis*, their relationship to the well-defined biovars is not known. *C. trachomatis* strains are sensitive to the action of sulfonamides and produce a glycogen-like material within the inclusion vacuole that stains with iodine. *C. psittaci* strains infect many avian species and mammals, causing such diseases as psittacosis, ornithosis, feline pneumonitis, and bovine abortion (59). Humans are infected secondarily from animals and develop pneumonia or systemic infection, including endocarditis. *C. psittaci* is resistant to the action of sulfonamides and produces inclusions that do not stain with iodine. *C. pneumoniae* has less than 10% DNA relatedness to the other species and has pear-shaped rather than round elementary bodies (EBs) (25, 26). It appears to be exclusively a human pathogen, although similar organisms have been isolated from horses and koalas. *C. pneumoniae* has been identified as the cause of a variety of respiratory tract diseases (pharyngitis, sinusitis, bronchitis, and pneumonia) and is distributed worldwide. It may also play a role in causing atherosclerotic cardiovascular disease. A fourth species, *C. pecorum*, has also been described (20), but its role as a pathogen is not clear and specialized reagents are required for its identification.

DESCRIPTION OF THE GENUS

Growth Cycle

C. trachomatis attaches to a heparan sulfate-like molecule on the surface of susceptible host cells (68). This molecule apparently functions as a bridge between a specific receptor on the surface of the epithelial cell and a receptor on the EB. Chlamydiae are ingested by susceptible host cells by a mechanism that is not yet completely defined but is similar to receptor-mediated endocytosis. The uptake process is directly influenced by the chlamydiae, and ingestion of chlamydiae is specifically enhanced (8). After attachment, the EB enters the cell in an endosome, within which the entire growth cycle is completed. The chlamydiae prevent phagolysosomal fusion. Once the EB (diameter, 0.25 to 0.35 μm) has entered the cell, it reorganizes into a reticulate body (diameter, 0.5 to 1 μm) that is richer in RNA than the EB. After approximately 8 h, the reticulate body begins dividing by binary fission. Approximately 18 to 24 h after infection, the reticulate bodies become EBs by a poorly understood reorganization or condensation process. The EBs are then released to initiate another cycle of infection. The EBs are specifically adapted for extracellular survival and are the infectious form of chlamydiae. The metabolically active and replicating form, the reticulate body, does not survive well outside the host cell and seems adapted for an intracellular milieu.

Antigenic Relationships

The chlamydiae possess group- (or genus-specific), species-specific, and type-specific antigens. Although the organisms are antigenically complex, only a few antigens play a role in diagnosis and pathogenesis. The group complement fixation (CF) antigen, shared by all members of the genus, is the lipopolysaccharide (LPS), with a ketodeoxyoctanoic acid as the reactive moiety. It may be analogous to the LPS of certain gram-negative bacteria (40). One-way cross-reactions have been reported between chlamydiae and some other bacteria, but these do not appear to influence serodiagnosis. The major outer membrane protein (MOMP) contains both species- and subspecies-specific antigens (9). The MOMP is responsible for most of the reactivity seen in the microimmunofluorescence (micro-IF) test, which was used to identify the original 15 serovars of *C. trachomatis* (63, 64). Recent studies in which monoclonal antibodies were used for serotyping have confirmed these originally described serovars and have also identified new serovars (32, 60). Studies involving DNA sequencing of the MOMP gene have localized the serotyping epitopes to the variable portions of the MOMP gene (58). A 60-kDa cysteine-rich structural protein has a highly immunogenic species-specific epitope (39). A 60-kDa heat shock protein that has sequence homology to analogous human genes may play an important role in inducing immunopathology (36). Multiple serovars of *C. psittaci* can be demonstrated by neutralization tests and by micro-IF (1, 18). Only one serovar of *C. pneumoniae* has been demonstrated.

CLINICAL SIGNIFICANCE

C. trachomatis is almost exclusively a human pathogen (49) and is the most common sexually transmitted bacterial agent. Within this species, serovars A, B, Ba, and C are associated with endemic trachoma, the most common preventable form of blindness, while serovars L1, L2, and L3 are associated with LGV. When sexual transmission of *C. trachomatis* biovars other than LGV is studied, serovars D through K are the major identifiable causes of nongonococcal urethritis in men and also cause epididymitis and may induce Reiter's syndrome (55). Proctitis and conjunctivitis occur in both men and women. In women, cervicitis, urethritis, endometritis, salpingitis, and perihepatitis result from chlamydial infection with these serovars. Salpingitis may produce tubal scarring, infertility, and ectopic pregnancy. The agent in the cervix may be transmitted to the neonate passing through the infected birth canal, and an eye disease (inclusion conjunctivitis of the newborn) and characteristic chlamydial pneumonia of infants may develop (4). Vaginal, pharyngeal, and enteric infections in neonates are also recognized.

Chlamydial genital tract infections have been associated with increased rates of transmission of human immunodeficiency virus (HIV) (65). This may occur either because chlamydia-induced inflammation results in the recruitment of CD4 lymphocytes into the genital tract (enhancing the number of HIV targets) or because chlamydia-induced inflammation stimulates HIV replication (enhancing transmission). Most chlamydial infections in women are clinically inapparent, and yet such infections are often associated with tubal damage. Thus, without empirical reasons for treatment, it is imperative that accurate laboratory diagnostic tests be used in screening programs aimed at controlling chlamydial infections and preventing their consequences in high-risk women.

Human psittacosis is a zoonosis usually contracted from exposure to an infected avian species. *C. psittaci* is ubiquitous among avian species, and infection in birds usually involves the intestinal tract. The organism is shed in the feces, contaminates the environment, and is readily spread by aerosols. *C. psittaci* is also common in domestic mammals. In some parts of the world, these infections have important economic consequences because *C. psittaci* causes a number of systemic and debilitating diseases in domestic mammals and, most importantly, can cause abortions (59). Human chlamydial infections resulting from exposure to infected domestic mammals do occur but seem to be relatively uncommon. There appears to be a greater risk to pregnant women who are exposed to infected farm animals.

C. pneumoniae, like *C. trachomatis*, appears to be a human infection without an animal reservoir (24). Seroepidemiological studies indicate that infections are very common worldwide. Age-specific prevalence and incidence rates suggest that infections are commonly acquired in later childhood, adolescence, and early adulthood, resulting in seroprevalences of 40 to 50% in the 30- to 40-year-old age group. Manifestations of infection include pharyngitis, bronchitis, and mild pneumonia (28). Within households, schools, and workplace environments and among military personnel in close living quarters, transmission occurs via respiratory secretions. In seroepidemiological studies, these infections have been linked with coronary artery disease as well as vascular disease at other sites. Following a demonstration of *C. pneumoniae*-like particles in atheromatous tissue by electron microscopy, *C. pneumoniae* genes and antigens have now been detected in atheromas. Rarely, the organism has been recovered in cultures of atheromatous tissue (47), and its possible etiologic role in atherosclerosis is currently under intense scrutiny.

COLLECTION, TRANSPORT, AND STORAGE

C. trachomatis is not a particularly labile organism. Maximal infectivity is achieved by keeping specimens cold and minimizing the time between specimen collection and processing in the laboratory. Swabs, scrapings, and small tissue samples should be forwarded to the laboratory in a special transport medium such as sucrose phosphate (2SP) or sucrose phosphate glutamate (SPG) supplemented with bovine serum, streptomycin, vancomycin, and nystatin. Because *Chlamydia* spp. are bacteria, the selection of antibiotics that can be used to prevent exogenous bacterial contamination is restricted. Broad-spectrum antibiotics such as tetracyclines, macrolides, or penicillin cannot be used. Aminoglycosides and fungicides are the mainstays and can be safely used. Chlamydial specimens should be refrigerated if they can be processed within 24 h after collection; otherwise, they should be frozen at −60°C.

C. psittaci strains are generally more stable. Some may persist in a contaminated environment for months without losing viability. The stability of *C. pneumoniae* has not been well studied, but 70% of the organisms remain viable after 24 h at 4°C (31).

When specimens are collected for enzyme immunoassay (EIA) or direct fluorescent-antibody (DFA) procedures, the descriptions and procedural instructions given in the product's package insert should be followed. When manufacturers supply swabs or specific transport media, they should be used, since the use of other materials may impair the sensitivity and/or specificity of the test.

For cytological studies, impression smears of tissues or scrapings of involved epithelial cell sites should be air dried and fixed appropriately (cold acetone or methanol for immunofluorescence, methanol for Giemsa stain, and heat for Macchiavello or Gimenez stain).

For diagnosis of most *C. trachomatis* infections in humans by cytology, culture, or antigen detection methods, samples should be collected by vigorous swabbing or scraping of the involved epithelial cell sites. Purulent discharges are inadequate and should be cleaned from the site before sampling is done. Appropriate sites include the conjunctiva for trachoma-inclusion conjunctivitis and the male anterior urethra (several centimeters into the urethra) or the cervix (within the endocervical canal) for genital infection. Because the trachoma biovar appears to infect only columnar or squamocolumnar cells, cervical specimens must be collected at the transitional zone or within the opening of the cervix. The organism can also infect the urethra of the female; organism recovery rates may be improved if a second sample is collected from the urethra and sent to the laboratory for testing in the same tube with the cervical sample.

Many different swab types can be used, but toxicity related to materials in swabs is not uncommon. It is useful to test swab types for toxicity in cell cultures or interference in nonculture assays when proprietary swabs are not provided by the manufacturer. As a general rule, swabs with wooden sticks should be avoided. Cotton, Dacron, and calcium alginate swabs may all be used successfully, although toxicity has been noted with specific lots of each. The cytobrush has also been used to collect endocervical specimens. It appears to collect more cells than swabs and has been associated in some investigators' experience with higher recovery rates of chlamydiae or higher rates of antigen detection by DFA (35). In other laboratories, there has been no advantage. If clinicians are well trained to collect adequate specimens with other swabs, the cytobrush will probably confer no particular advantage. However, for less well-trained personnel, the cytobrush may result in improved specimen quality.

For women with salpingitis, the samples may be collected by needle aspiration of the involved fallopian tube. Endometrial specimens may also yield the agent. In other clinical situations, the rectal mucosa, nasopharynx, and throat may be sampled. For infants with pneumonia, swabs may be collected from the posterior nasopharynx or the throat, although nasopharyngeal or tracheobronchial aspirates collected by intubation appear to be a superior source of the agent. For LGV, the likely specimens will be bubo pus, rectal or urethral swabbings, or biopsy samples.

For some nonculture tests, urine specimens are appropriate for diagnostic evaluation. For men, an effort should be made to obtain first-catch urine (the first 10 to 30 ml of urine). Specimens should be obtained at least 2 h after the last micturition, but it is not necessary to obtain the first urine specimen passed in the morning. Subsequent processing of the specimen will depend on the manufacturer's instructions. For some tests, 1 to 4 ml of urine is taken from the whole sample and processed further. With other tests, the entire urine specimen is processed. In either instance, it is typical to centrifuge the specimen, resuspend the sediment into the proprietary diluent, and follow the manufacturer's testing procedures for detection of chlamydial antigens or nucleotide sequences. First-catch urine specimens from men and women and vaginal swab specimens from women have been found to be the appropriate specimens for diagnosis of chlamydial infection by amplified nucleic acid tests (2, 12, 29, 52, 57).

Throat swabs are collected for *C. pneumoniae* detection. For detection of *C. psittaci* infections in humans (classic psittacosis), appropriate specimens include sputum and blood specimens. *C. psittaci* has been recovered from a variety of involved anatomic sites sampled by biopsy or at necropsy. For all culture methods, the sites sampled are likely to be contaminated and so the specimen should be collected into a medium that contains appropriate antibiotics to inhibit the growth of unwanted bacteria or fungi.

ISOLATION PROCEDURES

Biosafety Considerations

C. trachomatis is not considered a particularly dangerous pathogen to handle in the laboratory, but a number of laboratory-acquired infections, usually manifested as follicular conjunctivitis, have occurred. However, the LGV biovar is a more invasive organism, and severe cases of pneumonia have occurred when research workers were exposed to aerosols created by laboratory procedures such as sonication (6). *C. psittaci* must be considered a potentially dangerous organism to handle in the laboratory. For many years, it was a major cause of laboratory-acquired infections. These infections usually resulted from exposure to aerosols, but the stability of the organism in the environment is also a potential problem. This organism should not be handled in laboratories without appropriate containment facilities. Laboratory infections with *C. pneumoniae* have also occurred.

Specimen Processing

General guidelines for processing specimens are listed below. Fresh samples are preferred, but frozen material (−60°C) is acceptable.

Ocular and Genital Tract Specimens

For ocular and genital tract sites, the laboratory usually receives swabs in antibiotic-containing transport medium. The material should be refrigerated until it is inoculated into cell culture if inoculation can be accomplished in less than 24 h. Otherwise, it must be frozen at −60°C.

Bubo Pus

To prepare bubo pus, the viscous material is ground and then suspended in nutrient broth or cell culture medium to at least 20% by weight. Even when the pus is not viscous, dilution is advisable. If the bubo is not fluctuant, sterile saline may be injected and then aspirated for isolation attempts. The material should be tested for bacterial contaminants and inoculated into cell cultures.

Blood

The clot should be ground and beef heart broth or cell culture medium added to make a 10% suspension. The suspension is inoculated directly into cell culture. It is usually advisable to use several further dilutions as well, because the concentrated material may be toxic to the cells.

Sputum or Throat Washings

To prepare an emulsion of sputum or throat washings, sputum is suspended in 2 to 10 times (depending on its consistency) its volume of sterile antibiotic-containing broth (pH 7.2 to 7.4) or cell culture medium; it is emulsified thoroughly by shaking with glass beads in a sterile, tightly stoppered container. The emulsion is inoculated into the cell culture system after 1 to 2 h of treatment with antibiotics at room temperature. It may be advisable to centrifuge extracts for 20 to 30 min at 100 × *g* to remove coarse material.

Fecal Samples

Cloacal or rectal swabs, the droppings from caged birds, or fecal pellets are suspended in antibiotic broth or cell culture medium. The suspension is shaken thoroughly. After centrifugation at 300 × *g* for 10 min, the supernatant fluid is removed. It may be further diluted (1:2 and 1:20) with antibiotic solution and held for 1 h at room temperature before being inoculated into cell culture.

Tissue Samples

Frozen tissue is thawed in a refrigerator at about 4°C for 18 to 24 h. The specimen is weighed, minced with sterile scissors, and ground to a paste with a mortar and pestle or homogenizer. After the tissue has been ground thoroughly, the volume of antibiotic-containing diluent required to make a 10 to 20% emulsion is added and the suspension is thoroughly mixed. For cell culture, antibiotic-containing collection medium is used and 10^{-1} and 10^{-2} dilutions are inoculated.

Isolation in Cell Culture

All known chlamydiae grow in the yolk sac of the embryonated hen egg. However, if the inoculum is centrifuged, all chlamydiae (with some variability) appear to be able to grow in cell culture; psittacosis and LGV agents are capable of serial growth in cell culture without centrifugation. A number of direct cell lines have been used to support the growth of chlamydiae. It does not appear that any single cell line is markedly superior to others, since successful isolation has been performed with monkey kidney, HeLa, L, and McCoy cells, among others. McCoy and HeLa cells are most commonly used. There is less experience with *C. pneumoniae*. This organism grows poorly in McCoy and HeLa cells, especially in primary isolation from clinical specimens. HL cells and HEp-2 cells are more sensitive for the recovery of *C. pneumoniae* (16).

The recommended procedure for primary isolation of chlamydiae is cell culture. The most common technique involves inoculation of clinical specimens into cycloheximide-treated McCoy or other appropriate cells (48). The basic principle involves centrifugation of the inoculum onto the cell monolayer, incubation of the monolayer for 48 to 72 h, and staining. Use of fluorescein-conjugated monoclonal antibodies represents the most sensitive method for detecting *C. trachomatis* inclusions in cell culture (56) and also allows earlier detection of inclusions. Alternatively, iodine staining can be used. It is less expensive but also less sensitive. For *C. psittaci* and *C. pneumoniae*, the inclusions can be demonstrated with genus-specific monoclonal antibodies or by the Giemsa stain.

For the shell vial method, McCoy cells are plated onto 13-mm coverslips contained in 15-mm-diameter (1-dram [1 fluidram = 3.697 ml]) disposable glass vials. The cell concentration (approximately 1×10^5 to 2×10^5) is selected to give a light, confluent monolayer after 24 to 48 h of incubation at 37°C. For optimal results, the cells should be used within 24 to 72 h after they reach confluency.

The clinical specimens are shaken with glass beads before being used for inoculation. This procedure is safer and more convenient than sonication. The standard inoculation procedure involves removing medium from the cell monolayer and replacing it with the inoculum in a volume of 0.1 to 1 ml. The specimen is then centrifuged onto the cell monolayer at approximately 3,000 × *g* at room temperature for 1 h. The vials are held at 35°C for 2 h before the cells are washed or the medium is changed to medium containing 1 to 2 μg of cycloheximide per ml (this must be titrated for each batch used). The cells are incubated at 35°C for 48 to 72 h, and one coverslip is examined for inclusions by immunofluorescence, iodine staining, or Giemsa staining. The use of immunofluorescence can speed the process, since inclusions can clearly be seen (although they are smaller) at 24 h postinfection. Giemsa stain is more sensitive than iodine stain, but the microscopic evaluation is more difficult. Slide reading can be facilitated by examining the Giemsa-stained coverslip by dark-field microscopy.

If passage of positive material or blind passage of negative material is desired, the material should be passaged at 72 to 96 h postinoculation. The cell monolayer is disrupted by being shaken with glass beads on a Vortex mixer; the material is subjected to low-speed centrifugation to remove cell debris, and the supernatant is inoculated as described above. For symptomatic patients, at least 90% of specimens positive for *C. trachomatis* are identified in the first passage. In screening tests of asymptomatic patients, who often have a smaller amount of agent at the infected site, more of the positive specimens require passage for detection.

With trachoma, inclusion conjunctivitis, and the genital tract infections, the technique is as described above. For LGV, the aspirated bubo pus is diluted (10^{-1} and 10^{-2}) before inoculation. Second passages should always be made, because detritus from the inoculum may make it difficult to read the slides. For many *C. psittaci* isolation attempts, it may be convenient to lengthen the incubation period to 5 to 10 days before examining the coverslips for inclusions. These organisms do not require mechanical assistance for cell-to-cell infection (53). It has been suggested that repeating centrifugation at intervals during incubation may improve the recovery rates of *C. pneumoniae* (62).

Many laboratories processing large numbers of specimens use flat-bottom 48- or 96-well microtiter plates rather than vials (67). In this method, cells are plated onto coverslips or, more commonly, directly onto the plates. Processing and incubation are as described above, but microscopy is modified to use either long working objectives or inverted microscopes. This procedure offers considerable savings of reagents and time and is particularly useful when groups of mostly symptomatic patients are being screened. The microtiter technique may be less sensitive than the vial technique for screening largely asymptomatic groups of patients, who have less organism present.

Ongoing quality control is important in maintaining a sensitive and specific culture system. To test the validity of specimen collection, periodic evaluation of slides by DFA permits evaluation of the cellularity of specimens being obtained. To test the adequacy of specimen transport, periodic transport of specimens with known dilutions of chlamydia can be used to assess loss of viability or inclusion-forming units during transport. Daily inoculation of positive controls (known dilutions of chlamydia) is useful to determine the overall sensitivity of the cell culture system. Laboratories using the microtiter method should evaluate possible episodes of cross-contamination by reinoculation of any positive specimen occurring in wells adjacent to a high-titer positive specimen.

Yolk Sac Isolation

Although it is no longer generally used for evaluation of clinical specimens, the yolk sac is still used for preparing antigens for the micro-IF test. The specimen is held for 1 h at room temperature, and a 3.2-cm 22-gauge needle is used to inoculate 0.25 ml into the yolk sac. Before inoculation, the fertile eggs are incubated at 38.5 to 39°C in a moist atmosphere. The eggs to be used must be obtained from a flock fed an antibiotic-free diet. The eggs should be free from mycoplasmas. When they are 7 days old, the embryonated hen eggs are candled for viability, the locations of air sacs are marked, the shell is painted with tincture of iodine, and a hole is gently punched in the shell. The specimen is inoculated at a slight angle away from the embryo. After inoculation, the shell is again swabbed with iodine, and the hole is sealed (with glue or tape). The eggs are then incubated in a moist environment at 35°C and candled daily for 13 days. Eggs that die in the first 3 days after inoculation must be discarded. The yolk sacs of eggs that die thereafter are harvested. Harvesting entails painting the shell with iodine, cracking and removing the shell over the air sac, teasing away the shell and chorioallantoic membranes, and removing the yolk sac with forceps. Excess yolk material is stripped away. It is important that all instruments be sterile and that fresh instruments be used for each specimen. Impression smears are made and stained (Gimenez or the modified Macchiavello method). Tests to detect the growth of contaminating bacteria should be performed in thioglycolate broth. If the embryos are still viable at 13 days postinoculation, the eggs are chilled for several hours and the yolk sacs are harvested, ground in nutrient broth, and centrifuged lightly. The supernatant is passaged in another group of four 7-day-old embryonated hen eggs (1 ml of 50% yolk sac per egg). After two blind passages, attempts are terminated and the outcome is considered negative.

The generally acceptable criteria for positive isolation are the presence of EBs in the impression smears, serially transmissible egg death, the presence of group antigen in the yolk sac, and the absence of contaminating bacteria.

IDENTIFICATION

Since most laboratories now use cell culture isolation systems, the basic procedure for identification of chlamydiae involves demonstration of typical intracytoplasmic inclusions by appropriate immunofluoresence, iodine, or Giemsa staining procedures. Fluorescent-antibody staining provides both a morphological and an immunological means of identification and thus may be preferable for less experienced laboratories.

C. trachomatis strains can be serotyped by using type-specific and subspecies-specific batteries of monoclonal antibodies. These antibodies have been used in several assay formats, but the most readily adaptable, sensitive, and specific method appears to be the microwell typing system, in which inclusions in microtiter wells are stained with pools of type-specific and subspecies-specific monoclonal antibodies (60). Although serotyping of chlamydial strains may be of use in epidemiological studies, it is of little clinical use unless medicolegal issues are involved.

In addition to typing of *C. trachomatis* with commercially available monoclonal antibodies, other methods of typing have been developed. These include the use of restriction endonuclease patterns of PCR-amplified DNA and direct sequencing of the variable domains in the chlamydial MOMP. These variable regions include the peptides responsible for species, serovar, and serogroup specificities. Variability in the amino acid sequence of the variable-region peptides may predict antigenic variants (58). Since these tests were first applied, more subtypes have been identified, and it is likely that this process will continue, particularly if, as expected, these variants originate from immune selection. *C. pneumoniae* may be identified by use of commercially available species-specific monoclonal antibodies. Differentiation of *C. psittaci* and *C. pecorum* is a research procedure, since there are no commercially available reagents for this purpose.

DIRECT CYTOLOGICAL EXAMINATION

C. trachomatis infections of the conjunctiva, urethra, or cervix can be diagnosed by demonstrating typical intracytoplasmic inclusions on cytological examinations. The Giemsa stain was most often used in the past, but the more sensitive immunofluorescence procedures have now largely replaced it. Cytological testing to detect inclusions is particularly useful in diagnosing acute inclusion conjunctivitis of the newborn, in whom the sensitivity of this method exceeds 90%. The ability to detect intracellular diplococci in infants with gonococcal ophthalmia neonatorum is another benefit of this approach, and direct microscopy is obviously much faster than isolation procedures. Cytological testing is relatively insensitive (20 to 60% sensitivity) in diagnosing adult conjunctival and genital tract infections; therefore, other tests should be used in these situations.

Fluorescent-Antibody Technique

In the 1980s, fluorescein-conjugated monoclonal antibodies became available for cytological staining. Diagnostic tests involving these antibodies are based on detecting EBs in smears (Fig. 1), in contrast to previous cytological techniques, which detected inclusions (61). The early commercial DFA reagents were plagued with problems of cross-reactions with *Staphylococcus aureus* and other bacteria. These reagents have now been dramatically improved, however, and current experience indicates that the DFA test has approximately 75 to 85% sensitivity and 98 to 99% specificity compared with culture under conditions when both tests are performed under ideal circumstances (13).

The test requires a trained microscopist who can distinguish between fluorescing chlamydial particles and nonspecific fluorescence. Several DFA configurations are commercially available, as are a variety of monoclonal antibodies directed against MOMP or against LPS. Monoclonal antibodies to the LPS will stain all *Chlamydia* spp., but the quality of the fluorescence is somewhat mitigated by uneven distribution of LPS on the chlamydial particle (15). The anti-MOMP monoclonal antibodies are prepared against *C. trachomatis*; therefore, they are species specific and will not stain *C. psittaci* or *C. pneumoniae*. Further, the quality of fluorescence is better, because MOMP is evenly distributed on the chlamydial particle. Thus, if *C. trachomatis* is being

FIGURE 1 DFA test for *C. trachomatis* EBs.

sought, the anti-MOMP monoclonal antibodies are preferred. This procedure offers the possibility of rapid diagnosis, since the technique takes only 30 min to perform. A variation on this procedure involves centrifugation of the transport medium being used for other tests (cell culture or EIA) and preparation of a slide from the sediment. This is then stained with the fluorescent-antibody reagents. This is commonly used as a confirmatory test for a positive EIA result.

Giemsa Staining Technique

For Giemsa staining, the smear is air dried, fixed with absolute methanol for at least 5 min, and dried again. It is then covered with the diluted Giemsa stain (freshly prepared the same day) for 1 h. The slide is rapidly rinsed in 95% ethanol to remove excess dye and to enhance differentiation and then dried and examined microscopically. Longer staining periods (1 to 5 h) may be preferable with heavy tissue culture monolayers. EBs stain reddish purple. The initial bodies are more basophilic, staining bluish, as do most bacteria.

OTHER NONCULTURE DIAGNOSTIC TESTS

Enzyme Immunoassay

A number of commercially available products can detect chlamydial antigens in clinical specimens by EIA procedures (7, 11, 13, 14, 22, 34, 35, 51). These products use either monoclonal or polyclonal antibodies to detect chlamydial LPS, which is more soluble than the MOMP. Thus, these tests can theoretically detect all chlamydiae. However, they have not been extensively evaluated in the diagnosis of infections with *C. psittaci* or *C. pneumoniae* and are not approved for this purpose. Most EIAs take several hours to perform and are suitable for batch processing, thus allowing a laboratory to test many specimens.

The performance profiles of the commercially available EIAs vary considerably. Most EIAs are less sensitive than optimal culture systems in laboratories with expert technicians, although a few EIAs are about as sensitive as culture (13, 35, 51). Without confirmation, the tests have a specificity on the order of 97%. Therefore, they are not amenable to screening low-prevalence populations because of the low predictive value of a positive result in such groups. To address this problem, confirmatory tests have been developed by many manufacturers. In one of these assays, all positive results are repeated in the presence of a monoclonal antibody directed against the *Chlamydia*-specific epitope on the LPS. This results in blocking of the specific reactions but not of the false-positive results. The appropriate application of confirmatory tests increases the specificity to about 99.5% (34), reducing the number of false-positive tests in low-prevalence populations. However, the blocking confirmatory tests have been validated for cervical and urethral infections but have not been validated for use with specimens from many of the other anatomic sites that are commonly tested for presence of chlamydial antigen. Another approach to confirmation is to test a specimen by a second test based on a different principle, for example, a DFA based on MOMP detection to confirm an LPS-based EIA.

Nucleic Acid Probes

Many nucleic acid probes have been developed and evaluated by research laboratories. One commercially available probe test (PACE 2; Gen-Probe, Inc., San Diego, Calif.) utilizes DNA-RNA hybridization in an effort to increase sensitivity by detecting chlamydial RNA. Available data suggest that it is about as sensitive as the better antigen detection and cell culture methods and is relatively specific (14, 30).

TABLE 1 Relative sensitivities of culture and nucleic acid amplification assays

Test method	Sensitivity (%) of test in:			
	Males		Females	
	Urethral swab	Urine	Endocervical swab	Urine
Cell culture	51–86		52–88	
PCR (Amplicor-CT)		96–97	79–82	82–100
LCR (LCx-CT)	96–100	92–94	82–97	77–94
TMA (AMP-CT)		88–100	100	79–94

Amplified Nucleic Acid Tests

Three nucleic acid amplification methods are currently licensed for detection of *C. trachomatis* in clinical specimens: PCR (Amplicor *C. trachomatis* assay; Roche Molecular Systems, Branchburg, N.J.), the ligase chain reaction (LCR) (LCx *C. trachomatis* assay; Abbott Laboratories, Abbott Park, Ill.), and transcription-mediated amplification (TMA) (Gen-Probe Amplified *C. trachomatis* [AMP-CT] assay; Gen-Probe, Inc.). The principles for these assays are described in chapter 13. The PCR and LCR assays amplify nucleotide sequences on the cryptic plasmid, which is present in multiple copies in each *C. trachomatis* EB. The TMA reaction is directed against rRNA, which is also present in multiple copies. Theoretically, given the multiplicity of target sites for the amplification procedures being used, these techniques should be able to detect less than one EB. They can do so in purified suspensions of chlamydial particles; however, the actual sensitivity with clinical specimens is lower because of sampling problems and inhibition of the amplification reactions by factors in the clinical specimens (3, 5, 21, 38, 41, 42). Current data suggest that the PCR assay is more sensitive to inhibition than is either LCR or TMA. All assays appear to be highly specific if problems with cross-contamination of reactions are controlled carefully (44).

Clinical evaluations of the amplification methods (2, 3, 10, 12, 17, 21, 23, 27, 29, 38, 41–43, 46, 52, 54) have demonstrated that they are more sensitive than culture and the other nonculture methods (i.e., microscopy, immunoassays, probe assays [Table 1]). The assays can be used with first-voided urine samples as well as urethral and endocervical swab specimens. The ability to use urine specimens appears to be a major advantage for the amplification tests, because invasive collection methods are not required and specimens can be collected in settings other than traditional clinical or physician office settings. Vaginal swabs, collected by either the provider or the patient, can also be used, although there is less experience with these specimens (27, 57, 66). The amplification assays are rapidly becoming the tests of choice for diagnosis of chlamydial infection in routine clinical laboratories. However, when organisms are needed for further study, isolation in cell culture will continue to be used.

RAPID TESTS

It is clear that there is a strong need for a rapid diagnostic test for chlamydial infection. Many infections are asymptomatic or nonspecific in terms of symptoms and signs and thus are not empirically treated. Because effective single-dose therapy is now available for chlamydial infection, a point-of-care test would reduce the need for return visits and greatly improve efforts to control chlamydial infection. Unfortunately, the rapid tests that are currently available appear to be less sensitive than culture, and many of these assays have specificity problems as well. There are no independent evaluations which provide a basis to recommend any such test for routine use. Also of particular concern, point-of-care tests should not be used in a laboratory setting. Their ease of use does not justify accepting their poor performance profile. Suffice it to say that none of these procedures is as sensitive as chlamydial culture in expert hands. When culture is used as the gold standard, the sensitivity of the best rapid detection methods will be 75 to 85% (7). The sensitivities described in the package inserts provided by the manufacturers are often higher than these figures and represent favorable evaluations, often in comparison with an insensitive culture system. Even if the numbers in the package inserts were accurate, at this writing they would be outdated because of changes in the gold standard as noted below.

GOLD STANDARD

Initially, cell culture was considered to be a highly sensitive and specific assay for *C. trachomatis*. As further experience with cell culture was gained, some laboratorians estimated that the true sensitivity of culture was in the 75 to 85% range. This estimate was supported when antigen detection methods were developed, since there were a substantial number of antigen-positive and culture-negative specimens that could be confirmed as actually containing chlamydiae EB by DFA or by concurrence of multiple EIA results. Occasionally, repeat culture was positive, but more often alternative antigen detection methods yielded confirmatory results. These tests probably reflected nonviable chlamydiae in the specimens that died during transport and processing. Overall, however, the antigen detection methods were still less sensitive than culture. Thus, some package inserts that claimed 90% sensitivity were actually reflecting 90% compared to culture, which was only about 80%. The expansion of the gold standard to include multiple nonculture tests to differentiate true-positive results from culture-negative results was helpful in evaluating the antigen detection methods. However, when nucleic acid amplification tests were introduced, the use of antigen detection methods proved inadequate for this purpose because the nucleic acid amplification tests were actually far more sensitive than culture. Therefore, it became necessary to use alternate nucleic acid targets to confirm some of the culture-negative, nucleic acid-positive specimens. In many evaluations, the nucleic acid amplification tests detect 20 to 30% more positive specimens than could be detected by the earlier technology. The introduction of these tests also showed that there was considerably more variability in the sensitivity of culture from laboratory to laboratory than was true for the nucleic acid amplification tests.

However, it cannot be said that the nucleic acid amplification tests are a perfect gold standard, because none are 100% sensitive. This is probably due to the presence of inhibitors. Thus, at this writing, the gold standard for chlamydia diagnostics includes the most sensitive available nucleic acid amplification test (probably PCR [23, 42, 43, 46]) together with a sensitive culture to detect specimens (5 to 10% of all positive specimens) that are negative due to the presence of inhibitors. It is clear that in virtually all settings the nucleic acid amplification tests are the diagnostic tests of choice for urethral and cervical infections. They are far more sensitive than culture or the other nonculture diagnostic tests, and they are highly specific (>99.7%) and thus do not require confirmatory tests. The major disadvantages of these tests are that they are expensive compared with antigen detection methods and direct probes and experience with their use in eye or rectal specimens is limited. Since the treatment of diagnosed chlamydial infections prevents costly complications, it is likely that these more sensitive tests can still be justified as being cost-effective due to the increased number of cases being identified and treated. On the basis of performance, it is difficult to choose among the three amplification tests that are currently available. The PCR test is more likely to have its sensitivity reduced by inhibitors, but it is more suitable for batch processing and automation and thus will allow the laboratory to process more specimens. The TMA assay appears to be the most labor-intensive, and the LCR test has limited throughput. The following comments concerning antigen detection methods are intended as a guide for those who are doing chlamydia testing but cannot afford or do not have access to the nucleic acid amplification tests.

Advice on Use of Nonculture Tests

Of the many EIA and DFA procedures available for chlamydia diagnosis, relatively few have been adequately compared in large studies with direct head-to-head evaluation of performance. Therefore, it is difficult to confidently differentiate the performance of individual tests. In general, however, EIA has some false-positive reactions and usually requires expensive equipment, but it has the advantage of allowing bulk processing of specimens, which facilitates the screening of large numbers of patients. The introduction of blocking assays to confirm positive results has dramatically improved the specificity of the EIAs. Before that, both DFA and EIA procedures in expert hands typically resulted in 2 to 3% false-positive results, which meant that the predictive value of a positive test would be on the order of 50% in populations with a 2 to 3% prevalence and would be only about 60 to 70% in populations where infection rates were at the 5 to 6% level (as expected in many family-planning clinics nationwide). This low positive predictive value was bothersome to many clinicians and public health officials. It was also recognized that these procedures were less sensitive than culture (perhaps with a sensitivity of around 75 to 85% compared with culture).

What is very important here is that laboratorians choosing laboratory tests based on package inserts recognize that the quoted sensitivity figures for the antigen detection and the nucleic acid hybridization tests are overstated compared with the nucleic acid amplification tests. This simply reflects the evolution of this field, since the latter tests actually will detect 20 to 30% more positive specimens than can be detected by either culture or antigen detection methods. In reality, the older antigen detection tests thus could easily have sensitivities of less than 60% compared with nucleic acid amplification tests.

The DFA test has the advantage of allowing the microscopist to confirm the adequacy of the specimen. Since DFA is more labor-intensive than EIA, it is less well suited to processing large numbers of specimens. Anti-MOMP monoclonal antibodies provide superior staining of *C. trachomatis* EBs but will not detect the EBs of other species. Anti-LPS monoclonal antibodies will stain all chlamydiae but tend to be less bright and also to stain the particles unevenly (15). Most EIAs detect the LPS and thus should react with all chlamydial species. They have been widely studied only for *C. trachomatis* and therefore cannot be recommended for use in tests for *C. psittaci* or *C. pneumoniae* infections.

All nonculture tests have some advantages over culture. They are more rapid, and thus the results can be available in 30 min to 24 h. Because viability is not an issue, it is not necessary to maintain a cold chain. Specimens can be processed when cell culture is not available or when there are problems in transporting specimens to a laboratory. The one situation in which nonculture tests should not be used is when evidence of sexual abuse is being sought. False-positive results do occur with these tests if specimens are mishandled, and the tests have not been extensively evaluated on some of the specimens that are tested in cases of child abuse. Currently, it is imperative that culture be used to prove the existence of chlamydial infection for legal purposes. In most circumstances, nonculture method results are not admissible as evidence.

The diagnosis of *C. pneumoniae* infection represents a major challenge to clinical laboratories. There are no commercially available kits. Antigens for micro-IF tests and antibody for DFA tests can be purchased. The organism can be isolated in cell culture, but only with difficulty, since successful culture of this organism is poor in the most expert hands. A variety of procedures such as DNA hybridization, PCR, immunocytochemistry, and detection of circulating immune complexes of this organism have all been used in efforts to diagnose the infection. The sensitivity and specificity of these assays are unknown, and for all practical purposes they must be considered research procedures. For routine purposes, the best that can be recommended is to attempt to culture the organism with appropriate cells (HL or HEp-2 cells), recognizing that failure in cell culture certainly does not rule out infection, and to perform serological testing by micro-IF. Unfortunately, it appears that the laboratory diagnosis of *C. pneumoniae* infection will be limited to selected research laboratories or centers until some technological breakthrough is achieved.

The currently available nucleic acid amplification tests target nucleotide sequences specific to *C. trachomatis*. EIAs, which target chlamydial LPS, could be used to diagnose *C. pneumoniae* infection, but unfortunately, many false-positive results occur with the respiratory tract specimens that are likely to be tested for *C. pneumoniae*. DFA reagents are available, but their performance profiles have not been determined. PCR tests have been described for *C. pneumoniae*, but they are research procedures and are not commercially available.

SEROLOGICAL TESTS

The most widely used serological test for diagnosing chlamydial infections is the CF test. This test is useful in diagnosing psittacosis, in which paired sera often show fourfold or greater increases in titer. The same seems to be true for many *C. pneumoniae* infections. Approximately 50% of these infections are CF positive, although it may take 24 weeks to detect seroconversion (25). CF may also be useful in diagnosing LGV, since single titers greater than 1:64 are highly supportive of this clinical diagnosis in patients with a compatible clinical syndrome. With LGV, it is difficult to demonstrate rising titers since the nature of the disease is such that the patient is seen by the physician after the acute stage. Any titer above 1:16 is considered significant evidence of exposure to chlamydiae. The genus-specific and relatively insensitive CF test is not particularly useful in diagnosing trachoma, inclusion conjunctivitis, or the related genital tract infections, and it plays no role in diagnosing neonatal chlamydial infections.

The micro-IF method is a much more sensitive procedure for measuring antichlamydial antibodies. It may be used in diagnosing psittacosis, for which paired sera will show rising immunoglobulin G (IgG) titers. With LGV, it is again difficult to demonstrate rising titers, but single-point titers in patients with active cases usually show relatively high levels of IgM (>1:32) and IgG (≥1:2,000) antibody. Trachoma, inclusion conjunctivitis, and the genital tract infections may be diagnosed by the micro-IF technique if appropriately timed paired acute- and convalescent-phase sera can be obtained. However, it is often difficult to demonstrate rising antibody titers, particularly in sexually active people, because many of these individuals have chronic or repeat infections. Thus, the background rate of seroreactors in sexually transmitted disease clinics is >60%, making it particularly difficult to demonstrate seroconversion. In general, first attacks of chlamydial urethritis have been regularly associated with seroconversion. Individuals with systemic infection (epididymitis or salpingitis) usually have much higher antibody levels than do those with superficial infections, and women tend to have higher antibody levels than men.

Serological testing is particularly useful in diagnosing chlamydial pneumonia in neonates. In this case, high levels of IgM antibody are regularly found in association with disease (50). IgG antibodies are less useful, because the infants are being seen at a time when they have considerable levels of maternal IgG (all of these infections are acquired from the infected mother, who is almost always seropositive). It takes between 6 and 9 months for maternal antichlamydial antibodies to disappear. Infants older than 9 months may be tested for determination of the prevalence of chlamydial infection without the confounding effects of maternal antibody. Infants with inclusion conjunctivitis or respiratory tract carriage of chlamydiae without pneumonia usually have very low levels of IgM antibodies. Thus, a single IgM titer of >1:32 may support the diagnosis of chlamydial pneumonia.

C. pneumoniae TWAR infections are usually diagnosed by micro-IF. The diagnostic criterion has been (i) a fourfold rise in titer, (ii) an IgM titer of ≥1:16, or (iii) an IgG titer of ≥1:512 (24). IgG titers of >1:16 and <1:512 are considered evidence of prior infection but not necessarily recent infection.

The micro-IF technique uses many serovars of chlamydiae, and the procedure as simplified by Wang et al. (64) is recommended. Since serological testing is particularly useful in diagnosing neonatal infection and since the IgM antibody responses tend to be very serovar specific, the use of a single broadly reacting antigen will cause the test to miss at least 15 to 25% of the infections that other procedures can prove to be caused by chlamydiae or that would be positive by a multiple-antigen micro-IF. The single-antigen tests may involve either yolk sac suspensions of agent or identification of fluorescent inclusions in tissue monolayers. Serovars of the DEL serogroup are commonly chosen for this purpose.

Research workers should be warned that seroreactions specific for type A are, at least in the United States, liable to be spurious. These antibodies are usually transient and do not result in the persistent high levels of IgG antibodies that usually follow chlamydial infections.

EIA techniques that measure antichlamydial antibodies have been described. While most of these procedures have been successful in measuring IgG antibodies, they have not been as reliable in measuring IgM antibodies. Such tests are commercially available, but there is little published experience with them. The EIAs appear to be less sensitive than the micro-IF test and to miss some C-complex reactors, and they cannot be readily applied to IgM antibody. The procedure may be of some use in selected instances and for serosurveys in laboratories where micro-IF techniques are not available.

Single-point serological tests are of very little value in the diagnosis of uncomplicated lower genital tract infections, which represent the majority of tests. Although manufacturers may claim that their tests are specific for *C. trachomatis* and that titers of a specific level are diagnostic of current infection, neither of those claims is likely to be accurate. If the tests involve partially solubilized EBs for EIA or inclusion detection by IF, there is undoubtedly LPS present. The test will detect antibodies not only to *C. trachomatis* but also to *C. psittaci* or *C. pneumoniae*, because the LPS is a genus-specific antigen. Because of the high prevalence of antibody in high-risk populations, single positive results are seldom diagnostic for current genital infection. In most research evaluations, the positive predictive values have been on the order of 30 to 50%.

Procedure for the CF Test

The CF test may be performed in either the tube system or the microtiter system. Reagents should be standardized in the tube system, regardless of which test system will be used. The microtiter systems are most useful in screening large numbers of sera, but it is preferable to retest all positive sera in the tube system. Occasionally, sera giving titers in the range of 1:4 to 1:8 in the microdilution system are positive at 1:16 (taken as the significant level) in the tube system. Because guinea pigs may have naturally occurring chlamydial infections, the complement must be tested for antichlamydial antibodies.

All reagents are available commercially except for high-titer group antigen, which can be prepared as follows. Yolk sacs of 7-day-old embryonated hen eggs are inoculated with chlamydiae (e.g., psittacosis isolate 6BC) at a dose estimated to result in the death of about 50% of the inoculated eggs in 5 to 7 days. The eggs are candled daily, and those that die early are discarded. When the 50% death end point is approached, the remaining eggs (recently dead or live) are refrigerated for 3 to 24 h, and the yolk sacs are then harvested. If examination of random samples shows large numbers of particles, the yolk sacs are pooled. This preparation may be stored at −20°C until used for further processing. The yolk sacs are ground in a mortar with sterile sand. Beef heart broth (pH 7.0) is added to make a 20% suspension, and the material is cultured to determine whether it is free of bacterial contamination. The suspension is placed in a flask containing sterile glass beads and stored at 4°C for 3 to 6 weeks with daily shaking. It is then centrifuged at ca. 500 × *g* to remove coarse particles, transferred to a heavy sterile flask, and steamed at 100°C or immersed in boiling water for 30 min. After it has cooled, liquefied phenol is added to 0.5%. The antigen should then be refrigerated for at least 1 week before being used. It is stable for at least 1 year if it is not contaminated, and it should have an antigen titer of 1:256 or greater. A similar preparation from uninfected yolk sacs must be included as one of the controls.

Procedure for the Micro-IF Test

The micro-IF test is usually performed with chlamydial organisms grown in yolk sac. Tissue culture-grown agent can be used, but it may be necessary to concentrate the EBs and add some normal yolk sac to improve the contrast for microscopy. The individual yolk sacs are selected for EB richness and pretitrated to give an even distribution of particles. A 1 to 3% yolk sac suspension (in phosphate-buffered saline [pH 7.0]) is generally satisfactory. The antigens may be stored as frozen samples; after being thawed, they are mixed well on a Vortex mixer before use. Micro-IF antigens for research purposes are available through the Washington Research Foundation. The procedure is as follows. Antigen dots are placed on a slide in a specific pattern, with separate pen markings for each antigen. Each cluster of dots includes all of the antigenic types to be tested. The antigen dots are air dried and fixed on slides with acetone (15 min at room temperature). Slides may be stored frozen. They may sweat when thawed for use, but they can be conveniently dried (as can the original antigen dots) with the cool airflow of a hair dryer. Serial dilutions of serum (or tears or exudate) are placed on the different antigen clusters on the slides. The cluster of dots must be separated sufficiently to avoid running of serum from cluster to cluster. After the serum dilutions have been added, the slides are incubated for 0.5 to 1 h in a moist chamber at 37°C and then placed in a buffered saline wash for 5 min and in a second wash for 5 min. The slides are then dried and stained with fluorescein-conjugated anti-human immunoglobulin. Pretitrated conjugates in a known positive system are used to determine the appropriate working dilutions. This reagent may be prepared against any class of immunoglobulin being considered (IgA or secretory IgA for secretions, IgG, or IgM). Counterstains such as bovine serum albumin conjugated with rhodamine may be included. The slides are then washed twice more, dried, and examined by standard fluorescence microscopy. Use of a monocular tube is recommended to allow greater precision in determining the fluorescence of individual EB particles. The end points are read as the dilution giving bright fluorescence clearly associated with the well-distributed EBs throughout the antigen dot. Identification of the type-specific response is based on dilution differences reflected in the end points for different prototype antigens.

For each run of either CF or micro-IF, known positive and negative sera should always be included. These sera should always duplicate their titers as previously observed within the experimental (+1 dilution) error of the system.

ANTIMICROBIAL SUSCEPTIBILITY TESTING

Since strain-to-strain variation in antimicrobial susceptibility profiles and newly acquired drug resistance are both very infrequent among chlamydiae, susceptibility testing generally has little clinical utility. Among the most active drugs in vitro against *C. trachomatis* are tetracycline, doxycycline, erythromycin, azithromycin, rifampin, ofloxacin, and clindamycin. Therefore, the tetracyclines and macrolides have generally been the mainstays of therapy for infections due to chlamydiae.

Antimicrobial susceptibility testing for chlamydiae has not been standardized, and methodological differences doubtlessly contribute to different MICs reported from different laboratories. In general, organisms for testing are grown for at least two passages in antibiotic-free medium before being harvested for use in testing. An adjusted inoculum of ~100 inclusion-forming units per microtiter well is then used to infect antibiotic-free monolayers. After centrifugation of the inoculum onto the monolayer, serial dilutions of the test antibiotic can be added either immediately or at various time intervals over the next 24 h. After 48 h, fluorescein-conjugated monoclonal antibodies are used to identify the highest antibiotic dilution that prevents inclusion formation (MIC). Generally, monolayers are also disrupted and passaged to define the highest dilution that prevents viable chlamydiae from being detected in passage (MBC).

REFERENCES

1. **Banks, J., B. Eddie, M. Sung, N. Sugg, J. Schachter, and K. F. Meyer.** 1970. Plaque reduction technique for demonstrating neutralizing antibodies for *Chlamydia*. *Infect. Immun.* **2:**443–447.
2. **Bauwens, J. E., A. M. Clark, M. J. Loeffelholz, S. A. Herman, and W. E. Stamm.** 1993. Diagnosis of *Chlamydia trachomatis* urethritis in men by polymerase chain reaction assay of first-catch urine. *J. Clin. Microbiol.* **31:**3013–3016.
3. **Bauwens, J. E., A. M. Clark, and W. E. Stamm.** 1993. Diagnosis of *Chlamydia trachomatis* endocervical infections by a commercial polymerase chain reaction assay. *J. Clin. Microbiol.* **31:**3023–3027.
4. **Beem, M. O., and E. M. Saxon.** 1977. Respiratory-tract colonization and a distinctive pneumonia syndrome in infants infected with *Chlamydia trachomatis*. *N. Engl. J. Med.* **296:**306–310.
5. **Berg, E., G. Anestad, H. Moi, G. Storvold, and K. Skaug.** 1997. False-negative results of a ligase chain reaction assay to detect *Chlamydia trachomatis* due to inhibitors in urine. *Eur. J. Clin. Microbiol. Infect. Dis.* **16:**727–731.
6. **Bernstein, D. I., T. Hubbard, W. M. Wenman, B. L. Johnson, Jr., K. K. Holmes, H. Liebhaber, J. Schachter, R. Barnes, and M. A. Lovett.** 1984. Mediastinal and supraclavicular lymphadenitis and pneumonitis due to *Chlamydia trachomatis* serovars L1 and L2. *N. Engl. J. Med.* **311:** 1543–1546.
7. **Blanding, J., S. Aarnaes, V. Darrow, L. de la Maza, and E. Petersen.** 1995. The evaluation of the chlamydia optical immunoassay (OIA) for the direct detection of chlamydia in cervical specimens, p. 76. *In Program and Abstracts of the 35th Interscience Conference on Antimicrobial Agents and Chemotherapy*. American Society for Microbiology, Washington, D.C.
8. **Byrne, G. I., and J. W. Moulder.** 1978. Parasite-specified phagocytosis of *Chlamydia psittaci* and *Chlamydia trachomatis* by L and HeLa cells. *Infect. Immun.* **19:**598–606.
9. **Caldwell, H. D., and J. Schachter.** 1982. Antigenic analysis of the major outer membrane protein of *Chlamydia* spp. *Infect. Immun.* **35:**1024–1031.
10. **Carroll, K., W. Aldeen, M. Morrison, R. Anderson, D. Lee, and S. Mottice.** 1998. Evaluation of the Abbott LCx ligase chain reaction assay for detection of *Chlamydia trachomatis* and *Neisseria gonorrhoeae* in urine and genital swab specimens from a sexually transmitted disease clinic population. *J. Clin. Microbiol.* **36:**1630–1633.
11. **Chernesky, M., S. Castriciano, J. Sellors, I. Stewart, I. Cunningham, S. Landis, W. Seidelman, L. Grant, C. Devlin, and J. Mahony.** 1990. Detection of *Chlamydia trachomatis* antigens in urine as an alternative to swabs and cultures. *J. Infect. Dis.* **161:**124–126.
12. **Chernesky, M. A., H. Lee, J. Schachter, J. D. Burczak, W. E. Stamm, W. M. McCormack, and T. C. Quinn.** 1994. Diagnosis of *Chlamydia trachomatis* urethral infection in symptomatic and asymptomatic men by testing first-void urine in a ligase chain reaction assay. *J. Infect. Dis.* **170:** 1308–1311.
13. **Chernesky, M. A., J. B. Mahony, S. Castriciano, M. Mores, I. O. Stewart, S. F. Landis, W. Seidelman, E. J. Sargeant, and C. Leman.** 1986. Detection of *Chlamydia trachomatis* antigens by enzyme immunoassay and immunofluorescence in genital specimens from symptomatic and asymptomatic men and women. *J. Infect. Dis.* **154:** 141–148.
14. **Clarke, L. M., M. F. Sierra, B. J. Daidone, N. Lopez, J. M. Covino, and W. M. McCormack.** 1993. Comparison of the Syva MicroTrak enzyme immunoassay and Gen-Probe PACE 2 with cell culture for diagnosis of cervical *Chlamydia trachomatis* infection in a high-prevalence female population. *J. Clin. Microbiol.* **31:**968–971.
15. **Cles, L. D., K. Bruch, and W. E. Stamm.** 1988. Staining characteristics of six commercially available monoclonal immunofluorescence reagents for direct diagnosis of *Chlamydia trachomatis* infections. *J. Clin. Microbiol.* **26:** 1735–1737.
16. **Cles, L. D., and W. E. Stamm.** 1990. Use of HL cells for improved isolation and passage of *Chlamydia pneumoniae*. *J. Clin. Microbiol.* **28:**938–940.
17. **Crotchfelt, K., B. Pare, C. Gaydos, and T. Quinn.** 1998. Detection of *Chlamydia trachomatis* by the Gen-Probe AMPLIFIED *Chlamydia trachomatis* assay (AMP CT) in urine specimens from men and women and endocervical specimens from women. *J. Clin. Microbiol.* **36:**391–394.
18. **Eb, F., and J. Orfila.** 1981. Serotyping of "*Chlamydia psittaci*" by microimmunofluorescence test. *Ann. Microbiol. Paris* **132A:**81–96.
19. **Everett, K. D., and A. A. Andersen.** 1997. The ribosomal intergenic spacer and domain I of the 23S rRNA gene are phylogenetic markers for *Chlamydia* spp. *Int. J. Syst. Bacteriol.* **47:**461–473.
20. **Fukushi, H., and K. Hlrai.** 1992. Proposal of *Chlamydia pecorum* sp. nov. for *Chlamydia* strains derived from ruminants. *Int. J. Syst. Bacteriol.* **42:**306–308.
21. **Gaydos, C., M. Howell, T. Quinn, J. Gaydos, and K. McKee.** 1998. Use of ligase chain reaction with urine versus cervical culture for detection of *Chlamydia trachomatis* in an asymptomatic military population of pregnant and nonpregnant females attending Papanicolaou smear clinics. *J. Clin. Microbiol.* **36:**1300–1304.
22. **Gaydos, C. A., P. M. Roblin, M. R. Hammerschlag, C. L. Hyman, J. J. Eiden, J. Schachter, and T. C. Quinn.** 1994. Diagnostic utility of PCR-enzyme immunoassay, culture, and serology for detection of *Chlamydia pneumoniae* in symptomatic and asymptomatic patients. *J. Clin. Microbiol.* **32:**903–905.
23. **Goessens, W., J. Mouton, W. Van der Meijden, S. Deelen, T. Van Rijsoort-Vos, N. Den Toom, H. Verbraugh, and R. Verkooyen.** 1997. Comparison of three commercially available amplification assays, AMP CT, LCx and COBAS AMPLICOR, for detection of *Chlamydia trachomatis* in first-void urine. *J. Clin. Microbiol.* **35:** 2628–2633.
24. **Grayston, J. T.** 1989. *Chlamydia pneumoniae*, strain TWAR. *Chest* **95:**664–669.
25. **Grayston, J. T.** 1992. Infections caused by *Chlamydia pneumoniae* strain TWAR. *Clin. Infect. Dis.* **5:**757–761.
26. **Grayston, J. T., C.-C. Kuo, L. A. Campbell, and S.-P. Wang.** 1989. *Chlamydia pneumoniae* sp. nov. for *Chlamydia* sp. strain TWAR. *Int. J. Syst. Bacteriol.* **39:**88–90.
27. **Hook, E., K. Smith, C. Mullen, J. Stephens, L. Rinehardt, M. Pate, and H. Lee.** 1997. Diagnosis of genitourinary *Chlamydia trachomatis* infections by using the ligase chain reaction on patient-obtained vaginal swabs. *J. Clin. Microbiol.* **35:**2133–2135.
28. **Hyman, C. L., M. H. Augenbraun, P. M. Roblin, J. Schachter, and M. R. Hammerschlag.** 1991. Asymptom-

atic respiratory tract infection with *Chlamydia pneumoniae* TWAR. *J. Clin. Microbiol.* **29:**2082–2083.

29. **Jaschek, G., C. A. Gaydos, L. E. Welsh, and T. C. Quinn.** 1993. Direct detection of *Chlamydia trachomatis* in urine specimens from symptomatic and asymptomatic men by using a rapid polymerase chain reaction assay. *J. Clin. Microbiol.* **31:**1209–1212.
30. **Kluytmans, J., W. Goessens, J. Van Rijsoort-Vos, H. Niesters, and E. Stolz.** 1994. Improved performance of PACE 2 with modified collection system in combination with probe competition assay for detection of *Chlamydia trachomatis* in urethral specimens from males. *J. Clin. Microbiol.* **32:**568–570.
31. **Kuo, C. C., and J. T. Grayston.** 1988. Factors affecting viability and growth in HeLa 229 cells of *Chlamydia* sp. strain TWAR. *J. Clin. Microbiol.* **26:**812–815.
32. **Lampe, M. F., R. J. Suchland, and W. E. Stamm.** 1993. Nucleotide sequence of the variable domains within the major outer membrane protein gene from serovariants of *Chlamydia trachomatis*. *Infect. Immun.* **61:**213–219.
33. **Meyer, K. F.** 1967. The host spectrum of psittacosis-lymphogranuloma venereum (PL) agents. *Am. J. Ophthalmol.* **63**(Suppl.)**:**1225–1246.
34. **Moncada, J., J. Schachter, G. Bolan, J. Engelman, L. Howard, I. Mushahwar, G. Ridgway, G. Mumtaz, W. Stamm, and A. Clark.** 1990. Confirmatory assay increases specificity of the Chlamydiazyme test for *Chlamydia trachomatis* infection of the cervix. *J. Clin. Microbiol.* **28:** 1770–1773.
35. **Moncada, J., J. Schachter, G. Bolan, J. Nathan, M. A. Shafer, A. Clark, J. Schwebke, W. Stamm, T. Mroczkowski, Z. Seliborska, et al.** 1992. Evaluation of Syva's enzyme immunoassay for the detection of *Chlamydia trachomatis* in urogenital specimens. *Diagn. Microbiol. Infect. Dis.* **15:** 663–668.
36. **Morrison, R. P., R. J. Belland, K. Lyng, and H. D. Caldwell.** 1989. Chlamydial disease pathogenesis. The 57-kD chlamydial hypersensitivity antigen is a stress response protein. *J. Exp. Med.* **170:**1271–1283.
37. **Moulder, J. W.** 1984. Order Chlamydiales and family Chlamydiaceae, p. 729–739. *In* N. R. Krieg and J. G. Holt (ed.), *Bergey's Manual of Systematic Bacteriology*, vol. 1. The Williams & Wilkins Co., Baltimore, Md.
38. **Mouton, J., R. Verkooyen, W. Van der MeijDen, T. Van Rijsoort-Vos, W. Goessens, J. Kluytmans, S. Deelen, A. Luijendijk, and H. Verbrugh.** 1997. Detection of *Chlamydia trachomatis* in male and female urine specimens by using the amplified *Chlamydia trachomatis* test. *J. Clin. Microbiol.* **35:**1369–1372.
39. **Newhall, W. J., B. Batteiger, and R. B. Jones.** 1982. Analysis of the human serological response to proteins of *Chlamydia trachomatis*. *Infect. Immun.* **38:**1181–1189.
40. **Nurminen, M., M. Leinonen, P. Saikku, and P. H. Makela.** 1983. The genus-specific antigen of *Chlamydia*: resemblance to the lipopolysaccharide of enteric bacteria. *Science* **220:**1279–1281.
41. **Pasternack, R., P. Vuoriene, A. Kuukankorpi, T. Pitkajarvi, and A. Miettinen.** 1996. Detection of *Chlamydia trachomatis* infections in women by Amplicor PCR: comparison of diagnostic performance with urine and cervical specimens. *J. Clin. Microbiol.* **34:**995–998.
42. **Pasternack, R., P. Vuorinen, and A. Miettinen.** 1997. Evaluation of the Gen-Probe *Chlamydia trachomatis* transcription-mediated amplification assay with urine specimens from women. *J. Clin. Microbiol.* **35:**676–678.
43. **Pasternack, R., P. Vuorinen, T. Pitkajarvi, M. Koskela, and A. Miettinen.** 1997. Comparison of Manual Amplicor PCR, Cobas Amplicor PCR, and LCx assays for detection of *Chlamydia trachomatis* infection in women by using urine specimens. *J. Clin. Microbiol.* **35:**402–408.
44. **Peterson, E., V. Darrow, J. Blanding, S. Aarnaes, and L. de la Maza.** 1997. Reproducibility problems with the AMPLICOR PCR *Chlamydia trachomatis* test. *J. Clin. Microbiol.* **35:**957–959.
45. **Pudjiatmoko, H. Fukushi, Y. Ochiai, T. Yamaguchi, and K. Hirai.** 1997. Phylogenetic analysis of the genus *Chlamydia* based on 16S rRNA gene sequences. *Int. J. Syst. Bacteriol.* **47:**425–431.
46. **Puolakkainen, M., E. Hiltunen-Back, T. Reunala, S. Suhonen, P. Lanteenmake, M. Lehtinen, and J. Paavonen.** 1998. Comparison of performances of two commercially available tests, a PCR assay and a ligase chain reaction test, in detection of urogenital *Chlamydia trachomatis* infection. *J. Clin. Microbiol.* **36:**1489–1493.
47. **Ramirez, J. A.** 1996. Isolation of *Chlamydia pneumoniae* from the coronary artery of a patient with coronary atherosclerosis. The *Chlamydia pneumoniae*/Atherosclerosis Study Group. *Ann. Intern. Med.* **125:**979–982.
48. **Ripa, K. T., and P. A. Mardh.** 1977. Cultivation of *Chlamydia trachomatis* in cycloheximide-treated McCoy cells. *J. Clin. Microbiol.* **6:**328–331.
49. **Schachter, J.** 1978. Chlamydial infections. *N. Engl. J. Med.* **298:**428, 490, 540.
50. **Schachter, J., M. Grossman, and P. H. Azimi.** 1982. Serology of *Chlamydia trachomatis* in infants. *J. Infect. Dis.* **146:**530–535.
51. **Schachter, J., R. B. Jones, R. C. Butler, B. Rice, D. Brooks, B. Van Der Pol, M. Gray, and J. Moncada.** 1997. Evaluation of the Vidas Chlamydia test to detect and verify *Chlamydia trachomatis* in urogenital specimens. *J. Clin. Microbiol.* **35:**2102–2106.
52. **Schachter, J., W. E. Stamm, T. C. Quinn, W. W. Andrews, J. D. Burczak, and H. H. Lee.** 1994. Ligase chain reaction to detect *Chlamydia trachomatis* infection of the cervix. *J. Clin. Microbiol.* **32:**2540–2543.
53. **Schachter, J., N. Sugg, and M. Sung.** 1978. Psittacosis: the reservoir persists. *J. Infect. Dis.* **137:**44–49.
54. **Skulnick, M., R. Chua, A. Simor, D. Low, H. Khosid, S. Fraser, E. Lyons, E. Legere, and D. Kitching.** 1994. Use of the polymerase chain reaction for the detection of *Chlamydia trachomatis* from endocervical and urine specimens in an asymptomatic low prevalence population of women. *Diagn. Microbiol. Infect. Dis.* **20:**195–201.
55. **Stamm, W. E., L. A. Koutsky, J. K. Benedetti, J. L. Jourden, R. C. Brunham, and K. K. Holmes.** 1984. *Chlamydia trachomatis* urethral infections in men. Prevalence, risk factors, and clinical manifestations. *Ann. Intern. Med.* **100:** 47–51.
56. **Stamm, W. E., M. Tam, M. Koester, and L. Cles.** 1983. Detection of *Chlamydia trachomatis* inclusions in McCoy cell cultures with fluorescein-conjugated monoclonal antibodies. *J. Clin. Microbiol.* **17:**666–668.
57. **Stary, A., B. Najim, and H. H. Lee.** 1997. Vulval swabs as alternative specimens for ligase chain reaction detection of genital chlamydial infection in women. *J. Clin. Microbiol.* **35:**836–838.
58. **Stephens, R. S., E. A. Wagar, and G. K. Schoolnik.** 1988. High-resolution mapping of serovar-specific and common antigenic determinants of the major outer membrane protein of *Chlamydia trachomatis*. *J. Exp. Med.* **167:**817.
59. **Storz, J.** 1971. *Chlamydia and Chlamydia-Induced Diseases*. Charles C Thomas, Publisher, Springfield, Ill.
60. **Suchland, R. J., and W. E. Stamm.** 1991. Simplified microtiter cell culture method for rapid immunotyping of *Chlamydia trachomatis*. *J. Clin. Microbiol.* **29:**1333–1338.
61. **Tam, M. R., W. E. Stamm, H. H. Handsfield, R. Stephens, C. C. Kuo, K. K. Holmes, K. Ditzenberger, M.**

Krieger, and R. C. Nowinski. 1984. Culture-independent diagnosis of *Chlamydia trachomatis* using monoclonal antibodies. *N. Engl. J. Med.* **310:**1146–1150.

62. **Tjhie, J. H., R. Roosendaal, D. M. MacLaren, and C. M. Vandenbroucke-Grauls.** 1997. Improvement of growth of *Chlamydia pneumoniae* on HEp-2 cells by pretreatment with polyethylene glycol in combination with additional centrifugation and extension of culture time. *J. Clin. Microbiol.* **35:**1883–1884.
63. **Wang, S. P., and J. T. Grayston.** 1970. Immunologic relationship between genital TRIC, lymphogranuloma venereum, and related organisms in a new microtiter indirect immunofluorescence test. *Am. J. Ophthalmol.* **70:**367–374.
64. **Wang, S. P., J. T. Grayston, E. R. Alexander, and K. K. Holmes.** 1975. Simplified microimmunofluorescence test with trachoma-lymphogranuloma venereum (*Chlamydia trachomatis*) antigens for use as a screening test for antibody. *J. Clin. Microbiol.* **1:**250–255.
65. **Wasserheit, J. N.** 1994. Effect of changes in human ecology and behavior on patterns of sexually transmitted diseases, including human immunodeficiency virus infection. *Proc. Natl. Acad. Sci. USA* **91:**2430–2435.
66. **Wiesenfeld, H. C., R. P. Heine, A. Rideout, I. Macio, F. DiBiasi, and R. L. Sweet.** 1996. The vaginal introitus: a novel site for *Chlamydia trachomatis* testing in women. *Am. J. Obstet. Gynecol.* **174:**1542–1546.
67. **Yoder, B. L., W. E. Stamm, C. M. Koester, and E. R. Alexander.** 1981. Microtest procedure for isolation of *Chlamydia trachomatis*. *J. Clin. Microbiol.* **13:**1036–1039.
68. **Zhang, J. P., and R. S. Stephens.** 1992. Mechanism of *C. trachomatis* attachment to eukaryotic host cells. *Cell* **69:** 861–869.

*Rickettsia**

DAVID H. WALKER

58

TAXONOMY

DNA sequence data of the 16S rRNA, 17-kDa lipoprotein, citrate synthase, rickettsial outer membrane protein A (rOmpA), and rickettsial outer membrane protein B (rOmpB) genes have delineated the phylogeny of the genus *Rickettsia* (1, 2, 7, 31) (Fig. 1). The typhus group and spotted fever groups (SFG), defined originally by their distinctive lipopolysaccharide antigens, comprise the genus along with other species such as *R. bellii*, *R. felis*, and *R. canada*, which, as currently characterized, do not have phenotypes that fit so neatly into the phylogeny (22, 29, 30, 35) (Table 1). *Orientia* (formerly *Rickettsia*) *tsutsugamushi* diverges from the genus *Rickettsia* by approximately 10% in the 16S rRNA gene and differs greatly in its cell wall structure, having unrelated proteins and lacking lipopolysaccharide and peptidoglycan (21, 33) (Table 1). There is no consensus about the criteria that define the placement of two strains of *Rickettsia* into separate species, a situation that is most apparent in the SFG. The SFG contains bacteria that are generally recognized as human pathogens (*R. rickettsii*, *R. akari*, *R. conorii*, *R. africae*, *R. sibirica*, *R. japonica*, *R. honei*, and *R. australis*), as well as a rapidly growing list of organisms identified only in arthropods. Most of these species of indeterminant pathogenicity, including *R. montana*, *R. bellii*, *R. rhipicephali*, and *R. amblyommii*, are presumed to be nonpathogenic and are much more prevalent in ticks in the United States than is the pathogenic *R. rickettsii*. In Europe, *R. slovaca* has recently been proposed as a human pathogen but other rickettsiae (e.g., *R. helvetica* and *R. massiliae*) have not been associated with disease. According to some researchers, the criteria that have been applied to molecular phylogeny of other bacteria would define as few as three *Rickettsia* species in the SFG, namely, *R. akari*, *R. australis*, and all the rest lumped together as one, whereas tradition, geographic distribution, and clinical manifestations would place even closely related organisms such as *R. rickettsii* and *R. conorii* in separate species (Fig. 1; Table 2).

DESCRIPTION OF THE GENERA AND NATURAL HABITATS

Species of *Rickettsia* are small (0.3 to 0.5 μm by 1 to 2 μm), obligately intracellular bacteria of the alpha subdivision of the *Proteobacteria*, with a gram-negative cell wall structure that contains lipopolysaccharide, peptidoglycan, a major 135-kDa S-layer protein (rOmpB), a 17-kDa lipoprotein, and, for SFG rickettsiae, a surface-exposed protein (rOmpA) with a variable number of nearly identical tandem repeat units (35). *Rickettsia* spp. appear to be surrounded by an electron-lucent slime layer, reside free in the cytosol of their host cell, and are found in an arthropod host for at least a part of their life cycle, where they are maintained by transovarian transmission and/or cycles involving horizontal transmission to mammalian hosts (19) (Table 2).

Orienta tsutsugamushi (0.3 to 0.5 μm by 0.8 to 1.5 μm) has a major surface protein of 54 to 58 kDa as well as 110-, 80-, 46-, 43-, 39-, 35-, 28-, and 25-kDa surface proteins, but it lacks muramic acid, glucosamine, 2-keto-3-deoctulonic acid, and hydroxy fatty acids, suggesting the absence of lipopolysaccharide and peptidoglycan (33). Compared with *Rickettsia* spp., *Orientia* has a more plastic gram-negative cell wall with a thicker outer leaflet and thinner inner leaflet of the outer envelope and does not have a slime layer. *Orientia* resides free in the cytosol and is maintained in nature by transovarian transmission in trombiculid chiggers, which transmit the infection to humans during feeding as the larval stage (Table 2).

CLINICAL SIGNIFICANCE

In addition to Rocky Mountain spotted fever, rickettsialpox, murine typhus, flying squirrel-associated *R. prowazekii* infection, and cat flea-transmitted *R. felis* infection, which are indigenous to the United States, the potential for imported infections is significant for boutonneuse fever, African tick bite fever, murine typhus, scrub typhus, and even louse-borne typhus (4, 11–13, 29, 38, 41, 43). Other rickettsioses such as North Asian tick typhus, Flinders Island spotted fever, Japanese spotted fever, and Queensland tick typhus, either because of their geographic distribution and the infrequent travel in these areas or because of their incidence, are unlikely to be imported. Rocky Mountain spotted fever, louse-borne typhus, and scrub typhus are life-threatening illnesses even for young, previously healthy persons. Murine typhus, boutonneuse fever, and North Asian tick typhus can have a fatal outcome in patients who are elderly or have underlying diseases or other risk factors.

An average of 7 days after tick bite inoculation of rickett-

* This chapter contains information presented in chapter 56 by James G. Olson and Joseph E. McDade in the sixth edition of this Manual.

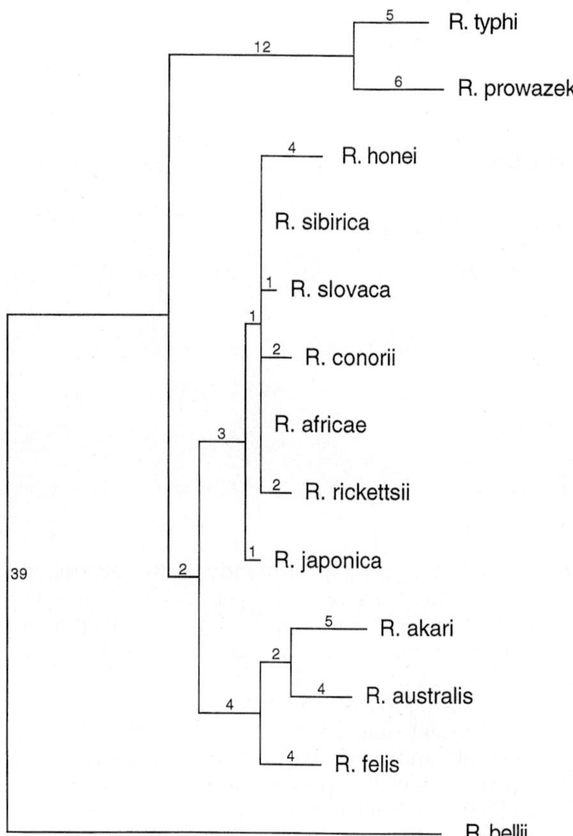

FIGURE 1 Unweighted maximum-parsimony tree prepared with PAUP 3.1 software, comparing a 324-nt segment of the *gltA* (citrate synthase) gene of known pathogenic rickettsiae. Values on the phylodendrogram represent branch lengths. I am grateful for Adrian Billings' preparation and analysis of this phylodendrogram. *Rickettsia bellii*, a presumed nonpathogen, is included for comparison.

siae, patients with Rocky Mountain spotted fever develop fever, severe headache, malaise, and myalgia, frequently accompanied by nausea, vomiting, and abdominal pain and sometimes by a cough (11, 12). Rash typically appears only after 3 to 5 days of illness. Rickettsiae infect the endothelial cells lining the blood vessels, frequently leading to increased vascular permeability and focal hemorrhages (9). In severe cases, rickettsial encephalitis with coma and seizures and noncardiogenic pulmonary edema are grave conditions that often presage death (37).

Rickettsialpox has been recognized mainly as an urban disease which is associated with a disseminated vesicular rash and an eschar at the location of rickettsial inoculation by the feeding mite (13). Although clinically it is a typical spotted fever rickettsiosis, no fatalities have been recorded.

Murine typhus causes rash in only slightly more than half of patients, cough and chest radiographic infiltrates suggesting pneumonia in many patients, and severe illness with seizures, coma, and renal and respiratory failure necessitating intensive care unit admission in 10% of hospitalized patients (4).

COLLECTION, TRANSPORT, AND STORAGE OF SPECIMENS

Blood should be collected as early as possible in the course of the illness. For the isolation of rickettsiae, blood should be obtained in a sterile heparin-containing vial before the patient is given antimicrobial agents that are active against rickettsiae (12, 17, 18). Heparinized blood is also useful during the acute stage of spotted fever rickettsiosis for immunocytologic detection of circulating endothelial cells containing rickettsiae (17). For isolation and immunocytologic diagnosis, blood should be stored temporarily at 4°C and processed as promptly as possible. If inoculation of cell culture or animals must be delayed for more than 24 h, plasma, buffy coat, or whole blood should be frozen rapidly and stored at −70°C or in liquid nitrogen. EDTA- or sodium citrate-anticoagulated blood collected in the acute state has been used effectively for the diagnosis of murine typhus, epidemic typhus, Japanese spotted fever, and scrub typhus by PCR (6, 28, 29, 32, 34, 43). If whole blood, plasma, or buffy coat cannot be processed for PCR within several days, it should be stored at −20°C or lower.

For serologic diagnosis, the initial blood sample is collected as early in the course of disease as possible and a second sample is collected after 1 or 2 weeks; if a fourfold rise in the antibody titer has not occurred, a third sample is collected 3 or 4 weeks after onset. The serum may be stored for several days at 4°C but should be stored frozen at −20°C or lower for longer periods to avoid degradation of the antibodies.

A 3-mm-diameter punch biopsy specimen of a skin lesion, preferably a maculopapule containing a petechia or the margin of an eschar, should be collected as soon as possible (11, 20, 36). Although treatment should not be delayed,

TABLE 1 Characteristics of *Rickettsia* spp. of the SFG and typhus group and *O. tsutsugamushi*

Organism	LPS[a]	PG[b]	rOmpA	rOmpB	17-kDa lipoprotein	56-kDa protein
SFG	S	+[c]	+	+	+	0[c]
Typhus group	T	+	0	+	+	0
R. canada	T	+	ND[d]	+	+	0
R. felis	ND	+	ND	+	+	0
R. bellii	B	+	0	ND	+	0
O. tsutsugamushi	0	0	0	0	0	+

[a] LPS, lipopolysaccharide; S, spotted fever group lipopolysaccharide present; T, typhus group lipopolysaccharide present; B, *bellii* type lipopolysaccharide present.
[b] PG, peptidoglycan.
[c] +, present; 0, absent.
[d] ND, not determined.

TABLE 2 Etiology, epidemiology, and ecology of rickettsial diseases

Organism	Disease	Geographic distribution	Typical mode of transmission to humans	Natural cycle
R. rickettsii	Rocky Mountain spotted fever	Western hemisphere	Tick bite	Transovarian in ticks and rodent-tick cycles
R. akari	Rickettsialpox	United States, Ukraine, Croatia, Korea	Mite bite	Transovarian in mites and mite-mouse cycles
R. conorii	Boutonneuse fever	Southern Europe, Africa, Middle East	Tick bite	Transovarian in ticks
R. africae	African tick bite fever	Eastern and southern Africa	Tick bite	Transovarian in ticks
R. sibirica	North Asian tick typhus	Northern Asia	Tick bite	Transovarian in ticks
R. japonica	Japanese spotted fever	Japan	Tick bite	Ticks
R. australis	Queensland tick typhus	Australia	Tick bite	Ticks
R. honei	Flinders Island spotted fever	Australia	Unknown	Unknown
R. prowazekii	Primary louse-borne typhus	Worldwide	Infected louse feces rubbed into broken skin or mucous membranes or inhaled as aerosol	Human-louse cycle; flying squirrel-flea and/or louse cycle
R. prowazekii	Brill-Zinsser disease	Worldwide	Recrudescence years after primary attack of louse-borne typhus	
R. typhi	Murine typhus	Worldwide	Infected flea feces rubbed into broken skin or mucous membranes or as aerosol	Rat-flea cycle; opposum-flea cycle
R. felis	Cat flea typhus	United States	Not known	Transovarian in cat fleas
O. tsutsugamushi	Scrub typhus	Japan, eastern Asia, northern Australia, west and southwest Pacific	Chigger bite	Transovarian in mites

it is best to take the specimen before the completion of a 24-h course of tetracycline or chloramphenicol. For immunohistologic detection of SFG or typhus group rickettsiae, the specimen can be snap-frozen for frozen sectioning or fixed in formaldehyde for the preparation of paraffin-embedded sections (9, 13, 20, 36–39). The former approach yields an answer more rapidly, but the latter is more convenient for shipping to a reference laboratory. Aseptically collected autopsy specimens, e.g., spleen and lung, are useful for rickettsial isolation; ideally, they are used fresh, or held for 24 h at 4°C or stored frozen at −70°C for longer periods, if they must be shipped to a public health or reference laboratory. Autopsy specimens can also be examined for the presence of rickettsiae by immunohistology or PCR.

ISOLATION PROCEDURES

Rickettsial isolation is performed in only a few laboratories. Cumbersome historic methods such as inoculation of adult male guinea pigs, mice, or the yolk sacs of embryonated chicken eggs have been supplanted by cell culture isolation methods except for isolation of *O. tsutsugamushi* by intraperitoneal inoculation of mice (12, 17, 18, 43). Vero, L-929, HEL, and MRC5 cells have been used in antibiotic-free media to isolate rickettsiae. The best results reported have been achieved with heparin-anticoagulated plasma or buffy coat collected from patients suspected to have boutonneuse fever prior to administration of antirickettsial therapy.

Samples containing 0.5 ml of clinical material mixed with 0.5 ml of tissue culture medium are inoculated as promptly as possible onto 3.7-ml shell vials with 12-mm round coverslips having a confluent layer of cells and centrifuged at 700 × *g* for 1 h at room temperature (17, 18). After removal of the inoculum, the shell vials are washed with phosphate-buffered saline and incubated with minimal essential medium containing 10% fetal calf serum in an atmosphere containing 5% CO_2 at 34°C. At 48 and 72 h, a coverslip is examined by immunofluorescence with antibodies against SFG and typhus group rickettsiae. Detection of four or more organisms is interpreted as a positive result. In France, this method has yielded a diagnosis in 59% of samples from patients with boutonneuse fever who had not been treated and had not developed antibodies to *R. conorii* before collection of the sample (17). Rickettsiae were detected after 48 h of growth in 82% of the positive samples. Standard (universal) precautions should be exercised, as is always appropriate for handling clinical specimens, and work should be performed in a laminar-flow biosafety hood with the investigator wearing gloves and gown. Although the quantity of rickettsiae in the cell culture is relatively small, aerosol, parenteral, and contact exposure should be avoided, as for mycobacteria, fungi, and viruses.

IDENTIFICATION OF RICKETTSIAL ISOLATES

Rickettsiae isolated in cell culture can be identified by indirect immunofluorescence with group-, species-, and strain-specific monoclonal antibodies in laboratories where they are available. In an increasing number of laboratories, rickettsial isolates are identified by molecular methods such as PCR amplification of genes that are genus specific (the genes encoding the 17-kDa protein, citrate synthase, or OmpB) or SFG specific (the gene encoding OmpA) followed by restriction fragment length polymorphism analysis (27). Determination of DNA sequences offers the opportunity to identify unique isolates that may represent novel strains or even species. Since *O. tsutsugamushi* is more distantly related to *Rickettsia* spp., it lacks all of the above genes but can be identified by PCR of the gene encoding the major immunodominant 56-kDa surface protein.

A well-established method for identifying the species of rickettsial isolates is microimmunofluorescence serotyping with mouse sera prepared precisely by intravenous inoculation with a substantial yet nonlethal dose of viable rickettsiae on days 0 and 7 and collection of the typing sera on day 10 (23). This rather cumbersome method requires propagation of large quantities of the isolate as well as the prototype strains to be compared for use as antigens for titer determination as well as for development of the typing sera. Thus, biohazard containment facilities and procedures are necessary.

DIRECT DETECTION IN CLINICAL SAMPLES BY IMMUNOLOGIC AND GENETIC METHODS

The diagnoses of Rocky Mountain spotted fever, boutonneuse fever, murine typhus, louse-borne typhus, and rickettsialpox have been established by immunohistochemical detection of rickettsiae in cutaneous biopsy specimens of rash and eschar lesions (9, 12, 13, 20, 36, 38, 39). Direct immunofluorescence staining with a fluorescein-conjugated polyclonal antiserum that is reactive with *R. rickettsii*, *R. conorii*, and *R. akari* has been applied successfully to frozen sections and formalin-fixed, paraffin-embedded sections of maculopapular rash lesions and eschars (Fig. 2). Monoclonal antibodies specific for either SFG or typhus group rickettsiae have been used to detect rickettsiae by immunoperoxidase staining in formalin-fixed, paraffin-embedded tissues from patients with Rocky Mountain spotted fever, boutonneuse fever, rickettsialpox, murine typhus, and louse-borne typhus as well as in tissues from animals experimentally infected with *R. australis*, *R. sibirica*, and *R. japonica*. The sensitivity and specificity of immunohistochemical detection of *R. rickettsii* in cutaneous biopsy specimens are 70 and 100%, respectively (12, 36). Eschar biopsy specimens can be used for a highly sensitive diagnosis of SFG rickettsioses.

Immunocytochemical detection of *R. conorii* in circulating endothelial cells has been accomplished by capture of the endothelial cells from blood samples with magnetic beads coated with a monoclonal antibody to a human endothelial cell surface antigen followed by immunofluorescent staining of the intracellular rickettsiae (17). Over a 6-year period, this method has achieved a sensitivity of 50% and a specificity of 94%. Rickettsiae were detected in 56% of untreated patients and in 29% of patients receiving antirickettsial treatment. *O. tsutsugamushi* has not been identified immunohistochemically in human tissue. In situ hybridization has not been used for the detection of rickettsiae in tissue samples.

PCR has been applied to the amplification of the DNA of *R. rickettsii*, *R. conorii*, *R. japonica*, *R. typhi*, *R. prowazekii*, *R. felis*, and *O. tsutsugamushi*, usually from peripheral blood, buffy coat, or plasma, but occasionally from fresh, frozen, or paraffin-embedded tissue (6, 28, 29, 32, 34, 43). For *Rickettsia* spp., the 17-kDa protein gene is the principal target, and the primers TTCTCAATTCGGTAAGGGC and ATATTGACCAGTGCTATTTC, which amplify a 246-bp DNA fragment, are used (29). The citrate synthase, 16S rRNA, and rOmpA genes have also been amplified diagnostically. For *O. tsutsugamushi*, the 56-kDa protein gene is the usual target of diagnostic PCR amplification for scrub typhus (32).

Molecular and immunohistochemical diagnostic testing, the most useful methods for establishing a diagnosis during the acute stage of illness when therapeutic decisions are critical, are available at this time, to the best of my knowledge, only in research laboratories.

SEROLOGIC TESTS

In most clinical microbiology laboratories, assays for antibodies to rickettsiae are the only tests performed. This situation is unfortunate for the patient with a life-threatening, acutely incapacitating rickettsial disease, because these assays are useful principally for serologic confirmation of the diagnosis in convalescence and usually do not provide information that is helpful in making critical therapeutic decisions during the acute illness. Patients who die of rickettsioses usually receive many antibiotics, none of which have antirickettsial activity owing in part to the lack of laboratory data providing clinical guidance for a rickettsial diagnosis. The earlier a diagnosis is established, the shorter the course of rickettsial illness after appropriate antirickettsial antibiotics are administered.

Serologic assays for the diagnosis of rickettsial infections in contemporary use include the "gold standard" indirect immunofluorescence assay (IFA), indirect immunoperoxidase assay, latex agglutination, enzyme immunoassay (EIA), *Proteus vulgaris* OX-19 and OX-2 and *Proteus mirabilis* OX-K strain agglutination, line blot, and Western immunoblotting (3–5, 8, 10, 12–15, 24, 26, 36, 42, 43). Only a portion of these assays are available as commercial kits or as assays performed in reference laboratories for some but not all, rickettsial diseases. Other serologic tests such as indirect hemagglutination, microagglutination, and complement fixation are no longer in general use.

The IFA contains all the rickettsial heat-labile protein antigens and group-shared lipopolysaccharide antigen and thus provides group-reactive serologic testing. Cumbersome cross-absorption has provided evidence for species-specific diagnoses by IFA and Western immunoblotting. IFA reagents are available commercially for SFG and typhus group rickettsiae from Integrated Diagnostics (Baltimore, Md.), MRL Diagnostics (Cypress, Calif.), and Bio-Mérieux, (Marcy L'Etoile, France), as well as for *O. tsutsugamushi* from Integrated Diagnostics. In cases of Rocky Mountain spotted fever, IFA detects antibodies at a diagnostic titer of ≥64. Effective antirickettsial treatment of this condition must be initiated by day 5 of illness to avoid a potentially fatal outcome. Other rickettsioses prevalent in the United States and Europe allow more leeway except in patients with particular risk factors for severe disease. For boutonneuse fever, a diagnostic IFA titer of ≥40 occurs in 46% of patients between days 5 and 9 of illness, in 90% between days 20 and 29, and in 100% thereafter (26). In murine typhus, diagnostic IFA titers are present in 50% of patients by the

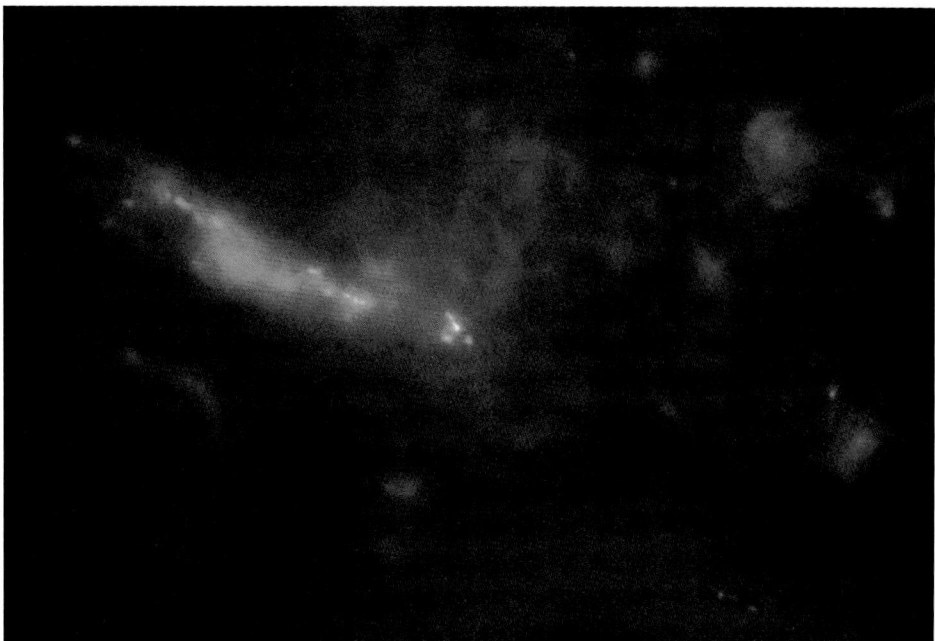

FIGURE 2 Direct immunofluorescence staining of skin biopsy specimens with anti-spotted fever group *Rickettsia* antibodies facilitates rapid diagnosis. Rickettsiae are present in the vessel wall.

end of the first week of illness and in nearly all patients by 15 days after onset (4). In areas where particular rickettsial diseases are endemic, a higher diagnostic cutoff titer is required. For example, for the IFA diagnosis of scrub typhus in patients residing in zones of endemic infection, an IFA titer to *O. tsutsugamushi* of ≥400 is 96% specific and 48% sensitive, with the sensitivity rising from 29% in the first week to 56% in the second week (3). Lowering the diagnostic cutoff titer to 100 raises the sensitivity only to 84% and reduces the specificity to 78%. These considerations are not as important when testing patients who have visited regions of endemic infection for only a short period.

Indirect immunoperoxidase assays for scrub typhus, murine typhus, boutonneuse fever, and presumably other rickettsioses yield results similar to IFA when the IgG diagnostic titer is set at 128 and the IgM titer is set at 32 (14). Advantages include the use of a more generally available light microscope rather than UV microscope and the production of a permanent slide result.

Latex agglutination test reagents for Rocky Mountain spotted fever are available in the United States only from Integrated Diagnostics. Latex beads coated with an extracted rickettsial protein-carbohydrate complex containing rickettsial lipopolysaccharide are agglutinated mainly by IgM antibodies, and there are reports of a sensitivity of 71 to 94% and a specificity of 96 to 99% (8). A diagnostic titer of 128 is often detected early in the second week of illness, by which time treatment should have already been started empirically.

EIAs have been developed in various formats including the use of antigens coated onto microtiter wells or immobilized on nitrocellulose or other sheets. Dot EIA kits for detecting antibodies against *R. rickettsii* and *R. typhi* are commercially available as Dip-S-Ticks from Integrated Diagnostics. They also have been developed, but are not available in the United States, for *O. tsutsugamushi* (14, 42). There are at present no publications in the peer-reviewed literature regarding the use of the dot EIA for the diagnosis of Rocky Mountain spotted fever. Compared with an IFA titer of ≥64 for the diagnosis of murine typhus, the dot EIA showed a sensitivity of 88% and specificity of 91% (14). The dot EIA for diagnosis of scrub typhus had sensitivities and specificities of only 80 and 77%, respectively, compared with 89 and 66%, respectively, at a cutoff titer of 128 (42). These assays make available diagnostic tools that do not require expensive, specialized equipment, but they suffer from all the limitations of serologic diagnosis that is achieved most often in the convalescent stage.

The assays that have been most widely used for the diagnosis of rickettsial diseases are agglutination of the OX-19 and OX-2 strains of *P. vulgaris* and the OX-K strain of *P. mirabilis*. These assays have been largely discredited owing to their low sensitivity and specificity (10, 36). Wherever possible, they should be replaced by more accurate serologic methods such as IFA and the indirect immunoperoxidase assay and others including recombinant protein antigens. For example, the recombinant 56-kDa surface protein of *O. tsutsugamushi* has been demonstrated to be effective for the diagnosis of scrub typhus (16). However, there are situations in developing countries where the choice is between the *Proteus* agglutination tests and none at all for the detection of important public health problems such as outbreaks of louse-borne typhus. In fact, the evidence leading to the recent recognition of some emerging infectious diseases such as Japanese spotted fever and Flinders Island spotted fever included *Proteus* agglutinating antibodies.

ANTIMICROBIAL SUSCEPTIBILITY

Data supporting the use of doxycycline or another tetracycline antibiotic as the drug of choice for the treatment of infections caused by *Rickettsia* spp. and *O. tsutsugamushi* and the use of chloramphenicol as an alternative drug have been derived principally from empirical experience and retrospective case studies. In addition to historic studies of the activity of antimicrobial agents against these obligately intracellular bacteria in infected animals and embryonated eggs, studies of the effects of antimicrobial agents in cell culture have supported the consideration of alternative drugs such as fluoroquinolones and josamycin for the treatment of boutonneuse fever (25). Except for the treatment of cases of scrub typhus in Thailand, which have not responded to doxycycline or chloramphenicol, and the treatment of rickettsial infection in pregnancy, there is little concern about antimicrobial susceptibility of these rickettsiae (25, 40). Antimicrobial susceptibility studies of rickettsiae are not routinely performed clinical laboratory tests.

INTERPRETATION AND REPORTING OF RESULTS

When reporting the results of an assay for antibodies in a single serum sample, the laboratorian seldom knows the duration of illness and whether the serum sample is from the acute or convalescent phase of infection. For sera that are nonreactive by dot EIA, by IFA at a dilution of 1:64, by the indirect immunoperoxidase assay at a dilution of 1:128, by latex agglutination at a dilution of 1:64, or by Weil-Felix *Proteus* agglutination at a titer of 1:160, the laboratory report should state that no antibodies were detected at the particular cutoff dilution, that negative results are expected in the acute stage of rickettsial illness, and that a second sample should be submitted to evaluate the possibility of seroconversion if no alternative diagnosis has been established. If paired acute- and convalescent-phase sera separated by an appropriate interval are available, they should be tested simultaneously. It is wise to test for all the rickettsial agents to which the patient is likely to have been exposed in the United States. SFG rickettsiae and *R. typhi* are the likely agents unless travel to an area with endemic scrub typhus has occurred. If the paired sera are negative, the report should state that the results do not support the diagnosis of rickettsial infection but that antibody synthesis is occasionally delayed, particularly in patients given early antirickettsial therapy. If a single serum sample contains an IFA antibody titer of ≥64, an IgM IFA titer of ≥1:32, an indirect immunoperoxidase antibody titer of ≥128, a latex agglutination titer of ≥64, or a Weil-Felix titer of ≥1:320, the laboratory report should state that antibodies reactive with the particular rickettsial antigen were detected at the measured titer, that the result provides supportive evidence for the diagnosis of the rickettsial disease, and that a convalescent-phase sample should be submitted to assess the possibility of seroconversion. If paired sera measured simultaneously show a fourfold or greater rise in titer, the report should state that the results strongly support the rickettsial diagnosis indicated by the tested antigen. If a significant titer was detected in the acute-phase sample but no rise or only a single doubling-dilution rise was measured, it should be stated that an additional later sample should be tested to look for a fourfold rise or fall in titer. The concept that recrudescent typhus could be distinguished from primary louse-borne typhus by the absence of IgM antibodies to *R. prowazekii* and of *Proteus* OX-19 agglutinating antibodies has been shown recently not to be the case (5). Western immunoblotting has been used by research laboratories to support a diagnosis with a particular species if antibodies react preferentially with rOmpA and/or rOmpB of that species. Cross-absorption with selected antigens can assist in distinguishing among infections with closely related species. The manufacturers of the dot EIA have recommended the interpretation that strongly reactive samples (three or four dots) may indicate the presence of a specific antibody response and that weakly reactive samples (one or two dots) are infrequent but possible in normal populations. Retesting 2 to 3 weeks later would establish the diagnosis if three or four dots develop in the convalescent-phase serum sample and should always be performed.

Isolation of a rickettsiae from blood or tissue may be interpreted as indicating an etiologic role. The level of identification of the isolate should be stated, whether identified only to a group containing particular organisms or to the species level.

Immunohistologic and immunocytologic diagnostic interpretation states the method, reactivity of the method (e.g., antibody reactive with SFG rickettsiae), and location of the antigen (e.g., in vascular endothelium and frequently in the adjacent vascular smooth muscle for *R. rickettsii*). Detection of three or more rickettsiae in vascular endothelium in biopsy specimens or four or more rickettsiae in captured circulating endothelial cells is diagnostic of rickettsial infection.

Interpretation of PCR results should state the target gene, the organisms that would be detected, and the presence or absence of a DNA product of a particular size. If a specific oligonucleotide probe or DNA sequencing confirmed the specificity of the identification, this result should be stated. A disclaimer should state the performance of positive and negative controls and the lack of evidence for but inability to exclude the possibility of DNA contamination. For negative immunohistologic, immunocytologic, and PCR results, it should always be stated that the failure to detect the agent does not exclude the diagnosis, along with data regarding the sensitivity and specificity of the assay in this laboratory and the effects of antirickettsial treatment on the sensitivity.

Special efforts should be made to establish the diagnosis of fatal cases including rickettsial isolation, immunohistologic testing, PCR, and serologic testing on samples collected at necropsy.

REFERENCES

1. **Anderson, B. E., G. A. McDonald, D. C. Jones, and R. L. Regnery.** 1990. A protective protein antigen of *Rickettsia rickettsii* has tandemly repeated, near-identical sequences. *Infect. Immun.* **58:**2760–2769.
2. **Anderson, B. E., R. L. Regnery, G. M. Carlone, T. Tzianabos, J. E. McDade, Z. Y. Fu, and W. J. Bellini.** 1987. Sequence analysis of the 17-kilodalton-antigen gene from *Rickettsia ricketsii*. *J. Bacteriol.* **169:**2385–2390.
3. **Brown, G. W., A. Shirai, C. Rogers, and M. G. Groves.** 1983. Diagnostic criteria for scrub typhus: probability values for immunofluorescent antibody and *Proteus* OXK agglutinin titers. *Am. J. Trop. Med. Hyg.* **32:**1101–1107.
4. **Dumler, J., J. P. Taylor, and D. H. Walker.** 1991. Clinical and laboratory features of murine typhus in south Texas, 1980 through 1987. *JAMA* **266:**1365–1370.
5. **Eremeeva, M. E., N. M. Balayeva, and D. Raoult.** 1994. Serological response of patients suffering from primary and recrudescent typhus: comparison of complement fixation reaction, Weil-Felix test, microimmunofluorescence, and immunoblotting. *Clin. Diagn. Lab. Immunol.* **1:**318–324.
6. **Furuya, Y., T. Katayama, Y. Yoshida, and I. Kaiho.** 1995. Specific amplification of *Rickettsia japonica* DNA from clinical specimens by PCR. *J. Clin. Microbiol.* **33:**487–489.

7. **Hackstadt, T., R. Messer, W. Cieplak, and M. G. Peacock.** 1992. Evidence for proteolytic cleavage of the 120-kilodalton outer membrane protein of rickettsiae: identification of an avirulent mutant deficient in processing. *Infect. Immun.* **60:**159–165.
8. **Hechemy, K. E., R. L. Anacker, R. N. Philip, K. T. Kleeman, J. N. MacCormack, S. J. Sasowski, and E. E. Michaelson.** 1980. Detection of Rocky Mountain spotted fever antibodies by a latex agglutination test. *J. Clin. Microbiol.* **12:**144–150.
9. **Horney, L. F., and D. H. Walker.** 1988. Meningoencephalitis as a major manifestation of Rocky Mountain spotted fever. *South. Med. J.* **81:**915–918.
10. **Kaplan, J. E., and L. B. Schonberger.** 1986. The sensitivity of various serologic tests in the diagnosis of Rocky Mountain spotted fever. *Am. J. Trop. Med. Hyg.* **35:**840–844.
11. **Kaplowitz, L. G., J. J. Fischer, and P. F. Sparling.** 1981. Rocky Mountain spotted fever: a clinical dilemma. *Curr. Clin. Top. Infect. Dis.* **2:**89–108.
12. **Kaplowitz, L. G., J. V. Lange, J. J. Fischer, and D. H. Walker.** 1983. Correlation of rickettsial titers, circulating endotoxin, and clinical features in Rocky Mountain spotted fever. *Arch. Intern. Med.* **143:**1149–1151.
13. **Kass, E. M., W. K. Szaniawski, H. Levy, J. Leach, K. Srinivasan, and C. Rives.** 1994. Rickettsialpox in a New York City hospital, 1980 to 1989. *N. Engl. J. Med.* **331:** 1612–1617.
14. **Kelly, D. J., C. T. Chan, H. Paxton, K. Thompson, R. Howard, and G. A. Dasch.** 1995. Comparative evaluation of a commercial enzyme immunoassay for the detection of human antibody to *Rickettsia typhi*. *Clin. Diagn. Lab. Immunol.* **2:**356–360.
15. **Kelly, D. J., P. W. Wong, E. Gan, and G. E. Lewis, Jr.** 1988. Comparative evaluation of the indirect immunoperoxidase test for the serodiagnosis of rickettsial disease. *Am. J. Trop. Med. Hyg.* **38:**400–406.
16. **Kim, I.-S., S.-Y. Seong, S.-G. Woo, M.-S. Choi, and W.-H. Chang.** 1993. High-level expression of a 56-kilodalton protein gene (*bor56*) of *Rickettsia tsutsugamushi* Boryong and its application to enzyme-linked immunosorbent assays. *J. Clin. Microbiol.* **31:**598–605.
17. **La Scola, B., and D. Raoult.** 1996. Diagnosis of Mediterranean spotted fever by cultivation of *Rickettsia conorii* from blood and skin samples using the centrifugation-shell vial technique and by detection of *R. conorii* in circulating endothelial cells: a 6-year follow-up. *J. Clin. Microbiol.* **34:** 2722–2727.
18. **Marrero, M., and D. Raoult.** 1989. Centrifugation-shell vial technique for rapid detection of Mediterranean spotted fever rickettsia in blood culture. *Am. J. Trop. Med. Hyg.* **40:**197–199.
19. **McDade, J. E., C. C. Shepard, M. A. Redus, V. F. Newhouse, and J. D. Smith.** 1980. Evidence of *Rickettsia prowazekii* infections in the United States. *Am. J. Trop. Med. Hyg.* **29:**277–284.
20. **Montenegro, M. R., S. Mansueto, B. C. Hegarty, and D. H. Walker.** 1983. The histology of "taches noires" of boutonneuse fever and demonstration of *Rickettsia conorii* in them by immunofluorescence. *Virchows Arch.* A **400:** 309–317.
21. **Oaks, E. V., R. M. Rice, D. J. Kelly, and C. K. Stover.** 1989. Antigenic and genetic relatedness of eight *Rickettsia tsutsugamushi* antigens. *Infect. Immun.* **57:**3116–3122.
22. **Philip, R. N., E. A. Casper, R. L. Anacker, J. Cory, S. F. Hayes, W. Burgdorfer, and C. E. Yunker.** 1983. *Rickettsia bellii* sp. nov.: a tick-borne rickettsia, widely distributed in the United States, that is distinct from the spotted fever and typhus biogroups. *Int. J. Syst. Bacteriol.* **33:**94–106.
23. **Philip, R. N., E. A. Casper, W. Burgdorfer, R. K. Gerloff, L. E. Hughes, and E. J. Bell.** 1978. Serologic typing of rickettsiae of the spotted fever group by microimmunofluorescence. *J. Immunol.* **121:**1961–1968.
24. **Raoult, D., and G. A. Dasch.** 1989. Line blot and western blot immunoassays for diagnosis of Mediterranean spotted fever. *J. Clin. Microbiol.* **27:**2073–2079.
25. **Raoult, D., and M. Drancourt.** 1991. Antimicrobial therapy of rickettsial diseases. *Antimicrob. Agents Chemother.* **35:**2457–2462.
26. **Raoult, D., S. Rousseau, B. Toga, C. Tamalet, H. Gallais, P. De Micco, and P. Casanova.** 1984. Diagnostic sérologique de la fièvre boutonneuse méditerranéenne. *Pathol. Biol.* **32:**791–794.
27. **Regnery, R. L., C. L. Spruill, and B. D. Plikaytis.** 1991. Genotypic identification of rickettsiae and estimation of intraspecies sequence divergence for portions of two rickettsial genes. *J. Bacteriol.* **173:**1576–1589.
28. **Sexton, D. J., S. S. Kanj, K. Wilson, G. R. Corey, B. C. Hegarty, M. G. Levy, and E. B. Breitschwerdt.** 1994. The use of a polymerase chain reaction as a diagnostic test for Rocky Mountain spotted fever. *Am. J. Trop. Med. Hyg.* **50:**59–63.
29. **Schriefer, M. E., J. B. Sacci, Jr., J. S. Dumler, M. G. Bullen, and A. F. Azad.** 1994. Identification of a novel rickettsial infection in a patient diagnosed with murine typhus. *J. Clin. Microbiol.* **32:**949–954.
30. **Schriefer, M. E., J. B. Sacci, Jr., J. A. Higgins, and A. F. Azad.** 1994. Murine typhus: updated roles of multiple urban components and a second typhus like rickettsia. *J. Med. Entomol.* **31:**681–685.
31. **Stothard, D. R., and P. A. Fuerst.** 1995. Evolutionary analysis of the spotted fever and typhus groups of *Rickettsia* using 16S rRNA gene sequences. *Syst. Appl. Microbiol.* **18:** 52–61.
32. **Sugita, Y., Y. Yamakawa, K. Takahashi, T. Nagatani, K. Okuda, and H. Nakajima.** 1993. A polymerase chain reaction system for rapid diagnosis of scrub typhus within six hours. *Am. J. Trop. Med. Hyg.* **49:**636–640.
33. **Tamura, A., N. Ohashi, H. Urakami, and S. Miyamura.** 1995. Classification of *Rickettsia tsutsugamushi* in a new genus, *Orientia* gen. nov., as *Orientia tsutsugamushi* comb. nov. *Int. J. Syst. Bacteriol.* **45:**589–591.
34. **Tzianabos, T., B. E. Anderson, and J. E. McDade.** 1989. Detection of *Rickettsia rickettsii* DNA in clinical specimens by using polymerase chain reaction technology. *J. Clin. Microbiol.* **27:**2866–2868.
35. **Vishwanath S.** 1991. Antigenic relationships among the rickettsiae of the spotted fever and typhus groups. *FEMS Microbiol. Lett.* **81:**341–344.
36. **Walker, D. H., M. S. Burday, and J. D. Folds.** 1980. Laboratory diagnosis of Rocky Mountain spotted fever. *South. Med. J.* **73:**1443–1447.
37. **Walker, D. H., C. G. Crawford, and B. G. Cain.** 1980. Rickettsial infection of pulmonary microcirculation: the basis for interstitial pneumonitis in Rocky Mountain spotted fever. *Hum. Pathol.* **11:**263–272.
38. **Walker, D. H., H.-M. Feng, S. Ladner, A. N. Billings, S. R. Zaki, D. J. Wear, and B. Hightower.** 1997. Immunohistochemical diagnosis of typhus rickettsioses using an anti-lipopolysaccharide monoclonal antibody. *Mod. Pathol.* **10:**1038–1042.
39. **Walker, D. H., F. M. Parks, T. G. Betz, J. P. Taylor, and J. W. Muehlberger.** 1989. Histopathology and immunohistologic demonstration of the distribution of *Rickettsia typhi* in fatal murine typhus. *Am. J. Clin. Pathol.* **91:** 720–724.
40. **Watt, G., C. Chouriyagune, R. Ruangweerayud, P. Watcharapichat, D. Phulsuksombati, K. Jongsakul, P. Teja-Isavadharm, D. Bhodhidatta, K. D. Corcoran, G. A.**

Dasch, and D. Strickman. 1996. Scrub typhus infections poorly responsive to antibiotics in northern Thailand. *Lancet* **348:**86–89.

41. **Watt, G., and D. Strickman.** 1994. Life-threatening scrub typhus in a traveler returning from Thailand. *Clin. Infect. Dis.* **18:**624–626.
42. **Weddle, J. R., T.-C. Chan, K. Thompson, H. Paxton, D. J. Kelly, G. Dasch, and D. Strickman.** 1995. Effectiveness of a dot-blot immunoassay of anti-*Rickettsia tsutsugamushi* antibodies for serologic analysis of scrub typhus. *Am. J. Trop. Med. Hyg.* **53:**43–46.
43. **Williams, W. J., S. Radulovic, G. A. Dasch, J. Lindstrom, D. J. Kelly, C. N. Oster, and D. H. Walker.** 1994. Identification of *Rickettsia conorii* infection by polymerase chain reaction in a soldier returning from Somalia. *Clin. Infect. Dis.* **19:**93–99.

*Coxiella**

THOMAS J. MARRIE AND DIDIER RAOULT

59

TAXONOMY

Coxiella burnetii has been placed in the γ subdivision of the class *Proteobacteria*, close to *Rickettsiella grylii*, *Legionella* spp., and *Francisella* spp., on the basis of comparison of the 16S rRNA-encoding gene sequences.

DESCRIPTION OF THE GENUS

C. burnetii is a pleomorphic coccobacillus with a gram-negative cell wall (3). It is an obligate intracellular microorganism measuring 0.2 by 0.7 μm. It does not stain with Gram stain but does stain with Gimenez stain. *C. burnetii* undergoes a developmental cycle in which there is a large-cell and a small-cell variant (40). The small-cell variant attaches to the host cell (usually a macrophage) and is ingested. *C. burnetii* develops within the phagolysosome, where the acid pH activates its metabolic enzymes. Following maturation to the large-cell variant, sporogenesis begins (40). Spore formation explains why *C. burnetii* is so successful as a pathogen. It can survive for up to 10 months at 15 to 20°C, for more than 1 month on meat in cold storage, and for more than 40 months in skim milk at room temperature (8).

C. burnetii undergoes phase variation akin to the smooth-to-rough transition of lipopolysaccarides of gram-negative bacteria (60). In nature and in laboratory animals, it exists in the phase I state, in which the organisms react with late-convalescent-phase (45 days) guinea pig sera and only slightly with early-convalescent-phase (21 days) sera (60). After numerous passages in cell culture or embryonated eggs, truncation of the lipopolysaccharide occurs, yielding the antigenic form, phase II. This phase variation is extremely important in the laboratory diagnosis of acute and chronic Q fever, as will be covered in a later section of this chapter.

NATURAL HABITATS

C. burnetii has been identified in arthropods, fish, birds, rodents, marsupials, and livestock (2). Indeed, it naturally infects more than 40 species (including 12 genera) of ticks on five continents (3). Lice, mites, and parasitic flies are also infected (43). Bandicoots, rats, rabbits, mice, porcupines, hedgehogs, tortoises, cattle, sheep, goats, dogs, swine, cats, camels, buffaloes, baboons, leopards, hyenas, chickens, ducks, geese, turkeys, pigeons, bats, and shrews have all been infected with this microorganism (30, 43).

CLINICAL SIGNIFICANCE

C. burnetii is the etiological agent of Q fever, an extremely common infection, which may occur in either the acute or the chronic form. Q fever is a zoonosis which is present worldwide except in New Zealand. In Nova Scotia, Canada, the overall seroprevalence of *C. burnetii* infection in humans is 14.8%, with seroprevalence rates increasing with age; for those 35 to 39 years of age the rate is 11.8%, while for those 70 to 75 years of age it is 66.7%.

Acute Q Fever

Up to half of *C. burnetii* infections are asymptomatic (13). However, acute Q fever has three distinct manifestations: (i) a self-limited febrile illness, (ii) pneumonia, and (iii) hepatitis. A study by Viciana et al. (67) in Spain found that 21% of 505 adults with fever for more than 1 week had Q fever. The manifestations of acute Q fever seem to vary from country to country. In Nova Scotia, Canada, pneumonia is the major manifestation of acute Q fever (50), while in France hepatitis is the predominant form of acute Q fever (64). Both pneumonia and hepatitis due to Q fever occur in the Basque region of Spain (35). At times the clinical picture of acute Q fever may be dominated by the involvement of organ systems other than those mentioned above. Aseptic meningitis and/or encephalitis complicate up to 1.3% of cases of acute Q fever (12). Uncommon manifestations of acute Q fever include bone marrow necrosis, hemophagocytosis, hemolytic anemia, lymphadenopathy mimicking lymphoma, transient hypoplastic anemia, splenic rupture, and erythema nodosum (5, 16). Q fever may also occur in the immunocompromised host, including human immunodeficiency virus-infected patients (51). Q fever complicating human pregnancy has been uncommonly documented, but it is probably more common than we recognize (6, 34, 49, 56, 61).

* This chapter contains information presented in chapter 56 by James G. Olson and Joseph E. McDade in the sixth edition of this Manual.

Chronic Q Fever

Chronic Q fever is the most serious form of *C. burnetii* infection. It almost always means endocarditis, but occasionally, infection of vascular grafts or aneurysms, osteomyelitis, hepatitis, and prolonged fever are manifestations (7). The most common manifestation of chronic Q fever is culture-negative endocarditis (7, 66). Q fever accounts for about 3% of all cases of endocarditis in England and Wales (46) and 15% of all cases of endocarditis in Marseille, France (21).

C. burnetii Infection in Domestic Animals

Cattle, sheep, and goats are the primary reservoirs of Q fever for humans. *C. burnetii* localizes to the uterus and mammary glands of infected animals (2). The organism undergoes reactivation during pregnancy, when it multiplies in the placenta and reaches extremely high numbers. In recent years infected parturient cats and dogs have been responsible for outbreaks of Q fever (35). *C. burnetii* has caused outbreaks of abortion in goats (2) and sheep (48).

Pregnant sheep are often used in neonatal research, and *Coxiella*-infected sheep brought into hospital laboratories or into the laboratories of research institutes have been responsible for outbreaks of Q fever in those institutes (9, 15, 24, 34, 41, 58).

Routes of Infection

Following parturition of an infected animal, the organism is aerosolized and is inhaled by susceptible individuals. Human volunteers who inhaled 1 infectious dose of *C. burnetii* had an incubation period of 16 days, whereas those who were exposed to 1,500 infectious doses had an incubation period of 10 days (63). Epidemiological studies suggest that ingestion of contaminated milk is a risk factor for Q fever (20, 32). Infection can occur via the percutaneous route since the crushing of an infected tick between the fingers resulted in Q fever (14). Intradermal inoculation and transfusion of contaminated blood have also resulted in Q fever (1). Vertical transmission in humans has been infrequently reported (19, 49). Person-to-person transmission is rare, but there have been a few cases (11, 19). Sexual transmission of *C. burnetii* has occurred in animals (29), and some investigators have suggested that this may be a route by which *C. burnetii* is transmitted in humans.

COLLECTION, TRANSPORT, AND STORAGE OF SPECIMENS

C. burnetii is highly infectious, and tissues from patients with Q fever should be processed under biosafety level 3 conditions, and then only by highly qualified personnel. *C. burnetii* can be isolated from blood and a variety of tissues, but this is not feasible in most laboratories. Since the organism can withstand very harsh environmental conditions, it is unlikely that the organism will die during transport to a suitable laboratory. Blood should be collected in tubes containing EDTA or sodium citrate (heparin interferes with PCR), and the leukocyte layer should be saved for PCR. Solid specimens should be frozen at −80°C until they are cultured. Most laboratories will depend on serological techniques to diagnose *C. burnetii* infection. For the diagnosis of acute Q fever, it is best that an acute-phase serum sample and a convalescent-phase serum sample collected 2 to 4 weeks later be tested. Serum samples from patients with Q fever processed under ordinary conditions present no hazard to laboratory workers.

There are three general approaches to the laboratory diagnosis of *C. burnetii* infection:

1. Direct detection of *C. burnetii* in tissue.
2. Isolation of *C. burnetii* from blood or from tissues.
3. Serological tests for the detection of antibodies to *C. burnetii* phase I and phase II antigens.

DIRECT DETECTION

C. burnetii can be identified in tissues by a direct immunofluorescence technique. This is of limited utility for the routine diagnosis of *C. burnetii* since, with the exception of heart valve tissue from patients with Q fever endocarditis, tissue specimens from patients with acute Q fever are not generally submitted to the laboratory. The major reason for this is that the illness is mild to moderate in severity and mortality is extremely unusual. Patients with Q fever endocarditis, however, do have high numbers of *C. burnetii* organisms in the affected valvular tissue. These can be demonstrated by direct immunofluorescence (52) or electron microscopy. Other techniques that can be used to detect *C. burnetii* in tissues include immunoperoxidase immunohistology (58) and capture enzyme-linked immunosorbent assays (ELISAs) or enzyme-linked immunofluorescence assays (10, 62).

PCR has successfully been used to detect DNA in cell cultures and clinical samples (59). Initially, PCR methods used specific hybridization of labeled DNA probes to nucleic acid amplified from clinical samples (22). These methods are very sensitive and specific but are available only in specialized research laboratories. The availability of *C. burnetii*-specific primers has allowed the development of a simple and reliable method for the detection of this bacterium, even in paraffin-embedded tissues (59). Furthermore, PCR has proven to be more sensitive than standard culture techniques for retrospective diagnosis with frozen samples and for the follow-up of patients treated for chronic Q fever (59). Fritz et al. (23) have used PCR to quantify the amount of *C. burnetii* in tissue. Primers derived from the *htpAB*-associated repetitive element (25) are especially useful. This element exists in at least 19 copies in the *C. burnetii* Nine Mile strain, phase I, genome, and PCR based on this gene is very sensitive.

ISOLATION

Isolation of *C. burnetii* must be done only in a biosafety level 3 containment facility due to its extreme infectivity. This microorganism can be isolated by inoculation of specimens into conventional cell cultures (e.g., Vero cells) (55), embryonated egg yolk sacs (45), or laboratory animals, such as mice or guinea pigs (26). The spleen of the inoculated animal is the most useful organ for the recovery of *C. burnetii*. Ground spleen extracts (0.2 to 0.5 ml of a 10% suspension) should be inoculated into embryonated eggs, which die 7 to 9 days later. These methods are used infrequently, but inoculation of animals remains helpful when the organism must be isolated from tissues contaminated with multiple bacteria or in order to obtain phase I *C. burnetii* antigens from phase II cells. The adaptation of a shell vial culture system from a commercially available method for virus culture has improved the isolation of intracellular bacteria, especially *C. burnetii* (33, 53, 55). Specimens are inoculated onto human embryonic lung fibroblasts grown on a 1-cm^2 coverslip within a small shell vial. The plasma and buffy coat from heparinized blood are diluted 1:2 with Eagle's minimal essential medium (EMEM). Tissue specimens are homogenized in phosphate-buffered saline (PBS) and diluted 1:2 in EMEM. Shell vials containing 12-mm-diameter round glass coverslips are seeded with 50,000 human embryonic lung cells in 1 ml of EMEM containing 10% fetal calf serum. The cells are incubated for 3 days at 37°C in an atmosphere containing 5% CO_2 until the monolayer is confluent. One milliliter of each homogenized specimen is placed into each of three shell vials. A 1-h centrifugation step (700 × *g* at 23°C) enhances the attachment and penetration of the bacteria into the cells. The supernatant is removed and the monolayer is washed twice with PBS. One milliliter of EMEM containing 10% fetal calf serum is added to each vial. After an incubation period of 6 days, *C. burnetii* is detected by microscopic examination after staining. It appears as short rods, which are not stained by the Gram staining method but which are visible after Gimenez staining. Confirmation of the presence of *C. burnetii* within the cells is performed by an indirect immunofluorescence assay with polyclonal or monoclonal anti-*C. burnetii* antibodies (53, 55). Positive cultures are passaged in cells several times to establish the isolated strain.

SEROLOGICAL TESTS

The microagglutination test (18, 43), the complement fixation test (17), the indirect immunofluorescent antibody (IFA) test (17, 42), and ELISA (68) have been used for the serological diagnosis of *C. burnetii* infection.

The IFA test is the serological test of choice for the diagnosis of both acute and chronic Q fever. The test is carried out by the procedure of Philip et al. (47) with purified whole-cell antigens at a concentration of 200 μg/ml. Both phase I and phase II cells are used. Each antigen (phase I and phase II cells) is diluted 1:2 with normal yolk sac (alternatively, serum samples can be diluted in PBS with 3% nonfat powdered milk to avoid nonspecific fixation of the antibodies), spotted onto slides, and fixed in acetone for 15 min at room temperature (approximately 20°C). The antigen spots are air dried and fixed in cold acetone for 15 min. Each serum sample is diluted 1:8 to 1:64 for screening for the presence of antibody. The diluted serum sample is added to each antigen spot. Known positive and negative control serum samples are included in each test. The antigen-serum sets are then overlaid with a 1:75 dilution of fluorescein isothiocyanate-conjugated antihuman polyvalent (γ, α, or μ chain specific) immunoglobulin or anti-immunoglobulin G (IgG)-, anti-IgA-, or anti-IgM-specific immunoglobulin and incubated for 30 min at 37°C in a moist chamber. The slides are then washed in PBS, rinsed in distilled water, and blotted dry. Coverslips are mounted onto the slides with glycerol mounting medium. The slides are immediately read with a microscope with a UV light source at a magnification of ×400. The endpoint is the highest dilution showing whole-cell fluorescence. If only screening dilutions are used, the titers of positive samples are then determined to the endpoint. All samples from a single patient should be run in parallel. The starting serum dilution to be used for testing by the IFA test depends on the level of background antibody in the test population and the antigen preparation. A starting dilution of 1:8 is generally used.

Serum samples from patients with Q fever endocarditis may cross-react with *Bartonella* spp. (31). For patients with a serological diagnosis of *Bartonella* endocarditis, the patient's sera should also be assayed for *C. burnetii* antibodies. The criteria given under Interpretation and Reporting of Results can be used to evaluate the results. Cross-reaction with other antigens is distinctly unusual. IgM and IgG antibody results can be confounded by the presence of rheumatoid factor; thus, a rheumatoid factor absorbent is used before determination of IgM and IgG titers (65).

With experimentally infected guinea pigs, ELISA was more sensitive than the IFA test. Antibodies against phase I whole cells were detected by day 9 following infection by ELISA, by day 16 by the IFA tests, and by day 20 by the complement fixation test. The ELISA for the diagnosis of Q fever has not been standardized, rendering comparison of titers from laboratory to laboratory impossible. There are no accepted criteria for the diagnosis of acute versus chronic Q fever by this test.

The complement fixation test is not as sensitive as the IFA test. Serum samples from about 20% of patients with acute Q fever are anticomplementary (34a). A prozone phenomenon may be present in serum samples from some patients with chronic Q fever. This could result in a false-negative test result unless the laboratory is aware of the possibility.

ANTIBIOTIC SUSCEPTIBILITIES

Antibiotic susceptibility testing of *C. burnetii* is difficult since this organism cannot be grown in axenic medium. Therefore, for purposes of antimicrobial susceptibility testing, three models of infection have been used: animals, chick embryos, and cell culture.

Huebner et al. (26) developed a guinea pig model for *C. burnetii* antibiotic susceptibility testing. Although in vivo assays are very important for the testing of antibiotic activity against *C. burnetii* (36), they are very expensive and are not readily available for every new antibiotic.

Antibiotics are injected into the yolk sac just after inoculation of the bacteria. The mean survival time of treated eggs compared to that of untreated ones determines antibiotic efficacy (36). This method is useful for testing the bacteriostatic activities of antibiotics. Using this method, Jackson (28) found that terramycin, aureomycin, and chloramphenicol were active against *C. burnetii*. Ormsbee (45), Ormsbee and Pickens (44), and Maurin et al. (37) improved the method by the addition of a complement fixation test. Rifampin, co-trimoxazole, and tetracyclines are bacteriostatic against *C. burnetii*. Penicillin, cephalothin, cycloserine, erythromycin, chloramphenicol, and clindamycin are ineffective. Pefloxacin and ofloxacin demonstrated activity against *C. burnetii* in this model (50).

Torres and Raoult (65) developed a shell vial assay with HEL cells for assessment of the bacteriostatic effects of antibiotics against *C. burnetii*. Amikacin and amoxicillin were not effective, ceftriaxone and fusidic acid were inconsistently active (65), while co-trimoxazole, rifampin, doxycycline, tetracycline, minocycline, and clarithromycin (38) as well as sparfloxacin and the quinolones PD 127,391 and PD 131,628 (27) were bacteriostatic. *C. burnetii* can establish a persistent infection in several cell lines (4), including L929 mouse fibroblasts and J774 or P388D1 murine macrophage-like cells. Infected cells can be maintained in continuous cultures for months (57). Raoult et al. (54), using P388D1 and L929 cells in which multiplication of infected cells was inhibited with cycloheximide during antibiotic challenges, showed that pefloxacin, rifampin, and doxycycline (54) as well as clarithromycin (38) are bacteriostatic. Hypothesizing that this lack of bactericidal activity was related to antibiotic inactivation by the low pH of the phagolysosomes in which *C. burnetii* is found, Raoult et al. (54) demonstrated that the addition of a lysosomotropic alkalinizing agent, chloroquine, to antibiotics improved the activities of doxycycline and pefloxacin, which then became bactericidal (39).

C. burnetii has developed resistance to ciprofloxacin when the organism is cultivated with increasing concentrations of this antibiotic due to a nucleotide mutation in the DNA gyrase subunit A gene (*gyrA*).

INTERPRETATION AND REPORTING OF RESULTS

By the IFA technique, a fourfold or greater rise in antibody titer between acute- and convalescent-phase serum samples is diagnostic of recent infection. In patients with acute Q fever, the titers of antibodies to the phase II antigen are always higher than the titers of antibodies to the phase I antigen. Indeed, in patients with acute Q fever the phase I antibody titer is usually ≤1 : 128 and requires up to 4 months to peak. Phase II antibody titers peak at 1 : 1,024 to 1 : 2,048 within 1 month of infection. IgM antibodies appear early and reach a peak at 16 weeks following the onset of symptoms, and 88% of individuals still have IgM antibodies at 32 weeks following the onset of symptoms (15).

If only a single serum sample is available, the minimum titer diagnostic of acute Q fever is 1 : 256 for antibody against the phase II antigen. Since *C. burnetii* IgM antibody persists for so long, a positive titer is not considered diagnostic of acute Q fever.

In patients with chronic Q fever (Q fever endocarditis), phase I antibody titers determined by the IFA technique are generally considerably higher than phase II antibody titers. It is not unusual for the sera of patients with Q fever endocarditis to have phase I antibody titers of ≥ 131,000. In the authors' experience, patients with Q fever endocarditis generally have phase I antibody titers of ≥1 : 8,192, while phase II antibody titers are usually two- to fourfold lower. Fournier et al. (21) have shown that a phase I *C. burnetii* IgG antibody titer of ≥1 : 800 by the IFA test is diagnostic of Q fever endocarditis. They suggested that the Duke criteria for the diagnosis of endocarditis be modified to include a phase I *C. burnetii* IgG antibody titer of ≥1 : 800 as a major criterion (21). Rarely in patients with chronic Q fever are the phase I and phase II antibody titers equal. Serial antibody testing is necessary to monitor the treatment of a patient with Q fever endocarditis. Antibody titers should fall with therapy. The authors recommend testing of patients with Q fever endocarditis once monthly for the first 6 months and then every 3 months thereafter. These patients generally require prolonged antibiotic therapy (up to 3 years). It is recommended that antibiotic therapy be continued until the phase I IgG antibody titer is ≤1 : 400 and the phase I IgA antibody titer is undetectable.

A phase I complement fixation titer of ≥1 : 200 is said to be diagnostic of Q fever endocarditis, although lower antibody titers have been found in patients with Q fever endocarditis (66).

We recognize the contributions of J. E. McDade and J. G. Olson, who wrote this chapter for the previous edition of the Manual.

REFERENCES

1. **Anonymous.** 1977. Editorial comment on Q fever transmitted by blood transfusion—United States. *Can. Dis. Weekly Rep.* **3:**210.
2. **Babudieri, B.** 1959. Q fever: a zoonosis. *Adv. Vet. Sci.* **5:** 81–182.
3. **Baca, O. G., and D. Paretsky.** 1983. Q fever and *Coxiella burnetii*: a model for host-parasite interactions. *Microbiol. Rev.* **47:**127–149.
4. **Baca, O. G., E. T. Akporiaye, A. S. Aragon, I. L. Martinez, M. V. Robles, and N. L. Warner.** 1981. Fate of phase I and phase II *Coxiella burnetii* in several macrophage-like tumor cell lines. *Infect. Immun.* **33:**258–266.
5. **Baumbach, A., B. Brehm, W. Sauer, G. Doller, and H. M. Hoffmeister.** 1992. Spontaneous splenic rupture complicating acute Q fever. *Am. J. Gastroenterol.* **87:** 1651–1653.
6. **Bental, T., M. Fejgin, A. Keysary, S. Rzotkiewicz, C. Oron, R. Nachum, Y. Beyth, and R. Lang.** 1995. Chronic Q fever of pregnancy presenting as *Coxiella burnetti* placentitis: successful outcome following therapy with erythromycin and rifampin. *Clin. Infect. Dis.* **21:**1318–1321.
7. **Brouqui, P., H. T. Dupont, M. Drancourt, Y. Berland, J. Etienne, C. Leport, F. Goldstein, P. Massip, M. Micoud, A. Bertrand, and D. Raoult.** 1993. Chronic Q fever: ninety-two cases from France; including 27 cases without endocarditis. *Arch. Intern. Med.* **153:**642–649.
8. **Christie, A. B.** 1974. Q fever, p. 876–891. *In* A. B. Christie (ed.), *Infectious Diseases, Epidemiology and Clinical Practice*. Churchill Livingstone, Edinburgh, United Kingdom.
9. **Curet, L. B., and J. C. Paust.** 1972. Transmission of Q fever from experimental sheep to laboratory personnel. *Am. J. Obstet. Gynecol.* **114:**566–568.
10. **Dackau, T.** 1993. Experimental studies on the development of an antigen-capture test (capture-ELIFA) for *Coxiella burnetii* in cow's milk as a possible alternative to animal studies. *Berl. Muench. Tieraerztl. Wochenschr.* **106**(3): 87–90.
11. **Deutch, D. L., and E. T. Peterson.** 1950. Q fever: transmission from one human being to others. *JAMA* **143:** 348–350.
12. **Drancourt, M., D. Raoult, B. Xeridat, L. Milandre, M. Nesri, and P. Dano.** 1991. Q fever meningoencephalitis in five patients. *Eur. J. Epidemiol.* **7:**134–138.
13. **Dupuis, G., J. Petite, O. Peter, and M. Vouilloz.** 1987. An important outbreak of human Q fever in a Swiss Alpine valley. *Int. J. Bacteriol.* **16:**282–287.
14. **Eklund, C. M., R. R. Parker, and D. B. Lackman.** 1947. Case of Q fever probably contracted by exposure to ticks in nature. *Public Health Rep.* **62:**1413–1416.
15. **Embil, J., J. C. Williams, and T. J. Marrie.** 1990. The immune response in a cat-related outbreak of Q fever as measured by the indirect immunofluorescence test and the enzyme-linked immunosorbent assay. *Can. J. Microbiol.* **36:**292–296.
16. **Estrov, Z., R. Bruck, and M. Shtalrid.** 1984. Histiocytic hemophagocytosis in Q fever. *Arch. Pathol. Lab. Med.* **108:** 7.
17. **Field, P. R., J. G. Hunt, and A. M. Murphy.** 1983. Detection and persistence of specific IgM antibody to *Coxiella burnetii* by enzyme-linked immunosorbent assay: a comparison with immunofluorescence and complement fixation tests. *J. Infect. Dis.* **148:**477–487.
18. **Fiset, P., R. A. Ormsbee, and R. Silberman.** 1969. A microagglutination technique for detection and measurement of rickettsial antibodies. *Acta Virol.* **13:**60–66.
19. **Fiset, P., C. L. Wisseman, Jr., and Y. El-Bataine.** 1975. Immunologic evidence of human fetal infection with *Coxiella burnetii*. *Am. J. Epidemiol.* **101:**65–69.
20. **Fishbein, D. B., and D. Raoult.** 1992. A cluster of *Coxiella burnetii* infections associated with exposure to vaccinated goats and their unpasteurized dairy products. *Am. J. Trop. Med. Hyg.* **47:**35–40.

21. **Fournier, P., J. P. Casalta, G. Habib, T. Messana, and D. Raoult.** 1996. Modification of the diagnostic criteria proposed by the Duke endocarditis service to permit improved diagnosis of Q fever endocarditis. *Am. J. Med.* **100:** 629–633.
22. **Frazier, M. E., L. P. Mallavia, J. E. Samuel, and O. G. Baca.** 1990. DNA probes for the identification of *Coxiella burnetii* strains. *Ann. N. Y. Acad. Sci.* **9:**411–417.
23. **Fritz, E., D. Thiele, H. Willems, and M. M. Wittenbrink.** 1995. Quantification of *Coxiella burnetii* by polymerase chain reaction (PCR) and a colorimetric microtiter plate by hybridization assay (CMHA). *Eur. J. Epidemiol.* **11:** 549–575.
24. **Hall, C. J., S. J. Richmond, E. O. Caul, N. H. Pearse, and I. A. Silver.** 1982. Laboratory outbreak of Q fever acquired from sheep. *Lancet* **i:**1004–1006.
25. **Hoover, T. A., M. H. Vodkin, and J. Williams.** 1992. A *Coxiella burnetii* repeated DNA element resembling a bacterial insertion sequence. *J. Bacteriol.* **174:**5540–5548.
26. **Huebner, R. J., G. A. Hottle, and E. B. Robinson.** 1948. Action of streptomycin in experimental infection with Q fever. *Public Health Rep.* **63:**357–362.
27. **Jabarit-Aldighieri, N., H. Torres, and D. Raoult.** 1992. Susceptibility of *Rickettsia conorii, R. rickettsii,* and *Coxiella burnetii* to PD 127, 391, PD 131, 628 pefloxacin, ofloxacin, and ciprofloxacin. *Antimicrob. Agents Chemother.* **36:** 2529–2532.
28. **Jackson, E. B.** 1951. Comparative efficacy of several antibiotics on experimental rickettsial infections in embryonated eggs. *Antibiot. Chemother.* **1:**231–241.
29. **Kruszewska, D., and S. K. Tyleswka-Wierzbanowska.** 1993. *Coxiella burnetii* penetration into the reproductive system of male mice, promoting sexual transmission of infection. *Infect. Immun.* **61:**4188–4195.
30. **Lang, G. H.** 1990. Coxiellosis (Q fever) in animals, p. 24–48. *In* T. J. Marrie (ed.), *Q Fever*, vol. 1. *The Disease.* CRC Press, Inc., Boca Raton, Fla.
31. **La Scola, B., and D. Raoult.** 1996. Serological cross-reactions between *Bartonella quintana, Bartonella henselae,* and *Coxiella burnetii. J. Clin. Microbiol.* **34:**2270–2274.
32. **Marmion, B. P., M. G. P. Stoker, C. B. V. Walker, and R. G. Carpenter.** 1956. Q fever in Great Britain—epidemiological information from a serological survey of healthy adults in Kent and East Anglia. *J. Hyg.* **54:**118–140.
33. **Marrero, M., and D. Raoult.** 1989. Centrifugation-shell vial technique for rapid detection of Mediterranean spotted fever rickettsia in blood culture. *Am. J. Trop. Med. Hyg.* **40:**197–199.
34. **Marrie, T. J.** 1993. Q fever in pregnancy: report of two cases. *Infect. Dis. Clin. Pract.* **2:**207–209.
34a. **Marrie, T. J.** Unpublished observation.
35. **Marrie, T. J., H. Durant, J. C. Williams, E. Mintz, and D. M. Waag.** 1988. Exposure to parturient cats: a risk factor for acquisition of Q fever in Maritime Canada. *J. Infect. Dis.* **158:**101–108.
36. **Maurin, M., and D. Raoult.** 1993. In vitro susceptibilities of spotted fever group rickettsiae and *Coxiella burnetii* to clarithromycin. *Antimicrob. Agents Chemother.* **37:** 2633–2637.
37. **Maurin, M., A. M. Benoliel, P. Bongrand, and D. Raoult.** 1992. Phagolysosomes of *Coxiella burnetii*-infected cell lines maintain an acid pH during persistent infection. *Infect. Immun.* **60:**5013–5016.
38. **Maurin, M., and D. Raoult.** 1993. Antimicrobial agents and intracellular pathogens, p. 153–179. *In* D. Raoult (ed.), *Current Concepts and Perspectives in Q Fever Treatment.* CRC Press, Inc., Boca Raton, Fla.
39. **Maurin, M., A. M. Benoliel, P. Bongrand, and D. Raoult.** 1992. Phagolysosomal alkalinization and the bactericidal effect of antibiotics: the *Coxiella burnetii* paradigm. *J. Infect. Dis.* **166:**1097–1102.
40. **McCaul, T. F., and J. C. Williams.** 1981. Developmental cycle of *Coxiella burnetii*: structure and morphogenesis of vegetative and sporogenic differentiations. *J. Bacteriol.* **147:**1063–1076.
41. **Meiklejohn, G., L. G. Reimer, P. S. Graves, and C. Helmick.** 1981. Cryptic epidemic of Q fever in a medical school. *J. Infect. Dis.* **144:**107–114.
42. **Murphy, A. M., and P. R. Field.** 1970. The persistence of complement fixing antibodies to Q fever (*Coxiella burnetii*) after infection. *Med. J. Aust.* **1:**1148–1150.
43. **Ormsbee, R. A.** 1965. Q fever Rickettsia, p. 1144–1160. *In* F. L. Horsfall and I. Tamm (ed.), *Viral and Rickettsial Infections of Man*, 4th ed. J. P. Lippincott Co., Philadelphia, Pa.
44. **Ormsbee, R. A., and E. G. Pickens.** 1951. Comparison by means of the complement-fixation test of the relative potencies of chloramphenicol, aureomycin, and terramycin in experimental Q fever infections in embryonated eggs. *J. Immunol.* **67:**437–448.
45. **Ormsbee, R. A.** 1952. The growth of *Coxiella burnetii* in embryonated eggs. *J. Bacteriol.* **63:**73–86.
46. **Palmer, S. R., and S. E. J. Young.** 1982. Q fever endocarditis in England and Wales, 1975–81. *Lancet* **ii:**1148–1149.
47. **Philip, R. N., E. A. Casper, R. A. Ormsbee, M. G. Peacock, and W. Burgdorfer.** 1976. Microimmunofluorescence test for the serological study of Rocky Mountain spotted fever and typhus. *J. Clin. Microbiol.* **3:**51–61.
48. **Polydorou, K.** 1981. Q fever in Cyprus: a short review. *Br. Vet. J.* **137:**470–477.
49. **Raoult, D., and A. Stein.** 1994. Q fever during pregnancy. A risk factor for women, fetuses and obstetricians. *N. Engl. J. Med.* **330:**371. (Letter.)
50. **Raoult, D., M. R. Yeaman, and O. G. Baca.** 1989. Susceptibility of *Coxiella burnetii* to pefloxacin and ofloxacin in ovo and cells. *Antimicrob. Agents Chemother.* **33:**621–623.
51. **Raoult, D., P. Brouqui, J. A. Gastraut, and B. Marchou.** 1992. Acute and chronic Q fever in patients with cancer. *Clin. Infect. Dis.* **14:**127–130.
52. **Raoult, D., J. C. Lauren, and M. Mutillod.** 1994. Monoclonal antibodies to *Coxiella burnetii* for antigenic detection in cell cultures and in paraffin embedded tissues. *Am. J. Clin. Pathol.* **101:**318–320.
53. **Raoult, D., H. Torres, and M. Drancourt.** 1991. Shell-vial assay: evaluation of a new technique for determining antibiotic susceptibility tested in 13 isolates of *Coxiella burnetii. Antimicrob. Agents Chemother.* **35:**2070–2077.
54. **Raoult, D., M. Drancourt, and G. Vestris.** 1990. Bactericidal effect of doxycycline associated with lysosomotropic agents in P388D1 cells. *Antimicrob. Agents Chemother.* **34:** 1512–1514.
55. **Raoult, D., G. Vestris, and M. Enea.** 1990. Isolation of 16 strains of *Coxiella burnetii* from patients using a sensitive centrifugation cell culture system and establishment of strains in HEL cells. *J. Clin. Microbiol.* **28:**2482–2484.
56. **Reichmann, N., R. Raz, A. Keysary, R. Goldwasser, and E. Faltau.** 1988. Chronic Q fever and severe thrombocytopenia in a pregnant woman. *Am. J. Med.* **85:**253–254.
57. **Roman, M. J., P. D. Coriz, and O. G. Baca.** 1986. A proposed model to explain persistent infection of host cells with *Coxiella burnetii. J. Gen. Microbiol.* **132:**1415–1422.
58. **Schmeer, N., W. Schmuck, W. Scheneider, et al.** 1987. Detection of *Coxiella burnetii* by the immunoperoxidase technique. *Mikrobiol. Hyg. Ser. A* **267:**67–73.
59. **Stein, A., and D. Raoult.** 1992. Detection of *Coxiella burnetii* by DNA amplification using polymerase chain reaction. *J. Clin. Microbiol.* **30:**2462–2466.
60. **Stoker, M. G. P., and P. Fiset.** 1956. Phase variation of

the Nine Mile and other strains of *Rickettsia burnetii*. *Can. J. Microbiol.* **2**:310–321.

61. **Syrucek, L., O. Sobeslavsky, and L. Gutvirth.** 1958. Isolation of *Coxiella burnetii* from human placentas. *J. Hyg. Epidemiol. Microbiol. Immunol.* **2**:29–35.
62. **Thiele, D., M. Karo, and H. Krauss.** 1992. Monoclonal antibody based capture Elisa/Elifa for detection of *Coxiella burnetii* in clinical specimens. *Eur. J. Epidemiol.* **8**:568–574.
63. **Tiggert, W. D., and A. S. Benenson.** 1956. Studies on Q fever in man. *Trans. Assoc. Am. Phys.* **69**:98–104.
64. **Tissot-Dupont, H., D. Raoult, P. Brouqui, F. Janbon, D. Peyramond, P.-J. Weiller, C. Chicheportiche, M. Nezri, and R. Poirier.** 1992. Epidemiologic features and clinical presentation of acute Q fever in hospitalized patients: 323 French cases. *Am. J. Med.* **93**:427–434.
65. **Torres, H., and D. Raoult.** 1993. In vitro activities of ceftriaxone and fusidic acid against 13 isolates of *Coxiella burnetii* determined using the shell vial assay. *Antimicrob. Agents Chemother.* **37**:491–494.
66. **Turck, W. P. G., G. Howitt, L. A. Turnberg, H. Fox, M. Longson, M. B. Matthews, and R. Das Gupta.** 1976. Chronic Q fever. *Q. J. Med.* **45**:193–217.
67. **Viciana, P., J. Pachon, J. A. Cuello, J. Palomino, M. E. Jimenez-Mejias, and J. M. Cisneros.** 1992. Fever of indeterminate duration in the community. A seven year study in the South of Spain, abstr. 683, p. 224. *In Program and Abstracts of the 32nd Interscience Conference on Antimicrobial Agents and Chemotherapy*. American Society for Microbiology, Washington, D.C.
68. **Waag, D., J. Chulay, T. Marrie, M. England, and J. Williams.** 1995. Validation of an enzyme immunoassay for serodiagnosis of acute Q fever. *Eur. J. Clin. Microbiol. Infect. Dis.* **14**:421–427.

*Ehrlichia**

J. STEPHEN DUMLER

60

TAXONOMY

Until recently, in vitro propagation of ehrlichiae was difficult or impossible. As a result, *Ehrlichia* species listed in *Bergey's Manual* are compiled as obligate intracellular bacteria with similar morphology in Giemsa-stained preparations, their host hematopoietic cell type, host mammalian species, geographic distribution of recognized infections, and vague serologic cross-reactivity (70). By these relatively host-defined criteria, *Ehrlichia* species are currently placed within the order *Rickettsiales* and in the family *Rickettsiaceae*.

Recent molecular phylogenetic analyses by using 16S rRNA gene and *groESL* operon nucleic acid sequence comparisons provide a more objective microbe-determined framework for characterization and indicate that three distinct clades exist among genera now designated as *Cowdria*, *Ehrlichia*, *Anaplasma*, *Neorickettsia*, and *Wolbachia* (2, 67). The accepted *Ehrlichia* species, *E. canis*, *E. phagocytophila*, *E. equi*, *E. sennetsu*, *E. risticii*, *E. chaffeensis*, *E. ewingii*, and *E. muris*, as well as the species incertae sedis *E. bovis*, *E. ovis*, *E. ondiri*, and *E. platys*, are admixed among these three clades; thus, taxonomic revision with renaming is likely to occur. The clades are currently designated *E. canis* genogroup, *E. phagocytophila* genogroup, and *E. sennetsu* genogroup, as shown in Fig. 1. This phylogenetic approach is further supported by serologic cross-reactions (24, 41), comparisons among major immunogenic surface proteins, and the cellular tropism of these bacteria.

DESCRIPTION OF THE GENUS

The genus *Ehrlichia*, first used in 1939 and formally designated by Moshkovski in 1945 to describe *E. canis*, are obligate intracellular gram-negative bacteria that infect and propagate most efficiently within cytoplasmic vacuoles, especially in mononuclear and granulocytic phagocytes (58, 67, 70). Within these cytoplasmic vacuoles, known to be endosomes for *E. chaffeensis* (12), microcolonies form clusters called morulae. Some species such as *E. sennetsu* grow as bacterial cells that maintain their individual vacuolar membranes when they undergo binary fission, and thus an intracellular aggregate or inclusion may not be identified by light microscopy. By ultrastructural analysis, two distinct morphologic forms may be identified: dense-core (or electron-dense) and reticulate (or electron-lucent) forms (55). Each of these forms is capable of binary fission; therefore, a developmental cycle has not been proven for ehrlichiae. Cell lysis is a feature of the infectious process and leads to the release of cell-free bacteria that may infect other competent cells. Release of the contents of vacuoles from living cells has also been proposed (13).

NATURAL HABITATS

Ehrlichiae are zoonotic agents that are transmitted to animals and humans most frequently after a tick bite for two of the genogroups and by ingestion of fish infested by ehrlichia-infected flukes for the other genogroup. *Wolbachia* species appear to be symbiotes of a broad range of arthropods. Thus, most species have the potential for vertebrate and invertebrate life stages. The tick vectors for species known to infect humans include members of the *Ixodes persulcatus* group (including *I. scapularis*, *I. pacificus*, and *I. ricinus*) for the *E. phagocytophila*-*E. equi*- human granulocytic ehrlichia (HGE) species (44, 57, 66), *Amblyomma americanum* (lone star tick) for *E. chaffeensis* (3), and *Rhipicephalus sanguineus* (brown dog tick) for *E. canis* (62). Although poorly studied, transovarial transmission in ticks does not appear to occur, and so *Ehrlichia* species depend upon high levels of bacteremia and in some cases persistent infection for enzootic maintenance (44, 62). Transstadial transmission in ticks allows ehrlichiae to be acquired from blood meals on naturally infected animals by the immature stages of ticks (larvae and nymphs), which can transmit the ehrlichiae to other mammalian hosts after molting to the next stage (nymph or adult). Humans are only inadvertently infected and represent an end-stage host for ehrlichiae. Natural maintenance of tick-borne ehrlichiae depends on the presence of appropriate tick vectors and mammalian hosts in the local environment.

Natural reservoirs that are known to exist for *E. chaffeensis* include both white-tailed deer (*Odocoileus virginianus*) and domestic dogs, as well as perhaps other animals that host *A. americanum* ticks (21, 43). The major reservoirs for the HGE agent are small mammals, especially the white-footed mouse (*Peromyscus leucopus*) in the eastern United States, although other small mammals such as chipmunks (*Tamias striatus*) and voles (*Clethrionomys gapperi*) are natu-

* This chapter contains information presented in chapter 57 by James G. Olson and Jacqueline E. Dawson in the sixth edition of this Manual.

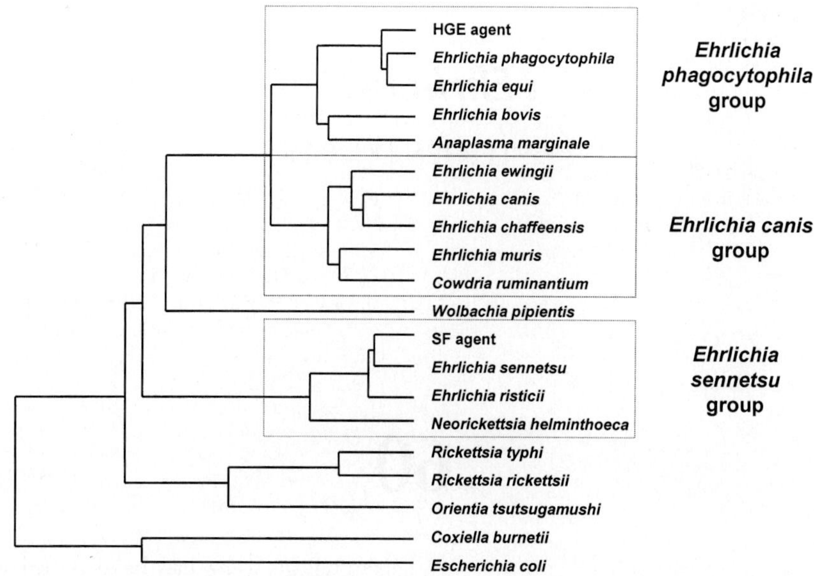

FIGURE 1 Phylogenetic tree depicting small-subunit (16S) rRNA gene sequences of *Ehrlichia* species and other genetically related bacteria. *Coxiella burnetii* and *Escherichia coli* are included for outgroup comparisons. Note the presence of three clades (boxes) that are represented as well-defined branches that contain the currently recognized *Ehrlichia* species.

rally infected and are frequent hosts to the immature stages of *I. scapularis* (66, 69). In Europe, red deer, sheep, cattle, and goats are persistently infected and serve as reservoirs. The reservoir for *E. sennetsu* is not known; however, epidemiological data suggests that consumption of raw fish was associated with sennetsu fever.

CLINICAL SIGNIFICANCE

Human Diseases

Human Monocytotropic Ehrlichiosis

The causative agent of human monocytotropic ehrlichiosis (HME) is *E. chaffeensis*, a monocytotropic ehrlichia that was first identified as a human pathogen in a patient with a severe febrile illness after sustaining tick bites in 1986 (46). More than 466 cases of HME were identified by the Centers for Disease Control and Prevention (CDC) between 1985 and 1996; however, serologic data compiled at a major commercial laboratory that performs serologic testing for *E. chaffeensis* includes more than 722 diagnostic serologic results between 1992 and 1995 alone, suggesting that HME occurs much more frequently than is reported (67). Passive and active case identification has revealed that clinically apparent HME occurs at least as frequently as Rocky Mountain spotted fever in Oklahoma, Georgia, Maryland, and North Carolina (67). Most cases are identified in the south central and southeastern United States, but infections have been increasingly identified in the mid-Atlantic region as well. Prospective evaluation of individuals with high rates of tick exposure shows that approximately 75% of seroconversions with antibody to *E. chaffeensis* are subclinical (34).

The median incubation period for HME is 9 days, and two-thirds of patients are males; the median age is 44 years (34). Patients typically present with high fever (97%), headache (81%), malaise (84%), and myalgia (68%), usually without other specific physical findings. Manifestations of gastrointestinal involvement (nausea, vomiting, or diarrhea), respiratory involvement (cough or pulmonary infiltrates), joint pain, or central nervous system involvement (stiff neck or confusion) are present in a substantial minority of patients. Rash is identified in only 36% and is only infrequently petechial. In spite of the nonspecific clinical symptoms and signs, laboratory findings are abnormal in at least 86% of patients; these findings include leukopenia (60 to 74%) with lymphopenia and neutropenia, thrombocytopenia (72%), and increased aspartate transaminase activities in serum (86 to 88%). Severe complications include a toxic shock-like syndrome with multiorgan failure, meningoencephalitis, diffuse alveolar damage associated with adult respiratory distress syndrome, and fulminant infections in patients immunocompromised by human immunodeficiency virus, high-dose corticosteroids, or organ transplantation (5, 29, 32, 47, 51, 60). The case fatality rate of approximately 2 to 3% would be higher if effective antimicrobial therapy were not available.

Human Granulocytotropic Ehrlichiosis

The causative agent of HGE, an ehrlichia that is virtually indistinguishable from the veterinary pathogens *E. phagocytophila* and *E. equi* by routine molecular and serologic methods (17, 24), causes an illness identical to *E. equi* and *E. phagocytophila* infection in horses and goats, respectively (10, 33, 45). HGE was first identified in 1990 in a patient from Wisconsin who sustained tick bites in an area where *E. chaffeensis* and its tick vector do not exist (7). As with HME, HGE is not a reportable illness in most states; thus, the true incidence and prevalence of the infection are unknown. However, prospective passive case collection in northwestern Wisconsin during 1990 through 1995 revealed a yearly incidence rate of 16 cases per 100,000 population, with peak rates identified as high as 58 cases per 100,000 population in some counties in 1995 (9). Since 1990, more than 350 cases of HGE were identified by the CDC, with more than half being found in southeastern New York State and nearly 40% being found in northwestern Wisconsin and northeastern Minnesota. Infected patients were identified in many other states and in several European countries (14, 25, 54, 65, 67). Subclinical infection is probably the norm, since nearly 14% of the population assessed in northwestern Wisconsin have antibodies indicative of prior infection (8). The tick vectors for HME and HGE coexist in the mid-Atlantic and southern New England states, as well as in the southern Midwest. Thus, both diseases can occur in these areas.

The illness has a median incubation period of 5 to 11 days after *Ixodes* spp. tick bites and occurs in patients with a median age of 43 to 60 years (1, 9). Twice as many men have the illness as women. Most patients present with high fever, myalgias, headache, and malaise; gastrointestinal, respiratory, musculoskeletal, or central nervous system involvement is found in fewer patients. Rash is observed in fewer than 11% of patients. Leukopenia, thrombocytopenia, and increased aspartate transaminase activities in serum are present in most patients. Severe complications of HGE include a septic shock-like illness with multiorgan failure, adult respiratory distress syndrome, and opportunistic infections (9, 37, 68). At least five deaths have been associated with HGE; at least three of these patients had opportunistic infections including *Candida* esophagitis, *Cryptococcus* pneumonia, invasive pulmonary aspergillosis, and herpes esophagitis (9, 37, 68).

Sennetsu Ehrlichiosis

Named after the Japanese term for mononucleosis, *Ehrlichia sennetsu* was first isolated from patients with suspected infectious mononucleosis in 1953 (48). This illness is rarely identified now. Patients develop a self-limited febrile illness with chills, headache, malaise, sore throat, anorexia, and generalized lymphadenopathy. Cases were identified only in Japan and possibly Malaysia. Laboratory findings include early leukopenia and atypical lymphocytes in the peripheral blood during early convalescence. No fatalities or severe complications have been reported.

COLLECTION, TRANSPORT, AND STORAGE OF SPECIMENS

Specimens that are obtained for diagnosis or confirmation of HME or HGE include EDTA- or acid citrate dextrose (ACD)-anticoagulated blood or cerebrospinal fluid (CSF) and serum. Because heparin has been associated with significant inhibition of thermostable polymerases, blood samples collected in this anticoagulant should be avoided. Currently, there are three methods of diagnosis during the acute phase of illness, when ehrlichiae are likely to be present in circulating peripheral blood or CSF leukocytes: (i) PCR amplification of *Ehrlichia* nucleic acids, (ii) detection of *Ehrlichia* morulae in the cytoplasm of infected leukocytes by using nonspecific Romanowsky stains (e.g., Giemsa or Wright) or by using specific immunocytologic or immunohistologic stains with *E. chaffeensis* or *E. phagocytophila* group antibodies, and (iii) culture of *Ehrlichia* species from blood or CSF. EDTA-anticoagulated blood is the most useful specimen for PCR and should be obtained during the acute phase of illness (20, 26, 36). Samples should be tested promptly, but if the blood is maintained at 4°C, it may still be possible to amplify nucleic acids several days to more than a week later. If delays beyond several days are anticipated and testing is still to be performed, the blood should be frozen at −20°C until used. There is less experience with collection and storage of CSF for PCR, but it is expected that similar conditions will yield appropriate results. PCR with serum or plasma is far less sensitive than with samples that contain infected leukocytes.

Peripheral blood smears or cytocentrifuge preparations of CSF cells should be prepared within several hours of obtaining the samples, since the leukocytes begin to degenerate rapidly. Once prepared, the air-dried blood smears and cytocentrifuge CSF preparations are stable at room temperature for months or years.

The culture conditions for *Ehrlichia* species are still being optimized. Currently the preferred specimen for culture is peripheral blood. Samples should be obtained by sterile venipuncture or lumbar puncture and submitted as soon as possible to the laboratory that will attempt culture. Usually, this requires overnight courier service, since culture is currently performed in only a few public health and research laboratories. Samples to be cultured should be maintained at approximately 4°C during shipping; it is important to avoid freezing, since that is likely to reduce the content of viable ehrlichiae. After cultivation, ehrlichia-infected cells may be stored frozen at −80°C for several months or in liquid nitrogen for longer periods. Storage of infected cells is best accomplished when more than 50 to 90% of the host cells are infected and is achieved by suspension of at least 10^6 cells per ml in tissue culture medium that contains 10% dimethyl sulfoxide and at least 30% fetal bovine serum.

ISOLATION PROCEDURES

E. chaffeensis and *E. canis*

E. chaffeensis has been isolated from peripheral blood of only six patients with HME, and *E. canis* has been isolated only once from an asymptomatic human (19, 20, 26, 53, 61). The most frequently used cell for primary isolation has been the canine histiocyte cell line, DH82; however, *E. chaffeensis* has been successfully cultivated in other cells including the human macrophage-like THP-1 cells, the fibroblast-like HEL-22 cells, and Vero cells (12, 13, 19). Isolation may be successful even when infected leukocytes are not observed on examination of peripheral blood. The usual format for isolation involves direct inoculation of whole blood or leukocyte fractions into flasks with a confluent layer of adherent cells or into flasks that contain approximately 2×10^5 to 1×10^6 nonadherent cells per ml of tissue culture medium. Macrophage-like cells that are highly phagocytic may be adversely affected by the presence of numerous erythrocytes; thus, it is recommended that either (i) cell confluency be reestablished after cultivation with erythrocyte-containing samples by addition of uninfected host cells, (ii) leukocytes be harvested after erythrocyte lysis (hypotonic lysis, $NHCl_4$ lysis, etc.), or (iii) leukocytes be fractionated from erythrocytes by density gradient centrifugation (e.g., Ficoll-Hypaque). Since *E. chaffeensis* may be present in a very small proportion of peripheral blood leukocytes, it is usually advisable to inoculate cultures with as many peripheral blood leukocytes as possible. This may be difficult owing to the leukopenia that often accompanies HME. The inoculum is allowed to interact with adherent host cells for several hours; the interaction is usually enhanced by incubation with rocking in a small volume of medium at 37°C. The inoculum may be removed if significant erythrocyte contamination is present; then the correct medium volume is reconstituted with fresh tissue culture medium. Since *Ehrlichia* species are bacteria, the medium must not contain antibiotics. The generation time of *E. chaffeensis* may be 8 h or more, and hence cultures must be maintained to allow a slow logarithmic or stable growth phase to avoid the host cells outgrowing the ehrlichiae. This may be accomplished by treating cells with inhibitors of eukaryotic cell division (e.g., cycloheximide or emetine), by irradiating the cells, or by simply reducing the concentration of fetal bovine serum.

The presence of infected cells is determined by sampling the medium (DH82 cells and THP-1 cells) or by lightly scraping part of the monolayer. These cells are examined by cytocentrifugation followed by application of Romanowsky or immunofluorescent stains for the presence of intracytoplasmic morulae or *E. chaffeensis* antigen (Fig. 2). Culture may require 1 month or more but has been achieved in as little as 1 week (20, 26, 61). Confirmation of the infectious agent is currently best achieved by PCR amplification with species-specific primers (2). Serologic analysis is useful but not specific, since *E. chaffeensis* shares antigens with *E. canis, E. ewingii, Cowdria ruminantium*, and some *E. phagocytophila* group ehrlichiae.

E. phagocytophila Group

The HGE agent has been successfully cultivated more often from human patients than has *E. chaffeensis, E. canis*, or *E. sennetsu* owing to the larger number of organisms that are present in peripheral blood in many infected patients. Isolation is best achieved in the human promyelocyte cell line HL60 and is rarely accomplished when ehrlichiae are not observed in peripheral blood smears. The optimal conditions for recovery of these bacteria have not been conclusively determined, but cultivation in HL60 cells has been achieved with or without the presence of granulocyte-differentiating chemicals (e.g., DMSO or retinoic acid) (36, 38). Because erythrocytes do not adversely affect the HL60 cells, direct inoculation of EDTA-anticoagulated blood is effective. Fractionation of blood into leukocytes by preparation of buffy coat or by isolation of granulocyte fractions by density gradient centrifugation is also effective (59). Ordinarily, 100 to 500 μl of blood that contains approximately 10^2 to 10^4 infected neutrophils is inoculated into a total of approximately 100-fold more uninfected HL60 cells that are in the exponential growth phase, and the cells are subsequently maintained at a concentration between 2×10^5 and 1×10^6 cells per ml of tissue culture medium.

Cultures are examined every 2 to 3 days by Romanowsky staining of cytocentrifuged preparations. Ehrlichial morulae appear as small aggregates of basophilic bacteria in the cytoplasm of the HL60 cells (Fig. 3). Since HL60 cells may contain a variety of cytoplasmic granules, immunocytologic testing can be very helpful. Cultures usually require between 5 and 10 days of cultivation before morulae are clearly identified, but infected cells may be detected as early as 3 days postinoculation. Definitive identification is achieved by PCR amplification with species-specific primers (17, 36, 52) or by sequence analysis of 16S rRNA genes that have been amplified by universal eubacterial PCR (17).

Ehrlichia sennetsu

E. sennetsu has been isolated from human peripheral blood and lymph node tissues by mouse inoculation (48). However, *E. sennetsu* is easily propagated in the murine macrophage-like cell line P388D$_1$ (48). It is identified by Romanowsky staining and PCR with species-specific oligonucleotide primers.

IDENTIFICATION

Romanowsky and Immunohistologic Identification

Patients with suspected HME or HGE should have Romanowsky-stained (Giemsa or Wright stain) peripheral blood or buffy coat leukocytes examined for the presence of ehrlichial morulae. This method is very insensitive and has been useful for identifying only about 1% of *E. chaffeensis*-infected patients and between 20 and 80% of patients with HGE (67, 68). Ordinarily, *E. chaffeensis* is detected predominantly in monocytes and *E. phagocytophila* group ehrlichiae are detected predominantly in neutrophils; however, patients with severe disease, with a large percentage of infected cells, may show ehrlichial morulae in atypical cells. Thus, the infected cell type may not absolutely identify the species responsible for the infection (46, 68). When present, ehrlichial morulae are small (1 to 3 μm in diameter), round to oval clusters of bacteria that stain basophilic to amphophilic with Romanowsky stains (Fig. 4). These clusters are present in the cytoplasm and have a stippled appearance owing to the presence of individual bacteria within the vacuole.

Immunohistologic methods may be used to identify *E. chaffeensis* and *E. phagocytophila* group ehrlichiae within human tissues, including bone marrow, liver, and spleen. An immunohistologic study of bone marrow detected *E. chaffeensis* in only 40% of specimens obtained during the active infection (27). Most immunohistologic studies have been performed with polyclonal antibodies that react with other *Ehrlichia* species. A monoclonal antibody may specifically detect *E. chaffeensis* in human tissues (74); however, these antibodies are not readily available except through research laboratories and the CDC.

PCR

PCR is an effective and rapid tool for identification of patients with HME and HGE. This test is available through research and commercial laboratories (e.g., Mayo Medical Laboratories, Rochester, Minn.) and the CDC. The majority of PCR methods are performed with ehrlichial 16S rRNA genes as target sequences for amplification. Several sets of primers that amplify nucleic acids from *E. chaffeensis* and the HGE agent are described, including nested sets that theoretically amplify *Ehrlichia* genus nucleic acids in one reaction followed by species-specific nucleic acids in the second stage reaction.

Ehrlichia chaffeensis

The most widely used PCR method for amplification of *E. chaffeensis* nucleic acids from clinical samples uses the HE1-HE3 primer set (4, 31, 63). This primer pair amplifies a 389-bp fragment that may be detected by simple nucleic acid staining (e.g., with ethidium bromide) after agarose gel electrophoresis or by Southern hybridization of the amplified products with an internal probe that is reported to increase the analytical sensitivity. The only clinical evaluations of *E. chaffeensis* PCR indicate that the HE1-HE3 system has a sensitivity of 79 to 100% compared with detection of *E. chaffeensis* or *E. canis* antibodies during convalescence; however, *E. chaffeensis* nucleic acids were frequently detected in patients who never developed antibodies, a finding of uncertain significance given the high degree of analytical specificity demonstrated with this system (4, 63). Similar results occur when using a nested PCR with broad-range *Ehrlichia* genus primers in an initial step followed by the HE1-HE3 primer pair (63). Other targets for PCR that have not been evaluated for clinical sensitivity or specificity in-

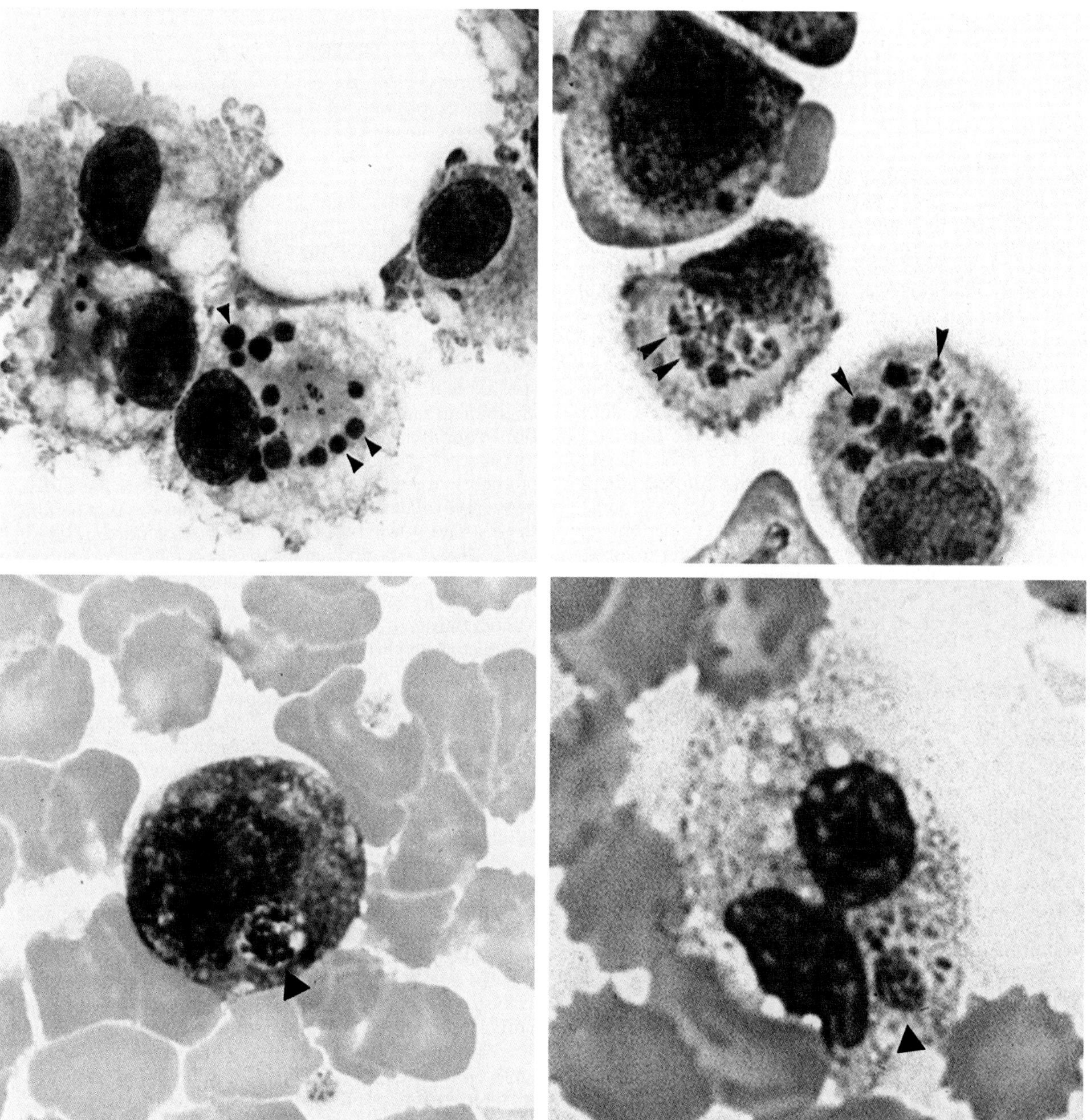

FIGURE 2 (Top left) *E. chaffeensis* cultured in the canine histiocyte cell line, DH82. Note the presence of basophilic, stippled, intracytoplasmic inclusions approximately 2 to 3 μm in diameter (arrows). The smaller intracytoplasmic granules may also be ehrlichial morulae (Romanowsky [Leukostat] stain; original magnification, ×1,000).

FIGURE 3 (Top right) HGE agent cultured in the human promyelocytic cell line, HL60. Note the presence of multiple basophilic, stippled, intracytoplasmic inclusions approximately 2 to 3 μm in diameter (arrows) (Romanowsky [Leukostat] stain; original magnification, ×1,000).

FIGURE 4 (Bottom) *E. chaffeensis* (A [left]) and the HGE agent (B [right]) in peripheral blood leukocytes. Note that the *E. chaffeensis* morula (arrow) is present in a monocyte (A) and that the HGE agent morula (arrow) is present in a neutrophil (B). Neutrophils are sometimes bilobed (pseudo-Pelger-Huet anomaly) in patients with HGE (Wright stain; original magnification, ×1,000).

clude the *groESL* operon, a variable-length repeated region of unknown significance that is present in *E. chaffeensis* (61, 64); the 120-kDa antigen gene that encodes an immunodominant antigen with tandemly repeated subunits that may vary among *E. chaffeensis* isolates; and the quinolinate synthase A gene, *nadA* (61, 76, 77).

Ehrlichia phagocytophila Group

Multiple PCR assays for detection of *E. phagocytophila* group ehrlichial nucleic acids, including the HGE agent, have been described (17, 30, 36, 52, 63). Most use regions of the 16S rRNA gene that are relatively specific to the group as targets for amplification. Since *E. phagocytophila*, *E. equi*, and the HGE agent differ by only 2 or 3 nucleic acids over the nearly 1,500-bp 16S rRNA gene, a specific PCR based on this gene cannot distinguish among these. The most frequently applied and evaluated method uses the primer set ge9f and ge10r, which amplify a 919-bp fragment, most often used as a single-stage reaction, with or without a hybridization probe to enhance sensitivity (17, 30). A popular alternative is the use of nested PCR with an outer set of primers that anneal to and amplify eubacterial 16S rRNA genes, followed by an internal PCR with *E. phagocytophila* group-specific primers (11, 63). To date, only one clinical evaluation to assess sensitivity and specificity has been performed; it compares the assay to a serologic standard and involves modifications to enhance sensitivity, including a proofreading thermostable polymerase and an alternative nucleic acid-binding dye detection (30). These modifications resulted in a 250-fold increase in analytical sensitivity such that <1 infected cell per μl of blood and fewer than 10 copies of *E. phagocytophila* group 16S rRNA genes could be detected. In the prospective evaluation, the PCR detected *E. phagocytophila* group nucleic acids in blood collected during the acute phase for six of seven patients who developed *E. phagocytophila* group antibodies in convalescence and correctly classified 10 suspected patients without seroconversions, for an overall clinical sensitivity of 86% and specificity of 100%. At least one PCR-positive patient from whom an *E. phagocytophila* group ehrlichia was isolated in cell culture never developed a detectable antibody response (1).

Limitations for Ehrlichial Diagnosis

As with all PCR methods, DNA amplicon contamination is a significant problem and should be controlled by use of careful technique, biochemical inactivation methods, and physical separation of PCR setup, amplification, and post-amplification analysis stages. False-positive reactions are a function of the users, primers, and test protocols. Careful selection of primers is required to avoid detection of sequences shared with unrelated organisms. For routine clinical use, nested PCR may be disadvantageous owing to the high potential for amplicon contamination and since one-stage PCRs seem to have very high analytical and clinical sensitivity. PCR is best performed on fresh samples obtained before antimicrobial therapy and early in the course of infection. Once therapy has been instituted, ehrlichial nucleic acids generally become undetectable within several days; however, some untreated patients may have *Ehrlichia* nucleic acids detected in blood for up to 30 days after the onset of illness, when all clinical manifestations have resolved (9, 25, 34, 60). Finally, PCR with 16S rRNA gene targets for *Ehrlichia* species has the potential to amplify sequences from closely related, albeit distinct species that might confound diagnosis (23). Thus, interpretation should include an evaluation of the patient's clinical status for the presence of an illness consistent with the known manifestations of either HME or HGE.

SEROLOGIC TESTS

Most cases of HME and HGE are diagnosed by retrospective serologic confirmation, and serology is the most sensitive method for diagnostic confirmation. Serologic testing for *E. chaffeensis* and *E. phagocytophila* is available through commercial laboratories (e.g., MRL, Highland Heights, Ky.) and public health laboratories. The most widely used test is the indirect fluorescent-antibody (IFA) test, which involves ehrlichia-infected cells fixed to glass slides. Ehrlichial antigens may be difficult to prepare and are available mostly through public health and research laboratories, although commercial production and distribution have begun (available through MRL). Immunoblot procedures are becoming increasingly popular because of the perception of increased specificity (15, 18, 24, 39, 71); all immunoblots should include an uninfected host cell control, since complete separation of ehrlichiae from infected cells is exceedingly difficult.

Currently, there is little standardization for any methods of ehrlichial serologic testing, and cutoff titers are dependent upon validation in individual laboratories that perform these assays. Owing partly to this lack of standardization and perhaps to the antigenic diversity of naturally occurring ehrlichiae, reproducibility of serologic results has been a problem. Although *Ehrlichia* spp. may possess some cross-reactive antigens, two distinct serologic tests are required to detect antibodies for *E. chaffeensis* and for the *E. phagocytophila* group ehrlichiae. The algorithm for serologic testing includes an initial screen at a dilution of 1:64 or 1:80 for antibodies to both *E. chaffeensis* and an *E. phagocytophila* group ehrlichia (often an HGE agent or *E. equi* strain). Reactive samples are then subjected to titer determination. Samples that react with both *E. chaffeensis* and *E. phagocytophila* group may be differentiated by titer determination or immunoblotting.

Ehrlichia chaffeensis IFA Test

E. chaffeensis antibodies are detected by an IFA test with *E. chaffeensis* Arkansas strain-infected DH82 canine macrophage-like cells. Serum is serially diluted starting at a dilution of 1:64. A positive reaction is detected by the demonstration of typical fluorescent intracytoplasmic ehrlichial morula morphology. It is important to identify the appropriate proportion of infected cells as determined by a positive control serum and the appropriate morphology for each antigen preparation to preclude false-positive interpretations. Prescreening for autoantibodies or routine removal of rheumatoid factors will lessen the risk of misinterpretation due to antibodies reactive with cellular components including nuclear and cytoplasmic antigens. A fourfold increase or decrease in antibody titer, with a peak titer or a single convalescent-phase titer of ≥64 in a patient with a consistent clinical history supports the diagnosis of HME. Antibody titers may be detected in a small proportion of subjects without HME owing to the presence of antigens that are highly conserved among bacterial species, including heat shock proteins (22, 71). Acute-phase sera should be obtained at the time of presentation with acute illness, and convalescent-phase sera are best obtained 3 to 6 weeks later (22).

The precise sensitivity and specificity of the IFA test for *E. chaffeensis* are not known but are assumed to be high because of a high degree of correlation of *E. chaffeensis* antibodies in patients with characteristic clinical findings (34).

Although immunoglobulin M (IgM) testing is routinely performed, no evaluation of its sensitivity or specificity in the confirmation of HME has been published. Previously, the serologically cross-reactive *E. canis* was used as a surrogate antigen; however, this serodiagnostic assay has a lower sensitivity than that obtained with *E. chaffeensis*, and its use should be discouraged (4). The role of immunoblotting in diagnosis is not well established; however, many patients with *E. chaffeensis* infection can be differentiated from patients with HGE by the demonstration of antibodies reactive with one or more of the 22-, 28-, 29-, and 120-kDa antigens of *E. chaffeensis* (15, 18). A recombinant 120-kDa protein that has been applied in a dot-blot method appears to offer a sensitive and specific serologic confirmation tool (75). Antibodies to *E. chaffeensis* have also been detected in patients diagnosed with Rocky Mountain spotted fever, Q fever, brucellosis, Lyme disease, and Epstein-Barr virus infections, suggesting that false-positive reactions do occur (22, 71). Antigenic diversity among isolates of *E. chaffeensis* is well described (19), but may not affect the detection of a polyclonal antibody response that is generated with human infection. Several reports have characterized patients with HME without antibody responses, even long after onset (31, 60). However, in the few cases in which *E. chaffeensis* infection has been most clearly proven by cultivation of the agent, patients who survived developed clear serologic reactions detected by IFA methods in convalescence (19, 20, 26, 61). Hypothetical reasons for the false-negative results include infection by antigenically diverse strains (unproven) and abrogation of antibody response by early therapy.

Ehrlichia phagocytophila Group IFA Test

The *E. phagocytophila* group includes three organisms, *E. phagocytophila*, *E. equi*, and the HGE agent, that cannot be distinguished by serologic reactions and probably represent a single species (2, 7, 24, 36, 39). Thus, IFA serologic testing is performed with any of these antigens. Previously, most testing was performed with neutrophils obtained from the blood of animals experimentally infected with *E. phagocytophila* or *E. equi* (7, 24, 45). Currently, the preferred method for testing human sera is the use of an HGE agent isolate propagated in the human HL60 promyelocyte cell line (6, 36, 50). It is now well known that antigenic diversity exists among *E. phagocytophila* group isolates, but it is unclear whether such diversity affects detection under clinical circumstances (6, 78). Most serologic diagnoses of HGE have been rendered by the demonstration of antibodies reactive with *E. equi*. Interpretation of immunofluorescent patterns is similar to that for *E. chaffeensis* and requires an experienced microscopist.

Sera should be screened at a single dilution (1:64 or 1:80) and, if reactive, should be diluted serially to determine the end-point titer. A serologic confirmation of the diagnosis is achieved when a fourfold rise in titer is demonstrated in convalescence with a minimum titer of 80 or when a single antibody titer of ≥80 is demonstrated in a patient with typical clinical features of HGE (1, 9). Approximately 25 to 45% of infected patients will have antibodies at the time of presentation (9); however, up to 14% of the population possess antibodies in some regions of heavy endemic infection, rendering this early serologic information less useful (8).

The sensitivity and specificity of the HGE serologic tests are not established, but both are believed to be high, because of good correlation between typical clinical cases and serologic reactions to *E. phagocytophila* group antigens (1, 9, 72). A role for IgM testing has been suggested when immunoblots are used (39), but it has not been clearly assessed by using IFA tests. An enzyme-linked immunosorbent assay (ELISA)-based method (56) and immunoblotting have been described (6, 24, 39, 71, 78), but their diagnostic utility is still being investigated. Immunoblotting may be used to differentiate between *E. phagocytophila* and *E. chaffeensis* infections by demonstration of antibodies to a major *E. phagocytophila* antigen of approximately 44 kDa in the sera of HGE patients (24, 71).

False-positive reactions have been observed in patients with other rickettsial infections, Q fever, and Epstein-Barr virus infections. Many patients with HGE develop antibodies that react with *Borrelia burgdorferi* by ELISA and demonstrate diagnostic IgG or IgM immunoblots (73). Although some patients have been demonstrated to have concurrent infection with the HGE agent and *B. burgdorferi*, the statistical probability that this mechanism accounts for most of these concurrent positive serologic results is very low (49, 71, 72).

ANTIBIOTIC SUSCEPTIBILITIES

Routine antimicrobial susceptibility testing of *Ehrlichia* isolates is unnecessary. These bacteria are maintained enzootically by transmission among ticks and feral mammalian reservoir hosts (3, 43, 52, 66, 69). The level of exposure of such vertebrate and invertebrate hosts to antimicrobial selection factors is very low, and thus antimicrobial resistance is very unlikely. Most patients with either HME or HGE become afebrile and show clinical improvement within 48 h of starting therapy with a tetracycline antibiotic, including doxycycline, the drug of choice (9, 34). Retrospective analysis of patients with HME has shown significantly higher efficacy for tetracyclines or chloramphenicol than for other broad-spectrum antimicrobial agents (34). In in vitro studies, tetracycline antibiotics are uniformly bactericidal for *Ehrlichia* species, whereas the MICs of chloramphenicol cannot be safely achieved in humans with HME or HGE (16, 42). In contrast, the most frequently used antibiotics for patients who have had recent tick bites, amoxicillin and ceftriaxone, and broad-spectrum antibiotics, such as other cephalosporins, aminoglycosides, and macrolides, that might be prescribed for undifferentiated fever are not effective for inhibition of ehrlichial growth in vitro. The rifamycins (rifampin and rifabutin) can achieve effective inhibition or killing of *Ehrlichia* species in vitro. Although the activity of ciprofloxacin is poor, trovofloxacin has a very low MIC for a human isolate of the *E. phagocytophila* group (42). The clinical efficacy of the rifamycins and trovafloxacin in vivo is not known.

Whereas persistent infections with *Ehrlichia* species may occur frequently in naturally and experimentally infected animals even after treatment with tetracycline (35, 40), persistence of ehrlichiae in humans has rarely been documented (28, 60). Therapy is usually highly effective at eliminating ehrlichiae from the blood of infected humans and allowing recovery.

INTERPRETATION AND REPORTING OF RESULTS

The current algorithm for identification and confirmation of infections by *Ehrlichia* species requires a complete evaluation of the history, physical examination, and laboratory results that will suggest the diagnosis. Before specific tests for etiologic determination are attempted, a decision concerning therapy should be made, since delays may lead to increased morbidity and perhaps mortality. At the time of acute illness and before institution of antiehrlichial therapy, EDTA-anticoagulated blood should be obtained for PCR amplification of *E. chaffeensis* and *E. phagocytophila* group ehrlichiae and considered for the possibility of in vitro cultivation. A peripheral blood or buffy coat smear should be examined for the presence of morulae that would confirm the presumptive diagnosis. Serum should be obtained and tested for antibodies reactive with *E. chaffeensis* or the *E. phagocytophila* group ehrlichiae, with an aliquot being saved for repeat testing when a convalescent-phase serum sample is obtained 3 to 6 weeks later.

The presence of intracytoplasmic inclusions within a leukocyte in peripheral blood might be due to the presence of overlying platelets, Döhle bodies, toxic granulations, nuclear fragments, other bacteria, yeasts or protozoa, inorganic materials, or granules of normal large granular lymphocytes or granulocytes. If the typical morphology of an *Ehrlichia* morula is observed, an assessment of the hematopoietic lineage and the percentage of cells that contain morulae should be made and reported. A report that identifies such structures should state only that structures consistent with *Ehrlichia* morulae have been identified and that definitive identification relies upon other specific laboratory evaluations.

A positive PCR result should be reported as such, indicating the presence of *E. chaffeensis* or *E. phagocytophila* group DNA, and it should be made clear that a positive PCR result is not equivalent to the culture of ehrlichiae from blood. A negative PCR result does not exclude the possibility of HME or HGE. Possible explanations for a false-negative PCR result include (i) an excessively long interval after the onset of clinical manifestations or tick bite until the blood sample was obtained, (ii) administration of antimicrobial therapy before collection of the sample, and (iii) the analytical and clinical sensitivities and specificities of the PCR assay used in the testing laboratory. Detection sensitivity limits should be stated as "xx copies/ml," "xx bacteria/ml," or "xx infected cells/ml," while clinical sensitivity data concerning the laboratory's clinical validation of the assay by using samples from proven patients with and without the disease should be readily available.

IFA serologic test results should be reported as the titer of antibodies determined to be reactive with *E. chaffeensis* or the *E. phagocytophila* group ehrlichiae, including the positive cutoff values determined in the laboratory. An interpretation should indicate whether the titers determined are considered "significant" or "positive" based on a fourfold increase or decrease or as single high-titer sera. Additionally, all interpretations should be made in the context of typical clinical and epidemiologic information. Immunoblot analyses should provide information about antibodies that react with specific antigens considered unique or diagnostic of infection with a single species of *Ehrlichia*.

REFERENCES

1. **Aguero-Rosenfeld, M. E., H. W. Horowitz, G. P. Wormser, D. F. McKenna, J. Nowakowski, J. Munoz, and J. S. Dumler.** 1996. Human granulocytic ehrlichiosis (HGE): a case series from a single medical center in New York State. *Ann. Intern. Med.* **125:**904–908.
2. **Anderson, B. E., J. E. Dawson, D. C. Jones, and K. H. Wilson.** 1991. *Ehrlichia chaffeensis*, a new species associated with human ehrlichiosis. *J. Clin. Microbiol.* **29:**2838–2842.
3. **Anderson, B. E., K. G. Sims, J. G. Olson, J. E. Childs, J. F. Piesman, C. M. Happ, G. O. Maupin, and B. J. B. Johnson.** 1993. *Amblyomma americanum*: a potential vector of human ehrlichiosis. *Am. J. Trop. Med. Hyg.* **49:** 239–244.
4. **Anderson, B. E., J. W. Summer, J. E. Dawson, T. Tzianabos, C. R. Greene, J. G. Olson, D. B. Fishbein, M. Olsen-Rasmussen, B. P. Hollowau, E. H. George, and A. F. Azad.** 1992. Detection of the etiologic agent of human ehrlichiosis by polymerase chain reaction. *J. Clin. Microbiol.* **30:**775–780.
5. **Antony, S. J., J. S. Dummer, and E. Hunter.** 1995. Human ehrlichiosis in a liver transplant recipient. *Transplantation* **60:**879–880.
6. **Asanovich, K. M., J. S. Bakken, J. E. Madigan, M. Aguero-Rosenfeld, G. P. Wormser, and J. S. Dumler.** 1997. Antigenic diversity of granulocytic *Ehrlichia* isolates from humans in Wisconsin and New York and a horse from California. *J. Infect. Dis.* **176:**1029–1034.
7. **Bakken, J. S., J. S. Dumler, S.-M. Chen, M. R. Eckman, L. L. Van Etta, and D. H. Walker.** 1994. Human granulocytic ehrlichiosis in the upper midwest United States. A new species emerging? *JAMA* **272:**212–218.
8. **Bakken, J. S., P. Goellner, S. Mattson, R. L. Tilden, K. Asanovich, J. Walls, and J. S. Dumler.** 1997. Seroprevalence of human granulocytic ehrlichiosis (HGE) among residents in northwestern Wisconsin, abstr. K57. *In Program and Abstracts of the 37th International Conference on Antimicrobial Agents and Chemotherapy*. American Society for Microbiology, Washington, D.C.
9. **Bakken, J. S., J. Krueth, C. Wilson-Nordskog, R. L. Tilden, K. Asanovich, and J. S. Dumler.** 1996. Clinical and laboratory characteristics of human granulocytic ehrlichiosis. *JAMA* **275:**199–205.
10. **Barlough, J. E., J. E. Madigan, E. DeRock, J. S. Dumler, and J. S. Bakken.** 1995. Protection against *Ehrlichia equi* is conferred by prior infection with the human granoulocytotropic ehrlichia (HGE agent). *J. Clin. Microbiol.* **33:** 3333–3334.
11. **Barlough, J. E., J. E. Madigan, E. DeRock, and L. Bigornia.** 1996. Nested polymerase chain reaction for detection of *Ehrlichia equi* genomic DNA in horses and ticks (*Ixodes pacificus*). *Vet. Parasitol.* **63:**319–329.
12. **Barnewell, R. E., Y. Rikihisa, and E. H. Lee.** 1997. *Ehrlichia chaffeensis* inclusions are early endosomes which selectively accumulate transferrin receptor. *Infect. Immun.* **65:** 1455–1461.
13. **Brouqui, P., M. L. Birg, and D. Raoult.** 1994. Cytopathic effect, plaque formation, and lysis of *Ehrlichia chaffeensis* grown on continuous cell lines. *Infect. Immun.* **62:** 405–411.
14. **Brouqui, P., J. S. Dumler, R. Lienhard, M. Brossard, and D. Raoult.** 1995. Human granulocytic ehrlichiosis in Europe. *Lancet* **346:**782–783.
15. **Brouqui, P., C. Lecam, J. Olson, and D. Raoult.** 1994. Serologic diagnosis of human monocytic ehrlichiosis by immunoblot analysis. *Clin. Diagn. Lab. Immunol.* **1:** 645–649.
16. **Brouqui, P., and D. Raoult.** 1992. In vitro antibiotic susceptibility of the newly recognized agent of ehrlichiosis in humans, *Ehrlichia chaffeensis*. *Antimicrob. Agents. Chemother.* **36:**2799–2803.
17. **Chen, S. M., J. S. Dumler, J. S. Bakken, and D. H. Walker.** 1994. Identification of a granulocytotropic *Ehrlichia* species as the etiologic agent of human disease. *J. Clin. Microbiol.* **32:**589–595.
18. **Chen, S. M., J. S. Dumler, H.-M. Feng, and D. H.**

Walker. 1994. Identification of the antigenic constituents of *Ehrlichia chaffeensis*. *Am. J. Trop. Med. Hyg.* **50:**52–58.

19. **Chen, S. M., X. J. Yu, V. L. Popov, E. L. Westerman, F. G. Hamilton, and D. H. Walker.** 1997. Genetic and antigenic diversity of *Ehrlichia chaffeensis*: comparative analysis of a novel human strain from Oklahoma and previously isolated strains. *J. Infect. Dis.* **175:**856–863.
20. **Dawson, J. E., B. E. Anderson, D. B. Fishbein, J. L. Sanchez, C. S. Goldsmith, K. H. Wilson, and C. W. Duntley.** 1991. Isolation and characterization of an *Ehrlichia* from a patient diagnosed with human ehrlichiosis. *J. Clin. Microbiol.* **29:**2741–2745.
21. **Dawson, J. E., and S. A. Ewing.** 1992. Susceptibility of dogs to infection with *Ehrlichia chaffeensis*, the causative agent of human ehrlichiosis. *Am. J. Vet. Res.* **53:** 1322–1327.
22. **Dawson, J. E., D. B. Fishbein, T. R. Eng, M. A. Redus, and N. R. Greene.** 1990. Diagnosis of human ehrlichiosis with the indirect fluorescent antibody test: kinetics and specificity. *J. Infect. Dis.* **162:**91–95.
23. **Dawson, J. E., C. K. Warner, V. Baker, S. A. Ewing, D. E. Stallknecht, W. R. Davidson, A. A. Kocan, J. M. Lockhart, and J. G. Olson.** 1996. *Ehrlichia*-like 16S rDNA sequence from wild white-tailed deer (*Odocoileus virginianus*). *J. Parasitol.* **82:**52–58.
24. **Dumler, J. S., K. M. Asanovich, J. S. Bakken, P. Richter, R. Kimsey, and J. E. Madigan.** 1995. Serologic cross-reaction among *Ehrlichia equi, Ehrlichia phagocytophila,* and human granulocytic ehrlichia. *J. Clin. Microbiol.* **33:** 1098–1103.
25. **Dumler, J. S., and J. S. Bakken.** 1996. Human granulocytic ehrlichiosis in Wisconsin and Minnesota: a frequent infection with the potential for persistence. *J. Infect. Dis.* **173:**1027–1030.
26. **Dumler, J. S., S. M. Chen, K. Asanovich, et al.** 1995. Isolation and characterization of a new strain of *Ehrlichia chaffeensis* from a patient with nearly fatal monocytic ehrlichiosis. *J. Clin. Microbiol.* **33:**1704–1711.
27. **Dumler, J. S., J. E. Dawson, and D. H. Walker.** 1993. Human ehrlichiosis: hematopathology and immunohistologic detection of *Ehrlichia chaffeensis*. *Hum. Pathol.* **24:** 391–396.
28. **Dumler, J. S., W. L. Sutker, and D. H. Walker.** 1993. Persistent infection with *Ehrlichia chaffeensis*. *Clin. Infect. Dis.* **17:**903–905.
29. **Dunn, B. E., T. P. Monson, J. S. Dumler, C. C. Morris, A. B. Westbrook, J. L. Duncan, J. E. Dawson, K. G. Sims, and B. E. Anderson.** 1992. Identification of *Ehrlichia chaffeensis* morulae in cerebrospinal fluid mononuclear cells. *J. Clin. Microbiol.* **30:**2207–2210.
30. **Edelman, D. C., and J. S. Dumler.** 1996. Evaluation of an improved PCR diagnostic assay for human granulocytic ehrlichiosis. *Mol. Diagn.* **1:**41–49.
31. **Everett, E. D., K. A. Evans, R. B. Henry, and G. McDonald.** 1994. Human ehrlichiosis in adults after tick exposure: diagnosis using polymerase chain reaction. *Ann. Intern. Med.* **120:**730–735.
32. **Fichtenbaum, C. J., L. R. Peterson, and G. J. Weil.** 1993. Ehrlichiosis presenting as a life-threatening illness with features of the toxic shock syndrome. *Am. J. Med.* **95:** 351–357.
33. **Fish, D., M. Papero, C. Gingrich-Baker, and R. T. Coughlin.** 1997. Natural and experimental infections of domestic sheep with the agent of human granulocytic ehrlichiosis, abstr. 75. *In Program and Abstracts of the Thirteenth Sesqui-Annual Meeting of the American Society for Rickettsiology.*
34. **Fishbein, D. B., J. E. Dawson, and L. E. Robinson.** 1994. Human ehrlichiosis in the United States, 1985 to 1990. *Ann. Intern. Med.* **120:**736–743.
35. **Foggie A.** 1951. Studies on the infectious agent of tick-borne fever in sheep. *J. Pathol. Bacteriol.* **63:**1–15.
36. **Goodman, J. L., C. Nelson, B. Vitale, J. S. Dumler, J. E. Madigan, T. J. Kurtti, and U. G. Munderloh.** 1996. Direct cultivation of the causative agent of human granulocytic ehrlichiosis. *N. Engl. J. Med.* **334:**262–263.
37. **Hardalo, C., V. Quagliarello, and J. S. Dumler.** 1995. Human granulocytic ehrlichiosis in Connecticut: report of a fatal case. *Clin. Infect. Dis.* **21:**910–914.
38. **Heimer, R., A. Van Andel, G. P. Wormser, and M. L. Wilson.** 1997. Propagation of granulocytic *Ehrlichia* spp. from human and equine sources in HL-60 cells induced to differentiate into functional granulocytes. *J. Clin. Microbiol.* **35:**923–927.
39. **IJdo, J. W., Y. Zhang, E. Hodzic, L. A. Magnarelli, M. L. Wilson, S. R. Telford III, S. W. Barthold, and E. Fikrig.** 1997. The early humoral response in human granulocytic ehrlichiosis. *J. Infect. Dis.* **176:**687–692.
40. **Iqbal, Z., and Y. Rikihisa.** 1994. Reisolation of *Ehrlichia canis* from blood and tissues of dogs after doxycycline treatment. *J. Clin. Microbiol.* **32:**1644–1649.
41. **Jongejan, F., L. A. Wassink, M. J. C. Thielemans, N. M. Perie, and G. Uilenberg.** 1989. Serotypes in *Cowdria ruminantium* and their relationship with *Ehrlichia phagocytophila* determined by immunofluorescence. *Vet. Microbiol.* **21:**31–40.
42. **Klein M. B., C. M. Nelson, and J. L. Goodman.** 1997. Antibiotic susceptibility of the newly cultivated agent of human granulocytic ehrlichiosis: promising activity of quinolones and rifamycins. *Antimicrob. Agents. Chemother.* **41:**76–79.
43. **Lockhart, J. M., W. R. Davidson, D. E. Stallknecht, J. E. Dawson, and E. W. Howerth.** 1997. Isolation of *Ehrlichia chaffeensis* from wild white-tailed deer (*Odocoileus virginianus*) confirms their role as natural reservoir hosts. *J. Clin. Microbiol.* **35:**1681–1686.
44. **MacLeod, J. R., and W. S. Gordon.** 1933. Studies in tick-borne fever of sheep. Transmission by the tick, *Ixodes ricinus*, with a description of the disease produced. *Parsitology* **25:**273–285.
45. **Madigan, J. E., P. J. Richter, R. B. Kimsey, J. E. Barlough, J. S. Bakken, and J. S. Dumler.** 1995. Transmission and passage in horses of the agent of human granulocytic ehrlichiosis. *J. Infect. Dis.* **172:**1141–1144.
46. **Maeda, K., N. Markowitz, R. C. Hawley, M. Ristic, D. Cox, and J. McDade.** 1987. Human infection with *Ehrlichia canis*, a leukocytic rickettsia. *N. Engl. J. Med.* **316:** 853–856.
47. **Marty, A. M., J. S. Dumler, G. Imes, H. P. Brusman, L. L. Smrkovski, and D. M. Frisman.** 1995. Ehrlichiosis mimicking thrombotic thrombocytopenic purpura. Case report and pathological correlation. *Hum. Pathol.* **26:** 920–925.
48. **Misao, T., and Y. Kobayashi.** 1954. Studies on infectious mononucleosis. I. Isolation of etiologic agent from blood, bone marrow, and lymph node of a patient with infectious mononucleosis by using mice. *Tokyo Iji Shinshi* **71:** 683–686.
49. **Nadelman, R. B., H. W. Horowitz, T.-C. Hsieh, J. M. Wu, M. Aguero-Rosenfeld, L. Schwartz, J. Nowakowski, S. Varde, and G. P. Wormser.** 1997. Simultaneous human granulocytic ehrlichiosis and Lyme borreliosis. *N. Engl. J. Med.* **337:**27–30.
50. **Nicholson, W. L., J. A. Comer, J. W. Sumner, C. Gingrich-Baker, R. T. Coughlin, L. A. Magnarelli, J. G. Olson, and J. E. Childs.** 1997. An indirect immunofluorescent assay using a cell culture-derived antigen for detection

of antibodies to the agent of human granulocytic ehrlichiosis. *J. Clin. Microbiol.* **35:**1510–1516.

51. **Paddock, C. D., D. P. Suchard, K. L. Grumbach, W. K. K. Hadley, R. L. Kerschmann, N. W. Abbey, J. E. Dawson, B. E. Anderson, K. G. Sims, J. S. Dumler, and B. G. Herndier.** 1993. Fatal seronegative ehrlichiosis in a patient with HIV infection. *N. Engl. J. Med.* **329:**1164–1167.
52. **Pancholi, P., C. P. Kolbert, P. D. Mitchell, K. D. Reed, J. S. Dumler, J. S. Bakken, and S. R. Telford III.** 1995. *Ixodes dammini* as a potential vector of human granulocytic ehrlichiosis. *J. Infect. Dis.* **172:**1007–1012.
53. **Perez, M., Y. Rikihisa, and B. Wen.** 1996. *Ehrlichia canis*-like agent isolated from a man in Venezuela: antigenic and genetic characterization. *J. Clin. Microbiol.* **34:**2133–2139.
54. **Petrovec, M., S. L. Furlan, T. A. Zupanc, F. Strle, P. Brouqui, V. Roux, and J. S. Dumler.** 1997. Human disease in Europe caused by a granulocytic *Ehrlichia*. *J. Clin. Microbiol.* **35:**1556–1559.
55. **Popov, V. L., S.-M. Chen, H.-M. Feng, and D. H. Walker.** 1995. Ultrastructural variation of cultured *Ehrlichia chaffeensis*. *J. Med. Microbiol.* **43:**411–421.
56. **Ravyn, M. D., J. L. Goodman, C. B. Kodner, D. K. Westad, L. A. Coleman, S. M. Engstrom, C. M. Nelson, and R. C. Johnson.** 1998. Immunodiagnosis of human granulocytic ehrlichiosis by using culture-derived human isolates. *J. Clin. Microbiol.* **36:**1480–1488.
57. **Richter, P. J., R. B. Kimsey, J. E. Madigan, et al.** 1996. *Ixodes pacificus* as a vector of *Ehrlichia equi*. *J. Med. Entomol.* **33:**1–5.
58. **Rikihisa, Y.** 1991. The tribe *Ehrlichieae* and ehrlichial diseases. *Clin. Microbiol. Rev.* **4:**286–308.
59. **Rikihisa, Y., N. Zhi, G. P. Wormser, B. Wen, H. W. Horowitz, and K. E. Hechemy.** 1997. Ultrastructural and antigenic characterization of a granulocytic ehrlichiosis agent directly isolated and stably cultivated from a patient in New York state. *J. Infect. Dis.* **175:**210–213.
60. **Roland, W. E., G. McDonald, C. W. Cauldwell, and E. D. Everett.** 1995. Ehrlichiosis—a cause of prolonged fever. *Clin. Infect. Dis.* **20:**821–825.
61. **Shore, G. M., S. M. Folk, D. C. Bartley, J. W. Sumner, and C. D. Paddock.** 1997. *Ehrlichia chaffeensis* infection in persons with HIV infection: clinical, microbiologic and epidemiologic features of three patients, abstr. 82. *In Program and Abstracts of the Thirteenth Sesqui-Annual Meeting of the American Society for Rickettsiology*.
62. **Smith, R. D., D. M. Sells, E. H. Stephenson, M. Ristic, and D. L. Huxsoll.** 1997. Development of *Ehrlichia canis*, causative agent of canine ehrlichiosis, in the tick *Rhipicephalus sanguineus* and its differentiation from a symbiotic rickettsia. *Am. J. Vet. Res.* **37:**119–126.
63. **Standaert, S. M., J. E. Dawson, W. Schaffner, J. E. Childs, K. L. Biggie, J. Singleton, Jr., R. R. Gerhardt, M. L. Knight, and R. H. Hutcheson.** 1995. Ehrlichiosis in a golf-oriented retirement community. *N. Engl. J. Med.* **333:**420–425.
64. **Sumner, J. W., K. G. Sims, D. C. Jones, and B. E. Anderson.** 1993. *Ehrlichia chaffeensis* expresses an immunoreactive protein homologous to the *Escherichia coli* GroEL protein. *Infect. Immun.* **61:**3536–3539.
65. **Sumption, K. J., D. J. M. Wright, S. J. Cutler, and B. A. S. Dale.** 1995. Human ehrlichiosis in the UK. *Lancet* **346:**1487–1488.
66. **Telford, S. R. III, J. E. Dawson, P. Katavolos, et al.** 1996. Perpetuation of the agent of human granulocytic ehrlichiosis in a deer tick-rodent cycle. *Proc. Natl. Acad. Sci. USA* **93:**6209–6214.
67. **Walker, D. H., and J. S. Dumler.** 1996. Emergence of ehrlichioses as human health problems. *Emerging Infect. Dis.* **2:**18–29.
68. **Walker, D. H., and J. S. Dumler.** 1997. Human monocytic and granulocytic ehrlichioses. Discovery and diagnosis of emerging tick-borne infections and the critical role of the pathologist. *Arch. Pathol. Lab. Med.* **121:**785–791.
69. **Walls, J. J., B. Greig, D. S. Neitzel, and J. S. Dumler.** 1997. Natural infection of small mammal species in Minnesota with the agent of human granulocytic ehrlichiosis. *J. Clin. Microbiol.* **35:**853–855.
70. **Weiss, E., and J. W. Moulder.** 1984. The rickettsias and chlamydias, p. 687–739. *In* N. R. Krieg and J. G. Holt (ed.), *Bergey's Manual of Determinative Bacteriology*, vol. 1. The Williams & Wilkins Co., Baltimore, Md.
71. **Wong, S. J., G. S. Brady, and J. S. Dumler.** 1997. Serological responses to *Ehrlichia equi*, *Ehrlichia chaffeensis*, and *Borrelia burgdorferi* in patients from New York state. *J. Clin. Microbiol.* **35:**2198–2205.
72. **Wormser, G., D. McKenna, M. Aguero-Rosenfeld, H. Horowitz, J. Munoz, J. Nowakowski, G. Gerina, P. Welch, H. Moorjani, T. Rush, G. Jacquette, A. Stankey, R. Falco, M. Rapoport, D. Ackman, J. Talarico, D. White, L. Frielander, R. Gallo, G. Brady, M. Mauer, S. Wong, R. Duncan, L. Kingsley, R. Taylor, G. Birkhead, D. Morse, and J. S. Dumler.** 1995. Human granulocytic ehrlichiosis—New York. *Morbid. Mortal. Weekly Rep.* **44:**593–595.
73. **Wormser, G. P., H. W. Horowitz, J. Nowakowski, et al.** 1997. Positive Lyme disease serology in patients with clinical and laboratory evidence of human granulocytic ehrlichiosis. *Am. J. Clin. Pathol.* **107:**142–147.
74. **Yu, X., P. Brouqui, J. S. Dumler, and D. Raoult.** 1993. Detection of *Ehrlichia chaffeensis* in human tissue by using a species-specific monoclonal antibody. *J. Clin. Microbiol.* **31:**3284–3288.
75. **Yu, X.-J., P. Crocquet-Valdes, L. C. Cullman, and D. H. Walker.** 1996. The recombinant 120-kilodalton protein of *Ehrlichia chaffeensis*, a potential diagnostic tool. *J. Clin. Microbiol.* **34:**2853–2855.
76. **Yu, X.-J., P. Crocquet-Valdes, and D. H. Walker.** 1997. Cloning and sequencing of the gene for a 120-kDa immunodominant protein of *Ehrlichia chaffeensis*. *Gene* **184:**149–154.
77. **Yu, X., J. F. Piesman, J. G. Olson, and D. H. Walker.** 1997. Geographic distribution of different genetic types of *Ehrlichia chaffeensis*. *Am. J. Trop. Med. Hyg.* **56:**679–680.
78. **Zhi, N., Y. Rikihisa, H. Y. Kim, G. P. Wormser, and H. W. Horowitz.** 1997. Comparison of major antigenic proteins of six strains of the human granulocytic ehrlichiosis agent by Western immunoblot analysis. *J. Clin. Microbiol.* **35:**2606–2611.

VIROLOGY

VOLUME EDITOR
ROBERT H. YOLKEN

SECTION EDITORS
DAVID A. LENNETTE, THOMAS F. SMITH, AND JOSEPH L. WANER

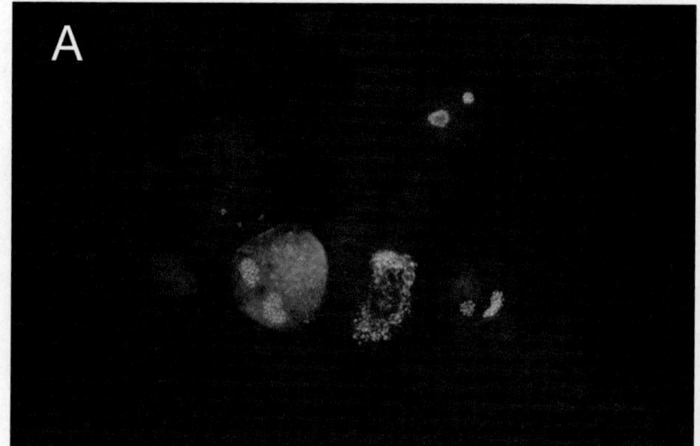

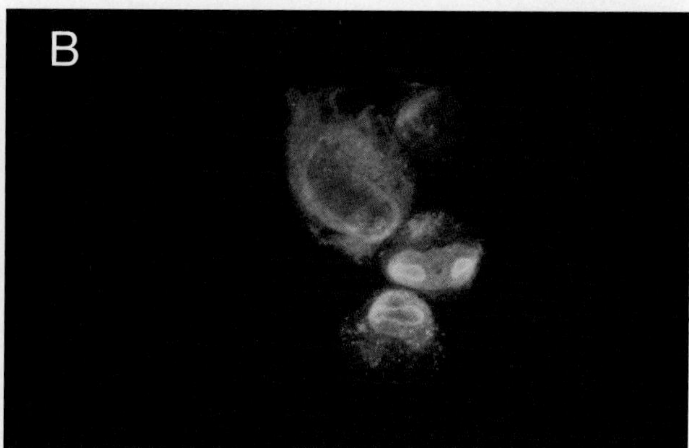

Immunofluorescent intranuclear cytomegalovirus inclusions in cultured human fetal lung cells as recognized by Z02 (A) and Z10 (B), two monoclonal antibodies of human origin (*J. Infect. Dis.* 159:436, 1989).

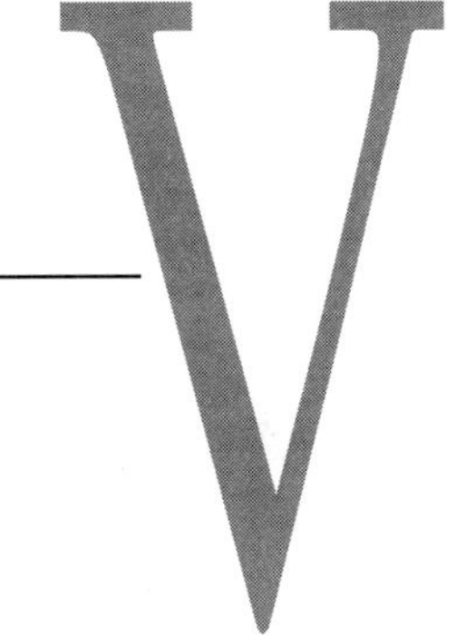

Taxonomy and Classification of Viruses

JOSEPH L. MELNICK

61

Viruses are separated into families on the basis of the type and form of the nucleic acid genome and the size, shape, substructure, and mode of replication of the virus particle. Within each family, classifications of genera and species depend on antigenicity in addition to other properties, particularly the base sequence homology.

Significant developments in classification and nomenclature of viruses are documented in the reports of the International Committee on Taxonomy of Viruses (ICTV), formerly the International Committee on Nomenclature of Viruses. These reports, published in 1971 (10), 1976 (3), 1979 (6), and 1982 (7), have dealt with viruses of humans, lower animals, insects, plants, bacteria, and fungi and have included summaries of the properties of those groups of viruses as related to their taxonomic placements. Recent decisions of the ICTV were summarized in an interim report published in 1989 (2) and in more definitive reports published in 1991 (5) and 1995 (9).

It seems probable that most of the major groups of viruses, particularly those infecting humans and the vertebrate animals of direct importance to humans, have been recognized. Many of the viruses have now been officially placed in families, genera, and species; within some families, subfamilies or subgenera or both have also been established. Although the focus of this chapter is on these families, progress also has been made with respect to the taxonomy of the viruses of other host groups. For a more detailed discussion of virus taxonomy, references 1 through 10 are recommended to the reader.

The ICTV has approved 73 families and groups of viruses. The kind and strandedness of the viral nucleic acid and the presence or absence of a lipoprotein envelope are the three key properties that form the basis for the classification of the 73 families and groups. These families and groups have been assigned to clusters, six of which infect vertebrates as shown in Fig. 1. Within these clusters, families are further classified on the basis of virion morphology and strategy of genomic replication.

In Table 1, properties of the major families of RNA-containing viruses of humans and other vertebrate animals are summarized; in Table 2, vertebrate viruses with a DNA genome are similarly treated. In Table 3, all of these families are listed along with the genera and individual viruses that may be of special concern for the viral diagnostic laboratory. Subfamilies are also included if they represent agents having direct or indirect bearing on human diseases. Thus, the family *Herpesviridae* includes subfamilies. Members recently added to this family include human herpesviruses which have not yet been placed in a genus. Since most of these viral agents are dealt with more fully in the other chapters of this section, the text that follows is confined to an explanation of and commentary on some examples from the tables, together with some notes about recent developments.

PICORNAVIRIDAE

The members of the family *Picornaviridae*, the smallest of the vertebrate viruses with RNA genomes, have been classed in five genera and several hundred species. One human picornavirus, echovirus type 22, remains unclassified.

Sixty-seven members of the genus *Enterovirus* are known to infect humans; these include polioviruses, coxsackieviruses of the A and B groups, echoviruses, and enterovirus serotypes that have been assigned sequential numbers rather than being placed in the echovirus or coxsackievirus subgroups (since the distinctions among these groups have been found to be less sharp than was recognized when these subdivisions were initially established).

More than 115 viruses infecting humans belong to the genus *Rhinovirus*. A third genus in the family is *Cardiovirus*, typified by encephalomyocarditis virus of mice, which may also (rarely) infect humans. A fourth genus, *Aphthovirus*, includes the economically important foot-and-mouth disease viruses of cattle.

After decades of investigation, hepatitis A virus has been classified as a picornavirus, genus *Hepatovirus*. Although it resembles enteroviruses in many respects, it differs in amino acid sequences and also in its greater resistance to thermal inactivation.

The picornavirus genome is one piece of linear, single-stranded, positive-sense RNA of low molecular weight (about 2.5×10^6). The RNA is infectious and serves as its own messenger for protein translation. The virion is about 27 nm in diameter; it contains 60 copies of each of the four major polypeptides. The enteroviruses and cardioviruses are acid stable and have a buoyant density in CsCl of about 1.34 g/cm^3; in contrast, the rhinoviruses and aphthoviruses are acid labile and have higher buoyant densities of about 1.4 g/cm^3. The base sequences of representative viral genomes have been determined, and the three-dimensional structure of the virion has been established.

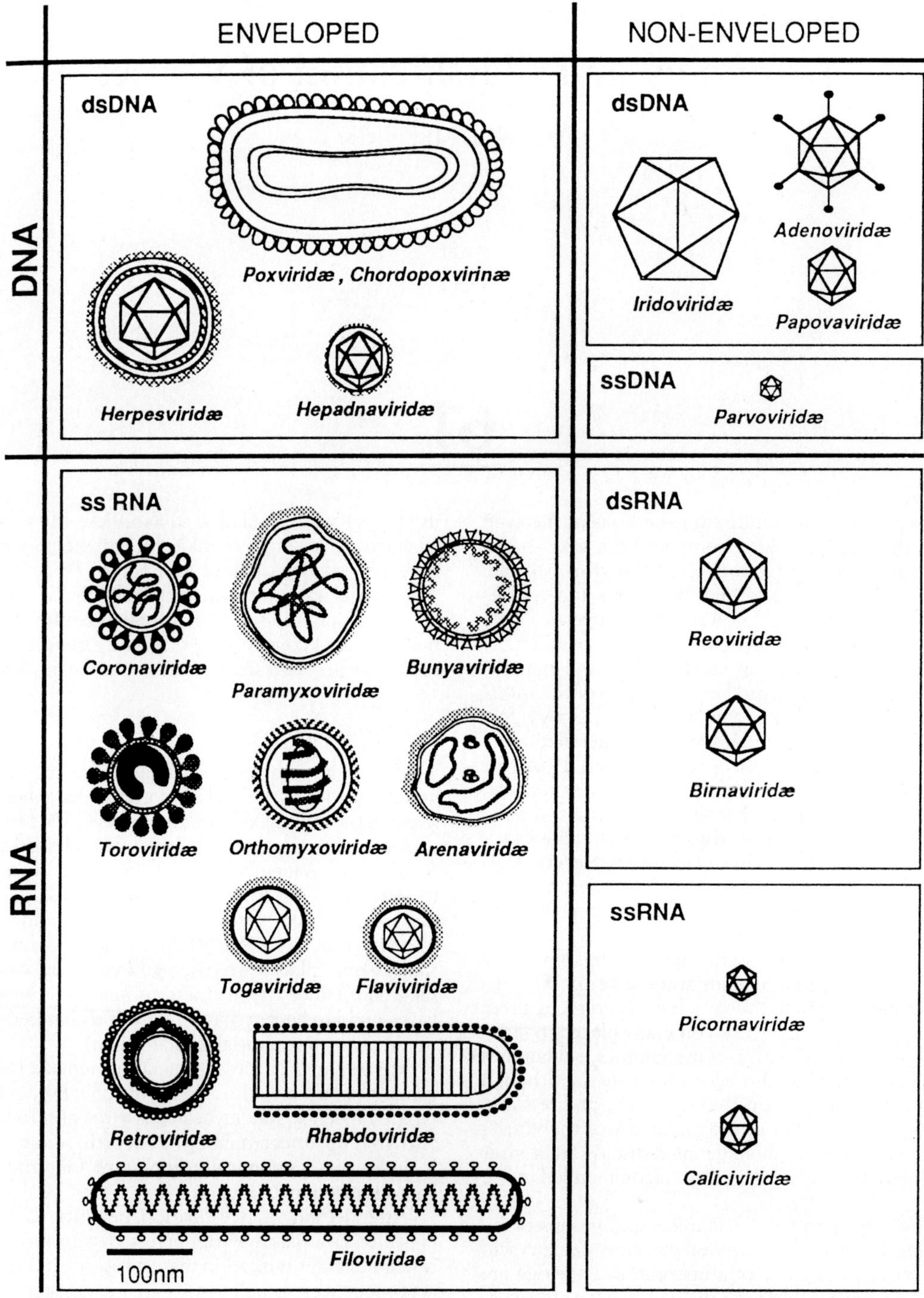

FIGURE 1 ICTV drawings of viruses in the common virus families of vertebrates. All the diagrams are drawn similarly: vertical lines separate enveloped and nonenveloped viruses, and horizontal lines separate DNA and RNA viruses. Within each of the resulting four sections, single-stranded (ss) and double-stranded (ds) genomes are indicated. As stated by the ICTV (5), "All the diagrams have been drawn approximately to the same scale to provide an indication of the relative sizes of the viruses; but this cannot be taken as definitive for the following reasons. (i) Different viruses within a family or genus may vary somewhat in size and shape. In general, the size and shape were taken from the type member of the taxon. (ii) Dimensions of some viruses are difficult to determine or only approximately known. (iii) Some viruses, particularly the larger enveloped ones, are pleomorphic. Only the outlines of most of the smallest viruses are given, with an indication of the icosahedral structure whenever appropriate. The large viruses are given schematically in surface outline, in section, or both, as seems most appropriate to display major morphological characteristics."

TABLE 1 Current classification of chief RNA-containing viruses of vertebrates

Characteristic	Classification													
Nucleic acid core	RNA													
Capsid symmetry	Icosahedral					Unknown or complex				Helical				
Virion: naked or enveloped	Naked				Enveloped	Enveloped				Enveloped				
Site of capsid assembly	Cytoplasm				Cytoplasm	Cytoplasm				Cytoplasm[a]				
Site of nucleocapsid envelopment					Plasma membrane[b]	Intracytoplasmic membranes		Plasma membrane		Plasma membrane				Intracytoplasmic membranes
Reaction to ether treatment	Resistant				Sensitive	Sensitive		Sensitive		Sensitive				Sensitive
No. of capsomeres	32	32	132	?	42									
Ribonucleoprotein helix diam (nm)							11–13			50	9–15	18	18	10–12
Virion diam (nm)	28–30	27–38	60–80	28–30	50–70	45–60	80–220	50–300	80–100	80 x 1,000	80–120	150–300	75 x 180	80–120
Size of nucleic acid in virion (kb/kbp)	7.2–8.4	7.4–7.7	16–27	7.2–7.9	9.7–11.8	9.5–12.5	20–30	10–14	7–11	19.1	10–13.6	16–20	13–16	11–21
Family	*Picornaviridae*	*Caliciviridae*	*Reoviridae*	*Astroviridae*	*Togaviridae*	*Flaviviridae*	*Coronaviridae*	*Arenaviridae*	*Retroviridae*	*Filoviridae*	*Orthomyxoviridae*	*Paramyxoviridae*	*Rhabdoviridae*	*Bunyaviridae*

[a] Capsid assembly of orthomyxoviruses occurs in the nucleus.
[b] Intracytoplasmic membranes for rubella virus.

TABLE 2 Current classification of the chief DNA-containing viruses of vertebrates

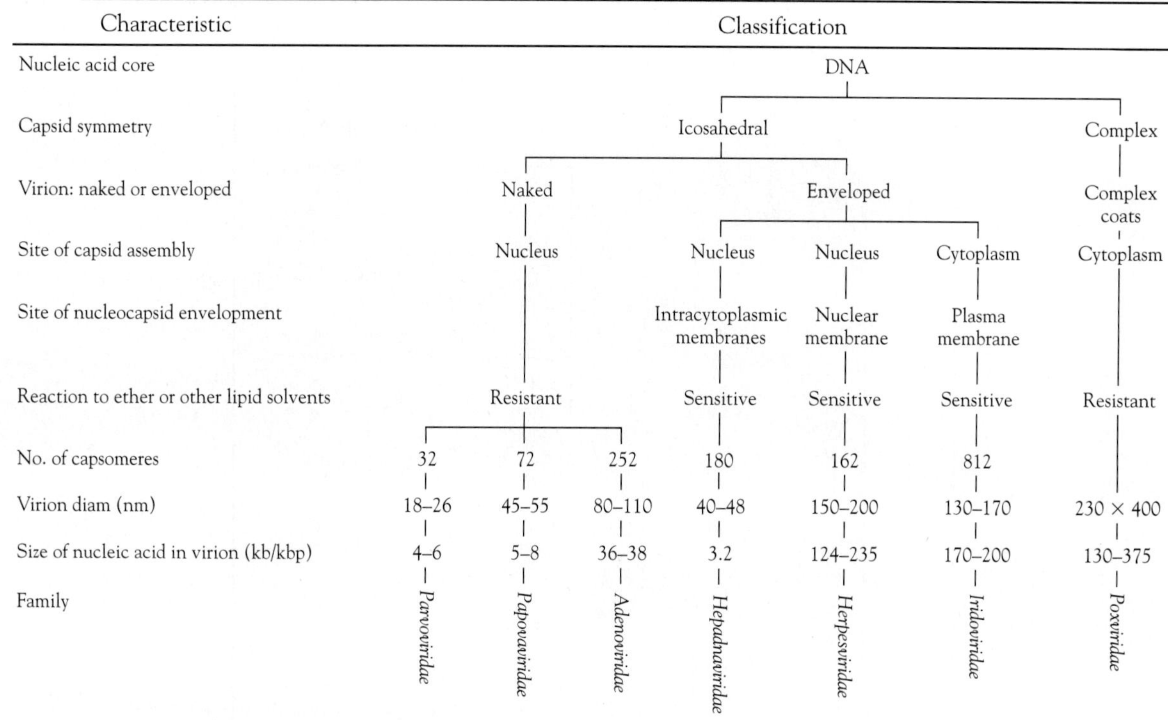

Characteristic	Classification						
Nucleic acid core	DNA	DNA	DNA	DNA	DNA	DNA	DNA
Capsid symmetry	Icosahedral	Icosahedral	Icosahedral	Icosahedral	Icosahedral	Icosahedral	Complex
Virion: naked or enveloped	Naked	Naked	Naked	Enveloped	Enveloped	Enveloped	Complex coats
Site of capsid assembly	Nucleus	Nucleus	Nucleus	Nucleus	Nucleus	Cytoplasm	Cytoplasm
Site of nucleocapsid envelopment				Intracytoplasmic membranes	Nuclear membrane	Plasma membrane	
Reaction to ether or other lipid solvents	Resistant	Resistant	Resistant	Sensitive	Sensitive	Sensitive	Resistant
No. of capsomeres	32	72	252	180	162	812	
Virion diam (nm)	18–26	45–55	80–110	40–48	150–200	130–170	230 × 400
Size of nucleic acid in virion (kb/kbp)	4–6	5–8	36–38	3.2	124–235	170–200	130–375
Family	*Parvoviridae*	*Papovaviridae*	*Adenoviridae*	*Hepadnaviridae*	*Herpesviridae*	*Iridoviridae*	*Poxviridae*

The diseases caused by picornaviruses range from paralytic poliomyelitis to aseptic meningitis, hepatitis, pleurodynia, myocarditis, skin rashes, and common colds; inapparent infection is very common. Different viruses may produce the same syndrome; on the other hand, a single picornavirus may cause several different syndromes. Strain differentiation among the polioviruses is of direct concern in public health and medical virology. In the years since 1951 (when the existence of three poliovirus serotypes became known), genomic differences within serotypes have been demonstrated, but the long-established strains used in the vaccines continue to confer excellent immunity against current wild strains.

CALICIVIRIDAE

Other recent additions to the taxonomic roll of RNA-containing viruses are the members of the families *Caliciviridae* and *Bunyaviridae*. The family *Caliciviridae* includes a number of viruses of pigs, cats, sea lions, and humans. Calicivirus particles have been observed in human feces in association with gastroenteritis. Norwalk virus, a widespread human agent causing acute epidemic gastroenteritis, is a calicivirus. Human caliciviruses have not yet been successfully adapted to tissue culture, but the Norwalk virus has been cloned and the capsid protein has been expressed in a baculovirus system to yield an abundance of nucleic acid-free shells that are similar in size and shape to those of Norwalk virus. These empty virus-like particles are proving useful in diagnosis and in epidemiologic studies. Other morphologically similar viruses associated with gastroenteritis and named according to the location of the outbreak include Hawaii, Montgomery, and Snow Mountain viruses, which seem to be separate serotypes of caliciviruses. Human hepatitis E virus is a calicivirus.

BUNYAVIRIDAE

Members of the *Bunyaviridae* form a family of more than 220 viruses, at least 145 of which belong to the *Bunyaviridae* supergroup of serologically interrelated arboviruses. With the taxonomic placement of this large group, the vast majority of the viruses of the classic arbovirus groupings, initially based on ecological properties and subdivided by serologic interrelationships, have been assigned to families on the basis of biophysical and biochemical characteristics. Human illness caused by Hantaan virus has been recognized in the Far East as Korean hemorrhagic fever, and a variant is known in Scandinavian and eastern European countries as epidemic nephropathy. The illness has been variously named "hemorrhagic fever with renal syndrome" or "muroid virus nephropathy." The agents of these diseases are now established as a genus, *Hantavirus*. The virus has a labile membrane and a tripartite single-stranded RNA genome. The most common natural hosts are mice (in Korea) and voles (in Europe). There have been several instances of infection of staff members handling laboratory rats infected with the virus, both in the Far East and more recently in Europe. Cases of human infection were reported from the southwestern United States in 1993, presenting as an adult respiratory distress syndrome. The hantavirus agent of this disease was named "Sin Nombre virus."

REOVIRIDAE

The RNA genome is single stranded in all of the virus families listed in Table 1 except the family *Reoviridae*, whose RNA is double stranded. Three serotypes within the genus *Reovirus* infect humans, monkeys, dogs, and cattle; in addition, at least five avian reoviruses are known.

Important human pathogens include Colorado tick fever

TABLE 3 Members of virus families, with emphasis on viruses that infect humans

Family	Genus	Common species
Picornaviridae	*Enterovirus*	Polioviruses
		Coxsackieviruses, group A
		Coxsackieviruses, group B
		Echoviruses
		Enteroviruses 68 through 71
		Viruses of other vertebrates
	Hepatovirus	Hepatitis A virus
		Hepatitis A virus of monkeys
	Cardiovirus	Encephalomyocarditis virus and mengovirus; mouse encephalomyelitis virus
	Rhinovirus	Virus types infecting humans
		Viruses of cattle
	Aphthovirus	Foot-and-mouth disease viruses of cattle and other cloven-hoofed animals
Caliciviridae	*Calicivirus*	Vesicular exanthema of swine virus
		Human hepatitis E virus
		Norwalk group of gastroenteritis viruses
Reoviridae	*Orthoreovirus*	Viruses of humans, monkeys, and lower vertebrates
		Viruses of birds
	Coltivirus	Colorado tick fever virus
	Orbivirus	17 subgroups, including Kemerovo virus of humans; also bluetongue virus of sheep and African horse sickness virus
	Rotavirus	Human rotaviruses
		Rotaviruses of many mammals, including SA-11 virus of monkeys and Nebraska calf diarrhea virus
Birnaviridae	*Birnavirus*	Infectious pancreatic necrosis virus of fish; infectious bursal disease virus of chickens
Togaviridae	*Alphavirus*	Sindbis virus and many other mosquito-borne viruses, including eastern, Venezuelan, and western equine encephalitis viruses and Semliki Forest virus
	Rubivirus	Rubella virus
Flaviviridae	*Pestivirus*	Viruses of cattle and pigs
	Flavivirus	Yellow fever virus and other mosquito-borne viruses, including viruses of dengue; of Japanese, Murray Valley, and St. Louis encephalitis; and of West Nile fever
		Tick-borne viruses, including viruses of Kyasanur Forest disease, Omsk hemorrhagic fever, European and Far Eastern tick-borne encephalitis of humans, and louping ill of sheep
		Viruses whose vectors are unknown
	Hepacivirus	Hepatitis C virus
Orthomyxoviridae	*Influenzavirus*	Influenza virus type A
		Influenza virus type B
		Influenza virus type C
Paramyxoviridae	*Paramyxovirus*	Human parainfluenza viruses, including Sendai virus
	Rubulavirus	Mumps virus
		Newcastle disease virus of fowl; viruses of other diseases of birds and mammals
	Morbillivirus	Measles virus
		Rinderpest virus of cattle
		Distemper virus of dogs
		Peste-des-petits-ruminants virus of sheep and goats
	Pneumovirus	Human respiratory syncytial virus
		Respiratory disease viruses of cattle and mice
Rhabdoviridae	*Vesiculovirus*	Vesicular stomatitis virus of horses, cattle, and pigs
	Lyssavirus	Rabies virus
		Lagos bat virus and others
Filoviridae	*Filovirus*	Marburg virus
		Ebola virus
Coronaviridae	*Coronavirus*	Human coronavirus
		Mouse hepatitis virus, infectious bronchitis virus of fowl, and other agents infecting pigs and other vertebrates

(Continued on next page)

TABLE 3 Members of virus families, with emphasis on viruses that infect humans (*Continued*)

Family	Genus	Common species
Bunyaviridae	*Bunyavirus*	Bunyamwera virus
		California encephalitis viruses
		La Crosse virus, other serologically cross-related groups, and several ungrouped viruses
	Phlebovirus	Sandfly fever viruses
		Other viruses of humans and lower animals, including Rift Valley fever virus of sheep and other ruminants, which may cause human disease
		Uukuniemi virus and 6 other agents, all belonging to same serogroup (infect rodents and ticks)
	Nairovirus	Crimean-Congo hemorrhagic fever virus
		Viruses of 5 other serogroups, including the virus of Nairobi sheep disease
	Hantavirus	Hantaan virus of hemorrhagic fever with renal syndrome
Retroviridae		
Oncovirinae	Type C oncovirus group	Sarcoma and leukemia viruses of mice, cats, cattle, birds, snakes and primates
	HTLV-BLV group	Human T-cell lymphotropic virus types 1 and 2
	Type B oncovirus group	Mammary tumor virus of mice (and humans?)
	Type D oncovirus group	Monkey (mammary tumor?) virus (Mason-Pfizer monkey virus)
Spumavirinae	*Spumavirus*	Syncytial and foamy viruses of humans, monkeys, cattle, and cats
Lentivirinae	*Lentivirus*	Human immunodeficiency virus (HIV)
		Visna, maedi, and progressive pneumonia viruses of sheep
Arenaviridae	*Arenavirus*	Lymphocytic choriomeningitis virus of mice
		Lassa fever virus
		Viruses of Tacaribe complex, including Junin and Machupo viruses of South American hemorrhagic fevers
Parvoviridae	*Erythrovirus*	Human parvovirus B19
	Parvovirus	Aleutian mink disease virus; viruses of rodents, pigs, cattle, cats, and dogs
	Dependovirus	Adeno-associated virus (adeno-satellite virus): humans (types 1–5); monkey (type 4); also of cattle, dogs, and birds
Papovaviridae	*Papillomavirus*	Human papillomaviruses (warts)
		Rabbit (Shope) papillomavirus
		Papillomaviruses of other mammals
	Polyomavirus	Polyomavirus of mice
		JC and BK viruses of humans
		Simian virus 40 of rhesus monkeys
		Lymphotropic virus of African green monkeys
		Viruses of mice, rabbits, and baboons
Adenoviridae	*Mastadenovirus*	Human adenoviruses
		Viruses of other mammals
	Aviadenovirus	Viruses of birds
Hepadnaviridae	*Hepadnavirus*	Human hepatitis B virus
		Hepatitis B viruses of woodchucks, ground squirrels, and ducks
Herpesviridae		
Alphaherpesvirinae	*Simplexvirus*	Human herpes simplex virus types 1 and 2
		Bovine mammillitis virus
		Herpes B virus of monkeys
	Varicellovirus	Varicella-zoster virus (human herpesvirus 3)
		Pseudorabies virus
	Unnamed	Equine rhinopneumonitis virus
		Marek's disease herpesvirus of fowl
		Herpesvirus saimiri and others, probably human herpesvirus 8
Betaherpesvirinae	*Cytomegalovirus*	Human cytomegalovirus (human herpesvirus 5)
	Muromegalovirus	Mouse cytomegalovirus
	Roseolovirus	Human herpesvirus 6
Gammaherpesvirinae	*Lymphocryptovirus*	Epstein-Barr virus (human herpesvirus 4)
Iridoviridae	*Iridovirus*	Iridescent insect viruses
		African swine fever virus (?)

(Continued on next page)

TABLE 3 (*Continued*)

Family	Genus	Common species
	Ranavirus	Frog viruses
	Piscinivirus	Fish viruses
Poxviridae		
Chordopoxvirinae (poxviruses of vertebrates)	*Orthopoxvirus*	Vaccinia virus
		Smallpox virus (variola)
		Poxviruses of lower animals
	Parapoxvirus	Orf virus and other viruses of ungulates
		Virus of milker's nodule
	Avipoxvirus	Fowlpox virus and other viruses of birds
	Capripoxvirus	Viruses of sheep and goats
	Leporipoxvirus	Myxoma virus of hares
		Fibroma viruses of rabbits and squirrels
	Suipoxvirus	Swinepox virus
	Yatapoxvirus	Yabapox and tanapox viruses
	Molluscipoxvirus	Molluscum contagiosum virus
Entomopoxvirinae		Poxviruses of insects

virus, genus *Coltivirus*, and the Kemerovo viruses, genus *Orbivirus*; other important orbiviruses are the bluetongue viruses of sheep and the viruses that cause African horse sickness.

The genus *Rotavirus* includes several viruses that infect humans as well as viruses of many other mammalian species, typified by simian virus SA-11 and Nebraska calf diarrhea virus. The human rotaviruses are recognized as causing a large proportion of the serious episodes of nonbacterial infantile diarrhea. Rotavirus gastroenteritis is one of the most common childhood illnesses throughout the world and is a leading cause of infant death in developing countries. These viruses also infect adults, particularly those in close contact with infants and children, but infected adults usually experience no symptoms or may have only minor illness.

RETROVIRIDAE

The family *Retroviridae* includes six genera, not only the RNA tumor viruses (type C retroviruses) but also the slowly growing lentiviruses of the maedi-visna group and the foamy virus group of agents (spumaviruses) that form syncytia in cell cultures. The human immunodeficiency viruses (HIV) associated with AIDS are lentiviruses.

Retroviruses characteristically have a reverse transcriptase (RNA-dependent DNA polymerase) within the virion. The genome is an inverted dimer of linear, single-stranded positive RNA. Replication of the viral RNA involves a DNA provirus that is integrated into host cellular DNA.

Endogenous members may be part of the germ line of vertebrate hosts, being inherited as Mendelian genes. The retrovirus genes may not be expressed, but they can be activated by physical and chemical agents, by superinfection with other retroviruses, and even by herpesviruses. It was through studies of retroviruses that the cellular oncogenes were recognized.

With some exceptions, retroviruses fall into host-species-specific groups of agents, including those that cause either leukemias or sarcomas, in avian, murine, or feline species. Other groups are murine mammary tumor virus and primate retroviruses.

The retroviruses have been divided into types according to morphologic, antigenic, and enzymatic differences. The type B retrovirus group includes the mouse mammary tumor virus. The type C retrovirus group includes mammalian, avian, and reptilian viruses. Members of the HTLV-BLV genus include human T-cell lymphotropic virus types 1 and 2, simian T-cell lymphotropic virus, and bovine leukemia virus. The type D group includes other viruses of monkeys.

Members of the *Spumavirus* genus, foamy viruses, do not induce tumors or cellular transformation but cause persistent asymptomatic infections in natural and experimental host animals. Foamy or syncytial viruses are known for a number of mammalian species, including humans.

The slow viruses of the maedi-visna group, which have been placed in the genus *Lentivirus*, are morphologically and chemically like other members of the family *Retroviridae* but do not induce tumors. Visna virus of sheep causes panleukoencephalitis. Serologically related viruses (variously designated maedi or progressive pneumonia viruses in different countries) cause interstitial pneumonitis.

Two types of the human lentivirus HIV have been recognized; type 1 is more widespread and more virulent. HIV is a completely exogenous virus, but after an individual is exposed to and infected by HIV, proviral DNA is integrated into the cellular DNA of infected cells. Numerous types of simian lentiviruses, related to HIV, have been isolated. The many different isolates of HIV exhibit considerable divergence, particularly in the gene that codes for viral envelope proteins. Visna virus, the prototype of the genus *Lentivirus*, is also known to undergo progressive antigenic variation in reaction to the host immune response during persistent infection.

PARVOVIRIDAE

All of the virus families shown in Table 2 have their DNA genomes in double-stranded form except for the members of the *Parvoviridae*, whose DNA is single stranded within the virion. Members of the family *Parvoviridae* are very small (Table 2). The size of the nucleic acid in the virion is relatively very small (4 to 6 kb) compared, for example, with the DNA of poxviruses (130 to 375 kbp). Some members display resistance to high temperatures (56°C for 60 min).

The family *Parvoviridae* encompasses viruses of numerous species of vertebrates, including humans. A member of the genus *Erythrovirus* is associated with disease in humans. This virus, parvovirus B19, causes a transient shutdown of erythrocyte production by killing the late erythroid progenitor cells. This shutdown presents particular problems for individuals already suffering from hemolytic anemias such as sickle cell anemia, causing aplastic crises.

A host range mutant of feline panleukopenia parvovirus, known as canine parvovirus, induces acute enteritis with leukopenia in young and adult dogs as well as myocarditis in puppies. Infections with this virus have reached enzootic proportions around the world.

Several serotypes of adeno-associated viruses, which belong to the genus *Dependovirus*, are known to infect humans, but they have not been shown to be associated with any human disease. Members of this genus cannot multiply in the absence of a replicating adenovirus that serves as a helper virus. The single-stranded DNA is present within the virion as either plus or minus complementary strands in separate particles. Upon extraction, the plus and minus DNA strands unite to form a double-stranded helix.

HEPADNAVIRIDAE

The name *Hepadnaviridae* reflects the DNA-containing genomes of its members and their replication within hepatocytes. Each of these viruses has a circular DNA genome that is double stranded except for a region of variable length that is single stranded. In the presence of appropriate substrates, DNA polymerase within the virion can complete the single-stranded region to its full length of 3,200 nucleotides.

Hepatitis B virus of humans and three similar viruses found in woodchucks, Beechey ground squirrels, and Pekin ducks share many basic features. All members of the family share antigens and have similar morphology and behavior in the infected host. Large amounts of excess viral coat protein are produced in the form of small 22-nm spherical and tubular particles (in the human virus, the antigen is known as hepatitis B surface antigen). The viruses replicate in the liver and are associated with acute and chronic hepatitis. More than 300 million persons are persistent carriers of the human virus and are at very high risk of developing chronic liver diseases, including cancer. The woodchuck hepatitis B virus also causes liver cancer in its natural host. Fragments of viral DNA may be found in the liver cancer cells of both species. Hepatitis D virus, or delta virus, is a subviral agent that can infect only cells that are already infected with hepatitis B virus. Hepatitis D virus is therefore a satellite virus.

RECENT DEVELOPMENTS

Up-to-date taxonomic information is now available through the ICTV site on the World Wide Web. The home page URL is http://www.ncbi.nlm.nih.gov/ICTV. This site provides access to virus taxonomy data and has links to the ICTV database and to the Index Virum, which has a comprehensive listing of families, genera, and species.

REFERENCES

1. **Andrewes, C. H., H. G. Pereira, and P. Wildy.** 1978. *Viruses of Vertebrates*, 4th ed. Macmillan Publishing Co., New York, N.Y.
2. **Brown, F.** 1989. The classification and nomenclature of viruses: summary of the results of meetings of the International Committee on Taxonomy of Viruses, Edmonton, Canada, 1987. *Intervirology* **30:**181–186.
3. **Fenner, F.** 1976. Classification and nomenclature of viruses: second report of the International Committee on Taxonomy of Viruses. *Intervirology* **7:**1–16.
4. **Fields, B. N., D. M. Knipe, R. M. Chanock, J. L. Melnick, B. Roizman, and T. P. Monath (ed).** 1990. *Virology*, 2nd ed. Raven Press, New York, N.Y.
5. **Francki, R. I. B., C. M. Fauquet, D. L. Knudson, and F. Brown.** 1991. Classification and nomenclature of viruses: fifth report of the International Committee on Taxonomy of Viruses. *Arch. Virol.* Suppl. 2, p. 1–450.
6. **Matthews, R. E. F.** 1979. Classification and nomenclature of viruses: third report of the International Committee on Taxonomy of Viruses. *Intervirology* **12:**129–296.
7. **Matthews, R. E. F.** 1982. Classification and nomenclature of viruses: fourth report of the International Committee on Taxonomy of Viruses. *Intervirology* **17:**1–199.
8. **Melnick, J. L.** 1966–1982. Summaries on viral taxonomy. *Prog. Med. Virol.*, vol. 6 through 28. (Published annually.)
9. **Murphy, F. A., C. M. Fauquet, D. H. L. Bishop, S. A. Ghabrial, A. W. Jarvis, G. P. Martelli, M. A. Mayo, and M. D. Summers.** 1995. Virus Taxonomy, sixth report of the International Committee on Taxonomy of Viruses. *Arch. Virol.* Suppl. 10, p. 1–586.
10. **Wildy, P.** 1971. Classification and nomenclature of viruses. First report of the International Committee on Nomenclature of Viruses. *Monogr. Virol.* **5:**1–81.

Algorithms for Detection and Identification of Viruses

ROBERT H. YOLKEN, DAVID A. LENNETTE,
THOMAS F. SMITH, AND JOSEPH L. WANER

62

Detection and accurate identification of viral infection are becoming increasingly important components of patient management and disease prevention. Viruses represent a biologically diverse group of human pathogens. This diversity poses a number of challenges for the laboratory attempting to provide an accurate diagnosis of a viral infection. For example, cultivation of viruses in cell culture remains the principal method of diagnosis in most clinical laboratories. However, the wide range of host cell tropism displayed by viral species results in large variations in the efficiency of cell culture for the diagnosis of different viral infections. In some cases, viruses do not replicate or produce detectable cytopathic effects in commonly available cell lines and other methods of "direct" diagnosis must be used. In addition, viral pathogens display variation in terms of the amounts of antigen shed into body fluids and the accessibility of these antigens to diagnostic immunoreagents. Similarly, viral agents vary greatly in terms of their ability to induce measurable host immune response following infection. These factors result in the different roles of the various immunological and microscopy-based assays in the clinical laboratory. Viral agents are more uniform in terms of the presence of nucleic acids. In theory, virtually any viral agent can be identified by the detection of viral DNA or RNA in body fluids, especially if nucleic acid amplification techniques such as PCR are employed. However, the applicability of these techniques is limited by the need for the appropriate reagents, expertise, and physical facilities necessary for the performance of these assays on a routine basis without the occurrence of false-positive and false-negative reactions.

Laboratory viral diagnosis attempts must be customized to take into account the needs of the patient, the capabilities of the laboratory, and the most likely potential etiologic agents. A summary of the utility of common assays for viral diagnosis is presented in Table 1. It is important to keep in mind that this table is intended only as a starting point; the reader should refer to the specific chapters for more detailed discussions. In addition, the individual context of specific assays must be taken into consideration; a "seldom useful" assay may be the method of choice under certain clinical or laboratory conditions in which the "generally useful" assay cannot be used. It should also be kept in mind that viral diagnosis is a rapidly changing field in terms of assay principles and the availability of specific reagents and diagnostic kits. The reader is encouraged to consult recent literature when presented with a diagnostic challenge.

TABLE 1 Methods for identification of viruses[a]

Virus	Applicability[b] of:					Comments
	Cell culture	Immunoassay	Microscopy	Nucleic acid	Immune response	
Adenovirus	A	A	B	C	B	Cell culture most useful for respiratory samples; enzyme immunoassay most widely used for fecal specimens; electron microscopy useful in suitably equipped laboratories for analysis of fecal samples
Arbovirus	C	D	C	B	A	CDC-NIH laboratory biosafety guidelines recommend biosafety level 2 to 4 containment facilities for cultivating arboviruses; electron microscopy may be useful in suitably equipped laboratories for the analysis of tissue samples; serological methods most widely used for diagnosis and epidemiological studies

(Continued on next page)

TABLE 1 Methods for identification of viruses[a] (*Continued*)

Virus	Applicability[b] of: Cell culture	Immunoassay	Microscopy	Nucleic acid	Immune response	Comments
Caliciviruses and related agents	C	B	A	B	C	Cell culture applicable to astroviruses but not to other agents; immunoassay potentially useful but requires specialized agents; electron microscopy useful in suitably equipped laboratories
Cytomegalovirus	A	D	B	B	A	Shell vial useful for rapid determination of viral replication; IgM antibodies useful for determining primary infection, especially in neonates; IgG antibodies useful for determination of susceptibility to primary infection and to viral reactivation in immunocompromised patients
Enteroviruses	A	D	D	A	C	Some strains cannot be passaged in routinely available cell lines; PCR is the method of choice for diagnosis of central nervous system infection
Epstein-Barr virus	D	D	B	B	A	In situ methods useful for diagnosis of virus-associated tumors; PCR can be useful for diagnosis of central nervous system infections; diagnosis generally made by detection of antibodies to defined viral components
Filoviruses and arenaviruses	B	C	B	B	A	Cell culture and other assays require appropriate biocontainment facilities; electron microscopy useful in suitably equipped laboratories
Hepatitis A virus	C	B	C	B	A	Detection of IgG and IgM class antibodies most useful as primary diagnostic test
Hepatitis B virus	D	A	B	B	A	Detection of specific viral antigens and antibodies allows for diagnosis and monitoring of the course of infection
Hepatitis C and G viruses	D	B	D	B	A	Serological methods most widely used for diagnosis and epidemiological studies; nucleic acid amplification methods useful if appropriate reagents and facilities are available
Hepatitis D virus	D	C	C	C	B	HDV diagnosis relevant only in the presence of hepatitis B infection; analysis of tissue obtained by liver biopsy may be required to demonstrate ongoing HDV replication
Hepatitis E virus	D	C	B	C	A	Electron microscopy useful in suitably equipped laboratories; diagnostic reagents available largely in specialized laboratories
Herpes simplex virus	A	B	A	B	B	Shell vial useful for rapid determination of viral replication; immunofluorescence microscopy useful for detection of viral antigens in skin lesions; PCR is the method of choice for diagnosis of central nervous system infection; serological methods generally used for determination of disease susceptibility
Herpesviruses 6, 7, and 8	C	C	C	B	C	Value of tissue culture varies with viral type. Not applicable to HHV-8; immunoassay is method of choice but is not generally available; microscopy is most useful for epidemiological studies

(*Continued on next page*)

TABLE 1 (*Continued*)

Virus	Applicability[b] of: Cell culture	Immunoassay	Microscopy	Nucleic acid	Immune response	Comments
Human immunodeficiency virus	B	B	D	A	A	Measurement of p24 core antigen useful for early diagnosis and monitoring; quantitative assessment of viral RNA is an important tool for monitoring the efficacy of antiviral therapy
Human papillomavirus	D	C	B	A	C	Detection of koilocytes and late structural antigens of the virus in tissue biopsy specimens useful for diagnosis; nucleic acid direct detection and amplification methods useful if appropriate reagents and facilities are available
Human parvoviruses	D	C	C	A	A	Nucleic acid direct detection and amplification methods useful if appropriate reagents and facilities are available; serological methods are most widely used for diagnosis and epidemiological studies; assays are not applicable in immunocompromised individuals
Human T-cell lymphotropic viruses	C	C	D	B	A	Serological methods are most widely used for diagnosis and epidemiological studies
Influenza viruses	A	A	A	C	B	Immunofluorescence and enzyme immunoassay of nasal wash specimens useful for rapid diagnosis; serological assays generally applied to epidemiological studies
Measles viruses	B	C	B	B	A	Serological assays useful for the determination of disease susceptibility and immune response to infection; PCR is the method of choice for diagnosis of central nervous system infection
Mumps virus	A	C	B	B	A	Immunofluorescence microscopy useful for the detection of viral antigens in respiratory secretions; PCR is the method of choice for diagnosis of central nervous system infection; serological assays useful for determination of disease susceptibility and immune response to infection
Parainfluenza viruses	A	C	A	C	C	Immunofluorescence of nasal wash specimens useful for rapid diagnosis
Polyomaviruses	D	D	C	A	D	In situ DNA hybridization used to detect virus in tissues; PCR used to detect JCV in cerebrospinal fluid and blood
Poxvirus	B	D	B	B	A	Value of tissue culture varies with viral type; electron microscopy useful in suitably equipped laboratories; serological assays generally useful but must be performed in a laboratory with appropriate reagents and expertise
Rabies virus	D	D	B	C	C	Cell culture useful for detection of viral antigens in brain tissue
Respiratory syncytial virus	A	A	A	C	C	Immunofluorescence microscopy useful for the detection of viral antigens in respiratory secretions
Rhinoviruses	A	C	C	C	D	Acid stability or other determination is required to distinguish them from enteroviruses in culture
Rotavirus	D	A	B	C	D	Electron microscopy useful in suitably equipped laboratories

(*Continued on next page*)

TABLE 1 Methods for identification of viruses[a] (*Continued*)

Virus	Applicability[b] of: Cell culture	Immunoassay	Microscopy	Nucleic acid	Immune response	Comments
Rubella virus	B	D	C	B	A	IgM antibodies useful for determining primary infection, especially in neonates; IgG antibodies useful for determining disease susceptibility and seroconversions in paired samples
Transmissible spongiform encephalopathy agents	D	D	C	D	D	Animal inoculation and other experimental techniques used in specialized laboratories
Varicella-zoster virus	A	D	A	C	B	Shell vial useful for rapid determination of viral replication; immunofluorescence useful for detection of skin lesions; serological methods useful for determination of susceptibility to infection

[a] "Cell culture" refers to cultivation of the virus directly from clinical samples, using cell lines and techniques which are generally available in diagnostic virology laboratories. "Immunoassay" refers to detection of viral antigens from clinical samples by solid-phase immunoassay techniques such as enzyme immunoassay (also known as enzyme-linked immunosorbent assay [ELISA]), particle agglutination assay, or radioimmunoassay. "Microscopy" refers to the detection of viral antigens by use of light or electron microscopic techniques. Light microscopic techniques include immunofluorescence, immunoperoxidase, and related methods. Electron microscopic techniques include the visualization of viral particles by negative staining or immunoelectron microscopic methods. "Nucleic acids" refers to the measurement of viral DNA or RNA extracted from clinical samples. The nucleic acid may be measured directly by hybridization or can be detected after amplification by PCR or other nucleic acid amplification methods. "Immune response" refers to the diagnosis of viral infection by the measurement of total or class-specific antibodies directed at the corresponding viral antigens. A variety of methods are used for the measurement of antibodies in blood and other body fluids. Specific methods for antibody measurement are presented in the individual chapters.

[b] A, test is generally useful for the indicated diagnosis; B, test is useful under certain circumstances or for the diagnosis of specific forms of infection, as delineated in the right-hand column and in the text of the individual chapters; C, test is seldom useful for generally diagnostic purposes but may be available in reference laboratories for epidemiological studies or for the diagnosis of unusual conditions; D, test is generally not used for laboratory diagnosis of infection.

Human Immunodeficiency Viruses*

JÖRG SCHÜPBACH

63

CLINICAL BACKGROUND

The human immunodeficiency viruses type 1 and 2 (HIV-1, HIV-2) are the causative agents of AIDS. AIDS is the end stage of a protracted pathogenic process in which the immune system of an infected person and its ability to control infections or malignant proliferative disorders are progressively destroyed.

Acute Retroviral Syndrome

The first clinical manifestations may appear a few days to a few weeks after infection with a transient condition frequently called *acute retroviral syndrome*. This syndrome is found in 50 to 70% of the infected patients and is characterized by clinical signs of immune activation and multisystem dysfunction. Patients frequently seek medical attention due to a flulike or infectious mononucleosis-like disease with fever, generalized lymphadenopathy, sore throat, arthralgia, myalgia, fatigue, rash, and/or weight loss. The rash consists of a maculopapular exanthema, especially of the trunk, with occasional transition into a papulovesicular appearance. Lesions of the oral mucosa, often aphthous, may also occur. Occasionally, diarrhea, pancreatitis, mild disturbance of hepatic functions, bacterial sepsis, thrombocytopenia, epiglottitis, lymphocytic alveolitis, or self-limiting neurological disorders like meningitis, encephalitis, polyneuropathy, or myelopathy may be found. Opportunistic infections normally seen only in advanced immunodeficiency, such as esophageal candidiasis, may be present. These symptoms typically resolve within 5 to 30 days.

Clinical Latency

Acute infection is followed by a long stage of disease-free clinical latency. Clinical latency is, however, not paralleled by viral latency, as demonstrated by high concentrations of HIV particles in plasma and, even more so, in lymphoid tissues (24, 50, 94, 140). That virus production in clinical latency is indeed very active has further been proven by the demonstration that the half-time of virus particles in plasma is only about 6 h and that one viral replication cycle takes about 2.6 days. About 10^{10} virus particles are produced, and eliminated, daily. Similarly, the turnover of productively infected $CD4^+$ T lymphocytes is high; half-time of this population has been estimated at 1.1 ± 0.4 days. In consequence, 35×10^6 $CD4^+$ cells are daily eliminated from the blood, amounting to 1.8×10^9 cells for the total body which must be daily replaced (67, 97, 148).

AIDS

The relentless production of HIV proteins, maintained by continuous viral replication in productively infected cells, and the ensuing elimination of host cells over many years finally lead to the destruction of the immune system, which is clinically manifested by the occurrence of opportunistic infections and tumors (Appendixes 1 and 2). In addition, infection of the central nervous system may lead to distinct HIV-associated diseases including the HIV-associated dementia complex, vacuolar myelopathy, and sensory neuropathy (109). The causative role of HIV in AIDS has been further corroborated by the demonstration that the virus load present in early infection and at later time points is highly associated with clinical outcome (71, 87).

Several disease classifications have been introduced since the first description of AIDS in 1981 (56). Some of these earlier classifications are still employed in the nonclinical research literature and shall therefore be briefly mentioned. The Centers for Disease Control and Prevention (CDC) 1985 classification used the descriptive terms *asymptomatic seropositive*, *lymphadenopathy-associated syndrome* (LAS), *lesser AIDS* (L-AIDS), and *AIDS*. The CDC 1986 classification and its 1987 revision used Groups I to IV for *acute infection*, *asymptomatic infection*, *persistent generalized lymphadenopathy*, and *other disease*, respectively, in conjunction with subgroups A to E which specify, in a group-dependent manner, absence or presence of pathological laboratory findings, constitutional or neurological conditions, secondary infections or cancers, or other HIV-associated conditions (4). The 1986 Walter Reed classification defined consecutive stages from WR0 (seronegative) to WR6, based on the absence or presence of chronic lymphadenopathy, $CD4^+$ T-cell counts above or below 400, reaction in delayed-type hypersensitivity tests, absence or presence of oral thrush or, respectively, opportunistic infections (111). The currently used CDC 93 classification (Table 1) is based on a combination of clinical and $CD4^+$ T-cell count categories which defines nine mutually exclusive stages (8).

* This chapter contains information presented in chapter 97 by Edward Barker and Susan W. Barnett in the sixth edition of this Manual.

TABLE 1 The CDC 93 classification[a]

CD4$^+$ T-cell category	Clinical category		
	A (asymptomatic, acute [primary] HIV or PGL)	B (symptomatic, not meeting conditions for A or C)	C (AIDS-indicator conditions)
1. ≥500/μl (≥29% of lymphocyte count)	A1	B1	C1
2. 200–499/μl (14–28% of lymphocyte count)	A2	B2	C2
3. <200/μl (<14% of lymphocyte count)	A3	B3	C3

[a] For clinical category definitions, see Appendixes 1 and 2.

AIDS Incubation Time

The median time to AIDS in untreated adult patients has been estimated at 10 to 11 years and is similar for homosexual men and drug addicts. Incubation time varies considerably. In the 5 to 10% *rapid progressors*, AIDS develops within 2 to 3 years after infection. On the other side of the spectrum, 5 to 10% of patients, the *nonprogressors*, are free of symptoms after 7 to 10 years and have stable CD4$^+$ T-cell counts, although these are significantly lower than those of uninfected controls. Data from large prospective cohort studies suggest that about 13% of HIV-positive homosexual men will remain AIDS-free for 20 years after seroconversion (88). In maternally transmitted pediatric infection, disease progression appears to follow a bimodal distribution, with a subgroup of children progressing rapidly to AIDS at a median age of approximately 5 months and 20% of infected children developing AIDS within 12 months (48). The mean time from birth to a stage of severe symptoms is estimated at 6.3 to 6.6 years (11, 105) and the time to death is estimated at 6.3 to 9.4 years (11). Based on 2,148 perinatally infected children, the mean durations of the stages of infection were 10 months for the symptom-free interval (stage N of the CDC 1994 pediatric classification [23]), 4 months for stage A (mild signs or symptoms), 65 months for stage B (moderate signs or symptoms), and 34 months for stage C (severe signs or symptoms). Though children thus usually develop moderate symptoms by the second year of life, they may not progress further for a long time (11) and as many as one-third are estimated to remain AIDS-free by 15 years of age in one study (105).

DESCRIPTION OF THE AGENTS

Primate Lentiviruses

HIV-1 and HIV-2 are members of the genus *Lentivirinae* of the family *Retroviridae*. They are enveloped positive-strand RNA viruses, with a diameter of about 110 nm. Infectious particles, or virions, contain two identical copies of single-stranded RNA of about 9 to 10 kb in length. These are surrounded by structural proteins forming the nucleocapsid and the matrix shell, to which a lipid envelope derived from the host cell membrane is attached. Viral glycoprotein oligomers which mediate adsorption to and penetration of the host cell membrane are inserted in this envelope (Fig. 1).

HIV-1, discovered in 1983 (12) and confirmed in the following year as being virologically and serologically associated with early and late stages of AIDS (53, 78, 108, 115, 127), is the more aggressive virus and responsible for the AIDS pandemic. HIV-2, identified in 1986 (29, 30), is apparently less pathogenic than HIV-1. Rates of heterosexual and mother-to-child transmission of HIV-2 are low, and latency dominates the clinical picture. Rarely, the virus may however cause AIDS (40, 81).

A group of related viruses, the simian immunodeficiency viruses (SIV), are distributed among various species of Old World monkeys and the chimpanzee (Fig. 2). It is thought that these primate lentiviruses may have arisen several millions of years ago in *Cercopithecus* monkeys. These viruses can be categorized into five major lineages, which include also the HIVs. Lineage 1 contains the various isolates of HIV-1, which can be classified into two groups, M (main) and O (outlier) (see below). It is evident that group M isolates (e.g., HIV-1/LAI) are more closely related to a chimpanzee isolate than to isolates of group O (e.g., HIV-1/ANT70). Lineage 2 contains the different isolates of HIV-2, which are closely related to viruses infecting sooty mangabeys (SIV_{sm}). This virus has also been naturally transmitted to macaques. An HIV-2 strain (HIV-2/ST) has been identified that differs less from its simian counterparts than it does from other human viruses. This, along with the fact that SIV infections in their natural simian host do not cause disease, has led to the conclusion that the HIV-1 and HIV-2 epidemics are both the result of simian-to-human cross-species transmission and thus represent zoonotic infections. Sequence comparisons indicate that such simian-to-human transmissions have occurred only relatively recently and on several different occasions (reviewed in reference 132).

HIV Groups and Subtypes

The extraordinary variability of HIV, due largely to rapid mutation and recombination, has led to the development and geographical distribution of distinctive groups and subtypes of viruses. In HIV-1, two groups, M and O, have been found. Group M is furthermore divided into subtypes A to J. Isolates of group O differ as much from each other as viruses from different subtypes of group M, but their limited number has so far precluded distinction of subtypes. In HIV-2, five subtypes (A to E) have been defined. HIV-1 subtype B viruses were responsible for the first epidemic in North America, Europe, and Australia and the metropolitan centers of other continents. Subtype E is the most prevalent in Thailand and Southeast Asia. Subtype F has been found in Brazil and Romania, and G is prevalent in Russia. Almost all HIV-1 subtypes are found in sub-Saharan Africa, with subtypes A, C, and D being the most prevalent in this continent. C is also frequent in India. Viruses of the M group, which are responsible for the AIDS pandemic, are rapidly spreading worldwide, whereas group O viruses are rarely isolated and virtually exclusively restricted to Gabon, Cameroon, or other countries located in the western part of equatorial Africa (132). Recent investigations indicate

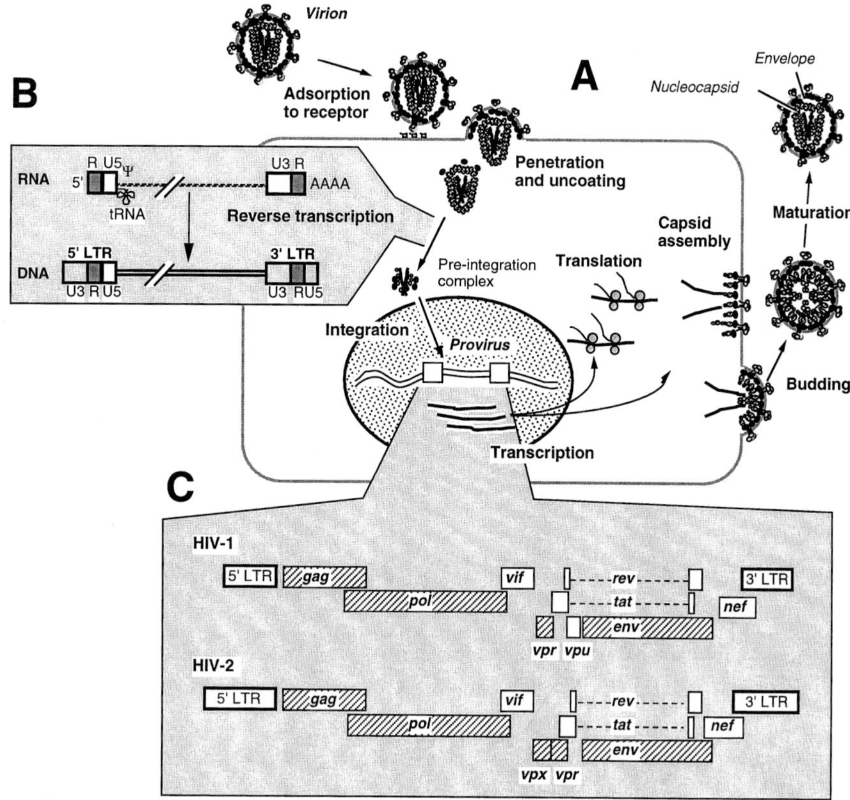

FIGURE 1 The HIV replication cycle. (A) Overview. (B) Reverse transcription. The retroviral genome contained in virions consists of RNA. Its characteristic features include terminal repeats (R), U5 (5′-untranslated), U3 (3′-untranslated), 3′-polyadenylation, a binding site for the reverse transcription primer $tRNA^{Lys3}$, and the encapsidation signal Ψ. During reverse transcription the viral RNA is reverse transcribed into double-stranded DNA and terminal sequences are partially duplicated in a way that leads to LTR composed of U3-R-U5. (C) Organization of the proviral genomes of HIV-1 and HIV-2. The genome codes for structural proteins and enzymes packaged into virions (hatched boxes) and accessory or regulatory proteins (open boxes) which are not packaged in significant amounts.

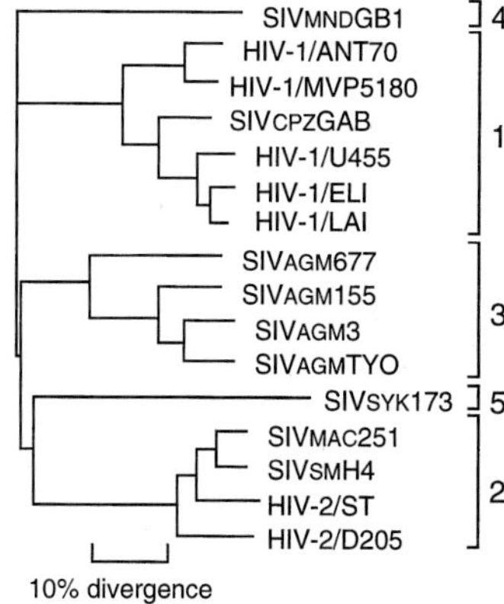

FIGURE 2 Phylogenetic tree of primate lentiviruses, derived from Pol protein sequences. Brackets on the right indicate the five major lineages. HIV-1/U455 is a group M/subtype A isolate. ELI is of subtype D and LAI of subtype B. ANT70 and MVP5180 represent group O. MND, mandrill; AGM, African green monkey; SYK, Sykes' monkey; SM, sooty mangabey (simplified from reference 132).

that substantial fractions of novel HIV-1 infections in various European countries are due to non-B subtypes, and this fraction is likely to grow in the future.

Full-length genome analysis indicates that HIV-1 subtypes A, B, C, and D are largely, if not entirely, distinguishable throughout the genome and show no clear evidence of intersubtype recombination. In contrast, all available sequences of subtypes E (from both Southeast Asia and Central Africa) and G are recombinant with subtype A; the nonrecombinant parental isolates of these subtypes have not yet been identified. Subtypes E and G, and some A/D recombinant HIV-1 isolates, have retained the cytoplasmic domain of gp41 from subtype A. Full-length sequences of subtypes F, H, I, and J are still unavailable. Some recombinants possess the matrix and core of one subtype and the outer envelope of another, functionally resembling pseudotypes (85). Evidence for superinfection and recombination has also been documented for HIV-2 (132).

Virus Stability, Safety Precautions, Disinfection, and Injuries

HIVs have been classified as agents of moderate risk. The risk of laboratory-acquired infection with these viruses stems primarily from contamination of the hands and mucous membranes of the eyes, nose, and mouth by infectious blood and other body fluids. There is no evidence that HIV is transmitted by the airborne route.

Strict adherence to the safety precautions outlined in more detail in section II, chapter 9, of this volume or available in a booklet from the World Health Organization (WHO) (7) is paramount in preventing nosocomial infections. Always wear good-quality gloves and a protective laboratory gown. Protect your eyes from spills. Use disposable unbreakable plasticware; never use glassware or other sharp or breakable objects. When sharp instruments cannot be avoided, protect your nondominant hand with a stainless steel chain mail or Kevlar glove.

Spills or contaminations of laboratory surfaces must be decontaminated immediately. Whenever possible, use a type 2 laminar flow biological safety cabinet (LFBSC) when handling any patient sample that may contain infectious virus. Use of an LFBSC is mandatory for virus isolation work. Centrifuges, including those used in laboratories that perform only serological testing, should be equipped with sealed centrifuge buckets. Research work with HIV and virus production require a designated biosafety level 3 laboratory with restricted access and a ducted exhaust-ventilation system which maintains negative air pressure and creates a directional airflow, as well as other safety measures.

HIVs are rapidly inactivated by detergents and disinfectants that are effective against other enveloped viruses. Otherwise, the virus is relatively stable. At autopsy, HIV was isolated up to 16.5 days postmortem from various tissues (47). Suspensions of the virus in protein-containing fluids or dried preparations are also relatively stable (141). At the optimum pH of 7.1, the half-life of the virus ranged from approximately 24 h at 37°C to no significant loss over 6 months at −75°C. Drying the virus on a glass surface or freezing caused a 5- to 12-fold and a 4- to 5-fold decrease of activity, respectively. The dried preparations, however, were about as stable as when stored in a buffered solution (141). In another study, 1 log of inactivation in culture fluid, seawater, sewage, and dechlorinated tap water (all sterile and kept at 16°C in the dark) required 1.3, 1.6, 2.9, and 1.8 days, respectively. After the first 4 days, the inactivation became even slower (1 long inactivation after 4.3, 2.6, 5.7, and 4.6 days, respectively). HIV was more stable than herpes simplex virus but less stable than poliovirus (117). These data are not meant to suggest that HIV transmission might occur by exposure to water, for which there is absolutely no basis. They should, however, make clear that caution when working with HIV and rapid disinfection of spills and contaminations is important.

The standard disinfectant recommended for contaminated surfaces is a hypochlorite solution with a concentration of 0.5% available chlorine (5 g/liter, 5,000 ppm). When working with HIV cultures and virus preparations, a higher concentration of 1% available chlorine is recommended (7, 145). Fresh 2% solutions of alkaline glutaraldehyde are effective, but care should be taken that they are not too dilute or have not become stale when used for disinfecting HIV associated with organic matter. A solution of iodine and detergent (2% Jodopax) will remove all detectable HIV-1 activity. In contrast, 70% industrial methylated spirit or 70% ethanol is ineffective in inactivating dried protein-rich spills of cell-free or cell-associated HIV within a reasonable length of time; complete inactivation requires up to 20 minutes (141, 144).

The risk of HIV infection following percutaneous needle-stick exposure to HIV-contaminated blood is estimated to be between 0.13 and 0.5%. The risk of infection by such accidents depends on the depth of the penetration (relative risk [RR] of percutaneous lesions, 16.1), visible contamination of the penetrating object with blood (RR, 5.2), prior use for an intravenous or intra-arterial injection (RR, 5.1), and the disease stage (respectively the viral load) of the index patient (RR, 6.4) (9).

Needle-stick or other puncture wounds, cuts, and skin contaminated by spills or splashes of specimen material should be thoroughly washed with soap and water and disinfected with a nonirritating disinfectant (cells of the immune system should not be attracted!). Bleeding from any wound should be encouraged. In case of a percutaneous penetration, an antiretroviral prophylactic treatment should be started *immediately*. Postexposure monotherapy with azidothymidine lowers the risk of infection by 80% (9). Currently, the recommended postexposure chemoprophylaxis consists of a triple combination, which includes two reverse transcriptase (RT) inhibitors and an efficient protease inhibitor. This should be given for at least 2, but no longer than 4, weeks. Chemoprophylaxis is not currently recommended when intact skin is exposed to blood or blood-containing body fluids.

The HIV Replication Cycle

An overview of HIV replication is given in Fig. 1A. Like all retroviruses, HIV particles contain a characteristic enzyme, RT. The enzyme is cleaved, and thereby activated, from a precursor protein by the action of another retroviral enzyme, the viral protease (PR). RT possesses three distinct enzymatic functions. It acts as an RNA-dependent DNA polymerase—the RT activity in the strict sense of the word—an RNase H, and a DNA-dependent DNA polymerase. After infection of a host cell, these different RT functions serve in turn to synthesize a cDNA of the viral RNA, to degrade RNA from the cDNA-RNA heteroduplex, and to duplicate the cDNA strand. Regulatory sequences present at both ends of the viral RNA (R-U5 at the 5′ end and U3-R at the 3′ end) are thereby complemented and partially duplicated in a manner that yields the so-called long terminal repeats (LTR). These contain U3-R-U5 and are located at both ends of the double-stranded viral DNA (Fig. 1B). This double-stranded DNA (dsDNA), which is still associated with some viral proteins in the so-called pre-integration complex, migrates into the nucleus where it is integrated into the host cell genome by a third specific retroviral enzyme, the integrase. The integrated retroviral DNA genome is called the provirus.

The genomic organization of HIV-1 and HIV-2 proviruses is shown in Fig. 1C. Like all retroviruses, HIVs possess the open reading frames (ORFs) *gag* and *env*, which code for structural proteins, namely, the precursor proteins of the viral capsid and the envelope, respectively, and *pol*, which codes for the enzymes. Additional overlapping ORFs code for the *trans*-acting transcriptional activator (Tat) and the regulator of viral expression (Rev), which are both essential for virus replication. Furthermore, both HIV types contain ORFs for several accessory or auxiliary proteins including, in the case of HIV-1, Vif, Vpr, Vpu, and Nef and, in the case of HIV-2, Vif, Vpx, Vpr, and Nef.

While host cell infection and provirus integration are largely mediated by the proteins carried in the virion, the production of viral RNA, structural proteins, and enzymes involves cellular enzymes associated with transcription and translation, but also a number of viral regulatory proteins, namely, Tat, Rev, Nef, and Vpr. Particles are assembled at the cell membrane and are, in a still immature and noninfec-

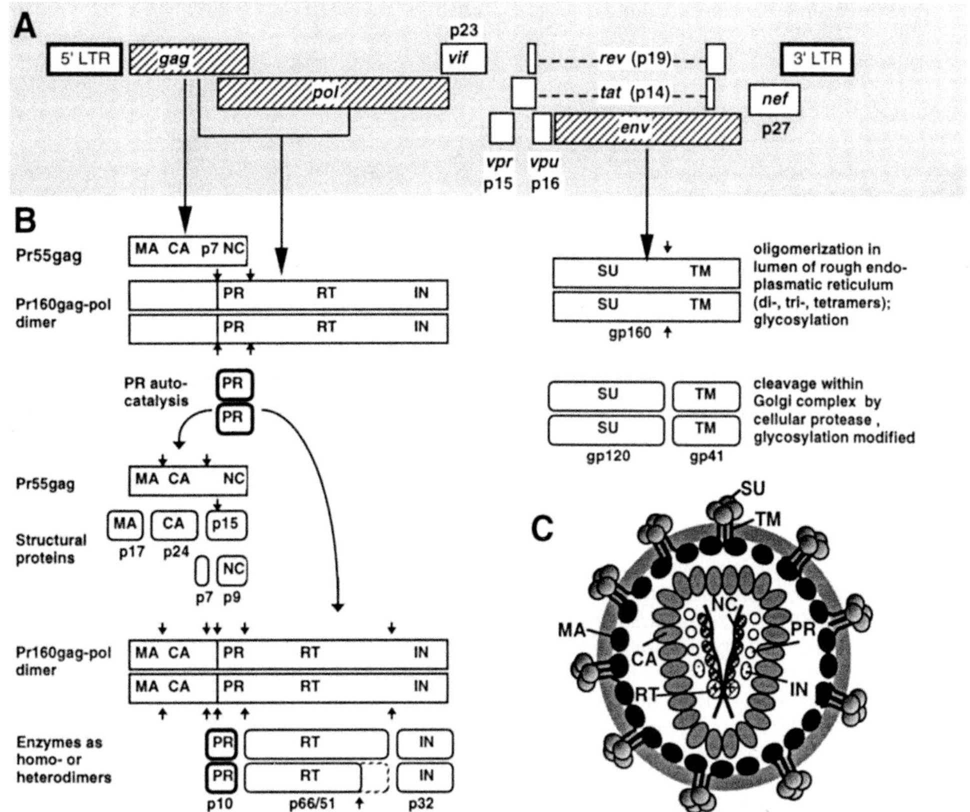

FIGURE 3 Translation of HIV-1 and particle composition. (A) Open reading frames of HIV-1. Open boxes denote ORFs of the accessory proteins Tat, Rev, Nef, Vif, Vpr, and Vpu which are directly translated into proteins of final size. Hatched boxes denote ORFs translated into precursor proteins. (B) Translational products of *gag*, *pol*, and *env*. The products of these genes are synthesized as polyprotein precursors. The principal Gag precursor $Pr55^{Gag}$ is cleaved by the viral protease (PR) into the matrix (MA) protein p17, the caspid (CA) protein p24, and a C-terminal protein p15 which is subsequently cleaved into p7 and the nucleocapsid (NC) p9. Cleavage of $Pr160^{Gag\text{-}Pol}$, which is produced by ribosomal frameshifting at the *gag-pol* junction, yields PR, RT, and the integrase (IN). All three enzymes remain dimerized after cleavage. RT first forms a homodimer, p66/66, which is subsequently modified into the heterodimer, p66/p51. The Env precursor gp160 is cleaved by a cellular protease into the surface (SU) protein gp120 and the smaller TM protein gp41. Tiny arrows indicate protease cleavage sites. (C) Protein composition of mature virions.

tious form, released by budding. For full maturation into infectious particles, the viral Gag and Gag-Pol precursor proteins must be cleaved by PR into the different subunit proteins. An overview of the different viral proteins and their position in the mature particle is given in Fig. 3.

Virus Entry

For infection of a host cell, the virion must bind to a membrane-located virus receptor which for the HIVs is the CD4 molecule (39, 73). CD4 is located on the surface of CD4-positive T lymphocytes, as well as on macrophage, dendritic, or other antigen-presenting cells. Interaction of the CD4-binding domain of the HIV surface glycoprotein, gp120, with CD4 induces a conformational change, whereupon the complex of CD4 and gp120 interacts with a coreceptor of the family of seven-transmembrane chemokine receptors (2, 45, 49, 51). These are G-protein-coupled signaling receptors which bind the chemokines that are involved in controlling activation and migration of various leukocytes to a site of infection. Langerhans cells (LC) or monocyte/macrophages exhibit the CCR5 chemokine receptor (formerly named CKR5) which permits infection by the M (macrophage)-tropic viruses of the non-syncytium-inducing (NSI) phenotype usually present in early infection (2, 45, 49). This interaction is inhibited by the natural ligands of CCR5, the β-chemokines RANTES, MIP-1α, and MIP-1β, whose identification as HIV suppressor factors led to the discovery of these long-sought coreceptors (31). In contrast, the coreceptor on $CD4^+$ T-cell lines is the CXCR4 molecule (formerly LESTR or fusin), which binds only T-cell tropic, syncytium-inducing (SI) isolates and whose natural ligand is the stroma-derived factor SDF-1 (13, 89). Primary $CD4^+$ T cells exhibit both coreceptors, CCR5 and CXCR4, and can thus be infected by both M- and T-tropic viruses.

Not all cells infectable with HIV, for example astrocytes, express detectable CD4. In these cells, galactosylceramide has been described as an alternative virus receptor for gp120. M cells of the enteric mucosa which may be involved in rectal infections are also negative for CD4, but positive for galactosylceramide (60, 84). Similarly, intestinal or vaginal epithelial cells, spermatozoa, and oligodendrocytes, all negative for CD4, may also be infectable via a galactosylceramide or related glycolipid receptor (1, 43, 137).

Virus Transmission and Establishment of Infection

The transmission of HIV is governed by the same basic principles as that of any other infectious agent. The probability of transmission depends on the closeness of contact with and the frequency of exposure to a source of infection and further on the infectious dose. HIV is predominantly transmitted by unprotected sexual intercourse, connatally from mother to child, or by parenteral inoculation. The efficacy of sexual transmission is significantly increased by the presence of coexisting genital infections which increase the number of infected cells in the genital secretions of the virus donor or the number of susceptible target cells when genital infection is present in the recipient. Moreover, local infection enhances immune activation, which favors virus replication.

Globally, the most frequent way of transmission is vaginal infection of women by unprotected sexual intercourse. Involvement of dendritic LC in vaginal infection was suggested in 1987 and subsequently substantiated by the demonstration that HIV-infected LC can be isolated from the skin of HIV-positive individuals (18) and are present at relatively high density in vaginal or male foreskin epithelia (68). LC and T-lymphocytes emigrating in vitro from human skin explants and forming tight conjugates were easily infectable with various primary or cell line-adapted isolates of HIV-1. Massive virus production was observed in conjugates, or even syncytia, composed of both memory T cells and LC, while LC alone released little virus (107). Studies with SIV in macaques demonstrated that free virus is able to penetrate the untraumatized vaginal epithelium and that the first cells infected are LC located in the vaginal epithelium (136). In addition to cell-free infection, virus may be transmitted by HIV-infected cells present in semen which may infect epithelial cells (139). Virus released from these cells may then infect dendritic cells or macrophages in the second line. Male genital infection may be mediated by LC present at relatively high density in the penile foreskin. Monocyte/macrophages present in the urethra might serve as alternative virus targets.

In rectal infection, a possible primary target of the virus is the intestinal M cells which are present at high frequency in the rectal mucosa, while dendritic cells were reported to be absent (3, 68, 119). M cells transport particulate antigenic material, such as bacteria or viruses, by endocytosis through the epithelial lining of the intestine and deliver them to lymphocytes, macrophages, and dendritic cells of the organized gut-associated lymphoid tissue located underneath. Mucosal explants from Peyer's patches of mice and rabbits demonstrated that HIV-1 particles adhered to the luminal membranes of M cells of both species and were endocytosed and delivered to intraepithelial spaces containing lymphocytes and macrophages (3). Alternatively, the virus might infect intestinal epithelial cells. In vitro infection of a human intestinal epithelial cell line which coexpresses CXCR4 and galactosylceramide, but not CD4, has been demonstrated (43). Presence of CXCR4 could favor infection by virulent T-tropic viruses, which might explain why receptive anal intercourse is associated with a faster progression to AIDS (101). In addition, high expression of other coreceptors, Bonzo/STRL33 in the small intestine and, respectively, BOB/GPR15 in the colon, has been observed (46).

Peroral infection has been documented in mother-to-child transmission involving breast-feeding and been implicated in some cases of transmission in which the only risk factor was receptive oral intercourse (118). In addition, recent studies with peroral inoculation of neonate macaques with SIV have demonstrated an efficiency of this route which, despite being 830 times lower than that of intravenous transmission, was 6,000-fold higher than rectal transmission (10).

Propagation of Infection and Generalization

LC are bone marrow-derived professional antigen-presenting cells (APC), which are positive for CD4, Fc gamma receptors, and HLA class II antigens and reside in many different tissues, including skin and all mucosal epithelia, except those of the urethra and the rectum (68). Upon contact with antigen they become activated and migrate by the afferent lymphatics to the regional lymph nodes, in order to present the antigen to T cells. HIV-infected LC by themselves appear not to replicate HIV well. However, if $CD4^+$ T cells are added to LC, very active virus replication is observed in vitro (25, 107, 150). Massive virus production has also been observed in multinucleated giant cells that exhibit dendritic cell markers and were found in mucosal surface of the nasopharyngeal adenoids of HIV-positive individuals (52). These observations suggest that during the close contact of dendritic cells and $CD4^+$ T cells required for antigen presentation, virus is activated from antigen-presenting cells and transmitted to the $CD4^+$ T cells, whence replication in conjugates of both cell types, or possibly even a fusion product of the two, is supported by mutual activation (Fig. 4). Such encounters leading to bursts of virus production may occur in the submucosal tissues of the viral entry ports themselves, in the afferent lymphatics, and, finally, in the mantle zone of the lymph node follicles, where the $CD4^+$ T cells reside. The availability of densely packed $CD4^+$ T cells in the absence of an efficient immune response results in large-scale virus production. In consequence, free virus particles, as well as virus-infected cells, can exit the lymph node by the efferent lymphatics and infect lymph nodes further downstream and enter the peripheral circulation. This process leads to generalized infection of all lymphoid tissues, as well as the central nervous system. Central nervous system infection is probably mediated by in-

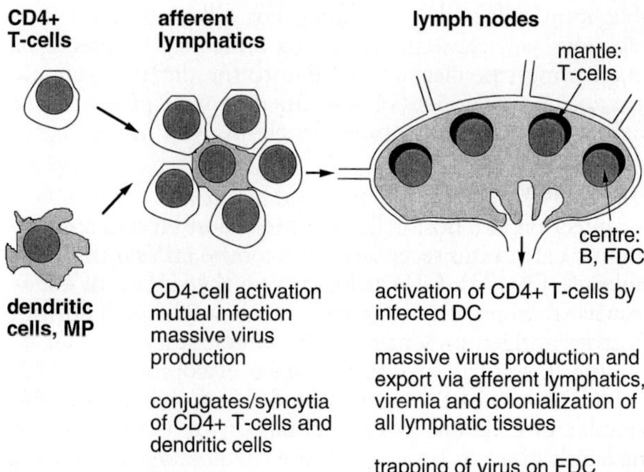

FIGURE 4 Propagation of HIV from the entry port to the lymphatics and the bloodstream. MP, macrophages; DC, dendritic cells; FDC, follicular dendritic cells.

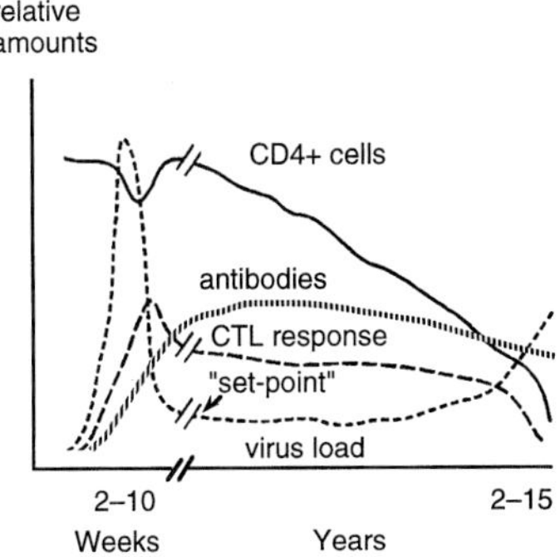

FIGURE 5 Virological and immunological parameters in the typical course of HIV infection (95).

fected cells of the monocyte/macrophage lineage which are known to possess the ability to cross the blood-brain barrier.

Acute Infection and Chronicity

Figure 5 summarizes the virological and immunological situation in acute and chronic infection. Hematogenic spread leads to infection of all lymphoid tissues in the body. Replication of HIV within the lymphatics causes, in the absence of a specific immune response, a rapid increase in production and release of viral particles and virus-infected cells. In the blood, this results in a concomitant burst in levels of cell-free or cell-associated infectious virus, particle-associated viral RNA, p24 antigen, and cell-associated DNA (28, 38, 57, 74, 103). The earliest virus population observed following HIV transmission is generally of the NSI phenotype and genotypically very homogeneous (44, 153), even after exposure to inocula of mixed NSI/SI phenotype (36). Lymph node biopsy performed close to acute infection shows germinal center hyperplasia with prominence of plasma cells in the cortical zones and a hyperplastic reticulum network of follicular dendritic cells and an abundance of B cells in the mantle zone and of $CD4^+$ T cells and interdigitating cells in the paracortex. Increased expression of interleukin 1 (IL-1), IL-2, IL-6, IL-10, tumor necrosis factor alpha (TNF-α), and gamma interferon (IFN-γ) is present (82). In the blood, severe primary HIV infection is characterized by an initial lymphopenia followed by $CD8^+$ lymphocytosis and inversion of the CD4/CD8 ratio. Subsequently, the $CD8^+$ count gradually returns to normal, whereas the CD4/CD8 ratio remains inverted because of a relatively low number of $CD4^+$ lymphocytes. Primary infection is followed by prolonged and severe cellular hyporesponsiveness to both mitogens and antigen (96, 134).

Viral levels decrease with the onset of the antiviral immune response, namely, the production of HIV-specific cytotoxic T lymphocytes (32, 74, 93) (Fig. 5). A reduced availability of infectable cells has also been proposed to be responsible for the decrease in virus load (102). Despite the absence of neutralizing antibodies at this timepoint, the humoral response, namely, antibody-dependent cellular cytotoxicity, also may contribute to virus load reduction (32).

After the reduction, concentrations of virus in the blood are stabilized on individually different levels, the so-called set-point or inflection point, which is strongly associated with disease outcome (65, 71, 87). The set-point is the equilibrium resulting from the interplay of viral, host cell, and immunological factors. This equilibrium is reached several months to 2 years after the acute phase. Thus, it may also be influenced by neutralizing antibodies which normally become detectable within this time. Viral titers in plasma change very little for a long time, which corresponds to clinical latency. During this time, the $CD4^+$ cell count decreases continuously at an individually characteristic rate. A marked increase in the level of viral RNA in plasma is seen only in advanced immunodeficiency, when the $CD4^+$ cell count has dropped to below 200.

The time to AIDS depends on age at the point of infection, with older patients whose immune system is impaired having a more rapid progression, indicating relevance of immunologic factors. Development of an increasingly complex viral quasispecies was found in nonprogressors, while rapid $CD4^+$ T-cell decline and AIDS were often associated with lower quasispecies complexity. This indirectly suggests that a strongly selective antiviral immune response is associated with a better prognosis in both adults (44, 86, 152) and children (54). Furthermore, a number of major histocompatibility complex-encoded genes have been identified which, alone or in combination, may positively or negatively affect disease progression (reviewed in reference 61). On the cellular level, resistance to infection by M-tropic viruses due to defects in the CCR5 coreceptor has been demonstrated (42, 135).

The common denominator of these prognostic factors is the extent by which the virus replicates in the host. Defects in coreceptors, a vigorous antiviral immune response, or an attenuated virus strain all contribute to restrict viral replication. On the other hand, immune activation, e.g., by chronic infections such as tuberculosis, enhances virus production. The resulting virus load after the establishment of equilibrium (i.e., the set-point) is thus the most important prognostic factor.

During the asymptomatic phase of the infection virus production in the lymphatics continues steadily (50, 94). Within the lymphoid tissues, virus is activated from latently infected $CD4^+$ T cells which are predominantly located in the mantle zone of follicles; macrophages may also be an important source of infectious virus (91). Released virus passes the follicular dendritic cell network. The follicular dendritic cell network has been shown to trap virus particles bound in immune complexes. Trapped virus remains infectious—even in the presence of neutralizing antibodies—and may thus infect T cells which migrate through the lymph node (63).

Virus Replication Dynamics

Effective antiretroviral drugs capable of rendering noninfectious most of the virus produced by virus-expressing cells have allowed to determine virus replication dynamics in various host cell compartments (Fig. 6). About 99% of virus production is thought to be maintained by productively infected lymphocytes in which the interval between infection, virus production, and cell death is a half-time of about 1 day. In order to keep the virus concentration in equilibrium, approximately 10^{10} virus particles must be released per day. The length of a replication cycle of acutely producing $CD4^+$ T cells was estimated at 2.6 days. Thirty-five million $CD4^+$ T cells are daily lost from the blood and must be replaced. In the whole body, this amounts to about 1.8×10^9 cells per day (67, 97, 98, 148).

In addition to the bulk virus production in acutely infected $CD4^+$ cells, latently infected $CD4^+$ cells and longer-lived cells such as macrophages or LC also contribute to virus production, but their share in untreated patients is about 1%. These proportions change when efficient antiret-

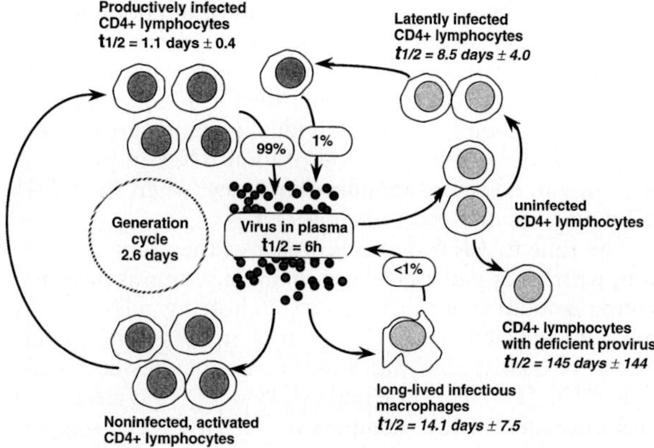

FIGURE 6 Kinetics of HIV production and elimination in vivo. Based on references 97 and 98.

roviral treatment blocks the acute replication cycle. In this phase, the longevity of these cell types with half-times on the order of weeks to, possibly, months necessitates continuation of aggressive therapy for several years. The outcome of these therapies is still uncertain.

DIAGNOSTIC ASPECTS OF HIV INFECTION

The two principal questions in HIV diagnostics are whether a person is infected and, if infected, how actively the virus is replicating. Susceptibility to antiretroviral drugs may evolve as another important question in the near future.

HIV infection can be detected by a variety of tests. Virus can be directly detected by assays for various viral components. These include proteins, which can be specifically assayed by immunological tests; RT, whose enzymatic activity can be detected by functional tests; and viral DNA or RNA, which can be identified by molecular tests. Most frequently, however, HIV infection is diagnosed by tests which assess whether an individual's immune system has produced an HIV-specific immune response. Since retroviruses are known to establish infections which persist for life, demonstration of an HIV-specific immune response, if it is consistent and directed against various different viral antigens, can be trusted to reflect ongoing infection. Thus, testing for HIV-specific antibodies is still the mainstay of HIV diagnostics, at least in adults. In infants, testing for virus components is clearly more reliable because of the potential transplacental transfer of antibodies from infected mothers to their offspring.

The diagnosis of HIV infection relies on commercially available test kits. Strong competition among the manufacturers and strict evaluation and control by the regulatory agencies of different countries have led to the availability of a number of excellent diagnostic products which are of high sensitivity and specificity, well standardized, and capable of providing a continuously high-quality standard of diagnostics in the user laboratory. They are frequently better and yield more consistent results than research procedures developed in the users' labs. Good commercial tests are therefore strongly recommended. Using unregistered tests for screening or for certain types of supplemental testing may even be unlawful in many countries.

Only very general descriptions of procedures will be given in the following sections, as commercial tests kits all contain detailed step-by-step instructions. For procedures which are not commercially available, the reader is directed to consult the referenced literature. The intent is to guide the reader through the multitude of available procedures and to discuss their points of strength and their weaknesses.

Diagnosis of HIV Infection

HIV Screening Tests

HIV-specific antibodies are produced within a few weeks after infection. The time to positivity in antibody tests (i.e., to seroconversion) depends on the infectious dose, the transmission mode, and the sensitivity of the antibody assay.

In a study based on first generation assays (see below), seroconversion was estimated to occur on average 45 days after infection; with 95% certainty the window period for 90% of individuals was less than 20 weeks (99). The use of other tests in reducing the average window period was estimated as follows: contemporary anti-HIV-1 or -2 enzyme immunoassays, −20.3 days (95% confidence interval [CI] range 8.0 to 32.5); p24 antigen and DNA PCR, −26.4 days (95% CI, 12.6 to 38.7); and RNA PCR, −31.0 days (95% CI, 16.7 to 45.3) (21). Thus, modern third-generation antibody screening assays should, on average, become positive 3 weeks after infection. The upper boundaries of the seroconversion interval in these more sensitive tests remain, however, undetermined.

There are numerous commercial HIV tests for screening, and it may be difficult to recognize the advantages and disadvantages of a particular test based on the information given by the manufacturer. An overview of different test formats and their properties is given in Fig. 7.

The most important kit formats used in HIV antibody screening are the indirect binding assay, the antibody capture assay, and the double-antigen sandwich assay. Indirect binding assays comprise the so-called "first-generation" enzyme-linked immunosorbent assays (ELISAs) which are based on purified viral lysate and "second-generation" tests based on recombinant antigen, usually representing Gag and TM. First-generation indirect binding assays are not restricted to ELISA but also include immunofluorescence and Western blots (WB) (immunoblots). Line immunoassays which use recombinant proteins may be categorized as second-generation indirect binding assays. Antibody capture assays usually employ recombinant proteins; their principle is that of an indirect binding assay which is reversed. Double-antigen sandwich assays (frequently also called third-generation assays) usually employ recombinant antigen. Particle agglutination, which may be considered a variant of a double antigen sandwich assay, is based on viral lysate. Although all of these different test formats detect antibodies, they vary in their precise diagnostic questions and answers. Indirect binding assays and antibody capture assays verify, by binding the sample's HIV-specific antibodies to an immunoglobulin-specific reagent, that a sample component reactive in such a test is in fact an immunoglobulin. In contrast, the identity of a component reactive in a double-antigen sandwich assay is not directly assessed and remains uncharacterized; the only information provided is that it is capable of linking solid-phase HIV antigen with liquid-phase tracer antigen.

The kit formats are affected in different ways by diagnostic variables. One possible problem is antigenic variation. The virus with which a patient is infected may exhibit proteins which vary considerably from the antigens used in the test. Consequently, the patient's antibodies may not bind efficiently to the test kit's antigen, and if they are present

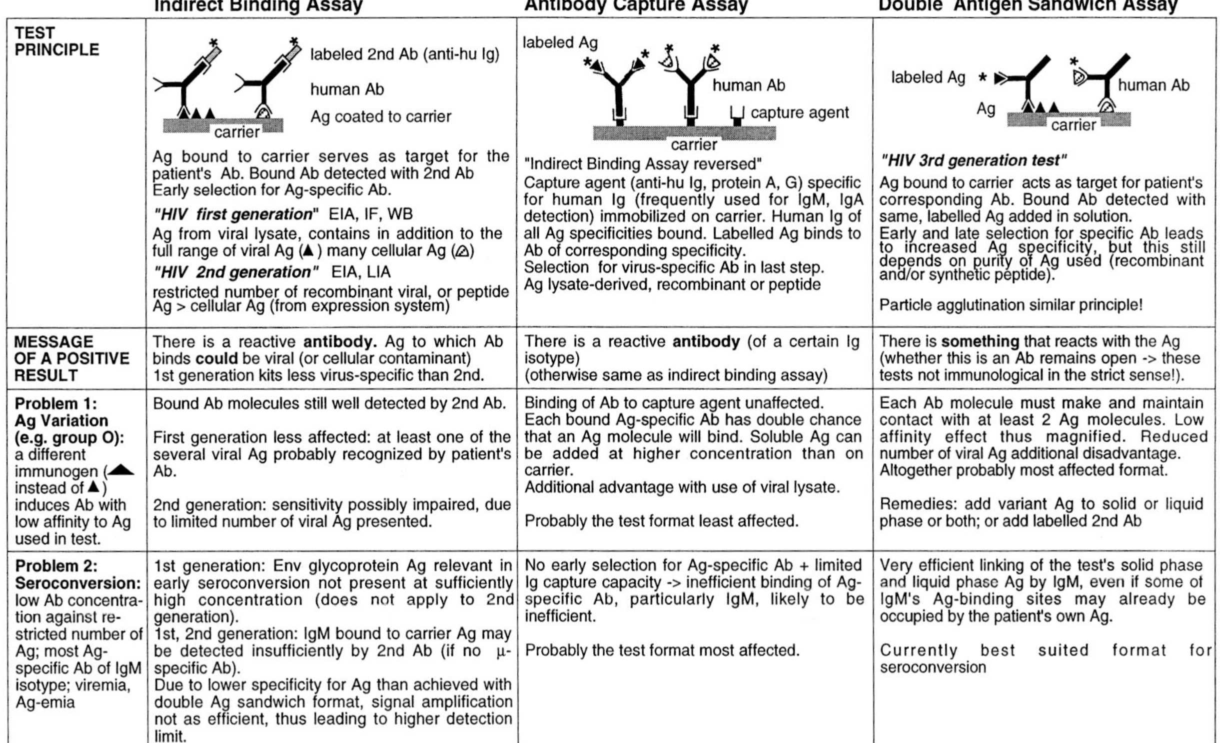

	Indirect Binding Assay	Antibody Capture Assay	Double Antigen Sandwich Assay
TEST PRINCIPLE	labeled 2nd Ab (anti-hu Ig) human Ab Ag coated to carrier carrier Ag bound to carrier serves as target for the patient's Ab. Bound Ab detected with 2nd Ab Early selection for Ag-specific Ab. ***"HIV first generation"*** EIA, IF, WB Ag from viral lysate, contains in addition to the full range of viral Ag (▲) many cellular Ag (◬) ***"HIV 2nd generation"*** EIA, LIA restricted number of recombinant viral, or peptide Ag > cellular Ag (from expression system)	labeled Ag human Ab capture agent carrier "Indirect Binding Assay reversed" Capture agent (anti-hu Ig, protein A, G) specific for human Ig (frequently used for IgM, IgA detection) immobilized on carrier. Human Ig of all Ag specificities bound. Labelled Ag binds to Ab of corresponding specificity. Selection for virus-specific Ab in last step. Ag lysate-derived, recombinant or peptide	labeled Ag Ag human Ab carrier ***"HIV 3rd generation test"*** Ag bound to carrier acts as target for patient's corresponding Ab. Bound Ab detected with same, labelled Ag added in solution. Early and late selection for specific Ab leads to increased Ag specificity, but this still depends on purity of Ag used (recombinant and/or synthetic peptide). Particle agglutination similar principle!
MESSAGE OF A POSITIVE RESULT	There is a reactive **antibody.** Ag to which Ab binds **could** be viral (or cellular contaminant) 1st generation kits less virus-specific than 2nd.	There is a reactive **antibody** (of a certain Ig isotype) (otherwise same as indirect binding assay)	There is **something** that reacts with the Ag (whether this is an Ab remains open -> these tests not immunological in the strict sense!).
Problem 1: Ag Variation (e.g. group O): a different immunogen (▲ instead of ▲) induces Ab with low affinity to Ag used in test.	Bound Ab molecules still well detected by 2nd Ab. First generation less affected: at least one of the several viral Ag probably recognized by patient's Ab. 2nd generation: sensitivity possibly impaired, due to limited number of viral Ag presented.	Binding of Ab to capture agent unaffected. Each bound Ag-specific Ab has double chance that an Ag molecule will bind. Soluble Ag can be added at higher concentration than on carrier. Additional advantage with use of viral lysate. Probably the test format least affected.	Each Ab molecule must make and maintain contact with at least 2 Ag molecules. Low affinity effect thus magnified. Reduced number of viral Ag additional disadvantage. Altogether probably most affected format. Remedies: add variant Ag to solid or liquid phase or both; or add labelled 2nd Ab
Problem 2: Seroconversion: low Ab concentration against restricted number of Ag; most Ag-specific Ab of IgM isotype; viremia, Ag-emia	1st generation: Env glycoprotein Ag relevant in early seroconversion not present at sufficiently high concentration (does not apply to 2nd generation). 1st, 2nd generation: IgM bound to carrier Ag may be detected insufficiently by 2nd Ab (if no μ-specific Ab). Due to lower specificity for Ag than achieved with double Ag sandwich format, signal amplification not as efficient, thus leading to higher detection limit.	No early selection for Ag-specific Ab + limited Ig capture capacity -> inefficient binding of Ag-specific Ab, particularly IgM, likely to be inefficient. Probably the test format most affected.	Very efficient linking of the test's solid phase and liquid phase Ag by IgM, even if some of IgM's Ag-binding sites may already be occupied by the patient's own Ag. Currently best suited format for seroconversion

FIGURE 7 Kit design and test performance of HIV screening tests. Synopsis of the most frequently used test formats, their principles, meaning of positive results, and performance in two typical problem situations. Ag, antigen; Ab, antibody; Ig, immunoglobulin; EIA, enzyme immunoassay; LIA, line immunoassay; WB, Western blot. Slightly modified from reference 121.

at low titer a false-negative result may be generated. This type of problem was first recognized after the discovery of HIV-2 when it was found that antibodies induced by HIV-2 were not well recognized by screening kits based solely on HIV-1 antigens. This led to the inclusion of HIV-2 components, usually of the transmembrane protein, into the kits. A similar problem was recognized when group O viruses were discovered (41, 58). Double-antigen sandwich assays are most affected by antigen variation, the reason being that in order to generate a positive result, antibodies must bind at least two antigen molecules. Double binding is unlikely if the kit antigen and the patient's antibodies do not strongly interact. In indirect binding assays and antibody capture assays, antibodies need only bind a single antigen molecule in order to generate a signal. The sensitivity of double-antigen sandwich assays was, however, relatively easily improved by inclusion of recombinant group O antigens into the solid and/or liquid phase.

Another typical problem situation is early seroconversion. Antibodies in this phase are restricted to a few viral proteins (usually envelope and p24), they are of low titer and low affinity, and the dominating immunoglobulin isotypes are immunoglobulin M (IgM) and possibly IgA. In addition, they may be partially saturated with HIV antigen, which is usually present at high concentrations. In this situation it is important that the test provide a high concentration of that antigen which is best recognized. This goal is more easily achieved with recombinant proteins than with viral lysate. Furthermore, the test must select for the few HIV-specific antibodies present in the bulk immunoglobulin. This is impossible with antibody capture assays, which bind immunoglobulins of all antigenic specificities. In addition, the test should detect IgM because, in the presence of antigenemia, its pentameric structure with a total of 10 antigen binding sites is most likely to still have several sites remaining accessible. The best assay in this situation is the double-antigen sandwich assay: it initially selects for HIV-specific antibodies (binding to solid phase), and it does not discriminate against non-IgG isotypes. The first test of this principle which went into diagnostic use is the particle agglutination assay, which was introduced in the mid-eighties, i.e., long before third-generation ELISAs were developed. This test, which uses viral lysate for antigen, performs remarkably well in seroconversion panels and, due to the broad spectrum of antigens present in the viral lysate, has in addition a broad detection range for antigenic variation (34, 147).

The practical relevance of these considerations is shown when the performance of different kits with seroconversion panels is compared. Among 25 different commercial kits compared by the Swiss Federal Office of Public Health on the basis of their performance on at least 15 different commercially available seroconversion panels, the 15 double-antigen sandwich assays were the most sensitive and occupied ranks 1 to 9, 12 to 14, 16, and 17. The six indirect binding assays occupied ranks 10, 15, 19, 21, 22, and 24, and the four antibody capture assays ranked at 11, 20, 23, and 25 (unpublished). Seroconversion panel comparisons also demonstrate the inferior sensitivity of immunofluorescence tests or WB, which rank together with other indirect antibody binding assays. Assessment of the performance in seroconversion panels followed by revocation of approval for the 10 to 20% least-sensitive kits is one of the most powerful instruments of regulatory agencies to guarantee a continuous further technical improvement of diagnostic tests for HIV (121).

In conclusion, for antibody screening in the laboratory one should use kits which detect antibodies to both HIV-1 and HIV-2, have documented good sensitivity to group M and O infections, and perform well in seroconversion panels. Reactive samples or those with results in a borderline zone have to be retested and, if repeatedly reactive, have to be submitted to confirmatory or supplemental testing.

Rapid Tests and Home Testing

Rapid tests are assays which can be performed with minimal or no laboratory equipment and yield results within 30 min. Such tests may be useful in certain situations, e.g., in assessing the risk of HIV transmission in needle-stick injuries and similar exposures to possibly HIV-contaminated materials, organ donations, or whenever a laboratory test result may not be available within due time. Rapid tests may be of different formats, including double-antigen sandwich, indirect binding, immunoglobulin capture, or agglutination assay. Some of them have good sensitivity and specificity. In more extensive seroconversion panel comparisons, the sensitivity of such tests seems, however, somewhat inferior to the most recent generation of ELISA-based tests (75, 80, 114). Therefore, the use of such tests should be restricted to emergency situations.

Many persons infected with HIV are not tested until they develop symptoms. Up to one-third of patients receive their HIV diagnosis within 2 months of progression to AIDS. The hope that such individuals would get tested earlier has led to the development of new testing strategies, some of which have already been approved by the Food and Drug Administration (FDA). Already approved are home test collection systems, where kits may be ordered by phone and are delivered by express courier. Blood is collected onto filter paper by finger pricking and sent to a designated laboratory for screening. If screening is reactive, supplemental tests can be performed on the same sample. Results, as well as personal counseling, are available by calling an information phone number. Such testing systems have a very good sensitivity and specificity, since testing remains in the hands of professionals. Collecting a sufficiently large specimen may be the biggest problem, which may affect 7 to 10% of the users. As an alternative, testing systems for other fluids, namely, oral fluids or urine, have also been approved by the FDA, despite the fact that their sensitivity cannot be evaluated by seroconversion panels. The observation that HIV-exposed seronegative individuals considered uninfected have a high frequency of HIV-reactive IgA in urine and that even 8% of supposedly unexposed controls exhibit such reactions presents certain problems regarding the specificity of such tests (83). It can also be expected that more problems would be encountered with true home testing kits in which all steps of the test have to be performed by the user. Such kits have therefore not yet been approved (19).

Supplemental Testing

Antibody

WB was introduced into HIV testing in 1984 (115, 127), was proposed for systematic confirmation of reactive ELISA results in 1985 (126), and has remained a principal confirmatory tool used worldwide. It has become clear that in comparison to other tests which were continuously improved, WB have remained first-generation kits which have some well-known flaws. Their sensitivity in seroconversion panels is clearly inferior to double-antigen sandwich tests, and they rank together with first-generation indirect antibody-binding ELISA. Furthermore, they are prone to detect cross-reactive antibodies not associated with HIV infection, which results in a high rate of indeterminate results.

One improvement, the use of recombinant proteins for the production of the strips, has been employed by a few manufacturers. When recombinant proteins are used instead of viral lysate, strips can be produced as line immunoassays in which the purified antigens are applied in separate bands to the membranes. Some of these tests have a better sensitivity and specificity than conventional WB and can discriminate between HIV-1 and HIV-2 infection. They still have a sizable rate of indeterminate results (106). This shows that indeterminate WB reactions are caused predominantly by antibodies that cross-react with HIV proteins rather than with cellular contaminants of the viral lysate. In another product, recombinant Env TM protein of HIV-2 has been added to strips otherwise produced with viral lysate, in order to improve detection of HIV-2 antibodies. While this format does improve detection of HIV-2 infections, a separate WB for HIV-2 is still needed to confirm the reaction.

WB is more prone to problems with carryover contamination than are the screening assays. The use of the very convenient multichannel troughs for incubation of the strips with the test sample presents a certain risk. Contamination with minute volumes of a strongly positive serum may lead to faint Env bands, even when the dilution is up to one million-fold. Intra-assay contamination can be ruled out by repeating the assay in an isolated test chamber. Repeat testing will not identify contamination of the specimen tube. Touching the wet inner side of a specimen tube lid with the gloved fingers may carry enough material to the lid of a subsequently opened tube to result in faint WB reactivity to Env antigens. The probability of such events depends on the share of strongly positive sera among the specimens tested by a laboratory and on how many times a specimen tube is opened. In order to minimize this risk, handling and testing samples from known HIV-positive individuals together with diagnostic samples should be avoided and gloves that have become contaminated with specimen must be changed immediately. It should also be recognized that samples with initial borderline results carry an increased risk of getting contaminated, since these tubes are opened repeatedly for supplemental testing. This results in a higher cumulative risk of contamination. Alarm bells should ring when a sample with borderline or low-positive results in screening has a faintly reactive WB. It may be an early seroconversion sample, but it may also be the result of contamination. The contamination problem is a strong reason why WB interpretation should follow the most stringent, and not the most sensitive, guidelines.

Indeterminate WB results have been described in patients with autoimmune disorders, in particular systemic lupus erythematosus, after infections with certain viruses including herpes simplex virus type 1 or cytomegalovirus, or after vaccination against influenza or rabies virus. For the latter, epitopes related to HIV have been implicated. Practically, such information is of little value and the origin of indeterminate WB reactions in individual patients usually remains obscure.

In spite of all these flaws, a WB with a "full-house" pattern of reactive antibodies probably remains the most convincing evidence for an HIV infection. In addition, WB may offer some information on whether the infection is caused by HIV-1 or HIV-2 (especially if the strips contain recombinant HIV-2 protein in addition to the viral lysate of HIV-1) and on the clinical stage of the infection (126). When reactive bands are few and their intensity low, interpretation is hazardous, however, and a diagnosis must not be based on WB alone.

WB interpretation guidelines. In an attempt to render WB more sensitive, the Association of State and Territorial Public Health Laboratory Directors and the Centers for Disease Control (ASTPHLD/CDC) issued interpretation recommendations which require antibody reaction (of undescribed intensity) to any two of three antigen bands including gp 120/160 (considered one antigen), gp41, and p24 (5). Since most of the gp160 and gp120 bands on WB are not due to the Env precursor or the SU protein but instead represent tetramers or trimers of gp41 (104), confirmed positivity established on reaction with gp120/gp160 and gp41 is most likely based on reaction with a single protein, TM, and thus inherently unsafe. The same is true for the very similar recommendations by the Consortium for Retrovirus Serology Standardization (CRSS), the only difference being that p24 may be replaced by p31 (*pol*). In the absence of other bands, this combination is, however, extremely rare and interpretation by CRSS is usually the same as that by ASTPHLD/CDC. Similarly, the WHO recommendation requests any two of gp160, gp120, and gp41 (6). This means practically that TM-reactive antibodies must be present at a concentration sufficient for detection of not only the strongest, but also the second-strongest TM band. The strongest TM band is usually the largest antigen, i.e., gp160, which migrates least in the sodium dodecyl sulfate-polyacrylamide gel electrophoresis (SDS-PAGE)-based separation of proteins and thus is the sharpest and best-detected band. Depending on the manufacturer, either gp120 or gp41 may be the second-strongest band. Due to varying degrees of glycosylation, gp41 migrates in SDS-PAGE as a very diffuse band. Reactive antibodies thus generate a signal that is much less well recognized than if the same antibodies bind to the sharp gp160 band.

Due to the propensity of WB to detect cross-reactive antibodies, a combination of Env and p24 bands is not sufficiently stringent for confirmation. WB analysis of 100 screening-negative but otherwise unselected Swiss blood donors showed isolated reaction with p24 in 9% and with gp120/160 in 3%, respectively. The likelihood of a chance combination leading to confirmed positivity in a normal donor would thus be $0.09 \times 0.03 = 0.0027$, i.e., 1 out of 370 (129). We and others (62) have observed several cases which satisfied the ASTPHLD/CDC criteria for WB positivity, kept this pattern essentially unchanged over years, but were negative in long-term follow up in all direct tests for HIV including virus culture, PCR for HIV DNA and RNA, and an antigen test of a sensitivity comparable to that of PCR (see below). Representative WB of a recent such case from our laboratory are shown in Fig. 8. In another such case, very low concentrations of particle-associated RT activity were detected in plasma and the activity was shown to be transmissible to fresh leukocytes in culture, thus suggesting an infectious agent undetectable in HIV-specific virus component tests (128).

More stringent interpretation criteria have been issued by the American Red Cross (ARC) and by the FDA. ARC

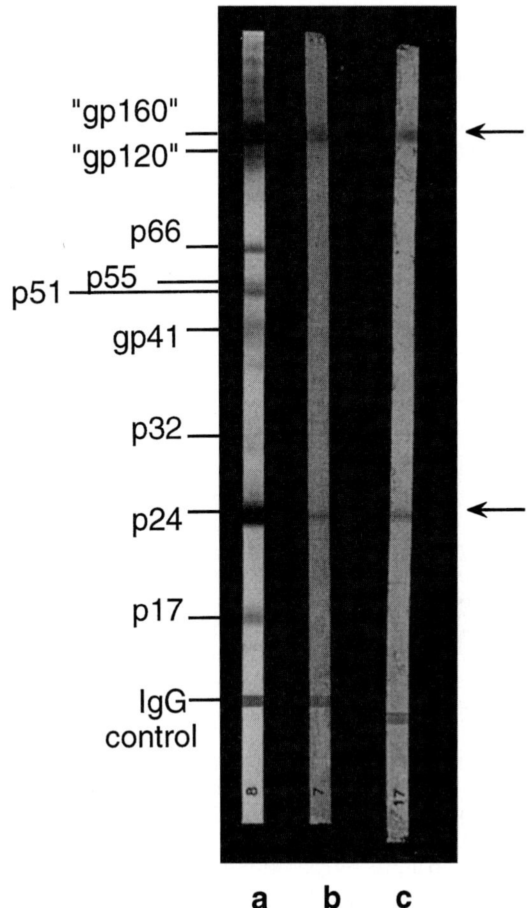

FIGURE 8 Example of false-positive Western blot interpretation according to ASTPHLD/CDC or CRSS guidelines. (a) Weakly positive control. (b) Sample of a healthy individual exhibiting weak reaction with gp160, gp120 (very weak), and p24. This sample was taken 3.5 months after an initial sample with the same pattern (not shown). (c) Sample of same individual taken 1 month after the initial sample. P24 antigen with signal-amplification-boosted ELISA was negative in all three plasma samples; PCR for viral DNA was negative in PBMC from samples b and c, and RNA was negative in plasma b. Culture with PBMC depleted of CD8$^+$ T cells from sample b was negative for p24 antigen and RT by PERT assay; this test was also negative with plasmas b and c.

requires at least one band each from Env, Gag, and Pol but does not specify the identity of these bands. The most stringent—but least sensitive—recommendation is by the FDA, which requires reactions with p24, p31, and Env.

In my opinion, only the most stringent interpretation guidelines are to be applied if a diagnosis of HIV infection is established by using WB as the only supplemental test. If some true cases of HIV infection are WB indeterminate by the FDA guidelines, this is of no concern as long as their WB patterns are suggestive of HIV infection. This is always the case if ASTPHLD/CDC interpretation would render these patterns positive. In all such cases, a safe diagnosis can be established based on supplemental tests for virus components. One has also to take into account that ASTPHLD/CDC criteria were established on the basis of a single commercial product, the Du Pont WB. Meanwhile, other valuable kits are available whose protein composition may differ. Guidelines established for one particular kit and with one particular sample cohort cannot be applied to other kits or populations from other geographical regions without careful reexamination of their validity.

Another attempt to make WB more sensitive in early infection is their use for detection of IgM. However, such testing lacks specificity. As detailed below, Gag-reactive antibodies of IgM, IgA, and IgG isotype are frequently detected by WB in serum of infants born to HIV-negative mothers. Therefore, many of these reactions appear due to common agents unrelated to HIV.

In order to avoid the practical and financial problems associated with WB, WHO has recommended alternative test strategies based on the use of at least two different screening tests (116). Large studies showed that such testing algorithms may yield results that are at least equivalent to the conventional testing algorithm in which all samples repeatedly reactive in a screening assay are submitted to WB testing. In one algorithm, reactive samples are submitted to another screening assay and only those samples with discrepant results are submitted to WB testing. As an alternative, initial screening is performed with two different tests and those with discrepancies are submitted to supplemental testing. Supplemental testing by WB can also be replaced without loss in sensitivity or specificity by a third screening assay (70, 77, 142, 146).

Given the further development of screening tests since the time these studies were done, such testing algorithms have become even more attractive. Particularly initial screening with two tests (which should ideally combine a double-antigen sandwich assay with either an indirect binding assay or an antibody capture assay) are bound to increase the sensitivity of the procedure still more. However, as mentioned above, this strategy does not establish whether an infection is due to HIV-1 or HIV-2 (see below). This question is of importance regarding the validity of results of sequence-based virus load determination or, respectively, the need for antiretroviral treatment. WB or, where available, a line or dot immunoassay will therefore frequently be done anyway. There are also some rapid tests which can discriminate between HIV-1 and HIV-2 infections.

Virus Components

In many cases, supplemental testing requires the use of tests for virus components. This applies to samples from patients presenting with signs, symptoms, or a history of an acute retroviral syndrome, as well as to all samples with indeterminate results in antibody testing. In addition, diagnosis of pediatric HIV infection is best established based on virus component tests. Virus components that can be assayed include the p24 antigen, viral DNA or RNA, and RT activity. In addition, the capability of the virus to replicate can be assessed by virus isolation in cell culture. This requires an HIV-specific virus component test for identification of virus released into the supernatant, usually an antigen test.

Commercially available diagnostic tests for these components include p24 antigen assays which are available from several companies. A commercial kit is available for PCR detection of HIV-1 DNA. Amplification-based tests for viral RNA are available from several manufacturers and currently include the polymerase chain reaction for reverse-transcribed RNA (RT-PCR), the nucleic acid sequence-based amplification (NASBA), and a signal-amplification procedure involving branched DNA probes (bDNA).

Antigen Tests

Antigen tests for p24 are easy to perform and diagnostically valuable in early infection, when antigen is usually present at high titers in the peripheral blood, while HIV-specific antibodies may still be undetectable or present at concentrations too low to permit a confirmed-positive diagnosis. The test principle consists of binding the p24 antigen present in a sample to p24-specific, usually monoclonal, capture antibodies which are coated onto a solid support. Unbound sample components are washed away and bound antigen is reacted with another p24-specific tracer antibody to which is conjugated an enzyme (horseradish peroxidase or alkaline phosphatase) capable of signal generation when combined with a suitable substrate (Fig. 9A). For confirmation of a reactive result, the sample must be subjected to a neutralization assay. This means that the antigen test is repeated in the presence of HIV-specific antibodies. These bind the antigen in immune complexes, thus preventing its detection in the test (Fig. 9B). The most advanced antigen test which has recently been approved by the regulatory agencies of several European countries detects not only groups M and O of HIV-1 very efficiently, but also HIV-2.

Antigen p24 measurement is frequently confronted with two principal confounders. One is the presence of p24-specific antibodies, which—as in the neutralization assay—complex the antigen, thus causing underdetection or false-negative results (Fig. 9B). This problem is exemplified in the course of early HIV infection during which the increase of antibody concentrations in serum or plasma leads to immune complexation of the antigen and a rapid decrease of its detectability. This may lead to a situation in which Western blots may still be inconclusive and the antigen test negative. The other problem is the presence of immunoglobulin-specific, rheumatoid-factor-like antibodies which may bridge the capture and the tracer antibody of an antigen test and thus cause overdetection or false-positive results (Fig. 9C). This type of problem is present when in the neutralization test the addition of HIV-specific antibodies to the test sample does not result in a higher degree of signal reduction than the addition of normal control antibodies.

Solutions to these problems proposed and introduced into routine testing were primarily aimed at improving detection of immune-complexed antigen. Acidification or base treatment leads to a significant, though incomplete, release of antigen, thus increasing the proportion of positives significantly. These treatments will, however, also release rheumatoid factors from preformed immunoglobulin-anti-immunoglobulin complexes, thus aggravating the problem

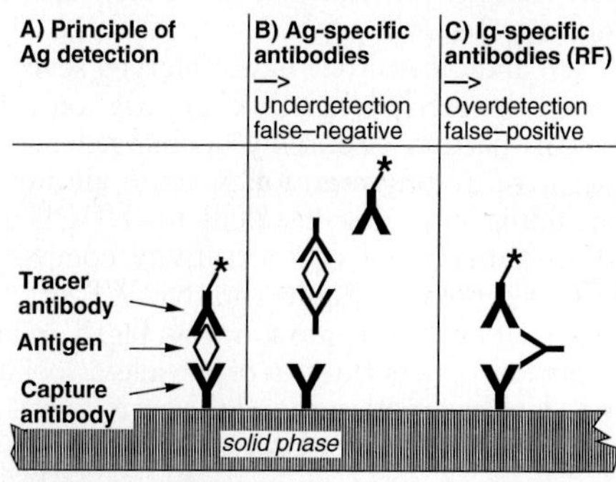

FIGURE 9 Principle of antigen testing and interference by antigen-specific or immunoglobulin-specific antibodies. For description, refer to text.

of false positivity (59). A third problem of antigen assays consists in their insufficient analytical and diagnostic sensitivity, which renders the practical use of these tests rather low when compared to molecular-based tests for viral RNA or DNA.

Recently, modifications at several steps of the antigen detection procedure have resulted in considerable improvements, however (Fig. 10A). First, boiling diluted serum for 5 min prior to antigen testing destroys the antigen-binding capacity of all antibodies, thus irreversibly eliminating both of the above interferences, while leaving the antigen in a condition permitting its detection by some, though not all, commercial assays (122). Moreover, use of plasma instead of serum and boosting the antigen assay with a simple signal amplification step rendered antigen detection in adult HIV-1 positive individuals as sensitive as a commercial RT-PCR kit for viral RNA quantification whose detection limit is about 200 copies/ml. This variant of antigen assay is thus of interest as a highly sensitive and specific, yet inexpensive diagnostic tool for both pediatric and adult HIV-1 infection

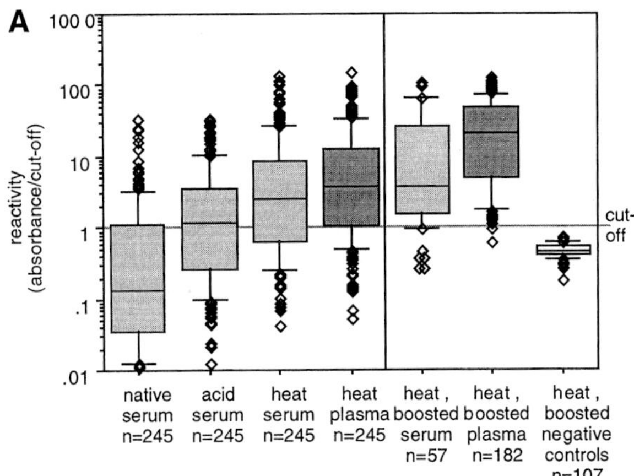

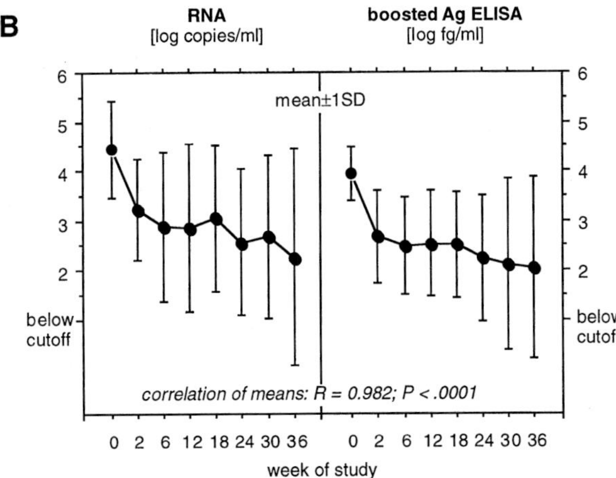

FIGURE 10 Improvements in p24 antigen detection and use of a signal-amplification-boosted p24 antigen ELISA of heat-denatured plasma for antiretroviral treatment monitoring. (A) Improvements achieved by various procedures involving the same cohort of serum or plasma samples from 245 HIV-positive patients at different stages of the infection. (B) Comparison of virus load testing by commercial RT-PCR and signal amplification-boosted antigen ELISA. Composed from references 15 and 125.

(79, 125). The same procedure can also be used as a quantitative test for antiretroviral treatment monitoring (see below).

Test for Viral RNA or DNA

As mentioned above, three different techniques for the sensitive detection of HIV RNA or DNA are presently available. In PCR, double-stranded DNA is denatured, a pair of HIV-specific primers is annealed to the separated viral DNA strands and these primers are extended by a heat-resistent DNA-dependent DNA polymerase (*Taq* polymerase). This procedure is continued for 30 to 40 cycles, each of which comprises a high-temperature denaturation, a low-temperature primer annealing, and an intermediate-temperature primer extension (DNA synthesis) element (76). If the starting material for PCR is RNA, a cDNA must first be generated by reverse transcription. This cDNA can then be amplified by the regular procedure (22). In the current commercial kit for HIV-1 group M genomic RNA, a 142-bp sequence from the *gag* gene is amplified and the double-stranded DNA product is analyzed by ELISA.

In NASBA, RNA is amplified in an isothermal multienzymatic procedure mediated by the enzymatic effects of RNA-dependent DNA polymerase (reverse transcriptase), RNase H, DNA-dependent DNA polymerase, and DNA-dependent RNA polymerase. This procedure thus mimicks the retroviral replication cycle (Fig. 1). The product of this procedure is RNA (72). A sequence from *gag* similar to that of the RT-PCR kit is amplified.

In the bDNA method, viral RNA is captured onto a solid surface by immobilized specific capture probes. Captured RNA is then reacted with "connector" probes which with one end hybridize to a series of short sequences of the *pol* region of the RNA and with the other end mediate fixation of branched DNA (bDNA) detector probes. These bDNA are then reacted with still other bDNA which hybridize to the first. Enzyme-labeled tracer probes are finally hybridized to all the branches, and the analysis is based on chemoluminescence (143). The procedure has been compared to a Christmas tree: the more branches it has, the more candles can be attached and the brighter is the light which emerges from a single tree. The principal difference of bDNA to PCR or NASBA is that there is no amplification of viral sequences and, in consequence, no carryover problem. What is called signal amplification is in fact a mere signal accumulation in which interacting molecular probes added to the reaction at predetermined high concentration are hybridized to captured viral RNA in an ordered process which results in the deposition of consecutive probe layers. The procedure is in fact comparable to an indirect antibody binding assay, where a first, antigen-specific antibody binds to the antigen and is then detected by second antibodies with specificity for the first. With this system, a greater degree of precision is achieved than with nucleic acid amplification techniques whose outcome depends on the efficacy of primer annealing in each cycle. Another important advantage of bDNA is the broad specificity, which is due to the use of about 40 different probes which cover most of the *pol* gene, the most conserved retroviral gene. The drawback of the method consists in its relatively high detection level, which must be compensated by large specimen volumes (2 ml of plasma).

These nucleic acid detection kits are primarily designated for the quantification of viral RNA. Depending on their detection level, some of them, in particular PCR, may also be suitable for diagnostic (qualitative) purposes. For

HIV-1 DNA or RNA, there is one commercial PCR kit. The NASBA procedure can be used for qualitative detection of HIV-1 RNA. Many diagnostic laboratories including ours have developed their own PCR methods, in particular for qualitative detection of viral DNA or RNA. Detailed step-by-step instructions for our own diagnostic procedures have been published (14). For RNA quantification, the use of commercial kits is preferable, due to a better comparability of results obtained in different laboratories.

The availability of commercial kits for the detection of HIV-1 RNA or DNA by sequence or signal amplification has rendered these tests attractive for laboratories with no background in molecular biology. The fact that under optimal circumstances a single gene copy can be detected by some of these tests has created a relatively uncritical attitude resulting in a degree of trust not yet justified in several aspects. More than antigen tests, molecular tests are sensitive to sequence variation resulting in false-negative results if inappropriate, i.e., not well conserved, sequences are used. Carryover contamination whose main source is amplified DNA, but which may also originate from other specimens, can also be a problem, in particular with PCR, and commercial products or systems must therefore have built-in carryover protection devices. In addition, precautionary measures are a must for all laboratories performing such tests (14).

An important factor in molecular testing is sample handling and sample preparation. Particle-associated RNA in plasma was claimed to be very unstable, demanding special expensive plasma preparation tubes (PPT) of a certain manufacturer and immediate separation of plasma from the cellular pellet before shipping the sample to the laboratory which performs the test. Independent investigators have not been able to confirm these claims. Their work indicates that HIV-1 RNA levels are stable (variance less than 0.3 log) up to 3 days after collection when stored either at room temperature or at 4°C as cell-free plasma in the EDTA-PPT tubes or even as EDTA anticoagulated whole blood in regular tubes. Comparison of paired HIV-1 positive plasma and serum specimens revealed that RNA quantitation was 20 to 65% lower in serum compared to plasma. EDTA plasma is thus the preferred specimen for these assays and provides the highest levels of RNA. EDTA-plasma that is prepared and frozen within 8 h of collection can thus be trusted to represent a good material for these tests. It can be thawed and frozen up to three times before RNA levels decrease significantly (55, 92, 131).

The maximal sensitivity of molecular tests is limited by sample size and sequence variation. The theoretical detection limit of the PCR is a single DNA molecule. However, 1 μg of genomic DNA, which contains the DNA of approximately 150,000 cells, corresponds to the number of PBMC contained in only about 75 μl of blood. Consequently, even with a detection limit of 1 provirus/μg of DNA, roughly 70,000 infected cells must be present in 5,000 ml of blood for PCR analysis to be positive. A detection limit of 10 copies per reaction is more realistic because of the Poisson distribution at very low copy numbers and the resulting reactions without any copy of HIV proviral DNA. Similarly, the sensitivity for the detection of particle-associated HIV RNA is limited by the efficiency of the reverse transcription step and by the volume of analyzed plasma. In order to achieve higher sensitivity, sample input is now frequently increased to milliliter plasma volumes (120). Further loss of sensitivity is due to sequence divergence of HIV-1 and HIV-2 and from the extensive sequence variation of HIV. Attempts to develop a unique pair of primers which allows PCR amplification from all HIV isolates have so far failed. Hence, in order to achieve a high sensitivity several pairs of primers are required, if both HIV types and all different subtypes are to be detected.

Comparative testing of different subtypes of HIV-1 indicated that results of first-generation test kits for quantification of viral RNA varied widely among subtypes other than B. In particular, RT-PCR was unable to detect subtype A in samples in which both bDNA and NASBA detected 10^4–10^5 RNA copies/ml. Recognition of subtype E, F, and G isolates was also impaired with the RT-PCR kit, though to a lesser degree. On the other hand, NASBA failed to detect subtype G even when the other two tests detected more than 10^5 copies. Subtype H was also underestimated. The test least affected was bDNA, which detected all isolates of subtypes A to H with copy estimates ranging from 17,000 to 600,000/ml (37). That bDNA is less impaired by sequence variation is certainly due to the use of the multitude of different *pol*-specific probes. A failure of some of these to hybridize to the target sequence has only a minor impact on overall signal generation from an individual RNA molecule than the misfit of a single primer used in the two amplification methods for target sequences.

The performance of the commercial RT-PCR kit has been significantly improved by addition of a "mix-in" primer pair. These primers amplify the same 142-nt sequence of *gag* as the primers of the ordinary kit, but due to some nucleotide substitutions hybridize better to subtypes A and E, the latter being a recombinant virus whose *gag* sequence originates from A (see above). These mix-in primers are just added to the reagents of the ordinary kit. Although results of company-independent systematic investigations are not yet available, the use of these mix-in primers is strongly recommended in view of the quickly increasing heterogeneity of virus subtypes in world regions previously dominated by subtype B. Adjustments to be implemented into RT-PCR kits in the near future will feature a novel downstream primer by which the amplified region of *gag* is slightly increased from 142 to 155 nt. These changes should further improve detection of divergent isolates by PCR.

The application of PCR to the detection of HIV at the screening level is currently precluded by the low level of automation, the lack of a pair of primers with the capability to amplify DNA from all HIV isolates, and occurrence of infected cells below the detection limit in some individuals. PCR is very helpful when serology fails to provide an answer. This applies in particular to specimens with borderline reactivity in screening assays or incomplete patterns on confirmatory WB, specimens from individuals with suspected acute phase disease, and babies of HIV-infected mothers.

Virus Isolation

For virus isolation, leukocytes are separated from anticoagulated blood samples by Ficoll centrifugation and cocultured with phytohemagglutinin-stimulated normal blood donor leukocytes. Culture supernatants are periodically assayed for viral antigen. Cultures usually become positive within 2 weeks, but culture times of up to 60 days are sometimes required (20, 66). The procedure has a sensitivity of about 90% over all stages, but the success rate is lower with samples from asymptomatic patients. In view of the fact that PCR for viral DNA or RNA as well as the signal amplification-boosted p24 antigen test both have diagnostic sensitivities of more than 96%, we have concluded that virus isolation is too inefficient, time-consuming, and costly for use as a routine diagnostic tool for HIV infection. The value of viral cultures is largely limited to samples in which the presence of indeterminate results is suggestive of infection with a retrovirus different from HIV.

PERT Assay

Particle-associated RT is a unique marker of infectious retrovirus particles. Measuring particle-associated RT activity with a sensitive procedure can be used as a general screening test for retroviruses. A family of novel tests collectively named product-enhanced RT (PERT) assays combine the broad detection range of RT tests with the high sensitivity of nucleic acid amplification procedures. PERT assays are based on the selective enhancement, by PCR or one of the various other nucleic acid amplification methods, of the cDNA product synthesized by the test sample's RT activity from an RNA template. A detailed overview of these procedures and detailed step-by-step instructions for a PCR-based PERT assay used in our laboratory have been published (17, 123). Assays based on this principle were also established by others (64, 133).

The PERT assay is 10^6 to 10^7 times more sensitive than a conventional RT test. The assay detects a variety of different retroviruses or RTs at a concentration corresponding to 1 nU of RT activity in the case of murine leukemia virus, which corresponds to 2.1×10^2 enzyme molecules or 3 to 11 particles (110). The PERT assay's sensitivity in fact rivals that of PCR for viral RNA, as demonstrated in HIV-1 infection. Testing of serial dilutions of HIV-1 by PERT assay and PCR for viral RNA indicated a detection level of 5 particles. With a 100-μl plasma sample, all of 30 untreated patients at different stages of HIV-1 infection were positive. In HIV-1 seroconversion panels, the PERT assay detected more positives than any other method including PCR for viral RNA. Importantly, the test's high sensitivity is not compromised by low specificity; the prevalence of elevated RT activity among 160 unselected blood donors was only 1.9% (16). Since the source of RT in these cases is unknown, no precise figure for the PERT assay's specificity can be given.

In conjunction with HIV diagnosis, the PERT assay is useful when a low $CD4^+$ lymphocyte count or indeterminate serological results, for example a Western blot positive according to ASTPHLD/CDC but indeterminate by FDA guidelines, suggest the presence of an HIV infection, possibly with an agent that is not well detected with current HIV-specific amplification methods. A negative result in the PERT assay renders an HIV infection very unlikely. If the PERT assay is positive, but HIV-specific PCR involving different genomic regions remains negative, identification and characterization of the suspected retroviral agent can be achieved with other recently developed procedures (33, 149).

Diagnosis of Pediatric HIV Infection

Diagnosis of HIV infection in babies born to HIV-positive mothers is complicated by the presence of HIV-specific IgG antibodies of maternal origin. IgG concentrations in term-born babies are as high as in their mothers. Since the half-life of IgG is about 3 weeks, HIV-specific maternal antibodies disappear slowly and traces may in some uninfected infants remain detectable by WB well beyond the 15 months given as an upper limit by most authors. We have observed traces of Env-reactive IgG in uninfected children of up to 22 months of age. These antibodies disappeared thereafter, and none of these children has since shown any sign of infection (130).

Since IgM and IgA isotypes are not subject to transplacental transport, their presence in the infant has been explored as a diagnostic marker. Detailed studies showed that Env-specific IgA antibodies have a good specificity, except in cord blood and during the first few days of life, when they are detectable in a high proportion of uninfected children, probably due to transplacental microtransfusion (100). After the newborn period, the specificity of Env-gp160-specific IgA was excellent. Diagnostic sensitivity in the first few months of life is, however, too low and a reliable diagnosis based on IgA reaction with gp160 is only possible after the first half year. IgM antibodies are predominantly directed against p24 and are of low specificity, since they are also produced in uninfected infants born to HIV-positive mothers and are even present in about 40% of control infants born to uninfected mothers. A further complication is the presence of IgG-reactive, rheumatoid-factor-like IgM or IgA which may also lead to false-positive results and which therefore requires quantitative removal of the IgG present in a sample, for example, by absorption with protein G-Sepharose (130). All this considered, serological diagnosis based on HIV-specific IgA or IgM is not recommended.

HIV infection in maternally exposed infants is best diagnosed with virus component tests. In pediatric HIV infection viral components are, on average, present at higher concentrations than in adult infection (124). Although virus culture is still regarded by some as a diagnostic "gold standard" for pediatric HIV infection, PCR for viral DNA or RNA is clearly more sensitive. Approximately one-third of maternally transmitted infections, probably those representing transmission in utero, can be detected within the first 10 days of life. In a few cases, DNA PCR from peripheral blood mononuclear cells may still be negative, when PCR for viral RNA in plasma is already positive. The rest, assumed to have become infected at birth, become PCR positive within the next 2 months. In Switzerland, babies with negative HIV results at birth are usually not retested before the age of 1 and 2 months. Using two different primer pairs and procedures published in detail (14), the prospective sensitivity of DNA-PCR in samples from infants older than 10 days has been 100% (85 positive out of 85 tested) in our laboratory.

The same sensitivity as with PCR is, however, also achieved with improved tests for p24 antigen (see above). Heat-mediated immune complex dissociation of samples and the use of a regular, unboosted antigen ELISA with a detection limit of about 2 pg/ml resulted in an overall diagnostic sensitivity of 96% (124). The combination of using plasma as a sample, heat-mediated immune complex dissociation and signal amplification-boosted p24 antigen ELISA with a detection limit of about 0.5 pg/ml increased the prospective sensitivity in infants older than 10 days to 100% (220 positive out of 220 samples tested; unpublished results of our laboratory; for method see reference 125). We have not seen a single sample positive by PCR for viral DNA or RNA, which would have been negative by the signal-boosted antigen assay. The high sensitivity of this antigen detection procedure has also been confirmed by others in a study of African samples (79). Used in combination, PCR and this antigen test permit independent detection of HIV infection in a single sample. Infection can then immediately be verified with a freshly drawn sample. A safe diagnosis of HIV infection can thus be established during the first few weeks and months of life.

Regarding specificity, very low levels of p24 (<1 pg/ml) may be present in the first days of life in infants who do not become infected. In some instances, this antigen was fully neutralizable and could be confirmed and neutralized in a second sample obtained a few weeks later, though its concentration was reduced (our unpublished observations). It is unclear whether such cases represent protein that is immune-complexed with maternal IgG and actively transported through the placenta, result from transplacental microtransfusion of maternal blood, or are the manifestation of a transient infection (112). It is important that a diagnosis of HIV infection in an infant is not exclusively based on antigen results from samples obtained in the first week of life.

Diagnosis of HIV-2 Infection

Screening tests, at least in several European countries, must demonstrate good sensitivity to HIV-2 on at least 200 different samples in order to receive approval by regulatory agencies. Detection of HIV-2 infection at the level of screening is therefore not a problem. In contrast, determining whether reactivity in screening is due to infection with HIV-1, HIV-2, or both may sometimes be difficult. On HIV-1 WB, sera from HIV-2-infected individuals frequently have strong reactions with Gag and Pol proteins when compared to Env. In particular, they may present with an unusually strong p32 (integrase) band. A suspected HIV-2 infection is further supported by reaction with the recombinant HIV-2 TM protein present on the products of some manufacturers. We have, however, occasionally seen a sample which did not react with this band, although HIV-2 infection was subsequently confirmed. The presence of isolated Gag bands on HIV-1 WB, or of strong reactivity against p24 and Gag precursors (p55, p43, p39) is not an indication of HIV-2 infection. Similarly, the presence of faint Gag-reactive bands on HIV-1 blots is usually not an indication for an HIV-2 WB.

Results of HIV-1 WB suggestive of HIV-2 infection should be confirmed by a WB produced from HIV-2 lysate or by tests employing specific recombinant proteins, e.g., a line immunoassay or a rapid test which differentiates between the two. If reaction to both HIV-1 and HIV-2 proteins is present at similar intensity, diagnostic PCR for both viruses will be necessary. HIV-2-infected, asymptomatic individuals, i.e., the overwhelming majority, have much lower viral loads than those infected with HIV-1. Virus culture for HIV-2 has only once been positive in our hands despite repeated attempts to isolate the virus from the half-dozen asymptomatic patients we have seen, even when $CD8^+$ T cells were removed prior to culturing and the highly sensitive PERT assay was used for monitoring of RT production.

Diagnostic Algorithms and General Considerations

A synopsis of the use of the various methods in HIV diagnostic testing of adults is shown in Fig. 11. It is based on the conclusion that the combination of two simple and relatively inexpensive procedures, antibody screening and antigen testing (especially with a procedure employing signal amplification), will not only detect virtually all untreated infections that can be diagnosed with molecular amplification methods, but also most of those that are missed by these molecular tests due to sequence variability or too-low levels of viral genome copies in the specimen.

It must be emphasized that HIV infection must never be established on the basis of a single sample, even if reactivity in screening has been confirmed by at least one supplemental test. The possibility that an error, for example, a sample mix-up or a contamination, might lead to a false-positive diagnosis dictates verification of all positive results in a second, freshly drawn sample. If the first sample presented with a low reactive result in screening and required different supplemental tests for confirmation, the supplemental tests

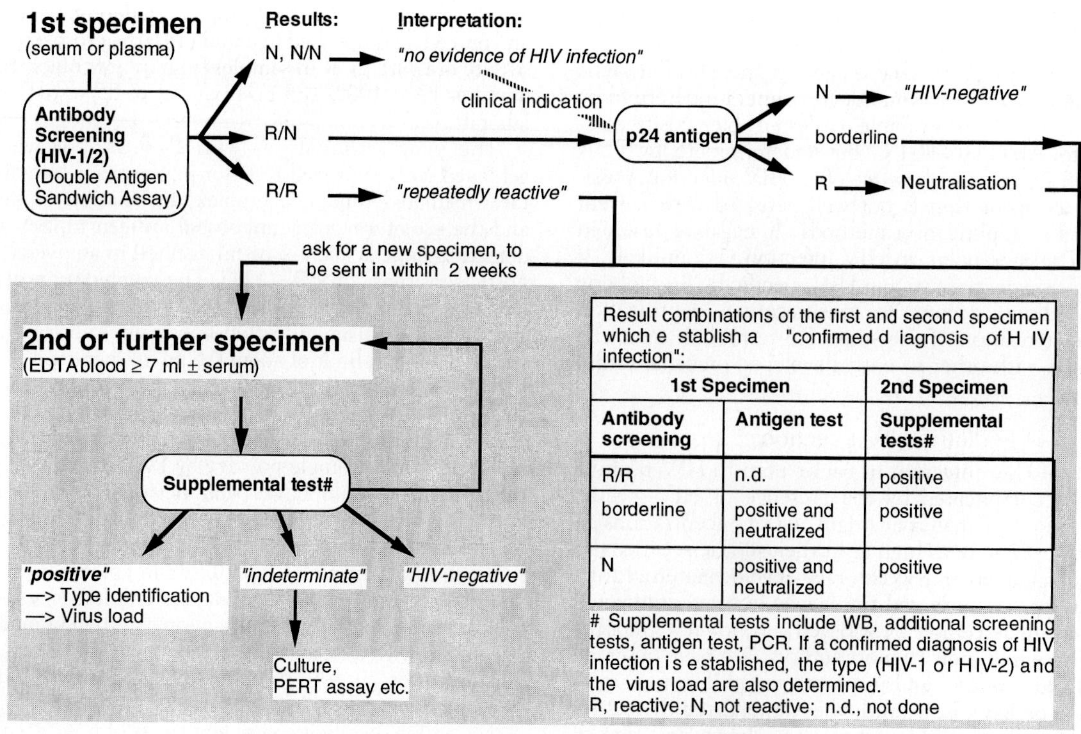

Result combinations of the first and second specimen which establish a "confirmed diagnosis of HIV infection":

1st Specimen		2nd Specimen
Antibody screening	**Antigen test**	**Supplemental tests#**
R/R	n.d.	positive
borderline	positive and neutralized	positive
N	positive and neutralized	positive

Supplemental tests include WB, additional screening tests, antigen test, PCR. If a confirmed diagnosis of HIV infection is established, the type (HIV-1 or HIV-2) and the virus load are also determined.
R, reactive; N, not reactive; n.d., not done

FIGURE 11 Diagnostic algorithms for adults.

should also be done on the second sample unless it is now clearly positive. Demonstration that the second sample has again the same low reactivity in screening is not sufficient verification.

Also, indeterminate results of different methods never add up to a positive result. For example, a borderline screening test plus a borderline WB with a pattern positive by ASTPHLD/CDC, but indeterminate by ARC or FDA criteria plus a reactive antigen test which cannot be confirmed by neutralization are not sufficient for a positive diagnosis. Testing must continue until clear-cut positive results are demonstrated.

When testing the first specimen, samples reactive in a screening test should be retested in a second, different screening assay. A more costly alternative is screening all samples by two different tests preferably performed in different runs, which increases the sensitivity in the early stage of infection and provides maximal protection against human error which is the most relevant source of false-positive or false-negative diagnosis. There is less need for the use of two different screening test kits if testing systems are used featuring automated positive sample identification from the bar-coded original test tube. Due to the high specificity of current test kits, a specimen reactive in two different screening tests is very unlikely to be a false positive and the tentative HIV-positive diagnosis can be verified with a freshly drawn sample, without a need for supplemental testing of the initial sample. Antigen screening should be performed liberally on all samples from patients with possible exposure to HIV, clinical signs of an acute retroviral syndrome, or discordant results of antibody screening or whenever absorbance values of these were elevated. Novel tests now available from some manufacturers combine antibody and antigen screening in a single assay and will once more render HIV screening more sensitive. The rate of false reactives in these tests remains to be seen. If antibody screening and antigen testing do not yield a clear result, a fresh sample, ideally an EDTA-anticoagulated blood sample, is demanded. This second sample, which permits all the different types of tests mentioned above, should come in with no further delay. There is no rational reason for a 3-month delay to diagnose an acute infection if it is suggested by the results of the first sample.

Assays performed on the second specimen are chosen according to the results of the first sample. Currently, a confirmatory laboratory should be able to perform a variety of supplemental tests in order to establish a confirmed diagnosis of HIV infection. A third positive screening assay, a positive WB according to FDA interpretation guidelines, a positive and neutralized antigen assay, or PCR for viral RNA or DNA may all be used alone or in combination to establish this diagnosis. Tests performed with the second sample should also establish the type of virus (HIV-1 or HIV-2) and the viral load, because this information is needed in order to assess whether an antiretroviral treatment should be given.

Viral Load Determination

Viral load determination is instrumental in several aspects of the clinical management of HIV infection. First, in early infection at the set-point, it serves to assess the likely course the infection will take. Based on the risk of progression, which depends on the viral load, appropriate treatment decisions can be made. The short-term efficacy of a specific antiretroviral treatment can then be assessed by measuring the reduction in viral concentrations achieved within the first 2 to 4 weeks after treatment initiation. Long-term efficacy is likely when viral levels continuously decrease below the level of detection and remain undetectable by the most sensitive assays.

Prognostic Value

Higher HIV RNA levels correlate with lower baseline $CD4^+$ counts, a more rapid decline in $CD4^+$ counts, and more rapid disease progression. Patients with more than 100,000 copies/ml of plasma within 6 months of seroconversion were 10-fold more likely to progress to AIDS over 5 years than those with fewer copies. Maintenance of <10,000 copies/ml in early HIV infection is associated with a decreased risk of progression to AIDS. However, in patients with more advanced disease, a low RNA count does not protect from progression; up to 30% of patients with <10,000 copies/ml progressed (35, 87, 90, 113, 151). Patients with advanced disease can present with high or low viral RNA titers.

As mentioned above, PCR, NASBA, and bDNA are valid procedures for viral load determinations. In plasma of most untreated patients viral RNA is detectable at all stages of disease. If RNA is undetectable in an untreated patient, this may reflect a very low virus load, as seen in long-term nonprogressors. However, the negative result may also be due to a virus subtype not well detected by the assay. In such cases, one should check the likelihood of an infection with an alternative subtype (A, E, F, or G) and verify that a procedure with good sensitivity to all the various subtypes was employed. Currently, the bDNA appears to be superior to other procedures in this respect, but future improvements of these might change this. A negative result in other virus component tests less affected by sequence variation supports a low load. Such alternative methods include the signal amplification-boosted p24 antigen assay and in particular the PERT assay which, being a functional test for RT activity, is completely independent of viral sequence. We have observed several subtype A infections in which RNA by the first-generation RT-PCR kit was undetectable but the antigen assay was positive and confirmed by neutralization. Use of the mix-in primers subsequently indicated 20,000 copies/ml of viral RNA in one such case, but still yielded a negative result in another.

Treatment Monitoring

Treatment monitoring assesses the short- and long-term treatment-induced reductions of the baseline viral load. Effective antiretroviral therapy significantly decreases HIV RNA levels in plasma within 1 week of initiation. No significant decrease within this period indicates absence of effect. Zidovudine monotherapy results in a median 0.7-log decrease in RNA levels in plasma within 2 weeks, which usually returns toward baseline by 6 months, indicating the outgrowth of a zidovudine-resistant viral quasispecies. Combinations of two nucleoside analog inhibitors of RT lead to more prominent reductions (-1.5 logs) which often persist for more than 1 year. Combination of two RT inhibitors with a protease inhibitor, so-called triple therapies, results in sustained reductions in plasma viral RNA (by 2 logs or more) which may last for prolonged periods. Treatment of patients in early disease with such combinations has resulted in a decrease in viral load that led to persistent nondetectability of viral RNA in plasma for more than 36 months, a slow decrease in PBMC-associated proviral DNA, and even decreasing titers of HIV-specific antibodies. Analysis of lymphoid tissues shows, however, that virus-expressing cells, not to mention provirus, are still detectable after prolonged periods. Interruption of the treatment regimen for very brief periods leads within a few days to the reappearance of virus in plasma to levels seen before initiation of the therapy.

Does the viral RNA concentration in plasma truly reflect the total body load, which is determined to more than 98% by the situation in the lymphoid tissues? These tissues have, in the efferent lymphatics, an outlet to the peripheral blood, and virus concentrations in plasma should thus more or less reflect the lymphoid tissue situation. The rapid decline of viral RNA in plasma observed after initiation of efficient antiretroviral combination therapy is in fact paralleled by a similar decline of virus load in lymphoid tissue (26). Specifically, in tonsillar tissue there was a rapid drop in mononuclear cells acutely producing virus, with a half-time of 0.9 days, which is comparable to the estimated half-time of 1.1 days of acutely infected $CD4^+$ T cells in the blood (67, 97, 98, 148). Viral RNA bound to follicular dendritic cells followed the decline with an initial half-time of 1.7 days (versus 0.6 days for virus in plasma). A phase of slower decay with half-times of 15 days for expressing cells and 14 days for follicular dendritic cell-bound virus then followed from day 2 onward. After 6 months of treatment, there were still infected cells and low levels of virus expression in a majority of patients (26). Ongoing low-level replication after 1 year of aggressive treatment has been confirmed by other groups who demonstrated the presence of unintegrated viral DNA (27). It thus appears that the current highly active antiretroviral treatment regimens are not 100% efficient in stopping viral replication—better drugs are needed.

Virus load studies under antiretroviral treatment have so far focused on effects in plasma and the lymphatics. Little is known about the impact of these regimens on HIV infection of the central nervous system and viral kinetics in the central nervous system have not been established.

RNA-based tests are currently viewed as the only feasible methods for viral load determination. These tests are, however, very expensive, which restricts their use. Our laboratory has therefore searched for alternatives. We have recently demonstrated that virus load monitoring can in many patients be done at considerably less expense with the signal-amplification-boosted p24 antigen assay (see above). In a study of 127 plasma samples taken at regular intervals from 23 patients with a $CD4^+$ cell count of less than 50 who received a defined antiretroviral treatment, the viral load was comparatively assessed by antigen assay and commercial quantitative RT-PCR (detection limit: 200 copies/ml). Overall detection during a median observation time of 25 weeks amounted to 75.6% for antigen and 73.6% for RT-PCR. The antigen detection limit was 0.2 pg/ml. Antigen was detectable in all 23 baseline samples, while RNA was undetectable in one. Antigen and RNA levels in 79 samples positive for both markers correlated with $R = 0.714$ ($P < 0.0001$). Average changes in levels of p24 and RNA at 8 timepoints correlated with $R = 0.982$ ($P < 0.0001$) (Fig. 10B). In individual patients, the two parameters behaved similarly, in certain cases virtually identically. In conclusion, the performance of this antigen detection procedure was comparable to commercial quantitative RT-PCR, thus providing a simple, high throughput alternative in monitoring the efficacy of antiretroviral treatment (15).

Drug Susceptibility Testing

The Achilles heel of any anti-infective agent is the development of resistance, in the case of the antiretroviral drugs used against HIV caused by mutations of the RT or the protease genes. Accumulation of at least three to four mutations in one viral gene is usually required before phenotypic resistance can be demonstrated in vitro. Since many of these resistance mutations affect different drugs resulting in cross-resistance, their detailed knowledge would be valuable for the design of treatment in individual patients. This is particularly true in view of the fact that viruses with resistance mutations are transmitted and may thus be present in patients prior to any antiretroviral treatment (69). A first commercial solution to the problem involves reverse hybridization of a biotinylated PCR fragment of the relevant part of the HIV-1 RT with short, immobilized oligonucleotide probes arranged on membrane strips similar to WB. These hybrids can then be detected via biotin-streptavidin coupling using a colorimetric system. Such line probe assays permit detection of various drug-selected variants in the HIV-1 RT gene (138). However, the test version currently sold does not include all RT inhibitors now in clinical use and not all of the relevant mutations. In addition, a strip for analysis of protease inhibitor resistance is not presently available. It can be assumed, however, that further versions of this system will be improved, that other solutions will be available from other manufacturers, and that commercial competition will result in less prohibitive prices. Drug susceptibility testing may thus in the future evolve as much a routine as in bacterial infection.

APPENDIX 1

Signs and Conditions Defining Category B

Symptomatic conditions in an HIV-infected adolescent or adult that are not included among conditions listed in clinical Category C and that meet at least one of the following criteria

(a) attributed to HIV infection or indicative of a defect in cell-mediated immunity

(b) considered by physicians to have a clinical course or to require management that is complicated by HIV infection

For example:

- Bacillary angiomatosis
- Candidiasis, oropharyngeal (thrush)
- Candidiasis, vulvovaginal; persistent, frequent, or poorly responsive to therapy
- Cervical dysplasia (moderate or severe)/cervical carcinoma in situ
- Constitutional symptoms, such as fever (38.5°C) or diarrhea >1 month
- Hairy leukoplakia, oral
- Herpes zoster (shingles), involving at least two distinct episodes or >1 dermatome
- Idiopathic thrombocytopenic purpura
- Listeriosis
- Pelvic inflammatory disease, particularly if complicated by tubo-ovarian abscess
- Peripheral neuropathy

APPENDIX 2

Signs and Conditions Defining Category C (AIDS Indicator Diseases)

- Candidiasis of bronchi, trachea, or lungs
- Candidiasis, esophageal
- Cervical cancer, invasive (added in 1993)
- Coccidioidomycosis, disseminated or extrapulmonary
- Cryptococcosis, extrapulmonary
- Cryptosporidiosis, chronic intestinal (>1 month's duration)
- Cytomegalovirus disease (other than liver, spleen, or nodes)
- Cytomegalovirus retinitis (with loss of vision)
- Encephalopathy, HIV-related
- Herpes simplex: chronic ulcer(s) (>1 month's duration); or bronchitis, pneumonitis, or esophagitis

- Histoplasmosis, disseminated or extrapulmonary
- Isosporiasis, chronic intestinal (>1 month's duration)
- Kaposi's sarcoma
- Lymphoma, Burkitt's (or equivalent term)
- Lymphoma, immunoblastic (or equivalent term)
- Lymphoma, primary, of brain
- *Mycobacterium avium* complex or *M. kansasii*, disseminated or extrapulmonary
- *Mycobacterium tuberculosis*, any site (pulmonary [added in 1993] or extrapulmonary)
- *Mycobacterium*, other species or unidentified species, disseminated or extrapulmonary
- *Pneumocystis carinii* pneumonia
- Pneumonia, recurrent (added in 1993)
- Progressive multifocal leukoencephalopathy
- *Salmonella* septicemia, recurrent
- Toxoplasmosis of brain
- Wasting syndrome due to HIV

REFERENCES

1. **Albright, A. V., J. Strizki, J. M. Harouse, E. Lavi, M. O'Connor, and F. Gonzales-Scarano.** 1996. HIV-1 infection of cultured adult oligodendrocytes. *Virology* **217:** 211–219.
2. **Alkhatib, G., C. Combadiere, C. C. Broder, Y. Feng, P. E. Kennedy, P. M. Murphy, and E. A. Berger.** 1996. CC CKR5: a RANTES, MIP-1alpha, MIP-1beta receptor as a fusion cofactor for macrophage-tropic HIV-1. *Science* **272:** 1955–1958.
3. **Amerongen, H. M., R. Weltzin, C. M. Farnet, P. Michetti, W. A. Haseltine, and M. R. Neutra.** 1991. Transepithelial transport of HIV-1 by intestinal M cells: a mechanism for transmission of AIDS. *J. Acquired Immune Defic. Syndr.* **4:**760–765.
4. **Anonymous.** 1987. Human immunodeficiency virus (HIV) infection codes. Official authorized addendum. ICD-9-CM (Revision No. 1). Effective January 1, 1988. *Morbid. Mortal. Weekly Rep.* **25:**1S–20S.
5. **Anonymous.** 1989. Interpretation and use of the western blot assay for serodiagnosis of human immunodeficiency virus type 1 infections. *Morbid. Mortal. Weekly Rep.* **38**(Suppl. 7)**:**1–7.
6. **Anonymous.** 1990. Acquired immunodeficiency syndrome (AIDS). Proposed WHO criteria for interpreting results from western blot assays for HIV-1, HIV-2, and HTLV-I/HTLV-II. *Weekly Epidemiol. Rec.* **65:**281–283.
7. **Anonymous.** 1991. *Biosafety Guidelines for Diagnostic and Research Laboratories Working with HIV. WHO AIDS Series, Volume 9.* World Health Organization, Geneva.
8. **Anonymous.** 1992. From the Centers for Disease Control and Prevention. 1993 revised classification system for HIV infection and expanded surveillance case definition for AIDS among adolescents and adults. *Morbid. Mortal. Weekly Rep.* **41:**(RR-17) 1–19.
9. **Anonymous.** 1995. Case-control study of HIV seroconversion in health-care workers after percutaneous exposure to HIV-infected blood—France, United Kingdom, and United States, January 1988–August 1994. *Morbid. Mortal. Weekly Rep.* **44:**929–933.
10. **Baba, T. W., A. M. Trichel, L. An, V. Liska, L. N. Martin, M. Murphey-Corb, and R. M. Ruprecht.** 1996. Infection and AIDS in adult macaques after nontraumatic oral exposure to cell-free SIV. *Science* **272:**1486–1489.
11. **Barnhart, H. X., M. B. Caldwell, P. Thomas, L. Mascola, I. Ortiz, H. W. Hsu, J. Schulte, R. Parrott, Y. Maldonado, and R. Byers.** 1996. Natural history of human immunodeficiency virus disease in perinatally infected children: an analysis from the Pediatric Spectrum of Disease Project. *Pediatrics* **97:**710–716.
12. **Barre-Sinoussi, F., J. C. Chermann, F. Rey, M. T. Nugeyre, S. Chamaret, J. Gruest, C. Dauguet, C. Axler-Blin, F. Vezinet-Brun, C. Rouzioux, W. Rozenbaum, and L. Montagnier.** 1983. Isolation of a T-lymphotropic retrovirus from a patient at risk for acquired immune deficiency syndrome (AIDS). *Science* **220:**868–871.
13. **Bleul, C. C., M. Farzan, H. Choe, C. Parolin, I. Clark-Lewis, J. Sodroski, and T. A. Springer.** 1996. The lymphocyte chemoattractant SDF-1 is a ligand for LESTR/fusin and blocks HIV-1 entry. *Nature (London)* **382:**829–833.
14. **Böni, J.** 1996. PCR detection of HIV. *Methods Mol. Biol.* **50:**93–107.
15. **Böni, J., M. Opravil, Z. Tomasik, M. Rothen, K. Bisset, P. Grob, R. Lüthy, and J. Schüpbach.** 1997. Simple monitoring of antiretroviral therapy with a signal-amplification-boosted HIV-1 P24 antigen assay with heat-denatured plasma. *AIDS* **11:**F47–F52.
16. **Böni, J., H. Pyra, and J. Schüpbach.** 1996. Sensitive detection and quantification of particle-associated reverse transcriptase in plasma of HIV-1-infected individuals by the product-enhanced reverse transcriptase (PERT) assay. *J. Med. Virol.* **49:**23–28.
17. **Böni, J., and J. Schüpbach.** Reverse transcriptase assay based on product enhancement for drug susceptibility assays. *In* D. Kinchington and R. F. Schinazi (ed.), *Antiviral Evaluation*, in press. Humana Press, Totowa, N.J.
18. **Braathen, L. R., G. Ramirez, R. O. Kunze, C. Mork, and O. Strand.** 1991. Latent infection of epidermal Langerhans cells in HIV-positive individuals. *Res. Virol.* **142:**119–121.
19. **Brodie, S., and P. Sax.** 1997. Novel approaches to HIV antibody testing. *AIDS Clin. Care* **9:**1–6.
20. **Burgard, M., M. J. Mayaux, S. Blanche, A. Ferroni, M. L. Guihard-Moscato, M. C. Allemon, N. Ciraru-Vigneron, G. Firtion, C. Floch, F. Guillot, E. Lachassine, M. Vial, C. Griscelli, C. Rouzioux, and the HIV Infection in Newborns French Collaborative Study Group.** 1992. The use of viral culture and p24 antigen testing to diagnose human immunodeficiency virus infection in neonates. *N. Engl. J. Med.* **327:**1192–1197.
21. **Busch, M. P., L. L. Lee, G. A. Satten, D. R. Henrard, H. Farzadegan, K. E. Nelson, S. Read, R. Y. Dodd, and L. R. Petersen.** 1995. Time course of detection of viral and serologic markers preceding human immunodeficiency virus type 1 seroconversion: implications for screening of blood and tissue donors. *Transfusion* **35:**91–97.
22. **Byrne, B. C., J. J. Li, J. Sninsky, and B. J. Poiesz.** 1988. Detection of HIV-1 RNA sequences by in vitro DNA amplification. *Nucleic Acids Res.* **16:**4165.
23. **Caldwell, M. B., M. J. Oxtoby, R. J. Simonds, M. L. Lindergren, and M. F. Rogers.** 1994. 1994 revised classification system for human immunodeficiency virus infection in children less than 13 years of age. *Morbid. Mortal. Weekly Rep.* **43**(RR-12)**:**1–10.
24. **Cameron, P. U., R. L. Dawkins, J. A. Armstrong, and E. Bonifacio.** 1987. Western blot profiles, lymph node ultrastructure and viral expression in HIV-infected patients: a correlative study. *Clin. Exp. Immunol.* **68:**465–478.
25. **Cameron, P. U., P. S. Freudenthal, J. M. Barker, S. Gezelter, K. Inaba, and R. M. Steinman.** 1992. Dendritic cells exposed to human immunodeficiency virus type-1 transmit a vigorous cytopathic infection to CD4+ T cells. *Science* **257:**383–387. (Erratum, **257:**1848.)
26. **Cavert, W., D. W. Notermans, K. Staskus, S. W. Wietgrefe, M. Zupancic, K. Gebhard, K. Henry, Z. Q. Zhang, R. Mills, H. McDade, J. Goudsmit, S. A. Danner, and A. T. Haase.** 1997. Kinetics of response in lymphoid tissues to antiretroviral therapy of HIV-1 infection. *Science* **276:** 960–964.

27. **Chun, T.-W.** 1997. Presented at the 11th Cent Gardes Meeting, Marnes-La-Coquette, France, 27 to 29 October, 1997.
28. **Clark, S. J., M. S. Saag, W. D. Decker, S. Campbell-Hill, J. L. Roberson, P. J. Veldkamp, J. C. Kappes, B. H. Hahn, and G. M. Shaw.** 1991. High titers of cytopathic virus in plasma of patients with symptomatic primary HIV-1 infection. *N. Engl. J. Med.* **324:**954–960.
29. **Clavel, F., D. Guetard, F. Brun-Vezinet, S. Chamaret, M. A. Rey, M. O. Santos-Ferreira, A. G. Laurent, C. Dauguet, C. Katlama, C. Rouzioux, D. Klatzmann, J. L. Champalimaud, and L. Montagnier.** 1986. Isolation of a new human retrovirus from West African patients with AIDS. *Science* **233:**343–346.
30. **Clavel, F., M. Guyader, D. Guetard, M. Salle, L. Montagnier, and M. Alizon.** 1986. Molecular cloning and polymorphism of the human immune deficiency virus type 2. *Nature (London)* **324:**691–695.
31. **Cocchi, F., A. L. De Vico, A. Garzino-Demo, S. K. Arya, R. C. Gallo, and P. Lusso.** 1995. Identification of RANTES, MIP-1 alpha, and MIP-1 beta as the major HIV-suppressive factors produced by CD8+ T cells. *Science* **270:**1811–1815.
32. **Connick, E., D. G. Marr, X. Q. Zhang, S. J. Clark, M. S. Saag, R. T. Schooley, and T. J. Curiel.** 1996. HIV-specific cellular and humoral immune responses in primary HIV infection. *AIDS Res. Hum. Retroviruses.* **12:** 1129–1140.
33. **Conrad, B., R. N. Weissmahr, J. Böni, R. Arcari, J. Schüpbach, and B. Mach.** 1997. A human endogenous retroviral superantigen as candidate autoimmune gene in type I diabetes. *Cell* **90:**303–313.
34. **Constantine, N. T., G. van der Groen, E. M. Belsey, and H. Tamashiro.** 1994. Sensitivity of HIV-antibody assays determined by seroconversion panels. *AIDS* **8:**1715–1720.
35. **Coombs, R. W., S. L. Welles, C. Hooper, P. S. Reichelderfer, R. T. D'Aquila, A. J. Japour, V. A. Johnson, D. R. Kuritzkes, D. D. Richman, S. Kwok, J. Todd, J. B. Jackson, V. De Gruttola, C. S. Crumpacker, and J. Kahn.** 1996. Association of plasma human immunodeficiency virus type 1 RNA level with risk of clinical progression in patients with advanced infection. *J. Infect. Dis.* **174:** 704–712.
36. **Cornelissen, M., G. Mulder-Kampinga, J. Veenstra, F. Zorgdrager, C. Kuiken, S. Hartman, J. Dekker, L. van der Hoek, C. Sol, R. Coutinho, and J. Goudsmit.** 1995. Syncytium-inducing (SI) phenotype suppression at seroconversion after intramuscular inoculation of a non-syncytium-inducing/SI phenotypically mixed human immunodeficiency virus population. *J. Virol.* **69:**1810–1818.
37. **Coste, J., B. Montes, J. Reynes, M. Peeters, C. Segarra, J. P. Vendrell, E. Delaporte, and M. Segondy.** 1996. Comparative evaluation of three assays for the quantitation of human immunodeficiency virus type 1 RNA in plasma. *J. Med. Virol.* **50:**293–302.
38. **Daar, E. S., T. Moudgil, R. D. Meyer, and D. D. Ho.** 1991. Transient high levels of viremia in patients with primary human immunodeficiency virus type 1 infection. *N. Engl. J. Med.* **324:**961–964.
39. **Dalgleish, A. G., P. C. Beverley, P. R. Clapham, D. H. Crawford, M. F. Greaves, and R. A. Weiss.** 1984. The CD4 (T4) antigen is an essential component of the receptor for the AIDS retrovirus. *Nature (London)* **312:** 763–767.
40. **D'Aquila, R. T.** 1996. Human immunodeficiency virus type 2: human biology of the other AIDS virus. *Curr. Clin. Top. Infect. Dis.* **16:**84–101.
41. **De Leys, R., B. Vanderborght, M. Vanden Haesevelde, L. Heyndrickx, A. van Geel, C. Wauters, R. Bernaerts, E. Saman, P. Nijs, B. Willems, H. Taelman, G. van der Groen, P. Piot, T. Tersmette, J. G. Huisman, and H. van Heuverswyn.** 1990. Isolation and partial characterization of an unusual human immunodeficiency retrovirus from two persons of west-central African origin. *J. Virol.* **64:** 1207–1216.
42. **Dean, M., M. Carrington, C. Winkler, G. A. Huttley, M. W. Smith, R. Allikmets, J. J. Goedert, S. P. Buchbinder, E. Vittinghoff, E. Gomperts, S. Donfield, D. Vlahov, R. Kaslow, A. Saah, C. Rinaldo, R. Detels, and S. J. O'Brien.** 1996. Genetic restriction of HIV-1 infection and progression to AIDS by a deletion allele of the CKR5 structural gene. *Science* **273:**1856–1862.
43. **Delézay, O., N. Koch, N. Yahi, D. Hammache, C. Tourres, C. Tamalet, and J. Fantini.** 1997. Co-expression of CXCR4/fusin and galactosylceramide in the human intestinal epithelial cell line HT-29. *AIDS* **11:**1311–1318.
44. **Delwart, E. L., H. W. Sheppard, B. D. Walker, J. Goudsmit, and J. I. Mullins.** 1994. Human immunodeficiency virus type 1 evolution in vivo tracked by DNA heteroduplex mobility assays. *J. Virol.* **68:**6672–6683.
45. **Deng, H., R. Liu, W. Ellmeier, S. Choe, D. Unutmaz, M. Burkhart, P. Di Marzio, S. Marmon, R. E. Sutton, C. M. Hill, C. B. Davis, S. C. Peiper, T. J. Schall, D. R. Littman, and N. R. Landau.** 1996. Identification of a major co-receptor for primary isolates of HIV-1. *Nature (London)* **381:**661–666.
46. **Deng, H., D. Unutmaz, V. KewalRamani, and D. Littman.** 1997. Expression cloning of new receptors used by simian and human immunodeficiency viruses. *Nature (London)* **388:**296–300.
47. **Douceron, H., L. Deforges, R. Gherardi, A. Sobel, and P. Chariot.** 1993. Long-lasting postmortem viability of human immunodeficiency virus: a potential risk in forensic medicine practice. *Forensic Sci. Int.* **60:**61–66.
48. **Downs, A. M., G. Salamina, and R. A. Ancelle-Park.** 1995. Incubation period of vertically acquired AIDS in Europe before widespread use of prophylactic therapies. *J. Acquired Immune Defic. Syndr. Hum. Retrovirol.* **9:** 297–304.
49. **Dragic, T., V. Litwin, G. P. Allaway, S. R. Martin, Y. Huang, K. A. Nagashima, C. Cayanan, P. J. Maddon, R. A. Koup, J. P. Moore, and W. A. Paxton.** 1996. HIV-1 entry into CD4+ cells is mediated by the chemokine receptor CC-CKR-5. *Nature (London)* **381:**667–673.
50. **Embretson, J., M. Zupancic, J. L. Ribas, A. Burke, P. Racz, K. Tenner-Racz, and A. T. Haase.** 1993. Massive covert infection of helper T lymphocytes and macrophages by HIV during the incubation period of AIDS. *Nature (London)* **362:**359–362.
51. **Feng, Y., C. C. Broder, P. E. Kennedy, and E. A. Berger.** 1996. HIV-1 entry cofactor: functional cDNA cloning of a seven-transmembrane, G protein-coupled receptor. *Science* **272:**872–877.
52. **Frankel, S. S., B. M. Wenig, A. P. Burke, P. Mannan, L. D. Thompson, S. L. Abbondanzo, A. M. Nelson, M. Pope, and R. M. Steinman.** 1996. Replication of HIV-1 in dendritic cell-derived syncytia at the mucosal surface of the adenoid. *Science* **272:**115–117.
53. **Gallo, R. C., S. Z. Salahuddin, M. Popovic, G. M. Shearer, M. Kaplan, B. F. Haynes, T. J. Palker, R. Redfield, J. Oleske, B. Safai, G. White, P. Foster, and P. D. Markham.** 1984. Frequent detection and isolation of cytopathic retroviruses (HTLV-III) from patients with AIDS and at risk for AIDS. *Science* **224:**500–503.
54. **Ganeshan, S., R. E. Dickover, B. T. Korber, Y. J. Bryson, and S. M. Wolinsky.** 1997. Human immunodeficiency virus type 1 genetic evolution in children with different rates of development of disease. *J. Virol.* **71:**663–677.

55. **Ginocchio, C. C., X. P. Wang, M. H. Kaplan, G. Mulligan, M. Cronin, D. Carroll, and J. Romano.** 1997. Effects of specimen collection, processing, and storage conditions on the stability of HIV-1 viral titers. *Fourth Conference on Retroviruses and Opportunistic Infections, Washington, DC. 22–26 January 1997*, p. 180, abstr. 624.
56. **Gottlieb, G. J., A. Ragaz, J. V. Vogel, A. Friedman-Kien, A. M. Rywlin, E. A. Weiner, and A. B. Ackerman.** 1981. A preliminary communication on extensively disseminated Kaposi's sarcoma in young homosexual men. *Am. J. Dermatopathol.* **3:**111–114.
57. **Graziosi, C., G. Pantaleo, L. Butini, J. F. Demarest, M. S. Saag, G. M. Shaw, and A. S. Fauci.** 1993. Kinetics of human immunodeficiency virus type 1 (HIV-1) DNA and RNA synthesis during primary HIV-1 infection. *Proc. Natl. Acad. Sci. USA* **90:**6405–6409.
58. **Gurtler, L. G., P. H. Hauser, J. Eberle, A. von Brunn, S. Knapp, L. Zekeng, J. M. Tsague, and L. Kaptue.** 1994. A new subtype of human immunodeficiency virus type 1 (MVP-5180) from Cameroon. *J. Virol.* **68:**1581–1585.
59. **Gutierrez, M., A. Vallejo, and V. Soriano.** 1995. Enhancement of HIV antigen detection after acid dissociation of immune complexes is associated with loss of specificity. *Vox Sang.* **68:**132–133. (Letter.)
60. **Harouse, J. M., S. Bhat, S. L. Spitalnik, M. Laughlin, K. Stefano, D. H. Silberberg, and F. Gonzalez-Scarano.** 1991. Inhibition of entry of HIV-1 in neural cell lines by antibodies against galactosyl ceramide. *Science* **253:** 320–323.
61. **Haynes, B. F., G. Pantaleo, and A. S. Fauci.** 1996. Toward an understanding of the correlates of protective immunity to HIV infection. *Science* **271:**324–328.
62. **Healey, D. S., and W. V. Bolton.** 1993. Apparent HIV-1 glycoprotein reactivity on western blot in uninfected blood donors. *AIDS* **7:**655–658.
63. **Heath, S. L., J. G. Tew, A. K. Szakal, and G. F. Burton.** 1995. Follicular dendritic cells and human immunodeficiency virus infectivity. *Nature (London)* **377:**740–744.
64. **Heneine, W., S. Yamamoto, W. M. Switzer, T. J. Spira, and T. M. Folks.** 1995. Detection of reverse transcriptase by a highly sensitive assay in sera from persons infected with human immunodeficiency virus type 1. *J. Infect. Dis.* **171:**1210–1216.
65. **Henrard, D. R., J. F. Phillips, L. R. Muenz, W. A. Blattner, D. Wiesner, M. E. Eyster, and J. J. Goedert.** 1995. Natural history of HIV-1 cell-free viremia. *JAMA* **274:** 554–558.
66. **Ho, D. D., T. Moudgil, and M. Alam.** 1989. Quantitation of human immunodeficiency virus type 1 in the blood of infected persons. *N. Engl. J. Med.* **321:**1621–1625.
67. **Ho, D. D., A. U. Neumann, A. S. Perelson, W. Chen, J. M. Leonard, and M. Markowitz.** 1995. Rapid turnover of plasma virions and CD4 lymphocytes in HIV-1 infection. *Nature (London)* **373:**123–126.
68. **Hussain, L. A., and T. Lehner.** 1995. Comparative investigation of Langerhans' cells and potential receptors for HIV in oral, genitourinary and rectal epithelia. *Immunology* **85:**475–484.
69. **Imrie, A., A. Beveridge, W. Genn, J. Vizzard, and D. A. Cooper.** 1997. Transmission of human immunodeficiency virus type 1 resistant to nevirapine and zidovudine. Sydney Primary HIV Infection Study Group. *J. Infect. Dis.* **175:** 1502–1506.
70. **Ittiravivongs, A., S. Likanonsakul, T. D. Mastro, S. Tansuphasawadikul, N. Young, T. Naiwatanakul, D. Kitayaporn, and K. Limpakarnjanarat.** 1996. Evaluation of a confirmatory HIV testing strategy in Thailand not using Western blot. *J. Acquired Immune Defic. Syndr. Hum. Retrovirol.* **13:**296–297. (Letter.)
71. **Jurriaans, S., B. Van Gemen, G. J. Weverling, D. Van Strijp, P. Nara, R. Coutinho, M. Koot, H. Schuitemaker, and J. Goudsmit.** 1994. The natural history of HIV-1 infection: virus load and virus phenotype independent determinants of clinical course? *Virology* **204:**223–233.
72. **Kievits, T., B. van Gemen, D. van Strijp, R. Schukkink, M. Dircks, H. Adriaanse, L. Malek, R. Sooknanan, and P. Lens.** 1991. NASBA isothermal enzymatic in vitro nucleic acid amplification optimized for the diagnosis of HIV-1 infection. *J. Virol. Methods* **35:**273–286.
73. **Klatzmann, D., E. Champagne, S. Chamaret, J. Gruest, D. Guetard, T. Hercend, J. C. Gluckman, and L. Montagnier.** 1984. T-lymphocyte T4 molecule behaves as the receptor for human retrovirus LAV. *Nature (London)* **312:** 767–768.
74. **Koup, R. A., J. T. Safrit, Y. Cao, C. A. Andrews, G. McLeod, W. Borkowsky, C. Farthing, and D. D. Ho.** 1994. Temporal association of cellular immune responses with the initial control of viremia in primary human immunodeficiency virus type 1 syndrome. *J. Virol.* **68:** 4650–4655.
75. **Kuun, E., M. Brashaw, and A. d. P. Heyns.** 1997. Sensitivity and specificity of standard and rapid HIV-antibody tests evaluated by seroconversion and non-seroconversion low-titre panels. *Vox Sang.* **72:**11–15.
76. **Kwok, S., D. H. Mack, K. B. Mullis, B. Poiesz, G. Ehrlich, D. Blair, A. Friedman-Kien, and J. J. Sninsky.** 1987. Identification of human immunodeficiency virus sequences by using in vitro enzymatic amplification and oligomer cleavage detection. *J. Virol.* **61:**1690–1694.
77. **Laleman, G., M. Kambale, I. Van Kerckhoven, N. Kapila, M. Konde, U. Selemani, P. Piot, and G. van der Groen.** 1991. A simplified and less expensive strategy for confirming anti HIV-1 screening results in a diagnostic laboratory in Lubumbashi, Zaire. *Ann. Soc. Belg. Med. Trop.* **71:** 287–294.
78. **Levy, J. A., A. D. Hoffman, S. M. Kramer, J. A. Landis, J. M. Shimabukuro, and L. S. Oshiro.** 1984. Isolation of lymphocytopathic retroviruses from San Francisco patients with AIDS. *Science* **225:**840–842.
79. **Lyamuya, E., U. Bredberg-Raden, A. Massawe, E. Urassa, G. Kawo, G. Msemo, T. Kazimoto, A. Ostborn, K. Karlsson, F. Mhalu, and G. Biberfeld.** 1996. Performance of a modified HIV-1 p24 antigen assay for early diagnosis of HIV-1 infection in infants and prediction of mother-to-infant transmission of HIV-1 in Dar es Salaam, Tanzania. *J. Acquired Immune Defic. Syndr. Hum. Retrovirol.* **12:** 421–426.
80. **Malone, J. D., E. S. Smith, J. Sheffield, D. Bigelow, K. C. Hyams, S. G. Beardsley, R. S. Lewis, and C. R. Roberts.** 1993. Comparative evaluation of six rapid serological tests for HIV-1 antibody. *J. Acquired Immune Defic. Syndr.* **6:**115–119.
81. **Marlink, R.** 1996. Lessons from the second AIDS virus, HIV-2. *AIDS* **10(7):**689–699. (Editorial.)
82. **Martin, D. J., L. Morris, C. M. Gray, S. F. Lyons, J. Murray, and P. Sonnenberg.** 1996. Analysis of a lymph node during HIV-1 seroconversion. *International Conference on AIDS (Canada), 7–12 July 1996.* **11(1):**268, abstr. Tu.A.2016.
83. **Mazzoli, S., D. Trabattoni, S. Caputo, S. Piconi, C. Ble, F. Meacci, S. Ruzzante, A. Salvi, F. Semplici, R. Longhi, M. Fusi, N. Tofani, M. Biasin, M. Villa, F. Mazzotta, and M. Clerici.** 1997. HIV-specific mucosal and cellular immunity in HIV-seronegative partners of HIV-seropositive individuals. *Nat. Med.* **3:**1250–1257.
84. **McAlarney, T., S. Apostolski, S. Lederman, and N. Latov.** 1994. Characteristics of HIV-1 gp120 glycoprotein binding to glycolipids. *J. Neurosci. Res.* **37:**453–460.

85. **McCutchan, F. E., M. O. Salminen, J. K. Carr, and D. S. Burke.** 1996. HIV-1 genetic diversity. *AIDS* **10:**S13–S20.
86. **McDonald, R. A., D. L. Mayers, R. C. Chung, K. F. Wagner, S. Ratto-Kim, D. L. Birx, and N. L. Michael.** 1997. Evolution of human immunodeficiency virus type 1 env sequence variation in patients with diverse rates of disease progression and T-cell function. *J. Virol.* **71:** 1871–1879.
87. **Mellors, J. W., C. R. Rinaldo, Jr., P. Gupta, R. M. White, J. A. Todd, and L. A. Kingsley.** 1996. Prognosis in HIV-1 infection predicted by the quantity of virus in plasma. *Science* **272:**1167–1170.
88. **Munoz, A., A. J. Kirby, Y. D. He, J. B. Margolick, B. R. Visscher, C. R. Rinaldo, R. A. Kaslow, and J. P. Phair.** 1995. Long-term survivors with HIV-1 infection: incubation period and longitudinal patterns of CD4+ lymphocytes. *J. Acquired Immune Defic. Syndr. Hum. Retrovirol.* **8:**496–505.
89. **Oberlin, E., A. Amara, F. Bachelerie, C. Bessia, J. L. Virelizier, F. Arenzana-Seisdedos, O. Schwartz, J. M. Heard, I. Clark-Lewis, D. F. Legler, M. Loetscher, M. Baggiolini, and B. Moser.** 1996. The CXC chemokine SDF-1 is the ligand for LESTR/fusin and prevents infection by T-cell-line-adapted HIV-1. *Nature (London)* **382:** 833–835.
90. **O'Brien, W. A., P. M. Hartigan, E. S. Daar, M. S. Simberkoff, and J. D. Hamilton.** 1997. Changes in plasma HIV RNA levels and CD4+ lymphocyte counts predict both response to antiretroviral therapy and therapeutic failure. *Ann. Intern. Med.* **126:**939–945.
91. **Orenstein, J., C. Fox, and S. Wahl.** 1997. Macrophages as source of HIV during opportunistic infections. *Science* **276:**1857–1861.
92. **Pachl, C., M. Saxer, T. Elbeik, M. Stempien, S. J. Fong, D. Kern, P. Sheridan, B. Hoo, D. Besemer, R. Kokka, et al.** 1993. Quantitation of HIV-1 RNA in plasma using a branched DNA (bDNA) signal amplification assay: evaluation of specimen collection and stability. *National Conference on Human Retroviruses and Related Infections (United States), 12–16 December 1993*, p. 110.
93. **Pantaleo, G., J. F. Demarest, H. Soudeyns, C. Graziosi, F. Denis, J. W. Adelsberger, P. Borrow, M. S. Saag, G. M. Shaw, R. P. Sekaly, and A. S. Fauci.** 1994. Major expansion of CD8+ T cells with a predominant V beta usage during the primary immune response to HIV. *Nature (London)* **370:**463–467.
94. **Pantaleo, G., C. Graziosi, J. F. Demarest, L. Butini, M. Montroni, C. H. Fox, J. M. Orenstein, D. P. Kotler, and A. S. Fauci.** 1993. HIV infection is active and progressive in lymphoid tissue during the clinically latent stage of disease. *Nature (London)* **362:**355–358.
95. **Pantaleo, G., C. Graziosi, and A. S. Fauci.** 1993. New concepts in the immunopathogenesis of human immunodeficiency virus infection. *N. Engl. J. Med.* **328:**327–335.
96. **Pedersen, C., E. Dickmeiss, J. Gaub, L. P. Ryder, P. Platz, B. O. Lindhardt, and J. D. Lundgren.** 1990. T-cell subset alterations and lymphocyte responsiveness to mitogens and antigen during severe primary infection with HIV: a case series of seven consecutive HIV seroconverters. *AIDS* **4:**523–526.
97. **Perelson, A. S., P. Essunger, Y. Z. Cao, M. Vesanen, A. Hurley, K. Saksela, M. Markowitz, and D. D. Ho.** 1997. Decay characteristics of HIV-1-infected compartments during combination therapy. *Nature (London)* **387:** 188–191.
98. **Perelson, A. S., A. U. Neumann, M. Markowitz, J. M. Leonard, and D. D. Ho.** 1996. HIV-1 dynamics in vivo: virion clearance rate, infected cell life-span, and viral generation time. *Science* **271:**1582–1586.
99. **Petersen, L. R., G. A. Satten, R. Dodd, M. Busch, S. Kleinman, A. Grindon, and B. Lenes.** 1994. Duration of time from onset of human immunodeficiency virus type 1 infectiousness to development of detectable antibody. *Transfusion* **34:**283–289.
100. **Petit, T., E. Gluckman, E. Carosella, Y. Brossard, O. Brison, and G. Socie.** 1995. A highly sensitive polymerase chain reaction method reveals the ubiquitous presence of maternal cells in human umbilical cord blood. *Exp. Hematol.* **23:**1601–1605.
101. **Phair, J., L. Jacobson, R. Detels, C. Rinaldo, A. Saah, L. Schrager, and A. Munoz.** 1992. Acquired immune deficiency syndrome occurring within 5 years of infection with human immunodeficiency virus type-1: the Multicenter AIDS Cohort Study. *J. Acquired Immune Defic. Syndr.* **5:**490–496.
102. **Phillips, A. N.** 1996. Reduction of HIV concentration during acute infection: independence from a specific immune response. *Science* **271:**497–499.
103. **Piatak, M., Jr., M. S. Saag, L. C. Yang, S. J. Clark, J. C. Kappes, K. C. Luk, B. H. Hahn, G. M. Shaw, and J. D. Lifson.** 1993. High levels of HIV-1 in plasma during all stages of infection determined by competitive PCR. *Science* **259:**1749–1754.
104. **Pinter, A., W. J. Honnen, S. A. Tilley, C. Bona, H. Zaghouani, M. K. Gorny, and S. Zolla-Pazner.** 1989. Oligomeric structure of gp41, the transmembrane protein of human immunodeficiency virus type 1. *J. Virol.* **63:** 2674–2679.
105. **Pliner, V., J. Weedon, and P. Thomas.** 1996. Estimation of long term survival to AIDS in perinatally infected children. *International Conference on AIDS (Canada), 7–12 July 1996.* **11(2):**140, abstr. We.C.3473.
106. **Pollet, D. E., E. L. Saman, D. C. Peeters, H. M. Warmenbol, L. M. Heyndrickx, C. J. Wouters, G. Beelaert, G. van der Groen, and H. Van Heuverswyn.** 1991. Confirmation and differentiation of antibodies to human immunodeficiency virus 1 and 2 with a strip-based assay including recombinant antigens and synthetic peptides. *Clin. Chem.* **37:**1700–1707.
107. **Pope, M., S. Gezelter, N. Gallo, L. Hoffman, and R. M. Steinman.** 1995. Low levels of HIV-1 infection in cutaneous dendritic cells promote extensive viral replication upon binding to memory CD4+ T cells. *J. Exp. Med.* **182:**2045–2056.
108. **Popovic, M., M. G. Sarngadharan, E. Read, and R. C. Gallo.** 1984. Detection, isolation, and continuous production of cytopathic retroviruses (HTLV-III) from patients with AIDS and pre-AIDS. *Science* **224:**497–500.
109. **Price, R. W.** 1996. Neurological complications of HIV infection. *Lancet* **348:**445–452.
110. **Pyra, H., J. Böni, and J. Schüpbach.** 1994. Ultrasensitive retrovirus detection by a reverse transcriptase assay based on product enhancement. *Proc. Natl. Acad. Sci. USA* **91:** 1544–1548.
111. **Redfield, R. R., D. C. Wright, and E. C. Tramont.** 1986. The Walter Reed staging classification for HTLV-III/LAV infection. *N. Engl. J. Med.* **314:**131–132.
112. **Rowland-Jones, S. L., and A. McMichael.** 1995. Immune responses in HIV-exposed seronegatives: have they repelled the virus? *Curr. Opin. Immunol.* **7:**448–455.
113. **Saag, M. S., M. Holodniy, D. R. Kuritzkes, W. A. O'Brien, R. Coombs, M. E. Poscher, D. M. Jacobsen, G. M. Shaw, D. D. Richman, and P. A. Volberding.** 1996. HIV viral load markers in clinical practice. *Nat. Med.* **2:**625–629.
114. **Samdal, H. H., B. G. Gutigard, D. Labay, S. I. Wiik, K. Skaug, and A. G. Skar.** 1996. Comparison of the sensitivity of four rapid assays for the detection of antibod-

ies to HIV-1/HIV-2 during seroconversion. *Clin. Diagn. Virol.* **7**:55–61.

115. **Sarngadharan, M. G., M. Popovic, L. Bruch, J. Schüpbach, and R. C. Gallo.** 1984. Antibodies reactive with human T-lymphotropic retroviruses (HTLV-III) in the serum of patients with AIDS. *Science* **224**:506–508.
116. **Sato, P. A., W. J. Maskill, H. Tamashiro, and D. L. Heymann.** 1994. Strategies for laboratory HIV testing: an examination of alternative approaches not requiring Western blot. *Bull. W. H. O.* **72**:129–134.
117. **Sattar, S. A., and V. S. Springthorpe.** 1991. Survival and disinfectant inactivation of the human immunodeficiency virus: a critical review. *Rev. Infect. Dis.* **13**:430–447.
118. **Schacker, T., A. C. Collier, J. Hughes, T. Shea, and L. Corey.** 1996. Clinical and epidemiologic features of primary HIV infection. *Ann. Intern. Med.* **125**:257–264.
119. **Schneider, T., R. Ullrich, and M. Zeitz.** 1996. The immunologic aspects of human immunodeficiency virus infection in the gastrointestinal tract. *Semin. Gastrointest. Dis.* **7**:19–29.
120. **Schockmel, G. A., S. Yerly, and L. Perrin.** 1997. Detection of low HIV-1 RNA levels in plasma. *J. Acquired Immune Defic. Syndr. Hum Retrovirol.* **14**:179–183.
121. **Schüpbach, J.** 1996. Licencing of diagnostic HIV kits—To keep a sensible standpoint in an area of permanent revolution. *Clin. Diagn. Virol.* **5**:137–146.
122. **Schüpbach, J., and J. Böni.** 1993. Quantitative and sensitive detection of immune-complexed and free HIV antigen after boiling of serum. *J. Virol. Methods* **43**:247–256.
123. **Schüpbach, J., and J. Böni.** 1993. Verfahren zum Nachweis reverser Transcriptase (Process for detecting reverse transcriptase). *PCT International Office Publication (WO 93/23560)*:1–118.
124. **Schüpbach, J., J. Böni, Z. Tomasik, J. Jendis, R. Seger, and C. Kind.** 1994. Sensitive detection and early prognostic significance of p24 antigen in heat-denatured plasma of human immunodeficiency virus type 1-infected infants. Swiss Neonatal HIV Study Group. *J. Infect. Dis.* **170**: 318–324.
125. **Schüpbach, J., M. Flepp, D. Pontelli, Z. Tomasik, R. Luthy, and J. Böni.** 1996. Heat-mediated immune complex dissociation and enzyme-linked immunosorbent assay signal amplification render p24 antigen detection in plasma as sensitive as HIV-1 RNA detection by polymerase chain reaction. *AIDS* **10**:1085–1090.
126. **Schüpbach, J., O. Haller, M. Vogt, R. Lüthy, H. Joller, O. Oelz, M. Popovic, M. G. Sarngadharan, and R. C. Gallo.** 1985. Antibodies to HTLV-III in Swiss patients with AIDS and pre-AIDS and in groups at risk for AIDS. *N. Engl. J. Med.* **312**:265–270.
127. **Schüpbach, J., M. Popovic, R. V. Gilden, M. A. Gonda, M. G. Sarngadharan, and R. C. Gallo.** 1984. Serological analysis of a subgroup of human T-lymphotropic retroviruses (HTLV-III) associated with AIDS. *Science* **224**: 503–505.
128. **Schüpbach, J., H. Pyra, J. Jendis, Z. Tomasik, and J. Böni.** 1996. Isolation of an in vitro transmissible agent with reverse transcriptase activity from a blood donor with a borderline-positive HIV-1 serology for more than five years. *Clin. Diagn. Virol.* **5**:197–203.
129. **Schüpbach, J., Z. Tomasik, and J. Böni.** 1990. Wide divergence of different HIV Western Blot (WB) interpretation standards in low-positive sera. *International Conference on AIDS, San Francisco, Calif. 20–24 June 1990.* **6**: 133, abstr. S.C.215.
130. **Schüpbach, J., Z. Tomasik, J. Jendis, J. Böni, R. Seger, and C. Kind.** 1994. IgG, IgM, and IgA response to HIV in infants born to HIV-1 infected mothers. Swiss Neonatal HIV Study Group. *J. Acquired Immune Defic. Syndr.* **7**:421–427.
131. **Sebire, K., K. McGavin, S. Land, and C. Birch.** 1996. Stability of HIV RNA in blood specimens. *Annu. Conf. Australas. Soc. HIV Med.* **8**(122):145.
132. **Sharp, P. M., D. L. Robertson, D. L. Gao, and B. H. Hahn.** 1994. Origins and diversity of human immunodeficiency viruses. *AIDS* **8**(Suppl. 1):S27–S42.
133. **Silver, J., T. Maudru, K. Fujita, and R. Repaske.** 1993. An RT-PCR assay for the enzyme activity of reverse transcriptase capable of detecting single virions. *Nucleic Acids Res.* **21**:3593–3594.
134. **Sinicco, A., G. Palestro, P. Caramello, D. Giacobbi, G. Giuliani, G. Paggi, M. Sciandra, and P. Gioannini.** 1990. Acute HIV-1 infection: clinical and biological study of 12 patients. *J. Acquired Immune Defic. Syndr.* **3**(3):260–265.
135. **Smith, M. W., M. Dean, M. Carrington, C. Winkler, G. A. Huttley, D. A. Lomb, J. J. Goedert, T. R. Obrien, L. P. Jacobson, R. Kaslow, S. Buchbinder, E. Vittinghoff, D. Vlahov, K. Hoots, M. W. Hilgartner, and S. J. Obrien.** 1997. Contrasting genetic influence of Ccr2 and Ccr5 variants on HIV-1 infection and disease progression. *Science* **277**:959–965.
136. **Spira, A. I., P. A. Marx, B. K. Patterson, J. Mahoney, R. A. Koup, S. M. Wolinsky, and D. D. Ho.** 1996. Cellular targets of infection and route of viral dissemination after an intravaginal inoculation of simian immunodeficiency virus into rhesus macaques. *J. Exp. Med.* **183**:215–225.
137. **Strizki, J. M., A. V. Albright, H. Sheng, M. O'Connor, L. Perrin, and F. Gonzalez-Scarano.** 1996. Infection of primary human microglia and monocyte-derived macrophages with human immunodeficiency virus type 1 isolates: evidence of differential tropism. *J. Virol.* **70**: 7654–7662.
138. **Stuyver, L., A. Wyseru, A. Rombout, C. Verhofstede, D. Rimland, R. F. Schinazi, and R. Rossau.** 1997. Line probe assay (LiPA) for the detection of drug-selected variants in the HIV-1 reverse transcriptase gene. *Int. Antiviral News* **5**:38–40.
139. **Tan, X., and D. M. Phillips.** 1996. Cell-mediated infection of cervix derived epithelial cells with primary isolates of human immunodeficiency virus. *Arch. Virol.* **141**: 1177–1189.
140. **Tenner-Racz, K., P. Racz, M. Bofill, A. Schulz-Meyer, M. Dietrich, P. Kern, J. Weber, A. J. Pinching, F. Veronese-Dimarzo, M. Popovic, D. Klatzmann, J. C. Gluckmann, and G. Janossy.** 1986. HTLV-III/LAV viral antigens in lymph nodes of homosexual men with persistent generalized lymphadenopathy and AIDS. *Am. J. Pathol.* **123**:9–15.
141. **Tjotta, E., O. Hungnes, and B. Grinde.** 1991. Survival of HIV-1 activity after disinfection, temperature and pH changes, or drying. *J. Med. Virol.* **35**:223–227.
142. **Urassa, W. K., U. Bredberg-Raden, E. Mbena, K. Palsson, E. Minja, R. A. Lema, K. Pallangyo, F. S. Mhalu, and G. Biberfeld.** 1992. Alternative confirmatory strategies in HIV-1 antibody testing. *J. Acquired Immune Defic. Syndr.* **5**(2):170–176.
143. **Urdea, M. S., J. C. Wilber, T. Yeghiazarian, J. A. Todd, D. G. Kern, S. J. Fong, D. Besemer, B. Hoo, P. J. Sheridan, R. Kokka, P. Neuwald, and C. A. Pachl.** 1993. Direct and quantitative detection of HIV-1 RNA in human plasma with a branched DNA signal amplification assay. *AIDS* **7**:S11–S14.
144. **van Bueren, J., D. P. Larkin, and R. A. Simpson.** 1994. Inactivation of human immunodeficiency virus type 1 by alcohols. *J. Hosp. Infect.* **28**:137–148.
145. **Van Bueren, J., R. A. Simpson, H. Salman, H. D. Farrelly, and B. D. Cookson.** 1995. Inactivation of HIV-1 by

chemical disinfectants: sodium hypochlorite. *Epidemiol. Infect.* **115:**567–579.

146. **van der Groen, G., I. Van Kerckhoven, G. Vercauteren, and P. Piot.** 1991. Simplified and less expensive confirmatory HIV testing. *Bull. W. H. O.* **69:**747–752.
147. **Vercauteren, G., G. Beelaert, and G. van der Groen.** 1995. Evaluation of an agglutination HIV-1 + 2 antibody assay. *J. Virol. Methods* **51:**1–8.
148. **Wei, X., S. K. Ghosh, M. E. Taylor, V. A. Johnson, E. A. Emini, P. Deutsch, J. D. Lifson, S. Bonhoeffer, M. A. Nowak, B. H. Hahn, M. S. Saag, and G. M. Shaw.** 1995. Viral dynamics in human immunodeficiency virus type 1 infection. *Nature (London)* **373:**117–122.
149. **Weissmahr, R. N., J. Schüpbach, and J. Böni.** 1997. Reverse transcriptase activity in chicken embryo fibroblast culture supernatants is associated with particles containing endogenous avian retrovirus EAV-0 RNA. *J. Virol.* **71:**3005–3012.
150. **Weissman, D., Y. Li, J. Ananworanich, L. J. Zhou, J. Adelsberger, T. F. Tedder, M. Baseler, and A. S. Fauci.** 1995. Three populations of cells with dendritic morphology exist in peripheral blood, only one of which is infectable with human immunodeficiency virus type 1. *Proc. Natl. Acad. Sci. USA* **92:**826–830.
151. **Welles, S. L., J. B. Jackson, B. Yen-Lieberman, L. Demeter, A. J. Japour, L. M. Smeaton, V. A. Johnson, D. R. Kuritzkes, R. T. D'Aquila, P. A. Reichelderfer, D. D. Richman, R. Reichman, M. Fischl, R. Dolin, R. W. Coombs, J. O. Kahn, C. McLaren, J. Todd, S. Kwok, and C. S. Crumpacker.** 1996. Prognostic value of plasma human immunodeficiency virus type 1 (HIV-1) RNA levels in patients with advanced HIV-1 disease and with little or no prior zidovudine therapy. *J. Infect. Dis.* **174:**696–703.
152. **Wolinsky, S. M., B. T. Korber, A. U. Neumann, M. Daniels, K. J. Kunstman, A. J. Whetsell, M. R. Furtado, Y. Cao, D. D. Ho, J. T. Safrit, and R. A. Koup.** 1996. Adaptive evolution of human immunodeficiency virus-type 1 during the natural course of infection. *Science* **272:**537–542.
153. **Zhu, T., H. Mo, N. Wang, D. S. Nam, Y. Cao, R. A. Koup, and D. D. Ho.** 1993. Genotypic and phenotypic characterization of HIV-1 patients with primary infection. *Science* **261:**1179–1181.

Human T-Cell Lymphotropic Virus Types I and II*

CHARLENE S. DEZZUTTI AND RENU B. LAL

64

CLINICAL BACKGROUND

Human T-cell lymphotropic virus (HTLV) type I (HTLV-I) is endemic in southern Japan, the Caribbean, Melanesia, sub-Saharan Africa, and Central and South America, with prevalence rates ranging from 5 to 27% in adult populations (16, 34). HTLV-II is endemic in several native Indian populations in the Americas and Pygmy tribes in Central Africa, with prevalence rates of 7% to 9% (13). In the United States, HTLV-I and -II prevalence ranges from 0.025% in asymptomatic blood donors to 7 to 49% among injecting drug users (IDU) and prostitutes (16). Nearly all HTLV-I-infected persons remain asymptomatic; only 1 to 4% of infected persons develop disease, with a mean time following infection of more than 40 years for the development of adult T-cell leukemia (ATL) and 10 years for the development of HTLV-associated myelopathy/tropical spastic paraparesis (HAM/TSP) (15, 34). HTLV-II has not yet been etiologically linked to any disease, though several cases of HTLV-II-infected individuals with peripheral neuropathy have been reported (13).

HTLV-I and -II infections are spread through sexual (male-to-female), vertical (mother-to-child), and parenteral (drug usage and blood transfusion) transmission (13, 16). Recent studies have shown that IDUs and sex with IDUs are the most important risk factors for HTLV-II transmission, even in a low-risk population such as blood donors (31). Because of the high risk of transfusion-related transmission of HTLV-I and -II (28), screening of volunteer blood donors has been implemented in Japan, the United States, Canada, several Caribbean countries, and several European countries (13, 16). These screening programs are identifying an increasing number of persons infected with HTLV-I and -II, resulting in lowered risk of transfusion-related transmission. The incidence rates of seroconversion associated with HTLV are estimated to be 1.09 per 100,000 persons per year, and the risk of transmitting HTLV infection by transfusing screened blood is estimated to be 1 in 641,000 in the United States (30).

COUNSELING

In the United States, blood donors whose serum specimens are repeatedly reactive by enzyme immunoassay (EIA) and confirmed as seropositive for HTLV-I and -II by additional tests, such as Western blot (WB) (immunoblot), are counseled and permanently deferred from donating blood (4). Blood donors with serum specimens that are repeatedly reactive on screening but not confirmed as seropositive for HTLV-I or -II (including false-positive and indeterminate EIA specimens) should also be notified and deferred if the same test result is obtained on two separate donations (4).

DISEASE ASSOCIATIONS

ATL

The diagnostic criteria for ATL includes a positive HTLV-I serology, presence of abnormal CD3+, CD4+, and CD25+ lymphocytes in the peripheral blood (with the exception of lymphoma), and presence of clonally integrated HTLV-I proviral DNA in CD4+ cells (34). The predominant clinical presentations of ATL are peripheral lymph node enlargement, hepatosplenomegaly, and skin lesions such as erythroderma and cutaneous nodules with subcutaneous infiltration of abnormal cells. Hypercalcemia is also frequently associated with ATL. The clinical subtypes of ATL range from smoldering type (mean survival time [MST] of >2 years), to chronic type (MST of 24 months), lymphoma type (MST of 10 months), and acute type (MST of 6 months) (32).

HAM/TSP

HAM/TSP is characterized by progressive and permanent lower extremity weakness, back pain, urinary incontinence, sensory disturbances, and gait disturbances (spasticity and hyperreflexia). HAM/TSP is often misdiagnosed as multiple sclerosis; however, HAM/TSP patients have anti-HTLV antibodies in their cerebrospinal fluid (CSF) and serum (15). In most cases, antibody titers and HTLV viral loads are higher in HAM/TSP patients than in ATL patients or asymptomatic carriers. Similar to ATL patients, HAM/TSP patients have abnormal lymphocytes (1 to 20% of total) and increased CD25+ cells in their circulation; however, the peripheral blood mononuclear cells (PBMCs) from HAM/TSP patients exhibit a high level of spontaneous proliferation in vitro, which is uncommon for ATL patients (15).

* This chapter contains information presented in chapter 98 by Helen Lee, John D. Burczak, and Jessie Shih in the sixth edition of this Manual.

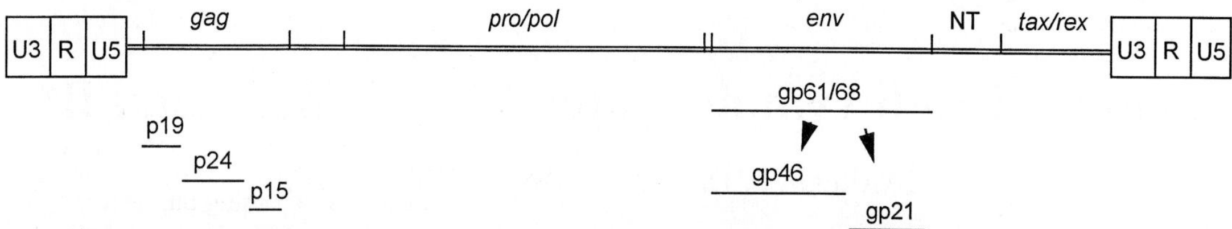

FIGURE 1 Organization of the HTLV genome. Homology between the gag proteins of HTLV-I and HTLV-II ranges from 56% for p19 to 83% for p24. Homology between gp46 for HTLV-I and -II is 61%, while the homology for gp21 is 84%. The gag and the env proteins are most immunogenic, and antibodies to these proteins are commonly detected by EIA and WB.

Other Diseases

Three other conditions have also been associated with HTLV-I infection: HTLV-I uveitis, HTLV-I-associated infective dermatitis, and HTLV-I-associated arthropathy (HAAP). HTLV-I uveitis is characterized by moderate to severe cellular infiltration in the eye and moderate retinal vasculitis (27). HTLV-I-associated infective dermatitis occurs primarily in infected children, and complications include crusted scabies, corneal opacities, chronic bronchiectasis, early death, and at times progression to ATL or HAM/TSP (23). HAAP is characterized by marked joint swelling, with occasional bone and joint lesions (29). Some data suggest that HTLV-I infection also causes Sjögren syndrome among infected persons in areas in which HTLV-I is endemic (29).

DESCRIPTION OF THE AGENTS

HTLV-I and -II are members of the *Oncovirinae* subfamily, different from the *Lentivirinae*, human immunodeficiency viruses types 1 and 2. HTLV-I and -II are typical C-type retroviruses; they contain an electron-dense, centrally located nuclear core, and they bud from the cell surface. Within the core, two positive-sense single-stranded RNA genomes are contained. Once a cell is infected, the RNA genome is converted by reverse transcriptase to DNA and integrates into the host genome. Both HTLV-I and -II have similar genomic organization (*gag*, *pro/pol*, *env*, pX, flanked by long terminal repeats [LTR]) and share approximately 60% of their nucleotide sequences (Fig. 1). The *gag* gene encodes for the structural proteins, p19, p24, and p15. The *pro/pol* genes encode for the protease and the reverse transcriptase, respectively. The *env* gene encodes for the transmembrane and external envelope glycoproteins, gp21 and gp46. The pX gene encodes for the spliced regulatory proteins tax and rex and three other open reading frames. The immunodominant regions of structural proteins and regulatory gene regions have been well characterized (25), and they are the basis for development of diagnostic assays for both detection and differentiation of HTLV-I and -II.

HTLV-I and -II Genetic Subtypes

The overall genome of HTLV is highly conserved; however, a greater nucleotide divergence in the LTR has been exploited for the development of restriction fragment length polymorphism (RFLP) testing methods to genotypically subtype both HTLV-I and -II (see Nucleic Acid Detection below). RFLP testing for HTLV-I shows that there is no correlation between HTLV-I subtypes and clinical outcomes, but subtypes are related to the geographical origin of the virus (20). There are three subtypes of HTLV-I, namely, cosmopolitan, African, and Melanesian subtypes (21). Further restriction digestion patterns subdivide the cosmopolitan subtype into subtypes A through D. Subtype A is found in Japan, the Caribbean basin, South Africa, India, Iran, Sakhalin, and South Africa, whereas subtype B is found predominantly in Japan, subtype C is in West Africa, and subtype D is in North Africa (38). Likewise, HTLV-II has two subtypes, IIa and IIb, which do not show specific geographic clustering but rather are present in specific risk populations (12, 13, 33). A third subtype, IIc, has recently been proposed based on the extended *tax* region, although genotypically it clusters with subtype IIa (8). Subtype IIa is commonly found among IDUs worldwide, whereas subtype IIb is found primarily among native Americans, except some native Brazilian tribes that have a predominance of subtype IIc (8). HTLV-II has also been further subtyped on the basis of additional restriction sites in the LTR (33). This genetic heterogeneity within HTLV-I and -II has provided valuable information on viral transmission and genetic markers of pathogenicity (13, 38).

LABORATORY DIAGNOSIS

Screening of blood donors for HTLV-I and -II has been implemented to prevent transfusion-related transmission (2, 3). The most common assays used for screening detect antibodies in serum or plasma. However, such assays detect only past exposure to the viruses. Direct detection of virus in body fluids can be achieved by assays for viral proteins or nucleic acids.

Serological Detection

Antibody responses to highly immunogenic regions of gag and env of HTLV-I and -II proteins can be measured in several ways. The major tests currently used for HTLV-I and -II are described in Table 1. The EIA is used as the primary screening assay, and WB is used as a confirmatory test.

The EIA is both simple and sensitive and generally uses purified HTLV-I-infected cell lysate to measure antibodies to HTLV-I and -II viral proteins. This rapid colorimetric test can be automated and performed on a large scale, and currently it is the method of choice for testing donated blood. However, the EIA cannot differentiate between an infection with HTLV-I or -II because of significant homology of structural proteins between the two viruses; hence, these screening assays are referred to as tests for HTLV-I/II (3). Comparative analysis of various commercial screening assays has revealed that sensitivity and specificity range from 93 to 100%, depending on the source of antigen used and the assay configuration (10, 19). Some screening assays fail

TABLE 1 Common serological, virological, and nucleic acid detection methods for HTLV-I/II

Detection method	Description
Serological	
Enzyme immunoassay (EIA)	Disrupted viral lysate or synthetic/recombinant antigens coat solid phase with subsequent addition of human serum. Antigen-specific antibodies bind, which is then detected by addition of enzyme-labeled anti-human immunoglobulin G antibodies. Good sensitivity, lacks specificity.
Western blot (WB)	Viral proteins are separated by electrophoresis and transferred to a membrane. Serum reacts with the membrane, and antibodies to individual proteins are identified. High sensitivity and specificity for individual gene products.
Virological	
Antigen capture	Microwell plates are coated with anti-gag polyclonal rabbit sera. Culture supernatant is added to the plates where the antigen is captured and detected with anti-HTLV^{gag} monoclonal antibody. High specificity. Quick and convenient.
Molecular	
Southern blot hybridization (SB)	Enzyme-restricted cellular DNA from PBMCs or cultured cells is electrophoresed and hybridized to an HTLV-I or HTLV-II probe. Good for evaluating monoclonal integration. Poor sensitivity at low proviral copy numbers.
PCR	Method of choice to detect and distinguish between HTLV-I and -II. Can be used to study proviral load and tissue distribution. High sensitivity and specificity.

to detect infection in low-titered sera from HTLV-II-infected individuals, resulting in transfusion-related transmission of HTLV-II (28). More recently, screening assays have been spiked with recombinant transmembrane protein r21e (Cambridge Biotech, Rockville, Md.), which enhances the sensitivity for detection of HTLV-II, or with added viral lysates from HTLV-II (Abbott Laboratories, Abbott Park, Ill.) to increase the sensitivity of HTLV-II detection (2). HTLV-I and -II do not cross-react with HIV.

The screening algorithm for HTLV testing is outlined in Fig. 2. If the initial screening EIA is positive, a repeat assay is performed. All repeatedly reactive specimens are further tested by a confirmatory WB (Fig. 3). If not confirmed by additional testing, the EIA results are considered false positives (18, 24). The diagnostic criteria, established by a U.S. Public Health Service Working Group, recommend that a specimen demonstrating antibodies to at least two gene products (*gag* and *env*) be considered positive (3, 4). Thus, a specimen demonstrating antibody reactivity to p24^{gag} and to gp46^{env} and/or gp61/68 should be considered seropositive for HTLV-I or -II. Specimens reacting with any of the bands but not satisfying the above criteria are designated indeterminate. Specimens with no immunoreactivity to any of the bands are considered negative for antibodies to HTLV-I and -II (EIA false-positive specimens).

Although the WB assays using purified viral lysates are highly sensitive for detecting p24^{gag} antibodies, they do not always detect antibodies to native envelope glycoproteins. Therefore, second-generation WB assays have been developed in which viral lysates have been "spiked" with recombinant p21e protein (Cambridge Biotech, Rockville, Md.) (Fig. 3). While this assay is extremely sensitive for detection of both HTLV-I and -II, it does not differentiate between HTLV-I and -II and it also gives many false-positive reactions, thereby requiring further testing with more-specific assays (18). To avoid these problems, a modified WB has been developed which contains type-specific recombinant proteins from the external glycoprotein of HTLV-I (rgp46^{I}) and HTLV-II (rgp46^{II}), as well as a truncated form of p21e (Genelabs Diagnostics, Ltd., Singapore) (Fig. 3). This assay not only serves as a confirmatory serologic test but also permits differentiation of infection between HTLV-I and -II (36). The modified WB has significantly improved specificity and is highly sensitive for most subtypes of HTLV-I and -II (36).

Specimens with reactivity to p24^{gag} and r21e, but no reactivity to either rgp46^{I} or rgp46^{II}, are referred to as HTLV-positive untypeable. PCR analysis of these untypeable specimens has identified the presence of HTLV-specific sequences (11, 36). A larger study of EIA-negative specimens (PCR positive for HTLV-II) has revealed that specimens containing low-titered antibodies to HTLV-I and -II can easily be missed by these tests (9). Both of the WB assays can give indeterminate results or show immunoreactivity to a single HTLV gene product and, therefore, not meet the criteria of seropositivity (18, 36). Antibody to gag proteins (p24, p19) is the most common indeterminate pattern that is observed in EIA-positive specimens. In some instances, when antibody to r21e is present, it may represent an early antibody response during seroconversion, and individuals with such reactivity should be retested (26). Typically, individuals with indeterminate WB profiles do not have risk factors for HTLV infection and are shown by PCR not to be infected with HTLV-I or -II (24). Such indeterminate WB results appear to represent antibodies to different viral and cellular antigens that cross-react with HTLV proteins (24). In contrast, recent studies from Africa have reported that specimens with indeterminate WB patterns could reflect infection with HTLV (11). Blood donors with indeterminate results should be deferred and their blood should be excluded for transfusion purposes.

Virus Isolation and Antigen Detection

Detection of viral particles from body fluids is the most direct way to demonstrate that an individual is infected with HTLV. However, virus antigen in body fluids is rarely detected because of the cell-associated nature of HTLV. Primary PBMC cultures do not always result in isolation; therefore, cocultivation with activated, allogeneic cells is required (1, 17). Briefly, mononuclear lymphocytes from the PBMCs or CSF of an infected person are stimulated with a mitogen, usually phytohemagglutinin (PHA), and then suspended in media containing recombinant interleukin-2. After 3 days, the cells are cocultivated with human, PHA-activated cord blood lymphocytes or PBMCs from an unin-

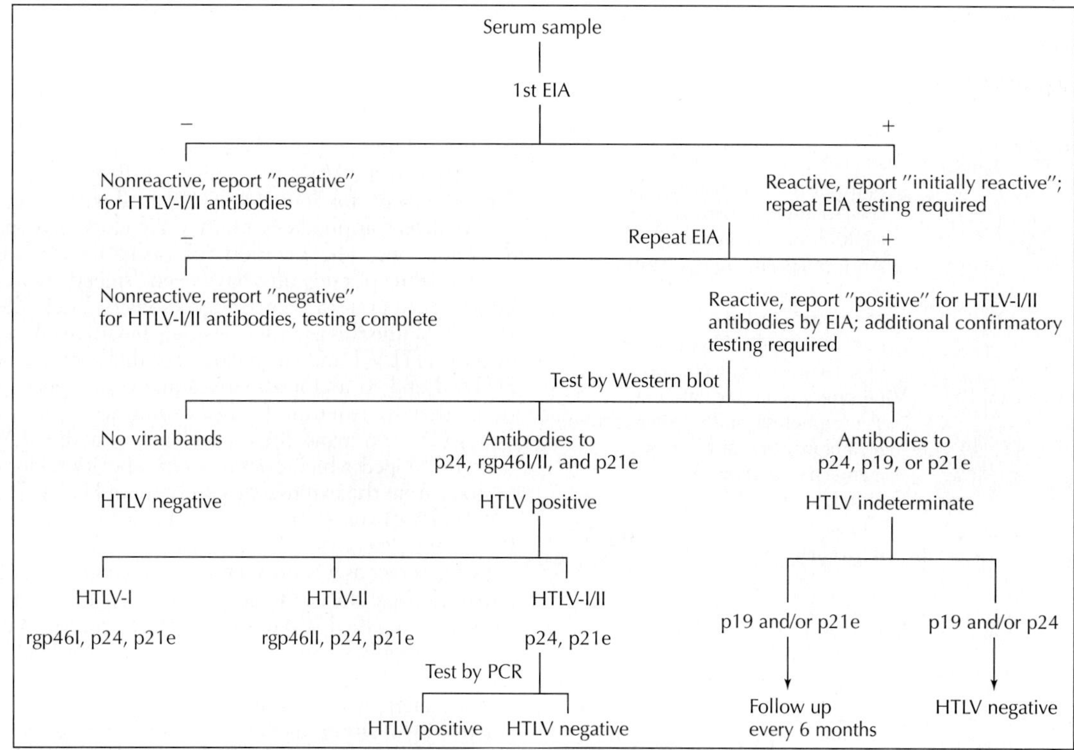

FIGURE 2 Serologic testing algorithm for the detection and confirmation of HTLV-I and HTLV-II infection. The serologic differentiation between HTLV-I and HTLV-II can be made if a WB 2.4 blot (Genelabs Diagnostic, Inc., Singapore) assay is used for confirmation. If the r21e WB (Cambridge Biotech, Rockville, Md.) is used for confirmation, a serotype differentiation between HTLV-I and -II cannot be made.

fected donor. Cultures are then replaced with fresh media every 3 to 5 days. The culture supernatants are monitored for the presence of virus by antigen capture assays (Cellular Products, Inc., Buffalo, N.Y., or Immunotech, Westbrook, Maine). These assays are highly specific for the detection of HTLV-I and -II gag antigens. Because of the cell-associated nature of HTLV, the cultures must often be maintained for several weeks, or even months, before viral gene expression can be detected.

Nucleic Acid Detection

After infection, the genome of HTLV-I and -II integrates in the DNA of the cell and is known as a provirus. Several techniques, including Southern blot hybridization and PCR, have been used to detect the HTLV proviruses in infected cells. PCR or reverse transcriptase PCR can be employed to detect virus expression and has been used to detect active virus replication in infected persons.

Southern blot hybridization of enzyme-digested DNA can identify viral sequences if large numbers of proviral copies are present in the sample. This assay detected HTLV-I in lymphoma cells and in cultured cells, and most importantly, it demonstrated the monoclonal integration of HTLV-I in tumor cells from ATL patients (37). However, because of its low sensitivity, requiring large numbers of HTLV-infected cells, Southern blot hybridization is not useful for detecting HTLV in PBMCs from asymptomatically infected persons.

PCR has become the reference method for determining infection status, testing the validity of serologic assays, distinguishing between HTLV-I and -II, and studying the in vivo viral load and tissue distribution. It also is valuable in characterizing serologically untypeable samples and in studying seroindeterminate or seronegative subjects with risks for HTLV infection. PCR is also useful for testing infants since their serostatus may not be a reliable indication of infection because of passively transferred maternal antibodies. Further, PCR is used for detecting infection during the period between exposure and seroconversion.

Two PCR procedures have been successfully used on PBMCs to confirm and differentiate between HTLV-I and -II infections. The first one uses HTLV consensus primers (e.g., *pol* SK110/111 and *tax* SK43/44) that allow amplification of both viruses; typing is achieved either by hybridizing the product to an HTLV-I-specific or HTLV-II-specific probe (Fig. 4) (14) or by specific restriction digestion patterns (35). A second approach employs type-specific primers and probes in separate amplifications (e.g., SK54/SK55, GAG49/GAG51 for HTLV-I; SK58/SK59, 2G1/2G4 for HTLV-II) (35). The PCR products can be detected with ^{32}P-end-labeled internal probes either by Southern blot hybridization or by liquid hybridization in which a radiolabeled probe is allowed to hybridize in solution. The products are then electrophoresed through a polyacrylamide gel and visualized by autoradiography of the gel. While the liquid hybridization is faster than Southern blotting, both methods have comparable sensitivities. Recently, a solid-phase nonradioactive EIA-based detection system has been developed which seems highly sensitive and specific for detection and differentiation of both HTLV-I and -II (7). In addition to

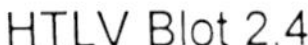

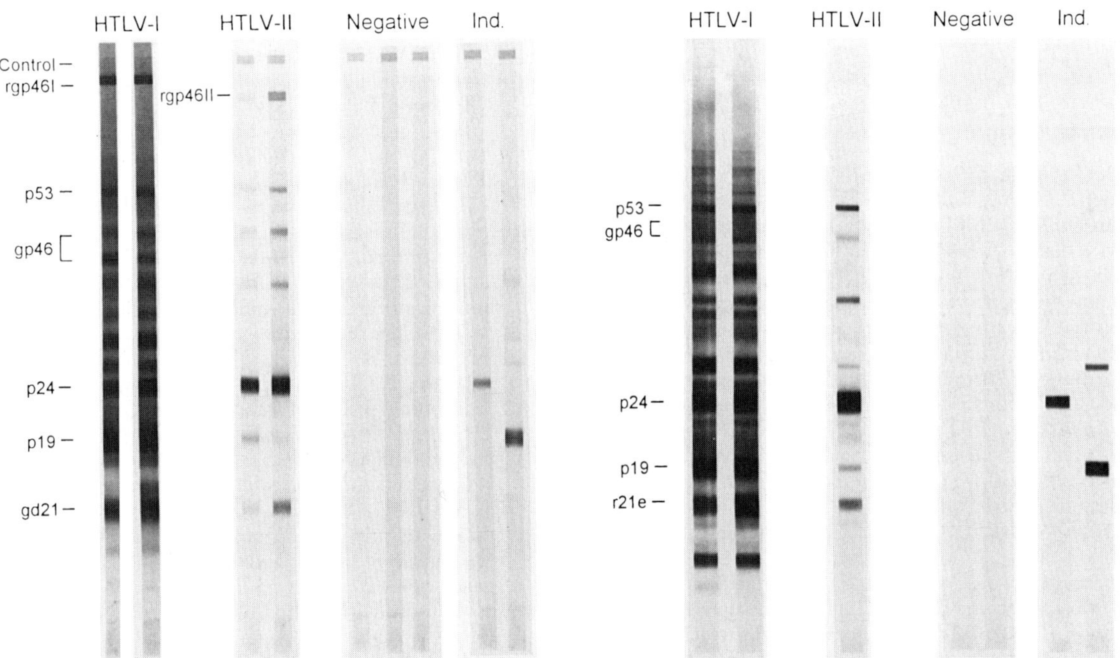

FIGURE 3 Western blot analysis of representative serum specimens. The left panel is the serum specimens run on the HTLV 2.4 blot (Genelabs Diagnostic, Inc.), and the right panel is the same specimens run on the HTLV r21e blot (Cambridge Biotech). (Note only one HTLV-II serum specimen was run on the r21e blot.)

typing and distinguishing the HTLV PCR product from other nonspecifically amplified material and enhancing the specificity of the assay, probing can also increase the sensitivity of the assay by identifying signals that are too weak to be seen on ethidium bromide-stained gels (5).

Different levels of PCR sensitivities have been reported for different study populations. Such variability may be due to several factors, including the efficiency of the primers, the amplification conditions, the quality of template, and the product detection system. The *pol* primers SK110/111 are most commonly used for detection and differentiation of HTLV-I and -II. Repeat testing of fresh lysates of PCR-negative samples and amplification by nested PCR, as well as 45-cycle amplification followed by enzyme-oligonucleotide detection, have increased the sensitivity of HTLV-I and -II detection (7, 14). However, the high sensitivity of PCR also increases the likelihood of false-positive results due to contamination of the reactions with target DNA from infected or previously amplified or cloned material; therefore, published recommendations to prevent contamination should be strictly followed (22).

Recently, PCR has also been used to genetically subtype HTLV-I and -II based on the LTR region. Restriction endonuclease digestion of PCR products and separation through an agarose gel with visualization of the bands by ethidium bromide allows for subtype determination (13, 21, 33).

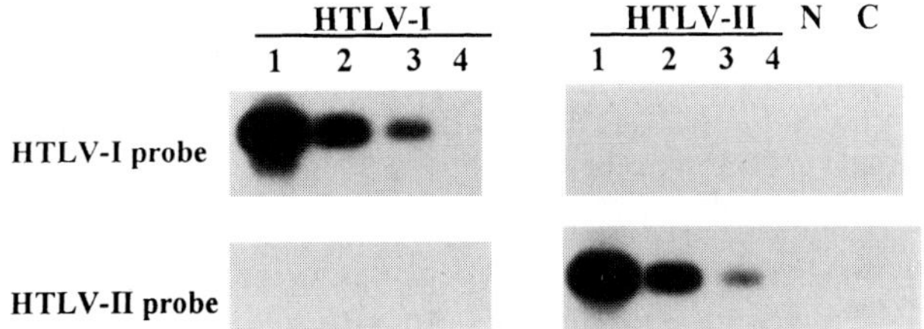

FIGURE 4 PCR amplification of HTLV-I and HTLV-II by pol primers (SK110/SK111) and detection by type-specific probes (SK112 for HTLV-I; SK188 for HTLV-II). Lanes: 1, HuT78 cell lysate containing 1,500 HTLV-I-(MT-2) or HTLV-II-(MoT) infected cells; 2, 150 HTLV-infected cells; 3, 2 HTLV-infected cells; and 4, zero HTLV-infected cells. N, HuT78 cell lysate; C, reagent control. (Reproduced with permission from W. Heneine and R. B. Lal, *Human T-Cell Lymphotropic Virus Type I*, John Wiley & Sons Limited, Sussex, England, 1996.)

RFLP subtyping has resulted in better understanding of the molecular epidemiology and the geographical distribution of virus-carrying populations and their movement in ancient times. RFLP subtyping has also resulted in further discrimination of HTLV by permitting viral fingerprint analysis for transmission studies.

REFERENCES

1. **Beilke, M. A.** 1992. Detection of HTLV-I in clinical specimens. *J. Virol. Methods* **40:**133–144.
2. **Busch, M. P., M. Laycock, S. H. Kleinman, J. W. Wages, M. Calabro, J. E. Kaplan, R. F. Khabbaz, and C. G. Hollingsworth.** 1994. The retrovirus epidemiology donor study. Accuracy of supplementary serologic testing for human T-lymphotropic virus types I and II in US blood donors. *Blood* **83:**1143–1148.
3. **Centers for Disease Control.** 1988. Licensure of screening tests for antibody to human T-lymphotropic virus type I. *Morbid. Mortal. Weekly Rep.* **37:**736–747.
4. **Centers for Disease Control and Prevention and the USPHS Working Group.** 1993. Guidelines for counseling persons infected with human T-lymphotropic virus type I (HTLV-I) and type II (HTLV-II). *Ann. Intern. Med.* **118:** 448–454.
5. **Dezzutti, C. S., P. P. Patel, S. M. Owen, W. M. Switzer, J. Meshulam, and R. B. Lal.** 1996. Sensitivity and specificity of a DNA PCR nonisotopic-based detection method for the confirmation of human T-lymphotropic virus types-I (HTLV-I) and -II (HTLV-II). *Clin. Diagn. Virol.* **6:** 103–110.
6. **Donegan, E., H. Lee, E. A. Operskalski, G. M. Shaw, S. H. Kleinman, M. P. Busch, C. E. Stevens, E. R. Schiff, M. J. Nowicki, C. G. Hollingsworth, and J. W. Mosely.** 1994. Transfusion transmission of retroviruses: human T-lymphotropic virus types I and II compared with human immunodeficiency virus type 1. *Transfusion* **34:**478–483.
7. **Dyster, L. M., L. Abbott, V. Bryz-Gornia, B. Poiesz, and L. D. Papsidero.** 1994. Microplate-based DNA hybridization assays for detection of human retroviral gene sequences. *J. Clin. Microbiol.* **32:**622–629.
8. **Eiraku, N., P. Novoa, M. C. Ferreira, C. Monken, R. Ishak, O. C. Ferreira, S. W. Zhu, R. Lorenco, P. Loureiro, N. Hammerschlak, S. Ijichi, and W. W. Hall.** 1996. Identification and characterization of a new and distinct molecular subtype of human T-cell lymphotropic virus type 2. *J. Virol.* **70:**1481–1492.
9. **Gallo, D., J. L. Diggs, and C. V. Hanson.** 1994. Evaluation of two commercial human T-cell lymphotropic virus Western blot (immunoblot) kits with problem specimens. *J. Clin. Microbiol.* **32:**2046–2049.
10. **Gallo, D., E. T. Yeh, E. S. Moore, and C. V. Hanson.** 1996. Comparison of four enzyme immunoassays for detection of human T-cell lymphotropic virus type 2 antibodies. *J. Clin. Microbiol.* **34:**213–215.
11. **Garin, B., S. Gosselin, G. de Thé, and A. Gessain.** 1994. HTLV-I/II infection in a high viral endemic area of Zaire, Central Africa: comparative evaluation of serology, PCR, and significance of indeterminate Western blot pattern. *J. Med. Virol.* **44:**104–109.
12. **Gessain, A., and G. de Thé.** 1996. What is the situation of human T cell lymphotropic virus type II (HTLV-II) in Africa? Origin and dissemination of genomic subtypes. *J. AIDS Hum. Retroviruses* **13**(Suppl. 1):s228–s235.
13. **Hall, W. W., R. Ishak, S. W. Zhu, P. Novoa, N. Eiraku, H. Takahashi, M. C. Ferreira, V. Azevedo, M. Ishak, O. C. Ferreira, C. Monken, and T. Kurata.** 1996. Human T lymphotropic virus type II (HTLV-II): epidemiology, molecular properties, and clinical features of infection. *J. AIDS Hum. Retroviruses* **13**(Suppl. 1):s204–s214.
14. **Heneine, W., R. F. Khabbaz, R. B. Lal, and J. E. Kaplan.** 1992. Sensitive and specific polymerase chain reaction assays for diagnosis of human T-cell lymphotropic virus type I (HTLV-I) and HTLV-II infections in HTLV-I/II seropositive individuals. *J. Clin. Microbiol.* **30:**1605–1607.
15. **Höllsberg, P., and D. A. Hafler.** 1993. Pathogenesis of diseases induced by human lymphotropic virus type I infection. *N. Engl. J. Med.* **328:**1173–1182.
16. **Kaplan, J. E., and R. F. Khabbaz.** 1993. The epidemiology of human T-lymphotropic virus types I and II. *Rev. Med. Virol.* **3:**137–148.
17. **Kitamura, H., D. L. Rudolph, C. Goldsmith, T. M. Folks, and R. B. Lal.** 1993. Isolation, characterization and transmission of human T-lymphotropic virus types I and II in cultures. *Curr. Microbiol.* **27:**355–360.
18. **Kleinman, S. H., J. E. Kaplan, R. F. Khabbaz, M. A. Calabro, R. Thomson, M. Busch, and The Retrovirus Epidemiology Donor Study Group.** 1994. Evaluation of a p21e-spiked Western blot (immunoblot) in confirming human T-cell lymphotropic virus type I or II infection in volunteer blood donors. *J. Clin. Microbiol.* **32:**603–607.
19. **Kline, R. L., T. Brothers, N. Halsey, R. Boulos, M. D. Lairmore, and T. C. Quinn.** 1991. Evaluation of enzyme immunoassay for antibody to human T-lymphotropic viruses type I/II. *Lancet* **337:**30–33.
20. **Komurian, F., F. Pelloquin, and G. de Thé.** 1991. In vivo genomic variability of human T-cell leukemia virus type I depends more upon geography than upon pathologies. *J. Virol.* **65:**3770–3778.
21. **Komurian-Pradel, F., F. Pelloquin, S. Sonoda, M. Osame, and G. de Thé.** 1992. Geographical subtypes demonstrated by RFLP following PCR in the LTR region of HTLV-I. *AIDS Res. Hum. Retroviruses* **8:**429–434.
22. **Kwok, S., and R. Higuchi.** 1989. Avoiding false positive results with PCR. *Nature (London)* **339:**237–238.
23. **La Grenade, L.** 1994. HTLV-I, infective dermatitis, and tropical spastic paraparesis. *Mol. Neurobiol.* **8:**147–153.
24. **Lal, R. B., D. L. Rudolph, J. E. Coligan, S. K. Brodine, and C. R. Roberts.** 1992. Failure to detect evidence of human T lymphotropic virus type-I and type-II in blood donors with isolated *gag* antibodies to HTLV-I/II. *Blood* **80:**544–550.
25. **Lal, R. B.** 1996. Delineation of immunodominant epitopes of human T-lymphotropic virus types I and II and their usefulness in developing serologic assays for detection of antibodies to HTLV-I and HTLV-II. *J. AIDS Hum. Retroviruses* **13**(Suppl. 1):s170–s178.
26. **Manns, A., E. L. Murphy, R. Wilks, G. Haynes, J. P. Figueroa, B. Hanchard, M. Barnett, J. Drummond, D. Waters, M. Cerney, J. R. Seals, S. S. Alexander, H. Lee, and W. A. Blattner.** 1991. Detection of early human T-cell lymphotropic virus type I antibody patterns during seroconversion among transfusion recipients. *Blood* **77:** 896–905.
27. **Mochizuki, M., A. Ono, E. Ikeda, N. Hikita, T. Watanabe, K. Yamaguchi, K. Sagawa, and K. Ito.** 1996. HTLV-I uveitis. *J. AIDS Hum. Retroviruses* **13**(Suppl. 1):s50–s56.
28. **Nelson, K. E., J. G. Donahue, A. Munoz, N. D. Cohen, P. M. Ness, A. Teague, V. A. Stambolis, D. H. Yawn, B. Callicott, H. McAllister, B. A. Reitz, H. Lee, H. Farzadegan, and C. G. Hollingsworth.** 1992. Transmission of retroviruses from seronegative donors by transfusion during cardiac surgery: a multicenter study of HIV-1 and HTLV-I/II infections. *Ann. Intern. Med.* **117:**554–559.
29. **Nishioka, K.** 1996. HTLV-I arthropathy and Sjögren syndrome. *J. AIDS Hum. Retroviruses* **13**(Suppl. 1):s57–s62.
30. **Schreiber, G. B., M. P. Busch, S. H. Kleinman, and J.**

J. Korelitz. 1996. The risk of transfusion-transmitted viral infections. The retrovirus epidemiology donor study. *N. Engl. J. Med.* **334:**1685–1690.

31. **Schreiber, G. B., E. L. Murphy, J. A. Horton, D. J. Wright, R. Garfein, H. C. Chien, and C. C. Nass.** 1997. Risk factors for human T-cell lymphotropic virus types I and II (HTLV-I and -II) in blood donors: the retrovirus epidemiology donor study. *J. AIDS Hum. Retroviruses* **14:** 263–271.
32. **Shimoyama, M., and The Lymphoma Study Group (1984–1987).** 1991. Diagnostic criteria and classification of clinical subtypes of adult T-cell leukemia-lymphoma. *Br. J. Haematol.* **79:**428–437.
33. **Switzer, W. M., D. Peiniazek, P. Swanson, H. H. Samdal, V. Soriano, R. F. Khabbaz, J. E. Kaplan, R. B. Lal, and W. Heneine.** 1995. Phylogenetic relationship and geographic distribution of multiple human T-cell lymphotropic virus type II subtypes. *J. Virol.* **69:**621–632.
34. **Tajima, K., and L. Cartier.** 1995. Epidemiological features of HTLV-I and adult T cell leukemia. *Intervirology* **38:** 238–246.
35. **Tuke, P. W., P. Luton, and J. A. Garson.** 1992. Differential diagnosis of HTLV-I and HTLV-II infections by restriction enzyme analysis of "nested" PCR products. *J. Virol. Methods* **40:**163–174.
36. **Varma, M., D. L. Rudolph, M. Knuchel, W. M. Switzer, K. G. Hadlock, M. Velligan, L. Chan, S. K. H. Foung, and R. B. Lal.** 1995. Enhanced specificity of truncated transmembrane protein for serologic confirmation of human T-cell lymphotropic virus type 1 (HTLV-1) and HTLV-2 infections by Western blot (immunoblot) assay containing recombinant envelope glycoproteins. *J. Clin. Microbiol.* **33:**3239–3244.
37. **Yamaguchi, K., M. Seiki, M. Yoshida, H. Nishimura, F. Kawano, and K. Takatsuki.** 1984. The detection of human T cell leukemia virus proviral DNA and its application for classification and diagnosis of T cell malignancy. *Blood* **63:** 1235–1240.
38. **Yamashita, M., E. Ido, T. Miura, and M. Hayami.** 1996. Molecular epidemiology of HTLV-I in the world. *J. AIDS Hum. Retroviruses* **13**(Suppl. 1):s124–s131.

Herpes Simplex Viruses

ANN M. ARVIN AND CHARLES G. PROBER

65

CLINICAL BACKGROUND

The common clinical manifestations of herpes simplex virus (HSV) infection have been recognized for centuries. With the development of methods for the laboratory isolation and characterization of HSV, two biologically distinct serotypes, HSV types 1 and 2 (HSV-1 and HSV-2), were identified. Furthermore, with the development and refinement of a variety of serologic techniques able to identify HSV infections, a better understanding of the epidemiology and pathogenesis of these infections in the human host has been achieved (7, 18, 101, 107). The prevalence of HSV-1 infections increases gradually from childhood, reaching 70 to 80% in later adult years, whereas HSV-2 infection is typically acquired as a sexually transmitted disease, so that its incidence begins to increase in adolescence (18, 107). The prevalence rates for HSV-2 infection range from about 15% to more than 50% in adults, depending on a variety of demographic variables (33, 49, 101). As with the other members of the herpesvirus group (varicella-zoster virus, Epstein-Barr virus, cytomegalovirus, human herpesvirus 6 [HHV-6], and HHV-7), initial infection with HSV results in the establishment of viral latency, with the potential for subsequent viral reactivation. The initial mucocutaneous infection caused by HSV-1 or HSV-2 is followed by latent infection of neuronal cells in the dorsal root ganglia (10, 42, 100). Subsequent viral reactivation is accompanied by viral excretion from the original mucocutaneous sites of infection, with or without the concomitant appearance of clinical signs and symptoms. HSV transmission can result from direct contact with infected secretions from a symptomatic or an asymptomatic host (21). Although previous infection with HSV-1 does not prevent infection upon exposure to HSV-2, preexisting HSV-1 immunity may modify the severity of HSV-2 infection, rendering it clinically mild or asymptomatic.

The classic presentation of primary HSV-1 infection is herpes gingivostomatitis, an infection of the oral mucosa resulting in extensive, painful vesicular lesions associated with a fever and marked submandibular lymphadenopathy. Recurrences of orolabial infections are referred to as fever blisters or cold sores. Other clinical manifestations of HSV-1 infection are conjunctivitis, keratitis, and herpetic whitlow. The most serious infection caused by HSV-1 is sporadic encephalitis, which occurs in older children and adults (78, 99, 110). This infection has a mortality rate of approximately 70% if untreated. The classic presentation of a primary HSV-2 infection is herpes genitalis, an infection characterized by the appearance of extensive, bilaterally distributed lesions in the genital area accompanied by fever, inguinal lymphadenopathy, and dysuria (21). Approximately 85% of cases of symptomatic primary genital HSV are caused by HSV-2, with the remaining cases being caused by HSV-1. Because genital HSV-1 infection is much less likely to produce recurrences, 99% of recurrent genital herpes is due to HSV-2 (21). The most serious consequence of genital HSV infection is neonatal herpes. Neonatal infection usually results from exposure of the infant to virus excreted by mothers at the time of vaginal delivery (4, 14, 112). Unfortunately, the majority (70%) of mothers who infect their neonates are experiencing asymptomatic genital infections at delivery (113). If the mother has a recurrent infection at delivery, the attack rate for the neonate is quite low, probably less than 5% (79). However, if the mother is experiencing a primary infection at delivery, the attack rate is probably greater than 50% (111). Neonates may present with infection localized to the skin, eyes, and mucosa or the central nervous system or may present with a disseminated infection. The mortality rate for untreated infants who develop disseminated infection exceeds 70% (113). Early institution of therapy can substantially reduce the morbidity and mortality of mucocutaneous infections and the mortality rates of disseminated and central nervous system infections (109, 111).

Many individuals with primary HSV-1 or HSV-2 infection do not manifest characteristic clinical disease. In fact, primary infections are often entirely asymptomatic. Similarly, despite the apparently universal establishment of latency, most individuals with past HSV infections do not experience symptomatic recurrences. Nevertheless, individuals who have had HSV-1 or HSV-2 infection are subject to asymptomatic reactivations associated with the isolation of infectious virus from oral or genital sites. Therefore, prevention of the transmission of HSV-1 and HSV-2 in the population is very difficult.

Because of the high prevalence of HSV infections in the general population, many patients who develop malignancy, an immunodeficiency such as AIDS, or other diseases that require immunosuppressive therapy may develop symptoms of HSV-1 or HSV-2 infection. These infections may be primary or may arise from reactivation of a past infection, and they may be associated with severe disease (93, 97). They can be locally invasive, causing extensive mucocutaneous necrosis, or they can spread to contiguous sites, causing deep tissue infections such as esophagitis or proctitis. Herpes infections in immunocompromised hosts can also result in viremia with dissemination to multiple organs, causing meningoencephalitis, pneumonitis, hepatitis, and coagulopathy. In addition to the susceptibility of classically immunosuppressed patients, some individuals with chronic skin diseases, particularly eczema, can experience severe primary HSV-1 infection, referred to as Kaposi's varicelliform eruption.

While a presumptive diagnosis of HSV infection can often be made on the basis of clinical findings, a definitive diagnosis is important in many circumstances. Appropriate laboratory testing allows the proper evaluation of mucocutaneous lesions in high-risk patients who are likely to benefit from specific antiviral therapy if the lesion is herpetic. Laboratory documentation of HSV infection also provides critical information for managing patients with disseminated disease or encephalitis. In addition, laboratory diagnosis is valuable for many patients with HSV infections that are not life-threatening. For example, proving that a genital lesion is caused by HSV-1 or HSV-2 facilitates counseling regarding the advisability of acyclovir therapy, the risk of recurrences, and the appropriate measures to reduce HSV transmission to contacts.

DESCRIPTION OF THE AGENT

HSV-1 and HSV-2, along with varicella-zoster virus, are the human herpesviruses that are classified in the alphaherpesvirus subfamily of herpesviruses (87). Important characteristics of this subfamily include a short replication cycle, production of lytic infection in tissue culture, and establishment of latency in sensory ganglia. Like other herpesviruses, HSV-1 and HSV-2 have icosahedral capsids consisting of 162 capsomeres surrounding a core that contains the viral DNA. HSV DNA is linear, double stranded, and relatively GC rich, with a molecular weight of 96×10^6. The viral genome consists of a long unique region and a short unique region, each of which is flanked by inverted-repeat regions. Extensive sequence homologies, involving about 40% of the genome, can be demonstrated between HSV-1 and HSV-2 DNAs. These homologies account for the antigenic cross-reactivity of the two serotypes and their other biological similarities. The overall pattern of nucleotide sequences composing HSV DNA is conserved, as are the nucleotide sequences of major regions of the genome. However, restriction endonuclease analysis demonstrates sufficient variability of cleavage sites among clinically unrelated isolates to permit the investigation of HSV transmission by molecular epidemiologic methods.

The phospholipid-rich viral envelope is acquired when the virion buds through regions of the nuclear membrane that have been modified by insertion of viral proteins. The complete virion has a diameter of between 110 and 120 nm. Tegument proteins have been identified between the capsid and the viral envelope. The HSV genome codes for more than 100 polypeptides, including a number of glycoproteins (designated glycoprotein A [gA] through gK), at least six capsid proteins, viral protein kinase, DNA polymerase, other enzymes, and DNA-binding proteins that are involved in viral replication (21, 87). The immediate-early proteins of the virus, such as ICP0 and ICP4, constitute products of the alpha genes of HSV that are involved in initiating the cascade by which the expression of HSV genes is regulated. With respect to the glycoproteins, gB and gD carry major epitopes to which neutralizing antibodies bind, and they appear to be involved in viral attachment to the target cell. gC binds to the cell surface complement receptor, C3b; gE and gI are involved in constituting the receptor for immunoglobulin that appears on infected-cell membranes. gB, gD, and gH also affect the movement of adsorbed virus from the surface into the cytoplasm of the cell. HSV gD has been identified as binding to a specific molecule on the cell membrane, designated HVEM (65). Although these and other functions of some HSV proteins have been defined or suggested, the understanding of specific effects on virus entry and virus-induced changes in mammalian cells remains limited. Because the host cell-derived viral envelope is phospholipid rich, the virus is readily inactivated by lipid solvents. Exposure to a pH of <4 and a temperature of >56°C maintained for 20.5 h also eliminates infectivity.

COLLECTION AND STORAGE OF SPECIMENS

HSV-1 and HSV-2 can be recovered from clinical specimens obtained by swabbing mucocutaneous lesions. In asymptomatic patients, virus may be recovered by swabbing mucocutaneous sites where lesions were observed previously. Cotton swabs are preferred for taking specimens for HSV culture; calcium alginate swabs can reduce viral recovery (24). Fresh vesicles, which contain a high concentration of virus, may be aspirated with a small-gauge (e.g., 25-gauge) needle attached to a tuberculin syringe. After aspiration, the surface of the vesicle is removed and a premoistened swab is used to absorb any remaining fluid. After vesicle fluid is collected, the base of the lesion is swabbed vigorously to recover infected epithelial cells. The swab specimens should be placed directly into 1 to 2 ml of viral transport medium (discussed in chapter 4) (98). Clinical specimens that might contain HSV can be effectively shipped to reference laboratories at ambient temperatures in Virocult transport tubes (Medical Wire and Equipment Co., Cleveland, Ohio). HSV can survive in these tubes for 2 to 3 days at 22°C, and the tubes are compact, enclosed, and resistant to breakage (47).

HSV can be isolated directly from cerebrospinal fluid (CSF) obtained from patients with meningitis, or it can be isolated from peripheral blood leukocytes in those with disseminated infection. Heparin can interfere with viral isolation and should not be used as an anticoagulant. HSV can also be isolated from homogenized sterile tissue specimens, such as brain tissue from patients with encephalitis (see chapter 5 for details). Trypsinizing the tissue may enhance the efficiency of virus isolation from such samples. HSV-2 can sometimes be isolated from urine samples obtained from patients with genital herpes complicated by urethritis or cystitis. Rectal swab specimens rarely yield HSV.

Rates of isolation of infectious HSV are highest if specimens are inoculated on the day they are taken; otherwise, careful attention must be given to conditions of transport and storage, which can affect the recovery of HSV. Specimens may be maintained at 4°C during transport and for up to 48 h (11, 116), but they must not be frozen at −20°C. See chapter 4 for additional information.

ISOLATION OF VIRUS

Viral culture is the most sensitive method for the laboratory diagnosis of HSV, and it also allows typing of the viral isolate. HSV-1 and HSV-2 cause typical cytopathic effects (CPE) in a wide variety of cell culture systems (30). Primary human embryonic cells and human diploid cell lines, such as MRC-5, are commonly used because they are commercially available and because other viruses can be isolated in these cell types. Primary rabbit kidney, mink lung, and rhabdomyosarcoma cells are particularly sensitive cell lines, especially for HSV isolation (51, 62). Continuous human or primate cell lines, such as HEp-2 and Vero cells, are somewhat less sensitive. The inoculation of two different cell lines in parallel can minimize the periodic variations in the sensitivity of different cell lines that are often difficult to avoid (16). The difference in the rates of recovery of HSV in two acceptable cell lines is less than 5% and is apparent with clinical specimens that contain low concentrations of virus. If primary cells are not used, the recovery of HSV is optimal when the cell lines are used at low passage numbers. Most procedures for HSV culture incorporate a 1-h adsorption at 36 to 37°C before incubation with a standard tissue culture medium such as Eagle's minimal essential medium supplemented with fetal calf serum and antibiotics.

The presence of HSV is detected by observing foci of enlarged, refractile cells in the monolayer; some clinical isolates also induce the formation of syncytia with multinucleated giant cells. Although the CPE induced by HSV-1 tends to be more diffuse throughout the monolayer than that induced by HSV-2, this observation is not sufficiently specific to permit the differentiation of the two virus types. The incubation time required to observe CPE depends on the concentration of virus in the sample and the condition of the tissue culture cells. With careful maintenance of tissue culture cells, samples with high concentrations of virus produce CPE within 18 to 24 h and samples containing low concentrations of virus should be identifiable as positive within 4 to 5 days. Cultures from oral or genital lesions can be expected to be positive within 3 days (16). In one study, CPE was observed within 4 days in more than 99% of genital tract specimens from women with asymptomatic HSV-2 reactivation (115). Addition of dexamethasone to the culture medium may hasten the appearance of viral CPE in standard tube cultures (114) or may increase the number of infected-cell foci that are visible, but it is not standard procedure (108).

The interval to virus identification can be shortened somewhat by preparing the tissue culture cells on removable glass coverslips and inoculating multiple cultures with each specimen. The coverslip is removed at intervals after inoculation, usually 24 and 48 h, and the monolayer is stained by using HSV antibodies labeled with fluorescein, biotinavidin complexes, staphylococcal protein A, or immunoperoxidase reagents (80, 91). Immunologic staining can reveal foci of virus-infected cells before the typical CPE is apparent. This immunologic approach has also been applied to regular tissue culture systems and to shell vial systems incorporating centrifugation of the specimen onto the monolayer (37). The yield for earlier viral diagnosis by these techniques depends on the specific tissue culture cell line used, the quality of the HSV-specific antibody reagents, and the viral inoculum in the clinical specimen (28, 45, 69, 76, 117). Typically, methods involving early immunologic staining at 24 h are not as sensitive as those involving standard tube cell cultures that are maintained for 5 to 7 days (29, 89, 114). In an alternative approach, the cells from one of the replicate cultures are lysed with detergent at intervals after inoculation, usually 24 and 48 h, and the supernatant is tested by an enzyme immunoassay method for HSV antigen detection. Another procedure that may shorten the interval to viral detection involves infection of cells in suspension followed by immunostaining (61). Earlier detection of HSV has also been accomplished by using HSV-specific DNA probes to demonstrate the presence of virus (32). The cumulative experience with early-detection methods used at 48 h compared with standard tube cultures indicates that the sensitivity with which HSV is identified in clinical specimens is maintained but not enhanced by the former. For clinical purposes, shortening the interval to virus isolation by 24 to 48 h is usually not critical. However, the fact that some of these procedures lend themselves to the semiautomated processing of specimens (Vitek Immune Diagnostic Assay System; Vitek Systems Inc., Hazelwood, Mo.) may be useful for large diagnostic laboratories (50). Simultaneous seeding of uninfected tissue culture cells along with the sample to be tested does not improve the detection of virus in the sample over that in standard shell vial culture methods, although the yield of infectious virus may be higher when assessed by plaque titer determination (48).

For mucocutaneous HSV infection, the success with which the laboratory can isolate the etiologic agent from clinical specimens depends substantially on the type of lesion being evaluated. For example, in one study, HSV was recovered from 94% of genital herpes lesions cultured during the vesicular stage, from 87% cultured during the pustular phase, and from 70% cultured during the ulcer stage but from only 27% cultured during the crusted stage (21, 66). The specific site of the infection also influences the success with which the virus is recovered. Examples include the observations that HSV-1 is rarely isolated from the CSF of patients with herpes encephalitis and that HSV-2 is more likely to be recovered from the usual site of lesion recurrences than from the cervix in women with asymptomatic reactivation of genital HSV-2 infection (4).

IDENTIFICATION OF THE VIRUS

It is important to confirm that CPE is due to HSV and not to varicella-zoster virus, cytomegalovirus, or nonspecific toxic changes. It is also often desirable to distinguish HSV serotypes. Although HSV serotypes have been differentiated in the past by biochemical and biological differences, the availability of HSV-specific monoclonal antibody reagents has facilitated the use of a simplified immunologic method of verifying and typing HSV isolates (9, 15, 38, 63). Identification of viral isolates with monoclonal antibodies has replaced inoculation of chicken embryo chorioallantoic membrane and guinea pig cells as well as neutralization endpoint and other immunologic procedures for differentiating HSV-1 and HSV-2 isolates. Although in theory a specific monoclonal antibody might not react with epitopes of the relevant viral protein as produced by all HSV strains, in practice it has been possible to develop reagents that are not significantly affected by this potential for antigenic variation. HSV typing with monoclonal antibody reagents is significantly more accurate than typing with polyclonal type-specific rabbit antisera. In a study performed in 1987, three pairs of commercially available monoclonal antibodies (Electro-Nucleonics, Inc.; Syva, Inc.; and Kallestad Laboratories, Inc.) tested in parallel performed satisfactorily (60). The specificity of the results corresponded closely with typing of isolates by restriction enzyme analysis, which defines the HSV type at the molecular level (9). Use of both HSV-1 and HSV-2 monoclonal antibody reagents makes strain differentiation part of the confirmation procedure.

Another approach to virus identification involves DNA-DNA hybridization in a dot blot system with cloned or synthetic DNA probes that are specific for unique nucleotide sequences of HSV-1 and HSV-2 (28, 75). Such methods are comparable to restriction endonuclease analysis in the specificity with which HSV types are distinguished and may become more widely used when better nonradioactive labeled probes are developed. The fact that HSV-1 is inhibited by antiviral agents such as bromovinyldeoxyuridine, to which HSV-2 strains are resistant, has also been exploited to differentiate HSV types.

DIRECT EXAMINATION

When mucocutaneous lesions are present, direct-detection methods can provide a rapid diagnosis of HSV infection. The most common method used for the direct detection of HSV in clinical specimens is direct immunofluorescence or immunoperoxidase staining of cells isolated from mucocutaneous lesions (9). These samples are best obtained by exposing the base of the lesion, removing cells with the blunt end of a cotton applicator stick, and immediately streaking the sample onto a glass slide. Since a negative result is reliable only if intact cells are transferred to the slide, the laboratory should confirm the adequacy of the specimen before processing it. With the use of fluorescein isothiocyanate-conjugated monoclonal antibodies to HSV to stain cytologic preparations of lesion scrapings, sensitivities are as high as 78 to 88% of those for tissue culture isolation, with relatively few false-positive reactions (38, 77, 95, 104). However, a sample for viral culture should be obtained when the lesion scraping is made, to allow confirmation of the direct-detection result, since both false-positive and false-negative results can occur with the immunofluorescence and immunoperoxidase staining methods. The Papanicolaou (Pap) stain or Tzanck test can be used to demonstrate cytologic changes in specimens obtained from suspected HSV lesions. The cytologic changes being sought include syncytial giant cells, "ballooning" cytoplasm, and Cowdry type A intranuclear inclusions. These pathologic examinations can be useful, inexpensive methods for evaluating patients with non-life-threatening illness. However, these methods are not specific for HSV and are much less sensitive than direct detection with immunologic reagents (21). Therefore, a negative Tzanck or Pap smear cannot be relied on to exclude the diagnosis of HSV in critical situations such as infections in newborns, pregnant women at term, patients with encephalitis, or immunosuppressed patients.

Direct detection of infected cells with immunologic reagents has been established as reliable for identifying virus-infected cells in brain tissue from patients with HSV encephalitis, but its sensitivity in this setting results from the fact that many cells harbor HSV. This method should not be extended to the analysis of other samples, such as testing cells from CSF of patients with encephalitis, attempting to detect HSV-infected cells in genital tract specimens from asymptomatic pregnant women, or examining cells in tracheal aspirate or bronchoalveolar lavage samples from immunocompromised patients with pneumonia.

Monoclonal antibodies capable of binding HSV proteins have also been used to enhance the detection of HSV antigens in clinical specimens by using enzyme-linked immunosorbent assays (ELISAs), immunoperoxidase assays, hemagglutination assays, or avidin-biotin enzyme conjugate assays (1, 2, 13, 20, 34, 64, 70, 72, 84, 95, 96). Most of these methods are applied to the detection of viral antigen in samples collected as described above for viral culture. The use of dual fluorescent probes allows the differentiation of HSV and varicella-zoster virus (12). Antigen detection may be enhanced by concentrating the sample by membrane filtration or by collecting the original sample in a special transport system (26, 86). The sensitivities of these methods compared with that of viral isolation range from 70 to 95%, with specificities of 65 to 95%. However, none of the antigen detection techniques has proved to be sensitive enough to detect the asymptomatic shedding of HSV (70, 103, 106). The sensitivities of commercial ELISAs for the detection of HSV antigens are also variable compared with viral culture (39). Direct comparisons of three commercial methods on culture-positive specimans revealed variations in sensitivity from 47 to 89% and variations in specificity from 85 to 100% (13). Antigen detection methods fail to identify viral proteins in specimans that contain low titers of infectious virus, which are revealed by the viral amplification that occurs after inoculation of tissue culture cells. Cross-reactivity with other herpesviruses does not affect the specificity of these assays.

Whereas methods that identify HSV proteins in the clinical sample are not likely to be improved sufficiently to permit the detection of asymptomatic HSV infection, the sensitivity of PCR appears to be adequate for this purpose (19, 41). Viral culture methods effectively amplify HSV by allowing viral replication. Similarly, PCR can amplify the "signal" of HSV DNA and has the potential to be much more sensitive than methods to detect viral proteins. Nevertheless, a negative PCR result does not exclude the diagnosis of HSV, because specimens obtained early in the clinical course of some infections may be negative and clinical specimens contain inhibitors of PCR (17, 41, 85). The inclusion of internal controls helps to improve the sensitivity and specificity of HSV PCR (68, 85). "Multiplex" PCR, using multiple primer pairs, can be used to distinguish HSV-1 from HSV-2 by further analysis of the PCR product by restriction enzyme digestion or DNA enzyme immunoassay (17); HSV can also be differentiated from other viral or bacterial pathogens present in the same clinical specimen (6, 46, 73). Options for nonradioactive probes, such as digoxigenin, may facilitate the use of HSV PCR in clinical diagnostic laboratories (82).

In genital herpes, PCR detects viral genome or genome fragments for several days after lesions become negative for infectious virus (19, 90). The clinical significance of the prolonged detection of HSV DNA is not known. Correlating PCR positivity and the risk of viral transmission to susceptible contacts and determining when PCR positivity is an indication for antiviral therapy is a subject of continuing clinical investigations (20). PCR can be made quantitative, and this modification may permit correlations with the presence of infectious virus (44). HSV PCR has potential value for testing CSF in patients with suspected herpes encephalitis (8, 40, 52, 71, 81, 88, 94, 99). HSV DNA was detected by PCR in CSF of 53 (98%) of 54 patients with biopsy-proven herpes encephalitis and was detected in all 18 CSF specimens obtained before brain biopsy from patients with proven herpes encephalitis (55). HSV PCR also has utility when clinical diagnosis is difficult, as illustrated by the detection of HSV in vitreous fluid and in unusual mucocutaneous lesions in AIDS patients (25, 58).

Direct viral detection by DNA hybridization with radiolabeled or biotinylated probes has also been evaluated for identifying HSV in pathologic specimens (31, 57, 105). These methods, as well as the use of electron microscopy, are sensitive for demonstrating infected cells in tissue sections but are not widely used in clinical laboratories.

SEROLOGIC DIAGNOSIS

The detection of immunoglobulin G (IgG) antibodies to HSV in serum means that the individual has been infected with HSV-1 or HSV-2 or both. Because these viruses cause persistent infection, the presence of HSV antibodies signifies that the individual harbors the virus in sensory ganglia and that the virus can be expected to reactivate intermittently. Assessing HSV immune status to document whether an individual is infected with HSV can be done by many serologic methods. Most methods are generally quite sensitive for detecting HSV IgG antibodies in individuals with past HSV infection regardless of whether the patient has had any recent signs of HSV disease. For most laboratories, HSV serologic testing is accomplished most efficiently by using commercial kits based on ELISA or latex agglutination procedures (27, 36). However, the extensive cross-reactivity between HSV-1 and HSV-2 makes it impossible to differentiate past HSV-1 from past HSV-2 infection by any of these methods, including microneutralization (35, 83, 101). Since physicians are not often aware of this problem, serologic reports that list HSV-1 and HSV-2 antibody titers separately are potentially misleading. As documented by Ashley et al. (6), currently licensed assays do not discriminate between infections with HSV-1 and HSV-2.

Recurrent HSV infections are not always accompanied by a significant rise in antibody titer. Quantitation of HSV IgG antibody titers is not helpful since titers may vary more than fourfold in the absence of viral reactivation. Therefore, serologic tests should not be used to diagnose recurrent HSV infections. Primary HSV infection can be documented by using any of the standard methods to show seroconversion with paired sera. However, just as cross-reactivity prevents the distinction of past HSV-1 from past HSV-2 infection, the serotype of HSV responsible for the seroconversion cannot be determined with commercially available serologic tests.

Testing for IgM antibodies does not improve the specificity of the serologic diagnosis in patients with clinical signs of HSV infection. HSV IgM assays cannot be used to distinguish primary from recurrent infections, because the host response to reactivation can also include IgM antibody production. In addition, the maintenance of quality control for HSV IgM antibody assays is very difficult and is complicated particularly by false-positive results, even when efforts are made to fractionate serum IgG and IgM before testing.

Testing for local production of HSV IgG in CSF samples can be used to document HSV encephalitis in some patients, but a 2- to 4-week interval may be required before positive results can be demonstrated (67). Therefore, serologic testing is not helpful in providing an early diagnosis to guide the use of antiviral therapy. There is no known diagnostic value in testing CSF for HSV IgM antibodies.

Serologic methods that circumvent the problem of cross-reactivity between HSV-1 and HSV-2 antibodies have been developed. Serum samples can be tested against HSV-1 and HSV-2 antigens by Western blotting (immunoblotting) to demonstrate reactivity with type-specific viral proteins (7). The fact that the gG protein of HSV-1 differs significantly from the HSV-2 homolog has also permitted the development of type-specific serologic assays to detect IgG and IgM antibodies (7, 12, 43, 59, 92, 101). Monoclonal antibody to HSV-2 gG is used either to capture the protein from an HSV-infected cell sonic extract in a solid-phase ELISA or to prepare immunoaffinity-purified HSV-2 gG for use as antigen in a dot blot assay. By using the capture ELISA method, antibodies to HSV-2 gG were detected in 96 to 98% of persons with previous episodes of culture-proved HSV-2 infections, with very few false-positive results (74, 101). Western blot analysis or assays detecting antibodies to HSV-2 gG can also be used to document primary HSV-2 infections, even in patients who have had previous infections caused by HSV-1 (7). Serologic testing by these methods confirms the unreliability of the clinical history of oral and genital lesions as an indicator of HSV-1 or HSV-2 infection (23, 33). Unfortunately, none of these HSV type-specific serologic tests has been developed for commercial use based upon a comparative analysis of sera shown to contain antibodies to HSV-2 by research methods or obtained from patients with HSV-2 infections that were confirmed virologically.

EVALUATION, INTERPRETATION, AND REPORTING OF RESULTS

Rapid Diagnostic Tests

Untreated encephalitis caused by HSV and HSV infections in neonates has mortality rates approximating 70% (113). In recent years, effective antiviral therapy has been developed for these life-threatening infections, resulting in the potential to reduce the mortality rates by at least 50% (109, 112). In addition, the course of severe mucocutaneous and disseminated HSV infections in immunosuppressed hosts can be favorably altered by antiviral chemotherapy (93). Furthermore, genital HSV infections, which are the cause of substantial morbidity, can now be effectively managed with acyclovir therapy; the severity of clinical attacks can be abrogated, and the frequency of recurrences can be diminished significantly (101). Thus, optimal patient management demands the availability of accurate diagnostic tests for HSV.

For non-life-threatening HSV infections, the availability of a diagnostic laboratory able to perform viral cultures is adequate. Since these infections can usually be recognized clinically, it is generally sufficient for a clinician to obtain virologic confirmation within several days of specimen submission. This can be accomplished readily with viral cultures. However, for life-threatening infections that mandate prompt antiviral therapy, an accurate and rapid diagnostic test for HSV must be used. The best currently available test is immunofluorescent staining of infected tissues. Patients with HSV encephalitis are more likely to have a favorable outcome if antiviral therapy is administered early in their infection (110). Since HSV encephalitis is difficult to diagnose clinically, brain biopsy may be the only way to demonstrate the etiology of the illness (110). Although antiviral therapy can be started before a definitive diagnosis is made, a positive rapid diagnostic test assures the clinician that optimal therapy has been initiated. A rapid diagnostic test for HSV also must be available to physicians involved with the treatment of newborn infants, because prompt therapy of newborns presenting with skin lesions as the only sign of an HSV infection usually has an excellent outcome. However, if the diagnosis and treatment of this infection are delayed, dissemination beyond the skin may soon follow and the outcome will be significantly worse (112).

Rapid diagnostic tests for HSV are not sensitive enough to permit the diagnosis of oral or genital HSV infections not associated with lesions, and the clinical use of these tests in these circumstances should be discouraged (103). As noted above, in clinical practice, HSV PCR results must be interpreted very carefully. False-positive as well as false-negative results complicate the application of PCR to clinical diagnosis, and antiviral therapy may interfere with HSV detection by PCR (3, 56, 102).

Isolate Typing

Although knowledge of the serotype of HSV responsible for the clinical infection is important epidemiologically, there are only a few situations in which a clinician needs this information. However, if isolates are not typed routinely, it is prudent to save the HSV isolate, at least until the clinician has been contacted, to be sure that typing is not desired. One situation in which it is mandatory to type HSV isolates is when the isolate is from the genital tract of a young child. A type 2 isolate recovered from the genital tract of a child should raise concern about the possibility of sexual abuse, whereas a type 1 isolate might be explained on the basis of autoinoculation from the oropharynx.

The type of HSV responsible for the infection can also have prognostic implications. For example, genital infections caused by HSV-1 are less likely to recur than are genital infections caused by HSV-2 (54), and HSV meningoencephalitis occurring in newborn infants is likely to be less severe if it is caused by HSV-1 (22).

Serology

Serologic tests for HSV that are routinely available cannot reliably differentiate antibodies to HSV-1 from antibodies to HSV-2. This fact underscores the futility of attempting to diagnose infections with either of these viruses serologically by using commercially available tests. Since most adults have had HSV-1 infection, often without any primary or recurrent symptoms, the serologic diagnosis of acute or past HSV-2 infection is not possible by available methods. Serologic tests can be used to diagnose a true primary HSV infection only if there is no HSV antibody in the acute-phase serum sample. In this circumstance, if antibody to HSV is present in the convalescent-phase serum sample, seroconversion can be diagnosed. However, because of the cross-reactivity between HSV-1 and HSV-2, the specific serotype of HSV responsible for the acute infection cannot be established without the use of one of the type-specific tests described above. It is important to recognize that recurrent infections with HSV cannot be diagnosed serologically. Although a rise in antibody titer might be evident, such rises may also be nonspecific or may represent a response to a recent exposure or infection with another herpesviruses, such as varicella-zoster virus.

Considering these limitations, laboratories using commercially available serologic kits should not attempt to report any type-specific HSV antibody titers. Laboratories should report only that serologic evidence of a prior or recent HSV infection is evident. In addition, because the assays detect cross-reacting antibodies, the practice of testing serum samples against both HSV-1 and HSV-2 antigens is not cost-effective for the patient or the laboratory. Until accurate methods are available, genital herpes will continue to be underdiagnosed (5, 53).

REFERENCES

1. **Adler-Storthz, K., C. Kendall, R. C. Kennedy, R. D. Henkel, and G. R. Dreesman.** 1983. Biotinavidin amplified enzyme immunoassay for detection of herpes simplex virus antigen in clinical specimens. *J. Clin. Microbiol.* **18:** 1329–1334.
2. **Amir, J., R. Straussberg, L. Harel, Z. Smetana, and I. Varsano.** 1996. Evaluation of a rapid enzyme immunoassay for the detection of herpes simplex virus antigen in children with herpetic gingivostomatitis. *Pediatr. Infect. Dis. J.* **15:**627–629.
3. **Ando, Y., H. Kimura, H. Miwata, T. Kudo, M. Shibata, and T. Morishima.** 1993. Quantitative analysis of herpes simplex virus DNA in cerebrospinal fluid of children with herpes simplex encephalitis. *J. Med. Virol.* **41:**170–173.
4. **Arvin, A. M., P. A. Henslelgh, C. G. Prober, D. S. Au, L. L. Yasukawa, A. E. Wittek, P. E. Palumbo, S. G. Paryanl, and A. S. Yeager.** 1986. Failure of anterpartum maternal cultures to predict the infant's risk of exposure to herpes simplex virus at delivery. *N. Engl. J. Med.* **315:** 796–800.
5. **Arvin, A. M., and C. G. Prober.** 1997. Herpes simplex virus type 2, a persistent problem. *N. Engl. J. Med.* **337:** 1158–1159.
6. **Ashley, R., A. Cent, V. Maggs, A. Nahmias, and L. Corey.** 1991. Inability of enzyme immunoassays to discriminate between infections with herpes simplex virus types 1 and 2. *Ann. Intern. Med.* **115:**520–526.
7. **Ashley, R. L., J. Militoni, F. Lee, A. Nahmias, and L. Corey.** 1988. Comparison of Western blot (immunoblot) and glycoprotein G-specific immunodot enzyme assay for detecting antibodies to herpes simplex virus types 1 and 2 in human sera. *J. Clin. Microbiol.* **26:**662–667.
8. **Aurelius, E., B. Johansson, B. Skoldenberg, and M. Forsgren.** 1993. Encephalitis in immunocompetent patients due to herpes simplex virus type 1 or 2 as determined by type-specific polymerase chain reaction and antibody assays of cerebrospinal fluid. *J. Med. Virol.* **39:**179–186.
9. **Balachandran, N., B. Franme, M. Chernesky, E. Kraisel, Y. Kouri, D. Garcia, C. Lavery, and W. E. Rawls.** 1982. Identification of typing of herpes simplex viruses with monoclonal antibodies. *J. Clin. Microbiol.* **16:**205–208.
10. **Baringer, J. R., and P. Swoveland.** 1973. Recovery of herpes simplex virus from trigeminal ganglions. *N. Engl. J. Med.* **288:**648–650.
11. **Bernard, D. L., K. Farnes, D. F. Richards, G. F. Croft, and F. B. Johnson.** 1986. Suitability of new chlamydia transport medium for transport of herpes simplex virus. *J. Clin. Microbiol.* **24:**692–695.
12. **Boucher, F. D., L. Y. Yasukawa, K. Kerns, M. Kastelein, A. M. Arvin, and C. G. Prober.** 1993. Detection of antibodies to herpes simplex virus type 2 with a mammalian cell line expressing glycoprotein gG-2. *Clin. Diagn. Virol.* **1:**29–38.
13. **Brinker, J. P., and J. E. Herrman.** 1995. Comparison of three monoclonal antibody-based enzyme immunoassays for detection of herpes simplex virus in clinical specimens. *Eur. J. Clin. Microbiol. Infect. Dis.* **14:**314–317.
14. **Brown, Z. A., S. Selke, J. Zeh, J. Kopelman, A. Maslow, R. L. Ashley, D. H. Watts, S. Berry, M. Herd, and L. Corey.** 1997. The acquisition of herpes simplex virus during pregnancy. *N. Engl. J. Med.* **337:**509–515.
15. **Brumback, B. G., P. G. Farthing, and S. N. Castellino.** 1993. Simultaneous detection of and differentiation between herpes simplex and varicella-zoster viruses with two fluorescent probes in the same test system. *J. Clin. Microbiol.* **31:**3260–3263.
16. **Callihan, D. R., and M. Menegus.** 1984. Rapid detection of herpes simplex virus in clinical specimens with human embryonic lung fibroblast and primary rabbit kidney cell cultures. *J. Clin. Microbiol.* **19:**563–565.
17. **Cassinotti, P., H. Mietz, and G. Siegl.** 1996. Suitability and clinical application of a multiplex nested PCR assay

for the diagnosis of herpes simplex virus infections. *J. Med. Virol.* **50:**75–81.

18. **Coleman, R. M., L. Pereira, P. D. Bailey, D. Dondero, C. Wickliffe, and A. J. Nahmias.** 1983. Determination of herpes simplex virus type-specific antibodies by enzyme-linked immunosorbent assay. *J. Clin. Microbiol.* **18:** 287–291.
19. **Cone, R. W., A. C. Hobson, Z. Brown, R. Ashley, S. Berry, C. Winter, and L. Corey.** 1994. Frequent detection of genital herpes simplex virus DNA by polymerase chain reaction among pregnant women. *JAMA* **272:** 792–796.
20. **Cone, R. W., P. D. Swenson, A. C. Hobson, M. Remington, and L. Corey.** 1993. Herpes simplex virus detection from genital lesions: a comparative study using antigen detection (HerpChek) and culture. *J. Clin. Microbiol.* **31:**1774–1776.
21. **Corey, L., and P. G. Spear.** 1986. Infections with herpes simplex viruses. *N. Engl. J. Med.* **314:**686–691, 749–757.
22. **Corey, L., E. F. Stone, R. J. Whitley, and K. Mohan.** 1988. Difference between herpes simplex virus type 1 and type 2 neonatal encephalitis in neurological outcome. *Lancet* **i:**1–4.
23. **Cowan, F. M., A. M. Johnson, R. Ashley, L. Corey, and A. Mindel.** 1996. Relationship between antibodies to herpes simplex virus (HSV) and symptoms of HSV infection. *J. Infect. Dis.* **174:**470–475.
24. **Crane, L. R., P. A. Gutterman, T. Chapel, and A. M. Lerner.** 1980. Incubation of swab materials with herpes simplex virus. *J. Infect. Dis.* **141:**531.
25. **Cunningham, E. T., Jr., G. A. Short, A. R. Irvine, J. S. Duker, and T. P. Margolis.** 1996. Acquired immunodeficiency syndrome-associated herpes simplex virus retinitis. Clinical description and use of a polymerase chain reaction-based assay as a diagnostic tool. *Arch. Ophthalmol.* **114:**834–840.
26. **Dascal, A., J. Chan-Thim, M. Morahan, J. Portnoy, and J. Mendelson.** 1989. Diagnosis of herpes simplex virus infection in a clinical setting by a direct antigen detection enzyme immunoassay kit. *J. Clin. Microbiol.* **27:**700–704.
27. **DeGirolami, P. C., J. Dakos, K. Eichelberger, and S. Biano.** 1988. Evaluation of a new latex agglutination method for detection of antibody to herpes simplex virus. *J. Clin. Microbiol.* **26:**1024–1025.
28. **Espy, M. J., and T. F. Smith.** 1988. Detection of herpes simplex virus in conventional tube cell cultures and in shell vials with a DNA probe kit and monoclonal antibodies. *J. Clin. Microbiol.* **26:**22–24.
29. **Espy, M. J., A. D. Wold, D. J. Jespersen, M. F. Jones, and T. F. Smith.** 1991. Comparison of shell vials and conventional tubes seeded with rhabdomyosarcoma and MRC-5 cells for the rapid detection of herpes simplex virus. *J. Clin. Microbiol.* **29:**2751–2753.
30. **Fayram, L., S. L. Aarnaes, E. M. Peterson, and L. M. de la Maza.** 1986. Evaluation of five cell types for the isolation of herpes simplex virus. *Diagn. Microbiol. Infect. Dis.* **5:**127–133.
31. **Forghani, B., K. W. Dupuis, and N. J. Schmidt.** 1985. Rapid detection of herpes simplex virus DNA in human brain tissue by in situ hybridization. *J. Clin. Microbiol.* **22:**656–658.
32. **Forman, M. S., C. S. Merz, and P. Charache.** 1992. Detection of herpes simplex virus by a nonradiometric spin-amplified in situ hybridization assay. *J. Clin. Microbiol.* **30:**581–584.
33. **Fleming, D. T., G. M. McQuillan, R. E. Johnson, A. J. Nahmias, S. O. Aral, F. K. Lee, and M. E. St. Louis.** 1997. Herpes simplex virus type 2 in the United States, 1976 to 1994. *N. Engl. J. Med.* **337:**1105–1111.
34. **Fung, J. C., J. Shanley, and R. C. Tilton.** 1985. Comparison of the detection of herpes simplex virus in direct clinical specimens with herpes simplex virus-specific DNA probes and monoclonal antibodies. *J. Clin. Microbiol.* **22:** 748–753.
35. **Garland, S. M., T. N. Lee, R. L. Ashley, L. Corey, and S. L. Sacks.** 1995. Automated microneutralization: method and comparison with western blot for type-specific detection of herpes simplex antibodies in two pregnant populations. *J. Virol. Methods* **55:**285–294.
36. **Gleaves, C. A., and J. D. Meyers.** 1988. Determination of patient herpes simplex virus immune status by latex agglutination. *J. Clin. Microbiol.* **26:**14Q2–14Q3.
37. **Gleaves, C. A., D. J. Wilson, A. D. Wold, and T. F. Smith.** 1985. Detection and serotyping of herpes simplex virus in MRC-5 cells by use of centrifugation and monoclonal antibodies 16 h postinoculation. *J. Clin. Microbiol.* **21:**29–32.
38. **Goldstein, L. C., L. Corey, J. K. McDougall, E. Tolentino, and R. C. Nowinski.** 1983. Monoclonal antibodies to herpes simplex viruses: use in antigenic typing and rapid diagnosis. *J. Infect. Dis.* **147:**829–837.
39. **Gonik, B., M. Seibel, A. Berkowitz, M. B. Woodin, and K. Mills.** 1991. Comparison of two enzyme-linked immunosorbent assays for detection of herpes simplex virus antigen. *J. Clin. Microbiol.* **29:**436–438.
40. **Guffond, T., A. Dewilde, P. E. Lobert, L. D. Caparros, D. Hober, and P. Wattre.** 1994. Significance and clinical relevance of the detection of herpes simplex virus DNA by the polymerase chain reaction in cerebrospinal fluid from patients with presumed encephalitis. *Clin. Infect. Dis.* **18:**744–749.
41. **Hardy, D. A., A. M. Arvin, L. L. Yasukawa, D. M. Lewinsohn, P. A. Hensleigh, and C. G. Prober.** 1990. The successful identification of asymptomatic genital herpes simplex infection at delivery using the polymerase chain reaction. *J. Infect. Dis.* **162:**1031–1035.
42. **Hill, T. J.** 1985. Herpes simplex virus latency, p. 201–206. *In* B. Roizman (ed.), *The Herpesviruses*, vol. 3. Plenum Publishing Corp., New York, N.Y.
43. **Ho, D. W., P. R. Field, W. L. Irving, D. R. Packham, and A. L. Cunningham.** 1993. Detection of immunoglobulin M antibodies to glycoprotein G-2 by Western blot (immunoblot) for diagnosis of initial herpes simplex virus type 2 genital infections. *J. Clin. Microbiol.* **31:** 3157–3164.
44. **Hobson, A., A. Wald, N. Wright, and L. Corey.** 1997. Evaluation of a quantitative competitive PCR assay for measuring herpes simplex virus DNA content in genital tract secretions. *J. Clin. Microbiol.* **35:**548–552.
45. **Hughes, J. H., D. R. Mann, and V. V. Hamparian.** 1986. Viral isolation versus immune staining of infected cell cultures for the laboratory diagnosis of herpes simplex virus infections. *J. Clin. Microbiol.* **24:**487–489.
46. **Jackson, R., D. J. Morris, R. J. Cooper, A. S. Bailey, P. E. Klapper, G. M. Cleator, and A. B. Tullo.** 1996. Multiplex polymerase chain reaction for adenovirus and herpes simplex virus in eye swabs. *J. Virol. Methods* **56:** 41–48.
47. **Johnson, F. B., R. W. Levitt, and D. F. Richards.** 1984. Evaluation of the Virocult transport tube for isolation of herpes simplex virus from clinical specimens. *J. Clin. Microbiol.* **20:**120–122.
48. **Johnson, F. B., G. Luker, and C. Chow.** 1993. Comparison of shell vial culture and the suspension-infection method for the rapid detection of herpes simplex viruses. *Diagn. Microbiol. Infect. Dis.* **16:**61–66.
49. **Johnson, R. E., A. J. Nahmias, L. S. Magder, F. K. Lee, C. A. Brooks, and C. B. Snowden.** 1989. A seroepidemi-

ologic survey of the prevalence of herpes simplex virus type 2 infection in the United States. *N. Engl. J. Med.* **321:**7–12.

50. **Johnston, S. L. G., S. Hamilton, R. Bindra, D. A. Hursh, and C. A. Gleaves.** 1992. Evaluation of an automated immunodiagnostic assay system for direct detection of herpes simplex virus antigen in clinical specimens. *J. Clin. Microbiol.* **30:**1042–1044.
51. **Johnston, S. L. G., K. Wellens, and C. S. Siegel.** 1990. Rapid isolation of herpes simplex virus by using mink lung and rhabdomyosarcoma cell cultures. *J. Clin. Microbiol.* **28:**2806–2807.
52. **Kimberlin, D. W., F. D. Lakeman, A. M. Arvin, C. G. Prober, L. Corey, D. A. Powell, S. K. Burchett, R. F. Jacobs, S. E. Starr, and R. J. Whitley.** 1996. Application of the polymerase chain reaction to the diagnosis and management of neonatal herpes simplex virus disease. National Institute of Allergy and Infectious Diseases Collaborative Antiviral Study Group. *J. Infect. Dis.* **174:** 1162–1167.
53. **Koutsky, L. A., C. E. Stevens, K. K. Holmes, R. L. Ashley, N. B. Kiviat, C. W. Critchlow, and L. Corey.** 1992. Underdiagnosis of genital herpes by current clinical and viral-isolation procedures. *N. Engl. J. Med.* **326:** 1533–1539.
54. **Lafferty, W. E., R. W. Coombs, J. Benedetti, C. Critchlow, and L. Corey.** 1987. Recurrences after oral and genital herpes simplex virus infection. Influence of site of infection and viral type. *N. Engl. J. Med.* **316:** 1444–1449.
55. **Lakeman, F. D., and R. J. Whitley.** 1995. Diagnosis of herpes simplex encephalitis: application of polymerase chain reaction to cerebrospinal fluid from brain-biopsied patients and correlation with disease. National Institute of Allergy and Infectious Diseases Collaborative Antiviral Study Group. *J. Infect. Dis.* **171:**857–863.
56. **Landry, M. L.** 1995. False-positive polymerase chain reaction results in the diagnosis of herpes simplex encephalitis. *J. Infect. Dis.* **172:**1641–1643.
57. **Langenberg, A., R. Zbanysek, J. Dragavon, R. Ashley, and L. Corey.** 1988. Detection of herpes simplex virus DNA from genital lesions by in situ hybridization. *J. Clin. Microbiol.* **26:**933–937.
58. **Langtry, J. A., L. S. Ostlere, D. A. Hawkins, and R. C. Staughton.** 1994. The difficulty in diagnosis of cutaneous herpes simplex virus infection in patients with AIDS. *Clin. Exp. Dermatol.* **19:**224–226.
59. **Lee, F. K., R. M. Coleman, L. Pereira, P. D. Bailey, M. Tatsumo, and A. J. Nahmias.** 1985. Detection of herpes simplex virus type 2-specific antibody with glycoprotein G. *J. Clin. Microbiol.* **22:**641–644.
60. **Lipson, S. M., T. E. Schutzbank, and K. Szabo.** 1987. Evaluation of three immunofluorescence assays for culture confirmation and typing of herpes simplex virus. *J. Clin. Microbiol.* **25:**391–394.
61. **Luker, G., C. Chow, D. F. Richards, and F. B. Johnson.** 1991. Suitability of infection of cells in suspension for detection of herpes simplex virus. *J. Clin. Microbiol.* **29:** 1554–1557.
62. **McCarter, Y. S., and A. Robinson.** 1997. Comparison of MRC-5 and primary rabbit kidney cells for the detection of herpes simplex virus. *Arch. Pathol. Lab. Med.* **121:** 122–124.
63. **Miller, M. J., and C. L. Howell.** 1983. Rapid detection and identification of herpes simplex virus in cell culture by a direct immunoperoxidase staining procedure. *J. Clin. Microbiol.* **18:**550–553.
64. **Miranda, Q. R., G. D. Bailey, A. S. Fraser, and H. J. Tenoso.** 1977. Solid-phase enzyme immunoassay for herpes simplex virus. *J. Infect. Dis.* **136**(Suppl.)**:** S304–S310.
65. **Montgomery, R. I., M. S. Warner, B. J. Lum, and P. G. Spear.** 1996. Herpes simplex virus-1 entry into cells mediated by a novel member of the TNF/NGF receptor family. *Cell* **87:**427–436.
66. **Moseley, R. C., L. Corey, D. Benjamin, C. Winter, and M. L. Remington.** 1981. Comparison of viral isolation, direct immunofluorescence, and indirect immunoperoxidase techniques for detection of genital herpes simplex virus infection. *J. Clin. Microbiol.* **13:**913–918.
67. **Nahmias, A. J., R. J. Whitley, A. N. Visintine, Y. Takei, C. A. Alford, and the Collaborative Antiviral Study Group.** 1982. Herpes simplex virus encephalitis: laboratory evaluations and their diagnostic significance. *J. Infect. Dis.* **145:**829–836.
68. **Nash, K. A., J. S. Klein, and C. B. Inderlied.** 1995. Internal controls as performance monitors and quantitative standards in the detection by polymerase chain reaction of herpes simplex virus and cytomegalovirus in clinical specimens. *Mol. Cell. Probes* **9:**347–356.
69. **Nerurkar, L. S., A. J. Jacob, D. L. Madden, and J. L. Sever.** 1983. Detection of genital herpes simplex infections by a tissue culture fluorescent-antibody technique with biotin-avidin. *J. Clin. Microbiol.* **17:**149–154.
70. **Nerurkar, L. S., M. Namba, C. Brashears, A. J. Jacob, Y. S. Lee, and J. L. Sever.** 1984. Rapid detection of herpes simplex virus in clinical specimens using a capture biotin-streptavidin enzyme-linked immunosorbent assay. *J. Clin. Microbiol.* **20:**109–114.
71. **Nicoll, J. A., S. Love, P. A. Burton, and P. J. Berry.** 1994. Autopsy findings in two cases of neonatal herpes simplex virus infection: detection of virus by immunohistochemistry, in situ hybridization and the polymerase chain reaction. *Histopathology* **24:**257–264.
72. **Ogburn, J. R., J. T. Hoffpauir, E. Cole, K. Hood, D. Michael, T. Nguyen, S. Raden, B. Raju, V. Reisinger, and P. E. Oefinger.** 1994. Evaluation of new transport medium for detection of herpes simplex virus by culture and direct enzyme-linked immunosorbent assay. *J. Clin. Microbiol.* **32:**3082–3084.
73. **Orle, K. A., C. A. Gates, D. H. Martin, B. A. Body, and J. B. Weiss.** 1996. Simultaneous PCR detection of *Haemophilus ducreyi*, *Treponema pallidum*, and herpes simplex virus types 1 and 2 from genital ulcers. *J. Clin. Microbiol.* **34:**49–54.
74. **Parkes, D. L., C. M. Smith, J. M. Rose, J. Brandis, and S. R. Coates.** 1991. Seroreactive recombinant herpes simplex virus type 2-specific glycoprotein G. *J. Clin. Microbiol.* **29:**778–781.
75. **Peterson, E. M., S. L. Aarnaes, R. N. Bryan, J. L. Ruth, and L. M. de la Maza.** 1986. Typing of herpes simplex virus with synthetic DNA probes. *J. Infect. Dis.* **153:** 757–762.
76. **Peterson, E. M., B. L. Hughes, S. L. Aarnaes, and L. M. de la Maza.** 1988. Comparison of primary rabbit kidney and MRC-5 cells and two stain procedures for herpes simplex virus detection by a shell vial centrifugation method. *J. Clin. Microbiol.* **26:**222–224.
77. **Pouletty, P., J. J. Chomel, D. Thouvenot, F. Catalan, V. Rabillon, and J. Kadouche.** 1987. Detection of herpes simplex virus in direct specimens by immunofluorescence assay using a monoclonal antibody. *J. Clin. Microbiol.* **25:** 958–959.
78. **Prober, C. G., and D. R. Enzmann.** 1996. Early diagnosis and management of herpes simplex encephalitis. *Pediatr. Infect. Dis. J.* **15:**387–388.
79. **Prober, C. C., W. M. Sullender, L. L. Yasukawa, D. S. Au, A. S. Yeager, and A. M. Arvin.** 1987. Low risk of

herpes simplex virus infections in neonates exposed to the virus at the time of vaginal delivery to mothers with recurrent herpes simplex virus infections. *N. Engl. J. Med.* **316:**240–244.

80. **Pruneda, R. C., and I. Almanza.** 1987. Centrifugation-shell vial technique for rapid detection of herpes simplex virus cytopathic effect in Vero cells. *J. Clin. Microbiol.* **25:**423–424.
81. **Puchhammer-Stoeckl, E., F. X. Heinz, M. Kundi, T. Popow-Kraupp, G. Grimm, M. M. Millner, and C. Kunz.** 1993. Evaluation of the polymerase chain reaction for diagnosis of herpes simplex virus encephalitis. *J. Clin. Microbiol.* **31:**146–148.
82. **Puchhammer, S. E., F. X. Heinz, and C. Kunz.** 1993. Evaluation of 3 nonradioactive DNA detection systems for identification of herpes simplex DNA amplified from cerebrospinal fluid. *J. Virol. Methods* **43:**257–266.
83. **Rawls, W. E.** 1985. Herpes simplex virus, p. 527–561. *In* B. Fields (ed.), *Virology*. Raven Press, New York, N.Y.
84. **Redfield, D. C., D. D. Richman, S. Albanil, M. N. Oxman, and C. M. Wahl.** 1983. Detection of herpes simplex virus in clinical specimens by DNA hybridization. *Diagn. Microbiol. Infect. Dis.* **1:**117–128.
85. **Revello, M. G., F. Baldanti, A. Sarasini, D. Zella, M. Zavattoni, and G. Gerna.** 1997. Quantitation of herpes simplex virus DNA in cerebrospinal fluid of patients with herpes simplex encephalitis by the polymerase chain reaction. *Clin. Diagn. Virol.* **7:**183–191.
86. **Richman, D. D., P. H. Cleveland, D. C. Redfield, M. N. Oxman, and C. M. Wahl.** 1984. Rapid viral diagnosis. *J. Infect. Dis.* **149:**298–310.
87. **Roizman, B.** 1995. Herpes simplex viruses and their replication, p. 2231–2296. *In* D. Knipe, B. Fields, and P. Howley (ed.), *Fields Virology*. Lippincott-Raven Press, Philadelphia, Pa.
88. **Rowley, A. H., R. J. Whitley, F. D. Lakeman, and S. M. Wolinsky.** 1990. Rapid detection of herpes simplex virus DNA in cerebrospinal fluid of patients with herpes simplex encephalitis. *Lancet* **335:**440–441.
89. **Rubin, S. J., and S. Rogers.** 1984. Comparison of culture set and primary rabbit kidney cell culture for the detection of herpes simplex virus. *J. Clin. Microbiol.* **19:** 920–922.
90. **Safrin, S., H. Shaw, G. Bolan, J. Cuan, and C. S. Chiang.** 1997. Comparison of virus culture and the polymerase chain reaction for diagnosis of mucocutaneous herpes simplex virus infection. *Sex. Transm. Dis.* **24:** 176–180.
91. **Salmon, V. C., R. B. Turner, M. J. Speranza, and J. C. Overall.** 1986. Rapid detection of herpes simplex virus in clinical specimens by centrifugation and immunoperoxidase staining. *J. Clin. Microbiol.* **23:**683–686.
92. **Sanchez-Martinez, D., S. Schmid, W. Whittington, D. Brown, W. C. Reeves, S. Chatterjee, R. J. Whitley, and P. E. Pellett.** 1991. Evaluation of a test based on baculovirus expressed glycoprotein G for detection of herpes simplex virus type-specific antibodies. *J. Infect. Dis.* **164:** 1196–1199.
93. **Saral, R.** 1988. Management of mucocutaneous herpes simplex virus infections in immunocompromised patients. *Am. J. Med.* **85**(2A)**:**57–60.
94. **Schlesinger, Y., P. Tebas, K. M. Gaudreault, R. S. Buller, and G. A. Storch.** 1995. Herpes simplex virus type 2 meningitis in the absence of genital lesions: improved recognition with use of the polymerase chain reaction. *Clin. Infect. Dis.* **20:**842–848.
95. **Schmidt, N. J., J. Dennis, V. Devlin, D. Callo, and J. Mills.** 1983. Comparison of direct immunofluorescence and direct immunoperoxidase procedures for detection of herpes simplex virus antigen in lesion specimens. *J. Clin. Microbiol.* **18:**445–448.
96. **Sewell, D. L. L., and S. A. Horn.** 1985. Evaluation of a commercial enzyme-linked immunosorbent assay for the detection of herpes simplex virus. *J. Clin. Microbiol.* **21:** 457–458.
97. **Shepp, D. H., B. A. Newton, P. S. Dandliker, N. Flournoy, and J. D. Meyers.** 1985. Oral acyclovir therapy for mucocutaneous herpes simplex virus infections in immunocompromised marrow transplant recipients. *Ann. Intern. Med.* **102:**783–785.
98. **Skinner, G. R., M. A. Billstrom, S. Randal, A. Ahmad, S. Patel, J. Davies, and A. Deane.** 1997. A system for isolation, transport and storage of herpes simplex viruses. *J. Virol. Methods* **65:**1–18.
99. **Skoldenberg, B.** 1996. Herpes simplex encephalitis. *Scand. J. Infect. Dis. Suppl.* **100:**8–13.
100. **Straus, S. E., J. F. Rooney, J. L. Sever, M. Seidlin, S. Nusinoff-Lehrman, and K. Cremer.** 1985. Herpes simplex virus infection: biology, treatment, and prevention. *Ann. Intern. Med.* **103:**404–419.
101. **Sullender, W. M., L. L. Yasukawa, M. Schwartz, L. Periera, P. A. Hensleigh, C. C. Prober, and A. M. Arvin.** 1988. Type specific antibodies to herpes simplex virus type 2 (HSV-2) glycoprotein G in pregnant women, infants exposed to maternal HSV 2 infections at delivery, and infants with neonatal herpes. *J. Infect. Dis.* **157:** 164–171.
102. **Troendle, A. J., G. J. Demmler, and G. J. Buffone.** 1993. Rapid diagnosis of herpes simplex virus encephalitis by using the polymerase chain reaction. *J. Pediatr.* **123:** 376–380.
103. **Verano, L., and F. J. Michalski.** 1995. Comparison of a direct antigen enzyme immunoassay, Herpchek, with cell culture for detection of herpes simplex virus from clinical specimens. *J. Clin. Microbiol.* **33:**1378–1379.
104. **Volpi, A., A. D. Lakeman, L. Pereira, and S. Stagno.** 1983. Monoclonal antibodies for rapid diagnosis and typing of genital herpes infections during pregnancy. *Am. J. Obstet. Gynecol.* **146:**813–815.
105. **Wang, J. Y., and K. T. Montone.** 1994. A rapid simple in situ hybridization method for herpes simplex virus employing a synthetic biotin-labeled oligonucleotide probe: a comparison with immunohistochemical methods for HSV detection. *J. Clin. Lab. Anal.* **8:**105–115.
106. **Warford, A. L., R. A. Levy, K. A. Rekrut, and E. Steinberg.** 1986. Herpes simplex virus testing of an obstetric population with an antigen enzyme-linked immunosorbent assay. *Am. J. Obstet. Gynecol.* **154:**21–28.
107. **Wentworth, B. B., and E. R. Alexander.** 1971. Seroepidemiology of infections due to members of the herpesvirus group. *Am. J. Epidemiol.* **94:**496–507.
108. **West, P. C., B. Aldrich, R. Hartwig, and C. J. Haller.** 1989. Increased detection of herpes simplex virus in MRC5 cells treated with dimethyl sulfoxide and dexamethasone. *J. Clin. Microbiol.* **27:**770–772.
109. **Whitley, R., A. M. Arvin, C. G. Prober, L. Corey, S. Burchett, S. Plotkin, et al.** 1991. A controlled trial comparing vidarabine with acyclovir in neonatal herpes simplex virus infection. *N. Engl. J. Med.* **324:**444–449.
110. **Whitley, R. J.** 1988. Herpes simplex virus infections of the central nervous system. A review. *Am. J. Med.* **85**(2A)**:**61–67.
111. **Whitley, R. J., and A. M. Arvin.** 1995. Herpes simplex virus infection, p. 354–372. *In* J. Remington and J. Klein (ed.), *Infectious Diseases of the Fetus and Newborn*, 4th ed. The W. B. Saunders Co., Philadelphia, Pa.
112. **Whitley, R. J., L. Corey, A. Arvin, F. D. Lakeman, C.**

V. Sumaya, P. F. Wright, L. M. Dunkle, R. W. Steele, S.-J. Soong, A. J. Nahmias, C. A. Alford, D. A. Powell, V. S. San Joaquin, and the NIAID Collaborative Antiviral Study Group. 1988. Changing presentation of herpes simplex virus infection in neonates. *J. Infect. Dis.* **158:**109–116.

113. **Whitley, R. J., A. J. Nahmias, A. M. Visintine, C. L. Fleming, and C. A. Alford.** 1980. The natural history of herpes simplex virus infection of mother and newborn. *Pediatrics* **66:**489–494.

114. **Woods, C. L., and R. D. Mills.** 1988. Effect of dexamethasone on detection of herpes simplex virus in clinical specimens by conventional cell culture and rapid 24-well plate centrifugation. *J. Clin. Microbiol.* **26:**1233–1235.

115. **Yeager, A. S., A. M. Arvin, and P. A. Hensleigh.** 1982. The validity of reporting results for herpes simplex virus after four days. *J. Reprod. Med.* **27:**447–448.

116. **Yeager, A. S., J. E. Morris, and C. C. Prober.** 1979. Storage and transport of cultures for herpes simplex virus, type 2. *Am. J. Clin. Pathol.* **72:**977–979.

117. **Zhao, L., M. L. Landry, E. S. Balkovic, and C. D. Hsiung.** 1987. Impact of cell culture sensitivity and virus concentration on rapid detection of herpes simplex virus by cytopathic effects and immunoperoxidase staining. *J. Clin. Microbiol.* **25:**1401–1405.

Human Cytomegalovirus*

RICHARD L. HODINKA

66

CLINICAL BACKGROUND

Cytomegalovirus (CMV) infections are common and usually asymptomatic; however, the incidence and spectrum of disease in newborns and in immunocompromised hosts establish this virus as an important human pathogen. CMV infections can be classified as being acquired before birth (congenital), at the time of delivery (perinatal), or later in life (postnatal). Similar to infections with other herpesviruses, primary infection with CMV results in the establishment of a persistent or latent infection. Reactivation of the virus can occur in response to different stimuli.

CMV infection has been detected in 0.2 to 2.5% of newborn infants and is the most common identified cause of congenital infection. Fewer than 5% of congenitally infected infants develop symptoms during the newborn period; possible manifestations range from severe disease with intrauterine growth retardation, jaundice, hepatosplenomegaly, petechiae, central nervous system abnormalities, and chorioretinitis to more limited involvement. Symptomatic infants may die of complications within the first months of life; more commonly, they survive but are neurologically damaged. It is now recognized that even congenitally infected infants who are asymptomatic at birth may develop hearing defects or learning disabilities later in life.

Newborns can also acquire infection at the time of delivery by contact with virus in the birth canal. Such infants begin to excrete virus at 3 to 12 weeks of age but usually remain asymptomatic. Thus far, it appears that such perinatally infected infants do not develop late neurologic sequelae of infection.

Most postnatal infections are acquired by close contact with individuals who are shedding virus. Since CMV has been detected in several body fluids, including saliva, urine, breast milk, tears, stool, vaginal and cervical secretions, blood, and semen, it is clear that transmission can occur in a variety of ways. Prolonged shedding of virus after congenital or acquired CMV infection contributes to the ease of virus spread. In addition, CMV can be transmitted by blood transfusion and organ transplantation.

The vast majority of children and adults who acquire CMV infection postnatally remain asymptomatic. In high-risk premature newborns infected as a result of blood transfusions, morbidity and mortality can be significant and hepatosplenomegaly, thrombocytopenia, atypical lymphocytosis, and hemolytic anemia have been described. Of children attending day care centers, 20 to 70% of those who enter as toddlers experience CMV infection over a 1- to 2-year period. Infection is usually asymptomatic, but the children may transmit CMV to their parents, posing a risk to an unborn fetus if the mother is pregnant at the time. In adults and adolescents, sexual transmission of CMV may occur. Symptoms in young adults include fever, lethargy, and atypical lymphocytosis that can mimic the symptoms caused by Epstein-Barr virus.

CMV infections are frequent and occasionally severe in children or adults with congenital or acquired defects of cellular immunity, such as patients with AIDS, cancer patients (particularly those with leukemia and lymphoma receiving chemotherapy), and recipients of organ transplants. Infections in these patients may be due to reactivation of latent virus or infection with exogenous virus, which may be introduced by blood transfusions or by the grafted organ. Symptoms tend to be most severe after primary infection; however, reactivation infection or reinfection in a severely immunocompromised host may also cause serious illness. The frequency and severity of CMV infection in organ transplant patients are variable and depend on the type of transplant, the source of the donated organ, the immune status of the recipient, and the duration of the immunosuppressive therapy. Symptoms in these patients include fever, leukopenia, thrombocytopenia, pneumonitis, hepatitis, retinitis, and encephalitis. Death may occur as a result of various complications, including bacterial and fungal superinfections. CMV infection, particularly when associated with pneumonitis, is an important cause of morbidity and mortality after bone marrow transplantation. In patients infected with human immunodeficiency virus, CMV is an important cause of fever, sight-threatening retinitis, encephalitis, and gastrointestinal infections including esophagitis, gastritis, and ulcerative colitis.

DESCRIPTION OF THE AGENT

CMV is a member of the family *Herpesviridae*, which includes Epstein-Barr virus, herpes simplex virus types 1 and 2, varicella-zoster virus, and human herpesvirus types 6, 7, and 8. Complete CMV particles have a diameter of 120 to

* This chapter contains information presented in chapter 72 by Richard L. Hodinka and Harvey M. Friedman in the sixth edition of this Manual.

200 nm and consist of a core containing double-stranded DNA, an icosahedral capsid, an amorphous tegument or matrix, and a surrounding phospholipid-rich envelope. Electron microscopic features of CMV include virions morphologically indistinguishable from those of other herpesviruses, a high ratio of defective viral particles, and the presence of spherical particles called dense bodies. Viral replication occurs in the nucleus of the host cell and involves the expression of immediate-early, early, and late classes of genes. The viral envelope is formed as assembled nucleocapsids bud from the inner surface of the nuclear membrane.

Molecular virologic techniques have been used to study variation among CMV strains. DNA-DNA reassociation kinetics analysis has shown that various CMV strains have considerable homology to AD-169, a standard laboratory strain; restriction endonuclease analysis has shown that DNAs from various strains have similar but distinctive fragment migration patterns (44). These studies suggest that CMV strains are closely related to each other, more so than are herpes simplex virus types 1 and 2. Antigenic heterogeneity among CMV strains has been detected in cross-neutralization and other serologic assays, but evidence for distinct serotypes is limited (90).

CMV is inactivated by a number of physical and chemical treatments, including heat (56°C for 30 min), low pH, lipid solvents, UV light, and cycles of freezing and thawing.

COLLECTION AND STORAGE OF SPECIMENS

Specimens for Virus Isolation

CMV can be isolated from a variety of body fluids; however, urine, throat washings, saliva, and anticoagulated whole blood (leukocytes) are most common for diagnostic purposes. Urine specimens should be clean-voided specimens. Because excretion of CMV in urine is intermittent, increased recovery of the virus is possible by processing more than one specimen. In the evaluation of immunocompromised patients, blood leukocyte cultures are particularly useful. Detection of CMV in leukocytes is often a better indicator of symptomatic CMV infection than is shedding of virus in the urine or respiratory secretions. Bronchial washings and biopsy and autopsy specimens, particularly of lungs, kidneys, spleen, liver, brain, and retinas, also can be processed for virus isolation. The details of specimen collection and processing are given in chapters 4 and 5. Since CMV loses infectivity when subjected to freezing and thawing, specimens for virus isolation should be kept at 4°C in an ice-water bath or refrigerator until they can be used to inoculate cultures, preferably within a few hours after collection. When prolonged transport times are unavoidable, infectivity is reasonably well preserved for at least 48 h at 4°C. If freezing the specimen is necessary, an equal volume of 0.4 M sucrose-phosphate added to the specimen helps preserve viral infectivity (41). All frozen specimens should be stored at −60 to −80°C or in liquid nitrogen. Complete loss of virus infectivity occurs if specimens are stored at −20°C.

Specimens for Direct Detection

Tissue specimens, respiratory secretions, urine sediment, cerebrospinal fluid (CSF), amniotic fluid, and peripheral blood leukocytes have been used for the direct detection of CMV antigens or nucleic acids. Plasma obtained from anticoagulated whole blood or serum obtained from clotted blood also can be used to detect CMV DNA in molecular amplification assays (66, 78). Impression smears, frozen sections, or formaldehyde-fixed and paraffin-embedded material can be used for in situ hybridization or histopathologic examination of tissue specimens.

Specimens for Serologic Testing

Single serum specimens are useful in screening for evidence of past infection with CMV and in identifying individuals at risk for CMV infection. This approach is especially helpful in testing sera from organ transplant donors and from donors of blood products that are to be administered to premature infants or bone marrow transplant patients. For the diagnosis of recent CMV infection, paired sera should be obtained at least 2 weeks apart when testing for immunoglobulin G (IgG) antibody. The acute-phase serum sample should be collected as soon as possible after onset of illness and tested simultaneously with the convalescent-phase serum sample. If congenital infection is suspected, both maternal and infant sera should be submitted. Detection of IgM in a single serum specimen may be beneficial, but laboratories performing these tests should be aware of the problems with such methods. Testing saliva for CMV-specific antibodies has been suggested as a noninvasive alternative to the collection of blood from children (1). In patients with CMV neurologic disease, CSF may be tested for viral antibody if paired with a serum specimen collected on the same date.

DIRECT EXAMINATION OF SPECIMENS

Histopathologic Testing

Characteristic large cells (cytomegalic cells) with basophilic intranuclear inclusions and, on occasion, eosinophilic cytoplasmic inclusions can be seen in routine sections of biopsy or autopsy material (Fig. 1). The nuclear inclusion has the appearance of an "owl's eye" because it is typically surrounded by a clear halo that extends to the nuclear membrane. Wright-Giemsa-, hematoxylin-eosin-, or Papanicolaou-stained lung or other biopsy specimens may demonstrate such cells. Although the presence of characteristic cytologic changes suggests CMV infection, virologic or serologic confirmation is suggested. Since CMV can infect tissues without producing morphologic changes, failure to find typical cytomegalic cells does not exclude the possibility of CMV infection.

Exfoliative Cytologic Testing

By using exfoliative cytologic techniques, a presumptive diagnosis of CMV can be made in 25 to 50% of cases of symptomatic congenital infection. Specimens from older infected individuals are rarely positive. Several fresh urine specimens should be submitted, since exfoliated cells disintegrate rapidly and may be shed only intermittently. Characteristic enlarged cells with prominent inclusions are seen in positive preparations. Exfoliative cytologic testing is most useful when virus isolation techniques are not available. This technique can be applied to other specimens, such as bronchoalveolar lavage fluid (92) and cervical secretions.

Immunofluorescence

Monoclonal antibodies to CMV can be used for the direct detection of CMV antigens by immunofluorescence tests on tissues obtained by biopsy or at autopsy (47, 87). Cytospin preparations of bronchoalveolar lavage specimens (58, 92), blood leukocytes (85, 86), and urine sediments (54) have also been examined in this manner. The sensitivity of the

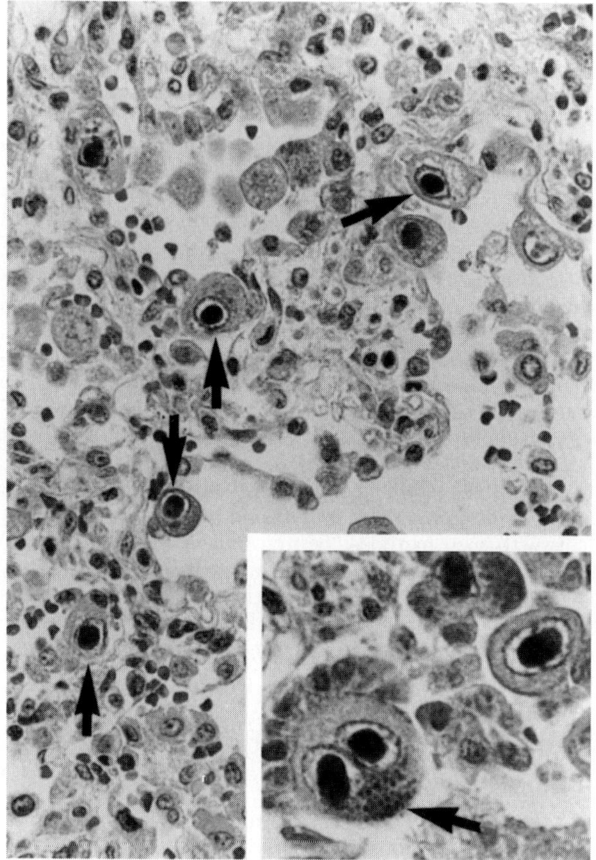

FIGURE 1 Fixed hematoxylin-eosin-stained lung tissue from a patient with interstitial pneumonia. Note the numerous giant cells that possess large intranuclear inclusions surrounded by characteristically clear halos (arrows). Less pronounced granular inclusions may also be present in the cytoplasm (inset). (Courtesy of Eduardo Ruchelli.)

assay is improved when mixtures of monoclonal antibodies are used (87). An advantage of immunofluorescence staining is its rapidity; results are available within several hours after tissue is obtained. For most specimens, this method is less sensitive than the shell vial culture technique described below, which has largely replaced tissue immunofluorescence as a rapid test for CMV diagnosis.

Antigenemia Assay

Within the last several years, considerable attention has been paid to the direct detection and quantitation of CMV from blood leukocytes (82, 83, 85, 86). A new procedure for the determination of CMV viremia has been developed, and it has been compared to conventional and shell vial culture isolation of CMV from blood. The CMV antigenemia assay has been shown to be a sensitive, specific, and rapid method for the early diagnosis of CMV infection, and it can be used for routine monitoring of patients at high risk for severe CMV disease. The test is relatively simple to perform and is based on immunocytochemical detection of the 65-kDa lower-matrix phosphoprotein (pp65) in the nuclei of peripheral blood leukocytes (Fig. 2). By using this assay, CMV can be detected before the onset of symptoms, and the viral load can be quantified to assist in predicting and differentiating CMV disease from asymptomatic infection (30, 51). The procedure has also been used to effectively evaluate the efficacy of antiviral therapy (32, 84) and to detect CMV in leukocytes of CSF from AIDS patients with infections of the central nervous system (73). The results of the antigenemia assay have been shown to correlate well with the quantitative detection of CMV DNA in leukocytes or plasma in molecular amplification assays (8, 29).

In the antigenemia assay, leukocytes (mainly polymorphonuclear leukocytes) are enriched from freshly collected whole blood by sedimentation with dextran. Alternatively, they can be isolated with Polymorphprep leukocyte separation medium (Nycomed Pharma AS, Majorstua, Norway), with comparable assay results (27). Any type of anticoagulated blood can be used, including blood collected in heparin, EDTA, sodium citrate, or acid citrate dextrose. The blood should be kept at 4°C during storage and transport and should be processed preferably within 6 h of collection for accurate and reliable quantitation of the virus load (52). A decrease in quantitative antigenemia levels after storage of blood specimens for 24 h has been described, although most positive specimens remain positive after this time (7, 52). Following sedimentation, the remaining erythrocytes are lysed with ammonium chloride, the granulocytes are counted, and a known number of cells are cytocentrifuged onto microscope slides. The cells are fixed and then permeabilized and stained with suitable monoclonal antibodies

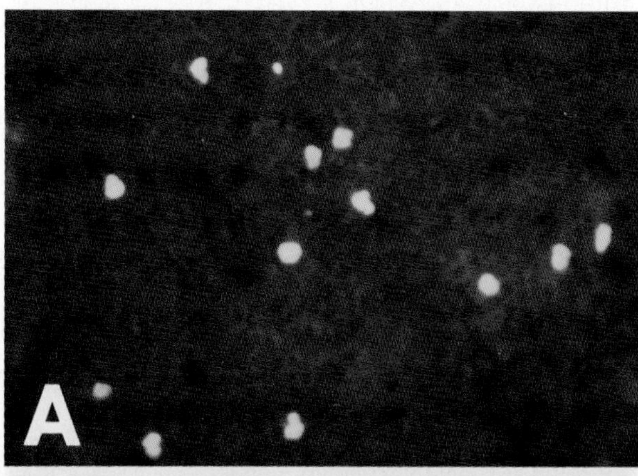

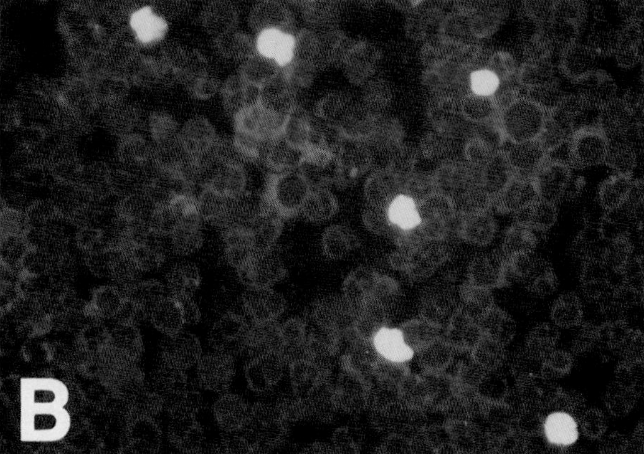

FIGURE 2 CMV antigen-positive polymorphonuclear leukocytes. Note the nuclear staining when a monoclonal antibody directed against pp65 is used. (A) Magnification, ×100; (B) magnification, ×400.

directed against CMV pp65. These processes are followed by incubation of the cells either with a horseradish peroxidase-labeled secondary antibody and a chromogen or with a fluorescein isothiocyanate-labeled conjugate diluted in a counterstain. Slides are read by microscopy at ×200 to ×400 magnification. Positive results are viewed as either homogeneous yellow-green fluorescence or a dark brown to red-brown color within the nuclei of infected cells. The results are usually expressed as the number of antigen-positive cells per total number of leukocytes evaluated. The procedure has the disadvantages of being labor-intensive and time-consuming; considerable time and effort are spent in isolating and counting cells, adjusting the cell concentration to 10^6/ml before preparing the slides for staining, and then reading the stained slides. Recently, a method for direct lysis of erythrocytes and subsequent isolation of leukocytes from whole blood has been described (39). This procedure allows for a shorter total assay time and the capability of processing more specimens. Commercial kits containing monoclonal antibodies and other reagents needed to perform the antigenemia assay are available (21, 53). Flow cytometry recently has been used in an attempt to automate the assay (46).

Electron Microscopy

The pseudoreplica method of electron microscopy can be used to detect CMV in urine and oral specimens of congenitally infected infants (56). Positive results can be obtained with almost all specimens that have infectivity titers of $\geq 10^4$ PFU/ml. An advantage of electron microscopy is its rapidity; also, stored or contaminated specimens that are unsuitable for isolation attempts can be examined. The main disadvantages of the technique are its relative insensitivity and the need for experienced personnel and expensive equipment.

Hybridization

Molecular dot blot hybridization techniques have been described for detection of the CMV genome in urine (12, 79) and peripheral blood leukocytes (57, 79). In situ hybridization has been used for the direct detection of CMV in formalin-fixed lung tissue (47, 62), Kaposi's sarcoma tissue (38), and cytospin preparations of bronchoalveolar lavage fluid (35, 92) and peripheral blood leukocytes (16, 81). Biotinylated or horseradish peroxidase-labeled CMV-specific DNA probe kits are commercially available. In situ hybridization has the advantage of being rapid and easy to read by light microscopy. However, current methods lack the sensitivity needed for routine use in clinical laboratories.

Molecular Amplification

PCR is currently the most widely used molecular method for the detection and quantification of CMV DNA and mRNAs. The sensitivity and specificity of PCR for diagnosis of active CMV infection have been evaluated (18, 43, 64, 75, 95). Amplification has been performed with a variety of primer pairs from the immediate-early antigen 1, major immediate-early antigen, glycoproteins B and H, the *Eco*RI D fragment, the *Hin*dIII X fragment, pp65, pp67, and the major capsid protein gene fragments. In several studies, the sensitivity of the assay was increased by amplifying genomic regions from both the immediate-early and the late CMV genes or by using nested primers to a single gene fragment. The use of both gene fragments enabled the detection of a variety of clinical isolates, indicating that strain variability is not a limiting factor for PCR diagnosis of CMV. PCR has been used to detect CMV DNA in a variety of clinical specimens from organ transplant recipients, patients with AIDS, and infants with congenital infection. It also has been used for the continued surveillance of immunocompromised patients and for evaluation of the therapeutic efficacy of antiviral drugs (31, 32, 83).

An unresolved issue with PCR for CMV diagnosis is whether the test can distinguish between active disease and asymptomatic infection or latency. CMV viremia is considered to be the best predictor of CMV disease, and CMV DNA has been successfully detected in peripheral blood leukocytes, plasma, or serum by PCR (31, 66, 75, 78, 83). However, the qualitative detection of CMV DNA in these specimens has been shown to have limited value in predicting symptomatic disease and in monitoring the success of antiviral therapy in immunocompromised patients. CMV DNA can be detected in blood by PCR in the absence of disease and antigenemia and can be found for weeks or months after successful therapy of symptomatic patients (3, 17, 32, 80). It has been demonstrated, however, that qualitative amplification of specific CMV mRNA transcripts that are expressed only during active infection may make it possible to identify the patients at greatest risk of developing symptomatic infection (4, 5, 37). At present, the clinical significance of results provided by qualitative PCR is unclear, but the method appears to be useful in certain settings. These include diagnosis of less common forms of CMV infection, such as detection of CMV in CSF of patients with encephalitis or polyradiculomyelitis; in urine, amniotic fluid, or fetal blood for diagnosis of congenital CMV infection; in the aqueous or vitreous humor in patients with CMV retinitis; and in blood of patients at high risk of severe infection, such as CMV donor-positive, recipient-negative transplant patients, so that antiviral therapy can be started early in the course of infection.

Quantitative and semiquantitative molecular assays for monitoring CMV DNA levels in blood have been developed and include target and signal amplification methods such as PCR, branched-chain technology, and a solution hybridization antibody capture assay (for reviews, see references 6 and 40). It has been shown that transplant and AIDS patients with active CMV disease have higher levels of CMV DNA and that a rapid rise in the CMV DNA copy number correlates with the presence of symptoms and drug failure during treatment (11, 19, 28, 29, 97). Also, Rasmussen et al. (72) have determined that quantitation of CMV DNA from peripheral blood leukocytes can be used to identify HIV-infected patients at risk for development of symptomatic CMV retinitis. It has also been determined that immunocompromised patients with CMV disease have more CMV DNA in either plasma or leukocyte fractions than do patients without disease but that the level of CMV DNA in leukocytes is higher than that in plasma (29, 98). Quantitation of CMV in plasma, therefore, may be less accurate for evaluating the risk of CMV disease progression and the efficacy of therapeutic drugs. Quantitative PCR methods for the estimation of CMV DNA levels in CSF and urine of CMV-infected patients have been described (25, 76), but more research is needed to assess the clinical relevance of quantitating CMV DNA from these specimens. It has been shown that the prognosis of congenital CMV infection may be directly related to the amount of CMV in the urine of an infected neonate and that quantitating CMV DNA in the CSF of AIDS patients may help determine if disorders of the central nervous system are attributed more to CMV than to the direct effects of human immunodeficiency virus or other opportunistic pathogens.

Other Direct Detection Methods

An enzyme-linked immunosorbent assay and a dot immunoperoxidase assay involving antisera to viral proteins have also been used for the direct detection of CMV from clinical specimens.

DETECTION IN CELL CULTURE

Processing of Specimens

Adjustment of urine specimens to pH 7.0 with 0.1 N NaOH or 0.1 N HCl is recommended to reduce toxicity to cell cultures. Centrifuging urine specimens to obtain sediment-enriched samples has been advocated but is usually unnecessary. Sediment-enriched urine samples from renal transplant recipients may produce toxicity more frequently than do uncentrifuged urine samples.

A number of procedures for obtaining peripheral blood leukocytes have been described. We have found density gradient centrifugation with either Ficoll-Hypaque (24, 42) or a mixture of sodium metrizoate and dextran 500 (PMN; Robbins Scientific, Sunnyvale, Calif.) to be most suitable for a clinical laboratory. Fresh blood collected in the presence of heparin, sodium citrate, acid citrate dextrose, or EDTA may be used. Both mononuclear cells and granulocytes are efficiently separated from erythrocytes in a single step. The procedure is rapid and easy to perform, and the reagents are commercially available. Compared with traditional sedimentation methods, the technique results in a greater number of virus isolates and an increased yield of infectious foci or plaques (42).

Respiratory, biopsy, autopsy, and other specimens are processed as described in chapter 5. All specimens are treated with antibiotics before inoculation of cell cultures. Portions of specimens not used to inoculate cell cultures should be mixed with equal volumes of 0.4 M sucrose-phosphate and frozen at −70°C or in liquid nitrogen; some infectivity may be preserved if further isolation attempts are necessary.

Cell Cultures

Human fibroblasts best support the growth of CMV and therefore are used for diagnostic purposes. Acceptable fibroblast cultures include those prepared from human embryonic tissues or foreskins and serially passaged diploid human fetal lung strains such as WI-38, MRC-5, or IMR-90. Diploid fibroblast cells should be used at a low passage number, since they may become less susceptible to CMV infection with increasing cell generations. Several of these fibroblast cell lines are commercially available. CMV can infect and replicate in certain human epithelial cells, but its growth is limited. CMV infection of nonhuman cells can occur but leads to abortive replication with expression of only immediate-early genes and proteins.

Isolation of Virus

Specimens to be tested are added in a volume of 0.2 ml to duplicate tubes of confluent fibroblasts maintained on Eagle minimal essential medium with 2% fetal bovine serum. Alternatively, the tubes are drained of medium, the inocula are absorbed for 1 h in a stationary position or by centrifugation at 700 × *g* for 45 min at 30 to 33°C (63), and then fresh medium is added. After inoculation, the tubes can be rolled or kept stationary at 37°C. At 24 h later, the medium is changed for tubes inoculated with urine or leukocyte specimens. Thereafter, and for other types of specimens, the medium is changed once a week or more frequently as the pH of the culture medium changes or if toxicity appears. When toxicity necessitates passage of the culture, cells rather than culture medium should be passaged, since CMV remains cell associated. Cells are removed by addition of 0.25% trypsin–0.1% EDTA to the monolayers and incubation at 37°C for approximately 1 min. When the cells detach, Eagle minimal essential medium with 2% fetal bovine serum is added, and the cells are used to inoculate fresh tubes. Tubes are examined for cytopathic effect (CPE) daily for the first 5 days and then twice a week for at least 4 weeks for most specimens (6 weeks for leukocyte specimens). Control, uninoculated cultures are handled in the same manner as those inoculated with clinical specimens.

The time of appearance and the extent of CPE depend on the amounts of virus present in specimens. In cultures inoculated with urine from a congenitally infected newborn, CPE may develop by 24 h and progress rapidly to involve most of the monolayer if the virus titer in the urine is extremely high. More commonly, foci of CPE, consisting of enlarged, rounded, refractile cells, appear during the first week and progression of CPE to surrounding cells proceeds slowly (Fig. 3). In cultures inoculated with urine or respiratory specimens from older individuals, CPE usually appears within 2 weeks. Leukocyte cultures may not become positive until after 3 to 6 weeks. The usual slow progression of CPE in cultures inoculated with clinical specimens is due, at least in part, to limited release of virus into extracellular fluid. With strains of CMV that have been serially passaged, including laboratory-adapted strains, greater amounts of extracellular virus are released and CPE progresses more rapidly.

For storage of fresh isolates, monolayers exhibiting CPE are treated with trypsin-EDTA and the cells obtained are suspended in Eagle minimal essential medium with 10% fetal bovine serum and 10% dimethyl sulfoxide and then frozen at −70°C. Infectivity can be better maintained for long periods by storage in liquid nitrogen.

Identification of Isolates

In many laboratories, CMV isolates are identified solely on the basis of characteristic CPE and host cell range. However, viruses such as adenovirus and varicella-zoster virus occasionally produce CPE indistinguishable from that of CMV. Suspected CMV isolates can be confirmed by an indirect immunofluorescence assay (IFA) with commercially available monoclonal or polyclonal antibodies. The appearance of typical nuclear fluorescence of infected cells indicates the presence of CMV.

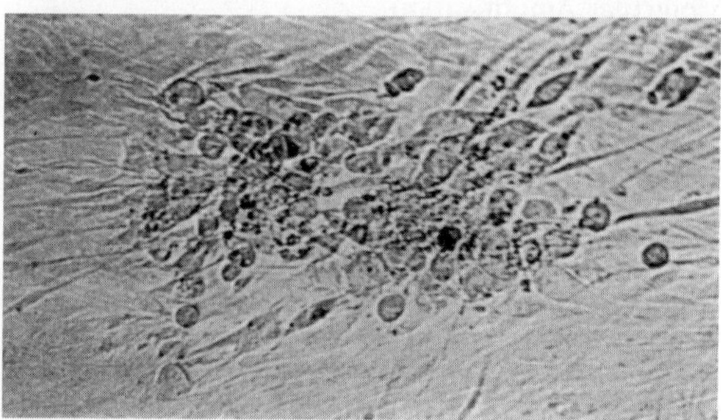

FIGURE 3 CPE produced by a CMV isolate in human skin fibroblasts 10 days postinoculation. Unstained preparation; magnification, ×100. (Courtesy of Sergio Stagno.)

Spin-Amplification Shell Vial Assay

The spin-amplification shell vial assay as described by Gleaves et al. (36) has gained wide acceptance as a rapid method for the detection of CMV in clinical specimens. The technique is based on the amplification of virus in cell cultures after low-speed centrifugation and detects viral antigens produced early in the replication of CMV before the development of CPE. Even low titers of virus present in specimens are easily amplified and rapidly detected within 24 h. Monoclonal antibodies are commercially available and have been used for the detection of CMV early antigens. In situ hybridization with commercially available DNA probes to CMV has also been used (34).

MRC-5 fibroblast cells are grown to confluency on 12-mm round coverslips in 1-dram (3.7-ml) shell vials and inoculated with 0.2 ml of specimen. Shell vials of MRC-5 cells can be obtained commercially or prepared in the laboratory. Monolayers should be inoculated within 1 week after preparation, since older monolayers demonstrate decreased sensitivity to CMV and increased toxicity (23). Pretreatment of the monolayers with dexamethasone, dimethyl sulfoxide, or these agents plus calcium may increase the sensitivity of the cells to CMV infection (93, 94), although other investigators have been unable to confirm these results (22). Two vials should be inoculated for urine, tissue, and bronchoalveolar lavage specimens, and three should be inoculated for blood specimens (67). Alternatively, disruption of purified leukocytes by sonication before their use in the shell vial assay may increase the sensitivity of CMV detection from blood (96). Increasing the frequency of blood collection and the volume of blood obtained also may enhance the diagnostic yield of the shell vial assay from this specimen (65). After inoculation, the vials are centrifuged at 700 × g for 40 min at 25°C and then 2.0 ml of Eagle minimum essential medium containing 2% fetal bovine serum and antibiotics is added. The cultures are incubated at 37°C for 16 to 24 h, fixed with acetone, and stained. A longer incubation time may be used, but the time should be determined by each laboratory on the basis of individual experience, reagents, and staining technique used and whether monolayers are purchased or prepared in the laboratory. Uninfected and CMV-infected monolayers are included as negative and positive controls, respectively. Mink lung (ML) cells, a nonhuman continuous cell line, have been shown to be comparable to MRC-5 fibroblasts for the detection of CMV in clinical specimens by shell vial culture (33, 55). A distinct advantage in using ML cells is that this cell line can be propagated and passaged in the laboratory for a long time without a decrease in susceptibility to CMV. Significantly less toxicity and an increase in the number of CMV-positive nuclei were also observed with ML cells. Our laboratory uses an IFA to detect the immediate-early antigen of CMV, with the E-13 mouse anti-CMV monoclonal antibody as the primary antiserum followed by a biotin-labeled goat anti-mouse antibody and avidin conjugated with fluorescein isothiocyanate. The monolayers are counterstained with Evans blue. Coverslips are scanned at ×200 to ×250 magnification, and specific staining is confirmed at ×400 to ×630. Positive cells contain apple green fluorescent nuclei against a red cytoplasmic background. Staining of immediate-early antigen appears as an even matte green fluorescence with specks of brighter green (Fig. 4A). Viral inclusions ("owl's eyes") may be visible in the nuclei (Fig. 4B).

The spin-amplification shell vial assay is a valuable adjunct to conventional virus isolation. It has the important features of being rapid, sensitive, and specific. However, skilled technical personnel and close attention to the quality of specimens, monolayers, and reagents are required for optimum performance. A modification of the shell vial assay to quantify CMV in blood and bronchoalveolar lavage specimens from transplant patients has been developed (10, 77). The quantitative method has been used to predict the outcome of CMV infection and to assess the effectiveness of antiviral treatment.

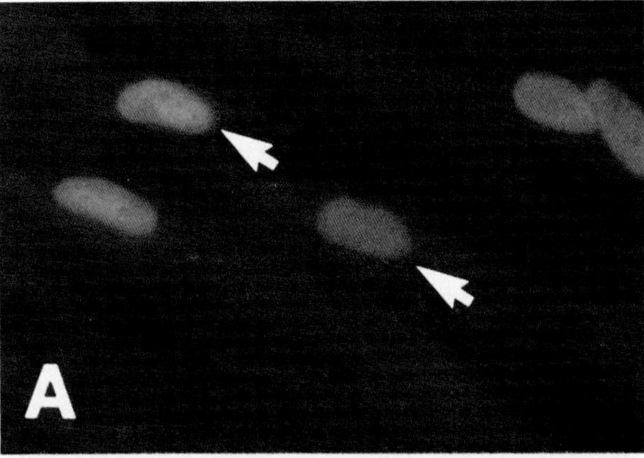

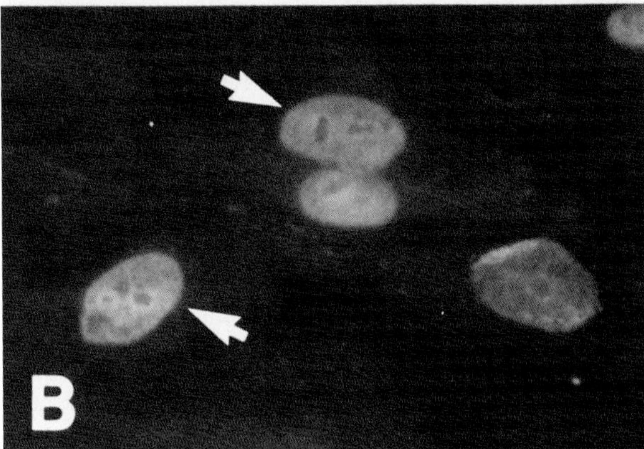

FIGURE 4 Demonstration of CMV early antigens in the nuclei (arrows) of infected MRC-5 cells following shell vial culture and IFA staining. Magnification, ×400.

SEROLOGIC DIAGNOSIS

A variety of tests are available for serodiagnosis of CMV infection. In deciding which test to perform, one should consider such factors as the patient population, cost, turnaround time, equipment needs, and ease of performance. The method that is chosen depends on the needs of individual laboratories. Overall, determination of a positive seroconversion remains a reliable means of diagnosing primary CMV infection, and the screening of blood and organ donors and recipients plays an important role in preventing the transmission of latent CMV to patients at high risk for severe CMV disease.

EIA

Over the last several years, enzyme immunoassays (EIA) have largely replaced other traditional methods for detecting antibodies to CMV. The main advantages of the EIA are that it is rapid, sensitive, and specific (59, 60, 68). In addition, multiple specimens can be handled daily. The EIA can be used effectively to determine the immune status of a patient (9, 20) and to detect significant rises in antibody titers (59). Kits that detect CMV IgG are available from a number of commercial sources. The kits are easy to use, and the manufacturers have provided detailed instructions. All of the materials necessary to perform the assay are included, and the reagents are stable with time. Some companies also provide a spectrophotometer and automated plate washer, which otherwise must be purchased separately at considerable expense. The development of robotics technology has led to the commercial availability of both fully automated and semiautomated EIA instruments, including sample dispensers, diluters, washers, and spectrophotometers with complete computer programming and generation of written reports.

Passive Latex Agglutination Test

The passive latex agglutination test provides a simple and rapid means of detecting antibodies to CMV in human sera and plasma. The method is highly sensitive and specific, and it may serve to determine the immune status of patients or blood donors (2, 45) or to satisfactorily detect significant antibody rises in paired sera (59, 60). Commercial kits are available. The procedure detects both IgG and IgM antibodies but does not differentiate between the two classes of immunoglobulins. The assay can be completed in 10 to 15 min and does not require extensive washes, long incubation times, or expensive equipment. The main disadvantages are that agglutination patterns can be difficult to discern and readings are subjective.

CF Test

The complement fixation (CF) test has been used for many years in clinical laboratories and is suitable for detecting rises in antibody titers. Reagents for the CF test are commercially available, and detailed procedures are described elsewhere (14, 49). The choice of antigen preparation for CF should depend in part on the purpose of the test. The CF test with glycine-extracted antigen is more sensitive for distinguishing seropositive from seronegative specimens (49), whereas the freeze-thawed antigen is slightly better for detecting fourfold or greater rises in titer (14). The method is technically demanding, requires rigid standardization, and has a long turnaround time. It is also less sensitive than other methods in detecting low levels of antibody. Therefore, it may be desirable to adopt an alternative system, such as EIA or a latex agglutination assay (see above), for routine diagnostic testing.

ACIF Test

The anticomplement immunofluorescence (ACIF) test is an immunofluorescence assay that detects CMV antibody (48, 71). The method is performed by incubating heat-inactivated serum with CMV-infected fibroblasts fixed to glass slides. CMV-specific antibody bound to the infected cells is detected by using complement and fluorescein-conjugated anticomplement antibodies. An important advantage of this assay over the CF test is its rapidity, since results can be available within 2 to 3 h. In addition, sera that are anticomplementary by the CF procedure can be tested by the ACIF test, and nonspecific cytoplasmic staining caused by binding of antibody to Fc receptors is avoided. Disadvantages of the ACIF test are that fewer specimens can be handled daily, the test requires cell culture facilities and an immunofluorescence microscope, and examination of slides requires considerable time and experience.

IFA

As an alternative to the ACIF test, the IFA can be performed (71). This test is slightly faster than the ACIF test but has the disadvantage that it should be performed on monolayers of infected cells grown on glass slides; these are more difficult to prepare than the cell suspensions used for making substrate slides in the ACIF test. In addition, specific nuclear fluorescence, which indicates a positive result, is sometimes difficult to distinguish from nonspecific cytoplasmic fluorescence. The latter occurs because CMV infection of fibroblasts induces a cytoplasmic Fc receptor that binds viral and nonviral IgG antibodies.

Several IFA systems for CMV antibody detection are commercially available. These include a solid-phase fluorescence immunoassay (trademarked as FIAX) in which CMV antigen and control antigen are absorbed onto solid surfaces. A single dilution of patient serum is applied to the solid surfaces, an anti-human IgG fluorescein conjugate is added, and the intensity of fluorescence is measured in a fluorometer (26). CMV-infected culture cells on glass slides and other IFA kits for measuring CMV antibodies are also available commercially.

CMV IgM Antibodies

Methods for measuring CMV IgM antibodies include IFA, EIA, and radioimmunoassays. The procedures are essentially the same as those used to detect IgG antibodies, except that anti-human IgM antibodies labeled with suitable markers are used. A recognized pitfall of CMV IgM assays is the occurrence of false-positive and false-negative reactions. False-positive reactions occur when sera contain unusually high levels of rheumatoid factor in the presence of specific CMV IgG (15). Rheumatoid factor is an Ig, usually of the IgM class, that reacts with IgG. It is produced in some rheumatologic, vasculitic, and viral diseases, including CMV infection. IgM rheumatoid factor forms a complex with IgG that may contain CMV-specific IgG. The CMV IgG binds to CMV antigen, carrying nonviral IgM with it. A test designed to detect IgM will produce a false-positive result. Therefore, it is important to test for rheumatoid factor and remove it if present when IgM antibodies are being measured. False-negative reactions occur if high levels of specific IgG antibodies competitively block the binding of IgM to CMV antigen. Separation of IgG and IgM fractions before testing decreases the incidence of both false-positive and false-negative results.

Rapid and simple methods for the removal of interfering rheumatoid factor and IgG molecules from serum have been developed. These include gel filtration, affinity chromatography, selective absorption of IgM to a solid phase, and removal of IgG by using hyperimmune anti-human IgG, staphylococcal protein A, or recombinant protein G from group G streptococci. Serum pretreatment methods are now incorporated within the procedures of commercially available immunofluorescence and EIA kits, which has resulted in more reliable IgM tests. More recently, reverse capture solid-phase IgM assays have been used as an alternative approach to avoiding false-positive or false-negative results. This method uses a solid phase coated with an anti-human IgM antibody to capture the IgM from a serum specimen, after which competing IgG antibody and immune complexes are removed by washing. The bound IgM antibody is then exposed to specific CMV antigen, and an enzyme-conjugated second antibody and substrate are added. The development and use of recombinantly derived CMV proteins as a source of antigenic substrate also have greatly improved the performance of IgM assays (50, 88).

Although the detection of CMV-specific IgM may be useful in the determination of recent or active infection, the results should be interpreted with caution. Because IgM does not cross the placenta, a positive result from a single serum specimen from an infected newborn is diagnostic. However, there may be a lack of or delay in production of IgM in the newborn. IgM antibody can appear in both primary and reactivated CMV infections and can persist for extended periods after a primary infection. This complicates the interpretation of test results, especially if a mother is positive for IgM during pregnancy. Also, patients with Epstein-Barr virus-induced infectious mononucleosis may produce heterotypic IgM responses, resulting in false-positive IgM results.

Other Serologic Tests

Immune adherence hemagglutination, indirect hemagglutination, and the neutralization test are other serologic tests used to measure CMV antibody.

INTERPRETATION OF RESULTS

Recovery of CMV from urine, respiratory secretions, or other body fluids within the first 3 weeks of life is the most sensitive and specific means of confirming the diagnosis of congenital infection. Urine is the preferred specimen because it contains greater amounts of virus, and the virus will therefore grow quickly in culture. Attempts to isolate and/or detect virus from blood and tissue of the infected newborn and from amniotic fluid and fetal tissue also can be made. Serologic tests are less useful because of transplacental passage of maternal antibody and technical problems with detection of CMV-specific IgM. A history of seroconversion from a negative to a positive IgG antibody response to CMV is diagnostic of primary infection and may be beneficial in evaluating a pregnant woman with symptoms of viral disease. Congenital infection should be suspected in infants with typical symptoms whose CMV titers persist at levels comparable to or sometimes higher than those of the mothers. Negative IgG titers in both mother and child exclude congenital CMV infection. Infants not previously tested but found to be excreting virus after 3 weeks of age may have either congenital or acquired infection. Standard serologic or virologic tests do not differentiate between these possibilities.

Interpretation of serologic tests performed on sera of patients 6 months of age or older is facilitated by the absence of passively acquired maternal antibody. If the initial serum specimen is negative for CMV antibodies and the second specimen is positive, a diagnosis of primary infection can be made. If a serum sample obtained early in an illness contains CMV antibodies and a second sample obtained several weeks later demonstrates a fourfold or greater rise in titer, a diagnosis of recent infection due to reactivation or reinfection can be made. Fourfold falls in titer are seldom observed early enough to be useful for laboratory diagnosis, since antibody levels tend to decline slowly over several months after infection. If acute- and convalescent-phase sera are both positive for CMV antibody but the antibody titer is unchanged, the result is interpreted as CMV infection at some time in the past. If the titers of the positive sera are high and the first specimen was obtained late in the illness, the results may indicate active infection, and appropriate specimens for viral isolation or direct detection should be obtained. Whenever possible, serologic diagnoses of CMV infection should be confirmed by virologic methods, particularly since fourfold fluctuations in CMV antibody titers have been noted in some apparently healthy seropositive individuals (91) and since immunocompromised hosts may not mount a normal immune response.

CMV serologic tests also play a significant role in the evaluation of an organ donor and recipient before transplantation. A seronegative recipient who receives an organ or blood products from a seropositive donor is at increased risk for developing primary CMV infection and serious disease. Knowing the serostatus of the donor and recipient is therefore important in determining the treatment or prophylaxis to be used and in considering the type of donor and blood products to be given. Serologic assays have limited utility in the screening of transplant recipients following transplantation.

In the immunocompromised host, virologic or serologic detection of CMV indicates active infection but does not establish whether the infection is responsible for symptomatic illness. CMV is ubiquitous, and there is a high rate of asymptomatic excretion in patients who never progress to disease. Reactivation of latent virus is also common, and other pathogens are simultaneously present in patients with overt disease. To implicate CMV as the cause of an illness, laboratory confirmation of active infection in an appropriate clinical setting is required. Routine surveillance for CMV, especially from urine, blood, and respiratory specimens, can identify transplant recipients and patients with human immunodeficiency virus infection at high risk for CMV disease (61, 69, 70, 74, 89). Detection of CMV in urine and respiratory specimens indicates active infection and the need to closely observe a patient so that appropriate medical management can be undertaken if disease develops. However, shedding of CMV in the urine and respiratory tract is common during asymptomatic infection and is usually not suggestive of more severe disease. When CMV is identified in peripheral blood leukocytes, the likelihood that the infection is symptomatic increases. However, asymptomatic viremia has also been described (13, 17) and is particularly common in patients with AIDS. The use of quantitative detection methods to predict which patients will progress to severe CMV disease is most beneficial for patient care. Detection of CMV in liver and particularly lung biopsy specimens must be interpreted with caution, since other pathogens (*Chlamydia trachomatis*, *Pneumocystis carinii*, and other bacteria or fungi) may also be present; when dual infection is documented, the relative importance of each pathogen in producing clinical illness may be difficult to determine.

The application of virologic methods, including conventional and shell vial culture, rapid direct-detection assays, and serologic testing, should be combined with clinical assessment of the patient to provide an accurate, reliable diagnosis of CMV infection and disease and to allow subsequent prompt, appropriate patient management and timely intervention with specific antiviral therapy. There is a particular need to differentiate CMV infection from graft rejection in transplant patients, since the administration of potent immunosuppressive anti-rejection drugs during active CMV infection can result in life-threatening disease.

REFERENCES

1. **Adler, S. P., and J. B. Wang.** 1996. Salivary antibodies to cytomegalovirus (CMV) glycoprotein B accurately predict

CMV infections among preschool children. *J. Clin. Microbiol.* **34:**2632–2634.

2. **Beckwith, D. G., D. C. Halstead, K. Alpaugh, A. Schweder, D. A. Blount-Fronefield, and K. Toth.** 1985. Comparison of a latex agglutination test with five other methods for determining the presence of antibody against cytomegalovirus. *J. Clin. Microbiol.* **21:**328–331.
3. **Bitsch, A., H. Kirchner, R. Dennin, J. Hoyer, L. Fricke, J. Steinhoff, K. Sack, and G. Bein.** 1993. Long persistence of CMV DNA in the blood of renal transplant patients after recovery from CMV infection. *Transplantation* **56:** 108–113.
4. **Bitsch, A., H. Kirchner, R. Dupke, and G. Bein.** 1992. Cytomegalovirus transcripts in peripheral blood leukocytes of actively infected transplant patients detected by reverse transcription-polymerase chain reaction. *J. Infect. Dis.* **167:**740–743.
5. **Blok, M. J., V. J. Goossens, S. J. V. Vanherle, B. Top, N. Tacken, J. M. Middeldorp, M. H. L. Christiaans, J. P. van Hooff, and C. A. Bruggeman.** 1998. Diagnostic value of monitoring human cytomegalovirus late pp67 mRNA expression in renal-allograft recipients by nucleic acid sequence-based amplification. *J. Clin. Microbiol.* **36:** 1341–1346.
6. **Boeckh, M., and G. Boivin.** 1998. Quantitation of cytomegalovirus: methodologic aspects and clinical applications. *Clin. Microbiol. Rev.* **11:**533–554.
7. **Boeckh, M., P., P. M. Woogerd, T. Stevens-Ayers, C. G. Ray, and R. A. Bowden.** 1994. Factors influencing detection of quantitative cytomegalovirus antigenemia. *J. Clin. Microbiol.* **32:**832–834.
8. **Boivin, G., J. Handfield, G. Murray, E. Toma, R. Lalonde, J. G. Lazar, and M. G. Bergerson.** 1997. Quantitation of cytomegalovirus (CMV) DNA in leukocytes of human immunodeficiency virus-infected subjects with and without CMV disease by using PCR and the SHARP signal detection system. *J. Clin. Microbiol.* **35:**525–526.
9. **Booth, J. C., G. Hannington, T. M. F. Bakir, H. Stern, H. Kangro, P. D. Griffiths, and R. B. Heath.** 1982. Comparison of enzyme-linked immunosorbent assay, radioimmunoassay, complement fixation, anticomplement immunofluorescence and passive haemagglutination techniques for detecting cytomegalovirus IgG antibody. *J. Clin. Pathol.* **35:**1345–1348.
10. **Buller, R. S., T. C. Bailey, N. A. Ettinger, M. Keener, T. Langlois, J. P. Miller, and G. A. Storch.** 1992. Use of a modified shell vial technique to quantitate cytomegalovirus viremia in a population of solid-organ transplant recipients. *J. Clin. Microbiol.* **30:**2620–2624.
11. **Chernoff, D. N., R. C. Miner, B. S. Hoo, L.-P. Shen, R. J. Kelso, D. Jekic-McMullen, J. P. Lalezari, S. Chou, W. L. Drew, and J. A. Kolberg.** 1997. Quantification of cytomegalovirus DNA in peripheral blood leukocytes by a branched-DNA signal amplification assay. *J. Clin. Microbiol.* **35:**2740–2744.
12. **Chou, S., and T. C. Merigan.** 1983. Rapid detection and quantitation of human cytomegalovirus in urine through DNA hybridization. *N. Engl. J. Med.* **308:**921–925.
13. **Cox, F., and W. T. Hughes.** 1975. Cytomegaloviremia in children with acute lymphatic leukemia. *J. Pediatr.* **87:** 190–194.
14. **Cremer, N. E., M. Hoffman, and E. H. Lennette.** 1978. Analysis of antibody assay methods and classes of viral antibodies in serodiagnosis of cytomegalovirus infection. *J. Clin. Microbiol.* **8:**152–159.
15. **Cremer, N. E., M. Hoffman, and E. H. Lennette.** 1978. Role of rheumatoid factor in complement fixation and indirect hemagglutination tests for immunoglobulin M antibody to cytomegalovirus. *J. Clin. Microbiol.* **8:**160–165.
16. **Dankner, W. M., J. A. McCutchan, D. D. Richman, K. Hirata, and S. A. Spector.** 1990. Localization of human cytomegalovirus in peripheral blood leukocytes by in situ hybridization. *J. Infect. Dis.* **161:**31–36.
17. **Delgado, R., C. Lumbreras, C. Alba, M. A. Pedraza, J. R. Otero, R. Gomez, E. Moreno, A. R. Noriega, and C. V. Paya.** 1992. Low predictive value of polymerase chain reaction for diagnosis of cytomegalovirus disease in liver transplant recipients. *J. Clin. Microbiol.* **30:**1876–1878.
18. **Demmler, G. J., G. J. Buffone, C. M. Schimbor, and R. A. May.** 1988. Detection of cytomegalovirus in urine from newborns by using polymerase chain reaction DNA amplification. *J. Infect. Dis.* **158:**1177–1184.
19. **Drouet, E., R. Colimon, S. Michelson, N. Fourcade, A. Niveleau, C. Ducerf, A. Boibieux, M. Chevallier, and G. Denoyel.** 1995. Monitoring levels of human cytomegalovirus DNA in blood after liver transplantation. *J. Clin. Microbiol.* **33:**389–394.
20. **Dylewski, J. S., L. Rasmussen, J. Mills, and T. C. Merigan.** 1984. Large-scale serological screening for cytomegalovirus antibodies in homosexual males by enzyme-linked immunosorbent assay. *J. Clin. Microbiol.* **19:**200–203.
21. **Erice, A., M. A. Holm, M. V. Sanjuan, D. L. Dunn, P. C. Gill, and H. H. Balfour, Jr.** 1995. Evaluation of CMV-vue antigenemia assay for rapid detection of cytomegalovirus in mixed-leukocyte blood fractions. *J. Clin. Microbiol.* **33:**1014–1015.
22. **Espy, M. J., A. D. Wold, D. M. Ilstrup, and T. F. Smith.** 1988. Effect of treatment of shell vial cell cultures with dimethyl sulfoxide and dexamethasone for detection of cytomegalovirus. *J. Clin. Microbiol.* **26:**1091–1093.
23. **Fedorko, D. P., D. M. Ilstrup, and T. F. Smith.** 1989. Effect of age of shell vial monolayers on detection of cytomegalovirus from urine specimens. *J. Clin. Microbiol.* **27:** 2107–2109.
24. **Ferrante, A., and Y. H. Thong.** 1980. Optimal conditions for simultaneous purification of mononuclear and polymorphonuclear leukocytes from human peripheral blood by the Hypaque-Ficoll method. *J. Immunol. Methods* **36:**109–117.
25. **Fox, J. C., P. D. Griffiths, and V. C. Emery.** 1992. Quantification of human cytomegalovirus DNA using the polymerase chain reaction. *J. Gen. Virol.* **73:**2405–2408.
26. **Friedman, H. M., N. B. Tustin, M. M. Hitchings, and S. A. Plotkin.** 1981. Comparison of complement fixation and fluorescent immunoassay (FIAX) for measuring antibodies to cytomegalovirus and herpes simplex virus. *Am. J. Clin. Pathol.* **76:**305–307.
27. **Garcia, A., J. Niubo, M. A. Benitez, M. Viqueira, and J. L. Perez.** 1996. Comparison of two leukocyte extraction methods for cytomegalovirus antigenemia assay. *J. Clin. Microbiol.* **34:**182–184.
28. **Gerdes, J. C., E. K. Spees, K. Fitting, J. Hiraki, M. Sheehan, D. Duda, T. Jarvi, C. Roehl, and A. D. Robertson.** 1993. Prospective study utilizing a quantitative polymerase chain reaction for detection of cytomegalovirus DNA in the blood of renal transplant patients. *Transplant. Proc.* **25:**1411–1413.
29. **Gerna, G., M. Furione, F. Baldanti, and A. Sarasini.** 1994. Comparative quantitation of human cytomegalovirus DNA in blood leukocytes and plasma of transplant and AIDS patients. *J. Clin. Microbiol.* **32:**2709–2717.
30. **Gerna, G., M. G. Revello, E. Percivalle, M. Zavattoni, M. Parea, and M. Battaglia.** 1990. Quantitation of human cytomegalovirus viremia by using monoclonal antibodies to different viral proteins. *J. Clin. Microbiol.* **28:**2681–2688.
31. **Gerna, G., D. Zipeto, M. Parea, E. Percivalle, M. Zavattoni, A. Gaballo, and G. Milanesi.** 1991. Early virus isolation, early structural antigen detection and DNA amplification by the polymerase chain reaction in

polymorphonuclear leukocytes from AIDS patients with human cytomegalovirus viraemia. *Mol. Cell. Probes.* **5:** 365–374.

32. **Gerna, G., D. Zipeto, M. Parea, M. G. Revello, E. Silini, E. Percivalle, M. Zavattoni, P. Grossi, and G. Milanesi.** 1991. Monitoring of human cytomegalovirus infections and ganciclovir treatment in heart transplant recipients by determination of viremia, antigenemia, and DNAemia. *J. Infect. Dis.* **164:**488–498.
33. **Gleaves, C. A., D. A. Hursh, and J. D. Meyers.** 1992. Detection of human cytomegalovirus in clinical specimens by centrifugation culture with a nonhuman cell line. *J. Clin. Microbiol.* **30:**1045–1048.
34. **Gleaves, C. A., D. A. Hursh, D. H. Rice, and J. D. Meyers.** 1989. Detection of cytomegalovirus from clinical specimens in centrifugation culture by in situ DNA hybridization and monoclonal antibody staining. *J. Clin. Microbiol.* **27:**21–23.
35. **Gleaves, C. A., D. Myerson, R. A. Bowden, R. C. Hackman, and J. D. Meyers.** 1989. Direct detection of cytomegalovirus from bronchoalveolar lavage samples by using a rapid in situ DNA hybridization assay. *J. Clin. Microbiol.* **27:**2429–2432.
36. **Gleaves, C. A., T. F. Smith, E. A. Shuster, and G. R. Pearson.** 1984. Rapid detection of cytomegalovirus in MRC-5 cells inoculated with urine specimens by using low-speed centrifugation and monoclonal antibody to an early antigen. *J. Clin. Microbiol.* **19:**917–919.
37. **Gozlan, J., J.-M. Saloed, C. Chouaid, C. Duvivier, O. Picard, M.-C. Meyohas, and J.-C. Petit.** 1993. Human cytomegalovirus (HCMV) late-mRNA detection in peripheral blood of AIDS patients: diagnostic value for HCMV disease compared with those of viral culture and HCMV DNA detection. *J. Clin. Microbiol.* **31:**1943–1945.
38. **Grody, W. W., K. J. Lewin, and F. Naeim.** 1988. Detection of cytomegalovirus DNA in classic and epidemic Kaposi's sarcoma by in situ hybridization. *Hum. Pathol.* **19:** 524–528.
39. **Ho, S. K. N., C.-Y. Lo, I. K. P. Cheng, and T.-M. Chan.** 1998. Rapid cytomegalovirus pp65 antigenemia assay by direct erythrocyte lysis and immunofluorescence staining. *J. Clin. Microbiol.* **36:**638–640.
40. **Hodinka, R. L.** 1998. The clinical utility of viral quantitation using molecular methods. *Clin. Diagn. Virol.* **10:** 25–47.
41. **Howell, C. L., and M. J. Miller.** 1983. Effect of sucrose phosphate and sorbitol on infectivity of enveloped viruses during storage. *J. Clin. Microbiol.* **18:**658–662.
42. **Howell, C. L., M. J. Miller, and W. J. Martin.** 1979. Comparison of rates of virus isolation from leukocyte populations separated from blood by conventional and Ficoll-Paque/Macrodex methods. *J. Clin. Microbiol.* **10:**533–537.
43. **Hsia, K., D. H. Spector, J. Lawrie, and S. A. Spector.** 1989. Enzymatic amplification of human cytomegalovirus sequences by polymerase chain reaction. *J. Clin. Microbiol.* **27:**1802–1809.
44. **Huang, E.-S., H. A. Kilpatrick, Y.-T. Huang, and J. S. Pagano.** 1976. Detection of human cytomegalovirus and analysis of strain variation. *Yale J. Biol. Med.* **49:**29–43.
45. **Hursh, D. A., A. D. Abbot, R. Sun, J. P. Iltis, D. H. Rice, and C. A. Gleaves.** 1989. Evaluation of a latex particle agglutination assay for the detection of cytomegalovirus antibody in patient serum. *J. Clin. Microbiol.* **27:** 2878–2879.
46. **Imbert-Marcille, B.-M., N. Robillard, A.-S. Poirier, M. Coste-Burel, D. Cantarovich, N. Milpied, and S. Billaudel.** 1997. Development of a method for direct quantification of cytomegalovirus antigenemia by flow cytometry. *J. Clin. Microbiol.* **35:**2665–2669.
47. **Jiwa, N. M., A. K. Raap, F. M. van de Rijke, A. Mulder, J. J. Weening, F. E. Zwaan, T. H. The, and M. van der Ploeg.** 1989. Detection of cytomegalovirus antigens and DNA in tissues fixed in formaldehyde. *J. Clin. Pathol.* **42:** 749–754.
48. **Kettering, J. D., N. J. Schmidt, D. Gallo, and E. H. Lennette.** 1977. Anti-complement immunofluorescence test for antibodies to human cytomegalovirus. *J. Clin. Microbiol.* **6:**627–632.
49. **Kettering, J. D., N. J. Schmidt, and E. H. Lennette.** 1977. Improved glycine-extracted complement-fixing antigen for human cytomegalovirus. *J. Clin. Microbiol.* **6:**647–649.
50. **Landini, M. P., T. Lazzarotto, G. T. Maine, A. Ripalti, and R. Flanders.** 1995. Recombinant mono- and polyantigens to detect cytomegalovirus-specific immunoglobulin M in human sera by enzyme immunoassay. *J. Clin. Microbiol.* **33:**2535–2542.
51. **Landry, M. L., and D. Ferguson.** 1993. Comparison of quantitative cytomegalovirus antigenemia assay with culture methods and correlation with clinical disease. *J. Clin. Microbiol.* **31:**2851–2856.
52. **Landry, M. L., D. Ferguson, S. Cohen, K. Huber, and P. Wetherill.** 1995. Effect of delayed specimen processing on cytomegalovirus antigenemia test results. *J. Clin. Microbiol.* **33:**257–259.
53. **Landry, M. L., D. Ferguson, T. Stevens-Ayers, M. W. A. de Jonge, and M. Boeckh.** 1996. Evaluation of CMV Brite kit for detection of cytomegalovirus pp65 antigenemia in peripheral blood leukocytes by immunofluorescence. *J. Clin. Microbiol.* **34:**1337–1339.
54. **Lucas, G., J. M. Seigneurin, J. Tamalet, S. Michelson, M. Baccard, J. F. Delagneau, and P. Deletoille.** 1989. Rapid diagnosis of cytomegalovirus by indirect immunofluorescence assay with monoclonal antibody F6b in a commercially available kit. *J. Clin. Microbiol.* **27:**367–369.
55. **MacKenzie, D., and L. C. McLaren.** 1989. Increased sensitivity for rapid detection of cytomegalovirus by shell vial centrifugation assay using mink lung cell cultures. *J. Virol. Methods* **26:**183–188.
56. **Macris, M. P., A. J. Nahmias, P. D. Bailey, F. K. Lee, A. M. Visintine, and A. W. Braun.** 1981. Electron microscopy in the routine screening of newborns with congenital cytomegalovirus infection. *J. Virol. Methods* **2:**315–320.
57. **Martin, D. C., D. A. Katzenstein, G. S. M. Yu, and M. C. Jordan.** 1984. Cytomegalovirus viremia detected by molecular hybridization and electron microscopy. *Ann. Intern. Med.* **100:**222–225.
58. **Martin, W. J., Jr., and T. F. Smith.** 1986. Rapid detection of cytomegalovirus in bronchoalveolar lavage specimens by a monoclonal antibody method. *J. Clin. Microbiol.* **23:** 1006–1008.
59. **Mayo, D. R., T. Brennan, S. P. Sirpenski, and C. Seymour.** 1985. Cytomegalovirus antibody detection by three commercially available assays and complement fixation. *Diagn. Microbiol. Infect. Dis.* **3:**455–459.
60. **McHugh, T. M., C. H. Casavant, J. C. Wilber, and D. P. Stites.** 1985. Comparison of six methods for the detection of antibody to cytomegalovirus. *J. Clin. Microbiol.* **22:** 1014–1019.
61. **Meyers, J. D., P. Lijungman, and L. D. Fisher.** 1990. Cytomegalovirus excretion as a predictor of cytomegalovirus disease after marrow transplantation: importance of cytomegalovirus viremia. *J. Infect. Dis.* **162:**373–380.
62. **Myerson, D., R. C. Hackman, and J. D. Meyers.** 1984. Diagnosis of cytomegaloviral pneumonia by in situ hybridization. *J. Infect. Dis.* **150:**272–277.
63. **Oefinger, P. E., R. M. Shawar, S. H. Loo, L. T. Tsai, and J. K. Arnett.** 1990. Enhanced recovery of cytomegalo-

virus in conventional tube cultures with a spin-amplified adsorption. *J. Clin. Microbiol.* **28:**965–969.
64. **Olive, D. M., M. Simsek, and S. Al-Mufti.** 1989. Polymerase chain reaction assay for detection of human cytomegalovirus. *J. Clin. Microbiol.* **27:**1238–1242.
65. **Patel, R., D. W. Klein, M. J. Espy, W. S. Harmsen, D. M. Ilstrup, C. V. Paya, and T. F. Smith.** 1995. Optimization of detection of cytomegalovirus viremia in transplantation recipients by shell vial assay. *J. Clin. Microbiol.* **33:** 2984–2986.
66. **Patel, R., T. F. Smith, M. Espy, R. H. Wiesner, R. A. F. Krom, D. Portela, and C. V. Paya.** 1994. Detection of cytomegalovirus DNA in sera of liver transplant recipients. *J. Clin. Microbiol.* **32:**1431–1434.
67. **Paya, C. V., A. D. Wold, D. M. Ilstrup, and T. F. Smith.** 1988. Evaluation of number of shell vial cell cultures per clinical specimen for rapid diagnosis of cytomegalovirus infection. *J. Clin. Microbiol.* **26:**198–200.
68. **Phipps, P. H., L. Gregoire, E. Rossier, and E. Perry.** 1983. Comparison of five methods of cytomegalovirus antibody screening of blood donors. *J. Clin. Microbiol.* **18:** 1296–1300.
69. **Pillay, D., A. A. Ali, S. F. Liu, E. Kops, P. Sweny, and P. D. Griffiths.** 1993. The prognostic significance of positive CMV cultures during surveillance of renal transplant recipients. *Transplantation* **56:**103–108.
70. **Pillay, D., H. Charman, A. K. Burroughs, M. Smith, K. Rolles, and P. D. Griffiths.** 1992. Surveillance for CMV infection in orthotopic liver transplant recipients. *Transplantation* **53:**1261–1265.
71. **Rao, N., D. T. Waruszewski, J. A. Armstrong, R. W. Atchison, and M. Ho.** 1977. Evaluation of anti-complementary immunofluorescence test in cytomegalovirus infection. *J. Clin. Microbiol.* **6:**633–638.
72. **Rasmussen, L., S. Morris, D. Zipeto, J. Fessel, R. Wolitz, A. Dowling, and T. C. Merigan.** 1995. Quantitation of human cytomegalovirus DNA from peripheral blood cells of human immunodeficiency virus-infected patients could predict cytomegalovirus retinitis. *J. Infect. Dis.* **171:** 177–182.
73. **Revello, M. G., E. Percivalle, A. Sarasini, F. Baldanti, M. Furione, and G. Gerna.** 1994. Diagnosis of human cytomegalovirus infection of the nervous system by pp65 detection in polymorphonuclear leukocytes of cerebrospinal fluid from AIDS patients. *J. Infect. Dis.* **170:**1275–1279.
74. **Salomn, D., F. Lacassin, M. Harzic, C. Leport, C. Perronne, F. Bricaire, F. Brun-Vezinet, and J.-L. Vilde.** 1990. Predictive value of cytomegalovirus viraemia for the occurrence of CMV organ involvement in AIDS. *J. Med. Virol.* **32:**160–163.
75. **Shibata, D., W. J. Martin, M. D. Appelman, D. M. Causey, J. M. Leedom, and N. Arnheim.** 1988. Detection of cytomegalovirus DNA in peripheral blood of patients with human immunodeficiency virus. *J. Infect. Dis.* **158:** 1185–1192.
76. **Shinkai, M., and S. Spector.** 1995. Quantitation of human cytomegalovirus (HCMV) DNA in cerbrospinal fluid by competitive PCR in AIDS patients with different HCMV central nervous system diseases. *Scand. J. Infect. Dis.* **27:** 559–561.
77. **Slavin, M. A., C. A. Gleaves, H. G. Schoch, and R. A. Bowden.** 1992. Quantification of cytomegalovirus in bronchoalveolar lavage fluid after allogeneic marrow transplantation by centrifugation culture. *J. Clin. Microbiol.* **30:** 2776–2779.
78. **Spector, S. A., R. Merrill, D. Wolf, and W. M. Dankner.** 1992. Detection of human cytomegalovirus in plasma of AIDS patients during acute visceral disease by DNA amplification. *J. Clin. Microbiol.* **30:**2359–2365.
79. **Spector, S. A., J. A. Rua, D. H. Spector, and R. McMillan.** 1984. Detection of human cytomegalovirus in clinical specimens by DNA-DNA hybridization. *J. Infect. Dis.* **150:** 121–126.
80. **Stanier, P., D. L. Taylor, A. D. Kitchen, N. Wales, Y. Tryhorn, and A. S. Tyms.** 1989. Persistence of cytomegalovirus in mononuclear cells in peripheral blood from blood donors. *Br. Med. J.* **299:**897–898.
81. **Stockl, E., T. Popow-Kraupp, F. X. Heinz, F. Muhlbacher, P. Balcke, and C. Kunz.** 1988. Potential of in situ hybridization for early diagnosis of productive cytomegalovirus infection. *J. Clin. Microbiol.* **26:**2536–2540.
82. **The, T. H., W. van der Bij, A. P. van den Berg, M. van der Giessen, J. Weits, H. G. Sprenger, and W. J. van Son.** 1990. Cytomegalovirus antigenemia. *Rev. Infect. Dis.* **12**(Suppl. 7)**:**S737–S744.
83. **The, T. H., M. van der Ploeg, A. P. van den Berg, A. M. Vlieger, M. van der Giessen, and W. J. van Son.** 1992. Direct detection of cytomegalovirus in peripheral blood leukocytes—a review of the antigenemia assay and polymerase chain reaction. *Transplantation* **54:**193–198.
84. **van den Berg, A. P., A. M. Tegzess, A. Scholten-Sampson, J. Schirm, M. van der Giessen, T. H. The, and W. J. van Son.** 1992. Monitoring antigenemia is useful in guiding treatment of severe cytomegalovirus disease after organ transplantation. *Transplant Int.* **5:**101–107.
85. **van der Bij, W., J. Schirm, R. Torensma, W. J. van Son, A. M. Tegzess, and T. H. The.** 1988. Comparison between viremia and antigenemia for detection of cytomegalovirus in blood. *J. Clin. Microbiol.* **26:**2531–2535.
86. **van der Bij, W., R. Torensma, W. J. van Son, J. Anema, J. Schirm, A. M. Tegzess, and T. H. The.** 1988. Rapid immunodiagnosis of active cytomegalovirus infection by monoclonal antibody staining of blood leukocytes. *J. Med. Virol.* **25:**179–188.
87. **Volpi, A., R. J. Whitley, R. Ceballos, S. Stagno, and L. Pereira.** 1983. Rapid diagnosis of pneumonia due to cytomegalovirus with specific monoclonal antibodies. *J. Infect. Dis.* **147:**1119–1120.
88. **Vornhagen, R., B. Plachter, W. Hinderer, T. H. The, J. van Zanten, L. Matter, C. A. Schmidt, H.-H. Sonneborn, and G. Jahn.** 1994. Early serodiagnosis of acute human cytomegalovirus infection by enzyme-linked immunosorbent assay using recombinant antigens. *J. Clin. Microbiol.* **32:**981–986.
89. **Walker, R. C.** 1991. The role of the clinical microbiology laboratory in transplantation. *Arch. Pathol. Lab. Med.* **115:** 299–305.
90. **Waner, J. L., and T. H. Weller.** 1978. Analysis of antigenic diversity among human cytomegaloviruses by kinetic neutralization tests with high-titered rabbit antisera. *Infect. Immun.* **21:**151–157.
91. **Waner, J. L., T. H. Weller, and S. V. Kevy.** 1973. Patterns of cytomegaloviral complement-fixing antibody activity: a longitudinal study of blood donors. *J. Infect. Dis.* **127:** 538–543.
92. **Weiss, R. L., G. W. Snow, G. B. Schumann, and M. E. Hammond.** 1990. Diagnosis of cytomegalovirus pneumonitis on bronchoalveolar lavage fluid: comparison of cytology, immunofluorescence, and in situ hybridization with viral isolation. *Diagn. Cytopathol.* **7:**243–247.
93. **West, P. G., B. Aldrich, R. Hartwig, and G. J. Haller.** 1988. Enhanced detection of cytomegalovirus in confluent MRC-5 cells treated with dexamethasone and dimethyl sulfoxide. *J. Clin. Microbiol.* **26:**2510–2514.
94. **West, P. G., and W. W. Baker.** 1990. Enhancement by calcium of the detection of cytomegalovirus in cells treated with dexamethasone and dimethyl sulfoxide. *J. Clin. Microbiol.* **28:**1708–1710.
95. **Wolf, D. G., and S. A. Spector.** 1992. Diagnosis of human

cytomegalovirus central nervous system disease in AIDS patients by DNA amplification from cerebrospinal fluid. *J. Infect. Dis.* **166:**1412–1415.

96. **Wunderli, W., M. K. Kagi, E. Gruter, and J. D. Auracher.** 1989. Detection of cytomegalovirus in peripheral leukocytes by different methods. *J. Clin. Microbiol.* **27:** 1916–1917.
97. **Zipeto, D., F. Baldanti, D. Zella, M. Furione, A. Cavicchini, G. Milanesi, and G. Gerna.** 1993. Quantification of human cytomegalovirus DNA in peripheral blood polymorphonuclear leukocytes of immunocompromised patients by the polymerase chain reaction. *J. Virol. Methods* **44:**45–56.
98. **Zipeto, D., S. Morris, C. Hong, A. Dowling, R. Wolitz, T. C. Merigan, and L. Rasmussen.** 1995. Human cytomegalovirus (CMV) DNA in plasma reflects quantity of CMV DNA present in leukocytes. *J. Clin. Microbiol.* **33:** 2607–2611.

Varicella-Zoster Virus

ANNE A. GERSHON, PHILIP LaRUSSA, AND SHARON P. STEINBERG

67

CLINICAL BACKGROUND

Varicella (chickenpox) and zoster represent different clinical manifestations of infection with the same agent, varicella-zoster virus (VZV). Varicella occurs most frequently in children and is characterized by a generalized vesicular exanthem often accompanied by fever. Zoster (shingles) usually occurs in adults or immunocompromised patients (including persons infected with human immunodeficiency virus, [HIV] and consists of a painful, circumscribed eruption of vesicular lesions with accompanying inflammation of associated dorsal root or cranial nerve sensory ganglia. Varicella is the primary infection with VZV, whereas zoster is a secondary infection due to reactivation of latent VZV in sensory ganglia. That zoster results from reactivation of latent virus rather than reintroduction of virus into the host is indicated by the following observations. (i) Zoster does not exhibit the seasonal prevalence seen with varicella (late winter and spring in temperate climates), nor does zoster frequently occur in parents who are often exposed to their own children with chickenpox. (ii) Latent VZV has been detected in sensory ganglia of autopsy specimens by PCR (60) and by in situ hybridization (10, 58). (iii) Molecular studies of VZV isolates from patients with zoster after either natural chickenpox or varicella vaccination have revealed that the viruses causing the primary infection and the subsequent zoster are the same (38, 86, 89). Studies after natural varicella or immunization indicate that reinfection and reactivation of VZV may occur in the absence of clinical symptoms (3, 34–36, 57, 91) and that second attacks of clinical varicella are infrequent but may occur (35, 44).

There are several situations in which providing a specific laboratory diagnosis of VZV infection is crucial. VZV infection may cause severe or fatal disease in individuals who are receiving immunosuppressive therapy or who have abnormalities in cell-mediated immune responses. Progressive, generalized varicella occurs in as many as 30% of children who acquire chickenpox while receiving chemotherapy and radiotherapy for cancer, and mortality in these cases has ranged from 7 to 28% (20, 21). In immunodeficient patients who have had varicella there is an increased risk of disseminated zoster, and in some studies mortality rates have been similar to those for varicella (57, 78). Providing a specific diagnosis of VZV infection in immunosuppressed patients or their contacts may guide in the administration of antiviral agents or passive immunization with varicella-zoster immune globulin (VZIG). Determining the immunity status (presence or absence of antibody) in high-risk immunocompromised individuals and in adults (who are also at some risk of developing severe varicella) exposed to VZV infection also guides in the management of these individuals. Live attenuated varicella vaccine was licensed for routine use in susceptible healthy persons in the United States in 1995, and determination of the immunity status is useful, particularly for adults with no history of varicella, since only about 25% of such individuals are actually susceptible to chickenpox. In addition, it is recognized that about 10% of vaccinated individuals may develop a "breakthrough" case of varicella caused by the wild-type (WT) virus, months to years after vaccination (29, 30, 43), since varicella vaccine does not provide 100% protection against subsequent infection. Although most cases of breakthrough varicella are mild, these patients may require diagnostic testing. It is important to provide a specific diagnosis of some of the less common manifestations of VZV infection, such as varicella pneumonia and encephalitic complications, particularly since antiviral drugs are now available. It is sometimes necessary to differentiate VZV infection from the vesicular eruptions caused by certain enteroviruses, bacterial agents, or hypersensitivity reactions, and also from generalized vesicular eruptions caused by herpes simplex virus (HSV). Diagnostic studies may clarify the cause of suspected reactions in the first days to weeks following varicella vaccination. Cutaneous pain in a dermatomal distribution in the absence of rash, termed zoster sine herpete, has been described, as well as encephalitis due to VZV in the absence of a skin rash (37, 55, 81).

VZV isolates that are resistant to acyclovir have been described, particularly in patients with underlying HIV infection who have received multiple courses of acyclovir for frequent recurrences of VZV infection (41, 56, 59, 66, 82). Methods to detect viruses resistant to acyclovir have not been standardized and are not widely used. Most VZVs are sensitive to 1.0 to 2.0 mg of acyclovir per ml (reported range 0.3 to 10.8 mg/ml) (2).

DESCRIPTION OF THE AGENT

VZV has the typical morphology of members of the family *Herpesviridae* and, along with HSV, is classified as an alphaherpesvirus. VZV has a DNA genome consisting of approximately 125,000 bp. The linear double-stranded genome ([80 ± 3] × 10^6 Da) consists of a 67 × 10^6-Da long unique DNA segment, U_L, flanked by terminal and internal repeats, and a 3.4 × 10^6-Da short unique sequence, U_S, flanked by internal and terminal repeats (16, 17, 84). The genome exists in a total of four isomers (two major isomers [95%] and two minor isomers [5%]) (11). The virion has a diameter of 150 to 200 nm and consists of an inner icosahedral capsid composed of 162 capsomeres, surrounded by a tegument, and an envelope composed of two or more membranes. The envelope contains essential lipid, and thus the infectivity of the virus is inactivated by lipid solvents (87). The virus produces approximately 30 structural and nonstructural proteins, including at least six glycoproteins, designated E, B, H, I, C, and L, which are at least partially analogous to the glycoproteins of HSV. The glycoproteins play roles in viral attachment to and penetration of host cells, and their recognition by the immune system of the host to these and other viral components results in humoral and cellular immunity to VZV. Immunity to nonstructural antigens undoubtedly also plays a role in host defense. To date, antigenic variation of VZV isolates has not been demonstrated, although minor strain differences can be demonstrated by restriction enzyme analysis of the viral genome (85). Restriction enzyme profiles of VZV isolates reveal the following: (i) there are no detectable differences between varicella and zoster isolates, (ii) the agent is remarkably stable after passage in vitro and in vivo, and (iii) epidemiologically unrelated strains may be differentiated with restriction enzymes. Multiple VZV strains are able to coexist in latent form in the same host. VZV DNA has partial homology to HSV, Epstein-Barr virus, equine herpesviruses, and pseudorabies viruses (28). VZV shares major antigens with herpesviruses that produce varicella-like disease in various simian species (15), and it appears to share minor antigens with HSV (73, 79).

COLLECTION, SHIPMENT, AND STORAGE OF SPECIMENS

Ideally, to make a laboratory diagnosis of VZV infection, the presence of the virus or one of its products should be demonstrated in tissues or fluids from the patient by using, for example, isolation in tissue culture, immunofluorescence (IF) staining, in situ hybridization, and/or PCR. Since VZV is not shed by asymptomatic patients, demonstration of its presence alone in affected tissues or fluids is diagnostic.

Specimens usually examined for VZV are smears of vesicular lesions, skin scrapings, vesicular fluid, and tissues obtained at autopsy. Obtaining smears from vesicular lesions (carefully ensuring that epithelial cells are included in the specimen by vigorous swabbing of the affected area) for IF staining should be attempted wherever feasible, since this procedure is more rapid and is often more sensitive than isolation in cell culture for detection of VZV (9, 14, 74, 94). Lung tissue is the autopsy tissue from which VZV is most frequently recovered. Although it is not yet available commercially, PCR has been used successfully for diagnosis of VZV infection from skin scrapings, vesicular fluid, respiratory secretions, buffy coat cells, and cerebrospinal fluid (CSF) (50–52, 68, 71). The virus has also been demonstrated by in situ hybridization (1, 81).

An acute-phase blood specimen should be taken as soon as possible after the onset of symptoms, to be tested in parallel with a convalescent-phase specimen collected 10 to 14 days later, in an effort to demonstrate a diagnostically significant increase in the VZV antibody titer or the presence of specific immunoglobulin M (IgM). The VZV immunity status is determined by testing a single blood specimen collected before or as soon as possible after exposure to VZV infection.

Smears of Cellular Material from Lesions

The use of smears of cellular material from lesions is a very successful method of identifying VZV quickly and rapidly distinguishing between VZV and HSV-1 and -2. Smears properly collected from the base of fresh vesicular lesions may be used for IF staining for the specific demonstration of VZV antigen in the infected epithelial cells. It is essential that the smears contain a large number of infected epithelial cells, and at least two smears (but preferably three) should be made to permit staining with conjugates to VZV and HSV. To obtain specimens, a sterile needle is used to lift off the top of a vesicle. A sterile swab moistened in sterile transport medium is then used to vigorously swab the base of the lesion, applying enough pressure to collect epithelial cells without causing bleeding. The swab should be used immediately to make smears on nonfluorescent slides, starting at the center of a 5-mm well on the slide and working in circles to the edge. (Slides with wells are commercially available.) The slides should be hand carried to the laboratory immediately for processing. If the slide cannot be delivered immediately, it should be air dried and then flooded with 0.5 ml of acetone. After the acetone evaporates, the slide can be refrigerated at 2 to 8°C for storage. For best results, the refrigeration time should be minimized.

The direct method of staining, with the use of fluorescein-conjugated mouse monoclonal antibodies to VZV or HSV glycoproteins available from commercial sources, is the most specific procedure (see below).

Depending upon the individual circumstances, it is optimal to obtain material for both IF staining and culture (see below). If insufficient material is available for both determinations, the material that is available may be submitted for IF or virus isolation only. Material should be placed in holding medium (see chapter 130) to be used for virus isolation. VZV is a very labile agent, however, so the time during which the specimen is kept in holding medium before being used for culture should be as short as possible.

Vesicular Fluids

Vesicular fluids collected into capillary pipettes, syringes, and/or swabs can be used for virus isolation attempts and electron microscopy but are unsatisfactory for IF staining. Fluids collected onto swabs and placed in holding medium may be used for virus isolation, although it is preferable to culture vesicular fluids without dilution. VZV in vesicular fluids is more stable than that on swabs or diluted into medium. Lesions present on skin for more than 4 days rarely yield infectious virus, but the fluids may give positive results by other techniques such as IF, electron microscopy, countercurrent immunoelectrophoresis (25), molecular hybridization with radioactive or biotinylated DNA and/or RNA probes (1, 24, 77), enzyme immunofiltration (8, 93), or PCR (6, 13, 26, 39, 40, 48–52, 61, 62, 68, 80).

Eventually PCR, a technique by which DNA is exponentially amplified so that it may be identified by molecular probes, is expected to become a standard method for demonstrating VZV infection, but at present it remains a research tool. Its particular value with regard to VZV is that the infectious virus is much more labile than its DNA, so that PCR is a much more sensitive method of demonstration of

VZV than is virus isolation. Another advantage for VZV is that it is possible to distinguish between vaccine-type and WT viruses by PCR and treatment of the amplification products with restriction enzymes, avoiding the step of virus isolation (51).

This PCR assay has proven useful to identify whether rashes are caused by vaccine or WT VZV and to investigate cases of possible vaccine reactions and transmission of vaccine virus to varicella-susceptible contacts. For example, rashes appearing within the first few weeks after immunization have been shown to be due to natural varicella rather than to the vaccine (18). This method has also been used to document the rare instances of spread of the vaccine-type virus from leukemic (39) and healthy (53, 69) vaccinees to other varicella-susceptible individuals.

Crusts from Lesions

Crusts do not yield infectious virus and are not suitable for IF staining or other specific antigen detection methods. If only crusts are available, they may be used for EM or one of the other methods described above such as PCR.

Lung, Liver, or Skin Tissue

Smears of autopsy tissue for IF staining are prepared by excising three or four pieces of autopsy tissue about 10 to 15 mm, holding the tissue with forceps, and gently pressing the cut surface to the clean area of a slide. A series of impressions is made over an area 30 to 40 mm long. Three or four slides should be prepared from each specimen. The slides are allowed to dry at room temperature for 15 to 20 min and then fixed in acetone for 10 min at room temperature and stained as described below. Suspensions of tissue are prepared for virus isolation as described in chapter 5.

IF staining on frozen sections of punch biopsy specimens from prevesicular or maculopapular skin lesions has also been used for the rapid and early diagnosis of VZV infections (63). This method is of limited usefulness for routine diagnosis, however, since it is obviously invasive.

Cerebrospinal Fluid and Blood (Buffy Coat)

Virus has been isolated from buffy coat cells (4, 19, 64, 65) and rarely from CSF (42) of immunologically normal and immunosuppressed patients. Demonstration of VZV in CSF by PCR appears to be more sensitive and useful than by culture (52, 70, 95). These materials should be promptly submitted to the laboratory as whole blood in sterile anticoagulant other than heparin, for example EDTA, and as undiluted CSF in a sterile tube, respectively.

Cytological Examination of Smears from Vesicular Lesions

Smears of cellular material collected from the base of vesicular lesions are prepared as described above. They are fixed with methanol and stained with buffered Giemsa stain at pH 7.0 to 7.2. Microscopic examination reveals the presence of multinucleated, giant epithelial cells with altered chromatin patterns (Fig. 1); these are characteristic of infection with either VZV or HSV.

Electron Microscopy

Vesicular fluids can be examined by EM. Crusts from lesions are ground in 1 or 2 drops of distilled water. When transportation of specimens to the laboratory presents a problem, heavy smears of fluids and crusts may be prepared on glass microscope slides and air dried; material from these smears is reconstituted in a drop of water for examination by EM.

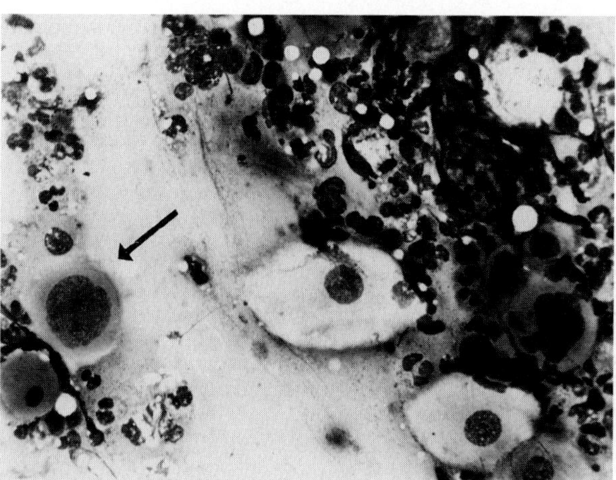

FIGURE 1 Giemsa-stained preparation of material from the base of a vesicular lesion. Magnification, ×160. Arrow indicates a giant cell with a folded nucleus characteristic of VZV or HSV.

Storage and Transport of Specimens

Specimens for virus isolation attempts should be inoculated into suitable cell cultures as soon as possible after collection. If inoculation must be delayed (realistically for no longer than 12 h), specimens may be transported or held on wet ice or in a refrigerator at 2 to 8°C. For longer holding periods, freezing at −70°C (or on dry ice) is required. Refrigeration is preferred for smears to be examined for viral antigen but is not necessary for smears to be examined for intranuclear inclusions or for specimens for PCR. Specimens from vesicular lesions may be infectious, and suitable precautions should be taken in packing and storage to protect postal and laboratory personnel.

ISOLATION AND IDENTIFICATION

Host Systems

Diploid human cell lines or primary human cell cultures are the most sensitive host system for isolation of VZV from clinical materials. Human fetal diploid kidney (HFDK) and human fetal diploid lung (HFDL) cells have been found to be highly satisfactory for primary isolation of VZV; these cells are available from commercial sources. Some laboratories have used human foreskin fibroblasts for isolation of VZV, but their sensitivity compared with that of HFDL cells is uncertain. Primary monkey kidney cells and embryonic guinea pig cells will support the growth of VZV but are less sensitive than HFDL cells. Cell cultures are initiated with Eagle minimal essential medium prepared in Hanks' or Earle's balanced salt solution base and supplemented with 10% heat-inactivated (56°C for 30 min) fetal bovine serum. Inoculated cell cultures are maintained in Eagle minimal essential medium prepared in Earle's balanced salt solution supplemented with 2% inactivated fetal bovine serum. Although this medium will maintain the cultures for 14 days without the need for a change of medium (a period usually sufficient for the development of a specific viral cytopathic effect [CPE]), a change of medium at least once a week is preferable.

Studies have shown that virus isolation, even in optimal cell culture systems, is less sensitive than IF staining or PCR

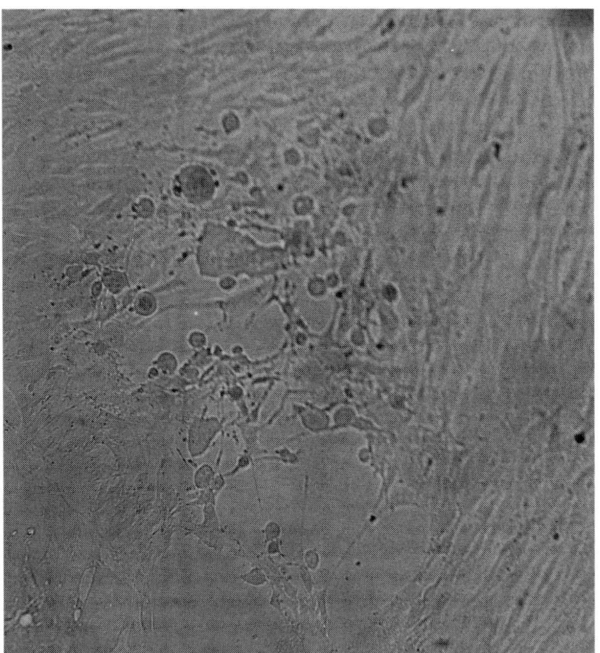

FIGURE 2 CPE of VZV in HFDK cells. Magnification, ×100. Uninfected cells seen on the periphery of the focus of CPE.

on lesion materials for diagnosis of VZV infection (5, 14, 25, 51, 74). The lability of viral infectivity in vesicular lesions and the strongly cell-associated nature of the virus probably both contribute to the difficulty of virus isolation.

VZV cannot be isolated in mouse or embryonated egg host cell systems.

Evidence of Infection in Cell Cultures

Figure 2 shows the characteristic CPE of VZV in HFDK cells. Initially, the CPE consists of small, discrete crescent-shaped foci of rounded and swollen refractile cells; in HFDK and HFDL cells, these may appear 2 to 14 days after inoculation of the cultures with clinical materials, but in most instances CPE is first apparent at 3 to 7 days. The foci of infected cells enlarge and may slowly involve much of the monolayer. The spread of infection can be accelerated by dispersing cells in the infected culture with trypsin (see below) and replanting them in growth medium in the same culture vessel.

Subpassage and Storage of Virus

Infectious VZV remains in close association with the host cell; therefore it is necessary to use virus-infected cells, rather than culture fluids, as an inoculum for serial propagation of the virus. Trypsin-dispersed infected cells are most suitable for subpassage of VZV. The medium is removed from cell cultures in which CPE involves approximately 50% of the cell sheet, and 1 ml of 0.25% trypsin solution is added to each tube culture. After the cells begin to round up (usually after 60 s at room temperature), most of the trypsin is removed and the small amount of residual trypsin is distributed over the monolayer; as soon as the cells detach from the glass surface, they are dispersed in the original volume of growth medium and inoculated into fresh cell cultures.

Virus in infected cells can be stored frozen if the viability of the cells is maintained through the use of a cryoprotective agent such as dimethyl sulfoxide in the freezing medium. Infected cells are dispersed with trypsin as described above and then suspended in Eagle minimal essential medium containing 10% heat-inactivated fetal bovine serum and 10% dimethyl sulfoxide. Infectious virus can be recovered after 18 months or more of storage at −70°C, but infectivity is preserved more effectively by storage of the infected cells in liquid nitrogen. High-titer cell-free virus prepared by sonic treatment of infected cells is stable for at least 5 years at −70°C in minimal essential medium with 10% sorbitol and 10% fetal bovine serum (75). In our experience, cell-free virus is stable for as long as 1 year when similarly frozen in Hanks' solution alone.

Identification of Isolates

Presumptive Identification

Presumptive identification of VZV may be made on the basis of a typical CPE, which is more focal and progresses more slowly than that of HSV. VZV may also be differentiated from HSV by its failure to produce a CPE in rabbit or hamster kidney cell cultures, in which HSV rapidly produces a CPE. The source of the specimen and the clinical manifestations of the illness in the patient should usually prevent confusion between VZV and human cytomegalovirus (CMV). However, if isolations are made from tissue specimens, it may be necessary to distinguish between these herpesviruses. VZV grows well in epithelial cells, whereas CMV generally produces a CPE only in human fibroblast cells. Production of CPE by CMV generally is slower and more focal than production of CPE by VZV. Furthermore, human CMV strains fail to produce CPE in primary monkey kidney cells, but after initial isolation VZV strains will generally do so. The preferred method of differentiation, however, is virus identification with monoclonal antibodies.

Specific Identification

Specific identification of VZV isolates is made by demonstrating their ability to react with a known positive antiserum. Monoclonal antibodies to VZV are available commercially, and their use has overcome problems previously encountered with immune VZV serum produced in animals. In the absence of monoclonal antibodies to VZV, acute- and convalescent-phase sera from a patient with a known case of varicella may be used. Identification is based upon the demonstration of a greater degree of IF reactivity of the isolate with the convalescent-phase serum sample than with the acute-phase sample. However, the use of human sera of uncertain antibody content for identification of viral isolates is not as reliable as the use of monoclonal antibodies. Human sera used for identification of VZV should be free from antibodies to the other human herpesviruses that must be distinguished from VZV, namely, HSV and CMV.

Specific identification of VZV isolates is accomplished most readily by IF staining by the direct method. An alternative method is indirect IF staining (see below) (88).

Antisera to VZV

The problems encountered in the production of VZV antisera have been related in large part to the strongly cell-associated nature of the virus, and various approaches have been used to produce adequately potent VZV antisera free from unwanted antibodies to host proteins; these methods include immunization of monkeys with virus grown in monkey kidney cell cultures, use of density gradient-purified virus for immunization of small animals, and immunization of rabbits made tolerant to human IgG. Hybridoma technology has been used to produce monoclonal antibodies of high potency and specificity (23, 88). Given the commercial availability and convenience of highly specific immune reagents for virus detection and identification, most clinical laboratories today are dependent upon their use. Commercial reagents, monoclonal antibodies for the most part, may be obtained as fluorescein-labeled immunoglobulins for use in direct IF staining or unlabeled for use in indirect IF staining.

IMMUNOFLUORESCENCE STAINING

Preparation of VZV Slides for IF Staining

Smears of VZV-infected cells are required for standardization of IF reagents, as positive controls when IF staining is used for virus detection in clinical materials or for identification of viral isolates, and as an antigen substrate for antibody assays.

The stock virus is subpassaged two to three times to increase infectivity by inoculating trypsinized infected cells from one culture into two cultures of uninfected cells. When cultures show a 3+ CPE at 24 h after inoculation, they are used for slide preparation. In some laboratories, the following technique has been used to control for nonspecific IF staining. The infected cells are dispersed with trypsin and mixed with trypsin-dispersed cells from two uninfected cultures. The inclusion of uninfected cells in the infected-cell smears controls for specificity of IF staining, since only roughly one-third of the cells in the smear should exhibit positive staining. In addition, uninfected cell controls are prepared from trypsinized uninfected cells of the same lot as those infected with VZV. The dispersed cells are suspended in 0.1 M phosphate-buffered saline (PBS) with 2% fetal bovine serum and sedimented by centrifugation at 1,000 × *g* for 5 min. The supernatant fluids are removed, and the packed cells are resuspended in PBS with 2% fetal bovine serum, using a volume of 0.01 ml per tube culture or 0.4 ml per 32-oz (ca. 0.95-liter) flask culture. Smears approximately 5 mm in diameter are made from this cell suspension by placing small drops (approximately 0.005 ml) on microscope slides or by using a cytospin apparatus. The smears are dried at room temperature, fixed with cold acetone for 10 min, and then dried at room temperature. They can be stored at −70°C until used. Before staining, the smears are ringed with a liquid embroidery pen, wax pencil, or diamond pen to retain the conjugate.

Standardization of Immune Reagents

Fluorescein-conjugated VZV immune conjugates (preferably monoclonal antibodies to VZV) should be tested against smears of VZV-infected cells to determine the appropriate "working dilution" for use in virus identification. Ideally, this should be determined in the user's laboratory, although commercially available labeled monoclonal antibodies are packaged in convenient plastic dropper bottles at working dilutions. If unlabeled VZV antibodies are to be used in indirect IF staining, optimal working dilutions of both the viral immune reagent and the conjugated antispecies immune reagent must be determined by preliminary block testing.

IF staining is done by either the direct or indirect method (see below) with dilutions of the reagent against smears of VZV-infected and uninfected cells, and the degree of specific IF is graded as 1+, 2+, 3+, and 4+. A reading of 4+ indicates glaring yellow-green fluorescence; 3+ indicates bright green but not glaring fluorescence; 2+ is dull green fluorescence; and 1+ and ± designate faint and questionable fluorescence, respectively. The working dilution of the reagent is the highest dilution giving specific staining of 4+ and showing no reactivity with uninfected control cells.

Direct IF Staining

If necessary, working dilutions of the immune conjugates are prepared in 0.1 M PBS (pH 7.3); otherwise, monoclonal antibodies supplied at working dilutions are used. Each of the conjugates is added to the specimen smear in a volume sufficient to cover the ringed area (ca. 0.05 ml). Positive and negative control slides for VZV and HSV should also be stained with each conjugate as a control on the reactivity and specificity of the conjugates. After addition of the conjugates, the slides are incubated in a humidified atmosphere at 18 to 25°C for 30 min and then rinsed twice in 0.01 M PBS (pH 7.2 to 7.5) (10 min for each rinse) and once in distilled water. They are allowed to air dry and are then mounted in buffered glycerol solution (9 parts glycerol and 1 part PBS [pH 7.2 to 7.5]) and covered with a coverslip.

Examination with a fluorescence microscope at ×100 to ×400 magnification should reveal specific staining of 3+ to 4+ intensity associated with both the cytoplasm and nucleus of the epithelial cells stained with the VZV conjugate and little or no staining in cells treated with the HSV conjugate (Fig. 3). Vesicular lesion specimens containing too few epithelial cells for definitive examination are reported as unsatisfactory rather than negative. In smears from vesicular skin lesions, positive specimens are defined as those that contain two or more cells with typical apple green fluorescence.

Identification of VZV isolated in cell cultures is performed by direct IF staining when the inoculated cultures show a 2+ viral CPE. Trypsin-dispersed cells from an infected tube culture (or infected cells mixed with those from two uninfected cultures of the same lot as described above) are suspended in 3 ml of PBS with 2% fetal bovine serum and sedimented by centrifugation at 1,000 × *g* for 5 min. Smears for IF staining are prepared on microscope slides from these cells as described above. Enough smears of each suspension are made to permit staining with both VZV and

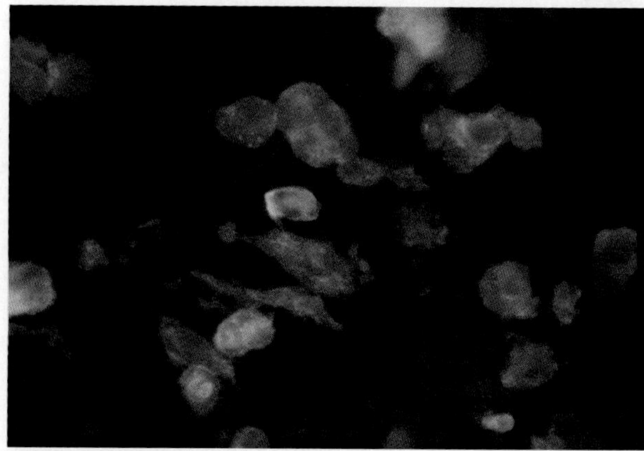

FIGURE 3 IF assay for the detection of VZV antigens. Nasopharyngeal wash was obtained from a patient with an active varicella infection and processed with a monoclonal antibody to VZV by using procedures described in the text.

HSV-1 and -2 conjugates, and smears from uninfected cultures are prepared similarly. The smears are fixed and stained as described above. Positive VZV and HSV control slides should be included in each run. Again, positive results are based upon staining of 3+ to 4+ intensity with the VZV conjugate, little or no staining with the HSV conjugate, and no staining with the uninfected control cells. If commercial reagents are used, there may be a background control stain such as Evans blue that will stain the uninfected cells a color easily distinguished from yellow-green fluorescence.

Indirect IF Staining

Unconjugated mouse monoclonal antibodies can be used for indirect detection of VZV in clinical specimens or for identification of virus isolated in cell culture (88), although direct detection as described above is simpler and preferable. It is essential when using the indirect method to use a conjugate against mouse Igs that is free from nonspecific reactivity with host tissues and host serum components in clinical specimens. This is determined by testing dilutions of the conjugate against infected and uninfected cell smears in the absence of intermediate mouse antibodies. The appropriate working dilutions of the VZV reagent and the anti-mouse globulin conjugate are determined by preliminary block titration.

The working dilution of the VZV monoclonal antibody is applied to the specimen smear; the specimen should also be stained with HSV antibodies as a control. Slides are processed as described above. Positive results are based upon 3+ to 4+ staining of the specimen with the VZV reagent and little or no staining with the HSV reagent.

Identification of VZV Isolates by Using Shell Vials

The shell vial technique is a combination technique involving virus isolation and early specific identification of virus with monoclonal antibody before the development of obvious CPE (72). It is a very convenient method for identification of VZV in clinical specimens. Its deficiency is that after a virus has been identified it is no longer viable, in contrast to standard virus isolation techniques, and cannot be saved or used to test for resistance to antiviral drugs. Therefore, some clinical laboratories inoculate both shell vials and standard cultures for virus isolation at the same time. This approach is also preferable since other viruses may be isolated in the tube cultures. Commercially available shell vials containing coverslips on which HFDL cells are growing in a monolayer are used. Swabs or vesicular fluids are diluted in approximately 1 ml of medium, and 0.2 ml is inoculated directly into shell vials from which medium has been removed and centrifuged for 40 min at 700 × *g* at room temperature. After centrifugation, 2 ml of maintenance medium is added to each vial. Uninfected vials are used as controls. Ideally, six vials are inoculated; three are incubated at 35 to 37°C for 24 h, and three are incubated under the same conditions for 72 h. At the appointed time, the vials are rinsed twice with 1 ml of PBS, with aspiration of PBS between washings. Monolayers are fixed by removing the medium, washing gently with PBS twice, and adding of 2 ml of cold acetone for 10 min. The coverslips are either stored at −70°C or washed with 1 ml of PBS for immediate use. For staining, one vial is incubated with 1 or 2 drops of commercial fluorescein-conjugated monoclonal antibody to VZV (already diluted to a working dilution as sold in the bottle) and another two vials are incubated with 1 drop each of fluorescein-conjugated monoclonal antibody to HSV-1 and -2 for 15 to 30 min at room temperature or 37°C. The vials are again washed with PBS twice and rinsed with distilled water once, and the coverslips are removed from the vials, air dried, and placed cell side down on microscope slides in mounting medium (phosphate-buffered glycerol [pH 7.2]). A coverslip is placed over the specimen, and the slides are examined as above by fluorescence microscopy. Positive results are based upon staining of 3+ to 4+ intensity with the VZV conjugate, little or no staining with the HSV conjugate, and no staining with the uninfected control cells. If all vials are negative after 24 h of incubation, the vials incubated for 72 h should be examined. Important controls to be included in each run include uninfected cultures with conjugate and known infected cultures with conjugate.

PCR

For the PCR assay for VZV, two primer pairs are used, one that generates a 222-bp fragment asymmetrically flanking a novel *Bgl*I restriction site that is present in Oka vaccine type VZV and approximately 15% of U.S. WT strains and another that generates a 350-bp fragment asymmetrically flanking a *Pst*I site that is present in all WT VZV strains but not in the Oka vaccine virus (51). Amplification products are digested with *Bgl*I and *Pst*I restriction enzymes. By examining the DNA fragments or patterns of the products of digestion, WT and vaccine-type viruses can be distinguished. The restriction fragment length polymorphisms are due to differences between circulating VZVs in the United States and Japan and are not reflective of attenuation of the vaccine virus. The molecular basis for attenuation of the Oka vaccine strain of VZV is unknown.

Electron Microscopy

A drop of the specimen is placed on a grid and blotted with filter paper. A drop of 3% phosphotungstic acid (prepared in distilled water buffered to neutrality with 1 N KOH) is then added and blotted. The specimen should be examined in an electron microscope as soon as possible. The demonstration of virus with typical morphology of herpesviruses (Fig. 4) identifies the etiological agent as a member of this group and distinguishes it from the vaccinia virus group, but it does not provide a specific diagnosis of VZV infection.

SEROLOGICAL METHODS

Serological procedures are used for laboratory diagnosis of varicella or zoster infections and also for determining the immunity status to varicella (presence or absence of VZV antibody) in certain individuals. Serodiagnosis is particularly useful for adults who have no history of varicella, since over 75% will have detectable VZV antibody and presumably therefore will have already experienced an episode of varicella (usually subclinical or without symptoms). Adults raised in countries with tropical climates are at increased risk of susceptibility to varicella compared to those from countries with temperate climates.

Serodiagnosis

The value of serological procedures for diagnosis of acute VZV infection is limited to some extent by the fact that heterotypic antibody titer rises to VZV may occur in certain patients with HSV infection who have experienced a prior infection with VZV. This would appear to be due to an antibody response to common antigens in the two viruses (73, 79).

In the past, the complement fixation (CF) test was the

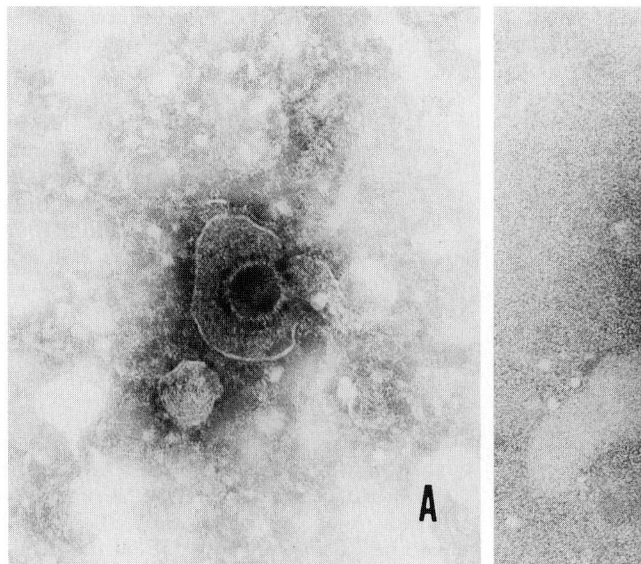

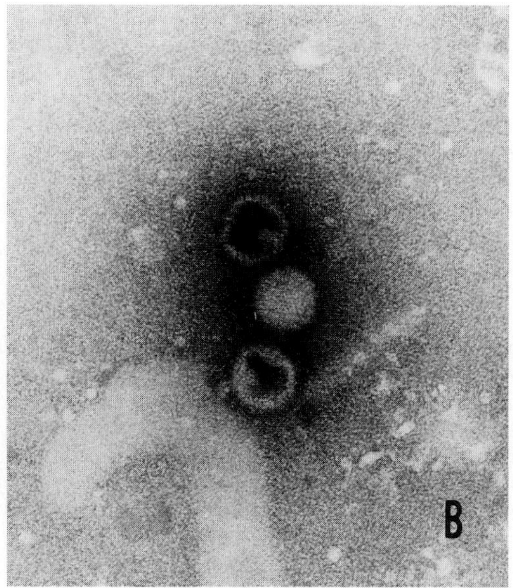

FIGURE 4 Electron micrograph of VZV in a preparation from a lesion swab. Magnification, ×80,000. (A) Enveloped virus; (B) naked nucleocapsids.

most widely used procedure for serodiagnosis of VZV infections. However, viral diagnostic laboratories are increasingly adopting enzyme immunoassays (EIAs) as their principal serological tool for viral diagnosis.

VZV antigens for EIA are available from commercial sources or can be prepared from infected HFDL or HFDK cultures. To prepare VZV antigen, cell cultures are inoculated with a high concentration of trypsin-dispersed, infected cells and harvested several days later, when they show advanced CPE. Glycine-buffered saline (0.043 M glycine, 0.15 M NaCl [pH 9]) is used to rinse infected monolayers, which are then scraped off the glass or plastic with a rubber policeman into approximately 1/20 of the original culture volume of fresh glycine-buffered saline and disrupted by sonication for 30 s at 2.2 to 2.6 A, and the antigen is clarified by centrifugation at 1,000 × *g* for 5 min at room temperature. Uninfected control antigen is prepared in the same manner. Antigens may be stored at −70°C.

For serodiagnosis of infection, acute- and convalescent-phase serum samples must be analyzed in the same test run. A fourfold or greater increase in IgG antibody titer between the acute- and convalescent-phase serum samples is considered diagnostically significant. In patients with varicella, antibodies are usually demonstrable within several days after onset of rash, and they reach a peak 2 to 3 weeks later. The antibody increase is usually more rapid in patients with zoster, and it is common for antibodies to be detectable at the time of onset of rash.

EIA

The technique for the EIA is described in detail in references 12, 22, and 31; however, a description of one EIA for VZV antibody follows (31). Tests are performed in microtiter plates marketed specifically for EIA procedures. Optimal dilutions of VZV and control antigens that clearly distinguish known positive and known negative control sera are determined. Ideally, optical densities (ODs) for positive control sera should be greater than the mean OD of control negative sera by at least 3 standard deviations. Wells are coated with an optimal dilution of VZV antigen or control antigen in 0.06 M bicarbonate buffer (pH 9.5) in a volume of 0.2 ml. After overnight incubation at 4°C, the unadsorbed antigen is removed by vacuum suction, the wells are washed with 0.01 M PBS (pH 7.3) containing 0.05% Tween 20, and protein adsorption sites are saturated by adding 0.35 ml of a 5% bovine albumin solution in PBS and incubating for 4 h at room temperature. The fluids are then aspirated, and the wells are washed with PBS. Serial twofold dilutions of serum are prepared with 0.05-ml microdilutions in wells coated with VZV antigen and with control antigen. (Alternatively a single dilution of serum such as 1:100 may be tested and the OD may then be compared to a panel of known negative, low, moderate, and high serum VZV antibody levels.) PBS (0.05 ml) is added to each well, and the wells are incubated overnight at room temperature. (Alternatively, a shorter incubation period of 1 to 5 h may be tried.) Controls include known positive and negative sera and wells incubated with diluent instead of serum. After the incubation with serum, the contents of the wells are aspirated, and the wells are washed three times with PBS. An optimal dilution of alkaline phosphatase-labeled antibodies to human IgG, prepared in PBS with 5% bovine serum albumin, is added in a volume of 0.1 ml, and the wells are incubated for 2 h at room temperature. The conjugate is then aspirated from the wells, and they are washed three times with PBS. The enzyme substrate, *p*-nitrophenylphosphate (1 mg/ml) in diethanolamine (10%) buffer (pH 9.8) with 10^{-3} M $MgCl_2$, is added in a volume of 0.1 ml, and after incubation at room temperature for 30 min the reaction is stopped by the addition of 0.05 ml of 3 N NaOH per well. The results should be read with an EIA reader, although it is possible to make a rough determination by visual inspection against a white background. The EIA may be used to identify IgG, IgA, or IgM antibodies against VZV.

A number of commercially marketed tests for measurement of VZV antibody by EIA are available and have been evaluated (7, 12, 54). In general, these tests are fairly specific; however, since they may lack sensitivity, they may result in some adults with immunity to varicella being misidentified as susceptible to chickenpox (7, 12). The main advantages of EIA are that it may be automated and that kits used for its performance are commercially available. It is more useful to screen individuals (especially adults) who might have had previous natural varicella than to identify persons who have responded to immunization.

Alternative methods which are applicable to the routine serodiagnosis of VZV infections are anticomplement immunofluorescence (ACIF) staining (27, 67), latex agglutination (LA) (32, 83), indirect immunofluorescence with fluorescent-antibody staining of membrane antigen in VZV-infected cells (FAMA) (90), and the immune adherence hemagglutination test (22). Neutralizing antibody to VZV can be assayed by plaque reduction techniques with cell-free virus obtained by sonic treatment of infected human diploid cells (76); however, this is primarily a research method rather than a diagnostic tool. For demonstration of antibodies after vaccination, the FAMA and LA assays are more sensitive than EIA (32, 83).

Determination of Immunity Status

A rapid and sensitive serological method is useful for determining past infection and presumed immunity to varicella. The CF test is not adequately sensitive for detection of antibody elicited by past infection, giving positive results in only 50% or fewer of individuals with a history of past varicella. EIA is more sensitive than CF, and demonstration of VZV antibody by this method is good evidence of prior infection with VZV (varicella). Both FAMA and LA have been used to determine immunity status, and the results have correlated well with resistance or susceptibility to infection in clinical settings. The FAMA method is somewhat cumbersome, requiring the use of live unifixed VZV-infected cells; however, its sensitivity and specificity make it ideal for determining immunity status.

FAMA Test

The FAMA test is performed as follows. Doubling dilutions of serum in PBS, beginning at 1:2 are made in a 96-well round bottom microtiter plate. Heat inactivation of serum is not required for this assay and should not be done since it may lead to nonspecific results. Cells infected with VZV are harvested when they exhibit 50 to 75% CPE. The medium is poured off the cultures, and the cells are scraped off the glass into any remaining medium and centrifuged at 700 × *g* for 2 min. The cells are taken up in PBS (about 1.5 ml/150-cm^2 flask), and dispersed in 0.025-ml aliquots into microtiter plates containing dilutions of serum. The cells are then incubated for 30 min at room temperature in a moist chamber. PBS is added to fill the well, and the plate is centrifuged at 1,000 × *g* at 4°C for 10 min, after which the PBS is removed by rapidly flipping the plate upside down (this can be done successfully with practice). The washing step is repeated. A working dilution of fluorescein-labeled anti-human IgG (0.025 ml) is added to each well, and the wells are again incubated for 30 min at room temperature. (This assay may also be used to measure specific VZV IgM antibody, in which case a fluorescein-labeled anti-human IgM conjugate is used.) The wells are washed twice, a drop of buffered glycerol (9 parts glycerol to 1 part PBS) is added to each well, and the cells are removed with an aspirator and placed on microscope slides. The cells are covered with a glass coverslip which is sealed with nail polish. The slides are then examined by fluorescence microscopy. The antibody titer is the highest dilution of serum yielding membrane fluorescence.

The sensitivity of this assay is believed to derive from the fact that live cells are used, which preserves the conformational structure of VZV glycoprotein antigens on the surface of infected cells. This structure is probably altered by fixation, which leads to decreased sensitivity for the detection of antibody. A modified FAMA assay in which cells are briefly fixed in dilute glutaraldehyde (0.075%) for 60 s at 0°C and stored at −70°C has, however, been described (92). The FAMA assay may be used to identify IgG, IgA, or IgM antibodies against VZV. The advantage of the FAMA test is its sensitivity; its disadvantages are that live-virus-infected cells are required and that it is technically rather difficult and cannot be automated.

ACIF Test

The ACIF test yields results comparable to FAMA and may be more convenient to perform (27, 67). This method avoids the nonspecific reactivity which may be encountered in indirect IF staining and permits examination of serum at dilutions as low as 1:2 and 1:4 (as do FAMA and LA). Smears of VZV-infected and uninfected cells are prepared as described above for IF staining, with fixation in cold acetone for 10 min. Smears may be stored frozen at −20°C for several months. Optimal dilutions of complement and conjugate are determined by box titrations of various dilutions of each reagent (diluted in Veronal-buffered saline [pH 7.2; 0.1 ionic strength]) against VZV-infected cells treated with appropriate dilutions of known positive and negative sera. Smears of VZV-infected and uninfected cells are treated with dilutions of heat-inactivated (56°C for 30 min) test serum diluted from 1:2 to 1:1,024 in 0.01 M PBS (pH 7.2) and incubated for 30 min at 37°C in a humidified chamber. After a 5-min rinse in PBS, an optimal dilution of cold guinea pig complement is added, and the slides are incubated for 45 min at 37°C in a humidified chamber. After a 5-min rinse in PBS, an optimal dilution of fluorescein-conjugated anti-guinea pig complement is added, and incubation is conducted for 30 min at 37°C in a moist chamber. After a 5-min rinse, the slides are air dried, mounted in 50% glycerol in PBS, and examined under UV illumination. As controls for the test, known positive and negative sera should be included in each test run. Serum specimens are tested against uninfected cells to control for the presence of antinuclear antibodies. The antibody titer is the highest dilution of serum yielding 3+ or 4+ fluorescence with infected cells but not with uninfected cells. The advantage of the ACIF test is its specificity; its disadvantages include the inability to automate the test, a high degree of training required to perform it, and the inability to distinguish between IgG and IgM against VZV.

Latex Agglutination Assay

The LA test makes use of commercially marketed emulsified latex particles coated with glycoproteins of VZV (33, 83). To perform a test, all reagents, which are stored at 4°C, are warmed to room temperature. Doubling dilutions of sera are made in 1-cm-diameter flat circles on a wax-coated 10-cm by 12-cm card supplied by the manufacturer, and the serum is spread evenly over the circle. A 0.025-ml drop of latex emulsion is added to each circle directly from the dropper bottle in which they are marketed. The card is briefly rotated by hand and placed on a mechanical rotator for 10 min at 90 to 110 rpm in a moist chamber. The circles are then examined for agglutination (obvious clumping of the latex particles) under a high-intensity desk-top lamp. For screening sera for immunity status, two dilutions are tested 1:4

and 1:50. A positive reaction in one or both wells is highly correlated with immunity to varicella. If possible, sera (particularly from adults) that are negative at screening dilutions should be retested at dilutions of 1:4 to 1:64 to avoid false-negative results due to prozone phenomena. False-positive reactions are rare (83). For testing acute- and convalescent-phase serum samples to diagnose VZV infection, doubling dilutions beginning at 1:4 can be used. Care must be taken with convalescent-phase specimens, to make certain that high antibody titers such as those greater than 1:4,096 are not missed due to a prozone effect. Thus, if a negative result is seen in a convalescent-phase serum specimen, the specimen should be retested with higher dilutions of serum. The chief advantages of the LA test are its simplicity, low cost, and the rapidity with which it may be performed (15 to 30 min). Its disadvantages are that it cannot be automated, it cannot be used to demonstrate VZV IgM, and the investigator must be certain of the appearance of agglutination of latex and must be aware of the prozone reactions which occur in 1 to 5% of sera, particularly those with high VZV antibody titers.

EVALUATION AND INTERPRETATION OF RESULTS

Clinical symptoms such as rash may be diagnostically deceiving; in one study, 13% of patients diagnosed as having zoster were found to have HSV infection on laboratory testing (47). Demonstration of VZV, specific antigen, or other viral products such as DNA in skin lesion material or autopsy tissue is diagnostic of active infection, since asymptomatic shedding, as occurs with some of the other herpesviruses such as HSV and CMV, is not known to occur. Demonstration of the presence of VZV IgM in serum is also highly suggestive of acute VZV infection.

Isolation of VZV is a relatively slow method and is often less sensitive than IF staining of lesion material or EM, since infectious virus persists for a shorter time in vesicles and is more labile than viral particles and antigens. The combination of virus isolation and early IF staining before the development of obvious CPE in shell vials is a practical alternative and provides significant information within 24 to 48 h. Other means of presumptive identification of isolates as VZV include the failure of VZV to multiply on rabbit or hamster kidney cells (in contrast to HSV) and the ability of VZV to propagate in primary monkey kidney cells and human epithelial cells (in contrast to human CMV). With the increasing availability of VZV-specific immune reagents from commercial sources, specific identification of isolates can be made readily by IF staining or other methods of antigen detection such as EIA. Pitfalls in the use of human sera for specific identification are indicated above.

Currently, the disadvantages of VZV PCR include false-positive reactions due to contamination of specimens with previously amplified VZV DNA (a problem common to PCR in general) and the unavailability of commercially marketed primers. Laboratories with potential VZV specimens amenable to PCR are encouraged to contact research laboratories, where this technique is being carried out until the assay becomes more generally available.

A fourfold or greater increase in IgG antibody titer to VZV antigen, in the absence of a similar rise to HSV antigen, is diagnostic of a current VZV infection. However, a high proportion (up to one-third) of individuals with primary HSV infections who have experienced a prior VZV infection show a heterotypic antibody response to VZV antigen, making a differential diagnosis between VZV and HSV infection difficult in the absence of clear-cut clinical findings. Thus, due to the characteristic clinical picture, it is more reliable to diagnose varicella than zoster by serological means. The best method of diagnosis of acute disease, including possible rashes associated with varicella vaccination, continues to be demonstration of the virus, its antigens, or its DNA.

Although negative results by FAMA, ACIF, LA, and EIA are reliable indicators of susceptibility to varicella, the occurrence of clinical varicella in a few individuals with low titers of VZV antibody demonstrated by FAMA and ACIF indicates that low levels of antibody demonstrable by these sensitive methods are not always a reliable indication of protection against clinical illness. This is particularly true for immunocompromised patients. Occasionally, second attacks of varicella occur (35, 44–46). Detection of antibody to VZV in serum of healthy individuals by FAMA has correlated with protection in up to 96% of persons in one study (35). More recently, similar accuracy with the LA assay has been demonstrated in healthy subjects (83). In general, to determine the immunity status to varicella, testing sera from immunocompromised persons for antibodies to VZV may be less reliable than simply asking the patient whether he or she had previous varicella. In contrast, testing serum from healthy individuals, particularly adults with no history of varicella, is a useful and reliable means of identifying persons susceptible or immune to varicella.

This work was supported in part by grant AI 24021 from NIH. We thank Jean McPhee for her critical review of the manuscript.

REFERENCES

1. **Annunziato, P., O. Lungu, A. Gershon, D. N. Silvers, P. LaRussa, and S. Silverstein.** 1997. *In situ* hybridization detection of varicella zoster virus in paraffin-embedded skin biopsy specimens. *Clin. Diagn. Virol.* **7:**69–76.
2. **Arvin, A., and A. Gershon.** 1996. Live attenuated varicella vaccine. *Annu. Rev. Microbiol.* **50:**59–100.
3. **Arvin, A., C. M. Koropchak, and A. E. Wittek.** 1983. Immunologic evidence of reinfection with varicella-zoster virus. *J. Infect. Dis.* **148:**200–205.
4. **Asano, Y., N. Itakura, Y. Hiroishi, S. Hirose, T. Nagai, T. Ozaki, T. Yazaki, Y. Yamanishi, and M. Takahashi.** 1985. Viremia is present in incubation period in nonimmunocompromised children with varicella. *J. Pediatr.* **106:** 69–71.
5. **Asano, Y., N. Itakura, Y. Hiroishi, S. Hirose, T. Ozaki, K. Okuno, T. Nagai, T. Yazaki, T. Yazaki, K. Yamanishi, and M. Takahashi.** 1985. Viral replication and immunologic responses in children naturally infected with varicella-zoster virus and in varicella vaccine. *J. Infect. Dis.* **152:**863–868.
6. **Baird, R. E., P. Daly, and M. Sawyer.** 1991. Varicella arthritis diagnosed by polymerase chain reaction. *Pediatr. Infect. Dis. J.* **12:**950–951.
7. **Balfour, H. H., C. K. Edelman, C. L. Dirksen, D. R. Palermo, C. S. Suarez, J. T. Kenala, and D. D. Crane.** 1988. Laboratory studies of acute varicella and varicella immune status. *Diagn. Microbiol. Infect. Dis.* **10:**149–158.
8. **Cleveland, P. H., and D. D. Richman.** 1987. Enzyme immunofiltration staining assay for immediate diagnosis of herpes simplex virus and varicella-zoster virus directly from clinical specimens. *J. Clin. Microbiol.* **25:**416–420.
9. **Coffin, S. E., and R. L. Hodinka.** 1995. Utility of direct immunofluorescence and virus culture for detection of varicella-zoster virus in skin lesions. *J. Clin. Microbiol.* **33:** 2792–2795.

10. **Croen, K. D., J. M. Ostrove, L. Y. Dragovic, and S. E. Straus.** 1988. Patterns of gene expression and sites of latency in human ganglia are different for varicella-zoster and herpes simplex viruses. *Proc. Soc. Natl. Acad. Sci.* **85:** 9773–9777.
11. **Davison, A. J.** 1991. Varicella-zoster virus. The fourteenth Fleming Lecture. *J. Gen. Virol.* **72:**475–486.
12. **Demmler, G., S. Steinberg, G. Blum, and A. Gershon.** 1988. Rapid enzyme-linked immunosorbent assay for detecting antibody to varicella-zoster virus. *J. Infect. Dis.* **157:**211–212.
13. **Dlugosch, D., A. M. Eis-Hubinger, J. P. Kleim, R. Kaiser, E. Bierhoff, and K. E. Schneweis.** 1992. Diagnosis of acute and latent varicella-zoster virus infections using the polymerase chain reaction. *J. Med. Virol.* **35:**136–141.
14. **Drew, W. L., and L. Mintz.** 1980. Rapid diagnosis of varicella-zoster virus infection by direct immunofluorescence. *Am. J. Clin. Pathol.* **73:**699–701.
15. **Dueland, A. N., J. R. Martin, M. Devlin, M. Wellish, R. Mahlingham, R. Cohrs, K. F. Soike, and D. Gilden.** 1992. Acute simian varicella infection. *Lab. Invest.* **66:**762–773.
16. **Dumas, A. H., J. L. M. C. Geelen, M. W. Weststrate, P. Werthein, and J. van der Noordaa.** 1981. *XbaI*, *PstI*, and *BglII* restriction enzyme maps of the two orientations of the varicella-zoster virus genome. *J. Virol.* **39:**390–400.
17. **Ecker, J. R., and R. W. Hyman.** 1982. Varicella zoster virus DNA exists as two isomers. *Proc. Natl. Acad. Sci. USA* **79:**156–160.
18. **Feder, H. M., P. LaRussa, S. Steinberg, and A. Gershon.** 1997. Clinical varicella following varicella vaccination: don't be fooled. *Pediatrics* **98:**897–899.
19. **Feldman, S., and E. Epp.** 1979. Detection of viremia during incubation period of varicella. *J. Pediatr.* **94:**746–748.
20. **Feldman, S., W. Hughes, and C. Daniel.** 1975. Varicella in children with cancer: 77 cases. *Pediatrics* **80:**388–397.
21. **Feldman, S., and L. Lott.** 1987. Varicella in children with cancer: impact of antiviral therapy and prophylaxis. *Pediatrics* **80:**465–472.
22. **Forghani, B., N. Schmidt, and J. Dennis.** 1978. Antibody assays for varicella-zoster virus: comparison of enzyme immunoassay with neutralization, immune adherence hemagglutination, and complement fixation. *J. Clin. Microbiol.* **8:**545–552.
23. **Forghani, B., N. Schmidt, C. K. Myoraku, and D. Gallo.** 1982. Serological reactivity of some monoclonal antibodies to varicella-zoster virus. *Arch. Virol.* **73:**311–317.
24. **Forghani, B., G. Yu, and J. Hurst.** 1991. Comparison of biotinylated DNA and RNA probes for rapid detection of varicella-zoster virus genome by in situ hybridization. *J. Clin. Microbiol.* **29:**583–591.
25. **Frey, H., S. Steinberg, and A. Gershon.** 1981. Varicella-zoster infections: rapid diagnosis by countercurrent immunoelectrophoresis. *J. Infect. Dis.* **143:**274–280.
26. **Furuta, Y., T. Takasu, S. Fukuda, C. Sato-Matsumura, Y. Inuyama, R. Hondo, and K. Nagashima.** 1992. Detection of varicella-zoster virus DNA in human geniculate ganglia by polymerase chain reaction. *J. Infect. Dis.* **166:** 1157–1159.
27. **Gallo, D., and N. J. Schmidt.** 1981. Comparison of anticomplement immunofluorescence and fluorescent antibody to membrane antigen test for determination of immunity status to varicella-zoster virus and for serodifferentiation of varicella-zoster and herpes simplex virus infections. *J. Clin. Microbiol.* **14:**539–543.
28. **Gelb, L.** 1990. Varicella zoster virus, p. 2011–2054. *In* B. N. Fields (ed.), *Virology*, 2nd ed. Raven Press, New York, N.Y.
29. **Gershon, A.** 1995. Varicella vaccine: its past, present, and future. *Pediatr. Infect. Dis. J.* **14:**742–744.
30. **Gershon, A.** 1995. Varicella-zoster virus: prospects for control. *Adv. Pediatr. Infect. Dis.* **10:**93–124.
31. **Gershon, A., H. Frey, S. Steinberg, M. Seeman, D. Bidwell, and A. Voller.** 1981. Enzyme-linked immunosorbent assay for measurement of antibody to varicella-zoster virus. *Arch. Virol.* **70:**169–172.
32. **Gershon, A., S. Steinberg, and P. LaRussa.** 1994. Detection of antibodies to varicella-zoster virus by latex agglutination. *Clin. Diagn. Virol.* **2:**271–277.
33. **Gershon, A., S. Steinberg, and P. LaRussa.** 1992. *Measurement of Antibodies to VZV by Latex Agglutination.* Society for Pediatric Research, Anaheim, Calif.
34. **Gershon, A. A., P. LaRussa, and S. Steinberg.** 1991. Live attenuated varicella vaccine: current status and future uses. *Semin. Pediatr. Infect. Dis.* **2:**171–178.
35. **Gershon, A. A., S. Steinberg, L. Gelb, and NIAID Collaborative Varicella Vaccine Study Group.** 1984. Clinical reinfection with varicella-zoster virus. *J. Infect. Dis.* **149:** 137–142.
36. **Gershon, A. A., S. Steinberg, and NIAID Collaborative Varicella Vaccine Study Group.** 1989. Persistence of immunity to varicella in children with leukemia immunized with live attenuated varicella vaccine. *N. Engl. J. Med.* **320:**892–897.
37. **Gilden, D. H., R. Wright, S. Schneck, J. M. Gwaltney, and R. Mahalingam.** 1994. Zoster sine herpete, a clinical variant. *Ann. Neurol.* **35:**530–533.
38. **Hayakawa, Y., S. Torigoe, K. Shiraki, K. Yamanishi, and M. Takahashi.** 1984. Biologic and biophysical markers of a live varicella vaccine strain (Oka): identification of clinical isolates from vaccine recipients. *J. Infect. Dis.* **149:** 956–963.
39. **Hughes, P., P. S. LaRussa, J. M. Pearce, M. L. Lepow, S. P. Steinberg, and A. Gershon.** 1994. Transmission of varicella-zoster virus from a vaccinee with underlying leukemia, demonstrated by polymerase chain reaction. *J. Pediatr.* **124:**932–935.
40. **Isada, N. B., D. P. Paar, M. Johnson, M. Evans, W. Holzgreve, F. Qureshi, and S. Straus.** 1991. *In utero* diagnosis of congenital varicella zoster infection by chorionic villus sampling and polymerase chain reaction. *Am. J. Obstet. Gynecol.* **165:**1727–1730.
41. **Jacobson, M. A., T. G. Berger, and S. Fikrig.** 1990. Acyclovir-resistant varicella-zoster virus infection after chronic oral acyclovir therapy in patients with the acquired immunodeficiency syndrome. *Ann. Intern. Med.* **112:** 187–191.
42. **Jemsek, J., S. B. Greenberg, L. Taber, D. Harvey, A. Gershon, and R. Couch.** 1983. Herpes zoster-associated encephalitis: clinicopathologic report of 12 cases and review of the literature. *Medicine* **62:**81–97.
43. **Johnson, C., T. Stancin, D. Fattlar, L. P. Rome, and M. L. Kumar.** 1997. A long-term prospective study of varicella vaccine in healthy children. *Pediatrics* **100:**761–766.
44. **Junker, A. K., E. Angus, and E. Thomas.** 1991. Recurrent varicella-zoster virus infections in apparently immunocompetent children. *Pediatr. Infect. Dis. J.* **10:**569–575.
45. **Junker, A. K., and P. Tilley.** 1994. Varicella-zoster virus antibody avidity and IgG-subclass patterns in children with recurrent chickenpox. *J. Med. Virol.* **43:**119–124.
46. **Junker, K., C. Avnstorp, C. Nielsen, and N. Hansen.** 1989. Reinfection with varicella-zoster virus in immunocompromised patients. *Curr. Probl. Dermatol.* **18:**152–157.
47. **Kalman, C. M., and O. L. Laskin.** 1986. Herpes zoster and zosteriform herpes simplex virus infections in immunocompetent adults. *Am. J. Med.* **81:**775–778.
48. **Kido, S., T. Ozaki, H. Asada, K. Higashi, K. Kondo, Y. Hayakawa, T. Morishima, M. Takahashi, and K. Yamanishi.** 1991. Detection of varicella-zoster virus (VZV) DNA

in clinical samples from patients with VZV by the polymerase chain reaction. *J. Clin. Microbiol.* **29:**76–79.

49. **Koropchak, C., G. Graham, J. Palmer, M. Winsberg, S. Ting, M. Wallace, C. Prober, and A. Arvin.** 1991. Investigation of varicella-zoster virus infection by polymerase chain reaction in the immunocompetent host with acute varicella. *J. Infect. Dis.* **163:**1016–1022.
50. **LaRussa, P., et al.** 1993. Diagnosis of VZV by PCR, abstr. 1026. *Society for Pediatric Research Annual Meeting.*
51. **LaRussa, P., O. Lungu, I. Hardy, A. Gershon, S. Steinberg, and S. Silverstein.** 1992. Restriction fragment length polymorphism of polymerase chain reaction products from vaccine and wild-type varicella-zoster virus isolates. *J. Virol.* **66:**1016–1020.
52. **LaRussa, P., S. Steinberg, and A. Gershon.** 1994. Diagnosis and typing of varicella-zoster virus (VZV) in clinical specimens by polymerase chain reaction (PCR), abstr. H61, p. 206. *In Program and Abstracts of the 34th Interscience Conference on Antimicrobial Agents and Chemotherapy.* American Society for Microbiology, Washington, D.C.
53. **LaRussa, P., S. Steinberg, F. Meurice, and A. Gershon.** 1997. Transmission of vaccine strain varicella-zoster virus from a healthy adult with vaccine-associated rash to susceptible household contacts. *J. Infect. Dis.* **176:**1072–1075.
54. **LaRussa, P., S. Steinberg, E. Waithe, B. Hanna, and R. Holzman.** 1987. Comparison of five assays for antibody to varicella-zoster virus and the fluorescent-antibody-to-membrane-antigen test. *J. Clin. Microbiol.* **25:**2059–2062.
55. **Lewis, G. W.** 1958. Zoster sine herpete. *Br. Med. J.* **1:** 418–421.
56. **Linnemann, C. C., K. K. Biron, W. G. Hoppenjans, and A. M. Solinger.** 1990. Emergence of acyclovir-resistant varicella zoster virus in an AIDS patient on prolonged acyclovir therapy. *AIDS* **4:**577–579.
57. **Locksley, R. M., N. Flournoy, K. M. Sullivan, and J. Meyers.** 1985. Infection with varicella-zoster virus after marrow transplantation. *J. Infect. Dis.* **152:**1172–1181.
58. **Lungu, O., P. Annunziato, A. Gershon, S. Stegatis, D. Josefson, P. LaRussa, and S. Silverstein.** 1995. Reactivated and latent varicella-zoster virus in human dorsal root ganglia. *Proc. Natl. Acad. Sci. USA* **92:**10980–10984.
59. **Lyall, E. G. H., M. M. Oglivie, N. M. Smith, and S. Burns.** 1994. Acyclovir resistant varicella zoster and HIV infection. *Arch. Dis. Child.* **70:**133–135.
60. **Mahalingham, R., M. Wellish, W. Wolf, A. N. Dueland, R. Cohrs, A. Vafai, and D. Gilden.** 1990. Latent varicella-zoster viral DNA in human trigeminal and thoracic ganglia. *N. Engl. J. Med.* **323:**627–631.
61. **Nahass, G. T., B. A. Goldstein, W. Zhu, U. Serfling, N. S. Penneys, and C. L. Leonardi.** 1992. Comparison of Tzanck, viral culture, and DNA diagnostic methods in detection of herpes simplex and varicella-zoster infection (PCR). *JAMA* **268:**2541–2544.
62. **Nishi, M., R. Hanashiro, S. Mori, K. Masuda, M. Mochizuki, and R. Hondo.** 1992. Polymerase chain reaction for the detection of the varicella-zoster genome in ocular samples from patients with acute retinal necrosis. *Am. J. Ophthalmol.* **114:**603–609.
63. **Olding-Stenkvist, E., and M. Grandien.** 1976. Early diagnosis of virus-caused vesicular rashes by immunofluorescence on skin biopsies. I. Varicella, zoster, and herpes simplex. *Scand. J. Infect. Dis.* **8:**27–35.
64. **Ozaki, T., T. Ichikawa, Y. Matsui, T. Kondo, T. Nagai, Y. Asano, K. Yamanishi, and M. Takahashi.** 1986. Lymphocyte-associated viremia in varicella. *J. Med. Virol.* **19:** 249–253.
65. **Ozaki, T., T. Ichikawa, Y. Matsui, T. Nagai, Y. Asano, K. Yamanishi, and M. Takahashi.** 1984. Viremic phase in nonimmunocompromised children with varicella. *J. Pediatr.* **104:**85–87.
66. **Pahwa, S., K. Biron, W. Lim, P. Swenson, M. Kaplan, N. Sadick, and R. Pahwa.** 1988. Continuous varicella-zoster infection associated with acyclovir resistance in a child with AIDS. *JAMA* **260:**2879–2882.
67. **Preissner, C., S. Steinberg, A. Gershon, and T. F. Smith.** 1982. Evaluation of the anticomplement immunofluorescence test for detection of antibody to varicella-zoster virus. *J. Clin. Microbiol.* **16:**373–376.
68. **Puchhammer-Stockl, E., T. Popow-Kraupp, F. Heinz, C. Mandl, and C. Kunz.** 1991. Detection of varicella-zoster virus DNA by polymerase chain reaction in the cerebrospinal fluid of patients suffering from neurological complications associated with chicken pox or herpes zoster. *J. Clin. Microbiol.* **29:**1513–1516.
69. **Salzman, M. B., R. Sharrar, S. Steinberg, and P. LaRussa.** 1997. Transmission of varicella-vaccine virus from a healthy 12 month old child to his pregnant mother. *J. Pediatr.* **131:**151–154.
70. **Sawyer, M., and Y. N. Wu.** 1993. Detection of varicella-zoster virus DNA by polymerase chain reaction in CSF of patients with VZV-related central nervous system complications, abstr. 1543. *In Program and Abstracts of the 36th Interscience Conference on Antimicrobial Agents and Chemotherapy.* American Society for Microbiology, Washington, D.C.
71. **Sawyer, M. H., Y. N. Wu, C. J. Chamberlin, C. Burgos, S. K. Brodine, W. A. Bowler, A. LaRocco, E. C. Oldfield, and M. R. Wallace.** 1992. Detection of varicella-zoster virus DNA in the oropharynx and blood of patients with varicella. *J. Infect. Dis.* **166:**885–888.
72. **Schirm, J., J. Meulenberg, G. Pastoor, P. C. Vader, and P. Schroder.** 1989. Rapid detection of varicella-zoster virus in clinical specimens using monoclonal antibodies on shell vials and smears. *J. Med. Virol.* **28:**1–6.
73. **Schmidt, N. J.** 1982. Further evidence for common antigens in herpes simplex and varicella-zoster virus. *J. Med. Virol.* **9:**27–36.
74. **Schmidt, N. J., D. Gallo, V. Devlin, J. D. Woodie, and R. W. Emmons.** 1980. Direct immunofluorescence staining for detection of herpes simplex and varicella-zoster virus antigens in vesicular lesions and certain tissue specimens. *J. Clin. Microbiol.* **12:**651–655.
75. **Schmidt, N. J., and E. H. Lennette.** 1976. Improved yields of cell-free varicella-zoster virus. *Infect. Immun.* **14:** 709–715.
76. **Schmidt, N. J., and E. H. Lennette.** 1975. Neutralizing antibody responses to varicella-zoster virus. *Infect. Immun.* **12:**606–613.
77. **Seidlin, M., H. E. Takiff, H. A. Smith, J. Hay, and S. Straus.** 1984. Detection of varicella-zoster virus by dot-blot hybridization using a molecularly cloned viral probe. *J. Med. Virol.* **13:**53–61.
78. **Shepp, D. H., P. S. Dandliker, and J. D. Meyers.** 1986. Treatment of varicella-zoster virus infection in severely immunocompromised patients: a randomized comparison of acyclovir and vidarabine. *N. Engl. J. Med.* **314:**208–212.
79. **Shiraki, K., T. Okuno, K. Yamanishi, and M. Takahashi.** 1982. Polypeptides of varicella-zoster virus (VZV) and immunological relationship of VZV and herpes simplex virus (HSV). *J. Gen. Virol.* **61:**255–269.
80. **Shoji, H., Y. Honda, I. Murai, Y. Sato, K. Oizumi, and R. Hondo.** 1992. Detection of varicella-zoster virus DNA by polymerase chain reaction in cerebrospinal fluid of patients with herpes zoster meningitis. *J. Neurol.* **239:**69–70.
81. **Silliman, C. C., D. Tedder, J. W. Ogle, J. Simon, B. K. Kleinschmidt-DeMasters, M. Manco-Johnson, and M. J. Levin.** 1993. Unsuspected varicella-zoster virus encephali-

tis in a child with acquired immunodeficiency syndrome. *J. Pediatr.* **123:**418–422.

82. **Smith, K., D. C. Kahlter, C. Davis, W. D. James, H. G. Skelton, and P. Angritt.** 1991. Acyclovir-resistant varicella zoster responsive to foscarnet. *Arch. Dermatol.* **127:** 1069–1071.
83. **Steinberg, S., and A. Gershon.** 1991. Measurement of antibodies to varicella-zoster virus by using a latex agglutination test. *J. Clin. Microbiol.* **29:**1527–1529.
84. **Straus, S. E., H. S. Aulakh, W. T. Ruyechan, J. Hay, T. A. Casey, G. F. Vande Woude, J. Owen, and H. A. Smith.** 1981. Structure of varicella-zoster virus DNA. *J. Virol.* **40:**516–526.
85. **Straus, S. E., J. Hay, H. Smith, and J. Owens.** 1983. Genome differences among varicella-zoster isolates. *J. Gen. Virol.* **64:**1031–1041.
86. **Straus, S. E., W. Reinhold, H. A. Smith, W. Ruyechan, D. Henderson, R. M. Blaese, and J. Hay.** 1984. Endonuclease analysis of viral DNA from varicella and subsequent zoster infections in the same patient. *N. Engl. J. Med.* **311:** 1362–1364.
87. **Takahashi, M.** 1983. Chickenpox virus. *Adv. Virus Res.* **29:**285–356.
88. **Weigle, K., and C. Grose.** 1983. Common expression of varicella-zoster viral glycoprotein antigens in vitro and in chickenpox and zoster vesicles. *J. Infect. Dis.* **148:** 630–638.
89. **Williams, D. L., A. Gershon, L. D. Gelb, M. K. Spraker, S. Steinberg, and A. H. Ragab.** 1985. Herpes zoster following varicella vaccine in a child with acute lymphocytic leukemia. *J. Pediatr.* **106:**259–261.
90. **Williams, V., A. Gershon, and P. Brunell.** 1974. Serologic response to varicella-zoster membrane antigens measured by indirect immunofluorescence. *J. Infect. Dis.* **130:** 669–672.
91. **Wilson, A., M. Sharp, C. Koropchak, S. Ting, and A. Arvin.** 1992. Subclinical varicella-zoster virus viremia, herpes zoster, and T lymphocyte immunity to varicella-zoster viral antigens after bone marrow transplantation. *J. Infect. Dis.* **165:**119–126.
92. **Zaia, J., and M. Oxman.** 1977. Antibody to varicella-zoster virus-induced membrane antigen: immunofluorescence assay using monodisperse glutaraldehyde-fixed target cells. *J. Infect. Dis.* **136:**519–530.
93. **Zeigler, T.** 1984. Detection of varicella-zoster viral antigens in clinical specimens by solid-phase enzyme immunoassay. *J. Infect. Dis.* **150:**149–154.
94. **Zirn, J. R., S. D. Tompkins, C. Huie, and C. R. Shea.** 1995. Rapid detection and distinction of herpesvirus infections by direct immunofluorescence. *J. Clin. Microbiol.* **33:** 724–728.
95. **Zoguereh, D. D., R. Saadoun, C. Zandotti, P. Cawston, and J. Moreau.** 1996. AIDS-related varicella zoster meningoencephalitis and radicular pain without cutaneous eruption. *AIDS* **10:**1604–1606.

Epstein-Barr Virus

EVELYNE T. LENNETTE

68

CLINICAL BACKGROUND

Epstein-Barr virus (EBV), the etiologic agent of infectious mononucleosis (IM), infects 80 to 90% of all adults worldwide. Primary infections occur during the first decade of life predominantly in areas with crowded living conditions and poor hygiene. Childhood infections are mostly asymptomatic, but 50 to 75% of delayed primary infections in young adults may be associated with classical IM, a self-limiting lymphoproliferative illness ranging from mild to severe (15).

Most cases of IM can be clinically diagnosed from the characteristic triad of fever, pharyngitis, and cervical lymphadenopathy generally lasting 1 to 4 weeks. In addition to elevated liver enzymes, lymphocytosis with prominent atypical lymphocytes is a common hematologic feature. Complications include splenomegaly, hepatitis, pericarditis, or central nervous system involvement. Rare fatal primary infections can occur in patients with histiocytic hemophagocytic syndrome, in immunologically incompetent patients, and in those with a genetic X-linked lymphoproliferative syndrome (13, 41). In 85 to 90% of IM patients, Paul-Bunnell heterophile antibody tests are positive; false positives may occur in 2 to 3% of patients and can be excluded only by EBV-specific serology. Specific laboratory diagnosis is also needed to differentiate the 10 to 15% of heterophile-negative EBV infections from mononucleoses induced by other agents such as cytomegalovirus, adenovirus, and *Toxoplasma gondii*. EBV-specific laboratory diagnosis is helpful in clinically atypical primary infections of adults and in mononucleoses of children with negative heterophile response.

Transmission of EBV requires salivary contact; airborne or blood-borne transmissions are not important routes of infection (15, 19). Familial transmission of EBV infections is common, as demonstrated by intrafamilial sharing of EBV strains (10). As with other herpesviruses, EBV causes a persistent, latent infection with intermittent reactivations. Infectious virus can be recovered from the oropharynx of the majority of seropositive, asymptomatic individuals, as well as from IM patients. The degree of shedding varies from person to person but remains constant for the same individual (43). Salivary EBV shedding in healthy individuals constitutes the primary means for person-to-person transmission. Infectious virus can be recovered from the immunosuppressed patients at greater frequency and at higher concentration (42). Due to the ubiquitousness of the virus in infected individuals, it has been difficult to ascertain the degree of morbidity attributable to EBV reactivations. While most reactivations are asymptomatic (18), there is evidence that they can be associated with severe, chronic diseases in rare instances (35).

In immunosuppressed patients, EBV-infected lymphoid cells are associated with a number of lymphoproliferative conditions, ranging from benign, polyclonal hyperplasias with no cytogenetic abnormalities to oligoclonal as well as monoclonal malignant lymphomas. The risk of posttransplant lymphoproliferative diseases increases with the intensity of immunosuppressive therapies during organ transplantations (14).

EBV has long been suspected of contributing to the tumorigenesis of Burkitt's lymphoma (BL), primarily a tumor of children in Africa and New Guinea, and nasopharyngeal carcinoma (NPC), an undifferentiated squamous carcinoma with particularly high incidence among southern Chinese (17). Viral antigens and genomes can be detected in both tumors (24, 29, 31, 47). Unusually high titers of antibodies to several antigens can be correlated with the patient's tumor burden. Serology can be helpful in the management and therapeutic monitoring of patients with either malignancy (17).

Based on the presence of EBV DNA, RNA, and clonality of the viral genome, there is now sufficient evidence to link EBV with B-cell lymphomas of patients with acquired and inherited immunodeficiencies (3, 45), with primary central nervous system lymphoma in AIDS patients (22), and with rare sinonasal angiocentric T-cell lymphomas of allograft recipients (25). EBV is consistently associated with about half of Hodgkin's lymphomas (40), with a small proportion of gastric carcinomas (37), and with carcinomas of the salivary glands and the lungs.

DESCRIPTION OF THE AGENT

As a member of the family *Herpesviridae*, EBV has the characteristic herpetic 120-nm enveloped morphology, with 162 capsomeres in icosahedral arrangement. Its double-stranded 172-kbp DNA exists both as a linear form in the mature virion and as a circular episomal form in latently infected cells. Its linear structure consists of a series of unique sequences alternating with internal repeat sequences, all sandwiched between two terminal repeat elements which are joined during circularization (4). Integration of viral into host chromosomal DNA occurs, but it is an irregular occurrence and not site specific.

In vivo, EBV infects primarily lymphoid cells of B lineage. Although it is known to infect other cell types, such as the nasopharyngeal epithelium of NPC patients, the tongue epithelium of patients with oral hairy leukoplakia, and the immature thymocytes of transplant recipients, there is no convincing evidence for EBV infections in the normal nasopharynx, tongue, and T lymphocytes of healthy individuals.

In vitro, EBV has been propagated only in B lymphocytes from human and subhuman primates. Although it shares common antigenic determinants with other EBV-like subhuman primate viruses and is closely related to human herpesvirus 8, EBV is antigenically distinct. It is unique among the herpesviruses in its ability to transform precursor and mature human B lymphocytes, converting them into lymphoblastoid lines capable of continuous growth in culture. Infected cells rarely produce infectious virus in vitro. Most transformed cell lines maintain the viral genome latently at a constant copy number per cell, with varying and restricted expression of the nuclear antigen complex (EBNA 1 to 6) and latent membrane proteins (LMP 1 and 2) (26). In addition to EBNA 1, all latently infected B cells contain high copy numbers of EBV-encoded RNAs, known as EBER1 and EBER2, which are nonpolyadenylated RNAs with unknown functions.

On the molecular level, EBV strains may now be classified into types A and B (sometimes referred as types 1 and 2) based on the polymorphism of their EBNA genes (1). Serologic and PCR investigations indicate that both types A and B have worldwide distribution, although type A appears to be more prevalent than type B (36). Dual infections with both types are not uncommon (38). Biologically, type A strains transform lymphocytes more efficiently than type B viruses (34). In immunosuppressed individuals, coinfection by multiple strains of EBV from exogenous sources as well as de novo recombinations can be readily demonstrated by both culture and PCR (9).

COLLECTION AND STORAGE OF SPECIMENS

Only a single acute-phase serum sample (1 to 5 ml) is generally needed for serodiagnosis. Convalescent serum collected 1 to 2 months after onset is occasionally needed for confirmation and interpretations. Aseptically collected serum can be stored at 5°C for several months. For long-term storage, freezing at −20°C is recommended.

For isolation of excreted virus, 5 to 10 ml of throat gargle collected in serum-free tissue culture medium or Hanks' balanced salts solution is satisfactory. Fetal bovine serum (2 to 5%) can then be added as a stabilizer, as well as antibiotics to suppress microbial growth. With serum additive, specimens can be held for 2 to 3 days with prompt refrigeration or frozen at −70°C for longer storage.

Tissues to be examined for viral nucleic acids and antigens are collected aseptically and refrigerated in saline or balanced salts solution. Suitable for this purpose are lymph nodes, spleen, liver, and biopsies of tumors. Fresh biopsies or thin (5 μm) cryosections, but not formalin-fixed tissues, may be examined for the presence of virus by direct immunostaining of specific EBV antigens. For the detection of EBV nucleic acid and PCR, fresh, frozen, or paraffin-embedded specimens are suitable.

Cerebrospinal fluid (CSF) is rarely useful for documentation of EBV-associated central nervous system disease during primary infection. Neither infectious virus nor a significant level of antibodies has been detected in CSF, although EBV DNA can be detectable by PCR in rare patients. CSF is useful, however, for diagnosis by PCR for EBV-associated brain tumors in immunosuppressed patients.

For detection of EBV in peripheral blood lymphocytes, 10 ml of heparinized (5 to 10 U/ml) blood is needed for culture or 3 to 5 ml of citrated blood for PCR. Blood specimens should be processed as soon as possible, although refrigeration is acceptable for up to 24 h.

DIRECT DETECTION

Electron Microscopy

Electron microscopy detection is not feasible, as EB virions are rarely present in infected tissues, where latency is the norm. One exception to this rule is EBV-infected tongue lesions of oral leukoplakia patients, in which high concentrations of mature virions can be readily demonstrated by electron microscopy (11).

Immunofluorescence

There are two main advantages to using immunofluorescence. The first is its rapidity (2 to 3 h); the second is the added possibility of combining immunofluorescence with histochemical staining to yield additional cytologic information to detect gene expressions on the cellular level, even in single cells. A number of investigational-use mouse monoclonal antibodies can be used for the detection of EBV-specific latent (EBNA 1, EBNA 2, and LMP-1) as well as lytic (viral capsid antigen [VCA], BZLF-1, early antigen-diffuse component [EA/D]) EBV antigens (8, 44). Expression of many of the viral proteins in infected cells depends on unknown host-regulated factors and is therefore variable. Of all the known viral-induced proteins, the latent EBNA complex (principally EBNA 1) is the most consistently present in all the EBV-associated lymphoproliferative diseases and tumors described. As a commercial anti-EBNA monoclonal diagnostic reagent is yet unavailable, carefully selected polyclonal human antiserum remains the most reliable source of reagents. EBNA can be readily detected in touch preparations or cryosections of needle biopsies, using the anticomplement indirect immunofluorescence (ACIF) staining technique with sensitivity of 1 to 2 genome equivalents (33). Commercially available mouse monoclonal anti-LMP-1 can be effectively used to detect EBV-infected Reed-Sternberg cells in Hodgkin's disease, in NPC tumors, and in posttransplant lymphoproliferative disorders. For the detection of lytically infected cells, such as those found in hairy oral leukoplakia lesions and in livers of transplant recipients undergoing primary EBV infections, commercially available mouse monoclonal anti-VCA and EA/D antisera can be very effective (Fig. 1).

Nucleic Acid Detection

For the clinical laboratory, the choice of which EBV nucleic acid procedures to use is dictated by the availability of specimens and the medical questions to be answered. In exchange for the rapidity of the immunofluorescence staining approach, the lengthier and more complex nucleic acid detections offer slightly higher sensitivity, especially in situations in which expression of specific proteins is uncertain. Any of the following procedures may be used to detect EBV in clinical samples: in situ hybridization on frozen or paraffin sections, cytohybridization on cell suspensions, dot blot hybridization, and Southern blot hybridization (5, 12, 40). The

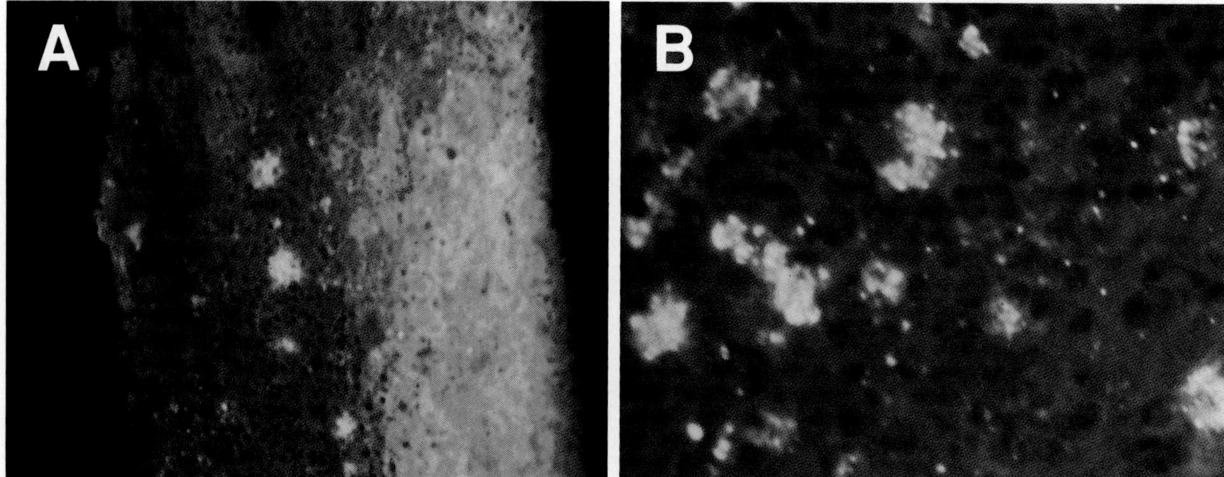

FIGURE 1 EBV EA/D-positive liver cryosection (panel A) and EBNA-positive lymph node (panel B), stained by ACIF.

first two methods require smaller amounts of tissue and can be combined with immunohistochemical staining; they are ideally suited for the detection of EBV in tumor tissues. The latter two involve DNA or RNA extraction and require larger samples but are useful where multiple analytic probes are needed.

PCR, however, has supplanted many of the procedures just mentioned by virtue of its efficacy and convenience in the clinical laboratory. Interpretation of PCR results can be problematic and unclear due to the persistent nature of EBV infection. For example, while a blood sample positive by PCR is indicative of a relatively high viral load in the peripheral blood (concentration of infected lymphocytes in healthy seropositive blood is below the detection limit of most PCR procedures), the increase may have no clinical significance. Previous reports showed that more than 80% of immunosuppressed patients have elevated numbers of EBV-infected peripheral blood lymphocytes, yet most are asymptomatic (42). In contrast, EBV-positive CSF of a human immunodeficiency virus-infected individual is significantly associated with primary central nervous system lymphoma (2). For unambiguous laboratory diagnosis of possible posttransplant EBV-associated lymphoproliferations or other malignancies, a positive PCR result should therefore be complemented by other laboratory data, such as in situ immunohistochemical detection of EBNA or EBERs in hyperplastic or neoplastic cells.

The sensitivity of PCR and hybridization assays can be maximized by the choice of probes. Two general-purpose probes are in wide use for EBV detection. The conserved *Bam*HI W region, coding for a long internal repeat sequence of EBNA 1, is present in multiple copies in EBV-infected cells. Probes based on gene fragments in this region have maximal sensitivity in DNA hybridization assays on clinical samples and in detection of PCR products (2, 39). For in situ hybridization assays, the *EBER1* and *EBER2* genes, each coding for a small RNA expressed in high (10^6 to 10^7) copy number, were found to be highly sensitive in detecting latently infected tissues and tumors (32). The abundance of the EBERs in infected tissues and the high concentration of PCR products have eliminated the need for radioactive probes.

For molecular epidemiologic surveys, PCR primer pairs complementary to the nonrandom polymorphic regions of *Bam*HI WYH and E regions can be used to study the distribution of major EBV types as well as intratype strains.

ISOLATION AND IDENTIFICATION OF VIRUS

EB viral isolation is diagnostically not practical for a combination of reasons. Few laboratories have ready access to freshly fractionated human fetal B lymphocytes, which are the only susceptible indicator cells for in vitro cultivation. In addition, with the exception of saliva or throat gargle specimens, infectious viruses are not present in the latently infected cells in the majority of the EBV-associated diseases. Finally, the standard cord blood lymphocyte transformation assay takes 2 to 4 weeks, too long to be clinically useful. For this assay, freshly fractionated human cord blood lymphocytes are inoculated with clarified and filtered saliva or throat gargle specimens and monitored weekly for 4 weeks. Necrosis of uninfected cultures is usually seen after 2 weeks, whereas virus-positive cultures should show clusters of large proliferating lymphoblastoid cells. Identification of the transforming agent is made by detecting EBNA in these cells by the ACIF procedure or by PCR as described in the Direct Detection section. For details of the transformation assay, please see the previous edition.

Identification of individual viral isolates is now possible by PCR on the basis of polymorphism of the EBNA 2 and 3 genes as mentioned above. In addition, the sizes of many of the EBNA protein family (EBNA 1 to 6) induced are strain dependent. Each isolate induces proteins with distinctive patterns in Western blotting, thus allowing the fingerprinting or EBNotyping of each virus (10).

SERODIAGNOSIS

Serologic testing is the method of choice for the diagnosis of primary infections (20). In patients with classical IM, a positive Paul-Bunnell heterophile antibody result is diagnostic and no further testing is necessary. Rapid qualitative agglutination or enzyme-linked immunoassay test kits for Paul-Bunnell heterophile antibodies are widely available and are effective for 80 to 85% of the IM patients. High levels of heterophile antibodies are seen during the first month of illness and decrease rapidly after week 4. The 3% false-positive rate for the Paul-Bunnell antibodies is mostly in individuals with low but persisting levels long after their primary illness (21). The false-negative rate (10 to 15%) is more frequent among young children than adolescents and adults. For these patients, EBV-specific serologic testing is needed.

Humoral response to primary EBV infections is rapid. Most patients have peak titers by the time they consult their physicians. Testing of paired sera is needed to show significant antibody changes in fewer than 20% of the cases. Effective laboratory diagnosis can generally be made on a single acute-phase serum sample by measuring antibodies to a panel of EBV-associated antigens. The level and spectrum of antibodies are sufficiently distinct in 90 to 95% of the cases to allow classification as to whether the patient (i) is still susceptible, (ii) has a current primary infection, (iii) has had a recent primary infection (within 2 to 3 months), (iv) had a past infection, or (v) may be having reactivated EBV infection (Table 1).

Antibodies to four antigen complexes can be measured, including VCA, EA/D, early antigen-restricted component (EA/R), and EBNA. In addition, differentiation of immunoglobulin G (IgG), IgM, and IgA subclasses to VCA may often be helpful for confirmatory purposes.

Anti-VCA

During the acute phase, both IgG-VCA and IgM-VCA are detectable. Whereas IgM-VCA disappears after 4 weeks, IgG-VCA declines to a lower level but persists for life. Lifelong neutralizing antibodies can also be detected early after onset. Complex neutralizing assays are rarely used to test immunity. As all patients with IgG-VCA also have neutralizing antibodies, anti-VCA antibodies accurately indicate immunity. In patients with BL and NPC, IgG-VCA is maintained at very high levels, usually 8 to 10 times the geometric mean titers of healthy adults. In NPC patients, high IgA-VCA titer and the presence of anti-LMP 2 antibodies are two outstanding EBV serologic features (28).

Anti-EA/D and EA/R

In the majority of patients, antibodies to EA/D show a transient rise in acute phase and are rarely detectable after 6 months. Transient anti-EA/R antibodies follow the disappearance of anti-EA/D and can be present for up to 2 years after onset (23). Moderate titers of both EA antibodies can reappear during EBV reactivation. With BL patients, IgG anti-EA/R are present at moderate to high levels, whereas NPC patients may have high IgG and IgA anti-EA/D titers.

Anti-EBNA

Antibodies to the EBNA complex, as measured by standard ACIF assay using Raji cells, are rarely present in the acute serum of patients with active infection. A gradual increase in EBNA antibodies occurs during the second to third month postinfection to near peak titers at 6 months, which are maintained for life. With severe immunosuppression, the anti-EBNA titers may gradually decrease but rarely disappear.

Anti-EBNA 1 to 6

It is now possible to measure antibody responses to individual EBNA components using transfected cell cultures (6). Following IM in healthy individuals, anti-EBNA 2 and -EBNA 6 antibodies increase transiently within the first 3 months. As anti-EBNA 2 antibodies wane and even disappear, anti-EBNA 1 antibodies emerge to reach peak titer between 6 and 12 months. In contrast, many patients with a chronic or complicated course of EBV primary infections have abnormal EBNA 1 to EBNA 2 titer ratios, primarily due to the persistence of EBNA 2. No clear associations can be made between the anti-EBNA 1 to 2 ratio and the duration or nature of illness. Anti-EBNA 1 is the dominant antibody component in serum as measured by the conventional ACIF using Raji cells (27). The significance of antibodies to other EBNA components is still under investigation.

The levels of each of the mentioned antibodies are usually lower in young patients. However, the profile does not differ with age. The exact titers to each antigen and the time needed to develop a full spectrum of antibodies vary widely between individuals. Also, many individuals may maintain EBV antibodies at high levels with or without reactivations (43). For these reasons, diagnosis based on "screening" titers is not feasible.

The optimal combination for EBV serology consists of measurement of IgG-VCA, IgG-EA, and EBNA. This combination allows the accurate classification of 90 to 95% of

TABLE 1 Serological profiles of EBV-associated syndromes

Antibody-antigen	Antibody presence[a]						
	Nonimmune	Infection			Reactive	BL	NPC
		Current primary	Recent primary	Past			
IgM-VCA[b]	−	+	−	−	−	−	−
IgG-VCA[c]	−	+	+	+	+	+ +	+ +
IgA-VCA[c]	−	+ or −	−	−	−	−	+ +
IgG-EA/D[d,e]	−	+	+	−	+ or −	−	+ +
IgA-EA/D[d]	−	−	−	−	Not known	−	+ +
IgG-EA/R[d]	−	+ or −	+ or −	−	+ or −	+ +	+ or −
Anti-EBNA[d]	−	−	Low	+	+	+	+ +
IgG-LMP2A/B[b,e]	−	−	−	−	−	−	+

[a] +, positive; −, negative.
[b] +, ≥1:10; −, <1:10.
[c] +, ≥1:20; −, <1:20.
[d] +, ≥1:5; −, <1:5.
[e] Present in 50 to 80% of patients.

the patients using a single specimen (see below). The inclusion of EBNA extends the time during which primary infections can be reliably diagnosed to 2 to 3 months. Diagnosis of primary infection should not rely on the detection of IgM-VCA. Both false-positive and false-negative results occur in IgM-VCA testing. The former is due to the presence of rheumatoid factor (16), while the latter results from late collection of serum samples.

Antibody Assays

There are a large number of serologic assays in use today. Commercially available kits are of two types: immunofluorescent assays (IFA) and enzyme-linked immunoassays (EIA). IFAs have fairly uniform performance characteristics as a group, principally because the cell substrates and their preparation are similar among suppliers. The performance of EIAs, on the other hand, is much more variable. Due to the plethora of antigen preparations used in the different kits, ranging from cell extracts to recombinant or fusion proteins to synthetic peptides, the reference criteria for interpretations established systematically for the immunofluorescence assays (Table 1) may not apply to all EIAs, even when the antigens are referred to by the same name. For example, EBNA is a complex of several large, native proteins as detected in the Raji cell by ACIF, whereas the same designation may be given to a single oligopeptide in an EIA assay. In general, there is good agreement between the IFA and EIA for VCA-IgG, fair agreement for the EBNA complex, and poor agreement for VCA-IgM and EA antibodies. In actual practice, the availability of more test choices has complicated, not simplified, serologic interpretations.

For the reference IFA test, the following are the most commonly used cell lines (21). (See the sixth edition of this Manual for details.)

For anti-VCA, either P3-HRl or B 95-8 is suitable. They are both virus producer cell lines, with 10 to 15% of the cells in the culture expressing VCA at any given time.

The Raji line is used for anti-EBNA tests; it expresses only the EBNA complex; VCA is absent and EA antigens are rarely detectable under normal culture conditions.

For EA/D, EA/R, Raji cells are treated with various chemicals, including tumor-promoting agents (46), iododeoxyuridine (7), and sodium butyrate (30) to express both antigens. As negative control, an EBV-negative cell line (BJAB, a B-lymphocyte line, or MOLT-4, a T-lymphoid line) must be included to exclude nonspecific antinuclear antibodies in some sera.

In the VCA-IFA procedure, acetone-fixed cells are incubated (30 min at 37°C) with fourfold dilutions of the patient's serum, followed with fluorescein isothiocyanate (FITC)-conjugated antiserum to the appropriate anti-human Ig subclasses (IgG, IgM, IgA).

Both EA/D and EA/R are present in acetone-fixed EA producing cells. Morphologically characteristic EA/D-positive cells appear as cells with diffuse, cytoplasmic speckled staining, often with a fine granular halo where the antigens have leaked out during fixation. EA/R, in contrast, is restricted to the cytoplasmic regions (probably Golgi apparatus) within the cells. Methanol fixation of the EA smears preferentially removes EA/R only; hence it can be used to prepare smears for the differentiation of the two antigens.

The more sensitive ACIF assay must be used to detect the low concentration of EBNA in EBV-transformed cells. Raji smears, fixed with a mixture of acetone and methanol, are incubated with the patient's serum. This is followed by successive 30-min incubations with EBV-negative complement (either pretested human or guinea pig) and appropriately FITC-conjugated anti-C3 antiserum. If human complement is used, FITC-anti β_1C/β_1A is preferable. The staining pattern is nuclear and should be present in all the cells.

INTERPRETATIONS

From the titers and profile of antibodies to VCA, EA, and EBNA in the acute phase serum, the patient can be classified as susceptible if anti-VCA is absent; with primary EBV infection if anti-VCA is present and anti-EBNA is absent; or immune with past infection if both anti-VCA and EBNA are present. Eighty percent of patients with active EBV infections produce anti-EA/D titers. These antibodies can be very useful as indicators of current or reactivated infections. In the absence of anti-EBNA, anti-EA confirms a primary infection. In the presence of anti-EBNA, anti-EA suggest a reactivated past infection.

IgM-VCA antibodies are present in approximately 85 to 90% of serum samples from IM patients submitted to our laboratory for EBV testing. Most of the 10 to 15% of serum samples that were IgM-VCA negative had low or undetectable levels of anti-EBNA, indicative of a primary infection within a recent 6 to 8 weeks. A second serum sample tested 4 to 6 weeks later would show a significant rise in anti-EBNA titers in all of the patients with primary disease. Hence, reliance on anti-EBNA instead of IgM-VCA effectively extends the acute phase of the illness. IgM-VCA titers found in the presence of elevated EBNA titers (e.g. >1:20) are of two types. The first is due to rheumatoid factors, which can be completely removed by absorption (16). The second includes infrequent sera with only anti-EBNA 2, indicative of a serum sample collected early during the acute phase before the appearance of EBNA 1. Differential anti-EBNA 1 and 2 testing or EBNA-Raji assays on paired sera (4 to 6 weeks apart) is usually helpful in this situation.

As with all serologic testing, significant changes in EBV antibodies can be demonstrated only with parallel assays. In general, the antibody titers to the various antigens are remarkably stable throughout an individual's lifetime. Significant changes in titers are seldom seen except during the early acute phase of the infection. Antibody level changes seen in EBV-associated tumors occur slowly and are seldom detectable at intervals shorter than 3 to 4 months. In patients with chronic conditions other than malignancies, profiles of EBV antibodies compatible with reactivated patterns are already established by the time most patients seek clinical diagnosis. Their EBV profiles do not undergo observable changes. Serial EBV serology on these patients is not needed.

REFERENCES

1. **Addlinger, H. K., H. Delius, U. K. Freese, J. Clark, and G. W. Bornkamm.** 1985. A putative transforming gene of Jijoye virus differs from that of Epstein-Barr prototypes. *Virology* **141:**221–228.
2. **Arribas, J. R., D. B. Clifford, C. J. Fichtenbaum, R. L. Roberts, W. G. Powderly, and G. A. Storch.** 1995. Detection of Epstein-Barr virus DNA in cerebrospinal fluid for diagnosis of AIDS-related central nervous system lymphoma. *J. Clin. Microbiol.* **33:**1580–1583.
3. **Cleary, M. L., R. F. Dorfman, and J. Skler.** 1986. Failure in immunological control of the virus infection: post transplant lymphomas, p. 163–181. *In* M. A. Epstein and B.

G. Achong (ed.), *The Epstein-Barr Virus: Recent Advances*. William Heinemann Medical Books, London.

4. **Dambaugh, T., K. Hennessy, S. Fennewald, and E. Kieff.** 1986. The virus genome and its expression in latent infection, p. 13–45. *In* M. A. Epstein and B. G. Achong (ed.), *The Epstein-Barr Virus: Recent Advances*. William Heinemann Medical Books, London.
5. **De Souza, Y. G., U. K. Freese, D. Greenspan, and J. S. Greenspan.** 1990. Diagnosis of Epstein-Barr virus infection in hairy leukoplakia by using nucleic acid hybridization and noninvasive techniques. *J. Clin. Microbiol.* **28:**2775–2778.
6. **Dillner, J., and B. Kallin.** 1988. The Epstein-Barr virus encoded proteins. *Adv. Cancer Res.* **50:**95–151.
7. **Gerber, P., and S. Lucas.** 1972. Epstein-Barr virus associated antigens activated in human cells by 5-bromodeoxyuridine. *Proc. Soc. Exp. Biol. Med.* **141:**431–435.
8. **Grasser, F. A., P. G. Murray, E. Kremmer, K. Klein, K. Remberger, W. Feiden, G. Reynolds, G. Niedobitek, L. S. Young, and N. Mueller-Lantzsch.** 1994. Monoclonal antibodies directed against the Epstein-Barr virus-encoded nuclear antigen 1 (EBNA1): immunohistologic detection of EBNA1 in the malignant cells of Hodgkin's disease. *Blood* **84:**3792–3798.
9. **Gratama, J. W., E. T. Lennette, B. Lonnqvist, M. A. Oosterveer, G. Klein, O. Ringden, and I. Ernberg.** 1992. Detection of multiple Epstein-Barr viral strains in allogeneic bone marrow transplant recipients. *J. Med. Virol.* **37:** 39–47.
10. **Gratama, J. W., M. A. P. Oosterveer, G. Klein, and I. Ernberg.** 1990. EBNA size polymorphism can be used to trace Epstein-Barr virus spread within families. *J. Virol.* **64:** 4703–4708.
11. **Greenspan, J. S., D. Greenspan, E. T. Lennette, D. I. Abrams, M. A. Conant, V. Petersen and U. K. Freese.** 1985. Replication of Epstein-Barr virus within the epithelial cells of oral "hairy" leukoplakia, an AIDS-associated lesion. *N. Engl. J. Med.* **313:**1564–1571.
12. **Greenspan, J. S., D. Greenspan, E. T. Lennette, D. I. Abrams, M. A. Conant, and V. H. Petersen.** 1985. Oral viral leukoplakia—a new AIDS-associated condition. *Adv. Exp. Med. Biol.* **187:**123–128.
13. **Grierson, H., and D. T. Purtillo.** 1987. Epstein-Barr virus infections in males with the X-linked lymphoproliferative syndrome. *Ann. Int. Med.* **106:**538–545.
14. **Hanto, D. W., G. Frizzera, K. J. Gajl-Peczalska, and R. L. Simmons.** 1985. Epstein-Barr virus, immunodeficiency and B cell lymphoproliferation. *Transplantation* **30:** 461–472.
15. **Henle, G., and W. Henle.** 1979. The virus as the etiologic agent of infectious mononucleosis, p. 197–307. *In* M. A. Epstein and B. G. Achong (ed.), *The Epstein-Barr Virus*. Springer Verlag KG, Berlin.
16. **Henle, G., E. T. Lennette, M. A. Alspaugh, and W. Henle.** 1979. Rheumatoid factor as a cause of positive reactions in tests for Epstein-Barr virus-specific IgM antibodies. *Clin. Exp. Immunol.* **36:**415–422.
17. **Henle, W., and G. Henle.** 1974. Epstein-Barr virus and human malignancies. *Cancer* **34:**1368–1374.
18. **Henle, W., and G. Henle.** 1980. Consequences of persistent Epstein-Barr virus infections, p. 3–9. *In* M. Essex, G. Todaro, and H. zur Hauzen (ed.), *Viruses in Naturally Occuring Cancers. Cold Spring Harbor Conferences on Cell Proliferation.* Cold Spring Harbor Laboratory, Cold Spring Harbor, N.Y.
19. **Henle, W., and G. Henle.** 1985. Epstein-Barr virus and blood transfusions, p. 201–209. *In* R. Y. Dodd and L. F. Baker (ed.), *Infection, Immunity and Blood Transfusion*. Alan R. Liss, Inc., New York.
20. **Henle, W., G. Henle, and C. A. Horwitz.** 1974. Epstein-Barr virus specific diagnostic tests in infectious mononucleosis. *Hum. Pathol.* **5:**551–565.
21. **Henle, W., G. Henle, and C. A. Horwitz.** 1979. Infectious mononucleosis and Epstein-Barr virus-associated malignancies, p. 441–470. *In* E. H. Lennette and N. J. Schmidt (ed.), *Diagnostic Procedures for Viral, Rickettsial and Chlamydial Infections*, 5th ed. American Public Health Association, Washington, D.C.
22. **Hochberg, F. H., G. Miller, R. T. Schooley, M. S. Hirsch, P. Feorino, and W. Henle.** 1983. Central-nervous-system lymphoma related to Epstein-Barr virus. *N. Engl. J. Med.* **309:**745–748.
23. **Horwitz, C. A., W. Henle, G. Henle, H. Rudnick, and E. Latts.** 1985. Long term serological follow-up of patients for Epstein-Barr virus after recovery from infectious mononucleosis. *J. Infect. Dis.* **151:**1150–1153.
24. **Huang, D. P., J. H. C. Ho, W. Henle, and G. Henle.** 1974. Demonstration of Epstein-Barr virus-associated nuclear antigen in nasopharyngeal carcinoma cells from fresh biopsies. *Int. J. Cancer* **14:**580–588.
25. **Jones, J. F., S. Shurin, C. Abramowsky, R. Tubbs, C. G. Sciotto, R. Wahl, J. Sands, D. Gottman, B. Z. Katz, and J. Sklar.** 1988. T-cell lymphomas containing Epstein-Barr viral DNA in patients with chronic Epstein-Barr virus infections. *N. Engl. J. Med.* **318:**733–740.
26. **Kieff, E., and D. Liebowitz.** 1990. Epstein-Barr virus and its replication, p. 1889–1920. *In* B. N. Fields and D. M. Knipe (ed.), *Virology*. Raven Press, New York, N.Y.
27. **Lennette, E. T., L. Rymo, M. Yadav, G. Masucci, K. Merk, L. Timar, and G. Klein.** 1993. Disease-related differences in antibody patterns against EBV-encoded nuclear antigens EBNA 1, EBNA 2 and EBNA 6. *Eur. J. Cancer* **11:**1584–1589.
28. **Lennette, E. T., G. Winberg, M. Yadav, G. Enblad, and G. Klein.** 1995. Antibodies to LMP2A/2B in EBV-carrying malignancies. *Eur. J. Cancer* **31A:**1875–1878.
29. **Lindahl, T., G. Klein, B. Johansson, and S. Singh.** 1974. Relationship between Epstein-Barr virus (EBV) DNA and the determined nuclear antigen (EBNA) in Burkitt's lymphoma biopsies and other lymphoproliferative diseases. *Int. J. Cancer* **13:**764–772.
30. **Luka, J., B. Kallin, and G. Klein.** 1979. Induction of the Epstein-Barr virus (EBV) cycle in latently infected cells by n-butyrate. *Virology* **94:**228–231.
31. **Nonoyama, M., C. H. Huang, J. S. Pagano, G. Klein, and S. Singh.** 1973. DNA of Epstein-Barr virus detected in tissue of Burkitt's lymphoma and nasopharyngeal carcinoma. *Proc. Nat. Acad. Sci. USA* **70:**3265–3268.
32. **Randhawa, P. S., R. Jaffe, A. J. Demitris, M. Nalesnik, T. E. Starzl, Y. Y. Chen, and L. M. Weiss.** 1992. Expression of Epstein-Barr virus-encoded small RNA (by the EBER-1 gene) in liver specimens from transplant recipients with post-transplantation lymphoproliferative disease. *N. Engl. J. Med.* **24:**1710–1714.
33. **Reedman, B. M., and G. Klein.** 1973. Cellular localization of an Epstein-Barr virus (EBV)-associated complement-fixing antigen in producer and non-producer lymphoblastoid cell lines. *Int. J. Cancer* **11:**499–520.
34. **Rickinson, A. B., L. S. Young, and M. Rowe.** 1987. Influence of the Epstein-Barr nuclear antigen EBNA 2 on the growth phenotype of virus-transformed B cells. *J. Virol.* **61:** 1310–1317.
35. **Schooley, R. T., R. W. Carey, G. Miller, W. Henle, R. Eastman, E. J. Mark, K. Kenyon, E. O. Wheeler, and R. Rubin.** 1986. Chronic Epstein-Barr virus infection associated with fever and interstitial pneumonitis. Clinical and serologic features and response to antiviral chemotherapy. *Ann. Int. Med.* **104:**636–643.
36. **Sculley, T. B., S. M. Cross, P. Borrow, and D. A. Cooper.**

1988. Prevalence of antibodies to Epstein-Barr virus nuclear antigen 2B in persons infected with the human immunodeficiency virus. *J. Infect. Dis.* **158:**186–192.

37. **Shibata, D., M. Tokunaga, Y. Uemura, E. Sato, S. Tanaka, and L. M. Weiss.** 1991. Association of Epstein-Barr virus with undifferentiated gastric carcinomas with intense lymphoid infiltration. *Am. J. Pathol.* **139:**469–474.
38. **Sixbey, J. W., P. Shirley, P. J. Chesney, D. M. Buntin, and L. Resnick.** 1989. Detection of a second widespread strain of Epstein-Barr virus. *Lancet* **ii:**761–765.
39. **Weiss, L. M., and L. A. Movahed.** 1989. In situ demonstration of Epstein-Barr viral genomes in viral-associated B cell lymphoproliferations. *Am. J. Pathol.* **134:**651–659.
40. **Weiss, L. M., L. A. Movahed, R. A. Warnke, and J. Sklar.** 1989. Detection of Epstein-Barr viral genomes in Reed-Sternberg cells of Hodgkin's disease. *N. Engl. J. Med.* **320:** 502–506.
41. **Wilson, E. R., A. Malluh, S. Stagno, and W. M. Crist.** 1981. Fatal Epstein-Barr virus-associated hemophagocytic syndrome. *J. Pediatr.* **98:**260–262.
42. **Yao, Q. Y., A. B. Rickinson, and M. A. Epstein.** 1985. In vitro analysis of the Epstein-Barr virus-host balance in long term renal allograft recipients. *Int. J. Cancer* **35:** 43–49.
43. **Yao, Q. Y., A. B. Rickinson, and M. A. Epstein.** 1985. A re-examination of the Epstein-Barr virus carrier state in healthy seropositive individuals. *Int. J. Cancer* **35:**35–42.
44. **Young, L. S., R. Lau, M. Rowe, G. Niedobitek, G. Packham, F. Shanahan, D. T. Rowe, D. Greenspan, J. S. Greenspan, A. B. Rickinson, and P. J. Farrell.** 1991. Differentiation-associated expression of the Epstein-Barr virus BZLF1 transactivator protein in oral hairy leukoplakia. *J. Virol.* **65:**2868–2874.
45. **Ziegler, J. L., W. L. Drew, R. C. Miner, L. Mintz, E. Rosenbaum, J. Gershow, E. T. Lennette, J. Greenspan, E. Shillitoe, J. Beckstead, C. Casavant, and K. Yamamoto.** 1982. Outbreak of Burkitt's-like lymphoma in homosexual men. *Lancet* **ii:**631–633.
46. **zur Hausen, H., F. J. O'Neill, U. K. Freese, and E. Hecker.** 1978. Persisting oncogenic herpesvirus induced by the tumour promoter TPA. *Nature* (London) **272:** 373–375.
47. **zur Hauzen, H., H. Schulte-Holthausen, G. Klein, W. Henle, G. Henle, P. Clifford, and L. Santesson.** 1970. EBV DNA in biopsies of Burkitt's tumours and anaplastic carcinomas of the nasopharynx. *Nature* (London) **228:** 1056–1058.

Human Herpesviruses 6, 7, and 8 and Herpes B Virus

JOHN A. STEWART, JOANNE L. PATTON, AND EVELYNE T. LENNETTE

69

HUMAN HERPESVIRUS 6

Clinical Background

Human Herpesvirus 6 and Childhood Disease

Roseola (exanthem subitum) is a common infectious disease of early childhood, characterized by an abrupt rise in temperature as high as 40°C followed in 2 to 4 days by a rapid drop in temperature that coincides with the appearance of an erythematous maculopapular rash that persists for 1 to 3 days. Physical findings that may occur before the rash appears are palpebral edema and suboccipital, postauricular, and cervical lymphadenopathy. Despite the fever, the illness is mild in most children unless complicated by convulsions (32, 49), but other neurologic symptoms and encephalitis occur, although they are rare. The rash may be either a patchy maculopapular exanthem similar to that seen with rubella or a more confluent eruption like that seen with measles. The skin lesions are not vesicular and appear first on the neck, behind the ears, and on the back; they may spread quickly to the rest of the body. The face and distal extremities are usually spared. The total illness lasts from 2 to 7 days and usually has no sequelae. A likely mode of transmission in childhood is by oral contact of a susceptible child with infected saliva or respiratory secretions of a family member. However, viral DNA has been detected in genital secretions (7), and sexual transmission is also possible.

Yamanishi et al. (58) were the first to isolate human herpesvirus 6 (HHV-6) from peripheral blood lymphocytes (PBL) of four children with roseola who also had a rise in HHV-6 antibody. These results verified the long-held belief, based on clinical features (8) and positive transmission studies in humans (reviewed in reference 7), that this "viral exanthemlike" illness was caused by a virus. HHV-6 has been confirmed as the causative agent of roseola by virus isolation (49), seroconversion (25), and PCR detection of HHV-6 DNA in cerebrospinal fluid (CSF) (32, 49) and PBL of children.

Population studies indicate that 90% of children become seropositive to HHV-6 between 6 and 24 months of age and that maternal antibodies appear to protect infants younger than 5 to 6 months of age from infection. Primary infection with HHV-6 takes the form of roseola (8) in 30% of children. Primary infection can also result in a rash without fever or a fever without rash. Of 243 febrile children younger than 3 years of age presenting at a hospital, HHV-6 was isolated from peripheral blood cells of 34 (14%) (42). Fever (mean 39.7°C), tympanic membrane inflammation, malaise, and irritability were found frequently. Serologic studies indicated that HHV-6 infection was primary in most children. A rash was noted or reported within a few days of the initial visit in 12 (35%) of the 34 HHV-6-positive children.

There is increasing recognition of the role of HHV-6 infection of the central nervous system (CNS) as a cause of neurologic complications (7). In a series of 21 roseola patients with generalized or focal seizures during their illness, HHV-6 DNA was amplified from the CSF of 6 of the 11 infants tested, including 3 with encephalitis (49). In another series of 10 patients with neurologic symptoms during the febrile phase of roseola, HHV-6 DNA was detected in the CSF of 9 (32). HHV-6 DNA was also detected in all CSF samples from eight children who had three or more febrile convulsions and were studied during their most recent seizure (32). Other studies indicate that the CNS may be a site of viral latency or persistence and suggest that recurrent febrile convulsions may be associated with reactivation of HHV-6 (7).

HHV-6 Infection and Adult Disease

Primary infection with HHV-6 is a rare event in adults, but syndromes that include lymphadenopathy, heterophile-negative mononucleosis-like illness, and hepatitis (25, 48) have occasionally been described. Steeper et al. (48) examined patients with mononucleosis-like illnesses who did not have Epstein-Barr virus (EBV) or human cytomegalovirus (HCMV) infection and found active HHV-6 infection in 8 of the 27 heterophile-negative patients. The clinical picture included a short febrile illness, mild cervical lymphadenopathy, elevations in liver enzyme levels suggestive of active viral hepatitis in two patients, and a prolonged febrile illness in a human immunodeficiency virus (HIV)-positive patient. Three similar patients with mononucleosis-like and/or hepatitis illnesses have been found to have acute HHV-6 infection (25).

HHV-6 activity has also been detected in organ recipients (most of whom are HHV-6 seropositive) following renal, cardiac, and bone marrow transplantation (7). After renal transplantation, about 50% of patients have an increase in antibody titer, viremia can be detected in a small number, and viral antigen has been detected in some rejected kidneys. No consistent association has been found between infection and organ rejection. Symptoms associated with HHV-6 reactivation or reinfection after marrow transplantation are malaise, fever and/or rash, leukopenia, interstitial pneumonitis, CNS involvement (seizures), and decreased bone marrow function (9, 27).

Initially, a number of studies reported a higher prevalence of immunofluorescence assay (IFA) antibody to HHV-6 in patients with connective tissue diseases (e.g., sarcoidosis), lymphomas, lymphoid hyperplasia, and immunosuppression or -deficiency (7). However, more sensitive assays have shown that the actual seropositive rate for the healthy population exceeds 90% (40, 45). Thus, the studies showing an increased seroprevalence rate for patients with certain diseases probably indicate that the patients have higher antibody titers to HHV-6 but the prevalence of infection is not increased compared with that in controls. Higher antibody titers to a number of viruses are also found in patients with connective tissue diseases, leukemia, lymphoid hyperplasia, HIV infection, and chronic fatigue syndrome. This observation may reflect a polyclonal B-cell stimulation or even increased reactivation of latent viruses, such as HHV-6, in patients with these diseases.

Description of the Agent

General Properties

After its discovery in 1986, HHV-6 was quickly recognized as a unique member of the family *Herpesviridae* that is serologically (44) and genetically (22, 35) distinct from the other herpesviruses. HHV-6 DNA is clearly distinct from the DNA of the other human herpesviruses, herpes simplex virus types 1 and 2 (HSV-1 and HSV-2), varicella-zoster virus, HCMV, and EBV, by both restriction endonuclease digestion and nucleic acid hybridization (35). However, HHV-6 does appear to have a biologic similarity to the other members of the herpesvirus family in its ability to survive in a latent form in the human host. The virus envelope encloses an icosahedral capsid of 162 capsomeres, with a core containing a double-stranded DNA genome of 161 to 170 kb (34). HHV-6 is inactivated by ether and lipid solvents. Cell-free virus does not survive cycles of freezing and thawing unless stored in a protein-rich environment, such as skim milk medium. More than 20 polypeptides ranging in size from 30 to 220 kDa are found in solubilized cells (3) or purified virions (57). One of these, a 101-kDa polypeptide, is strongly reactive on Western immunoblot analysis with both HHV-6-positive human sera and a murine monoclonal antibody. Reactivity to this polypeptide is valuable in diagnostic testing since it is a specific marker for HHV-6 infection.

HHV-6 Strain Groups

HHV-6 (strain GS) was first isolated from a patient with a lymphoproliferative disorder (44). Additional isolates of importance came from patients with AIDS in Uganda (strain U1102) and Zaire (strain Z29). As independent isolates of HHV-6 were obtained and compared, it became clear that they formed two groups that differed in molecular and biological properties (1, 7, 22). Differences in restriction site polymorphisms that extend across the genome have been able to classify all isolates into two groups. However, the nucleotide sequence identity for several regions of the viral genome is very high, ranging from 94 to 96% between the variant groups. It was only after much debate that a decision was made to formally recognize GS and U1102-like viruses as HHV-6 variant A and Z29-like viruses as HHV-6 variant B (1). The biological differences in the two variants extend to the clinical level as well, with almost all HHV-6 isolates from roseola and related febrile illnesses found to be variant B (HHV-6B) (16). Both variants have been isolated from immunocompromised individuals. Variant A (HHV-6A) has recently been isolated during an acute febrile illness of infants in Zambia (29), but it has been detected more frequently in patients with Kaposi's sarcoma, AIDS, and CFS than has variant B (17). No serologic method to distinguish the immune response to the variants has been described.

Collection and Storage of Specimens

In acute illness, most isolates of HHV-6 have been obtained from PBL samples. Successful isolation is most frequent from the PBL of roseola patients in the febrile stage before rash appears and nears zero after 4 days of rash. Heparinized blood samples should be collected aseptically, and the mononuclear cells should be purified on Ficoll gradients. For best results, cultures should be set up within 24 h of blood collection. Freezing mononuclear cells for later isolation is not advised because the virus is highly labile and survives freeze-thaw cycles poorly. Although the DNA of HHV-6 is frequently found in PBL and saliva of normal adults, the virus is infrequently isolated from PBL of these adults. Detection of the virus or DNA in saliva or respiratory secretions in acute illness has not been evaluated.

Detection of Viral Nucleic Acid

Cloned fragments of HHV-6 DNA can be used to detect the genome in situ or by Southern blot hybridization assays (7). A number of primer and probe sequences have been developed to perform diagnostic PCR assays. The PCR has been successfully used to detect HHV-6 DNA from (i) the blood, saliva, and CSF of roseola patients (32, 49); (ii) the blood of patients with AIDS and lymphoproliferative disorders; (iii) the blood and tissue specimens of immunosuppressed patients (9, 13, 27); and (iv) the blood and saliva of healthy seropositive adults and children. There is insufficient information from quantitation studies to correlate the amount of HHV-6 DNA with clinical manifestations. Some of the primer sequences described are useful for discrimination between HHV-6A and HHV-6B and do not react with the closely related human herpesvirus 7 (HHV-7).

The rate of DNA detection in healthy seropositive controls varies widely from study to study, reflecting differences in the number of PBL sampled, the primer pairs used, and the number of cycles performed in the assays. Because positive PCR findings can result from the presence of only a few copies of HHV-6 DNA in circulating lymphocytes or tissue samples, measurement of the amount of DNA detected is needed to correctly assess the role of HHV-6 infection in the disease states being investigated (13). More baseline studies in normal individuals in the general population are needed to help evaluate positive results.

Virus Isolation

HHV-6 has been isolated from the peripheral blood by primary culture of mononuclear cells and by cocultivation of these cells with either stimulated cord blood lymphocytes (CBL) or adult PBL (35). Isolation rates are higher with CBL. After isolation, some strains are able to grow in continuous lymphocyte cell lines. For cocultivation studies, mononuclear cells are purified from fresh human cord blood on Ficoll gradients and stimulated to blast formation by culturing for 1 to 3 days with 0.002% phytohemagglutinin (PHA), and 5% interleukin-2 in growth medium (RPMI 1640 with 10% fetal calf serum, 0.01 mg of hydrocortisone per ml, and antibiotics). The cord cells are cocultivated with an equal volume of mononuclear cells from patients, incubated at 37°C in 5% CO_2, observed twice weekly for cytopathic effects, and assayed for the appearance of HHV-6 antigen by the anticomplement immunofluorescence test (ACIF) or IFA after 7 to 10 days. All cell cultures are passaged every 7 to 10 days into CBL freshly stimulated with PHA in growth media.

Identification

Large balloon-like cells may appear after cocultivation with CBL, suggesting that infection is present. However, such cells may also appear in the absence of infection, and therefore immunologic tests are needed to confirm infection. IFA and the ACIF test, performed with well-characterized human sera, have been used to document HHV-6 isolation but do not differentiate HHV-6 from HHV-7. It is preferable to use commercially available monoclonal antibodies to HHV-6 or in situ hybridization with HHV-6-specific probe sequences to exclude HHV-7 and give precise, HHV-6 variant-specific identification. Monoclonal antibodies to the other HHV types should not react with HHV-6-infected cells. Some of the isolates from saliva initially identified as HHV-6 (41) have been subsequently identified as HHV-7 with HHV-7-specific reagents (7).

Serologic Diagnosis

A variety of serologic assays for HHV-6, including IFA, ACIF, enzyme immunoassay (EIA), immunoblotting, and neutralization, are in use. All these assays are potentially sensitive and specific enough to evaluate samples from clinical studies and detect a rise in antibody titer. However, they are not as useful as virus isolation or DNA detection methods for establishing an early diagnosis of HHV-6 infection because immunoglobulin M (IgM) antibody does not appear until 5 to 7 days after onset and IgG does not appear until 7 to 10 days after onset. The serologic diagnosis of recent HHV-6 infection is based on finding a fourfold or greater increase in the IFA or ACIF titer or a significant increase in EIA values between acute- and convalescent-phase sera. Seroconversion in paired serum specimens usually indicates a primary infection with HHV-6. However, when IFA or the ACIF test is used, both of which are less sensitive than the EIA, seroconversion may be difficult to distinguish from a rising titer in a person with virus reactivation. Serologic studies of childhood illnesses helped establish that primary infection with HHV-6 occurs in children with roseola (58). Serologic studies are of the greatest use in epidemiologic studies and prospective studies of the role of HHV-6 in various diseases. Future studies of this type must take into account the partial cross-reaction found between HHV-6 and HHV-7 (56) and the difficulty in distinguishing the serologic response to the two HHV-6 variants.

The effects of reactivation upon antibody production are not yet defined. Rising or elevated HHV-6 IgG titers have been found in patients actively infected with HCMV and EBV (18, 26), but the relative role of each virus in the illness was not clear. Complete removal of HCMV IgG reactivity from five serum samples (from patients who had a primary HCMV infection and a rise in the HHV-6 IgG titer) had no effect on the HHV-6 titer of four, but the fifth had an eightfold drop in the HHV-6 IgG titer (26). Two adults with acute febrile illnesses had IgG present in baseline samples and still developed HHV-6 IgM (18). Thus, IgM is produced in both primary and reactivated HHV-6 infections and may be detected by both EIA and IFA. In addition, major rises in the IgG titer may accompany primary HCMV or EBV infections.

IFA

One widely used serologic procedure for HHV-6 is IFA. As IFAs have become more sensitive, their estimation of antibody prevalence in the general population has risen to >90% (7). With the discovery that HHV-6 (GS) can be cultivated efficiently in several T-cell lines, such as HSB-2, the IFA became easier to perform and more reproducible.

ACIF Assay

To avoid the strong nonspecific fluorescent staining of CBL frequently observed with the IFA, an ACIF test was adopted that greatly reduced nonspecific fluorescence and gave a stronger signal with positive cells. This assay has been found to be highly specific for HHV-6 and to have minimal cross-reactivity with the other HHVs (35). The ACIF test has been effectively used in detecting the antibody response of roseola patients (58) and in seroprevalence studies.

The ACIF test is performed by adding heat-inactivated serum specimens to wells on slides containing acetone-fixed HHV-6 (GS or Z29)-infected cells. After incubation and washing steps, either guinea pig complement or a human serum containing complement that does not have detectable antibodies to HHV-6 at the working dilution is added. After further incubation and washing steps, complement fixation is detected by addition of fluorescein-labeled goat anti-human C3 reagent. Characteristically, cytoplasmic fluorescence is somewhat granular whereas nuclear fluorescence is solid and bright.

EIA

Several EIA methods that use antigen prepared from purified virions from infected cell culture medium (45) or HHV-6-infected whole-cell lysates (6, 40) have been described. To perform an EIA for antibody to HHV-6, Saxinger et al. (45) prepared antigen by disruption of virions or infected HSB-2 cells in a Tris (pH 8), Triton X-100, 0.6M NaCl buffer. The clarified lysate was diluted to a concentration of 0.5 μg/100μl and used to coat microtiter plates. Other methods of preparing EIA antigen involve harvesting infected cells in buffers from pH 7.4 to 9.6, disrupting the cells by freeze-thaw cycles and/or sonication, and usually coating microtiter plates in sodium carbonate buffer (pH 9.6). After another washing cycle, antigen-coated plates are incubated with serum dilutions and thoroughly washed with buffer containing detergent. Bound antibody-antigen complex is detected with enzyme-conjugated anti-human IgG reagents and their appropriate substrates. The specificity of the EIA reaction has been documented by preincubation of sera with soluble HHV-6, HSB-2 control, HCMV, EBV, HSV, and VZV antigens. The other herpesvirus antigens showed no competitive cross-reactivity with IgG antibodies to HHV-6 (45), whereas the HHV-6-adsorbing antigens reduced binding to HHV-6 by more than 90% and failed to reduce significantly the titer to any of the other five HHVs (40, 45). In addition to its specificity, the EIA is highly sensitive, with 94 to 97% of people older than 2 years of age demonstrating EIA reactivity to HHV-6.

Other Serologic Procedures

Other tests used to detect HHV-6 antibodies include immunoblotting, immunoprecipitation, and neutralization. The immunoblotting and immunoprecipitation assays (3, 57) are key procedures in the detailed analysis of the individual polypeptides and proteins involved in the immune response to HHV-6. Neutralization has been less widely used.

Interpretation of Results

Detection of virus or DNA from the peripheral blood of a patient is the best indicator of active HHV-6 infection but does not distinguish primary infection from reactivation of latent infection. The results of serologic tests are more difficult to interpret. The presence of specific HHV-6 IgM is an indication of active infection, but low levels of IgM may also be found during reactivation or reinfection (18). Demonstration of a fourfold rise in the IFA or ACIF antibody titer in a young child with a febrile rash illness confirms the diagnosis of roseola with HHV-6 infection. However, in older children and adults, a concurrent rise in the level of antibody to HCMV or EBV has been reported quite frequently in connection with a rise in HHV-6 antibody titer. When serologic evidence of dual infection is obtained, the relative importance of each pathogen in producing illness may be difficult to ascertain. To confirm HHV-6 involvement in disease, the virus should be isolated from the peripheral blood or a tissue sample of an involved organ, and active or recent infection should be established by serologic tests on paired serum specimens (7). If the virus cannot be cultivated, PCR of serum or the affected tissue or in situ immunohistochemistry should be performed, and these assays should be correlated with serologic tests on paired serum specimens. Caution is also needed in interpreting seroprevalence studies. A positive result in adequately controlled tests indicates infection at some undetermined time in the past, but false-negative results can be obtained with insensitive procedures. In addition, the potentially confounding role of HHV-7 producing cross-reactive antibodies must be considered.

HUMAN HERPESVIRUS 7

Clinical Background

The role of HHV-7 in human disease processes is largely unknown. The only clinical association has been with a roseola-like illness in young children from whom HHV-7 was isolated but HHV-6 was not (50). The finding that HHV-7 can be isolated from the saliva of 75% of healthy adults (5, 19) suggests that it may be transmitted by contact with oral secretions.

Description of the Agent

HHV-7 (RK) was first isolated in 1989 by Frenkel et al. (20) from PBL of a 25-year-old healthy man after activation of his CD4$^+$ T cells. Lymphocytes infected with the RK strain exhibited a cytopathic effect that consisted of enlarged ballooning cells and syncytium formation. No virus was recovered from unactivated cells. Typical icosahedral herpesvirus particles were observed in infected cultures by electron microscopy. The particles had a distinct tegument layer around the capsid, appearing similar to HHV-6. The DNA of HHV-7 (RK) did not hybridize with large probes from HSV, EBV, VZV, or HCMV, but some HHV-6 DNA probes cross-hybridized. Thus, the RK strain was more closely related to HHV-6A and HHV-6B than to any of the other HHVs, but it was shown to be clearly distinct by restriction endonuclease analysis (20).

HHV-7 can be shown to be immunologically distinct from HHV-6 by Western immunoblot assays with human serum specimens and MAb (19). Seroconversions to HHV-6 and HHV-7 have been observed as distinct and separate events. Additional studies with some MAb derived from HHV-6A also indicated limited antigenic similarity to HHV-7. MAb to two proteins of HHV-6A reacted with many or all of the HHV-7 isolates tested, but four other HHV-6 MAb failed to react with any of the HHV-7 strains (4, 5, 56). IFA and EIA have shown that HHV-7 is a highly prevalent virus that infects children somewhat later than HHV-6 (6).

Collection and Storage of Specimens

Heparinized blood samples should be collected aseptically, and the mononuclear cells should be purified on Ficoll gradients. The cells are usually cocultivated with PHA-stimulated CBL. For best results, cultures should be set up within 24 h of blood collection.

Detection of Viral Nucleic Acid

An HHV-7-specific DNA clone which displays no cross-reactions to either variant of HHV-6 has been identified. This clone can be used in HHV-7-specific tissue assays by in situ hybridization methods (5). HHV-7-specific PCR primers have been developed from the sequence of a DNA fragment of HHV-7 (JI). These primers amplify HHV-7 DNA but do not amplify the DNA from any of the other known human herpesviruses, including 12 HHV-6 strains (4).

Virus Isolation

HHV-7 can be isolated from saliva and PBL and propagated in PHA-stimulated CBL and PBL by essentially the same procedures employed for HHV-6. Because HHV-7 may reactivate HHV-6 which is latent in PBL, CBL are the preferred cells. Saliva specimens are diluted 1:3 with lymphocyte growth medium (RPMI 1640, 10% fetal calf serum, 32 U of interleukin-2 per ml, antibiotics) and centrifuged at 2,000 × g. The supernatant is passed through a 0.45-μm-pore-size filter and then inoculated into two or three individual PHA-stimulated CBL cultures by centrifugal enhancement. Ficoll-purified PBL are cocultivated with at least two individual PHA-stimulated CBL cultures. All cell cultures are incubated at 37°C in 5% CO_2, observed twice a week for cytopathic effects, and passaged weekly into freshly PHA-stimulated CBL in growth medium.

Virus Identification

Cytopathic effects may be induced in CBL by HHV-7 or HHV-6. Specific HHV-7 reagents, such as PCR primers (4) and cloned DNA fragments (5), or DNA restriction endonuclease cleavage patterns (5, 20) must be used. To distinguish these agents, specific MAb may also be used for this purpose.

Serological Diagnosis

The human immune response to HHV-7 can be measured by IFA, EIA, and immunoblot assays with HHV-7-infected cells as the antigen source (4, 5, 56). Two teams differentiated the immune response to HHV-7 from that to HHV-6 by studying sequential serum specimens obtained from young children (51, 56). They noted that seroconversion to HHV-7, detected by IFA, occurred independently of seroconversion to HHV-6 (most children were already positive to HHV-6). Torigoe et al. (51) noted that 12 of 20 children with antibody to HHV-6 in the acute phase of HHV-7 infections had a significant increase in the HHV-6 titer. High titers to HHV-6 did not protect them from subsequent HHV-7 infection. Tanaka et al. also found an increase in the HHV-6 IgG titer in children with HHV-6 antibodies (from a previous HHV-6 infection) during a primary HHV-7 infection (50). Some children with seroconversion to HHV-6 during an episode of roseola illness have also been shown to have an increase in antibody titer to HHV-7. This finding may indicate some immune response to cross-reactive epitopes of these viruses as well as reactivation of the initially infecting virus.

Antigenic cross-reactivity has also been examined by antigen adsorption of homologous and heterologous antibody before testing the residual antibody of each specimen by HHV-6B and HHV-7 EIAs (5). Most cord blood and adult serum specimens contain antibody to both viruses by EIA. HHV-6B and HHV-7 antigens adsorbed 10 to 30% of the antibody activity of the heterologous virus but adsorbed far more activity of the homologous virus (5). With this additional evidence that cross-reactive epitopes are present with these viruses, an adsorption step may be necessary to determine specific titers to each virus when infected cells are used as antigens.

Interpretation of Results

The isolation of HHV-7, or detection of HHV-7 DNA, from saliva, PBL, and other tissue sites indicates that virus is present but does not indicate whether a given illness is due to active HHV-7 infection. Many oral infections are asymptomatic and persistent, and it is not known what type of disease, other than a roseola-like illness, may be caused by primary infection. However, isolation of HHV-7 in high titer from a diseased tissue and convincing epidemiologic correlation of that illness with HHV-7 might provide evidence that HHV-7 might be the etiologic agent.

The results of serologic tests are also difficult to interpret. Demonstration of a significant rise in HHV-7 antibody titer in a young child or an adult with stable or negative HHV-6 titers (with no evidence of another pathogen) would indicate that active infection may be present. When serologic evidence of dual infection is obtained, the relative importance of each pathogen in producing illness may be difficult to ascertain. Some caution is also needed in interpreting seroprevalence studies until the nature of the cross-reaction with HHV-6 is more completely investigated and HHV-7 specific tests are available.

HUMAN HERPESVIRUS 8

Clinical Background

Knowledge of the natural history and the biology of HHV-8, the newest member of the family *Herpesviridae*, is currently limited but is increasing rapidly. Although a viral etiology for Kaposi's sarcoma (KS) was postulated in the 1970s, it took several decades until Chang et al., using representational difference analysis, discovered HHV-8 in KS tissues (11). Classical KS is a rare malignancy that occurs primarily in Mediterranean and Eastern European adults (12, 36), but it can occur in children, as exemplified by the patient originally described by Kaposi (28). Endemic KS, on the other hand, is common in sub-Saharan equatorial Africa (Uganda, Zaire, Rwanda, and Burundi have the highest prevalence) and accounts for up to 10 to 17% of all adult malignancies. There is an equal incidence in males and females, and the incidence is age related, increasing from puberty to adulthood (59). In the United States, KS affects primarily HIV-1-infected homosexual men (up to 25% developed KS during the 1980s, which represented a 20,000-fold risk) but only rarely affects HIV-1-infected hemophiliacs, children, or HIV-1-negative transplant recipients.

Clinically, KS is a vasocutaneous, multifocal tumor of uncertain histogenesis and complex histopathology. It evolves in stages, from benign proliferation to aggressive and invasive spindle cell sarcoma. Late-stage skin lesions consist of a mixture of spindle cells, endothelial cells, infiltrating lymphocytes, dendritic cells, mast cells, and macrophages. In immunosuppressive-drug-associated KS, the development and progression of the tumor can be reversed upon withdrawal of the drug, suggesting a dependence on an impaired host immune status.

HHV-8 DNA can be detected in virtually all forms of KS lesions by PCR, including the classical Mediterranean KS, HIV-1-negative African endemic KS, posttransplantation KS, and AIDS-related KS (12). About half of HIV-related KS patients and 35% of HIV-1-infected individuals have detectable HHV-8 sequences in $CD19^+$ B cells in the peripheral blood by PCR; the presence of these sequences presages the progression to KS and correlates with the development of tumor within 5 years in 75% of individuals (54). HHV-8 DNA sequences can also be detected in patients with multicentric Castleman's disease (12) and primary effusion lymphoma (PEL) (formerly known as body cavity-based lymphoma) (12). Both are rare B-cell proliferative conditions associated with HIV-1-immune disorders.

Information on the clinical syndrome associated with HHV-8 primary infection is very incomplete. In 50 HIV-1-negative Zambian infants experiencing their first febrile episode (some with respiratory symptoms), HHV-8 was detected by PCR in 8% of the blood samples and persisted for longer than 3 months (29). Serologic testing was not performed in this study to document primary infection.

Description of the Agent

Gene sequence information indicates that HHV-8 (also known as KS-associated herpesvirus) is a member of the gamma-2 herpesviruses of the *Rhadinovirus* genus (37). HHV-8 is closely related to herpesvirus saimiri and EBV, both of which are associated with lymphoproliferative diseases: herpesvirus saimiri with a fulminant T-cell disorder of squirrel monkeys and EBV with Burkitt's lymphoma.

In vivo, HHV-8 infects several cell types. DNA is detectable in PEL cells (12), which have a clonal Ig gene rearrangement but lack surface Ig or B-cell antigens, and in endothelial and spindle cells in nodular KS lesions (12). In these three cell types, HHV-8 establishes persistent, latent infection with expression of latent antigens detectable immunohistochemically as nuclear, punctate staining (43). HHV-8 sequences are also found in $CD19^+$ peripheral B cells (2). Only PEL cells can be propagated without loss of the latent viral genomes. These cells can be induced (by sodium butyrate or phorbol esters) (36) to generate typical herpesvirus virions, visible by electron microscopy.

Collection and Storage of Specimens

Body fluids and biopsy specimens should be collected aseptically and refrigerated immediately; tissues should be held in saline or a viral transport medium. Suitable specimens include skin lesions, various lymphoid and organ tissues, whole blood or bone marrow (with anticoagulant), saliva, and seminal fluid. Fresh, frozen, and paraffin-embedded tissues are also suitable specimens for nucleic acid detection procedures.

Direct Examination and Identification

Viral isolation by available cell culture systems is not possible at present. In vasoformative spindle cells of PCR-positive KS lesions, typical herpesvirus virions were infrequently observed by electron microscopy, as were eosinophilic intranuclear viral inclusions by light microscopy (38). HHV-8 infection is most reliably indicated by detection of the genome in various tissues and in B cells of peripheral blood by PCR (2). The original and the most widely used primers are specific for the highly conserved 233-bp region of the KS330Bam fragment. These primers have a 97% sensitivity and specificity when used on KS lesions. In situ hybridization can be performed on solid tissues (38).

Latently and lytically expressed nuclear antigens can be detected by IFA in infected cells by using sera from KS patients (33) or by immunohistochemical staining of paraffin sections with affinity-purified human antibodies (43). These developmental procedures gave excellent staining of PEL cells and sections of 10 tumor samples.

Serologic Diagnosis

A large number of HHV-8-specific serologic assays have been investigated, including indirect IFA, ACIF, EIA, and immunoblotting with a variety of antigens, including native, recombinant, and peptide antigens, which give highly variable results. Because of this lack of consensus among the tests, the seroepidemiology of HHV-8 infection has been confusing. The results of various assays suggest that more than 80% of the KS patients, irrespective of geographic origin or HIV-1 infection, are HHV-8 seropositive. These assays also indicate that among the HIV-1-infected population, HHV-8 prevalence is highest in HIV-1-positive homosexual males, is intermediate in intravenous drug users and heterosexual subjects, and lowest in hemophiliacs and children. However, different assays give disparate data on the rate of seropositivity attached to each risk group. The largest disagreement regards the seroprevalence of the general population, which ranges from 0 to 25% (21, 31, 33). However, given the known prevalence of KS in Africa before the HIV-1 outbreak, coupled with the increasing number of reports of HHV-8 DNA detected in subjects not at risk for HIV-1 infection, HHV-8 clearly infects individuals in the general population with a yet to be determined prevalence. More importantly, there is sufficient evidence to conclude that HHV-8 infection is primarily, though not exclusively, sexually transmitted (12). In the general population, there is no recognized disease(s) associated with HHV-8 infection. Although HHV-8 and EBV have genomic homology, serologic cross-reactions between the two have not been reported. The following brief descriptions of the various assays should be taken as work in progress. Information on the utility of each procedure is still accumulating, and the efficacy of each remains to be determined.

MIFA

MAb-enhanced IFA (MIFA) is a three-step IFA test used to differentially measure antibodies to the lytic and latent antigen complex expressed in the BCBL-1 lymphoma cell line after treatment with a phorbol ester. In this assay, the cell preparation is incubated with patient serum, then with mouse monoclonal anti-human IgG antiserum, and finally with fluorescein-conjugated anti-mouse reagent. All cells express the characteristic punctate nuclear antigen, but only 20 to 30% of them express the cytoplasmic lytic antigens. The microscopist can readily classify serum reactions as anti-latent and/or anti-lytic. All infected individuals have anti-lytic antibodies, but anti-latent antibodies are rarely present in the general population. In contrast, all of the African KS patients and nearly all HIV-1-infected KS patients have both anti-lytic and anti-latent antibodies by MIFA.

IFA and ACIF

Anti-latent antibodies are the main antibodies measured by the IFA procedure. The primary difficulty reported with this assay is the high background reaction in assays with PEL cell lines that contain both EBV and HHV-8 (12, 36, 37). This problem necessitates laborious serum absorption with EBV-infected cells or the use of a higher cutoff dilution, which decreases the sensitivity. Another solution to this problem involves preparation of cell nuclei followed by the three-step ACIF assay (31). However, this procedure does not allow detection of anti-cytoplasmic antibodies, which may be the major reactants in some sera.

Immunoblotting

The immunoblot assay can detect antibodies to both the lytic and latent antigens. Reactions to latent antigens are apparent as a doublet of 226 and 234 kDa; this doublet is present in 80% of KS patients but only 17% of HIV-1-infected homosexual males (21). When this procedure was used, seroconversion to the latent antigens was detected in 52% of the HIV-1-infected males before the appearance of KS. Testing for anti-lytic antibodies by this procedure has been reported on a limited number of patients (36).

EIA with Defined Antigens

Recombinant protein of the HHV-8 capsid-related (lytic) antigen from open reading frame 65 (ORF 65) (47) and peptides corresponding to a fragment of the minor capsid protein from ORF 26 have been evaluated by EIA (15). The sensitivities of first-generation tests with these defined reagents appear to be lower than those of tests with cell-derived antigens.

Interpretation of Results

Most of the discussion given for the interpretation of HHV-7 applies to HHV-8 as well. There is insufficient information on the natural history of HHV-8 and the efficacy of the laboratory tests to allow clinically meaningful interpretations. The significance of HHV-8 DNA in tissues of subjects not at risk for HIV-1 infection is unclear, in that very few such individuals develop KS and the pathophysiology associated with the virus in this population is unknown. The same can be said of serologic evidence of infection. The only situation where HHV-8 laboratory results may be of help is finding HHV-8 DNA in the peripheral blood of HIV-1-infected homosexual males, where the data are sufficient to indicate a risk of KS tumor development.

B VIRUS

Clinical Background

B virus, or cercopithecine herpesvirus 1 (formerly called herpesvirus simiae), is indigenous to Old World monkeys, such as rhesus (*Macaca mulatta*), cynomolgus (*Macaca fascicularis*), and other Asiatic monkeys of the genus *Macaca*. As the simian counterpart of HSV, B virus causes subclinical infections as well as dermal, oral, eye, and genital lesions in monkeys. Whitley (55) and Weigler (52) have reviewed the biology of B virus and the importance of the virus to humans because of its ability to cause life-threatening CNS infections. The virus can be transmitted by monkey bites, by direct or indirect contact with saliva, by aerosols to the eye, or even by contact with some monkey cell cultures that are widely used in the virus laboratory (53).

After an incubation period of a few days to 1 month or more, an infected person may show localized redness and vesicles and may have pain at the site of virus inoculation. Vesicles on the mucous membranes, pneumonia, diarrhea, abdominal pain, pharyngitis, and lymphocytic pleocytosis have been reported. In almost all untreated symptomatic cases, a frequently fatal ascending myelitis and encephalopathy occur; most infected individuals who survive are left with severe brain damage (39). Although the risk of disease with B virus appears to be low (on the basis of the small number of known cases compared with the thousands of macaque contacts yearly), human infection is a potential hazard of working with Old World monkeys, and precautionary measures to protect workers from infection are critical (24). Detection of four human cases in Florida in 1987 (24), two cases in Michigan in 1989 (14), and a recent case in Atlanta emphasizes this need.

Description of the Agent

B virus is similar to HSV in morphologic features and size and is inhibited by antiviral agents that suppress DNA synthesis (55). An enveloped herpesvirus, it is sensitive to lipid solvents, acidic pH, and detergent solutions. There is an antigenic relationship between HSV and B virus, so that antisera to B virus will neutralize both viruses equally well whereas antisera to HSV will neutralize homologous virus at much higher titers than it will neutralize B virus (55). The extent of the cross-reaction is enhanced by complement. B virus appears hardier than HSV; it may survive for 7 days at 37°C and for weeks at 4°C and is very stable when stored at −70°C. The virus can be isolated in a number of cell lines, including primary rabbit kidney and vervet monkey cells and established lines such as HeLa or BSC1. Rhesus monkey kidney cells readily support the growth of B virus, whereas HSV isolates grow poorly in these cells. The cytopathic effect produced by B virus in many cell lines is quite similar to that produced by HSV, and specific serologic or molecular procedures are needed to identify B virus. The virus can be successfully grown in a number of animal systems as well.

Safety

Because of the potential hazards of B virus infections, guidelines for preventing infection in monkey handlers have been established (10, 24) and caution should be exercised by laboratory workers in processing specimens suspected of containing B virus. Laboratory assistance in investigating such specimens can be obtained from the National Institutes of Health B Virus Resource Laboratory, Viral Immunology Center, Georgia State University, Atlanta, Ga., phone (404) 651-0808, or from the Virus Reference Laboratories, Inc., San Antonio, Tex., phone (210) 615–2061.

Collection and Storage of Specimens

Vesicular fluid of lesions, swabs from the oropharynx, conjunctiva, and skin lesions, or skin biopsy specimens from affected areas can be used for the diagnosis of B virus infection. The cotton tips of the applicators used to swab the lesions should be broken off into screw-cap vials containing 2 ml of tryptose phosphate broth with 0.5% gelatin or another viral transport medium that contains protein (skim milk or veal infusion broth). Specimens for virus isolation should be kept cold (4 to 8°C) at all times (but not frozen) and promptly shipped to the appropriate laboratory. Inquiries can be directed to the Centers for Disease Control and Prevention, phone (404) 639-3311 [(404) 639-2888 at night].

Virus Isolation and Serological Procedures

Since B virus propagation should be handled under biosafety level 4 conditions, laboratory investigation of specimens from patients or monkeys suspected of having B virus infection is best referred to experienced laboratories equipped to handle B virus cultures. Rapid diagnosis of infection has been greatly facilitated by the development of a PCR assay to detect B virus DNA in clinical samples (46). The serologic diagnosis of recent B virus infection is complicated by the extensive cross-reactivity between HSV and B virus (52). Adequate testing requires the demonstration of at least a fourfold rise in "specific antibody titer" against B virus in paired serum specimens. Specific antibody assays such as immunoblotting (14, 23) or an EIA for specific antibodies by using adsorption procedures (14, 30) are currently available in only a few reference laboratories equipped to handle B virus. In B-virus-infected patients, a rise in titer against HSV may frequently be measured along with an increase in titer to B virus. An increase in antibody is usually observed 10 to 14 days after the onset of illness but may be greatly delayed if the patient is treated with an antiviral medication such as acyclovir.

REFERENCES

1. **Ablashi, D. V., H. Agut, Z. Berneman, G. Campadelli-Fiume, D. Carrigan, L. Ceccerini-Nelli, B. Chandran, S. Chou, H. Collandre, R. Cone, T. Danbaugh, S. Dewhurst, D. DiLuca, L. Foa-Tomasi, B. Fleckenstein, N. Frenkel, R. Gallo, U. Gompels, C. Hall, M. Jones, G. Lawrence, M. Martin, L. Montangnier, F. Neipel, J. Nicholas, P. Pellett, A. Razzaque, G. Torrelli, B. Thomson, S. Salahuddin, L. Wyatt, and K. Yamanishi.** 1993. Human herpesvirus-6 strain groups: a nomenclature. *Arch. Virol.* **129:**363–366.
2. **Ambroziak, J. A., D. J. Blackbourn, B. G. Herndier, R. G. Glogau, J. H. Gullett, A. R. McDonald, E. T. Lennette, and J. A. Levy.** 1995. Herpes-like sequences in HIV-infected and uninfected Kaposi's sarcoma patients. *Science* **268:**582–583.
3. **Balachandran, N., S. Tirawatnapoong, B. Pfeiffer, D. V. Ablashi, and S. Z. Salahuddin.** 1991. Electrophoretic analysis of human herpesvirus 6 polypeptides immunoprecipitated from infected cell with human sera. *J. Infect. Dis.* **163:**29–34.
4. **Berneman, Z. N., D. V. Ablashi, G. Li, M. Eger-Fletcher, M. S. Reitz, Jr., C.-H. Hung, I. Brus, A. L. Komaroff, and R. Gallo.** 1992. Human herpesvirus 7 is a T-lymphotropic virus and is related to, but significantly different from, human herpesvirus 6 and human cytomegalovirus. *Proc. Natl. Acad. Sci. USA* **89:**10552–10556.
5. **Black, J. B., T. F. Schwarz, J. L. Patton, K. Kite-Powell, P. E. Pellett, S. Wiersbitsky, R. Bruns, C. Muller, G. Jager, and J. A. Stewart.** 1996. Evaluation of immunoassays for detection of antibodies to human herpesvirus 7. *Clin. Diagn. Lab. Immunol.* **3:**79–83.
6. **Black, J. B., N. Inoue, K. Kite-Powell, S. Zaki, and P.**

E. Pellett. 1993. Frequent isolation of human herpesvirus 7 from saliva. *Virus Res.* **29:**91–98.

7. **Braun, D. K., G. Dominguez, and P. E. Pellett.** 1997. Human herpesvirus 6. *Clin. Microbiol. Rev.* **10:**521–567.
8. **Breese, B. B.** 1941. Roseola infantum (exanthema subitum). *N. Y. State J. Med.* **41:**1854–1859.
9. **Carrigan, D. R., W. R. Drobyski, S. K. Russler, M. A. Tapper, K. K., Knox, and R. C. Ash.** 1991. Interstitial pneumonitis associated with human herpesvirus 6 infection after marrow transplantation. *Lancet* **338:**147–149.
10. **Centers for Disease Control.** 1987. Guidelines for prevention of Herpesvirus simiae (B virus) infection in monkey handlers. *Morbid. Mortal. Weekly Rep.* **36:**680–682, 687–689.
11. **Chang, Y., E. Cesarman, M. S. Pessin, F. Lee, J. Culpepper, D. M. Knowles, and P. S. Moore.** 1994. Identification of herpesvirus-like DNA sequences in AIDS-associated Kaposi's sarcoma. *Science* **266:**1865–1869.
12. **Chang, Y., and P. S. Moore.** 1996. Kaposi's sarcoma (KS)-associated herpesvirus and its role in KS. *Infect. Agents Dis.* **5:**215–222.
13. **Cone, R. W., R. C. Hackman, M.-L. W. Huang, R. A. Bowden, J. D. Meyers, M. Metcalf, J. Zeh, R. Ashley, and L. Corey.** 1993. Human herpesvirus 6 in lung tissue from patients with pneumonitis after bone marrow transplantation. *N. Engl. J. Med.* **329:**156–161.
14. **Davenport, D. S., D. R. Johnson, G. R. Holmes, D. A. Jewett, S. C. Ross, and J. K. Hilliard.** 1994. Diagnosis and management of human B virus (*Herpesvirus simiae*) infections in Michigan. *Clin. Infect. Dis.* **19:**33–41.
15. **Davis, D. A., R. W. Humphrey, F. M. Newcomb, T. R. O'Brien, J. J. Goedert, S. E. Straus, and R. Yarchoan.** 1997. Detection of serum antibodies to a Kaposi's sarcoma-associated herpesvirus-specific peptide. *J. Infect. Dis.* **175:**1071–1079.
16. **Dewhurst, S., B. Chandran, K. McIntyre, K. Schnabel, and C. B. Hall.** 1992. Phenotypic and genetic polymorphisms among human herpesvirus-6 isolates from North American infants. *Virology* **190:**490–493.
17. **Di Luca, D., P. Mirandola, T. Ravaioli, B. Bigoni, and E. Cassai.** 1996. Distribution of HHV-6 variants in human tissues. *Infect. Agents Dis.* **5:**203–214.
18. **Fox, J. D., P. Ward, M. Briggs, W. Irving, T. G. Stammers, and R. S. Tedder.** 1990. Production of IgM antibody to HHV6 in reactivation and primary infection. *Epidemiol. Infect.* **104:**289–296.
19. **Frenkel, N., and E. Roffman.** 1996. Human herpesvirus 7, p. 2609–2622. *In* B. N. Fields, D. M. Knipe, and P. M. Howley (ed.), *Field's Virology*. Lippincott-Raven Publishers, Philadelphia, Pa.
20. **Frenkel, N., E. C. Schirmer, L. S. Wyatt, G. Katsafanas, E. Roffman, R. M. Danovich, and C. H. June.** 1990. Isolation of a new herpesvirus from human CD4 + T cells. *Proc. Natl. Acad. Sci. USA* **87:**748–752.
21. **Gao, S.-J., L. Kingsley, D. R. Hoover, T. J. Spira, C. R. Rinaldo, A. Saah, J. Phair, R. Detels, P. Parry, Y. Chang, and P. S. Moore.** 1996. Seroconversion to antibodies against Kaposi's sarcoma-associated herpesvirus-related latent nuclear antigens before the development of Kaposi's sarcoma. *N. Engl. J. Med.* **335:**233–241.
22. **Gompels, U. A., J. Nicholas, G. Lawrence, M. Jones, B. J. Thomson, and M. E. Martin.** 1995. The DNA sequence of human herpesvirus-6: structure, coding content, and genome evolution. *Virology* **209:**29–51.
23. **Heberling, R. L., and S. S. Kalter.** 1987. A dot-immunobinding assay on nitrocellulose with psoralen inactivated *Herpesvirus simiae* (B virus). *Lab. Anim. Sci.* **37:**304–308.
24. **Holmes, G. P., L. E. Chapman, J. A. Stewart, S. E. Straus, J. K. Hilliard, D. S. Davenport, and the B Virus Working Group.** 1995. Guidelines for the prevention and treatment of B-virus infections in exposed persons. *Clin. Infect. Dis.* **20:**421–439.
25. **Irving, W. L., J. Chang, D. R. Raymond, R. Dunstan, P. Grattan-Smith, and A. L. Cunningham.** 1990. Roseola infantum and other syndromes associated with acute HHV-6 infection. *Arch. Dis. Child.* **65:**1297–1300.
26. **Irving, W. L., V. M. Ratnamohan, L. C. Hueston, J. R. Chapman, and A. L. Cunningham.** 1990. Dual antibody rises to cytomegalovirus and human herpesvirus type 6: frequency of occurrence in CMV infections and evidence for genuine reactivity to both viruses. *J. Infect. Dis.* **161:**910–916.
27. **Kadakia, M. P., W. B. Rybka, J. A. Stewart, J. L. Patton, F. R. Stamey, M. Elsawy, P. E. Pellet, and J. A. Armstrong.** 1996. Human herpesvirus 6: infection and disease following autologous and allogeneic bone marrow transplantation. *Blood* **87:**5341–5354.
28. **Kaposi, M.** 1872. Idiopatisches multiples Pigmentsarkom der Haut. *Arch. Dermatol. Syphilis* **4:**265–273.
29. **Kasolo, F. C., E. Mpabalwani, and U. A. Gompels.** 1997. Infection with AIDS-related herpesviruses in human immunodefiency virus-negative infants and endemic childhood Kaposi's sarcoma in Africa. *J. Gen. Virol.* **78:**847–855.
30. **Katz, D., J. K. Hilliard, R. Eberle, and S. L. Liper.** 1986. ELISA for detection of group-common and virus-specific antibodies in human and simian viruses. *J. Virol. Methods* **14:**99–109.
31. **Kedes, D. H., E. Operskalski, M. Busch, R. Kohn, J. Flood, and D. Ganem.** 1996. The seroepidemiology of human herpesvirus 8 (Kaposi's sarcoma-associated herpesvirus): distribution of infection in KS risk groups and evidence for sexual transmission. *Nat. Med.* **2:**918–924.
32. **Kondo, K., H. Nagafuji, A. Hata, C. Tomomori, and K. Yamanishi.** 1993. Association of human herpesvirus 6 infection of the central nervous system with recurrence of febrile convulsions. *J. Infect. Dis.* **167:**1197–2000.
33. **Lennette, E. T., D. J. Blackbourn, and J. A. Levy.** 1996. Antibodies to human herpesvirus type 8 in the general population and in Kaposi's sarcoma patients. *Lancet* **348:**858–861.
34. **Lindquester, G. J., N. Inoue, R. D. Allen, J. W. Castelli, F. R. Stamey, T. R. Dambaugh, J. J. O'Brian, R. M. Danovich, N. Frenkel, and P. E. Pellett.** 1996. Restriction endonuclease mapping and molecular cloning of the human herpesvirus 6 variant B strain Z29 genome. *Arch. Virol.* **141:**367–379.
35. **Lopez, C., P. Pellett, J. Stewart, C. Goldsmith, K. Sanderlin, J. Black, D. Warfield, and P. Feorino.** 1988. Characteristics of human herpesvirus-6. *J. Infect. Dis.* **157:**1271–1273.
36. **Miller, G., M. O. Rigsby, L. Heston, E. Grogan, R. Sun, C. Metroka, J. A. Levy, S.-J. Gao, Y. Chang, and P. S. Moore.** 1996. Antibodies to butyrate-inducible antigens of Kaposi's sarcoma-associated herpesvirus in patients with HIV-1 infection. *N. Engl. J. Med.* **334:**1292–1297.
37. **Moore, P. S., S.-J. Gao, G. Dominguez, E. Cesarman, O. Lungu, D. M. Knowles, R. Garber, P. E. Pellett, D. J. McGeoch, and Y. Chang.** 1996. Primary characterization of a herpesvirus agent associated with Kaposi's sarcoma. *J. Virol.* **70:**549–558.
38. **Orenstein, J. M., S. Alkan, A. Blauvelt, K. T. Jeang, M. D. Weinstein, D. Ganem, and B. Herndier.** 1997. Visualization of human herpesvirus type 8 in Kaposi's sarcoma by light and transmission electron microscopy. *AIDS* **11:**F35–F45.
39. **Palmer, A. E.** 1987. B virus, *Herpesvirus simiae*: historical perspectives. *J. Med. Primatol.* **16:**99–130.

40. **Parker, C. A., and J. M. Weber.** 1993. An enzyme-linked immunosorbent assay for the detection of IgG and IgM antibodies to human herpesvirus type 6. *J. Virol. Methods* **41:**265–276.
41. **Pietroboni, G. R., G. B. Harnett, M. R. Bucens, and R. W. Honess.** 1988. Antibody to human herpesvirus 6 in saliva. *Lancet* **i:**1059.
42. **Pruksananonda, P., C. B. Hall, R. A. Insel, K. McIntyre, P. E. Pellet, C. E. Long, K. C. Schnabel, P. H. Pincus, F. R. Stamey, T. R. Danbaugh, and J. A. Stewart.** 1992. Primary human herpesvirus 6 infection in young children. *N. Engl. J. Med.* **326:**1445–1450.
43. **Rainbow, L., G. M. Platt, G. R. Simpson, R. Sarid, S.-J. Gao, H. Stoiber, C. S. Herrington, P. S. Moore, and T. F. Schulz.** 1997. The 222- to 234-kilodalton latent nuclear protein (LNA) of Kaposi's sarcoma-associated herpesvirus (human herpesvirus 8) is encoded by orf 73 and is a component of latency-associated nuclear antigen. *J. Virol.* **71:** 5915–5921.
44. **Salahuddin, S. Z., D. V. Ablashi, P. D. Markham, S. F. Josephs, S. Sturzenegger, M. Kaplan, G. Halligan, P. Biberfeld, F. Wong-Staal, B. Kramarsky, and R. C. Gallo.** 1986. Isolation of a new virus, HBLV, in patients with lymphoproliferative disorders. *Science* **234:**596–601.
45. **Saxinger, C., H. Polesky, N. Eby, S. Grufferman, R. Murphy, G. Tegtmeier, V. Parekh, S. Memon, and C. Hung.** 1988. Antibody reactivity with HBLV (HHV-6) in U.S. populations. *J. Virol. Methods* **21:**199–208.
46. **Scinicariello, F., R. Eberle, and J. K. Hilliard.** 1993. Rapid detection of B virus (herpesvirus simiae) DNA by polymerase chain reaction. *J. Infect. Dis.* **168:**747–750.
47. **Simpson, G. R., T. F. Schulz, D. Whitby, P. M. Cook, C. Boshoff, L. Rainbow, M. R. Howard, S. J. Gao, R. A. Bohenzky, P. Simmonds, C. Lee, A. de Ruiter, A. Hatzakis, R. S. Tedder, I. V. Weller, R. A. Weiss, and P. S. Moore.** 1996. Prevalence of Kaposi's sarcoma associated herpesvirus infection measured by antibodies to recombinant capsid protein and latent immunofluorescence antigen. *Lancet* **348:**1133–1138.
48. **Steeper, T. A., C. A. Horwitz, D. V. Ablashi, S. Z. Salahuddin, C. Saxinger, R. Saltzman, and B. Schwartz.** 1990. The spectrum of clinical and laboratory findings resulting from human herpesvirus-6 in patients with mononucleosis-like illnesses not resulting from Epstein-Barr virus or cytomegalovirus. *Am. J. Clin. Pathol.* **93:**776–783.
49. **Suga, S., T. Yoshikawa, Y. Asano, T. Kozawa, T. Nakashima, I. Kobayashi, T. Yazaki, H. Yamamoto, Y. Kajita, T. Ozaki, Y. Nishimura, T. Yamanaka, A. Yamada, and J. Imanishi.** 1993. Clinical and virological analyses of 21 infants with exanthem subitum (roseola infantum) and central nervous system complications. *Ann. Neurol.* **33:** 597–603.
50. **Tanaka, K., T. Kondo, S. Torigoe, S. Okeda, T. Mukai, and K. Yamanishi.** 1994. Human herpesvirus 7: another causal agent for roseola (exanthem subitum). *J. Pediatr.* **125:**1–5.
51. **Torigoe, S., T. Kumamoto, W. Koide, K. Taya, and K. Yamanishi.** 1995. Clinical manifestations associated with human herpesvirus 7 infection. *Arch. Dis. Child.* **72:** 518–519.
52. **Weiger, B. J.** 1992. Biology of B virus in macaque and human hosts: a review. *Clin. Infect. Dis.* **14:**555–567.
53. **Wells, D. L., S. L. Lipper, J. K. Hilliard, J. A. Stewart, G. P. Holmes, K. L. Herrmann, M. P. Kiley, and L. B. Schonberger.** 1989. *Herpesvirus simiae* contamination of primary rhesus monkey cell cultures: CDC recommendations to minimize risks to laboratory personnel. *Diagn. Microbiol. Infect. Dis.* **12:**333–336.
54. **Whitby, D., M. R. Howard, M. Tenant-Flowers, N. S. Brink, A. Copas, C. Boshaoff, T. Hatzioannou, F. E. Suggett, D. M. Aldam, A. S. Denton, R. F. Miller, I. V. D. Weller, R. A. Weiss, R. S. Tedder, and T. F. Schulz.** 1995. Detection of Kaposi's sarcoma-associated herpesvirus (KSHV) in peripheral blood of HIV-infected individuals and progression to Kaposi's sarcoma. *Lancet* **346:**799–802.
55. **Whitley, R. J.** 1996. Cercopithecine herpesvirus 1 (B virus), p. 2623–2635. *In* B. N. Fields, D. M. Knipe, and P. M. Howley (ed.), *Field's Virology*. Lippincott-Raven Publishers, Philadelphia, Pa.
56. **Wyatt, L. S., W. J. Rodriguez, N. Balachandran, and N. Frenkel.** 1991. Human herpesvirus 7: antigenic properties and prevalence in children and adults. *J. Virol.* **65:** 6260–6265.
57. **Yamamato, M., J. B. Black, J. A. Stewart, C. Lopez, and P. Pellett.** 1990. Identification of a nucleocapsid protein as a specific serological marker of human herpesvirus 6 infection. *J. Clin. Microbiol.* **28:**1957–1962.
58. **Yamanishi, K., T. Okuno, K. Shiraki, M. Takahashi, T. Kondo, Y. Asano, and T. Kurata.** 1988. Identification of human herpesvirus 6 as a causal agent for exanthem subitum. *Lancet* **i:**1065–1067.
59. **Ziegler, J. L.** 1993. Endemic Kaposi's sarcoma in Africa and local volcanic soils. *Lancet* **342:**1348–1351.

Influenza Viruses

THEDI ZIEGLER AND NANCY J. COX

70

CLINICAL BACKGROUND

Epidemiology

Influenza is a highly contagious, acute respiratory disease which may spread rapidly and pervasively through a population. Epidemics and pandemics (global epidemics) of influenza have been documented for centuries. Based on antigenic differences in the nucleoprotein (NP) and the matrix protein (M), influenza viruses are grouped into types A, B, and C. Influenza A viruses are further classified into subtypes according to the properties of their major membrane glycoproteins, the hemagglutinin (HA) and the neuraminidase (NA). A total of 15 HA subtypes and 9 neuraminidase subtypes have been identified so far, all of which can be identified among influenza viruses resident in aquatic birds. However, documented epidemics and pandemics of influenza A among humans since 1889 appear to have been caused by viruses with HAs of only the H1, H2, and H3 subtypes, which have appeared cyclically. Epidemiologic, serologic, and virologic evidence suggests that H2 viruses emerged in approximately 1889, H3 viruses emerged in 1899, H1 emerged in 1918, H2 emerged in 1957, H3 emerged in 1968, and H1 emerged in 1977. In general, epidemics caused by type A viruses alternate with those caused primarily by type B viruses. Influenza C viruses typically cause localized outbreaks of mild upper respiratory tract infection in children and young adults.

In regions with temperate climates, influenza viruses cause epidemics almost every year, and many of them are associated with considerable morbidity and mortality. Epidemics typically occur from December to March and from May through August in temperate regions of the northern and southern hemispheres, respectively. Influenza seasonality in tropical and subtropical climates is less well defined; however, influenza viruses may circulate in these areas throughout the year, with peak activity in the summer months or in rainy seasons. During a community-wide influenza epidemic, there may be a sudden increase in visits to clinics, physicians' offices, or hospital emergency rooms. High attack rates in schools and residential institutions are common. Epidemics in a community generally last 3 to 8 weeks.

Annual vaccination with trivalent inactivated vaccine is now the primary measure for the control of influenza. In the United States, the two antiviral drugs amantadine and rimantadine have been licensed for prevention and treatment of infections caused by influenza A viruses. There is now considerable interest in both new influenza vaccines and antiviral agents, particularly the live attenuated influenza virus vaccines and the NA inhibitors, as additional measures for the prevention and control of influenza. More detailed information about influenza epidemiology, prevention, and control is available in references 1 and 7.

Disease Manifestations

Influenza often begins after an incubation period of 1 to 4 days with sudden onset of fever that may be accompanied by sore throat, dry cough, headache, myalgia, malaise, or anorexia. A fever of 38 to 40°C lasting from 1 to 5 days is common. Most signs and symptoms resolve within a week; however, cough and malaise may persist. The spectrum of illness ranges from asymptomatic infection or mild pharyngitis to pneumonia with fatal outcome. Otitis media is a common complication of influenza in children. The most severe complications contributing to the mortality associated with influenza are lower respiratory tract infections, which may present as primary viral pneumonia, mixed viral and bacterial pneumonia, or secondary bacterial pneumonia. For more detailed information on the clinical presentation of influenza, see references 1 and 7.

Transmission

Influenza virus replicates in the columnar epithelial cells of the respiratory tract. From there, the virus gains access to respiratory secretions and is spread by small-particle aerosols expelled into the air during sneezing, coughing, and speaking. Transmission may also occur by direct contact. There is no firm evidence for reintroduction of influenza viruses from latently or persistently infected individuals.

CHARACTERISTICS OF THE VIRUSES

Influenza A and B viruses are enveloped viruses with five internal nonglycosylated proteins (NP, M, and three polymerases) and three integral membrane proteins (HA, NA, and M2 or NB). Influenza A and B viruses cannot be distinguished morphologically. Virus particles are pleomorphic, usually roughly spherical, and 80 to 120 nm in diameter after multiple passages. Elongated filamentous forms have been noted after a single passage. The most striking morphologic feature of influenza A and B viruses is a surface layer of spike-like projections, 10 to 14 nm long and 4 to 6 nm in diameter, formed by HA and NA. Viral nucleocapsids have helical symmetry and are 30 to 110 nm long. Influenza C viruses have a reticular surface structure.

Influenza A and B viruses contain eight single-stranded RNA segments that are complementary to mRNA (i.e., negative sense) and that encode at least 10 polypeptides, of which 8 are structural viral proteins (see above) and 2 are found in infected cells (NS1 and NS2). Terminal 3′ and 5′ nucleotides in each segment are believed to form panhandle structures important in the recognition of viral RNA by the viral polymerase proteins.

The three largest RNA segments encode polymerase proteins, designated PB1, PB2, and PA, that synthesize the RNAs necessary for virus replication and associate with the NP and viral RNA as a replication complex. PB1 and PB2 are involved in initiation and elongation functions during transcription of the mRNA, and the PA protein is probably involved in replication of viral RNA. The HA was named for its role in the agglutination of erythrocytes and is encoded by RNA segment 4. It is responsible for virus attachment, virus penetration, and membrane fusion. HA is synthesized as a single polypeptide of approximately 550 amino acids that is subsequently cleaved into two polypeptide chains, HA1 and HA2, by host cell proteases. Viruses with uncleaved HA can bind to host cells but cannot cause fusion and are not infectious. The functional HA exists as a homotrimer. X-ray crystallographic studies have revealed that the HA trimer has a globular head domain and a fibrous stem domain. The variable HA1 polypeptide makes up the globular head region and is folded into a β-sheet structure and loops which surround the conserved receptor binding pocket. Five overlapping antigenic regions have been identified in the globular head domain. The fibrous stem region, which is proximal to the viral membrane, is composed primarily of residues from HA2 but also contains residues from HA1. This stem region consists of three helices twisting around each other as a triple coiled-coil structure which stabilizes the HA trimer. The HA is anchored in the membrane at its C-terminal end. Neutralizing antibodies directed against the HA play a crucial role in immunity to influenza infection, and variation in this molecule allows the virus to evade preexisting immunity from previous infection or immunization.

RNA segment 5 codes for the NP, which plays a structural role in viral ribonucleoprotein formation, is involved in replication, and, in its phosphorylated form, possesses kinase activity. Although NP is targeted by cytotoxic T lymphocytes that recognize conserved or cross-reacting epitopes, immunization with NP provides limited protection from virus infection.

The glycoprotein NA is encoded by RNA segment 6 and is present in patches on the surface of the virus. NA cleaves terminal sialic acid residues from oligosaccharide chains. NA activity may allow penetration of the virus through the mucus layer to epithelial cells in the respiratory tract and removes sialic acid from virus and infected cells to prevent self-aggregation and permit the release of virus from infected cells. The NA is synthesized and is present in virions as a single polypeptide chain anchored in the membrane at the N-terminal end. Functional NA exists as a homotetramer and appears as a mushroom-shaped spike after release from virus particles by detergent. The three-dimensional structure of the molecule reveals that the NA is composed of a tetrameric globular head and a long filamentous tail. The globular head consists of mainly β-sheet structure containing the sialidase catalytic site surrounded by variable antigenic loops. Antibodies to NA do not completely neutralize virus infectivity except at very high concentrations, but they do restrict virus replication and attenuate illness.

RNA segment 7 encodes the viral membrane proteins M1 and M2 of influenza A viruses. The highly conserved, type-specific M1 membrane is the most abundant protein in virus particles and is located under the lipid envelope of the virus. This protein has a structural function, is involved in the control of viral RNA polymerase activity, and participates in virus assembly by interacting with both HA and NP. Although antibodies to M1 protein are found after infection or vaccination with influenza virus and although an epitope for recognition of M1 protein by cytotoxic T cells has been demonstrated, the significance of M protein in immunity to influenza virus is uncertain. The M2 protein of influenza A viruses is encoded by a second open reading frame in RNA segment 7. A spliced mRNA transcript codes for this 97-amino-acid integral membrane protein, which shares 9 amino acids at its N-terminal end with the M1 protein. M2 is found in large amounts in infected cells but in only small amounts in mature virus. It is a proton channel that performs essential functions in viral uncoating and maturation. The functional form of the protein is a tetramer with approximately 24 N-terminal amino acids in the extracellular domain, a 19-amino-acid hydrophobic transmembrane domain, and a 54-amino-acid intracellular domain. Single amino acid changes in the transmembrane domain of the M2 protein confer resistance to the antiviral drugs amantadine and rimantadine. Antibodies to the M2 protein are found in postinfection serum of humans and ferrets, but the role of the M2 protein in immunity is unknown. RNA segments 6 and 7 of influenza A and B viruses encode different proteins. The NB protein of influenza B virus, which corresponds functionally to the M2 protein, is encoded by RNA segment 6 (the NA gene). CM2, the corresponding protein of influenza C viruses, is also encoded by RNA 6 (the M gene for influenza C viruses).

RNA segment 8 codes for two nonstructural proteins, NS1 and NS2 (recently renamed NEP), that are translated from an uninterrupted and a spliced mRNA transcript, respectively. These proteins share 9 amino acids at their N termini, and both are phosphorylated in infected cells. NS1 is synthesized in large amounts early in infection, whereas NS2 appears later. Both proteins accumulate in the nucleus.

Although influenza C viruses are similar to influenza A and B viruses, they contain seven RNA segments and possess only one surface glycoprotein, which contains hemagglutinating, esterase, and fusion activities. Influenza C viruses have no NA activity, and their receptor-binding specificity differs from that of influenza A and B viruses.

Influenza virus nomenclature includes the type of influenza virus, the host of origin for nonhuman strains, the geographic origin, the strain number, and the year of isolation. An antigenic description of the HA and NA of influenza A viruses is given in parentheses after the year of isolation. For example, A/Hong Kong/1/68 (H3N2) and A/USSR/90/77 (H1N1) are prototype strains for the A(H3N2) and A(H1N1) subtypes, respectively.

Two distinct types of antigenic variation occur in influenza viruses and allow them to evade preexisting immunity. The first is antigenic shift, which involves the appearance of a new subtype of influenza A virus containing a novel HA or novel HA and NA that are immunologically distinct from those of viruses circulating previously. This abrupt change in antigenicity has been associated with pandemics, as occurred in 1957 with the emergence of the Asian (H2N2) virus and in 1968 with the emergence of the Hong Kong (H3N2) strain. The second type of antigenic variation is antigenic drift, which is more gradual and occurs through the accumulation of point mutations in the HA and NA within a subtype, resulting in the inability of antibody to previous strains to neutralize the mutant virus. This type of antigenic variation is responsible for periodic epidemics. Antigenic heterogeneity within a subtype is detected by hemagglutination inhibition (HAI) and NA inhibition tests, as well as by other serological techniques. This antigenic heterogeneity is reflected in genetic changes that can be detected by sequencing the genes encoding the HA and NA. For more detailed information on the molecular biology of influenza viruses, see references 6, 7, and 21.

LABORATORY DIAGNOSIS

Laboratory diagnosis of influenza virus infections should benefit the patient from whom the clinical specimen has been obtained and provide useful information to the treating physician. If a laboratory result is available early during the course of infection, the patient may benefit from specific antiviral treatment with amantadine or rimantadine. A diagnostic result obtained soon after the onset of illness also may help prevent spread of the virus to contacts. This is particularly important when the patient lives with individuals susceptible to severe complications of influenza infection, such as immunocompromised individuals, the elderly, or persons with severe underlying cardiac or pulmonary diseases. In such situations, the persons at risk might be protected by antiviral prophylaxis. Rapid recognition of influenza outbreaks in nursing homes or hospitals can help prevent spread of the virus in these settings. Laboratory diagnosis of influenza virus infections is also the foundation of global surveillance of influenza. Viruses isolated from clinical specimens may be antigenically and genetically characterized in specialized laboratories, and the epidemic spread of new antigenic variants is monitored through this global influenza surveillance network. This information provides the basis for annually selecting appropriate influenza virus strains to be included in trivalent inactivated vaccines. Thus, an influenza virus isolated from a clinical sample collected anywhere in the world may be selected as a vaccine strain.

Several techniques are suitable for laboratory diagnosis of influenza virus infections. Isolation and propagation of the virus in cell cultures or in embryonated hen eggs followed by characterization of the virus by HAI testing and demonstration of a fourfold or greater increase in specific antibody titers between acute- and convalescent-phase sera are standard techniques. Although these methods are highly sensitive and specific, their clinical value is limited because several days to several weeks may be required to obtain a result. A diagnostic result can be obtained more rapidly by the direct detection of viral antigens or viral nucleic acids in clinical specimens. In some instances, the sensitivity of these methods may be inferior to that of standard virus isolation or serologic testing, but the early availability of laboratory results increases the clinical usefulness of rapid procedures. Rapid culture assays combine the high sensitivity of standard virus isolation and the speed of direct methods for the diagnosis of viral infections.

Collection, Transport, and Storage of Specimens

The timing and quality of specimen collection greatly affect laboratory results. Clinical specimens should be taken early, preferably within 3 days of symptom onset. Nasopharyngeal or throat swabs alone or combined, nasopharyngeal aspirates, and nasal washes are useful specimens for virus culture and for the direct detection of viral antigens or nucleic acids. Bronchoalveolar lavage and tracheal aspirate specimens may be considered if clinically warranted.

The infectivity of viruses is stabilized by placing clinical specimens in a suitable transport medium. Tryptose phosphate broth, veal infusion broth, cell culture medium, and sucrose phosphate buffer, all supplemented with 0.5% bovine serum albumin or 0.1% gelatin, antibiotics, and antimycotics, are appropriate transport media (15). Virus infectivity is relatively well preserved if specimens are stored at 4°C in these liquids. After collection, specimens should be shipped to the laboratory without delay and should be refrigerated at all times. The samples should be stored at −70°C immediately after collection if laboratory processing cannot take place by 3 to 4 days after collection. Immediate transport of the specimen to the laboratory and prompt processing are mandatory if the infection is to be diagnosed by the detection of viral antigens in exfoliated epithelial cells by fluorescent-antibody staining.

Isolation of Influenza Viruses in Cell Culture

Primary monkey kidney cells and the Madin-Darby canine kidney cell line (MDCK) (CCL 34; American Type Culture Collection, Rockville, Md.) are most commonly used for the isolation and propagation of influenza viruses. MDCK cells support the growth of influenza A, B, and C viruses when 1 to 2 μg of trypsin per ml is added to the maintenance medium to sustain multiple cycles of replication (24). L-1-Tosylamide-2-phenylethyl chloromethyl ketone (TPCK)-treated trypsin is recommended because of its greater stability at physiologic temperatures. Vero cells (13) and MRC-5 human diploid embryonic lung fibroblasts (8) also support the growth of influenza viruses. A recent study compared the sensitivity of Vero and MRC-5 cells to that of MDCK cells (29). Over a 16-month period, 63 of 746 respiratory specimens were culture positive for influenza A in MDCK cells, 45 were positive in Vero cells, and 36 were positive in MRC-5 cells. A human melanoma cell line highly susceptible to influenza C viruses has been reported (27).

For standard virus isolation, cell culture tubes are seeded with approximately 10^5 MDCK cells in growth medium containing 5 to 10% fetal bovine serum. The tubes are incubated at 37°C, and before the cells are completely confluent, the growth medium is removed, the cell sheet is washed with Hanks' buffer or serum-free medium to remove nonspecific inhibitors present in serum, and then serum-free maintenance medium is added. For inoculation, the medium is removed, 100 to 300 μl of specimen is added to each of two or three tubes, and the tubes are incubated at 34°C in a stationary rack for approximately 2 h. The inoculate is aspirated and replaced by maintenance medium containing TPCK-trypsin. Alternatively, 100 to 300 μl of clinical specimen is inoculated directly into maintenance medium containing TPCK-trypsin, and the medium is changed the following day.

Some influenza viruses destroy the cell sheet within a few days after inoculation. However, in the absence of cytopathic effect, cultures should be tested by the hemadsorption or hemagglutination test at 2- to 3-day intervals (17). A blind passage of negative cultures after 10 to 14 days of incubation may increase the sensitivity of virus isolation.

Isolation of Influenza Viruses in Embryonated Hen Eggs

Allantoic and amniotic cavities of embryonated chicken eggs are inoculated with fresh clinical material. It has been found that 10- to 11-day-old embryonated eggs are optimal for recovery of influenza A and B viruses, while 7- to 8-day-old embryonated eggs are preferred for influenza C viruses. After inoculation, the eggs are incubated at 33 to 34°C for 2 to 3 days for influenza A and B viruses and approximately 5 days for influenza C viruses (17). After one or two passages, most influenza A and B viruses will grow efficiently in the allantoic cavity, but influenza C virus grows only in the amniotic cavity. The presence of influenza viruses in egg fluids is detected by the hemagglutination test.

Some influenza viruses grow to relatively high titers in eggs or cell cultures, and care must be taken to avoid cross-contamination when harvesting infected cultures or eggs. Whenever possible, cell cultures or eggs should be inoculated in a different area of the laboratory from the area used for harvesting of virus-positive material. If this is impossible, fresh clinical specimens should be inoculated before positive cultures or eggs are processed. The work area must be disinfected with organic solvents such as 70% ethanol between procedures. Influenza virus-containing material is inactivated by autoclaving.

Identification and Characterization of Influenza Viruses

Influenza viruses generally can agglutinate human type O, guinea pig, turkey, or chicken erythrocytes. However, influenza C viruses do not agglutinate guinea pig cells, and therefore hemagglutination tests should be performed with both chicken and guinea pig cells. Influenza C viruses and some low-passage influenza A virus isolates may rapidly elute from erythrocytes at room temperature; therefore, the cells should be allowed to settle at 4°C for 1 to 2 h (17). The HAI test with specific antisera is used to identify the hemagglutinating virus. It is important to exclude other hemagglutinating agents, such as mumps and parainfluenza viruses, which also grow in eggs and cell cultures. Typing, subtyping, and further antigenic characterization of influenza viruses is done by HAI (Table 1). Cell culture-grown viruses can be identified by FA or immunoperoxidase staining of cells with specific antibodies.

Detection of Influenza Viruses by Rapid Culture Assays

Early identification of influenza viruses, before microscopically visible cytopathic effect occurs, is possible by using immunologic staining of infected cell cultures with specific antibodies. For rapid culture assays, MDCK cells are grown in 24-well cell culture plates or in shell vials. These culture dishes are suitable for centrifuged inoculation, which increases the sensitivity of influenza virus isolation (33). Clinical specimens are inoculated in duplicate, and the cultures are centrifuged at 700 × *g* for 30 to 60 min and incubated at 35°C in a 5% CO_2 atmosphere. After 18 to 72 h, the medium is removed and the cells are washed twice with phosphate-buffered saline (PBS) and fixed with acetone (80% [vol/vol] in PBS for plastic plates) or methanol. Virus antigens are then detected by FA or immunoperoxidase staining with type-specific antibodies. The sensitivities of rapid culture assays vary from approximately 60 to 100% compared to those of standard virus isolation (12, 26, 35).

A rapid culture assay for the simultaneous type- and subtype-specific detection of influenza A and B viruses has recently been introduced (47). Clinical specimens were inoculated into duplicate wells of 24-well cell culture plates seeded with MDCK cells, centrifuged at 700 × *g* for 45 min, and incubated overnight (approximately 14 to 16 h) at 36°C in a 5% CO_2 atmosphere. Specific virus antigens were detected after acetone fixation by immunoperoxidase staining. Two pools of monoclonal antibodies (MAbs) (41) were used to subtype influenza viruses. Pool A contained two MAbs to the NP of influenza A virus, and pool B contained one MAb to the HA and one to the NP of influenza B virus. Two MAbs which recognize conserved epitopes on the denatured HA1 and HA2 subunits of A/Victoria/3/75 (31) were used to discriminate between H3 and "non-H3," i.e., H1 subtypes. A new panel of subtype-specific MAbs has been evaluated recently (37). Of six MAbs tested with 22 influenza A reference viruses, two reacted exclusively with H3 viruses and four reacted exclusively with H1 viruses. With a combination of pools A and B and these new MAbs, 200 recent isolates were typed and subtyped and 63 isolates were correctly identified as type A (H1N1), 95 were identified as type A (H3N2), 41 were identified as type B, and 1 was identified as a mixture of influenza A and B viruses.

Detection of Infected Cells in Clinical Specimens by FA Staining

Detection of infected, exfoliated epithelial cells in respiratory specimens is a rapid and sensitive method for the labora-

TABLE 1 HAI test with World Health Organization influenza virus reagents from the 1998 to 1999 collection

Reference antigen	Type- and subtype-specific sheep antiserum[a]			
	A/BJ/262/95	A/Sydney/05/97	B/BJ/184/93	B/BJ/243/97
A/Beijing/262/95 (H1N1)	**2,560**[b]	80	10	<10
A/Sydney/05/97 (H3N2)	<10	**640**[b]	40	<10
B/Beijing/184/93	<10	<10	**320**[b]	10
B/Beijing/184/93 Ether treated	<10	<10	**2,560**[b]	80
B/Beijing/243/97	<10	<10	40	**1,280**[b]
B/Beijing/243/97 Ether treated	<10	<10	320	**5,120**[b]

[a] Sheep sera are treated with receptor-destroying enzyme. Values are reciprocals of the highest serum dilution that inhibits hemagglutination.

[b] Homologous titers between antigens and their corresponding antisera.

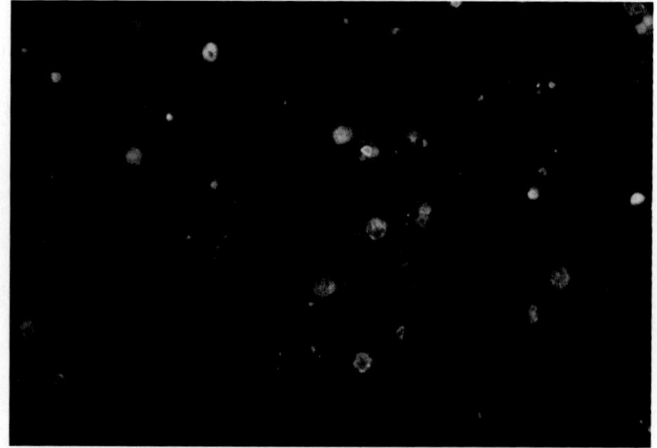

FIGURE 1 Immunofluorescence assay for the detection of influenza A virus antigen. A nasopharyngeal wash specimen was obtained from a patient with an active influenza A infection and processed with a MAb to influenza A virus by procedures described in the text.

tory diagnosis of respiratory virus infections. Epithelial cells are washed free of contaminating mucus, fixed, and stained with specific, well-characterized MAbs, some of which are commercially available (22, 23, 34). When specimens are collected properly and refrigerated at all times, epithelial cells are handled carefully, and the results are read by an experienced microscopist with a good fluorescence microscope, the sensitivity of this technique compares well with that of standard virus isolation. Nonspecific fluorescence from contaminating mucus can be reduced by treating the specimens with dithiothreitol (39) or *N*-acetylcysteine (25) and by centrifuging the cells through Percoll (39). An example of FA staining of a clinical sample is presented in Fig. 1.

Detection of Influenza Virus Antigens by Immunoassays

Sensitive and specific radioimmunoassays, enzyme immunoassays (EIAs), and fluoroimmunoassays for the detection of respiratory virus antigens in clinical samples have been developed by several laboratories. These assays can produce a result within a few hours, but their sensitivity is inferior to that of standard virus isolation. However, specimens in which virus infectivity has been inactivated due to inappropriate storage or transportation may be positive and these assays are less labor-intensive than virus culture.

A rapid EIA specific for influenza A virus, which produces a result in 15 to 20 min, is available commercially (16, 30, 38, 42). In this test, antigens in clinical specimens are trapped on a membrane and reacted with a type-specific MAb and with an anti-mouse enzyme-conjugate and substrates. A positive result is indicated by a colored triangle visible on the membrane. As few as 20 infected cells or approximately 2,000 infectious virus particles can yield a positive result. This test is particularly suitable for the rapid identification of outbreaks in nursing homes, hospitals, or schools.

Molecular Methods for the Detection, Identification, and Characterization of Influenza Viruses

Molecular methods are now applied widely in the diagnosis of influenza virus infections as well as in the characterization of influenza virus isolates. Molecular methods offer several advantages over other laboratory methods. Abundant sequence information derived from isolates collected over several decades and from many geographic regions is now available. These data were necessary for selecting conserved target sequences to allow the identification of all isolates within a subtype. An appropriate choice of nucleotide sequences also allows assays to discriminate between subtypes or even between strains within a subtype. The genetic analysis of a large number of influenza viruses isolated throughout the world each year provides information for a timely update of molecular reagents if required. With currently available technology, the design and synthesis of new molecular probes are more practical than the preparation of updated specific MAbs on a regular basis.

Influenza viruses in clinical specimens can be identified by molecular hybridization (14). Virus particles were solubilized by treating nasopharyngeal aspirates with proteinase K. The released viral nucleic acids were extracted, precipitated, denatured, spotted onto nylon membranes, and immobilized by drying the membranes in a vacuum oven. After prehybridization, ^{32}P-labeled probes consisting of cloned P, NP, and M genes of influenza virus type A were added and the filters were incubated at 37°C for 66 h. After unbound probe was removed by extensive washing, bound probe was detected by autoradiography. The sensitivity of this assay is approximately 1 pg of viral RNA. Appropriate storage of the clinical specimens at −70°C is critical for high assay sensitivity. Under optimal conditions, this assay detected viral RNA in specimens from approximately 75% of patients with documented influenza virus infections.

The reverse transcriptase PCR (RT-PCR) method is now an important tool for the detection of influenza viruses in clinical specimens and in the genetic characterization of influenza virus isolates. Viral nucleic acids are extracted from clinical specimens, allantoic fluid of embryonated hen eggs, or cell culture material by using guanidium thiocyanate (2) or commercial kits. Complementary DNA is synthesized by in vitro reverse transcription of viral RNA primed either by specific synthetic oligonucleotides matching known nucleotide sequences on the viral genes or by random hexamers. This complementary DNA is then amplified with specific primers and DNA polymerase. Finally, the amplified product is detected by any of the numerous methods developed for this purpose.

Subtype-specific detection of influenza A virus in throat swabs has been performed by combining primers specific for the genes encoding H1 and H3 HA (44). The specific primer pairs were selected to amplify a segment approximately 150 bp longer for H3 than for H1. This allowed easy identification of the subtype, based on the migration pattern of the amplified products in agarose gel electrophoresis after staining of the gels with ethidium bromide. The specimens were subjected to 25 cycles of amplification, and if no bands of the appropriate size were visible in the gel, a fraction of the amplified material was amplified for 25 additional cycles. The assay detected 1 to 5 PFU, and all 17 culture-positive gargling fluids were positive by PCR. Six culture-negative samples were negative by PCR, and no cross-reaction was observed with H2N2 viruses or type B viruses.

In another study (5), primers were chosen from conserved, type-specific regions of the NS gene of influenza virus types A, B, and C. After reverse transcription of viral RNA, cDNA was amplified for 40 cycles. The product was electrophoresed in agarose gels, transferred to nylon membranes by Southern blotting, hybridized with a ^{32}P-labeled oligonucleotide probe specific for the amplified product, and detected by autoradiography. The virus type could be determined by the length of the amplified product. Primer pairs and oligonucleotide probes were highly type specific, and no amplified products were observed when nucleic acids from a variety of other respiratory pathogens were tested. Subpicogram amounts of viral RNA were detected by this assay, and for clinical samples, the results of the PCR assays corresponded well to those of virus isolation and FA staining. This assay was compared with culture in tertiary rhesus monkey kidney cells and with direct detection of viral antigens by FA staining in a prospective study of 434 respiratory specimens obtained from a children's hospital during a 5-month period (4). Only type A influenza viruses were detected. Twenty-one specimens were positive by all three methods. Two additional samples tested positive by PCR and by virus culture but remained negative by FA staining. Another two samples that were positive by PCR were negative by the other techniques, and two culture-positive specimens were negative by PCR.

The superiority of RT-PCR over virus culture was demonstrated by using serial nasal wash specimens collected from nine volunteers experimentally infected with influenza virus type A (3). Of the 90 specimens collected over a period of 10 days, 37 were positive by RT-PCR and 26 were positive by virus isolation in MDCK cells. For specimens collected on day 4 postinfection or later, RT-PCR was more sensitive than virus culture; however, three culture-positive specimens collected 3 days after infection were negative by RT-PCR.

More recently, a multiplex RT-PCR which allows the type- and subtype-specific identification of currently circulating human influenza viruses has been developed (43). With three sets of oligonucleotide primers, it was possible to identify the NP gene of influenza A virus, the NS gene of influenza B virus, the HA genes of influenza A virus subtypes H1 and H3, and the NA gene of influenza A virus subtypes N1 and N2. cDNA was synthesized in a reaction mixture containing primers for H1, H3, N1, N2, and B/NS. The product of this reaction was split in two aliquots for amplification. To one part, oligonucleotide primers specific for H1, H3, and B/NS were added, and to the other part, primers specific for N1 and N2 were added. After 40 cycles of amplification, specific products were identified in agarose gels after staining with ethidium bromide. Unfortunately, the number of samples tested was too small to allow conclusions about the potential for routine use.

A type- and subtype-specific multiplex nested RT-PCR format has been evaluated on 619 specimens collected during the 1995 to 1996 influenza season in England (10). Nasal and throat swabs were analyzed by PCR and by virus culture in primary monkey kidney and MDCK cells. RNA was extracted from 100 μl of sample and reverse transcribed with random hexamer primers. Oligonucleotide primer sets specific for H1, H3, and B HAs were selected for two rounds of PCR amplification so that they could be used under similar conditions in one reaction tube (46). After 35 cycles of amplification with a set of outer primers, 2 μl of the reaction mixture was amplified for another 35 cycles with a set of nested primers (11). The virus type and subtype were identified by amplicon size in ethidium bromide-stained agarose gels. Influenza viruses were found in 270 of the 619 specimens. Of those, 176 were positive by virus culture and by PCR, 72 were positive by PCR only, and 24 were positive by culture only. Both methods agreed on the type and subtype identified. This multiplex RT-PCR appears promising for the direct detection and partial characterization of influenza viruses from large numbers of clinical specimens.

PCR combined with endonuclease restriction analysis has been applied to the genetic characterization of influenza viruses. For this technique, oligonucleotide primers are designed to amplify a product that contains unique restriction enzyme cleavage sites. This method can discriminate between two separate genetic lineages of influenza A (H3N2) viruses which circulate simultaneously during an influenza season (9, 48); can determine the genetic stability of cold-adapted, reassortant live vaccine strains (18); and allows rapid identification of drug-resistant influenza isolates (19).

Serologic Methods in Influenza Diagnosis

Although serologic methods rarely produce a result early during the course of an influenza virus infection, they often can establish the diagnosis if other methods fail. The complement fixation test (CF), HAI, the neutralization test (NT), and EIA are the most widely used assays in serodiagnosis and seroepidemiologic studies of influenza. CF detects type-specific antibodies to NP but is relatively insensitive in detecting diagnostic rises in titer between acute- and convalescent-phase sera. HAI and NT are type, subtype, and even strain specific and can be used to identify the antigenic variant causing the infection. Both HAI and NT are useful in measuring the immunogenicity of vaccines and in determining whether preexisting antibodies derived from natural infection or from vaccination may protect an individual from infection with circulating epidemic viruses. Nonspecific inhibitors of hemagglutination found in some human or animal sera can cause false-positive results in the HAI test, but methods are available to remove these inhibitors (17, 36). The source of antigen can affect results obtained by HAI, since significant increases in titer are more often detected with cell culture-derived antigens than with egg-grown preparations (28, 32).

The specificity of EIA is influenced by the selection of the antigen and the conjugate to different isotypes of immunoglobulins. Detection of immunoglobulin M- or A-class antibodies collected early after the onset of disease may provide a diagnosis of the infection (20, 40).

Drug Susceptibility Tests

Recent increased use of antiviral drugs for the prophylaxis and treatment of infections caused by influenza A virus has made testing of isolates for drug resistance more important than in the past. The conventional assay for drug sensitivity testing is the highly sensitive and accurate plaque reduction assay. Assays which allow the testing of large numbers of specimens are EIAs which measure the synthesis of viral proteins in the presence or absence of the drug under study and restriction analysis of PCR-amplified viral nucleic acids (19).

CONCLUSIONS

With the wide range of diagnostic tests available, each laboratory must choose the methods which best fit the daily routine. Techniques that are continuously used in a laboratory and for which quality assurance procedures are well established are the most reliable. Standardized reagents should be used to achieve a high level of test reproducibility. Culture-independent tests for the detection of viral antigens or nucleic acids should be used if a result must be obtained rapidly for clinical or epidemiologic reasons. For early detection of antigenic variants or completely new subtypes and for the surveillance of their spread in the human population, it is important that laboratories continue to isolate influenza viruses and submit the isolates to specialized laboratories for antigenic and genetic analyses. For example, a combination of diagnostic techniques was used to screen and subtype large numbers of specimens submitted for the laboratory diagnosis of H5N1 infections during the 1997 outbreak in Hong Kong. Many clinical samples were screened for type A influenza viruses by rapid commercially available EIAs or IFA tests. MAbs and PCR primers specific for H5 HA were used for the rapid identification of H5N1-positive samples (45). Cell culture or serologic testing was used to confirm the H5N1 infection, and the sensitivity and specificity of these rapid methods were high, although EIA appeared more sensitive than direct immunofluorescence. Rapid diagnosis of H5N1 influenza in hospital patients was used for initiation of early antiviral therapy, for early isolation of infected patients, and for identification and investigation of contacts. Viruses were subsequently sent to reference laboratories for complete antigenic and genetic characterization. This recent example clearly illustrates that by combining rapid methods with conventional cell culture, large numbers of specimens can be efficiently screened. This approach was useful for patient management; for reducing uncertainty among patients, health care workers, and the public; and for obtaining viruses for analysis.

REFERENCES

1. **Betts, R. F.** 1995. Influenza virus, p. 1546–1567. *In* G. L. Mandell, J. E. Bennett, and P. Dolin (ed.), *Principles and Practice of Infectious Diseases*. Churchill Livingstone, Inc., New York, N.Y.
2. **Boom, R., C. J. A. Sol, M. M. M. Salimans, C. L. Jansen, P. M. E. Wertheim-van Dillen, and J. van der Noordaa.** 1990. Rapid and simple method for purification of nucleic acids. *J. Clin. Microbiol.* **28:**495–503.
3. **Cherian, T., L. Bobo, M. C. Steinhoff, R. A. Karron, and R. H. Yolken.** 1994. Use of PCR-enzyme immunoassay for identification of influenza A virus matrix RNA in clinical samples negative for cultivable virus. *J. Clin. Microbiol.* **32:**623–628.
4. **Claas, E. C. J., A. J. van Milaan, M. J. W. Sprenger, M. Ruiten-Stuiver, G. I. Arron, P. H. Rothbarth, and N. Masurel.** 1993. Prospective application of reverse transcriptase polymerase chain reaction for diagnosing influenza infections in respiratory samples from a children's hospital. *J. Clin. Microbiol.* **31:**2218–2221.
5. **Claas, E. C. J., M. J. W. Sprenger, G. E. M. Kleter, R. van Beek, W. G. V. Quint, and N. Masurel.** 1992. Type-specific identification of influenza viruses A, B, and C by the polymerase chain reaction. *J. Virol. Methods* **39:**1–13.
6. **Cox, N. J., and C. A. Bender.** 1995. The molecular epidemiology of influenza viruses. *Semin. Virol.* **6:**359–370.
7. **Cox, N. J., and Y. Kawaoka.** 1998. Orthomyxoviruses: influenza, p. 385–433. *In* B. W. J. Mahy and L. Collier (ed.), *Topley and Wilson's Microbiology and Microbial Infections*, vol. 1. Arnold, London, United Kingdom.
8. **De Ona, M., S. Melon, P. de la Iglesia, F. Hidalgo, and A. F. Verdugo.** 1995. Isolation of influenza virus in human lung embryonated fibroblast cells (MRC-5) from clinical samples. *J. Clin. Microbiol.* **33:**1948–1949.
9. **Ellis, J. S., C. J. Sadler, P. Laidler, H. Rebelo de Andrade, and M. C. Zambon.** 1997. Analysis of influenza A H3N2 strains isolated in England during 1995–1996 using polymerase chain reaction restriction. *J. Med. Virol.* **51:** 234–241.
10. **Ellis, J. S., D. M. Fleming, and M. C. Zambon.** 1997. Multiplex reverse transcription-PCR for surveillance of influenza A and B viruses in England and Wales in 1995 and 1996. *J. Clin. Microbiol.* **35:**2076–2082.
11. **Ellis, J. S., P. Chakraverty, and J. P. Clewley.** 1995. Genetic and antigenic variation in the haemagglutinin of recently circulating human influenza A (H3N2) viruses in the United Kingdom. *Arch. Virol.* **140:**1889–1904.
12. **Espy, M. J., T. F. Smith, M. W. Harmon, and A. P. Kendal.** 1986. Rapid detection of influenza virus by shell vial assay with monoclonal antibodies. *J. Clin. Microbiol.* **24:**677–679.
13. **Govorkova, E. A., N. V. Kaverin, L. V. Gubareva, B. Meignier, and R. G. Webster.** 1995. Replication of influenza A viruses in a green monkey kidney continuous cell line (Vero). *J. Infect. Dis.* **172:**250–253.
14. **Havlickova, M., A. Z. Pljusnin, and B. Tumova.** 1990. Influenza virus detection in clinical specimens. *Acta Virol.* **34:**446–456.
15. **Johnson, F. B.** 1990. Transport of viral specimens. *Clin. Microbiol. Rev.* **3:**120–131.
16. **Johnston, S. L. G., and H. Bloy.** 1993. Evaluation of a rapid enzyme immunoassay for detection of influenza A virus. *J. Clin. Microbiol.* **31:**142–143.
17. **Kendal, A. P., J. J. Skehel, and M. S. Pereira.** 1982. *Concepts and Procedures for Laboratory-Based Influenza Surveillance*. Centers for Disease Control, Atlanta, Ga.
18. **Klimov, A. I., and N. J. Cox.** 1995. PCR restriction analysis of genome composition and stability of cold-adapted reassortant live influenza vaccines. *J. Virol. Methods* **52:** 41–49.
19. **Klimov, A. I., E. Rocha, F. G. Hayden, P. A. Shult, L. F. Roumillat, and N. J. Cox.** 1995. Prolonged shedding of amantadine-resistant influenza A viruses by immunodeficient patients: detection by polymerase chain reaction-restriction analysis. *J. Infect. Dis.* **172:**1352–1355.
20. **Koskinen, P., T. Vuorinen, and O. Meurman.** 1987. Influenza A and B virus IgG and IgM serology by enzyme immunoassays. *Epidemiol. Infect.* **99:**55–64.
21. **Lamb, R. A., and R. M. Krug.** 1996. Orthomyxoviridae: the viruses and their replication, *In* B. N. Fields, D. M. Knipe, P. M. Howley, et al. (ed.), *Fields Virology*, 3rd ed. Lippincott-Raven Publishers, Philadelphia, Pa.
22. **Leonardi, G. P., H. Leib, G. S. Birkhead, C. Smith, P. Costello, and W. Conron.** 1994. Comparison of rapid detection methods for influenza A virus and their value in health-care management of institutionalized geriatric patients. *J. Clin. Microbiol.* **32:**70–74.
23. **McDonald, J. C., and P. Quennec.** 1993. Utility of a respiratory virus panel containing a monoclonal antibody pool for screening of respiratory specimens in nonpeak respiratory syncytial virus season. *J. Clin. Microbiol.* **31:** 2809–2811.
24. **Meguro, H., J. D. Bryant, A. E. Torrence, and P. F. Wright.** 1979. Canine kidney cell line for isolation of respiratory viruses. *J. Clin. Microbiol.* **9:**175–179.
25. **Miller, H. R., P. H. Phipps, and E. Rossier.** 1986. Reduction of nonspecific fluorescence in respiratory specimens by pretreatment with *N*-acetylcysteine. *J. Clin. Microbiol.* **24:**470–471.
26. **Mills, R. D., K. J. Cain, and G. L. Woods.** 1989. Detection of influenza virus by centrifugal inoculation of MDCK cells and staining with monoclonal antibodies. *J. Clin. Microbiol.* **27:**2505–2508.
27. **Nishimura, H., K. Sugawara, F. Kitame, K. Nakamura, N. Katsushima, H. Moriuchi, and Y. Nymazaki.** 1989. A human melanoma cell line highly susceptible to influenza C virus. *J. Gen. Virol.* **70:**1653–1661.
28. **Pyhälä, R., L. Pyhälä, M. Valle, and K. Aho.** 1987. Egg-grown and tissue-culture-grown variants of influenza A

(H3N2) virus with special attention to their use as antigens in seroepidemiology. *Epdemiol. Infect.* **99:**745–753.

29. **Reina, J., V. Fernandez-Baca, I. Blanco, and M. Munar.** 1997. Comparison of Madin-Darby canine kidney cells (MDCK) with a green monkey continuous cell line (Vero) and human lung embryonated cells (MRC-5) in the isolation of influenza A virus from nasopharyngeal aspirates by shell vial culture. *J. Clin. Microbiol.* **35:**1900–1901.
30. **Ryan-Poirier, K. A., J. M. Katz, R. G. Webster, and Y. Kawaoka.** 1992. Application of Directigen FLU-A for the detection of influenza A virus in human and nonhuman specimens. *J. Clin. Microbiol.* **30:**1072–1075.
31. **Sanchez-Fauquier, A., N. Villanueva, and J. A. Melero.** 1987. Isolation of cross-reactive, subtype-specific monoclonal antibodies against influenza virus HA1 and HA2 hemagglutinin subunits. *Arch. Virol.* **97:**251–265.
32. **Schild, G. C., J. S. Oxford, J. C. de Jong, and R. G. Webster.** 1983. Evidence for host-cell selection of influenza virus antigenic variants. *Nature* (London) **303:** 706–709.
33. **Seno, M., Y. Kanamoto, S. Takao, N. Takei, S. Fukuda, and H. Umisa.** 1990. Enhancing effect of centrifugation on isolation of influenza virus from clinical specimens. *J. Clin. Microbiol.* **28:**1669–1670.
34. **Spada, B., K. Biehler, P. Chegas, J. Kaye, and M. Riepenhoff-Talty.** 1991. Comparison of rapid immunofluorescence assay to cell culture isolation for the detection of influenza A and B viruses in nasopharyngeal secretions from infants and children. *J. Virol. Methods* **33:**305–310.
35. **Stokes, C. E., J. J. Bernstein, S. A. Kyger, and F. G. Hayden.** 1988. Rapid diagnosis of influenza A and B by 24-h fluorescent focus assays. *J. Clin. Microbiol.* **26:** 1263–1266.
36. **Subbarao, E. K., Y. Kawaoka, K. Ryan-Poirier, M. L. Clements, and B. R. Murphy.** 1992. Comparison of different approaches to measuring influenza A virus-specific hemagglutination inhibition antibodies in the presence of serum inhibitors. *J. Clin. Microbiol.* **30:**996–999.
37. **Tkacova, M., E. Vareckova, I. C. Baker, J. M. Love, and T. Ziegler.** 1997. Evaluation of monoclonal antibodies for subtyping of currently circulating human type A influenza viruses. *J. Clin. Microbiol.* **35:**1196–1198.
38. **Todd, S. J., L. Minnich, and J. L. Waner.** 1995. Comparison of rapid immunofluorescence procedure with TestPack RSV and Directigen FLU-A for diagnosis of respiratory syncytial virus and influenza A virus. *J. Clin. Microbiol.* **33:**1650–1651.
39. **Ukkonen, P., and I. Julkunen.** 1987. Preparation of nasopharyngeal secretions for immunofluorescence by one-step centrifugation through Percoll. *J. Virol. Methods* **15:** 291–301.
40. **Vikerfors, T., G. Lindegren, M. Grandien, and J. van der Logt.** 1989. Diagnosis of influenza A virus infections by detection of specific immunoglobulins M, A, and G in serum. *J. Clin. Microbiol.* **27:**453–458.
41. **Walls, H. H., M. W. Harmon, J. J. Slagle, C. Stockskale, and A. P. Kendal.** 1986. Characterization and evaluation of monoclonal antibodies developed for typing influenza and influenza B viruses. *J. Clin. Microbiol.* **23:**240–245.
42. **Waner, J. L., S. J. Todd, H. Shalaby, P. Murphy, and L. V. Wall.** 1991. Comparison of Directigen FLU-A with viral isolation and direct immunofluorescence for the rapid detection and identification of influenza A virus. *J. Clin. Microbiol.* **29:**479–482.
43. **Wright, K. E., G. A. R. Wilson, D. Novosad, C. Dimock, D. Tan, and J. M. Weber.** 1995. Typing and subtyping of influenza viruses in clinical samples by PCR. *J. Clin. Microbiol.* **33:**1180–1184.
44. **Yamada, A., J. Imanishi, E. Nakajima, K. Nakajima, and S. Nakajima.** 1991. Detection of influenza viruses in throat swab by using polymerase chain reaction. *Microbiol. Immunol* **35:**259–265.
45. **Yuen, K. Y., P. K. S. Chan, M. Peiris, D. N. C. Tsang, T. L. Que, K. F. Shortridge, P. T. Cheung, W. K. To, E. T. F. Ho, R. Sung, A. F. B. Cheng, and members of the H5N1 study group.** 1998. Clinical features and rapid viral diagnosis of human disease associated with avian influenza A H5N1 virus. *Lancet* **351:**467–471.
46. **Zhang, W., and D. H. Evans.** 1991. Detection and identification of human influenza viruses by the polymerase chain reaction. *J. Virol. Methods* **33:**165–189.
47. **Ziegler, T., H. Hall. A. Sanchez-Fauquier, W. C. Gamble, and N. J. Cox.** 1995. Type- and subtype-specific detection of influenza viruses in clinical specimens by rapid culture assay. *J. Clin. Microbiol.* **33:**318–321.
48. **Zou, S.** 1997. A practical approach to genetic screening for influenza virus variants. *J. Clin. Microbiol.* **35:**2623–2627.

Parainfluenza Viruses

JOSEPH L. WANER

71

CLINICAL BACKGROUND

The four parainfluenza viruses (PIVs) of humans cause upper respiratory disease in children and adults. PIV type 1 (PIV-1) is the principal cause of laryngotracheobronchitis (croup), although PIV-2, PIV-3, and other infectious agents may also cause this disorder. The average number of hospitalizations per year due to croup has been reported to be 41,000; biennial epidemics of PIV-1 were associated with 18,000 excess hospitalizations for croup, while PIV-2 played a minor role in croup hospitalizations (21). Nevertheless, types 1 and 2 behave similarly, although type 2 generally produces milder illness. The most severe illness caused by PIV-1 and -2 occurs in children less than 5 years of age. Type 3 infection produces the most severe illness in infants less than 1 year old. PIV-3 is second only to respiratory syncytial virus (RSV) in importance as a cause of bronchiolitis and pneumonia in infants (3, 5, 11, 23). Type 4 consists of two antigenic subgroups, A and B, and causes mild upper respiratory disease, but it is rarely encountered when only isolation in cell culture is used for diagnosis. Reinfections with PIVs are common but are generally less severe clinically than primary infections (3, 12). PIV infections in older children and adults are more likely to be asymptomatic or to result in mild disease resembling the common cold syndrome (30). Aside from causing respiratory disease, PIV-3 can also be isolated from spinal fluids of patients with symptoms of meningeal infection (27) and for prolonged periods from adults without acute symptoms (15). Genetic variations and antigenic subgroups exist among the PIVs, but these variations have not been shown to have biological implications or to affect the choice of the diagnostic methods used.

PIV-1 and -2 occur in alternate-year patterns, tending to produce epidemics in the autumn and early winter (4, 13). Characteristically, PIV-1 is associated with epidemics of acute respiratory illness in odd-numbered years. Type 3 is predominantly endemic and displays little or no seasonality. PIVs are transmitted via infected respiratory secretions through close person-to-person contact and aerosols. The viruses remain viable on surfaces for several hours (2) but rapidly lose their infectivity on hands (1); PIVs are readily inactivated by heat and detergents. Laboratory-associated infections should not occur if careful laboratory practices are followed. Vaccines are being developed and immune therapy is being investigated, but neither is currently available.

DESCRIPTION OF THE VIRUS

PIVs belong to the family *Paramyxoviridae*. PIV-1 and PIV-3 belong to the genus *Paramyxovirus*, while PIV-2, PIV-4A, and PIV-4B belong to the genus *Rubulavirus*. The viruses have a helical symmetry and single-stranded, nonsegmented RNA genomes with negative polarity. Virions have envelopes obtained by budding from the host cell cytoplasmic membrane. PIVs have six structural proteins, although coding strategies and the total number of gene products may differ between the paramyxoviruses (6). The HN (hemagglutinin-neuraminidase) and F (fusion) proteins are found in the envelope and are glycosylated. The HN protein is larger than the F protein and is necessary for adsorption to the host cell. After adsorption, the F protein mediates virion entry into the cell. The F protein is also responsible for cell-to-cell spread, manifested morphologically in cell cultures as syncytia. The remaining structural proteins are the large nucleocapsid protein, the nucleoprotein, the phosphoprotein, and the matrix protein.

Common antigens are shared by the four PIVs, mumps virus, Newcastle disease virus, Sendai virus (PIV-1 of mice), bovine PIV-3, and simian virus 5. Isolates of human PIVs can be distinguished according to type with specific antisera, particularly monoclonal antibodies (MAbs) (29).

COLLECTION AND STORAGE OF SPECIMENS

The object of specimen collection for the diagnosis of PIV infection is to obtain secretions from the respiratory tract. Efforts should also be made to obtain cellular material, particularly if direct procedures for viral identification are to be attempted. PIV-3 may be excreted for 3 to 10 days following primary infection, but it may be excreted for shorter intervals after secondary infections (5). Nevertheless, the greatest quantity of virus is excreted early in the course of illness, making the prompt collection of specimens critical for the efficient isolation of virus.

Collection of specimens is most commonly accomplished with a wash of the nasopharynx. However, respiratory secretions may be aspirated with a suction device without the addition of a wash. A convenient and effective adaptation of the method described by Hall and Douglas (16) is recommended. The nasopharynx is vigorously swabbed with a Dacron swab on a flexible aluminum or plastic shaft to loosen mucus and cellular material. Approximately 2 ml of sterile saline is then introduced into the nasopharynx through small tubing attached to a 5-ml syringe; a convenient source of tubing is a Butterfly-22 infusion set. The wash and swab are placed together in 1.5 ml of transport medium and are carried to the laboratory on wet ice. Alternatively, a swab may be inserted into the back of the nasopharynx, held in place for 1 min, and rolled on wells of hydrophobic slides to transfer the cells. The latter procedure works best when experienced personnel routinely do specimen collection.

Adults and older children may resist nasopharyngeal (NP) washes due to the discomfort associated with the procedure. Throat or NP swabs may be used alone but are generally not as effective as NP washes, particularly for antigen detection. The swab should be placed in the transport medium, and the specimen should be taken promptly on wet ice to the laboratory. Specimens should be held at 4°C and should not be frozen if processing will be accomplished within 48 h of collection. A sample (approximately 0.3 ml) should be stored at −70°C for possible use in reevaluating the specimen or for future reference.

Investigations concerning optimum specimen collection methods for nucleic acid amplification techniques have not been reported. Specimens may be obtained by washing or swabbing and may be frozen for long periods if necessary. In either case, the RNA must be extracted from the specimen before analysis. It is likely that the much greater sensitivity of amplification techniques will allow less rigid criteria to be exercised in specimen collection and handling.

Transport medium should consist of a buffered salt solution (pH 7.0) containing a protein-stabilizing agent and antibiotics. In this laboratory, a medium consisting of tryptic soy broth with 0.5% gelatin, gentamicin (50 μg/ml), chloramphenicol (5.0 μg/ml), and amphotericin B (2.0 μg/ml) is used.

ISOLATION IN CELL CULTURE

Primary human embryonic kidney cells and primary monkey kidney (PMK) cells are the most sensitive cells used for the isolation of PIVs by culture. NCI-H292 is a continuous line of mucoepidermoid cells that may also be used for the isolation of PIVs (18). PIV isolates may be adapted to grow in other continuous cell lines (Vero, HEp-2, LLC-MK2, and HeLa cells), but these are not recommended for use in the isolation of virus from clinical specimens. Other viruses that may be present as pathogens in the respiratory tract replicate in PMK cell cultures, which should be an essential component of the laboratory's isolation protocol; primary rhesus monkey cells are recommended. Tubes of uninfected PMK cell cultures are maintained on Eagle minimal essential medium (MEME) with 5% newborn calf serum and are held at 35°C. Cultures are refed every 4 to 5 days until use but should not be used after 10 days after receipt of the cultures.

Before inoculation of cell cultures, specimen material is vigorously mixed, the collection swab is pressed against the side of the container to express fluid, and the swab is discarded. The maintenance medium is removed from two PMK cell cultures, and the cultures are washed twice with Hank's balanced salt solution (HBSS). Each tube is inoculated with 0.2 ml of the specimen, and the cultures are absorbed at 37°C. The inoculum is removed after 1 h, and the cultures are washed once with serum-free medium containing trypsin (SFM) and are refed with SFM. Cultures are incubated in a roller drum at 35°C; stationary incubation is also satisfactory. In our experience, medium containing serum may delay hemadsorption (HAd) of PIVs for 1 to 3 days and may also diminish the degree of HAd seen. A suitable SFM consists of 50 ml of medium 199, 46 ml of MEME, 3 ml of 100× vitamins for MEME, 0.5 ml of glucose (50% solution), 1 ml of glutamine (200 mM), 0.1 ml of trypsin (0.025%), 50 mg of gentamicin per ml, and 2 mg of amphotericin B per ml; the medium 199 and MEME should be buffered with HEPES. Cultures that are refed every 4 days may be maintained on SFM for 10 to 14 days.

Cultures are observed daily for cytopathic effect (CPE) to detect not only PIVs but also other viruses that may have been in the specimen and that may replicate in PMK cells. In our experience, approximately 50% of PIV isolates show a CPE at between 4 and 5 days after inoculation. The CPEs of the PIVs may range from unrecognizable to destructive, depending on the PIV type and the isolate. Typically, PIV-1 is identified by HAd before a CPE appears (Fig. 1b); the CPE consists of small rounded cells that are often difficult to discern as a CPE. The CPE of PIV-2 is often syncytial (Fig. 1c); PIV-3 may show "bridging" of the infected monolayer (Fig. 1d). Degeneration of the entire monolayer often characterizes the CPE of PIV-4.

The detection of a PIV (or other hemadsorbing virus) in cell culture following the appearance of a CPE is confirmed by HAd. However, HAd may be detected before an identifiable CPE is detected and may be used as an inexpensive rapid method for the detection of hemadsorbing viruses, including PIVs. More than 50% of the PIV-1 and PIV-3 isolates hemadsorb by 48 h after inoculation (22). A convenient strategy is examination of cultures for HAd 24 h after inoculation and at 48-h intervals thereafter; cultures should also be examined for HAd at the earliest sighting of a CPE. Guinea pig erythrocytes (RBCs) are washed four times with HBSS and are prepared as a 4% solution that may be stored at 4°C for 3 to 4 days. The medium from the cultures to be tested is removed and 1 ml of cold HBSS is added to each tube, followed by the addition of 0.2 ml of a 0.4% solution of RBCs prepared in cold HBSS from the stock solution. The tubes are first incubated at 4°C for 30 min, viewed, and reincubated at room temperature for 30 min; influenza virus should hemadsorb at 4°C and room temperature, whereas PIVs generally hemadsorb only at 4°C. The temperature differences seen are associated with degrees of HAd and are not absolute reactions. Uninfected culture tubes of the same lot number as those inoculated should be hemadsorbed at the same time to control for the presence of hemadsorbing monkey viruses in the cell cultures. Human PIVs are more likely to hemadsorb in a diffuse pattern (Fig. 1b); monkey viruses often hemadsorb in clusters. Virus proteins may adhere to the glass, particularly on the edges of monolayers, resulting in RBC adsorption to the glass in the absence of visible cellular material. If HAd is not seen the RBCs may be poured off and the cultures may be washed with HBSS, refed with SFM, and incubated until the next HAd attempt.

Cells may be scraped from an inoculated tube as early as 48 h after inoculation and prepared for immunofluorescence (IF) as described below. IF is more sensitive than HAd and results in a specific diagnosis. The cells are stained with a pool of MAbs to the PIVs or with MAbs to each type. The remaining inoculated cultures should be retained in case the IF procedure is falsely negative or to identify a possible dual infection. In the absence of a CPE and if HAd is not performed, laboratories may routinely stain cultures 7 to 10 days after inoculation and finalize the results.

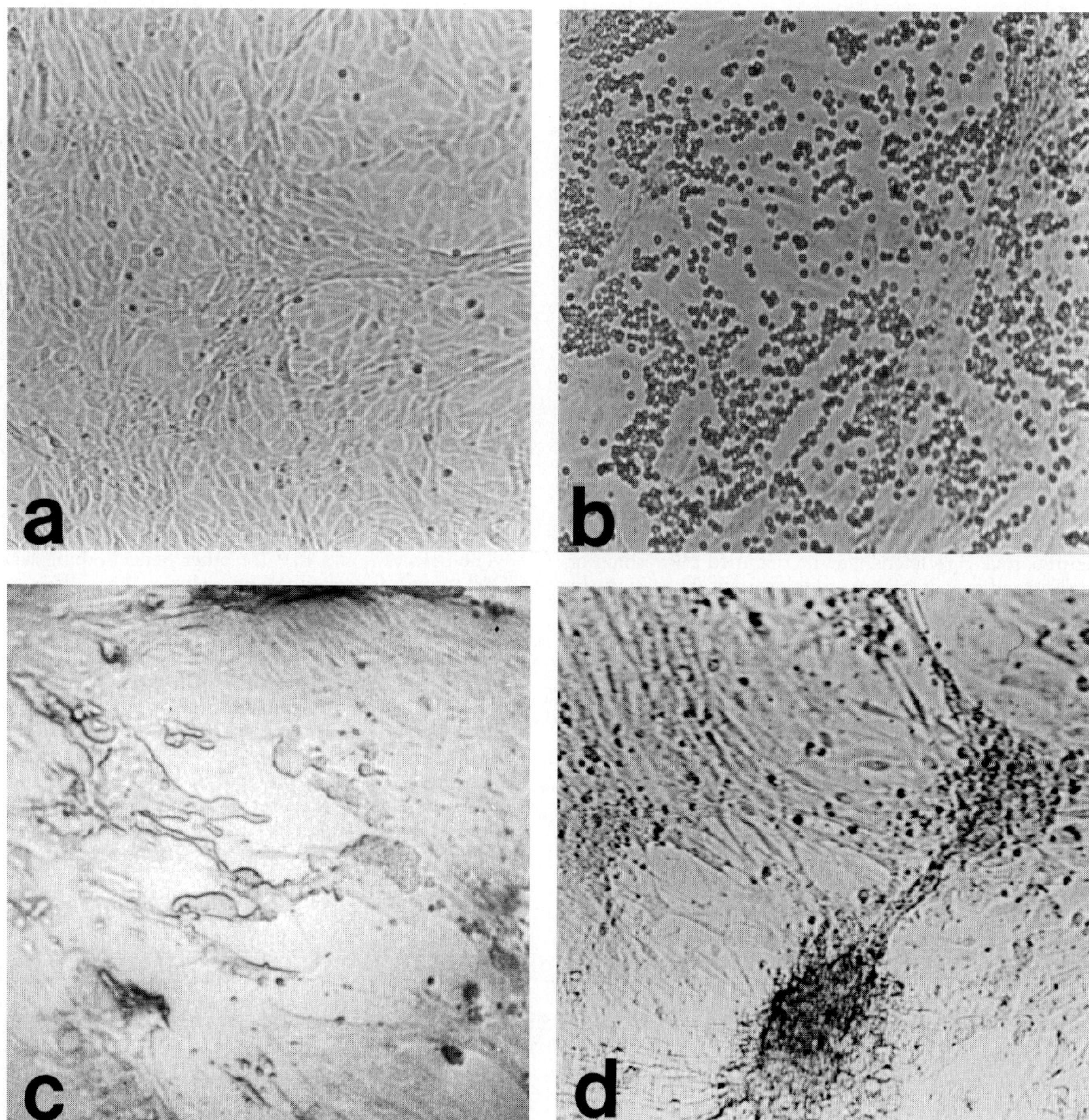

FIGURE 1 HAd of PIV-1 and cytopathic effect of PIV-2 and PIV-3 in primary rhesus monkey kidney cell cultures. (a) Uninfected cells; (b) HAd of PIV-1; (c) CPE of PIV-2; (d) CPE of PIV-3.

DETECTION OF ANTIGEN

IF

The most commonly used method of detecting PIV antigens directly in patient specimens or in infected cell cultures is by direct or indirect IF (Fig. 2) (29, 31). MAbs to all four human PIVs may be purchased as individual reagents or as a PIV pool.

For direct examination of cells obtained from NP washes, specimens should be obtained as described above; the nasopharynx should be swabbed prior to washing to obtain increased numbers of NP cells. Cells in the specimen are washed with phosphate buffered saline (PBS; pH 7.0) until the mucus is virtually removed, which usually requires one to three washes. The cells are resuspended in 0.25 ml of PBS, and 10 to 20 μl of the cell suspension is applied to 8-mm wells circumscribed on eight-well enamel-coated glass slides (Cell-Line Associates, Newfield, N.J.). The wells are examined at ×100 magnification to assess the numbers of cells and the morphologies of the cells present. Specimens yielding fewer than an average of 20 columnar epithelial cells per well should be rejected; squamous epithelial cells are unsatisfactory. The slides are air dried, fixed in cold acetone for 10 min, dipped three times in distilled H_2O to rinse the slides, and air dried before staining. Slides may be stored with a desiccating agent for several months at −70°C.

Cells sufficient for the preparation of 20 or more wells are usually obtained. The specimen can be comprehensively examined by staining three or four wells each with antibodies to the common respiratory viruses of the season, i.e., RSV, influenza types A and B, adenovirus, and PIVs. MAbs

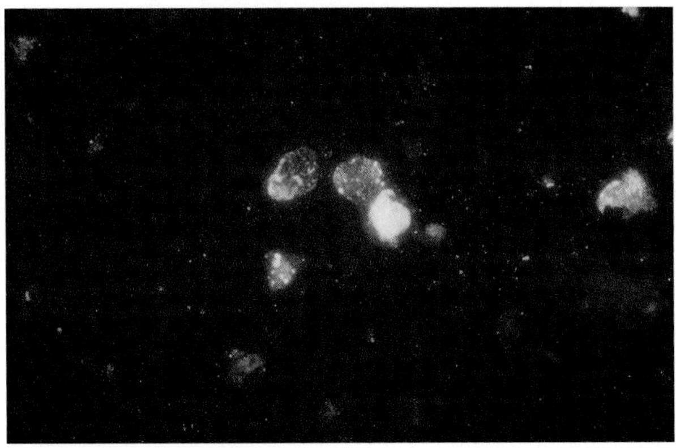

FIGURE 2 Indirect IF reaction with antigen-positive cells from an NP wash with a pool of MAbs to PIV-1, -2, and -3.

to these viruses are the immune reagents of choice and are commercially available. A pool of MAbs to PIVs may be applied to the specimen; application of the antibodies to four to six wells provides a good expectation of sensitive and specific results. Conventional staining protocols usually require more than a total of 60 min of incubation time. A rapid IF format reported for RSV and influenza virus that requires 20 min for completion after specimen preparation may also be used for the detection of PIVs (26). The detection of a PIV without knowledge of the type is sufficient for clinical purposes and may be done rapidly with less expense by using the pool; if desired, specific typing may be done later.

Shell Vial Assay

Centrifugation of a specimen onto a monolayer of susceptible cells and subsequent staining of the monolayer for a viral antigen(s) provides a rapid and sensitive assay for the detection of PIVs (25). Susceptible cell lines growing on coverslips contained in shell vials may be purchased. Alternatively, cell cultures may be passaged in the laboratory onto coverslips in shell vials. When the monolayer is approximately 90% confluent, 0.2 ml of a specimen is inoculated into duplicate vials containing 0.2 ml of medium. Virus and uninfected controls should be included in each centrifugation run. After the vials are centrifuged at 700 × *g* for 45 min at ambient temperature, the inoculum is aspirated and the cultures are overlaid with medium; SFM is not required. Following 2 days of incubation at 37°C, the coverslips are removed from the vials and prepared for IF as described above; additional cultures may be prepared for staining at 4 days after inoculation. The coverslips may be reacted with a pool of MAbs to the PIVs or with an MAb to one type of PIV. Coverslips are screened at a magnification of ×200, and positive cells are confirmed at a magnification of ×400.

EIA

PIV antigens may be identified in infected cell cultures or clinical specimens by enzyme immunoassay (EIA) (24), which is comparable in specificity to IF but slightly less sensitive than IF (14). Time-resolved fluoroimmunoassay may be more sensitive than EIA or IF (17). Commercial test kits are not available in the United States, but EIA may be constructed from reagents purchased as single components or prepared locally. PIV antigens and control antigens may be obtained from infected cell cultures. Chapter 12 of this Manual and the publications cited therein should be referred to for the preparation of EIA.

DETECTION OF NUCLEIC ACID

PCR is the most promising molecular technique that may be amenable to the routine diagnosis of PIV infections. Reports of studies that have used PCR to detect PIVs in clinical specimens should be consulted to choose primers and to determine the experimental protocol. The detection of the single-stranded RNA genome of PIVs requires use of the reverse transcription-PCR (RT-PCR) technique. RNA is extracted from specimens and reverse transcribed to make cDNA. Primers for highly conserved sequences of the NH gene have been successfully used to detect PIV-1 (7) and PIV-3 (19) in clinical specimens. Similarly, sequences of the 5′ noncoding region of the F gene were used as primers to detect PIV-3 by RT-PCR. The sequences of the primers and target nucleic acid were sufficiently similar to those of PIV-1 that PIV-1 and PIV-3 could be detected (10). However, differentiation of virus type was not possible by the procedure.

Diversity among isolates of PIV-3 has also been studied by using RT-PCR to amplify sequences in a hypervariable region of the F gene; the virus isolates examined were grown in cell culture before the analysis (20). The amplified sequences were identified by EIA with a nonisotopically labeled RNA probe. There are numerous other variations to detection protocols, but the use of nonisotopic labels is a pragmatic necessity for the clinical laboratory.

Molecular methods have not been routinely applied to the detection of PIVs. The common use of nucleic acid amplification for the detection of PIVs is hampered by the complexity of the assays, cost, and lack of specific treatment for PIV infections to justify the expense. There is also a lack of comprehensive studies comparing RT-PCR with other rapid techniques. The introduction of a molecular test into the laboratory should be accompanied by established predictive values of the test and knowledge of the clinical significance of the lower detection limit. It is also prudent to devise an algorithm for the use of the RT-PCR test in conjunction with more traditional diagnostic methods.

SEROLOGY

The common tests used for the detection of antibodies to the PIVs are complement fixation (CF), hemagglutination-inhibition (HI), IF, neutralization, and EIA. Some antigens are shared among the PIVs and between the PIVs and other paramyxoviruses, notably, mumps virus. Cross-reactions are therefore common in serological tests. Heterotypic responses may also occur in patients, making a specific serological diagnosis of a PIV infection difficult. Immunoglobulin M (IgM) antibodies to each of the PIVs may be detected by EIA or IF, and IgM antibodies generally show fewer heterologous responses than IgG antibodies (8, 28).

HI and CF tests have been the standard serological tests, but they have been replaced in most laboratories by EIA. EIA is generally considered more sensitive than HI or CF; the CF test, however, is more specific than HI or EIA. The neutralization test (9) is also very specific but is cumbersome to perform and is not amenable to routine use in most laboratories. Published experience with the IF-antibody test is sparse, but the procedure should be considered by laboratories with expertise in IF.

Blood samples are obtained and are allowed to clot, and

the sera are collected following centrifugation at low speed. Tests for IgG antibodies should be performed simultaneously with paired sera taken during the acute phase of illness and at least 2 weeks later. If IgM antibody is to be assayed, IgG should be removed from the serum by adsorption onto latex beads coated with anti-IgG or by column chromatography; kits are available commercially. PIV antigens for use in CF or HI tests may be purchased. Alternatively, antigens may be prepared from infected cell cultures. These antigens may also be used in locally constructed EIAs. A cell culture infected with a PIV may be prepared as antigen for IF-antibody tests by conventional procedures (8, 29).

EIA

Chapter 12 and the references cited therein should be referred to for the means of construction of EIA. Soluble antigen is prepared in alkaline buffer, and the mixture is incubated overnight at 4°C in wells of 96-well microdilution plates; comparable wells are prepared with control antigen. The wells are washed with PBS containing 0.5% bovine serum albumin (BSA) and 0.05% Tween 20. Sera are serially diluted in the PBS–BSA–Tween 20 buffer, and the dilutions are added to PIV- and control antigen-treated wells. Following incubation for 1 h at 37°C, the wells are washed three times and an anti-human IgG–enzyme conjugate (peroxidase is recommended) prepared in the PBS–BSA–Tween 20 buffer is added; controls include positive and negative sera, wells without a test serum but with conjugate, and wells without a test serum or conjugate. The plates are incubated for an additional hour at 37°C and washed. An appropriate substrate is added, and the quantity of the developed color is measured spectrophotometrically. Commonly, patient sera are reported as positive when their absorbance values are a minimum of 2 standard deviations above a control value or after the absorbance values are plotted on a dose-response curve obtained with a reference pool of sera. A critical ratio of the absorbance values of an acute-phase serum sample and a convalescent-phase serum sample is sometimes obtained to determine whether the difference is significant.

HI

Antigens for the HI test may be purchased or prepared from infected cell cultures. Antigen must be carefully titrated with guinea pig RBCs for hemagglutination before use in the test. The highest dilution of antigen that shows partial agglutination of the RBCs is the endpoint. The endpoint dilution is divided by 8 to arrive at the dilution of antigen required to provide 4 U of hemagglutinin.

Sera must be treated before testing to remove nonspecific inhibitors and agglutinins. Equal volumes of receptor-destroyer enzyme and serum (0.1 ml is recommended) are incubated together overnight at 37°C. After inactivation at 56°C for 30 min, the serum is incubated with 0.2 ml of 15% guinea pig RBCs for 1 h at 4°C; the RBCs are removed by centrifugation. The serum dilution at this point is 1:4.

Serial twofold dilutions of the treated serum are made in microtiter wells with PBS as a diluent. Four units of antigen are added to each well, and the reactants are mixed. Antigen, antibody, RBC, and serum controls must be included. In each test, twofold dilutions of the antigen should be made such that 4, 2, 1, 0.5, and 0.25 U of antigen are evaluated for HA activity. A reference serum with a known antibody titer is tested to control for specificity and sensitivity; an erythrocyte control consists of RBCs incubated only with PBS, and serum controls consisting of 1:8 dilutions of each serum sample to be tested are incubated only with PBS.

The reaction mixtures are incubated for 1 h at room temperature, followed by the addition of 0.4% guinea pig RBCs to each well. The incubation is continued at room temperature until RBC buttons are distinct in the RBC and serum control wells. Hemolysis or agglutination indicates nonspecific reactions associated with the RBCs and/or the serum. The 4- and 2-U antigen control wells should show complete agglutination, the 1-U well should show partial agglutination, and the 0.5- and 0.25-U wells should not show agglutination. The endpoint is the highest dilution of a serum sample that completely inhibits agglutination, as evidenced by a complete RBC button in the well.

EVALUATION OF TEST RESULTS

The isolation of virus or the identification of viral antigen in a clinical specimen is the most valuable information to be conveyed to a clinician. PIVs are rarely present in healthy individuals, and their presence in the context of disease is diagnostic. A policy of immediately reporting virus isolation or a positive result for antigen detection by telephone is recommended. The quality of a specimen should also be a consideration in the reporting of results, particularly negative results. A negative result obtained with a poor specimen may have a low negative predictive value. In such instances this information should be conveyed to the clinician.

The length of time required to identify the replication of PIV in cell cultures usually compromises the usefulness of virus isolation in patient management. Efforts should therefore be made to use rapid techniques to identify PIV antigen directly in clinical specimens or in infected cell cultures; direct IF and the shell vial method are the recommended rapid tests. The identification of a PIV without designation of type is sufficient because type-specific therapies are not available.

Antibody determinations are used primarily to make a retrospective diagnosis or to obtain seroepidemiological data on PIV infection in a community. Since reinfection is common, the presence of antibody per se is of little value in evaluating protective immune status. Seroconversion or an increase in the antibody titer in the convalescent-phase serum specimen of fourfold or greater over that in the acute-phase serum specimen is diagnostic of recent infection. A fourfold diminution of the antibody titer or the presence of IgG antibody in a single serum specimen does not have diagnostic significance. The possible presence of maternal antibody and the immature status of the immune system in infants less than 6 months old make serology unreliable for this age group. Heterologous antibody responses in patients make serological typing of PIVs unreliable. Although IgM antibody shows a less heterologous response than IgG antibody, experiences with IgM tests vary considerably and do not support the use of the test for obtaining a reliable diagnosis. Serology is therefore of little value in obtaining a diagnosis of acute infection.

REFERENCES

1. **Ansari, S. A., S. Springthorpe, S. A. Sattar, S. Rivard, and M. Rahman.** 1991. Potential role of hands in the spread of respiratory viral infections: studies with human parainfluenza virus 3 and rhinovirus 14. *J. Clin. Microbiol.* **29:**2115–2119.
2. **Brady, M. T., J. Evans, and J. Cuartas.** 1990. Survival

and disinfection of parainfluenzaviruses on environmental surfaces. *Am. J. Infect. Control* **18:**18–23.

3. **Chanock, R. M., J. A. Bell, and R. H. Parrott.** 1961. Natural history of parainfluenza virus infection, p. 126–137. *In* M. Pollard (ed.), *Perspectives in Virology*, vol. 2. Burgess Publishing Co., Minneapolis, Minn.
4. **Chanock, R. M., and P. H. Parrott.** 1965. Acute respiratory disease in infancy and childhood: present understanding and prospects for prevention. *Pediatrics* **36:**21–39.
5. **Chanock, R. M., R. H. Parrott, K. M. Johnson, A. Z. Kapikian, and J. A. Bell.** 1963. Myxoviruses: parainfluenza. *Am. Rev. Respir. Dis.* **88:**152–166.
6. **Collins, R. M., R. M. Chanock, and K. McIntosh.** 1996. Parainfluenza viruses, p. 1205–1241. *In* B. N. Fields (ed.), *Virology*. Raven Press, New York, N.Y.
7. **Fan, J., and K. J. Henrickson.** 1996. Rapid diagnosis of human parainfluenza virus type 1 infection by quantitative reverse transcription-PCR-enzyme hybridization assay. *J. Clin. Microbiol.* **34:**1914–1917.
8. **Fedova, D., J. Novotny, and I. Kubinova.** 1992. Serological diagnosis of parainfluenza virus infections: verification of the sensitivity and specificity of the haemagglutination-inhibition (HI), complement fixation (CF), immunofluorescence (IFA) tests and enzyme immunoassay (ELISA). *Acta Virol.* **36:**304–312.
9. **Frank, A. L., J. Puck, B. J. Hughes, and T. R. Cate.** 1980. Microneutralization test for influenza A and B and parainfluenza 1 and 2 viruses that uses continuous cell lines and fresh serum enhancement. *J. Clin. Microbiol.* **12:** 426–432.
10. **Gilbert, L. L., A. Dakhama, B. M. Bone, E. E. Thomas, and R. G. Hegele.** 1996. Diagnosis of viral respiratory tract infections in children by using a reverse transcription-PCR panel. *J. Clin. Microbiol.* **34:**140–143.
11. **Glezen, W. P., and F. W. Denny.** 1973. Epidemiology of acute lower respiratory disease in children. *N. Engl. J. Med.* **288:**498–505.
12. **Glezen, W. P., A. L. Frank, L. H. Taber, and J. A. Kasel.** 1984. Parainfluenza virus type 3: seasonality and risk of infection and reinfection in young children. *J. Infect. Dis.* **150:**851–857.
13. **Glezen, W. P., F. A. Loda, and F. W. Denny.** 1982. Parainfluenza viruses, p. 441–454. *In* A. S. Evans (ed.), *Viral Infections of Humans. Epidemiology and Control.* Plenum Publishing Corp., New York, N.Y.
14. **Grandien, M., C.-A. Petterson, P. S. Gardner, A. Linde, and A. Stanton.** 1985. Rapid viral diagnosis of acute respiratory infections: comparison of enzyme-linked immunosorbent assay and the immunofluorescent technique for detection of viral antigens in nasopharyngeal secretions. *J. Clin. Microbiol.* **22:**757–760.
15. **Gross, P. A., R. H. Green, and M. G. M. Curnen.** 1973. Persistent infection with parainfluenza type 3 virus in man. *Am. Rev. Respir. Dis.* **108:**894–898.
16. **Hall, C. B., and R. G. Douglas, Jr.** 1975. Clinically useful method for the isolation of respiratory syncytial virus. *J. Infect. Dis.* **131:**1–5.
17. **Hierholzer, J. C., P. G. Bingham, R. A. Coombs, K. H. Johansson, L. J. Anderson, and P. E. Halonen.** 1989. Comparison of monoclonal antibody time-resolved fluoroimmunoassay with monoclonal antibody capture-biotinylated detector enzyme immunoassay for respiratory syncytial virus and parainfluenza virus antigen detection. *J. Clin. Microbiol.* **27:**1243–1249.
18. **Hierholzer, J. C., E. Castells, G. G. Banks, J. A. Bryan, and C. T. McEwen.** 1993. Sensitivity of NCI-H292 human lung mucoepidermoid cells for respiratory and other human viruses. *J. Clin. Microbiol.* **31:**1504–1510.
19. **Karron, R. A., J. L. Froehlich, L. Bobo, R. B. Belshe, and R. H. Yolken.** 1994. Rapid detection of parainfluenza virus type 3 RNA in respiratory specimens: use of reverse transcription-PCR-enzyme immunoassay. *J. Clin. Microbiol.* **32:**484–488.
20. **Karron, R. A., K. L. O'Brien, J. L. Froehlich, and V. A. Brown.** 1993. Molecular epidemiology of a parainfluenza type 3 virus outbreak on a pediatric ward. *J. Infect. Dis.* **167:**1441–1445.
21. **Marx, A., T. J. Torok, R. C. Holman, M. J. Clarke, and L. J. Anderson.** 1997. Pediatric hospitalizations for croup (laryngotracheobronchitis): biennial increases associated with human parainfluenza virus 1 epidemics. *J. Infect. Dis.* **176:**1423–1427.
22. **Minnich, L. L., and C. G. Ray.** 1987. Early testing of cell cultures for detection of hemadsorbing viruses. *J. Clin. Microbiol.* **25:**421–422.
23. **Parrott, R. H., A. J. Vargosko, H. W. Kim, J. A. Bell, and R. M. Chanock.** 1962. Acute respiratory diseases of viral etiology. III. Myxoviruses: parainfluenza. *Am. J. Public Health* **52:**907–917.
24. **Sarkkinen, H. K., P. E. Halonen, and A. A. Salmi.** 1981. Type-specific detection of parainfluenza viruses by enzyme immunoassay and radioimmunoassay in nasopharyngeal specimens of patients with acute respiratory disease. *J. Gen. Virol.* **56:**49–58.
25. **Schirm, J., D. S. Luijt, G. W. Pastoor, J. M. Mandema, and F. P. Schroder.** 1992. Rapid detection of respiratory viruses using mixtures of monoclonal antibodies on shell vial cultures. *J. Med. Virol.* **38:**147–151.
26. **Todd, S. J., L. Minnich, and J. L. Waner.** 1995. Comparison of rapid immunofluorescence procedure with TestPack RSV and Directigen FLU-A for diagnosis of respiratory syncytial virus and influenza A virus. *J. Clin. Microbiol.* **33:**1650–1651.
27. **Vreede, R. W., H. Schellekens, and M. Zuijderwijk.** 1992. Isolation of parainfluenza virus type 3 from cerebrospinal fluid. *J. Infect. Dis.* **165:**1166.
28. **Vuorinen, T., and O. Meurman.** 1989. Enzyme immunoassays for detection of IgG and IgM antibodies to parainfluenza types 1, 2 and 3. *J. Virol. Methods* **23:**63–70.
29. **Waner, J. L., N. J. Whitehurst, T. Downs, and D. G. Graves.** 1985. Production of monoclonal antibodies against parainfluenza 3 virus and their use in diagnosis by immunofluorescence. *J. Clin. Microbiol.* **22:**535–538.
30. **Wenzel, R. P., D. P. McCormick, and W. E. Beam, Jr.** 1972. Parainfluenza pneumonia in adults. *JAMA* **221:** 294–295.
31. **Wong, D. T., R. C. Welliver, K. R. Riddlesberger, M. S. Sun, and P. L. Ogra.** 1982. Rapid diagnosis of parainfluenza virus infection in children. *J. Clin. Microbiol.* **16:** 164–167.

Respiratory Syncytial Virus

DEBRA A. TRISTRAM AND ROBERT C. WELLIVER

72

CLINICAL BACKGROUND

Epidemiology

Respiratory syncytial virus (RSV) is the most common viral agent causing lower respiratory tract illness in infancy. Outbreaks of RSV infections occur worldwide, with striking epidemics noted in temperate climates in the winter and early spring. In the tropics, epidemics occur during the rainy seasons. Outbreaks usually span approximately 2 to 5 months. Within this period, the majority of cases usually occur within a 1- to 2-month peak (41). Although several investigators have attempted to delineate the climatic conditions responsible for the appearance of RSV, its persistence for several months, and its subsequent disappearance for an approximately equal number of months, no one has been able to clearly establish a link between climate and epidemics (19). While all age groups are susceptible to RSV infections, the majority of hospitalizations for RSV disease occur in 2- to 6-month-old children. Admission rates for bronchiolitis and pneumonia can reach as high as 24/1,000 in young infants experiencing primary RSV infection. Males are slightly more likely to experience severe RSV disease, as are infants from industrialized areas and infants exposed to parental cigarette smoke (45). Both a greater number of siblings and attendance at day care also increase the risk of infection with RSV (29).

By the first year of life, 50% of all infants experience a primary RSV infection; by 2 years, nearly all have contracted RSV disease (5, 63). Reinfections are common, despite the presence of RSV-specific local and systemic antibodies and neutralizing antibody (22). Nosocomial spread of RSV on pediatric wards is an annual problem encountered by hospital infection control personnel (13).

Disease Manifestations

Common syndromes due to RSV include bronchiolitis and pneumonia. The former is a wheezing-associated illness preceded by 3 to 5 days of upper respiratory tract symptoms. Wheezing and thoracic hyperinflation are prominent. Patients with pneumonia also present after several days of upper respiratory tract symptoms, and crackles are heard on auscultation of the chest. Frequently, the two syndromes overlap. For healthy patients, although illness from RSV disease can be severe, recovery is usual. Among infants and children hospitalized with lower respiratory tract disease due to RSV, mortality rates are relatively low, i.e., usually less than 1% in otherwise healthy hosts (15). However, among patients with respiratory or cardiac compromise or immune system dysfunction, mortality rates as high as 37% have been reported, although 3 to 5% is probably a more accurate estimate (52). Significant morbidity and mortality may occur in RSV infection of the elderly. Outbreaks producing lower respiratory tract disease in nursing homes (16) and institutions for the mentally retarded (17) have been reported.

Another manifestation of RSV disease in infants is apnea, with or without associated respiratory symptoms. Various studies since the early 1960s have determined the incidence of RSV-associated apnea to be between 16 and 20% (11). Infants with significant risk for apnea include premature infants, young infants (usually <6 weeks old), and infants with a history of apnea of prematurity.

Transmission

Virus transmission has been documented to occur most commonly through contact with infected droplets, most often in fomites. RSV can survive for up to 6 h on environmental surfaces and is most infectious when applied directly to the mucosal surface of the eye or nose by infected hands or objects. Airborne transmission, except by close, direct contact with an infected person, is uncommon. Schools or day care provide ideal settings for the spread of virus to susceptible individuals.

DESCRIPTION OF THE VIRUS

Morphology

RSV has been assigned to the family *Paramyxoviridae*, although morphologic and antigenic differences distinguish RSV from other members of the paramyxovirus family. RSV has a smaller nucleocapsid (13 to 14 nm in diameter) and lacks neuraminidase and a hemagglutinin (56). Thus, RSV has been assigned a separate genus, *Pneumovirus*, within the family *Paramyxoviridae*. It shares this genus with the pneumonia virus of mice and with bovine, ovine, and caprine RSV. Although there are no further members of this genus as yet, antibody studies of other species have demonstrated naturally occurring RSV antibody. This suggests that there may be other viruses related to human RSV and capable of producing disease in other species that have not yet been recovered and identified.

RSV is a small, single-stranded, negative-sense RNA virus. Its genome is linear, with a molecular mass of about 5×10^6 Da (46). Single RSV particles are pleomorphic, ranging in size from 100 to 350 nm (6). Each particle is bounded by a cellular membrane that has 12- to 15-nm spikes composed of F and G glycoproteins on the outer surface at regular intervals. The spherical virion is composed of a lipid bilayer membrane containing an RNA nucleocapsid. The RNA is a nonsegmented helical structure with a periodicity of 65 to 70 nm in a herringbone pattern and appears to be similar to the nucleoproteins of other paramyxoviruses when viewed by negative-staining electron microscopy (12).

Biochemistry

Analysis of the nucleotide sequence of RSV has allowed the accurate identification of RSV proteins encoded by the genome. At least 10 specific protein products have been identified thus far (12, 32). The structural proteins are N, P, and L in the nucleocapsid; F and G on the surface of the viral envelope; and M and M2 in the viral envelope. SH (formerly 1A) may be a third integral membrane protein, but it is also expressed on the surfaces of RSV-infected cells. Two nonstructural proteins, formerly designated 1B and 1C, are now called NS1 and NS2.

The first two protein products encoded by the RSV genome reading from the 3′ to the 5′ end are NS1 and NS2. NS1 is slightly acidic, while NS2 is basic (69).

The N protein is intermediate in size and serves as the major structural protein for the nucleocapsid, while P and L are most likely involved in transcription and replication (46). Monoclonal antibodies raised against N stain intracytoplasmic inclusion bodies in an immunofluorescence assay (72). P is heavily phosphorylated, unlike the other RSV proteins, and is relatively acidic (60). In an immunofluorescence assay, monoclonal antibodies to P also stain intracytoplasmic inclusion bodies (72). The L protein is very large (250 kDa) and relatively hydrophobic. Because of its size and its location in the nucleocapsid, L is believed to be the viral RNA-dependent RNA polymerase (46).

The viral envelope contains several proteins: matrix (M), a 22-kDa protein (M2), and the surface glycoproteins F and G. The M protein is present in detergent-solubilized cores but not in nucleocapsids, suggesting that it is similar to other matrix proteins found in enveloped RNA viruses (46). It is most likely hydrophobic and basic, as suggested by its reduced amino acid sequence (9, 60). The exact location and function of the second putative matrix protein, M2, are not known. M2 is highly basic and hydrophilic and is expressed on the surfaces of infected cells, as determined by immunofluorescence studies (58). F and G are two large glycosylated proteins found on the surface of the viral envelope; they are important immunogens during RSV infection.

The G glycoprotein is highly glycosylated; the protein component is relatively small (32 kDa) compared to the mature, fully processed glycoprotein (85 kDa) (76). It has an unusually high content of serine and threonine, to which the O-linked carbohydrate side chains are attached (76). The function of G protein seems to be host cell adsorption, analogous to the hemagglutinin protein of parainfluenza viruses.

RSV strains can be separated antigenically into two subgroups, A and B. The G glycoprotein seems to have the greatest variation in amino acid sequences in the two RSV subgroups. Comparisons between the G ectodomains of two subgroup A viruses showed a 94% homology, while subgroup B (strain 18537) showed 47% divergence from the subgroup A reference strain (35). The central region, containing cysteine residues and flanking amino acid sequences, was the only region conserved among the strains. In contrast, the F glycoprotein is highly conserved, and antibody to F protein cross-reacts with both A- and B-group F protein (34).

The F glycoprotein has been identified as the fusion protein by studies with monoclonal antibodies (72). F glycoprotein is one of the major components of the projections on the outer surface of the virion and one of the major immunogens of RSV (24). After glycosylation, the F protein is proteolytically cleaved in the infected cell prior to virion assembly. The two subunits F1 and F2 are linked by a disulfide bridge (71). Although direct evidence is not available, it is possible that, similar to what occurs in other paramyxoviruses, posttranslational enzymatic cleavage is required for the formation of infectious viral particles (14).

COLLECTION AND STORAGE OF SPECIMENS

Samples of nasopharyngeal secretions recovered by nasal washing or direct aspiration are two or three times more likely to yield RSV in cell culture than specimens obtained by swabs (47). Nasopharyngeal aspirates apparently result in greater recovery of epithelial cells than do washes or swabs, and so aspirates should be more effective for immunofluorescence assays, in which antigen is detected on the surface of exfoliated cells. Aspirates are also superior to swabs in enzyme immunoassays (EIAs) (1).

Nasal wash specimens are obtained by placing a 1-oz (28.350-g) tapered rubber bulb syringe containing 5 to 7 ml of sterile saline solution into and occluding the nostril and then rapidly squeezing and releasing the bulb. Fluid recovered in the bulb is emptied into a container containing transport medium. Nasopharyngeal aspirates are best obtained by attaching a size 5 or 8 French polyethylene pediatric feeding tube to a DeLee collection trap, passing the tube into the nasopharynx, and applying suction (approximately 15 to 25 lb/in^2) by wall suction or with a manual suction pump. Optimal results are achieved by suctioning through both nostrils. Recovery of secretions is greater if transport medium is rinsed through the feeding tube into the specimen trap (1, 38). Swab specimens should be collected by carefully and thoroughly swabbing the nasopharynx and placing the swab into a vial containing transport medium.

Specimens need not be placed directly into cell culture at the bedside but should be placed on wet ice before transport to the laboratory to maintain optimal recovery of RSV in cell culture. The transport medium should include a physiologic salt solution and a protein stabilizer such as 0.5% bovine serum albumin or 0.5% gelatin. Since the use of Hanks' balanced salt solution has been reported to decrease the absorbance in an RSV EIA, this solution may not be optimal (27), but several others in common use are acceptable.

RSV is rapidly destroyed at 55°C, and as much as 90% of cell culture infectivity is lost when virus is kept at 37°C for 24 h. Mailing specimens to the laboratory or transporting them at room temperatures can be expected to result in substantial loss of cell culture infectivity. Therefore, all specimens to be analyzed by cell culture or immunofluorescence (in which cellular viability must be maintained) should be transported at refrigerator temperature or on wet ice. Samples for EIAs may be transported at ambient temperatures without loss of reactivity. Approximately 50% of infectivity is lost after a single freeze-thaw cycle. Therefore, freezing should be avoided, but if samples must be stored at refrigerator temperatures for more than 1 day, rapid freezing and holding the virus at −70°C will maintain the titer of virus for at least several months (26). The addition of sucrose or glycerin to the storage medium may enhance viral survival while the virus is frozen. RSV is denatured rapidly at low pH and survives optimally at pH 7.5 (26).

DIRECT EXAMINATION

Immunofluorescence

Immunofluorescence techniques to detect RSV antigens were first applied to cells maintained in vitro and infected with the virus. The characteristic fluorescence in cytoplasm was observed as early as the second day following inoculation of cell cultures. More recently, indirect immunofluorescence techniques have been applied to exfoliated nasopharyngeal epithelial cells present in samples of secretions obtained from patients with RSV infection (21). Several acceptable commercial kits that use both direct immunofluorescence and indirect immunofluorescence techniques for the detection of RSV antigen in respiratory secretions have been developed (8, 10). One review (40) discussed 12 studies in which direct fluorescent-antibody tests were compared with culture and 19 studies in which indirect fluorescent-antibody tests were compared with culture for the detection of RSV infection. With either technique, the sensitivity of the immunofluorescence assay in comparison to culture was usually above 80% and was as high as 97%. The specificity was generally greater than 90%. It should be noted that for all antigen detection techniques (including the EIAs described below), the actual sensitivity is probably greater than that of cell culture. Specimens exposed to temperatures that render RSV unrecoverable from cell culture may still be positive by antigen detection techniques. Similarly, samples obtained later in the course of clinical illness may not contain recoverable virus but may still be positive by antigen detection techniques (38). Indirect immunofluorescence techniques may have a slightly greater sensitivity for detecting RSV (usually ≥95%) than direct fluorescent-antibody tests do (40). Specificities are also generally somewhat higher with indirect fluorescent-antibody tests. Numerous variables can affect the results of either assay, including method of collection of secretions, time during the course of illness when samples were obtained, and use of fresh versus frozen samples. Therefore, comparing separate studies that use different methods is difficult. In any case, reliable results with immunofluorescence tests are available within a few hours of obtaining specimens, and many laboratories have replaced cell culture with antigen detection techniques for establishing a diagnosis of RSV infection.

The preparation of samples for immunofluorescence testing is critical for obtaining optimal results. Samples of respiratory secretions obtained either by washing or by direct aspiration are suspended in growth medium. Excess mucus is removed by 1 to 2 min of vortexing. Particularly tenacious mucus can be broken up by the addition of an equal volume of dimercaptoethanol or *N*-acetylcysteine before vortexing (49). Several cycles of centrifugation at 300 to 500 × *g* may be useful in removing mucus. The sediment containing exfoliated cells is then spotted onto microscope slides, air dried, and fixed for 10 min in cold acetone. Teflon-coated slides containing 13-mm-diameter wells have been specifically produced for this purpose, although standard microscope slides are sufficient. Anti-RSV antibodies and fluorescein-conjugated anti-bovine immunoglobulins are available either in commercially available kits or individually. The first antibody should be incubated with cells on slides for 15 to 30 min and then adequately washed. A similar incubation period should be used for fluorescein-conjugated antibodies, again with careful rinsing. Slides are then examined under ×400 magnification with a fluorescence microscope (8, 10, 65).

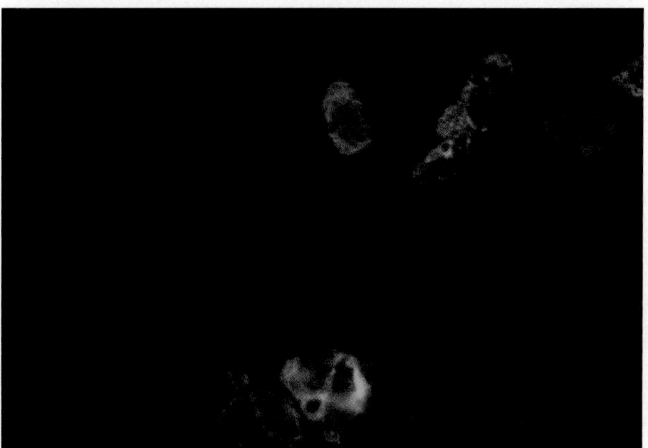

FIGURE 1 Assay for RSV antigens. Nasal wash samples were collected from patients, processed, and reacted with a monoclonal antibody as described in the text.

A satisfactory specimen should have more than 100 cells on the slide. Specific RSV fluorescence is within the cell and is characterized by granular fluorescence on the cell surface or larger inclusionlike fluorescence within the cytoplasm. Most newer commercial kits involve monoclonal antibodies against surface glycoproteins and the nucleocapsid proteins, which are responsible for membrane and cytoplasmic fluorescence, respectively. Polyclonal sera have also been used in commercial kits. A representative immunofluorescence reaction is depicted in Fig. 1.

EIAs

Over the past few years, EIA has probably become the most frequently used method of antigen detection for RSV. A review of 20 studies in which EIAs were used to detect RSV antigen showed sensitivities of ≥90% in 8 and specificities of ≥90% in 13 of the studies (40). While some investigators have found immunofluorescence assays to be slightly more accurate than EIAs (59), the observed differences are generally fairly minor, and EIAs have other advantages in comparison to immunofluorescence techniques. First, intact respiratory tract cells are not required for EIA, and EIAs are often positive when suboptimal handling of specimens has resulted in the inactivation of culturable virus (18, 47). Therefore, specimen handling requirements are not as strict as those associated with culture or immunofluorescence assays. Other advantages include the technical simplicity of the EIAs, objective end points, the potential for automation, and assay times as short as 15 to 20 min (25).

EIAs generally use plastic microtiter trays as the solid phase. More recently, EIAs that use a membrane filter to absorb the viral antigen present in clinical specimens have been employed. In these assays, a colored reaction product appears bound to the membrane. These tests have internal controls that must be visible for the test to be valid (57, 65, 67). In our experience and in the experience of at least some others, these membrane immunoassays have reduced accuracy in comparison to the immunofluorescence assay and EIAs noted above (57). Freezing and thawing of specimens appear to increase the sensitivity of some of the membrane EIAs. These procedures, however, are time-consuming and tend to override the advantage of a rapid test.

As with immunofluorescence assays, adequate preparation of clinical specimens is essential for optimum results in an EIA. Mucus should be broken up or removed by repeated pipetting, sonication, and vortexing of specimens or by the addition of *N*-acetylcysteine to specimens. Sonication and treatment with detergents have been reported to increase signals in EIA, presumably by releasing antigens from the cells (28, 59). Since some antigen is probably present in the fluid phase of secretions, whole secretions can be expected to give higher EIA signals than either washed cells alone or secretions from which the cells have been removed by centrifugation.

False-positive results are a particular problem in EIAs. These results should be excluded by using appropriate blocking antibodies if several clinical specimens are positive by EIA but negative by cell culture (8, 40, 64). Both immunofluorescence assays and EIAs can be applied to cell cultures, often revealing the presence of viral antigens before cytopathic effects (CPE) are present (8).

PCR

Although not yet commercially available, PCR technology has been applied to the detection of RSV. Both clinical samples (20, 53) and RSV-infected cell culture material (20, 23) have provided sufficient RNA for proliferation and detection by reverse transcription-PCR (RT-PCR). As expected, RT-PCR was more likely to detect the presence of RSV in clinical samples than were the parallel comparison tests involving IFA or a modified shell vial method (20). PCR has also been used to discriminate between RSV subgroups A and B in culture (23) and may provide a useful alternative to subgrouping RSV with monoclonal antibodies in the future.

For most clinical situations, the use of rapid fluorescence methods is less expensive and sufficient for the diagnosis of RSV. For the present, RT-PCR should be reserved for complicated respiratory cases where conventional methods, such as IFA, have failed to determine the etiology. As PCR technology becomes more widely available and less expensive, it may ultimately replace currently used techniques in the clinical arena.

CULTIVATION OF THE VIRUS

Recovery of Cell Culture

Standard cell culture infectivity is a useful method for recovering RSV from clinical specimens. Specimens obtained by direct aspiration into polyethylene catheters or recovered by nasal washes are superior to swabs and, interestingly, to aspirates of tracheal secretions (66). RSV grows best in human epithelial cell lines such as HEp-2 and HeLa cells. The A549 human epithelial cell line seems somewhat less sensitive for recovery of RSV. A variety of primary monkey kidney and human fibroblast cell lines are also useful for recovery of RSV but are not as sensitive as human epithelial cell lines. Nevertheless, it has been estimated that up to 20% of RSV strains will not be recovered if human epithelial cell lines alone are used (4), although this is not our experience. A combination of human epithelial cell lines, primary monkey kidney cell lines, and human fibroblasts seems optimal for virus recovery. There is considerable variation in sensitivity among lots of the same cell line and a decrease in sensitivity of cell lines as they are maintained by multiple passages (4, 66). Sensitivity may also differ for the same cells grown in different media (37).

Several different culture media are adequate for the growth of RSV. The addition of glutamine (43) and calcium (61) appears to be necessary for optimal growth and development of CPE. Growth of RSV is enhanced if monolayers of cells are inoculated when they are approximately 50 to 75% confluent (54). Growth at 36°C is equivalent to growth at 33°C (4). CPE usually appear between days 3 and 7 in culture. Large syncytia composed of fused cells with eosinophilic granules within the cytoplasm are characteristic (Fig. 2). However, growth may occur without the development of syncytia, and as many as 26% of isolates of RSV will be recovered only by repeated passage of previously inoculated cells. This is best accomplished by scraping monolayers and adsorbing the recovered cells on a fresh monolayer for 1 h before adding maintenance medium. Subtype B strains of RSV (see below) may develop CPE more slowly than subtype A strains.

Continued passage of large inocula of RSV or passage of temperature-sensitive mutants at nonpermissive temperatures may result in persistent infection of cell lines. CPE is not obvious, and the amount of cell-free virus is diminished (55).

The shell vial technique has been used with several viruses, including RSV (62). In the study by Smith et al. (62), 0.2-ml aliquots of clinical specimens were added directly to shell vials and then centrifuged at 700 × *g* and 32°C for 60 min. Overall, the recovery rates of RSV in shell vials are similar to those of conventional tube cultures. However, of 46 specimens that were eventually positive for CPE, 43 were already positive at 16 h and the other 3 were positive at 40 h by the shell vial assay. In conventional tube cultures,

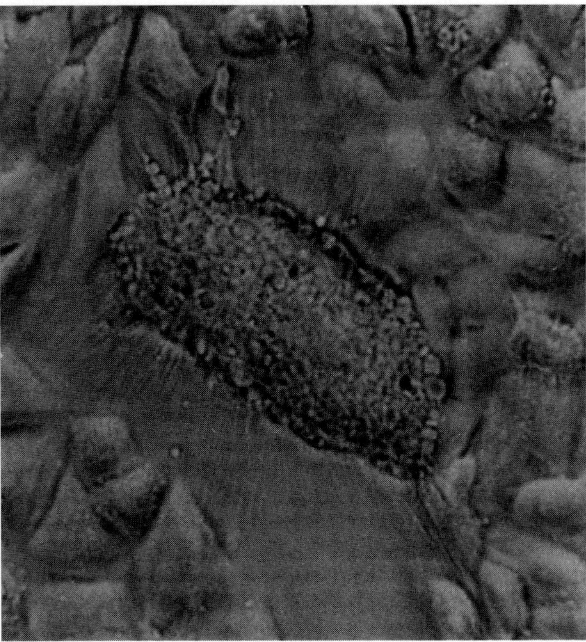

FIGURE 2 Syncytium formation by RSV in human lung epithelial cells.

CPE was first observable at day 2 at the earliest, with a median of 4.5 days. Of 147 clinical specimens that were originally negative for RSV by direct immunofluorescence, 6 were positive after 16 h of incubation in shell vials. The shell vial technique identified RSV in 16 of 17 specimens that were positive by EIA and in an additional 3 specimens that were negative by EIA.

The use of shell vials appears to slightly increase the sensitivity of culture methods for detection of RSV and greatly increases the speed at which isolates are detected. However, the increased time and effort required for centrifugation of specimens preclude the use of shell vials for screening large numbers of clinical specimens for RSV.

It is arguable whether antigen detection techniques such as immunofluorescence and EIA should replace cell culture as the standard against which other methods of detection should be tested. For the single purpose of comparison with methods that will be developed in the future, the immunofluorescence assay, EIA, and culture are reasonably similar in sensitivity and specificity, while antigen detection techniques have a considerable advantage in being less time-consuming. However, laboratories interested in detecting any viral pathogen in a given specimen (as opposed to simply ruling in or ruling out RSV) should continue to use cell culture at least as an adjunct to RSV, since viruses other than RSV may be recovered from 5 to 25% of specimens submitted for diagnosis of RSV infection (7).

Subtyping of Viruses

In the past, all RSV strains have been considered to be of a single serotype in that human neutralizing antisera recognize all strains with relatively equal efficiency. Nevertheless, different strains may have detectable differences in the antigenic makeups of individual viral proteins. Application of panels of monoclonal antibodies to different RSV strains allows classification of these strains into two subtypes, based largely on differences in the G glycoprotein (3). Strains of RSV can be broadly divided into subgroup A (characterized by the Long and A2 strains) and subgroup B (characterized by strain 18537). Nucleotide and amino acid sequencing analyses indicate that the F glycoproteins of each subgroup are 53% antigenically related and have 89% amino acid sequence homology (34). In contrast, the G glycoproteins of group A and group B strains are 5% antigenically related and have 53% amino acid sequence homology (36). Retrospective analyses have indicated that these strains have existed for decades and that they circulate concurrently during RSV epidemics in all areas of the world. Infections due to one subtype or the other can cluster geographically or temporally.

The significance of this antigenic variation remains unclear. Infection with a subgroup A virus tends to induce good cross-reactive antibody responses against subgroup B viruses, while primary infection with a subgroup B virus induces lesser cross-reactive responses to subtype A strains. However, once children are primed by a group A infection, reinfection with either virus induces heterologous rises in neutralizing antibody titers (50). While no definitive study has been completed, there is currently no indication that reinfection with a heterologous strain is accompanied by any greater severity of illness than reinfection with a homologous strain (51). While epidemiologically important, the identification of subtypes of RSV has not yet entirely explained the frequency with which RSV reinfections occur.

IDENTIFICATION OF ISOLATES

The appearance of characteristic syncytia in cell culture (Fig. 2) is, in many laboratories, considered adequate to establish the presence of RSV. Parainfluenza or measles virus would be expected to produce syncytia only very rarely on the HEp-2, A549, or Vero cell lines used for RSV. However, while ours may not be a general practice, our virology laboratory routinely performs immunofluorescence assays on all cell cultures showing CPE (an educated guess is made as to which virus is present) to confirm the identity of isolates.

SEROLOGIC METHODS

Neutralization Tests for RSV Antibody

Standard neutralization assays are useful in the diagnosis of RSV infection. Neutralization assays performed in test tubes are somewhat more laborious and less precise than plaque reduction or microneutralization assays performed in plastic microtiter plates. A microneutralization assay performed in 96-well microtiter trays is probably the most widely used neutralization assay currently (2). It may be necessary to carry out neutralization assays with both subtype A and subtype B strains, since the use of subtype B strains may give slightly lower neutralizing titers than do subtype A strains with the same antisera.

Neutralizing antibody titers usually increase by 10 days after the onset of acute illness, reach a peak at 20 to 30 days, and decline substantially over the following year. Reinfections result in a more rapid increase in titer and a higher peak titer. However, up to 40% of subjects with documented RSV infection, particularly infants, do not develop increases in neutralizing titer following infection (16). The addition of complement to assay wells may enhance the observed titers (39).

Immunofluorescence Antibody Testing

Immunofluorescence techniques with commercially available antisera are useful for the diagnosis of RSV infection in all age groups (70, 73). Responses in the immunoglobulin M (IgM), IgG, and IgA isotypes are readily detectable, both in serum and in nasopharyngeal secretions.

In primary infection, IgM responses are detectable 5 to 9 days after the onset of symptoms and persist for several weeks. With secondary infection in childhood, responses are of a somewhat greater magnitude but do not appear to occur earlier than 4 days after the onset of symptoms. In adults, who probably have had multiple infections, IgM is first detectable at about the same time and also persists for several weeks. Significant increases in RSV IgG antibody titers occur 2 to 4 weeks after the onset of symptoms due to primary infection but are greatly accelerated following secondary infection in infancy. Levels of serum IgA antibody remain relatively low following primary infection but are also enhanced following secondary infection. In one small study, significant increases in RSV IgM antibody were noted in 13% of eight infants younger than 3 months of age with RSV infection and in 50 and 71% of infants 3 to 6 months and 6 to 12 months of age, respectively, at the time of RSV infection (73).

False-positive IgM responses may be present in the first month of life as a result of antibody formation against maternal RSV-specific IgG present in the serum of the infant. These complexes bind to RSV antigen used as targets in either EIA or the immunofluorescence assay, but they also react with anti-IgM antibodies.

RSV infection can also be documented by significant increases in RSV-specific IgG antibody in immunofluorescence assays. Fourfold or greater increases may occur more commonly with primary infection in infants older than 6 months (73).

Titers obtained by immunofluorescence assays for each of the isotypes correlate well with neutralizing-antibody responses. The peak in neutralizing-antibody response correlates most closely with the IgG response detected by immunofluorescence but is attained earlier. Neutralizing titers, especially those measured with the addition of complement, are appreciably higher than those measured by immunofluorescence (39). Titers detected by immunofluorescence also correlate well with complement fixation titers but appear earlier and also have the advantage of making diagnosis of infection with a single serum specimen possible by identification of an IgM-specific response (48).

Antibody EIAs

Several investigators have used EIAs to detect antibody responses to RSV in various isotypes. In primary infection, IgM responses generally first appear in serum on days 5 to 8 following the onset of illness and persist for several weeks, similar to IgM responses determined by immunofluorescence. Hornsleth and colleagues (31) were able to detect RSV-specific IgM responses by EIA in 21 of 26 infants and young children judged to have primary infection. Meurman et al. (48) found that five (63%) of eight patients younger than 6 months at the time of infection produced detectable IgM antibodies whereas all patients older than 12 months had detectable IgM responses. RSV-specific IgM responses can also be used to identify infection in elderly individuals who are presumably undergoing recurrent RSV infection (70).

EIAs can also be used to document significant increases in RSV-specific IgG antibody titers. Meurman et al. (48) found significant increases in IgG antibody titers in 24 of 26 infants and young children with RSV infection. The only two patients who failed to develop positive responses were <4 months of age at the time of infection. Other investigators have found diagnostic serologic responses in approximately 50% of infants 1 to 3 months of age and in 85 to 95% of older infants with primary RSV infection. In various studies, titers measured by EIAs correlated well with those measured by immunofluorescence (48), complement fixation (68), and neutralizing antibody (16). Immunofluorescence assays are slightly more sensitive than EIA (46, 66), while both are more sensitive than complement fixation assays (48, 68, 70).

EIAs have also been used to detect RSV-specific IgA antibodies in serum and secretions (48, 74) and RSV-specific IgE responses (74, 75).

EIAs that use a variety of different antigen sources have been developed. These sources include RSV-infected cells grown directly in microtiter plates and fixed with acetone or ethanol; infected cells grown in tissue culture flasks, collected, and then adsorbed to microtiter plates by desiccation (66); virus grown in cell culture and recovered by freezing and thawing of cells before being adsorbed to plates by overnight incubation at 4°C (67); and virus partially purified by centrifugation over sucrose gradients, diluted in carbonate buffer, and adsorbed to plates overnight at 4°C (75). Plates can also be incubated first with capture antibodies adsorbed overnight at 4°C before incubation with viral antigen (70). In our experience, use of purified virus is necessary to reduce the background absorbance readings sufficiently to allow detection of low titers of antibody. The use of desiccated infected cells as antigen has been associated with the development of a prozone phenomenon, in which negative responses are found at lower serum dilutions and positive responses are found at higher dilutions (68).

Although the immunofluorescence assay is probably somewhat more sensitive than EIA for detecting antibody, the EIA techniques are nevertheless accurate, somewhat easier to perform, and amenable to automation. Therefore, they are probably the method of choice for measuring RSV antibody responses. EIAs have also been used to detect RSV-specific antibody responses in IgG subclasses (30) as well as antibody to specific viral proteins (33). Target proteins are purified by affinity chromatography.

Immunoblot Assays

Antibody responses to individual RSV proteins can be measured by immunoblotting (33, 42). Virus should be partially purified on sucrose gradients and separated by sodium dodecyl sulfate-polyacrylamide gel electrophoresis under reducing conditions on 9% polyacrylamide gels. Viral proteins are then electroblotted onto nitrocellulose membranes.

Fusion Inhibition Antibody

RSV-immune sera contain high titers of antibody to the fusion protein. However, most of this antibody is not functional, in that it does not inhibit fusion of membranes by the virus. Specific antifusion antibody reactivity can be detected and may be of some importance in studying natural immunity as well as in studies of the development of effective vaccines (42).

Summary

Neutralizing antibody (and perhaps fusion-inhibiting antibody) is the only antibody that correlates with protection against reinfection with RSV. In addition, neutralization assays are as sensitive as other assays for detecting seroconversion to RSV. Therefore, they will remain irreplaceable as investigative tools. Nevertheless, immunofluorescence and, particularly, EIA techniques are much more rapidly performed, are approximately as accurate as neutralization assays for detecting increases in antibody titer, and afford the capability of rapid serologic diagnosis by demonstrating the presence of IgM-specific antibody. Therefore, immunofluorescence assays and EIAs may eventually replace neutralization assays in the serologic diagnosis of RSV infection. However, serologic diagnostic techniques are less sensitive than cell culture isolation and rapid diagnostic techniques generally for the diagnosis of RSV infection, and no serologic assay has been standardized or has achieved wide acceptance as a useful diagnostic method for detection of RSV infection. Immunoblot assays and fusion inhibition antibody assays are basically research techniques at this point.

EVALUATION AND REPORTING

With proper obtaining and handling of specimens, the rapid diagnostic tests have reasonable sensitivity, often greater than that of cell culture, for the detection of RSV. Nevertheless, false-negative results by rapid diagnostic methods or cell culture can be expected in a small percentage of cases, and negative tests or cultures should never be interpreted as excluding the possibility of RSV infection. In particular, seriously ill children with highly characteristic illnesses in the peak period of RSV epidemics should not necessarily have antiviral therapy withheld on the basis of a negative test result.

When properly performed, rapid diagnostic tests have high specificity for RSV. The specificity of cell culture is probably even higher. Nevertheless, it seems wise for any laboratory to confirm rapid diagnostic test results at least occasionally by cell culture or by another antigen detection assay to avoid false-positive reports.

Prompt reporting of positive test results may assist clinicians in discontinuing unnecessary forms of therapy or in isolating infected individuals, thereby preventing nosocomial spread of infection.

REFERENCES

1. **Ahluwalia, G., J. Embree, P. McNicol, B. Law, and G. W. Hammond.** 1987. Comparison of nasopharyngeal aspirate and nasopharyngeal swab specimens for respiratory syncytial virus diagnosis by cell culture, indirect immunofluorescence assay, and enzyme-linked immunosorbent assay. *J. Clin. Microbiol.* **25:**763–767.
2. **Anderson, L. J., J. C. Hierholzer, P. G. Bingham, and Y. O. Stone.** 1985. Microneutralization test for respiratory syncytial virus based on an enzyme immunoassay. *J. Clin. Microbiol.* **22:**1050–1052.
3. **Anderson, L. J., J. C. Hierholzer, Z. Tsou, et al.** 1985. Antigenic characterization of respiratory syncytial virus strains with monoclonal antibodies. *J. Infect. Dis.* **151:** 626–633.
4. **Arens, M. Q., Z. M. Swierkosz, R. R. Schmitt, P. Armstrong, and K. A. Rivetna.** 1986. Enhanced isolation of respiratory syncytial virus in cell culture. *J. Clin. Microbiol.* **23:**800–802.
5. **Beem, M.** 1987. Repeated infections with respiratory syncytial virus. *J. Immunol.* **98:**1115–1122.
6. **Bertaiume, L., J. Joncas, and V. Pavilanis.** 1974. Comparative structure, morphogenesis and biological characteristics of the respiratory syncytial (RS) virus and the pneumonia virus of mice (PVM). *Arch. Gesamte Virusforsch.* **45:** 39–51.
7. **Blanding, J. G., M. G. Hoshiko, and H. R. Stutman.** 1989. Routine viral culture for pediatric respiratory syncytial specimens submitted for direct immunofluorescence testing. *J. Clin. Microbiol.* **27:**1438–1440.
8. **Bromberg, K., G. Tannis, and B. Daidone.** 1991. Early use of indirect immunofluorescence for the detection of respiratory syncytial virus in HEp-2 cell culture. *Am. J. Clin. Pathol.* **96:**127–129.
9. **Cash, P., C. R. Pringle, and C. M. Preston.** 1979. The polypeptides of human respiratory syncytial virus: products of cell-free protein synthesis and post-translational modifications. *Virology* **92:**375–384.
10. **Cheeseman, S. H., L. T. Pierik, D. Leombruno, K. E. Spinos, and K. McIntosh.** 1986. Evaluation of a commercially available direct immunofluorescence staining reagent for the detection of respiratory syncytial virus in respiratory secretions. *J. Clin. Microbiol.* **24:**155–156.
11. **Church, N. R., N. G. Anas, C. B. Hall, and J. G. Brooks.** 1984. Respiratory syncytial virus-related apnea in infants. *Am. J. Dis. Child.* **138:**247–250.
12. **Collins, P. L., Y. T. Huang, and G. W. Wertz.** 1984. Identification of a tenth mRNA of respiratory syncytial virus and assignment of polypeptides to the 10 viral genes. *J. Virol.* **49:**572–578.
13. **Ditchburn, R. K., J. McQuillin, P. S. Gardner, and S. D. M. Court.** 1971. Respiratory syncytial virus in hospital cross-infection. *Br. Med. J.* **3:**671–733.
14. **Dubovi, E. J., J. D. Geratz, and R. R. Tidwell.** 1983. Enhancement of respiratory syncytial virus-induced cytopathology by trypsin, thrombin, and plasmin. *Infect. Immun.* **40:**351–358.
15. **Eriksson, M., M. Forsgren, S. Sjoberg, M. von Sydow, and S. Wolontis.** 1983. Respiratory syncytial virus identification in young hospitalized children: identification of risk patients and prevention of nosocomial spread by rapid diagnosis. *Acta Paediatr. Scand.* **72:**47–51.
16. **Falsey, A., and E. E. Walsh.** 1992. Humoral immunity to respiratory syncytial virus in the elderly. *J. Med. Virol.* **36:** 39–43.
17. **Finger, F., L. J. Anderson, R. C. Dicker, B. Harrison, R. Doan, A. Downing, and L. Corey.** 1987. Epidemic respiratory syncytial virus infection in institutionalized young adults. *J. Infect. Dis.* **155:**1335–1339.
18. **Flander, R. T., P. D. Lindsay, R. Chairez, T. A. Brawner, M. L. Kumar, P. D. Swenson, and K. Bromberg.** 1986. The evaluation of clinical specimens for the presence of respiratory syncytial virus antigen using an enzyme immunoassay. *J. Med. Virol.* **19:**1–9.
19. **Florman, A. L., and L. C. McLaren.** 1988. The effect of altitude and weather on the occurrence of outbreaks of respiratory syncytial virus infections. *J. Infect. Dis.* **158:** 1401–1402.
20. **Freymuth, F., G. Eugene, A. Vabret, J. Petitjean, E. Gennetay, J. Brouard, J. F. Dunamel, and B. Guillois.** 1995. Detection of respiratory syncytial virus by reverse transcription-PCR and hybridization with a DNA enzyme immunoassay. *J. Clin. Microbiol.* **33:**3352–3355.
21. **Gardner, P. S., and J. McQuillin.** 1968. Application of immunofluorescent antibody technique in rapid diagnosis of respiratory syncytial virus infection. *Br. Med. J.* **3:** 340–343.
22. **Glezen, W. P., L. H. Taber, A. L. Frank, and J. A. Kasel.** 1986. Risk of primary infection and reinfection with respiratory syncytial virus. *Am. J. Dis. Child.* **140:**543–546.
23. **Gottschalk, J., R. Zbinden, L. Kaempf, and I. Heinzer.** 1997. Discrimination of respiratory syncytial virus subgroups A and B by reverse transcription-PCR. *J. Clin. Microbiol.* **34:**41–43.
24. **Gruber, C., and S. Levine.** 1983. Respiratory syncytial virus polypeptides. III. The envelope-associated proteins. *J. Gen. Virol.* **64:**825–832.
25. **Halstead, D. C., S. Todd, and G. Fritch.** 1990. Evaluation of five methods for respiratory syncytial virus detection. *J. Clin. Microbiol.* **28:**1021–1025.
26. **Hambling, M. H.** 1964. Survival of the respiratory syncytial virus during storage under various conditions. *Br. J. Exp. Pathol.* **45:**647–655.
27. **Hendry, R. M., and K. McIntosh.** 1982. Enzyme-linked immunosorbent assay for detection of respiratory syncytial virus infection: development and description. *J. Clin. Microbiol.* **16:**324–328.
28. **Hendry, R. M., L. T. Pierik, and K. McIntosh.** 1986. Comparison of washed nasopharyngeal cells and whole nasal secretions for detection of respiratory syncytial virus antigens by enzyme-linked immunosorbent assay. *J. Clin. Microbiol.* **23:**383–384.
29. **Holberg, C. J., A. L. Wright, F. D. Martinez, C. G. Ray, L. M. Taussig, and M. D. Lebowitz.** 1991. Risk factors for respiratory syncytial virus-associated lower respiratory illnesses in the first year of life. *Am. J. Epidemiol.* **133:** 1135–1151.
30. **Hornsleth, A., N. Bech-Thomsen, and B. Friis.** 1985. Detection of RS-virus IgG-subclass-specific antibodies: variation according to age in infants and small children and the diagnostic value in RS-virus-infected small infants. *J. Med. Virol.* **16:**329–335.
31. **Hornsleth, A., B. Friis, P. C. Grauballe, and P. A. Krasilnikof.** 1984. Detection by ELISA of IgA and IgM antibod-

ies in secretion and IgM antibodies in serum in primary lower respiratory syncytial virus infection. *J. Med. Virol.* **13:**149–161.

32. **Huang, Y. T., P. L. Collins, and G. W. Wertz.** 1982. The genome of respiratory syncytial virus is a negative-stranded RNA that codes for at least seven mRNA species. *J. Virol.* **43:**150–157.
33. **Jimenez, H. B., H. M. Keir, and P. Cash.** 1987. Immunoblot analysis of human antibody response to respiratory syncytial virus infection. *J. Gen. Virol.* **68:**1267–1275.
34. **Johnson, P. R., and P. L. Collins.** 1988. The fusion glycoproteins of human respiratory syncytial virus of subgroups A and B: sequence conservation provides a structural basis for antigen relatedness. *J. Gen. Virol.* **69:**2623–2628.
35. **Johnson, P. R., R. A. Olmsted, G. A. Prince, B. R. Murphy, D. W. Alling, E. E. Walsh, and P. L. Collins.** 1987. Antigenic relatedness between glycoproteins of human respiratory syncytial virus subgroups A and B: evaluation of the contributions of F and G glycoproteins to immunity. *J. Virol.* **61:**3163–3166.
36. **Johnson, P. R., M. K. Spriggs, R. A. Olmsted, and P. L. Collins.** 1987. The G glycoprotein of human respiratory syncytial virus of subgroups A and B: extensive sequence diversions between antigenically related proteins. *Proc. Natl. Acad. Sci. USA* **84:**5625–5629.
37. **Jordan, W. S., Jr.** 1962. Growth characteristics of respiratory syncytial virus. *J. Immunol.* **88:**581–590.
38. **Kaul, A., R. Scott, M. Gallagher, M. Scott, J. Clement, and P. L. Ogra.** 1978. Respiratory syncytial virus infection: rapid diagnosis in children by use of indirect immunofluorescence. *Am. J. Dis. Child.* **132:**1088–1090.
39. **Kaul, T. N., R. C. Welliver, and P. L. Ogra.** 1981. Comparison of fluorescent-antibody, neutralizing antibody and complement-enhanced neutralizing antibody assays for detection of serum antibody to respiratory syncytial virus. *J. Clin. Microbiol.* **13:**957–962.
40. **Kellog, J. A.** 1991. Culture vs. direct antigen assays for detection of microbial pathogens from lower respiratory tract specimens suspected of containing the respiratory syncytial virus. *Arch. Pathol. Lab. Med.* **115:**451–458.
41. **Kim, H. W., J. O. Arrobio, C. D. Brandt, B. C. Jeffries, G. Pyles, J. L. Reid, R. M. Chanock, and R. H. Parrott.** 1973. Epidemiology of respiratory syncytial virus infection in Washington, DC. I. Importance of the virus in different respiratory tract disease syndromes and temporal distribution of infection. *Am. J. Epidemiol.* **98:**216–225.
42. **Levine, S., A. Dajani, and R. Klaiber-Franco.** 1988. The response of infants with bronchiolitis to the proteins of respiratory syncytial virus. *J. Gen. Virol.* **69:**1229–1239.
43. **Marquez, A., and G. D. Hsiung.** 1967. Influence of glutamine on multiplication and cytopathic effect of respiratory syncytial virus. *Proc. Soc. Exp. Biol. Med.* **124:**95–99.
44. **Masters, H. B., B. J. Bate, C. Wren, and B. A. Lauer.** 1988. Detection of respiratory syncytial virus antigen in nasopharyngeal secretions by Abbott Diagnostics enzyme immunoassay. *J. Clin. Microbiol.* **26:**1103–1105.
45. **McConnochie, K. M., and K. J. Roghmann.** 1989. Wheezing at 8 and 13 years: changing importance of bronchiolitis and passive smoking. *Pediatr. Pulmonol.* **6:**138–146.
46. **McIntosh, K., and R. M. Chanock.** 1990. Respiratory syncytial virus, p. 963–1074. In B. N. Fields and D. M. Knipe (ed.), *Fields Virology*. Raven Press, New York, N.Y.
47. **McIntosh, K., R. M. Hendry, M. L. Fahnestock, and L. T. Pierik.** 1982. Enzyme-linked immunosorbent assay for the detection of respiratory syncytial virus infection: application to clinical samples. *J. Clin. Microbiol.* **16:**329–333.
48. **Meurman, O., O. Ruuskanen, H. Sarkkinen, P. Hanninen, and P. E. Halonen.** 1984. Immunoglobulin class specific antibody response in respiratory syncytial virus infection measured by enzyme immunoassay. *J. Med. Virol.* **14:**67–72.
49. **Millar, H. R., P. H. Phipps, and E. Rossier.** 1986. Reduction of nonspecific fluorescence in respiratory specimens by pre-treatment with n-acetylcysteine. *J. Clin. Microbiol.* **24:**470–471.
50. **Muelenear, P. M., F. W. Henderson, V. G. Heming, E. E. Walsh, L. J. Anderson, J. A. Prince, and B. R. Murphy.** 1991. Group-specific serum antibody responses in children with primary and recurrent respiratory syncytial virus infections. *J. Infect. Dis.* **164:**15–21.
51. **Mufson, M. A., R. B. Belshe, C. Orvell, and E. Norrby.** 1987. Subgroup characteristics of respiratory syncytial virus strains recovered from children with two consecutive infections. *J. Clin. Microbiol.* **25:**1535–1539.
52. **Navas, L., E. Wang, V. De Carvãlho, and J. Robinson.** 1992. Improved outcome of respiratory syncytial virus infection in a high-risk hospitalized population of Canadian children. *J. Pediatr.* **121:**348–354.
53. **Paton, A., J. Paton, A. Lawrence, P. Goldwater, and R. Harris.** 1992. Rapid detection of respiratory syncytial virus in nasopharyngeal aspirates by reverse transcription and polymerase chain reaction amplification. *J. Clin. Microbiol.* **30:**901–904.
54. **Pons, M. W., A. L. Lambert, D. M. Lambert, and O. M. Rochovansky.** 1983. Improvement of respiratory syncytial virus replication in actively growing HEp-2 cells. *J. Virol. Methods* **7:**217–221.
55. **Pringle, C. R., P. V. Shirodaria, and P. E. Cash.** 1978. Initiation and maintenance of persistent infection by respiratory syncytial virus. *J. Virol.* **28:**199–211.
56. **Richman, A. V., F. A. Pedreia, and N. M. Tauraso.** 1971. Attempts to demonstrate hemagglutination and hemadsorption by respiratory syncytial virus. *Appl. Microbiol.* **21:**1099–1100.
57. **Rothbarth, P. H., M.-C. Hermus, and P. Schrijnemakers.** 1991. Reliability of two new test kits for rapid diagnosis of respiratory syncytial virus infection. *J. Clin. Microbiol.* **29:**824–826.
58. **Routledge, E. G., J. McQuillan, A. C. R. Samson, and G. L. Toms.** 1985. The development of monoclonal antibodies to respiratory syncytial virus and their use in diagnosis by indirect immunofluorescence. *J. Med. Virol.* **15:**305–320.
59. **Sarkkinen, H. K., P. E. Halonen, P. P. Arestila, and A. A. Salmi.** 1981. Detection of respiratory syncytial, parainfluenza type 2 and adenovirus antigens by radioimmunoassay and enzyme immunoassay on nasopharyngeal specimens from children with acute respiratory disease. *J. Clin. Microbiol.* **13:**258–265.
60. **Satake, M., S. Elango, and S. Venkatesan.** 1984. Sequence analysis of the respiratory syncytial virus phosphoprotein gene. *J. Virol.* **52:**991–994.
61. **Shahrabadi, M. S., and P. W. K. Lee** 1988. Calcium requirement for syncytium formation in HEp-2 cells by respiratory syncytial virus. *J. Clin. Microbiol.* **26:**139–141.
62. **Smith, M. C., C. Creutz, and Y. T. Huang.** 1991. Detection of respiratory syncytial virus in nasopharyngeal secretions by shell vial technique. *J. Clin. Microbiol.* **29:**463–465.
63. **Suto, T., N. Yano, M. Ikeda, M. Miyamoto, S. Takai, S. Shigeta, Y. Hinuma, and N. Ishida.** 1965. Respiratory syncytial virus infection and its serologic epidemiology. *Am. J. Epidemiol.* **82:**211–224.
64. **Swierkosz, E. M., R. Flander, L. Melvin, J. D. Miller, and M. W. Kline.** 1989. Evaluation of the Abbott TEST PACK RSV enzyme immunoassay for detection of respiratory syncytial virus in nasopharyngeal swab specimens. *J. Clin. Microbiol.* **27:**1151–1154.

65. **Thomas, E. E., and L. E. Book.** 1991. Comparison of two rapid methods for detection of respiratory syncytial virus (Test Pack RSV and Ortho Elisa) with direct immunofluorescence and virus isolation for the diagnosis of pediatric RSV infection. *J. Clin. Microbiol.* **29:**632–635.
66. **Treuhaft, M. W., J. M. Soukup, and B. J. Sullivan.** 1985. Practical recommendations for the detection of pediatric respiratory syncytial virus infections. *J. Clin. Microbiol.* **22:** 270–273.
67. **Van Beers, D., M. DeFoor, L. DiCesare, and C. Vandenveld.** 1991. Evaluation of a commercial enzyme and immunomembrane filter assay for detection of respiratory syncytial virus in clinical specimens. *Eur. J. Clin. Microbiol. Infect. Dis.* **10:**1073–1076.
68. **Vaur, L., H. Agut, A. Jarbarg-Cheon, G. Prud'homme, J. C. Nicolas, and F. Bricout.** 1986. Simplified enzyme-linked immunosorbent assay for specific antibodies to respiratory syncytial virus. *J. Clin. Microbiol.* **24:**596–599.
69. **Venkatesan, S., N. Elango, M. Satake, E. Camargo, and R. M. Chanock.** 1984. Organization and expression of respiratory syncytial virus genome, p. 31–44. *In* R. Lerner and R. M. Chanock (ed.), *Modern Approaches to Vaccines*. Cold Spring Harbor Laboratory, Cold Spring Harbor, N.Y.
70. **Vikerfors, T., M. Grandian, M. Johansson, and C.-A. Pettersson.** 1988. Detection of an immunoglobulin M response in the elderly for early diagnosis of respiratory syncytial virus infection. *J. Clin. Microbiol.* **26:**808–811.
71. **Walsh, E. E., M. W. Brandriss, and J. J. Schlesinger.** 1985. Purification and characterization of the respiratory syncytial virus fusion protein. *J. Gen. Virol.* **66:**409–415.
72. **Walsh, E. E., and J. Hrushka.** 1983. Monoclonal antibodies to respiratory syncytial virus proteins: identification of the fusion protein. *J. Virol.* **47:**171–177.
73. **Welliver, R. C., T. N. Kaul, T. I. Putnam, M. Sun, K. Riddlesberger, and P. L. Ogra.** 1980. The antibody response to primary and secondary infection with respiratory syncytial virus: kinetics of class-specific responses. *J. Pediatr.* **96:**808–813.
74. **Welliver, R. C., M. Sun, D. Rinaldo, and P. L. Ogra.** 1985. Respiratory syncytial virus-specific IgE responses following infection: evidence for a predominantly mucosal response. *Pediatr. Res.* **19:**420–424.
75. **Welliver, R. C., D. T. Wong, M. Sun, E. Middleton, Jr., R. S. Vaughan, and P. L. Ogra.** 1981. The development of respiratory syncytial virus-specific IgE and the release of histamine in nasopharyngeal secretions after infection. *N. Engl. J. Med.* **305:**841–846.
76. **Wertz, G. W., P. L. Collins, Y. T. Huang, C. Gruber, S. Levine, and L. A. Ball.** 1985. Nucleotide sequence of the G protein gene of human respiratory syncytial virus reveals an unusual type of viral membrane protein. *Proc. Natl. Acad. Sci. USA* **82:**4075–4079.

Measles Virus

AIMO A. SALMI

73

DESCRIPTION OF THE VIRUS

Measles virus belongs to the family *Paramyxoviridae* and is a member of the genus *Morbillivirus* (8). Other well-characterized members of this genus are rinderpest virus of cattle and distemper virus of dogs. Members of this genus have recently been isolated from different carnivores, including seals (4). The only natural hosts of measles virus are humans and primates, but it has been adapted to grow in rodents as well. Measles virus is monotypic, but small biological antigenic variations at the epitope level have been described (27). The variation is based on genetic variability in virus genes (23). Such variations have no effect on protective immunity, since measles infection still provides a lifelong immunity against reinfection.

The main biochemical and structural features of measles virus are similar to those of other members of the family *Paramyxoviridae*. Its genetic information is carried by a single-stranded linear RNA that sediments at 50S to 52S, has a molecular weight of about 5×10^6, and is approximately 16,000 ribonucleotides in length. The enveloped measles virions are pleomorphic and 100 to 250 nm in diameter. The envelope is composed of a cell-derived lipid bilayer from which two types of viral glycoproteins protrude. They are seen by electron microscopy as surface projections of 9 to 15 nm.

The measles virus is composed of six major structural polypeptides, three of which are associated with the envelope. The two protruding glycoproteins, the hemagglutinin (H) and fusion (F) proteins, are the most important antigens inducing protective antibodies. Most of the neutralizing antibodies are against the H protein; antibodies against the F protein inhibit the spread of measles virus in tissue and have some neutralizing capacity as well. The third virus protein associated with the envelope and lining its inner surface is the hydrophobic matrix (M) protein. The helical nucleocapsid enclosed in the envelope is composed of the RNA genome surrounded by the major internal protein, the nucleoprotein (N). Two minor proteins associated with the nucleocapsid core are the polymerase (phospho; P) protein and the large (L) protein, both of which are involved with the RNA polymerase function of the virion. T-cell immunity to these internal proteins also plays a role in protection.

Measles virus is labile and can be readily inactivated with chemicals affecting the lipid envelope. It is also sensitive to heat inactivation; its infectivity can be maintained for years by storage at $-70°C$ but not at $-20°C$. In contrast, measles virus antigens are relatively stable; hemagglutinating antigens and antigens to be used for enzyme immunoassay (EIA) can be stored at 4°C for months without significant loss of antigenic activity.

CLINICAL BACKGROUND

Measles virus causes an acute, generalized infection that until recently has been one of the most common viral diseases of childhood worldwide (8, 15). The typical epidemiologic pattern of rapidly spreading outbreaks is most often observed in springtime (3). Epidemic peaks coincide with the school year in developed countries. Measles epidemics at 2- to 5-year intervals were common in densely populated countries before the licensure of measles vaccine. Now the goal of the expanded global program for immunization is to eliminate measles entirely. Extensive immunization of children has eliminated indigenous measles in some countries (22). Occasional cases or small epidemics of measles have been observed in vaccinated populations in developed countries (2, 16), but most of the infected individuals have been unvaccinated. In developing countries, measles elimination programs have been less successful until now. Measles incidence has, however, decreased in all parts of the world, and the decrease is clearly associated with the increase of vaccination coverage. The eradication of measles can ultimately be reached, although it seems to take a longer time than initially estimated. Measles is rarely fatal in North America and Europe, but mortality can be as high as 20% in developing countries. Poor nutrition and suboptimal hygienic conditions are contributing factors. Measles is still a disease of early childhood in developing countries, but vaccination programs may change the epidemiologic pattern in the future.

Measles is spread from an infected person to a susceptible one, mainly via aerosol. Virus is excreted late during the 9- to 12-day incubation period, and the patient continues to be infectious until early convalescence. The primary site of infection is the mucosal cells of the respiratory tract. The infection spreads to local lymph nodes, and viremia is established. Circulating virus is found in T cells, B cells, and monocytes. Virus spreads to other susceptible organs during the viremic phase. Virus has been found in lung, gut, bile duct, bladder, skin, and lymphoid organs (14).

The prodromal symptoms of measles are similar to those of other upper respiratory tract infections: running nose, sneezing, cough, and fever. Redness of eyes and photophobia are also early symptoms. Koplik's spots on the mouth epithelium, which usually appear after the prodromal symptoms, are the hallmark of the clinical signs of measles. At the time of the viremia, a typical macular or maculopapular exanthem appears. It is first observed in forehead and neck and spreads later to the trunk and upper extremities and finally to lower extremities. High fever at the time of rash onset is characteristic. Patients are infectious a few days before the onset of rash and continue to excrete virus until the rash has disappeared. If no complicating sequelae appear, the disease disappears in 1 to 2 weeks after the onset of rash. If the infection is severe, total recovery may take weeks.

Changes in electroencephalograms are seen in about 50% of patients with uncomplicated measles, indicating central nervous system (CNS) involvement. The number of lymphocytes in the cerebrospinal fluid (CSF) is also frequently increased in measles patients. Although measles virus can replicate in brain cells, changes observed in the CNS are likely due to autoimmune reactions.

Measles virus rarely causes an acute encephalitis, but postinfectious encephalomyelitis has been reported to occur in about 0.1% of patients. Measles virus readily causes persistent infection in vitro and may also establish persistence in vivo, especially in the CNS. A rare complication of measles is subacute sclerosing panencephalitis (SSPE), which occurs at a frequency of about 1/1,000,000. Patients with SSPE, most often boys, usually have a history of an uneventful measles infection early in life. After a latent period of 1 to 10 years, a progressive neurologic disease develops that is lethal within a few years. Virologically, a persistent, defective infection progresses in the CNS of these patients.

Persistent measles virus infection has also been suspected in other chronic autoimmune diseases. Patients with multiple sclerosis as well as those with systemic lupus erythematosus have consistently been found to have elevated levels of measles antibodies. This finding does not necessarily indicate any role of the virus in the etiology or pathogenesis of these diseases but may reflect polyclonal activation of B cells known to occur during the course of these diseases. Paget's disease of bone, otosclerosis, and Crohn's disease, chronic inflammation of the bowel, have also been associated with measles virus infection.

Variants of clinical measles have been observed. Atypical measles may occur in persons previously immunized if the immunity after vaccination was only partial. In such patients, the rash may be hemorrhagic or vesicular and develops first in extremities. Enlargement of lymph nodes and spleen is frequently seen. Such atypical cases may be difficult to diagnose clinically. Diarrhea is often a prominent sign of measles patients in developing countries. Measles may be unusually severe in patients in whom T-cell functions are impaired. These patients frequently develop giant-cell pneumonia and severe involvement of other organ systems. Measles inclusion body encephalitis is an often fatal clinical syndrome in immunocompromised patients.

A diagnosis of measles is usually obvious from the clinical symptoms, especially in light-skinned individuals. However, recognizing measles rash on the background of a dark skin may be difficult. Laboratory diagnosis by specific virologic tests is necessary to confirm the clinical diagnosis in all atypical cases. Even typical measles patients may not be properly diagnosed clinically by physicians who have not previously seen measles patients. Since small measles epidemics are still found even in vaccinated populations in Europe and North America, specific laboratory confirmation is always an important addition to the clinical evaluation of patients suspected of having measles virus infection.

COLLECTION AND STORAGE OF SPECIMENS

The success rate for isolation of measles virus from clinical specimens is low. It has been isolated from the nasopharyngeal and conjunctival specimens during the prodrome and early-rash illness and from stool and urine specimens during late illness. Although the CNS is frequently involved in the pathogenetic process of measles, virus isolation from CSF is rarely successful. Specimens for virus isolation are taken early during the acute phase of the infection by using standard procedures, refrigerated (but not frozen), and transported to the virus laboratory in fewer than 2 days. Since the infectivity of measles virus is labile, the transport medium should contain protein to stabilize the infectivity. Buffered media supplemented with bovine serum albumin or fetal calf serum are good for this purpose.

Direct demonstration of measles virus antigen in infected cells is successful more often than virus isolation, since large amounts of virus antigens accumulate in infected cells. Therefore, a specimen for antigen detection should have a high number of infected cells. The best specimen for this purpose is nasopharyngeal secretion collected by a mucus extractor with a mucus trap of the type commonly used in infectious disease wards. The collected mucus is refrigerated and sent immediately to the laboratory for direct immunofluorescence or antigen detection by immunoassay. Virus antigen may also be detected in circulating leukocytes. Heparinized blood is sent refrigerated to the virus laboratory for this examination.

A single serum specimen is sufficient for the demonstration of virus-specific immunoglobulin M (IgM) antibodies, provided that it has been taken within 4 to 5 weeks of the onset of measles. Sputum can also be used for detection of virus-specific IgM. Intrathecal measles virus antibody synthesis, which occurs in all SSPE patients, many multiple sclerosis patients, and some measles patients, can be demonstrated by titrating antibodies in both serum and CSF. For that purpose, paired serum and CSF specimens are taken on the same day and sent to the virus laboratory. Immunoglobulins are more labile in CSF than in serum and require refrigerated transport of paired specimens to the laboratory.

Serologic diagnosis can also be based on demonstration of a significant increase in antibody titer in paired serum specimens. The first specimen should be taken as soon as possible after the onset of the disease. The second specimen can be taken as early as 7 days but preferably 10 to 14 days after the first specimen.

Testing of paired acute- and convalescent-phase serum specimens is especially important for the diagnosis of patients who have been immunized against measles but who subsequently become infected. Such patients usually have a record of measles immunization and often have detectable but low titers of IgG antibodies to measles virus in their acute-phase serum specimens. The acute-phase sera do not, however, have detectable IgM antibodies, but acute- and convalescent-phase paired sera show diagnostic rises in IgG measles virus-specific antibody titers.

DIRECT EXAMINATION

Typical paramyxoviruslike viruses may be seen in clinical specimens from measles patients by using the electron microscope. However, since all members of the family *Paramyxoviridae* are similar morphologically, no specific viral diagnosis can be made by such an examination. Measles virus-infected cells are typically multinucleated and are formed by fusion of a large number of infected cells. Such cells are pathognomonic for measles, and their presence in throat washings or peripheral blood mononuclear cells can be used as an indication of measles infection. Eosinophilic inclusions are found in the cytoplasms or nuclei of infected cells. The inclusions represent accumulated viral nucleocapsid material and are considered to be diagnostic in SSPE patients.

Although histologic examination may aid in the diagnosis of measles, specific diagnosis requires a direct demonstration of virus antigens in the cells. This can be done by immunofluorescence staining of tissue cells obtained from patients (7). The most useful substrate for staining is cells from nasopharyngeal secretions, peripheral blood, and urine sediment. Virus antigen can also be found in skin biopsy samples obtained during the rash. For immunofluorescence, the specimen is spread on a glass slide, air dried, and fixed in ice-cold acetone for 10 min. Fixed slides can be stored frozen, preferably at −70°C.

The fixed cells are stained for measles virus antigens by hyperimmune antiserum or monoclonal antibodies to the N or P protein and fluoresceinated secondary antibodies specific for the primary antibodies. Both primary and secondary antisera for measles virus staining are commercially available. Standard staining conditions commonly used in immunofluorescence staining should be employed. The stained samples are examined for a specific staining pattern that is typically cytoplasmic; late during the infectious cycle and in chronic measles such as SSPE, it may also be intranuclear. Measles virus-infected cells, especially late during the infectious cycle, contain a large mass of virus antigens. Especially prominent are the N and P antigens, which can be seen in small spots or as large fluorescing bodies in the cytoplasm. For reference purposes, cells infected with a laboratory strain of measles virus should be included as a positive control.

Direct demonstration of viral antigens by radioimmunoassay or enzyme immunoassay (EIA) has been used for rapid diagnosis of respiratory virus infections. Nasopharyngeal specimens without fixation can be directly used in such tests. Although a few nanograms of measles virus antigen per milliliter can be detected by EIA (25), such an antigen assay has not been widely used in diagnostic laboratories and is not commercially available.

Hybridization tests for measles virus RNA in tissues have been used in research laboratories (6) but have not been commonly used in diagnostic laboratories. PCR is a sensitive method for direct demonstration of measles virus RNA in plasma samples, nasopharyngeal secretions, and peripheral blood mononuclear cells (10, 12, 17). The sensitivity and specificity of different variants of PCR assays are comparable to those of virus isolation and IgM assays. Results with larger test series with clinical samples and commercial PCR assays have not yet been published.

ISOLATION OF VIRUS

Measles virus can be isolated from patients during the prodromal state, at the time of the rash, and for a few days afterwards. Since the success rate for virus isolation is low (24), this approach cannot be used as the primary means for the laboratory diagnosis of measles infection. Virus isolation is more important for the characterization of measles in patients with poor or delayed antibody responses, which occur in many patients with atypical measles.

Although tissue culture-adapted laboratory strains of measles virus grow readily in a number of continuous cell lines of human or primate origin, virus strains from measles patients are more difficult to cultivate. The best cells for virus isolation are primary human fetal kidney cells. Since such cells are not generally available, primary monkey kidney cells are the second choice. These cells can be prepared from monkey kidney tissue, if available in the virus laboratory, or may be obtained from commercial sources. Primary human amniotic cells have also been used to isolate virus strains from patients, but the success rate is lower than with primary kidney cells. B95-8 cells (distributed by the American Type Culture Collection), which are marmoset lymphocytes transformed by Epstein-Barr virus, have been shown to support the growth of naturally occurring strains of measles virus (13). This cell line is a good choice for measles virus isolation from clinical specimens.

The cytopathic effect (CPE) appears late after the inoculation of a measles virus-containing sample. The inoculated cultures should be observed for typical CPE for at least 2 weeks. Two types of CPE may be observed in the cultures: (i) spindle-shaped, light-reflecting single cells that increase in number when the infection advances and (ii) multinucleated giant cells (syncytia) that increase in size during the culture time. The type of CPE depends on the multiplicity of infection, the virus strain, and the cells used to propagate the virus.

In chronic measles infections (i.e., in SSPE patients), the virus is defective and cell associated and cannot be isolated by ordinary techniques (11). Instead, cocultivation of patient brain or peripheral blood cells with susceptible cell lines is required. The procedure may take a few weeks and requires many passages of the cell mixture before the CPE appears or antigens can be demonstrated in the coculture. Virus isolated by the cocultivation technique may remain cell associated.

IDENTIFICATION OF VIRUS

Methods

The finding that the CPE caused by the isolated virus is syncytial suggests that the isolated virus has a fusion protein. This observation, combined with the clinical information, justifies the suspicion that the isolated virus may be measles virus. A preliminary test that can easily be done is hemadsorption with monkey erythrocytes, preferably from African green monkeys. However, this test is not specific for measles virus. Proper identification of the virus causing the CPE requires use of specific antisera.

A hyperimmune animal antiserum specific for measles virus, monoclonal antibodies specific for the internal polypeptides (N, P, and M), or a mixture of different monoclonal antibodies can be used to identify the isolated virus. Both hyperimmune sera and monoclonal antibodies can be purchased from commercial sources. The most convenient identification test is direct immunofluorescence with specific antisera. Cells with CPE are scraped off, spread on a glass slide, and fixed in ice-cold acetone for 10 min. Staining with measles virus-specific antibodies and fluoresceinated secondary antibodies is done by standard procedures. Fluorescence of typical intracellular inclusions stained with the specific antiserum identifies the isolated virus. Staining with a serum specimen taken from a hyperimmunized animal before the immunization should be used, if possible, as a negative control. Virus antigen in infected cells can also be identified by a specific EIA for measles virus antigens (25).

SEROLOGIC DIAGNOSIS

The presence of specific antibodies in a single serum specimen indicates past or present measles infection or vaccination. Demonstration of a significant increase of specific antibody titers in a serum pair taken at a 7- to 14-day interval is the basis of the diagnosis of an acute infection. As a rapid virus diagnosis method, demonstration of virus-specific IgM antibodies in only one specimen is the method of choice. In all serologic tests, known positive and negative controls should be included in the series.

HI

The hemagglutination inhibition (HI) test is based on the ability of measles virus H protein to bind to monkey erythrocytes. If the H protein is in a dimeric form or in a larger particle such as the measles virion, erythrocytes form aggregates that can easily be seen. Specific antibodies inhibit this aggregation, the phenomenon on which the HI antibody test is based.

Preparation of the HI Antigen

The antigen for the HI test is available commercially but can also be easily prepared in a virus laboratory. Continuous cell lines known to give a high yield of measles virus, such as Vero, CV-1, or HeLa, should be used. Since measles virus is homotypic, any virus strain can be used for hemagglutinin preparation. When the CPE is spread throughout the cell layer, the culture is harvested. Because a large amount of H protein is found both in the cellular membranes and in released virus, whole cultures can be harvested and used for antigen preparation. The material is frozen and thawed five times and centrifuged at 10,000 × *g* for 20 min; the supernatant is divided into smaller portions and stored at −20°C. The hemagglutinating ability of the antigen can be increased a minimum of fourfold by treatment with Tween 80 and ether (18).

The hemagglutination is measured by titration on round-bottom microtiter plates by using erythrocytes from Old World monkeys such as African green or rhesus monkeys. To 0.025-ml volumes of twofold antigen dilutions, 0.5% monkey erythrocytes are added, and the plates are incubated for 1 h at 37°C. The last dilution giving a clear agglutination contains 1 hemagglutinating unit (HAU) of measles antigen. All reagents are diluted in phosphate-buffered saline (PBS). If the erythrocytes aggregate spontaneously, then the dilutions are made in PBS supplemented with 0.2 to 1% bovine serum albumin.

HI Test

Human sera frequently contain nonspecific inhibitors of hemagglutination. Such inhibitors can be removed by adding an equal volume of 25% kaolin in PBS and incubating it for 20 min at room temperature. The mixture is then centrifuged, and the supernatant, which represents a 1:2 dilution of the original serum, can be stored at −20°C. Some human sera agglutinate monkey erythrocytes and must be absorbed with an equal volume of 50% monkey erythrocytes for at least 4 h at 4°C.

For the HI test, twofold dilutions of serum specimens starting with a 1:2 or 1:4 dilution are made on microtiter plates, using a volume of 0.025 ml, and 4 HAU of measles antigen is added in a volume of 0.025 ml. After 1 h of incubation at room temperature, 0.05 ml of 0.5% monkey erythrocytes is added; the plates are then shaken and incubated at 37°C for 1 h. The agglutination pattern is read, and the HI titer is determined as the last dilution inhibiting agglutination. As a control, the hemagglutinating measles virus antigen is backtitrated to make sure that the amount of hemagglutinin is 4 HAU in the test.

EIA

Measles antibodies can also be measured by EIA. EIA test kits for measles virus antibodies are commercially available, but such tests can also be set up in any virus laboratory. Measles virus antigen is available from commercial sources and can also be prepared by using standard laboratory virus strains and continuous cell lines supporting virus growth. The cells are maintained in Eagle minimal essential medium without or with 2% fetal bovine serum and are infected with a high multiplicity of infectious virus. When the CPE has spread throughout the cell monolayer, the supernatant and the infected cells are harvested separately and processed for antigens.

Infected cells contain a large amount of the N, P, and H proteins and lesser amounts of M, F, and L proteins. For practical purposes, a crude antigen prepared from infected cells is satisfactory for measuring an increase in the level of IgG antibodies and determining the immunity status of the patient. If the antigen is used in the IgM assays, purified virus should be used.

Preparation of EIA Antigen

For preparation of the crude cellular antigen, the infected cells are washed three times with cold PBS and resuspended in 10-fold-diluted PBS. The cells are disrupted with powerful ultrasonic equipment or in a tightly fitting Dounce homogenizer. The debris is removed by low-speed centrifugation in an ordinary tabletop refrigerated centrifuge at 500 × *g* for 15 min. The particulate material in the supernatant is pelleted in an ultracentrifuge at 80,000 × *g* for 2 h. The pellet is resuspended in a small volume of PBS. The resuspension might require a vigorous homogenization. The amount of protein in the antigen is determined, and the antigen is divided into smaller portions and stored frozen, preferably at −70°C. Storage at −20°C is acceptable, but the antigen tends to aggregate, especially if the storage temperature occasionally rises above −20°C.

Purification of Measles Virus

Measles virus for use as EIA antigen is purified from supernatants of infected cells collected at the time when the CPE has spread to 75 to 100% of the cells. After the supernatant has been clarified by centrifugation at 10,000 × *g* for 20 min, it can be stored for a few days at 4°C before further purification. The supernatant is then concentrated 10- to 20-fold in a hollow fiber or membrane concentration apparatus. To the concentrated supernatant, NaCl and α-D-methylmannoside are added to final concentrations of 2 mol/liter and 4%, respectively. These additives reduce the nonspecific binding of cellular debris to the virions. After 30 min on ice, the supernatant is layered onto a step gradient consisting of 10 ml of 18% potassium tartrate and 5 ml of

36% potassium tartrate in a buffer consisting of 0.2 M glycine, 0.2 M NaCl, 20 mM Tris, and 2 mM EDTA (pH 7.8) (GNTE buffer). The gradients are centrifuged at 80,000 × g for 90 min. The virus material at the 18 to 36% interface is collected, diluted with GNTE buffer to a tartrate concentration of less than 18%, and layered on a 24-ml linear 18 to 36% potassium tartrate gradient prepared in the GNTE buffer. The gradients are centrifuged at 80,000 × g for 3 h or overnight. The virus band is collected, diluted in GNTE, and pelleted at 80,000 × g for 30 min. The virus is suspended in PBS and stored at −70°C.

EIA for Measles Virus Antibodies

Flat-bottom microtiter plates are first coated with crude antigen or purified virus material. The plates should be of a special EIA type or of reliable tissue culture-treated plastic. For coating, the antigen is diluted in PBS or 50 mM carbonate buffer (pH 9.6) to a concentration giving the best binding of specific antibodies. This concentration should be determined experimentally by checkerboard titration, but a concentration of 5 to 50 μg/ml for a crude lysate antigen or 0.5 to 5 μg/ml for purified virions is a good guess for a proper coating concentration. A 0.1-ml volume of the diluted antigen is added to each well in the microtiter plate, which is then incubated overnight at room temperature or at 4°C. Blocking of all remaining protein-binding sites on the plastic plate is done by incubating the wells for 1 to 2 h with 0.1 ml of EIA incubation buffer, consisting of PBS supplemented with 0.5% bovine serum albumin and 0.5% Tween 20.

Serum dilutions are made in two- or fourfold series in EIA incubation buffer, starting from a dilution of 1:50 to 1:200. Dilutions can be made with a multichannel pipette directly on the antigen-coated plates. Incubation with the serum dilutions is for 1 h at 37°C or for 2 h at room temperature, after which the plates are washed three times with washing buffer (PBS supplemented with 0.1% Tween 20).

The next step is addition of enzyme-labeled antibodies that recognize human immunoglobulins. The antibodies can be specific for human IgG, which is the major immunoglobulin class of antibodies during measles convalescence and in immune individuals. For demonstration of a titer increase in a specimen pair or of the immunity status of an individual, the antibody can also be specific for all human immunoglobulins. Incubation with the labeled antibodies is for 1 h at 37°C or for 2 h at room temperature, after which the plates are washed as described above. The final step in the assay is incubation of the plates with the substrate solution. The composition of the substrate depends on the enzyme coupled to the antihuman antibodies. For example, a reliable substrate for horseradish peroxidase is hydrogen peroxide (6 mmol/liter) and *o*-phenylenediamine (17 mmol/liter) in phosphate (50 mmol/liter)-citrate (20 mmol/liter) buffer (pH 5.5).

Titers of the serum specimens can be determined from the absorbance values of the different serum dilutions by criteria established in the laboratory. As in other serologic tests, a fourfold increase in antibody titer can be considered proof of a recent virus infection. Since there are no official standards of EIA, the series should always include known positive and negative serum specimens.

Simplified antibody tests based on EIA, which can be used in developing countries, have also been described (5).

IgM Determinations

The presence of IgM antibodies in a serum specimen indicates an early phase of an immune response. Nearly 100% of serum specimens taken during acute measles infection or in early convalescence are positive for measles virus-specific IgM antibodies (21, 29). Since an IgM determination can normally be made in less than 24 h in the laboratory, this test can be used for rapid virologic diagnosis of an acute measles infection. The main pitfall of an ordinary IgM test is the possibility of nonspecific positive reaction mainly due to rheumatoid factor interference (28, 29). Therefore, determination of rheumatoid factor should be included in an ordinary IgM antibody test in order to exclude false-positive results.

Physical separation of IgM and IgG and subsequent antibody tests of the fractions were earlier used for measles-specific IgM determination. Such methods are laborious and are not in general use. Instead, specific antibodies that recognize the μ chain of human IgM binding to measles virus antigen are widely used in different tests.

IgM determination by fluorescent-antibody techniques requires measles virus-infected fixed cells, fluoresceinated antibodies specific to human IgM, and a microscope equipped with a UV light source and proper fluorescence filters. Any laboratory strain of measles virus can be used to infect a continuous cell line. Cells left uninfected should also be prepared and used as negative controls. Infected and control cultures are washed three times with PBS, fixed in ice-cold acetone for 10 min, and air dried. Fixed cells can be stored for a couple of months at −20°C without a significant loss of antigenicity. Slides taken from cold storage should first be brought to room temperature and then rinsed in PBS. The serum specimen to be tested is incubated on antigen slides at 37°C in a moist chamber for 30 min, and the slide is washed three times in PBS. A predetermined dilution of fluorescein-labeled antibodies to human IgM (μ chain specific) is added to the slide and incubated for 30 min at 37°C. After three more washings with PBS, the slides are sealed with coverslips and examined under a fluorescence microscope.

Other immunoassays offer more objective means of IgM determination. Although radioimmunoassay (1) is reliable, EIA has replaced it because of the hazards associated with the use of radioactive material. Measles virus-specific IgM antibodies can be measured by direct EIA as described above for IgG antibodies except that specific antibodies for human μ chain tagged with an enzyme are used for detection of IgM antibodies bound to measles antigen on the solid phase. Testing of only one serum dilution is sufficient for IgM determination. The best dilution depends on the technical requirements of the system used, but a dilution of 1:50 to 1:200 is generally optimal.

Since many human serum specimens have IgM antibodies capable of binding to cellular proteins, it is necessary to simultaneously test sera against antigens prepared from infected and noninfected cells or to use highly purified virions. Another pitfall in the direct IgM EIA is the nonspecific reaction due to IgM-class rheumatoid factor, which binds to IgG. Such binding of the indicator antibodies to IgM-class rheumatoid factor that is attached to measles virus-specific IgG gives a false-positive reaction. Therefore, if the level of rheumatoid factor is elevated in the serum specimen, the IgM test results are not reliable. Such specimens should be absorbed with heat-aggregated human immunoglobulins or latex particles coated with human IgG prior to testing (29).

The problems with rheumatoid factor can be avoided if the order of reagents in the IgM test is reversed (28). In this system (often referred to as reverse, or capture, EIA), the first layer coated to the solid phase consists of antibodies to human IgM (μ specific; commercially available). The second step is incubation of the test specimens on the solid phase, which results in the binding of IgM to the solid phase. The presence of IgM antibodies specific for measles virus can be detected in two ways. In one approach, purified virus is added to the solid phase, and the bound virus is detected by specific antibodies conjugated with an enzyme marker. If the antibodies are used unconjugated, an extra layer of conjugated antibodies specific for the animal species used to produce the measles virus-specific antiserum is required (28). The second approach is use of purified measles virus directly labeled with an enzyme (26).

It is easy to recognize negative and strongly positive serum specimens. Difficulties arise when the absorbance reading is only slightly elevated. The best way to decide the cutoff level for positivity in such cases is to test a large number of randomly selected serum specimens likely to be IgM negative and determine the mean and the standard deviation, which can then be used to determine the 95% probability level of true IgM positivity. After this standardization has been performed, known IgM-negative sera can be used as reference for the cutoff level.

Other Serologic Tests

A number of other tests have been used to detect antibodies to measles virus in a serum specimen or an increase in the titer of a serum pair. Indirect immunofluorescence tests for IgG and IgM antibodies are still practical alternatives. These tests should be done according to the protocol used for immunofluorescence tests for other viral antibodies. Research laboratories have measured antibodies to different measles virus polypeptides by immunoprecipitation of radiolabeled virus proteins and Western immunoblotting (9, 20), but such tests are better suited for qualitative assessment of the immune response to each of the viral polypeptides than for quantitative measurement of the immune response. The neutralization and hemolysis inhibition tests can be used for diagnostic tests, since they measure antibodies of direct biological significance. Information about immunity obtained with these tests may be important if epidemics of measles infection appear in a vaccinated population.

Neutralization

The neutralization test generally correlates with immunity, since it measures antibodies capable of inhibiting virus growth in vitro. It is more cumbersome than most of the other antibody tests, since it is based on the inhibition of measles virus growth in cell culture. The test requires no special equipment beyond the ordinary cell culture facility. Stock measles virus is diluted to contain 100 50% tissue culture infective doses per 0.1 ml. Equal amounts of serially diluted serum specimen and the diluted virus are incubated together at 4°C for 60 min. A 0.2-ml volume of this mixture is added to each of three to six tissue culture tubes and incubated at 37°C until CPE appears in half of the control tubes with 1 50% tissue culture infective dose of virus alone. The titer is determined to be the dilution at which the CPE is inhibited in more than half of the tubes. The neutralization tests can also be done in microtiter format, which is more practical for titer determination of a large number of specimens.

HLI Test

The hemolysis inhibition (HLI) test measures the presence of antibodies inhibiting hemolysis caused by the F protein of measles virus. However, since the expression of hemolytic activity requires that virus particles be anchored to erythrocytes via the hemagglutinin, antibodies to the H protein also interfere with the hemolysis reaction. Because the HLI antibodies are effective in inhibiting virus spread in tissues, their measurement is relevant, especially if there is a measles outbreak in a vaccinated population (19).

Antigen used in the HLI test should have a large amount of F protein. Since the level of F protein can vary from one preparation to another, the best cell-virus combination for preparing such an antigen should be experimentally determined. Infected cells in a 10% suspension or 10- to 20-times-concentrated supernatant of virus-infected cells are the starting material for preparing the hemolyzing antigen. The material is disrupted by five cycles of freezing and thawing or by vigorous sonication. The hemolyzing activity of the antigen is determined by adding 0.1 ml of washed 10% green monkey erythrocytes to a twofold dilution series of 0.4 ml hemolysing antigen in PBS. After 3 h of incubation at 37°C, the erythrocytes are centrifuged at 1,000 × g for 10 min, and the A_{540} of the supernatant is measured. An antigen dilution giving an absorbance of about 0.5 is selected as the working dilution.

For the HLI test, 0.2 ml of the working dilution of the hemolyzing antigen is added to equal volumes of serial twofold dilutions of the serum specimen. After 1 h of incubation at room temperature, 0.1 ml of a 10% suspension of monkey erythrocytes is added. After incubation for 3 h at 37°C, the erythrocytes are centrifuged and the optical density of the supernatant is read. The HLI titer of the serum is the dilution giving at least 50% reduction of hemolysis as calculated from the control hemolysis with added PBS but without serum specimen.

EVALUATION AND INTERPRETATION OF RESULTS

Isolation of measles virus indicates active virus replication in the patient and is the basis for a specific virologic diagnosis. Negative results for virus isolation do not exclude measles virus infection, since the sensitivity of the isolation method is low. Careful timing of specimens and testing of more than one specimen are important for successful virus isolation. Cocultivation of cells from SSPE patients results in virus isolation in only a small percentage of cases. Therefore, negative virus isolation results for these patients do not exclude the diagnosis of SSPE.

HI is one of the best methods for determining the immunity status of an individual, since it is easy to perform and the presence of HI antibodies is known to correlate with protective immunity. HI titers of 1/10 or higher are considered protective against secondary infection, but the lower limit of protection clearly depends on the sensitivity of the test system used. The presence of neutralizing antibodies also correlates well with protective immunity, but the neutralization test is more cumbersome and less often done. EIA measures antibodies to all viral components and can be used as a sensitive test to determine whether an individual has been infected with measles virus. There are rare individuals, however, who are strongly positive in EIA but have only low levels of HI or neutralizing antibodies. It is not clear whether such individuals are protected against reinfection. EIA is the most sensitive and becomes positive in most patients already at the time of rash. HI and neutralization tests are less sensitive and become positive 1 to 2 days later than the EIA.

All the serologic tests described above can be used to demonstrate a significant increase of antibody level in a serum pair. A fourfold or greater increase indicates an acute measles infection. If the first serum specimen is taken during the first 2 days of the rash and the second one is taken a minimum of 7 days later, a significant increase in antibody titer can usually be demonstrated. This is true for patients with ordinary measles, but patients with impaired immunity may synthesize only a low amount of antibodies, and thus no significant increase would be demonstrated in a specimen pair taken at an interval of a few days. An increase may still be seen if the serum specimens are taken a few weeks apart.

A diagnostic serologic test for SSPE patients is the demonstration of intrathecal measles virus-specific antibody synthesis. This can be shown by calculating the CSF/serum titer ratio. The normal ratio is about 1/200 to 1/500, but in SSPE patients, it is from 1/5 to 1/50. Such a low ratio indicates intrathecal antibody synthesis, provided that ratios of other viral antibodies, e.g., adenovirus antibodies, are not reduced.

Demonstration of virus-specific IgM antibodies is the best rapid diagnostic test. All patients with ordinary measles have IgM antibodies in specimens taken late during the rash and at least until 4 to 6 weeks later. The tests can still be negative during the first 3 days after the onset of rash. Only low levels of IgM antibodies are seen in some SSPE patients early after the onset of the disease (30). The only pitfall of the ordinary measles IgM tests is nonspecific positive results due to rheumatoid factor and occasional binding of IgM to nonviral cellular antigens. If these possibilities are excluded, e.g., by using a reverse IgM assay, the test can be very reliable as a rapid diagnostic test.

REFERENCES

1. **Arstila, P., T. Vuorimaa, K. Kalimo, P. Halonen, M. Viljanen, K. Granfors, and P. Toivanen.** 1977. A solid phase radioimmunoassay for IgG and IgM antibodies against measles virus. *J. Gen. Virol.* **34:**167–176.
2. **Atkinson, W. L., W. A. Orenstein, and S. Krugman.** 1992. The resurgence of measles in the United States. *Annu. Rev. Med.* **43:**451–463.
3. **Black, F. L.** 1997. Measles, p. 507–529. *In* A. S. Evans and R. A. Kaslow (ed.), *Viral Infections of Humans: Epidemiology and Control*, 4th ed. Plenum Medical Book Co., New York.
4. **Blixenkorne-Möller, M., V. Svansson, M. Appel, J. Krogsrud, P. Have, and C. Örvell.** 1992. Antigenic relationship between field isolates of morbilliviruses from different carnivores. *Arch. Virol.* **123:**279–294.
5. **Condorelli, F., and T. Ziegler.** 1993. Dot immunobinding assay for simultaneous detection of specific immunoglobulin G antibodies to measles virus, mumps virus, and rubella virus. *J. Clin. Microbiol.* **31:**717–719.
6. **Fournier, J. G., M. Tardieu, P. Lebon, O. Robain, G. Ponsot, S. Rozenblatt, and M. Bouteille.** 1985. Detection of measles virus RNA in lymphocytes from peripheral blood and brain perivascular infiltrates of patients with subacute sclerosing panencephalitis. *N. Engl. J. Med.* **313:**910–915.
7. **Fulton, R. E., and P. J. Middleton.** 1975. Immunofluorescence in diagnosis of measles infections in children. *J. Pediatr.* **86:**17–22.
8. **Griffin, D. E., and W. J. Bellini.** 1996. Measles virus, p. 1267–1312. *In* B. N. Fields, D. M. Knipe, and P. M. Howley (ed.), *Fields Virology*, 3rd ed. Lippincott-Raven Publishers, Philadelphia, Pa.
9. **Hankins, R. W., and F. L. Black.** 1986. Western blot analysis of measles virus antibody in normal persons and in patients with multiple sclerosis, subacute sclerosing panencephalitis, or atypical measles. *J. Clin. Microbiol.* **24:**324–329.
10. **Jin, L., A. Richards, and D. W. Brown.** 1996. Development of a dual target-PCR for detection and characterization of measles virus in clinical specimens. *Mol. Cell. Probes* **10:**191–200.
11. **Katz, M., and H. Koprowski.** 1973. The significance of failure to isolate infected viruses in cases of SSPE. *Arch. Gesamte Virusforsch.* **41:**390–393.
12. **Kawashima, H., T. Mori, K. Takekuma, A. Hoshika, M. Hata, and T. Nakayama.** 1996. Polymerase chain reaction detection of the hemagglutinin gene from an attenuated measles vaccine strain in the peripheral mononuclear cells of children with autoimmune hepatitis. *Arch. Virol.* **141:**877–884.
13. **Kobune, F., H. Sakata, and A. Sugiura.** 1990. Marmoset lymphoblastoid cell as a sensitive host for isolation of measles virus. *J. Virol.* **64:**700–705.
14. **Moench, T. R., D. E. Griffin, C. R. Obriecht, A. J. Vaisberg, and R. T. Johnson.** 1988. Acute measles in patients with and without neurological involvement: distribution of measles virus antigen and RNA. *J. Infect. Dis.* **158:**433–442.
15. **Morgan, E. M., and F. Rapp.** 1977. Measles virus and its associated diseases. *Bacteriol. Rev.* **41:**636–666.
16. **Mouallem, M., E. Friedman, R. Pauzner, and Z. Farfel.** 1987. Measles epidemic in young adults: clinical manifestations and laboratory analysis in 40 patients. *Arch. Intern. Med.* **147:**1111–1113.
17. **Nakayama, T., T. Mori, S. Yamaguchi, S. Sonoda, S. Asamura, R. Yamashita, Y. Takeuchi, and T. Urano.** 1995. Detection of measles virus genome directly from clinical samples by reverse transcriptase-polymerase chain reaction and genetic variability. *Virus Res.* **35:**1–16.
18. **Norrby, E.** 1962. Hemagglutination by measles virus. IV. A simple procedure for production of high potency antigen for hemagglutination-inhibition (HI) tests. *Proc. Soc. Exp. Biol. Med.* **111:**814–818.
19. **Norrby, E., G. Enders-Ruckle, and V. ter Meulen.** 1975. Differences in the appearance of antibodies to structural components of measles virus after immunization with inactivated and live virus. *J. Infect. Dis.* **132:**262–269.
20. **Norrby, E., C. Örvell, B. Vandvik, and D. J. Cherry.** 1981. Antibodies against measles virus polypeptides in different disease conditions. *Infect. Immun.* **34:**718–724.
21. **Pedersen, I. R., A. Antonsdottir, T. Evald, and C. H. Mordhorst.** 1982. Detection of measles IgM antibodies by enzyme linked immunosorbent assay (ELISA). *Acta Pathol. Microbiol. Scand.* **90:**153–160.
22. **Peltola, H., O. P. Heinonen, M. Valle, M. Paunio, M. Virtanen, V. Karanko, and K. Cantell.** 1994. The elimination of indigenous measles, mumps, and rubella from Finland by a 12-year, two-dose vaccination program. *N. Engl. J. Med.* **331:**1397–1402.
23. **Rota, J. S., J. L. Heath, P. A. Rota, G. E. King, M. L. Celma, J. Carabana, M. R. Fernandez, D. Brown, L. Jin, and W. J. Bellini.** 1996. Molecular epidemiology of measles virus: identification of pathways of transmission and implications for measles elimination. *J. Infect. Dis.* **173:**32–37.
24. **Sakaguchi, M., Y. Yoskikawa, K. Yamanouchi, K. Takeda, and T. Sato.** 1986. Characteristics of fresh isolates of wild measles virus. *Jpn. J. Exp. Med.* **56:**61–67.
25. **Salmi, A., and G. Lund.** 1984. Immunoassays for measles virus nucleocapsid antigen: effect of antigen-antibody complexes. *J. Gen. Virol.* **65:**1655–1663.
26. **Salonen, J., R. Vainionpää, and P. Halonen.** 1986. Assay

of measles virus IgM and IgG class antibodies by use of peroxidase labelled viral antigens. *Arch. Virol.* **91:**93–106.

27. **Sheshberadaran, H., S.-N. Chen, and E. Norrby.** 1983. Monoclonal antibodies against five structural components of measles virus. I. Characterization of antigenic determinants on nine strains of measles virus. *Virology* **128:** 341–353.
28. **Tuokko, H.** 1984. Comparison of non-specific reactivity in indirect and reverse immunoassays for measles and mumps immunoglobulin M antibodies. *J. Clin. Microbiol.* **20:**972–979.
29. **Tuokko, H., and A. Salmi.** 1983. Detection of IgM antibodies to measles virus by enzyme immunoassay. *Med. Microbiol. Immunol.* **171:**187–198.
30. **Ziola, B., P. Halonen, and G. Enders.** 1986. Synthesis of measles virus-specific IgM antibodies and IgM-class rheumatoid factor in relation to clinical onset of subacute sclerosing panencephalitis. *J. Med. Virol.* **18:**51–59.

Mumps Virus

ELLA M. SWIERKOSZ

74

CLINICAL BACKGROUND

Mumps is an acute, usually self-limited, systemic illness characterized most commonly by bilateral or unilateral parotitis accompanied by high fever and fatigue, although up to one-third of infections may be asymptomatic. Extra-salivary gland manifestations include meningitis, encephalitis, orchitis, oophoritis, polyarthritis, and pancreatitis. Nephritis, thyroiditis, mastitis, prostatitis, hepatitis, thrombocytopenia, and deafness have been reported as rare manifestations of mumps infection (2). Recently, Ni et al. (43) have presented molecular evidence supporting the role of mumps in the etiology of endocardial fibroelastosis. Humans are the only natural host of mumps virus. Infection confers long-lasting immunity to clinical disease (2). Most cases of mumps occur in children and teenagers aged 5 to 19 years (6). In 1996, 751 cases of mumps were reported in the United States, a >99% decrease since licensure of the live, attenuated mumps vaccine in 1967 (6).

The incubation period of the virus ranges from 14 to 25 days, with an average of 16 to 18 days. Transmission is by droplet, with primary viral replication occurring in the upper respiratory mucosal epithelium (18). A live, attenuated mumps vaccine in a trivalent form combined with live, attenuated vaccines against rubella and measles is administered to children at 12 to 15 months of age and a second dose is administered at 4 to 6 or 11 to 12 years of age (5). Despite the availability of mumps vaccine, outbreaks continue to occur in vaccinated and unvaccinated populations (7, 53).

DESCRIPTION OF AGENT

Mumps virus is a member of the genus *Rubulavirus* in the family *Paramyxoviridae* (42). In addition to mumps virus, the paramyxoviruses include Newcastle disease virus and the parainfluenza viruses. Like other paramyxoviruses, mumps virus is a pleomorphic, enveloped virus that is between 100 and 600 nm in diameter and that contains a helical nucleocapsid composed of negative-sense, single-stranded RNA and three nucleocapsid-associated proteins (L, NP, and P). The involvement of both the P and the L proteins in RNA-dependent RNA polymerase activity is postulated. Two surface glycoproteins, the fusion (F) and hemagglutinin-neuraminidase (HN) proteins, project from the lipid envelope and are visualized as spikes by electron microscopy. The HN protein, which has both hemagglutinating and neuraminidase activities, mediates adsorption of the virus to host cells, while the F glycoprotein mediates fusion of lipid membranes, allowing penetration of the nucleocapsid into the cell. The F glycoprotein is also responsible for mediating hemolysis of erythrocytes. Antibody against the HN protein neutralizes viral infectivity. A third membrane-associated protein, called the M, or matrix, protein is believed to mediate assembly of the virion along the inner surface of the virus-modified host cell membrane. An additional gene is believed to code for a small hydrophobic (SH) protein that may also be associated with membranes (63). Only one antigenic type of mumps virus has been detected by hemagglutination-inhibition (HI) or neutralization assays. Antigenic differences among mumps virus strains have been demonstrated with HN-specific monoclonal antibody (51). Analysis of the SH gene sequence has also revealed differences among mumps virus strains (31, 56). Moreover, strain-dependent differences in cytopathology and neurovirulence have been described (37). Immunologic cross-reactivity and RNA sequence homology have been demonstrated with parainfluenza virus types 2 and 4 (20, 24, 29, 30, 45, 57). Mumps virus infectivity is destroyed by organic solvents, nonionic detergents, heat, oxidizing agents, and formalin treatment (42). Mumps virus, like other paramyxoviruses, is relatively unstable and loses its infectivity when it is stored for longer than 4 h in protein-free medium (12).

The first in vitro cultivation of mumps virus was in chick embryos (33), and the virus was subsequently successfully cultivated in tissue culture derived from chick embryos and in mammalian cell cultures (16).

SPECIMEN SELECTION

Laboratory diagnosis of mumps is achieved by viral isolation, detection of viral antigen, detection of the viral genome by reverse transcriptase PCR (RT-PCR), or serologic testing. Mumps virus can be isolated from saliva from 9 days before and up to 8 days after the onset of symptoms (18, 61), from urine for up to 2 weeks postonset (62), from the cerebrospinal fluid (CSF) of patients with meningitis (61), and from swabs of the area around Stensen's duct (61). Viremia has rarely been detected (28, 46). By RT-PCR, the mumps virus genome has been amplified from nasopharyngeal aspirates and swabs, throat swabs, saliva, CSF, and urine (1, 3, 23).

Specimens should be obtained early in the course of illness, when the virus titer is highest. Swab specimens, aspirates, and saliva should be placed in a viral transport medium containing a buffered salt solution, protein, pH indicator, and antibiotics. Specimens should be kept cold (2 to 8°C) if they are transported within 1 day of collection. If they are not processed within 1 day of collection, specimens should be frozen at −70°C or colder.

For serologic diagnosis, acute- and convalescent-phase blood samples should be submitted. Acute-phase blood should be collected as soon as possible after the onset of symptoms, while convalescent-phase blood should be collected 14 or more days postonset. Mumps virus-specific immunoglobulin M (IgM) can be measured in a single serum specimen. For patients with meningitis, antibody titers in CSF and in a serum specimen collected at the same time as the CSF should be determined (11, 40, 52, 59). A single serum specimen is used to assess immune status. Mumps virus-specific IgM can be detected in saliva 1 to 5 weeks after the onset of illness (47). The use of whole blood spotted onto filter paper was shown to be a convenient, accurate alternative to the use of blood obtained by venipuncture for determination of immunity to mumps virus (8).

DETECTION OF VIRAL ANTIGEN AND VIRAL NUCLEIC ACID

Hierholzer et al. (19) applied a time-resolved fluoroimmunoassay for the detection of mumps virus antigen in clinical specimens, but this technique has not gained widespread use. Direct immunofluorescence (IF) of cells of the respiratory tract and CSF has been used for the rapid detection of mumps virus and is readily adaptable to a routine diagnostic laboratory (4, 35, 39). PCR has been applied to the detection of the mumps virus genome in clinical samples (1, 3, 23).

VIRUS ISOLATION

Mumps virus can be cultured in primary and continuous cells lines as well as in embryonated chicken eggs. In the diagnostic virology laboratory, commercially available primary rhesus monkey kidney (RhMK) and human neonatal kidney (HNK) cells are commonly used (41). Virus can be isolated from saliva 9 days before and up to 8 days after the onset of parotitis (18, 61). Viruria can be detected up to 2 weeks after the onset of symptoms (62). Virus can also be recovered from the CSF during meningitis (61).

Cell culture tubes are incubated at 35 to 37°C and are examined by low-power microscopy (magnification, ×40 to ×100) on a daily basis for the first week and every third or fourth day thereafter for a total of 14 days. The appearance of multinucleated giant cells suggests a paramyxovirus, but a cytopathic effect (CPE) may not appear or may be very subtle. Primary monkey kidney cells may contain endogenous viruses that produce syncytia. For detection of viral growth in the absence of a CPE, the hemadsorption test is performed with guinea pig erythrocytes (GP-RBCs) at days 5 to 7 and day 14 postinoculation (54). For the hemadsorption test, the cell culture medium is removed from the culture tube and approximately 0.5 ml of a 0.4 to 0.5% suspension of GP-RBCs in phosphate-buffered saline (pH 7.2) is added. Cell culture tubes are refrigerated for 20 min on their sides to allow the GP-RBCs to cover the cell monolayer. Cell culture tubes are examined microscopically for the presence of small or large clumps of GP-RBCs adhering to the monolayer. Uninfected control tubes are tested in parallel with the inoculated tubes to rule out the nonspecific adsorption of erythrocytes and to detect endogenous simian paramyxoviruses. Hemadsorption-positive cultures can be typed by IF staining (see below).

IDENTIFICATION OF VIRUS

Identification of hemadsorption-positive isolates by IF is rapid and technically simple (25, 26). Mumps virus-specific monoclonal antibodies are commercially available. Cells from hemadsorption-positive tubes can be stained directly, or a second-passage culture showing maximal CPE or hemadsorption can be used. Other methods of identification of mumps virus isolates include the complement fixation (CF), HI, hemadsorption-inhibition, and neutralization tests (36, 41, 50, 55). Crude antigen prepared from infected cell culture tubes is used in a microtiter CF test (50). Immune serum for the HI test must be pretreated with the receptor-destroying enzyme of *Vibrio cholerae* or with periodate to remove nonspecific inhibitors of agglutination. Nonspecific hemagglutinins must be removed by absorption with packed erythrocytes (RBCs). Immune serum should also be tested with parainfluenza viruses to identify heterologous reactions (41, 55). The hemadsorption-inhibition assay is less sensitive than the HI test but is technically simpler to perform (41).

SEROLOGIC DIAGNOSIS

Traditional serologic diagnosis is based on the demonstration of a significant rise in titer between acute- and convalescent-phase sera. An acute-phase serum sample should be collected at the onset of symptoms, and convalescent-phase serum should be collected a minimum of 2 weeks later. A more timely diagnosis can be obtained by measuring the IgM antibody titer in acute-phase serum. The immune status of an individual can be determined by measurement of the IgG titer in a single serum sample. The mumps skin test is not a reliable measure of immune status. Both false-positive and false-negative results occur, and application of the skin test antigen to an immune individual can stimulate antibody rises in serum, thus causing interpretive errors (2).

CF Test

The CF test has been used for several decades for the serologic diagnosis of mumps. Both S and V antigens, which correspond to the NP and HN virus proteins, respectively, should be tested for the effective detection of seroconversions (10, 17, 21). In the CF test, serum antibodies to mumps antigen will form complexes which bind or "fix" guinea pig complement. This depletes complement, preventing binding of complement to the indicator system (sheep RBCs and antibody to sheep RBCs) and subsequent lysis of the sheep RBCs. In the absence of mumps virus-specific antibody, complement will bind to the indicator system, causing lysis of the sheep RBCs. Because the CF test is extremely labor-intensive and difficult to standardize, it has largely been replaced by other serologic tests. The CF test is performed as described previously (50). Antigens for the CF test are available commercially.

HI Test

Viral hemagglutinins on the virus surface bind to receptors of RBCs of certain species. In the case of mumps virus, GP-

RBCs are used. Hemagglutination refers to the lattice that is formed between RBCs and virus. The lattice can be seen at the bottom of a test tube or microtiter well as clumping of RBCs. The HI test is based on the ability of mumps virus antibody to inhibit virus-mediated hemagglutination. Twofold serial dilutions of patient serum are incubated with a constant amount of mumps virus hemagglutinin followed by the addition of GP-RBCs. The highest dilution of serum exhibiting inhibition of hemagglutination is the endpoint. Patient serum must be pretreated to remove nonspecific inhibitors and nonspecific agglutinins. The HI procedure is identical to that described above for the identification of viral isolates (55).

Neutralization Assays

Neutralization assays measure the ability of serum antibody to inhibit viral infectivity as measured by the absence of a viral CPE or hemadsorption in cell cultures. Neutralization assays can be performed with RhMK, HNK, or primary chick embryo cell culture tubes or in microtiter plates seeded with Vero cells (13, 27, 36). The microtiter plate procedures conserve reagents and patient sera, and the results correlate well with those obtained by the tube test. The neutralization test is labor-intensive and relatively costly and is rarely used.

IF Test

The IF test allows the detection of both IgG and IgM antibodies to mumps virus. Serial dilutions of patient serum are applied to microscope slide wells containing acetone-fixed, infected cells. IgG and IgM are detected by using fluorescein isothiocyanate-conjugated anti-human IgG or IgM. Stained slides are observed under a fluorescence microscope. The highest dilution of serum showing intracytoplasmic fluorescence is the endpoint. Slides containing uninfected cells should be prepared as a control for nonspecific fluorescence. A solid-phase immunofluorescence assay (FIAX; Wampole, Cranbury, N.J.) is available for measurement of the IgG titer to mumps virus. It is intended for determination of immune status from single serum samples. The IF test is performed routinely in many diagnostic laboratories.

ELISA

A number of microplate enzyme-linked immunosorbent assay (ELISA) procedures that measure IgG and IgM antibody titers to mumps virus have been described (9, 14, 34, 38, 44, 48, 49, 58). The antigens used include whole virus, sonicated virus, purified HN (V) and NP (S) antigens, and peroxidase-labeled antigens. Commercial ELISA kits are available from a number of suppliers (9). ELISA has supplanted most other serologic tests.

Hemolysis-in-Gel Test

The hemolysis-in-gel test (13) is based on the principle that mumps virus antigen coated onto RBCs is lysed by specific antibody in the presence of complement. It has been replaced in favor of less tedious assays.

CSF and Salivary Antibody

IgG and IgM antibody titers can be measured in the CSF of patients with meningitis. Titers in CSF have been measured by ELISA, and by the HI, CF, hemolysis-inhibition, and mixed hemadsorption tests (11, 40, 52, 59). Mumps virus-specific IgM has been detected in saliva from patients with acute cases of mumps by an antibody-capture radioimmunoassay (47).

EVALUATION AND INTERPRETATION OF RESULTS

Isolation of mumps virus or detection of the mumps virus antigen or genome from CSF, respiratory specimens, or urine establishes a diagnosis of mumps. The serologic diagnosis of mumps is problematic because of the cross-reactions between mumps virus and parainfluenza viruses (22, 32, 44). Paired serum specimens exhibiting fourfold or greater rises in titer against mumps virus should be tested against the parainfluenza viruses in the absence of parotitis. If a rise in titer against one or more parainfluenza viruses is observed, it is not possible to make a definitive diagnosis of mumps without a compatible clinical picture.

Serologic testing by the CF test should include testing for both V and S antigens (10, 17). Early work describing the CF test demonstrated that antibody to the S antigen arose earlier and more rapidly in patients with acute cases of mumps and that lower levels of or absent S antibody in the presence of V antibody was a sign of long-past infection (17). A more recent study of 40 patients with mumps demonstrated that V antibody appeared earlier than S antibody in 14 patients, while S antibody appeared earlier in only 2 patients (10). Therefore, for maximal sensitivity, both antigens should be used. Because antibodies measured by the CF test may disappear over time, a negative CF test result is not a reliable indicator of susceptibility to infection. Moreover, cross-reactivity with parainfluenza viruses may occur by this assay.

Assays for IgM are useful for the diagnosis of acute mumps, since cross-reactions between mumps and parainfluenza viruses have not been observed for IgM antibody (14, 38, 60). However, IgM assays false positive because of rheumatoid factor and IgM assays false negative because of high levels of IgG occur (49). IgM capture ELISA (14, 34, 49) is very sensitive and specific and can be used to diagnose current mumps virus infection. IgM antibody, measured by IgM capture ELISA, was present in all patients with mumps by the fifth day of illness, and peak IgM titers were reached at 1 week of illness and persisted for at least 6 weeks (14, 49).

The ELISA has a high sensitivity compared to that of the neutralization assay and is suited for determination of immune status, although cross-reactions with other paramyxoviruses also occur (15, 34). ELISA is more sensitive than the CF and HI tests for the detection of low levels of antibodies (48). For the diagnosis of acute mumps virus infections, significant titer rises may be more difficult to detect by ELISA than by the CF test because of the early appearance of antibody by ELISA (38).

In cases of mumps virus meningitis, mumps virus-specific IgG is found in CSF and confirms the diagnosis. The CF and HI tests are relatively insensitive for the detection of antibody in CSF compared to the ELISA (11, 40, 52, 59). IgG is present in CSF within a few days after the onset of disease and peaks at 7 to 10 days (59).

REFERENCES

1. **Afzal, M. A., J. Buchanan, J. A. Dias, M. Cordeiro, M. L. Bentley, C. A. Shorrock, and P. D. Minor.** 1997. RT-PCR based diagnosis and molecular characterization of mumps viruses derived from clinical specimens collected during the 1996 mumps outbreak in Portugal. *J. Med. Virol.* **52:**349–353.
2. **Baum, S. G., and N. Litman.** 1995. Mumps virus, p. 1496–1501. *In* G. L. Mandell, J. E. Bennett, and R. Dolin

(ed.), *Mandell, Douglas, and Bennett's Principles and Practice of Infectious Diseases*, 4th ed. Churchill Livingstone, New York, N.Y.

3. **Boriskin, Y. S., J. C. Booth, and A. Yamada.** 1993. Rapid detection of mumps virus by the polymerase chain reaction. *J. Virol. Methods* **42:**23–32.
4. **Boyd, J. F., and V. Vince-Ribaric.** 1973. The examination of cerebrospinal fluid cells by fluorescent antibody staining to detect mumps antigen. *Scand. J. Infect. Dis.* **5:**7–15.
5. **Centers for Disease Control and Prevention.** 1997. Recommended childhood immunization schedule—United States, 1997. *Morbid. Mortal. Weekly Rep.* **46:**35–40.
6. **Centers for Disease Control and Prevention.** 1997. Status report on the childhood immunization initiative: reported cases of selected vaccine-preventable diseases—United States, 1996. *Morbid. Mortal. Weekly Rep.* **46:**665–671.
7. **Cheek, J. E., R. Baron, H. Atlas, D. L. Wilson, and R. D. Crider, Jr.** 1995. Mumps outbreak in a highly vaccinated school population. Evidence for large-scale vaccination failure. *Arch. Pediatr. Adolesc. Med.* **149:**774–778.
8. **Condorelli, F., G. Scalia, A. Stivala, R. Gallo, A. Narino, C. M. Battaglini, and A. Castro.** 1994. Detection of immunoglobulin G to measles virus, rubella virus, and mumps virus in serum samples and in microquantities of whole blood dried on filter paper. *J. Virol. Methods* **49:**25–36.
9. **Doern, G. V., L. Robbie, and R. St. Amand.** 1997. Comparison of the Vidas and Bio-Whittaker enzyme immunoassays for detecting IgG reactive with varicella-zoster virus and mumps virus. *Diagn. Microbiol. Infect. Dis.* **28:**31–34.
10. **Freeman, R., and M. H. Hambling.** 1980. Serological studies on 40 cases of mumps virus infection. *J. Clin. Pathol.* **33:**28–32.
11. **Fryden, A., H. Link, and E. Norrby.** 1978. Cerebrospinal fluid and serum immunoglobulin and antibody titers in mumps meningitis and aseptic meningitis of other etiology. *Infect. Immun.* **21:**852–861.
12. **Ginsberg, H. S.** 1988. Paramyxoviruses, p. 239–259. *In* R. Dulbecco and H. S. Ginsberg (ed.), *Virology*, 2nd ed. J. B. Lippincott Co., Philadelphia, Pa.
13. **Grillner, L., and J. Blomberg.** 1976. Hemolysis-in-gel and neutralization tests for determination of antibodies to mumps virus. *J. Clin. Microbiol.* **4:**11–15.
14. **Gut, J. P., C. Spiess, S. Schmitt, and A. Kirn.** 1985. Rapid diagnosis of acute mumps infection by a direct immunoglobulin M antibody capture enzyme immunoassay with labeled antigen. *J. Clin. Microbiol.* **21:**346–352.
15. **Harmsen, T., M. C. Jongerius, C. W. Van Der Zwan, A. D. Plantinga, C. A. Kraaijeveld, and G. A. M. Berbers.** 1992. Comparison of a neutralization enzyme immunoassay and an enzyme immunoassay for evaluation of immune status of children vaccinated for mumps. *J. Clin. Microbiol.* **30:**2139–2144.
16. **Henle, G., and F. Deinhardt.** 1955. Propagation and primary isolation of mumps virus in tissue culture. *Proc. Soc. Exp. Biol. Med.* **89:**556–560.
17. **Henle, G., S. Harris, and W. Henle.** 1948. The reactivity of various human sera with mumps complement fixation antigens. *J. Exp. Med.* **88:**133–147.
18. **Henle, G., W. Henle, K. K. Wendell, and P. Rosenberg.** 1948. Isolation of mumps virus from human being with induced apparent or inapparent infections. *J. Exp. Med.* **88:**223–232.
19. **Hierholzer, J. C., P. G. Bingham, E. Castells, and R. A. Coombs.** 1993. Time-resolved fluoroimmunoassays with monoclonal antibodies for rapid identification of parainfluenza type 4 and mumps virus. *Arch. Virol.* **130:**335–352.
20. **Ito, Y., M. Tsurudome, M. Hishiyama, and A. Yamada.** 1987. Immunological interrelationships among human and non-human paramyxoviruses revealed by immunoprecipitation. *J. Gen. Virol.* **68:**1289–1297.
21. **Jensik, S. C., and S. Silver.** 1976. Polypeptides of mumps virus. *J. Virol.* **17:**363–373.
22. **Julkunen, I.** 1984. Serological diagnosis of parainfluenza virus infections by enzyme immunoassay with special emphasis on purity of viral antigens. *J. Med. Virol.* **14:**177–187.
23. **Kashiwagi, Y., H. Kawashima, K. Takekuma, A. Hoshika, T. Mori, and T. Nakayama.** 1997. Detection of mumps genome directly from clinical samples and a simple method for genetic differentiation of the Hosino vaccine strain from wild strains of mumps virus. *J. Med. Virol.* **52:**195–199.
24. **Kawano, M., H. Bando, T. Yuasa, K. Kondo, M. Tsurudome, H. Komada, M. Nishio, and Y. Ito.** 1990. Sequence determination of the hemagglutinin-neuraminidase (HN) gene of the human parainfluenza type 2 virus and the construction of a phylogenetic tree for HN proteins of all the paramyxoviruses that are infectious to humans. *Virology* **174:**308–313.
25. **Keller, E. W.** 1992. Detection and identification of viruses by immunofluorescence, p. 8.9.1–8.9.10. *In* H. D. Isenberg (ed.), *Clinical Microbiology Procedures Handbook*. American Society for Microbiology, Washington, D.C.
26. **Keller, E. W.** 1992. Preparation of cell spots for immunofluorescence, p. 8.10.1–8.10.9. *In* H. D. Isenberg (ed.), *Clinical Microbiology Procedures Handbook*. American Society for Microbiology, Washington, D.C.
27. **Kenny, M. T., K. L. Albright, and R. P. Sanderson.** 1970. Microneutralization test for the determination of mumps antibody in Vero cells. *Appl. Microbiol.* **20:**371–373.
28. **Kilham, L.** 1948. Isolation of mumps virus from the blood of a patient. *Proc. Soc. Exp. Biol. Med.* **69:**99–100.
29. **Komada, H., E. Klippmark, C. Örvell, R. E. Randall, Y. Ito, and E. Norrby.** Immunological relationships between parainfluenza virus type 4 and other paramyxoviruses studied by use of monoclonal antibodies. *Arch. Virol.* **116:**277–283.
30. **Kondo, K., H. Bando, M. Kawano, M. Tsurudome, H. Komada, M. Nishio, and Y. Ito.** 1990. Sequencing analyses of comparison of parainfluenza virus type 4A and 4B NP protein genes. *Virology* **174:**1–8.
31. **Künkel, U., G. Driesel, U. Henning, E. Gerike, H. Willers, and E. Schreier.** 1995. Differentiation of vaccine and wild mumps viruses by polymerase chain reaction and nucleotide sequencing of the SH gene. *J. Med. Virol.* **45:**121–126.
32. **Lennette, E. H., F. W. Jensen, R. W. Guenther, and R. L. Magoffin.** 1963. Serologic responses to para-influenza viruses in patients with mumps virus infection. *J. Lab. Clin. Med.* **61:**780–788.
33. **Leymaster, G. R., and T. G. Ward.** 1947. Direct isolation of mumps virus in chick embryos. *Proc. Soc. Exp. Biol. Med.* **65:**346–348.
34. **Linde, G. A., M. Granstrom, and C. Örvell.** 1987. Immunoglobulin class and immunoglobulin G subclass enzyme-linked immunosorbent assays compared with microneutralization assay for serodiagnosis of mumps infection and determination of immunity. *J. Clin. Microbiol.* **25:**1653–1658.
35. **Lindeman, J., W. K. Muller, J. Versteeg, G. T. A. M. Bots, and A. C. B. Peters.** 1974. Rapid diagnosis of meningoencephalitis, encephalitis. Immunofluorescent examination of fresh and in vitro cultured cerebrospinal fluid cells. *Neurology* **24:**143–148.
36. **Lipson, S. M.** 1992. Neutralization test for the identification and typing of viral isolates, p. 8.14.1–8.14.8. *In* H. D.

Isenberg (ed.), *Clinical Microbiology Procedures Handbook.* American Society for Microbiology, Washington, D.C.

37. **Merz, D. C., and J. S. Wolinsky.** 1981. Biochemical features of mumps virus neuraminidases and their relationship with pathogenicity. *Virology* **114:**218–227.
38. **Meurman, O., P. Hanninen, R. V. Krishna, and T. Ziegler.** 1982. Determination of IgG- and IgM-class antibodies to mumps virus by solid-phase enzyme immunoassay. *J. Virol. Methods* **4:**249–257.
39. **Minnich, L., and C. G. Ray.** 1980. Comparison of direct immunofluorescent staining of clinical specimens for respiratory virus antigens with conventional isolation techniques. *J. Clin. Microbiol.* **12:**391–394.
40. **Morishima, T., M. Miyazu, T. Ozaki, S. Isomura, and S. Suzuki.** 1980. Local immunity in mumps meningitis. *Am. J. Dis. Child.* **134:**1060–1064.
41. **Mufson, M. A.** 1989. Parainfluenza viruses, mumps virus, Newcastle disease virus, p. 669–691. *In* N. J. Schmidt and R. W. Emmons (ed.), *Diagnostic Procedures for Viral, Rickettsial, and Chlamydial Infections*, 6th ed. American Public Health Association, Washington, D.C.
42. **Murphy, F. A.** 1996. Viral taxonomy, p. 33–34. *In* B. N. Fields, P. M. Knipe, P. M. Howley, R. M. Chanock, J. L. Melnick, T. P. Monath, B. Roizman, and S. E. Straus (ed.), *Fields Virology*, 3rd ed. Lippincott-Raven, Philadelphia, Pa.
43. **Ni, J., N. E. Bowles, Y.-H. Kim, G. Demmler, D. Kearney, T. J. Bricker, and J. Towbin.** 1997. Viral infection of the myocardium in endocardial fibroelastosis: molecular evidence for the role of mumps virus as an etiologic agent. *Circulation* **95:**133–139.
44. **Nicolai-Scholten, M. E., R. Ziegelmaier, F. Behrens, and W. Hopken.** 1980. The enzyme-linked immunosorbent assay (ELISA) for determination of IgG and IgM antibodies after infection with mumps virus. *Med. Microbiol. Immunol.* **168:**81–90.
45. **Örvell, C., R. Rydbeck, and A. Love.** 1986. Immunological relationships between mumps virus and parainfluenza viruses studied with monoclonal antibodies. *J. Gen. Virol.* **67:**1929–1939.
46. **Overman, J. R.** 1958. Viremia in human mumps virus infections. *Arch. Intern. Med.* **102:**354–356.
47. **Perry, K. H., D. W. G. Brown, J. V. Parry, S. Panday, D. Pipkin, and A. Richards.** 1993. Detection of measles, mumps, and rubella antibodies in saliva using antibody capture radioimmunoassay. *J. Med. Virol.* **40:**235–240.
48. **Popow-Kraupp, T.** 1981. Enzyme-linked immunosorbent assay (ELISA) for mumps virus antibodies. *J. Med. Virol.* **8:**79–88.
49. **Sakata, H., M. Tsurudome, M. Hishiyama, Y. Ito, and A. Sugiura.** 1985. Enzyme-linked immunosorbent assay for mumps IgM antibody: comparison of IgM capture and indirect IgM assay. *J. Virol. Methods* **12:**303–311.
50. **Schmidt, N., and R. W. Emmons.** 1989. General principles of laboratory diagnostic methods for viral, rickettsial and chlamydial infections, p. 21–28. *In* N. J. Schmidt and R. W. Emmons (ed.), *Diagnostic Procedures for Viral, Rickettsial and Chlamydial Infections*, 6th ed. American Public Health Association, Washington, D.C.
51. **Server, A. C., D. C. Merz, M. N. Waxham, and J. S. Wolinsky.** 1982. Differentiation of mumps virus strains with monoclonal antibody to the HN glycoprotein. *Infect. Immun.* **35:**179–186.
52. **Sharief, M. K., and E. J. Thompson.** 1990. A sensitive ELISA system for the rapid detection of virus specific IgM antibodies in the cerebrospinal fluid. *J. Immunol. Methods* **130:**19–24.
53. **Sosin, D. M., S. L. Cochi, R. A. Gunn, C. E. Jennings, and S. R. Preblud.** 1989. Changing epidemiology of mumps and its impact on university campuses. *Pediatrics* **84:**779–784.
54. **Swenson, P. D.** 1992. Detection of viruses by hemadsorption, p. 8.8.1–8.8.5. *In* H. D. Isenberg (ed.), *Clinical Microbiology Procedures Handbook.* American Society for Microbiology, Washington, D.C.
55. **Swenson, P. D.** 1992. Hemagglutination inhibition test for the identification of influenza viruses, p. 8.12.1–8.12.11. *In* H. D. Isenberg (ed.), *Clinical Microbiology Procedures Handbook.* American Society for Microbiology, Washington, D.C.
56. **Takeuchi, K., K. Tanabayashi, M. Hishiyama, A. Yamada, and A. Sugiura.** 1991. Variations of nucleotide sequences and transcription of the SH gene among mumps virus strains. *Virology* **181:**364–366.
57. **Tanabayashi, K., K. Takeuchi, M. Hishiyama, A. Yamada, M. Tsurudome, Y. Ito, and A. Sugiura.** 1990. Nucleotide sequence of the leader and nucleocapsid protein gene of mumps and epitope mapping with the in vitro expressed nucleocapsid protein. *Virology* **177:**124–130.
58. **Ukkonen, P., M. L. Granstrom, and K. Penttinen.** 1981. Mumps-specific immunoglobulin M and G antibodies in natural mumps infection as measured by enzyme-linked immunosorbent assay. *J. Med. Virol.* **8:**131–142.
59. **Ukkonen, P., M. L. Granstrom, J. Rasanen, E. M. Salonen, and K. Penttinen.** 1981. Local production of mumps IgG and IgM antibodies in the cerebrospinal fluid of meningitis patients. *J. Med. Virol.* **8:**257–265.
60. **Ukkonen, P., O. Vaisanen, and K. Penttinen.** 1980. Enzyme-linked immunosorbent assay for mumps and parainfluenza type 1 immunoglobulin G and immunoglobulin M antibodies. *J. Clin. Microbiol.* **11:**319–323.
61. **Utz, J. P., J. A. Kasel, H. G. Cramblett, C. F. Szwed, and R. H. Parrott.** 1957. Clinical and laboratory studies of mumps. I. Laboratory diagnosis by tissue-culture technics. *N. Engl. J. Med.* **257:**497–502.
62. **Utz, J. P., C. F. Szwed, and J. A. Kasel.** 1958. Clinical and laboratory studies of mumps. II. Detection and duration of excretion of virus in urine. *Proc. Soc. Exp. Biol. Med.* **99:**259–261.
63. **Wolinksy, J. S.** 1996. Mumps virus, p. 1243–1265. *In* B. N. Fields, D. M. Knipe, P. M. Howley, R. M. Chanock, J. L. Melnick, T. P. Monath, B. Roizman, and S. E. Straus (ed.), *Fields Virology*, 3rd ed. Lippincott-Raven, Philadelphia, Pa.

Rubella Virus

MAX A. CHERNESKY AND JAMES B. MAHONY

75

CLINICAL BACKGROUND

Rubella virus is found only in human populations and causes rubella (German measles). Postnatal rubella is transmitted chiefly through direct contact with nasopharyngeal secretions or through contact with droplets of these secretions. The peak incidence of infection occurs in the late winter and early spring. Subclinical infection is common. The periods of maximum communicability appear to be the few days before and 5 to 7 days after the onset of the rash. Volunteer studies indicate the presence of rubella virus in nasopharyngeal secretions from 7 days before to 14 days after the onset of the rash. Infants with congenital rubella may continue to shed virus in nasopharyngeal secretions and urine for 1 year or more and may transmit infection to susceptible contacts. Virus can be isolated from the nasopharynx at 6 months of age in approximately 10 to 20% of these patients.

Before the widespread use of rubella vaccine, rubella was an epidemic disease with 6- to 9-year cycles; the majority of cases occurred in children. Currently, the incidence of rubella in North America has declined by more than 99% from the incidence in the prevaccine era. Although the risk of acquiring rubella has declined sharply in all age groups, including adolescents and young adults, a greater percentage of the cases are in young, unvaccinated adults in settings in which young adults are grouped together. Recent serologic surveys have indicated that 10 to 20% of young adults are susceptible to rubella. The degree of susceptibility in young adults is due predominantly to underutilization of vaccine in this population rather than to waning immunity in immunized persons.

The incubation period for postnatal rubella ranges from 10 to 21 days and is usually 16 to 18 days. It is usually a mild disease characterized by an erythematous maculopapular discrete rash, postauricular and suboccipital lymphadenopathy, and slight fever. Some 25 to 50% of infections are asymptomatic. Transient polyarthralgia and polyarthritis occur occasionally in children but are extremely common in older individuals. Encephalitis and thrombocytopenia are rare complications.

The most commonly described anomalies associated with congenital rubella are ophthalmologic (cataracts, microphthalmia, glaucoma, and chorioretinitis), cardiac (patent ductus arteriosus, peripheral pulmonary artery stenosis, and atrial or ventricular septal defects), auditory (sensorineural deafness), and neurologic (microcephaly, meningoencephalitis, and mental retardation). Infants with congenital rubella frequently are growth retarded and have radiolucent bone disease, hepatosplenomegaly, thrombocytopenia, jaundice, and purpura-like skin lesions ("blueberry muffin" appearance).

Antibodies to the virus appear as the rash fades (Fig. 1), and initially both immunoglobulin G (IgG) and IgM antibodies can be detected. Antibodies of the IgM class generally do not persist beyond 4 to 5 weeks after onset of illness, but IgG antibodies usually persist throughout life. Reinfection with the virus can occur, but it is almost always asymptomatic and can be detected only by a rise in the level of IgG antibodies. The risk of fetal damage resulting from rubella reinfection during pregnancy is negligible. The attenuated virus vaccines induce production of IgM and IgG antibodies similar to that observed with natural infections, except that the titers produced by the vaccine are somewhat lower. Reinfection rates with wild virus are greater among vaccinees than among persons previously infected under natural conditions.

Reliable laboratory technology has been developed for (i) determination of immunity to rubella, (ii) diagnosis of postnatal rubella, and (iii) diagnosis of congenital rubella. Because antibody responses are rapid and specific and virus isolation procedures are slow and expensive, serologic procedures are usually performed for disease diagnosis (the exception is virus isolation for a diagnosis of congenitally infected newborn).

DESCRIPTION OF THE GENUS

Rubella virus is classified as a rubivirus and is a member of the family *Togaviridae*, which also contains the arthropod-borne alphaviruses and flaviviruses as well as members of the genus *Pestivirus*. Classification is based on morphologic, antigenic, and physicochemical properties. Only one type or species of rubella virus has been recognized so far, and it is immunologically distinct from all other known viruses. The virus possesses three major structural proteins: two glycoproteins, E1 (58,000 Da) and E2 (42,000 to 47,000 Da), are associated with the envelope, and nucleocapsid protein C (33,000 Da) is found internally. The virus is spherical, with a diameter of 60 to 70 nm, and contains a dense central core surrounded by a lipid bilayer. Replication of viral RNA

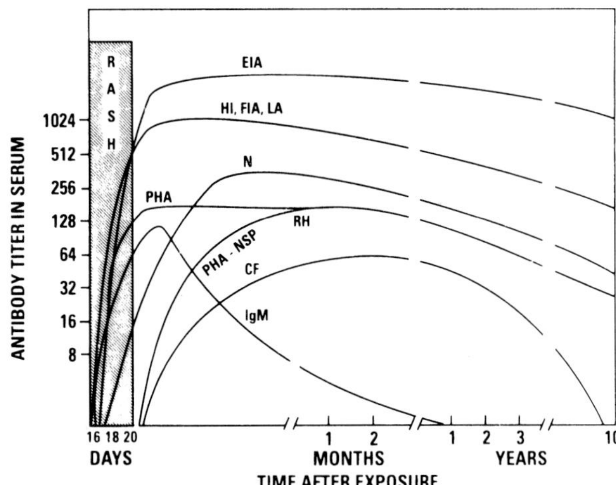

FIGURE 1 Antibody response after rubella virus infection. FIA, fluorescence immunoassay; N, neutralization; NSP, nonstructural protein.

and synthesis of protein occur in the cytoplasm of the cell, and the virus matures by budding into cytoplasmic vesicles or from the marginal plasma membrane. The virus is destroyed by lipid solvents or trypsin but not by freezing-thawing or ultrasonification.

ISOLATION AND IDENTIFICATION

A wide variety of cell types are susceptible to infection by rubella virus. For primary isolation of rubella virus from clinical specimens, however, primary African green monkey kidney (AGMK), Vero, or RK-13 cell cultures are recommended. Isolation of rubella virus in primary cultures of AGMK cells has been considered the standard method (15). Rubella virus is detected in this cell type by interference with the cytopathic effects (CPE) of a challenge virus. Virus isolation in AGMK is carried out as follows. Four tubes containing cell monolayers are drained of medium. A 0.2-ml volume of the specimen is inoculated into each tube and allowed to adsorb for 1 h at 35 to 36°C. A 1.5-ml volume of maintenance medium (Eagle basal medium with 2% inactivated fetal bovine serum) is then added to each tube, and the tubes are incubated in stationary racks at 35 to 36°C for 10 days. Four uninoculated AGMK cell cultures serve as controls. At the end of the incubation period, the tubes are examined for CPE. If none is found, two inoculated and two control tubes are challenged with 100 to 1,000 50% tissue culture infective doses of a challenge virus. The viruses most commonly used as the challenge agent for rubella virus isolation in AGMK cells are echovirus type 11 or coxsackievirus A9. Tubes containing challenge virus are read 3 or 4 days after challenge. The presence of rubella virus is indicated by complete destruction of the control cells and little or no CPE in the inoculated tubes. Absolute identification of the isolate requires specific neutralization of the interference with rubella antibody.

Specimens with low concentrations of rubella virus may produce little or partial interference in the culture tubes initially inoculated. The culture fluids may have to be passaged to demonstrate the virus. Fluid from the cultures that were not challenged should be inoculated into an additional four tubes of AGMK cells. Control tubes are also used. All these tubes should be incubated for an additional 7 to 8 days. Two inoculated tubes and two control tubes are then challenged with echovirus type 11 and observed for CPE. The absence of interference with echovirus cytopathogenicity on passage of fluid from tubes that did not initially demonstrate interference confirms the absence of an interfering agent. If virus is not found after one such passage, it is rarely found by further passages.

Some laboratories use RK-13 or Vero cells for isolation of rubella virus. In these cell systems, rubella virus produces CPE; however, the CPE is not always clear on primary isolation, and cell culture fluids may have to be passaged several times for full detection of virus. These cell systems, however, do offer the advantage of direct neutralization for identification of an isolate. Furthermore, an indirect immunofluorescence staining method has been shown to be specific and sensitive for identifying rubella virus isolates in these cells (16).

Fresh unfrozen tissue specimens may be of particular value in attempts to isolate virus from fetal tissues and organs. A convenient method is to explant a minced tissue fragment with growth medium and allow sufficient time for the outgrowth of cells. When the cells have formed monolayers, the extracellular fluids can be harvested and tested for the presence of an interfering agent as described above. This method of rubella virus isolation is more sensitive than the method in which tissue extracts of homogenates of ground tissue are used.

Rubella virus can be specifically neutralized with rubella antiserum prepared in rabbits. Such antisera are available from several commercial sources. Immune-rabbit serum is diluted to contain 4 U of neutralizing antibody. A healthy preimmune (rubella antibody-free)-rabbit serum is diluted similarly for the control titer determination. The media from the two companion, unchallenged cultures containing the interfering agent are pooled, and serial 10-fold dilutions (undiluted to 10^{-6} diluted) are made in maintenance medium; 0.1-ml samples of each dilution are inoculated into three culture tubes. The 10^{-1}, 10^{-2}, and 10^{-3} dilutions are also combined with equal volumes of the prediluted rubella antiserum and of the prediluted healthy-rabbit serum. After 1 h of incubation at 35°C, 0.2 ml of each mixture is inoculated into each of three AGMK tubes. The tubes are incubated at 35 to 36°C for 7 to 8 days, challenged with echovirus type 11, and observed for the development of enterovirus CPE. Destruction of the AGMK monolayers inoculated with the isolate dilution containing between 10 and 100 50% tissue culture infective doses plus the immune-rabbit serum but not of those inoculated with the healthy-rabbit serum indicates that the isolate is rubella virus.

DETECTION OF AMPLIFIABLE NUCLEIC ACID

Reverse trascription-PCR (RT-PCR) has been successfully used to amplify RNA extracted from chorionic villi removed by biopsy from the fetus in utero (9). The technique uses rubella virus-specific oligonucleotide primers to reverse transcribe a cDNA, which is then amplified by PCR and detected by Southern blotting. Nested RT-PCR can be used for prenatal and postnatal diagnosis of congenital rubella (3). RT-PCR amplification of a 185-bp product (external R2 and R7 oligonucleotides) and a 143-bp product (internal pair of RII and R8C oligonucleotides) within the E1 open reading frame of the rubella virus genome can be performed on clinical tissue. Compared to culture of the virus, RT-

PCR can be made highly diagnostic for congenitally acquired rubella by the testing of lens aspirates. RT-PCR is also useful for detecting rubella virus RNA in products of abortion and prenatally acquired amniotic fluid and chorionic villus biopsy specimens. The use of these amplification techniques is generally limited to research or reference laboratories.

SEROLOGIC TESTING

Serologic techniques for the detection of antibodies to rubella virus provide the approach of choice for laboratory diagnosis of acute and congenital rubella infections and for the determination of rubella immune status. The methods currently available include passive hemagglutination (PHA), radial hemolysis (RH) in gel, latex agglutination (LA), hemagglutination inhibition (HI), complement fixation (CF), enzyme immunoassay (EIA), and indirect fluorescent antibody test (IFA), as well as other, less popular approaches and a variety of rubella-specific IgM antibody assays. It is not yet fully understood which of this myriad of serologic techniques for measuring rubella IgG antibodies best approximates immunity to reinfection or disease in the fetus.

Investigation of the pregnant patient who has been in contact with another person with rubella presents a challenge for a rapid and accurate serologic diagnosis. If the patient develops a rash or other clinical signs of infection, a serum specimen should be collected at that time and paired with a second serum specimen collected 5 or more days later. The two specimens are investigated in parallel (same test, same day). A fourfold or greater rise in HI or CF antibodies together with clinical symptoms is diagnostic of recent infection. Alternatively, a significant change in optical densities or binding ratios of the sera in an EIA would be diagnostic. Seroconversion in any patient is conclusive for recent rubella virus infection. If EIA is available for rubella IgM testing, a single serum sample collected between days 3 and 21 after onset of rash usually yields a positive diagnosis (5). Patients without clinical symptoms but with rising titers to rubella virus (with the first serum sample containing antibodies) pose a special problem. They may have a primary infection or reinfection with an anamnestic antibody boost. To confirm these cases, a rubella IgM determination may be performed. Measurement of rubella IgG avidity (8) by EIA or coupled with urea treatment of the sera (18) may help determine the presence of primary infection or reinfection or the approximate time of infection in the asymptomatic pregnant patient. A third type of problem case involves patients whose sera are collected several days after the infection, when all serologic indicators are at a plateau (Fig. 1); testing for IgM may be helpful. Serologic examination of the suspected contacts may also be helpful in these situations.

Serologic investigation of a suspected case of congenital rubella could involve several approaches. One approach is to make serial determinations of rubella HI or solid-phase immunoassay (SPIA) antibodies during the first 6 months of life; persistence of the titer in the infant during this time (Fig. 2) is highly suggestive of congenital rubella. As a second approach, the demonstration of rubella virus-specific IgM antibody in infant serum during the neonatal period is diagnostic of congenital rubella. A third approach is to perform immunoblotting and peptide EIA (20) on sera collected from suspected patients in the neonatal period (11), looking for reduced bands to E1 and E2 proteins (11).

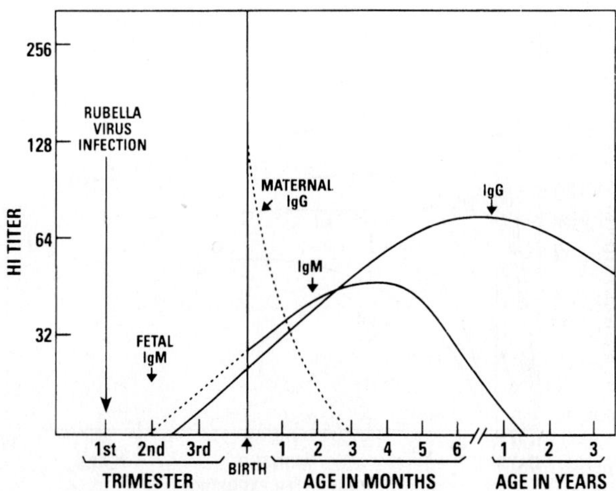

FIGURE 2 Antibody responses in an infant congenitally infected with rubella virus.

TEST PROCEDURES

Passive Hemagglutination

PHA represents a rapid, inexpensive way of screening for rubella immunity. PHA to nonstructural proteins (Fig. 1) parallels CF and neutralization responses after infection, whereas PHA structural protein responses are more closely aligned with HI and SPIA. Both antibodies remain measurable for years after infection or immunization as an index of immunity. PHA employs erythrocytes stabilized with formaldehyde-pyruvic aldehyde that have been sensitized with rubella virus antigen. The erythrocytes agglutinate in the presence of specific rubella antibody. To perform the test, phosphate buffer is added to V-bottom microwells. Specimens, as well as positive and negative controls, are added and mixed, and the sensitized cells are then added. A row of erythrocytes without rubella antigen is used as a control, which allows more objective scoring of results. A button of erythrocytes signifies the absence of antibody (susceptibility to rubella), whereas a dispersed settling of erythrocytes indicates a positive reaction (immunity to rubella).

Radial Hemolysis

RH is widely used in Europe and can be used to screen large numbers of serum samples by preparing plates in advance and storing them at 4°C. We have successfully used the method of Russell et al. (14). Freshly drawn sheep erythrocytes are washed with glucose-gelatin-Veronal buffer, treated with 2.5 mg of trypsin (Difco Laboratories, Detroit, Mich.) per ml in glucose-gelatin-Veronal buffer for 1 h at room temperature, and sensitized with rubella hemagglutinating antigen (Flow Laboratories, McLean, Va.; 240 hemagglutination units [HAU] per ml) in HEPES-saline-albumin-gelatin buffer (pH 6.2) for 1 h at 4°C. Sensitized erythrocytes (0.15 ml of a 50% suspension) are mixed with 0.4 ml of guinea pig complement (diluted 1:3) and reincubated. All sera are tested in control plates containing unsensitized erythrocytes to monitor nonspecific hemolysis. Zones of hemolysis in control plates may range from 3.5 to 5 mm in diameter. Zone diameters of >5 mm are taken to indicate immunity.

Latex Agglutination

Rapid LA tests are used predominantly for immunity screening. The tests incorporate antigen-coated latex particles and may be performed on a card or in a tray. Agglutination is particularly useful for the processing of small numbers of specimens.

Hemagglutination Inhibition

Since the original description of the HI test for rubella virus (17), several modifications have been introduced. These include the choice of indicator erythrocytes (6), optimal pH of reagents (7), methods for removal of nonspecific inhibitors from sera (9), methods for preparation of the antigen (15), and duration of incubation of antigen with the sera (13). The test is conveniently performed in disposable plastic or vinyl V-bottom microtiter plates. The titer of the rubella hemagglutinating antigen is determined each time the test is performed. Control cups containing no antigen are included. Before the HI test is performed, nonspecific inhibitors of hemagglutination (10) and nonspecific agglutinins must be removed from the sera. Known positive and negative control sera are treated similarly. The antigen titer is determined in a separate section of the plate by using doubling dilutions. The hemagglutination pattern is read after 1 h at 4°C. The highest dilution of serum that completely inhibits hemagglutination is taken as the end-point or rubella titer.

Complement Fixation

The CF test is performed by a standard technique (19).

Enzyme Immunoassay

EIA kits are commercially available from a number of North American and European suppliers and have been developed for rubella IgG and IgM.

All of the commercially available EIAs are solid-phase capture assays in which microplate wells, beads, or filters are used to measure antibodies to envelope and/or capsid proteins. Most of these assays are performed in 2 h or less and are low in cost. Automation is built into some EIAs (1), whereas others are manual. Most of the tests are quantitative or semiquantitative and incorporate several positive and negative controls.

Indirect Fluorescent-Antibody Assay

The IFA test for rubella antibody, in which chronically infected LLC-MK_2 cell cultures were used as the solid-phase antigen, was first described in 1962 (4). Other acutely infected cell systems or even purified rubella antigens have since been used for the rubella IFA test. For the classic IFA test, acutely infected cells are grown either on Leighton tube coverslips or in culture flasks, trypsinized, and deposited on slides to form smears. The cytoplasm of cells infected with rubella virus contains rubella antigens. These antigens are used to detect specific antibodies by the indirect method, in which an anti-human globulin conjugated to fluorescein isothiocyanate is used. The technique is rapid and relatively inexpensive and allows quantitation of IgG and IgM antibodies; however, IFA results are read visually with a fluorescence microscope and are open to subjective interpretation. Alternatively, a soluble rubella antigen immobilized on an opaque plastic surface has been used in an IFA test called FIAX. The antigen-sensitized surface is allowed to react in a two-step precedure with the serum and the fluorescein-labeled conjugate, and the resulting fluorescent signal is measured objectively with a fluorometer. The intensity of the fluorescence signal correlates with the titer of rubella antibody.

Other assays for detecting rubella antibody include mixed hemadsorption, time-resolved fluoroimmunoassay, silver-enhanced gold-labeled immunosorbent assay, rubella-IgG-peptide EIA (20), and nonreducing rubella immunoblotting (21). These tests have not gained widespread usage.

IgM Antibody Detection

Rubella-specific IgM antibodies can be detected by sucrose density gradient fractionation followed by HI, EIA, or IFA. Density gradient centrifugation entails diluting the test serum 1:3 in phosphate-buffered saline and adsorbing it with pigeon erythrocytes. After removal of the erythrocytes, the serum is placed on a gradient that is constructed by layering the various sucrose solutions in phosphate-buffered saline in a 5-ml cellulose nitrate tube (37, 33, 28, 24, 18, and 12% [wt/vol], as determined by refractometer readings). Before the test serum is layered, the gradient is allowed to equilibrate by overnight diffusions at 4°C. The specimen is carefully laid on top of the gradient and then centrifuged for 16 to 18 min at 150,000 × g. The bottom of the tube is carefully punctured with a needle-type fraction collector, and 10 to 20 fractions are collected (0.3 ml [about 20 drops] per fraction). Fractions 2 to 4 usually contain IgM, fractions 6 to 9 contain IgG, and the top two fractions contain nonspecific inhibitors of hemagglutination. Alternatively, other Ig separation techniques such as gel filtration, staphylococcal protein A absorption, quaternary aminoethyl-Sephadex chromatography, and 2-mercaptoethanol destruction have been used with variable success. Commercial EIAs for testing whole sera for rubella IgM are available. These EIAs usually involve a pretreatment step or use anti-IgM capture antibody on the solid phase and Fab antibody fragments as the indicator reagent to eliminate false-positive results for rheumatoid factor. These assays have high levels of sensitivity and specificity (2, 5).

Lymphocyte Transformation

A rubella virus-specific lymphocyte transformation assay that uses cryopreserved mononuclear cells has been developed (12). A negative rubella virus-specific lymphocyte transformation response in a seropositive child 3 years of age or younger is highly suggestive of congenitally acquired rubella.

INTERPRETATION AND REPORTING

Confirmation of clinical rubella requires the demonstration of a fourfold rise in antibody titers in paired sera or of the presence of rubella virus-specific IgM. There is considerable variability in the antibody titers maintained during life, and a firm diagnosis cannot be made on the basis of the absolute titer of a single serum sample. Because of day-to-day variations in the results of tests, paired sera must be tested in parallel. Differences in IgM titers in paired sera tested on different days may reflect test-to-test variation rather than a true change in antibody concentration. This consideration is especially important when paired sera are collected from pregnant women who have not experienced clinical illness. Judgments about therapy should be withheld until the sera have been reexamined in parallel. Sera positive for rubella IgM in EIA should be examined for rheumatoid factor to rule out a false-positive result.

Whenever possible, EIA responses should be converted to HI antibody equivalence, which has been routinely used to determine immunity, expressed as international units (IU). Currently advisory groups suggest that between 10 and

15 IU represents immunity to rubella in the majority of cases, where a dilution of 1:8 in the HI test is equivalent to 15 IU.

Patients without detectable antibodies are usually susceptible to infection by rubella virus; however, a small percentage of adults may not have detectable antibodies and yet are immune. Neutralizing antibodies at low dilutions can usually be detected in the sera of these patients. The lack of serologic responses to rubella virus vaccine in women who do not have detectable antibodies is often due to low levels of neutralizing antibodies. With the HI test described above, the first dilution in the test is 1:8. A patient serum sample that is positive only at 1:8 should be retested to rule out a possible false-positive reaction.

Testing for Immune Status

Qualitative, quantitative, and semiquantitative tests are used to determine the immune status. The package insert of commercial kits should be followed regarding the threshold (or cutoff) point for defining immunity and the units for reporting results. In reporting the results, one should indicate which assay was used. The physician must be provided with the threshold value to define the immune status and interpret the test result. The report should include quantitative units or contain the words "positive" or "negative." If the manufacturer defines an equivocal zone around the threshold value of the test, marginal results should be annotated. Laboratories are advised to establish a definitive procedure for dealing with the issue of equivocal results (additional testing by another method, additional specimens for assay, physician notification, etc.).

Where there is no history of exposure or possible infection, the presence of antibody at or above the threshold level is evidence of previous immunization or exposure to rubella virus.

Diagnosis of Rubella

The system for reporting the results of diagnostic tests relates to the test used and the manufacturer's recommendation in the package insert. The report of a qualitative IgM antibody test should be either "positive for IgM antibody" (IgM antibody present) or "negative for IgM antibody" (IgM antibody not detected). For quantitative IgG tests, the results should be reported in quantitative units as international units per milliliter. The generic and proprietary names of the test must be provided. Interpretation should accompany the results. For example, the presence of rubella-specific IgM antibody is evidence of a current or recent infection. Detection of changes in IgG titer requires following the manufacturer's recommendation for interpretation of a significant change in antibody concentration between acute- and convalescent-phase specimens. If a traditional sequential-dilution test such as HI is used, a fourfold or greater rise in antibody titer between the acute- and convalescent-phase specimens is evidence of a current or recent infection.

Diagnosis of Congenital Rubella

The same tests used for diagnosing clinical rubella are used for congenital rubella, and the reports of results of testing are similar. However, the interpretation may be different. Because maternal IgM antibodies do not generally pass the placental barrier, the presence of IgM in the neonatal circulation is evidence of congenital infection. The absence of IgM antibody does not rule out congenital infection. Contamination of cord blood with maternal blood negates the use of this specimen for testing. If infection of the fetus occurs in the first trimester of pregnancy, 90% of infected babies will have detectable circulating IgM antibody; if infection occurs very late in pregnancy, the rate is much lower.

Because IgG antibodies pass the placental barrier, most IgG antibody in cord or neonatal blood will be of maternal origin and the concentration will have significantly declined in the 6-month sample from the neonate. If it was produced as a result of congenital infection, high levels of antibodies will be measured at 6 months.

REFERENCES

1. **Abbott, G. G., J. W. Safford, R. G. MacDonald, M. C. Craine, and R. R. Applegren.** 1990. Development of automated immunoassays for immune status screening and serodiagnosis of rubella virus infection. *J. Virol. Methods* **27:** 227–240.
2. **Best, J., S. Palmer, P. Morgan-Capner, and J. Hodgson.** 1984. A comparison of Rubazyme-M and MACRIA for the detection of rubella-specific IgM. *J. Virol. Methods* **8:** 99–109.
3. **Bosma, T. J., K. M. Corbett, M. B. Eckstein, S. O'Shea, P. Vijayalakshmi, J. E. Banatvala, K. Morton, and J. M. Best.** 1995. Use of PCR for prenatal and postnatal diagnosis of congenital rubella. *J. Clin. Microbiol.* **33:**2881–2887.
4. **Brown, G. C., H. F. Maassab, J. A. Veronelli, and T. J. Francis.** 1964. Rubella antibodies in human serum: detection by the indirect fluorescent-antibody technique. *Science* **145:**943–945.
5. **Chernesky, M. A., L. Wyman, J. B. Mahony, S. Castriciano, J. T. Unger, J. W. Safford, and P. S. Metzel.** 1984. Clinical evaluation of the sensitivity and specificity of a commercially available enzyme immunoassay for detection of rubella virus-specific immunoglobulin M. *J. Clin. Microbiol.* **20:**400–404.
6. **Gupta, J. D., and J. D. Harley.** 1970. Use of formalinized sheep erythrocytes in the rubella hemagglutination-inhibition test. *Appl. Microbiol.* **20:**843–844.
7. **Gupta, J. D., and V. J. Peterson.** 1971. Use of a new buffer system with formalinized sheep erythrocytes in the rubella hemagglutination-inhibition test. *Appl. Microbiol.* **21:** 749–750.
8. **Hedman, K., and S. A. Rousseau.** 1989. Measurement of avidity of specific IgG for verification for recent primary rubella. *J. Med. Virol.* **27:**288–292.
9. **Ho-Terry, L., G. M. Terry, and P. Londesborough.** 1990. Diagnosis of foetal rubella virus infection by polymerase chain reaction. *J. Gen. Virol.* **71:**1607–1611.
10. **Liebhaber, H.** 1970. Measurement of rubella antibody by hemagglutination inhibition. II. Characteristics of an improved HAI test employing a new method for removal of nonimmunoglobulin HA inhibitors from serum. *J. Immunol.* **104:**826–834.
11. **Meitsch, K., G. Enders, J. S. Wolinsky, R. F. Faber, and B. Pustowoit.** 1997. The role of rubella-immunoblot and rubella-peptide-EIA for the diagnosis of the congenital rubella syndrome during the prenatal and newborn periods. *J. Med. Virol.* **51:**280–283.
12. **O'Shea, S., J. Best, and J. E. Banatvala.** 1992. A lymphocyte transformation assay for the diagnosis of congenital rubella. *J. Virol. Methods* **37:**139–148.
13. **Pattison, J. R., D. S. Dane, and J. E. Mace.** 1975. Persistence of specific IgM after natural infection with rubella virus. *Lancet* **i:**185–187.
14. **Russell, S. M., S. R. Benjamin, M. Briggs, M. Jenkins, P. P. Mortimer, and S. B. Payne.** 1978. Evaluation of the single radial hemolysis (SRH) technique for rubella antibody measurement. *J. Clin. Pathol.* **31:**521–526.
15. **Schmidt, N. J., and E. H. Lennette.** 1966. Rubella comple-

ment fixing antigens derived from the fluid and cellular phases of infected BHK-21 cells: extraction of cell-associated antigen with alkaline buffers. *J. Immunol.* **97:** 815–821.

16. **Schmidt, N. J., E. H. Lennette, J. D. Woodie, and H. H. Ho.** 1966. Identification of rubella virus isolates by immunofluorescent staining, and a comparison of the sensitivity of three cell culture systems for recovery of virus. *J. Lab. Clin. Med.* **68:**502–509.
17. **Stewart, G. L., P. D. Parkman, H. E. Hopps, R. D. Douglas, J. P. Hamilton, and H. M. Meyer, Jr.** 1967. Rubellavirus hemagglutination-inhibition test. *N. Engl. J. Med.* **276:**554–557.
18. **Thomas, H. I. J., and P. Morgan-Capner.** 1991. Rubella-specific IgG avidity: a comparison of methods. *J. Virol. Methods* **31:**219–228.
19. **U. S. Public Health Service.** 1965. *Standardized Diagnostic Complement Fixation Method and Adaptation to Micro Test.* U.S. Public Health Service Public Health monograph 74. U.S. Government Printing Office, Washington, D.C.
20. **Wolinsky, J. S., M. McCarthy, O. Allen-Cannady, W. T. Moore, R. Jin, S.-N. Cao, A. E. Lovett, and D. Simmons.** 1991. Monoclonal antibody-defined epitope map of expressed rubella virus protine domains. *J. Virol.* **65:** 3986–3994.
21. **Zhang, T., C. A. Mauracher, L. A. Mitchell, and A. Tingle.** 1992. Detection of rubella virus-specific immunoglobulin G (IgG), IgM and IgA antibodies by immunoblot assays. *J. Clin. Microbiol.* **30:**824–830.

Adenoviruses

GÖRAN WADELL, ANNIKA ALLARD, AND JOHN C. HIERHOLZER

76

CLINICAL BACKGROUND

Adenoviruses have been recovered from virtually every organ system of humans and have been associated with many clinical syndromes (Table 1). Adenovirus illnesses are endemic throughout the year and occur in all age groups, although they are most common among school-aged children, for whom approximately 50% of the infections are asymptomatic. Adenoviruses cause localized outbreaks of respiratory disease in the winter and spring, outbreaks of swimming pool-associated pharyngoconjunctival fever (PCF) in the summer, and epidemic keratoconjunctivitis (EKC) associated with industrial eye trauma or ophthalmologic procedures at any time of the year. Adenoviruses cause 5 to 15% of cases of gastroenteritis in infants and preschool children (4, 50, 51, 56). Epidemics of acute respiratory disease that can occur whenever new military recruits are housed together are now preventable by active immunization with the appropriate serotypes in enteric-coated capsules (48). Of the 51 candidate serotypes presently described, the most common are types 1 to 8, 11, 12, 21, 31, 35, 37, 40, and 41 (1–4, 11, 12a, 14, 16, 20, 21, 25, 39, 42, 44, 51, 54, 60–62).

Upper respiratory illness caused by adenoviruses can take the form of pharyngitis or tonsillitis and occurs chiefly in infants and young children. It is associated primarily with types 1 to 7 (11, 42, 44). Findings include coryza, fever, cough, exudate on the pharyngeal walls, a granular appearance of the mucosa, and tender, enlarged cervical nodes. A notable feature of infection with types 1, 2, 5, and 6 is the persistence of virus in a latent state in adenoidal and tonsillar tissues in about 50% of infected children. Another epidemiologically important feature is the excretion of virus in the stool for many months without recurrence of symptoms (16).

Lower respiratory illness, including bronchitis, bronchiolitis, and pneumonia, often complicates adenovirus infection. Severe pneumonia, sometimes fatal, occurs in infants and children (rarely in adults) and is caused mostly by types 3, 4, 7, and 21 (11, 39, 42, 44–46). Extrapulmonary signs such as kidney and liver involvement and encephalomeningitis can occur, especially in infants and immunocompromised patients, and in such patients the generalized disease usually has a fatal outcome (20). Some children who recover from type 3, 7, or 21 pneumonia have residual lung disease. A cough syndrome similar to whooping cough has been reported in children following type 5 and rarely type 1 to 3 infection (21).

PCF is characterized by fever, pharyngitis, conjunctivitis, and cervical lymphadenopathy, often with headache, diarrhea, and rash. Typical illness with follicular conjunctivitis is generally evident 5 to 6 days after exposure, with infected individuals shedding virus for about 10 days. Types 1 to 7 are usually implicated in these infections (42, 44).

Sporadic cases of keratoconjunctivitis are caused by many adenoviruses, but EKC is caused by types 8, 19a, and 37 (20, 59, 62). This severe eye disease becomes apparent after an 8- to 10-day silent incubation period. The initial onset of follicular conjunctivitis with preauricular lymphadenopathy can be accompanied by headache, malaise, and, depending on the serotype, mild upper respiratory illness. After 1 to 2 weeks with these symptoms, subepithelial corneal keratitis develops and may persist for an extended period. Contaminated tonometers, ophthalmic wash solutions, hands of medical personnel, and towels are the vehicles by which ocular infections are spread to susceptible persons; thus, most cases of EKC in nonindustrial communities are spread iatrogenically. Spread of adenoviruses in eye clinics can be eliminated, however, by triaging patients, separating patients and staff, thorough handwashing, using unit dosage eyedrops, avoiding invasive procedures on patients with EKC, and properly disinfecting equipment and surfaces. In industrial settings with high levels of airborne particulates, EKC outbreaks have resulted from eye-fomite-eye transmission. Trauma to the corneal epithelium is required for initiating virus infection, particularly with type 8. In type 19a- or 37-associated EKC, infection can spread to the eye from respiratory or genital sites (19, 21, 54).

Acute hemorrhagic conjunctivitis and acute hemorrhagic cystitis are both sometimes caused by type 11 and rarely by type 21, and the virus is readily recovered from eye secretions or urine as appropriate (10, 21).

Adenovirus infections in immunocompromised patients (those with immune deficiencies, including AIDS; those undergoing kidney, liver, or marrow transplants; and those receiving cancer chemotherapy) pose a major problem and are often fatal (20, 30). Adenoviruses cause generalized illness in perhaps 10% of these patients; virus has been recovered from the brain, throat, leukocytes, lung, urine, stool, cerebrospinal fluid, kidney, liver, and pancreas (10, 20, 21, 25, 60).

TABLE 1 Adenovirus infections and serotypes involved

Syndrome	Signs and symptoms	Serotype(s) involved:	
		Frequently	Infrequently
Upper respiratory illness	Coryza, pharyngitis, fever, tonsillitis, diarrhea	1–3, 5, 7	4, 6, 11, 18, 21, 29, 31
Lower respiratory illness	Bronchitis, pneumonia, fever, coryza, cough	3, 4, 7, 21	1, 2, 5, 35
Pertussis syndrome	Paroxysmal cough, vomiting, fever, upper respiratory illness	5	1, 2, 3
Acute respiratory disease	Tracheobronchitis, fever, myalgia, coryza, pneumonia	4, 7	3, 14, 21, 35
PCF	Pharyngitis, conjunctivitis, fever, coryza, headache, diarrhea, rash, cervical lymphadenopathy	3, 4, 7	1, 11, 14, 16, 19, 37
EKC	Keratitis, headache, preauricular nodes, coryza, pharyngitis, diarrhea	8, 37	3, 4, 7, 10, 11, 19, 21
Acute hemorrhagic conjunctivitis	Chemosis, follicles, subconjunctival hemorrhage, preauricular nodes, fever	11	2–8, 14, 15, 19, 37
Cystitis	Cystitis (usually hemorrhage), fever, pharyngitis	11	7, 21, 34, 35
Immunocompromised host disease	Diarrhea, rash, upper respiratory illness, pneumonia, hepatitis, cystitis, otitis media	1, 2, 5, 11, 34, 35, 43, 44, 48, 49	4, 7–10, 13, 15–17, 19–23, 25–33, 37–39, 42, 45–47, 50, 51
Gastroenteritis (infant)	Diarrhea, fever, nausea, vomiting, mild upper respiratory illness	31, 40, 41	1, 2, 12–17, 21, 25, 26, 29
Central nervous system disease	Meningitis, encephalitis, Reye's syndrome	7	3, 32
Venereal disease	Ulcerative genital lesions, urethritis, cervicitis	2, 37	1, 5, 7, 11, 18, 19, 31

Gastroenteritis and related syndromes have been associated with adenovirus infection in infants and children (21, 44, 50). Types 40 and 41 and, to a lesser extent, types 2 and 31 cause acute gastroenteritis (4, 12, 17, 18, 26, 29, 30, 33, 50, 51).

Neurologic disease, usually as part of multisystem disease, is sometimes caused by adenoviruses, with type 7 infection being particularly severe. Reye's syndrome is infrequently associated with the childhood serotypes, especially type 3. Types 1 to 3, 6, 7, 12, and 32 have been isolated from cerebrospinal fluid or brain tissue (21, 44).

Serotypes 2, 19a, and 37 have been recovered from herpes-like genital lesions, often associated with orchitis, cervicitis, or urethritis. Other syndromes have also been described (19, 21, 44). Finally, adenoviruses are often incriminated in nosocomial transmission. This is not surprising, because they cause 10% of the pneumonia cases in hospitalized children, intensive supportive therapy is required for these patients, adenoviruses are shed for long periods in the stool and are transmissible via both fomites and aerosolized droplets, and the viruses can readily infect respiratory and ocular tissues of other patients and of susceptible hospital personnel (11, 16, 42, 44, 46, 50, 56).

DESCRIPTION OF THE AGENT

Human adenoviruses are nonenveloped, double-stranded DNA viruses of the family *Adenoviridae*, genus *Mastadenovirus*. They are 70 to 90 nm in diameter and icosahedral, and they comprise 10 structural proteins with molecular weights of 5,000 to 120,000. They have a buoyant density in cesium chloride of 1.33 to 1.34 g/cm^3 and a molecular weight by sedimentation coefficient of 170 $\times$ 10^6 to 175 $\times$ 10^6.

Adenoviruses replicate in the cell nucleus and tend to be host species specific. The viruses produce characteristic cytopathic effects (CPE) that are accompanied by accumulation of multiple antigenic components and organic acids in the host cell culture fluids. All human adenoviruses possess genus-specific antigenic determinants on the hexon capsomeres. The capsid proteins of adenoviruses are arranged in an icosahedron with 20 triangular faces and 12 vertices. Each virion contains 240 hexons and 12 pentons. The hexons are dispersed on the triangular faces and edges, and the pentons are located in the vertices of the icosahedron. Each penton consists of a base (or vertex capsomere) and a fiber which is a rod-like outward projection with a terminal knob. The length of the fiber shaft is characteristic for the members of each subgenus. Inside the capsid is a single molecule of linear, double-stranded DNA with a molecular weight of 20 $\times$ 10^6 to 24 $\times$ 10^6. The G+C base composition of the genome for the different human adenoviruses ranges from 47 to 60% (38, 53, 54).

Crude suspensions of most adenoviruses are stable for prolonged periods at −20 to −100°C at pH 6 to 9. Infectious virus is rapidly inactivated at 56°C and by exposure to 0.25% sodium dodecyl sulfate, free chlorine at 0.5 μg/ml, UV irradiation, or 1:400 to 1:4,000 dilutions of formalin. The agents are not affected by treatment with ether or chloroform, and they can be readily lyophilized without special precautions. The lyophilized viruses appear to retain their infectivity indefinitely at 4 or −10°C or colder.

Classification

Adenoviruses have been isolated from every species of the placental mammals, marsupials, birds, and amphibians that have been studied. Human adenoviruses are now classified into six subgenera, A to F. Adenoviruses were originally classified by Rosen according to their hemagglutinating properties, and this classification was extended by Hierholzer in 1973 (19a) (Table 2). The enteric adenoviruses display a hardly discernible agglutination of rat erythrocytes (RBC) that is similar to the property of the members of subgenus A (13). In 1967, Huebner introduced a classification system based on oncogenic properties. More recently, the size of the structural polypeptides of the virion (58) and the DNA homology of the viral genome have been used to group all known human adenoviruses into six subgenera (58). The human adenoviruses have served as a model for oncogenicity in newborn hamsters. The subgenus A adenoviruses induced tumors in most newborn hamsters within 2 months after inoculation. Subgenus B and E adenoviruses induced tumors in a few animals after 4 to 18 months. Subgenus C, D, and F adenoviruses can transform a rat cell in vitro. Analysis of the apparent molecular mass of virion polypeptides by sodium dodecyl sulfate-polyacrylamide gel electrophoresis provided more detailed information on the relationship between human adenoviruses (58) (Table 3).

The conclusive classification of viruses should be based on differences in nucleotide sequence between the genomes of the different viruses. The DNA homology of adenoviruses has been studied by hybridization techniques, DNA restriction analysis, and nucleotide sequencing. These techniques confirm the assignment of the 51 human adenovirus serotypes into six subgenera.

Members belonging to the genus *Mastadenovirus* have common epitopes on the hexons. A subgenus is defined by a DNA homology of more than 50% between members within a subgenus and less than 20% between members of different subgenera. The serotype is defined by quantitative neutralization with hyperimmune sera. The ratio of homologous to heterologous neutralization titer must be greater than 16:1. The designation "recombinant" should be used only when the two parent genomes have been identified. An evolutionary variant is one in which genetic alteration was generated via insertion or intragenomic recombination in progeny of the same strain. A genomic cluster is a group of genome types that are significantly more closely related to each other than to any other genome type. The genome type denotes a distinct viral entity within a genomic cluster as identified by DNA restriction analysis. A strain is defined as the progeny of each wild-type isolate (3, 21, 24, 26, 38, 53, 54, 58).

Subgenus A

Types 12, 18, and 31 are distinctly different from each other in both polypeptide patterns and genome composition. All can be isolated from the stools of healthy humans. Type 31 has frequently been isolated from immunocompromised hosts and children with diarrhea (50).

Subgenus B

Two distinct clusters of DNA homology are seen after DNA restriction. The first, B:1, consists of types 3, 7, 16, 21, and 51, which are associated primarily with outbreaks of respiratory disease but can also cause a systemic infection including diarrhea. They account for one-third of all adenovirus isolates that have been typed and reported to the World Health Organization. The second cluster, B:2, consists of types 11, 14, 34, and 35. They cause persistent infections of the urinary tract. However, types 14 and 11 are also associated with outbreaks of respiratory disease (42, 58).

Subgenus C

Types 1, 2, 5, and 6 display DNA homology of 98% in pairwise comparison. They represent 59% of all adenovirus isolates reported to the World Health Organization. They can persist for years in lymphoid tissue and are intermittently shed into stools.

Subgenus D

Subgenus D consists of more than 30 serotypes, many of which are characterized by a tropism for the eye. Serotypes 8, 19a, and 37 are associated with EKC and sporadic keratoconjunctivitis.

TABLE 2 Subdivision of the human adenoviruses by HA properties[a]

Subgroup	Serotypes	HA subgroup	HA titers with RBC from:
A	12, 18, 31	3B[b]	Rat (incomplete)
B	3, 7, 11, 16, 34, 35	1A	Monkey
	14, 21, 51	1B[c]	Monkey
C	1, 2, 5, 6	3A	Rat (incomplete)
D	8, 9, 37	2A	Rat, mouse, human, guinea pig, dog
	10, 19, 26, 27, 36, 38, 39	2B	Rat, mouse, human
	13, 43	2C	Rat, mouse, human, monkey
	15, 22, 23, 30, 44, 45, 46, 47	2D	Rat, mouse, monkey
	17, 24, 32, 33, 42, 50	2E	Rat, mouse
	20, 25, 28, 29	2F[c]	Rat (atypical), monkey
E	4	3A	Rat (incomplete)
F	40, 41	3A[c]	Rat (atypical)

[a] Adapted from references 21 and 24.
[b] Very low HA titers.
[c] Moderate HA titers.

TABLE 3 Properties of human adenovirus serotypes of subgenera A to F[a]

Subgenus	Serotype(s)	DNA: Homology (%) Intrageneric	DNA: Homology (%) Intergeneric	DNA: G + C content (%)	DNA: No. of *Sma*I fragments[b]	Apparent mol mass of major internal polypeptides (kDa): V	VI	VII	Length of fibers (nm)	Oncogenicity in newborn hamsters	Tropism symptoms
A	12, 18, 31	48–69	8–20	48	4–5	51.0–51.5, 46.5–48.5[c]	25.5–26.0	18	28–31	High (tumors in most animals in 4 mo)	Cryptic enteric infection
B1	3, 7, 16, 21	89–94	9–20	51	8–10	53.5–54.5	24	18	9–11	Weak (tumors in few animals in 4–18 mo)	Respiratory disease
B2	14,[d] 11, 34, 35										Persistent kidney infections
C	1, 2, 5, 6	99–100	10–16	58	10–12	48.5	24	18.5	23–31	None	Persistent respiratory disease in lymphoid tissue
D	8–10, 13, 15, 17, 19, 20, 22–30, 32, 33, 36, 37, 38, 39, 42–47[e]	94–99	4–17	58	14–18	50.0–50.5[f]	23.2	18.2	12–13	None	Keratoconjunctivitis
E	4		4–23	58	16–19	48	24.5	18	17	None	Conjunctivitis Respiratory diseasse
F	40, 41	62–69	15–22	52	9–12	46.0–48.5	25.5	17.5	28–33	None	Infantile diarrhea

[a] Adapted from references 53–55 and 58.
[b] The restricted DNA fragments were analyzed on 0.8 to 1.2% agarose slab gels. DNA fragments smaller than 400 bp were not resolved.
[c] Polypeptide V of type 31 was a single band of 48 kDa.
[d] Members of subgenus B are divided into two clusters of DNA homology based on pronounced differences in DNA restriction sites.
[e] Only polypeptide analysis and/or DNA RE analysis has been performed with types 32 to 39 and types 42 to 47.
[f] Polypeptides V and VI of type 8 showed apparent molecular masses of 45 and 22 kDa, respectively. Polypeptide V of type 30 showed an apparent molecular mass of 48.5 kDa.

Subgenus E

Type 4 is the only serotype; however, two distinctly different genomic clusters represented by the type 4 prototype and the type 4 genome type have been recognized. Serotype 4 has been associated with epidemic follicular conjunctivitis and respiratory disease (53).

Subgenus F

Types 40 and 41 are fastidious, with impaired replication in established epithelial cell lines. These two enteric adenoviruses are associated with infantile diarrhea of long duration (13, 50, 58).

Antigenic Components

Replication of adenoviruses is accompanied by excess formation of antigenic components, which are liberated into the culture medium as soluble antigens. These proteins are complex structures that carry many antigenic determinants; in particular, the hexons, vertex capsomeres, and fibers possess distinct type- and subgroup-specific antigens. The type-specific determinants on the hexon and fiber are exposed on the surface of the virion and give rise to serum neutralization (SN) antibodies. In addition, the fiber is a strong hemagglutinin and thus elicits hemagglutination inhibition (HI) antibodies. The genus-specific antigen is the principal determinant on the hexon but resides on the internal part of the capsid and thus is not exposed externally and does not elicit protective antibodies. The vertex capsomere is the toxic cell detachment factor seen in overinoculated cultures. Additional determinants on these components evoke heterotypic SN and HI antibody responses. These determinants are mostly subgroup specific, although intersubgroup relationships may exist (38, 54).

The complete agglutination of monkey and rat RBC by adenoviruses of subgroups B and D is associated with intact virus particles and three forms of soluble hemagglutinins. The complete soluble forms consist of dodecons (groups of 12 pentons), dimers of pentons, and dimers of fibers (38). The partial agglutination of rat RBC seen with subgroup C viruses is due to the relative excess of monomeric pentons and fibers in cell culture fluids (52). These soluble antigens, however, produce complete agglutination of rat RBC in the presence of a heterotypic subgroup C antiserum in the test diluent (24, 38, 44, 54). Thus, the adenovirus components have specific biological properties and serological reactivities, which form the basis of many laboratory tests.

COLLECTION AND STORAGE OF SPECIMENS

Adenoviruses are stable and are readily recovered from obvious sites of infection. Nasopharyngeal swabs or aspirates, nasal swabs or aspirates, swabs of eye exudates, stool or rectal swabs, urine, urethral or cervical swabs, and biopsy or autopsy tissues are all adequate specimens as dictated by the patient's symptoms. Viral detection rates are greatly enhanced by proper collection of specimens early in the disease and by prompt cold or frozen shipment to the laboratory. Details of collection of respiratory, conjunctival, rectal, and other specimens are described in chapter 4.

Paired blood samples are needed to establish or confirm a diagnosis by serologic methods. The first specimen should be collected as soon as possible after the onset of symptoms, and the second should be collected 2 to 4 weeks later. After clotting, serum is separated under sterile conditions and stored at −10 to −20°C.

DIRECT EXAMINATION

Many methods have been used for the direct detection of adenoviruses in clinical materials, and research in this area is still keen because of the ongoing need to quickly and accurately diagnose a viral infection. Electron microscopy (EM) and immunoelectron microscopy (IEM) have been the principal means of identifying adenoviruses in clinical materials. In one procedure, tissue sections obtained at biopsy or autopsy are fixed, stained, and examined for inclusions or "crystalline" arrays of mature virions in the cell nucleus. In another method, specimens of respiratory secretions, urine, or stool (as 10 to 20% extracts) are clarified and observed directly by pseudoreplica negative-stain EM. Sensitivity is increased by concentrating the specimen (for throat or nasal washes, bronchial aspirates, and urine) by ultracentrifugation or membrane ultrafiltration. Sensitivity is further increased by IEM, in which the specimen (whether concentrated or not) is incubated with a hyperimmune antiserum or a human convalescent-phase serum before the grids are prepared for EM; aggregates of virus particles then indicate both the viral morphology and a specific reaction with the serum used. The first method has proven useful for diagnosis in tissue samples and for pathologic studies. The pseudoreplica method has been highly useful for diagnosis of adenovirus gastroenteritis (12, 33). Solid-phase IEM, in which hyperimmune adenovirus-specific immunoglobulin G (IgG) is adsorbed to the EM grid coated with *Staphylococcus aureus* protein, permits identification of adenovirus from crude preparations (47).

For immunofluorescence assay (IFA) examination, cells in unfrozen specimens are washed, resuspended in phosphate-buffered saline (PBS), fixed on slides in acetone, and reacted with antihexon or antivirion serum and antiglobulin conjugate (see chapter 5). Dense nuclear and stipled cytoplasmic staining are positive reactions for adenoviruses. A sensitive extension of IFA is the time-resolved fluoroimmunoassay (TR-FIA), in which a purified adenovirus monoclonal antibody (MAb) is used as capture antibody in plastic wells, the specimen is added to the wells, and a europium-labeled adenovirus MAb is used as the detector antibody. The specific fluorescence of the sample is measured by a fluorometer after a time delay to allow the autofluorescence to decay (21, 23).

For antigen detection by enzyme immunoassay (EIA), a polyclonal capture antibody is adsorbed to the plates and then antigens or specimens, a second polyclonal antibody (detector) from a different animal species, enzyme-conjugated antispecies antibody, and the substrate/color system are added in order (see chapter 12). The sensitivity is increased by using MAbs at the detector antibody position and further increased by using MAbs at both positions in the assay (21, 23, 33).

Radioimmunoassay (RIA) is equal in sensitivity and ease of performance to EIA but carries the problem of disposal of the radioactive wastes produced. RIA has been used to detect adenoviruses in respiratory secretions and stool specimens (36) Counterimmunoelectrophoresis (CIE) is a convenient test for detecting adenoviruses in toxic and environmental samples but is not as sensitive as EIA. CIE has identified adenovirus antigens in swimming pool water, serum specimens, ophthalmic drops used in eye clinics, and stool specimens (21, 29).

ISOLATION OF VIRUS

All of the human adenoviruses except types 40 and 41 replicate and produce CPE in continuous human cell lines of epithelial origin such as HeLa, KB, A549, or HEp-2; primary human embryonic kidney (HEK) cells; human embryonic lung fibroblasts (HELF, WI38, MRC-5); and other embryonic fibroblast cells as well. Different strains of types 40 and 41 display unpredictable replication in the aforementioned cells but grow to consistent (but low) titers in tertiary cynomolgus monkey kidney cells (14), the Graham 293 adenovirus type 5-transformed secondary HEK cell line, and HEp-2 cells under special conditions (21, 24). For cultivating adenoviruses, Eagle minimal essential medium supplemented with 2% heat-inactivated fetal calf serum and antibiotics is satisfactory as a maintenance medium. Infected cells become enlarged, rounded, and very refractile and aggregate into irregular clusters typical of adenovirus CPE (4, 11, 12, 16, 18, 26).

Preparation of the specimen for isolation is important. Respiratory and urine specimens are treated with antibiotics and clarified by low-speed centrifugation for 3 min to remove cells, fibers, and other debris. Stool specimens are brought to 10 to 20% suspensions with PBS or maintenance medium, shaken with glass beads if necessary, and clarified by centrifugation for 30 min. Biopsy or autopsy tissue specimens are minced into small fragments with sterile surgical scissors and then homogenized in a glass tissue grinder or sterile mortar with a sand abrasive and 5 ml of PBS or maintenance medium. A 10 to 20% suspension is made in this manner and then clarified by low-speed centrifugation. Blood monocytes are prepared for culture by applying 3 ml of heparinized blood cells on a Ficoll-Hypaque gradient. The cells are washed and resuspended in RPMI medium with 20% fetal calf serum to a final concentration of 1.5×10^6 cells/ml. Portions (0.5 ml) of the cell suspensions are then placed on human embryonic fibroblast feeder monolayers for cocultivation.

Specimens are inoculated onto cell cultures as soon as possible after they are received. Undiluted test material (0.4 to 0.5 ml) is inoculated into one or two cell culture tubes, adsorbed for 1 h at ambient temperature, overlaid with 1 ml of maintenance medium, and incubated at 35 to 36°C either stationary or on a roller drum. Several uninoculated tubes of each cell type used should be incubated and observed for evidence of nonspecific cellular degeneration and for eventual use as negative controls in identity tests. Sometimes, inoculation of a clinical specimen, especially stool, blood, and urine, leads to transient or irreparable toxic effects on the cell culture. Such toxicity is apparent within 24 h but can be minimized by washing the cell cultures or at least decanting the inoculum after the 1-h adsorption period. All cultures, including blind passages, should be read for CPE twice a week, fed with fresh maintenance medium as required, and subpassaged once after 2 weeks (for HEK and fibroblast cells) or three times at weekly intervals (for continuous epithelial cells), so that all cultures are held and read for at least 28 days. This regimen will yield the highest isolation rates. For identification, degeneration should progress until all the cells are affected (4+ CPE) in order to obtain sufficient yields of soluble antigens, hemagglutinins, and infectious virus to identify the isolate. Soluble antigen yields are highest in HEp-2 or KB cells; infectious virus yields are highest in HEK cells for types 1 to 39 and 42 to 51 and in Graham 293 cells for types 40 and 41.

A highly practical improvement in adenovirus isolation is the shell vial technique (15, 49). In this procedure, the cell monolayer is established on coverslips, the clinical specimen is added, and the culture is incubated for 1 or 2 days; IFA tests on the coverslip with anti-hexon MAb or with other antisera determine the presence or absence of adenovirus. Sensitivity can be increased by a brief centrifugation of the inoculated cultures (15).

IDENTIFICATION OF VIRUS

Grouping Tests

All of the tests used for direct detection are also used to identify an isolate as an adenovirus. IEM, IFA, RIA, TR-FIA, and PCR are solely genus-specific tests. CIE, EIA, and DNA or PCR assays are genus specific but can be made type specific if selected antisera, MAbs, DNA fragments, or restriction fragment length polymorphism PCR products are used, as appropriate. Restriction enzyme (RE) analysis can be made type specific if several REs are used; however, the prototype strains are rarely encountered. It is apparent, therefore, that the test procedure selected is determined by the level of typing desired. In general, IFA, EIA, TR-FIA, complement fixation (CF), or latex agglutination is used to classify an isolate as an adenovirus; agglutination with monkey, human, and rat RBC is used to place the virus into a subgroup; and then HI and SN tests with selected antisera are used to determine the serotype.

The genus-specific IFA, EIA, TR-FIA, and CF test are based on reactions of soluble hexons in the culture fluids and antihexon serum or hexon-specific MAb (21). Procedures for IFA and EIA are described in chapters 5 and 12; the CF test is described below under Serological Diagnosis. The test system used depends on convenience; all will easily identify hexons in cell cultures.

Typing Tests

Adenovirus serotyping is based on neutralization, but HI is more convenient (21, 24, 44, 54). In laboratories unable to procure fresh RBC for HA and HI tests, the only typing method available is SN. In this case, antisera to types 1 to 8, 11, 21, 35, and 37 should be routinely included unless epidemiological or clinical data for the isolate suggest the use of a smaller set of sera (Table 1).

HI Test

Microtiter HA and HI tests are performed in either flexible or hard plastic U-plates. Serial twofold dilutions (1:2 to 1:4,096) of the isolate in 0.05-ml volumes are prepared in plain PBS diluent, in PBS with 1% type 4 antiserum (for subgroup C strains), and in PBS with 1% type 6 antiserum (for subgroup E). (The type 4 and 6 animal antisera are required for adenoviruses giving incomplete HA patterns. The sera should have titers of at least 1:320, be heat inactivated at 56°C for 30 min, and be absorbed with rat RBC. The absorption is performed by adding 0.1 ml of RBC for every 1.0 ml of a 1:10 dilution of serum, incubating the mixture overnight at 4°C, and pelleting the cells by centrifugation at $1,800 \times g$ for 5 min at 4°C.)

RBC are collected and stored in Alsever solution. Monkey and rat RBC must be handled gently and used within 4 days of collection; immediately before use, the RBC are washed and adjusted to 0.4% in PBS. An equal volume of 0.4% rhesus or vervet monkey RBC is now added to one set of duplicate PBS diluent dilutions, and rat RBC are added to the others. The same volume of each RBC suspension is added to two separate wells containing 0.05 ml of each type of diluent to serve as cell controls. The plates are then covered with tape, shaken gently, and incubated in a 37°C water bath for 1 h. After this time, the RBC control wells should exhibit complete sedimentation and a teardrop pattern when the plates are tilted slightly. An HA titer is defined as the reciprocal of the highest dilution of virus that shows complete HA; the dilution end point is then considered to contain 1 HA unit per 0.05 ml. The pattern of HA titers with monkey, human, and rat RBC in the PBS diluent and with rat RBC in the heterotypic serum diluent thus defines the subgroup to which the isolate belongs (Table 2) (21, 24).

For the HI test, the typing antisera are heat inactivated and absorbed with the appropriate RBC as described above for type 4 and 6 immune sera. The antisera are diluted serially in 0.025-ml amounts in PBS diluent, and the virus at 4 HA units/0.025 ml (i.e., the HA titer divided by 8) is added per well. For a subgroup C or E isolate, antiserum dilutions are prepared in the appropriate heterotypic serum diluent as described above. The mixtures are agitated briefly and incubated at ambient temperature for 1 h before the appropriate RBC suspension is added (at 0.05 ml/well). A backtitration, i.e., serial twofold dilutions of the test antigen dose (0.05 ml in 0.05 ml of PBS or heterotypic serum diluent as appropriate), and cell controls are included in each test. The plates are incubated in the 37°C water bath for 1 h. After this time, the first four serial dilutions of the backtitration should exhibit a complete HA pattern, thus indicating that the proper antigen dose was used in the test. The isolate is identified by the typing serum which completely inhibits HA to or near the known homologous titer of the antiserum. Cross-reactions may be observed within antisera of the same subgroup; these are discussed below under Interpretation. Further characterization of the isolate may be obtained by SN tests.

SN Tests

SN tests are readable with definitive results and are the closest approximation that the laboratory has to the human serum response following infection; however, they are not as convenient to run as HA and HI tests. Three types of SN test can be carried out: the 7-day test in epithelial cell cultures, the 3-day test in monkey kidney cells, and microneutralization tests (11, 16, 21, 26, 44).

Conventional 7-day SN tests may be carried out with HEp-2, A549, HeLa, HEK, or Graham 293 cells. The virus isolate must be subjected to titer determination for infectivity in the cells to be used in the test, by preparing serial 10-fold dilutions of virus in Hanks balanced salt solution (HBSS) and inoculating the tubes in triplicate with 0.1 ml of dilution. After 7 days of incubation at 36°C, the end point (or titer) is read by CPE and is considered to be 1 50% tissue culture infective dose ($TCID_{50}$) of virus/0.1 ml. Since the slow and inconsistent development of CPE at high dilutions of an adenovirus culture tends to obscure the end point, a working dilution of virus which has a titer of 100 $TCID_{50}$ per 0.1 ml is used. Type-specific antisera are then selected for the SN test, heat inactivated at 56°C for 30 min, and diluted in HBSS in a twofold series from 1:10 to 1:1,280 (or slightly beyond the homologous titer of each antiserum). For the SN step, 0.3 ml of virus dilution is mixed with 0.3 ml of each antiserum dilution, incubated at ambient temperature for 1 h, and inoculated onto fresh cell cultures in triplicate at 0.2 ml/tube. Uninoculated cell controls and a back titration, consisting of a 10-fold dilution series from the working dilution used in the test, are included in the test. The tubes are incubated, fed, and read as usual, with the final reading taken at 7 days. The back titration should show CPE ending around the second dilution. As in HI, the virus type is indicated by inhibition (of CPE) to or near the homologous titer of an antiserum. The antibody end point is thus defined as the reciprocal of the highest dilution of serum which completely neutralizes the CPE.

The most widely used SN procedure is the 3-day test in primary rhesus MK cell cultures. This test does not measure inhibition of infectivity but, rather, measures inhibition of the viral toxicity induced by the vertex capsomere. If MK cells are not available, the test can be done in established MK lines, such as Vero, LLC-MK2, or BSC-1. To determine the challenge dose of virus to be used in the test, 0.1 ml of each serial twofold dilution (1:1 to 1:128) prepared in maintenance medium is inoculated into three cell cultures which each contain 1 ml of maintenance medium. The mixture is incubated at 35 to 36°C and the degree of CPE is read at 3 days. The highest dilution of virus producing 1+ to 2+ CPE (i.e., with 25 to 50% of the cell sheet being affected) in the cells at 3 days is considered the end point, and the virus dose to be used in the SN test is 1 dilution back from this end point. As above, the selected antisera are heat inactivated, diluted serially to encompass the known homologous antibody titer of each, mixed with an equal volume (0.3 ml) of the isolate dilution, and incubated at ambient temperature for 1 h. Then, 0.2 ml of each virus-serum mixture is inoculated onto fresh cells in triplicate. Uninoculated cell control tubes and three virus control tubes, containing 0.1 ml of the working dilution used in the test, are included. The tubes are incubated, fed, and read as usual, with the final reading being taken at 3 days. At this time, the virus controls should show 1+ to 2+ CPE; the virus type is indicated by inhibition of CPE to or near the homologous titer of an antiserum.

Microneutralization tests can be done in secondary rhesus monkey kidney cells, Vero cells, and HEp-2 cells. In the Vero test, the virus titer is determined by using flat-bottomed 96-well plates in replicas of six, with the virus being serially diluted in growth medium by an automatic diluter with flame-sterilized loops, manually with a multichannel pipettor, or automatically with a programmable diluter and disposable tips. Then, 0.05 ml of a Vero cell suspension at 175,000 cells/ml is dropped into all the wells, including the cell control wells. The plate is gently shaken, sealed with sterile tape or a lid, incubated at 35 to 36°C for 5 days, and read by staining with a crystal violet-formaldehyde solution. The end point is the highest dilution of virus showing 0 to 1+ staining (i.e., 4+ to 3+ CPE) in 5 days. SN tests then utilize serial dilutions of heat-inactivated antisera made with sterile diluting equipment as above, 2 U of virus (1 dilution back from the end point) per well, and the cell suspension. The plates are sealed, incubated, and stained as described above. Cell controls and a virus back titration should be included. The test is read visually for uninfected (stained) cells, and the antibody end point is defined as above. Types 40 and 41 have peculiar features that separate them from the other adenoviruses in terms of growth and identification in cell cultures; reviews concerning the enteric adenoviruses should be consulted for details of these specialized procedures (4, 12, 21, 26, 51, 56).

SEROLOGICAL DIAGNOSIS

Serodiagnosis is accomplished with an acute-phase and convalescent-phase serum pair collected at an interval of 2 to 4 weeks. The timing for collection of the convalescent-phase serum is not critical if the acute-phase serum was taken early in the illness. Because of the ubiquity of the adenoviruses and the numerous cross-reactions between related serotypes, seroconversion involving a fourfold or greater rise in antibody titer is necessary to document infection. Adenovirus infection can be documented by a genus-reactive test such as CF or EIA, either of which can include the adenovirus antigen as part of a battery of antigens. For illnesses in which adenoviruses play an important role, such as acute respiratory distress, EKC, or PCF, genus-reactive tests can be followed by type-specific tests to pinpoint the serotype involved, or the type-specific test alone can be carried out for the serotypes usually involved (16).

CF Test

The CF test is the most widely used and best-standardized serological test for adenovirus infection. The test antigen is commercially available or is easily made by propagating a common serotype in HEp-2 or KB cells and harvesting by three freeze-thaw cycles 2 or 3 days after 4+ CPE is obtained. The supernatant fluid after clarification serves as the CF antigen, which is tested for potency by block titer determinations against a reference human or animal antiserum. Alternatively, the sensitivity of the CF test can be improved by using a semipurified hexon preparation. The adenovirus CF antigen is stable and group specific, enabling it to detect all 51 human serotypes plus intermediate and atypical strains with equal reliability. Furthermore, it can be part of a battery of a dozen or more viral antigens tested simultaneously, thereby making the test cost-effective and efficient in terms of labor and materials. The main disadvantage of the CF test is its low sensitivity. A pool of antigens from adenovirus type 7 (subgenus B), adenovirus type 5 (subgenus C), and adenovirus type 4 (subgenus E) can enhance the sensitivity of the CF test. Although CF titers are highly reproducible among tests and among laboratories, they detect infection in only 50 to 70% of cases in general and in fewer than 50% of cases in young children and in adenovirus-immunized military recruits (21, 36, 45, 48).

EIA

EIA is much more sensitive than CF and is becoming increasingly used in diagnostic laboratories (36). Good reagents and automated EIA readers are now commercially available. The test can be carried out in either of two ways. In the first, a common adenovirus (e.g., type 2, 4, or 7) is cultured to produce a high titer of soluble antigens as for the CF antigen. After clarification and dialysis against an alkaline buffer, the supernatant fluid is added to each well of 96-well microtiter plates and incubated overnight at 4°C to prepare the solid-phase antigen. A purified or semipurified hexon preparation is preferable for this step because cellular and medium proteins, as well as the type-specific soluble components (fiber, dodecon, etc.), would be removed. After three washes with PBS containing 0.5% gelatin and 0.15% Tween 20, serial dilutions (in PBS-gelatin-Tween) of the patient's paired sera (1:200 to 1:25,600) are added to parallel rows and the reaction is incubated at 37°C for 1.5 h. After another three washes, commercially available anti-human IgG-peroxidase conjugate at about a 1:1,000 dilution in PBS-gelatin-Tween is added. The plates are placed at 37°C for 1 h, washed, and developed for color (see chapter 12).

In the second procedure, ammonium sulfate-precipitated IgG from an adenovirus antiserum in alkaline buffer is attached to each well of a plate for the solid phase, to serve as the capture antibody. After the antibody is washed, antigen (either crude or purified as described above) is added and incubated at 37°C for 1.5 h. The plates are again washed, and serial dilutions of the patient's paired sera (the detector antibody) are added. The patient's sera must be diluted (1:200 to 1:25,600) in PBS-gelatin-Tween solution containing 1.5% heat-inactivated normal serum of the capture antibody species; this procedure greatly reduces the nonspecific background color. After another incubation at 37°C for 1.5 h and subsequent washing, the anti-human IgG-peroxidase conjugate is added and the mixture is incubated at 37°C for 1 h. The plates are then washed and the substrate is added as above.

Both procedures are highly sensitive and can be made quite reproducible if adequate care is taken throughout. Controls should include negative virus (cell controls), reagent controls, and positive and negative human sera. The background absorption in a well-devised test should be negligible; in most EIA readers, it is automatically subtracted from the test serum readings.

HI Test

HI and SN tests are more sensitive than CF, and they measure increases in type-specific antibody levels. Although some reagents are commercially available, most laboratories prepare their own stocks of the common adenovirus serotypes for use as HA antigens or infectious virus in HI and SN tests (20, 24, 45, 54). Human serum specimens are treated for HI tests by heat inactivation (56°C for 30 min) and removal of nonspecific agglutinins by absorption with 50% suspensions of rat or rhesus RBC, as appropriate. The sera are then diluted 1:8 to 1:1,024 in the microtiter plate, leaving 0.025 ml in each well. A virus suspension diluted to contain 4 HA units/0.025 ml is added to each well, mixed gently, and incubated at ambient temperature for 1 h. Then 0.05 ml of RBC suspension is added per well, and the plate is agitated, sealed with tape, and incubated in a 37°C water bath for 1 h. A virus backtitration, serum controls, and cell controls should be included in the test. The end point (serum titer) is the highest dilution of serum completely inhibiting agglutination by 4 HA units of virus.

SN Tests

SN tests are performed as described above. Acute- and convalescent-phase serum specimens are inactivated at 56°C for 30 min and serially diluted (1:4 to 1:512) in maintenance medium in sterile tubes, leaving 0.3 ml of each dilution in the tubes. To each tube is added 0.3 ml of the dilution of seed virus. The tubes are shaken and incubated at ambient temperature for 1 h, and 0.2 ml of each virus-serum mixture is then added to each of two cell cultures. A virus control is made with a 1:2 dilution of the working virus dilution used in the test and is inoculated at 0.2 ml per tube; a backtitration is made with four serial 10-fold dilutions of the working virus dilution and is inoculated at 0.1 ml per tube. Uninoculated or sham-inoculated tubes serve as cell controls. Occasionally, known positive and negative sera should be included in the test as a check on the entire system. The cultures are read daily, and the test is concluded when 32 to 320 $TCID_{50}$/0.1 ml is apparent in the virus backtitration. The highest serum dilution in which both tubes show no adenovirus CPE is considered the end point.

Alternatively, the 3-day test in MK cells or a micro-SN test such as in Vero cells may be carried out by using the same principles. In both tests, cell controls and a virus backtitration step should be included. The micro-SN test is ideal for serum surveys because a large number of tests can be carried out in a single run, with little cost in cells, media, and supplies. Also, the test is read visually for uninfected (stained) cells. A fourfold or greater increase in titer between the acute- and convalescent-phase serum samples is indicative of a type-specific seroconversion (21, 45, 54).

Preparation of Hyperimmune Sera

Purified virions can be obtained after centrifugation of infected cells disrupted by sonication on discontinuous CsCl gradients followed by equilibrium centrifugation. The final contamination of host cell proteins amounted to 0.0006% (57).

Provided that *Cercopithecus aethiops* or *Cynomologus* RBC can be obtained, hemadsorption at 37°C followed by several washes with PBS at 37°C and a final elution at 4°C will yield highly purified virions and dodecons. They can then be separated by differential centrifugation due to their distinctly different S values (700 and 60, respectively). This method can be preferentially used on type 3, 7, and 16 members of subgenus B.

Preimmunization sera must be secured. A 25-μg sample of purified virions in Freund's complete adjuvant injected intramuscularly in rabbits followed 6 weeks later by an intravenous injection of 10 μg of purified virions will, after an additional week, yield high-titer sera (25,000 to 100,000 measured by enzyme-linked immunosorbent assay).

For diagnostic purposes, preimmune and hyperimmune sera must be used in parallel since rabbits can be naturally infected by adenoviruses, enteroviruses, reovirus, herpesviruses, and other viruses that cross-react with their human counterparts.

MOLECULAR TECHNIQUES FOR VIRUS IDENTIFICATION

Preparation of Viral DNA

Infected cells are a more abundant and feasible source of viral DNA than are purified virions. The infected cell monolayer can be lysed, when more than 50% of the cells show CPE, by addition of 0.6% sodium dodecyl sulfate. Proteinase K is then added to 100 μg/ml and incubated for 60 min at 37°C. Finally, NaCl is added to 1 M. The lysate is gently mixed and stored overnight at 4°C. Centrifugation at 17,000 × *g* for 30 min will bring down cellular DNA. The supernatant is collected and RNases A and T1 are added to a final concentration of 30 μg/ml and 80 U, respectively. The RNase preparations should have been preincubated at 80°C for 30 min. Then proteinase K is added again, and the mixture is incubated for 4 h at 37°C. The viral DNA is then extracted three times with phenol-ether and precipitated with 2 volumes of ethanol at −20°C. This procedure will yield viral DNA of sufficient quantity and quality to perform DNA RE analysis. However, the preparation will contain sheared cellular DNA (27). The procedure of Shinagawa et al. (43) will yield adenovirus DNA of higher purity. This method is based on the fact that the terminal protein is covalently linked to the linear viral DNA. The phenol extraction is performed before proteinase K digestion. The terminal protein is then denaturated, and the DNA-protein complex will be trapped at the phenol/aqueous interface. This procedure can be performed on a microscale in Eppendorf tubes.

DNA preparation for PCR analysis should be as simple as possible to minimize the risk of contamination. Direct amplification from the heated supernatant from an infected tissue culture tube can be performed. Clinical specimens require some extraction. Most commercial kits use the chaotropic properties of guanidine isothiocyanate combined with a nuclease binding or DNA binding matrix. Alkali treatment is a simple procedure for handling clinical specimens. The specimen is diluted in 20 mM HEPES (pH 7.3)–NaOH to a final concentration of 0.5 mM and incubated for 15 min at 37°C. The mixture is neutralized by addition of an equal amount of HCl mixture. A high concentration of NaCl will result. The mixture should therefore be diluted 10-fold in distilled water, and a 10-μl sample is used for template DNA in the PCR performed at a final volume of 50 μl. Two-step nested PCR assays are useful for direct detection of adenoviruses in many kinds of clinical specimens. Detailed protocols are available in reference 5 (Table 4). An additional primer pair from the P2 region of the hexon has been published (22). Further, Saitoh-Inagawa et al. used primers from the P1 and P2 regions of the hexon to design a nested PCR that could detect adenoviruses of subgenera B, C, D, E, and F (41).

Direct Detection of Adenovirus DNA

The fastidious nature of enteric adenoviruses has posed a challenge to investigators attempting to develop molecular techniques for the direct detection of types 40 and 41. Specific probes have been identified (9) for use in direct identification of viruses in stool specimens (17, 31, 33, 37). Up to 10^{11} virus particles can be shed per g of feces. Therefore, viral DNA can be extracted from stools to allow RE analysis of DNA (58). RE analysis with the 5′CCC GGG-specific

TABLE 4 Oligonucleotide primers for general detection of adenoviruses

General primer position	Name	Sequence	Amplimer length and annealing temp	Reference
18858–18883	hex1885deg	5′-GCC (C/G)CA (G/A)TG G(G/T)C (T/A)TA CAT GCA CAT C-3′	301 bp, 55°C	Modified from 7
19158–19136	hex1913deg	5′-CAG CAC (G/C)CC ICG (A/G)AT GTC AAA-3′		
18931–18955	nehex1893deg	5′-GCC CG(C/T) GC(A/C) ACI GAI AC(G/C) TAC TTC-3′	171 bp, 55°C	Modified from 6
19075–19103	nehex1905deg	5′-CC(C/T) AC(A/G) GCC AGI GT(A/G) (A/T)AI CG(A/C) (A/G)C(C/T) TTG TA-3′		
21592–21617	A2H-pcr 4R	5′-ATG ACT TTT GAG GTG GAT CCC ATG GA-3′	134 bp, 52°C	35
21726–21703	A2H-pcr 1	5′-GCC GAG AAG GGC GTG CGC AGG TA-3′		

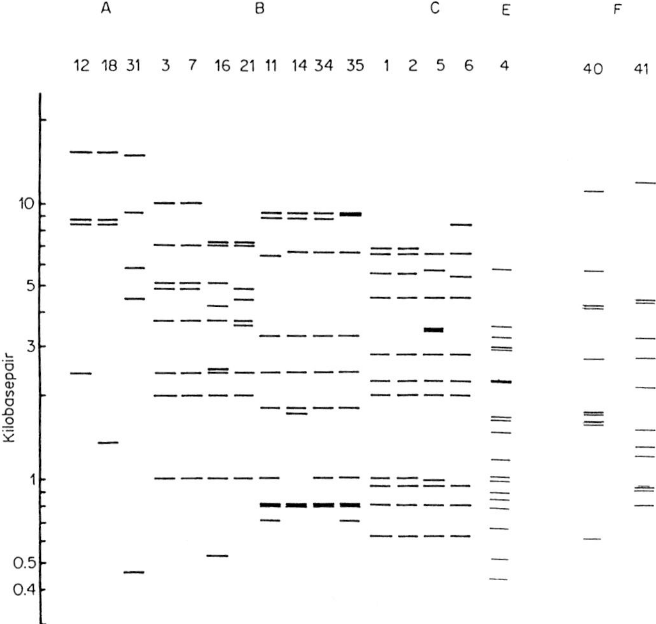

FIGURE 1 Schematic presentation of the *Sma*I DNA RE patterns of all the human adenovirus prototypes of subgenera A, B, C, E, and F.

*Sma*I provides information on subgenus origin and allows the identification of most adenovirus types (55) (Fig. 1 and 2). Access to a catalog of DNA restriction patterns of adenovirus prototypes 1 to 41 provides a means of identification of unknown adenovirus strains (3). The use of RE analysis has revealed the genetic diversity within each adenovirus serotype (58). Li et al. (34) detected 17 and 19 genome types of adenovirus types 3 and 7, respectively, by using 12 REs. A suggestion for a time-saving pathway for genome type identification is given in Fig. 3.

The prototype strains are as a rule no longer circulating. However, an unknown strain can frequently be typed by comparing its restriction patterns for several REs with the patterns of the prototype strains.

PCR for Detection of Adenoviruses

The appearance of PCR technology has offered both opportunities and challenges. It is now possible to detect noncultivatable adenoviruses directly in clinical specimens. However, it was a challenge to design PCR probes that allowed amplification of all human adenoviruses. Highly conserved nucleotide sequences were identified in the hexon gene that allowed attempts to perform a general adenovirus PCR assay (7, 32, 35). Nested two-step PCR was developed to enhance the efficacy of PCR performed directly on clinical specimens such as stools (6). This method can also be used to detect pollution of water, provided that adequate extraction methods are used (40).

Information on the subgenus origin of an unidentified adenovirus amplimer can be obtained by using primers flanking the VA RNA regions (40). Typing of adenoviruses can be performed by PCR followed by restriction fragment length polymorphism analysis with the obtained amplimer. Allard et al. (8) could type adenovirus types 40 and 41, whereas Saitoh-Inagawa et al. (41) could identify the etio-

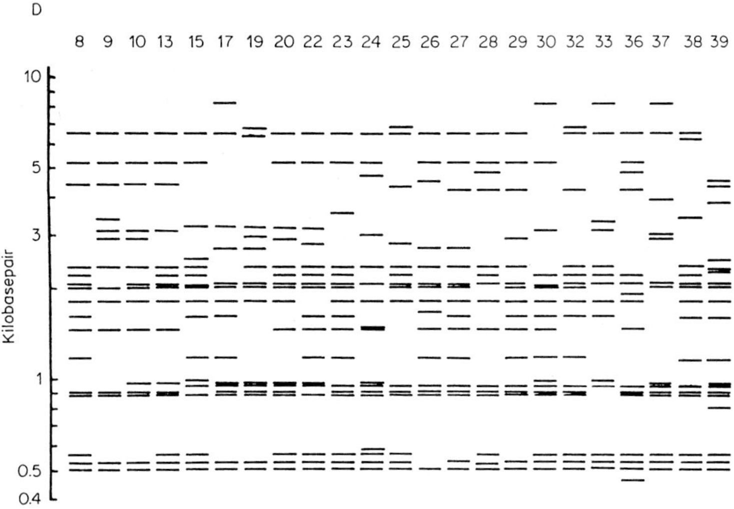

FIGURE 2 Schematic presentation of *Sma*I DNA RE patterns obtained after cleavage of DNA from adenovirus prototypes belonging to subgenus D.

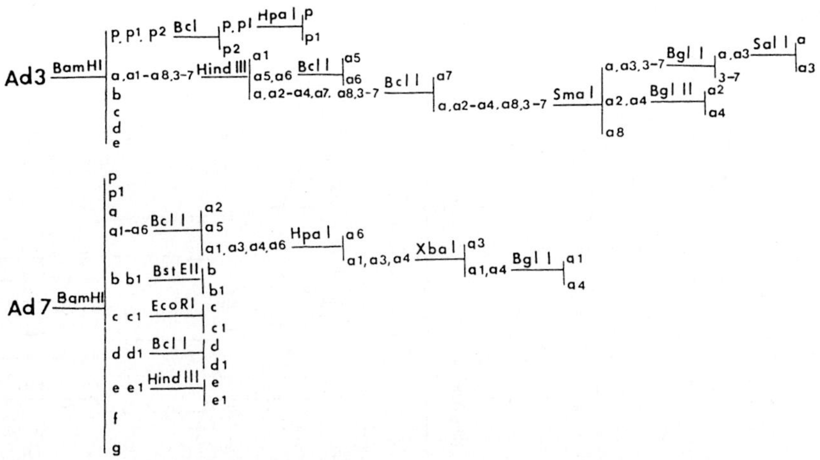

FIGURE 3 Pathways for genome type identification of adenovirus types 3 and 7. These pathways are the most economical and time-saving methods. For instance, all the strains of type 7 were analyzed first with *Bam*HI. The RE patterns were compared with known data (2, 3, 34, 53, 55). Five genome types, 7p, 7p1, 7a, 7f, and 7g, could be directly identified from their unique patterns. The remaining strains could be allocated to different smaller groups, for example, a1 to a6. After the second RE, *Bcl*I, was used, two other genome types, 7a2 and 7a5, could be identified. The remaining strains could be further analyzed with the third RE, *Hpa*I. Type 7a6 could then be identified. The procedure was continued until the last genome type was identified.

logical agents of adenovirus conjunctivitis. Type-specific primers for types 8, 31, 40, and 41 have been described (5). These serotypes can thus be typed by type-specific PCR. The general primer pair first published in 1990 from the P1 region of the hexons was based on the then available hexon sequences from adenoviruses of subgenus C and F (7). It is now evident that PCR assays with these primers suffer from low sensitivity for detection of members of subgenus B. Allard has recently developed a general PCR assay based on degenerate sequences specific for hexon genes; these sequences are preferred (5) (Table 4).

EVALUATION, INTERPRETATION, AND REPORTING OF RESULTS

IFA, CF, EIA, and TR-FIA for antigen identify all human adenoviruses by the group-specific hexon-antihexon reaction, whereas PCR recognizes adenoviruses by detecting common nucleotide sequences in the hexon gene (5–7, 22, 35). All five tests perform well for this task, but each has limitations. HI and SN tests, being type specific, are subject to interpretative problems arising from the multitude of antigenic cross-reactions that occur among the human adenoviruses (12a, 14, 20, 21, 24, 26, 28, 44, 45, 54, 61). For instance, all three viruses in subgroup A (Table 2) cross-react in SN tests. Types 12 and 18 exhibit a bilateral cross between themselves, and type 31 antisera cross-react with type 12 and 18 viruses. Among subgroup B viruses, the most significant reciprocal cross-reactions observed in both HI and SN tests are among types 7, 11, and 14 and between types 3 and 7. Types 34 and 35 are not readily discernible by HI but are identified by SN. The subgroup C viruses are devoid of any cross-reactions except in occasional antisera.

The major HI and SN cross-reactions in subgroup D do not always coincide, and so this subgroup presents the greatest difficulties in serotyping. Types 8 and 9, types 10, 19, and 37, types 13, 38, and 39, types 15, 22, and 42, types 20 and 47, types 24, 32, 33, and 46, and types 29 and 45 are not easily distinguishable by HI but are readily typed by SN. Conversely, types 15, 23, and 29 are clearly identified by HI but are closely related by SN. Other crosses in either test are unilateral and have low titers.

A notable reciprocal intergroup cross-reaction, seen only in the SN test, occurs between type 4 (in subgroup E) and type 16 (in subgroup B). Type 4 also crosses with types 40 and 41 of subgroup F. Type 40 is difficult to distinguish from type 41 by HI but can be distinguished by carefully constructed SN tests, EIA with MAbs, DNA hybridization probes, and RE analyses (33, 51). Similarly, isolates with restriction enzyme patterns different from the prototype are the rule rather than the exception, and these "DNA variants" appear to be common for all serotypes (2, 3, 21, 30, 34, 46, 51, 53, 54, 60). Thus, RE patterns with selected enzymes are often part of the laboratory study of clinical isolates and have epidemiological value. Serotyping can by definition be performed only by serological methods. RE analyses performed with several enzymes can as a rule support and extend the typing by defining genome types (34, 58). Analysis based on single RE patterns is not a substitute for serotyping.

For serological tests, a significant (fourfold or greater) rise in antibody titer between the acute- and convalescent-phase sera is required for diagnosis or confirmation of infection. Consequently, the tests cannot be performed until late in the convalescent period, when the results are of less clinical importance than during the acute illness. Nevertheless, the results may be of epidemiological importance or of clinical interest in establishing an association between an unusual illness and adenovirus infection. Since CF and EIA detect antibody stimulated by infection with any human adenovirus, they are valuable only as screening tests for adenovirus infection; they will not yield information on the infecting serotype. Also, CF is less sensitive than the HI and SN tests, especially in younger children and in patients with superficial infections such as conjunctivitis, and the EIA is not yet standardized. For both tests, reagent controls (complement, hemolysin, etc., for CF; diluent, enzyme, etc., for EIA), antigen controls and backtitration, and positive and negative human serum controls should be included for proper interpretation of results.

The HI and SN tests are more sensitive provided that the infecting serotype is included as an antigen. Rises in titers of antibody to heterotypic adenoviruses may occur with both the HI and SN tests in as many as 25% of adult infections, generally between types of the same HA subgroup (21). For these reasons, serological tests on individual patients cannot be considered to establish the infecting serotype in the absence of virus isolation or epidemiological factors.

Whether a patient's illness is due to adenovirus infection is a more difficult question. Many adenovirus infections are asymptomatic and persistent. In infants, antibody may not develop until months after the onset of infection. Isolation of an adenovirus, and even serological evidence of infection, may be coincidental to a disease caused by infection with a different agent. On the other hand, isolation of an adenovirus (especially to high titer) from a diseased organ or its secretions, or previous epidemiological association of the patient's syndrome with a particular adenovirus, is considered valid evidence that the adenovirus is the etiological agent of the illness.

REFERENCES

1. **Abzug, M. J., and M. J. Levin.** 1991. Neonatal adenovirus infection: four patients and review of the literature. *Pediatrics* **87:**890–896.
2. **Adrian, T., M. Becker, J. C. Hierholzer, and R. Wigand.** 1989. Molecular epidemiology and restriction site mapping of adenovirus 7 genome types. *Arch. Virol.* **106:**73–84.
3. **Adrian, T., G. Wadell, J. C. Hierholzer, and R. Wigand.** 1986. DNA restriction analysis of adenovirus prototypes 1 to 41. *Arch. Virol.* **91:**277–290.
4. **Albert, M. J.** 1986. Enteric adenoviruses. *Arch. Virol.* **88:** 1–17.
5. **Allard, A.** 1995. PCR for the detection of adenoviruses, p. 357–366. In Y. Becker and G. Darai (ed.), *Frontiers of Virology. PCR: Protocols for Diagnosis of Human and Animal Virus Diseases.* Springer-Verlag GmbH, Heidelberg, Germany.
6. **Allard, A. K., B. Albinsson, and G. Wadell.** 1992. Detection of adenoviruses in stools from healthy persons and patients by two-step polymerase chain reaction. *J. Med. Virol.* **37:**149–157.
7. **Allard, A. K., R. Girones, P. Juto, and G. Wadell.** 1990. Polymerase chain reaction for detection of adenoviruses in stools. *J. Clin. Microbiol.* **28:**2659–2667.
8. **Allard, A. K., A. Kajon, and G. Wadell.** 1994. Simple procedure for discrimination and typing of enteric adenoviruses after detection by polymerase chain reaction. *J. Med. Virol.* **44:**250–257.
9. **Allard, A. K., G. Wadell, K. M. Evander, and G. K. K. Lindman.** 1985. Specific properties of two enteric adenovirus 41 clones, mapped within the E1A region. *J. Virol.* **54:** 145–150.
10. **Ambinder, R. F., W. Burns, M. Forman, P. Charache, R. Arthur, W. Beschorner, G. Santos, and R. Saral.** 1986. Hemorrhagic cystitis associated with adenovirus infection in bone marrow transplantation. *Arch. Intern. Med.* **146:** 1400–1401.
11. **Brandt, C. D., H. W. Kim, A. J. Vargosko, et al.** 1969. Infections in 18,000 infants and children in a controlled study of respiratory tract disease. I. Adenovirus pathogenicity in relation to serologic type and illness syndrome. *Am. J. Epidemiol.* **90:**484–500.
12. **Brown, M., M. Petric, and P. J. Middleton.** 1984. Diagnosis of fastidious enteric adenoviruses 40 and 41 in stool specimens. *J. Clin. Microbiol.* **20:**334–338.

12a. **de Jong, J. C., A. G. Wermenbol, M. W. Verweij-Uijterwaal, K. W. Slaterus, P. Wertheim-van Dillen, G. J. J. van Doornum, S. H. Khoo, and J. C. Hierholzer.** Adenoviruses from human immunodeficiency virus-infected patients, including two new candidate serotypes 50 and 51 of subgenus D and B1, respectively. *J. Infect. Dis.*, in press.

13. **de Jong, J. C., R. Wigand, A. H. Kidd, G. Wadell, J. G. Kapsenberg, C. J. Muzerie, A. G. Wermenbol, and R. G. Firtzlaff.** 1983. Candidate adenovirus 40 and 41: fastidious adenovirus from human infantile stool. *J. Med. Virol.* **11:** 215–231.
14. **de Jong, J. C., R. Wigand, G. Wadell, et al.** 1981. Adenovirus 37: identification and characterization of a medically important new adenovirus type of subgroup D. *J. Med. Virol.* **7:**105–118.
15. **Espy, M. J., J. C. Hierholzer, and T. F. Smith.** 1987. The effect of centrifugation on the rapid detection of adenovirus in shell vials. *Am. J. Clin. Pathol.* **88:**358–360.
16. **Fox, J. P., C. E. Hall, and M. K. Cooney.** 1977. The Seattle virus watch. VII. Observations of adenovirus infections. *Am. J. Epidemiol.* **105:**362–386.
17. **Hammond, G., C. Hannan, T. Yeh, K. Fischer, G. Mauthe, and S. E. Straus.** 1987. DNA hybridization for diagnosis of enteric adenovirus infection from directly spotted human fecal specimens. *J. Clin. Microbiol.* **25:** 1881–1885.
18. **Hammond, G. W., G. Mauthe, J. Joshua, and C. K. Hannan.** 1985. Examination of uncommon clinical isolates of human adenoviruses by restriction endonuclease analysis. *J. Clin. Microbiol.* **21:**611–616.
19. **Harnett, G. B., P. A. Phillips, and M. M. Gollow.** 1984. Association of genital adenovirus infection with urethritis in men. *Med. J. Aust.* **141:**337–338.

19a. **Hierholzer, J. C.** 1973. Further subgrouping of the human adenoviruses by differential hemagglutination. *J. Infect. Dis.* **128:**541–550.

20. **Hierholzer, J. C.** 1992. Adenoviruses in the immunocompromised host. *Clin. Microbiol. Rev.* **5:**262–274.
21. **Hierholzer, J. C.** 1995. Adenoviruses, p. 169–188. *In* E. H. Lennette, D. A. Lennette, and E. T. Lennette (ed.), *Diagnostic Procedures for Viral, Rickettsial and Chlamydial Infections*, 7th ed. American Public Health Association, Washington, D.C.
22. **Hierholzer, J. C., P. E. Halonen, P. O. Dahlen, P. G. Bingham, and M. M. McDonough.** 1993. Detection of adenovirus in clinical specimens by polymerase chain reaction and liquid-phase hybridization quantitated by time-resolved fluorometry. *J. Clin. Microbiol.* **31:**1886–1891.
23. **Hierholzer, J. C., K. H. Johansson, L. J. Anderson, C. J. Tsou, and P. E. Halonen.** 1987. Comparison of monoclonal time-resolved fluoroimmunoassay with monoclonal capture-biotinylated detector enzyme immunoassay for adenovirus antigen detection. *J. Clin. Microbiol.* **25:** 1662–1667.
24. **Hierholzer, J. C., Y. O. Stone, and J. R. Broderson.** 1991. Antigenic relationships among the 47 human adenoviruses determined in reference horse antisera. *Arch. Virol.* **121:** 179–197.
25. **Hierholzer, J. C., R. Wigand, L. J. Anderson, T. Adrian, and J. W. Gold.** 1988. Adenoviruses from patients with AIDS: a plethora of serotypes and a description of 5 new serotypes of subgenus D (types 43–47). *J. Infect. Dis.* **158:** 804–813.
26. **Hierholzer, J. C., R. Wigand, and J. C. de Jong.** 1988. Evaluation of human adenoviruses 38, 39, 40, and 41 as new serotypes. *Intervirology* **29:**1–10.

27. **Hirt, B.** 1967. Selective extraction of polyoma DNA from infected mouse cell cultures. *J. Mol. Biol.* **26:**365–369.
28. **Hyypiä, T.** 1985. Detection of adenovirus in nasopharyngeal specimens by radioactive and nonradioactive DNA probes. *J. Clin. Microbiol.* **21:**730–733.
29. **Jacobsson, P. Å., M. E. Johansson, and G. Wadell.** 1979. Identification of an enteric adenovirus by immunoelectroosmophoresis (IEOP) technique. *J. Med. Virol.* **3:**307–312.
30. **Johansson, M. E., M. Brown, J. C. Hierholzer, A. Thorner, H. Ushijima, and G. Wadell.** 1991. Genome analysis of adenovirus type 31 strains from immunocompromised and immunocompetent patients. *J. Infect. Dis.* **163:** 293–299.
31. **Kidd, A. H., E. H. Harley, and M. J. Erasmus.** 1985. Specific detection and typing of adenovirus type 40 and 41 in stool specimens by dot-blot hybridization. *J. Clin Microbiol.* **22:**934–939.
32. **Kidd, A. H., M. Jönsson, D. Garwicz, A. E. Kajon, A. G. Wermenbol, M. W. Verweij, and J. C. deJong.** 1996. Rapid subgenus identification of human adenovirus isolates by a general PCR. *J. Clin. Microbiol.* **34:**622–627.
33. **Leite, J. P., H. G. Pereira, R. S. Azeredo, and H. G. Schatzmayr.** 1985. Adenoviruses in faeces of children with acute gastroenteritis in Rio de Janeiro, Brazil. *J. Med. Virol.* **15:**203–209.
34. **Li, Q.-G., Q.-J. Zeng, Y-H. Liu, and G. Wadell.** 1996. Molecular epidemiology of adenovirus types 3 and 7 isolated from children with pneumonia in Beijing. *J. Med. Virol.* **49:**170–177.
35. **McDonough, M., O. Kew, and J. Hierholzer.** 1993. PCR detection of human adenoviruses, p. 389–393. *In* D. H. Persing, T. F. Smith, F. C. Tenover, and T. J. White (ed.), *Diagnostic Molecular Microbiology: Principles and Applications.* American Society for Microbiology, Washington, D.C.
36. **Meurman, O., O. Ruuskanen, and H. Sarkkinen.** 1983. Immunoassay diagnosis of adenovirus infections in children. *J. Clin. Microbiol.* **18:**1190–1195.
37. **Niel, C., S. A. Gomes, J. P. Leite, and H. G. Pereira.** 1986. Direct detection and differentiation of fastidious and nonfastidious adenoviruses in stools by using a specific nonradioactive probe. *J. Clin. Microbiol.* **24:**785–789.
38. **Norrby, E.** 1969. The structural and functional diversity of adenovirus capsid components. *J. Gen. Virol.* **5:**221–236.
39. **Pinto, A., R. Beck, and T. Jadavji.** 1992. Fatal neonatal pneumonia caused by adenovirus type 35. *Arch. Pathol. Lab. Med.* **116:**95–99.
40. **Puigh, M., J. Jofre, F. Lucena, A. Allard, G. Wadell, and R. Girones.** 1994. Detection of adenovirus and enterovirus in polluted waters by nested PCR amplification. *Appl. Microbiol.* **60:**2963–2970.
41. **Saitoh-Inagawa, W., A. Oshima, K. Aoki, N. Itoh, K. Isobe, E. Uchio, S. Ohno, H. Nakajima, K. Kara, and H. Ishiko.** 1996. Rapid diagnosis of adenoviral conjunctivitis by PCR and restriction fragment length polymorphism analysis. *J. Clin. Microbiol.* **34:**2113–2116.
42. **Schmitz, H., R. Wigand, and W. Heinrich.** 1983. Worldwide epidemiology of human adenovirus infections. *Am. J. Epidemiol.* **117:**455–466.
43. **Shinagawa, M., A. Matsuda, T. Ishigama, H. Goto, and G. Sato.** 1983. A rapid and simple method for preparation of adenovirus DNA from infected cells. *Microbiol. Immunol.* **27:**817–822.
44. **Sohier, R., Y. Chardonnet, and M. Prunieras.** 1965. Adenoviruses: status of current knowledge. *Prog. Med. Virol.* **7:**253–325.
45. **Stalder, H., J. C. Hierholzer, and M. N. Oxman.** 1977. New human adenovirus (candidate adenovirus type 35) causing fatal disseminated infection in a renal transplant recipient. *J. Clin. Microbiol.* **6:**257–265.
46. **Straube, R. C., M. A. Thompson, R. B. van Dyke, et al.** 1983. Adenovirus type-7b in a childrens hospital. *J. Infect. Dis.* **147:**814–819.
47. **Svensson, L., G. Wadell, I. Uhnoo, M. Johansson, and C.-H. VonBonsdorff.** 1983. Cross-reactivity between enteric adenoviruses and adenovirus type 4. Analysis of epitopes by solid phase immune electron microscopy. *J. Gen. Virol.* **64:**2517–2520.
48. **Takafuji, E. T., J. C. Gaydos, R. G. Allen, and F. H. Top.** 1979. Simultaneous administration of live, enteric-coated adenovirus types 4, 7, and 21 vaccines: safety and immunogenicity. *J. Infect. Dis.* **140:**48–53.
49. **Trabelsi, A., B. Pozzetto, A. D. Mbida, F. Grattard, A. Ros, and O. G. Gaudin.** 1992. Evaluation of four methods for rapid detection of adenovirus. *Eur. J. Clin. Microbiol. Infect. Dis.* **11:**535–539.
50. **Uhnoo, I., G. Wadell, L. Svensson, and M. Johansson.** 1984. Importance of enteric adenoviruses Ad40 and Ad41 in acute gastroenteritis in infants and young children. *J. Clin. Microbiol.* **20:**365–372.
51. **van der Avoort, H. G., A. G. Wermenbol, T. P. Zomerdijk, J. A. Kleijne, J. A. van Asten, P. Jensma, A. D. Osterhaus, A. H. Kidd, and J. C. de Jong.** 1989. Characterization of fastidious adenovirus types 40 and 41 by DNA restriction enzyme analysis and by neutralizing monoclonal antibodies. *Virus Res.* **12:**139–158.
52. **Wadell, G.** 1969. Hemagglutination with adenovirus serotypes belonging to Rosen's subgroups II and III. *Proc. Soc. Exp. Biol. Med.* **132:**413–421.
53. **Wadell, G.** 1984. Molecular epidemiology of human adenoviruses. *Curr. Top. Microbiol. Immunol.* **110:**191–220.
54. **Wadell, G.** 1988. *Adenoviridae*: the adenoviruses, p. 284–300. *In* E. H. Lennette, P. Halonen, and F. A. Murphy (ed.), *Laboratory Diagnosis of Infectious Diseases: Principles and Practice,* vol. II. *Viral, Rickettsial, and Chlamydial Diseases.* Springer-Verlag, New York, N.Y.
55. **Wadell, G.** 1987. Adenoviruses, p. 251–274. *In* A. J. Zuckerman, J. E. Banatvala, and J. E. Pattison (ed.), *Principles and Practices of Clinical Virology*. John Wiley & Sons, Inc., New York, N.Y.
56. **Wadell, G., A. Allard, M. Johansson, L. Svensson, and I. Uhnoo.** 1994. Enteric adenoviruses, p. 519–545. *In* A. Z. Kapikian (ed.), *Virus Infections of the Gastrointestinal Tract,* 2nd ed. Marcel Dekker, Inc., New York, N.Y.
57. **Wadell, G., M. L. Hammarskjöld, and T. Varsanyi.** 1973. Incomplete virus particles of adenovirus type 16. *J. Gen. Virol.* **20:**287–302.
58. **Wadell, G., M. L. Hammarskjöld, G. Winberg, T. Varsanyi, and G. Sundell.** 1980. Genetic variability of adenoviruses. *Ann. N. Y. Acad. Sci.* **354:**16–42.
59. **Warren, D., K. E. Nelson, J. A. Farrar, E. Hurwitz, J. Hierholzer, E. Ford, and L. J. Anderson.** 1989. A large outbreak of epidemic keratoconjunctivitis: Problems in controlling nosocomial spread. *J. Infect. Dis.* **160:** 938–943.
60. **Webb, D. H., A. F. Shields, and K. H. Fife.** 1987. Genomic variation of adenovirus type 5 isolates recovered from bone marrow transplant recipients. *J. Clin. Microbiol.* **25:** 305–308.
61. **Wigand, R., N. Sehn, J. C. Hierholzer, J. C. de Jong, and T. Adrian.** 1985. Immunological and biochemical characterization of human adenoviruses from subgenus B. I. Antigenic relationships. *Arch. Virol.* **84:**63–78.
62. **Wishart, P. K., C. James, M. S. Wishart, and S. Darougar.** 1984. Prevalence of acute conjunctivitis caused by chlamydia, adenovirus, and herpes simplex virus in an ophthalmic casualty department. *Br. J. Ophthalmol.* **68:**653–655.

Rhinoviruses

MARIE L. LANDRY

77

CLINICAL BACKGROUND

The rhinovirus group derives its name from the predominant site of its replication and symptomatology, the nose. The rhinovirus group constitutes the major virus group associated with the acute respiratory illness known as the common cold. The average person suffers two to five colds per year, and one-third to one-half of these are due to rhinoviruses. Although the common cold is generally a trivial illness, it is acutely disabling. The cost of the common cold in terms of days lost from work, cold remedies, and analgesics is in the billions of dollars.

In 1930 it was first recognized that the common cold was caused by a "filtrable agent" (20). With the development of cell culture techniques in the 1950s, rhinovirus was first isolated (4, 50, 52). Use of the more sensitive human embryonic lung cell culture and growth conditions that mimicked those of the nose led to the isolation of a number of different serologic types in the 1960s. In 1967 serotypes 1A to 55 were designated, in 1971 serotypes 56 to 89 were designated, and in 1987 serotypes 90 to 100 were designated (33).

In temperate zones, rhinovirus infections peak in September and show a second peak in the spring, yet they continue to cause colds throughout the summer. Prevalent serotypes change from year to year, with multiple types circulating in a given area at any time. A minority of serotypes appear to be responsible for a majority of illnesses. Earlier studies suggested that serotypes with lower numbers were being gradually replaced by serotypes with higher numbers or strains that could not be typed. It was postulated that this situation represented either recirculation of a large number of antigenically stable types or antigenic drift. More recent studies of rhinovirus strains have found that most isolates have already been identified (33, 43). Nevertheless, antigenic variants have been detected for several serotypes and can be induced in the laboratory (49, 55).

Rhinovirus infections are spread from person to person by virus-contaminated respiratory secretions. Although transmission of rhinovirus colds among adult volunteers can be interrupted with the use of products such as virucidal tissues, the exact mode of transmission of rhinoviruses has been the subject of some controversy. Studies with volunteers have shown that inoculation of virus into the nose or conjunctiva is the most efficient way to initiate infection (21). Rhinovirus is present in highest titers in the nose and commonly contaminates the hands of infected persons. Some investigators have found that the virus can be transmitted to others by hand-to-hand contact, followed by self-inoculation of virus into the nose or conjunctiva (6, 30). Nevertheless, a recent study found that rhinovirus transmission, at least in adults, occurred primarily by the aerosol route (19).

From studies with volunteers, the incubation period for rhinoviruses after inoculation has been found to be 2 or 3 days. The peak of virus shedding coincides with acute rhinitis. Virus may become undetectable by 4 or 5 days or may be present in low titers for up to 2 weeks. Nasal epithelial cells are infected and are shed into nasal mucus. However, the symptoms of rhinovirus infection are produced in part by chemical mediators of inflammation (31, 45). Symptoms persist for 7 days on average and include profuse watery discharge, nasal congestion, sneezing, headache, mild sore throat, cough, and little or no fever. Psychological stress appears to increase both the susceptibility to rhinovirus infection and the development of clinical symptoms (16), whereas exposure to a cold environment does not (23).

Infection of the lower respiratory tract can also occur (28), especially in the very young (54), the elderly (46), and those with chronic illnesses (39) or underlying pulmonary disease (15). In fact, the clinical manifestations of rhinovirus infections in hospitalized children are indistinguishable from those caused by respiratory syncytial virus (37). Rhinovirus infections have been shown to exacerbate chronic bronchitis and asthma, and a fatal case in an asthmatic infant, with isolation of virus from lung and blood postmortem, has been reported (40). The mechanism of rhinovirus-induced airway hyperresponsiveness is currently the subject of intensive study (24, 29). Rhinoviruses have also been associated with otitis media and sinusitis (57). Immunity is type specific and correlates best with the local production of immunoglobulin A (IgA) (10, 14).

DESCRIPTION OF THE AGENT

The *Picornaviridae* family is comprised of five genera, including three that are pathogenic for humans: *Enterovirus*, *Hepatovirus*, and *Rhinovirus*. The rhinovirus virion consists of a nonenveloped icosahedral nucleocapsid, 20 to 27 nm in diameter, with 60 protomeric units consisting of four protein subunits, VP1, VP2, VP3, and VP4. These structural polypeptides are obtained by posttranslational cleavage of a large polypeptide precursor (3). VP1, VP2, and VP3 reside on the exterior of the virus and make up its protein coat. VP4 resides inside the protein shell of the virion. The virion nucleic acid is single-stranded, positive-sense RNA, approximately 7,200 nucleotides in length, with a molecular mass of 2.4×10^6 Da. Rhinovirus genomes have been sequenced and have been found to show 45 to 62% homology with poliovirus genomes (13). Rhinovirus replicates in the cytoplasm of infected cells, producing infectious virions that sediment at a buoyant density of 1.40 g/liter in cesium chloride. Empty capsids and particles lacking one or more structural polypeptides are also produced. Infectious and noninfectious particles are immunologically distinct (42).

As they have no lipid envelope, rhinoviruses are resistant to inactivation by organic solvents, such as ether, chloroform, ethanol, and 5% phenol. Although rhinoviruses are relatively thermostable, heating at 50 to 56°C progressively decreases infectivity, as virions become empty capsids. Rhinoviruses are differentiated from enteroviruses by their loss of infectivity upon exposure to pH 3 for 3 h at room temperature. After mild acid inactivation (pH 5), two types of particles, A particles, which lack VP4, and B particles, which lack both VP4 and RNA, are formed.

At present, 100 rhinovirus serotypes have been designated on the basis of neutralization tests. There is no group antigen, but by use of high-titered hyperimmune rabbit and guinea pig antisera, cross-reactions between antigenic types have been detected (17). As a result, 50 serotypes have been categorized into 16 subgroups (49). Treatment with low pH, heat, or 2 M urea also produces virus particles that react with heterologous antisera (42).

X-ray crystallography and cryoelectron microscopy studies have found that the large depressions, or "canyons," found on each of the 60 protomeric units are sites for cell receptor binding (48, 53). Conformational changes in the canyon floor can be produced by certain antiviral agents, thus inhibiting virus attachment to cells or virus uncoating (38, 51).

Rhinoviruses can be divided into three groups based on binding to cell receptors (1, 59). Intercellular adhesion molecule 1 (ICAM-1) is the cell receptor for the majority (major group) of rhinoviruses, or approximately 90% of the serotypes. ICAM-1 is a member of the immunoglobulin supergene family and may be expressed on the surface of many different cells, including those that are active in respiratory tract immune responses (60). The natural ligand for ICAM-1 is lymphocyte function-associated antigen (LFA-1), and since the binding sites for LFA-1 and rhinovirus overlap, rhinovirus may block ICAM-1–LFA-1 binding on leukocytes and disrupt local airway immune responses. It has been postulated that this process may be a factor in the pathogenesis of secondary viral or bacterial respiratory tract infections (27). Less is known about the minor-group receptor, which has been tentatively identified as a 120-kDa cell surface protein of unknown function. Rhinovirus serotype 87 appears to utilize neither the major-group nor the minor-group receptor.

Based on antiviral susceptibility, rhinoviruses have been divided into two groups, A and B, which do not coincide with receptor classifications. Rather, serotypes within each group show sequence homologies with VP1 and the antiviral binding site (5).

COLLECTION AND STORAGE OF SPECIMENS

In natural infections, rhinovirus can be isolated from 1 day before to 6 days after the onset of cold symptoms but is shed in highest concentrations on day 1 or 2 of illness. Since rhinovirus is excreted in highest titers from the nose, nasal rather than throat specimens should be obtained for virus isolation. Likewise, sputum is a low-yield specimen for the isolation of rhinovirus. Comparisons of nasal wash, nasal swab, throat gargle, and throat swab specimens for the isolation of rhinovirus from clinical specimens revealed nasal wash to be the best (3, 8, 14). Nasal wash specimens are obtained as follows. Tilt the patient's head backward and instill 1 ml of sterile phosphate-buffered saline into one of the nostrils. Ask the patient to lean forward and allow the washing to drip into a sterile petri dish or other collection container. Repeat with the other nostril until each nostril has been washed with 5 ml of phosphate-buffered saline. Transfer the washings into a sterile container with an equal volume of viral transport media (VTM) containing antibiotics; the inclusion of phenol red in VTM allows the detection of an acid pH, which would adversely affect the isolation of rhinovirus.

If a nasal wash specimen cannot be obtained, a combination of a nasal or nasopharyngeal swab specimen and a throat swab specimen should be collected. The swabs should be immersed in a vial containing 2 ml of VTM.

Specimens should be transported promptly to the laboratory. Best results are obtained with rapid inoculation of cell cultures; however, specimens can be kept for 24 to 48 h at 4°C in VTM at a neutral pH. If longer delays are necessary, specimens should be frozen at −70°C and thawed just prior to inoculation. Freezing does not appear to be detrimental to virus recovery (8).

DIRECT EXAMINATION

Due to the large number of rhinovirus serotypes and the lack of a group antigen, it has been difficult to develop tests for the direct detection of viral antigen in clinical specimens. Enzyme immunoassays (EIAs) with polyclonal antisera to two different human rhinoviruses have been developed for the detection of rhinovirus directly in clinical specimens and after overnight amplification in cell cultures (18). A number of stock viruses of different serotypes were cross-reactive to various degrees in these EIA systems. However, when clinical specimens from volunteers infected with homologous virus were tested, correlations with virus isolation were disappointing: 89% for culture-amplified and 67% for direct EIA techniques. Subsequently, an EIA-based receptor binding system utilizing biotinylated soluble ICAM-1 for detection of the major subgroup of rhinoviruses was developed; tests with stock viruses revealed a detection limit of 10^3 50% tissue culture infective doses ($TCID_{50}$) (41).

Since a high degree of homology exists in the 5′-noncoding regions of picornavirus genomes, recent emphasis has been placed on nucleic acid detection methods. However, cross-reactions between enteroviruses and rhinoviruses can occur. In situ hybridization has been useful in localizing rhinovirus replication in the respiratory tract for research studies (7). Unfortunately, hybridization techniques have been relatively insensitive for the detection of rhinovirus in nasal washings (2, 12).

PCR has shown the most promise for direct detection. With an initial reverse transcriptase step to generate cDNA, PCR can detect picornaviruses in clinical material with a sensitivity equivalent to or greater than that of culturing (25, 36, 47). With the use of appropriate primers, rhinovirus can also be differentiated from enterovirus based on the sizes of their respective PCR products by simple gel electrophoresis (47). Unfortunately, primers that are able to distinguish rhinovirus from enterovirus may not be the most sensitive for the detection of rhinovirus in clinical specimens (36). Another approach consists of PCR followed by liquid-phase hybridization and quantitative adsorption of hybrids onto microtiter wells (32). This method makes use of primers found to be highly sensitive for picornavirus detection, followed by a hybridization step specific for rhinoviruses. Although promising, these amplification techniques remain research tools at present.

ISOLATION OF VIRUS

Cell Culture

Rhinoviruses are best isolated in sensitive cell culture systems and grow only in cells of human or monkey origin. Although rhinoviruses were originally isolated in primary monkey kidney cells, these cells have not been consistent in yielding a broad range of isolates. The use of sensitive human embryonic lung fibroblast (HELF) strains has provided superior results. Rhinoviruses were originally separated into M and H strains based on their ability to replicate in monkey and human cells (M strains replicate in both monkey and human cells, whereas H strains replicate only in human cells). However, this distinction is no longer used, since H strains can be adapted to grow in monkey cells.

The most commonly used cells in clinical laboratories are HELF strains WI-38 and MRC-5. WI-38 cells are significantly more sensitive than MRC-5 cells (8), but MRC-5 cells are more commonly available in clinical laboratories. Human embryonic kidney cells can also support rhinovirus replication. Several HeLa cell clones, such as HeLa M, Ohio HeLa, HeLa H, HeLa R-19, and HeLa I cells, support the replication of rhinoviruses to high titers and have been used in research studies and to prepare rhinovirus antigens (1, 3, 8). A human fetal tonsil cell line was initially reported to be more sensitive than MRC-5 and HeLa cells for rhinovirus isolation (26). However, HeLa I cells were recently found to be more sensitive than WI-38, MRC-5, fetal tonsil, HeLa H, or HeLa M cells for the recovery of rhinovirus from clinical specimens (8). Unfortunately, different lots of normally sensitive cell lines have been found to vary over 100-fold in sensitivity to rhinovirus (11); the reasons for this variation are not known. Therefore, for optimal results, simultaneous use of several sensitive systems is recommended.

After inoculation, cultures are incubated in a standard cell culture medium, such as Eagle's minimum essential medium with 2% fetal calf serum and antibiotics, at a neutral pH. It is important that culture conditions mimic those of the nose; cultures should be incubated at 33°C with continuous rotation in a roller drum to provide aeration of the monolayer. Cytopathic effect (CPE) can be observed as early as 24 to 48 h after inoculation and is often detected by day 4. Passage of infected HeLa cell cultures may be necessary for some isolates before CPE is apparent. Cellular changes are easier to read in fibroblasts and are often detected earlier in these cells than in epithelial cell lines. Both large and small rounded, refractile cells with pyknotic nuclei are observed in foci that also contain cellular debris (Fig. 1). Rhinovirus CPE is similar to enterovirus CPE but may sometimes be confused with nonspecific changes. The CPE progress over a 2- or 3-day period, with the degree of cellular change depending on the serotype and the inoculum dose. It should be noted that rhinovirus CPE can regress or that virus may become inactivated if left too long. Therefore, cultures should be promptly passaged. Passage is also necessary to increase virus titers prior to the performance of identification tests.

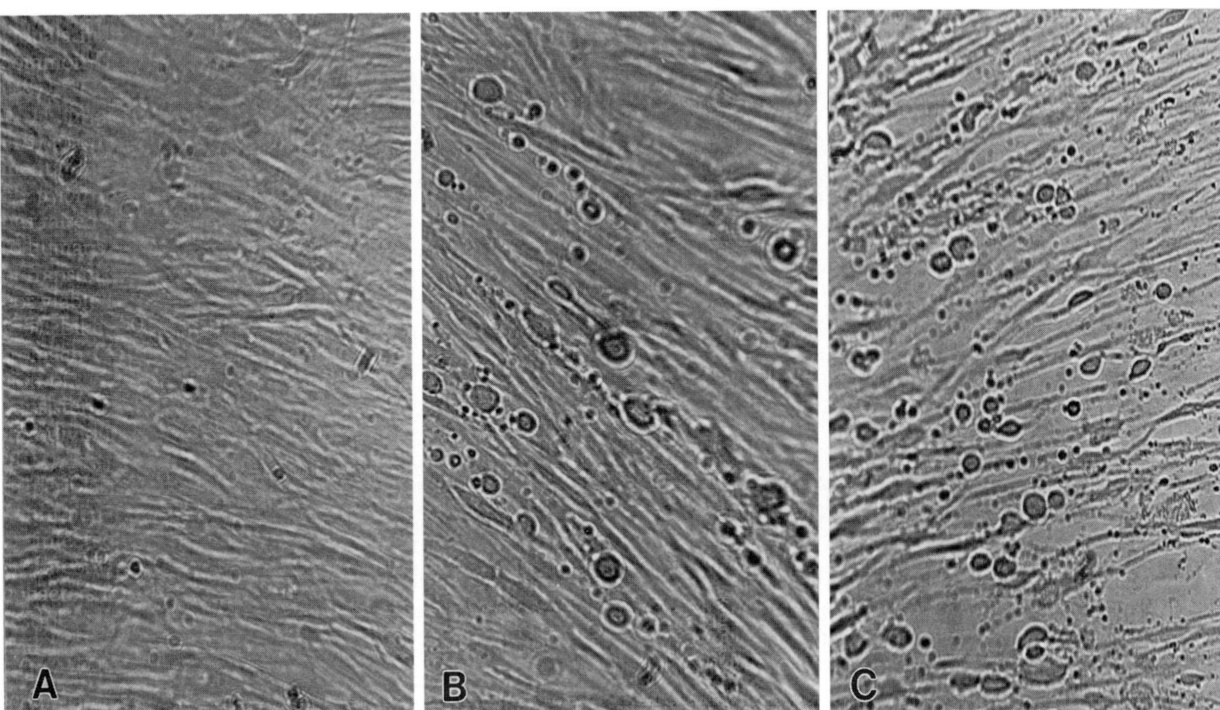

FIGURE 1 Rhinovirus CPE in HELF. (A) Uninfected cells. (B) Early focus of rhinovirus CPE. (C) More advanced rhinovirus CPE. Magnification, ×100.

HELF cell cultures should be observed for 14 days, with refeeding at 7 days to increase recovery of virus. HeLa cell cultures can be observed for only up to 7 or 8 days, when passage becomes necessary due to nonspecific cell degeneration and rounding.

Organ Culture

Organ cultures of human fetal nasal epithelium or trachea have been used to isolate rhinoviruses not grown in standard cell cultures. For optimal recovery, both organ cultures and standard cell culture systems are necessary. Due to the limited supply of fetal material, however, this method is not widely used. Details of the procedure have been reviewed elsewhere (3). In brief, pieces of nasal epithelium or trachea are incubated in culture tubes at 33°C in a roller drum, examined daily for ciliary activity, and monitored for pH changes. If rhinovirus is replicating, ciliary activity ceases within 5 to 7 days. Virus can be harvested in supernatant fluids and passaged to fresh organ cultures or cell cultures.

IDENTIFICATION OF VIRUS

A presumptive diagnosis of a rhinovirus isolate is made by the appearance and progression of characteristic CPE in the appropriate clinical setting. Further identification of a virus isolate requires confirmation of the properties of rhinovirus, such as sensitivity to temperature and an acid pH and resistance to lipid solvents. Prior to the performance of these tests, passage of isolates is necessary to obtain a minimum titer of 10^3 $TCID_{50}$/ml. For routine viral diagnostic laboratories, these tests are sufficient (Fig. 2). Since 100 rhinovirus serotypes have been identified and no group antigen has

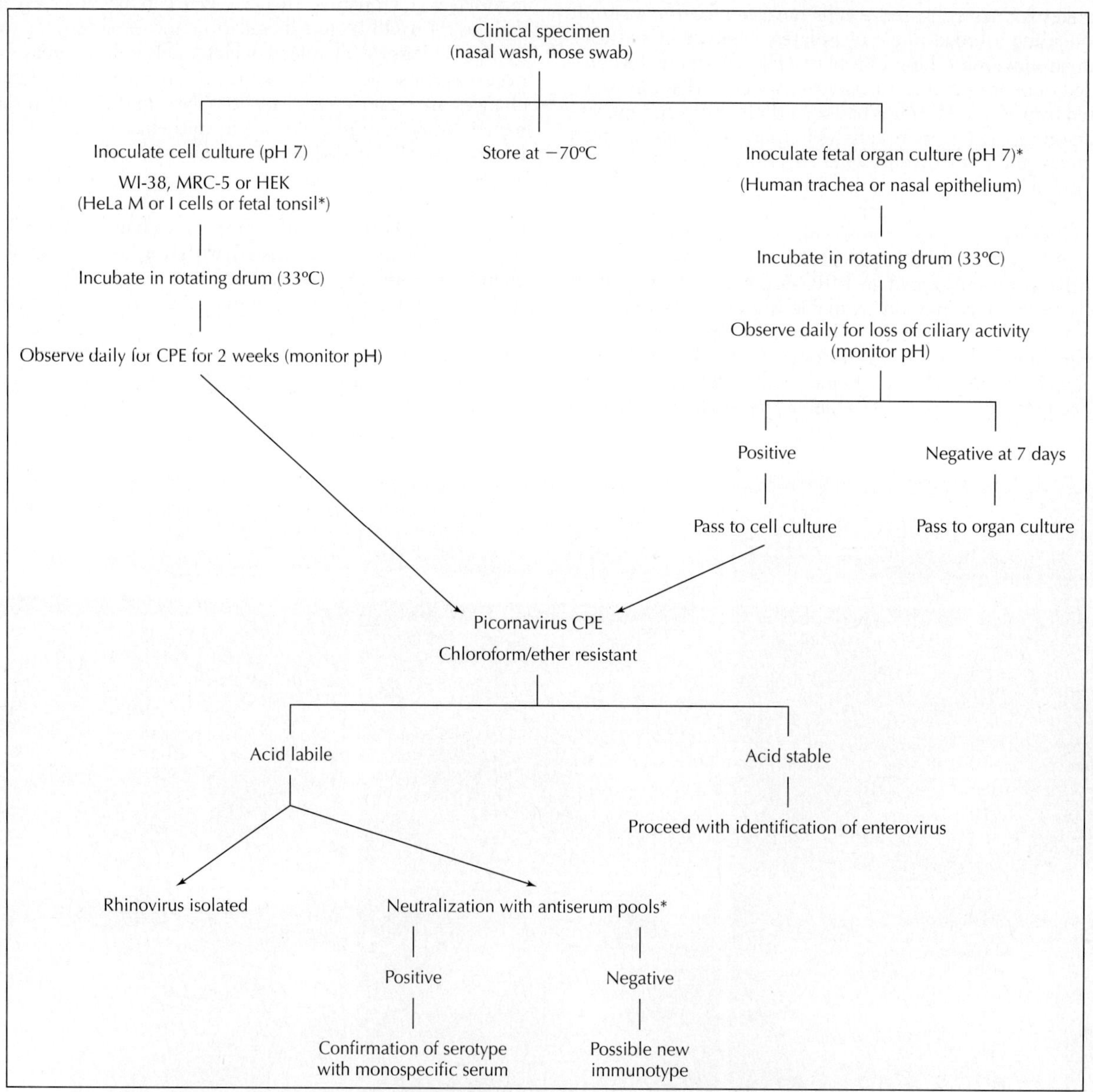

FIGURE 2 Flow scheme for the isolation and identification of rhinovirus. Techniques usually reserved for the research laboratory are marked by an asterisk. HEK, human embryonic kidney cells.

been found, specific serotype identification by neutralization is very time-consuming and costly and is not routinely available, even in research settings. Further confirmation of the identity of presumptive rhinovirus isolates may be obtained by genotypic analysis in research laboratories but is otherwise not available.

Acid pH Stability

Rhinoviruses are sensitive to a low pH, whereas enteroviruses are stable. Thus, a reduction in virus titer by 2 to 3 $\log_{10}$ $TCID_{50}$ can be expected upon exposure of rhinovirus to a low pH. First, prepare two solutions of a buffer, such as HEPES, one at pH 3.0 and one at pH 7.0. Add 0.2 ml of unknown virus suspension to 1.8 ml of pH 3.0 HEPES and 0.2 ml of virus to 1.8 ml of pH 7.0 HEPES. Keep the mixtures at room temperature for 3 h; then adjust the pH to 7.0, make serial dilutions of the mixtures, and inoculate the dilutions into cell cultures. If the unknown virus is a rhinovirus, a minimum 2 $\log_{10}$ reduction in virus titer should be evident in the acid-treated sample. A known rhinovirus and a known enterovirus should be treated in a similar fashion as controls.

Resistance to Lipid Solvents

Since rhinoviruses lack a lipid envelope, they are resistant to treatment with lipid solvents, such as chloroform or ether, and infectivity titers should not be affected. Add 0.1 ml of chloroform to 1 ml of isolate, shake the mixture vigorously for 10 min, and centrifuge the mixture at $1,000 \times g$ for 5 to 10 min. Remove the top (or aqueous) phase, prepare serial dilutions, and inoculate the dilutions into cell cultures. Alternatively, add 0.2 ml of diethyl ether to 0.8 ml of isolate in a stoppered tube and shake the mixture vigorously. Allow the mixture to react at room temperature for 1 to 2 h; shake the tube intermittently. Transfer the mixture into an open glass petri dish in a fume hood and allow the ether to evaporate. Prepare serial dilutions and inoculate them into cell cultures.

An equal volume of unknown virus should be processed in a similar manner but not treated with chloroform or ether. A known picornavirus and a chloroform-sensitive virus, such as herpes simplex virus, should also be included as controls. The picornavirus should be unaffected, and the herpes simplex virus should be completely inactivated.

Temperature Sensitivity

Since rhinoviruses grow best at 33°C, they can be distinguished from enteroviruses by inoculation of serial dilutions of the unknown virus and incubation of one set of cultures at 33°C and a replicate set of cultures at 37°C. The onset of CPE should be more rapid and the titer of virus obtained should be higher at the lower temperature.

Neutralization Tests

Specific identification of rhinoviruses by serotyping is an expensive and labor-intensive procedure that is rarely performed. Hyperimmune antisera for types 1A to 100 are available through the American Type Culture Collection. Intersecting serum pools similar to those used for enterovirus identification have been prepared, and isolates are usually tested in a microneutralization procedure to conserve reagents. Serotype confirmation is then performed with monospecific antiserum. Neutralization generally involves the neutralization of 30 to 100 $TCID_{50}$ of virus-induced CPE by 20 U of antiserum. Nontypeable isolates are occasionally found. Detailed procedures are described elsewhere (3).

Other Tests

EIAs that can detect rhinovirus antigens in cell cultures have been developed (18). Nucleic acid hybridization techniques can also be used for the identification of rhinovirus isolates in cell cultures (2); however, cross-reactions with enteroviruses can occur. When appropriate primers are used, PCR can distinguish rhinoviruses from enteroviruses and has been found to be equivalent to acid sensitivity testing in accuracy and cheaper in terms of reagent costs (9). PCR has also been used successfully to type a limited number of serotypes (56).

SEROLOGIC DIAGNOSIS

Although detection of an increase in antibody to rhinovirus in natural infections may detect many infections not diagnosed by virus isolation (35), the number of possible serotypes makes blind serologic testing impractical at present. However, if a virus isolate has been recovered, the patient's serum can be tested against that isolate.

The standard serologic assay to measure antibody in serum or nasal wash specimens is the neutralization test (22). For maximum sensitivity, a low challenge dose (3 to 30 $TCID_{50}$) should be used. Plaque reduction neutralization has also been used. Complement fixation detects heterotypic antibody responses to rhinoviruses and enteroviruses and does not parallel neutralization results. Hemagglutination inhibition has also been used but is not as sensitive as neutralization, and not all rhinoviruses react with erythrocytes.

EIAs with human rhinovirus (HRV)-EL and HRV-2 antigens have been used to detect serum and nasal IgG and IgA in volunteers inoculated with these two viruses (10). The EIAs were 100 to 10,000 times more sensitive than neutralization. The problem of detecting antibodies to multiple serotypes in natural infections has not been addressed.

ANTIVIRAL SUSCEPTIBILITY

Many antiviral agents show activity against rhinoviruses in the laboratory, yet inadequate drug delivery to the site of infection has reduced clinical benefit in patients. Thus, treatment of rhinovirus infections is still experimental. Recent studies have included intranasal administration of soluble ICAM-1 in rhinovirus-infected volunteers, use of either intranasal ipratropium bromide (an anticholinergic agent) or zinc gluconate lozenges in natural colds, or administration of antiviral and antimediator agents in combination (31, 34, 44, 58). The usefulness of these approaches requires further study and validation.

EVALUATION, INTERPRETATION, AND REPORTING OF RESULTS

The laboratory diagnosis of rhinovirus infection is currently based upon the isolation of virus with characteristic CPE in cell systems sensitive for isolation, such as HELF, human embryonic kidney, and HeLa cells. Incubation at 33°C and rotation of cultures provide optimal conditions for virus replication. Differentiation of rhinoviruses from enteroviruses, with which their CPE can be confused, is based primarily on acid stability testing of isolates. Rhinoviruses are inactivated by pH 3 to 5, whereas enteroviruses are unaffected. Sensitivity to temperature and resistance to organic solvents are additional features of rhinovirus isolates. Specific identification of rhinovirus serotypes by neutralization tests is reserved for epidemiologic or research studies.

At present in the clinical laboratory, rhinoviruses are rarely specifically sought and optimal conditions for rhinovirus isolation are not generally used. Since there is no treatment, specimens from outpatients with the common cold are rarely cultured. Rather, rhinoviruses are isolated when the clinical diagnosis is influenza or respiratory syncytial virus. However, if specific therapy becomes available, this situation will change.

Serologic assays for antibody to rhinovirus are also not performed outside the research setting but can provide useful information in studies of viral pathogenesis and immunity.

Because of the tremendous economic cost of rhinovirus infections, much work is being done to understand their pathogenesis and develop treatment. Thus, the development of rapid and accurate diagnostic tests in the research setting should prove useful to the clinical laboratory in the near future.

REFERENCES

1. **Abraham, G., and R. J. Colonno.** 1984. Many rhinovirus serotypes share the same cellular receptor. *J. Virol.* **51:** 340–345.
2. **Al-Nakib, W., G. Stanway, M. Forsyth, P. J. Hughes, J. W. Almond, and D. A. Tyrrell.** 1986. Detection of human rhinoviruses and their molecular relationships using cDNA probes. *J. Med. Virol.* **20:**289–296.
3. **Al-Nakib, W., and D. A. J. Tyrrell.** 1988. Picornaviridae: rhinoviruses—common cold viruses, p. 723–742. *In* E. H. Lennette, P. Halonen, and F. A. Murphy (ed.), *Laboratory Diagnosis of Infectious Diseases: Principles and Practice*, vol. 2. Springer-Verlag, New York, N.Y.
4. **Andrewes, C. H., D. M. Chaproneiri, A. E. H. Gompels, H. G. Pereira, and A. T. Roden.** 1953. Propagation of common cold virus in tissue cultures. *Lancet* **i:**546–547.
5. **Andries, K., B. Dewindt, J. Snoeks, L. Wouters, H. Moereels, P. J. Lewis, and P. A. Janssen.** 1990. Two groups of rhinoviruses revealed by a panel of antiviral compounds present sequence divergence and differential pathogenicity. *J. Virol.* **64:**1117–1123.
6. **Ansari, S. A., V. S. Springthorpe, S. A. Sattar, S. Rivard, and M. Rahman.** 1991. Potential role of hands in the spread of respiratory viral infections: studies with human parainfluenza virus 3 and rhinovirus 14. *J. Clin. Microbiol.* **29:**2115–2119.
7. **Arruda, E., T. R. Boyle, B. Winther, D. C. Pevear, J. M. Gwaltney, Jr., and F. G. Hayden.** 1995. Localization of human rhinovirus replication in the upper respiratory tract by in situ hybridization. *J. Infect. Dis.* **171:** 1329–1333.
8. **Arruda, E., C. E. Crump, B. S. Rollins, A. Ohlin, and F. G. Hayden.** 1996. Comparative susceptibilities of human embryonic fibroblasts and HeLa cells for isolation of human rhinoviruses. *J. Clin. Microbiol.* **34:**1277–1279.
9. **Atmar, R. L., and P. R. Georghiou.** 1993. Classification of respiratory tract picornavirus isolates as enteroviruses or rhinoviruses by using reverse transcription-polymerase chain reaction. *J. Clin. Microbiol.* **31:**2544–2546.
10. **Barclay, W. S., and W. Al-Nakib.** 1987. An ELISA for the detection of rhinovirus specific antibody in serum and nasal secretion. *J. Virol. Methods* **15:**53–64.
11. **Brown, P. K., and D. A. J. Tyrrell.** 1964. Experiments on the sensitivity of strains of human fibroblasts to infection with rhinovirus. *Br. J. Exp. Pathol.* **45:**571–578.
12. **Bruce, C. B., W. Al-Nakib, J. W. Almond, and D. A. J. Tyrrell.** 1989. Use of synthetic oligonucleotide probes to detect rhinovirus RNA. *Arch. Virol.* **105:**179–187.
13. **Callahan, P. L., S. Mizutani, and R. J. Colonno.** 1985. Molecular cloning and complete sequence determination of RNA genome of human rhinovirus type 14. *Proc. Natl. Acad. Sci. USA* **82:**732–736.
14. **Cate, T. R., R. B. Couch, and K. M. Johnson.** 1964. Studies with rhinovirus in volunteers; production of illness, effect of naturally acquired antibody, and demonstration of a protective effect not associated with serum antibody. *J. Clin. Invest.* **43:**56–67.
15. **Chidekel, A. S., C. L. Rosen, and A. R. Bazzy.** 1997. Rhinovirus infection associated with serious lower respiratory illness in patients with bronchopulmonary dysplasia. *Pediatr. Infect. Dis. J.* **16:**43–47.
16. **Cohen, S., and D. A. J. Tyrrell.** 1991. Psychological stress and susceptibility to the common cold. *N. Engl. J. Med.* **325:**606–612.
17. **Couch, R. B.** 1996. Rhinoviruses, p. 713–734. *In* B. N. Fields, D. M. Knipe, and P. M. Howley (ed.), *Fields Virology*, 3rd ed. Raven Press, New York, N.Y.
18. **Dearden, C. J., and W. Al-Nakib.** 1987. Direct detection of rhinoviruses by an enzyme-linked immunosorbent assay. *J. Med. Virol.* **23:**179–189.
19. **Dick, E. C., L. C. Jennings, K. A. Mink, C. D. Wartgow, and S. L. Inhorn.** 1987. Aerosol transmission of rhinovirus colds. *J. Infect. Dis.* **156:**442–448.
20. **Dochez, A. R., G. S. Shibley, and K. C. Mills.** 1930. Studies of the common cold. IV. Experimental transmission of the common cold to anthropoid apes and human beings by means of a filtrable agent. *J. Exp. Med.* **52:** 701–716.
21. **Douglas, R. G., Jr.** 1970. Pathogenesis of rhinovirus common colds in human volunteers. *Ann. Otol. Rhinol. Laryngol.* **79:**563–571.
22. **Douglas, R. G., Jr., W. F. Fleet, T. R. Cate, and R. B. Couch.** 1968. Antibody to rhinovirus in human sera. I. Standardization of a neutralization test. *Proc. Soc. Exp. Biol. Med.* **127:**497–502.
23. **Douglas, R. G., Jr., K. M. Lindgren, and R. B. Couch.** 1968. Exposure to cold environment and rhinovirus common cold. Failure to demonstrate effect. *N. Engl. J. Med.* **127:**497–502.
24. **Einarsson, O., R. B. Geba, M. Landry, Z. Zhu, and J. A. Elias.** 1996. Stimulation of interleukin-11 *in vivo* and *in vitro* by respiratory viruses and induction of airways hyperresponsiveness. *J. Clin. Invest.* **97:**915–924.
25. **Gama, R. E., P. R. Horsnell, P. J. Hughes, C. Northm, C. B. Bruce, W. Al-Nakib, and G. Stanway.** 1989. Amplification of rhinovirus specific nucleic acids from clinical material using the polymerase chain reaction. *J. Med. Virol.* **28:**73–77.
26. **Geist, F. C., and F. G. Hayden.** 1985. Comparative susceptibilities of strain MRC-5 human embryonic lung fibroblast cells and the Cooney strain of human fetal tonsil cells for isolation of rhinoviruses from clinical specimens. *J. Clin. Microbiol.* **22:**455–456.
27. **Gern, J. E., B. Joseph, D. M. Galagan, W. R. Borcherding, and E. C. Dick.** 1996. Rhinovirus inhibits antigen-specific T cell proliferation through an intercellular adhesion molecule-1-dependent mechanism. *J. Infect. Dis.* **174:** 1143–1150.
28. **Gern, J. E., D. M. Galagan, N. N. Jarjour, E. C. Dick, and W. W. Busse.** 1997. Detection of rhinovirus RNA in lower airway cells during experimentally induced infection. *Am. J. Respir. Crit. Care Med.* **155:**1159–1161.
29. **Grunberg, K., M. C. Timmers, H. H. Smits, E. P. de**

Klerk, E. C. Dick, W. J. Spaan, P. S. Hienstra, and P. J. Sterk. 1997. Effect of experimental rhinovirus colds on airway hyperresponsiveness to histamine and interleukin-8 in nasal lavage in asthmatic subjects in vivo. *Clin. Exp. Allergy* **27:**36–45.

30. **Gwaltney, J. M., Jr., P. B. Moskalski, and J. O. Hendley.** 1978. Hand-to-hand transmission of rhinovirus colds. *Ann. Intern. Med.* **88:**463–467.
31. **Gwaltney, J. M., Jr.** 1992. Combined antiviral and antimediator treatment of rhinovirus colds. *J. Infect. Dis.* **166:** 776–782.
32. **Halonen, P., E. Rocha, J. Hierholzer, B. Holloway, T. Hyypia, P. Hurskainen, and M. Pallansch.** 1995. Detection of enteroviruses and rhinoviruses in clinical specimens by PCR and liquid-phase hybridization. *J. Clin. Microbiol.* **33:**648–653.
33. **Hamparian, V. V., R. J. Colonno, M. K. Cooney, E. C. Dick, J. M. Gwaltney, Jr., J. H. Hughes, W. S. Jordan, Jr., A. Z. Kapikian, W. J. Mogabgab, A. Monto, C. A. Phillips, R. R. Rueckert, J. H. Schieble, E. J. Stott, and D. A. J. Tyrrell.** 1987. A collaborative report: rhinoviruses—extension of the numbering system from 89 to 100. *Virology* **159:**191–192.
34. **Hayden, F. G., L. Diamond, P. B. Wood, D. C. Korts, and M. T. Wecher.** 1996. Effectiveness and safety of intranasal ipratropium bromide in common colds. *Ann. Intern. Med.* **125:**89–97.
35. **Hendley, J. O., J. M. Gwaltney, Jr., and W. S. Jordan, Jr.** 1969. Rhinovirus infections in an industrial population. IV. Infections within families of employees during two fall peaks of respiratory illness. *Am. J. Epidemiol.* **89:**184–196.
36. **Johnston, S. L., G. Sanderson, P. K. Pattemore, S. Smith, P. G. Vardin, C. B. Bruce, P. R. Lambden, D. A. J. Tyrrell, and S. T. Holgate.** 1993. Use of polymerase chain reaction for diagnosis of picornavirus infection in subjects with and without respiratory symptoms. *J. Clin. Microbiol.* **31:**111–117.
37. **Kellner, G., T. Popow-Kraupp, M. Kundi, C. Binder, and C. Kunz.** 1989. Clinical manifestations of respiratory tract infections due to respiratory syncytial virus and rhinoviruses in hospitalized children. *Acta. Paediatr. Scand.* **78:** 390–394.
38. **Kim, K. H., P. Willingman, Z. X. Gong, M. J. Kremer, M. S. Chapman, I. Minor, M. A. Oliveira, M. G. Rossmann, K. Andries, G. D. Diana, E. J. Dutko, M. A. McKinlay, and D. C. Pevear.** 1993. A comparison of the antirhinoviral drug binding pocket in HRV14 and HRV1A. *J. Mol. Biol.* **230:**206–225.
39. **Krilov, L., L. Pierik, E. Keller, K. Mahan, D. Watson, M. Hirsch, V. Hamparian, and K. McIntosh.** 1986. The association of rhinoviruses with lower respiratory tract disease in hospitalized patients. *J. Med. Virol.* **19:**345–352.
40. **Las Heras, J., and V. L. Swanson.** 1983. Sudden death of an infant with rhinovirus infection complicating bronchial asthma: case report. *Pediatr. Pathol.* **1:**319–323.
41. **Last-Barney, K., S. D. Marlin, E. J. McNally, C. Cahill, D. Jeanfavre, R. B. Faanes, and V. J. Merluzzi.** 1991. Detection of major group rhinoviruses by soluble intercellular adhesion molecule-1 (sICAM-1). *J. Virol. Methods* **35:**255–264.
42. **Longberg-Holm, K., and F. H. Yin.** 1973. Antigenic determinants of infective and inactivated human rhinovirus type 2. *J. Virol.* **12:**114–123.
43. **Monto, A. S., E. R. Bryan, and S. Ohmit.** 1987. Rhinovirus infections in Tecumseh, Michigan: frequency of illness and number of serotypes. *J. Infect. Dis.* **156:**43–49.
44. **Mossad, S. B., M. L. Macknin, S. V. Medendorp, and P. Mason.** 1996. Zinc gluconate lozenges for treating the common cold. *Ann. Intern. Med.* **125:**81–88.
45. **Naclerio, R. M., D. Proud, L. M. Lichtenstein, A. Kagey-Sobotka, J. O. Hendley, and J. M. Gwaltney, Jr.** 1988. Kinins are generated during experimental rhinovirus colds. *J. Infect. Dis.* **157:**133–142.
46. **Nicholson, K. G., J. Kent, V. Hammersley, and E. Cancio.** 1996. Risk factors for lower respiratory complications of rhinovirus infections in elderly people living in the community: prospective cohort study. *BMJ* **313:**1119–1123.
47. **Olive, D. M., S. Al-Mufti, W. Al-Mulla, M. A. Khan, A. Pasca, G. Stanway, and W. Al-Nakib.** 1990. Detection and differentiation of picornaviruses in clinical samples following genomic amplification. *J. Gen. Virol.* **71:** 2141–2147.
48. **Olson, N. H., P. R. Kolatkar, M. A. Oliveira, R. H. Cheng, J. M. Greve, A. McClelland, T. S. Baker, and M. G. Rossman.** 1993. Structure of a human rhinovirus complexed with its receptor molecule. *Proc. Natl. Acad. Sci. USA* **90:**507–511.
49. **Patterson, L. J., and V. V. Hamparian.** 1997. Hyperantigenic variation occurs with human rhinovirus type 17. *J. Virol.* **71:**1370–1374.
50. **Pelon, W., W. J. Mogabgab, I. A. Phillips, and W. E. Pierce.** 1957. A cytopathogenic agent isolated from naval recruits with mild respiratory illness. *Proc. Soc. Exp. Biol. Med.* **94:**262–267.
51. **Pevear, D. C., M. J. Fancher, P. J. Felock, M. G. Rossmann, M. S. Miller, G. Diana, A. M. Treasurywala, M. A. McKinlay, and F. J. Dutko.** 1989. Conformational change in the floor of the human rhinovirus canyon blocks adsorption to HeLa cell receptors. *J. Virol.* **63:**2002–2007.
52. **Price, W. H.** 1956. The isolation of a new virus associated with respiratory clinical disease in humans. *Proc. Natl. Acad. Sci. USA* **42:**892–896.
53. **Rossman, M. G., E. Arnold, J. W. Erickson, E. A. Frankenberger, J. P. Griffith, H. J. Hecht, J. E. Johnson, G. Kramer, M. Luo, A. G. Mosser, R. R. Rueckert, B. Sherry, and G. Vriend.** 1985. Structure of a human common cold virus and functional relationship to other picornaviruses. *Nature* **317:**145–153.
54. **Schmidt, H. J., and R. J. Fink.** 1991. Rhinovirus as a lower respiratory tract pathogen in infants. *Pediatr. Infect. Dis. J.* **10:**700–702.
55. **Stott, E. J., and M. Walker.** 1969. Antigenic variation among strains of rhinovirus type 51. *Nature* **224:** 1311–1312.
56. **Torgersen, H., T. Skern, and D. Blaas.** 1989. Typing of human rhinoviruses based on sequence variations in the 5′ non-coding region. *J. Gen. Virol.* **70:**3111–3116.
57. **Turner, R. B., W. S. Cail, J. O. Hendley, F. G. Hayden, W. J. Doyle, J. V. Sorrentino, and J. M. Gwaltney, Jr.** 1992. Physiologic abnormalities in the paranasal sinuses during experimental rhinovirus colds. *J. Allergy Clin. Immunol.* **90:**474–478.
58. **Turner, R. B., M. T. Wecker, G. Pohl, T. J. Witek, Jr., S. Marlin, E. McNally, and F. G. Hayden.** 1997. Efficacy of soluble ICAM-1 (sICAM) for prevention of rhinovirus infection and illness, abstr. H-85. *In Program and Abstracts of the 37th Interscience Conference on Antimicrobial Agents and Chemotherapy*. American Society for Microbiology, Washington, D.C.
59. **Uncapher, C. R., C. M. DeWitt, and R. J. Colonno.** 1991. The major and minor group receptor families contain all but one human rhinovirus serotype. *Virology* **180:**814–817.
60. **Winther, B., J. M. Greve, J. M. Gwaltney, Jr., D. J. Innes, J. R. Eastham, A. McClelland, and J. O. Hendley.** 1997. Surface expression of intercellular adhesion molecule 1 on epithelial cells in the human adenoid. *J. Infect. Dis.* **176:** 523–525.

Enteroviruses

HARLEY A. ROTBART

78

CLINICAL BACKGROUND

The enteroviruses (EVs) are among the most common and most important viral pathogens of humans (10, 39). The paralytic potential of the polioviruses, the prototypic EVs, was recognized as early as the 14th century B.C., as illustrated in Egyptian art. Summer epidemics of paralytic poliomyelitis ravaged the United States through the 1950s. Since the introduction of vaccines in the late 1950s and early 1960s, much of the developed world is now virtually free of poliovirus infections. Ongoing efforts by the World Health Organization toward global eradication within the next decade have led to dramatic results in Africa, Asia, and other former regions of endemicity (7, 8).

Control of poliovirus infections in much of the world has focused attention on the nonpoliovirus EVs (NPEVs), which include the coxsackieviruses, echoviruses, and newer numbered EVs (Table 1). In the United States alone, the NPEVs are estimated to cause 5 to 10 million symptomatic infections annually (76). In temperate climates, these infections occur during the summer and fall months; young children are the most common victims, as both the incidence and the severity of NPEV infections vary inversely with the patient's age. In addition to the actual diseases that they cause, the EVs are of great concern because they mimic other pathogens. Distinguishing EV infections from those due to common bacteria and other viruses on clinical grounds alone is often difficult (10). Hence, unnecessary treatment for other infections is frequently instituted during EV infections.

The EVs are responsible for a wide array of clinical diseases affecting many organ systems (Table 2). It is important to note that no disease is uniquely associated with any specific EV serotype and that no serotype is uniquely associated with any one disease (10, 39, 54, 67). This is true even of paralytic poliomyelitis, which has been associated with numerous NPEV serotypes (19, 39). For that reason, it is sufficient in most circumstances to speak of diseases that "EVs cause" and to diagnose "an EV" in the laboratory without necessarily specifying or identifying the particular serotype. Certain clinical syndromes are indeed more likely to be caused by one or a few serotypes (see below), but significant overlap exists among the serotypes and the diseases that they cause.

Most EV infections are asymptomatic (10, 39). The most common symptomatic manifestation of EV infection is a nonspecific febrile illness with or without a rash. This so-called viral syndrome is one of the most numerically important causes of fever among children. When accompanied, as it often is, by upper respiratory tract symptoms, the "summer cold" is indistinguishable from the same illness caused by rhinoviruses (fellow picornaviruses) in the fall and winter months. By far the most vexing clinical EV syndrome that a physician encounters is aseptic meningitis. The EVs are the most common cause of meningitis in the United States (68). In young infants with the disease, clinical criteria used to distinguish EV meningitis from that due to bacteria and herpes simplex virus are unreliable. As a result, even though EV meningitis is generally benign in outcome and no specific therapy is currently available, thousands of children annually are hospitalized and treated with unnecessary antibiotics and antiherpes medications because of the fear that a case of meningitis is not due to an EV (12, 68). Additional acute clinical EV syndromes of significance include encephalitis, poliomyelitis (particularly due to the polioviruses), myocarditis (particularly due to coxsackievirus group B), hemorrhagic conjunctivitis (particularly due to serotypes coxsackievirus group A24 and enterovirus type 70), hand-foot-mouth syndrome, Bornholm disease (pleurodynia), and overwhelming neonatal sepsis (particularly due to the echoviruses and group B coxsackieviruses). The last syndrome is thought to be due to perinatal transmission, either transplacentally or during birth, from mother to infant. Despite the name EV, enteric disease is not a prominent manifestation, although diarrhea and vomiting may be significant manifestations of certain outbreaks of "summer flu" due to the EVs. Hepatitis A virus (HAV) was formerly known as EV 72 but has since been reclassified in its own genus of picornaviruses and is, appropriately, no longer considered an EV (48); typical EV clinical syndromes have not been associated with HAV infections (HAV is discussed separately in chapter 81 of this Manual). Mild hepatitis, almost always in association with other more significant findings, is common during infection with many EV serotypes.

In addition to the well-recognized acute EV diseases, EVs have been implicated in several chronic illnesses, including juvenile-onset diabetes mellitus, chronic fatigue syndrome, dermatomyositis, polymyositis, congenital hydrocephalus, and amyotrophic lateral sclerosis. Evidence for these associations has been obtained largely from serologic or nucleic

TABLE 1 EV serotypes

Subgroup	Serotypes
Poliovirus	1–3
Coxsackieviruses A	1–22, 24[a]
Coxsackieviruses B	1–6
Echovirus	1–9, 11–27, 29–31[a]
Numbered EVs	68–71

[a] Coxsackievirus A23, echoviruses 10 and 28, and EV 72 have been reclassified (48).

acid hybridization studies; definitive proof is lacking, and confirmatory studies remain to be done.

Persistent EV infections occur in agammaglobulinemic patients; manifestations almost always include meningoencephalitis (38). Half of all patients with persistent EV meningoencephalitis have concomitant dermatomyositis or polymyositis. These observations confirm the important role of antibody in EV clearance, an unusual phenomenon, because most other viruses are contained largely by cell-mediated immunity. A syndrome of late-onset muscular atrophy and pain occurs in individuals who suffered paralytic poliomyelitis 20 to 40 years previously (15); evidence for persistent or latent infection in these individuals has been conflicting.

Recently, an antiviral compound with broad reactivity for the EVs was advanced to clinical trials (78); other such compounds are in development. The availability of specific antiviral therapy for the EVs will make accurate and efficient diagnostic methods even more imperative.

DESCRIPTION OF THE AGENTS

The EVs comprise more than 60 distinct serotypes (48) within the family *Picornaviridae* ("pico" meaning small and "rna" indicating RNA). The traditional taxonomic subgroups of EVs (Table 1) are based on the patterns of replication of the individual serotypes in various host cells and tissues (see below and Table 3) (39, 40). Like other picornaviruses, EVs are small (27- to 30-nm diameter; 1.34-g/ml buoyant density) and consist of a simple viral capsid and a single strand of positive (message)-sense RNA. EVs are acid and ether stable and grow optimally at core body temperature (36 to 37°C). The capsid contains four proteins (VP1 through VP4) arranged in 60 repeating protomeric units of an icosahedron (reviewed in references 67 and 71). Variations within capsid proteins VP1 through VP3 are responsible for the antigenic diversity among the EVs; neutralization sites are most densely clustered on VP1. VP4 is not present on the viral surface; rather, it is closely associated with the RNA core, functioning as an anchor to the viral capsid. Destabilization of VP4 results in viral uncoating (see below) (71). The atomic structures of two poliovirus serotypes, types 1 and 3, have been resolved by computerized crystallographic studies, which reveal a deep cleft or canyon in the center of each protomeric unit into which the specific cellular receptor for the EVs fits when the virus encounters a susceptible host cell (23).

The encapsidated RNA of the human EVs is approximately 7.4 kb long and serves as a template for both viral protein translation and RNA replication, the latter accomplished via a double-stranded replicative-intermediate form of RNA (71). A single reading frame begins at approximately nucleotide 740 from the 5′ end and terminates at approximately nucleotide 7370, leaving 740 bases at the 5′ end and 70 bases at the 3′ end [just upstream from a poly(A) tail] untranslated; these untranslated sequences are involved in viral regulatory activities, such as replication and translation. A single polyprotein is translated from the open reading frame. Posttranslational modification is accomplished by virus-encoded proteases and results in generation of the four capsid proteins as well as the enzymes necessary for replication and translation.

Although genetic differences in the capsid coding regions result in the wide variety of EV serotypes, great similarities exist among the genomes of many of the EVs in a number of other regions along the RNA, including the untranslated sequences at the 5′ and 3′ ends; these homologous regions have been exploited for the nucleic acid diagnostic tests discussed below (13, 66). Echoviruses 22 and 23 appear genetically dissimilar from the other EVs and may ultimately, like HAV, require reclassification (26).

TABLE 2 Most common and/or most important clinical syndromes proven to be caused by EVs

Organ system	Disease
Neurologic	Aseptic meningitis, encephalitis, poliomyelitis
Respiratory	Common cold, stomatitis–herpangina–hand-foot-mouth syndrome, pharyngitis, tonsillitis, rhinitis, pleurodynia (Bornholm disease)
Cardiovascular	Myocarditis, pericarditis
Miscellaneous	Febrile exanthematous illness, neonatal sepsis

COLLECTION AND STORAGE OF SPECIMENS

The EVs are quite stable in liquid environments, able to survive for many weeks in water, body fluids, and sewage. This characteristic results from a combination of thermostability in the presence of divalent cations, acid stability, and the absence of a lipid envelope. Cerebrospinal fluid, serum or whole blood, and urine may be submitted to the laboratory in their original collection tubes; rectal or throat swabs or nasal wash specimens are best transported and stored in viral transport medium (see chapter 4 of this Manual). Viral infectivity for cell cultures is preserved for long periods (years) at −70°C and probably at −20°C as well. Stability for shorter periods (weeks) at 4°C is acceptable. Viral infectivity may decrease at room temperature over days to weeks. Hence, specimens "suboptimally" stored in hematology or chemistry laboratories may still be adequate for EV isolation. Some small loss of viral titer occurs with each freeze-thaw; hence, multiple freeze-thaw cycles should be avoided, and original specimens should be divided into aliquots if repeat testing is anticipated.

Specimens for PCR detection of enteroviral RNA (see below) should be handled in such a way as to preserve viral capsid integrity, thus protecting the target EV RNA molecule from the ubiquitous nucleases in body fluids. The addition of RNase inhibitor substances, such as vanadyl ribonucleoside complex or placental RNase inhibitor, to specimens prior to freezing may protect the RNA of the relatively few virions that are lysed during the freeze-thaw process.

Sera for antibody testing are best collected at both acute and convalescent stages of the infection (separated by 2 to

TABLE 3 Susceptibilities of commonly used cell lines for isolation of EVs[a]

Cell line	Polioviruses	Coxsackieviruses		EVs
		Type A	Type B	
Monkey kidney				
Rhesus	+ + +	+	+ + +	+ + +
Cynomolgus	+ + + +	+	+ + +	+ + +
Buffalo green (BGM)	+ + +	+	+ + + +	+ +
Human				
HeLa	+ + +	+	+ + +	+
Kidney (HK)	+ + +	+	+ +	+ + +
WI-38	+ +	+ +	+	+ + +
Embryonic lung (HELF)	+ + +	+ +	+	+ + +
MRC-5	+ + +	+	+	+ + +
Rhabdomyosarcoma (RD)	+ + +	+ + +	+	+ + +
HEp-2	+ + +	+	+ + +	+

[a] Relative susceptibilities: +, minimally susceptible; + + + +, maximally susceptible.

4 weeks), frozen at −20°C, thawed, and then tested simultaneously.

DIRECT EXAMINATION

There are many compelling reasons for seeking a rapid direct diagnostic assay for the EVs. Isolation of EVs in cell cultures and recognition of cytopathic effects (see below) require a high level of expertise and may be quite labor-intensive. Some EV serotypes, particularly within coxsackievirus group A, do not grow at all in cell cultures (24, 30, 35, 45, 46, 58, 79, 80). Of greater significance, 25 to 35% of specimens from patients with characteristic EV infections are negative in cell cultures (11) because of antibody neutralization in situ; inadequate collection, handling, and processing of the samples; or insensitivity intrinsic to the cell lines used. Suckling mouse inoculation, a technique too cumbersome to be widely available, improves the yield somewhat (24, 30, 45–47). EVs that do grow in cell cultures may do so slowly. Reported mean isolation times for EVs from cerebrospinal fluid range from 3.7 to 8.2 days (11, 27, 47, 80); EVs from other sites, where viral titers are higher, often grow more rapidly (21, 47, 50, 80).

Electron microscopy for EV detection has little to no application in clinical laboratory practice. The only clinical specimen that has a high enough concentration of EVs to reach detectability by electron microscopy is feces (80). As noted earlier, the EVs are rarely causes of significant gastroenteritis. Hence, fecal samples are usually solid, making detection of EVs difficult. Additionally, the presence of EVs in feces is, in and of itself, of little diagnostic import, as asymptomatic shedding may follow true infection for many weeks to months (see Evaluation and Interpretation of Results below). Other specimens could be concentrated to enhance electron microscopic detection of the EVs, but this process would contribute little to what can be learned more easily with other direct viral assays and viral isolation.

The absence of a widely shared antigen has hampered the development of immunoassays for the EVs (22). The greatest success has been obtained with assays limited to a particular subgroup of EV serotypes, e.g., group B coxsackieviruses, which have an antigen in common (83). Reports of polyclonal antibodies (61) and monoclonal antibodies (5, 75, 82, 84, 85) that cross-react with multiple EV serotypes are promising, but further testing is required to determine the clinical relevance of those observations. These reagents have been applied to serotyping of EV isolates (see below), but with the exception of a single report of a monoclonal antibody specific for echovirus 11 (49), the utility of these reagents for direct detection of EVs in clinical specimens has not been demonstrated. The epitope for one such antibody has been localized to nine residues of VP1 (72).

cDNA probes derived from cloned sequences of the EVs have been prepared and demonstrated to detect multiple EV serotypes in dot blot hybridization experiments (66). Although EVs were readily detected in body fluids during reconstruction experiments, the sensitivity in actual clinical specimens was only 33% or less. RNA probes for the EVs are more sensitive (66) but still not of clinical utility in detecting cerebrospinal fluid infections. The limiting variable in all of these hybridization-based assays is undoubtedly the low titer of EVs in many specimens, particularly cerebrospinal fluid from patients with aseptic meningitis, which may be as low as 1 to 10 titratable virions per ml (80).

The most promising development in direct detection of the EVs has been the application of PCR (3, 33, 63, 64–66, 69, 70). Three general strategies have been used: "universal" detection of many or all serotypes; "serotype-specific" or "group-specific" detection of a limited number of serotypes; and "strain-specific" detection of variations within a single serotype. Universal detection of the EVs by PCR will be discussed in this section. A potentially important application of group-specific EV PCR is the discrimination of polioviruses from the NPEVs in clinical specimens (1, 17, 32). Strain-specific PCR is of use mainly for the study of the genetic shifts and drifts of individual EV strains and the study of specific molecular virulence determinants (62).

Three well-characterized sets of PCR primers and probes for the universal detection of the EVs are shown in Fig. 1 (9, 25, 65). All are directed at highly conserved regions of the 5′ noncoding region of the viral genome. One of these primer sets (65) was tested against 66 EV serotypes and found to amplify 60 of the serotypes tested (coxsackievirus A15 was not available for testing); only coxsackieviruses A11, A17, and A24 and echoviruses 16, 22, and 23 failed to be amplified with these reagents (86). Subsequently, other investigators used these same primers and probes successfully to identify coxsackieviruses A11, A15, A17, and A24 and echovirus 16 but confirmed that echoviruses 22 and 23 were not reactive (29). The last two serotypes, as noted above,

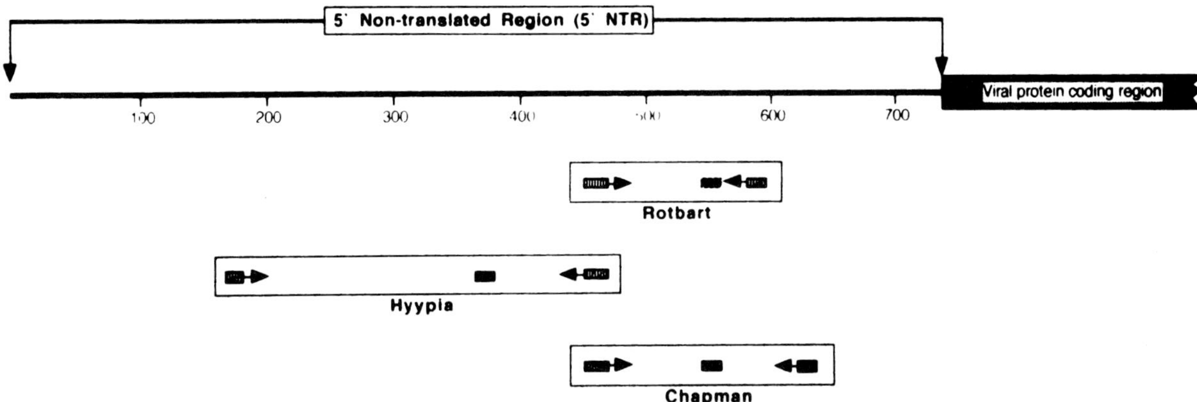

FIGURE 1 Locations, within the 5′ nontranslated region of the EV genomes, of the three most completely studied primer and probe combinations for PCR (9, 25, 65).

are atypical of other EVs and may require reclassification (26). EV PCR with these and other primer-probe sets has been tested in clinical settings by many investigators and found to be consistently more sensitive than culturing and virtually 100% specific (3, 52, 56, 66, 69, 70, 73).

Specimens to be studied by PCR must be treated to extract the target EV RNA from the material and remove potentially inhibitory substances, such as proteins and lipids. PCR testing of untreated body fluids is unsuccessful, as is simple heat treatment; this is true whether the fluids tested are relatively "pristine," such as cerebrospinal fluid and serum, or more proteinaceous, such as nasal washes or feces. The most common extraction techniques use either phenol-chloroform-sodium dodecyl sulfate or guanidinium thiocyanate (64). All solutions are prepared in diethyl pyrocarbonate-treated water (to minimize RNase contamination of water and glassware), and reactions are carried out in the presence of RNase inhibitors. Following extraction, reverse transcription of the EV RNA is accomplished with the downstream primer and any of several commercially available reverse transcriptases. PCR itself is performed with *Taq* polymerase in an automated thermal cycler for 30 to 35 cycles of denaturation, annealing, and extension. Detection of the amplified product can be performed by any of several conventional techniques that use a confirmatory hybridization step with the oligomeric probe molecule, including ethidium bromide-stained agarose gels with confirmatory Southern hybridization, dot blot hybridization, and microtiter plate hybridization assay. The wide array of reported conditions for EV PCR extraction, reverse transcription, amplification, and detection have been reviewed (64). The nucleotide dUTP and the enzyme uracil *N*-glycosylase should be used in all PCRs (36), and other standardized precautions should also be taken to minimize the risk of carryover contamination from one experiment to another (see chapter 13 of this Manual).

Recently, a kit containing many of the above-noted components, including a previously reported primer-probe set (65), was developed and tested in the clinical setting. A 5-h, microtiter plate-based format, the kit was demonstrated to perform better than cell culturing in diagnosing EV aseptic meningitis (3, 31, 34, 69, 70) and neonatal EV infection (2). The assay is applicable to cerebrospinal fluid, blood, urine, throat, nasopharyngeal, and rectal specimens (3, 69). Because the technique can be performed in a few hours, it has the potential of having a dramatic impact on the quality and cost of patient management (12, 74).

A quantitative EV PCR has been reported (37) and may find applicability with the development of antiviral therapy for the EVs. Nested and seminested PCR assays also have been reported for the EVs and have demonstrated high sensitivity (55). Great caution must be exercised with these approaches because of the increased opportunity for carryover contamination inherent in multiple tube-opening and manipulation steps; false-positive results are likely.

ISOLATION OF VIRUS

The original subclassification of the EVs was based on the ability of individual serotypes to grow in various cell culture and animal systems. Hence, coxsackievirus group A serotypes were characteristically able to replicate in suckling mice, with resultant diffuse myositis and flaccid paralysis. However, these viruses were not readily grown in tissue culture cells derived from monkey or human tissues. In contrast, group B coxsackieviruses grow readily in tissue cultures of both simian and human origins as well as in suckling mice; the pathology in the latter differs from that of group A coxsackieviruses in that the myositis with B serotypes is more focal and direct infection of brain, myocardium, pancreas, and liver also occurs. Neither group of coxsackieviruses is pathogenic for monkeys. The echoviruses were defined by their ability to grow only in simian-derived tissue culture cells but not at all in animal systems. The polioviruses grow most prolifically in cells of human and simian origins and in monkeys; they do not grow in murine models. Since these original distinctions were observed, they have been significantly blurred by the identification of new strains and new tissue culture cell lines, resulting in crossover patterns of EV growth. For that reason, recently discovered serotypes have been numbered (EVs 68 to 71) (40, 44).

Isolation of EVs in tissue cultures remains the "gold standard" for diagnosis. The commercial availability of increasing numbers and types of continuous cell lines has provided numerous options for routine EV culturing. The general susceptibilities of commonly used cell lines for the EVs are summarized in Table 3; a quick glance at that table shows that no single cell line is optimal for all EV serotypes. Monkey kidney cell lines, the traditional first choice for EV isolation, have good sensitivity for the polioviruses, group B coxsackieviruses, and echoviruses, whereas human diploid fibroblasts, such as WI-38 and HELF (human embryonic lung fibroblasts), have higher yields for group A coxsackieviruses. RD cells, derived from a human rhabdomyosarcoma, are the most sensitive for detection of group A coxsackieviruses but fail with most group B coxsackieviruses; RD cells are notoriously difficult to work with in the laboratory, with rapid overgrowth and cell degeneration, and detection of EV growth frequently requires blind passages. For ease of use, most laboratories use a combination of a continuous monkey kidney cell line, such as CMK (cynomolgus monkey kidney), with a human diploid fibroblast line (such as WI-38, MRC-5, or HELF). Studies have shown improved yield and rapidity of EV detection with the addition of BGM (Buffalo green monkey kidney) and RD cells, albeit associated with greater cost and complexity (11, 14). Duplicate tubes of each cell line do not appear to significantly improve viral isolation, with the possible exception of isolation in rhesus monkey kidney cells (11). If enough cell lines are used, the patterns of growth in each by a single EV isolate may accurately predict the subclassification of the isolate (24, 28) although the clinical value of that information is limited. Primary human amnion cells have proven useful for isolation of many EV serotypes, including the group A coxsackieviruses (79); the difficulty in preparing and maintaining these cells, however, has resulted in their disuse. Centrifugation-enhanced inoculation (shell vial assay) combined with monoclonal antibodies reduces the time for detection of enteroviruses in cell cultures (5).

Preparation of clinical samples for inoculation into cell cultures was previously reviewed (30, 45, 46, 58). Feces are suspended (10 to 20% final concentration) in a tube of sterile saline containing glass beads. Vigorous shaking and subsequent settling of the emulsified feces are followed by low-speed centrifugation of the supernatant for about 15 min. Antibiotics are added at concentrations comparable to those in viral transport media (see chapter 5 of this Manual), and a longer low-speed (or shorter high-speed) centrifugation is performed. The resultant supernatant is inoculated directly onto cell cultures. An identical procedure may be performed for the following specimens: rectal swabs in viral transport media, throat swabs in viral transport media, and nasal or pharyngeal washes. Swabs should be squeezed out against the sides of the collection tube and discarded rather than broken off into the media, as swab components may be toxic to cells. Specimens already in transport media containing antibiotics need not be retreated following the initial centrifugation. Cerebrospinal fluid, serum, and urine need no pretreatment and may be inoculated directly onto cell cultures. Serum and urine tend to be more toxic to cells and often require a change of the culture media within 24 h of inoculation. Occasionally, EVs may be antibody bound in serum or cerebrospinal fluid and detectable only following acid dissociation, procedures for which have been presented elsewhere in detail (41, 45). Preparation of body tissues from biopsy or autopsy for EV isolation are as described for viral culturing in general in chapter 5 of this Manual.

Although it is the most sensitive method for laboratory diagnosis of coxsackievirus group A infection, isolation of EVs in suckling mice is rarely performed any longer because of the difficulties of the technique and of animal maintenance. This method has been reviewed elsewhere (47).

IDENTIFICATION OF THE AGENTS

As noted above, the determination of the specific serotype of infecting EVs is often unnecessary because the diseases caused by the EVs are not serotype specific. In most circumstances, therefore, it is adequate and useful for the diagnostic laboratory to report the presence of an EV without further detail. The most common exception to this principle is in pediatrics, where distinguishing between vaccine strain polioviruses and nonpolioviruses is critical to interpretation of viral culture results. During the first 2 years of life, children are repeatedly immunized with trivalent oral poliovirus vaccine (Sabin strains), whose components, like all EVs, may be shed from the throat for 1 to 2 weeks and in the feces for several weeks to months. Hence, isolates from those two sites must be identified as either nonpoliovirus or poliovirus serotypes, with the latter presumed to be of vaccine origin unless unusual clinical circumstances suggest wild-type infection. Vaccine poliovirus has only rarely been recovered from cerebrospinal fluid or blood (20, 41); further characterization of EV isolates from those sites is thus less important. Distinguishing between polioviruses and NPEVs can be accomplished by two methods, one proven and one experimental. The standard method uses neutralization of the isolate with a pool of antisera directed against the three poliovirus serotypes (24). Successful inhibition of growth by the antisera confirms the poliovirus identity of the isolate, whereas failure to neutralize an isolate with typical cytopathic effects implies the presence of an NPEV. The neutralization method, as previously detailed, uses a fixed titer of virus (typically 100 50% tissue culture infective doses) and pooled antipoliovirus sera (each at a final dilution of 20 U) (24). The experimental method uses a set of PCR primers that is specific for the three poliovirus serotypes; the PCR assay is performed on the culture-passaged isolate and accurately discriminates between polioviruses and NPEVs (1, 17, 32). This latter method has the potential for being simpler and more rapid than viral neutralization for distinguishing between vaccine strains of poliovirus and disease-causing NPEVs, particularly as PCR assays become more user-friendly (see above). Recent recommendations regarding poliovirus immunization may obviate the need to distinguish between poliovirus and NPEV serotypes because inactivated vaccine preparations will be used increasingly in the youngest infants (57).

Further identification of an NPEV to specific serotype is useful under certain circumstances. Indeed, the very principle that most clinical manifestations of EV infections are not serotype specific was historically established by serotyping studies. Epidemiologic studies of patterns of EV infections require knowledge of specific serotypes (18, 51), as do descriptions of unusual clinical manifestations, such as poliomyelitis due to NPEVs (19) and pandemic hemorrhagic conjunctivitis (18, 77). Only via serotyping will new EVs be discovered, as was the case most recently with the higher-number EVs; this task may become more definitive with molecular methods (13, 32, 40, 44, 51, 62). As noted above, an approximation as to the subgroup of an isolate can be accomplished by analysis of the cell lines infected by an isolate (28); plaque morphology may give additional clues as to serotype within a subgroup (24). The gold standard for EV serotype determination, however, continues to be the use of intersecting pools of lyophilized antisera, as established by Lim and Benyesh-Melnick (LBM pools) (42, 43). Each isolate can be screened against 16 antisera with 8 pools or against 25 antisera with 10 pools. A checkerboard analysis localizes the isolate to a single serotype designation on the basis of the pattern of neutralization with the intersecting serum pools. Microtiter plate neutralization works equally well and saves significant quantities of serum reagents. The LBM pools are available in limited supplies from the World Health Organization.

Broadly reactive and serotype-specific EV monoclonal antibodies have been developed (5, 72, 75, 82, 84) and applied to tissue culture confirmation by immunofluorescence. Preliminary studies have indicated that these reagents, used singly and in pools, may find an important role in serotype identification. Immunofluorescence is a more rapid, simpler procedure than traditional neutralization-based serotyping, and the supply of monoclonal antibodies is unlimited.

SEROLOGIC DIAGNOSIS

Serologic testing, like immunoassays, has had only a limited role in EV diagnosis because of the great diversity of EV serotypes and the lack of a single common antigen. If the specific serotype of an infecting EV is known or suspected, e.g., in community-wide outbreaks, confirmatory immunoglobulin G (IgG) serologic testing can be performed on individual patients to document a rise in antibody titer from the acute to the convalescent phase of infection, thus providing useful epidemiologic information; little actual benefit accrues to the patient. When an EV is recovered from the feces or throat of a patient with unusual clinical manifestations, the etiologic role of the EV may be more firmly established by documenting a fourfold rise in antibody titer to that serotype in paired acute- and convalescent-phase sera. Serosurveys of populations for past exposure to specific EVs have been performed by testing for antibody in single serum specimens; such studies may be useful for retrospective disease associations, such as with EVs and diabetes mellitus (4) or dilated cardiomyopathy (53). Those kinds of studies are subject to many types of sampling bias and therefore are of limited value. In the usual scenario, when a patient presents with meningitis or other acute manifestations of illness and an EV is suspected, serologic testing is not a practical option.

Three traditional types of antibody determinations have been applied to the EVs: neutralization, complement fixation, and hemagglutination inhibition. Neutralizing antibodies rise early in infection with the EVs and persist for many years or for life. They may be assessed in standard tube dilutions or with microtiter plates; in either format, a fixed quantity of a single serotype of EV is inoculated onto cells in the presence of serial dilutions of the patient's serum (30, 45, 46, 58). Ideally, acute- and convalescent-phase sera are tested in parallel simultaneously. The rapid appearance of serum neutralizing antibodies following EV infection may make it difficult to document a fourfold rise in titer with convalescence. Complement fixation antibody assays are of much less utility, as these antibodies are transient (weeks to months) and broadly cross-reactive among EV serotypes, i.e., nonspecific. Historically, these assays were successfully applied only in testing for infection with the polioviruses. Only about a quarter to a third of all EV serotypes agglutinate erythrocytes, making hemagglutination inhibition of minimal usefulness; this type of antibody is also cross-reactive among EV serotypes and hence nonspecific.

Coxsackievirus group B IgM assays, which take advantage of the shared antigen among the six coxsackievirus group B serotypes and the early appearance of the IgM class of antibodies, have appeared promising (6, 16, 59). Although the IgM response measured in these assays may be nonspecific, i.e., a response to a non-coxsackievirus group B EV may result in a positive assay, the nonspecificity may actually make this test more broadly reflective of recent exposure to any of numerous EV serotypes; cross-reactivity with non-EV pathogens causing infection has not been thoroughly studied. Many patients in the reported studies had positive IgM assays but were found negative for EV infection by culturing, making the IgM assays either more sensitive or less specific than traditional culture diagnosis. These IgM tests are not yet widely available, and clinical experience with them remains limited. Attempts to use more broadly reactive EV antigens in IgM assays have met with technical shortcomings (59, 60).

EVALUATION AND INTERPRETATION OF RESULTS

The concept of permissive versus nonpermissive sites of infection is critical to the interpretation of EV assays. The nasopharynx and the gastrointestinal tract are permissive sites of infection; i.e., EVs have ready access to these sites and may remain as "colonizers" for weeks to months. Detection of EVs by virus isolation or PCR at these sites must be interpreted cautiously, because their presence alone does not establish causality of the illness in question. The EV in the feces of a patient today may be leftover shedding from an infection that occurred weeks ago and may have nothing to do with the meningitis the patient presents with currently. Indeed, virtually 100% of patients with EV aseptic meningitis have detectable EV in feces (50), but most persons shedding EV in feces at any particular time are asymptomatic. Feces are thus the most sensitive and least specific site for detecting true EV-associated illness. Since the shedding period in the nasopharynx after EV infection is shorter than that in feces, the specificity of an EV isolate from the nasopharynx for true causality of current symptoms is better than that with feces but far short of a definitive association. Further complicating the evaluation of results from these two body sites in young children is the frequent administration of live attenuated oral poliovirus vaccine in the first years of life. Most EV isolates from feces and nasopharynges of young children that are encountered by the diagnostic virology laboratory are, in fact, vaccine strain poliovirus. Reporting an EV isolate in this setting without specifying poliovirus versus NPEV can lead the physician to wrongly discontinue antibiotics or antiherpes therapy in the belief that an EV etiology has been established.

In contrast, the central nervous system, bloodstream, and genitourinary tract are nonpermissive sites of EV infection; i.e., detection of virus in specimens from these sites implies true invasive infection and a high likelihood of association with current illness. Rare reports of coinfections of the cerebrospinal fluid by bacteria and EVs have appeared (81). In these patients, the bacterium-associated clinical sequelae dominated. That is, the patients were clinically suspected of having bacterial meningitis, and the virus was isolated incidentally; the patients were sick enough that identification of a virus before identification of the bacterium would have been unlikely to dissuade the clinician from continued use of antibiotics. In the much more common situation, where the clinical presentation is typical of viral meningitis, coinfection with a clinically "silent" bacterium would be extraordinarily unlikely. Hence, identification of an EV from a nonpermissive site in a patient with a clinically compatible illness is usually sufficient evidence for establishing EV causality. The distinction between polioviruses and NPEVs in specimens from nonpermissive sites is less important, since vaccine strains of poliovirus rarely have been reported in such specimens and, in those rare instances, may actually be causing the illness in question (20, 41).

The utilities and shortcomings of serologic assays are described above. In general, results of a single serologic assay are uninterpretable except perhaps for IgM tests, which remain to be standardized and more widely tested. Commercially available serologic or immunoassay panels for the EVs are, in general, derived from only limited numbers of serotypes and lack standardization or published quality controls.

REFERENCES

1. **Abraham, R., T. Chonmaitree, J. McCombs, B. Prabhakar, P. T. Lo Verde, and P. L. Ogra.** 1993. Rapid detection of poliovirus by reverse transcription and polymerase chain amplification: application for differentiation between poliovirus and nonpoliovirus enteroviruses. *J. Clin. Microbiol.* **31:**395–399.
2. **Abzug, M. J., M. Loeffelholz, and H. A. Rotbart.** 1995. Diagnosis of neonatal enterovirus infection by polymerase chain reaction. *J. Pediatr.* **126:**447–450.
3. **Andreoletti, L., N. Blassel-Damman, A. Dewilde, L. Vallee, R. Cremer, D. Hober, and P. Wattre.** 1998. Comparison of use of cerebrospinal fluid, serum, and throat swab specimens in diagnosis of enteroviral acute neurological infection by a rapid RNA detection PCR assay. *J. Clin. Microbiol.* **36:**589–591.
4. **Barrett-Conner, E.** 1985. Is insulin-dependent diabetes mellitus caused by coxsackievirus B infection? A review of the epidemiologic evidence. *Rev. Infect. Dis.* **7:**207–215.
5. **Baurlet, T., J. Gharbi, S. Omar, M. Aouni, and B. Pozzetto.** 1998. Comparison of rapid culture method combining an immunoperoxidase test and a group specific anti-VP1 monoclonal antibody with conventional virus isolation techniques for routine detection of enteroviruses in stools. *J. Med. Virol.* **54:**204–209.
6. **Bell, E. J., R. A. McCartney, D. Basquill, and A. K. R. Chaudhuri.** 1986. μ-Antibody capture ELISA for the rapid diagnosis of enterovirus infections in patients with aseptic meningitis. *J. Med. Virol.* **19:**213–217.
7. **Centers for Disease Control.** 1996. Progress toward poliomyelitis eradication—Africa, 1996. *Morbid. Mortal. Weekly Rep.* **46:**321–325.
8. **Centers for Disease Control.** 1995. Progress toward global eradication of poliomyelitis. *Morbid. Mortal. Weekly Rep.* **45:**565–568.
9. **Chapman, N. M., S. Tracy, C. J. Gauntt, and U. Fortmueller.** 1990. Molecular detection and identification of enteroviruses using enzymatic amplification and nucleic acid hybridization. *J. Clin. Microbiol.* **28:**843–850.
10. **Cherry, J. D.** 1998. Enteroviruses: coxsackieviruses, echoviruses, and polioviruses, p. 1787–1838. *In* R. D. Feigin and J. D. Cherry (ed.), *Textbook of Pediatric Infectious Diseases,* 4th ed. The W. B. Saunders Co., Philadelphia, Pa.
11. **Chonmaitree, T., C. Ford, C. Sanders, and H. L. Lucia.** 1988. Comparison of cell cultures for rapid isolation of enteroviruses. *J. Clin. Microbiol.* **26:**2576–2580.
12. **Chonmaitree, T., M. A. Menegus, and K. R. Powell.** 1982. The clinical relevance of CSF viral culture. A two-year experience with aseptic meningitis in Rochester, New York. *JAMA* **247:**1843–1847.
13. **Currey, K. M., and B. A. Shapiro.** 1997. Higher order structures of coxsackievirus B nontranslated region RNA. *Curr. Top. Microbiol. Immunol.* **223:**169–190.
14. **Dagan, R., and M. A. Menegus.** 1986. A combination of four cell types for rapid detection of enteroviruses in clinical specimens. *J. Med. Virol.* **19:**219–228.
15. **Dalakas, M. C., J. L. Sever, D. L. Madden, N. M. Papadopoulos, I. C. Shekarchi, P. Albrecht, and A. Krezlewicz.** 1984. Late postpoliomyelitis muscular atrophy: clinical, virologic, and immunologic studies. *Rev. Infect. Dis.* **6:**S562–S567.
16. **Dorries, R., and V. Ter Meulen.** 1983. Specificity of IgM antibodies in acute human coxsackievirus B infections, analyzed by indirect solid phase enzyme immunoassay and immunoblot technique. *J. Gen. Virol.* **64:**159–167.
17. **Eggers, D., L. Pasamontes, M. Ostermayer, and K. Bienz.** 1995. Reverse transcription multiplex PCR for differentiation between polio- and enteroviruses from clinical and environmental samples. *J. Clin. Microbiol.* **33:**1442–1447.
18. **Gjoen, K. V., and A. L. Bruce.** 1997. Specific detection of coxsackie viruses A by the polymerase chain reaction. *Clin. Diagn. Virol.* **8:**183–188.
19. **Grist, N. R., and E. J. Bell.** 1984. Paralytic poliomyelitis and nonpolio enteroviruses: studies in Scotland. *Rev. Infect. Dis.* **6:**S385–S386.
20. **Gutierrez, K. M., and M. J. Abzug.** 1990. Vaccine-associated poliovirus meningitis in children with ventriculoperitoneal shunts. *J. Pediatr.* **117:**424–427.
21. **Herrmann, E. C., Jr., D. A. Person, and T. F. Smith.** 1972. Experience in laboratory diagnosis of enterovirus infections in routine medical practice. *Mayo Clin. Proc.* **47:**577–586.
22. **Herrmann, J. E., R. M. Hendry, and M. F. Collins.** 1979. Factors involved in enzyme-linked immunoassay of viruses and evaluation of the method for identification of enteroviruses. *J. Clin. Microbiol.* **10:**210–217.
23. **Hogle, J. M., M. Chow, and D. J. Filman.** 1985. Three dimensional structure of poliovirus at 2.9 A resolution. *Science* **229:**1358–1365.
24. **Hsiung, G. D.** 1973. Enteroviruses, p. 54–67. *In* G. D. Hsiung (ed.), *Diagnostic Virology.* Yale University Press, New Haven, Conn.
25. **Hyypiä, T., P. Auvinen, and M. Maaronen.** 1989. Polymerase chain reaction for human picornaviruses. *J. Gen. Virol.* **70:**3261–3268.
26. **Hyypiä, T., C. Horsnell, M. Maaronen, M. Khan, N. Kalkkinen, P. Auvinen, L. Kinnunen, and G. Stanway.** 1992. A distinct picornavirus group identified by sequence analysis. *Proc. Natl. Acad. Sci. USA* **89:**8847–8851.
27. **Jarvis, W. R., and G. Tucker.** 1981. Echovirus type 7 meningitis in young children. *Am. J. Dis. Child.* **135:**1009–1012.
28. **Johnston, S. L. G., and C. S. Siegel.** 1990. Presumptive identification of enteroviruses with RD, HEp-2, and RMK cell lines. *J. Clin. Microbiol.* **28:**1049–1050.
29. **Kao, S.-Y., T. M. Niemiec, M. J. Loeffelholz, B. Dale, and H. A. Rotbart.** 1995. Direct and uninterrupted RNA amplification of enteroviruses with colorimetric microwell detection. *Clin. Diagn. Virol.* **3:**247–257.
30. **Kapsenberg, J. G.** 1988. Picornaviridae: the enteroviruses (polioviruses, coxsackieviruses, echoviruses), p. 692–722. *In* E. H. Lennette, P. Halonen, and F. A. Murphy (ed.), *Laboratory Diagnosis of Infectious Diseases: Principles and Practice.* Springer-Verlag, New York, N.Y.
31. **Kessler, H. H., B. Sanker, H. Rabenau, A. Berger, A. Vince, C. Lewinski, B. Weber, K. Pierer, O. Stuenzer, E. Marth, and H. W. Doern.** 1997. Rapid diagnosis of enterovirus infection by a new one-step reverse transcription-PCR assay. *J. Clin. Microbiol.* **35:**976–977.
32. **Kilpatrick, D. R., B. Nottay, C. F. Yang, S. J. Yank, E. Da Silva, S. Penaranda, M. Pallansch, and O. Keu.** 1998. Serotype-specific identification of polioviruses by PCR using primers containing mixed-base or deoxyinosine residues at positions of codon degeneracy. *J. Clin. Microbiol.* **36:**352–357.
33. **Kuan, M. M.** 1997. Detection and rapid differentiation of

human enteroviruses following genomic amplification. *J. Clin. Microbiol.* **35:**2598–2601.

34. **Lina, B., B. Pozzetto, L. Andreoletti, et al.** 1996. Multicenter evaluation of a commercially available PCR assay for diagnosing enterovirus infection in a panel of cerebrospinal fluid specimens. *J. Clin. Microbiol.* **34:**3002–3006.
35. **Lipson, S. M., R. Walderman, P. Costello, and K. Szabo.** 1988. Sensitivity of rhabdomyosarcoma and guinea pig embryo cell cultures to field isolates of difficult-to-cultivate group A coxsackieviruses. *J. Clin. Microbiol.* **26:** 1298–1303.
36. **Longo, M. C., M. S. Berninger, and J. L. Hartley.** 1990. Use of uracil DNA glycosylase to control carry-over contamination in polymerase chain reactions. *Gene* **93:** 125–128.
37. **Martino, T. A., M. J. Sole, L. Z. Penn, C. C. Liew, and P. Liu.** 1993. Quantitation of enteroviral RNA by competitive polymerase chain reaction. *J. Clin. Microbiol.* **31:** 2634–2640.
38. **McKinney, R. E., S. L. Katz, and C. M. Wilfert.** 1987. Chronic enteroviral meningoencephalitis in agammaglobulinemic patients. *Rev. Infect. Dis.* **9:**334–356.
39. **Melnick, J. L.** 1990. Enteroviruses: polioviruses, coxsackieviruses, echoviruses, and newer enteroviruses, p. 549–605. *In* B. N. Fields and D. M. Knipe (ed.), *Virology*. Raven Press, New York, N.Y.
40. **Melnick, J. L.** 1996. My role in the discovery and classification of the enteroviruses. *Annu. Rev. Microbiol.* **50:**1–24.
41. **Melnick, J. L., R. O. Proctor, A. R. Ocampo, A. R. Diwan, and E. Ben-Porath.** 1966. Free and bound virus in serum after administration of oral poliovirus vaccine. *Am. J. Epidemiol.* **84:**329–342.
42. **Melnick, J. L., V. Rennick, B. Hampil, N. J. Schmidt, and H. H. Ho.** 1973. Lyophilized combination pools of enterovirus equine antisera: preparation and test procedures for the identification of field strains of 42 enteroviruses. *Bull. W.H.O.* **48:**263–268.
43. **Melnick, J. L., N. J. Schmidt, B. Hampil, and H. H. Ho.** 1977. Lyophilized combination pools of enterovirus equine antisera: preparation and test procedures for the identification of field strains of 19 group A coxsackievirus serotypes. *Intervirology* **8:**172–181.
44. **Melnick, J. L., I. Tagaya, and H. Von Magnus.** 1974. Enteroviruses 69, 70, and 71. *Intervirology* **4:**369–370.
45. **Melnick, J. L., H. A. Wenner, and C. A. Phillips.** 1979. Enteroviruses, p. 471–534. *In* E. H. Lennette and N. J. Schmidt (ed.), *Diagnostic Procedures for Viral, Rickettsial and Chlamydial Infections*, 5th ed. American Public Health Association, Washington, D.C.
46. **Melnick, J. L., H. A. Wenner, and L. Rosen.** 1964. The enteroviruses, p. 194–242. *In* E. H. Lennette and N. J. Schmidt (ed.), *Diagnostic Procedures for Viral and Rickettsial Diseases*, 3rd ed. American Public Health Association, Inc., Washington, D.C.
47. **Menegus, M. A.** Enteroviruses, p. 943–947. *In* A. Balows, W. J. Hausler, Jr., K. L. Herrmann, H. D. Isenberg, and H. J. Shadomy (ed.), *Manual of Clinical Microbiology*, 5th ed. American Society for Microbiology, Washington, D.C.
48. **Miller, M. J.** 1997. Viral taxonomy. *Clin. Infect. Dis.* **25:** 18–20.
49. **Minnich, L., E. Brown, R. Ashley, C. Andreou, D. Hirsch, E. Yanek, S. Oliver, W. Giles, and S. Maxwell.** 1993. *Abstr. 9th Annu. Clin. Virol. Symp.*, p. 50.
50 **Mintz, L., and W. L. Drew.** 1980. Relation of culture site to the recovery of nonpolio enteroviruses. *Am. J. Clin. Pathol.* **74:**324–326.
51. **Muir, P., V. Kammerer, K. Korn, M. N. Mulders, T. Poyry, B. Weissbrich, R. Kandoff, G. M. Cleator, and A. M. Van Loon.** 1998. Molecular typing of enteroviruses: current status and future requirements. The European Union Concerted Action on Virus Meningitis and Encephalitis. *Clin. Microbiol. Rev.* **11:**202–227.
52. **Muir, P., F. Nicholson, M. Jhetam, S. Neogi, and J. E. Banatvala.** 1993. Rapid diagnosis of enterovirus infection by magnetic bead extraction and polymerase chain reaction detection of enterovirus RNA in clinical specimens. *J. Clin. Microbiol.* **31:**31–38.
53. **Muir, P., A. J. Tilzey, T. A. H. English, F. Nicholson, M. Signy, and J. E. Banatvala.** 1989. Chronic relapsing pericarditis and dilated cardiomyopathy: serological evidence of persistent enterovirus infection. *Lancet* **i:** 804–807.
54. **Muir, P., and A. M. Van Loon.** 1997. Enterovirus infection of the central nervous system. *Intervirology* **40:** 153–166.
55. **Nicholson, F., G. Meetoo, S. Aiyar, J. E. Banatuala, and P. Muir.** 1994. Detection of enterovirus RNA in clinical samples by nested polymerase chain reaction for rapid diagnosis of enterovirus infection. *J. Virol. Methods* **48:** 155–166.
56. **Olive, D. M., S. Al-Mufti, W. Al-Mulla, M. A. Khan, A. Pasca, G. Stanway, and W. Al-Nakib.** 1990. Detection and differentiation of picornaviruses in clinical samples following genomic amplification. *J. Gen. Virol.* **71:** 2141–2147.
57. **Peter, G. (ed.).** 1997. *Red Book: Report of the Committee on Infectious Diseases*, 24th ed., p. 15–21. American Academy of Pediatrics, Elk Grove Village, Ill.
58. **Phillips, C. A.** 1980. Enteroviruses and reoviruses, p. 823–828. *In* E. H. Lennette, A. Balows, W. J. Hausler, Jr., and J. P. Truant (ed.), *Manual of Clinical Microbiology*, 3rd ed. American Society for Microbiology, Washington, D.C.
59. **Pozzetto, B., O. G. Gaudin, M. Aouni, and A. Ros.** 1989. Comparative evaluation of immunoglobulin M neutralizing antibody response in acute-phase sera and virus isolation for the routine diagnosis of enterovirus infection. *J. Clin. Microbiol.* **27:**705–708.
60. **Reigel, F., F. Burkhardt, and U. Schilt.** 1985. Cross-reactions of immunoglobulin M and G antibodies with enterovirus-specific viral structural proteins. *J. Hyg.* **95:**469–481.
61. **Romero, J., J. R. Putnak, and E. Wimmer.** 1986. The use of poliovirus proteins VP3 and 2C as group antigens for the detection of enteroviral infections by indirect immunofluorescence, abstr. 967. *Pediatr. Res.* **20:**319.
62. **Romero, J. R., C. Price, and J. J. Dunn.** 1997. Genetic divergence among the group B coxsackieviruses. *Curr. Top. Microbiol. Immunol.* **223:**97–152.
63. **Romero, J. R., and H. A. Rotbart.** 1993. PCR detection of the human enteroviruses, p. 401–406. *In* D. H. Persing, T. F. Smith, F. C. Tenover, and T. J. White (ed.), *Diagnostic Molecular Microbiology: Principles and Applications*. American Society for Microbiology, Washington, D.C.
64. **Romero, J. R., and H. A. Rotbart.** 1994. PCR-based strategies for the detection of human enteroviruses, p. 341–374. *In* G. D. Ehrlich and S. J. Greenberg (ed.), *PCR-Based Diagnostics in Infectious Disease*. Blackwell Scientific Publications, Boston, Mass.
65. **Rotbart, H. A.** 1990. Enzymatic RNA amplification of the enteroviruses. *J. Clin. Microbiol.* **28:**438–442.
66. **Rotbart, H. A.** 1991. Nucleic acid detection systems for enteroviruses. *Clin. Microbiol. Rev.* **4:**156–168.
67. **Rotbart, H. A. (ed.).** 1995. *Human Enterovirus Infections*. ASM Press, Washington, D.C.
68. **Rotbart, H. A.** 1995. Meningitis and encephalitis, p. 271–289. *In* H. A. Rotbart (ed.), *Human Enterovirus Infections*. ASM Press, Washington D.C.
69. **Rotbart, H. A., A. Ahmed, S. Hickey, R. Dagan, G. H. McCracken, R. T. Whitley, J. F. Modlin, M. Cascino,**

J. F. O'Connell, M. A. Menegus, and D. Blum. 1997. Diagnosis of enterovirus infection by polymerase chain reaction of multiple specimen types. *Pediatr. Infect. Dis. J.* **16:**409–411.

70. **Rotbart, H. A., M. H. Sawyer, S. Fast, C. Lewinski, N. Murphy, E. F. Keyser, J. Spadoro, S.-Y. Kao, and M. Loeffelholz.** 1994. Diagnosis of enteroviral meningitis by using PCR with a colorimetric microbial detection assay. *J. Clin. Microbiol.* **32:**2590–2592.
71. **Rueckert, R. R.** 1990. Picornaviruses and their replication, p. 507–548. *In* B. N. Fields and D. M. Knipe (ed.), *Virology*. Raven Press, New York, N.Y.
72. **Samuelson, A., M. Forsgren, and M. Sallberg.** 1995. Characterization of the recognition site and diagnostic potential of an enterovirus group-reactive monoclonal antibody. *Clin. Diagn. Lab. Immunol.* **2:**385–386.
73. **Sawyer, M. H., D. Holland, N. Aintablian, J. D. Connor, E. F. Keyser, and N. J. Waecker, Jr.** Diagnosis of enteroviral central nervous system infection by polymerase chain reaction during a large community outbreak. *Pediatr. Infect. Dis. J.*, in press.
74. **Schlesinger, Y., M. N. Sawyer, and G. A. Storch.** 1994. Enteroviral meningitis in infancy: potential role for polymerase chain reaction in patient management. *Pediatrics* **94:**157–162.
75. **Schnurr, D., S. Yagi, and V. Devlin.** 1993. *Abstr. 9th Annu. Clin. Virol. Symp.*, p. 66.
76. **Strikas, R. A., L. J. Anderson, and R. A. Parker.** 1986. Temporal and geographic patterns of isolates of nonpolio enterovirus in the United States, 1970–1983. *J. Infect. Dis.* **153:**346–351.
77. **Wadia, N. H., S. M. Katrak, V. P. Misra, P. N. Wadia, K. Miyamura, K. Hashimoto, T. Ogino, T. Hikiju, and R. Kono.** 1983. Polio-like motor paralysis associated with acute hemorrhagic conjunctivitis in an outbreak in 1981 in Bombay, India: clinical and serologic studies. *J. Infect. Dis.* **147:**660–668.
78. **Weiner, L. B., H. A. Rotbart, D. C. Gilbert, F. G. Hayden, J. H. Mynhardt, D. C. Dwyer, H. Trocha, J. M. Rogers, and M. A. McKinlay.** 1997. Treatment of enterovirus meningitis with pleconaril (VP63843), an antipicornaviral agent. *In Program and Abstracts of the 37th Interscience Conference on Antimicrobial Agents and Chemotherapy*.
79. **Wenner, H. A., and M. F. Lenahan.** 1961. Propagation of group A coxsackie viruses in tissue cultures. *Yale J. Biol. Med.* **34:**421–438.
80. **Wilfert, C. M., and J. Zeller.** 1985. Enterovirus diagnosis, p. 85–107. *In* L. M. de la Maza and E. M. Peterson (ed.), *Medical Virology IV*. Lawrence Erlbaum Associates, Publishers, Hillsdale, N.J.
81. **Wright, H. T., R. M. McAllister, and R. Ward.** 1962. "Mixed" meningitis: reports of a case with isolation of Haemophilus influenzae type b and echovirus type 9 from the cerebrospinal fluid. *N. Engl. J. Med.* **267:**142–144.
82. **Yagi, S., D. Schnurr, and J. Lin.** 1992. Spectrum of monoclonal antibodies to coxsackievirus B-3 includes type- and group-specific antibodies. *J. Clin. Microbiol.* **30:** 2498–2501.
83. **Yolken, R. H., and V. M. Torsch.** 1980. Enzyme-linked immunosorbent assay for detection and identification of coxsackie B antigen in tissue cultures and clinical specimens. *J. Med. Virol.* **6:**45–52.
84. **Young, S. A., B. Strong, and R. Radloff.** 1993. *Abstr. 9th Annu. Clin. Virol. Symp.*, p. 67.
85. **Yousef, G. E., I. N. Brown, and J. F. Mowbray.** 1987. Derivation and biochemical characterization of an enterovirus group-specific monoclonal antibody. *Intervirology* **28:** 163–170.
86. **Zoll, G. J., W. J. G. Melchers, H. Kopecka, G. Jambroes, H. J. A. Van Der Poel, and J. M. D. Galama.** 1992. General primer-mediated polymerase chain reaction for detection of enteroviruses: application for diagnostic routine and persistent infections. *J. Clin. Microbiol.* **30:**160–165.

Rotaviruses

MARY L. CHRISTENSEN

79

DESCRIPTION OF ROTAVIRUSES

Rotaviruses are major causes of gastroenteritis in the young of many animal species including humans. Rotaviruses were discovered in the 1970s by electron microscopic (EM) examination of patients' specimens and were called "rotaviruses" because of their wheel-like appearance. Like other viruses that cause gastroenteritis in humans, rotaviruses are fastidious and are difficult to grow in routine cell cultures unless special techniques are used. Rotaviruses are in the family *Reoviridae*, whose members possess a double layer of icosahedral shells approximately 70 nm in diameter. They contain a core of double-stranded RNA. The rotavirus double-stranded RNA genome consists of 11 gene segments, which can be separated by polyacrylamide gel electrophoresis (5). Due to the segmentation of the genome, reassortment of genes can occur during coinfection of a cell with two different rotavirus types.

Three of the gene segments that code for three major rotavirus antigens are of particular interest (5). Gene segment 6 codes for VP6, the major inner core structural protein (9). VP6 is responsible for the group specificity of rotaviruses, which are divided into groups A through E. Human rotaviruses belong to group A, B, or C. Group A is the most common and most extensively studied rotavirus that infects humans; viruses in this group also infect several animal species. Human group A rotaviruses are subdivided into subgroups I and II. The subgroup specificity is also determined by VP6.

Gene segment 7, 8, or 9, depending on the strain of rotavirus, codes for VP7. VP7 is the major outer capsid protein, which is glycosylated. It is responsible for the G serotype specificity of group A viruses. The term "G" stands for glycosylated. Four major G serotypes, 1 through 4, that infect humans are well recognized and characterized. G serotype 2 has subgroup I specificity, whereas G serotypes 1, 3, and 4 have subgroup II specificity. Serotype 1 is the most prevalent G serotype infecting humans worldwide, although serotypes 2, 3, and 4 are also prevalent and are seen worldwide. Other G serotypes that infect humans include types 6, 8, 9, 10, and 12 (2, 10, 11, 18, 20, 25).

Gene segment 4 codes for VP4, a protease-sensitive outer capsid protein with hemagglutination properties. In electron micrographs, VP4 appears as cylindrical spikes radiating from the virion surface. It is responsible for the P serotype specificity of group A viruses. The term "P" stands for "protease sensitive." The P serotypes infecting humans include 1A, 1B, 2A, 3, 4, 5, and 8 (11, 16, 21). The P serotypes are independent of the G serotypes. However, the most commonly seen associations of G and P serotypes are an association of G serotypes 1, 3, and 4 with P serotype 1A and an association of G serotype 2 with P serotype 1B. These common types and their association have important implications for the development of rotavirus vaccines (11, 19).

Of particular interest is the nonstructural protein, NSP-4, which has an enterotoxin-like activity. This protein alone can induce diarrhea within hours of administration to mice, without the presence of rotavirus virions (1).

CLINICAL SIGNIFICANCE

Viral gastroenteritis is the second most common clinical disease occurring in developed countries; it is exceeded only by viral upper respiratory tract illness. Rotaviruses are the major cause of viral gastroenteritis in infants and young children in both developed and developing countries. In developing countries, approximately 125 million cases of rotavirus infection occur annually, with an estimated 873,000 deaths. In the United States, approximately three million cases occur each year, with 150 deaths (19). Infants and young children aged 6 months to 3 years exhibit the most severe disease. Healthy full-term neonates may become infected with the virus but are usually asymptomatic or have only mild disease (12). This may be due to protection by maternal antibody in serum and colostrum, as well as by nonspecific protective factors in colostrum. Rotaviruses occasionally cause gastroenteritis in the elderly, especially those living in nursing and retirement homes. Crowding of individuals and declining cellular and humoral immunity are contributing factors. Other causes of viral gastroenteritis, especially in the pediatric population, include enteric adenoviruses, astroviruses, coronaviruses, and caliciviruses. Norwalk and Norwalk-like viruses, which are members of the *Calicivirus* family, are a major cause of gastroenteritis in older children, adolescents, and adults, as well as in younger children (see chapter 80).

Gastroenteritis caused by group A rotaviruses occurs in all parts of the world. The majority of rotavirus infections occurring worldwide in infants and children are caused by group A rotaviruses. In countries that have temperate climates, group A rotavirus epidemics occur yearly during the colder months of the year, although endemic or sporadic cases may occur during the other months. During the winter months in temperate zones, nearly 50% of all pediatric gastroenteritis is due to rotavirus infection. Rotaviruses may be spread more easily in winter due to low indoor relative humidity, which may contribute to aerosolization of the virions, thus promoting its spread (3). Crowding indoors may also be a contributing factor. In tropical countries, group A rotavirus infection usually occurs endemically throughout the year, although in some countries minor increases in rotavirus diarrhea have been reported during the dry season.

Group B rotaviruses have been found primarily in China, where they have caused major epidemics, especially of adults (5). However, children and neonates can also develop symptomatic group B rotavirus infection. Group B viruses have rarely been seen outside mainland China. Group C rotaviruses cause gastroenteritis in both children and adults. Although they have occurred worldwide, they have been seen only sporadically or in small outbreaks (15).

Rotavirus infection is spread mainly by the fecal-oral route, although additional spread by the respiratory route has been suggested. The virus infects primarily the mature enterocytes, which are the epithelial cells on the tips of the villi of the small intestine. After an incubation period of about 1 to 2 days, the onset of rotavirus gastroenteritis is sudden, with vomiting and diarrhea, fever, occasionally abdominal pain, and even respiratory symptoms (5). Loss of fluids and electrolytes due to vomiting and diarrhea can lead to severe dehydration, hospitalization, and even death, especially in infants and very young children. Treatment consists primarily of fluid and electrolyte replacement, either orally or intravenously. Like most viral infections, rotavirus infection is self-limiting. Infection and rotavirus shedding can occur in all age groups, although infections by group A viruses are usually asymptomatic in older children and adults. Nosocomial infections are frequent and can account for up to 50% of the cases of rotavirus infection in hospitals if strict infection control measures are not undertaken. Transmission of the virus may be difficult to control, since 10^{10} or more virions per g of stool may be shed by patients, while less than 10 focus-forming units of virus can initiate an infection (5).

Rotavirus reinfection in the same individual usually involves different serotypes from those found in the primary infection. Antibody that develops after infection may persist for as long as 6 months; antibodies can either protect individuals from reinfection or reduce the severity of reinfection (5).

Several different types of rotavirus vaccines have been evaluated in clinical trials. They are still in the developmental and evaluation stages. The aim of a rotavirus vaccine is not to prevent infection or even mild illness but to prevent severe disease that can lead to dehydration and electrolyte imbalance (19). To date, the rotavirus vaccines tested have been live, attenuated vaccines that are administered by the oral route, similar to the live polio vaccine. Vaccines that have been evaluated in humans include vaccines developed from bovine rotaviruses, those developed from rhesus monkey rotavirus (RRV), and human-RRV reassortants. In the last instance, a quadrivalent vaccine that contains one RRV with a G serotype 3 specificity and three human-RRV reassortants with G serotype specificities of types 1, 2, and 4 has been developed and evaluated. These are the most common serotypes causing disease. Another aim is to have a vaccine that is compatible with the live, oral polio vaccine, so that the two vaccines can be administered together following accepted immunization protocols.

COLLECTION, TRANSPORT, AND STORAGE OF SPECIMENS

For the direct detection of rotavirus, stool specimens should be collected during the acute phase of the illness, preferably the first 3 to 5 days of illness. Specimens should be placed directly into clean plastic or glass screw-cap jars or cups for submission to the laboratory. The specimen container should not contain any preservatives, detergents, or metal ions. In addition, the container should not contain viral transport media or tissue culture media. These media may contain fetal bovine serum or other sera, which may contain inhibitors or antibodies to rotavirus. All of these substances could interfere with enzyme immunoassays (EIAs) and latex agglutination (LA) tests. In addition, adding specimens to viral transport medium could dilute out the specimen beyond the limits of detection of viral particles.

Liquid stool specimens from pediatric patients in diapers can be obtained in several ways. Liquid diarrheal stool can be prevented from being absorbed into a diaper either by placing a disposable diaper, inside out, on an infant or by placing a layer of plastic wrap inside a clean diaper. Alternatively, a clean pediatric urine bag can be placed over the anal area to collect very watery stool. Liquid stool soaked in a diaper can be removed by pressing a cotton swab into the diaper until the swab is *well saturated* with stool. A saturated swab will take up 0.1 to 0.15 ml of fluid. If this method is used, it is recommended that two or three swabs be submitted at one time, so that sufficient stool material can be eluded from the swabs into the EIA or LA buffer used in the initial stool-processing step. However, rectal swabs per se should not be submitted, since sufficient virions may not be present on the rectal swab for detection.

Specimens should be transported and stored at 4°C. For long-term storage, specimens should be frozen undiluted between −20 and −60°C and not repeatedly frozen and thawed.

DETECTION OF ROTAVIRUSES

Since rotaviruses are difficult to propagate in cell culture, other detection methods have been developed and used. Three diagnostic methods can be easily carried out in diagnostic laboratories and on large numbers of specimens, often without specialized equipment. These are the EIA, the rapid membrane EIA, and the LA test. These three tests are antibody-based tests that utilize antigen-antibody reactions. A number of commercial EIA, membrane EIA, and LA kits that detect group A rotaviruses are available (Table 1).

EIAs

Commercially available EIAs are three-layer double-antibody sandwich assays. They may utilize one of several modifications, and they vary in several respects. First, either polyclonal or monoclonal antibodies may be used for the capture and detector antibody systems, although some of the assays

TABLE 1 General characteristics of commercial rotavirus tests

Test	Kit name (manufacturer)	Type of antibody[a]	Negative control beads, tubes, or wells	Form for final reading	Total incubation time (min)
EIA	IDEIA Rotavirus (Dako)	Polyclonal/polyclonal	No	Microtiter	70
	Pathfinder (Kallestad)	Polyclonal/monoclonal	No	Tube, microtiter	75
	Rotaclone (Meridian)	Monoclonal/monoclonal	No	Microtiter	70
	Rotazyme II (Abbott)	Polyclonal/polyclonal	No	Tube	150
	Vidas Rotavirus (bioMérieux)	Polyclonal/monoclonal	Yes	Reagent strip	30
EIA, rapid	Test Pack Rotavirus (Abbott)	Polyclonal/monoclonal-polyclonal mixture	No	Reaction disk	7
	ImmunoCard Rota. STAT (Meridian)	Monoclonal/polyclonal	No	Line on device	10
	ImmunoCard Rotavirus (Meridian)	Polyclonal/polyclonal	No	Circle on card	6
LA	Diarlex Rota-Adeno (Orion)	Polyclonal	Yes	Latex beads	2
	Meritec-Rotavirus (Meridian)	Polyclonal	Yes	Latex beads	5
	Murex Rotavirus Latex (Murex)	Polyclonal	Yes	Latex beads	17
	Slidex Rota-kit 2 (bioMérieux)	Polyclonal	Yes	Latex beads	7–12
	Virogen Rotatest (Wampole)	Polyclonal	Yes	Latex beads	17

[a] For EIA, capture antibody/detector antibody; for LA test, antibody on latex.

use polyclonal antibodies for both. Second, either microtiter wells, larger wells, test tubes, or reagent strips are used for the reaction mixtures. A standard laboratory spectrophotometer can be used to read the tubes, whereas a microtiter reader is needed for the microtiter wells. Companies may furnish computerized spectrophotometers to read tubes or microtiter plates. One company also provides a specific color chart for visual readings. Some manufacturers do suggest that visual readings can be carried out. However, with low-level positive or borderline readings, spectrophotometric readings and mathematical calculations of cutoff values based on the manufacturer's directions are recommended. One company's automated instrument reads the amount of fluorescence from a fluorescent enzyme substrate. EIA readings may be considered semiquantitative, since positive readings will range from high-level to low-level readings. Thus, more information on the amount of viral antigen being excreted can be obtained from an EIA than from a membrane EIA or LA test, which are read qualitatively as "positive" or "negative." EIAs are also useful when large numbers of specimens are to be run at one time. EIAs are usually run at ambient temperature. One company (Meridian) manufactures a rotavirus group EIA, an adenovirus type 40 and 41 EIA, and an adenovirus group EIA, all of which have the same format and can be run concomitantly on diarrheal stools from gastroenteritis patients.

Membrane EIA

Simple, fast, easy-to-read qualitative membrane EIAs are also commercially available and require very little equipment. In these tests, a stool suspension and the necessary reagents are added to a small reaction disk or test card. The results are easily read visually after 7 to 10 min of total incubation time at ambient temperature. A plus (+) sign, a colored line, or a colored circle will appear if the specimen is positive. Positive controls are built into each system to determine if the test was carried out correctly. No special equipment or expertise is needed, and these EIAs are sensitive and specific (4). Membrane EIAs can be run in less than 30 min total hands-on time and are useful for running one or several rotavirus tests at one time. This type of test can be used in small-volume hospital laboratories, as stat tests in large-volume hospital laboratories, or in physicians' offices.

LA Tests

LA tests have the advantages of requiring very little equipment and being very rapid (they are usually completed within 30 min at ambient temperature). All of the LA test kits contain both test latex particles coated with anti-rotavirus serum and control latex particles coated with nonimmune serum or globulin. Most LA tests have a high level of specificity (5, 8, 13, 22), due in part to the incorporation in the test procedure of the negative control latex particles. LA tests are usually not as sensitive as EIAs (5, 6, 13, 17, 22). The sensitivity of LA tests is adequate for use with specimens taken early in infection, when large amounts of virus are being excreted. However, the sensitivity tends to be lower than that of EIAs for specimens taken late in infection, when significantly fewer virions are being excreted. Like the membrane EIA, LA tests are useful for running one or several rotavirus tests at one time. They are good for laboratories with low-volume rotavirus testing or for stat testing in laboratories that normally use EIAs for their high-volume rotavirus testing. One company (Orion Diagnostica) manufactures a combination kit containing reagents for both rotavirus and enteric adenovirus testing.

Additional Test Criteria

There are additional criteria to take into consideration when choosing among the standard EIA, the membrane EIA, and the LA test. The total incubation times of the standard EIAs can range from 75 min to 2 h or more, which is significantly longer than is needed to report the results of LA tests. However, the actual hands-on-time for EIA is significantly shorter than the total incubation times. EIAs are usually more sensitive than LA tests (5, 7, 8, 12, 13, 17, 22), although this criterion can vary from manufacturer to manufacturer. Monoclonal antibody-based kits appear to be more sensitive than polyclonal antibody-based kits (5, 7, 8, 12, 13, 17, 22). Kits that contain negative control wells or beads tend to be more specific, since they minimize false-positive reactions (7). However, neither the commercially available LA tests nor the EIAs detect group B or C rotaviruses, and some assays do not detect certain group A serotypes (17).

All of the commercially available standard EIAs, membrane EIAs, and LA tests should be carried out as specified by the manufacturers. Quality control standards specified in the kits should be adhered to. Positive and negative controls are provided in the kits and should be used as instructed by the manufacturers.

PCR

Several PCR techniques for detecting and typing rotaviruses have been developed in research laboratories but are not available for routine use. A highly sensitive PCR procedure for detecting group A rotaviruses in stools has been developed (24). In this procedure, viral RNA is extracted and purified from stools and the inhibitory substances in the stools are removed. The resultant RNA is used in a reverse transcriptase reaction to produce complementary DNA (cDNA), which is then amplified by PCR. The same set of primers are used for both the reverse transcriptase step and the PCR step, with directed primers to rotavirus gene 6, which codes for the group-specific antigen. These primers consist of the first 20 bases of gene 6 for primer 1, and a 25-base segment between bases 234 and 259 for primer 2. As few as 500 genomic copies of purified rotavirus RNA can be detected in this manner. Rotavirus RNA can be detected experimentally in fecal samples at dilutions of 1,000- to 10,000-fold beyond the limits of detection by EIA.

A PCR technique has also been developed for typing six of the group A rotaviruses, with type-specific primers derived from six variable regions on gene 9 (14). In addition, PCR techniques have been developed to identify gene 4 (VP4) types (10) and to detect group B and group C rotaviruses.

Electron Microscopy

Before the availability of EIAs and LA tests, rotaviruses were detected by EM, and this method is still being used by some laboratories. The EM method has several advantages. It is relatively rapid, especially when a small number of samples are evaluated. EM can detect both group A and non-group A rotaviruses, as well as other enteric viruses. However, it has several disadvantages. (i) It requires the use of expensive equipment. (ii) It may be less sensitive than EIA. (iii) When a large number of specimens are run at once, EM can be slower and more tedious than other methods now available. The EM procedure for detecting rotaviruses and other enteric viruses in stools has been described previously (6), and more information on detecting diarrheic viruses is available in chapter 80.

Culture

Culture of human rotaviruses is usually not done in diagnostic laboratories, since the virus is found in large quantities in stool specimens and can be rapidly detected by antigen detection tests. Only a minority of the virions in a specimen are infectious to cell cultures. However, some research laboratories have cultivated rotaviruses by using various manipulations, including pretreating specimens with trypsin, adding low levels of trypsin to cell culture maintenance medium, and rolling the cell cultures (5). By these methods, the virus can be propagated in primary kidney cells or lines of kidney cells from various species of monkeys. Cytopathic effect can usually be observed after several passages and may consist of cell fusion, rounding, granularity, lysis, and sloughing. Viruses from patient specimens may grow better in primary cells but can then be passaged in the cell lines (5, 23).

SEROLOGY

Detection of virus in stools is the major approach used for diagnosing rotavirus gastroenteritis in the routine diagnostic laboratory. Blood or serum is usually not submitted, since serological testing for diagnosing rotavirus gastroenteritis is not usually done in diagnostic laboratories. Serological studies involving EIA, radioimmunoassay, and other methods have been carried out primarily in research laboratories (i) for typing or grouping of new isolates or (ii) for epidemiologic purposes (5).

EVALUATION, INTERPRETATION, AND REPORTING OF RESULTS

EIAs

Certain standard EIA results can be read visually. With one kit, patient results and control results can be compared to a color chart provided with the kit. With several other kits, patient results can be compared to the color development of the positive and negative controls. All EIAs can also be read spectrophotometrically, with results being considered positive if they are greater than a cutoff value specified by the manufacturer. One company's kit has a "gray zone" in which the specimen spectrophotometric readings that are within 10% of the cutoff value are considered suspect. These tests should be repeated, preferably with a new specimen from the patient. With all kits, all controls should fall within the criteria specified by the manufacturer; if they do not, the test should be repeated. Spectrophotometric readings are recommended for accuracy, especially with low-level or borderline specimens.

Due to the wide variation in the composition of the stool specimens being tested, it is possible that some specimens contain a substance(s) which may bind nonspecifically in the EIAs, giving low-level false-positive test results, near the cutoff value. Low-level positive results could also be the result of (i) low levels of rotavirus antigen being excreted or (ii) submission of insufficient, minute amounts of stool specimen on a swab or in a container. If the quantity of stool submitted is smaller than that specified by the manufacturer of the kit being used, it is recommended that this be recorded for additional information if a low-level positive, "suspect," or negative result is obtained. It is recommended that the spectrophotometric cutoff value and gray zone, if applicable, be reported along with the spectrophotometric reading of the patient's specimen. This information, along with the quantity of specimen submitted, if inadequate, is useful information for the physician in deciding if an additional specimen should be sent for testing.

The limit of sensitivity of EIA is about 10^6 virions per ml of stool. Thus, negative results would be obtained with stool specimens containing fewer virions. The rotavirus EIAs, as well as the membrane EIAs and the LA tests, detect inactive virus particles and viral antigen, as well as live rotavirus particles.

Membrane EIAs

The membrane EIAs are read visually. Depending on the brand of kit, a plus (+) sign, a colored line, or a colored circle indicates a positive reaction and shows that the test was carried out correctly. A minus (−) sign or the lack of a colored line or colored circle in the test area indicates a negative reaction. Built-in positive controls in all of the tests will indicate if the test was carried out properly and if the reagents performed satisfactorily. These results can be reported as "positive for rotavirus" or "negative for rotavirus," respectively.

As with the EIAs, membrane EIAs may give a negative result if there are low levels of rotavirus antigen that are below the limits of detection, which is in the range of 10^6 to 10^7 virions per ml of stool. The package inserts of each test specify the limits of sensitivity in terms of virion numbers. It is suggested that when reporting results, the limits of sensitivity of the test be included with the test results, especially with negative results. Negative results may also be obtained if inadequate amounts of specimen were submitted or if the specimens were diluted before the initial test procedure. Inadequate amounts of stool sample or dilution of stool before it is received in the laboratory should be recorded along with a negative result, so that this information can be given to the physician, along with a request for a new specimen.

LA Tests

The LA tests are also read visually. The positive rotavirus control reagent should cause agglutination of the test latex particles coated with antirotavirus serum. A patient specimen is positive if it agglutinates the test latex but does not agglutinate the negative control latex. A patient specimen is negative if the test latex particles and the negative control latex particles do not agglutinate. These results can be reported as "positive for rotavirus" and "negative for rotavirus," respectively.

A patient specimen agglutinating both the test latex and the negative control latex contains nonspecific agglutinins. The specimen may be a true negative, or the nonspecific agglutinins may be masking any agglutination of the test latex caused by rotavirus particles in the specimen. When nonspecific agglutination occurs, the test should be repeated on a new dilution of the original specimen or, preferably, on a new specimen. If nonspecific agglutination persists, the specimen should be tested by an EIA method or by the membrane EIA.

Due to the incorporation of the negative control latex, the LA tests are highly specific, usually approaching 100% specificity in most studies. The limits of specificity of the LA tests are approximately 10^7 virions per g of stool. It is suggested that the limits of sensitivity of the test be included with the test results, especially when negative results are reported.

REFERENCES

1. **Ball, J. M., P. Tian, C. Q. Zeng, A. Morris, and M. K. Estes.** 1996. Age-dependent diarrhea is induced by a viral nonstructural glycoprotein. *Science* **272:**101–104.
2. **Beards, G. M., U. Desselberger, and T. H. Flewett.** 1989. Temporal and geographical distributions of human rotavirus serotypes, 1983 to 1988. *J. Clin. Microbiol.* **27:** 2827–2833.
3. **Brandt, C. D., H. W. Kim, W. J. Rodriguez, J. O. Arrobio, B. C. Jefferies, and R. H. Parrott.** 1982. Rotavirus gastroenteritis and weather. *J. Clin. Microbiol.* **16:** 478–482.
4. **Chernesky, M., S. Castriciano, J. Mahony, M. Spiewak, and L. Schaeffer.** 1988. Ability of TESTPACK ROTAVIRUS enzyme immunoassay to diagnose rotavirus gastroenteritis. *J. Clin. Microbiol.* **26:**2459–2461.
5. **Christensen, M. L.** 1989. Human viral gastroenteritis. *Clin. Microbiol. Rev.* **2:**51–89.
6. **Christensen, M. L., and C. Howard.** 1991. Viruses causing gastroenteritis, p. 950–958. *In* A. Balows, W. J. Hausler, Jr., K. L. Herrmann, H. D. Isenberg, and H. J. Shadomy (ed.), *Manual of Clinical Microbiology*, 5th ed. American Society for Microbiology, Washington, D.C.
7. **Cromien, J. L., C. A. Himmelreich, R. I. Glass, and G. A. Storch.** 1987. Evaluation of new commercial enzyme immunoassay for rotavirus detection. *J. Clin. Microbiol.* **25:** 2359–2362.
8. **Dennehy, P. H., D. R. Gauntlett, and W. E. Tente.** 1988. Comparison of nine commercial immunoassays for the detection of rotavirus in fecal specimens. *J. Clin. Microbiol.* **26:**1630–1634.
9. **Estes, M. K., B. B. Mason, S. Crawford, and J. Cohen.** 1984. Cloning and nucleotide sequence of the simian rotavirus gene 6 that codes for the major inner capsid protein. *Nucleic Acids Res.* **12:**1875–1887.
10. **Gentsch, J. R., R. I. Glass, P. Woods, V. Gouvea, M. Gorziglia, J. Flores, B. K. Das, and M. K. Bhan.** 1992. Identification of group A rotavirus gene 4 types by polymerase chain reaction. *J. Clin. Microbiol.* **30:**1365–1373.
11. **Gentsch, J. R., P. A. Woods, M. Ramachandran, B. K. Das, J. P. Leite, A. Alfieri, R. Kumar, M. K. Bhan, and R. I. Glass.** 1996. Review of G and P typing results from a global collection of rotavirus strains: implications for vaccine development. *J. Infect. Dis.* **174**(Suppl. 1)**:**S30–S36.
12. **Giaquinto, C., G. Errico, E. Ruga, I. Naso, and R. D'Elia.** 1986. Evaluation of ELISA test for rotavirus diagnosis in neonates *J. Pediatr.* **109:**565–566.
13. **Gilchrist, M. J. R., T. S. Bretl, K. Moultney, D. R. Knowlton, and R. L. Ward.** 1987. Comparison of seven kits for detection of rotavirus in fecal specimens with a sensitive, specific enzyme immunoassay. *Diagn. Microbiol. Infect. Dis.* **8:**221–228.
14. **Gouvea, V., R. I. Glass, P. Woods, K. Taniguchi, H. F. Clark, B. Forrester, and Z.-Y. Fang.** 1990. Polymerase chain reaction amplification and typing of rotavirus nucleic acid from stool specimens. *J. Clin. Microbiol.* **28:**276–282.
15. **Gouvea, V., J. R. Allen, R. I. Glass, Z.-Y. Fang, M. Bremont, J. Cohen, M. A. McCrae, L. J. Saif, P. Sinarachatanant, and E. O. Caul.** 1991. Detection of group B and C rotaviruses by polymerase chain reaction. *J. Clin. Microbiol.* **29:**519–523.
16. **Gunasena, S., O. Nakagomi, Y. Isegawa, E. Kaga, T. Nakagomi, A. D. Steele, J. Flores, and S. Ueda.** 1993. Relative frequency of VP4 gene alleles among human rotaviruses recovered over a 10-year period (1982–1991) from Japanese children with diarrhea. *J. Clin. Microbiol.* **31:** 2195–2197.
17. **Mathewson, J. J., D. K. Winsor, Jr., H. L. DuPont, and S. L. Secor.** 1989. Evaluation of assay systems for the detection of rotavirus in stool specimens. *Diagn. Microbiol. Infect. Dis.* **12:**139–141.
18. **Matson, D. O., M. K. Estes, J. W. Burns, H. B. Greenberg, K. Taniguchi, and S. Urasawa.** 1990. Serotype variation of human group A rotaviruses in two regions of the USA. *J. Infect. Dis.* **162:**605–614.
19. **Midthun, K. J., and A. Z. Kapikian.** 1996. Rotavirus vaccines: an overview. *Clin. Microbiol. Rev.* **9:**423–434.
20. **Midthun, K., J. Valdesuso, A. Z. Kapikian, Y. Hoshino, and K. Y. Green.** 1989. Identification of serotype 9 human rotavirus by enzyme-linked immunosorbent assay with monoclonal antibodies. *J. Clin. Microbiol.* **27:**2112–2114.
21. **Steele, A. D., D. Garcia, J. Sears, G. Gerna, O. Nakagomi, and J. Flores.** 1993. Distribution of VP4 gene

alleles in human rotaviruses by using probes to the hyper-divergent region of the VP4 gene. *J. Clin. Microbiol.* **31:** 1735–1740.

22. **Thomas, E. E., M. L. Puterman, E. Kawano, and M. Curran.** 1988. Evaluation of seven immunoassays for detection of rotavirus in pediatric stool samples. *J. Clin. Microbiol.* **26:**1189–1193.
23. **Ward, R. L., D. R. Knowlton, and M. J. Pierce.** 1984. Efficiency of human rotavirus propagation in cell culture. *J. Clin. Microbiol.* **19:**748–753.
24. **Wilde, J., J Eiden, and R. Yolken.** 1990. Removal of inhibitory substances from human fecal specimens for detection of group A rotaviruses by reverse transcriptase and polymerase chain reaction. *J. Clin. Microbiol.* **28:** 1300–1307.
25. **Woods, P. A., J. Gentsch, V. Gouvea, L. Mata, A. Simhon, M. Santosham, Z.-S. Bai, S. Urasawa, and R. I. Glass.** 1992. Distribution of serotypes of human rotavirus in different populations. *J. Clin. Microbiol.* **30:** 781–785.

Caliciviruses, Astroviruses, and Other Diarrheic Viruses

MARTIN PETRIC

80

CLINICAL BACKGROUND

Gastroenteritis viruses have been recognized as major human pathogens for almost the past three decades. They comprise a broad group of agents which includes members of the families *Reoviridae* (rotavirus), *Adenoviridae* (enteric adenoviruses), *Caliciviridae* (Norwalk group viruses and caliciviruses), *Astroviridae* (astrovirus), and *Coronaviridae* (coronavirus and torovirus, which are now classified into the order *Nidovirales*) (10). Although virtually all of these agents were first recognized in the 1970s, the major advances until recently were in our knowledge of rotaviruses, which were not only the most commonly recognized agents but also the most amenable to investigation due to their distinct morphology, nucleic acid composition, and growth in cell culture (6). This chapter addresses the gastroenteritis viruses other than rotaviruses, which are discussed in chapter 79.

Caliciviruses

Based on the genomic sequences, the human caliciviruses are currently considered to comprise three distinct genogroups, the Norwalk virus group, the Snow Mountain agent (SMA) group, and the Sapporo virus group. Based on their morphology, these agents have also been called small round structured viruses (SRSV) and, in the case of the Sapporo virus group, typical caliciviruses (36).

Human caliciviruses were the first viral agents to be associated with gastroenteritis. By applying immunoelectron microscopy (IEM) to fecal specimens of volunteers infected with the stool filtrates from a gastroenteritis outbreak from Norwalk, Ohio, 27-nm virus particles were visualized in 1972 and the agent was designated the Norwalk virus. Based on studies of outbreaks and studies of volunteers, the clinical features of the Norwalk virus were found to include nausea, vomiting, diarrhea, abdominal cramps, headache, and fever (37). The illness has a mean incubation period of 24 h and a duration of 12 to 48 h. It may be severe in debilitated and elderly patients, although asymptomatic infections have been documented. Norwalk virus outbreaks have occurred in institutions, cruise ships, restaurants, and the family setting (38). The source of infection in outbreaks, which occur throughout the year, is likely to be contaminated food or water, and secondary spread can occur. Antibody response is detectable after infection and is protective for a limited period. Based on serological studies, the virus has a worldwide distribution (37) and even has an impact on military operations, as in the case of the Desert Shield virus (49).

A number of viruses morphologically similar to the Norwalk virus have been variously called Norwalk-like viruses or SRSVs. The association of these agents with gastroenteritis has been established in outbreak and volunteer studies (37). These viruses cause an illness clinically similar to that due to Norwalk virus and have similar epidemiological features. There is, however, serological evidence that the SMA viruses are acquired earlier in life than Norwalk virus itself (36). Drinking water has recently been conclusively documented as a vehicle for virus transmission (5). Many SRSVs belong to the SMA genogroup, although some belong to the Norwalk genogroup.

Viruses with typical calicivirus morphology, first found in 1976 in stool specimens from symptomatic patients, received their name based on their morphologic similarity to the feline calicivirus (12, 50). The four human calicivirus strains identified to date have been designated UK 1 through UK 3 and Sapporo virus (12). These viruses, having typical calicivirus morphology, are currently classified in the Sapporo genogroup (13). Evidence that these are pathogens came from studies of gastroenteritis outbreaks that were associated with excretion of calicivirus in the stools and were followed by seroconversion. Clinical features of calicivirus-associated gastroenteritis are diarrhea and vomiting, generally without fever. The illness has been reported to last 1 to 11 days and to have an incubation period of 48 to 72 h (12). Symptomatic infections occur in infants and young children, but geriatric outbreaks have also been documented. Infections occur throughout the year but show an increased incidence in the winter months. The virus is transmitted in institutional settings and through vehicles of contaminated food and water (6). The virus occurs worldwide, and virtually the entire population is seropositive by the age of 4 years (12).

Astroviruses

Astroviruses, which are detected in stool specimens by electron microscopy (EM), were first associated with gastroenteritis in 1975 (43). Astroviruses which are not antigenically related to the human pathogens have also been detected in a number of animal species (43). There are at least seven distinct serotypes of human astrovirus (44). The association of astroviruses with gastroenteritis was determined as a result of investigations of outbreaks of mild gastroenteritis, prospective studies, and studies of infection in volunteers (27, 43). Clinical symptoms, which generally last up to 3 days, include vomiting, abdominal pain, fever, and diarrhea. The diarrhea has been known to continue for 7 to 14 days and to be accompanied by virus excretion (43). The disease is most common in infants and young children, although asymptomatic infections have been noted (25, 49). Symptomatic illness occurs more rarely and with diminished symptoms in adults (11). The incubation period is estimated to be 3 to 4 days, and secondary spread is common (40, 49).

Enteric Adenoviruses

Although adenoviruses have been cultured from stool specimens of children with gastroenteritis almost since their discovery, it was only when abundant fecal shedding was detected by EM that they were considered etiologic agents of this disease (11, 21). A subset of these adenoviruses which could not be isolated in conventional cell cultures were referred to as fastidious enteric adenoviruses (17). These were shown to belong to types 40 and 41, which could be propagated in Graham 293 cells or Chang conjunctival cells. The role of enteric adenoviruses in gastroenteritis was definitively demonstrated in prospective studies, where they were found to account for 59% of the adenoviruses detected in stools and were the only detectable agent associated with 7% of cases of diarrhea (17). The distinguishing clinical symptoms of infection with these viruses were prolonged diarrhea and low-grade fever, with or without vomiting, which could last for more than 14 days. Secondary spread among children is common. The virus is a common cause of pediatric gastroenteritis (11, 17), with infections being most common in infants younger than 2 years. Asymptomatic shedding has been reported (6, 17, 42). Enteric adenovirus infections occur year-round, and there is an increased incidence in the warmer months (11).

Coronaviruses and Toroviruses

Although coronaviruses such as transmissible gastroenteritis virus and toroviruses such as Breda virus are major gastrointestinal pathogens of animals, human agents resembling these viruses have been only sporadically associated with cases of gastrointestinal illness (11, 56). The detection of human torovirus-like particles in patients with gastroenteritis was first reported in 1984, and these agents were shown to be associated with acute and persistent diarrhea in children and to be potentially important nosocomial pathogens (4, 31, 41). Seroconversion following infection has been demonstrated by IEM and hemagglutination inhibition assays with virus purified from stool specimens (19, 31). Since these viruses have not been reproducibly isolated in cell culture and reference antisera are not routinely available, their detection is generally limited to EM examination of patient specimens.

Small Round Viruses and Other Agents

Viral particles ranging from 25 to 30 nm in diameter have been found in stool specimens from patients with gastroenteritis. These have been termed small round viruses or "picorna-parvo-like agents" based on their morphology. They could represent enteroviruses or phages, and their role in gastroenteritis has not been well established. Certain agents such as the Aichi strain have been successfully grown in cell culture and have been shown to be antigenically unique agents associated with gastroenteritis (61). Picobirnavirus, another small virus reported to be associated with an outbreak of diarrhea in Brazil, has a defined double-stranded RNA genome of two segments. Such small round agents are currently under investigation and are proving to be novel agents of gastroenteritis (6, 10a, 11).

DESCRIPTION OF THE AGENTS

Morphology and Structure

Most reports on the structure of gastroenteritis viruses have been based on negative contrast electron microscopy. A short description of the characteristic features of the morphology of each of these agents is therefore presented.

The human caliciviruses include both the typical caliciviruses and the atypical caliciviruses consisting of the SRSVs (36). The typical 35-nm-diameter caliciviruses (Fig. 1A) have well-defined scalloped edges and 32 cup-shaped depressions over the surface of the virion, which makes for easy, unambiguous identification (50). In contrast, the SRSVs (Norwalk-like viruses), while having a similar diameter to that of calicivirus (or smaller), have less well-defined and more fuzzy edges, which are particularly distinct if the particles are penetrated by stains (Fig. 1B). The Norwalk virus, measuring 27 nm in diameter, is reported to have a somewhat indistinct, rough outer edge (37).

Astrovirises (Fig. 1C) have smooth edges with the characteristic five- or six-pointed star in the center of the 28- to 30-nm particle. The star shape, which is believed to be due to shallow hollows in the viral surface where stain is differentially deposited, may be apparent in only a fraction of the particles (50).

Small round viruses (Fig. 1D) lack the structural features noted for the above agents. They are 25 to 30 nm in diameter and have smooth outlines.

Adenoviruses (Fig. 1E) are icosahedral structures, 70 to 75 nm in diameter, which can be readily recognized by EM and are easily differentiated from rotaviruses, which have a similar size but a different arrangement of capsomerers (51).

Coronaviruses and toroviruses are unique among the human gastroenteritis agents in that they are enveloped viruses with helical symmetry (Fig. 1F). This feature has made the definitive detection of these agents in stool specimens by EM problematic. The distinct elongated peplomeres of the coronaviruses distinguish them from toroviruses, whose peplomere fringe is less distinct, as shown in Fig. 1G (19, 30, 40). Toroviruses also tend to assume a rod- or kidney-shaped configuration. These viruses are 100 to 150 nm in diameter.

Physical-Chemical Characteristics

Recent advances have provided new insights into the physical-chemical nature of the viruses described above. The salient features of the nucleic acid and protein composition of these agents are summarized in Table 1.

Antigenic Characteristics

Antigenic homology exists among the viruses in each group. While limited cross-reactivity between the caliciviruses of the Norwalk virus and the SMA genogroups has been documented (13), enzyme-linked immunosorbent assays (ELISAs) based on the respective recombinant capsid antigens are type specific and the Sapporo group is antigenically distinct (36). Enteric adenovirus types 40 and 41 can be specifically recognized by monoclonal antibodies and differentiated from other adenoviruses with which they share the adenovirus antigen (58). Astroviruses exist as seven distinct

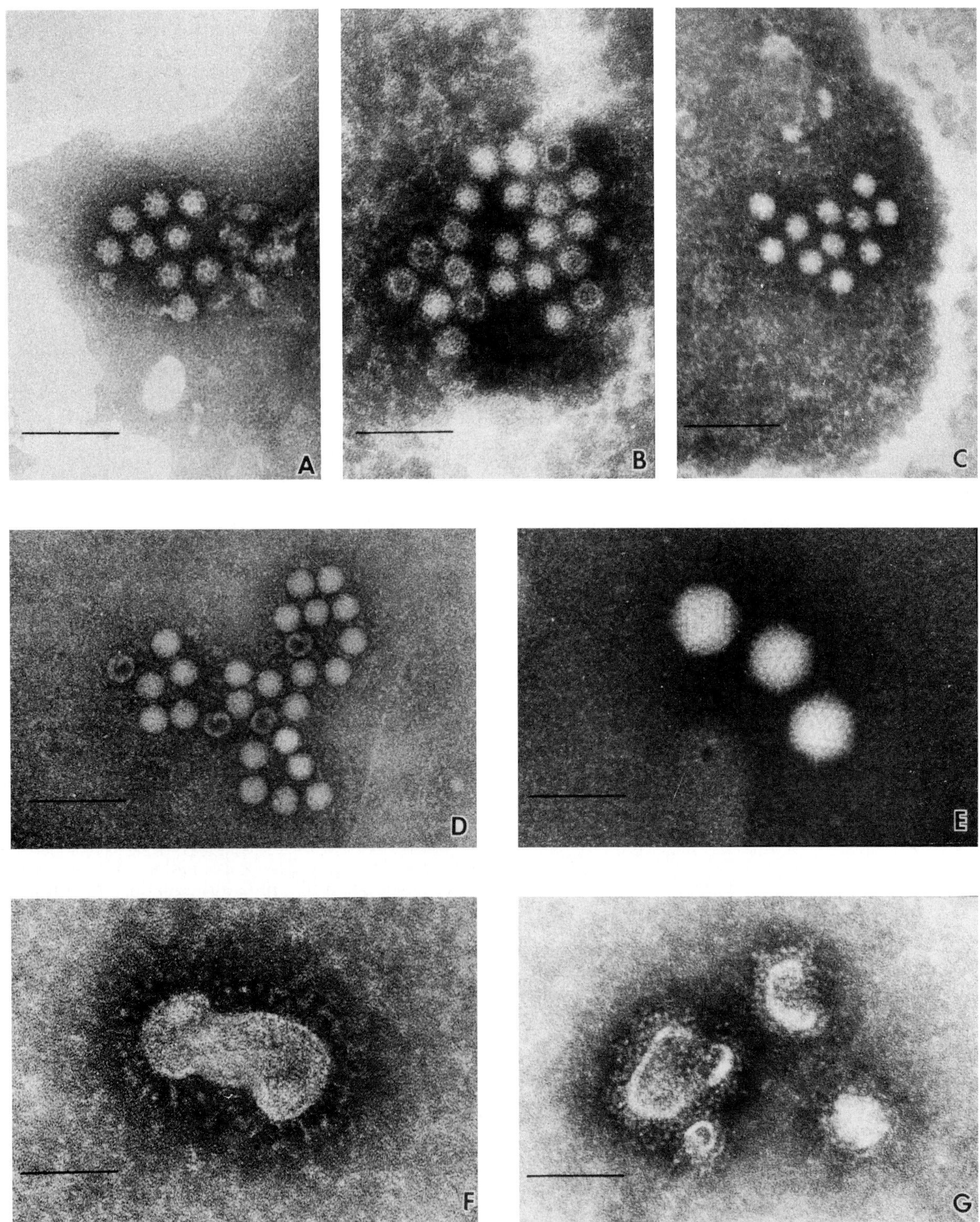

FIGURE 1 Gastroenteritis viruses. (A) Calicivirus. (B) Norwalk-like virus. (C) Astrovirus. (D) Small round virus. (E) Adenovirus. (F) Coronavirus. (G) Torovirus-like particle. Bars, 100 nm.

TABLE 1 Nucleic acid and protein composition of gastroenteritis viruses

Virus	Nucleic acid		Major structural proteins		
	Type[a]	Genome size (kb)	ORFs	Function[b]	Size(s) (kDa)
Calicivirus	ssRNA	8	3	Capsid	59–65
Norwalk	ssRNA	8	3	Capsid	56.6
Norwalk-like	ssRNA	8	3	Capsid	59
Astrovirus	ssRNA	7	3	Capsid	30, 29, 21
Adenovirus	dsDNA	30	30[c]	Hexon	120
				Penton	80
				Fiber	40
Coronavirus[d]	ssRNA	30	5	N	50–60
				E1	20–30
				E2	180–200
				E3	120–140
Torovirus[e]	ssRNA	25	5	N	18
				M	20
				S	75–90
				HE	65

[a] ss, single stranded; ds, double stranded.
[b] N, nucleocapsid; E, envelope; M, membrane; S, spike (peplomere); HE, hemagglutinin-esterase.
[c] mRNAs are extensively spliced (29).
[d] Based on the animal coronavirus genome (28).
[e] Based on the Berne virus genome (30).

serotypes. However, they do possess cross-reactive antigens, since a group-specific monoclonal antibody to five serotypes of human astroviruses has been developed (26). Cross-reactivity of the human torovirus-like particles with the calf torovirus, the Breda virus, has been reported (40). The antigenic features of these viruses have important implications for the design of tests to diagnose viruses directly and for serological assays.

Genetics

The nucleic acid sequences of at least part of the genomes of all the recognized gastroenteritis viruses are now known. The cloning and sequencing of the Norwalk virus genome and that of related viruses have allowed for major progress in our understanding of the human caliciviruses (34, 45). The single-stranded RNA genome of Norwalk virus has an open reading frame (ORF) coding for the polymerase at the 5′ end, a capsid ORF in the 3′ half of the genome, and an ORF at the extreme 3′ end which has as yet no known function. The polymerase sequence is of interest since it has sufficient heterogeneity to allow sequence-specific subtyping of the human caliciviruses (3, 34). Sequencing the genome of the astrovirus has led to the creation of the family *Astroviridae* (32, 54). The genome possesses three ORFs, of which ORF 3 (at the 3′ end) codes for the capsid proteins. A subgenomic RNA corresponding to the 3′ end of the astrovirus genome has been shown to code for a precursor protein, which is cleaved into three capsid proteins (9, 54). The genome of the enteric adenovirus 40 has been completely sequenced (15), and defined sequences of enteric adenovirus 41 have been reported (1, 23). There is also evidence of homology between the genomes of the human and calf toroviruses (19, 39).

SPECIMEN COLLECTION AND STORAGE

Specimens should be collected as soon as the gastroenteritis is diagnosed and ideally within the first 48 h of illness. Specimens collected after 1 week of illness may yield negative results either because the virus shedding has decreased or because the virus is complexed with coproantibody. Stool specimens of between 1 and 10 g are generally placed into plastic or glass jars without preservatives or transport media. Liquid specimens can be collected by being scraped from a diaper with a wooden tongue depressor. Alternatively, the diaper can be lined with a plastic wrap to capture a portion of the watery stool. Rectal swabs are discouraged, since they often do not contain an adequate quantity of virus for direct EM observation. Ileostomy contents are acceptable specimens, as are postmortem segments of the bowel and their contents.

Gastroenteritis viruses are relatively stable and preserve well at 4°C for up to 1 week. For prolonged storage, specimens can be frozen at −70°C, although this may be deleterious for EM detection of virus (48). Serological diagnosis of gastroenteritis virus is generally performed in a research setting, and tests are not commercially available. Acute and convalescent-phase sera are, however, valuable in the performance of IEM or ELISA based on recombinant antigens when studying an outbreak (36).

DIRECT EXAMINATION BY EM

EM still lends itself to gastroenteritis virus diagnosis for a number of reasons. The viruses are generally easily recognizable due to their distinct morphology and are present at above threshold concentrations for detection by EM. This has the advantage that the specimens can be examined with a minimum degree of processing. Moreover, the quantity of virus ($>10^6$ particles/g) generally corresponds to active infection and not asymptomatic shedding. Since the infections caused by gastroenteritis viruses have relatively similar symptoms, the broad-spectrum approach offered by EM is best suited for their diagnosis. The virus in stool specimens is stable and can readily be transported. The EM approach is best when used to examine no more than 30 specimens per day. For larger numbers, such as would occur in investigations of outbreaks or research-oriented efforts, EM may prove suboptimal.

Procedure

A 10 to 20% stool suspension is prepared by resuspending the specimen in either distilled water or a 1% ammonium acetate solution with a pipette. The specimen is then applied to a copper EM grid, 300 to 400 mesh size, which is coated with Formvar (polyvinyl formol) reinforced by carbon shadowing. This is best performed over a 50-mm-diameter petri dish containing a 42.5-mm diameter Whatman filter. After approximately 1 min, the specimen is removed from the grid with a fragment of filter paper. If the specimen is particularly viscous, the grid may be washed with a drop of the ammonium acetate solution or distilled water. A drop of 2% phosphotungstic acid (pH 7) is then applied to the grid for 10 to 30 s and removed by blotting with a fragment of filter paper. The dried grid is then placed under a short-wavelength UV light at 900 W/cm^2 for 10 min to inactivate any viruses and examined by EM (18, 51).

This method covers the general approach; however, a number of variations are acceptable. The grid may be touched to the virus suspension made on a Parafilm square. The times of exposure of the grid to the specimen may be varied over a considerable range. Washing of the grid with a drop of ammonium acetate before staining may be used to remove nonviral debris.

Concentration of Specimens

While stool samples are generally processed directly, specimen concentration should be considered in suspected calicivirus outbreaks or when the specimen was collected outside the period of maximum excretion. Concentration can be performed by ultracentrifugation or by agar diffusion. By using the Beckman Airfuge with the EM-90 rotor, the specimen can be deposited directly on the EM grid (18). The clarified stool suspension prepared as outlined above is deposited into the sector well of the rotor, and a Formvar- and carbon-coated grid is placed in the peripheral depression. After centrifugation at 90,000 rpm for 30 min, the grids are removed and processed as outlined above. If larger quantities of virus are to be concentrated, a conventional ultracentrifuge with a swinging-bucket rotor may be used. Centrifugation at 100,000 × *g* for 1 h at 4°C will deposit virtually all viruses (16). The supernatant is discarded, and the well-drained pellet is resuspended in distilled water and processed as outlined above. When ultracentrifugation is used, it is important to clarify the stool suspension by either filtration or low-speed centrifugation to avoid excessive quantities of debris, which may obscure the virus particles.

The resuspended stool specimen can also be subjected to agar diffusion to concentrate the virus particles (18). The specimen is placed on a small block of 1% agar or agarose made up in distilled water, and the grid is floated on the surface of the drop. The preparation is kept at room temperature until the drop is absorbed into the agar, at which time the grid is removed and processed for EM as described above. This procedure not only concentrates virus particles but also removes excessive quantities of salts, which diffuse into the agarose. Such salts in the specimen may lead to crystal or precipitate formation on the grid and interfere with the detection of viruses.

IEM

IEM, which is based on the principle that antibodies which develop in response to infection will clump virus particles, played a pivotal role in the establishment of gastroenteritis viruses as pathogens (37). Antisera can be acute- and convalescent-phase patient sera, pooled human serum globulin, or hyperimmune animal antibodies specifically prepared with purified virus antigens. The IEM procedure involves incubation of the stool suspension with an equal volume of reference antiserum for 1 h at 37°C (18). The immune complexes, collected by centrifugation for 30 min at 15,000 × g, are subjected to negative-contrast EM as outlined above. A simplified version of this technique, called solid-phase IEM, involves coating the EM grid with antibody to the virus (18). This can be either a reference antibody or an immune serum globulin. The virus particles in the specimen applied to this grid will be preferentially captured by the immobilized antibody. Virus can also be specifically concentrated by incorporating reference antibody into the agar block described above. In this case, the EM grid is placed on the agar block and the serum specimen drop is placed on the grid. The antibody diffuses through the grid and forms immune complexes of virus on the grid surface. Alternatives to these approaches involve reacting the virus suspension with antibody labeled with colloidal gold. This facilitates the detection of virus and subviral particles that would not have been apparent on preliminary examination of the specimen by EM.

In addition to enhancing the sensitivity with which these agents can be detected in patient specimens, IEM has been applied to the typing of these viruses, as in the case of the caliciviruses and the Norwalk-like viruses (13). IEM continues to be the most basic approach to demonstrate the immunospecific reactivity of a virus particle and the convalescent-phase serum of the patient, such as for the human torovirus (19).

Examination of Grids by EM

The stained, disinfected grids are examined by EM with voltages of 60 to 100 kV. A grid can first be examined at a low scanning magnification of ×1,000 to ×3,000 to determine if it is acceptable for further examination. Grids which are opacified by excess debris or on which no stained material can be detected are inappropriate, and new grids should be prepared with appropriately altered concentrations of the specimen. Grid fields which show a modest amount of granular staining are then examined at ×40,000 to ×50,000 magnification. Under these conditions, the larger viruses are easily seen and even the smallest viruses are approximately 1 to 2 mm in diameter. To be effective, the microscope must be set to maximum resolving power at the high magnification with a high degree of contrast. The fine-structure features used to identify caliciviruses and especially astroviruses require a resolution of approximately 1 nm.

Virus particles present in the grid field are most readily detected in areas of moderate background staining, where they appear as lighter structures surrounded by a dark contrasting background as shown in Fig. 1. The most definitive of the spherical structures are the adenoviruses, whose icosahedral capsids are readily discerned and even the capsomeres are resolved in well-prepared specimens. Among the smaller viruses, the typical caliciviruses with their scalloped edges and well-defined cup-like depressions are readily identified. As shown in Fig. 1A, they may exhibit several distinct orientations. The astroviruses have smooth edges and a comparatively less well-defined morphology, but a distinct star is evident in at least a subset of particles, as shown in Fig. 1C. The atypical caliciviruses such as the Norwalk-like viruses also have a defined morphology. The capsomeres appear larger and grouped around a central core. Accordingly, such viruses have been called at times "mini-reo" or "mini-rota," since particles with stain-penetrated centers appear to have capsomeres arranged around a central core (51). Norwalk virus has been described as being smaller, measuring 27 nm in diameter (37). Finally, nonstructured particles described as small round viruses, whose significance is still in question, are also visualized, as shown in Fig. 1D.

Among the nonspherical particles, the coronaviruses form pleomorphic structures with well-delineated dumbbell-shaped peplomeres or spikes. Generally, the peplomeres form a dark halo around the enveloped capsid. Torovirus-like particles have a less well-defined peplomere fringe. A proportion of these are kidney shaped, while others have well-established darker-staining regions in the center of the particle, as seen in Fig. 1G. Detection of these particles by EM is less definitive than that of the spherical structured viruses, and there is a need for readily available, alternative immunospecific diagnostic tests to confirm the diagnosis. All particles lacking well-defined features, such as are present in adenoviruses or typical caliciviruses, can pose diagnostic dilemmas if seen as individual particles. When such particles are visualized as clumps or clusters, confidence in identification is enhanced.

In addition to the above-described, well-recognized virus particles, several other structures are visualized in stool specimens. These include the obvious flagella, pili, and bacteria, as well as cell wall components, cell membrane blebs, and bacteriophages. The bacteriophages may pose problems since they may be confused for viruses, especially if their tails are sheared off. Experienced electron microscopists can readily discriminate between these structures and accepted viruses. For those not familiar with EM detection of viruses, a set of reference grids containing stained preparations of the different viruses should be requested from a reference laboratory. Since different microscopes have unique features of resolution, such grids often prove very useful in recognizing the morphology of the viruses in a specific microscope.

IMMUNOSPECIFIC ANTIGEN ASSAYS

Most immunospecific assays for gastroenteritis viruses were developed for rotavirus because of its antigenicity and ease of purification. A limited number of immunospecific assays are available for adenoviruses, and developments in this area are expected with the availability of reference monoclonal antibodies (58). A commercial assay kit, containing positive and negative controls and protocols, has been marketed under the name Adenoclone Type 40/41 (Cambridge Bioscience, Worcester, Mass.). This kit, which is also available to detect adenovirus group antigen, should be considered, since adenoviruses other than types 40 and 41 are involved in the etiology of gastroenteritis (17). There have been reports that some ELISA formats do not detect all enteric adenoviruses (57). An alternative to ELISA is the commercially available group-specific latex agglutination assay, Adenolex (Orion Diagnostica, Helsinki, Finland), with its obvious advantage of speed and simplicity. This has evolved into a new version called Diarlex for the detection of both adenovirus and rotavirus.

Immunospecific tests of the ELISA or radioimmunoassay format, utilizing convalescent-phase human serum, have been described for most of the gastroenteritis viruses. With limited availability of reagents, these tests were applicable only in the research settings or reference laboratories. Immunoassays for the detection of Norwalk-like viruses had been impractical for routine use, since the source of antigen was limited to stool collected in outbreaks or volunteer studies (25). The recent cloning and expression of the calicivirus capsid proteins have allowed the production of reference antigens and antibody reagents to develop well-standardized ELISAs for direct diagnosis of the virus and for serologic testing (6, 35, 36). An ELISA has also been described for the detection of the typical calicivirus antigen and antibody (55). Monoclonal antibodies to astroviruses have been developed and used in the ELISA format (26). Finally, by using the Breda virus hyperimmune antiserum, human torovirus can be detected by ELISA (40). The progress that has been made in the cloning and expression of viral genomes means that defined recombinant antigens are becoming available. These will allow the commercial production of comprehensive panels of immunodiagnostic reagents for standardized detection of these viruses.

ISOLATION IN CELL CULTURE

The fastidious enteric adenoviruses were first identified because they failed to grow in conventional cell cultures (11, 17). Specific cell lines, such as Graham 293 lung fibroblasts, transformed with the 5′ end of the adenovirus genome, do promote the growth of these agents and are the cell line of choice. All astrovirus serotypes grow in HEK or LLC-MK_2 cell cultures in the presence of 10 μg of trypsin per ml (43). Neither the calicivirus group nor the human torovirus and coronavirus agents have been reproducibly propagated in cell cultures (11). While growth in culture has a major impact in terms of investigation of the virus, it generally takes time and is not considered sufficiently rapid to contribute substantially to the management of disease. It is, however, valuable in the preparation of diagnostic reagents and in the characterization of the virus pathogens.

ASSAYS BASED ON THE VIRAL GENOME

Identification of Fastidious Enteric Adenovirus Types 40 and 41 by Restriction Endonuclease Digestion of Genomic DNA

In the early studies on the characterization of enteric adenoviruses, these agents were found to have restriction sites that on digestion generated fragments with unique sizes that could be visualized by polyacrylamide gel electrophoresis (59). Such an approach was found to be more faithful in characterizing the enteric adenovirus after one passage in cell culture than was serum neutralization after repeated passages (7). In the latter approach, a much smaller quantity of conventional adenovirus, which may be present due to a presumed earlier infection, could quickly outgrow the enteric adenovirus and result in inaccurate typing of the agent causing the illness. Among the restriction endonucleases, *Sma*I proved effective in identifying adenovirus types 40 and 41. DNA can also be extracted from adenoviruses present in the stool specimen. After clarification of the stool suspension, the virus is precipitated with polyethylene glycol and the DNA is extracted and digested with *Sma*I (8).

Dot Blot Assays

By using the cloned restriction fragment Ad 41 *Bgl*II-D as a probe, adenovirus types 40 and 41 can be detected directly from patient specimens in a dot blot hybridization assay. The stool specimen, clarified by centrifugation, is spotted onto a nitrocellulose membrane, which is then treated with 1 M NaOH to disrupt the virus and denature the DNA (24). Alternatively, the DNA may be extracted from the clarified specimen and spotted onto the nitrocellulose membrane.

Astroviruses have been detected by dot blot hybridization with a cDNA probe from an internal region of astrovirus type 1. This proved more sensitive than EM diagnosis and was in fact able to detect astrovirus among specimens considered to be small round viruses (60). When a dot blot procedure with an RNA probe was compared with EIA, it was clear that while the former could detect virus at greater dilutions, it was in practice a less sensitive method (53).

By using cDNA probes specific for the 3′ end of the Berne virus genome, torovirus in human stool specimens was successfully detected by dot blot hybridization (39). This is an important finding since torovirus-like particles are difficult to detect by EM with the same certainty as icosehedral viruses.

PCR

The application of PCR technology to the detection of gastroenteritis viruses has now been reported for most gastroenteritis viruses. The application of reverse transcription-PCR (RT-PCR) to the detection of caliciviruses was first described for the Norwalk virus (33) and subsequently for the other atypical caliciviruses (22). It was further shown that these viruses could be genotyped by using RT-PCR followed by Southern blotting or dot blotting (3, 47).

The RT-PCR procedure generally involves the extraction of the RNA from the virus preparation, reverse transcription, and PCR and detection of the amplicons. The approach of Jiang et al. (33) is most commonly used, although other approaches have proven successful (3, 47). The primers are directed to the polymerase 3D region of these viruses. A very successful set of primers corresponding to nucleotides 4754 to 4876 of the Norwalk virus genome has been reported to detect the atypical caliciviruses and was also used to detect typical and atypical caliciviruses (3, 46). In the RT-PCR procedure, the virus is extracted form the stool suspension with Freon and concentrated by polyethylene glycol precipitation. The RNA is extracted from the virus pellet with phenol-chloroform after digestion with proteinase K in the presence of 1.25% cetyltrimethylammonium bromide. The RT-PCR approach, considered 100 times more sensitive than dot blot hybridization of the genomic RNA, was able to detect virus in stool specimens to a dilution of 10^{-4}. Sequencing of amplicon products of RT-PCR on several distinct atypical caliciviruses serotyped by IEM allowed the design of primers and probes for the genotyping and subtyping of these agents (3). By using the digoxigenin-labeled probes, caliciviruses from institutional and community outbreaks can be readily subtyped (47). Amplicons can also be sequenced to characterize the viruses further.

RT-PCR assays reported for astroviruses have a format similar to those used for caliciviruses. Virus RNA is extracted from the stool specimen by the polyethylene glycol-cetyltrimethylammonium bromide procedure (33). The primers, which allow the detection of seven serotypes, are from the 3' terminus of the genome between nucleotides 6797 and 6709 of human astrovirus type 2. The 89-nucleotide amplicons are detected by electrophoresis on agarose gels and stained with ethidium bromide. This assay, which is more costly and time-consuming than ELISA, is substantially more sensitive (52).

PCR has been applied to the diagnosis of adenoviruses in stool specimens (1, 2). Group-specific primers corresponded to sequences of the adenovirus type 2 hexon gene used in the PCR result in the production of an amplicon of approximately 300 bases for adenovirus serotypes 1 to 47. For the diagnosis of enteric adenoviruses, the amplicons are then digested with restriction endonuclease *Taq*I, which makes a single cut at nucleotide 191 of the amplicon and results in two fragments of 191 and 110 bp (2).

RT-PCR has been applied to the diagnosis of human and bovine toroviruses by using primers from the 3' noncoding region of the Berne virus genome (19, 20). These developments are important since these viruses are more difficult to diagnose by EM and do not grow in cell culture.

INTERPRETATION OF RESULTS

In all studies, the presence of virus in the stool specimen has correlated statistically with gastrointestinal illness. However, it must be borne in mind that a variable number of gastroenteritis virus infections will be asymptomatic, as, for example, in studies on astrovirus and torovirus gastroenteritis (27, 31, 52). To some extent, the less sensitive EM plays an important role in that it requires a higher virus concentration in the stool specimen, which is more likely to be consistent with the disease process (21). However, EM is, by the same logic, a suboptimal method to monitor shedding of the virus, which may have an adverse effect on containment of virus infections. Nevertheless, EM remains a fundamental and comprehensive method for the detection of the gastroenteritis viruses. Cell culture is relatively sensitive but is generally too slow to provide meaningful results in what are usually self-limiting infections which spread rapidly. It does, however, provide a valuable standard against which to compare other methods. Unfortunately, neither the caliciviruses nor the toroviruses can be diagnosed by cell culture. Immunospecific assays provide rapid results with adequate sensitivity and can, in certain instances (Adenolex), be available on a rapid-testing basis. They has been shown to have excellent potential in that they are relatively simple to perform and at present are relatively free of problems. However, development of commercial immunospecific assays is progressing slowly. Nucleic acid probes and PCR technology show a great deal of promise, especially with agents such as the caliciviruses. While these approaches have the highest sensitivity, the implications of asymptomatic gastrointestinal virus shedding have yet to be fully established. On the other hand, this method has great potential for the detection of viruses in environmental specimens and may in the long run have a major effect on the burden of viral gastroenteritis originating from food and water sources (5).

REFERENCES

1. **Allard, A., R. Girones, P. Juto, and G. Wadell.** 1990. Polymerase chain reaction for detection of adenoviruses in stool specimens. *J. Clin. Microbiol.* **28:**2659–2667.
2. **Allard, A., A. Kajon, and G. Wadell.** 1994. Simple procedure for discrimination and typing of enteric adenoviruses after detection by polymerase chain reaction. *J. Med. Virol.* **44:**250–257.
3. **Ando, T., S. S. Monroe, J. R. Gentsch, Q. Jin, D. C. Lewis, and R. I. Glass.** 1995. Detection and differentiation of antigenically distinct small round-structured viruses

(Norwalk-like viruses) by reverse transcription-PCR and Southern hybridization. *J. Clin. Microbiol.* **33:**64–71.

4. **Beards, G. M., J. Green, C. Hall, and T. H. Flewett.** 1984. An enveloped virus in stools of children and adults with gastroenteritis that resembles the Breda virus of calves. *Lancet* **i:**1050–1051.
5. **Beller, M., A. Ellis, S. Lee, M. Drebot, S. Jenkerson, E. Funk, M. Sobsey, O. Simmons, S. S. Munroe, T. Ando, J. Noel, M. Petric, J. Middaugh, and J. Spika.** 1997. Outbreak of viral gastroenteritis due to a contaminated well: international consequences. *JAMA* **278:**563–568.
6. **Blacklow, N. R., and H. B. Greenberg.** 1991. Viral gastroenteritis. *N. Engl. J. Med.* **325:**252–264.
7. **Brown, M., M. Petric, and P. J. Middleton.** 1984. Diagnosis of fastidious enteric adenoviruses 40 and 41 in stool specimens. *J. Clin. Microbiol.* **20:**334–338.
8. **Buitenwerf, J., J. J. Lowrens, and J. C. de Jong.** 1985. A simple and rapid method for typing adenoviruses 40 and 41 without cultivation. *J. Virol. Methods* **10:**39–44.
9. **Carter, M. J., and M. M. Wilcox.** 1996. The molecular biology of astroviruses. *Arch. Virol.* **12**(Suppl.)**:**277–285.
10. **Cavanagh, D.** 1997. *Nidovirales:* a new order comprising *Coronaviridae* and *Arteriviridae*. *Arch. Virol.* **142/3:**629–633.

10a. **Chandra, R.** 1997. Picobirnavirus, a novel group of undescribed viruses of mammals and birds. *Acta Virol.* **41:** 59–62.

11. **Christiansen, M. L.** 1989. Human viral gastroenteritis. *Clin. Microbiol. Rev.* **2:**51–89.
12. **Cubitt, W. D.** 1987. The candidate caliciviruses. *Ciba Found. Symp.* **128:**127–143.
13. **Cubitt, W. D., N. R. Blacklow, J. E. Herrmann, N. A. Nowak, S. Nakata, and S. Chiba.** 1987. Antigenic relationships between human caliciviruses and Norwalk virus. *J. Infect. Dis.* **156:**806–814.
14. **Cubitt, W. D.** 1996. Historical background and classification of caliciviruses and astroviruses. *Arch. Virol.* **12**(Suppl.)**:**225–235.
15. **Davidson, A. J., E. A. Telford, M. S. Watson, K. McBride, and V. Mautner.** 1993. The DNA sequence of adenovirus type 40. *J. Mol. Biol.* **234:**1308–1316.
16. **Davies, H. A..** 1982. Electron microscopy and immune electron microscopy for detection of gastroenteritis viruses, p. 37–49. *In* D. A. J. Tyrrell and A. Z. Kapikian (ed.), *Virus Infections of the Gastrointestinal Tract*. Marcel Dekker, Inc., New York, N.Y.
17. **de Jong, J. C., R. Weigand, A. H. Kidd, G. Waddell, J. G. Kapsenberg, C. J. Muzerie, A. G. Wermenbol, and R. G. Firtzlaff.** 1983. Candidate adenoviruses 40 and 41: fastidious adenoviruses from human infant stool. *J. Med. Virol.* **11:**215–231.
18. **Doane, F., and N. Anderson.** 1987. Methods for preparing specimens for electron microscopy, p. 14–31. *In Electron Microscopy in Diagnostic Virology*. Cambridge University Press, New York, N.Y.
19. **Duckmanton, S., B. Luan, J. Devenish, R. Tellier, and M. Petric.** 1997. Characterization of human torovirus from faecal specimens. *Virology* **239:**158–168.
20. **Duckmanton, L., S. Carmen, E. Nagy, and M. Petric.** 1998. Detection of bovine toroviruses from fecal specimens by reverse transcriptase-polymerase chain reaction. *J. Clin. Microbiol.* **36:**1266–1270.
21. **Flewett, T. H.** 1976. Diagnosis of enteritis viruses. *Proc. R. Soc. Med.* **69:**693–696.
22. **Green, J., J. P. Norcott, D. Lewis, C. Arnold, and D. W. G. Brown.** 1993. Norwalk-like viruses: demonstration of genomic diversity by polymerase chain reaction. *J. Clin. Microbiol.* **31:**3007–3012.
23. **Grydsuk, J. D., E. Fortsas, M. Petric, and M. Brown.** 1996. Common epitope on protein VI of enteric adenoviruses from subgenus A-F. *J. Gen. Virol.* **77:**1811–1819.
24. **Hammond, G., C. Hannan, T. Yeh, K. Fischer, G. Mauthe, and S. E. Straus.** 1987. DNA hybridization for diagnosis of enteric adenovirus infection from directly spotted human fecal specimens. *J. Clin. Microbiol.* **25:** 1881–1885.
25. **Hedberg, C. W., and M. T. Osterholm.** 1993. Outbreaks of food-borne and waterborne viral gastroenteritis. *Clin. Microbiol. Rev.* **6:**199–210.
26. **Herrmann, J. E., R. W. Hudson, D. M. Perron-Henry, J. B. Kurtz, and N. R. Blacklow.** 1988. Antigenic characteristics of astrovirus serotypes and development of astrovirus specific monoclonal antibodies. *J. Infect. Dis.* **158:** 182–185.
27. **Herrmann, J. E., D. N. Taylor, P. Echeverria, and N. R. Blacklow.** 1991. Astroviruses as a cause of gastroenteritis in children. *N. Engl. J. Med.* **324:**1757–1760.
28. **Holmes, K. V.** 1990. Coronaviridae and their replication, p. 841–856. *In* B. N. Fields, D. M. Knipe, R. M. Chanock, M. S. Hirsch, J. L. Melnick, T. P. Monath, and B. Roizman (ed.), *Virology*, 2nd ed. Raven Press, New York, N.Y.
29. **Horowitz, M. S.** 1990. Adenoviruses and their replication, p. 1679–1721. *In* B. N. Fields, D. M. Knipe, R. M. Chanock, M. S. Hirsch, J. L. Melnick, T. P. Monath, and B. Roizman (ed.), *Virology*, 2nd ed. Raven Press, New York, N.Y.
30. **Horzinek, M. C., M. Weiss, and J. Ederveen.** 1987. *Toroviridae:* a proposed new family of enveloped RNA viruses. *Ciba Found. Symp.* **128:**162–191.
31. **Jamieson, F., E. Wang, C. Bain, J. Good, L. Duckmanton, and M. Petric.** 1998. Human torovirus: a new nosocomial gastrointestinal pathogen. *J. Infect. Dis.* **178:**1263–1269.
32. **Jiang, B., S. S. Monroe, E. V. Koonin, S. E. Stine, and R. I. Glass.** 1993. RNA sequence of astrovirus: distinctive genomic organization and a putative retroviral-like ribosomal frame shifting signal that directs the viral replicase synthesis. *Proc. Natl. Acad. Sci. USA* **90:**10539–10543.
33. **Jiang, X., J. Wang, D. Graham, and M. Estes.** 1992. Detection of Norwalk virus in stool by polymerase chain reaction. *J. Clin. Microbiol.* **30:**2529–2534.
34. **Jiang, X., M. Wang, K. Wang, and M. Estes.** 1993. Sequence and genomic organization of Norwalk virus. *Virology* **195:**51–61.
35. **Jiang, X., D. Cubitt, J. J. Treanor, J. Hu, X. Dai, D. O. Matson, and L. K. Pickering.** 1995. Development of an EIA to detect MX strain, a human calicivirus in the Snow Mountain agent genogroup. *J. Gen. Virol.* **76:**2739–2747.
36. **Jiang, X., D. O. Matson, W. D. Cubitt, and M. Estes.** 1996. Genetic and antigenic diversity of human caliciviruses (HuCVs) using RT-PCR and new EIAs. *Arch Virol.* **12**(Suppl.)**:**251–262.
37. **Kapikian, A. Z., and R. M. Chanock.** 1990. Norwalk group viruses, p. 671–693. *In* B. N. Fields, D. M. Knipe, R. M. Chanock, M. S. Hirsch, J. L. Melnick, T. P. Monath, and B. Roizman (ed.), *Virology*, 2nd ed. Raven Press, New York, N.Y.
38. **Kaplan, J. E., G. W. Gary, R. C. Baron, N. Singh, L. B. Schonberger, R. Feldman, and H. B. Greenberg.** 1982. Epidemiology of Norwalk gastroenteritis and the role of Norwalk virus in outbreaks of acute non-bacterial gastroenteritis. *Ann. Intern. Med.* **96:**756–761.
39. **Koopmans, M., A. Herrewegh, and M. Horzinek.** 1991. Diagnosis of torovirus infection. *Lancet* **337:**859.
40. **Koopmans, M., M. Petric, R. L. Glass, and S. S. Monroe.** 1993. Enzyme-linked immunosorbent assay reactivity of torovirus-like particles in fecal specimens from humans with diarrhea. *J. Clin. Microbiol.* **31:**2738–2744.

41. **Koopmans, M., E. S. M. Goosen, A. A. M. Lima, I. T. McAuliffe, J. P. Nataro, L. J. Barrett, R. I. Glass, and R. L. Guerrant.** 1997. Association of torovirus with acute and persistent diarrhea in children. *Pediatr. Infect. Dis. J.* **16:**504–507.
42. **Kotloff, K. L., G. A. Losonsky, J. G. Morris, S. S. Wasserman, N. Singh-Naz, and M. M. Levine.** 1989. Enteric adenovirus infection and childhood diarrhea: an epidemiologic study in three clinical settings. *Pediatrics* **84:**219–225.
43. **Kurtz, J. B., and T. W. Lee.** 1987. Astroviruses: human and animal. *Ciba Found. Symp.* **128:**92–107.
44. **Kurtz, J. B., and T. W. Lee.** 1994. Prevalence of human astrovirus serotypes in the Oxford region 1976–1992. *Epidemiol. Infect.* **112:**187–193.
45. **Lambden, P. R., E. O. Caul, C. R. Ashley, and I. Clarke.** 1993. Sequence and genome organization of a human small round structured (Norwalk-like) virus. *Science* **259:** 516–518.
46. **Le Guyader, F., M. K. Estes, M. E. Hardy, F. H. Neil, J. Green, D. W. G. Brown, and R. L. Atmar.** 1996. Evaluation of a degenerate primer for the PCR detection of human caliciviruses. *Arch. Virol.* **141:**225–235.
47. **Levett, P. N., M. Gu, B. Luan, M. Fearon, J. Stubberfield, F. Jamieson, and M. Petric.** 1996. Longitudinal study of molecular epidemiology of small round-structured viruses in a pediatric population. *J. Clin. Microbiol.* **34:**1497–1501.
48. **Lew, J., C. W. Lebaron, R. I. Glass, T. Torok, P. M. Griffin, J. G. Wells, D. D. Juranek, and S. P. Wahlquist.** 1990. Recommendations for collection of laboratory specimens associated with outbreaks of gastroenteritis. *Morbid. Mortal. Weekly Rep.* **39:**RR14.
49. **Lew, J. F., A. Z. Kapikian, X. Jiang, M. K. Estes, and K. Y. Green.** 1994. Molecular characterization and expression of the capsid protein of a Norwalk-like virus recovered from a Desert Shield troop with gastroenteritis. *Virology* **200:** 319–325.
50. **Madeley, C. R.** 1979. Comparison of the features of astroviruses and caliciviruses by electron microscopy. *J. Infect. Dis.* **139:**519–523.
51. **Middleton, P. J., M. Szymanski, and M. Petric.** 1977. Viruses associated with acute gastroenteritis in young children. *Am. J. Dis. Child.* **131:**733–737.
52. **Mitchell, D. K., S. S. Monroe, X. Jiang, D. O. Matson, R. I. Glass, and L. K. Pickering.** 1995. Virologic features of an astrovirus diarrhea outbreak in a daycare center revealed by reverse transcriptase-polymerase chain reaction. *J. Infect. Dis.* **172:**1437–1444.
53. **Moe, C. L., J. R. Allen, S. S. Monroe, H. E. Gary, C. D. Humphrey, J. E. Herrmann, N. R. Blacklow, C. Caracamo, M. Koch, K. H. Kim, and R. Glass.** 1991. Detection of astrovirus in pediatric stool specimens by immunoassay and RNA probe. *J. Clin. Microbiol.* **29:**2390–2395.
54. **Monroe, S. S., B. Jiang, S. E. Stine, M. Koopmans, and R. I. Glass.** 1993. Subgenomic RNA sequence of the human astrovirus supports classification of *Astroviridae* as a new family of RNA viruses. *J. Virol.* **67:**3611–3614.
55. **Nakata, S., M. E. Estes, and S. Chiba.** 1988. Detection of human calicivirus antigen and antibody by enzyme-linked immunosorbent assays. *J. Clin. Microbiol.* **26:**2001–2005.
56. **Payne, C. M., C. G. Ray, V. Borduin, L. L. Minich, and M. D. Lebowitz.** 1987. An 8 year study of viral agents of acute gastroenteritis in humans: ultrastructural observations and seasonal distribution with a major emphasis on corona-like particles. *Diagn. Microbiol. Infect. Dis.* **5:** 39–54.
57. **Scott-Taylor, T., G. Ahluwalia, B. Klisko, and G. Hammond.** 1990. Prevalent enteric adenovirus variant not detected by commercial monoclonal antibody enzyme immunoassay. *J. Clin. Microbiol.* **28:**2797–2801.
58. **Singh-Naz, N., W. J. Rodriguez, A. H. Kidd, and C. D. Brandt.** 1988. Monoclonal antibody enzyme-linked immunosorbent assay for specific identification and typing of subgroup F adenovirus. *J. Clin. Microbiol.* **26:**297–300.
59. **Wadell, G., A. Allard, M. Johansson, M. Svensson, and I. Unhoo.** 1987. Enteric adenoviruses. *Ciba Found. Symp.* **128:**63–101.
60. **Willcocks, M. M., M. J. Carter, J. G. Silcock, and C. R. Madeley.** 1991. A dot-blot hybridization procedure for the detection of astrovirus in stool samples. *Epidemiol. Infect.* **107:**405–410.
61. **Yamashita, T., K. Sakae, Y. Ishihara, S. Isomura, and E. Utagawa.** 1993. Prevalence of newly isolated cytopathic small round virus (Aichi strain) in Japan. *J. Clin. Microbiol.* **31:**2938–2943.

Hepatitis A Virus*

JINHUA XIANG AND JACK T. STAPLETON

81

CLINICAL BACKGROUND

Hepatitis A, previously called infectious hepatitis, is caused by hepatitis A virus (HAV). HAV infection accounts for 20 to 25% of clinically apparent hepatitis cases worldwide (118), usually occurring in people between 5 and 30 years of age. The Centers for Disease Control and Prevention estimates that 143,000 cases of acute hepatitis A occur in the United States each year (43). HAV infection leads to approximately 80 deaths and to an estimated cost of 200 million dollars in medical care and lost productivity annually in the United States. Worldwide, the annual incidence of HAV infection exceeds 1.4 million cases, resulting in an estimated cost of 1.5 to 3 billion dollars (43). HAV is transmitted predominantly by the fecal-oral route, usually following contact with an index case or during travel to an underdeveloped area where the virus is endemic. Nonetheless, approximately 40% of U.S. patients with hepatitis A do not identify any apparent risk factor (27). In the United States, a number of factors associated with the acquisition of HAV have been identified; these include exposure to an infected household member, homosexual intercourse, illicit intravenous drug use, and exposure of children and caretakers in day-care facilities to individuals incubating or in the early phases of HAV infection. Poor sanitary and hygienic conditions and international travel promote the transmission of the virus (118). Common-source outbreaks related to food handlers and transmission through ingestion of bivalve shellfish have led to large-scale outbreaks of hepatitis A (27, 78). Transmission of HAV by contaminated blood or blood products is rare but is well documented (47). Outbreaks and sporadic cases of hepatitis A have been observed among hemophilia patients receiving factor VII preparations (62, 73, 85). With reverse transcription (RT)-PCR methods, HAV RNA was found in the pooled plasma used to prepare the factor VIII, in the purified factor VIII, and in acute-phase sera from infected individuals (73). These specific factor VIII concentrates had been treated by a virucidal (solvent-detergent) method that proved ineffective in inactivating nonenveloped viruses (73, 97).

The clinical course of hepatitis A can range from a mild, anicteric illness to severe, prolonged hepatitis with jaundice. Inapparent or anicteric hepatitis occurs in over 90% of infected children under the age of 5; thus, very few HAV-infected children have recognized illness (reviewed in references 34, 42, and 120). However, the rate of clinically apparent hepatitis among adults with HAV infection is about 75%. In developing countries, HAV is endemic, and virtually all individuals are infected early in life. However, as developing regions of the world improve their overall level of sanitation, the acquisition of HAV occurs at an older age, when symptomatic infection is more likely. Consequently, although the overall rate of HAV infection decreases, the incidence of clinically apparent disease paradoxically increases.

The incubation period for hepatitis (the time between exposure to HAV and the onset of clinical symptoms or biochemical evidence of liver disease) may range from 15 to 50 days; however, the mean duration is 28 days (42). It appears that the incubation period is inversely related to the inoculum of virus (42, 46). A short prodomal or preicteric phase, varying from several days to more than 1 week, often precedes the onset of jaundice. This phase may be characterized by fever, fatigue, malaise, myalgia, anorexia, nausea, and vomiting. The icteric phase of HAV infection may begin with the appearance of dark, golden brown urine due to bilirubinemia, followed one to several days later by pale stool and yellowish discoloration of the mucous membranes, conjunctivae, sclera, and skin (42, 46, 120). The duration of hepatitis A is variable, but clinical and biochemical indicators of hepatitis usually resolve within 4 to 8 weeks of the onset of illness (28). HAV antigen and RNA have been detected in feces with immunoassays and RT-PCR methods, respectively. Study of individuals with acute HAV infection and the use of animal models of HAV infection have shown that HAV can be detected in feces within 10 days prior to the onset of jaundice, and this finding can persist for up to 3 months, even after the alanine aminotransferase (ALT) levels have returned to normal (64, 137). Thus, it appears that fecal shedding of HAV can last for months after the resolution of symptoms, and this shedding may serve as a source of transmission of the virus in the community (137). Figure 1 summarizes the timing of fecal shedding and clinical events and the timing of the detection of HAV-specific antibodies (described below).

Hepatitis A does not cause chronic liver disease, although several complications can accompany HAV infection. A cholestastic form of hepatitis characterized by fever,

* This chapter contains information presented in chapter 90 by Jean B. Cederna and Jack T. Stapleton in the sixth edition of this Manual.

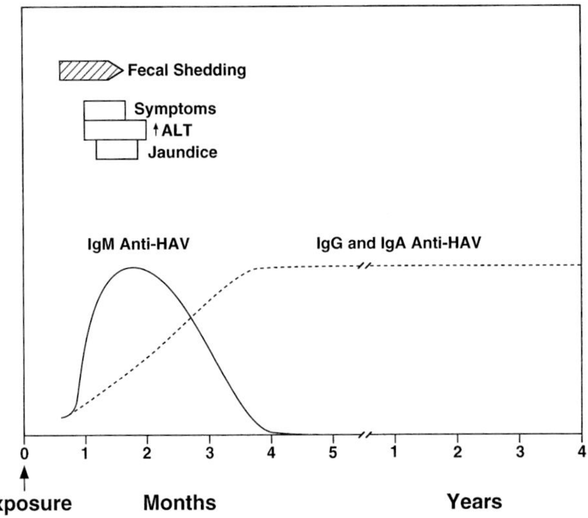

FIGURE 1 Summary of fecal shedding and anti-HAV IgM, IgG, and IgA antibody levels in relationship to exposure and clinical findings following infection with HAV. With highly sensitive RT-PCR methods, HAV RNA may be detected for several weeks after resolution of the symptoms of acute hepatitis A (see the text).

pruritus, prolonged jaundice, and weight loss has been described, and symptoms may last for more than 6 months (38). Skin rash, including urticaria (17), cryoglobulinemia (50), Guillain-Barré syndrome (11), meningoencephalitis (7), renal failure (11), and hematologic (41) and cardiovascular (37) complications have all been reported to accompany HAV infection. Hepatitis A relapse, or biphasic hepatitis A, is not uncommon (12, 36, 52), and in one study, up to 10% of patients hospitalized for acute hepatitis A suffered a second episode of hepatitis following release from the hospital (121).

Fulminant hepatitis is a relatively uncommon entity, but HAV infection accounts for approximately 5 to 20% of all cases (70). Fulminant hepatitis is characterized by increasing severity of jaundice, deterioration in liver function, drowsiness, fetor hepaticus, and eventually encephalopathy and coma (96). Hepatitis A has an overall fatality rate of approximately 0.15 death per 1,000 cases. However, a recent study (43) reported 381 deaths per 115,000 cases, for a fatality rate of 3.3 deaths per 1,000 cases. Over 70% of the deaths in this study occurred in adults over 49 years old, and in this age group, the fatality rate was 27 deaths per 1,000 cases (2.7%) (43). In cases of fulminant hepatitis A, liver transplantation has been successfully performed (20, 92). Because 60% of patients with fulminant hepatitis A recover without transplantation, including those with grade 4 hepatic encephalopathy, it is difficult to select patients for transplantation (reviewed in references 110 and 115). One case of recurrent HAV infection in a transplanted liver with an associated acute elevation in transaminase levels has been described (32).

The clinical symptoms of and laboratory findings for hepatitis A are similar to those found in other types of viral hepatitis and, unfortunately, therefore cannot be used to distinguish one form of hepatitis from another. The levels of serum aspartate aminotransferase and ALT rise abruptly, with peak levels ranging from less than 300 to greater than 3,000 IU/liter. In most cases, the aspartate aminotransferase and ALT levels are greater than 500 IU/liter (28). The magnitude of serum aminotransferase levels does not correlate well with the degree of liver cell damage.

Prevention of HAV infection requires hygienic measures, including the sanitary disposal of human waste and the maintenance of adequate standards for the purity of drinking water. HAV infection from contaminated drinking water or contaminated shellfish may be prevented by chemical or heat inactivation of the virus (42, 54). In addition, it is clear that anti-HAV antibody is critical and sufficient by itself to prevent reinfection (reviewed in reference 134). Passive immunization with pooled human serum immunoglobulins (Ig) is one way to protect individuals either following known exposure to HAV or prior to exposure in a setting in which HAV infection is endemic or epidemic (134). Pre- or postexposure immunization with Ig is approximately 90% effective in preventing HAV infection (134). Recipients of Ig have very low levels of detectable anti-HAV antibodies (112), indicating that vaccines that elicit comparable levels of anti-HAV antibodies should confer similar levels of protection (109, 112). Passive prophylaxis with Ig within the first 2 weeks following exposure to HAV may reduce icteric illness but may not necessarily prevent infection (134). This process is called passive-active immunization.

Several formalin-inactivated, cell culture-derived HAV vaccines have been developed (reviewed in reference 115). These vaccines are highly immunogenic, with greater than 90% of individuals developing detectable anti-HAV antibodies following immunization (30, 115). The duration of the presence of anti-HAV antibody following immunization appears to be greater than 5 years (30), and mathematical modeling of the measured rates of antibody decay suggests that protective levels of antibody should be present for greater than 10 years in most vaccinees (30). Immunogenicity trials and field trials of formalin-inactivated, cell culture-derived HAV vaccine preparations have demonstrated a high degree of efficacy in eliciting neutralizing antibody and preventing both disease and seroconversion in situations in which HAV infection is endemic (5, 23, 51, 77, 129, 132). These inactivated vaccine preparations are very well tolerated, with the major side effect being pain at the injection site (39, 45, 56, 77, 129). Active immunization in the United States has been targeted for individuals at the highest risk of hepatitis A, such as day-care center workers, travelers to less-developed regions, persons with hemophilia, food handlers, intravenous drug abusers, and homosexual men. However, it is likely that universal childhood vaccination will be required to result in a major impact on the overall rate of hepatitis A (69). Presently, the high cost of production of inactivated HAV vaccines and the moderate level of morbidity associated with hepatitis A preclude serious consideration of universal childhood vaccination.

Live attenuated HAV vaccines, particularly the H2 strain developed in China, are under development (74, 107, 136). The H2 strain has been administered to thousands of volunteers in China (74) and may well be an effective alternative to formalin-inactivated vaccines. Unfortunately, problems with this approach have limited its application in developed countries. Since there is no marker for attenuation, there is no readily available method to test this vaccine for reversion to virulence. In addition, if the virus is overattenuated, it can become incapable of replicating in the human host (reviewed in reference 115). Consequently, this vaccine is unlikely to be widely used outside of China or the developing world in the near future. A great deal of research is being directed toward identifying the molecular mechanisms responsible for attenuation; thus, this approach may ultimately prove widely successful. It is also possible to produce recombinant HAV subviral particles, and these are immunogenic in small animals (76, 116). However, it is not yet clear if there are sufficient advantages of these vaccines over formalin-inactivated HAV vaccines to lead to their further development.

DESCRIPTION OF THE AGENT

HAV is a member of the *Picornaviridae*. It was initially classified as enterovirus 72, but subsequent determinations of its nucleotide and amino acid sequences and proteolytic processing cascade resulted in its reclassification as a new genus, hepatovirus (Table 1). The icosahedral, nonenveloped virion has a diameter of 27 to 28 nm (21, 133), a buoyant density of 1.32 to 1.35 g/cm^3 in cesium chloride, and a sedimentation coefficient of 156S (14, 68). Like other picornaviruses, HAV has a positive-sense RNA genome (13, 84, 128). Viral particles appear to assemble as pentameric precursors which sediment at 14S in sucrose gradients (1, 116). Twelve pentamers assemble in a concentration-dependent manner into empty capsids (approximately 59S to 76S) (68, 106, 116).

The HAV genome is about 7,478 nucleotides long and contains a single long open reading frame which begins 735 bases from the 5′ end. The 5′ nontranslated region (5′ntr) directs translation by use of an internal ribosomal entry site (8, 13, 48). The 5′ntr comprises 10% of the total genome. A short 3′ nontranslated region (3′ntr) has been poorly characterized. The single open reading frame encodes a polyprotein which undergoes cotranslational, viral protease-mediated cleavage into nonstructural and structural proteins (as proposed in Fig. 2). The structural protein precursor (P1, based on the nomenclature of Rueckert and Wimmer [102]) is a 98,000-Da protein (1, 116, 134) which appears to be cleaved from the remainder of the polyprotein by the viral 3C protease region (44, 104). The remaining polyprotein is cleaved by the 3C protease region into four proteins, VP0 (1AB), VP3 (1C), VP1 (1D), and PX (1D precursor). HAV structural proteins range in size from 27,000 to 42,000 Da, and the PX protein can be removed from virions by treatment with exogenous proteinases (10, 117, 124). In other picornaviruses, a fourth polypeptide (VP4 [1A]) results from the cleavage of VP0 into VP2 and VP4. This cleavage is thought to occur during RNA encapsidation and may be catalyzed by RNA. Although VP4 has not been conclusively demonstrated in HAV, two groups have demonstrated that the HAV 1B immunoreactive protein found in empty capsids migrates more slowly (by an estimated 2,500 Da) than the 1B protein found in infectious virions (1, 61), supporting the presence of a small VP4 (1A) molecule which is cleaved from 1B during the encapsidation of viral RNA.

The stability of HAV appears to exceed that of all known picornaviruses. HAV is partially resistant to heat and is still infectious after 10 to 12 h at 60°C (94). Inactivation of HAV suspended in buffered saline occurs after 4 min at 70°C and immediately at 85°C. The virus is also stable under

TABLE 1 *Picornaviridae* family

Characteristic	Hepatovirus	Enterovirus	Rhinovirus	Cardiovirus	Aphthovirus
Major members	Human and primate HAV	Poliovirus, echovirus, coxsackievirus	Human and animal rhinoviruses	Encephalomyocarditis virus	Foot-and-mouth disease virus
No. of serotypes	1	>70	>110	1	7
Hosts	Humans, other primates	Humans, other vertebrates	Humans, other vertebrates	Humans, other vertebrates, rodents	Most cloven-hoofed animals
Optimal growth temp (°C)	36–37	36–37	33–34	36–37	36–37
Stability at:					
60°C	Stable	Labile	Labile	Labile	Labile
pH 3	Stable	Stable	Labile	Stable	Labile
pH 6	Stable	Stable	Becoming stable	Stable	Labile
Structural protein sizes (kDa)					
VP1 (1D)	28.1	33.5	31.7	23.3	32.4
VP2 (1B)	24.8	30	29	24.7	28.5
VP3 (1C)	27.8	26.4	25.1	24.3	26.2
VP4 (1A)	2.5	7.4	7.2	8.5	7.2
PX	42	NP[a]	NP	NP	NP
RNA[b]					
G+C content (%)	38	46	39	49	52
5′ntr[c]	735	741	678	205	1,200
3′ntr[c]	64	72	47	120	93

[a] NP, not present.
[b] RNAs were from representative strains from each genus.
[c] Number of nucleotides in addition to those in the poly(A) tail.

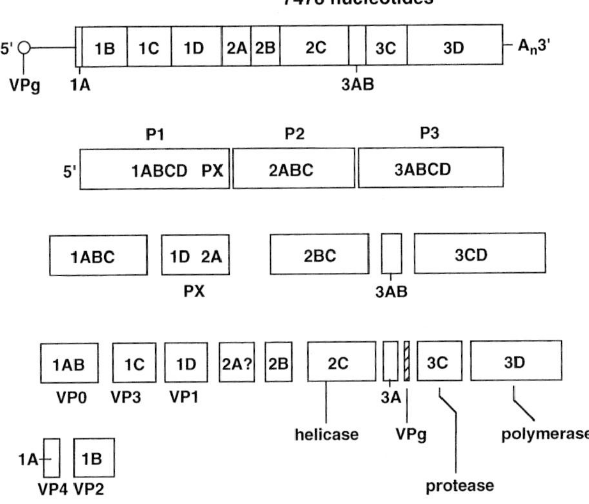

FIGURE 2 Proposed proteolytic cascade for HAV. The HAV genomic RNA is depicted on the top line, with its 5′ VPg-linked protein, 5′ntr, long single open reading frame, 3′ntr, and polyadenylated 3′ end (A_n3'). The single long open reading frame is cleaved into structural proteins (VP0, VP3, VP1, and PX) and nonstructural proteins (2B, 2C, 3A, 3B, 3C, and 3D). The HAV 3C protease has been shown to be responsible for the cleavage of 1C-1D, 1D-2A, 2A-2B, 2C-3A, 3A-3B, 3B-3C, and 3C-3D. The mechanism of cleavage of 1A-1B and the ultimate fate of 2A have not been determined. Nonstructural proteins with known functions are identified (protease, polymerase, and VPg). There are sequence homologies among picornavirus nucleoside triphosphate binding domains on the HAV 2C protein, and it is believed that 2C has a helicase function.

extremes of pH (42). HAV is generally stable at pH 3 (103). Although variable results have been reported, HAV is generally inactivated by a pH greater than 10 (Table 1). HAV is resistant to treatment with ethyl ether and chloroform, presumably because it lacks a lipid-containing envelope. Hypochlorous acid at a concentration of 1 mg/liter is generally sufficient to inactivate HAV within 30 min. Infectivity can also be abolished by sodium hypochlorite, iodine, and potassium permanganate, but chloramine-T and peracetic acid do not inactivate the virus (42).

HAV has only one serotype and does not react with an enterovirus-specific monoclonal antibody or cDNA probes (101). Human HAV strains can be grouped into four genotypes (I, II, III, and VII), and HAV strains unique to simians belong to three additional genotypes (IV, V, and VI) (98, 99). The nucleotide sequences in the P1-encoding regions vary between these genotypes by 15 to 25% (98). Despite this variation, there is good evidence that most, if not all, human strains of HAV are closely related antigenically (63, 66, 115). Simian strains of HAV recovered from old-world monkeys share antigenic sites with human HAV strains and are thus detected by immunoassays with polyclonal antibodies (2, 66, 109). However, these strains demonstrate antigenic differences from human HAV strains at specific neutralization epitopes within the single, immunodominant HAV antigenic neutralization site (2, 67, 114). Since neutralizing polyclonal antibodies cross-react with simian strains, it is believed that inactivated and attenuated vaccines produced from a genotype I (human) strain should provide protection against all relevant human and simian HAV strains (108, 109).

HAV antigenic structure has been partially characterized by evaluating neutralizing monoclonal antibodies for their ability to bind virions and subviral particles and by characterizing spontaneously occurring mutants which escape neutralization by these monoclonal antibodies. HAV contains a major immunodominant neutralization site (114) which involves amino acid residues on viral structural proteins 1D and 1C (VP1 and VP3) (83, 90, 91). Although several of these neutralization epitopes are present on 14S pentameric subviral particles, at least one neutralization epitope is formed only when the 14S particles assemble into empty capsids (116). These antibody binding sites appear to be conformationally dependent, since disruption of the virus by detergents largely destroys antigenicity and individual capsid proteins do not react with neutralizing monoclonal antibodies (116, 133). In addition to the antigenic regions on VP1 and VP3, distinct conformationally dependent epitopes involving VP1 and VP2 and a nonconformationally dependent epitope involving VP1 have also been identified (81, 91).

Early studies demonstrated that HAV utilizes a specific cell receptor that is present on a wide variety of cell lines of mammalian origin (40, 111). Viral binding is strictly calcium dependent (40, 111), and attachment does not appear to be altered by mutations conferring resistance to neutralizing monoclonal antibodies (111). Recently, Kaplan and colleagues identified a mucin-like protein on monkey kidney cells which appears to specifically bind HAV (57). Following transfection of this protein into nonsusceptible murine Ltk^- cells, HAV attachment and productive infection were demonstrated (57). A human mucin-like protein homolog apparently has been identified recently (20a).

NATURAL HOSTS

Hepatitis A produces disease in humans, chimpanzees, macaque monkeys, owl monkeys, stump-tailed monkeys, and several species of South American marmosets. Disease in nonhuman primates is usually milder than that in humans, although HAV or viral antigen generally can be detected in serum, liver, bile, and feces. Other primates do not develop clinical infection with HAV. On occasion, monkeys appear to have anti-HAV antibodies shortly after they are captured, suggesting a nonhuman reservoir for HAV (9, 42, 66).

A great deal of information regarding the virologic and immunologic aspects of HAV infection has been learned from experimental hepatitis A in nonhuman primates. Several virus strains have been used in these primate models. Initial studies done at the National Institutes of Health and the Centers for Disease Control and Prevention used the MS-1 and Phoenix strains of HAV to experimentally infect marmosets (42). Animals developed elevated enzyme levels 3 to 4 weeks following intravenous or oral inoculation with the virus. HAV antigen was detected in feces during the acute phase of the illness, and animals developed anti-HAV antibody by the time aminotransferase levels were elevated. High concentrations of antibody persisted during convalescence (Fig. 1). Fecal shedding of HAV by experimentally infected chimpanzees has been studied in several laboratories with human strains MS-1 and HM-175 (42). In general, shedding of HAV by chimpanzees is neither as prolonged nor as intense as that by marmosets; thus, chimpanzees have not been a major source of viral antigen for other studies.

HAV replication is readily detected in the livers of experimentally infected nonhuman primates. *Saguinus mystax* marmosets were injected with the CR326 strain of HAV, and animals were sacrificed at 3- to 4-day intervals. Infectious virus was detected in the liver during the first week of infection, 2 weeks or more prior to the onset of hepatitis. Large amounts of antigen were harvested from the liver for use in complement fixation and immunoadherence hemagglutination assays (reviewed in reference 42). Immunofluorescence and immunoelectron microscopy (IEM) were used to identify HAV in the livers of experimentally infected nonhuman primates. However, since the advent of tissue culture propagation of HAV, primate models are not used as a source of antigen for serologic testing.

Chimpanzees experimentally infected with HAV may have circulating immune complexes in their sera (75). These circulating immune complexes are predominantly IgG directed against HAV. HAV RNA specific for the VP1 and VP3 regions was detected in the immune complexes by PCR, suggesting that infectious virus was present. These immune complexes may be involved in the pathogenesis of some of the clinical complications of HAV described above (e.g., urticaria, cryoglobulinemia, skin rash, arthritis, and renal disease).

HAV IDENTIFICATION

Direct examination for hepatitis A is impractical because HAV particles are shed in very low concentrations and may be obscured by other particulate matter. However, IEM can overcome these obstacles and was the first technique used to identify HAV (21). IEM can distinguish particulate antigens from other, morphologically similar particles by depositing antibody on the surface of the particles, which may be visualized or identified by labeled secondary antibodies and by the formation of immune aggregates. Even though this technique is useful, it is time-consuming and expensive and requires an experienced microscopist. New techniques have replaced this technique as a diagnostic tool, although a combination of conventional IEM and solid-phase IEM can be used to identify HAV in stool and cell culture extracts (49).

Although HAV from clinical specimens can be propagated in cell cultures (see below), growth is slow and unpredictable, and several months of blind passages are usually required before viral antigen can be detected. Consequently, isolation of virus in cell cultures is not a practical tool for identifying HAV from clinical specimens.

Because HAV is highly antigenic, a variety of serologic methods have been developed for identifying HAV antigen. Radioimmunoassay (RIA) techniques were among the first methods established to identify HAV antigen (42, 105). Unlabeled anti-HAV antibody preparations (usually sera obtained from early-convalescent-phase patients) is bound to the plastic surface of a microtiter well, test samples are applied, and ^{125}I-labeled anti-HAV IgG is added to detect bound HAV. The test is considered positive for HAV if the ratio of counts per minute detected by gamma scintillation counting is greater than or equal to 2.1 times the mean counts per minute for negative control samples. Enzyme-linked immunoabsorbent assay or enzyme immunoassay (EIA) techniques have largely replaced RIA techniques for the detection of HAV antigen. EIA substitutes an enzyme-conjugated antibody probe for the radionuclide-conjugated antibody probe of the RIA. Horseradish peroxidase or alkaline phosphatase may be used to label the secondary antibodies. Hydrolysis of the substrate occurs when HAV is present and can be measured visually or spectrophotometrically. Antigen detection can be enhanced by use of a nitrocellulose membrane as a high-capacity solid-phase material for the nonspecific capture of antigen (82). The nitrocellulose-EIA method can be used to detect as little as 1 ng of HAV protein, which corresponds to 1.5×10^4 viral particles (82).

Hepatitis A may also be detected by molecular hybridization of HAV RNA with cloned HAV cDNA (95, 122). Hybridization is approximately 10-fold more sensitive than IEM or RIA, and specificity can be enhanced by purifying HAV from clinical specimens by use of an immunoaffinity step with anti-HAV monoclonal antibodies (54). HAV-specific single-stranded RNA probes have been used in dot blot hybridization tests to detect HAV in environmental samples (139). Radioactive and nonradioactive RNA probes are generated by in vitro transcription of HAV templates inserted in a plasmid vector. HAV RNA is purified from samples by proteinase K digestion, followed by phenol-chloroform extraction and ethanol precipitation (55). Hybridization with RNA probes is generally performed at a higher stringency than is that with cDNA probes.

RT-PCR has proven to be a useful tool for identifying HAV from clinical specimens. With the immunoaffinity step described for cDNA-RNA hybridization, specificity is enhanced to the point at which the method can be used for fecal specimens (55). RNA may be extracted from immunoaffinity-purified virus by proteinase K digestion, phenol-chloroform extraction, and ethanol precipitation. Alternatively, heating the samples to 95°C following immunoaffinity purification releases sufficient quantities of viral RNA from the capsids to allow subsequent RT. HAV RNA is converted to cDNA by RT, and cDNA is amplified by PCR with a thermostable DNA polymerase. With this method, products can be detected by ethidium bromide staining in agarose gels and by Southern transfer or dot blotting with oligonucleotide probes to detect HAV-specific sequences (55).

Strain comparison has been accomplished by sequence analysis of cDNA amplified by PCR. Genotypic differences are detected by comparing the sequences of the PCR products from feces-derived or cell culture-adapted HAV isolates. As noted above, sequence analysis of geographically diverse isolates has categorized virus strains into seven subgroups based on RNA sequence similarities (55, 98). These subgroups of HAV are indistinguishable by commercial EIA and RIA methods but vary by 15 to 25% in their RNA sequences. The conservation of HAV antigenicity suggests that the antigenic site plays a critical role in the life cycle of the virus (90, 91, 111, 114).

COLLECTION, TRANSPORT, AND STORAGE OF SPECIMENS

Standard separation and storage of sera allow accurate serologic results to be obtained for both anti-HAV IgM and total anti-HAV antibody. Antibody titers are stable and anti-HAV levels in lots of Ig do not decrease significantly during storage at 4°C for more than 3 weeks; however, repetitive freezing and thawing of sera may lead to a diminution in titers (112, 113).

Samples of feces may contain HAV antigen if collected during the 2 weeks prior to illness or several days after the onset of symptoms (Fig. 1). Under unusual circumstances, fecal virus shedding may be protracted, especially in infants (100, 137). Twenty percent fecal slurries or 50% saliva samples are prepared with phosphate-buffered saline containing 0.02% sodium azide. These specimens can be stored at

−70°C for more than 6 months without a significant loss of antigenicity or antibody titers (113). Liver biopsy specimens may also be obtained for the detection of HAV particles by immunofluorescence or IEM. Saliva and bile may also be collected for antibody testing (see below). To preserve infectivity, HAV must be stored at 4°C or frozen at −20 to −70°C. When HAV is stored at 4°C, infectivity is reduced only 0.5 $\log_{10}$ unit after 16 weeks; titers remain stable at both −20 and −70°C for over 6 months (105).

ISOLATION PROCEDURES

HAV is very difficult to isolate and propagate in vitro. Even when well adapted to cell cultures, HAV takes several days to weeks to reach maximal titers. Initial in vitro propagation of HAV was done with freshly extracted primary adult marmoset hepatocyte cultures (93). Hepatocyte-like epithelial cell outgrowth appeared at 7 days. It was later discovered that primary African green monkey cells could be used to grow HAV. Once HAV has adapted to growth in cell cultures, it is capable of replicating in a variety of primate cell lines and, under certain circumstances, nonprimate mammalian cell lines (18). Multiple human and nonhuman primate cell lines are frequently used to propagate HAV; these include fetal rhesus monkey kidney cells (FrhK-4 and -6) (22, 93), human diploid embryonic lung fibroblasts (25, 29, 33), hepatocyte-derived cells (PLC/PRF/5 and HepG2) (29), and LLC-MK2, Vero, MRC-5, CaCo2, and other transformed cell lines (133). HAV has been isolated in cell cultures from human and experimentally infected nonhuman primate liver, bile, feces, and sera. Viral antigen yields in the most productive systems are no more than 100 ng/ml. Total viral particle counts are estimated to be about 100-fold higher than the infectious titer. However, following adaptation to growth in cell cultures, this ratio diminishes considerably (68, 105).

HAV ANTIBODY DETECTION

Commercially available assays for anti-HAV IgM are the methods of choice for establishing the diagnosis of acute hepatitis A. To identify total anti-HAV antibody, a competition immunoassay which tests the ability of test sera to compete with labeled anti-HAV antibody (either radiolabeled or enzyme linked) for binding to antigen attached to the solid phase is usually used. To identify acute infection, an IgM-specific antibody assay is required (Fig. 1). The most commonly used anti-HAV IgM method is a solid-phase antibody capture immunoassay. The solid phase is coated with anti-human IgM. The presence of antibody to HAV in the captured IgM from the test serum is indicated by the sequential binding of HAV and labeled anti-HAV reagents (122). Results are usually evaluated by comparison with a cutoff value that is determined from positive and negative controls supplied by the manufacturer. Almost all hepatitis A patients are anti-HAV IgM positive at the onset of symptoms and IgM negative 6 months following infection.

Several methods have been developed to evaluate sera for HAV-neutralizing activity. All use cell culture-adapted virus which is incubated with complement-depleted sera prior to virus titration in cell cultures. Neutralizing activity is determined by a 50 or 90% reduction in virus foci or by a 50% reduction in the tissue culture infective dose. Because HAV is generally not cytopathic in cell cultures, novel approaches to determining viral infectious titers have been developed. Methods that use RIA or EIA to detect virus growth in a terminal-dilution microtiter assay have been described (24), as have modifications of a more standard plaque assay (65). This radioimmunofocus assay requires 7 to 14 days of incubation of HAV-infected cell monolayers overlaid with agarose. The agarose is gently removed, the cells are fixed with acetone, and foci of HAV replication are detected with ^{125}I-labeled anti-HAV IgG. Variations of these methods have also been described (59). Because of the labor intensity of and time involved in these assays (generally 2 to 3 weeks per assay), these methods are not practical for general use. Quantitation of neutralizing activity in sera is generally determined by one of two methods. Following incubation of a known inoculum of HAV with serial dilutions of sera, the dilution of sera which inhibits the growth of virus by 50 or 90% is determined (neutralization titer). Alternatively, a single dilution of antibody (or sera) is incubated with serial dilutions of virus inocula, and the $\log_{10}$ reduction in HAV infectivity is calculated. The former method is more widely used.

Saliva and urine provide convenient sources of test material, particularly for children or in epidemiologic studies. Anti-HAV IgM antibodies can be reliably detected by EIA in the saliva of patients with acute or recent hepatitis A but not in the saliva of patients without a recent HAV infection (86–88). Anti-HAV IgM persists for 2 to 4 months. The ratio of anti-HAV IgM to anti-HAV IgG correlates closely with the interval from the onset of infection. Anti-HAV IgA and IgG can also be detected in the saliva of persons with hepatitis A or in those who have recovered from an HAV infection (87). The role of anti-HAV IgA in preventing infection is unclear, as salivary and fecal IgA antibodies do not exhibit neutralizing activity following experimental and natural HAV infections (113).

Another approach that has been evaluated for diagnostic serologic testing uses a hemagglutinin inhibition assay (19, 119). Virus-specific hemagglutination of various species of erythrocytes has been demonstrated for HAV. This activity is blocked by anti-HAV IgG and IgM antibodies and is not affected by inactivation of HAV infectivity by 0.03% β-propiolactone (19, 119). Thus, methods other than EIA may be used for the diagnosis of recent HAV infection.

IMMUNOLOGIC ASPECTS OF HEPATITIS A

It is clear that antibody to HAV is critical and sufficient by itself to prevent reinfection (133); however, several lines of evidence indicate a potential role for cell-mediated immunity in the clearance of HAV from hepatocytes and in HAV pathogenesis (26, 126, 127). HAV persistently infects cells in vitro and does not cause a direct cytopathic effect (42). Peak virus shedding in feces and peak viremia in experimental HAV infection occur before the development of symptoms (42, 64). Anti-HAV antibody is almost always present at the time of symptoms, and in the unusual cases in which it is not, gamma interferon is detectable prior to seroconversion (138). All of these data indirectly suggest that cell-mediated immune destruction of HAV-infected hepatocytes leads to hepatitis.

Among the potential mediators of cell-mediated immunity, it appears that antibody-dependent cellular cytotoxicity does not occur in HAV infection (31). Conflicting reports about the presence (60) or absence of natural killer cell responses to HAV-infected cells exist (28).

Cell-mediated cytotoxicity has been demonstrated to be important in the immune response to HAV infection (31). Virus-specific cytotoxic T cells develop in the course of

HAV infection, as measured by a microcytotoxicity assay of peripheral blood lymphocytes in infected patients (126, 127, 135). Clonal analysis identified antigen-specific $CD8^+$ T lymphocytes in liver biopsies obtained during acute HAV infection (26), implicating these cells as being responsible for the destruction of infected hepatocytes (26). Nearly 50% of liver-derived T-cell clones displayed HAV-specific cytotoxicity, compared with <1% of peripheral blood lymphocyte clones, further supporting the role of cytolytic T cells in the pathogenesis of acute hepatitis A (26). Both nonstructural (58) and structural (135) HAV proteins appear to elicit HAV-specific cytolytic T cells.

Evaluation of patients with acute HAV infection for the presence of cytokines demonstrated increased levels of interleukin-1α, interleukin-1β, interleukin-6, and tumor necrosis factor alpha in serum (123), suggesting that these may be related to disease activity and thus may play some role in hepatocyte injury (123). The human MxA protein is a new specific marker for type I interferon activity both in vitro and in vivo. In one study of patients with acute hepatitis A, 10 of 10 patients had detectable MxA protein during the first 2 weeks of clinical symptoms (53). The MxA protein may originate from interferon-exposed and subsequently damaged hepatocytes (53).

Finally, circulating immune complexes are usually detected in acute HAV infection (125). IgM immune complexes are significantly more common than IgG immune complexes and appear to result in higher ALT levels and increased levels of serum bilirubin (125). In one study, 95.6% of patients with acute hepatitis A had demonstrable circulating immune complexes (125).

SUSCEPTIBILITY TO ANTIVIRAL AGENTS

A variety of compounds which have antiviral activity against picornaviruses or other classes of viruses have been evaluated for activity against HAV. The antipicornavirus drug Disoxaril (WIN 51711) inhibits the uncoating of a number of human picornaviruses but was found not to have any effect on the H141 strain of HAV and to have only a modest inhibitory effect on three other strains when tested at high concentrations (130). Highly charged antiviral compounds, such as protamine and carrageenan, have specific inhibitory effects on HAV replication in cell cultures, although the mechanism of action has not been characterized (6, 35). Ribavirin and amantadine have in vitro antiviral activity at concentrations achievable in vivo (15, 131). No clinical trials of these antiviral drugs have been reported.

Recent crystallization of the HAV 3C protease (4, 16) has led to the identification of potential HAV protease inhibitors (72). A peptidyl monofluoromethyl ketone has been shown to inhibit HAV 3C protease in vitro and to inhibit HAV replication ex vivo (79); hence, specific HAV therapy may soon be feasible. In addition, the HAV 3C protease is inhibited by zinc, like other picornavirus 3C proteases (71, 89). Since zinc therapy has been shown to be effective for common colds, presumably due to inhibition of the rhinovirus 3C protease (80), there is rationale for studying zinc therapy for HAV. At this time, there are no data on this therapy.

INTERPRETATION OF DIAGNOSTIC ASSAYS

Evaluation of IgM and total Ig to HAV by EIA provides the diagnosis of acute or past infection with hepatitis A. Anti-HAV IgM is almost always present in serum at the time of symptoms from hepatitis A and may be present for several months after the acute illness (Fig. 1). Therefore, anti-HAV IgM antibody can be used to make a diagnosis of recent HAV infection (28, 42). Although it is often called the anti-HAV IgG test, the total anti-HAV Ig assay also measures IgM and IgA antibodies to HAV. The total anti-HAV Ig assay is positive during acute hepatitis A and remains positive indefinitely (42, 46). The pattern of a positive total anti-HAV Ig test and a negative anti-HAV IgM test indicates that the patient has had a previous infection with HAV and is protected against reinfection. However, an exogenous source of anti-HAV antibody in the patient may result in a positive total anti-HAV Ig assay. For example, patients who have had recent transfusions, newborn infants (in the first 6 months of life), and frequent recipients of intravenous Ig may have received enough circulating anti-HAV antibody for it to be detected by the EIA (46). Although the sera of Ig recipients was not found to contain detectable levels of anti-HAV antibody when older commercial immunoassays were used (112, 133), current assays may identify anti-HAV antibody in the recipients of intravenous Ig regularly administered for immunologic disorders (3).

REFERENCES

1. **Anderson, D. A., and B. C. Ross.** 1990. Morphogenesis of hepatitis A virus: isolation and characterization of subviral particles. *J. Virol.* **64:**5284–5289.
2. **Balayan, M. S.** 1992. Natural hosts of hepatitis A virus. *Vaccine* **10**(Suppl. 1)**:**S27–S31.
3. **Ballas, Z. K., and J. A. Hudson.** 1993. Hepatitis A, B, and C seroconversion in patients receiving intravenous immunoglobulin (IVIG). *J. Allergy Clin. Immunol.* **91:**148.
4. **Bergmann, E. M., S. C. Mosmann, M. M. Chernaia, B. A. Malcolm, and M. N. James.** 1997. The refined crystal structure of the 3C gene product from hepatitis A virus: specific proteinase activity and RNA recognition. *J. Virol.* **71:**2436–2448.
5. **Binn, L. N., W. H. Bancroft, S. M. Lemon, R. H. Marchwicki, J. W. LeDuc, C. J. Trahan, E. C. Staley, and C. M. Keenan.** 1986. Preparation of a prototype hepatitis A virus vaccine from infected cell culture. *J. Infect. Dis.* **153:** 749–756.
6. **Biziagos, E., J. M. Crance, J. Passagot, and R. Deloince.** 1987. Effect of antiviral substances on hepatitis A virus replication in vitro. *J. Med. Virol.* **22:**57–66.
7. **Bromberg, K., D. N. Newhall, and G. Peter.** 1982. Hepatitis A and meningoencephalitis. *JAMA* **247:**815.
8. **Brown, E. A., S. P. Day, R. W. Jansen, and S. M. Lemon.** 1991. Genetic variability within the 5′ nontranslated region of hepatitis A virus RNA. Implications for secondary structure and function. *J. Hepatol.* **13**(Suppl. 4)**:** S138–S143.
9. **Brown, E. A., R. W. Jansen, and S. M. Lemon.** 1989. Characterization of a simian hepatitis A virus (HAV): antigenic and genetic comparison with human HAV. *J. Virol.* **63:**4932–4937.
10. **Cederna, J. B., D. Klinzman, J. McLinden, P. L. Winokur, and J. T. Stapleton.** 1993. Unpublished data.
11. **Chio, F., Jr., and A. A. Bakir.** 1992. Acute renal failure in hepatitis A. *Int. J. Artif. Organs* **15:**413–416.
12. **Chiriaco, P., C. Guadalupi, M. Armigliato, F. Bortolotti, and G. Realdi.** 1986. Polyphasic course of hepatitis type A in children. *J. Infect. Dis.* **153:**378–379.
13. **Cohen, J. I., J. R. Ticehurst, R. H. Purcell, A. Buckler-White, and B. M. Baroudy.** 1987. Complete nucleotide sequence of wild-type hepatitis A virus: comparison with

different strains of hepatitis A virus and other picornaviruses. *J. Virol.* **61:**50–59.

14. **Coulepis, A. G., S. A. Locarnini, E. G. Westaway, G. A. Tannock, and I. D. Gust.** 1982. Biophysical and biochemical characterization of hepatitis A virus. *Intervirology* **18:**107–127.
15. **Crance, J. M., E. Biziagos, J. Passagot, H. Van Cuyck-Gandre, and R. Deloince.** 1990. Inhibition of hepatitis A virus replication in vitro by antiviral compounds. *J. Med. Virol.* **31:**155–160.
16. **Dinakarpandian, D., B. Shenoy, M. Pusztai-Carey, B. A. Malcolm, and P. R. Carey.** 1997. Active site properties of the 3C proteinase from hepatitis A virus (a hybrid cysteine/serine protease) probed by Raman spectroscopy. *Biochemistry* **36:**4943–4948.
17. **Dollberg, S., Y. Berkun, and E. Gross-Kieselstein.** 1991. Urticaria in patients with hepatitis A virus infection. *Pediatr. Infect. Dis. J.* **10:**702–703.
18. **Dotzauer, A., S. M. Feinstone, and G. Kaplan.** 1994. Susceptibility of nonprimate cell lines to hepatitis A virus infection. *J. Virol.* **68:**6064–6068.
19. **Dubois, D. R., L. N. Binn, P. L. Summers, R. L. Timchak, D. A. Barvir, R. H. Marchwicki, and K. H. Eckels.** 1990. Preparation of noninfectious hepatitis A virus hemagglutinin for detecting hemagglutination inhibition antibodies. *J. Virol. Methods* **28:**299–304.
20. **Fagiuoli, S., G. Shah, H. I. Wright, and D. H. Van Thiel.** 1993. Types, causes, and therapies of hepatitis occurring in liver transplant recipients. *Dig. Dis. Sci.* **38:**449–456.

20a. **Feinstone, S.** Personal communication.

21. **Feinstone, S. M., A. Z. Kapikian, and R. H. Purcell.** 1973. Hepatitis A: detection by immune electron microscopy of a virus like antigen associated with acute illness. *Science* **182:**1026–1028.
22. **Flehmig, B.** 1981. Hepatitis A virus in cell culture. II. Growth characteristics of hepatitis A virus in Frhk-4/R cells. *Med. Microbiol. Immunol.* **170:**73–81.
23. **Flehmig, B., U. Heinricy, and M. Pfisterer.** 1989. Immunogenicity of a killed hepatitis A vaccine in seronegative volunteers. *Lancet* **i:**1039–1041.
24. **Flehmig, B., M. Ranke, T. Berthold, and H. J. Gerth.** 1979. A solid phase radioimmunoassay for detection of IgM antibodies to hepatitis A virus. *J. Infect. Dis.* **140:**169–175.
25. **Flehmig, B., A. Vallbracht, and G. Wurster.** 1981. Hepatitis A virus in cell culture. III. Propagation of hepatitis A virus in human embryo kidney and human embryo fibroblasts. *Med. Microbiol. Immunol.* **170:**83–89.
26. **Fleischer, B., S. Fleischer, K. Maier, K. H. Wiedmann, and A. Vallbracht.** 1990. Clonal analysis of infiltrating T lymphocytes in liver tissue in viral hepatitis A. *Immunology* **69:**14–19.
27. **Francis, D. P., S. C. Hadler, T. J. Prendergast, E. Peterson, M. M. Ginsberg, C. Lookabaugh, J. R. Holmes, and J. E. Maynard.** 1984. Occurrence of hepatitis A, B, and non-A/non-B in the United States. CDC Sentinel County Hepatitis Study 1. *Am. J. Med.* **76:**69–74.
28. **Friedman, L. S., and J. L. Dienstag.** 1984. The disease and its pathogenesis, p. 55–79. *In* R. J. Gerety (ed.), *Hepatitis A*. Academic Press Ltd., London, England.
29. **Frosner, G. G., F. Deinhardt, R. Scheid, V. Gauss-Muller, N. Holmes, V. Messelberger, G. Siegl, and J. J. Alexander.** 1979. Propagation of human hepatitis A virus in a hepatoma cell line. *Infection* **7:**303–305.
30. **Fujiyama, S., K. Odoh, M. Tanaka, I. Kuramoto, and K. Tomita.** 1997. Evaluation of the timing of the booster injection after a primary vaccination against hepatitis A. *J. Gastroenterol. Hepatol.* **12:**172–175.
31. **Gabriel, P., A. Vallbracht, and B. Flehmig.** 1986. Lack of complement-dependent cytolytic antibodies in hepatitis A virus infection. *J. Med. Virol.* **20:**23–31.
32. **Gane, E., R. Sallie, M. Saleh, B. Portmann, and R. Williams.** 1995. Clinical recurrence of hepatitis A following liver transplantation for acute liver failure. *J. Med. Virol.* **45:**35–39.
33. **Gauss-Muller, V., G. G. Frosner, and F. Deinhardt.** 1981. Propagation of hepatitis A virus in human embryo fibroblasts. *J. Med. Virol.* **7:**233–239.
34. **Gerety, R. J. (ed.).** 1984. *Hepatitis A*. Academic Press Ltd., London, England.
35. **Girond, S., J. M. Crance, H. Van Cuyck-Gandre, J. Renaudet, and R. Deloince.** 1991. Antiviral activity of carrageenan on hepatitis A virus replication in cell culture. *Res. Virol.* **142:**261–270.
36. **Glikson, M., E. Galun, R. Oren, R. Tur-Kaspa, and D. Shouval.** 1992. Relapsing hepatitis A. Review of 14 cases and literature survey. *Medicine* (Baltimore) **71:**14–23.
37. **Gordon, S. C., A. S. Patel, R. J. Veneri, K. A. Keskey, and S. M. Korotkin.** 1989. Case report: acute type A hepatitis presenting with hypotension, bradycardia, and sinus arrest. *J. Med. Virol.* **28:**219–222.
38. **Gordon, S. C., K. R. Reddy, L. Schiff, and E. R. Schiff.** 1984. Prolonged intrahepatic cholestasis secondary to acute hepatitis A. *Ann. Intern. Med.* **101:**635–637.
39. **Goubau, P., V. Van Gerven, A. Safary, A. Delem, J. Knops, E. D'Hondt, F. E. André, and J. Desmyter.** 1992. Effect of virus strain and antigen dose on immunogenicity and reactogenicity of an inactivated hepatitis A vaccine. *Vaccine* **10**(Suppl. 1)**:**S114–S118.
40. **Grace, K., E. Amphlett, S. Day, S. Lemon, D. Sangar, D. J. Rowlands, and B. E. Clarke.** 1991. *In vitro* translation of hepatitis A virus subgenomic RNA transcripts. *J. Gen. Virol.* **72:**1081–1086.
41. **Gundersen, S. G., A. Bjoerneklett, and J. N. Bruun.** 1989. Severe erythroblastopenia and hemolytic anemia during a hepatitis A infection. *Scand. J. Infect. Dis.* **21:**225–228.
42. **Gust, I. D., and S. M. Feinstone.** 1988. *Hepatitis A*. CRC Press, Inc., Boca Raton, Fla.
43. **Hadler, S. C.** 1991. *Viral Hepatitis and Liver Disease*, p. 14–20. Williams & Wilkins, Baltimore, Md.
44. **Harmon, S. A., W. Updike, X.-Y. Jia, D. F. Summers, and E. Ehrenfeld.** 1992. Polyprotein processing in *cis* and in *trans* by hepatitis A virus 3C protease cloned and expressed in *Escherichia coli*. *J. Virol.* **66:**5242–5247.
45. **Hoke, C. H., Jr., L. N. Binn, J. E. Egan, R. F. DeFraites, P. O. Macarthy, B. L. Innis, K. H. Eckels, D. Dubois, E. D'Hondt, M. H. Sjogren, R. Rice, J. C. Sadoff, and W. H. Bancroft.** 1992. Hepatitis A in the US Army: epidemiology and vaccine development. *Vaccine* **10**(Suppl. 1)**:**S75–S79.
46. **Hollinger, F. B., and A. P. Glombicki.** 1990. Hepatitis A virus, p. 1383–1399. *In* G. L. Mandell, Jr., R. G. Douglas, and J. E. Bennett (ed.), *Principles and Practice of Infectious Diseases*. Churchill Livingstone, New York, N.Y.
47. **Hollinger, F. B., and J. Ticehurst.** 1990. Hepatitis A virus, p. 631–667. *In* B. N. Fields and D. M. Knipe (ed.), *Virology*. Raven Press, Ltd., New York, N.Y.
48. **Hsieh, S. Y., P. Y. Yang, and Y. F. Liaw.** 1997. Cloning and characterization of the extreme 5′-terminal sequences of the RNA genomes of GB virus C/hepatitis G virus. *Proc. Natl. Acad. Sci. USA* **94:**3206–3210.
49. **Humphrey, C. D., E. H. Cook, Jr., and D. W. Bradley.** 1990. Identification of enterically transmitted hepatitis virus particles by solid phase immune electron microscopy. *J. Virol. Methods* **29:**177–188.
50. **Inman, R. D., M. Hodge, M. E. A. Johnston, J. Wright, and J. Heathcote.** 1986. Arthritis, vasculitis, and cryoglo-

bulinemia associated with relapsing hepatitis A virus infection. *Ann. Intern. Med.* **105:**700–703.

51. **Innis, B. L., R. Snitbhan, P. Kunasol, T. Laorakpongse, W. Poopatanakool, S. Suntayakorn, T. Suknantapong, A. Safary, and J. W. Boslego.** 1992. Field efficacy trial of inactivated hepatitis A vaccine among children in Thailand. *Vaccine* **10**(Suppl. 1)**:**S159. (Extended abstract.)
52. **Jacobson, I. M., B. J. Nath, and J. L. Dienstag.** 1985. Relapsing viral hepatitis type A. *J. Med. Virol.* **16:** 163–169.
53. **Jakschies, D., R. Zachoval, R. Muller, M. Manns, K. U. Nolte, H. K. Hochkeppel, M. A. Horisberger, H. Deicher, and P. Von Wussow.** 1994. Strong transient expression of the type I interferon-induced MxA protein in hepatitis A but not in acute hepatitis B and C. *Hepatology* **19:**857–865.
54. **Jansen, R. W., J. E. Newbold, and S. M. Lemon.** 1985. Combined immunoaffinity cDNA-RNA hybridization assay for detection of hepatitis A virus in clinical specimens. *J. Clin. Microbiol.* **22:**984–989.
55. **Jansen, R. W., G. Siegl, and S. M. Lemon.** 1990. Molecular epidemiology of human hepatitis A virus defined by an antigen-capture polymerase chain reaction method. *Proc. Natl. Acad. Sci. USA* **87:**2867–2871.
56. **Just, M., and R. Berger.** 1992. Reactogenicity and immunogenicity of inactivated hepatitis A vaccines. *Vaccine* **10**(Suppl. 1)**:**S110–S113.
57. **Kaplan, G., A. Totsuka, P. Thompson, T. Akatsuka, Y. Moritsugu, and S. M. Feinstone.** 1996. Identification of a surface glycoprotein on African green monkey kidney cells as a receptor for hepatitis A virus. *EMBO J.* **15:** 4286–4296.
58. **Karayiannis, P., S. O'Rourke, J. Waters, R. Watts, and H. C. Thomas.** 1994. Studies of cytotoxic T lymphocyte activity in tamarins with acute hepatitis A virus infection, p. 155–157. *In* K. Nishioka, H. Suzuki, S. Mishiro, and T. Oda (ed.), *Viral Hepatitis and Liver Disease*. Springer-Verlag, Tokyo, Japan.
59. **Krah, D. L., R. D. Amin, D. R. Nalin, and P. J. Provost.** 1991. A simple antigen-reduction assay for the measurement of neutralizing antibodies to hepatitis A virus. *J. Infect. Dis.* **163:**634–637.
60. **Kurane, I., L. N. Binn, W. H. Bancroft, and F. A. Ennis.** 1985. Human lymphocyte responses to hepatitis A virus-infected cells: interferon production and lysis of infected cells. *J. Immunol.* **135:**2140–2144.
61. **Kusov, Y. Y., Y. A. Kazachkov, G. K. Dzagurov, G. A. Khozinskaya, M. S. Balayan, and V. Gauss-Müller.** 1992. Identification of precursors of structural proteins VP1 and VP2 of hepatitis A virus. *J. Med. Virol.* **37:**220–227.
62. **Lemon, S. M.** 1995. Hepatitis A virus and blood products: virus validation studies. *Blood Coagulation Fibrinolysis* **6:** s20–s22.
63. **Lemon, S. M., and L. N. Binn.** 1983. Antigenic relatedness of two strains of hepatitis A virus determined by cross-neutralization. *Infect. Immun.* **42:**418–420.
64. **Lemon, S. M., L. N. Binn, R. Marchwicki, P. C. Murphy, L. H. Ping, R. W. Jansen, L. V. S. Asher, J. T. Stapleton, D. W. Taylor, and J. W. LeDuc.** 1990. In vivo replication and reversion to a wild type of a neutralization-resistant antigenic variant of hepatitis A virus. *J. Infect. Dis.* **161:** 7–13.
65. **Lemon, S. M., L. N. Binn, and R. H. Marchwicki.** 1983. Radioimmunofocus assay for quantitation of hepatitis A virus in cell culture. *J. Clin. Microbiol.* **17:**834–839.
66. **Lemon, S. M., S. F. Chao, R. W. Jansen, L. N. Binn, and J. W. LeDuc.** 1987. Genomic heterogeneity among human and nonhuman strains of hepatitis A virus. *J. Virol.* **61:**735–742.
67. **Lemon, S. M., R. W. Jansen, and E. A. Brown.** 1992. Genetic, antigenic and biological differences between strains of hepatitis A virus. *Vaccine* **10**(Suppl. 1)**:**S40–S44.
68. **Lemon, S. M., R. W. Jansen, and J. E. Newbold.** 1985. Infectious hepatitis A particles produced in cell culture consist of three distinct types with different buoyant densities in CsCl. *J. Virol.* **54:**78–85.
69. **Lemon, S. M., and J. T. Stapleton.** 1994. Prevention of hepatitis A, p. 61–79. *In* A. J. Zuckerman and H. C. Thomas (ed.), *Viral Hepatitis*. Churchill Livingstone, London, England.
70. **Ludmerer, K. M., and J. M. Kissane.** 1984. Fulminant hepatic failure in a 21-year old man. *Am. J. Med.* **76:** 718–724.
71. **Malcolm, B. A., S. M. Chin, D. A. Jewell, J. R. Stratton-Thomas, K. B. Thudium, R. Ralston, and S. Rosenberg.** 1992. Expression and characterization of recombinant hepatitis A virus 3C proteinase. *Biochemistry* **31:**3358–3363.
72. **Malcolm, B. A., C. Lowe, S. Shechosky, R. T. McKay, C. C. Yang, V. J. Shah, R. J. Simon, J. C. Vederas, and D. V. Santi.** 1995. Peptide aldehyde inhibitors of hepatitis A virus 3C proteinase. *Biochemistry* **34:**8172–8179.
73. **Mannucci, P. M., S. Gdovin, A. Gringeri, M. Colombo, A. Mele, N. Schinaia, N. Ciavarella, S. U. Emerson, and R. H. Purcell.** 1994. Transmission of hepatitis A to patients with hemophilia by factor VIII concentrates treated with organic solvent and detergent to inactivate viruses. The Italian Collaborative Group. *Ann. Intern. Med.* **120:** 1–7.
74. **Mao, J.** 1990. Development of live, attenuated hepatitis A vaccine (H2-strain). *Vaccine* **8:**523–524.
75. **Margolis, H. S., and O. V. Nainan.** 1990. Identification of virus components in circulating immune complexes isolated during hepatitis A virus infection. *Hepatology* **11:** 31–37.
76. **McLinden, J., J. Stapleton, and E. Rosen.** 1991. Anti-HAV neutralizing antibodies made to antigens produced by recombinant baculoviruses, p. 239–244. *In* H. Ginsberg, F. Brown, R. A. Lerner, and R. Chanock (ed.), *Vaccines 91: Modern Approaches to New Vaccines*. Cold Spring Harbor Laboratory Press, Cold Spring Harbor, N.Y.
77. **McMahon, B. J., J. Williams, L. Bulkow, M. Snowball, R. Wainwright, M. Kennedy, and D. Krause.** 1995. Immunogenicity of an inactivated hepatitis A vaccine in Alaska native children and native and non-native adults. *J. Infect. Dis.* **171:**676–679.
78. **Melnick, J. L.** 1982. Classification of hepatitis A virus as enterovirus type 72 and of hepatitis B virus as hepadnavirus type 1. *Intervirology* **18:**105–106.
79. **Morris, T. S., S. Frormann, S. Shechosky, C. Lowe, M. S. Lall, V. Gauss-Muller, R. H. Purcell, S. U. Emerson, J. C. Vederas, and B. A. Malcolm.** 1997. In vitro and ex vivo inhibition of hepatitis A virus 3C proteinase by a peptidyl monofluoromethyl ketone. *Bioorg. Med. Chem.* **5:** 797–807.
80. **Mossad, S. B., M. L. Macknin, S. V. Medendorp, and P. Mason.** 1996. Zinc gluconate lozenges for treating the common cold. A randomized, double-blind, placebo-controlled study. *Ann. Intern. Med.* **125:**81–88.
81. **Murphy, P., L. H. Ping, and S. M. Lemon.** 1993. Peptide scanning demonstrates the presence of a linear epitope located near the carboxy terminus of VP1 of hepatitis A virus, abstr. 14, p. 102. *In 8th International Symposium on Viral Hepatitis and Liver Disease*.
82. **Nadala, E. C. B., and P. C. Loh.** 1990. A nitrocellulose-enzyme immunoassay method for the detection of hepatitis A virus. *J. Virol. Methods* **28:**155–164.
83. **Nainan, O. V., M. A. Brinton, and H. S. Margolis.** 1992.

Identification of amino acids located in the antibody binding sites of human hepatitis A virus. *Virology* **191**:984–987.

84. **Najarian, R., D. Caput, and W. Gee.** 1985. Primary structure and gene organization of human hepatitis A virus. *Proc. Natl. Acad. Sci. USA* **82**:2627–2631.
85. **Normann, A., J. Graff, A. Gerritzen, H.-H. Brackmann, and B. Flehmig.** 1992. Detection of hepatitis A virus RNA in commercially available factor VIII preparation. *Lancet* **340**:1232–1233.
86. **O'Farrell, B. J., E. Rajan, S. S. Albloushi, M. G. Courtney, J. Fielding, and A. G. Shattock.** 1997. The reliability of saliva as a sample for the detection of hepatitis A immunoglobulins under various sampling conditions. *Clin. Diagn. Virol.* **7**:153–157.
87. **Parry, J. V., K. R. Perry, S. Panday, and P. P. Mortimer.** 1989. Diagnosis of hepatitis A and B by testing saliva. *J. Med. Virol.* **28**:255–260.
88. **Perry, K. R., J. V. Parry, E. M. Vandervelde, and P. P. Mortimer.** 1992. The detection in urine specimens of IgG and IgM antibodies to hepatitis A and hepatitis B core antigens. *J. Med. Virol.* **38**:265–270.
89. **Petithory, J. R., F. R. Masiarz, J. F. Kirsch, D. V. Santi, and B. A. Malcolm.** 1991. A rapid method for determination of endoproteinase substrate specificity: specificity of the 3C proteinase from hepatitis A virus. *Proc. Natl. Acad. Sci. USA* **88**:11510–11514.
90. **Ping, L.-H., R. W. Jansen, J. T. Stapleton, J. I. Cohen, and S. M. Lemon.** 1988. Identification of an immunodominant antigenic site involving the capsid protein VP3 of hepatitis A virus. *Proc. Natl. Acad. Sci. USA* **85**: 8281–8285.
91. **Ping, L.-H., and S. M. Lemon.** 1992. Antigenic structure of human hepatitis A virus defined by analysis of escape mutants selected against murine monoclonal antibodies. *J. Virol.* **66**:2208–2216.
92. **Pons, J. A.** 1995. Role of liver transplantation in viral hepatitis. *J. Hepatol.* **22**:146–153.
93. **Provost, P. J., and M. R. Hilleman.** 1979. Propagation of human hepatitis A virus in cell culture in vitro. *Proc. Soc. Exp. Biol. Med.* **160**:213–221.
94. **Provost, P. J., B. S. Wolanski, W. J. Miller, O. L. Ittensohn, W. J. McAleer, and M. R. Hilleman.** 1975. Physical, chemical and morphological dimensions of human hepatitis A virus strain CR326. *Proc. Soc. Exp. Biol. Med.* **148**: 532–539.
95. **Purcell, R. H., J. H. Hoofnagle, J. Ticehurst, and J. L. Gerin.** 1989. Hepatitis viruses, p. 957–1065. *In* N. J. Schmidt and R. Emmons (ed.), *Diagnostic Procedures for Viral, Rickettsial, and Chlamydial Infections*, 6th ed. American Public Health Association, Washington, D.C.
96. **Rakela, J., S. M. Lange, J. Ludwig, and W. P. Baldus.** 1985. Fulminant hepatitis: Mayo Clinic experience with 34 cases. *Mayo Clin. Proc.* **60**:289–292.
97. **Robertson, B. H., D. Friedberg, A. Normann, J. Graff, B. Flehmig, and D. Shouval.** 1994. Sequence variability of hepatitis A virus and factor VIII associated hepatitis A infections in hemophilia patients in Europe. An update. *Vox Sang.* **46**:39–45.
98. **Robertson, B. H., R. W. Jansen, B. Khanna, A. Totsuka, O. V. Nainan, G. Siegl, A. Widell, H. S. Margolis, S. Isomura, K. Ito, T. Ishizu, Y. Moritsugu, and S. M. Lemon.** 1992. Genetic relatedness of hepatitis A virus strains recovered from different geographical regions. *J. Gen. Virol.* **73**:1365–1377.
99. **Robertson, B. H., B. Khanna, O. V. Nainan, and H. S. Margolis.** 1991. Epidemiologic patterns of wild-type hepatitis A virus determined by genetic variation. *J. Infect. Dis.* **163**:286–292.
100. **Rosenblum, L. S., M. E. Villarino, O. V. Nainan, M. E. Melish, S. C. Hadler, P. P. Pinsky, W. R. Jarvis, C. E. Ott, and H. S. Margolis.** 1991. Hepatitis A outbreak in a neonatal intensive care unit: risk factors for transmission and evidence of prolonged viral excretion among preterm infants. *J. Infect. Dis.* **164**:476–482.
101. **Rotbart, H. A.** 1989. Human enterovirus infections: molecular approaches to diagnosis and pathogenesis, p. 243–264. *In* B. L. Semler and E. Ehrenfeld (ed.), *Molecular Aspects of Picornavirus Infection and Detection*. American Society for Microbiology, Washington, D.C.
102. **Rueckert, R. R., and E. Wimmer.** 1984. Systematic nomenclature of picornavirus proteins. *J. Virol.* **50**: 957–959.
103. **Scholz, E., U. Heinricy, and B. Flehmig.** 1989. Acid stability of hepatitis A virus. *J. Gen. Virol.* **70**: 2481–2485.
104. **Schultheiss, T., Y. Y. Kusov, and V. Gauss-Muller.** 1994. Proteinase 3C of hepatitis A virus (HAV) cleaves the HAV polyprotein P2-P3 at all sites, including VP1/2A and 2A/2B. *Virology* **198**:275–281.
105. **Siegl, G.** 1984. The biochemistry of hepatitis A virus, p. 9–32. *In* R. J. Gerety (ed.), *Hepatitis A*. Academic Press Ltd., London, England.
106. **Siegl, G., and G. G. Frosner.** 1978. Characterization and classification of virus particles associated with hepatitis A. I. Size, density, and sedimentation. *J. Virol.* **26**:40–47.
107. **Sjogren, M. H., R. H. Purcell, K. McKee, L. Binn, P. Macarthy, J. Ticehurst, S. Feinstone, J. Caudill, A. See, C. Hoke, W. Bancroft, and E. D'Hondt.** 1992. Clinical and laboratory observations following oral or intramuscular administration of a live attenuated hepatitis A vaccine candidate. *Vaccine* **10**:S135–S138.
108. **Stapleton, J. T.** 1992. Passive immunization against hepatitis A. *Vaccine* **10**:S45–S47.
109. **Stapleton, J. T.** 1995. Host immune response to hepatitis A virus. *J. Infect. Dis.* **171**:s9–s14.
110. **Stapleton, J. T.** 1998. Hepatitis A. *In* S. Spector (ed.), *Hepatitis Viruses*, in press. Humana Press, Totowa, N.J.
111. **Stapleton, J. T., J. Frederick, and B. Meyer.** 1991. Hepatitis A virus attachment to cultured cell lines. *J. Infect. Dis.* **164**:1098–1103.
112. **Stapleton, J. T., R. Jansen, and S. M. Lemon.** 1985. Neutralizing antibody to hepatitis A virus in immune serum globulin and in the sera of human recipients of immune serum globulin. *Gastroenterology* **89**:637–642.
113. **Stapleton, J. T., D. K. Lange, J. W. LeDuc, L. N. Binn, R. W. Jansen, and S. M. Lemon.** 1991. The role of secretory immunity in hepatitis A virus infection. *J. Infect. Dis.* **163**:7–11.
114. **Stapleton, J. T., and S. M. Lemon.** 1987. Neutralization escape mutants define a dominant immunogenic neutralization site on hepatitis A virus. *J. Virol.* **61**:491–498.
115. **Stapleton, J. T., and S. M. Lemon.** 1997. New vaccines against hepatitis A, p. 571–585. *In* M. M. Levine, G. C. Woodrow, J. B. Kaper, and G. S. Cobon (ed.), *New Generation Vaccines*. Marcel Dekker, Inc., New York, N.Y.
116. **Stapleton, J. T., V. Raina, P. L. Winokur, K. Walters, D. Klinzman, E. Rosen, and J. H. McLinden.** 1993. Antigenic and immunogenic properties of recombinant hepatitis A virus 14S and 70S subviral particles. *J. Virol.* **67**: 1080–1085.
117. **Stapleton, J. T., E. Rosen, D. Klinzman, and J. McLinden.** 1993. Protease digestion of hepatitis A virus proteins present in recombinant subviral particles, abstr. 3, p. 99. *In 8th International Symposium on Viral Hepatitis and Liver Disease*.
118. **Strader, D. B., and L. B. Seeff.** 1996. New hepatitis A vaccines and their role in prevention. *Drugs* **51**:359–366.

119. **Summers, P. L., D. R. Dubois, W. Houston Cohen, P. O. Macarthy, L. N. Binn, M. H. Sjogren, R. Snitbhan, B. L. Innis, and K. H. Eckels.** 1993. Solid-phase antibody capture hemadsorption assay for detection of hepatitis A virus immunoglobulin M antibodies. *J. Clin. Microbiol.* **31:**1299–1302.
120. **Tabor, E.** 1984. Clinical presentation of hepatitis A, p. 47–53. *In* R. J. Gerety (ed.), *Hepatitis A*. Academic Press Ltd., London, England.
121. **Tanno, H., O. H. Fay, J. A. Fojman, and J. Palazzi.** 1988. Biphasic form of hepatitis A virus infection: a frequent variant in Argentina. *Liver* **7:**53–57.
122. **Ticehurst, J. R., S. M. Feinstone, T. Chestnut, N. C. Tassopoulos, H. Popper, and R. H. Purcell.** 1987. Detection of hepatitis A virus by extraction of viral RNA and molecular hybridization. *J. Clin Microbiol.* **25:**1822–1829.
123. **Torre, D., C. Zeroli, M. Giola, G. Ferrario, G. P. Fiori, G. Bonetta, and R. Tambini.** 1994. Serum levels of interleukin-1 alpha, interleukin-1 beta, interleukin-6, and tumor necrosis factor in patients with acute viral hepatitis. *Clin. Infect. Dis.* **18:**194–198.
124. **Totsuka, A., H. Yamamoto, and Y. Moritsugu.** 1993. Proteolytic cleavage sites in hepatitis A virus polyprotein, abstr. 4, p. 99. *In 8th International Symposium on Viral Hepatitis and Liver Disease*.
125. **Tsai, J. F., H. S. Margolis, J. E. Jang, M. S. Ho, W. Y. Chang, M. Y. Hsieh, Z. Y. Lin, and J. H. Tsai.** 1996. Increased IgM class circulating immune complexes in acute hepatitis A virus infection. *Clin. Immunol. Immunopathol.* **78:**291–295.
126. **Vallbracht, A., P. Gabriel, K. Maier, F. Hartmann, and B. Flehmig.** 1986. Cell-mediated cytotoxicity in hepatitis A virus infection. *Hepatology* **6:**1308–1314.
127. **Vallbracht, A., K. Maier, Y. D. Stierhof, K. H. Wiedmann, B. Flehmig, and B. Fleischer.** 1989. Liver-derived cytotoxic T cells in hepatitis A virus infection. *J. Infect Dis.* **160:**209–217.
128. **Weitz, M., B. M. Baroudy, W. L. Maloy, J. R. Ticehurst, and R. H. Purcell.** 1986. Detection of a genome-linked protein (VPg) of hepatitis A virus and its comparison with other picornaviral VPgs. *J. Virol.* **60:**124–130.
129. **Werzberger, A., B. Mensch, B. Kuter, L. Brown, J. Lewis, R. Sitrin, W. Miller, D. Shouval, B. Wiens, G. Calandra, J. Ryan, P. Provost, and D. Nalin.** 1992. A controlled trial of a formalin-inactivated hepatitis A vaccine in healthy children. *N. Engl. J. Med.* **327:**453–457.
130. **Widell, A.** 1988. Hepatitis A virus virological studies. Ph.D. dissertation. University of Lund, Lund, Sweden.
131. **Widell, A., B. G. Hansson, B. Oberg, and E. Nordenfelt.** 1986. Influence of twenty potentially antiviral substances on in vitro multiplication of hepatitis A virus. *Antiviral Res.* **6:**103–112.
132. **Wiedermann, G., F. Ambrosch, H. Kollaritsch, H. Hofmann, C. Kunz, E. D'Hondt, A. Delem, F. E. André, A. Safary, and J. Stéphenne.** 1990. Safety and immunogenicity of an inactivated hepatitis A candidate vaccine in healthy adult volunteers. *Vaccine* **8:**581–584.
133. **Winokur, P. L., J. H. McLinden, and J. T. Stapleton.** 1991. The hepatitis A virus polyprotein expressed by a recombinant vaccinia virus undergoes proteolytic processing and assembly into virus-like particles. *J. Virol.* **65:**5029–5036.
134. **Winokur, P. L., and J. T. Stapleton.** 1992. Immunoglobulin prophylaxis for hepatitis A. *Clin. Infect. Dis.* **14:**580–586.
135. **Wunschmann, S., A. Vallbracht, B. Flehmig, P. Winokur, D. Klinzman, and J. T. Stapleton.** Cytolytic T lymphocyte epitopes are present on hepatitis A virus structural proteins. *In* M. Rizzeto (ed.), *Viral Hepatitis and Liver Disease*, in press.
136. **Xiang, J. H., Y. Y. Cao, G. L. Zhong, D. J. Zhou, and D. X. Dong.** 1997. Culture of rapid growth-adapted hepatitis A virus Lu8 strain. *Chin. J. Biol.* **10:**12–15.
137. **Yotsuyanagi, H., K. Koike, K. Yasuda, K. Moriya, Y. Shintani, H. Fujie, K. Kurokawa, and S. Iino.** 1996. Prolonged fecal excretion of hepatitis A virus in adult patients with hepatitis A as determined by polymerase chain reaction. *Hepatology* **24:**10–13.
138. **Zachoval, R., M. Kroener, M. Brommer, and F. Deinhardt.** 1990. Serology and interferon production during the early phase of acute hepatitis A. *J. Infect. Dis.* **161:**353–354.
139. **Zhou, Y.-J., M. K. Estes, X. Jiang, and T. G. Metcalf.** 1991. Concentration and detection of hepatitis A virus and rotavirus from shellfish by hybridization tests. *Appl. Environ. Microbiol.* **57:**2963–2968.

Hepatitis B and D Viruses

F. BLAINE HOLLINGER AND JULES L. DIENSTAG

82

CLINICAL AND EPIDEMIOLOGIC FEATURES

Viral hepatitis is primarily a disease of the liver that is caused by a number of well-characterized viruses, including hepatitis B virus (HBV) and HDV. The clinical features of hepatitis B are extremely variable. In most acutely infected patients, inapparent (subclinical) hepatitis develops without symptoms or jaundice. Other patients acquire symptoms without jaundice (anicteric hepatitis), while jaundice with symptoms (icteric hepatitis) occurs in approximately 25 to 35% of those infected with HBV. Symptoms may range from mild and transient to severe and prolonged. Patients may recover completely, be overwhelmed by fulminant hepatitis and die (<1.5% of hospitalized patients), or become chronically infected.

Hepatitis B

The incubation period of acute hepatitis B ranges from 6 to 16 weeks in most patients. The incubation period may be shortened by a large inoculum and infection by the percutaneous route; it may be prolonged by physicochemical alteration of HBV (UV irradiation, heat, or storage at room temperature), coinfection with HCV (51), or administration of high-titer anti-hepatitis B surface antigen (HBsAg) antibody (anti-HBs) to HBV-infected persons shortly after exposure. Variations in host response can also lead to differences in the incubation period.

The prodromal or preicteric phase of hepatitis B tends to be more insidious and prolonged than that of hepatitis A, lasting from 1 to 2 weeks in 80% of patients. It is frequently characterized by malaise, low-grade fever (<39.5°C), fatigability, myalgia, blunting of olfactory and gustatory senses, anorexia, nausea, and vomiting. Weight loss of 1 to 5 kg is common, as is right upper quadrant discomfort or pain associated with hepatomegaly. Physical examination reveals a tender, enlarged liver.

The icteric phase of acute viral hepatitis is often accompanied by the appearance of dark urine followed shortly thereafter by the development of clinical jaundice. With the emergence of jaundice, symptoms tend to improve, and fever usually subsides. The icteric phase lasts, on average, about 1 month. In 10 to 20% of patients infected with HBV, extrahepatic manifestations of the disease develop, most of them believed to be mediated by virus-specific immune complex injury. These include a serum sickness-like syndrome, acute necrotizing vasculitis (polyarteritis nodosa), and membranous glomerulonephritis.

Biochemical tests of liver disease, such as an elevated alanine aminotransferase (ALT) level, are essential for the clinical diagnosis of acute hepatitis B. Other liver enzymes are not as helpful. The total bilirubin concentration is usually less than 10 mg/dl but may occasionally exceed 20 mg/dl. A prolongation of the prothrombin time may reflect early and potentially serious derangements of liver function and may portend a poor outcome.

The factors that determine outcome or chronicity remain largely unknown. In general, the frequency of clinically overt forms of hepatitis B increases with age, whereas the likelihood of becoming chronically infected decreases. Infection in the perinatal period leads to chronicity without symptoms in about 85% of neonates born to HBsAg carrier mothers whose sera contain high concentrations of virus, as manifested by the presence of hepatitis B e antigen (HBeAg) or HBV DNA. In contrast, the rates of transmission and progression to chronicity are dramatically reduced in infants born to mothers whose virus loads are low. In infants 1 year of age, the incidence of development of a persistent infection following acute disease falls to 26%, and by 3 years of age, the incidence is as low as 8%. The potential for chronicity in immunocompetent adults ranges from 1 to 4%, but symptoms are more common during the acute infection.

HLA class I- and II-restricted cytotoxic T lymphocytes (CTLs) appear to play a major role in facilitating viral clearance during acute HBV infection and in the pathogenesis of hepatocellular injury by recognizing HBV nucleocapsid epitopes expressed on the surfaces of infected hepatocytes. Patients with chronic hepatitis B usually are devoid of or deficient in HLA class I- and II-restricted CTLs directed against these epitopes (9). In transgenic mice that accumulate high concentrations of HBV large-envelope polypeptide (HBsAg) within the endoplasmic reticulum (see Description of the Agent below), liver cell injury leads to chronic active hepatitis and hepatocellular carcinoma (16), but a role for HBsAg-directed CTLs in humans with hepatitis B has not been demonstrated.

Pathologic features of acute hepatitis B include both degenerative and regenerative parenchymal changes that lead to lobular disarray. During recovery, regenerative changes predominate; however, in some patients, confluent necrosis, which is potentially progressive and fatal, may occur. Histologic examination is useful for distinguishing among acute viral hepatitis, chronic hepatitis, and cirrhosis. Chronic hepatitis B is associated with hepatocellular carcinoma, especially in males living in Asia and Africa. The incidence of death from liver cancer and cirrhosis increases as a direct function of age; however, cirrhosis is not always a requirement for the development of hepatocellular cancer due to HBV infection.

Hepatitis B is transmitted by percutaneous exposure to blood, blood products, and blood-contaminated instruments. Intimate contact, especially sexual contact, and perinatal spread from mother to newborn are the two other common modes of HBV transmission. Approximately one-third of cases of acute hepatitis B in the United States occur in the absence of a recognized mode of transmission.

Antiviral therapy with interferon or nucleoside analogs that inhibit reverse transcriptase is effective in suppressing viral replication by converting chronic replicative HBV infection into a nonreplicative or repressed state, resulting in a sustained virologic response in 30 to 40% of patients (14, 89). After liver transplantation, HBV reinfection of the new liver is universal, resulting in significant HBV-induced liver injury in a number of these patients. Histologic features of fibrosing cholestatic hepatitis develop in some patients, leading to early graft loss (58). Hepatitis B immune globulin (HBIG) or antiviral therapy appears to modulate these outcomes (69).

Hepatitis D

HDV, previously called the delta agent, is a defective RNA virus that requires concomitant HBV infection for its own replication and expression. In the United States, most cases of hepatitis D are observed primarily in populations frequently exposed to blood-contaminated needles and blood products, such as injection drug users and hemophiliacs; secondary cases have been recorded in sexual partners of drug users, and such cases can amplify the spread of HDV within population groups other than those recognized as being at high risk for HDV infection. In Mediterranean countries, person-to-person spread, including household contact, is an important mode of transmission. Sustained epidemics of clinically severe acute hepatitis D have been observed in South American populations with high HBV carrier rates (76).

Because HDV infection can become established only in persons with HBV infection, acquisition of acute hepatitis D can occur simultaneously with acute HBV infection (coinfection), or HDV infection can become superimposed upon an already established chronic HBV infection (superinfection). Acute coinfection with both HBV and HDV usually causes an acute illness indistinguishable from acute HBV infection alone except that the likelihood of fulminant hepatitis can be as high as 5%. A biphasic course is sometimes observed during coinfection. HDV infection does not increase the rate of chronicity of acute hepatitis B, and complete recovery is the rule. The importance of HDV infection lies in its ability to convert an asymptomatic or mild, chronic HBV infection into fulminant or more severe and rapidly progressive disease. In HBV carriers who experience HDV superinfection, chronic HDV infection leading to severe chronic hepatitis and cirrhosis is the rule unless the patient succumbs to fulminant hepatitis (24, 76). Limited success has been achieved in treating chronic hepatitis D patients with alpha interferon. High-dose, long-term therapy is required, but relapses are common after therapy is stopped (18, 48). Patients with hepatitis D who have hepatic decompensation are candidates for liver transplantation, the outcome of which is better than that for patients with chronic hepatitis B alone (69).

PROCESSING OF SPECIMENS FOR HBV AND HDV AND OCCUPATIONAL SAFETY GUIDELINES

Except for HBV DNA, HDV RNA, and hepatitis delta antigen (HDAg), the stability of serologic markers that develop following HBV or HDV infection eliminates the need for extraordinary collection and storage procedures if bacterial contamination is minimized. Serum or plasma should be separated from blood samples within 24 h and stored at 2 to 8°C if testing is to take place within 5 days. Should longer delays be anticipated, the processed specimens must be frozen. The addition of a bacteriostatic agent to the samples is rarely indicated. Should this become necessary, a final concentration of 0.01% thimerosal, 0.1% sodium azide, or 25 to 50 μg of gentamicin sulfate per ml is preferred. Because heparinized or severely hemolyzed blood may occasionally cause false-positive enzyme immunoassay (EIA) responses, such samples should be avoided.

For nucleic acid analysis, samples should be processed within 6 h and either tested within 24 h or stored at −70°C or lower. Plasma recovered from blood collected in tubes containing EDTA (lavender-top tubes) or in tubes containing anticoagulant citrate dextrose (ACD; yellow-top tubes) is preferred for genome amplification techniques (e.g., PCR). Conversely, heparinized plasma is considered unacceptable, because heparin binds to DNA (2) and interferes with *Taq* polymerase-mediated PCR (33), causing false-negative results. Heparin also inhibits reverse transcription (33, 88). Should heparinized samples be the only material available for HBV DNA or HDV RNA analysis, the deproteinized sample should be treated with heparinase I (0.004 units/μl) in 0.005 M Tris-HCl (pH 7.6) containing 0.001 M $CaCl_2$. For HDV RNA, RNase inhibitor and dithiothreitol must also be added at concentrations of 0.5 units/μl and 0.0006 M, respectively. After 2 h at 20 to 25°C, the sample may be used directly for PCR-based amplification (2, 33, 44).

Processed samples or unseparated blood can be shipped at ambient temperatures by overnight carrier if delivery is expected to be made within 24 h. However, sensitivity and safety are best achieved by shipping these samples in Styrofoam boxes containing at least 5 kg of dry ice, which should maintain samples in a frozen state for at least 72 h when the ambient temperature is <98°F (ca. 37°C). In accordance with the provisions cited in the Interstate Shipment of Etiologic Agents (*Code of Federal Regulations*, Title 42, Part 72), etiologic samples can be shipped by passenger-carrying or cargo aircraft if the volume is no more than 50 ml and is accompanied with the proper documentation (Shipper's Declaration of Dangerous Goods) and a UN Hazard Class 6.2 label. Volumes between 50 ml and 4 liters also can be shipped, but only on cargo aircraft with a "Cargo Aircraft Only" label. The infectious material must be wrapped in sufficient absorbent material to retain all the sample should breakage occur and placed in the inner container of a double mailing canister. Each container should be sealed with vinyl plastic tape, placed in an insulated Styrofoam mailing carton, and covered with dry ice. Up to 400 lb of dry ice can be used, but the package must be sent as freight if it weighs more than 150 lb. Excess space is filled with bubble wrap,

Styrofoam peanuts, or other filler. Although HBV and HDV serologic markers are stable for years at −70°C (−30°C for antibodies), repetitive freezing and thawing may lead to substantial losses in concentration.

Laboratory personnel should regard all specimens collected from hepatitis B patients as potentially dangerous. The Occupational Safety and Health Administration (OSHA) standards for occupational exposure to blood-borne pathogens (29 *Code of Federal Regulations* 1910.1030) are designed to provide protection to employees exposed to blood and other potentially infectious materials. Compliance is mandatory. At the core of the standard is the concept of universal precautions, which mandate that all human blood and certain human body fluids be treated as if they are known to be infectious for human immunodeficiency virus (HIV), HBV, or other blood-borne pathogens. OSHA mandates that all employees who have an occupational exposure be offered hepatitis B vaccine at no cost. OSHA standards and additional safety recommendations can be found in the literature (5, 54, 91).

Ideally, the use of needles or other sharps should be avoided whenever possible; when used, they should be placed in puncture-resistant sharps containers and incinerated or autoclaved before being discarded. All other materials should be placed in discard pans and autoclaved at 121°C for 20 min. A 1 to 10% commercial bleach solution (0.05 to 0.5% sodium hypochlorite), prepared fresh each week to avoid deterioration, is effective against most, if not all, human viruses and is the treatment of choice for disinfection. An exposure time of 15 min is recommended, although the presence of organic material (e.g., serum) may impair the response. Thus, large volumes of disinfectant relative to the volumes of virus-containing materials should be used to inactivate viruses effectively. Because hypochlorites may be corrosive to many metals, the solutions should not be allowed to remain in contact with such materials for more than 10 min. It is safe to autoclave bleach at a final dilution of 1:100. Alternative recommended means of inactivating HBV include 2.0% aqueous alkalinized glutaraldehyde (pH 8.4) and 1% Wescodyne.

HBV

Description of the Agent

HBV is the prototype agent for a new family of DNA viruses designated *Hepadnaviridae*. Related viruses are found in woodchucks, ground squirrels, Peking ducks, and tree squirrels. Features shared by these viruses include virion size and ultrastructure; distinctive polypeptide and antigenic compositions; comparable DNA sizes, structures, and genetic organizations; and a unique mechanism of viral DNA replication. Recently, separate genera for the mammalian and avian hepadnaviruses have been proposed because of differences in their molecular biology.

Ultrastructural examination of particles observed in the sera of patients with HBV infection reveals three distinct morphologic entities in various proportions (Fig. 1). The more numerous forms (by a factor of 10^4 to 10^6) are the small, pleomorphic, spherical, noninfectious particles measuring 17 to 25 nm in diameter (mean diameter, 20 nm). Particle counts of 10^{13} have been detected in some sera. Tubular or filamentous forms of various lengths, but with diameters similar to those of the small particles, also are observed. A third particle, the hepatitis B virion, is a complex double-shelled particle with a diameter of approximately 42 to 47 nm. Originally designated the Dane particle, it consists of an outer shell or lipid-containing envelope, approximately 7 nm in thickness, that surrounds an electron-dense inner core having a diameter of 25 to 27 nm. The sera of infected patients may contain as many as 10^{10} infectious virions per ml. The terminology used to describe the various antigens and antibodies associated with HBV is given in Table 1. The complex antigen found on the surface of HBV and comprising the 20-nm-diameter spherical particles and tubular forms is called HBsAg. Previous designations included the Australia or Au antigen and the hepatitis-associated antigen. The envelope or HBsAg proteins are represented by three HBV-encoded polypeptides sometimes designated the small (or major), middle, and large proteins of HBsAg. The major or small protein is encoded by the S region of the S gene and consists of a 226-amino-acid polypeptide (24,000 Da) and its glycosylated form (27,000 Da). The middle protein is encoded by the pre-S2 and S regions of the S gene and contains an additional glycosylation site in the pre-S2 region. The large polypeptide consists of 389 to 400 amino acids encoded by the pre-S1, pre-S2, and S regions of the S gene of the HBV genome but generally lacks the pre-S2 glycosylation site.

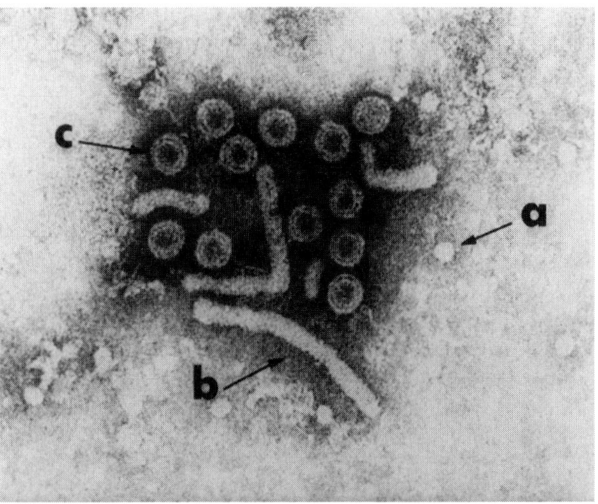

FIGURE 1 Electron micrograph of serum showing the presence of three distinct morphologic entities: a, 17- to 25-nm-diameter pleomorphic, spherical particles; b, tubular or filamentous forms with diameters similar to those of the small particles; c, 42- to 47-nm-diameter double-shelled spherical particles representing the hepatitis B virion (Dane particle). Magnification, ×105,600. Purified preparations of the pleomorphic, spherical HBsAg particles (a), plasma derived or genetically engineered, are used in human hepatitis B vaccines.

Analysis has revealed that one antigenic specificity, designated *a*, is common to all HBsAg preparations. In addition, there are two sets of allelic determinants, *d* or *y* and *w* or *r*. Thus, there are four principal subtypes of HBsAg: *adw*, *ayw*, *adr*, and *ayr*. Because of antigenic heterogeneity in the *w* determinant, there are 10 major serotypes of HBV. The predominant subtype found in North America is *adw*; *ayw* is the second most common. HBV subtypes do not change after infection; therefore, subtype determination can be helpful in tracing infection from one source to another.

The 20-nm-diameter particles primarily contain only S-region-encoded sequences and have average buoyant densities of 1.18 g/cm^3 in CsCl and 1.16 g/cm^3 in sucrose, a

TABLE 1 Nomenclature for viral hepatitis B

Term	Abbreviation	Description
Hepatitis B virus	HBV	42-nm-diam double-shelled particle that consists of a 7-nm-diam outer shell and 27-nm-diam inner core. Core contains a small, circular, partially double-stranded DNA molecule and DNA polymerase activity. Originally called the Dane particle. This is the prototype for the family *Hepadnaviridae*.
Hepatitis B surface antigen	HBsAg	Complex antigen found on surface of HBV and on 20-nm-diam particles and tubular forms. Formerly designated Australia (Au) antigen or hepatitis-associated antigen (HAA).
Hepatitis B core antigen	HBcAg	Antigen associated with 27-nm-diam core of HBV.
Hepatitis B e antigen	HBeAg	Antigen closely associated with nucleocapsid of HBV. Also found as soluble protein in serum.
Antibodies to HBsAg, HBcAg, and HBeAg	Anti-HBs, anti-HBc, and anti-HBe, respectively	Specific antibodies produced in response to their respective antigens.

molecular weight of 3.7×10^6 to 4.6×10^6, and a sedimentation coefficient that ranges from 39S to 54S. The low buoyant densities of these particles reflect the presence of lipids, which are presumably of cell membrane origin (20). The tubular forms contain mostly small and middle-sized polypeptides, while the lipid-containing envelope of HBV is replete with all S gene products.

The complete virion has a buoyant density of about 1.22 g/cm^3 in CsCl and consists of an envelope of HBsAg, an internal core or nucleocapsid that contains core proteins with hepatitis B core antigen (HBcAg) and HBeAg specificities, and a small (3,200-bp), circular, partially double-stranded DNA molecule with a molecular weight of 1.6×10^6 (79). The HBV genome is partially double stranded because of incomplete extension of the positive-sense strand by the endogenous DNA polymerase enzyme incorporated within the virion. Because some HBV particles may contain no DNA while others contain genomes with single-stranded gaps of different lengths, the buoyant densities of the nucleocapsids in CsCl can range from 1.30 to 1.36 g/cm^3 (35). Antibodies to HBsAg (anti-HBs), HBcAg (anti-HBc), and HBeAg (anti-HBe) are produced in response to their respective antigens.

HBcAg and HBeAg have different antigenic specificities. The core protein is a polypeptide with a molecular size of 22,000 Da that is encoded by the C gene of HBV. The precore sequence within the C gene is important for expression and secretion of a polypeptide with HBeAg specificity. Proteolytic cleavage of the core protein results in truncated forms of HBeAg that have molecular sizes of approximately 17,000 Da and that appear to lack the viral DNA-binding domain. HBeAg either circulates freely in the blood as a soluble protein or is bound to albumin, α_1-antitrypsin, or immunoglobulin. It is a reliable marker for the presence of intact virions and thus for infectivity. A mutation at the end of the precore region leading to a translational stop codon yields a variant that is unable to produce HBeAg: such precore mutants may contribute to the pathogenesis of chronic hepatitis B and fulminant hepatitis. Other HBV gene mutations have been observed in the core, core promoter, envelope, and polymerase regions. The envelope protein variants may become relevant if they are able to escape vaccine-induced anti-HBs or lead to failure of HBIG therapy after transplantation.

The stability of HBV does not always coincide with that of HBsAg. Immunogenicity and antigenicity, but not infectivity, are retained after exposure to ether, acid (pH 2.4 for at least 6 h), and heat (98°C for 1 min, 60°C for 10 h); however, inactivation may be incomplete under these conditions if the concentration of virus is excessively high. Exposure of HBsAg to 0.25% sodium hypochlorite for 3 min destroys antigenicity and infectivity. Infectivity in serum is lost after direct boiling for 2 min, autoclaving at 121°C for 20 min, or exposure to dry heat at 160°C for 1 h. More recent studies have shown that HBV is inactivated by exposure to sodium hypochlorite (500 mg of free chlorine per liter) for 10 min, 0.1 to 2% aqueous glutaraldehyde, Sporicidin (pH 7.9), 70% isopropyl alcohol, 80% ethyl alcohol at 11°C for 2 min, Wescodyne diluted 1:213, or combined β-propiolactone, UV irradiation, and solvent-detergent mixtures [tri(*n*-butyl)phosphate and Triton X-100] (4, 28, 36, 61). HBV retains infectivity when stored at 30 to 32°C for at least 6 months and when frozen at −20°C for 15 years.

Direct Examination

Although not applicable to rapid, large-scale screening of HBV infections by clinical laboratories, immunofluorescence, in situ hybridization, immunohistochemistry, and thin-section electron microscopy have been used extensively to examine pathologic specimens for the presence of HBV-associated antigens or particles (3, 8, 21, 31, 50, 64). Indeed, nonisotopic in situ detection methods for the simultaneous analysis of HBV-related nucleic acids and antigens in paraffin-embedded liver tissue are providing important insights into the relationship between HBV DNA replication and gene expression at the single-cell level (25, 26). Within different hepatocytes, HBsAg is localized exclusively in the cytoplasm, whereas HBcAg is usually detected in the nucleus. Cytoplasmic HBcAg can also be demonstrated, especially during active replication of the virus. Detection of complete virions in the liver is uncommon; however, HBcAg-containing capsids are occasionally observed in the nuclei of hepatocytes.

The techniques used for immunoperoxidase or immunofluorescence staining are well known. As a general rule, immunofluorescence staining of cryostat sections is superior to the use of paraffin sections. However, cryostat sections are not always available, and cellular outlines are better resolved in uniformly cut paraffin sections than in frozen sections. Reduction of nonspecific background staining of formalin-fixed sections can be achieved by treating tissue with 0.1% trypsin for 2 to 6 h at 37°C before staining. In situations in which autologous antibody might bind to cell-associated antigen, cryostat sections can be treated for 5 min with 0.1 M glycine-HCl buffer (pH 1.2) before specific antibody is added.

Recently, biotin-streptavidin systems have been introduced for detecting viral antigens in cells or in tissues. This methodology offers a number of advantages over other immunodiagnostic clinical techniques: (i) the binding of streptavidin to biotin is extremely rapid and essentially irreversible because of the high affinity constant ($>10^{15}$ M^{-1}) that exists between these two proteins (affinity constants of antibody for most antigens are generally 10^6-fold lower); (ii) sensitivity is enhanced, even when highly diluted primary antibody is used, because the four binding sites on avidin permit amplification of the response; (iii) formalin-fixed, paraffin-embedded histologic sections, smears, and frozen sections can be examined by conventional light microscopy; and (iv) background staining is greatly reduced.

The avidin-biotin-labeled horseradish peroxidase complex (ABC) procedure of Hsu and associates (29, 30) is highly sensitive and specific. Briefly, formalin-fixed tissue sections are incubated at 37°C for 12 to 16 h, deparaffinized, and hydrated through xylene and a graded alcohol series. The fixation process should use a buffered formalin, not exceeding 4% formaldehyde, that is sufficient to maintain the integrity of the tissue without destroying the antigenic determinants being evaluated. The sections are exposed sequentially to a primary antibody, a biotinylated antispecies immunoglobulin G (IgG), and Vectastain ABC reagent (Vector Laboratories, Burlingame, Calif.). Next, the tissue antigen is localized by incubating the sections in freshly prepared peroxidase substrate solution. After each step of the staining procedure, slides are rinsed with 10 mM phosphate-buffered saline (PBS; pH 7.6). Sections should not be allowed to dry out during the staining procedure; therefore, a humidified chamber is recommended for incubations. If the antigen concentration is low, the substrate incubation step may be lengthened to achieve maximal staining. If nonspecific staining occurs, it can be reduced by incubating the sections for 20 min with diluted normal serum prepared from the species in which the secondary antibody is made. Many mammalian tissues contain endogenous peroxidase. If this problem exists, sections may be incubated for 30 min in 0.3% hydrogen peroxide in methanol either before primary antibody is added or, for those situations in which the antigenic determinant may be destroyed by hydrogen peroxide, before the ABC reagent step.

We have detected HBsAg and HBcAg in liver tissue by an enhanced biotin-streptavidin method (26) that uses a mouse anti-HBs monoclonal antibody and a rabbit anti-HBc polyclonal antibody, respectively, and a commercially available immunodetection kit (StrAviGen Super Sensitive Alkaline Phosphatase Kit; BioGenex Laboratory, Ramon, Calif.). This kit uses an alkaline phosphatase-conjugated streptavidin and a chromogenic substrate solution (naphthol phosphate substrate and fast red chromogen) for localization of tissue antigens.

Paraffin-embedded liver tissue can also be evaluated by in situ hybridization with a digoxigenin-labeled DNA probe and a digoxigenin detection system (25, 26). Digoxigenin is preferred over biotin for several reasons. Endogenous biotin (but not digoxigenin) is present in liver tissue and often results in high levels of background staining (56, 90). In addition, biotin has a high binding affinity for HBsAg (86). Finally, digoxigenin-labeled probes are comparable in sensitivity to radiolabeled probes (23). Probes representing the complete 3.2-kb genomic DNA of HBV and a suitable negative-control DNA preparation are labeled with digoxigenin-dUTP by random priming (19) with a DNA labeling and detection kit (Boehringer Mannheim Biochemical Co., Indianapolis, Ind.). The probes are chemically stable and can be used for extended periods. Before hybridization, deparaffinized and rehydrated sections are rendered permeable by sequential treatment with acid, heat, and proteinase K. Washing of the sections at room temperature in PBS containing glycine will stop the proteinase K digestion, and RNA is removed by digestion with RNase A. The sections are prehybridized and then overlaid with the appropriate digoxigenin-labeled probe. A coverslip is placed over each section, and the probe and tissue DNAs are denatured in situ by heating them at 95°C for 4 min. After quenching on ice, the hybridization reaction is carried out at 42°C for 12 to 16 h. Following removal of the coverslips, the digoxigenin-labeled hybrids are detected with an antidigoxigenin alkaline phosphatase conjugate and an enzyme substrate-chromogen solution. The color reaction is stopped with Tris-EDTA buffer (pH 8.0). For the simultaneous detection of HBV DNA and antigens, in situ hybridization with two different chromogens (red and blue-purple) is carried out after completion of the immunohistochemical procedure. Neither method interferes with or significantly reduces the sensitivity or specificity of the other method; however, too strong an opposing signal could mask or reduce the other signal. Amplification of virus-specific HBV DNA by PCR in paraffin-embedded tissue can facilitate the detection of low-copy-number DNA present in a sample if this is followed by in situ hybridization (45). Conversely, PCR can be used to directly detect HBV DNA in paraffin-embedded liver tissue when optimal DNA extraction techniques are used (12). However, extraction from frozen tissues is less difficult to achieve and is still preferred.

Cell Cultures and Animal Models

Despite recent evidence for the growth of HBV in primary cultures of healthy adult or fetal human hepatocytes (22, 57, 66), serial propagation over a prolonged period has not been accomplished. Still, the use of stably transfected cell lines provides a model of HBV replication, even though the life cycle is incomplete and only low concentrations of virus are produced. Chimpanzees and other high-order primates are highly susceptible to experimental induction of hepatitis B but are not routinely available (1). The pattern of infection is similar to that observed in humans except that the disease is clinically milder. Nevertheless, the chimpanzee model has played an essential role in studies of viral inactivation, vaccine safety and efficacy, disinfection kinetics, infectivity determinations and immunopathology, and in seroepidemiologic investigations. Because of its limited role as a model for studying viral replication or evaluating antiviral agents, it is being replaced by other animal systems such as the woodchuck, Peking duck, and transgenic mouse (49).

Serologic Identification of Hepatitis B Antigens, Antibodies, and Virus

A number of serologic techniques with different degrees of sensitivity and specificity have been developed for the detection of HBV antigens and their specific antibodies (Table 2). These radioimmunoassay (RIA) or EIA methods rely on the sandwich principle or are competitive binding immunoassays (Table 3). Readers interested in detailed information concerning the purification of hepatitis B-associated antigens, preparation of HBV-specific antiserum, and discontinued assays of historical interest such as agarose gel diffusion, discontinuous counterimmunoelectrophoresis, rheophor-

TABLE 2 U.S. licensed or approved manufacturers of hepatitis B assays

Assay	Manufacturer[a]	
	RIA	EIA
HBsAg	1, 4	1, 2, 3, 4
Anti-HBs	1, 4	1, 4
Anti-HBc	1, 4	1, 3, 4
IgM Anti-HBc	1, 4	1, 4
HBeAg	1, 4	1, 4
Anti-HBe	1, 4	1, 4
HBV DNA	1	

[a] Manufacturers: 1, Abbott Laboratories; 2, Sanofi Diagnostics; 3, Ortho Diagnostics Systems; 4, Sorin/Incstar Corp.

esis, complement fixation, reverse passive latex agglutination, and reverse passive hemagglutination are referred to the third edition of this Manual. The procedure for HBV-associated DNA polymerase is detailed in the fourth edition of this Manual.

EIA

The EIA technique is at least as sensitive as RIA and is the favored method. Improvements in the test have reduced the number of repeatably false-positive reactions, and specificity is almost comparable to that of RIA. Table 2 lists those commercial companies that manufacture licensed qualitative third-generation EIAs for the detection of HBV serologic markers, and Table 3 gives the principles of the procedures. EIA kits have longer shelf lives than RIA kits (6 to 15 months versus 2 months). Specific details of the assays can be obtained from the package insert that accompanies each kit, and it is imperative that these instructions be followed explicitly.

Diagnostic EIA products licensed to detect HBsAg (Table 4) follow a generic protocol with a number of minor variations that do not appear to alter the sensitivity or specificity of the assay significantly (except for those procedures with an abbreviated incubation period). Nuances in the various EIA procedures include sample incubation, either simultaneously (one step) with conjugated anti-HBs or consecutively (two step); variation in incubation or color development ranging from 30 min to overnight; use of polystyrene beads or microwells; use of monoclonal versus polyclonal anti-HBs; and selection of alkaline phosphatase instead of horseradish peroxidase for the enzyme-conjugated antibody. These assays are capable of detecting HBsAg at a level of approximately 0.25 to 0.5 ng/ml.

In one scenario, HBsAg is detected by mixing human test serum or plasma with enzyme-conjugated anti-HBs in the presence of a polystyrene bead or microplate well coated with anti-HBs. In each of the assays, appropriate positive and negative controls must be included to ensure the validity of the assay. Trays are sealed with an adhesive cover, and incubation is allowed to proceed overnight at room temperature. During the incubation period, HBsAg binds to the antibody-coated solid phase and also combines with the enzyme-labeled antibody to form an anti-HBs–antigen–enzyme-conjugated anti-HBs sandwich. The contents of the wells are aspirated, and the reaction trays are washed. A chromogenic substrate is added, resulting in the development of a measurable colored reaction product. After a 30-min incubation, the enzyme reaction is arrested with either sulfuric acid or sodium hydroxide, depending on the substrate being used, and the sample is read in a spectrophotometer at the appropriate optical density. Test samples (S) giving absorbance values equal to or greater than the calculated cutoff value (C) are considered reactive for HBsAg. An alternative method of determining positivity is to divide S by C. Thus, any specimen with an S/C ratio of $\geq$1.0 is considered reactive for HBsAg. Within limits, there is a direct correlation between the magnitude of the S/C ratio and the concentration of HBsAg in the specimen; however, the sizes of the various HBsAg-containing particles and the surface area of the support system restrict the working range to between 0.25 ng/ml and 1 μg/ml, above which level saturation (a plateau) is reached. Because sera from many carriers have HBsAg concentrations that range from 50 to 300 μg/ml, the sample must be diluted until a value that falls within the working range of the assay is obtained if quantitation of HBsAg becomes necessary.

Depending on the assay, final readings should be made within 30 to 120 min after the addition of acid or base to the reaction tray. The control blank used to calibrate the instrument should be reused whenever prolonged interruptions occur or if color develops in the blank. Care should be taken to avoid splashing specimens or reagents outside of wells or high up on the rim of the reaction tray, for such splashes may not be removed in subsequent washing and could cause false-positive test results. Sodium azide poisons

TABLE 3 Principles of procedures used in various hepatitis B assays

Serologic assay	Principle of procedure (RIA or EIA)	Type of support system	Adsorbed reagent	Label or conjugate
HBsAg	Sandwich	Bead, well	Anti-HBs	Anti-HBs
HBeAg	Sandwich	Bead, well	Anti-HBe	Anti-HBe
Anti-HBs	Sandwich	Bead, well	HBsAg	HBsAg
IgM anti-HBc	Sandwich (modified)[a]	Bead, well	Anti-IgM	Anti-HBc
Anti-HBc	Competitive binding[b]	Bead, well	HBcAg	Anti-HBc[b]
Anti-HBe	Competitive binding[c]	Bead, well	Anti-HBe	Anti-HBe

[a] IgM-specific anti-HBc that is immunologically bound to an anti-IgM-coated (μ-chain-specific) bead is detected by adding recombinant DNA-derived HBcAg and then the appropriate anti-HBc label or conjugate.

[b] The anti-HBc EIA from Ortho Diagnostic Systems is a sandwich assay in which the label or conjugate is murine monoclonal antibodies specific for human IgG and IgM.

[c] Anti-HBe in the test sample and adsorbed anti-HBe compete for a standardized amount of HBeAg added to the reaction well before the addition of anti-HBe label or conjugate.

TABLE 4 Comparison of commercial EIAs for detection of HBsAg[a]

Manufacturer	Support system	Adsorbed anti-HBs	Anti-HBs conjugate	Sample vol (μl)
Abbott Laboratories	Beads	MM	MM-HRP	200
Genetic Systems Corp.	Wells	MM	MM-HRP	200
Organon Teknika Corp.	Wells	GP	Chimpanzee-AP	200
Ortho Diagnostic Systems	Wells	MM	MM-HRP	200
Sorin/Incstar Corp.[b]	Wells	MM	Sheep-HRP	100

[a] MM, murine monoclonal antibody, GP, guinea pig; HRP, horseradish peroxidase; AP, alkaline phosphatase.
[b] Unlicensed product for research use only; not for use in diagnostic procedures.

the enzyme substrate; therefore, this reagent should not be present in the wash solution. As with the RIA procedure, the wash step is a critical part of the assay. If any delivery port is clogged or dispenses wash solution erratically, reproducibility and precision will suffer. Application of trace amounts of silicone grease to the tube dispensers used to wash beads keeps the water from adhering to the metal and facilitates the washing process. Substitutions for recommended wash solutions should be avoided. For example, phosphate inhibits alkaline phosphatase and could lower the optical density, whereas Tris buffer may increase alkaline phosphatase activity (82).

Repeatably reactive HBsAg results that cannot be confirmed as positive are highly unusual. Nevertheless, the seriousness of the diagnosis, with its attendant medical, social, and economic repercussions, mandates that a confirmatory test be attempted on all repeatably positive specimens. This can be approached in one of two ways: (i) specimens may be tested with another licensed HBsAg assay, or (ii) a blocking or inhibition assay can be performed to see whether unlabeled anti-HBs will specifically inhibit the reaction. The detection of anti-HBc in the absence of anti-HBs also corroborates a positive HBsAg result. Low-level reactivity, e.g., S/C ratios of <1.5, must always be viewed with suspicion. Partially heparinized plasma can cause low-level false-positive HBsAg reactions. This often can be corrected by the addition of thrombin to the sample or by storing the sample at 2 to 8°C for 48 h before retesting. Heparin may appear in the blood of patients on hemodialysis who are given heparin prior to dialysis, in bedridden patients being given heparin to prevent thrombophlebitis, and in patients with heparin locks.

Erroneous interpretations also can be avoided by ensuring that the negative control samples are comparable to the test specimen. Thus, tests for HBsAg in fluids of low density, such as cerebrospinal fluid, should use "normal" (healthy) cerebrospinal fluid (or comparable low-density material) as the control. In general, protein-deficient specimens and recalcified plasma result in higher background levels, thereby altering the cutoff values.

In an emergency, the solid-phase EIA may be modified to provide an answer within 45 min. Although sensitivity is approximately fivefold less than that of the regular assay, the number of positive specimens likely to be missed should be relatively small. To further reduce the number of false-negative values, at the expense of increasing the number of false-positive reactions, the cutoff value can be reduced to 1.5 times the value for the negative control (or an S/C ratio of 0.75). Ultimately, verification of a positive reaction by the regular procedure will be necessary.

Solid-phase EIA for the detection of anti-HBs is similar in principle to HBsAg detection except that the specimen is incubated with polystyrene beads (Ausab EIA; Abbott Laboratories, Abbott Park, Ill.) or in microtiter wells (Sorin/Incstar Corp., Stillwater, Minn.; for research use only) that have been coated with HBsAg subtypes *ad* and *ay*. Anti-HBs bound to the fixed HBsAg is detected with a complex consisting either of biotin-labeled human HBsAg and horseradish peroxidase-conjugated rabbit antibiotin or of horseradish peroxidase-conjugated human HBsAg. An absorbance value that is equal to or exceeds the cutoff value or an S/C ratio of ≥1.0 indicates the presence of anti-HBs in the sample.

Recently, Abbott Laboratories has released a licensed anti-HBs quantitation panel for monitoring HBsAg vaccinees. The standards are assayed with the EIA or RIA anti-HBs kits. The panel consists of five vials containing 0, 15, 40, 75, and 150 mIU of human polyclonal anti-HBs per ml based on the World Health Organization (WHO) Anti-HBs Reference Preparation. Specimens are tested in the same assay, and the results are compared to a standard curve generated from the quantitation panel data. Test samples whose values exceed the highest standard are diluted with a specimen dilution buffer and retested. Although results are usually equivalent to those obtained with the WHO Reference Preparation in the RIA (see below), the results for individual specimens may vary. The lower limit of detection for anti-HBs when this quantitative panel is used is 1 mIU/ml. Sorin/Incstar Corp. also has a panel of six standards that can be used for research purposes only, i.e., not for diagnostic procedures.

Three commercial anti-HBc EIA kits are licensed in the United States (Table 2). Two of the kits are competitive binding EIAs (Abbott Laboratories and Sorin/Incstar) in which anti-HBc from the test sample competes with a constant amount of horseradish peroxidase-conjugated human anti-HBc for a limited number of binding sites on beads (Abbott) or in wells (Sorin) that have been coated with recombinant DNA-derived HBcAg. Within limits, the amount of anti-HBc present in the sample is inversely proportional to the amount of color development. Results are compared to a calculated cutoff value. An alternative method for reporting results in competitive binding assays is to compute a cutoff-to-sample (or C/S) ratio. In this way, any result that is ≥1.0 is considered positive, as it is for direct-binding "sandwich" assays in which an S/C ratio is calculated. (As an aid to remembering the correct order of the letters, think of S for sandwich and C for competitive.)

The other commercial EIA kit for anti-HBc (Ortho Diagnostic Systems) uses the sandwich principle, in which the specimen is incubated in microtiter wells coated with HBcAg. Bound anti-HBc is detected with horseradish peroxidase-conjugated murine monoclonal antibodies specific for human IgG and IgM. In this direct reacting (sandwich) assay, higher optical densities are recorded in reactive samples; thus, an S/C ratio is calculated to achieve positive results of ≥1.0.

Two licensed EIA kits are available for the detection of IgM-specific anti-HBc (Table 2). To measure IgM-specific anti-HBc in serum or plasma, the EIA IgM anti-HBc test uses a modified sandwich technique in which anti-HBc of the IgM class is removed or "captured" from the serum by anti-human IgM (μ-chain specific) bound to polystyrene beads. The subsequent addition of recombinant DNA-derived HBcAg results in the attachment of the antigen to any IgM anti-HBc that has combined with the solid-phase anti-human IgM. The sandwich is completed following the addition of radiolabeled anti-HBc. In this assay, 10 μl of test serum is diluted 1:1,071 (Abbott Laboratories) or 1:4,000 (Sorin/Incstar) and then incubated for 1 h at 40°C with a polystyrene bead coated with antibody specific for human IgM (μ-chain specific). During this interval, IgM anti-HBc is captured by the beads. After the liquid is removed and the beads are washed, HBcAg and horseradish peroxidase-conjugated human anti-HBc are added to the bead to which IgM-specific anti-HBc may be immunologically bound. After another incubation period (room temperature for 18 to 22 h or 45°C for 3 h), the beads are rewashed and transferred to tubes, in which color development occurs in the presence of the enzyme substrate. Next, the reaction is stopped, and the intensity of the color is measured with a spectrophotometer. The absorbance is proportional to the quantity of IgM-specific anti-HBc present in the sample. A cutoff value is determined; specimens giving absorbance values equal to or greater than the calculated cutoff value or having S/C ratios of ≥1.0 are considered positive for IgM antibodies to HBcAg.

Two commercial kits are available for the detection of HBeAg and anti-HBe (Table 2). The tests are performed with the same kit but use different assay principles (sandwich principle for the HBeAg and competitive binding for the anti-HBe procedure). In the direct-reacting (sandwich) HBeAg test of Abbott, polystyrene beads coated with human anti-HBe are added to 200 μl of test samples, and incubation proceeds for 18 to 22 h at 15 to 30°C. After the beads are washed, anti-HBe conjugate is added and incubation continues at 40°C for 2 h. After an additional wash step, substrate solution is added and samples are incubated for 30 min at 15 to 30°C. The reaction is stopped with acid, and absorbance values are determined. Absorbance values are increased when HBeAg is present in the serum. A positive reaction is one with a value equal to or greater than the cutoff value or with an S/C ratio of ≥1.0. The test for anti-HBe is a modified competitive binding assay in which anti-HBe in 50 μl of the test serum competes with anti-HBe-coated beads for a standardized amount of recombinant DNA HBeAg. Sealed trays containing the serum and beads are incubated for 18 to 22 h at 15 to 30°C, and then the beads are washed. Next, anti-HBe conjugate is added and incubation is continued for 2 h at 40°C. If anti-HBe is present in the test sample, less HBeAg will be available to bind to the bead, and therefore, less anti-HBe conjugate will be immunologically coupled. Within limits, the larger the amount of anti-HBe in the specimen, the lower the absorbance value. Specimens with absorbances equal to or less than the cutoff value are considered reactive for anti-HBe, as in other competitive binding assays. For this assay, a C/S ratio is computed so that values of ≥1.0 will signify the presence of anti-HBe in the test sample.

RIA

Although EIA has replaced RIA as the most popular method for detecting the various serologic markers of hepatitis B, the RIA technique continues to be the standard to which all other assays are compared. RIA kits for HBV (Table 2) are currently offered by Abbott Laboratories and Sorin/Incstar Corp. Detailed procedures for performing these assays are included with each kit. Each run must be validated on the basis of conditions set forth by the manufacturer.

The concepts of the procedures for commercial RIA tests for HBsAg, total anti-HBc, IgM anti-HBc, HBeAg, and anti-HBe are identical to the EIA tests described previously. The reader is directed to the sixth edition of this Manual for a more detailed description of these specific methods.

With the advent of hepatitis B (HBsAg) vaccine, the need for precision and accuracy in quantifying anti-HBs has become more important. Solid-phase RIA for the detection of anti-HBs is similar in principle to HBsAg detection, except that the specimen is incubated with polystyrene beads coated with human HBsAg, subtypes *ad* and *ay*. To permit results that can be expressed in milli-international units per milliliter, Hollinger et al. (27) have modified the RIA. Anti-HBs concentrations are based on the First International WHO Reference Preparation for HBIG (lot 26.1.77) provided by the International Laboratory for Biological Standards, Central Laboratory of The Netherlands Red Cross Transfusion Services. An arbitrary value of 50 IU (50,000 mIU) of anti-HBs has been assigned to this product. The WHO anti-HBs reference preparation is reconstituted in 0.5 ml of sterile, pyrogen-free water, and the mixture is allowed to equilibrate overnight at 2 to 8°C. It is then diluted in normal recalcified human plasma to contain 125 mIU/ml. To determine the number of milli-international units per milliliter of a sample, an S/R ratio is computed as follows: (sample cpm − negative-control mean cpm)/(reference cpm − negative control mean cpm). Determination of the regression of the S/R ratio (Fig. 2) on the anti-HBs concentration for the WHO Reference Preparation (0.1 to 500 mIU/ml) by using the computer nonlinear regression program BMDP3R (15) yielded the following formula: mIU/ml $= 130.75\ (e^{0.66765(S/R)} - 1)$ (reciprocal of dilution). The lower limit of detection for anti-HBs is 1.5 mIU/ml when this procedure is used. Samples whose anti-HBs concentrations exceed 500 mIU/ml can be diluted 10-fold in normal recalcified human plasma and retested. To conserve the WHO Reference Preparation, the laboratory should procure a large batch of human serum or recalcified plasma containing polyclonal anti-HBs and determine its relationship to the WHO Reference Preparation (diluted to 125 mIU/ml) by using the S/R ratio. The exponent in the formula must be adjusted proportionally to conform with the alternative laboratory reference standard. For example, if the S/R relationship between the laboratory standard and the WHO Reference Preparation is 0.500, the exponent in the formula (0.66765) must be reduced by a factor of 0.5. Conversely, an S/R ratio of 1.5 would increase the exponent by a factor of 1.5. Once this adjustment is made, the laboratory reference standard can be substituted for the WHO Reference Preparation. The laboratory standard (stored at −30°C) should be periodically reevaluated to verify its accuracy against the WHO reference reagent, which can be aliquoted and stored at −70°C. As with the EIAs, quantitative determination of anti-HBs also can be done by using a panel of commercial standards (see EIA section above).

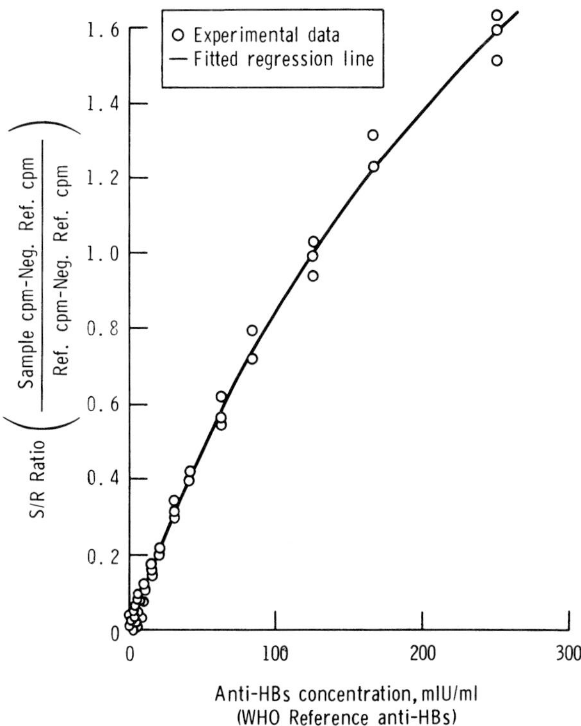

FIGURE 2 RIA standard curve for anti-HBs showing regression of the *S/R* ratio on the anti-HBs concentration (from reference 27). For the regression equation, see text.

Dot Blot Hybridization Techniques

Although hybridization procedures are beyond the scope of most clinical laboratories (42), an awareness of their availability is desirable. Human serum and tissue can be analyzed for HBV DNA sequences by dot hybridization techniques (52, 70–72, 92). In this technique, the HBV DNA in the sample is immobilized on a nitrocellulose or nylon membrane and is hybridized to a radioactive probe. Typically, sample preparation consists of mixing the serum with alkali to lyse the HBV and separate the DNA strands. After addition of the alkaline serum to the manifold in which the filter membrane is held, vacuum is applied. The DNA strands (and protein) bind to the membrane forming the dot. In order to fix the DNA to the membrane, nitrocellulose filters are baked, and nylon filters are exposed to UV light. The hybridization mixture consists of a buffer solution with the ^{32}P-labeled probe (typically, a recombinant cloned HBV DNA labeled to a specific activity of 2×10^8 to 4×10^8 cpm/μg of DNA). To reduce nonspecific binding of the probe to the membrane, Denhardt solution (0.1% bovine serum albumin, 0.1% Ficoll, 0.1% polyvinylpyrrolidone) and an excess of sheared, denatured, nonhomologous DNA are included in the hybridization mixture. The specificity of the hybridization reaction depends on the temperatures used for hybridization and washing and on the composition of the reagents used in these steps. After hybridization, the filter is washed, dried, and autoradiographed. This method is capable of visually detecting 0.1 to 1.0 pg (28,000 to 280,000 genomic equivalents) of HBV DNA sequences within 24 h, with a 2- to 10-fold increase after 5 days of autoradiography. Similar hybridization studies can be performed by using DNA extracted from small portions of frozen biopsy specimens.

Quantitation Hybridization Techniques

Commercial kits that do not require PCR are available for the quantitation of HBV DNA in serum or plasma. Although these techniques do not achieve the sensitivity of quantification methods based on PCR amplification, they may be useful in monitoring the status of HBV infection.

A commercial liquid-phase molecular hybridization assay for the detection and quantitation of HBV DNA in serum (37) has recently become available for research purposes (Abbott Hepatitis B Viral DNA; Abbott Laboratories). The assay can be performed only with serum, and lipemic serum should be clarified by centrifugation prior to use. Specimens may be stored for up to 14 days at 2 to 8°C; otherwise, they should be frozen. Multiple freezing-thawing cycles should be avoided. Nucleases of microbial or human origin may degrade the sample. Thus, extra care must be taken to avoid contamination with nucleases on the skin or on surfaces handled by humans, and pipette tips should be autoclaved before use to destroy nuclease activity. The serum specimen being tested is solubilized to expose the HBV genome and is then incubated with a ^{125}I-labeled HBV DNA probe at 65°C for 18 h for hybridization to the HBV DNA in the test specimen. The mixture is loaded onto a disposable plastic column for elution of hybrid molecules from the unhybridized ^{125}I-HBV probe. The eluate is counted for 10 min in a gamma counter, and the counts are reported as total counts. The cutoff value is derived by multiplying the mean of the positive control values by 0.015 and adding this number to the mean for the negative control values. Samples with net counts within 10% of the cutoff value should be retested. The assay can detect as few as 4×10^4 HBV molecules, or about 0.15 pg of HBV DNA, a sensitivity that is equivalent to that of filter hybridization (60, 93).

The Chiron Amplex-HBV assay (Fig. 3) is a sandwich nucleic acid hybridization method for the quantitative detection of HBV DNA in human serum (84, 85). It is available for research use only (not for use in diagnostic procedures). In this assay, synthetic oligodeoxyribonucleotides containing unique primary segments designed to hybridize to the minus-sense strand of HBV DNA are covalently attached to a secondary fragment through branch points. These target probes hybridize to HBV DNA and to complementary synthetic fragments bound to a solid phase. On another level, the secondary fragments of the target probe direct the binding of multiple copies of synthetic branched DNA amplifier molecules that contain repeated nucleotide sequences that hybridize with enzyme-modified alkaline phosphatase-labeled probes. The detection scheme relies on alkaline phosphatase-catalyzed chemiluminescence emission from a dioxetane substrate, and the results are recorded as luminescence counts on a plate luminometer (Fig. 3). Light emissions are proportional to the amount of HBV DNA present in each specimen, and HBV DNA is quantitated by comparing light emission values in the test specimen against those obtained on standards. As few as 700,000 HBV DNA equivalents per ml can be detected with this assay.

Another kit for the quantitation of HBV DNA, the Digene Hybrid Capture system, has a dynamic range of 3 million HBV DNA copies (10 pg) to 600 million HBV DNA copies (2 ng) per ml. The assay requires 50 μl of serum. The addition of alkali to the sample causes the virions to lyse and the DNA strands to separate. The single-stranded HBV DNA is hybridized to a full-length RNA probe, and the hybrid is captured onto the surface of a tube coated with

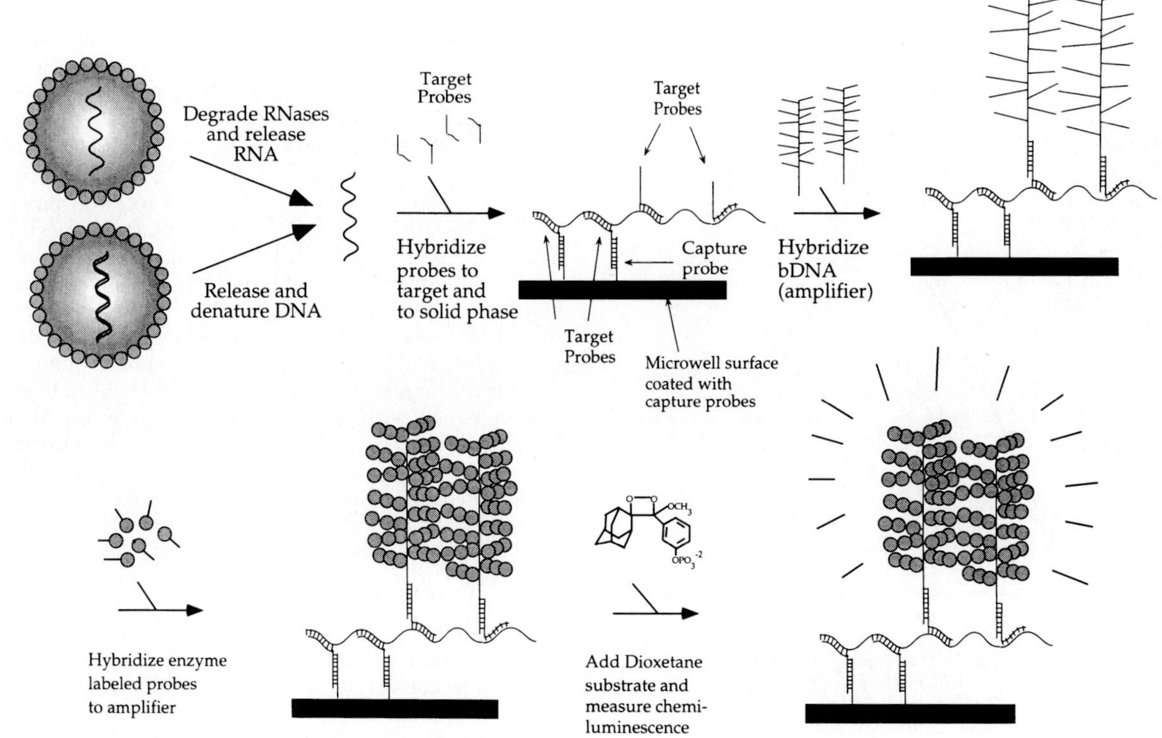

FIGURE 3 Chiron branched DNA (bDNA) signal amplification assay. (© 1993 Chiron Corporation.)

an anti-RNA–DNA antibody. A second antibody that is conjugated to alkaline phosphatase is allowed to bind to the immobilized complex. Chemiluminescent signals proportional to the amount of HBV DNA are produced by the action of the alkaline phosphatase on a substrate.

PCR Assay

Recently, the PCR assay, which makes possible the detection of as few as 10 HBV DNA molecules per ml, has been used for amplification of HBV DNA in serum (83). This assay is 100 to 1,000 times more sensitive than the dot hybridization technique for detecting HBV DNA. Synthetic oligonucleotide primers that are complementary to a conserved sequence on the genome that will be amplified are prepared. The procedure allows denaturation of the DNA to separate the strands of the DNA duplex that contains the target region, annealing of the primers to their complementary regions, and extension of the primers. The discovery of a thermostable enzyme isolated from *Thermus aquaticus*, called *Taq* DNA polymerase, has increased the specificity of the reaction by allowing extension to take place at an elevated temperature. Denaturation, annealing, and extension constitute a cycle and are accomplished by varying the temperature for each reaction. The products of the previous cycle act as templates for succeeding cycles, resulting in an exponential doubling of the DNA. Thus, for every 20 cycles, the target region is amplified about a millionfold, and a second round of 20 cycles with a different pair of primers results in $>10^{12}$ amplification. Alternatively, the second round of amplification may be replaced by a sensitive detection method such as hybridization to a labeled probe.

A number of PCR procedures for detecting HBV DNA in serum have been described (40, 83). Viral DNA can be purified from serum by proteinase K digestion, phenol and chloroform extraction, and precipitation with ethanol, following which the DNA is redissolved in water. Amplification is carried out in a DNA thermal cycler with primers that anneal to highly conserved sequences of the HBV genome. Descriptions of the PCR procedure and guidelines to guard against contamination can be found in references 17, 32, 38, 43, 53, and 77.

Interpretation of Test Results in Hepatitis B Disease

Successful detection of HBV serologic markers depends not only on the relative sensitivity of the test procedures but also on the availability of experienced personnel who comprehend the idiosyncrasies of the procedure and are meticulous in their performance of the test. For example, most nonrepeatably reactive specimens result from improper washing of beads or wells (see EIA above), contamination of counting tubes or holders with radioactive material, or cross-contamination of nonreactive specimens with droplets from highly positive samples.

Provided that all procedural details are observed, the final evaluation and interpretation of any test result will be determined by the specificity of the reagents used. It is important for the diagnostic virologist to appreciate the difficulties encountered by commercial companies in preparing quality reagents and automating immunoassays. The preparation of specific polyclonal antibody or the use of monoclonal antibodies has dramatically improved the sensitivities and specificities of these assays, as has the production of HBV antigens by recombinant DNA technology. Confirmatory testing of specimens by blocking assays or specificity testing with a reference antigen or antiserum also assists in the validation of a laboratory result.

The marked increase in the sensitivity of the PCR assay for HBV DNA compared with that of the RIA or EIA for HBsAg should not imply that an equivalent increase in the number of HBV-infected persons will be realized. Experience indicates that practically all patients with acute and chronic hepatitis B have HBsAg concentrations that are detectable by conventional assays; thus, the use of methods for detecting HBV DNA is usually unnecessary, and such methods should be reserved for specific indications such as monitoring treatment with interferon. It is noteworthy, however, that HBV DNA has been detected rarely in the sera and/or livers of some HBsAg-negative patients with or without other HBV serologic markers (34, 39, 41, 59, 81). It has also been reported that some hepatitis B vaccine nonresponders may have low-level HBV infection (78), which may account for their nonresponsiveness. Finally, PCR is so sensitive that HBV DNA can be detected in the livers of some patients who have recovered completely from their infections.

As shown in Fig. 4 and summarized in Table 5, the presence of HBsAg in serum indicates active HBV infection, either acute or chronic. In a typical acute HBV infection, HBsAg will be detected 2 to 4 weeks before the ALT level becomes abnormal and 3 to 5 weeks before symptoms or jaundice develops. The presence of HBV DNA precedes the appearance of HBsAg in the serum. Anti-HBc, primarily of the IgM class, usually appears when the ALT level begins to increase. The presence of IgM-specific anti-HBc at a relatively high titer (>1:1,000) is evidence of an acute infection. These elevated titers decline regardless of whether the disease resolves or becomes chronic. Figure 5 illustrates the typical serologic pattern that occurs in a patient who becomes chronically infected. It should be recognized that sera from 5 to 15% of chronic hepatitis B patients may be positive by the IgM anti-HBc assay during reactivation of their disease, although the IgM-specific anti-HBc levels are generally low, e.g., near the cutoff level for the test.

Because the total-anti-HBc test is invariably positive when HBsAg is present in a clinically ill patient (see Fig. 4 and Table 5 for rare exceptions to this statement), this test can be used to validate the HBsAg reaction. Tests with discordant results should always be repeated (see Table 6 for examples of discordant or unusual profiles). In perhaps 5 to 10% of patients with acute hepatitis B (especially those with fulminant disease) and more frequently during early convalescence, HBsAg may be undetectable in serum. Examination of these sera for IgM-specific anti-HBc may help in establishing the correct diagnosis (see caveat above concerning detection of IgM-specific anti-HBc in chronic hepatitis B patients during reactivation of disease). In the absence of anti-HBc and HBsAg, past or present hepatitis B disease can almost always be excluded (see above for exceptions). In contrast, the presence of anti-HBc alone is plausi-

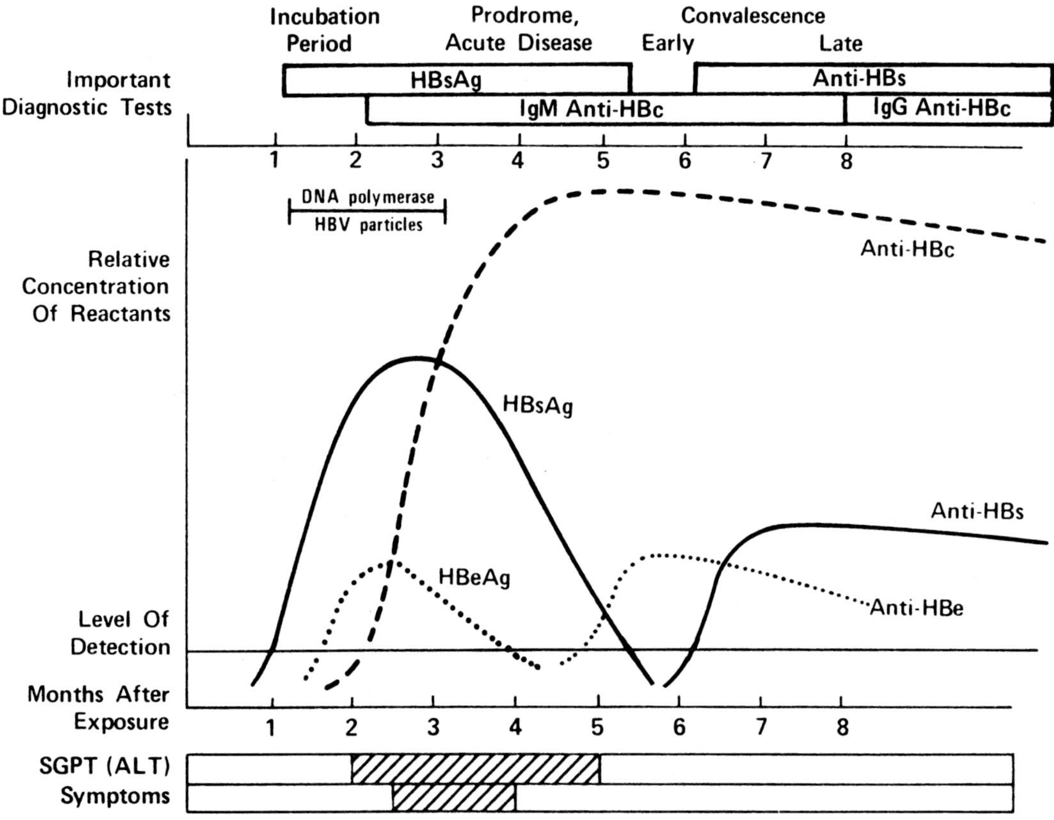

FIGURE 4 Serologic and clinical patterns observed during acute HBV infection. SGPT, serum glutamic pyruvic transaminase.

TABLE 5 Interpretation of HBV serologic markers in patients with hepatitis

Assay result			Interpretation
HBsAg	Anti-HBs	Anti-HBc	
Positive	Negative	Negative	Early acute HBV infection. Confirmation is required to exclude nonrepeatable or nonspecific reactivity (see text).
Positive	(±)[a]	Positive	HBV infection, either acute or chronic. Differentiate with IgM anti-HBc (see text for exceptions). Determine level of replicative activity (infectivity) with HBeAg or HBV DNA.
Negative	Positive	Positive	Indicates previous HBV infection and immunity to hepatitis B.
Negative	Negative	Positive	Possibilities include HBV infection in remote past, "low-level" HBV carrier, "window" between disappearance of HBsAg and appearance of anti-HBs, or false-positive reaction. Investigate with IgM anti-HBc and/or challenge with HBsAg vaccine (see text). When present, anti-HBe helps validate anti-HBc reactivity.
Negative	Negative	Negative	Another infectious agent, toxic injury to liver, disorder of immunity, hereditary disease of liver, or disease of biliary tract.
Negative	Positive	Negative	Vaccine-type response.

[a] ±, anti-HBs is usually absent in this situation, but may occasionally be present.

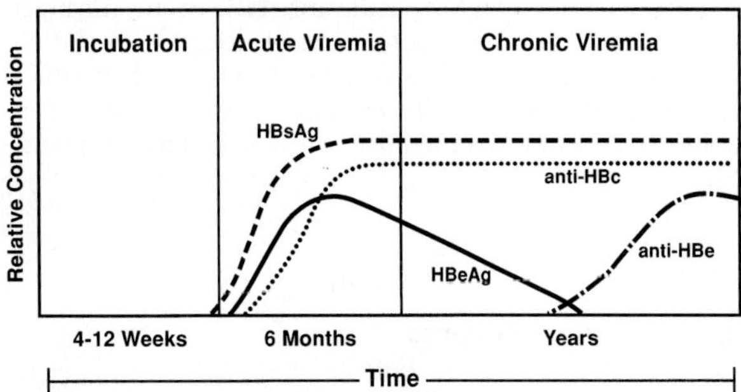

FIGURE 5 Typical sequence of serologic markers in patients with acute hepatitis B who develop persistent infection after exposure to HBV.

ble evidence for an active HBV infection in a small percentage of patients. This relationship is not infallible, however, because some patients who have recovered from hepatitis B with the development of anti-HBs and anti-HBc may eventually lose their anti-HBs, resulting in a solitary anti-HBc response. Challenging a patient displaying this profile with HBsAg vaccine leads to an anamnestic response 2 weeks later (anti-HBs level, >20 mIU/ml), whereas the HBsAg-negative carrier will fail to respond in this time interval.

Chronic hepatitis B patients may be tested for HBsAg, anti-HBc, or HBV DNA to determine their levels of HBV replication and their potential for enhanced infectivity. HBsAg-positive specimens contain high concentrations of HBV DNA in contrast to anti-HBc-positive samples, in which the number of hepatitis B virions is markedly reduced. As anticipated, HBsAg-positive patients are more likely to transmit hepatitis B sexually, percutaneously, or perinatally. HBeAg seroconversion to anti-HBe, with loss of HBV DNA, is a desirable objective in the treatment of hepatitis B with antiviral agents such as interferon.

Antibody to HBsAg becomes detectable usually immediately after, but sometimes several weeks after, the disappearance of HBsAg. It is believed that anti-HBs is produced much earlier but is not observed as a result of the formation of immune complexes in the presence of excess HBsAg. Antibody to HBsAg, with or without anti-HBc, specifies immunity against reinfection. Anti-HBs without anti-HBc develops in persons who receive hepatitis B vaccine (which contains only HBsAg), and levels of ≥10 mIU/ml are considered protective. It has been proposed that detection of anti-HBc, not detection of anti-HBs, be used as a screening test to determine susceptibility to HBV for the purpose of recommending hepatitis B vaccination. Depending on the circumstances, passive transfer of anti-HBs or anti-HBc may be observed in patients receiving clotting factors, after immunoglobulin administration, or in neonates of mothers with current or past hepatitis B. Since blood donations are pretested for HBsAg and total anti-HBc, passive transfer of antibodies following transfusions of blood is unlikely unless the donor has been vaccinated (donors are not tested for anti-HBs). Recognition of these possibilities will avoid an erroneous diagnosis of HBV exposure or infection, because passive antibodies disappear gradually over 3 to 6 months, while actively produced antibodies are remarkably stable over many years.

Subtyping of specimens by the clinical laboratory provides additional information to the clinician or hospital epidemiologist, because the mutually exclusive subdeterminants are virus specific and not host determined. This fact can be helpful in determining the source of infection or can provide epidemiologic evidence for relatedness among

TABLE 6 Discordant or unusual hepatitis B serologic profiles requiring further evaluation

HBsAg positive/anti-HBc negative
HBsAg, anti-HBs, and anti-HBc positive
Anti-HBs or anti-HBc positive only
HBsAg negative/HBeAg positive
Positive for HBeAg and anti-HBe
Anti-HBc negative/IgM anti-HBc positive

patients. Sequencing a segment of the HBV genome also can be used to determine the source of an infection, but this method is available only as a research tool.

HDV

Description of Agent

HDV is an unclassified, roughly spherical, subviral satellite of HBV with an average diameter that ranges from 36 to 43 nm (67, 80). A nucleocapsid of about 19 nm (versus 27 nm for HBV) is encapsidated by HBsAg. The nucleocapsid contains multiple copies of delta antigen (both the large and the small antigens), which are the only HDV RNA-encoded proteins, and a 1.7-kb RNA genome. The HDV genome is a single-stranded, covalently closed circle of single polarity (positive stranded) with viroidlike protein-coding regions (62, 80, 87). The large delta antigen acts to suppress viral replication, while the small antigen supports it. HDV assumes the HBsAg subtype of the HBV present in the host. Although intracellular HDV replication has been accomplished without HBV in in vitro systems, assembly of intact HDV virions and pathogenicity in vivo require the helper function of HBV to support the replication of HDV (67, 80).

Extensive base pairing of the RNA genome of HDV yields substantial internal complementarity, resulting in an unbranched rodlike structure that is reminiscent of viroids or plant RNA satellite viruses. In tissue, RNA molecules of both polarities, sometimes existing as multimers of the 1.7-kb RNA, are detected. The various forms are consistent with a rolling-circle model of replication. The genome is nonhomologous with HBV DNA. Both the genome and the complementary antigenome can function as a ribozyme that can lead to self-cleavage and ligation. HDAg, a phosphoprotein that is nonglycosylated and that may bind to the HDV genome, is the product of the only open reading frame (ORF 5) on the antigenomic strand of HDV. It consists of two proteins, a 195-amino-acid 24-kDa protein and a larger, 214-amino-acid 27-kDa protein (80). The virus particle has a buoyant density in CsCl of 1.25 g/cm^3 and a sedimentation coefficient that is intermediate between those of HBsAg and intact HBV particles. It is inactivated by formalin under conditions similar to those that inactivate HBV.

Direct Examination

Because HDAg is rarely detectable in serum, even when the serum is known to be infectious, and because antibodies to HDV (anti-HDV) are present indefinitely in patients or experimental animals with chronic HDV infection, liver biopsy with immunohistochemical staining for intrahepatic HDAg is a reliable way to demonstrate ongoing HDV replication. However, these methodologies are not practical for adoption as rapid screening tests by clinical laboratories. The anti-HDV probe, to which fluorescein or peroxidase is conjugated, is usually derived from serum or plasma that contains a high titer of anti-HDV and a low level of anti-HBc. Thus, the anti-HBc reactivity can be reduced substantially or eliminated entirely by dilution. However, an anti-HDV-negative, anti-HBc-positive control probe should be used in parallel with the anti-HDV probe to validate the anti-HDV specificity of staining. Controls for other sources of nonspecificity, including autoantibodies to nuclear antigens, should be incorporated into procedures for immunohistochemical staining. With these techniques, investigators have shown that the HDAg localizes primarily to the liver cell nucleus and rarely can be detected in the cytoplasm. Although frozen cryostat sections are preferable, HDAg is stable to formalin fixation and paraffin embedding. Therefore, HDAg can be studied in stored paraffin-embedded tissue after digestion of the section with trypsin or pronase (11).

Serologic Identification of Hepatitis D Antigens, Antibodies, and Virus

Anti-HDV has been identified and quantitated primarily by RIA or EIA (11, 65). Tests for anti-HDV require a source of HDAg. Previously, the HDAg had been obtained from HDAg-positive human (postmortem) or chimpanzee liver or serum. Recently, a more reliable source has become available in the form of HDAg-positive woodchuck liver. HDAg can be extracted from human liver only with strong dissociating agents such as 6 M guanidine hydrochloride or 8 M urea. When liver tissue is obtained from experimentally infected chimpanzees or woodchucks at the peak of intrahepatic HDAg expression, i.e., before the appearance of anti-HDV, antigen can be harvested by simple aqueous extraction. Although HDAg is rarely detectable in the sera of patients with acute HDV infection, occasionally the amount of antigen present is sufficient to serve as a source of antigen for diagnostic testing.

Serum containing anti-HDV can be obtained from patients or experimental animals with acute or chronic HDV infection. As mentioned above, anti-HBc reactivity, invariably present in anti-HDV-positive serum, is relatively low in serum samples with a high level of anti-HDV activity. Thus, residual anti-HBc activity can be diluted out, and HBsAg is removed by ultracentrifugation.

RIA

A commercial RIA for anti-HDV is available for diagnostic purposes (Abbott Anti-Delta; Abbott Laboratories). The test is a competitive binding RIA in which anti-HDV in the test serum competes with ^{125}I-labeled human anti-HDV for woodchuck liver-derived HDAg coating a solid-phase polystyrene bead. In this assay, 100 μl of ^{125}I-labeled anti-HDV and 100 μl of serum or plasma to be tested are delivered to a reaction well, and an HDAg-coated bead is added. Appropriate negative and positive control samples are incorporated into each test run, and the trays are incubated for 18 to 22 h at room temperature. After incubation, liquid is aspirated from the wells and the beads are washed with distilled or deionized water, transferred to tubes, and assayed in a gamma counter. Samples with a count rate equal to or below the cutoff value are considered reactive for anti-HDV; counts above the cutoff range are considered negative. A C/S ratio of $\geq$1.0 is also considered positive. The manufacturer provides specific guidelines to determine whether a test is valid.

HDAg can be detected by solid-phase sandwich RIA as described by Rizzetto et al. (65). The test is based on the binding of HDAg in serum to anti-HDV adherent to a solid phase, followed by incubation with an ^{125}I-labeled IgG anti-HDV probe. Because HDAg always circulates within an HBsAg-encapsidated particle, detection of HDAg requires detergent disruption (with 0.5% Tween 80, Nonidet P-40, or deoxycholate) of the virion to expose the internal, otherwise sequestered antigen. Adding to the difficulty of HDAg detection is the transient nature of HDV antigenemia occurring during early infection. This simple solid-phase RIA for HDAg can be modified for detection of anti-HDV in a competitive binding RIA. A standardized quantity of HDAg is added to beads coated with anti-HDV. Anti-HDV from the test serum or plasma competes with a constant amount of ^{125}I-labeled anti-HDV for the HDAg immunologically bound to the beads. A ≥50% reduction in the net counts per minute compared to the counts per minute in a negative control is evidence for the presence of anti-HDV in the sample. Measurement of anti-HDV titers is achieved by diluting the serum and determining the dilution that inhibits binding of ^{125}I-anti-HDV by 50%.

Acute HDV infection is accompanied by an early, transient anti-HDV response predominantly of the IgM class (74). An antibody class capture, solid-phase RIA for IgM anti-HDV is available outside the United States. The methodology for this technique is analogous to that for the detection of IgM-specific anti-HBc, and interested readers are referred to the hepatitis B EIA section above, in which details of this assay are provided. Since IgM anti-HDV persists in chronic infection and may exist at a high titer in patients with severe acute hepatitis D (74), the presence of IgM anti-HDV does not distinguish between acute and chronic HDV infection.

EIA

A commercial EIA for anti-HDV based on the configuration described above for the commercial RIA (10) is available for diagnostic purposes (Abbott Anti-Delta EIA; Abbott Laboratories). Similarly, RIA techniques for the detection of HDAg have been applied to the detection of HDAg by EIA, and the same limitation (transient nature of the antigenemia during early acute infection) applies (11).

Western Blot

HDAg can be detected by Western blotting (immunoblotting). More sensitive than RIA and EIA, blotting is reactive in more than 70% of patients with chronic hepatitis D (6). Because of its technical sophistication, Western blotting has not been adapted for routine clinical diagnosis; instead, it remains a research tool confined to a small number of research laboratories.

Hybridization Techniques

A noninvasive approach for detecting HDV RNA in serum has been made possible with the recent availability of cloned cDNA probes (13, 63, 68, 75). The cDNA probe for HDV-associated RNA is incubated with serum, and HDV RNA is identified by dot blot hybridization analysis. This technique remains limited to a small number of research laboratories but holds promise as a simple, noninvasive test for the diagnosis of chronic HDV infection. Techniques for detection of HDV RNA in hepatic tissue by in situ hybridization with ^{125}I and nonradioactive probes have been developed as well (46, 55). Like dot hybridization techniques for the detection of HDV RNA in serum, these techniques remain the domain of specialized research laboratories. Finally, HDV RNA also can be detected by riboprobe hybridization; this is one of the most sensitive assays for HDV infection, reactive in >80% of infected patients (73).

PCR Assay

The most sensitive method for the detection of HDV RNA relies on amplification by PCR. The basic approach is the same as that outlined above for the detection of HBV DNA except that a reverse transcriptase step is required to obtain DNA complementary to HDV RNA in serum or liver tissue (47, 94). A nonradioisotopic PCR assay has been described as well (7). These approaches are not routinely available but are confined to specialized research laboratories.

Interpretation of Test Results

Infection with HDV can occur in the presence of acute or chronic HBV infection. The duration of HBV infection determines the duration of HDV infection. The presence of HDV infection can be identified by demonstrating intrahepatic HDAg by immunohistochemical staining or, more practically, anti-HDV seroconversion (a rise in titer of anti-HDV or de novo appearance of IgM-specific anti-HDV, which is detectable only briefly, if at all). Because IgM-specific anti-HDV is transient in acute HDV infection and IgG anti-HDV is often undetectable once HBsAg disappears, retrospective serodiagnosis of acute, self-limited, simultaneous HBV and HDV infections is difficult.

In contrast to patients with acute HBV infection, patients with chronic HBV infection can support HDV replication indefinitely. This can happen when acute HDV infection occurs in the presence of a nonresolving acute HBV infection. More commonly, acute HDV infection becomes chronic when it is superimposed on an underlying chronic HBV infection (Fig. 6). In such cases, the HDV superinfection appears as a clinical exacerbation or as an episode resembling acute viral hepatitis in someone already chronically infected with HBV. In the past, events resembling acute hepatitis in an HBV carrier or a patient with chronic hepatitis B were attributed to superimposed hepatitis C or to the natural history of the disease, e.g., reactivation of HBV. A portion of such episodes, however, represents acute superinfection with HDV.

When a patient presents with acute hepatitis and has HBsAg and anti-HDV in the serum, determination of the immunoglobulin class of anti-HBc is helpful in differentiating coinfection from superinfection. Although IgM-specific anti-HBc does not distinguish absolutely between acute and chronic HBV infections (see above), its presence is a presumptive indicator of recent infection, and its absence is a reliable indicator of infection in the remote past. Thus, in simultaneous acute HBV and HDV infections, IgM-specific

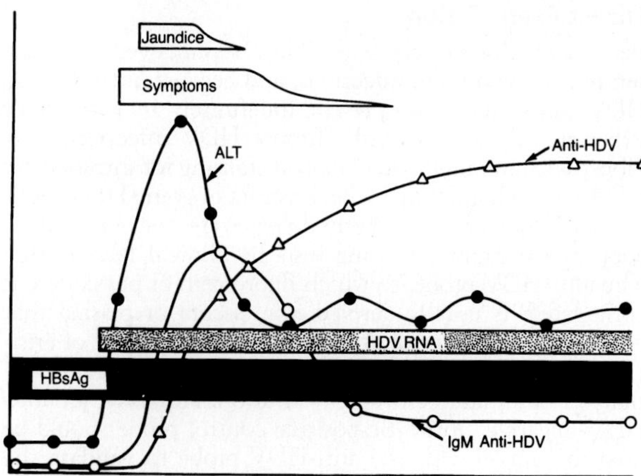

FIGURE 6 Typical serologic course of acute HDV superinfection in an HBsAg carrier (from reference 27a).

anti-HBc is detectable, whereas in acute HDV infection superimposed upon chronic HBV infection, anti-HBc is primarily of the IgG class. A high titer of anti-HDV (>1:1,000) is indicative of ongoing viral replication in a patient with chronic HDV infection.

As noted above, cDNA tests for the presence of HDV-associated RNA will be useful in the future for determining the presence of ongoing HDV replication and relative infectivity. HDV RNA appears early in the course of the disease, continues during the symptomatic stage of illness, and disappears when the disease resolves. In chronic HDV infection, HDV RNA persists in most, but not all, patients, and its presence correlates with the detection of HDAg in the livers of these individuals (Fig. 6). Currently, probes for this marker are restricted to a limited number of research laboratories.

This effort was supported in part by the Eugene B. Casey Foundation.

REFERENCES

1. **Barker, L. F., J. E. Maynard, R. H. Purcell, J. H. Hoofnagle, K. R. Berquist, and W. T. London.** 1975. Viral hepatitis, type B, in experimental animals. *Am. J. Med. Sci.* **270:**189–195.
2. **Beutler, E., T. Gelbart, and W. Kuhl.** 1990. Interference of heparin with the polymerase chain reaction. *BioTechniques* **9:**166.
3. **Blum, H. E., A. Figus, A. T. Haase, and G. N. Vyas.** 1985. Laboratory diagnosis of hepatitis B virus infection by nucleic acid hybridization analyses and immunohistologic detection of gene products. *Dev. Biol. Scand.* **59:** 125–139.
4. **Bond, W. W., M. S. Favero, N. J. Petersen, and J. W. Ebert.** 1983. Inactivation of hepatitis B virus by intermediate-to-high-level disinfectant chemicals. *J. Clin. Microbiol.* **18:**535–538.
5. **Bond, W. W., N. J. Petersen, and M. S. Favero.** 1977. Viral hepatitis B: aspects of environmental control. *Health Lab. Sci.* **14:**235–252.
6. **Buti, M., R. Esteban, R. Jardi, F. Rodriguez-Frias, J. Casacuberta, J. I. Esteban, E. Allende, and J. Guardia.** 1989. Chronic delta hepatitis: detection of hepatitis delta virus in serum by immunoblot and correlation with other markers of delta viral replication. *Hepatology* **10:**907–910.
7. **Cariani, E., A. Ravaggi, M. Pouti, G. Mantero, A. Albertini, and D. Primi.** 1992. Evaluation of hepatitis delta virus RNA levels during interferon therapy by analysis of polymerase chain reaction products with a nonradioisotopic hybridization assay. *Hepatology* **15:**685–689.
8. **Chan, V. T. W., and J. O. McGee.** 1990. Non-radioactive probes; preparation, characterization and detection, p. 59–70. *In* J. M. Polak and J. O. McGee (ed), *In Situ Hybridization: Principles and Practice*. Oxford University Press, Oxford, United Kingdom.
9. **Chisari, F. V.** 1997. Immunobiology and pathogenesis of viral hepatitis, p. 405–415. *In* M. Rizzetto, R. H. Purcell, J. L. Gerin, and G. Verme (ed.), *Viral Hepatitis and Liver Disease*, Proceedings of IX Triennial International Symposium on Viral Hepatitis and Liver Disease. Edizioni Minerva Medica, Turin, Italy.
10. **Crivelli, O., M. Rizzetto, C. Lavarini, A. Smedile, and J. L. Gerin.** 1981. Enzyme-linked immunosorbent assay for detection of antibody to the hepatitis B surface antigen-associated delta antigen. *J. Clin. Microbiol.* **14:** 173–177.
11. **Crivelli, O., J. W. K. Shih, and M. Rizzetto.** 1983. Methods for detection of the delta antigen and antibody in liver and serum, p. 121–126. *In* G. Verme, F. Bonino, and M. Rizzetto (ed.), *Viral Hepatitis and Delta Infection*. Alan R. Liss, Inc., New York, N.Y.
12. **de Lamballerie, X., F. Chapel, C. Vignoli, and C. Zandotti.** 1994. Improved current methods for amplification of DNA from routinely processed liver tissue by PCR. *J. Clin. Pathol.* **47:**466–467.
13. **Denniston, K. J., B. H. Hoyer, A. Smedile, F. V. Wells, J. Nelson, and J. L. Gerin.** 1986. Cloned fragment of the hepatitis delta virus RNA genome: sequence and diagnostic application. *Science* **232:**873–875.
14. **Dienstag, J. L., R. P. Perrillo, E. R. Schiff, M. Bartholomew, C. Vicary, and M. Rubin.** 1995. A preliminary trial of lamivudine for chronic hepatitis B infection. *N. Engl. J. Med.* **333:**1657–1661.
15. **Dixon, W. J., and M. B. Brown.** 1979. *BMDP-79*. University of California Press, Berkeley.
16. **Dunsford, H. A., S. Sell, and F. V. Chisari.** 1990. Hepatocarcinogenesis due to chronic liver cell injury in hepatitis B virus transgenic mice. *Cancer Res.* **50:**3400–3407.
17. **Erlich, H. A.** 1989. *PCR Technology: Principles and Applications for DNA Amplification*. Stockton Press, New York, N.Y.
18. **Farci, P., A. Mandas, A. Coiana, M. E. Lai, V. Desmet, P. Van Eyken, Y. Gibo, L. Caruso, S. Scaccabarozzi, D. Criscuolo, J.-C. Ryff, and A. Balestrieri.** 1994. Treatment of chronic hepatitis D with interferon alfa-2a. *N. Engl. J. Med.* **330:**88–94.
19. **Feinberg, A. P., and B. Vogelstein.** 1983. A technique for radiolabeling DNA restriction endonuclease fragments to high specific activity. *Anal. Biochem.* **132:**6–13.
20. **Gavilanes, F., J. M. Gonzalez-Ros, and D. L. Peterson.** 1982. Structure of hepatitis B surface antigen. *J. Biol. Chem.* **257:**7770–7777.
21. **Gowans, E. J., A. R. Burrel, B. P. Jilbert, and B. P. Marmion.** 1985. Cytoplasmic (but not nuclear) hepatitis B virus core antigen reflects HBV DNA synthesis at the level of the infected hepatocyte. *Intervirology* **24:** 220–225.
22. **Gripon, P., C. Diot, and C. Guguen-Guillouzo.** 1993. Reproducible high level infection of cultured adult human hepatocytes by hepatitis B virus: effect of polyethylene glycol on adsorption and penetration. *Virology* **192:** 534–540.
23. **Guo, K. J., and D. S. Bowden.** 1991. Digoxigenin-labeled probes for the detection of hepatitis B virus DNA in serum. *J. Clin. Microbiol.* **29:**506–509.
24. **Hadziyannis, S. J.** 1997. Review: hepatitis delta. *J. Gastroenterol. Hepatol.* **12:**289–298.
25. **Han, K. H., F. B. Hollinger, C. A. Noonan, H. Solomon, G. B. G. Klintmalm, R. M. Genta, and B. Yoffe.** 1993. Southern-blot analysis and simultaneous *in situ* detection of hepatitis B virus-associated DNA and antigens in patients with end-stage liver disease. *Hepatology* **18:** 1032–1036.
26. **Han, K. H., F. B. Hollinger, C. A. Noonan, and B. Yoffe.** 1992. Simultaneous detection of HBV-specific antigens and DNA in paraffin-embedded liver tissue by immunohistochemistry and in situ hybridization using a digoxigenin-labeled probe. *J. Virol. Methods* **37:**89–97.
27. **Hollinger, F. B., E. Adam, D. Heiberg, and J. L. Melnick.** 1981. Response to hepatitis B vaccine in a young adult population, p. 451–466. *In* W. Szmuness, H. J. Alter, and J. E. Maynard (ed.), *Viral Hepatitis*, 1981 International Symposium. *Proceedings of the Third International Symposium on Viral Hepatitis and Liver Disease*. The Franklin Institute Press, Philadelphia, Pa.

27a. **Hoofnagle, J. H.** 1989. Type D (delta) hepatitis. *JAMA* **261:**1321–1325.

28. **Horowitz, B., R. Bonomo, A. M. Prince, S. N. Chin, B. Brotman, and R. W. Shulman.** 1992. Solvent/detergent-treated plasma: a virus-inactivated substitute for fresh frozen plasma. *Blood* **79:**826–831.

29. **Hsu, S.-M., L. Raine, and H. Fanger.** 1981. Use of avidin-biotin-peroxidase complex (ABC) in immunoperoxidase techniques: a comparison between ABC and unlabeled antibody (PAP) procedures. *J. Histochem. Cytochem.* **29:**577–580.

30. **Hsu, S.-M., L. Raine, and H. Fanger.** 1981. A comparative study of the peroxidase-antiperoxidase method and an avidin-biotin complex method for studying polypeptide hormones with radioimmunoassay antibodies. *Am. J. Clin. Pathol.* **75:**734–738.

31. **Huang, S., H. Minassian, and J. D. More.** 1976. Application of immunofluorescent staining on paraffin sections improved by trypsin digestion. *Lab. Invest.* **35:**383–390.

32. **Innis, M. A., D. H. Gelfand, J. J. Sninsky, and T. H. White.** 1990. *PCR Protocols: a Guide to Methods and Applications*. Academic Press, Inc., San Diego, Calif.

33. **Izraeli, S., C. Pfleiderer, and T. Lion.** 1991. Detection of gene expression by PCR amplification of RNA derived from frozen heparinized whole blood. *Nucleic Acids Res.* **19:**6051.

34. **Kaneko, S., R. H. Miller, S. M. Feinstone, M. Unoura, K. Kobayashi, N. Hattori, and R. H. Purcell.** 1989. Detection of serum hepatitis B DNA in patients with chronic hepatitis using the polymerase chain reaction assay. *Proc. Natl. Acad. Sci. USA* **86:**312–316.

35. **Kaplan, P. M., E. C. Ford, R. H. Purcell, and J. L. Gerin.** 1976. Demonstration of subpopulations of Dane particles. *J. Virol.* **17:**885–893.

36. **Kobayashi, H., M. Tsuzuki, K. Koshimizu, H. Toyama, N. Yoshihara, T. Shikata, K. Abe, K. Mizuno, N. Otomo, and T. Oda.** 1984. Susceptibility of hepatitis B virus to disinfectants or heat. *J. Clin. Microbiol.* **20:** 214–216.

37. **Kuhns, M., V. Thiers, A. Courouce, J. Scotto, P. Tiollais, and C. Brechot.** 1984. Quantitative detection of HBV DNA in human serum, p. 665–666. *In* G. N. Vyas, J. L. Deinstag, and J. H. Hoofnagle (ed.), *Viral Hepatitis and Liver Disease*. Grune and Stratton, Orlando, Fla.

38. **Kwok, S., and R. Higuchi.** 1989. Avoiding false positives with PCR. *Nature (London)* **339:**237–238.

39. **Lai, M. E., P. Farci, A. Figus, A. Balestrieri, M. Arnone, and G. N. Vyas.** 1989. Hepatitis B virus DNA in the serum of Sardinian blood donors negative for the hepatitis B surface antigen. *Blood* **73:**17–19.

40. **Larzul, D., F. Guigue, J. J. Sninsky, D. H. Mack, C. Brechot, and J. L. Guesdon.** 1988. Detection of hepatitis B virus sequences in serum by using *in vivo* enzymatic amplification. *J. Virol. Methods* **20:**227–237.

41. **Liang, T. J., H. E. Blum, K. Hasegawa, H. Takahashi, E. Galun, and J. R. Wands.** 1991. Detection and transmission of low-level hepatitis B-related virus in HBsAg-negative patients, p. 684–687. *In* F. B. Hollinger, S. M. Lemon, and H. S. Margolis (ed.), *Viral Hepatitis and Liver Disease*. The Williams & Wilkins Co., Baltimore, Md.

42. **Lin, H. J.** 1989. Biochemical detection of hepatitis B virus constituents. *Adv. Clin. Chem.* **27:**143–199.

43. **Lin, H. J., N. Shi, M. Mizokami, and F. B. Hollinger.** 1992. Polymerase chain reaction assay for hepatitis C virus RNA using a single tube for reverse transcription and serial rounds of amplification with nested primer pairs. *J. Med. Virol.* **38:**220–224.

44. **Lin, H. J., T. Tanwandee, and F. B. Hollinger.** 1997. Improved methods for quantification of human immunodeficiency virus type 1 RNA and hepatitis C virus RNA in blood using spin column technology and chemiluminescent assays of PCR products. *J. Med. Virol.* **51:**46–63.

45. **Long, A. A., P. Komminoth, E. Lee, and H. J. Wolfe.** 1993. Comparison of indirect and direct in-situ polymerase chain reaction in cell preparations and tissue sections. *Histochemistry* **99:**151–162.

46. **Lopez-Talavera, J., M. Buti, J. Casacuberta, H. Allende, R. Jardi, R. Esteban, and J. Guardia.** 1993. Detection of hepatitis delta virus RNA in human liver tissue by nonradioactive in situ hybridization. *J. Hepatol.* **17:**199–203.

47. **Madejón, A., I. Castillo, J. Bartolomé, M. L. Campillo, J. C. Porres, A. Moreno, and V. Carreño.** 1990. Detection of HDV-RNA by PCR in serum of patients with chronic HDV infection. *Hepatology* **11:**381–384.

48. **Malaguarnera, M., S. Restuccia, G. Pistone, P. Ruello, I. Giugno, and B. A. Trovato.** 1996. A meta-analysis of interferon-alpha treatment of hepatitis D virus infection. *Pharmacotherapy* **16:**609–614.

49. **Marion, P. L., C. Trepo, K. Matsubara, and P. M. Price.** 1990. Experimental models in hepadnavirus research: report of a workshop, p. 866–874. *In* F. B. Hollinger, S. M. Lemon, and H. S. Margolis (ed.), *Viral Hepatitis and Liver Disease*. The Williams & Wilkins Co., Baltimore, Md.

50. **Mason, A., M. Wick, H. White, and R. Perrillo.** 1993. Hepatitis B virus replication in diverse cell types during chronic hepatitis B virus infection. *Hepatology* **18:** 781–789.

51. **Mimms, L. T., J. W. Mosley, F. B. Hollinger, R. D. Aach, C. E. Stevens, M. Cunningham, D. V. Vallari, L. H. Barbosa, and G. J. Nemo.** 1993. Effect of concurrent acute infection with hepatitis C virus on acute hepatitis B virus infection. *Br. Med. J.* **307:**1095–1097.

52. **Morace, G., K. von der Helm, W. Jilg, and F. Deinhardt.** 1985. Detection of hepatitis B virus DNA in serum by a rapid filtration-hybridization assay. *J. Virol. Methods* **12:** 235–242.

53. **Mullis, K. B., and F. A. Faloona.** 1987. Specific synthesis of DNA in vitro via a polymerase catalyzed chain reaction. *Methods Enzymol.* **155:**335–350.

54. **National Committee for Clinical Laboratory Standards.** 1989. *Protection of Laboratory Workers from Infectious Disease Transmitted by Blood, Body Fluids, and Tissue: Tentative Guideline*, document M29-T. National Committee for Clinical Laboratory Standards, Villanova, Pa.

55. **Negro, F., F. Bonino, A. Di Bisceglie, J. Hoofnagle, and J. Gerin.** 1989. Intrahepatic markers of hepatitis delta virus infection: a study by *in situ* hybridization. *Hepatology* **10:**916–920.

56. **Niedobitek, G., T. Finn, H. Herbst, and H. Stein.** 1989. Detection of viral genomes in the liver by *in situ* hybridization using ^{35}S-bromodeoxyuridine- and biotin-labeled probes. *Am. J. Pathol.* **134:**633–639.

57. **Ochiya, T., T. Tsurimoto, K. Ueda, K. Okubo, M. Shiozawa, and K. Matsubara.** 1989. An *in vitro* system for infection with hepatitis B virus that uses primary human fetal hepatocytes. *Proc. Natl. Acad. Sci. USA* **86:** 1875–1879.

58. **O'Grady, J. G., H. M. Smith, S. E. Davies, H. M. Daniels, P. T. Donaldson, K. C. Tan, B. Portmann, G. J. Alexander, and R. Williams.** 1992. Hepatitis B virus reinfection after orthotopic liver transplantation. Serological and clinical implications. *J. Hepatol.* **14:**104–111.

59. **Paterlini, P., G. Gerken, F. Khemeny, D. Franco, A. D'Errico, W. Grigioni, J. Wands, M. Kew, E. Pisi, P. Tiollais, and C. Brechot.** 1991. Primary liver cancer in HBsAg-negative patients: a study of HBV genome using the polymerase chain reaction, p. 605–610. *In* F. B. Hollinger, S. M. Lemon, and H. S. Margolis (ed.), *Viral Hepa-*

titis and Liver Disease. The Williams & Wilkins Co., Baltimore, Md.

60. **Pontisso, P., M. G. Ruvaletto, G. Fattovich, L. Chemello, G. Morsica, L. Brollo, V. Matteotti, and A. Alberti.** 1989. Serum HBV-DNA in anti-HBe positive patients detected by filter and liquid phase hybridization assays. *Mol. Cell. Probes* **3:**245–249.
61. **Prince, A. M., W. Stephan, and B. Brotman.** 1983. *β*-Propiolactone/ultraviolet irradiation: a review of its effectiveness for inactivation of virus in blood derivatives. *Rev. Infect. Dis.* **5:**92–107.
62. **Purcell, R. H., and J. L. Gerin.** 1996. Hepatitis delta virus, p. 2819–2830. *In* B. N. Fields and D. M. Knipe (ed.), *Virology*. Raven Press, New York, N.Y.
63. **Rashoffer, R., M. Buti, R. Esteban, R. Jardi, and M. Roggendorf.** 1988. Demonstration of hepatitis D virus RNA in patients with chronic hepatitis. *J. Infect. Dis.* **157:**191–195.
64. **Ray, M. B.** 1979. *Hepatitis B Virus Antigens in Tissue*. University Park Press, Baltimore, Md.
65. **Rizzetto, M., J. W. Shih, and J. L. Gerin.** 1980. The hepatitis B virus-associated *δ* antigen: isolation from liver, development of solid-phase radioimmunoassays for *δ* antigen and anti-*δ* and partial characterization of *δ* antigen. *J. Immunol.* **125:**318–324.
66. **Rumin, S., P. Gripon, J. Le Seyec, M. Corral-Debrinski, and C. Guguen-Guillouzo.** 1996. Long-term productive episomal hepatitis B virus replication in primary cultures of adult human hepatocytes infected in vitro. *J. Viral Hepatitis* **3:**227–238.
67. **Ryu, W.-S., M. Bayer, and J. Taylor.** 1992. Assembly of hepatitis delta virus particles. *J. Virol.* **66:**2310–2315.
68. **Saldanha, J., F. di Blasi, C. Blas, J. Velosa, F. M. Ramalho, V. di Marco, I. Mora, M. C. de Moura, V. Carreno, A. Craxi, H. C. Thomas, and J. Monjardino.** 1989. Detection of hepatitis delta virus RNA in chronic liver disease. *J. Med. Virol.* **9:**23–28.
69. **Samuel, D., R. Muller, G. Alexander, L. Fassati, B. Ducot, J.-P. Benhamou, H. Bismuth, and Investigators of the European Concerted Action on Viral Hepatitis Study.** 1993. Liver transplantation in European patients with the hepatitis B surface antigen. *N. Engl. J. Med.* **329:**1842–1847.
70. **Scotto, J., M. Hadchouel, C. Hery, J. Yvart, P. Tiollais, and C. Brechot.** 1983. Detection of hepatitis B virus DNA in serum by a simple spot hybridization technique: comparison with results for other viral markers. *Hepatology* **3:**279–284.
71. **Shafritz, D. A., and S. J. Hadziyannis.** 1984. Hepatitis B virus DNA in liver and serum, viral antigens and antibodies, virus replication, and liver disease activity in patients with persistent hepatitis B virus infection, p. 80–90. *In* F. V. Chisari (ed.), *Advances in Hepatitis Research*. Mason Publishing USA, Inc., New York, N.Y.
72. **Shimizu, Y., S. Ida, T. Matsukura, and T. Yuasa.** 1984. Determination of hepatitis B virus DNA in serum by molecular hybridization. *Microbiol. Immunol.* **28:**1117–1123.
73. **Smedile, A., K. F. Bergmann, B. M. Baroudy, F. V. Wells, R. H. Purcell, F. Bonino, M. Rizzetto, and J. L. Gerin.** 1990. Riboprobe assay for HDV RNA: a sensitive method for the detection of the HDV genome in clinical serum samples. *J. Med. Virol.* **30:**20–24.
74. **Smedile, A., C. Lavarini, O. Crivelli, G. Raimondo, M. Fassone, and M. Rizzetto.** 1982. Radioimmunoassay detection of IgM antibodies to the HBV-associated delta (*δ*) antigen: clinical significance in *δ* infection. *J. Med. Virol.* **9:**131–138.
75. **Smedile, A., M. Rizzetto, K. Denniston, F. Bonino, F. Wells, G. Verme, F. Consolo, B. Hoyer, R. H. Purcell, and J. L. Gerin.** 1986. Type D hepatitis: the clinical significance of hepatitis D virus RNA in serum as detected by a hybridization-based assay. *Hepatology* **6:**1297–1302.
76. **Smedile, A., M. Rizzetto, and J. L. Gerin.** 1994. Advances in hepatitis D virus biology and disease. *Prog. Liver Dis.* **12:**157–175.
77. **Sninsky, J. J.** 1991. Application of the polymerase chain reaction to the detection of viruses, p. 799–805. *In* F. B. Hollinger, S. M. Lemon, and H. S. Margolis (ed.), *Viral Hepatitis and Liver Disease*. The Williams & Wilkins Co., Baltimore, Md.
78. **Takahashi, H., J. T. Liang, H. E. Blum, M. Zeniya, K. Fujise, H. Kameda, and J. R. Wands.** 1991. Identification of low-level hepatitis B viral genome in hepatitis B vaccine nonresponders in Japan, p. 779–781. *In* F. B. Hollinger, S. M. Lemon, and H. S. Margolis (ed.). *Viral Hepatitis and Liver Disease*. The Williams & Wilkins Co., Baltimore, Md.
79. **Takahashi, T., S. Nakagawa, T. Hashimoto, K. Takahashi, M. Imai, Y. Miyakawa, and M. Mayumi.** 1976. Large-scale isolation of Dane particles from plasma containing hepatitis B antigen and demonstration of a circular double-stranded DNA molecule extruding directly from their cores. *J. Immunol.* **117:**1392–1397.
80. **Taylor, J. M.** 1996. Hepatitis delta virus and its replication, p. 2809–2818. *In* B. N. Fields and D. M. Knipe (ed.), *Virology*. Raven Press, New York, N.Y.
81. **Thiers, V., E. Nakajima, D. Kremsdorf, D. Mack, H. Schellekens, F. Driss, A. Goudeau, J. Wands, J. Sninsky, P. Tiollais, and C. Brechot.** 1988. Transmission of hepatitis B from hepatitis B-seronegative subjects. *Lancet* **ii:**1273–1276.
82. **Tijssen, P.** 1985. *Practice and Theory of Enzyme Immunoassays*. Elsevier Science Publishers, Amsterdam, The Netherlands.
83. **Ulrich, P. P., R. A. Bhat, B. Seto, D. Mack, J. Sninsky, and G. N. Vyas.** 1989. Enzymatic amplification of hepatitis B virus DNA in serum compared with infectivity testing in chimpanzees. *J. Infect. Dis.* **160:**37–43.
84. **Urdea, M. S.** 1989. Synthesis and characterization of branched DNA (bDNA) for the direct and quantitative detection of CMV, HBV, HCV, and HIV. *Clin. Chem.* **39:**725–726.
85. **Urdea, M. S., J. A. Running, T. Horn, J. Clyne, L. L. Ku, and B. D. Warner.** 1987. A novel method for the rapid detection of specific nucleotide sequences in crude biological samples without blotting or radioactivity; application to the analysis of hepatitis B virus in human serum. *Gene* **61:**253–264.
86. **Van den Oord, J. J., F. Facchetti, C. De Wolf-Peeters, and V. J. Desmet.** 1989. Binding of biotin to hepatitis B surface antigen: a possible pitfall in immunohistochemistry. *J. Histochem. Cytochem.* **37:**551–554.
87. **Wang, K.-S., W.-L. Choo, A. J. Weiner, J.-H. Ou, R. C. Najarian, R. M. Thayer, G. T. Mullenbach, K. J. Denniston, J. L. Gerin, and M. Houghton.** 1986. Structure, sequence and expression of the hepatitis delta (*δ*) viral genome. *Nature (London)* **323:**508–513.
88. **Willems, M., H. Moshage, F. Nevens, J. Fevery, and S. H. Yap.** 1993. Plasma collected from heparinized blood is not suitable for HCV-RNA detection by conventional RT-PCR assay. *J. Virol. Methods* **42:**127–130.
89. **Wong, D. K., A. M. Cheung, K. O'Rourke, C. D. Naylor, A. S. Detsky, and J. Heathcote.** 1993. Effect of alpha-interferon treatment in patients with hepatitis B e antigen-positive chronic hepatitis B: a meta-analysis. *Ann. Intern. Med.* **119:**312–323.
90. **Wood, G. S., and R. Warnke.** 1981. Suppression of endogenous avidin-binding activity in tissues and its rele-

vance to biotin-avidin detection systems. *J. Histochem. Cytochem.* **29:**1196–1204.

91. **World Health Organization.** 1993. *Laboratory Biosafety Manual,* 2nd ed. World Health Organization, Geneva, Switzerland.
92. **Yoffe, B., D. K. Burns, H. S. Bhatt, and B. Combes.** 1990. Extrahepatic hepatitis B virus DNA sequences in patients with acute hepatitis B infection. *Hepatology* **12:** 187–192.
93. **Zarski, J. P., M. Kuhns, L. Berck, F. Degos, S. W. Schalm, P. Tiollais, and C. Brechot.** 1989. Comparison of a quantitative standardized HBV-DNA assay and a classical spot hybridization test in chronic active hepatitis B patients undergoing antiviral therapy. *Res. Virol.* **140:** 283–291.
94. **Zignego, A. L., P. Dény, C. Féray, A. Ponzetto, P. Gentilini, P. Tiollais, and C. Bréchot.** 1990. Amplification of hepatitis delta virus RNA by polymerase chain reaction: a tool for viral detection and cloning. *Mol. Cell. Probes* **4:** 43–51.

Hepatitis C and G Viruses

JUDITH C. WILBER

83

HEPATITIS C VIRUS

Clinical Background

Hepatitis C virus (HCV) is the major cause of parenterally transmitted non-A, non-B hepatitis. Antibody to HCV is found in more than 80% of patients with well-documented non-A, non-B hepatitis. The worldwide prevalence of HCV is 0.2 to 2% among blood donors and up to 80% among intravenous drug users. Most HCV infections are transmitted by transfusion and other parenteral means such as sharing of needles, occupational exposure to blood, and hemodialysis. Perinatal transmission and sexual transmission are relatively infrequent. Apparent household transmission may be attributed to sharing of blood-contaminated instruments such as razors and toothbrushes. However, for close to half of individuals with HCV infection the route of transmission is unknown (6). HCV infection becomes chronic in more than 80% of patients and is often asymptomatic even when liver damage is discernible on biopsy (13, 85). Significant liver disease may occur regardless of clinical symptoms, alanine aminotransferase (ALT) levels, HCV genotypes, and viral load. Hepatitis C is the most common liver disease currently seen in clinical practice. Many patients remain asymptomatic for decades. Lack of symptoms and minor liver enzyme elevations are typical of HCV infection and cannot be taken as evidence of lack of progression; liver biopsy is generally recommended to help assess disease activity and stage the severity of fibrosis (95). Chronic HCV is characterized by fluctuating ALT levels (39) and recognizable changes in liver histology, leading to cirrhosis in about 20% of patients. Once cirrhosis is established, the patient is at risk of decompensation, liver failure requiring transplantation, or hepatocellular carcinoma. The incidence of hepatocellular carcinoma in HCV-infected individuals in the United States is 3 to 5% per year.

Therapy with alpha interferon has been approved by the U.S. Food and Drug Administration (FDA) and can eliminate the virus (28). However, fewer than half of HCV-infected individuals respond to treatment, and relapse is common (45). Ribavirin in combination with alpha interferon was also approved recently, and it appears that the sustained response rate is higher than that achieved with interferon alone.

Description of the Agent

HCV is a small, enveloped, positive-sense, single-stranded RNA virus. The genome has approximately 9,400 nucleotides containing a single large open reading frame that spans almost the entire genome and codes for a polyprotein of 3011 amino acids (55). It is distantly related to both the animal pestiviruses and human flaviviruses, which have similar genetic and polypeptide organizations. Although there is little homology between HCV and any other known viral sequences, there is a 45 to 49% homology with pestivirus sequences in the 5′ terminal untranslated region (5′ UTR), while the hydrophobicity profile of the polyprotein is closer to that of the flaviviruses (22). The putative organization of the virus is shown in Fig. 1.

HCV shows significant sequence diversity throughout the genome. Comparison of sequences has led to the description of a number of viral types (16, 19, 36, 75, 78, 89, 90, 96), which may differ by as much as 33% throughout the genome. The 5′ UTR is the most conserved, while the envelope region is the most variable. Currently, differentiation of genotypes is done by nucleotide sequencing, differential reverse transcriptase PCR (RT-PCR), RT-PCR with type-specific probes, restriction fragment length polymorphism (RFLP) analysis, and serotyping. These techniques have been used in the 5′ UTR (63), the core region (78), and the NS5 region (36, 89). Nomenclature is currently confusing, since new types were named by each investigator. However, there is a consensus for naming HCV genotypes according to the convention proposed by Simmonds et al. (88, 89). Genotype 1a is common in the United States, while genotype 1b is most prevalent in Japan and Europe, followed by genotypes 2 and 3. Type 3 is most common in individuals who acquire the disease through drug abuse. HCV type 4 is predominant throughout the Middle East and parts of Africa and has a high prevalence in the population in Egypt (17). Genotype 5a is predominant among infected blood donors from areas in South Africa (18), while genotype 6 is found in Hong Kong and Southeast Asia (73). Proposed genotypes 7, 8, and 9, also found in Southeast Asia, are closely related to genotype 6 and may someday be classified as type 6 subtypes (74).

It remains to be seen whether genotyping of HCV is important clinically. Genotype 1b infection may be typified by a high viral load and may be less responsive to interferon treatment than other genotypes. Whether genotype 1b is associated with more severe liver injury is unclear because of confounding factors such as duration of infection and mode of transmission (87). Patients with cirrhosis who were

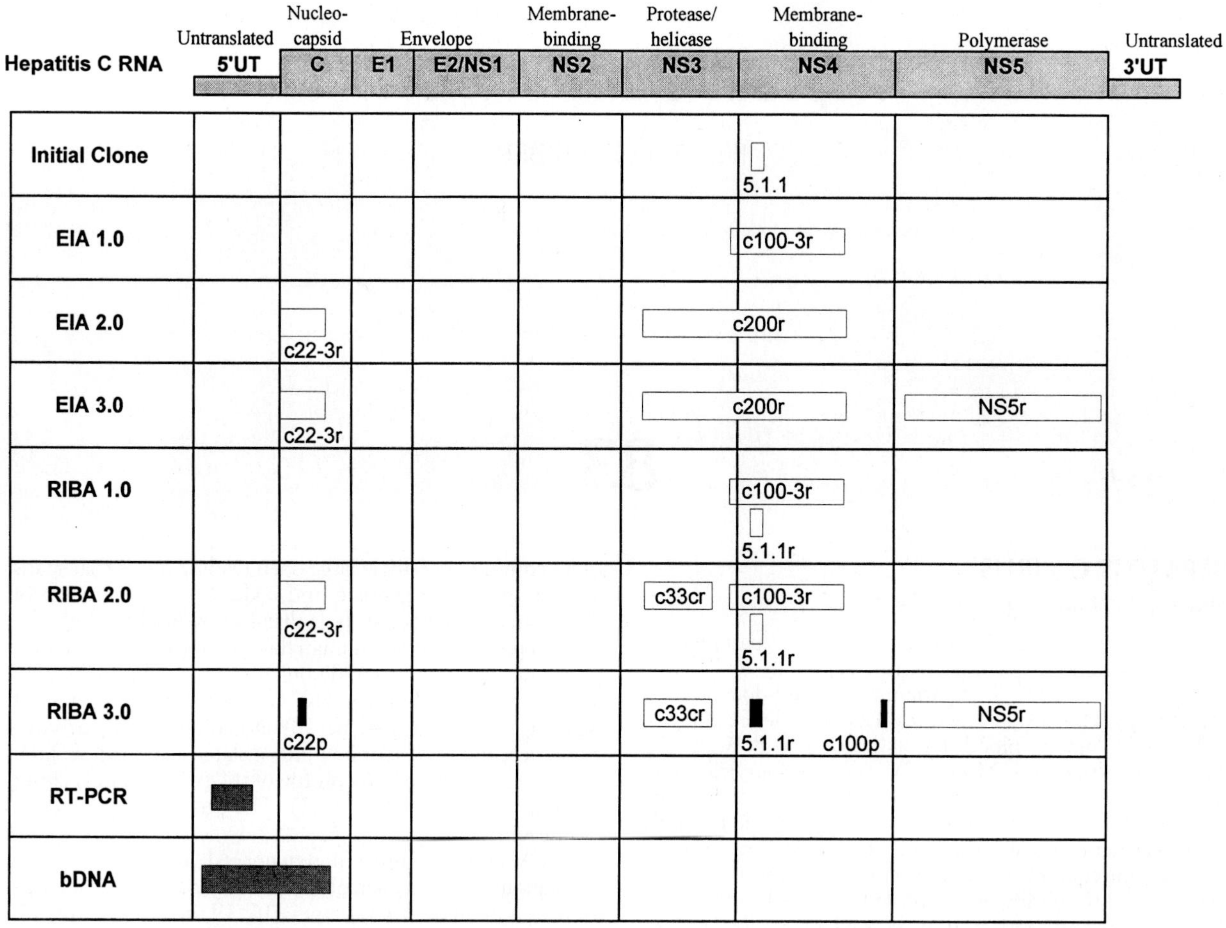

Hepatitis C RNA	Untranslated 5'UT	Nucleo-capsid C	Envelope E1	E2/NS1	Membrane-binding NS2	Protease/ helicase NS3	Membrane-binding NS4	Polymerase NS5	Untranslated 3'UT
Initial Clone							5.1.1		
EIA 1.0							c100-3r		
EIA 2.0		c22-3r					c200r		
EIA 3.0		c22-3r					c200r	NS5r	
RIBA 1.0							c100-3r 5.1.1r		
RIBA 2.0		c22-3r				c33cr	c100-3r 5.1.1r		
RIBA 3.0		c22p				c33cr	5.1.1r c100p	NS5r	
RT-PCR	■								
bDNA	■	■							

FIGURE 1 Map of the putative functional regions of the HCV genome and derivations of the recombinant HCV antigens. Also shown are the recombinant and synthetic antigens used in serologic assays, the region used most commonly for RT-PCR primers, and the areas where target probes are located for bDNA signal amplification. 5′ UT, 5′ UTR. Symbols: □, recombinant peptides; ■, synthetic peptides; ▒, region for probes and/or primers.

infected with genotype 1 or 2 had a similar prognosis and similar rates of progression to hepatocellular carcinoma, while patients infected with more than one genotype showed the most unfavorable course of disease (8).

Discovery of the Agent

Once serologic tests for hepatitis A and B were developed and hepatitis B testing was instituted for the screening of blood donors in the early 1970s, it was clear that at least one other agent was responsible for transfusion-associated hepatitis (41, 58). Serum from implicated donors was capable of transmitting disease to chimpanzees, and studies with infected chimpanzees revealed that the agent was a small, enveloped virus that was probably related to the flaviviruses (10). For more than a decade, conventional methods failed to isolate the virus in cell culture, to visualize it by electron microscopy, or to find specific antibodies or antigens for use in diagnostic tests.

Finally, cloning of the viral genome led to an antigen with which the first diagnostic tests could be developed and to the viral nucleic acid sequence from which numerous antigens, nucleic acid probes, and the phylogenetic relationships could be derived (21, 55). A large volume of plasma from a chimpanzee infected with contaminated factor XIII concentrate was ultracentrifuged, and all of the nucleic acid was extracted from the pellet. Random primers were used to copy the nucleic acid into cDNA fragments, which were cloned. Clone 5-1-1 was found to produce a polypeptide reactive with antibody from patients with non-A, non-B hepatitis. By using clone 5-1-1 as a hybridization probe, overlapping clones were found and were ligated together to form the gene fragment C100. A resulting recombinant antigen, c100-3, was used to develop the first screening test for transfusion-associated non-A, non-B hepatitis (60). Numerous antigens have now been identified and incorporated into serologic assays.

Serologic Tests

The c100-3 antigen was first used in a radioimmunoassay to determine whether this newly identified antigen would indeed detect antibody specific for an agent of transfusion-transmitted non-A, non-B hepatitis (60). This assay was used to test a coded panel of sera from the National Institutes of Health that had proved all previous putative non-A, non-B hepatitis agents incorrect (1). All but one of the non-A, non-B hepatitis-positive serum samples were detected, and the one sample that was missed was obtained from a patient in the acute phase of the disease. There were no false-positive results and no discordant results for duplicate samples included in the panel. The c100-3 antigen was then used by Ortho Diagnostic Systems and Chiron Corporation to develop a microwell enzyme immunoassay (EIA), which was approved for use by FDA in May 1990. HCV antibody testing was immediately instituted in all voluntary blood collection agencies in the United States as a part of routine donor screening. A bead-based EIA with the same antigen was manufactured by Abbott Laboratories, and it was approved for use in July 1990.

These first-generation HCV EIAs were reactive for 80 to 90% of patients who developed chronic non-A, non-B hepatitis following transfusion. However, antibody is not detected in the earliest stages of infection (3). The window of seronegativity is 10 to 15 weeks in some cases, but antibody may not appear for 6 to 12 months in a small number of other cases. Antibody to c100-3 generally disappears from patients whose infections resolve, although this may take years.

New serologic tests were developed when additional reactive recombinant antigens that would increase the sensitivity of the HCV antibody tests were found. Multiple-antigen EIAs (EIA-2) were approved by FDA in 1992. The new antigens incorporated into the assays are c22-3 from the nucleocapsid (core) region and c33c from the nonstructural region NS3. c33c was combined with c100-3 to form a single expression protein from NS3 and NS4 called c200. The additional antigens allow the earlier detection of antibody to HCV and the identification of greater numbers of patients with acute and chronic non-A, non-B hepatitis than was possible by the first-generation assays (20, 72, 98). About 10 to 30% more HCV antibody-positive individuals are detected by the second-generation assays. A third version of HCV EIA (EIA-3) incorporates an antigen from the NS5 region and new configurations of the antigens in EIA-2 (Fig. 1). The performances of EIA-1, EIA-2, and EIA-3 were compared (99) for routine blood donor screening (99,394 donations were tested by EIA-1, 167,999 donations were tested by EIA-2, and 262,090 donations were tested by EIA-3) and with serial samples from nine patients with documented acute posttransfusion HCV infection. Eight (0.01%) repeat donors previously negative by EIA-1 were found to be positive by EIA-2 and were confirmed to be positive by a four-antigen strip immunoassay and/or by detection of HCV RNA. The specificities of EIA-1, EIA-2, and EIA-3 were 99.8, 99.7, and 99.7%, respectively. For the nine patients who acquired HCV posttransfusion, HCV antibody was detected at the same time by EIA-2 and EIA-3 in seven patients and 63 and 77 days earlier by EIA-3 than by EIA-2 in two patients.

The immunoglobulin M (IgM) response has not been found to be useful for the detection of an early antibody response and may be absent, late, or persistent after HCV infection (104). HCV-specific IgM can be detected at any time during the course of HCV infection (12). In one evaluation, 79% of patients with chronic HCV infection were found to be anti-core HCV IgM positive, and detection of anti-HCV IgM seemed to be associated with viral replication and biochemical evidence of hepatic necrosis (69). All anti-HCV IgM-positive patients had detectable HCV RNA. Of 84 patients with positive results for anti-core HCV IgM antibody, 59 (70.2%) had abnormal ALT levels. The level of anti-core HCV IgM was significantly higher in those with abnormal ALT levels, but there was no difference in the levels of anti-core HCV IgM in those with chronic hepatitis versus those with cirrhosis.

As with other immunoassays, screening of low-risk populations yields a large number of false-positive reactions. A strip immunoassay (SIA; RIBA SIA [RIBA-1]; Chiron Corporation) was developed as a supplemental test to help distinguish HCV-specific antibody from nonspecific reactivity. Reactivity by RIBA-1 gave an additional indication that the reactivity by EIA was specific for HCV antibody and correlated with infectivity when testing donors implicated in the transmission of non-A, non-B hepatitis (35, 98). The Abbott Laboratories reference laboratory used a neutralization or blocking assay and has developed other nitrocellulose strip-based assays used in research.

A four-antigen SIA (the RIBA HCV 2.0 SIA [RIBA-2]) was approved for use by FDA in June 1993. RIBA-2 incorporates antigens 5-1-1 from *Escherichia coli*, c100-3 and c22-3 from yeast, c33c from *E. coli*, and superoxide dismutase (SOD). A specimen is considered positive if there are reactions with two or more bands representing at least two different gene regions with intensities equal to or greater than that for the weak IgG control ($\geq 1+$) and there is no reaction with the SOD band. If the specimen reacts with bands from only one gene region, it is considered indeterminate (15). A specimen is also considered indeterminate if it reacts with the SOD band in addition to HCV antigens with $\geq 1+$ reactivity. The absence of HCV antigen bands with $\geq 1+$ reactivity or a strip with an SOD band alone is considered negative. In one study (59), HCV RNA was detected in 127 of 140 (91%) RIBA-2-positive donations (81, 91, and 96% of donations with two, three, and four reactive bands, respectively), 5 of 88 (5.7%) indeterminate donations, and 0 of 66 (0%) RIBA-2-negative donations.

Many blood specimens that are reactive by multiple-antigen EIAs have indeterminate reactions by RIBA-2. Most of these exhibit immunoreactivity to c22-3 only (93). The RIBA 3.0 SIA (RIBA-3) was developed to resolve the status of samples with indeterminate reactions by RIBA-2 (82). In RIBA-3, the c100-3 and c22-3 bands are synthetic peptides, while c33c and a new band representing the NS5 region are recombinant proteins (5-1-1 is not included). The synthetic peptides help avoid nonspecific cross-reactivity and provide increased sensitivity. For HCV RNA-positive individuals, the sensitivity of RIBA-3 is significantly higher than that of RIBA-2 (99.5 versus 93.3%; $P = 0.0005$) (27). This is not caused by inclusion of the NS5 antigen but is caused by the higher sensitivities of the c33 and c100 antigens (RIBA-2; 94.3 and 62.6%, respectively; RIBA-3, 99.5 and 88.6%, respectively). Replacement of the c22 and c100 recombinant proteins by synthetic peptides significantly reduced nonspecific reactivity against these antigens (27, 82).

Direct Tests

Since no routine culture methods are available, detection of viral RNA in serum is used as a marker for the virus itself. Quantification of viral RNA may be useful in monitoring the course of disease and the effectiveness of antiviral treatment. Many of the early studies for determination of the specificity of HCV antibody tests relied on retrospective analysis of the transmission of HCV infection through infected units of blood. Eighty to 90% of donors who were RIBA positive transmitted non-A, non-B hepatitis to recipients (38). Some individuals with true HCV antibody may have recovered from the infection. Detection of HCV RNA is accomplished by amplification methods such as RT-PCR (11, 44, 46, 48, 100, 101) or branched-DNA (bDNA) signal amplification (4, 31, 97). More than 90% of RIBA-positive specimens are also positive for HCV RNA, corresponding to the infectivity noted in transfusion studies.

RT-PCR transcribes a portion of extracted viral RNA into DNA and amplifies the number of DNA molecules to a detectable level through the use of primers, enzymes, and temperature cycling. Most laboratories use primers from the 5′ UTR of the HCV genome because it is the most conserved, region. Many different RT-PCR methods are being used in research laboratories, along with numerous methods for detection of the amplified product. For example, many researchers use two-stage nested PCR to increase the sensitivity enough that only ethidium bromide staining is necessary to detect the bands on the gel, thus avoiding the use of radioactive probes. However, the second round of amplification is not necessary to achieve the sensitivity and it may lead to contamination (46, 49, 101). Use of a labeled HCV-specific probe to detect the PCR product increases both the sensitivity and the specificity, and nonradioactive labels are now available (40, 46). A commercial RT-PCR for the detection of HCV RNA (Amplicor HCV; Roche Molecular Systems) is based on a single, combined reverse transcription and amplification reaction, uses biotinylated primers, and detects amplification products in a horseradish peroxidase-avidin colorimetric system in microwell plates with a specific nucleic acid probe. Amplicor uses uracil-*N*-glycosylase (UNG) to aid in the prevention of carryover contamination. It has clinical sensitivity and specificity equivalent to those of nested RT-PCR (46).

A test for HCV RNA should be requested when an individual has reactive or indeterminate HCV serology with or without specific clinical symptomatology and altered liver enzyme levels, and it is a potential tool for the follow-up of patients with HCV infection. According to the 1997 National Institutes of Health Consensus Statement on Management of Hepatitis C (77), if a RIBA test is positive, the patient can benefit from testing for HCV RNA by PCR, the result of which will indicate whether the patient has ongoing HCV viremia. A single positive assay for HCV RNA by PCR confirms infection; unfortunately, a single negative assay does not prove that the patient is not viremic or has recovered from hepatitis C. Follow-up testing for ALT levels and perhaps repeating the test for HCV RNA in the future may be needed. It should be noted, however, that not all laboratories perform RT-PCR for HCV RNA correctly. Eighty-six laboratories participated in a collaborative study (26) and tested a coded panel of four HCV RNA-positive plasma samples including a weakly positive plasma sample, six HCV RNA-negative plasma samples, and two dillution series of plasma containing HCV RNA genotype 1 and 3 standards. The 86 laboratories submitted 136 sets of results. Ninety-nine were assayed by a PCR developed in-house, 28 were assayed by the commercial Amplicor assay, and 9 were assayed by other amplification methods. Twenty-two data sets (16%) had faultless results, 39 (29%) missed the weakly positive sample only, and 75 data sets (55%) had false-positive and/or false-negative results. Participants that used the commercial RT-PCR test had a sufficient quality score somewhat more often than investigators that used assays developed in-house (64 versus 45%; $P = 0.11$). The UNG system in the commercial RT-PCR test did not prevent five laboratories from generating false-positive results for the six HCV RNA-negative samples.

Several methods have been developed for the quantitative measurement of HCV RNA; these are based on signal or target amplification. bDNA signal amplification (97) was developed as a quantitative method (Quantiplex HCV RNA 1.0 [bDNA-1]; Chiron Corporation). The second version of the bDNA assay (Quantiplex HCV RNA 2.0 [bDNA-2]; Chiron Corporation), introduced in 1995, achieved equivalent quantification of genotypes 1 through 6 (31). By this technique, 50 μl of serum is placed directly in the well of a 96-well plate. Proteinase K and detergent are added in a reagent that also contains target oligonucleotide probes. These probes include a set of 5 target probes, each of which hybridizes to a portion of the HCV RNA and to capture probes in the well, and another set of 18 target probes that mediate hybridization of the RNA to synthetic bDNA amplifier molecules. All of the probes are located in the 5′ UTR and core regions of the HCV genome (Fig. 1). Each bDNA molecule then hybridizes 45 alkaline phosphatase-labeled probes. The complex is incubated with a chemiluminescent substrate, dioxetane, and the light emitted is measured in a luminometer and compared to that on a standard curve to determine the level of RNA in the sample. The standards for bDNA analysis were developed with purified and independently quantified viral RNA transcripts of genotypes 1 through 6 (23). Target amplification methods include dilutional analysis, competitive PCR, and a noncompetitive method (Amplicor Monitor; Roche Molecular Systems) which uses an internal standard that serves to assess the overall efficiency of the system. The dynamic range of bDNA analysis is reported to be 2×10^5 to 1.2×10^8 genome equivalents/ml (31), and that of the Amplicor Monitor assay is reported to be 1×10^3 to 1×10^6 copies/ml (24). However, independent parallel studies have shown that the values obtained by the Amplicor Monitor assay are 10- to 40-fold lower than the values obtained by bDNA analysis (50, 56).

The accuracies of the different methods for the quantification of HCV in plasma were determined with samples from individuals infected with different genotypes and by using RNA transcripts of predetermined concentrations (52). Significant differences in the efficiency of detection of genotypes 1, 2, and 3 were observed for the bDNA-1 and Amplicor Monitor assays, whereas the bDNA-2 assay and the nested PCR at the limiting dilution were able to quantify genotypes with equal sensitivities. By quantifying RNA transcripts of different genotypes, the sensitivities of the Amplicor Monitor assay for sequences of the type 2 and type 3 transcripts were estimated to be 11 and 8%, respectively, of those achieved for genotype 1. Differences in the efficiency of quantification should be taken into account in future investigations of the relationship between genotype and viral load.

A novel fluorescent EIA for the detection and quantification of serum HCV core protein has been developed (80) and is available in Japan. Core protein levels appear to correlate well with HCV RNA levels.

Genotyping

HCV genotypes may be investigated by a variety of laboratory methods that target different parts of the HCV genome and that have various degrees of technical difficulty. Common methods are RT-PCR with type-specific primers from the core region, hybridization of amplified 5′ noncoding region to type-specific probes, RFLP analysis of the NS5 region, identification of type-specific antibodies against epitopes of the NS4 region by EIA or SIA, and sequence analysis of the 5′ noncoding region, the core region, or the NS5 region. Generally concordant results are found by the available methods (34, 47, 63, 78). Concordant results among

EIA, hybridization of type-specific probes, and type-specific PCR were more likely when the type-specific PCR revealed only a single HCV genotype (42). Type-specific hybridization and EIA usually recognized the genotype producing the strongest DNA band in samples in which type-specific PCR suggested a mixed infection. Sequencing is commonly used to determine the genotype when the results of other methods are discordant (84).

Collection, Storage, and Handling of Samples

HCV antibody assays use either serum or plasma. For HCV RNA detection and quantification, the specimen of choice is sterile serum, although plasma may also be used. Plasma may be collected in tubes containing EDTA, acid citrate dextrose, sodium citrate, or other anticoagulants. Heparin should be avoided if PCR studies are planned because it inhibits DNA polymerase. Viral RNA is vulnerable to degradation by high levels of proteinases and RNase in blood, although it appears to be somewhat protected as long as the virion is intact (14). It is very important to remove the serum or plasma from the cellular blood components as soon as possible to avoid viral degradation by granulocytes (25, 29). The separated serum or plasma should be refrigerated or frozen within 4 to 6 h of collection. Storage at −80°C is recommended because a significant loss of HCV RNA has been observed after storage at −20°C (51). Specimens should be kept cold after thawing. Although repeated freezing and thawing does not appear to cause a significant decrease in virus levels, it is very important to control the conditions between freezes.

Selection of Tests and Interpretation

Diagnosis of HCV infection is currently achieved by detecting specific antibody by EIAs and SIAs that use antigens derived from the cloning of the HCV genome. If both antibody tests are positive, there is a high likelihood that the patient is infected. Liver enzyme levels should be followed, and biopsy should be considered. Detection of HCV RNA in patient specimens demonstrates active HCV infection. Prior to seroconversion, the viral load reaches peak levels long before the ALT peak is seen (4). After seroconversion, serum virus levels may become extremely low, often below the limit of detection of qualitative RT-PCR for HCV RNA. Therefore, if the serology tests (EIA and SIA) are positive, a negative RT-PCR result should not be used to rule out HCV infection and should be followed up by further testing at a later date. Tests for HCV RNA may also be used to help diagnose cases of HCV infection if the SIA result is indeterminate. Positive antibody test results with repeatedly negative RNA test results may represent a resolved infection, which occurs in only 10 to 20% of patients with HCV infection.

There are several reasons why HCV RNA detection and quantification could be useful in evaluating patients:

1. Diagnosis of acute infection. High levels of HCV RNA are detectable before seroconversion. Follow-up antibody tests should be reactive within 2 weeks to 6 months.
2. Evaluation of patients with chronic hepatitis who are negative for antibody to HCV or have indeterminate results. Patients who are immunocompromised or who are on hemodialysis may have low or undetectable levels of specific antibody.
3. Evaluation of HCV infection in individuals whose ALT levels are normal.
4. Monitoring of antiviral therapy.
   a. Patients with a sustained response to alpha interferon therapy have lower pretreatment levels of HCV RNA than nonresponders (62, 67, 68, 70, 79, 94, 103). This can be used to help set expectations prior to therapy. In addition, individuals with higher HCV RNA levels may benefit from different treatment regimens.
   b. Unchanged HCV RNA levels during treatment may indicate the need to alter the course of therapy.
   c. A sustained loss of detectable HCV RNA in serum may indicate a response to treatment.
   d. Further clinical studies to provide an understanding of the course of HCV disease will be facilitated by the ability to follow HCV RNA levels.

For individuals chronically infected with HCV, it may be of interest to determine the genotype of the infecting virus. It is not clear whether different outcomes are associated with different genotypes, but genotype 1b may be less amenable than the other genotypes to interferon therapy.

Serologic assays for HCV antibody are the key elements in preventing transmission of HCV through the blood supply and in diagnosing HCV infection. Qualitative and quantitative assays for HCV RNA facilitate the monitoring of viremia throughout the course of disease, selection and adjustment of treatment protocols, and evaluation of the efficacy of therapy. Serologic and direct viral assays provide the basis for continuing studies on the epidemiology, natural history, progression, and treatment of HCV infection.

HEPATITIS G VIRUS

Clinical Background

Although cases of posttransfusion hepatitis and sporadic and fulminant hepatitis (54) have been reported, most people infected with hepatitis G virus (HGV) are asymptomatic, and it is not clear that any significant disease is associated with HGV infection (53). Although high levels of HGV RNA are found in the blood, the liver is not a significant site of replication (83). HGV RNA is only rarely detected in patients with elevated transaminase levels of unknown etiology (86). The mode of transmission appears to be parenteral, and individuals infected with HGV are commonly coinfected with HCV, hepatitis B virus (HBV), and, less commonly, human immunodeficiency virus. Many studies have shown that infection with HGV does not alter the severity of HCV or HBV infection, the course of disease caused by HCV or HBV, or the response to therapy for HCV or HBV infection (32, 61, 71, 81). High-titer maternal viremia and mode of delivery are closely associated with mother-to-infant transmission of HGV, and the infection usually becomes persistent in infants (65). However, as in the findings from several studies of adult transfusion recipients, no association between HGV infection and clinical or biochemical signs of hepatitis or extrahepatic disease has been seen (102).

Prevalence

The prevalence of HGV in blood donors and transfusion recipients was examined by testing for HGV RNA in serum samples collected between 1972 and 1995 from 357 transfusion recipients, 157 controls who did not receive transfusions, 500 randomly selected volunteer blood donors, and

230 donors of blood received by HGV-infected patients (2). Of the 79 patients with transfusion-associated hepatitis, 63 (80%) were infected with HCV and 3 had preexisting HCV and the cause of their acute hepatitis could not be determined; of the remaining 13 patients, 3 had acute HGV infection, and no agent was identified in 10 patients. Six of the 63 patients (10%) with HCV infection were also infected with HGV. The ALT levels paralleled the levels of HCV RNA but not those of HGV RNA. The three patients infected only with HGV had mild hepatitis (the mean peak ALT level was 198 U/liter; none had jaundice). There were 35 HGV infections among the 357 transfusion recipients; only 3 had hepatitis with HGV as the sole viral marker. One of the 157 controls and 7 of the 500 randomly selected blood donors (1.4%) had detectable HGV RNA. In all eight instances in which a transfusion recipient had acute HGV infection after transfusion and samples from all donors could be tested, at least one HGV-positive donor was identified.

Serum samples from the Centers for Disease Control and Prevention surveillance study of acute viral hepatitis were tested for HGV RNA (5). Samples were from patients in four U.S. counties who presented with acute hepatitis from 1985 to 1986 or 1991 to 1995. HGV RNA was detected in 4 of 45 (9%) patients with non-A to non-E hepatitis, 23 of 116 (20%) patients with hepatitis C, 25 of 100 (25%) patients with hepatitis A, and 32 of 100 (32%) patients with hepatitis B. The clinical characteristics of the acute illness were similar for patients with HGV infection alone and those with hepatitis A, B, or C with or without HGV infection. During a follow-up period of 1 to 9 years, chronic hepatitis did not develop in any of the patients with HGV infection alone, but 75% were persistently positive for HGV RNA, as were 87% of those with both hepatitis C and HGV infection.

The ability to measure HGV anti-E2 antibody has made it possible to determine the epidemiologic history of infection. For example, the prevalence of anti-E2 antibody was 3.0 to 8.1% in volunteer blood donors, 34.0% in plasmapheresis donors, 85.2% in intravenous drug users, and 13.3% in West African subjects, all of whom tested negative by RT-PCR (33).

Discovery of the Agent

Some cases of hepatitis associated with blood transmission are not attributable to hepatitis A through E viruses. In searching for other viruses associated with liver disease, a new blood-borne virus was identified by two different groups: GBV-C (37) and HGV (66). GBV was named for the surgeon whose serum led to the identification of the viral sequence. His serum was inoculated into tamarins, from which three viruses, designated GBV-A, GBV-B, and GBV-C, were eventually cloned, sequenced, and identified. GBV-A and GBV-B are tamarin viruses; the GBV-C sequence was used to identify a human virus possibly associated with non-A to non-E hepatitis. HGV was identified from the plasma of a patient with chronic hepatitis by sequence-independent single-primer amplification (66). Extension from an immunoreactive DNA clone yielded the entire genome. GBV-C and HGV are different subtypes of the same virus.

Since the term "GBV-C" does not follow naming conventions and it is unknown whether "HGV" is a significant cause of hepatitis, the virus has not yet been named officially. For simplicity, this chapter uses the term HGV.

Description of the Agent

HGV is a single-stranded RNA virus with a genome of 9,392 nucleotides encoding a polyprotein of 2,873 amino acids (66). The virus was placed in the family *Flaviviridae* and was found to be closely related to GB virus C (GBV-C) and distantly related to HCV. The organization is similar to that of other members of the family *Flaviviridae*, with structural regions at the 5′ end and nonstructural regions at the 3′ end.

Genotypes

The 5′ UTR sequences of 33 HGV-positive samples obtained from different geographic areas were determined by RT-PCR and dideoxy chain termination sequencing, the alignment of sequences, estimation of the number of nucleotide substitutions per site, and construction of phylogenetic trees (76, 91). The 5′ UTR of HGV was found to be heterogeneous, with 70.9 to 99.5% homology. Three distinct phylogenetic branches were observed consistently in all phylogenetic trees. GBV-C is the prototype for one branch, the first isolate of HGV is the prototype for another branch, and there is a branch consisting of isolates from Asia (57). RFLP analysis with *Scr*FI and *Bsm*FI for genotype-specific restriction sites has been described for use in the genotyping of HGV (76).

Serologic Tests

EIAs with the HGV E2 envelope antigen produced in CHO cells have been developed to test for antibodies to this protein in human sera. Most anti-E2-positive patients are HGV RNA negative and vice versa, indicating an inverse correlation of these two viral markers (33, 64, 92).

Direct Tests

Like HCV, HGV has not been successfully grown in cell culture. Specific antigen detection has not been reported. Direct detection of the virus depends on the detection of HGV RNA, which is accomplished by RT-PCR. Primers and probes have been described for the 5′ UTR, NS3, and NS5a regions (7, 9, 30, 43). Parallel testing with two PCR primer sets may eliminate false-negative results attributable to the genetic heterogeneity of the virus.

Collection and Storage of Samples

The stability of HGV has not been studied extensively. The methods used for the collection and storage of HCV should be adequate because HGV is an enveloped RNA virus related to HCV.

Selection of Tests and Interpretation of Results

Acute and chronic infection can be diagnosed by detection of HGV RNA in serum. Recovery appears to be associated with the disappearance of RNA and the appearance of HGV E2 antibody.

REFERENCES

1. **Alter, H. J.** 1991. Descartes before the horse: I clone, therefore I am: the hepatitis C virus in current perspective. *Ann. Intern. Med.* **115:**644–649.
2. **Alter, H. J., Y. Nakatsuji, J. Melpolder, J. Wages, R. Wesley, J. W. Shih, and J. P. Kim.** 1997. The incidence of transfusion-associated hepatitis G virus infection and its relation to liver disease. *N. Engl. J. Med.* **336:**747–754.
3. **Alter, H. J., R. H. Purcell, J. W. Shih, J. C. Melpolder, M. Houghton, Q.-L. Choo, and G. Kuo.** 1989. Detection of antibody to hepatitis C virus in prospectively followed

transfusion recipients with acute and chronic non-A non-B hepatitis. *N. Engl. J. Med.* **321**:1494–1500.

4. **Alter, H. J., R. Sanchez-Pescador, M. S. Urdea, J. C. Wilber, R. J. Lagier, A. M. Di Bisceglie, J. W. Shih, and P. D. Neuwald.** 1995. Evaluation of branched DNA signal amplification for the detection of hepatitis C virus RNA. *J. Viral Hepatitis* **2**:121–132.
5. **Alter, M. J., M. Gallagher, T. T. Morris, L. A. Moyer, E. L. Meeks, K. Krawczynski, J. P. Kim, and H. S. Margolis.** 1997. Acute non-A-E hepatitis in the United States and the role of hepatitis G virus infection. Sentinel Counties Viral Hepatitis Study Team. *N. Engl. J. Med.* **336:** 741–746.
6. **Alter, M. J., S. C. Hadler, F. N. Judson, A. Mares, W. J. Alexander, P. Y. Hu, and J. K. Miller.** 1990. Risk factors for acute non-A, non-B hepatitis in the United States and association with hepatitis C infection. *JAMA* **264:** 2231–2235.
7. **Andonov, A., R. Chaudhary, H. Jacobsen, and C. Sauder.** 1998. Comparison of six sets of PCR primers from two different genomic regions for amplification of GB virus C/hepatitis G virus RNA. *J. Clin. Microbiol.* **36**:286–289.
8. **Benvegnu, L., P. Pontisso, D. Cavalletto, F. Noventa, L. Chemello, and A. Alberti.** 1997. Lack of correlation between hepatitis C virus genotypes and clinical course of hepatitis C virus-related cirrhosis. *Hepatology* **25**:211–215.
9. **Bhardwaj, B., K. Qian, J. Detmer, M. Mizokami, J. A. Kolberg, M. S. Urdea, G. Schlauder, J. M. Linnen, J. P. Kim, G. L. Davis, and J. Y. Lau.** 1997. Detection of GB virus-C/hepatitis G virus RNA in serum by reverse transcription polymerase chain reaction. *J. Med. Virol.* **52:** 92–96.
10. **Bradley, D. W., K. A. McCaustland, E. H. Cook, C. A. Schable, J. W. Ebert, and J. E. Maynard.** 1985. Posttransfusion non-A non-B hepatitis in chimpanzees: physiochemical evidence that the tubule-forming agent is a small, enveloped virus. *Gastroenterology* **88**:773–779.
11. **Bréchot, C.** 1993. Polymerase chain reaction for the diagnosis of hepatitis B and C viral hepatitis. *J. Hepatol.* **17**(Suppl. 3):S35–S41.
12. **Brillanti, S., M. Foli, P. Perini, C. Masci, M. Miglioli, and L. Barbara.** 1991. Long-term persistence of IgM antibodies to HCV in chronic hepatitis C. *Hepatology* **14:** 969–974.
13. **Brillanti, S., S. Gaiani, M. Miglioli, M. Foli, C. Masci, and L. Barbara.** 1993. Persistent hepatitis C viraemia without liver disease. *Lancet* **341**:464–465.
14. **Busch, M. P., J. C. Wilber, P. Johnson, L. Tobler, and C. S. Evans.** 1992. Impact of specimen handling and storage on detection of hepatitis C virus RNA. *Transfusion* **32:** 420–425.
15. **Busch, M. P., L. Tobler, S. Quan, J. C. Wilber, P. Johnson, A. Polito, E. Steane, A. Zola, C. Bahl, M. Nelles, and S. R. Lee.** 1993. A pattern of 5-1-1 and c100-3 only on hepatitis C virus (HCV). *Transfusion* **33**:84–88.
16. **Cha, T. A., E. Beall, B. Irvine, J. Kolberg, D. Chien, G. Kuo, and M. S. Urdea.** 1992. At least five related, but distinct hepatitis C viral genotypes exist. *Proc. Natl. Acad. Sci. USA* **89**:7144–7148.
17. **Chamberlain, R. W., N. J. Adams, A. A. Saeed, P. Simmonds, and R. M. Elliott.** 1997. Complete nucleotide sequence of a type 4 hepatitis C virus variant, the predominant genotype in the Middle East. *J. Gen. Virol.* **78:** 1341–1347.
18. **Chamberlain, R. W., N. J. Adams, L. A. Taylor, P. Simmonds, and R. M. Elliott.** 1997. The complete coding sequence of hepatitis C virus genotype 5a, the predominant genotype in South Africa. *Biochem. Biophys. Res. Commun.* **236**:44–49.
19. **Chan, S.-W., F. McOmish, E. C. Holmes, B. Dow, J. F. Peutherer, E. Follett, P. L. Yap, and P. Simmonds.** 1992. Analysis of a new hepatitis C virus type and its phylogenetic relationship to existing variants. *J. Gen. Virol.* **73:** 1131–1141.
20. **Chemello, L., D. Cavalletto, P. Pontisso, F. Bortolotti, C. Donada, V. Donadon, M. Frezza, P. Casarin, and A. Alberti.** 1993. Patterns of antibodies to hepatitis C virus in patients with chronic non-A, non-B hepatitis and their relationship to viral replication and liver disease. *Hepatology* **17**:179–182.
21. **Choo, Q.-L., G. Kuo, A. J. Weiner, L. R. Overby, D. W. Bradley, and M. Houghton.** 1989. Isolation of a cDNA clone derived from a blood-borne non-A, non-B viral hepatitis genome. *Science* **244**:359–364.
22. **Choo, Q.-L., K. H. Richman, J. H. Han, K. Berger, C. Lee, C. Dong, C. Gallegos, D. Coit, A. Medina-Selby, P. J. Barr, A. J. Weiner, D. W. Bradley, G. Kuo, and M. Houghton.** 1991. Genetic organization and diversity of the hepatitis C virus. *Proc. Natl. Acad. Sci. USA* **88:** 2451–2455.
23. **Collins, M. L., C. Zayati, J. J. Detmer, B. Daly, J. A. Kolberg, T.-A. Cha, B. D. Irvine, J. Tucker, and M. S. Urdea.** 1995. Preparation and characterization of RNA standards for use in quantitative branched DNA hybridization assays. *Anal. Biochem.* **226**:120–129.
24. **Colucci, G., and K. Gutekunst.** 1997. Development of a quantitative PCR assay for monitoring HCV viraemia levels in patients with chronic hepatitis C. *J. Viral Hepatitis* **4**(Suppl. 1):75–78.
25. **Cuypers, H. T. M., D. Bresters, N. Winkel, H. W. Reesink, A. J. Weiner, M. Houghton, C. L. van der Poel, and P. N. Lelie.** 1992. Storage conditions of blood samples and primer selection affect the yield of cDNA polymerase chain reaction products of hepatitis C virus. *J. Clin. Microbiol.* **30**:3220–3224.
26. **Damen, M., H. T. Cuypers, H. L. Zaaijer, H. W. Reesink, W. P. Schaasberg, W. H. Gerlich, H. G. Niesters, and P. N. Lelie.** 1996. International collaborative study on the second EUROHEP HCV-RNA reference panel. *J. Virol. Methods* **58**:175–185.
27. **Damen, M., H. L. Zaaijer, H. T. M. Cuypers, H. Vrielink, C. L. van der Poel, H. W. Reesink, and P. N. Lelie.** 1995. Reliability of the third-generation recombinant immunoblot assay for hepatitis C virus. *Transfusion* **35:** 745–749.
28. **Davis, G. L., L. A. Balart, E. R. Schiff, K. Lindsay, H. C. Bodenheimer, R. P. Perrillo, W. Carey, I. M. Jacobson, J. Payne, J. L. Dienstag, D. H. Van Thiel, C. Tamburro, J. Lefkowitch, J. Albrecht, C. Meschievitz, T. J. Ortego, A. Gibas, and the Hepatitis Interventional Therapy Group.** 1989. Treatment of chronic hepatitis C with recombinant interferon alfa. *N. Engl. J. Med.* **321:** 1501–1505.
29. **Davis, G. L., J. Y. N. Lau, M. S. Urdea, P. D. Neuwald, J. C. Wilber, K. Lindsay, R. P. Perrillo, and J. Albrecht.** 1994. Quantitative detection of hepatitis C virus RNA with a solid-phase signal amplification method: definition of optimal conditions for specimen collection and clinical application in interferon-treated patients. *Hepatology* **19:** 1337–1341.
30. **de Medina, M., G. O. Perez, G. Hess, E. R. Schiff, K. R. Reddy, L. J. Jeffers, J. P. Pennell, B. Leclerq, M. Hill, V. Schluter, and M. Ashby.** 1998. Prevalence of hepatitis C and G virus infection in chronic hemodialysis patients. *Am. J. Kidney Dis.* **31**:224–226.
31. **Detmer, J., R. Lagier, J. Flynn, C. Zayati, J. Kolberg, M. Collins, M. Urdea, and R. Sanchez-Pescador.** 1996. Accurate quantification of hepatitis C virus (HCV) RNA

from all HCV genotypes by using branched-DNA technology. *J. Clin. Microbiol.* **34:**901–907.
32. **Dickson, R. C., K. P. Qian, and J. Y. Lau.** 1997. High prevalence of GB virus C/hepatitis G virus infection in liver transplant recipients. *Transplantation* **63:**1695–1697.
33. **Dille, B. J., T. K. Surowy, R. A. Gutierrez, P. F. Coleman, M. F. Knigge, R. J. Carrick, R. D. Aach, F. B. Hollinger, C. E. Stevens, L. H. Barbosa, G. J. Nemo, J. W. Mosley, G. J. Dawson, and I. K. Mushahwar.** 1997. An ELISA for detection of antibodies to the E2 protein of GB virus C. *J. Infect. Dis.* **175:**458–461.
34. **Dixit, V., S. Quan, P. Martin, D. Larson, M. Brezina, R. DiNello, K. Sra, J. Y. N. Lau, D. Chien, J. Kolberg, A. Tagger, G. Davis, A. Polito, and G. Gitnick.** 1995. Evaluation of a novel serotyping system for hepatitis C virus: strong correlation with standard genotyping methodologies. *J. Clin. Microbiol.* **33:**2978–2983.
35. **Ebeling, F., R. Naukkarinen, and J. Leikola.** 1990. Recombinant immunoblot assay for hepatitis C virus antibody as predictor of infectivity. *Lancet* **335:**982–983.
36. **Enomoto, N., A. Takada, T. Nakao, and T. Date.** 1990. There are two major types of hepatitis C virus in Japan. *Biochem. Biophys. Res. Commun.* **170:**1021–1025.
37. **Erker, J. C., J. N. Simons, A. S. Muerhoff, T. P. Leary, M. L. Chalmers, S. M. Desai, and I. K. Mushahwar.** 1996. Molecular cloning and characterization of a GB virus C isolate from a patient with non-A-E hepatitis. *J. Gen. Virol.* **77**(Pt. 11)**:**2713–2720.
38. **Esteban, J. I., A. Gonzales, J. M. Hernandez, L. Viladomiu, C. Sanchez, J. C. Lopez-Talavera, G. Martin-Vega, X. Vidal, R. Esteban, and J. Guardia.** 1991. Evaluation of antibodies to hepatitis C virus in a contemporary study of transfusion-associated hepatitis. *N. Engl. J. Med.* **232:**1107–1112.
39. **Farci, P., H. J. Alter, D. Wong, R. H. Miller, J. W. Shih, B. Jett, and R. H. Purcell.** 1991. A long-term study of hepatitis C virus replication in non-A, non-B hepatitis. *N. Engl. J. Med.* **325:**98–104.
40. **Farma, E., E. Boeri, P. Bettini, C. M. Repetto, J. McDermott, F. B. Lillo, and O. E. Varnier.** 1996. Single-step PCR in molecular diagnosis of hepatitis C virus infection. *J. Clin. Microbiol.* **34:**3171–3174.
41. **Feinstone, S. M., A. Z. Kapikian, R. H. Purcell, H. J. Alter, and P. V. Holland.** 1975. Transfusion-associated hepatitis not due to viral hepatitis type A or B. *N. Engl. J. Med.* **292:**767–770.
42. **Forns, X., M. D. Maluenda, F. X. Lopez-Labrador, S. Ampurdanes, E. Olemdo, J. Costa, P. Simmonds, J. M. Sanchez-Tapias, M. T. Jimenez de Anta, and J. Rodes.** 1996. Comparative study of three methods for genotyping hepatitis C virus strains in samples from Spanish patients. *J. Clin. Microbiol.* **34:**2516–2521.
43. **Forns, X., D. Tan, H. J. Alter, R. H. Purcell, and J. Bukh.** 1997. Evaluation of commercially available and in-house reverse transcription-PCR assays for detection of hepatitis G virus or GB virus C. *J. Clin. Microbiol.* **35:** 2698–2702.
44. **Garson, J. A., R. S. Tedder, M. Briggs, P. Tuke, J. A. Glazebrook, A. Trute, D. Parker, J. A. J. Barbara, M. Contreras, and S. Aloysius.** 1990. Detection of hepatitis C viral sequences in blood donations by "nested" polymerase chain reaction and prediction of infectivity. *Lancet* **335:** 1419–1422.
45. **Garson, J. A., S. Brillanti, C. Ring, P. Perini, M. Miglioli, and L. Barbara.** 1992. Hepatitis C viraemia rebound after "successful" interferon therapy in patients with chronic non-A, non-B hepatitis. *J. Med. Virol.* **37:**210–214.
46. **Gerken, G., P. Pontisso, M. Roggendorf, M. G. Rumi, P. Simmonds, C. Trepo, S. Zeuzem, and G. Colucci.** 1996. Clinical evaluation of a single reaction, diagnostic polymerase chain reaction assay for the detection of hepatitis C virus RNA. *J. Hepatol.* **24:**33–37.
47. **Gish, R. G., K. P. Qian, S. Quan, Y. L. Xu, I. Pike, A. Polito, R. DiNello, and J. Y. N. Lau.** 1997. Concordance between hepatitis C virus serotyping assays. *J. Viral Hepatitis* **4:**421–422.
48. **Gretch, D., W. Lee, and L. Corey.** 1992. Use of aminotransferase, hepatitis C antibody, and hepatitis C polymerase chain reaction RNA assays to establish the diagnosis of hepatitis C virus infection in a diagnostic virology laboratory. *J. Clin. Microbiol.* **30:**2145–2149.
49. **Gretch, D. R., J. J. Wilson, R. L. Carithers, C. dela Rosa, J. H. Han, and L. Corey.** 1993. Detection of hepatitis C virus RNA: comparison of one-stage polymerase chain reaction (PCR) with nested-set PCR. *J. Clin. Microbiol.* **31:**289–291.
50. **Hadziyannis, E., M. W. Fried, and F. S. Nolte.** 1997. Evaluation of two methods for quantitation of hepatitis C virus RNA. *Mol. Diagn.* **2:**39–46.
51. **Halfon, P., H. Khiri, V. Gerolami, M. Bourliere, J. M. Feryn, P. Reynier, A. Gauthier, and G. Cartouzou.** 1996. Impact of various handling and storage conditions on quantitative detection of hepatitis C virus RNA. *J. Hepatol.* **25:** 307–311.
52. **Hawkins, A., F. Davidson, and P. Simmonds.** 1997. Comparison of plasma virus loads among individuals infected with hepatitis C virus (HCV) genotypes 1, 2, and 3 by Quantiplex HCV RNA assay versions 1 and 2, Roche Monitor Assay, and an in-house limiting dilution method. *J. Clin. Microbiol.* **35:**187–192.
53. **Haydon, G. H., L. M. Jarvis, K. J. Simpson, P. C. Hayes, and P. Simmonds.** 1997. The clinical significance of the detection of hepatitis GBV-C RNA in the serum of patients with fulminant, presumed viral, hepatitis. *J. Viral Hepatitis* **4:**45–49.
54. **Heringlake, S., S. Osterkamp, C. Trautwein, H. L. Tillman, K. Boker, S. Muerhoff, I. K. Mushahwar, G. Hunsmann, and M. P. Manns.** 1996. Association between fulminant hepatic failure and a strain of GBV virus C. *Lancet* **348:**1626–1629.
55. **Houghton, M., A. Weiner, J. Han, G. Kuo, and Q.-L. Choo.** 1991. Molecular biology of the hepatitis C viruses: implications for diagnosis, development and control of viral disease. *Hepatology* **14:**381–388.
56. **Jacob, S., D. Baudy, E. Jones, X. Lizhe, A. Mason, F. Regenstein, and R. Perrillo.** 1997. Comparison of quantitative HCV RNA assays in chronic hepatitis C. *Am. J. Clin. Pathol.* **107:**362–367.
57. **Katayama, K., S. Fukushi, C. Kurihara, N. Ishiyama, H. Okamura, F. B. Hoshino, and A. Oya.** 1997. New variant groups identified from HGV isolates. *Arch. Virol.* **142:** 1021–1028.
58. **Koretz, R. L., S. Ritman, and G. L. Gitnick.** 1973. Post-transfusion hepatitis in recipients of blood screened by newer assays. *Lancet* **ii:**694–696.
59. **Krajden, M., J. Zhao, C. Bourke, V. Scalia, P. Gill, and W. Lau.** 1996. Detection of hepatitis C virus by PCR in second-generation enzyme immunoassay-seropositive blood donors by using matched pairs of fresh frozen plasma and pilot tube sera. *J. Clin. Microbiol.* **34:**2191–2195.
60. **Kuo, G., Q.-L. Choo, H. J. Alter, G. L. Gitnick, A. G. Redeker, R. H. Purcell, T. Miyamura, J. L. Dienstag, M. J. Alter, C. E. Stevens, G. E. Tegtmeier, F. Bonino, M. Colombo, W.-S. Lee, C. Kuo, K. Berger, J. R. Shuster, L. R. Overby, D. W. Bradley, and M. Houghton.** 1989. An assay for circulating antibodies to a major etiologic virus of human non-A, non-B hepatitis. *Science* **244:** 362–364.

61. **Lau, J. Y., K. Qian, J. Detmer, M. L. Collins, E. Orito, J. A. Kolberg, M. S. Urdea, M. Mizokami, and G. L. Davis.** 1997. Effect of interferon-alpha and ribavirin therapy on serum GB virus C/hepatitis G virus (GBV-C/HGV) RNA levels in patients chronically infected with hepatitis C virus and GBV-C/HGV. *J. Infect. Dis.* **176:**421–426.
62. **Lau, J. Y. N., G. L. Davis, J. Kniffen, K.-P. Qian, M. S. Urdea, C. S. Chan, M. Mizokami, P. D. Neuwald, and J. C. Wilber.** 1993. Significance of serum hepatitis C virus RNA levels in chronic hepatitis C. *Lancet* **341:**1501–1504.
63. **Lau, J. Y. N., G. L. Davis, L. E. Prescott, G. Maertens, K. L. Lindsay, K. Qian, M. Mizokami, P. Simmonds, and The Hepatitis Interventional Therapy Group.** 1996. Distribution of hepatitis C virus genotypes determined by line probe assay in patients with chronic hepatitis C seen at tertiary referral centers in the United States. *Ann. Intern. Med.* **124:**868–876.
64. **Lefrere, J., P. Loiseau, J. Maury, J. Lasserre, M. Mariotti, N. Ravera, J. Lerable, G. Lefevre, L. Morand-Joubert, and R. Girot.** 1997. Natural history of GBV-C/hepatitis G virus infection through the follow-up of GBV-C/hepatitis G virus-infected blood donors and recipients studied by RNA polymerase chain reaction and anti-E2 serology. *Blood* **90:**3776–3780.
65. **Lin, H. H., D. S. Chen, P. J. Chen, M. H. Chang, D. P. Liu, K. Y. Yeh, and J. H. Kao.** 1998. Mother-to-infant transmission of GB virus C/hepatitis G virus: the role of high-titered maternal viremia and mode of delivery. *J. Infect. Dis.* **177:**1202–1206.
66. **Linnen, J., J. J. Wages, Z. Y. Zhang-Keck, K. E. Fry, K. Z. Krawczynski, H. Alter, E. Koonin, M. Gallagher, M. Alter, S. Hadziyannis, P. Karayiannis, K. Fung, Y. Nakatsuji, J. W. Shih, L. Young, M. J. Piatak, C. Hoover, J. Fernandez, S. Chen, J. C. Zou, T. Morris, K. C. Hyams, S. Ismay, J. D. Lifson, J. P. Kim, et al.** 1997. Molecular cloning and disease association of hepatitis G virus: a transfusion-transmissible agent. *Science* **271:**505–508.
67. **Magrin, S., A. Craxi, C. Fabiano, L. Marino, G. Fiorentino, O. Lo Iacono, R. Volpes, V. Di Marco, P. Almasio, A. Vaccaro, M. S. Urdea, J. C. Wilber, C. Bonura, F. Gianguzza, V. Capursi, S. Filiberti, L. Stuyver, and L. Pagliaro.** 1996. HCV viremia is more important than genotype as a predictor of response to interferon in Sicily (Southern Italy). *J. Hepatol.* **25:**583–590.
68. **Magrin, S., A. Craxi, C. Fabiano, R. G. Simonetti, G. Fiorentino, L. Marino, O. Diquattro, V. Di Marco, O. Loiacono, R. Volpes, P. Almasio, M. S. Urdea, P. Neuwald, R. Sanchez-Pescador, J. Detmer, J. C. Wilber, and L. Pagliaro.** 1994. Hepatitis C viremia in chronic liver disease: relationship to interferon-α or corticosteroid treatment. *Hepatology* **19:**273–279.
69. **Martinelli, A. L. C., D. Brown, H.-B. Braun, G. Michel, and G. M. Dusheiko.** 1996. Quantitative assessment of hepatitis C virus RNA and IgM antibodies to hepatitis C core in chronic hepatitis C. *J. Hepatol.* **24:**21–26.
70. **Martinot-Peignoux, M., P. Marcellin, M. Pouteau, C. Castelnau, N. Boyer, M. Poliquin, C. Degott, I. Descombes, V. Le Breton, V. Milotova, J. P. Benhamou, and S. Erlinger.** 1995. Pretreatment serum hepatitis C virus RNA levels and hepatitis C virus genotype are the main and independent prognostic factors of sustained response to interferon alfa therapy in chronic hepatitis C. *Hepatology* **22:**1050–1056.
71. **McHutchison, J. G., O. V. Nainan, M. J. Alter, A. Sedghi-Vaziri, J. Detmer, M. Collins, and J. Kolberg.** 1997. Hepatitis C and G co-infection: response to interferon therapy and quantitative changes in serum HGV-RNA. *Hepatology* **26:**1322–1327.
72. **McHutchison, J. G., J. L. Person, S. Govindarajan, B. Valinluck, T. Gore, S. R. Lee, M. Nelles, A. Polito, D. Chien, R. DiNello, S. Quan, G. Kuo, and A. G. Redeker.** 1992. Improved detection of hepatitis C virus antibodies in high-risk populations. *Hepatology* **15:**19–25.
73. **Mellor, J., E. A. Walsh, L. E. Prescott, L. M. Jarvis, F. Davidson, P. L. Yap, P. Simmonds, and International HCV Collaborative Study Group.** 1996. Survey of type 6 group variants of hepatitis C virus in Southeast Asia by using core-based genotyping assay. *J. Clin. Microbiol.* **34:**417–423.
74. **Mizokami, M., T. Gojobori, K.-I. Ohba, K. Ikeo, X.-M. Ge, T. Ohno, E. Orito, and J. Y. N. Lau.** 1996. Hepatitis C virus types 7, 8 and 9 should be classified as type 6 subtypes. *J. Hepatol.* **24:**622–624.
75. **Mori, S., N. Kato, A. Yagyu, T. Tanaka, Y. Ikeda, B. Petchclai, P. Chiewsilp, T. Kurimura, and K. Shimotohno.** 1992. A new type of hepatitis C virus in patients in Thailand. *Biochem. Biophys. Res. Commun.* **183:**334–342.
76. **Mukaide, M., M. Mizokami, E. Orito, K. Ohba, T. Nakano, R. Ueda, K. Hikiji, S. Iino, S. Shapiro, N. Lahat, Y. M. Park, B. S. Kim, T. Oyunsuren, M. Rezieg, M. N. Al-Ahdal, and J. Y. Lau.** 1997. Three different GB virus C/hepatitis G virus genotypes. Phylogenetic analysis and a genotyping assay based on restriction fragment length polymorphism. *FEBS Lett.* **407:**51–58.
77. **National Institutes of Health.** 1997. *Management of Hepatitis C*, p. 1–41. NIH consensus statement. vol. 15. National Institutes of Health, Bethesda, Md.
78. **Okamoto, H., Y. Sugiyama, S. Okada, K. Kurai, Y. Akahane, Y. Sugai, T. Tanaka, K. Sato, F. Tsuda, Y. Miyakawa, and M. Mayumi.** 1992. Typing hepatitis C virus by polymerase chain reaction with type-specific primers: application to clinical surveys and tracing infectious sources. *J. Gen. Virol.* **73:**673–679.
79. **Orito, E., M. Mizokami, T. Nakano, H. Terashima, O. Nojiri, K. Sakakibara, M. Mizuno, M. Ogino, M. Nakamura, Y. Matsumoto, K.-I. Miyata, and J. Y. N. Lau.** 1994. Serum hepatitis C virus RNA level as a predictor of subsequent response to interferon-a therapy in Japanese patients with chronic hepatitis C. *J. Med. Virol.* **44:**410–414.
80. **Orito, E., M. Mizokami, T. Tanaka, J. Y. N. Lau, K. Suzuki, M. Yamauchi, Y. Ohta, A. Hasegawa, S. Tanaka, and M. Kohara.** 1996. Quantification of serum hepatitis C core virus core protein level in patients chronically infected with different hepatitis C virus genotypes. *Gut* **39:**876–880.
81. **Pawlotsky, J. M., D. Dhumeaux, I. K. Mushahwar, C. J. Soussy, E. S. Zafrani, J. Remire, F. Darthuy, A. Bastie, S. M. Desai, G. Germanidis, M. Pellerin, A. S. Muerhoff, and F. Roudot-Thoraval.** 1998. GB virus C (GBV-C) infection in patients with chronic hepatitis C. Influence on liver disease and on hepatitis virus behaviour: effect of interferon alfa therapy. *J. Med. Virol.* **54:**26–37.
82. **Pawlotsky, J.-M., A. Fleury, V. Choukroun, L. Deforges, F. Roudot-Thoraval, P. Aumont, J. Duval, and D. Dhumeaux.** 1994. Significance of highly positive c22-3 "indeterminate" second-generation hepatitis C virus (HCV) recombinant immunoblot assay (RIBA) and resolution by third-generation HCV RIBA. *J. Clin. Microbiol.* **32:**1357–1359.
83. **Pessoa, M. G., T. L. Wright, H. M. Hassoba, M. Collins, J. Kolberg, J. Detmer, and N. A. Terrault.** 1998. Quantitation of hepatitis G and C viruses in the liver: evidence that hepatitis G virus is not hepatotropic. *Hepatology* **27:**877–880.
84. **Prescott, L. E., A. Berger, J. M. Pawlotsky, P. Conjeevaram, I. Pike, and P. Simmonds.** 1997. Sequence analysis of hepatitis C virus variants producing discrepant results

with two different genotyping assays. *J. Med. Virol.* **53:** 237–244.

85. **Puoti, C., A. Magrini, T. Stati, P. Rigato, F. Montagnese, P. Rossi, L. Aldegheri, and S. Resta.** 1997. Clinical, histological, and virological features of hepatitis C virus carriers with persistently normal or abnormal alanine transaminase levels. *Hepatology* **26:**1393–1398.
86. **Sarrazin, C., G. Herrmann, W. K. Roth, J. Lee, S. Marx, and S. Zeuzem.** 1997. Prevalence and clinical and histological manifestation of hepatitis G/GBV-C infections in patients with elevated aminotransferases of unknown etiology. *J. Hepatol.* **27:**276–283.
87. **Serfaty, L., O. Chazouilleres, A. Poujol-Robert, L. Morand-Joubert, C. Dubois, Y. Chretien, R. E. Poupon, J. C. Petit, and R. Poupon.** 1997. Risk factors for cirrhosis in patients with chronic hepatitis C virus infection: results of a case-control study. *Hepatology* **26:**776–779.
88. **Simmonds, P., A. Alberti, H. J. Alter, F. Bonino, D. W. Bradley, C. Bréchot, J. T. Brouwer, S.-W. Chan, K. Chayama, et al.** 1994. A proposed system for the nomenclature of hepatitis C viral genotypes. *Hepatology* **19:** 1321–1324.
89. **Simmonds, P., E. C. Holmes, T.-A. Cha, S.-W. Chan, F. McOmish, B. Irvine, E. Beall, P. L. Yap, J. Kolberg, and M. S. Urdea.** 1993. Classification of hepatitis C virus into six major genotypes and a series of subtypes by phylogenetic analysis of the NS-5 region. *J. Gen. Virol.* **74:** 2391–2399.
90. **Simmonds, P., F. McOmish, P. L. Yap, S.-W. Chan, C. K. Lin, G. Dusheiko, A. A. Saeed, and E. C. Holmes.** 1993. Sequence variability in the 5′ non-coding region of hepatitis C virus: identification of a new virus type and restrictions on sequence diversity. *J. Gen. Virol.* **74:** 661–668.
91. **Smith, D. B., N. Cuceanu, F. Davidson, L. M. Jarvis, J. L. Mokili, S. Hamid, C. A. Ludlam, and P. Simmonds.** 1997. Discrimination of hepatitis G virus/GBV-C geographical variants by analysis of the 5′ non-coding region. *J. Gen. Virol.* **78:**1533–1542.
92. **Tacke, M., S. Schmolke, V. Schlueter, S. Sauleda, J. I. Esteban, E. Tanaka, K. Kiyosawa, H. J. Alter, U. Schmitt, G. Hess, B. Ofenloch-Haehnle, and A. M. Engel.** 1997. Humoral immune response to the E2 protein of hepatitis G virus is associated with long-term recovery from infection and reveals a high frequency of hepatitis G virus exposure among healthy blood donors. *Hepatology* **26:** 1626–1633.
93. **Tobler, L. H., M. P. Busch, J. Wilber, R. DiNello, S. Quan, A. Polito, R. Kochesky, C. Bahl, M. Nelles, and S. R. Lee.** 1994. Evaluation of indeterminate c22-3 reactivity in volunteer blood donors. *Transfusion* **34:**130–134.
94. **Toyoda, H., S. Nakano, T. Kumada, I. Takeda, K. Sugiyama, T. Osada, S. Kiriyama, E. Orito, and M. Mizokami.** 1996. Comparison of serum hepatitis C virus RNA concentration by branched DNA probe assay with competitive reverse transcription polymerase chain reaction as a predictor of response to interferon-alpha therapy in chronic hepatitis C patients. *J. Med. Virol.* **48:**354–359.
95. **Trivedi, M.** 1997. Newly diagnosed hepatitis C. Lack of symptoms doesn't mean lack of progression. *Postgrad. Med.* **102:**95–98.
96. **Tsukiyama-Kohara, K., M. Kohara, K. Yamaguchi, N. Maki, A. Toyoshima, K. Miki, S. Tanaka, N. Hattori, and A. Nomoto.** 1991. A second group of hepatitis C viruses. *Virus Genes* **5:**243–254.
97. **Urdea, M. S.** 1993. Synthesis and characterization of branched DNA (bDNA) for the direct and quantitation detection of CMV, HBV, HCV, HIV. *Clin. Chem.* **39:** 725–726.
98. **van der Poel, C. L., H. T. M. Cuypers, H. W. Reesink, A. J. Weiner, S. Quan, R. Di Nello, J. J. P. van Boven, I. Winkel, D. Mulder-Folkerts, P. J. Exel-Oehlers, W. Schaasberg, A. Leentvaar-Kuypers, A. Polito, M. Houghton, and P. N. Lelie.** 1991. Confirmation of hepatitis C virus infection by new four-antigen recombinant immunoblot assay. *Lancet* **337:**317–319.
99. **Vrielink, H., H. W. Reesink, P. J. van den Burg, H. L. Zaaijer, H. T. Cuypers, P. N. Lelie, and C. L. van der Poel.** 1997. Performance of three generations of anti-hepatitis C virus enzyme-linked immunosorbent assays in donors and patients. *Transfusion* **37:**845–849.
100. **Weiner, A. J., G. Kuo, D. W. Bradley, F. Bonino, G. Saracco, C. Lee, J. Rosenblatt, Q.-L. Choo, and M. Houghton.** 1990. Detection of hepatitis C viral sequences in non-A, non-B hepatitis. *Lancet* **335:**1–3.
101. **Wilber, J. C., P. J. Johnson, and M. S. Urdea.** 1993. Reverse-transcriptase PCR for hepatitis C virus RNA, p. 327–331. *In* D. H. Persing, T. F. Smith, F. C. Tenover, and T. J. White (ed.), *Diagnostic Molecular Microbiology: Principles and Applications*. American Society for Microbiology, Washington, D.C.
102. **Woelfle, J., M. J. Lentze, E. Schreier, K. M. Keller, and T. Berg.** 1998. Persistent hepatitis G virus infection after neonatal transfusion. *J. Pediatr. Gastroenterol. Nutr.* **26:** 402–407.
103. **Yuki, N., N. Hayashi, A. Kasahara, H. Hagiwara, T. Takehara, M. Oshita, K. Katayama, H. Fusamoto, and T. Kamada.** 1995. Pretreatment viral load and response to prolonged interferon-α course for chronic hepatitis C. *J. Hepatol.* **22:**457–463.
104. **Zaaijer, H. L., L. T. Mimms, H. T. Cuypers, H. W. Reesink, C. L. van der Poel, S. Taskar, and P. N. Lelie.** 1993. Variability of IgM response in hepatitis C virus infection. *J. Med. Virol.* **40:**184–187.

Hepatitis E Virus

JOHN R. TICEHURST

84

Hepatitis E virus (HEV) is a small, nonenveloped, spherical, positive-strand RNA virus (Fig. 1 and 2) and the only known agent of enterically transmitted (ET) non-A, non-B (NANB) hepatitis (ET-NANB hepatitis). Like all recognized hepatitis viruses, HEV appears to be a unique and important agent of acute disease worldwide (Fig. 3). Hepatitis E is a self-limited illness (Fig. 4) that varies in severity, with an unusually high frequency of fulminant disease among pregnant women. *Pregnant health-care professionals, including laboratory workers, should be excluded from potential contact with HEV.*

Hepatitis E has not been considered endemic in the United States because the few reported cases followed travel in known areas of endemicity such as Africa, Asia, and Mexico, and because outbreaks of ET hepatitis have always been attributed to hepatitis A virus (HAV). New studies, however, have shown that HEV infected domestic swine in Illinois (56) and two men who lived in Minnesota and Tennessee; only the latter had recently traveled from the United States, to Mexico, where he could have acquired the virus (47, 68). These three "United States" ("US") viruses are genetically similar to each other but distinct from HEV prototypes (thus representing one of two putative North American genotypes, with at least one additional genotype for Africa and Asia; Fig. 5). While the impact of "US" strains has not yet been determined, HEV should be suspected after recent travel in a region of known endemicity and considered when there is no evidence for another cause of acute hepatitis (47).

Many current laboratory methods for detecting HEV infections appear to be analytically sensitive and specific, but their clinical use, to aid diagnosis, is not straightforward. Assays for HEV RNA are not commercially available anywhere, and the predictive value of a negative result (NPV) is very low. Assays for antibodies to HEV (anti-HEV) are not commercially available in the United States; those sold elsewhere detect antibodies directed against antigens representing Mexican and African-Asian strains. Certain testing is available from the U.S. Centers for Disease Control and Prevention (CDC) (see "Collection, Transport, and Storage of Specimens" and "Assays for Detecting Anti-HEV").

DESCRIPTION OF THE AGENT

History

Soon after HAV and hepatitis B virus (HBV) were identified during the 1970s, it became apparent that there were additional NANB agents of viral hepatitis. In industrialized countries, NANB hepatitis was usually associated with blood transfusion and other forms of parenteral transmission. Thus, most references to NANB hepatitis in American literature more precisely described parenterally transmitted NANB hepatitis (PT-NANB hepatitis). The vast majority of PT-NANB hepatitis cases have been associated with hepatitis C virus since its identification in 1989 (13). The other recognized PT-NANB agent, hepatitis D virus, always requires active HBV replication.

It was also recognized that epidemics of ET hepatitis occurred in southern Asia and other developing regions. The first such epidemic involved 29,000 cases in Delhi, India, during 1955 and 1956 and resulted from contamination of a major water supply with raw sewage (3, 61). An etiologic agent was not isolated, so it was thought that HAV caused the outbreak. However, differences from hepatitis A (Table 1) were clues that another agent was involved. In 1980, Khuroo (43) and Wong et al. (see reference 61) demonstrated that the Delhi epidemic and other epidemics were associated with at least one unidentified agent of ET-NANB hepatitis.

In 1983, Balayan et al. (9) identified a viral agent of ET-NANB hepatitis that was subsequently named hepatitis E virus (HEV) and shown to have been a worldwide human pathogen for many years (3, 5, 6, 12, 13, 61, 66). The identity of HEV was independently established in 1990, when its genome was molecularly cloned by Reyes et al. (66). To date, there is only one recognized serotype of HEV, but strains from different epidemics and sporadic cases have distinguishing properties. Hepatitis E should be used to refer only to disease caused by HEV because HEV may not be the only cause of ET-NANB hepatitis (see "Evidence for Additional Agents of ET Hepatitis") (3, 27, 32).

Taxonomy

Although HEV was formerly classified in the family *Caliciviridae*, genus *Calicivirus* (25), the Executive Committee of the International Committee on Taxonomy of Viruses has approved its removal to an unassigned genus of "hepatitis E-like viruses" (59a) because certain characteristics distinguish HEV from typical caliciviruses (10, 60). For example, analysis of amino acid sequences determined that HEV, rubella virus (family *Togaviridae*, genus *Alphavirus*), and beet necrotic yellow vein virus (family *Togaviridae*, genus *Furovirus*) could represent a distinct category among a "super-

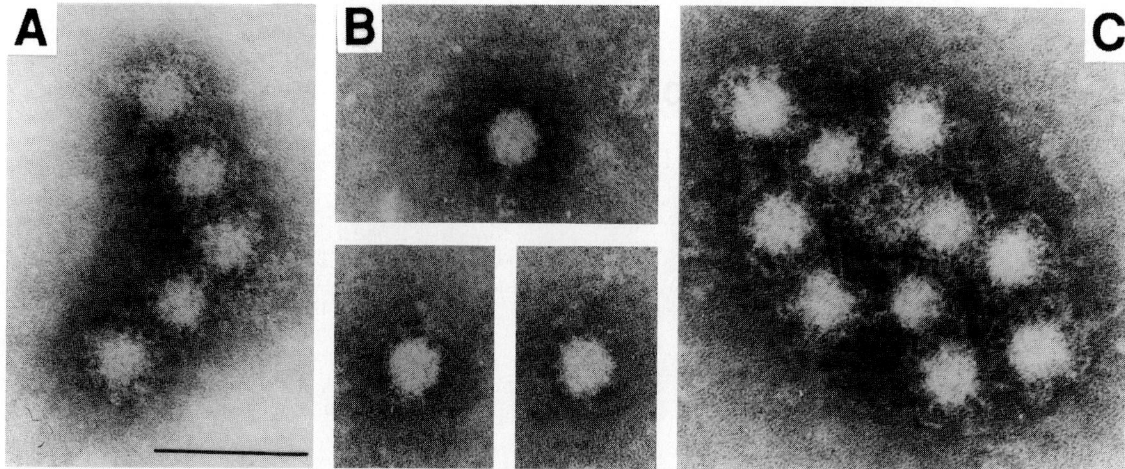

FIGURE 1 HEV particles in bile from an HEV Mexico 86-infected monkey, detected by IEM. Antibody coating (Ab) was semiquantitatively rated as 0 (none) to 4+ (heavy). Bar, 100 nm. Reagent Mexican serum containing a high concentration of anti-HEV (45) was used to screen for virus-like particles (A: 5-particle complex with 4+ Ab) that were then identified as HEV by masked testing with paired sera from an HEV Burma 82-infected monkey (B: preinoculation serum, which should not yield antibody-coated HEV particles—3 separated particles with 0 to 1+ Ab; C: acute-phase serum, which should yield heavily coated HEV particles—11-particle complex with 4+ Ab). This bile was subsequently shown to contain HEV RNA and infectious HEV (51, 57, 75); such specimens can be a reagent HEV source for IEM to detect anti-HEV (e.g., A and C indicate high-level anti-HEV, whereas B demonstrates little or no anti-HEV). (Modified from a figure in reference 75.)

group" of alpha-like viruses (44). Additional distinguishing characteristics are discussed in the legend to Fig. 2 and the following sections.

Characteristics of Virus Particles

HEV particles in feces or bile are nearly spherical and ≈29 nm in diameter, smaller than typical caliciviruses and slightly larger than picornaviruses (Fig. 1) (13, 73, 74). HEV particles are probably icosahedral, with a surface structure that is much more subtle than the distinctive cup-like indentations on caliciviruses ("calici" stands for chalice) (5, 9, 25, 61, 73, 75). Electron-dense particles in hepatocytes have been observed during infection but have not been immunologically identified as HEV (73). Partially purified HEV particles sedimented at 183S and had a buoyant density of 1.29 g/cm^3 in potassium tartrate-glycerol (13), like certain caliciviruses (25).

Resistance and Inactivation

Little is known about the resistance of HEV. While there are no published descriptions of its inactivation, HEV particles must survive the pH range of the gastrointestinal tract (60) and were intact when prepared from lyophilized feces and morphologically resistant to trichlorotrifluorothane (73–75). HEV may be labile in dense hyperosmolar solutions (sucrose or CsCl) or during storage between −120 and 8°C, although it is more stable at lower temperatures (19). An Indian strain was reported to be more resistant to changes in temperature (18). Successful efforts to control HEV outbreaks have included chlorination of water supplies. Most laboratories assume that HEV is destroyed by iodinated disinfectants or autoclaving.

Genome

HEV has a small, positive-strand RNA genome with distinctive characteristics (11, 34, 66, 68, 70). The prototype nucleotide and amino acid sequences, which represent HEV strain Burma 82, are markedly dissimilar from those of other viruses (Fig. 2) (44, 70). The genome is nearly 7,200 nucleotides (nt) long, with short noncoding regions at each end. Its 5′ terminus is capped, like those of most eukaryotic mRNAs but unlike the 5′ termini of picornaviral and typical caliciviral genomes (to which a small, virus-encoded protein, VPg, is covalently linked), suggesting that translation and replication of HEV RNA may be regulated by mechanisms different from those of typical caliciviruses. Detectable HEV RNAs in liver tissue included molecules of approximately 7,500 nt (genome), 3,700 nt, and 2,000 nt; these were polyadenylated and appeared to be 3′ coterminal (70).

At least three open reading frames (ORF) are used. ORF1 is thought to encode nonstructural proteins and several antigenic epitopes. ORF2 encodes the major capsid protein and at least one immunogenic epitope. The function of ORF3 is not known, but it encodes at least one antigenic epitope (33, 87, 88); such an ORF is not found in typical caliciviral genomes (25). Although HEV ORF1 and ORF2 resemble those of caliciviruses with regard to organization, size, and genomic location, HEV does not have a 3′-terminal ORF like that of typical caliciviruses. HEV proteins are not well characterized (Fig. 2).

Differences between Strains

Among strains for which nucleotide sequences have been determined, only HEV strain Mexico 86 and the "US" strains were collected in the Western hemisphere, and their genomes are distinct from each other and from those of the relatively homogeneous African-Asian group (Fig. 5) (34, 56, 68, 76). When sequences of Mexican and Asian strains are compared, nucleotide identities are approximately 75% for ORF1, 81% for ORF2, and 91% for ORF3; corresponding amino acid identities are 84, 93, and 87%. In contrast, the

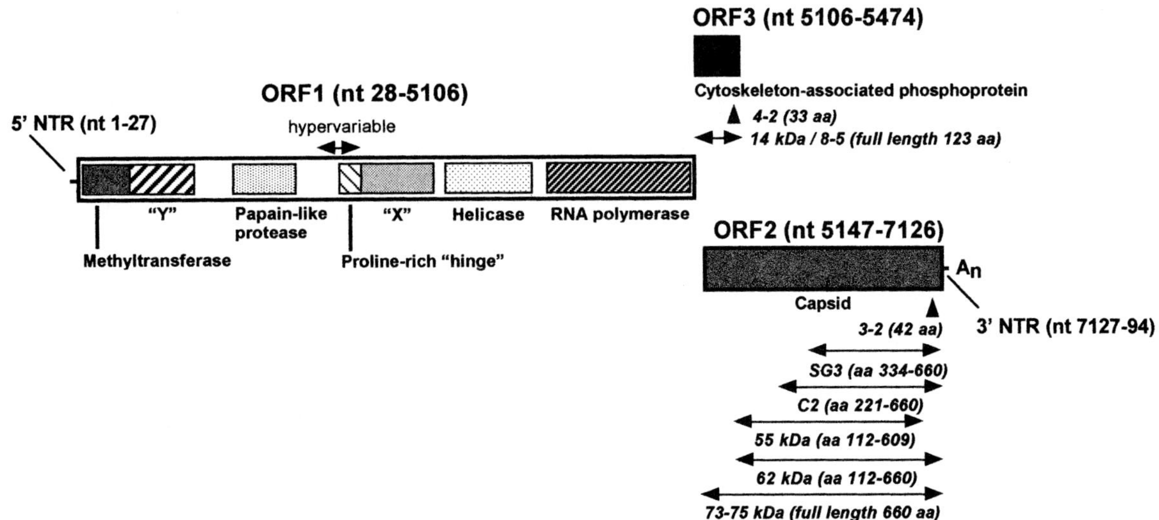

FIGURE 2 Diagram of the positive-strand RNA genome of HEV. Nucleotide positions are based on those of the HEV Burma 82 genome, which is 7,194 nt long before a 3′ polyadenylated tail of several hundred nucleotides (A_n) (70). Short 5′- and 3′-nontranslated regions (NTR) surround three ORF. ORF1 and ORF3 overlap by 1 nt, ORF1 and ORF2 are separated by 41 nt, and ORF2 and ORF3 overlap by 328 nt. Hypervariable sequences (nt 2011 to 2325) are approximately 56% identical between Mexican and Asian strains, resulting in extensive amino acid (aa) differences (11, 34, 76). Based on amino acid domains that have limited similarity to those of other viruses, ORF1 is thought to encode nonstructural proteins: putative functions are indicated below domains (shaded and cross-hatched) in the ORF1 rectangle; several domains of unknown function were identified by similarity with those of rubella virus ("Y," proline-rich "hinge," and "X"), beet necrotic yellow vein virus ("Y"), and alphaviruses ("X") (44, 66). The 5′ termini of ORF2 and ORF3 encode hydrophobic domains that suggest signal activity (60). ORF2 encodes (i) the probable major capsid protein (≈20-nm, capsid-like particles were formed when 55-, 62-, or 73- to 75-kDa proteins [double-headed arrows] were produced in insect cells) with a highly basic N-terminal domain that could participate in genome encapsidation; (ii) immunogenic epitopes (55- and 62-kDa proteins induced protective immunity in monkeys; protein C2 induced partial immunity); and (iii) epitopes, some of which appear to be conformation dependent, that react with acute- or convalescent-phase antibodies (SG3, 55-kDa, 62-kDa, 73- to 75-kDa, C2, and other proteins; short C-terminal polypeptide 3-2 [arrowhead]) (33, 49, 50, 60, 64, 65, 68, 70, 77, 79, 81, 85–87, 89). The function of ORF3 is not known, but its expression and immunogenicity were implied when antibodies to C-terminal polypeptide 4-2 were detected in postinfection sera (3-2 and 4-2 were the first immunoreactive domains to be identified) (87); more recently, full-length protein (14-kDa/8-5) expression in insect cells led to its use in assays for anti-HEV (33), and expression of a phosphoprotein in animal cell cultures led to its putative association with the cytoskeleton (88). Postinfection sera have also reacted with peptides representing ORF1 domains, especially those at the C terminus of the putative RNA polymerase (40), and other ORF2 and ORF3 domains (not shown) (24, 41). (Adapted from similar figures in references 11, 44, and 87.)

sequences of Burma 82 and Pakistan 87 are highly similar (93 to 99% nucleotide and 99 to 100% amino acid identities for the three ORF), except for a hypervariable region of ORF1 (Fig. 2). Reactivity in most immunoassays has not been affected by the geographic origins of antigens or antibodies (13, 45, 52, 65, 73, 79, 82, 87), but the effect of relatively distinct strains has not yet been fully determined (18, 27, 47, 56, 68).

Growth in Cell Culture

Intensive efforts to isolate HEV in cell cultures date to the Delhi epidemic of 1955 and 1956 (73). Among several reports of in vitro propagation since 1989, encouraging results have been described: cocultivation of kidney or liver cells from HEV-infected cynomolgus monkeys (*Macaca fascicularis*); with FRhK4 continuous rhesus monkey kidney cells, leading to a cytopathic effect (CPE) after 25 passages (7, 28); CPE after passage of fibroblast-adapted HEV in A549 human lung carcinoma cells (35); and persistent low-level replication, without CPE, in primary cynomolgus monkey hepatocytes or in PLC/PRF/5 human hepatocellular carcinoma cells that were inoculated with feces or bile containing HEV (55, 71). Negative-strand HEV RNA detection was used as a criterion for replication during two of these studies (28, 71). However, these results have not been reproduced in other laboratories.

NATURAL AND EXPERIMENTAL HOSTS

Human are not the only hosts for HEV. Anti-HEV have been detected in sera from wild-caught rhesus monkeys (*Macaca mulatta*), cynomolgus monkeys, and rodents and

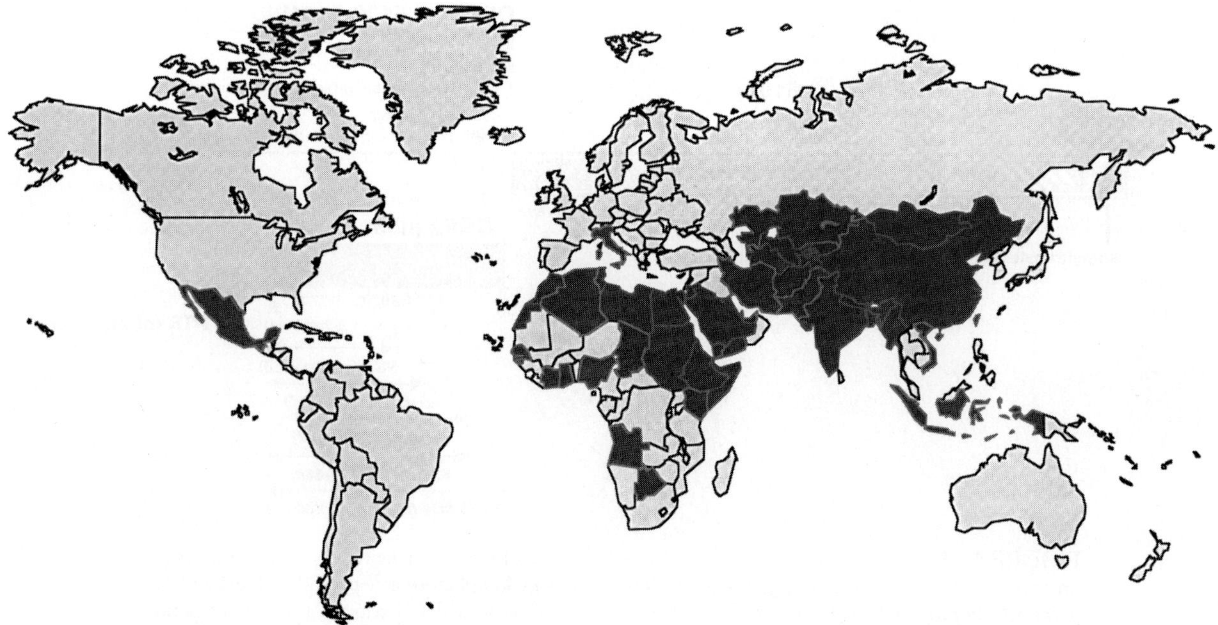

FIGURE 3 Worldwide distribution of hepatitis E. Dark shading indicates countries in which outbreaks have been recognized or in which HEV of the African-Asian and Mexican genotypes (see Fig. 5) has been associated with >25% of sporadic non-A, non-B, non-C hepatitis. This map is similar to figures in references 60 to 62 and was modified from slide 66 in a CDC presentation on the Internet (http://www.cdc.gov/ncidod/diseases/hepatitis/slideset/httoc.htm) by adding Gambia (45), Ghana (61), Italy (15), Tunisia (16), and Vietnam (23). Patterns of distribution vary within countries and are associated with inadequate public sanitation. The detected prevalence of anti-HEV IgG has been lower than expected in areas of endemicity but higher than expected in areas where outbreaks have not been recognized (8, 60, 62, 72). While these data suggest that HEV infections may occur (without a high frequency of anti-HEV IgM) in additional countries on every continent, high variability in the specificity and sensitivity of anti-HEV IgG assays (Table 2) (54) makes it impossible at this time to draw accurate conclusions about the overall prevalence of HEV infection. Furthermore, the worldwide impact of "US" strains (see Fig. 5) (47, 56, 68) is not yet known.

from domestic chickens and swine (22, 39, 56, 60, 75, 80). Although it is not known if all such animals were infected with HEV or with an unrecognized but antigenically similar agent, some pigs were viremic and had histologic evidence of hepatitis (22, 56) and rhesus monkeys with naturally acquired anti-HEV were partially protected from experimental infection (80).

Experimentally infected animals have yielded valuable data for understanding the pathogenesis of hepatitis E and have been essential sources of anti-HEV, virus, and HEV antigens in liver tissue (HEVAg). Most such infections have been in primates, especially cynomolgus and rhesus monkeys and chimpanzees (*Pan troglodytes*) (5, 9, 13, 45, 51, 61, 73, 75, 76, 79, 81, 82). Other studies have used domestic piglets (*Sus scrofa domestica*), rats, or lambs (7, 8, 39, 60).

HEPATITIS E

Clinical Significance

HEV is responsible for much of the viral hepatitis in regions of endemicity: individuals can be affected by large epidemics, focal outbreaks, or sporadic disease (in India, approximately 60% of sporadic hepatitis) (5, 7, 13, 17, 61, 74, 82). Fulminant hepatitis E is unusual except in pregnant women, in whom the mortality rate has been 10 to 20% and highest during the third trimester (43, 61). HEV is a recognized threat for military personnel, even those from areas of endemicity (2, 82, 83). All Americans should be considered at risk for infection with HEV (2). The clinical significance of "US" strains (47, 56, 68) is not yet known.

Epidemiology

Outbreaks and epidemics are often associated with fecal contamination of drinking water (Table 1) (61, 74). Although children are affected (37, 69), hepatitis E is predominantly a disease of young adults, especially males (13, 43, 61). The increase in anti-HEV prevalence during young adulthood (see below) suggests an element of sexual transmission (60). It is not known if the high frequency of fulminant hepatitis E in pregnant women is due to epidemiologic or pathogenic factors (see, "Pathogenesis" and "Symptoms and Signs"). One study suggested that mother-to-infant transmission of HEV was common (42), a finding that was not observed during experimental infection (80). The role of nonhuman hosts (see above) in HEV transmission has not been determined.

Regions of endemicity are located in most of Africa, central and southern Asia, and Mexico (Fig. 3) where anti-HEV prevalence has been unexpectedly low and without a substantial increase after age 30 (7, 29, 41, 45, 60–62, 73). Anti-HEV were detected in only 25% of 12- to 48-year-old

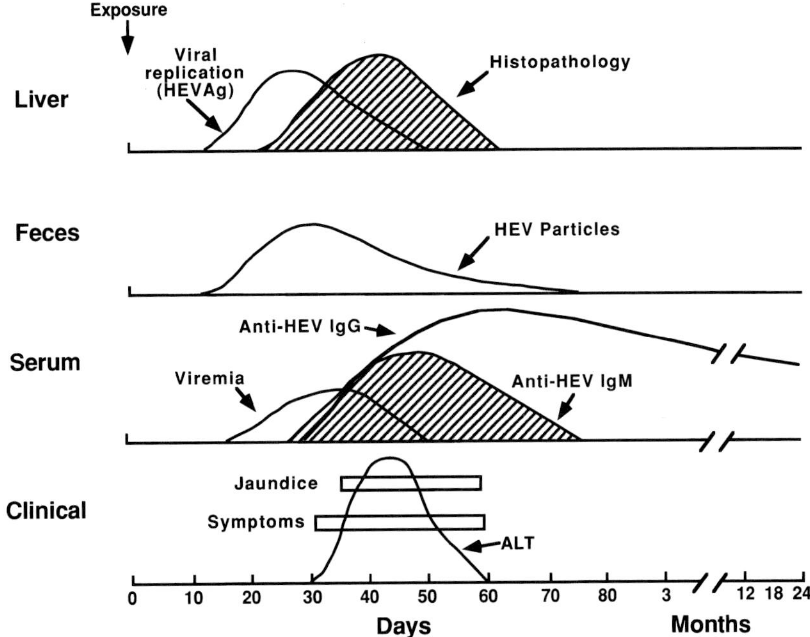

FIGURE 4 Diagram of a typical human case of hepatitis E, with somewhat speculative (because detailed knowledge of natural history is limited) virologic, histopathologic, serologic, and clinical events. Although some of these patterns are based on findings from experimentally infected animals (9, 13, 51, 75, 76, 79, 81, 82), humans generally have a longer incubation period (here, 37 days from exposure to development of jaundice) and more severe disease (among nonhumans, only swine develop overt signs such as jaundice). The earliest recognized evidence of infection is viral replication in the liver, detected as HEVAg by IF microscopy, HEV particles by IEM, or HEV RNA by PCR (see Table 3) (45, 51, 75). The liver is the only known site of HEV replication; release of progeny virions from hepatocytes into bile leads to HEV excretion (HEV particles in feces, detected by RT-PCR, IEM, or inoculation of susceptible animals) (57, 74, 75). Viremia (detected by PCR) is also thought to reflect HEV release from the liver (76). Histopathologic changes, anti-HEV, and signs and symptoms develop as HEV replication wanes, but HEV may still be detectable during clinical illness (57, 74). Curves for antibodies (anti-HEV IgG and anti-HEV IgM) appear to vary with reagent antigens used in assays (see Table 2; Fig. 2) (49, 54): anti-HEV IgG has been detected in more late-convalescence patients by EIAs based on large ORF2 proteins than by IEM, IF blocking, or other EIAs (14, 17, 30, 45, 54, 75, 79, 81, 86, 87). Anti-HEV IgG develops rapidly after anti-HEV IgM, is usually present at high levels when jaundice appears, typically reaches peak concentrations before convalescence (reciprocal titers of 10^3 to 10^5 at 2 to 4 weeks after hepatitis onset), and then rapidly decreases to levels that remain detectable for ≥1 year in most patients (3, 14, 26, 30, 60). Anti-HEV IgA may develop and diminish in a pattern similar to that of anti-HEV IgM (17). The ALT concentration in serum is the usual marker for biochemical evidence of hepatitis; some hosts have bimodal ALT elevations, with the first increase during the incubation period (51, 60, 75, 79). (Adapted from similar figures in reference 60.)

persons in the Kathmandu Valley of Nepal, where summer-long epidemics occur every few years, and in 16, 24, 28, and 31% of persons during the second through fifth decades, respectively (21). Similar results were obtained in both 1982 and 1992 in west central India, where no epidemics occurred during the 10-year interval; anti-HAV prevalence was ≥95% among persons ≥6 years old (6). To explain low anti-HEV prevalence and disease predominance among young adults when other enteric viruses infect young children, possibilities include low HEV circulation in the environment, high proportion of subclinical infections among children, or loss of protective immunity.

Epidemics have not been recognized in the United States, Canada, South America, Europe, Japan, New Zealand, or Australia; nearly all patients with hepatitis E have recently traveled to or emigrated from a region of endemicity (2, 47, 68, 73). Among individuals from nonepidemic regions who do not have clearly defined risk factors, the prevalence of reactivity in assays for anti-HEV immunoglobulin G (IgG) typically ranges from 1 to 21%, usually much higher than expected. Such prevalence has been reported, for example, for California, Maryland, South America, and southern Europe (7, 26, 65, 72, 87). The specificity of such reactivity has been questioned by studies that compared different assays (54, 72, 75), but some Americans were shown to carry antibodies that neutralized the infectivity of HEV for cynomolgus monkeys (72). Furthermore, while anti-HEV were not detected among patients with sporadic NANB hepatitis in CDC "sentinel counties" studies (1), two American men with sporadic hepatitis E were infected with "US" strains; one of them probably acquired the virus in the United States. Genotype-specific reagents helped to

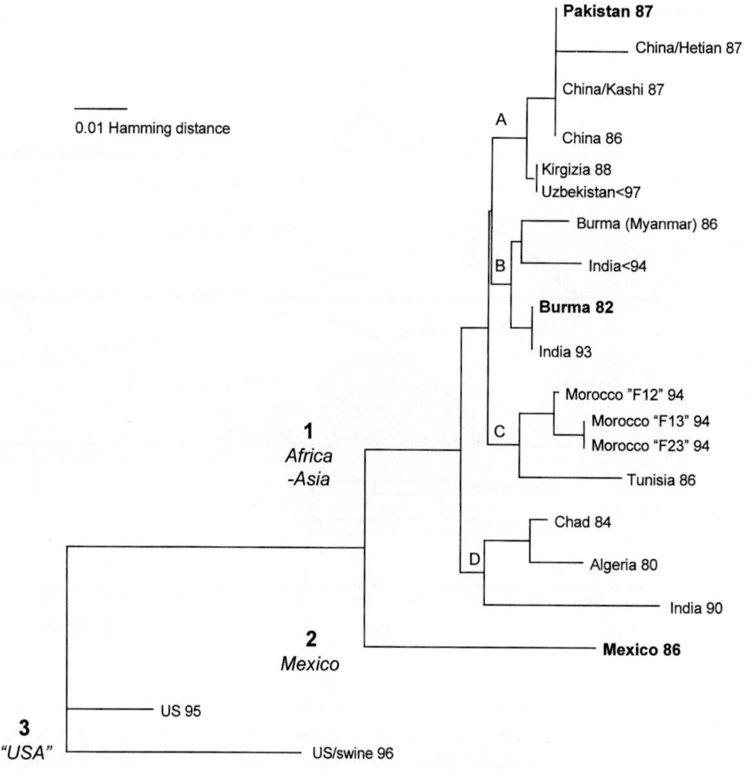

FIGURE 5 Phylogenetic tree of nucleotide sequences of 20 representative HEV strains, designated by nation and year of origin, except for strains Uzbekistan<97 and India<94 (< indicates the year submitted to GenBank because collection date was not specified). China 87 strains are distinguished by city names, F designations are for three patients from a Moroccan epidemic, and US/swine 96 was collected from pigs (16, 56). Bold type indicates prototype strains Pakistan 87 (often called Sar-55), Burma 82, and Mexico 86 (also referred to as Mexico-14 or Telixtac-14) (34, 70, 76). From top to bottom, GenBank accession numbers are M80581, L08816, L25595, D11092, AF010417, AF010422, D10330, X98292, M73218, X99441, AF010418, AF010419, AF010420, AF010421, AF001275, AF001276, U22532, M74506, AF03537, and AF011921 (68, 83). The phylogenetic tree was kindly prepared by Oliver Laeyendecker (Department of Medicine, Johns Hopkins University) from 155-nt sequences representing a conserved ORF1-ORF3-ORF2 overlap region (Fig. 2) (16, 31). The Hamming distance (bar) (0.01 is ≈1% nucleotide difference) between any two sequences is the total length of horizontal lines connecting them on the tree. This tree indicates three putative genotypes (1, 2, and 3; "USA" is in quotation marks because a third, genetically similar "US" strain could have been acquired in Mexico [68]) and four geographically based subgroups within genotype 1: A, central Asia; B, southeastern Asia; C, northwest Africa; and D, Africa-India. In the text, "US" designates strains from the United States that could have been acquired elsewhere, whereas the two strains in this figure were likely to have been acquired in the United States. There may be an additional subgroup or genotype representing five Chinese strains (84) for which the ORF1-ORF3-ORF2 sequence has not been reported. These and similar data suggest that there has been little mutational pressure on African and Asian strains for at least 10 years (1980 to 1990). The Hamming distances between African-Asian, Mexican, and US strains suggest, as does epidemiologic information, that HEV has infected people for many years (60, 61). Other epidemiologic data indicate that HEV was introduced to southern Africa and southwestern Asia by immigrants from southeastern Asia (32, 60); however, phylogenetic analysis of ORF2 and ORF3 grouped strain India 90 with HEV from southeastern Asia (56).

associate HEV with their disease (47, 68). Thus, HEV may cause sporadic hepatitis in certain individuals or populations within nonepidemic regions or may infect with limited pathogenicity due to strain, host, or environmental factors. HEV does not appear to be a major cause of fulminant hepatitis in people from regions of nonendemicity (46, 48). Like any virus, HEV may also have antigenic "relatives" that infect worldwide or in discrete locations with as-yet-undetermined manifestations (72). For accurate determination of seroprevalence, it is important to use assays (Table 2) that are clinically sensitive (i.e., detect antibodies to all HEV strains that cause hepatitis E in the studied population) and specific (i.e., yield negative results in the absence of hepatitis E).

Pathogenesis

During natural infection, HEV gains access to the body via oral ingestion. The mechanism by which HEV reaches the

TABLE 1 Comparison of viral hepatitis E and hepatitis A[a]

Similarities
Worldwide distribution with epidemic and sporadic cases
Prevalence of antiviral antibodies increases with age
Fecal-oral transmission
Low potential for transmission by transfusion or other parenteral modes
Chronic disease not recognized
Transmissible to nonhuman primates
Differences (hepatitis E)
Nonuniform distribution: outbreaks recognized only in southern and central Asia, Africa, and Mexico
Anti-HEV prevalence much lower than expected in regions of endemicity (approximately 3 to 30%) and much higher than expected where outbreaks have not been recognized (up to 21%) (26, 60, 62, 72, 87)
Slightly longer incubation period: mean of 40 days, range of 2–8 weeks
Cholestasis more prominent
High (10–20%) mortality among pregnant women, particularly during third trimester
Clinically apparent secondary cases unusual
Endemic hepatitis E predominantly a disease of young adults
Concentrations of anti-HEV usually highest during the acute phase and early convalescence phase (3, 5, 14, 26, 54, 73)
Anti-HEV IgG detectable in nearly all patients when they initially present with hepatitis
Transmissible to swine (7, 56)

[a] For other details, see reviews such as references 7, 8, 60, and 61.

liver, its only known site of replication in primates, is not known. HEV replication in the cytoplasm of hepatocytes is usually the first detectable event during experimental infection, before hepatocellular changes and long before inflammatory changes and biochemical evidence of hepatitis (Fig. 4) (45, 51, 75). Progeny virus is probably released from hepatocytes to the gallbladder (by an unknown mechanism) and then excreted into the feces. Viremia is approximately concurrent with fecal HEV excretion (76). Although a study suggested that HEV was also present in the kidneys (7), the origin, duration, and diagnostic significance of nonenterohepatic HEV are not yet known. In general, in vivo concentrations of HEV appear to be very low. HEV is predominantly excreted during the incubation period and early acute phase, usually at very low levels: 12 of 13 PCR-positive specimens had a titer of $<10^6$ genomes per g of feces (9, 57, 74, 75).

Because anti-HEV and hepatitis develop concurrently, some consider hepatitis E to be an immunopathologic disease, wherein viral damage to hepatocytes may be minimal but host responses to infected cells result in hepatitis (13, 51, 73, 75). The pathogenesis of fulminant hepatitis E in pregnant women is not understood (see reference 61 for a hypothesis related to the Shwartzman phenomenon).

Symptoms and Signs

Most patients have a moderately severe but self-limited illness (Fig. 4) that cannot be distinguished from other forms of acute hepatitis. A prodrome may occur (14, 74). Acute-phase symptoms can include jaundice, anorexia, abdominal pain, nausea, vomiting, fever, and pruritus (9, 13, 61). Jaundice, the cardinal sign of acute viral hepatitis, can be manifested as yellow skin, scleral icterus, dark urine, or clay-colored feces. Nonspecific signs include fever, hepatomegaly, and abdominal tenderness. HEV infections occur subclinically or without jaundice (14): subclinical-to-clinical ratios were estimated to be 7:1 for an outbreak in Pakistan and 2:1 in Nepal, a nation with high endemicity (21, 52). While such ratios are not well characterized, especially as they relate to age, milder infections are probably more frequent in children. In animal studies, there appears to be a correlation between inoculum size and disease severity (52, 81).

During acute hepatitis E, patients may have elevated concentrations in serum of alanine aminotransferase (ALT), aspartate aminotransferase, bilirubin, and alkaline phosphatase. None of these is specific, but elevated alkaline phosphatase levels can reflect biliary obstruction, which can histopathologically distinguish hepatitis E. Although liver biopsy is rarely indicated, two patterns of HEV-associated histopathologic changes have been observed: (i) obstructive or cholestatic changes, thought to be characteristic of hepatitis E, and (ii) nonspecific changes found in all forms of acute viral hepatitis (43, 61). In the first pattern, the most distinctive features are a pseudoglandular arrangement of hepatocytes around distended bile canaliculi and bile stasis because of casts in canaliculi or casts in hepatocytes. Obstructive changes have been prominent in pregnant women, with or without fulminant disease. Pregnant women with fulminant hepatitis also have had a high incidence of disseminated intravascular coagulation (Kane [see reference 61]).

Patient Management, Infection Control, and Prevention

As with other forms of acute viral hepatitis, care is supportive because there are no specific modes of therapy. Guidelines for isolation have not been established (7), but feces and serum from a newly ill patient should be considered biohazardous until proven otherwise. Pregnant women should be prohibited from laboratories studying HEV and should avoid contact with patients or their specimens Health-care workers have been infected with HEV, and there has been a nosocomial outbreak (67). Recent identification of natural infections in swine (22, 56) raises the possibility of iatrogenic transmission via xenotransplantation.

Outbreaks have been controlled by instituting or restoring public sanitation measures. These typically include coincident chlorination of and elimination of fecal contamination from water supplies. Avoidance of potentially contaminated water and raw foods is the only measure for protecting individuals against infection because there is no effective immunoprophylaxis.

Naturally or passively acquired anti-HEV have protected or partially protected nonhuman primates from experimental hepatitis E (52, 73, 79, 80). There is some evidence for partial protection of humans in epidemic settings via naturally acquired anti-HEV, but this effect has not been observed for a population with a high level of endemicity (14, 52). Immune globulin from the United States and Europe has not prevented hepatitis E in certain travelers (2), and there is inconclusive evidence for protection by immune globulin prepared in regions of endemicity (60). Promising efforts to develop an HEV vaccine have used recombinant DNA (recDNA) technology for expressing ORF2 proteins (Fig. 2) (50, 79, 81, 89), which induced protection in cynomolgus and rhesus monkeys (64, 77, 78). The possibility of a Jennerian vaccine has been raised by the identification of porcine HEV strains (22, 56).

TABLE 2 Immunoassays for detecting anti-HEV in serum[a]

Type of: Antigen	Detection	Result	Method	Reagent antigen(s) (source)	Anti-HEV detected	Clinical: Sensitivity (%)	Clinical: Specificity[b] (%)	Practicality
recDNA	Indirect	Qualitative or semiquantitative	ORF2 protein EIA	ORF2, large, i.e., 55–75 kDa (baculovirus-infected cells)	IgG IgM	High (96–98) High	High (93–98) High?	High
		Qualitative or semiquantitative	Polypeptide EIA	ORF2, ORF3, "mosaic" (*Escherichia coli*)	IgG IgM IgA	Mod (67–91) Low–high? Mod?	High (95–100) High? High?	High
		Qualitative	Western blot	ORF2, ORF3 (*E. coli* or baculovirus-infected cells)	IgG IgM	Mod–high (83–98) Low–high?	Low–high (79–98) Mod–high?	Mod
		Qualitative or semiquantitative	Peptide EIA	ORF1, ORF2, ORF3 (peptide synthesizer)	IgG IgM	Low (15–57) Mod?	Low–high (84–100) Mod?	Very high
Native[c]	Blocking	Qualitative or semiquantitative	IF microscopy	HEVAg (frozen liver)	Total	Mod?	High?	Mod
	Direct	Semiquantitative	IEM	HEV particles (feces, bile, or liver)	Total IgM	High? High?	High? Mod?	Very low

[a] All solid-phase methods, except for traditional IEM (immune complexes formed in suspension); in solid-phase IEM, grids are coated with protein A, anti-IgG, or anti-IgM to capture immune complexes (36). "Mosaic" polypeptide EIA uses a bacterial protein in which five HEV epitopes (three representing ORF2 and one each representing ORF3 of HEV strains Mexico 86 and Burma 82) are inserted (30). Quantitative data for sensitivity and specificity are from Mast et al. (54); qualitative estimates are based on other studies (3–5, 17, 20, 29, 30, 49, 58, 60, 72, 75, 79, 81, 87). Mod, moderate. It appears that certain assays based on capsid protein (ORF2 protein EIA, mosaic polypeptide EIA, IEM) are the most sensitive (30, 54, 75, 79, 81). Similarly, a Western blot assay with reagent ORF2 protein appeared to be more sensitive than one with ORF3 protein (33). Sensitivity and specificity for detecting IgM depend on assay configuration; e.g., if test sera are overdiluted, the assay will be insensitive during the acute phase, and if they are underdiluted, the assay may yield a positive result long after infection (a biologically true-positive, clinically false-positive result) (26, 60, 87).

[b] None of the assays has detected reactivity during infections with other hepatitis viruses or during other liver diseases. However, the specificity of recDNA-based assays is not completely understood: reactivity has been detected in healthy individuals from areas of nonendemicity and where epidemics of hepatitis E have not been reported (54, 62, 72). Thus, PPV will vary greatly and will be very low in low-prevalence populations. However, identification of infections with "US" strains of HEV may lead to different concepts (47, 56, 68).

[c] Technical capability and reagent antigens are available at a few research institutions. HEVAg-containing liver tissue is usually from experimentally infected cynomolgus monkeys. IF microscopy also uses fluorescein-conjugated anti-HEV IgG as a reagent; a few convalescent-phase sera have been identified as good sources of anti-HEV IgG (45, 51).

COLLECTION, TRANSPORT, AND STORAGE OF SPECIMENS

If a diagnostic assay becomes widely available, acute-phase serum (or perhaps plasma) will probably be the necessary and sufficient specimen. For now, a general rule for suspected hepatitis E is to collect specimens early and often. Storage should be as cold as possible, avoiding freezes and thaws. Preillness specimens are ideal if exposed contacts are identified. These approaches are recommended because (i) levels of anti-HEV are usually highest before convalescence, (ii) HEV may be labile and is predominantly excreted at very low concentrations during early illness, and (iii) clinical specimens are needed for validating research methods. For transportation, solid CO_2 (dry ice, −70°C) is usually the most practical freezing medium. The vapor phase of liquid N_2 (−120°C) is preferred for specimens suspected of containing HEV (19). Biohazard identification labels should be used on packages thought to contain HEV (feces and preacute- or acute-phase sera) or other agents of disease. U.S.-bound shipments of HEV need an importation permit from the CDC.

Acute-phase serum is often the only available specimen. Preexposure serum is rarely stored but might be part of an institutional collection (5) or obtained before travel. Serum collected during convalescence can be useful for detecting anti-HEV IgG. Storage at 4°C is probably acceptable for several days, and storage at −20°C will preserve anti-HEV, but ≤−70°C should be used when viremia is suspected. If a specimen is collected for testing by the CDC (see "Assays for Detecting Anti-HEV"), >1 ml of serum should be stored in a plastic cryovial for overnight shipment on ice packs (4°C).

Feces should be collected early in the disease, at least during the first week of jaundice. Specimens should be stored at ≤−70°C; −120°C is preferred for specimens suspected of containing HEV (19). Lyophilization preserves HEV particles (74), but its effects on particle concentration and infectivity are not known.

Liver biopsy is rarely indicated during hepatitis E. If tissue is available (because of appropriate indications or death), virus or HEVAg may be detectable (48, 51). Obstructive histopathologic changes (see "Symptoms and Signs") would support a diagnosis of hepatitis E. Tissue should be kept at 4°C by perfusion with iced saline and processed quickly. For detecting virus, tissue should be cut into cubes of ≤0.5 cm^3, immediately frozen, and stored at ≤−70°C; −120°C is preferred. For immunofluorescence (IF) microscopy, tissue cubes should be placed in frozen-tissue embedding medium and then stored at ≤−70°C. For light or electron microscopy, standard fixation methods should be used (51, 75).

ASSAYS FOR DETECTING ANTI-HEV

Tests for the diagnosis of acute hepatitis E, if they become readily available in the United States, will probably detect anti-HEV IgM in acute-phase serum or plasma by use of recDNA-based polypeptide antigens in an enzyme immunoassay (EIA) format. EIAs that use antigens based on the prototype Burmese and Mexican HEV strains are sold elsewhere (Fig. 2 and 5). Alternatively, certain IgG reactivities that appear to be acute-phase specific (24, 49) might be useful for diagnosis. Several assay formats have been used for the qualitative detection of anti-HEV IgG, IgM, or IgA; semiquantitative titers have been determined by serial 4- or 10-fold dilution of test serum (Table 2). The clinical utility of any IgM assay is highly dependent on its ability to yield positive results at the presentation of illness and negative results after a reasonably short period of convalescence; such performance, which respectively and partially measures clinical sensitivity and specificity, has not been extensively characterized for any anti-HEV IgM assay. Anti-HEV IgG EIA results from patients, especially in seroprevalence studies, must be interpreted with caution because positive results do not indicate when infection occurred and may not be clinically specific; negative results could be clinically false, with anti-HEV having waned to levels that are no longer detectable by one or more assay formats (54, 60, 62, 72) (see "Epidemiology" and "Interpretation and Reporting of Test Results"). Older methods that use native HEVAg are valuable but are cumbersome and are performed at only a few research institutions.

The Food and Drug Administration has not approved any HEV assays for use in the United States, and I do not know of any in-house anti-HEV assays (developed and validated by a clinical laboratory for the population that it serves). recDNA-based EIA testing for anti-HEV is available without charge at the CDC (see "Collection, Transport, and Storage of Specimens"); "research-use-only" results cannot be legally used for diagnosis or management of patients (53). For further information, please contact the Hepatitis Branch, CDC, by calling (404) 639-3048 or sending a fax message to (404) 639-1538.

As understanding of HEV prevalence (particularly with regard to genotype-specific seroreactivity) increases and as data accumulate for rapid assays, it might be appropriate to consider two-step testing (like that used for detecting antibodies to hepatitis C virus, human immunodeficiency virus, and *Borrelia burgdorferi*) in settings where the likelihood of HEV infection is low. Typically, the first step is chosen for rapidity and high sensitivity, while the second, more clinically specific, step is chosen to increase positive predictive value (PPV). Unless the clinical specificity of the second step approaches 100%, its results should be considered supplemental rather than confirmatory. For detecting anti-HEV, the first step would almost certainly be an EIA. Second-step candidates would include Western blotting, IF blocking, immune electron microscopy (IEM), and reactivity blocking ("neutralization") EIAs for anti-HEV and, for acute-phase testing, assays for HEV RNA.

Assays Based on recDNA Technology

Recent efforts have yielded EIAs in which solid-phase reagent antigens bind anti-HEV in diluted test serum; binding is then detected by enzyme-labeled antibodies to human γ chains or IgG, μ chains or IgM, or IgA (17). Solid phases include microtiter plates and Western blot strips. Most antigens include the C termini of proteins encoded by ORF2 and ORF3 (Fig. 2). ORF2 antigens appear to yield higher sensitivity than those from ORF3, especially for detecting IgM (33, 87) or convalescent-phase IgG (54). ORF1 antigens have the potential to distinguish anti-HEV induced by an infection from anti-HEV induced by a nonreplicating vaccine (40, 60). Detailed procedures are not described below because commercially available kits include instructions, research methods change, and all assays use standard EIA techniques. Because specificity and sensitivity have not been fully established, seroepidemiologic concepts based on these assay results, especially for anti-HEV IgG, may not be accurate (54, 62, 72).

ORF2 Protein EIA

ORF2 protein EIAs detect anti-HEV IgM and IgG by use of a reagent antigen(s) of 55 to 75 kDa expressed in baculovirus-infected cells from complete or 5′-truncated ORF2 (Fig. 2) (50, 79, 81, 89). Testing of sera and plasma from experimentally infected primates demonstrated a high correlation with IEM and sensitivity higher than that of polypeptide EIAs (79, 81). Temporal patterns of anti-HEV responses during outbreaks were similar to those detected by polypeptide EIAs, but IgG reactivity increased (as a geometric mean titer) during the first 2 weeks of the acute phase and then persisted (3, 14, 54). These assays appear to be at least as accurate as any other format for detecting anti-HEV (Table 2) (54) and can probably detect IgM and IgG antibodies developed during human infection with the "US" strains of HEV (56).

Polypeptide EIA

Polypeptide EIAs use a reagent antigen of HEV polypeptide fused with a bacterial protein. For example, kits with ORF2 and ORF3 antigens are available in Asia from Diagnostic Biotechnology (Genelabs) and in Europe from Abbott Laboratories; the former use HEV polypeptides 3-2(M), 4-2(M), and 4-2(B), while the latter use SG3 and 8-5 (M and B designate sequences representing HEV strains Mexico 86 and Burma 82, respectively) (Table 2 and Fig. 2). Antigen SG3 appeared to increase the sensitivity for detecting anti-HEV IgM or IgG (87). In general, anti-HEV IgM and IgA were less frequently detected than anti-HEV IgG, which usually persisted but at lower concentrations than during the acute phase (17, 58, 87). The HEV strain US 95-infected patient developed IgG, but not IgM, against polypeptides representing Asian-African and Mexican strains (47).

Western Blot

Western blots (immunoblots) have been used in research studies for detecting anti-HEV IgG and IgM (37, 49, 65). For reagent antigen, most have used electrophoretically separated lysates of genetically engineered cells that express one HEV polypeptide, usually representing ORF2 and often fused with a bacterial protein. Two Western blot assays for anti-HEV IgG did not appear to perform as accurately as ORF2 EIAs in a blind study (54). Western blot sensitivity for convalescent-phase IgG decreased when certain ORF2 protein epitopes were present but not in a reactive conformation (49); such proteins might be useful for detecting acute-phase-specific anti-HEV.

Peptide EIA

Peptide EIAs have been developed by use of synthetic peptides with sequences that are included in the 3-2 and 4-2 antigens or that correspond to putative nonstructural proteins or central portions of the ORF2 protein (Fig. 2). These assays identified antibodies, predominantly IgG, in sera from geographically diverse HEV infections; results correlated well with those from Western blotting and IF microscopy (29, 40, 41, 82). Peptides might enable discrimination among infections with African-Asian, Mexican, and "US" strains by exploiting sequence differences in the C termini of ORF2 and ORF3 proteins. For example, EIAs with peptides representing antigens 4-2 (Fig. 2) and 3-2 with a 6-amino-acid, N-terminal extension were developed: in two patients infected with "US" strains of HEV, IgM antibodies from both and IgG antibodies from one were detected only with the peptides that represented strain US 95 sequences (41, 68).

Assays with Native HEV Antigens as Reagents

Available quantities of HEV have been insufficient for rapid, practical assays. IEM and IF microscopy were crucial to early understanding of HEV infections and are specific when correctly performed (Table 2). However, each requires reagents that are difficult to obtain, a special microscope, training, and intensive labor. IEM and IF microscopy have been valuable for epidemiology, for studying experimental infections (45, 75), and for supplementing selected results from recDNA-based EIAs.

IEM

IEM involves mixing of test serum and reagent virus to form immune complexes of antibody-coated virus particles. The anti-HEV concentration can be semiquantitatively determined by rating the coating of antibodies (Fig. 1) or by serial 10-fold dilution (75). While "staple-like" coating suggests the presence of IgM (5), the antibody class can be more accurately and rapidly identified by solid-phase IEM, in which immune complexes are captured on grids coated with anti-IgM, anti-IgG, or *Staphylococcus aureus* protein A (36). Please see references 5 and 73 for more details.

IF Microscopy

IF microscopy detects anti-HEV in a blocking format: antibodies in test sera interfere with the binding of fluorescein-conjugated anti-HEV IgG to reagent HEVAg in frozen liver tissue (45). Sera are rated as 0 (no blocking), ± (partial), or + (blocking) (75), or a titer is determined by serial twofold dilution. Results are obtained more rapidly than with IEM.

EIA and Radioimmunoassay

EIAs and radioimmunoassays have been described (with reagent HEV particles from feces, bile, or cell cultures) but not reproduced (7, 73).

Neutralization

Neutralization of HEV has been observed by mixing test serum and reagent HEV before inoculating cell cultures (55, 71) or susceptible monkeys (77). Available evidence suggests that these systems detect neutralizing antibodies, at least some of which are directed against epitopes expressed by the ORF2 protein. Although neither system is practical (in particular, cultures must be kept for approximately 2 weeks before they are assayed by amplification of any replicated HEV RNA), they may lead to a valuable assay for antibodies that correlate with immunity.

ASSAYS FOR DETECTING HEV

As noted above, HEV is a distinct pathogen. Its nucleotide and amino acid sequences are unique among those that are known. Nonspecific amplification of DNA from viruses or other sources has not been reported with HEV oligonucleotides. Similarly, HEV antigens are not known to cross-react with antigens of other agents.

HEV concentrations in feces, serum, liver, and bile appear to be highest before and during the first week of jaundice (Fig. 4). Such concentrations are usually too low, however, for detection of viral antigens by immunoassay or HEV RNA by direct hybridization (51, 57, 68), and there are no practical methods for isolating the virus in cell cultures. There are no commercial assays for detecting HEV. It is unlikely that any such assays will be developed because they are difficult to develop and perform, NPV is low, and assays for anti-HEV IgM are promising (see Table 5), unless two-step testing is necessary (see "Assays for Detecting Anti-HEV") or recent findings lead to the recognition of HEV as an important human or veterinary pathogen in developed countries (47, 56, 68). Among current research methods (see Table 3), preferred assays detect HEV via reverse transcription of RNA and amplification of cDNA by PCR.

Detection of HEV RNA, HEV Particles, or HEVAg

PCR

PCR is analytically sensitive and appears to be analytically and clinically specific, but its clinical sensitivity is only moderate because HEV concentrations are low and because most viral replication and excretion take place before the onset of jaundice (Fig. 4 and Table 3). HEV RNA has been detected in feces, serum, bile, and liver during natural or experimental infections (11, 20, 51, 57, 60, 76, 83) and in cell cultures (7, 55, 71). When serial fecal specimens from an outbreak were assayed by PCR, HEV was detected in 29% of 39 specimens (representing 5 of 11 patients) and most often within the first 7 days of icterus but as late as 16 days (57); similarly, 46% of 166 single fecal specimens had detectable HEV RNA, with a higher yield during the first week of illness and when specimens were transported to the laboratory at −120°C (19). In a study of 67 patients with sporadic hepatitis E, HEV was detected more often in serum than in feces (93 versus 67% of patients) and more frequently during the second week of illness than during the first week (20). Viremia usually follows a temporal pattern like that of HEV excretion in feces (69) but has been detected as long as 39 to 112 days after the onset of illness (20, 59). Occasionally, acute-phase feces or sera have had detectable HEV RNA without anti-HEV IgM, so PCR can be used to identify HEV infections in seronegative patients (19, 20, 52). However, isolated PCR-positive results should always be regarded carefully, even when the possibility of in-laboratory contamination is low.

RNA has been purified from specimens by several techniques, including chemical extraction (phenol or guanidinium isothiocyanate and phenol), adsorption (silica powder), or affinity capture (4, 11, 20, 51, 57). In one version of affinity capture PCR (AC/PCR), microcentrifuge tubes are coated with anti-human IgM, washed, incubated with reagent (acute-phase serum), washed, incubated with 100 μl of 5% (wt/vol) fecal suspension, and then washed before PCR (11). A similar method, in which immune complexes are formed and then captured, yielded results similar to those obtained with chemically extracted RNA (57).

Many different oligonucleotides have been successfully used for priming the amplification of HEV cDNA. The primer sets shown in Table 4, which represent conserved sequences, have sensitively detected African, Asian, and

TABLE 3 Detecting HEV[a]

Method	Detects	Specimens	HEV reagent(s) or method	Analytical sensitivity[b,c]	Practicality[c]
PCR (or AC/PCR)	HEV RNA	Feces, serum, bile, liver	Oligonucleotides (for AC/PCR, serum with anti-HEV)	Very high	Moderate
IEM	HEV particles	Feces, bile, liver	Paired sera: negative (preinoculation) and positive (infection) for anti-HEV	Low	Very low
IF microscopy	HEVAg	Liver	Fluorescein-conjugated anti-HEV IgG	Low?	Low
Animal inoculation[d]	Infectious HEV	Feces, bile, liver[e]	Assay for HEV or anti-HEV	High	Very low

[a] All methods appear to be analytically and clinically specific for HEV; thus, PPV is very high when illness is consistent with hepatitis E. PCR (reverse transcription followed by amplification of cDNA) is the only amplification technique that has been reported for HEV. AC/PCR has been described in several studies (11, 51, 57, 83).

[b] A total of $10^{6.7}$ genomes, as detected by PCR, corresponded to 10^6 cynomolgus monkey 50% infectious doses of HEV Pakistan 87 (81); a similar method detected as few as 20 molecules of cloned HEV Mexico 86 cDNA (57). Concentrations of HEV in serum are generally thought to be lower than those in feces; one patient was reported to have 5×10^3 genomes per ml of serum (68). The analytical sensitivity of IEM is $\approx 10^6$ particles/ml, much lower than that of AC/PCR (51, 57). The rating for IF microscopy is based on few data comparing it with PCR (51).

[c] Clinical sensitivity and NPV are low because HEV replication wanes or ceases in many patients before jaundice develops. Practicality reflects specimen availability, technical difficulty, cost, and NPV.

[d] Cell culture isolation has been reported (7, 28, 35, 55, 71) but, even if confirmed, will be impractical unless nearly all strains propagate and unless rapid methods are developed for detecting replication.

[e] Potential sources of infectious HEV include serum (induced hepatitis in chimpanzees and tamarins, but these animals were not tested for evidence of HEV replication; Purcell et al. [cited in reference 73]) and kidney (monkey kidney was reported as a culture inoculum [7]).

TABLE 4 Oligonucleotide primers for detecting HEV RNA via synthesis and amplification of cDNA[a]

Region	Type of primer[b]	Orientation	Nucleotide positions	Sequence (5′ to 3′)[c]	Amplicon (bp)	Reported use(s)
ORF2	Outer	Sense	6578–6597	GC**C** GAG TA**T** GAC CAG **T**CC AC	530	Sensitive detection and sequencing of African, Asian, and Mexican strains (no data for amplification of "US" strains) (57, 83, 87)
		Antisense	7127–7108	A**CA** ACT CCC G**A**G TTT TAC C**C**		
	Inner	Sense	6650–6668	AAT GT**T** GC**G** AC**C** GG**C** GC**G** C	448	
		Antisense	7097–7078	TAA G**G**C GCT GAA G**C**T CAG C**G**		
ORF2	Outer	Sense	6578–6600	GC**C** GAG TAY GAC CAG **T**CC AC**T** TA	530	Detection and sequencing of porcine US strain (56)
		Antisense	7127–7105	A**YA** ACT CCC G**A**G TTT TAC C**C**A CC		
	Inner	Sense	6645–6667	T**G** G**G**K AAT GTW GC**G** ACY GG**C** GC**G**	441	
		Antisense	7085–7063	G**C**T CAG C**G**A **C**AG TWG A**C**T GRA A**A**		
ORF1-ORF3-ORF2	Outer	Sense	4989–5009	**T**GG ***G***CT CGT **T**CA TAA CCT **G**AT	339	Sequencing of North African and Central Asian strains (16)
		Antisense	5327–5307	GGT TGG TTG GAT GAA TAT AGG		
	Inner	Sense	4996–5019	GT **T**CA TAA CCT **G**AT TGG CAT GCT **A**	312	
		Antisense	5307–5284	G GGA **TT**G CGA AGG GCT GAG AAT CA		
ORF1	Outer	Sense	34–54	GCC CAT CAG TTT ATT AAG GCT	342	Detection of viremia in Egyptians (nested) (69) and Americans (outer primers) and sequencing of "US" strains (68)
		Antisense	375–358	CTG AAC ATC ***C***CG ***G***CC ***G***AC		
	Inner	Sense	55–74	CCT GGC AT**C** ACT ACT GC**T** AT	266	
		Antisense	320–301	TCA TTT ATT GAG CGG GGA TG		

[a] Selected from among many that have been successful for reverse transcription and amplification (via PCR, to date) because they represent conserved sequences among African, Asian, and Mexican strains and because they enabled sensitive detection of African-Asian and Mexican strains or detection of "US" strains. It is not known if any primers amplify all HEV strains with a sensitivity appropriate for clinical use. Methods should be optimized, with particular attention to annealing temperatures, e.g., 1 or 2 min at 42°C (16, 56) versus 30 s at 53°C (68). Nucleotide positions and sequences are relative to those of the HEV Burma 82 sense (positive-strand) genome or its antisense complement (70) (GenBank accession no. M73218).

[b] Although each set has been used for nested amplification, with outer antisense primers also having been used for cDNA synthesis, I would avoid two rounds of PCR in a clinical laboratory, instead performing single-round amplification followed by direct hybridization with a labeled probe. No such methods have been reported, but probes were described for hybridization after nested PCR with the first set of ORF2 primers (nt 6782 to 6801, 5′ TCT TTC TGG GAG GCA GGC AC 3′; the four underlined nucleotides are different in HEV strain US 95) (87) or with the ORF1 primers (nt 133 to 278) (69). An inner primer might also work as a probe.

[c] HEV Burma 82 sequences, with two exceptions: (i) ORF1-ORF3-ORF2 primers represent HEV Pakistan 87, so that the outer sense fourth base (G) differs (76), and (ii) bold italicized bases in the ORF1 outer antisense primer differ (68). Bold, underlined bases are those known to differ in HEV strain US 95 (68). The two sets of ORF2 primers are nearly identical, except for the inner antisense primers (which overlap for 8 nt) and, in the second set, for degenerate positions (designated as Y for C and T, K for G and T, W for A and T, and R for A and G).

Mexican strains (16, 57, 87) or successfully amplified "US" strains (47, 56, 68), but it is not yet known if any particular set will amplify all HEV strains with the consistent sensitivity desired for clinical use. The hypervariable region of ORF1 (Fig. 2) should be avoided, except for studying sequence variability (11).

IEM

IEM enables visual identification of HEV in feces, bile, or liver but is insensitive and requires reagent sera and a trained, patient observer (5, 12, 51, 74, 75). It is highly specific when the microscopist knows how to recognize typical HEV particles and when reagent paired sera are used. The morphologic characteristics of HEV are not sufficiently distinct for distinguishing it from other viruses and objects likely to be present, such as HAV and other picornaviruses, Norwalk and other caliciviruses, parvoviruses, and bacteriophages (61, 73). To identify HEV with certainty, IEM must be performed with paired sera (Fig. 1 and Table 3). A solid-phase method, which uses grids coated with protein A or anti-immunoglobulin to capture immune complexes (see above), appeared to be more sensitive than traditional IEM (36).

IF Microscopy

IF microscopy with labeled anti-HEV IgG reagent detects and can semiquantitatively estimate the concentration of HEVAg in frozen liver tissue (45, 51). HEVAg have not been characterized, but their presence coincides with HEV that is detectable in liver and bile by IEM and PCR (48, 51). In addition, fluorescence can be blocked by adsorption of the reagent IgG with C2, a recDNA-based ORF2 protein (Fig. 2) (63).

EIA and Radioimmunoassay

EIAs and radioimmunoassays with labeled anti-HEV reagent have been reported but not confirmed (7, 60, 73).

Detection of Infectious HEV

There are no routine methods for isolating HEV in clinical laboratories. Researchers usually detect and propagate HEV by inoculating susceptible animals. Reports of isolating HEV from feces or bile in cell cultures suggested that it was present at a low level and devoid of CPE (7, 55, 71, 73); culture methods must be enhanced to become practical.

CLINICAL LABORATORY TESTING

Precise conclusions about a particular patient may not be possible with current assays unless their performance is carefully established by the testing laboratory. The likelihood of identifying an acute, recent, or past infection may be enhanced, however, if several concepts are considered. First, detection of HEV in a clinical specimen nearly always indicates acute infection (predominantly late incubation or first week of jaundice), but a negative result does not rule out hepatitis E because many patients do not have detectable HEV. Second, anti-HEV IgM (or IgA) identifies acute or recent infection, usually within 6 to 9 months of exposure. The absence of these antibodies does not rule out acute hepatitis E because many patients in outbreaks have had negative results with current polypeptide EIAs. Third, total anti-HEV or anti-HEV IgG are the only viral markers that currently are detectable in nearly all acutely infected patients, but they do not define when infection occurred. Anti-HEV levels are usually highest during acute hepatitis or early convalescence, so seroconversion (increase in antibody concentration between acute and late convalescent phases) rarely occurs. In addition, the absence of anti-HEV does not rule out past infection because IgG directed against certain reagent HEV antigens can decline to undetectable levels. Fourth, because the specificity of recDNA-based assays for anti-HEV is not completely understood, a positive anti-HEV result should be interpreted with caution for a low-risk individual, such as an American with no history of travel to a region of endemicity. Some of these concepts may change as data accumulate.

To make a diagnosis of HEV infection, it must be suspected (47). For patients in the United States, hepatitis E is suggested by two travel scenarios: a visit to a region of endemicity when previous exposure to HEV was unlikely or emigration from a country where HEV is endemic. Hepatitis E is more likely if a hepatitis outbreak was occurring in the region of travel.

Testing Algorithms

Testing should be performed on the basis of clinical indications: diagnosis of acute hepatitis E, diagnosis of hepatitis E during convalescence, or past infection with HEV. Criteria from the CDC are appropriate for considering if a specimen should be tested for anti-HEV: the patient should have had a discrete onset of illness with jaundice or with a serum ALT concentration at least 2.5-fold higher than the upper reference-range value and negative results for anti-HAV IgM, anti-HBc (hepatitis B core) IgM, and anti-HCV in acute-phase serum (53). Additional history and laboratory data can exclude other causes of hepatitis, including microorganisms (such as HDV, Epstein-Barr virus, cytomegalovirus, dengue viruses, yellow fever virus, leptospiras, or *Coxiella burnetii*), drugs (such as ethanol, anesthetics, or antimicrobial agents), tumor, autoimmunity, or gallbladder disease.

For diagnosis of acute hepatitis E, serum and feces are most likely to be available. It is more practical to test serum than feces, particularly because it is more likely to yield diagnostic results. An accurate assay for anti-HEV IgM is the method of choice: positive results usually indicate acute HEV infection (supplemental testing is probably not necessary), but patients with acute hepatitis E have been anti-HEV IgM negative (Table 5). Alternatively, serum or feces can be assayed for HEV RNA by PCR in a laboratory with extensive experience in amplification techniques (to minimize the possibility of a false-positive result due to contamination): PPV is very high but NPV is lower than that for anti-HEV IgM assays. Although testing for both anti-HEV and HEV RNA provides the most information (Tables 5 and 6), it is more practical to test first for anti-HEV and then for HEV RNA if anti-HEV IgM is not detected. *For diagnosis of hepatitis E during convalescence,* serum should be tested in an assay for anti-HEV IgG that detects long-lasting antibodies (54); depending on the interval since illness, anti-HEV IgM or, rarely, HEV RNA might be detectable (20, 59). Testing of paired sera is unlikely to yield evidence of seroconversion unless a preexposure sample happens to be available; to compare semiquantitative titers of anti-HEV IgG, each specimen must be tested with the same assay, preferably by the same laboratory and in the same run. *For diagnosis of past infection,* serum should be tested with an assay for long-lasting anti-HEV IgG.

Interpretation and Reporting of Test Results

Interpretation is not difficult when a patient has jaundice, biochemical evidence of hepatitis, and detectable HEV and anti-HEV IgM: the diagnosis is icteric hepatitis E (Tables 5 and 6). Similar data without jaundice could represent an-

TABLE 5 Interpretation of clinical signs and laboratory data for acute hepatitis and other manifestations of HEV infection (African, Asian, or Mexican strains)[a]

Diagnostic indication	Jaundice	Elevated ALT	Virologic findings	PPV	NPV
Icteric hepatitis E[b]	+	+	Anti-HEV IgM, acute phase (majority of patients) *OR*	Moderate to high	Moderate
			HEV in acute-phase feces, serum, liver, or bile *OR*	Very high	Very low
			Increase in anti-HEV concentration during late acute phase or during convalescence (rare finding) *OR*	High	Low
			Anti-HEV during acute phase or during convalescence *AND* not detected preexposure (rare specimen)	High	Very high
Anicteric hepatitis E[c]	–	+	Same as icteric		
Acute subclinical infection[c]	–	–	HEV in feces or serum ± anti-HEV IgM	High	Low
Recent infection[c]	–	–	Anti-HEV IgM	Moderate to high[b]	Low
Possible acute hepatitis E[d]	+	+	Acute-phase anti-HEV, IgG or total (or IgM-like, as detected by IEM)	Low to moderate	Low
Past infection[e]	–	–	Anti-HEV, IgG or total	Low to high	Moderate

[a] Elevated ALT represents elevated serum ALT level or other biochemical evidence of hepatitis. PPV varies directly with assay specificity and with the prevalence of HEV infection in the population to which the patient belongs. NPV varies directly with assay sensitivity and inversely with prevalence. Predictive value ratings in this table reflect those in the literature, including a recent multicenter study of the performance of anti-HEV IgG assays (54). Although not yet determined, interpretation of data is likely to be similar for infections with "US" strains, especially if reagents are known to be reactive with the infecting strain (47, 56, 68).

[b] Anti-HEV IgM detected in an assay intended to detect only that analyte or by testing of the IgM fraction in an assay for total anti-HEV (5); predictive values are critically affected by assay configuration, especially with regard to a solid-phase capture reagent (usually HEV antigen or anti-μ chain) and the dilution of test serum. The serum IgA response to HEV may be similar to that of IgM (17). The method for detecting HEV is nearly always PCR. PPV is greatly affected by the quality assurance program of a laboratory (i.e., ability to prevent specimen contamination from amplicons or other specimens); for NPV, see Table 3, footnote c.

[c] Could represent prodrome, so patient should be monitored for later progression to icteric hepatitis E.

[d] PPV varies with assay specificity and with population seroprevalence; diagnosis is more likely if there is no evidence of other causes of hepatitis and if illness follows first exposure to HEV.

[e] Cannot determine when infection occurred. For low to high PPV, see footnote *d*. For moderate NPV, the absence of anti-HEV IgG does not mean that an individual was never infected because anti-HEV may wane to undetectable levels, particularly with certain assay formats (see Table 2 and text) (54).

icteric hepatitis E or subclinical infection, depending on the presence of other symptoms and signs. A patient with only anti-HEV IgM most likely has acute hepatitis E but could have had a recent infection with a persistent IgM response followed by a second liver disease. Possible acute hepatitis E is represented by anti-HEV (total, IgG, or IgM-like, as determined by IEM) only when the patient has a low probability of past exposure and no evidence for another agent; this finding alone is less likely to indicate acute hepatitis E for patients from areas of endemicity. In an apparently healthy individual with a history of NANB hepatitis, detection only of total anti-HEV or anti-HEV IgG may represent past infection; however, this result could also represent an incubating HEV infection or a false-positive result. Finally, acute and recent infections may not have detectable HEV or anti-HEV IgM (but are almost certain to have detectable total anti-HEV or anti-HEV IgG), and past infections may not have any HEV markers. Each laboratory should prepare result-reporting text (Table 6) according to the population that it serves and the performance of its assays.

TABLE 6 Reporting of results

Specimen	Assay for:	Report if assay result is: Positive	Report if assay result is: Negative
Serum	Anti-HEV IgM	Anti-HEV IgM detected: consistent with current or recent HEV infection	Anti-HEV IgM not detected: consider other causes of hepatitis; if HEV infection strongly suspected, test for anti-HEV IgG, HEV RNA, or IgM to another HEV genotype
	Anti-HEV IgG	Anti-HEV IgG detected: evidence of infection but cannot determine when infection occurred; if acute hepatitis E suspected, consider testing for anti-HEV or HEV RNA	Anti-HEV IgG not detected: no evidence of infection (with HEV genotypes represented by reagent antigens in the assay); if acute hepatitis E suspected, consider testing for anti-HEV IgM or HEV RNA
Serum, feces, or liver	HEV RNA	HEV RNA detected: evidence of current infection	HEV RNA not detected but cannot exclude current HEV infection

EVIDENCE FOR ADDITIONAL AGENTS OF ET HEPATITIS

In the United States, a significant proportion of sporadic hepatitis is "non-ABCDE"; frequent association with HEV "US" strains is not likely because anti-HEV IgG, regardless of the infecting strain, should have been detected by the assays that identified the cases as "non-E" (1, 47, 56, 68). In other settings, where enteric transmission occurs regularly, many patients have hepatitis but no evidence for acute infection with known viruses, including HEV or HAV. Examples have been reported as sporadic disease in Egypt, Ethiopia, India, Peru, Saudi Arabia, Tajikistan, and Uzbekistan (32, 38). A Siberian epidemic may have been caused by an antigenically distinct HEV-like agent (27), but another candidate, with the suggested name of hepatitis F virus, was not subsequently recognized as an agent of ET hepatitis. While some such disease might be identified as hepatitis E by highly sensitive assays, Arankalle et al. (3) used an ORF2 protein EIA to conclude that a 1987 epidemic in the Andaman Islands, India, was non-A, non-E. Such data will probably lead to the discovery of at least one more agent of ET hepatitis or a new serotype of HAV or HEV.

This chapter is dedicated to Mikhail Balayan (discoverer of HEV, distinguished virologist, gracious host, and friend) and to Alice and Robert Ticehurst (who introduced me to microbiology). I thank Mike Balayan, George Dawson, Howard Fields, Paul Kwo, Charlie Longer, Eric Mast, X. J. Meng, Bob Purcell, George Schlauder, Sergei Tsarev, Hélène van Cuyck-Gandré, and Patrice Yarbough for unpublished data, manuscripts, or helpful discussions. I also thank the colleagues at the Food and Drug Administration and Johns Hopkins for continuing to educate me in laboratory medicine and, in particular, Steve Gutman for enthusiastic support. Expert technical contributions at Johns Hopkins were most appreciated: clerical work by Jean Mehsling, photography for Fig. 1 by Norm Barker, graphics for Fig. 4 by Rick Tracy (and for Fig. 3 by Tom O'Brien, a generous slidemaker at CDC), and sequence analysis for Fig. 5 by Oliver Laeyendecker.

REFERENCES

1. **Alter, M. J., M. Gallagher, T. T. Morris, L. A. Moyer, E. L. Meeks, K. Krawczynski, J. P. Kim, and H. S. Margolis.** 1997. Acute non-A-E hepatitis in the United States and the role of hepatitis G virus infection. Sentinel Counties Viral Hepatitis Study Team. *N. Engl. J. Med.* **336:** 741–746.
2. **Anonymous.** 1993. Hepatitis E among U.S. travelers, 1989–1992. *Morbid. Mortal. Weekly Rep.* **42:**1–4.
3. **Arankalle, V. A., M. S. Chadha, S. A. Tsarev, S. U. Emerson, A. R. Risbud, K. Banerjee, and R. H. Purcell.** 1994. Seroepidemiology of water-borne hepatitis in India and evidence for a third enterically-transmitted hepatitis agent. *Proc. Natl. Acad. Sci. USA* **91:**3428–3432.
4. **Arankalle, V. A., L. P. Chobe, J. Jha, M. S. Chadha, K. Banerjee, M. O. Favorov, T. Kalinina, and H. Fields.** 1993. Aetiology of acute sporadic non-A, non-B hepatitis in India. *J. Med. Virol.* **40:**121–125.
5. **Arankalle, V. A., J. Ticehurst, M. A. Sreenivasan, A. Z. Kapikian, H. Popper, K. M. Pavri, and R. H. Purcell.** 1988. Aetiological association of a virus-like particle with enterically transmitted non-A, non-B hepatitis. *Lancet* **i:** 550–554.
6. **Arankalle, V. A., S. A. Tsarev, M. S. Chadha, D. W. Alling, S. U. Emerson, K. Banerjee, and R. H. Purcell.** 1995. Age-specific prevalence of antibodies to hepatitis A and E viruses in Pune, India, 1982 and 1992. *J. Infect. Dis.* **171:**447–450.
7. **Balayan, M. S.** 1993. Hepatitis E virus infection in Europe: regional situation regarding laboratory diagnosis and epidemiology. *Clin. Diagn. Virol.* **1:**1–9.
8. **Balayan, M. S.** 1997. Epidemiology of hepatitis E virus infection. *J. Viral Hepatitis* **4:**155–165.
9. **Balayan, M. S., A. G. Andzhaparidze, S. S. Savinskaya, E. S. Ketiladze, D. M. Braginsky, A. P. Savinov, and V. F. Poleschuk.** 1983. Evidence for a virus in non-A, non-B hepatitis transmitted via the fecal-oral route. *Intervirology* **20:**23–31.
10. **Berke, T., B. Golding, X. Jiang, D. W. Cubitt, M. Wolfaardt, A. W. Smith, and D. O. Matson.** 1997. Phylogenetic analysis of the caliciviruses. *J. Med. Virol.* **52:** 419–424.
11. **Bi, S. L., M. A. Purdy, K. A. McCaustland, H. S. Margolis, and D. W. Bradley.** 1993. The sequence of hepatitis E virus isolated directly from a single source during an outbreak in China. *Virus Res.* **28:**233–247.
12. **Bradley, D., A. Andjaparidze, E. H. Cook, Jr., K. McCaustland, M. Balayan, H. Stetler, O. Velazquez, B. Robertson, C. Humphrey, M. Kane, and I. Weisfuse.** 1988. Aetiological agent of enterically transmitted non-A, non-B hepatitis. *J. Gen. Virol.* **69:**731–738.
13. **Bradley, D. W.** 1990. Hepatitis non-A, non-B viruses become identified as hepatitis C and E viruses. *Prog. Med. Virol.* **37:**101–135.
14. **Bryan, J. P., S. A. Tsarev, M. Iqbal, J. Ticehurst, S. Emerson, A. Ahmed, J. Duncan, A. R. Rafiqui, I. A. Malik, R. H. Purcell, and L. J. Legters.** 1994. Epidemic hepatitis E in Pakistan: patterns of serologic response and evidence that antibody to hepatitis E virus protects against disease. *J. Infect. Dis.* **170:**517–521.
15. **Cacopardo, B., R. Russo, W. Preiser, F. Benanti, G. Brancati, and A. Nunnari.** 1997. Acute hepatitis E in Catania (eastern Sicily) 1980–1994. The role of hepatitis E virus. *Infection* **25:**313–316.
16. **Chatterjee, R., S. Tsarev, J. Pillot, P. Coursaget, S. U. Emerson, and R. H. Purcell.** 1997. African strains of hepatitis E virus that are distinct from Asian strains. *J. Med. Virol.* **53:**139–144.
17. **Chau, K. H., G. J. Dawson, K. M. Bile, L. O. Magnius, M. H. Sjogren, and I. K. Mushahwar.** 1993. Detection of IgA class antibody to hepatitis E virus in serum samples from patients with hepatitis E virus infection. *J. Med. Virol.* **40:**334–338.
18. **Chauhan, A., J. B. Dilawari, U. Kaur, N. K. Ganguly, S. Bushnurmath, and Y. K. Chawla.** 1994. Atypical strain of hepatitis E virus (HEV) from north India. *J. Med. Virol.* **44:**22–29.
19. **Chobe, L. P., M. S. Chadha, K. Banerjee, and V. A. Arankalle.** 1997. Detection of HEV RNA in faeces by RT-PCR during the epidemics of hepatitis E in India (1976–1995). *J. Viral Hepatitis* **4:**129–133.
20. **Clayson, E. T., K. S. A. Myint, R. Snitbhan, D. W. Vaughn, B. L. Innis, L. Chan, P. Cheung, and M. P. Shrestha.** 1995. Viremia, fecal shedding, and IgM and IgG responses in patients with hepatitis E. *J. Infect. Dis.* **172:** 927–933.
21. **Clayson, E. T., M. P. Shrestha, D. W. Vaughn, R. Snitbhan, K. B. Shrestha, C. F. Longer, and B. L. Innis.** 1997. Rates of hepatitis E virus infection and disease among adolescents and adults in Kathmandu, Nepal. *J. Infect. Dis.* **176:**763–766.
22. **Clayson, E. T., R. Snitbhan, M. Ngarmpochana, D. W. Vaughn, and M. P. Shrestha.** 1996. Evidence that the hepatitis E virus (HEV) is a zoonotic virus: detection of natural infections among swine, rats, and chickens in an area endemic for human disease, p. 329–335. *In* Y. Buisson, P. Coursaget, and M. Kane (ed.), *Enterically-Transmitted Hepatitis Viruses*. La Simarre, Joué-les-Tours, France.

23. **Corwin, A. L., H. B. Khiem, E. T. Clayson, K. S. Pham, T. T. Vo, T. Y. Vu, T. T. Cao, D. Vaughn, J. Merven, T. L. Richie, M. P. Putri, J. He, R. Graham, F. S. Wignall, and K. C. Hyams.** 1996. A waterborne outbreak of hepatitis E virus transmission in southwestern Vietnam. *Am. J. Trop. Med. Hyg.* **54:**559–562.
24. **Coursaget, P., N. Depril, Y. Buisson, C. Molinie, and R. Roue.** 1994. Hepatitis type E in a French population: detection of anti-HEV by a synthetic peptide-based enzyme-linked immunosorbent assay. *Res. Virol.* **145:**51–57.
25. **Cubitt, D., D. W. Bradley, M. J. Carter, S. Chiba, M. K. Estes, L. J. Saif, F. L. Schaffer, A. W. Smith, M. J. Studdert, and H. J. Thiel.** 1995. Caliciviridae, p. 359–363. *In* F. A. Murphy, C. M. Fauquet, D. H. L. Bishop, S. A. Ghabrial, A. W. Jarvis, G. P. Martelli, M. A. Mayo, and M. D. Summers (ed.), *Virus Taxonomy: Classification and Nomenclature of Viruses. Sixth Report of the International Committee on Taxonomy of Viruses (Archives of Virology,* Supplement 10). Springer-Verlag, Vienna, Austria.
26. **Dawson, G. J., K. H. Chau, C. M. Cabal, P. O. Yarbough, G. R. Reyes, and I. K. Mushahwar.** 1992. Solid-phase enzyme-linked immunosorbent assay for hepatitis E virus IgG and IgM antibodies utilizing recombinant antigens and synthetic peptides. *J. Virol. Methods* **38:**175–186.
27. **Doroshenko, N. V., T. G. Smolina, G. K. Zairov, and V. M. Stakhanova.** 1989. Serologic proof of the existence of different types of non-A, non-B hepatitis with fecal-oral mechanism of transmission. *Vopr. Virusol.* **2:**164–167. (In Russian.)
28. **Dzagurov, G. K., V. V. Kupriianov, and M. S. Balaian.** 1997. Replication of hepatitis E virus in FRhK-4 cell culture. *Vopr. Virusol.* **42:**63–66. (In Russian.)
29. **Favorov, M. O., Y. E. Khudyakov, H. A. Fields, N. S. Khudyakova, N. Padhye, M. J. Alter, E. Mast, L. Polish, T. L. Yashina, D. M. Yarasheva, G. G. Onischenko, and H. S. Margolis.** 1994. Enzyme immunoassay for the detection of antibody to hepatitis E virus (anti-HEV) based on synthetic peptides. *J. Virol. Methods* **46:**237–250.
30. **Favorov, M. O., Y. E. Khudyakov, E. E. Mast, T. L. Yashina, C. N. Shapiro, N. S. Khudyakova, D. L. Jue, G. G. Onischenko, H. S. Margolis, and H. A. Fields.** 1996. IgM and IgG antibodies to hepatitis E virus (HEV) detected by an enzyme immunoassay based on an HEV-specific artificial recombinant mosaic protein. *J. Med. Virol.* **50:**50–58.
31. **Felsenstein, J.** 1989. PHYLIP—phylogeny inference package (version 3.56). *Cladistics* **5:**164–166.
32. **Ghabrah, T. M., G. T. Stickland, S. Tsarev, P. Yarbough, P. Farci, R. Engle, S. Emerson, and R. Purcell.** 1995. Acute viral hepatitis in Saudi Arabia: seroepidemiological analysis, risk factors, clinical manifestations, and evidence for a sixth hepatitis agent. *Clin. Infect. Dis.* **21:**621–627.
33. **He, J., A. W. Tam, P. O. Yarbough, G. R. Reyes, and M. Carl.** 1993. Expression and diagnostic utility of hepatitis E virus putative structural proteins expressed in insect cells. *J. Clin. Microbiol.* **31:**2167–2173.
34. **Huang, C.-C., D. Nguyen, J. Fernandez, K. Y. Yun, K. E. Fry, D. W. Bradley, A. W. Tam, and G. R. Reyes.** 1992. Molecular cloning and sequencing of the Mexico isolate of hepatitis E virus (HEV). *Virology* **191:**550–558.
35. **Huang, R., N. Nakazono, K. Ishii, D. Li, O. Kawamata, R. Kawaguchi, and Y. Tsukada.** 1995. Hepatitis E virus (87A strain) propagated in A549 cells. *J. Med. Virol.* **47:** 299–302.
36. **Humphrey, C. D., E. H. Cook, Jr., and D. W. Bradley.** 1990. Identification of enterically transmitted hepatitis virus particles by solid phase immune electron microscopy. *J. Virol. Methods* **29:**177–188.
37. **Hyams, K. C., M. A. Purdy, M. Kaur, M. C. McCarthy, M. A. Hussain, A. El-Tigani, K. Krawczynski, D. W. Bradley, and M. Carl.** 1992. Acute sporadic hepatitis E in Sudanese children: analysis based on a new Western blot assay. *J. Infect. Dis.* **165:**1001–1005.
38. **Hyams, K. C., P. O. Yarbough, S. Gray, J. Callahan, E. Gotuzzo, J. Gutierrez, P. B. Vasquez, C. G. Hayes, and D. M. Watts.** 1996. Hepatitis E virus infection in Peru. *Clin. Infect. Dis.* **22:**719–720.
39. **Karetnyi, Y. V., D. I. Dzhumalieva, R. K. Usmanov, I. P. Titova, Y. I. Litvak, and M. S. Balayan.** 1993. Probable involvement of rodents in the spread of hepatitis E. *J. Microbiol. Epidemiol. Immunol.* **4:**52–56.
40. **Kaur, M., K. C. Hyams, M. A. Purdy, K. Krawczynski, W. M. Ching, K. E. Fry, G. R. Reyes, D. W. Bradley, and M. Carl.** 1992. Human linear B-cell epitopes encoded by the hepatitis E virus include determinants in the RNA-dependent RNA polymerase. *Proc. Natl. Acad. Sci. USA* **89:**3855–3858.
41. **Khudyakov, Y. E., N. S. Khudyakova, D. L. Jue, T. W. Wells, N. Padhya, and H. A. Fields.** 1994. Comparative characterization of antigenic epitopes in the immunodominant region of the protein encoded by open reading frame 3 in Burmese and Mexican strains of hepatitis E virus. *J. Gen. Virol.* **75:**641–646.
42. **Khuroo, M. S., S. Kamili, and S. Jameel.** 1995. Vertical transmission of hepatitis E virus. *Lancet* **345:**1025–1026.
43. **Khuroo, M. S.** 1980. Study of an epidemic of non-A, non-B hepatitis. Possibility of another human hepatitis virus distinct from post-transfusion non-A, non-B type. *Am. J. Med.* **68:**818–824.
44. **Koonin, E. V., A. E. Gorbalenya, M. A. Purdy, M. N. Rozanov, G. R. Reyes, and D. W. Bradley.** 1992. Computer-assisted assignment of functional domains in the nonstructural polyprotein of hepatitis E virus: delineation of an additional group of positive-strand RNA plant and animal viruses. *Proc. Natl. Acad. Sci. USA* **89:**8259–8263.
45. **Krawczynski, K., and D. W. Bradley.** 1989. Enterically transmitted non-A, non-B hepatitis: identification of virus-associated antigen in experimentally infected cynomolgus macaques. *J. Infect. Dis.* **159:**1042–1049.
46. **Kuwada, S. K., V. M. Patel, F. B. Hollinger, H. J. Lin, P. O. Yarbough, R. H. Wiesner, D. Kaese, and J. Rakela.** 1994. Non-A, non-B fulminant hepatitis is also non-E and non-C. *Am. J. Gastroenterol.* **89:**57–61.
47. **Kwo, P. Y., G. G. Schlauder, H. A. Carpenter, P. J. Murphy, J. E. Rosenblatt, G. J. Dawson, E. E. Mast, K. Krawczynski, and V. Balan.** 1997. Acute hepatitis E by a new isolate acquired in the United States. *Mayo Clin. Proc.* **72:**1133–1136.
48. **Lau, J. Y. N., R. Sallie, J. W. Fang, P. O. Yarbough, G. R. Reyes, B. C. Portmann, G. Mieli-Vergani, and R. Williams.** 1995. Detection of hepatitis E virus genome and gene products in two patients with fulminant hepatitis E. *J. Hepatol.* **22:**605–610.
49. **Li, F., J. Torresi, S. A. Locarnini, H. Zhuang, W. Zhu, X. Guo, and D. A. Anderson.** 1997. Amino-terminal epitopes are exposed when full-length open reading frame 2 of hepatitis E virus is expressed in Escherichia coli, but carboxy-terminal epitopes are masked. *J. Med. Virol.* **52:** 289–300.
50. **Li, T. C., Y. Yamakawa, K. Suzuki, M. Tatsumi, M. A. Razak, T. Uchida, N. Takeda, and T. Miyamura.** 1997. Expression and self-assembly of empty virus-like particles of hepatitis E virus. *J. Virol.* **71:**7207–7213.
51. **Longer, C. F., S. L. Denny, J. D. Caudill, T. A. Miele, L. V. S. Asher, K. S. A. Myint, C.-C. Huang, W. F. Engler, J. W. LeDuc, L. N. Binn, and J. R. Ticehurst.** 1993. Experimental hepatitis E: pathogenesis in cynomol-

gus macaques (*Macaca fascicularis*). *J. Infect. Dis.* **168:** 602–609.

52. **Longer, C. F., J. E. Elliot, J. D. Caudill, L. N. Binn, J. P. Bryan, M. Iqbal, B. L. Innis, E. T. Clayson, M. P. Shrestha, S. A. Tsarev, H. Y. Zhang, and J. Ticehurst.** 1996. Observations on subclinical hepatitis E virus (HEV) infection and protection against reinfection, p. 362–371. *In* Y. Buisson, P. Coursaget, and M. Kane (ed.), *Enterically-Transmitted Hepatitis Viruses*. La Simarre, Joué-lès-Tours, France.
53. **Mast, E. E.** 1997. Personal communication.
54. **Mast, E. E., M. J. Alter, P. V. Holland, and R. H. Purcell.** 1998. Evaluation of assays for antibody to hepatitis E virus by a serum panel. Hepatitis E Virus Antibody Serum Panel Evaluation Group. *Hepatology* **27:**857–861.
55. **Meng, J., P. Dubreuil, and J. Pillot.** 1997. A new PCR-based seroneutralization assay in cell culture for diagnosis of hepatitis E. *J. Clin. Microbiol.* **35:**1373–1377.
56. **Meng, X. J., R. H. Purcell, P. G. Halbur, J. R. Lehman, D. M. Webb, T. S. Tsareva, J. S. Haynes, B. J. Thacker, and S. U. Emerson.** 1997. A novel virus in swine is closely related to the human hepatitis E virus. *Proc. Natl. Acad. Sci. USA* **94:**9860–9865.
57. **Miele, T. A., H. Y. Zhang, J. D. Caudill, R. W. Jansen, C. F. Longer, J. F. Duncan, I. Hussain, A. Ahmed, M. Iqbal, I. A. Malik, L. J. Legters, G. R. Reyes, D. W. Bradley, S. M. Lemon, and J. R. Ticehurst.** 1995. Unpublished data.
58. **Mushahwar, I. K., G. J. Dawson, K. M. Bile, and L. O. Magnius.** 1993. Serological studies of an enterically transmitted non-A, non-B hepatitis in Somalia. *J. Med. Virol.* **40:**218–221.
59. **Nanda, S. K., I. H. Ansari, S. K. Acharya, S. Jameel, and S. K. Panda.** 1995. Protracted viremia during acute sporadic hepatitis E virus infection. *Gastroenterology* **108:** 225–230.

59a. **Pringle, C. R.** 1998. Viral taxonomy—San Diego 1998. *Arch. Virol.* **143:**1449–1459.

60. **Purcell, R. H.** 1996. Hepatitis E virus, p. 2831–2843. *In* B. N. Fields, D. M. Knipe, P. M. Howley, R. M. Chanock, J. L. Melnick, T. P. Monath, B. Roizman, and S. E. Straus (ed.), *Fields Virology*, 3rd ed. Lippincott-Raven, Philadelphia, Pa.
61. **Purcell, R. H., and J. R. Ticehurst.** 1988. Enterically transmitted non-A, non-B hepatitis: epidemiology and clinical characteristics, p. 131–137. *In* A. J. Zuckerman (ed.), *Viral Hepatitis and Liver Disease*. Alan R. Liss, Inc., New York, N.Y.
62. **Purcell, R. H., and S. A. Tsarev.** 1996. Seroepidemiology of hepatitis E, p. 153–166. *In* Y. Buisson, P. Coursaget, and M. Kane (ed.), *Enterically-Transmitted Hepatitis Viruses*. La Simarre, Joué-lès-Tours, France.
63. **Purdy, M. A., D. Carson, K. A. McCaustland, D. W. Bradley, M. J. Beach, and K. Krawczynski.** 1994. Viral specificity of hepatitis E virus antigens identified by fluorescent antibody assay using recombinant HEV proteins. *J. Med. Virol.* **44:**212–214.
64. **Purdy, M. A., K. A. McCaustland, K. Krawczynski, J. Spelbring, G. R. Reyes, and D. W. Bradley.** 1993. Preliminary evidence that a *trpE*-HEV fusion protein protects cynomolgus macaques against challenge with wild-type hepatitis E virus (HEV). *J. Med. Virol.* **41:**90–94.
65. **Purdy, M. A., K. A. McCaustland, K. Krawczynski, A. Tam, M. J. Beach, N. C. Tassopoulos, G. R. Reyes, and D. W. Bradley.** 1992. Expression of a hepatitis E virus (HEV)-*trpE* fusion protein containing epitopes recognized by antibodies in sera from human cases and experimentally infected primates. *Arch. Virol.* **123:**335–349.
66. **Reyes, G. R., M. A. Purdy, J. P. Kim, K.-C. Luk, L. M. Young, K. E. Fry, and D. W. Bradley.** 1990. Isolation of a cDNA from the virus responsible for enterically transmitted non-A, non-B hepatitis. *Science* **247:**1335–1339.
67. **Robson, S. C., S. Adams, N. Brink, B. Woodruff, and D. Bradley.** 1992. Hospital outbreak of hepatitis E. *Lancet* **339:**1424–1425. (Letter.)
68. **Schlauder, G. G., G. J. Dawson, J. C. Erker, P. Y. Kwo, M. F. Knigge, D. L. Smalley, J. E. Rosenblatt, S. M. Desai, and I. K. Mushahwar.** 1998. The sequence and phylogenetic analysis of a novel hepatitis E virus isolated from a patient with acute hepatitis reported in the United States. *J. Gen. Virol.* **79:**447–456.
69. **Schlauder, G. G., G. J. Dawson, I. K. Mushahwar, A. Ritter, R. Sutherland, A. Moaness, and M. A. Kamel.** 1993. Viraemia in Egyptian children with hepatitis E virus infection. *Lancet* **341:**378. (Letter.)
70. **Tam, A. W., M. M. Smith, M. E. Guerra, C.-C. Huang, D. W. Bradley, K. E. Fry, and G. R. Reyes.** 1991. Hepatitis E virus (HEV): molecular cloning and sequencing of the full-length viral genome. *Virology* **185:**120–131.
71. **Tam, A. W., R. White, P. O. Yarbough, B. J. Murphy, C. P. McAtee, R. E. Lanford, and T. R. Fuerst.** 1997. In vitro infection and replication of hepatitis E virus in primary cynomolgus macaque hepatocytes. *Virology* **238:** 94–102.
72. **Thomas, D. L., P. O. Yarbough, D. Vlahov, S. A. Tsarev, K. E. Nelson, A. J. Saah, and R. H. Purcell.** 1997. Seroreactivity to hepatitis E virus in areas where the disease is not endemic. *J. Clin. Microbiol.* **35:**1244–1247.
73. **Ticehurst, J.** 1991. Identification and characterization of hepatitis E virus, p. 501–513. *In* F. B. Hollinger, S. M. Lemon, and H. S. Margolis (ed.), *Viral Hepatitis and Liver Disease*. The Williams & Wilkins Co., Baltimore, Md.
74. **Ticehurst, J., T. J. Popkin, J. P. Bryan, B. L. Innis, J. F. Duncan, A. Ahmed, M. Iqbal, I. Malik, A. Z. Kapikian, L. J. Legters, and R. H. Purcell.** 1992. Association of hepatitis E virus with an outbreak of hepatitis in Pakistan: serologic responses and pattern of virus excretion. *J. Med. Virol.* **36:**84–92.
75. **Ticehurst, J., L. L. Rhodes, Jr., K. Krawczynski, L. V. Asher, W. F. Engler, T. L. Mensing, J. D. Caudill, M. H. Sjogren, C. H. Hoke, Jr., J. W. LeDuc, D. W. Bradley, and L. N. Binn.** 1992. Infection of owl monkeys (*Aotus trivirgatus*) and cynomolgus monkeys (*Macaca fascicularis*) with hepatitis E virus from Mexico. *J. Infect. Dis.* **165:** 835–845.
76. **Tsarev, S. A., S. U. Emerson, G. R. Reyes, T. S. Tsareva, L. J. Legters, I. A. Malik, M. Iqbal, and R. H. Purcell.** 1992. Characterization of a prototype strain of hepatitis E virus. *Proc. Natl. Acad. Sci. USA* **89:**559–563.
77. **Tsarev, S. A., T. S. Tsareva, S. U. Emerson, S. Govindarajan, M. Shapiro, J. L. Gerin, and R. H. Purcell.** 1994. Successful passive and active immunization of cynomolgus monkeys against hepatitis E. *Proc. Natl. Acad. Sci. USA* **91:**10198–10202.
78. **Tsarev, S. A., T. S. Tsareva, S. U. Emerson, S. Govindarajan, M. Shapiro, J. L. Gerin, and R. H. Purcell.** 1997. Recombinant vaccine against hepatitis E: dose response and protection against heterologous challenge. *Vaccine* **15:** 1834–1838.
79. **Tsarev, S. A., T. S. Tsareva, S. U. Emerson, A. Z. Kapikian, J. Ticehurst, W. London, and R. H. Purcell.** 1993. ELISA for antibody to hepatitis E virus (HEV) based on complete open-reading frame-2 protein expressed in insect cells: identification of HEV infection in primates. *J. Infect. Dis.* **168:**369–378.
80. **Tsarev, S. A., T. S. Tsareva, S. U. Emerson, M. K. Rippy,**

P. Zack, M. Shapiro, and R. H. Purcell. 1995. Experimental hepatitis E in pregnant rhesus monkeys: failure to transmit hepatitis E virus (HEV) to offspring and evidence of naturally acquired antibodies to HEV. *J. Infect. Dis.* **172:** 31–37.

81. **Tsarev, S. A., T. S. Tsareva, S. U. Emerson, P. O. Yarbough, L. J. Legters, T. Moskal, and R. H. Purcell.** 1994. Infectivity titration of a prototype strain of hepatitis E virus (HEV) in cynomolgus monkeys. *J. Med. Virol.* **43:** 135–142.

82. **Uchida, T., T. T. Aye, X. Ma, F. Iida, T. Shikata, M. Ichikawa, T. Rikihisa, and K. M. Win.** 1993. An epidemic outbreak of hepatitis E in Yangon of Myanmar: antibody assay and animal transmission of the virus. *Acta Pathol. Jpn.* **43:**94–98.

83. **van Cuyck-Gandré, H., H. Y. Zhang, S. A. Tsarev, N. J. Clements, S. J. Cohen, J. D. Caudill, Y. Buisson, P. Coursaget, R. L. Warren, and C. F. Longer.** 1997. Characterization of hepatitis E virus (HEV) from Algeria and Chad by partial genome sequence. *J. Med. Virol.* **53:** 340–347.

84. **Wu, J. C., I. J. Sheen, T. Y. Chiang, W. Y. Sheng, Y. J. Wang, C. Y. Chan, and S. D. Lee.** 1998. The impact of traveling to endemic areas on the spread of hepatitis E virus infection: epidemiological and molecular analyses. *Hepatology* **27:**1415–1420.

85. **Yarbough, P. O.** 1996. Assay development of diagnostic tests for IgM and IgG antibody to hepatitis E virus, p. 294–296. *In* Y. Buisson, P. Coursaget, and M. Kane (ed.), *Enterically-Transmitted Hepatitis Viruses*. La Simarre, Joué-lès-Tours, France.

86. **Yarbough, P. O.** 1997. Advances in hepatitis E. *Curr. Opin. Infect. Dis.* **10:**398–401.

87. **Yarbough, P. O., A. W. Tam, K. Gabor, E. Garza, R. A. Moeckli, I. Palings, C. Simonsen, and G. Reyes.** 1994. Assay development of diagnostic tests for hepatitis E, p. 367–370. *In* K. Nishioka, H. Suzuki, S. Mishiro, and T. Oda (ed.), *Viral Hepatitis and Liver Disease*. Springer-Verlag, Tokyo, Japan.

88. **Zafrullah, M., M. H. Ozdener, S. K. Panda, and S. Jameel.** 1997. The ORF3 protein of hepatitis E virus is a phosphoprotein that associates with the cytoskeleton. *J. Virol.* **71:** 9045–9053.

89. **Zhang, Y., P. McAtee, P. O. Yarbough, A. W. Tam, and T. Fuerst.** 1997. Expression, characterization, and immunoreactivities of a soluble hepatitis E virus putative capsid protein species expressed in insect cells. *Clin. Diagn. Lab. Immunol.* **4:**423–428.

Human Papillomavirus*

NANCY B. KIVIAT

85

STRUCTURE AND NOMENCLATURE

The papillomaviruses constitute one of the two genera of the family *Papovaviridae*. These viruses are naked icosahedral capsids composed of 72 capsomeres 45 to 55 nm in diameter with a double-stranded supercoiled circular DNA genome of approximately 8,000 bp (16). The papillomaviruses are currently classified as a genus within the family *Papovaviridae* (44); however, as more has been learned about the structure and function of the virus, there is a growing consensus that these viruses should be classified as subfamilies rather than as a genus of *Papovaviridae*. Within the genus *Papillomavirus*, a large number of species-specific papillomaviruses have been identified, including those which infect humans (human papillomaviruses [HPVs]), cows, deer, dogs, monkeys, rabbits, and horses, among others (8, 37). Over the last decade, it has also become clear that there are many different types of HPV. Two HPVs were originally classified as being of the same or different "types" on the basis of the amount of DNA homology that they share, as demonstrated by reassociation kinetics. Currently, nucleotide sequencing is the "gold standard" for establishing the amount of homology present. If the DNA sequences of the E6, E7, and L1 open reading frames (ORFs) of two HPVs demonstrate less than 90% homology, they are classified as being distinct types. If between 2 and 10% DNA divergence is present, then the two viruses are considered subtypes of the same HPV type, while variants have less than 2% divergence (36). More than 70 different types of HPV have been identified from clinical specimens collected from humans throughout the world (56). As more and more clinical samples are analyzed, it is becoming apparent that a large number of subtypes and variants exist for each type of virus (13, 95, 100).

As discussed below, specific types of HPV tend to show some tissue tropism, and depending on the type of epithelium infected, HPV types are often referred to as "cutaneous" or "mucosal" types of HPV. In general, cutaneous types infect keratinizing epithelium, while mucosal HPVs (such as the genital tract HPVs) infect nonkeratinizing epithelium. Over the last decade, most attention has focused on the more than 30 sexually transmitted HPVs (designated "genital" types) and their role in the pathogenesis of genital tract epithelial cancers. Recently, there has been considerable interest in cutaneous HPV types, which may play a role in the pathogenesis of nonmelanoma skin cancers. It is also becoming apparent that different variants confer different potentials for malignancy. This may help explain why many women are infected with "oncogenic" types of HPV but only a few develop cancer.

Detailed descriptions of the organization of the viral genome have appeared elsewhere (8). Briefly, the papillomavirus genome consists of an upstream regulatory region, an "early region," which encodes the proteins necessary for viral DNA replication and transformation (ORFs E6, E7, E1, E2, E4, E5, E3, and E8), and a "late region" (ORFs L1 and L2), which encodes viral structural proteins, including the major capsid proteins necessary for productive viral replication. ORFs of particular interest in genital types of HPV are in the early regions and include the E6 and E7 ORFs. These ORFs are important in transformation. In the oncogenic genital HPV types but not in the nononcogenic genital types, these ORFs encode proteins that interfere with normal cellular tumor suppressor proteins. E6 of the oncogenic (but not of the nononcogenic) genital types of HPV has been shown to bind to and increase the level of degradation of p53, while E7 binds to and antagonizes the function of the retinoblastoma tumor suppressor protein (pRB) (8, 29, 68). In nonmalignant genital lesions the virus is episomal, while some integrated virus appears to be present in most invasive HPV-related genital tract cancers (56). Very little is known about the specifics of transformation of cutaneous HPVs.

PATHOGENESIS, NATURAL HISTORY, AND TRANSMISSION

It is well established that HPVs induce epithelial cell proliferation and that replication of HPV is tightly linked to squamous epithelial cell differentiation, with capsids being produced only in terminally differentiated squamous cells. For this reason, traditional techniques for culturing viruses cannot be used for HPV. The only animal model now available involves transplantation of HPV-infected tissue to the renal subscapular area of athymic nude mice (53).

Since the virus cannot be propagated, serologic assays were difficult to develop, and thus, relatively little is known

* This chapter contains information presented in chapter 95 by Nancy B. Kiviat and Laura A. Koutsky in the sixth edition of this Manual.

about the natural history and transmission of these infections. However, the recent successful in vitro production of virus-like particles (produced with, for example, baculovirus vectors) has allowed the development of sensitive and specific HPV type-specific serologic assays.

Transmission of cutaneous HPV types is direct or via fomites, while transmission of genital types is thought to be primarily through sexual contact (51). Several investigators have reported that approximately two-thirds of the partners of women with clinically diagnosed warts also have or develop such a pathology within several months (73). Transmission from mothers to children during childbirth rarely results in laryngeal papillomatosis (18).

HPV infects stratified squamous, metaplastic squamous, and columnar epithelia. The virus appears to first gain access to the lower portion of the epithelium in areas of local trauma and there infects basal epithelial cells (45, 85, 103). Reexpression of virus also has been noted to occur in areas of epithelial trauma. For example, laryngeal warts frequently develop near tracheotomy sites, and genital warts develop at the edges of areas of laser ablation (77, 82). Infection results in focal areas of hyperplasia of all layers of the epithelium. The majority of HPV infections are self-limited, but it is now clear that in a subset of genital HPV infections malignant tumors develop (69). As noted above, recent data suggest that certain types of HPV may also play a role in the pathogenesis of nonmelanomatous skin cancers (including squamous and basal cell cancers) (26).

ANATOMIC DISTRIBUTION

Specific types of HPV tend to infect different types of epithelia and produce different clinical and pathological manifestations (Table 1). However, tissue tropism is not completely site specific. For example, HPV types 6 and 11 infect both the genital tract and the larynx, and while HPV type 16 (HPV-16) generally infects the genital tract, the virus has been detected at nongenital sites, for example, in periungual lesions (30, 34, 63, 67).

Cutaneous HPV Infection

Infection with HPV types 1 to 4 is thought to occur almost universally during childhood or adolescence and is generally self-limited without consequence. Some types of HPV that infect the nongenital or keratinizing epithelium have been detected primarily among patients with epidermodysplasia verruciformis or other forms of immunosuppression (56). Recent data suggest that infection with such types is in fact more widely distributed but difficult to detect in persons with normal immune systems. A number of novel types of HPV have recently been described in both neoplastic and nonneoplastic skin lesions (26, 54), and as discussed below, their role in nonmelanoma skin cancers is now being examined. An unusual form of cutaneous HPV infection usually associated with HPV-7 also occurs in meat handlers.

Mucosal HPV Infection

Mucosal HPVs primarily infect the anogenital tract epithelium, but these HPV types can also be found in the oral mucosa, conjunctiva, and respiratory tract. Genital tract HPV infection is thought to be the most common sexually transmitted viral infection in the United States (51). Current evidence suggests that more than 50% of sexually active adults have been infected with a genital HPV (50). Some infections, for example, genital warts, can easily be identified by the clinician, others can be identified only by microscopy, while others are detected only through the use of assays for HPV DNA. The prevalence of HPV infection, whether it is diagnosed clinically, by microscopy, or by molecular assays, varies significantly with the age, gender, and sexual behavior of the specific population (19).

Genital warts occur on the vulva, vagina, cervix, penis, and anus. Descriptions of genital warts can be found even in ancient Greek writings (73); however, only recently has it become clear that a number of different sexually transmitted viruses are responsible for these lesions. In addition, over the last 10 years we have learned that the flat lesions, seen by gynecologists with the aid of a colposcope after applica-

TABLE 1 Common HPV types, sites of infection, clinical manifestations, and association with invasive cancers

HPV type	Site infected	Clinical manifestation	Association with malignancy
Cutaneous			
1	Soles of feet	Deep plantar warts	None
2–4	Hands, arms	Common warts	None
7	Hands, arms	Butcher's warts	None
5, 8, 9, 12, 14, 15, 17, 19–25, 36, 37, 38	Forehead, arms, trunk	Flat, macular warts and neoplastic lesions primarily in patients with epidermodysplasia verruciformis	Over 30% of epidermodysplasia verruciformis patients infected with types 5, 8, 14, 17, and 20 develop malignancy
26–29, 34	Forehead, arms, trunk	Common flat warts	Frequent, especially in immunosuppressed patients; Bowen's disease
Mucosa			
6, 11	Anogenital epithelium larynx, upper respiratory tract, conjunctiva, and oral cavity	Papillomatosis primarily laryngeal, also in upper respiratory tract; condylomata; intraepithelial neoplasia	Rare, Buschke Löwenstein tumors
42–44	Anogenital epithelium	Condylomata; intraepithelial neoplasia	Rare
31, 33, 35, 51, 52	Anogenital epithelium	Condylomata; intraepithelial neoplasia	Occasionally
16, 18, 45, 56	Anogenital epithelium	Condylomata; intraepithelial neoplasia	Most frequently of all types

tion of acetic acid, are related to the typical genital warts seen on the vulva and penis. Women and men with clinically visible papillary warts frequently also have such flat warts.

Association with Malignancy

In addition to being a common sexually transmitted disease, genital infection with HPV is of considerable importance because specific types of genital HPVs play a major role in the pathogenesis of epithelial cancers of the female and male genital tracts (51, 56). Over the last decade a number of case-control and cohort studies have convincingly demonstrated that specific types of HPV are the causal agents of at least 90% of cervical cancers (70). The genital HPVs are commonly referred to as being of "high/intermediate" or "low" risk, depending on the frequency with which they are present in cancers. The most common types conferring a high/intermediate risk include HPV types 16, 18, 31, 33, 35, 45, 51, 52, and 56; HPV types 6, 11, 42, 43, and 44 are considered to confer a low risk because they are almost never associated with malignancy (58). The lack of a serologic assay has made it difficult to estimate the risk of malignancy conferred by infection with oncogenic types of HPV. Several cohort studies examining the risk of development of cervical intraepithelial neoplasia (CIN) grade 2 and/or 3 in relationship to HPV type have been reported (10, 52). In one study of cytologically negative women attending a sexually transmitted disease (STD) clinic, the cumulative incidence of CIN grade 2 and/or 3 at 2 years was 38% among women in whom oncogenic HPV type 16 or 18 was detected by Southern transfer hybridization at some time during the study. After adjusting for the presence of HPV, factors that were independently associated with the development of CIN grade 2 and/or 3 included serologic evidence of *Chlamydia trachomatis* infection and a positive culture for *Neisseria gonorrhoeae* (52). Whether the risk for the development of CIN grade 2 and/or 3, the lesion thought to be the precursor of invasive cancer, will be similar in other populations is unknown. Laboratory-based studies have provided an explanation for the association between infection with intermediate-risk types of HPV and malignancy. As mentioned above, intermediate- but not low-risk types of genital HPV produce oncoproteins (designated E6 and E7) that bind to normal tumor suppressor proteins p53 and pRB. This interaction is thought to be central to carcinogenesis (68).

Several hypotheses have been put forth to explain why only a minority of women infected with HPV-16 go on to develop cervical cancer. A number of studies have examined the role of cofactors such as smoking or birth control methods in the development of malignancy (7). Furthermore, some data suggest that the many different HPV-16 variants that have been documented to occur with variable frequency in all populations have different biological behaviors (14, 93, 98, 101). In vitro and in vivo data suggest that certain HPV variants may in fact alter the risk of clinical disease (1, 31, 41, 55, 62, 79, 99). Of particular interest is a recent report of an association between an HPV-16 variant with a base pair change at nucleotide 83 with invasive cervical cancer (102). Additionally, we found that women in Seattle infected with certain HPV-16 variants were at greater risk of the development of CIN grade 2 and/or 3 (99). Similar findings were also found with regard to the risk of development of anal carcinoma in situ among men who have sex with men (97).

In patients with epidermodysplasia verruciformis, a rare autosomal dominant genetic disorder of cellular immunity, or in patients with iatrogenic immunosuppression, cutaneous infection with HPV types is commonly associated with malignancy. At least 30% of patients with epidermodysplasia verruciformis and many patients with renal transplants have been reported to develop HPV-related cancers of the skin, especially in sun-exposed areas (37, 80, 103). The roles of various types of HPV in the pathogenesis of nonmelanoma squamous and basal cell cancers in those without immune dysfunction are now under investigation by a number of researchers (2, 5, 23, 24, 26, 27, 43, 54, 61, 64, 87, 104). However, the epidemiology and molecular biology of HPV in the development of such cancers are largely undefined.

PREVALENCE OF HPV INFECTION

The prevalence of HPV infection varies with the diagnostic method used (clinical examination, microscopic examination, detection of HPV DNA with or without amplification of DNA), the age, and the sexual behavior of the population tested. Since the virus cannot be cultured, the development of an assay for the detection of antibodies to specific types of HPV in serum has been difficult. Recently, however, several groups have engineered the production of HPV type-specific capsids or virus-like particles which are now beginning to be used as the antigen targets for serologic assays in natural history studies (11). At present, however, we know relatively little about the lifetime risk of infection with genital types of HPV. It appears that the time to the development of antibodies to HPV-16 is slow. In a study of women with incident HPV-16 infection, the median time to the development of HPV-16-specific antibodies was 1 year (12).

As with other STDs, evidence of current infection including the presence of genital warts, cytologic or microscopic evidence of cervical HPV infection, and detection of HPV DNA is most frequently detected among sexually active young women between 15 and 25 years of age. Manifestations of productive HPV infections such as warts and HPV-associated squamous intraepithelial lesions of the cervix, common shortly after women become sexually active, are only rarely detected in menopausal and postmenopausal women, perhaps reflecting immunity (19). There appears to have been a marked increase in the age-adjusted incidence of genital warts beginning during the 1950s and 1970s, as was seen with several other STDs. In the early 1990s it was estimated that about 1% of men and women in the United States between the ages of 15 and 49 years had clinically evident genital warts (diagnosed with the unaided eye) (19).

As described above, characteristic changes caused by HPV can be seen in Pap smears or in tissue biopsy specimens. The prevalence of HPV infection detected cytologically appears to be about 2%, with a range of from 0.7 to 3% (22, 65, 81). Among women attending STD clinics, 8 to 13% had Pap smears that showed signs of HPV infection (28). In contrast to the apparent rise in the prevalence of clinically diagnosed warts over the last 20 years, Pap smears have not shown a similar increase in the prevalence of HPV-associated changes. However, a review of Pap smears in Kuopio, Finland, in 1985 and 1986 showed the prevalence of HPV-related changes to be 3% in 1985, with 7% of women with an initially negative cytology having HPV-related changes seen on a Pap smear 1 year later (89). Whether the increase in clinically diagnosed genital warts is due to increased awareness of disease or whether the absence of such an increase in koilocytosis reflects changes in the cytologic classification schemes that have occurred over the last 15 years is unclear.

Recent studies that have used very sensitive PCR-based methods suggest that most adults in whom HPV DNA is detected in genital tract samples do not have clinical or morphologic evidence of HPV infection (4, 17, 21, 32, 33, 49, 66, 70, 76, 83, 90, 93, 94). The rate of detection of HPV DNA in women under 40 years of age with normal cytology has been reported to range from 1.5 to close to 50%, with most studies reporting prevalences of greater than 15%. The prevalence of the intermediate-risk HPV types in normal smears is considerably lower, ranging from 2.9 to 30%. The reported prevalence of HPV and specific types of HPV DNA are lower among older women. In addition to true differences in prevalence, the technical factors that might result in various levels of detection have been discussed above.

DIAGNOSIS OF HPV INFECTION

Since HPV cannot be cultured, a variety of other methods have been used to detect infection.

Clinical and Colposcopic Examination

The use of clinical examination for the detection of genital HPV is convenient but extremely insensitive and nonspecific. Only the larger, primarily papillary lesions can be identified. The majority of genital HPV infections, especially those of the cervix, are flat and invisible to the unaided eye (75). Many such cervical lesions become visible on colposcopic examination, especially if colposcopy is performed after application of acetic acid to the cervical epithelium. However, among women who have not been preselected on the basis of cytology and who are at high risk for STDs (including HPV infection), colposcopy lacks specificity, and compared to molecular tests, colposcopy is insensitive (74). Recent data suggest that subclinical infection with cutaneous HPV types is also exceedingly common (5).

Microscopic Examination of Exfoliated Cell Samples (Pap Smears) or Tissue Biopsy Specimens

Squamous cells infected with HPV frequently show a variety of changes, with some morphologic features being associated with infection with specific types or groups of HPV. In genital tract infections, the most characteristic HPV-related change is perinuclear clearing, with an increase in the density of the surrounding rim of the cytoplasm (48, 84). Cells exhibiting such changes are referred to as koilocytes and can be seen in both exfoliated cell samples and in tissue biopsy specimens. Other changes that are frequently present in HPV-infected cells include changes in the shapes and sizes of both the cytoplasm and the nucleus and changes in the amount and distribution of the nuclear chromatin. Abnormalities of keratinization are frequently present, but they are often subtle. While most pathologists will agree on the diagnosis of HPV infection in those genital tract biopsy specimens or smears when all such changes are clearly present, several studies have shown that there is poor intra- and interobserver reproducibility for the diagnosis of HPV infection (47). Furthermore, compared to detection with DNA probes, microscopic diagnosis is insensitive.

Immunocytochemistry

Detection of late structural antigens with polyclonal antibodies raised against Shope papillomavirus allows confirmation of the presence of HPV on characteristic tissue biopsy specimens. The assay is specific but insensitive because in many cases only small amounts of late structural proteins are present (86), and it is rarely used today.

Electron Microscopy

Although electron microscopic identification of HPV in either cellular scrapings or tissue is possible, this approach is costly and time-consuming and has low sensitivity due to the limited sample size. Furthermore, as with clinical or microscopic examination, one is unable to determine the specific type of HPV present.

Detection of Specific Types of HPV DNA by DNA Hybridization

HPV DNA sequences can be detected by hybridization technology with either DNA or RNA probes directed against specific types of HPV DNA. A number of different hybridization techniques have been used, including Southern blotting, dot blotting, sandwich assays, hybridization in solution, or in situ hybridization. These techniques can be performed with fresh, frozen, or fixed tissue or exfoliated cell samples from which DNA can be extracted. The sensitivities of such assays, which are the gold standard for the diagnosis of HPV infection, can be increased by target amplification, for example, by PCR, the ligase chain reaction, nucleic acid sequence-based amplification, or signal amplification. The most sensitive approach has been hybridization performed in conjunction with one of these amplification techniques (60, 72), with hybridization incorporating ultrasensitive PCR methods theoretically allowing detection of one copy of HPV DNA in an assay which uses 1% of the collected material per reaction (57). Each of these techniques has advantages and disadvantages, and the choice of method used depends on the information desired, the expertise of the laboratory personnel performing the test, and the turnaround time required for a result. Nevertheless, the only U.S. Food and Drug Administration (FDA)-approved test for the detection of HPV from the cervix (swabs) or from biopsy tissue is the Digene Hybrid Capture system by a chemiluminescence assay for the qualitative detection of DNA of low- and high-risk types of the virus. While a summary of each technique is presented below, the reader is referred to other sources for further detailed descriptions of these various assays (chapter 13).

In Situ Hybridization

In situ hybridization can be performed with tissue or with filters. While filter in situ hybridization was used in early studies of HPV, this approach has largely been abandoned due to problems with both specificity and sensitivity. Tissue-based in situ hybridization (15, 40, 71) offers the advantages of providing hybridization while conserving morphology and may allow one to determine whether HPV is integrated or episomal in nature (78, 96). In addition to the detection of specific HPV types with a reported sensitivity of approximately 25 copies, it is also possible to detect gene-specific transcripts by in situ hybridization (88). However, this assay is labor-intensive and is not appropriate for the routine analysis of large numbers of specimens. While most low-grade HPV-related lesions of the cervix (CIN grade 1) are positive, many CIN grade 2 and 3 lesions are not. A number of researchers have used this in conjunction with PCR to achieve increased sensitivity (3, 72). Currently, however, although in situ hybridization by PCR has been reported, this technique has not been widely adapted. In general, in situ hybridization is an important research tool in the study of HPV.

STH and DH (Hybridization without Prior Amplification of HPV DNA)

Prior to the development of PCR-based assays, Southern transfer hybridization (STH) or dot blot hybridization (DH) was widely used for the detection of HPV DNA (59). For STH, DNA must be extracted, purified, fragmented by use of restriction enzymes, electrophoresed, transferred to filters, denatured, and hybridized with HPV-specific probes. To achieve maximum sensitivity, multiple DNA (RNA) probes were used, frequently under conditions of various stringencies, to detect as many of the HPV types of interest as possible. The filters were generally stripped and then reprobed with a different set of type-specific HPV probes. Although nonradiolabeled probes can be used in performing this technique, the use of radiolabeled DNA probes increases the sensitivity approximately 10-fold over that obtained with nonradiolabeled probes (20). From 0.1 to 0.01 HPV genome copies per cell are generally detectable with radiolabeled probes (25). DH is similar to STH but does not include the electrophoresis and fragmentation steps.

The advantage of STH was the fact that it offered specificity because it employed visualization of the specific banding patterns associated with specific types of viruses. Furthermore, it is relatively sensitive. In addition, by lowering the stringency of the hybridization, it is possible to screen for uncharacterized HPV types. This assay was widely used in early studies of the prevalence of HPV, but it has several major drawbacks. The assay is very time-consuming and labor-intensive, and highly trained personnel are required to perform the technique in a standardized manner. The turnaround time is usually weeks to months, depending on the number of rounds of hybridization performed. The processing, hybridization, and probing techniques for this assay vary considerably from laboratory to laboratory, and since even minor changes in protocol can alter test results, reproducibility is less than optimal. Furthermore, the reading of STH blots is often extremely difficult and not highly reproducible. Brandsma et al. (6) showed that interlaboratory variation was substantial for the performance of Southern blotting, with the level of interlaboratory agreement varying between 67 and 97% for HPV positivity and between 50 and 92% for HPV type specificity. Factors that have the potential to affect the test outcome include the way in which the genital epithelium is sampled (biopsy versus smear, direct scraping versus vaginal wash), the amount of DNA used in the assay, the number and types of specific probes used, the stringency of the washes, and the number of rounds of hybridization performed, in addition to the reading of the filters. This technique still has some specific applications in research settings, such as confirming the presence of viral integration into host DNA.

DH is considerably less difficult to perform. In DH assays purified cellular DNA is fixed in the form of a "dot" onto the membrane without prior electrophoresis (46). The membrane filters are then probed with DNA or RNA probes to detect specific HPV DNA sequences. Nonspecific staining is a problem since no specific banding pattern is present, as is the case for STH. Although early assays with DNA probes presented problems with high background, several commercially available assays that use RNA probes and that target the genital types of HPV originally appeared in this format and had extremely good specificities, with sensitivities similar to that of STH (46). Dot blot assays offered several important advantages over STH. In addition to being relatively easy to perform, they are very reproducible and a large number of specimens can be processed at one time with a 1-day turnaround time, compared to 2 to 3 days for STH (25, 38, 56, 83).

Solution hybridization is the basis of a commercially available, FDA-approved assay (Digene Hybrid Capture System) with full-length RNA probes to 14 different HPV types. In this assay, denatured patient sample is reacted with long single-stranded RNA probes which are grouped into high/intermediate-risk types (types 16, 18, 31, 33, 35, 45, 51, 52, 56) and low-risk types (types 6, 11, 42, 43, and 44). The DNA-RNA hybrids formed by in-solution hybridization are "captured" by immobilized alkaline phosphatase-conjugated antibodies onto the DNA-RNA hybrids. The detection of the antibody-hybrid complexes is achieved with a chemiluminescence detection system. The assay can detect as few as 1,000 copies of HPV DNA.

HPV DNA Detection Assays Combining Amplification of HPV DNA and Hybridization

The addition of amplification of HPV DNA by PCR prior to hybridization allows a significant increase in sensitivity (38).

A number of different primers and procedures for PCR have been described. The sensitivity of this technique for the detection of HPV and the specific types of HPV varies not only with the specific primers and probes used but also with the specific procedures used. One approach is to first amplify HPV DNA with consensus primers designed to facilitate the amplification of a broad spectrum of HPV types by targeting the well-conserved L1 or E1 ORF of the HPV genome (25, 38). The PCR products generated from such primers are then applied to a membrane (as a dot or in a fashion similar to that used for the Southern blotting procedure) and hybridized with labeled DNA or RNA type-specific probes. While a detailed discussion of the different primer sets that have been described is beyond the scope of this chapter, the choice of primers to be used is of considerable importance. For example, if the target DNA is damaged, as is frequently the case in older paraffin-embedded biopsy specimens or on Pap smears, primers designed to produce smaller amplification products offer the greatest sensitivity. If one is searching for uncharacterized HPV types, increasing the degeneracy of the primers will broaden the spectrum of detectable HPVs, although the likelihood of amplifying non-HPV DNA sequences will also increase (38). Currently, the most often used approach is to use a general or consensus primer pair directed at the conserved L1 ORF. The most commonly used primer sets include sets of consensus primers: MY09-MY11 (91) and GP5-GP6 (92). Currently, the latest versions of the MY09-MY11 primers, which encompass a 450-bp region, are able to detect many different types of HPV with relatively consistent sensitivities. Typing can be done by digesting amplicons with specific restriction endonucleases and subsequent electrophoresis; however, most efficient is the use of oligonucleotide probe-based detection (91). Well-characterized primers and probes for typing can currently be purchased, and it is anticipated that a PCR assay for the detection of HPV will be commercially available in the near future.

Detection of variants of the different HPV types has recently become of considerable interest in research settings given the likelihood that different variants have different biologic behaviors. While sequencing of the specific regions of the HPV genome can be used to detect variants, this is expensive and thus may not be appropriate for the analysis of large numbers of samples. A more cost-effective approach is prescreening by PCR-based single-stranded conformational polymorphism (PCR-SSCP) analysis to classify molecular variants based on the SSCP patterns. Variants that show different SSCP patterns can then be sequenced to determine sequence variation (100). Another approach is to use lineage-specific hybridization (10), a technique that was developed for the rapid assignment of HPV-16 variants to one of five previously identified phylogenetic HPV-16 lineages (42).

PCR-based detection of HPV DNA offers greatly increased sensitivity, but several potential pitfalls have been identified, the most important being the possibility for contamination either from the clinic or from the laboratory. Contamination from HPV plasmids, PCR products, or sample-to-sample transfer has been reported. The following are some anticontamination precautions that are common in laboratories processing large numbers of specimens by PCR: preparation of a master mixture of reaction reagents in a sterile biosafety hood, the use of positive displacement pipets or plugged pipet tips for all amplification reactions, and the routine inclusion of negative control samples consisting of a known number of HPV-negative K562 cells through all of the sample preparation steps. The last procedure allows one to assess laboratory technique and check for interspecimen contamination. In addition, sample preparation, PCR amplification, and PCR product analyses should all be done in separate areas with equipment and glassware that are specifically dedicated to that task. If plasmids are present in the laboratory, contamination with plasmid DNA can be reduced by using anticontamination primers. These primers flank the cloning side of the plasmid so that in case of contamination, no PCR product is produced under standard conditions (4, 93). Lastly, 10% of randomly selected positive specimens and 5% of randomly selected negative specimens should be tested. We have also found that regular interlaboratory comparisons with other laboratories that regularly test large numbers of specimens are useful.

COLLECTION OF SPECIMENS

A number of different collection media have been described, and several are commercially available (56). The ideal collection medium allows one to proceed to hybridization without extensive manipulation of the clinical specimen. This is of considerable importance in avoiding specimen contamination, especially when amplifying DNA prior to hybridization. Care therefore must be taken to collect specimens in a medium that is free of reagents that inhibit amplification. It is preferable that collection media also have a relatively long shelf life, be stable at room temperature or with minimal refrigeration, and inactivate infectious agents.

There has been a good deal of debate as to how to best collect samples from the female genital tract for the detection of HPV DNA by hybridization. During the period when STH was being widely used, some researchers advocated performing vaginal washing rather than direct sampling of the cervix (9). This was thought to increase the amount of HPV collected for hybridization. While vaginal washing did increase the amount of virus collected, the additional HPV DNA collected primarily reflects vaginal infection rather than cervical disease. Since the cervix is the primary site of interest, the usefulness of collecting vaginal HPV DNA is unclear. With the widespread addition of DNA amplification to hybridization assays, the question of whether an adequate amount of HPV DNA can be obtained from directed cervical sampling has become moot. On the other hand, even by PCR technology, it is difficult to get an adequate number of cells from the more keratinized epithelium of the external genitalia of men and women (39).

SEROLOGIC DETECTION OF HPV

Even by an assay as sensitive as PCR, it is likely that we are detecting only current infections and possibly a portion of latent infections. Although problems were encountered during early attempts to develop sensitive and type-specific serologic assays, considerable progress has been made since virus-like particles (capsids) that are produced by cloning HPV in vaccinia virus or baculovirus with expression of capsids containing configurationally correct L1 and L2 epitopes (35) have become available.

It appears that development of type-specific antibodies can be detected in the majority of women during the 12- to 15-month period following an incident HPV infection. The relationship between the presence of such antibodies and the development of disease is now being examined. It is now clear that antibodies are produced; it is not known whether infection with HPV and specific types of HPV produces long-lasting antibodies at levels that will be readily detectable. Preliminary data suggest that antibodies are detectable for at least up to 10 to 15 years after the time of the initial detection of HPV DNA (51a). It is also hoped that specific serologic markers that allow us to identify women at risk for the development of invasive disease can be developed.

REPORTING AND INTERPRETATION OF RESULTS

At present, with our very limited understanding of the natural history, means of transmission, and risk of development of malignancy associated with HPV infection, the relevance of detecting HPV DNA is unclear. Similarly, the clinical implications of a negative test are not clear at present. As discussed above, oncogenic types of genital tract HPV DNA are detectable in many young sexually active men and women, but only a subset will probably ever develop HPV-related cancer. Furthermore, the meaning of a negative test result is difficult to assess, since we know little about the likelihood of misclassification due to intermittent shedding of virus or due to problems with sampling or the reproducibilities of even the most sensitive assays such as PCR. Furthermore, at present, treatment of genital tract pathology is based on morphology rather than on the detection of specific types of HPV, and therefore, the clinical impact of the detection of HPV DNA is unclear. However, given the central role of specific types of HPV in the pathogenesis of cancer, it is clear that the detection of HPV DNA will play a role in cervical cancer control in the future, either as an adjunct to cytology in assessing which women need further workup or close follow-up or perhaps as a primary screening method for certain populations. The results of a number of several large population-based studies examining the utility of testing for HPV will likely appear within the next several years.

Lastly, it is important to realize that a positive testing result for HPV offers no definitive proof that sexual assault has occurred either in children or in adults, nor can we determine at present the source or indicate the time of origin of a current infection.

REFERENCES

1. **Bavin, P. J., P. G. Walker, and V. C. Emery.** 1993. Sequence microheterogeneity in the long control region of clinical isolates of human papillomavirus type 16. *J. Med. Virol.* **39:**267–272.
2. **Berkhout, R. J., L. M. Tieben, H. L. Smits, J. N. Bavinck, B. J. Vermeer, and J. ter Schegget.** 1995. Nested PCR approach for detection and typing of epidermodysplasia verruciformis-associated human papillomavirus types in cutaneous cancers from renal transplant recipients. *J. Clin. Microbiol.* **33:**690–695.
3. **Bernard, H. U., S. Y. Chan, M. M. Manos, C. K. Ong, L. L. Villa, H. Delius, C. L. Peyton, H. M. Bauer, and C. M. Wheeler.** 1994. Identification and assessment of known and novel human papillomaviruses by polymerase chain reaction amplification, restriction fragment length polymorphisms, nuleotide sequence, and phylogenetic algorithms. *J. Infect. Dis.* **170:**1077–1085.
4. **Beyer-Finkley, E., H. Pfister, and F. Girardi.** 1990. Anticontamination primers to improve specificity of polymerase chain reaction in human papillomavirus screening. *Lancet* **335:**1289–1290.
5. **Boxman, I. L., R. J. Berkhout, L. H. Mulder, M. C. Wolkers, J. N. Bouwes-Bavinck, B. J. Vermeer, and J. ter Schegget.** 1997. Detection of human papillomavirus DNA in plucked hairs from renal transplant recipients and healthy volunteers. *J. Invest. Dermatol.* **108:**712–715.
6. **Brandsma, J., R. D. Burk, W. D. Lancaster, H. Pfister, and M. H. Schiffman.** 1989. Interlaboratory variation as an explanation for varying prevalence estimates of human papillomavirus infection. *Int. J. Cancer* **43:**260–262.
7. **Briton, L. A.** 1992. Epidemiology of cervical cancer—overview, p. 3–24. *In* N. Munoz, F. X. Bosch, K. V. Shah, and A. Meheus (ed.), *The Epidemiology of Cervical Cancer and Human Papillomavirus*. IARC Scientific Publications No. 119. International Agency for Research on Cancer, Lyon, France.
8. **Broker, T. R., and M. Botchan.** 1986. Papillomaviruses: retrospectives and prospectives. *Cancer Cells* **4:**17–36.
9. **Burk, R. D., A. S. Kadish, S. Calderin, and S. L. Romney.** 1986. Human papillomavirus infection of the cervix detected by cervicovaginal lavage and molecular hybridization: correlation with biopsy results and Papanicolaou smear. *Am. J. Obstet. Gynecol.* **154:**982–989.
10. **Campion, M. J., D. J. McCance, J. Cuzick, and A. Singer.** 1986. Progressive potential of mild cervical atypia: prospective cytological, colposcopic, and virological study. *Lancet* **ii:**237–240.
11. **Carter, J. J., G. C. Wipf, M. E. Hagensee, B. McKnight, L. A. Habel, S.-K. Lee, J. Kuypers, N. Kiviat, J. R. Daling, L. A. Koutsky, D. H. Watts, K. K. Holmes, and D. A. Galloway.** 1995. Use of human papillomavirus type 6 capsids to detect antibodies in people with genital warts. *J. Infect. Dis.* **172:**11–18.
12. **Carter, J. J., L. A. Koutsky, G. C. Wipf, N. D. Christensen, S.-K. Lee, J. Kuypers, N. Kiviat, and D. A. Galloway.** 1996. The natural history of human papillomavirus type 16 capsid antibodies among a cohort of university women. *J. Infect. Dis.* **174:**927–936.
13. **Chan, S. Y., H. U. Bernard, C. K. Ong, S. P. Chan, B. Hofmann, and H. Delius.** 1992. Phylogenetic analysis of 48 papillomavirus types and 28 subtypes and variants: a showcase for the molecular evolution of DNA viruses. *J. Virol.* **66:**5714–5725.
14. **Chan, S. Y., L. Ho, C. K. Ong, V. Chow, B. Drescher, M. Durst, J. ter Meulen, L. Villa, F. Luande, H. N. Mgaya, and H. U. Bernard.** 1992. Molecular variants of human papillomavirus type 16 from four continents suggest ancient pandemic spread of the virus and its coevolution with humankind. *J. Virol.* **66:**2057–2066.
15. **Chapman, W. B., A. T. Lorincz, G. D. Willett, V. C. Wright, and R. J. Kurman.** 1993. Evaluation of two commercially available in situ hybridization kits for detection of human papillomavirus DNA in cervical biopsies: comparison to Southern blot hybridization. *Mod. Pathol.* **6:** 73–79.
16. **Coggin, J. R., and H. zur Hausen.** 1979. Workshop on papillomaviruses and cancer. *Cancer Res.* **39:**545–546.
17. **Coll-Seck, A., M. A. Faye, C. W. Critchlow, A. D. Mbaye, J. Kuypers, G. Woto-Gaye, C. Langley, E. B. De, K. K. Holmes, and N. B. Kiviat.** 1994. Cervical intraepithelial neoplasia and human papillomavirus infection among Senegalese women seropositive for HIV-1 or HIV-2 or seronegative for HIV. *Int. J. STD AIDS* **5:**189–193.
18. **Corbitt, G., A. P. Zarod, J. R. Arrand, M. Longson, and W. T. Farrington.** 1988. Human papillomavirus (HPV) genotypes associated with laryngeal papilloma. *J. Clin. Pathol.* **41:**284–288.
19. **Critchlow, C. W., and L. A. Koutsky.** 1995. Epidemiology of human papillomavirus infection, p. 53–81. *In* A. Mindel, (ed.), *Genital Warts: Human Papillomavirus Infection*. Edward Arnold, London, United Kingdom.
20. **Crum, C. P., G. Nuovo, D. Friedman, and S. V. Silverstein.** 1988. A comparison of biotin and isotope-labeled ribonucleic acid probes for in situ detection of HPV 16 ribonucleic acid in genital precancers. *Lab. Invest.* **58:** 354–359.
21. **Czegledy, J., K. O. Rogo, M. Evander, and G. Wadell.** 1992. High-risk human papillomavirus types in cytologically normal cervical scrapes from Kenya. *Med. Microbiol. Immunol.* **180:**321–326.
22. **de Brux, J., G. Orth, O. Croissant, B. Cochard, and M. Ionesco.** 1983. Condylomatous lesions of the cervix uteri: development in 2466 patients. *Bull. Cancer* **70:**410–422.
23. **de Jong Tieben, L. M., R. J. Berkhout, H. L. Smits, J. N. Bouwes-Bavinck, B. J. Vermeer, F. J. van der Woude, and J. ter Schegget.** 1995. High frequency of detection of epidermodysplasia verruciformis-associated human papillomavirus DNA in biopsies from malignant and premalignant skin lesions from renal transplant recipients. *J. Invest. Dermatol.* **3:**367–371.
24. **Delius, H., B. Saegling, K. Bergmann, V. Shamanin, and E.-M. de Villiers.** 1998. The genomes of three of four novel HPV types, defined by differences of their L1 genes, show high conservation of the E7 gene and the URR. *Virology* **240:**359–365.
25. **de Villiers, E.-M.** 1992. Hybridization methods other than PCR: an update, p. 111–120. *In* N. Munoz, F. X. Bosch, K. V. Shah, and A. Meheus (ed.), *The Epidemiology of Cervical Cancer and Human Papillomavirus*. IARC Scientific Publications No. 119. International Agency for Research on Cancer, Lyon, France.
26. **de Villiers, E.-M.** 1998. Human papillomavirus infections in skin cancers. *Biomed. Pharmacother.* **52:**26–33.
27. **de Villiers, E.-M., D. Lavergne, K. McLaren, and E. C. Benton.** 1997. Prevailing papillomavirus types in non-melanoma carcinomas of the skin in renal allograft recipients. *Int. J. Cancer* **73:**356–361.
28. **Drake, M., G. Medley, and H. Mitchell.** 1987. Cytological detection of human papillomavirus infection. *Obstet. Gynecol. Clin. N. Am.* **14:**431–450.
29. **Dyson, N., P. M. Howley, K. Munger, and E. Harlow.** 1989. The human papillomavirus-16 E7 oncoprotein is able to bind to the retinoblastoma gene product. *Science* **243:** 934–937.
30. **Eliezri, Y. D., S. J. Silverstein, and G. J. Nuovo.** 1990. Occurrence of human papillomavirus type 16 DNA in cu-

taneous squamous and basal cell neoplasms. *J. Am. Acad. Dermatol.* **23:**836–842.

31. **Ellis, J. R. M., P. J. Keating, J. Baird, E. F. Hounsell, D. V. Renouf, M. Rowe, M. F. Hopkins, M. E. Duggan-Keen, J. S. Bartholomew, L. S. Young, and P. L. Stern.** 1995. The association of an HPV-16 oncogene variant with HLA-B7 has implications for vaccine design in cervical cancer. *Nat. Med.* **1:**464–470.
32. **Engels, H., A. Nyongo, M. Temmerman, W. G. V. Quint, E. van Marck, and W. J. Eylenbosch.** 1992. Cervical cancer screening and detection of genital HPV-infection and chlamydial infection by PCR in different groups of Kenyan women. *Ann. Soc. Belge. Med. Trop.* **72:**53–62.
33. **Fairley, C. K., S. Chen, S. N. Tabrizi, K. Leeton, M. A. Quinn, and S. M. Garland.** 1992. The absence of genital human papillomavirus DNA in virginal women. *Int. J. STD AIDS* **3:**414–417.
34. **Forslund, O., P. Nordin, K. Andersson, B. Stenquist, and B. G. Hansson.** 1997. DNA analysis indicates patient-specific human papillomavirus type 16 strains in Bowen's disease on fingers and in archival samples from genital dysplasia. *Br. J. Dermatol.* **136:**678–682.
35. **Galloway, D. A.** 1992. Serological assays for the detection of HPV antibodies, p. 147–161. *In* N. Munoz, F. X. Bosch, K. V. Shah, and A. Meheus (ed.), *The Epidemiology of Human Papillomavirus and Cervical Cancer.* IARC Scientific Publications No. 119. International Agency for Research on Cancer, Lyon, France.
36. **Galloway, D. A., and J. K. McDougall.** Biology of genital human papillomaviruses. *In* K. K. Holmes, P.-A. Mardh, P. F. Sparling, and P. J. Wiesner (ed.), *Sexually Transmitted Diseases,* 3rd ed., in press. McGraw-Hill Book Co., New York, N.Y.
37. **Gissmann, L.** 1984. Papillomaviruses and their association with cancer in animals and in man. *Cancer Surv.* **3:** 162–181.
38. **Gravitt, P. E., and M. M. Manos.** 1992. Polymerase chain reaction-based methods for the detection of human papillomavirus DNA, p. 121–133. *In* N. Munoz, F. X. Bosch, K. V. Shah, and A. Meheus (ed.), *The Epidemiology of Human Papillomavirus and Cervical Cancer.* IARC Scientific Publications No. 119. International Agency for Research on Cancer, Lyon, France.
39. **Grussendorf-Conen, E. I., E.-M. de Villiers, and L. Gissman.** 1986. Human papillomavirus genomes in penile smears of healthy men. *Lancet* 2 **ii:**1092.
40. **Hames, B. D., and S. J. Higgins (ed.).** 1985. *Nucleic Acid Hybridisation: a Practical Approach.* IRL Press, Oxford, United Kingdom.
41. **Hecht, J. L., S. Kadish, G. Jiang, and R. D. Burk.** 1995. Genetic characterization of the human papillomavirus (HPV) 18 E2 gene in clinical specimens suggests the presence of a subtype with decreased oncogenic potential. *Int. J. Cancer* **60:**369–376.
42. **Ho, L., S. Chan, R. D. Burk, B. C. Das, K. Fujinaga, J. P. Icenogle, T. Kahn, N. Kiviat, W. Lancaster, P. Mavromara, S. Mitrani-Rosenbaum, B. Norrild, M. R. Pillai, J. Stoerker, K. Syrjaenen, S. Syrjaenen, S. Tay, L. L. Villa, C. M. Wheeler, A. Williamson, and H. Bernard.** 1993. The genetic drift of human papillomavirus type 16 is a means of reconstructing prehistoric viral spread and the movement of ancient human populations. *J. Virol.* **67:** 6413–6423.
43. **Hopfl, R., G. Bens, U. Wieland, A. Petter, B. Zelger, P. Fritsch, and H. Pfister.** 1997. Human papillomavirus DNA in non-melanoma skin cancers of a renal transplant recipient: detection of a new sequence related to epidermodysplasia verruciformis associated types. *J. Invest. Dermatol.* **108:**53–56.
44. **Howley, P. M.** 1996. Papillomaviridae: the viruses and their replication, p. 2045–2076. *In* B. N. Fields, D. M. Knipe, P. M. Howley, R. M. Chanock, J. L. Melnick, T. P. Monath, B. Roizman, and S. E. Straus (ed.), *Fields Virology,* vol. 2, 3rd ed. Lippincott-Raven Publishers, Philadelphia, Pa.
45. **Jenson, A. B., R. J. Kurman, and W. D. Lancaster.** 1987. Tissue effects of and host response to human papillomavirus infection. *Obstet. Gynecol. Clin. N. Am.* **14:**397–406.
46. **Kiviat, N., L. Koutsky, C. Critchlow, D. Galloway, D. Vernon, M. Peterson, P. McElhose, S. Pendras, C. Stevens, and K. Holmes.** 1990. Comparison of Southern transfer hybridization and dot filter hybridization for detection of cervical human papillomavirus infection with types 6, 11, 16, 18, 31, 33, and 35. *Am. J. Clin. Pathol.* **94:** 561–565.
47. **Kiviat, N. B., C. W. Critchlow, and R. J. Kurman.** 1992. Reassessment of the morphological continuum of cervical intraepithelial lesions: does it reflect different stages in the progression to cervical carcinoma?, p. 59–66. *In* N. Munoz, F. X. Bosch, K. V. Shah, and A. Meheus (ed.), *The Epidemiology of Cervical Cancer and Human Papillomavirus.* IARC Scientific Publications No. 119. International Agency for Research on Cancer, Lyon, France.
48. **Kiviat, N. B., L. A. Koutsky, C. W. Critchlow, A. T. Lorincz, A. P. Cullen, J. Brockway, and K. K. Holmes.** 1992. Prevalence and cytologic manifestations of HPV types 6, 11, 16, 18, 31, 33, 35, 42, 43, 44, 45, 51, 52, and 56 among 500 consecutive women. *Int. J. Gynecol. Pathol.* **11:**197–203.
49. **Kjaer, S. K., and E. Lynge.** 1989. Incidence, prevalence and time trends of genital HPV infection determined by clinical examination and cytology, p. 113–124. *In* N. Munoz, F. X. Bosch, and O. M. Jensen (ed.), *Human Papillomavirus and Cervical Cancer.* IARC Scientific Publications No. 94. International Agency for Research on Cancer, Lyon, France.
50. **Koutsky, L. A., and N. B. Kiviat.** Human papillomavirus infections. *In* K. K. Holmes, P.-A. Mardh, P. F. Sparling, and P. J. Wiesner (ed.), *Sexually Transmitted Diseases,* 3rd ed., in press. McGraw-Hill Book Co., New York, N.Y.
51. **Koutsky, L. A., D. A. Galloway, and K. K. Holmes.** 1988. Epidemiology of genital human papillomavirus infection. *Epidemiol. Rev.* **10:**122–163.

51a. **Koutsky, L. A., D. A. Galloway, and N. B. Kiviat.** Unpublished data.

52. **Koutsky, L. A., K. K. Holmes, C. W. Critchlow, C. E. Stevens, J. Paavonen, A. M. Beckmann, T. A. DeRouen, D. A. Galloway, D. Vernon, and N. B. Kiviat.** 1992. A cohort study of the risk of cervical intraepithelial neoplasia grade 2 or 3 in relation to human papillomavirus infection. *N. Engl. J. Med.* **327:**1272–1278.
53. **Kreider, J. W.** 1987. Susceptibility of various human tissues to transformation in vivo with human papillomavirus type 11. *Int. J. Cancer* **39:**459.
54. **Leigh, I. M., and M. T. Glover.** 1995. Skin cancer and warts in immunosuppressed renal transplant recipients. *Recent Results Cancer Res.* **139:**69–86.
55. **Londesborough, P., L. Ho, G. Terry, J. Cuzick, C. Wheeler, and A. Singer.** 1996. Human papillomavirus (HPV) genotype as a predictor of persistence and development of high grade lesions in women with minor cervical abnormalities. *Int. J. Cancer* **69:**364–368.
56. **Lorincz, A.** 1995. Human papillomaviruses, p. 465. *In* E. H. Lennette, D. A. Lennette, and E. T. Lennette (ed.), *Diagnostic Procedures for Viral, Rickettsial, and Chlamydial Disease,* 7th ed. American Public Health Association, Washington, D.C.
57. **Lorincz, A.** 1996. Molecular methods for the detection of

human papillomavirus infection. *Obst. Gynecol. Clin. N. Am.* **23:**707–730.

58. **Lorincz, A. T., R. Reid, A. B. Jenson, M. D. Greenberg, W. Lancaster, and R. J. Kurman.** 1992. Human papillomavirus infection of the cervix: relative risk associations of fifteen common anogenital types. *Obstet. Gynecol.* **79:** 328–337.
59. **Lorincz, A. T.** 1990. Human papillomavirus detection tests, p. 953–959. *In* K. K. Holmes, P.-A. Mardh, P. F. Sparling, P. J. Wiesner, W. Cates, S. M. Lemon, and W. E. Stamm (ed.), *Sexually Transmitted Diseases*, 2nd ed. McGraw-Hill Book Co., New York, N.Y.
60. **Manos, M. M., Y. Ting, D. K. Wright, A. J. Lewis, T. R. Broker, and S. M. Wolinsky.** 1989. The use of polymerase chain reaction amplification for the detection of genital human papillomavirus, p. 209–214. *In* M. Furth and M. Greaves (ed.), *Cancer Cells*, vol. 7. *Molecular Diagnostics of Human Cancer*. Cold Spring Harbor Laboratory Press, Cold Spring Harbor, N.Y.
61. **Mansat-Krzyzanowska, E., J. Dantal, M. Hourmant, P. L. Litous, J. P. Soulillou, and B. Dr'eno.** 1997. Frequency of mucosal HPV DNA detection (types 6/11, 16/18, 31/35/51) in skin lesions of renal transplant patients. *Transplant. Int.* **10:**137–140.
62. **May, M., X. P. Dong, F. Stubenrauch, P. G. Fuchs, and H. Pfister.** 1994. The E6/E7 promoter of extrachromosomal HPV16 DNA in cervical cancers escapes from cellular repression by mutation of target sequences for YY1. *EMBO J.* **13:**1460–1466.
63. **McGrae, J. D., Jr., C. E. Greer, and M. M. Manos.** 1993. Multiple Bowen's disease of the fingers associated with human papilloma virus type 16. *Int. J. Dermatol.* **32:** 104–107.
64. **McGregor, J. M., R. J. Berkhout, M. Rozycka, J. ter Schegget, J. N. Bouwes-Bavinck, L. Brooks, and T. Crook.** 1997. p53 mutations implicate sunlight in post-transplant skin cancer irrespective of human papillomavirus status. *Oncogene* **15:**1737–1740.
65. **Meisels, A., and C. Morin.** 1986. Flat condyloma of the cervix: two variants with different prognosis, p. 115–119. *In* R. Peto and H. zur Hausen (ed.), *Viral Etiology of Cervical Cancer*. Banbury Report No. 21. Cold Spring Harbor Laboratory Press, Cold Spring Harbor, N.Y.
66. **Melkert, P. W. J., E. Hopman, A. van den Brule, E. K. J. Risse, P. J. van Diest, O. P. Bleker, T. Helmerhorst, M. I. Schipper, C. J. L. M. Meijer, and J. M. M. Walboomers.** 1993. Prevalence of HPV in cytomorphologically normal cervical smears, as determined by the polymerase chain reaction, is age-dependent. *Int. J. Cancer* **53:**919–923.
67. **Moy, R. L., and M. B. Quan.** 1991. The presence of human papillomavirus type 16 in squamous cell carcinoma of the proximal finger and reconstruction with a bilobed transposition flap. *J. Dermatol. Surg. Oncol.* **17:**171–175.
68. **Munger, K., M. Scheffner, J. M. Huibregtse, and P. M. Howley.** 1992. Interactions of HPV E6 and E7 oncoproteins with tumor suppressor gene products, p. 197–217. *In* A. J. Levine (ed.), *Tumor Suppressor Genes, the Cell Cycle and Cancer* (L. M. Franks, ed., *Cancer Surveys*, vol. 1). Cold Spring Harbor Laboratory Press, Cold Spring Harbor, N.Y.
69. **Munoz, N., and F. X. Bosch.** 1992. HPV and cervical cancer: review of case-control and cohort studies, p. 251–262. *In* N. Munoz, F. X. Bosch, K. V. Shah, and A. Meheus (ed.), *The Epidemiology of Cervical Cancer and Human Papillomavirus*. IARC Scientific Publications No. 119. International Agency for Research on Cancer, Lyon, France.
70. **Munoz, N., F. X. Bosch, S. de Sanjose, L. Fafur, I. Izarzugaza, M. Gili, P. Viadiu, C. Navarro, C. Martos, N. Ascunce, L. C. Gonzalez, J. M. Kaldor, E. Guerrero, A. Lorincz, M. Samtamaria, P. Alonso de Ruiz, N. Aristizabal, and K. Shah.** 1992. The causal link between human papillomavirus and invasive cervical cancer: a population-based case-control study in Colombia and Spain. *Int. J. Cancer* **52:**743–749.
71. **Nagai, N., G. Nuovo, D. Friedman, and C. P. Crum.** 1987. Detection of human papillomavirus nucleic acids in genital precancers with the in situ hybridization technique. *Int. J. Gynecol. Pathol.* **6:**366–379.
72. **Nuovo, G. J., P. MacConnell, A. Forde, and P. Delvenne.** 1991. Detection of human papillomavirus DNA in formalin-fixed tissues by in situ hybridization after amplification by polymerase chain reaction. *Am. J. Pathol.* **139:**847–854.
73. **Oriel, J. D.** 1971. Natural history of genital warts. *Br. J. Vener. Dis.* **47:**1–13.
74. **Paavonen, J., C. E. Stevens, P. Wolner-Hanssen, C. W. Critchlow, T. DeRouen, N. Kiviat, L. A. Koutsky, W. E. Stamm, L. Corey, and K. K. Holmes.** 1988. Colposcopic manifestations of cervical and vaginal infections. *Obstet. Gynecol. Surv.* **43:**373–381.
75. **Paavonen, J., L. A. Koutsky, and N. Kiviat.** 1990. Cervical neoplasia and other STD-related genital and anal neoplasias, p. 561–592. *In* K. K. Holmes, P.-A. Mardh, P. F. Sparling, P. J. Wiesner, W. Cates, S. M. Lemon, and W. E. Stamm (ed.), *Sexually Transmitted Diseases*, 2nd ed. McGraw-Hill Book Co., New York, N.Y.
76. **Pao, C. C., C.-Y. Lin, J.-S. Maa, C.-H. Lai, S.-Y. Wu, and Y.-K. Soong.** 1990. Detection of human papillomaviruses in cervicovaginal cells using polymerase chain reaction. *J. Infect. Dis.* **161:**113–115.
77. **Papay, F., B. Wood, and M. Coulson.** 1988. Squamous cell papilloma at the tracheooesophageal puncture stoma. *Arch. Otolaryngol. Head Neck Surg.* **144:**564–568.
78. **Park, J. S., R. J. Kurman, T. D. Keissis, and K. V. Shah.** 1991. Comparison of peroxidase-labeled DNA probes with radioactive RNA probes for detection of human papillomaviruses by in situ hybridization in paraffin sections. *Mod. Pathol.* **4:**81–85.
79. **Parkin, D. M., E. Laara, and C. S. Muir.** 1988. Estimates of the worldwide frequency of sixteen major cancers in 1980. *Int. J. Cancer* **41:**184–197.
80. **Pfister, H., A. Gasseenmairer, F. Nurnberger, and G. Stuttgen.** 1983. HPV 5 DNA in a carcinoma of an epidermodysplasia verruciformis patient infected with various human papillomavirus types. *Cancer Res.* **43:**1436–1441.
81. **Rakoczy, P., G. Sterret, J. Kulski, D. Whitaker, L. Hutchison, J. McKenzie, and E. Pixley.** 1990. Time trends in the prevalence of human papillomavirus infections in archival Papanicolaou smears: analysis by cytology, DNA hybridization, and polymerase chain reaction. *J. Med. Virol.* **32:**10–17.
82. **Reid, R., and M. D. Greenberg.** 1991. Human papillomavirus related diseases of the vulva. *Clin. Obstet. Gynecol.* **34:**630–650.
83. **Schiffman, M. H., H. M. Bauer, A. T. Lorincz, M. M. Manos, J. C. Byrne, A. G. Glass, D. M. Cadell, and P. M. Howley.** 1991. A comparison of Southern blot bybridization and polymerase chain reaction methods for the detection of human papillomavirus DNA. *J. Clin. Microbiol.* **29:**573–577.
84. **Schneider, A., and L. Koutsky.** 1992. Natural history and epidemiological features of genital HPV infection, p. 25–52. *In* N. Munoz, F. X. Bosch, K. V. Shah, and A. Meheus (ed.), *The Epidemiology of Cervical Cancer and Human Papillomavirus*. IARC Scientific Publications No. 119. International Agency for Research on Cancer, Lyon, France.
85. **Schneider, A., T. Oltersdorf, and V. Schneider.** 1987. Distribution pattern of human papilloma virus 16 genome

in cervical neoplasia by molecular in situ hybridization of tissue sections. *Int. J. Cancer* **39:**717–721.

86. **Shah, K. V.** 1990. Biology of human genital tract papillomaviruses, p. 425–431. *In* K. K. Holmes, P.-A. Mardh, P. F. Sparling, and P. J. Wiesner (ed.), *Sexually Transmitted Diseases*. McGraw-Hill Book Co. New York, N.Y.
87. **Shamanin, V., H. zur Hausen, D. Lavergne, D. M. Proby, I. M. Leigh, C. Neumann, H. Hamm, M. Goos, U.-F. Haustein, E. G. Jung, G. Plewig, H. Wolff, and E.-M. de Villiers.** 1996. Human papillomavirus infections in nonmelanoma skin cancers from renal transplant recipients and nonimmunosuppressed patients. *J. Natl. Cancer Inst.* **88:**802–811.
88. **Stoler, M. H.** 1993. In situ hybridization: a research technique or routine diagnostic test? *Arch. Pathol. Lab. Med.* **117:**478–481.
89. **Syrjanen, K., M. Hakama, S. Saarikoski, M. Vayrynen, M. Yliskoski, S. Syrjanen, V. Kataja, and O. Castren.** 1990. Prevalence, incidence, and estimated life-time risk of cervical human papillomavirus infection in a nonselected Finnish female population. *Sex. Transm. Dis.* **17:**15–19.
90. **ter-Meulen, J., H. C. Eberhardt, J. Luande, H. N. Mgaya, J. Chang-Clause, H. Mtiro, M. Mhina, P. Kashaija, S. Ockert, X. Yu, G. Mienhardt, L. Gissmann, and M. Pawlita.** 1992. Human papillomavirus (HPV) infection, HIV infection and cervical cancer in Tanzania, East Africa. *Int. J. Cancer* **51:**515–521.
91. **Ting, Y., and M. M. Manos.** 1990. Detection and typing of genital human papillomaviruses, p. 356. *In* D. H. Gelfand, T. White, M. A. Innis, and J. J. Sninsky (ed.), *PCR Protocols: A Guide to Methods and Applications*. Academic Press, Inc., San Diego, Calif.
92. **van den Brule, A. J., C. J. Meijer, V. Bakels, P. Kenemans, and J. M. Walboomers.** 1990. Rapid detection of human papillomavirus in cervical scrapes by combined general primer-mediated and type-specific polymerase chain reaction. *J. Clin. Microbiol.* **28:**2739–2743.
93. **van den Brule, A. J., E. C. Claas, M. du Maine, W. J. Melchers, T. Helmerhorst, W. G. Quint, J. Lindeman, C. J. Meijer, and J. M. Walboomers.** 1989. Use of anticontamination primers in the polymerase chain reaction for the detection of human papillomavirus genotypes in cervical scrapes and biopsies. *J. Med. Virol.* **29:**20–27.
94. **van Doornum, G. J. J., C. Hooykaas, L. H. J. Juffermans, S. M. G. A. van der Lans, and M. M. D. van der Linden.** 1992. Prevalence of human papillomavirus infections among heterosexual men and women with multiple sexual partners. *J. Med. Virol.* **37:**13–21.
95. **Van Ranst, M., J. B. Kaplan, and R. D. Burk.** 1992. Phylogenetic classification of human papillomaviruses: correlation with clinical manifestations. *J. Gen. Virol.* **73:** 2653–2660.
96. **Wolber, R. A., and P. B. Clement.** 1991. In situ DNA hybridization of cervical small cell carcinoma and adenocarcinoma using biotin-labeled human papillomavirus probes. *Mod. Pathol.* **4:**96–100.
97. **Xi, L. F., C. W. Critchlow, C. M. Wheeler, L. A. Koutsky, D. A. Galloway, J. Kuypers, J. P. Hughes, S. E. Hawes, C. Surawicz, G. Goldbaum, K. K. Holmes, and N. B. Kiviat.** Risk of anal carcinoma in situ in relation to human papillomavirus type 16 variants. *Cancer Res.*, in press.
98. **Xi, L. F., G. W. Demers, L. A. Koutsky, N. B. Kiviat, J. Kuypers, D. H. Watts, K. K. Holmes, and D. A. Galloway.** 1995. Analysis of human papillomavirus type 16 variants indicates establishment of persistent infection. *J. Infect. Dis.* **172:**747–755.
99. **Xi, L. F., L. A. Koutsky, D. A. Galloway, J. Kuypers, J. P. Hughes, C. M. Wheeler, K. K. Holmes, and N. B. Kiviat.** 1997. Genomic variation of human papillomavirus type 16 and risk for high grade cervical intraepithelial neoplasia. *J. Natl. Cancer Inst.* **89:**796–802.
100. **Xi, L. F., G. W. Demers, N. B. Kiviat, J. Kuypers, A. M. Beckmann, and D. A. Galloway.** 1993. Sequence variation in non-coding region of HPV type 16 detected by single strand conformation polymorphism analysis. *J. Infect. Dis.* **168:**610–617.
101. **Yamada, T., M. Manos, J. Peto, C. E. Greer, N. Munoz, F. X. Bosch, and C. M. Wheeler.** 1997. Human papillomavirus type 16 sequence variation in cervical cancers: a worldwide perspective. *J. Virol.* **71:**2463–2472.
102. **Zehbe, I., E. Wilander, H. Delius, and M. Tommasino.** 1998. Human papillomavirus 16 E6 variants are more prevalent in invasive cervical carcinoma than the prototype. *Cancer Res.* **58:**829–833.
103. **zur Hausen, H.** 1989. Papillomaviruses as carcinoma viruses, p. 1–26. *In* G. Klein (ed.) *Advances in Viral Oncology*. Raven Press, New York, N.Y.
104. **zur Hausen, H.** 1996. Papillomavirus infections—a major cause of human cancers. *Biochim. Biophys. Acta* **1288:**55–78.

Polyomaviruses

EUGENE O. MAJOR

86

CLINICAL BACKGROUND

Diseases associated with infection with the human polyomaviruses JC virus (JCV) and BK virus (BKV) occur mostly in immunocompromised adults, indicating a reactivation of a latent infection. JCV was isolated from brain tissue of a Hodgkin's lymphoma patient with the demyelinating disease progressive multifocal leukoencephalopathy (PML). Although virus particles resembling polyomaviruses have been associated with lesions in the white matter of PML patients, it was not until JCV was consistently isolated from numerous other PML patients' brain tissues that JCV was considered the etiologic agent of PML (63, 65, 69, 81). The virus lytically infects the oligodendrocyte in the white matter of the brain, which results in focal or multifocal plaques of demyelination. Such lesions can be demonstrated by magnetic resonance imaging or computerized tomography scans, as seen in Fig. 1, which also demonstrates the essential elements of the histopathology of PML. The clinical outcome most frequently seen in PML patients is hemiparesis or motor dysfunction, visual deficits such as cortical blindness or hemianopsia, and progressive dementia or cognitive impairment (9, 53, 69). Although JCV is tumorigenic in hamsters and owl and squirrel monkeys (49, 82), it has not been consistently associated with human neoplasms. However, JCV genomic DNA and T protein were identified in a human oligoastroglioma (68). BKV has been associated with kidney infections, particularly in renal transplant patients such as the original patient, who suffered ureteral stenosis (22, 33). BKV infection has also been associated with renal infections in bone marrow transplant patients (15). However, BKV has not been specifically identified as the etiologic agent in these infections.

There have also been reports of pancreatitis in a limited number of BKV-infected patients (6, 20). BKV DNA has been found in a human adenoma, pancreatic islet cells, and an insulinoma. Genomic sequences have also been found in gliomas and other tumors in the brain (26). It is not known whether BKV plays any role in the etiology of these tumors. BKV has not been associated with central nervous system infections such as encephalitis or demyelination.

On the basis of seroepidemiologic studies, the general population appears to be susceptible to human polyomavirus infections. Serum conversion occurs at ages 5 to 8 in almost 80% of the population worldwide (2, 3, 17, 32, 46, 64). Many individuals maintain antibody titers to one or the other of the viruses, sometimes both, throughout their lives. It is not clear in all cases whether these titers represent recurrent infection or reactivation of a latent infection. The nature of the primary BKV or JCV infection is also not known. Since both viruses can be excreted in the urine, however, even under conditions of no apparent disease, it is assumed that the kidney can be infected at some early stage following viral contact. For JCV, however, lymphoid tissues such as bone marrow and spleen have also been identified as sites for initial and/or latent infection (36, 43, 50). Tonsillar stromal cells as well as $CD34^+$ hematopoietic stem cells have been shown to be susceptible to JCV infection in culture (60) as well as in situ, suggesting that this tissue may be the initial site of JCV infection (61).

BKV can be detected in the urine of individuals following bone marrow and renal transplantation as well as in the urine of healthy individuals (5, 8, 23, 39). There is also a report indicating that a relatively large number of human immunodeficiency virus type 1 (HIV-1)-seropositive individuals shed BKV in their urine (55). Analysis of antibody of BKV from graft recipients revealed a relatively high incidence of infection in this population, i.e., 25% with primary infection and 21% with viral reactivation (3). These studies also revealed that primary infection could arise from the donor organ. The presence of virus, however, does not predict poor graft survival or illness in the host.

JCV has been associated with infection of the oligodendrocyte, the myelin-producing cell in the white matter in the human brain, leading to PML. JCV is not currently associated with any other pathological condition. Viral antigen or viral DNA is always present in lesions of the white matter normally identified from biopsy or autopsy tissues. Use of immunocytochemistry or in situ DNA hybridization confirms the presence of JCV in brain tissue and therefore establishes the diagnosis of PML in patients whose clinical history and neuroradiological signs are consistent with PML (1, 19, 25, 74). These assays also provide evidence that JCV can be present in B cells in the bone marrow and spleens of infected individuals (43). JCV DNA has also been identified in peripheral blood lymphocytes (PBLs) and cerebrospinal fluid (CSF) by PCR analysis (34, 76, 77, 79). Although the exact nature of primary infection is not known, it appears that JCV can establish latency in lymphoid organs and upon immune suppression can be reactivated in lym-

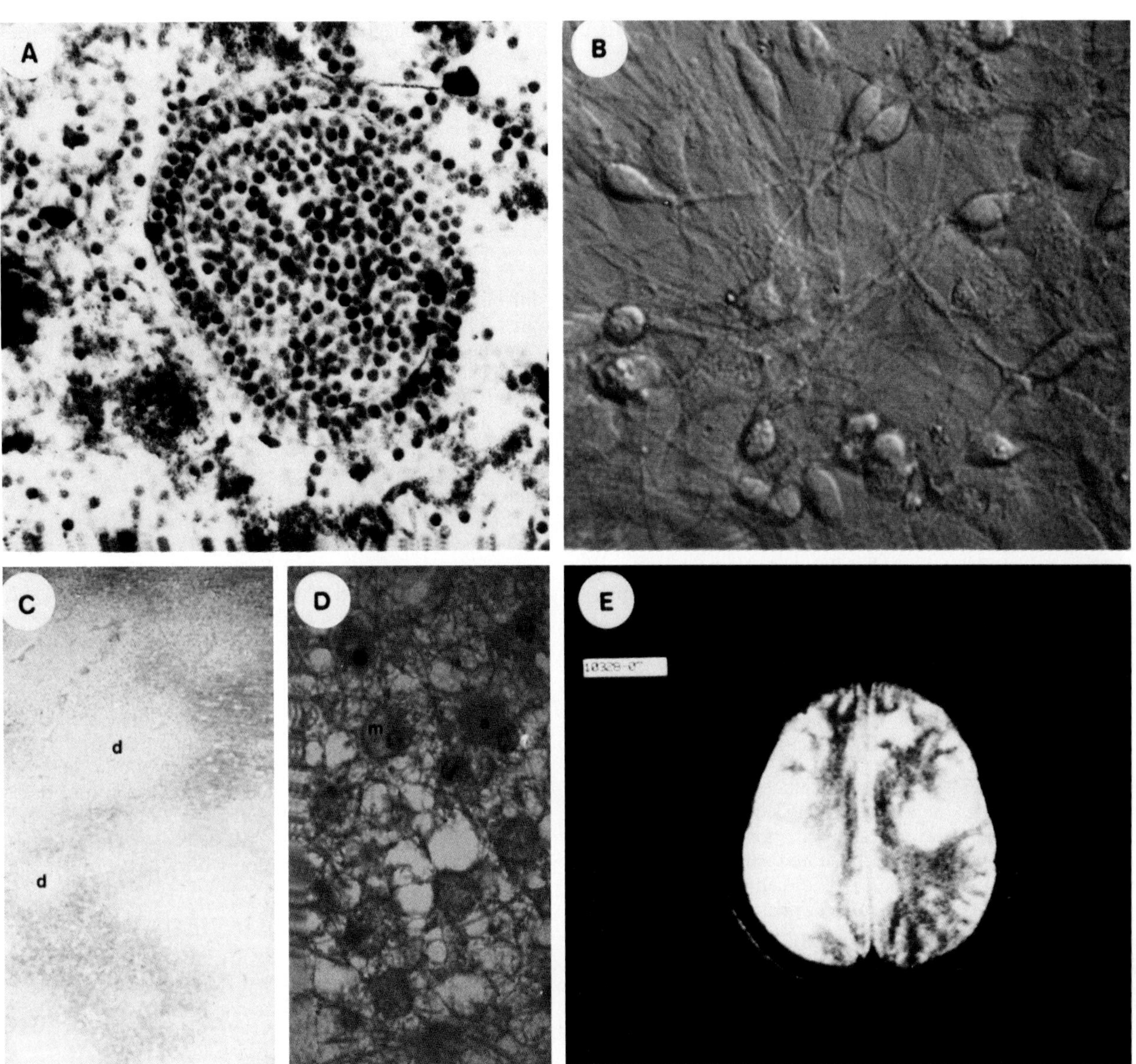

FIGURE 1 Representation of the major elements in the pathogenesis of PML. (A) Electron micrograph of brain tissue from a PML patient showing the assembly of JCV particles in the nucleus of an infected oligodendrocyte. (B) Human fetal neuroglial cells in culture demonstrating the morphological heterogeneous population of cells. (C) Luxol fast blue stain of the white matter with demyelinated plaque lesions in a patient with PML. d, area of myelination. (D) Hematoxylin stain of lesion showing the presence of a macrophage (m) and an astrocyte (a). (E) Magnetic resonance image of PML-affected brain with lesions of the subcortical white matter.

phocytes and travel to the brain. JCV-infected B lymphocytes in PBLs and brain tissue have been described (50, 77). The recognition of JCV-induced PML in transplant and cancer patients has been rare in the past, with only several hundred cases reported each year in the United States. However, PML occurs in approximately 5% of all AIDS patients, among whom thousands of cases of PML are reported worldwide each year (12, 13, 80). PML may be the presenting illness in patients with AIDS or may occur later in the course of the disease. To date there are no predictive laboratory tests for PML in terms of either CD4 levels or the detection of JCV in the peripheral blood. The increased awareness and diagnosis of PML in this patient group have alerted laboratories and clinicians to consider PML in non-AIDS patients as well.

DESCRIPTION OF THE AGENTS

Both JCV and BKV were described in 1971. They were isolated from a cell culture made from inoculations of urine from one patient and brain tissue from another patient into a human fetal kidney cell culture and a brain cell culture, respectively (33, 65). These viruses were classified in the genus *Polyomavirus* of the family *Papovaviridae* because of their architecture (icosahedral) and size (40-nm diameter) and because of the physical and genetic makeup of their double-stranded DNA genomes (63). Both viruses have the ability to hemagglutinate human type O erythrocytes, unlike simian virus 40. Virion particles are assembled in the nucleus from capsid proteins VP1, VP2, and VP3. VP1 is the external protein used for attachment to a presumed glycoprotein cell receptor and is responsible for the virion's ability to agglutinate human type O erythrocytes. Treatment of cells with neuraminidase eliminates or greatly reduces virus infectivity. Antibodies to VP1 neutralize infection and prevent hemagglutination. VP2 and VP3 are internal to the virion particle and presumably assist in assembly by ionic bonding to the nucleotides of the viral genome.

DNA sequence analysis of BKV and JCV showed an approximately 75% homology between the two at the DNA level and 68% homology at the amino acid level (30). The most significant differences in the viral genomes were in the noncoding nucleotide sequences responsible for viral DNA replication and transcription. These nucleotides exist as tandem repeats located directly between the regions coding for the multifunctional nonstructural T proteins and the three structural capsid proteins. These regulatory sequences are responsible for the rather limited cellular host range of JCV (primarily human glial cells) and the less restricted host range of BKV (epithelial cells of human and nonhuman primate origin as well as other cell types) (11, 27, 31, 53, 54). It appears that during replication these sequences are subject to substantial rearrangements both in vivo and in vitro (24, 30, 58, 59).

SPECIMENS: BODY FLUIDS AND TISSUES

Relevant body fluids for analysis include urine, blood, and CSF. BKV is most frequently detected in urine. Whether the sample is to be used for future PCR assays, virus isolation, or other tests, the urine can be stored at −80°C for long periods. Processing of urine involves centrifugation at approximately 1,000 × *g* to collect cells and then at high speeds (100,000 × *g*) to pellet the virus from the urine. Cell or virus pellets obtained by high-speed centrifugation can then be extracted for nucleic acid analysis or suspended in neutral pH buffer for virus isolation. These samples can be used for hemagglutination assays of human type O erythrocytes (22, 23) or for inoculation of susceptible cell cultures. Direct immunofluorescence examination of cells pelleted from urine has also been described (40).

Blood can be collected in either citrate buffer or heparin since organic solvent extraction should be used to prepare the DNA template. Buffy coats of PBLs can be prepared by using a Ficoll-Hypaque or comparable separation medium. CSF can be collected and stored at −80°C. Blood should be kept at room temperature until processing, which should be done within 24 h. CSF and PBLs can be processed for viral DNA by standard phenol-chloroform extraction procedures. Nucleic acid samples are quantitated by UV spectroscopy and are used as templates for PCR analysis. They can be kept at 4°C for long periods in a Tris buffer with 0.01 M EDTA. DNA can be frozen as well, but freeze-thaw cycles may damage the DNA sufficiently that it does not give consistent results by PCR. A summary of the most frequently collected clinical samples and virus assays is presented in Table 1.

JCV is most frequently detected in situ in infected brain tissues from suspected PML patients. Samples are often brain biopsy or autopsy specimens that are either formalin fixed and paraffin embedded or frozen. Tissue sections can also be processed for antigen detection by using antibodies to the virion capsid VP1 protein. Several mouse monoclonal antibodies to the nonstructural viral T protein have been used for the detection of JCV or BKV infection (35, 48, 56, 73). No commercial source for monoclonal antibodies which distinguish the primate polyomaviruses is currently available. Tissue sections from bone marrow or kidney biopsy specimens can be processed in a similar manner. Bone marrow aspirates should be centrifuged prior to plating onto gelatin-coated slides, air dried, and fixed in paraformaldehyde at 4°C prior to hybridization with a JCV probe.

DIAGNOSIS OF POLYOMAVIRUS INFECTIONS

Hemagglutination inhibition assays form the basis of routine serologic testing for the presence of antibody against both

TABLE 1 Laboratory selection and appropriate assays for virus identification

Specimen	Virus identified				
	Virus isolation[a]	Hemagglutination	PCR[b]	Antigen detection[c]	DNA hybrid[d]
Body fluids					
Urine	BKV, JCV	BKV, JCV	BKV, JCV		BKV, JCV[e]
Blood (lymphocytes)		JCV	JCV		
CSF		JCV	BKV, JCV		
Tissues[f]					
Brain	JCV		BKV, JCV	JCV	JCV
Kidney	BKV, JCV	BKV, JCV	BKV, JCV	BKV, JCV	BKV, JCV
Marrow		JCV	JCV	JCV	JCV
Tonsil			JCV		

[a] Most permissive cell cultures are derived from human fetal kidney for BKV and fetal brain for JCV. An established cell line of fetal astrocytes, SVG (45), is equally efficient for JCV isolation.

[b] Primer pair selection for genome amplification is made from conserved regions around the coding and noncoding sequences.

[c] Antibody to either the viral T protein or the capsid protein VP1 is used in immunofluorescence and immunocytochemistry assays (30, 41, 48, 61).

[d] Radioactive or biotin-labeled probes are used for the in situ DNA hybridization test. Biotin-labeled probes distinguish between JCV and BKV and detect active viral replication.

[e] Pelleted uroepithelial cells are targets for hybridization.

[f] Tissue sections may routinely be formalin fixed and paraffin embedded. Frozen sections are also useful for in situ DNA hybridization (1, 35). Either embedded or frozen sections can be extracted for DNA templates for testing by PCR.

BKV and JCV. Also, an enzyme-linked immunosorbent assay for the detection of immunoglobulin M antibody has been developed for these polyomaviruses (47, 48). Serology is generally not helpful in the diagnosis of acute infections, since the majority of the population demonstrates antibodies from previous exposure or reactivation of infection. There is little evidence that a rise in antibody titers is an indication of acute infection. Serology, however, does play an important role in establishing the epidemiology of the spread of human polyomaviruses and has contributed information on the worldwide distributions of both JCV and BKV (4, 51, 53, 62).

VIRUS ISOLATION

With the availability of antibody and DNA probes for BKV and JCV, virus isolations are not routinely done. The most susceptible cell types that support virus multiplication are primary cultures derived from human embryonic tissues. BKV grows well in human embryonic kidney cells and epithelial cells and also forms plaques on these cells. The enlargement of nuclei and the gradual but continual peeling of cells in the monolayer are evidence of a viral cytopathic effect. Some virus is shed into the cell culture medium, while a portion of the virus remains cell associated. Freeze-thaw cycles assist in releasing virus that can be detected by hemagglutination assays.

JCV grows best in human fetal brain cultures and multiplies in the astrocyte and the precursor oligodendroglial cell. JCV does not infect neurons in culture or in the brain. Even under optimum conditions with a sufficient viral inoculum, JCV growth takes weeks, and multiple passages are sometimes required before progeny virus can be detected. The viral cytopathic effect is subtle and is observed as translucent cells with large nuclei that begin to shed from the culture layer. Virus is not shed into the medium, and therefore, treatment of cell lysates with a nonionic detergent such as sodium deoxycholate is necessary for sample preparation for the hemagglutination assay. As an alternative to primary cultures from human fetal brain, an established human fetal cell line, SVG, is susceptible to JCV productive infection and grows readily in the laboratory (52).

NUCLEIC ACID TECHNIQUES

Tissue sections have also been analyzed successfully by using in situ DNA hybridization, as demonstrated in Fig. 2. There are several reports on the advantages of DNA hybridization over antigen detection in terms of specificity and sensitivity (1, 5, 21, 70). In one of these assays, the DNA probe used was biotin labeled. Although they are not as sensitive at detecting very low copy numbers of JCV, biotin-labeled probes detect as few as 100 copies, which is sufficient for diagnostic use with clinical tissue samples. This hybridization assay measures DNA replication, an earlier event in the life cycle of viral multiplication than virion capsid formation. It is possible that some cells are infected but do not produce sufficient antigen for immunocytochemical tests. DNA hybridization can also be used to identify these cells. Use of gelatin-coated or sialinated-treated slides may improve the adherence of the tissues for immunocytochemistry or hybridization. Biopsy of other tissues such as bone marrow and bone marrow aspirates has been reported previously (43, 50). Figure 2 shows cells in a bone marrow biopsy specimen that give a positive signal upon hybridization with a biotin-labeled probe for JCV DNA.

Application of nucleic acids extracted from clinical samples to membrane filters is also in common use for virus detection. Extracted nucleic acid samples either can be directly blotted onto a filter (dot blot procedures) or can be electrophoresed through agarose gels and then blotted onto a filter (Southern procedures). Radiolabeled viral genomic probes can be used to identify the DNA of either virus. These methods are routinely used in laboratories, but their completion requires several days and they employ labeled probes with relatively high specific activities, e.g., 10^8 dpm/μg of [^{32}P]DNA. Under these conditions, it can be difficult to differentiate BKV and JCV owing to their nucleotide sequence homologies.

PCR of Urine Samples

The use of PCR and other nucleic acid amplification techniques results in increased sensitivity. However, there are difficulties with the interpretation of a positive result. Since both BKV and JVC are excreted in urine and appear in kidney tissue under normal as well as pathological conditions, PCR has been used to detect viral genomes in urine in a number of studies (7, 29, 45, 55, 57). Essentially, both viruses can be found in approximately 10% of pregnant women, 30% of samples from patients with renal tumors, bone marrow and renal transplant recipients, and 40 to 70% of older individuals and individuals who are infected with HIV-1. The high rate of shedding of viral particles in the urine negates the utility of these assays for the diagnosis of acute infections (10, 28).

PCR Analysis of Blood and CSF

The pathogenesis of JCV infection leading to demyelination in the brain suggests viral latency in the kidney and lymphoid cells in the bone marrow, spleen, or lymph nodes. Upon reactivation due to weakened immune surveillance, JCV becomes associated with PBLs, most notably the B cells. Evidence for the presence of JCV DNA in PBLs comes from examination of a large number of PML patients (71, 77). JCV DNA has also been detected in a large number of CSF samples from PML patients with or without AIDS but not in non-PML patients (16, 38, 78, 79). There have been several reports of PCR detection of JCV DNA in the brain tissue of PML patients, as expected, and one report of the detection of JCV in B cells in the brains of PML patients (38, 66, 75). A summary of the percentage of JCV-positive blood and CSF samples from immune-suppressed and non-immune-suppressed PML patients is shown in Fig. 2. It is noteworthy that approximately 5% of healthy individuals have JCV DNA in their peripheral circulation. It appears in Fig. 2 that the B lymphocyte identified by flow cytometry gives rise to the PCR signal in blood samples.

EVALUATION AND INTERPRETATION OF RESULTS

The number of immune-suppressed individuals will continue to increase owing to neoplastic diseases, AIDS, and therapies requiring immune suppression of renal, bone marrow, heart, and other graft recipients. Since serology is not a principal tool for the diagnosis of infections caused by human polyomaviruses, the detection of viral proteins or nucleic acids is essential. Also, virus isolation for the detection of either BKV or JCV is very time-consuming and is prone to false-negative results. Since BKV is associated with renal infections, identification of virus in urine by nucleic acid hybridization or immunocytochemistry for viral pro-

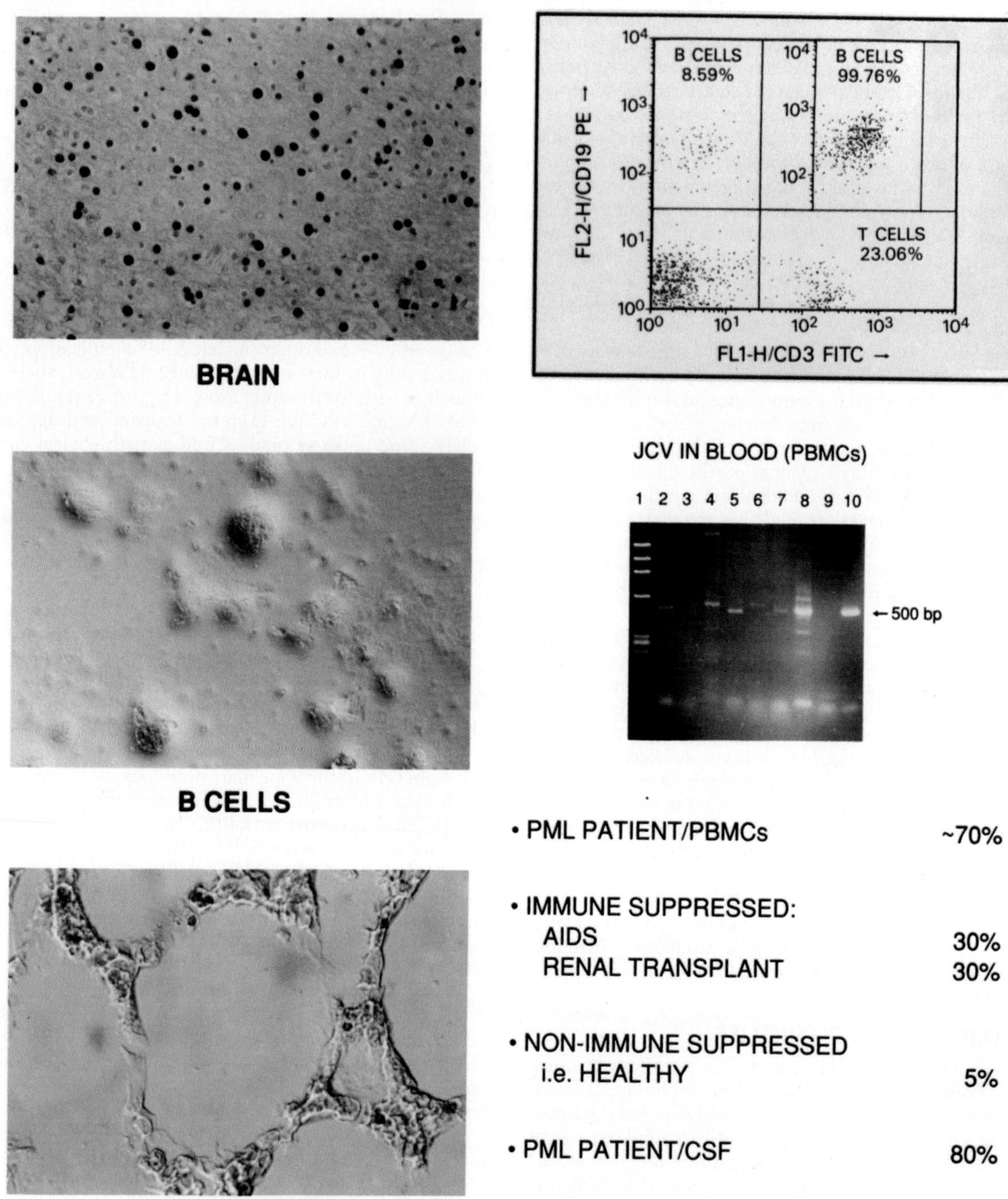

FIGURE 2 Summary of the detection of JCV DNA in tissues and the percentage of clinical samples that test PCR positive for JCV DNA. Photomicrographs on the left show brain and bone marrow biopsy tissue and B lymphocytes with positive signals following in situ DNA hybridization with a biotin-labeled probe for JCV DNA. Panels on the right are graphic demonstrations. The top panel shows the separation of peripheral lymphocytes by using flow cytometry indicating >99% purity of B lymphocytes collected by fluorescence-activated cell sorter gating on a CD19 fluorescence marker (*y* axis) separated from CD3 cells (*x* axis). FITC, fluorescein isothiocyanate; PE, phycoerythrin. The middle panel shows the results of PCR analysis of DNA templates made from sorted cells run on an agarose gel and stained with ethidium bromide. The lower panel shows the results of PCR analysis from many studies as the percentage of samples from PML and non-PML individuals positive for JCV DNA PBMCs, peripheral blood mononuclear cells.

teins is useful. Brain tissue is still needed for the diagnosis of JCV-induced PML. In situ DNA hybridization is the most reliable assay for detection of the presence of JCV in brain tissue and has proven to be more specific and more sensitive than immunocytochemistry. The list of samples routinely collected for the detection of these viruses and the most appropriate assays performed with these samples are presented in Table 1.

For patients with suspected PML for whom a brain biopsy is not appropriate or possible, the presence of JCV DNA in CSF along with radiographic findings in an immunodeficient patient may strongly suggest a diagnosis of PML. Currently, PCR analysis of CSF for the detection of JCV DNA is 80% sensitive and has a high degree of specificity (almost 95%). The use of noninvasive procedures, i.e., PCR of CSF, to analyze samples for the diagnosis of viral infections in the nervous system will be helpful, although it is subject to some false-negative results.

THERAPEUTIC STRATEGIES FOR POLYOMAVIRUS INFECTION

There is currently no accepted treatment for JCV and BKV infections and only anecdotal accounts of therapies for JCV-induced PML. Recent reviews describe in detail these attempts at therapy (51, 53). Among the compounds tested, nucleoside analogs, particularly cytosine arabinoside (ara-C), have been used to treat a large number of PML patients. Reports have not shown a consistent positive response, but for a few patients, treatment seems to have produced some improvement in cognitive ability and motor function (18, 67). One report on treatment with cytarabine and alpha interferon in combination described a marked improvement in the clinical course of disease (72). However, the use of nucleoside analogs in patients with impaired immunity is difficult to manage. A clinical trial protocol with ara-C in PML patients with AIDS has been conducted through the AIDS Clinical Trial Group, ACTG 243. Laboratory data indicate that ara-C blocks JCV replication but is not toxic to human fetal glial cells in culture (51) or to a human fetal glial cell line persistently infected with JCV (41). In the AIDS Clinical Trial Group study, ara-C was administered intrathecally or intravenously for 6 months only to patients with biopsy-proven cases of PML. The presence and concentration of virus in peripheral blood and CSF were monitored by PCR. Clinical improvement was the goal of the study. This trial enrolled 64 patients and represented the first controlled treatment trial for PML. The clinical data, however, indicated that ara-C administered either intravenously or intrathecally did not improve the clinical outcome of PML in the AIDS patients enrolled in the trial (37). Camptothecin, a drug that interferes with viral replication by inhibition of topoisomerase, may be effective in cell culture experiments (44). This drug may also have activity against BKV.

A number of cases of remission of PML have been documented both clinically and neuroradiologically, in some cases essentially without therapeutic intervention (14). Reversal of clinical symptoms has been found and resolution of plaque lesions has been seen by magnetic resonance imaging. It is therefore possible that treatment may help prevent further virus dissemination to the brain and/or slow or block viral multiplication in the white matter. Whether remyelination can occur in patients with PML to reverse clinical symptoms remains to be fully tested.

The mechanisms that protect individuals who have JCV in their peripheral circulation from developing PML or who are long-term survivors of or in remission from the clinical course of PML are under investigation. Studies of the importance of cellular immune reactivity to JCV infection need emphasis and may help to explain susceptibility to the development of PML.

REFERENCES

1. **Aksamit, A., J. L. Sever, and E. O. Major.** 1986. Progressive multifocal leukoencephalopathy: JC virus detection by in situ hybridization compared with immunocytochemistry. *Neurology* **36:**499–504.
2. **Andrews, C., K. Shah, R. Daniel, M. Hirsch, and R. Rubin.** 1988. A serologic investigation of BK virus and JC virus infections in recipients of renal allografts. *J. Infect. Dis.* **158:**176–181.
3. **Andrews, C. A., R. Daniel, and K. Shah.** 1983. Serologic studies of papovavirus infections in pregnant women and renal transplant recipients, p. 133–141. *In* J. L. Sever and D. L. Madden (ed.), *Polyomaviruses and Human Neurological Disease*. Alan R. Liss, Inc., New York, N.Y.
4. **Aoki, N., M. Mori, K. Kato, Y. Sakamoto, K. Noda, M. Tajima, and H. Shimada.** 1996. Antibody against synthetic multiple antigen peptides (MAP) of JC virus capsid protein (VP1) without cross reaction to BK virus: a diagnostic tool for progressive multifocal leukoencephalopathy. *Neurosci. Lett.* **205:**111–114.
5. **Arthur, R., A. Beckmann, C. L. Chou, R. Saral, and K. Shah.** 1985. Direct detection of the human papovavirus BK in urine of bone marrow transplant recipients: comparison of DNA hybridization with ELISA. *J. Med. Virol.* **16:** 29–36.
6. **Arthur, R., K. Shah, S. Baust, G. Santos, and R. Saral.** 1986. Association of BK viruria with hemorrhagic cystitis in recipients of bone marrow transplants. *N. Engl. J. Med.* **315:**230–234.
7. **Arthur, R. A., S. Dagostin, and K. Shah.** 1989. Detection of BK virus and JC virus in urine and brain tissue by the polymerase chain reaction. *J. Clin. Microbiol.* **27:** 1174–1179.
8. **Arthur, R. A., K. V. Shah, P. Charache, and R. Saral.** 1988. BK and JC virus infections in recipients of bone marrow transplants. *J. Infect. Dis.* **158:**563–569.
9. **Åstrom, K.-E., E. L. Mancall, and E. P. Richardson, Jr.** 1958. Progressive multifocal leukoencephalopathy. *Brain* **81:**93–127.
10. **Azizzi, A.** 1996. Human polyomaviruses DNA detection in peripheral blood leukocytes from immunocompetent and immunocompromised individuals. *J. Neurovirol.* **6:** 411–416.
11. **Beckman, A., and K. V. Shah.** 1983. Propagation and primary isolation of JCV and BKV in urinary epithelial cell cultures, p. 3–14. *In* J. L. Sever and D. L. Madden (ed.), *Polyomaviruses and Human Neurological Diseases*. Alan R. Liss, Inc., New York, N.Y.
12. **Berger, J. R., B. Kaszovitz, M. J. Post, and G. Dickinson.** 1987. Progressive multifocal leukoencephalopathy associated with human immunodeficiency virus infection. A review of the literature with a report of sixteen cases. *Ann. Intern. Med.* **107:**78–87.
13. **Berger, J. R., G. Scott, J. Albrecht, A. Belman, C. Tornatore, and E. O. Major.** 1992. Progressive multifocal leukoencephalopathy in HIV-1 infected children. *AIDS* **6:** 837–841.
14. **Berger, J. R., and L. Mucke.** 1988. Prolonged survival and partial recovery in AIDS-associated progressive multifocal leukoencephalopathy. *Neurology* **38:**1060–1065.
15. **Bogdanovic, G., P. Ljungman, F. Wang, and T. Dallianis.** 1996. Presence of human polyomavirus DNA in the pe-

ripheral circulation of bone marrow transplant patients with and without hemorrhagic cystitis. *Bone Marrow Transplant.* **17:**573–576.

16. **Brouqui, P., C. Bollet, J. Delmont, and A. Bourgeade.** 1992. Diagnosis of progressive multifocal leukoencephalopathy by PCR detection of JC virus from CSF. *Lancet* **339:** 1182.
17. **Brown, P., T. Tsai, and D. C. Gajdusek.** 1975. Seroepidemiology of human papovaviruses: discovery of virgin populations and some unusual patterns of antibody prevalence among remote peoples of the world. *Am. J. Epidemiol.* **102:** 331–340.
18. **Buckman, R., and E. Wiltshaw.** 1976. Progressive multifocal leukoencephalopathy successfully treated with cytosine arabinoside. *Br. J. Haematol.* **34:**153–154.
19. **Budka, H., and K. Shah.** 1983. Papovavirus antigens in paraffin section of PML brains, p. 299–309. *In* J. L. Sever and D. L. Madden (ed.), *Polyomaviruses and Human Neurological Diseases*. Alan R. Liss, Inc., New York, N.Y.
20. **Cheeseman, S., P. Black, R. Rubin, K. Cantell, and M. Hirsch.** 1980. Interferon and BK papovavirus—clinical and laboratory studies. *J. Infect. Dis.* **141:**157–161.
21. **Chesters, P. M., J. Heritage, and D. J. McCance.** 1983. Persistence of DNA sequences of BK virus and JC virus in normal human tissues and in diseased tissues. *J. Infect. Dis.* **147:**676–682.
22. **Coleman, D. V., S. D. Gardner, and A. M. Field.** 1973. Human polyomavirus infection in renal allograft recipients. *Br. Med. J.* **3:**371–375.
23. **Coleman, D. V., M. R. Wolfendale, R. A. Daniel, N. K. Dhanjal, S. D. Gardner, P. E. Gibson, and A. M. Field.** 1980. A prospective study of human polyomavirus infection in pregnancy. *J. Infect. Dis.* **142:**1–8.
24. **Dörries, K.** 1984. Progressive multifocal leukoencephalopathy: analysis of JC virus DNA from brain and kidney tissue. *Virus Res.* **1:**25–38.
25. **Dörries, K., R. T. Johnson, and V. Ter Meulen.** 1979. Detection of polyoma virus DNA in PML-brain tissue by (in situ) hybridization. *J. Gen. Virol.* **42:**49–57.
26. **Dörries, K., G. Loeber, and J. Meixensbarger.** 1987. Association of polyomaviruses JC, SV40, and BK with human brain tumors. *Virology* **160:**268–270.
27. **Feigenbaum, L., K. Khalili, E. O. Major, and G. Khoury.** 1987. Regulation of the host range of human papovavirus JCV. *Proc. Natl. Acad. Sci. USA* **84:**3695–3698.
28. **Ferrante, P., R. Caldarelli-Stefano, E. Omodeo-Zorini, A. E. Cagni, L. Cocchi, F. Suter, and R. Maserati.** 1997. Comprehensive investigation of the presence of JC virus in AIDS patients with and without progressive multifocal leukoencephalopathy. *J. Med. Microbiol.* **52:**235–242.
29. **Flægstad, T., A. Sundsfjord, R. R. Arthur, M. Pedersen, T. Traavik, and S. Subramani.** 1991. Amplification and sequencing of the control regions of BK and JC virus from human urine by polymerase chain reaction. *Virology* **180:** 553–560.
30. **Frisque, R., G. Bream, and M. Cannella.** 1984. Human polyomavirus JC virus genome. *J. Virol.* **51:**458–469.
31. **Gardner, S., E. Mackenzie, C. Smith, and A. Porter.** 1984. Prospective study of the human polyomaviruses BK and JC and cytomegalovirus in renal transplant recipients. *J. Clin. Pathol.* **37:**578–586.
32. **Gardner, S. D.** 1973. Prevalence in England of antibody to human polyomavirus (BK). *Br. Med. J.* **1:**77–78.
33. **Gardner, S. D., A. M. Field, D. V. Coleman, and B. Hulme.** 1971. New human papovavirus (BK) isolated from urine after renal transplantation. *Lancet* **i:**1253–1257.
34. **Gibson, P., W. Knowles, J. Hand, and D. Brown.** 1993. Detection of JC virus DNA in cerebrospinal fluid of patients with progressive multifocal leukoencephalopathy. *J. Med. Virol.* **39:**278–281.
35. **Greenlee, J., and P. M. Keeney.** 1986. Immunoenzymatic labelling of JC papovavirus T antigen in brains of patients with progressive multifocal leukoencephalopathy. *Acta Neuropathol.* **71:**150–153.
36. **Grinnel, B. W., B. L. Padgett, and D. L. Walker.** 1983. Distribution of nonintegrated DNA from JC papovavirus in organs of patients with progressive multifocal leukoencephalopathy. *J. Infect. Dis.* **147:**669–675.
37. **Hall, C. D., U. Dafni, D. Simpson, D. Clifford, P. Wetherill, B. Cohen, J. McArthur, H. Hollander, C. Yainnoutsos, E. Major, L. Millar, J. Timponse, and the ACTG 243 Team.** 1998. Failure of cytosine arabinoside therapy of human immunodeficiency virus type 1 associated progressive multifocal leukoencephalopathy. *N. Engl. J. Med.* **338:**1345–1351.
38. **Hammarin, A. L., G. Bogdanovic, V. Svedhem, R. Pirskkanen, L. Morfeldt, and M. Grandien.** 1991. Amplification of JC virus DNA from brain and cerebrospinal fluid of patients with progressive multifocal leukoencephalopathy. *Neurology* **41:**1967–1971.
39. **Hogan, F., E. Borden, J. McBain, B. L. Padgett, and D. Walker.** 1980. Human polyomavirus infections with JC virus and BK virus in renal transplant patients. *Ann. Intern. Med.* **92:**373–378.
40. **Hogan, T. F., B. L. Padgett, D. L. Walker, E. C. Borden, and J. A. McBain.** 1980. Rapid detection and identification of JC virus and BK virus in human urine by using immunofluorescence microscopy. *J. Clin. Microbiol.* **11:** 178–183.
41. **Hou, J., and E. O. Major.** 1998. The efficacy of nucleoside analogues against JC virus multiplication in a persistently infected human astroglial cell line. *J. Neurovirol.* **4:** 451–456.
42. **Houff, S. A., D. Katz, C. Kufta, and E. O. Major.** 1989. A rapid method for in situ hybridization for viral DNA in brain biopsies from patients with acquired immunodeficiency syndrome (AIDS). *AIDS* **3:**843–845.
43. **Houff, S. A., E. O. Major, D. Katz, C. Kufta, J. Sever, S. Pittaluga, J. Roberts, J. Gitt, N. Saini, and W. Lux.** 1988. Involvement of JC virus-infected mononuclear cells from the bone marrow and spleen in the pathogenesis of progressive multifocal leukoencephalopathy. *N. Engl. J. Med.* **318:**301–305.
44. **Kerr, D., C. Chang, J. Gordon, M. Bjornsti, and K. Khalili.** 1993. Inhibition of human neurotropic virus (JCV) DNA replication in glial cells by camptothecin. *Virology* **196:**612–618.
45. **Kitamura, T., Y. Aso, N. Kuniyoshi, K. Hara, and Y. Yogo.** 1990. High incidence of urinary JC virus infection in non-immunocompromised older patients. *J. Infect. Dis.* **161:**1128–1133.
46. **Knight, R. S., N. M. Hyman, S. D. Gardner, P. E. Gibson, M. M. Esiri, and C. P. Warlow.** 1988. Progressive multifocal leukoencephalopathy and viral antibody titres. *J. Neurol.* **235:**458–461.
47. **Knowles, W., P. Gibson, J. Hand, and D. Brown.** 1992. An M-antibody capture radioimmunoassay for detection of JC virus-specific IgM. *J. Virol. Methods* **40:**95–106.
48. **Knowles, W., I. Sharp, L. Efstratiou, J. Hand, and S. Gardner.** 1991. Preparation of monoclonal antibodies to JC virus and their use in the diagnosis of progressive multifocal leukoencephalopathy. *J. Med Virol.* **34:**127–131.
49. **London, W. T., S. A. Houff, D. L. Madden, D. A. Fuccillo, M. Gravell, W. C. Wallen, A. E. Palmer, J. L. Sever, B. L. Padgett, D. L. Walker, G. M. ZuRhein, and T. Ohashi.** 1978. Brain tumors in owl monkeys inoculated

with a human polyomavirus (JC virus). *Science* **201:** 1246–1249.

50. **Major, E. O., K. Amemiya, G. Elder, and S. A. Houff.** 1990. Glial cells of the human developing brain and B cells of the immune system share a common DNA binding factor for recognition of the regulatory sequences of the human polyomavirus, JCV. *J. Neurosci. Res.* **27:**461–471.
51. **Major, E. O., and B. L. Cufman.** 1997. Viral induced demyelination leading to progressive multifocal leukoencephalopathy; the involvement of both immune and nervous system target cells, p. 305–321. *In* J. Remington and P. K. Peterson (ed.), *In Defense of the Brain: the ImmunoPathogenesis of CNS Infections*. Blackwell Science, Cambridge, United Kingdom.
52. **Major, E. O., A. E. Miller, P. Mourrain, R. Traub, E. De Widt, and J. L. Sever.** 1985. Establishment of a line of human glial cells that supports JC virus multiplication. *Proc. Natl. Acad. Sci. USA* **82:**1257–1261.
53. **Major, E. O., K. Amemiya, C. Tornatore, S. Houff, and J. R. Berger.** 1992. Pathogenesis and molecular biology of progressive multifocal leukoencephalopathy, the JC virus-induced demyelinating disease of the human brain. *Clin. Microbiol. Rev.* **5:**49–73.
54. **Major, E. O., and D. A. Vacante.** 1989. Human fetal astrocytes in culture support the growth of the neurotropic human polyomavirus, JCV. *J. Neuropathol. Exp. Neurol.* **48:**425–436.
55. **Markowitz, B., H. Thompson, J. Mueller, J. Cohen, and W. Dynan.** 1993. Incidence of BK virus and JC virus viruria in human immunodeficiency virus infected and uninfected subjects. *J. Infect. Dis.* **167:**13–20.
56. **Marshall, J., A. Smith, and S. Cheng.** 1991. Monoclonal antibody specific for BK virus large T antigen allows discrimination among the different papovaviral large T antigens. *Oncogene* **6:**1673–1676.
57. **Marshall, W., A. Telenti, J. Proper, A. Aksamit, and T. Smith.** 1991. Survey of urine from transplant recipients for polyomaviruses JC and BK using the polymerase chain reaction. *Mol. Cell. Probes* **5:**125–128.
58. **Martin, J. D., D. M. King, J. M. Slauch, and R. J. Frisque.** 1985. Differences in regulatory sequences of naturally occurring JC virus variants. *J. Virol.* **53:**306–311.
59. **Miyamura, T., A. Furuno, and K. Yoshiike.** 1985. DNA rearrangement in the control region for early transcription in a human polyomavirus JC host range mutant capable of growing in human embryonic kidney cells. *J. Virol.* **54:** 750–756.
60. **Monaco, M. C. G., W. J. Atwood, M. Gravell, C. S. Tornatore, and E. O. Major.** 1996. JC virus infection of hematopoietic progenitor cells, primary B lymphocytes, and tonsillar stromal cells: implications for viral latency. *J. Virol.* **70:**7004–7012.
61. **Monaco, M. C. G., P. N. Jensen, J. Hou, L. C. Durham, and E. O. Major.** Detection of JC virus DNA in human tonsil tissue: evidence for site of initial viral infection. *J. Virol.*, in press.
62. **Neel, J. V., E. O. Major, A. A. Awa, T. Glover, and A. Burgess.** 1996. Rogue type chromosomal damage in lymphocytes is associated with infection with the human polyomavirus JCV: an hypothesis. *Proc. Natl. Acad. Sci. USA* **93:**2690–2695.
63. **Padgett, B. L., C. M. Rogers, and D. L. Walker.** 1977. JC virus, a human polyomavirus associated with progressive multifocal leukoencephalopathy: additional biological characteristics and antigenic relationships. *Infect. Immun.* **15:**656–662.
64. **Padgett, B. L., and D. L. Walker.** 1973. Prevalence of antibodies in human sera against JC virus, an isolate from a case of progressive multifocal leukoencephalopathy. *J. Infect. Dis.* **127:**467–470.
65. **Padgett, B. L., G. ZuRhein, D. Walker, R. Echroade, and B. Dessel.** 1971. Cultivation of papova-like virus from human brain with progressive multifocal leukoencephalopathy. *Lancet* **i:**1257–1260.
66. **Perrons, C. J., J. D. Fox, S. B. Lucas, N. S. Brink, R. S. Tedder, and R. F. Miller.** 1996. Detection of polyomaviral DNA in clinical samples from immunocompromised patients: correlation with clinical disease. *J. Infect.* **32:** 205–209.
67. **Portegies, P., P. R. Algra, C. E. M. Hollar, J. M. Prins, P. Reiss, J. Valk, and J. Lange.** 1991. Response to cytarabine in progressive multifocal leukoencephalopathy in AIDS. *Lancet* **337:**680–681.
68. **Rencic, A., J. Gordon, J. Otte, M. Curtis, A. Kovatich, P. Zoltick, K. Khalili, and D. Andrews.** 1996. Detection of JC virus DNA sequence and expression of the viral oncoprotein, tumor antigen, in brain of immunocompetent patient with oligoastrocytoma. *Proc. Natl. Acad. Sci. USA* **93:**7352–7357.
69. **Richardson, E. P., Jr.** 1961. Progressive multifocal leukoencephalopathy. *N. Engl. J. Med.* **265:**815–823.
70. **Schmidbauer, M., H. Budka, and K. V. Shah.** 1990. Progressive multifocal leukoencephalopathy (PML) in AIDS and in the pre-AIDS era. A neuropathological comparison using immunocytochemistry and in situ DNA hybridization for virus detection. *Acta Neuropathol.* **80:**375–380.
71. **Schneider, E., and K. Dorries.** 1993. High frequency of polyomavirus infection in lymphoid cell preparations after allogeneic bone marrow transplantation. *Transplant. Proc.* **25:**1271–1273.
72. **Steiger, M., G. Tarnsby, S. Gabe, J. McLaughlin, and A. Schapira.** 1993. Successful outcome of progressive multifocal leukoencephalopathy with cytarabine and interferon. *Ann. Neurol.* **33:**407–411.
73. **Stoner, G. L., C. F. Ryschkewitsch, D. L. Walker, and H. D. Webster.** 1986. JC papovavirus large tumor (T)-antigen expression in brain tissue of acquired immune deficiency syndrome (AIDS) and non-AIDS patients with progressive multifocal leukoencephalopathy. *Proc. Natl. Acad. Sci. USA* **83:**2271–2275.
74. **Stoner, G. L., D. Soffer, C. F. Ryschkewitsch, D. L. Walker, and H. D. Webster.** 1988. A double-label method detects both early (T-antigen) and late (capsid) proteins of JC virus in progressive multifocal leukoencephalopathy brain tissue from AIDS and non-AIDS patients. *J. Neuroimmunol.* **19:**223–236.
75. **Telenti, A., A. J. Aksamit, J. Proper, and T. F. Smith.** 1990. Detection of JC virus DNA by polymerase chain reaction in patients with progressive multifocal leukoencephalopathy. *J. Infect. Dis.* **162:**858–861.
76. **Telenti, A., W. Marshall, A. Aksamit, J. Smilack, and T. Smith.** 1992. Detection of JC virus by polymerase chain reaction in cerebrospinal fluid from two patients with progressive multifocal leukoencephalopathy. *Eur. J. Clin. Microbiol. Infect. Dis.* **11:**253–254.
77. **Tornatore, C., J. Berger, S. Houff, B. Curfman, K. Meyers, D. Winfield, and E. Major.** 1992. Detection of JC virus DNA in peripheral lymphocytes from patients with and without progressive multifocal leukoencephalopathy. *Ann. Neurol.* **31:**454–462.
78. **Vago, L., P. Clinque, E. Sala, M. Nebuloni, R. Caldarelli, S. Racca, P. Ferrante, G. Trabottoni, and G. Costanzi.** 1996. JCV-DNA and BKV-DNA in the CNS tissue and CSF of AIDS patients and normal subjects. Study of 41 cases and review of the literature. *J. Acquired Immune Defic. Syndr. Hum. Retrovirol.* **12:**139–146.
79. **Weber, T., R. Turner, S. Frye, J. Haas, E. Schielke, W.**

Luke, W. Luer, K. Felgenhauer, and G. Hunsmann. 1994. Specific diagnosis of progressive multifocal leukoencephalopathy by polymerase chain reaction. *J. Infect. Dis.* **169:** 1138–1141.

80. **Wiley, C. A., M. Grafe, C. Kennedy, and J. A. Nelson.** 1988. Human immunodeficiency virus (HIV) and JC virus in acquired immune deficiency syndrome (AIDS) patients with progressive multifocal leukoencephalopathy. *Acta Neuropathol.* **76:**338–346.

81. **ZuRhein, G. M.** 1969. Association of papovavirions with a human demyelinating disease (progressive multifocal leukoencephalopathy). *Prog. Med. Virol.* **11:**185–247.

82. **ZuRhein, G. M.** 1983. Studies of JC virus-induced nervous system tumors in the Syrian hamster: a review, p. 205–221. *In* J. L. Sever and D. L. Madden (ed.), *Polyomavirus and Human Neurological Diseases*. Alan R. Liss, Inc., New York, N.Y.

Human Parvoviruses*

MARIALUISA ZERBINI AND MONICA MUSIANI

87

TAXONOMY

The *Parvoviridae* family consists of small, unenveloped, icosahedral single-stranded DNA (ssDNA) viruses of many animal species. It includes two subfamilies, the *Densovirinae*, members of which infect insects, and the *Parvovirinae*, members of which infect vertebrates. The *Parvovirinae* subfamily is divided into three genera: *Dependovirus*, *Parvovirus*, and *Erythrovirus* (11). Members of the genus *Dependovirus* (e.g., adeno-associated virus) are defective and require helper viruses for their own replication. Some adeno-associated virus types have been recovered from human specimens but have not been conclusively considered the causative agents of human diseases (10). Members of the genus *Parvovirus*, some of which are of veterinary interest, replicate without a helper virus in many animal species. Members of the *Erythrovirus* genus, which replicate in erythroid progenitor cells without a helper virus, include nonhuman primate parvoviruses and erythrovirus B19 (B19V; human parvovirus B19).

Human parvovirus B19 was first found by Cossart et al. in 1975 (27), when a nonspecific result was observed during the screening of blood donors for hepatitis B surface antigen by counterimmunoelectrophoresis. Immune electron microscopy of the blood unit, labeled B19, revealed viral particles classified as parvovirus-like on the basis of size and morphology. B19 is the only parvovirus that is a human pathogen and is associated with several defined clinical syndromes; it is therefore the subject of this chapter.

DESCRIPTION OF THE AGENT

B19 virions, as observed by electron microscopy, are icosahedral and have a diameter of approximately 26 nm. The viral particles are unenveloped and contain genetic material consisting of ssDNA. Complete virions have a molecular mass of 5.5×10^6 to 6.2×10^6 Da and a buoyant density of 1.39 to 1.42 g/cm^3 in CsCl. They do not appear to contain lipids or carbohydrates, and no enzymatic functions have been demonstrated in association with B19 viral particles. The physical properties contribute to viral resistance to heat, solvent, and detergent treatments (21).

B19 capsids are made of two polypeptides, the VP1 (83-kDa) and the VP2 (58-kDa) proteins, which represent about 4 and 96%, respectively, of the capsid proteins (69). B19 capsids contain an ssDNA genome of about 5,600 nucleotides. Plus and minus strands are packaged in separate particles in equivalent numbers and, after extraction, the complementary strands may hybridize to form double-stranded DNA (10).

Comparison of the sequences of two different isolates of B19 (Au and Wi) (12, 83) showed homology of 99.2%, and further studies confirmed that the B19 genome is relatively stable (31, 36, 42, 57). In B19 genomes, all protein-coding regions cluster along the plus DNA strand. There are two large open reading frames (ORFs), which together span almost the entire genome in the plus strand, as well as two smaller ORFs. Nine overlapping transcripts have been identified in infected cells, and the initiation of all of the transcripts starts at a single left-hand-side promoter localized at map unit 6 (P6) (67). A single transcript from the major left-hand ORF is translated into nonstructural protein(s), while four overlapping transcripts from the major right-hand ORF are translated into the VP1 and the smaller VP2 structural proteins. Moreover, four transcripts from the smaller ORFs are translated into 11- and 7.5-kDa proteins, whose biological properties have not yet been determined.

The major nonstructural protein, NS1, with a molecular mass of 71 kDa, binds to cellular DNA, transactivates the P6 promoter, and is cytotoxic for mammalian cells (52); the involvement of NS1 in B19 DNA replication has been suggested. Antigenic domains are localized in the carboxy-terminal region of NS1 (93). The VP1 and VP2 capsid proteins, from the same reading frame, are identical, except that VP1 contains 227 additional amino acids at the amino terminus. This VP1 unique region is on the exterior of the capsid and contains multiple neutralizing epitopes (78). Neutralizing epitopes have also been mapped to VP2 and to the junction region of VP1 and VP2 (79). Most of the neutralizing epitopes in the VP1 unique region appear to be linear; in contrast, those in VP2 are mainly conformational.

In vivo parvovirus B19 has a limited host range, and its replication requires mitotically active cells. Permissive B19 target cells are human erythroid progenitor cells. In the erythroid lineage, susceptibility to B19 infection increases with differentiation from erythroid progenitors BFU-E (burst-forming unit–erythroid) to erythroblasts (89). The B19 cel-

* This chapter contains information presented in chapter 84 by J. R. Pattison in the sixth edition of this Manual.

lular receptor is a neutral glycosphingolipid of the erythrocyte membrane, called globoside, which is the P antigen of the P blood group system (15). B19 antireceptor seems to be located within the VP2 capsid protein (1a). The cellular receptor P antigen is expressed not only on mature erythrocytes and erythroid progenitors but also on megakaryocytes and endothelial, placental, fetal liver, myocardial, and kidney cortical cells. B19 has been shown to be cytotoxic for erythroid progenitor cells. Moreover, in nonpermissive cells, virus cytotoxicity can also be found as a result of the selective expression of the nonstructural protein gene, leading to cell death by apoptosis. The typical cytopathic effect shown by B19-infected erythroid precursor cells consists of large intranuclear inclusion bodies with peripheral condensation of chromatin (lantern cells) and cytoplasmic vacuolization, features typical of apoptosis. Electron microscopy also reveals swollen mitochondria, pseudopoda extension, and parvovirus particles in crystalline arrays in the nucleus and cytoplasm.

CLINICAL SIGNIFICANCE

Epidemiology

Parvovirus B19 is distributed worldwide and is a common cause of human infection. B19 infection can occur in any month of the year in sporadic or epidemic form. In temperate climates, however, epidemic manifestations are more common in late winter, spring, and early summer, with epidemic peaks every 2 to 4 years. B19 epidemics are mainly associated with two of the major clinical manifestations of the infection, erythema infectiosum (EI) and transient aplastic crisis (TAC).

The prevalence of immunoglobulin G (IgG) antibodies against B19 structural proteins increases with age. In Europe and the United States, about 15% of 5-year-old children have detectable IgG and approximately 50% of 5- to 20-year-old subjects are seropositive. In the adult population, seropositivity increases up to 60 to 70%, and more than 80% of the elderly population has detectable IgG (2, 24, 53). The incidence of B19 infection has been studied directly with healthy blood donors. In a study of English blood donors, the incidence of viremia, with antigens detected by countercurrent immunoelectrophoresis, was estimated to be 1 in 24,000 (25), but recent studies performed with the very sensitive PCR showed that B19 viremia could be detected in approximately 1 in 3,300 English blood donors (51) tested during a nonepidemic period or 1 in 167 Japanese blood donors tested during a period of a minor epidemic (97).

Virus transmission generally occurs by the respiratory route through respiratory secretions and saliva droplets. Transmission takes place frequently among household and school contacts during outbreaks of B19 infection (77), with high risks being associated with close contact between infected and susceptible individuals for a prolonged time. Parvovirus B19 infection can also be transmitted from mother to fetus through the transplacental route and may lead to nonimmune hydrops or fetal death. Moreover, B19 can be transmitted parenterally via blood or blood products obtained from donors who were bled during the viremic phase of B19 infection. B19 DNA has been detected by PCR in batches of albumin, factor VIII, factor IX, clotting factor concentrates, and immunoglobulins. Hemophiliacs were found to be infected with B19 after receiving dry heat-treated or steam-treated factors VIII and IX or solvent- or detergent-treated clotting factors (8, 96).

Disease Manifestations

Parvovirus B19 infection can occur totally asymptomatically or with mild nonspecific symptoms. However, infection also can lead to numerous clinical manifestations ranging from acute self-limiting diseases to sometimes chronic illnesses. The course of B19 infection has been analyzed in experimental studies.

Experimental B19 Infection

In two studies with human volunteers (5, 73), 12 normal volunteers (8 seronegative and 4 seropositive) were infected by intranasal instillation of saline dilutions of sera containing B19 particles. All but one of the eight seronegative subjects became viremic. The virus was first detected 6 days after inoculation, with peaks on days 8 and 9 and viral titers comparable to those observed both in natural infection in blood donors and in aplastic crises (about 10^{11} genome copies/ml). Concurrently with viremia, the virus was also detected in nasal washes and gargle specimens. In viremic patients, high titers of specific IgM antibodies developed during the second week after inoculation, and IgG antibodies appeared at the end of the second week and early in the third week. Of the four seropositive volunteers inoculated with B19, only one, who had traces of IgG antibodies detected before inoculation, developed low-grade viremia, followed by an early increase in IgM and IgG antibodies; these findings suggested that reinfection can occur. In the group of seronegative volunteers infected with B19, infection became clinically overt at two quite distinct times after inoculation. The first phase of illness occurred at the end of the first week, with pyrexia and nonspecific symptoms, including headache, myalgia, chills, and itching. A second phase of illness could be identified after an incubation period of 17 to 18 days, with symptoms typical of B19 infection: erythematous rash and arthralgias (5). During the second week after inoculation, as a consequence of B19 infection, hematologic changes were observed. The most impressive finding was the absence of reticulocytes, followed by a slight but significant decrease in the hemoglobin level, together with a transient decrease in the levels of neutrophils, lymphocytes, and platelets (Fig. 1).

EI

The most common clinical manifestation caused by parvovirus B19 consists of an exanthematous illness of childhood, EI, also known as fifth disease. These two names, together with slapped-cheek disease, are well known as a childhood disease first recognized to be caused by B19 in 1983 during an outbreak in a primary school in London, England (6, 7). The mean incubation period for EI is estimated to be approximately 17 to 19 days. Prodromal symptoms may include low-grade fever, headache, and various degrees of conjunctivitis, upper-respiratory-tract complaints, cough, myalgia, nausea, and diarrhea. Normally, the rash, which is likely to be immune complex mediated, first appears on the face. The often confluent maculopapular erythema on the cheeks and the relative perioral pallor provide the slapped-cheek appearance. The subsequent eruption becomes bilaterally symmetric on the arms, legs, and trunk but only rarely on the palms and soles, has a reticular or lacy pattern, and lasts for about 1 week. The rash can wax and wane for about 3 weeks and can reappear in relation to a rise in body temperature (fever, heat, exercise, and sunlight exposure). The differential clinical diagnosis includes rubella, other viral or bacterial exanthems, and allergy.

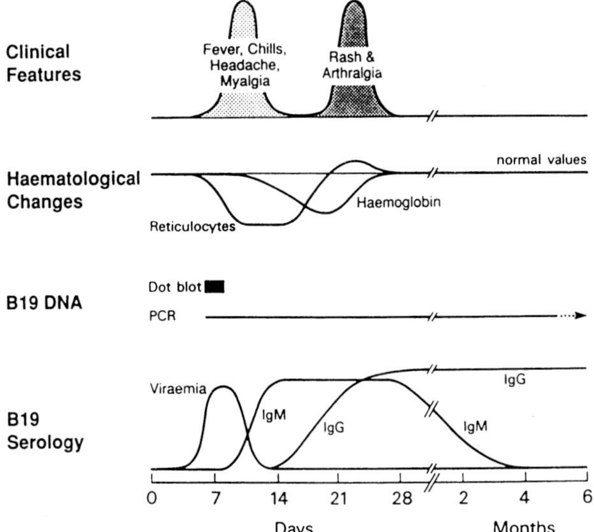

FIGURE 1 Clinical features, hematologic changes, presence of B19 DNA, and serological findings associated with B19 infection in a normal individual (reprinted from *Blood Reviews* [18] with permission of the publisher).

Joint Illness

Two large studies in 1985 reported the relationship between B19 and arthropathy (76, 95). Joint involvement can occur as a consequence of B19 infection in the presence or absence of a cutaneous rash. B19 arthritis is uncommon in children (less than 10% of cases) and can be mild and of a short duration. Joint symptoms have been reported in 50 to 80% of adults, especially women, frequently in the absence of a rash. B19-associated arthritis, which is likely to be immune complex mediated, is typically polyarticular and symmetric. The involved joints include the proximal interphalangeal joints of the hands and feet and, less frequently, the wrists, elbows, knees, and ankles. The joint pain can be accompanied by swelling, warmth, erythema, and stiffness. The symptoms usually disappear after several weeks, but in some cases they can recur or can persist for months or even years (64). Although some patients with B19 arthropathy meet the American Rheumatism Association criteria for a diagnosis of rheumatoid arthritis and criteria for juvenile chronic arthritis, recent studies are still not in agreement about the role of parvovirus B19 in the etiopathogenesis of rheumatoid arthritis and juvenile chronic arthritis (46, 66, 88, 90a).

Aplastic Crises

TAC is an acute self-limited erythropoietic arrest that is common to chronic hemolytic disorders and is characterized by the abrupt onset of severe anemia associated with a decrease in reticulocytes in peripheral blood. In 1981, B19 was found to cause TAC in children with sickle cell anemia (72). After its first description, B19-associated TAC was found in a wide range of patients with underlying chronic hemolytic anemias and in patients with erythroid "stress" (18). During TAC, viremia is often present; reticulocytes in the peripheral blood are absent, and the bone marrow is characterized by the absence of erythroid precursors. Severe anemia is associated with thrombocytopenia, granulocytopenia, or pancytopenia. B19-induced aplastic crisis can also be associated with flu-like symptoms, gastroenteritis, pallor, dyspnea, weakness, lethargy, and confusion. Rash manifestations appear to be rare. Congestive heart failure and bone marrow necrosis may develop, and the illness can be life threatening (41). Aplastic crisis generally occurs as a single episode in the life of a patient and, although severe, is self-limited because of the appearance of a specific immune response. In some cases, TAC may require hospitalization and prompt treatment with blood transfusion.

B19 and Pregnancy

Parvovirus B19 infection was recognized in 1984 (18a, 47a) as a potential hazard to the fetus. The rate of transplacental transmission of B19, estimated at between 25 and 33%, can result in fetal hydrops, which can occur 1 to 12 weeks after maternal symptomatic or asymptomatic infection. B19-associated hydrops, which represents 16 to 18% of all idiopathic nonimmune hydrops, most often resolves spontaneously, with the delivery of apparently normal infants; however, B19 hydrops can lead to fetal loss at an incidence of between 1.66% and 9% (39, 40, 75). B19-associated fetal hydrops and fetal loss appear to be the results of viral replication in erythroid precursors, leading to the interruption of erythrocyte production, severe anemia, and congestive heart failure. B19 DNA has been found in myocardial cells (54), and myocarditis can also contribute to fetal damage. The great majority of cases of fetal hydrops and fetal loss occur in the second trimester. Fetal B19 infections do not commonly cause congenital abnormalities, but cases of infants born with chronic anemia have been described (16). Rare cases of other congenital anomalies associated with B19 infection have also been described and include meconium peritonitis (99), eye malformations, multiple structural defects, myocardial infarction, splenic calcifications, and hydrocephalus.

B19 Infection in Immunocompromised Patients

Parvovirus B19 may be an important pathogen in immunocompromised patients, such as patients with congenital immunodeficiency syndrome or AIDS, organ transplant recipients, patients with lymphoproliferative disorders, and patients with other malignancies. In chronically infected immunocompromised patients, B19 viremia can persist at a very low titer for several months or even years (17, 33). However, B19 clinical manifestations seem to be associated mainly with chronic medium- to high-titer viremia or recurrent increases in viral titer ($>10^4$ genome copies/μl) (1, 63). Persistent B19 infection in immunocompromised patients may lead to chronic bone marrow failure with selective aplasia of erythrocyte precursors, resulting in severe chronic anemia, most often without immune system-mediated symptoms such as rash and/or arthralgias. Immunoglobulin treatment of immunocompromised patients, chronically infected with parvovirus B19, has been effective in clearing the virus from circulation in some cases. In other cases it has been used to ameliorate the clinical course of persistent B19 infections.

B19 Infection and Atypical Clinical Manifestations

Several unusual clinical conditions also have been described in concomitance with B19 infection. These include hematologic disorders, such as hemophagocytic syndrome, transient erythroblastopenia of childhood, idiopathic thrombocytopenic purpura, and acquired chronic pure erythrocyte aplasia. Vasculitis, neurologic diseases, hepatobiliary tract disorders, cardiovascular manifestations, renal diseases, and respiratory disorders also have been described in association with B19 infection. However, the scarcity of data concerning these conditions does not allow the role of B19 in these conditions to be established (92).

LABORATORY DIAGNOSIS

Parvovirus B19 is difficult to cultivate in vitro. As primary cell cultures for the propagation of B19, samples of human bone marrow (68), fetal liver, erythroid leukemic cells, cord blood, and normal peripheral blood have been used. In these cultures stimulated with the hormone erythropoietin, B19 replication is limited to a fraction of the cell population. Several attempts have been made to replicate B19 in continuous cell cultures, especially in erythroleukemic cell lines. Up to now, B19 has been propagated in only three cell lines: the megakaryocytoblastoid cell lines UT7 (84) and MB02 (58) and the erythroleukemic cell line JK1 (90). In primary cultures and in the cell lines, B19 replicates at low levels, and none of these systems is suitable for routine virus isolation and propagation. Since parvovirus B19 cannot be grown routinely in vitro, parvovirus B19 infection is generally diagnosed either by direct detection of B19 antigens or DNA in clinical specimens or by serologic tests.

COLLECTION AND STORAGE OF SPECIMENS

Serum Samples

Serum samples are the most practical specimens for the detection of B19 antigens, genome, and antibodies. They should be collected as soon as possible after disease onset. Blood specimens should be drawn in sterile tubes and transported in an adequate volume to the laboratory in accordance with standard safety procedures. Serum specimens can be stored for short periods at 4°C until use; they should be frozen at −20°C for antibody detection or at −70°C for virus detection. Serum for PCR must be stored in such a way as to avoid any contact with B19 probes and B19 viremic serum samples.

Cellular and Tissue Samples

Bone marrow aspirates, cord blood samples, amniotic fluid cells, and biopsy specimens of placenta and fetal tissues are used for B19 genome detection by in situ hybridization or PCR. Amniotic fluids should be directly drawn in test tubes, while bone marrow and cord blood samples should be aspirated into test tubes containing an anticoagulant solution (sodium citrate, EDTA, or heparin). Heparin should be avoided if a cellular sample is going to be processed for PCR. Bone marrow and cord blood samples to be processed for PCR should be collected by centrifugation on Ficoll gradients. Amniotic fluid cells can be processed by simple centrifugation. Cellular specimens for in situ hybridization should be smeared or centrifuged onto pretreated or silane-treated glass slides, fixed with 4% paraformaldehyde in phosphate-buffered saline, and dehydrated with ethanol washes. Air-dried specimens can be stored for at least 4 months at 4°C. Paraffin-embedded or frozen fetal tissue sections can also be used for B19 DNA detection by in situ hybridization, while for PCR, fresh or freshly frozen specimens are recommended.

DIRECT DETECTION

Parvovirus B19 can be detected in blood about 6 days after infection, reaching high peaks of viremia in 2 to 3 days (5). In acute infections, high-titer viremia has been shown to last about 1 week; then the viral titer decreases and viral DNA can be detected for several months only by PCR (62). In TAC, clinical presentation is coincident with the high-titer viremia phase; in EI or B19-associated arthropathy, clinical manifestations appear later, when viremias are present at lower titers. In fetal hydrops, B19 is detected principally inside cells from cord blood and amniotic fluid. Moreover, in cord blood serum and in amniotic fluid, B19 is detected mainly by PCR; in 50% of respective maternal sera, the virus can still be present at low titers (102). Patients chronically infected with B19 mainly show variable-titer viremias, although clinical manifestations are generally associated with medium- to high-titer viremias (1, 63).

Dot Blot Hybridization Assay

In the dot blot hybridization assay, serum samples are filtered or spotted onto nylon membranes, alkali denaturated, neutralized, digested with proteolytic enzymes, and fixed to the membrane. Several protocols for hybridization with minor modifications have been described. These protocols generally involve a brief prehybridization reaction followed by the hybridization reaction with the labeled B19 probe. To detect B19 DNA, ss- and dsDNA probes and ssRNA probes have been used. Probes can be obtained from cloned B19 DNA fragments, from PCR amplification of desired sequences, or from synthetically produced oligonucleotides (9, 22, 29, 74, 101) and nowadays digoxigenin is extensively used as label.

In dot blot hybridizations, digoxigenin-labeled probes are detected by reaction with antidigoxigenin Fab fragments conjugated with enzymes (alkaline phosphatase or peroxidase), which can then be detected by colorimetric or chemiluminescent reactions (43, 61). In colorimetric detection, a colored precipitate is formed at the enzyme site on the membrane; in chemiluminescent detection, light is emitted by the chemiluminescent substrate during the enzymatic reaction. The photons emitted are then detected by X-ray films, ultrasensitive Polaroid films, or luminometers. One advantage of chemiluminescent detection is that X-ray or photographic films give a permanent record of the results, while membranes stained with chromogenic substrates can lose color differentiation. Moreover, membranes used with chemiluminescent substrates can be rehybridized several times, as chemiluminescent detection does not alter the color of the membranes.

The limit of detection with colorimetric substrates is 0.1 to 0.05 pg of parvovirus B19 DNA homologous to the probe, while the limit of detection with chemiluminescent substrates is 50 to 20 fg of DNA, with RNA probes or longer DNA probes offering the highest sensitivity. Since 1 pg of B19 DNA corresponds to approximately 10^5 B19 genome copies and since, during the acute phase of B19 infections, viremia can reach titers of 10^{11} to 10^{14} particles/ml, the sensitivity of the dot blot hybridization assay is appropriate for detecting medium- to high-titer viremias. Additionally, the possibility of testing pools of serum samples by dot blot hybridization makes this technique particularly suitable for large-scale screenings (98, 103).

Microwell Hybridization Assay

A microwell hybridization assay has been developed to detect human parvovirus DNA in serum samples. A digoxigenin-labeled RNA probe is used to recognize B19 DNA-specific sequences, and a second, biotin-labeled probe is used to capture the hybrids in streptavidin-coated wells. Digoxigenin labeling is detected by an immunoenzymatic reaction with a chemiluminescent substrate. The chemiluminescent microwell hybridization assay is generally more sensitive than dot blot hybridization (47).

In Situ Hybridization Assay

In situ hybridization is a successful method for the localization of B19 DNA inside individual cells with the preservation of cellular and tissue morphology. In situ hybridization has been used for the detection of B19 DNA in bone marrow cells and fetal cells and tissues, being helpful in the diagnosis of B19 infections and particularly in the study of the pathogenesis of B19-associated diseases. The probes used for in situ hybridization to detect B19 DNA have been obtained either from synthetic oligonucleotides or from cloned DNA fragments. Synthetic oligonucleotides, because of their small size, have good penetration properties, and the fact that they are single stranded rules out the possibility of annealing with complementary strands in the hybridization solution. Cloned probes, which are usually longer, have the advantage of being more highly labeled and of recognizing more of the target DNA, resulting in a stronger signal.

For B19 probes, either isotopic or nonisotopic labels, such as biotin or digoxigenin (38, 55, 65), have been used. Digoxigenin-labeled probes have proved very sensitive and specific for the detection of the B19 genome, while biotinylated probes have sometimes proved nonspecific (65).

In the in situ hybridization assay, digoxigenin-labeled probes are immunoenzymatically revealed by use of antidigoxigenin Fab fragments labeled with alkaline phosphatase or with peroxidase and colorimetric substrates. The final colored product precipitated at the site of the reaction can be observed under an ordinary light microscope. The need for objective analysis by digital imaging and for increased sensitivity has led to the development of new methods, such as chemiluminescence in situ hybridization, in which the light emitted from the hybridized probes is quantified and localized with a high-performance luminometer connected to an optical microscope and to a personal computer (60).

PCR

The PCR assay is the most sensitive diagnostic tool for detecting B19 DNA. Small aliquots of serum samples and cellular or tissue samples can be used. Serum samples can be tested without pretreatment in order to avoid cross-contamination. However, serum pretreatment to partially purify DNA and to inactivate *Taq* polymerase inhibitors also can be used (34). For cellular or tissue samples, sample lysis and/or DNA purification is required. PCR for B19 DNA has been performed with two types of assays: single-step PCR and nested PCR. Several oligonucleotide pairs amplifying various regions of the genome have been used successfully for both single-step and nested PCRs, since the B19 genome is very stable (20, 23, 30, 49, 59, 71, 80). More recently, several PCR-enzyme immunoassays (EIAs) were developed to detect B19 DNA (32, 100). These assays include a single-step PCR and identification of the amplified product by a capture hybridization assay in microwells, with immunoenzymatic detection of the captured hybrids. The colorimetric reaction of the detector system is automatically measured with a spectrophotometer, thus permitting an objective evaluation of the result. An assay for the quantitation of parvovirus B19 DNA in serum samples has also been developed in a PCR-EIA format (competitive PCR assay) (37). For this quantitative assay, an internal standard competitor which differs from the original genome sequence in a short mutagenized fragment has been constructed. Target and internal standard sequences are coamplified by the same set of primers and labeled with digoxigenin during the amplification reaction. The different amplicons are detected in two separate hybridization reactions with biotinylated probes specific for the original and mutagenized sequences. The different hybrids are captured in streptavidin-coated microtiter wells and detected immunoenzymatically. A good level of sensitivity has been achieved, with an exact quantitative evaluation over the range of 10^2 to 10^5 genome copies.

SEROLOGY

Serological procedures to detect antibodies against B19 structural proteins are commercially available and are routinely used to diagnose recent B19 infections and to determine immune status. In immunocompetent hosts, specific IgM antibodies develop during the second week after viral infection and are detectable for up to 4 to 6 months and sometimes longer. In patients with aplastic crises, IgM appears several days after the onset of clinical symptoms; in patients with EI or joint illness, IgM is already present at the appearance of the rash or joint symptoms. Moreover, B19 IgM can be detected in 50% of maternal sera at the time of clinical diagnosis of fetal hydrops, while in the fetal sera IgM is rarely found. In immunocompetent hosts, specific IgG antibodies appear several days following IgM and persist for years. Their presence is a sign of past infection. IgG gives protective immunity, but reinfections have been described in the presence of a low level of specific IgG. In immunocompromised patients, B19-specific immune responses may be normal, altered, or even absent. Therefore, serological investigation is not the main tool for diagnosing B19 infection in these patients.

The development of serological tests for the detection of B19 antibodies has been hampered by the limited availability of native antigens, since the isolation of viral particles as a source of antigens relies on the detection of viremic blood units by screening of blood donors. In recent years, several efforts have been made to obtain synthetic (35, 48) and recombinant B19 structural proteins VP1 and VP2 to overcome the shortage of B19 antigens. Recombinant parvovirus B19 structural proteins have been expressed in several systems, both prokaryotic and eukaryotic; these include *Escherichia coli* cells transformed with recombinant plasmids expressing B19 peptides as fusion proteins (56, 87); Chinese hamster ovary cells transfected with a recombinant plasmid expressing B19 antigens (45), COS-7 mammalian cells transfected with hybrid vector B19-SV40 cells (26), and *Spodoptera frugiperda* insect cells infected with B19 recombinant baculoviruses (13, 44). Recently, recombinant B19 nonstructural protein NS1 was also expressed in both prokaryotic and eukaryotic systems (50, 93).

RIA

Radioimmunoassay (RIA) has been used to detect both IgM and IgG antibodies against parvovirus B19. RIA is presently used mainly to detect specific IgM antibodies, and detection is based on the antibody capture principle (IgM antibody capture RIA [MACRIA]). In MACRIA, anti-human IgM (μ chain specific) antibody is adsorbed to a solid phase, and IgM from patient sera is captured. Specific B19 IgM is then quantitated by the addition of B19 antigen, followed by an anti-B19 monoclonal antibody and a radiolabeled detection antibody (4). The results of MACRIA are expressed in terms of arbitrary RIA units.

EIAs

EIAs have been developed as a nonisotopic alternative to RIA (3, 81). Several kits are now commercially available for both IgM and IgG detection. Some of these kits use synthetic peptides corresponding to part of the B19 structural proteins VP1 and VP2. Others use baculovirus-expressed structural proteins or *E. coli*-expressed B19 structural proteins. In these kits, IgM antibodies are mainly detected with a capture EIA format, while IgG antibodies are generally detected with an indirect enzyme-linked immunosorbent assay format with antigen coated to a solid phase. Evaluations of commercial test kits for the detection of B19 IgM by EIAs have shown that recombinant antigen-based EIAs have higher specificity and sensitivity than synthetic peptide antigen EIAs (19, 91).

Other assays have been used to study B19 immune responses. These assays include immunocapture EIA with native antigens, indirect EIA with prokaryotically expressed VP1 antigen, and baculovirus-expressed VP2 or a mixture of baculovirus-expressed VP1 and VP2.

EIA has also been used to measure IgG avidity. In the avidity assay, patient antibodies are first allowed to bind to an immobilized antigen, after which the low-avidity antibodies are eluted with a denaturing agent. The remaining antigen-bound IgG is quantified immunoenzymatically (85). Recently, EIA was also used to study the differential IgG responses to B19 conformational and linear epitopes of VP1 and VP2 with native and denatured antigens (86).

Immunofluorescence

B19-specific IgM or IgG can be detected by indirect immunofluorescence with commercial assays. In these assays, insect cells infected with a recombinant baculovirus expressing VP1 antigen are used as B19 antigen-positive cells. Glass slides onto which insect cells expressing VP1 are fixed are incubated with human sera to be tested. Bound human antibodies are detected with fluorescein isothiocyanate-conjugated anti-human IgG or IgM antibodies (14). To avoid false-positive IgM results, sera to be tested for IgM antibodies must be pretreated in order to avoid the presence of rheumatoid factor or to prevent competition from IgG antibodies.

Western Blot

Western blot assays are commercially available and allow the evaluation of the antibody response against distinct B19 structural proteins. For these assays, recombinant or native B19 antigens are electrophoresed in denaturing gels and then transferred to nitrocellulose membranes. Antigens immobilized on membranes are exposed to human sera, followed by an enzyme-linked secondary antibody; finally, a colorimetric substrate is used to visualize the immunoreactive bands (70, 82). Western blots are not suitable for the routine serological diagnosis of B19, since they are more expensive than EIAs, they require a subjective interpretation of the results, and they are not applicable for the screening of a large number of samples.

Capture Hemadherence Assay

The capacity of human parvovirus B19 to agglutinate human or monkey erythrocytes was recently used to develop IgG or IgM antibody capture hemadherence assays. In these assays, IgM and IgG captured on microtiter plates are revealed by the addition of B19 native or recombinant antigen, and erythrocytes are used as the detector system (28, 94). These assays are sensitive and simple to perform. They have therefore been proposed as an alternative to other immunological assays for parvovirus B19 diagnosis.

INTERPRETATION AND REPORTING OF THE RESULTS

A laboratory diagnosis of B19 infection is required, since the infection has been associated with a wide variety of clinical manifestations. A diagnostic protocol must consider both the type of pathology and the type of patient. Diagnostic methods for detecting the presence of parvovirus B19 and for investigating the specific immune response must be considered in detail (Table 1).

Antigen detection by counterimmunoelectrophoresis (82a), immunoelectron microscopy (27), and RIA-EIA (3, 26a) was used in the first studies to detect B19, but these have been replaced by more sensitive and specific techniques, most of them suitable for screening numerous specimens. These mainly consist of dot blot immunoassay for B19 antigen detection (37a) and hybridization assays and PCR for B19 DNA detection. Dot blot immunoassay has proved to be a practical assay for large-scale screening of serum samples. It can be performed in 4 h and has a sensitivity comparable to or slightly higher than that achieved by dot blot hybridization. Nucleic acid hybridization assays and PCR are the most common methods used to detect the presence of B19. Dot blot hybridization assay has an average sensitivity of 10^4 genome copies and is suited to the detection of medium- to high-titer viremias. Most patients with aplastic crises have titers of viremia $>10^5$ B19 particles/ml at the time of clinical presentation, so this method is useful for confirming TAC. In situ hybridization is able to detect the presence of B19 DNA in a single infected cell; the genome copy number in an average B19-infected erythroid cell is about 8×10^3. This technique also provides information about the morphologic context of the specific tissue and the cells involved in the infection. In situ hybridization is mainly used for the diagnosis of B19 infections in patients

TABLE 1 Main diagnostic approaches for clinical manifestations associated with B19 infection

Clinical manifestation(s)	Direct detection	Antibody detection	Clinical specimens
EI		IgM	Serum
Joint illness		IgM	Serum
Aplastic crisis	DNA by dot blot hybridization assay		Serum
B19 and pregnancy	DNA by PCR (mother); DNA by hybridization assays and PCR (fetus)	IgM (mother); IgM (fetus)	Serum (mother); serum and/or cord blood cells (fetus)
B19 infection in immunocompromised patient	DNA by hybridization assays and PCR		Serum and/or bone marrow cells

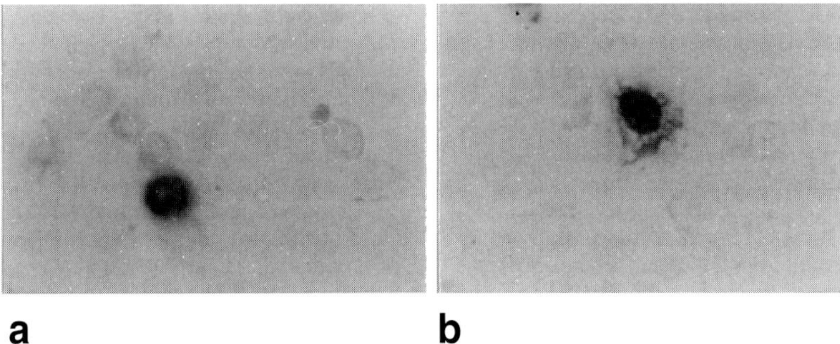

FIGURE 2 In situ hybridization assay for the detection of B19 DNA with a digoxigenin-labeled probe. Smears of cells from bone marrow aspirate (a) and amniotic fluid (b) show clear-cut nuclear positivity (reprinted from the *Journal of Clinical Microbiology* [102] with permission of the publisher).

with hematologic disorders and in hydropic fetuses by analysis of bone marrow cells and fetal specimens (Fig. 2). In some cases, in situ hybridization has proved positive in the absence of viremias detectable by dot blot hybridization and PCR.

Several PCR assays with an average sensitivity of 10 to 100 genome copies have been developed. PCR is the most sensitive technique for detecting B19 DNA in body fluids and extracted tissue and cell samples. PCR is technically demanding and not suitable for the screening of numerous samples; it also presents a risk of laboratory contamination. It is therefore not recommended as a routine test. PCR is mainly used to detect very low-titer viremias found in the course of persistent B19 infection in immunocompromised patients, in the convalescent phase of acute infection, and in fetal B19 infections. PCR is also suitable for the diagnosis of B19 infection in maternal sera and fetal sera at the time of clinical diagnosis of fetal hydrops. PCR allows blood products to be screened for the presence of B19 DNA. A recently developed quantitative PCR allows the clearance of parvovirus B19 to be monitored, the viral load in the course of persistent or recurrent infections to be monitored, and the efficacy of immunoglobulin therapy to be evaluated.

Serological diagnosis of recent infection is generally achieved by IgM capture assays in both RIA and EIA formats. IgM detection is the main tool for the diagnosis of EI and B19-associated arthropathies, since clinical manifestations appear when high-titer viremias are no longer detectable but the specific immune response has already been mounted. Specific IgM can be detected in over 90% of cases of EI and B19-associated arthropathies during the symptomatic phase. In fetal hydrops, anti-B19 IgM in maternal sera is a sign of recent infection, although at the time of clinical diagnosis of fetal hydrops, it can found in 50% of cases. The finding of anti-B19 IgM in fetal blood is also a sign of fetal infection, but its absence cannot exclude B19 infection. In immunocompromised patients, IgM detection provides evidence of a recent B19 infection, but in these patients, the serological response can be reduced or even absent. Therefore, if serological tests for B19 antibodies are inconclusive, viral detection methods may be the correct choice for a prompt diagnosis.

B19 IgG antibodies are mainly detected by indirect EIA, and their presence indicates a past infection. However, seroconversion to IgG between paired sera is a sign of a recent infection. In infants, the presence of specific IgG at 1 year of age is considered to be of retrospective diagnostic value for fetal or neonatal B19 infection.

REFERENCES

1. **Abkowitz, J. L., K. W. Brown, R. W. Wood, N. L. Kovach, S. W. Green, and N. S. Young.** 1997. Clinical relevance of parvovirus B19 as a cause of anemia in patients with human immunodeficiency virus infection. *J. Infect. Dis.* **176:**269–273.

1a. **Agbandje-McKenna, M., and M. G. Rossmann.** 1997. The structure of human Parvovirus B19. Receptor interaction. *Monogr. Virol.* **20:**11.

2. **Anderson, L. J.** 1987. Role of parvovirus B19 in human disease. *Pediatr. Infect. Dis. J.* **6:**711–718.

3. **Anderson, L. J., C. Tsou, R. A. Parker, T. L. Chorba, H. Wulff, P. Tattersall, and P. P. Mortimer.** 1986. Detection of antibodies and antigens of human parvovirus B19 by enzyme-linked immunosorbent assay. *J. Clin. Microbiol.* **24:**522–526.

4. **Anderson, M. J., L. R. Davis, S. E. Jones, and J. R. Pattison.** 1982. The development and use of an antibody capture radioimmunoassay for specific IgM to a human parvovirus-like agent. *J. Hyg.* **88:**309–324.

5. **Anderson, M. J., P. G. Higgins, L. R. Davis, J. S. Willman, S. E. Jones, I. M. Kidd, J. R. Pattison, and D. A. J. Tyrrel.** 1985. Experimental parvoviral infections in humans. *J. Infect. Dis.* **152:**257–265.

6. **Anderson, M. J., S. E. Jones, S. P. Fisher-Hoch, E. Lewis, S. M. Hall, C. L. R. Bartlett, B. J. Cohen, P. P. Mortimer, and M. S. Pereira.** 1983. Human parvovirus, the cause of erythema infectiosum (fifth disease)? *Lancet* **i:**1378.

7. **Anderson, M. J., E. Lewis, I. M. Kidd, S. M. Hall, and B. J. Cohen.** 1984. An outbreak of erythema infectiosum associated with human parvovirus infection. *J. Hyg. Camb.* **93:**85–93.

8. **Azzi, A., S. Ciappi, K. Zakrzewska, M. Morfini, G. Mariani, and P. M. Mannucci.** 1992. Human parvovirus B19 infection in haemophiliacs first infused with two high purity, virally attenuated factor VIII concentrates. *Am. J. Hematol.* **39:**228–230.

9. **Azzi, A., K. Zakrzewska, G. Gentilomi, M. Musiani, and M. Zerbini.** 1990. Detection of B 19 parvovirus infections by a dot blot hybridization assay using a digoxigenin-labelled probe. *J. Virol. Methods* **27:**125–134.

10. **Berns, K. I.** 1996. Parvoviridae: the viruses and their replication, p. 2173–2197. *In* B. N. Fields, D. M. Knipe, and P. M. Howley (ed.), *Fields Virology*, 3rd ed. Raven Press, New York, N.Y.

11. **Berns, K. I., M. Bergoin, M. Bloom, M. Lederman, N. Muzyczka, G. Siegl, J. Tal, and P. Tattersall.** 1995. Parvoviridae. *Arch. Virol.* **10**(Suppl.)**:**169–175.

12. **Blundell, M. C., C. Beard, and C. R. Astell.** 1987. In vitro identification of a B19 parvovirus promoter. *Virology* **157:**534–538.
13. **Brown, C. S., M. M. M. Salimans, M. H. M. Noteborn, and H. T. Weiland.** 1990. Antigenic parvovirus B19 coat proteins VP1 and VP2 produced in large quantities in a baculovirus expression system. *Virus Res.* **15:**197–212.
14. **Brown, C. S., M. J. A. W. M. Van Bussel, A. L. M. Wassenaar, A. M. W. van Elsacker-Niele, H. T. Weiland, and M. M. M. Salimans.** 1990. An immunofluorescence assay for the detection of parvovirus B19 IgG and IgM antibodies based on recombinant viral antigen. *J. Virol. Methods* **29:**53–62.
15. **Brown, K. E., S. M. Anderson, and N. S. Young.** 1993. Erythrocyte P antigen: cellular receptor for B19 parvovirus. *Science* **262:**114–117.
16. **Brown, K. E., S. W. Green, J. Antunez de Mayolo, J. A. Bellanti, S. D. Smith, T. J. Smith, and N. S. Young.** 1994. Congenital anaemia after transplacental B19 parvovirus infection. *Lancet* **343:**895–896.
17. **Brown, K. E., and N. S. Young.** 1995. Persistent parvovirus B19 infection. *Rev. Med. Microbiol.* **6:**246–256.
18. **Brown, K. E., and N. S. Young.** 1995. Parvovirus B19 infection and hematopoiesis. *Blood Rev.* **9:**176–182.
18a. **Brown, T., A. Anand, L. D. Ritchie, J. P. Clewley, and T. M. S. Reid.** 1984. Intrauterine parvovirus infection associated with hydrops fetalis. *Lancet* **ii:**1033.
19. **Bruu, A. L., and S. A. Nordbø.** 1995. Evaluation of five commercial tests for detection of immunoglobulin M antibodies to human parvovirus B19. *J. Clin. Microbiol.* **33:**1363–1365.
20. **Cassinotti, P., M. Weitz, and G. Siegl.** 1993. Human parvovirus B19 infections: routine diagnosis by a new nested polymerase chain reaction assay. *J. Med. Virol.* **40:**228–234.
21. **Clewley, J. P.** 1984. Biochemical characterization of a human parvovirus. *J. Gen. Virol.* **65:**241–245.
22. **Clewley, J. P.** 1985. Detection of human parvovirus using a molecularly cloned probe. *J. Med. Virol.* **15:**173–181.
23. **Clewley, J. P.** 1989. Polymerase chain reaction assay of parvovirus B19 DNA in clinical specimens. *J. Clin. Microbiol.* **27:**2647–2651.
24. **Cohen, B. J., and M. M. Buckley.** 1988. The prevalence of antibody to human parvovirus B19 in England and Wales. *J. Med. Microbiol.* **25:**151–153.
25. **Cohen, B. J., A. M. Field, S. Gudnadottir, S. Beard, and J. A. J. Barbara.** 1990. Blood donor screening for parvovirus B19. *J. Virol. Methods* **30:**233–238.
26. **Cohen, B. J., A. M. Field, J. Mori, K. E. Brown, J. P. Clewley, J. St. Amand, and C. R. Astell.** 1995. Morphology and antigenicity of recombinant B19 parvovirus capsids expressed in transfected COS-7 cells. *J. Gen. Virol.* **76:**1233–1237.
26a. **Cohen, B. J., P. P. Mortimer, and M. S. Pereira.** 1983. Diagnostic assays with monoclonal antibodies for the serum parvovirus-like virus (SPLV). *J. Hyg.* **91:**113–130.
27. **Cossart, Y. E., A. M. Field, B. Cant, and D. Widdows.** 1975. Parvovirus-like particles in human sera. *Lancet* **i:**72–73.
28. **Cubel, R. C., A. C. R. Alferes, B. J. Cohen, and J. P. Nascimento.** 1994. Application to immunoglobulin M capture hemadherence assays of hemagglutination of monkey erythrocytes by native and recombinant human parvovirus B19 antigen. *J. Clin. Microbiol.* **32:**1997–1999.
29. **Cubie, H., J. Grzybowski, C. da Silva, L. Duncan, T. Brown, and N. M. Smith.** 1995. Synthetic oligonucleotide cocktails as probes for detection of human parvovirus B19. *J. Virol. Methods* **53:**91–102.
30. **Durigon, E. L., D. D. Erdman, G. W. Gary, M. A. Pallansch, T. J. Torok, and L. J. Anderson.** 1993. Multiple primer pairs for polymerase chain reaction (PCR) amplification of human parvovirus B19 DNA. *J. Virol. Methods* **44:**155–165.
31. **Erdman, D., E. Durigon, Q. Y. Wang, and L. J. Anderson.** 1996. Genetic diversity of human parvovirus B19: sequence analysis of the VP1/VP2 gene from multiple isolates. *J. Gen. Virol.* **7:**2767–2774.
32. **Erdman, D. D., E. L. Durigon, and B. P. Holloway.** 1994. Detection of human parvovirus B19 DNA PCR products by RNA probe hybridization enzyme immunoassay. *J. Clin. Microbiol.* **32:**2295–2298.
33. **Frickhofen, N., and N. S. Young.** 1989. Persistent parvovirus B19 infections in humans. *Microb. Pathog.* **7:**319–327.
34. **Frickhofen, N., and N. S. Young.** 1991. A rapid method of sample preparation for detection of DNA viruses in human serum by polymerase chain reaction. *J. Virol. Methods* **35:**65–72.
35. **Fridell, E., B. J. Cohen, and B. Wahren.** 1991. Evaluation of a synthetic peptide enzyme-linked immunosorbent assay for immunoglobulin M to human parvovirus B19. *J. Clin. Microbiol.* **29:**1376–1381.
36. **Gallinella, G., S. Venturoli, G. Gentilomi, M. Musiani, and M. Zerbini.** 1995. Extent of sequence variability in a genomic region coding for capsid proteins of B19 parvovirus. *Arch. Virol.* **140:**1119–1125.
37. **Gallinella, G., M. Zerbini, M. Musiani, S. Venturoli, G. Gentilomi, and E. Manaresi.** 1997. Quantitation of parvovirus B19 DNA sequences by competitive PCR: differential hybridization of the amplicons and immunoenzymatic detection on microplate. *Mol. Cell. Probes* **11:**127–133.
37a. **Gentilomi, G., M. Musiani, M. Zerbini, G. Gallinella, S. Venturoli, and E. Manaresi.** 1997. Dot immunoperoxidase assay for the detection of parvovirus B19 antigens in serum samples. *J. Clin. Microbiol.* **35:**1575–1578.
38. **Gentilomi, G., M. Zerbini, M. Musiani, G. Gallinella, D. Gibellini, S. Venturoli, M. C. Re, S. Pileri, C. Finelli, and M. La Placa.** 1993. In situ detection of B19 DNA in bone marrow of immunodeficient patients using a digoxigenin labelled probe. *Mol. Cell. Probes* **7:**19–24.
39. **Gratacós, E., P. J. Torres, J. Vidal, E. Antolin, J. Costa, M. T. Jimenez de Anta, V. Carach, P. Alonso, and A. Fortuny.** 1995. The incidence of human parvovirus B19 infection during pregnancy and its impact on perinatal outcome. *J. Infect. Dis.* **171:**1360–1363.
40. **Hall, C. J.** 1994. Parvovirus B19 infection in pregnancy. *Arch. Dis. Child.* **71:**4–5.
41. **Harris, J. W.** 1992. Parvovirus B19 for the hematologist. *Am. J. Hematol.* **39:**119–130.
42. **Hemaur, A., A. von Poblotzki, A. Gigler, P. Cassinotti, G. Siegl, H. Wolf, and S. Modrow.** 1996. Sequence variability among different B19 isolates. *J. Gen. Virol.* **77:**1781–1785.
43. **Hicks, K. E., S. Beard, B. J. Cohen, and J. P. Clewley.** 1995. A simple and sensitive DNA hybridization assay used for the routine diagnosis of human parvovirus B19 infection. *J. Clin. Microbiol.* **33:**2473–2475.
44. **Kajigaya, S., H. Fujii, A. Field, S. Anderson, S. Rosenfeld, L. J. Anderson, T. Shimada, and N. S. Young.** 1991. Self assembled B19 parvovirus capsids, produced in a baculovirus system, are antigenically and immunogenically similar to native virions. *Proc. Natl. Acad. Sci. USA* **88:**4646–4650.
45. **Kajigaya, S., T. Shimada, S. Fujita, and N. S. Young.** 1989. A genetically engineered cell line that produces

empty capsids of B19 (human) parvovirus. *Proc. Natl. Acad. Sci. USA* **86:**7601–7605.
46. **Kerr, J. R., J. P. Cartron, M. D. Curran, J. E. Moore, J. R. M. Elliot, and R. A. B. Mollan.** 1995. A study of the role of parvovirus B19 in rheumatoid arthritis. *Br. J. Rheumatol.* **34:**809–813.
47. **Kim, E. C., E. L. Durigon, D. D. Erdman, and L. J. Anderson.** 1994. Chemiluminescent microwell hybridization assay for direct detection of human parvovirus B19 DNA. *J. Virol. Methods* **50:**349–354.
47a. **Knott, P. D., G. A. C. Welply, and M. J. Anderson.** 1984. Serologically proved intrauterine infection with parvovirus. *Br. Med. J.* **289:**1033–1034.
48. **Koch, W. C.** 1995. A synthetic parvovirus B19 capsid protein can replace viral antigen in antibody capture enzyme immunoassay. *J. Virol. Methods* **55:**67–82.
49. **Koch, W. C., and S. P. Adler.** 1990. Detection of human parvovirus B19 DNA by using the polymerase chain reaction. *J. Clin. Microbiol.* **28:**65–69.
50. **Leruez-Ville, M., I. Vassias, C. Pallier, A. Cecille, U. Hazan, and F. Morinet.** 1997. Establishment of a cell line expressing human parvovirus B19 non-structural protein from an inducible promoter. *J. Gen. Virol.* **78:**215–219.
51. **McOmish, F., P. L. Yap, A. Jordan, H. Hart, B. J. Cohen, and P. Simmonds.** 1993. Detection of parvovirus B19 in donated blood: a model system for screening by polymerase chain reaction. *J. Clin. Microbiol.* **31:** 323–328.
52. **Momoeda, M., S. Wong, M. Kawase, N. S. Young, and S. Kajigaya.** 1994. A putative nucleoside triphosphate-binding domain in the nonstructural protein of B19 parvovirus is required for cytotoxicity. *J. Virol.* **68:** 8443–8446.
53. **Morbidity and Mortality Weekly Report.** 1989. Risks associated with human parvovirus B19 infection. *Morbid. Mortal. Weekly Rep.* **38:**81–97.
54. **Morey, A. L., J. W. Keeling, H. J. Porter, and K. A. Fleming.** 1992. Clinical and histopathological features of parvovirus B19 infection in the human fetus. *Br. J. Obstet. Gynaecol.* **99:**566–574.
55. **Morey, A. L., H. J. Porter, J. W. Keeling, and K. A. Fleming.** 1992. Non-isotopic in situ hybridization and immunophenotyping of infected cells in the investigation of human fetal parvovirus infection. *J. Clin. Pathol.* **45:** 673–678.
56. **Morinet, F., L. D'Auriol, J. D. Tratschin, and F. Galibert.** 1989. Expression of the human parvovirus B19 protein fused to protein A in Escherichia coli. Recognition by IgM and IgG antibodies in human sera. *J. Gen. Virol.* **70:**3091–3097.
57. **Morinet, F., J. D. Tratschin, Y. Perol, and G. Siegl.** 1986. Comparison of 17 isolates of the human parvovirus B19 by restriction enzyme analysis. *Arch. Virol.* **90:** 165–172.
58. **Munshi, N. C., S. Zhou, M. J. Woody, D. A. Morgan, and A. Srivastava.** 1993. Successful replication of parvovirus B19 in the megakaryocytic leukemia cell line MB-02. *J. Virol.* **67:**562–566.
59. **Musiani, M., A. Azzi, M. Zerbini, D. Gibelli, S. Venturoli, K. Zakrzewska, M. C. Re, G. Gentilomi, G. Gallinella, and M. La Placa.** 1993. Nested polymerase chain reaction assay for the detection of B19 parvovirus DNA in human immunodeficiency virus patients. *J. Med. Virol.* **40:**157–160.
60. **Musiani, M., A. Roda, M. Zerbini, G. Gentilomi, P. Pasini, G. Gallinella, and S. Venturoli.** 1996. Detection of parvovirus B19 DNA in bone marrow cells by chemiluminescence in situ hybridization. *J. Clin. Microbiol.* **34:** 1313–1316.
61. **Musiani, M., M. Zerbini, D. Gibellini, G. Gentilomi, S. Venturoli, G. Gallinella, E. Ferri, and S. Girotti.** 1991. Chemiluminescence dot blot hybridization assay for detection of B19 parvovirus DNA in human sera. *J. Clin. Microbiol.* **29:**2047–2050.
62. **Musiani, M., M. Zerbini, G. Gentilomi, M. Plazzi, G. Gallinella, and S. Venturoli.** 1995. Parvovirus B19 clearance from peripheral blood after acute infection. *J. Infect. Dis.* **172:**1360–1363.
63. **Musiani, M., M. Zerbini, G. Gentilomi, G. Rodorigo, D. De Rosa, D. Gibellini, S. Venturoli, and G. Gallinella.** 1995. Persistent B19 parvovirus infections in haemophilic HIV-1 infected patients. *J. Med. Virol.* **46:** 103–108.
64. **Naides, S. J., L. L. Scharosch, F. Foto, and E. J. Howard.** 1990. Rheumatologic manifestations of human parvovirus B19 infection in adults. *Arthritis Rheum.* **33:**1297–1308.
65. **Nascimento, J. P., N. F. Hallam, A. M. Field, J. P. Clewley, K. E. Brown, and B. J. Cohen.** 1991. Detection of B19 parvovirus in human fetal tissue by in situ hybridization. *J. Med. Virol.* **33:**77–82.
66. **Nikkari, S., A. Roivainen, P. Hannonen, T. Mottonen, R. Luukkainen, T. Yli-Jama, and P. Toivanen.** 1995. Persistence of parvovirus B19 in synovial fluid and bone marrow. *Ann. Rheum. Dis.* **54:**597–600.
67. **Ozawa, K., J. Ayub, H. Yu-Shu, G. Kurtzman, T. Shimada, and N. Young.** 1987. Novel transcription map for the B19 (human) pathogenic parvovirus. *J. Virol.* **61:** 2395–2406.
68. **Ozawa, K., G. Kurtzman, and N. Young.** 1986. Replication of the B19 parvovirus in human bone marrow cell cultures. *Science* **233:**883–886.
69. **Ozawa, K., and N. S. Young.** 1987. Characterization of capsid and noncapsid proteins of B19 parvovirus propagated in human erythroid bone marrow cell cultures. *J. Virol.* **61:**2627–2630.
70. **Palmer, P., C. Pallier, M. Leruez-Ville, M. Deplanche, and F. Morinet.** 1996. Antibody response to human parvovirus B19 in patients with primary infection by immunoblot assay with recombinant proteins. *Clin. Diagn. Lab. Immunol.* **3:**236–238.
71. **Patou, G., D. Pillay, S. Myint, and J. Pattison.** 1993. Characterization of a nested polymerase chain reaction assay for detection of parvovirus B19. *J. Clin. Microbiol.* **31:**540–546.
72. **Pattison, J. R., S. E. Jones, J. Hodgson, L. R. Davis, J. M. White, J. E. Stroud, and L. Murtaza.** 1981. Parvovirus infections and hypoplastic crisis in sickle-cell anaemia. *Lancet* **i:**664–665.
73. **Potter, C. G., A. C. Potter, C. S. Hatton, H. M. Chapel, M. J. Anderson, J. R. Pattison, D. A. Tyrrel, P. G. Higgins, J. S. Willman, H. F. Parry, and P. M. Cotes.** 1987. Variations of erythroid and myeloid precursors in the marrow and peripheral blood of volunteer subjects infected with human parvovirus (B19). *J. Clin. Invest.* **79:**1486–1492.
74. **Prato, C., T. Paper, and F. Morinet.** 1991. Use of M13 single stranded DNA digoxigenin labelled probe for detection of human parvovirus B19 viraemia. *J. Virol. Methods* **34:**227–231.
75. **Public Health Laboratory Service Working Party on Fifth Disease.** 1990. Prospective study of human parvovirus (B19) infection in pregnancy. *Br. Med. J.* **300:** 1166–1170.
76. **Reid, D. M., T. Brown, T. S. M. Reid, J. A. N. Rennie, and C. J. Eastmond.** 1985. Human parvovirus-associated arthritis: a clinical and laboratory description. *Lancet* **i:** 422–424.
77. **Rice, P. S., and B. J. Cohen.** 1996. A school outbreak

of parvovirus B19 infection investigated using salivary antibody assays. *Epidemiol. Infect.* **116:**331–338.

78. **Rosenfeld, S. J., K. Yoshimoto, S. Kajigaya, S. Anderson, N. S. Young, A. Field, P. Warrener, G. Bansal, and M. S. Collet.** 1992. Unique region of the minor capsid protein of human parvovirus B19 is exposed on the virion surface. *J. Clin. Invest.* **89:**2023–2029.
79. **Saikawa, T., S. Anderson, M. Momoeda, S. Kajigaya, and N. S. Young.** 1993. Neutralizing linear epitopes of B19 parvovirus cluster in the VP1 unique and VP1-VP2 junction regions. *J. Virol.* **67:**3004–3009.
80. **Salimans, M. M. M., S. Holsappel, F. M. van de Rijke, N. M. Jiwa, A. K. Raap, and H. T. Weiland.** 1989. Rapid detection of human parvovirus B19 DNA by dot-hybridization and the polymerase chain reaction. *J. Virol. Methods* **23:**19–23.
81. **Salimans, M. M. M., M. J. A. W. M. Van Bussel, C. S. Brown, and W. J. M. Spaan.** 1992. Recombinant parvovirus B19 capsids as a new substrate for detection of B19 specific IgG and IgM antibodies by an enzyme-linked immunosorbent assay. *J. Virol. Methods* **39:**247–258.
82. **Schwartz, T. F., M. Roggendorf, and F. Deinhardt.** 1988. Human parvovirus B19, ELISA and immunoblot assay. *J. Virol. Methods* **20:**155–168.

82a. **Serjeant, G. R., J. M. Topley, K. Mason, B. E. Serjeant, J. R. Pattison, S. E. Jones, and R. Mohamed.** 1981. Outbreak of aplastic crises in sickle cell anaemia associated with parvovirus-like agent. *Lancet* **ii:**595–597.

83. **Shade, R. O., M. C. Blundell, S. F. Cotmore, P. Tattersall, and C. R. Astell.** 1986. Nucleotide sequence and genome organization of human parvovirus B19 isolated from the serum of a child during aplastic crisis. *J. Virol.* **58:**921–936.
84. **Shimomura, S., N. Komatsu, N. Frickhofen, S. Anderson, S. Kajigaya, and N. S. Young.** 1992. First continuous propagation of B19 parvovirus in a cell line. *Blood* **79:** 18–24.
85. **Söderlund, M., C. S. Brown, B. J. Cohen, and K. Hedman.** 1995. Accurate serodiagnosis of B19 parvovirus infections by measurement of IgG avidity. *J. Infect. Dis.* **171:**710–713.
86. **Söderlund, M., C. S. Brown, W. J. M. Spaan, L. Hedman, and K. Hedman.** 1995. Epitope type-specific IgG responses to capsid proteins VP1 and VP2 of human parvovirus B19. *J. Infect. Dis.* **172:**1431–1436.
87. **Söderlund, M., K. E. Brown, O. Meurman, and K. Hedman.** 1992. Prokaryotic expression of a VP1 polypeptide antigen for diagnosis by a human parvovirus B19 antibody enzyme immunoassay. *J. Clin. Microbiol.* **30:**305–311.
88. **Söderlund, M., R. von Essen, J. Haapasaari, U. Kiistala, O. Kiviluoto, and K. Hedman.** 1997. Persistence of parvovirus B19 DNA in synovial membranes of young patients with or without chronic arthropathy. *Lancet* **349:** 1063–1065.
89. **Takahashi, T., K. Ozawa, K. Takahashi, S. Asano, and F. Takaku.** 1990. Susceptibility of human erythropoietic cells to B19 parvovirus in vitro increases with differentiation. *Blood* **75:**603–610.
90. **Takahashi, T., K. Ozawa, K. Takahashi, Y. Okuno, Y. Muto, F. Takaku, and S. Asano.** 1993. DNA replication of parvovirus B19 in a human erythroid leukemia cell line (JK-1) in vitro. *Arch. Virol.* **131:**201–208.

90a. **Takahashi, Y., C. Murai, S. Shibata, Y. Munakata, T. Ishii, K. Ishii, T. Saitoh, T. Sawai, K. Sugamura, and T. Sasaki.** 1998. Human parvovirus B19 as a causative agent for rheumatoid arthritis. *Proc. Natl. Acad. Sci. USA* **95:**8227–8232.

91. **Tolfvenstam, T., U. Rudén, and K. Broliden.** 1996. Evaluation of serological assays for identification of parvovirus B19 immunoglobulin M. *Clin. Diagn. Lab. Immunol.* **3:**147–150.
92. **Torok, T. H.** 1997. Unusual clinical manifestations reported in patients with parvovirus B19 infection. *Monogr. Virol.* **20:**61–92.
93. **von Poblotzki, A., A. Gigler, B. Lang, H. Wolf, and S. Modrow.** 1995. Antibodies to parvovirus B19 NS-1 protein in infected individuals. *J. Gen. Virol.* **76:** 519–527.
94. **Wang, Q. Y., and D. D. Erdmann.** 1995. Development and evaluation of capture immunoglobulin G and M hemadherence assay using human type O erythrocytes and recombinant parvovirus B19 antigen. *J. Clin. Microbiol.* **33:**2466–2467.
95. **White, D. G., P. P. Mortimer, D. R. Blake, A. D. Woolf, B. J. Cohen, and P. A. Bacon.** 1985. Human parvovirus arthropathy. *Lancet* **i:**419–421.
96. **Yee, T. T., B. J. Cohen, K. J. Pasi, and C. A. Lee.** 1996. Transmission of symptomatic parvovirus B19 infection by clotting factor concentrate. *Br. J. Haematol.* **93:**457–459.
97. **Yoto, Y., T. Kudoh, K. Haseyama, N. Suzuki, T. Oda, T. Katoh, T. Takahashi, S. Sekiguchi, and S. Chiba.** 1995. Incidence of human parvovirus B19 DNA detection in blood donors. *Br. J. Haematol.* **91:**1017–1018.
98. **Yoto, Y., T. Kudoh, K. Haseyama, N. Suzuki, Y. Matsunaga, and S. Chiba.** 1995. Large-scale screening for human parvovirus B19 DNA in clinical specimens by dot blot hybridization and polymerase chain reaction. *J. Med. Virol.* **47:**438–441.
99. **Zerbini, M., G. A. Gentilomi, G. Gallinella, R. Morandi, S. Calvi, B. Guerra, and M. Musiani.** 1998. Intrauterine parvovirus B19 infection and meconium peritonitis. *Prenat. Diagn.* **18:**599–606.
100. **Zerbini, M., D. Gibellini, M. Musiani, S. Venturoli, G. Gallinella, and G. Gentilomi.** 1995. Automated detection of digoxigenin-labelled B19 parvovirus amplicons by a capture hybridization assay. *J. Virol. Methods* **55:**1–9.
101. **Zerbini, M., M. Musiani, D. Gibellini, G. Gentilomi, S. Venturoli, G. Gallinella, and M. La Placa.** 1993. Evaluation of strand-specific RNA probes visualized by colorimetric and chemiluminescent reactions for the detection of B19 parvovirus DNA. *J. Virol. Methods* **45:**169–178.
102. **Zerbini, M., M. Musiani, G. Gentilomi, S. Venturoli, G. Gallinella, and R. Morandi.** 1996. Comparative evaluation of virological and serological methods in prenatal diagnosis of parvovirus B19 fetal hydrops. *J. Clin. Microbiol.* **34:**603–608.
103. **Zerbini, M., M. Musiani, S. Venturoli, G. Gallinella, D. Gibellini, G. Gentilomi, and M. La Placa.** 1990. Rapid screening for B19 parvovirus DNA in clinical specimens with a digoxigenin-labeled DNA hybridization probe. *J. Clin. Microbiol.* **28:**2496–2499.

Rabies Virus

JEAN S. SMITH

88

CLINICAL BACKGROUND

Rabies is a fatal infection of the central nervous system acquired most often through virus-contaminated saliva transmitted by the bite of a rabid animal. In areas of the world where rabies in dogs is poorly controlled and antirabies treatments are unavailable or are of poor quality, the number of human deaths from rabies is estimated to be between 35,000 and 50,000 annually (34). In contrast, there are on average two human deaths from rabies each year in the United States (15). Vaccination and control programs for domestic dogs (1) and the widespread use of rabies immune globulin and potent vaccines for human postexposure treatment (33) have been very successful at preventing disease. However, these successes do not minimize the importance of rabies to public health in the United States. Rabies is endemic in a variety of wild species (7,124 cases were diagnosed in 1996 [13]), and the risk of disease transmission to humans and domestic animals necessitates expenditures that exceed $300 million annually for rabies control programs (18). One to two million animal bites per year are treated by physicians in the United States (25). Fortunately, only a small proportion of these bites involves a risk of rabies infection. The most important function of a rabies laboratory is to rapidly and accurately identify rabies-infected animals so that appropriate rabies preventive measures can be initiated. In addition to diagnostic responsibilities, the rabies laboratory often performs virus typing for epidemiological investigations. The increased use of oral baiting of wildlife with rabies vaccines to create immune barriers to prevent or slow the spread of new or established outbreaks (17) creates a need for more precise identification of the virus variants involved in cases of rabies.

DESCRIPTION OF THE AGENT

The rabies virion contains a single-stranded, negative-sense RNA genome of approximately 12,000 nucleotides encoding five proteins from an equal number of monocistronic mRNAs (27). Electron microscopy has shown that the virus particle has the characteristic structure of members of the family *Rhabdoviridae*; it is a rigid, bullet-shaped virus, approximately 180 nm in length and 75 nm in diameter. The external surface of the virus consists of a lipid bilayer envelope derived from the host cell plasma membrane and of transmembrane glycoprotein spike-like projections encoded by the virus. The surface glycoprotein (or G protein) is thought to bind specifically to cellular receptors and to confer the neurotropism observed in infected animals. On the inner surface of the viral envelope, closely associated with the membrane-bound G protein, is a second membrane or matrix protein thought to play a role in virus budding. The internal, nucleocapsid core of the virus particle is a helix of RNA associated with a phosphorylated nucleoprotein (or N protein), a nucleocapsid-associated phosphoprotein, and a transcriptase protein. By analogy with vesicular stomatitis virus, the rhabdovirus whose biochemistry is known in the most detail, this RNA-N protein (RNP) complex is thought to function in the transcription and replication of the virion RNA.

The N and G proteins play important roles in diagnosis and treatment. The G protein is responsible for the induction and binding of neutralizing antibodies. Vaccines containing only the G protein, either as a purified viral protein or as a recombinant DNA-derived protein, can confer protective immunity to lethal infection with rabies virus (32). Detection of antibodies to this protein is used to assess vaccine efficacy (6). Accumulations of viral RNP form the intracytoplasmic inclusions that are diagnostic of rabies virus infection (20) and can be observed directly by histopathologic means (the Negri body) or indirectly by their reaction with antiserum to the RNP complex or antibodies specific for the N protein. Distinctive variants of rabies virus can be identified by reaction with panels of monoclonal antibodies (MAbs) directed to the N protein (24) or by patterns of nucleotide substitution identified by genetic analysis of the N protein gene (28).

COLLECTION AND STORAGE OF SPECIMENS

Safety Recommendations for Specimen Collection

All material collected for rabies diagnosis should be considered infectious, and appropriate handling and shipping precautions should be taken (4). Preexposure rabies immunization is recommended for veterinarians, animal control personnel, and diagnosticians (3). Those assisting in the removal of the brain from an animal suspected of having rabies should wear heavy rubber gloves, a face shield, and protective clothing.

Animal Rabies Samples

Examination of brain tissue is the only reliable method of rabies diagnosis. Because of the potential for false-negative results in some clinically rabid animals (10), intravitam diagnosis of rabies in animals is not recommended. Spread of virus from the central nervous system to peripheral nerves and tissues is irregular, and neither the presence nor the absence of antibodies is a reliable indicator of infection.

Wild animals that have attacked and bitten a human or a domestic animal and stray or unwanted domestic animals involved in an unprovoked biting incident are always considered potentially rabid. These animals should be killed at once, and the brain should be submitted to a state or local public health laboratory for testing. Because recent epidemiological data suggest that bite transmission of rabies virus may occur during seemingly insignificant physical contact with bats, rabies testing of bats is recommended even in the absence of a demonstrable bite or scratch, if there is a reasonable probability that such contact occurred (e.g., a sleeping individual awakens to find a bat in the room, an adult witnesses a bat in the room with a previously unattended child, mentally challenged person, or intoxicated individual).

Because rabies is relatively uncommon in domestic animals in the United States, an apparently normal, healthy dog, cat, or ferret involved in a human bite can be confined by its owner and observed for 10 days. Unless the animal develops signs suggestive of rabies during this period, it need not be killed and tested for rabies, and no antirabies biologic agents are required for the person bitten. No dog, cat, or ferret held for the quarantine period has ever been implicated in a human death from rabies in the United States. In areas outside the United States, where rabies is endemic in dogs, antirabies treatment often is begun at the time of the bite exposure but is terminated if the biting animal remains healthy during the quarantine period.

Small rodents (such as squirrels, hamsters, mice, and rats) and lagomorphs (rabbits and hares) are almost never found to be infected with rabies. Testing of these animals is evaluated on a case-by-case basis by the state or local health department.

Circumstances may dictate what method of euthanasia is used, but unnecessary damage to the head of the animal should be avoided. Large animals should be decapitated, and only the head should be submitted for testing. In most states, this service is provided by contract with local veterinarians or animal control officials. Small animals, such as bats, can be submitted intact. Specimens should be placed in a suitable watertight container that is tightly sealed. This container, with absorbent material, then should be placed in a large, watertight, insulated container and refrigerated with cold packs. Overnight transit to a state or local diagnostic laboratory should be arranged. For longer transit times, freezing of the sample on dry ice is recommended. Alternatively, suspension of approximately 1.5-mm^2 pieces of brain samples in 50% glycerine-saline will stabilize the virus in samples shipped on wet ice or cold packs. (Do not freeze samples stored in glycerine-saline.)

Because antirabies treatment is usually delayed pending the results of laboratory tests, the sample should be processed immediately. Brain tissue for confirmatory tests can be stored for 1 month or longer at −20°C (freezers with automatic defrost cycles should not be used for specimen or reagent storage). Rabies virus samples are viable indefinitely at −70°C or below.

Most laboratories receive animal heads and must remove the brain for testing. For all animals, a negative determination can be made only by examining portions of the brain stem, cerebellum, and hippocampus. This requirement necessitates the cumbersome and often dangerous removal of the brain from the cranium. Care must be taken to protect laboratory workers against displaced bone fragments and brain tissue and fluids during this operation and also to prevent cross-transfer of material to subsequent specimens. Some laboratories now use a coring technique to remove brain tissue through the foramen magnum of animals for which rabies is highly suspected (reservoir species, such as skunks, raccoons, foxes, and coyotes) or to facilitate brain tissue removal from larger, difficult to handle animals, such as horses, cows, and goats. Core sampling not only reduces risk to laboratory workers inherent in the necropsy procedure but also eliminates the necessity for instruments which, if not thoroughly decontaminated, could transfer infected material to other samples. Videos depicting traditional and coring methods are available from the state health departments in Austin, Tex., and Sacramento, Calif., and from the National Laboratory Training Network, Nashville, Tenn. With both methods, no tissue from the sample should be discarded until all tests are complete.

A clinical laboratory occasionally examines specimens that have been handled improperly during transit or that are partially decomposed because of a delay before the animals were found. Positive results for these samples are reliable, but the dependability of negative results varies with the method used for diagnosis (antigen detection is more sensitive than isolation for decomposed samples) and the strain of virus infecting the animal (14). As a general rule, a negative finding is reliable if the condition of the brain tissue is such that intact portions of the brain stem, cerebellum, and hippocampus can be removed from the cranium and thin, uniform touch impressions for antigen detection can be made from each section.

Preservation of tissues by fixation in formalin is not recommended for rabies diagnosis. A number of procedures have been developed for the examination of formalin-fixed brain tissue (11, 31), but they are not in widespread use. Forwarding of samples to reference laboratories for testing may significantly delay the results.

Human Rabies Samples

Although human rabies is an extremely rare disease in the United States (15), rabies should be considered a possible diagnosis in cases of viral encephalitis of unknown etiology. An early diagnosis, although unlikely to affect patient outcome, often reduces the number of potential exposures to the virus during contact with the patient and permits the identification of persons who are candidates for rabies prophylaxis. Samples of saliva, cutaneous nerves, or other tissues can be tested for the presence of infectious virus, viral nucleic acid, or viral antigen. Antibodies in the serum of an unvaccinated individual also suggest a rabies virus infection. Methods for collecting these samples are indicated in Appendix 1. Because not all tissue samples are positive in every case of human rabies (15), every diagnosis should include tests of skin biopsy, saliva, and serum samples. Cerebrospinal fluid should be included if the patient has received antirabies treatment. If all tests are negative and rabies is still suspected, additional samples should be tested later in the clinical course.

Corneal epithelium, while positive for rabies virus antigen in some patients, is difficult to sample correctly, especially from comatose patients, and is no longer recommended as a suitable diagnostic sample. Rabies virus has been isolated from the spinal fluid of some patients, but such isolation tends to occur very late in the clinical course, if at all. Because of the rarity of the disease and the lack of effective treatment, a brain biopsy is not indicated. However, biopsy samples negative for herpesvirus encephalitis should be tested for evidence of rabies virus infection.

The postmortem diagnosis of rabies is made by examination of brain tissue. Portions of the medulla (brain stem), cerebellum, and hippocampus should be frozen and shipped on dry ice to a public health laboratory. Preservation of tissues by fixation in formalin is not recommended for rabies diagnosis.

DIRECT EXAMINATION OF CLINICAL SAMPLES FOR RABIES VIRUS ANTIGEN

The direct fluorescent-antibody (DFA) test for rabies virus antigen in brain tissue is the preferred test for rabies diagnosis (8, 29–31) because of its sensitivity and specificity, the speed and ease with which it may be performed, and the economy of its reagents. Fluorescein isothiocyanate (FITC)-labeled antirabies virus antibody conjugates can be prepared against whole rabies virions or purified RNP or as a mixture of MAbs reactive with the N protein. These preparations are available commercially (BBL Microbiology Systems, Cockeysville, Md.; Centocor Inc., Malvern, Pa.; Chemicon International Inc., Temecula, Calif.; and Pasteur Diagnostics, Paris, France). Control material for specific adsorption (normal and rabies virus-infected brain suspensions) is available from both the Lansing, Mich., and the Kansas City, Kans., public health rabies laboratories.

DFA Test

Rabies virus in the brains of infected animals produces intracytoplasmic inclusions of various shapes (dust-like particles <1 μm in diameter and/or large, round to oval masses and strings 2 to 10 μm in diameter). When specifically stained with an FITC-labeled antibody, these inclusions appear smooth, with very bright margins and a somewhat less intensely stained central area (Fig. 1). Staining is graded by intensity (+4, a glaring, apple green brilliance; +1, dull but still noticeably apple green) and by the amount of antigen present in a tissue impression (+3 to +4, a massive green infiltration of large inclusions and dust-like particles in every area of the impression; +1 to +2, isolated small inclusions in only a few microscopic fields).

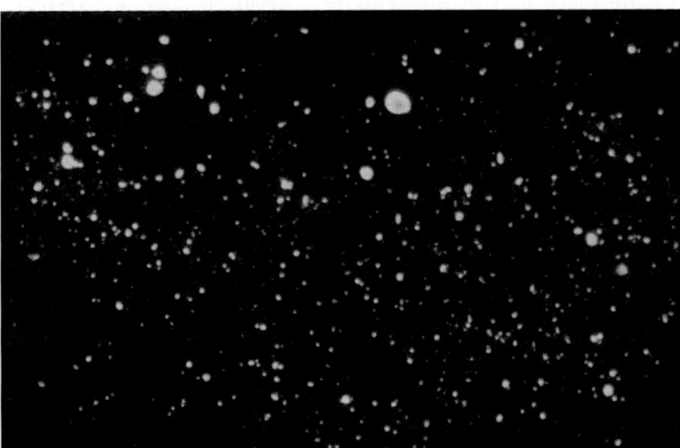

FIGURE 1 Brain tissue from a rabies virus-infected bat stained with FITC-labeled antirabies antibody. Photograph taken by Wallis M. Velleca.

Thin tissue impressions are made by lightly touching cut sections from each of the three areas of the brain sampled (medulla, cerebellum, and hippocampus) to clean microscope slides. For medium-sized animals (e.g., carnivores), each side of the brain is tested separately, for a total of six impressions per test. Adequate sampling of large animals, e.g., horses and cows, requires 12 impressions, as each hemisphere is tested in duplicate. The brains of small animals, such as bats, can be tested in cross section for a total of three impressions. Before being stained, impressions are air dried for 10 to 15 min and fixed in acetone at −20°C for 1 to 4 h or overnight. After removal from the acetone, the slides are allowed to air dry for 10 to 15 min.

A new technique (7) under evaluation in several laboratories fixes rabies slides by brief heating (ca. 1 min) in a precalibrated microwave. Early tests have shown the slides to work as well for immunofluorescence as acetone-fixed material when the staining procedure is modified to include a dilute detergent with the antirabies virus reagent. In addition to speed, the microwave procedure has the advantage of eliminating the problem of discarding acetone as a hazardous waste material.

Each test should include slides made from known positive and negative animals. The positive control slide serves as a sensitivity control for the antirabies virus conjugate, and the negative control slide is used to detect nonspecific staining or adherence of aggregates of labeled antibodies, which may be mistaken for rabies virus antigen. Slides should be prepared in advance, stored at −70°C, and fixed at the time of the test. Unfixed slides are stable for at least 1 month.

Each impression is reacted with FITC-conjugated antirabies virus antibody for 30 min at 37°C in a humidified chamber. Slides are then rinsed and mounted with a phosphate-buffered glycerol mounting medium (pH 8.0 to 8.5). A standard fluorescence microscope with appropriate filters (e.g., excitation at 450 to 490 nm with a dichromatic beam splitter and barrier filter at 510 to 520 nm) is used to observe fluorescing rabies virus antigen in infected tissues, typically at a magnification of ×400 to ×1,000. Slides from each half brain are read independently, preferably by different technicians, and the results are recorded and compared.

Quality Control in the DFA Test

Almost all DFA tests should be unequivocally positive or negative. Repeat tests are necessary only if (i) the antigen accumulations or inclusions stain with diminished intensity compared to the control slide or the inclusions are of an atypical morphology or (ii) the antigen is found in $<10\%$ of the microscopic fields (+1 distribution) or the antigen distribution is unusual (e.g., antigen is found in the hippocampus only). In these situations, slides should be remade from the reserved brain tissue taken at necropsy, and the test should be repeated with a second anti-rabies virus reagent prepared with antibody from a different source and rabies adsorption controls prepared from normal and rabies virus-infected brains. Samples negative with both reagents in both adsorption suspensions in the repeat test are reported as negative. Rabies virus-positive samples should stain with both anti-rabies virus reagents diluted in a normal brain suspension. No staining should be seen with reagents diluted in an infected brain suspension. When only one reagent yields positive results, the sample must be reported as inconclusive or nondiagnostic for rabies. The sample should then be tested by an alternative test for rabies (virus isolation or reverse transcription [RT]-PCR). Discordant results between two reagents in the repeat test should be extremely rare, and the sample should be submitted to a national or regional reference laboratory for confirmation of the observation. Reagent staining that is the result of a nonspecific reaction can be found in tissue stained with both normal and infected brain adsorption controls. When only one reagent reacts in this manner and no staining is observed with the second reagent, the sample is reported as negative. When both reagents show nonspecific staining, there is the risk that specific staining present in the tissue may be masked. The sample must be reported as nondiagnostic, and an alternative test must be performed. When a rabies test is nondiagnostic, postexposure treatment recommendations must be based on clinical and epidemiological evaluations of the animal and its history.

The source of most nonspecific staining is improper washing, which leaves dried reagent on the slides. Mishandling of the reagent by repeated freeze-thaw cycles may also leave aggregates of immunoglobulin and dissociated FITC that are difficult to remove, even with extended washing. Aliquots of the reagent should be stored at −70°C. The working stock of the conjugate should be stored at +4°C and discarded after 1 week. If necessary, aggregates can be removed by filtration or centrifugation at 10,000 × *g* for 20 min. (Note that adsorption with rabies virus-infected brain tissue does not always control for nonspecific adherence of aggregates of FITC-labeled anti-rabies virus antibody and may contribute to nonrecognition of the problem by specifically removing the antibody aggregates.)

A less frequent source of nonspecific or undesired staining is the capture of immunoglobulins in the reagent by Fc receptors on contaminating gram-positive cocci in the sample or infiltrating immune cells in response to an infection other than rabies in the animal (e.g., distemper). Because these receptors are isotype and species specific (12) and different reagents contain different antibody preparations, this type of nonspecific staining will usually be recognized in repeat tests with two reagents from different sources. The staining often fades rapidly, has an atypical morphology, and is difficult to reproduce in repeat tests. If available, staining with an FITC-conjugated normal antibody (of the same isotype and species as your reagent) will confirm the presence of Fc receptors in the test tissue. The use of an anti-rabies virus reagent at too concentrated of a dilution may exacerbate the problem of binding to Fc receptors.

Each new lot of an anti-rabies virus conjugate should be titrated in twofold dilutions to determine its effective limit. At the optimum dilution, antigen in a positive control slide will stain with a glaring, apple green brilliance (+4 staining intensity), and no background or nonspecific fluorescence will be observed in negative tissue. It is very important that slides used for conjugate evaluation contain the small, dust-like rabies virus inclusions along with the larger string-like inclusions. Detection of the dust-like particles requires a stronger dilution of the conjugate and thus is a more stringent evaluation of the reagent. To ensure test sensitivity, the working dilution of the conjugate should be made at least twofold more concentrated than the last dilution which stained the small inclusions with +4 intensity. The working dilution should be determined after any filtration step and checked for conjugate diluted both in phosphate-buffered saline–0.75% bovine serum albumin and in mouse or rabbit brain adsorption suspensions.

Atypical and/or sparse staining may also be the result of cross contamination of negative samples with small amounts of brain material from a strongly positive sample. A contamination problem is usually not recognized until rabies virus antigen is seen in the brain of an animal for which a diagnosis of rabies is unusual or unexpected (e.g., a vaccinated domestic animal or a rodent) or until an increase in the number of samples in which antigen is present in only one area of the brain is seen. The contamination may arise during several steps in the diagnostic procedure. All necropsy instruments should be autoclaved, and a separate set should be used for each animal to be necropsied. Although it may seem primitive, the use of hammers, chisels, and large butcher knives may be preferable to the use of saws for opening the cranium. The former instruments are relatively inexpensive and can be maintained in sufficient quantities so that a separate instrument is used for each animal. If used, Stryker saws or bone saws cleaned in a cold sterilant between uses should always be considered a possible source of contaminating material. Cold sterilants are effective for surface decontamination only, and while they may inactivate rabies virus, they do not always denature rabies virus antigen in adherent tissue. Deposition of this antigen on subsequent samples may result in false-positive test results. When tissue is removed for slide preparation, care should be taken to avoid areas of the brain that may have been penetrated by saws. If the entire brain is not saved for confirmatory testing, precautions against contamination should be taken in removing brain sections for storage. Petri dishes or ointment tins are preferable to test tubes for tissue storage so that individual areas of the brain are not in contact with each other. If possible, slides from each test animal should be fixed in individual containers. The acetone should be replaced after the preparation of each set of slides, and the jars should be cleaned and autoclaved. Rabies virus-infected tissue also accumulates in the vessels used for acetone fixation of slides and can be a source of false-positive test results.

Problems with nonspecific staining and cross contamination can be recognized more readily if the record of test results for each sample includes the amounts of rabies virus antigen observed in slides made from the brain stem, cerebellum, and hippocampus. The observation of antigen in only one section of the brain (especially the hippocampus) is unusual and should elicit repeat testing of the sample and a great deal of interest in the laboratory.

Although standardized procedures for DFA tests exist, a recent survey of rabies laboratories in the United States (23) revealed the use of potentially deleterious modifications that may reduce the sensitivity of the standard test.

The modification most likely to compromise a diagnosis is the failure to include in each test slides made from the medulla or brain stem. Although rabies virus antigen is normally distributed throughout all areas of the brain of an infected animal, rabies virus-specific inclusions are found only in the brain stem in a small number of cases. Additionally, even when rabies antigen is present in all areas of the brain, the amount of staining is often larger in the brain stem, leading to a more confident diagnosis. An uneven distribution of antigen in the infected brain is a frequent observation in larger animals, and a strong argument could be made that tests of horses and cows can be considered nondiagnostic without the inclusion of the brain stem or medulla. For example, a +4 antigen distribution was seen in all areas of the brains of 684 of 688 rabid skunks (99%) diagnosed in Texas from 1989 to 1992. In contrast, a uniform antigen distribution was seen in only 12 of 41 rabid horse brains (29%) tested during this same time period (23).

Fixation for less than 1 h and at temperatures greater

than 4°C results in less brilliant and possibly incomplete staining. In emergency situations, a positive diagnosis can be made by examination of slides fixed for shorter intervals. A second test of slides fixed for longer intervals should be used to confirm a negative diagnosis.

Mounting at a pH of >8 enhances the intensity of fluorescence of fluorescein compounds. Mounting agents should be stabilized with phosphate buffers, since the instability of carbonate-buffered mounting agents can be particularly deleterious to MAb reagents (9).

The pH of rinse buffers should be 7.6 to 7.8.

Slides should be examined at ×10 ocular and ×40 to ×63 objective magnifications. Lower magnifications may not be sufficient for all stained rabies virus antigenic forms to be easily observed.

All laboratories should participate in national rabies virus proficiency testing (available through the Wisconsin Laboratory of Hygiene, Madison). Additionally, every laboratory should have the capability for a periodic evaluation of the sensitivity and specificity of their DFA test, either within the laboratory or through the services of a national or regional reference laboratory. Each confirmatory test should include DFA-positive and -negative sample controls. Isolation of virus by inoculation of mice or cell culturing is the most commonly used confirmatory test, but the use of RT-PCR is increasing. In addition to the conditions already specified (atypical or sparse staining not clarified in a repeat test), a confirmatory test should be performed when (i) rabies is diagnosed in a multiply vaccinated domestic animal or a wild animal not normally associated with rabies (e.g., a small rodent) or (ii) a larger sample size is needed (e.g., to confirm a negative test result for a brain sample from a large animal, such as a horse or cow).

DFA Test of Skin Biopsy

Serial frozen sections of skin biopsy samples (3 to 6 μm thick) are fixed in cold acetone for 10 min, air dried for 10 min, and stained with DFA as detailed above. Rabies virus-specific intracytoplasmic inclusions may be seen in the cutaneous nerves surrounding the hair shaft. Serial sections should show antigen throughout the nerve fiber. Only rarely is antigen seen in contiguous tissue.

Other Tests for Rabies Virus Antigen

Histologic stains for Negri bodies (26), although fast, inexpensive, and specific, will detect only 50 to 80% of DFA-positive samples. This lack of sensitivity severely limits their usefulness, except in situations where the DFA test is unavailable. Enzyme-linked immunosorbent assays (ELISA) (2) are more sensitive, more economical alternatives to histologic methods for laboratories without fluorescence microscopes. However, these tests lack the specificity gained from direct observation of fluorescent rabies virus intracytoplasmic inclusions, and the relatively high cutoff between negative and positive responses somewhat diminishes their sensitivity as compared with DFA.

ISOLATION OF RABIES VIRUS

Cell Culture

Rabies virus is poorly cytopathic. Evidence of virus growth is provided by DFA detection of viral antigen in acetone-fixed cell monolayers. As observed in our laboratory and others, murine neuroblastoma (MNA) cells are the most sensitive cells for street rabies virus strains. These cells are available from Biowhittaker, Walkersville, Md. A similar cell line (CCL 131) may be obtained from the American Type Culture Collection, Manassas, Va. These cells prefer an acidic medium with increased vitamins, which may be prepared from commercially available stocks. Eagle's minimum essential medium (EMEM; Gibco Laboratories, Grand Island, N.Y.) should be supplemented with an additional 2× vitamins, 2× glutamine, and 10% fetal bovine serum. Each new lot of bovine serum should be checked for inhibitors of rabies virus. Penicillin (100 U/ml), streptomycin (100 μg/ml), and amphotericin B (0.25 μg/ml) also should be added. The final concentration of sodium bicarbonate should be 0.75 mg/ml. This medium is optimized for cell growth in closed-flask cultures. Open-flask cultures or cell culture slides (e.g., for virus isolation) should be incubated in an atmosphere of 0.5% CO_2 at 37°C and 90% humidity. Higher CO_2 levels require a higher concentration of sodium bicarbonate in the medium.

Brain material for virus isolation is prepared in EMEM as a 20% suspension of the medulla, cerebellum, and hippocampus. After centrifugation at 500 × *g* for 10 min, 0.5 ml of the supernatant is added to a suspension of 2×10^6 MNA cells in 1.5 ml of EMEM. The cells and virus are incubated for 1 h at 37°C. Unless there is obvious evidence of bacterial contamination of the sample, the inoculum may be left on the cells and the cell suspension may be divided for incubation as flask cultures or slide or plate cultures. Saliva samples for virus isolation are diluted 1:3 into media with antibiotics, vortexed vigorously, frozen and thawed once, and centrifuged at 500 to 1,000 × *g* for 20 min. The supernatant (0.5 ml) is inoculated as described above.

After 40 to 48 h of culturing, the slides (or plates) are fixed in cold (−20°C) acetone for 5 min and examined by the DFA test. Most samples positive in the DFA test are positive for virus isolation at this time. Flask cultures of samples with an expected low initial infectivity or cultures used for the confirmation of negative results are given fresh medium after 3 days, and culturing is continued for an additional 3 to 4 days. At this time, the primary flask culture is trypsinized and used to prepare new slide cultures. There is no need to include supernatant from the primary culture. The secondary slide cultures are incubated for 3 to 4 h (to allow the cells to attach to the slides) or overnight, and the slides are examined by the DFA test as described above. Samples which are negative upon examination of these secondary cultures are considered negative.

Virus Isolation by Mouse Inoculation

A 20% suspension of approximately 0.3 g of tissue from the medulla, cerebellum, and hippocampus is prepared in phosphate-buffered saline containing a protein stabilizer (such as 0.75% bovine serum albumin fraction V). Penicillin (500 U/ml) and streptomycin (2 mg/ml) are also added to prevent animal death from bacterial contamination of the tissue suspension. Five weanling mice or two families of suckling mice are inoculated intracerebrally with a 1:2 dilution of centrifuged suspension (500 × *g* for 5 min) and observed daily for 30 days for signs of rabies (trembling, humping, paralysis, or prostration). A 7- to 20-day incubation period is expected in mice inoculated with street rabies virus preparations, but longer incubation periods are sometimes observed. Virus can be detected by the DFA test in the brains of inoculated mice well in advance of the appearance of clinical signs or death. An earlier diagnosis can be made if extra mice are inoculated and their brains are examined at daily intervals postinoculation.

DETECTION OF VIRAL RNA BY MOLECULAR TECHNIQUES

Because the diagnosis of rabies is made late in the clinical course, after an accumulation of virus in the brain, enhanced sensitivity through RT-PCR is not needed for rabies diagnosis. The greater expense of RT-PCR than of immunofluorescence makes it unlikely that the procedure will gain widespread use as a routine test, even though there are several potential applications to rabies virus testing. Primers 10g (CTACAATGGATGCCGAC; RT and amplification) and 304 (TTGACGAAGATCTTGCTCAT; amplification), located at positions 66 and 1533, respectively (5), will amplify all of the variants of rabies virus known to be present in the United States (20a). For RT-amplification of smaller products and increased sensitivity when RNA is limited or degraded, primers at position 1157 (109BT, GAGAAGGAACTTCAGGA; and 509, GAGAAAGAACTTCAAGA) can be used with primer 304. However, this region is less well conserved across all rabies virus variants, and two separate reactions are usually required to achieve the sensitivity necessary when RNA is limited. The sensitivity of a primary RT-PCR should be equal to or higher than that of an isolation test and must be determined empirically before RT-PCR is used routinely. Nested PCR should be unnecessary for routine samples but is helpful for samples in which RNA is present in extremely small quantities (e.g., samples taken antemortem in suspected cases of human rabies).

VIRUS TYPING

Both MAbs (24) and nucleotide sequence analysis (28) have been used in epidemiological studies, where the precise identification of a rabies virus variant can provide information about patterns of disease transmission. MAb typing is performed as an indirect immunofluorescence test with an FITC-conjugated antimouse immunoglobulin. Touch impression slides from brain material used for the diagnostic test can be used directly for typing if rabies virus antigen is found in 75 to 100% of microscopic fields. Alternatively, the virus must be amplified in cell cultures. A panel of seven antibodies with known patterns of reactivity (21) is available from Chemicon International. This panel includes an antibody that distinguishes rabies from nonrabies viruses in the genus *Lyssavirus*. Any sample found positive for rabies virus by a standard diagnostic test in the United States should be found positive with this MAb. Any negative finding obtained with this MAb should be reported to the Centers for Disease Control and Prevention, and the sample should be submitted for confirmatory testing. Other antibodies in the panel will help to identify rabies virus variants commonly circulating in animal reservoirs for rabies in different areas of the United States and can be useful in the early identification of new outbreaks of rabies. Some variants of rabies virus are not easily distinguished by MAb typing, and differentiation of these viruses requires nucleotide sequence analysis of the products of RT-PCR (16). Analysis may be performed by use of restriction digestion patterns, use of specific primers, or direct comparison of nucleotides.

SEROLOGY

The sensitivity and specificity of the different assay methods for rabies virus antibody vary greatly (22). The suitability of a particular method is determined by the purpose for which the results are intended. Since the surface G protein is the most important protein for conferring immunity to lethal infection with rabies virus, assays of vaccine immunogenicity should measure antibody to this protein. Most commonly, neutralizing antibody is measured, but G-protein-specific ELISA are also applicable. Diagnostic tests should be able to detect any antibody present, regardless of the viral protein that induced it, and ELISA with whole-virus immunosorbents are the most sensitive assays available.

All persons tested 2 to 4 weeks after completion of the recommended schedule for preexposure or postexposure rabies prophylaxis demonstrate an antibody response to rabies virus, and no treatment failures have been documented in the United States (3). Therefore, it is not necessary to document seroconversion to vaccination unless the patient is immunocompromised. Serology may be useful, however, for persons who are at continued risk and who are scheduled to receive booster doses of vaccine 6 months to 2 years after preexposure immunization. A booster dose of vaccine is unnecessary for patients with sustained levels of antibody to rabies virus.

Neutralization Test

The standard test for antibody to G protein measures the ability of a serum to neutralize a challenge inoculum, usually indicated by a reduction in the number of fluorescent-antibody-stained microscopic foci of infected cells. There are several modifications of this procedure (22).

First, an appropriate inoculum of the challenge virus standard strain of rabies virus is determined by serial dilution. Tenfold increments are prepared in eight-well Lab-tek slides, resulting in a final volume of 0.1 ml/well. An equal volume of MNA cells (50,000 to 100,000 cells) in EMEM (see above) is added. After 20 h of incubation, infected cells are stained by the fluorescent-antibody technique. At an ocular magnification of $\times 160$, approximately 50 microscopic fields may be observed in each well of an eight-well slide. One infectious unit of virus is that contained in the virus dilution at which 50% of the observed fields contain one or more infected cells (50% focus-forming dose [FFD_{50}]). In a rabies virus antibody titration, each serum dilution receives 32 to 100 FFD_{50} of virus. The antibody titer is the reciprocal of the serum dilution that reduces the challenge virus to one FFD_{50} (97 to 99% virus reduction). The number of international units of rabies virus antibody in a test serum is determined by comparison with a titration of a rabies virus reference serum standard included in each test. Serum drawn 2 to 4 weeks postvaccination should contain 0.5 international unit of antibody (approximately equivalent to complete neutralization of the challenge virus with a 1:25 dilution of serum). Booster doses at 6-month or 2-year intervals are required if a 1:5 serum dilution fails to completely neutralize the challenge virus.

If large serosurveys are anticipated, it is possible to perform all titrations with microtiter plates and to detect changes in virus concentration by ELISA. This method permits automation of all pipetting, spectrophotometric reading of color development, and titer calculation by computer analysis of data.

ELISA

Although not yet in wide use, several ELISAs for the determination of antibodies have been developed. An ELISA based on whole virus as the immunosorbent is one of the most sensitive assay methods available. Using such an assay, Savy and Atanasiu (19) were able to detect anti-rabies virus immunoglobulin M antibody very early in the clinical course of three human rabies cases and well before neutralizing antibodies could be detected. If estimates of vaccine immunogenicity are required, the immunosorbent should contain only the G protein. Simple methods for the purification of the G protein have been published (12), and materials for a G-protein-specific ELISA are available in kit form from Diagnostics Pasteur. Although extensive comparative trials have not been conducted, data suggest that the G-protein-specific ELISA is a reliable and simple alternative to the neutralization test.

APPENDIX 1
Collection of Samples for Diagnosis of Rabies in Humans

A diagnosis of rabies should be considered for patients with signs or symptoms of encephalitis or myelitis. The course of the illness, additional history, and laboratory tests for other, more common causes can determine if samples specific for rabies virus should be collected. The following instructions should be used to collect samples only after a consultation with your state health department and with the Rabies Laboratory at the Centers for Disease Control and Prevention.

Patient history

Please provide information on the clinical history of the patient and provide the name and phone number of the physician who should be contacted with the results.

Samples

All samples should be considered potentially infectious. Test tubes and other sample containers must be securely sealed (tape around the cap will ensure that the containers do not open during transit). If immediate shipment is not possible, samples should be stored frozen at −20°C or below. Samples should be shipped frozen on dry ice overnight in watertight primary containers and leak-proof secondary containers that meet the guidelines of the International Air Transport Association. The Rabies Laboratory at the Centers for Disease Control and Prevention should be telephoned at the time of shipment and given information on the mode of shipment, expected arrival time, and courier tracking number.

Saliva

Using a sterile eyedropper pipette, collect saliva and place it in a small sterile container that can be sealed securely. No preservatives or additional material should be added. Laboratory tests to be performed include the detection of rabies virus RNA (by RT-PCR of extracted nucleic acids) and isolation of infectious virus in cell cultures. Tracheal aspirates and sputum are not suitable for rabies virus tests.

Neck biopsy

A section of skin 5 to 6 mm in diameter should be taken from the posterior region of the neck at the hairline. The biopsy specimen should contain a minimum of 10 hair follicles and should be of a sufficient depth to include the cutaneous nerves at the base of the follicle. Place the specimen on a piece of sterile gauze moistened with sterile water in a sealed container. Do not add preservatives or additional fluids. Laboratory tests to be performed include RT-PCR and immunofluorescence staining for viral antigen in frozen sections of the biopsy.

Serum and cerebrospinal fluid

At least 0.5 ml of serum or cerebrospinal fluid should be collected; no preservatives should be added. Do not use whole blood. If no vaccine or rabies immune serum has been given, the presence of antibody to rabies virus in the serum is diagnostic, and tests of cerebrospinal fluid are unnecessary. Antibody to rabies virus in cerebrospinal fluid, regardless of the immunization history, suggests a rabies virus infection. Laboratory tests for antibody include indirect immunofluorescence and virus neutralization.

Brain biopsy

The rarity of rabies and the lack of an effective treatment make the collection of a brain biopsy unwarranted; however, biopsy samples negative for herpesvirus encephalitis should be tested for evidence of rabies virus infection. Place the biopsy in a sealed sterile container. Do not add preservatives or additional fluids. Laboratory tests to be performed include RT-PCR and immunofluorescence staining for viral antigen in touch impressions.

Postmortem diagnosis of rabies is made by immunofluorescence staining of viral antigen in touch impressions of brain tissue. Portions of the medulla (brain stem), cerebellum, and hippocampus should be frozen and shipped on dry ice to a public health laboratory. Preservation of tissues by fixation in formalin is not recommended for rabies diagnosis.

REFERENCES

1. **Beran, G. W.** 1991. Urban rabies, p. 427–443. *In* G. M. Baer (ed.), *The Natural History of Rabies*, 2nd ed. CRC Press, Inc., Boca Raton, Fla.
2. **Bourhy, H., and P. Perrin.** 1996. Rapid rabies enzyme immunodiagnosis (RREID) for rabies antigen detection, p. 105–113. *In* F. X. Meslin, M. M. Kaplan, and H. Koprowski (ed.), *Laboratory Techniques in Rabies*, 4th ed. World Health Organization, Geneva, Switzerland.
3. **Centers for Disease Control.** 1991. Rabies prevention—United States, 1991: recommendations of the Immunization Practices Advisory Committee (ACIP). *Morbid. Mortal. Weekly Rep.* **40:**1–19.
4. **Centers for Disease Control and National Institutes of Health.** 1988. *Biosafety in Microbiological and Biomedical Laboratories*. U.S. Government Printing Office, Washington, D.C.
5. **Conzelmann, K. K., J. H. Cox, L. G. Schneider, and H. J. Thiel.** 1990. Molecular cloning and complete nucleotide sequence of the attenuated rabies virus SAD B19. *Virology* **175:**485–499.
6. **Cox, J. H., B. Dietzschold, and L. G. Schneider.** 1977. Rabies virus glycoprotein. II. Biological and serological characterization. *Infect. Immun.* **16:**754–759.
7. **Davis, C., S. Neill, and P. Raj.** 1997. Microwave fixation of rabies specimens for fluorescent antibody testing. *J. Virol. Methods* **68:**177–182.
8. **Dean, D. J., W. A. Abelseth, and P. Atanasiu.** 1996. The fluorescent antibody test, p. 88–93. *In* F. X. Meslin, M. M. Kaplan, and K. Koprowski (ed.), *Laboratory Techniques in Rabies*, 4th ed. World Health Organization, Geneva, Switzerland.
9. **Durham, T. M., J. S. Smith, F. L. Reid, C. T. Hale-Smith, and M. B. Fears.** 1986. Stability of immunofluorescence reactions produced by polyclonal and monoclonal antibody conjugates for rabies virus. *J. Clin. Microbiol.* **24:**301–303.
10. **Fekadu, M., and J. H. Shaddock.** 1984. Peripheral distribution of virus in dogs inoculated with two strains of rabies virus. *Am. J. Vet. Res.* **45:**724–729.
11. **Hamir, A. N., and G. Moser.** 1994. Immunoperoxidase test for rabies: utility as a diagnostic test. *J. Vet. Diagn. Investig.* **6:**148–152.
12. **Herrmann, J. E.** 1995. Immunoassays for the diagnosis of infectious diseases, p. 110–122. *In* P. R. Murray, E. J. Baron, M. A. Pfaller, F. C. Tenover, and R. H. Yolken (ed.), *Manual of Clinical Microbiology*, 6th ed. American Society for Microbiology, Washington, D.C.
13. **Krebs, J. W., T. W. Strine, J. S. Smith, D. L. Noah, C. E. Rupprecht, and J. E. Childs.** 1997. Rabies surveillance in the United States during 1996. *J. Am. Vet. Med. Assoc.* **211:**1525–1539.

14. **Lewis, V. J., and W. L. Thacker.** 1974. Limitations of deteriorated tissue for rabies diagnosis. *Health Lab. Sci.* **11:** 8–12.
15. **Noah, D. L., C. L. Drenzek, J. S. Smith, J. W. Krebs, L. A. Orciari, J. Shaddock, D. Sanderlin, S. Whitfield, M. Fekadu, J. G. Olson, C. E. Rupprecht, and J. E. Childs.** 1998. Epidemiology of human rabies in the United States, 1980 to 1996. *Ann. Intern. Med.* **128:**922–930.
16. **Rohde, R. E., S. U. Neill, K. A. Clark, and J. S. Smith.** 1998. Molecular epidemiology of rabies epizootics in Texas. *Clin. Diagn. Virol.* **8:**209–217.
17. **Rupprecht, C. E., C. A. Hanlon, M. Niezgoda, J. R. Buchanan, D. Diehl, and H. Koprowski.** 1993. Recombinant rabies vaccines: efficacy assessment in free-ranging animals. *Onderstepoort J. Vet. Res.* **60:**463–468.
18. **Rupprecht, C. E., J. S. Smith, J. Krebs, M. Niezgoda, and J. E. Childs.** 1996. Current issue in rabies prevention in the United States: health dilemmas, public coffers, private interests. *Public Health Rep.* **111:**400–407.
19. **Savy, V., and P. Atanasiu.** 1978. Rapid immunoenzymatic technique for titration of rabies antibodies IgG and IgM. *Dev. Biol. Stand.* **40:**247–253.
20. **Schneider, L. G., B. Dietzschold, R. E. Dierks, W. Matthaeus, P. J. Enzmann, and K. Strohmaier.** 1973. Rabies group-specific ribonucleoprotein antigen and a test system for grouping and typing of rhabdoviruses. *J. Virol.* **11:** 748–755.
20a. **Smith, J.** Unpublished data.
21. **Smith, J. S.** 1989. Rabies virus epitopic variation: use in ecologic studies. *Adv. Virus Res.* **36:**215–253.
22. **Smith, J. S.** 1991. Rabies serology, p. 235–252. *In* G. M. Baer (ed.), *The Natural History of Rabies*, 2nd ed. CRC Press, Inc., Boca Raton, Fla.
23. **Smith, J. S.** 1995. Rabies virus, p. 997–1003. *In* P. R. Murray, E. J. Baron, M. A. Pfaller, F. C. Tenover, and R. H. Yolken (ed.), *Manual of Clinical Microbiology*, 6th ed. American Society for Microbiology, Washington, D.C.
24. **Smith, J. S., and A. A. King.** 1996. Monoclonal antibodies for the identification of rabies and non-rabies lyssaviruses, p. 145–156. *In* F. X. Meslin, M. M. Kaplan, and H. Koprowski (ed.), *Laboratory Techniques in Rabies*, 4th ed. World Health Organization, Geneva, Switzerland.
25. **Sosin, D. M., J. J. Sacks, and R. W. Sattin.** 1992. Causes of nonfatal injuries in the United States. *Accid. Anal. & Prev.* **24:**685–687.
26. **Sureau, P., P. Ravisse, and P. E. Rollin.** 1991. Rabies diagnosis by animal inoculation, identification of Negri bodies, or ELISA, p. 203–217. *In* G. M. Baer (ed.), *The Natural History of Rabies*, 2nd ed. CRC Press, Inc., Boca Raton, Fla.
27. **Tordo, N.** 1996. Characteristics and molecular biology of the rabies virus, p. 28–52. *In* F. X. Meslin, M. M. Kaplan, and H. Koprowski (ed.), *Laboratory Techniques in Rabies*, 4th ed. World Health Organization, Geneva, Switzerland.
28. **Tordo, N., D. Sacramento, and H. Bourhy.** 1996. The polymerase chain reaction (PCR) technique for diagnosis, typing and epidemiological studies of rabies, p. 157–170. *In* F. X. Meslin, M. M. Kaplan, and H. Koprowski (ed.), *Laboratory Techniques in Rabies*, 4th ed. World Health Organization, Geneva, Switzerland.
29. **Trimarchi, C. V., and J. Debbie.** 1991. The fluorescent antibody in rabies, p. 219–233. *In* G. M. Baer (ed.), *The Natural History of Rabies*, 2nd ed. CRC Press, Inc., Boca Raton, Fla.
30. **Velleca, W. M., and F. T. Forrester.** 1981. *Laboratory Methods for Detecting Rabies*. U.S. Government Printing Office, Washington, D.C.
31. **Webster, W. A., and G. A. Casey.** 1988. Diagnosis of rabies infection, p. 201–223. *In* J. B. Campbell and K. M. Charlton (ed.), *Rabies*. Kluwer Academic Publishers, Boston, Mass.
32. **Wiktor, T. J., R. I. Macfarlan, K. J. Reagan, B. Dietzschold, P. J. Curtis, W. H. Wunner, M. P. Kieny, R. Lathe, J. P. Lecocq, M. Mackett, et al.** 1984. Protection from rabies by a vaccinia virus recombinant containing the rabies virus glycoprotein gene. *Proc. Natl. Acad. Sci. USA* **81:**7194–7198.
33. **World Health Organization.** 1992. WHO Expert Committee on Rabies, Eighth Report. *WHO Tech. Rep. Ser.* **824:** 1–84.
34. **World Health Organization.** 1996. *World Survey of Rabies 30 for the Year 1994*. World Health Organization, Geneva, Switzerland.

Arboviruses

THEODORE F. TSAI

89

EPIDEMIOLOGIC AND CLINICAL BACKGROUND

The arboviruses (arthropod-borne viruses) are a taxonomically heterogeneous group of more than 500 viruses that share common modes of vector-borne transmission (13, 14, 32, 34, 39). The *International Catalogue of Arboviruses* (22) also includes certain taxonomically related zoonotic viruses that are spread directly from animals without the agency of a vector. Most arboviruses are transmitted between specific arthropod vectors and vertebrate hosts, e.g., birds and small mammals, in which infections typically are asymptomatic. In contrast, infections occurring in animals to which the virus has not adapted a parasitic relationship often result in various degrees of illness or in death.

Approximately 150 of the recognized arboviruses cause illness in humans; however, the approach to laboratory diagnosis is greatly simplified by considering the possibilities in light of the patient's history of travel and/or exposure (13, 14, 32). Although some arboviruses, such as the dengue viruses, are virtually cosmopolitan, others have a more limited geographic distribution in which they have adapted to specific vectors and intermediate animal hosts. By considering the known incubation periods of the principal arboviral infections in the context of the itinerary of places and circumstances under which infection may have been acquired, the differential diagnosis can be narrowed considerably.

The epidemiologic and clinical characteristics of medically important arboviruses are summarized in Table 1. More comprehensive descriptions can be found elsewhere (13, 14, 32, 39). Current information on arboviral outbreaks and transmission patterns can be obtained from state health departments, from the worldwide web at www.who.org/programmes/emc/news.htm and www.cdc.gov/travel/travel.html, and from the listserv promed (send e-mail message to majordomo@usa.health net.org [without a subject heading] subscribe promed⟨sender's e-mail address⟩).

The majority of arboviral infections result in simple febrile illnesses that cannot be distinguished clinically from other common viral infections. Clinical features that characterize acute arboviral fevers include a sudden onset of debilitating symptoms; extreme headache, myalgia, and lumbar pain; relatively rapid resolution (e.g., within 24 to 48 h for Oropouche and sandfly fever); and for some infections (e.g., some cases of Colorado tick fever and dengue), a recrudescent course of fever and symptoms. Lymphadenopathy may be prominent in West Nile fever. Several important arboviruses (e.g., dengue and Sindbis viruses) also produce a rash, but these exanthems are not distinctive, and even when cases have occurred in epidemic proportions, dengue outbreaks have been incorrectly characterized as epidemics of influenza or measles. Several alphaviruses, e.g., Sindbis, chikungunya, Mayaro, and Ross River viruses, produce an acute viral syndrome with polyarthritis and exanthem that must be differentiated clinically from rubella, hepatitis A and B, parvoviral, and mycoplasmal infections, among other diseases.

Neurotropic arboviruses such as the viruses of St. Louis, Murray Valley, Western, and Japanese encephalitis (JE) cause aseptic meningitis or encephalitis in only a minority of infected persons; most infections are asymptomatic or lead to a mild illness, sometimes with headache. Pathologically, global involvement of cortical, subcortical, and brain stem structures and spinal cord myelitis is typical; consequently, various neurologic presentations are possible, with combinations of coma, weakness, cerebellar and extrapyramidal movement disorders, cranial palsies, and other manifestations of bulbar dysfunction and myelitis.

Hantaviruses, cosmopolitan rodent-borne *Bunyaviridae* spread directly from infected rodent urine and secretions, are linked with three clinical syndromes. Hantaan, Seoul, and Dobrava viruses cause hemorrhagic fever with renal syndrome, an acute pantropic infection marked by diffuse capillary dysfunction, acute renal insufficiency due to interstitial nephritis, vascular instability, and hemorrhagic manifestations (40). In Scandinavia and western Europe, Puumula virus causes a similar but milder form of the disease, nephropathia epidemica, typified by a febrile grippe and clinically insignificant renal insufficiency and rarely with more serious systemic illness. Sin Nombre and New York viruses cause a pattern of capillary leakage limited to the lungs and produce acute pulmonary edema, thrombocytopenia, and shock, with death in 50% of patients (23, 24, 51). A similar pulmonary syndrome is produced by Bayou and related viruses; but in addition, proteinuria and myositis are components of the illness (40, 44a). Unlike the other hantaviruses, which do not spread from person to person, Laguna Negra and Andes viruses have been implicated in outbreaks with interhuman transmission, including physicians caring for patients (49). Although Sin Nombre viral antigen is found in lung

TABLE 1 Arboviral and zoonotic viral infections by geographic area, mode of transmission, and clinical syndrome[a]

Location and virus	Febrile illness			Meningo-encephalitis	Hemorrhagic fever	Other
	Nondescript	With rash	With arthritis			
North America						
Mosquito borne						
Cache Valley				○		
California encephalitis				○		
Dengue 1–4		●			●	Hepatitis
EEE				○		
Everglades (VEE type II)				○		
Jamestown Canyon				○		Respiratory symptoms
Keystone				○		
LaCrosse				●		
StLE				●		
Snowshoe hare				○		
Tensaw				○		
Trivittatus				○		Respiratory symptoms
VEE (sylvatic subtypes 1D and 1E)	○			○		Pneumonitis
Western equine encephalitis				●		Perinatal illness after congenital third-trimester infection
Sand fly borne						
Vesicular stomatitis (New Jersey and Indiana)	○			○		Respiratory illness
Tick borne						
Colorado tick fever	●			○	○	
Powassan				○		
Salmon River	○					
Zoonoses						
Lymphocytic choriomeningitis	○			○	○	Pneumonia, parotitis, orchitis, arthritis; congenital infection-CNS malformation
Bayou, Black Creek Canal						Noncardiogenic pulmonary edema, nephrosis, myositis
Modoc				○		
New York, Sin Nombe						Noncardiogenic pulmonary edema
Rabies				○		
Rio Bravo	○			○		Pneumonia, orchitis
Seoul						Interstitial nephritis
Unknown mode of transmission						
Borna						Psychiatric illness?
Central and South America						
Mosquito borne						
Bussuquara	○					
Cache Valley	○					
Catu	○					
Cotia	○					
Dengue 1–4		●		○	●	Hepatitis, perinatal illness after congenital third-trimester infection

(Continued on next page)

TABLE 1 (*Continued*)

Location and virus	Febrile illness			Meningo-encephalitis	Hemorrhagic fever	Other
	Nondescript	With rash	With arthritis			
EEE				○		
Fort Sherman	○					
Group C viruses (Apeu, Caraparu, Itaqui, Madrid, Marituba, Murutucu, Nepuyo, Oriboca, Ossa, Restan)	○					
Guama	○					
Guaroa	○			?		Hepatitis
Ilheus	○			○		
Mayaro		●	●			
Mucambo (VEE type IIIA)	○			○		
Piry	○					
Rocio				●		
StLE	○			○		
Tacaiuma	○					Two cases with concurrent malaria were fatal
Tonate (VEE type IIIB)	○					
Tucunduba				○		
VEE (epizootic subtypes IABC)	●			●		Abortion, CNS malformation after first-trimester infection
VEE (sylvatic subtypes 1D, 1E, and 1F)	○			○		Pneumonitis
Western equine encephalitis				●		
Wyeomyia	○					
Xingu	○					Hepatitis?
YF	●				●	Hepatitis
Sand fly and/or midge borne						
Alenquer	○					
Candiru	○					
Chagres	○					
Changuinola	○					
Morumbi	○					
Oropouche	●	○		○		
Punta Toro	○					
Serra Norte	○					
Vesicular stomatitis (New Jersey and Indiana)	○			○		
Vesicular stomatitis (Alagoas)				○		
Zoonoses						
Andes, Laguna Negra						Noncardiogenic pulmonary edema, nephrosis
Guanarito				○	●	
Junin				○	●	Fatal congenital infection
Machupo				○	●	
Rabies				○		
Rio Bravo	○			○		Pneumonia, orchitis
Sabia					○[b]	
Unknown mode of transmission						
Borna						Psychiatric illness?

(*Continued on next page*)

TABLE 1 Arboviral and zoonotic viral infections by geographic area, mode of transmission, and clinical syndrome[a] (*Continued*)

Location and virus	Febrile illness			Meningo-encephalitis	Hemorrhagic fever	Other
	Nondescript	With rash	With arthritis			
Europe						
Mosquito borne						
Batai	○			○		
Inkoo	○			○		Respiratory illness
Sindbis (Ockelbo)	●	●	●			
Snowshoe hare				○		
Tahyna	●			○		Respiratory illness
West Nile	○	○	○	●		
Sand fly borne						
Sandfly fever (Naples)	●					
Sandfly fever (Sicilian)	●					
Toscana	●			●		
Tick borne						
Bhanja	○			○		
Central European encephalitis[c]	●			●		Hepatitis, thrombocytopenia
Congo-Crimean hemorrhagic fever					●	
Dhori				○[b]		
Kemerovo				○		
Lipovnik				○		
Louping ill				○		
Thogoto	○			○		Hepatitis, optic neuritis
Tribec				○		
Zoonoses						
Erve				○		Thunderclap headache
Lymphocytic choriomeningitis	●			●	○	Pneumonia, arthritis, orchitis, parotitis; congenital infection-CNS malformation
Dobrava	○				○	Interstitial nephritis, pantropic
Puumula	●			○	○	Interstitial nephritis, myocarditis
Rabies				○		
Seoul	○				○	Interstitial nephritis, pantropic
Unknown mode of transmission						
Borna						Psychiatric illness?
Asia						
Mosquito borne						
Batai	○			○		
Beijng				●		
Chandipura	○			○		
Chikungunya		●	●	○	○	
Dengue 1–4	●	●		○	●	Hepatitis common; perinatal illness after third-trimester infection
JE				●		Abortion after congenital first- and second-trimester infection
Kunjin		○	○	○		

(*Continued on next page*)

TABLE 1 *(Continued)*

Location and virus	Febrile illness			Meningo-encephalitis	Hemorrhagic fever	Other
	Nondescript	With rash	With arthritis			
Semliki forest (MeTri)				○		
Sindbis	●	●	●	○	○	
Snowshoe hare				○		
Tahyna	●			○		Respiratory illness
West Nile	●	●	●	○		Hepatitis, pancreatitis
Yunnan	○					
Zika		●				
Sand fly borne						
Chandipura	○			○		
Sandfly fever (Naples)	●					
Sandfly fever (Sicilian)	●					
Tick borne						
Alma-Arasan	○					
Banna				●		
Congo-Crimean hemorrhagic fever					●	
Dhori				○[b]		
Ganjam	○					
Issyk-kul	○					
Karshi	○					
Kemerovo				○		
Kyasanur Forest				●	●	Pneumonia, retinitis
Negishi				○		
Omsk hemorrhagic fever				●	●	Pneumonia
Powassan				○		
Tamdy	○					
Russian spring-summer encephalitis				●		
Syr-Darya Valley		○				
Wanowrie				○	○	
Zoonoses						
Hantaan					●	Pantropic, interstitial nephritis
Lymphocytic choriomeningitis	○			○		Pneumonia, arthritis, orchitis, parotitis; congenital infection-CNS malformation
Rabies				○		
Seoul					●	Pantropic, interstitial nephritis
Unknown mode of transmission						
Borna						Psychiatric illness?
Africa						
Mosquito borne						
Babanki	●	●	●			
Bangui		○				
Banzi	○					
Bhanja	○			○		
Bunyamwera		●		○		
Bwamba		●		○		
Chikungunya		●	●	○	○	

(Continued on next page)

TABLE 1 Arboviral and zoonotic viral infections by geographic area, mode of transmission, and clinical syndrome[a] (*Continued*)

Location and virus	Febrile illness			Meningo-encephalitis	Hemorrhagic fever	Other
	Nondescript	With rash	With arthritis			
Dengue 1–4	●	●		○	●	Hepatitis; perinatal illness after congenital third-trimester infection
Germiston		○		○		
IgboOra			○			
Ilesha		●		○	○	
Koutango		○				
Lebombo	○					
Ngari				○		
Nyando	○					
O'nyong-nyong		●	●			
Orungo	●					
Pongola			○			
Rift Valley Fever	●			●	●	Hepatitis, retinitis
Semliki Forest	○			○		
Shokwe	○					
Shuni	○					
Sindbis		●	●		○	
Spondweni		○				
Tahyna	●			○		Respiratory illness
Tataguine		●				
Usutu		○				
Wesselsbron	○					Hepatitis
West Nile	●	●	●	●		Hepatitis
YF	●				●	Hepatitis, pancreatitis
Zika		○				
Sand fly borne						
Chandipura	○			○		
Sandfly fever (Naples)	●					
Sandfly fever (Sicilian)	●					
Tick borne						
Abadina	○					
Bhanja	○			○		
Congo-Crimean hemorrhagic fever					●	
Dhori				○[b]		
Dugbe	○			○		
Nairobi sheep disease	○					
Quaranfil	○			○		
Thogoto	○			○		Hepatitis, optic neuritis
Zoonoses						
Dakar bat	○					
Duvenhage				○		
Lassa				○	●	Pantropic; abortion, hearing loss
Lymphocytic choriomeningitis	○			○	○	Pneumonia, arthritis, orchitis, parotitis; congenital infection-CNS malformation
Mokola				○		
Monkeypox		●				
Rabies				○		
Tanapox		○				

(*Continued on next page*)

TABLE 1 *(Continued)*

Location and virus	Febrile illness			Meningo-encephalitis	Hemorrhagic fever	Other
	Nondescript	With rash	With arthritis			
Unknown mode of transmission						
Ebola (Zaire, Sudan, Ivory Coast)		●			●	Pantropic; abortion
Kasokero	○					
LeDantec				○		
Marburg		●				Pantropic
Australia and Oceania						
Mosquito borne						
Barmah Forest			●			Glomerulonephritis
Dengue 1–4	●	●				Hepatitis; perinatal illness after congenital third-trimester infection
Edge Hill			○			
GanGan			○			
JE				○		
Kokobera			○			
Kunjin			○	○		
Murray Valley				●		
Ross River		●	●	○		Glomerulonephritis
Sepik	○					
Sindbis	○	○	○			
Trubanaman	○					
Zoonoses						
Ballina				○		
Equine morbillivious						Fatal pneumonia

[a] Adapted from reference 8. Key: ○, rare, sporadic; ●, frequent, epidemic. Only arboviruses causing illness after natural infection are listed; viruses causing illness after laboratory exposure only are indicated by footnote.
[b] Illness reported only after laboratory-acquired infection.
[c] Also transmitted by ingestion of infected milk products.

endothelial cells, thus far, neither the virus nor the genomic sequences have been detected in bronchoalveolar fluid, and no laboratory or human-to-human cases have been reported.

Viscerotropic infection in yellow fever (YF), in some cases of dengue, and in certain other arboviral infections may result in hepatitis and jaundice, accounting for 5 to 10% of clinically diagnosed cases of viral hepatitis in areas where the diseases are epidemic (27). Generalized hemorrhage and multisystem organ failure are the end results of fulminant YF and dengue hemorrhagic fever, mimicking malaria, leptospirosis, and the viral hemorrhagic fevers produced by Lassa and other arenaviruses, the filoviruses Ebola and Marburg viruses, and Congo-Crimean hemorrhagic fever virus. Although YF and dengue do not pose a risk for person-to-person nosocomial transmission, the other viruses are proven hazards to hospital and laboratory workers (see chapter 90) (9, 35).

Except for the hemorrhagic fevers addressed in chapter 90 of this Manual, specific therapy of arboviral infections is unavailable. Consequently, the rationale for promptly establishing a laboratory diagnosis of an arboviral infection is to hasten confirmation of other treatable conditions and to assist public health officials in identifying arboviral infections with epidemic potential.

DESCRIPTION OF THE AGENTS

Viruses adapted to arthropod vectors occur in several taxonomic families, but the majority are RNA viruses in the families *Togaviridae* (formerly group A arboviruses), *Flaviviridae* (formerly group B arboviruses), *Bunyaviridae*, *Reoviridae*, and *Rhabdoviridae* (Table 2) (34, 39). The majority are enveloped viruses and are unstable in the environment. The *Orbiviridiae*, *Bunyaviridae*, and *Orthomyxoviridae* contain multiple genomic segments and may undergo reassortment. Complete nucleotide sequences or sequences of certain genomic segments have been determined for a few arboviruses, facilitating production of synthetic antigens for diagnosis and as candidate vaccines. Important antigenic determinants have been elucidated for the most important arboviruses, and viral and group-specific monoclonal antibodies are available for taxonomic and diagnostic purposes.

Most arboviruses elaborate hemagglutinins that aggregate goose, chick, and/or human group O erythrocytes. Hemagglutination (HA) occurs optimally within a narrow and specific pH range, a property that may aid in virus identification. In general, serologic cross-relationships are most evident in hemagglutination-inhibition (HI) and binding assays, e.g., enzyme-linked immunosorbent assays (ELISAs) and immunofluorescent-antibody (IFA) tests, and occur to a lesser extent in complement fixation (CF) tests. These broad antigenic relationships can be refined in viral neutral-

TABLE 2 Taxonomic and physical characteristics of arboviruses and certain zoonotic viruses

Family: virus	No. of arboviruses causing human disease/no. of arboviruses recognized	Genome	No. of genomic segments	Virion size (nm)	Morphology
Togaviraidae: alphaviruses	16/31	Positive single-stranded RNA	1	60	Spherical, enveloped
Flaviviridae: flaviviruses	31/62	Positive single-stranded RNA	1	40–50	Spherical, pleomorphic, enveloped
Bunyaviridae: bunyaviruses, phleboviruses, nairoviruses, hantaviruses	71/263	Negative and ambisense single-stranded RNA	3	80–120	Spherical, pleomorphic, enveloped
Reoviridae: orbiviruses, coltiviruses	10/198	Double-stranded RNA	10/12	60–100	Spherical, nonenveloped
Rhabdoviridae: lyssaviruses, vesiculoviruses	10/38	Negative single-stranded RNA	1	60–85 by 180	Bullet shaped, enveloped
Arenaviridae: arenaviruses	6/16	Ambisense single-stranded RNA	2	50–300	Spherical, pleomorphic
Filoviridae: filoviruses	5/5	Negative single-stranded RNA	1	80 by 14,000	Tubular, filamentous
Orthomyxoviridae: Thogoto-like viruses	2/2	Negative single-stranded RNA	6/7	90–120	Pleomorphic, enveloped
Poxviridae: orthopoxviruses, yatapoxviruses, unassigned	3/30	Double-stranded DNA		200–400	Pleomorphic, enveloped
Others	4				

ization tests that differentiate individual viruses and even more specific subtype relationships through ratios of homologous and heterologous N-antibody titers. Genomic sequence divergence among strains of a single virus in separate geographic locations differentiates "viral topotypes," which apparently result from the isolation and evolutionary divergence of these strains in distinct ecologic niches. Topotypic differences for populations of JE, YF, dengue, West Nile, eastern equine encephalitis (EEE), Oropouche, Snowshoe hare, and LaCrosse viruses, among others, have been described, and such genetic changes have been linked to differences in clinical expression of infections with Sindbis, Venezuelan equine encephalomyelitis (VEE), Oropouche, and St. Louis encephalitis (StLE) viruses.

Most arboviruses can be cultivated in a variety of primary and continuous cell lines, including primary duck and chick embryo cells, primary hamster kidney cells, C6/36 *Aedes albopictus* and AP61 *Aedes pseudoscutellaris* mosquito cell lines, and Vero, LLC-MK_2, BHK-21, CER, SW13, and PK cell lines. The rapidity and pattern of cytopathic effects (CPEs) vary in each virus-cell system; e.g., primary duck and BHK-21 cells are rapidly destroyed by most arboviruses, and replication in monkey kidney cell lines is generally slower. AP61 and C6/36 cells exhibit nearly universal susceptibility to the arboviruses, including the dengue viruses, which grow comparatively poorly in continuous monkey kidney cell lines. The mosquito cell lines, generally incubated at 28°C, exhibit little or no CPE, and evidence of viral replication must be sought by immunofluorescence (IF) or other means. Some flaviviruses form cell syncytia in these lines. The majority of arboviruses are lethal for suckling (2- to 3-day-old) mice, which exhibit signs of illness, paralysis, and death within days to 2 weeks after intracerebral inoculation. Some field isolates exhibit virulence for mice only after adaptation through blind passage.

COLLECTION AND STORAGE OF SPECIMENS

Few primary diagnostic laboratories can justify arboviral isolation and identification as a service, and most laboratories should focus on the appropriate collection of specimens for referral to a reference laboratory. Most arboviruses produce a brief, low level of viremia in humans, and it is only by chance that a viral isolate can be recovered from blood in these instances. However, certain arboviruses, notably the viruses of dengue, YF, chikungunya, and VEE and of Ross River, Oropouche, and sandfly fevers, produce a sufficiently high level of viremia ($>10^{3.5}$/ml) and viremia of sufficient duration (ca. 5 to 7 days after the onset of fever) that humans serve as hosts for epidemic transmission. For YF, this represents the urban, *Aedes aegypti*-borne form of the disease. From the perspective of the clinical laboratory, these infections can be diagnosed by isolating virus from blood obtained during the acute phase of illness or by detecting genomic sequences by reverse transcriptase PCR (RT-PCR) (see below). For example, VEE viral titers in blood are maintained from $10^{3.8}$ to $10^{5.7}$ through at least the final 4 days of illness and virus can be recovered through the 8th day of illness (1). Viral isolates from the blood of patients with YF fever and O'nyong-nyong have been recovered up to the 6th day after onset. Viruses causing encephalitis usually can be recovered from blood only during the preneuroinvasive phase of illness, and then they are usually recovered only by chance (39). The virus of Colorado tick fever infects bone marrow erythrocytic precursors, leading to infection of the erythrocyte for its lifetime; virus can be recovered from blood obtained several weeks after clinical recovery, and infection has been transmitted through transfusion.

Viral isolates can be recovered by biopsy or at autopsy from the viscera of patients with acute YF, dengue hemorrhagic fever, or other viscerotropic arboviral infections and from brain or cerebrospinal fluid (CSF) of patients with central nervous system (CNS) infection. Brain samples should be taken from several areas, including the cortex, brain nuclei, cerebellum, and brain stem. Neurotropic arboviruses sometimes can be isolated from CSF obtained by lumbar puncture during the acute stages of encephalitis or aseptic meningitis. In the few clinical evaluations that have been published, RT-PCR has been variably sensitive in detecting arboviral genomic sequences in CSF (12, 37, 47). Alphaviruses rarely have been isolated from skin lesions, the joint fluids of patients with acute polyarthritis, and the upper respiratory tracts of 7 to 40% of patients with acute VEE. Under certain circumstances, arboviruses or their antigens have been detected in urine, milk, semen, and vitreous fluid. Clinical laboratories sometimes receive arthropods for viral isolation. These samples can be referred in the same manner as tissues to a reference laboratory, where they are ground, often in pools, for viral isolation or antigen detection.

A plan for dividing available tissues or fluids for viral isolation, electron microscopy, and assays for the direct detection of antigen and genomic sequences should be devised. Tissues should be collected aseptically and rapidly transported to the laboratory in viral transport medium or on a moist sponge. If the aliquot for viral isolation can be processed within 24 to 48 h, it can be maintained at 4°C; otherwise, the sample should be immediately frozen at −70°C in a mechanical freezer or stored on dry ice. Samples for virus isolation should be kept frozen continuously, avoiding freeze-thaw cycles, which inactivate virus. The aliquot for electron microscopy should be minced and placed directly in glutaraldehyde. Autolytic changes occur rapidly, and tissues should be fixed as quickly as possible. To prepare sections for immunohistochemical examination, a portion of the sample should be either fixed in buffered formalin or, preferably, embedded in freeze medium and frozen. Touch preparations are less reliable. Aliquots for antigen detection by other means and for PCR should be frozen at −70°C. Samples should be shipped by express mail in double, sealed containers following Interstate Commerce Commission (ICC) regulations. Frozen samples should be shipped separately on dry ice. International shipments may require import and/or customs permits and clearances.

Serologic studies are best done by comparing antibody titers in serum samples drawn during the first week of illness and 2 to 3 weeks later. A single serum specimen may be sufficient for the diagnosis of certain arboviral infections for which immunoglobulin M (IgM) assays are available. Detection of virus-specific IgM in CSF is a sensitive and highly specific approach to diagnosing CNS infection. Both CSF and serum samples should be tested. IgM capture ELISAs for the arboviral encephalitis transmitted in the United States are offered by several reference laboratories. Serum and CSF samples should be collected aseptically, stored either refrigerated or frozen, and transported according to ICC regulations. Freeze-thaw cycles may reduce antibody titers and should be avoided. Blood or serum blotted onto filter paper and dried may be suitable for some serologic assays.

No specific procedures for patient preparation are required. Ribavirin, chloroquine, rimantadine, amantadine, and other weak bases inhibit replication of some arboviruses and may interfere with their isolation. The isolation of certain arboviruses could be inhibited in patients treated with alpha or gamma interferon or other immunomodulators. Some preparations of gamma globulin, including preparations for intravenous use, may contain arboviral antibodies and could interfere with the isolation of arboviruses from patient specimens or with arboviral serologic procedures.

DIRECT EXAMINATION

Clinical application and experience with direct detection methods for arboviruses generally have been limited, and specimens should be evaluated in parallel by conventional viral isolation and serologic procedures. When tissue is available, direct examination by electron microscopy can rapidly provide evidence of an arboviral infection. Experienced observers can identify virions morphologically, often to the level of a viral family, in thin tissue sections. Visualization of togaviruses in brain tissue helped establish a diagnosis of EEE in some reported cases. Virions may be absent, however, from autopsy tissues of patients who died after a prolonged course of illness and from whom infection had previously been cleared.

Immunohistochemical staining of peripheral blood mononuclear cells or tissue sections has been successful in detecting arboviral antigens in CSF and brain specimens from encephalitis patients; in the viscera of patients with YF, dengue, and other viscerotropic infections; and in the joint fluids of patients with acute arthritis (11, 15, 17). Dengue virus, JE virus, and other flaviviruses infect and replicate in mononuclear cells, and their detection in the peripheral blood or CSF is a highly sensitive although somewhat laborious approach to rapid and specific diagnosis. In one study, IF detection of JE virus-infected mononuclear cells in CSF was only 58% sensitive, but the assay could be completed in 2 to 3 h, and in some cases, antigen-bearing cells were present before intrathecal antiviral antibodies were detectable (16). Infected peripheral mononuclear cells also have been observed in JE patients with recrudescent symptoms after their previous recovery from acute infection, indicating the possibility of latent infection and recurrent viremia (38, 42). Monoclonal antibodies specific to many medically important arboviruses are available, and for more obscure arboviruses, hyperimmune mouse antibodies can be used. Antibodies and information on their working dilutions can be obtained from the Centers for Disease Control and Prevention (CDC) and other reference laboratories. Although trypsinized, formalin-fixed tissues are suitable for examination by the IFA test, frozen sections are generally preferred because trypsinization procedures have not been standardized for all arboviruses and because success varies with the duration of formalin fixation. Viral RNA has been detected by in situ hybridization in archived formalin-fixed and paraffin-embedded tissues as well as in fresh tissues from patients with YF, dengue, hantaviral, and other hemorrhagic fevers (33).

Antigen capture ELISAs have been developed for several arboviruses; however, the formation of immune antibody-virus complexes in dengue and YF has interfered with the detection of viral antigens in viremic blood (30, 31). Although complexes can be chemically dissociated, the assays have not been shown to be clinically useful. The detection threshold of antigen capture ELISAs for StLE and JE viruses (ca. $10^{4.0}$ PFU/ml) has been sufficiently sensitive for their application in the epidemiologic surveillance of infected arthropod vectors (46).

Reverse transcription PCR procedures have been described for the detection of numerous arboviruses; however, few have been evaluated clinically (2, 10, 12, 18, 19, 25, 28, 36, 37, 41, 44, 47, 50). Thus far, PCR has found a more important role in viral identification than in direct detection from clinical specimens. Prospective PCR evaluation of clinical samples from suspected dengue patients obtained at their initial presentation was 95% sensitive and 95% specific, which is nearly equal to the sensitivity of viral isolation when the most sensitive techniques of mosquito and mosquito cell culture inoculation were used (21, 44, 50). However, the sensitivity of PCR for the diagnosis of Ross River fever was related inversely to the presence and level of virus-specific antibody: while 38% of samples with low or negative antibody titers were PCR positive, no samples with high antibody levels were positive (41). PCR amplification of viral genomic sequences in skin lesions proved to be more sensitive than viral isolation in the diagnosis of acute Ockelbo (Sindbis virus) infection (17). Although PCR analysis of CSF appears to be highly sensitive for the diagnosis of CNS infections due to herpesviruses, enteroviruses, and other neurotropic agents, clinical evaluations of PCR assays for the diagnosis of arboviral CNS infections have been limited. In the cases of tick-borne encephalitis (TBE) and JE, PCR seems less sensitive than IgM capture serology, but a nested PCR was 62% sensitive in identifying cases of Toscana encephalitis (12, 37, 47). Genomic sequences of California serogroup bunyaviruses (e.g., LaCrosse and Jamestown Canyon viruses) have been detected in CSF from isolated patients. A universally applicable set of PCR conditions for the amplification of arboviral cDNA has been proposed to facilitate specimen processing (26).

VIRAL ISOLATION

Many of the medically important arboviruses have caused infections in laboratory workers, occasionally in outbreaks. The pathogenesis of infections acquired from aerosols created by pipetting and other procedures may differ from that of natural infection, with the possibility of direct CNS invasion through the olfactory epithelium. On the basis of this experience, the joint CDC-National Institutes of Health (NIH) laboratory biosafety manual recommends biosafety level 2 to 4 containment facilities for laboratory work with arboviruses (9, 35). Arboviruses should be handled in certified laminar-flow hoods in rooms whose air is exhausted directly through HEPA filters and is not commingled with air from other laboratory areas (single-pass air). In addition, laboratory staff should be immunized with available arboviral vaccines. Laboratories that process CNS specimens from patients with encephalitis should consider immunizing staff with rabies vaccine as well.

Tissues, fluids, and serum collected in the acute phase of illness should be inoculated into cultures of several cell lines, including C6/36 or AP61 mosquito cells, a monkey kidney cell line such as Vero or LLC-MK_2, BHK-21 or CER cells, and, if available, primary duck embryo cells and 2- to 4-day-old suckling mice. Intrathoracic inoculation of uninfected *Toxorhynchites* mosquitoes is the most sensitive system for the isolation of dengue viruses. Ideally, serum specimens should be inoculated neat and in 10^{-1} and 10^{-2} dilutions to avoid the prozone effects due to viral autointerference and viral antibodies present in the specimen. Tissues should be ground with a mortar and pestle and diluted similarly on a weight-to-volume basis with a protein- and antibiotic-containing medium, e.g., phosphate-buffered saline with 0.75% bovine serum albumin and 1% gentamicin. After adsorption to the drained cell monolayer, cell cultures are fed with medium and are observed daily or more often for signs of a CPE. Small flasks (25 cm^2), tubes, or coverslips in shell vials may be used. Viral growth in C6/36 and AP61 cells does not reliably produce a CPE, and these cells must be examined for viral replication by the IFA test or other means. When medium from infected cultures is harvested for passage, fetal calf serum should be added to a final concentration of 20 to 40% before the medium is frozen at −70°C. The effect of spin amplification on the isolation of arboviruses has not been clinically evaluated.

Intracerebrally inoculated mice (one litter of six to eight mice for each dilution) should be observed twice daily for up to 2 weeks for signs of illness and death. Ill and dead mice should be frozen at −70°C until the infected organs can be passaged in cell culture. When a bunyaviral etiology is suspected, it is prudent to harvest livers as well, because certain bunyaviruses replicate to higher titers in mouse liver than in mouse brain.

VIRAL IDENTIFICATION

While the identification of viral isolates previously has depended on their antigenic characterization, increasingly PCR is used because the procedure is equally quick and, in conjunction with sequence analysis of the PCR product, can provide even more specific identification of the isolates than ELISA, IF, or other rapid immunologically based assays. PCR-based assays that amplify conserved sequences among medically important alphaviruses, bunyaviruses, or flaviviruses permit the assignment of an unknown virus within a broad taxon and, with sequence analysis of amplified products, their precise identification. Such omnibus primers have been reported for alpha- and flaviviruses and for certain groups of bunya- and reoviruses (10, 12, 25, 36). Moreover, sequence analysis rapidly can describe strain relationships of potential epidemiologic importance.

Viral isolates established in cell culture are most easily identified antigenically by immunohistochemical or IFA examination with a series of polyvalent (NIH grouping fluids) or broadly reactive monoclonal antibodies. The reactivity of an unknown virus with 1 of the 30 arboviral grouping fluids (produced in mice as hyperimmune ascitic fluids against four or more viruses) permits its broad placement within that group of viruses. The unknown is further identified by its reactivity against a panel of monovalent antibodies representing viruses in the group (Fig. 1). Alternatively, monoclonal antibodies reactive against antigens common to the flaviviruses, alphaviruses, or other taxonomic groups may be used. Often, however, IFA reactions among antibodies to related viruses overlap, and identification by cross-neutralization, the most specific means of serologic identification, is indicated.

Viral identification by cross-neutralization is best done if the unknown virus is first adapted to produce plaques in a cell culture system. Initially, a unidirectional plaque neutralization test is done with reference antisera to viruses most closely related to the unknown against their homologous viruses and the unknown (see below). The ratios of homologous and heterologous titers are examined (with fourfold differences defined as significant) to determine the relationship of the unknown to the other viruses. Definitive identification necessitates production of an immune serum against the unknown and bidirectional tests. Viruses that can be differentiated by fourfold differences in neutralization titer in both directions are considered distinct (homologous and heterologous titers of both antibodies differ by more than fourfold). Virus pairs that show a fourfold difference in one direction only (only one of the two antibodies differs

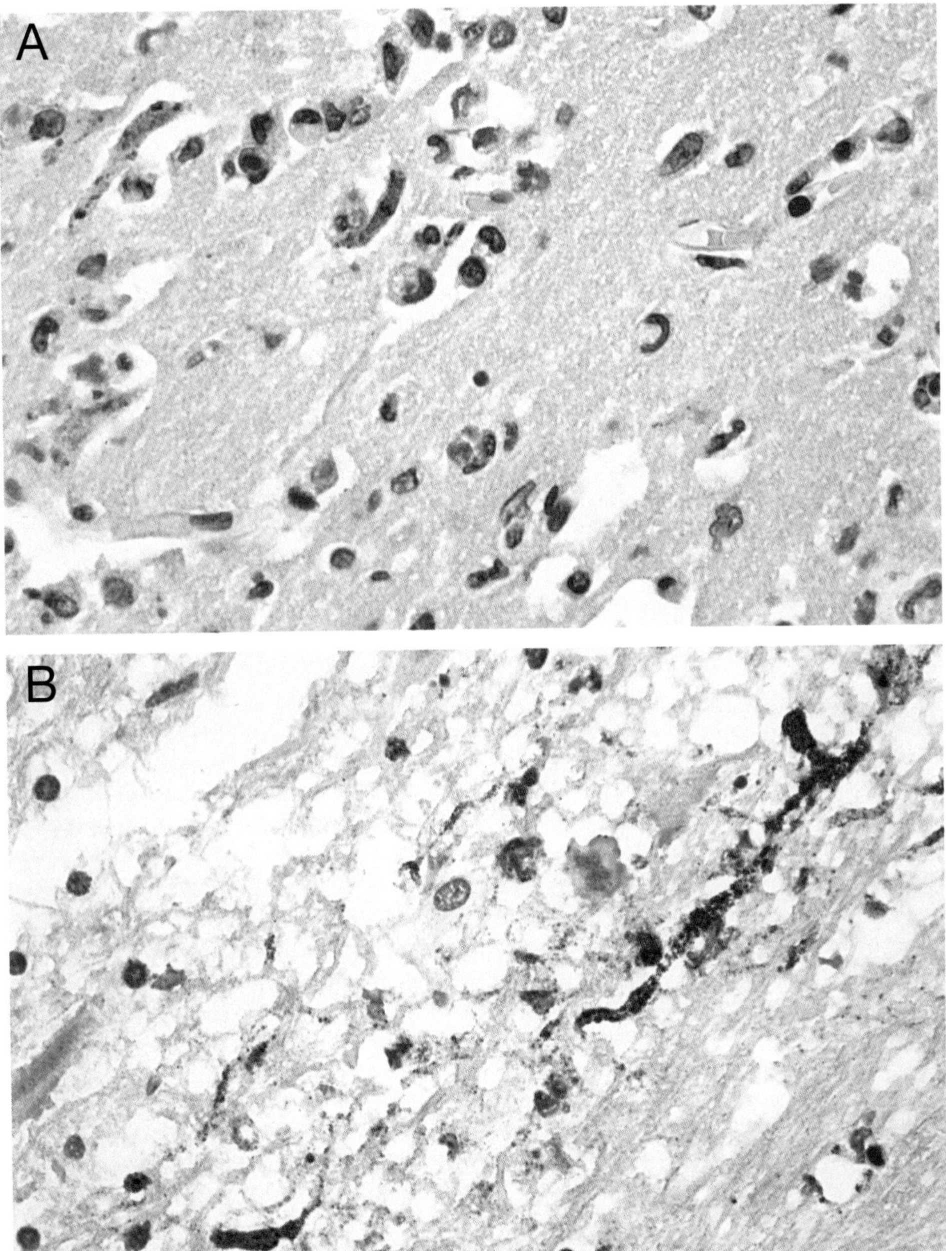

FIGURE 1 (A) Immunostained neurons in brain cortex of a fatal LaCrosse encephalitis case (immunoalkaline phosphatase staining; naphthol fast red substrate with light hematoxylin counterstain; original magnification, ×158) (W. J. Shieh, T. F. Tsai, C. E. Downs, and S. Zaki, unpublished data); (B) immunostaining in necrotic areas of brain cortex in a fatal case of eastern equine encephalomyelitis (immunoalkaline phosphatase staining; naphthol fast red substrate with light hematoxylin counterstain; original magnification, ×158) (W. J. Shieh, P. Greer, J. Guarner, and S. Zaki, unpublished data).

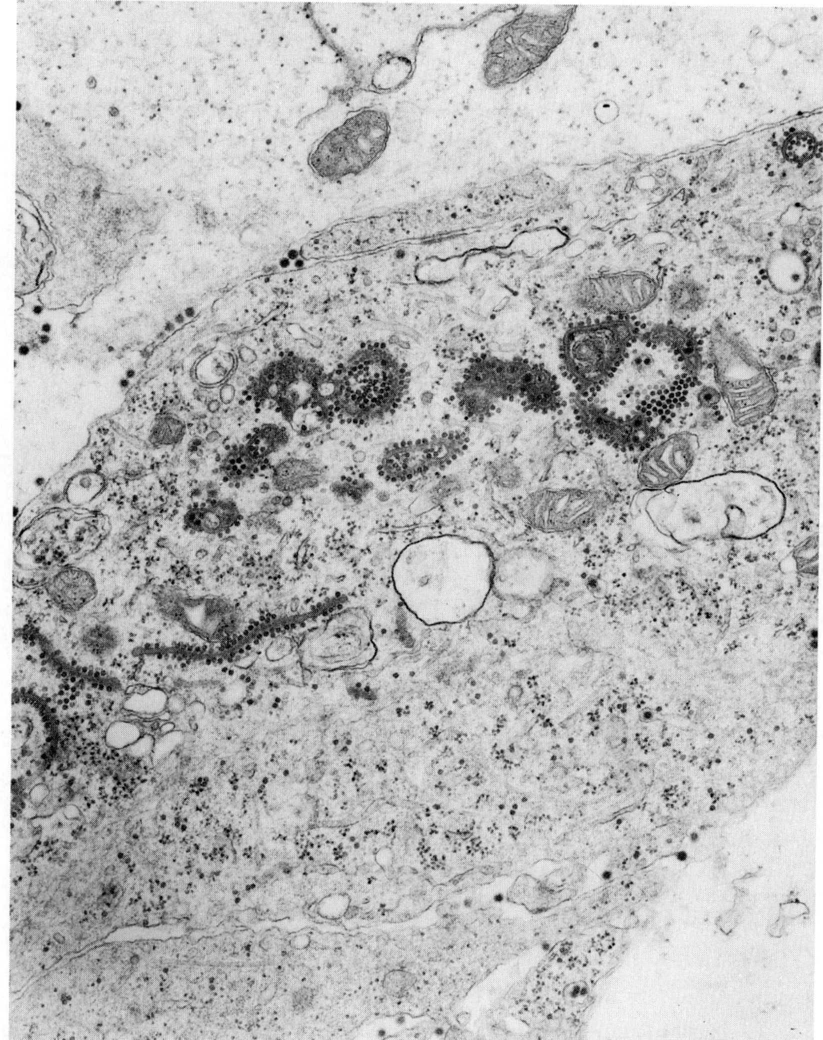

FIGURE 2 *Togaviridae*: alphavirus. EEE virus in mouse brain at 48 h postinfection. Viral nucleocapsids average 28 to 30 nm in diameter and lie within the cytoplasmic matrix and upon electron-dense membranous structures. Enveloped virions are seen passing through the plasma membrane and average 55 to 60 nm in diameter.

by more than fourfold in its homologous and heterologous neutralization titers) are considered subtypes of the same virus. The comparative reactivities of monoclonal antibodies against individual viruses in more convenient binding assays generally have confirmed or supported this classical approach.

When IFA screening with broadly reactive antibodies fails to place an unknown virus within a group of arboviruses, morphologic examination of the unknown by negative-stain electron microscopy can rapidly categorize the virus within a taxon. Virions generally can be found in cell culture medium or directly in clinical specimens that have infectivity titers of 10^6/ml. Although most pathology laboratories do not routinely prepare negatively stained grids, examination of thin sections of infected cell cultures can often be arranged. Cells or mouse brain infected with EEE (Fig. 2), StLE (Fig. 3), and LaCrosse (Fig. 4) viruses are shown in thin sections as examples of the morphologic appearance of an alphavirus, a flavivirus, and a bunyavirus, respectively.

SEROLOGY

In most circumstances, laboratory confirmation of arboviral infections still relies on serologic procedures. The classic serologic tests, HI and CF, have gradually been replaced in diagnostic laboratories by IgM capture ELISA. The former two still find use in reference laboratories for differentiating certain arboviral infections. Complete descriptions of arboviral serologic procedures are given in the *Manual of Clinical Laboratory Immunology* (45) and other sources (6).

ELISA

The antibody capture format for detecting IgM in serum or CSF is more sensitive and specific than indirect methods of IgM detection (3–7, 43, 47a). Among patients with dengue infections, virus-specific IgM can be detected in the sera of 90 to 95% of patients by the 6th day after the onset of illness (47a). Among patients with CNS infections due to flaviviruses, alphaviruses, or bunyaviruses, 40% of patients generally have detectable IgM in combinations of serum

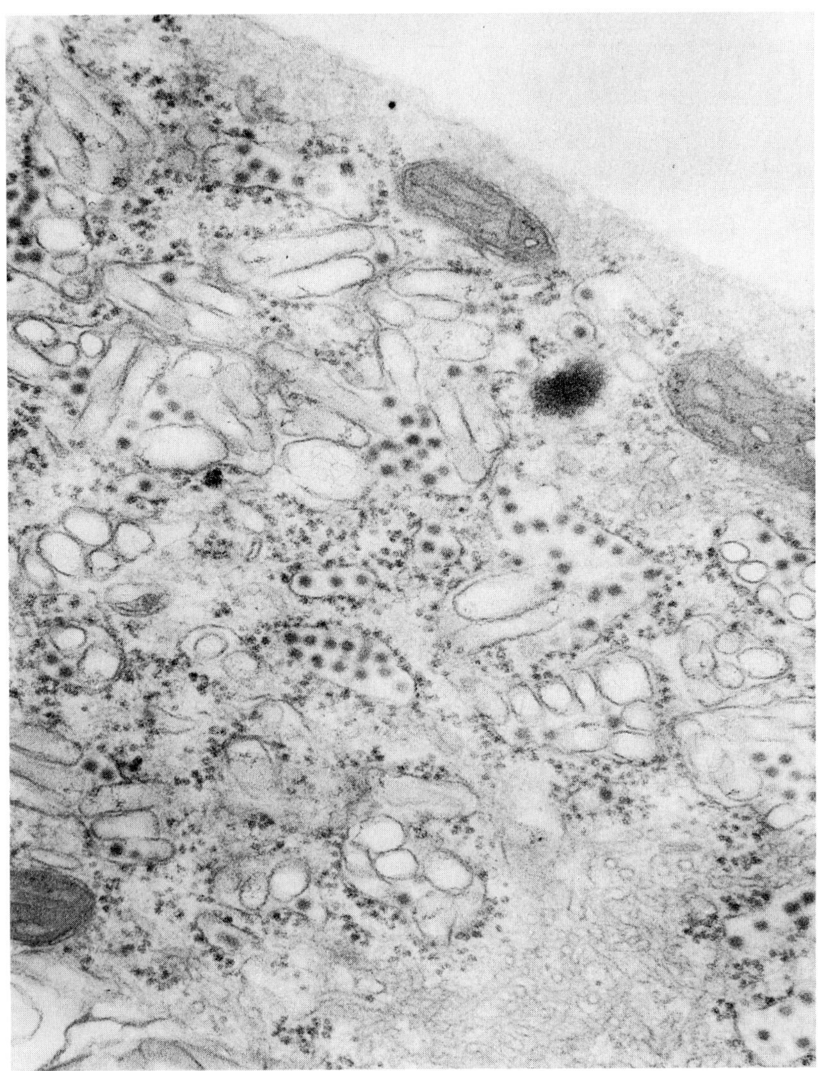

FIGURE 3 *Flaviviridae*: flavivirus. StLE virus-infected cell cultures. Enveloped viral particles accumulate within the cisternae of the endoplasmic reticulum. Cylindrical and round membranous structures are seen within the endoplasmic reticulum at the sites of viral accumulation.

and/or CSF by day 4 postonset and nearly all patients have detectable IgM by 10 days postonset (approximately 10% cumulative positivity with each postonset day) (3, 7). The presence of virus-specific IgM in CSF reflects intrathecal antibody production and is considered diagnostic of recent CNS infection. In serum, a declining level of virus-specific IgM can be detected for months and up to a year postonset in some patients, reducing the diagnostic specificity of the test (42). Therefore, a positive IgM result for a single serum sample is considered only presumptive evidence of recent infection. An analogous IgA capture ELISA for Ross River polyarthritis was shown to be better suited for the diagnosis of recent infection, because the level of virus-specific IgA declined more rapidly than that of IgM (8). Arboviral IgG antibodies are detected by an indirect sandwich method.

Heterologous reactions to antigenically related viruses are a vexing problem in areas where several related viruses cocirculate. Cross-reactions between dengue viruses and JE virus or between YF virus and the numerous flaviviruses that circulate in West Africa frequently produce overlapping values that may be uninterpretable. The specificity of IgM capture ELISA is somewhat better than that of HI, but further improvements have been sought by calculating ratios of absorbance to two or more antigens or by examining the areas under the absorbance curves over several serum dilutions (20).

Numerous schemes have been devised to define the threshold of a positive or significant ELISA absorbance value (20). Some laboratories define a positive reaction in multiples (units) of the absorbance of a weak positive specimen, an approach that controls plate-to-plate variations in specimen reactivity. An alternative approach is to define the threshold absorbance as a multiple (e.g., 5 standard deviations) above the mean absorbance of samples from a population of uninfected persons. A simple multiple of two times the absorbance of a negative control generally produces a conservative interpretation, exceeding 5 standard deviations above the mean for the samples with negative results.

Bedside membrane dot blot and immunochromato-

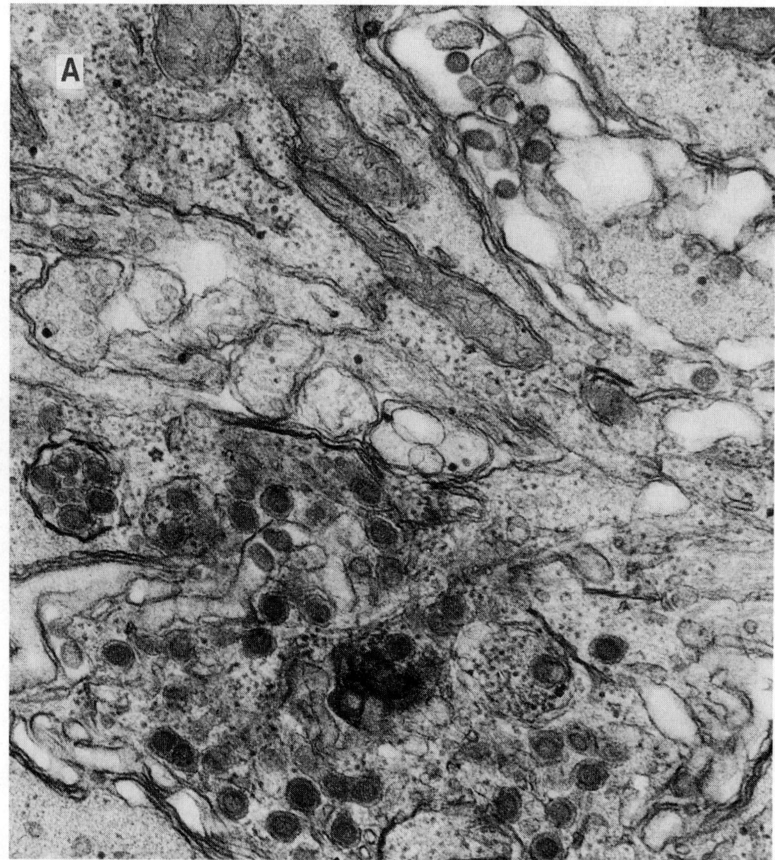

FIGURE 4 *Bunyaviridae*: bunyavirus. LaCrosse virus-infected mouse brain. (A) Virions are seen within cisternae of Golgi complex, endoplasmic reticulum, and vesicles of a neuron. Virus particles measure 90 to 105 nm in diameter.

graphic tests for the rapid diagnosis of dengue and JE exhibit adequate sensitivity, specificity, and simplicity that they can be used in primary care hospitals or outpatient facilities. Further clinical evaluations are needed, but such kits may bring the capacity for serologic diagnosis within the reach of a wider range of laboratories and medical care facilities in developed and developing countries (48).

HI

For the arboviruses that hemagglutinate erythrocytes, i.e., *Flaviviridae*, *Bunyaviridae*, alphaviruses, and certain *Rhabdoviridae*, the HI test is a convenient screening serologic procedure. HI antibody titers rise rapidly within the first week after the onset of illness and are long-lived, persisting at low levels for decades in some instances. These kinetics are consistent with the mixed IgM and IgG isotype distribution of HI antibodies. The use of gander erythrocytes is preferred, although chick and trypsinized human O erythrocytes have also been used. Inactivated sucrose-acetone extracts of infected mouse brains provide a high-titer source of antigen; for viruses that do not propagate to a high titer in mouse brain, infected-cell-culture antigens are used. For each virus, HA is optimal within a narrow pH range of less than half a pH unit. Before the HI test is performed, a preliminary HA test is completed in which the specific pH optimum and the antigen titer are determined.

Nonspecific inhibitors of HA present in some sera are removed preferably by acetone extraction. Serum samples are conventionally tested at 1:10 and at further twofold dilutions to the endpoint. Fourfold changes between acute- and convalescent-phase samples are diagnostic of recent infection; a titer of >1:80 may be interpreted as presumptive evidence of recent infection; a titer of >2,560 is evidence of a recent secondary antibody response to flaviviral infection.

The HI test is highly sensitive in confirming an infection when pairs of serum samples obtained at adequately timed intervals are available, but it is considerably less useful when applied to a single serum sample. Furthermore, HI antibodies tend to be broadly reactive, recognizing common epitopes within antigenic groups or complexes. Although a primary infection may lead to a specific antibody response, repeated infections with related viruses produce an increasing dominance of heterologous antibodies that yield undifferentiated elevated titers of antibodies to a variety of related viruses, rendering the HI test result uninterpretable.

The HI test is often used in epidemiologic surveys because of the broad reactivity and the longevity of HI antibodies and because the procedure is robust. Capillary blood samples collected on filter paper and dried can be stored for short periods without refrigeration, mailed, and tested after reconstitution. The procedure is not limited by species-specific reagents and can be used for wildlife and animal surveys, which are often a component of field studies.

Indirect Immunofluorescence

Some laboratories find indirect immunofluorescence to be a convenient procedure that also allows the differentiation

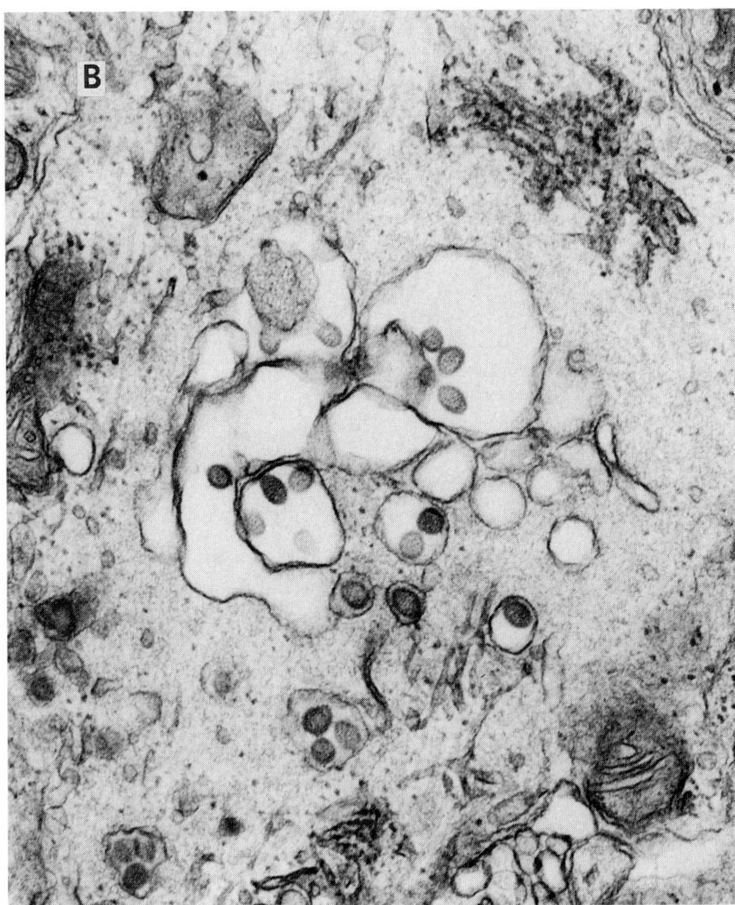

FIGURE 4 (*Continued*) (B) Virions budding into or accumulating in a Golgi complex.

of IgG and IgM responses. Infected cells fixed onto microscope slides with multiple wells are the usual antigen substrate. A multivalent slide with EEE, Western equine encephalitis, StLE, and LaCrosse virus-infected cells and uninfected control cells is commercially available. Positive and negative human control samples are also supplied when slides are purchased in kit form. Anti-human IgG and IgM fluorescein isothiocyanate conjugates are commercially available, but they should be titrated to ascertain their optimal working dilutions. To conserve antigen, serum samples (1:16 dilution) and CSF (neat) can be screened and then tested in further twofold dilutions to the endpoint only if positive. Positive IgM reactions should be verified as specific by ruling out the presence of rheumatoid factor (serum IgM antibodies directed against IgG).

Immunofluorescent IgM antibodies become detectable within a few days after the onset of illness, and IgG antibodies appear shortly thereafter. Immunofluorescent IgG antibodies are long-lived, paralleling the longevity of HI and neutralizing antibodies. Fourfold changes are diagnostic of recent infection, and in some circumstances, single or stable elevated titers (>1:128) may indicate recent infection. The sensitivity and specificity of the indirect fluorescent-antibody and HI tests are similar. Cross-reactions among the flaviviruses, e.g., between StLE and dengue viruses, occasionally present a problem in interpretation, usually for patients who had resided previously in Asia or Latin America.

CF Test

The CF test is moderately specific and is often used to narrow the definition of a heterologous HI antibody response. The half-life of CF antibodies is 2 to 3 years, and the test can be used as an imprecise measure of recent infection. Thus, some laboratories use the HI test to screen samples and the CF test to define the recency and specificity of infection. Some arboviruses, such as the Colorado tick fever virus and the orbiviruses, do not hemagglutinate erythrocytes, and the CF test is then used for primary diagnosis. Because the test is relatively insensitive, it should be used in combination with some other procedure. Fourfold changes are diagnostic of recent infection, and in some circumstances, a single or stable elevated titer of 1:32 may be accepted as presumptive evidence of recent infection.

CF antibody titers generally rise slowly after infection, often peaking as late as 6 weeks after the onset of illness. Convalescent-phase serum samples should be obtained 2 to 3 months after the onset of illness to ensure against missing a late-rising CF antibody response. Some individuals fail to produce detectable CF antibodies, and advanced age may be associated with a blunted, delayed, or undetectable response. In one study of mostly elderly StLE patients, a CF antibody response could not be detected in 20% of patients.

Neutralization

The neutralization test is the most specific of the common serologic procedures and is used principally to sort out the heterologous reactions observed in other assays. The presence of viral neutralizing antibodies is also considered the best evidence of protective immunity, and response to immunization is usually monitored by following neutralizing antibody levels. Neutralizing antibodies generally become detectable within the first week after the onset of illness, peak in the following 2 weeks, and decay slowly, persisting for years and often over a lifetime. Reexposures and infections with related viruses may stimulate an accelerated secondary response. Although the neutralizing antibody response is relatively specific, repeated infections with related viruses produce a progressively broader heterologous immune response, with the possible extension of cross-protection in some instances. Often, these extensive heterologous reactions cannot be resolved with cross-neutralization tests.

Infectious virus is used in the neutralization test; consequently, the procedure should be performed only in laboratories capable of working safely at the appropriate biosafety level. Neutralizing antibodies are best quantitated in a plaque reduction assay, in which dilutions of heat-inactivated serum are mixed with a fixed dose of virus and exogenous complement. The 50% endpoint is calculated by probit analysis, or the highest serum dilution inhibiting 80 to 90% of the infectious virus dose observed in virus control wells is accepted as the endpoint. Serum samples generally are diluted 1:5, and with the addition of an equal volume of virus, the initial test dilution is 1:10. Fourfold changes in titer are considered diagnostic of recent infection, and in some circumstances, a single or stable elevated titer (>1:80) can be interpreted as presumptive evidence of recent infection.

The neutralizing capacity of a serum sample can also be measured by testing a single dilution of the serum against a series of virus dilutions. The result is expressed as the serum's log neutralization index.

Other Procedures

As stated previously, heterologous serologic reactions in patients who have had repeated arboviral infections are difficult to sort out even after all available conventional tests have been exhausted. In one attempt to improve specificity, the narrow reactivity provided by viral monoclonal antibodies has been adapted to a serologic test by combining test sample and virus-specific monoclonal antibody in a competitive ELISA (4). Virus-specific antibodies present in the test sample block binding of the monoclonal antibody conjugate to viral antigen, thus reducing absorbance. Synthetic antigens, expressed as polyproteins that include areas of the envelope glycoprotein or that are produced by proteolytic cleavage, have provided some differentiation of flaviviral antibody responses in ELISAs, by immunohistochemical staining of expressed antigen on cell surfaces, or by Western blotting (immunoblotting). Although these techniques may be applicable to population surveys, their discriminatory powers for clinical diagnostic purposes require further confirmation.

EVALUATION AND INTERPRETATION OF TEST RESULTS

Unlike herpesviruses, adenoviruses, and other viruses that produce persistent or latent infections, nearly all human arboviral infections are acute and are terminated by viral clearance. Thus, the recovery of an arbovirus from an ill patient is virtually diagnostic. However, rare subacute, progressive, or recrudescent infections and experimental models of persistent infection have been reported for Russian spring-summer encephalitis, West Nile fever, and JE. One study found circulating JE virus-infected peripheral mononuclear cells in patients who had experienced a recrudescence of symptoms months after recovery, and in another study subacute CNS infection was suggested (38, 42). Many other arboviruses and related zoonotic viruses, e.g., hantaviruses and other *Bunyaviridae*, arenaviruses, *Rhabdoviridae*, and orbiviruses, also produce persistent infections of animals, but it is unknown whether infections with these and related viruses (other than rabies) can be established as persistent or latent infections in humans.

The effect of human immunodeficiency virus (HIV) infection and the resulting immunodeficiency on the clinical course of arboviral infections is unknown. In a series of StLE outbreaks, HIV-infected persons have been at higher risk for acquiring illness but have had no more serious a clinical illness or poorer outcome (29). Although AIDS in Africa and Asia is occurring in areas where numerous pathogenic arboviruses are also transmitted, no studies have reported on their occurrence as opportunistic infections.

Serologic results should be interpreted in view of the epidemiologic history of exposure and the immunization history of the patient. Vaccines for YF, JE, and TBE are commercially available in the United States or abroad; and experimental vaccines for Kayasunar Forest disease, Argentine hemorrhagic fever, hemorrhagic fever with renal syndrome, and Rift Valley fever may be accessible in some circumstances. A vaccination history should be sought, because evidence of immunization might mitigate against certain diagnoses and because vaccine-induced antibodies can interfere with the interpretation of serologic test results. The influence of HIV-associated immunosuppression on the serologic response to arboviral infections is unknown; however, results for immunosuppressed patients should be interpreted with caution. Some HIV-infected patients without clinical evidence of immunosuppression have responded normally to YF vaccine. Hepatitis C virus has recently been identified as a *Flaviviridae*; however, there are no serologic cross-reactions in either direction between hepatitis C virus (in a new-generation ELISA) and arthropod-borne flaviviruses.

REFERENCES

1. **Bowen, G. S., and C. H. Calisher.** 1977. Virological and serological studies in Venezuelan equine encephalomyelitis in humans. *J. Clin. Microbiol.* **4:**22–27.
2. **Brown, T. M., G. J. Chang, D. B. Cropp, K. E. Robbins, and T. F. Tsai.** 1994. Detection of yellow fever virus by polymerase chain reaction. *Clin. Diagn. Virol.* **2:**41–51.
3. **Burke, D. S., A. Nisalak, M. A. Ussery, T. Laorakpongse, and S. Chantavibul.** 1985. Kinetics of IgM and IgG responses to Japanese encephalitis virus in human serum and cerebrospinal fluid. *J. Infect. Dis.* **151:**1093–1099.
4. **Burke, D. S., A. Nisalak, and M. K. Gentry.** 1987. Detection of flavivirus antibodies in human serum by epitope blocking immunoassay. *J. Med. Virol.* **23:**165–173.
5. **Calisher, C. H., V. P. Berardi, D. J. Muth, and E. E. Buff.** 1986. Specificity of immunoglobulin M and G antibody responses in humans infected with eastern and western equine encephalitis viruses: application to rapid serodiagnosis. *J. Clin. Microbiol.* **23:**369–372.
6. **Calisher, C. H., B. J. Beaty, and R. E. Shope.** Arboviruses. *In* E. H. Lennette, D. A. Lennette, and E. T. Lennette (ed.), *Diagnostic Procedures for Viral, Rickettsial and Chlamydial*

ment, ranging from mild irritability and lethargy to abnormalities in gait, tremors of the upper extremities, and, in severely ill patients, coma, delirium, and convulsions, occurs in more than half the patients. During the second week of illness, clinical improvement may begin or complications may develop. Complications include extensive petechial hemorrhages, oozing from puncture wounds, melena, and hematemesis. These manifestations of capillary damage and thrombocytopenia do not result in life-threatening blood loss. However, hypotension and shock may develop, often in combination with serious neurologic signs, among the 15% of patients who die. Survivors begin to show improvement by the third week. Recovery is slow; weakness, fatigue, and mental difficulties may last for weeks, and a significant proportion of patients relapse with a "late neurologic syndrome," which includes headache, cerebellar tremor, and cranial nerve palsies. In contrast to Lassa fever, clinical laboratory studies are frequently useful. Total leukocyte counts usually fall to 1,000 to 2,000 cells/mm^3, although the differential remains normal. Platelet counts fall precipitously, usually to 25,000 to 100,000/mm^3 and occasionally lower. Routine clotting parameters are usually normal or slightly deranged, but patients with severe cases show evidence of disseminated intravascular coagulation.

Marburg and Ebola virus infections are clinically similar, although the frequencies of reported signs and symptoms vary. Following incubation periods of 4 to 16 days, onset is sudden and is marked by fever, chills, headache, anorexia, and myalgia. These signs are soon followed by nausea, vomiting, sore throat, abdominal pain, and diarrhea. When first examined, patients are usually overtly ill, dehydrated, apathetic, and disoriented. Pharyngeal and conjunctival injection are usual. Within several days, a characteristic maculopapular rash over the trunk, petechiae, and mucous membrane hemorrhages appears. Gastrointestinal bleeding, accompanied by intense epigastric pain, is common, as are petechiae and bleeding from puncture wounds and mucous membranes. Shock develops shortly before death, often 6 to 16 days after the onset of illness. Abnormalities in coagulation parameters include fibrin split products and prolonged prothrombin and partial thromboplastin times, suggesting that disseminated intravascular coagulation is a terminal event. Clinical laboratory studies usually reveal profound leukopenia early, followed by a rapid rise in association with secondary bacteremia. Platelet counts decline to 50,000 to 100,000/mm^3 during the hemorrhagic phase.

DESCRIPTION OF THE AGENTS

Arenaviridae

The family *Arenaviridae* comprises 19 named viruses which share unique morphologic and physiochemical characteristics. Antigenic relationships are established mainly on the basis of broadly reactive antibody binding assays, historically the complement fixation (CF) test (6) and more recently the indirect fluorescent-antibody (IFA) test (59) and the enzyme-linked immunosorbent assay (ELISA). Both serologic and phylogenetic analyses of viral RNA divide the arenaviruses into two complexes. The LCM or Old World complex includes LCM virus and the Lassa viruses, including a number of apparently benign Lassa-like strains from Mozambique, Zimbabwe, and the Central African Republic. On the basis of RNA sequence homologies, these are unique viruses rather than substrains of Lassa virus. All have been isolated from rodents of the family *Muridae*. The Tacaribe or New World complex includes Tacaribe, Junin, Machupo, Amapari, Parana, Latino, Pichinde, Tamiami, Flexal, Guanarito, Sabia, Oliveros, Whitewater Arroyo, and Pirital viruses. All New World complex viruses have been isolated from rodents of the family *Cricetidae* or, for Tacaribe virus, from bats. The Old and New World complexes are distantly related; only when very high-titer antisera are used can cross-reactions be observed in binding assays. Monoclonal antibodies with specificities for structural proteins of arenaviruses suggest that the N protein is the group-reactive determinant whereas the envelope glycoproteins (G1 and G2) are responsible for type specificity (3, 4).

The morphology of arenaviruses is distinctive in thin-section electron microscopy (42) and was the basis for first associating LCM virus with Machupo virus and ultimately associating these viruses with all the viruses in the present family. Individual virions are pleomorphic and range in size from 60 to 280 nm (mean, 110 to 130 nm). A unit membrane envelops the structure and is covered with club-shaped, 10-nm projections. No symmetry has been discerned. The most prominent and distinctive feature of these virions is the presence of different numbers of electron-dense particles (usually 2 to 10), which may be connected by fine filaments. These particles, 20 to 25 nm in diameter, are identical to host cell ribosomes by biochemical and oligonucleotide analysis. Three major virion structural proteins are usually found (4). Two are glycosylated, G1 (50,000 to 72,000 Da) and G2 (31,000 to 41,000 Da), which constitute the virion envelope and spikes and which both serve as highly type-specific neutralization targets. The third, the N protein (63,000 to 72,000 Da), is clearly associated with the virion RNA and is considered the nucleocapsid protein. The N protein in intact cells or virions is not accessible to antibody but can readily be detected in acetone-fixed cells by immunofluorescence. Nucleocapsids can be isolated by treatment of intact virions with detergent. Liberated nucleocapsids are 10 nm in diameter and range to 450 nm long. Two size classes of closed or circular nucleocapsid have been identified, 640 and 1,300 nm in diameter. Small, 3- to 4-nm-diameter beaded strands can also be resolved. Some arenaviruses elaborate a soluble protein, antigenically related to the N protein, into supernatant fluids of infected cell cultures. The group-reactive arenavirus antigen measured in the CF and IFA tests and ELISA is associated with the nucleocapsid N protein. No hemagglutinins have been found.

Four RNA species with distinct oligonucleotide fingerprints can be isolated from intact arenavirus virions. Two species are virus specific: the small (S) RNA (22S), which codes for N and GPC, the precursor of G1 and G2, and the large (L) RNA (31S), which codes for the viral polymerase and the Z protein, a putative regulatory element (5). The 28S and 18S species, isolated in different proportions depending on external conditions, are ribosomal.

Arenaviruses mature by budding at the cytoplasmic membrane, and host proteins are incorporated into the virion envelope. Vero cells infected with each of the viruses contain distinctive intracytoplasmic inclusion bodies. Immunohistochemistry with monoclonal antibodies shows that these intracytoplasmic inclusions are immunoreactive with anti-N but not anti-G1 or anti-G2 antibody. All arenaviruses are readily inactivated by ethyl ether, chloroform, sodium deoxycholate, and acidic media (pH less than 5). β-Propiolactone (55) and gamma irradiation (14) are both reported to inactivate arenavirus infectivity while preserving reactivity in standard serologic tests.

Filoviridae

The filoviruses, Marburg virus and Ebola virus, have a common morphology and similar genomic organization and complement of structural proteins (30). Marburg and Ebola virus virion RNA is nonsegmented, negative, and single-stranded (NNS RNA), 19.1 kb, long, and 4.0 × 10^6 to 4.5 × 10^6 Da. The viral genomes are linearly arranged in a manner consistent with other NNS-RNA viruses. A substantial degree of similarity to the paramyxoviruses, especially in the nucleocapsid and polymerase genes, was noted. However, comparison with other filovirus protein sequences confirms that filoviruses are distinct. Furthermore, filoviruses are sufficiently distinct by ultrastructural and serologic criteria to warrant separate taxonomic status as members of the family *Filoviridae* (23, 31).

The viral particles are very large, typically 790 to 970 nm long and consistently 80 nm in diameter. Bizarre structures of widely different lengths, sometimes exceeding 14,000 nm, as well as branching, circular, or "6" shapes, probably resulting from coenvelopment of multiple nucleocapsids during budding, are frequently found in negatively stained preparations (Fig. 1) (15, 41).

Marburg and Ebola viruses have at least seven virus-specific structural proteins, expressed from seven genes (23). For Ebola virus, the ribonucleoprotein complex contains L (180 kDa), N (104 kDa), VP30 (30 kDa), and VP35 (35 kDa) in loose association. L is an RNA-dependent RNA polymerase, and VP35 may play a role similar to the P protein of paramyxoviruses and rhabdoviruses. GP (125 kDa) is the major spike protein; VP40 (a matrix protein) plus VP24 make up the remaining protein content of the multilayered envelope (31, 49). The GP of Ebola virus and that of Marburg virus can be differentiated by the presence or absence of N- and O-linked glycans. When grown in Vero or MA-104 cells, GP of Marburg virus is totally devoid of terminal sialic acid whereas that of Ebola virus has abundant (2-3)-linked sialic acid. A region of the GP of both viruses has a high degree of homology to the immunosuppressive protein of oncogenic retroviruses. Phylogenetic analysis of GP genes from filoviruses clearly separates Marburg and Ebola viruses and, furthermore, defines two distinct lineages for Marburg virus (51) and four Ebola-virus subtypes (52).

Despite their unusual morphologic properties, Marburg and Ebola viruses resemble the arenaviruses and other lipid-enveloped viruses in being susceptible to lipid solvents, β-propiolactone (55), formaldehyde, UV light, and gamma radiation (14). These viruses are stable at room temperature for several hours but are inactivated by incubation at 60°C for 1 h.

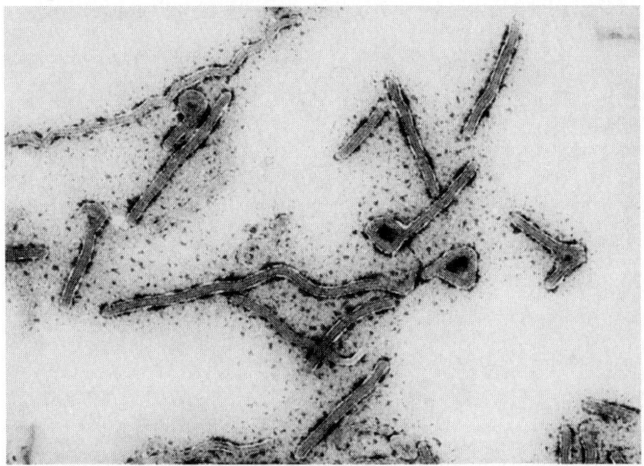

FIGURE 1 Electron micrograph of Ebola virus (Reston strain). Filamentous particles, 80 nm in diameter with 50-nm cores and different lengths, some >10,000 nm, are evident. Negative strain (sodium phosphotungstate) of supernatant fluids from MA-104 cells. Magnification, ×15,787. (Courtesy of T. W. Geisbert.)

COLLECTION AND STORAGE OF SPECIMENS

For virus isolation, serum, heparinized plasma, or, less ideally, whole blood should be collected during the acute, febrile stages of illness and frozen on dry ice or in liquid nitrogen vapor. Throat wash and urine specimens should also be collected and mixed with an equal volume of buffered diluent containing serum proteins to stabilize viral infectivity prior to freezing. Storage at higher temperatures (above −40°C) will lead to rapid losses in infectivity. Lassa virus is successfully obtained from most acute-phase serum samples and throat washings obtained within several weeks of onset; it is isolated less frequently from urine. Junin virus is usually recoverable from serum for a period of 3 to 10 days after onset and from throat washings for a similar period, but it is rarely recovered from urine. Machupo virus is recovered from only one in five acute-phase serum samples and even less frequently from throat washings or urine. LCM virus may be recovered from acute-phase serum samples obtained during the first week after onset, but it is rarely, if ever, recovered from throat washings or urine specimens. LCM virus may also be isolated from cerebrospinal fluid during the period of meningeal involvement and from the brain at autopsy. Marburg and Ebola viruses are usually recovered from acute-phase serum samples; various specimens including throat washings, urine, soft tissue effusates, semen, and anterior eye fluid have yielded these viruses, even when the specimens were obtained late in convalescence. Lassa, Machupo, Junin, Marburg, and Ebola viruses are all readily isolated from the spleen, lymph nodes, liver, and kidney obtained at autopsy, but rarely, if ever, from brain or other central nervous system tissues. Notably, Lassa virus is usually isolated from the placentas of infected pregnant women. Specimens collected for viral isolation are also suitable for testing by antigen capture ELISA; maintenance at −20°C for periods up to several weeks is adequate for antigen preservation. Impression smears of infected tissues, prepared as described in the next section, may be fixed by immersion in cold acetone and stored frozen for viral antigen staining by the IFA test. Formaldehyde-fixed tissues and paraffin-embedded blocks are also suitable for immunohistochemical identification of viral antigens.

Blood obtained in early convalescence for serodiagnosis may be infectious despite the presence of antibodies, and it should be handled accordingly (8–10). Maintenance of samples at −20°C or below is sufficient to preserve antibody titers and antigenicity, but lower temperatures are required to preserve infectivity. Certain anticoagulants should be avoided: citrate interferes with the IFA test, both citrate and oxalate cause nonspecific cytopathic effects in Vero and MA-104 cells used for virus isolation, and EDTA can interfere with some ELISA techniques. Heparinized plasma or serum samples are best.

Manipulation of these specimens and tissues, including sera obtained from convalescent patients, may pose a serious biohazard and should be minimized outside a maximum-containment laboratory. Current recommendations in the United States are that such samples be manipulated only at the BSL-4 containment level (8–10). At a minimum, barrier nursing procedures should be implemented and personnel caring for the patient and handling diagnostic specimens should wear disposable caps, gowns, shoe covers, surgical gloves, and face masks (preferably full-face respirators equipped with high-efficiency particulate air [HEPA] filters) (9). Gloves should be disinfected immediately if they come in direct contact with infected blood or secretions. All disposable and reusable equipment should be placed directly in a suitable disinfectant solution, such as sodium hypochlorite, phenolic detergent, or a solution of quaternary ammonium compounds. Reusable equipment can then be sterilized. Glass equipment (e.g., microscope slides, microhematocrit tubes, syringes) poses a significant hazard also; substitutes should be found for all glass equipment, with the exception of Vacutainer tubes for blood collection. Use of Vacutainer tubes is considered safer than use of syringes and needles, which must be disassembled before their contents are transferred to another tube. Procedures which generate aerosols (e.g., trituration and centrifugation) should be minimized and performed only if additional protective equipment, such as a flexible plastic film isolator capable of maintaining negative pressure and HEPA-filtered exhaust, is available. For specialized procedures, the infectivity of samples may be greatly reduced, if not totally inactivated, by the addition of Triton X-100, and may be safely tested by serologic or antigen capture assays in the field. Heating to 60°C for 1 h will render diagnostic specimens noninfectious and is acceptable for measurement of heat-stable substances such as electrolytes, blood urea nitrogen, and creatinine. When the equipment is available, sterilization by ^{60}Co γ-irradiation is the preferred method. Extraction of RNA from infectious samples by using guanidinium thiocyanate should be conducted in a laminar-flow hood.

For all testing of infectious material, samples should be packaged in accordance with current recommendations (7) and forwarded, after consultation, to one of the following laboratories that maintain BSL-4 facilities and a diagnostic capability for these agents:

1. Centers for Disease Control and Prevention
   Special Pathogens Branch
   Division of Viral and Rickettsial Diseases
   Center for Infectious Diseases
   Atlanta, GA 30333
   Phone: (404) 639-1115. Fax: (404) 639-1118
2. U.S. Army Medical Research Institute of Infectious Diseases
   Headquarters, Fort Detrick
   Frederick, MD 21702-5011
   Phone: (301) 619-2833. Fax: (301) 610-4625
3. Center for Applied Microbiology and Research
   Special Pathogens Unit
   Salisbury
   Porton Down, Wiltshire SP4 OJG
   England
   Phone: 0980-610391. Fax: 0980-611093
4. National Institute for Virology
   Private Bag X4
   Sandringham,
   Johannesburg,
   South Africa
   Phone: 27-11-882-9910. Fax: 27-11-882-0596

DIRECT EXAMINATION

Electron Microscopy

Marburg and Ebola viruses have been successfully visualized directly by electron microscopy of both heparinized blood and urine obtained during the febrile period as well as of tissue culture supernatant fluids. These materials are processed by immediate fixation with 0.5% glutaraldehyde followed by low-speed centrifugation. Virions are then sedimented at 12,000 × *g* for 15 min, resuspended in 1/100 of the original sample volumes, and placed on Formvar-carbon coated electron microscopy grids, which are then negatively stained with 1% phosphotungstic acid for 30 s and examined. The combination of the size and shape of the virions is sufficiently characteristic to allow a morphologic diagnosis of filovirus (15, 41), even when the isolate is a new entity, such as EBO-R (24). These virions are differentiated and identified as Marburg or Ebola virus by immunoelectron microscopy techniques (16–18) (Fig. 2). These immunoelectron microscopy techniques also work well for diagnosis of arenavirus infections, although the morphology of the virions is less striking. Retrospective examination of ultrathin sections of formalin-fixed tissues obtained from patients at autopsy have occasionally revealed typical Marburg or Ebola virus or arenavirus particles (17). EBO-R particles can also be identified in inoculated culture cells (Fig. 3).

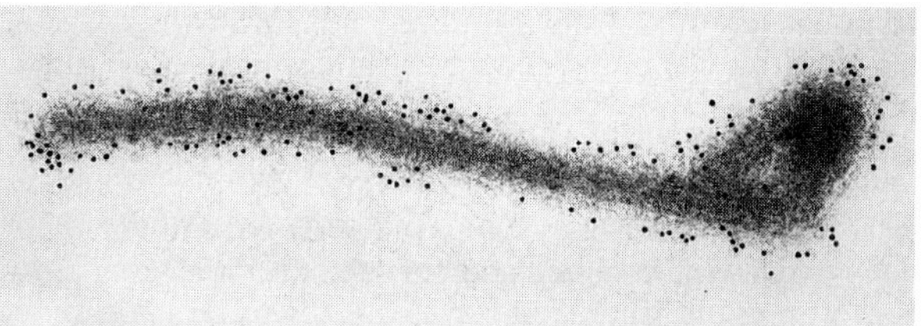

FIGURE 2 Immunoelectron microscopic staining of Ebola virus (Reston strain) when incubated with polyclonal guinea pig anti-Ebola serum followed by anti-guinea pig IgG labelled with gold spheres. Magnification, ×58,310. (Courtesy of T. W. Geisbert.)

Immunohistochemistry

Direct immunofluorescent-antibody (DFA) and IFA staining of impression smears or air-dried suspensions of the liver, spleen, or kidney have been used successfully to detect cytoplasmic inclusion bodies associated with Marburg virus in-

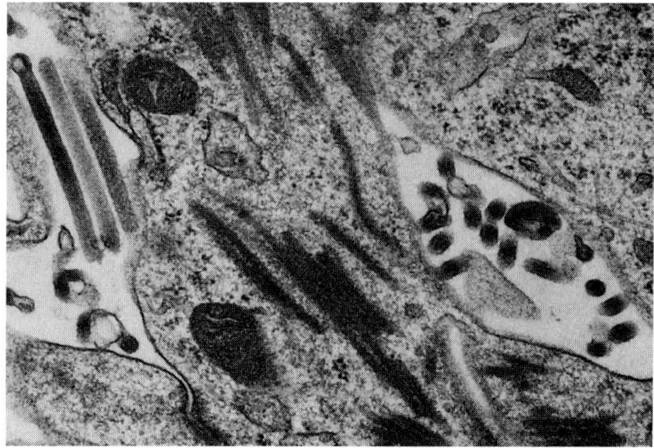

FIGURE 3 Thin section of infected MA-104 cells, showing Ebola virus virions budding into intracytoplasmic vacuoles in longitudinal and cross section and intracytoplasmic inclusions formed by nucleocapsids. Magnification, ×26,730. (Courtesy of T. W. Geisbert.)

fection; clumps of Marburg virus antigen have also been observed by DFA examination of infected, dried, citrated blood smears. This approach was successfully adapted to the diagnosis of EBO-R in impression smears from blood, tissues, and nasal turbinates, as it was to the detection of Junin virus-infected cells in peripheral blood and urinary sediment. The development of immunohistochemical techniques for detection of filovirus and arenavirus antigens in formalin-fixed tissues has recently advanced to the point that their results are far more satisfactory than those of IFA examination of frozen, acetone-fixed sections (11, 12, 22). Obtaining frozen sections for diagnosis is rarely worth the biohazard incurred, especially since the threshold sensitivity for detection exceeds 6 $\log_{10}$ PFU per g. For filoviruses, paraffin blocks of tissues are sectioned and mounted on silane-coated slides. They are deparaffinized, hydrated, digested with protease, and stained for the presence of viral antigens with cocktails of murine monoclonal antibodies (22, 24). Biotinylated horse anti-mouse antiserum is then reacted, and the product is developed with a streptavidin-alkaline phosphatase system. Substitution of other chromogens can further increase sensitivity while reducing background (11). Recently, remarkable success was reported in the application of immunohistochemistry to demonstration of Ebola virus antigens in formalin-fixed skin biopsy specimens obtained from Ebola virus patients in Zaire (60).

Genome Detection

Experimental systems for in situ nucleic acid hybridization of VHF genomes have been developed, especially for LCM (53) and Ebola (56) viruses. These methods may eventually find application in the clinical setting but not as primary diagnostic tools. For Ebola virus (56), plasmids for sequences in viral NP, GP, VP30, and VP35 were used. Tissue sections from experimentally infected animals were deparaffinized, rinsed in ethanol, and sequentially treated with protease buffer, washed, rinsed, and air dried. Riboprobes, diluted to 1 μg/ml in hybridization buffer, were heated to 65°C for 10 min, 50 μl was applied to each section, and the samples were incubated at 50°C for 3 h. Slides were washed with 2× SSC (1× SSC is 0.15 M NaCl plus 0.015 M sodium citrate), blocked with 5% normal sheep serum, and incubated with polyclonal sheep anti-digoxigenin Fab fragments conjugated to alkaline phosphatase. Following overnight storage at 40°C, the chromogenic substrate nitroblue tetrazolium (NBT) and 5-bromo-4-chloro-3-indolyl phosphate (BCIP) were added. The slides were washed and counterstained with Nuclear Fast Red. This procedure is now being adapted to detect genomes of Lassa virus and has shown success, but it has not yet been field tested.

In contrast, reverse transcriptase PCR (RT-PCR) assay has become a very useful tool for the rapid, definitive diagnosis of most VHF infections. By using RT-PCR, Ebola virus genome was detected in 12 of the first 14 blood samples obtained from the 1995 outbreak in Zaire within hours of arrival in the laboratory (45, 60). Within several days, sequences were available for the PCR products, confirming the identity of the agent as the EBO-Z strain. PCR also facilitated the diagnosis of Ebola virus in EBO-R outbreaks in quarantined primates in 1989, 1992, and 1996 (48). Protocols which maximize detection are usually based on conserved sequences, such as the L gene or N, while discrimination and phylogeny are based on the more variable GP region. The sensitivity of RT-PCR for Ebola virus strains approaches that of conventional isolation. However, it must be remembered that the volume of clinical sample which is actually tested in the PCR well is quite small, usually 2 μl; therefore, the concentration of infectious virions in the clinical material must exceed 500/ml to ensure a positive PCR signal. The role of early antibodies as potential inhibitors of RT-PCR versus conventional isolation are unknown.

RT-PCR has also been evaluated in a small series of serum samples from Lassa fever patients in West Africa (54). The sensitivity of PCR relative to conventional viral isolation was 0.82, and the specificity was 0.68. PCR was positive for more of the disease course than was isolation, perhaps because of its greater sensitivity in the presence of the early antibodies associated with acute Lassa fever. These results predict good success for the detection of Lassa virus in tissue samples obtained at autopsy, but this has never been field tested. Likewise, various strategies for RT-PCR have been devised to detect Junin virus RNA in clinical materials (38, 39). Some of these are reputed to be far more sensitive than conventional isolation procedures, especially in the presence of antibody. Any method which promises to be a reliable substitute for procedures which entail manipulation of infectious BL-4 virus deserves attention.

ISOLATION OF VIRUS

The best general method currently available for isolation of Marburg and Ebola viruses and the pathogenic arenaviruses is the inoculation of appropriate cell cultures (usually Vero cells) followed by IFA or other immunologically specific testing of the inoculated cells for the presence of viral antigens at intervals. Especially for EBO-R and EBO-S, MA-104 cells (a fetal rhesus monkey kidney cell line) are more sensitive than Vero cells. Supernatant fluids should be collected for backtitration and confirmatory testing, as detailed below. Primary isolations in cell cultures have been routinely used for years to obtain Lassa, Machupo, Junin, and Marburg viruses and EBO-Z from field-collected materials. Vero cell inoculation should also work for LCM virus, but intracranial (i.c.) inoculation of weanling mice is still regarded as the most sensitive established indicator of LCM virus (21). EBO-S has also been isolated by Vero cell inoculation, but less reliably, since several blind passages are usually required; SW-13 and MA-104 cells are more sensitive. Other cell lines, including human diploid lung (MRC-5) and BHK-21 cells, also work. Although historically Machupo and Junin viruses were isolated by i.c. inoculation of newborn hamsters and mice, respectively, Vero cells are approximately as sensitive and are far less cumbersome to manage in BL-4 containment. Furthermore, Vero cells permit isolation and identification, usually within 1 to 5 days, a significant advantage over the use of animals, since 7 to 20 days of incubation is required for illness to develop in the animals.

Clinical specimens and clarified tissue homogenates (usually 10% [wt/vol]) are diluted in a suitable maintenance medium, such as Eagle's minimal essential medium with Earle's salts and 2% heat-inactivated calf serum, and adsorbed in small volumes to cell monolayers grown in suitable vessels, such as tissue culture T-25 flasks or 60-mm petri dishes. It is important to test higher dilutions of these specimens as well as more concentrated material, since autointerference (probably from defective interfering particles present in lower dilutions) may totally inhibit viral replication as measured by the IFA test, ELISA, or plaque formation at lower dilutions. Following adsorption, sufficient maintenance medium is added to maintain the cells for 7 days. Inoculation of replicate vessels permits destructive testing of cells at frequent intervals. Cells inoculated with high-titer samples contain antigen within 1 to 2 days of inoculation, whereas cells inoculated with low-titer material may require up to 7 days to accumulate detectable antigen. If no antigen is detected by 7 days, the sample is considered negative, but supernatant fluids should be blind-passaged to confirm the absence of virus. When EBO-S is suspected, the requirement for blind passage is anticipated and supernatant fluids are harvested and passed at 3- to 5-day intervals; cells are usually stained in "real time" to accelerate the identification process. To confirm the presence and identity of the virus, supernatant fluids are tested for evidence of viral replication by plaque formation or by antigen capture ELISA or RT-PCR techniques. Cocultivation of Hypaque-Ficoll-separated peripheral blood leukocytes with susceptible cells has increased the isolation frequency of Junin virus. Cocultivation of lymphocytes from spleens of experimentally infected animals has yielded Lassa virus late in convalescence, even after neutralizing antibody has appeared. The technique merits systematic development for the remaining arenavirus and filovirus pathogens.

Although adequate cell culture systems exist for the isolation of LCM virus, most isolations to date have been obtained in mice. Weanling mice, 3 to 4 weeks old, are inoculated i.c. with undiluted samples. Care must be taken to use mice from a colony known to be free of LCM virus. Since the "high-dose" phenomenon of viral interference is occasionally a problem, a dilution of each sample (perhaps 1:100) is usually also inoculated into a second group of mice. Many LCM virus isolates produce a characteristic convulsive disease within 5 to 7 days, which is nearly pathognomonic. Brains from dead mice may be used to prepare CF or ELISA antigens or may be subjected to IFA staining to obtain presumptive identification. Clarified mouse brain may also be used as antigen for confirmatory testing by neutralization or RT-PCR.

Animal inoculations are recommended for primary isolation of the other arenaviruses and for Marburg and Ebola viruses only when cell cultures are not available and when adequate biocontainment facilities exist to maintain the animals. Newborn mice (1 to 3 days old) are highly susceptible to Junin virus inoculated i.c.; newborn hamsters are believed to be more sensitive to Machupo virus. For the SAHF viruses, particularly Junin virus, young adult guinea pigs inoculated either i.c. or peripherally have been used. Guinea pigs die 7 to 18 days after Junin virus inoculation. Most LCM virus strains are also lethal for guinea pigs. Strain 13 guinea pigs are exquisitely sensitive to most Lassa virus strains and uniformly die 12 to 18 days after inoculation; outbred Hartley strain guinea pigs are somewhat less susceptible. The pathogenicity of virulent Lassa virus strains for outbred Swiss albino mice inoculated i.c. seems to vary with different sources; mice should not be seriously considered for Lassa virus isolations. Marburg virus and the EBO-Z and EBO-S strains of Ebola virus produce febrile responses in guinea pigs 4 to 10 days after inoculation; however, none of these viruses kills guinea pigs consistently on primary inoculation and only EBO-Z has been adapted to uniform lethality by sequential guinea pig passages. EBO-Z is usually pathogenic for newborn mice inoculated i.c., but EBO-S, EBO-R, and Marburg virus are not.

IDENTIFICATION OF VIRUS

Typing Antisera

Detection of viral antigens in infected tissue culture cells (usually Vero or MA-104) permits a presumptive diagnosis, provided that the serologic reagents have been tested against all the reference arenaviruses and filoviruses expected in a given laboratory, thus permitting an interpretation of viral cross-reactions. Virus isolates in cell culture supernatant fluids or tissue homogenates are presumptively or specifically identified by their reactivity with diagnostic antisera in various serologic tests (see below). Specific polyclonal antisera are prepared in adult guinea pigs, hamsters, rats, or mice inoculated intraperitoneally with infectious virus. Rhesus and cynomolgus monkeys that are convalescent from experimental infections are also reasonable sources for larger quantities of immune sera. Diagnostic antisera produced by single injection of infectious virus are less cross-reactive and usually have higher titers than those produced by multiple injections of inactivated antigens. To further reduce the induction of extraneous antibodies, inoculum virus should be derived from tissues or cells homologous to the species being immunized; likewise, the virus suspension should be stabilized with homologous serum or serum proteins. Sera produced for use in the CF, DFA, and IFA tests and ELISA should be collected 30 to 60 days after inoculation; sera for neutralization tests should be collected later. All sera must be rigorously tested for the presence of live virus before being removed from a maximum-containment system.

Production and use of specific murine monoclonal antibodies with fine specificities for N and GP epitopes of LCM virus, Junin virus (50), and other arenaviruses have been reported, and monoclonal antibodies for Lassa and Marburg viruses and EBO-Z, EBO-S, and EBO-R with similar potential exist. Reference reagents for Lassa, Machupo, Marburg, and Ebola viruses are not generally available; hyperimmune mouse ascitic fluids for LCM, Junin, and Tacaribe viruses are available from the National Institutes of Health, Research Resources Branch.

Immunofluorescence Procedures

To process infected cells for DFA examination and presumptive identification, inoculated cell monolayers are dispersed by trypsinization (0.05% trypsin with 0.02% EDTA) for 10 min at 37°C, diluted in phosphate-buffered saline (PBS) containing 10% calf serum, and centrifuged at 400 $\times$ *g* for 10 min. The cell pellet is washed by resuspension in PBS, centrifugation, and resuspension in PBS to a final concentration of 10^6 cells per ml. Small drops (10 to 20 μl each) of cell suspensions are placed onto circular areas of specially prepared epoxy-coated slides that were cleaned previously by immersion in ethanol followed by polishing to remove residual oily deposits. These "spot slides" are air dried, fixed in acetone at room temperature for 10 min, and either stained immediately or stored frozen at -70°C. Although acetone fixation greatly reduces the number of infectious intracellular viruses, spot slides prepared in this manner should still be considered infectious and handled accordingly. Recently, gamma irradiation has been used to render spot slides noninfectious (14), with no diminution in fluorescent-antigen intensity. Alternatively, infected cells may be biologically inactivated with β-propiolactone (55). Gamma irradiation is recommended if the appropriate equipment is available.

For DFA tests, specific immune globulin conjugated to fluorescein is diluted to a working concentration predetermined by box titration and flooded onto the infected cells, which are then incubated at room temperature for 30 min in a moist chamber. Evans blue is sometimes added (0.005%) to the conjugate as a counterstain. After incubation, the slides are washed by immersion in PBS for two

10-min periods, dipped in water to remove salts, dried by evaporation, and mounted under coverslips in PBS-glycerol (pH 7.8). Specific viral fluorescence is characterized as intense, punctate to granular aggregates confined to the cytoplasm of infected cells. Specific MBG and EBO fluorescence may include large, bizarrely shaped aggregates up to 10 μm across. Nonspecific fluorescence is rarely a problem in DFA procedures for these viruses. Detection of Marburg, Ebola, Lassa, and LCM virus antigens by the DFA test is usually considered sufficient for a definitive diagnosis, although Lassa and LCM viruses cross-react at low levels in this test. Detection of Junin or Machupo virus antigens by the DFA test constitutes a presumptive diagnosis, since these viruses can be reliably distinguished from each other only by neutralization tests. IFA formats for viral detection are more cumbersome and cross-reactive but can be used if direct conjugates are unavailable. Immunohistochemical techniques for detecting arenaviruses (11) and filoviruses (12, 22) with a variety of chromogens can also be applied.

Complement Fixation Test

The CF test was routinely used in early investigations for the detection and presumptive identification of the arenaviruses and Marburg virus. However, this test is rarely used now, since reliable, simplified, and more sensitive immunofluorescence procedures (described above) have been developed. Detailed instructions for performing the CF test for arenaviruses are available (6), and the method can be applied to Marburg and Ebola viruses as well.

Antigen Capture ELISA

Recent development of an antigen capture ELISA for quantitative detection of arenavirus and filovirus antigens in viremic sera and tissue culture supernatants has facilitated the early detection and identification of these agents (34, 43). These tests reliably detect antigens in samples inactivated by either β-propiolactone or irradiation; therefore, they can be conducted safely without elaborate containment facilities. The threshold sensitivities for these assays are approximately 2.1 to 2.5 $\log_{10}$ PFU per ml, and so they are sufficiently sensitive to detect antigen in most acute-phase VHF viremias and to detect viruses in the concentrations present in throat wash and urine samples. The antigen capture ELISA developed for Ebola virus serves as a generic model for antigen capture ELISAs for both the arenavirus and filovirus groups (34). Substitution of a monoclonal antibody of high avidity and appropriate specificities for polyclonal sera generally increases the sensitivities and specificities of these antigen capture ELISAs. However, monoclonal antibodies with broad cross-reactivity (57) are potentially useful for the development of a general pan-arenavirus detector system.

Genome Analysis

As described above, RT-PCR has been developed for detection of the arenavirus and filovirus pathogens (LCM, Lassa, Junin, Ebola, and Marburg viruses) as well as many of the nonpathogenic strains. The acquisition of a reaction product facilitates sequence analysis and rapid definitive identification of the isolate. This approach is rapidly replacing identification methods based on serologic criteria.

SEROLOGIC DIAGNOSIS

Indirect Fluorescent-Antibody Test

Until recently, the IFA test was widely regarded as the most practical single method for documenting recent infections with Marburg and Ebola viruses and the arenaviruses, and it is still widely used. Preparation of spot slides with infected Vero cells is identical to the procedure described above. Some refinements to enhance reproducibility and quality between spot slide lots have been suggested (13). Although monovalent spot slides are usually desired and are prepared with cells optimally infected with a single virus, polyvalent spot slides can also be prepared by mixing cells infected with different viruses selected from these or other taxonomic groups which have similar geographic distributions (28). Test sera are diluted serially, usually in twofold or fourfold increments, starting at 1:10 or 1:16. Infected cells (and uninfected control cells) are incubated with serum dilutions, washed, reincubated with appropriate fluorescein-conjugated anti-globulin (or specific anti-immunoglobulin M [IgM] or IgG), washed, mounted, and observed. End point determination is very subjective. Most experienced observers consider the end point to be the highest dilution producing typical cytoplasmic fluorescence clearly positive relative to uninfected cells. Although it is possible to obtain reproducible end points within individual laboratories, discrepancies in titers determined by different laboratories are common and probably relate to variations in interpretation, epi-illumination intensity, filtration systems, and fluorescein conjugates. There is general agreement that use of oil immersion objectives increases background, leading to lower apparent end points. For Ebola virus antibodies, backgrounds may be sufficiently high that 1:64 is adopted as the cutoff titer (13). Antibodies measured by the IFA test are usually the first to appear, often becoming detectable within the first few days of hospitalization for Lassa virus, within 10 days of onset for Marburg and Ebola viruses, and somewhat later for Junin and Machupo viruses. The presence of specific IgM antibodies or a rising IFA titer permits a presumptive diagnosis of acute infection (58). IgM antibodies measured by IFA decline to undetectable titers within several months, while IgG antibodies, which are thought to compete with IgM in IFA tests, persist for at least several years.

Complement Fixation Test

The CF test is rarely used now because it is inferior to the IFA test for both the arenavirus and filovirus infections.

Neutralization Tests

As described above, reliable tests for measuring neutralizing antibody to Marburg and Ebola viruses are not currently available. For the arenaviruses, plaque reduction tests with Vero cells are generally used. For measuring neutralizing antibody to Lassa and LCM viruses, which are both difficult to neutralize and are poor inducers of this antibody, test sera are diluted, usually 1:10, in medium containing 10% guinea pig serum as a complement source and mixed with serial dilutions of challenge virus. Titers are expressed as a $\log_{10}$ neutralization index, defined as ($\log_{10}$ PFU in control) − ($\log_{10}$ PFU in test serum). For Junin and Machupo viruses, the more conventional serum dilution-constant virus format is normally used, although the constant serum-virus dilution format is equally useful for distinguishing among strains. Neutralizing-antibody responses require weeks to months to evolve but persist for years. Performance of these tests is restricted to laboratories equipped to handle the infectious viruses.

Acute-phase sera from Lassa fever patients frequently contain both infectious virus and IFA and CF antibodies. In survivors, neutralizing antibodies to Lassa virus first appear very late in convalescence (6 weeks or later), long after the viremia has disappeared. This pattern of early IFA and delayed neutralizing-antibody response is similar for LCM virus infections. Neutralizing antibodies against Junin and Machupo viruses become detectable 3 to 4 weeks after onset, soon after the termination of viremia. For Marburg and Ebola viruses, as for Lassa virus, the antibody evolves late (27); while these antibodies are thought to be important in protection against reinfection, their role in resolution of acute infections is less firmly established (26).

ELISA for Detection of IgG and IgM Antibodies

ELISA procedures for Lassa-specific IgG and IgM have been developed (43) and successfully used on field-collected human sera. When this ELISA is used in combination with the Lassa antigen capture ELISA described above, virtually all Lassa fever patients can be specifically diagnosed within hours of hospital admission. As with the antigen capture ELISA, success of the antibody ELISA is critically dependent on highly avid, purified capture antibodies or globulins. A simplification of this procedure, which entails the use of infected Vero cell lysate as the antigen, diluted in SerDil and adsorbed directly to the microtiter plate wells, has been developed for Ebola virus. Test sera are serially diluted, initially 1:16, and incubated with antigen in a format analogous to the antigen capture ELISA described above. Following incubation, washing, and addition of rabbit anti-human serum, color development is measured by the horseradish peroxidase-ABTS system. Samples are considered positive if the optical density at 410 nm exceeds the mean plus 3 standard deviations for the normal serum controls. This procedure can be further modified to detect virus-specific IgM by coating the plates with anti-human IgM followed by test serum dilutions and cell lysate antigens and then using the antigen capture protocol. These developmental procedures have worked well with animals experimentally infected with Lassa and Ebola viruses, but the IgM ELISA has been less successful for Junin virus. A simplification of the ELISA plate procedure substituting filter paper discs has been reported (29); it appears to sacrifice some sensitivity and precision in comparison with the more established procedures but may find application in a field setting. All of these developmental assays are sufficiently robust to warrant field testing. If successful, IgG and IgM ELISAs will probably replace the more subjective IFA tests as the serologic tests of choice (33).

Western Blotting

Western blotting is feasible for demonstrating antibodies to arenaviruses and filoviruses. However, it has never been applied systematically or routinely to diagnosis, although it was proposed as a confirmatory test to supplement the IFA test for filovirus antibodies (13). Detection of the nucleocapsid (N) band plus either VP30 or VP24 was taken as diagnostic. The Western blotting procedure was further refined by miniaturization, using the Phast system sodium dodecyl sulfate-polyacrylamide gel electrophoresis and transblot apparatus (Phast Western blot [PWB] system). It was found that 10 to 15% gradient gels provided the best results and that the optimum amount of protein loaded per lane was 50 ng. A dilution of 1:200 ensured the detection of all positive samples and absence of background staining. In the PWB system, VP30 and VP24 were rarely seen; therefore, a sole band (N) was taken as positive. When skim milk (0.5%) was added to the serum diluent to reduce background, specific reaction with N alone correlated closely with IFA test positivity. All Ebola virus-positive sera tested from earlier outbreaks and experimentally infected primates were positive in this test. There remain problematic sera that test positive in the IFA test (at 1:64 or greater) that test negative by PWB, raising the suspicion that other, serologically related but distinct filoviruses may be circulating.

Other Serologic Tests

Other serologic tests have been applied to diagnosis. Gel diffusion tests have been used for arenaviruses, but those tests detect antibodies directed primarily against nucleocapsid and are less sensitive than the IFA test or even the CF test; therefore, gel diffusion tests have little application in modern diagnosis. Another test developed for Lassa virus (and antibodies) is a reversed passive-hemagglutination (and inhibition) test involving Lassa virus antibody-coated erythrocytes which agglutinate in the presence of viral antigen (20). The test has not gained widespread acceptance, perhaps because meticulous care is required to obtain satisfactory antibody-erythrocyte conjugates. For Ebola virus, a radioimmunoassay, using ^{125}I-labeled staphylococcal protein A, was successfully used on many human and animal sera and discriminates the EBO-Z and EBO-S strains (47). However, it is considered too labor-intensive to find general use in the diagnostic laboratory. PWB (described above) holds promise as a confirmatory test for the filovirus IFA test and may be adapted for use with the arenaviruses as well. All of these alternative tests are too cumbersome to be adopted as the primary serologic screening method. Western immunoblotting and radioimmunoassay procedures are used in specialized laboratories to determine the fine specificities of monoclonal antibodies and occasionally to confirm the results of serosurveys based on ELISA or the IFA test. With experience, the proper roles for these alternate procedures in the routine diagnosis of Marburg and Ebola virus and arenavirus infections will be established.

EVALUATION AND INTERPRETATION OF RESULTS

Early diagnosis of arenavirus and filovirus infection is desirable since specific immune plasma and appropriately selected antiviral drugs are often effective when treatment is initiated soon after onset. Early recognition of these infections should also trigger strict isolation procedures to prevent spread of the disease to patient contacts. In areas where specific viruses are endemic, the index of suspicion is often high and experienced clinicians may be remarkably accurate in rendering an accurate diagnosis of fully developed cases on clinical grounds alone. However, even in these areas, specific virologic and serologic tests are required to confirm clinical impressions, since many other diseases, including malaria, typhoid, rickettsiosis, idiopathic thrombocytopenia, and viral hepatitis, may masquerade as an arenavirus or filovirus infection. While the availability of inactivated antigen spot slides for IFA tests in field hospitals has facilitated the diagnosis, based on seroconversion by IFA, timely diagnosis requires a means of detecting infectious virus or antigen in the field. The antigen capture ELISA holds promise to detect clinically relevant concentrations of virus in β-propiolactone-inactivated sera, body fluids, and tissues, as convincingly demonstrated in EBO-R-infected primates (24, 34, 48).

PCR assays may eventually eliminate almost all need to isolate infectious virus to establish a definitive diagnosis, and thus they will reduce the need for BL-4 biocontainment.

In the interim, however, detection of viral antigens by DFA tests in Vero cells inoculated with patient specimens will continue to be important in establishing a definitive diagnosis. Inoculation of tissue cultures for DFA examination and isolation of these viruses should not be conducted outside a maximum-containment laboratory, with the exception of LCM virus, which may be handled at a lower containment level (10). Identification by a DFA test yields a definitive diagnosis, except for Junin and Machupo viruses, which are reliably discriminated from each other only by the neutralization test or more sophisticated tools of molecular virology. Quantitative cross-testing by the DFA test can discriminate among other virus strains that cross-react by the DFA test, such as Lassa virus with LCM virus and EBO-Z with EBO-S. For virus isolates originating from areas where the geographic distributions of related viruses overlap, it is essential that quantitative DFA testing be done and desirable that identification be confirmed by neutralization tests when available. The ability to amplify viral genomes from infected tissues, and even from formalin-fixed tissues, and to sequence the reaction products may well eclipse serologic methods of identification and classification of arenaviruses (2) and filoviruses (52).

While interpretation of serologic data is usually facilitated by the generally restricted geographic ranges of these viruses, the ranges do overlap and occasionally IFA and CF data are ambiguous. Investigations spanning several decades (1) have shown the simultaneous development of CF antibodies against Junin and LCM virus antigens in patients in the AHF-endemic zone clinically diagnosed with cases of AHF, including some from whose acute-phase blood Junin virus was isolated. This fact creates serious difficulties in reaching a definite diagnosis not heretofore encountered with other arenavirus infections of humans; as a result, epidemiologic evaluation of data may be faulty. The geographic distributions of Junin and Machupo viruses certainly overlap that of LCM virus in South America. In Africa the distribution of Lassa virus may overlap those of the apparently less virulent virus strains from rodents in Zimbabwe, Mozambique, and the Central African Republic, which cross-react strongly with Lassa virus by IFA testing, thus confusing the interpretation of serologic data from African surveys. The extent to which heterologous arenavirus infection and/or reinfection broadens antibody specificity has not been systematically evaluated for any of the available serologic tests. For Ebola virus, IFA tests have been sensitive and specific in detecting seroconversions and acutely convalescent individuals in the midst of an outbreak. However, the IFA test may have yielded misleading results when applied to population-based serosurveys; a significant proportion of human and primate sera are reactive by IFA testing even when there is no clinical or epidemiological evidence of previous infection with known filoviruses. Despite these potential problems, the experience to date has been that in the midst of outbreaks caused by Marburg or Ebola virus or the arenaviruses, identifications of the etiologic agents by DFA and IFA testing have been clear and unambiguous, especially when the diagnoses were confirmed by neutralization tests.

Because of the biohazard, virus isolation data for these viruses is usually available only retrospectively. Marburg virus and EBO-Z are usually isolated from acute-phase serum samples, while EBO-S is isolated less often, perhaps because of the need for blind passage. In the past, opportunities to isolate some of these viruses may have been missed by use of newborn mice as the primary detection system. Lassa virus is usually recovered from acute-phase sera of hospitalized patients soon after admission, frequently in the presence of specific IgM antibody. Junin, Machupo, and LCM viruses are recovered less frequently, and diagnosis is usually based on seroconversion. The IFA and ELISA responses are the earliest for all these viruses, being detectable 7 to 10 days after onset for Lassa and LCM viruses, 10 to 14 days for Marburg and Ebola viruses, 12 to 17 days for Junin virus, and 17 to 30 days for Machupo virus. The CF antibodies evolve several days after the IFA response. The presence of specific IgM antibodies detected by IFA is indicative of recent infection, since IgM-IFA or IgM-ELISA titers persist for less than 3 months. The presence of specific IgM-IFA titers in the cerebrospinal fluid of LCM patients constitutes a definitive diagnosis. For all the arenavirus and filovirus pathogens, a rising IgM or IgG titer constitutes a strong presumptive diagnosis. Since IgM titers, as well as CF titers, do not persist for long, a decreasing titer suggests a recent infection which occurred perhaps several months previously.

For Lassa fever patients, a detectable IFA or ELISA response does not necessarily signal imminent recovery; viremia frequently persists, and patients die after an IFA response is detected. For Junin, LCM, Marburg, and Ebola virus infections, the appearance of antibodies detectable by IFA coincides with the disappearance of viremia and with recovery. In Machupo virus infection, IFA titers appear even later, 1 week or more after the crisis has passed. For the arenaviruses, neutralizing antibodies appear much later in convalescence than do IFA or CF antibodies. The filoviruses are notoriously poor inducers of neutralizing antibody. The reasons for these poor neutralizing-antibody responses are thought to be related to the high degree of glycosylation and to the presence of a possibly immunosuppressive epitope in the GP (membrane) protein. For Ebola virus, the production of a secreted, truncated virion surface glycoprotein has been speculated to act as an immunologic decoy or antibody sink during acute infection.

Neutralizing antibodies against arenaviruses persist for long periods, perhaps for life, and thus provide the most reliable basis for determining the minimum resistance of a population to reinfection. The role of neutralizing antibody in acute recovery is less clear. The protective efficacy of passively administered immune plasma is believed to be a function of neutralizing-antibody titers, and plasma should be selected on this basis, especially for Lassa fever, since protective efficacy is predicted by neutralizing-antibody titers and not by IFA testing (25). A similar correlation has been made for Ebola virus protective immunity, although passively administered IgG with very high neutralizing-antibody titers conferred only partial protection to experimentally infected primates (26). Among the group-specific antibody tests for arenaviruses, ELISA-based assays are widely believed to provide a more objective method than fluorescence (33). IgM capture ELISA and antigen capture ELISA are rapidly becoming routine.

The highest priority for future development is refinement of the available diagnostic tools to permit definitive virus identifications in the field. PCR-based assays will add another dimension to the capability of field laboratories to diagnose acute disease almost in real time. Proper tailoring of primers should permit the design of tests with the proper degree of specificity. The emergence of two new arenavirus pathogens, Guanarito and Sabia, as well as EBO-R, Whitewater Arroyo, and Pirital viruses in the past decade, serves as a reminder that broadly reactive, grouping reagents are still required to augment the newly evolving tools of

PCR and capture ELISAs based on extremely specific monoclonal antibodies and gene sequences. An investment in rapid diagnosis should result in more timely intervention with effective treatment regimens, and through implementation of appropriate public health measures may reduce the dissemination of these highly virulent viral pathogens.

REFERENCES

1. **Ambrosio, A. M., M. R. Feuillade, G. S. Gamboa, and J. I. Maiztegui.** 1994. Prevalence of lymphocytic choriomeningitis virus infection in a human population in Argentina. *Am. J. Trop. Med. Hyg.* **50:**381–386.
2. **Bowen, M. D., C. J. Peters, et al.** 1996. The phylogeny of new world (Tacaribe complex) arenaviruses. *Virology* **219:**285–290.
3. **Buchmeier, M. J., H. A. Lewicki, O. Tomori, and M. B. A. Oldstone.** 1981. Monoclonal antibodies to lymphocytic choriomeningitis and Pichinde viruses: generation, characterization, and cross-reactivity with other arenaviruses. *Virology* **113:**73–85.
4. **Buchmeier, M. J., and B. S. Parekh.** 1987. Protein structure and expression among arenaviruses. *Curr. Top. Microbiol. Immunol.* **133:**41–58.
5. **Buchmeier, M. J., J. C. S. Clegg, M. Y. Franze-Fernandez, D. Kolakofsky, C. J. Peters, and P. J. Southern.** 1995. *Arenaviridae. Arch. Virol.* (Suppl. 10)**:**319–323.
6. **Casals, J.** 1977. Serologic reactions with arenaviruses. *Medicina (Buenos Aires)* **37**(Suppl. 3)**:**59–68.
7. **Centers for Disease Control.** 1980. Interstate shipment of etiologic agents. *Fed. Regist.* **45:**48626–48629.
8. **Centers for Disease Control.** 1988. Management of patients with suspected viral hemorrhagic fever. *Morbid. Mortal. Weekly Rep.* **37**(Suppl. 3)**:**1–16.
9. **Centers for Disease Control.** 1995. Update. Management of patients with suspected viral hemorrhagic fever—United States. *Morbid. Mortal. Weekly Rep.* **44:** 475–479.
10. **Centers for Disease Control and National Institutes of Health.** 1993. *Biosafety in Microbiology and Biomedical Laboratories.* HHS Publication (CDC) 93–8395. U.S. Government Printing Office, Washington, D.C.
11. **Connolly, B. M., A. B. Jenson, C. J. Peters, S. J. Geyer, J. F. Barth, and R. A. McPherson.** 1993. Pathogenesis of Pichinde virus infection in strain 13 guinea pigs: an immunocytochemical, virologic, and clinical chemistry study. *Am. J. Trop. Med. Hyg.* **49:**10–23.
12. **Connolly, B. M., K. E. Steele, K. J. Davis, T. W. Geisbert, W. M. Kell, N. K. Jaax, and P. B. Jahrling.** 1999. Pathogenesis of experimental Ebola virus infection in guinea pigs. *J. Infect. Dis.* **179**(Suppl.)**:**S203–S217.
13. **Elliott, L. H., S. P. Bauer, G. Perez-Oronoz, and E. S. Lloyd.** 1993. Improved specificity of testing methods for filovirus antibodies. *J. Virol. Methods* **43:**85–100.
14. **Elliott, L. H., J. B. McCormick, and K. M. Johnson.** 1982. Inactivation of Lassa, Marburg, and Ebola viruses by gamma irradiation. *J. Clin. Microbiol.* **16:**704–708.
15. **Geisbert, T. W., and P. B. Jahrling.** 1995. Differentiation of filoviruses by electron microscopy. *Virus Res.* **39:** 129–150.
16. **Geisbert, T. W., and N. K. Jaax.** 1997. Marburg hemorrhagic fever: report of a case studied by immunohistochemistry and electron microscopy. *Ultrastruct. Pathol.* **22:**3–17.
17. **Geisbert, T. W., and P. B. Jahrling.** 1990. Use of immunoelectron microscopy to show Ebola virus during the 1989 United States epizootic. *J. Clin. Pathol.* **43:**813–816.
18. **Geisbert, T. W., P. B. Jahrling, M. A. Hanes, and P. M. Zack.** 1992. Association of Ebola-related Reston virus particles and antigen with tissue lesions of monkeys imported to the United States. *J. Comp. Pathol.* **106:** 137–152.
19. **Georges-Courbot, M. C., A. Sanchez, C. Y. Lu, S. Baize, E. Leroy, J. Lansout-Soukate, C. T'eve-B'enissan, A. J. Georges, S. G. Rtappier, S. R. Zaki, R. Swanepoel, P. A. Leman, P. E. Rollin, C. J. Peters, S. T. Nichol, and T. G. Ksiazek.** 1997. Isolation and phylogenetic characterization of Ebola viruses causing different outbreaks in Gabon. *Emerging Infect. Dis.* **3:**59–62.
20. **Goldwasser, R. A., L. H. Elliott, and K. M. Johnson.** 1980. Preparation and use of erythrocyte-globulin conjugates to Lassa virus in reversed passive hemagglutination and inhibition. *J. Clin. Microbiol.* **11:**593–599.
21. **Hotchin, J., and E. Sikora.** 1975. Laboratory diagnosis of lymphocytic choriomeningitis. *Bull. W. H. O.* **52:** 555–558.
22. **Jaax, N, K., K. J. Davis, T. W. Geisbert, A. P. Vogel, G. P. Jaax, M. Topper, and P. B. Jahrling.** 1996. Lethal experimental infection of rhesus monkeys with Ebola-Zaire (Mayinga) virus by the oral and conjunctival route of exposure. *Arch. Pathol. Lab. Med.* **120:**140–155.
23. **Jahrling, P. B., H. Dieter-Klenk, A. Sanchez, M. P. Kiley, C. J. Peters, and R. Swanepoel.** 1995. *Filoviridae. Arch. Virol.* (Suppl. 10)**:**319–323.
24. **Jahrling, P. B., T. W. Geisbert, D. W. Dalgard, E. D. Johnson, T. G. Ksiazek, W. C. Hall, and C. J. Peters.** 1990. Preliminary report: isolation of Ebola virus from monkeys imported to USA. *Lancet* **335:**502–505.
25. **Jahrling, P. B., and C. J. Peters.** 1984. Passive antibody therapy of Lassa fever in cynomolgus monkeys. *Infect. Immun.* **44:**528–533.
26. **Jahrling, P. B., T. W. Geisbert, J. B. Geisbert, J. R. Swearengen, M. Bray, N. K. Jaax, J. W. Huggins. J. W. LeDuc, and C. J. Peters.** 1999. Evaluation of immune globulin and recombinant interferon á-2b for treatment of experimental Ebola virus infections. *J. Infect. Dis.* **179**(Suppl.)**:**S224–S234.
27. **Jahrling, P. B., T. W. Geisbert, N. K. Jaax, M. A. Hanes, T. G. Ksiazek, and C. J. Peters.** 1996. Experimental infection of cynomolgus macaques with Ebola-Reston filoviruses from the 1989–1990 U.S. epizootic. *Arch. Virol.* (Suppl. 11)**:**115–134.
28. **Johnson, K. M., L. H. Elliott, and D. L. Heymann.** 1981. Preparation of polyvalent viral immunofluorescent intracellular antigens and use in human serosurveys. *J. Clin. Microbiol.* **14:**527–529.
29. **Kalter, S. S., R. L. Heberling, J. D. Barry, and P. Y. Tian.** 1995. Detection of Ebola-Reston (filoviridae) virus antibody by dot-immunobinding assay. *Lab. Anim. Sci.* **45:** 523–525.
30. **Kiley, M. P., E. T. W. Bowen, G. A. Eddy, M. Isaacson, K. M. Johnson, J. B. McCormick, F. A. Murphy, S. R. Pattyn, D. Peters, O. W. Prozesky, R. L. Regnery, D. I. H. Simpson, W. Slenczka, P. Sureau, G. Van der Groen, P. A. Webb, and H. Wulff.** 1982. Filoviridae: taxonomic home for Marburg and Ebola viruses? *Intervirology* **18:** 24–32.
31. **Kiley, M. P., N. J. Cox, L. H. Elliott, A. Sanchez, R. Defries, M. J. Buchmeier, D. D. Richman, and J. B. McCormick.** 1988. Physiochemical properties of Marburg virus: evidence for three distinct virus strains and their relationship to Ebola virus. *J. Gen. Virol.* **69:**1957–1967.
32. **Kilgore, P. E., C. J. Peters, et al.** 1995. Prospects for the control of Bolivian Hemorrhagic fever. *Emerging Infect. Dis.* **3:**97–100.
33. **Ksiazek, T. G., P. E. Rollin, A. J. Williams, D. S. Bressler, M. L. Martin, R. Swanepoel, F. J. Burt, P. A. Lemon, A. K. Rowe, R. Mukunu, A. Sanchez, and C. J. Peters.** 1999. Clinical virology of Ebola hemorrhagic fever (EHF)

virus: virus, virus antigen, and IgG and IgM findings among EHF patients in Kikwit, Democratic Republic of Congo, 1995. *J. Infect. Dis.* **179**(Suppl.)**:**S177–S187.

34. **Ksiazek, T. G., P. E. Rollin, P. B. Jahrling, E. Johnson, D. W. Dalgard, and C. J. Peters.** 1992. Enzyme immunosorbent assay for Ebola virus antigens in tissues of infected primates. *J. Clin. Microbiol.* **30:**947–950.
35. **Lederberg, J., R. E. Shope, and S. C. Oals, Jr. (ed.).** 1992. *Emerging Infections. Microbial Threats to Health in the United States.* National Academy Press, Washington, D.C.
36. **Le Guenno, B., P. Formenty, M. Wyers, P. Gounon, F. Walker, and C. Boesch.** 1995. Isolation and partial characterisation of a new strain of Ebola virus. *Lancet* **345:** 1271–1274.
37. **Lehmann-Grube, F.** 1971. Lymphocytic choriomeningitis virus. *Virol. Monogr.* **10:**1–173.
38. **Lozano, M. E., D. Enria, et al.** 1995. Rapid diagnosis of Argentine hemorrhagic fever by reverse transcriptase PCR-based assay. *J. Clin. Microbiol.* **33:**1327–1332.
39. **Lozano, M. E., D. M. Posik, et al.** 1997. Characterization of arenaviruses using a family-specific primer set for RT-PCR amplification and RFLP analysis. Its potential use for detection of uncharacterized arenaviruses. *Virus Res.* **49:** 79–89.
40. **Martini, G. A.** 1971. Marburg virus disease. Clinical syndrome, p. 1–9. *In* G. A. Martini and R. Siegert (ed.), *Marburg Virus Disease.* Springer-Verlag, New York, N.Y.
41. **Murphy, F. A., G. Van der Groen, S. G. Whitfield, and J. V. Lange.** 1978. Ebola and Marburg virus morphology and taxonomy, p. 61–84. *In* S. R. Pattyn (ed.), *Ebola Virus Haemorrhagic Fever.* Elsevier/North Holland Biomedical Press, Amsterdam, The Netherlands.
42. **Murphy, F. A., and S. G. Whitfield.** 1975. Morphology and morphogenesis of arenaviruses. *Bull. W. H. O.* **52:** 409–419.
43. **Niklasson, B. S., P. B. Jahrling, and C. J. Peters.** 1984. Detection of Lassa virus antigens and Lassa-specific IgG and IgM by enzyme-linked immunosorbent assay. *J. Clin. Microbiol.* **20:**239–244.
44. **Peters, C. J., M. Buchmeier, P. Rollin, and T. G. Ksiazek.** 1996. Arenaviruses, p. 1521–1551. *In* B. N. Fields, D. M. Knipe, P. M. Howley et al. (ed.), *Fields' Virology.* Lippencott-Raven, Philadelphia, Pa.
45. **Peters, C. J.** 1996. Emerging infections—Ebola and other filoviruses. *West. J. Med.* **164:**36–38.
46. **Peters, C. J.** 1997. Viral hemorrhagic fevers, p. 779–799. *In* N. Nathanson (ed.), *Viral Pathogenesis.* Lippincott-Raven Publishers, Philadelphia, Pa.
47. **Richman, D. D., P. H. Cleveland, J. B. McCormick, and K. M. Johnson.** 1983. Antigenic analysis of strains of Ebola virus: identification of two Ebola virus serotypes. *J. Infect. Dis.* **147:**268–271.
48. **Rollin, P. E., R. J. Williams, D. S. Bressler, S. Pearson, M. Cottingham, G. Pucak, A. Sanchez, S. G. Trappier, R. L. Peters, P. W. Greer, S. Zaki, T. Demarcus, K. Hendricks, M. Kelley, D. Simpson, T. W. Geisbert, P. B. Jahrling, C. J. Peters, and T. G. Ksiazek.** 1999. Ebola-Reston virus among quarantined nonhuman primates recently inported from the Philippines to the United States. *J. Infect. Dis.* **179**(Suppl.)**:**S108–S114.
49. **Sanchez, A., M. P. Kiley, B. P. Holloway, and D. D. Auperin.** 1993. Sequence analysis of the Ebola virus genome: organization, genetic elements, and comparison with the genome of Marburg virus. *Virus Res.* **29:**215–240.
50. **Sanchez, A., D. Y. Pifat, R. H. Kenyon, C. J. Peters, J. B. McCormick, and M. P. Kiley.** 1989. Junin virus monoclonal antibodies: characterization and cross-reactivity with other arenavirues. *J. Gen. Virol.* **70:**1125–1132.
51. **Sanchez, A, S. G Trappier, U. Stroher, S. T. Nichol, M. D. Bowen, and H. Feldmann.** 1998. Variation in the glycoprotein and VP35 genes of Marburg virus strains. *Virology* **240:**138–146.
52. **Sanchez, A., S. G, Trappier, B. W. Mahy, C. J. Peters, and S. T. Nichol.** 1996. The virion glycoproteins of Ebola virus are encoded in two reading frames and are expressed through transcriptional editing. *Proc. Natl. Acad. Sci. USA* **93:**3602–3607.
53. **Southern, P. J., and M. B. A. Oldstone.** 1986. Molecular anatomy of viral infection: study of viral nucleic acid sequences and proteins in whole body sections, p. 147–156. *In* M. B. A. Oldstone (ed.), *Concepts in Viral Pathogenesis II.* Springer-Verlag, New York, N.Y.
54. **Trappier, S. G., A. L. Conaty, B. B. Farrar, D. D. Auperin, J. B. McCormick, and S. P. Fisher-Hoch.** 1993. Evaluation of the polymerase chain reaction for diagnosis of Lassa virus infection. *Am. J. Trop. Med. Hyg.* **49:**214–221.
55. **Van der Groen, G., and L. H. Elliott.** 1982. Use of betapropiolactone-inactivated Ebola, Marburg, and Lassa intracellular antigens in immunofluorescent antibody assay. *Ann. Soc. Belg. Med. Trop.* **62:**49–54.
56. **Vogel, P., B. Connolly, D. Abplanalp, T. W. Geisbert, W. M. Kell, P. B. Jahrling, and N. K. Jaax.** 1997. Pathology of experimental Ebola-Zaire (Mayinga) virus infection transmitted to guinea pigs by oral, conjunctival, and tonsillar routes. *Cell Vision* **4:**298–307.
57. **Weber, E. L., and M. J. Buchmeier.** 1988. Fine mapping of a peptide sequence containing an antigenic site conserved among arenaviruses. *Virology* **164:**30–38.
58. **Wulff, H., and K. M. Johnson.** 1979. Immunoglobulin M and G responses measured by immunofluorescence in patients with Lassa or Marburg virus infections. *Bull. W. H. O.* **57:**631–635.
59. **Wulff, H., J. V. Lange, and P. A. Webb.** 1978. Interrelationships among arenaviruses measured by indirect immunofluorescence. *Intervirology* **9:**344–350.
60. **Zaki, S. R., and P. H. Kilmarx.** 1997. Ebola virus hemorrhagic fever, p. 299–312. *In* C. R. Horsburgh and A. M. Nelson (ed.), *Pathology of Emerging Infections.* American Society for Microbiology, Washington, D.C.

Poxviruses Infecting Humans*

SUSAN L. ROPP, JOSEPH J. ESPOSITO, VLADIMIR N. LOPAREV, AND GREGORY J. PALUMBO

91

CLINICAL EPIDEMIOLOGIC PERSPECTIVE

This chapter focuses on poxvirus infections of humans. Description of the taxonomic structure of the family *Poxviridae* (14), reviews of poxvirus characteristics (4, 5, 8, 11, 18, 24, 27, 41, 59, 61), and protocols for various laboratory diagnostic methods (17, 19, 26, 43–46) have been published.

All known poxviruses in nature at the present time that infect humans cause sporadic zoonoses except for molluscum contagiosum virus (MCV) (48, 50), which is transmitted strictly between humans. The zoonotic poxviruses include members of the genera *Orthopoxvirus* (monkeypox virus [32], cowpox virus [3], and the vaccinia virus subspecies buffalopox virus [13, 38]), *Parapoxvirus* (Orf, milker's nodule, sealpox, and papulosa stomatitis viruses [48, 52]), and *Yatapoxvirus* (tanapox, Yaba monkey tumor, and Yaba-like disease viruses [31, 34, 55]). Orf virus and MCV infections are the most common poxvirus infections worldwide; dermatologic lesions often can be readily identified, and so laboratory confirmation is not usually needed (24, 48, 50, 52).

Two human orthopoxviruses not in nature are vaccinia virus, certain strains of which were used for human vaccination to globally eradicate smallpox, and variola virus, the etiologic agent of smallpox (12, 24, 25, 27, 41). Since the early 1980s, vaccinia virus, and certain other poxviruses have been used for development of recombinant viruses expressing a variety of proteins, including vaccine immunogens (4, 18, 41, 52, 61).

GENERAL DESCRIPTION OF THE AGENTS

Morphology

All poxviruses described in this chapter belong to the family *Poxviridae*, subfamily *Chordopoxviridae* (14). Virions are large and brick shaped (orthopoxviruses, yatapoxviruses, or molluscipoxviruses) or ovoid (parapoxviruses). Virions range in length from 220 to 450 nm and in width and depth from 140 to 260 nm. All poxviruses contain a core, which in conventional negatively stained thin sections appears dumbbell shaped and is surrounded by a complex series of membranes. In negatively stained sections, lateral bodies of undefined function occupy the space between the outer membrane and the bar of the dumbbell. Recently, cryoelectron microscopy has indicated a different morphology in which the core is a sphere within the sphere of the outer membrane and lateral bodies are not present; this may be a dehydration effect of negative staining (41).

Virus particles contain about half of the 200 viral genome-encoded proteins, including structural proteins and a virtually complete system for primary transcription of viral genes (41). The genome, which is within a nucleoprotein complex (nucleosome) inside the core, consists of a single linear molecule of double-stranded DNA composed, depending on the strain, of about 130 to 375 kbp of DNA that is covalently closed at each end to form hairpin-like telomeres. Complete genome DNA sequences have been reported for vaccinia virus Copenhagen strain (28, 29) (GenBank accession no. M35027); for variola virus strains Bangladesh-1975 (35, 36) (GenBank accession no. L22579), India-1967 (57, 58) (GenBank accession no. X69198), and Garcia-1966 (GenBank accession no. Y16780); and for MCV (56) (GenBank accession no. U60315).

During virus replication (41), virion morphogenesis begins in the cytoplasm as the viral outer membrane initiates from cisternae of the intermediate compartment between the endoplasmic reticulum and the Golgi stacks. The cisternal membrane becomes interspersed with viral proteins, elongates into a crescent-shaped spicule-coated membrane, and encloses the nucleoprotein to form a spherical immature virus particle. The bilayer surface membrane of the particle differentiates, with one layer becoming the outer membrane and the other becoming the core membrane, thereby forming an intracellular mature virion (IMV), formerly called intracellular naked virion.

A small portion of IMVs may be further processed to acquire a bilayer tegument of Golgi cisternal membrane interspersed with viral proteins. The intracellular enveloped IMV then exits the cell (exocytosis) by fusing the outermost lipoprotein layer with the plasma membrane and releasing the IMV within a single lipoprotein layer (envelope); this is called the extracellular enveloped virion. IMVs and extracellular enveloped virions are mature infectious particles with distinct surface antigenic properties and apparently different cellular attachment receptors and mechanisms of cell entry. Both mechanisms, however, result in uncoating of the particle, release of the viral contents into the cell, and initiation of virus-controlled transcription for

* This chapter contains information presented in chapter 100 by Joseph J. Esposito and Robert F. Massung in the sixth edition of this Manual.

early-class protein synthesis, which precedes the production of crescents and immature particles.

Differentiating Features

DNA restriction endonuclease assays and DNA sequencing are the most precise methods for poxvirus genus, species, strain, and variant identification and differentiation (13, 16, 22, 23, 34, 49). The G + C contents of orthopoxviruses, yatapoxviruses, MCV, and parapoxviruses are ~33, ~32, ~60, and ~63%, respectively. More recently developed methods of identification include PCR amplification of various genome DNA segments followed by restriction endonuclease assay of the amplicons (30, 33, 39, 40, 53). The Appendix provides a stepwise protocol for PCR analysis of the gene for the hemagglutinin (HA) protein of orthopoxviruses to exemplify the procedure.

Histopathologic testing, electron microscopy, determination of virus growth features, and antigenic testing have also been used for differentiating poxviruses (8, 12, 13, 16, 20–22, 26, 31, 34, 38, 62). Poxviruses grow in the cytoplasm, producing basophilic or B-type inclusions (virus factories or viroplasm), which represent the site of virus replication. Certain species, e.g., the orthopoxvirus cowpox virus, produce acidophilic inclusions or A-type inclusions, which are proteinaceous deposits detectable with stains such as Giemsa and hematoxylin-eosin. Depending on the strain, A-type inclusions may (V^+) or may not (V^-) contain virions. Although electron microscopy can distinguish between orthopoxvirus and parapoxvirus morphology, it cannot differentiate between species; selected serologic, biological, and DNA-based assays must be used.

Poxvirus genera can usually be identified and differentiated by virus neutralization tests (NT) with hyperimmune reference sera (8, 17, 19, 43–46). However, within a given genus, poxviruses are closely related antigenically, and so it is sometimes difficult to identify the infecting species. *Orthopoxvirus* is the only poxvirus genus whose members produce an HA antigen detectable by hemadsorption and hemagglutination assays with erythrocytes of chickens selected to be suitable for such tests. Inhibition of hemagglutination and hemadsorption by patient serum is an indicator of orthopoxvirus infection (17, 19, 43–46); antibodies persist for 1 to 5 years after infection.

Orthopoxviruses are the only human poxviruses that produce pocks (62) on the chorioallantoic membrane (CAM) of fertile chicken eggs; therefore, pock morphology is useful for species and variant differentiation. Parapoxviruses, yatapoxviruses, and MCV do not form pocks on the CAM, although avipoxviruses, leporipoxviruses, and capripoxviruses do so.

Orthopoxviruses

The genus *Orthopoxvirus* contains four species that infect humans: variola virus, monkeypox virus, vaccinia virus, and cowpox virus. A Global Commission of the World Health Organization (WHO) declared smallpox eradicated in December 1979, and the declaration was sanctioned by the World Health Assembly in May 1980 (25). Human monkeypox, a zoonotic smallpox-like disease caused by monkeypox virus in rainforest countries of Africa, is now regarded as the most serious human poxvirus infection (32). Ectromelia (syn. mousepox) virus is an orthopoxvirus that has been implicated in various human infections (65); however, such reports are not well founded because the virus can be a notorious contaminant of laboratory mice (10), which are used for diagnostics.

Variola Virus

Variola virus has a strict human host range and no animal reservoir; it was transmitted between humans by aerosol or contact (25). Variola major virus strains produced a severe prodrome, fever, prostration, and rash. A toxemia or other form of systemic shock led to case fatality rates of up to 30%, with secondary attack rates among unvaccinated contacts within households of 30 to 80%. Variola minor virus strains (alastrim, amass, or kaffir viruses) produced less severe infection and case fatality rates of less than 1%, although secondary attack rates among unvaccinated contacts within households also ranged from 30 to 80%. DNA and biological data have indicated that European and South American alastrim variola minor viruses are very similar to each other but distinct from the so-called African variola minor viruses (e.g., strain Somalia 1977), which probably are attenuated variants of variola major virus (12, 35, 37). The last naturally occurring smallpox case occurred in Somalia in October 1977, although a fatal laboratory-associated infection with variola major virus occurred at the University of Birmingham, England, in August 1978 (24, 25).

Naturally acquired ordinary smallpox progressed from an oropharyngeal enanthem to a dermal exanthem, a skin rash that developed through stages of macule, papule, vesicle, and pustule (25). A noticeably higher density of the lesions appeared on the face and extremities than on the trunk; thus, the lesions were centrifugally distributed. Severe chickenpox rash caused by varicella-zoster virus had often been misdiagnosed as smallpox, but chickenpox rash is uniformly distributed and rarely appears on the palms and soles. Smallpox rarely developed without a rash, but it was sometimes misdiagnosed as acute leukemia, meningococcemia, or idiopathic thrombocytopenic purpura.

Variola major smallpox was differentiated into four main clinical types: (i) ordinary smallpox (90% of cases) produced viremia, fever, prostration, and rash; (ii) modified smallpox (5% of cases) produced a mild prodrome with few skin lesions in previously vaccinated people; (iii) flat smallpox (5% of all cases) produced slowly developing focal lesions with generalized infection and a ~50% fatality rate; and (iv) hemorrhagic smallpox (<1% of cases) induced bleeding into the skin and the mucous membranes and was invariably fatal within a week of onset. A discrete type of the ordinary form resulted from alastrim variola minor virus infection (25).

Monkeypox Virus

A review describing human monkeypox is available (32). Monkeypox was first recognized by Von Magnus in Copenhagen in 1958 as an exanthem of primates in captivity. Later, the disease was seen in other captive animals, including primates in zoos and animal import centers. Human monkeypox was first reported in 1970 in the Democratic Republic of Congo (DRC; formerly Zaire). Serosurveys and virologic investigations in the 1980s in the DRC by the WHO indicated that monkeys are sporadically infected, as are humans; that three-fourths of cases, mainly in children under 15 years of age, were from animal contact; that vaccinia virus vaccination has about 85% protective efficacy; that monkeypox virus has a broad host range, including squirrels (*Funisciurus* spp. and *Heliosciurus* spp.); and that human monkeypox has a secondary attack rate of 9% among unvaccinated contacts within households (i.e., it is much less transmissible than smallpox). Since 1970, the disease has been seen in the DRC, Liberia, Ivory Coast, Sierra Leone, Nigeria, Benin, Cameroon, and Gabon; most cases have been in the DRC, which has a population of about

30 million (338 cases were discovered prospectively during WHO intensified monkeypox surveillance in Zaire from 1981 to 1986). Human monkeypox was recently reported from the DRC, mainly in children under 15. Based on reported monkeypox onset dates in a largely retrospective study complicated by a concurrent outbreak of chickenpox, about 250 serosubstantiated monkeypox cases occurred among 0.5 million people in 78 villages from February 1996 to October 1997. About three-fourths of the cases appeared to result from human-to-human transmission; however, the secondary attack rate of 8% among unvaccinated contacts within households appeared to be about the same as in the 1981 to 1986 surveillance (6, 7, 42, 63, 64).

The clinical appearance of human monkeypox is much like that of smallpox, with fever, a centrifugally distributed vesiculopustular rash (including on the palms and soles), respiratory distress, and, in some cases, death from systemic shock. Like variola virus, monkeypox virus appears to enter through skin abrasions or the mucosa of the upper respiratory tract, where it produces an enanthem and cough. During primary viremia, the virus migrates to regional lymph nodes, and during secondary viremia, it is disseminated throughout the body and the skin rash appears. During prodrome, lymphadenopathy (generally inguinal) with fever and headache are common. Individual skin lesions develop through stages of macule, papule, vesicle, and pustule. Sequelae involve secondary infections, permanent scarring and pitting at the sites of the lesions, and sometimes alopecia and corneal opacities.

Virologic identification and differentiation of monkeypox virus are used to confirm infection. Generally, virus isolation in cell culture and/or CAMs and genome DNA restriction analysis are performed; however, several recently developed PCR techniques for type-specific identification of virus directly from lesions, which do not require virus propagation, have become available (see Appendix). In contrast, identification of infection by using case-patient serum is difficult because of the close antigenic relationship of orthopoxviruses (2, 21, 27) and because the efficacy of commonly used tests (e.g., NT and hemagglutination inhibition assays) ranges from 50 to 95%. No reliable, fully sensitive, type-specific serologic test to retrospectively identify orthopoxvirus infections has yet been developed for routine use.

Vaccinia Virus

Vaccinia virus infections are not generally regarded as naturally occurring, although vaccinee-to-cattle and cattle-to-human transmissions have occurred on farms during smallpox mass vaccination campaigns. Vaccinia virus, which was used mainly for vaccination against smallpox, protects against other orthopoxviruses. Routine smallpox vaccination of civilians stopped worldwide by 1980. In the United States, the Advisory Committee on Immunization Practices recommends as a safeguard that laboratory and health care workers at high risk for infection be vaccinated within 10 years of potential exposure. The vaccine is contraindicated in persons with eczema and other immunocompromising conditions. Treatment for herpesvirus and certain other infections constitutes misuse of smallpox vaccine. In the United States, the Centers for Disease Control and Prevention (CDC) Drug Service provides a potency-tested licensed vaccine after approval of a formal request by the administering physician; vaccinia immunoglobulin is also available to treat postvaccine side effects. The National Immunization Program at CDC provides clinical advice on human poxvirus infections.

Serious complications rarely occur when generally healthy persons are vaccinated with vaccinia virus strains recommended by the WHO and authorized in the country of use. Presently in the United States, the New York Board of Health strain (the viral component in the Wyeth Dryvax licensed vaccine) is used. Side effects, which are rare, include postvaccine encephalitis and encephalopathy, severe skin reactions including eczema vaccinatum, progressive vaccinia (vaccinia necrosum), generalized vaccinia, and certain autoinoculation complications, including ocular involvement (24–27, 48).

Sporadic outbreaks of the vaccinia virus subspecies buffalopox virus that involve transmission between milking buffalo, cattle, and humans have been reported, mainly in India but also in Egypt, Bangladesh, Pakistan, and Indonesia. Vaccinia-like lesions have been observed on the animals' teats and the milkers' hands; milk is infectious. Biological data and limited DNA analyses of isolates from an outbreak in India in 1985 suggest that buffalopox virus may be derived from vaccinia virus strains transmitted from humans to livestock during the smallpox vaccination era (13, 27).

Cowpox Virus

Cowpox, sometimes a rare occupational infection of humans, can be acquired by contact with infected cows; more often, other animals, e.g., infected rats, pet cats, and zoo and circus elephants, have been sources of the disease. Cowpox virus is a rather diverse species and has been isolated from humans and a variety of animals in Europe and adjoining regions of Asia (3). A recent serosurvey of wild animals in Great Britain found orthopoxvirus antibodies in a portion of bank and field voles and wood mice collected, which is consistent with small rodents being reservoir hosts for cowpox virus (2). Lesions in humans occur mainly on the fingers, with reddening and swelling; autoinoculation of other parts of the body may occur, and systemic severe infections have been reported. The skin lesions are likened to those of a primary vaccinia virus vaccination: the site becomes papular, and in 4 to 5 days a vesicle develops; healing takes about 3 weeks (1, 24, 26, 27).

Yatapoxviruses

The three members of the genus *Yatapoxvirus*, tanapox virus (TPV), Yaba-like disease virus of monkeys (YLDV), and Yaba monkey tumor virus (YMTV), are serologically related (55). DNA maps of TPV and YLDV are extremely similar, suggesting they are the same agent; however, these DNA maps are markedly different from YMTV DNA maps, even though the three DNAs cross-hybridize extensively (34). The epidemiology and natural history of yatapoxviruses are poorly understood. YMTV and YLDV infections have occurred in animal handlers (55); however, TPV is the main naturally occurring human pathogen in the genus (24, 26). Tanapox is an endemic zoonosis of equatorial Africa that is thought to be transmitted mechanically to humans by biting insects, especially during the rainy season (31). TPV and YLDV infections in humans consist of a brief fever followed by the development of firm, elevated, round, necrotic maculopapular nodules that are distinct from the vesiculopustular lesions of orthopoxviruses. Generally, few lesions develop, and these are found primarily on the skin of the upper arms, face, neck, or trunk (26). Symptoms include a low-grade fever, backache, and headache before lesions appear. Lesions umbilicate without pustulation during recovery from infection; they usually heal in 2 to 4 weeks. YMTV produces epidermal histiocytomas, tumor-like masses of histiocytic polygonal mononuclear cell infiltrates that advance to suppurative inflammatory sites.

Parapoxviruses

Three different parapoxvirus diseases occur in humans (26, 52), generally as occupational, nonsystemic infections: milker's nodule (in dairy cattle, the disease is termed pseudocowpox or paravaccinia), Orf (in sheep and goats, the disease has been referred to as Orf, contagious ecthyma, contagious pustular dermatitis, contagious pustular stomatitis, or sore mouth), and papulosa stomatitis (in calves and beef cattle, the disease is termed bovine papular stomatitis).

Parapoxvirus infections are transmitted to humans by direct contact with infected livestock through abraded skin on the hands and fingers, and ocular autoinoculation sometimes occurs (26, 48). Milker's nodule usually occurs as a single reddened hemispheric papule that matures to a purplish, smooth, firm nodule up to 2 cm in size; the lesions usually are not painful and can persist for about 6 weeks. Human Orf virus infection is usually found on the fingers, hands, and arms but may also be found on the face and neck; fever and swelling of draining lymph nodes may be present, and the lesions often ulcerate and are painful. Autoinoculation of the eye may lead to serious sequelae (48), including corneal opacity and secondary infection. Contact with (e.g., skinning) certain wild animals, including deer, reindeer, chamois, and Japanese serow, has also been a source of human parapoxvirus infection; technicians handling grey seals have contracted sealpox virus (52).

Molluscipoxviruses

MCV is the sole member of the genus *Molluscipoxvirus*, and restriction endonuclease mapping of isolates suggests there are two or three subtypes (50). MCV appears to have a human-restricted host range and does not grow readily in culture.

Molluscum contagiosum occurs worldwide as a contact disease in children or as a sexually transmitted disease in adults (24, 26, 48). In children and teenagers, the lesions generally appear on the trunk, limbs (except the palms and soles), and face, where there may be ocular involvement. Infection is usually transmitted by direct or indirect skin contact, such as among wrestlers or in public baths and swimming pools. When molluscum contagiosum is transmitted sexually among teenagers and adults, the lesions are mostly on the lower abdomen, pubis, inner thighs, and genitalia. Lesions are pearly, flesh colored, raised, firm, umbilicated nodules that measure about 5 mm in diameter. The lesions tend to disseminate by autoinoculation. MCV is an opportunistic pathogen in approximately 15% of AIDS patients in the United States. Two predominant MCV subtypes, MCVI and MCVII, have been detected in a limited number of samples examined by restriction pattern and base sequence analyses, but no correlation of subtype with disease syndrome or geographic distribution has been confirmed (48, 50). A rapid PCR and amplicon restriction fragment length polymorphism analysis using skin lesion material has been described for differentiating the MCV subtypes (47).

COLLECTION, HANDLING, AND STORAGE OF SPECIMENS

In the United States and its territories, a suspected case of smallpox should be immediately reported to the appropriate state or territorial health department. After the health department reviews the case and if smallpox still is suspected, it should be immediately reported to the WHO Collaborating Center for Smallpox and Other Poxvirus Infections, Poxvirus Section, Division of Viral and Rickettsial Diseases, National Center for Infectious Diseases, CDC, Atlanta, GA 30333. CDC has appropriate secure containment facilities for storage and work with variola virus and appropriate laboratories for examining other human poxviruses. In the United States and territories, other routine poxvirus diagnostic specimens, including suspected Orf virus and MCV samples, generally should be examined through private diagnostic laboratories or local governmental health laboratories.

Basic procedures for collecting clinical specimens can be found in chapter 4. It is extremely important not to cross contaminate samples (i.e., to use one sample per container) and to collect a large enough specimen to permit effective testing, including by cell culture and PCR. Suitable specimens for virologic tests of most suspected poxvirus infections are at least two to four scabs and/or vesicular fluid samples; it is important to try to include cellular material at the base of vesicles if skin biopsy specimens are obtained. Preferably, vesicular fluid is collected from each single lesion as a droplet on a glass microscope slide and air dried without being smeared. Each slide is stored in an individual plastic slide holder to avoid cross contamination. Alternatively, the fluid from separate lesions is collected in separate capillary tubes or on separate sterile dry swabs. It cannot be overemphasized that it is vital to store lesion samples of a given patient separately from each other (dual varicella and monkeypox infections have been detected in this manner) and from those of other patients to avoid cross contamination. Autopsy specimens for virus isolation, including portions of skin, liver, spleen, lung, and/or kidney, should be frozen; formalin-fixed tissue is suitable for histopathologic study.

After the appropriate laboratory has given approval for the specimens to be sent, the specimens should be placed in an appropriate biosafe container (e.g., glass vials should not be used; plastic vials or bottles or slide holders are preferred containers for specimens). So-called transport fluid or glycerol should not be used to send poxvirus specimens. Specimens collected from patients with poxvirus infections can be stored at 4°C for a short time, but −20 to −70°C should be used for long-term storage. Changes in the pH of specimens, such as those caused when dry-ice vapors enter containers, can be avoided by using proper closures with a gasket and by sealing the vials with Parafilm. A metal, plastic, or paperboard outer container, appropriately sealed, should be used. International, U.S., and local packing and shipping regulations must be followed.

LABORATORY DIAGNOSTIC METHODS

Earlier versions of this chapter (17, 45) have included extensive comments on factors affecting a confident diagnosis of poxvirus infection, particularly conditions of samples and preparation of certain reagents (15, 17, 45, 51).

Virologic Methods

The Poxvirus Section at CDC uses mainly a combination of methods, including electron microscopy, virus growth in cell culture and/or on the CAMs of 12-day-old chicken embryos, and DNA assay, for identifying and differentiating poxviruses. Various PCR protocols have been developed for poxviruses (30, 33, 39, 40, 53), and one for the HA gene of orthopoxviruses is described in the Appendix. Various other laboratory protocols for poxvirus diagnostics, including recent methods of DNA restriction analysis, have been detailed in previous editions of this Manual and elsewhere (17, 19, 26, 43–46).

Serologic Methods

When virus specimens are not available, antibody assessment by the NT or other methods may be the only way to attempt to define the etiology of the disease; generally, serum specimens are used. There is no one routine immunologic test that defines a person's degree of protection against a poxvirus infection. Protection is genetically defined and requires a concert of cell-mediated and humoral immune responses. The presence of neutralizing antibodies generally indicates recovery from an infection, not always protection from future infection. Neutralizing antibodies against variola, monkeypox, cowpox, or vaccinia viruses are often detectable as early as 6 days after infection or vaccinia virus vaccination; the efficacy of the NT using various origin animal and human sera has been from 50 to 95%. Neutralizing antibodies have been detected up to 20 years after vaccinia virus vaccination or natural infection with other human orthopoxviruses (25).

The primary focus of serologic methods used at CDC is the assay of antibodies against human orthopoxviruses; for this purpose, the virus NT, the hemagglutination inhibition assay, and the Western blot assay are the main methods. Various techniques for poxvirus serologic testing used at CDC are detailed elsewhere (8, 9, 17, 19, 26, 43–46, 54).

The Western blot assay is performed essentially as described by Towbin et al. (60) and uses various antigens including purified virus and concentrates of culture fluid from infected cells maintained under medium that contains 1% or no serum supplement. Because MCV cannot be readily grown in culture, no routine serologic test is available, and serologic testing for parapoxviruses is not performed at CDC: these infections are readily diagnosed clinically, often with the aid of histopathologic testing performed by a local diagnostic facility.

In the NT, a fourfold rise in antibody titer between serum samples drawn during the acute and convalescent phases is usually considered diagnostic of poxvirus infection. When only one serum specimen is available from one phase of infection, confirmation of a clinical diagnosis may be difficult to impossible. Because orthopoxviruses are closely related, serum cross-absorption tests, such as those performed by immunofluorescent-antibody or immunodiffusion methods, have been used with variable success with patient and animal serum. Orthopoxvirus antigen cross-absorption assays have been performed using hyperimmune animal sera (20, 21) and in serosurveys for animal or human monkeypox infection (32, 45, 46). False-positive results should be ruled out by using appropriate control sets of sera of known provenance.

Serologic Tests for Milker's Nodule, Orf, Tanapox, and Molluscum Contagiosum

Serologic methods used at CDC to help confirm parapoxvirus infections have included enzyme-linked immunosorbent assays (ELISAs) (9) and Western blot assays that use various antigen preparations. Serologic testing for TPV infection by standard ELISA (9) with antigens obtained from concentrates of infected cell culture, by an indirect immunofluorescent-antibody test, and by NT has been moderately effective. Optimally, serum should be collected at the time of actual disease and 3 to 5 weeks or more after the presumed onset date. Presently, there is no routine serologic test for MCV infection because the virus cannot be readily propagated in culture for antigen production.

APPENDIX 1

This appendix describes a method for extracting DNA (see also references 15 and 17) from lesional material suitable for PCR and a summary of the PCR method used for the orthopoxvirus HA gene region (53).

Preparation of Poxvirus DNA from Clinical Samples

Viral DNA was extracted from clinical samples by using the NucleoSpin C&T Kit (Machery-Nagel GmBH & Co.) and a slightly modified manufacturer's protocol as follows.

1. Homogenize one to four scabs in 100 μl of phosphate-buffered saline (PBS; 0.1 M NaCl plus 0.01 M sodium phosphate [pH 7.4]) either by freeze-thawing and sonication or by disruption with a microcentrifuge tube mortar and pestle (Kontes, Vineland, N.J.).
2. Digest proteins in half of the homogenate enzymatically in 180 μl of T1 buffer plus 50 μl of proteinase K (provided in the NucleoSpin Kit). Incubate for 3 h at 56°C or overnight at 37°C; gently mix periodically.
3. Further treat DNA-protein complexes by adding 200 μl of B3 buffer, which contains guanidine chloride, and incubate the mixture at 70°C for 10 min.
4. Adsorb virus DNA onto the affinity resin provided in the kit after mixing 210 μl of 100% ethanol with the digest-guanidine mixture and applying the mixture to a NucleoSpin column attached to a vacuum manifold (Promega, Madison, Wis.).
5. Wash the resin-absorbed DNA three times by drawing through the column 500 μl of B5 buffer (provided in the kit).
6. Remove excess fluid from the resin by centrifugation of the column at 6,000 $\times$ g for 1 min.
7. Elute DNA from the resin in the column by placing the column into a 1.5 ml microcentrifuge tube, add 100 μl of deionized distilled H_2O to the resin, and incubate the tube with the resin column for 5 min at 70°C.
8. Collect the eluate by centrifugation at 6,000 $\times$ g for 5 min, and then repeat steps 7 and 8.
9. Combine the eluates, which contain the DNA.

Orthopoxvirus HA-PCR assay

Two preferred PCR methods are sometimes needed to verify othopoxvirus strains from lesion specimens and are described in detail in reference 53. One method uses a set of 10 species-specific primer pairs. The second, summarized below, has been used to identify and differentiate orthopoxviruses by producing amplicons with a consensus sequence primer pair to amplify HA DNA from New World, North American orthopoxviruses (raccoon, skunk, and vole poxviruses) and another pair to amplify HA DNA from Old World, Eurasian-African orthopoxviruses (variola, vaccinia, cowpox, monkeypox, camelpox, ectromelia mousepox, and gerbilpox viruses). Amplicons produced with either pair are digested with *RsaI* or *TaqI*, and then the digest fragments are resolved by gel electrophoresis. This HA PCR and restriction fragment length polymorphism procedure is performed as follows.

1. Prepare template DNA from virions or infected tissue cultures as described in reference 17 or from lesion specimens as summarized above.
2. Prepare the reaction mixture in a total volume of 100 μl containing 200 μM each deoxynucleoside triphosphate, 50 mM KCl, 10 mM Tris-hydrochloride buffer (pH 8.3), 2.5 mM $MgCl_2$, 60 ng of each primer, 50 ng of template DNA, and 2.5 U of *Taq* polymerase (Boehringer Mannheim). To amplify Eurasian-African orthopoxvirus DNA, use 60 ng each of HA consensus primers EACP1 (5′-ATGACACGATTGCCAATAC) and EACP2 (5′-CTAGACTTTGTTTTCTG). To amplify North American orthopoxvirus DNA, use 60 ng each of HA consensus primers NACP1 (5′-ACGATGTCGTATACTTTGAT) and NACP2 (5′-GAAACAACTCCAAATATCTC).

3. Cycle the reaction mixtures 25 times through denaturation at 94°C for 1 min, annealing at 55°C for 2 min, and elongation at 72°C for 3 min.

4. Analyze 15 μl of the reaction mixture by electrophoresis with 3% NuSieve-GTG agarose and 1% SeaKem-GTG agarose gels (FMC BioProducts, Rockland, Maine).

5. Visualize and photograph the DNA. The primer pair EACP1-EACP2 and Eurasian-African strains produce amplicons of the following sizes: variola virus, 942 bp; vaccinia virus, 948 bp; camelpox virus, 960 bp; monkeypox virus, 942 bp; ectromelia virus, 846 bp; cowpox virus, 942 bp; and gerbilpox virus, 960 bp. The primer pair NACP1-NACP2 and North American strains produce amplicons of the following sizes: raccoon poxvirus, 652 bp; skunk poxvirus, 658 bp; and volepox virus, 580 bp.

6. To differentiate the viruses add 5 U of either endonuclease *Taq*I or *Rsa*I (New England Biolabs) to 30 μl of reaction product solution, incubate the mixture for 2 h at 37°C for *Rsa*I or 65°C for *Taq*I, and use gel electrophoresis as in step 4 to resolve the digest fragments and determine the fragment sizes. *Taq*I digestion of the Eurasian-African orthopoxvirus HA amplicons will produce fragments of the following sizes: variola virus, 536 and 406 bp; vaccinia virus, 451, 295, 105, and 97 bp; camelpox virus, 474, 331, 90, and 75 bp; monkeypox virus, 451, 220, 105, 91, and 75 bp; ectromelia virus, 343, 220, 111, 97, and 75 bp; cowpox virus, 303, 289, 115, 96, and 91 bp; and gerbilpox virus, 342, 331, 97, 80, 75, and 35 bp. *Rsa*I digests of the North American orthopoxvirus HA amplicons will produce fragments of the following sizes: raccoon poxvirus, 194, 192, 153, and 113 bp; skunk poxvirus, 264, 202, 113, 71, and 8 bp; and volepox virus, 467, and 113 bp.

REFERENCES

1. **Baxby, D., M. Bennett, and B. Getty.** 1994. Human cowpox 1969–93: a review based on 54 cases. *Br. J. Dermatol.* **131:**598–607.
2. **Bennett, M., A. J. Crouch, M. Begon, B. Duffy, S. Feore, R. M. Gaskell, D. F. Kelly, C. M. McCracken, L. Vacary, and D. Baxby.** 1997. Cowpox in British voles and mice. *J. Comp. Pathol.* **116:**35–44.
3. **Bennett, M., C. J. Gaskill, D. Baxby, R. M. Gaskill, D. F. Kelly, and J. Naidoo.** 1990. Feline cowpox virus infection. A review. *J. Small Anim. Pract.* **14:**167–173.
4. **Binns, M. M., and G. L. Smith.** 1992. *Recombinant Poxviruses.* CRC Press, Inc., Boca Raton, Fla.
5. **Buller, R. M. L., and G. J. Palumbo.** 1991. Poxvirus pathogenesis. *Microbiol. Rev.* **55:**80–122.
6. **Centers for Disease Control and Prevention.** 1997. Human monkeypox—Kasai Oriental, Zaire, 1996–1997. *Morbid. Mortal. Weekly Rep.* **46:**304–307.
7. **Centers for Disease Control and Prevention.** 1997. Human monkeypox—Kasai Oriental, Kasai Oriental, Democratic Republic of Congo, February 1996–October 1997. *Morbid. Mortal. Weekly Rep.* **46:**1168–1171.
8. **Cole, G. A., and R. V. Blanden.** 1982. Immunology of poxviruses. *Compr. Immunol.* **9:**1–19.
9. **Conroy, J. M., R. W. Stevens, and K. E. Hechemy.** 1991. Enzyme immunoassay, p. 87–92. *In* A. Balows, W. J. Hausler, K. L. Herrmann, H. D. Isenberg, and H. J. Shadomy (ed.), *Manual of Clinical Microbiology*, 5th ed. American Society for Microbiology, Washington, D.C.
10. **Dick, E. J., C. L. Kittell, H. Meyer, P. L. Farrar, S. L. Ropp, J. J. Esposito, R. M. L. Buller, H. Neubauer, Y. H. Kang, and A. E. McKee.** 1996. Mousepox outbreak in a laboratory mouse colony. *Lab. Anim. Sci.* **46:**602–611.
11. **Dumbell, K. R.** 1989. Poxviruses, p. 395–427. *In* J. Porterfield (ed.), *Andrews' Viruses of Vertebrates*, 5th ed. Bailliere Tindall, London, United Kingdom.
12. **Dumbell, K. R., and F. Huq.** 1986. The virology of variola minor. Correlation of laboratory tests with the geographic distribution and human virulence of variola isolates. *Am. J. Epidemiol.* **123:**403–415.
13. **Dumbell, K. R., and M. Richardson.** 1993. Virological investigations of specimens from buffaloes affected by buffalopox in Maharashtra State, India between 1985 and 1987. *Arch. Virol.* **128:**257–267.
14. **Esposito, J. J., D. Baxby, D. N. Black, S. Dales, G. Darai, K. R. Dumbell, R. R. Granados, W. K. Joklik, G. McFadden, B. Moss, R. W. Moyer, D. J. Pickup, A. J. Robinson, and D. N. Tripathy.** 1995. Poxviridae, p. 79–91. *In* F. A. Murphy, C. M. Fauquet, D. H. L. Bishop, S. A. Gabrial, A. W. Jarvis, G. P. Martelli, M. A. Mayo, and M. D. Summers (ed.), *Virus Taxonomy. Classification and Nomenclature of Viruses. Sixth Report of the International Committee on Taxonomy of Viruses.* Springer-Verlag, New York, N.Y.
15. **Esposito, J. J., R. Condit, and J. F. Obijeski.** 1981. The preparation of orthopoxvirus DNA. *J. Virol. Methods* **2:**175–179.
16. **Esposito, J. J., and J. C. Knight.** 1985. Orthopoxvirus DNA: a comparison of restriction profiles and maps. *Virology* **143:**230–251.
17. **Esposito, J. J., and R. F. Massung.** 1995. Poxvirus infections in humans, p. 1131–1138. *In* P. R. Murray, F. Tenover, E. J. Baron, M. A. Pfaller, and R. H. Yolken (ed.), *Manual of Clinical Microbiology*, 5th ed., American Society for Microbiology, Washington, D.C.
18. **Esposito, J. J., and F. A. Murphy.** 1989. Infectious recombinant vectored virus vaccines. *Adv. Vet. Sci. Comp. Med.* **33:**195–247.
19. **Esposito, J. J., and J. H. Nakano.** 1992. Human poxviruses, p. 643–668. *In* E. H. Lennette (ed.), *Laboratory Diagnosis of Viral Infections*, 2nd ed. Marcel Dekker, Inc., New York, N.Y.
20. **Esposito, J. J., J. F. Obijeski, and J. H. Nakano.** 1977. Serological relatedness of monkeypox, variola, and vaccinia viruses. *J. Med. Virol.* **1:**35–47.
21. **Esposito, J. J., J. F. Obijeski, and J. H. Nakano.** 1977. The virion and soluble antigen proteins of variola, monkeypox, and vaccinia viruses. *J. Med. Virol.* **1:**95–110.
22. **Esposito, J. J., J. F. Obijeski, and J. H. Nakano.** 1978. Orthopoxvirus DNA: strain differentiation by electrophoresis of restriction endonuclease fragmented virion DNA. *Virology* **89:**53–66.
23. **Esposito, J. J., J. F. Obijeski, and J. H. Nakano.** 1985. Can variola viruses be derived from monkeypox virus? An investigation based on DNA mapping. *Bull. W. H. O.* **63:**695–703.
24. **Fenner, F.** 1996. Poxviruses, p. 2673–2702. *In* B. N. Fields, D. Knipe, and P. Howley (ed.), *Fields' Virology*, 3rd ed. Raven Press, New York, N.Y.
25. **Fenner, F., D. A. Henderson, I. Arita, Z. Jezek, and I. Ladnyi.** 1988. *Smallpox and Its Eradication.* World Health Organization, Geneva.
26. **Fenner, F., and J. H. Nakano.** 1988. Poxviridae: the poxviruses, p. 177–207. *In* E. H. Lennette, P. Halonen, and F. A. Murphy (ed.), *Laboratory Diagnosis of Infectious Diseases*, vol. 2. *Viral, Rickettsial, and Chlamydial Diseases.* Springer-Verlag, New York, N.Y.
27. **Fenner, F., R. Wittek, and K. R. Dumbell.** 1989. *The Orthopoxviruses.* Academic Press, Inc., New York, N.Y.
28. **Goebel, S. J., G. P. Johnson, M. E. Perkus, S. W. Davis, J. P. Winslow, and E. Paoletti.** 1990. The complete DNA sequence of vaccinia virus. *Virology* **179:**247–266.
29. **Goebel, S. J., G. P. Johnson, M. E. Perkus, S. W. Davis,**

J. P. Winslow, and E. Paoletti. 1990. The complete DNA sequence of vaccinia virus. *Virology* **179:**517–563. (Appendix.)

30. **Ibrahim, M. S., J. J. Esposito, P. B. Jahrling, and R. S. Lofts.** 1997. The potential of 5′ nuclease PCR for detecting a single-base polymorphism in *Orthopoxvirus*. *Mol. Cell. Probes* **11:**143–147.
31. **Jezek, Z., I. Arita, M. Szczeniowski, K. M. Paluku, R. Kalisa, and J. H. Nakano.** 1985. Human tanapox in Zaire: clinical and epidemiological observations on cases confirmed by laboratory studies. *Bull. W. H. O.* **63:** 1027–1035.
32. **Jezek, Z., and F. Fenner.** 1988. Human monkeypox. *Monogr. Virol.*, **17:**1–140.
33. **Knight, J. C., R. F. Massung, and J. J. Esposito.** 1995. Polymerase chain reaction identification of smallpox virus, p. 297–302. *In* Y. Becker and G. Darai (ed.), *Diagnosis of Human Viruses by Polymerase Chain Reaction Technology*, 2nd ed. Springer-Verlag KG, Berlin, Germany.
34. **Knight, J. C., F. J. Novembre, D. R. Brown, C. S. Goldsmith, and J. J. Esposito.** 1989. Studies on Tanapox virus. *Virology* **172:**116–124.
35. **Massung, R. F., J. J. Esposito, L. Liu, Q. Jin, T. R. Utterback, J. C. Knight, L. Aubin, T. E. Yuran, J. M. Parsons, V. N. Loparev, N. A. Selivanov, K. F. Cavallaro, A. R. Kerlavage, B. W. J. Mahy, and J. C. Venter.** 1993. Potential virulence determinants in terminal regions of variola smallpox virus. *Nature* **366:**748–751.
36. **Massung, R. F., L.-I. Liu, J. Qi, J. C. Knight, T. E. Yuran, A. R. Kerlavage, J. M. Parsons, J. C. Venter, and J. J. Esposito.** 1994. Analysis of the complete genome of smallpox variola major virus strain Bangladesh-1975. *Virology* **201:**215–240.
37. **Massung, R. F., V. N. Loparev, J. C. Knight, A. V. Totmenin, V. E. Chizhikov, J. M. Parsons, P. F. Safronov, V. V. Gutorov, S. N. Shchelkunov, and J. J. Esposito.** 1996. Terminal region sequence variations in variola virus DNA. *Virology* **221:**291–300.
38. **Mathew, T.** 1987. *Advances in Medical and Veterinary Virology, Immunology and Epidemiology: Cultivation and Immunological Studies on Pox Group of Viruses with Special Reference to Buffalo Pox Virus.* Thajema Publishers, New Delhi, India.
39. **Meyer, H., M. Pfeffer, and H.-J. Rziha.** 1994. Sequence alterations within and downstream of the A-type inclusion protein genes allow differentiation of Orthopoxvirus species by polymerase chain reaction. *J. Gen. Virol.* **75:** 1975–1981.
40. **Meyer, H., S. L. Ropp, and J. J. Esposito.** 1998. Poxviruses, p. 199–211. *In* A. Warnes and J. Stephenson (ed.), *Methods in Molecular Medicine: Diagnostic Virology Protocols.* Humana Press, Totowa, N.J.
41. **Moss, B.** 1996. *Poxviridae* and their replication, p. 2637–2671. *In* B. N. Fields, D. M. Knipe, and P. M. Howley (ed.), *Fields' Virology*, 3rd ed. Raven Press, New York, N.Y.
42. **Mukinda, V. B. K., G. Mwema, M. Kilundu, D. L. Heymann, A. S. Khan, and J. J. Esposito.** 1997. Re-emergence of human monkeypox in Zaire in 1996. *Lancet* **349:** 1449–1450.
43. **Nakano, J. H.** 1978. Comparative diagnosis of poxvirus diseases, p. 267–339. *In* E. Kurstak and C. Kurstak (ed.), *Comparative Diagnosis of Viral Diseases*, vol. 1. Academic Press, Inc., New York, N.Y.
44. **Nakano, J. H.** 1979. Poxviruses, p. 257–308. *In* E. H. Lennette and N. J. Schmidt (ed.), *Diagnostic Procedures for Viral, Rickettsial, and Chlamydial Infections*, 5th ed. American Public Health Association, Inc., Washington, D.C.
45. **Nakano, J. H.** 1985. Poxviruses, p. 733–741. *In* E. H. Lennette, A. Balows, W. J. Hausler, Jr., and H. J. Shadomy (ed.), *Manual of Clinical Microbiology*, 4th ed. American Society for Microbiology, Washington, D.C.
46. **Nakano, J. H., and J. J. Esposito.** 1989. Poxviruses, p. 224–265. *In* N. J. Schmidt and R. W. Emmons (ed.), *Diagnostic Procedures for Viral, Rickettsial, and Chlamydial Infections*, 6th ed. American Public Health Association, Inc., Washington, D.C.
47. **Nunez, A., J. M. Funes, M. Agromayor, M. Moratilla, A. J. Varas, J. L. Lopez-Estebaranz, M. Esteban, and A. Martin-Gallardo.** 1996. Detection and typing of molluscum contagiosum virus in skin lesions by using a simple lysis method and polymerase chain reaction. *J. Med. Virol.* **50:**342–349.
48. **Pepose, J. S., and J. J. Esposito.** 1996. *Molluscum contagiosum*, Orf, and vaccinia virus ocular infections in humans, p. 846–856. *In* J. S. Pepose, G. N. Holland, and K. R. Wilhelmus (ed.), *Ocular Infection and Immunity.* Mosby-Year Book, Inc., St. Louis, Mo.
49. **Porter, C. D., and L. C. Archard.** 1992. Characterization by restriction mappings of three subtypes of molluscum contagiosum virus. *J. Med. Virol.* **38:**1–6.
50. **Porter, C. D., N. W. Blake, J. J. Cream, and L. C. Archard.** 1992. *Molluscum contagiosum* virus, p. 233–257. *In* D. Wright and L. C. Archard (ed.), *Molecular and Cell Biology of Sexually Transmitted Diseases*, Chapman & Hall, London, United Kingdom.
51. **Rice, C. M., C. A. Franke, J. H. Strauss, and D. E. Hruby.** 1985. Expression of Sindbis virus structural proteins via recombinant vaccinia virus: synthesis, processing, and incorporation into mature sindbis virus. *J. Virol.* **56:** 227–239.
52. **Robinson, A. J., and D. J. Lyttle.** 1992. Parapoxviruses: their biology and potential as recombinant vaccine vectors, p. 285–327. *In* M. M. Binns and G. L. Smith (ed.), *Recombinant Poxviruses.* CRC Press, Inc., Boca Raton, Fla.
53. **Ropp, S. L., Q. Jin, J. C. Knight, R. F. Massung, and J. J. Esposito.** 1995. PCR strategy for identification and differentiation of smallpox and other orthopoxviruses. *J. Clin. Microbiol.* **33:**2069–2076.
54. **Rosebrock, J. A.** 1991. Labeled-antibody techniques: fluorescent, radioisotopic, immunochemical, p. 79–86. *In* A. Balows, W. J. Hausler, K. L. Herrmann, H. D. Isenberg, and H. J. Shadomy (ed.), *Manual of Clinical Microbiology*, 5th ed. American Society for Microbiology, Washington, D.C.
55. **Rouhandeh, H.** 1988. Yaba virus, p. 1–15. *In* G. Darai (ed.), *Virus Diseases in Laboratory and Captive Animals.* Martinus Nijhoff, Boston, Mass.
56. **Senkevich, T. G., E. V. Koonin, J. J. Bugert, G. Darai, and B. Moss.** 1997. The genome of Molluscum contagiosum virus: analysis and comparison with other poxviruses. *Virology* **233:**19–42.
57. **Shchelkunov, S. N., S. S. Marennikova, V. M. Blinov, S. M. Resenchuk, A. V. Totmenin, V. E. Chizhikov, V. V. Gotorov, P. F. Sanfronov, R. K. Kurmanov, and L. S. Sandakhchiev.** 1993. Entire coding sequence of the variola virus. *Dokl. Akad. Nauk* **328:**629–632.
58. **Shchelkunov, S. N., R. F. Massung, and J. J. Esposito.** 1995. Comparison of the genome DNA sequences of Bangladesh-1975 and India-1967 variola viruses. *Virus Res.* **36:** 107–118.
59. **Smith, G. L.** 1993. Vaccinia virus glycoproteins and immune evasion. *J. Gen. Virol.* **74:**1725–1740.
60. **Towbin, H., T. Staehelin, and J. Gordon.** 1979. Electrophoretic transfer of proteins from SDS-PAGE to nitrocellulose sheets: procedure and some applications. *Proc. Natl. Acad. Sci. USA* **76:**4350–4354.
61. **Turner, P. C., and R. W. Moyer, (ed.).** 1990. Poxviruses. *Curr. Top. Microbiol. Immunol.* **163:**1–211.

62. **Westwood, J. C. N., P. H. Phipps, and E. A. Boulter.** 1957. The titration of vaccinia virus on the chorioallantoic membrane of the developing chick embryo. *J. Hyg.* **52:** 123–139.

63. **World Health Organization.** 1996. Monkeypox, Zaire. *Weekly Epidemiol. Rec.* **71:**326.

64. **World Health Organization.** 1996. Monkeypox, Zaire. *Weekly Epidemiol. Rec.* **72:**101–108.

65. **Zheng, Z. M., S. Specter, J. H. Zhang, H. Friedman, and W. P. Zhu.** 1992. Further characterization of the biological and pathogenic properties of erythromelalgia-related poxviruses. *J. Gen. Virol.* **73:**2011–2019.

Transmissible Spongiform Encephalopathies

DAVID M. ASHER

92

The transmissible spongiform encephalopathies (TSEs) comprise a group of at least three infectious diseases of humans and four infectious diseases of animals (Table 1)—diseases with roughly similar clinical courses and histopathologic findings (63). All are caused by similar unique pathogenic agents. The TSEs have been called "slow" infections—a term coined by Sigurdsson (168) to describe infectious diseases with long incubation periods and protracted clinical courses (months or years), fatal outcomes, pathologic findings restricted to a single organ system, and a limited range of susceptible hosts. The term "prion" was suggested as a designation for the pathogenic agents (154) in recognition of their association with at least one important protein. However, since the actual molecular structure of the pathogens remains unknown and disputed (39), they are called simply "TSE agents" in this review.

EPIDEMIOLOGY

Kuru was the most common cause of death in women of the Fore language group of Papua New Guinea in the 1950s and early 1960s and also affected many children of both sexes over the age of 4 years and a few men (65). The disease has almost completely disappeared among the Fore and has not affected anyone born after 1960 (108). This peculiar epidemiologic pattern suggests that the infection was naturally transmitted only by cannibalism, which ended in the late 1950s, and implies that the incubation period may be as short as 4 years or longer than 35 years.

Creutzfeldt-Jakob disease (CJD) (105) is an uncommon cause of dementia, affecting an estimated one per million per year or less in most populations studied, although frequencies in several isolated areas are more than 30 times higher (128). Males and females are affected in approximately equal numbers (23). The natural mechanisms of transmission for most cases of CJD—often called "sporadic" CJD (sCJD)—are not yet understood. A growing number of iatrogenic cases of CJD (iCJD) (Table 2) have been recognized (19, 21, 63): contaminated surgical instruments (143, 192), cortical electrodes (10), corneal transplants (56), dural grafts (35, 36, 54, 98, 124, 173, 197), and human pituitary hormones (19, 41, 62, 87, 125) have been implicated as the sources of iCJD in young people. (By experimentally transmitting CJD to animals, it was confirmed that at least one batch of growth hormone and an electrode remained contaminated years after their last use in humans [68, 69].) Incubation periods for iCJD as short as 14 months and longer than 20 years have been reported (Table 2).

Two instances of married couples with CJD (99, 129), two cases in neuropathology technicians (137, 169), and single cases in a neurosurgeon (64), a pathologist (77), and an oral surgeon (9) have been described. However, the empirical risk for medical personnel and for other contacts of CJD patients appears to be low.

Familial TSEs have an autosomal dominant pattern of occurrence. In tissues of subjects with familial TSEs, infectious agents with the same properties as TSE agents found in patients with sporadic and iatrogenic cases can be demonstrated. The fatal familial insomnia (FFI) syndrome differs from other TSEs in that although the disease has been transmitted from brain tissues of patients to rodents (43, 176), attempts to transmit the disease to monkeys have not succeeded (21).

The outbreak of bovine spongiform encephalopathy (BSE or "mad cow" disease) beginning in the United Kingdom in the mid-1980s has affected more than 170,000 cattle, apparently infected by accidental incorporation into cattle feed of contaminated meat- and bone meal-containing renderings of scrapie-infected sheep and later of cattle (16, 189). The epidemic appears to have peaked in late 1992, probably due to a ban on the feeding of ruminant proteins to cattle that began in the summer of 1988. (A similar precautionary ban was introduced in the United States in 1997.) Several continental European countries have also had smaller numbers of cases of BSE in native cattle. Early on, the BSE outbreak raised fears that a scrapie agent, having crossed one "species barrier" from sheep into cattle and later affecting other ungulates and domestic cats, might have broadened its range of susceptible hosts to include humans (3). This dread event seems to have occurred and is the most plausible explanation for a unique new variant of Creutzfeldt-Jakob disease (vCJD) among more than 20 adolescents and young adults, first reported in 1996 in the United Kingdom and France (38, 191). The appearance of a previously unrecognized variant of CJD with unique clinical and pathological features in a young age group sharing no apparent common risk factor except for their probable exposure to products potentially contaminated with the BSE agent suggests strongly that the BSE agent caused vCJD. Findings that both vCJD and naturally and experimentally

TABLE 1 TSEs of humans and animals

Disease	Naturally infected hosts
Creutzfeldt-Jakob disease	Humans
Sporadic CJD	
Iatrogenic CJD	
Familial CJD	
New-variant CJD	
Gerstmann-Sträussler-Scheinker syndrome	Humans
Kuru	Humans
Bovine spongiform encephalopathy	Cattle, zoo ungulates, zoo felines, domestic cats
Chronic wasting disease	American deer, elk
Scrapie	Sheep, goats
Transmissible mink encephalopathy	Mink

transmitted BSE stimulate the accumulation of abnormal proteins with an unusual glycosylation pattern (85) and transmit to mice a TSE with the same profile of neuropathologic lesions (27) provide additional evidence incriminating the BSE agent as the source of vCJD. The specific vehicle for transmission of vCJD has not been identified, but meat or a meat product, possibly contaminated with bovine neural tissue, seems most likely. The magnitude of the outbreak of vCJD in the United Kingdom cannot be predicted with confidence yet (44). A more modest increase in the diagnosis of sCJD has also been noted in the general population and among dairy workers in the United Kingdom (45); it is not clear whether this results from an increased prevalence of sCJD or from improved case finding. Neither BSE nor vCJD has been recognized in the United States in spite of active surveillance programs coordinated by the U.S. Department of Agriculture (52) and the Centers for Disease Control and Prevention (88, 165).

Scrapie is an important disease of sheep in the United Kingdom and on the European continent and has become increasingly common in American sheep in recent years (195). No epidemiologic evidence has implicated scrapie as a source of human CJD.

Transmissible mink encephalopathy (TME), last recognized in the United States in 1985, is postulated to have resulted from feeding contaminated beef to mink (122), and cattle were found to be susceptible to a variety of strains of scrapie from U.S. sheep (46); however, a survey of brains of more than 6,000 U.S. cattle with a variety of neurologic abnormalities (52) detected no evidence of naturally occurring TSE. Nothing is known about the origin of a scrapie-like chronic wasting disease (CWD) affecting both captive and wild American elk, white-tail deer, and mule deer in Colorado and Wyoming (170, 194); no link with scrapie has been established.

TABLE 2 Iatrogenic transmission of CJD by products of human origin

Product	No. of patients	Incubation time	
		Mean	Range
Cornea	2	17 mo	16–18 mo
Dura mater graft	47	7.4 yr	1.3–16 yr
Pituitary extract			
Growth hormone	>95[a]	12 yr	5–30 yr
Gonadotrophin	4	13 yr	12–16 yr

[a] 16 cases among ca. 8,000 estimated recipients in the United States.

CLINICAL PICTURE AND COURSE OF ILLNESS

Kuru (65) is characterized by progressive loss of coordination, cerebellar ataxia of the extremities and trunk, and a variety of signs of brain stem degeneration. There is little clinical evidence of cerebral cortex involvement and no frank dementia. Most patients have the shivering tremors that gave kuru its name in the Fore language. Convulsive seizures and myoclonic jerks have not been observed. Patients become progressively incapacitated and usually die from pneumonia, infected decubitus ulcers with septicemia, or accidental burns within a year of onset. The disease has never been recognized outside Papua New Guinea.

CJD was first described more than 70 years ago (105). sCJD typically affects middle-aged adults, although iatrogenically infected young adults and older adolescents have been described (17). The disease usually begins insidiously with vague complaints of sensory disturbance—particularly visual—or confusion. Patients become progressively demented, sometimes quite rapidly over only a few weeks. Most patients eventually have repetitive myoclonic jerking movements of the extremities and may have generalized "startle" myoclonus as well. Rigidity and pathologic cortical-release reflexes appear as the cerebral gray matter degenerates. A variety of other neurologic abnormalities, including convulsions and asymmetric weakness and spasticity that may suggest a space-occupying lesion, occur less commonly. Most patients die less than a year after onset, although a few patients survive much longer (21). Death usually results from pneumonia or one of the other complications to which patients with terminal neurologic diseases are subject. Remission of CJD has been claimed but never well documented. In many series of CJD, about 10% of patients have a family history of presenile dementia. Gerstmann-Sträussler-Scheinker syndrome (GSS) is an extremely rare familial spongiform encephalopathy with progressively severe cerebellar ataxia and relatively later onset of dementia (127). It may be considered a variant of familial CJD (fCJD). The new vCJD differs from typical sCJD in the clinical picture and course of illness as well as in the age at onset (Table 3) (191). Scrapie, TME, CWD, and BSE (and TSEs of cats and exotic ungulates attributed to exposure to BSE agent) resemble the human TSEs to some degree in clinical picture, clinical course, and histopathologic findings.

Patients with FFI (66, 117, 131, 132, 138), which is also extremely rare, have progressively severe insomnia and dysautonomia as well as ataxia, myoclonus, and other signs resembling those of CJD and GSS.

PATHOLOGY

The spongiform encephalopathies are all characterized by marked involvement of the central nervous system (CNS), which is most severe in the gray matter although there may be secondary loss of myelin and white matter involvement as well. The characteristic histopathologic feature is spongiform degeneration of the neuropil with neuronal vacuolation and loss of neurons (8, 29, 33, 110). It was the spongy

TABLE 3 Clinical and histopathological features of patients with new-variant CJD and typical sporadic CJD[a]

Clinical feature	New-variant CJD (10 patients)	Sporadic CJD (185 patients)
Age at death (yr), median (range)[b]	29 (19–41)	65
Duration of illness (mo), median (range)[b]	12 (8–23)	4
Presenting sign(s)	Abnormal behavior, dysesthesia	Dementia
Later signs	Dementia, ataxia, myoclonus	Ataxia, myoclonus
Periodic complexes on EEG	None	Most
% with PRNP codon 129 Met/Met	100	83
Histopathologic changes	Vacuolation, neuronal loss, astrocytosis, amyloid plaques (100%)	Vacuolation, neuronal loss, astrocytosis, amyloid plaques (~15%)
% with "florid" PrP plaques[c]	100	0
PrP glycosylation pattern	BSE-like[d]	Not BSE-like

[a] Modified from reference 191.
[b] Median age and duration for v-CJD, average for typical sporadic CJD.
[c] Dense plaques, pale periphery, surrounded by vacuolated cells.
[d] "Type 4" PrP (85) with excess of high-molecular-mass glycoform.

appearance of the cerebral gray matter that gave the group of diseases its name (71). Neuronal loss is accompanied by proliferation and hypertrophy of fibrillary astrocytes. The cerebellum is prominently involved in patients with kuru, GSS, and vCJD, with marked loss of Purkinje and granule cells. Some degree of cerebellar degeneration also occurs in patients with other types of CJD. Amyloid plaques are universally present in the brains of patients with GSS, very common in the brains of those with kuru (at least 70% of cases), and occasionally found in the brains of those with CJD (about 15% of cases); they are most often seen in the cerebellum but occur elsewhere as well. Brains of patients with vCJD have consistently contained peculiar amyloid plaques surrounded by daisy-like rings of vacuoles—termed "florid" plaques (110, 191); florid plaques are also common in brains of cervids with CWD (170) but have been rare in CJD patients (173) other than those with vCJD. It may be significant that florid plaques were also prominent in the brains of cynomolgus monkeys experimentally infected with the BSE agent (113) but not in the brains of cattle with naturally transmitted BSE. Inflammatory cells and changes of primary demyelination are notably lacking in the brains of patients with TSE. Patients with FFI have had selective atrophy of the anteroventral and medial-dorsal thalamic nuclei; only a few patients affected with FFI had spongiform changes in the cerebral cortex, and none had plaques.

An abnormal protein, relatively resistant to protease digestion, accumulates in the brains of patients with TSEs. The protein was first recognized morphologically by negative-stain electron microscopy as "scrapie-associated fibrils" (SAF) (134, 135) and later by sodium dodecyl sulfate-polyacrylamide gel electrophoresis as a unique band of protein with an apparent molecular mass of 27 to 30 kDa (14). The protein, designated PrP27-30 (130), was found to be a sialoglycoprotein (15) consisting of 55 amino acids (139) with attached carbohydrates, a neuraminic acid (15), and an inositol (172). Particularly in disease of long duration, this protein (most often referred to as "prion" protein [PrP]) is present in the amyloid plaques noted above—amorphous accumulations of proteinaceous material that demonstrates characteristic birefringence under polarized light when stained with Congo red. Antibodies prepared against PrP do not react with the amyloid plaques found in Alzheimer's disease and vice versa (151). Even in brains without plaques, immunostaining often reveals extracellular accumulations of PrP in subependymal and periventricular areas (49) and in the Golgi apparatus or endoplasmic reticulum of neurons (151).

The PrPs of various species are similar in amino acid sequence and antigenicity but are not identical (13). They are derived from larger precursor proteins of 253 amino acids, originally designated PrP33-35 (136), and later designated "control" PrP (PrP^{C}) in normal animals and PrP^{Sc} or PrP^{CJD} in animals with scrapie and CJD, respectively. To reduce confusion, since PrP^{Sc} and PrP^{CJD} generated in animals of the same species are identical to each other and to their protease-sensitive precursor PrP^{C} in amino acid sequence, some authorities prefer to call them protease-resistant PrP (PrP-res) and protease-sensitive PrP (PrP-sen), respectively. Since the amino acid sequences of PrP-sen and PrP-res are identical (145), the change in protease resistance must result in posttranslational alteration, the nature of which is still not fully understood. The conversion of PrP-sen to PrP-res is accompanied by a shift from a predominantly alpha-helical structure to a predominantly beta-sheet conformation (7, 150, 155, 162, 163). One model proposed that PrP-sen probably contained four alpha-helical structures (94); however, further analysis suggested that the folded 110-amino-acid domain where most known point mutation sites lie contains a two-stranded antiparallel beta-sheet and three alpha-helices (158). The connection between changes in folding of PrP and the infectious agents of the spongiform encephalopathies is under investigation. PrP-sen, secreted at the surface membranes of a variety of normal cells and rapidly catabolized by cells (34), is apparently not essential for normal life, although several subtle alterations of neurologic function have been observed in mice not expressing PrP (2). Mice not expressing PrP (PrP-null mice) are not susceptible to infection with TSE agents (30, 184).

PATHOGENESIS AND NATURAL TRANSMISSION

Most studies investigating the pathogenesis of the spongiform encephalopathies have been conducted with natural and experimental scrapie (57, 58, 79–82). The agent appears to enter the body through the integument; in sheep the intact intestinal tract may be a portal of entry as well. The agent appears to replicate first in local lymph nodes draining the portal of entry. Later it replicates in the spleen and other lymphoid organs throughout the body. Recent studies with immunodeficient mice and lymphocyte-reconstituted PrP-deficient transgenic mice suggest that lymphoid cells (180), specifically B lymphocytes (107), may be needed for a TSE agent to spread through the circulation to the CNS. The scrapie agent may also ascend peripheral nerves to enter the spinal cord directly (104), without involvement of lymphoid tissues. In any event, the TSE agents appear in the CNS only relatively late in the course of experimental infections initiated by the subcutaneous route, which is presumed to mimic natural disease most closely. In cattle with experimental orally transmitted BSE, agent has been found only in the CNS, trigeminal and dorsal root ganglia, eyes, and distal ileum (186), although bone marrow has been tentatively implicated as well. Infectious TSE agent has been found in several nonneural tissues and in cerebrospinal fluid (CSF) of patients dying of CJD (21); the tissue distribution and amounts of agent present during the prolonged incubation periods of TSEs in humans are not known.

Three authorities reported finding the TSE agent in blood of patients with CJD (119, 174, 175) as well as in humans without CJD (120); other studies failed to confirm those findings (21, 72). Epidemiologic studies found no convincing evidence that exposure to human blood or blood products constituted a risk factor for acquiring CJD (60, 88, 157). However, blood of some animals experimentally infected with TSEs was found to contain agent, probably in cellular elements (32, 111, 118). Patients with vCJD had a more prominent expression of PrP-res in lymphoid tissues than did those with sCJD; because of concern that pathogenesis of vCJD may differ from that of sCJD, potential infectivity of blood in subjects with that condition is under investigation. In no TSE have antibodies or cell-mediated immune response to the infectious agents been detected, nor has interferon been found.

Pregnant women with kuru or CJD have not transmitted the disease to their children (63). TME has also not been passed from infected mink to their offspring (123). Scrapie has not been transmitted from affected rodents to offspring in utero, although sheep can apparently be infected with scrapie in utero as well as by contact with affected animals after birth (51, 96). Cow-to-calf transmission does not appear to be a major factor in maintaining the current epidemic of BSE in the United Kingdom (42, 55, 190) but is suspected to occur; milk seems an unlikely vehicle for cow-to-calf transmission (179).

HOST GENETICS

CJD has long been recognized to occur in families (6); in most series, 5 or 10% of CJD patients have a family history of presenile dementia. Pedigrees of fCJD generally suggest an autosomal dominant mode of inheritance: the disease occurs without skipping generations and affects approximately half the siblings of patients, both males and females in equal numbers. GSS also shows an autosomal dominant pattern of inheritance (90). The genetic basis for fCJD and GSS appears to reside in a series of mutations in the gene coding for the PrP precursor protein, designated the PRNP gene, on the short arm of human chromosome 20. PRNP has an open reading frame of 759 nucleotides (253 codons), in which more than 10 point mutations and a variety of insertions have been linked to fCJD or GSS (155).

The importance in spongiform encephalopathies of the gene encoding PrP in animals was noted for experimental scrapie and later for CJD in mice (31, 188); the sinc gene, long known to control incubation periods of scrapie incubation in mice (97), was found to be closely linked if not identical to the PrP gene, and a similar close linkage was found between the PrP-encoding and scrapie incubation-period genes of sheep (95). In mice of some genotypes infected with certain strains of scrapie agent, the incubation periods were so long as to exceed the life span of the animal, producing a phenotype resistant to disease although not to inapparent infection (53).

The important role of the PrP gene in susceptibility to TSEs (possibly including the species barrier), incubation periods, and pathogenesis has been further clarified by a series of elegant studies with transgenic mice (155). Mice are ordinarily resistant to hamster-adapted strains of scrapie; however, when a portion of the PrP gene sequence from hamsters was engineered into mice, they acquired susceptibility to those strains and the agent recovered from mice had hamster-adapted biological properties (156). Increased expression in mice of an engineered PrP gene bearing a mutation similar to one found in most patients with GSS caused a disease resembling scrapie (92), and "serial" transmission of disease to hamsters and transgenic mice, although not to conventional mice, via relatively large amounts of brain tissue was claimed (91); a similar complex neurologic disease was also observed in mice expressing abnormal amounts of wild-type PrP (187). As noted above, PrP-null mice—not expressing PrP—were resistant to scrapie disease and to infection with TSE agent (30, 164, 185). Taken together, these findings convincingly demonstrate, among other things, that an animal must express PrP to be infected with a TSE agent and that the presence of wild-type PrP genes, the level of PrP transgene expression, and the sequence of the transgene can profoundly influence experimental TSE (181). (They have not convinced skeptics that PrP-res alone, whether generated by uninfected animals ov-

TABLE 4 Point mutations in PRNP gene associated with TSEs[a]

Codon	Normal amino acid	Mutant amino acid	Type of spongiform encephalopathy
178	Asp	Asn	fCJD
180	Val	Ile	fCJD
200[b]	Glu	Lys	fCJD
208	His	Arg	fCJD
210	Val	Ile	fCJD
232	Met	Arg	fCJD
102[b]	Pro	Leu	GSS
105	Pro	Leu	GSS
117	Ala	Val	GSS
145	Tyr	Stop[c]	GSS
198	Phe	Ser	GSS
217	Gln	Arg	GSS
129	Met or Val	Met or Val	fCJD/178Asn + 129Val FFI/178Asn + 129Met
117	Ala	Ala	?None[c]
124	Gly	Gly	?None
232	Met	Arg	?None

[a] Some information kindly provided by L. Cervenakova.

[b] The largest numbers of familial spongiform encephalopathies were associated with these mutations.

[c] Stop, stop codon/amber mutant; ?None, possible normal polymorphism.

erexpressing abnormal transgenes or extracted from tissues of TSE-infected conventional animals, is a self-replicating pathogen causing a TSE [39, 61].)

Owen et al. discovered an abnormal restriction endonuclease pattern in the PRNP genes of affected members in a family with typical autosomal dominant fCJD (147); Goldgaber et al. found that patients from other families with fCJD lacked that abnormality (76), suggesting that other mutations might also be involved. Owen et al. soon learned that their mutation was a large insertion of about 150 bases (146) in a region of five normal octapeptide tandem repeats between codons 51 and 91 of the PRNP gene (coding for six extra repeats there). Several other insertions in the octapeptide repeat region from 51 to 91, besides the six-octapeptide insertion first discovered, have also been associated with fCJD and GSS (73).

Hsaio et al. found a single nucleotide change in codon 102 of the PRNP gene (102^{Leu}, changing the encoded amino acid from proline to leucine) linked to GSS (90). Goldgaber et al. identified another point mutation in PRNP at codon 200 (200^{Lys}) that cosegregated with fCJD (75). 102^{Leu} and 200^{Lys} are the two most common point mutations associated with familial spongiform encephalopathies, but other point mutations (see Table 4 and Fig. 1) have also been found.

FFI was first described in a large northern Italian kindred and later in several others (66, 117, 131–133, 138). A protease-resistant PrP was detected in the brains of patients with FFI, although its cleavage product was slightly smaller than that of PrP found in CJD and GSS patients (138). In patients with FFI, a mutation was found in the PRNP gene at codon 178 (178^{Asn}), which was identical to that found in some kindreds with fCJD. However, the two groups of patients differed in PRNP sequences at another codon on the abnormal allele, codon 129 (a codon encoding methionine in some normal subjects and valine in others); FFI patients had 129^{Val} linked to 178^{Asn}, while fCJD patients had 129^{Met} (74, 132). It remains unknown how the same point mutation in one codon of a gene might interact with otherwise normal polymorphic nucleotides in another codon of the same gene to produce different clinical illnesses. As noted, FFI was not successfully transmitted to primates in several attempts (21), although two independent transmissions to mice were reported (43, 176).

Patients with iCJD and sCJD were much more often homozygous at codon 129 of the PRNP gene (>90%) than were subjects in the general population (about 50%) (50, 149), suggesting that homozygotes are more susceptible to CJD infection than are heterozygotes—although heterozygosity at that locus was found in some subjects with CJD. One series suggested that 129 Val homozygotes were overrepresented among subjects with iCJD but not those with sCJD (112). In a small series of patients with sporadic CJD, valine homozygotes were reported to have more pathologic charges in deep gray matter and methionine homozygotes were found to be more affected in the cerebral cortex (116). Thus far, all patients with vCJD to be genotyped were homozygotic for PRNP 129 Met (191). In addition to the methionine-valine polymorphism at codon 129 and a methionine-arginine polymorphism at codon 232 in normal subjects, there are other normal polymorphisms in the PRNP gene at codons 117 and 124 (silent differences, where both variants encode the same amino acid) and in the 51-to-91 octapeptide repeat region, where both deletions and short insertions of less than five extra repeats have been detected in healthy subjects (63). Recently, a new PRNP polymorphism—Glu or Lys at codon 219—was reported in Japan; each of 85

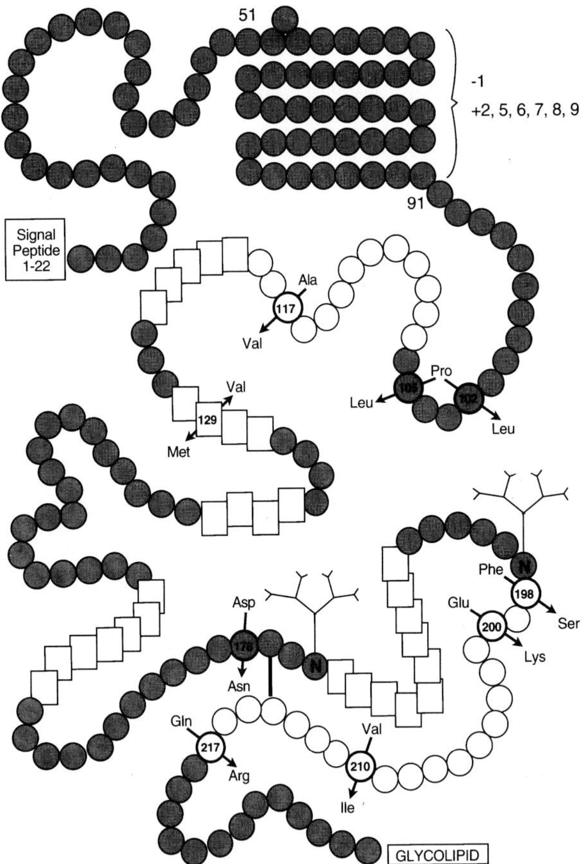

FIGURE 1 Schematic diagram of PrP, the prion protein, found in brains of humans and animals with TSEs. The 230-amino-acid backbone of PrP is depicted with the random turn and coil indicated by gray circles, the alpha-helix indicated by open circles, and the beta-sheet indicated by open rectangles. Cysteine residues 179 and 214 are linked by a disulfide bond, and sugar groups are attached to asparagines at positions 181 and 197. Important posttranslational modifications include the N-terminal cleavage of a 22-amino-acid signal peptide and replacement of a C-terminal 23-residue sequence by a glycophosphatidyl inositol, via which the protein is anchored to the cell membrane. Sites of several point mutations, insertions and deletions—some associated with disease and several found in normal subjects—are indicated by arrows and the bracket. Reprinted from reference 18 with permission of the publisher.

patients with sCJD was homozygous for Glu at codon 219, although some 12% of healthy Japanese subjects were heterozygous (167).

It should be noted that not all subjects with point mutations in the PRNP gene have expressed the disease, even in affected families. Penetrance appears to be quite high for GSS in family members with the 102^{Leu} mutation and for fCJD in those with the 178^{Asn} mutation and, when projected into advanced age, for the 200^{Lys} mutation (37, 171). Two healthy octogenarians having the 210^{Ile} mutation in a CJD-affected kindred have been described (152). Several members with the 178^{Asn} mutation in families with FFI also survived past the age of 60 years without showing signs of illness (66). It is not known if such unaffected family members bearing mutations in the PRNP gene have "inapparent" infections, perhaps due to exceptionally long incubation periods, or have escaped infection. Whatever the explanation, variations in the expression of disease must be kept in mind when dealing with unaffected family members.

INFECTIOUS AGENTS

The agents of the spongiform encephalopathies are unique in their physical properties. They are all experimentally transmissible to a variety of animals including monkeys and rodents (21). Although a variety of cell cultures have been infected with TSE agents (100, 153, 161), their use has been limited because the cells have displayed no cytopathic effects and the agents propagated to much lower titers in cultures than in brain tissue. Most studies characterizing the properties of TSE agents have used strains of scrapie agent adapted to mice and hamsters, which have incubation periods as short as 60 days and high infectivity titers in the brain (103).

The infectious agents display extreme resistance to physical inactivation by heat and by ionizing and UV radiation, as well as to chemical inactivation by a wide array of substances that destroy most viruses. This behavior, plus the fact that the agents show significant decrease in titers of infectivity after exposure to proteases (40) and other treatments that denature or degrade proteins (154, 155), has convinced many authorities they are probably replicating proteins devoid of nucleic acid (67, 78, 115, 155). Prusiner (154) suggested that these novel agents be called "prions" in recognition of their protein component and in anticipation that they would be found to lack nucleic acids. He and others preferring the all-protein hypothesis have emphasized that the aberrant physical behavior of the agents is inconsistent with properties of nucleic acids and that infectivity has seldom if ever been separated from the prion protein, which they propose to be the infectious agent itself (154, 155). Copious evidence supporting the prion hypothesis has been thoroughly reviewed by Prusiner, its originator and nomenclator (155), and the recent awarding of a Nobel Prize to him attests to the wide acceptance that his theory enjoys.

Other authorities remain unconvinced by the prion hypothesis (39) and skeptical of the evidence marshaled by its proponents for the following reasons. (i) Reinterpretation of irradiation-inactivation kinetic studies suggested that the presence of a small nucleic acid genome has not been excluded (160). (ii) No confirmed studies have demonstrated the physical size of the infectivity-bearing agent to be smaller than that of a small virus (70). (iii) No studies have convincingly demonstrated that a purified protein, uncontaminated with some nucleic acid from an infected host (102), contains the self-replicating agent of a spongiform encephalopathy. (iv) In several experimental systems, the kinetics of PrP-res formation failed to correlate with kinetics of infectivity (47, 114, 121, 141, 196). (v) The prion hypothesis has not yet satisfactorily explained the phenomenon of strain-like behavior by the spongiform encephalopathy agents. Various "strains" of the scrapie agent have properties (such as incubation period, distribution of histopathologic lesions, and presence or absence of visible amyloid-plaque formation) that "breed" true on passage in inbred mice (26, 61), and those properties have occasionally undergone sudden changes resembling the mutations that occur in the genomes of conventional pathogens. The molecular basis for such strain-like biological behavior is easily understood if the agents have small nucleic acid genomes but not if they consist entirely of a ubiquitous host-encoded protein like PrP, posttranslationally modified but without changes in normal primary amino acid structure.

Proponents of the prion hypothesis have put forth a variety of ingenious additional hypotheses to explain how proteins might transmit self-replicating information not encoded in their primary amino acid sequences (2); perhaps the most appealing is that differences in folding of PrP may be self-replicating through "template-directed" formation of a complex between molecules of PrP-res and PrP-sen induced to assume a specific and unique protease-resistant pathogenic conformation (126). (An additional factor, postulated to be a chaperone protein termed protein X, is proposed to play a role as well [100, 183].) There is limited experimental evidence supporting the hypothesis; two different strains of TME agent propagated in the same host species (hamsters) stimulated the accumulation of two different types of PrP-res, displaying different proteinase-K-cleavage sites (11); a similar finding was reported with an FFI agent (182). Self-propagation of differences in proteins is not without precedent: two stable characteristics, heritable through the cytoplasm, have been attributed to self-propagating conformational differences in proteins of fungi (89, 126), although such proteins are not known to be infectious. Skeptics, concerned that conformational differences in protein folding cannot account for the large number of strains of TSE agent—at least 20 for scrapie (39)—maintain that the TSE agents more probably contain small nucleic acid genomes (160) that remain to be discovered. Virus-like structures have been observed in sections of TSE brain tissues (48, 142), and tiny putatively virus-like particles were recently described in extracts of TSE tissues (148); however, such particles have never been convincingly associated with infectivity, and no unique nonhost nucleic acids have been identified in infectious materials. Thus, after more than 25 years of controversy, the nature of the TSE agents remains disputed.

LABORATORY DIAGNOSIS

The TSEs are generally diagnosed during life by their typical constellations of clinical findings. CJD should be suspected in a middle-aged patient (or in a younger person with a history of possible iatrogenic transmission or presenting in a setting suggestive of vCJD) having progressive dementia and myoclonic jerks. Later in disease, the electroencephalogram (EEG) frequently shows typical periodic high-voltage complexes on a slow and disorganized background (5). Periodic discharges have not been found in EEGs of patients with vCJD, which show only diffuse slowing (191).

Hematologic studies and clinical chemistries are unrevealing. The CSF often contains moderately increased amounts of protein, which is not diagnostic; the cell content of the CSF is normal. Two-dimensional electrophoresis and isoelectric focusing of CSF in gels followed by silver staining revealed the presence of two abnormal polypeptides (designated polypeptides 130 and 131) in CSF of most (although not all) patients with confirmed CJD but only rarely in those with Alzheimer's disease (12, 84, 198). The polypeptides have been identified as "14-3-3" protein (93)—a normal protein abundant in neurons and playing some role in the stabilization of other proteins. The 14-3-3 protein is not related to PrP. The finding of 14-3-3 protein in CSF was not specific for CJD; it was also common in CSF specimens from some patients with acute viral encephalitides and recent cerebral infarcts. In practice, the usual diagnostic problem is to differentiate between CJD and Alzheimer's disease, and the presence of 14-3-3 proteins in CSF militates against the latter. Finding the 14-3-3 protein in CSF was of some help in confirming the diagnosis of vCJD (193). Its value early in the course of CJD is not yet known. Immunoassay for 14-3-3 proteins in CSF is currently available only in research laboratories. The protein has not been detected in the serum of patients with CJD (93).

Definitive laboratory diagnosis of TSE can be made only from brain tissue. Histopathologic examination by a skilled and experienced neuropathologist remains the standard by which other tests must be judged (8, 29). In addition to evaluation of spongiform change in sections stained with hematoxylin and eosin, stains for astrocytes (immunostains for glial fibrillary acidic protein) and, especially, for PrP-res help in the diagnosis (33, 110). Immunostaining of PrP-res may be enhanced by pretreating sections with formic acid (106) or autoclaving (83, 177). A recent report suggested that detection of PrP-res in lymphoid tissues may provide early diagnosis of scrapie in sheep (140, 166); possible diagnosis of vCJD from tonsil biopsy specimens has been suggested (86). The demonstration of PrP-res in brains of patients with progressive dementia by Western immunoblotting has been especially useful in confirming the diagnosis of spongiform encephalopathy (20) and is probably more sensitive than immunohistochemical staining of tissue sections (110). Unfortunately, at present the techniques for detecting PrP-res remain available only by special arrangement with research laboratories. Well-characterized antibodies and improved methods have been described (101). A monoclonal antibody that reacts with PrP-res but not PrP-sen (109) may eventually facilitate the detection of PrP-res by allowing selective affinity binding without the need for protease digestion.

Inoculation of brain tissue suspensions intracerebrally into susceptible animals with induction of typical spongiform encephalopathy is diagnostic but extremely time-consuming and expensive; for example, squirrel monkeys, perhaps the most consistently susceptible to experimental CJD agent among commercially available animals (4), must be observed for at least 3 years before a transmission attempt is considered tentatively negative. Most attempts to transmit disease to rodents from patients with well-documented cases of sCJD have been unsuccessful. Attempts at primary transmission to animals have sometimes been confusing because of problems with contamination in laboratories where the agents of spongiform encephalopathies are studied.

LABORATORY SAFETY

Although, as discussed above, the risk to laboratory personnel of accidental infection with spongiform encephalopathy agents appears to be very low, potentially contaminated tissues should be handled with caution because of the uniformly fatal outcome of the diseases, the extreme resistance of the etiologic agents to disinfection, and the difficulty of detecting their presence (28). The introduction of universal precautions into medical laboratories responsible for testing of human tissues and body fluids (144) may reduce the risk of accidental infection with the spongiform encephalopathy agents. Whenever possible, disposable materials should be used and discarded carefully, if possible by incineration, by laboratories handling potentially contaminated specimens. Although the spongiform encephalopathy agents may not be completely destroyed by heat, even at very high temperatures (22), titers of infectivity are reduced markedly by heating (159); at least 2 h in the stream autoclave at ≥132°C is currently recommended to decontaminate objects that withstand such treatment. The infectivity titers of spongiform encephalopathy agents are also reduced substantially by exposure to 5.25% sodium hypochlorite (undiluted household chlorine bleach) (178) and sodium hydroxide (24) (2 M or stronger is often recommended). A commercial phenolic disinfectant was reported to be very effective in inactivating the scrapie agent (59) but is not currently available.

The same formic acid treatment reported to improve immunostaining of PrP-res and other amyloids in tissue sections significantly reduces the infectivity of TSE agents as well (25); such treatment is now used by most pathology laboratories handling cases of potential TSE. Protocols for safely obtaining and processing tissues from cases of TSE are available through the Internet. (The College of American Pathologists provides such a protocol through its site on the World Wide Web at http://www.cap.org/html/publications/cjd.html.) A standard operating procedure for safe handling of materials potentially contaminated with TSE agents that is suitable for use by microbiology laboratories has been made available by the Office of Environmental Health and Safety of the University of California at San Francisco (http://www.ehs.ucsf.edu/manuals/BSM/appendix%20L.html#appendixL2). A regimen of postexposure prophylaxis, based on conclusions of studies of experimental pathogenesis of TSEs and of chemical treatments known to inactivate TSE agents, was recently recommended (1) but has not been validated.

REFERENCES

1. **Aguzzi, A., and J. Collinge.** 1997. Post-exposure prophylaxis after accidental prion inoculation. *Lancet* **350:** 1519–1520.
2. **Aguzzi, A., and C. Weissmann.** 1997. Prion research: the next frontiers. *Nature* **389:**795–798.
3. **Asher, D. M.** 1991. Slow viral infections of the central nervous system, p. 145–166. *In* W. M. Scheld, R. J. Whitley, and D. T. Durack (ed.), *Infections of the Central Nervous System*. Raven Press, New York, N.Y.
4. **Asher, D. M.** 1993. Transmission of human spongiform encephalopathies to experimental animals: comparison of the chimpanzee and squirrel monkey. *Dev. Biol. Stand.* **80:** 9–13.
5. **Asher, D. M.** 1997. Slow viral infections of the human nervous system, p. 199–221. *In* W. M. Scheld, R. J. Whitley, and D. T. Durack (ed.), *Infections of the Central Nervous System*. Raven Press, New York, N.Y.
6. **Asher, D. M., C. L. Masters, D. C. Gajdusek, and C. J. Gibbs, Jr.** 1983. Familial spongiform encephalopathies, p. 273–291. *In* S. Kety, L. Rowland, R. Sidman, and S. Matthysse (ed.), *Genetics of Neurological and Psychiatric Disorders*. Raven Press, New York, N.Y.
7. **Baldwin, M. A., K. M. Pan, J. Nguyen, Z. W. Huang, D. Groth, A. Serban, M. Gasset, I. Mehlhorn, R. J. Fletterick, F. G. Cohen, and S. B. Prusiner.** 1994. Spectroscopic characterization of conformational differences between PrPc and PrPsc—an alpha-helix to beta-sheet transition. *Philos. Trans. R. Soc. London Sect. B* **343:** 435–441.
8. **Bell, J. E., and J. W. Ironside.** 1993. Neuropathology of spongiform encephalopathies in humans. *Br. Med. Bull.* **49:**738–777.
9. **Berger, J. R., and N. J. David.** 1993. Creutzfeldt-Jakob disease in a physician—a review of the disorder in health care workers. *Neurology* **43:**205–206.
10. **Bernoulli, C., J. Siegfried, G. Baumgartner, F. Regli, T.**

Rabinowics, D. C. Gajdusek, and C. J. Gibbs, Jr. 1977. Danger of accidental person-to-person transmission of Creutzfeldt-Jakob disease by surgery. *Lancet* **i:**478–479.

11. **Bessen, R. A., D. A. Kocisko, G. J. Raymond, S. Nandan, P. T. Lansbury, and B. Caughey.** 1995. Non-genetic propagation of strain-specific properties of scrapie prion protein. *Nature* **375:**698–700.
12. **Blisard, K., L. Davis, M. Harrington, J. Lovell, M. Kornfeld, and M. Berger.** 1990. Pre-mortem diagnosis of Creutzfeldt-Jakob disease by detection of abnormal cerebrospinal fluid proteins. *J. Neurol. Sci.* **99:**75–81.
13. **Bode, L., M. Pocchiari, H. Gelderblom, and H. Diringer.** 1985. Characterization of antisera against scrapie-associated fibrils (SAF) from affected hamster and cross-reactivity with SAF from scrapie-affected mice and from patients with Creutzfeldt-Jakob disease. *J. Gen. Virol.* **66:**2471–2478.
14. **Bolton, D. C., M. P. McKinley, and S. B. Prusiner.** 1982. Identification of a protein that purifies with the scrapie prion. *Science* **218:**1309–1311.
15. **Bolton, D. C., R. K. Meyer, and S. B. Prusiner.** 1985. Scrapie PrP 27–30 is a sialoglycoprotein. *J. Virol.* **53:** 596–606.
16. **Bradley, R., and J. W. Wilesmith.** 1993. Epidemiology and control of bovine spongiform encephalopathy (BSE). *Br. Med. Bull.* **49:**932–959.
17. **Brown, P.** 1990. Iatrogenic Creutzfeldt-Jakob disease. *Aust. N. Z. J. Med.* **20:**633–635.
18. **Brown, P.** 1994. The "brave new world" of transmissible spongiform encephalopathy (infectious cerebral amyloidosis). *Mol. Neurobiol.* **8:**79–87.
19. **Brown, P., L. Cervenáková, L. G. Goldfarb, W. R. McCombie, R. Rubenstein, R. G. Will, M. Pocchiari, J. F. Martinez-Lage, C. Scalici, C. Masullo, G. Graupera, J. Ligan, and D. C. Gajdusek.** 1994. Iatrogenic Creutzfeldt-Jakob disease—an example of the interplay between ancient genes and modern medicine. *Neurology* **44:**291–293.
20. **Brown, P., M. Coker-Vann, K. Pomeroy, M. Franko, D. M. Asher, C. J. Gibbs, Jr., and D. C. Gajdusek.** 1986. Diagnosis of Creutzfeldt-Jakob disease by Western blot identification of marker protein in human brain tissue. *N. Engl. J. Med.* **314:**547–551.
21. **Brown, P., C. J. Gibbs, Jr., P. Rodgers-Johnson, D. M. Asher, M. P. Sulima, A. Bacote, L. G. Goldfarb, and D. C. Gajdusek.** 1994. Human spongiform encephalopathy: the NIH series of 300 cases of experimentally transmitted disease. *Ann. Neurol.* **35:**513–529.
22. **Brown, P., P. P. Liberski, A. Wolff, and D. C. Gajdusek.** 1990. Resistance of scrapie infectivity to steam autoclaving after formaldehyde fixation and limited survival after ashing at 360°C: practical and theoretical implications. *J. Infect. Dis.* **161:**467–472.
23. **Brown, P., M. A. Preece, and R. G. Will.** 1992. Friendly fire in medicine—hormones, homografts, and Creutzfeldt-Jakob disease. *Lancet* **340:**24–27.
24. **Brown, P., R. Rohwer, and D. Gajdusek.** 1984. Sodium hydroxide disinfection of Creutzfeldt-Jakob disease virus. *N. Engl. J. Med.* **310:**727.
25. **Brown, P., A. Wolff, and D. C. Gajdusek.** 1990. A simple and effective method for inactivating virus infectivity in formalin-fixed tissue samples from patients with Creutzfeldt-Jakob disease. *Neurology* **40:**887–890.
26. **Bruce, M. E.** 1993. Scrapie strain variation and mutation. *Br. Med. Bull.* **49:**822–838.
27. **Bruce, M. E., R. G. Will, J. W. Ironside, I. McConnell, D. Drummond, A. Suttie, L. McCardle, A. Chree, J. Hope, C. Birkett, S. Cousens, H. Fraser, and C. J. Bostock.** 1997. Transmissions to mice indicate that 'new variant' CJD is caused by the BSE agent. *Nature* **389:**498–501.
28. **Budka, H., A. Aguzzi, P. Brown, J. M. Brucher, O. Bugiani, J. Collinge, H. Diringer, F. Gullotta, M. Haltia, J.-J. Hauw, J. W. Ironside, H. A. Kretzschmar, P. L. Lantos, C. Masullo, M. Pocchiari, W. Schlote, J. Tateishi, and R. G. Will.** 1995. Tissue handling in suspected Creutzfeldt-Jakob disease (CJD) and other human spongiform encephalopathies (prion diseases). *Brain Pathol. (Zurich)* **5:** 319–322.
29. **Budka, H., A. Aguzzi, P. Brown, J. M. Brucher, O. Bugiani, F. Gullotta, M. Haltia, J.-J. Hauw, J. W. Ironside, K. Jellinger, H. A. Kretzschmar, P. L. Lantos, C. Masullo, W. Schlote, J. Tateishi, and R. O. Weller.** 1995. Neuropathological diagnostic criteria for Creutzfeldt-Jakob disease (CJD) and other human spongiform encephalopathies (prion diseases). *Brain Pathol. (Zurich)* **5:**459–466.
30. **Büeler, H., A. Aguzzi, A. Sailer, R. A. Greiner, P. Autenried, M. Aguet, and C. Weissmann.** 1993. Mice devoid of PrP are resistant to scrapie. *Cell* **73:**1339–1347.
31. **Carlson, G. A., D. T. Kingsbury, P. A. Goodman, S. Coleman, S. T. Marshall, S. DeArmond, D. Westaway, and S. B. Prusiner.** 1986. Linkage of prion protein and scrapie incubation time genes. *Cell* **46:**503–511.
32. **Casaccia, P., A. Ladogana, X. G. Xi, and M. Pocchiari.** 1989. Levels of infectivity in the blood throughout the incubation period of hamsters peripherally injected with scrapie. *Arch. Virol.* **108:**145–149.
33. **Castellani, R., P. Parchi, J. Stahl, S. Capellari, M. Cohen, and P. Gambetti.** 1996. Early pathologic and biochemical changes in Creutzfeldt-Jakob disease: study of brain biopsies. *Neurology* **46:**1690–1693.
34. **Caughey, B., R. E. Race, D. Ernst, M. J. Buchmeier, and B. Chesebro.** 1989. Prion protein biosynthesis in scrapie-infected and uninfected neuroblastoma cells. *J. Virol.* **63:** 175–181.
35. **Centers for Disease Control and Prevention.** 1997. Creutzfeldt-Jakob disease associated with cadaveric dura mater grafts—Japan, January 1979–May 1996. *Morbid. Mortal. Weekly Rep.* **46:**1066–1069.
36. **Centers for Disease Control and Prevention.** 1998. Creutzfeldt-Jakob disease associated with cadaveric dura mater grafts—Japan, January 1979–May 1996. *JAMA* **279:** 11–12.
37. **Chapman, J., J. Ben-Israel, Y. Goldhammer, and A. D. Korczyn.** 1994. The risk of developing Creutzfeldt-Jakob disease in subjects with the PRNP gene codon 200 point mutation. *Neurology* **44:**1683–1686.
38. **Chazot, G., E. Broussolle, C. Lapras, T. Blattler, A. Aguzzi, and N. Kopp.** 1996. New variant of Creutzfeldt-Jakob disease in a 26-year-old French man. *Lancet* **347:** 1181. (Letter.)
39. **Chesebro, B.** 1998. BSE and prions: uncertainties about the agent. *Science* **279:**42–43.
40. **Cho, H. J.** 1980. Requirement of a protein component for scrapie infectivity. *Intervirology* **14:**213–216.
41. **Cochius, J. I., N. Hyman, and M. M. Esiri.** 1992. Creutzfeldt-Jakob disease in a recipient of human pituitary-derived gonadotrophin—a second case. *J. Neurol. Neurosurg. Psychiatry* **55:**1094–1095.
42. **Collee, J. G., and R. Bradley.** 1997. BSE: a decade on—part 2. *Lancet* **349:**715–721.
43. **Collinge, J., M. S. Palmer, K. C. Sidle, I. Gowland, R. Medori, J. Ironside, and P. Lantos.** 1995. Transmission of fatal familial insomnia to laboratory animals. *Lancet* **346:** 569–570.
44. **Cousens, S. N., E. Vynnycky, M. Zeidler, R. G. Will, and P. G. Smith.** 1997. Predicting the CJD epidemic in humans. *Nature* **385:**197–198.
45. **Cousens, S. N., M. Zeidler, T. F. Esmonde, R. De Silva, J. W. Wilesmith, P. G. Smith, and R. G. Will.** 1997.

Sporadic Creutzfeldt-Jakob disease in the United Kingdom: analysis of epidemiological surveillance data for 1970–96. *Br. Med. J.* [*Clin. Res.*] **315:**389–395.

46. **Cutlip, R. C., J. M. Miller, R. E. Race, A. L. Jenny, J. B. Katz, H. D. Lehmkuhl, B. M. Debey, and M. M. Robinson.** 1994. Intracerebral transmission of scrapie to cattle. *J. Infect. Dis.* **169:**814–820.
47. **Czub, M., H. R. Braig, and H. Diringer.** 1988. Replication of the scrapie agent in hamsters infected intracerebrally confirms the pathogenesis of an amyloid-inducing virosis. *J. Gen. Virol.* **69:**1753–1756.
48. **David-Ferreira, J. F., K. L. David-Ferreira, C. J. Gibbs, Jr., and J. A. Morris.** 1968. Scrapie in mice: ultrastructural observations in the cerebral cortex. *Proc. Soc. Exp. Biol. Med.* **28:**313–320.
49. **DeArmond, S. J., M. P. McKinley, R. A. Barry, M. B. Braunfeld, J. R. McColloch, and S. B. Prusiner.** 1985. Identification of prion amyloid filaments in scrapie-infected brain. *Cell* **41:**221–235.
50. **Deslys, J. P., D. Marce, and D. Dormont.** 1994. Similar genetic susceptibility in iatrogenic and sporadic Creutzfeldt-Jakob disease. *J. Gen. Virol.* **75:**23–27.
51. **Detwiler, L. A.** 1992. Scrapie. *Rev. Sci. Technol.* **11:**491–537.
52. **Detwiler, L. A.** 1997. Update on BSE contingency plan. *J. Am. Vet. Assoc.* **211:**837.
53. **Dickinson, A. G., H. Fraser, and G. W. Outram.** 1979. Scrapie incubation time can exceed natural lifespan. *Nature* **256:**732–733.
54. **Diringer, H., and H. R. Braig.** 1989. Infectivity of unconventional viruses in dura mater. *Lancet* **i:**439–440.
55. **Donnelly, C. A., A. C. Ghani, N. M. Ferguson, R. M. Anderson, N. M. Ferguson, C. A. Donnelly, M. E. Woolhouse, and R. M. Anderson.** 1997. Recent trends in the BSE epidemic. The epidemiology of BSE in cattle herds in Great Britain. II. Model construction and analysis of transmission dynamics. *Nature* **389:**903.
56. **Duffy, P., G. Collins, A. G. Devoe, B. Streeten, and D. Cohen.** 1974. Possible person-to-person transmission of Creutzfeldt-Jakob disease. *N. Engl. J. Med.* **290:**693.
57. **Eklund, C. M., W. J. Hadlow, and R. C. Kennedy.** 1963. Some properties of the scrapie agent and its behavior in mice. *Proc. Soc. Exp. Biol. Med.* **112:**974–979.
58. **Eklund, C. M., R. C. Kennedy, and W. J. Hadlow.** 1967. Pathogenesis of scrapie virus infection in the mouse. *J. Infect. Dis.* **117:**15–22.
59. **Ernst, D. R., and R. E. Race.** 1993. Comparative analysis of scrapie agent inactivation methods. *J. Virol. Methods* **41:**193–201.
60. **Esmonde, T. F. G., R. G. Will, J. M. Slattery, R. Knight, R. Harries Jones, R. Desilva, and W. B. Matthews.** 1993. Creutzfeldt-Jakob disease and blood transfusion. *Lancet* **341:**205–207.
61. **Farquhar, C. F., R. A. Somerville, and M. E. Bruce.** 1998. Straining the prion hypothesis. *Nature* **391:**345–346.
62. **Fradkin, J. E., L. B. Schonberger, J. L. Mills, W. J. Gunn, J. M. Piper, D. K. Wysowski, R. Thomson, S. Durako, and P. Brown.** 1991. Creutzfeldt-Jakob disease in pituitary growth hormone recipients in the United States. *JAMA* **265:**880–884.
63. **Gajdusek, D. C.** 1996. Infectious amyloids. Subacute spongiform encephalopathies as transmissible cerebral amyloidoses, p. 2851–2900. *In* B. N. Fields and D. M. Knipe (ed.), *Virology*. Raven Press, New York, N.Y.
64. **Gajdusek, D. C., C. J. Gibbs, Jr., K. Earle, G. J. Dammin, W. C. Schoene, and H. R. Tyler.** 1974. Transmission of subacute spongiform encephalopathy to the chimpanzee and squirrel monkey from a patient with papulosis maligna of Köhlmeyer-Degos. *Excerpta Med. Int. Congr. Ser.* **319:**390–392.
65. **Gajdusek, D. C., and V. Zigas.** 1957. Degenerative disease of the central nervous system in New Guinea: epidemic occurrence of "kuru" in the native population. *N. Engl. J. Med.* **257:**974–978.
66. **Gambetti, P., R. Petersen, L. Monari, M. Tabaton, L. Autilio Gambetti, P. Cortelli, P. Montagna, and E. Lugaresi.** 1993. Fatal familial insomnia and the widening spectrum of prion diseases. *Br. Med. Bull.* **49:**980–994.
67. **Gibbons, R. A., and G. D. Hunter.** 1967. Nature of the scrapie agent. *Nature* **215:**1041–1043.
68. **Gibbs, C. J., Jr., D. M. Asher, P. W. Brown, J. E. Fradkin, and D. C. Gajdusek.** 1993. Creutzfeldt-Jakob disease infectivity of growth hormone derived from human pituitary glands. *N. Engl. J. Med.* **328:**358–359.
69. **Gibbs, C. J., Jr., D. M. Asher, A. Kobrine, H. L. Amyx, and D. C. Gajdusek.** 1994. Transmission of Creutzfeldt-Jakob disease to a chimpanzee by electrodes contaminated during neurosurgery. *J. Neurol. Neurosurg. Psychiatry* **57:**757–758.
70. **Gibbs, C. J., Jr., and D. C. Gajdusek.** 1971. Transmission and characterization of the agents of spongiform virus encephalopathies: kuru, Creutzfeldt-Jakob disease, scrapie and mink encephalopathy. *Res. Publ. Assoc. Res. Nerv. Ment. Dis.* **49:**383–410.
71. **Gibbs, C. J., Jr., D. C. Gajdusek, D. M. Asher, M. P. Alpers, E. Beck, P. M. Daniel, and W. B. Matthews.** 1968. Creutzfeldt-Jakob disease (spongiform encephalopathy): transmission to the chimpanzee. *Science* **161:**388–389.
72. **Godec, M. S., D. M. Asher, W. E. Kozachuk, C. L. Masters, J. U. Rubi, J. A. Payne, D. J. Rubi Villa, E. E. Wagner, S. I. Rapoport, and M. B. Schapiro.** 1994. Blood buffy coat from Alzheimer's disease patients and their relatives does not transmit spongiform encephalopathy to hamsters. *Neurology* **44:**1111–1115.
73. **Goldfarb, L. G., P. Brown, and D. C. Gajdusek.** 1992. The molecular genetics of human transmissible spongiform encephalopathy, p. 139–153. *In* S. B. Prusiner, J. Collinge, J. Powell, and B. Anderton (ed.), *Prion Diseases of Humans and Animals*. Ellis Horwood Ltd., Chichester, United Kingdom.
74. **Goldfarb, L. G., R. B. Petersen, M. Tabaton, P. Brown, A. C. LeBlanc, P. Montagna, P. Cortelli, J. Julien, C. Vital, W. W. Pendelbury, M. Haltia, P. R. Wills, J.-J. Hauw, P. E. McKeever, L. Monari, B. Schrank, G. D. Swergold, L. Autilio-Gambetti, D. C. Gajdusek, E. Lugaresi, and P. Gambetti.** 1992. Fatal familial insomnia and familial Creutzfeldt-Jakob disease: disease phenotype determined by a DNA polymorphism. *Science* **258:**806–808.
75. **Goldgaber, D., L. G. Goldfarb, P. Brown, D. M. Asher, W. T. Brown, W. S. Lin, J. W. Teener, S. M. Feinstone, R. Rubenstein, R. J. Kascsak, J. W. Boellard, and D. C. Gajdusek.** 1989. Mutations in familial Creutzfeldt-Jakob disease and Gerstmann-Sträussler-Scheinker's syndrome. *Exp. Neurol.* **106:**204–206.
76. **Goldgaber, D., J. W. Teener, L. G. Goldfarb, D. M. Asher, P. W. Brown, S. Feinstone, and D. C. Gajdusek.** 1988. No Msp 1 polymorphism in the open reading frame of the PrP gene in patients with familial Creutzfeldt-Jakob disease. *Alzheimer Dis. Assoc. Disord.* **2:**311.
77. **Gorman, D. G., D. F. Benson, D. G. Vogel, and H. V. Vinters.** 1992. Creutzfeldt-Jakob disease in a pathologist. *Neurology* **42:**463.
78. **Griffith, J. S.** 1967. Self-replication and scrapie. *Nature* **215:**1043–1044.
79. **Hadlow, W. J., R. C. Kennedy, T. A. Jackson, H. W. Whitford, and C. C. Boyle.** 1974. Course of experimental

scrapie virus infection in the goat. *J. Infect. Dis.* **129:** 559–567.

80. **Hadlow, W. J., R. C. Kennedy, and R. E. Race.** 1982. Natural infection of Suffolk sheep with scrapie virus. *J. Infect. Dis.* **146:**657–664.

81. **Hadlow, W. J., R. C. Kennedy, R. E. Race, and C. M. Eklund.** 1980. Virologic and neurohistologic findings in dairy goats affected with natural scrapie. *Vet. Pathol.* **17:** 187–199.

82. **Hadlow, W. J., R. E. Race, R. C. Kennedy, and C. M. Eklund.** 1979. Natural infection of sheep with scrapie virus, p. 3–12. *In* S. B. Prusiner and W. J. Hadlow (ed.), *Slow Transmissible Diseases of the Nervous System*, vol. 2. Academic Press, Inc., New York. N.Y.

83. **Haritani, M., Y. I. Spencer, and G. A. H. Wells.** 1994. Hydrated autoclave pretreatment enhancement of prion protein immunoreactivity in formalin-fixed bovine spongiform encephalopathy-affected brain. *Acta Neuropathol. (Berlin)* **87:**86–90.

84. **Harrington, M. G., C. R. Merril, D. M. Asher, and D. C. Gajdusek.** 1986. Abnormal proteins in the cerebrospinal fluid of patients with Creutzfeldt-Jakob disease. *N. Engl. J. Med.* **315:**279–283.

85. **Hill, A. F., M. Desbruslais, S. Joiner, K. C. L. Sidle, I Gowland, J. Collinge, L. J. Doey, and P. Lantos.** 1997. The same prion strain causes vCJD and BSE. *Nature* **389:** 448–450, 526.

86. **Hill, A. F., M. Zeidler, J. Ironside, and J. Collinge.** 1997. Diagnosis of new variant Creutzfeldt-Jakob disease by tonsil biopsy. *Lancet* **349:**99–100.

87. **Hintz, R., M. MacGillivray, A. Joy, and R. Tintner.** 1985. Fatal degenerative neurological disease in patients who received pituitary-derived human growth hormone. *Morbid. Mortal. Weekly Rep.* **34:**359–366.

88. **Holman, R. C., A. S. Khan, E. D. Belay, and L. B. Schonberger.** 1996. Creutzfeldt-Jakob disease in the United States, 1979–1994: using national mortality data to assess the possible occurrence of variant cases. *Emerg. Infect. Dis.* **2:**333–337.

89. **Horwich, A. L., and J. S. Weissman.** 1997. Deadly conformations—protein misfolding in prion disease. *Cell* **89:** 499–510.

90. **Hsiao, K., H. F. Baker, T. J. Crow, M. Poulter, F. Owen, J. D. Terwilliger, D. Westaway, J. Ott, and S. B. Prusiner.** 1989. Linkage of a prion protein missense variant to Gerstmann-Sträussler syndrome. *Nature* **338:**342–345.

91. **Hsiao, K. K., D. Groth, M. Scott, S. L. Yang, H. Serban, D. Raff, D. Foster, M. Torchia, S. J. DeArmond, and S. B. Prusiner.** 1994. Serial transmission in rodents of neurodegeneration from transgenic mice expressing mutant prion protein. *Proc. Natl. Acad. Sci. USA* **91:**9126–9130.

92. **Hsiao, K. K., M. Scott, D. Foster, D. F. Groth, S. J. DeArmond, and S. B. Prusiner.** 1990. Spontaneous neurodegeneration in transgenic mice with mutant prion protein. *Science* **250:**1587–1590.

93. **Hsich, G., K. Kenney, C. J. Gibbs, K. H. Lee, and M. G. Harrington.** 1996. The 14-3-3 brain protein in cerebrospinal fluid as a marker for transmissible spongiform encephalopathies. *N. Engl. J. Med.* **335:**924–930.

94. **Huang, Z. W., J. M. Gabriel, M. A. Baldwin, R. J. Fletterick, S. B. Prusiner, and F. E. Cohen.** 1994. Proposed three-dimensional structure for the cellular prior protein. *Proc. Natl. Acad. Sci. USA* **91:**7139–7143.

95. **Hunter, N., J. D. Foster, A. G. Dickinson, and J. Hope.** 1989. Linkage of the gene for the scrapie-associated fibril protein (PrP) to the Sip gene in Cheviot sheep. *Vet. Rec.* **124:**364–366.

96. **Hunter, N., J. D. Foster, W. Goldmann, M. J. Stear, J. Hope, and C. Bostock.** 1996. Natural scrapie in a closed flock of Cheviot sheep occurs only in specific PrP geno types. *Arch. Virol.* **141:**809–824.

97. **Hunter, N., J. Hope, I. McConnell, and A. G. Dickinson.** 1987. Linkage of the scrapie-associated fibril protein (PrP) gene and Sinc using congenic mice and restriction fragment length polymorphism analysis. *J. Gen. Virol.* **68:** 2711–2716.

98. **Janssen, R. B., and L. B. Schonberger.** 1991. Creutzfeldt-Jakob disease from allogeneic dura: a review of risks and safety. *J. Oral Maxillofac. Surg.* **49:**274–275.

99. **Jellinger, K., F. Seitelberger, W.-D. Heiss, and W. Holczabek.** 1972. Konjugale Form der subakuten spongiöse Enzephalopathie (Jakob-Creutzfeldt Erkrankung). *Wien Klin. Wochenschr.* **84:**245–249.

100. **Kaneko, K., L. Zulianello, M. Scott, C. M. Cooper, A. C. Wallace, T. L. James, F. E. Cohen, and S. B. Prusiner.** 1997. Evidence for protein X binding to a discontinuous epitope on the cellular prion protein during scrapie prion propagation. *Proc. Natl. Acad. Sci. USA* **94:** 10069–10074.

101. **Kascsak, R. J., R. Fersko, D. Pulgiano, R. Rubenstein, and R. I. Carp.** 1997. Immunodiagnosis of prion disease. *Immunol. Invest.* **26:**259–268.

102. **Kellings, K., S. B. Prusiner, and D. Riesner.** 1994. Nucleic acids in prion preparations—unspecific background or essential component? *Philos. Trans. R. Soc. London Ser. B* **343:**425–430.

103. **Kimberlin, R. H., and C. A. Walker.** 1977. Characteristics of a short incubation model of scrapie in the golden hamster. *J. Gen. Virol.* **34:**295–304.

104. **Kimberlin, R. H., and C. A. Walker.** 1988. Pathogenesis of experimental scrapie. *Ciba Found. Symp.* **135:**37–62.

105. **Kirschbaum, W. R.** 1968. *Jakob-Creutzfeldt Disease*. American Elsevier, New York, N.Y.

106. **Kitamoto, T., K. Ogomori, J. Tateishi, and S. B. Prusiner.** 1987. Formic acid pretreatment enhances immunostaining of cerebral and systemic amyloids. *Lab. Invest.* **57:**230–236.

107. **Klein, M. A., R. Frigg, E. Flechsig, A. J. Raeber, U. Kalinke, H. Bluethmann, F. Bootz, M. Suter, R. M. Zinkernagel, and A. Aguzzi.** 1997. A crucial role for B cells in neuroinvasive scrapie. *Nature* **390:**687–690.

108. **Klitzman, R. L., M. P. Alpers, and D. C. Gajdusek.** 1984. The natural incubation period of kuru and the episodes of transmission in three clusters of patients. *Neuroepidemiology* **3:**3–20.

109. **Korth, C., B. Stierli, P. Streit, M. Moser, O. Schaller, R. Fischer, W. Schulz-Schaeffer, H. Kretzschmar, A. Raeber, U. Braun, F. Ehrensperger, S. Hornemann, R. Glockshuber, R. Riek, M. Billeter, K. Wuthrich, and B. Oesch.** 1997. Prion (PrPSc)-specific epitope defined by a monoclonal antibody. *Nature* **390:**74–77.

110. **Kretzschmar, H. A., J. W. Ironside, S. J. DeArmond, and J. Tateishi.** 1996. Diagnostic criteria for sporadic Creutzfeldt-Jakob disease. *Arch. Neurol.* **53:**913–920.

111. **Kuroda, Y., C. J. Gibbs, Jr., H. L. Amyx, and D. C. Gajdusek.** 1983. Creutzfeldt-Jakob disease in mice: persistent viremia and preferential replication of virus in low-density lymphocytes. *Infect. Immun.* **41:**154–161.

112. **Laplanche, J. L., N. Delasnerie-Laupretre, J. P. Brandel, J. Chatelain, P. Beaudry, A. Alperovitch, and J.-M. Launay.** 1994. Molecular genetics of prion diseases in France. *Neurology* **44:**2347–2351.

113. **Lasmézas, C. I., J. P. Deslys, R. Demalmay, K. T. Adjou, F. Lamoury, D. Dormont, O. Robain, J. Ironside, and J. J. Hauw.** 1996. BSE transmission to macaques. *Nature* **381:**743–744.

114. **Lasmézas, C. I., J. P. Deslys, O. Robain, A. Jaegly, V. Beringue, J. M. Peyrin, J. G. Fournier, J.-J. Hauw, J.**

Rossier, and D. Dormont. 1997. Transmission of the BSE agent to mice in the absence of detectable abnormal prion protein. *Science* **275:**402–405.

115. **Lewin, P.** 1972. Scrapie: an infective peptide? *Lancet* **i:** 748.
116. **MacDonald, S. T., K. Sutherland, and J. W. Ironside.** 1996. Prion protein genotype and pathological phenotype studies in sporadic Creutzfeldt-Jakob disease. *Neuropathol. Appl. Neurobiol.* **22:**285–292.
117. **Manetto, V., R. Medori, P. Cortelli, P. Montagna, P. Tinuper, A. Baruzzi, G. Rancurel, J.-J. Hauw, J. J. Vanderhaeghen, P. Mailleux, O. Bugiani, F. Tagliavini, C. Bouras, N. Rizzuto, E. Lugaresi, and P. Gambetti.** 1992. Fatal familial insomnia—clinical and pathologic study of five new cases. *Neurology* **42:**312–319.
118. **Manuelidis, E. E., E. J. Gorgacz, and L. Manuelidis.** 1978. Viremia in experimental Creutzfeldt-Jakob disease. *Science* **200:**1069–1071.
119. **Manuelidis, E. E., J. H. Kim, J. R. Mericangas, and L. Manuelidis.** 1985. Transmission to animals of Creutzfeldt-Jakob disease from human blood. *Lancet* **ii:**896–897.
120. **Manuelidis, E. E., and L. Manuelidis.** 1993. A transmissible Creutzfeldt-Jakob disease-like agent is prevalent in the human population. *Proc. Natl. Acad. Sci. USA* **90:** 7724–7728.
121. **Manuelidis, L., W. Fritch, and Y. G. Xi.** 1997. Evolution of a strain of CJD that induces BSE-like plaques. *Science* **277:**94–98.
122. **Marsh, R. F.** 1990. Bovine spongiform encephalopathy in the United States. *J. Am. Vet. Med. Assoc.* **196:**1677.
123. **Marsh, R. F., and R. P. Hanson.** 1979. On the origin of transmissible mink encephalopathy, p. 451–460. *In* S. B. Prusiner and W. J. Hadlow (ed.), *Slow Transmissible Diseases of the Nervous System.* Academic Press, Inc., New York, N.Y.
124. **Marx, R. E., and E. R. Carlson.** 1991. Creutzfeldt-Jakob disease from allogeneic dura: a review of risks and safety. *J. Oral Maxillofac. Surg.* **49:**272–274.
125. **Masson, C., I. Delalande, J. P. Deslys, D. Henin, C. Falletbianco, D. Dormont, and D. Leys.** 1991. Creutzfeldt-Jakob disease after pituitary-derived human growth hormone therapy—two cases with valine 129 homozygous genotype. *Neurology* **44:**179–180.
126. **Masters, C. L., and K. Beyreuther.** 1997. Spongiform encephalopathies. Tracking turncoat prion proteins. *Nature* **388:**228–229.
127. **Masters, C. L., D. C. Gajdusek, and C. J. Gibbs, Jr.** 1981. Creutzfeldt-Jakob disease virus isolation from the Gerstmann-Sträussler syndrome, with an analysis of the various forms of amyloid deposition in the virus-induced spongiform encephalopathies. *Brain* **104:**559–588.
128. **Masters, C. L., J. O. Harris, D. C. Gajdusek, C. J. Gibbs, Jr., C. Bernoulli, and D. M. Asher.** 1979. Creutzfeldt-Jakob disease: patterns of world wide occurrence and the significance of familial and sporadic clustering. *Ann. Neurol.* **5:**177–188.
129. **Matthews, W. B.** 1975. Epidemiology of Creutzfeldt-Jakob disease in England and Wales. *J. Neurol. Neurosurg. Psychiatry* **38:**210–213.
130. **McKinley, M. P., D. C. Bolton, and S. B. Prusiner.** 1983. A protease-resistant protein is a structural component of the scrapie prion. *Cell* **35:**57–62.
131. **Medori, R., P. Montagna, H. J. Tritschler, A. Leblanc, P. Cortelli, P. Tinuper, E. Lugaresi, and P. Gambetti.** 1992. Fatal familial insomnia—a second kindred with mutation of prion protein gene at codon-178. *Neurology* **42:**669–670.
132. **Medori, R., and H. J. Tritschler.** 1993. Prion protein gene analysis in 3 kindreds with fatal familial insomnia (FFI)—codon-178 mutation and codon-129 polymorphism. *Am. J. Hum. Genet.* **53:**822–827.
133. **Medori, R., H. J. Tritschler, A. Leblanc, F. Villare, V. Manetto, H. Y. Chen, R. Xue, S. Leal, P. Montagna, P. Cortelli, P. Tinuper, P. Avoni, M. Mochi, A. Baruzzi, J.-J. Hauw, J. Ott, E. Lugaresi, L. Autilio-Gambetti, and P. Gambetti.** 1992. Fatal familial insomnia, a prion disease with a mutation at codon-178 of the prion protein gene. *N. Engl. J. Med.* **326:**444–449.
134. **Merz, P. A., R. A. Somerville, H. M. Wisniewski, and K. Iqbal.** 1981. Abnormal fibrils from scrapie-infected brain. *Acta Neuropathol. (Berlin)* **54:**63–74.
135. **Merz, P. A., R. A. Somerville, H. M. Wisniewski, L. Manuelidis, and E. E. Manuelidis.** 1983. Scrapie-associated fibrils in Creutzfeldt-Jakob disease. *Nature* **306:** 474–476.
136. **Meyer, R. K., M. P. McKinley, K. A. Bowman, M. B. Braunfeld, R. A. Barry, and S. B. Prusiner.** 1986. Separation and properties of cellular and scrapie prion proteins. *Proc. Natl. Acad. Sci. USA* **83:**2310–2314.
137. **Miller, D. C.** 1988. Creutzfeldt-Jakob disease in histopathology technicians. *N. Engl. J. Med.* **318:**853–854.
138. **Monari, L., S. G. Chen, P. Brown, P. Parchi, R. B. Petersen, J. Mikol, F. Gray, P. Cortelli, P. Montagna, B. Ghetti, L. G. Goldfarb, D. C. Gajdusek, E. Lugaresi, P. Gambetti, and L. Autilio-Gambetti.** 1994. Fatal familial insomnia and familial Creutzfeldt-Jakob disease—different prion proteins determined by a DNA polymorphism. *Proc. Natl. Acad. Sci. USA* **91:**2839–2842.
139. **Multhaup, G., H. Diringer, H. Hilmert, H. Prinz, J. Heukeshoven, and K. Beyreuther.** 1985. The protein component of scrapie-associated fibrils is a glycosylated low molecular weight protein. *EMBO J.* **4:**1495–1501.
140. **Muramatsu, Y., A. Onodera, M. Horiuchi, N. Ishiguro, and M. Shinagawa.** 1994. Detection of PRP (SC) in sheep at the preclinical stage of scrapie and its significance for diagnosis of insidious infection. *Arch. Virol.* **134:** 427–432.
141. **Muramoto, T., T. Kitamoto, J. Tateishi, and I. Goto.** 1993. Accumulation of abnormal prion protein in mice infected with Creutzfeldt-Jakob disease via intraperitoneal route—a sequential study. *Am. J. Pathol.* **143:** 1470–1479.
142. **Narang, H. K., D. M. Asher, K. L. Pomeroy, and D. C. Gajdusek.** 1987. Abnormal tubulovesicular particles in brains of hamsters with scrapie. *Proc. Soc. Exp. Biol. Med.* **184:**504–509.
143. **Nevin, S., W. H. McMenemy, D. Behrman, and D. P. Jones.** 1960. Subacute spongiform encephalopathy: a subacute form of encephalopathy attributed to vascular dysfunction (spongiform cerebral atrophy). *Brain* **83:** 519–564.
144. **Occupational Safety and Health Administration and U.S. Department of Labor.** 1991. Occupational exposure to bloodborne pathogens: final rule. 29 CFR Part 1910.1030. *Fed. Regist.* **56:**64175–64182.
145. **Oesch, B., D. Westaway, M. Wälchli, M. P. McKinley, S. H. B. Kent, R. Aebersold, R. A. Barry, P. Tempst, D. B. Teplow, L. E. Hood, S. B. Prusiner, and C. Weissman.** 1985. A cellular gene encodes scrapie PrP 27–30 protein. *Cell* **40:**735–746.
146. **Owen, F., M. Poulter, R. Lofthouse, J. Collinge, T. J. Crow, D. Risby, H. F. Baker, R. M. Ridley, K. Hsiao, and S. B. Prusiner.** 1989. Insertion in prion protein gene in familial Creutzfeldt-Jakob disease. *Lancet* **i:**51–52.
147. **Owen, F., M. Poulter, R. Lofthouse, T. J. Crow, D. Risby, H. F. Baker, and R. M. Ridley.** 1988. A rare Msp1 polymorphism in the human prion gene in a family with

a history of early onset dementia. *Neurosci. Lett. Suppl.* **32:**S53.

148. **Özel, M., and H. Diringer.** 1994. Small virus-like structure in fractions from scrapie hamster brain. *Lancet* **343:** 894–895.
149. **Palmer, M. S., A. J. Dryden, J. T. Hughes, and J. Collinge.** 1991. Homozygous prion protein genotype predisposes to sporadic Creutzfeldt-Jakob disease. *Nature* **352:** 340–342.
150. **Pan, K. M., M. Baldwin, J. Nguyen, M. Gasset, A. Serban, D. Groth, I. Mehlhorn, Z. W. Huang, R. J. Fletterick, F. E. Cohen, and S. B. Prusiner.** 1993. Conversion of alpha-helices into beta-sheets features in the formation of the scrapie prion proteins. *Proc. Natl. Acad. Sci. USA* **90:**10962–10966.
151. **Piccardo, P., J. Safar, M. Ceroni, D. C. Gajdusek, and C. J. J. Gibbs.** 1990. Immunohistochemical localization of prion protein in spongiform encephalopathies and normal tissue. *Neurology* **40:**518–522.
152. **Pocchiari, M., M. Salvatore, F. Cutruzzola, M. Genuardi, C. T. Allocatelli, C. Masullo, G. Macchi, G. Alema, S. Galgani, Y. G. Xi, R. Petraroli, M. C. Silvestrini, and M. Brunori.** 1993. A new point mutation of the prion protein gene in Creutzfeldt-Jakob disease. *Ann. Neurol.* **34:**802–807.
153. **Priola, S. A., B. Caughey, R. E. Race, and B. Chesebro.** 1994. Heterologous PrP molecules interfere with accumulation of protease-resistant PrP in scrapie-infected murine neuroblastoma cells. *J. Virol.* **68:**4873–4878.
154. **Prusiner, S. B.** 1982. Novel proteinaceous infectious particles cause scrapie. *Science* **216:**136–144.
155. **Prusiner, S. B.** 1997. Prion diseases and the BSE crisis. *Science* **278:**245–251.
156. **Prusiner, S. B., M. Scott, D. Foster, K.-M. Pan, D. Groth, C. Mirenda, M. Torchia, S. L. Yang, D. Serban, G. A. Carlson, P. C. Hoppe, D. Westaway, and S. J. DeArmond.** 1990. Transgenetic studies implicate interactions between homologous PrP isoforms in scrapie prion replication. *Cell* **63:**673–686.
157. **Ricketts, M. N., N. R. Cashman, E. E. Stratton, and S. ElSaadany.** 1997. Is Creutzfeldt-Jakob disease transmitted in blood? *Emerg. Infect. Dis.* **3:**155–163.
158. **Riek, R., S. Hornemann, G. Wider, M. Billeter, R. Glockshuber, and K. Wuthrich.** 1996. NMR structure of the mouse prion protein domain PrP (121–321). *Nature* **382:**180–182.
159. **Rohwer, R. G.** 1984. Virus-like sensitivity of scrapie agent to heat inactivation. *Science* **223:**600–602.
160. **Rohwer, R. G.** 1991. The scrapie agent: "a virus by any other name." *Curr. Top. Microbiol. Immunol.* **172:** 195–232.
161. **Rubenstein, R., D. Hui, R. Race, W. Ju, C. Scalici, M. Papini, R. Kascsak, and R. Carp.** 1994. Replication of scrapie strains in vitro and their influence on neuronal functions, p. 331–337. *In* J. Bjornsson, R. I. Carp, A. Love, and H. M. Wisniewski (ed.), *Slow Infections of the Central Nervous System.* New York Academy of Sciences, New York, N.Y.
162. **Safar, J., P. P. Roller, D. C. Gajdusek, and C. J. Gibbs, Jr.** 1993. Conformational transitions, dissociation, and unfolding of scrapie amyloid (prion) protein. *J. Biol. Chem.* **268:**20276–20284.
163. **Safar, J., P. P. Roller, D. C. Gajdusek, and C. J. Gibbs, Jr.** 1993. Thermal stability and conformational transitions of scrapie amyloid (prion) protein correlate with infectivity. *Protein Sci.* **2:**2206–2216.
164. **Sailer, A., H. Bueler, M. Fischer, A. Aguzzi, and C. Weissmann.** 1994. No propagation of prions in mice devoid of PrP. *Cell* **77:**967–968.
165. **Schonberger, L. B.** 1998. New variant Creutzfeldt-Jakob disease and bovine spongiform encephalopathy. *Infect. Dis. Clin. North Am.* **12:**111–121.
166. **Schreuder, B. E. C., L. J. van Keulen, M. E. Vromans, J. P. Langeveld, and M. A. Smits.** 1996. Preclinical test for prion diseases. *Nature* **381:**563.
167. **Shibuya, S., J. Higuchi, R. W. Shin, J. Tateishi, and T. Kitamoto.** 1998. Protective prion protein polymorphisms against sporadic Creutzfeldt-Jakob disease. *Lancet* **351:** 419.
168. **Sigurdsson, B.** 1954. Observations on three slow infections of sheep. *Br. Med. J.* [*Clin. Res.*] **110:**255–270, 307–322, 341–354.
169. **Sitwell, L., B. Lach, E. Atack, and D. Atack.** 1988. Creutzfeldt-Jakob disease in histopathology technicians. *N. Engl. J. Med.* **318:**854.
170. **Spraker, T. R., M. W. Miller, E. S. Williams, D. M. Getzy, W. J. Adrian, G. G. Schoonveld, R. A. Spowart, K. I. O'Rourke, J. M. Miller, and P. A. Merz.** 1997. Spongiform encephalopathy in free-ranging mule deer (Odocoileus hemionus), white-tailed deer (Odocoileus virginianus) and Rocky Mountain elk (Cervus elaphus nelsoni) in northcentral Colorado. *J. Wildl. Dis.* **33:**1–6.
171. **Spudich, S., J. A. Mastrianni, M. Wrensch, R. Gabizon, Z. Meiner, I. Kahana, H. Rosenmann, E. Kahana, and S. B. Prusiner.** 1995. Complete penetrance of Creutzfeldt-Jakob disease in Libyan Jews carrying the E200K mutation in the prion protein gene. *Mol. Med.* **1:**607–613.
172. **Stahl, N., D. R. Borchelt, K. Hsiao, and S. B. Prusiner.** 1987. Scrapie prion protein contains a phosphatidylinositol glycolipid. *Cell* **51:**229–240.
173. **Takashima, S., J. Tateishi, Y. Taguchi, and H. Inoue.** 1997. Creutzfeldt-Jakob disease with florid plaques after cadaveric dural graft in a Japanese woman. *Lancet* **350:** 865–866. (Letter.)
174. **Tamai, Y., H. Kojima, R. Kitajima, F. Taguchi, Y. Ohtani, T. Kawaguchi, S. Miura, M. Sato, and Y. Ishihara.** 1992. Demonstration of the transmissible agent in tissue from a pregnant woman with Creutzfeldt-Jakob disease. *N. Engl. J. Med.* **327:**649.
175. **Tateishi, J.** 1985. Transmission of Creutzfeldt-Jakob disease from human blood and urine into mice. *Lancet* **ii:** 1074.
176. **Tateishi, J., P. Brown, T. Kitamoto, Z. M. Hoque, R. Roos, R. Wollman, L. Cervenakova, and D. C. Gajdusek.** 1995. First experimental transmission of fatal familial insomnia. *Nature* **376:**434–435.
177. **Tateishi, J., and T. Kitamoto.** 1993. Developments in diagnosis for prion diseases. *Br. Med. Bull.* **49:**971–979.
178. **Taylor, D. M.** 1996. Exposure to, and inactivation of, the unconventional agents that cause transmissible degenerative encephalopathies, p. 105–118. *In* H. Baker and R. M. Ridley (ed.), *Methods in Molecular Medicine: Prion Diseases.* Humana Press, Totowa, N.J.
179. **Taylor, D. M., C. E. Ferguson, C. J. Bostock, and M. Dawson.** 1995. Absence of disease in mice receiving milk from cows with bovine spongiform encephalopathy. *Vet. Rec.* **136:**592.
180. **Taylor, D. M., I. McConnell, and H. Fraser.** 1996. Scrapie infection can be established readily through skin scarification in immunocompetent but not immunodeficient mice. *J. Gen. Virol.* **77:**1595–1599.
181. **Telling, G. C., T. Haga, M. Torchia, P. Tremblay, S. J. DeArmond, and S. B. Prusiner.** 1996. Interactions between wild-type and mutant prion proteins modulate neurodegeneration in transgenic mice. *Genes Dev.* **10:** 1736–1750.
182. **Telling, G. C., P. Parchi, S. J. DeArmond, P. Cortelli, P. Montagna, R. Gabizon, J. Mastrianni, E. Lugaresi, P.**

Gambetti, and S. B. Prusiner. 1996. Evidence for the conformation of the pathologic isoform of the prion protein enciphering and propagating prion diversity. *Science* **274:**2079–2082.

183. **Telling, G. C., M. Scott, J. Mastrianni, R. Gabizon, M. Torchia, F. E. Cohen, S. J. DeArmond, and S. B. Prusiner.** 1995. Prion propagation in mice expressing human and chimeric PrP transgenes implicates the interaction of cellular PrP with another protein. *Cell* **83:**79–90.
184. **Weissmann, C., H. Büeler, M. Fischer, and M. Aguet.** 1993. Role of the PrP gene in transmissible spongiform encephalopathies. *Intervirology* **35:**164–175.
185. **Weissmann, C., H. Bueler, M. Fischer, A. Sauer, and M. Aguet.** 1994. Susceptibility to scrapie in mice is dependent on PrPc. *Philos. Trans. R. Soc. London Ser. B* **343:**431–433.
186. **Wells, G. A., S. A. Hawkins, R. B. Green, A. R. Austin, I. Dexter, Y. I. Spencer, M. J. Chaplin, M. J. Stack, and M. Dawson.** 1998. Preliminary observations on the pathogenesis of experimental bovine spongiform encephalopathy (BSE): an update. *Vet. Rec.* **142:**103–106.
187. **Westaway, D., S. J. DeArmond, J. Cayetanocanlas, D. Groth, D. Foster, S.-L. Yang, M. Torchia, G. A. Carlson, and S. B. Prusiner.** 1994. Degeneration of skeletal muscle, peripheral nerves, and the central nervous system in transgenic mice overexpressing wild-type prion proteins. *Cell* **76:**117–129.
188. **Westaway, D., P. A. Goodman, C. A. Mirenda, M. P. McKinley, G. A. Carlson, and S. B. Prusiner.** 1987. Distinct prion proteins in short and long scrapie incubation period mice. *Cell* **51:**651–662.
189. **Wilesmith, J. W.** 1993. Epidemiology of bovine spongiform encephalopathy and related diseases. *Arch. Virol.* **S7:**245–254.
190. **Wilesmith, J. W., G. A. Wells, J. B. Ryan, D. Gavier-Widen, and M. M. Simmons.** 1997. A cohort study to examine maternally-associated risk factors for bovine spongiform encephalopathy. *Vet. Rec.* **141:**239–243.
191. **Will, R. G., J. W. Ironside, M. Zeidler, S. N. Cousens, K. Estibeiro, A. Alperovitch, S. Poser, M. Pocchiari, A. Hofman, and P. G. Smith.** 1996. A new variant of Creutzfeldt-Jakob disease in the UK. *Lancet* **347:** 921–925.
192. **Will, R. G., and W. B. Matthews.** 1982. Evidence for case-to-case transmission of Creutzfeldt-Jakob disease. *J. Neurol. Neurosurg. Psychiatry* **45:**235–238.
193. **Will, R. G., M. Zeidler, P. Brown, M. Harrington, K. H. Lee, and K. L. Kenney.** 1996. Cerebrospinal-fluid test for new-variant Creutzfeldt-Jakob disease. *Lancet* **348:** 955.
194. **Williams, E. S., and S. Young.** 1980. Chronic wasting disease of mule deer: a spongiform encephalopathy. *J. Wildl. Dis.* **16:**89–98.
195. **Wineland, N. E., L. A. Detwiler, and M. D. Salman.** 1998. Epidemiologic analysis of reported scrapie in sheep in the United States: 1,117 cases (1947–1992). *J. Am. Vet. Med. Assoc.* **212:**713–718.
196. **Xi, Y. G., L. Ingrosso, A. Ladogana, C. Masullo, and M. Pocchiari.** 1992. Amphotericin-B treatment dissociates in vivo replication of the scrapie agent from PrP accumulation. *Nature* **356:**598–601.
197. **Yamada, M., Y. Itoh, N. Suematsu, M. Matsushita, and E. Otomo.** 1997. Panencephalopathic type of Creutzfeldt-Jakob disease associated with cadaveric dura mater graft. *J. Neurol. Neurosurg. Psychiatry* **63:**524–527.
198. **Yun, M., W. Wu, L. Hood, and M. Harrington.** 1992. Human cerebrospinal fluid protein database—edition 1992. *Electrophoresis* **13:**1002–1013.

MYCOLOGY

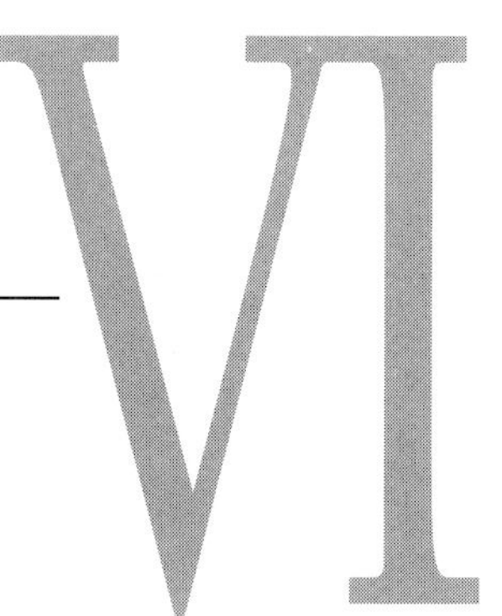

VOLUME EDITOR
MICHAEL A. PFALLER

SECTION EDITOR
ROBERT A. FROMTLING

(continued)

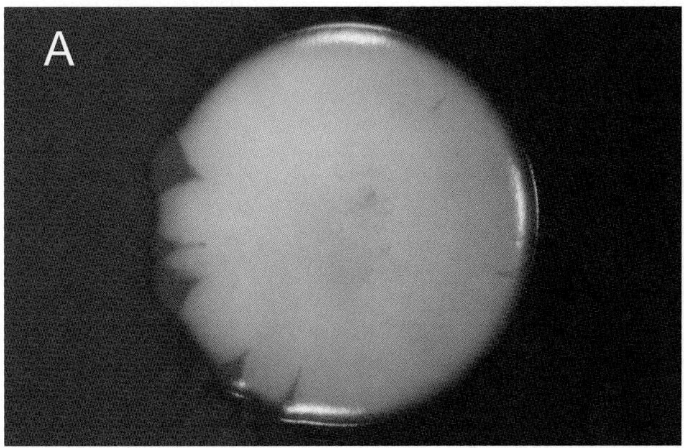

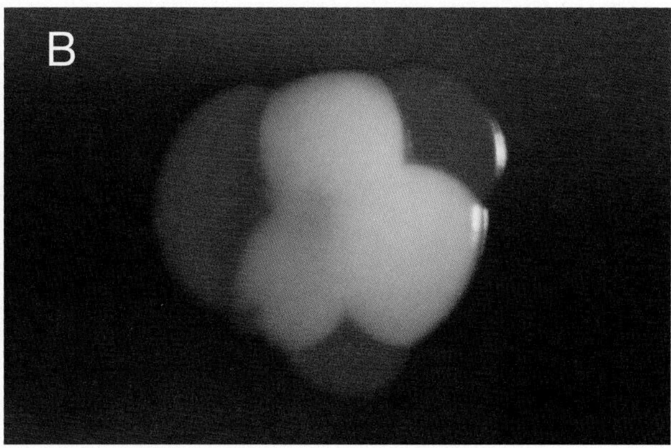

High-frequency phenotypic switching between the "white" and the "opaque" (red) phase in *Candida albicans* strain WO-1 *(photograph courtesy of David R. Soll, University of Iowa).*

Taxonomy, Classification, and Morphology of the Fungi

DENNIS M. DIXON, JUDITH C. RHODES, AND ROBERT A. FROMTLING

93

Mycology now is part of the microbiological mainstream; fungi have become a serious public health hazard (14). Clinical mycology techniques, including the recent standardization of in vitro susceptibility testing of yeasts (9) (see chapter 126), have advanced significantly in the past decade. Application of these techniques should be included in the routine tests of each hospital and clinical microbiology laboratory (7). The list of opportunistic fungal pathogens—"the emerging fungal threat"—is increasing at an impressive rate that is related to the expanding size of the immunocompromised patient population (14). The clinical laboratory technologist must be able to recognize an increasingly large group of potential fungal pathogens. Organisms once thought to be "contaminants" are now confirmed pathogens in immunocompromised patients. In addition, there is a critical need to recognize that even though a given isolate may not be a documented fungal pathogen in the textbooks, its isolation from a normally sterile site and its ability to grow at 37°C require that it be considered a possible pathogen. With few exceptions, all of the fungi that infect humans can grow at 37°C. Beyond this, it is difficult to specifically identify traits or factors associated with virulence in the pathogenic fungi.

Mycological identification can be challenging and occasionally frustrating because of the importance placed upon morphology and the need to become familiar with certain structures and terms. However, investing a small amount of time to learn a few basic structures and principles of classification can result in the ability to recognize and properly identify many medically important fungi.

TAXONOMY, CLASSIFICATION, AND MORPHOLOGY

Fungi were among the first microorganisms recognized because some of the fruiting structures, e.g., mushrooms, are large enough to be seen without a microscope. The word "mycology," in fact, is derived from *mykes*, the Greek word for mushroom. Fungi were initially classified with the plants, and much of the botanical influence is still seen, even though the organisms have been transferred to a separate, fifth kingdom on the basis of cell structure (Table 1). The nomenclature of the fungi is governed by the International Code of Botanical Nomenclature (adopted by the 15th International Botanical Congress, Tokyo, 1993). Morphology retains an important role in the identification of most fungi. This places demands upon the observer to become familiar with the organisms through experience. Morphology is more important for the identification of moulds than of yeasts, but even with the latter, morphology on a medium such as cornmeal agar is a key first step in the identification process.

Fungi are extremely successful organisms, as evidenced by their ubiquity in nature. They are an important component in the energy cycle, where they function as decomposers. Thus, fungi are valuable as saprophytes in nature. Of the estimated 250,000 species, fewer than 150 are known to be primary pathogens of humans. The infection of humans seems to be an accident of nature, since it represents a "dead end" for the fungus; i.e., most fungal infections are not contagious but are acquired through exposure to a point source in nature, where the organism exists as a saprophyte. This fact has practical implications in the laboratory and is why moulds, in particular, should be manipulated in a biological safety cabinet.

Fungi are eukaryotic, chemoheterotrophic organisms with cell walls containing chitin and/or cellulose. They may be unicellular or multicellular, although there is a tendency for fungi to be multicellular and multinucleate. The body of a fungus is termed a thallus. Fungi can be grouped simply on the basis of morphology as either yeasts or moulds (for a discussion of "mould" versus "mold," see reference 4). A yeast can be defined morphologically as a cell that reproduces by budding, a process whereby a progenitor cell pinches off a portion of itself to produce a progeny cell. In this connotation, yeasts are generally unicellular and produce circular, restricted, pasty, or mucoid colonies. In contrast, moulds are multicelled, filamentous forms of fungi consisting of thread-like filaments termed hyphae that interweave to form a mat-like structure termed a mycelium. The resulting colonies often are described as "fuzzy." Many medically important fungi, such as *Blastomyces dermatitidis* and *Histoplasma capsulatum*, can exist in each of these two morphologies and thus are termed "dimorphic." When additional forms are present, the term "polymorphic" is applied (Fig. 1).

Fungi reproduce by the formation of spores, which may be either asexual (involving mitosis only) or sexual (involving meiosis; preceded by fusion of the protoplasm and nuclei of two cells). Asexual spores are of two general types: sporangiospores and conidia (Fig. 2). Sporangiospores are asexual spores produced within a containing structure (sporangium);

TABLE 1 Simplified taxonomic scheme illustrating major groups of Kingdom Fungi (Myceteae) in which medically important fungi are classified[a]

Taxonomic designation	Representative genera	Human disease
Phylum: Zygomycota		
Class: Zygomycetes		
Order: Mucorales	*Rhizopus*, *Mucor*, *Rhizomucor*, *Absidia*, *Cunninghamella*, *Saksenaea*	Zygomycosis; opportunistic in patients with diabetes, leukemia, severe burns, or malnutrition; rhinocerebral infections
Order: Entomophthorales	*Basidiobolus*, *Conidiobolus*	Zygomycosis; subcutaneous infections
Phylum: Ascomycota		
Class: Ascomycetes		
Order: Saccharomycetales	*Saccharomyces*, *Pichia* (teleomorphs of some *Candida* spp.)	Numerous mycoses
Order: Onygenales	*Arthroderma* (teleomorphs of *Trichophyton* and *Microsporum* spp.)	Dermatophytoses
	Ajellomyces (teleomorphs of *Histoplasma* and *Blastomyces* spp.)	Systemic mycoses
Order: Eurotiales	Teleomorphs of some *Aspergillus* and *Penicillium* spp.	Aspergillosis; penicillosis; hyalohyphomycosis
Order: Microascales	*Pseudallescheria boydii* (teleomorph of *Scedosporium apiospermum*)	Mycetoma; hyalohyphomycosis
Order: Pyrenomycetes	*Nectria*, *Gibberella* (teleomorphs of many *Fusarium* spp.)	Mycotic keratosis; hyalohyphomycosis
Class: Archiascomycetes		
Order: Pneumocystidales	*Pneumocystis carinii*[b]	Pneumonia
Phylum: Basidiomycota		
Class: Basidiomycetes		
Order: Agaricales	*Amanita*, *Agaricus*	Mushroom poisoning from consumption of poisonous species (e.g., *Amanita* spp.)
Order: Tremellales	*Filobasidiella* (teleomorphs of *Cryptococcus neoformans*)	Cryptococcosis
Form group[c]: Deuteromycota		
Class: Deuteromycetes		
Order: Cryptococcales	Imperfect yeasts: *Candida*, *Cryptococcus*, *Trichosporon*, *Malassezia*	Numerous mycoses
Order: Moniliales		
Family: Moniciliaceae	*Epidermophyton*, *Coccidioides*, *Paracoccidioides*, *Sporothrix*, *Aspergillus*	Numerous mycoses
Family: Dematiaceae	*Phialophora*, *Fonsecaea*, *Exophiala*, *Wangiella*, *Cladophialophora*, *Bipolaris*, *Exserohilum*, *Alternaria*	Chromoblastomycosis; mycetoma; phaeohyphomycosis
Order: Sphaeropsidales	*Phoma*	Phaeohyphomycosis

[a] Modified from information in reference 1.
[b] See reference 3.
[c] This form group or phylum and all of its taxa are form taxa.

they are characteristic of the lower fungi classified in the Zygomycetes, such as *Rhizopus* and *Mucor* spp. Typically, these fungi have broad, sparingly septate hyphae. Conidia are asexual spores that are borne naked, as evidenced in *Aspergillus* and *Penicillium* spp. and the dermatophytes. The conidial fungi are classified together as the Deuteromycetes (Fungi Imperfecti). Sexual spores result from meiosis (Fig. 3). The meiotic nuclei are packaged into cells that function as spores. These spores and their mode of production serve as the basis for taxonomic grouping.

One fungus can produce both sexual and asexual spores. Specialized structures (fruiting bodies, or fructifications) may be associated with either sexual or asexual spores. Information on these fruiting bodies is summarized in Table 2. Recognition of a particular fruiting structure can be a useful step in the identification process. Determination of the type of spore is critical to establishing both the type of fruiting structure and the ultimate identification of the fungus.

The Zygomycetes produce zygospores (Fig. 3) that are rarely seen in the clinical laboratory, since most of the medically important species are heterothallic; that is, two different strains of compatible mating types are required for the production of sexual spores. The higher fungi are represented by the classes Ascomycetes, Basidiomycetes, and Deuteromycetes. The sexual spore of the Ascomycetes is the ascospore, characterized by its production within a containing sac (ascus). The sexual spore of the Basidiomycetes is the basidiospore, characterized by extrusion from a club-shaped structure (basidium). The Deuteromycetes produce no known sexual spores. They are included with the higher fungi because they are presumed to represent the conidial stages of Ascomycetes and, more rarely, Basidiomycetes that

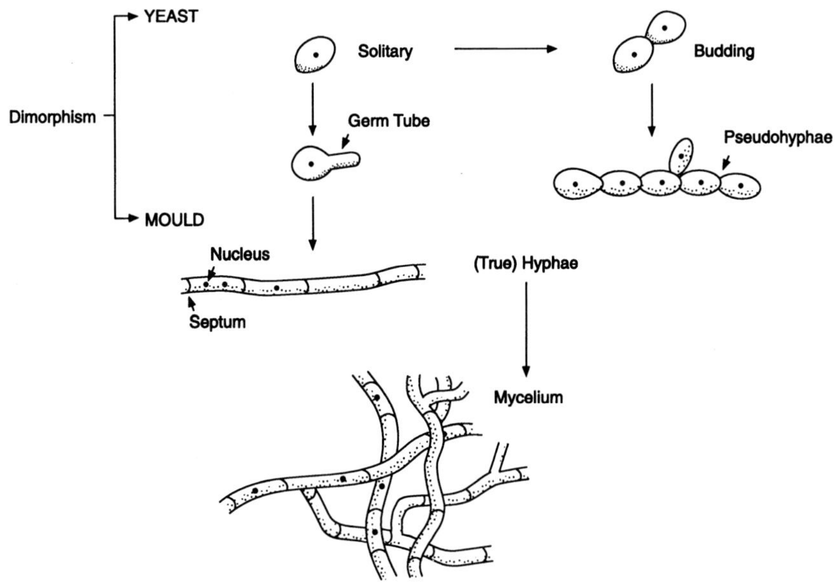

FIGURE 1 Simplified representations of the fungal thallus. Figure courtesy of J. Shockey, Merck Research Laboratories.

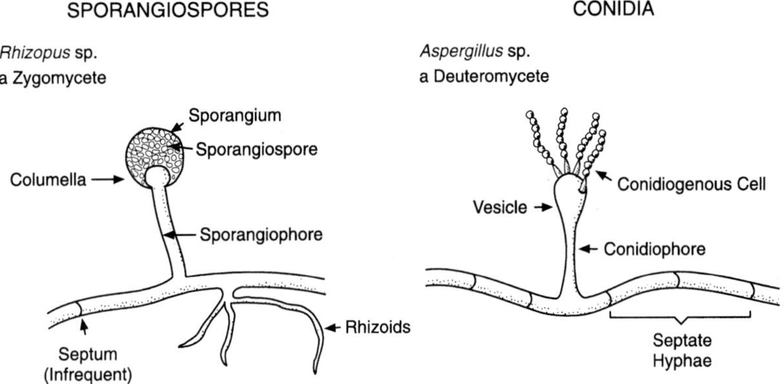

FIGURE 2 Stylized representation of two kinds of asexual fungal spores. Figure courtesy of J. Shockey, Merck Research Laboratories.

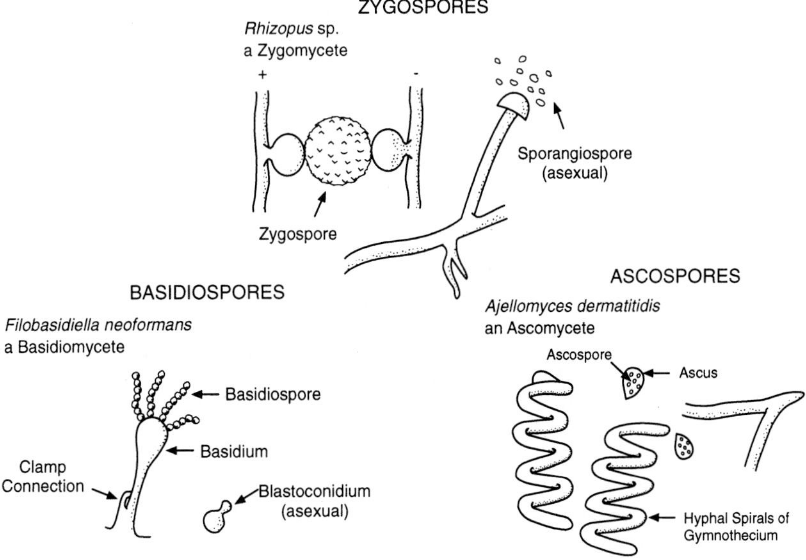

FIGURE 3 Stylized representation of three kinds of asexual fungal spores, using medically important examples. Figure courtesy of J. Shockey, Merck Research Laboratories.

TABLE 2 Fruiting structures helpful in classifying some medically important fungi

Fruiting structure	Characteristics	Taxonomic group	Representative genera
Sexual (ascomata)		Ascomycota	*Chaetomium*, *Leptosphaeria*
Perithecium	Spherical or flask-shaped ascoma with opening		
Cleistothecium	Spherical ascoma; no opening	Ascomycota	*Pseudallescheria*, *Emericella*, *Ajellomyces*,[a] *Arthroderma*[a]
Asexual (conidiomata)			
Pycnidium	Spherical or flask-shaped conidioma, usually with opening	Deuteromycota	*Hendersonula (Nattrassia)*, *Phoma*, *Pyrenochaeta*
Synnema	Rope-like tangle of conidiophores, usually with apical fertile region	Deuteromycota	*Graphium*
Sporodochium	Clump or conidiophores	Deuteromycota	*Fusarium*, *Epicoccum*

[a] The term "gymnothecium" occasionally is used to refer to the characteristic, loosely woven cleistothecium produced by these genera.

have lost the ability to produce sexual spores. Certain Deuteromycetes may never have had the ability to produce sexual spores. Since sexual spores hold taxonomic precedence, the Deuteromycetes represent a provisional taxonomic group.

Designation of a given spore as sexual or asexual is dependent largely upon knowledge of the life cycle of the fungus (to determine whether the spore is the result of meiosis or mitosis) and recognition of the characteristic morphology of the spore. Of particular importance with the conidial fungi is the complication imposed by finding that the sexual stage of a fungus has been named on the basis of its conidial (asexual) form. For example, *Blastomyces dermatitidis* was named in 1898 on the basis of its asexual characteristics: a fungus (*myces*) that reproduced by budding (*Blasto*) recovered from a patient with dermatitis (*dermatitidis*). The fungus grows as a yeast in tissue (37°C) and as a mould in culture (25°C), and it produces lateral solitary spores meeting the definition of conidia. In 1968, the fungus was found

TABLE 3 Groupings of conidia based on ontogeny

Conidial group	Characteristic	Representative genera
Thallic development	Hyphal tip ceases to elongate; wall growth depolarizes. Entire segment begins to differentiate, and cell wall growth occurs by thickening process.	
Arthroconidia	Thallic production whereby hyphal segments fragment into individual cells delimited by prior development of septum. All other modes of ontogeny listed below are modifications of blastic productions.	*Coccidioides*, *Geotrichum*
Blastic development	Essentially a budding process whereby localization (polarization) of growth occurs at region of mother cell that "blows out" to give rise to conidium.	
Blastoconidia	Conidium originates as blown-out portion of mother cell. Developing cell is recognizable before being delimited by septum. Daughter cell may separate completely or remain attached to form chains.	*Candida*, *Cryptococcus*, and most other yeasts; *Cladophialophora*
Phialoconidia	Blastic production from tubular, often flask-shaped conidiogenous cell (phialide) that does not increase in length or width.	*Aspergillus*, *Fusarium*, *Lecythophora*, *Malassezia*, *Penicillium*, *Phialophora*
Annelloconidia	Blastic production from flask-shaped conidiogenous cell (annellide) that extends via percurrent growth (inner layers grow through outer layers) and often tapers.	*Exophiala*, *Phaeoannellomyces*, *Scedosporium*, *Scopulariopsis*
Poroconidia	Blastic production through channel in cell wall of conidiogenous cell.	*Alternaria*, *Bipolaris*, *Curvularia*, *Drechslera*, *Exserohilum*
Sympoduloconidia	Successive blastic conidial production characterized by continued growth of conidiogenous cell to one side of base of conidium. Typically results in zigzag or distorted ampulliform appearance of conidiogenous cell. Poroconidia of *Curvularia*, *Drechslera*, *Bipolaris*, and *Exserohilum* spp. are produced on sympodial conidiophores.	*Sporothrix*, *Dactylaria*
Aleurioconidia	Older but useful term describing conidia that typically have broad bases of attachment to conidiogenous cell and separate by lysis of conidiogenous hyphal walls, leaving remnant attached to conidium as annular frill. *Epidermophyton*, *Microsporum*, and *Trichophyton* spp. now are recognized to produce conidia by a thallic process, and their conidia are now termed holothallic conidia. *Blastomyces*, *Chrysosporium*, and *Histoplasma* spp. produce holoblastic conidia.	*Blastomyces*, *Chrysosporium*, *Histoplasma*, *Epidermophyton*, *Microsporum*

to complete a life cycle by mating with an opposite mating type to yield a diploid zygote that undergoes meiosis to yield ascospores. Since *B. dermatitidis* was the name chosen to describe the entity known only in the asexual form, a new name, *Ajellomyces dermatitidis*, was chosen for the ascomycetous form. The form isolated in clinical microbiology laboratories is *B. dermatitidis*, and this name is retained for that description. However, we now know that *B. dermatitidis* represents the conidial form of an ascomycete; the asexual form of a conidial fungus is known as the anamorph, and the sexual form is known as the teleomorph. The entire fungus is collectively termed the holomorph. The name of the teleomorph also serves as the name of the holomorph.

The Deuteromycetes can be segregated into the Blastomycetes, Coelomycetes, and Hyphomycetes. The Blastomycetes contain anamorphs that reproduce by budding; the Coelomycetes contain moulds that produce conidia within a cavity of fungal tissue referred to as a conidioma (e.g., pycnidium [Table 2]); the Hyphomycetes contain moulds that produce conidia without fruiting structures or with synnemata (Table 2) or that produce only sterile hyphae. The Hyphomycetes are often further described as being either dematiaceous (darkly pigmented) or hyaline (nonpigmented), although these terms may be used to describe any fungus. Useful separations among the Deuteromycetes are made on the basis of morphology and ontogeny of the conidia and conidiogenous cells (cells that produce conidia). Conidia may develop either by a blastic process (budding) or by a thallic process (fragmentation). A summary of some different types of conidiogenesis is presented in Table 3. Since different fungi can produce conidia that appear similar, it is often helpful to study a variety of microscopic fields in order to evaluate the mode of development of the conidium from the conidiogenous cell.

The term "yeast" is not a formal taxon; therefore, the use of this term can vary among mycologists. Some mycologists restrict this term to a specific group of Ascomycetes that produce ascospores in a free ascus, are primarily unicellular, and reproduce asexually by either budding (e.g., *Saccharomyces* spp.) or fission (e.g., *Schizosaccharomyces* spp.). By using this reasoning, fungi which have budding morphologies without the characteristically borne ascospores are termed "yeast-like." For example, although *B. dermatitidis* reproduces by budding and has a teleomorph that produces ascospores, the ascus is contained in a fruiting-body morphology, i.e., is not free. Thus, "yeast" would be used by those following strict taxonomic usage and "yeast-like" would be used by those using a morphological definition.

LABORATORY PROCEDURES

Basic bacteriological techniques may be used when working with fungi in the laboratory. However, since fungi have longer generation times than most bacteria, cultures must be kept longer and provisions must be made to prevent media from excessive drying. This can be done by pouring plates with more media than bacteriological plates, sealing them with paraffin tape, incubating them in moist chambers, or using tubed media where possible.

Yeasts can be manipulated in the laboratory in much the same way as bacteria. Moulds, however, require some specialized procedures. Inflexible, straight needles rather than loops are generally preferred, and colonies are transferred by cutting a small portion of growth to be used as a point inoculum. If there is sufficient spore production, moulds may be streaked for isolation with a standard bacteriological loop. Using a straight needle to select portions of a mould inoculum before streaking it across a plate is useful in separating mixed cultures. To separate fungi mixed with bacteria, cultures can be streaked on media containing antibacterial antibiotics. If this fails, 1 drop of a broth or saline suspension of the mixed culture can be used to inoculate each of four tubes of Sabouraud broth (1.0 ml), to which is added in series either 1, 2, 3, or 4 drops of concentrated HCl (5).

Microscopy is an important step in the identification of fungi. Bright-field optics and a magnification of about ×500 are sufficient to resolve the features of medically important fungi mounted in lactophenol (for pigmented fungi) or lactophenol cotton blue (Poirrier's blue; for unpigmented fungi). (Note: phenol is listed as a hazardous chemical; solutions containing phenol should be prepared, stored, and used in an approved chemical safety cabinet.) Often, however, critical evaluation of conidial ontogeny requires greater magnification (×1,000). Some structures, such as the annellations present on annellides or the collarettes present on phialides, are easier to distinguish with phase-contrast optics. Fluorescent brighteners (calcofluor white) used in conjunction with a UV light source and the proper filter combination are useful not only for detecting fungi in clinical material but also for examining conidial ontogeny. In one study, optimal results were obtained with a 330- to 380-μm excitation filter, a 420-μm barrier filter, and a 515-W eyepiece side-absorption filter (13).

Specimen mounts for microscopic examination of moulds include teased, mashed, and slide culture preparation. The simplest mount is the teased preparation. Sterile, straight dissecting needles are used to remove a portion of growth that is teased apart in 95% ethanol; a drop of lactophenol cotton blue is added, and the mount is sealed with a coverslip. A modification of the teased preparation involves cutting a small section of growth and the uppermost surface of adherent medium from the plate and mashing this in a drop of mounting medium on a slide by using a coverslip. In more critical studies to determine conidial ontogeny, it may be necessary to set up a slide culture. However, the slide culture procedure should be limited to organisms of low virulence; if it is used with dimorphic fungi, special safety precautions must be defined and rigidly followed. The procedure requires sterile glass slides and coverslips and a sterile moist chamber. It is convenient to autoclave a supply of glass petri dishes containing U-shaped bent glass rods, slides, and coverslips. A square of sporulation agar (potato glucose, cornmeal, cereal) smaller than the coverslip is then cut out of the agar plate and placed on the slides within the petri dish. The edges of the agar are then inoculated, and the coverslip is placed on top of the agar. The result is a glass incubation chamber that is kept moist by the addition of water; the fungus should grow on both glass surfaces in contact with the agar. Thus, it is possible to remove the coverslip for mounting in lactophenol on a fresh slide and, after removal of the agar block, to place a drop of lactophenol cotton blue and another coverslip on the original slide. Any of the preparations described above can be kept as reference slides after being sealed with nail polish or permount.

The taxonomy of the medically important yeasts is based not only upon morphology but also upon extensive physiological characterization as used in clinical bacteriology. Commercial products are available to assist in detecting the key physiological reactions necessary to identify these organisms (see chapter 94). Although not as important as in the taxonomy of the yeasts, certain physiological reactions and special tests can be helpful in the identification of the moulds.

LABORATORY SAFETY

Biosafety must be a top priority in any clinical laboratory (2, 8, 11, 12). All clinical laboratory personnel should be trained in the principles of biosafety and should know how to follow established safety procedures when working with any potential human pathogen. The reader is referred to the American Society for Microbiology publication *Laboratory Safety: Principles and Practices* (2) for detailed information on this important subject. Additional information on the safe collection, transport, and storage, as well as appropriate handling and processing of clinical specimens that may contain pathogenic fungi, is outlined in chapters 4 and 5 of this Manual.

STOCK CULTURES

Stock cultures of fungi are an essential source of material for quality control organisms, for reference cultures to be used in comparative identification, for production of known metabolites, and for teaching collections. Several methods of preserving fungal cultures have been reported (6, 10); these vary according to the organisms represented; the size of the collection; and considerations of cost, practicality, and personal preference. Two of the simplest methods involve either freezing actively growing agar slant cultures at −10°C (caution: *Epidermophyton* spp. and many Zygomycetes may not survive freezing) or preparing sterile-water suspensions of cultures. For the latter method, cultures are grown on potato glucose agar until mature (several days to 2 weeks) and mycelium, spores, or yeast cells are scraped or washed from the surface of slants with sterile distilled water and a pipette (6). The resulting fungal suspensions can be sealed in sterile vials to prevent evaporation and stored at room temperature. A time-tested but less commonly used technique is to cover an agar slant culture of a fungus with sterile mineral oil. For long-term preservation, preparation of lyophilized cultures and storage of cultures at −70°C or in liquid nitrogen are well-established procedures (10), but they require expensive equipment. However, cultures stored by these techniques may be kept for many years without loss of viability or alteration of biochemical or morphological characteristics.

CONCLUSION

The descriptions, procedures, and guidelines outlined in chapters 93 through 102 of this Manual represent the current knowledge in specialized areas of medical mycology that are relevant for specialists working in clinical microbiology. In addition to the cited literature, a list of selected references appears at the end of this chapter for those interested in learning more about basic and medical mycology and related applications. The American Society for Microbiology, the Centers for Disease Control and Prevention, and several universities frequently conduct workshops and training programs in medical mycology, including specialty courses in clinical mycology. Information on these programs may be found in *ASM News* and in the newsletters of the Medical Mycological Society and the International Society for Human and Animal Mycology. The reader also is referred to the Mycology Website http://fungus.utmb.edu/ for further information on fungi and valuable links to additional mycology websites.

REFERENCES

1. **Alexopoulos, C. J., C. W. Mims, and M. Blackwell.** 1996. *Introductory Mycology*, 4th ed. John Wiley & Sons, Inc., New York, N.Y.
2. **Fleming, D. O., J. H. Richardson, J. J. Tulis, and D. Vesley (ed.).** 1995. *Laboratory Safety: Principles and Practices*, 2nd ed. ASM Press, Washington, D.C.
3. **Haase, G.** 1997. *Pneumocystis carinii* Delanoe & Delanoe (1912) has been placed in the Archiascomycetales, a class of Ascomycota. *Infect. Immun.* **65:**4365–4366.
4. **Illman, W. I.** 1970. On the use of mould versus mold for mycelial fungus. *Mycologia* **62:**1214.
5. **McGinnis, M. R.** 1980. *Laboratory Handbook of Medical Mycology*. Academic Press, Inc., New York, N.Y.
6. **McGinnis, M. R., A. A. Padhye, and L. Ajello.** 1974. Storage of stock cultures of filamentous fungi, yeasts, and some aerobic actinomycetes in sterile distilled water. *Appl. Microbiol.* **28:**218–222.
7. **Merz, W. G.** 1994. The clinical mycology laboratory: meeting the challenges of the 90s. *Infect. Dis. Clin. Pract.* **3**(Suppl. 2)**:**560–567.
8. **National Academy of Sciences of the USA.** 1989. *Biosafety in the Laboratory: Prudent Practices for the Handling and Disposal of Infectious Materials*. National Academy Press, Washington, D.C.
9. **National Committee for Clinical Laboratory Standards.** 1997. *Reference Method for Broth Dilution Antifungal Susceptibility Testing for Yeasts: Approved Standard*. NCCLS document M27A. National Committee for Clinical Laboratory Standards, Wayne, Pa.
10. **Pasarell, L., and M. R. McGinnis.** 1992. Viability of fungal cultures maintained at −70°C. *J. Clin. Microbiol.* **30:**1000–1004.
11. **Richmond, J. Y., and R. W. McKinney (ed.).** 1993. *Biosafety in the Microbiological and Biomedical Laboratories*, 3rd ed. DHSS publication (CDC) 93-8395. U.S. Government Printing Office, Washington, D.C.
12. **Salkin, I. F., and R. Gershon.** 1992. Biohazards and safety, p. 14.1.1–14.1.6. *In* H. D. Isenberg (ed.), *Clinical Microbiology Procedures Handbook*. American Society for Microbiology, Washington, D.C.
13. **Salkin, I. F., M. R. McGinnis, M. J. Dykstra, and M. G. Rinaldi.** 1988. *Scedosporium inflatum*, an emerging pathogen. *J. Clin. Microbiol.* **26:**498–503.
14. **Sternberg, S.** 1994. The emerging fungal threat. *Science* **266:**1632–1634.

SELECTED REFERENCES FOR FURTHER STUDY

1. **Beneke, E. S., and A. L. Rogers.** 1995. *Medical Mycology and Human Mycoses*. Star Publishing Co., Belmont, Calif.
2. **Hawksworth, D. L., P. M. Kirk, B. C. Sutton, and D. N. Pegler.** 1995. *Ainsworth & Bisby's Dictionary of the Fungi*, 8th ed. CAB International, Kew, Surrey, United Kingdom.
3. **Kane, J., R. Summerbell, L. Sigler, S. Krajden, and G. Land.** 1997. *Laboratory Handbook of Dermatophytes*. Star Publishing Co., Belmont, Calif.
4. **Kendrick, B.** 1985. *The Fifth Kingdom*. Mycologue Publications, Waterloo, Ontario, Canada.
5. **Kwon-Chung, K. J., and J. E. Bennet.** 1992. *Medical Mycology*. Lea & Febiger, Philadelphia, Pa.
6. **Larone, D. H.** 1995. *Medically Important Fungi: a Guide to Identification*. ASM Press, Washington, D.C.
7. **St. Germain, G., and R. Summerbell.** 1996. *Identifying Filamentous Fungi: a Clinical Laboratory Handbook*. Star Publishing Co., Belmont, Calif.

Algorithms for Detection and Identification of Fungi

WILLIAM G. MERZ AND GLENN D. ROBERTS

94

Rapid, accurate diagnosis of fungal infections is crucial for guiding early, appropriate antifungal therapies. This is critical since cultures may take days to weeks to become positive. Delays in the initiation of appropriate therapy, unfortunately, often correlate with poor outcomes. Issues specifically relating to specimen procurement and specimen processing for fungal culture are addressed in chapter 5. Isolation and identification of fungi in culture are addressed for each organism group in the respective chapters. The purpose of this chapter is to present non-culture-based assays that can be performed directly with clinical specimens. These specific approaches include direct microscopic examination, antigen detection, detection of fungus-specific metabolites, detection of cell wall components, and detection of fungus-specific nucleic acids. These assays, however, *never* replace proper culturing since none is 100% sensitive or specific.

DIRECT EXAMINATION

Direct examination of specimens for detection of fungal elements should be performed in all clinical laboratories by trained personnel since specialized equipment and reagents are not necessary. A definitive diagnosis of many mycotic infections can be made when fungal elements specific for certain fungi are pathognomonic of infection. Some examples include the detection of *Histoplasma capsulatum* in blood or bone marrow, detection of cysts of *Pneumocystis carinii*, and detection of the presence of *Blastomyces dermatitidis* and *Coccidioides immitis* by direct examination.

Detection of specific fungal elements, which are part of our normal flora or the environment, may be crucial in making a decision as to whether a specific fungus that has been recovered is a contaminant or an opportunistic pathogen. Detection of wide, wavy hyphae morphologically compatible with the agent of zygomycosis is necessary for specific diagnosis of the acute fulminant infection in the patient with diabetes mellitus in acidosis. A culture positive for *Rhizopus* may be a contaminant or a pathogen, and prevention of a delay in time of initiation of aggressive antifungal therapy and surgical procedures is crucial. Other, similar important examples include *Aspergillus* or the agents of hyalohyphomycosis and phaeohyphomycosis, in which the detection of hyphae in a clinical specimen is strongly associated with the presence of disease.

In addition, the detection of specific fungal elements allows the laboratory to add specialized media or to use an increased incubation time for optimal recovery of fungi. Flagging of cultures with a positive direct examination for *Blastomyces dermatitidis*, *Coccidiodes immitis*, or *Histoplasma capsulatum* has permitted recovery of these pathogens by extending the incubation period beyond the laboratory's normal incubation time.

However, limitations and potential problems with direct examinations must be considered. First, a negative direct examination *never* rules out a fungal infection. The sensitivity varies by anatomical site, the amount of specimen examined, the number of organisms, the type of patient, and the quality of the examiner. Second, false-positive findings do occur, unfortunately. Lysed lymphocytes in an India ink preparation of a cerebrospinal fluid (CSF) sample have been mistaken for *Cryptococcus neoformans*, collagen fibers have been mistaken for "fungal elements," fat droplets have been confused with budding yeast cells, and fibers from swabs have been called zygomycetous hyphae, etc. Equivocal findings should always be reviewed by more than one reader, or a second procedure should be performed to aid in this type of problem. A false-positive direct examination usually is more harmful than a false-negative direct examination!

Since direct examinations are less sensitive than cultures, cultures should be performed with specimens and direct examinations should be performed only if a sufficient volume is provided. Like all policies, exceptions exist; a positive direct examination of a mouth lesion specimen suspected of being candidiasis may be more important than a positive culture.

A number of stains or procedures can be used to detect fungal elements by direct examination of clinical specimens (Table 1). Each method has its own advantages and disadvantages. The wet prep, KOH, calcofluor, Gram stain, Wright stain, Giemsa stain, and monoclonal fluorescent-antibody assays for the detection of *Pneumocystis carinii* are often performed in clinical laboratories.

Papanicolaou staining is usually performed in a cytopathology laboratory, and periodic acid-Schiff staining and methenamine silver staining are usually performed by pathology laboratories. Laboratory personnel may occasionally be called upon to aid in interpretation, so familiarity with these staining procedures may be helpful.

TABLE 1 Methods available for direct microscopic detection of fungal elements in clinical specimens

Method (reference)	Use	Time required	Advantages	Disadvantages
Alcian blue staining	Detection of *C. neoformans* in CSF	2 min	When positive in CSF, it is diagnostic.	Not commonly used; like India ink, does not detect all cases.
Calcofluor white staining (9, 14)	Detection of fungi including *P. carinii*	1 min	Can be mixed with KOH; detects fungi rapidly due to bright fluorescence.	Requires fluorescence microscope; background fluorescence is prominent, but fungi exhibit more intense fluorescence. Vaginal secretions are difficult to interpret.
Giemsa staining	Examination of bone marrow and peripheral blood smear	15 min	Detects intracellular *H. capsulatum*.	Detection is usually limited to *H. capsulatum*.
Giemsa staining and rapid modifications	Examination of induced sputum and bronchoscopy specimens	13 min	Detects intracystic bodies and trophozoites of *P. carinii*.	Does not stain cysts and does stain organisms other than *P. carinii*.
Gram staining	Detection of bacteria	3 min	Is commonly performed with most clinical specimens submitted for bacteriology and will detect most fungi, if present.	Some fungi stain well; however, others, e.g., *Cryptococcus* spp., stain weakly in some instances and exhibit only stippling. Common Gram-stained artifacts appear as yeast cells.
India ink treatment	Detection of *C. neoformans* in CSF	1 min	When positive in CSF, is diagnostic of meningitis.	Negative in many cases of meningitis; not reliable.
Potassium hydroxide treatment	Clearing of specimen to make fungi more readily visible	5 min; if clearing is not complete, an additional 5 to 10 min is necessary	Rapid detection of fungal elements.	Experience required since background artifacts are often confusing. Clearing of some specimens may require an extended time.
Methylene blue treatment	Fungi in skin scrapings	2 min	Usually added to KOH; provides contrast for detection of elements.	Background staining of cells makes reading of results difficult.
Methenamine silver staining	Detection of fungi in histologic section	1 h	Best stain for detection of fungal elements.	Requires a specialized staining method that is not usually readily available to microbiology laboratories.
Papanicolaou staining	Examination of secretions for presence of malignant cells	30 min	Cytotechnologist can detect fungal elements.	Requires specialized staining and reader familiar with this stain.
Periodic acid-Schiff staining	Detection of fungi	20 min; 5 additional min needed if counterstaining is used	Stains fungal elements well; hyphae and yeasts can be readily distinguished.	*Blastomyces dermatitidis* appears pleomorphic. Periodic acid-Schiff stain-positive artifacts can appear as yeast cells.
Toluidine blue staining	Examination of induced sputum and bronchial specimens for *P. carinii*	25 min	Detects the cyst walls of *P. carinii* as a purple color.	The background stains. It does stain other fungi.

(Continued on next page)

TABLE 1 (*Continued*)

Method (reference)	Use	Time required	Advantages	Disadvantages
Fluorescent monoclonal antibody treatment (19)	Examination of induced sputum and bronchial specimens for *P. carinii*	45 min	Detects the cysts of *P. carinii*.	Specific for *P. carinii*.
Wright staining	Examination of bone marrow or peripheral blood smears	7 min	Detects intracellular *H. capsulatum*.	Detection is usually limited to *H. capsulatum*.

Fungi, as a group, exhibit great diversity and polymorphism. This is exemplified by the various morphologies and structures which are seen in pathologic tissue. However, recognition of these diverse structures in clinical specimens can provide a very specific identification of many fungal pathogens or at least a definable list of possible other pathogens. The characteristic fungal elements seen in clinical specimens are presented in Fig. 1, which is organized by anatomic site, and in Table 2, which is organized by fungal structure. Most fungi appear the same in tissue as they do in other clinical specimens. Figures 2 to 31 illustrate these fungal elements seen in clinical specimens.

TABLE 2 Characteristic fungal elements seen by direct examination of clinical specimens

Morphologic fungal element found	Organism(s)	Diam range (μm)	Characteristic features
Yeast forms	*Histoplasma capsulatum*	2–5	Small; oval to round budding cells; often found clustered within histocytes; difficult to detect when present in small numbers; often intracellular; Fig. 2 and 3
Yeast forms	*Sporothrix schenckii*	2–6	Small; oval to round to cigar shaped; single or multiple buds present; uncommonly seen in clinical specimens; Fig. 4
Yeast forms	*Cryptococcus neoformans*	2–15	Cells vary in size; usually spherical but may be football shaped; buds usually single and "pinched off"; capsule may or may not be evident; rarely, pseudohyphal forms with or without capsule may be seen; Fig. 5–8
Yeast forms	*Blastomyces dermatitidis*	8–15	Cells usually large and spherical, double refractile; buds usually single, but several may remain attached to parent cells; buds connected by broad base; Fig. 9 and 10
Yeast forms	*Paracoccidioides brasiliensis*	5–60	Cell usually large and surrounded by smaller buds around periphery ("mariner's wheel" appearance); smaller cells (2–5 μm) that resemble *H. capsulatum* may be present; buds have "pinched off" appearance; Fig. 11 and 12
Yeast forms (fission)	*Penicillium marneffei*	3	Fission yeast, not budding yeast; Fig. 31
Cysts and trophozoites	*Pneumocystis carinii*	5–12 (cysts)	Cysts are round to cup shaped, possibly with four intracystic bodies; trophozoites are free smaller stages; Fig. 26 and 27

(*Continued on next page*)

TABLE 2 Characteristic fungal elements seen by direct examination of clinical specimens (*Continued*)

Morphologic fungal element found	Organism(s)	Diam range (μm)	Characteristic features
Spherules	*Coccidioides immitis*	10–200	Spherules vary in size; some contain endospores, others are empty. Adjacent spherules may resemble *B. dermatitidis*; endospores may resemble *H. capsulatum* but show no evidence of budding. Spherules may produce multiple germ tubes if direct preparation is kept in moist chamber for ≥24 h; hyphae may be found in cavitary lesions; Fig. 13 and 14
"Sporangium"	*Rhinosporidium seeberi*	6–300	Large, thick-walled sporangia containing sporangiospores; mature sporangia are larger than spherules of *Coccidioides immitis*.
Yeast forms and pseudohyphae or true hyphae	*Candida* spp.	3–4 (yeast forms) 5–10 (pseudohyphae)	Cells usually exhibit single budding; pseudohyphae, when present, are constricted at ends and remain attached like links of sausage; true hyphae, when present, have parallel walls and are septate; Fig. 15 and 16
Yeast forms and hyphae	*Malassezia furfur*	3–8 (yeast forms) 5–10 (pseudohyphae)	Short, curved hyphal elements usually present along with round yeast cells that retain their spherical shapes in compacted cluster; Fig. 17
Wide nonseptate hyphae	Zygomycetes: *Mucor* spp., *Rhizopus* spp., and other genera	10–30	Hyphae are large, ribbon-like, often fractured or twisted. Occasionally, septa may be present, branching usually at right angles. Smaller hyphae overlap those of *Aspergillus* spp., particularly *Aspergillus flavus*; Fig. 18 to 20
Hyaline septate hyphae	Dermatophytes; skin and nails	3–15	Hyaline septate hyphae commonly seen; chains of arthroconidia may be present; Fig. 21
Hyaline septate hyphae	Hair	3–15	Arthroconidia on periphery of hair shaft that produce sheaths indicate ectothrix infection. Arthroconidia formed by fragmentation of hyphae within hair shaft indicate endothrix infection. Long hyphal filaments or channels within hair shaft indicate favus hair infection.
Hyaline septate hyphae	*Aspergillus* spp.	3–12	Hyphae are septate and exhibit dichotomous, 45° angle branching; larger hyphae, often disturbed, may resemble those of zygomycetes; Fig. 22 to 24
Hyaline septate hyphae	*Geotrichum* spp.	4–12	Hyphae and rectangular arthroconidia are present and are sometimes rounded. Irregular forms may be present; Fig. 25
Hyaline septate hyphae	*Pseudallescheria boydii* (cases other than mycetoma)	3–12	Hyphae are septate and are impossible to distinguish from those of other hyaline molds, e.g., *Aspergillus* spp.
Hyaline septate hyphae	*Fusarium* spp.	3–12	Hyphae are septate and are impossible to distinguish from those of other hyaline molds, e.g., *Aspergillus* spp.

(*Continued on next page*)

TABLE 2 (*Continued*)

Morphologic fungal element found	Organism(s)	Diam range (μm)	Characteristic features
Dematiaceous septate hyphae	*Bipolaris* spp., *Curvularia* spp., *Exserohilum* spp., *Exophiala* spp., *Phialophora* spp., *Wangiella dermatitidis*, *Xylohypha bantiana*, *Phaeoannellomyces werneckii*	2–6 1.5–5	Dematiaceous polymorphous hyphae are seen; budding cells with single septa and chains of swollen rounded cells may be present. Occasionally, aggregates may be present when infection is caused by *Phialophora* and *Exophiala* spp.; Fig. 30
Sclerotic bodies	*Cladosporium carrionii*, *Fonsecaea compacta*, *Fonsecaea pedrosoi*, *Phialophora verrucosa*, *Rhinocladiella acquaspersa*	5–20	Brown, round to pleomorphic, thick-walled cells with transverse septa. Commonly, cells contain two fission plates that form tetrads of cells. Occasionally, branched septate hyphae may be found in addition to sclerotic bodies. Fig. 26
Granules	*Acremonium falciforme*, *Acremonium kilense*, *Acremonium recifei*	200–300	White, soft granules without cement-like matrix
Granules	*Curvularia geniculata*, *Curvularia lunata*	500–1,000	Black, hard grains with cement-like matrix at periphery
Granules	*Aspergillus nidulans*	65–160	White, soft granules without cement-like matrix
Granules	*Exophiala jeanselmei*	200–300	Black, soft granules, vacuolated, without cement-like matrix, made of dark hyphae and swollen cells
Granules	*Fusarium* spp.	200–500	White, soft granules without cement-like matrix
Granules	*Fusarium moniliforme*, *Fusarium solani*	300–600	
Granules	*Leptosphaeria* spp.	400–600	Black, hard granules; cement-like matrix; periphery composed of polygonal swollen cells and center composed of hyphal network
Granules	*Madurella grisea*	350–500	Black, soft granules without cement-like matrix; periphery composed of polygonal swollen cells and a center composed of a hyphal network
Granules	*Madurella mycetomatis*	200–900	Black to brown hard granules of two types: (i) rust brown, compact, and filled with cement-like matrix and (ii) deep brown, filled with numerous vesicles, 6–14 μm in diam, cement-like matrix in periphery, and central area of light-colored hyphae
Granules	*Neotestudina rosatti*	300–600	White, soft granules with cement-like matrix at periphery
Granules	*Pseudallescheria boydii*	200–300	White, soft granules composed of hyphae and swollen cells at periphery in cement-like matrix
Granules	*Pyrenochaeta romeroi*	300–600	Black, soft granules composed of polygonal swollen cells at periphery; cement-like matrix

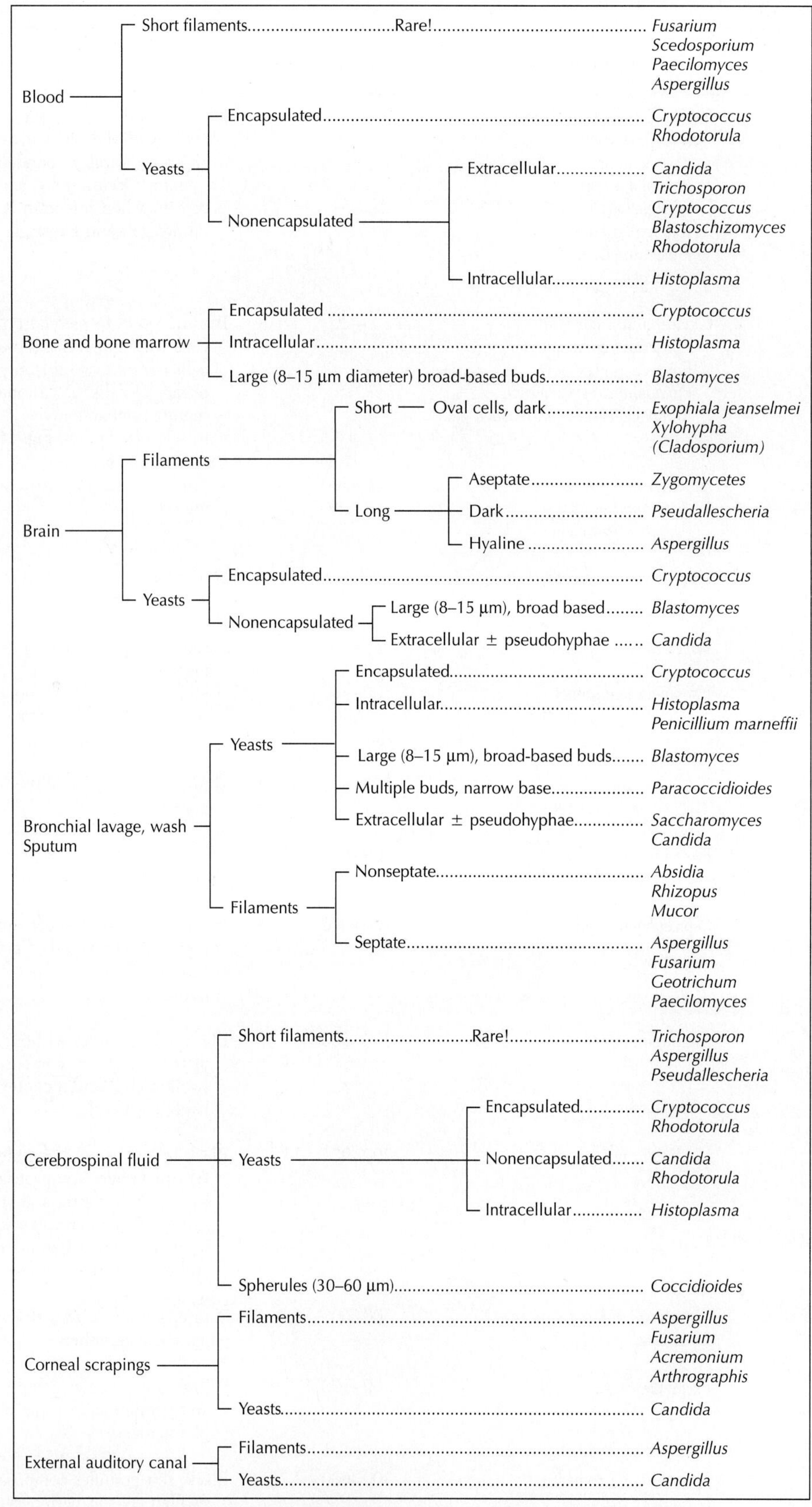

FIGURE 1 Fungal elements detected by microscopic examination. The figure is compliments of Kevin Hazen and is reprinted from *Essential Procedures for Clinical Microbiology* (11a).

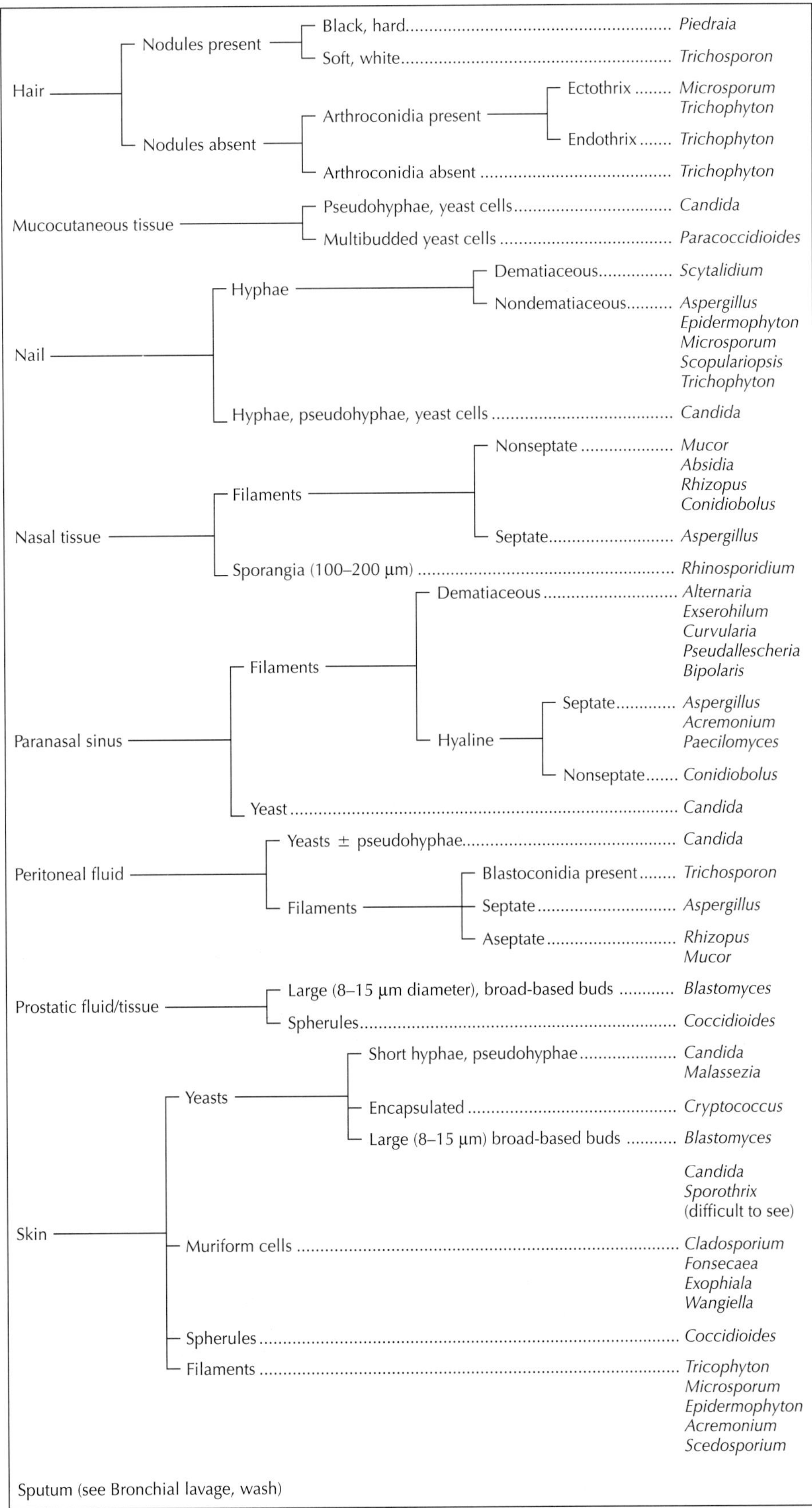

FIGURE 1 *(Continued)*

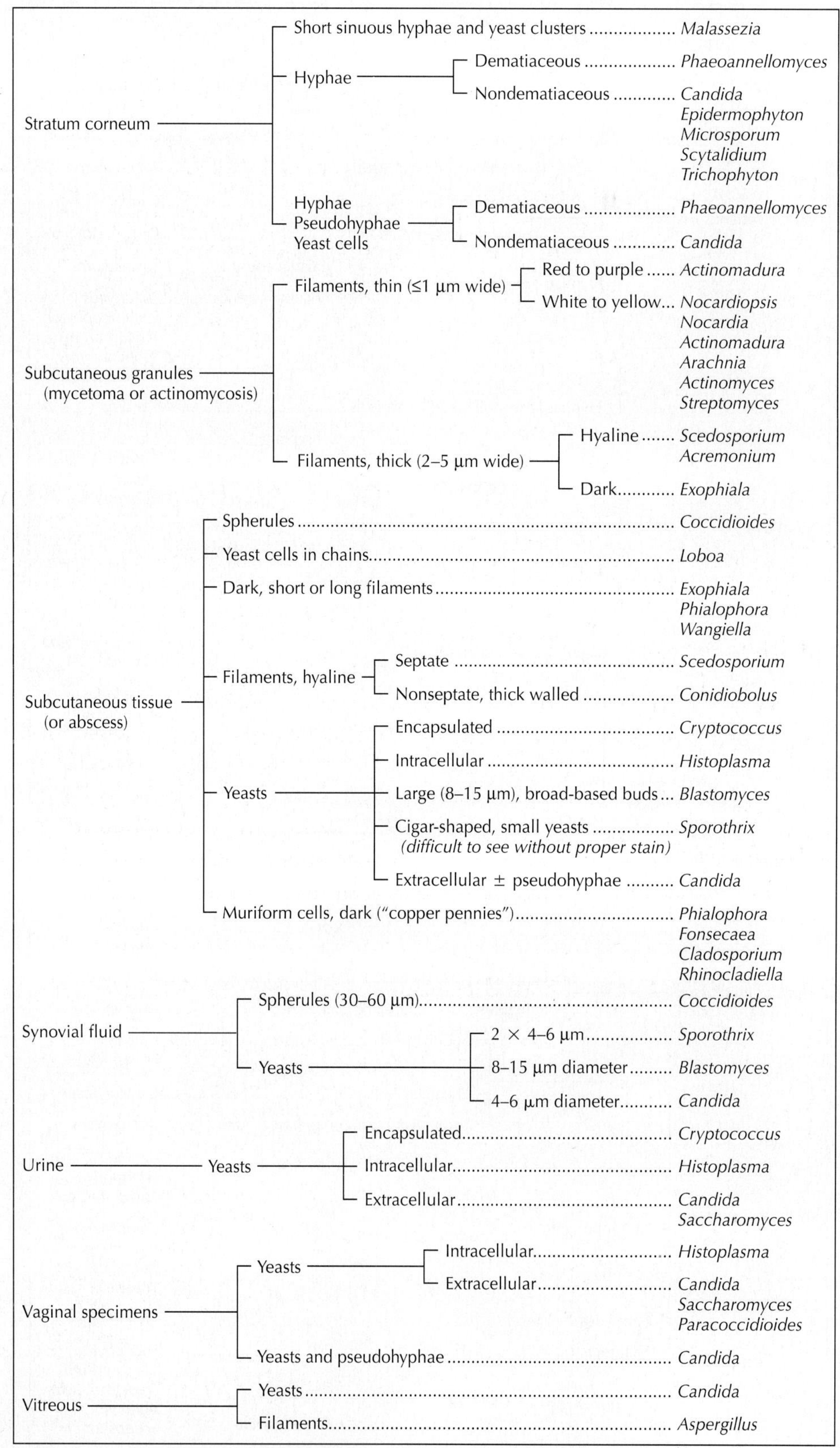

FIGURE 1 *(Continued)*

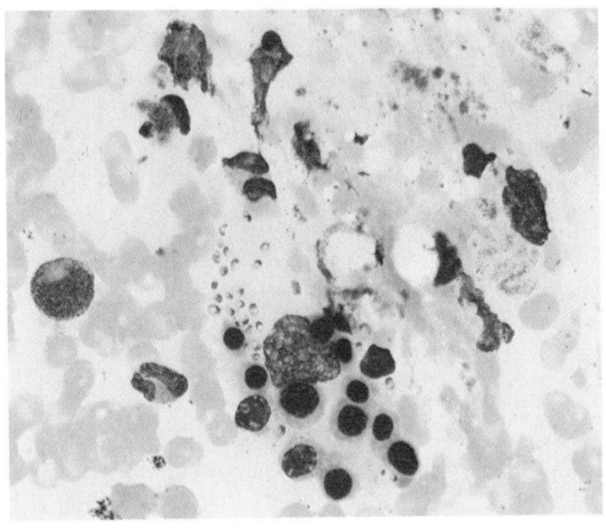

FIGURE 2 *H. capsulatum* in bone marrow. Small intracellular yeast cells are apparent in this Wright-Giemsa preparation. Magnification, ×1,852.

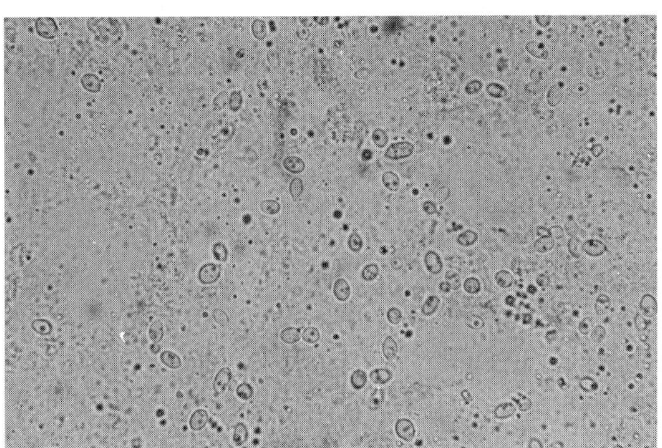

FIGURE 3 Numerous small budding yeast cells of *H. capsulatum* present in sputum as seen by bright-field microscopy. Magnification, ×1,852.

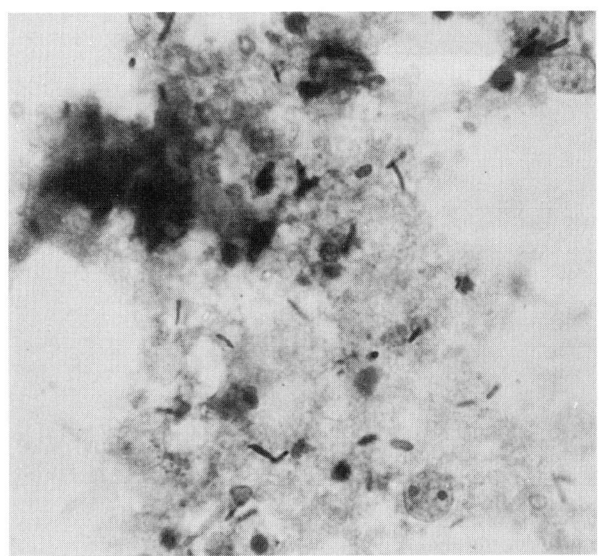

FIGURE 4 Periodic acid-Schiff stain of exudate from a cutaneous ulcer, showing numerous elongated yeast cells (cigar bodies) of *Sporothrix schenckii*. Magnification, ×1,915.

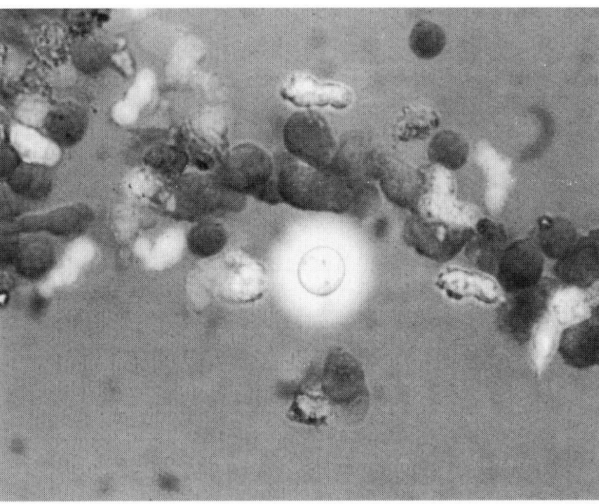

FIGURE 5 India ink preparation of CSF showing a single encapsulated, spherical yeast cell of *C. neoformans*. Magnification, ×2,385.

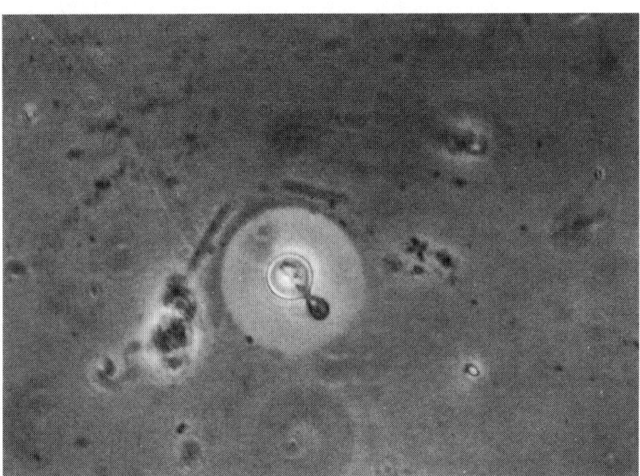

FIGURE 6 Phase-contrast photomicrograph of *C. neoformans* in sputum. Note the spherical yeast cell with a "narrow-necked" bud attached. Magnification, ×2,385.

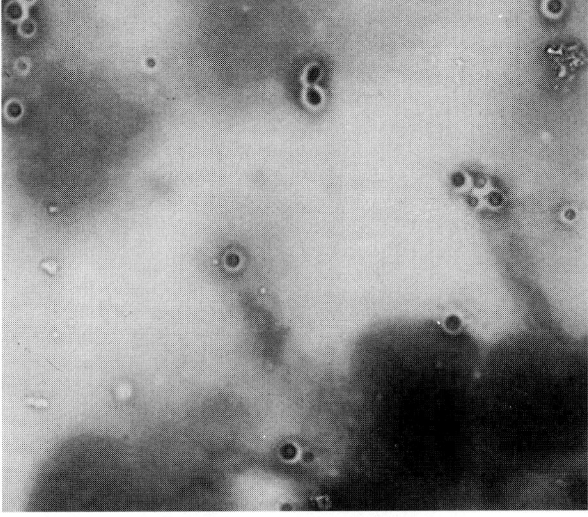

FIGURE 7 Periodic acid-Schiff stain of sputum, showing spherical yeast cells of *C. neoformans*. Note the presence of a capsule and the variation in sizes of cells. Magnification, ×1,590.

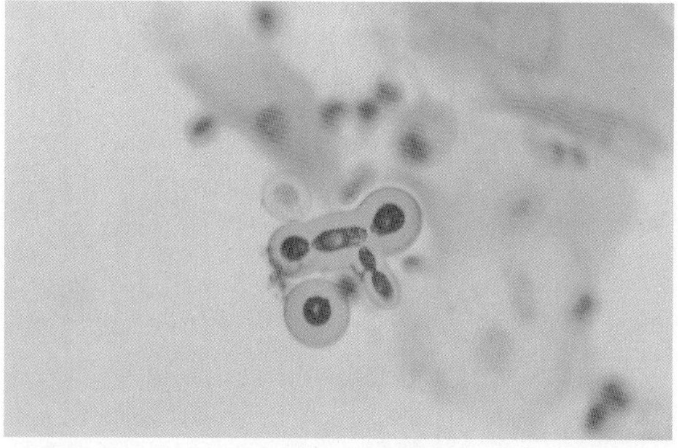

FIGURE 8 Papanicolaou stain of sputum showing the rare pseudohyphal form of *C. neoformans*. Note the capsule surrounding all cells. Magnification, ×2,210.

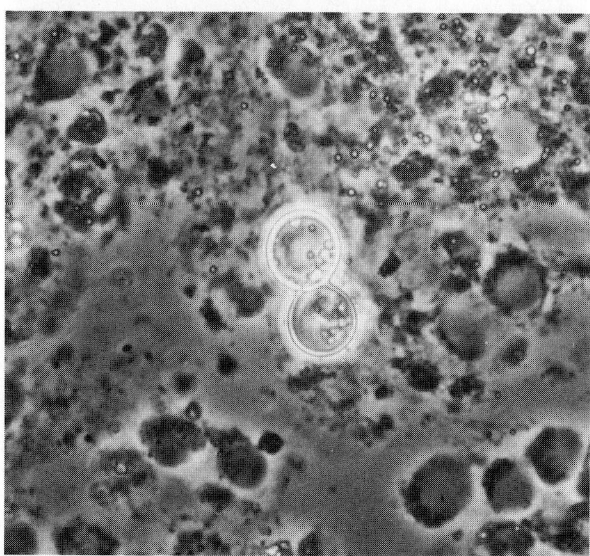

FIGURE 9 Phase-contrast photomicrograph of *B. dermatitidis* in sputum. The presence of a large, broad-based, budding yeast cell with a "double-contoured" wall is characteristic. Magnification, ×3,040.

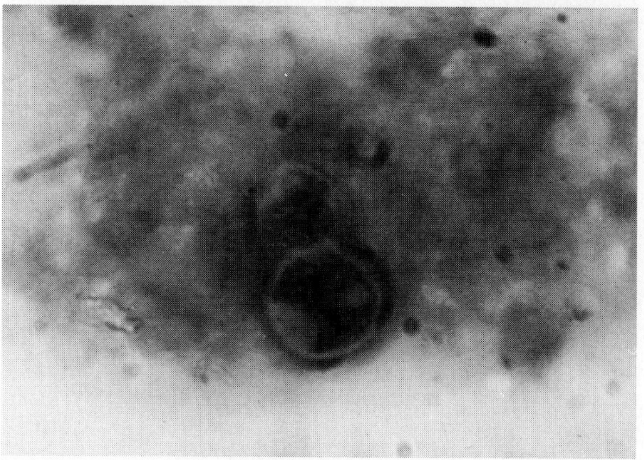

FIGURE 10 Gram stain of *B. dermatitidis* yeast form in sputum. Magnification, ×1,852.

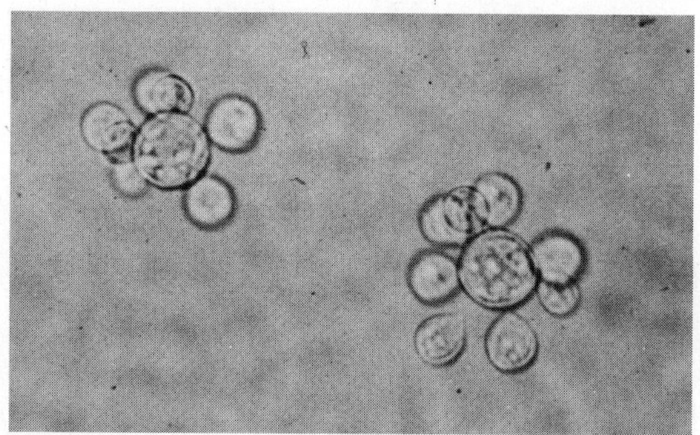

FIGURE 11 Bright-field photomicrograph of *Paracoccidioides brasiliensis*, showing multiple budding yeast cells resembling mariner's wheels. Magnification, ×1,590.

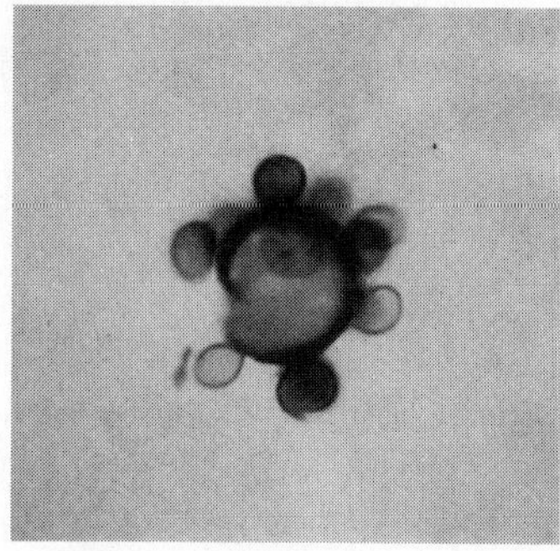

FIGURE 12 Methenamine silver stain of *P. brasiliensis* yeast form. Magnification, ×980.

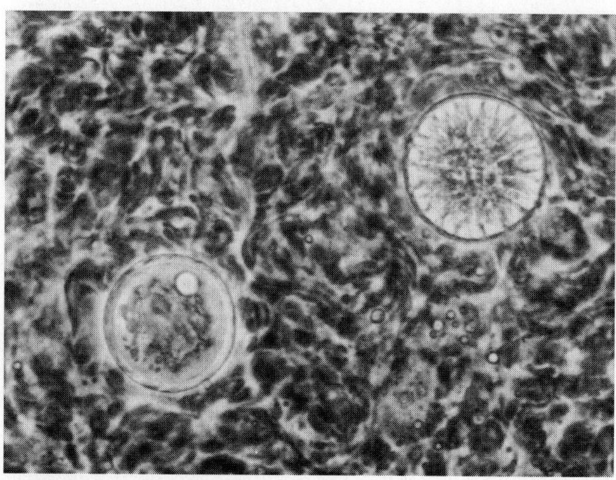

FIGURE 13 Phase-contrast photomicrograph of *Coccidioides immitis* spherules in sputum. Note the absence of endospores and the presence of cleavage furrows on one spherule. Magnification, ×2,400.

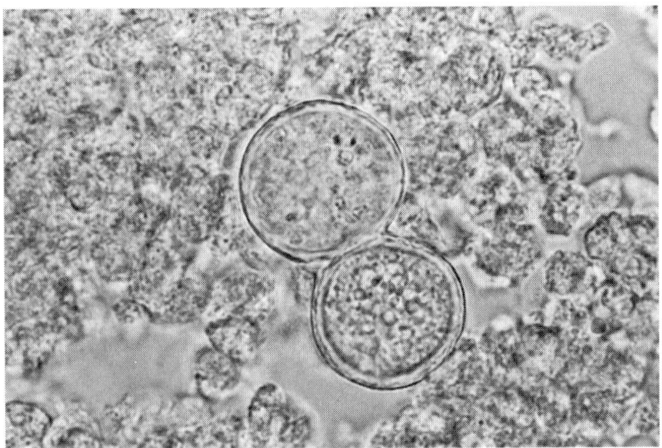

FIGURE 14 Bright-field photomicrograph of two adjacent spherules of *Coccidioides immitis* that morphologically resemble *B. dermatitidis*. Note the presence of endospores in one spherule. Magnification, ×1,228.

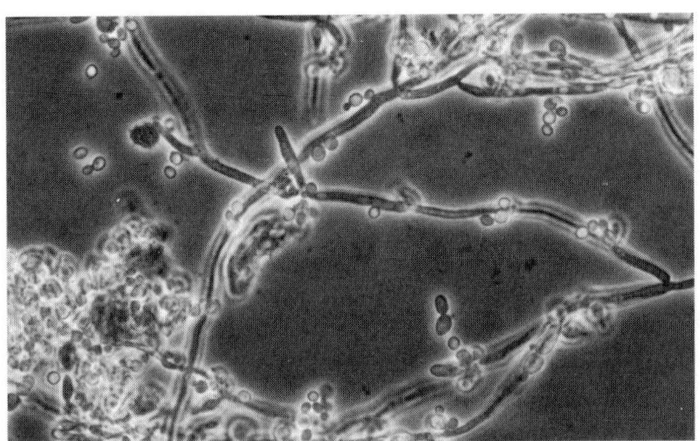

FIGURE 15 Phase-contrast photomicrograph of a *Candida* sp. in peritoneal fluid. Note the presence of blastoconidia and pseudohyphae characteristic of the genus. Magnification, ×1,493.

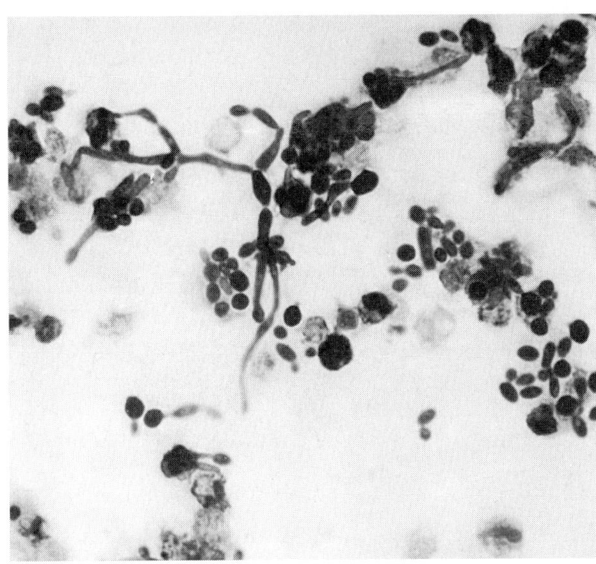

FIGURE 16 Periodic acid-Schiff stain of a *Candida* sp. Magnification, ×1,390.

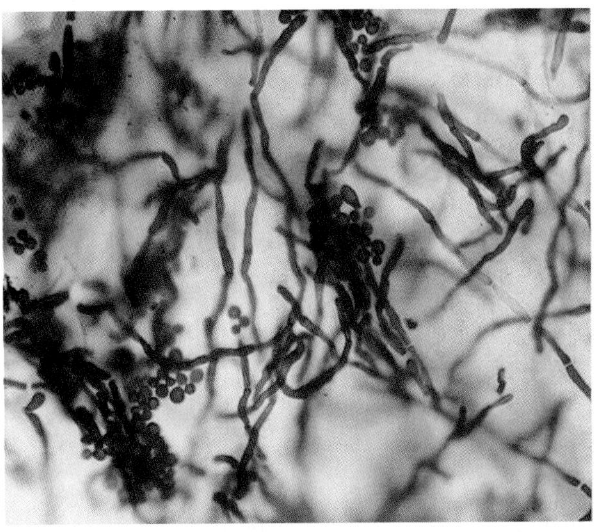

FIGURE 17 Periodic acid-Schiff stain of skin showing hyphal and yeast elements characteristic of *Malassezia furfur*. Magnification, ×1,590.

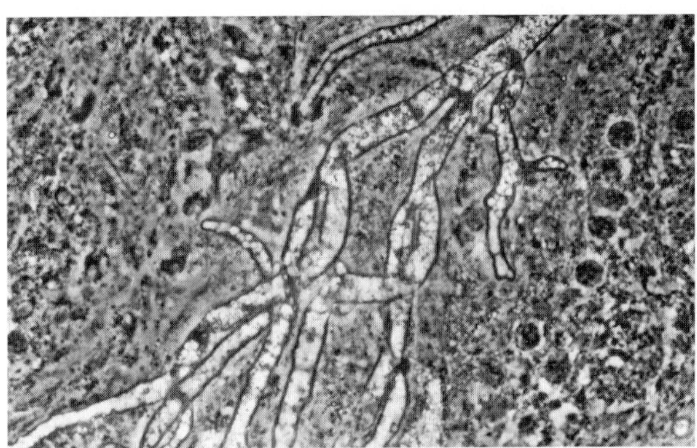

FIGURE 18 Phase-contrast photomicrograph of wound exudate, showing large, aseptate, twisted hyphae characteristic of a zygomycete. Magnification, ×1,493.

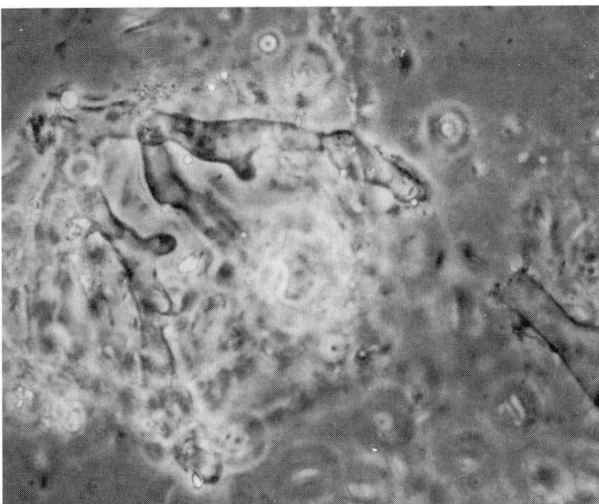

FIGURE 19 Phase-contrast photomicrograph showing fractured pieces of large aseptate hyphae characteristic of a zygomycete. Magnification, ×1,990.

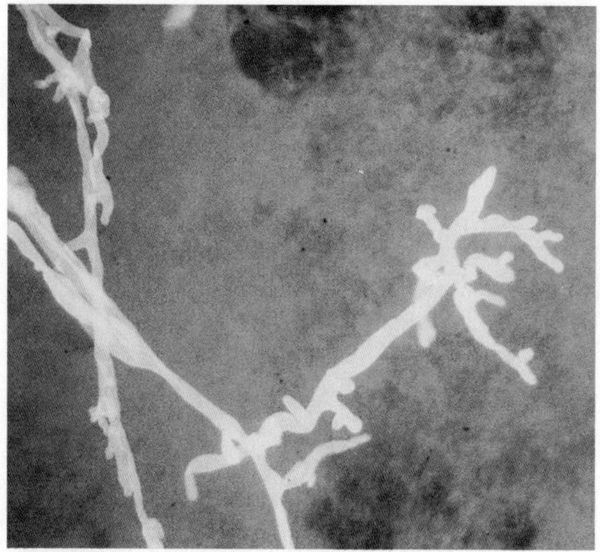

FIGURE 20 Calcofluor white stain of sputum showing characteristic hyphae of a zygomycete. Magnification, ×928.

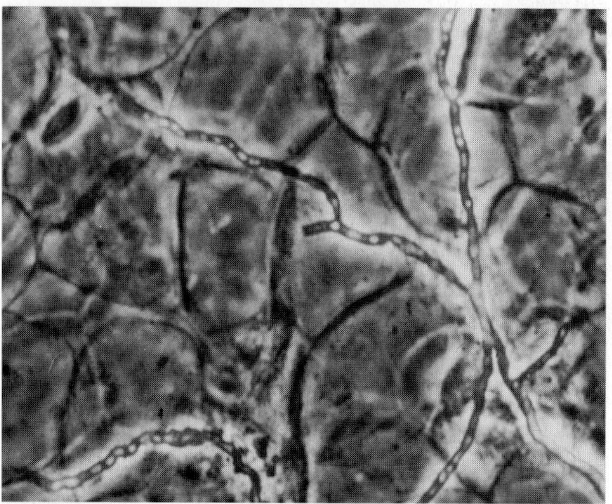

FIGURE 21 Phase-contrast photomicrograph of hyphae of a dermatophyte intertwined with squamous cells. Magnification, ×1,535.

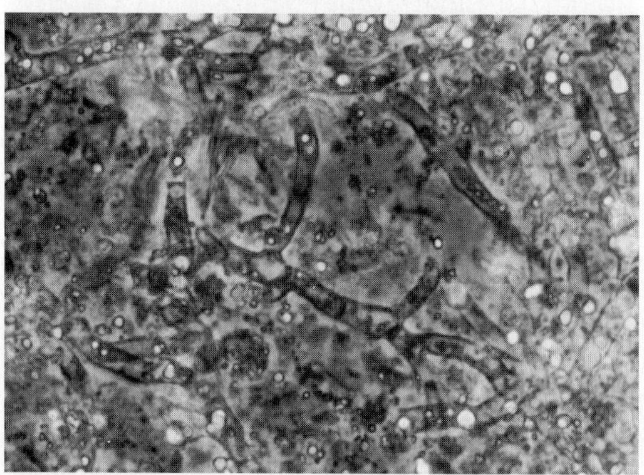

FIGURE 22 Phase-contrast photomicrograph of exudate from lung tissue, showing septate hyphae. An *Aspergillus* sp. was recovered in culture. Magnification, ×3,040.

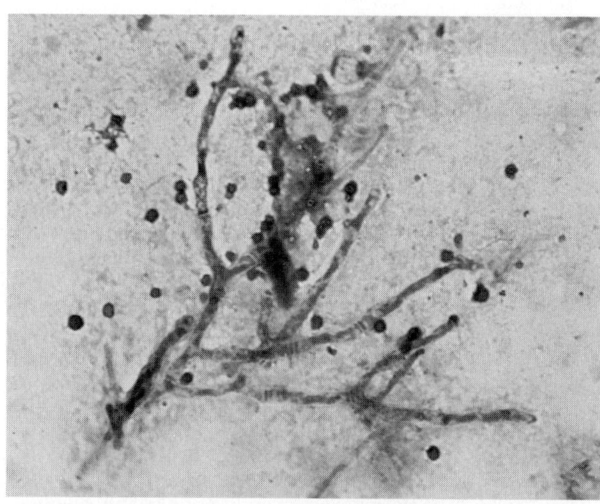

FIGURE 23 Gram stain sputum, showing dichotomously branching, septate hyphae consistent with those of an *Aspergillus* sp. Magnification, ×1,860.

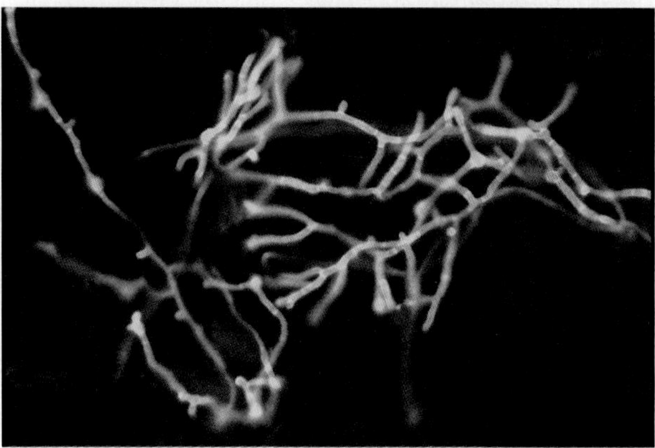

FIGURE 24 Calcofluor white stain of hyphae characteristic of an *Aspergillus* sp. Magnification, ×1,200.

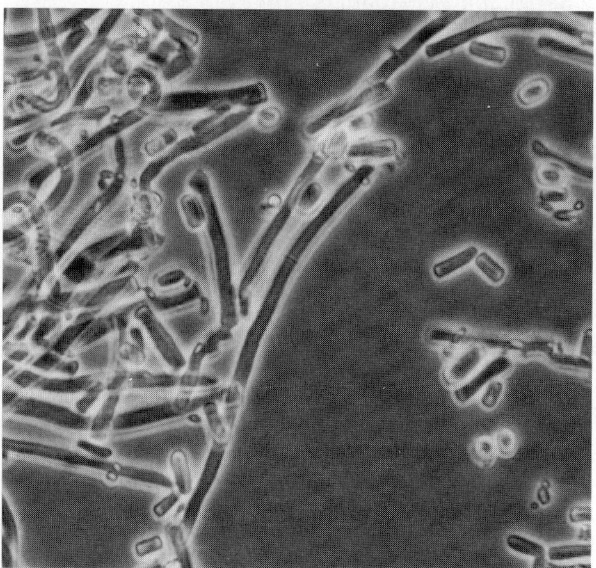

FIGURE 25 Phase-contrast photomicrograph showing hyphae and arthroconidia in sputum. A *Geotrichum* sp. was recovered in culture. Magnification, ×1,597.

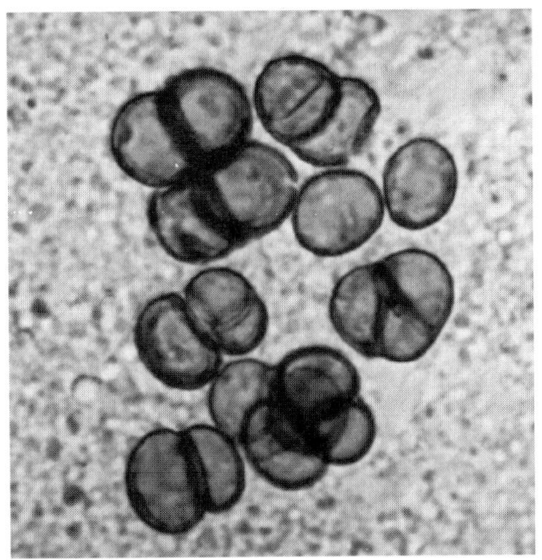

FIGURE 26 KOH preparation of sclerotic cells in tissue that are characteristic of the tissue form of the etiologic agents of chromoblastomycosis. Magnification, ×1,535.

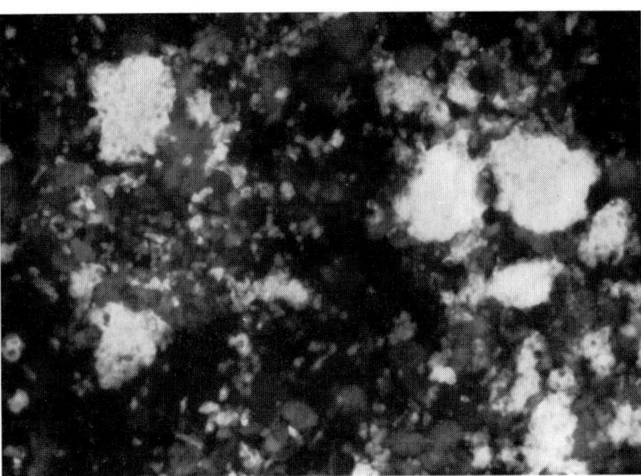

FIGURE 29 Monoclonal fluorescent-antibody stain of *P. carinii* in an induced sputum specimen. Magnification, ×1,200.

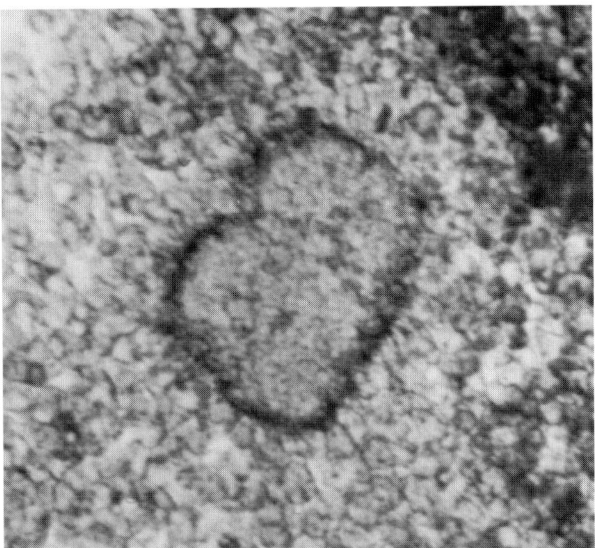

FIGURE 27 KOH preparation of a granule found in wound exudate that is characteristically seen in mycetoma. Magnification, ×500.

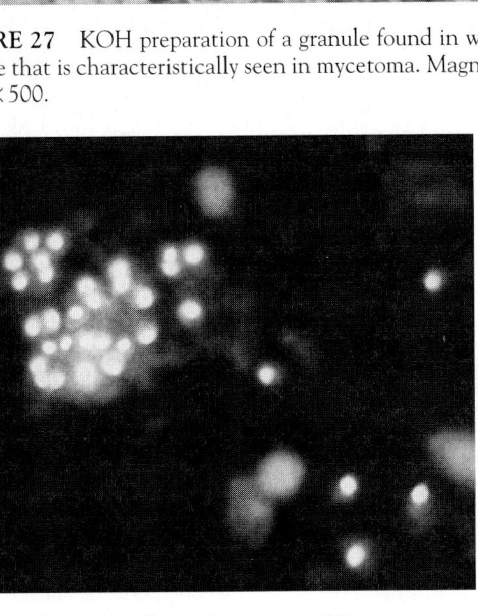

FIGURE 28 Calcofluor white stain of *P. carinii* cysts in an induced sputum specimen. Magnification, ×1,589.

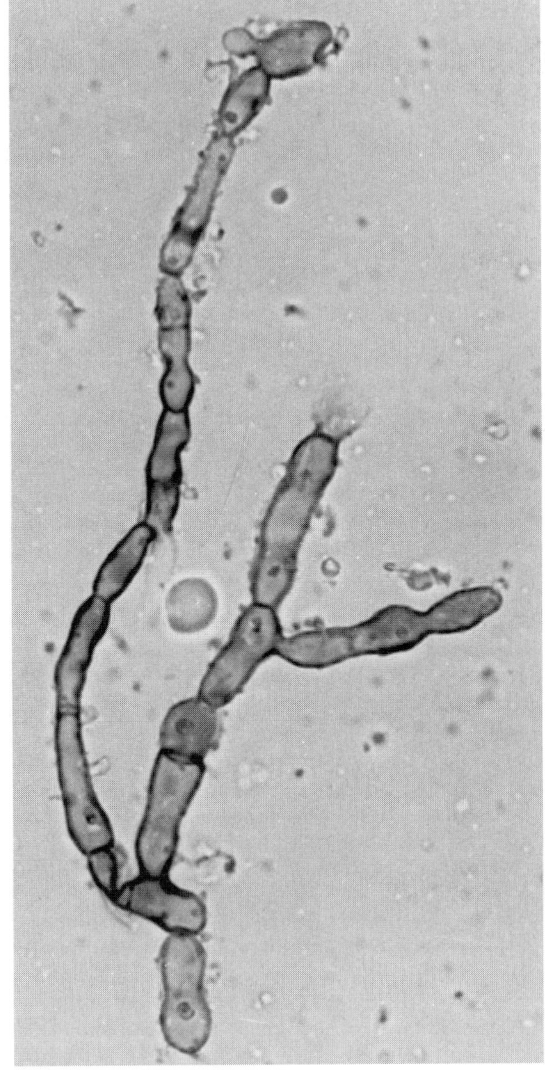

FIGURE 30 KOH stain of dematiaceous hyphae in an aspirate of a subcutaneous cyst. Magnification, ×2,000.

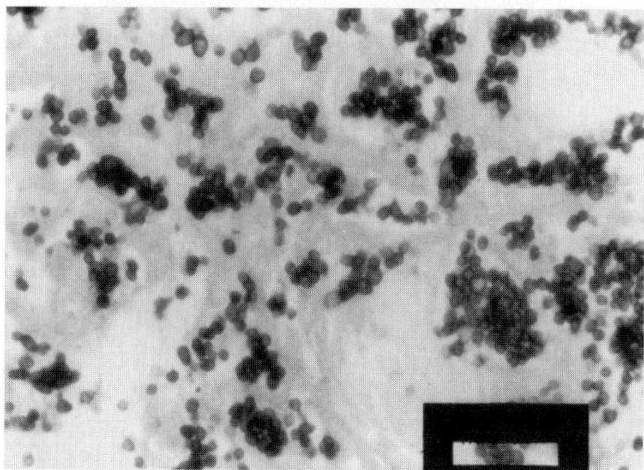

FIGURE 31 Methenamine silver staining of fission yeast cells of *Penicillium marneffei*. Bar, 25 μm. Picture compliments of C. R. Cooper.

ANTIGEN DETECTION

Cryptococcosis Antigen

Detection of cryptococcal antigen for the diagnosis of progressive cryptococcal infections is probably the best antigen detection assay for the diagnosis of any infectious disease.

The polysaccharide capsule that is detected is produced in large quantities and becomes dissolved in body fluids, e.g., CSF and serum. Temporally, antigen detection may precede the detection of viable organisms in CSF and positive cultures of CSF. Although there are serologic differences among *Cryptococcus neoformans* isolates due to the presence of different surface epitopes, there is sufficient cross-reactivity to detect antigen from all serotypes. Sensitivities vary primarily by patient population, stage or duration of infection, and assay methodology. When performed properly, there should be very few false-positive results. False-positive results do occur; some are specific for the type of assay performed, and some are generic. Sera from patients with invasive infections with *Trichosporon beigelii* will react with the anticryptococcal antibodies due to the production of a cross-reacting polysaccharide. There may be false-negative results, and these are mostly due to the extent of infection: single focal lesions, e.g., pulmonary lesions, may not produce a significant quantity of antigen in serum for detection. False-negative results for patients with disseminated or progressive infections are less frequent, although they sometimes occur and are difficult to explain.

Latex agglutination kits are commercially available (Murex, Meridian, Wampole, and Immunomycologics), and they are reliable, being both sensitive and specific when performed by following strict procedures and when the results are read and interpreted by trained personnel (13). Advantages include the following: the assays are easy to perform, they can be performed with CSF and serum specimens, they do not require special equipment, and the technology is familiar to most personnel. Potential problems with the latex tests include (i) the need for subjective reading of agglutination, (ii) the need for pretreatment to improve sensitivity and specificity, and (iii) the need for meticulous control of factors that cause false-positive results.

The sensitivity of latex assays may be as high as 99% (13). False-negative results are assumed to be due to a low concentration of the polysaccharide antigen or due to a prozone effect at high antigen concentrations. Treatment of CSF by boiling or treatment with pronase to destroy any protein that might bind or block the antigen-antibody reaction may increase the sensitivity and the titer of the antigen. More importantly, however, pretreatment of serum with pronase or boiling of CSF may destroy rheumatoid factor or other proteins that might contribute to a false-positive reaction. These potential false-positive reactions can be detected with control latex beads coated only with normal globulins. Agar and the syneresis fluid on agar produce false-positive reactions that are not destroyed by pronase (1). In addition, platinum wire loops may cause false-positive reactions (10). Therefore, it is critical that a CSF specimen be aliquotted for antigen testing before processing for culture is performed. Additionally, DF-1, a fastidious, gram-negative, nonfermenting bacterium, has caused false-positive results with CSF samples, as has *Trichosporon beigelii* (13).

An enzyme immunoassay (EIA) is also commercially available (Meridian) for the detection of cryptococcal polysaccharide antigen (5). It is a sandwich EIA. Advantages include the following: (i) the endpoint is objective, (ii) the assay does not require pretreatment of specimens, and (iii) analytically, the assay is more sensitive than latex assays. Limitations are (i) the need for an EIA instrument for reading and interpretation of the results for some specimens, and (ii) the fact that, per assay, the EIA is more expensive, expecially when the titer of a sample must be determined. Although the prozone effect should not occur, there have been specimens that were negative when they were used undiluted but positive when they were used at a dilution of 1:20 or higher (16a).

Titering of specimens for the retrieval of semiquantitative data can be helpful in some circumstances. A higher titer usually correlates with worse disease. In the future and with more data, the titer may be one criterion to be used to choose the chemotherapeutic regimen or determine the need for hospitalization for individual patients. Titers in CSF can also be helpful in monitoring therapy when the titers are tested over appropriate intervals (at least 2 weeks). This is necessary since the antigen, a complex heteropolysaccharide, is not cleared rapidly. When comparing titers, it is best if the titration assays are performed at the same time, with the same reagents, and by the same individual.

A big challenge for the clinical laboratory is the return of a patient (usually a patient with AIDS) who has had previous cryptococcal meningitis and presents with a new central nervous system event which could be cryptococcal relapse or some other infection or noninfectious disease. Since AIDS patients rarely, if ever, clear the antigen, they will be positive even in the absence of active infection. Titers may be helpful, but the definitive decision often depends on the results of culture of the CSF.

Histoplasmosis

In 1986, Wheat et al. (34) described a radioimmunoassay that was capable of detecting a heat-stable polysaccharide antigen of *Histoplasma capsulatum* in serum, urine, or bronchoalveolar lavage fluid.

Since that time, numerous publications have documented experience with the test. In one series, 195 patients having clinical or laboratory evidence of histoplasmosis were studied for the presence of antigenemia or antigenuria. Antigen was detected in 92, 21, and 39% of patients with disseminated, chronic pulmonary, and self-limited histoplasmosis, respectively (35). Histoplasma antigen was present in 41.6% of 12 patients having histoplasma meningitis.

Furthermore, antigen was found in 1 of 11 patients with coccidioidal meningitis (32). Histoplasma antigen was detected in 70.3% of the bronchoalveolar washings of 27 histoplasmosis patients with AIDS. *Histoplasma capsulatum* was recovered from 88.9% of the patients. Antigenemia and antigenuria were detected in 92.6 and 88.5% of the patients, respectively (30). Twenty-six cases of disseminated or self-limited histoplasmosis among children 18 years of age or younger were reviewed to assess the usefulness of the histoplasma antigen test in the pediatric population. Antigenuria was detected in 20 patients with progressive disease who were treated with amphotericin B. Antigen levels decreased and correlated with clinical improvement (4). It has been shown that the results of therapy can be followed since the level of antigenuria decreases during therapy and increases during relapses in immunocompromised patients (31).

The specificity of the histoplasma antigen test was questioned in 1989 when 16% of patients with blastomycosis had positive test results (33). Another false-positive histoplasma antigen test result for a patient with blastomycosis was reported and suggested that care should be taken in interpreting the results of antigen-based tests since cross-reactivity may occur (6). Recently, Wheat et al. (29) evaluated the method for cross-reactivity using urine samples from patients with other disseminated fungal infections. Not surprisingly, histoplasma antigen was found in 63.1% (12 of 19), 88.9% (8 of 9), and 94.4% (17 of 18) of patients with blastomycosis, paracoccidioidomycosis, and *Penicillium marneffei* infection, respectively. The investigators emphasized that the cross-reactivity of the test does not detract from its value for rapid diagnosis and in fact may be useful diagnostically, since antifungal therapy is essentially the same, depending on the severity of the clinical picture (29).

The recent development of an assay with a monoclonal antibody to a 69- to 70-kDa antigen used in an enzyme-linked immunosorbent assay format appears to offer promise of a more specific assay (7). The overall sensitivity was 71.4%, and the specificity was 98% for healthy controls and 85.4% for those with chronic fungal infections. The Histoplasmosis Antigen Test is available only through the Histoplasmosis Reference Laboratory (1001 West 10th Street, OPW 441, Indianapolis, IN 46202).

Candidiasis

Cell wall mannan and mannoproteins have been considered for use as diagnostic markers of invasive candidiasis. In the healthy host, anticandida antibodies have made these compounds virtually unavailable for detection, and mannan antigen is rapidly cleared from serum, if it is present in detectable amounts. Theoretically, the immunocompromised patient should not produce specific antibody, and one study has reported promising results with an assay that could separate patients who were colonized from those who had invasive candidiasis (3).

In addition to cell wall antigen, cytoplasmic antigens have been used as diagnostic and prognostic markers for candidiasis. Enolase has been evaluated as an antigenic marker by a multicenter study group (27). The overall sensitivity was 75% (18 of 24) for patients with neoplastic disease, 85% (11 of 13) for patients proven with deep-tissue infection, and 64% (7 of 11) for patients with fungemia. The overall specificity was 96%. It appears that enolase detection may precede positive blood cultures by several days (8, 17). However, this assay is not commercially available.

For some years, a latex agglutination test (CANDTEC, Ramco Laboratories, Inc., Houston, Tex.) has been available. The study design of the investigations probably explains the multitude of results generated by various centers. In general, the specificity of the test appears to be low, and many patients without candidiasis have positive test results (23).

An excellent discussion of the detection of *Candida* antigen was written by Walsh and Chanock (26); however, none of the assays except the latex test are commercially available.

CHEMICAL DETECTION

Fungus-Specific Metabolites

The detection of fungus-specific metabolites has the potential to be a powerful approach for the diagnosis and management of fungal infections. Rapid detection of the metabolites by a quantifiable chemical assay with sera could be extremely useful for diagnosis. Changes in the concentrations during therapy should reflect increases or decreases in fungal metabolism and correlate with therapeutic failures or successes, respectively (28). Two fungal polyols, D-arabinitol and D-mannitol, have been documented to be produced in vitro and also in vivo during infection. None of these assays is commercially available.

D-Arabinitol has been shown to be a fungus-specific metabolite produced by some *Candida* species: *C. albicans*, *C. tropicalis*, *C. parapsilosis*, and *C. pseudotropicalis*. One approach is to determine the D-arabinitol/L-arabinitol ratio in urine samples (2, 15). The isomers are separated and quantitated by gas-liquid chromatography with or without mass spectrometry. The sensitivity of the method is approximately 88%.

The second approach is to determine a serum D-arabinitol/creatine ratio, with the D-arabinitol being quantitated by an isomer-specific enzymatic assay (27). The sensitivity was 70% overall and 80% for D-arabinitol-producing species. The specificity was 86%, with 19 of 40 patients with false-positive results having probable cases of candidiasis.

D-Mannitol, another fungal polyol, is also produced by some but not all pathogenic fungi. Therefore, detection of D-mannitol can be used as a fungal screening test or, more importantly, as a marker for the monitoring of therapy. Studies with a patient with *Cryptococcus neoformans* meningitis support the potential role of this metabolite for monitoring this important human infection (36). Cloning of the fungal D-mannitol dehydrogenase gene has been performed and should provide sufficient enzyme for use in a clinical laboratory assay (22).

Structural Components

Another non-culture-based method for use in the diagnosis of fungal infections is the detection of a component of certain fungal cell walls, (1–3)-β-D-glucan, in serum (20). The basis of this assay is that a *Limulus* coagulation cascade has a second pathway that is very sensitive and specific for (1–3)-β-D-glucan, a moiety of the cell walls of many but not all pathogenic fungi. Detection of this fungal structural component, therefore, is not specific for a single fungal species but is specific for several fungal species, including *Aspergillus* and *Candida* species; *Cryptococcus neoformans*, however, is not detected by this assay. The format is a chemical assay with a chromogenic endpoint read on a spectrophotometer. The assay is quantitative, with sensitivity to a concentration of 1.0 pg.

Clinical evaluations have yielded a sensitivity of between

84.4 and 100% and a specificity of 88% for the diagnosis of candidemia (21). This assay also has the potential to be used for the diagnosis of aspergillosis. With a very small sample size, a sensitivity of 100% was documented (18).

NUCLEIC ACID DETECTION

The most immediate need for nucleic acid detection methods is for the immunocompromised patient group. Fungal infections usually have a sudden onset, progress rapidly, and are often fatal unless treatment is initiated very early during the course of the infection. Unfortunately, serologic tests are of little value since these patients are rarely able to produce antibodies due to their suppressed immune system but also due to the rapid progression of infection. Cultures often require several days before a diagnosis can be made and are often of little diagnostic value until after the disease has progressed. The direct microscopic examination of clinical specimens, including biopsy specimens, is essentially the only means available for rapid diagnosis. The sensitivity, however, is often low and is dependent on the experience of the person observing the specimen. Thus, the need for some non-culture-based detection system is apparent. Little emphasis has been placed in this area; however, some work offers promise.

Nucleic acid detection requires some form of amplication method, whether PCR or another system, to produce enough nucleic acid for detection. Some assays are limited since only a single copy of target nucleic acid may be present in an organism.

Furthermore, the number of fungal cells present in a clinical specimen may also be limited. This is extremely important in respiratory tract specimens, which have a heterogeneous fungal population. The low copy number and the small organism load make it difficult even for an optimized amplification system to detect the nucleic acid of a causative agent in a clinical specimen. DNases and RNases that degrade the nucleic acid of fungal cells may be present. In addition, inhibitors of the amplification steps are often present in clinical specimens, and these may block the ability to detect fungal nucleic acid. It might appear that these problems are insurmountable, but they are not. Promise for eliminating this adverse variable appears to be related to specimen processing. Better concentration and purification of the nucleic acid in clinical specimens will almost certainly lead to better detection of fungal nucleic acid in clinical specimens. Promising work has already begun in the area of molecular detection of fungal infections (11, 12, 16, 22, 24, 25), but the methods are available only in academic centers where investigational programs are located. In addition, the costs associated with the use of nucleic acid amplification diagnostic tests are prohibitive. However, the potential for their use in the laboratory diagnosis of fungal diseases offers great promise. More work must be done to enhance the sensitivity and reduce the costs of these important tests.

REFERENCES

1. **Boom, W. H., D. J. Piper, K. L. Ruoff, and M. J. Ferro.** 1985. New cause for false-positive results with the cryptococcal antigen test by latex agglutination. *J. Clin. Microbiol.* **22:**856–857.
2. **Christensson, B., T. Wiebe, C. Pehrson, and L. Larsson.** 1997. Diagnosis of invasive candidiasis in neutropenic children with cancer by determination of D-arabinitol/L-arabinitol ratios in urine. *J. Clin. Microbiol.* **35:**636–640.
3. **DeBernardis, F., C. Girmenia, M. Boccanera, D. Adrian, P. Martino, and A. Cassone.** 1993. Use of a monoclonal antibody in a dot immunobinding assay for detection of a circulating mannoprotein of *Candida* sp. in neutropenic patients with invasive candidiasis. *J. Clin. Microbiol.* **31:** 3142–3146.
4. **Fojtasek, M. F., M. B. Kleiman, P. Connolly-Stringfield, R. Blair, and L. J. Wheat.** 1994. The histoplasma antigen assay in disseminated histoplasmosis in children. *Pediatr. Infect. Dis. J.* **13:**801–805.
5. **Gade, W., S. W. Hinnefeld, L. S. Babcock, P. Gilligan, W. Kelly, K. Wait, D. Greer, M. Pinilla, and R. L. Kaplan.** 1991. Comparison of the PREMIER cryptococcal antigen enzyme immunoassay and the latex agglutination assay for detection of cryptococcal antigens. *J. Clin. Microbiol.* **29:**1616–1619.
6. **Garner, J. A., and D. Kernodle.** 1995. False-positive *Histoplasma* antigen test in a patient with pulmonary blastomycosis. *Clin. Infect. Dis.* **21:**1054.
7. **Gomez, B. L., J. I. Figueroa, A. J. Hamilton, B. L. Ortiz, M. A. Robledo, A. Restrepo, and R. J. Hay.** 1997. Development of a novel antigen detection test for histoplasmosis. *J. Clin. Microbiol.* **35:**2618–2622.
8. **Gutierrez, J., C. Maroto, G. Piedrola, E. Martin, and J. A. Perez.** 1993. Circulating *Candida* antigens and antibodies: useful markers of candidemia. *J. Clin. Microbiol.* **31:** 2550–2552.
9. **Hageage, G. J., and B. J. Harrington.** 1984. Use of calcofluor white in clinical mycology. *Lab. Med.* **15:**109–112.
10. **Heelan, J. S., L. Corpus, and N. Kessimian.** 1991. False positive reactions in the latex agglutination test for *Cryptococcus neoformans* antigen. *J. Clin. Microbiol.* **29:**1260–1261.
11. **Hopfer, R. L., P. Walden, S. Setterquist, and W. E. Hughsmith.** 1993. Detection and differentiation of fungi in clinical specimen using polymerase chain reaction (PCR) amplification and restriction enzyme analysis. *J. Med. Vet. Mycol.* **31:**65–75.

11a. **Isenberg, H. D. (ed. in chief).** 1998. *Essential Procedures for Clinical Microbiology*. ASM Press, Washington, D.C.

12. **Kan, V. L.** 1993. Polymerase chain reaction for the diagnosis of candidemia. *J. Infect. Dis.* **168:**779–783.
13. **Kaufman, L., and E. Reiss.** 1992. Serodiagnosis of fungal diseases, p. 506–528. *In* N. R. Rose, E. C. DeMacario, J. L. Fahey, H. Friedman, and G. M. Penn (ed.), *Manual of Clinical Laboratory Immunology*, 4th ed. American Society for Microbiology, Washington, D.C.
14. **Kim, Y. K., S. Parulekar, P. K. Yu, R. J. Pisani, T. F. Smith, and J. P. Anhalt.** 1990. Evaluation of calcofluor white stain for detection of *Pneumocystis carinii*. *Diagn. Microbiol. Infect. Dis.* **13:**307–310.
15. **Lehtonen, L., V.-J. Anttila, T. Ruutu, J. Salonen, J. Nikoskelainen, E. Eerola, and P. Ruutu.** 1996. Diagnosis of disseminated candidiasis by measurement of urine D-arabinitol/L-arabinitol ratio. *J. Clin. Microbiol.* **34:**2175–2179.
16. **Makimura, K., S. Y. Murayama, and H. Yamaguchi.** 1994. Detection of a wide range of medically important fungi by polymerase chain reaction. *J. Med. Microbiol.* **40:**358–364.

16a. **Merz, W. G.** Unpublished data.

17. **Mitsutake, K., T. Miyazaki, T. Tashiro, Y. Yamamoto, H. Kakeya, T. Otsubo, S. Kawamura, M. A. Hossain, T. Noda, Y. Hirakata, and S. Kohno.** 1996. Enolase antigen, mannan antigen, Cand-Tec antigen, and β-glucan in patients with candidemia. *J. Clin. Microbiol.* **34:**1918–1921.
18. **Miyazaki, T., S. Kohno, K. Mitsutake, S. Maesaki, K. Tanaka, N. Ishikawa, and K. Hara.** 1995. Plasma (1→3) β-D-glucan and fungal antigenemia in patients with candi-

demia, aspergillosis, and cryptococcosis. *J. Clin. Microbiol.* **33:**3115–3118.

19. **Ng, L., N. A. Virani, R. E. Chaisson, D. M. Yajko, H. T. Sphar, K. Cabrian, N. Rollins, P. Charache, M. Krieger, W. K. Hadley, and P. C. Hopewell.** 1990. Rapid detection of *Pneumocystis carinii* using a direct fluorescent monoclonal antibody stain. *J. Clin. Microbiol.* **28:** 2228–2233.
20. **Obayashi, T., H. Tamura, S. Tanaka, M. Ohki, S. Takahashi, M. Arai, M. Masuda, and T. Kawai.** 1985. A new chromogenic endotoxin-specific assay using recombined *Limulus* coagulation enzyme and its clinical applications. *Clin. Chem. Acta* **149:**55–65.
21. **Obayashi, T., M. Yoshida, T. Mori, H. Goto, A. Yasuoka, H. Iwasaki, H. Teshima, S. Kohno, and A. Horiuchi.** 1995. Plasma (1→3) β-D-glucan measurement in diagnosis of invasive deep mycosis and fungal febrile episodes. *Lancet* **345:**17–20.
22. **Perfect, J. R., T. H. Rude, B. Wong, T. Flynn, V. Chaturvedi, and W. Niehaus.** 1996. Identification of a *Cryptococcus neoformans* gene that directs expression of the cryptic *Saccharomyces cerevisiae* mannitol dehydrogenase gene. *J. Bacteriol.* **178:**5257–5261.
23. **Petri, M. G., J. Konig, H. P. Moecke, H. J. Gramm, H. Barkow, P. Kujath, R. Denhart, H. Schafer, N. Meyer, P. Kalmar, P. Thulig, J. Muller, and H. Lode.** 1997. Epidemiology of invasive mycosis in ICU patients: a prospective multicenter study in 435 non-neutropenic patients. *Intensive Care Med.* **23:**317–325.
24. **Reddy, L. V., A. Kumar, and V. P. Kurup.** 1993. Specific amplication of *Aspergillus fumigatus* DNA by polymerase chain reaction. *Mol. Cell. Probes* **7:**121–126.
25. **Sandhu, G. S., B. C. Kline, L. Stockman, and G. D. Roberts.** 1995. Molecular probes for diagnosis of fungal infections. *J. Clin. Microbiol.* **33:**2913–2919.
26. **Walsh, T. J., and S. J. Chanock.** 1997. Laboratory diagnosis of invasive candidiasis: a rationale for complementary use of culture and nonculture-based detection systems. *Int. J. Infect. Dis.* **1**(Suppl. 1)**:**S11–S19.
27. **Walsh, T. J., J. W. Hathorn, J. D. Sobel, W. G. Merz, V. Sanchez, J. M. Maret, H. R. Buckley, M. A. Pfaller, R. Schaufele, C. Sliva, E. Navarro, J. Lecciones, P. Chandrasekar, J. Lee, and P. A. Pizzo.** 1991. Detection of circulating *Candida* enolase by immunoassay in patients with cancer and candidiasis. *N. Engl. J. Med.* **324:**1026–1031.
28. **Walsh, T. J., W. G. Merz, J. W. Lee, R. Schaufele, T. Sein, P. O. Whitcomb, M. Ruddel, J. Wingard, W. Burns, A. Switchenko, T. Goodman, and P. A. Pizzo.** 1995. Diagnosis and therapeutic monitoring of invasive candidiasis by rapid enzymatic detection of D-arabinitol. *Am. J. Med.* **99:**164–172.
29. **Wheat, J., H. Wheat, P. Connolly, M. Kleiman, K. Supporapinyo, K. Nelson, R. Bradsher, and A. Restrepo.** 1997. Cross-reactivity in *Histoplasma capsulatum* variety *capsulatum* antigen assays of urine samples from patients with endemic mycoses. *Clin. Infect. Dis.* **24:**1169–1171.
30. **Wheat, L. J., P. Connolly-Stringfield, B. Williams, K. Connolly, M. Bartlett, and M. Durkin.** 1992. Diagnosis of histoplasmosis in patients with the acquired immunodeficiency syndrome by detection of *Histoplasma capsulatum* polysaccharide antigen in bronchoalveolar lavage fluid. *Am. Rev. Respir. Dis.* **145:**1421–1424.
31. **Wheat, L. J., P. Connolly-Stringfield, R. Blair, K. Connolly, T. Garringer, and B. P. Katz.** 1991. Histoplasmosis relapse in patients with AIDS: detection using *Histoplasma capsulatum* variety *capsulatum* antigen levels. *Ann. Intern. Med.* **115:**936–941.
32. **Wheat, L. J., R. B. Kohler, R. P. Tewari, M. Garten, and M. L. French.** 1989. Significance of histoplasma antigen in the cerebrospinal fluid of patients with meningitis. *Arch. Intern. Med.* **149:**302–304.
33. **Wheat, L. J., P. Connolly-Stringfield, R. B. Kohler, P. T. Frame, and M. R. Gupta.** 1989. *Histoplasma capsulatum* polysaccharide antigen in diagnosis and management of disseminated histoplasmosis in patients with acquired immunodeficiency syndrome. *Am. J. Med.* **87:**396–400.
34. **Wheat, L. J., R. B. Kohler, and R. P. Tewari.** 1986. Diagnosis of disseminated histoplasmosis by detection of *Histoplasma capsulatum* antigen in serum and urine specimens. *N. Engl. J. Med.* **314:**83–88.
35. **Williams, B., M. Fojtasek, P. Connolly-Stringfield, and L. S. Wheat.** 1994. Diagnosis of histoplasmosis by antigen detection during an outbreak in Indianapolis, IN. *Arch. Pathol. Lab. Med.* **118:**1205–1208.
36. **Wong, B., J. R. Perfect, S. Beggs, and K. A. Wright.** 1990. Production of the hexitol D-mannitol by *Cryptococcus neoformans* in vitro and in rabbits with experimental meningitis. *Infect. Immun.* **58:**1664–1670.

Candida, *Cryptococcus*, and Other Yeasts of Medical Importance

NANCY G. WARREN AND KEVIN C. HAZEN

95

NATURAL HABITAT AND CLINICAL SIGNIFICANCE

Yeasts are ubiquitous in our environment, being found on fruits, vegetables, and other plant materials. Some live as normal inhabitants in and on our bodies. Therefore, they may be found in specimens without having any clinical significance. Yeasts are considered opportunistic pathogens and may be cultured from specimens of patients debilitated in some fashion, e.g., by hormone imbalance or by the administration of immunosuppressive agents. Diseases such as AIDS and others which cause a diminution or depletion of the immunological system also are predisposing factors for yeast infections. Endocarditis caused by yeasts has been associated with the use of nonsterile equipment by drug addicts. Fungemia may occur when indwelling catheters are not changed or removed at frequent intervals; it also has been reported in infants supported by lipid-supplemented hyperalimentation (19).

Yeasts are by far the most common fungi isolated from human patients. The decision as to the significance of their presence in a specimen ultimately rests with the physician, but accurate, complete information from the laboratory is essential for a reasonable conclusion to be made. Taking careful note of such information as the type of specimen (e.g., closed, normally sterile sites rather than sputum or urine), the number of specimens from the same patient positive for the same organism, and the number of colonies grown are all critical pieces of information.

CHARACTERISTICS OF YEASTS

Yeasts are unicellular, eukaryotic, budding cells and are generally round to oval or, less often, elongate or irregular in shape. They multiply principally by the production of blastoconidia (buds). When blastoconidia are produced one from the other in a linear fashion without separation, a structure termed a pseudohypha is formed. Under certain circumstances some yeasts may produce true septate hyphae. Such circumstances are associated with the reduction of oxygen, e.g., in host tissues or as submerged colonies in agar medium, at the bottom of broth media in a test tube or in the presence of 5 to 10% CO_2.

Cultures of yeasts are moist, creamy, or glabrous to membranous in texture. Several produce a capsule which makes the colony mucoid. With rare exceptions aerial hyphae are not produced. Colonies may be hyaline or brightly colored or may be darkly pigmented due to the presence of melanins. The latter group, found in the family Dematiaceae, is discussed in chapter 101 and is not discussed here. Dimorphic fungal pathogens possessing a yeast phase in tissue are likewise discussed in other chapters.

Although there are many genera and hundreds of yeast species, only a relatively few produce disease in humans and animals. They generally are identified (classified) by observing the macroscopic and microscopic features mentioned above. Usually, biochemical tests also are required for definitive identification to the species level. In most instances the pathogenic yeasts are found in the Deuteromycetes or Fungi Imperfecti, that is, fungi which do not exhibit a sexual or teleomorphic state in culture.

Yeasts also may be classified by their method of sexual reproduction into the Ascomycetes and Heterobasidiomycetes. A few genera may produce a sexual state on standard mycological media over time. In some instances it may be necessary to identify the teleomorphic state of a yeast culture. This is best accomplished by submitting it to a reference laboratory for further study.

DIRECT EXAMINATION

The appropriate examination of a clinical specimen is essential prior to proper processing of the material. Additionally, it often will aid the laboratorian and the physician in a preliminary identification, either ruling in or ruling out certain pathogenic yeasts. Certain methods are universal to the preliminary observation of fungi in a specimen, e.g., Gram staining or Calcofluor or 20% KOH treatment. However, other methods such as the use of India ink for the demonstration of a capsule are used for yeasts only. This method is used with cultures and specimens of urine, cerebrospinal fluid, etc., which have been centrifuged. It generally is not useful with primary specimens such as sputum or other material which does not allow the even distribution of the ink. It must be remembered that if 20% KOH is used on a preparation, neither India ink nor Gram stain may subsequently be added.

In performing the microscopic examination of a specimen for yeasts, structures that may aid in identification may be observed: (i) size and shape of the organism, (ii) mode of attachment of a bud(s), (iii) presence or absence of a

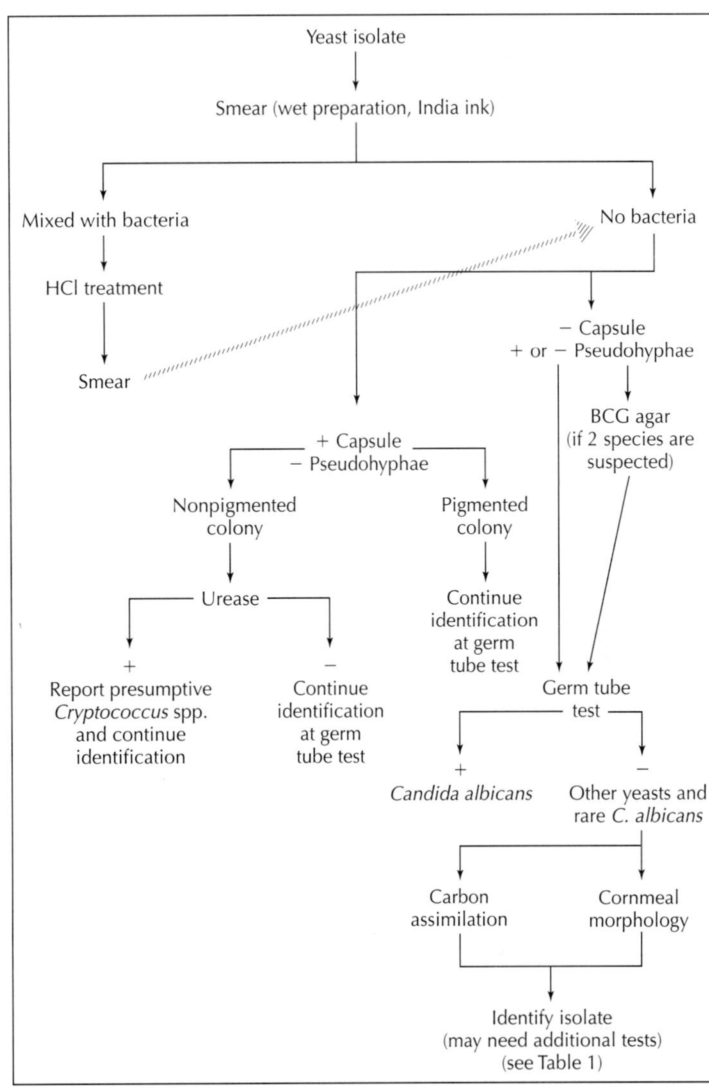

FIGURE 1 Scheme for identification of yeasts from clinical specimens.

capsule, (iv) thickness of the cell wall, (v) presence of pseudohyphae, and (vi) presence of arthroconidia. Other unusual structures also should be noted.

IDENTIFICATION

A scheme for yeast identification is presented in Fig. 1. When viewed as a general guideline, it offers a basic approach to yeast identification, but it also allows flexibility for adaptation to individual laboratory situations. The morphologic and physiologic properties of the most commonly encountered yeasts in clinical specimens are found in Table 1. Particularly salient characteristics of individual yeasts will be reemphasized in the sections dealing with specific yeast genera. A sound, systematic approach to yeast identification cannot be stressed enough. With the numerous yeast identification systems available today, most yeast species can be identified easily; however, repeat testing sometimes is necessary and morphologic characteristics on cornmeal or similar agars should be mandatory.

Macroscopic Characteristics of Yeasts

Most yeasts (*Malassezia furfur* being an exception) grow well on common mycological and bacteriological media. Growth is usually detected in 48 to 72 h, and subcultures or laboratory-adapted strains may grow more rapidly. Colonies have a smooth to wrinkled, creamy appearance; some pigment may be observed initially or may intensify with age. Heavily encapsulated yeasts will give a very moist, mucoid appearance.

The ability of yeasts to grow at 37°C is a very important characteristic. Most pathogenic species grow readily at 25 and 37°C, while saprophytes usually fail to grow at the higher temperature. Additionally, some yeast species, e.g., *Candida albicans*, will grow in the presence of cycloheximide (Actidione) found in Mycosel, Mycobiotic, and similar agars, while most other yeasts, including *Cryptococcus neoformans*, will be inhibited.

Pellicle growth on the surface of liquid media such as Sabouraud glucose broth or malt extract broth has been used in the past to assist with yeast identification. More recent evidence suggests that this characteristic can be variable; however, as an ancillary test, it may be helpful with identifying *Candida tropicalis* and *Candida krusei*.

Microscopic Characteristics of Yeasts

Upon isolation of a suspected yeast from clinical specimens the first examination made should be a wet preparation of

TABLE 1 Cultural and biochemical characteristics of yeasts frequently isolated from clinical specimens[a]

Species	Growth at 37°C	Pellicle in broth	Pseudo- or true hyphae	Chlamydospores	Germ tubes	Capsule, India ink	Assimilation of [b]:												Fermentation of:						Urease	KNO_3 utilization	Phenol oxidase	Ascospores
							Glucose	Maltrose	Sucrose	Lactose	Galactose	Melibiose	Cellobiose	Inositol	Xylose	Raffinose	Trehalose	Dulcitol	Glucose	Maltrose	Sucrose	Lactose	Galactose	Trehalose				
Candida abicans	+	−	+	+	+	−	+	+	+*	−	+	−	−	−	+	−	+	−	F	F	−	−	F	F	−	−	−	−
C. catenulata	+*	−	+	−	−	−	+	+	−	−	+	−	−	−	+	−	−	−	F*	−	−	−	−	−	−	−	−	−
C. famata	+	−	−	−	−	−	+	+	+	+*	+	+	+	−	+	+	+	+*	W	−	W	−	−	W	−	−	−	−*
C. glabrata	+	−	−	−	−	−	+	−	−	−	−	−	−	−	−	−	+	−	F	−	−	−	−	F	−	−	−	−
C. guilliermondii	+	−	+	−	−	−	+	+	+	−	+	+	+	−	+	+	+	+	F	−	F	−	F*	F	−	−	−	−*
C. kefyr	+	−	+	−	−	−	+	−	+	+	+	−	+*	−	+*	+	−*	−	F	−	F	F*	F	−	−	−	−	−
C. krusei[c]	+	+	+	−	−	−	+	−	−	−	−	−	−	−	−	−	−	−	F	−	−	−	−	−	+*	−	−	−*
C. lambica	+*	+	+	−	−	−	+	−	−	−	−	−	−	−	+	−	−	−	F	−	−	−	−	−	−	−	−	−*
C. lipolytica[c]	+	+	+	−	−	−	+	−	−	−	−	−	−	−	−	−	−	−	−	−	−	−	−	−	+	−	−	−*
C. lusitaniae[d]	+	−	+	−	−	−	+	+	+	−	+	−	+	−	+	−	+	−	F	−	F	−	F	F	−	−	−	−*
C. parapsilosis[e]	+	−	+	−	−	−	+	+	+	−	+	−	−	−	+	−	+	−	F	−	−	−	−	−	−	−	−	−
C. pintolopesii[g]	+	−	−	−	−	−	+	−	−	−	−	−	−	−	−	−	−	−	F	−	−	−	−	−	−	−	−	−
C. rugosa	+	−	+	−	−	−	+	−	−	−	+	−	−	−	+*	−	−	−	−	−	−	−	−	−	−	−	−	−
C. tropicalis[d,e]	+	+	+	−[f]	−	−	+	+	+	−	+	−	+	−	+	−	+	−	F	F	F	−	F*	F*	−	−	−	−
C. zeylanoides	−	−*	+	−	−	−	+	−	−	−	−*	−	−*	−	−	−	+	−	−	−	−	−	−	−	−	−	−	−
Cryptococcus neoformans	+	−	R	−	−	+	+	+	+	−	+	−	+	+	+	+*	+	+	−	−	−	−	−	−	+	−	+	−
Cryptococcus albidus	−*	−	−	−	−	+	+	+	+	+*	+*	+	+	+	+	+	+	+*	−	−	−	−	−	−	+	+	−	−
Cryptococcus laurentii	+*	−	−	−	−	+	+	+	+	+	+	+*	+	+	+	+*	+	+	−	−	−	−	−	−	+	−	−	−
Cryptococcus luteolus	−	−	−	−	−	+	+	+	+	−	+	+	+	+	+	+	+	+	−	−	−	−	−	−	+	−	−	−
Cryptococcus terreus	−*	−	−	−	−	+	+	+*	−	+*	+*	−	+	+	+	−	+	−*	−	−	−	−	−	−	+	+	−	−
Cryptococcus uniguttulatus	−	−	−	−	−	+	+	+	+	−	−*	−	−*	+	+	+*	−*	−	−	−	−	−	−	−	+	−	−	−
Rhodotorula glutinus	+	−	−	−	−	−*	+	+	+	−	+*	−	+	−	+	+	+	−	−	−	−	−	−	−	+	+	−	−
Rhodotorula rubra	+	−	−	−	−	−*	+	+	+	−	+	−	+*	−	+	+	+	−	−	−	−	−	−	−	+	−	−	−
S. cerevisiae	+	−	−*	−	−	−	+	+	+	−	+	−	−	−	−	+	+*	−	F	F	F	−	F	F*	−	−	−	+
H. anomala	+*	−	−	−	−	−	+	+	+	−	+	−	+	−	+	−	+	−	F	F*	F	−	F	−	−	+	−	+
Geotrichum candidum[h]	−*	+	+	−	−	−	+	−	−	−	+	−	−	−	+	−	−	−	−	−	−	−	−	−	−	−	−	−
B. capitatus	+	+	+	−	−	−	+	−	−	−	+	−	−	−	−	−	−	−	−	−	−	−	−	−	−	−	−	−
P. wickerhamii[h]	+	−	−	−	−	−	+	−	−	−	+	−	−	−	−	−	+	−	−	−	−	−	−	−	−	−	−	−

[a] +, positive reaction; −, negative reaction; *, strain variation; R, rare; F, the sugar is fermented (i.e., gas is produced); W, weak fermentation. Based on data from Barnett et al. (7) and Kreger-van Rij (49).
[b] +, Growth greater than that of the negative control. [c] *C. lipolytica* assimilates erythritol; *C. krusei* does not. Maximum growth temperatures 43 to 45°C for *C. krusei* and 33 to 37°C for *C. lipolytica*.
[d] *C. lusitaniae* assimilates rhamnose; *C. tropicalis* usually does not. [e] *C. parapsilosis* assimilates L-arabinose; *C. tropicalis* usually does not.
[f] Rare strains of *C. tropicalis* produce teardrop-shaped chlamydospores. [g] *C. pintolopesii* is a thermophilic yeast capable of growth at 40 to 42°C. [h] Not yeasts but may be confused with several yeast genera.

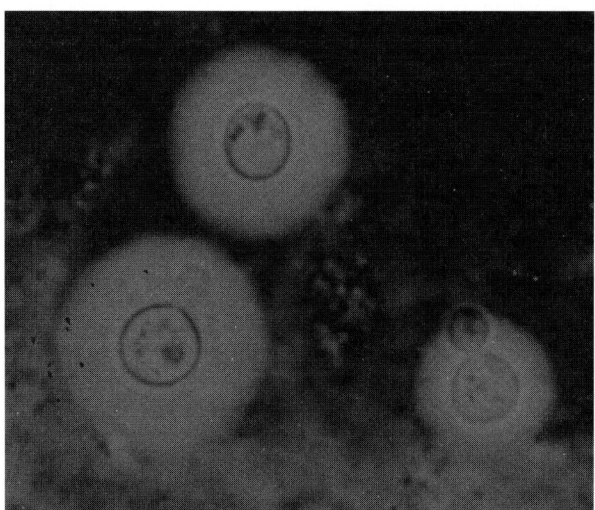

FIGURE 2 India ink preparation of *Cryptococcus neoformans*. Magnification, ×400. (Courtesy of E. S. Jacobson.)

a colony. This provides an initial clue to the organism's identity. A small amount of growth is emulsified in a drop of sterile distilled water and is examined microscopically with a reduced light source. Observations should include size and shape of the yeast, the method of bud attachment, and the presence or absence of pseudohyphae, true hyphae, or arthroconidia. Any round or slightly oval budding yeast for which rare or no pseudohyphae are seen in this preparation should be examined further for the presence of a capsule.

The same wet preparation used for the initial microscopic examination can be used for an India ink examination. A small drop of India ink is added close to the edge of the coverslip and is allowed to diffuse under it. The preparation then can be examined for the presence of encapsulated yeasts (Fig. 2). The outline of the yeast cell, surrounded by a clear area which is the mucopolysaccharide capsule, will be obvious against a dark India ink background. False-positive preparations usually are the result of contaminated ink or artifacts, which can exhibit ragged edges. Capsular size cannot be used for identification purposes because this characteristic may be influenced by culture age, medium composition, and strain variation. The presence of a capsule does not automatically ensure that the yeast is *C. neoformans* because other cryptococci, *Rhodotorula* spp., and rare *Candida* spp. will produce capsules. In practice, any nonpigmented, round, encapsulated yeast recovered from cerebrospinal fluid should be considered *C. neoformans* until proven otherwise.

Purity of Cultures

Before any additional physiologic tests are performed, it is essential to ensure that one has a pure culture. A Gram stain of the culture can verify purity, but often, bacterial contamination can be detected during the wet preparation examination. If the culture is mixed with bacteria, the isolate should be inoculated onto a blood agar plate and individual colonies should be picked or, alternatively, treated with hydrochloric acid (Fig. 1). The HCl procedure is performed by inoculating a colony into three tubes of Sabouraud glucose broth (each containing 5 ml of broth). A capillary pipet is used to add 4 drops of 1 N HCl to the first tube, 2 drops to the second tube, and 1 drop to the third tube. After incubation at 25°C for 24 to 48 h, 0.1 ml of each broth is subcultured onto fresh Sabouraud glucose agar plates.

It is possible that more than one yeast species will be recovered from a clinical specimen, especially if the specimen is from a normally nonsterile site (107). Careful attention to colonial morphology and microscopic characteristics can offer clues to the presence of a mixed population. Subculturing of individual isolates onto additional media can be helpful (107), and the use of CHROMagar (see below) may delineate the presence of more than one yeast species.

Morphology Studies

While examination of a wet preparation gives a primary indication of the yeast involved, more extensive study of morphology on cornmeal agar or other, similar agars will offer the opportunity to correlate morphologic characteristics with the results of biochemical tests. Microscopic examination should reveal thick-walled chlamydospores of *C. albicans* or other structures of the other yeasts (Table 2). Special attention also should be given to the size and shape of the pseudohyphae and the arrangement of blastoconidia along the pseudohyphae. Figure 3 illustrates several of the morphologic characteristics. The use of known control organisms can ensure the quality of the medium and can offer the opportunity to compare the morphologies of known standard organisms with those of the organisms in the test culture in question. Experience is needed to detect some of the more subtle characteristics, and these findings should be considered preliminary, i.e., one of the first steps in complete yeast identification.

TABLE 2 Microscopic appearance of several yeasts and yeastlike fungi

Organism	Pseudohyphae	True hyphae	Blastoconidia	Arthroconidia	Annelloconidia	Chlamydospores	Ascospores
B. capitatus	×	×	×		×		
C. albicans	×	×	×			×	
Other *Candida* spp.	×[a]	×[a]	×				×[a]
Cryptococcus spp.			×				
Geotrichum spp.		×		×			
Hansenula spp.	×[a]		×				×
Rhodotorula spp.			×				
Saccharomyces spp.	×[a]		×				×
Trichosporon spp.	×	×	×	×			

[a] Strain variation.

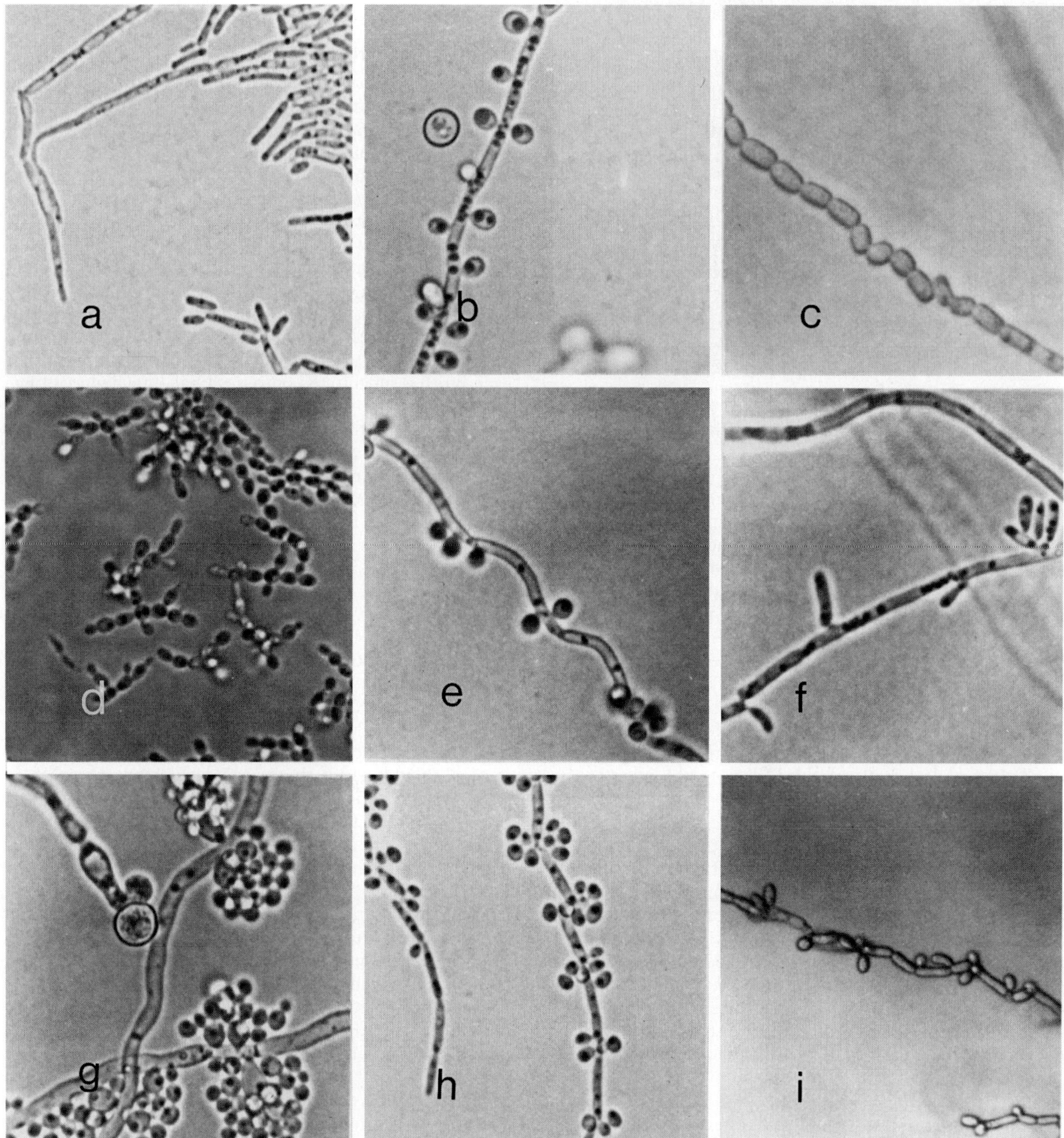

FIGURE 3 Morphologic features of some yeast and yeastlike organisms on cornmeal agar at 24 to 48 h of growth at ambient temperature. (a) *Candida krusei*: extremely elongated, rarely branched pseudohyphae; few blastoconidia. (b) *Candida tropicalis*: blastoconidia formed at septa and between septa. (c) *Geotrichum candidum*: arthroconidia. (d) *Candida guilliermondii*: chains of blastoconidia forming sparse pseudohyphae in a young culture. (e) *Candida lusitaniae*: short, distinctly curved pseudohyphae with blastoconidia formed at and occasionally between septa. (f) *Blastoschizomyces capitatus*: true hyphae, annelloconidia resembling arthroconidia. (g) *Candida albicans*: blastoconidia, chlamydospores, true hyphae, and pseudohyphae. (h) *Candida parapsilosis*: elongated, delicately curved pseudohyphae with blastoconidia at the septae. (i) *Trichosporon* spp.: blastoconidia formed at the corners of arthroconidia. Magnification, ×370. (Courtesy of B. A. Davis.)

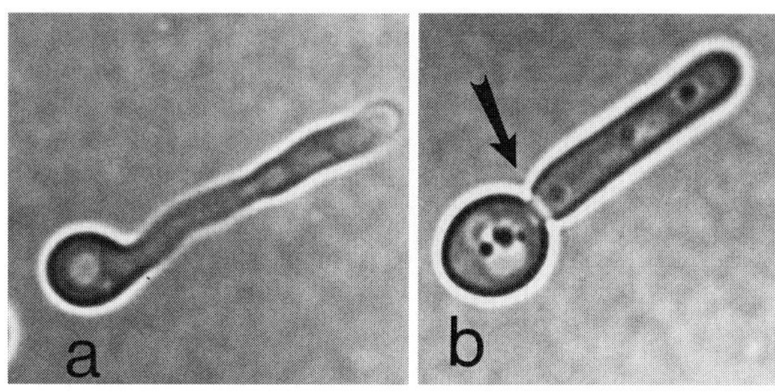

FIGURE 4 Germ tube test. (a) Germ tube formation of *C. albicans*. (b) Blastoconidial germination with constriction (arrow) of *C. tropicalis* not seen with true germ tubes of *C. albicans*. Magnification, ×400. (Courtesy of B. A. Davis.)

Germ Tube Test

One of the most valuable and simplest tests for the rapid presumptive identification of *C. albicans* is the germ tube test (Fig. 4a). The test is considered presumptive because not all isolates of *C. albicans* will be germ tube positive and false-positive results may be obtained, especially with *C. tropicalis*, despite the use of well-trained staff to perform the test (20). Microscopic observation of the preparation will reveal that the short hyphal initials produced by *C. albicans* are not constricted at the junction of the blastoconidium and germ tube. Frequently, so many *C. albicans* blastoconidia produce germ tubes that the germ tubes become entwined with each other, producing clumps of cells. *Candida tropicalis* also can produce hyphal initials, but the blastoconidia are larger than those of *C. albicans*, and there is a definite constricture where the hyphal initial joins a blastoconidium (Fig. 4b). In addition to using a known culture of *C. albicans* as a positive test control, negative controls for *C. tropicalis* and *Candida glabrata* also should be included. Optimum conditions are obtained by using colonies grown on Sabouraud glucose agar or blood agar at 30°C for 24 to 48 h. The test is performed by inoculating several colonies into the test substrate (such as fetal bovine serum) and incubating the suspension at 37°C for 3 h. When *C. tropicalis* produces germ tube-like structures, the proportion of cells within the population is less than 15%. The preparation should not be incubated at 37°C for longer than 4 h because other hypha-producing yeasts will begin to germinate after this time.

Ascospore Formation

Several yeasts recovered from clinical specimens may be present in their teleomorphic (sexual) state. In order to enhance the production of ascospores, cultures should be inoculated onto media such as Fowell's acetate agar or V-8 juice agar, incubated at room temperature for 2 to 5 days, and examined by wet preparation for the presence of ascospores within asci. Some mycologists prefer to use special stains to detect ascospores. The Ziehl-Neelsen stain routinely used in mycobacteriology can be used if needed; however, most ascospores can easily be detected in a drop of sterile distilled water. Ascospore production in *Saccharomyces cerevisiae* is evidenced by the presence of one to four globose spores (Fig. 5c); *Hansenula anomala* produces one to four hat-shaped spores (Fig. 5a). Ascospore formation is a very useful tool for the identification of isolates that are difficult to identify (Table 3).

Phenol Oxidase Test

The phenol oxidase test is a screening procedure that detects the ability of *C. neoformans* to produce phenol oxidase on substrates containing caffeic acid. The most frequently used medium is "birdseed" agar (containing niger or thistle seeds) and a number of formulations described by several investigators have shown various degrees of success. Apparently, test performance is related to the glucose content of the medium; the more glucose in the medium, the less likely a valid test result will be obtained. When *C. neoformans* is subcultured on the medium, colonies turn a dark brown in 2 to 5 days. Because of the wide variation in medium formulations, the test must be subjected constantly to quality control measures. Some laboratories advocate the use of birdseed agar as part of the primary plating of respiratory samples for culture for the early detection of *C. neoformans* isolates.

Urease Test

The urease test detects a yeast's ability to produce the enzyme urease. In the presence of suitable substrates, urease splits urea, producing ammonia, which raises the pH and which causes a color shift in the phenol red indicator from amber to pinkish red. The urease test aids in the identification of *Cryptococcus* spp. and *Rhodotorula* spp., which are all urease positive. Most strains of *Trichosporon* spp. are positive, while *Geotrichum* spp. and *Blastoschizomyces capitatus* are negative. Nearly all *Candida* spp. encountered in clinical specimens are urease negative, exceptions being *Candida lipolytica* and some strains of *C. krusei*.

Carbohydrate Assimilation Tests

The mainstay of yeast identification to the species level is the carbohydrate assimilation test (Table 1), which measures the ability of a yeast to utilize a specific carbohydrate as the sole source of carbon in the presence of oxygen. Several reliable commercially available kits (such as the API 20C AUX system [bioMérieux SA, Marcy l'Etoile, France] and BBL Minitek Yeast Set [Becton Dickinson Microbiology Systems, Sparks, Md.]) and automated and semiautomated systems are on the market today that make the classical method of Wickerham and Burton (103) unnecessary for routine clinical isolates.

Nitrate Assimilation Test

The rationale behind the nitrate assimilation test is similar to that behind the carbon assimilation test. It tests the ability of a yeast to utilize nitrate as a sole nitrogen source. While it is not necessary to perform nitrate assimilation studies with every yeast isolate, this information can be helpful with certain groups of yeasts. The test is most beneficial when trying to identify *Cryptococcus*, *Rhodotorula*, and *Hansenula* spp.

Carbohydrate Fermentation Tests

Fermentative yeasts recovered from clinical specimens produce carbon dioxide and alcohol; therefore, the production of gas and not a pH shift is indicative of fermentation. Rarely are fermentation studies needed to identify most of the commonly isolated yeasts if the mycologist is familiar with typical morphology on cornmeal agar. The test is most helpful in differentiating the various species of *Candida*; *Cryptococcus* and *Rhodotorula* spp. are nonfermentative.

Rapid Identification of Yeasts

Rapid identification of yeasts provides timely information to physicians for patient management. This is particularly true given the recognition that various yeast species (such as *Candida krusei*, *C. parapsilosis*, *C. lusitaniae*, *C. tropicalis*, and *Cryptococcus neoformans*) are inherently or potentially

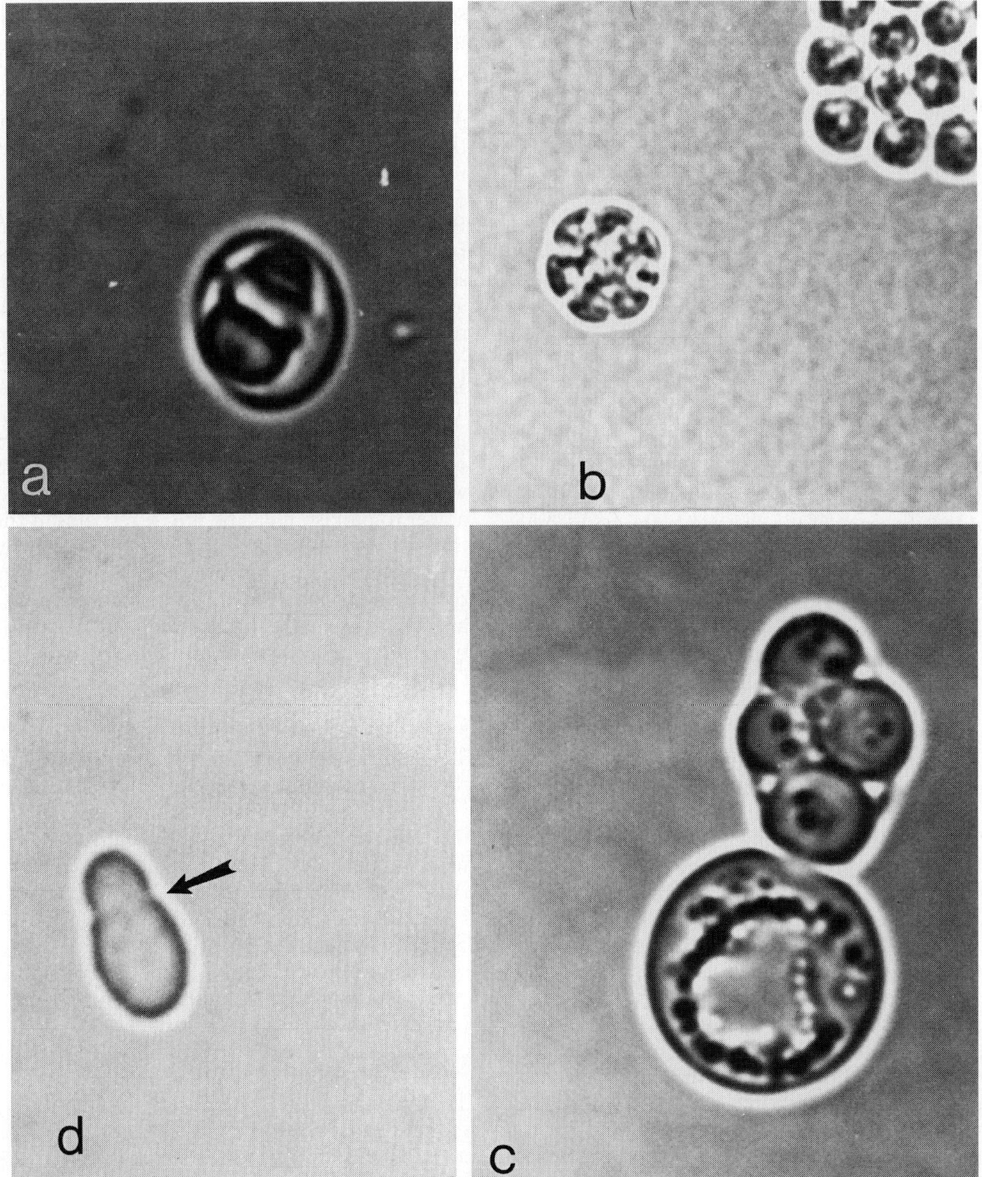

FIGURE 5 Diagnostic features of selected yeasts. (a) Ascus of *H. anomala* containing hat-shaped ascospores. (b) Sporangium of *P. wickerhamii* containing sporangiospores. (c) *S. cerevisiae* with vegetative cell and ascus containing four globose ascospores. (d) Bottle-shaped, budding yeast demonstrating phialoconidium and collarette (arrow) of *M. furfur*. Magnification, ×1,000. (Courtesy of B. A. Davis.)

resistant to amphotericin B or the newer azole agents (30, 99). Institution of effective antifungal therapy as early as possible can only improve patient outcome.

While single tests which discriminate between two species or which confirm a presumptive identification have been developed, rapid (same-day) tests that apply to a broad range of species have only recently become available. At best, the tests that identify multiple species are limited to the more common species seen in the clinical laboratory. Examples of such tests are the Microscan Yeast Identification Panel (Baxter-Microscan, West Sacramento, Calif.) and IDS RapID Yeast Plus (Innovative Diagnostic Systems, Norcross, Ga.) (69, 91).

Rapid tests that provide definitive or presumptive identification within the same day (<24 h) of colony formation are divided into those that are either specific for a single species, are limited to a few species, or apply to multiple genera (Table 4). In general, the tests listed within group 1 of Table 4 are presumptive and confirmation of the identification is needed.

Preformed enzymes provide one system for the identification of multiple species with a single test panel. Such tests may be acutely affected by incubation temperature (38) and are effectively limited to the identification of the more common yeast species isolated in the clinical laboratory. However, detection of specific exoenzymes can be extremely use-

TABLE 3 Appearance of asci or ascospores of ascomycetous yeasts[a]

Anamorphic spp.	Previous synonym or obsolete name	Teleomorph (alternative spp.)	Hetero- or homothallic	Ascospores
Blastoschizomyces capitatus	*Geotrichum capitatum* *Trichosporon capitatum*	*Dipodascus capitatus*	Hetero	4/ascus, hyaline ellipsoidal, with slimy sheath when released
Candida cifferii		*Stephanomyces ciferrii*	Hetero	1–4/ascus, helmet or hat shaped
Candida famata	*Torulopsis candida*	*Debaryomyces hansenii*	Homo	1–2/ascus, spherical with warts[b]
Candida guilliermondii		*Pichia guilliermondii* (*Yamadazyma guilliermondii*)	Hetero	Variable
Candida kefr	*Candida pseudotropicalis*, *Candida macedoniensis*	*Kluyveromyces marxianus* var. *marxianus*	Homo	1–4/ascus, crescent to reniform, agglutinates on MEA[c]
Candida krusei		*Issatchenkia orientalis*	Homo	1–2/ascus, spherical[d]
Candida lipolytica		*Saccharomycopsis lipolytica*	Hetero	1–4/ascus, spherical to hat-shaped protuberance on one or two ends
Candida lusitaniae	*Candida obtusa*, *Candida parapsilosis* var. *obtusa*	*Clavispora lusitaniae*	Hetero	1–4/ascus, clavate on MEA
Candida norvegensis		*Pichia norvegensis*	Homo	1–4/ascus, hat shaped on acetate agar
Candida pintolopesii	*Candida slooffii*	*Saccharomyces telluris*	Homo	1–2/ascus, spherical to ovoid, rough to spiny
Candida pelliculosa		*Hansenula anomala*	Hetero	1–4/ascus, hat shaped
Candida pulcherrima		*Metschnikowia pulcherrima*	Hetero	1–2/ascus, from chlamydospore, spherical with peduncle
Candida utilis		*Hansenula jadinii*	Homo	1–4/ascus, hat shaped on MEA
		Saccharomyces cervisiae	Homo	1–4/ascus, spherical or short ellipsoidal (on acetate agar)

[a] Modified from Hazen (37).
[b] Difficult to see.
[c] MEA, malt extract agar.
[d] Difficult to induce.

TABLE 4 Rapid tests (<24 h) available for presumptive or definitive identification of yeasts following colony formation

Test name		
Group 1 (for single species)[a]	Group 2 (for several species)	Group 3 (for multiple genera)
Albicans-Sure (*C. albicans*)	CandiSelect	AMS-Yeast Biochemical Card
Albicans ID (*C. albicans*)	Candida check	Microbial Identification System (MIDI)
Albistrip (*C. albicans*)	CHROMagar	Microscan Rapid Yeast ID
BactiCard Candida (*C. albicans*)	Fungiscreen H	Quantum II
Bichrolatex Albicans (*C. albicans*)		RapID Yeast Plus System
Fluoroplate (*C. albicans*)		
Germ tube (*C. albicans*)		
Rapidec albicans (*C. albicans*)		
C. albicans screen (Murex CA 50) (*C. albicans*)		
Bichrolate krusei (*C. krusei*)		
Caffeic acid disk (*C. neoformans*)		

[a] Name of species given within parentheses.

ful for resolution of the confusion between two or three possible species. In particular, several rapid tests are available for this purpose, particularly for the detection of *C. albicans* (e.g., the *C. albicans* screen [Carr-Scarborough Microbiologicals, Decatur, Ga.] and the Albistrip [Lab M Ltd., Bury, United Kingdom]). These tests are excellent for confirmation of a germ tube-positive organism such as *C. albicans* and could be used in place of more long-term identification tests for this purpose. Use of these tests for confirmation purposes can provide a financial savings to the clinical laboratory. Both tests depend on the production of two enzymes (proline aminopeptidase and β-galactosaminadase) instead of a single enzyme (β-galactosaminadase), which could otherwise lead to spurious results (90).

Several media have been formulated to provide presumptive identification of one or two yeast species on the basis of colony characteristics. Recently, CHROMagar *Candida* (CHROMagar France, Paris, France [distributed in the United States by Hardy Diagnostics, Santa Maria, Calif.]) has been introduced. This medium allows the differentiation of more than 10 species and is marketed for the presumptive identification of *C. albicans*, *C. tropicalis*, and *C. krusei*. Colony identification is based on the differential release of chromogenic breakdown products from various substrates following differential exoenzyme activity. It is important to recognize that the identifications are presumptive. Evidence suggests that variation in colony appearance occurs among the species (8, 70). The directions of the manufacturer must be strictly followed, as is the case in any rapid test based on exoenzyme activity. Incubation time and temperature significantly affect the appearance of the colony. The medium is especially useful for the detection of mixed yeast infections in blood and for resolving identification problems.

Troubleshooting Difficult Identifications

Laboratories will encounter yeast isolates that do not easily fit into a specific species, particularly when commercial identification systems are used. Key features help separate troublesome organisms from others. For example, urease production separates basidiomycetous yeasts from ascomycetous yeasts. Maximum growth temperature, cycloheximide resistance, and the ability to assimilate cellobiose, inositol, or trehalose are helpful. For more difficult identifications, use of traditional auxanographic methods but with carbon source-impregnated disks on yeast carbon base agar plates may provide the most accurate assimilation information. Fermentation tests should also be considered.

Maintenance of Yeast Cultures

Well-characterized yeast isolates should be retained for use as quality control organisms to ascertain the performance of media and to provide examples of known positive and negative biochemical and morphological reactions. Yeasts can be maintained easily in a culture collection by heavily inoculating a tube of sterile distilled water with a 48- to 72-h-old yeast culture grown on Sabouraud glucose agar. The yeast suspension should remain viable for at least 2 years if the cap on the tube is tightened securely and the tube is stored at room temperature. To retrieve the culture, 1 to 2 drops of the suspension is removed aseptically from the tube with a sterile capillary pipet and the suspension is inoculated onto Sabouraud glucose agar.

ORGANISMS RESEMBLING YEASTS

Occasionally, organisms such as moulds, algae, etc., may grow on mycologic media and produce colonies which resemble those produced by yeasts. However, careful attention to morphologic characteristics will differentiate them from each other. The following are several examples of such organisms which are recovered from clinical specimens and which superficially can be confused with yeasts.

Genus *Geotrichum*

Members of the genus *Geotrichum* may be confused with yeasts because they produce a white to cream-colored, mealy, subsurface colony on fungal media. Occasionally, an aerial mycelium may be produced, giving a colony which superficially resembles *Coccidioides immitis*. Microscopic examination reveals septate, hyaline hyphae which break into arthroconidia upon maturation (Fig. 3c). No other structures are observed. *Geotrichum candidum* may be separated from *Trichosporon* spp. by carbohydrate assimilation tests and the lack of urease and blastoconidium production. *Geotrichum* spp. occasionally may be isolated from patient specimens, but rarely is it considered a pathogen except in extremely debilitated individuals.

Genus *Ustilago*

The genus *Ustilago* represents a heterobasidiomycetous fungus which is parasitic on the seeds and flowers of many cereals and grasses. It may be inhaled and therefore may be isolated from sputum specimens. The colonies are slowly growing and, when young, are moist, compact, and white. With age, short hyphae are produced and the colonies become velvety or powdery. Microscopically, the cells are irregular and yeastlike or elongate and spindle shaped and may resemble arthroconidia. With the production of short hyphae, clamp connections are formed. Physiologically, most isolates are nitrate positive and have a carbohydrate assimilation test pattern similar to that of *Cryptococcus albidus*.

Black Yeasts

Occasional isolates of *Sporothrix schenckii*, *Aureobasidium pullulans*, and agents of phaeohyphomycosis initially produce white to tan yeastlike colonies on primary isolation media. Identification methods for these organisms are quite different from yeast identification methods and are discussed in chapter 101.

Genus *Prototheca*

Prototheca is a ubiquitous achlorophyllous alga that lives on decaying organic matter and that rarely produces disease in humans and animals (46, 76). Human infection usually involves the skin and underlying tissues or olecranon bursa. Systemic protothecosis with algaemia is an extremely rare manifestation (11). *Prototheca wickerhamii* is recovered most often from human specimens, while *Prototheca zopfii* usually is associated with infections in animals. Colonies are white to cream colored, yeastlike, and dull or moist to mucoid in appearance. The optimal growth temperature is 30°C, and growth is inhibited by medium containing cycloheximide. Microscopically, the cells are variable in size and shape and do not bud (Fig. 5b). Asexual reproduction is by release of sporangiospores from sporangia. Generally, sporangia of *P. zopfii* (14 to 16 μm) are larger than those of *P. wickerhamii* (7 to 13 μm), but this characteristic can be influenced by environmental conditions. Cells of *P. wickerhamii* are round, while most strains of *P. zopfii* will exhibit cells which are oval to cylindrical in shape. Carbon assimilation studies can be used for identification purposes. Both species assimilate glucose and galactose; additionally, *P. wickerhamii* assimilates trehalose. Members of the genus *Prototheca* are nonfermentative (74).

CHARACTERISTICS OF SELECTED MEDICALLY IMPORTANT YEAST GENERA

Genus *Blastoschizomyces*

Blastoschizomyces capitatus, a newly proposed combination for *Blastoschizomyces pseudotrichosporon* and *Trichosporon capitatum* (83), has recently been recognized as an emerging cause of invasive fungal disease in leukemic patients (64) and patients with endocarditis (73). It is widely distributed in nature and occasionally has been recovered as part of the normal skin flora. Disseminated disease usually is associated with immunosuppressive conditions (5). Macroscopically, colonies are glabrous with radiating edges, white to cream colored, and shiny. Microscopically, isolates produce true hyphae, pseudohyphae, and annelloconidia resembling arthroconidia (Fig. 5f). On the basis of morphologic features alone, *B. capitatus* can be difficult to separate from *Trichosporon* spp. and physiologic tests are needed. *B. capitatus* is nonfermentative and can be separated from *Trichosporon* spp. by growth on Sabouraud glucose agar at 45°C and on cycloheximide-containing agar at room temperature and by its failure to hydrolyze urea. At least one author has suggested that *B. capitatus* should be considered a member of the genus *Geotrichum* (21).

Genus *Candida*

The heterogeneous genus *Candida* belongs to the family Cryptococcaceae within the Deuteromycetes (Fungi Imperfecti). The genus contains approximately 200 species. This number is not immutable. Technological advances that affect apparent taxonomic relationships will continually result in reassignments of the present species and the discovery of new species. These advances may also lead to the designation of new genera.

Candida is a form genus. As such, the taxonomic relationship of the species within the genus is not well defined. Teleomorphs of several genera have been demonstrated for different species of *Candida*. The teleomorphic genera include *Clavispora*, *Debaryomyces*, *Issatchenkia*, *Kluyveromyces*, and *Pichia*. This large number of teleomorphic relationships demonstrates that the genus *Candida* is a mixture of unrelated species. One reason for the wide variety of species is due to the definition of *Candida*. The genus designation is used for any asexual yeast which does not have one of the following features: (i) acetic acid production; (ii) visually detectable red, pink, or orange pigments; (iii) arthroconidia; (iv) unipolar or bipolar budding on a broad base; (v) blastoconidia formed on sympodulae; (vi) buds formed on stalks; (vii) needle-shaped terminal conidia; (viii) triangular cells; (ix) enteroblastic-basipetal budding usually with mucoid colonies and the ability to grow on inositol as a sole carbon source; and (x) ballistoconidia (49).

The genus *Candida* no longer contains species that are positive for diazonium blue B (DBB), which is associated with yeasts having a basidiomycetous affinity (such as *Cryptococcus* spp.). DBB-positive organisms (e.g., *Candida humicola*, *Candida curvata*, *Candida diffluens*, and *Candida scottii*) have been reassigned to either the *Cryptococcus* genus or the *Rhodotorula* genus.

Another change in species epithets includes the controversial fusion of *Candida stellatoidea* with *C. albicans*. *Candida claussenii* and *Candida langeronii* have also been merged into *C. albicans* (104). Genetic evidence supporting the fusion of *C. stellatoidea* indicates that two types (designated types I and II) of *C. stellatoidea* exist (78). Type II, which does not assimilate sucrose, appears to be a sucrose-negative mutant of *C. albicans* (56). A definitive association of type I *C. stellatoidea* with *C. albicans* has not been established.

Candida species are ubiquitous yeasts, being found on many plants and as part of the normal flora of the alimentary tracts of mammals and mucocutaneous membranes of humans (68). Essentially all areas of the gastrointestinal (GI) tract of humans can harbor *Candida*. The overall carriage rate in healthy individuals has been estimated to reach 80%, but this value is likely an underestimate due to methodologic problems associated with the detection of low levels of yeasts in GI specimens. The most commonly isolated species (50 to 70% of yeast isolates) from the GI tracts of humans is *C. albicans*, followed by *C. tropicalis*, *C. parapsilosis*, and *C. glabrata*. Mixed yeast infections can be obtained, and the laboratory should have a method for detecting mixed infections, such as CHROMagar as described above.

C. glabrata is regarded as a symbiont of humans and can routinely be isolated from the oral cavity and the genitourinary, alimentary, and respiratory tracts of most individuals. As an agent of serious infection, it has been associated with endocarditis (15), meningitis (2), and multifocal, disseminated disease (41). It is often recovered from urine specimens and has been estimated to account for as many as 21% of urinary yeast isolates (29).

Candida spp. can be present in clinical specimens as a result of environmental contamination, colonization, or actual disease processes. An accurate diagnosis requires proper handling of clinical material. For example, a few *C. albicans* cells will multiply rapidly in sputum left at room temperature, giving the inaccurate impression that large numbers of yeasts are present.

Candida spp. that are part of the normal flora can invade tissue and produce a life-threatening pathology in patients whose immune defenses have been altered by disease or iatrogenic intervention. *C. albicans* is the species most commonly isolated from nearly all forms of candidiasis (68). Contributing to its high degree of association with disease is its high prevalence in the healthy population, as described above. In addition, *C. albicans* appears to possess a number of virulence factors that may promote successful parasitism. These attributes include relatively rapid germination upon seeding of tissue from the bloodstream (39), protease production (55), surface integrinlike molecules for adhesion to extracellular matrix proteins (34, 96), a complement protein binding receptor (13, 31), phenotypic switching (89), and surface variation and hydrophobicity (40). These attributes have recently been reviewed (14, 18). Only *C. tropicalis* appears to be more virulent than *C. albicans* when it is present in patients with leukemia or lymphoreticular malignant disease (105). Other medically important *Candida* spp. include *C. catenulata*, *C. ciferrii*, *C. guilliermondii*, *C. haemulonii*, *C. kefyr*, *C. krusei*, *C. lipolytica*, *C. lusitaniae*, *C. norvegensis*, *C. parapsilosis*, *C. pulcherrima*, *C. rugosa*, *C. utilis*, *C. viswanathii*, and *C. zeylanoides* (37, 79). This list is not exclusive because other rare agents will certainly be added in the future. The species that are emerging as opportunistic pathogens include *C. lipolytica*, *C. lusitaniae*, and *C. krusei*. These three species have been isolated from patients with fungemia. *C. lusitaniae*, which is generally an organism with a low level of virulence, may be either innately or potentially resistant to amphotericin B (35). *C. krusei* isolates appear to be susceptible to ketoconazole but not to fluconazole

(106). An extensive review of the genus and of the diseases produced by *Candida* spp. has been presented by Odds (68). Regardless of the species, a single isolate of *Candida* from blood should be considered significant whether it comes from an immunocompromised or an immunocompetent patient (24). Taken together with the reported rate of 10% for nosocomial bloodstream infections caused by *Candida* species (6), it is evident that *Candida* fungemia represents a serious patient management problem.

Oral candidiasis is considered a defining illness for AIDS. It may be present in patients in the prodromal stages of AIDS or may accompany late stages of AIDS (CD4 T-cell count of <400 cells/μl) (71, 95). Oral candidiasis is a marker for esophageal candidiasis in patients in the late stages of AIDS (95). Mucocutaneous forms of candidiasis are often related to defects in cell-mediated immunity, while systemic spread is generally associated with neutropenia (22, 28). Thus, despite the presence of oral or esophageal candidiasis, the systemic spread of *Candida* in AIDS patients is uncommon. When it occurs, systemic spread is associated with a drop in the neutrophil count (23).

Sullivan et al. (92, 93) have recommended that the new species *Candida dubliniensis* be established for particular isolates of *C. albicans* that exhibit unusual phenotypic characteristics, such as abundant chlamydospore production, resistance to fluconazole, lack of intracellular β-glucosidase, and poor growth at 42°C. The establishment of this new taxon is controversial, although molecular evidence suggests that this organism may be distinct (93). The organism has been recovered from the oral cavities of human immunodeficiency virus (HIV)-infected patients.

There is a serotype preference of the organisms causing oral candidiasis in AIDS and other immunocompromised patients. While the distributions of serotypes A and B are approximately equal in healthy individuals, serotype B is more prevalent in immunocompromised patients (12). The importance of this observation is unclear. However, serotype B isolates are physiologically different from serotype a isolates in that serotype B isolates exhibit greater karyotype variability and are more likely to develop resistance to flucytosine (3, 4).

The blastoconidia of *Candida* spp. vary in shape from round to oval to elongate. Occasional initial isolates, especially from patients receiving antimicrobial agents, may be highly pleomorphic. Asexual reproduction is by multilateral budding, and a true mycelium may be present. If sexual reproduction occurs, the yeasts are classified in their teleomorphic state. The appearance of pseudohyphae and the attachment of blastoconidia are important characteristics to be observed when identifying *Candida* spp. Figure 3 illustrates these morphologic features. Observation of germ tubes and chlamydospores is also helpful in identifying *C. albicans*. Growth on fungal media can be detected as early as 24 h; however, colonies usually are visible in 48 to 72 h as white to cream-colored or tan colonies. They are creamy in texture and may become more membranous and convoluted with age. Occasionally, initial isolates of *C. albicans* on Sabouraud glucose agar are wrinkled or rugose but revert to smooth colonies on subculture. In our experience, many isolates of *C. albicans* produce colonies with "feet" (i.e., colonies with short marginal extensions) on blood agar, while other yeasts do not. These colonies should not be used to perform germ tube tests because of their obvious hyphal or pseudohyphal morphology. Most *Candida* spp. grow well aerobically at 25 to 30°C, and many will grow at 37°C or above. Several species of *Candida*, most notably, *C. albicans*, are diploid (80, 102). These species apparently have lost the ability to undergo meiosis.

Carbon assimilation and occasionally fermentation studies are needed to differentiate the species (Table 1), but rapid confirmation tests for particular species are becoming available (see Rapid Identification of Yeasts above). Of the *Candida* spp. usually recovered from clinical specimens, *C. guilliermondii* is the only one to assimilate dulcitol, and *C. kefyr* (previously *C. pseudotropicalis*) assimilates lactose. The assimilation of rhamnose can be helpful in separating *C. lusitaniae* from the biochemically similar but rhamnose-negative variants of *C. tropicalis* (86). For atypical isolates of *C. lusitaniae*, which can be confused with *C. tropicalis*, good growth on Trichophyton agar #1 with biotin but weak growth on vitamin-free medium indicates *C. tropicalis* (94). Certain rare strains of *C. tropicalis* may assimilate cellobiose weakly and may exhibit an assimilation pattern similar to that of *C. parapsilosis*. The inclusion of arabinose is helpful, since *C. parapsilosis* readily assimilates this carbohydrate, while most strains of *C. tropicalis* do not. Urease generally is not produced, nor is KNO_3 utilized by the *Candida* species listed in Table 1.

Genus *Cryptococcus*

The genus *Cryptococcus* contains many species, six of which are noted in Table 1. Of these, *C. neoformans* is considered the only human pathogen, although *Cryptococcus albidus* (42, 50) and a few others rarely have been implicated in disease in severely debilitated individuals (36). *Cryptococcus* is a round to oval yeastlike fungus ranging greatly in size, from 3.5 to 8 μm or more in diameter with a single bud and a narrow neck between parent and daughter cells (Fig. 2). Unusually large yeast cells (up to 60 μm) have been observed, and this size appears to be associated with higher incubation temperatures (61). Occasionally, several buds may be seen; rarely, pseudohyphae are observed. The cell wall is quite fragile, and it is not unusual to find collapsed or crescent-shaped cells, especially in stained tissue sections. Cells are characterized by the presence of a mucopolysaccharide capsule that varies from a wide halo to a nearly undetectable, lighter zone around the cells, depending on the strain and the medium used. Use of India ink with wet preparations or the mucicarmine stain for mucopolysaccharide with fixed tissue preparations may be helpful in elucidating the capsule. Colonies typically are mucoid due to the presence of capsular material, become dry and duller with age, and exhibit a wide range of colors (cream, tan, pink, yellow). The color may darken with age. Strains possessing only a slight capsule may appear to be similar to colonies of *Candida*. All members of the genus produce urease, utilize various carbohydrates, and are nonfermentative.

C. neoformans was the first serious fungal pathogen of humans to be identified as a heterobasidiomycetous yeast. Mating studies (52) have demonstrated two separate mating pairs, depending on the serotype. At least four serotypes of *C. neoformans* have been identified: serotypes A, B, C, and D. Serotypes A and D were found to produce the teleomorphic state *Filobasidiella neoformans*, and serotypes B and C produce the teleomorph originally named *Filobasidiella bacillispora* (54). The latter species was found to be identical to *C. neoformans* var. *gattii* (97). Although there are certain differences besides serotype, e.g., utilization of creatinine and certain dicarboxylic acids, temperature tolerance, and virulence for mice, all cryptococci are now considered to be varieties of *F. neoformans*, and all are known to produce disease. Standard laboratory tests do not differentiate among the serotypes. However, media for separating serotypes A and D from serotypes B and C have been recommended, but these media are not commercially available (57, 84).

The different serotypes of *C. neoformans* also exhibit epidemiologic differences (9). *C. neoformans* var. *neoformans* serotypes A and D are the most common worldwide, with the highest prevalence of serotype a being seen in Japan and in tropical and subtropical areas such as Southeast Asia, Brazil, Australia, and Southern California. Serotype B is much more prevalent than serotype C, and the majority of serotype C isolates have been found in Southern California (53).

C. neoformans was first detected in the environment in the late 19th century when Sanfelice recovered the yeast from peach juice. Since then, however, *C. neoformans* var. *neoformans* has been most frequently associated with aged pigeon (and other bird) droppings and soils contaminated with these droppings. The yeast usually is not found in fresh droppings but is most evident in the bird excreta that has accumulated over long periods of time on window ledges, vacant buildings, and other roosting sites. (53). It has only been recently that the environmental habitat of *C. neoformans* var. *gattii* has been identified. Recovery of *C. neoformans* var. *gattii* serotype B from the environment coincides with the flowering of the river red gum tree (*Eucalyptus camaldulensis*). Likewise, the global distribution of cryptococcal disease due to *C. neoformans* var. *gattii* correlates with the distribution of this tree (25).

Initial cryptococcal infection begins by inhalation of the fungus into the lungs, usually followed by hematogenous spread to the brain and meninges. Involvement of the skin, bones, and joints is seen, and *C. neoformans* is often cultured from the urine of patients with disseminated infection. In patients without HIV infection, cryptococcosis, particularly cryptococcal meningitis, usually is seen in association with underlying conditions such as lupus erythematosus, sarcoidosis, leukemia, lymphomas, and Cushing's syndrome.

Cryptococcosis is one of the AIDS-defining diseases. Patients with cryptococcosis and serologic evidence of HIV infection are considered to have AIDS. In nearly 45% of AIDS patients, cryptococcosis was reported as the first AIDS-defining illness. Because none of the presenting signs or symptoms of cryptococcal meningitis (such as headache, fever, and malaise) are sufficiently characteristic to distinguish it from other infections that occur in patients with AIDS, determination of cryptococcal antigen titers and culturing of blood and cerebrospinal fluid are useful in making a diagnosis (16).

All species of *Cryptococcus* are nonfermentative aerobes. Separation of *Cryptococcus* species is based on the assimilation of various carbohydrates and KNO_3 (Table 1). *C. neoformans* may be distinguished from other species of *Cryptococcus* by these biochemical studies, as well as growth at 37°C, which may be seen with *C. albidus* and *Cryptococcus laurentii*. *C. neoformans* may be differentiated from other yeasts and from other species of *Cryptococcus* by its production of brown colonies on birdseed agar, although with occasional isolates (particularly serotype C isolates) the production of phenol oxidase may have to be induced. Differentiation from the genus *Rhodotorula*, which also forms a capsule, produces urease, and is nonfermentative, usually is accomplished by noting the utilization of inositol (Table 1) and the absence of carotenoid pigments characteristically present in *Rhodotorula*. *C. neoformans* can be distinguished from other nondematiaceous yeasts in fixed tissue by the use of a Fontana-Masson stain, which will detect melanin precursors in the cell wall.

Genus *Hansenula*

Two species in the genus *Hansenula* have been reported to cause disease in humans. *Hansenula anomala* has been associated with catheter-related infections (1, 48, 67), and *Hansenula polymorpha* has been recovered from the mediastinal lymph nodes of a child with chronic granulomatous disease (65). Variations in colony morphology may cause confusion with *Cryptococcus* and *Candida* spp. The texture may be smooth to wrinkled, and the color may be white, cream, or tan. Microscopically, multilateral budding cells are observed. Pseudohyphae and true hyphae have been reported as characteristics of the genus; however, they have not been observed with the two species presented here. Individual species are either homothallic or heterothallic. Although *H. anomala* is heterothallic, the diploid form is the one usually recovered from clinical specimens. The asci contain one to four hat-shaped spores (Fig. 5a). All members of the genus are nitrate positive. Carbohydrate assimilation and fermentation studies are needed to identify the individual species (51).

Genus *Malassezia*

Seven species of *Malassezia* have been recovered from human specimens and include *M. furfur*, *M. globosa*, *M. obtusa*, *M. pachydermatis*, *M. restricta*, *M. slooffiae*, and *M. sympodialis* (33). The most common clinical species is *M. furfur*. This species includes the previously named species *Pityrosporum ovale* and *Pityrosporum orbiculare*. Recent karyotype analysis suggests that the different cell morphologies seen with *M. furfur* are associated with alterations of its seven chromosomes (43). No teleomorphic state has been described; however, cell wall structure and a positive DBB staining reaction suggest that this form genus may be closely related to the Basidiomycetes (87). *M. furfur* is the agent of the superficial disease pityriasis versicolor (previously named tinea versicolor). It has been documented to cause catheter-associated sepsis related to hyperalimentation with lipid emulsions in neonates and immunocompromised patients (19, 45, 63). Pneumonia may be present in the septic picture for all age groups (63). In addition, *M. furfur* has been reported from patients with peritonitis in which the patients received continuous peritoneal dialysis (98) and is implicated as a possible cause or an associated agent in seborrheic dermatitis, dandruff, atopic dermatitis, and confluent and reticulate papillomatosis (63, 81). However, Ingham and Cunningham (45) note that the etiologic significance of *M. furfur* in these diseases is controversial. Cutaneous infections caused by *Malassezia* species are treatable with a wide number of agents. Relapse rates are high for patients treated with topical agents, and prophylactic use of oral agents (itraconazole or ketoconazole) may be necessary to prevent relapses. Catheter-associated disease is best treated by removal of the catheter and, if necessary, with systemic antifungal agents (19, 77).

M. furfur is normally a commensal organism of human skin. *M. pachydermatis*, which is typically found on animals, rarely has been reported as a cause of sepsis, particularly in low-birth-weight children receiving lipid emulsions through a central venous catheter (85). Two isolates of *M. sympodialis* from human sources have been reported (88). The role of this organism in human disease may be underestimated because of its similarity to *M. furfur* in routine identification tests used in the clinical laboratory (see below).

Culture of routine skin scrapings for the diagnosis of pityriasis versicolor is not usually necessary, and the appearance on direct examination of the clinical material is usually characteristic. The clinical laboratory should be prepared to isolate M. *furfur* from patients with fungemia or other serious infections. M. *furfur* is an obligate lipophile, requiring long-chain fatty acids (C_{12} to C_{24}) for growth (Table 4). M. *pachydermatis*, in contrast, is not an obligate lipophile. Initial cultures of M. *furfur* from blood specimens may result in tiny colonies on solid media or weak growth in broth cultures. Upon subculture to media without lipid supplementation, no growth will be seen.

Lipid supplementation is usually accomplished by overlaying the medium with several drops of sterile olive oil. Alternate media, such as Sabouraud glucose agar with olive oil and Tween 80 incorporated into the agar and GYP-S agar (glucose-yeast extract-peptone agar plus olive oil, Tween 80, and glycerol monostearate), devised by Faergemann (27) work well and offer the opportunity for colony quantitation. Other media for supporting *Malassezia* growth have been developed (10, 60).

After incubation at 35 to 37°C under normal atmospheric conditions, growth usually appears as creamy colonies in 2 to 4 days. Microscopically, *Malassezia* species appear in culture as small, bottle-shaped, budding yeasts (Fig. 5d). Hyphal forms may also be observed in tissue. Careful observation (which is facilitated with differential interference contrast) will reveal that the junction between the bud and the mother cell (which is described as a reduced phialide with a collarette) is rather broad and is not as constricted in appearance as it is in *Candida* species. Routine biochemical testing for the identification of *Malassezia* spp. usually is not attempted. However, organisms that are identified as C. *lipolytica* (glucose, glycerol, and sorbitol positive) with the API 20C AUX system (bioMérieux SA, Marcy l'Etoile, France) may actually be M. *pachydermatis* (63). In this case, morphology is helpful. Identification to the genus level is accomplished by demonstrating typical microscopic and macroscopic morphologies and good growth at 37°C but no or poor growth at 25°C. Growth on Sabouraud glucose agar with and without lipid additives allows separation of M. *furfur* and M. *sympodialis* from M. *pachydermatis*. It should be noted that C. *glabrata* can behave like M. *furfur*. In this case, morphology must be obtained. To distinguish M. *furfur* from M. *sympodialis*, both of which are obligate lipophiles and grow as phialidic yeasts in young cultures, the organisms should be subcultured onto media overlaid with either oleic acid or Tween 80. *Malassezia* spp. are nonfermentative and urease positive.

Genus *Pichia*

The teleomorphic genus *Pichia* encompasses several species of *Candida* (for example, C. *lambica* and C. *guilliermondii*). Generally, the anamorphic (asexual) state is the one recovered from clinical specimens, because mating studies usually are needed to produce the teleomorphic (sexual) form. The biochemical and physiological reactions of the teleomorph should be identical to those of the anamorph, as listed in Table 1. *Pichia anomala* is the teleomorph of H. *anomala*.

Genus *Rhodotorula*

Rhodotorula spp. are normal inhabitants of moist skin and can be recovered from such environmental sources as shower curtains, bathtub grout, and toothbrushes (17). In rare instances *Rhodotorula* spp. have been reported to cause septicemia (72), meningitis (75), systemic infection (82), and sepsis related to complications from indwelling central venous catheters (47).

Rhodotorula spp. share many similar physiologic and morphologic properties with *Cryptococcus* spp. Both are round to oval-shaped, multilateral budding yeasts with capsules, produce urease, and fail to ferment carbohydrates. *Rhodotorula* spp. differ from cryptococci by their inability to assimilate inositol and their obvious carotenoid pigment.

Genus *Saccharomyces*

S. *cerevisiae* is the most common species of the genus recovered in the clinical laboratory. Usually thought to be nonpathogenic, occasionally it has been reported to cause thrush, vulvovaginitis (17), and fungemia (26, 37).

Multilateral budding yeast cells are round to oval, and short rudimentary (occasionally well-developed) pseudohyphae may be formed. Ascospore production can be enhanced easily by growing the yeast on Fowell's acetate agar for 2 to 5 days at room temperature. Asci contain one to four round, smooth ascospores (Fig. 5c). Other physiologic properties are listed in Table 1. Assimilation of raffinose by S. *cerevisiae* is noteworthy. Very few yeasts encountered in the clinical laboratory utilize this carbon source, and when this is observed, S. *cerevisiae* should be considered.

Genus *Torulopsis*

By general consensus among most mycologists the genus *Torulopsis* has been combined with the genus *Candida* (7, 66, 108). Refer to earlier discussions in the section on *Candida* above for information about C. *glabrata* and other species.

Genus *Trichosporon*

The genus *Trichosporon* has recently undergone extensive taxonomic reevaluation (32). Distinct morphologic and physiologic patterns of invasive clinical, superficial clinical, and environmental isolates have been recognized among isolates of *Trichosporon beigelii* (59). Partial sequencing of the 26S RNA, in addition to studies of ultrastructure, DNA, and ubiquinone systems, has led researchers to recommend a revision of the genus to include a large number of species possessing marked ecological preferences (32). deHoog and Guarro (21) recognize five *Trichosporon* spp. pathogenic for humans: T. *asahii*, T. *cutaneum*, T. *inkin*, T. *mucoides*, and T. *ovoides*. The two species involved with deep fungal infections are T. *asahii* and T. *mucoides*. T. *asahii* infections often present with hematogenous dissemination, while T. *mucoides* has been recovered from patients with central nervous system disease. The other three species, T. *cutaneum* (T. *beigelii*), T. *inkin*, and T. *ovoides*, are more difficult to distinguish and have been casually grouped as the T. *cutaneum* (or T. *beigelii*) complex. The true nature of the invasive capability of *Trichosporon* spp. was not recognized until 1970 (81). Disseminated disease due to *Trichosporon* is uncommon but is increasingly reported (58, 62). Infection in the immunocompromised host, especially granulocytopenic patients, frequently produces a fatal disease that is refractory to amphotericin B therapy (44, 100, 101). See chapter 100 for a discussion of superficial *Trichosporon* infections.

Trichosporon spp. belong to the family Cryptococcaceae and have basidiomycetous affinities. They produce blastoconidia of various shapes, well-developed hyphae, pseudohyphae, and arthroconidia (Fig. 3j). In cases in which a *Trichosporon* isolate produces only a few blastoconidia, differentiation from *Geotrichum* spp. may be difficult. Inoculation of malt extract broth at room temperature will encourage blastoconidia production in *Trichosporon* spp., usu-

TABLE 5 Pertinent characteristics of selected *Trichosporon* spp.[a]

Trichosporon species	Assimilation of: L-Rhamnose	Melibiose	Raffinose	Ribitol	Xylitol	L-Arabinitol	Galactitol	Growth at 37°C	Urease
T. asahii	+	–	–	V	V	+	–	+	+
T. cutaneum	+	+	+	+	+	+	–	–	+
T. inkin	–	–	–	–	–	–	–	+	+
T. mucoides	+	+	+	+	+	+	+	+	+
T. ovoides	+	–	V	–	V	–	–	+	+

[a] +, positive reaction; –, negative reaction; V, strain variation.

ally within 48 to 72 h. Table 5 lists some pertinent characteristics of selected *Trichosporon* spp. Growth usually is observed within 1 week on solid media, and young colonies are cream colored, smooth, and shiny, later becoming dry, membranous, and cerebriform. Most *Trichosporon* spp. are nonfermentative.

REFERENCES

1. **Alter, S. J., and J. Farley.** 1994. Development of *Hansenula anomala* infection in a child receiving fluconazole therapy. *Pediatr. Infect. Dis. J.* **13:**158–159.
2. **Anhalt, E., J. Alvarez, and R. Bert.** 1986. *Torulopsis glabrata* meningitis. *South. Med. J.* **79:**916.
3. **Asakura, K., S.-I. Iwaguchi, M. Homma, T. Sukai, K. Higashide, and K. Tanaka.** 1991. Electrophoretic karyotypes of clinically isolated yeasts of *Candida albicans* and *C. glabrata*. *J. Gen. Microbiol.* **137:**2531–2538.
4. **Auger, P., C. Dumas, and J. Joly.** 1979. A study of 666 strains of *Candida albicans*: correlation between serotype and susceptibility to 5-fluorocytosine. *J. Infect. Dis.* **139:** 590–594.
5. **Baird, D. R., M. Harris, R. Menon, and R. Stoddart.** 1985. Systemic infection with *Trichosporon capitatum* in two patients with leukemia. *Eur. J. Clin. Microbiol.* **4:** 62–64.
6. **Banerjee, S. N., T. G. Emori, D. H. Culver, R. P. Gaynes, W. R. Jarvis, T. Horan, J. R. Edwards, J. Tolson, T. Henderson, W. J. Martone, and The National Nosocomial Infections Surveillance System.** 1991. Secular trends in nosocomial primary bloodstream infections in the United States, 1980–1989. *Am. J. Med.* **91**(Suppl. 3B)**:**86S–89S.
7. **Barnett, J. A., R. W. Payne, and D. Yarrow.** 1983. *Yeasts: Characteristics and Identification*. Cambridge University Press, Cambridge, United Kingdom.
8. **Baumgartner, C., A. Freydiere, and Y. Gile.** 1996. Direct identification and recognition of yeast species from clinical material by using Albicans ID and CHROMagar Candida plates. *J. Clin. Microbiol.* **34:**454–456.
9. **Bennett, J. E., K. J. Kwon-Chung, and D. H. Howard.** 1977. Epidemiological differences among serotypes of *Cryptococcus neoformans*. *Am. J. Epidemiol.* **105:**582–586.
10. **Bezjak, V., T. M. Al-Nakib, and R. Chandy.** 1989. New oil-free media for *Malassezia furfur* (*Pityrosoporum orbiculare*), abstr. F-51, p. 466. *In Abstracts of the 89th Annual Meeting of the American Society for Microbiology 1989*. American Society for Microbiology, Washington, D.C.
11. **Boyd, A. S., M. Langley, and L. E. King.** 1995. Cutaneous manifestation of *Prototheca* infections. *J. Am. Acad. Dermatol.* **32:**758–764.
12. **Brawner, D. L., G. L. Anderson, and K. Y. Yuen.** 1992. Serotype prevalence of *Candida albicans* from blood culture isolates. *J. Clin. Microbiol.* **30:**149–153.
13. **Calderone, R. A., L. Linehan, E. Wadsworth, and A. L. Sandberg.** 1988. Identification of C3d receptors on *Candida albicans*. *Infect. Immun.* **56:**252–258.
14. **Calderone, R. A., and P. C. Braun.** 1991. Adherence and receptor relationship of *Candida albicans*. *Microbiol. Rev.* **55:**1–20.
15. **Carmody, T. J., and K. K. Kane.** 1986. *Torulopsis* (*Candida*) *glabrata* endocarditis involving a bovine pericardial xenograft heart valve. *Heart Lung* **15:**40–42.
16. **Chuck, S. L., and M. A. Sande.** 1989. Infections with *Cryptococcus neoformans* in the acquired immunodeficiency syndrome. *N. Engl. J. Med.* **321:**794–799.
17. **Cooper, B. H., and M. Silva-Hutner.** 1985. Yeasts of medical importance, p. 526–541. *In* E. H. Lennette, A. Balows, W. J. Hausler, Jr., and H. J. Shadomy (ed.), *Manual of Clinical Microbiology*, 4th ed. American Society for Microbiology, Washington, D.C.
18. **Cutler, J. E.** 1991. Putative virulence factors of *Candida albicans*. *Annu. Rev. Microbiol.* **45:**187–218.
19. **Danker, W. M., S. A. Spector, J. Fierer, and C. E. Davis.** 1987. *Malassezia* fungemia in neonates and adults: complication of hyperalimentation. *Rev. Infect. Dis.* **9:**743–753.
20. **Dealler, S. F.** 1991. *Candida albicans* colony identification in 5 minutes in a general microbiology laboratory. *J. Clin. Microbiol.* **29:**1081–1082.
21. **deHoog, G. S., and J. Guarro.** 1995. *Atlas of Clinical Fungi*. Centraalbureau voor Schimmelcultures, Delft, The Netherlands.
22. **Domer, J. E., and R. I. Kehrer.** 1993. Introduction to *Candida*: systemic candidiasis, p. 49–116. *In* J. W. Murphy, H. Friedman, and M. Bendinelli (ed.), *Fungal Infections and Immune Responses*. Plenum Press, New York, N.Y.
23. **Drouhet, E., and B. Dupont.** 1991. Candidosis in heroin addicts and AIDS: new immunologic data on chronic mucocutaneous candidosis, p. 61–72. *In* E. Tümbay, H. P. R. Seeliger, and O. Ang (ed.), Candida *and Candida Mycosis*. Plenum Press, New York, N.Y.
24. **Edwards, J. E., Jr., and S. G. Filler.** 1992. Current strategies for treating invasive candidiasis: emphasis on infections in nonneutropenic patients. *Clin. Infect. Dis.* **14**(Suppl. 1)**:**S106–S113.
25. **Ellis, D. H., and T. J. Pfeiffer.** 1990. Natural habitat of *Cryptococcus neoformans* var. *gattii*. *J. Clin. Microbiol.* **28:** 1642–1644.
26. **Eschete, M. L., and B. C. West.** 1980. *Saccharomyces cerevisiae* septicemia. *Arch. Intern. Med.* **140:**1539.
27. **Faergemann, J.** 1984. Quantitative culture of *Pityrosporum orbiculare*. *Int. J. Dermatol.* **23:**330–333.
28. **Filler, S. G., and J. E. Edwards, Jr.** 1993. Chronic mucocutaneous candidiasis, p. 117–133. *In* J. W. Murphy, H. Friedman, and M. Bendinelli (ed.), *Fungal Infections and Immune Responses*. Plenum Press, New York, N.Y.
29. **Frye, K. R., J. M. Donovan, and G. W. Drach.** 1988. *Torulopsis glabrata* urinary infections: a review. *J. Urol.* **139:**1245–1249.
30. **Galgiani, J. N., J. Reiser, C. Brass, A. Espinel-Ingroff, M. A. Gordon, and T. M. Kerkering.** 1987. Comparison of relative susceptibilities of *Candida* species to three antifungal agents as determined by unstandardized methods. *Antimicrob. Agents Chemother.* **31:**1343–1347.
31. **Gilmore, B. J., E. M. Retsinas, J. S. Lorenz, and M. K. Hostetter.** 1988. An iC3b receptor on *Candida albicans*:

structure, function, and correlates for pathogenicity. *J. Infect. Dis.* **257:**38–46.

32. **Guého, E., M. T. Smith, G. S. de Hoog, G. Billon-Grand, R. Christen, and W. H. Batenburg-van der Vegte.** 1992. Contributions to a revision of the genus *Trichosporon. Antonie Leeuwenhoek J. Microbiol. Serol.* **61:** 289–316.
33. **Guilot, J., and E. Guého.** 1995. The diversity of *Malassezia* yeasts confirmed by rRNA sequence and nuclear DNA comparisons. *Antonie Leeuwenhoek J. Microbiol. Serol.* **67:**297–314.
34. **Gustafson, K. S., G. M. Vercellotti, C. M. Bendel, and M. K. Hostetter.** 1991. Molecular mimicry in *Candida albicans. J. Clin. Invest.* **87:**1896–1902.
35. **Hadfield, T. L., M. B. Smith, R. E. Winn, M. G. Rinaldi, and C. Guerra.** 1987. Mycoses caused by *Candida lusitaniae. Rev. Infect. Dis.* **9:**1006–1012.
36. **Hajjeh, R. A., M. E. Brandt, and R. W. Pinner.** 1995. Emergence of cryptococcal disease: epidemiologic perspectives 100 years after its discovery. *Epidemiol. Rev.* **17:** 303–320.
37. **Hazen, K. C.** 1995. New and emerging yeast pathogens. *Clin. Microbiol. Rev.* **8:**462–478.
38. **Hazen, K. C., and B. W. Hazen.** 1987. Temperature-modulated physiological characteristics of *Candida albicans. Microbiol. Immunol.* **31:**497–508.
39. **Hazen, K. C., D. L. Brawner, M. H. Riesselman, J. E. Cutler, and M. A. Jutila.** 1991. Differential adherence of hydrophobic and hydrophilic *Candida albicans* yeast cells to mouse tissues. *Infect. Immun.* **59:**907–912.
40. **Hazen, K. C., and P. M. Glee.** 1995. Cell surface hydrophobicity and medically important fungi. *Curr. Top. Med. Mycol.* **6:**1–31.
41. **Hickey, W. F., L. H. Sommerville, and F. J. Schoen.** 1983. Disseminated *Candida glabrata*: report of a uniquely severe infection and a literature review. *Am. J. Clin. Pathol.* **80:**724–727.
42. **Horowitz, I. D., E. A. Blumburg, and L. Krevolin.** 1993. *Cryptococcus albidus* and mucormycosis empyema in a patient receiving hemodialysis. *South. Med. J.* **86:** 1070–1072.
43. **Howell, S. A., C. Quin, and G. Midgeley.** 1993. Karyotypes of oval cell forms of *Malassezia furfur. Mycoses* **36:** 263–266.
44. **Hoy, J., K.-C. Hsu, K. Rolston, R. L. Hopfer, M. Luna, and G. P. Bodey.** 1986. *Trichosporon beigelii* infection: a review. *Rev. Infect. Dis.* **8:**959–967.
45. **Ingham, E., and A. C. Cunningham.** 1993. *Malassezia furfur. J. Med. Vet. Mycol.* **31:**265–288.
46. **Kaplan, W.** 1978. Protothecosis and infections caused by morphologically similar green algae, p. 218–232. *In The Black and White Yeasts.* Pan American Health Organization Publication 356, Proceedings of the IV International Conference on Mycoses. Pan American Health Organization, Washington, D.C.
47. **Kiehn, T. E., E. Gorey, A. E. Brown, F. F. Edwards, and D. Armstrong.** 1992. Sepsis due to *Rhodotorula* related to use of indwelling central venous catheters. *Clin. Infect. Dis.* **14:**841–846.
48. **Klein, A. S., G. T. Tortora, R. Malowitz, and W. H. Greene.** 1988. *Hansenula anomala*: a new fungal pathogen. *Arch. Intern. Med.* **148:**1210–1213.
49. **Kreger-Van Rij, N. J. W. (ed).** 1984. *The Yeasts, a Taxonomic Study*, 3rd ed. Elsevier Science Publishers B. V., Amsterdam, The Netherlands.
50. **Krumholz, R. A.** 1972. Pulmonary cryptococcosis. A case due to *Cryptococcus albidus. Am. Rev. Respir. Dis.* **105:** 421–424.
51. **Kurtzman, C. P.** 1984. Genus 11. *Hansenula* H. et P. Sydow, p. 165–213. *In* N. J. W. Kreger-van Rij (ed.), *The Yeasts, a Taxonomic Study*, 3rd ed. Elsevier Science Publishers B. V., Amsterdam, The Netherlands.
52. **Kwon-Chung, K. J.** 1975. A new genus, *Filobasidiella*, the perfect state of *Cryptococcus neoformans. Mycologia* **67:** 1197–1200.
53. **Kwon-Chung, K. J., and J. E. Bennett.** 1992. *Medical Mycology*, p. 397–446. Lea & Febiger, Philadelphia, Pa.
54. **Kwon-Chung, K. J., J. E. Bennett, and T. S. Theodore.** 1978. *Cryptococcus bacillisporus* sp. nov. serotype B-C of *Cryptococcus neoformans. Int. J. Syst. Bacteriol.* **28:** 616–620.
55. **Kwon-Chung, K. J., D. Lehman, C. Good, and P. T. Magee.** 1985. Genetic evidence for the role of extracellular proteinase in virulence of *Candida albicans. Infect. Immun.* **49:**571–575.
56. **Kwon-Chung, K. J., J. B. Hicks, and P. N. Lipke.** 1990. Evidence that *Candida stellatoidea* type II is a mutant of *Candida albicans* that does not express sucrose-inhibitable α-glucosidase. *Infect. Immun.* **58:**2804–2808.
57. **Kwon-Chung, K. J., I. Polacheck, and J. E. Bennett.** 1982. Improved diagnostic medium for separation of *Cryptococcus neoformans* var. *neoformans* (serotypes A and D) and *Cryptococcus neoformans* var. *gattii* (serotypes B and C). *J. Clin. Microbiol.* **15:**535–537.
58. **Leblond, V., O. Saint-Jean, A. Datry, G. Lecso, C. Frances, S. Bellefigh, M. Gentilini, and J. L. Binet.** 1986. Systemic infections with *Trichosporon beigelii* (*cutaneum*). *Cancer* **58:**2399–2405.
59. **Lee, J. W., G. A. Melcher, M. G. Rinaldi, P. A. Pizzo, and T. J. Welsh.** 1990. Patterns of morphologic variation among isolates of *Trichosporon beigelii. J. Clin. Microbiol.* **28:**2823–2827.
60. **Leeming, J. P., and F. H. Notman.** 1987. Improved methods for isolation and enumeration of *Malassezia furfur* from human skin. *J. Clin. Microbiol.* **25:**2017–2019.
61. **Love, G. L., G. D. Boyd, and D. L. Greer.** 1985. Large *Cryptococcus neoformans* isolated from brain abscess. *J. Clin. Microbiol.* **22:**1068–1070.
62. **Manzella, J. P., I. J. Berman, and M. D. Kubrika.** 1982. *Trichosporon beigelii* fungemia and cutaneous dissemination. *Arch. Dermatol.* **118:**343–345.
63. **Marcon, M. J., and D. A. Powell.** 1992. Human infections due to *Malassezia* spp. *Clin. Microbiol. Rev.* **5:** 101–119.
64. **Martino, P., M. Venditti, A. Micozzi, G. Morace, L. Polonelli, M. P. Mantovani, M. C. Petti, V. L. Burgio, C. Santini, P. Serra, and F. Mandelli.** 1990. *Blastoschizomyces capitatus*: an emerging cause of invasive fungal disease in leukemia patients. *Rev. Infect. Dis.* **18:**579–582.
65. **McGinnis, M. R., D. H. Walker, and J. D. Folds.** 1980. *Hansenula polymorpha* infection in a child with chronic granulomatous disease. *Arch. Pathol. Lab. Med.* **104:** 290–292.
66. **McGinnis, M. R., and M. G. Rinaldi.** 1997. Selected medically important fungi and some common synonyms and obsolete names. *Clin. Infect. Dis.* **25:**15–17.
67. **Neumeister, B., M. Rockemann, and R. Marre.** 1992. Fungaemia due to *Candida pelliculosa* in a case of acute pancreatitis. *Mycoses* **35:**309–310.
68. **Odds, F. C.** 1988. Candida *and Candidosis*, 2nd ed. Bailliere Tindall, London, United Kingdom.
69. **Pfaller, M. A., T. Preston, M. Bale, F. P. Koontz, and B. A. Body.** 1988. Comparison of the Quantum II, API Yeast Ident and AutoMicrobic Systems for identification of clinical yeast isolates. *J. Clin. Microbiol.* **26:** 2054–2058.
70. **Pfaller, M. A., A. Houston, and S. Coffman.** 1996. Application of CHROMagar Candida for rapid screening of

clinical specimens for *Candida albicans*, *Candida tropicalis*, *Candida krusei*, and *Candida* (*Torulopsis*) *glabrata*. *J. Clin. Microbiol.* **34:**58–61.

71. **Phelan, J. A., B. R. Saltzman, G. H. Friedland, and R. S. Klein.** 1987. Oral findings in patients with acquired immunodeficiency syndrome. *Oral Surg.* **64:**50–56.
72. **Pien, F. D., R. L. Thompson, D. Deye, and G. D. Roberts.** 1980. *Rhodotorula* septicemia: two cases and a review of the literature. *Mayo Clin. Proc.* **55:**258–260.
73. **Polacheck, I., I. F. Salkin, R. Kitzes-Cohen, and R. Raz.** 1992. Endocarditis caused by *Blastoschizomyces capitatus* and taxonomic review of the genus. *J. Clin. Microbiol.* **30:**2318–2322.
74. **Pore, R. S.** 1985. *Prototheca* taxonomy. *Mycopathologia* **90:**129–139.
75. **Pore, R. S., and J. Chen.** 1976. Meningitis caused by *Rhodotorula*. *Sabouraudia* **14:**331–335.
76. **Pore, R. S., E. A. Barnett, W. C. Barnes, et al.** 1983. *Prototheca* ecology. *Mycopathologia* **81:**49–62.
77. **Redline, R. W., S. S. Redline, B. Boxerbaum, and B. B. Dahms.** 1985. Systemic *Malassezia furfur* infections in patients receiving intralipid therapy. *Hum. Pathol.* **16:** 815–822.
78. **Rikkerink, E. H. A., B. B. Magee, and P. T. Magee.** 1990. Genomic structure of *Candida stellatoidea*: extra chromosomes and gene duplication. *Infect. Immun.* **58:** 949–954.
79. **Rinaldi, M. G.** 1993. Biology and pathogenicity of *Candida* species, p. 1–20. *In* G. P. Bodey (ed.), *Candidiasis: Pathogenesis, Diagnosis and Treatment*. Raven Press, New York, N.Y.
80. **Rine, J., W. Hansen, E. Hardeman, and R. W. Davis.** 1983. Targeted selection of recombinant clones through gene dosage effects. *Proc. Natl. Acad. Sci. USA* **80:** 6750–6754.
81. **Ring, J., D. Abeck, and K. Neuber.** 1992. Atopic eczema: role of microorganisms on the skin surface. *Allergy* **47:** 265–269.
82. **Rusthoven, J. J., R. Feld, and P. J. Tuffnell.** 1984. Systemic infection by *Rhodotorula* spp. in the immunocompromised host. *J. Infect.* **8:**244–246.
83. **Salkin, I. F., M. A. Gordon, W. M. Samsonoff, and C. L. Rieder.** 1985. *Blastoschizomyces capitatus*, a new combination. *Mycotaxon* **22:**373–380.
84. **Salkin, I. F., and N. J. Hurd.** 1982. New medium for differentiation of *Cryptococcus neoformans* serotype pairs. *J. Clin. Microbiol.* **15:**169–171.
85. **Sanguinetti, V., M. P. Tampieri, and L. Morganti.** 1984. A survey of 120 isolates of *Malassezia* (*Pityrosporum*) *pachydermatis*. *Mycopathologia* **85:**93–95.
86. **Schlitzer, R. L., and D. G. Ahearn.** 1982. Characterization of atypical *Candida tropicalis* and other uncommon clinical yeast isolates. *J. Clin. Microbiol.* **15:**511–516.
87. **Simmons, R. B., and D. G. Ahearn.** 1987. Cell wall ultrastructure and DBB reaction of *Sporopachydermia quercuum*, *Bullera tsugae* and *Malassezia* spp. *Mycologia* **79:** 38–43.
88. **Simmons, R. B., and E. Guého.** 1990. A new species of *Malassezia*. *Mycol. Res.* **94:**1146–1149.
89. **Soll, D. R.** 1992. High-frequency switching in *Candida albicans*. *Clin. Microbiol. Rev.* **5:**183–203.
90. **Spicer, A. D., and K. C. Hazen.** 1992. Rapid confirmation of *Candida albicans* identification by combination of two presumptive tests. *Med. Microbiol. Lett.* **1:**284–289.
91. **St.-Germain, G., and D. Beauchesne.** 1991. Evaluation of the Microscan Rapid Yeast Identification Panel. *J. Clin. Microbiol.* **29:**2296–2299.
92. **Sullivan, D., K. Haynes, J. Bille, P. Boerlin, L. Rodero, S. Lloyd, M. Henman, and D. Coleman.** 1997. Widespread geographic distribution of oral *Candida dubliniensis* strains in human immunodeficiency virus-infected individuals. *J. Clin. Microbiol.* **35:**960–964.
93. **Sullivan, D. J., T. J. Westerneng, K. A. Haynes, D. E. Bennett, and D. C. Coleman.** 1995. *Candida dubliniensis* sp. nov.: phenotypic and molecular characterization of a novel species associated with oral candidosis in HIV-infected individuals. *Microbiology* **141:**1507–1521.
94. **Summerbell, R. C.** 1992. *Candida lusitaniae* confirmed by a simple test, abstr. F90, p. 513. *In Abstracts of the 92nd General Meeting of the American Society for Microbiology 1992*. American Society for Microbiology, Washington, D.C.
95. **Tavitian, A., J.-P. Raufman, and L. E. Rosenthal.** 1986. Oral candidiasis as a marker for esophageal candidiasis in the acquired immunodeficiency syndrome. *Ann. Intern. Med.* **104:**54–55.
96. **Tronchin, G., J. P. Bouchara, V. Annaix, R. Robert, and J. M. Senet.** 1991. Fungal cell adhesion molecules in *Candida albicans*. *Eur. J. Epidemiol.* **7:**23–33.
97. **Vanbreuseghem, R., and M. Takashio.** 1970. An atypical strain of *Cryptococcus neoformans* (San Felice) Vuillemin 1894. II. *C. neoformans* var *gattii* var. nov. *Ann. Soc. Belge. Med. Trop.* **50:**695–702.
98. **Wallace, M., H. Bagnall, D. Glen, and S. Averill.** 1979. Isolation of lipophilic yeasts in "sterile" peritonitis. *Lancet* **ii:**956.
99. **Walsh, T. J., and A. Pizzo.** 1988. Treatment of systemic fungal infections: recent progress and current problems. *Curr. J. Clin. Microbiol. Infect. Dis.* **7:**460–475.
100. **Walsh, T. J., G. P. Melcher, M. G. Rinaldi, J. Lecciones, D. A. McGough, P. Kelly, J. Lee, D. Callender, M. Rubin, and P. A. Pizzo.** 1990. *Trichosporon beigelii*, an emerging pathogen resistant to amphotericin B. *J. Clin. Microbiol.* **28:**1616–1622.
101. **Watson, K. C., and S. Kallichurum.** 1970. Brain abscess due to *Trichosporon cutaneum*. *J. Med. Microbiol.* **3:** 191–193.
102. **Whelan, W. L., and K. J. Kwon-Chung.** 1988. Auxotrophic heterozygosities and the ploidy of *Candida parapsilosis* and *Candida krusei*. *J. Med. Vet. Mycol.* **26:**163–171.
103. **Wickerham, L. J., and K. A. Burton.** 1948. Carbon assimilation tests for the classification of yeasts. *J. Bacteriol.* **56:**363–371.
104. **Wickes, B. L., J. B. Hicks, W. G. Merz, and K. J. Kwon-Chung.** 1992. The molecular analysis of synonymy among medically important yeasts within the genus *Candida*. *J. Gen. Microbiol.* **138:**901–907.
105. **Wingard, J. R., J. D. Dick, W. G. Merz, G. R. Sanford, R. Saral, and W. H. Burns.** 1982. Differences in virulence of clinical isolates of *Candida tropicalis* and *Candida albicans* in mice. *Infect. Immun.* **37:**833–836.
106. **Wingard, J. R., W. G. Merz, M. G. Rinaldi, T. R. Johnson, J. E. Karp, and R. Saral.** 1991. Increase in *Candida krusei* infection among patients with bone marrow transplantation and neutropenia treated prophylactically with fluconazole. *N. Engl. J. Med.* **325:**1274–1277.
107. **Yamane, N., and Y. Saitoh.** 1985. Isolation and detection of multiple yeasts from a single clinical sample by use of Pagano-Levin agar medium. *J. Clin. Microbiol.* **21:** 276–277.
108. **Yarrow, D., and S. A. Meyer.** 1978. Proposal for amendment of the diagnosis of the genus *Candida* Berkhout mon. cons. *Int. J. Syst. Bacteriol.* **28:**611–615.

Pneumocystis

W. KEITH HADLEY AND VALERIE L. NG

96

DESCRIPTION OF THE AGENT

Pneumocystis carinii is a unicellular eukaryotic organism with a tropism for growth on respiratory surfaces of mammals (95, 113, 116, 125). Although originally classified with the protozoa, recent evidence suggests that *P. carinii* is more phylogenetically related to fungi (28, 87, 94, 107, 110, 113). *P. carinii* and fungi have similar cyst wall ultrastructures, have mitochondria with lamellar cristae (protozoan mitochondria have tubular cristae), and have cyst forms containing intracystic bodies resembling those of ascospores formed by the ascomycetes (94, 95, 113). The 16S rRNA subunit of *P. carinii* is most homologous with that of ascomycetes (27, 109, 110) while the 5S rRNA is most homologous with that of primitive zygomycetes (123). The β-tubulin gene is 89 to 91% homologous with that of the filamentous fungi (24, 25). The protein synthesis elongation factor, EF-3, and thymidylate synthase of *P. carinii* are most homologous with those of ascomycetes, and thymidylate synthase and dihydrofolate reductase activities are on two separate proteins (in contrast, protozoa produce a single bifunctional protein) (26, 28). A 6.8-kb fragment of mitochondrial DNA that encodes apocytochrome B; NADH dehydrogenase subunits 1, 2, 3, and 6; cytochrome oxidase subunit II; and a small subunit of rRNA have an average similarity of 60% with fungi (but only 20% with protozoa) (87, 110).

In contrast with the above, *P. carinii* has a number of features that are atypical for fungi. Ergosterol, the sterol found in the membranes of most fungi, has not been detected in pneumocystis, perhaps explaining the clinical inefficacy of commonly used antifungal agents that are dependent on binding to or inhibiting synthesis of ergosterol (i.e., amphotericin B or imidazole and triazole antifungal agents, respectively) (28, 51, 89). Cholesterol is the major sterol in *P. carinii*, and a variety of unusual sterols seemingly unique to *P. carinii* have been identified (51). *P. carinii* does not grow continuously in in vitro culture. It contains only two copies of the genes encoding 16S-like rRNA (hundreds of copies of this gene are present in most fungi), and the cell wall of the trophic form is fragile and flexible (instead of tough and rigid as commonly present in the cell walls of vegetative yeasts) (107).

Both sexual and asexual life cycles have been proposed for *Pneumocystis* (94). Pneumocystis cells consist of up to eight ovoid to fusiform intracystic bodies (spores) within a cyst (spore coat), or as free trophic forms (1.5 to 5 μm in diameter) with small nuclei (0.5 to 1.0 μm) and flexible membranes. The precyst (sporocyst) has a larger nucleus and a rigid wall.

Since *P. carinii* cannot be propagated continuously in host cell-free (axenic) culture systems, study of the organism in vivo is limited to analysis of specimens either directly obtained from infected mammals or cocultured with feeder cells. Rat-derived pneumocystis, cocultured with mammalian lung-derived cells, has been the most successful system and therefore the system most studied (3, 4, 103). Short-term host cell-free culture systems that maintain metabolism and may increase numbers of pneumocystis cells over several days have been developed recently. Although viability can and has been measured by incorporation of radiolabel from a substrate into its product (20, 22), enumeration of pneumocystis (a polymorphic organism which is strongly self-adherent as well as adherent to host cells) and determination of viability remain problematic for all currently used *P. carinii* culture systems (3, 52, 59).

Animal models of *P. carinii* infection have been highly predictive of human response to infection, therapy, and prophylaxis. The corticosteroid-treated latently infected rat model, developed by Frankel, has been used to study therapeutic or prophylactic agents prior to human trials (31). The transtracheal-inoculated corticosteroid-treated rat model allows a more uniform infection with standardized inocula (5, 104). Other models include immunodeficient mice (nude mouse, *scid* mouse, T-cell-deficient mouse) and other mammals.

There is emerging molecular biology-based evidence that different varieties, and possibly different species, of pneumocystis exist. Although pneumocystis strains recovered from rats, humans, and other mammals are morphologically indistinguishable, differences in surface antigens, karyotypes, and nucleic acid sequences of a variety of cloned genes can be demonstrated (39, 61, 68, 101). There is evidence that rats can be simultaneously infected with two different strains of pneumocystis (23). Based on DNA sequences obtained from multiple animal sources, it has been proposed that *P. carinii* be subgrouped into *P. carinii* f. sp. carinii (rat prototype, or Pc1), *P. carinii* f. sp. ratti (rat variant, or Pc2), *P. carinii* f. sp. hominis (human, or Pc3), *P. carinii* f. sp. mustelae (ferret), *P. carinii* f. sp. muris (mouse), *P. carinii* f. sp. eaui (horse), *P.*

carinii f. sp. suis (pig), and *P. carinii* f. sp. oryctolagi (rabbit) (1, 107). The genetic differences supporting this proposed classification of *P. carinii* may be useful for tracking the epidemiology of pneumocystis (60) and must be considered when designing therapeutic drugs or diagnostic reagents.

The natural reservoir of *P. carinii* remains unknown. Infection of multiple animal species with *P. carinii* suggests that it is widespread in the environment (43, 45), and recent studies have demonstrated *P. carinii* DNA sequences in spores found in air samples (117). Although airborne transmission of *P. carinii* between rats has been convincingly demonstrated (42, 47), it is unlikely that infected rodents serve as a zoonotic reservoir for human infection, since rat-derived *P. carinii* strains are genetically distinct from those of humans (101, 108).

P. CARINII INFECTION

The respiratory tract is thought to be the portal of entry for *P. carinii*, since the apparent primary infection is in the lung. Although the infectious form of *P. carinii* is not known, the freshly released intracystic body or the small trophic form is approximately the same size (i.e., 1 to 3 μm) as other pulmonary pathogens that are successfully spread deep into the lung via aerosolization (i.e., tubercle bacillus). Despite reported cases of of middle ear infection by *P. carinii* (32, 56, 97, 105, 122), there is no evidence for nasopharyngeal colonization by *P. carinii* in humans. Clinical conditions associated with *P. carinii* are listed in Table 1.

The cellular events surrounding *P. carinii* infection, although not clearly defined, suggest a major role for the major surface glycoprotein of *P. carinii*, gpA. gpA is a high-mannose glycoprotein that mediates binding of *P. carinii* trophic forms to alveolar epithelial cells (65, 88), with adherence further facilitated by host fibronectin. gpA, by virtue of its high mannose content, binds to alveolar macrophages through their cell surface mannose receptors. gpA also binds to SP-A (128), a major lectin-like apoprotein of surfactant (93) and augments SP-A's ability to inhibit surfactant phospholipid secretion by host type II alveolar epithelial cells in vitro (66). Treatment of experimental *P. carinii* infection with anti-gpA antibodies ameliorates or prevents infection (33).

The pathology of *P. carinii* pneumonia in humans bears similarities to that observed for the corticosteroid-mediated immunosuppressed experimental rat model system (44, 120). Attachment of *P. carinii* trophozoites to the type 1 pneumocyte is followed by diffuse alveolar injury and leakage of exudate through the basement membrane. Adherent clusters of *P. carinii* of various stages accumulate in the alveoli concomitant with a small mononuclear infiltration, a decrease in surfactant phospholipids, and edema, thickening, and fibrosis of the alveolar septa. There is impaired gas exchange and altered lung compliance. Hypoxemia, increased alveolar-arterial oxygen gradient, respiratory alkalosis, and reduced vital capacity and diffusing capacity (or "alveolar-capillary block") usually occur. A temporary worsening of hypoxemia is often observed following initial appropriate therapy. *P. carinii* can occasionally be found within a noncaseating granuloma in the lung. Pneumocystis infection may spread directly from the lung to the pleural space and adjacent lymph nodes, and hematogenous spread can occur to highly vascular organs. Extrapulmonary pneumocystosis has occurred in lymph nodes, spleen, liver, bone marrow, endocrine organs, gastrointestinal and genitourinary tracts, heart, eyes, and ears (78, 80, 90, 112).

TABLE 1 Clinical conditions associated with *P. carinii* pneumonia

Prematurity of infant
Malnutrition, protein and caloric (marasmus)
Corticosteroid therapy
Cytotoxic therapy
Advanced malignancy
Immunosuppressive therapy
Preparation for organ transplantation
Cushing's syndrome
Hodgkin's disease
Non-Hodgkin's lymphoma
Chronic lymphocytic leukemia
Solid tumors
Congenital immunodeficiency
HIV-I infection and/or AIDS
Old age

The high seroprevalence of antipneumocystis antibodies present at a young age in humans has led to the assumption that *P. carinii* infection in immunosuppressed adults and older children is caused by reactivation of presumably latent disease. The following evidence, however, suggests that newly acquired infection can occur and that reactivation of latent infection may not necessarily account for all cases of *P. carinii* pneumonia. First, epidemic-like clusters of *P. carinii* pneumonia have occurred in either immunodeficient or immunocompetent adults in different geographical regions (18, 30, 49, 102). (There is insufficient evidence, however, that person-to-person transmission occurs for humans [6, 69], and routine isolation of patients with *P. carinii* pneumonia is not currently recommended.) Second, highly sensitive detection methods (i.e., monoclonal antibodies or nucleic acid amplification techniques, such as PCR) have failed to detect latent infection in immunocompetent humans (72, 73, 84, 117). Third, immune reconstitution of immunodeficient mice with naturally acquired *P. carinii* not only rid them of infection, but residual *P. carinii* could not be detected in their lungs and their disease did not recur following CD4+ lymphocyte depletion and corticosteroid treatment (17). These findings were supported by similar observations of spontaneous *P. carinii* clearance within one year in the lungs of 75% of rats (i.e., no "residual" organisms detectable by histology or PCR) with corticosteroid-induced *P. carinii* pneumonia (115). Lastly, both fluorescent monoclonal antipneumocystis antibodies and PCR detection methods have failed to detect *P. carinii* in the lungs of AIDS patients without *P. carinii* pneumonia (73).

P. carinii pneumonia in marasmic children is observed primarily in countries with limited socioeconomic development where protein and calorie malnutrition occurs. The clinical onset of *P. carinii* pneumonia in the marasmic child can be subtle, often heralded by poor feeding and signs of upper respiratory infection. After 1 to 2 weeks, respiratory distress becomes apparent, and approximately 25% of such infants will die if untreated. Those who survive usually have a subsequent 4- to 6-week course of a febrile illness. A profuse lymphocytic plasma cell infiltrate is characteristic of and unique to pneumocystosis in the marasmic, malnourished child of less than 4 months of age (114).

P. carinii pneumonia in nonmarasmic infants, whether

resulting from primary congenital immunodeficiency, treatment of malignancy, organ transplantation, or human immunodeficiency virus type 1 (HIV-1) infection, also has an insidious onset. Clinical signs include fever, intercostal retractions accompanying respirations, respiratory distress and cyanosis, and crackling rales. *P. carinii* pneumonia in infants with perinatally acquired HIV-1 infection is seldom manifest before 3 to 6 months of age. In contrast to that in the HIV-1 infected adult, the CD4+ lymphocyte count at time of diagnosis of *P. carinii* pneumonia in the infant perinatally infected with HIV-1 is often more than 450/mm^3 (43).

P. carinii pneumonia in older children and adults typically presents with shortness of breath, fever, and a nonproductive cough. In HIV-1-infected individuals, these symptoms may last for weeks to months before the symptoms become severe enough for medical attention. Respiratory distress is usually apparent and manifested by tachypnea and tachycardia. A chest X-ray usually shows bilateral diffuse infiltrates extending from the hilar region but may appear normal or, rarely, show nodules or cavitation. There is often increased lung uptake of gallium^{67} (15, 44, 120, 121). The CD4+ lymphocyte count has proven to be a useful predictor of opportunistic pneumonia in the HIV-1-infected adult, with *P. carinii* pneumonia more likely to occur at CD4+ counts ≤200/mm^3.

DIAGNOSIS OF *P. CARINII* PNEUMONIA

Diagnosis of *P. carinii* pneumonia, at present, is dependent on the morphologic identification of the organism. The organism can be detected in a variety of respiratory specimens, i.e., sputum, induced sputum, tracheal aspirate fluid, bronchoalveolar lavage (BAL) fluid, tissue obtained by transbronchial biopsy (TBBx), cellular material obtained by bronchial brush, pleural fluid, and tissue obtained by open thorax lung biopsy. The microbiology laboratory is equipped to process these specimens to diagnose a variety of opportunistic infections.

The diagnostic yield of the various specimens is critically dependent on the underlying disease of the patient, the expertise of the staff evaluating the patient and obtaining the specimen, and the expertise of the laboratory staff for processing and examining the specimen. For AIDS patients, 80% of *P. carinii* pneumonia diagnoses can be made from induced sputum specimens (74). In contrast, for patients with an underlying immunosuppression other than AIDS, *P. carinii* is only rarely observed in induced sputum and diagnosis is dependent on examination of specimens obtained by bronchoscopy or biopsy (44, 46, 121, 126). The difference in diagnostic yield of induced sputum specimens has been attributed to a presumed higher burden of *P. carinii* in AIDS patients. For infants and young children who are unable to produce sputum, tracheal aspirate fluid, open thorax lung biopsy, or respiratory specimens obtained by a special pediatric bronchoscopy service must be used for diagnosis (9, 46).

At San Francisco General Hospital, AIDS patients selected to undergo further laboratory evaluation for *P. carinii* pneumonia must meet the following criteria: (i) belong to a group at risk for HIV transmission or other cause of immunodeficiency, (ii) exhibit respiratory symptoms, and (iii) have objective evidence of lung disease (at least one of the following: abnormal chest X-ray film, reduced diffusing capacity for carbon monoxide, and/or abnormal lung uptake of gallium^{67} citrate) (74). Restricting laboratory evaluation for *P. carinii* pneumonia to only those patients with a reasonable pretest probability of having the disease, as determined by respiratory medicine physicians, is cost-effective (124). Laboratory evaluation of induced sputa is not useful as a screening test for occult *P. carinii* pneumonia in asymptomatic HIV-1-infected patients (58).

SPECIMEN REQUIREMENTS AND PROCESSING

Induced Sputum

Sputum induction does not require expensive equipment or a physician's participation, and the patient experiences little discomfort and rarely experiences any complication. Sputum induction is best done in a centralized facility by pulmonary function laboratory technicians, respiratory therapists, or specially trained assistants. The induction facility should have adequate air changes, negative pressure ventilation, and respirators to protect personnel from other pathogens which may be concomitantly present (e.g., tuberculosis). Alternatively, sputum inductions can be done within a chamber with HEPA-filtered exhaust.

For induced sputum specimens, adequate preparation of the patient is of utmost importance. Vigorous brushing of the teeth, tongue, and gums with a toothbrush and normal saline for 5 to 10 minutes before sputum induction, followed by thorough rinsing, is critical to remove as much cellular debris of oral origin as possible. Toothpaste should not be used, as it can interfere with subsequent processing and staining of the specimen. Deep inhalation of nebulized 3% sodium chloride solution by the patient will result in osmotic accumulation of fluid in and irritation of the respiratory passages with subsequent coughing and expectoration of bronchoalveolar contents. The induced sputum specimen is usually mucoid and translucent in appearance; only rarely is it purulent. When pneumocystis clumps are present, they are 0.1 to 0.2 mm in diameter and cream to light tan in appearance. In early studies of induced sputum for diagnosis of pneumocystis pneumonia, the sputum was smeared directly (8, 86). This proved less sensitive than procedures using mucolysis and concentration of the specimen (57, 74).

In the laboratory, the induced sputum specimen is mucolyzed by the addition of an equal volume of freshly made 0.0065 M dithiothreitol (Stat-Pak Sputolysin, Caldon-Biotech, Carlsbad, Calif.; diluted to the manufacturer's specifications) or 0.5% *N*-acetyl-L-cysteine and incubation on a rotary shaker at 35°C with intermittent vigorous vortexing until the specimen is almost completely liquified (complete liquification will completely disperse the pneumocystis and make microscopic detection difficult). The mostly liquified specimen is concentrated by centrifugation at 1,300 × *g* for 5 min and the sediment is smeared on glass slides, which are then air dried and heat fixed (74). Prolonged heat fixation (i.e., 7 to 10 passes through the hottest portion of a Bunsen burner flame) is important in fixing the material to the slide, since most of the natural cellular adhesins are removed during mucolysis. Slides containing fixed material are then stained (see below) and examined microscopically for the presence of pneumocystis.

BAL

Bronchoscopy is performed by a pulmonary physician and requires special facilities in the event that emergency resuscitation of the patient is necessary; the facility must also provide adequate ventilation to protect personnel from other respiratory pathogens. The procedure uses a fiberoptic bronchoscope to examine the respiratory tract (9, 12, 81). A Ballard catheter has also been used to obtain BAL specimens with high diagnostic yield (13, 64).

To obtain lavage fluid, the bronchoscope is wedged into a segmental bronchus, and 100 to 150 ml of 0.75% saline is used to flush the alveoli in the lung segment attached to the bronchus; approximately 50 to 60 cm^2 of lavage fluid is usually recovered. Site-directed BAL may increase diagnostic yield in certain patients (14, 127). Fluid obtained by bronchoalveolar lavage is liquid, does not need mucolysis, and is easily concentrated by centrifugation (74). The centrifuged pellet is used to make smears on glass slides, which are fixed in absolute methanol or acetone while the specimen is still moist. After air drying and heat fixation, slides can be stained and microscopically examined for pneumocystis.

TBBx

The TBBx is obtained during bronchoscopy by using a cutting tool passed through the fiberoptic bronchoscope to punch through the bronchial wall to obtain adjacent lung tissue. The TBBx procedure can, on occasion, result in serious complications to the patient, including hemorrhage and pneumothorax.

If a TBBx is obtained, the biopsy should be collected on Telfa or sterile gauze, barely moistened with nonbacteriostatic saline and folded around the TBBx. It is important to keep the specimen moist but not wet; excess saline will dilute tissue adhesins such that touch imprints will wash away during staining. The specimen should be kept moist in a small sterile container with a tightly fitted lid. If handled sterilely, the specimen can first be used to make imprint or touch preparations on clean, alcohol-flamed and cooled slides, and the remainder can be ground or minced and subjected to various microbiological cultures. If the biopsy tissue is large enough, touch preparations can be made from additional sterilely cut surfaces. The touch preparations should be fixed in absolute methanol or acetone while still moist; slides should be air dried and heat fixed before being stained. Alternatively the biopsy can be ground in a tissue grinder and smears can be made on microscope slides, fixed, and stained (10).

Open Thorax Lung Biopsy

This procedure involves obtaining a lung biopsy after the chest has been surgically opened (11). The biopsy can be visually directed to a lung lobe or segment involved by the disease process. The biopsy specimen should be handled by the operating room staff as described above for TBBx. The specimen for microbiological examination must not be placed in saline or fixative, which would preclude examination of touch preparations or microbiological culture.

Other Specimens Derived from the Respiratory Tract

On occasion, pneumocystis can be detected in a variety of specimens obtained from the respiratory tract, including spontaneously produced sputum (which may be principally saliva, since the patient with pneumocystosis usually has a nonproductive cough), fluid obtained by tracheobronchial aspiration (perhaps the only means of sampling young children who cannot produce sputum or for intubated patients), fluid obtained by bronchial wash (obtained by washing the bronchial wall without wedging the bronchoscope in a bronchus), or specimens obtained by bronchial brushing (55). Spontaneously derived sputum and tracheobronchial aspiration fluid should be treated as described for induced sputum, whereas bronchial wash fluid and bronchial brushing can be handled as described for bronchoalveolar lavage fluid. None of the above-mentioned specimens have as high a diagnostic yield as induced sputum or specimens obtained by bronchoscopy (i.e., lavage and/or biopsy).

DIAGNOSTIC YIELD OF INDUCED SPUTUM AND BRONCHOSCOPY-DERIVED SPECIMENS

In studies performed at San Francisco General Hospital, *P. carinii* is detected in approximately 55% of all induced sputa obtained from individuals suspected of *P. carinii* pneumonia and meeting the aforementioned clinical criteria. The sensitivity of induced sputum (i.e., detection of *P. carinii* in induced specimens from patients ultimately diagnosed with *P. carinii* pneumonia) is approximately 75 to 80%, whereas the sensitivity of BAL is virtually 100% (8, 12). Although earlier studies suggested that TBBx might be the most sensitive diagnostic specimen, the experience at San Francisco General Hospital spanning 1990 to 1994 suggests that examination of BAL fluid has the same sensitivity as examination of TBBx touch preparations. All stains (e.g., Giemsa, rapid Giemsa-like, toluidine blue, Gomori methenamine silver, immunofluorescent, Gram-Weigert, calcofluor) have comparable sensitivities for the detection of *P. carinii* (21, 76, 79, 106). By definition, the specificity of either induced sputum or BAL fluid for *P. carinii* pneumonia is 100% (i.e., there are no false-positive results).

The 75 to 80% sensitivity of induced sputum for the diagnosis of *P. carinii* pneumonia indicates that this diagnostic test has a 20 to 25% false-negative rate. One study demonstrated that 50.5% of patients whose induced sputa lacked *P. carinii* had *P. carinii* detected in specimens obtained by follow-up bronchoscopy (41).

The following algorithm was devised for evaluation of patients suspected of *P. carinii* pneumonia and seen at San Francisco General Hospital (Fig. 1). Induced sputum is the primary specimen obtained for evaluation because of the ease of obtaining the specimen on an outpatient basis by nonphysician staff with little attendant patient morbidity. Bronchoscopy with BAL and/or transbronchial biopsy is reserved for those patients whose induced sputum specimens lack pneumocystis or who are unable to produce an induced sputum specimen (77).

OTHER DIAGNOSTIC MODALITIES

Although useful for epidemiological studies, serological assays to detect anti-pneumocystis antibodies have not been clinically useful to aid in the diagnosis of pneumocystis pneumonia (83, 85). Likewise, antigen capture assays for pneumocystis antigen have not proven clinically useful.

Nucleic acid amplification of pneumocystis-specific genes has generated a lot of interest as to their potential for diagnosis of *P. carinii* infection. Most studies have convincingly demonstrated that PCR-based methods are more sensitive than conventional microscopic examination of stained specimens for the detection of *P. carinii* (29, 62, 67, 82, 91, 111), but such PCR-based methods are currently more labor-intensive, expensive, and time-consuming than conventional staining and microscopic examination of specimens. Furthermore, although PCR-based diagnostic testing was more sensitive, it was less specific than conventional microscopy-based methods (i.e., *P. carinii* was detected when clinical disease was not apparent) (2, 29, 91). Since the

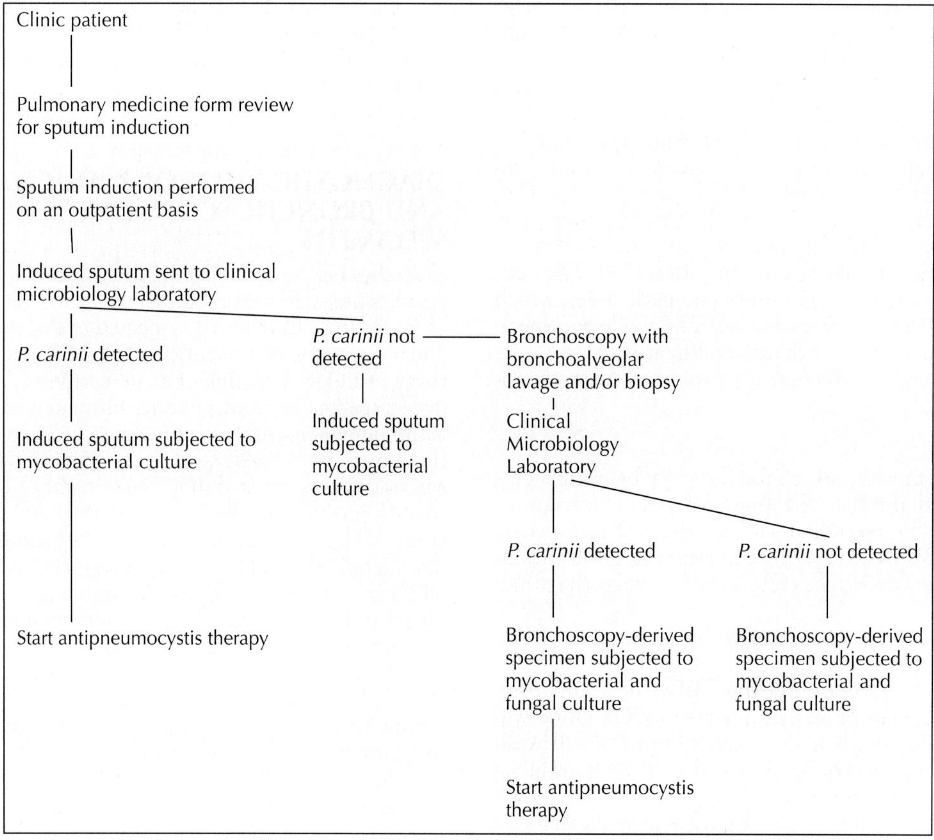

FIGURE 1 Algorithm for evaluation of patient suspected of having *P. carinii* pneumonia.

current microscopy-based method has been convincingly demonstrated to produce results concordant with clinical diagnosis and patient therapy and subsequent clinical course, the current higher cost and longer turnaround times for PCR-based results limit its clinical utility (48).

STAINING CHARACTERISTICS OF PNEUMOCYSTIS

A variety of stains have been used for the identification of pneumocystis. The pneumocystis cyst wall contains sugars commonly present in chitin and yeast glucan polymers (71); thus, stains commonly used to detect fungi (e.g., periodic acid-Schiff, Gomori's methenamine silver, toluidine blue, calcofluor) have been used for the identification of pneumocystis (7, 21, 35, 37, 70, 79, 106). In addition to cyst wall staining, two focal thickenings ("double commas") in the cyst wall apparently unique to pneumocystis also stain with these stains. The role of these focal thickenings is unknown.

Giemsa and rapid Giemsa-like stains do not stain the cell wall and instead stain the nuclei of the cellular stages purple and the cytoplasm light blue; the location of the cell wall is readily apparent by the clear negative stain (8, 10, 12, 16, 21, 74). Direct fluorescein-conjugated monoclonal anti-pneumocystis antibodies used for immunofluorescent staining stain the walls of the trophic forms and cysts (21, 34, 76, 79).

The staining characteristics, advantages, and disadvantages to the various stains used for the detection of pneumocystis are shown in Fig. 2 and discussed in Table 2.

Quantification of the burden of pneumocystis from any of the above-mentioned specimens is problematic because (i) disease may occur in discrete regions of the lung not readily accessible to sputum induction or lavage, (ii) individual patients will exert variable efforts to produce an induced sputum specimen, (iii) the quantity of fluid aspirated back after BAL will differ between patients, (iv) trophic forms and cysts in induced sputum specimens may be difficult to detect and enumerate depending on the degree of mucolysis and stain used, and (v) clumps of pneumocystis from different patients (either in BAL fluid or mucolyzed, induced sputum) can be widely variable in size. Attempts to quantify organism load in response to appropriate antipneumocystis therapy has thus been problematic (3).

The microbiology laboratory at San Francisco General Hospital receives approximately 400 induced sputum specimens and 120 BAL fluids annually for evaluation for the presence of pneumocystis or other pulmonary pathogens. The rapid Giemsa-like stain is used for diagnosis because of the low cost, ease, and rapidity of the stain and capacity to show the trophic forms and nucleated structures within cysts (precysts and intracystic bodies). This stain also permits judgement of specimen quality by demonstration of host alveolar macrophages. In addition, the distinctive Giemsa-stained morphologic appearance of *Cryptococcus neoformans*, *Histoplasma capsulatum*, *Strongyloides stercoralis* larvae, and *Toxoplasma gondii* permit rapid diagnosis of pulmonary infections caused by these pathogens which may not

TABLE 2 Comparison of stains used to detect *P. carinii*[a]

Stain (reference)	Time to perform stain	Cyst wall	T and IB	Advantages	Disadvantages
Giemsa (7)	30–60 min	Unstained. Cyst wall appears as a clear (unstained) ring around intracystic bodies.	Nuclei stain red-purple. Cytoplasm stains light blue.	Inexpensive. Stain simple to perform. Stains cells in all *P. carinii* stages. Stains most other pathogens (e.g., bacteria, parasites, fungi). Stains host cells.	Experienced reader required to distinguish *Pneumocystis* clumps from stained host cells in background.
Rapid Giemsa-like stains (e.g., Diff-Quik) (57, 74, 76, 79)	<5 min				
Fluorescein-conjugated monoclonal antibody (direct fluorescent-antibody stain) (34, 57, 76, 79)	30 min	Stains and fluoresces apple green. Cyst contents unstained (i.e., appear black). Fold in the cyst wall sometimes apparent.	Stained. Appears as a small polygon outlined in fluorescent apple green. Nuclei not stained.	Easy for an experienced reader to screen. Immuno-fluorescent staining is sensitive and specific.	Requires fluorescent microscope. Reagent is expensive.
Methenamine silver (Gomori/Grocott) (37, 70, 79, 99)	6–24 h (conventional), 1–2 h (rapid)	Stains brown to black. Cyst wall thickenings (double comma) and fold in the cyst wall stain dark brown to black.	Unstained.	Easy to screen for cysts.	Prolonged staining time (conventional). Moderate cost (time). Strong acid used. T and IB unstained. Host cells unstained.
Toluidine blue O (35, 79)	1–6 h	Stains violet to purple. Cyst wall thickenings (double comma) and fold in the cyst wall stain darker violet to purple.	Unstained.	Easy to screen for cysts.	Prolonged staining time (conventional). Moderate cost (time). Strong acid used. T and IB unstained. Host cells unstained.
Calcofluor white (7, 106)	<5 min	Stains blue-white or green depending on filter. Cyst wall and thickenings intensely fluorescent.	Unstained.	Cysts fluoresce brilliantly. Stain simple to perform. Inexpensive (time).	Requires fluorescent microscope. Strong alkali used. T and IB unstained. Also stains fungi; needs experienced reader to distinguish morphology of *Pneumocystis* cysts from other fungi.
Gram-Weigert	<5 min	Unstained.	IB stain purple. T faintly visible.	Commonly available in cytopathology labs.	Faint staining overcome by experienced observer.
Papanicolaou (99)	1–6 h	Unstained.	IB stain purple. T faintly visible.	Commonly available in cytopathology labs.	Faint staining overcome by experienced observer.

[a] T, trophic forms; IB, intracystic bodies.

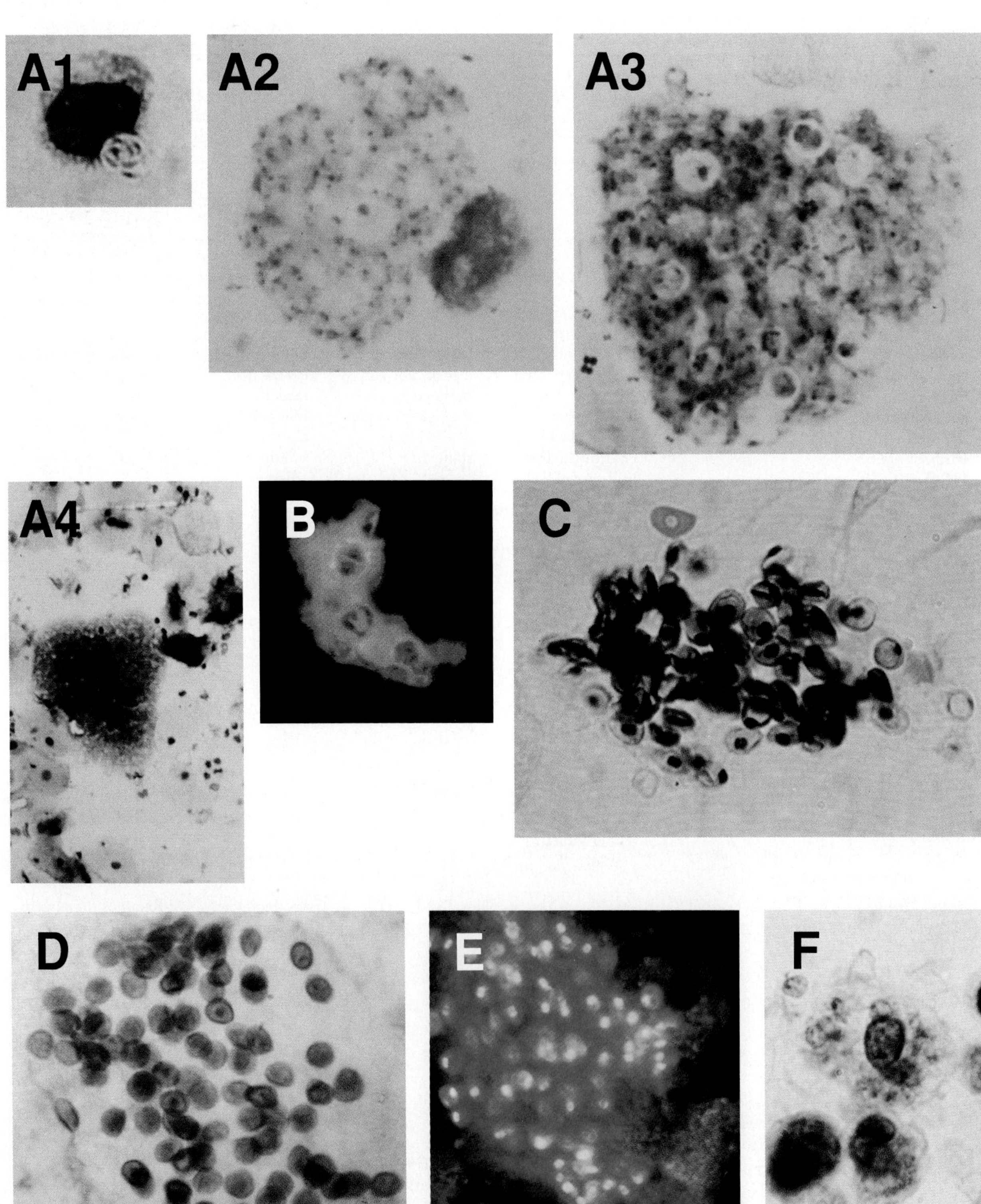
A1
A2
A3
A4
B
C
D
E
F

be detected with other stains (74, 77). Because background host cells will also stain, training and expertise in interpreting cellular elements in Giemsa-stained preparations is required. Laboratories with a lower volume of pneumocystis specimens may prefer to use immunofluorescent staining or one of the other stains described in Table 2.

ORGANIZATION OF THE CLINICAL MICROBIOLOGY LABORATORY FOR DIAGNOSIS OF *P. CARINII* PNEUMONIA

The clinical microbiology laboratory often receives specimens for the diagnosis of a variety of opportunistic infections by either direct stain or culture; this same specimen can also be used to diagnose *P. carinii* pneumonia. By use of rapid processing and staining techniques, a laboratory diagnosis of *P. carinii* pneumonia can usually be made within a few hours. Stat specimen processing is not necessary because pneumocystis trophozoites and cysts remain clearly identifiable in specimens collected at least three to four days after appropriate anti-pneumocystis therapy has been instituted (100). If *P. carinii* pneumonia is clinically suspected, treatment should be initiated without awaiting laboratory confirmation.

The algorithm adopted by each individual hospital for the diagnosis of PCP will depend upon the (i) age of the population seen, (ii) primary disease process which predisposes to *P. carinii* pneumonia, (iii) number of patients who may have *P. carinii* pneumonia, (iv) number of physicians and facilities to perform bronchoscopy, and (v) availability of inpatient or clinic facilities.

The algorithm presented earlier (Fig. 1) is in use at San Francisco General Hospital, where the majority of the patients who receive a diagnosis of *P. carinii* pneumonia have AIDS. In addition to pneumocystis, other pulmonary pathogens may be concomitantly present. For this reason, if an induced sputum sample contains pneumocystis, it will also be subjected to mycobacterial culture since a specimen obtained from the normally sterile lower respiratory tract of the patient under consideration will not be obtained. Fungal cultures are not performed on induced sputa because *Candida* spp. and environmental fungi are found, and disseminating fungal pathogens are usually not recovered (74). Recovery of bacterial pathogens from induced sputum specimens is virtually identical to that recovered from spontaneously produced sputum (74, 77). If an induced sputum specimen lacks pneumocystis, the patient undergoes bronchoscopy and BAL fluid is obtained. The fluid is examined for pneumocystis and also subjected to culture for fungi and mycobacteria (77).

THERAPY

Intravenous trimethoprim-sulfamethoxazole (TMP/SMX) is usually the first treatment selected for patients with acute *P. carinii* pneumonia, since oral TMP/SMX can be given after the patient has responded favorably. Only a few patients, however, are able to complete the TMP/SMX regimen because of the high frequency of side effects. Parenteral pentamidine isethionate has been used for primary therapy or as an alternate drug if TMP/SMX is too toxic. Pentamidine may also be quite toxic and not tolerated. Aerosolized and inhaled pentamidine have fewer side effects than TMP/SMX but are less effective. Other therapeutic agents or combinations [i.e., dapsone with trimethoprim, clindamycin with primaquine, atovaquone (BW566C80), and trimetrexate] have been used for mild to moderately severe acute *P. carinii* pneumonia, although they may be less effective (96, 118, 119).

Examination of respiratory specimens obtained during or after completion of therapy to determine therapeutic effectiveness and risk of relapse is not recommended. One study demonstrated that detection of *P. carinii* in BAL fluid obtained on day 21 of therapy was associated with an increased risk of relapse (19). Other studies, however, have demonstrated persistence of *P. carinii* in BAL fluid and lack of clinical correlation with relapse or death in the majority of patients who were successfully treated for *P. carinii* pneumonia (92, 100).

PROPHYLAXIS

As a consequence of more aggressive immunosuppressive therapy for malignancies, transplant recipients, and HIV-infected patients (<200 CD4+ cells/mm^3), there is a large population at risk for the development of primary (first episode) and secondary (recurrent) *P. carinii* pneumonia. With identification of these risk groups, randomized trials of various therapeutic agents for prophylaxis have been studied (38, 98, 118). TMP/SMX (160 to 180 mg daily) has proven more effective than aerosolized pentamidine (300 mg monthly) for prevention of *P. carinii* pneumonia in HIV-infected adults, even though pentamidine has fewer side effects and may be considered most useful for patients who cannot tolerate TMP/SMX (53, 54). Dapsone or dapsone/pyrimethamine are also effective. Extrapulmonary pneumocystosis has been documented for patients who had received prophylaxis with either aerosolized pentamidine or with systemic therapy (78).

The widespread use of prophylaxis against *P. carinii* infection especially in the HIV-1-infected population has decreased but not eradicated clinically apparent infections

FIGURE 2 *P. carinii* life stages observed in Giemsa and rapid Giemsa-like stained clinical specimens (magnification, × 1,000 unless stated). (A) Rapid Giemsa-like (Diff-Quik) stains of induced sputum. (A1) Single mature cyst (8 μm) containing eight fusiform, intracystic bodies with purple nuclei and light blue cytoplasm. Note clear unstained wall of cyst at its periphery. Cyst is attached to alveolar macrophage. (A2) Thin clump of mostly small trophic forms (2 to 3 μm) with small, purple nuclei and light blue cytoplasms. One precyst with large nucleus and clear (unstained) wall is visible. (A3) Thick clump with precysts and cysts with varying numbers of intracystic bodies and trophic forms overlying each other. (A4) Thick clump (×250) with overlying *P. carinii* cells of various stages. Note squamous epithelial cells and other host cells in mucolyzed concentrate. (B) Direct fluorescent-antibody stain of induced sputum. Note apple-green fluorescein stain on wall and wall fold of cyst. Structures inside cyst are unstained (black). Trophic forms which are confluent are stained on surface. (C) Gomori's methenamine silver stain (Grocott) of BAL fluid. Cyst walls and thickenings (double comma) are stained black. Trophic forms in clump are not stained. (D) Toluidine blue O stain of BAL fluid. Cyst walls and thickenings (double comma) are stained purple. Trophic forms in clump are not stained. (E) Calcofluor stain of BAL fluid. Cyst walls with thickenings (double comma) are highly fluorescent (color varies with barrier filter). Trophic forms may be lightly stained. (F) Papanicolaou's stain of pleural fluid. Pneumocystis trophic forms are phagocytized by macrophage. Nuclei are dark, and cytoplasm is green.

(40). This may result in a reduction of the need for diagnostic services. Recurrent infections, often restricted to the lung apices, are more common in individuals receiving aerosolized pentamidine prophylaxis. In contrast, recurrent infection is less commonly observed in individuals receiving TMP/SMX prophylaxis. Difficulty in identifying pneumocystis by microscopic examination of respiratory specimens from individuals receiving prophylaxis has been reported (11, 50), although altered morphology or staining characteristics of pneumocystis has not been observed by others (63, 75).

REFERENCES

1. **Anonymous.** 1994. Revised nomenclature for *Pneumocystis carinii*. *J. Eukaryot. Microbiol.* **41:**121S–122S.
2. **Armbruster, C., L. Pokieser, and A. Hassl.** 1995. Diagnosis of *Pneumocystis carinii* pneumonia by bronchoalveolar lavage in AIDS patients. Comparison of Diff-Quik, fungifluor stain, direct immunofluorescence test and polymerase chain reaction. *Acta Cytol.* **39(6):**1089–1093.
3. **Armstrong, M. Y. K., and M. T. Cushion.** 1994. In vitro cultivation, p. 3–24. *In* P. D. Walzer (ed.), Pneumocystis carinii *Pneumonia*. Marcel Dekker, Inc., New York.
4. **Bartlett, M. S., R. Eichholtz, and J. W. Smith.** 1985. Antimicrobial susceptibility of *Pneumocystis carinii* in culture. *Diagn. Microbiol. Infect. Dis.* **3:**381–387.
5. **Bartlett, M. S., J. A. Fishman, M. M. Dirkin, S. F. Queener, and J. W. Smith.** 1990. *Pneumocystis carinii*: improved models to study efficacy of drugs for treatment or prophylaxis of pneumocystis pneumonia in the rat. *Exp. Parasitol.* **70:**100–106.
6. **Bartlett, M. S., S. H. Vermund, R. Jacobs, P. J. Durant, M. M. Shaw, J. W. Smith, X. Tang, J. J. Lu, B. Li, S. Jin, and C. H. Lee.** 1997. Detection of *Pneumocystis carinii* DNA in air samples: likely environmental risk to susceptible persons. *J. Clin. Microbiol.* **35:**2511–2513.
7. **Baselski, V. S., M. K. Robison, L. W. Pifer, and D. R. Woods.** 1990. Rapid detection of *Pneumocystis carinii* in bronchoalveolar lavage samples by using Cellufluor staining. *J. Clin. Microbiol.* **28:**393–394.
8. **Bigby, T. D., D. Margolskee, J. L. Curtis, P. F. Michael, D. Sheppard, W. K. Hadley, and P. C. Hopewell.** 1986. The usefulness of induced sputum in the diagnosis of *Pneumocystis carinii* pneumonia in patients with the acquired immunodeficiency syndrome. *Am. Rev. Respir. Dis.* **133:** 515–518.
9. **Birriel, J. A., J. A. Adams, M. A. Saldana, K. Mavunda, S. Goldfinger, D. Vernon, B. Holzman, and R. M. McKay.** 1991. Role of flexible bronchoscopy and bronchoalveolar lavage in the diagnosis of pediatric acquired immunodeficiency syndrome-related pulmonary diseases. *Pediatrics* **87:**897–899.
10. **Blumenfeld, W., E. Wagar, and W. K. Hadley.** 1984. Use of transbronchial biopsy for diagnosis of opportunistic pulmonary infections in acquired immunodeficiency syndrome (AIDS). *Am. J. Clin. Pathol.* **81:**1–5.
11. **Bonfils-Roberts, E. A., A. Nickodem, and T. F. Nealon.** 1990. Retrospective analysis of the efficacy of open lung biopsy in acquired immunodeficiency syndrome. *Ann. Thorac. Surg.* **49:**115–117.
12. **Broaddus, C., M. D. Dake, M. S. Stulbarg, W. Blumenfeld, W. K. Hadley, A. J. A. Golden, and P. C. Hopewell.** 1985. Bronchoalveolar lavage and transbronchial biopsy for the diagnosis of pulmonary infections in the acquired immunodeficiency syndrome. *Ann. Intern. Med.* **102:** 747–752.
13. **Bustamante, E. A., and H. Levy.** 1994. Sputum induction compared with bronchoalveolar lavage by Ballard catheter to diagnose *Pneumocystis carinii* pneumonia. *Chest* **105(3):** 816–822.
14. **Cadranel, J., K. Gillet-Juvin, M. Antoine, F. Carnot, P. Reynaud, A. Parrot, M. F. Carette, C. Mayaud, and D. Israel-Biet.** 1995. Site-directed bronchoalveolar lavage and transbronchial biopsy in HIV-infected patients with pneumonia. *Am. J. Respir. Crit. Care Med.* **152(3):** 1103–1106.
15. **Centers for Disease Control.** 1986. Update: acquired immunodeficiency syndrome—United States. *Morbid. Mortal. Weekly Rep.* **35:**757–766.
16. **Chagas, C.** 1909. Nova tripanozomiaze humana. *Mem. Inst. Oswaldo Cruz* **1:**159–218.
17. **Chen, W., F. F. Gigliotti, and A. G. Harmsen.** 1993. Latency is not an inevitable outcome of infection with *Pneumocystis carinii*. *Infect. Immun.* **61:**5406–5409.
18. **Chusid, M. J., and K. A. Heyrman.** 1978. An outbreak of *Pneumocystis carinii* pneumonia at a pediatric hospital. *Pediatrics* **62:**1031–1035.
19. **Colangelo, G., R. P. Baughman, M. N. Dohn, and P. T. Frame.** 1991. Follow-up bronchoalveolar lavage in AIDS patients with *Pneumocystis carinii* pneumonia. *Am. Rev. Respir. Dis.* **143:**1067–1071.
20. **Comley, J. C. W., R. J. Mullin, L. A. Wolfe, M. H. Hanlon, and R. Ferone.** 1991. A microculture screening assay for the primary in vitro evaluation of drugs against *Pneumocystis carinii*. *Antimicrob. Agents Chemother.* **35:**1965–1974.
21. **Cregan, P., A. Yamamoto, A. Lum, T. VanDerHeide, M. MacDonald, and L. Pulliam.** 1990. Comparison of four methods for rapid detection of *Pneumocystis carinii* in respiratory specimens. *J. Clin. Microbiol.* **28:**2432–2436.
22. **Cushion, M. T., and D. Ebbets.** 1991. Growth and metabolism of *Pneumocystis carinii* in axenic culture. *J. Clin. Microbiol.* **28:**1385–1394.
23. **Cushion, M. T., J. Zhang, M. Kaselis, D. Giuntoli, S. L. Stringer, and J. R. Stringer.** 1993. Evidence for two genetic variants of *Pneumocystis carinii* coinfecting laboratory rats. *J. Clin. Microbiol.* **31:**1217–1223.
24. **Dyer, M., F. Volpe, C. J. Delves, N. Somia, S. Burns, and J. G. Scaife.** 1992. Cloning and sequence of a β-tubulin cDNA from *Pneumocystis carinii*: possible implications for drug therapy. *Mol. Microbiol.* **6:**991–1001.
25. **Edlind, T. D., M. S. Bartlett, G. A. Weinberg, G. N. Prah, and J. W. Smith.** 1992. The β-tubulin gene from rat and human isolates of *Pneumocystis carinii*. *Mol. Microbiol.* **6:**3365–3373.
26. **Edman, J. C., U. Edman, M. Cao, B. Lundgren, J. A. Kovacs, and D. V. Santi.** 1989. Isolation and expression of the *Pneumocystis carinii* dihydrofolate reductase gene. *Proc. Natl. Acad. Sci. USA* **86:**8625–8629.
27. **Edman, J. C., J. A. Kovacs, H. Masur, D. V. Santi, H. J. Elwood, and M. L. Sogin.** 1988. Ribosomal RNA sequences show *Pneumocystis carinii* to be a member of the fungi. *Nature (London)* **334:**519–522.
28. **Edman, J. C., and M. L. Sogin.** 1994. Molecular phylogeny of *Pneumocystis carinii*, p. 91–105. *In* P. D. Walzer (ed.), Pneumocystis carinii *Pneumonia*, 2nd ed. Marcel Dekker, Inc., New York.
29. **Elvin, K.** 1994. Laboratory diagnosis and occurrence of *Pneumocystis carinii*. *Scand. J. Infect. Dis. Suppl.* **94:**1–34.
30. **Fenelon, L. E., C. T. Keane, M. Bakir, and I. J. Temperley.** 1985. A cluster of *Pneumocystis carinii* infections in children. *Br. Med. J.* **291:**1683.
31. **Frenkel, J. K., J. T. Good, and J. A. Schultz.** 1966. Latent pneumocystis infection of rats, relapse and chemotherapy. *Lab. Invest.* **15:**1559–1577.
32. **Gherman, C. R., R. R. Ward, and M. L. Bassis.** 1988. *Pneumocystis carinii* otitis media and mastoiditis as the ini-

tial manifestation of the acquired immunodeficiency syndrome. *Am. J. Med.* **85:**250–252.

33. **Gigliotti, F., and W. T. Hughes.** 1988. Passive immunoprophylaxis with specific monoclonal antibody confers partial protection against *Pneumocystis carinii* pneumonitis in animal models. *J. Clin. Invest.* **81:**1666–1668.
34. **Gill, V. J., G. Evans, F. Stock, J. E. Parrillo, H. Masur, and J. A. Kovacs.** 1987. Detection of *Pneumocystis carinii* by fluorescent-antibody stain using a combination of three monoclonal antibodies. *J. Clin. Microbiol.* **25:**1837–1840.
35. **Gosey, L. L., R. M. Howard, F. G. Witebsky, F. P. Ognibene, T. C. Wu, V. J. Gill, and J. D. MacLowry.** 1985. Advantages of modified toluidine blue O stain and bronchoalveolar lavage for the diagnosis of *Pneumocystis carinii* pneumonia. *J. Clin. Microbiol.* **22:**803–807.
36. **Grimes, M. M., J. D. LaPook, M. H. Bar, H. S. Wasserman, and A. Dwork.** 1987. Disseminated *Pneumocystis carinii* infection in a patient with acquired immunodeficiency syndrome. *Hum. Pathol.* **18:**307–308.
37. **Grocott, R. G.** 1955. A stain for fungi in tissue sections and smears using Gomori's methenamine-silver nitrate technique. *Am. J. Clin. Pathol.* **25:**975–979.
38. **Hardy, W. D., J. Feinberg, D. M. Finkelstein, M. E. Power, W. He, C. Kaczka, P. T. Frame, M. Holmes, H. Waskin, R. J. Fass, W. G. Powderly, R. T. Steigbigel, A. Zuger, R. S. Holtzman, for the AIDS Clinical Trials Group.** 1992. A controlled trial of trimethoprim-sulfamethoxazole or aerosolized pentamidine for secondary prophylaxis of *Pneumocystis carinii* pneumonia in patients with acquired immunodeficiency syndrome. *N. Engl. J. Med.* **327:**1842–1848.
39. **Hong, S.-T., P. E. Steele, M. T. Cushion, P. D. Walzer, S. L. Stringer, and J. R. Stringer.** 1990. *Pneumocystis carinii* karyotypes. *J. Clin. Microbiol.* **28:**1785–1795.
40. **Hoover, D. R., A. J. Saah, H. Bacellar, J. Phair, R. Detels, R. Anderson, R. A. Kaslow, for the Multicenter AIDS Cohort Study.** 1993. Clinical manifestations of AIDS in the era of pneumocystis prophylaxis. *N. Engl. J. Med.* **329:**1922–1926.
41. **Huang, L., F. M. Hecht, J. D. Stansell, R. Montanti, W. K. Hadley, and P. C. Hopewell.** 1995. Suspected *Pneumocystis carinii* pneumonia with a negative induced sputum examination. Is early bronchoscopy useful? *Am. J. Respir. Crit. Care Med.* **151**(6)**:**1866–1871.
42. **Hughes, W. T.** 1982. Natural mode of acquisition for de novo infection with *Pneumocystis carinii*. *J. Infect. Dis.* **145:** 842–848.
43. **Hughes, W. T.** 1987. Pneumocystis carinii *Pneumonitis*, vol. 1, p. 57–69. CRC Press Inc, Boca Raton, Fla.
44. **Hughes, W. T.** 1987. Pneumocystis carinii *Pneumonitis*, vol. 2, p. 1–15. CRC Press Inc., Boca Raton, Fla.
45. **Hughes, W. T.** 1987. Pneumocystis carinii *Pneumonitis*, vol. 1, p. 97–104. CRC Press, Boca Raton, Fla.
46. **Hughes, W. T.** 1994. Clinical manifestations in children, p. 319–329. *In* P. D. Walzer (ed.), Pneumocystis carinii *Pneumonia*, 2nd ed. Marcel Dekker, Inc., New York.
47. **Hughes, W. T., D. L. Bartley, and B. S. Smith.** 1983. A natural source of infection due to *Pneumocystis carinii*. *J. Infect. Dis.* **147:**595.
48. **Ieven, M., and H. Goossens.** 1997. Relevance of nucleic acid amplification techniques for diagnosis of respiratory tract infections in the clinical laboratory. *Clin. Microbiol. Rev.* **10:**242–256.
49. **Jacobs, J. L., D. M. Libby, R. A. Winters, D. M. Gelmont, E. D. Fried, B. J. Hartman, and J. Laurence.** 1991. A cluster of *Pneumocystis carinii* pneumonia in adults without predisposing illnesses. *N. Engl. J. Med.* **324:**246–250.
50. **Jules-Elysee, K. M., D. E. Stover, M. B. Zaman, E. M. Bernard, and D. A. White.** 1990. Aerosolized pentamidine: effect on diagnosis and presentation of *Pneumocystis carinii* pneumonia. *Ann. Intern. Med.* **112**(10)**:**750–757.
51. **Kaneshiro, E. S.** 1998. The lipids of *Pneumocystis carinii*. *Clin. Microbiol. Rev.* **11:**27–41.
52. **Kaneshiro, E. S., Y.-P. Wu, and M. T. Cushion.** 1991. Assays for testing *Pneumocystis carinii* viability. *J. Protozool.* **38:**85S–87S.
53. **Kaplan, J. E., H. Masur, K. K. Holmes, M. M. McNeil, L. S. Schonberger, T. R. Navin, D. L. Hanson, P. A. Gross, H. W. Jaffe, and the USPHS/IDSA Prevention of Opportunistic Infections Working Group.** 1995. USPHS/IDSA guidelines for the prevention of opportunistic infections in persons infected with human immunodeficiency virus: introduction. *Clin. Infect. Dis.* **21**(Suppl.1)**:** S1–S11.
54. **Kaplan, J. E., H. Masur, K. K. Holmes, C. M. Wilfert, R. Sperling, S. A. Baker, C. B. Trapnell, K. A. Freedberg, D. Cotton, W. G. Powderly, H. W. Jaffe, and the USPHS/IDSA Prevention of Opportunistic Infections Working Group.** 1995. USPHS/IDSA guidelines for the prevention of opportunistic infections in persons infected with human immunodeficiency virus: an overview. *Clin. Infect. Dis.* **21**(Suppl. 1)**:**S12–S31.
55. **Karpel, J. P., D. Prezant, D. Appel, and G. Bezahler.** 1986. Endotracheal lavage for the diagnosis of *Pneumocystis carinii* pneumonia in intubated patients with acquired immune deficiency syndrome. *Crit. Care Med.* **14:**741.
56. **Kohan, D., S. G. Rothstein, and N. L. Cohen.** 1988. Otologic disease in patients with acquired immunodeficiency syndrome. *Ann. Otol. Rhinol. Laryngol.* **97:**636–640.
57. **Kovacs, J. A., V. L. Ng, H. Masur, G. Leoung, W. K. Hadley, G. Evans, H. C. Lane, F. P. Ognibene, J. Shelhamar, J. E. Parrillo, and V. J. Gill.** 1988. Diagnosis of *Pneumocystis carinii* pneumonia: improved detection in sputum with use of monoclonal antibodies. *N. Engl. J. Med.* **318:** 589–593.
58. **Kvale, P. A., N. I. Hansen, N. Markowitz, M. J. Rosen, M. C. Jordan, L. Meiselman, J. Glassroth, L. B. Reichman, J. M. Wallace, J. D. Stansell, P. C. Hopewell, and the Pulmonary Complications of HIV Infection Study Group.** 1994. Routine analysis of induced sputum is not an effective strategy for screening persons infected with human immunodeficiency virus for Mycobacterium tuberculosis or *Pneumocystis carinii*. Pulmonary Complications of HIV Infection Study Group. *Clin. Infect. Dis.* **19**(3)**:**410–416.
59. **Lapinsky, S. E., D. Glencross, N. G. Car, J. M. Kallenbach, and S. Zwi.** 1991. Quantification and assessment of viability of *Pneumocystis carinii* organisms by flow cytometry. *J. Clin. Microbiol.* **29:**911–915.
60. **Lee, C.-H., J. Helweg-Larsen, X. Tang, S. Jin, B. Li, M. S. Bartlett, J.-J. Lu, B. Lundgren, J. D. Lundgren, M. Olsson, S. B. Lucas, P. Roux, A. Cargnel, C. Atzori, O. Matos, and J. W. Smith.** 1998. Update on *Pneumocystis carinii* f. sp. hominis typing based on nucleotide sequence variations in internal transcribed spacer regions of rRNA genes. *J. Clin. Microbiol.* **36:**734–741.
61. **Lee, C.-H., J.-J. Lu, M. S. Bartlett, M. M. Durkin, T.-H. Liu, J. Wang, B. Jiang, and J. W. Smith.** 1993. Nucleotide sequence variation in *Pneumocystis carinii* strains that infect humans. *J. Clin. Microbiol.* **31:**754–757.
62. **Leibovitz, E., H. Pollack, T. Moore, J. Papellas, L. Gallo, K. Krasinski, and W. Borkowsky.** 1995. Comparison of PCR and standard cytological staining for detection of *Pneumocystis carinii* from respiratory specimens from patients with or at high risk for infection by human immunodeficiency virus. *J. Clin. Microbiol.* **33:**3004–3007.
63. **Levine, S. J., H. Masur, V. J. Gill, I. Feuerstein, A. F. Suffredini, D. Brown, H. C. Lane, R. Yarchoan, J. H.**

Shelhamer, and F. P. Ognibene. 1991. Effect of aerosolized pentamidine prophylaxis on the diagnosis of *Pneumocystis carinii* pneumonia by induced sputum examination in patients infected with the human immunodeficiency virus. *Am. Rev. Respir. Dis.* **144:**760–764.

64. **Levy, H.** 1994. Comparison of Ballard catheter bronchoalveolar lavage with bronchoscopic bronchoalveolar lavage. *Chest* **106(6):**1753–1756.
65. **Limper, A. H., S. T. Pottratz, and W. J. Martin II.** 1991. Modulation of *Pneumocystis carinii* adherence to cultured lung cells by a mannose-dependent mechanism. *J. Lab. Clin. Med.* **118:**492–499.
66. **Lipshik, G. Y., J. F. Tremi, S. D. Moore, and M. F. Beers.** 1998. *Pneumocystis carinii* glycoprotein A inhibits surfactant phospholipid secretion by rat alveolar type II cells. *J. Infect. Dis.* **177:**182–187.
67. **Lu, J. J., C. H. Chen, M. S. Bartlett, J. W. Smith, and C. H. Lee.** 1995. Comparison of six different PCR methods for detection of *Pneumocystis carinii*. *J. Clin. Microbiol.* **33:** 2785–2788.
68. **Lundgren, B., R. Cotton, J. D. Lundgren, J. C. Edman, and J. A. Kovacs.** 1990. Identification of *Pneumocystis carinii* chromosomes and mapping of five genes. *Infect. Immun.* **58:**1705–1710.
69. **Lundgren, B., K. Elvin, L. P. Rothman, I. Ljungstrom, C. Lidman, and J. D. Lundgren.** 1997. Transmission of Pneumocystis carinii from patients to hospital staff. *Thorax* **52:**422–424.
70. **Mahan, C. T., and G. E. Sale.** 1978. Rapid methenamine silver stain for pneumocystis and fungi. *Arch. Pathol. Lab. Med.* **102:**351–352.
71. **Matsumoto, Y., S. Matsuda, and T. Tegoshi.** 1989. Yeast glucan in the cyst wall of *Pneumocystis carinii*. *J. Protozool.* **36:**21S–22S.
72. **Matusiewicz, S. P., R. J. Fergusson, A. P. Greening, G. K. Crompton, and S. M. Burns.** 1994. *Pneumocystis carinii* in bronchoalveolar lavage fluid and bronchial washings. *Br. Med. J.* **308:**1206–1207.
73. **Millard, P. R., and A. R. Heryet.** 1988. Observations favoring *Pneumocystis carinii* pneumonia as a primary infection: a monoclonal antibody study on paraffin sections. *J. Pathol.* **154:**365–370.
74. **Ng, V. L., I. Gartner, L. A. Weymouth, C. D. Goodman, P. C. Hopewell, and W. K. Hadley.** 1989. The use of mucolysed induced sputum for the identification of pulmonary pathogens associated with human immunodeficiency virus infection. *Arch. Pathol. Lab. Med.* **113:**488–493.
75. **Ng, V. L., S. M. Geaghan, G. Leoung, S. Shiboski, J. Fahy, L. Schnapp, D. M. Yajko, P. C. Hopewell, and W. K. Hadley.** 1993. Lack of effect of prophylactic aerosolized pentamidine on the detection of *Pneumocystis carinii* in induced sputum or bronchoalveolar lavage specimens. *Arch. Pathol. Lab. Med.* **117(5):**493–496.
76. **Ng, V. L., N. A. Virani, R. E. Chaisson, D. M. Yajko, H. T. Sphar, K. Cabrian, N. Rollins, P. Charache, M. Krieger, W. K. Hadley, and P. C. Hopewell.** 1990. Rapid detection of *Pneumocystis carinii* using a direct fluorescent monoclonal antibody stain. *J. Clin. Microbiol.* **28:** 2228–2233.
77. **Ng, V. L., D. Yajko, and W. K. Hadley.** 1993. Update on laboratory tests for the diagnosis of pulmonary disease in HIV-1-infected individuals. *Semin. Respir. Inf.* **8(2):** 86–95.
78. **Ng, V. L., D. M. Yajko, and W. K. Hadley.** 1997. Extrapulmonary pneumocystosis. *Clin. Microbiol. Rev.* **10:** 401–418.
79. **Ng, V. L., D. M. Yajko, L. W. McPhaul, I. Gartner, B. Byford, C. D. Goodman, P. S. Nassos, C. A. Sanders, E. L. Howes, G. Leoung, P. C. Hopewell, and W. K. Hadley.** 1990. Evaluation of an indirect fluorescent-antibody stain for detection of *Pneumocystis carinii* in respiratory specimens. *J. Clin. Microbiol.* **28:**975–979.
80. **Northfelt, D. W., M. J. Clement, and S. Safrin.** 1990. Extrapulmonary pneumocystosis: clinical features in human immunodeficiency virus infection. *Medicine* **69:** 392–398.
81. **Ognibene, F. P., J. Shelhamer, V. Gill, A. M. Macher, D. Loew, M. M. Parker, E. Gelman, A. S. Fauci, J. E. Parrillo, and H. Masur.** 1984. The diagnosis of *Pneumocystis carinii* pneumonia in patients with the acquired immunodeficiency syndrome using segmental bronchoalveolar lavage. *Am. Rev. Respir. Dis.* **129:**929–932.
82. **Olsson, M., K. Elvin, C. Lidman, S. Lofdahl, and E. Linder.** 1996. A rapid and simple nested PCR assay for the detection of *Pneumocystis carinii* in sputum samples. *Scand. J. Infect. Dis.* **28(6):**597–600.
83. **Peglow, S. L., A. G. Smulian, M. J. Linke, C. L. Pogue, S. Nurre, J. Crisler, J. Phair, J. W. M. Gold, D. Armstrong, and P. D. Walzer.** 1990. Serologic responses to specific *Pneumocystis carinii* antigens in health and disease. *J. Infect. Dis.* **161:**296–306.
84. **Peters, S. E., A. E. Wakefield, K. Sinclair, P. R. Millard, and J. M. Hopkin.** 1992. A search for *Pneumocystis carinii* in post-mortem lungs by DNA amplification. *J. Pathol.* **166:**195–198.
85. **Pifer, L. L., W. T. Hughes, S. Stago, and D. Woods.** 1978. *Pneumocystis carinii* infection: evidence for high prevalence in normal and immunosuppressed children. *Pediatrics* **61:**35–41.
86. **Pitchenik, A. E., P. Ganjei, A. Torres, D. A. Evans, E. Rubin, and H. Baier.** 1986. Sputum examination for the diagnosis of *Pneumocystis carinii* pneumonia in the acquired immunodeficiency syndrome. *Am. Rev. Respir. Dis.* **133:** 226–229.
87. **Pixley, F. J., A. E. Wakefield, S. Baerji, and J. M. Hopkin.** 1991. Mitochondrial gene sequences show fungal homology for *Pneumocystis carinii*. *Mol. Microbiol.* **5:**1347–1351.
88. **Pottratz, S. T., J. Paulsrud, J. S. Smith, and W. J. Martin.** 1991. *Pneumocystis carinii* attachment to cultured lung cells by pneumocystis gp 120, a fibronectin binding protein. *J. Clin. Invest.* **88:**403–407.
89. **Ragan, M. A.** 1989. Biochemical pathways and the phylogeny of the eukaryotes. *In* B. Fernholm, K. Bremer, and H. Jornwall (ed.), *The Hierarchy of Life*. Elsevier Science Publishers, Amsterdam.
90. **Raviglione, M. C.** 1990. Extrapulmonary pneumocystosis: the first 50 cases. *Rev. Infect. Dis.* **12:**1127–1138.
91. **Ribes, J. A., A. H. Limper, M. J. Espy, and T. F. Smith.** 1997. PCR detection of *Pneumocystis carinii* in bronchoalveolar lavage specimens: analysis of sensitivity and specificity. *J. Clin. Microbiol.* **35:**830–835.
92. **Roger, P. M., F. Vandenbos, P. Pugliese, F. De Salvador, J. Durant, Y. Le Fichoux, and P. Dellamonica.** 1998. Persistence of *Pneumocystis carinii* after effective treatment of *P. carinii* pneumonia is not related to relapse or survival among patients infected with Human Immunodeficiency Virus. *Clin. Infect. Dis.* **26:**509–510.
93. **Rooney, S. A., S. L. Young, and C. R. Mendelson.** 1994. Molecular and cellular processing of lung surfactant. *FASEB J.* **8:**957–967.
94. **Ruffolo, J. J.** 1994. *Pneumocystis carinii* cell structure, p. 25–43. *In* P. D. Walzer (ed.), Pneumocystis carinii *Pneumonia*, 2nd ed. Marcel Dekker, Inc., New York.
95. **Ruffolo, J. J., M. T. Cushion, and P. D. Walzer.** 1989. Ultrastructural observations on life cycle stages of *Pneumocystis carinii*. *J. Protozool.* **36:**53S–54S.
96. **Safrin, S.** 1994. New developments in the management of *Pneumocystis carinii* disease, p. 95–112. *In* P. Volberding

and M. A. Jacobson (ed.), *AIDS Clinical Review 1993/1994*. Marcel Dekker, Inc., New York.

97. **Sandler, E. D., J. M. Sandler, a. P. E. LeBoit, and B. M. Wenig.** 1990. *Pneumocystis carinii* otitis media in AIDS: a case report and review of the literature regarding extrapulmonary pneumocystosis. *Otolaryngology* **103:**817–821.
98. **Schneider, M. M. E., A. I. M. Hoepelman, J. Karel, M. E. Schattenkerk, T. L. Nielson, Y. van der Graaf, J. P. H. J. Frissen, I. M. E. van der Ende, A. F. P. Kolsters, J. C. C. Borleffs, and and the Dutch AIDS Treatment Group.** 1992. A controlled trial of aerosolized pentamidine or trimethoprim-sulfamethoxazole as primary prophylaxis against *Pneumocystis carinii* pneumonia in patients with human immunodeficiency virus infection. *N. Engl. J. Med.* **327:**1836–1841.
99. **Schumann, G. B., and J. J. Swensen.** 1991. Comparison of Papanicolaou's stain with Gomori methenamine silver (GMS) stain for cytodiagnosis of *Pneumocystis carinii* in bronchoalveolar lavage (BAL) fluid. *Am. J. Clin. Pathol.* **95:**583–586.
100. **Shelhamer, J. H., F. P. Ognibene, A. M. Macher, C. Tuazon, R. Steiss, D. Longo, J. A. Kovacs, M. M. Parker, C. Natanson, H. C. Lane, A. S. Fauci, J. E. Parrillo, and H. Masur.** 1984. Persistence of *Pneumocystis carinii* in lung tissue of acquired immunodeficiency syndrome patients treated for pneumocystis pneumonia. *Am. Rev. Respir. Dis.* **130:**1161–1165.
101. **Sinclair, K., A. E. Wakefield, S. Benerji, and J. M. Hopkin.** 1991. *Pneumocystis carinii* organisms derived from rat and human hosts are genetically distinct. *Mol. Biochem. Parasitol.* **45:**183–184.
102. **Singer, C., D. Armstrong, P. P. Rosen, and D. Schottenfeld.** 1975. *Pneumocystis carinii* pneumonia: a cluster of eleven cases. *Ann. Intern. Med.* **82:**772–777.
103. **Sloand, E.** 1993. The challenge of *Pneumocystis carinii* culture. *J. Eukaryot. Microbiol.* **40:**188–195.
104. **Smith, J. W., M. S. Bartlett, and S. F. Queener.** 1994. Development of models and their use to discover new drugs for therapy and prophylaxis of *Pneumocystis carinii* pneumonia, p. 487–509. *In* P. D. Walzer (ed.), Pneumocystis carinii *Pneumonia*, 2nd ed. Marcel Dekker, Inc., New York.
105. **Smith, M. A., L. S. Hirschfield, G. Zahtz, and F. P. Siegal.** 1988. *Pneumocystis carinii* otitis media. *Am. J. Med.* **85:**745–746.
106. **Stratton, N., J. Hryniewicki, S. L. Aarnaes, G. Tan, L. M. de la Maza, and E. M. Peterson.** 1991. Comparison of monoclonal antibody and calcofluor white stains for the detection of *Pneumocystis carinii* from respiratory specimens. *J. Clin. Microbiol.* **29:**645–647.
107. **Stringer, J. R.** 1996. *Pneumocystis carinii*: what is it, exactly? *Clin. Microbiol. Rev.* **9:**489–498.
108. **Stringer, J. R., S. L. Stringer, J. Zhang, R. Baughman, A. G. Smulian, and M. L. Cushion.** 1993. Molecular genetic distinction of *Pneumocystis carinii* from rats and humans. *J. Eukaryot. Microbiol.* **40:**733–741.
109. **Stringer, S. L., K. Hudson, M. A. Blase, P. D. Walzer, M. T. Cushion, and J. R. Stringer.** 1989. Sequence from ribosomal RNA of *Pneumocystis carinii* compared to those of four fungi suggests an ascomycetous affinity. *J. Protozool.* **36:**14S–16S.
110. **Stringer, S. L., J. R. Stringer, M. A. Blase, P. D. Walzer, and M. T. Cushion.** 1989. *Pneumocystis carinii*: sequence from ribosomal RNA implies a close relationship with fungi. *Exp. Parasitol.* **68:**450–461.
111. **Tang, X., M. S. Bartlett, J. W. Smith, and C. H. Lee.** 1997. A single-tube nested PCR for *Pneumocystis carinii* f. sp. hominis. *J. Clin. Microbiol.* **35:**1597–1599.
112. **Telzak, E. E., R. J. Cote, J. W. M. Gold, S. W. Campbell, and D. Armstrong.** 1990. Extrapulmonary *Pneumocystis carinii* infections. *Rev. Infect. Dis.* **12:**380–386.
113. **ul-Haque, A., S. B. Plattner, R. T. Cook, and M. N. Hart.** 1987. *Pneumocystis carinii* taxonomy as viewed by electron microscopy. *Am. J. Clin. Pathol.* **87:**504–510.
114. **Vanek, J., and O. Jirovec.** 1952. Parasitic pneumonia: interstitial plasma cell pneumonia of premature infants caused by *Pneumocystis carinii*. *Zentralbl. Bakteriol.* **158:** 120–127.
115. **Vargas, S. L., W. T. Hughes, A. E. Wakefield, and H. S. Oz.** 1995. Limited persistence in and subsequent elimination of *Pneumocystis carinii* from the lungs after *P. carinii* pneumonia. *J. Infect. Dis.* **172:**506–510.
116. **Vavra, J., and K. Kucera.** 1970. *Pneumocystis carinii* Delanoe: its ultrastructure and ultrastructural affinities. *J. Protozool.* **17:**463–483.
117. **Wakefield, A. E.** 1996. DNA sequences identical to *Pneumocystis carinii* f. sp. carinii and *Pneumocystis carinii* f. sp. hominis in samples of air spora. *J. Clin. Microbiol.* **34:**1754–1759.
118. **Walker, R. S., and H. Masur.** 1994. Current regimens of therapy and prophylaxis, p. 439–466. *In* P. D. Walzer (ed.), Pneumocystis carinii *Pneumonia*, 2nd ed. Marcel Dekker, Inc., New York.
119. **Walzer, P. D.** 1994. Development of new anti-*Pneumocystis carinii* drugs, p. 511–543. *In* P. D. Walzer (ed.), Pneumocystis carinii *Pneumonia*, 2nd ed. Marcel Dekker, Inc., New York.
120. **Walzer, P. D.** 1994. Pathogenic mechanisms, p. 251–265. *In* P. D. Walzer (ed.), Pneumocystis carinii *Pneumonia*, 2nd ed. Marcel Dekker, Inc., New York.
121. **Walzer, P. D., D. P. Perl, D. J. Krogstead, P. G. Rawson, and M. G. Schultz.** 1974. *Pneumocystis carinii* pneumonia in the United States: epidemiologic, diagnostic and clinical features. *Ann. Intern. Med.* **80:**83–93.
122. **Wasserman, L., and P. Haghighi.** 1992. Otic and ophthalmic pneumocystosis in acquired immunodeficiency syndrome. *Arch. Pathol. Lab. Med.* **116:**500–503.
123. **Watanabe, J., H. Hori, K. Tanabe, and Y. Nakamura.** 1989. Phylogenetic association of *Pneumocystis carinii* with the "Rhizopoda/Myxomycota/Zygomycota group" indicated by comparison of 5S ribosomal RNA sequences. *Mol. Biochem. Parasitol.* **32:**163–167.
124. **Wehner, J. H., W. A. Jensen, C. M. Kirsch, F. T. Kagawa, and A. C. Campagna.** 1994. Controlled utilization of induced sputum analysis in the diagnosis of *Pneumocystis carinii* pneumonia. *Chest* **105**(6)**:**1770–1774.
125. **Yoshida, Y.** 1989. Ultrastructural studies of *Pneumocystis carinii*. *J. Protozool.* **36:**53–60.
126. **Young, L. S.** 1984. Clinical aspects of pneumocystosis in man: epidemiology, clinical manifestations, diagnostic approaches, and sequelae, p. 139–174. *In* P. D. Walzer (ed.), Pneumocystis carinii *Pneumonia*, 2nd ed. Marcel Dekker, Inc., New York.
127. **Yung, R. C., A. B. Weinacker, D. J. Steiger, T. R. Miller, E. J. Stern, C. J. Salmon, D. N. Chernoff, M. G. Luistro, S. Kuntz, and J. A. Golden.** 1993. Upper and middle lobe bronchoalveolar lavage to diagnose *Pneumocystis carinii* pneumonia. *Am. Rev. Respir. Dis.* **148:** 1563–1566.
128. **Zimmerman, P. E., D. R. Voelker, F. X. McCormack, and W. J. Martin.** 1992. The 120 kD surface glycoprotein of *Pneumocystis carinii* is a ligand for surfactant protein A. *J. Clin. Invest.* **86:**143–149.

Aspergillus, Fusarium, and Other Opportunistic Moniliaceous Fungi

LYNNE SIGLER AND MICHAEL J. KENNEDY

97

NATURAL HABITAT AND CLINICAL SIGNIFICANCE

The opportunistic moniliaceous (hyaline or brightly colored) moulds produce a varied spectrum of clinical conditions and constitute a phylogenetically diverse group of common to rare fungi that typically occur as saprobes in soil, in air, or on plant litter or as facultative plant pathogens. Some of them, especially members of the genus *Aspergillus*, may be recovered from specimens without having any clinical significance. Others are isolated infrequently enough to challenge the diagnostic proficiency of the laboratory, and critical assessment is required to evaluate the significance of their recovery. While several of the genera treated in this chapter include species having either brightly colored or dark (phaeoid) spores, the emphasis is on those fungi that grow in tissue in the form of hyaline or lightly colored, septate hyphal elements.

In addition to the rising incidence of infection caused by well-recognized species of the genus *Aspergillus*, there has been a concomitant increase in the numbers of infections caused by other species, historically thought of as laboratory contaminants or harmless saprobes. The spectrum of disease caused by hyaline moulds is diverse, is largely determined by the local and general immunologic and physiologic state of the host, and may be symptomatic or asymptomatic. In most instances, the portal of entry for fungal propagules is either through a break in the epidermis or by way of the lungs. Exceptions to this include introduction into the body by means of contaminated surgical instruments, intraocular lens, prosthetic devices, or other contaminated materials or solutions associated with surgery or routine health care.

Although these opportunistic moulds can grow in most body tissues and fluids, colonization or invasion is commonly associated with subcutaneous soft tissue and mucous membranes. Individuals whose resistance is lowered as a result of a severe debilitating disease or immunosuppressive therapy typically suffer from invasive pulmonary or paranasal sinus infection, but in some instances, the infecting fungus may spread to surrounding tissues or disseminate to virtually any organ. Fungemia is uncommon. Noninvasive forms of infection also have been noted in debilitated individuals as well as in individuals with apparently normal defense mechanisms. In such cases, the fungus colonizes a preexisting cavity in the lungs such as an ectatic bronchus, a tuberculous cavity, or a lung cyst. Other clinical syndromes usually occurring in immunocompetent individuals include chronic sinusitis, onychomycosis, subcutaneous abscess, mycotic keratitis or otomycosis, and allergic manifestations including bronchopulmonary mycosis and sinusitis in atopic patients.

DISEASE TERMINOLOGY

The use of the term aspergillosis to define infections caused by species of *Aspergillus* is well established, but the practice of coining disease names based on the genus of fungus involved is disadvantageous for infections caused by uncommon or rare fungal pathogens. The wide variety of fungi involved makes it difficult to place the organisms into accessible groups, and problems arise when fungus names are changed. To avoid unnecessary name changes for disease names based on the genus of the fungus involved, two major disease groups have been proposed: hyalohyphomycosis and phaeohyphomycosis (3). Although the groups encompass similar clinical spectra, they are distinguished by the presence in tissue of septate hyphal filaments without (hyalohyphomycosis) or with (phaeohyphomycosis) pigmentation or melanin in the cell wall; however, there has been some confusion over use of the terms. If melanin pigmentation in tissue is the primary criterion for inclusion under the broad umbrella of phaeohyphomycosis, several fungi which are dark colored in vitro should be excluded from this group, since they grow as hyaline elements in tissue. Species of the genus *Scedosporium*, for instance, form pigmented conidia in vitro and hyaline hyphae in tissue that are indistinguishable from those of *Aspergillus* species. Similarly, the black mould *Nattrassia mangiferae* (*Scytalidium dimidiatum*) usually forms hyaline or lightly pigmented hyphal elements in tissue. Although special stains (e.g., the Masson-Fontana silver stain) may help to detect melanin in fungal elements in tissue, the results are not always decisive. Some fungi with variable pigmentation, such as *Sporothrix schenckii*, may stain faintly or inconsistently (81). In practice, the terms are more often used to denote infections caused by either moniliaceous or dematiaceous fungi. For example, a subcommittee of the International Society for Human and Animal Mycology (ISHAM) redefined phaeohyphomycosis as infection caused by a dematiaceous fungus (113). Although the term hyalohyphomycosis was proposed initially to be complementary to phaeohyphomycosis and was not intended to replace well-established disease names such as aspergillosis, the ISHAM subcommittee recommended its use only for infections caused by "*unusual* hyaline pathogens." Instead, they suggested that fungal diseases be named by providing a specific description of the pathology and naming the causative agent, e.g., subcutaneous cyst caused by fungus X.

ETIOLOGIC AGENTS

The number of moniliaceous fungal species that have been reported to cause opportunistic infections in humans and animals is increasing, and it is beyond the scope of this chapter to describe them all. The reader is referred to several reference manuals (25, 32, 60, 80, 83, 162). A continuing and vexing problem is that verification of the authenticity of reports cannot be done if the fungus is inadequately described and illustrated and if case isolates are not sent for deposit in culture collections. This chapter describes in detail the medically important species of the genus *Aspergillus* (see Table 2) and provides salient colonial and microscopic characteristics of the more common species of *Fusarium* and other currently recognized moniliaceous opportunists (see Tables 3 through 5).

Collection, Transport, Storage, and Processing of Specimens

Clinical specimens from patients with suspected mycosis are to be collected with prudence and transported to the laboratory and processed as soon as possible by using the standard procedures described in chapters 4 and 5 of this Manual. Because of the diverse clinical manifestations, various sites may need to be examined for fungal elements. Biopsy material, transtracheal aspirates, and sputum samples collected in the early morning all may be useful specimens for the isolation and detection of hyaline moulds, as are infected nails. Swabs taken from mucous membranes and skin lesions are generally of little help in diagnosing infections caused by these fungi, and their use is not recommended unless duplicate specimens are taken. The reliability in determining whether an isolate is a possible pathogen is increased if the two specimens contain the same organism. Blood cultures are of little use in the isolation of *Aspergillus* species (173), but *Pseudallescheria boydii* or *Fusarium* species may be reliably detected (105, 134).

Media for isolation usually contain antibacterial agents such as chloramphenicol either alone or in combination with gentamicin, penicillin, or streptomycin. Opportunistic moulds are variably sensitive to cycloheximide, so media containing this selective agent should be used cautiously. For optimum recovery, the specimen should be inoculated onto several types of media and incubated at 28 to 30°C. Suspicious isolates should be tested for their ability to grow at 37°C.

Significance of Isolation

Although the majority of saprobic and plant pathogenic moulds are not considered pathogenic and appear unlikely to be able to adapt to or take advantage of risk factors that predispose the host to opportunistic infection, those capable of growing at or near body temperature must be considered to have latent pathogenic capability. The diversity of fungi capable of colonizing or invading human tissue has increased dramatically in recent years, as reflected by new reports of proven infection. Moreover, certain fungi are isolated often enough to be suspicious for pathogenic potential. Still, there is a need for definitive evidence of infection due to a normally saprobic mould. The laboratory procedure for confirming fungal etiology includes (i) detection in the specimen of hyphal elements which are compatible with the morphology of the isolated mould, (ii) isolation of several colonies of a fungus or isolation of the same fungus from a repeat specimen, (iii) accurate identification of the isolated mould, and (iv) confirmation of the mould's ability to grow at or near body temperature. Species of *Aspergillus*, *Fusarium*, or *Scedosporium* isolated from all deep tissues or body fluids must be considered colonizers or potential invasive pathogens. No fungal isolate should be discarded as a contaminant without thorough examination of the clinical specimen. Quality control measures to ensure that isolation media are not contaminated and the inspection of the slant or plate to evaluate where the fungus is growing relative to where the specimen was placed may also be important in evaluating whether an isolate is involved in disease. Close communication between mycologists and physicians also is essential, especially for rare or unusual opportunists.

Taxonomy and Identification

The opportunistic moniliaceous moulds are distributed throughout the kingdom Fungi and belong to genera of the Ascomycotina, Basidiomycotina, and Fungi Imperfecti (also called Deuteromycotina). The Fungi Imperfecti is a special division or "form" division comprising fungi for which no meiotic stage (teleomorph or sexual stage) is known as well as fungi which are mitotic stages (anamorphs, asexual stages) of ascomycetes and basidiomycetes. Today the phylogenetic relationships between many anamorphs and higher fungi are known by discovery of teleomorphs or are inferred by comparison of nucleic acids. While this knowledge is extremely important in understanding fungal biology, proposals to abandon use of the Fungi Imperfecti and anamorphic names have met with resistance in medical mycology, in which the majority of fungi recovered from specimens are anamorphs. Although teleomorphs occasionally are isolated in culture, they may be difficult to obtain by routine culture methods. The Fungi Imperfecti includes both yeasts (unicellular growth) and moulds (filamentous growth) and is divided into three form classes: (i) Blastomycetes, including unicellular organisms reproducing by budding or fission and sometimes producing hyphae (yeasts and yeast-like fungi; see chapter 95), (ii) Hyphomycetes, and (iii) Coelomycetes. Reproduction in mould fungi is characterized by the production of conidia, which are reproductive propagules produced following mitotic division of the nucleus. Conidia are formed when the nucleus migrates into the propagule from a specialized cell called a conidiogenous cell. The conidiogenous cell(s) may be borne on an erect simple or branched structure known as a conidiophore (Hyphomycetes) or within a specialized fruiting body called a conidioma (Coelomycetes).

Most of the pathogenic moulds are classified in the Hyphomycetes. Identification of hyphomycetes is based on morphology of the conidia and the mechanisms by which conidia are formed (conidiogenesis). Three basic tools are necessary for practical observation of these features. (i) An ocular micrometer is essential for determining sizes of conidia or sexual spores when present. Identification of moulds often requires comparison with published taxonomic descriptions in which size is often a key criterion for species distinction. (ii) A dissecting microscope with magnification up to ×60 and basal illumination is useful for the examination of colonies in plates or tubes for the presence of conidia in chains or slimy heads, specialized structures such as hülle cells, sclerotia, conidiomata, or sexual fruiting bodies forming under the aerial mycelium or embedded in the agar. (iii) Microscopic mounts which allow observation of how a fungus forms its conidia also are necessary. Slide culture preparations are excellent for many fungi (60), but conidial structures of some species of *Aspergillus* or *Penicillium* may not be typical in slide culture conditions, and tease or tape mounts are preferred (69, 125, 126).

Morphologic features of importance for the identification of conidial fungi include (i) conidium size and shape and pattern of septation, (ii) color of conidia and conidiophore, whether light (hyaline or moniliaceous) or dark (dematiaceous), (iii) developmental aspects of conidiogenesis, including nature of the conidiogenous cell, (iv) mechanism of conidium liberation or dehiscence, and (v) structure of the conidioma (if present). Differences in conidial shape and septation are useful characters for preliminary distinction and have traditionally been used for grouping conidial fungi (known as Saccardo spore groups) (115). Conidia may be single celled (amerosporae) or may have one (didymosporae) or more septa (phragmosporae). If a fungus produces both nonseptate and septate conidia, the conidia are often referred to as micro- and macroconidia. Conidia also vary in shape, being long and narrow (scolecosporae), as in *Fusarium* species, spirally coiled (helicosporae), or star shaped (staurosporae). Development of a conidium may occur by conversion of an existing cell or several cells (thallic-arthric) or may involve new wall building or blowing out of a portion of the wall (blastic). Conidiogenesis usually occurs at a particular location on a conidiogenous cell. If development occurs at a site that remains fixed and gives rise to more than one conidium, then the site is stable or determinate. If development occurs at new points on the conidiogenous cell (or axis), then the site is unstable or indeterminate. New sites may occur on an axis which lengthens (progressive) or shortens (retrogressive). The conidiogenous cell produces a single conidium or multiple conidia. Sympodial development involves the development of a single conidium at successive sites on a lengthening axis. Conidiogenous cells which are specialized to produce multiple conidia include the phialide and annellide. Conidia are produced successively (serially) and develop in slimy masses or in chains, with the youngest at the base of the chain (basipetal). Although it is sometimes difficult to differentiate between the two types of cells, the annellide elongates and sometimes narrows during the formation of each new conidium, leaving an often imperceptible series of rings or scars on the conidiogenous cell. Scrutiny of the cell with an oil immersion objective may be necessary to make this distinction. Conidia may also form in acropetal chains, with the youngest conidium at the tip of the chain. Distinction between acropetal and basipetal chains may be revealed by comparison of the size and wall morphologies of the top and bottom conidia of the chain. The youngest conidium is recognizable by its smaller size, lighter color if the conidia are pigmented, and differences in wall ornamentation if the conidia are roughened. Some conidiogenous cells form multiple conidia simultaneously over the surface of the swollen cell. When mature, conidia detach by fission of a double septum (schizolytic dehiscence) or by sacrifice of a supporting cell (rhexolytic dehiscence) either by fracture of a thin-walled region of the supporting cell or by lysis. Lytic dehiscence involves enzymatic disintegration of the supporting cell(s) and typically occurs in the dermatophytes and related fungi.

The presence of different spore states can make identification difficult. Subculture from the different states is necessary to confirm that the associated states belong to the same fungus and that the isolate is not contaminated. Different conidial states are called synanamorphs, and moulds having more than one independent stage are called pleomorphic and occasionally polymorphic fungi. Some moulds have associated yeast stages, while others form conidiomata in which the conidia are the same or different from conidia formed on simple conidiophores. Conidiomatal structures include sporodochia (conidiophores borne crowded on a compact mass of hyphae or a hyphal stroma) (e.g., *Fusarium* species), synnemata (conidiophores aggregated into a compound stalk) (e.g., *Graphium* state of *P. boydii*), and pycnidia (conidiogenous cells formed inside a round or oval fruiting body) (e.g., *Nattrassia mangiferae*). Expression of a synanamorph may be influenced by the agar medium used and may be lost upon repeated subculture.

ASPERGILLUS SPECIES

Aspergillosis now is considered the second most common fungal infection requiring hospitalization in the United States. In patients with positive fungus cultures, *Aspergillus* species are the second most common isolate after *Candida* species, but positive cultures alone may not indicate a pathogenic process (43). While some reports indicate that, when isolated, aspergilli are significant in only 10% of cases (164), others suggest that for patients with risk factors predisposing them to invasive fungal disease, multiple positive cultures are strongly suggestive of invasive aspergillosis (13). Infections may be primary or secondary, and the infections vary in severity and clinical course (7, 13, 98, 133). The clinical manifestations (Table 1) are largely determined by the local or general immunologic and physiologic state of the host, but various forms of the disease may integrate and overlap (13, 72, 98, 133). Risk factors for invasive aspergillosis include granulocytopenia in leukemic patients, neutropenia following bone marrow or organ transplantation, and high-dose corticosteroid or cytotoxic drug therapy (13, 72, 105, 133). Pulmonary aspergillosis is becoming a more common complication in patients with AIDS, but collectively, more cases have been reported in patients with other risk factors including drug-induced neutropenia, treatment with corticosteroids, and smoking of marijuana (10, 11, 28, 44, 96, 133).

Direct Examination

Assessment of the pathologic importance of any species of *Aspergillus* isolated from clinical specimens can be difficult, even with positive radiologic or computed tomographic findings, because aspergilli are routinely isolated from respiratory, cutaneous, or other specimens. It is imperative to determine clinical significance by (i) demonstrating hyphae in fresh clinical material and (ii) isolating heavy growth from a single specimen or the same species from multiple specimens.

Hyphal elements and the details of hyphal morphology of aspergilli may be observed readily in routine KOH preparations without or with a fluorescent compound such as calcofluor white (105) or in tissue section with fungal stains. *Aspergillus* hyphae will stain also with hematoxylin and

TABLE 1 Classification of *Aspergillus* infection[a,b]

I. Disease in the healthy host
  A. Toxicosis or mycotoxicosis
    1. Ingestion of mycotoxins
    2. Ingestion of other metabolites
  B. Allergic manifestations
    1. Allergic asthma
    2. Allergic rhinitis
    3. Allergic sinusitis
    4. Extrinsic allergic alveolitis
    5. Hypersensitivity pneumonitis
    6. Allergic bronchopulmonary aspergillosis
  C. Superficial or noninvasive infections
    1. Cutaneous infection
    2. Otomycosis
    3. Sinusitis
    4. Saprophytic bronchopulmonary aspergillosis
    5. Tracheobronchitis
  D. Invasive infection
    1. Single organ
    2. Multiple organs (disseminated)
II. Infection associated with tissue damage or foreign body
  A. Keratitis and endophthalmitis
  B. Burn wound infection
  C. Osteomyelitis
  D. Prosthetic valve endocarditis
  E. Vascular graft infection
  F. Aspergilloma (fungus ball)
  G. Empyema and pleural aspergillosis
  H. Peritonitis
III. Infection in the compromised host
  A. Primary cutaneous aspergillosis
  B. Sino-orbital infection
  C. Pulmonary aspergillosis
    1. Invasive tracheobronchitis
    2. Chronic necrotizing pulmonary aspergillosis
    3. Acute invasive pulmonary aspergillosis
  D. Central nervous system aspergillosis
  E. Invasive (disseminated) aspergillosis
  F. Gastrointestinal infarction (rare)

[a] Modified from Bodey and Vartivarian (13).
[b] Patients infected with other fungi discussed in this chapter may present with similar clinical syndromes, and the structures of these fungi in tissue may resemble those of *Aspergillus* species.

eosin if the tissue is properly fixed, is not understained with hematoxylin, and is not necrotic. Viable hyphae are often basophilic to amphophilic, whereas hyphae in macerated or necrotic tissue tend to be eosinophilic (19). The appearance of *Aspergillus* hyphae may vary with the type of infection. In acute invasive aspergillosis (see Fig. 2), aspergilli typically are seen as hyaline, septate hyphae that are 3 to 6 μm in diameter, branch dichotomously at acute (45°) angles, and have smooth parallel walls with no or slight constrictions at the septa (19). In invasive aspergillosis, hyphae proliferate extensively throughout the tissue, often in parallel or radial arrays. Aspergilli colonizing pulmonary cavitary lesions grow as tangled masses of hyphae and in chronic infection may exhibit atypical hyphal features such as swellings measuring up to 12 μm in diameter and/or absence of conspicuous septa. When hyphal elements typical of aspergilli are present in histologic sections, a presumptive diagnosis can be made, but culture is required for confirmation. Hyphae of other moulds, such as *Fusarium* species or *P. boydii*, may resemble those of aspergilli both in their propensity to grow in the lumens of blood vessels and in their formation of dichotomously branched hyphae. Fluorescent-antibody techniques also demonstrate problems in differentiating among the same fungi, and efforts are ongoing to make the tests more specific and widely available (63). The presence of typical conidial heads or ascomata in lung cavities or in the ear canal aids in the diagnosis and may allow a presumptive identification of the fungus. Especially if *Aspergillus niger* is the cause of infection, calcium oxalate crystals also may be found in respiratory specimens (13, 145). Free conidia may resemble structures such as yeast cells or cysts of *Pneumocystis carinii*, when stained with Gomori's methenamine silver stain, which masks the conidium color, but conidia of the aspergilli are often roughened. Distorted and broader hyphae may be mistaken for those of zygomycetes, but the hyphae of the latter are generally broader (up to 15 μm), have nonparallel walls which often appear collapsed and acutely twisted, and are infrequently septate (19).

Immunodiagnosis and Metabolite Detection

Immunologic tests have long been used as important aids in the diagnosis of various clinical forms of aspergillosis (98, 133, 141). This is especially true for diagnosis of patients with aspergilloma, in which a high percentage demonstrate immunoglobulin G (IgG) precipitating antibodies (80, 133), and for patients with allergic bronchopulmonary aspergillosis, for which diagnostic criteria include positive skin test reactions to *Aspergillus* antigens and elevated levels of IgE and specific IgE and IgG precipitating antibodies to *Aspergillus* species in serum (65, 71, 72, 80). The detection of circulating antibodies or *Aspergillus* antigens has also helped to define the etiology of infection in patients yielding negative cultures, in patients in whom certain forms of aspergillosis are masked by or mistaken for other diseases, and in patients in whom two or more fungi were found to coexist (47, 68, 78, 175). While such tests are extremely important, especially for the rapid diagnosis of invasive aspergillosis when early treatment is required to resolve a potentially fatal form of the disease (112, 133), our ability to detect these infections early is still quite limited (106).

Detection of Antibody

The detection of antibody in serum or other body fluids and reactivity in skin tests is, to some degree, dependent upon the purity, chemical nature, and uniqueness of the antigen preparation used (78). Extracts from the whole mycelium, metabolic products secreted into the medium during the growth of *Aspergillus* spp., purified antigens, and more recently, recombinantly expressed and purified antigens have all been used in serologic tests and immunoassays. Although such antigen preparations are available commercially, standardized antigens are still not widely available. As reviewed by Kurup and Kumar (78), two of the major reasons for the lack of standardized antigens are that (i) antigen preparations are highly variable and (ii) antigens show various degrees of cross-reactivity. Work is ongoing to address these issues and to find ways to express, purify, and prepare improved antigen preparations (e.g., see references 50, 56, 98, 104, 191, and 192).

Several serologic tests with disparate sensitivities have been developed to detect circulating antibodies. As noted above, these have proven valuable in aiding diagnosis, especially of allergic aspergillosis and aspergilloma, but they are less useful in the diagnosis of invasive disease in patients with little or no humoral response. Immunodiffusion remains the most widely used technique, primarily because it is simple and easy to perform (78), but it lacks sensitivity and gives no quantitative information on antibody concentrations. A micromodification of Wadsworth's agar gel diffusion against a pool of antigens was found to correlate well with other methods (78). Other tests which have achieved some success for the diagnosis of aspergillosis include enzyme-linked immunosorbent assay (ELISA), biotin-avidin-linked immunosorbent assay (BALISA), radioimmunoassay (RIA), and indirect immunofluorescence (141). Of these, various ELISAs are the most amenable to the clinical laboratory. While in some cases these assays can be highly sensitive, reliable, and versatile, their routine use in many clinical laboratories has been limited by interlaboratory discrepancies in results and by immunological responses leading to false-positive results for some patient groups (10, 78). The reasons for this vary but are primarily due to the ubiquitous nature of aspergilli (leading to high background antibody titers), the lack of ability of immunocompromised patients to mount diagnostic humoral immune responses, cross-reactivities between different fungi and even bacteria, and the selection of *Aspergillus* antigens used (70, 78, 106). One study aimed at improving standardization of serodiagnosis evaluated various commercial and homemade antigen preparations in a multihospital setting (121). The data showed that most discrepancies in results were most likely related to differences in the nature of the antigen preparations and that the Paragon System, a new immunoelectrophoresis system, was a reliable technique requiring only small amounts of serum and having a turnaround time (24 to 48 h) shorter than those of competitive methods. Other factors of note are that some antigens have limited binding specificity and bind only to certain immunoglobulin classes or isotypes within those classes (79) and that the ELISA may not be sensitive enough to detect relatively low levels of antigen-specific IgE or subclasses of IgG (71, 77, 78).

Detection of Antigen

Demonstrable antibodies against aspergilli may be absent from patients with immunosuppression (38, 195), and detection of antibody may be limited by antifungal therapy or by the acute and fulminant course of some *Aspergillus* infections (16, 38, 188, 195). Kurup and Kumar (78) reviewed several studies which found various degrees of success in detecting specific antibodies to aspergilli in the sera of patients with invasive disease. In patients with invasive infection, antigen detection may be helpful in establishing an early, accurate diagnosis (7, 61, 112). As well, monitoring of the levels of circulating antigens may be useful for the management of such patients, especially those with immunosuppression or underlying hematologic malignancies (118, 165). However, at least one report comparing multiple antibody and antigen detection methods suggests that while currently available antibody assays for the serodiagnosis of invasive disease are inadequate, antigen detection tests appear to be highly specific but lack sufficient sensitivity to be of practical use in the clinical laboratory (89).

A variety of tests for the detection of soluble antigens of *Aspergillus* spp. in the serum, urine, or other body fluids and even within host phagocytic cells have been developed (111, 118, 124, 195). Of these, RIA, ELISA and BALISA, latex agglutination, and immunoblotting have been the most commonly used methods (51, 57, 70, 76, 170, 196). These methods may provide sensitivity sufficient to allow early diagnosis in some cases (78, 112, 180), but few are commercially available (178). A latex agglutination test, Pastorex Aspergillus (Sanofi Diagnostics Pasteur, Marnes-La-Coquette, France), has been evaluated in several hospital and clinical laboratories (10, 31, 53, 110, 132, 183) with a variety of specimens, including serum, urine, sputum, and pulmonary fluids. Results show that the test lacks sensitivity and specificity compared with results of ELISA and that a low level of false-positive results (~6%) occurs in patients with no evidence of invasive disease. While this kit appears to be too insensitive for use in the diagnosis of invasive aspergillosis in the early stages, it may contribute to diagnosis and management when cultures remain negative and serial samples are obtained (183). Modifications of these techniques are being evaluated in efforts to improve assay sensitivity. The development of immunologic tests using monoclonal antibodies and previously undescribed antigens for the detection of *Aspergillus* antigenemia hold promise for rapid antigen detection for early diagnosis and greater sensitivity (52). Methods for the detection of antigenemia have recently been summarized by Kurup and Kumar (78). Regardless of the test used, success in detecting antigenemia is directly related to the frequency of monitoring of samples (50, 186, 191). As with the detection of antibody, false-negative results in antigen assays may be ascribed, in part, to antifungal therapy, the course of infection, and the timing of sample collection (180).

Skin Tests

Skin test reactivity to *Aspergillus* antigen extracts is used for patients with suspected allergic bronchopulmonary aspergillosis (ABPA), atopic dermatitis, or allergic asthma sensitized to aspergilli (31, 104). Two types of reaction are observed: type I (immediate) and type II (Arthrus). Type I reactions are cutaneous weal-and-flare reactions that occur within 15 to 20 min of skin test challenge, while type II reactions develop ~4 to 10 h after skin testing and last longer. A delayed-type skin reaction also may be present in some patients, particularly those with hypersensitivity pneumonitis (78). Skin prick and/or intradermal tests, which have received much recent attention for the diagnosis of allergic conditions (e.g., see reference 22), make use of various fungal allergens (22, 78). Using the Pharmacia CAP system (a new solid-phase immunoassay), Crameri and coworkers (22, 104) showed that recombinant allergens that can be produced as highly pure proteins performed better than commercial *A. fumigatus* extracts and may contribute significantly to the improvement in (and automation of) the diagnosis of ABPA.

Detection of Fungal Metabolites

Another way of diagnosing aspergillosis in the absence of culture is to demonstrate a distinctive metabolic product in the fluids or tissues of infected patients. Several species of *Aspergillus* produce large amounts of the 6-carbon polyol mannitol in culture, and infected animals with invasive disease have been shown to have high body fluid and/or tissue mannitol levels (106). Routine use of this diagnostic approach has been hampered by the need for complex analytical methods such as multidimensional gas chromatography (GC) and combined GC-mass spectrometry (106).

Molecular Techniques

Because the infection is associated with a high rate of mortality in immunocompromised patients, rapid diagnosis of invasive aspergillosis continues to be a serious problem for the clinician. This has led to a continued search for improved direct and indirect tests which are specific and reproducible in routine laboratory practice and which allow a rapid and reliable diagnosis. The serious nature of the disease frequently leads to the early initiation of therapy, but this action may impede obtaining an accurate diagnosis for patients in whom suspected aspergillosis has not been unequivocally confirmed by both culture and histopathology. The sensitivity and specificity of molecular techniques make them attractive as alternative methods for the early diagnosis of invasive aspergillosis, but they are still experimental. The techniques appear to be highly sensitive and specific (35, 114, 159, 193), even when blood cultures, serologic assays, and other examinations detect no pathogens (59, 181), and results can be obtained on the same day (159). PCR-based assays appear to be amenable to the clinical laboratory. Oligonucleotide primers that specifically amplify DNA from *Aspergillus* species have been developed, and several studies have demonstrated both the utility and validity of PCR for the laboratory diagnosis of invasive disease (35, 59, 100, 114, 159, 182). These and other data show that some primers are highly sensitive and specific, detecting as little as 1 pg of genomic DNA. Similar studies aimed at detecting aspergillosis by PCR have also shown a high degree of correlation (93 to 99%) between culture and PCR results (35, 114, 159, 193).

Molecular Typing, Taxonomic Classification, and Epidemiology

Historically, genetic fingerprinting and epidemiologic studies have been hampered by the lack of simple, reproducible typing methods. Better knowledge of the genetics of aspergilli and the advent of more user friendly methods for the preparation and manipulation of DNA (12) now allow detailed analyses. Studies show that probes that are species and isolate specific can be developed and that molecular techniques are useful in detection-identification systems and for epidemiologic studies. Genetic fingerprinting of aspergilli by restriction fragment length polymorphism (RFLP) analysis of genomic DNA has been shown to provide a measure of strain relatedness and of the nosocomial origin of aspergillosis cases (16, 24, 27, 29, 41, 84, 86, 101). Similar results have been obtained with randomly amplified polymorphic DNA (RAPD) typing patterns (8, 15, 100) and Southern blots probed with the rRNA gene (160) or nonribosomal genomic sequences (50). PCR has also been adapted for the fingerprinting of aspergilli by using single primers, alone or in combination, with arbitrary (88) or repetitive (42, 177) DNA sequences. Loudon et al. (88) used PCR to amplify polymorphic DNA patterns from 19 *A. fumigatus* isolates from six patients with aspergilloma and showed that some but not all primers gave good discrimination between isolates. In that study, typeability and reproducibility compared favorably with results obtained by immunoblot fingerprinting and *Xba*I-generated RFLP analysis of the same isolates, but RAPD typing was found to be less labor-intensive. Furthermore, their results suggested that aspergillomas sometimes contain isolates of more than one type. van Belkum and coworkers (177) found that PCR amplification of repetitive DNA motifs allowed discrimination of *Aspergillus* species, and by using a primer deduced from a prokaryotic repeat motif, they could type *A. fumigatus* isolates originating from different patients or from different anatomical sites.

Aspergillus Taxonomy and Identification

The genus *Aspergillus* comprises anamorphic (mitotic) species with known or presumed connections to the family Trichocomaceae of the Ascomycotina. Because early monographic treatments (131) included teleomorphic (meiotic) features within descriptions of *Aspergillus* species, a practice inconsistent with the International Code of Botanical Nomenclature, problems have arisen in the nomenclature of some well-known species. Experts in the field have attempted to rectify outstanding problems and have compiled a list of names in current use in the family Trichocomaceae. The list includes 185 species of *Aspergillus* and 65 associated teleomorphs (45). About 20 taxa have been reliably reported from human or animal infection (80), and of these, *A. fumigatus*, *A. flavus*, and *A. niger* are the most common pathogenic species worldwide (80, 133, 136). When isolated on media such as Sabouraud dextrose agar (SDA), aspergilli tend to reproduce in the asexual form. Subculture to standard Czapek-Dox, Czapek-Dox with added glucose (20 to 30%), and 2% malt extract agar (131) or on modifications of these media (69) allows comparison of colonial and microscopic features with those given in monographs and taxonomic keys and stimulates development of a teleomorph (32, 69, 115, 131). Some species are osmophilic and grow poorly on media with low concentrations of sugar.

Because the large number of species within the genus makes identification to the species level difficult even for the experienced microbiologist, the aspergilli were placed into distinct, accessible groups (131). More recent treatments of *Aspergillus* have formally defined the groups as sections within subgenera (32, 69). A key to the representative species within each group is provided in Fig. 1, and the diagnostic features of several aspergilli are described in Table 2. Although aspergilli are usually identified on the basis of conidial characteristics, the presence of sexual structures (cleistothecia and ascospores; Fig. 4) allows ready identification of species that have teleomorphs in the genera *Eurotium*, *Emericella*, and *Neosartorya*. Teleomorphic species are described under these names in Table 2.

Both macroscopic and microscopic characters are required for the identification of *Aspergillus* species. Colony growth rates, obverse and reverse colors, texture, topography, and the presence of exudate droplets or diffusible pigments should be recorded after 7 days on identification media (32, 69, 115). Isolates not immediately identifiable should be retained longer for the possible development of ascomata or other structures that may be helpful in the identification of an isolate. Differences in size, color, and wall ornamentation of various structures, the shape and size of vesicles, and the arrangement of metulae and phialides are important microscopic features. An upright stipe or conidiophore arises either directly from the vegetative hyphae or from a specialized hyphal cell called a foot cell, is usually nonseptate, and varies in color, length, and wall ornamentation in different species. The stipe terminates in a swollen cell, called a vesicle (Fig. 1, 4, 18, and 19), which is globose, subglobose, hemispherical, pyriform (pear shaped), or clavate. Either the entire vesicle or a portion of it is covered with phialides, which form the conidia. Phialides arise simultaneously directly from the vesicle (uniseriate; Fig. 1 and 18), from the intermediate series of cells called metulae (biseriate; Fig. 1 and 19), or by a combination of both processes, as occurs in *A. flavus* (Fig. 1). Examination of a colony under a dissecting microscope allows observation of conidial chains to determine whether they are borne in a single column (columnar) or whether the columns are split, with some arising at right angles to the stipe (radiate). The conidia are typically ellipsoidal or globose and vary in size, color, and wall markings depending upon the species. Scle-

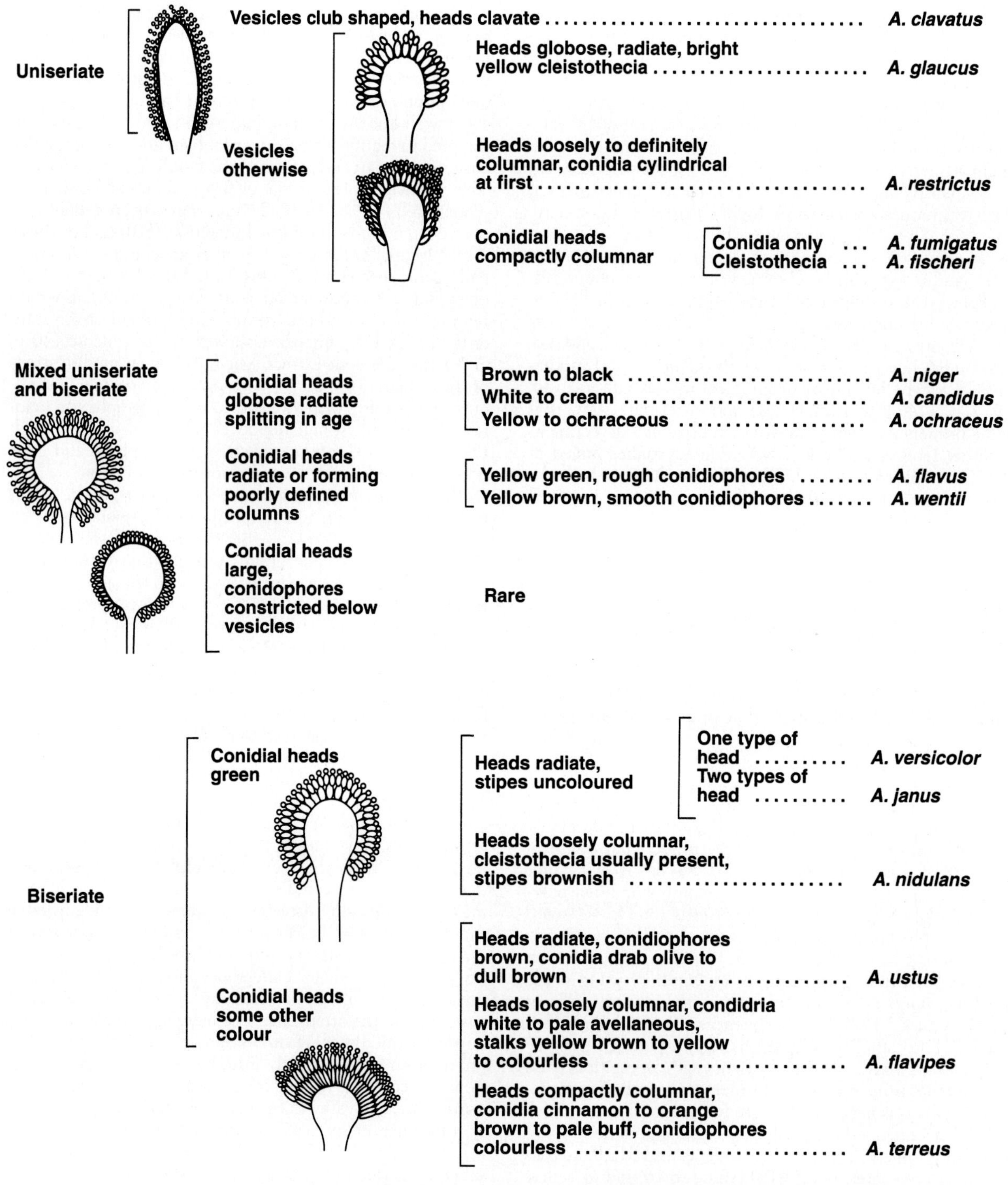

Uniseriate	Vesicles club shaped, heads clavate		A. clavatus
	Vesicles otherwise	Heads globose, radiate, bright yellow cleistothecia	A. glaucus
		Heads loosely to definitely columnar, conidia cylindrical at first	A. restrictus
		Conidial heads compactly columnar — Conidia only	A. fumigatus
		Conidial heads compactly columnar — Cleistothecia	A. fischeri
Mixed uniseriate and biseriate	Conidial heads globose radiate splitting in age	Brown to black	A. niger
		White to cream	A. candidus
		Yellow to ochraceous	A. ochraceus
	Conidial heads radiate or forming poorly defined columns	Yellow green, rough conidiophores	A. flavus
		Yellow brown, smooth conidiophores	A. wentii
	Conidial heads large, conidophores constricted below vesicles	Rare	
Biseriate	Conidial heads green	Heads radiate, stipes uncoloured — One type of head	A. versicolor
		Heads radiate, stipes uncoloured — Two types of head	A. janus
		Heads loosely columnar, cleistothecia usually present, stipes brownish	A. nidulans
	Conidial heads some other colour	Heads radiate, conidiophores brown, conidia drab olive to dull brown	A. ustus
		Heads loosely columnar, condidria white to pale avellaneous, stalks yellow brown to yellow to colourless	A. flavipes
		Heads compactly columnar, conidia cinnamon to orange brown to pale buff, conidiophores colourless	A. terreus

FIGURE 1 Key to the representative species within "group series" of *Aspergillus*. (Reprinted with permission from reference 115.)

rotia are firm, fruiting body-like structures composed of swollen hyphal cells but lacking internal spores. Hülle cells are globose or variable in shape and have thick and highly refractive walls (Fig. 4). They commonly occur near the center of a colony immersed in the vegetative mycelium where their presence may be indicated by droplets of exudate. Hülle cells are often associated with cleistothecial ascomata such as in *Emericella* species (Fig. 4; Table 2). Cleistothecia have outer walls composed of interwoven hyphae and interiors filled randomly with asci and ascospores. The shape, color, size, and wall features of both ascomata and ascospores are important characters for differentiating teleomorphs of *Aspergillus* species. Sterile variants of aspergilli are occasionally isolated from specimens and may sometimes appear highly atypical. The more common variant is white and felty, but glabrous cerebriform variants occur rarely and

TABLE 2 Characteristics of some medically important *Aspergillus* species grown on identification media[a]

Section[b] and species	Seriation		Colony color	Microscopic features[c]	Comment	Selected references[d]
	Uniseriate	Biseriate				
Fumigati						
A. fumigatus	+		Dark blue-green to grayish turquoise; slate gray with age; reverse, variable; variants white or yellowish white (Fig. 3)	Conidiophore mostly up to 300 μm long and 5–8 μm wide, smooth, uncolored or greenish; vesicle dome shaped, 20–30 μm in diam, phialides on upper half only; head strongly columnar; conidia subglobose to globose, occasionally ellipsoidal, smooth to echinulate, 2–3.5 μm in diam	Distinguished by blue-green colonies, growth at 45°C and columnar heads with single layer of phialides. Sterile white fast growing or glabrous cerebriform slowly growing variants may be confirmed by thermotolerance and exoantigen test. Cosmopolitan airborne mould often found in compost piles, soil of potted plants; most common pathogen	13, 25, 32, 60, 69, 80, 115, 133, 136, 157, 167
Neosartorya fischeri (anamorph, *A. fischerianus*)	+		White to gray green; exudate uncolored or pale brown	Conidiophores and conidial heads and conidia as for *A. fumigatus*; cleistothecia globose, mostly 150–350 μm; creamy white, ascospores rough walled with two crests, 5–8 μm long; three varieties distinguished by ascospore morphologies (Fig. 18)	Conidial characteristics and thermotolerance strongly similar to *A. fumigatus*, but colonies usually whiter with fewer conidial heads; rarely reported as a pathogen; some clinical isolates reported as *N. fischeri* have been reidentified as *Neosartorya pseudofischeri*	25, 32, 80, 115, 122, 166
Flavi						
A. flavus	+[e]	+	Yellow to dark yellowish green	Conidiophore mostly 400–850 μm long and 20 μm wide, roughened, uncolored; vesicle subglobose or globose, 25–45 μm in diam; loosely radiate or splitting into columns in age; conidia globose or ellipsoidal, roughened, 3–6 μm in diam	Toxigenic[f]; brown to black sclerotia sometimes present; growth usually enhanced at 37°C; heads vary in size and seriation; colony color may be influenced by culture medium additives such as yeast extract; second most common human pathogen	32, 69, 80, 115, 133, 136, 192

(*Continued on next page*)

TABLE 2 Characteristics of some medically important *Aspergillus* species grown on identification media[a] *(Continued)*

Section[b] and species	Seriation		Colony color	Microscopic features[c]	Comment	Selected references[d]
	Uniseriate	Biseriate				
Nigri,	+[e]					
A. niger		+	Black with white margin and yellow surface mycelium; reverse, uncolored or pale yellow	Conidiophore 400–3,000 μm long and 15–20 μm wide, smooth, uncolored to brownish near tip; vesicle globose, 30–75 μm in diam; radiate and then splitting into columns in age; conidia globose with thick walls, brownish black, roughened, 4–5 μm in diam	Frequent cause of otomycosis; sometimes associated with intracavitary colonization, especially in diabetics	25, 32, 69, 80, 115, 133, 136, 145, 162
Versicolores						
A. versicolor		+	Green to gray-green or tan with patches of pink or yellow; reverse, variable and often deep red	Conidiophore 200–400 μm long and 5 μm wide, smooth, uncolored, yellowish or pale brown; vesicle ovate to elliptical, 9–16 μm in diam, head radiate to loosely columnar; conidia globose, echinulate, 2.5–3 μm in diam; hülle cells globose (Fig. 19)	Toxigenic; distinguished by slowly growing, greenish tan or variably colored colonies, and small biseriate vesicles. Conidial heads of *A. sydowii* are similar but colonies are blue-green. Reduced structures resembling penicilli are sometimes present	25, 32, 60, 69, 80, 115, 162
A. sydowii		+	Blue-green often resembling *Penicillium* spp.	Conidiophore 150–350 μm long and 3–8 μm wide, smooth, thick walled, uncolored or pale brown; vesicle globose or elliptical, 7–13 μm in diam, head radiate; conidia globose, very rough, 2.5–4 μm in diam; reduced structures resembling penicilli common	Distinguished from *A. versicolor* by slowly growing blue-green colonies; diminutive heads resembling penicilli are common	25, 32, 60, 69, 80, 115, 162

Terrei,					
A. terreus	+	Tan to cinnamon brown, rarely orange-brown; reverse, yellow or tan	Conidiophore 100–250 μm long and 4.5–6 μm wide, smooth, uncolored; vesicle dome shaped, 10–16 μm in diam; phialides on upper half; head columnar; conidia globose or subglobose, smooth, 2 μm in diam; solitary single-celled conidia commonly formed, sessile on submerged hyphae	Cinnamon brown colonies, columnar heads, and solitary accessory conidia are highly distinctive	25, 32, 68, 69, 80, 115, 176
Nidulantes					
Emericella nidulans (anamorph, *A. nidulans*)	+	Dark green if mainly conidial; buff to purplish brown if cleistothecial; reverse, deep red to purple	Conidiophore 70–150 μm long and 3–6 μm wide, smooth, brown; vesicle hemispherical, 8–12 μm in diam; phialides on upper part, columnar; conidia globose, rough, 3–4 μm in diam; cleistothecia reddish brown, globose, 100–250 μm, hülle cells globose; ascospores lenticular with two longitudinal crests, ~5 μm long, reddish purple (Fig. 4)	Toxigenic; distinguished by reddish brown cleistothecia, abundant hülle cells, reddish purple ascospores with two crests, short, brown conidiophores and "stout" metulae	25, 32, 69, 80, 115, 162
Emericella quadrilineata	+	Olive green to grayish purple; reverse, purple	Conidial heads, ascocarps, and hülle cells similar to those of *E. nidulans*. Ascospores also similar but have two major and two minor equatorial crests	Distinguished from *E. nidulans* by four crests on ascospores	25, 69, 115, 127
Flavipedes					
A. flavipes	+	White with patches of yellow or pale grayish buff; reverse, yellow to golden brown	Conidiophore 150–400 μm long and 4–8 μm wide, smooth to roughened, uncolored to pale brown; vesicle subglobose, 10–20 μm in diam; radiate to loosely columnar; conidia globose, smooth, 2–3 μm in diam; cleistothecia and hülle cells rarely produced	Distinguished from *A. terreus* by more slowly growing colonies, metulae usually formed over entire vesicle and radiate to loosely columnar heads	69, 115

(Continued on next page)

TABLE 2 Characteristics of some medically important *Aspergillus* species grown on identification media[a] *(Continued)*

Section[b] and species	Seriation		Colony color	Microscopic features[c]	Comment	Selected references[d]
	Uniseriate	Biseriate				
Usti						
A. ustus		+	Brownish gray or olive-gray; reverse, yellow; dull reddish or purplish	Conidiophore 75–400 μm long and 4–7 μm wide, smooth, becoming brown; vesicle globose or subglobose, 7–16 μm in diam; fertile over upper two-thirds; radiate to loosely columnar; conidia globose, rough, 3–4.5 μm in diam; irregular hülle cells often present	Distinguished by dull gray-green colonies, small vesicles, brown conidiophores, and irregularly shaped hülle cells when present	25, 32, 60, 69, 80, 115, 187
A. deflectus		+	Slowly growing, becoming mouse gray with pinkish margins or patches of yellow	Conidiophore 40–125 μm long and 2.5–3.5 μm wide, smooth, reddish brown; vesicle hemispherical, 5–7 μm in diam, typically bent at right angle to stipe; phialides on upper surface, columnar; conidia globose, 3–3.5 μm in diam; smooth to roughened; hülle cells sometimes present	Distinguished by vesicle bent almost at right angle to stipe; rarely reported as pathogen in humans and dogs	25, 55
Aspergillus						
Eurotium spp. (anamorphs, *A. glaucus* and other spp.)	+		Deep green mixed with bright yellow or red; reverse, uncolored or pale yellow	Conidiophore 200–350 μm long and 7–12 μm wide, smooth, uncolored to pale brown; vesicle globose, 15–30 μm in diam; conidial heads large, radiate; conidia subglobose, echinulate, 5 μm in diam, cleistothecia thin walled, yellow, globose, 75–150 μm, ascospores smooth or roughened, with furrow and rounded or frilled crests	Formerly called *glaucus* group; osmophilic, reproduction enhanced on high-sugar media; growth poor at 37°C; species difficult to distinguish by features of conidial heads, but readily identified by ascospore morphology. *E. repens*, *E. ruber*, and *E. amstelodami* rarely reported as pathogens. *E. umbrosus*, reported as cause of farmer's lung, is another name for *E. herbariorum* (anamorph, *A. glaucus*)	25, 32, 65, 69, 80, 115, 162

Restricti						
A. restrictus	+		Dull olive green to brownish green, very slowly growing	Conidiophore 80–200 μm long and 4–8 μm wide, smooth or roughened, uncolored; vesicle hemispherical, 8–20 μm in diam, phialides on upper third, head columnar; conidia cylindrical to ellipsoidal, roughened, 4–7 μm long and 3–4 μm wide	May be confused with *A. fumigatus* but differs by very slow growth on routine media, slightly enhanced growth on high-sugar media, no growth at 37°C; cylindrical conidia developing in long, adherent columns	25, 32, 69, 80, 115
Candidi						
A. candidus	+[e]	+	White to cream	Conidiophore mostly 200–500 μm long and 7–10 μm wide, smooth to roughened, uncolored; vesicle globose or subglobose, 17–35 μm in diam; fertile over entire surface; radiate; conidia globose, smooth, 3–4 μm in diam; reddish purple sclerotia sometimes present	Distinguished from all colored aspergilli by white, slowly growing colonies; from *A. niveus* by larger vesicles, metulae covering entire surface and absence of teleomorph; predominantly biseriate, sometimes uniseriate on smaller heads	25, 32, 69, 80, 115

[a] Modified from previous versions of this chapter with data from references 32 and 69.
[b] Modern concepts have replaced group names with subgenera and sections (69); refer to reference (45) for names in common use.
[c] Refer to the section *Aspergillus* Taxonomy and Identification in the text for descriptions of terms.
[d] Refer to reference manuals by De Hoog and Guarro (25), Domsch et al. (32), Kane et al. (60), Klich and Pitt (69), Kwon-Chung and Bennett (80), Onions et al. (115), or St.-Germain and Summerbell (162) for species descriptions and illustrations.
[e] Predominantly biseriate.
[f] Only species producing potent toxins are noted as toxigenic, but other species may produces toxins of lesser significance.

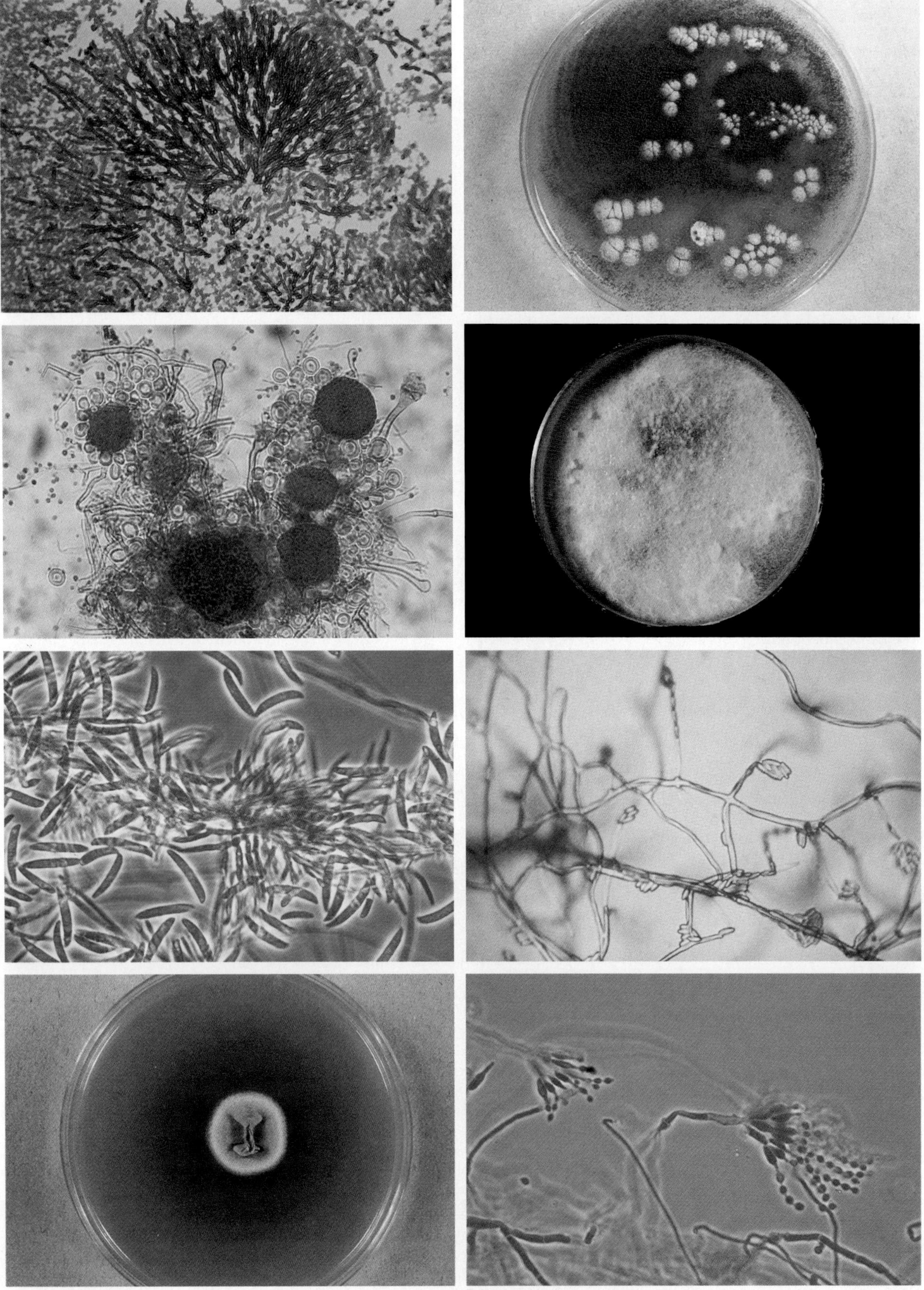

may not be recognized as aspergilli (Fig. 3) (157). A sterile white mould which grows at 45°C, especially if it is isolated from respiratory specimens of a patient with chronic infection, may be considered suspicious for *A. fumigatus*. Exoantigen tests are useful for the identification to the genus level and, in the case of *A. fumigatus*, to the species level (144).

OTHER MONILIACEOUS MOULDS

Features of some opportunistic moniliaceous fungi are described in Table 3.

Fusarium and *Cylindrocarpon* Species

Fusarium species are cosmopolitan soil saprobes and facultative plant pathogens that can cause infection or toxicosis in humans and animals (108). Infections that have been reported include keratitis, onychomycosis, colonization of burned or necrotic skin of wounds or ulcers, sinusitis, and infection of the deeper tissues including mycetoma (see chapter 102 of this Manual), endophthalmitis, peritonitis, endocarditis, osteomyelitis, arthritis, and subcutaneous and brain abscesses (48, 60, 80, 108, 136). An increased incidence of disseminated infection often with a fatal outcome has been seen in patients with prolonged neutropenia due to therapy for leukemia or lymphoma or following bone marrow transplantation (48, 75, 80, 93, 108, 134, 168, 179). Cutaneous lesions, fungemia, rhinocerebral involvement, pneumonia, or all of these are common clinical findings of disseminated fusarial infection (48, 108, 128, 134), and biopsy of skin lesions may be helpful in establishing a diagnosis. In contrast to the low rate of recovery of *Aspergillus* species in blood cultures in cases of invasive aspergillosis, there is a high rate of recovery (~60%) from blood of patients with disseminated fusarial infection (80, 119, 134).

In direct examination, the hyphae of *Fusarium* species resemble those of aspergilli or *Scedosporium* species in size (3 to 6 μm in width), septation, branching pattern, and predilection for vascular invasion. Dichotomous branching is common, branches are often constricted at their sites of origin from the parent hyphae (19), and hyphae may show areas of collapse. Swellings or chlamydospore-like structures may be found, especially in vascular lesions (19), and conidia are rarely found in human or animal infection (37, 119). Immunohistologic methods may help to distinguish between infections caused by some hyaline moulds, but cross-reactivity is problematic (48, 63). A definitive diagnosis requires isolation and identification of the fungus; serologic tests are not in common use (48).

The distinguishing features of the three most common pathogenic species are summarized in Table 4. Considerable proficiency is required to identify other species of *Fusarium* with certainty, and a reference laboratory should be consulted. Although fusaria grow well on most mycologic media, the medium can profoundly influence the colonial topography, color, and conidium development, and use of a rich medium to maintain isolates can result in cultural variation and loss of ability to produce macroconidia. Identification schemes usually require observation of growth rates, the colors of the colony's obverse and reverse sides, the color of conidial masses, and microscopic features on media such as potato dextrose agar and tap water agar supplemented with either sterilized carnation leaves or potassium chloride (108, 109).

Relatives of *Fusarium* species, *Cylindrocarpon* species are also cosmopolitan soil- and plant-associated fungi which are recovered occasionally as contaminants from specimens. Rare cases of keratitis and mycetoma have been documented (25, 198).

Acremonium, Lecythophora, Phialemonium, and *Phaeoacremonium* Species

The genus *Acremonium*, formerly called *Cephalosporium*, includes approximately 100 species associated with soil, insects, sewage, rhizospheres of plants, and other environmental substrates. Teleomorphs are included in the ascomycetous genera *Nectria* and *Emericellopsis*, among others (32). Most reports of infection due to *Acremonium* species are cases of mycetoma (see chapter 102), onychomycosis, keratitis, and colonization of soft contact lens (80, 136). Reliable reports of invasive infection are rare. Pulmonary disease in a boy with chronic granulomatous disease; granuloma with erosion of the hard palate, maxilla, and mandible; meningitis; cerebritis in an intravenous drug user; prosthetic valve endocarditis; osteomyelitis following trauma; arthritis; esophagitis; and fungemia (66, 80, 140, 158, 169) have been documented. While it is not too difficult to recognize members of the genus, identification to the species level is very difficult, and many reports of infection are based on unidentified species (80). Species of *Acremonium* grow well on SDA, and some species can tolerate cycloheximide. *Acremonium kiliense* (Fig. 13) the most common medically important species, produces cylindrical conidia and solitary hyaline chlamydospores, especially on oatmeal agar. *Acremonium recifei* also produces chlamydospores, but its conidia are sickle shaped or slightly curved. Colonies of *Acremonium strictum*, a common soil and occasional airborne fungus, are moist and pale salmon colored and resemble those of *Lecythophora hoffmannii*; *A. strictum* can be isolated from blood

FIGURE 2 (row 1, left) Section of lung showing dichotomously branched hyphae of *Aspergillus* in invasive aspergillosis. Hematoxylin-eosin staining was used.

FIGURE 3 (row 1, right) An atypical isolate of *Aspergillus fumigatus* described in reference 157. This slowly growing glabrous, cerebriform colony began to demonstrate growth typical of that of *A. fumigatus* after 3 months in culture.

FIGURE 4 (row 2, left) *Emericella* (*Aspergillus*) *nidulans* showing *Aspergillus* heads, cleistothecia, and hülle cells.

FIGURE 5 (row 2, right) Colony of *Fusarium solani* on potato flake agar after 2 weeks. (Reprinted with permission of Deanna A. Sutton and The Williams & Wilkins Co.)

FIGURE 6 (row 3, left) Macroconidia of *Fusarium solani* stained with lactofuchsin.

FIGURE 7 (row 3, right) Chains of microconidia produced by *Fusarium verticillioides* (*Fusarium moniliforme*) on potato flake agar. (Courtesy of Deanna A. Sutton and The Williams & Wilkins Co.)

FIGURE 8 (row 4, left) Colony of *Penicillium marneffei* showing diffusing red pigment on Sabouraud dextrose agar after 7 days. Note that a few *Penicillium* species produce diffusible red pigments.

FIGURE 9 (row 4, right) Compact biverticillate penicillus of *Penicillium marneffei*.

TABLE 3 Key features of some opportunistic moniliaceous fungi

Genus	Key features	Etiologic agents	Comments	Selected reference(s)
Acremonium	Colonies slowly growing (usually <3 cm in diam in 10 days), often white, cottony, fasciculate (spikey), glabrous or moist and pink or salmon colored. Conidiogenous cells solitary, slender (ca. 2 μm wide), mostly unbranched, awl-shaped (needle-shaped) phialides. Conidia one celled, straight or curved, in slimy masses (Fig. 13)	*A. alabamense*, *A. falciforme*, *A. kiliense*, *A. potronii*, *A. receifei*, *A. curvulum*, *A. strictum*, *Acremonium* spp.	Differs from *Fusarium* by slow growth rate, narrower hyphae (mostly <2 μm in width), and more slender and needle-like phialides. Compare with *Lecythophora*, *Phaeoacremonium*, *Phialemonium*	25, 32, 39, 60, 66, 80, 136, 140, 162
Acrophialophora	Colonies fast growing, growth enhanced at 37°C, yellowish white, darkening to grayish brown. Conidiophores brown, seta-like. Conidiogenous cells flask-shaped phialides borne near the tip of conidiophores or on vegetative hyphae. Conidia in long chains, one celled, lemon shaped, smooth or roughened	*A. fusispora*	Compare with *Paecilomyces*. Single report of keratitis	25
Aphanoascus	Colonies moderately fast growing, yellowish white, granular; cycloheximide tolerant. A homothallic ascomycete forming globose cleistothecia containing roughened ascospores; associated with a *Chrysosporium* anamorph consisting of terminal one-celled aleurioconidia and alternate arthroconidia	*A. fulvescens*	Compare with *Chrysosporium* and dermatophytes	60, 80
Arthrographis	Colonies slowly growing, growth enhanced at 37°C, initially yellowish white, and yeast-like, becoming hyphal and tan, cycloheximide tolerant. Conidiophores dendritic (tree-like), bearing lateral branches. Arthroconidia formed by fragmentation of branches or of undifferentiated hyphae	*A. kalrae*	Compare *Sctyalidium hyalinum*, *Onychocola*, *Hormographiella*	66, 120, 151, 152
Aureobasidium	Colonies wet, pale salmon or pink, usually darkening in age to black. For microscopic features see description in chapter 101	*A. pullulans*	Differs from *Lecythophora hoffmannii* and *Acremonium strictum* by absence of distinct phialides	25
Beauveria	Colonies slow to moderately fast growing, yellowish-white. Conidiogenous cells solitary, in whorls or in sporodochia, basally swollen, proliferating sympodially at the tip in a zigzag (geniculate) fashion. Conidia one celled, subglobose	*B. alba* (also called *Engyodontium album*), *B. bassiana*	Compare *Sporothrix*	25, 66, 95, 138
Chaetomium	Colonies fast growing, yellowish green to gray. Conidia absent or formed from phialides. Ascomata perithecia bearing coiled, straight, branched brown or indistinct setae. Ascospores lemon shaped, brown, smooth (Fig. 15)	*C. strumarium*, *C. atrobrunneum*, *C. globosum*	*C. strumarium* and *C. atrobrunneum* show enhanced growth at 42°C, but *C. globosum* fails to grow at this temp	2, 25, 49, 60, 194

Chrysosporium	Colonies slow to moderately fast growing, yellowish white. Conidia single celled smooth to roughened aleurioconidia formed sessile or at the ends or on the sides of unswollen stalks. Arthroconidia sometimes present	*C. parvum* (see *Emmonsia* spp.) or unidentified species; see also *Aphanoascus fulvescens*	Reports of infection by unnamed species are difficult to evaluate because the isolates are not described well enough to confirm etiology	60, 85? (see text), 163, 174
Cylindrocarpon	Colonies fast growing, yellowish-white, tan, orange or purple, felty or cottony. Conidiogenous cells awl-shaped phialides with a single opening, solitary, in branched structures or in sporodochia (conidiophores borne crowded on a compact mass of hyphae). Macroconidia straight or curved, with rounded ends, multicelled; microconidia one or two celled. Chlamydospores sometimes present	*Cylindrocarpon destructans*, *C. cyanescens*, *C. lichenicola*	Distinguished from *Fusarium* by the more rounded shape of the basal cells of the macroconidia	25, 80, 198
Emmonsia	Colonies yellowish white to buff. Aleurioconidia single celled smooth to roughened, formed sessile or at the ends or on the sides of swollen stalks. Dimorphic, forming thick-walled swollen cells called adiaspores in vitro at maximum growth temp	*E. crescens*, *E. parva*	Distinguished from *Blastomyces* and *Histoplasma* by exoantigen tests, DNA probe, absence of budding cells; differs from *Chrysosporium* by swollen stalks	25, 34, 60, 146–148
Fusarium	About 100 species grouped into sections. Colonies fast growing (>7 cm in diam after 10 days); obverse and reverse colors white, cream to orange, tan, brown, carmine red, reddish brown, pink, purple, or blue to blue-green; texture felty or cottony or sparse and wet looking. Conidiogenous cells awl-shaped phialides with one (monophialide) or more than one opening (polyphialide). Phialides solitary, in branched structures or in sporodochia (conidiophores borne crowded on a compact mass of hyphae). Conidia of two types that are common or rare depending on the species. Macroconidia multicelled, with two to five septa, fusiform or sickle shaped, often with a distinct notched basal cell. Macroconidia produced in the aerial mycelium less typical than those produced in sporodochia. Microconidia oval, globose, ellipsoidal, clavate or reniform (kidney shaped), one or two celled, and borne in slimy heads or in short chains in the aerial mycelium. Chlamydospores sometimes present; solitary, in chains or in clusters (Fig. 5–7)	*Fusarium solani*, *F. oxysporum*, and *F. verticillioides* (*F. moniliforme*) are most common (Table 4); *F. anthophilum*, *F. chlamydosporum*, *F. dimerum*, *F. napiforme*, *F. nygamai*, *F. proliferatum*, *F. roseum*, and *F. sacchari* are rarely reported	Differs from *Acremonium* by faster-growing colonies; broader, more robust hyphae and phialides; and usually by presence of macroconidia. Many species are toxigenic	25, 32, 48, 60, 75, 80, 93, 108, 109, 119, 134, 136, 168, 179
Hormographiella	Colonies fast growing, white, amber to tan, woolly, cycloheximide sensitive. Conidiophores short, bearing short fertile branches. Arthroconidia schizolytic, thin walled, single celled, often adherent around the conidiophore. Sclerotia sometimes present	*H. aspergillata*, *H. verticillata*	Differs from *A. kalrae* by cycloheximide sensitivity, fast growth rate	25, 66, 149, 184

(*Continued on next page*)

TABLE 3 Key features of some opportunistic moniliaceous fungi *(Continued)*

Genus	Key features	Etiologic agents	Comments	Selected reference(s)
Lecythophora	Colonies white to salmon, moist or fasciculate (spikey), or tan darkening to black in patches. Conidiogenous cells adelophialides (short, stumpy phialides without a basal septum), as well as awl-shaped phialides. *L. mutabilis* forms brown chlamydospores, while *L. hoffmannii* does not. See also chapter 101 of this Manual	*L. hoffmannii, L. mutabilis*	Differs from *Acremonium* and *Phaeoacremonium* by predominance of adelophialides. Hyphal elements in tissue are usually reported as hyaline	25, 39, 92, (see text under *Scytalidium*)
Myceliophthora	Colonies fast growing, thermophilic, cinnamon brown. Conidia pale brown, roughened, single-celled aleurioconidia formed on swollen stalks	*M. thermophila*	Differs from *Chrysosporium* by swollen stalks	14, 60
Onychocola	Colonies restricted, raised, yellowish white to grayish white, cycloheximide tolerant. Conidia one- or two-celled cylindrical or swollen arthroconidia forming in adherent chains, detaching by fracture of thin-walled cells. Brown knobby setae often present (Fig. 12)	*O. canadensis*	Differs from *S. hyalinum* and *Hormographiella* by adherent chains, slow growth and cycloheximide tolerance	25, 60, 150
Paecilomyces	About 40 species grouped into two sections. Section *Paecilomyces* includes the thermotolerant *P. variotii* and anamorphs of *Byssochlamys* and *Thermoascus* with fast-growing yellowish brown, buff, white, or orange colonies. Section *Isarioidea* includes *P. lilacinus* and species that are more slowly growing with white, reddish gray, violet, or brightly colored colonies. Conidiogenous cells phialides formed on verticillately branched conidiophores. Conidia single celled, in chains. Ascospores of *T. crustaceus* are orange brown, rough walled (Fig. 10, 11, and 20)	*P. lilacinus, P. variotii* are most common (see Table 5); *P. marquandii, P. javanicus, Thermoascus crustaceus*	Differs from *Penicillium* by colonies in colors other than bright green or blue-green and by the basally swollen phialides that taper toward the neck and that are bent away from the main axis An isolate of *P. viridis* from human infection was reidentified as *P. variotii*. Compare with *Acrophialophora*	17, 25, 32, 44, 66, 80, 94, 116, 136, 139, 162, 172, 190
Penicillium	About 200 species divided into four subgenera according to conidiophore branching. Colonies moderately fast growing, powdery, green to blue green, rarely other colors. Conidiophores erect, with one to three levels of branching. Conidiogenous cell phialides borne on the stipes or on branches called metula. Conidia globose or ellipsoidal, smooth to roughened, in chains. Sclerotia and ascomata sometimes present. *P. marneffei* distinguished by reddish brown vegetative hyphae, golden yellow to pale green aerial hyphae, and red diffusible pigment; compact biverticillate or irregular penicilli on short, roughened conidiophores and growth at 37°C in a yeast-like form (Fig. 8 and 9)	*P. marneffei* (true pathogen) *P. brevicompactum, P. chrysogenum, P. citrinum, P. commune, P. decumbens, P. purpurogenum, P. spinulosum*, and unidentified species	Exoantigen test useful for identification of *P. marneffei*, a member of the subgenus Biverticillium. Other species may produce red diffusible pigments but fail to convert to yeast-like form. Many species toxigenic	4, 5, 20, 25, 26, 32, 33, 40, 45, 54, 62, 64, 66, 80, 87, 99, 117, 125, 126, 136, 143, 162, 197

Phaeoacremonium	Colonies white, tan, or grayish brown. Conidiogenous cells solitary unbranched or branched awl-shaped phialides often arising from hyphal strands. Conidia single celled, curved, rarely straight, in slimy masses. See chapter 101 of this Manual for further description	*P. parasiticum*, *P. inflatipes*	Accommodates *Phialophora parasitica* and several other species intermediate between *Acremonium* and *Phialophora*	23, 25, 92 (see text under *Scytalidium*)
Phialemonium	Colonies yellowish to green. Conidiogenous cells adelophialides (short, stumpy phialides without a basal septum), as well as awl-shaped phialides. See also chapter 101 of this Manual	*P. curvatum*, *P. obovatum*	Compare *Acremonium* and *Lecythophora*	39
Schizophyllum	Colonies fast growing, growth enhanced at 37°C, white, woolly or cottony, cycloheximide sensitive. Conidia absent. Hyphae bearing clamp connections and short, thin, pegs or spicules; both may be absent. Clamped isolates usually develop fan-shaped, gilled mushrooms on sporulation media after 3 to 6 wk (Fig. 16, 17, and 23)	*S. commune*	Clinical picture resembles aspergillosis and clampless isolates resemble aspergilli by histopathology. *S. commune* may be the cause of sinusitis attributed to *Myriodontium keratinophilum* and *Chrysosporium* sp. (see text)	6, 21, 85, 90, 135, 149, 153, 154
Scopulariopsis	Colonies white, buff, gray-brown to black. Conidiogenous cells annellides formed on branched conidiophores with one or two levels of branching. Conidia one celled, globose or ellipsoidal, in chains. *S. brevicaulis* distinguished by buff or tan, granular colonies, thick-walled smooth to coarsely roughened conidia that are truncate at the base and rounded or pointed at the tip and measure 5–8 μm wide by 5–7 μm long. Ascospores of *Microascus* species are orange, lens or half-moon shaped, and released in a cirrus (a long adherent column) from a short-necked ascocarp (Fig. 21)	*S. brevicaulis*, *S. candida*, *S. brumptii*, *Microascus cinereus*, *Microascus cirrosus*	*S. candida* differs from *S. brevicaulis* in having smooth conidia and white colonies. *S. brumptii* differs from *Scedosporium* species by the conidia produced in chains rather than in slimy masses. *Microascus* species differ from *Chaetomium* species by the orange ascospores produced in cirri from short-necked ascomata	1, 9, 25, 32, 46, 60, 66, 73, 74, 91, 97, 107, 123, 129, 162, 189
Scytalidium	Colonies rapidly growing (>8 cm in diam by 7–10 days), yellowish white or black, dense, cottony or woolly, cycloheximide sensitive. Conidia one- or two-celled arthroconidia formed by schizolytic fragmentation of branched hyphae varying in width from 2–10 μm in diam. Hyphae and arthroconidia of *S. hyalinum* are hyaline to pale yellow; those of *S. dimidiatum* are light to dark brown. Pycnidial conidia of *Nattrassia mangiferae* stage are initially hyaline and then develop median brown band (Fig. 14 and 22)	*S. hyalinum*, *S. dimidiatum* (synanamorph is known as *Nattrassia mangiferae* or, formerly, *Hendersonula toruloidea*)	Isolates reported as *S. lignicola* from human infection have been reidentified as *S. dimidiatum*. *S. lignicola* differs from *S. dimidiatum* in colonial and microscopic features and should not be considered a synonym, as has been suggested in the literature	25, 60, 92, 102, 137, 151, 156, 162
Sporothrix	Colonies of *S. cyanescens* moderately fast growing, white to lavender, red diffusible pigment often present; cycloheximide sensitive. Conidiophores solitary, forming conidia sympodially on small denticles on sides or at tips. Primary conidia bear one to three secondary conidia; brown pigmented sessile conidia absent	*S. cyanescens* (also called *Cerinosterus cyanescens*) (for description of *S. schenckii*, see chapter 101)	Affinity of *S. cyanescens* is closer to smuts than to other species of *Cerinosterus*. *S. schenckii* differs in being dimorphic and in forming brown sessile conidia	25, 155, 171

TABLE 4 Morphological features of the three commonly isolated *Fusarium* spp.[a]

Characteristic	*F. solani*	*F. oxysporum*	*F. verticillioides* (*F. moniliforme*[b])
Colonies on potato dextrose agar after 4 days at 25°C	3–3.5 cm in diam, creamy white with cream slimy areas, developing blue-green to bluish brown colors, never orange, reverse uncolored, rarely violet (Fig. 5)	4.5–6.5 cm in diam; creamy white, often with purple or violet tints, sporodochia cream to orange, slimy, reverse uncolored to dark blue or purple	4.5–6.5 cm in diam; white, peach to purple, sporodochia orange, reverse uncolored to dark purple
Phialides	Mono, long, slender, sometimes verticillately branched	Mono, short, stout, mostly unbranched	Mono, long, branched and unbranched
Microconidia	Cylindrical to oval, nonseptate	Oval to kidney shaped, single celled, in heads	Oval to club shaped with flattened base, mostly single celled, in chains[c] or in heads (Fig. 7)
Macroconidia	Mostly three-septate (one to five septate), 28–42 by 4–6 μm, slightly curved, rounded at each end or basal cell notched (Fig. 6).	Mostly three (or up to five) septate moderately curved, 27–60 by 3–4.5 μm, pointed at each end	Present or rare, three to five (or up to seven) septate, sickle shaped to almost straight, 30–60 by 3–4 μm, basal cell foot shaped
Chlamydospores[d]	Present, formed singly and in pairs, commonly produced	Present, formed singly and in pairs, usually abundant	Absent

[a] Modified from previous versions of this chapter with data from references 32 and 109.
[b] *F. verticillioides* is preferred over the name *F. moniliforme*, which has a broader concept.
[c] Best observed on carnation leaf agar or KCl medium (109).
[d] Best observed on carnation leaf agar or in sterile distilled water (109).

and can sporulate in tissue (140). The genera *Lecythophora* and *Phialemonium* are distinguished from *Acremonium* by their formation of short, stumpy phialides without basal septa (called adelophialides), in addition to the more awl-shaped phialides (39), but these distinctions are not always readily observed. Colonies of *Lecythophora mutabilis* darken as brown-pigmented chlamydospores develop in older cultures, but the development of these structures may be influenced by the culture medium. The genus *Phaeoacremonium* includes *Phaeoacremonium parasiticum* and some other species associated with human infection and has been distinguished from *Acremonium* by its pigmented vegetative hyphae and conidiophores (23). Although these genera are treated with the dematiaceous medically important fungi (see chapter 101), colonies are often white, salmon, or yellowish to greenish but may darken with age to brown depending upon the species.

Beauveria, Metarhizium, and *Sporothrix* Species

Beauveria bassiana and *Metarhizium anisopliae* are soil fungi well known as insect pathogens. *B. bassiana*, *Beauveria alba* (also known as *Engyodontium album*), and *M. anisopliae* have been identified as agents of keratitis (18, 66, 95, 138). Evidence that *B. bassiana* is an invasive human pathogen is doubtful because in the only reported case, the isolated mould was described as having greenish colonies and had microscopic features inconsistent with those of *B. bassiana* (66). Conidia of *Metarhizium* are produced from phialides, while species of *Beauveria* and *Sporothrix* have solitary conidia borne sympodially. *Sporothrix schenckii* is a well-known dimorphic pathogen described in chapter 101 of this Manual. It forms sessile pigmented conidia in addition to hyaline conidia. *Sporothrix cyanescens* (also known as *Cerinosterus cyanescens*) is isolated infrequently as a contaminant from blood, skin, or respiratory specimens but has been reported as the cause of nodular lung lesions in a heart transplant patient (155, 171).

Chaetomium Species

A member of the Ascomycotina, the genus *Chaetomium* comprises almost 300 species characterized by the formation of perithecial ascomata (fruiting bodies having an opening) usually covered with hairs or setae and containing brown somewhat lemon-shaped ascospores with one or two germ pores. Three species are confirmed to cause human infection; reports involving other species have not been validated. *Chaetomium globosum* occurs commonly as a contaminant or as a rare agent of onychomycosis (60), but its propensity to cause deep infection is not confirmed (2, 49). Yeghen et al. (194) used immunohistochemical staining to confirm that *Chaetomium* and not *Aspergillus* was the cause of infection in their leukemic patient, but their illustrations and thermotolerance of the case isolate are suggestive of *Chaetomium atrobrunneum* rather than *C. globosum*. Only *Chaetomium strumarium* and *Chaetomium atrobrunneum* are reliably reported from infections involving the brain (2).

Chrysosporium, Emmonsia, Myriodontium, and *Myceliophthora* Species

Members of the genera *Chrysosporium*, *Emmonsia*, *Myriodontium*, and *Myceliophthora* produce solitary, usually single-celled conidia which are called aleurioconidia because of their lytic method of conidium dehiscence (60). Members of the first three genera are related to the dermatophytes and the dimorphic pathogens, sharing with them a tolerance of cycloheximide and having teleomorphs in the ascomycete order Onygenales (60, 146). *Emmonsia* species, formerly placed in the genus *Chrysosporium*, cause adiaspiromycosis mainly in rodents and occasionally in humans and are biologically related to *Blastomyces* and *Histoplasma* (147, 148). *Emmonsia* species are dimorphic, and the infection is named after the tissue form, which is a large thick-walled, chlamydospore-like, nonreproducing spore called an adiaspore. Two species are distinguished by their maximum growth temperatures and the different sizes of their adiaspores (147, 148). Most reports of human pulmonary infection concern *Emmonsia crescens*, which has a maximum growth temperature of ~37°C and larger adiaspores (often 100 μm or more in diameter). In most instances, the fungus is not cultured but is recognized from histopathology alone (148). *Emmonsia parva* was reported from disseminated infection in a patient with AIDS (34), but other reports concerning this species are not reliably documented. The adiaspores of *E. parva* are smaller (usually 10 to 25 μm in diameter), and the maximum growth temperature is ~40°C. The validity of *Chrysosporium* species as etiologic agents is questionable, since in the few reports of infection (85, 163, 174), the isolated organism has not been identified to the species level or described well enough to confirm the etiology. *Myriodontium keratinophilum* and *Chrysosporium* species were reported to cause sinusitis (85, 90). However, it seems likely that the fungi involved were misidentified *Schizophyllum commune*, an emerging agent of sinusitis. The hyphal spicules of the latter species could be confused with the stalks of the former two species (60). Although the osteomyelitis infection described by Stillwell et al. (163) has been reported in several subsequent papers as being caused by *E. parva*, the original investigators neither mentioned this species nor reported the presence of adiaspores. Cutaneous mycosis caused by *Aphanoascus fulvescens*, an ascomycete with a *Chrysosporium* anamorph, has been reliably documented (60, 80). Species of *Chrysosporium* and the similar genus *Geomyces*, as well as *M. keratinophilum*, are occasional contaminants of respiratory and cutaneous specimens (60). Members of the genus *Myceliophthora* produce aleurioconidia similar to those of onygenalean fungi, but they have affinities within the order Sordariales. Disseminated infection in a leukemic patient was caused by the thermophilic species *M. thermophila* (14).

Paecilomyces Species

Species of *Paecilomyces* occur worldwide as soil saprophytes, insect parasites, and agents of biodeterioration. *Paecilomyces lilacinus* is a well-documented agent of eye infection, with manifestations including keratitis, endophthalmitis, corneal ulcer, and orbital granuloma (66, 80, 161). Predisposing factors include the use of extended-wear contact lenses, implantation of inadequately sterilized lenses, and the use of topical corticosteroids before the onset of clinically apparent keratitis (80, 161). *Paecilomyces variotii* has been isolated from several patients with endocarditis following valve replacement (58, 66, 80). Cutaneous and subcutaneous infection, pulmonary infection, pyelonephritis, sinusitis, cellulitis, peritonitis, and fungemia have been reported in both immunocompetent and immunosuppressed patients (17, 30, 66, 94, 172, 190). Surgery, prosthetic implants and the use of contaminated solutions or lotions are risk factors predisposing patients to infection since the conidia of both species are relatively resistant to most sterilization techniques (17, 32, 94, 116, 136). Fungal elements in tissue are hyaline, septate, and about 2 to 4 μm wide and have parallel walls or show swellings. The colonial and morphologic features of medically important *Paecilomyces* species (Fig. 10, 11, and 20) are described in Table 5.

Penicillium Species

Members of the genus *Penicillium* are the ubiquitous blue-green moulds that are among the most common of all laboratory contaminants and that can be isolated easily from respiratory specimens and body surfaces. Like its close relative *Aspergillus*, the genus *Penicillium* comprises anamorphic (mitotic) species with known or presumed connections to the family Trichocomaceae (45). The only true pathogen is *Penicillium marneffei*, a member of the subgenus *Biverticillium* (87), now the third most common cause of disseminated opportunistic infection in patients with AIDS in parts of southeast Asia (33, 185). The species is unique among the penicillia in being dimorphic and forming in tissue a unicellular yeast-like organelle that reproduces by planate division. It is endemic in southeast Asia and southern China, where it is associated with four species of bamboo rat but is rarely isolated from soil (4, 20, 33). Infections are more common in immunosuppressed than immunocompetent hosts and are usually disseminated with multiple organ involvement including lung, liver, and skin. A potential for laboratory-acquired infection was demonstrated by the individual who first described *P. marneffei* and who developed a small nodule after accidentally puncturing his finger while inoculating laboratory rodents (142). The fungus can usually be isolated from characteristic skin lesions, blood, or bone marrow (33), and presumptive diagnosis may be made by demonstration of the yeast-like cells of *P. marneffei* in smears or biopsy specimens especially from these sites. The yeast-like cells are oval or cylindrical and 3 to 6 μm in length and may have a cross wall. They may be difficult to distinguish from the yeast cells of *Histoplasma capsulatum*, especially when they are within phagocytes, but the latter may show evidence of budding rather than planate division, and they stain with specific fluorescent-antibody conjugates of *H. capsulatum*. Although an exoantigen test showed efficacy, other serodiagnostic tests for penicilliosis marneffei are still under development (62, 64, 143, 197).

Other species of *Penicillium* have been implicated in human infection, but the validity of many reports has been questioned (136). Although *Penicillium* species grow over a wide range of temperatures (from 5 to 45°C), many species are completely or strongly inhibited at 37°C and thus have a low potential for causing human infection. Even repeated isolation of a *Penicillium* species from patient specimens does not necessarily indicate an etiologic role unless the isolate is accompanied by typical fungal elements in tissue specimens or smears of lesional exudates (136). Other factors that should be considered when assessing the significance of repeated isolation include the isolation of any other fungal species, the patient's possible exposure to airborne conidia, and a diagnosis of bronchiectasis, since conidia may remain viable for prolonged periods without invasion or colonization (80). Nonetheless, several species have been reported to cause peritonitis, urinary tract infection, endocarditis, lung infection, fungemia, and disseminated infection (5, 25, 26, 40, 66, 80). The role of penicillia in allergy and hypersensitivity pneumonitis is well established (54, 117). The identification of penicillia is a complex task requiring growth of an isolate on a variety of media at different temperatures and careful microscopic examination (125, 126).

TABLE 5 Morphologic features of selected *Paecilomyces* species[a]

Characteristic	*P. lilacinus*	*P. marquandii*	*P. variotii*
Colonies on potato dextrose agar after 7 days at 25°C	3–3.5 cm in diam, white becoming dull red or reddish gray,[b] cottony, reverse colorless or vinaceous (Fig. 11)	2 cm in diam, violet brown[b] with white margin, cottony, often with radial folds, reverse yellow, slight yellow diffusible pigment	7–8 cm in diam, yellowish to olive-brown, powdery (Fig. 10)
Thermotolerance	Strongly restricted at 37°C	No growth at 37°C	Reported up to 50°C, but many isolates show no growth above 40°C
Conidiophores	Rough walled, pigmented yellow or purple, metulae densely clustered, bearing whorls of two to four phialides (verticillate), rarely synnematous (Fig. 20)	Smooth walled, hyaline, verticillately branched, metulae with two to four phialides, often forming loose synnemata	Verticillately or irregularly branched, metulae bearing two to seven phialides
Phialides	Taper abruptly to narrow neck, about 1 μm wide	Taper abruptly to narrow neck, about 1 μm wide	Phialides robust, tapering gradually to form long neck about 2 μm wide
Conidia	Smooth to rough, ellipsoidal to fusiform, hyaline to vinaceous in mass, 2.5–3 by 2–2.2 μm	Smooth to slightly rough, ellipsoidal to fusiform, hyaline to purple in mass, 3–3.5 by 2–2.2 μm	Variable in size and shape, mostly 3.2–5 by 2–4 μm or up to 15 μm long, ellipsoidal to cylindrical smooth, hyaline to yellow-brown
Solitary conidia	Absent	Present, thin walled, often in submerged mycelium	Terminal or intercalary, brown, thick walled

[a] Modified from previous versions of this chapter with data from references 32 and 139.
[b] Color names from Kornerup and Wanscher (71a).

Czapek yeast extract agar, malt extract agar, and 25% glycerol nitrate agar and incubation at 5, 25, and 37°C should be used. The use of SDA alone is not recommended.

Scedosporium Species

Scedosporium species are soil-, manure-, and water-inhabiting moulds with virulence and clinical spectra remarkably similar to those of *Aspergillus*. The two species known to cause human and animal infection are *Scedosporium apiospermum*, the anamorph of the ascomycete *P. boydii*, and *Scedosporium prolificans*. The characteristic features of these species are described in chapter 101 of this Manual. The similarities between species of *Aspergillus* and *Scedosporium* both in their spectra of clinical syndromes and their appearance in tissue have led to their mention in this chapter, even though species of *Scedosporium* are darkly pigmented in culture. In tissue sections, the hyphae of *Scedosporium* species are hyaline, septate, branched, and hematoxylinophilic and can be reliably distinguished from the hyphae of the aspergilli and other hyaline moulds only by direct immunofluorescence. Occasionally, conidia which are pale brown and ovoid or cylindrical are formed, generally in fungus balls or in the sinuses (66); their presence allows presumptive identification. Culture and serologic analysis are

FIGURE 10 (row 1, left) Colony of *Paecilomyces variotii* on potato-dextrose agar after 7 days.
FIGURE 11 (row 1, right) Colony of *Paecilomyces lilacinus* on potato dextrose agar after 14 days.
FIGURE 12 (row 2, left) Culture of three different isolates of *Onychocola canadensis* after 5 weeks on Mycosel agar.
FIGURE 13 (row 2, right) Colony of *Acremonium kiliense* on Sabouraud dextrose agar after 9 days.
FIGURE 14 (row 3, left) Colony of *Scytalidium hyalinum* on Sabouraud dextrose agar after 7 days.
FIGURE 15 (row 3, right) Colony of *Chaetomium strumarium* showing yellowish surface mycelium and diffusing pink pigment on cornmeal agar after 5 weeks.
FIGURE 16 (row 4, left) Monokaryotic (clampless) hyphae of *Schizophyllum commune* in pulmonary fungus ball. Gomori methenamine silver stain was used.
FIGURE 17 (row 4, right) Dikaryotic culture of *Schizophyllum commune* showing development of gilled fruiting bodies on potato dextrose agar after 7 weeks.

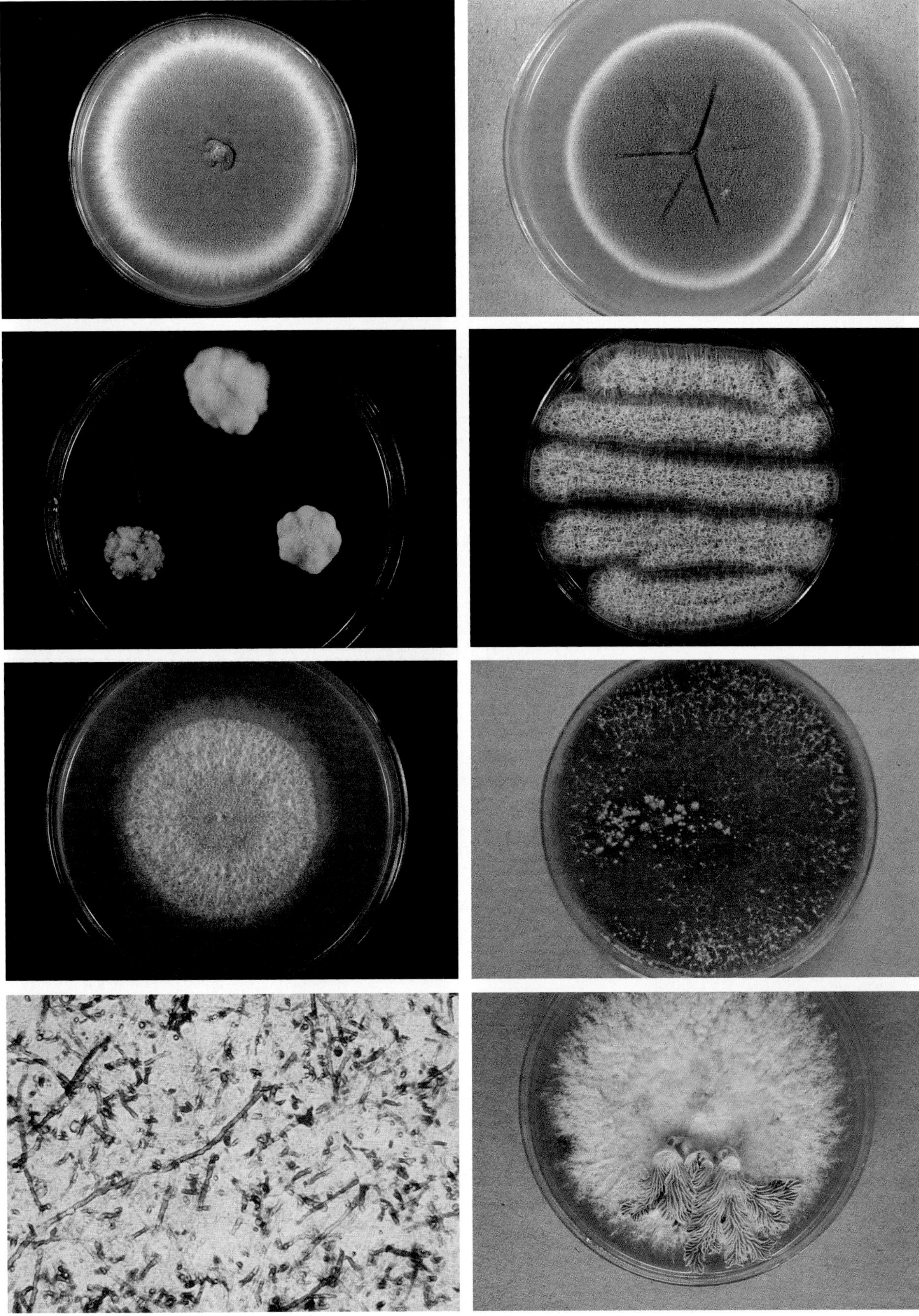

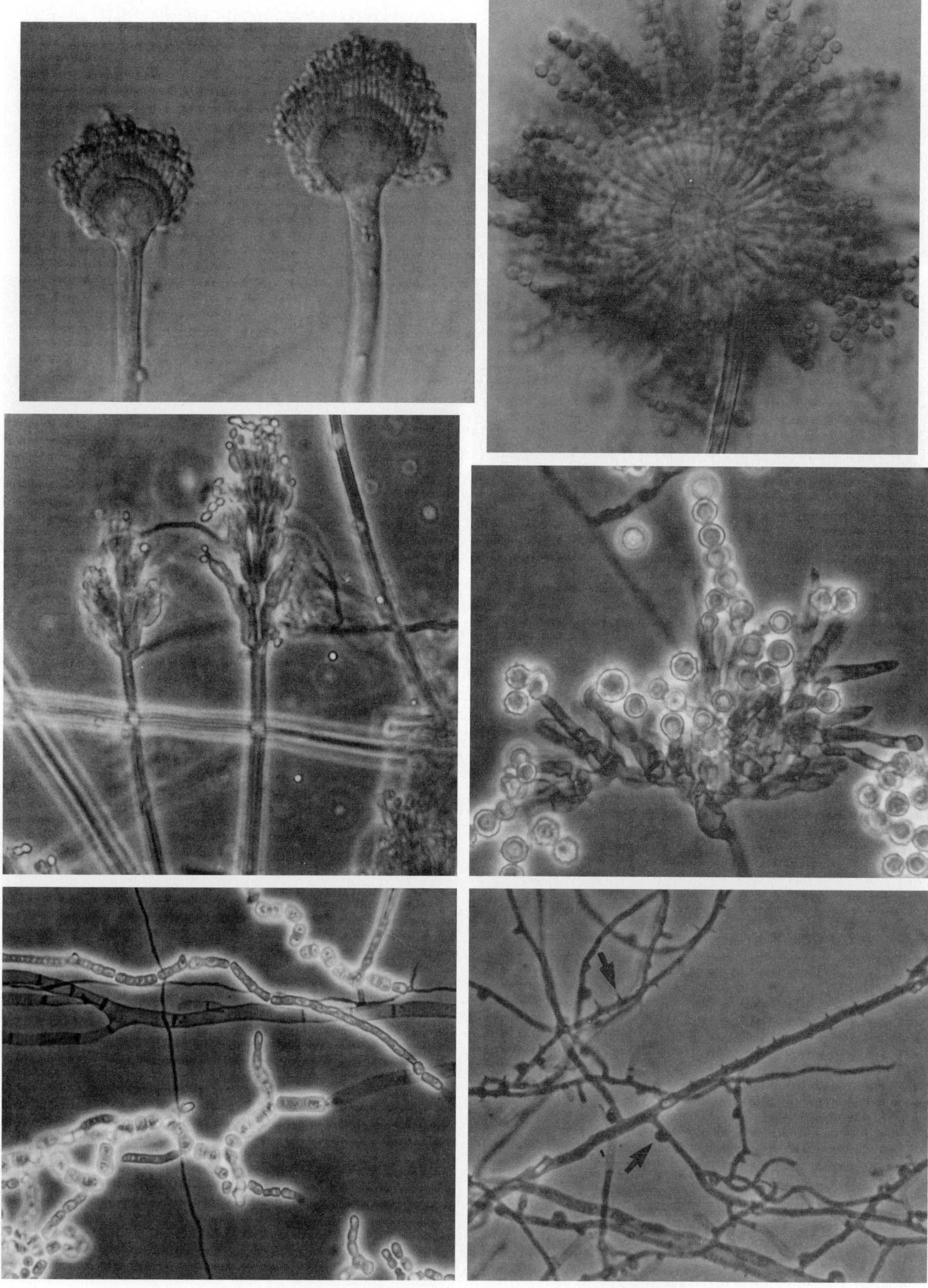

still necessary to establish the diagnosis, especially since aspergilli and *P. boydii* have been found to coexist in the same infection (136).

Scopulariopsis Species

Members of the genus *Scopulariopsis* are common soil fungi and agents of deterioration, especially of cellulosic substrates. The genus *Scopulariopsis* contains both brightly colored and dark species (103), some of which have teleomorphs in the genus *Microascus* of the Microascaceae (1, 32). Darkly pigmented species which form synnemata in culture are classified in the closely related genus *Cephalotrichum* (also known as *Doratomyces*). Of the 30 species known, only a few are reliably reported from human infections. Species causing onychomycosis include *Scopulariopsis brevicaulis*, by far the most important as both pathogen and regular contaminant, *Scopulariopsis candida, Microascus cirrosus* and *Microascus cinereus* (60); reports of onychomycosis concerning other species have not been validated. Like species of *Fusarium* and *Paecilomyces variotii, S. brevicaulis* may colonize necrotic tissue, but *Scopulariopsis* species are rarely invasive. *S. brevicaulis* has been recovered from otomycosis, keratitis, prosthetic valve endocarditis, subcutaneous tissue, and bone (66, 97, 123); *S. candida* caused invasive sinonasal infection (73); unidentified species were reported to cause pneumonia and invasive infection in leukemic patients (107, 189); and *S. brumptii* was isolated from lung nodules in an intravenous drug user with hypersensitivity pneumonitis (46). *M. cirrosus* and *M. cinereus* have caused invasive infection in immunosuppressed patients (74, 91), and the latter has been found together with *Aspergillus* in the lung and maxillary sinus (9, 82). *Scopulariopsis* species grow well on all laboratory media and are strongly or moderately resistant to cycloheximide. Dematiaceous *Scopulariopsis* species are difficult to identify, and a reference laboratory should be consulted. A recent report describes a new genus and species for a mould with features suggestive of a *Microascus* (129).

Scytalidium, Onychocola, and *Arthrographis* Species

Scytalidium hyalinum and *Scytalidium dimidiatum* are closely related fungi (102, 137) and are best known as agents of superficial infection, mainly causing onychomycosis of the toenails (see chapter 101 of this Manual) (60, 102). In tissue, hyphae of both species are hyaline, pale yellow, or, rarely, brown, in the case of *S. dimidiatum*. Although invasive infections are rare, a recent review (156) indicated that *S. hyalinum* has been the cause of subcutaneous infection in one patient, while *S. dimidiatum* was the cause of sinusitis, subcutaneous abscesses, mycetoma, facial lesions, endophthalmitis, or fungemia in nine patients with histories of diabetes, chronic obstructive lung disease, granulocytopenia, or immunosuppression. *S. dimidiatum* has also caused deep infection of the lymph node and toe in a patient with AIDS (92). A phialidic fungus was isolated from the sinus of the same patient and identified as *Lecythophora hoffmannii*; however, the isolate proved to be a species of *Phaeoacremonium*. Another arthroconidial hyphomycete rarely causing onychomycosis or infections of the glabrous skin is *Onychocola canadensis* (150). Described initially on the basis of 5 isolates from Canada, more than 30 human isolates of the fungus have been recorded from New Zealand, Australia, Europe, and the United Kingdom (148a). The thermotolerant arthroconidial fungus *Arthrographis kalrae* is a rare opportunist recovered from skin, lung, and a corneal ulcer (120, 151, 152). Because initial growth is often yeast-like, an isolate may not be recognized as a pleomorphic mould and may be subjected to tests commonly used for yeast identification.

Schizophyllum commune and Other Basidiomycetes

Allergic reactions due to inhalation of mushroom spores (54) and mycetismus due to the ingestion of mushrooms have frequently been reported, but the incidence of human infections by members of the Basidiomycotina is rare. Several reports have described the isolation of *Schizophillum commune* from various anatomical sites including brain, lung, hard and soft palate, and possibly nail in both immunocompetent and immunosuppressed patients (135, 149). The fungus is being recognized as a significant cause of allergic pathologies including sinusitis, allergic bronchopulmonary mycosis, and bronchial mucoid impaction, a type of hypersensitivity reaction to *S. commune* hyphae (6, 21, 149, 153, 154) (see also discussion under *Chrysosporium*). Hyphae in tissue are narrow (3 to 6 μm wide) or are broader (up to 10 μm) and somewhat irregular. The hyphae in tissue or culture may be recognized as belonging to a basidiomycete if clamp connections are present at the septa; if characteristic pegs or spicules are present, the hyphae are typical of *S. commune* (Fig. 23). However these structures may be absent and the hyphae then resemble those of *Aspergillus* species or other moulds (6, 149, 153) (Fig. 16). Antibody and antigen tests and *Aspergillus*-specific fluorescent-antibody staining have been recommended as aids in the differential diagnosis (135), and the identification of atypical isolates may require specialized techniques (153). Species of *Coprinus* also have been rarely implicated in invasive infection with evidence of hyphal filaments by histopathology. *Coprinus cinereus* or its anamorph *Hormographiella aspergillata* was the cause of a fatal lung infection in a leukemic patient and of endocarditis in a patient following valve replacement (66, 184). Some basidiomycetes and species of smuts (Ustilaginaceae, Tilletiaceae) are commonly isolated from respiratory specimens, and their significance is difficult to evaluate (149, 151). Repeat isolation and the presence of fila-

FIGURE 18 (top left) Uniseriate conidial heads of *Neosartorya fischeri* var. *spinosa*. Magnification, ×610.

FIGURE 19 (top right) Biseriate conidial head of *Aspergillus versicolor*. Magnification, ×770.

FIGURE 20 (middle left) Verticillate conidiophore of *Paecilomyces lilacinus* bearing whorls of phialides. Magnification, ×750.

FIGURE 21 (middle right) Rough-walled conidia in chains formed on annellides in *Scopulariopsis brevicaulis*. Note the branched conidiogenous apparatus. Magnification, ×580.

FIGURE 22 (bottom left) Hyphae dividing by schizolytic dehiscence to form arthroconidia in *Scytalidium hyalinum*. Magnification, ×460.

FIGURE 23 (bottom right) *Schizophyllum commune* in slide culture preparation showing clamp connections and narrow pegs or spicules. Magnification, ×580.

ments in sputum have implicated *Coprinus micaceus* and the thermotolerant *Sporotrichum pruinosum*, the anamorph of *Phanerochaete chrysosporium* (36, 67, 149), a species being investigated for its utility in biodegradation. *Tilletiopsis minor* caused subcutaneous infection in an immunosuppressed patient (130), but meningitis attributed to a species of *Ustilago* has not been confirmed (66).

REFERENCES

1. **Abbott, S. P., L. Sigler and R. S. Currah.** 1998. *Microascus brevicaulis* sp. nov., the teleomorph of *Scopulariopsis brevicaulis*, supports placement of *Scopulariopsis* with the Microascaceae. *Mycologia* **90:**297–302.
2. **Abbott, S. P., L. Sigler, R. McAleer, D. A. McGough, M. G. Rinaldi, and G. Mizell.** 1995. Fatal cerebral mycoses caused by the ascomycete *Chaetomium strumarium*. *J. Clin. Microbiol.* **33:**2692–2698.
3. **Ajello, L.** 1986. Hyalohyphomycosis and phaeohyphomycosis: two global disease entities of public health importance. *Eur. J. Epidemiol.* **2:**243–251.
4. **Ajello, L., A. A. Padhye, S. Sukroongreung, C. H. Nilakul, and S. Tantimavanic.** 1995. Occurrence of *Penicillium marneffei* infections among wild bamboo rats in Thailand. *Mycopathologia* **131:**1–8.
5. **Alvarez, S.** 1990. Systemic infection caused by *Penicillium decumbans* in a patient with acquired immunodeficiency syndrome. *J. Infect. Dis.* **162:**283.
6. **Amitani, R., K. Nishimura, A. Niimi, H. Kobayashi, R. Nawada, T. Murayama, H. Taguchi, and F. Kuze.** 1996. Bronchial mucoid impaction due to the monokaryotic mycelium of *Schizophyllum commune*. *Clin. Infect. Dis.* **22:**146–148.
7. **Andriole, V. T.** 1996. *Aspergillus* infections: problems in diagnosis and treatment. *Infect. Agents Dis.* **5:**47–54.
8. **Aufauvre-Brown, A., J. Cohen, and D. W. Holden.** 1992. Use of randomly amplified polymorphic DNA markers to distinguish isolates of *Aspergillus fumigatus*. *J. Clin. Microbiol.* **30:**2991–2993.
9. **Aznar, C., C. de Bievre, and C. Guiguen.** 1989. Maxillary sinusitis from *Microascus cinereus* and *Aspergillus repens*. *Mycopathologia* **105:**93–97.
10. **Batisse, D., M. Eliaszewicz, F. Dromer, O. Ronin, and B. Dupont.** 1997. *Aspergillus* antigen (AA) detection in the diagnosis of invasive aspergillosis in HIV-infected patients, abstr. D-127, p. 106. *In Program and Abstracts of the 37th Interscience Conference on Antimicrobial Agents and Chemotherapy*. American Society for Microbiology, Washington, D.C.
11. **Bedi, R. S.** 1994. Allergic bronchopulmonary aspergillosis: review of 20 cases. *Indian J. Chest Dis. Allied Sci.* **36:**181–186.
12. **Bir, N., A. Paliwal, K. Muralidhar, P. Reddy, and P. U. Sarma.** 1995. A rapid method for the isolation of genomic DNA from *Aspergillus fumigatus*. *Prep. Biochem.* **25:**171–181.
13. **Bodey, G. P., and S. Vartivarian.** 1989. Aspergillosis. *Eur. J. Clin. Infect. Dis.* **8:**413–437.
14. **Bourbeau, P., D. A. McGough, H. Fraser, N. Shah, and M. G. Rinaldi.** 1992. Fatal disseminated infection caused by *Myceliophthora thermophila*, a new agent of mycosis: case history and laboratory characteristics. *J. Clin. Microbiol.* **30:**3019–3023.
15. **Buffington, J., R. Reporter, B. A. Lasker, M. M. McNeil, J. M. Lanson, L. A. Ross, L. Mascola, and W. R. Jarvis.** 1994. Investigation of an epidemic of invasive aspergillosis: utility of molecular typing with the use of random amplified polymorphic DNA probes. *Pediatr. Infect. Dis. J.* **13:**386–393.
16. **Caillot, D., C. Durand, O. Casasnovas, J. F. Couaillier, A. Bernard, M. Buisson, E. Solary, A. Brachet, B. Cuisenier, and A. Bonnin.** 1995. Invasive pulmonary aspergillosis in neutropenic patients. Analysis of a series of 36 cases: contribution of thoracic scanners and itraconazole. *Ann. Med. Interne Paris* **146:**84–90.
17. **Castro, L. G. M., A. Salebian, and M. N. Sotto.** 1990. Hyalohyphomycosis by *Paecilomyces lilacinus* in a renal transplant patient and a review of human *Paecilomyces* species infections. *J. Med. Vet. Mycol.* **28:**15–26.
18. **Cepero de Garcia, M. C., M. L. Arboleda, F. Barraquer, and E. Grose.** 1997. Fungal keratitis caused by *Metarhizium anisopliae*. *J. Med. Vet. Mycol.* **35:**361–363.
19. **Chandler, F. W., and J. C. Watts.** 1987. *Pathologic Diagnosis of Fungal Infections*. American Society of Clinical Pathologists, Inc., Chicago, Ill.
20. **Chariyalertsak, S., P. Vanittanakom, K. E. Nelson, T. Sirishanthana, and N. Vanittanakom.** 1996. *Rhizomys sumatrensis* and *Cannomys badius*, new natural animal hosts of *Penicillium marneffei*. *J. Med. Vet. Mycol.* **34:**105–110.
21. **Clark, S., C. K. Campbell, A. Sandison, and D. I. Choa.** 1996. *Schizophyllum commune*: an unusual isolate from a patient with allergic fungal sinusitis. *J. Infect.* **32:**147–150.
22. **Crameri, R., J. Lidholm, G. Menz, H. Gronlund, and K. Blaser.** 1996. Automated serology with recombinant allergens. A feasibility study. *Adv. Exp. Med. Biol.* **409:**111–116.
23. **Crous, P. W., W. Gams, M. J. Wingfield, and P. S. van Wyk.** 1996. *Phaeoacremonium* gen. nov. associated with wilt and decline diseases of woody hosts and human infections. *Mycologia* **88:**786–796.
24. **Debeaupuis, J.-P., J. Sarfati, V. Chazalet, and J.-P. Latage.** 1997. Genetic diversity among clinical and environmental isolates of *Aspergillus fumigatus*. *Infect. Immun.* **65:**3080–3085.
25. **De Hoog, G. S., and J. Guarro.** 1995. *Atlas of Clinical Fungi*. Centraalbureau voor Schimmelcultures, Baarn, The Netherlands.
26. **De La Camara, R., I. Pinilla, E. Munoz, B. Buendia, J. L. Steegman, and J. M. Fernandez-Ranada.** 1996. *Penicillium brevicompactum* as the cause of necrotic lung ball in an allogenic bone marrow transplant patient. *Bone Marrow Transplant.* **18:**1189–1193.
27. **Denning, D. W., K. V. Clemons, L. H. Hanson, and D. A. Stevens.** 1990. Restriction endonuclease analysis of total cellular DNA of *Aspergillus fumigatus* isolates of geographically and epidemiologically diverse origin. *J. Infect. Dis.* **162:**1151–1158.
28. **Denning, D. W., S. E. Follansbee, M. Scolaro, S. Norris, H. Edelstein, and D. A. Stevens.** 1991. Pulmonary aspergillosis in the acquired immunodeficiency syndrome. *N. Engl. J. Med.* **324:**654–662.
29. **Denning, D. W., G. S. Shankland, and D. A. Stevens.** 1991. DNA fingerprinting of *Aspergillus fumigatus* isolates from patients with aspergilloma. *J. Med. Vet. Mycol.* **29:**339–342.
30. **Dharmasena, F. M., G. S. R. Davies, and D. Catovsky.** 1985. *Paecilomyces variotii* pneumonia complicating hairy cell leukemia. *Br. Med. J.* **290:**967–968.
31. **Disch, R., G. Menz, K. Blaser, and R. Crameri.** 1995. Different reactivity to recombinant *Aspergillus fumigatus* allergen I/a in patients with atopic dermatitis or allergic asthma sensitized to *Aspergillus fumigatus*. *Int. Arch. Allergy Immunol.* **108:**89–94.
32. **Domsch, K. H., W. Gams, and T.-H. Anderson.** 1980. *Compendium of Soil Fungi*. IHW-Verlag, Eching, Germany. (Reprinted in 1993.)

33. **Duong, T. A.** 1996. Infection due to *Penicillium marneffei*, an emerging pathogen: review of 155 reported cases. *Clin. Infect. Dis.* **23:**125–130.
34. **Echavarria, E., E. L. Cano, and A. Restrepo.** 1993. Disseminated adiaspiromycosis in a patient with AIDS. *J. Med. Vet. Mycol.* **31:**91–97.
35. **Einsele, H., H. Hebart, G. Roller, J. Loffler, I. Rothenbofer, C. A. Muller, R. A. Bowden, J. Van Burik, D. Engelhard, L. Kanz, and U. Schumacher.** 1997. Detection and identification of fungal pathogens in blood using molecular probes. *J. Clin. Microbiol.* **35:**1353–1360.
36. **Emmons, C. W.** 1954. Isolation of *Myxotrichum* and *Gymnoascus* from lungs of animals. *Mycologia* **46:**334–338.
37. **Frelier, P. F., L. Sigler, and P. E. Nelson.** 1985. Mycotic pneumonia caused by *Fusarium moniliforme* in an alligator. *J. Med. Vet. Mycol.* **23:**399–402.
38. **Fujita, S., M. Hasegawa, N. Shintani, and S. Koizumi.** 1995. Fluctuations in serum antigens and antibodies in a patient with primary cutaneous aspergillosis associated with acute leukemia. *Kansenshogaku Zasshi* **69:**218–222.
39. **Gams, W., and M. R. McGinnis.** 1983. *Phialemonium*, a new anamorphic genus intermediate between *Phialophora* and *Acremonium*. *Mycologia* **75:**977–987.
40. **Gelfand, M. S., F. Hammond Cole, Jr., and R. C. Baskin.** 1990. Invasive pulmonary penicilliosis: successful therapy with amphotericin B. *South. Med. J.* **83:**701–704.
41. **Girardin, H., J.-P. Latage, T. Srikantha, B. Morrow, and D. R. Soll.** 1993. Development of DNA probes for fingerprinting *Aspergillus fumigatus*. *J. Clin. Microbiol.* **31:** 1547–1554.
42. **Girardin, H., J. Sarfati, F. Traore, J. Dupouy-Camet, F. Derouin, and J. P. Latge.** 1994. Molecular epidemiology of nosocomial invasive aspergillosis. *J. Clin. Microbiol.* **32:** 684–690.
43. **Goodwin, S. D., J. Fiedler-Kelly, T. H. Grasela, W. A. Schell, and J. R. Perfect.** 1992. A nationwide survey of clinical laboratory methodologies for fungal infections. *J. Med. Vet. Mycol.* **30:**153–160.
44. **Gradon, J. D., J. G. Timpone, and S. M. Schnittman.** 1992. Emergence of unusual opportunistic pathogens in AIDS: a review. *Clin. Infect. Dis.* **15:**134–157.
45. **Greuter, W.** 1993. NCU-2. *Names in Current Use in the families Trichocomaceae, Cladoniaceae, Pinaceae and Lemnaceae.* Koeltz Scientific Books, Konigstein, Germany.
46. **Grieble, H. G., J. W. Rippon, N. Maliwan, and V. Daun.** 1975. *Scopulariopsis* and hypersensitivity pneumonitis in an addict. *Ann. Intern. Med.* **83:**326–329.
47. **Griffin, T. D., J. P. McFarland, and W. C. Johnson.** 1991. Hyalohyphomycosis masquerading as squamous cell carcinoma. *J. Cutan. Pathol.* **18:**116–119.
48. **Guarro, J., and J. Gene.** 1995. Opportunistic fusarial infections in humans. *Eur. J. Clin. Microbiol. Infect. Dis.* **14:** 741–754.
49. **Guarro, J., L. Soler, and M. G. Rinaldi.** 1995. Pathogenicity and antifungal susceptibility of *Chaetomium* species. *Eur. J. Clin. Microbiol. Infect. Dis.* **14:**613–618.
50. **Haynes, K. A., P. Tuinstra, T. A. Hughes, L. M. Wijnands, T. R. Rogers, and A. K. Allen.** 1996. Purification and characterization of a 93 kDa *Aspergillus fumigatus* antigen with diagnostic potential. *J. Med. Vet. Mycol.* **34:** 421–426.
51. **Haynes, K. A., J. P. Latge, and T. R. Rogers.** 1990. Detection of *Aspergillus* antigens associated with invasive infection. *J. Clin. Microbiol.* **28:**2040–2044.
52. **Hetherington, S. V., S. Henwick, D. M. Parham, and C. C. Patrick.** 1994. Monoclonal antibodies against a 97-kilodalton antigen from *Aspergillus flavus*. *Clin. Diagn. Lab. Immunol.* **1:**63–67.
53. **Hopwood, V., E. M. Johnson, J. M. Cornish, A. B. Foot, E. G. Evans, and D. W. Warnock.** 1995. Use of the Pastorex *Aspergillus* antigen latex agglutination test for the diagnosis of invasive aspergillosis. *J. Clin. Pathol.* **48:** 210–213.
54. **Horner, W. E., A. Helbling, J. E. Salvaggio, and S. B. Lehrer.** 1995. Fungal allergens. *Clin. Microbiol. Rev.* **8:** 161–179.
55. **Jang, S. S., T. E. Dorr, E. L. Biberstein, and A. Wong.** 1986. *Aspergillus deflectus* infection in four dogs. *J. Med. Vet. Mycol.* **24:**95–104.
56. **Jensen, H. E., D. Stynen, J. Sarfati, and J. P. Latge.** 1993. Detection of galactomannan and the 18 kDa antigen from *Aspergillus fumigatus* in serum and urine from cattle with systemic aspergillosis. *Zentralbl. Veterinarmed. B* **40:** 397–408.
57. **Johnson, T. M., V. P. Kurup, A. Resnick, R. C. Ash, J. N. Fink, and J. Kalbfleisch.** 1989. Detection of circulating *Aspergillus fumigatus* antigen in bone marrow transplant patients. *J. Clin. Lab. Med.* **114:**700–707.
58. **Kalish, S. B., and R. Goldschmidt.** 1982. Infective endocarditis caused by *Paecilomyces variotii*. *J. Clin. Pathol.* **78:** 249–252.
59. **Kanda, Y., H. Akiyama, Y. Onozawa, T. Motegi, S. Yamagata-Murayama, and H. Yamaguchi.** 1997. *Aspergillus* endocarditis in a leukemia patient diagnosed by a PCR assay. *Kansenshogaku Zasshi* **71:**269–272.
60. **Kane, J., R. Summerbell, L. Sigler, S. Krajden, and G. Land.** 1997. *Laboratory Handbook of Dermatophytes*. Star Publishing Company, Belmont, Calif.
61. **Kappe, R., A. Schulze-Berge, and H. G. Sonntag.** 1996. Evaluation of eight antibody tests and one antigen test for the diagnosis of invasive aspergillosis. *Mycoses* **39:**13–23.
62. **Kaufman, L., P. G. Standard, S. A. Anderson, M. Jalbert, and B. L. Swisher.** 1995. Development of specific fluorescent-antibody test for tissue form of *Penicillium marneffei*. *J. Clin. Microbiol.* **33:**2136–2138.
63. **Kaufman, L., P. G. Standard, M. Jalbert, and D. Kraft.** 1997. Immunohistologic identification of *Aspergillus* spp. and other hyaline fungi by using polyclonal fluorescent antibodies. *J. Clin. Microbiol.* **35:**2206–2209.
64. **Kaufman, L., P. G. Standard, M. Jalbert, P. Kantipong, K. Kimpakarnjanarat, and T. D. Mastro.** 1996. Diagnostic antigenemia tests for penicilliosis marneffei. *J. Clin. Microbiol.* **34:**2503–2505.
65. **Kaukonen, K., J. Savolainen, M. Nermes, M. Viander, and E. O. Terho.** 1997. IgE antibody response against *Aspergillus umbrosus* in farmer's lung disease. *Int. Arch. Allergy Immunol.* **112:**313–316.
66. **Kennedy, M. J., and L. Sigler.** 1995. *Aspergillus, Fusarium* and other moniliaceous fungi, p. 765–790. *In* P. R. Murray, E. J. Baron, M. A. Pfaller, F. C. Tenover, and R. H. Yolken (ed.), *Manual of Clinical Microbiology*, 6th ed. American Society for Microbiology, Washington, D.C.
67. **Khan, Z. U., H. S. Randhawa, T. Kowshik, S. N. Gaur, and G. A. de Vries.** 1988. The pathogenic potential of *Sporotrichum pruinosum* isolated from the human respiratory tract. *J. Med. Vet. Mycol.* **26:**145–151.
68. **Kimura, M., S. I. Udagawa, A. Shoji, H. Kume, M. Iimori, T. Satou, and S. Hashimoto.** 1990. Pulmonary aspergillosis due to *Aspergillus terreus* combined with staphylococcal pneumonia and hepatic candidiasis. *Mycopathologia* **111:**47–53.
69. **Klich, M. A., and J. I. Pitt.** 1988. *A Laboratory Guide to Common Aspergillus Species and Their Teleomorphs*. Commonwealth Scientific and Industrial Research Organization, North Ryde, Australia.
70. **Knight, F., and D. W. R. Mackenzie.** 1992. *Aspergillus* antigen latex test for diagnosis of invasive aspergillosis. *Lancet* **339:**188.

71. **Knutsen, A. P., P. S. Hutcheson, K. R. Mueller, and R. G. Slavin.** 1990. Serum immuno-globulins E and G anti-*Aspergillus fumigatus* antibody in patients with cystic fibrosis who have allergic bronchopulmonary aspergillosis. *J. Lab. Clin. Med.* **116:**724–727.

71a. **Kornerup, A., and J. H. Wanscher.** 1983. *Methuen Handbook of Colour.* Eyre Methuen Ltd., London, United Kingdom.

72. **Krasnick, J., R. Patterson, and M. Roberts.** 1995. Allergic bronchopulmonary aspergillosis presenting with cough variant asthma and identifiable source of *Aspergillus fumigatus. Ann. Allergy Asthma Immunol.* **75:**344–346.

73. **Kriesel, J. D., E. E. Adderson, W. M. Gooch III, and A. T. Pavia.** 1994. Invasive sinonasal disease due to *Scopulariopsis candida*: case report and review of *Scopulariopsis. Clin. Infect. Dis.* **19:**317–319.

74. **Krisher, K. K., N. B. Holdridge, M. M. Mustafa, M. G. Rinaldi, and D. A. McGough.** 1995. Disseminated *Microascus cirrosus* infection in a pediatric bone marrow transplant patient. *J. Clin. Microbiol.* **33:**735–737.

75. **Krulder, J. W., R. W. Brimicombe, P. W. Wijermans, and W. Gams.** 1996. Systemic *Fusarium nygamai* infection in a patient with lymphoblastic non-Hodgkin's lymphoma. *Mycoses* **39:**121–123.

76. **Kurup, V. P.** 1986. Enzyme-linked immunosorbent assay in the detection of specific antibodies against *Aspergillus* in patient sera. *Zentralbl. Bakteriol. Mikrobiol. Hyg. Reihe A* **261:**509–516.

77. **Kurup, V. P.** 1988. Production and characterization of a murine monoclonal antibody to *Aspergillus fumigatus* antigen having IgG- and IgE-binding activity. *Int. Arch. Allergy Appl. Immunol.* **86:**400–406.

78. **Kurup, V. P., and A. Kumar.** 1991. Immunodiagnosis of aspergillosis. *Clin. Microbiol. Rev.* **4:**439–456.

79. **Kurup, V. P., M. Ramasamy, P. A. Greenberger, and J. N. Fink.** 1988. Isolation and characterization of a relevant *Aspergillus fumigatus* antigen with IgG and IgE binding activity. *Int. Arch. Allergy Appl. Immunol.* **86:**176–182.

80. **Kwon-Chung, K. J., and J. E. Bennett.** 1992. *Medical Mycology.* Lea & Febiger, Philadelphia, Pa.

81. **Kwon-Chung, K. J., W. B. Hill, and J. E. Bennett.** 1981. New, special stain for histopathological diagnosis of Cryptococcosis. *J. Clin. Microbiol.* **13:**383–387.

82. **Lacey, J.** 1986. *Microascus cinereus* (Emile-Weil & Gaudin) Curzi: a human pathogen? *Mycopathologia* **96:**137–142.

83. **Larone, D.** 1995. *Medically Important Fungi,* 3rd ed. American Society for Microbiology, Washington, D.C.

84. **Leenders, A., A. Van Belkum, S. Janssen, S. De Marie, J. Kluytmans, J. Wielenga, B. Lowenberg, and H. Verbrugh.** 1996. Molecular epidemiology of apparent outbreak of invasive aspergillosis in a hematology ward. *J. Clin. Microbiol.* **34:**345–351.

85. **Levy, F. E., J. T. Larson, E. George, and R. H. Maisel.** 1991. Invasive *Chrysosporium* infection of the nose and paranasal sinuses in an immunocompromised host. *Otolaryngol. Head Neck Surg.* **104:**384–388.

86. **Lin, D. M., P. F. Lehmann, B. H. Hamory, A. A. Padhye, E. Durry, R. W. Pinner, and B. A. Lasker.** 1995. Comparison of three typing methods for clinical and environmental isolates of *Aspergillus fumigatus. J. Clin. Microbiol.* **33:**1596–1601.

87. **LoBuglio, K. F., and J. W. Taylor.** 1995. Phylogeny and PCR identification of the human pathogenic fungus *Penicillium marneffei. J. Clin. Microbiol.* **33:**85–89.

88. **Loudon, K. W., J. P. Burnie, A. P. Coke, and R. C. Matthews.** 1993. Application of polymerase chain reaction to fingerprinting *Aspergillus fumigatus* by random amplification of polymorphic DNA. *J. Clin. Microbiol.* **31:**1117–1121.

89. **Manso, E., M. Montillo, G. DeSio, S. D'Amico, G. Discepoli, and P. Leoni.** 1994. Value of antigen and antibody detection in the serological diagnosis of invasive aspergillosis in patients with hematological malignancies. *Eur. J. Clin. Microbiol. Infect. Dis.* **13:**756–760.

90. **Maran, A. G. D., K. Kwong, L. J. R. Milne, and D. Lamb.** 1985. Frontal sinusitis caused by *Myriodontium keratinophilum. Br. Med. J.* **290:**207.

91. **Marques, A. R., K. J. Kwon-Chung, S. M. Holland, M. L. Turner, and J. I. Gallin.** 1995. Suppurative cutaneous granulomata caused by *Microascus cinereus* in a patient with chronic granulomatous diseases. *Clin. Infect. Dis.* **20:**110–114.

92. **Marriott, D. J., K. H. Wong, E. Azner, J. L. Harkness, D. A. Cooper, and D. Muir.** 1997. *Scytalidium dimidiatum* and *Lecythophora hoffmannii*: unusual causes of fungal infections in patients with AIDS. *J. Clin. Microbiol.* **35:**2949–2952.

93. **Martino, P., R. Gastaldi, R. Raccah, and C. Girmania.** 1994. Clinical patterns of *Fusarium* infections in immunocompromised patients. *J. Infect.* **28**(Suppl. 1)**:**7–15.

94. **Marzec, A., L. G. Heron, R. C. Pritchard, R. H. Butcher, H. R. Powell, A. P. S. Disney, and F. A. Tosolini.** 1993. *Paecilomyces variotii* in peritoneal dialysate. *J. Clin. Microbiol.* **31:**2392–2395.

95. **McDonnell, P. J., T. P. Werblin, L. Sigler, and W. R. Green.** 1985. Mycotic keratitis due to *Beauveria alba. Cornea* **3:**213–216.

96. **Meyohas, M. C., P. Roux, J. L. Poirot, J. L. Meynard, and J. Frottier.** 1994. Aspergillosis in acquired immunodeficiency syndrome. *Pathol. Biol. Paris* **42:**647–651.

97. **Migrino, R. Q., G. S. Hall, and D. L. Longworth.** 1995. Deep tissue infections caused by *Scopulariopsis brevicaulis*: report of a case of prosthetic valve endocarditis and review. *Clin. Infect. Dis.* **21:**672–674.

98. **Miller, W. T.** 1996. Aspergillosis: a disease with many faces. *Semin. Roentgenol.* **31:**52–66.

99. **Mok, T., A. P. Koehler, M. Y. Yu, D. H. Ellis, P. J. Johnson, and N. W. R. Wickham.** 1997. Fatal *Penicillium citrinum* pneumonia with pericarditis in a patient with acute leukemia. *J. Clin. Microbiol.* **35:**2654–2656.

100. **Mondon, P., M. P. Brenier, E. Coursange, B. Lebeau, P. Ambroise-Thomas, and R. Grillot.** 1997. Molecular typing of *Aspergillus fumigatus* strains by sequence-specific DNA primer (SSDP) analysis. *FEMS Immunol. Med. Microbiol.* **17:**95–102.

101. **Moody, S. F., and B. M. Tyler.** 1990. Use of nuclear DNA restriction fragment length polymorphisms to analyze the diversity of the *Aspergillus flavus* group: *A. flavus, A. parasiticus,* and *A. nomius. Appl. Environ. Microbiol.* **56:**2453–2461.

102. **Moore, M. K.** 1992. The infection of human skin and nail by *Scytalidium* species, p. 1–42. *In* M. Borgers, R. Hay, and M. G. Rinaldi (ed.), *Current Topics in Medical Mycology.* Springer-Verlag, New York, N.Y.

103. **Morton, F. J., and G. Smith.** 1963. The genera *Scopulariopsis* Bainier, *Microascus* Zukal, and *Doratomyces* Corda. *In Mycological Papers No.* 86. Commonwealth Mycological Institute, Kew, Surrey, England.

104. **Moser, M., R. Crameri, E. Brust, M. Suter, and G. Menz.** 1994. Diagnostic value of recombinant *Aspergillus fumigatus* allergen I/a for skin testing and serology. *J. Allergy Clin. Immunol.* **93:**1–11.

105. **Musial, C. A., F. R. Cockerill III, and G. D. Roberts.** 1988. Fungal infections of the immunocompromised host: clinical and laboratory aspects. *Clin. Microbiol. Rev.* **1:**349–364.

106. **National Institute of Allergy and Infectious Diseases.** 1994. *NIAID Workshop on Molecular and Immunologic Ap-*

proaches to the Diagnosis and Treatment of Systemic Mycoses: Summary. National Institute of Allergy and Infectious Diseases, Bethesda, Md.

107. **Neglia, J. P., D. D. Hurd, P. Ferrieri, and D. C. Snover.** 1987. Invasive *Scopulariopsis* in the immunocompromised host. *Am. J. Med.* **83:**1163–1166.
108. **Nelson, P. E., M. C. Dignani, and E. J. Anaissie.** 1994. Taxonomy, biology and clinical aspects of *Fusarium* species. *Clin. Microbiol. Rev.* **7:**479–504.
109. **Nelson, P. E., T. A. Toussoun, and W. F. O. Marasas.** 1983. Fusarium *Species: an Illustrated Manual of Identification*. Pennsylvania State University Press, State College.
110. **Niki, Y.** 1996. Sero-diagnosis for pulmonary aspergillosis—its utility in early diagnosis. *Rinsho Byori* **44:** 518–523.
111. **Niki, Y., K. Hashiguchi, and R. Soejima.** 1994. Invasive pulmonary aspergillosis diagnosed by antigen detection in urine. *Chest* **105:**1304. (Letter.)
112. **Niki, Y., K. Hashiguchi, S. Tamada, K. Yoshida, S. Sugimura, M. Nakajima, O. Moriya, N. Okimoto, and R. Soejima.** 1994. A case of *Aspergillus niger* pneumonia cured with an early diagnosis. *Kansenshogaku Zasshi* **68:** 788–791.
113. **Odds, F., T. Arai, A. F. DiSalvo, E. G. V. Evans, R. J. Hay, H. S. Randhawa, M. G. Rinaldi, and T. J. Walsh.** 1992. Nomenclature of fungal diseases: a report and recommendations from a subcommittee of the International Society for Human and Animal Mycology (ISHAM). *J. Med. Vet. Mycol.* **30:**1–10.
114. **Ohgoe, K., S. Miyanishi, M. Aihara, and S. Matsuo.** 1997. Significance of *Aspergillus fumigatus* rDNA detected by polymerase chain reaction in diagnosis of pulmonary aspergillosis. *Kansenshogaku Zasshi* **71:**507–512.
115. **Onions, A. H. S., D. Allsopp, and H. O. W. Eggins.** 1981. *Smith's Introduction to Industrial Mycology*. Edward Arnold, London, United Kingdom.
116. **Orth, B., R. Frei, P. H. Itin, M. G. Rinaldi, B. Speck, A. Gratwohl, and A. F. Widmer.** 1996. Outbreak of invasive mycoses caused by *Paecilomyces lilacinus* from a contaminated skin lotion. *Ann. Intern. Med.* **125:**799–806.
117. **Park, H. S., K. S. Jung, S. O. Kim, and S. J. Kim.** 1994. Hypersensitivity pneumonitis induced by *Penicillium expansum* in a home environment. *Clin. Exp. Allergy* **24:** 383–385.
118. **Patterson, T. F., P. Miniter, J. E. Patterson, J. M. Rappeport, and V. T. Andriole.** 1995. *Aspergillus* antigen detection in the diagnosis of invasive aspergillosis. *J. Infect. Dis.* **171:**1553–1558.
119. **Perfect, J. R., and W. A. Schell.** 1996. The new fungal opportunists are coming. *Clin. Infect. Dis.* **22:**(Suppl. 2): S112–S118.
120. **Perlman, E. M., and L. Binns.** 1997. Intense photophobia caused by *Arthrographis kalrae* in a contact lens wearing patient. *Am. J. Ophthalmol.* **123:**547–549.
121. **Persat, F., M. Gari-Toussaint, B. Lebeau, M. Cambon, H. Raberin, A. Addo, S. Picot, M. A. Piens, A. Blancard, M. Mallie, J. M. Bastide, and R. Grillot.** 1996. Specific antibody detection in human aspergillosis: a GEMO (Group d'Etude des Mycoses Opportunistes) multicentre evaluation of a rapid immunoelectrophoresis method (Paragon). *Mycoses* **39:**427–432.
122. **Peterson, S. W.** 1992. *Neosartorya pseudofischeri* sp. nov. and its relationship to other species in *Aspergillus* section *Fumigati*. *Mycol. Res.* **96:**547–554.
123. **Phillips, P., W. S. Wood, G. Phillips, and M. G. Rinaldi.** 1989. Invasive hyalohyphomycosis caused by *Scopulariopsis brevicaulis* in a patient undergoing allogenic bone marrow transplant. *Diagn. Microbiol. Infect. Dis.* **12:** 429–432.
124. **Pierard, G. E., J. Arrese-Estrada, C. Pierard-Franchimont, A. Thiry, and D. Stynen.** 1991. Immunohistochemical expression of galactomannan in the cytoplasm of phagocytic cells during invasive aspergillosis. *Am. J. Clin. Pathol.* **96:**373–376.
125. **Pitt, J. I.** 1979. *The Genus* Penicillium *and Its Teleomorphic States* Eupenicillium *and* Talaromyces. Academic Press, London, United Kingdom.
126. **Pitt, J. I.** 1988. *A Laboratory Guide to Common Penicillium Species*, 2nd ed. Commonwealth Scientific and Industrial Research Organisation, North Ryde, Australia.
127. **Polachek, I., A. Nagler, E. Okon, P. Drakos, J. Plaskowitz, and K. J. Kwon-Chung.** 1992. *Aspergillus quadrilineatus*, a new causative agent of fungal sinusitis. *J. Clin. Microbiol.* **30:**3290–3293.
128. **Prins, C., P. Chavez, K. Tamm, and C. Hauser.** 1995. Ecthyma gangrenosum-like lesions: a sign of disseminated *Fusarium* infection in the neutropenic patient. *Clin. Exp. Dermatol.* **20:**428–430.
129. **Rajendran, C.** 1997. *Ascosubramania* gen. nov., and its *Fonsecaea*-like anamorph causing chromoblastomycosis in India. *J. Med. Vet. Mycol.* **35:**335–339.
130. **Ramani, R., R. T. Kahn, and V. Chaturvedi.** 1997. *Tilletiopsis minor*: a new etiologic agent of human subcutaneous mycosis in an immunocompromised patient. *J. Clin. Microbiol.* **35:**2992–2995.
131. **Raper, K. B., and D. I. Fennell.** 1965. *The Genus* Aspergillus. The Williams & Wilkins Co., Baltimore, Md.
132. **Rath, P. M., R. Oeffelke, K. D. Muller, and R. Ansorg.** 1996. Non-value of *Aspergillus* antigen detection in bronchoalveolar lavage fluids of patients undergoing bone marrow transplantation. *Mycoses* **39:**367–370.
133. **Richardson, M. D.** 1998. *Aspergillus* and *Penicillium* species, p. 281–312. *In* L. Ajello and R. Hay (ed.), *Topley & Wilson's Microbiology and Microbial Infections*, 9th ed., vol. 4. Edward Arnold, London, United Kingdom.
134. **Richardson, S. E., R. M. Bannatyne, R. C. Summerbell, J. Milliken, R. Gold, and S. S. Weitzman.** 1988. Disseminated fusarial infection in the immunocompromised host. *Rev. Infect. Dis.* **10:**1171–1181.
135. **Rihs, J. D., A. A. Padhye, and C. B. Good.** 1996. Brain abscess caused by *Schizophyllum commune*: an emerging basidiomycete pathogen. *J. Clin. Microbiol.* **34:**1628–1632.
136. **Rippon, J. W.** 1988. *Medical Mycology: The Pathogenic Fungi and the Pathogenic Actinomycetes*, 3rd ed. The W.B. Saunders Co., Philadelphia, Pa.
137. **Roeijmans, H. J., G. S. De Hoog, C. S. Tan, and M. J. Figge.** 1997. Molecular taxonomy and GC/MS of metabolites of *Scytalidium hyalinum* and *Nattrassia mangiferae* (*Hendersonula toruloidea*). *J. Med. Vet. Mycol.* **35:**181–188.
138. **Sachs, S. W., J. Baum, and C. Mies.** 1985. *Beauveria bassiana* keratitis. *Br. J. Ophthalmol.* **69:**548–550.
139. **Samson, R. A.** 1974. *Paecilomyces* and some allied hyphomycetes. *Studies Mycol.* **6:**1–117.
140. **Schell, W. A., and J. R. Perfect.** 1996. Fatal, disseminated *Acremonium strictum* infection in a neutropenic host. *J. Clin. Microbiol.* **34:**1333–1336.
141. **Schonheyder, H.** 1987. Pathogenic and serological aspects of pulmonary aspergillosis. *Scand. J. Infect. Dis. Suppl.* **51:**1–62.
142. **Segretain, G.** 1959. *Penicillium marneffei* n. sp. agent d'une mycose du systeme reticuloendothelial. *Mycopathologia* **11:**327–353.
143. **Sekhon, A. S., J. S. K. Li, and A. K. Garg.** 1982. Penicilliosis marneffei: serological and exoantigen studies. *Mycopathologia* **77:**51–57.
144. **Sekhon, A. S., P. G. Standard, L. Kaufman, A. K. Garg,**

and P. Cifuentes. 1986. Grouping of *Aspergillus* species with exoantigens. *Diagn. Immunol.* **4:**112–116.

145. **Severo, L. C., G. R. Geyer, N. da Silvo Porto, M. B. Wagner, and A. T. Londero.** 1997. Pulmonary *Aspergillus niger* intracavitary colonization. Report of 23 cases and a review of the literature. *Rev. Iberoam. Micol.* **14:**104–110.
146. **Sigler, L.** 1993. Perspectives on Onygenales and their anamorphs by a traditional taxonomist, p. 161–168. *In* D. R. Reynolds and J. W. Taylor (ed.), *The Fungal Holomorph: a Consideration of Mitotic, Meiotic and Pleomorphic Speciation.* CAB International, Wallingford, United Kingdom.
147. **Sigler, L.** 1996. *Ajellomyces crescens* sp. nov., taxonomy of *Emmonsia* species, and relatedness with *Blastomyces dermatitidis* (teleomorph *Ajellomyces dermatitidis*). *J. Med. Vet. Mycol.* **34:**303–314.
148. **Sigler, L.** 1998. Agents of adiaspiromycosis, p. 571–583. *In* L. Ajello and R. Hay (ed.), *Topley & Wilson's Microbiology and Microbial Infections,* 9th ed., vol. 4. Edward Arnold, London, United Kingdom.

148a. **Sigler, L.** Unpublished data.

149. **Sigler, L., and S. P. Abbott.** 1997. Characterizing and conserving diversity of filamentous basidiomycetes from human sources. *Microbiol. Cult. Coll.* **13:**21–27.
150. **Sigler, L., S. P. Abbott, and A. Woodgyer.** 1994. New records of nail and skin infection due to *Onychocola canadensis* and description of its teleomorph *Arachnomyces nodosetosus* sp. nov. *J. Med. Vet. Mycol.* **32:**275–285.
151. **Sigler, L., and J. W. Carmichael.** 1976. Taxonomy of *Malbranchea* and some other Hyphomycetes with arthroconidia. *Mycotaxon* **4:**349–488.
152. **Sigler, L., and J. W. Carmichael.** 1983. Redisposition of some fungi referred to *Oidium microspermum* and a review of *Arthrographis*. *Mycotaxon* **18:**495–507.
153. **Sigler, L., L. De La Maza, G. Tan, K. N. Egger, and R. K. Sherburne.** 1995. Diagnostic difficulties caused by a nonclamped *Schizophyllum commune* isolate in a case of fungus ball of the lung. *J. Clin. Microbiol.* **33:**1979–1983.
154. **Sigler, L., S. Estrada, N. A. Montealegre, E. Jaramillo, M. Arango, C. De Bedout, and A. Restrepo.** 1997. Maxillary sinusitis caused by *Schizophyllum commune* and experience with treatment. *J. Med. Vet. Mycol.* **35:**365–370.
155. **Sigler, L., J. L. Harris, D. M. Dixon, A. L. Flis, I. R. Salkin, M. Kemna, and R. M. Duncan.** 1990. Microbiology and potential virulence of *Sporothrix cyanescens*, a fungus rarely isolated from blood and skin. *J. Clin. Microbiol.* **28:**1009–1015.
156. **Sigler, L., R. C. Summerbell, L. Poole, M. Wieden, D. A. Sutton, M. G. Rinaldi, M. Aguirre, G. W. Estes, and J. N. Galgiani.** 1997. Invasive *Nattrassia mangiferae* infections: case report, literature review, therapeutic and taxonomic appraisal. *J. Clin. Microbiol.* **35:**433–440.
157. **Sigler, L., M. A. Viviani, U. Magrini, R. Epis, V. Fregoni, A. Grancini, and A. Pastorini.** 1997. Systemic lymphonodal aspergillosis in an immunocompetent male: a case of difficult diagnosis caused by an atypical isolate, abstr. P396. *In Abstracts of the International Society for Human and Animal Mycology.*
158. **Simon, G., G. Rakoczy, J. Galgoczy, T. Verebely, and J. Bokay.** 1991. *Acremonium kiliense* in oesophagus stenosis. *Mycoses* **34:**257–260.
159. **Spreadbury, C., D. Holden, A. Aufauvre-Brown, B. Bainbridge, and J. Cohen.** 1993. Detection of *Aspergillus fumigatus* by polymerase chain reaction. *J. Clin. Microbiol.* **31:**615–621.
160. **Spreadbury, C. L., B. W. Bainbridge, and J. Cohen.** 1990. Restriction fragment length polymorphisms in isolates of *Aspergillus fumigatus* probed with part of the intergenic spacer region from the ribosomal RNA gene complex of *Aspergillus nidulans*. *J. Gen. Microbiol.* **136:**1991–1994.
161. **Starr, M. B.** 1987. *Paecilomyces lilacinus* keratitis: two case reports in extended wear contact lens wearers. *CLAO J.* **13:**95–101.
162. **St.-Germain, G., and R. Summerbell.** 1996. *Identifying Filamentous Fungi.* Star Publishing Co., Belmont, Calif.
163. **Stillwell, W. T., B. D. Rubin, and J. L. Axelrod.** 1984. *Chrysosporium*, a new causative agent in osteomyelitis. *Orthopedics* **184:**190–192.
164. **Stimlan, C. V., D. E. Dines, R. F. Rodgers-Sullivan, G. D. Roberts, and W. C. Sheehan.** 1980. Respiratory tract *Aspergillus*—clinical significance. *Minn. Med.* **63:**25–30.
165. **Stynen, D.** 1994. Specific antigens and antibodies in invasive aspergillosis. *Pathol. Biol. Paris* **42:**683–687.
166. **Summerbell, R. C., L. de Repentigny, C. Chartrand, and G. St.-Germain.** 1992. Graft-related endocarditis caused by *Neosartorya fischeri* var. *spinosa*. *J. Clin. Microbiol.* **30:**1580–1582.
167. **Summerbell, R. C., S. Krajden, and J. Kane.** 1989. Potted plants in hospitals as reservoirs of pathogenic fungi. *Mycopathologia* **106:**13–22.
168. **Summerbell, R. C., S. E. Richardson, and J. Kane.** 1988. *Fusarium proliferatum* as an agent of disseminated infection in an immunocompromised patient. *J. Clin. Microbiol.* **26:**82–87.
169. **Szombathy, S. P., M. G. Chez, and R. M. Laxer.** 1988. Acute septic arthritis due to *Acremonium*. *J. Rheumatol.* **15:**714–715.
170. **Talbot, G. H., M. H. Weiner, S. L. Gerson, M. Provencher, and S. Hurwitz.** 1987. Sero-diagnosis of invasive aspergillosis in patients with hematologic malignancy: validation of the *Aspergillus fumigatus* antigen radioimmunoassay. *J. Infect. Dis.* **155:**12–27.
171. **Tambini, R., C. Farina, R. Fiocchi, B. Dupont, E. Gueho, G. Delvecchio, F. Mamprin, and G. Gavezzeni.** 1996. Possible pathogenic role for *Sporothrix cyanescens* isolated from lung lesion in a heart transplant patient. *J. Med. Vet. Mycol.* **34:**195–198.
172. **Tan, T. Q., A. K. Ogden, J. Tillman, G. J. Demmler, and M. G. Rinaldi.** 1992. *Paecilomyces lilacinus* catheter-related fungemia in an immunocompromised patient. *J. Clin. Microbiol.* **30:**2479–2483.
173. **Telenti, A., and G. D. Roberts.** 1989. Fungal blood cultures. *Eur. J. Clin. Microbiol. Infect. Dis.* **8:**825–831.
174. **Toshniwal, R., S. Goodman, S. A. Ally, V. Ray, C. Bodino, and C. A. Kallick.** 1986. Endocarditis due to *Chrysosporium* species: a disease of medical progress? *J. Infect. Dis.* **153:**638–639.
175. **Treger, T. R., D. W. Bisscher, M. S. Bartlett, and J. W. Smith.** 1985. Diagnosis of pulmonary infection caused by *Aspergillus*: usefulness of respiratory cultures. *J. Infect. Dis.* **153:**638–639.
176. **Tritz, D. M., and G. L. Woods.** 1993. Fatal disseminated infection with *Aspergillus terreus* in immunocompromised hosts. *Clin. Infect. Dis.* **16:**118–122.
177. **van Belkum, A., W. G. V. Quint, B. E. de Pauw, W. J. G. Melchers, and J. F. Meis.** 1993. Typing of *Aspergillus* species and *Aspergillus fumigatus* isolates by interrepeat polymerase chain reaction. *J. Clin. Microbiol.* **31:**2502–2505.
178. **Van Cutsem, J., L. Meulemans, F. Van Gerven, and D. Stynen.** 1990. Detection of circulating galactomannan by Pastorex *Aspergillus* in experimental invasive aspergillosis. *Mycoses* **33:**61–69.
179. **Vativarian, S. E., E. J. Anaissie, and G. P. Bodey.** 1993. Emerging fungal pathogens in immunocompromised patients: classification, diagnosis and management. *Clin. Infect. Dis.* **17**(Suppl. 2):S487–S491.

180. **Verweij, P. E., E. C. Dompeling, J. P. Donnelly, A. V. Schattenberg, and J. F. Meis.** 1997. Serial monitoring of *Aspergillus* antigen in the early diagnosis of invasive aspergillosis. Preliminary investigations with two examples. *Infection* **25:**86–89.
181. **Verweij, P. E., J. P. Latge, A. J. Rijs, W. J. Melchers, B. E. De-Pauw, J. A. Hoogkamp-Korstanje, and J. F. Meis.** 1995. Comparison of antigen detection and PCR assay using bronchoalveolar lavage fluid for diagnosing invasive pulmonary aspergillosis in patients receiving treatment for hematological malignancies. *J. Clin. Microbiol.* **33:**3150–3153.
182. **Verweij, P. E., J. F. Meis, J. Sarfati, J. A. Hoogkamp-Korstanje, J.-P. Latge, and W. J. Melchers.** 1996. Genotypic characterization of sequential *Aspergillus fumigatus* isolates from patients with cystic fibrosis. *J. Clin. Microbiol.* **34:**2595–2597.
183. **Verweij, P. E., A. J. Rijs, B. E. De-Pauw, A. M. Horrevorts, J. A. Hoogkamp-Korstanje, and J. F. Meis.** 1995. Clinical evaluation and reproducibility of the Pastorex *Aspergillus* antigen latex agglutination test for diagnosing invasive aspergillosis. *J. Clin. Pathol.* **48:**474–476.
184. **Verweij, P. E., M. Van Kasteren, J. Van de Nes, G. S. De Hoog, B. E. De Pauw, and J. F. G. M. Meis.** 1997. Fatal pulmonary infection caused by the basidiomycete *Hormographiella aspergillata*. *J. Clin. Microbiol.* **35:**2675–2678.
185. **Viviani, M. A., and A. M. Tortorano.** 1998. *Penicillium marneffei*, p. 399–419. L. Ajello and R. Hay (ed.), *Topley & Wilson's Microbiology and Microbial Infections*, 9th ed., vol. 4. Edward Arnold, London, United Kingdom.
186. **Weiner, M. H.** 1980. Antigenemia detected by radioimmunoassay in systemic aspergillosis. *Ann. Intern. Med.* **92:** 793–796.
187. **Weiss, L. M., and W. A. Thiemke.** 1983. Disseminated *Aspergillus ustus* infection following cardiac surgery. *Am. J. Clin. Pathol.* **80:**408–411.
188. **Wheat, L. J.** 1986. The role of the serologic diagnostic laboratory and the diagnosis of fungal disease, p. 43–68. *In* G. A. Sarosi and S. F. Davies (ed.), *Fungal Diseases of the Lung*. Grune and Stratton, Inc., New York, N.Y.
189. **Wheat, L. J., M. Bartlett, M. Ciccarelli, and J. W. Smith.** 1984. Opportunistic *Scopulariopsis* pneumonia in an immunocompromised host. *South. Med. J.* **77:**1608–1609.
190. **Williamson, P. R., K. J. Kwon-Chung, and J. J. Gallin.** 1992. Successful treatment of *Paecilomyces variotii* infection in a patient with chronic granulomatous disease and a review of *Paecilomyces* species infections. *Clin. Infect. Dis.* **14:**1023–1026.
191. **Wilson, E. V., V. M. Hearn, and D. W. R. Mackenzie.** 1987. Evaluation of a test to detect circulating *Aspergillus fumigatus* antigen in a survey of immunocompromised patients with proven or suspected invasive disease. *J. Med. Vet. Mycol.* **25:**365–374.
192. **Witzig, R. S., D. L. Greer, and N. E. Hyslop, Jr.** 1996. *Aspergillus flavus* mycetoma and epidural abscess successfully treated with itraconazole. *J. Med. Vet. Mycol.* **34:** 133–137.
193. **Yamakami, Y., A. Hashimoto, I. Tokimatsu, and M. Nasu.** 1996. PCR detection of DNA specific for *Aspergillus* species in serum of patients with invasive aspergillosis. *J. Clin. Microbiol.* **34:**2464–2468.
194. **Yeghen, T., L. Fenelon, C. K. Campbell, D. W. Warnock, A. V. Hoffbrand, H. G. Prentice, and C. C. Kibbler.** 1996. *Chaetomium* pneumonia in patient with acute myceloid leukemia. *J. Clin. Pathol.* **49:**184–186.
195. **Young, R. C., and J. E. Bennett.** 1971. Invasive aspergillosis. Absence of detectable antibody response. *Am. Rev. Respir. Dis.* **104:**710–716.
196. **Yu, B., Y. Niki, and D. Armstrong.** 1990. Use of immunoblotting to detect *Aspergillus fumigatus* antigen in sera and urines of rats with experimental invasive aspergillosis. *J. Clin. Microbiol.* **28:**1575–1579.
197. **Yuen, K. Y., S. S. Wong, D. N. Tsang, and P. Y. Chau.** 1994. Serodiagnosis of *Penicillium marneffei* infection. *Lancet* **344:**444–445.
198. **Zoutman, D. E., and L. Sigler.** 1991. Mycetoma of the foot caused by *Cylindrocarpon destructans*. *J. Clin. Microbiol.* **29:**1855–1859.

Rhizopus, Rhizomucor, Absidia, and Other Agents of Systemic and Subcutaneous Zygomycoses

MALCOLM D. RICHARDSON AND GILLIAN S. SHANKLAND

98

TAXONOMY

The term zygomycosis embraces deep or subcutaneous mycoses, namely, mucormycosis and the entomophthoramycoses, caused by fungi belonging to various genera of the class *Zygomycetes*. The entomophthoramycoses are subdivided into basidiobolomycosis and conidiobolomycosis (7).

MUCORMYCOSIS

Definition

The term mucormycosis is used to refer to infections due to molds belonging to the order *Mucorales*. These organisms can cause rhinocerebral, pulmonary, gastrointestinal, cutaneous, or disseminated infections in predisposed individuals. The different clinical forms are often associated with particular underlying conditions. In most cases, mucormycosis occurs in patients already receiving treatment because of another disease. For this reason, it may not be immediately recognized.

Mucormycosis is an uncommon, frequently fatal fungal infection which rarely arises in otherwise healthy people. An underlying disease, for example, diabetes mellitus, is almost always present. Mucormycosis appears stereotypically in different anatomical sites: paranasal, rhino-orbital, rhinocerebral, cerebral, pulmonary, and gastrointestinal regions and the soft tissue of the extremities. It can also appear as disseminated disease.

Geographic Distribution

Mucormycosis is distributed worldwide.

Causative Organisms and Their Habitats

Many different organisms have been implicated in mucormycosis, but the most common causes of human infection are *Rhizopus arrhizus* and then *Rhizopus microsporus* var. *rhizopodiformis*. Other, less frequent etiological agents, but for which a major pathogenic role for humans has been established, include *Absidia corymbifera*, *Apophysomyces elegans*, *Cunninghamella bertholletiae*, *Mucor* species, *Rhizomucor pusillus*, and *Saksenaea vasiformis*. These molds are ubiquitous and thermotolerant and can be isolated in large numbers from soil or decomposing organic matter, such as leaves, fruit, and bread. Their spores are often airborne.

Nosocomial outbreaks of mucormycosis are not as common as hospital-related *Aspergillus* infections but have been reported for leukemic patients. Nosocomial cutaneous infections with *R. microsporus* var. *rhizopodiformis* have been traced to contaminated dressings and wooden tongue depressors used as immobilizing splints in a neonatal intensive care unit (14).

The major risk factors predisposing individuals to mucormycosis include uncontrolled diabetes mellitus, other forms of metabolic acidosis, burns, and malignant hematological disorders. Treatment is seldom of benefit unless these underlying conditions can be corrected.

Pathogenesis

The *Mucorales* are opportunistic fungi capable of causing acute, rapidly developing, and often fulminant infections in the compromised host (2, 19, 20). Major risk factors include ketoacidosis, lymphoma, leukemia, neutropenia, corticosteroid or other long-term immunosuppressive therapies, and desferrioxamine therapy of dialysis patients with aluminum or iron overload. To date, there have been only a few reported infections associated with AIDS; therefore, this disease does not appear to be a significant risk factor (23). Trauma to the skin, including severe burns, intravenous catheters, intravenous drug abuse, or even an insect bite, may also result in infection in the compromised host.

The pathogenesis of mucormycosis is unclear. Although the infection is undoubtedly exogenous, possible sources have only occasionally been suggested, e.g., adhesive dressings, air conditioning filter units, and food. Cutaneous trauma may be an underestimated event in the initiation of many cases of mucormycosis. However, most infections follow inhalation of spores that have been released into the air, and the lungs and nasal sinuses are common sites of infection. The most common predisposing illness for gastrointestinal infection is severe malnutrition or disruption of the gastrointestinal mucosa.

The infectious propagule responsible for the establishment of zygomycosis is unproven. Many studies have suggested that sporangiospores are responsible; others have indicated that small hyphal fragments initiate disease. Since sporangiospores of mucoraceous fungi are both uncommon in air and readily contained by phagocytic cells normally found in pulmonary tissues, it is possible that in some cases, especially when trauma is the associated factor, hyphal fragments are the infectious propagule.

Usually, mucormycosis develops first in the nasal mucosa or in the sinuses and then spreads to involve the soft parts of the orbit and the brain. However, the extent of disease appears to be host dependent, and not all patients with paranasal mucormycosis ultimately develop rhinocerebral mucormycosis. The infection does not normally progress in patients who have disease limited to the paranasal sinuses and who have undergone extensive surgery or treatment with amphotericin B. Thus, host factors may be as important as treatment in determining the outcome of paranasal mucormycosis. In other cases, the pulmonary vessels are affected, resulting in infarction and parenchymatous necrosis. Less often, infection follows ingestion or traumatic inoculation of organisms into the skin. Invasion of the intestinal blood vessels can cause extensive necrosis, and if the fungus enters the cutaneous blood vessels, there may be involvement of all the layers of the skin.

Clinical Manifestations

Detailed reviews of the clinical types of mucormycosis are given in references 2, 11, 16, 19, 20, 23, and 24. Mucormycosis is an opportunistic infection and is seldom seen in individuals with an intact immune system. Various forms are recognized; each is associated with particular underlying conditions. Like the etiological agents of aspergillosis, the causative organisms of mucormycosis have a predilection for vascular invasion, causing thrombosis, infarction, and necrosis of tissue. The clinical hallmark of mucormycosis is the rapid onset of necrosis and fever. In most cases, progress is rapid and death follows unless treatment is initiated. The anatomical distribution of lesions appears to correlate to a certain degree with defined predisposing conditions, e.g., craniofacial involvement in individuals with diabetic acidosis, pulmonary and disseminated infections in patients with acute leukemia, and gastrointestinal and cutaneous lesions following local trauma. Indeed, cutaneous infections have possibly replaced craniofacial and pulmonary diseases as the prevalent clinical manifestation of mucormycosis, a change mirrored by the emergence of *R. microsporus* var. *rhizopodiformis* (as *R. rhizopodiformis* in many cases) as a significant pathogen.

Rhinocerebral Mucormycosis

The term rhinocerebral or craniofacial mucormycosis is used to describe infection which begins in the paranasal sinuses and then spreads to involve the orbit, face, palate, or brain. The term should be used only when there is documented brain involvement in addition to involvement of sinuses alone or involvement of both sinuses and orbit, respectively. It is not clear whether paranasal and rhino-orbital mucormycoses are simply rhinocerebral mucormycosis in evolution or whether the extent to which mucormycosis progresses beyond the paranasal sinuses to involve the orbit and the brain is dependent on the host response. Rhinocerebral mucormycosis is most commonly seen in individuals with acidosis, particularly those with uncontrolled diabetes mellitus, but it also occurs in leukemic patients and organ transplant recipients. It is a common clinical form of mucormycosis and is often fatal within 1 week of onset if left untreated.

The initial symptoms include unilateral headache, nasal or sinus congestion or pain, and serosanguinous nasal discharge. Fever is also common. Most patients are not seen during the initial stage of local nasal and sinus infection. Two-thirds or more are lethargic or comatose by the time of their examination.

The primary sites of infection are the nasal turbinates; infection results in a florid acute inflammatory reaction and extensive necrotizing sinusitis. Cavenous sinus thrombosis and pituitary infarction are commonly seen in fatal cases. If the infection spreads into the orbit, periorbital or perinasal swelling will progress to induration and discoloration. Ptosis, proptosis, dilatation and fixation of the pupil, and loss of vision may occur. Drainage of black pus from the eye is a useful diagnostic sign. From the orbit infection may spread into the brain, leading to frontal lobe necrosis and abscess formation. These features result from invasion of the fungus through the cribriform plate.

Mucormycosis arising in association with chronic maxillary or frontal sinusitis results in unilateral manifestations, such as nasal secretion of blood-tinged mucus, facial and orbital pain, palpebral ptosis, and involvement of the hard palate, which becomes gray or blackish and ulcerates. X rays reveal opacification of the sinus where the infection is located.

If the infection spreads into the palate, a black necrotic lesion is often found. This is an important diagnostic sign. Necrotic lesions may also be found on the nasal mucosa. Nasal septum or palate perforation is frequent.

The cerebrospinal fluid (CSF) findings are nonspecific. The protein concentration may be slightly increased, but the glucose concentration is usually normal. There may be modest mononuclear pleocytosis. CSF cultures are sterile.

The radiological findings are nonspecific but are useful in delineating the extent of the infection. Diffuse craniofacial bone destruction is typical. Computed tomography (CT) and magnetic resonance (MR) scans are helpful in defining the extent of bone and soft tissue destruction but are more useful in planning surgical intervention than in establishing a diagnosis. CT scans of the head often reveal sinus opacification, but other changes are minimal, even when there is massive orbital infection. MR scanning may be preferred for diabetic patients, for whom CT contrast agents may be contraindicated.

Pulmonary Mucormycosis

Pulmonary mucormycosis is seldom diagnosed during life. Mucormycosis may develop in the lungs as a result of aspiration of infectious material, following inhalation, or from hematogenous or lymphatic spread during dissemination. Most cases occur in leukemic patients undergoing remission induction treatment. Pulmonary infiltrates develop, with infarction of focal areas of lung. The clinical signs are those of bronchitis, pneumonia, and thrombosis. Necrosis of the parenchyma leads to cavitation; the bronchi may be perforated, resulting in hemoptysis. If the infection is left untreated, hematogenous dissemination to other organs, particularly the brain, will often occur. The infection is fatal within 2 to 3 weeks.

The most common presentation is unremitting fever and the development or progression of lung infiltrates despite broad-spectrum antibacterial treatment. Hemoptysis and pleuritic chest pain are uncommon but, when present, are helpful in suggesting a fungal infection. However, there are no characteristic symptoms or signs to distinguish mucormycosis from aspergillosis.

The chest radiographic findings are nonspecific, but the most common finding is focal or diffuse infiltrates that progress to consolidation, cavitation, or wedge-shaped peripheral lesions representing hemorrhagic infarction. Pleural effusion is uncommon.

Gastrointestinal Mucormycosis

Mucormycosis limited to the gastrointestinal tract is rare. It has usually been encountered in malnourished infants or children. Lesions are most common in the stomach, colon, and ileum. It is seldom diagnosed during life. Frequently associated diseases include amoebic colitis, pellagra, malnutrition, and kwashiorkor.

The symptoms are varied and depend on the site affected. Nonspecific abdominal pain and hematemesis are typical. Necrotic ulcers develop, and peritonitis follows if intestinal perforation occurs. Intestinal mucormycosis is a fulminant illness ending in death within several weeks due to bowel infarction, sepsis, or hemorrhagic shock.

Cutaneous Mucormycosis

Cutaneous mucormycosis is a particular problem in infected patients with burns, in whom spread to underlying tissue is common. The initial signs include fever, swelling, and changes in the appearance of the burn wound. The development of severe underlying tissue necrosis and infarction in a burn patient should suggest the diagnosis.

Mucormycotic gangrenous cellulitis can follow other forms of trauma to the skin. In diabetic or immunosuppressed patients, cutaneous lesions may arise at an insulin injection site or a catheter insertion site. More massive trauma, such as open fractures or crash injuries, has been present in other patients. Necrotizing cutaneous mucormycosis has occurred in patients who have had contaminated surgical dressings applied to their skin.

Cutaneous lesions resembling ecthyma gangrenosum may develop following hematogenous dissemination of the fungus in immunosuppressed patients. The lesions begin as erythematous, indurated painful cellulitis and evolve into ulcers covered with a black eschar.

Disseminated Mucormycosis

Disseminated mucormycosis may follow any of the four forms of mucormycosis described so far, but it is usually seen in neutropenic patients with pulmonary infection. Less commonly, dissemination occurs from the gastrointestinal tract, burns, or other cutaneous lesions. The most common site of spread is the brain, but metastatic necrotic lesions have also been found in the spleen, heart, and other organs. Disseminated mucormycosis is usually diagnosed after the patient has died of the infection. Occasionally, metastatic cutaneous lesions permit an earlier diagnosis.

Cerebral infection following hematogenous dissemination is distinct from the rhinocerebral form of mucormycosis. It results in abscess formation and infarction. Patients present with sudden onset of focal neurological deficits or coma. Investigation of the CSF is unhelpful; protein, glucose, and cell abnormalities are nonspecific and cultures are sterile. CT and MR scans are useful in locating the lesions.

Other Forms of Mucormycosis

Isolated mucormycotic brain lesions have been reported for a number of individuals, particularly parenteral drug abusers, in whom the typical presentation is localized cerebral lesions. The infection presents as a rapid deterioration in neurological status.

Other unusual focal forms of mucormycosis include endocarditis, osteomyelitis, and pyelonephritis.

Mucormycosis in Association with Desferrioxamine Administration

There is a clear association between desferrioxamine use (for the treatment of iron overload) and the development of mucormycosis. Most of the reported cases have involved rhinocerebral disease (reviewed in reference 19). Desferrioxamine is a siderophore derived from *Streptomyces pilosus*. Siderophores are high-affinity iron chelators used by microorganisms to concentrate iron for bioavailability. A number of fungi require iron for growth, and it appears that the fungi responsible for mucormycosis can utilize the iron bound to desferrioxamine. The fact that desferrioxamine is removed by renal clearance means that its circulating time is prolonged in patients on dialysis, possibly increasing the risk for these patients.

Mucormycosis in AIDS

A total of 28 human immunodeficiency virus (HIV)-positive patients with mucormycosis have been reported (reviewed in reference 23). The risk factor for HIV infection was known in 22 of these patients, namely, sexual transmission in 6 patients and intravenous drug abuse in 16. It is presumed that intravenous drug injection was the portal of entry for fungal propagules. The most prevalent clinical presentations of mucormycosis in the intravenous drug-abusing HIV-positive patients appeared to be cerebral, cutaneoarticular, and renal (accounting for 88% of presentations in total).

Differential Diagnosis

Rhinocerebral mucormycosis is a dramatic and distinctive condition, but it can be confused with cavernous sinus thrombosis, bacterial orbital cellulitis, or rhinocerebral aspergillosis or pseudallescheriosis. The clinical manifestations of pulmonary mucormycosis cannot be distinguished from those of gram-negative bacterial pneumonia, aspergillosis, or pseudallescheriosis.

Essential Investigations and Their Interpretation

Because mucormycosis is such an aggressive infection, early diagnosis is essential for successful treatment (2). It is, however, often difficult to obtain suitable and timely specimens.

Collection and Transport of Specimens

If there is any suspicion of mucormycosis, a diligent search for clues that would help to establish a specific microbiological diagnosis should be initiated without delay. The most useful clue is the presence of a black necrotic eschar either in the nasopharynx or on the palate. This eschar or material sloughing from it may be mistaken for clotted blood. Material from the eschar and underlying tissue should be obtained by biopsy or curette and transported to the laboratory as quickly as possible.

Direct Microscopy

A definitive diagnosis of mucormycosis is best achieved by direct histopathological examination and culturing. Biopsies of pulmonary, rhinocerebral, and cutaneous lesions and scrapings of necrotic mucocutaneous lesions are appropriate specimens.

The necrotic material should be gently broken apart and mounted in a few drops of 20% (wt/vol) potassium hydroxide (KOH). Typical wide, nonseptate hyphae with right-angled branching may be seen. Demonstration of mycelial elements in the correct clinical setting constitutes strong evidence for mucormycosis. If the KOH preparation is unrevealing, surgical biopsy or debridement of necrotic material should be done. Any material obtained should be examined with KOH and stained with methenamine silver (Grocott's modification; GMS) and hematoxylin and eosin (H&E) (see below). If fungal elements are seen, further biopsy specimens should be obtained. The rapid progression of untreated mucormycosis allows no delays in diagnostic efforts.

The microscopic demonstration of *Mucorales* in clinical material taken from necrotic lesions is more significant than the isolation of these organisms in cultures. However, different species cannot be distinguished from each other morphologically. These organisms can be distinguished from other molds, such as *Aspergillus*, due to their characteristic broad, nonseptate filaments with right-angled branching. Compared to *Aspergillus*, zygomycetes are larger, do not have parallel walls with 45° angle branching, and do not radiate from a single point in tissues. Furthermore, agents of mucormycosis stain poorly with periodic acid-Schiff (PAS) but stain well with H&E. Negative microscopic examinations do not eliminate the possibility of mucormycosis even if a portion of necrotic tissue has been examined carefully.

Central nervous system involvement in rhinocerebral mucormycosis may suggest the presence of the etiological agent in CSF. However, agents of mucormycosis have not been isolated from CSF. In cases of suspected pulmonary mucormycosis, biopsy material or material from fine-needle percutaneous aspiration should be examined. Sputum culturing is rarely helpful. Metastatic skin lesions, if present, may allow a diagnosis to be made without performance of a lung biopsy. In isolated cases, fungal elements have been seen in bronchoalveolar lavage fluid and isolated in cultures. Intestinal mucormycosis is usually a rapidly progressive disease ending in death in a few days. In almost all cases, the diagnosis is not suspected until histological examination of gangrenous tissue obtained at surgery or autopsy reveals fungi. Antemortem diagnosis is difficult. In suspected cases, the demonstration of fungi in gastric aspirates or feces may be useful.

Histopathology

Biopsy specimens or scrapings from oral lesions are most satisfactory for histological examination and culturing. Demonstration of the fungus in tissue is diagnostic of disease, but culturing must be done to determine the specific etiological agent. Mucoraceous fungi are readily seen with H&E stain and GMS stain. Another useful stain is cresyl fast violet, which stains zygomycete walls brick red and other fungi blue or purple.

Hyphal elements of mucoraceous fungi consist of broad, twisted, ribbon-like hyphae, which are variable in width (up to 50 μm) and which often are devoid of cytoplasm and have collapsed walls (Fig. 1). True septa are not present, although wrinkles and folds in the cell wall may appear to be septa unless the microscope is focused up and down on the apparent boundary. Hyphal walls vary in thickness. Branches often occur at an angle of 90° from the main hyphal trunk (Fig. 2). The side branches may be much narrower than the main hyphal trunk. Mucoraceous fungi can be mistaken for sclerosed capillaries or nematodes and may also be confused with empty spherules of *Coccidioides immitis* in regions of endemicity. The small amount of fungus present in tissue sections and the oblique angles at which they are cut make their identification by histological morphology alone difficult. In some tissues, hyphae and hyphal fragments

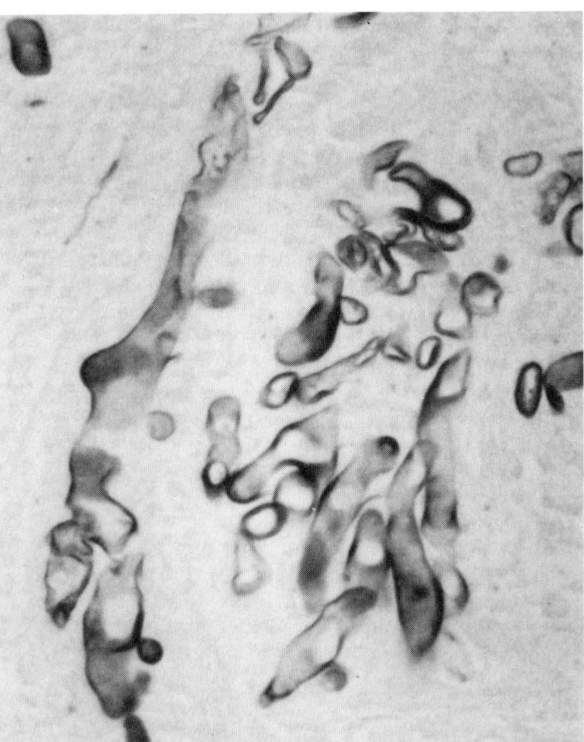

FIGURE 1 Hyphae of *R. arrhizus* in an H&E-stained section of soft palate from a patient with rhinocerebral mucormycosis. Note the irregular shapes and diameters of the hyphae. Magnification, ×400.

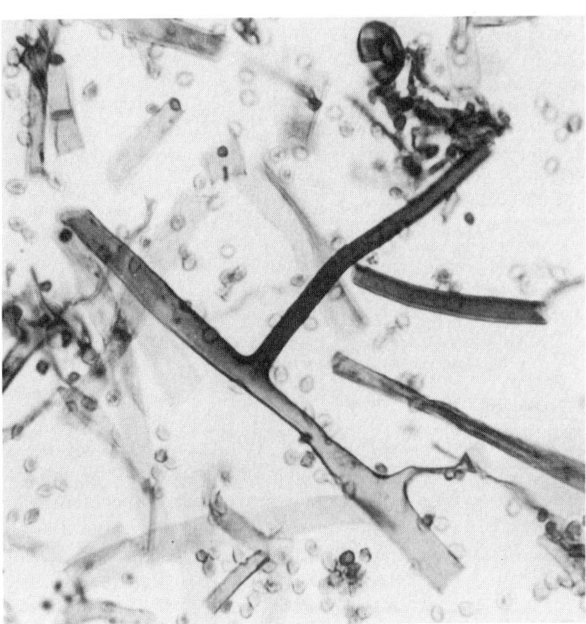

FIGURE 2 Hyphae of *R. arrhizus* in a PAS-stained section of an agar block from a glucose-peptone culture. Note the difference in the widths of the hyphal fragments and a narrow lateral hypha growing at a 90° angle from the main hyphal trunk. Magnification, ×370.

may appear to be septate and constricted at prominent septations. Often, hyphae may have terminal bulbous swellings and lateral oval to spherical structures.

The pathology does not vary with the site of infection. Gangrene involvement is common. Surfaces show massive hemorrhage with recent emboli, and in older lesions, the appearance is putty-like. The tissue reaction is not consistent. In some cases, no cellular response is seen, but usually there are various degrees of edema and necrosis with neutrophil accumulation, plasma cells, and some giant cells. The acute reaction shows diffuse infiltration of polymorphonuclear leukocytes. Eosinophils are not often seen. Tissues often exhibit a suppurative reaction but may show granulomatous changes. The characteristic feature is the involvement of blood vessels, with mucoraceous fungi invading the walls of arteries and causing thrombosis and necrosis of the adjacent tissues. The lumens and walls of blood vessels often contain hyphae, chlamydoconidia, fibrin, and inflammatory cells.

Another pertinent feature is the presence of spherical to ovoid, 15- to 30-μm-diameter, thick-walled, hyaline chlamydospores. Chlamydospores of mucoraceous fungi stain well with PAS and H&E but stain either poorly or not at all with GMS. Because of fixation and processing of tissues, the chlamydospore cytoplasm can retract from the plasma membrane, creating an artificial clear space between the condensed cytoplasm and the thick, rigid cell walls. Some chlamydospores stain entirely; others can appear as empty rings. Chlamydospores are seen in the vicinity of mucoraceous hyphae. Detached chlamydoconidia can resemble the yeast-form cells of *Blastomyces dermatitidis* or the immature spherules and arthroconidia of *C. immitis*. In pulmonary mucormycosis, chlamydospores are most often observed in alveolar spaces, the lumens of bronchioles, and the visceral pleura. In cutaneous mucormycosis, chlamydoconidia may be seen within necrotic tissue on or near a wound surface.

Immunohistochemical methods of staining can be useful in the diagnosis of infections with mucoraceous fungi and in their separation from other agents of fungal disease. Tissue sections can be deparaffinized, treated with a 1% trypsin solution (pH 8.0) for 1 h at 37°C, and examined by direct immunofluorescence with specific fluorescent-antibody conjugates to the major species. Alternatively, permanent preparation can be made by staining tissue sections by immunoperoxidase techniques with polyvalent antibodies specific for the major species. The specificity and activity of these antibodies can be assessed by staining sections of agar blocks cut from seeded cultures in which the fungus grows three dimensionally throughout the agar. However, the supply of these antibodies is currently limited to specialized or reference laboratories.

Culturing

Isolation of the causative agents of mucormycosis has been achieved for only a small proportion of cases, but specimens should be sent for culturing if the clinician suspects mucormycosis. Because the *Mucorales* are common contaminants, isolation of these organisms from sputum, aspirated material from sinuses, or bronchial washings must be interpreted with caution. However, if the patient is diabetic or immunosuppressed, the isolation should not be ignored. The agents of mycormycosis can be grown on most laboratory media, but glucose-peptone agar (glucose, 4%; mycologic peptone, 1%; agar, 2%) or 4% malt extract agar (malt extract, 4%; agar, 2%) is recommended because typical morphology can be demonstrated. Media containing cycloheximide should not be used because cycloheximide inhibits the growth of these fungi. Small portions of biopsy material should be point inoculated onto glucose-peptone agar. Swab cultures of the nose or palate are usually negative and are not recommended. Cultures should be incubated at room temperature and at 37°C. Tissue material should not be homogenized, as this procedure kills viable hyphal elements of mucoraceous fungi. Refrigeration may also reduce the viability of some of these agents.

Serological Tests

No commercially available serological tests for mucormycosis are available at present. However, agar gel double-diffusion and enzyme-linked immunosorbent assay formats have been developed and evaluated for a few patients. It is unlikely that these tests are going to be appropriate for fulminating infections. The development of infection-specific antigens and monoclonal antibodies together with oligonucleotide primers and probes may facilitate the early diagnosis of mucormycosis in the future. For a contemporary review of the role and utility of serological tests in mucormycosis, see the review by Hopwood and Evans (10).

General Description of Fungi Most Likely To Be Isolated and Basis of Identification

The descriptions given below contain morphological terms specific to mucoraceous fungi. A glossary of terms is given in the Appendix.

Identification of most zygomycetes is based primarily on the morphology of the sporangia, i.e., arrangement and number of sporangiospores, shape, color, presence or absence of columellae and apophyses, and presence or absence of rhizoids. Growth temperature studies can also be especially helpful in identifying and differentiating members of the genera *Rhizopus*, *Rhizomucor*, and *Absidia*. The *Mucorales* are characterized by the production of nonseptate hyphae. However, septa occasionally are formed in older cultures. Some genera produce rhizoids, root-like anchors (Fig. 3), which are connected by hyphae called stolons. The *Mucorales* reproduce asexually by producing spores in sporangia, which are borne on sporangiophores. In some genera, the

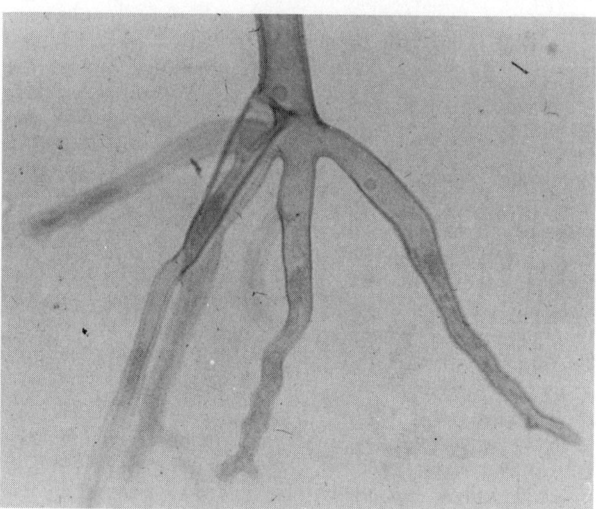

FIGURE 3 Typical formation of rhizoids which are characteristic of *Rhizopus* and *Rhizomucor* and to some extent also of *Absidia*. Magnification, ×400.

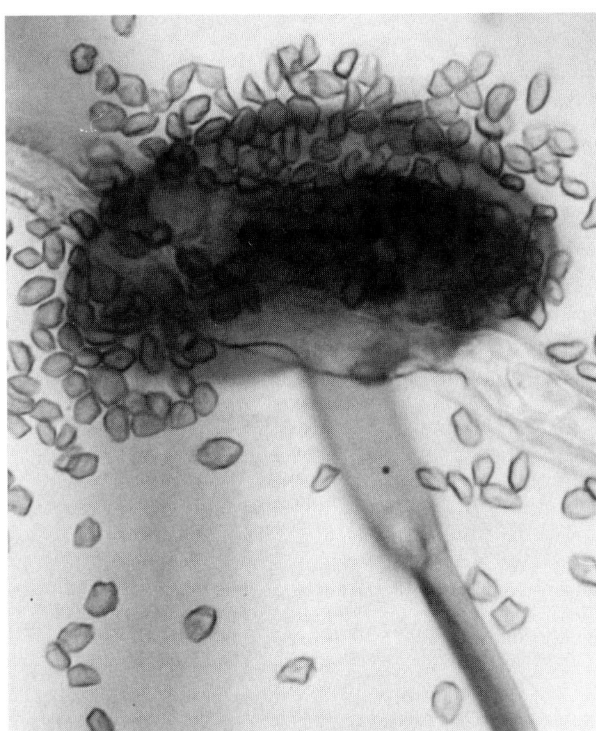

FIGURE 4 Sporangium, apophysis, and sporangiospores of *R. arrhizus* (NCPF 2634). Note the rhomboidal and lemon-shaped sporangiospores with striae (wrinkles) on the surface. Magnification, ×336.

sporangiophore swells where it meets the sporangium, forming the structure called an apophysis (Fig. 4). Typically, a sporangium is a globose swelling at the apex of a sporangiophore. The sporangium contains a central, variously shaped collumella, which is separated from the spore-containing sac by a membrane. The cytoplasm of the sporangium is cleaved into hundreds of sporangiospores during maturation (Fig. 4). In addition, some genera of *Mucorales* produce small sporangia called sporangioles. Finally, a few genera, for example, *Cunninghamella*, produce sporangia which contain a single spore; these are called conidia. Sexual reproduction in the *Mucorales* is characterized by the formation of zygospores. However, determining the presence of zygospores is not part of a routine laboratory identification scheme.

Several excellent monographs and laboratory manuals on the taxonomy and detailed identification of zygomycete fungi have been published (5, 6, 9, 11, 13, 17, 18, 21). The interested worker is referred to these sources to complement the features highlighted here and for routine isolates not corresponding to the descriptions given below.

Description of Causative Agents

The descriptions of the causative agents of zygomycoses given below are based almost entirely on their asexual characteristics. These are as follows:

1. Type and number of sporangiospores.
2. Structure containing the sporangiospores.
3. Structure supporting the sporangiophore.
4. Presence or absence of branching in the sporangiophore.
5. Shape of the columella.
6. Presence or absence of rhizoids and their location in relation to the sporophore or stolon.

Spore containers are named according to the number of reproductive elements they hold, e.g.:

1. A sporangium contains many spores.
2. A merosporangium contains moderate numbers of spores.
3. A sporangiola contains one to a few spores.

The key morphological characteristics of the hyphae which typify the zygomycetes are the internodes and the rhizoids. An internode is a runner (or stolon) which runs between contact points on the substrate; rhizoids are root-like hyphae growing within the substrate. Further classification of the zygomycetes can be based on the presence of branched or unbranched sporangiophores at or between the internodes, the presence or absence of rhizoids, and the maximum temperature for growth. The differentiation of these fungi to the species level is difficult, but a scheme of identification based on a combination of asexual morphology and biochemical characteristics has made it more feasible for the clinical laboratory. The descriptions given below are based on the colony appearance and microscopic morphology of individual isolates (some deposited in the National Culture Collection of Pathogenic Fungi, Mycology Reference Laboratory, Public Health Laboratory, Bristol, United Kingdom) cultured on 4% malt agar as a primary isolation medium and subcultured on glucose-peptone agar without the addition of cycloheximide. The maximum incubation temperature is indicated, assuming that primary isolation plates of clinical specimens from suspected cases of fungal infection are routinely incubated at a range of temperatures, e.g., 28, 37, and 45°C.

Rhizopus arrhizus (*Rhizopus oryzae*)

Found in soil, decaying fruit and vegetables, animal feces, and old bread, *R. arrhizus* is the most prevalent agent of mucormycosis. Approximately 60% of all the culturally proven cases of human mucormycosis and nearly 90% of the rhinocerebral cases are caused by *R. arrhizus*. Less commonly, it has been isolated from other sites. Pneumonia and sinusitis (with or without extension to the orbits, face, or brain) are associated with diabetic ketoacidosis, hematological malignancy, and treatment with iron chelation therapy or corticosteroids. Soft tissue infection can develop after traumatic injury, and nosocomial outbreaks related to contaminated adhesive tape have been reported.

Colony Morphology

R. arrhizus forms a fast-growing, white cottony colony at 28°C, filling a 9-cm-diameter petri dish within 2 to 3 days and reaching up to about 8 mm in height. The fungus can grow at temperatures of up to 45°C if routine primary isolation plates are incubated at this temperature. Colonies tend to collapse, becoming brownish gray to blackish gray, depending on the amount of sporulation. Growth is inhibited by cycloheximide.

Microscopic Morphology

The single most useful characteristic in identifying the genus *Rhizopus* is the presence of simple sporangiophores borne singly or in groups opposite rhizoids (Fig. 5). Broad, nonseptate hyphae are seen in *R. arrhizus*. Sporangiophores are up to 3,500 μm long and 18 μm wide, smooth walled, nonseptate, and simple, with a single axis or branched, and

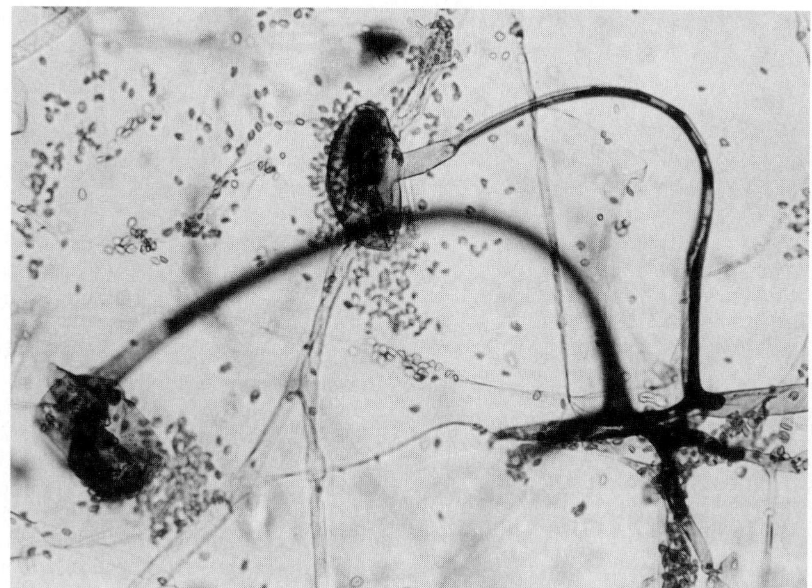

FIGURE 5 *R. arrhizus* (NCPF 2634). Note the simple sporangiosphores borne singly opposite rhizoids. Some sporangia have collapsed, and the sporangial wall has dissolved. Magnification, ×400.

they arise from stolons opposite brownish rhizoids, usually in groups of three or more. Grayish black sporangia are globose, often with a flattened base, powdery in appearance, and up to 200 μm in diameter. Columellae are ellipsoidal on a truncate base, mouse gray, and up to 130 μm long. Sporangiospores vary in shape and size, having a rhomboidal lemon shape with ridges on the surface.

Rhizopus microsporus var. *rhizopodiformis*

The second most common species associated with mucormycosis, *R. microsporus* var. *rhizopodiformis* causes nearly 15% of all culturally proven cases of the disease in humans. The organism is isolated mainly from cutaneous lesions, some of which have been associated with semiocclusive wound dressings and the use of Elastoplast bandages to cover surgical wounds (reviewed in reference 11). Contaminated wooden tongue depressors used as splints reportedly caused an outbreak of nosocomial infections with *R. microsporus* var. *rhizopodiformis* in a neonatal intensive care unit (14). Rhinocerebral disease is rarely caused by this organism.

Colony Morphology

Colonies range from gray to dark grayish brown.

Microscopic Morphology

Rhizoids are hyaline to subhyaline. Sporangiophores are shorter (maximum length, 1,000 μm) than those of *R. arrhizus* and are produced singly or in groups of up to four (Fig. 6). Sporangia average 100 μm in diameter. Columellae are pyriform or somewhat elongated, with distinct angular apophyses (Fig. 7). Sporangiospores (4 to 6 μm) are subglobose to slightly rhomboidal, with a smooth or finely spinulose surface. The fungus is thermotolerant, growing well at up to 50°C.

Rhizopus microsporus var. *microsporus*

R. microsporus var. *microsporus* is an emerging pathogen and has been reliably identified in two patients with cutaneous infections and for whom amputation of the affected area was required (26).

Colony Morphology

R. microsporus var. *microsporus* may be distinguished from other related pathogenic species by growth at 46°C but not at 50°C.

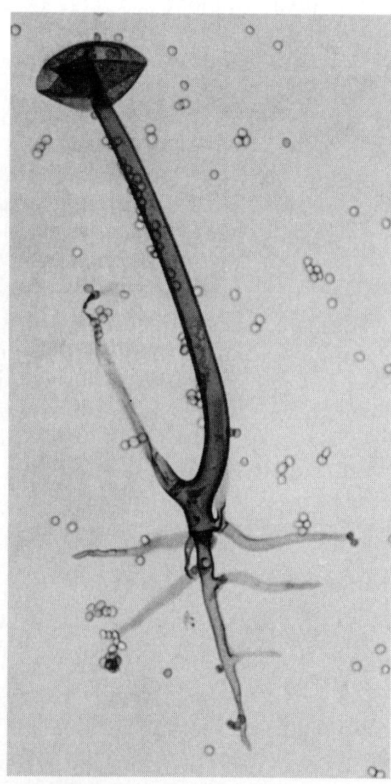

FIGURE 6 *R. microsporus* var. *rhizopodiformis* (NCPF 2955). Note the short sporangiophore compared with that of *R. arrhizus* and the branched rhizoids. Magnification, ×400.

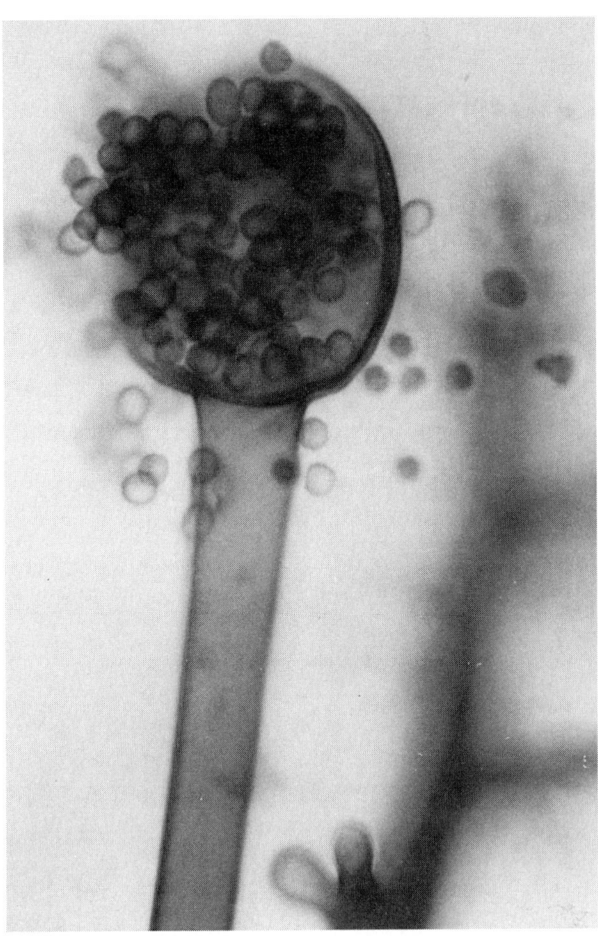

FIGURE 7 *R. microsporus* var. *rhizopodiformis* (NCPF 2955). Note the partially dissolved sporangial wall, smooth-walled globose to subglobose sporangiospores, and angulated, truncated apophysis. Magnification, ×400.

Microscopic Morphology

The sporangiophores of *R. microsporus* var. *microsporus* are angular to broadly ellipsoidal, striated, and up to 6.5 μm long.

Rhizomucor pusillus

R. pusillus is found in decaying fruits and vegetables and in soil. Very few reports of human disease have been published. *R. pusillus* has been isolated from immunocompromised patients with pulmonary, rhinofacial, and disseminated infections and occasionally from patients with cutaneous infections and endocarditis. This fungus can also cause mycotic abortions in cows, horses, and pigs.

Colony Morphology

The organism grows rapidly and is initially white, turning dark smoke gray or brown as sporulation occurs. Colony texture is floccose to woolly. Growth is inhibited by cycloheximide. The maximum growth temperature of 54 to 58°C is a useful distinguishing feature.

Microscopic Morphology

R. pusillus forms broad, sparsely septate hyaline hyphae. Sporangiophores are mainly monopodially branched and anchored to the substratum by short rhizoids (Fig. 8). Sporangia are globose and dark brown and measure up to 100 μm in diameter. *Rhizomucor* differs from *Rhizopus* by forming sporangia without apophyses. Columellae are subglobose to pyriform. The sporangium wall dissolves to leave a collar around the sporangiophore. Globose to subglobose hyaline sporangiospores are released (3 to 5 μm in diameter).

Absidia corymbifera

A. corymbifera is an infrequent agent of mucormycosis in humans. It is found worldwide in soil, compost, and decaying vegetation. Documented cases include meningitis in an immunocompetent patient following a perforating head injury, cutaneous infection in an immunocompetent patient, and renal infection in an AIDS patient. Infection is most probably acquired by inhalation of sporangiospores. *A. corymbifera* is the only species of the genus *Absidia* pathogenic for humans and is also an agent of bovine mycotic abortions.

Colony Morphology

A. corymbifera forms rapidly growing colonies that quickly fill a petri dish. It grows well at 25 to 45°C; some isolates can grow at 50°C. The very high colonies are light gray to grayish brown. The reverse is colorless to very slightly yellow or buff with age. A colony may originate from stolons between rhizoids or from finely branched aerial hyphae. *A. corymbifera* does not grow in the presence of cycloheximide.

Microscopic Morphology

A. corymbifera forms broad (often 10 μm or more), sparsely septate hyphae with stolons and internodal rhizoids. Sporangiophores are hyaline to light gray and branched simply or in a corymbiform pattern. Sporangia are pyriform, 100 to 150 μm in diameter, and hyaline when young but

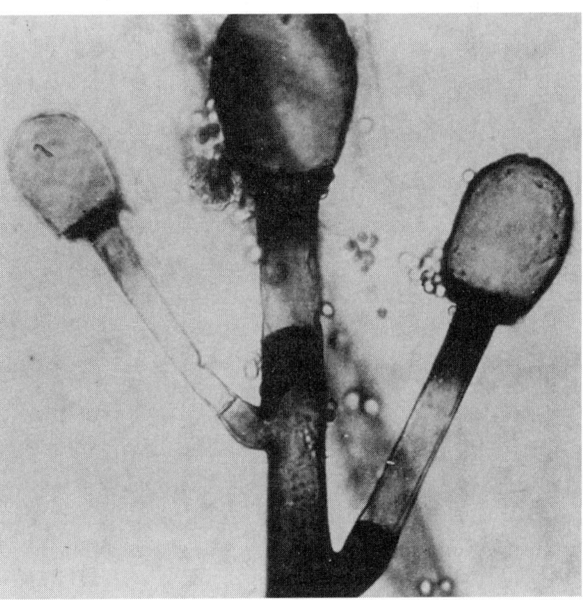

FIGURE 8 *R. pusillus*. Note the monopodially branched sporangiophores, pyriform columellae, and small sporangiospores. A collarette can be seen around the sporangiophore. Magnification, ×400. (Reprinted with permission of Kaminski's Teaching Slides on Medical Mycology, Adelaide Children's Hospital, Adelaide, Australia.)

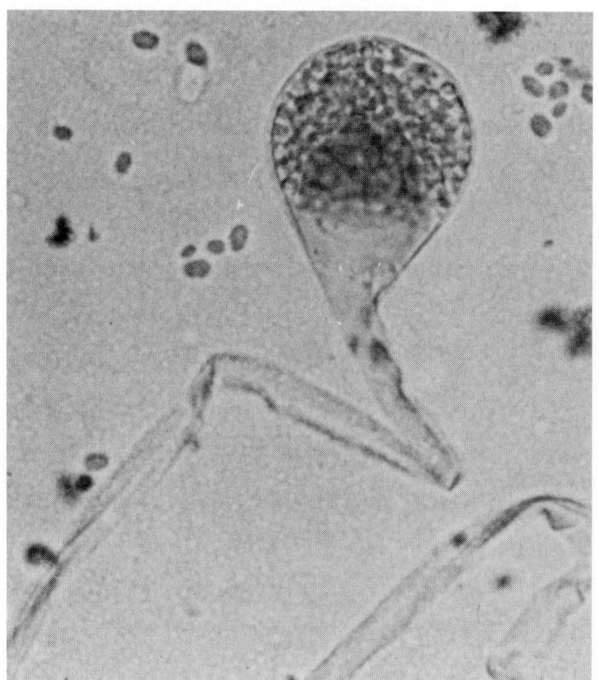

FIGURE 9 A. *corymbifera*. Note the relatively fine sporangiophore, pyriform sporangium, hemispherical columella, and long, conical apophysis. Sporangiospores vary in morphology from globose to long ellipsoidal. Magnification, ×400.

grayish brown to greenish beige with age (Fig. 9). A swollen apophysis is seen at the point where the sporangiophore merges with the sporangium. Sporangia are 20 to 80 μm in diameter, erect, hyaline to slightly brownish, pyriform, and fragile. Columellae are hemispherical to short ovoidal. Sporangiospores have a greenish yellow tinge and are variable in shape and size, with dimensions ranging from 3.2 to 3.9 by 3.1 to 3.5 μm to a long ellipsoidal shape of 4.1 to 4.9 by 2.3 to 2.9 μm.

Cunninghamella bertholletiae

In the genus *Cunninghamella*, only the species C. *bertholletiae* has been verified as a human pathogen (11). C. *bertholletiae* is widely distributed in soil and decaying vegetation and animal matter and has been recovered from cheese and Brazil nuts. Infection is acquired by inhalation of conidia. Mating reactions have been very important in delineating *Cunninghamella* species.

Colony Morphology

C. *bertholletiae* grows very fast, filling a petri dish within 2 to 3 days. Colonies are initially white, becoming dark gray and powdery with development. The reverse is colorless to buff. Primary isolates can grow at temperatures of up to 42°C. The organism is sensitive to cycloheximide.

Microscopic Morphology

The sporangiophores of C. *bertholletiae* are up to 20 μm wide and straight, with verticillate or single branches. Vesicles are subglobose to pyriform, with terminal ones being up to 40 μm and lateral ones being 10 to 30 μm in diameter. Sporangiola are globose (7 to 11 μm in diameter) or ellipsoidal (9 to 13 by 6 to 10 μm), verrucose or short echinulate, and hyaline when single but brownish when in a mass (Fig. 10). C. *bertholletiae* grows optimally at 25 to 30°C; the maximum temperature tolerated is 50°C.

Saksenaea vasiformis

S. *vasiformis* is widespread in tropical soils and is a known agent of subcutaneous zygomycosis. Infection is acquired by traumatic implantation of the fungus. This infection generally occurs in previously healthy people who have sustained traumatic injury, such as head or scalp trauma, burns, insertion of an arterial catheter, or a tattoo (4). Such patients have recovered after surgical debridement and treatment with amphotericin B or removal of the arterial catheter. An intact immune response in these patients was probably a major factor in determining successful outcome.

At least 14 cases of invasive infection in both immunocompromised and immunocompetent individuals have been reported. Most patients have presented with necrotic skin lesions, although it is not clear whether these were primary lesions or a manifestation of disseminated infection. Disseminated infection is rapidly fatal. S. *vasiformis* is a rare cause of rhinocerebral mucormycosis. One case in an immuno-

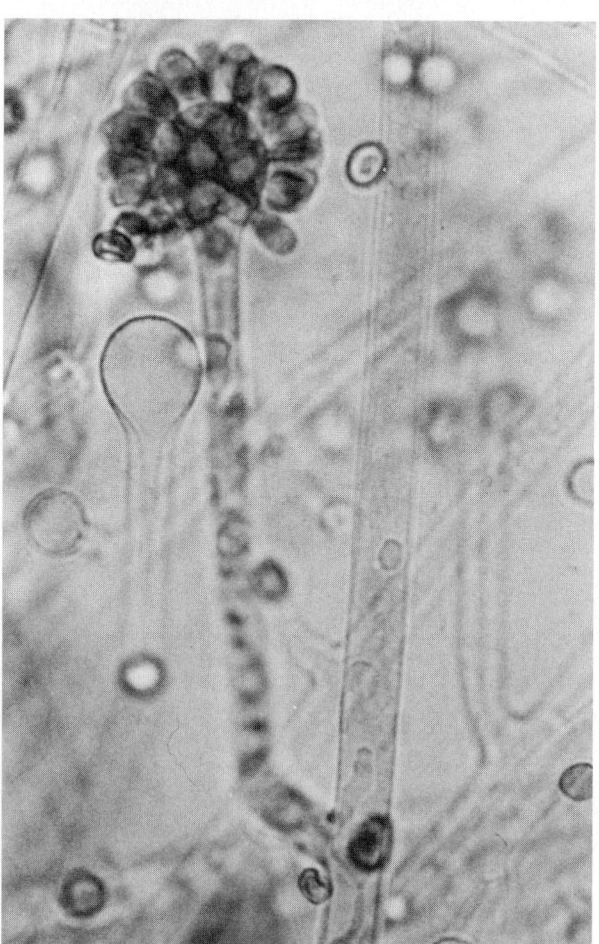

FIGURE 10 C. *bertholletiae*. Note the single sporangiophore branching off a main hyphal trunk and the subglobose to pyriform vesicle bearing ellipsoidal sporangiola. Magnification, ×400. (Reprinted with permission of Kaminski's Teaching Slides on Medical Mycology, Adelaide Children's Hospital, Adelaide, Australia.)

compromised child and one case in an adult have been reported. Both cases were fatal.

Colony Morphology

Colonies of *S. vasiformis* grow rapidly and are downy and white, with no reverse pigment.

Microscopic Morphology

S. vasiformis forms broad, nonseptate hyphae and flask-shaped sporangia (Fig. 11) with a distinct spherical venter (that portion of a phialide that lies between the base of a phialide and the condiogenous locus) and a long neck, arising singly or in pairs from dichotomously branched, darkly pigmented rhizoids. The collumellae are prominent and dome shaped. Small, oblong sporangiospores, 1 to 2 by 3 to 4 μm in size, are discharged through the neck of the sporangia following the dissolution of an apical mucilaginous plug.

Laboratory identification may be difficult or delayed because of the failure of the mold to sporulate on primary isolation media or on subsequent subcultures on potato dextrose agar. Sporulation may be stimulated by the use of nutrient-deficient media, such as cornmeal-glucose-sucrose-yeast extract agar. See reference 17 for the sporulation procedure.

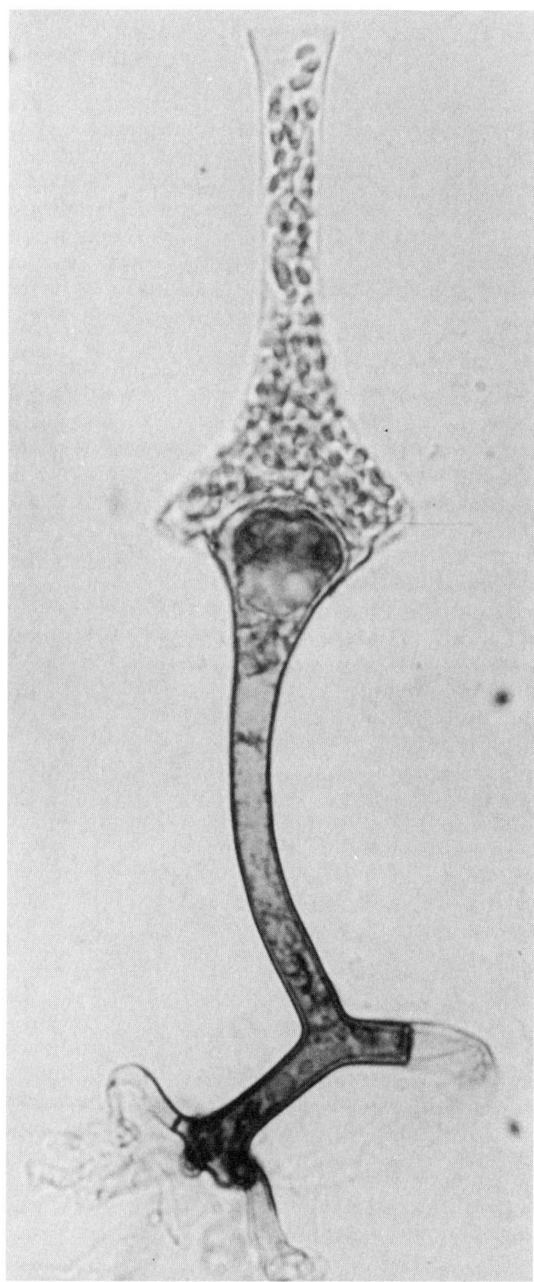

FIGURE 11 *S. vasiformis*. Note the flask-shaped sporangium with a distinct, globose columella and small, smooth, elongated sporangiospores. Magnification, ×400. (Reprinted with permission of Kaminski's Teaching Slides on Medical Mycology, Adelaide Children's Hospital, Adelaide, Australia.)

Mucor Species

Mucor species are infrequently the causative agents of mucormycosis. The genus contains 49 recognized species, many of which are widespread in the environment. However, few species have been recovered from well-documented cases of mucormycosis, and infections due to members of this genus are rare.

Identification of *Mucor* species beyond the generic level is difficult because the pathogenic species lack distinctive characteristics. Emerging pathogens within the *Mucor* genus are *Mucor circinelloides* and *Mucor ramosissimus* (25). Very few cases of human disease have been associated with *M. circinelloides*; to date, these have been limited to cutaneous infections. Very few cases of human disease caused by *M. ramosissimus* have been reported. Cases may be underreported due to inaccurate or incomplete identification of the invading organism. *M. ramosissimus* has been associated with peritoneal dialysis-associated peritonitis, septic arthritis, and mucocutaneous and rhinocerebral diseases.

Colony Morphology

Mucor species are rapidly growing organisms. Colonies are initially white and cottony but become gray to brown as sporulation occurs. *Mucor* species are inhibited by the concentration of cycloheximide usually incorporated in routine isolation media. Most species grow poorly, if at all, at 37°C.

Microscopic Morphology

The genus *Mucor* can be differentiated from the genera *Absidia*, *Rhizopus*, and *Rhizomucor* by the absence of stolons and rhizoids. *Mucor* species produce simple or sympodially branching sporangiophores from nonseptate hyphae. There is no swelling where the sporangiophore and the sporangium merge (Fig. 12). The gray-brown sporangia themselves are globose, have columellae, and contain globose to ellipsoidal sporangiospores.

Apophysomyces elegans

A. elegans was originally found in soil samples from a mango orchard in India. Subsequently, 14 human cases of mucormycosis resulting from traumatic implantation or contamination of burns with this organism were described (3, 4). In most patients, there was no apparent underlying risk factor. Localized invasion may progress rapidly, leading to necrotizing fasciitis and death, especially if the patient is treated for a bacterial rather than a fungal infection. *Apophysomyces* species closely resemble *Absidia* species in morphology.

Colony Morphology

A. elegans grows rapidly. Colonies are initially white, becoming creamy white to buff with age and downy, with no

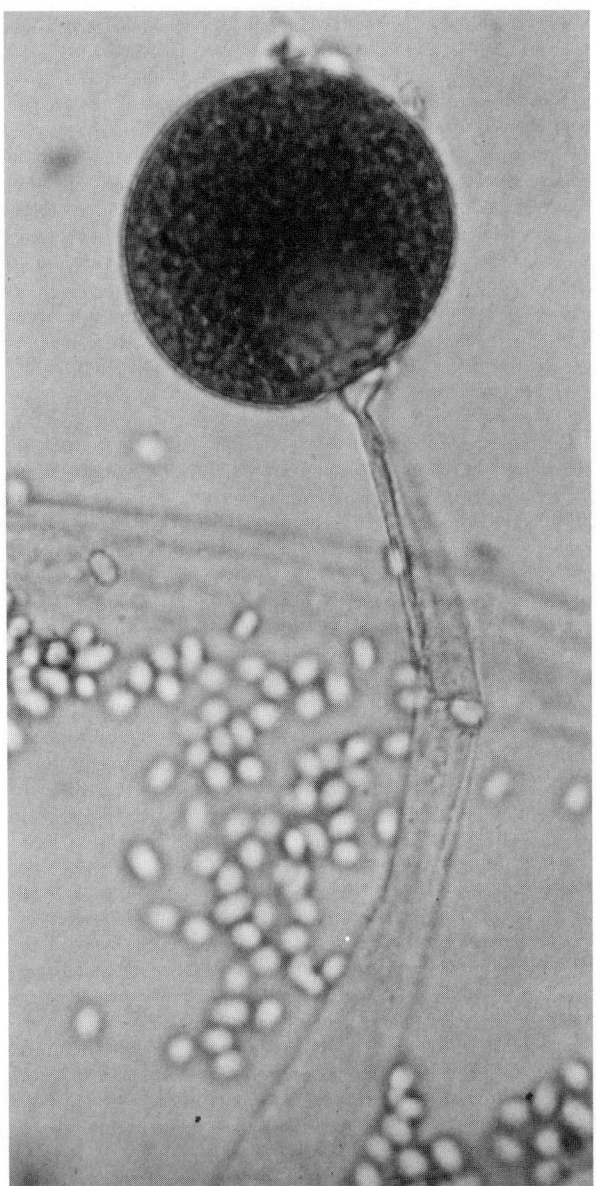

FIGURE 12 *Mucor* species. Note the globose sporangium containing small sporangiospores on a simple sporangiophore. Magnification, ×400. (Reprinted with permission of Kaminski's Teaching Slides on Medical Mycology, Adelaide Children's Hospital, Adelaide, Australia.)

reverse pigment. The organism grows well at temperatures of up to 42°C. The growth of *A. elegans* is not inhibited by cycloheximide.

Microscopic Morphology

A. elegans does not sporulate on routine mycological media; it forms only broad, nonseptate hyphae. Characteristic identifying features include sporangiophores arising singly from aerial hyphal segments. Thin-walled, hyaline, light grayish brown rhizoids are produced opposite sporangiophores. A foot cell (resembling that seen with *Aspergillus* species) is present at the union of the sporangiophores and the surrounding hyphae. Sporangia are pyriform (20 to 50 μm in diameter) and have prominent funnel- or wine glass-shaped apophyses and hemispherical columellae produced singly at the tip of each sporangiophore. Sporangiospores are smooth, mostly oblong (5.4 to 8.0 by 4.0 to 5.7 μm), occasionally globose, and light brown.

Rare Causes of Mucormycosis

Rare causes of mucormycosis include *Cokeromyces recuvatus*, *Syncephalastrum racemosum*, and *Mortierella* species.

Treatment and Antifungal Susceptibility

Amphotericin B is the drug of choice for mucormycosis. There are a number of reports of the successful use of liposomal amphotericin B (AmBisome; Nexstar Pharmaceuticals) for the treatment of rhinocerebral and cutaneous mucormycoses (1, 7, 12, 15). The use of liposomal amphotericin B allows the delivery of high doses of amphotericin B without significant infusion-related reactions or nephrotoxicity. Another lipid formulation of amphotericin B, amphotericin B colloidal dispersion (Amphotec or Amphocil; Sequus Pharmaceuticals Inc.), has also been used effectively for the treatment of rhinocerebral mucormycosis (22). Amphotericin B lipid complex (Abelcet; The Liposome Company) in combination with granulocyte colony-stimulating factor has been used to treat disseminated mucormycosis in a neutropenic patient (8).

The necessity for the prompt administration of amphotericin B (and radical debridement of affected tissue) does not allow antifungal susceptibility tests to be performed, and they are not necessary. Other antifungal drugs (ketoconazole, fluconazole, and itraconazole) have no role in the management of mucormycosis.

ENTOMOPHTHORAMYCOSES (SUBCUTANEOUS PHYCOMYCOSIS AND SUBCUTANEOUS ZYGOMYCOSIS)

Conidiobolomycosis

Definition

Conidiobolomycosis is a chronic mycosis affecting the subcutaneous tissues. It originates in the nasal sinuses and spreads to the adjacent subcutaneous tissues of the face, causing disfigurement.

Geographic Distribution

Coniodiobolomycosis occurs mainly in the tropical rain forests of Africa, South America, Central America, and Southeast Asia.

Causative Organism and Its Habitat

Conidiobolus coronatus (*Entomophthora coronata*) lives as a saphrophyte in soil humus and on decomposing plant matter in moist, warm climates. It can also parasitize certain insects. The disease is most common among adult males, particularly those living or working in tropical rain forests. Infection is acquired through inhalation of spores or through their introduction into the nasal cavities by soiled hands.

Clinical Manifestations

C. coronatus infection generally begins with unilateral involvement of the nasal mucosa. The most common nasal symptom is obstruction, but frequent nose-bleeds can occur and are evidence of the development of a nasal polyp in the anterior region of the inferior turbinate. Subcutaneous nodules then develop in the nasal and perinasal regions and may be associated with epidermal lesions.

The spread of the infection is slow but relentless. The infection is usually confined to the face, and the development of gross facial swelling involving the forehead, periorbital region, and upper lip is very distinctive. As a rule, the lesions are firmly attached to the underlying tissue, although the bone is spared. The skin remains intact. Spread to the lymph nodes has been reported.

Differential Diagnosis

Even if, in advanced cases, the diagnosis is obvious from the clinical appearance, mycological and histological examinations are essential for confirmation.

Essential Investigations and Their Interpretation

Microscopy

Microscopic examination of smears or tissue from the nasal mucosa reveals broad, nonseptate, thin-walled mycelial filaments.

Culturing

Tissue obtained by biopsy or curettage should be cultured. Positive cultures are difficult to obtain, and the pathologic material must be inoculated on the largest possible number of media; the media should be incubated at 25 to 35°C to enhance the growth of *C. coronatus*.

Colony morphology. Colonies of *C. coronatus* grow rapidly; are flat, cream colored, and glabrous; and become radially folded and covered by a fine, powdery, white surface mycelium and condiophores. The lid of the petri dish soon becomes covered with conidia, which are forcibly discharged by the conidiophores. The colony may become tan to brown with age.

Microscopic morphology. Condiophores are simple, forming solitary, terminal conidia which are spherical, 10 to 25 μm in diameter, and single celled and which have a prominent papilla. Conidia may also produce hair-like appendages called villae. Conidia germinate either to produce single or multiple hyphal tubes which may also become conidiophores bearing secondary conidia or to produce multiple short conidiophores, each bearing a small secondary conidium (6).

Histopathology

Biopsy specimens show fibroblastic proliferation and an inflammatory reaction with lymphocytes, plasma cells, histiocytes, eosinophils, and giant cells. Broad, thin-walled hyphae with occasional septa branched at right angles are seen. The Splendore-Hoeppli phenomenon may be seen.

Treatment and Antifungal Susceptibility

Treatment of *C. coronatus* infection is difficult, but patients often respond to oral itraconazole (200 to 400 mg/day) or ketoconazole (200 to 400 mg/day). Amphotericin B has also been used. Treatment should be continued for at least 1 month after the lesions have cleared. The long-term prognosis is highly variable.

Saturated potassium iodide solution is useful for patients in developing countries because of its ease of administration and low cost. The starting dose is 1 ml three times daily, and the dose is increased to up to 4 to 6 ml three times daily as tolerated. Treatment must be continued for at least 1 month after the lesions have disappeared. Allergic reactions and gastrointestinal intolerance are common complications, and relapse is common even after successful initial treatment.

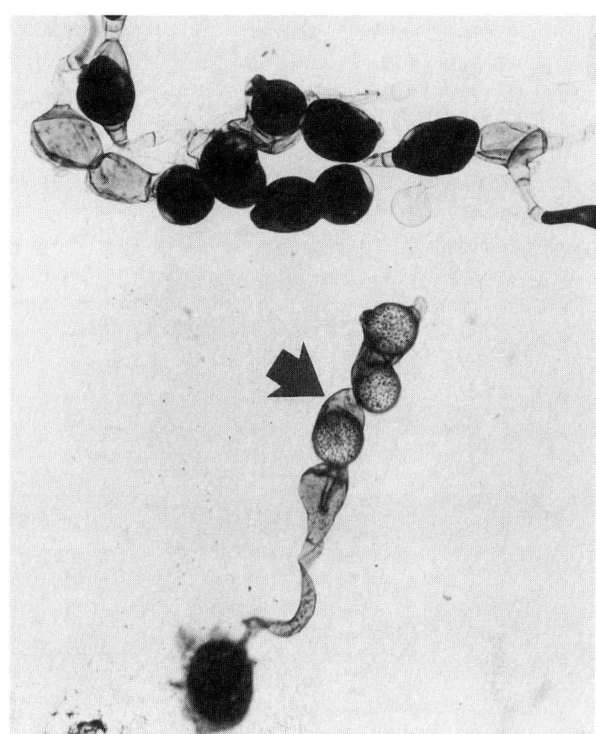

FIGURE 13 Zygospores of *B. ranarum* showing beak-like appendages (arrow). Magnification, ×400.

Surgical resection of infected tissue is seldom successful; it may hasten the spread of infection.

Basidiobolomycosis

Definition

Basidiobolomycosis is a chronic subcutaneous infection of the trunk and limbs.

Geographic Distribution

Basidiobolomycosis is encountered chiefly in the tropical regions of East Africa, West Africa, Indonesia, and India.

Causative Organism and Its Habitat

The most widely held view is that *Basidiobolus ranarum* is the sole agent causing the disease and that *Basidiobolus meristosporus* and *Basidiobolus haptosporus* are only synonyms of the former; however, not all authors are of this opinion.

B. ranarum has been isolated from the guts of frogs, toads, and lizards that had apparently swallowed infected insects. It has also been isolated from ants and decaying plant matter.

It is still uncertain how the disease is acquired and what the length of incubation is. Inoculation through a thorn prick or an insect bite has been suggested, as has contamination of a wound or other abrasion. The infection is most common in children.

Clinical Manifestations

The subcutaneous swelling that characterizes the disease is usually localized to the back of the shoulders and to the arms, but it may also be found on the buttocks and thighs.

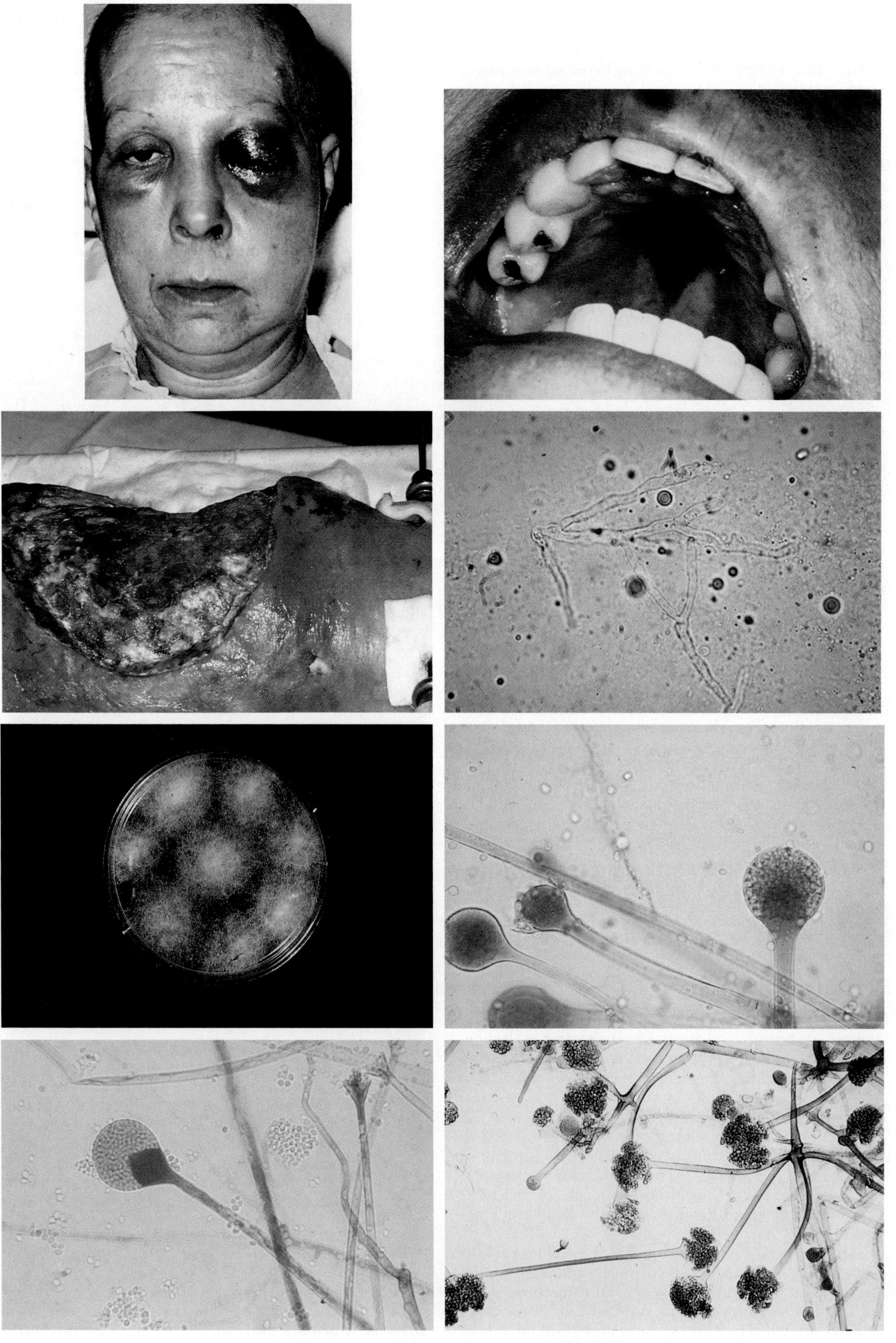

The initial swelling may be fast or slow in onset, and it is hard and painless. The spread is slow but relentless, and a large mass which is attached to the skin but not the underlying tissue is formed (unlike that in *C. coronatus* infection). The infection causes disfigurement, but the skin covering the lesions does not ulcerate. Lymphatic obstruction may occur and can result in massive lymphoedema.

There is no functional impairment as long as the joints are not blocked by the volume of the swelling. The underlying bone and joints are not affected by the disease.

Differential Diagnosis

The disease can be diagnosed with confidence on the basis of appearance and the results of the mycological and particularly the histological examinations. Basidiobolomycosis closely resembles soft tissue sarcoma. Mycetoma has the same degree of induration as basidiobolomycosis, but the presence of draining sinuses, fixation to underlying structures, and extension to bone seen with mycetoma make the distinction relatively easy. Bacterial cellulitis is much more acute and painful than cellulitis associated with zygomycosis. All of these conditions can be reliably distinguished from zygomycosis by biopsy and culturing of the lesions.

Essential Investigations and Their Interpretation

Specimens must be taken from the subcutaneous tissue when the infection is seen as nodules, which develop into massive, firm, indurated swellings. The nodules are freely movable over the underlying muscle but are attached to the skin, which is hyperpigmented but not ulcerated.

Microscopy

Direct microscopy reveals wide, irregular hyphae or hyphal fragments with few septa.

Culture

Specimens should be cultured on Sabouraud dextrose agar at 30°C. Identifiable colonies should be obtained in less than 1 week.

Colony morphology. Colonies grow moderately fast at 30°C; are flat, yellowish gray, and glabrous; and become radially folded and covered by a fine, powdery, white surface mycelium. Satellite colonies are often formed by germinating conidia ejected from the primary colony.

Microscopic morphology. Large, vegetative hyphae (8 to 20 μm in diameter) that form round, smooth, thick-walled zygospores (20 to 50 μm in diameter) with two closely appressed beak-like appendages are characteristic (Fig. 13). Two types of asexual spores, primary and secondary, are formed. Primary spores are globose, one celled, and solitary and are forcibly discharged from a sporophore. The sporophore has a distinct swollen area just below the spore that actively participates in the discharge of the spore. Secondary spores are clavate and one celled and are passively released from a sporophore. The sporophore is not swollen at the base. The apex of the passively released spore has a knob-like adhesive tip. These spores may function as sporangia, producing several sporangiospores. See reference 6 for additional details.

Histopathology

The histopathological features of basidiobolomycosis are very similar to those of conidiobolomycosis.

Treatment and Antifungal Susceptibility

The treatment of choice appears to be saturated potassium iodide solution. In some cases, co-trimoxazole has been found to be more effective than potassium iodide. The recommended dose is two tablets three times daily (each tablet contains 400 mg of sulfamethoxazole and 80 mg of trimethoprim). As with potassium iodide solution, treatment should be continued for 1 month after the lesions have cleared. Oral ketoconazole (400 mg/day) has sometimes been successful, but amphotericin B has seldom been helpful. Susceptibility testing is not appropriate.

If a patient has an enlarged, useless limb resistant to

FIGURE 14 (row 1, left) Rhinocerebral mucormycosis. Infection has spread into the orbit, causing thrombosis, infarction, and necrosis of tissue. The black discharge from the nose is a typical sign. (From M. D. Richardson, D. W. Warnock, and C. K. Campbell, *Slide Atlas of Fungal Infection. Systemic Fungal Infections*, Blackwell Science Ltd., Oxford, United Kingdom, 1995.)

FIGURE 15 (row 1, right) Oral lesion in rhinocerebral mucormycosis (from M. D. Richardson, D. W. Warnock, and C. K. Campbell, *Slide Atlas of Fungal Infection. Systemic Fungal Infections*, Blackwell Science Ltd., Oxford, United Kingdom, 1995).

FIGURE 16 (row 2, left) Cutaneous mucormycosis in a burn (from M. D. Richardson, D. W. Warnock, and C. K. Campbell, *Slide Atlas of Fungal Infection. Systemic Fungal Infections*, Blackwell Science Ltd., Oxford, United Kingdom, 1995).

FIGURE 17 (row 2, right) Microscopic appearance of necrotic material from a case of mucormycosis, showing the typical broad, nonseptate hyphae with right-angled branching (from M. D. Richardson, D. W. Warnock, and C. K. Campbell, *Slide Atlas of Fungal Infection. Systemic Fungal Infections*, Blackwell Science Ltd., Oxford, United Kingdom, 1995).

FIGURE 18 (row 3, left) *Absidia corymbifera* culture (from M. D. Richardson, D. W. Warnock, and C. K. Campbell, *Slide Atlas of Fungal Infection. Systemic Fungal Infections*, Blackwell Science Ltd., Oxford, United Kingdom, 1995).

FIGURE 19 (row 3, right) *Absidia corymbifera* sporing structures (from M. D. Richardson, D. W. Warnock, and C. K. Campbell, *Slide Atlas of Fungal Infection. Systemic Fungal Infections*, Blackwell Science Ltd., Oxford, United Kingdom, 1995).

FIGURE 20 (row 4, left) Microscopic appearance of *Mucor* species.

FIGURE 21 (row 4, right) Microscopic appearance of *Rhizopus microsporus* var. *rhizopodiformis* (from M. D. Richardson, D. W. Warnock, and C. K. Campbell, *Slide Atlas of Fungal Infection. Systemic Fungal Infections*, Blackwell Science Ltd., Oxford, United Kingdom, 1995).

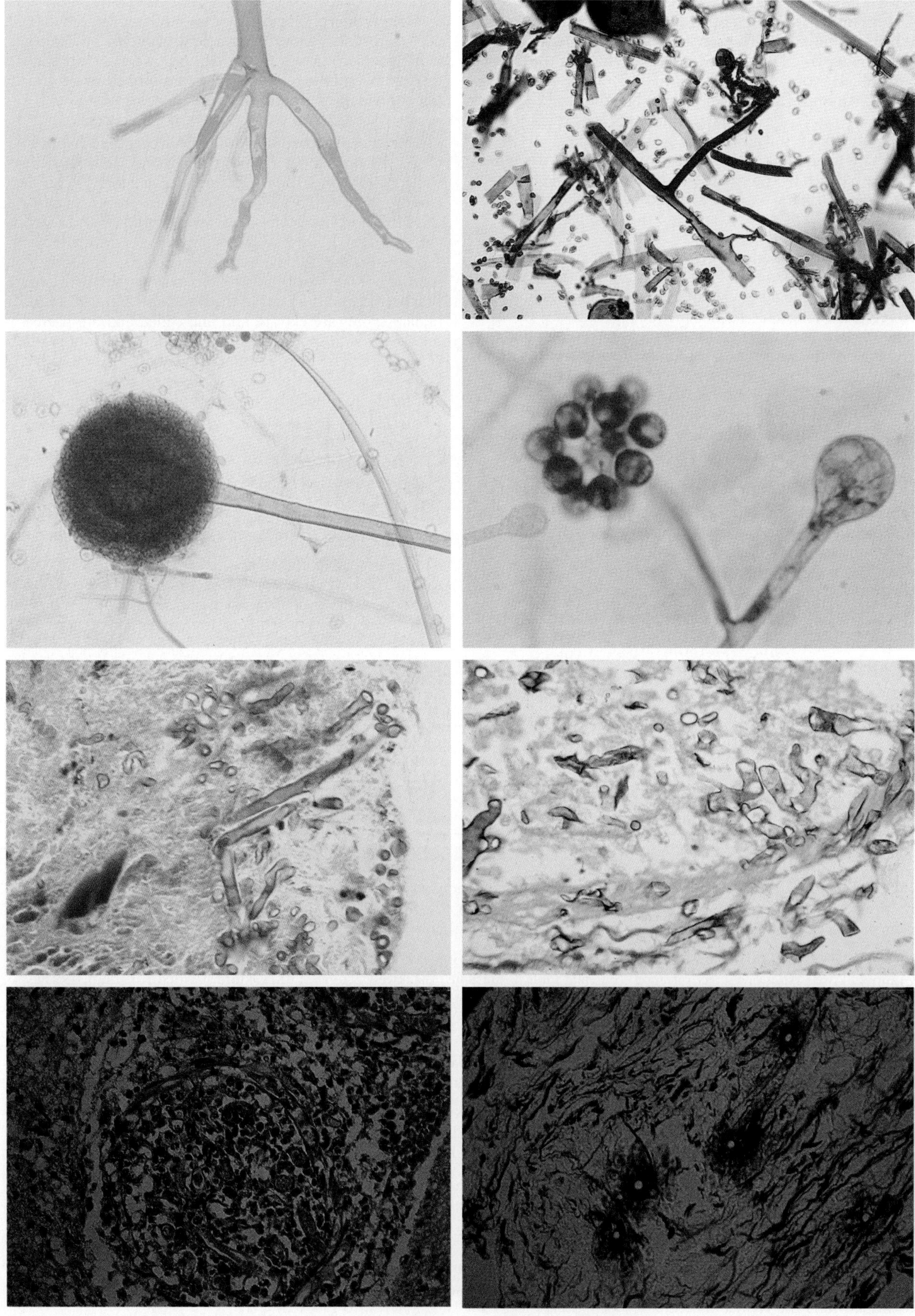

medical treatment, amputation should be considered to forestall bacterial superinfection.

ILLUSTRATIONS

Figures 14 through 29 illustrate infectious lesions and morphological and histopathological characteristics of several important agents of zygomycosis.

APPENDIX 1

Glossary of Terms

This glossary includes specific terms used to describe morphological structures of agents of zygomycosis (for detailed mycological glossaries and definitions, see references 3, 4, and 7).

Apophysis: a swelling; the term is applied to the swelling of a sporangiophore immediately below the columella

Collar: an annulus of sporangial wall remnants at the tip of a sporangiophore

Collarette: a small collar

Columella: a dome-like structure at the tip of a sporangiophore

Pyriform: pear shaped

Rhizoid: a short, branching hypha that resembles a root

Sporangium: a sac-like structure in which the entire internal contents are cleaved into asexual spores

Sporangiolum: a small sporangium producing a small number of sporangiospores

Sporangiophore: a specialized hypha upon which a sporangium develops

Sporangiospore: an asexual spore produced within a sporangium

Sporophore: any structure that bears spores

Stolon: a runner or horizontal hypha from which new hyphae, rhizoids, sporangiophores, or any combination of these structures arises

Zygospore: a resting spore resulting from the fusion of two gametangia

REFERENCES

1. **Berenguer, J., P. Munoz, F. Parras, V. Fernandez-Baca, T. Hernandez-Sampelayo, and E. Bouza.** 1994. Treatment of deep mycoses with liposomal amphotericin B. *Eur. J. Clin. Microbiol. Infect. Dis.* **13:**504–507.
2. **Boelaert, J. R.** 1994. Mucormycosis (zygomycosis): is there news for the clinician? *J. Infect.* **28:**1–6.
3. **Caceres, A. M., C. Sardinas, C. Marcano, R. R. Guevara, J. Barros, G. Bianchi, V. Rosario, R. Balza, M. Silva, M. Redondo, and M. Nunez.** 1997. *Apophysomyces elegans* limb infection with a favourable outcome: case report and review. *Clin. Infect. Dis.* **25:**331–332.
4. **Chakrabart, A., P. Kumar, A. A. Padhye, L. Chatha, S. K. Singh, A. Das, J. D. Wig, and R. N. Kataria.** 1997. Primary cutaneous zygomycosis due to *Saksenaea vasiformis* and *Apophysomyces elegans*. *Clin. Infect. Dis.* **24:**580–583.
5. **de Hoog, G. S., and J. Guarro.** 1995. *Atlas of Clinical Fungi.* Centraalbureau voor Schimmelcultures, Baarn and Delft, The Netherlands/Universitat Rovira i Virgili, Reus, Spain.
6. **de Vroey, C.** 1989. Identification of agents of subcutaneous mycoses, p. 111–139. *In* E. G. V. Evans and M. D. Richardson (ed.), *Medical Mycology: a Practical Approach.* IRL Press, Oxford, England.
7. **Fisher, E. W., A. Toma, P. H. Fisher, and A. D. Cheesman.** 1991. Rhinocerebral mucormycosis: use of liposomal amphotericin B. *J Laryngol. Otol.* **105:**575–577.
8. **Gonzalez, C. E., D. R. Couriel, and T. J. Walsh.** 1997. Disseminated zygomycosis in a neutropenic patient: successful treatment with amphotericin B lipid complex and granulocyte colony-stimulating factor. *Clin. Infect. Dis.* **24:** 192–196.
9. **Goodman, N. L., and M. G. Rinaldi.** 1991. Agents of zygomycosis, p. 674–692. *In* A. Balows, W. J. Hausler, Jr., K. L. Herrmann, H. D. Isenberg, and H. J. Shadomy (ed.), *Manual of Clinical Microbiology*, 5th ed. American Society for Microbiology, Washington, D.C.
10. **Hopwood, V., and E. G. V. Evans.** 1991. Serological tests in the diagnosis and prognosis of fungal infection in the compromised patient, p. 312–353. *In* D. W. Warnock and M. D. Richardson (ed.), *Fungal Infection in the Compromised Patient*, 2nd ed. John Wiley & Sons, Chichester, England.
11. **Kwon-Chung, K. J., and J. E. Bennett.** 1992. Mucormycosis, p. 524–559. *In Medical Mycology*. Lea & Febiger, Philadelphia, Pa.
12. **Lim, K. K. T., M. J. Potts, D. W. Warnock, N. B. N.**

FIGURE 22 (row 1, left) Rhizoids of *Rhizopus*.

FIGURE 23 (row 1, right) Hyphae of *Rhizopus oryzae* in a PAS-stained section of an agar block of a glucose-peptone culture.

FIGURE 24 (row 2, left) Microscopic appearance of *Rhizopus* species.

FIGURE 25 (row 2, right) Microscopic appearance of *Cunninghamella* species.

FIGURE 26 (row 3, left) Histological appearance of mucormycosis in H&E-stained section of soft palate from a patient with rhinocerebral mucormycosis.

FIGURE 27 (row 3, right) Histological appearance of mucormycosis. The hyphae show nondichotomous, irregular branching. (From M. D. Richardson, D. W. Warnock, and C. K. Campbell, *Slide Atlas of Fungal Infection. Systemic Fungal Infections*, Blackwell Science Ltd., Oxford, United Kingdom, 1995.)

FIGURE 28 (row 4, left) Histological appearance of mucormycosis in an H&E-stained section of brain. The tissue reaction shows necrosis and nonspecific inflammation.

FIGURE 29 (row 4, right) Histopathological appearance of entomophthoramycosis in submucosa of nose caused by *Conidiobolus coronatus*. Note the marked Splendore-Hoeppli phenomenon surrounding the fungal elements.

Ibrahim, E. M. Brown, and C. J. Burns-Cox. 1994. Another case report of rhinocerebral mucormycosis treated with liposomal amphotericin B. *Clin. Infect. Dis.* **18:** 653–654.

13. **McGinnis, M. R.** 1980. *Laboratory Handbook of Medical Mycology*. Academic Press, Inc., New York, N.Y.
14. **Mitchell, S. J., J. Gray, M. E. I. Morgan, M. D. Hocking, and G. M. Durbin.** 1996. Nosocomial infection with *Rhizopus microsporus* in pre-term infants: association with wooden tongue depressors. *Lancet* **348:**441–443.
15. **Munckhof, W., R. Jones, F. A. Tosolini, A. Marzec, P. Angus, and M. L. Grayson.** 1993. Cure of *Rhizopus* sinusitis in a liver transplant recipient with liposomal amphotericin B. *Clin. Infect. Dis.* **16:**183.
16. **Parfrey, N. A.** 1986. Improved diagnosis and prognosis of mucormycosis. A clinicopathologic study of 33 cases. *Medicine* **65:**113–123.
17. **Rhodes, J. C., and K. J. Kwong-Chung.** 1989. Identification of agents of systemic mycoses, p. 141–170. *In* E. G. V. Evans and M. D. Richardson (ed.), *Medical Mycology: a Practical Approach*. IRL Press, Oxford, England.
18. **Scholer, H. J., E. Muller, and M. A. A. Schipper.** 1983. Mucorales, p. 3–59. *In* D. H. Howard (ed.), *Fungi Pathogenic for Humans and Animals. Part A. Biology*. Marcel Dekker, Inc., New York, N.Y.
19. **Skahan, K. J., B. Wong, and D. Armstrong.** 1991. Clinical manifestations and management of mucormycosis in the compromised patient, p. 153–190. *In* D. W. Warnock and M. D. Richardson (ed.), *Fungal Infection in the Compromised Patient*, 2nd ed. John Wiley & Sons, Chichester, England.
20. **Smith, J. M. B.** 1989. The Phycomyces, p. 115–169. *In Opportunistic Mycoses of Man and Other Animals*. C.A.B. International Mycologic Institute, Wallingford, England.
21. **Sutton, D. A., A. W. Fothergill, and M. G. Rinaldi.** 1998. *Guide to Clinically Significant Fungi*. Williams & Wilkins, Baltimore, Md.
22. **Tkatch, L. S., S. Kusne, and D. Eibling.** 1993. Successful treatment of zygomycosis of the paranasal sinuses with surgical debridement and amphotericin B colloidal dispersion. *Am. J. Otolaryngol.* **14:**249–253.
23. **Van den Saffele, J. K., and J. R. Boelaert.** 1996. Zygomycosis in HIV-positive patients: a review of the literature. *Mycoses* **39:**77–84.
24. **Walsh, T. J., M. R. Rinaldi, and P. A. Pizzo.** 1993. Zygomycosis of the respiratory tract, p. 149–170. *In* G. A. Sarosi and S. F. Davies (ed.), *Fungal Diseases of the Lung*, 2nd ed. Raven Press, New York, N.Y.
25. **Weitzman, I., and P. Della-Latta.** 1997. Emerging zygomycotic agents. *Clin. Mycol. Newsl.* **19:**81–85.
26. **West, B. C., A. D. Oberle, and K. J. Kwon-Chung.** 1995. Mucormycosis caused by *Rhizopus microsporus* var. *microsporus*: cellulitis in the leg of a diabetic patient cured by amputation. *J. Clin. Microbiol.* **33:**3341–3344.

Histoplasma, Blastomyces, Coccidioides, and Other Dimorphic Fungi Causing Systemic Mycoses

DAVISE H. LARONE, THOMAS G. MITCHELL, AND THOMAS J. WALSH

99

Fungal dimorphism may be defined as growth of a mould form in the natural environment or in the laboratory at 25 to 30°C and as growth in the yeast or spherule form in tissues or when incubated on enriched media at 37°C (7, 47, 75, 86, 94). The dimorphic fungi that cause endemic systemic mycoses are *Histoplasma capsulatum* var. *capsulatum*, *Histoplasma capsulatum* var. *duboisii*, *Blastomyces dermatitidis*, *Coccidioides immitis*, and *Paracoccidioides brasiliensis*. These fungi also have been termed primary or systemic fungal pathogens. In the environment, they all produce a filamentous or mycelial form with hyaline, branching, septate hyphae. The conidia or hyphae of *B. dermatitidis*, *P. brasiliensis*, and both varieties of *H. capsulatum* convert to budding yeast cells in tissue or on enriched media at 37°C in the laboratory. *C. immitis* produces spherules in tissue or in vitro under the appropriate conditions. Temperature is a critical variable in inducing dimorphism in these fungi. The mycelial form at 25 to 30°C undergoes morphological conversion to the yeast or spherule form at 37°C. *B. dermatitidis* and *P. brasiliensis* may convert to their yeast forms in response to temperature alone (58). *H. capsulatum* requires elevated temperatures and the presence of reducing conditions, such as free thiol groups from cysteine (53). The conversion of *C. immitis* from arthroconidia to spherules requires changes in temperature, CO_2 content, and nutrients (9).

Although *Penicillium marneffei* and *Sporothrix schenckii* are regarded as dimorphic fungi, which cause disseminated infection, these organisms will be discussed elsewhere (see chapters 97 and 101, respectively). The term "dimorphism" may be more broadly defined to encompass morphological transformations of other fungi, such as *Candida albicans*, *Wangiella dermatitidis*, and *Phialophora verrucosa* (as well as other fungi causing chromoblastomycosis) (86, 94).

TAXONOMY AND MYCOLOGY

Dimorphic fungi causing systemic mycoses are assigned to the form class *Deuteromycetes*. The names *H. capsulatum* var. *capsulatum*, *H. capsulatum* var. *duboisii*, *B. dermatitidis*, *C. immitis*, and *P. brasiliensis* designate the anamorphs (asexual stage) of these fungi. The teleomorphs (sexual stage) of *H. capsulatum* var. *capsulatum*, *H. capsulatum* var. *duboisii*, and *B. dermatitidis* are classified in the subdivision of *Ascomycotina* and the family *Gymnoascaceae* (44–46, 48, 54, 55). The teleomorphs of *C. immitis* and *P. brasiliensis* are not known.

H. capsulatum Darling 1906

The name *H. capsulatum* was suggested by the appearance of the yeast cells within macrophages of a patient who had died of an infection thought to be due to a protozoan (11). Despite its name, which was based on early descriptions of the histopathological lesions, *H. capsulatum* is neither a protozoan nor encapsulated. The fungus was first cultured from the blood of an infected child (13). The sexual stage or teleomorph of *H. capsulatum* was demonstrated by Kwon-Chung et al. (44, 45) and was named *Emmonsiella capsulata*. The new term *Ajellomyces capsulatus* was proposed by McGinnis and Katz (57) on taxonomic grounds.

H. capsulatum grows at 25 to 30°C on Sabouraud glucose agar (SGA) as a white to buff colony within 6 to 8 weeks. The mycelium is characterized by hyphae with slender conidiophores and spherical or pyriform tuberculate and non-tuberculate macroconidia measuring 8 to 16 μm in diameter. Finely roughened macroconidia of 2 to 5 μm in diameter may be abundant in fresh clinical isolates.

When the mould phase of *H. capsulatum* is incubated at 37°C on enriched medium, such as brain heart infusion (BHI) agar with blood and cysteine, conidia will germinate and convert to yeast cells. After subculture, blastoconidia that are ovoid to spherical and that measure 2 to 4 μm in diameter develop. This same yeast morphology is present in tissue. Although *H. capsulatum* now should be technically termed *Histoplasma capsulatum* var. *capsulatum*, the former term will be retained throughout this chapter for simplicity.

H. capsulatum var. *duboisii* Drouhet 1957

Originally designated *Histoplasma duboisii* by Vanbreuseghem, this organism was later recognized by Drouhet as a variant of *H. capsulatum* and is thus designated *H. capsulatum* var. *duboisii* (76). Mating studies have confirmed that *H. capsulatum* and *H. capsulatum* var. *duboisii* are variants of the same species (48). The in vitro morphological features of the mycelial and yeast phases of *H. capsulatum* var. *duboisii* are virtually identical to those of *H. capsulatum* (70). In vivo, however, *H. capsulatum* var. *duboisii* develops larger, thick-walled, oval yeast cells 10 to 15 μm in diameter. This organism will hereafter be referred to as *H. capsulatum* var. *duboisii*.

B. dermatitidis Gilchrist et Stokes 1898

B. dermatitidis was originally isolated from a cutaneous lesion (19). The teleomorph of *B. dermatitidis* was identified as

Ajellomyces dermatitidis (54, 55). At 25 to 30°C, *B. dermatitidis* grows as a mould with conidia and septate hyphae usually within 14 days; some strains grow more slowly. The mould form of *B. dermatitidis* produces abundant conidia from aerial hyphae and lateral conidiophores. These conidia are spherical, ovoid, or pyriform in shape and 2 to 10 μm in diameter, resembling the macroconidia of *H. capsulatum*. However, unlike the macroconidia of *H. capsulatum*, the conidia of *B. dermatitidis* are smooth. Thick-walled chlamydospores 7 to 18 μm in diameter also may be observed in *B. dermatitidis*. Colonies usually require 2 or more weeks for full development. On enriched media at 37°C, *B. dermatitidis* grows as a yeast with colonies that are folded, pasty, and moist. The yeast cells of *B. dermatitidis* in vitro or in tissue are thick walled and spherical; they produce single buds with a characteristically broad base of attachment between the bud and parent cell.

C. immitis Rixford et Gilchrist 1896

The life cycle of *C. immitis* involves the development of hyphae, arthroconidia, and spherules. In native soil or on routine laboratory culture, *C. immitis* produces branching, septate hyphae and arthroconidia that usually develop in alternate hyphal cells. As the arthroconidia mature, the hyphal cells between them disintegrate and the arthroconidia are released as unicellular structures. The arthroconidia are characteristically barrel shaped, measuring approximately 3 by 6 μm, and often bear remnants of cell wall material from the disrupted adjacent hyphal cells. Hyphae appear within 3 to 5 days, but arthroconidia may not be apparent until 10 days. In tissue or on special media, the arthroconidia become spherical, enlarge, and develop into spherules that may contain endospores. Spherules range in size up to 80 μm. At maturity, the spherules rupture to release the endospores, which may themselves develop into spherules.

P. brasiliensis (Splendore) Almeida 1930

P. brasiliensis at 25 to 30°C initially produces a nonspecific mycelial colony that may later bear a variety of conidia (e.g., chlamydospores, arthroconidia, and single conidia) (73). In tissue or on enriched media at 37°C, the characteristic yeast form develops. The budding yeast cells are globes to pyriform; they may become quite large (10 to 30 μm in diameter), produce numerous small buds (2 to 10 μm), and resemble a mariner's wheel or pilor wheel.

SYSTEMIC MYCOSES DUE TO DIMORPHIC FUNGI

Systemic fungal infections have become increasingly important problems with the advent of new and expanding populations of immunocompromised patients (5, 15, 25, 27, 37, 38, 47, 83, 98, 100–104). Improved transportation and mobility of contemporary society no longer restrict the presentation of histoplasmosis, blastomycosis, coccidioidomycosis, and paracoccidioidomycosis to their respective areas of endemicity. Newer advances in antifungal therapy have expanded therapeutic options and reduced the toxicity of treatments for these mycoses (30, 34, 41, 99), hence increasing the importance of an accurate microbiologic diagnosis. A basic understanding of the pathogenesis, epidemiology, and clinical manifestations of the systemic mycoses caused by the dimorphic fungi will permit a better approach to laboratory identification and clinical diagnosis (Table 1).

Pathogenesis

In most cases, human systemic mycoses due to the dimorphic fungi are initiated when aerosolized conidia are inhaled (37). For *H. capsulatum* and *P. brasiliensis*, the conidia are initially contained by alveolar macrophages, which are modulated by T lymphocytes, resulting in localized granulomatous inflammation (12, 61, 80, 82). By comparison, a combined acute (pyogenic) and chronic (mononuclear or macrophage) inflammatory response often is observed with *C. immitis* and *B. dermatitidis* (3, 22). More than 95% of cases of histoplasmosis, coccidioidomycosis, and paracoccidioidomycosis are estimated to be self-limiting and produce minimal symptoms. In most cases, the only evidence of infection is the development of an immune response, which is manifested by conversion to a positive delayed-type skin reaction and the production of specific precipitins and complement-fixing antibodies (60, 81). The small percentage of these episodes that advance to progressive pulmonary infection or clinically overt disseminated infection is often associated with predisposing risk factors, particularly underlying defects in cell-mediated immunity.

Epidemiology and Clinical Manifestations

Histoplasmosis

H. capsulatum has been isolated from soil with high nitrogen concentrations, especially those related to droppings of starlings, chickens, and bats (20). Outbreaks of pulmonary histo-

TABLE 1 General epidemiologic features of the primary mycoses

Feature	Mycosis			
	Histoplasmosis	Blastomycosis	Coccidioidomycosis	Paracoccidioidomycosis
Saprobic form (<35°C) with hyaline septate hyphae	Yes	Yes	Yes	Yes
Tissue form	Yeasts	Yeasts	Spherules	Yeasts
High infection rate in areas of endemicity	Yes	?	Yes	Yes
≥90% of infections are initiated via respiratory tract	Yes	Yes	Yes	Yes
≥90% of infections are asymptomatic	Yes	?	Yes	Yes
≥90% of infections are self-limiting	Yes	?	Yes	Yes
≥90% of infections involve immunocompetent hosts	Yes	Yes	Yes	Yes
Approximate % of males among patients with disease	80–90	50–90	75–90	95

plasmosis have been associated with exposure to these reservoirs (21, 76, 80, 90). *H. capsulatum* is found principally along the Ohio, Mississippi, and St. Lawrence rivers but is found in other areas of the United States and throughout the world (3, 24, 33, 101, 102).

The clinical manifestations of histoplasmosis may be classified according to site (pulmonary, extrapulmonary, or disseminated infection), by duration of infection (acute, subacute, and chronic), and by pattern of infection (primary versus reactivation). Primary acute pulmonary histoplasmosis may develop in a healthy, immunocompetent host who is exposed to a heavy inoculum (21). Yeast cells of *H. capsulatum* may be observed on direct examination of sputum.

Histoplasmosis may reactivate years later in isolated tissues, particularly the central nervous system, adrenal glands, mucocutaneous surfaces, and other sites (50, 68, 85, 102, 105). This pattern of histoplasmosis, which often occurs in elderly and immunocompromised patients, must be differentiated from other mycoses, tuberculosis, or neoplastic disease (35, 101). Tissue from any of these sites may be submitted for culture and histopathologic studies.

Disseminated histoplasmosis may develop in immunocompromised patients with cellular immunodeficiencies, especially AIDS patients and solid-organ transplant recipients (1, 25, 27, 75). However, disseminated histoplasmosis of infancy may develop in otherwise apparently healthy infants less than 2 years of age. Specimens for culture include blood, urine, bone marrow, and sputum. Patients with AIDS and disseminated histoplasmosis may have multiple cutaneous lesions. Biopsy and culture of these cutaneous lesions may reveal *H. capsulatum*. Disseminated histoplasmosis may be found in multiple mucosal and deep tissue sites (8, 18, 29, 62, 71, 84, 85, 96).

African Histoplasmosis

African histoplasmosis is caused by *H. capsulatum* var. *duboisii* and is limited to equatorial Africa between 20°N and 10°S, which includes Gabon, Uganda, and Kenya. African histoplasmosis is distinguished from histoplasmosis due to *H. capsulatum* var. *capsulatum* by (i) larger, thick-walled yeast cells (10 to 15 μm in diameter) in tissue biopsy specimens, (ii) diminished pulmonary involvement, (iii) greater frequency of skin and bone lesions, and (iv) pronounced giant cell formation (16, 42, 76). Isolated lesions may develop in the cutaneous and subcutaneous tissues or bone. Another presentation is multiple, disseminated lesions that may involve the skin, subcutaneous tissues, bone, lymph nodes, or abdominal organs.

Blastomycosis

Human and canine cases of blastomycosis occur principally in the Ohio and Mississippi river valleys but are not limited to these regions (10, 17, 61). *B. dermatitidis* has been isolated from riverbank soil and beaver dams associated with outbreaks of blastomycosis (39, 40). Although the disease is commonly known as North American blastomycosis, it has been reported from other continents, although only rarely (6, 59).

B. dermatitidis may cause self-limited or localized pulmonary lesions. Chronically progressive blastomycosis may involve one or more organs, most commonly the lungs, followed by the skin, genitourinary tract, bone, or central nervous system in immunocompromised patients (3, 61, 87).

Sputum samples, bronchial lavage fluid, or lung biopsy specimens may be submitted for microscopy and culture. Sputum collected to identify malignant cells in patients with chronic pulmonary infiltrates may reveal unsuspected yeast cells of *B. dermatitidis*. Lung biopsy may reveal a pyogranulomatous reaction with marked fibrosis. Cutaneous lesions may be ulcerative or verrucous and resemble a variety of chronic infections or skin cancer. Biopsy demonstrates pseudoepitheliomatous hyperplasia, acanthosis, and intraepidermal and dermal abscesses containing blastoconidia of *B. dermatitidis*. Osteomyelitis develops in up to one-third of patients with disseminated blastomycosis. The genitourinary tract, especially the prostate and epididymis, is another target of *Blastomyces*. Urine collected for culture after prostate massage may also reveal *B. dermatitidis*. Meningitis due to blastomycosis is uncommon and difficult to diagnose by culture of lumbar cerebrospinal fluid; recovery of *B. dermatitidis* may be improved with culture of ventricular or cisternal fluid (43).

Coccidioidomycosis

C. immitis is distributed in the arid soil of regions of the southwestern United States and northwestern Mexico, Argentina, and other areas of Central and South America (65, 88). Drought followed by heavy rains or dust cloud-generating events such as construction or earthquakes can cause outbreaks of coccidioidomycosis in areas of endemicity (66, 79). Clinical manifestations of coccidioidomycosis have been classified in three general groups: (i) initial pulmonary infection, which is usually self-limiting, (ii) pulmonary complications, and (iii) extrapulmonary disease (4, 8, 83, 106). Primary infections in healthy hosts usually resolve spontaneously without antifungal therapy. However, primary pulmonary infection, particularly in immunocompromised patients, may evolve into one of several complications: pulmonary nodules, thin-walled cavities, progressive pneumonia, pyopneumothorax, and bronchopleural fistula. Dissemination to extrapulmonary sites may result in cutaneous and soft-tissue infection, osteomyelitis, arthritis, and meningitis. Cerebrospinal fluid, other body fluids, and biopsy specimens of tissues infected with *C. immitis* may be submitted to the clinical microbiology laboratory for microscopic examination and culture.

Paracoccidioidomycosis

P. brasiliensis is restricted to Central and South America, but within this vast area, the endemicity varies considerably (5, 52, 56, 72). More than 95% of patients who progress to symptomatic paracoccidioidomycosis are males, possibly because of estrogen-mediated inhibition of mycelium-to-yeast transformation (74, 89). Paracoccidioidomycosis may be considered to have three patterns of infection: acute pneumonia, chronic pneumonia, and disseminated infections (92). These infections may be further classified as primary infection or reactivation. Fever, cough, sputum production, chest pain, dyspnea, hemoptysis, malaise, and weight loss may occur with pneumonia and disseminated infection. Extrapulmonary lesions often develop on the face and oral mucosa. Other sites include lymph nodes, spleen, liver, bone, central nervous system, gastrointestinal tract, and adrenal glands.

COLLECTION, TRANSPORT, AND STORAGE OF SPECIMENS

Methods of collection, transport, and storage of specimens are detailed in chapter 4. Most specimens from patients with suspected endemic mycoses are sputum, bronchoalveolar lavage, transtracheal aspirate, or lung biopsy specimens. Several aspects of collection and transport of specimens are particularly relevant to the dimorphic fungi. Sputum is often contaminated with bacteria, saprophytic yeasts endogenous to the oral cavity, and airborne conidia of saprophytic moulds. Care must be taken to transport, process, and properly culture such contaminated specimens promptly to avoid overgrowth by more rapidly growing bacteria or saprophytic fungi. If clinical specimens are mailed, they may be shipped at room temperature.

Blastomycosis and coccidioidomycosis may cause suppurative cutaneous and visceral lesions. Specimens consisting of pus or exudate should be collected by aspiration, whenever possible. Swabs should be avoided, but when they are used to collect specimens, they should be transported directly to the laboratory, preferably in commercial transport systems to prevent drying. Normally sterile fluids and tissues should also be transported promptly to the laboratory, especially if their collection required an invasive procedure. Extreme care should be given to such specimens because the repetition of an invasive procedure to replace a lost or damaged specimen subjects the patient to further discomfort and risk of complications. Tissue should be divided and submitted for histopathologic and mycologic examinations. Where available and appropriate, special tissue stains should be requested, such as the Grocott-Gomori methenamine silver (GMS), periodic acid-Schiff (PAS), and Giemsa stains.

BIOSAFETY

The conidia of the mycelial form of dimorphic fungi are highly infectious and are easily transmissible by aerosolization. The arthroconidia of *C. immitis* have a high propensity for airborne transmission. The yeast forms of dimorphic fungi in tissue are also infectious if aerosolized (e.g., during specimen processing) and inhaled or accidentally injected by direct percutaneous inoculation. Laboratory-acquired infections due to the systemic dimorphic fungi have been well documented (98). Overall, laboratory-acquired fungal infections are more common than bacterial, parasitic, and chlamydial infections and are second only to viral infections (69). Coccidioidomycosis and histoplasmosis constituted 46% of these fungal infections.

All plating of specimens and study of cultures should be performed within a biosafety cabinet (see chapter 9). Plates with a suspicious hyaline mould should be opened only in a biosafety cabinet and should be handled with extreme care. Slants are preferable to plates for the isolation of dimorphic fungi. Slants are safer, require less space, and are more resistant to desiccation during protracted incubation. However, plates are appropriate for the initial recovery of dimorphic fungi from lysis-centrifugation blood cultures. Shrink seals are advised for plates in order to prevent accidental opening and to retard drying. If colonies of dimorphic fungi, such as *C. immitis*, are identified on plates, they should subsequently be sealed with tape in the biosafety cabinet, properly decontaminated, and disposed of. Slide cultures should *not* be set up for an isolate suspected of being a systemic dimorphic fungus.

LABORATORY DIAGNOSIS

General Guidelines

The dimorphic fungi that cause systemic mycoses are identified by direct microscopic examination of specimens, by isolation and characterization of the fungus in cultures, by use of specific DNA probes, or by demonstration of specific exoantigens produced in culture (78) (Tables 2 and 3). The systemic dimorphic fungi produce hyaline, septate hyphae at 25 to 30°C in the laboratory. The conidia or hyphae of

TABLE 2 Characteristics of dimorphic fungi causing systemic infection

Anamorph (teleomorph)	Ecology	Mycelial form	Tissue form
H. capsulatum (A. capsulatus)	Alkaline soil, bird and bat guano; Ohio, Missouri, and Mississippi river valleys	Hyphae, globose microconidia, 3–5 μm in diam; tuberculate and nontuberculate macroconidia (8–16 μm)	Small oval yeasts; 2–4 μm in diam
H. capsulatum var. *duboisii (A. capsulatus)*	Central Africa	Hyphae, microconidia, tuberculate and nontuberculate macroconidia identical to those of *H. capsulatum*	Thick-walled yeasts; narrow-based budding; 10–15 μm in diam
B. dermatitidis (A. dermatitidis)	Riverbanks?; Ohio and Mississippi river valleys	Hyphae and oval, pyriform, to globose terminal and lateral conidia (2–10 μm)	Thick-walled yeasts; wide-based singly budding; 8–15 μm in diam
C. immitis	Soil; semiarid regions of southwestern United States; Mexico, Central and South America	Hyphae and arthroconidia (3–6 μm)	Spherules (20–60 μm in diam) containing endospores 2–4 μm in diam
P. brasiliensis	Soil?; Central and South America	Hyphae; rare oval to globose terminal and lateral microconidia; intercalary chlamydospores	Thick-walled multiply budding yeasts; 15–30 μm in diam

TABLE 3 Summary of methods for microbiological identification of dimorphic fungi that cause systemic mycoses

Direct microscopic examination
- Wet preparations of fresh clinical specimens[a]
  - Calcofluor white or KOH
  - Combination of calcofluor white and KOH

Preparations of fixed specimens
- Wright or Giemsa stain (especially of bone marrow aspirates or buffy coat smears to detect *H. capsulatum* within monocytes or macrophages)
- Cytopathology (*B. dermatitidis* or *H. capsulatum* or the spherules of *C. immitis*) by Papanicolaou staining methods
- Indirect fluorescent-antibody staining
- Staining of a paraffin-embedded clot section of bone marrow aspirate (with H&E, PAS, GMS, Giemsa, and Wright stains), especially for *H. capsulatum*
- Histopathologic examination of paraffin-embedded tissue specimens (with H&E, PAS, GMS, Giemsa, and Wright stains)

Culture
- Nonsterile specimens
  - Primary isolation on media[b] containing antibacterial antibiotics (e.g., chloramphenicol, gentamicin, streptomycin, or penicillin) with and without cycloheximide to inhibit saprophytic fungi
  - Yeast extract agar with concentrated ammonium hydroxide (inhibits the growth of *Candida* spp. but not the systemic dimorphic fungi)
  - Cultures incubated at 30°C under aerobic conditions
  - Tubes or plates to be held for 4–8 wk or longer[c]
- Sterile specimens[d]
  - Primary isolation on media[b]
  - Cultures incubated at 30°C under aerobic conditions
  - Subculture suspicious mycelial colonies to promote sporulation[e]
  - Tubes or plates to be held for 4–8 wk or longer[c]
- Conversion of mycelial form to yeast form

Exoantigen identification
- Detection of cell-free antigens produced by the mycelium from cultures

Nucleic acid probes
- Identification of cultured isolates

[a] Touch preparations of freshly resected tissues may also be stained with calcofluor white.
[b] Such as blood agar, BHI agar, inhibitory mould agar, SGA, enriched broth, and BHI broth.
[c] Subculture suspicious colonies. Laboratories in regions of endemicity may also consider incubating cultures directly at 37°C.
[d] Tissues should be minced or homogenized before plating. Mincing is preferable to homogenization.
[e] Potato-dextrose agar or SGA.

most isolates of *B. dermatitidis*, *P. brasiliensis*, and both varieties of *H. capsulatum* will convert to budding yeast cells in tissue or on enriched media at 37°C in the laboratory. Mycelium-to-yeast conversion appears to be more reliable at 37°C than at 35°C. Conversion from the mycelial to the yeast form usually requires 7 to 14 days or longer. During the early phases of conversion a mixture of mycelial and yeast forms is found. *C. immitis* produces spherules in vitro under the appropriate conditions; however, this conversion is not a routine procedure in most clinical microbiology laboratories.

On routine culture at 25 to 30°C in the laboratory, the five species of dimorphic fungi discussed in this chapter grow as moulds and produce colonies that may be indistinguishable from each other as well as many saprophytic species. Detection of circulating antibodies and fungal antigens in serum or other normally sterile body fluids of infected patients is useful in establishing a clinical diagnosis of certain endemic mycoses, particularly coccidioidomycosis and histoplasmosis (60, 81). The reader is referred to the *Manual of Clinical Laboratory Immunology* for complete coverage of serologic tests (35).

Direct Examination

Careful direct microscopic examination of specimens may provide rapid presumptive diagnosis of a systemic mycosis, which is advantageous since these dimorphic fungi tend to grow slowly. Fresh, wet preparations of sputum, centrifuged cerebrospinal fluid, or urine, pus, skin scrapings, tissue impression smears, and similar specimens should be examined directly with calcofluor white, KOH, or both (26). Calcofluor white is an exceptionally valuable stain for the direct visualization of fungi in specimens.

Sputum may be concentrated and stained directly with Wright or Giemsa stain to detect *H. capsulatum* within monocytes or macrophages. Patients with pulmonary mycoses due to dimorphic fungi may have chronic pulmonary infiltrates resembling lung cancer. Papanicolaou staining methods used by cytopathologists are valuable for detection of the spherules of *C. immitis* and the yeast cells of *B. dermatitidis* and *H. capsulatum* (77). Indeed, routine Papanicolaou staining of sputum from patients with suspected endemic pulmonary mycoses may be an effective method of rapid diagnosis.

Bone marrow aspirates, buffy coat smears, and peripheral blood smears are valuable for the early detection of *H. capsu-*

latum in patients with disseminated histoplasmosis. Giemsa or Wright stain reveals the yeast cells within circulating monocytes or tissue macrophages. Staining of a paraffin-embedded clot section of bone marrow aspirate with PAS, GMS, Giemsa, and Wright stains is another method that allows the detection of *H. capsulatum* in granulomas (97).

Touch preparations of bone marrow biopsy specimens, lymph nodes, and other tissues are an efficient means of detecting fungi in these tissues. The same group of special stains, as well as calcofluor white, may be applied to slides to which the freshly cut surface of a tissue specimen has been pressed, dried, and fixed with heat or ethanol. Immunohistologic methods with fluorescent antibody, immunoperoxidase, and gold-silver staining are performed in a few specialized laboratories (32).

Culture

Several considerations pertain to the culture of systemic dimorphic fungi. As indicated previously, nonsterile specimens, such as sputum or skin, are often contaminated with bacteria and saprophytic fungi that can overgrow the slower-growing dimorphic fungi. Therefore, primary isolation media should contain antibacterial antibiotics (e.g., chloramphenicol, gentamicin, streptomycin, or penicillin) and cycloheximide to inhibit saprophytic fungi. Media without cycloheximide should also be included because this compound inhibits many opportunistic pathogens, such as *Cryptococcus neoformans*, *Candida* spp., *Aspergillus* spp., and zygomycetes. Alternatively, such specimens can be plated on yeast extract agar to which a drop of concentrated ammonium hydroxide is allowed to diffuse from the edge of the plate; this inhibits the growth of *Candida* species but not the systemic dimorphic fungi (84).

Normally sterile specimens may be inoculated directly onto blood agar, BHI agar, inhibitory mould agar, SGA, and enriched broth such as BHI broth. Tissues should be minced or homogenized before plating. All cultures for systemic dimorphic fungi should be incubated at 25 to 30°C under aerobic conditions. Since tubes or plates are to be held for 4 to 8 weeks or longer, the incubator should be well humidified to prevent desiccation of the agar. Culture tubes are preferable; however, if plates are used, 25 ml of agar should be used per plate. Lids should be fastened with shrink seals or two tabs of tape to prevent accidental opening. Laboratories in the regions of endemicity may also consider incubating cultures simultaneously at 37°C.

Exoantigen Identification

The mycelial forms that are suspected of being *H. capsulatum*, *B. dermatitidis*, *C. immitis*, or *P. brasiliensis* require confirmation of identification. The exoantigen technique is a simple diagnostic method that detects the presence of cell-free antigens, known as exoantigens, which are produced by the mycelial-form cultures. A specific exoantigen detected in the aqueous extract of a mycelial-form culture may identify any of the systemic dimorphic fungi (Table 4). This procedure is relatively rapid and is applicable to nonsporulating cultures. Exoantigens are demonstrated by immunodiffusion of specific antigens in either a concentrated aqueous extract of the colony on solid medium or the supernatant of a broth culture of the isolate. Reference antisera identify specific antigens in the isolate and the control antigen.

Methods for the detection of exoantigens have been developed by Kaufman and Standard (36). To test a culture on solid medium, the mature slant culture is overlaid with a solution of Merthiolate (1:5,000) at room temperature.

TABLE 4 Species-specific exoantigens for the identification of systemic dimorphic fungal pathogens

Feature	Exoantigen(s)[a]
H. capsulatum	h, m
B. dermatitidis	A
C. immitis	HS, F, HL
P. brasiliensis	1, 2, 3

[a] Exoantigens are detected by precipitin lines of identity in immunodiffusion tests of concentrated culture supernatants versus reference antigens and antisera (27).

After overnight incubation, the fluid is aspirated and a 5-ml sample is concentrated 50-fold (Minicon B-15; Amicon Corp.) or is tested unconcentrated for *C. immitis*. The concentrate is placed on a microimmunodiffusion well opposite reference antigens and antisera. Note that antiserum is placed in the center well 1 h before the control antigens and concentrate are added to the adjacent wells. The microimmunodiffusion plate is incubated for 24 h at room temperature, the template is removed, the surface of the agarose plate is washed and covered with distilled water, and the plate is read over indirect light for lines of identity (Fig. 1). Any line of identity with control antigen-antibody is significant.

Some isolates produce more readily detectable antigen when grown in liquid medium at 25°C for 3 or more days. For this procedure, one or more 30-ml BHI cultures are established in 125-ml flasks, which are incubated on a gyratory shaker at 150 rpm. After 3 days, all or a portion of the culture is removed and 1% Merthiolate is added to give a final concentration of 1:5,000. The Merthiolate-treated sample is shaken for another day and centrifuged. Five-milliliter samples of the supernatant are concentrated 10- and 25-fold as described above and are tested for the presence of specific exoantigen. Note than *C. immitis* does not require concentration. If 3-day cultures are unproductive, concentrated culture supernatants from older cultures may be tested.

Nucleic Acid Probes

A recent advancement in the identification of dimorphic fungi from cultures is the development of nucleic acid probes. Probes for the identification of *H. capsulatum*, *B. dermatitidis*, and *C. immitis* are commercially available in a nonisotopic kit format (AccuProbe; Gen-Probe Inc., San Diego, Calif.). The procedure takes approximately 1 h and consists of three major steps:

1. Sample preparation. A suspension of the test organism in the mould or yeast phase is sonicated to lyse the fungal cells and release target rRNA. It is then heat inactivated to ensure death of the isolate.
2. Hybridization. The organism lysate is incubated with a DNA probe labeled with acridinium ester. The probe hybridizes with the target rRNA (if present), forming a stable double-stranded hybrid. The acridinium ester is in a protected position in the double-stranded hybrid of a positive sample but remains exposed if target rRNA is not present.
3. Selection and detection. Selection reagent is added to hydrolyze acridinium ester on single, unhybridized strands of the probe. The solution tube is placed in a luminometer, into which hydrogen peroxide and sodium hydroxide are injected. In the presence of intact acridinium ester, bound in the DNA probe-target rRNA hybrid, chemiluminescence

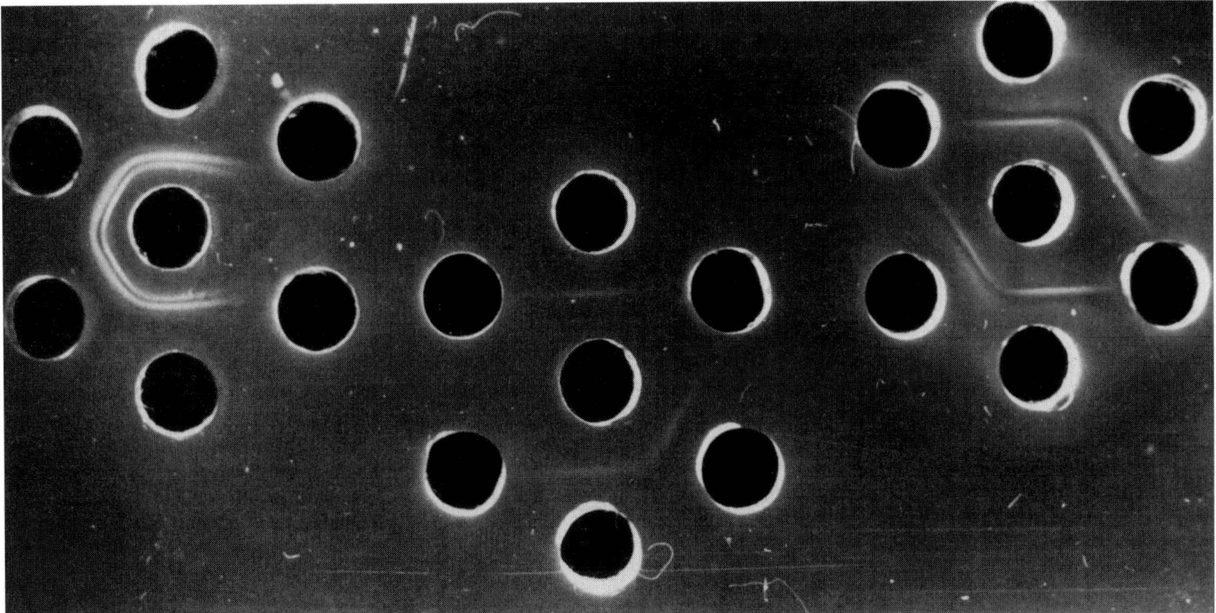

FIGURE 1 Lines of identity for exoantigens in agarose microimmunodiffusion plate.

occurs instantaneously and is measured by the luminometer. The amount of light generated is proportional to the amount of target nucleic acid in the test suspension. A predetermined number of relative light units must be obtained for a test to be considered positive.

Studies with *H. capsulatum* have shown that isolates of any age cultured on any medium may be used successfully with the AccuProbe system (28, 31, 63). Dark-colored fungi sometimes produce false-positive results that may be due to chemiluminescence of pigments such as melanin. Because the dimorphic fungi do not produce deep pigments, dark colonies need not be tested, and the potential problem can be avoided.

Although the probe method is more expensive to perform than exoantigen testing, the probes offer the advantages of early testing of very young cultures, rapid processing, easy interpretation of results, and a high level of accuracy for the identification of *H. capsulatum*, *B. dermatitidis*, and *C. immitis* (64, 91).

Laboratory Identification of Specific Dimorphic Fungi

H. capsulatum

Direct examination of specimens for *H. capsulatum* is best accomplished with special stains. The budding yeast cells of *H. capsulatum* (2 to 4 μm) on a calcofluor white or KOH preparation of sputum may be too small for reliable detection and may be confused with *Candida glabrata*, which is similar in size and shape and which often colonizes the human oropharynx (Fig. 2 and 3). The small yeast cells of *H. capsulatum* are frequently observed within the cytoplasm of macrophages. In contrast, the yeast cells of *C. glabrata* are seldom found within macrophages. Nevertheless, the only reliable methods of distinguishing between these two species are culture and indirect fluorescent-antibody staining. Giemsa and hematoxylin and eosin (H&E) stains reveal the intracellular yeasts of *H. capsulatum* more readily, especially in sputum, blood smears, bone aspirates, and biopsy specimens. The GMS stain delineates the yeast cells but not the cellular detail of the host inflammatory cells.

Histopathologic examination of paraffin-embedded specimens with H&E and PAS stains reveals that *H. capsulatum* elicits a granulomatous inflammatory response. Different patterns of inflammation may be evident, depending on the duration and severity of infection. Large numbers of the tiny yeasts pack the cytoplasm of macrophages in acute pulmonary or disseminated histoplasmosis (Fig. 4). The yeast cells of *H. capsulatum* must be distinguished from cells of the intracellular parasites *Leishmania donovani* and *Toxoplasma gondii*. *L. donovani* contains a kinetoplast, which is not pres-

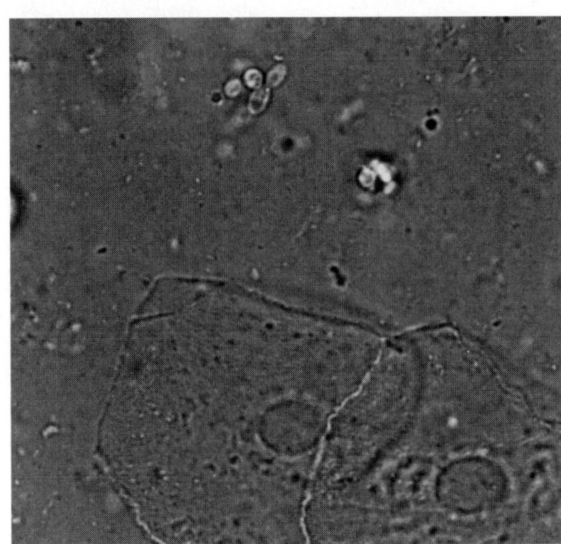

FIGURE 2 KOH wet mount of sputum showing blastoconidia of *H. capsulatum* adjacent to epithelial cells. Original magnification, ×400.

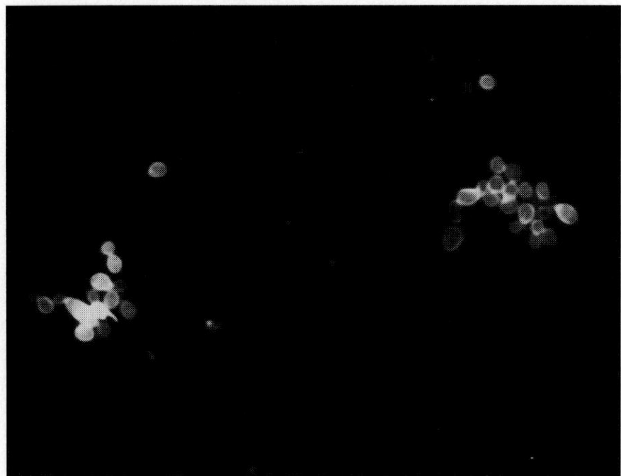

FIGURE 3 Calcofluor white wet mount of sputum showing blastoconidia of *H. capsulatum*. Original magnification, ×400.

ent in the yeast cells of *H. capsulatum*. The tachyzoites of *T. gondii* are not stained with the GMS stain.

H. capsulatum should also be distinguished histologically from the small form of *B. dermatitidis*, the endospores and young spherules of *C. immitis*, the very similar cells of *Penicillium marneffei*, and the yeast cells of *Cryptococcus neoformans*. Yeast cells of *B. dermatitidis* have a broader base of attachment between the bud and parent cell than do those of *H. capsulatum*. The presence of spherules of various sizes distinguishes *C. immitis* in tissue. *P. marneffei* cells reproduce via septation rather than via budding (see chapter 97). Alcian blue or Mayer mucicarmine stain will stain the polysaccharide capsule of *C. neoformans* but will not stain *H. capsulatum*, which lacks a capsule.

Culture of specimens infected with *H. capsulatum* at 25 to 30°C reveals a fluffy, slowly growing colony with an aerial mycelium that varies in color from white to buff to brown (2, 49). During early growth of the mycelial culture, spherical to oval to pyriform microconidia (2 to 5 μm in diameter) are present. These microconidia may be sessile on the sides of hyphae and attached to short lateral conidiophores. With continued growth, the mould develops slender conidiophores and characteristic globose and pyriform, tuberculate and nontuberculate macroconidia measuring 8 to 16 μm in diameter (Fig. 5). Since these macroconidia may resemble those of the saprophytic genus *Sepedonium*, a suspicious isolate must be converted to the yeast form, be shown to produce the h or m exoantigen, or give a positive reaction when tested with a specific nucleic acid probe to identify it as *H. capsulatum*. Furthermore, *H. capsulatum* grows on media with cycloheximide at 25 to 30°C, but the monomorphic *Sepedonium* spp. are inhibited. *Chrysosporium* spp. develop conidia that resemble those of *H. capsulatum*; however, *Chrysosporium* spp. are not dimorphic, do not produce exoantigens, and do not react with *Histoplasma*-specific probes. The *Chrysosporium* state of *Renispora flavissima* may also resemble the mycelium of *H. capsulatum*.

Conversion of the mycelial form of *H. capsulatum* to the yeast form is performed by incubating the mycelial culture

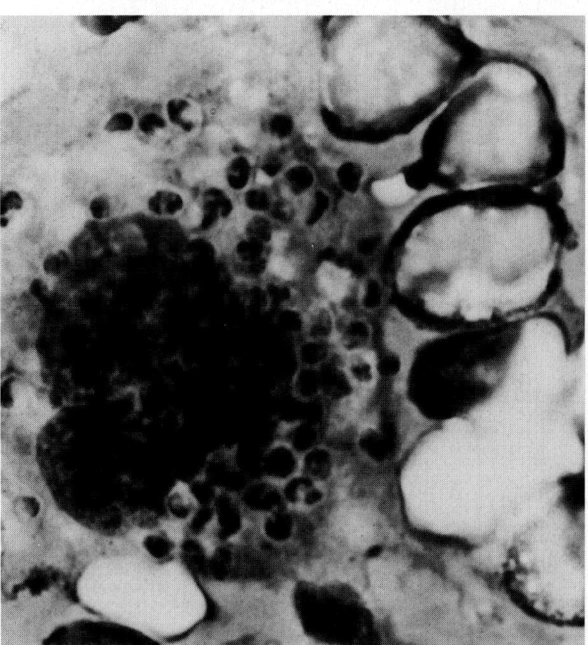

FIGURE 4 Bone marrow aspirate with macrophage containing numerous blastoconidia of *H. capsulatum*. Giemsa stain; original magnification, ×1,000.

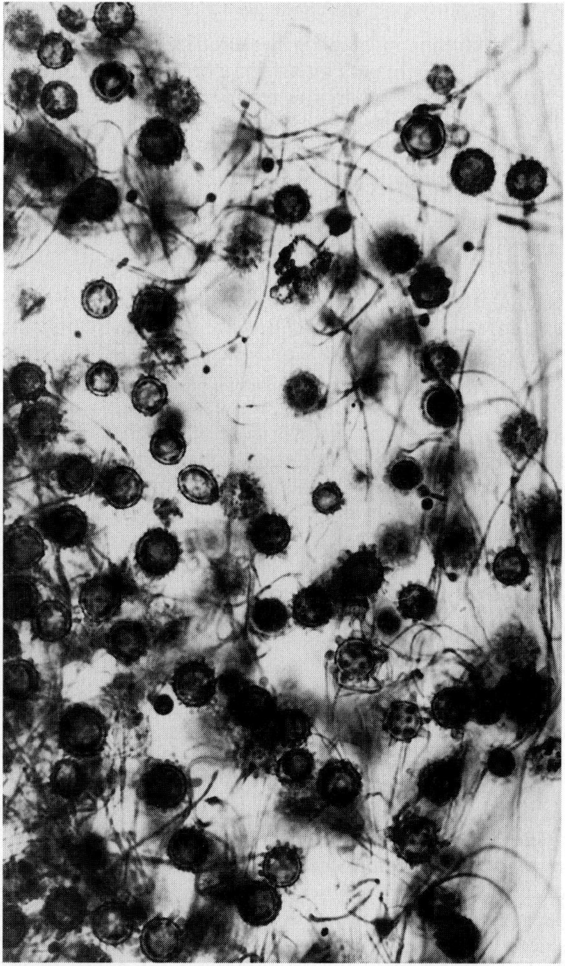

FIGURE 5 Mycelial phase of *H. capsulatum* demonstrating tuberculate and nontuberculate macroconidia. Original magnification, ×400.

at 37°C on enriched medium, such as BHI agar with cysteine. This conversion may be difficult but can be performed best at 37°C instead of 35°C. When the mycelium is incubated at 37°C, spherical to oval budding yeast cells (2 to 5 μm in diameter) develop. Hyphal cells may form buds directly or develop enlarged, transitional cells that subsequently begin to bud (Fig. 6). The microconidia also may convert to budding yeast cells. Complete conversion is rarely achieved, but the presence of a mixture of typical yeast cells with hyphal elements is sufficient to confirm the identification. Yeast cells of *H. capsulatum* in vitro or in vivo are small and ellipsoidal, approximately 1 to 3 by 3 to 5 μm. This conversion usually requires at least 7 to 10 days. Such yeast cells may also be isolated directly on blood agar plates or other enriched media incubated at 37°C. Buds are often formed at the smaller end of ellipsoidal yeast cells and are attached by a narrow connection.

The lysis-centrifugation technique (Isolator; Wampole Laboratories, Cranbury, N.J.) is by far the most effective method of recovering *H. capsulatum* from blood specimens (51, 67, 107). The tube in which the blood is collected for culture contains a mixture (saponin, propylene glycol, sodium polyanetholesulfonate, and EDTA) that lyses leukocytes, prevents coagulation, and inhibits complement. After the tube is centrifuged at 3,000 × *g* for 30 min, the supernatant is withdrawn from the tube and the concentrate is transferred via a pipette from the bottom of the tube to a culture medium. A variety of media may be used, including inhibitory mould agar, SGA, BHI agar, or chocolate agar plates. *H. capsulatum* may be isolated as a mixture of yeast cells and hyphae directly from lysis-centrifugation blood cultures, which are routinely incubated at 35°C. Over the years biphasic media have been relatively successful in recovering *H. capsulatum*. *H. capsulatum* has also been fortuitously isolated from blood inoculated into Middlebrook broth selective for acid-fast bacilli, i.e., BACTEC 13A medium (23).

H. capsulatum var. *duboisii*

H. capsulatum var. *duboisii* differs reliably from *H. capsulatum* var. *capsulatum* only in its tissue form. Direct examination of purulent material or tissue biopsy specimens (usually skin, lymph nodes, or both) treated with calcofluor white or KOH reveals large, thick-walled, budding yeasts of *H. capsulatum* var. *duboisii* that measure 10 to 15 μm in diameter. The spherical to ellipsoidal yeast cells in infected tissue are found within the abundant multinucleate giant cells in a fibrogranulomatous inflammatory reaction (Fig. 7). Retraction of the cytoplasm of the phagocytes from the yeasts produces an artifactual "capsule" on H&E staining. With GMS stain, the narrow attachment between the buds and yeasts creates a figure eight or double-cell budding configuration. The yeast cells may occasionally be connected in short chains. *H. capsulatum* var. *duboisii* is distinguishable from *B. derma-*

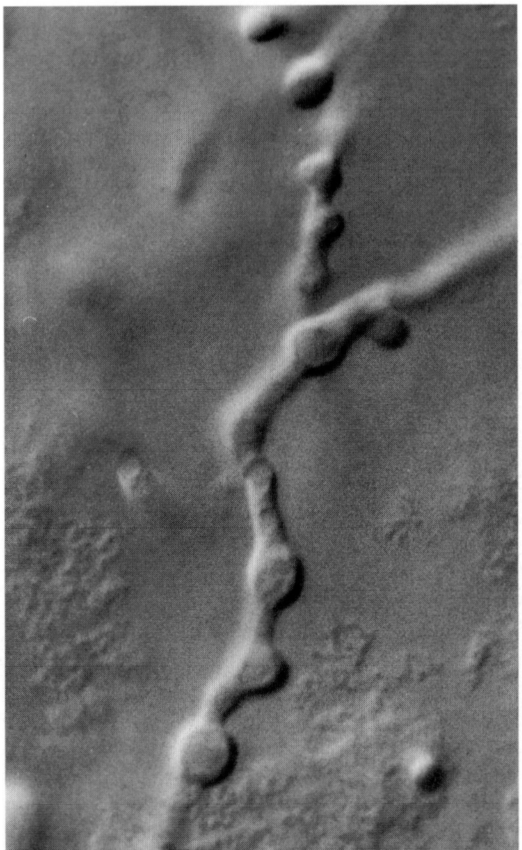

FIGURE 6 Transitional phase of *H. capsulatum* during conversion from mycelial phase to yeast phase at 35°C. Original magnification, ×400.

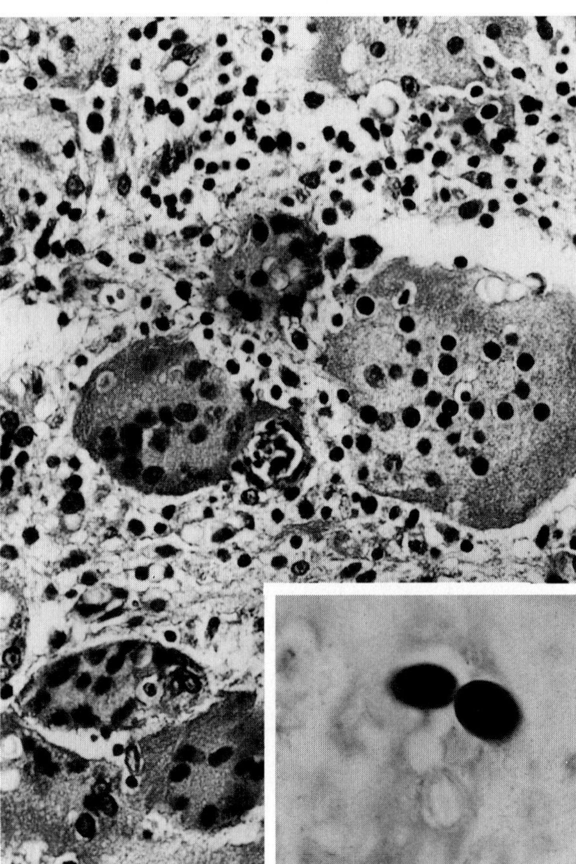

FIGURE 7 Bone biopsy specimen showing multinucleate giant cells and intracytoplasmic blastoconidia of *H. capsulatum* var. *duboisii*. Original magnification, ×250. Bone biopsy revealing budding yeast of *H. capsulatum* var. *duboisii* (methenamine silver stain). Original magnification, ×1,250.

titidis in tissue by the presence of narrow-based budding in the former and broad-based budding in the latter. Moreover, the abundance of many intracellular thick-walled yeasts in numerous multinucleate giant cells is more typical of *H. capsulatum* var. *duboisii* than of *B. dermatitidis*.

The colonial morphology and microscopic appearance of the mould form of *H. capsulatum* var. *duboisii* grown at 25 to 30°C are the same as those of *H. capsulatum*, including the typical microconidia and macroconidia. Distinction between the in vitro yeast phases of *H. capsulatum* var. *duboisii* and *H. capsulatum* var. *capsulatum* may be difficult. When the mould is incubated at 37°C, the fungus converts to yeast cells that are similar in size and shape to those of *H. capsulatum* var. *capsulatum*, especially in early cultures (70). Thus, histopathologic documentation of the characteristic tissue forms of *H. capsulatum* var. *duboisii* is a critical step for establishing the laboratory diagnosis of this organism.

B. dermatitidis

Direct calcofluor white or KOH mounts of sputum, exudates, and tissues can demonstrate the yeast cells of *B. dermatitidis*, which are large, spherical, and thick walled and measure approximately 8 to 15 μm in diameter (Fig. 8 and 9). The yeast cells bud singly and have a wide base of attachment between the bud and the parent yeast cell. The bud of *B. dermatitidis* often attains the same size as the parent yeast before becoming detached. Infected tissues stained with GMS will reveal these characteristic yeast forms (Fig. 10).

When specimens are cultured at 25 to 30°C, *B. dermatitidis* initially produces a fluffy white colony on routine mycologic media. Some strains develop tan, glabrous colonies without conidia, and others may produce light brown colonies with concentric rings. The mould form of *B. dermatitidis* produces conidia 2 to 10 μm in diameter that are located on long or short terminal or lateral hyphal branches (Fig. 11). These conidia are typically spherical, ovoid, or pyriform in shape. Thick-walled chlamydospores 7 to 18 μm in diameter may also be observed in older cultures. The colony and conidia resemble those of *Chrysosporium* spp. and may not be distinguishable from an early culture of *H. capsulatum* having only hyphae, conidiophores, and microconidia. The identification is confirmed by conversion to the yeast form by growth at 37°C, a positive test with a nucleic acid probe, or detection of exoantigen A. However, confirmation of culture identification is probably not necessary if a tissue diagnosis of blastomycosis is also established.

At 37°C, the yeast form grows as a white to light brown, wrinkled colony. In vitro or in tissue, the yeast cells of *B. dermatitidis* are thick walled and spherical; they produce single buds with a characteristically wide base of attachment between the bud and the parent cell. The microscopic morphology of *B. dermatitidis* isolates may vary. A small form produces yeast cells in tissue resembling *H. capsulatum* (76).

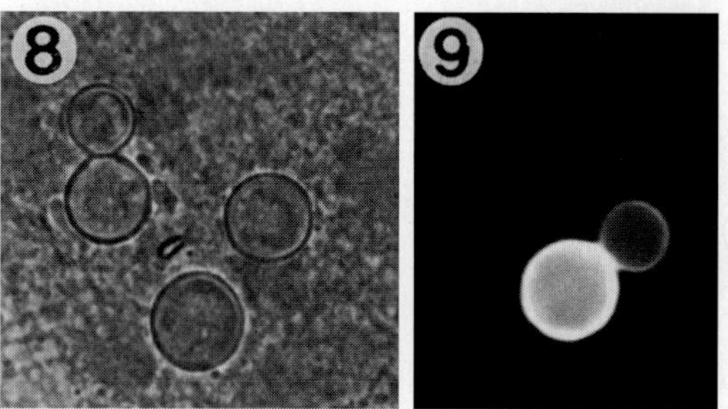

FIGURE 8 KOH wet mount of sputum showing budding yeast of *B. dermatitidis*. Original magnification, ×400.

FIGURE 9 Calcofluor white wet mount of sputum showing budding yeast of *B. dermatitidis*. Original magnification, ×400.

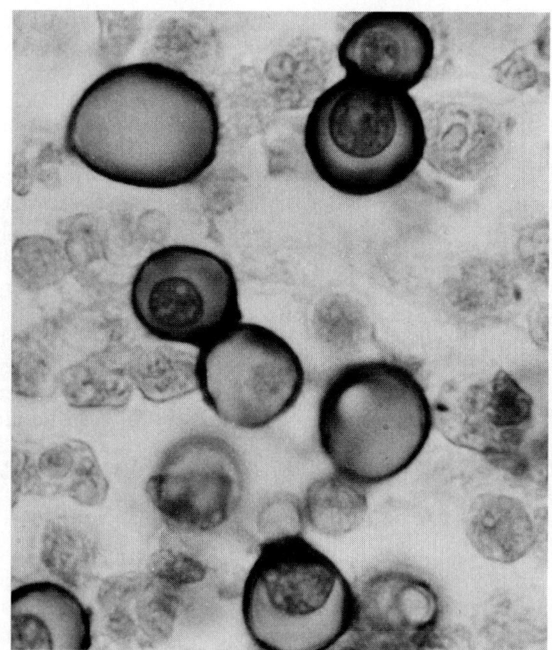

FIGURE 10 Lung biopsy specimen demonstrating blastoconidia of *B. dermatitidis* (GMS stain). Original magnification, ×1,250.

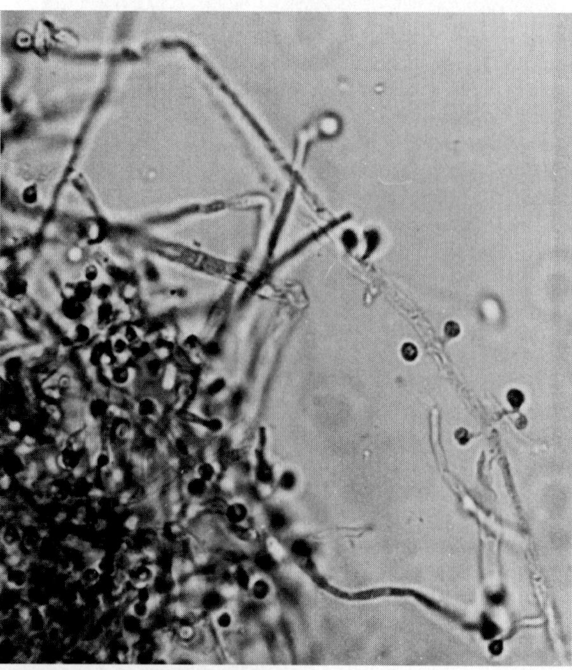

FIGURE 11 Mycelial phase of *B. dermatitidis*. Original magnification, ×400.

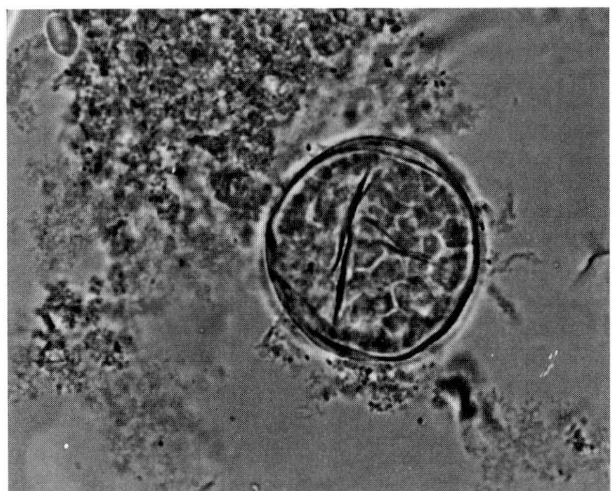

FIGURE 12 KOH wet mount of sputum showing spherule of *C. immitis* Original magnification, ×400.

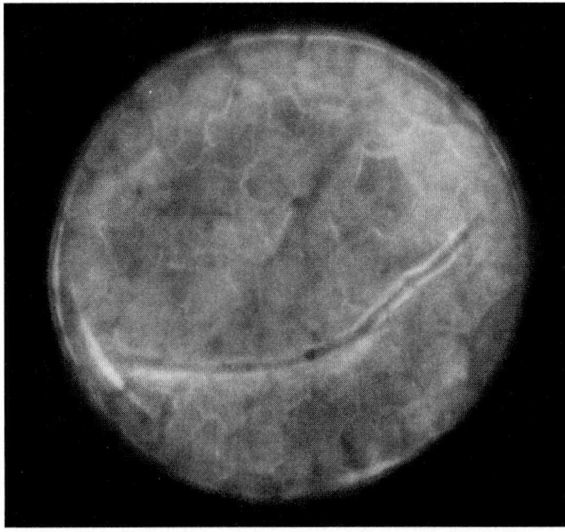

FIGURE 14 Calcofluor white wet mount of sputum showing spherule of *C. immitis*. Original magnification, ×400.

Although most of these small forms of *B. dermatitidis* possess the characteristic features of broadly attached buds, cells with narrow attachments may be observed. Rarely, hyphae are also seen in tissue along with yeast cells of *B. dermatitidis*.

C. immitis

Because of the risks to laboratory personnel when working with the mould form of *C. immitis*, direct examinations of sputum, exudates, and tissue are highly recommended. Mature spherules are thick walled, usually 20 to 60 μm in diameter, and are easily recognized on wet mounts with KOH or calcofluor white (Fig. 12 to 15). Larger spherules may measure up to 80 μm in diameter. Endospores (2 to 4 μm) can be observed in intact or recently disrupted spherules. During maturation, spherules undergo progressive endosporulation. Immature or smaller spherules (10 to 20 μm in diameter) lacking endospores may resemble phagocytic cells, artifacts, or other fungi. Mature spherules rupture to release the endospores. Hyphae may develop in chronic cavitary and granulomatous lesions of pulmonary coccidioidomycosis or in a pleural space with a low CO_2 content (14). Hyphal forms of *C. immitis* have also been found in cerebrospinal fluid (95).

The histopathology of coccidioidomycosis presents a

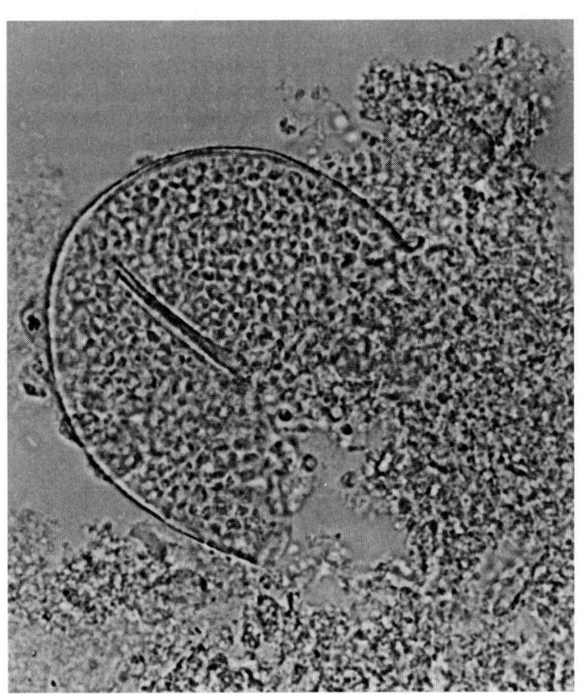

FIGURE 13 KOH wet mount of sputum showing disrupted spherule and endospores of *C. immitis*. Original magnification, ×400.

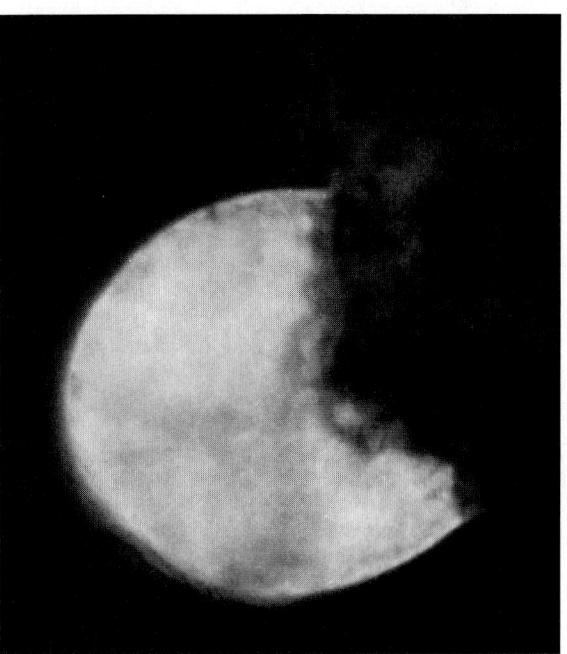

FIGURE 15 Calcofluor white wet mount of sputum showing disrupted spherule and faintly visible endospores of *C. immitis*. Original magnification, ×400.

variable inflammatory response ranging from an acute pyogenic to a chronic granulomatous reaction. This variability may be due to an acute inflammatory reaction to endospores after the rupture of spherules. A granulomatous response is observed in association with intact spherules. Spherules of *C. immitis* are easily identified in tissue by routine staining with H&E, GMS, and PAS stains, particularly the last one (Fig. 16). Endospores within the spherules of infected tissue may be observed histologically by H&E and PAS stains.

Endospores and small spherules may be confused with atypical forms of *B. dermatitidis* and nonbudding yeasts of *H. capsulatum*, *P. brasiliensis*, *C. glabrata*, and *C. neoformans*. *Prototheca wickerhamii* may resemble small spherules, and *Rhinosporidium seeberi* may simulate larger spherules of *C. immitis*. Some pollen grains found in sputum may also resemble spherules.

Specimens suspected of containing *C. immitis* should be cultured on slants instead of plates. *C. immitis* grows readily on conventional media at 25 to 30°C usually within 1 week as a floccose colony composed of hyaline, septate hyphae with arthroconidia (Fig. 17). The pigmentation and texture of colonies are highly variable. Colors range from buff to yellow to tan; the texture may be floccose to powdery, depending on the degree of fragmentation of the hyphae into arthroconidia. Slide cultures should *not* be set up for isolates suspected of being *C. immitis*.

The arthroconidia of *C. immitis* develop initially in the lateral hyphal branches and are thick-walled, barrel-shaped cells 2 to 4 by 3 to 6 μm that alternate with empty, thin-walled disjunctor cells. As the walls of these disjunctor cells deteriorate, the arthroconidia become detached and dispersed. The mycelium of *C. immitis* must be distinguished from those of other genera that produce hyphae and arthroconidia, including *Malbranchea*, *Uncinocarpus*, *Arthroderma*, *Auxarthron*, *Geotrichum*, and *Oidiodendron*.

Conversion of the mould form of *C. immitis* to the tissue form is not routinely performed in clinical microbiology laboratories, although a synthetic broth can be used to generate viable endospores (9). An agar medium for cultivation of spherules may also be used for rapid in vitro conversion and identification of *C. immitis* (93). Alternatively, spherules may be produced by intraperitoneal injection of hyphae and arthroconidia into laboratory animals in approved facilities. However, nucleic acid probe analysis and demonstration of exoantigen HS production are the safest and fastest methods of confirmation.

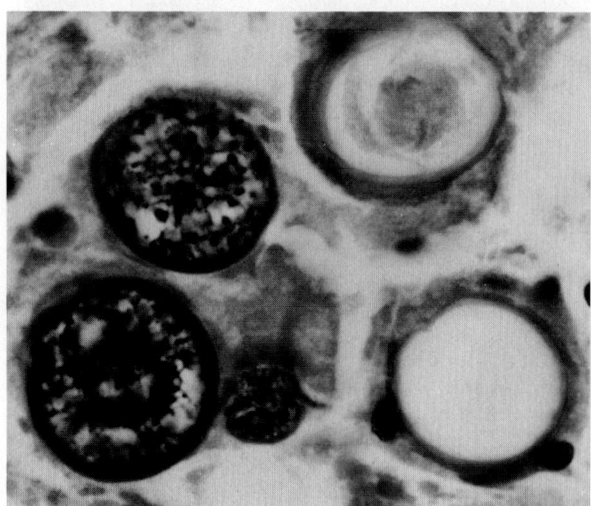

FIGURE 16 Lung biopsy specimen demonstrating empty spherules and spherules filled with endospores of *C. immitis* (PAS stain). Original magnification, ×469.

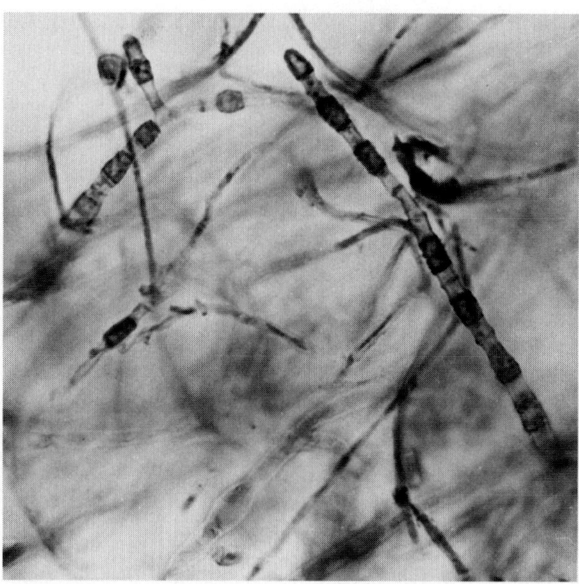

FIGURE 17 Mycelial phase of *C. immitis* demonstrating hyphae with thick-walled arthroconidia alternating with thin-walled disjunctor cells on potato dextrose agar at 25°C. Original magnification, ×400.

P. brasiliensis

P. brasiliensis may be identified by direct examination of sputum, bronchoalveolar lavage, pus from draining lymph nodes, scrapings from an ulcer, or tissue biopsy specimens. A wet mount of such material may reveal variations of the characteristic thick-walled pilot wheel or mariner's wheel configuration of the *P. brasiliensis* yeast form (Fig. 18 and 19). The parent yeast cell measures 15 to 30 μm in diameter, whereas the buds are 2 to 10 μm in diameter and have a narrow base of attachment. Some yeast cells may measure as much as 60 μm in diameter. The presence of multiple budding distinguishes this yeast from *C. neoformans* and *B. dermatitidis*. Histopathologic examination by H&E, GMS, and PAS staining of tissue infected with *P. brasiliensis* reveals a pyogranulomatous process with infiltrating polymorphonuclear leukocytes, mononuclear cells, macrophages, and

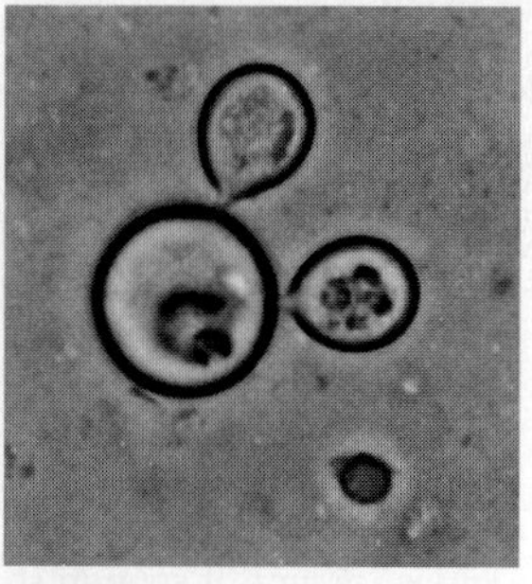

FIGURE 18 KOH wet mount of sputum showing blastoconidia of *P. brasiliensis*. Original magnification, ×400.

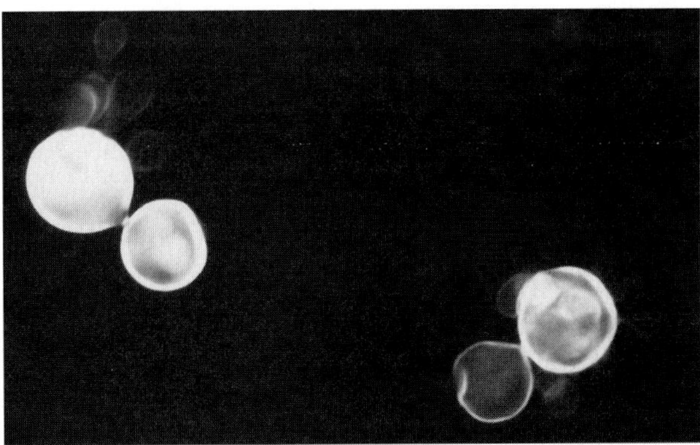

FIGURE 19 Calcofluor white wet mount of sputum showing blastoconidia of *P. brasiliensis*. Original magnification, ×400.

multinucleate giant cells. Singly budding forms that resemble *B. dermatitidis* are occasionally observed; however, the multiple budding forms seen elsewhere in the specimen distinguish *P. brasiliensis* from *B. dermatitidis*.

At 25 to 30°C, isolates of *P. brasiliensis* grow slowly and produce colonies that vary in gross morphology, ranging from glabrous, brown colonies to wrinkled, floccose, beige or white colonies. Primary isolation is improved on yeast extract agar (73). The mould form of *P. brasiliensis* may require growth for several weeks before conidia develop. These conidia may be absent to infrequent. When present, the microconidia appear laterally along the hyphae and may resemble those of *B. dermatitidis*. Chlamydoconidia may predominate in the mycelium. Rectangular arthroconidia and intercalary chlamydospores may also be produced (Fig. 20). Since the microscopic features of the mycelial form of *P. brasiliensis* are not specific, conversion to the yeast form or detection of specific antigen is necessary for definitive identification.

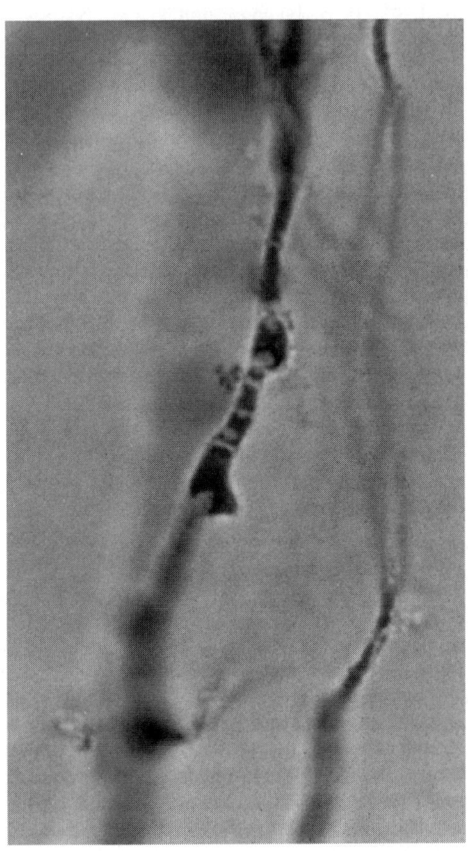

FIGURE 20 Mycelial phase of *P. brasiliensis*. Original magnification, ×400.

When the hyphae are incubated at 35 to 37°C on BHI or Kelley medium, the yeast form develops slowly. The yeast colony is folded, friable, and white to gray and consists of singly and multiply budding cells. The multiply budding yeast cells demonstrate the characteristic mariner's wheel configuration, similar to that seen in tissue. The parent yeast cell measures 10 to 25 μm in diameter, and the progeny buds, which are narrowly attached, are up to 10 μm in diameter.

REFERENCES

1. **Ampel, N. M.** 1996. Emerging disease issues and fungal pathogens associated with HIV infection. *Emerg. Infect. Dis.* **2:**109–116.
2. **Berliner, M.** 1968. Primary subcultures of *Histoplasma capsulatum*. 1. Macro- and micromorphology of the mycelial phase. *Sabouraudia* **6:**111–118.
3. **Bradsher, R. W.** 1996. Histoplasmosis and blastomycosis. *Clin. Infect. Dis.* **22**(Suppl. 2)**:**S102–S111.
4. **Bronnimann, D. A., and J. N. Galgiani.** 1989. Coccidioidomycosis. *Eur. J. Clin. Microbiol. Infect. Dis.* **8:**466–473.
5. **Brummer, E., E. Castaneda, and A. Restrepo.** 1993. Paracoccidioidomycosis: an update. *Clin. Microbiol. Rev.* **6:** 89–117.
6. **Carman, W. F., J. A. Frean, H. H. Crewe-Brown, G. A. Culligan, and C. N. Young.** 1989. Blastomycosis in Africa. *Mycopathologia* **107:**25–32.
7. **Cole, G. T., and S. H. Sun.** 1985. Arthroconidium-spherule-endospore transformation in *Coccidioides immitis*, p. 281–333. *In* P. J. Szaniszlo (ed.), *Fungal Dimorphism with Emphasis on Fungi Pathogenic for Humans*. Plenum Press, New York, N.Y.
8. **Collins, M. H., B. Jiang, J. M. Croffie, S. K. Chong, and C. H. Lee.** 1996. Hepatic granulomas in children. A clinicopathologic analysis of 23 cases including polymerase chain reaction for histoplasma. *Am. J. Surg. Pathol.* **20:** 332–338.
9. **Converse, J. L.** 1956. Effect of physico-chemical environment on spherulation of *Coccidioides immitis* in a chemically defined medium. *J. Bacteriol.* **72:**784–792.
10. **Cote, E., S. C. Barr, C. Allen, and E. Eaglefeather.** 1997. Blastomycosis in six dogs in New York state. *J. Am. Vet. Med. Assoc.* **210:**502–504.
11. **Darling, S. T. A.** 1906. A protozoan general infection producing pseudotubercles in the lungs and focal necrosis in the liver, spleen, and lymph nodes. *JAMA* **46:** 1283–1285.
12. **Davies, S. F.** 1988. Diagnosis of pulmonary fungal infections. *Semin. Respir. Infect.* **3:**162–171.
13. **de Monbreun, W. A.** 1934. The cultivation and cultural characteristics of Darling's *Histoplasma capsulatum*. *Am. J. Trop. Med. Hyg.* **14:**93–135.
14. **Dolan, M. J., C. P. Lattuda, G. P. Melcher, R. Zellmer, R. Allendoerfer, and M. G. Rinaldi.** 1992. Coccidioides immitis presenting as a mycelial pathogen with empyema and hydropneumothorax. *J. Med. Vet. Mycol.* **30:**249–255.
15. **Dixon, D. M., M. M. McNeil, M. L. Cohen, B. G. Gellin, and J. R. La Montagne.** 1996. Fungal infections: a growing threat. *Public Health Rep.* **111:**226–235.

16. **Drouhet, E.** 1989. African histoplasmosis. *Bailliere's Clin. Trop. Med. Communicable Dis. Int. Pract. Res.* **4:**221–247.
17. **Furcolow, M. L., J. F. Busey, R. W. Menges, et al.** 1970. Prevalence and incidence studies of human and canine blastomycosis. II. Yearly incidence studies in three states, 1960–1967. *Am. J. Epidemiol.* **92:**121–131.
18. **Gerber, M. E., J. D. Rosdeutscher, A. M. Seiden, and T. A. Tami.** 1995. Histoplasmosis: the otolaryngologist's perspective. *Laryngoscope* **105:**919–923.
19. **Gilchrist, T. C., and W. R. Stokes.** 1898. A case of pseudo-lupus vulgaris caused by a *Blastomyces*. *J. Exp. Med.* **3:**53–78.
20. **Goodman, N. L., and H. W. Larsh.** 1967. Environmental factors and growth of *Histoplasma capsulatum* in soil. *Mycopathol. Mycol. Appl.* **33:**145.
21. **Goodwin, R. A., J. E. Loyd, and R. M. Des Prez.** 1981. Histoplasmosis in normal hosts. *Medicine* **60:**231.
22. **Graham, A. R., R. E. Sobonya, D. A. Bronnimann, and J. N. Galgiani.** 1988. Quantitative pathology of coccidioidomycosis in acquired immunodeficiency syndrome. *Hum. Pathol.* **19:**800–806.
23. **Graham, D. R., C. Drake, and J. E. Barenfanger.** 1996. Recovery of *Histoplasma capsulatum* from BACTEC TB media. *J. Clin. Microbiol.* **34:**208–209.
24. **Gurney, J. W., and D. J. Conces.** 1996. Pulmonary histoplasmosis. *Radiology* **199:**297–306.
25. **Hadley, S., and A. W. Karchmer.** 1995. Fungal infections in solid organ transplant recipients. *Infect. Dis. Clin. N. Am.* **9:**1045–1074.
26. **Hageage, G. J., and B. J. Harrington.** 1984. Use of calcofluor white in clinical mycology. *Lab. Med.* **15:**109–112.
27. **Hajjeh, R. A.** 1995. Disseminated histoplasmosis in persons infected with human immunodeficiency virus. *Clin. Infect. Dis.* **21**(Suppl. 1)**:**S108–S110.
28. **Hall, G. S., K. Pratt-Rippin, and J. A. Washington.** 1992. Evaluation of a chemiluminescent probe assay for identification of *Histoplasma capsulatum* isolates. *J. Clin. Microbiol.* **30:**3003–3004.
29. **Halline, A. G., M. Maldonado-Lutomirsky, J. W. Ryoo, A. Pau, and K. Pursell.** 1997. Colonic histoplasmosis in AIDS: unusual endoscopic findings in two cases. *Gastrointest. Endosc.* **45:**199–204.
30. **Hood, S., and D. W. Denning.** 1996. Treatment of fungal infection in AIDS. *J. Antimicrob. Chemother.* **37**(Suppl. B)**:**71–85.
31. **Huffnagle, K. E., and R. M. Gander.** 1993. Evaluation of Gen-Probe's *Histoplasma capsulatum* and *Cryptococcus neoformans* AccuProbes. *J. Clin. Microbiol.* **31:**419–421.
32. **Jensen, H. E., H. C. Schonheyder, M. Hotchi, and L. Kaufman.** 1996. Diagnosis of systemic mycoses by specific immunohistochemical tests. *APMIS* **104:**241–258.
33. **Johnson, P. C., and G. A. Sarosi.** 1989. Community-acquired fungal pneumonias. *Semin. Respir. Infect.* **4:**56–63.
34. **Kauffman, C. A.** 1996. Role of azoles in antifungal therapy. *Clin. Infect. Dis.* **2:**S148–S153.
35. **Kaufman, L., J. A. Kovacks, and E. Reiss.** 1997. Clinical immunomycology, p. 585–604. *In* N. R. Rose, E. Conway de Macario, J. D. Folds, H. C. Lane, and R. M. Nakamura (ed.), *Manual of Clinical Laboratory Immunology*, 5th ed. ASM Press, Washington, D.C.
36. **Kaufman, L., and P. G. Standard.** 1987. Specific and rapid identification of medically important fungi by exoantigen detection. *Annu. Rev. Microbiol.* **41:**209–225.
37. **Khardori, N.** 1989. Host-parasite interaction in fungal infections. *Eur. J. Clin. Microbiol. Infect. Dis.* **8:**331–351.
38. **Kirkland, T. N., and J. Fierer.** 1996. Coccidioidomycosis: a reemerging infectious disease. *Emerg. Infect. Dis.* **2:** 192–199.
39. **Klein, B. S., J. M. Vergeront, A. F. DiSalvo, L. Kaufman, and J. P. Davis.** 1987. Two outbreaks of blastomycosis along rivers in Wisconsin. Isolation of *Blastomyces dermatitidis* from riverbank soil and evidence of its transmission along waterways. *Am. Rev. Respir. Dis.* **136:**1333–1338.
40. **Klein, B. S., J. M. Vergeront, R. J. Weeks, U. N. Kumar, G. Mathai, B. Varkey, L. Kaufman, R. W. Bradsher, J. F. Stoebig, and J. P. Davis.** 1986. Isolation of *Blastomyces dermatitidis* in soil associated with a large outbreak of blastomycosis in Wisconsin. *N. Engl. J. Med.* **314:**529–534.
41. **Klepser, M. E., and T. B. Klepser.** 1997. Drug treatment of HIV-related opportunistic infections. *Drugs* **53:**40–73.
42. **Kotloff, K. L., P. A. Vial, J. W. R. Young, and A. G. Smith.** 1987. *Histoplasma duboisii* infection in a Liberian girl. *Pediatr. Infect. Dis. J.* **6:**202–205.
43. **Kravitz, G. R., S. F. Davies, M. R. Eckman, et al.** 1981. Chronic blastomycotic meningitis. *Am. J. Med.* **71:** 501–505.
44. **Kwon-Chung, K. J., R. J. Weeks, and H. W. Larsh.** 1974. Studies on *Emmonsiella capsulata* (*Histoplasma capsulatum*). II. Distribution of the two mating types in 13 endemic states of the United States. *Am. J. Epidemiol.* **99:**44–49.
45. **Kwon-Chung, K. J.** 1972. Sexual stage of Histoplasma capsulatum. *Science* **175:**326.
46. **Kwon-Chung, K. J.** 1973. Studies on *Emmonsiella capsulata*. I. Heterothallism and development of the ascocarp. *Mycologia* **65:**109–121.
47. **Kwon-Chung, K. J., and J. E. Bennett.** 1992. *Medical Mycology*. Lea & Febiger, Philadelphia, Pa.
48. **Kwon-Chung, K. J.** 1975. Perfect state (*Emmonsiella capsulata*) of the fungus using large-form African histoplasmosis. *Mycologia* **67:**980.
49. **Larone, D. H.** 1995. *Medically Important Fungi, a Guide to Identification*, 3rd ed. ASM Press, Washington, D.C.
50. **Livas, I. C., P. S. Nechay, and W. M. Nauseef.** 1995. Clinical evidence of spinal and cerebral histoplasmosis twenty years after renal transplantation. *Clin. Infect. Dis.* **20:**692–695.
51. **Lyons, R., and G. Woods.** 1995. Comparison of the BacT/Alert and Isolator blood culture systems for recovery of fungi. *Am. J. Clin. Pathol.* **103:**660–662.
52. **Mann, B. J., B. W. Baylis, S. J. Urbanski, A. P. Gibb, and H. R. Rabin.** 1996. Paracoccidioidomycosis: case report and review. *Clin. Infect. Dis.* **23:**1026–1032.
53. **Maresca, B., and G. S. Kobayashi.** 1989. Dimorphism in *Histoplasma capsulatum*: a model for the study of cell differentiation in pathogenic fungi. *Microbiol. Rev.* **53:**186–209.
54. **McDonough, E. S., and A. L. Lewis.** 1967. *Blastomyces dermatitidis*: production of the sexual stage. *Science* **156:** 528–529.
55. **McDonough, E. S., and A. L. Lewis.** 1968. The ascigerous stage of *Blastomyces dermatitidis*. *Mycologia* **60:**76–83.
56. **McEwen J. G., A. M. Garcia, B. L. Ortiz, S. Botero, and A. Restrepo.** 1995. In search of the natural habitat of *Paracoccidioides brasiliensis*. *Arch. Med. Res.* **26:**305–306.
57. **McGinnis, M. R., and B. Katz.** 1979. *Ajellomyces* and its synonym *Emmonsiella*. *Mycotaxon* **8:**157–164.
58. **Medoff, G., A. Painter, and G. S. Kobayashi.** 1987. Mycelial- to yeast-phase transitions of the dimorphic fungi *Blastomyces dermatitidis* and *Paracoccidioides brasiliensis*. *J. Bacteriol.* **169:**4055–4060.
59. **Mercantini, R., R. Marsella, D. Moretto, P. Mercantini, L. Balus, A. Mastroianni, and C. Ferraro.** 1995. Macroscopic and microscopic characteristics of an African *Blastomyces dermatitidis* strain. *Mycoses* **38:**477–480.
60. **Mitchell, T. G.** 1988. Serodiagnosis of mycotic infections, p. 303–323. *In* B. B. Wentworth (ed.), *Diagnostic Procedures for Mycotic and Parasitic Infections*. American Public Health Association, Washington, D.C.
61. **Mitchell, T. G.** 1992. Blastomycosis, p. 1898–1906. *In* R.

D. Reigin and J. D. Cherry (ed.), *Textbook of Pediatric Infectious Diseases*, 3rd ed. The W. B. Saunders Co., Philadelphia, Pa.

62. **Nittayananta, W., P. Kumplanont, S. Srisintorn, P. Akkayanont, S. Chungpanich, R. Teanpaisan, M. Chareonwatanan, and T. Nuntanaranont.** 1997. Oral histoplasmosis associated with candidiasis in HIV-infected patients: a report of two cases. *Br. Dent. J.* **182:**309–312.
63. **Padhye, A. A. G. Smith, D. McLaughlin, P. G. Standard, and L. Kaufman.** 1992. Comparative evaluation of a chemiluminescent DNA probe and an exoantigen test for rapid identification of *Histoplasma capsulatum*. *J. Clin. Microbiol.* **30:**3108–3111.
64. **Padhye, A. A., G. Smith, P. G. Standard, D. McLaughlin, and L. Kaufman.** 1994. Comparative evaluation of chemiluminescent DNA probe assays and exoantigen tests for rapid identification of *Blastomyces dermatitidis* and *Coccidioides immitis*. *J. Clin. Microbiol.* **32:**867–870.
65. **Pappagianis, D.** 1988. Epidemiology of coccidioidomycosis. *Curr. Top. Med. Mycol.* **2:**199–238.
66. **Pappagianis, D.** 1994. Marked increase in cases of coccidioidomycosis in California: 1991, 1992, and 1993. *Clin. Infect. Dis.* **19**(Suppl. 1)**:**S14–S18.
67. **Paya, C. V., G. D. Roberts, and F. R. Cockerill III.** 1987. Laboratory methods for the diagnosis of disseminated histoplasmosis: clinical importance of the lysis-centrifugation blood culture technique. *Mayo Clin. Proc.* **62:**480–485.
68. **Peddi, V. R., S. Hariharan, and M. R. First.** 1996. Disseminated histoplasmosis in renal allograft recipients. *Clin. Transplant.* **10:**160–165.
69. **Pike, R. M.** 1979. Laboratory-associated infections: incidence, fatalities, cases, and prevention. *Annu. Rev. Microbiol.* **33:**41–66.
70. **Pine, L., E. Drouhet, and G. Reynolds.** 1964. A comparative morphological study of the yeast phases of *Histoplasma capsulatum* and *Histoplasma duboisii*. *Sabouraudia* **3:** 211–224.
71. **Randhawa, H. S., S. Chaturvedi, Z. U. Khan, V. P. Chaturvedi, S. K. Jain, R. C. Jain, and G. Bazaz-Malik.** 1995. Epididymal histoplasmosis diagnosed by isolation of *Histoplasma capsulatum* from semen. *Mycopathologia* **131:** 173–177.
72. **Restrepo, A.** 1985. The ecology of *Paracoccidioides brasiliensis*: a puzzle still unresolved. *Sabouraudia* **23:**323–334.
73. **Restrepo, A., and I. Correa.** 1973. Comparison of two culture media for primary isolation of *Paracoccidioides brasiliensis* from sputum. *Sabouraudia* **10:**260–265.
74. **Restrepo, A., M. E. Salazar, L. E. Cano, E. P. Stover, D. Feldman, and D. A. Stevens.** 1984. Estrogens inhibit mycelium-to-yeast transformation in the fungus *Paracoccidioides brasiliensis*: implications for resistance of females to paracoccidioidomycosis. *Infect. Immun.* **46:**346–353.
75. **Rippon, J. W.** 1980. Dimorphism in pathogenic fungi. *Crit. Rev. Microbiol.* **8:**49–97.
76. **Rippon, J. W.** 1988. *Medical Mycology. The Pathogenic Fungi and the Pathogenic Actinomycetes*, 3rd ed., p. 1–797. The W. B. Saunders Co., Philadelphia, Pa.
77. **Sanders, J. S., G. A. Sarosi, D. J. Nollett, and J. L. Thompson.** 1977. Exfoliative cytology in the rapid diagnosis of pulmonary blastomycosis. *Chest* **72:**193–196.
78. **Sandu, G. S., B. C. Kline, L. Stockman, and G. D. Roberts.** 1995. Molecular probes for diagnosis of fungal infections. *J. Clin. Microbiol.* **33:**2913–2919.
79. **Schneider, E., R. A. Hajjeh, R. A. Spiegel, R. W. Jibson, E. L. Harp, G. A. Marshall, R. A. Gunn, M. M. McNeil, R. W. Pinner, R. C. Baron, R. C. Burger, L. C. Hutwagner, C. Crump, L. Kaufman, S. E. Reef, G. M. Feldman, D. Pappagianis, and S. B. Werner.** 1997. A coccidioidomycosis outbreak following the Northridge, California, earthquake. *JAMA* **277:**904–908.
80. **Schwarz, J.** 1981. *Histoplasmosis*, Plenum Press, New York, N.Y.
81. **Segal, G. P.** 1987. Serodiagnostic procedures in the systemic mycoses. *Semin. Respir. Med.* **9:**136–144.
82. **Singer-Vermes, L. M., E. Burger, M. F. Franco, M. M. Di-Bacchi, M. J. Mendes-Giannini, and V. L. Calich.** 1989. Evaluation of the pathogenicity and immunogenicity of seven *Paracoccidioides brasiliensis* isolates in susceptible inbred mice. *J. Med. Vet. Mycol.* **27:**71–82.
83. **Singh, V. R., D. K. Smith, J. Lawerence, P. C. Kelly, A. R. Thomas, B. Spitz, and G. A. Sarosi.** 1996. Coccidioidomycosis in patients infected with human immunodeficiency virus: review of 91 cases at a single institution. *Clin. Infect. Dis.* **23:**563–568.
84. **Smith, C. D., and N. L. Goodman.** 1975. Improved culture method for the isolation of *Histoplasma capsulatum* and *Blastomyces dermatitidis* from contaminated specimens. *Am. J. Clin. Pathol.* **62:**276–280.
85. **Smith, M. B., V. J. Schnadig, P. Zaharopoulos, and C. Van Hook.** 1997. Disseminated *Histoplasma capsulatum* infection presenting as genital ulcerations. *Obstet. Gynecol.* **89:**842–844.
86. **Soll, D. R.** 1985. *Candida albicans*, p. 167–195. *In* P. J. Szaniszlo (ed.), *Fungal Dimorphism with Emphasis on Fungi Pathogenic for Humans*. Plenum Press, New York, N.Y.
87. **Steck, W. D.** 1989. Blastomycosis. *Dermatol. Clin.* **7:** 241–250.
88. **Stevens, D. A. (ed.).** 1980. *Coccidioidomycosis*. Plenum Press, New York, N.Y.
89. **Stevens, D. A.** 1989. The interface of mycology and endocrinology. *J. Med. Vet. Mycol.* **27:**133–140.
90. **Stobierski, M. G., C. J. Hospedales, W. N. Hall, B. Robinson-Dunn, D. Hock, and D. A. Sheill.** 1996. Outbreak of histoplasmosis among employees in a paper factory—Michigan, 1993. *J. Clin. Microbiol.* **34:**1220–1223.
91. **Stockman, L., K. A. Clark, J. M. Hunt, and G. D. Roberts.** 1993. Evaluation of commercially available acridinium ester-labeled chemiluminescent DNA probes for culture identification of *Blastomyces dermatitidis*, *Coccidioides immitis*, *Cryptococcus neoformans*, and *Histoplasma capsulatum*. *J. Clin. Microbiol.* **31:**845–850.
92. **Sugar, A. M.** 1988. Paracoccidioidomycosis. *Infect. Dis. Clin. N. Am.* **2:**913–924.
93. **Sun, S. H., M. Huppert, and K. R. Vukovich.** 1976. Rapid in vitro conversion and identification of *Coccidioides immitis*. *J. Clin. Microbiol.* **3:**186–190.
94. **Szaniszlo, P. J., and J. L. Harris (ed.).** 1985. *Fungal Dimorphism with Emphasis on Fungi Pathogenic for Humans*. Plenum Press, New York, N.Y.
95. **Wages, D. S., L. Helfend, and H. Finkle.** 1995. *Coccidioides immitis* presenting as a hyphal form in a ventriculoperitoneal shunt. *Arch. Pathol. Lab. Med.* **119:**91–93.
96. **Wagner, J. D., C. D. Prevel, and R. Elluru.** 1996. *Histoplasma capsulatum* necrotizing myofasciitis of the upper extremity. *Ann. Plast. Surg.* **36:**330–333.
97. **Walsh, T. J., R. Catchatourian, and H. Cohen.** 1983. Disseminated histoplasmosis complicating bone marrow transplantation. *Am. J. Clin. Pathol.* **79:**509–511.
98. **Walsh, T. J., and P. A. Pizzo.** 1988. Nosocomial fungal infections: a classification for hospital-acquired fungal infections and mycoses arising from endogenous flora or reactivation. *Annu. Rev. Microbiol.* **42:**517–545.
99. **Walsh, T. J., J. Hiemenz, and E. Anaissie.** 1996. Recent progress and current problems in treatment of invasive fungal infections in neutropenic patients. *Infect. Dis. Clin. N. Am.* **10:**365–400.

100. **Wheat, J.** 1995. Endemic mycoses in AIDS: a clinical review. *Clin Microbiol. Rev.* **8:**146–159.
101. **Wheat, L. J.** 1988. Systemic fungal infections: diagnosis and treatment. I. Histoplasmosis. *Infect. Dis. Clin. N. Am.* **2:**841–859.
102. **Wheat, L. J.** 1989. Diagnosis and management of histoplasmosis. *Eur. J. Clin. Microbiol. Infect. Dis.* **8:**480–490.
103. **Wheat, L. J., P. Connolly-Stringfield, B. Williams, K. Connolly, R. Blair, M. Bartlett, and M. Durkin.** 1992. Diagnosis of histoplasmosis in patients with acquired immunodeficiency syndrome by detection of Histoplasma capsulatum polysaccharide antigen in bronchoalveolar lavage fluid. *Am. Rev. Respir. Dis.* **145:**1421–1424.
104. **Wheat, L. J., T. G. Slama, J. A. Horton, et al.** 1982. Risk factors for disseminated or fatal histoplasmosis. Analysis of a large urban outbreak. *Ann. Intern. Med.* **96:** 159–163.
105. **Wheat, L. J., B. E. Batteiger, and B. Sathapatayavongs.** 1990. *Histoplasma capsulatum* infections of the central nervous system. A clinical review. *Medicine* **69:**244–260.
106. **Williams, P. L., R. Johnson, D. Pappagianis, H. Einstein, U. Slager, F. T. Koster, J. J. Eron, and J. Morrison.** 1992. Vasculitic and encephalitic complications associated with Coccidioides immitis infection of the central nervous system in humans: report of 10 cases and review. *Clin. Infect. Dis.* **14:**673–682.
107. **Wilson, M. L., T. E. Davis, S. Mirrett, J. Reynolds, D. Fuller, S. D. Allen, K. K. Flint, F. Koontz, and L. B. Reller.** 1993. Controlled comparison of the BACTEC high-blood-volume fungal medium, BACTEC Plus 26 aerobic blood culture bottle, and 10-milliliter Isolator blood culture system for detection of fungemia and bacteremia. *J. Clin. Microbiol.* **31:**865–871.

Trichophyton, Microsporum, Epidermophyton, and Agents of Superficial Mycoses*

JULIUS KANE AND RICHARD C. SUMMERBELL

100

TAXONOMY

The etiologic agents of dermatophytosis are classified, along with some nonpathogenic relatives, in three anamorphic genera: *Trichophyton, Microsporum,* and *Epidermophyton.* Those dermatophytes capable of reproducing sexually, i.e., producing ascomata with asci and ascospores, are classified in the teleomorphic genus *Arthroderma* (77) in the family *Arthrodermataceae* of the order *Onygenales* (14), phylum *Ascomycota.* The recorded connections between the teleomorphic and anamorphic states of the dermatophytes and dermatophytoids (dermatophyte-like nonpathogens in the same anamorphic genera [68]) are given in Table 1. Most sexually reproducing dermatophytes are associated with soil or with animals that, in nature, burrow or make dens in soil (70).

NATURAL HABITAT

Dermatophytes are keratinophilic fungi which are capable of invading the keratinous tissues of living animals. They are grouped into three categories on the basis of host preference and natural habitat (Table 2) (2). Anthropophilic species almost exclusively infect humans; animals are rarely infected. Geophilic species are soil-associated organisms, and soil per se or soilborne keratinous debris (e.g., shed hairs and molted feathers) is a source of infection for humans as well as other animals. Zoophilic species are essentially pathogens of nonhuman mammals or birds, although animal-to-human transmission is not uncommon. This grouping may be helpful in determining the source of infection; e.g., human infections caused by *Microsporum canis* are often the result of contact between susceptible children and stray kittens (40). Clinical species identification of dermatophytes assists in controlling infections whose source may be a family pet.

Some dermatophytes, e.g., *Trichophyton rubrum,* are cosmopolitan, whereas others, e.g., *Trichophyton concentricum,* are geographically limited (54). *T. concentricum* is found only in the Pacific Islands and regions in Southeast Asia and Central and South America.

CLINICAL MANIFESTATIONS

The dermatophytoses (tinea or ringworm) are defined as fungal infections of the keratinized tissues (hair, nails, skin, etc.) of humans, other mammals, and birds by dermatophytes (a term properly restricted to pathogenic members of the genera *Epidermophyton, Microsporum,* and *Trichophyton* [4]). Cutaneous infections resembling dermatophytoses may be caused by yeasts or by unrelated filamentous fungi that are normally saprobes or plant pathogens; these infections are referred to as opportunistic dermatomycoses (80).

Tissue invasion is normally cutaneous; dermatophytes are usually unable to penetrate deeper tissues as a result of nonspecific inhibitory factors in serum (38), inhibition of fungal keratinases (16), and other immunological barriers (82). Infection may range from mild to severe as a consequence of the reaction of the host to the metabolic products of the fungus, the virulence of the infecting strain, the anatomic location of the infection, and local environmental factors. Occasionally, subcutaneous tissue may be invaded, e.g., in Majocchi's granuloma, kerion, mycetomalike processes (10, 83), or, more rarely, a generalized systemic infection (8).

Anatomic Location

Infections caused by dermatophytes are named according to the anatomic location involved, e.g., tinea barbae (beard and moustache), tinea capitis (scalp, eyebrows, and eyelashes), tinea corporis (face, trunk, and major limbs), tinea cruris (groin, perineal, and perianal areas), tinea pedis (soles and toe webs), tinea manuum (palms), and tinea unguium (nails). Different dermatophyte species may produce clinically identical lesions; conversely, a single species may infect many anatomic sites.

Tinea barbae, usually caused by zoophilic fungi, e.g., *Trichophyton verrucosum* and granular forms of *Trichophyton mentagrophytes,* is typically highly inflamed and may present as acute pustular folliculitis that can progress to suppurative boggy lesions (kerion). A less severe form that appears as dry, erythematous, scaly lesions also occurs. Tinea capitis may vary from highly erythematous, patchy, scaly areas with dull gray hair stumps to highly inflamed lesions with folliculitis, kerion formation, alopecia, and scarring. *Trichophyton tonsurans* and *M. canis* are the most common agents (54). Favus (tinea favosa), usually caused by *Trichophyton schoenleinii* and rarely caused by *Trichophyton violaceum* or *Microsporum gypseum,* is a chronic infection of the scalp and glabrous skin characterized by the formation of cup-shaped crusts resembling honeycombs (scutula). Tinea corporis, which can be caused by any dermatophyte, is classically manifested as circular, erythematous lesions with scaly, raised, active, often vesicular borders. Chronic lesions on the trunk and extremities usually are caused by *T. rubrum.* Tinea cruris ("jock itch"), usually caused by *T. rubrum* or *Epidermophyton floccosum,* typically appears as scaly, erythematous to tawny brown, bilateral and asymmetric lesions extending down to the inner thigh and exhibiting a sharply marginated border frequently studded with small vesicles. Tinea pedis varies in appearance; the most common manifestation is maceration, peeling, itch-

* This chapter contains information presented in chapter 65 by Irene Weitzman, Julius Kane, and Richard C. Summerbell in the sixth edition of this Manual.

TABLE 1 Teleomorph-anamorph states of dermatophytes and similar species[a]

Anamorph	Teleomorph
Trichophyton spp.	*Arthroderma* spp.
T. ajelloi	*A. uncinatum*
T. flavescens	*A. flavescens*
T. gloriae	*A. gloriae*
T. mentagrophytes	*A. benhamiae*
	A. vanbreuseghemii
T. simii	*A. simii*
T. terrestre	*A. quadrifidum*
	A. insingulare
	A. lenticularum
T. vanbreuseghemii	*A. gertleri*
Microsporum spp.	
M. amazonicum	*A. borellii*
M. boullardii	*A. corniculatum*
M. cookei	*A. cajetani*
M. canis	*A. otae*
M. gypseum	*A. fulvum*
	A. incurvatum
	A. gypseum
M. nanum	*A. obtusum*
M. persicolor	*A. persicolor*
M. racemosum	*A. racemosum*
M. vanbreuseghemii	*A. grubyi*
Microsporum sp.	*A. cookiellum*

[a] Data are from reference 39. Species lacking teleomorphs (e.g., *E. floccosum*) are not included in the table.

TABLE 2 Grouping of dermatophytes on the basis of host preference and natural habitat[a]

Anthropophilic	Geophilic	Zoophilic
Epidermophyton floccosum	*Microsporum* spp.	*Microsporum* spp.
Microsporum spp.	*M. fulvum*	*M. canis*
M. audouinii	*M. gypseum*	*M. equinum*
M. ferrugineum	*M. nanum*	*M. gallinae*
Trichophyton spp.	*M. persicolor*	
T. concentricum	*M. praecox*	*Trichophyton* spp.
T. gourvilii	*M. racemosum*	*T. equinum*
T. kanei	*M. vanbreuseghemii*	*T. mentagrophytes* var. *erinacei*
T. krajdenii	*Trichophyton* spp.	*T. mentagrophytes* var. *mentagrophytes* (granular)
T. megninii	*T. vanbreuseghemii*	*T. sarkisovii*
T. mentagrophytes (velvety)[b]		*T. simii*
T. raubitschekii		*T. verrucosum* var. *verrucosum*
T. rubrum		*T. verrucosum* var. *autotrophicum*
T. schoenleinii		
T. soudanense		
T. tonsurans		
T. violaceum		
T. yaoundei		

[a] Normally nonpathogenic, soil-associated dermatophytoids such as *T. terrestre* and *M. cookei* are not included in this table.

[b] Anthropophilic *T. mentagrophytes* isolates have often been called *T. mentagrophytes* var. *interdigitale* or *T. interdigitale*. The former, however, is an invalid name under the International Code of Botanical Nomenclature, and the latter, pending type studies, remains a synonym of *T. mentagrophytes*.

ing, and painful fissuring between the fourth and fifth toes. An acute inflammatory condition with vesicles and pustules and a hyperkeratotic chronic infection of the sole ("moccasin foot") are other manifestations. *T. mentagrophytes* frequently causes the more inflammatory type of infections, whereas *T. rubrum* usually causes the more chronic type. Tinea unguium, most often caused by *T. rubrum*, usually appears as thickened, deformed, friable, discolored nails with accumulated subungal debris or as white patches in the superficial or proximal-subungual portions of the nail.

Transmission and Contagion

Anthropophilic fungi usually are transmitted by close human contact or indirectly by sharing of clothes, combs, brushes, towels, bedsheets, etc. Tinea capitis is highly contagious and may spread rapidly within a family, institution, or school. Transmission of tinea cruris is associated with the sharing of clothing, towels, and sanitary facilities. The transmission of tinea pedis and tinea unguium is controversial (58, 80). Recently, acquisition of chronic *T. rubrum* tinea pedis has been suggested to require a dominant autosomal susceptibility gene (85). Geophilic infections involve transmission from soil to humans or other mammals. Outbreaks originating from infected soil with secondary human-to-human transmission have been reported (6). Infections caused by zoophilic species result from animal-to-human contact (cats, dogs, cattle, laboratory animals, etc.) or from indirect transmission involving fomites. The fungi may then be transmitted among humans to a limited extent, especially in institutions (64).

Detection

Patients with suspected tinea capitis may be examined with a Wood's lamp (filtered UV light peak of 365 nm) in a darkened room for the presence of bright green fluorescent hairs. Such hairs, considered Wood's light positive, typically occur in the small spored ectothrix type of hair invasion caused by *Microsporum audouinii*, *M. canis*, and *Microsporum ferrugineum*. Hairs infected with *T. schoenleinii* may show a dull green color (56).

A Wood's lamp can also be used to differentiate between dermatophytosis and nonfungal skin conditions that may be similar clinically, e.g., erythrasma. In erythrasma, the skin fluoresces orange to coral red, whereas in dermatophytosis, the skin is not fluorescent.

Direct microscopic examination of skin, hair, and nails is the most rapid method of determining fungal etiology and may be accomplished by examining the clinical material in 10% potassium hydroxide (KOH) or 10% sodium hydroxide (NaOH), 25% NaOH with 5% glycerin, or calcofluor white (57).

LABORATORY METHODS

Collection and Transport of Specimens

Whenever feasible, aseptic technique should be used to minimize contamination. Sufficient clinical material for direct microscopic examination and culture should be collected. The following equipment should be available for collection and transport of specimens: sterile nail clippers, scissors, forceps for epilation of hairs, sterile scalpel blades and/or curettes, sterile gauze squares, 70% alcohol for disinfection, sterile water for cleaning of painful areas, and clean pill packets or clean paper envelopes to contain and transport the clinical specimens. Black photographic paper may be useful for collecting and better visualizing scrapings. Closed tubes are not recommended for specimens, since they retain moisture, which may result in an overgrowth of contaminants. Disposable brushes have been recommended for the collection of specimens from the scalp or fur of animals (43).

Hairs from the scalp should be epilated with sterile forceps. If the specimen is Wood's light positive, epilate only fluorescent hairs. In favus, the scutulum at the mouth of the hair follicle is suitable for culture and microscopic examination. Hairs invaded by endothrix fungi may need to be dug out with the tip of a sterile scalpel blade because the hairs often break off at scalp level, making them difficult to grasp with forceps. Rubbing with a sterile moistened swab has been successful with pediatric patients (25). After disinfection with alcohol or cleansing with sterile water, active borders of skin lesions should be scraped with a scalpel to collect epidermal scales. In vesicular tinea pedis, the tops of the vesicles can be removed with sterile scissors for direct examination and culture. Substitution of vesicle fluid for these often heavily colonized vesicle tops is not recommended. Nails should be disinfected with alcohol gauze squares. The most desirable material for culture in typical subungual onychomycosis is the waxy subungual debris, which contains the fungal elements. The highest proportion of viable elements for culturing is often found close to the juncture of the nail bed. In order to remove contaminating saprobic fungi and bacteria, the crumbly debris directly underneath the nail near the tips is removed with the scalpel before material is collected for culture. If the dorsal nail plate is diseased, scrape and discard the outer surface before removing underlying material for culture.

Direct Microscopic Examination

Nail clippings should be aseptically cut into smaller fragments and, where possible, pounded with a heavy object while still inside their collection packet in order to release friable, flaky material containing the greatest amount of dermatophyte inoculum. Skin or nail scrapings, nail fragments, or hair roots are placed in 1 or 2 drops of one of the above-mentioned KOH or NaOH solutions on a clean glass slide. A coverslip is placed on top, and the preparation is heated gently (short of boiling) by being passed rapidly over a Bunsen burner three or four times and then allowed to sit at room temperature for a few minutes for clearing. The exact time needed will depend on the concentration of hydroxide used, the thickness of specimen fragments, and the exact amount of heat imparted by contact with the flame. Clearing is evident to the naked eye as a pronounced decrease in the opacity of the scraping. Alternatively, a slide warmer set at 51 to 54°C may be used to heat the slides for 1 h (37). Laboratories using 10% KOH or NaOH solution for skin may find that nail scrapings may require a stronger alkali solution (up to 25% KOH or NaOH). Fungi may also be demonstrated by use of calcofluor white (57) or other glucan-binding fluorescent dyes such as Congo red (37). All preparations should be examined under low power and confirmed under high power.

TABLE 3 Hair invasion by dermatophytes on the human host

Ectothrix	Endothrix	Favic
T. megninii	*T. gourvilii*	*T. schoenleinii*[a]
T. mentagrophytes	*T. soudanense*	
T. verrucosum	*T. tonsurans*	
M. audouinii[b]	*T. violaceum*	
M. canis[b]	*T. yaoundei*	
M. ferrugineum[b]		
M. fulvum		
M. gypseum		
M. praecox		

[a] Species giving dull green fluorescence under a Wood's light.
[b] Species giving bright green fluorescence under a Wood's light.

Skin and nails infected with dermatophytes may reveal one or more of the following: hyaline hyphal fragments; septate, often branched hyphae; and chains of arthroconidia (Fig. 1).

The appearance of infected hairs depends on the invading dermatophyte species. Hyphae invade the hairs, and arthroconidia are formed by fragmentation of these hyphae. The appearance and locations of the arthroconidia may suggest the infecting genera or species (Table 3), as may the sizes (56). Three main types of colonizations (ectothrix, endothrix, and favic) are observed by the direct microscopic examination. The terms "ectothrix" and "endothrix" refer to the location of the arthroconidia in relation to the hair shaft.

In ectothrix colonization, arthroconidia appear as a mosaic sheath around the hair or as chains on the surface of the hair shaft (Fig. 2). In *M. canis*, *M. audouinii*, and *M. ferrugineum* infections, colonized hairs fluoresce green under a Wood's lamp; other ectothrix infections (Table 3) are nonfluorescent. Endothrix hair invasion is observed as chains of arthroconidia filling the insides of shortened hair

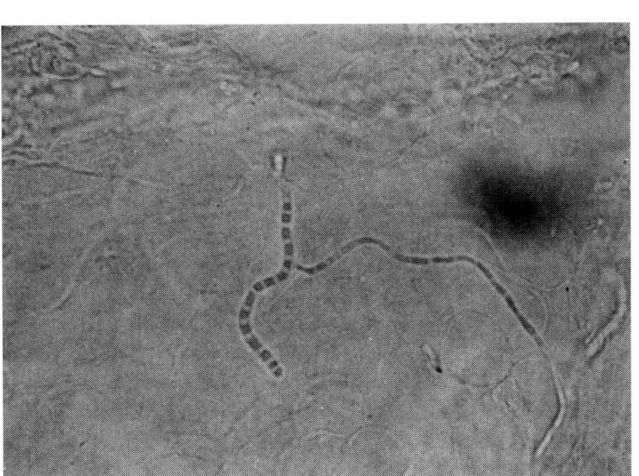

FIGURE 1 Dermatophyte hyphae in skin scraping. NaOH mount. Magnification, ×400.

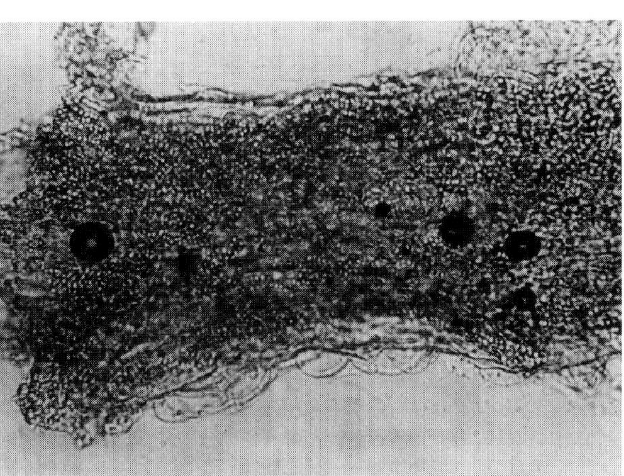

FIGURE 2 *M. audouinii*, ectothrix type of hair invasion. Magnification, ×400.

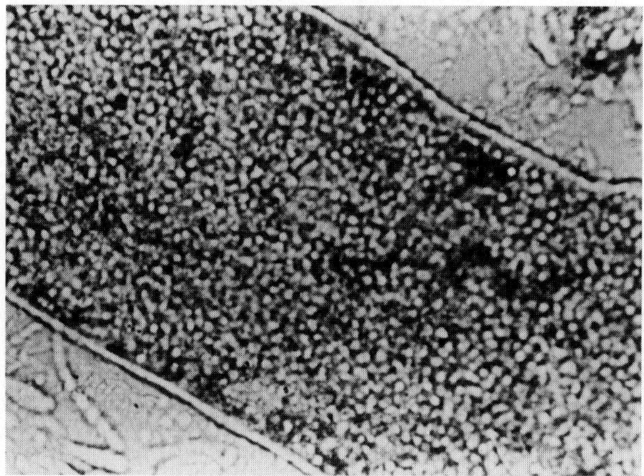

FIGURE 3 *T. tonsurans*, endothrix type of hair invasion. Magnification, ×1,000.

stubs (Fig. 3). Hairs are Wood's lamp negative. In favic hairs, hyphae, air bubbles, or tunnels and fat droplets are observed in the intrapilar area (Fig. 4). These hairs are dull green under a Wood's lamp. In general, all infected hairs show hyphae within the hair shaft at some time during the course of infection, usually during the early stages.

Isolation Media

The most common media used for the isolation of dermatophytes are Sabouraud glucose agar (SDA) (pH 5.6) and Emmons' modification of SDA, with less glucose (2% instead of 4%) and a pH between 6.8 and 7.0, paired with SDA containing chloramphenicol and cycloheximide to inhibit bacterial and saprobic fungal contamination (available commercially as, for example, Mycobiotic agar [Difco Laboratories, Detroit, Mich.; Remel, Lenexa, Kans.]) or Mycosel [BBL Microbiology Systems, Cockeysville, Md.]). SDA with chloramphenicol (Remel, Difco), inhibitory mould agar (BBL), and Littman oxgall agar (Difco, Remel) are recommended for the isolation of cycloheximide-sensitive fungi that cause clinical infections resembling dermatophytosis (57). The addition of gentamicin is recommended for specimens heavily contaminated with bacteria (71). SDA with cycloheximide, chloramphenicol, and gentamicin (CCG) is routinely used as an isolation medium in some laboratories (37).

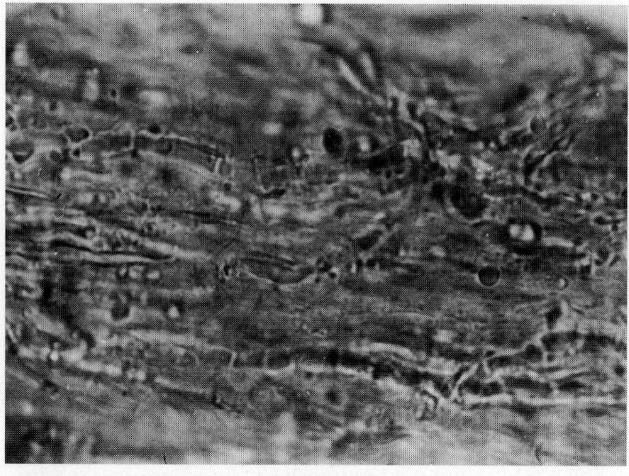

FIGURE 4 Hair from a patient with favus infected with *T. schoenleinii*. Magnification, ×1,000.

Additional and alternative media may be used. For example, Casamino Acids (Difco; vitamin-free)–erythritol–albumin agar medium plus CCG may be used for filament-positive skin and nail specimens, especially from body sites where *Candida* overgrowth may be a problem (e.g., groin and fingernails). This medium (available as Candida Inhibitory Agar from Biomedia Unlimited, Toronto, Ontario, Canada) prevents the suppression of dermatophyte growth in vitro by *Candida albicans*, *Candida parapsilosis*, and related biotin-requiring yeasts (18). Dermatophyte species with vitamin requirements may grow poorly on it, and it is always used in combination with a cycloheximide-containing SDA. For specimens from patients from regions where cattle are commonly raised, SDA plus CCG can be replaced by bromcresol purple (BCP)-milk solids-yeast extract agar plus CCG (BCPMSYE) (available commercially from Biomedia). This medium enhances growth and reveals the characteristic casein hydrolysis of *T. verrucosum* (7, 36), in addition to permitting the normal outgrowth of other dermatophytes. Some laboratories use potato flake agar plus chloramphenicol and cycloheximide (available commercially, e.g., from Hardy Media, Santa Maria, Calif.) instead of SDA, since the former medium accelerates red pigment production in *T. rubrum* and promotes typical conidiation.

Another primary isolation medium which may be used is dermatophyte test medium (DTM; available commercially from Difco and Remel). This selective medium screens for the presence of dermatophytes in heavily contaminated material (from feet, nails, etc.). The growth of dermatophytes causes a rise in pH, thus changing the phenol red indicator from yellow to red (72). The use of DTM should be combined with morphological study, since fungi other than dermatophytes can grow and turn the medium red (45, 60). Rapid sporulating medium (Bacti Lab, Mountain View, Calif.) is similar in principle to DTM but has a pH indicator that turns from yellow to blue-green, making the red reverse pigment of typical *T. rubrum* discernible (7). Another related medium, dermatophyte indicator medium (DIM) (61), has recently been shown to give false-positive results with fewer fungi than DTM (61). Most of the fungi giving false-positive reactions are strongly morphologically dissimilar to dermatophytes (61). Like DTM, DIM gives positive results for dermatophytes, normally nonpathogenic dermatophytoids such as *Trichophyton ajelloi*, and closely related, nonpathogenic arthrodermataceous fungi such as *Chrysosporium georgiae* (61); therefore, positive reactions cannot be treated as an indicator of pathogenicity. DTM gives false-negative results with some *Microsporum* isolates (48), while DIM gives false-negative results with some isolates of *T. verrucosum* (61).

Cultures on primary isolation medium are routinely incubated at 25 to 30°C and are examined weekly for up to 4 weeks. Two weeks suffices for all dermatophytes if BCPMSYE is being used to detect *T. verrucosum*, since this species may take more than 14 days to produce noticeable colonies on SDA, but it will usually be noticeable within 4 to 7 days on BCPMSYE.

IDENTIFICATION

Identification of the dermatophyte species is often based on (i) colony characteristics in pure culture on SDA and (ii) microscopic morphology. These criteria alone, however, may be insufficient, since colonial appearance may vary or be similar for different species. Characteristic pigmentation may fail to appear, and isolates, especially *Trichophyton* spp., may not sporulate. Special media may be required to stimulate pigment production; it may be necessary to use sporulation and physiologic tests in conjunction with morphology to identify the species correctly.

Colony Characteristics

In observing gross colony morphology, note the colors of the surface and the reverse of the colony, the texture of the surface (powdery, granular, woolly, cottony, velvety, or glabrous), the topography (elevation, folding, margins, etc.), and the rate of growth.

Microscopic Morphology

Microscopic morphology, especially the appearance and arrangement of the conidia (macroconidia or microconidia) and other structures, may be determined with teased mounts or slide culture preparations mounted in lactophenol cotton blue (LCB), in lactophenol aniline blue (phenol, an ingredient of LCB and lactophenol aniline blue, is listed as a hazardous chemical; therefore, solutions containing phenol should be prepared, stored, and used in an approved chemical safety cabinet), or in more permanent mounting fluids (75). Sometimes a special medium such as cornmeal or cornmeal-glucose agar, potato-glucose agar, SDA plus 3 to 5% NaCl (30, 35), pablum cereal agar (37), rapid sporulating agar (7), or lactrimel agar (11, 28) may be required to stimulate sporulation.

Physiologic Tests

In Vitro Hair Perforation Test

The in vitro hair perforation test distinguishes between atypical isolates of *T. mentagrophytes* and *T. rubrum* (5). It may also be used to make other distinctions such as *M. canis* versus *Microsporum equinum* (53). Hairs exposed to *T. mentagrophytes* and *M. canis* show wedge-shaped perforations perpendicular to the hair shaft (a positive test result), whereas *T. rubrum* and *M. equinum* do not form these perforating structures.

Place short strands of human hair in petri dishes and autoclave the dishes at 121°C for 10 min; add 25 ml of sterile distilled water and 2 or 3 drops of 10% sterilized yeast extract. Inoculate these plates with several fragments of the test fungus that has been grown on SDA; incubate the plates at 25°C, and examine them at regular intervals over a period of 21 days. Hairs may be examined microscopically for perforations by removing a few segments and placing them in a drop of LCB mounting fluid. Gently heating the mounts aids in the detection of the fungus.

Special Nutritional Requirements

Nutritional tests aid in the routine identification of *Trichophyton* species that seldom produce conidia or that resemble each other morphologically (20). Certain species have distinctive nutritional requirements, whereas others do not. The method uses a casein basal medium that is vitamin-free (*Trichophyton* agar 1 [T1]) to which various vitamins are added, i.e., inositol (T2), thiamine and inositol (T3), thiamine (T4), and nicotinic acid (T5), and an ammonium nitrate basal medium (T6) to which histidine is added (T7). These media are available commercially in dehydrated form from Difco and in prepared form from Remel. A small fragment (about the size of the head of a pin) from the culture to be tested is placed on the surface of the basal medium (controls) and the media containing the vitamin and amino acid additives. Care must be taken to avoid transferring agar from the fungus inoculum to the nutritional media. Cultures are incubated at room temperature (or 37°C if *T. verrucosum* is suspected) and read after 7 and 14 days. The amount of growth is graded from 0 to 4+. Commonly observed reactions are summarized in Table 4.

TABLE 4 Dermatophyte nutritional responses as elucidated by *Trichophyton* agars[a]

Species	Response by vitamin tests					Response by amino acid tests	
	1 Vitamin free	2 Inositol	3 Thiamine + inositol	4 Thiamine	5 Nicotinic acids	6 Amino acid free	7 Histidine
M. gallinae[b]						4	4
T. concentricum, 50%	4	4	4	4	4		
T. concentricum, 50%	2	2	4	4	2		
T. equinum var. *equinum*	0	0	0	0	4		
T. equinum var. *autotrophicum* (New Zealand, Australia)	4	4	4	4	4		
T. megninii						0	4
T. soudanense	v	v	v	v	v	v	v
T. tonsurans	1	1	4	4	1	4	4
T. verrucosum var. *autotrophicum*	4	4	4	4	4		
T. verrucosum var. *verrucosum*, 84%	1	2	4	2	1		
T. verrucosum var. *verrucosum*, 16%	1	1	4	4	1	4	4
T. violaceum	1	1	4	4	1	4	4

[a] Only the growth responses for organisms with growth factor requirements and the selected organism which must be most closely compared with them are included in this table. The numbers in the table body indicate the relative degree of growth according to the traditional 1+ to 4+ visually approximated scale: 0, no growth; 1, slight growth, strongly nutrient-deprived colony morphology (very sparse, subsurface colonial growth only or colony diameter strongly reduced compared to that of the Sabouraud agar control); 2, partially stimulated growth but still significantly suppressed compared to that of the control; 4, growth comparable to that of the control (the table includes no 3+ reactions); v, variable.

[b] Blank spaces in the chart indicate growth responses which are not customarily examined but which are insignificantly different from control growth responses on Sabouraud agar.

TABLE 5 Important characteristics of clinically isolated *Trichophyton* species[a]

Species	Colony on SDA	Microscopic morphology	Comments[b]
T. ajelloi	Cream or orange-tan; flat; powdery; reverse is blackish purple, sometimes nonpigmented; rapid growth	Microconidia rare; macroconidia numerous, fusiform to cylindrical, thick walled, multiseptate, 5–12 cells long, with widely separated cellular compartments (Fig. 5)	Geophilic species; rarely pathogenic
T. concentricum	Beige, brown, or reddish; elevated and convoluted; glabrous to velvety; no undersurface color; slow growth	Micro- and macroconidia usually absent; chlamydospores may be present	Geographically restricted (certain indigenous peoples in Southeast Asia, Oceania, and tropical Americas); 50% of isolates are stimulated by thiamine; others are autotrophic
T. equinum	Cream colored; flat; fluffy; reverse is yellow becoming reddish brown; rapid growth	Elongate, clavate or subglobose, stalked microconidia; macroconidia rare, similar to those of *T. mentagrophytes*	Requires nicotinic acid; autotrophic variety has been described (65)
T. fischeri	White; velvety to cottony; reverse is brownish red to wine red; closely resembles *T. rubrum*	Copious pyriform and subglobose microconidia along unbranched hyphae, macroconidia long and sinuous, cylindrical to clavate; thin antheridiumlike hyphal projections often produced	Nonpathogenic; features similar to those of *T. rubrum* except isolation normally from site free of dermatophytosis (e.g., repeatedly KOH-negative lesion); no red undersurface pigment on CEAA (29); many dichotomous branches in colony margin on BHI (37); always heavily conidiating
T. gourvilii	Pink to red; heaped up; convoluted; glabrous; becoming velvety; slow growth	Typical *Trichophyton*-type microconidia usually found	No special nutritional requirements
T. kanei	White; velvety to granular; reverse is brownish red to wine red	Macroconidia predominant, cylindrical to clavate, often with T-shaped bases; microconidia absent; arthroconidia small, mostly cylindrical, pyriform when formed terminally	Urease test weakly positive; in vitro hair test negative; growth restricted on BCPMSG and no pH change within 7 days
T. krajdenii	Surface cottony white with golden yellow margin; reverse golden yellow; diffusible yellow pigment often produced (Fig. 18a)	Pyriform to subglobose microconidia rare to moderately abundant; macroconidia rare; nodular bodies common	Contains nonmating isolates formerly considered *T. mentagrophytes* var. *nodulare* (invalid name) (34); urease positive; perforates hair in vitro; grows at 37°C; growth on BCPMSG shows alkalinity within 7–10 days
T. megninii	Pink to rose; radially folded; suedelike; reverse is wine red	Pyriform to clavate microconidia; macroconidia rare, similar to those of *T. rubrum*	Requires L-histidine; urease positive

T. mentagrophytes	White, cream, tan, yellowish, or pink; flat; powdery, granular (Fig. 18b), or velvety; reverse is light tan, yellow, red, or reddish brown; sometimes produces diffusible melanoid pigment; rapid growth	Globose to pyriform microconidia in clusters or singly along hyphae; clavate macroconidia present in some strains (Fig. 6); helically coiled hyphal appendages ("spirals") and antlerlike hyphae observed	Urease positive; perforates hair in vitro; grows at 37°C; growth profuse on BCPMSG, with alkalinity within 7 days. *T. mentagrophytes* var. *erinacei*, from hedgehogs and affected persons, is urease negative and has a yellow colony reverse
T. raubitschekii	Buff; raised center with radial grooves; velvety to granular; reverse is blood red	Microconidia clavate, globose, or subglobose, sessile or on short stalks along unbranched hyphae; macroconidia abundant on primary isolation; thin, elongate with blunt ends, 5–9 cells (Fig. 7)	Urease positive; in vitro hair perforation test negative; growth restricted on BCPMSG and no pH change within 7 days
T. rubrum	White; velvety, seldom powdery (Fig. 18c); reverse is wine red (Fig. 18d), sometimes yellow, orange, or with diffusible melanoid pigment; growth and color variants are described elsewhere (84)	Pyriform microconidia rare to abundant (sometimes absent), usually along unbranched hyphae, macroconidia absent to rare, thin, cylindrical to clavate in granular cultures (Fig. 8)	Urease test negative; in vitro hair perforation test negative; red undersurface pigment on CEAA except in yellow and hyaline variants (18); restricted on BCPMSG with no pH change within 7 days; monopodial marginal hyphae on BHI (37); should be differentiated from *T. raubitschekii* (33) and *T. fischeri* (29)
T. sarkisovii	Sandy brown to fulvous; leathery, folded; reverse is cinnamon; produces diffusible cinnamon pigment	Clavate microconidia up to 10 μm long; macroconidia not found; chlamydospores in chains similar to those of *T. verrucosum* but up to twice as large (to 17 μm as opposed to ≤9 μm)	Isolated only from Bactrian camels in central Asia; no vitamin requirement
T. schoenleinii	White to tan; heaped and convoluted; glabrous or waxy, becoming velvety on subculture; reverse lacks pigment; slow growth	Micro- and macroconidia rarely seen; chlamydospores often numerous; hyphal tips often show "nailhead" morphology and branch to form antlerlike structures (favic chandeliers)	Autotrophic for vitamins, which differentiates it from *T. verrucosum* var. *verrucosum*
T. simii	White to pale buff; flat or slightly convoluted; powdery; reverse is straw to salmon colored; rapid growth	Numerous macroconidia; some fragment or develop swellings resembling chlamydospores; pyriform microconidia and spirals may be found	Physiological reactions are as *T. mentagrophytes*; normally distinguished by mating studies
T. soudanense	Yellow-orange (like apricots) to wine red; flat with convolutions; suedelike texture; fringed (eyelash) periphery; reverse is yellow, orange-yellow, or red	Pyriform microconidia rare; macroconidia very rare; reflexive branching characteristic	Growth stimulated at 37°C (79)
T. terrestre	White, pale yellow, or red; flat, granular to downy; reverse is pale yellow, yellowish brown, or red; rapid growth	Microconidia clavate to pyriform, single or clustered, short, intermediate, or fully extended to attain size of macroconidia; clavate to cylindrical, thin walled, 2–6 cells (Fig. 9)	Geophilic; normally nonpathogenic; usually no growth at 37°C; must be differentiated from *T. mentagrophytes*

(Continued on next page)

TABLE 5 Important characteristics of clinically isolated *Trichophyton* species[a] (*Continued*)

Species	Colony on SDA	Microscopic morphology	Comments[b]
T. tonsurans	Color varies with isolate (yellow, cream, white, pink, brown, gray, etc.); convoluted; raised or flat; velvety to powdery (Fig. 18e); reverse is dark brown to mahogany red or vivid yellow (Fig. 18f)	Clavate to elongate microconidia; some swollen into balloon forms and attached to branched conidiophores by short stalks (Fig. 10); macroconidia rare	Stimulated by thiamine
T. vanbreuseghemii	Buff colony; leathery; finely grainy; reverse whitish or pale yellow	Abundant macroconidia with cells of uneven length, tending to fragment into single cells; microconidia small, boxy	Geophilic; very rare in clinical laboratory; physiological reactions as for *T. mentagrophytes*
T. verrucosum	Cream, tan, or ocher; flat, shield shaped, or convoluted; glabrous to finely velvety surface; slow growth	Microconidia uncommon, pyriform to subglobose; macroconidia rare, "rat-tail" shaped; chlamydospores usually numerous, symmetrical and in chains (Fig. 11), especially from culture at 37°C on BCPMSYE	All strains from human and bovine sources require thiamine; most require inositol as well; growth stimulated at 37°C, differentiating species from *T. schoenleinii*; growth and clear halo within 6 days on BCPMSYE (36); *T. verrucosum* var. *autotrophicum*, from sheep, does not require vitamins
T. violaceum	Violet or lavender, rarely white; heaped and convoluted; glabrous or velvety; purple (rarely white) undersurface; slow growth	Micro- and macroconidia usually lacking; asymmetrically inflated chlamydospores may be found (37)	Growth and sporulation stimulated by thiamine
T. yaoundei	Buff or light yellow developing brown pigment diffusing into medium; glabrous, leathery; flat, becoming heaped and folded; reverse is light tan; slow growth	Pyriform microconidia rare; macroconidia not found; chlamydospores seen	Geographically limited to Africa or to persons with African ancestry; growth slightly stimulated on thiamine and inositol

[a] Adapted from Weitzman and colleagues (76, 80) and Kane et al. (37).
[b] CEAA, Casamino Acids-erythritol-albumin agar; BCPMSG, BCP-milk solids-glucose agar; BCPMSYE, BCP-milk solids-yeast extract; BHI, brain heart infusion agar.

TABLE 6 Important characteristics of pathogenic *Epidermophyton* and *Microsporum* species[a]

Species	Colony on SDA	Microscopic morphology	Comments[b]
E. floccosum	Yellowish green to khaki; flat to radially folded; powdery to velvety; yellow-brown on reverse; white tufts common on surface of older cultures; slow growth	Abundant, widely clavate, smooth-walled macroconidia, 20–40 by 6–8 μm, single or in clusters, with 0–4 septa (Fig. 12); chlamydospores common in older cultures	Invades skin, nails, and rarely, hair (62); no microconidia
M. audouinii	Grayish white, cream to tan; flat, spreading; velvety; light salmon pink to light reddish brown on reverse; moderate growth	Usually no conidia, but if present, microconidia pyriform, macroconidia fusiform, beaked, often with a constriction and with few septa at irregular intervals (Fig. 13); apiculate terminal chlamydospores are most characteristic feature; pectinate hyphae may be present	Prepubertal tineal capitis and tinea corporis; poor growth and brownish discoloration of rice grains; does not perforate hair in vitro (53)
M. canis	White to pale buff (Fig. 18); woolly; yellow-orange to orange-brown reverse; rarely nonpigmented on reverse; rapid growth	Numerous fusiform macroconidia with thick walls and up to 15 septa; 18–125 by 5–25 μm, with asymmetric knobbed apex (Fig. 14); few microconidia	Good growth and sporulation on rice grains; perforates hair in vitro (53). *M. canis* var. *distortum* has macroconidia distorted, bizarrely shaped
M. cookei	Yellowish to reddish tan; flat; powdery, granular, or downy; dark purple-red on reverse; rapid growth	Macroconidia numerous, some resembling those of *M. gypseum*, but most with thicker walls (1–5 μm) and widely separately cellular compartments (Fig. 15) macroconidia abundant	Geophilic species; rarely pathogenic
M. equinum	White, pale buff to pale salmon; folding; velvety to finely powdery; buff to salmon on reverse	Macroconidia infrequent on SDA, elliptical to fusiform, 18–60 by 5–15 μm, 2–4 cells; thick walls may resemble those of *M. canis*	Macroconidia stimulated by niger seed medium 8 agar (32); does not perforate hair in vitro (53); growth on rice grains resembles that of *M. audouinii* (1)
M. ferrugineum	Yellowish to rust colored; folded; waxy; white, velvety variants found in Balkans (55); very slow grower	Usually no conidia; numerous chlamydospores, irregular hyphae, and long, straight, coarse hyphae with prominent septa ("bamboo hyphae")	Geographically restricted to parts of Africa, Asia, and Eastern Europe; light yellow colonies on Lowenstein-Jensen medium differentiate it from dark, reddish brown colonies of *T. soudanense* (73, 79)
M. gallinae	White tinged with pink; slightly folded, downy; raspberry red diffusing pigment on reverse; rapid to moderate growth	Macroconidia fairly abundant, blunt tipped, sometimes curved, 6–8 by 15–50 μm, 2–10 cells; cell walls usually smooth, sometimes echinulate; pyriform microconidia	Conidia stimulated by yeast extract or thiamine in medium

(*Continued on next page*)

TABLE 6 Important characteristics of pathogenic *Epidermophyton* and *Microsporum* species[a] *(Continued)*

Species	Colony on SDA	Microscopic morphology	Comments[b]
M. *gypseum* complex (M. *gypseum*, M. *fulvum*, and M. *boullardii*)	Pale buff, rosy buff to light cinnamon, white border; flat; powdery, granular to floccose; buff to reddish brown on reverse; rapid growth	Abundant macroconidia, 25–60 by 7.5–15 μm; ellipsoidal to fusiform, up to 6 septa, thin walled (Fig. 16); microconidia moderately abundant	Perforates hair in vitro; definitive identification of species is obtained by mating tester strains on appropriate media to induce teleomorph (51, 81) or by examining colonial and microscopic features on Takashio's medium (17)
M. *nanum*	Cream to buff; powdery reddish brown on reverse; moderate growth	Abundant obovate to clavate macroconidia, 10.5–30 by 6.5–13 μm, usually 2 cells; microconidia few to moderately abundant	Grows more slowly than members of M. *gypseum* complex; must be differentiated from *Trichothecium roseum*
M. *persicolor*	Yellowish buff becoming peach to pink; flat; powdery to downy; reddish brown on reverse; rapid growth	Abundant microconidia, spherical to pyriform (few clavate), stalked, borne mostly in grapelike clusters but also singly along the sides of hyphae; thin-walled macroconidia (Fig. 17) often smooth; spiral hyphae common	Perforates hair in vitro; resembles T. *mentagrophytes*; can be differentiated on BCPMSG (35); rough-walled macroconidia on SDA–3% NaCl (35); peach- to rose-colored colonies on cereal agar (49); absence of good growth at 37°C (35) with rare exceptions
M. *praecox*	Cream to yellowish tan; folded; powdery; pale yellow to orange on reverse; moderate growth	Numerous long fusiform macroconidia, some with apical appendages, 40–90 by 7–17 μm, 2–8 septa, thin walled; microconidia absent	Does not perforate human hair in vitro (78)
M. *racemosum*	White, cream, or buff; flat; finely granular; dark purple-red on reverse; rapid growth	Macroconidia abundant, fusiform to elliposidal, 41–77 by 9 μm, 3–8 septa, moderately thick walls; numerous microconidia mostly stalked and produced in grapelike clusters	Macroconidia resembling those of M. *gypseum*
M. *vanbreuseghemii*	Pink to deep rose, light buff, or yellowish; flat; coarsely granular to downy; cream to pale yellow on reverse; rapid growth	Abundant cylindrofusiform macroconidia 43.7–87.5 μm, thicked walled, up to 12 septa, with widely spaced cellular compartments; numerous pyriform to obovate microconidia borne singly along sides of hyphae	

[a] Adapted from Weitzman et al. (76, 80) and Kane et al. (37).
[b] BCPMSG, BCP-milk solids-glucose agar; SDA, Sabouraud glucose agar.

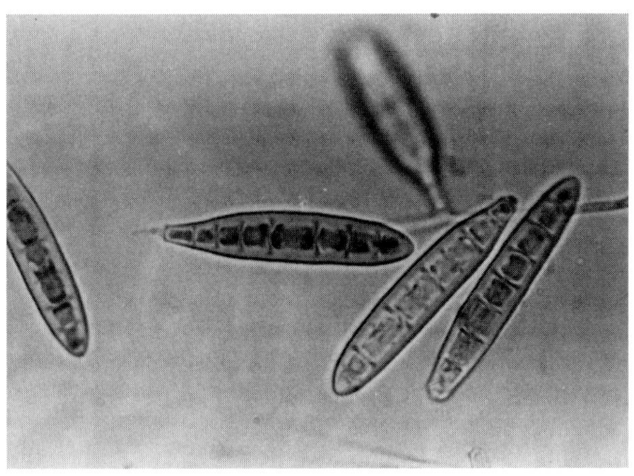

FIGURE 5 Smooth-walled macroconidia of *Trichophyton ajelloi*. Magnification, ×400.

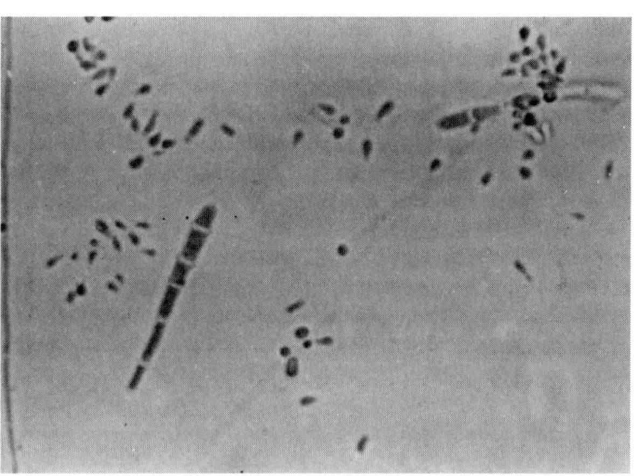

FIGURE 8 Long, narrow macroconidium and clavate to pyriform microconidia of *T. rubrum*. Magnification, ×400.

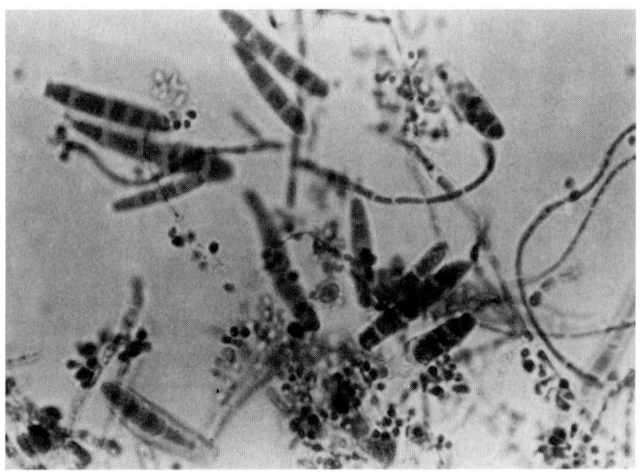

FIGURE 6 Macroconidia and microconidia *T. mentagrophytes* on SDA–5% NaCl. Magnification, ×400.

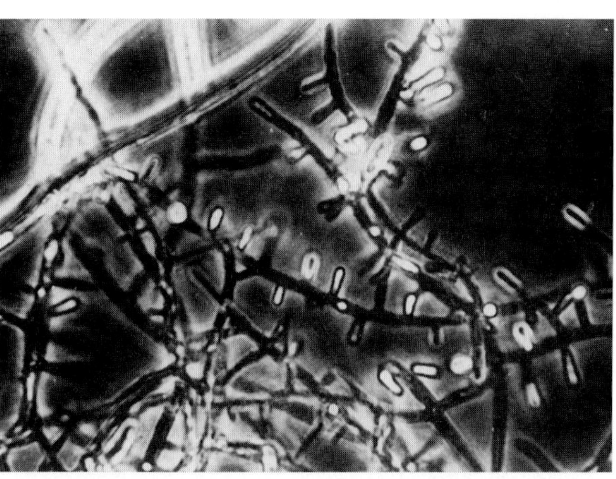

FIGURE 9 Clavate macroconidium, microconidia, and intermediate conidia of *T. terrestre*. Phase-contrast microscopy. Magnification, ×400.

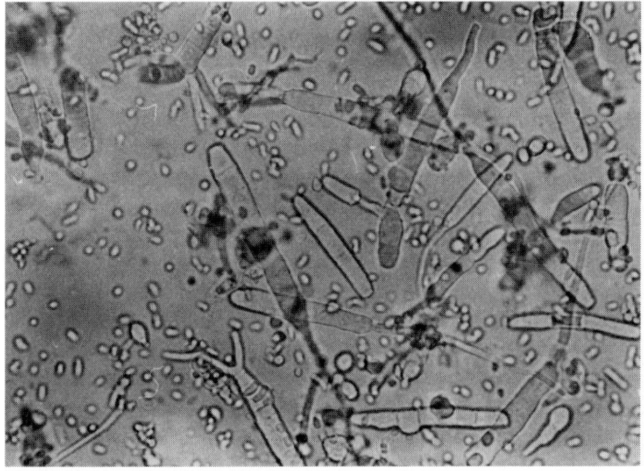

FIGURE 7 Smooth-walled macroconidia of *T. raubitschekii* from primary isolate on SDA. Magnification, ×400.

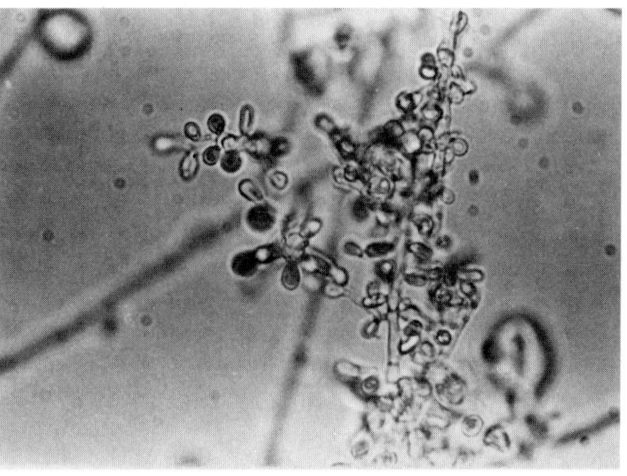

FIGURE 10 Microconidia with typical refractile cytoplasm of *T. tonsurans*. Magnification, ×400.

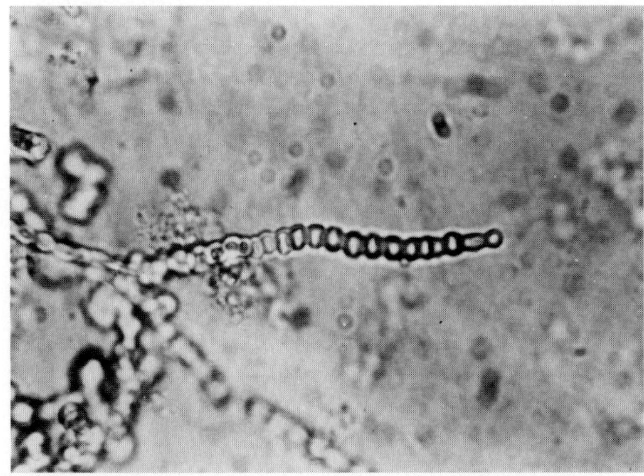

FIGURE 11 Characteristic chlamydospores produced by *T. verrucosum* or BCPMSYE. Magnification, ×400.

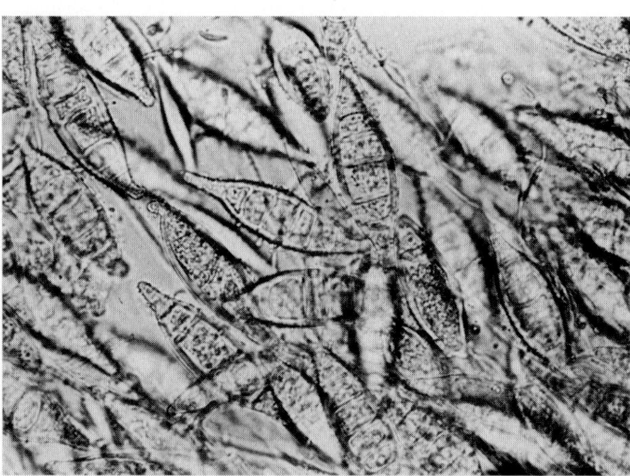

FIGURE 14 Macroconidia of *M. canis* with rough thick walls. Magnification, ×400.

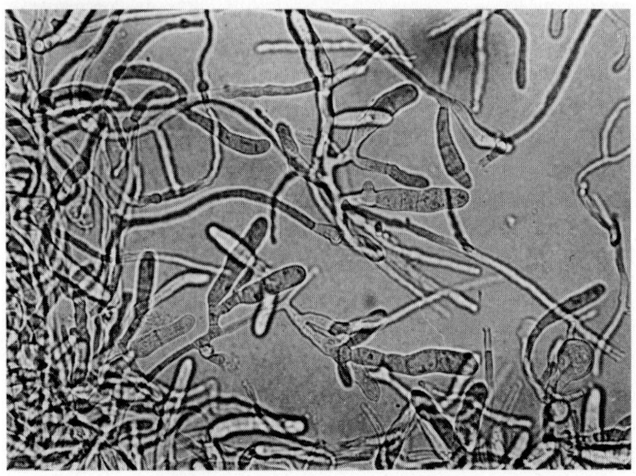

FIGURE 12 Macroconidia of *E. floccosum* on SDA. Note the absence of microconidia. Magnification, ×400.

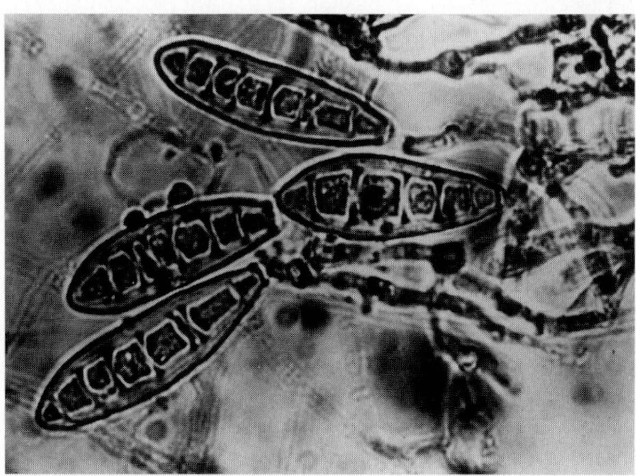

FIGURE 15 Macroconidia of *M. cookei*, showing thick walls and pseudosepta. Magnification, ×400.

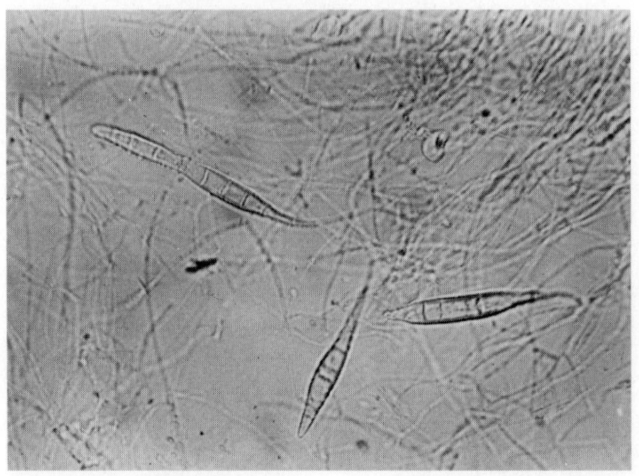

FIGURE 13 Macroconidia of *M. audouinii* on SDA–3% NaCl. Magnification, ×400.

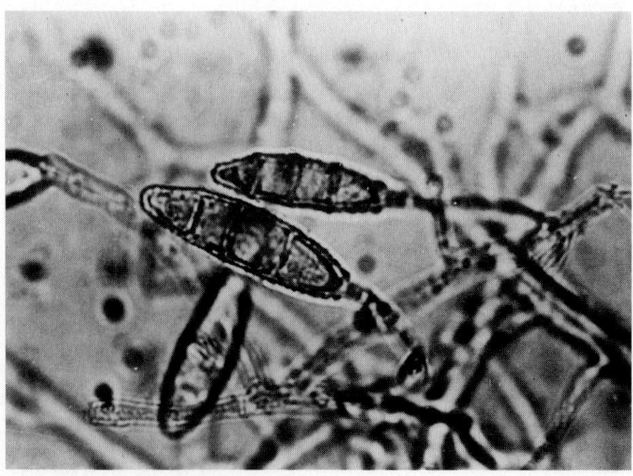

FIGURE 16 Macroconidia of *M. gypseum*. Magnification, ×400.

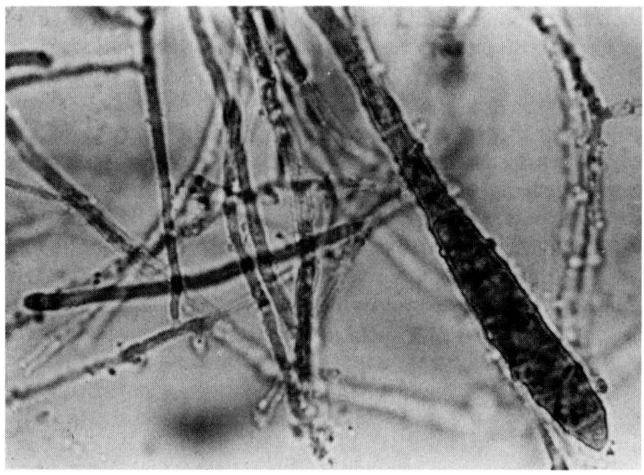

FIGURE 17 Rough-walled macroconidium of M. *persicolor* on SDA–3% NaCl. Magnification, ×1,000.

Urea Hydrolysis

The ability to hydrolyze urea provides additional data that can be used to aid in the differentiation of *T. rubrum* (urease negative) from *T. mentagrophytes* (typically urease positive) and *T. rubrum* from *Trichophyton raubitschekii* (urease positive) (59, 63). Christensen urea agar and broth may both be used; the broth appears to be the more sensitive of these alternatives (31). After the urea medium is inoculated, it is incubated at 25 to 30°C for up to 7 days. The tubes should be examined every 2 to 3 days for the color change from orange or pale pink to purple-red that indicates the presence of urease, a positive test result. Negative and positive controls should always be done on new batches of these media.

Growth on BCPMSG Medium

BCP-milk solids-glucose (BCPMSG) medium is available commercially as Dermatophyte Differential Agar (Biomedia) and Dermatophyte Milk Agar (Hardy). The type of growth (profuse versus restricted) and a change in the pH indicator (BCP) indicating alkalinity are especially useful for differentiating *T. rubrum* from *T. mentagrophytes* and *T. mentagrophytes* from *Microsporum persicolor* (35, 69). *T. rubrum* shows restricted growth and produces no alkaline reaction on BCPMSG medium, whereas *T. mentagrophytes* typically shows profuse growth and an alkaline reaction. Although *M. persicolor* shows profuse growth, it does not result in an alkaline reaction. Other tests for differentiating *T. mentagrophytes* from *M. persicolor* are described elsewhere (49).

Cultures to be tested are inoculated onto slants of BCPMSG medium and are examined for pH change and growth characteristics at the end of a 7-day incubation at 25°C. A color change from pale blue to violet-purple indicates an alkaline reaction.

Growth on Polished Rice Grains

Unlike most dermatophytes, *M. audouinii* grows poorly on rice grains and produces a brownish discoloration of the rice (13). *M. equinum* has been reported to have a growth pattern resembling that of *M. audouinii* (1). This is a useful test for differentiating these species from *M. canis* and from other dermatophytes that typically grow and sporulate on rice grains. It may be especially useful in areas where *M. audouinii* is still endemic, e.g., Africa, or where immigration from such areas is reintroducing it.

The medium is prepared in 12-ml flasks by mixing 1 part raw unfortified rice grains and 3 parts water (13) or 8.0 g of rice grains and 125 ml of distilled water. Autoclave the rice-water mixture at 15 lb/in^2 for 15 min. Inoculate the surface of the rice, and incubate the sample for 2 weeks at 25 to 30°C.

Temperature Tolerance and Temperature Enhancement

Tests for temperature tolerance and enhancement are useful for differentiating *T. mentagrophytes* from *Trichophyton terrestre* (50), *T. mentagrophytes* from *M. persicolor* (35), *T. verrucosum* from *T. schoenleinii* (56), and *Trichophyton soudanense* from *M. ferrugineum* (79). At 37°C, *T. mentagrophytes* shows good growth, whereas *T. terrestre* does not grow and *M. persicolor* generally grows poorly or not at all (a single atypical isolate with good growth has recently been obtained); growth of *T. verrucosum* and *T. soudanense* is enhanced, but that of *T. schoenleinii* and *M. ferrugineum* is not.

Inoculate two slants of SDA with an equivalent fragment of the culture. Incubate the slants at room temperature (25 to 30°C) and at 37°C. Compare the growth at both temperatures when mature colonies appear at room temperature. Appropriate controls are recommended and should be compared first.

Molecular Techniques

Some molecular methods for distinguishing *Trichophyton* species have recently been described (42, 46, 47). For example, the arbitrary primer 5′-ACCCGACCTG-3′ gives different results with *T. rubrum*, *T. mentagrophytes*, and *T. tonsurans* (42). Restricted total cellular DNA may also be used to distinguish *T. rubrum* and *T. mentagrophytes* (47). Such methods may be of particular value with extremely atypical isolates.

DESCRIPTION OF ETIOLOGIC AGENTS

Identification of dermatophytes in the routine clinical laboratory is based on the anamorph, i.e., the asexual state seen in culture, rather than on the teleomorph (sexual form). Characteristic features of dermatophyte species are presented in Tables 5 and 6. These tables also include data on some similar but rarely or never pathogenic *Microsporum* and *Trichophyton* species, which must be distinguished from pathogenic species.

Two types of hyaline conidia may be produced by the dermatophytes: large multicellular, smooth or rough, thin- or thick-walled macroconidia and smaller unicellular, smooth-walled microconidia. The three genera are grouped according to the presence or absence of these two types of conidia and the appearance of the surface of the macroconidia, i.e., rough versus smooth. However, this rigid morphologic distinction has become a morphologic continuum based on overlapping characteristics (52). Identification of these species is based on the microscopic appearance and arrangement of the conidia (Fig. 5 through 17), colonial morphology on SDA (Fig. 18), and physiologic tests (Table 7).

Trichophyton Species

Macroconidia have smooth thin to thick walls, are variable in shape (clavate, fusiform to cylindrical), vary in number of septa (1 to 12) and in size (8 to 86 by 4 to 14 μm), and are borne singly or in clusters. Microconidia, which are usually present and more numerous than macroconidia, may be globose, pyriform, or clavate and are borne singly or in grapelike clusters. Although the production of microconidia is more characteristic of this genus, three lineages producing macroconidia but lacking microconidia have been described: *Trichophyton* (*Keratinomyces*) *longifusum* (3, 19), *Trichophyton kanei* (67), and a variant form of *T. tonsurans* (52). Some species such as *T. schoenleinii* rarely produce conidia, and nonsporulating isolates of normally conidial species, especially *T. rubrum*, may be encountered.

Microsporum Species

Microsporum species produce macroconidia and microconidia that may be rare or numerous, depending on the species and the substrate. The distinguishing characteristic is the macroconidium, which is typically rough walled (varying from minutely to strongly roughened). Macroconidia also vary in shape (obovate, fusiform to cylindrofusiform), number of septa (1 to 15), size (6 to 160 by 6 to 25 μm), and width of the cell wall. Microconidia are pyriform or clavate and usually are arranged singly along the sides of the hyphae. *Microsporum* species invade skin, hair, and rarely, nails. Although morphologic species distinction is usually based on colonies grown on SDA, Takashio's medium may be used specifically for the presumptive distinction of the biological (teleomorphic) species within the *M. gypseum* complex on the basis of colonial and microscopic features (17). These species are otherwise distinguishable only by mating or molecular testing.

Epidermophyton Species

In *Epidermophyton* species, microconidia are lacking; only smooth-walled, broadly clavate macroconidia are produced. They have one to nine septa, are 20 to 60 μm long by 4 to 13 μm wide, and are borne singly or in clusters of two or three. *E. floccosum* is the only pathogen (the genus has only two species); it invades skin, nails, and rarely, hair (62).

SUPERFICIAL MYCOSES

In the superficial mycoses, the causative fungi colonize the cornified layers of the epidermis or the suprafollicular portion of the hair. There is little tissue damage, and a cellular response from the host generally is lacking. The diseases are largely cosmetic in impact, involving changes in the pigmentation of the skin (tinea versicolor or tinea nigra) or the formation of nodules along the distal hair shaft (black piedra and white piedra).

In contrast to agents of the dermatophytoses, the etiologic agents are diverse and unrelated.

Tinea versicolor (Pityriasis versicolor)

Tinea versicolor is an infection of the stratum corneum caused by a group of closely similar lipophilic yeast species of the *Malassezia furfur* complex. Members of this complex infecting human skin were often treated until recently as a single species, but it has been shown by molecular, physiologic, and serotyping studies that they are separate (23). The complex includes *M. furfur* (synonyms, *Pityrosporum furfur* and *Pityrosporum ovale* pro parte), *Malassezia sympodialis*, *Malassezia globosa* (probable synonym, *Pityrosporum orbiculare*), *Malassezia restricta*, *Malassezia slooffiae*, and *Malassezia obtusa* (23). In routine clinical reporting, referring to these organisms as members of the *M. furfur* complex is sufficient.

Tinea versicolor lesions appear as scaly, discrete or concrescent, hypopigmented or hyperpigmented (fawn, yellow-brown, brown, or red) patches chiefly on the neck, torso, and limbs. The infection is largely cosmetic, becoming apparent when the skin fails to tan normally. The disease has a worldwide distribution; it is common in temperate zones and is very prevalent in the tropics. *M. furfur* and related yeasts are found on the normal skin and elicit disease only under conditions, local or systemic, that favor the overgrowth of the organism.

The *M. furfur* complex has been associated with folliculitis (9), obstructive dacryocystitis (55), systemic infections in patients receiving intralipid therapy (15), and seborrheic dermatitis, especially in patients with AIDS (21). Two excellent reviews of human infections caused by *Malassezia* spp. and characteristics of the genus have recently been published (26, 44).

Direct Examination

The fungi are observed readily when scrapings are mounted in 10% KOH plus ink (12), 25% NaOH plus 5% glycerin, calcofluor white, or Kane's formulation (glycerol, 10 ml; Tween 80, 10 ml; phenol, 2.5 g; methylene blue, 1.0 g; distilled water, 480 ml). The presence of short, septate, occasionally branching filaments 2.5 to 4 μm in diameter and of variable lengths along with clusters of small, unicellular, oval or round budding yeast cells (Fig. 19) with a collarette between mother and daughter cells (budding is phialidic) averaging 4 μm (up to 8 μm) in size is diagnostic.

Isolation and Culture

Culture is not essential for identification unless the findings of direct microscopic examination are atypical or unless full species determination is desired for research purposes. Also, *M. furfur* complex members are part of the normal flora of the skin, and a positive culture does not indicate infection. The species require exogenous lipid and do not grow on routine mycology media. If culture is desired, scrapings may be inoculated onto SDA plus cycloheximide and chloramphenicol (Mycosel; BBL), Mycobiotic agar (Difco), or Littman oxgall agar (Difco, Remel), overlaid with sterile olive oil (we recommend Gallo or Pompeian), and incubated at 32°C. Leeming's medium, which uses whole milk as a major lipid source, is superior to at least some olive oil media for primary isolation (41). Growth of the yeasts is slow; colonies

FIGURE 18 (a) *Trichophyton krajdenii*, SDA, 12 days, showing typical bright yellow pigmentation. (b) Zoophilic *T. mentagrophytes* (mating tester strain of *Arthroderma vanbreuseghemii*), 14 days. (c) *T. rubrum*, SDA, 10 days, surface showing cottony white mycelium. (d) *T. rubrum*, SDA, 10 days, reverse showing typical red pigment. (e) *T. tonsurans*, SDA, 14 days, surface showing low velvety texture, mixed white and brownish mycelium. (f) *T. tonsurans*, SDA, 14 days, reverse showing mixture of mahogany red-brown and sulfur yellow coloration. (g) *M. canis*, SDA, 10 days, relatively flat colony showing pale striate margin and yellowish pigment near colony center. (h) Brown filaments of *P. werneckii* in NaOH mount of scraping from tinea nigra. Magnification, ×400.

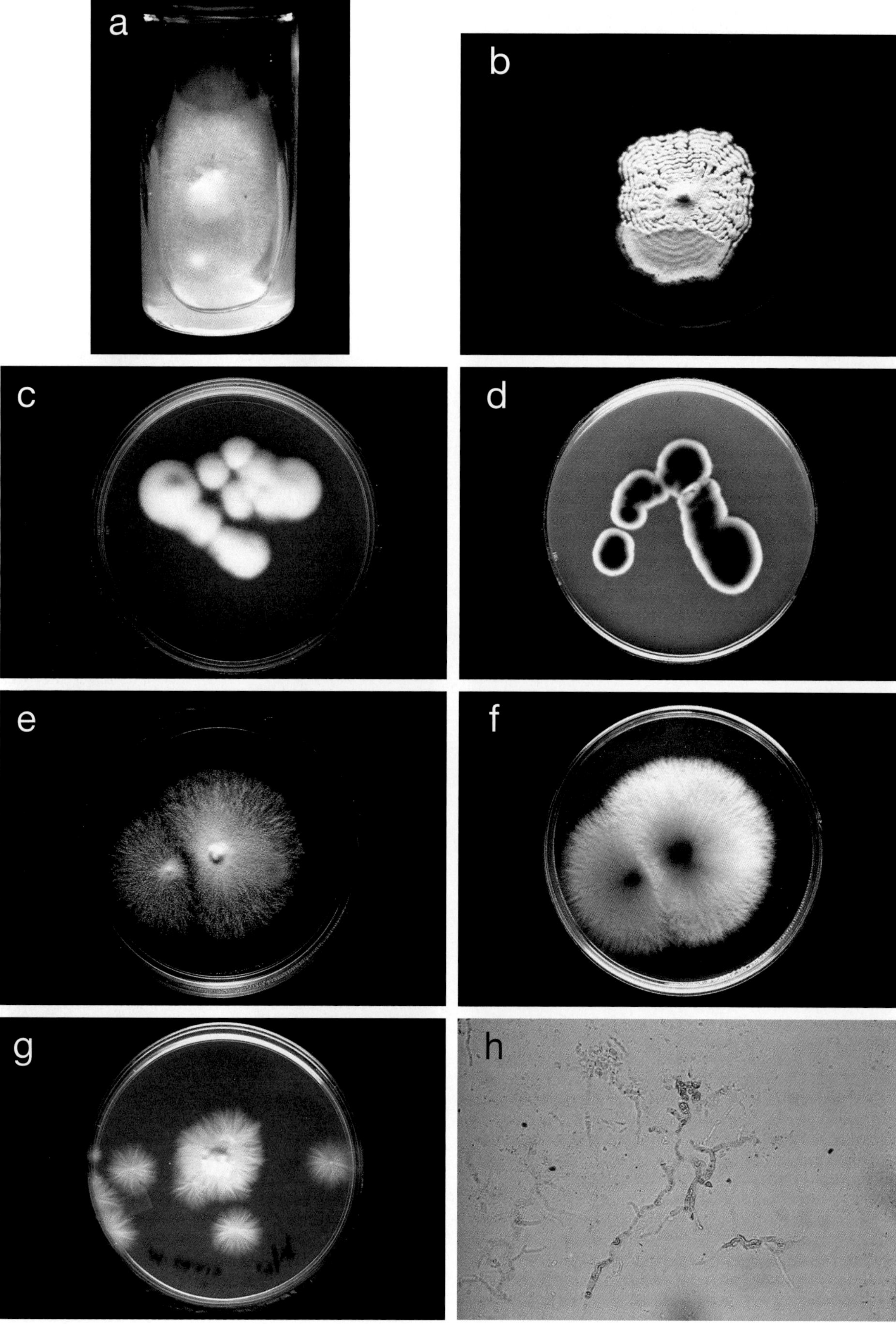
a
b
c
d
e
f
g
h

TABLE 7 Sequence of procedures for identification of dermatophytes in pure culture[a]

1. Examine colony for colors of surface and reverse, topography, texture, and rate of growth. Proceed to step 2.
2. Prepare tease mounts and search for identifying microscopic morphology, especially presence, appearance, and arrangement of macroconidia and microconidia (consult Fig. 5 to 18 and Tables 5 and 6). If results are inconclusive, proceed to step 3.
3. Prepare slide cultures or transparent tape mounts and examine for characteristic morphology as indicated above if tease mounts do not provide sufficient information. Consider special media if sporulation is absent (potato-glucose agar, lactrimel, SDA with 3–5% NaCl). At the same time, proceed to step 4.
4. Perform as many of the following physiologic and other special tests as necessary for identification.
   a. Urease (ensure culture is bacteria-free!)
   b. Nutritional requirements if a *Trichophyton* sp. is suspected.
   c. Growth on rice grains if a *Microsporum* sp. is suspected.
   d. In vitro hair perforation test.
   e. Temperature tolerance and/or optimum temperature of growth.
   f. Special differentiation media, e.g., BCP milk solids-glucose to distinguish *T. mentagrophytes* from *M. persicolor* (35), *T. rubrum* from *T. mentagrophytes* (69) and *T. megninii* (37), and *M. equinum* from *M. canis* (37); Lowenstein-Jensen or BCP-milk solids-glucose to distinguish *T. soudanense* from *M. ferrugineum* (37, 79).
   g. Mating or molecular studies (to be performed in reference laboratories).

[a] It may be necessary to incubate cultures on brain heart infusion agar or similar media to ensure the absence of antibiotic-resistant bacterial contamination before proceeding to step 4. Procedures are adapted from Weitzman and colleagues (76, 80) and Kane et al. (37).

are cream colored, glossy, and raised (Fig. 20), later becoming dull, dry, and tan to brownish. Only budding yeast cells generally appear in culture (Fig. 21).

Tinea Nigra

Tinea nigra is characterized by the appearance, primarily on the palms of the hands and less commonly on the dorsa of the feet, of flat, sharply marginated, brownish black, nonscaly macules.

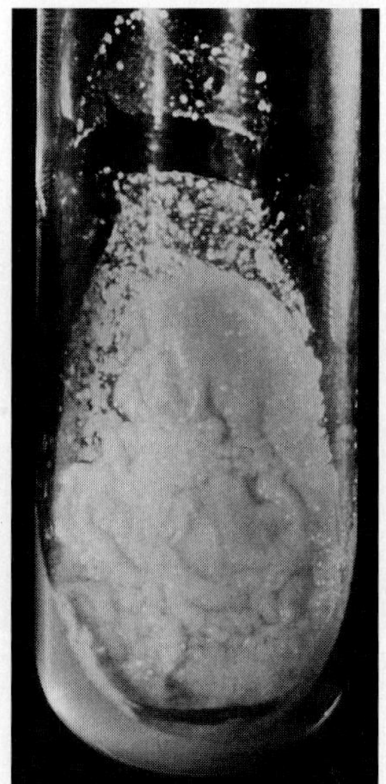

FIGURE 20 Culture of *M. furfur* on Littman oxgall agar overlaid with olive oil.

The disease, almost always caused by *Phaeoannellomyces werneckii*, is most common in tropical areas (55) and has been contracted occasionally in coastal areas in and near the southeastern United States (74). Cases diagnosed outside the area of endemicity have resulted from travel to the tropical regions of the Americas or the Caribbean islands (55).

Direct Microscopic Examination

Microscopic examination of skin scrapings in KOH or NaOH reveals numerous light brown, frequently branching septate filaments 1.5 to 5 μm in diameter (Fig. 18h); short, sinuous filaments; and budding cells, some of which are septate.

Isolation

On SDA with or without antibiotics *P. werneckii* grows slowly and usually appears within 2 to 3 weeks as moist,

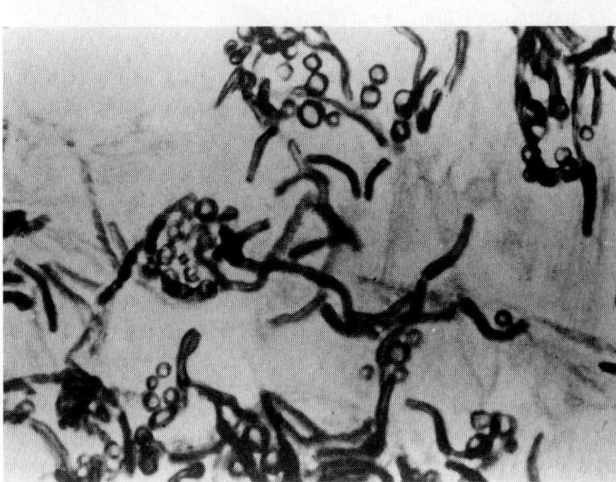

FIGURE 19 *M. furfur* in skin scrapings from a lesion of tinea versicolor (Kane's stain). Magnification, ×1,000.

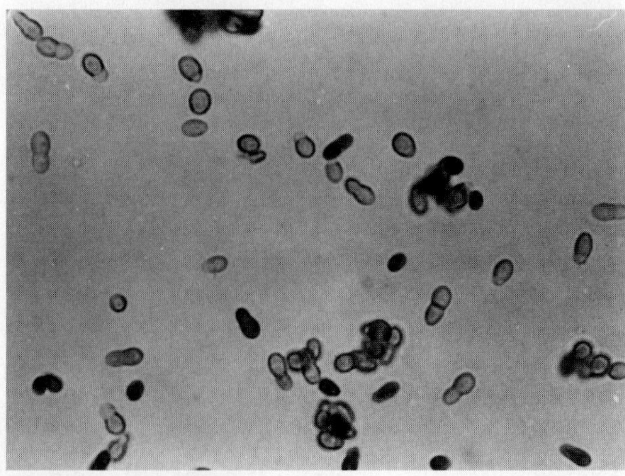

FIGURE 21 Microscopic appearance of *M. furfur* yeast cells on Littman oxgall agar overlaid with olive oil. Magnification, ×400.

shiny olive to greenish black yeastlike colonies. The micromorphology of *P. werneckii* is described in chapter 101.

Black Piedra

Black piedra is a fungal infection of the scalp hair, less commonly of the beard or moustache, and rarely of axillary or pubic hairs. The disease is characterized by the presence of discrete, hard, gritty, dark brown to black nodules adhering firmly to the hair shaft (Fig. 22). It is found mostly in tropical regions in Africa, Asia, and Central and South America. Humans as well as primates are infected.

The etiologic agent in humans is *Piedraia hortae*, an ascomycete whose nodules serve as ascostromata containing locules that harbor the asci and ascospores.

Direct Microscopic Examination

Hair fragments containing the nodules are mounted in 25% NaOH or KOH, heated gently, and carefully squashed without breaking the coverslip (the nodules are very hard). The squashed preparation of a mature nodule should reveal compact masses of dark, septate hyphae around the surface of the hair and round to oval asci containing hyaline, curved, fusiform, aseptate ascospores that bear one or more appendages.

Isolation, Culture, and Identification

SDA with chloramphenicol and SDA with chloramphenicol and cycloheximide should be used for isolation. Some reports have indicated that cycloheximide may be inhibitory; however, others have used this antibiotic successfully.

Colonies are very slow growing, are dark brown to black, and are heaped in the center with a flat periphery. A dark brown to black, short, aerial mycelium eventually covers the young glabrous colony. Some colonies produce a reddish brown diffusible pigment on the agar. Microscopic examination reveals only highly septated dark hyphae and swollen intercalary cells. Conidia and ascospores are usually not found on routine mycological media.

White Piedra

White piedra is a fungal infection of the hair shaft characterized by the presence of soft white, yellowish, beige, or greenish nodules found chiefly on facial, axillary, or genital hairs

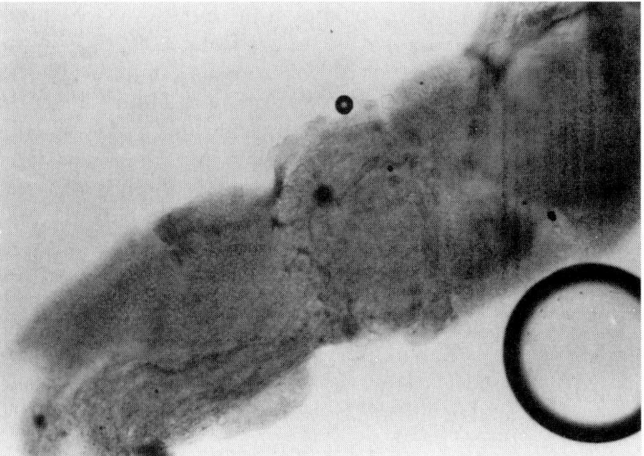

FIGURE 23 White piedra nodule on hair from the groin. Magnification, ×1,000.

(Fig. 23) and less commonly on the scalp, eyebrows, and eyelashes. Nodules may be discrete or more often coalescent, forming an irregular transparent sheath.

The infection occurs sporadically in North America and Europe and more commonly in South America, Africa, and the Orient (55). Although white piedra is an uncommon infection, genital white piedra is more frequent in certain populations (27, 66).

Microscopic examination of hairs containing the adherent nodules mounted in 10% KOH or 25% NaOH–5% glycerin and squashed under a coverslip will reveal intertwined hyaline septate hyphae, hyphae breaking up into oval or rectangular arthroconidia 2 to 4 μm in diameter (Fig. 24), occasional blastoconidia, and bacteria that may surround the nodule as a zooglea.

The isolates were formerly described as *Trichosporon beigelii* or *Trichosporon cutaneum* but are now correctly identified in most cases as *Trichosporon ovoides* (causes scalp hair white piedra) and *Trichosporon inkin* (causes most cases of pubic white piedra) (24). As with *M. furfur*, they form a complex of difficult-to-identify species whose distinction is not known to have strong clinical implications; they may thus be reported as members of the *T. cutaneum* complex or the *T. beigelii* complex. The latter name has nomenclatural

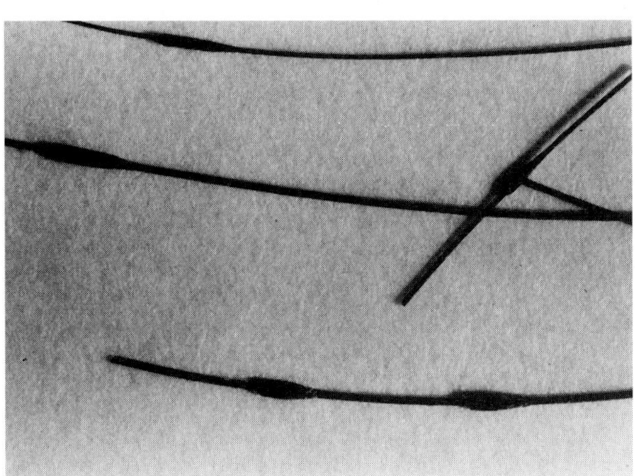

FIGURE 22 Black piedra nodules on scalp hair. NaOH mount. Magnification, ×100.

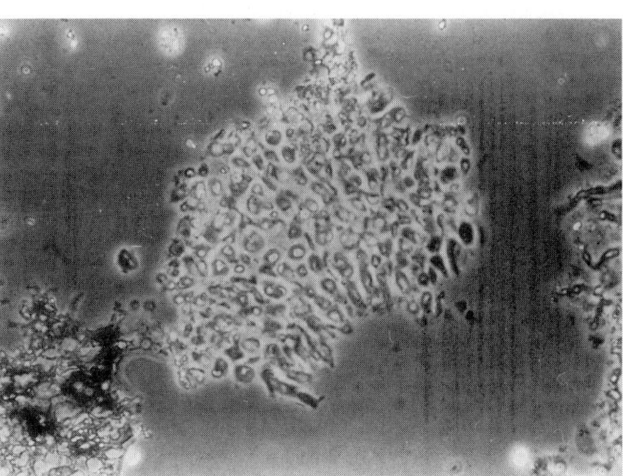

FIGURE 24 Arthroconidia from a crushed nodule of white piedra. Magnification, ×1,000.

problems (22) and may soon drop from currency. The causal agents of white piedra may be readily isolated on SDA with chloramphenicol or other isolation media containing antibacterial antibiotics. The isolation medium should not contain cycloheximide, since this drug is inhibitory to some of the species. Growth is rapid, yielding white to cream-colored colonies that exhibit a variety of colonial morphologies depending on the species. A description of the genus and characteristics of the species are given in papers by Gueho et al. (22, 24).

REFERENCES

1. **Aho, R.** 1987. Mycological studies on *Microsporum equinum* isolated in Finland, Sweden and Norway. *J. Med. Vet. Mycol.* **25:**255–260.
2. **Ajello, L.** 1960. Geographic distribution and prevalence of the dermatophytes. *Ann. N. Y. Acad. Sci.* **89:**30–38.
3. **Ajello, L.** 1968. A taxonomic review of the dermatophytes and related species. *Sabouraudia* **6:**147–159.
4. **Ajello, L.** 1974. Natural history of the dermatophytes and related fungi. *Mycopathol. Mycol. Appl.* **53:**93–110.
5. **Ajello, L., and L. K. Georg.** 1957. In vitro cultures for differentiating between atypical isolates of *Trichophyton mentagrophytes* and *Trichophyton rubrum*. *Mycopathol. Mycol. Appl.* **8:**3–7.
6. **Alsop, J., and A. P. Prior.** 1961. Ringworm infection in a cucumber greenhouse. *Br. Med. J.* **1:**1081–1083.
7. **Aly, R.** 1994. Culture media for growing dermatophytes. *J. Am. Acad. Dermatol.* **31:**S107–S108.
8. **Araviysky, A. N., R. A. Aravivysky, and G. A. Eschkov.** 1975. Deep generalized trichophytosis. *Mycopathologia* **56:** 47–65.
9. **Back, O., J. Faergemann, and R. Hornquist.** 1985. *Pityrosporum* folliculitis: a common disease of the young and middle-aged. *J. Am. Acad. Dermatol.* **12:**56–61.
10. **Barson, W. J.** 1985. Granuloma and pseudogranuloma of the skin due to *Microsporum canis*. *Arch. Dermatol.* **121:** 895–897.
11. **Borelli, D.** 1962. Medios caseros para micologia. *Arch. Venez. Med. Trop. Parasitol. Med.* **4:**301–310.
12. **Cohen, M. M.** 1954. A simple procedure for staining tinea versicolor (*M. furfur*) with fountain pen ink. *J. Invest. Dermatol.* **22:**9–10.
13. **Conant, N. F.** 1936. Studies on the genus *Microsporum*. I. Cultural studies. *Arch. Dermatol.* **33:**665–683.
14. **Currah, R. S.** 1985. Taxonomy of the Onygenales: Arthrodermataceae, Gymnoascaceae, Myxotrichaceae and Onygenaceae. *Mycotaxon* **24:**1–216.
15. **Danker, W. M., S. A. Spector, J. Fierer, and C. E. Davis.** 1987. *Malassezia* fungemia in neonates and adults: complication of hyperalimentation. *Rev. Infect. Dis.* **9:**743–753.
16. **Dei Cas, E., and A. Vernes.** 1986. Parasitic adaptation of pathogenic fungi to mammalian hosts. *Crit. Rev. Microbiol.* **13:**173–218.
17. **DeMange, C., N. Contet-Andonneau, M. Kombila, M. Miegeville, M. Berthonneau, C. DeVroey, and G. Percebois.** 1992. *Microsporum gypseum* complex in man and animals. *J. Med. Vet. Mycol.* **30:**301–308.
18. **Fischer, J. B., and J. Kane.** 1974. The laboratory diagnosis of dermatophytosis complicated with *Candida albicans*. *Can. J. Microbiol.* **20:**167–182.
19. **Florian, E., and J. Galgoczy.** 1964. *Keratinomyces longifusus* sp. nov. from Hungary. *Mycopathol. Mycol. Appl.* **24:** 73–80.
20. **Georg, L. K., and L. B. Camp.** 1957. Routine nutritional tests for the identification of dermatophytes. *J. Bacteriol.* **74:**113–121.
21. **Groisser, D., E. J. Bottone, and M. Lebwohl.** 1989. Association of *Pityrosporum orbiculare* (*Malassezia furfur*) with seborrheic dermatitis in patients with acquired immunodeficiency syndrome (AIDS). *J. Am. Acad. Dermatol.* **20:** 770–773.
22. **Guého, E., G. S. de Hoog, and M. T. Smith.** 1992. Neotypification of the genus *Trichosporon*. *Antonie Leeuwenhoek* **61:**285–288.
23. **Guého, E., G. Midgley, and J. Guillot.** 1996. The genus *Malassezia* with description of four new species. *Antonie Leeuwenhoek* **69:**337–355.
24. **Guého, E., M. T. Smith, G. S. de Hoog, G. Billon-Grand, R. Christen, and W. H. Batenburg-van der Vegte.** 1992. Contributions to a revision of the genus *Trichosporon*. *Antonie Leeuwenhoek* **61:**289–316.
25. **Head, E. S., J. C. Henry, and E. M. MacDonald.** 1984. The cotton swab; technic for the culture of dermatophyte infections: its efficacy and merit. *J. Am. Acad. Dermatol.* **11:**797–801.
26. **Ingham, E., and A. C. Cunningham.** 1993. *Malassezia furfur*. *J. Med. Vet. Mycol.* **31:**265–288.
27. **Kalter, D. C., J. A. Tschen, P. L. Cernoch, M. E. McBrid, J. Sperber, S. Bruce, and J. E. Wolf, Jr.** 1986. Genital white piedra: epidemiology, microbiology, and therapy. *J. Am. Acad. Dermatol.* **14:**982–993.
28. **Kaminski, G. W.** 1985. The routine use of modified Borelli's lactrimel (MBLA). *Mycopathologia* **91:**57–59.
29. **Kane, J.** 1977. *Trichophyton fischeri* sp. nov.: a saprophyte resembling *Trichophyton rubrum*. *Sabouraudia* **15:**231–241.
30. **Kane, J., and J. B. Fischer.** 1975. The effect of sodium chloride on the growth and morphology of dermatophytes and some other keratolytic fungi. *Can. J. Microbiol.* **21:** 742–749.
31. **Kane, J., and J. B. Fischer.** 1976. The differentiation of *Trichophyton rubrum* from *T. mentagrophytes* by use of Christensen's urea broth. *Can. J. Microbiol.* **17:**911–913.
32. **Kane, J., A. Padhye, and L. Ajello.** 1982. *Microsporum equinum* in North America. *J. Clin. Microbiol.* **16:**943–947.
33. **Kane, J., I. F. Salkin, I. Weitzman, and C. Smitka.** 1981. *Trichophyton raubitschekii* sp. nov. *Mycotaxon* **13:**259–266.
34. **Kane, J., J. A. Scott, R. C. Summerbell, and B. Diena.** 1992. *Trichophyton krajdenii* sp. nov.: an anthropophilic dermatophyte. *Mycotaxon* **40:**307–316.
35. **Kane, J., L. Sigler, and R. C. Summerbell.** 1987. Improved procedures for differentiating *Microsporum persicolor* from *Trichophyton mentagrophytes*. *J. Clin. Microbiol.* **25:**2449–2452.
36. **Kane, J., and C. Smitka.** 1978. Early detection and identification of *Trichophyton verrucosum*. *J. Clin. Microbiol.* **8:** 740–747.
37. **Kane, J., R. C. Summerbell, L. Sigler, S. Krajden, and G. Land.** 1997. *Laboratory Handbook of Dermatophytes and Other Filamentous Fungi from Skin, Hair and Nails*. Star Publishing Co., Belmont, Calif.
38. **King, R. D., H. A. Khan, J. C. Foye, J. H. Greenberg, and H. E. Jones.** 1975. Transferrin, iron and dermatophytes. Serum dermatophyte inhibitory component definitively identified as unsaturated transferrin. *J. Lab. Clin. Med.* **86:** 204–212.
39. **Kwon-Chung, K. J., and J. E. Bennett.** 1992. *Medical Mycology*, p. 105–161. Lea & Febiger, Philadelphia, Pa.
40. **Lawson, G. T. N., and W. J. McLeod.** 1957. *Microsporum canis*—an intensive outbreak. *Br. Med. J.* **2:**1159–1160.
41. **Leeming, J., and F. Notman.** 1987. Improved methods for isolation and enumeration of *Malassezia furfur* from human skin. *J. Clin. Microbiol.* **25:**2017–2019.
42. **Liu, D., S. Coloe, J. Pedersen, and R. Baird.** 1996. Use of arbitrarily primed polymerase chain reaction to differentiate *Trichophyton* dermatophytes. *FEMS Microbiol. Lett.* **136:**147–150.

43. **Mackenzie, D. W. R.** 1963. "Hairbrush diagnosis" in detection and eradication of nonfluorescent scalp ringworm. *Br. Med. J.* **2:**363–365.
44. **Marcon, M. J., and D. A. Powell.** 1992. Human infections due to *Malassezia* spp. *Clin. Microbiol. Rev.* **5:**101–119.
45. **Merz, W. G., C. L. Berger, and M. Silva-Hutner.** 1970. Media with pH indicators for the isolation of dermatophytes. *Arch. Dermatol.* **102:**545–547.
46. **Mitchell, H. T., W. A. Hutchins, R. C. Summerbell, and P. F. Lehmann.** 1994. Investigation of species allied to *Trichophyton rubrum* by using isoenzymes and random amplified polymorphic DNA (RAPD), abstr. F-93, p. 604. *In Abstract of the 94th General Meeting of the American Society for Microbiology 1994.* American Society for Microbiology, Washington, D.C.
47. **Mochizuki, T., M. Uehara, T. Menon, and S. Ranganathan.** 1996. Minipreparation of total cellular DNA is useful as an alternative molecular marker of mitochondrial DNA for the identification of *Trichophyton mentagrophytes* and *Trichophyton rubrum*. *Mycoses* **39:**31–35.
48. **Moriello, K. A., and D. J. Deboer.** 1991. Fungal flora of the haircoat of cats with and without dermatophytosis. *J. Med. Vet. Mycol.* **29:**285–292.
49. **Padhye, A. A., F. Blank, P. J. Koblenzer, S. Spatz, and L. Ajello.** 1973. *Microsporum persicolor* infection in the United States. *Arch. Dermatol.* **108:**561–562.
50. **Padhye, A. A., and J. Carmichael.** 1971. The genus *Arthroderma* Berkeley. *Can. J. Bot.* **49:**1525–1540.
51. **Padhye, A. A., A. S. Sekhon, and J. W. Carmichael.** 1973. Ascocarp production by *Arthroderma* and *Nannizzia* species on keratinous and nonkeratinous media. *Sabouraudia* **11:**109–114.
52. **Padhye, A. A., I. Weitzman, and E. Domenech.** 1994. An unusual variant of *Trichophyton tonsurans* var. *sulfureum*. *J. Med. Vet. Mycol.* **32:**147–150.
53. **Padhye, A. A., C. N. Young, and L. Ajello.** 1980. Hair perforation as a diagnostic criterion in the identification of *Epidermophyton*, *Microsporum* and *Trichophyton* species, p. 115–120. *In Superficial Cutaneous and Subcutaneous Infections.* Scientific publication no. 396. Pan American Health Organization, Washington, D.C.
54. **Rippon, J. W.** 1985. The changing epidemiology and emerging patterns of dermatophyte species. *Curr. Top. Med. Mycol.* **1:**209–234.
55. **Rippon, J. W.** 1988. *Medical Mycology: the Pathogenic Fungi and the Pathogenic Actinomycetes*, 3rd ed., p. 154–168. The W. B. Saunders Co., Philadelphia, Pa.
56. **Rippon, J. W.** 1988. *Medical Mycology: the Pathogenic Fungi and the Pathogenic Actinomycetes*, 3rd ed., p. 169–275. The W. B. Saunders Co., Philadelphia, Pa.
57. **Robinson, B. E., and A. A. Padhye.** 1988. Collection transport and processing of clinical specimens, p. 11–32. *In* B. B. Wentworth (ed.), *Diagnostic Procedures for Mycotic and Parasitic Infections*, 7th ed. American Public Health Association, Washington, D.C.
58. **Rosenthal, S. A.** 1974. The epidemiology of tinea pedis, p. 515–526. *In* H. M. Robinson, Jr. (ed.), *The Diagnosis and Treatment of Fungal Infections.* Charles C Thomas, Publisher, Springfield, Ill.
59. **Rosenthal, S. A., and H. Sokolsky.** 1965. Enzymatic studies with pathogenic fungi. *Dermatol. Int.* **4:**72–79.
60. **Salkin, I. F.** 1973. Dermatophyte test medium: evaluation with nondermatophytic pathogens. *Appl. Microbiol.* **26:** 134–137.
61. **Salkin, I. F., A. A. Padhye, and M. E. Kemna.** 1997. A new medium for presumptive identification of dermatophytes. *J. Clin. Microbiol.* **35:**2660–2662.
62. **Sberna, F., V. Farella, V. Geti, F. Taviti, G. Agostini, P. Vannini, B. Knopfel, and E. M. Difonzo.** 1993. Epidemiology of dermatophytoses in the Florence area of Italy: 1985–1990. *Mycopathologia* **122:**153–162.
63. **Sequeira, H., J. Cabrita, C. DeVroey, and C. Wuytack-Raes.** 1991. Contributions to our knowledge of *Trichophyton megninii*. *J. Med. Vet. Mycol.* **29:**417–418.
64. **Shah, P.C., S. Krajden, J. Kane, and R. C. Summerbell.** 1988. Tinea corporis caused by *Microsporum canis*: report of a nosocomial outbreak. *Eur. J. Epidemiol.* **4:**33–38.
65. **Smith, J. M. B., R. D. Jolly, L. K. George, and M. D. Connole.** 1968. *Trichophyton equinum* var. *autotrophicum*: its characteristics and geographic distribution. *Sabouraudia* **6:**296–304.
66. **Stenderup, A., H. Schonheyder, P. Ebbesen, and M. Melbye.** 1986. White piedra and *Trichosporon beigelii* carriage in homosexual men. *J. Med. Vet. Mycol.* **24:**401–406.
67. **Summerbell, R. C.** 1987. *Trichophyton kanei*, sp. nov. a new anthropophilic dermatophyte. *Mycotaxon* **28:**509–523.
68. **Summerbell, R. C., A. Li, and R. Haugland.** 1997. What constitutes a functional species in the asexual dermatophytes? *Microbiol. Cult. Coll.* **13:**29–37.
69. **Summerbell, R. C., S. A. Rosenthal, and J. Kane.** 1988. Rapid method for differentiation of *Trichophyton rubrum*, *Trichophyton mentagrophytes*, and related dermatophyte species. *J. Clin. Microbiol.* **26:**2279–2282.
70. **Tanaka, S., R. C. Summerbell, R. Tsuboi, T. Kaaman, T. Matsumoto, and T. L. Ray.** 1992. Advances in dermatophytes and dermatophytosis. *J. Med. Vet. Mycol.* **30**(Suppl. 1)**:**29–39.
71. **Taplin, D.** 1965. The use of gentamicin in mycology. *J. Invest. Dermatol.* **45:**549–550.
72. **Taplin, D., N. Zaias, G. Rebell, and H. Blank.** 1969. Isolation and recognition of dermatophytes on a new medium (DTM). *Arch. Dermatol.* **99:**203–209.
73. **Vanbreuseghem, R., and R. Zaman.** 1963. Contributions a l'identification du *Trichophyton* (*Langeronia*) *soudanense* et du *Trichophyton ferrugineum*. *Ann. Soc. Belge Med. Trop.* **3:**259–270.
74. **Van Velsor, H., and H. Singletary.** 1964. Tinea nigra palmaris. *Arch. Dermatol.* **90:**59–61.
75. **Weeks, R. J., and A. A. Padhye.** 1982. A mounting medium for permanent preparations of micro-fungi. *Mykosen* **25:**702–704.
76. **Weitzman, I., and J. Kane.** 1991. Dermatophytes and agents of superficial mycoses, p. 601–616. *In* A. Balows, W. J. Hausler, Jr., K. L. Herrmann, H. D. Isenberg, and H. J. Shadomy (ed.), *Manual of Clinical Microbiology*, 5th ed. American Society for Microbiology, Washington, D.C.
77. **Weitzman, I., M. R. McGinnis, A. A. Padhye, and L. Ajello.** 1986. The genus *Arthoderma* and its later synonym *Nannizzia*. *Mycotaxon* **25:**505–518.
78. **Weitzman, I., and S. McMillen.** 1980. Isolation in the United States of a culture resembling *M. praecox*. *Mycopathologia* **70:**181–186.
79. **Weitzman, I., and S. A. Rosenthal.** 1984. Studies in the differentiation between *Microsporum ferrugineum* Ota and *Trichophyton soudanense* Joyeaux. *Mycopathologia* **84:**95–101.
80. **Weitzman, I., S. A. Rosenthal, and M. Silva-Hutner.** 1988. Superficial and cutaneous infections caused by molds: dermatomycoses, p. 33–97. *In* B. B. Wentworth (ed.), *Diagnostic Procedures for Mycotic and Parasitic Infections*, 7th ed. American Public Health Association, Washington, D.C.
81. **Weitzman, I., and M. Silver-Hutner.** 1967. Non-keratinous agar media as substrates for the ascigerous state in certain members of the Gymnoascaceae pathogenic for man and animals. *Sabouraudia* **5:**335–339.
82. **Weitzman, I., and R. C. Summerbell.** 1995. The dermatophytes. *Clin. Microbiol. Rev.* **8:**240–259.

83. **West, B. C., and K. J. Kwon-Chung.** 1980. Mycetoma caused by *Microsporum audouinii*. *Am. J. Clin. Pathol.* **73:** 447–454.
84. **Young, C. N.** 1972. Range of variation among isolates of *Trichophyton rubrum*. *Sabouraudia* **10:**164–170.
85. **Zaias, N., A. Tosti, G. Rebell, R. Morelli, F. Bardazzi, H. Bieley, M. Zaiac, B. Glick, B. Paley, M. Allevato, and R. Baran.** 1996. Autosomal dominant pattern of distal subungual onychomycosis caused by *Trichophyton rubrum*. *J. Am. Acad. Dermatol.* **34:**302–304.

Bipolaris, Exophiala, Scedosporium, Sporothrix, and Other Dematiaceous Fungi

WILEY A. SCHELL, IRA F. SALKIN, LESTER PASARELL, AND MICHAEL R. McGINNIS

101

TAXONOMY, DESCRIPTION, AND NATURAL HABITATS

Dematiaceous fungi are characterized by the presence of a brown to black color in the cell walls of their vegetative cells, conidia, or both, which results in colonies that range from olive or gray to black. The dark pigmentation of the majority of medically important fungi is caused by the deposition of dihydroxynaphthalene melanin formed via pentaketide metabolism. These ubiquitous and cosmopolitan fungi are pathogens of plants and saprobes of soil and decaying matter, but they occasionally cause infections in humans and animals (26, 41, 49, 63). In medical mycology, dematiaceous fungi often are thought of as being exclusively hyphomycetes, but some ascomycetes, basidiomycetes, coelomycetes, and zygomycetes also are dematiaceous. Recently, it has been suggested that the term "dematiaceous" is a misnomer, and the term "phaeoid" has been suggested as a replacement (92).

CLINICAL SIGNIFICANCE

Mycotic infections caused by dematiaceous fungi include mycetoma (see chapter 102), chromoblastomycosis, phaeohyphomycosis, and sporotrichosis, and they have been found in normal and compromised hosts. Typically they are initiated by inoculation with the etiologic agent through abrasion or penetrating injury. However, cases of sinusitis and some cases of pulmonary or disseminated infection are initiated by inhalation of conidia from the environment. Chromoblastomycosis is a chronic, localized cutaneous to subcutaneous opportunistic mycosis, characterized by the presence of muriform (sclerotic) bodies in infected tissue (Fig. 26 in chapter 94). By definition, mature muriform bodies have intersecting cross walls, but those of earlier developmental stages have only one septum or none. Muriform bodies result as vegetative growth occurs without the elongation process found in hyphae. Division of these bodies takes place by splitting along their septal planes. The finding of muriform bodies in cutaneous or subcutaneous tissue is pathognomonic for chromoblastomycosis, although they very rarely can be seen in other mycotic infections as well (109). In some cases, dematiaceous hyphae are also seen. Three fungal species account for virtually all cases of chromoblastomycosis. Because all agents of chromoblastomycosis form muriform bodies that are similar in appearance, the identity of the fungus involved in a particular case cannot be determined by its tissue morphology; the fungus must be cultured and identified.

In contrast to chromoblastomycosis, phaeohyphomycosis is characterized by the presence in tissue of dematiaceous yeastlike cells, pseudohyphae, or hyphae or any combination of these forms. The name "phaeohyphomycosis" is not restricted to hyphomycetes; it encompasses all fungi having dematiaceous cells in infected tissue, regardless of the taxonomic classification of the etiologic agent. The hyphae observed in clinical specimens may be regular and uniform in diameter or irregular in shape with many swollen cells. Although most agents of phaeohyphomycosis form dark cells in infected tissue, it should be noted that certain fungi, particularly species of the genera *Alternaria, Bipolaris,* and *Curvularia,* often appear to be hyaline in tissue due to meager formation of melanin yet are considered agents of phaeohyphomycosis because they are manifestly dematiaceous when grown in culture. Furthermore, use of the Masson-Fontana stain (64) reveals the presence of melanin in the cell walls of these fungi within tissue sections. Phaeohyphomycosis (2, 41) encompasses a spectrum of opportunistic mycoses that ranges from purely cosmetic afflictions to fatal cerebral infections, and can be caused by more than 100 species of fungi. As with chromoblastomycosis, the identities of etiologic agents of phaeohyphomycosis cannot be determined from microscopic examination of clinical specimens. These fungi must be grown on laboratory culture media before they can be identified. The most common phaeohyphomycosis syndromes include allergic fungal sinusitis, keratitis, and subcutaneous infection. Subcutaneous infections commonly present as either a cyst or diffuse lesion, are chronic, and usually remain localized.

Sporotrichosis, caused by *Sporothrix schenckii,* typically is a cutaneous to subcutaneous chronic infection that may undergo lymphatic spread. Musculoskeletal involvement and disseminated infection are rare, and nasal and pulmonary infections following inhalation of conidia have been documented (17, 19, 48, 63). In addition, many infections have been transmitted by animals (5, 107, 109). Sporotrichosis is included in this chapter because the etiologic agent is dematiaceous in culture and because the presence of melanin can be demonstrated within yeast cell walls in tissue by using the Masson-Fontana stain. Certain dematiaceous fungi also have been documented as etiologic agents of mycetoma (see chapter 102).

COLLECTION, TRANSPORT, PROCESSING, AND EXAMINATION OF SPECIMENS

General guidelines for the collection, processing, and examination of specimens are provided in chapters 4, 5, and 94. The most frequently submitted specimens for the recovery of dematiaceous fungi include aspirates, scrapings, and surgical tissue. Swabs are not an effective means of specimen collection and should be avoided when possible. Transport media should not be used unless specimens can be easily retrieved in their entirety. Specimens must not be allowed to become desiccated before being processed. Specimen portions that are necrotic, purulent, or caseous should be selected for microscopic examination and inoculation onto isolation media. Tissue specimens should be minced with scalpels into 0.5 to 1.0-mm pieces and inoculated directly to culture media. Tissue homogenizers should not be used, because some moulds do not have regularly septate (compartmentalized) hyphae and thus can be easily killed by homogenization. Most dematiaceous opportunists will grow on media containing cycloheximide, but media without cycloheximide also must be included.

Most of the currently available antifungal drugs have little efficacy for infections caused by dematiaceous fungi. However, if the infecting agent is known to be a dematiaceous fungus, certain therapeutic approaches which offer an improved outcome in some cases can be used. For this reason, it is essential that when fungal cells are detected by microscopic examination of clinical specimens, they be evaluated for the presence of melanin under bright-field illumination. The amount of melanin present may be slight; therefore, it is imperative that the microscope illumination be correctly adjusted by the Köhler technique (86). In laboratories that use fluorescence microscopy, bright-field examination of a positive field can be accomplished without moving the slide by blocking light from the UV lamp, sliding the fluorescence filters out of the light path, and turning on the incandescent bulb. In addition, it must be noted that heavily melanized fungal cells such as muriform bodies and granules may not be reliably detected with calcofluor white. Therefore, when chromoblastomycosis or mycetoma is suspected, examination of clinical specimens by bright-field microscopy is required. An alternative method for demonstrating the presence of melanin is the use of the Masson-Fontana stain. In sporotrichosis, the number of yeast cells in clinical specimens typically is very small, and their sizes and shapes are not distinctive. As a result, KOH examination of culture-positive specimens usually gives a negative result. However, in tissue sections that have been treated with diastase and stained by either the Gomori or periodic acid-Schiff technique, foci of host response to the fungus will be apparent, and scattered cells of *S. schenckii* often can be seen within these foci. Fluorescent-antibody-specific conjugates have been developed for *S. schenckii* but are available only at certain reference laboratories (58).

IDENTIFICATION

To help ensure that a mould is in pure culture, it may be isolated by transferring hyphal tips or individual germinating conidia or by streaking the organism onto plated culture medium containing antibacterial agents and subsequently isolating individual colonies for subculture to a similar medium (76). Ascertaining the purity of the isolate is important because many of the opportunistic dematiaceous pathogens are pleomorphic, meaning that a single isolate can produce conidia of more than one kind or by more than one mechanism. For an accurate identification, it must be known whether the various types of conidia present in a culture were formed by a single pleomorphic fungus or were due to the presence of more than one fungus. The identification of dematiaceous fungi (10, 26, 28, 37, 38, 49, 76, 129) ultimately rests upon their microscopic morphologies and to a lesser extent upon their colony morphologies and physiologic characteristics (Table 1). Morphologic evaluations are normally based upon cultures that have been grown on a medium such as potato dextrose agar or cornmeal dextrose agar at 25 to 30°C for approximately 2 weeks. It is essential to study the microscopic and gross characteristics of young as well as fully mature colonies. Many microscopic fields must be examined to observe variant as well as predominant features. The importance of conidium development in defining the anamorphic genera of dematiaceous fungi makes it essential to determine how a particular fungus forms its conidia. Slide culture preparations (76) with potato dextrose agar or cornmeal dextrose agar are ideal for determining conidiogenesis (slide culture preparations should be opened or dismantled only with a biological safety cabinet if the isolate is a possible *S. schenckii* or *Cladophialophora bantiana* strain; these species pose a risk of pulmonary infection). These nutritionally minimal media usually stimulate the formation of spores. If a suspected pathogen does not produce spores under such conditions, exposure to a naked incandescent light bulb for several days in a 12-h-light, 12-h-dark cycle while the fungus is growing on a medium such as 2% water agar, V-8 juice agar, potato dextrose agar, cornmeal dextrose agar, moistened sterile wooden sticks, or moistened filter paper may stimulate sporulation. Other sporulation induction techniques include exposing the isolate to UV light (310 to 410 nm), growing the isolate at high and low temperatures; growing it on hay infusion agar, soil extract agar, or cereal agar; or lyophilizing and reviving it. For the identification of certain fungi, it may be helpful to demonstrate physiologic phenomena such as thermotolerance, gelatin liquefaction, or resistance to cycloheximide. When such studies are used, it is important to include controls that will demonstrate the viability of the inoculum.

A modern nomenclature that addresses the complex reproductive cycle of fungi and facilitates the discussion of their identification has gained acceptance during the past 20 years (16). The term "anamorph" is used to characterize an asexual reproductive structure or form produced by a fungus. Some fungi seen in the clinical laboratory produce more than one anamorph. For example, the pathogen *Scedosporium apiospermum*, which forms a distinctive anamorph (the *Scedosporium* anamorph) consisting of solitary annellated conidiogenous cells (see Fig. 8a), may exhibit an additional anamorph typical of the genus *Graphium* (see Fig. 8c). When a single fungus produces more than one anamorph, the term "synanamorph" is used to designate any of the concurrently existing forms. In the present example, the *Graphium* form is a synanamorph of *S. apiospermum* (and vice versa). In addition, some isolates of *S. apiospermum* have the ability to produce a sexual form that is characterized by the formation of ascocarps, within which the sexually recombinant ascospores arise. The sexual form of a fungus is referred to as the "teleomorph." The teleomorph formed by most clinical strains of *S. apiospermum* is *Pseudallescheria*

TABLE 1 Diagnostic features of selected medically important dematiaceous fungi

Genus	Diagnostic characteristics
Alternaria	Colonies rapidly growing, cottony, gray to black. Conidiophores erect, dark, septate, simple or branched. Conidia muriform, obclavate, with beak (tapering apex), darkly pigmented, smooth or rough, sometimes solitary, usually in simple or branched acropetal chains. Fig. 1a. Compare to *Bipolaris, Curvularia, Exserohilum,* and *Helminthosporium*. (26, 37, 38, 49, 76)
Aureobasidium	Colonies smooth, moist, yellow, white, cream, light pink, or light brown, finally becoming black from development of arthroconidia (in a *Scytalidium* synanamorph). Conidiogenous cells undifferentiated from hyphae; intercalary, terminal, or arising as short lateral branches. Conidia hyaline, smooth, ellipsoidal, variable in shape and size; one celled, often producing secondary blastoconidia. Large, dark, one-to two-celled, thick-walled arthroconidia (i.e., the *Scytalidium* synanamorph) usually present. Differs from *Hormonema* spp. by conidia arising in synchrony. Differs from *Phaeococcomyces* spp. by the lack of dematiaceous yeast cells. Fig. 4a. Compare to *Hormonema, Scytalidium*. (25, 37, 38, 49)
Bipolaris	Colonies rapidly growing, woolly, gray to black. Conidiophores dark, erect, simple or branched, septate, geniculate due to sympodial development. Conidia multiseptate, cylindrical to oblong, dark; septal walls thickened, hilum slightly protruding. Fig. 1c. Compare to *Curvularia, Drechslera, Exserohilum, Helminthosporium*. (3, 26, 49, 80, 93)
Chaetomium	Colonies rapidly growing, fluffy, initially hyaline becoming olive-green to brown. Perithecia forming on surface of substratum; dark brown to black, globose to flask shaped, ostiolate; with distinctive elongate, hairlike hyphae arising from exterior. Asci clavate, dissolving upon maturity. Eight ascospores of *C. globosum* per ascus, lemon shaped, one celled, brown. Fig. 9a and b. Compare to *Coniothyrium, Lasiodiplodia, Phoma*. (32, 49, 129)
Cladophialophora	Colonies slow to moderate in growth rate, velvety, olivaceous gray to black; growth on cycloheximide; gelatin hydrolysis negative (rarely weak). Hyphae and conidia pale to mid brown; conidial scars not markedly dark; conidia one celled. *C. carrionii* with short, lateral or terminal conidiophores bearing infrequently branched, long chains of conidia that tend to not disarticulate completely; conidia ca. 5 μm long, elliptical, bilaterally symmetrical, mainly uniform in size and shape; growth up to 37°C. Fig. 3a. *C. bantiana* conidiophores hyphalike, poorly differentiated, pale brown. Conidia occurring in very long, sparsely branched chains that are poorly differentiated from conidiophore and vegetative hyphae. *C. bantiana* now includes isolates previously classified as *Xylohypha emmonsii*. Isolates of *C. bantiana* from cerebral lesions exhibit growth at 40°C; some isolates (those previously classified as *X. emmonsii*) limited to subcutaneous infection do not grow above 37°C. Conidia of *C. bantiana* measure 2 to 2.5 by 4 to 7 μm. Fig. 2c and d. Compare to *Cladosporium*. (26, 47, 49, 78, 91, 125)
Cladosporium	Colonies rapidly growing, velvety or cottony, olive-gray to olive-brown or black. Conidiophores dark, erect, long, often septate and branching. Conidia one celled (several celled in some species), smooth or rough, with dark prominent hila, occurring in long, fragile, profusely branched acropetal chains. Conidia at branch points of chains are usually shield shaped. Usually no growth at 37°C; gelatin hydrolysis usually positive. Fig. 3b and c. Compare to *Fonsecaea, Cladophialophora*. (26, 37, 38, 47, 49, 76, 129)
Coniothyrium	Colonies of *C. fuckelii* moderate in growth rate, floccose, hyaline becoming mid to dark brown. Pycnidia globose, averaging 200 to 300 μm, brown, three to five cell layers thick, unilocular, with ostiole. Conidia one celled, ellipsoidal, guttulate, smooth, brown at maturity, 1.5 to 2.5 by 3 to 4.5 μm. Phialides ampulliform, 4 to 6 by 3 to 4.5 μm. Distinguished from *Phoma* by brown conidia. Fig. 9c and d. Compare to *Chaetomium, Phoma, Pleurophoma, Pleurophomopsis*. (60, 121)
Curvularia	Colonies rapidly growing, woolly, gray to grayish black or brown. Conidiophores dark, erect, geniculate owing to sympodial development. Conidia multiseptate, usually curved, with central cell larger and darker than end cells; thickness of septa and outer cell wall approximately the same; hilum dark. Fig. 1b. Compare to *Alternaria, Bipolaris, Drechslera, Exserohilum*. (26, 37, 38, 49, 76)
Dactylaria	Colonies flat, olivaceous-gray to brown, usually with Bordeaux red-diffusible pigment on Emmons modified Sabouraud glucose agar. Conidiophores hyaline, erect, occasionally geniculate owing to sympodial development. Conidia two celled, cylindrical to oblong, dark, released by rhexolytic dehiscence. One-celled, globose, phialoconidia may be present in young colonies. *D. constricta* var. *gallopava* grows at 45°C; inhibited on media containing cycloheximide; gelatin positive in >21 days; pathogenic for humans and fowl. *D. constricta* var. *constricta* does not grow at 45°C; grows on media containing cycloheximide; rapidly gelatin positive; not known to be pathogenic. Fig. 2a. Compare to *Scolecobasidium*. (26, 29, 49, 104)

(*Continued on next page*)

TABLE 1 Diagnostic features of selected medically important dematiaceous fungi (*Continued*)

Genus	Diagnostic characteristics
Exophiala	Colonies usually yeastlike when young (from presence of *Phaeoannellomyces* synanamorph), becoming mouldlike with age, pale brown to black. Conidiophores hyaline to subhyaline, hyphalike or distinct. Conidiogenous cells annellides. Conidia one celled (three celled in *E. salmonis*), hyaline to pale brown, accumulating in balls at apices of the annellides. *E. castellanii* is characterized by poorly differentiated conidiogenous cells having inconspicuous annellations; no growth at 40°C. *E. jeanselmei* annellides tapering to a narrow apex; grows up to ca. 37°C, no growth at 40°C; assimilates KNO_3. Two varieties of *E. jeanselmei* exist: *E. jeanselmei* var. *jeanselmei* bears well-developed, erect, lageniform to cylindrical annellides; *E. jeanselmei* var. *lecanii-corni* bears annellations arising directly from hyphae. *E. moniliae* exhibits swollen annellides terminating in a very long annellated apex; assimilates KNO_3. *E. spinifera* forms distinct spinelike, multicellular conidiophores bearing annellides that are lageniform to cylindrical, tapering to a long, annellated apex; assimilates KNO_3. Fig. 5a to g. Compare to *Phaeoannellomyces*, *Phaeococcomyces*, *Rhinocladiella*, *Wangiella*. (26, 25, 28, 39, 55, 73–76, 87)
Exserohilum	Colonies rapidly growing, woolly, gray to black. Conidiophores dark, erect, geniculate owing to sympodial development. Conidia multiseptate, cylindrical to oblong, dark, with strongly protruding hila. Fig. 1d. Compare to *Bipolaris*, *Drechslera*, *Helminthosporium*. (3, 26, 49, 80, 93)
Fonsecaea	Colonies slow growing, velvety, olivaceous black. Conidiophores pale to mid brown, usually erect, apically swollen owing to compact sympodial development. Conidia one celled, pale to mid brown; primary conidia functioning as sympodial conidiogenous cells to produce secondary conidia. Tertiary conidia form similarly. *Cladosporium*, *Phialophora*, or *Rhinocladiella* synanamorphs may be present. *F. compacta* is differentiated from *F. pedrosoi* by conidia that are subglobose, broadly attached, and arranged in compact conidial heads. Both species grow at 37°C. Fig. 3d. Compare to *Cladosporium*, *Rhinocladiella*. (26, 76, 81)
Hormonema	Colonies smooth, moist; yellow, white, cream, light pink, or light brown, finally becoming black from development of arthroconidia. Conidiogenous cells undifferentiated from hyphae; intercalary, terminal, or arising as short lateral branches. Conidia hyaline, smooth, ellipsoidal, variable in shape and size; one celled, often producing secondary blastoconidia. Large, dark, one-to-two-celled, thick-walled arthroconidia (i.e., a *Scytalidium* anamorph) usually present. Differs from *Aureobasidium* spp. by conidia arising successively. Differs from *Phaeococcomyces* spp. by the lack of dematiaceous yeast cells. Fig. 4b. Compare to *Aureobasidium*, *Scytalidium*. (25, 37, 38, 49)
Lasiodiplodia	Colonies rapidly growing, cottony with abundant aerial mycelium, gray to black. Pycnidia variable in shape, large, up to 5,000 μm wide, five to seven layers thick, stromatic with ostiole, sometimes setose, forming within 1 to 3 weeks. Conidia initially one celled, elliptical and hyaline; mature conidia two celled, dark brown, and longitudinally striate, 20 to 30 by 10 to 15 μm. Annellides cylindrical and hyaline, sometimes branched. Fig. 10a to c. Compare to *Coniothyrium*, *Nattrassia*, *Phoma*. (49, 96)
Lecythophora	Colonies of moderate growth rate, waxy to slimy, pink to salmon or reddish, often with a central brown area in isolates that form chlamydoconidia. Phialides intercalary, cylindrical to lageniform; often with distinct collarette, periclinal wall thickenings, tip greater than 1.2 μm in diameter, tip conically tapering. Conidia one celled, smooth-walled, hyaline, cylindrical to allantoid, accumulating in slimy balls. Fig. 7a and b. Compare to *Acremonium*, *Hyphozyma*, *Phialemonium*, *Phialophora*. (44, 49, 61)
Nattrassia	Colonies of *N. magniferae* rapidly growing; hyaline initially, becoming brownish black. The *S. dimidiatum* synanamorph almost always present. Pycnidia develop within 1 to 2 months, are variable in shape, several layers thick and up to 500 μm wide, stromatic, and ostiolate. Conidia initially hyaline, one celled; mature conidia two to three celled and centrally dark colored, 12 to 13 by 4.5 to 5 μm. Phialides are lageniform and hyaline. Fig. 10d and e. Compare to *Coniothyrium*, *Lasiodiplodia*, *Phoma*. (57, 122)
Phaeoacremonium	Colonies moderate in growth rate, initially cream, with dark brown patches developing, eventually entirely brown. *P. parasiticum* produces phialides of variable length, some isolates forming extremely long phialides swollen near their bases, with prominent cell wall encrustations; conidia elliptical to cylindrical, often curved. This species was previously classified as *Phialophora parasitica*. Compare to *Phialophora*, *Acremonium*, *Sporothrix*. (21, 26, 42)
Phaeoannellomyces	Colonies mucoid, slow-growing, smooth, yeastlike, pale brown to black. Yeast cells are annellides, one celled in *P. elegans*, subhyaline to pale brown; pseudohyphae may be formed; hyphae and conidiophores absent but may be produced by associated synanamorphs. *P. elegans* usually occurs as a synanamorph associated with *Exophiala* spp. *P. werneckii* differs by having large two-celled (and one-celled) yeast annellides, with prominent accumulation of broad annellations (scars). Fig. 4e and f. Compare to *Exophiala*, *Phaeococcomyces*, *Wangiella*. (75, 82)
Phaeococcomyces	Colonies mucoid, slow-growing, smooth, yeastlike, pale brown to black. Yeasts one celled, subhyaline to pale brown, formed as multilateral holoblastic conidia; annelloconidia are not formed. Pseudohyphae may be formed; hyphae and conidiophores absent but may be produced by associated synanamorphs. Often produce synanamorphs when grown on cornmeal agar or potato dextrose agar. *P. exophialae* usually occurs as a synanamorph associated with *Wangiella dermatitidis*. Fig. 4d. Compare to *Exophiala*, *Phaeoannellomyces*, *Wangiella*. (22, 25, 82)

(*Continued on next page*)

TABLE 1 (*Continued*)

Genus	Diagnostic characteristics
Phialemonium	Colonies moderate in growth rate, flat, moist, white, becoming yellowish, with a yellow-green diffusing pigment for *P. obovatum*. Conidiophores hyaline, hyphalike. Intercalary and distinct phialides without obvious collarettes arising from hyphae at the agar surface or occasionally from short aerial hyphae. Conidia one celled, hyaline, smooth-walled, aggregated into slimy balls, obovate to allantoid. In contrast to *Lecythophora* spp., the conidiiferous pegs arising from the hyphae are cylindrical, often 1 μm or less in diameter at the tip. Fig. 7c. Compare to *Acremonium, Hyphozyma, Lecythophora, Phialophora*. (44, 61)
Phialophora	Colonies moderate in growth rate, cottony to velvety, olive-gray to black. Conidiophores (if present) usually short, pale brown. Conidiogenous cells phialides with distinct collarettes. Conidia one celled, hyaline to pale brown, accumulating as balls at the apices of the phialides. *P. repens* produces intercalary phialides without basal septa, or phialides cylindrical to slightly lageniform with a delicate collarette; phialides rarely in branched clusters; conidia cylindric, curved. *P. richardsiae* produces phialides of variable size and shape; some phialides long with flaring, flattened, saucer-shaped collarettes; conidia of two shapes (globose conidia from phialides with flattened, saucer-shaped collarettes; cylindrical, often curved conidia from phialides of varying length with inconspicuous collarettes). *P. verrucosa* produces flask-shaped phialides with cup-shaped, dark, often deep, collarettes; conidia elliptical. The species previously classified as *P. parasitica* is reclassified as *Phaeoacremonium parasiticum*. Fig. 6. Compare to *Lecythophora, Phialemonium*. (26, 28, 37, 38, 44, 49, 50, 129)
Phoma	Colonies slow growing, dark gray to olive-brown. Pycnidia globose, subglobose, or pyriform; brown to black; superficial or immersed; ostiolate. Conidia hyaline, one celled, ovoid to cylindrical, arising from phialides. Fig. 9e and f. Compare to *Coniothyrium, Nattrassia, Pyrenochaeta, Pleurophoma, Pleurophomopsis*. (32, 33, 89, 121)
Rhinocladiella	Colonies moderate in growth rate, velvety, olive-black. Conidiophores pale to mid brown, erect, sympodial, usually bearing distinct crowded scars. Conidia one celled, fusiform to obovate, pale brown, with a flat basal scar. Conidia occur along the conidiophore. *R. atrovirens* can exhibit a *Phaeoannellomyces elegans* synanamorph. Fig. 2b. Compare to *Exophiala, Fonsecaea, Ramichloridium, Sporothrix*. (37, 38, 110)
Scedosporium	Colonies very rapidly growing, cottony, smoky-gray to dark brown. Conidiophores hyaline, short or long. Predominant conidiogenous cells are hyaline annellides with or without swollen bases; characterized by prominent bulging annellations. Conidia one celled, obovate, truncate, subhyaline to light black, single or in balls. *S. prolificans* differs from *S. apiospermum* by having conidiogenous cells with prominent swollen bases; and by most isolates failing to grow on media containing cycloheximide. Fig. 8a and b. Compare to *Pseudallescheria, Scopulariopsis*. (35, 67, 79, 106)
Scytalidium	Colonies rapidly growing, woolly, hyaline initially, becoming gray to brownish black (colonies of *S. hyalinum* remain hyaline). Hyphae form chains of one- to two-celled arthroconidia that are hyaline or pale brown to brown, subglobose to ellipsoidal. May occur as synanamorph with *Aureobasidium* spp., *Hormonema* spp., and *Nattrassia mangiferae*. Some mycologists consider *S. lignicola* to be a synonym of *S. dimidiatum*; others consider *S. lignicola* to be distinct on the basis of its production of hyaline arthroconidia only, in conjunction with brown chlamydospores, while *S. dimidiatum* produces only dark arthroconidia. Fig. 4c. Compare to *Aureobasidium, Hormonema*. (76, 114, 117, 122, 129)
Sporothrix	Colonies of typical clinical isolates of *S. schenckii* initially cream, smooth, moist, yeastlike; gradually turning brown in irregular patches; becoming velvety to lanose as aerial hyphae develop. Conidiophores elongate, compactly sympodial, with swollen apex; bearing one-celled, hyaline, elliptical to obovate conidia in a rosette fashion. Dissimilar conidia arise directly from the vegetative hyphae and are dematiaceous, thick-walled, oval (rarely triangular), one celled. Grows as a yeast at 37°C. Fig. 7d to g. Compare to *Rhinocladiella, Phaeoacremonium*. (23, 30, 76, 115)
Wangiella	Colonies slow-growing, initially yeastlike (from presence of *Phaeococcomyces* synanamorph), smooth, viscous, pale brown to black, becoming filamentous to velvety. Conidiophores hyphalike, subhyaline to pale brown. Conidiogenous cells phialides without distinct collarettes, intercalary or lateral from hyphae. Phialides cylindrical with rounded apices. Conidia one celled, subglobose to elliptical or obovoid, subhyaline to pale brown, accumulating in balls or slipping down the conidiogenous cells. Annellidic synanamorph (*Exophiala*) often present. Grows at 40°C; does not assimilate KNO_3. Fig. 5h and i. Compare to *Exophiala, Phaeoannellomyces, Phaeococcomyces, Phialophora*. (39, 73, 90, 118)

boydii (see Fig. 8d). Finally, the term "holomorph" is used to encompass the whole fungus, inclusive of all of its forms. In this example, the whole fungus (holomorph) consists of the *P. boydii* teleomorph and the *Scedosporium* and *Graphium* synanamorphs. Because sexual structures are considered to be taxonomically more significant than asexual structures, the classification of a fungus must be based upon its teleomorph when the latter is known. As a result, the name used for the teleomorph is also used for the holomorph. Problems may arise in certain anamorph-teleomorph connections when a teleomorph is known to have more than one anamorph or when a single anamorph is associated with several different teleomorphs. For example, *S. apiospermum* is one anamorph that is produced by several species of the teleomorphic genera *Pseudallescheria* and *Petriella*. For that reason, it would be incorrect to use the name *P. boydii* for an isolate of *S. apiospermum* that failed to develop the *P. boydii* teleomorph in culture. In the clinical laboratory, a given isolate should be named according to the morph(s) actually present. Laboratorians are cautioned that as they strive for mycologic accuracy, they must ensure that laboratory reports are completely clear regarding the possible clinical significance of an isolate if a new or less familiar name is used.

Several dematiaceous pathogens have no known teleomorph but do have multiple synanamorphs. Because each of the synanamorphs of a pleomorphic fungus may be referred to by a separate name, the identification process for such fungi can be confusing. A widely accepted approach to this problem is to base the name of an isolate upon the single anamorph that is judged to be the most distinctive, conspicuous, and stable. An accompanying synanamorph may then be referred to, if needed, by a genus-level name. In the case of the pleomorphic pathogen *Fonsecaea pedrosoi* (see Fig. 3d), for example, the synanamorph upon which the identification is based is a compactly sympodial conidiophore which apically produces a series of conidia that in turn give rise to a second series of conidia; similarly, a third series may be formed. This form is the *F. pedrosoi* synanamorph. In addition, a *Rhinocladiella* (sympodial) synanamorph, a *Phialophora* (phialide) synanamorph, and a *Cladosporium* synanamorph may be seen, but these are not essential to the identification of an isolate as *F. pedrosoi* (81).

The black yeast-like fungi form one group whose members are at times extremely difficult and frustrating to identify. The genera *Phaeococcomyces* and *Phaeoannellomyces* were established (22, 25, 82) to accommodate synanamorphs that exhibit dematiaceous budding yeasts, and occasional short pseudohyphae or toruloid hyphal elements. Black yeasts usually constitute one synanamorph of pleomorphic fungi. They are recognized by their brown or black, usually mucoid, yeast-like colonies. One of the most frequently isolated black yeasts in the clinical laboratory is the *Phaeoannellomyces* synanamorph associated with *Exophiala jeanselmei*. When the yeastlike isolates of this fungus are transferred from initial isolation media to potato dextrose agar or cornmeal agar, hyphae and the typical conidiogenous cells and conidia of *E. jeanselmei* rapidly become evident. The assumption that a black yeast, regardless of whether the colony is initially dematiaceous, should be identified as *Aureobasidium pullulans* is incorrect.

Sterile isolates represent a second group of medically important fungi that are especially difficult to identify. They commonly are referred to as members of the form-order Mycelia Sterilia. Some of these fungi cause phaeohyphomycosis and mycetoma. When sterile dematiaceous fungi are isolated, the induction of conidia or fruiting bodies should be attempted as previously discussed. The cultures should be kept for several weeks before being discarded. With time, some of these fungi may develop, either in the agar or at the colony surface, structures such as ascocarps, pycnidia, or synnemata, which produce spores or conidia. When fruiting bodies (structures within which propagules are formed) are present, the first step is to determine whether they are ascocarps (sexual reproduction) or pycnidia (asexual reproduction). Ascomycetes, such as *Chaetomium* and *Leptosphaeria* spp., are recognized by the presence of ascocarps within which asci and ascospores are formed (asci often dissolve at maturity and may be visible only in immature ascocarps). If the fruiting bodies are pycnidial, they contain conidia rather than ascospores, and the isolate is then likely to be a member of the sphaeropsidales. Several agents of phaeohyphomycosis, such as *Coniothyrium fuckelii*, *Lasiodiplodia theobromae*, *Phoma* spp., *Pleurophoma* spp., and *Pleurophomopsis* spp., are pycnidial.

Alternaria spp.

Species of *Alternaria* (Fig. 1a) have been documented in phaeohyphomycotic infections of bone, cutaneous tissue, ears, eyes, paranasal sinuses, and the urinary tract (128, 131). An *Alternaria* sp. and *Alternaria alternata* (synonym, *A. tenuis*) are the only well-documented human pathogens in this genus. The *Alternaria* anamorph of *Pleospora infectoria* has been reported to be a pathogen of humans but has not been documented convincingly. *Alternaria* isolates are difficult to identify beyond the genus level. If an isolate must be identified to species, it should be sent to a specialist.

Aureobasidium spp.

A. pullulans (Fig. 4a) has been implicated as an agent of phaeohyphomycosis in humans and other animals, having been isolated from cultures of nail, skin, peritoneal fluid, spleen, and subcutaneous tissue (15, 18, 43, 51, 99, 105). *Aureobasidium* species are often confused with *Hormonema* species. In *Hormonema* species, conidia arise in a basipetal succession from either hyaline or dematiaceous, hyphalike conidiogenous cells (Fig. 4b). In contrast, *A. pullulans* produces conidia in a synchronous manner (25). Because several authors have illustrated *Hormonema* spp. under the name *Aureobasidium*, it may be that some cases of infection ascribed to *A. pullulans* were actually caused by misidentified isolates of *Hormonema* spp.

Bipolaris spp.

Several species of *Bipolaris* (Fig. 1c), including *B. australiensis*, *B. hawaiiensis*, and *B. spicifera*, have caused meningitis, paranasal sinusitis, subcutaneous, eye, and pulmonary infections (80). At least one species of *Drechslera*, *D. biseptata*, has been shown to be an opportunistic pathogen (130). Species of *Drechslera*, *Exserohilum*, and *Helminthosporium* frequently had been confused in the past with *Bipolaris* species, but subsequent taxonomic studies (3, 80) established useful criteria for separating species of these genera.

Chaetomium spp.

Chaetomium species (Fig. 9a and b) have been associated with infections of the blood, lungs, brain, skin, and nails in both healthy and immunocompromised patients (6, 119, 136). Colonization of bone marrow transplant patients has also been reported. In some cases, *C. globosum* and *C. strumarium* were specifically identified. When species identification is needed, isolates should be sent to a reference laboratory.

Cladophialophora spp.

The genus *Cladophialophora* Borelli (1980) has been reintroduced and redefined to accommodate the transfer of certain species previously classified in other genera, including *Cladosporium* and *Xylohypha* (24). The more notable species in *Cladophialophora* are *C. carrionii* (formerly *Cladosporium carrionii*) and *C. bantiana* (formerly known under the now synonymous binomials of *Cladosporium bantianum*, *Xylohypha bantiana*, *Cladosporium trichoides*, and *Xylohypha emmonsii*). These phylogenetic relationships were inferred on the basis of results of partial sequencing of large-subunit rRNA (69). *C. bantiana* (Fig. 2c and d) is a neurotropic mould that has caused dozens of cases of cerebral phaeohyphomycosis (31) and may also be involved in cutaneous and subcutaneous infections (56, 91). Since there is evidence suggesting that the organism can gain entrance via a pulmonary route, isolates should be handled with extreme care in a biological safety cabinet. *C. carrionii* (Fig. 3a) is a leading

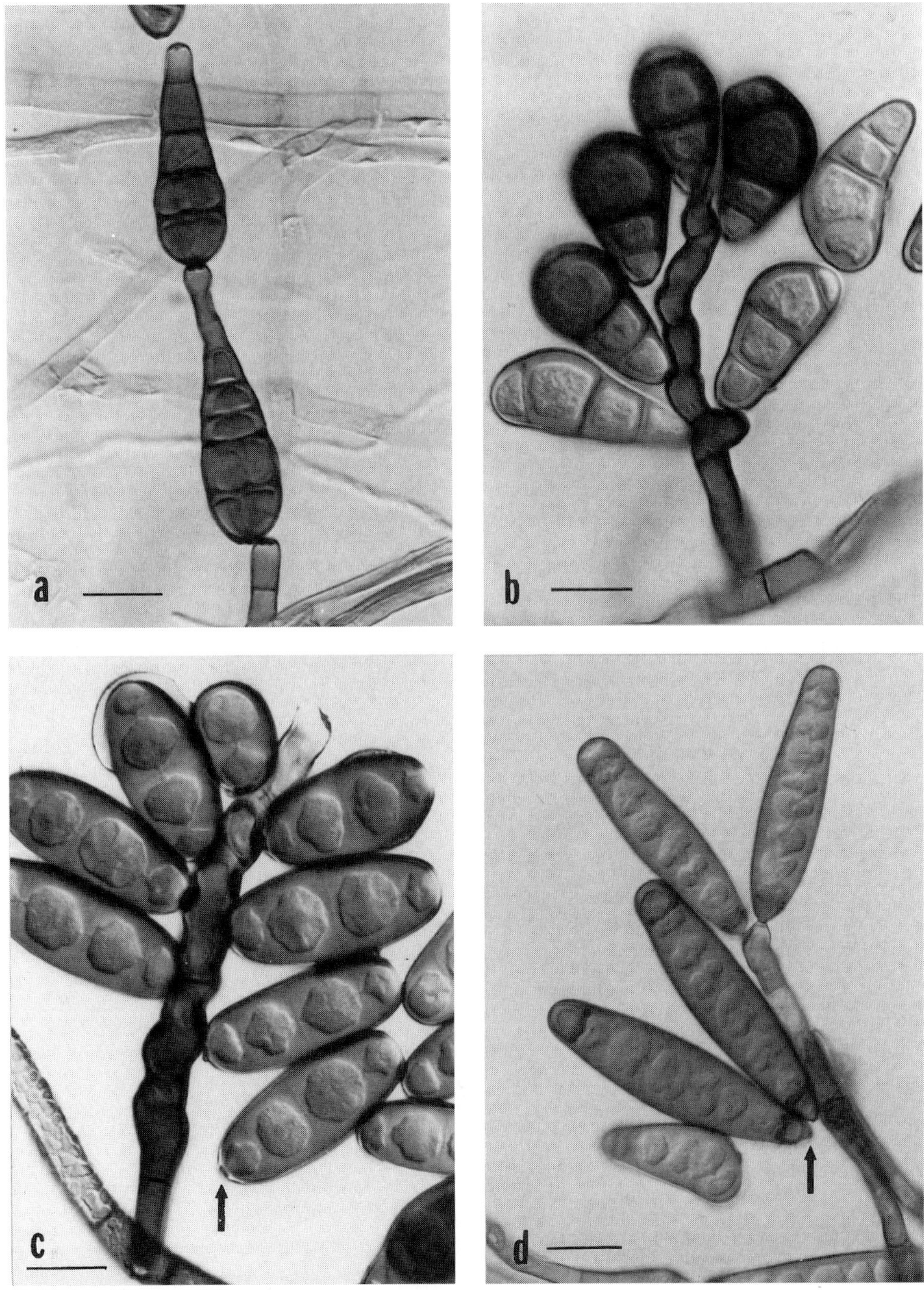

FIGURE 1 (a) *Alternaria* spp. Muriform conidia with tapering apices (beaks) arise in chains from the conidiophore. (b) *Curvularia* spp. Curved conidia develop from a geniculate conidiophore. (c) *Bipolaris spicifera*. The hilum (arrow) of each conidium protrudes only slightly. (d) *Exserohilum rostratum*. Each conidium has a strongly protruding hilum (arrow). Bars, ca. 10 μm.

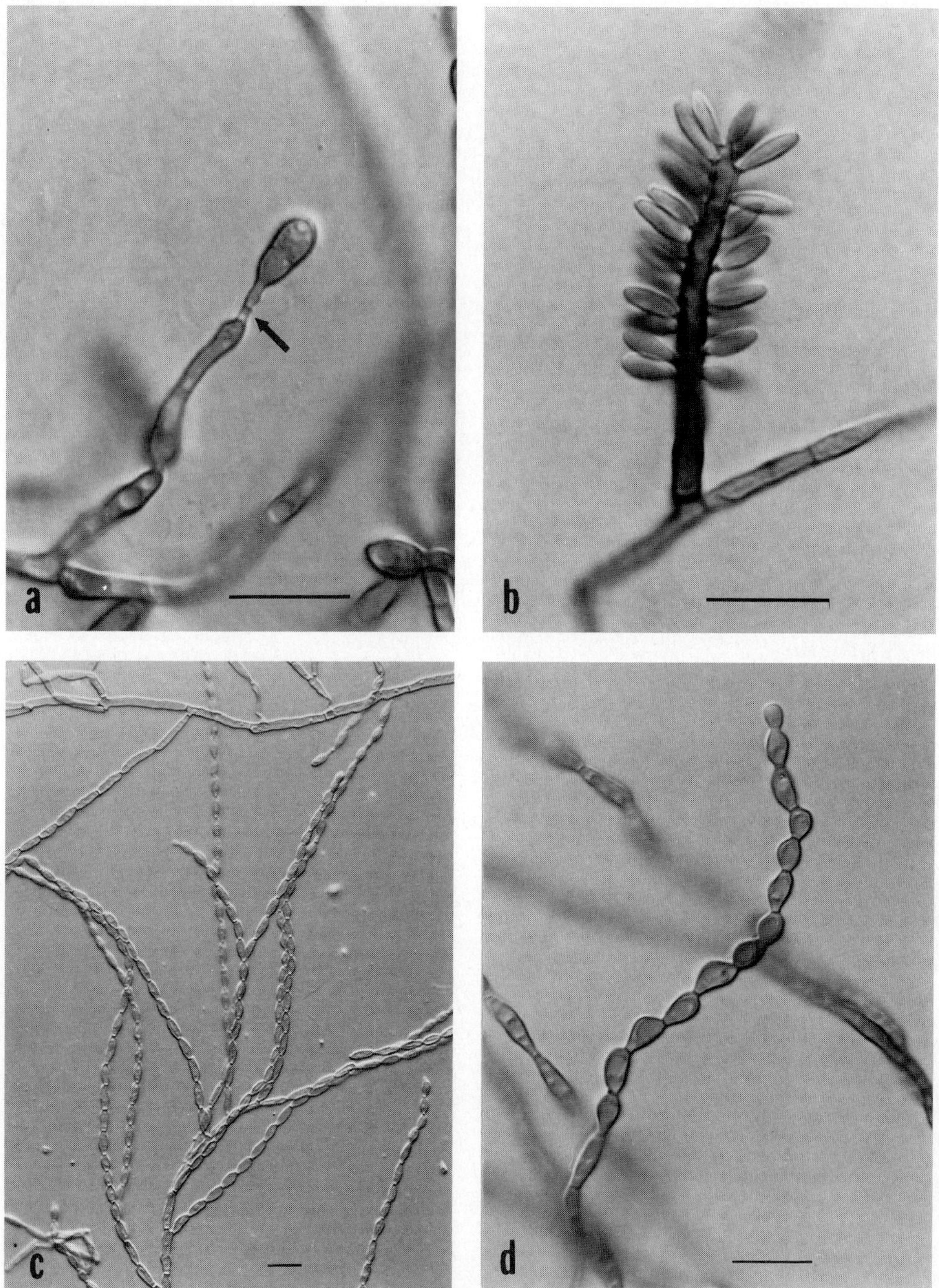

FIGURE 2 (a) *Dactylaria constricta.* A two-celled conidium is attached to the conidiophore by a narrow denticle (arrow). (b) *Rhinocladiella aquaspersa.* Numerous one-celled conidia arise from elongated sympodial conidiophores. (c and d) *Cladophialophora bantiana.* Long, sparsely branching chains of blastoconidia arise from poorly differentiated hyphae. Bars, ca. 10 μm.

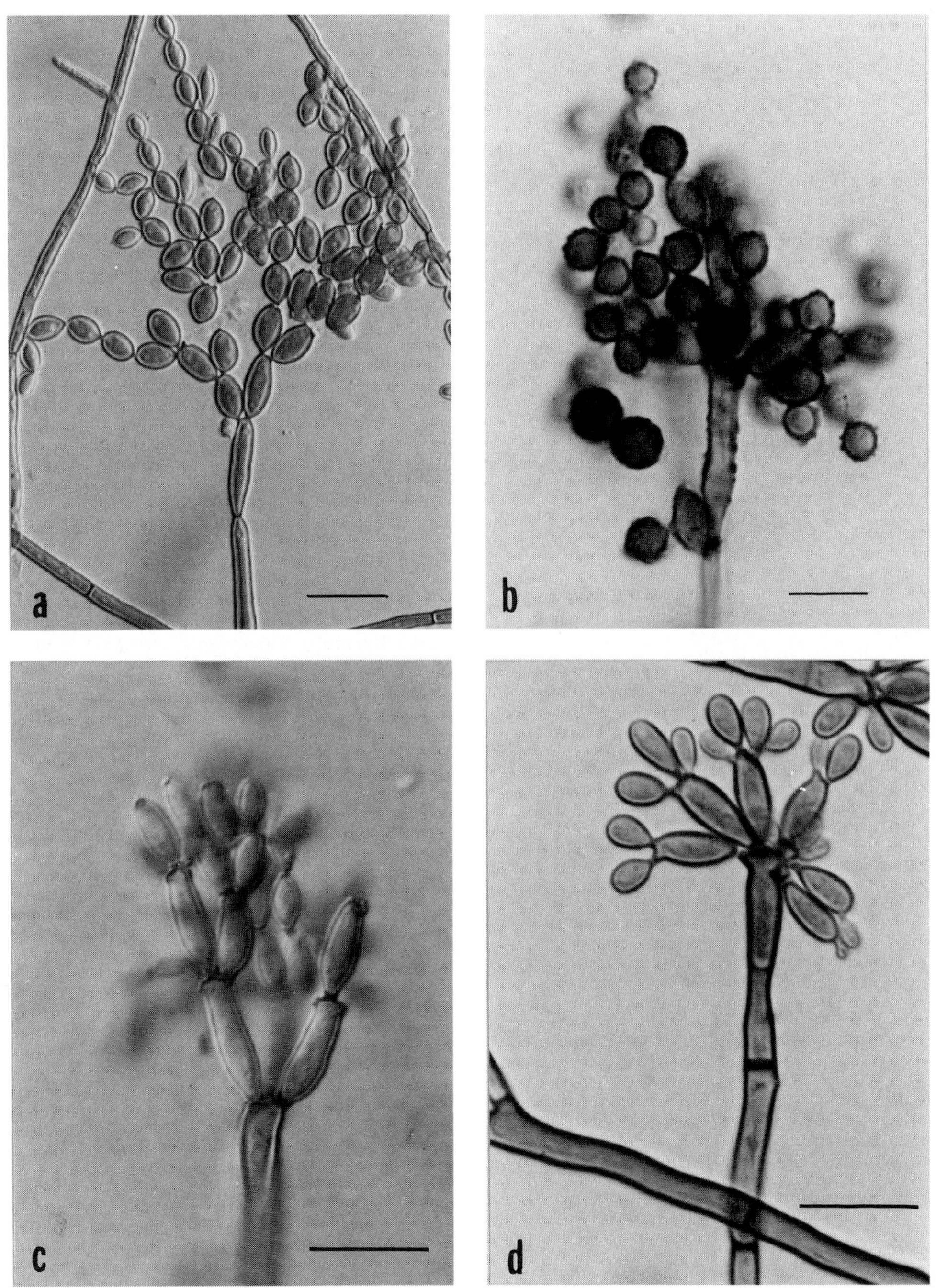

FIGURE 3 (a) *Cladophialophora carrionii*. Sparsely branched long chains of blastoconidia develop from an erect conidiophore. (b) *Cladosporium sphaerospermum*. Conidia are mostly spherical to subglobose and in very fragile, highly branched chains. (c) *Cladosporium cladosporioides*. Smooth conidia show prominent hila (scars) and are in highly branched fragile chains; shield-shaped cells are numerous. (d) *Fonsecaea pedrosoi*. Two to four series of conidia arise at the apex of a sympodial conidiophore. Bars, ca. 10 μm.

agent of chromoblastomycosis in Africa, Australia, and Madagascar (40, 109).

Cladosporium spp.

Cladosporium species have been found in cutaneous, subcutaneous, and eye infections (49, 66, 108). Species of *Cladosporium*, especially *C. cladosporioides* and *C. sphaerospermum* (Fig. 3b and c), are among the most common dematiaceous mould contaminants in the clinical laboratory.

Coniothyrium spp.

C. fuckelii (Fig. 9c and d) has been recovered from a healthy host with cutaneous phaeohyphomycosis (111), a leukemic patient with liver infection (60), and a heart transplant patient with cutaneous infection. This species is very similar to *Microsphaeropsis olivacea*; taxonomic problems between these taxa need to be addressed.

Curvularia spp.

As a group, *Curvularia* species (Fig. 1b) are leading agents of fungal sinusitis and keratitis and may cause endocarditis, mycetoma, pulmonary infection, and subcutaneous phaeohyphomycosis as well (101, 135). *C. geniculata*, *C. lunata*, *C. pallescens*, *C. senegalensis*, and *C. verruculosa* have been specifically identified from infections. Work by Ellis (37, 38) should be consulted if a *Curvularia* isolate must be identified to species.

Dactylaria spp.

D. constricta var. *gallopava* (Fig. 2a) has been documented as an etiologic agent of disseminated infections in immunocompromised humans as well as the cause of epizootic encephalitis in flocks of turkeys and chickens (62, 68, 113). This name was proposed (29) as a new combination for the two previously described dematiaceous hyphomycetes *D. gallopava* and *Scolecobasidium constrictum*. The two varieties of *D. constricta* are differentiated on the basis of physiologic characteristics and pathogenicity in experimental animals (104). Some workers have suggested recognizing the two varieties as distinct species as well as placing them in the genera *Ochroconis* and *Scolecobasidium*.

Exophiala spp.

E. jeanselmei (Fig. 5a to c) is a leading etiologic agent of subcutaneous phaeohyphomycosis and has also caused mycetoma and peritonitis (120). *Exophiala moniliae* (Fig. 5f) and *E. spinifera* (Fig. 5d and e) also have been reported as agents of phaeohyphomycosis (9, 71). *E. werneckii* has been renamed *Phaeoannellomyces werneckii* (82) and is discussed under the genus *Phaeoannellomyces*. The colony morphology of *Exophiala* species is varied. Most isolates initially grow in a yeast form (*Phaeoannellomyces* synanamorph), which is succeeded by a hyphal *Exophiala* synanamorph. As a result, colonies are moist and yeastlike at first, becoming velvety to woolly with age. Some isolates that are predominantly the *Phaeoannellomyces* synanamorph of *E. jeanselmei* may remain yeastlike. Conidiophores of *Exophiala* spp. are dematiaceous, simple or hyphalike. The conidia are one-celled in most species and accumulate in balls at the apices of the annellides. With careful study using the oil immersion objective, annellations (rings) usually can be seen at the apices of the annellides.

Exserohilum spp.

Phaeohyphomycosis of skin, subcutaneous tissue, and nasal sinuses caused by species of *Exserohilum* has been documented (7, 53, 80, 88). *Exserohilum* (Fig. 1d) contains three recognized opportunistic pathogens: *E. longirostratum*, *E. mcginnisii*, and *E. rostratum*. Members of the genus *Exserohilum* have been confused previously with species of *Bipolaris*, *Drechslera*, and *Helminthosporium*, but taxonomic studies have clarified the distinctions (3, 80).

Fonsecaea spp.

F. compacta and *F. pedrosoi* are the only species in the genus, and both can cause chromoblastomycosis. *F. pedrosoi* is the leading agent worldwide, while *F. compacta* is extremely rare. *F. pedrosoi* also can cause phaeohyphomycosis (41, 77, 84). *Fonsecaea* isolates are pleomorphic. They are characterized by the development of one-celled primary conidia that form on erect, dark, compactly sympodial conidiophores. These primary conidia in turn become conidiogenous cells and form secondary one-celled conidia. This process usually results in only two or three levels of conidia (in contrast to *Cladosporium* spp.), and constitutes the distinctive morphology of the genus (Fig. 3d). A second kind of conidial development results in structures similar to the form seen in the genus *Rhinocladiella* and is referred to as a *Rhinocladiella* synanamorph (incorrectly called *Acrotheca*-like). Yet another synanamorph may be observed in which the conidia occur as branching chains, similar to those found in the genus *Cladosporium* (a *Cladosporium* synanamorph). *Fonsecaea* spp. also may produce phialides with collarettes bearing balls of one-celled conidia that are typical of the genus *Phialophora* (a *Phialophora* synanamorph). Because of this pleomorphic nature, earlier studies of *F. pedrosoi* and *F. compacta* had placed these species in the genera *Phialophora* and *Rhinocladiella*.

Lasiodiplodia theobromae

L. theobromae (syn. *Botryodiplodia theobromae*) (Fig. 10a to c), is a well-documented cause of keratitis following injury to the cornea (98, 108). Rare cases of subcutaneous infection have also been reported (70).

Lecythophora spp.

L. hoffmannii (Fig. 7a and b) and *L. mutabilis* have been found in patients with subcutaneous phaeohyphomycosis, endocarditis, and peritonitis (100). The genus *Lecythophora* was reintroduced for two species that previously had been described in the genus *Phialophora*. *Lecythophora* differs from *Phialophora* in part by the frequent lack of a septum at the base of the phialide. The microscopic morphology of *Lecythophora* spp. can be very similar to that of *Phialemonium* spp. *Lecythophora* differs from *Phialemonium* in part by forming colonies that are pink to salmon or reddish when young. *L. hoffmannii* and *L. mutabilis* are distinguished from each other by the absence and presence of brown chlamydoconidia, respectively. Detailed descriptions (44, 61) should be consulted for the identification of isolates, and the use of a reference laboratory is recommended.

Nattrassia mangiferae

N. mangiferae (Fig. 10d and e) is a pycnidial fungus, previously known as *Hendersonula toruloidea*, that can cause phaeohyphomycosis of the skin and nails (116). The associated synanamorph *Scytalidium dimidiatum* is the form that is first isolated in the clinical laboratory, and if a special medium such as sterile banana slices is used, the *N. mangiferae* anamorph sometimes forms after incubation for 2 months.

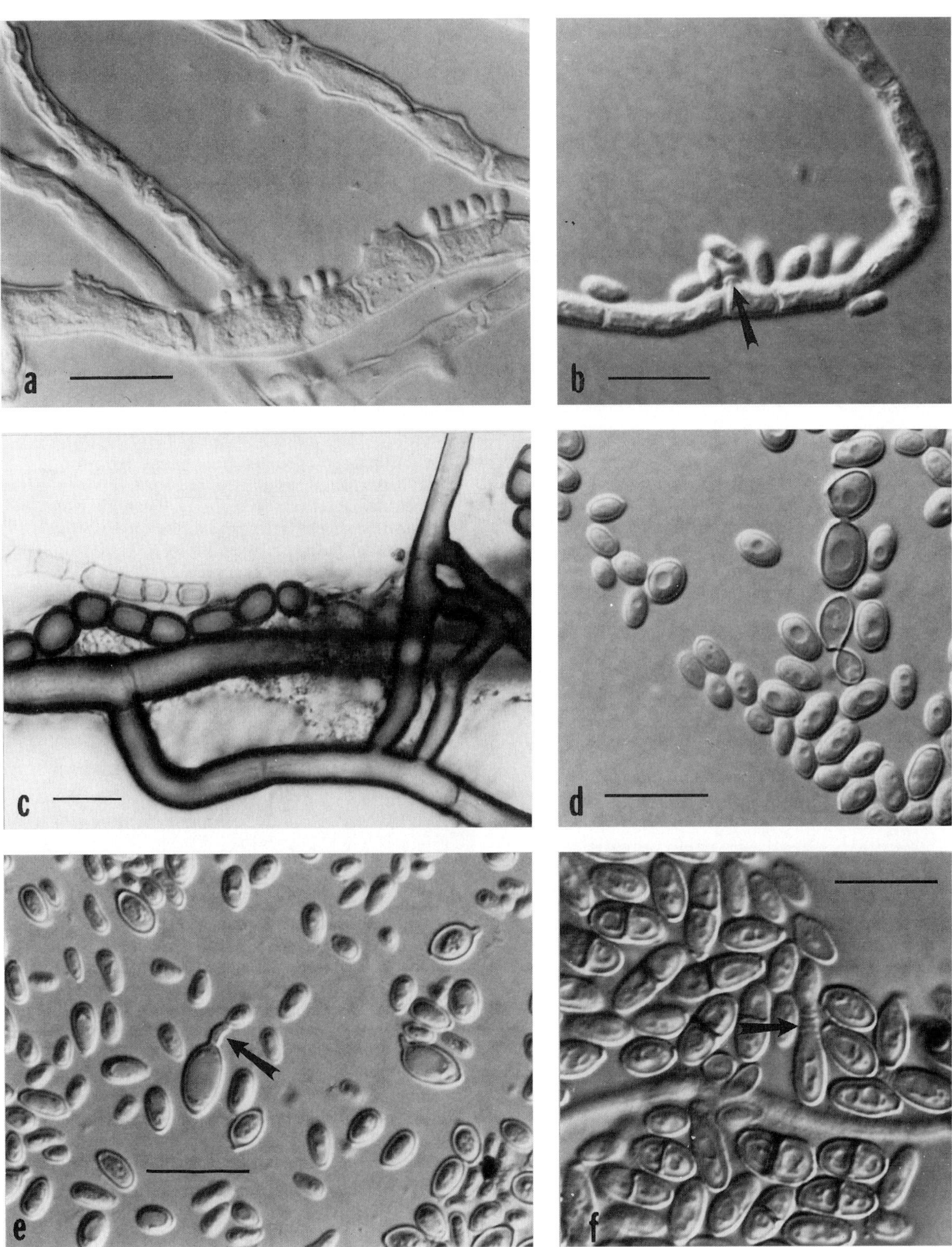

FIGURE 4 (a) *Aureobasidium pullulans.* Conidia develop in a synchronous manner, each from its own locus. (b) *Hormonema* sp. Conidia develop in a sequential manner from a single locus (arrow). (c) *Scytalidium dimidiatum.* Conidial chains consist of one- or two-celled arthroconidia. (d) *Phaeococcomyces* sp. Blastoconidia arise singly from various sites along the cell wall. (e) *Phaeoannellomyces elegans.* Yeasts are one-celled annellides with long, narrow zones of annellations (arrow). (f) *Phaeoannellomyces werneckii.* Yeasts are one- to two-celled annellides with broad, prominent annellations (arrow). Bars, ca. 10 μm.

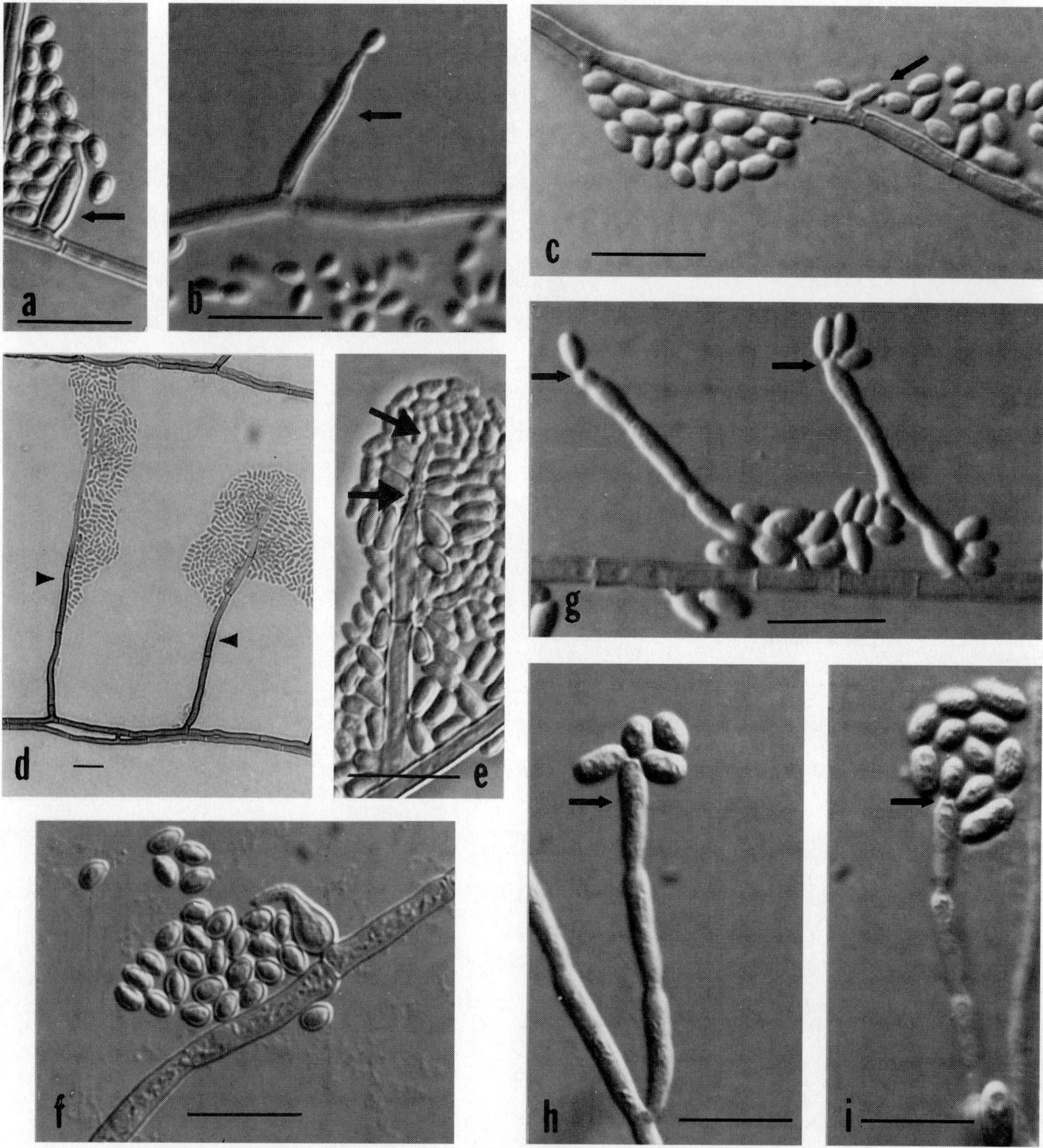

FIGURE 5 (a and b) *Exophiala jeanselmei* var. *jeanselmei*. Annellides (arrows) are well developed and lageniform to cylindrical. (c) *Exophiala jeanselmei* var. *lecanii-corni*. Annellations (arrow) arise directly from hyphae. (d and e) *Exophiala spinifera*. Conidiophores (arrows) are multicellular and spine-like, the annellated region of annellides (arrows) becomes very long. (f) *Exophiala moniliae*. Annellides are swollen at the base. (g) *Exophiala castellanii*. Annellides have inconspicuous annellations (arrows). (h and i) *Wangiella dermatitidis*. One-celled conidia arise from phialides (arrows) that lack collarettes. Bars, ca. 10 μm.

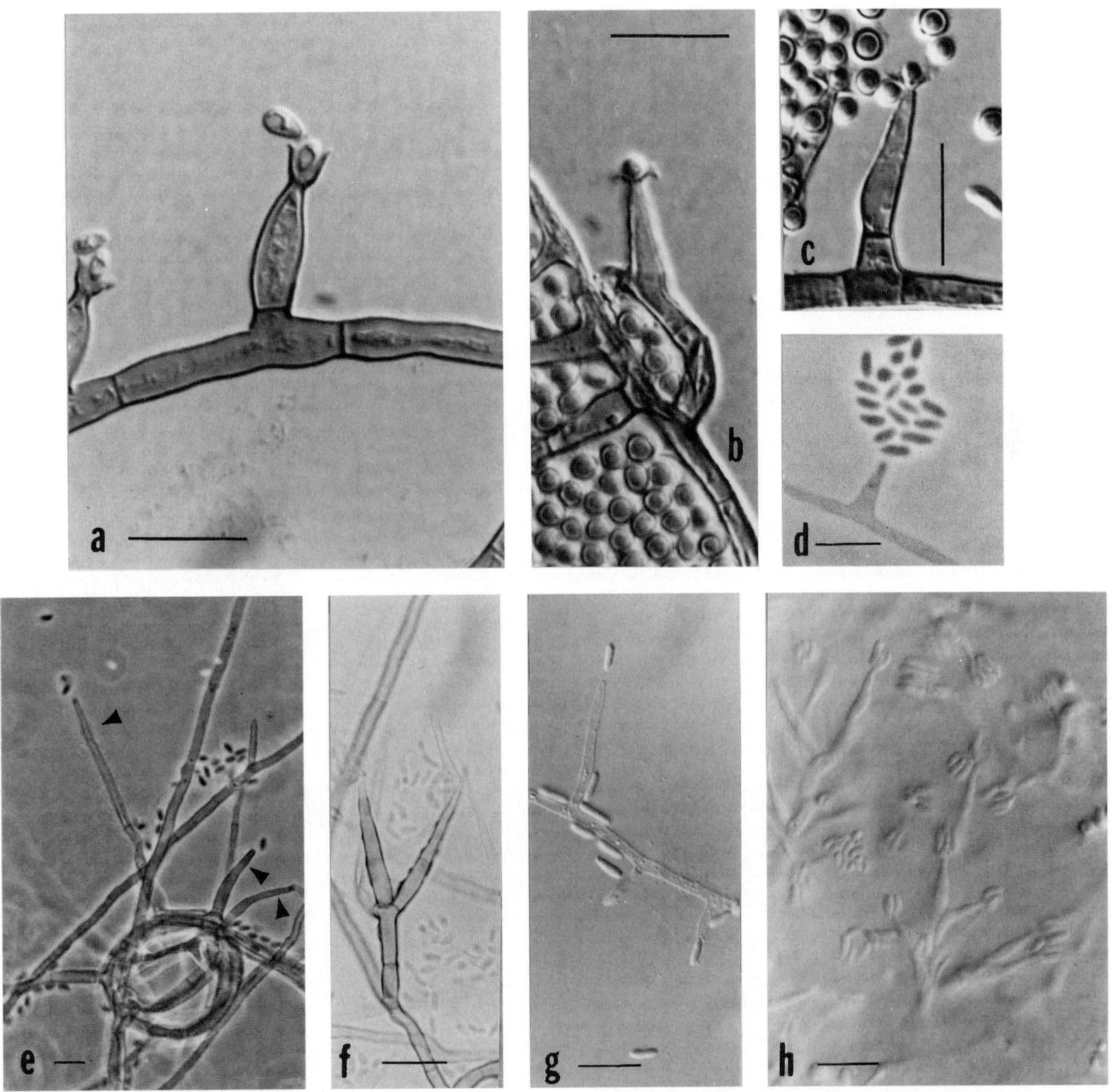

FIGURE 6 (a) *Phialophora verrucosa*. A deep cup-shaped collarette at the apex of the phialide is characteristic. (b and c) *Phialophora richardsiae*. The species is characterized by phialides with flattened collarettes bearing spherical conidia. (d) *Phialophora richardsiae*. Other phialides have inconspicuous collarettes and form cylindrical conidia. (e and f) *Phaeoacremonium parasiticum* (formerly *Phialophora parasitica*). Phialides (arrows) are short to extremely long, sometimes with dark encrustations of the cell wall. Collarettes are inconspicuous, not flaring; conidia are curved to cylindrical. (g and h) *Phialophora repens*. Phialides vary in length, are lageniform to cylindrical, are sometimes sinuous, and rarely occur in branched clusters. Collarettes are subtle to absent. Conidia are cylindrical and often curved. Bars, ca. 10 μm.

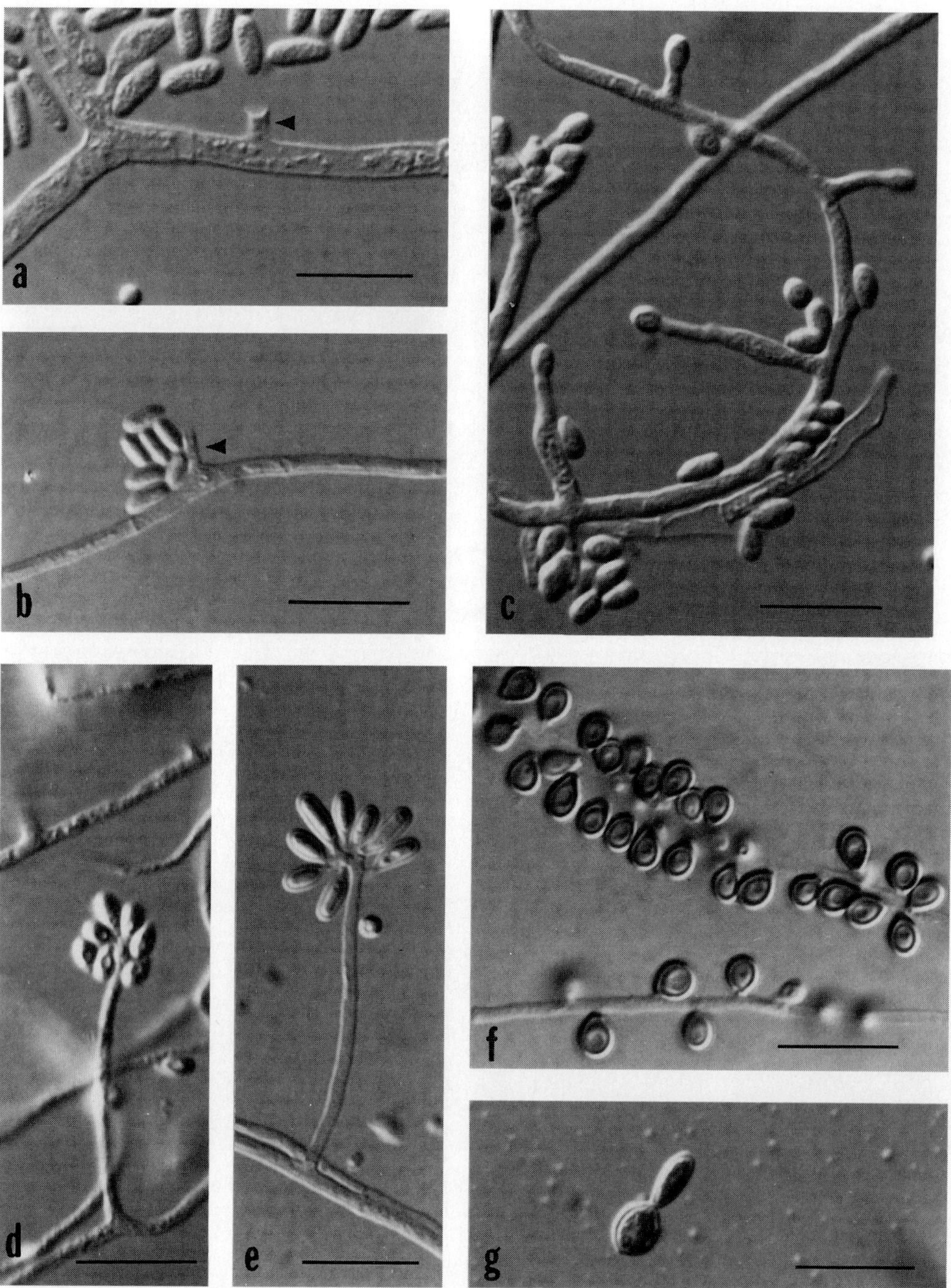

FIGURE 7 (a and b) *Lecythophora hoffmannii*. Phialides (arrows) are very short, often conically tapering, and with collarettes; the basal septum usually is absent. (c) *Phialemonium* species. Phialides are cylindrical to lageniform and without collarettes. (d to g) *Sporothrix schenckii*. Solitary conidia on denticles arise from sympodial conidiophores (d and e). Thick-walled dematiaceous conidia arise along vegetative hyphae (f). Yeast synanamorph (g). Bars, ca. 10 μm.

Phaeoannellomyces spp.

P. werneckii (syn. *Cladosporium werneckii*, *Exophiala werneckii*) and *P. elegans* are known agents of phaeohyphomycosis (2, 41, 77). The genus *Phaeoannellomyces* was created to accommodate black yeasts that are characterized by the development of yeast cells that function as annellides (82). *P. werneckii* is classified in the blastomycete genus *Phaeoannellomyces* because the two-celled yeast anamorph is stable, distinctive, unique in appearance, and well represented in isolates of the species. *Phaeoannellomyces elegans* (Fig. 4e), which is a synanamorph associated with *E. jeanselmei*, is distinguished from *P. werneckii* (Fig. 4f) by its formation of one-celled annellated yeast cells.

Phaeococcomyces spp.

The genus *Phaeococcomyces* (Fig. 4d) contains black yeasts that form holoblastic conidia from various points on the parent cell (multilateral), in contrast to the annellidic process seen in *Phaeoannellomyces* spp. Most clinical isolates are *Phaeococcomyces exophialae*, which usually give rise gradually to the accompanying hyphomycete synanamorph *Wangiella dermatitidis*. *Phaeococcomyces*, which was originally named *Phaeococcus* (22, 25), contains additional species that are distinguished from each other primarily by morphologic criteria.

Phialemonium spp.

The genus *Phialemonium* contains three species, two of which (*P. curvatum* and *P. obovatum*) are known to cause phaeohyphomycosis. Reported cases involve subcutaneous cysts, disseminated infection, endocarditis, and peritonitis (44, 61, 112). The microscopic morphology of *Phialemonium* (Fig. 7c) is morphologically intermediate between those of the genera *Acremonium* and *Phialophora* and is very similar to that of the genus *Lecythophora*. Colonies are white, with some strains having a diffusible yellow-green pigment or a faint vinaceous hue. Detailed descriptions (44, 61) should be consulted for the identification of isolates, and the use of a reference laboratory is recommended.

Phialophora spp.

P. verrucosa (Fig. 6a) is a leading cause of chromoblastomycosis in North America, second only to *Fonsecaea pedrosoi*. It is also an etiologic agent of phaeohyphomycosis, as are *P. bubakii*, *P. repens* (Fig. 6g and h), and *P. richardsiae* (Fig. 6b to d) (50, 95). Other reported infections include endocarditis, keratitis, osteomyelitis, atypical eumycetoma, and opportunistic infections in AIDS patients (34, 126, 127). Two additional agents of phaeohyphomycosis that were previously described as *Phialophora* species have been transferred to the genus *Lecythophora* (*L. hoffmannii* and *L. mutabilis*) (44). This reclassification was necessary because the phialides, collarettes, and hyphae of these fungi are hyaline and because the phialides are short and intercalary with conically tapering tips which exhibit periclinal wall thickenings and which exceed 1.2 μm in diameter. *Phialophora parasitica* (Fig. 6e and f), an agent of phaeohyphomycosis (42, 52), has been reclassified as *Phaeoacremonium parasiticum* (21).

Phoma spp.

P. eupyrena, *P. minutella*, *P. minutispora*, *P. oculo-hominis*, *P. sorghina*, and several *Phoma* isolates (Fig. 9e and f) which were not identified to species have been documented as etiologic agents of phaeohyphomycotic infections involving cutaneous and subcutaneous tissues, lungs, corneas, and sinuses (8, 97, 138), as well as the agents of hypersensitivity pneumonitis. Because species identification of members of this genus is extremely difficult, isolates should be referred to reference laboratories if detailed identification is needed.

Rhinocladiella spp.

R. aquaspersa (Fig. 2b), previously known as *Acrotheca aquaspersa*, has only rarely been reported as causing chromoblastomycosis; these cases were from Brazil and Mexico (110). *R. atrovirens* has caused cerebral phaeophyphomycosis in an AIDS patient (27), and similar infections (14) have been attributed to *Ramichloridium mackenziei* (a dematiaceous hyphomycete that is very similar in appearance to *R. obovoideum* and which may eventually be proven to be congeneric with *Rhinocladiella*). In addition to the sympodial anamorph that characterizes the genus *Rhinocladiella*, an annellidic anamorph (as seen in *Exophiala* spp.) and a phialidic anamorph (as seen in *Wangiella* spp.) may be present.

Scedosporium spp.

S. apiospermum (Fig. 8a), previously known as *Monosporium apiospermum*, is an anamorph of *Pseudallescheria boydii* (a fungus once classified as *Petriellidium boydii* and *Allescheria boydii*) (Fig. 8d) (79). Several species of ascomycetes in addition to *Pseudallescheria boydii* may produce an *S. apiospermum* anamorph. Historically, this fungus has been known as the main cause of fungal mycetoma in North America, but in developed countries it is now seen more often as an agent of phaeohyphomycosis, infecting paranasal sinuses, eyes, joints, subcutaneous tissue, lungs, and brain (11, 20, 45, 54, 63, 124). In such cases, it grows in the form of hyphae that look like those produced by *Aspergillus* and *Fusarium* spp. *S. prolificans* (syn. *S. inflatum*) (Fig. 8b) is an opportunistic pathogen that has been isolated numerous times from bone and soft tissue infections (67, 132, 133), as well as from cutaneous infection and fungemia (12, 46). The fungus may disseminate from the initial site of inoculation to visceral organs in immunocompromised individuals (4, 85, 94). The conidiogenous cells of *S. prolificans* may appear to proliferate sympodially; this, however, is an artifact (35).

Scytalidium spp.

S. dimidiatum (Fig. 4c), a synanamorph of the pycnidial fungus *Nattrassia mangiferae*, is a documented pathogen of nails and skin (36, 65, 83) and rarely of subcutaneous tissue (102, 116). *S. hyalinum* similarly causes nail and skin infections and has caused subcutaneous infection as well (137). *S. hyalinum* is not a dematiaceous species but has been classified in the genus *Scytalidium*. A recent study suggests that *S. hyalinum* may be a melanin-lacking mutant that is conspecific with *Nattrassia mangiferae* (103). *S. lignicola* has been reported to be a cause of phaeohyphomycosis; its taxonomy, however, is contested. Some mycologists consider *S. lignicola* to be a synonym of *S. dimidiatum* (122). Others consider the two to be distinct species but point out that infections previously attributed to *S. lignicola* were instead caused by misidentified isolates of *S. dimidiatum* (57). In either case, it is agreed that only *S. hyalinum* and *S. dimidiatum* are known to be pathogenic. Several descriptions should be consulted for the identification of *Scytalidium* spp. (26, 114, 122).

Sporothrix spp.

The etiologic agent of sporotrichosis was originally described as *S. schenckii* but later was erroneously transferred

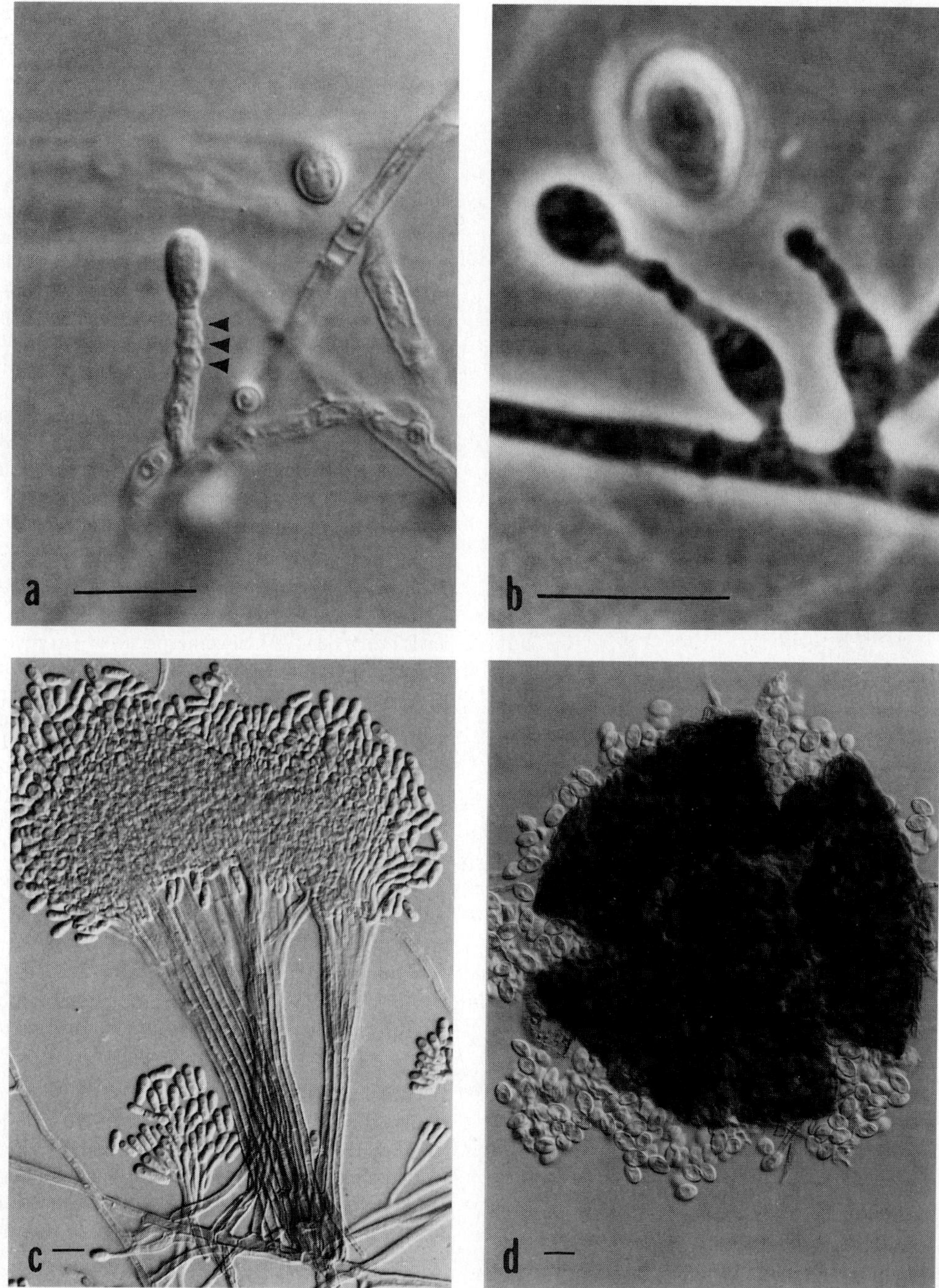

FIGURE 8 (a) *Scedosporium apiospermum.* Annellides are characterized by accentuated annellations (arrows). (b) *Scedosporium prolificans.* Annellides are characterized by swollen bases. (c) *Graphium* species. Conidiophores consist of fused hyphae bearing terminal annellides. (d) *Pseudallescheria boydii.* The globose ascocarp ruptures to release football-shaped (ellipsoidal) ascospores. Bars, ca. 10 μm.

to the genus *Sporotrichum*. *Sporotrichum* species are basidiomycetous fungi that are neither dimorphic nor pathogenic for humans or other animals. Of the more than one dozen species of *Sporothrix* described, only *S. schenckii* (Fig. 7d to g) is a proven pathogen. *S. cyanescens*, distinctive for its purple-blue diffusible pigment, can be recovered from clinical specimens, but animal studies have not shown it to be pathogenic (23, 115, 123). To identify an isolate as *S. schenckii*, one must demonstrate that it undergoes dimorphism, i.e., that the mould can be transformed into a stable yeast at elevated temperature. To do so, the isolate must be subcultured on an enriched medium such as brain-heart infusion agar, chocolate agar, or brain-heart infusion broth containing 0.1% agar and grown under 5% CO_2 at 35 to 37°C. Occasional isolates can be difficult to convert and may require multiple subcultures and extended incubation. In some

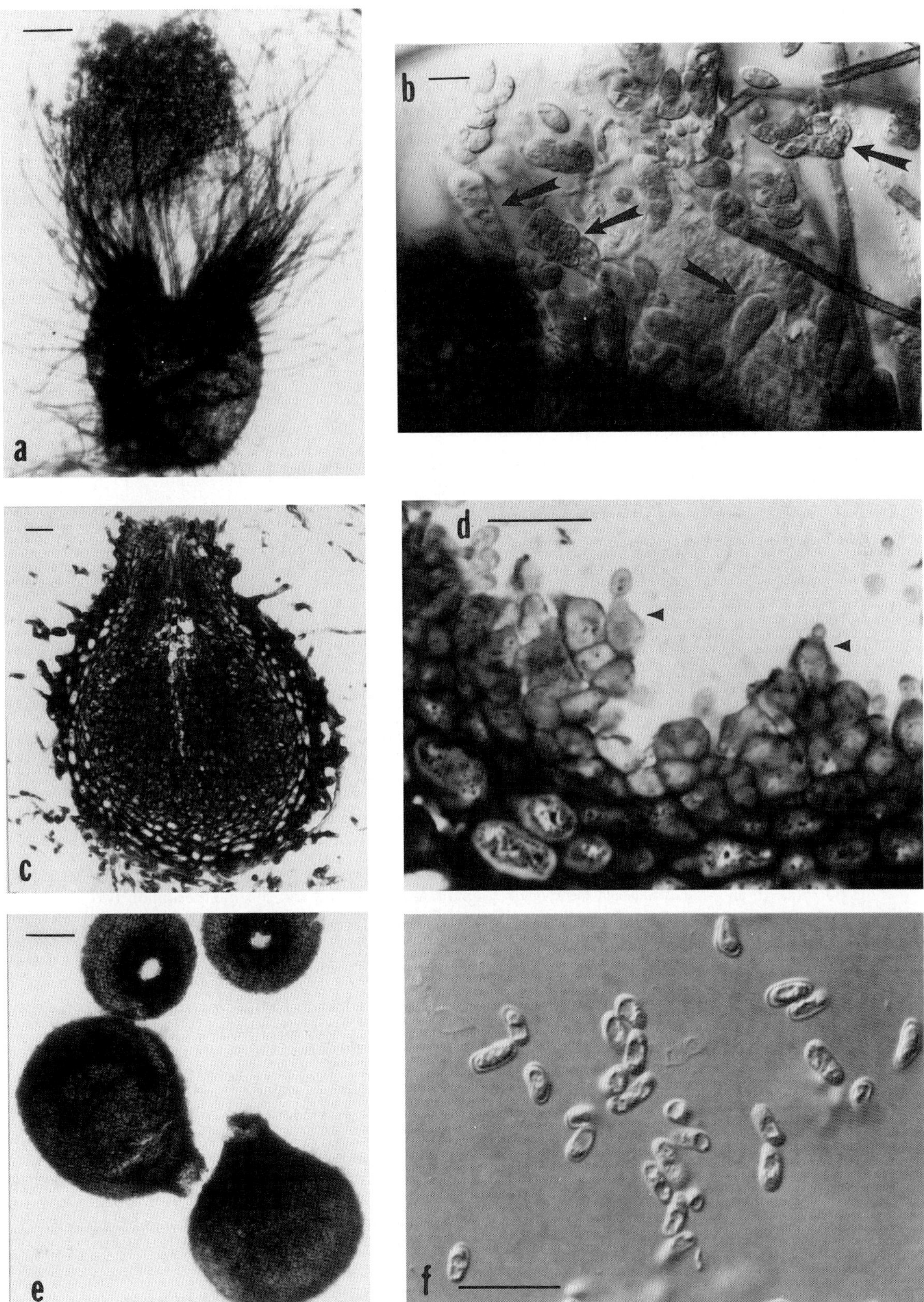

FIGURE 9 (a) *Chaetomium globosum*. Ascocarps are characterized by flexous, upwardly oriented hairlike hyphae. Bar, ca. 50 μm. (b) *Chaetomium globosum*. Lemon-shaped, dark ascospores form within asci (arrows). Bar, ca. 10 μm. (c) *Coniothyrium fuckelii* vertical section. Bar, ca. 10 μm. The pycnidium is globose and ostiolate. (d) *Coniothyrium fuckelii*. Phialides (arrows) give rise to conidia that are brown at maturity. Bar, ca. 10 μm. (e) *Phoma* species. Pycnidia are subglobose and ostiolate. Bar, ca. 50 μm. (f) *Phoma* species. One-celled phialoconidia are hyaline. Bar, ca. 10 μm.

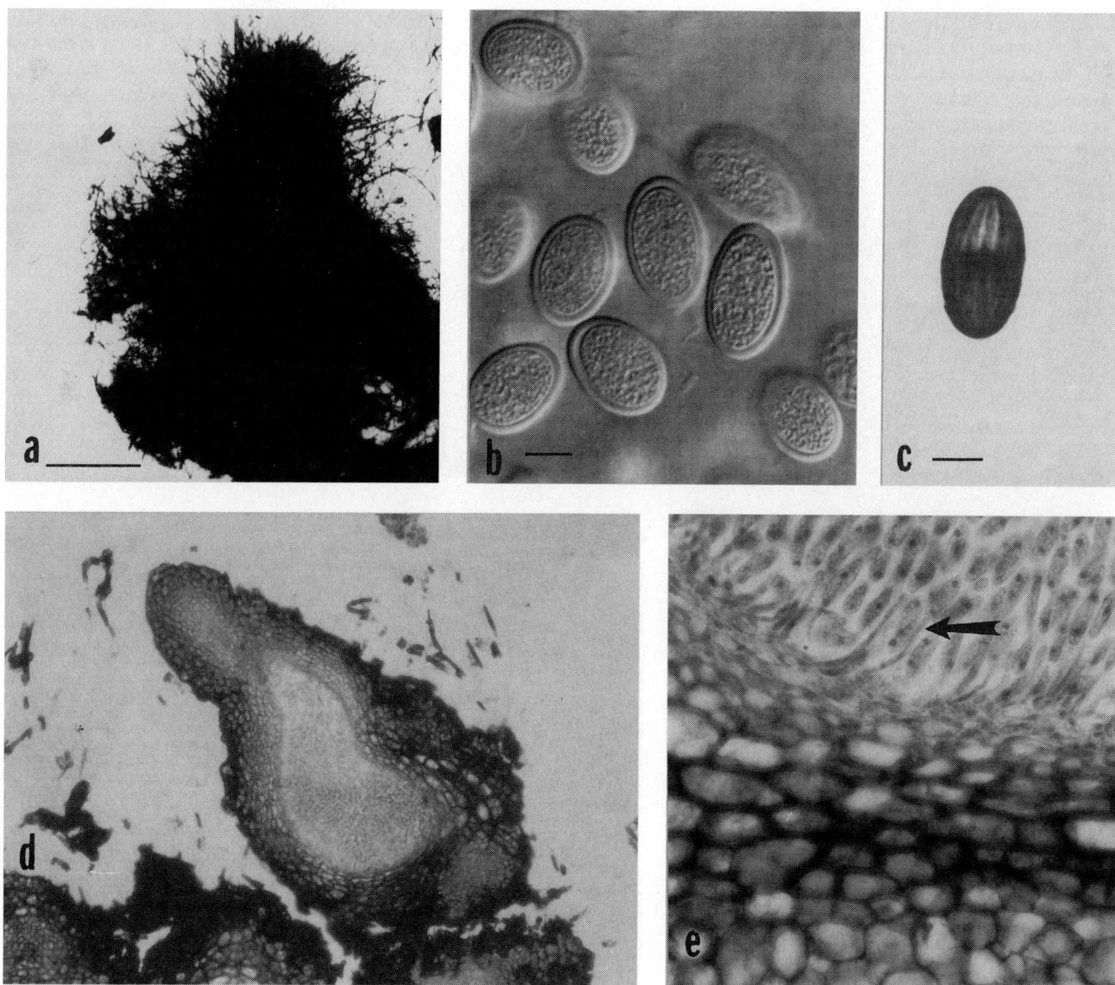

FIGURE 10 (a) *Lasiodiplodia theobromae*. Pycnidia are ostiolate and typically pyriform. Bar, ca. 300 μm. (b and c) *Lasiodiplodia theobromae*. Conidia are one celled and hyaline, becoming two celled, dark, and striate at maturity. Bar, ca. 10 μm. (d and e) *Nattrassia mangiferae* vertical sections. Pycnidia are variably shaped. Conidia arise from phialides (arrow).

isolates, conversion may be limited to small portions of the colony. Environmental as well as clinical isolates of *S. schenckii* will form the yeast phase when grown on appropriate media at 37°C. Isolates of *Sporothrix* sp. which were recovered from environmental sources such as sphagnum moss and which lacked the dematiaceous thick-walled conidia (Fig. 7f) have been shown to be avirulent in mice (30). Although an ascomycete teleomorph has been connected to environmental isolates of *Sporothrix* sp., no teleomorph has been found for isolates of *S. schenckii* recovered from infections of humans.

Wangiella spp.

W. dermatitidis (Fig. 5h and i) is an agent of phaeohyphomycosis that typically causes infections of cutaneous and subcutaneous tissue. Infections of the eye, brain, and joints have also been documented (1, 72, 134). Isolates are found in sputum and stool specimens but are considered to be clinically insignificant. *W. dermatitidis* is pleomorphic in that most isolates initially grow in a yeast form (*Phaeococcomyces* synanamorph) with development of toruloid hyphae, which is succeeded by the hyphal *W. dermatitidis* synanamorph. In addition to the typical phialides, some conidiogenous cells possess a group of slightly raised, truncate protrusions at their apices that occur as a result of polyblastic development. Furthermore, annellides of the kind seen in *Exophiala* also are produced rarely. This occasional presence of annellides has led some mycologists to propose a recombination as *E. dermatitidis*. However, the genus *Wangiella* was created because the phialides without collarettes which are the predominant and distinctive feature of *W. dermatitidis* could not be accommodated in any existing genus (73). Results from partial sequencing of large-subunit rRNA have not yet resolved this question (69).

SEROLOGIC AND MOLECULAR BIOLOGY-BASED TESTS

There are few serologically based tests applicable to the dematiaceous fungi. A latex agglutination test is commercially available (Immuno-Mycologics Inc., Norman, Okla.) for detecting antibodies to *Sporothrix schenckii*, but despite one study (13) that reported the sensitivity and specificity to be 90 to 94% and 95 to 100%, respectively, the test has not been used widely. The remaining serologic tests consist of fluorescent-antibody conjugates for differential staining of histologic sections (58) and the exoantigen test for identification of cultures (59, 93). None of these reagents are commercially available; they are available only at certain reference laboratories (e.g., Centers for Disease Control and Prevention, Atlanta, Ga.). Investigation into the molecular identification of dematiaceous fungi is under way but is currently limited to taxonomic research; no commercial applications are available.

ANTIBIOTIC SUSCEPTIBILITIES

Antifungal susceptibility testing of dematiaceous fungi can be performed in the research setting by various methods, but it is not widely conducted in clinical laboratories because a standard method for these fungi has not been established. Collaborative susceptibility studies of opportunistic moulds are under way, however, and standardized testing eventually may become available. Sporotrichosis can be treated effectively with orally administered itraconazole or terbinafine, and many infections will respond to potassium iodide or fluconazole. Infections with other dematiaceous fungi, however, have historically been difficult to manage. Surgical excision, when feasible, has been the most consistently effective treatment option, but the newer antifungal compounds itraconazole and terbinafine have been effective in many cases and now have become drugs of choice. Voriconazole also appears to be promising for infections caused by dematiaceous fungi.

EVALUATION, INTERPRETATION, AND REPORTING OF RESULTS

Determining whether a particular dematiaceous fungus is involved in a disease process can be difficult at times because most of these fungi are occasionally recovered from clinical specimens as contaminants. Documentation of a dematiaceous fungus as the etiologic agent of a mycotic infection includes sound evidence that an infection exists, that the suspected etiologic agent is seen in clinical specimens, that the morphology of the fungus in the clinical specimens is compatible with the suspected etiologic agent, and that the recovered fungus is identified properly. The repeated recovery of a suspected etiologic agent, especially from more than one anatomic site, is highly significant. The ability of the suspected etiologic agent to grow on media at 37°C may serve as corroborative evidence of its potential to cause infection. Isolation of a dematiaceous fungus from a normally sterile body site is suspicious and should not be quickly dismissed as contamination, particularly if colonies are numerous or if more than one culture vessel shows growth. If isolated from a nonsterile pulmonary specimen such as sputum or bronchial lavage fluid, a well-documented opportunist from a genus such as *Fonsecaea*, *Cladophialophora*, or *Dactylaria* (not often seen as contaminants) also should be assessed carefully as a possibly significant finding.

More than 100 species of dematiaceous fungi have caused infection in humans, and many of these are relatively rare. However, few clinicians are familiar with the ecology of these fungi and the infections they sometimes cause. For this reason, laboratory reports should include interpretations when possible, and the laboratory director or designee should initiate a discussion of potentially significant findings with physicians. Compilations are available which (as of their publication dates) referenced all known opportunistic fungal pathogens, and these can be valuable aids in interpreting mycology results (26, 49, 76). Infections caused by dematiaceous fungi are being diagnosed increasingly among healthy as well as compromised patients. Concurrently, the expanding diversity of etiology within this group of fungi is becoming apparent. As more is learned about the epidemiology and pathogenicity of these fungi and as our ability to treat these infections improves, it will become increasingly important for the clinical laboratory to provide accurate examinations, identifications, and interpretations to clinicians.

REFERENCES

1. **Ajanee, N., M. Alam, K. Holmberg, and J. Khan.** 1996. Brain abscess caused by *Wangiella dermatitidis*: case report. *Clin. Infect. Dis.* **23:**197–198.
2. **Ajello, L.** 1975. Phaeohyphomycosis: definition and etiology. *Pan Am. Health Org. Sci. Publ.* **304:**126–133.
3. **Alcorn, J. L.** 1983. Generic concepts in *Drechslera, Bipolaris* and *Exserohilum*. *Mycotaxon* **17:**1–86.
4. **Alvarez, M., B. Lopez Ponga, C. Rayon, J. Garcia Gala, M. C. Roson Porto, M. Gonzalez, J. V. Martinez-Suarez, and J. L. Rodriguez-Tudela.** 1995. Nosocomial outbreak caused by *Scedosporium prolificans (inflatum)*: four fatal cases in leukemic patients. *J. Clin. Microbiol.* **33:** 3290–3295.
5. **Amaya Tapia, A., E. Uribe Jimenez, R. Diaz Perez, M. A. Covarrubias Velasco, D. Diaz Santana Bustamante, G. Aguirre Avalos, and A. Rodriguez Toledo.** 1996. Esporotricosis cutanea transmitida por mordedura de tejon. *Med. Cutanea Ibero-Latino-Americana* **24:**87–89.
6. **Anandi, V., T. J. John, A. Walter, J. C. Shastry, M. K. Lalitha, A. A. Padhye, L. Ajello, and F. W. Chandler.** 1989. Cerebral phaeohyphomycosis caused by *Chaetomium globosum* in a renal transplant recipient. *J. Clin. Microbiol.* **27:**2226–2229.
7. **Aquino, V. M., J. M. Norvell, K. Krisher, and M. M. Mustafa.** 1995. Fatal disseminated infection due to *Exserohilum rostratum* in a patient with aplastic anemia: case report and review. *Clin. Infect. Dis.* **20:**176–178.
8. **Baker, J. G., I. F. Salkin, P. Forgacs, J. H. Haines, and M. E. Kemna.** 1987. First report of subcutaneous phaeohyphomycosis of the foot caused by *Phoma minutella*. *J. Clin. Microbiol.* **25:**2395–2397.
9. **Barba-Gomez, J. F., J. Mayorga, M. R. McGinnis, and A. Gonzalez-Mendoza.** 1992. Chromoblastomycosis caused by *Exophiala spinifera*. *J. Am. Acad. Dermatol.* **26:** 367–370.
10. **Barron, G. L.** 1968. *The Genera of Hyphomycetes from Soil.* The Williams & Wilkins Co., Baltimore, Md.
11. **Bart, P. A., G. Greub, A. Cometta, and J. Bille.** 1996. *Scedosporium apiospermum* osteomyelitis in a neutropenic patient. *J. Mycol. Med.* **6:**178–181.
12. **Bouza, E., P. Munoz, L. Vega, M. Rodriguez-Creixems, J. Berenguer, and A. Escudero.** 1996. Clinical resolution of *Scedosporium prolificans* fungemia associated with reversal of neutropenia following administration of granulocyte colony-stimulating factor. *Clin. Infect. Dis.* **23:**192–193.
13. **Bulmer, S. O., L. Kaufman, W. Kaplan, D. W. McLaughlin, and D. E. Kraft.** 1973. Comparative evaluation of five serological methods for the diagnosis of sporotrichosis. *Appl. Microbiol.* **26:**4–8.
14. **Campbell, C. K., and S. S. A. Al-Hedaithy.** 1993. Phaeohyphomycosis of the brain caused by *Ramichloridium mackenziei* sp. nov. in Middle Eastern countries. *J. Med. Vet. Mycol.* **31:**325–332.
15. **Caporale, N. E., L. Calegari, D. Perez, and E. Gezuele.**

1996. Peritoneal catheter colonization and peritonitis with *Aureobasidium pullulans*. *Perit. Dial. Int.* **16:**97–98.

16. **Carmichael, J. W.** 1979. Cross-reference names for pleomorphic fungi, p. 31–41. *In* B. Kendrick (ed.), *The Whole Fungus*. National Museums of Canada, Ottawa, Canada.
17. **Castrejon, O. V., M. Robles, and O. E. Zubieta Arroyo.** 1995. Fatal fungemia due to *Sporothrix schenckii*. *Mycoses* **38:**373–376.
18. **Clark, E. C., S. M. Silver, G. E. Hollick, and M. G. Rinaldi.** 1995. Continuous ambulatory peritoneal dialysis complicated by *Aureobasidium pullulans* peritonitis. *Am. J. Nephrol.* **15:**353–355.
19. **Clay, B. M., and V. K. Anand.** 1996. Sporotrichosis: a nasal obstruction in an infant. *Am. J. Otolaryngol.* **17:** 75–77.
20. **Cremer, G., and P. Boiron.** 1966. Epidemiology and biology of *Scedosporium* species. *J. Mycol. Med.* **6:**165–171.
21. **Crous, P. W., W. Gams, M. J. Wingfield, and P. S. van Wyk.** 1996. *Phaeoacremonium* gen. nov. associated with wilt and decline disease of woody hosts and human infections. *Mycologia* **88:**786–796.
22. **de Hoog, G. S.** 1979. Nomenclatural notes on some black yeast-like hyphomycetes. *Taxonomy* **28:**347–348.
23. **de Hoog, G. S., and G. A. de Vries.** 1973. Two new species of *Sporothrix* and their relations to *Blastobotrys nivea*. *Antonie Leeuwenhoek J. Microbiol. Serol.* **39:** 515–520.
24. **de Hoog, G. S., E. Gueho, F. Masclaux, A. H. Gerrits van den Ende, K. J. Kwon-Chung, and M. R. McGinnis.** 1995. Nutritional physiology and taxonomy of human-pathogenic *Cladosporium-Xylohypha* species. *J. Med. Vet. Mycol.* **33:**339–347.
25. **de Hoog, G. S., and E. J. Hermanides-Nijhof.** 1977. The black yeasts and allied hyphomycetes. *Stud. Mycol.* **15:** 100–173.
26. **de Hoog, G. S., J. Guarro, C. S. Tan, R. G. F. Wintermans, and J. Gene.** 1995. Pathogenic fungi and common opportunists, p. 1–243. *In* G. S. de Hoog and J. Guarro (ed.), *Atlas of Clinical Fungi*. Centraalbureau voor Schimmelcultures, Baarn, The Netherlands.
27. **del Palacio-Hernanz, A., M. K. Moore, C. K. Campbell, A. del Palacio-Perez-Medel, and R. del Castillo-Cantero.** 1989. Infection of the central nervous system by *Rhinocladiella atrovirens* in a patient with acquired immunodeficiency syndrome. *J. Med. Vet. Mycol.* **27:**127–130.
28. **Dixon, D. M., and A. Polak-Wyss.** 1991. The medically important dematiaceous fungi and their identification. *Mycoses* **34:**1–18.
29. **Dixon, D. M., and I. F. Salkin.** 1986. Morphologic and physiologic studies of three dematiaceous pathogens. *J. Clin. Microbiol.* **24:**12–15.
30. **Dixon, D. M., I. F. Salkin, R. A. Duncan, N. J. Hurd, J. H. Haines, M. E. Kemna, and F. B. Coles.** 1991. Isolation and characterization of *Sporothrix schenckii* from clinical and environmental sources associated with the largest U.S. epidemic of sporotrichosis. *J. Clin. Microbiol.* **29:** 1106–1113.
31. **Dixon, D. M., and T. J. Walsh.** 1989. Infections due to *Xylohypha bantiana* (*Cladosporium trichoides*). *Rev. Infect. Dis.* **11:**515–525.
32. **Domsch, K. H., W. Gams, and T. H. Anderson.** 1980. *Compendium of Soil Fungi*, vol. I and II. Academic Press, Inc., New York, N.Y.
33. **Dooley, D. P., M. L. Beckius, B. S. Jeffrey, C. K. McAllister, W. H. Radentz, A. R. Feldman, M. G. Rinaldi, S. R. Bailey, and J. H. Keeling.** 1989. Phaeohyphomycotic cutaneous disease caused by *Pleurophoma* in a cardiac transplant patient. *J. Infect. Dis.* **159:**503–507.
34. **Duggan, J. M., M. D. Wolf, and C. A. Kauffman.** 1995. *Phialophora verrucosa* infection in an AIDS patient. *Mycoses* **38:**215–218.
35. **Dykstra, M. J., I. F. Salkin, and M. R. McGinnis.** 1990. An ultrastructural comparison of conidiogenesis in *Scedosporium apiospermum*, *Scedosporium inflatum*, and *Scopulariopsis brumptii*. *Mycologia* **81:**896–904.
36. **Elewski, B. E.** 1996. Onychomycosis caused by *Scytalidium dimidiatum*. *J. Am. Acad. Dermatol.* **35:**336–338.
37. **Ellis, M. B.** 1971. *Dematiaceous Hyphomycetes*. Commonwealth Mycological Institute, Kew, England.
38. **Ellis, M. B.** 1976. *More Dematiaceous Hyphomycetes*. Commonwealth Mycological Institute, Kew, England.
39. **Espinel-Ingroff, A., P. R. Goldson, M. R. McGinnis, and T. M. Kerkering.** 1988. Evaluation of proteolytic activity to differentiate some dematiaceous fungi. *J. Clin. Microbiol.* **26:**301–307.
40. **Esterre, P., A. Andriantsimahavandy, E. R. Ramarcel, and J.-L. Pecarrere.** 1996. Forty years of chromoblastomycosis in Madagascar: a review. *Am. J. Trop. Med. Hyg.* **55:**45–47.
41. **Fader, R. C., and M. R. McGinnis.** 1988. Infections caused by dematiaceous fungi: chromoblastomycosis and phaeohyphomycosis. *Infect. Dis. Clin. North Am.* **2:** 925–938.
42. **Fincher, R. M. E., J. F. Fisher, A. A. Padhye, L. Ajello, and J. C. H. Steele, Jr.** 1988. Subcutaneous phaeohyphomycotic abscess caused by *Phialophora parasitica* in a renal allograft recipient. *J. Med. Vet. Mycol.* **26:**311–314.
43. **Franco, A., I. Aranda, M. J. Fernandez, M. A. Arroyo, F. Navas, D. Albero, and J. Olivares.** 1996. Chromomycosis in a European renal transplant recipient. *Nephrol. Dial. Transplant.* **11:**715–716.
44. **Gams, W., and M. R. McGinnis.** 1983. *Phialemonium*, a new anamorph genus intermediate between *Phialophora* and *Acremonium*. *Mycologia* **75:**977–987.
45. **Garcia-Arata, M. I., M. J. Otero, M. Zomeno, M. A. de la Figuera, M. C. de las Cuevas, and M. Lopez-Brea.** 1996. *Scedosporium apiospermum* pneumonia after autologous bone marrow transplantation. *Eur. J. Clin. Microbiol. Infect. Dis.* **15:**600–603.
46. **Gillum, P. S., A. Gurswami, and J. W. Taira.** 1997. Localized cutaneous infection by *Scedosporium prolificans* (*inflatum*). *Int. J. Dermatol.* **36:**297–299.
47. **Gonzales, M. S., B. Alfonso, D. Seckinger, A. A. Padhye, and L. Ajello.** 1984. Subcutaneous phaeohyphomycosis caused by *Cladosporium devriesii*. *Sabouraudia* **22:** 427–432.
48. **Gori, S., A. Lupetti, M. Moscato, M. Parenti, and A. Lofaro.** 1997. Pulmonary sporotrichosis with hyphae in a human immunodeficiency virus-infected patient—a case report. *Acta Cytol.* **41:**519–521.
49. **Guarro, J., G. S. de Hoog, M. J. Figueras, and J. Gene.** 1995. Rare opportunistic fungi, p. 243–668. *In* J. Guarro, G. S. de Hoog, M. J. Figueras, and J. Gene (ed.), *Atlas of Clinical Fungi*. Centraalbureau voor Schimmelcultures, Baarn, The Netherlands.
50. **Hironaga, M., K. Nakano, I. Yokoyama, and J. Kitajima.** 1989. *Phialophora repens*, an emerging agent of subcutaneous phaeohyphomycosis in humans. *J. Clin. Microbiol.* **27:** 394–399.
51. **Hirsch, B. E., B. F. Farber, J. F. Shapiro, and S. Kennelly.** 1996. Successful treatment of *Aureobasidium pullulans* prosthetic hip infection. *Infect. Dis. Clin. Pract.* **5:** 205–207.
52. **Hood, S. V., C. B. Moore, J. S. Cheesbrough, A. Mene, and D. W. Denning.** 1997. Atypical eumycetoma caused by *Phialophora parasitica* successfully treated with itraconazole and flucytosine. *Br. J. Dermatol.* **136:**953–956.
53. **Hsu, M. M., and Y.-Y. Lee.** 1993. Cutaneous and subcu-

taneous phaeohyphomycosis caused by *Exserohilum rostratum*. *J. Am. Acad. Dermatol.* **28:**340–344.

54. **Ichikawa, T., M. Saiki, S. Tokunaga, and T. Saida.** 1997. *Scedosporium apiospermum* skin infection in a patient with nephrotic syndrome. *Acta Dermato-Venereol.* **77:**172–173.
55. **Iwatsu, T., K. Sishimura, and M. Makoto.** 1984. *Exophiala castellanii* sp. nov. *Mycotaxon* **20:**307–314.
56. **Jacyk, W. K., J. H. Du Bruyn, N. Holm, H. Gryffenberg, and V. O. Karusseit.** 1997. Cutaneous infection due to *Cladophialophora bantiana* in a patient receiving immunosuppressive therapy. *Br. J. Dermatol.* **136:** 428–430.
57. **Kane, J., R. Summerbell, L. Sigler, S. Krajden, and G. Land.** 1997. *Laboratory Handbook of Dermatophytes: a Clinical Guide and Laboratory Manual of Dermatophytes and Other Filamentous Fungi from Skin, Hair, and Nails.* Star Publishing Co., Belmont, Calif.
58. **Kaplan, W., and A. G. Ochoa.** 1963. Application of the fluorescent antibody technique to the rapid diagnosis of sporotrichosis. *J. Lab. Clin. Med.* **62:**835–841.
59. **Kaufman, L., P. Standard, and A. Padhye.** 1980. Serologic relationships among isolates of *Exophiala jeanselmei* (*Phialophora jeanselmei*, *P. gouferotii*) and *Wangiella dermatitidis*. *Pan Am. Health Org. Sci. Publ.* **396:**252–258.
60. **Kiehn, T. E., B. Polsky, E. Punithalingam, F. F. Edwards, A. E. Brown, and D. Armstrong.** 1987. Liver infection caused by *Coniothyrium fuckelii* in a patient with acute myelogenous leukemia. *J. Clin. Microbiol.* **25:** 2410–2412.
61. **King, D., L. Pasarell, D. M. Dixon, M. R. McGinnis, and W. G. Merz.** 1993. A phaeohyphomycotic cyst and peritonitis caused by *Phialemonium* species and a reevaluation of its taxonomy. *J. Clin. Microbiol.* **31:**1804–1810.
62. **Kralovic, S. M., and J. C. Rhodes.** 1995. Phaeohyphomycosis caused by *Dactylaria* (human dactylariosis): report of a case with review of the literature. *J. Infect.* **31:** 107–113.
63. **Kwon-Chung, K. J., and J. E. Bennett.** 1992. *Medical Mycology*. Lea & Febiger, Philadelphia, Pa.
64. **Kwon-Chung, K. J., W. B. Hill, and J. E. Bennett.** 1981. New, special stain for histopathological diagnosis of cryptococcosis. *J. Clin. Microbiol.* **13:**383–387.
65. **Little, M. G., and M. L. Hammond.** 1995. *Scytalidium dimidiatum* in Australia. *Australas. J. Dermatol.* **36:** 204–205.
66. **Lopez, C., L. Ramos, G. Weisburd, S. Margasin, and R. Ramirez.** 1997. Feohifomicosis causada por *Cladosporium cladosporioides*. *J. Med. Microbiol.* **46:**699–703.
67. **Malloch, D., and I. F. Salkin.** 1984. A new species of *Scedosporium* associated with osteomyelitis in humans. *Mycotaxon* **21:**247–255.
68. **Mancini, M. C., and M. R. McGinnis.** 1992. *Dactylaria* infection of a human being: pulmonary disease in a heart transplant recipient. *J. Heart Lung Transplant.* **11:** 827–830.
69. **Masclaux, F., E. Gueho, G. S. de Hoog, and R. Christen.** 1995. Phylogenetic relationships of human-pathogenic *Cladosporium (Xylohypha)* species inferred from partial LS rRNA sequences. *J. Med. Vet. Mycol.* **33:**327–338.
70. **Maslen, M. M., T. Collis, and R. Stuart.** 1996. *Lasiodiplodia theobromae* isolated from a subcutaneous abscess in a Cambodian immigrant to Australia. *J. Med. Vet. Mycol.* **34:**279–283.
71. **Matsumoto, T., K. Nishimoto, K. Kimura, A. A. Padhye, L. Ajello, and M. R. McGinnis.** 1984. Phaeohyphomycosis caused by *Exophiala moniliae*. *Sabouraudia* **22:** 17–26.
72. **Matsumoto, T. T., T. Matsuda, M. R. McGinnis, and L. Ajello.** 1993. Clinical and mycological spectrum of *Wangiella dermatitidis* infections. *Mycoses* **36:**145–155.
73. **McGinnis, M. R.** 1978. Human pathogenic species of *Exophiala*, *Phialophora*, and *Wangiella*. *Pan Am. Health Org. Sci. Publ.* **356:**35–59.
74. **McGinnis, M. R.** 1978. Taxonomy of *Exophiala jeanselmei* (Langeron) McGinnis and Padhye. *Mycopathologia* **65:** 79–87.
75. **McGinnis, M. R.** 1979. Taxonomy of *Exophiala werneckii* and its relationship to *Microsporum mansonii*. *Sabouraudia* **17:**145–154.
76. **McGinnis, M. R.** 1980. *Laboratory Handbook of Medical Mycology*. Academic Press, Inc., New York, N.Y.
77. **McGinnis, M. R.** 1983. Chromoblastomycosis and phaeohyphomycosis: new concepts, diagnosis and mycology. *Am. Acad. Dermatol.* **8:**1–16.
78. **McGinnis, M. R., D. Borelli, A. A. Padhye, and L. Ajello.** 1986. Reclassification of *Cladosporium bantianum* in the genus *Xylohypha*. *J. Clin. Microbiol.* **23:**1148–1151.
79. **McGinnis, M. R., A. A. Padhye, and L. Ajello.** 1982. *Pseudallescheria* Negroni et Fischer, 1943, and its later synonym *Petriellidium* Malloch. *Mycotaxon* **14:**94–102.
80. **McGinnis, M. R., M. G. Rinaldi, and R. E. Winn.** 1986. Emerging agents of phaeohyphomycosis: pathogenic species of *Bipolaris* and *Exserohilum*. *J. Clin. Microbiol.* **24:** 250–259.
81. **McGinnis, M. R., and W. A. Schell.** 1980. The genus *Fonsecaea* and its relationship to the genera *Cladosporium*, *Phialophora*, *Ramichloridium*, and *Rhinocladiella*, p. 215–224. *In Proceedings of the 5th International Conference on the Mycoses: Superficial, Cutaneous, and Subcutaneous Infections*. Pan American Health Organization, Washington, D.C.
82. **McGinnis, M. R., W. A. Schell, and J. Carson.** 1985. *Phaeoannellomyces* and the Phaeoannellomycetaceae, new dematiaceous Blastomycete taxa. *Sabouraudia* **23:** 179–188.
83. **Midgley, G., and M. K. Moore.** 1996. Nail infections. *Dermatol. Clin.* **14:**41–49.
84. **Morris, A., W. A. Schell, D. McDonagh, S. Chafee, and J. R. Perfect.** 1995. *Fonsecaea pedrosoi* pneumonia and *Emericella nidulans* cerebral abscesses in a bone marrow transplant patient. *Clin. Infect. Dis.* **21:**1346–1348.
85. **Nenoff, P., U. Gutz, K. Tintelnot, A. Bosse-Henck, M. Mierzwa, J. Hofmann, L. C. Horn, and U. F. Haustein.** 1996. Disseminated mycosis due to *Scedosporium prolificans* in an AIDS patient with Burkitt lymphoma. *Mycoses* **39:**461–465.
86. **Oldham, A. D.** 1988. Care and use of the microscope, p. 574–578. *In* B. B. Wentworth (ed.), *Diagnostic Procedures for Mycotic and Parasitic Infections*. American Public Health Association, Washington, D.C.
87. **Padhye, A. A.** 1978. Comparative study of *Phialophora jeanselmei* and *P. gougerotii* by morphological, biochemical, and immunological methods. *Pan Am. Health Org. Sci. Publ.* **356:**60–65.
88. **Padhye, A. A., L. Ajello, M. A. Wieden, and K. K. Steinbronn.** 1986. Phaeohyphomycosis of the nasal sinuses caused by a new species of *Exserohilum*. *J. Clin. Microbiol.* **24:**245–249.
89. **Padhye, A. A., R. W. Gutekunst, D. J. Smith, and E. Punithalingam.** 1997. Maxillary sinusitis caused by *Pleurophomopsis lignicola*. *J. Clin. Microbiol.* **35:**2136–2141.
90. **Padhye, A. A., M. R. McGinnis, and L. Ajello.** 1978. Thermotolerance of *Wangiella dermatitidis*. *J. Clin. Microbiol.* **8:**424–426.
91. **Padhye, A. A., M. R. McGinnis, L. Ajello, and F. W. Chandler.** 1988. *Xylohypha emmonsii* sp. nov., a new agent of phaeohyphomycosis. *J. Clin. Microbiol.* **26:**702–708.

92. **Pappagianis, D., and L. Ajello.** 1994. Dematiaceous—a mycologic misnomer? *J. Med. Vet. Mycol.* **32:**319–321.
93. **Pasarell, L., M. R. McGinnis, and P. G. Standard.** 1990. Differentiation of medically important isolates of *Bipolaris* and *Exserohilum* with exoantigens. *J. Clin. Microbiol.* **28:** 1655–1657.
94. **Pickles, R. W., D. E. Pacey, D. B. Muir, and W. H. Merrell.** 1996. Experience with infection by *Scedosporium prolificans* including apparent cure with fluconazole therapy. *J. Infect.* **33:**193–197.
95. **Pitrak, D. L., E. W. Koneman, R. C. Estupinan, and J. Jackson.** 1988. *Phialophora richardsiae* in humans. *Rev. Infect. Dis.* **10:**1195–1203.
96. **Punithalingham, E.** 1976. *Botryodiplodia theobromae*. *CMI Descriptions of Pathogenic Fungi and Bacteria*, no. 519. Commonwealth Mycological Institution, Kew, England.
97. **Rai, M. K.** 1989. *Phoma sorghina* infections in human beings. *Mycopathologia* **105:**167–170.
98. **Rebell, G., and R. K. Forster.** 1976. *Lasiodiplodia theobromae* as a cause of keratomycoses. *Sabouraudia* **14:**155–170.
99. **Redondo-Bellon, P., M. Idoate, M. Rubio, and J. Ignacio Herrero.** 1997. Chromoblastomycosis produced by *Aureobasidium pullulans* in an immunosuppressed patient. *Arch. Dermatol.* **133:**663–664.
100. **Rinaldi, M. G., E. L. McCoy, and D. F. Winn.** 1982. Gluteal abscess caused by *Phialophora hoffmannii* and review of the role of this organism in human mycoses. *J. Clin. Microbiol.* *16:*181–185.
101. **Rinaldi, M. G., P. Phillips, J. G. Schwartz, R. E. Winn, G. R. Holt, F. W. Shagets, J. Elrod, G. Nishioka, and T. B. Aufdemorte.** 1987. Human *Curvularia* infections. Report of five cases and review of the literature. *Diagn. Microbiol. Infect. Dis.* **6:**27–39.
102. **Rockett, M. S., S. C. Gentile, K. H. Zygmunt, and C. J. Gudas.** 1996. Subcutaneous phaeohypomycosis caused by *Scytalidium dimidiatum* in the foot of an immunosuppressed host. *J. Foot Ankle Surg.* **35:**350–354.
103. **Roeijmans, H. J., G. S. de Hoog, C. S. Tan, and M. J. Figge.** 1997. Molecular taxonomy and GC/MS of metabolites of *Scytalidium hyalinum* and *Nattrassia mangiferae* (*Hendersonula toruloidea*). *J. Med. Vet. Mycol.* **35:** 181–188.
104. **Salkin, I. F., and D. M. Dixon.** 1987. *Dactylaria constricta*: description of two varieties. *Mycotaxon* **29:**377–381.
105. **Salkin, I. F., J. A. Martinez, and M. E. Kemna.** 1986. Opportunistic infection of the spleen caused by *Aureobasidium pullulans*. *J. Clin. Microbiol.* **23:**828–831.
106. **Salkin, I. F., M. R. McGinnis, M. J. Dykstra, and M. G. Rinaldi.** 1988. *Scedosporium inflatum*, an emerging pathogen. *J. Clin. Microbiol.* **26:**498–503.
107. **Saravanakumar, P. S., P. Eslami, and F. A. Zar.** 1996. Lymphocutaneous sporotrichosis associated with a squirrel bite: case report and review. *Clin. Infect. Dis.* **23:** 647–648.
108. **Schell, W. A.** 1986. Oculomycosis caused by dematiaceous fungi, p. 105–109. *In Proceedings of the VI International Conference on the Mycoses*. Pan American Health Organization, Washington, D.C.
109. **Schell, W. A.** 1997. Agents of chromoblastomycosis and sporotrichosis, p. 315–336. *In* L. Ajello and R. Hay (ed.), *Topley & Wilson's Microbiology and Microbial Infections*, vol. 4. *Mycology*. Edward Arnold, London, England.
110. **Schell, W. A., M. R. McGinnis, and D. Borelli.** 1983. *Rhinocladiella aquaspersa*, a new combination for *Acrotheca aquaspersa*. *Mycotaxon* **17:**341–348.
111. **Schell, W. A., and J. R. Perfect.** 1993. *Coniothyrium fuckelii*, a species in need of a genus: second case of human infection, abstr. F-34. *In Abstracts of the 93rd General Meeting of the American Society for Microbiology 1993*. American Society for Microbiology, Washington, D.C.
112. **Schonheyder, H. C., H. E. Jensen, W. Gams, O. Nyvad, P. Van Nga, B. Aalbaek, and J. Stenderup.** 1996. Late bioprosthetic valve endocarditis caused by *Phialemonium* aff. *curvatum* and *Streptococcus sanguis*: a case report. *J. Med. Vet. Mycol.* **34:**209–214.
113. **Sides, E. H., J. D. Benson, and A. A. Padhye.** 1991. Phaeohyphomycotic brain abscess due to *Ochroconis gallopavum* in a patient with malignant lymphoma of a large cell type. *J. Med. Vet. Mycol.* **29:**317–322.
114. **Sigler, L., and J. W. Carmichael.** 1976. Taxonomy of *Malbranchea* and some other hyphomycetes with arthroconidia. *Mycotaxon* **4:**349–488.
115. **Sigler, L., J. L. Harris, D. M. Dixon, A. L. Flis, I. F. Salkin, M. Kemna, and R. A. Duncan.** 1990. Microbiology and potential virulence of *Sporothrix cyanescens*, a fungus rarely isolated from blood and skin. *J. Clin. Microbiol.* **28:**1009–1015.
116. **Sigler, L., R. C. Summerbell, L. Poole, M. Wieden, D. A. Sutton, M. G. Rinaldi, M. Aguirre, G. W. Estes, and J. N. Galgiani.** 1997. Invasive *Nattrassia mangiferae* infections: case report, literature review, and therapeutic and taxonomic appraisal. *J. Clin. Microbiol.* **35:**433–440.
117. **Sigler, L., and C. J. K. Wang.** 1990. *Scytalidium circinatum* sp. nov., a hyphomycete from utility poles. *Mycologia* **82:** 399–404.
118. **St. Germain, G., and R. Summerbell.** 1996. *Identifying Filamentous Fungi*. Star Publishing Co., Belmont, Calif.
119. **Stiller, M. J., S. Rosenthal, R. C. Summerbell, J. Pollack, and A. Chan.** 1992. Onychomycosis of the toenails caused by *Chaetomium globosum*. *J. Am. Acad. Dermatol.* **26:**775–776.
120. **Sudduth, E. J., A. J. Crumbley, and W. E. Farrar.** 1992. Phaeohyphomycosis due to *Exophiala* species: clinical spectrum of disease in humans. *Clin. Infect. Dis.* **15:** 639–644.
121. **Sutton, B. C.** 1980. *The Coelomycetes: Fungi Imperfecti with Pycnidia Acervuli and Stromata*. Robert MacLehose & Co., Ltd., Glasgow, Scotland.
122. **Sutton, B. C., and B. J. Dyko.** 1989. Revision of *Hendersonula*. *Mycol. Res.* **93:**466–488.
123. **Tambini, R., C. Farina, R. Fiocchi, B. Dupont, E. Gueho, G. Delvecchio, F. Mamprin, and G. Gavazzeni.** 1996. Possible pathogenic role of *Sporothrix cyanescens* isolated from a lung lesion in a heart transplant patient. *J. Med. Vet. Mycol.* **34:**195–198.
124. **Tekavec, J., E. Mlinaric-Missoni, and V. Babic-Vazic.** 1997. Pulmonary tuberculosis associated with invasive pseudallescheriasis. *Chest* **111:**508–511.
125. **Tintelnot, K., P. von Hunnius, G. S. de Hoog, A. Polak-Wyss, E. Gueho, and F. Masclaux.** 1995. Systemic mycosis caused by a new *Cladophialophora* species. *J. Med. Vet. Mycol.* **33:**349–354.
126. **Turiansky, G. W., P. M. Benson, L. C. Sperling, P. Sau, I. F. Salkin, M. R. McGinnis, and W. D. James.** 1995. *Phialophora verrucosa*: a new cause of mycetoma. *J. Am. Acad. Dermatol.* **32:**311–315.
127. **Uberti-Foppa, C., L. Fumagalli, N. Gianotti, A. M. Viviani, R. Vaiani, and E. Gieho.** 1995. First case of osteomyelitis due to *Phialophora richardsiae* in a patient with HIV infection. *AIDS* **9:**975–976.
128. **Viviani, M. A., A. M. Tortorano, G. Laria, A. Giannetti, and G. Bignotti.** 1986. Two new cases of cutaneous alternariosis with a review of the literature. *Mycopathologia* **96:**3–12.
129. **Wang, C. J. K.** 1990. Microfungi, p. 1–356. *In* C. J. K. Wang and R. A. Zabel (ed.), *Identification Manual for*

Fungi from Utility Poles in the Eastern United States. American Type Culture Collection, Rockville, Md.

130. **Washburn, R. G., D. W. Kennedy, M. G. Begley, D. K. Henderson, and J. E. Bennett.** 1988. Chronic fungal sinusitis in apparently normal hosts. *Medicine (Baltimore)* **67:**231–247.
131. **Wiest, P. M., K. Wiese, M. R. Jacobs, A. B. Morrissey, T. I. Abelson, W. Witt, and M. M. Lederman.** 1987. *Alternaria* infection in a patient with acquired immune deficiency syndrome: case report and review of invasive *Alternaria* infections. *Rev. Infect. Dis.* **9:**799–803.
132. **Wilson, C. M., E. J. O'Rourke, M. R. McGinnis, and I. F. Salkin.** 1990. *Scedosporium inflatum*: clinical spectrum of a newly recognized pathogen. *J. Infect. Dis.* **161:** 102–107.
133. **Wood, G. M., J. G. McCormack, and D. B. Muir.** 1992. Clinical features of human infection with *Scedosporium inflatum*. *Clin. Infect. Dis.* **14:**1027.
134. **Woollons, A., C. R. Darley, S. Pandian, P. Arnstein, J. Blackee, and J. Paul.** 1996. Phaeohyphomycosis caused by *Exophiala dermatitidis* following intra-articular steroid injection. *Br. J. Dermatol.* **135:**475–477.
135. **Yau, Y. C., J. de Nanassy, R. C. Summerbell, A. G. Matlow, and S. E. Richardson.** 1994. Fungal sternal wound infection due to *Curvularia lunata* in a neonate with congenital heart disease: case report and review. *Clin. Infect. Dis.* **19:**735–740.
136. **Yeghen, T., L. Fenelon, C. K. Campbell, D. W. Warnock, A. V. Hoffbrand, H. G. Prentice, and C. C. Kibbler.** 1996. *Chaetomium* pneumonia in patient with acute myeloid leukaemia. *J. Clin. Pathol.* **49:**184–186.
137. **Zaatari, G. S., R. Reed, and R. Morewessel.** 1984. Subcutaneous hyphomycosis caused by *Scytalidium hyalinum*. *Am. J. Clin. Pathol.* **82:**252–256.
138. **Zaitz, C., E. M. Heins-Vaccari, R. S. de Freitas, G. L. H. Arria-Gada, L. Ruiz, S. A. S. Totoli, A. C. Marques, G. G. Rezze, H. Muller, H. Valente, and C. S. Lacaz.** 1997. Subcutaneous phaeohyphomycosis caused by *Phoma cava*. Report of a case and review of the literature. *Rev. Inst. Med. Trop. Sao Paulo* **39:**43–48.

Fungi Causing Eumycotic Mycetoma

ARVIND A. PADHYE AND MICHAEL R. McGINNIS

102

DEFINITION OF THE INFECTION

A mycetoma (plural, mycetomata) (35) is a localized, chronic, noncontagious, granulomatous infection involving cutaneous and subcutaneous tissues and eventually, in some cases, bones. Mycetomata are generally confined to either the feet or the hands but occasionally affect sites such as the back, shoulders, buttocks, and, rarely, the scalp. The lesions contain granulomas and abscesses that suppurate and drain through sinus tracts. The pus contains sclerotia (granules, grains) (34) that vary from approximately 0.2 to over 5 mm in diameter. The size, color, shape, and internal architecture of the sclerotia vary with the species of agent, sometimes suggesting the specific etiology. Both filamentous fungi and actinomycetes are known to cause mycetomata. Mycetomata caused by actinomycetes are called actinomycotic mycetomata, and those incited by filamentous fungi are referred to as eumycotic mycetomata. The disease occurs worldwide and is more commonly seen in humans than in lower animals. Only a few authentic cases of mycetoma involving dogs, horses, and goats have been described in the literature (2, 10, 25, 30).

OCCURRENCE OF CAUSAL AGENTS IN NATURE

The causal agents of eumycotic mycetoma are saprophytes that live on organic debris associated with soil. The various causal agents have been isolated from either soil or plant material (1, 4, 20, 27). Using specific isolation media and techniques, Segretain (48) and Segretain and Mariat (51) showed that *Leptosphaeria senegalensis* and *Leptosphaeria tompkinsii* could be recovered from about 50% of the dry thorns of *Acacia* trees that were examined, particularly those that had been stained by mud during the rainy season. *Neotestudina rosatii* has been isolated from sandy ground (31), and *Madurella mycetomatis* has been recovered from soil and anthills (47, 55). *Acremonium* spp., *Curvularia* spp., *Aspergillus nidulans*, *Aspergillus flavus*, and *Pseudallescheria boydii* frequently have been isolated from soil. Borelli (6) isolated *Madurella grisea* from soil in Venezuela.

MODE OF INFECTION AND SYMPTOMS

A mycetoma develops after a traumatic injury by items such as contaminated thorns, splinters, fish scales or fins, snake bites, insect bites, farm implements, and knives. The development of mycetoma after accidental implantation of the etiologic agent during surgery (43) and in a renal transplant recipient (21) has been reported as well. The initial lesion is often characterized by a feeling of discomfort and pain at the point of inoculation. Weeks or months later, the subcutaneous tissue at the site of inoculation becomes indurated, abscesses develop, and sinuses may drain to the surface. The lesions are characterized by swelling, suppurating abscesses, granulomas, and sinuses from which serosanguinous fluid containing sclerotia (granules) is discharged. The mycetoma develops slowly beneath thick fibrosclerous tissue. The subsequent phase of proliferation involves the invasion of muscles and intramuscular layers. The granulomatous lesions can extend as deep as bone, where severe bone destruction, formation of small cavities, and the occurrence of complete remodeling can occur. Early osteolytic damage includes loss of the cortical margin and external erosion of the bone. As the infection progresses, blood, lymphatic vessels, and nerves may be damaged. Frequently, secondary bacterial infections and osteomyelitis producing total bone destruction occur. Pain is often associated with the development of multiple fistulae.

Regardless of the etiologic agent involved, the causal organisms develop in the form of soft or hard, compact mycelial masses (sclerotia), historically known as granules or grains, within the infected tissue. The hallmark of a mycetoma is a sclerotium (granule) composed of nonconidiating mycelium that may or may not be embedded in a cement-like matrix. These structures frequently contain host tissue. Weathered et al. (57) described the cement in *M. mycetomatis* as being an amorphous, electron-dense material with areas containing variably sized membrane-bound vesicular inclusions. Some of the host material, especially at the periphery of the granule, provides a protective barrier for the fungus against antifungal agents and humoral immunologic responses, such as antibodies.

Mycetoma develops mainly among people such as field workers, farmers, and fishermen, who are in contact with contaminated materials. Even though the prevalence of mycetomata is much higher in males than in females owing to increased exposure of the former, women and children who walk barefoot also are vulnerable to infection.

Fungus balls, or fungomata, caused by *Aspergillus* species,

Coccidioides immitis, or *P. boydii* and other fungi in preexisting lung cavities, are inappropriately called mycetomas (22). In the absence of well-organized sclerotia, they should be referred to as fungus balls, aspergillomas, or coccidioidomas (32). Similarly, mycelial aggregates formed by dermatophytes in cutaneous-subcutaneous tissues differ in many respects from the sclerotia of mycetoma. They differ by lacking granule ontogeny, a distinct surrounding Splendore-Hoeppli reaction, and the entry of the fungus from ruptured hair follicles into deeper tissue following rupture. Such infections caused by dermatophytes are best referred to as pseudomycetomata rather than mycetomata (3).

GEOGRAPHIC DISTRIBUTION OF EUMYCOTIC MYCETOMA

Eumycotic mycetomata occur in people living primarily in tropical to hot temperate zones. They frequently are reported from countries near the Tropic of Cancer, but they also occur beyond this area. Numerous cases have been described from Africa, Asia, South America, and Central America. Mycetomata are not seen as commonly in the United States as in tropical countries. A survey of the literature from 1979 to 1992 revealed that not more than 10 cases of eumycotic mycetoma had been reported in the United States. However, one of us (A.A.P.) has studied three cases of black grain eumycotic mycetomata among Mexican immigrants to the United States. The causal agents were identified as *M. mycetomatis* in one case and *M. grisea* in two cases. Lack of familiarity with these agents because of their rare occurrence in the United States can cause delay in their proper identification.

CLIMATIC CONDITIONS

Climate has a definite influence on the prevalence and distribution of mycetomata. Rivers that flood each year during the wet season in many countries of Africa and Asia influence the distribution of the causal agents. Rainfall also aids the spread of the etiologic agents on organic matter (16).

COLLECTION AND EXAMINATION OF GRANULES

Because all of the agents of eumycotic mycetoma are soil or plant saprophytes, some of which can be encountered as contaminants of clinical specimens, their etiologic role in mycetomata must be established carefully. A definitive diagnosis is based on the demonstration of sclerotia in tissue or sinuses and the repeated isolation of the causal fungus from sclerotia aspirated from preferably unopened sinuses.

Pus, exudate, or biopsy material should be examined for the presence of sclerotia (granules), which vary in size from 0.2 to 5 mm or more and are usually detectable with the naked eye. Their color, internal architecture, size, and shape give a fair indication of the identity of the etiologic agent. Actinomycotic and eumycotic mycetomata are differentiated by the examination of crushed granules stained with Gram stain. Actinomycotic granules are composed of gram-positive, interwoven, thin filaments, 0.5 to 1.0 μm in diameter, as well as coccoid and bacillary forms. Granules of eumycotic agents, on the other hand, are composed of broad, interwoven, septate hyphae, 2 to 5 μm in diameter, with many bizarrely shaped swollen cells up to 15 μm in diameter, especially at the periphery of the granules. In many species, the granules also contain a cement-like material.

To maximize the chances of obtaining pure cultures of the etiologic agents, granules from eumycotic mycetomata should be washed several times with saline containing antibacterial antibiotics such as penicillin and streptomycin. The granules then should be cultured on several petri dishes of Sabouraud glucose agar (SGA; Difco Laboratories, Detroit, Mich.) containing chloramphenicol (50 mg/liter) and SGA containing chloramphenicol and cycloheximide (500 mg/liter each). Plates should be incubated at 25 and 37°C. All plates should be observed at 48-h intervals. Because many of the fungi that cause eumycotic mycetoma grow slowly, petri dishes should be incubated for 6 weeks before being discarded as negative. Identification of the isolated fungus is based on gross colony morphology and pigmentation, the morphology of its conidiophores, conidiogenous cells, and conidia, and the mechanism of conidiogenesis. Since certain species (*M. grisea*, *M. mycetomatis*, *N. rosatii*, *Pyrenochaeta mackinnonii*, and *Pyrenochaeta romeroi*) do not sporulate readily, sporulation media and physiologic tests, such as those for carbohydrate and nitrate utilization, must be used for identification.

ETIOLOGIC AGENTS AND THEIR CLASSIFICATION

The various species known to cause eumycotic mycetoma are discussed below. Of these species, 5 belong to the division Ascomycota, and 20 are classified under the Deuteromycota (Fungi Imperfecti) (Table 1).

TABLE 1 Etiologic agents of eumycotic mycetoma

Etiologic agent	Reference(s)
Ascomycota	
Emericella nidulans (*Aspergillus nidulans*)	29
Leptosphaeria senegalensis	31
Leptosphaeria tompkinsii	18
Neotestudina rosatii	49
Pseudallescheria boydii	37
Deuteromycota	
Acremonium falciforme	23, 38
Acremonium kiliense	23
Acremonium recifei	23, 30
Aspergillus flavus	58
Curvularia geniculata	10
Curvularia lunata	29, 30
Corynespora cassicola	30
Cylindrocarpon destructans	17, 59
Exophiala jeanselmei	36, 42
Fusarium moniliforme	30, 31
Fusarium solani var. *coeruleum*	31, 35, 54
Fusarium solani var. *minus*	35
Madurella grisea	6, 26, 28, 29, 51
Madurella mycetomatis	6, 26, 31
Phaeoacremonium inflatipes	14, 15
Phialophora verrucosa	56
Plenodomas avramii	8
Polycytella hominis	12
Pseudochaetosphaeronema larense	9, 44
Pyrenochaeta mackinnonii	7, 44
Pyrenochaeta romeroi	5, 44, 50

CHARACTERISTICS OF GRANULES IN TISSUE

The granules of eumycotic mycetomata are composed of septate mycelial filaments that are at least 2 to 4 μm in diameter. The mycelium may be distorted and bizarre in form and size, and the cell walls of the fungi, especially toward the periphery of the granules, are thickened. Vesicles are frequently present, especially at the periphery of the granules. The mycelium of the granules may or may not be embedded in a cement-like substance, depending on the species involved. Often the granules elicit an immunologic response, known as the Splendore-Hoeppli reaction (antigen-antibody) (13, 35). This reaction is seen histologically in the form of a deposit of eosinophilic material around the granule.

Depending on the etiologic agent involved, the granules are white to yellow-brown to black and range from 200 μm to 5 mm in diameter. The color gives some indication of the species involved. Most textbooks on medical mycology mention a definitive relationship between the color of the granules and the causal species.

The causal agents that produce hyaline mycelia and conidia generally produce white granules in tissue, whereas *M. mycetomatis* and several other phaeoid fungi form black granules in tissue. It is believed that melanin, host protein, and dark debris result in the dark color of these granules. Melanin is a low-molecular-weight compound that is anchored to extracellular proteins. The precursor for the extracellular production of melanin is typically 1,8-dihydroxynaphthalene (34, 35). Generally, fungi that produce pigmented mycelia and/or conidia have dark granules in tissue. There are several exceptions to this rule. For example, hyaline fungi such as *Acremonium kiliense* and *Fusarium solani* var. *coeruleum* have been described in the literature as producing black granules in tissue (23, 54). Likewise, phaeoid etiologic agents such as *Phaeoacremonium inflatipes* and *P. boydii* produce white granules in tissue (14, 15, 27, 37). Although the gross and microscopic characteristics of the granules provide insight into the identity of the etiologic agent or a particular group to which it belongs, definitive identification of the etiologic agent should be based on repeated isolation of the same fungus from several granules and on colonial features, microscopic characteristics of conidia and conidiophores, and mechanism of conidiogenesis. The characteristics of the granules formed by each of the causal species are summarized in Table 2.

DESCRIPTION OF THE MORE PREVALENT ETIOLOGIC AGENTS

The etiologic agents described below are species that are isolated most commonly from human or lower-animal mycetoma. The physiologic characteristics of the five species most commonly isolated from eumycotic mycetoma are summarized in Table 3. In the United States, cases of eumycotic mycetoma are not common. Among the cases studied, the following species, in diminishing order of frequency, were isolated: *P. boydii*, *Acremonium falciforme*, *M. mycetomatis*, *M. grisea*, and *Exophiala jeanselmei*.

Acremonium falciforme

Three *Acremonium* species (*A. falciforme*, *A. kiliense*, and *Acremonium recifei*) are known to cause mycetoma. *A. falciforme* is the second most common cause of mycetoma in the United States. It was found to be an agent of eumycotic

TABLE 2 Gross characteristics of granules of eumycotic mycetoma agents

Kind of granule in tissue and species	Texture	Size range (mm)	Cement-like matrix
White grain			
Acremonium falciforme	Soft	0.2–0.5	Absent
Acremonium kiliense	Soft	0.2–0.5	Absent
Acremonium recifei	Soft	0.2–0.5	Absent
Emericella nidulans	Soft	1.0–2.0	Absent
Aspergillus flavus	Soft	0.2–0.5	Absent
Cylindrocarpon cyanescens	Soft	0.2–0.3	Absent
Cylindrocarpon destructans	Soft	0.2–0.5	Absent
Fusarium moniliforme	Soft	0.2–0.5	Absent
Fusarium solani	Soft	0.2–0.6	Absent
Neotestudina rosatii	Soft	0.5–1.0	Present, peripheral
Phaeoacremonium inflatipes	Soft	0.5–1.0	Absent
Polycytella hominis	Soft	0.5–1.0	Absent
Pseudallescheria boydii	Soft	0.5–1.0	Absent
Black grain			
Corynespora cassicola	Hard	0.2–0.5	Absent
Curvularia geniculata	Hard	0.5–1.0	Present, peripheral
Curvularia lunata	Hard	0.5–1.0	Present, peripheral
Exophiala jeanselmei	Soft	0.2–0.3	Absent
Leptosphaeria senegalensis	Hard	0.5–2.0	Present, peripheral
Leptosphaeria tompkinsii	Hard	0.5–2.0	Present, peripheral
Madurella grisea	Soft	0.3–0.6	Present, peripheral
Madurella mycetomatis	Hard	0.5–5.0	Present, homogeneous
Phialophora verrucosa	Soft	0.5–1.0	Absent
Plenodomus avramii	Soft	0.5–0.8	Absent
Pseudochaetosphaeronema larense	Soft	0.2–0.5	Absent
Pyrenochaeta mackinnonii	Soft	0.2–0.5	Absent
Pyrenochaeta romeroi	Soft	0.2–0.6	Absent

TABLE 3 Physiologic characteristics of some causal agents of eumycotic mycetoma

Etiologic agent	Utilization of:								Starch hydrolysis	Protease activity	Optimum growth temp (°C)
	Galactose	Glucose	Lactose	Maltose	Sucrose	Asparagine	KNO_3	$(NH_4)_2SO_4$			
A. falciforme	+	+	−	+	+	+	+	+	−	+	30
E. jeanselmei	+	+	−	+	+	+	+	+	+	−	30
M. grisea	+	+	−	+	+	+	+	+	+	+	25
M. mycetomatis	+	+	+	+	−	+	+	+	+	+	37
P. boydii	+	+	−	−	+	+	+	+	−	+	30

mycetoma in the San Francisco Bay area of California (23). It was also reported as the cause of mycetoma in a renal transplant recipient (21) and as the etiologic agent of mycetoma in a patient from New York (38).

The granules of *A. falciforme* are white to pale yellow, soft, and 0.2 to 0.5 mm in diameter. They are composed of slender, polymorphic, septate hyphae that are 1.5 to 2.0 μm in diameter and have irregular bulbous swellings and peripheral cementing material. In tissue sections, the granules resemble those produced by *P. boydii*. Therefore, the diagnosis should be based not only on the morphology of the granules in tissue but also on the isolation and identification of the causal agent.

Colonies of *A. falciforme* on SGA grow slowly, reaching 60 to 65 mm in 2 weeks. They are downy and gray-brown and become gray-violet. The reverse of the colony develops a violet-purple pigment. The hyphae are hyaline, septate, smooth, branched, and 1.5 to 2.5 μm in diameter. They bear erect, undifferentiated, unbranched, repeatedly septate conidiophores. The conidia are borne at the tip of phialidic conidiogenous cells, where they accumulate in mucoid clusters. The conidia are allantoid, slightly curved, and nonseptate to monoseptate. They measure 7.0 to 8.5 by 2.7 to 3.2 μm (Fig. 1). The intercalary or, rarely, terminal chlamydospores are smooth, thick walled, and 5 to 8 μm in diameter.

The other two species, *A. kiliense* and *A. recifei*, are not known to cause mycetoma as frequently as *A. falciforme*. Their granules are similar in morphology to those of *A. falciforme* and cannot be differentiated from each other or from those produced by *P. boydii*. When isolated, *A. kiliense* develops pinkish orange, glabrous colonies with coremia. Conidia are broadly elliptical to cylindrical and nonseptate, occurring in gleoid masses at the tips of lateral, long, tapering phialides with vestigial collarettes. Chlamydospores are present. Colonies of *A. recifei* are white to pinkish buff and moist to glabrous. Their conidiophores are branched, bearing long, tapering phialides. Conidia are claviform and nonseptate to monoseptate.

Curvularia geniculata

Curvularia geniculata is the etiologic agent of mycetoma in dogs in the United States (10). Its granules are black to dark brown, firm, and 0.5 to 1.0 mm or more in diameter. In tissue sections, the granules are spherical, ovoid, or irregularly shaped and are often surrounded by a zone of epithelioid cells. The periphery of the granules is a dense, interwoven mass of dematiaceous mycelium and thick-walled, chlamydospore-like cells embedded in a cement-like substance. The interior of the granules is vacuolar and consists of a loose network of septate hyphal filaments.

In culture, *C. geniculata* develops a floccose to downy, olive-gray to black colony. Microscopically, the dematiaceous, septate hyphae bear solitary, geniculate conidiogenous cells (Fig. 2). The conidia are without protruding hila. They are smooth walled, predominently five celled, and curved; the swollen median cell is pale to dark brown, in contrast to the lighter end cells.

Curvularia lunata

Curvularia lunata has been described as an etiologic agent of mycetoma among humans in Senegal and Sudan (29, 51). Its granules resemble those of *C. geniculata* in their morphologic characteristics. In culture, *C. lunata* produces geniculate conidiophores that are sympodial in their development. Conidia are without protruding hila. They are smooth and predominently four celled; the penultimate cell is pale to dark brown (Fig. 3).

Exophiala jeanselmei

E. jeanselmei is known as an agent of eumycotic mycetoma in India (52, 53), Malaya, Thailand (45), Argentina (41), and the United States (42). *E. jeanselmei* produces granules in host tissue that are brown to black, irregular in shape, and fragile. Detached portions or fragments of the granules often are found within giant cells. When extruded through sinuses, the granules often look like worm cases (vermiform) because of their elongated shapes and irregular surfaces. In tissue sections, they appear as hollow structures or as sinuous bands that are vermiform. The external surface is composed of brown, thick-walled hyphae and thick-walled chlamydospore-like cells. The granules are free of cement-like material. Within the hollow granules, smaller, degenerated hyphal fragments with leukocytes and giant cells may be seen.

Initially, the colonies of *E. jeanselmei* may be yeast-like and black, gradually spreading, becoming raised or dome shaped, and 20 to 25 mm in diameter. Microscopically, yeast-like cells are produced by solitary annellidic conidiogenous cells that are one celled (*Phaeoannellomyces* synanamorph). After 2 weeks on SGA, the colonies are covered with short aerial hyphae. At this stage, the colonies are mousy gray to olive-gray, with an olive-black reverse. The septate mycelium is sometimes toruloid, branched, and pale brown. The conidiophores are partially differentiated from the vegetative hyphae, solitary, branched or unbranched, smooth walled, and pale brown. The tips of the conidiogenous cells are closely annellated, cylindrical, obclavate, smooth walled, pale brown to black, and elongate as a result of successive conidial formation. The conidia, which aggregate in masses at the tips of annellides, tend to slide down the conidiophore or along the hyphae. The smooth conidia are exogenous, nonseptate, subglobose, and ellipsoidal to cylindrical, measuring 1.5 to 2.8 μm in diameter (Fig. 4).

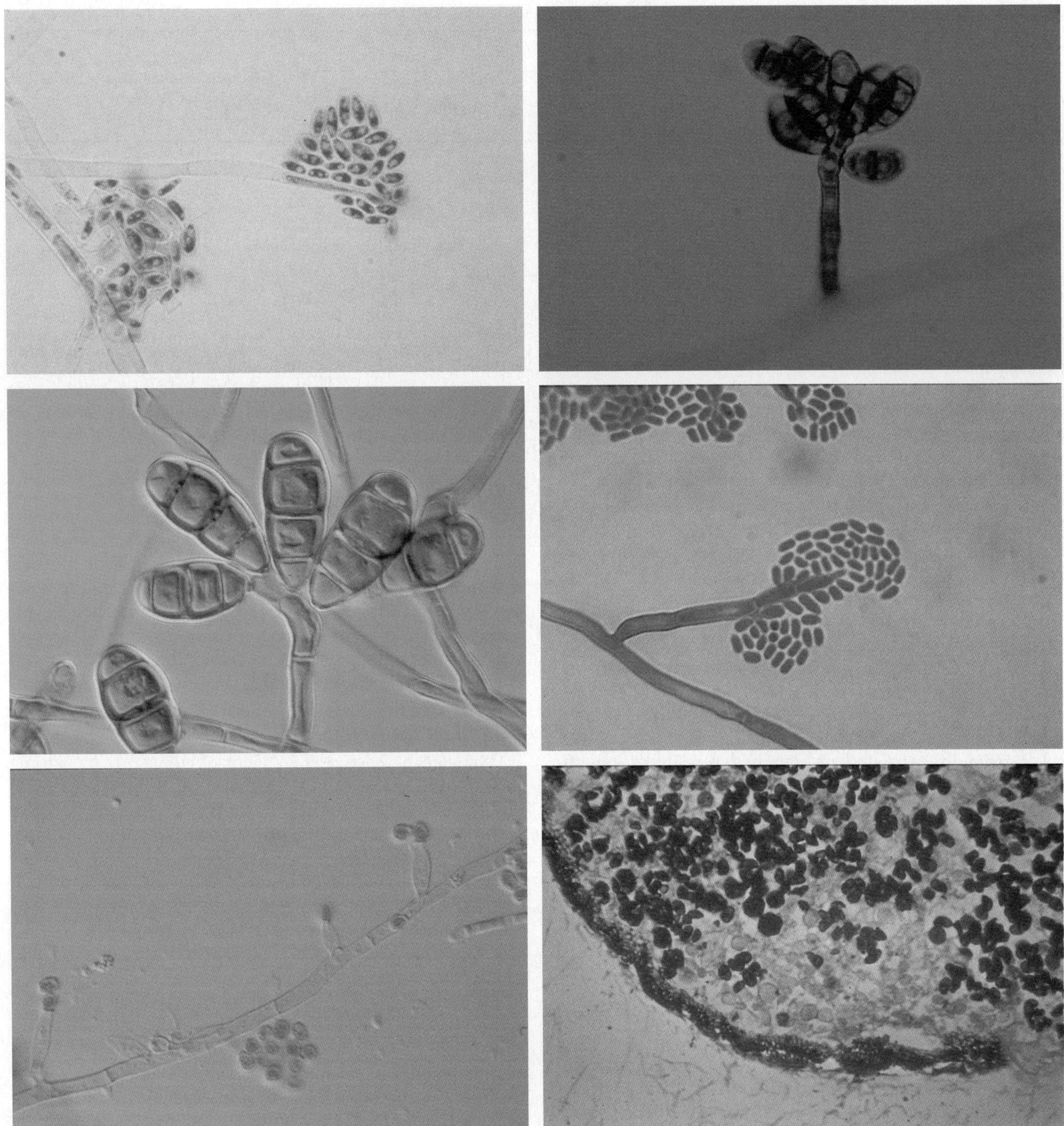

FIGURE 1 (top left) *A. falciforme*. Slide culture on SGA showing erect, septate conidiophore, phialidic conidiogenous cell, and slightly curved conidia. Magnification, ×160.

FIGURE 2 (top right) *C. geniculata*. Slide culture on potato dextrose agar showing geniculate conidiogenous cell and septate, curved conidia. Magnification, ×160.

FIGURE 3 (middle left) *C. lunata*. Geniculate conidiogenous cell bearing smooth, predominantly four-celled conidia. Magnification, ×160.

FIGURE 4 (middle right) *E. jeanselmei*. Lateral, septate conidiophore bearing closely annellated conidiogenous cells producing smooth, nonseptate, ellipsoidal to cylindric conidia. Magnification, ×160.

FIGURE 5 (bottom left) *M. mycetomatis*. Slide culture on soil extract agar showing lateral phialides and globose conidia. Magnification, ×250.

FIGURE 6 (bottom right) *N. rosatii*. Cross section of an ascocarp showing an ascomatal wall of interwoven hyphae and containing dark asci and ascospores. Magnification, ×250.

Leptosphaeria senegalensis

L. senegalensis and *L. tompkinsii* cause mycetoma in the northern tropical zone of West Africa, especially Senegal and Mauritania, and in India. The granules of the two species are indistinguishable from each other. They are black, 0.5 to 2.0 mm in size, and firm to hard. In tissue sections, the granules are round to polylobulated, with large vesicles. At the periphery, the mycelium is embedded in a black, cement-like substance. The central portion of each granule consists of a loose network of hyphae.

In culture, *L. senegalensis* and *L. tompkinsii* grow rapidly and produce gray-brown colonies. On cornmeal agar, both species produce ascostroma that are nonostiolate, scattered, immersed or superficial, globose to subglobose, black, and covered with brown, flexuous hyphae. The asci are numerous, eight spored, clavate to cylindrical, and double walled. The major difference between the two species is found in the ascospores, which differ in size, shape, septation, and the nature of the gelatinous sheath that surrounds them (18, 19).

Madurella grisea

M. grisea occurs as an etiologic agent of black grain mycetoma in South America, India, Africa, North America, and Central America (28, 30). In the United States, five cases caused by *M. grisea* have been described (11, 39). Two new cases of mycetoma caused by *M. grisea* among Mexican immigrants were diagnosed during 1996.

The granules are black, 0.3 to 0.6 mm in diameter, and soft to firm. In tissue sections, the granules are oval, lobulated or kidney shaped (reniform), and sometimes vermiform. They are composed of a dense network of hyphae weakly pigmented in the center and brown to blackish brown in the peripheral region as the result of the presence of a brown, cement-like interstitial material.

In culture, *M. grisea* forms slowly growing velvety colonies that are cerebriform, radially furrowed or smooth, and dark gray to olive-brown to black. The reverses of the colonies are black. In old cultures, a red-brown diffusible pigment is produced by many isolates. Microscopically, the hyphae are septate, light to dark brown, 1 to 3 μm in diameter, and nonsporulating. Chlamydospores rarely are observed. Large moniliform hyphae 3 to 5 μm in diameter are often present. Some isolates of *M. grisea* have been described as producing abortive or fertile pycnidia (33, 50). Such isolates are indistinguishable from *P. mackinnonii* (7, 46).

Madurella mycetomatis

The granules produced by *M. mycetomatis* are reddish brown to black. They may reach 5 mm or more in diameter and are firm to hard. In tissue sections, the granules are compact, variable in size and shape, and frequently multilobulated. They are composed of hyphae that are 1.2 to 5.0 μm in diameter and that terminate in enlarged hyphal cells at the periphery of the granules, which measure 12 to 15 μm in diameter. The cell wall pigment is minimal, but hyphal cells contain brown particles. The hyphae are embedded in a conspicuous brown matrix that is characteristic of *M. mycetomatis*. Some granules are vesicular and more regular in size and shape. The vesicles are predominantly visible in the peripheral zone in a dense, brown, cement-like matrix.

In culture, *M. mycetomatis* shows wide variation. Colonies grow slowly and are initially white, becoming olivaceous, yellow, or brown, flat or dome shaped, and velvety to glabrous, with a characteristic brown diffusible pigment. On nutritionally deficient media, sclerotia 750 μm in diameter develop. These are black and consist of undifferentiated polygonal cells. On SGA, the mycelium is sterile. On nutritionally poor media, such as soil extract or hay infusion agar, about 50% of the isolates produce round to pyriform conidia 3 to 4 μm in diameter from the tips of phialides. The phialides are long and tapering, often with inconspicuous collarettes. They range from 3 to 15 μm in length. Occasionally, two or three phialides may arise from a lateral branch (Fig. 5).

M. mycetomatis grows better at 37°C than at 30°C, whereas *M. grisea* grows better at 30°C than at 37°C. The ability of *M. mycetomatis* isolates to grow at temperatures as high as 40°C serves as a useful diagnostic criterion for distinguishing them from *M. grisea* isolates. *M. mycetomatis* is slowly proteolytic and utilizes glucose, maltose, and galactose but not sucrose. It utilizes potassium nitrate, ammonium sulfate, asparagine, and urea and hydrolyzes starch. *M. grisea*, on the other hand, is weakly proteolytic and assimilates glucose, maltose, and sucrose but not lactose (Table 3).

Neotestudina rosatii

The granules of *N. rosatii* are white to brownish white, 0.5 to 1.0 mm in diameter, and soft. In tissue sections, the granules appear to be polyhedral to subregular and consist of hyphae which are embedded in the peripheral cement-like material. The granules manifest an eosinophilic border. The central portion of each granule consists of more or less disintegrated mycelium and chlamydospores. Mycetoma caused by *N. rosatii* has been described in Australia, Cameroon, Guinea, Senegal, and Somalia (31, 49).

In culture, colonies of *N. rosatii* grow slowly, attaining diameters of 25 to 28 mm in 2 weeks, and have an aerial mycelium that is grayish black to brownish black. On potato-carrot or cornmeal agar incubated at 30°C, most of the ascomata are submerged. The ascostromal walls are smooth and are surrounded by interwoven brown to hyaline hyphae. The eight-spored asci, 12 to 35 by 10 to 25 μm, are scattered in the central part of the ascostroma and are globose to subglobose, thick walled, and bitunicate, becoming evanescent as ascospores mature (Fig. 6). Ascospores vary in size (9.0 to 12.5 by 4.5 to 8.0 μm) and shape, ranging from ellipsoidal to bicampanulate, asymmetrical, or slightly curved, are constricted at the median transverse septum, and have smooth brown walls.

Pseudallescheria boydii (Anamorph: *Scedosporium apiospermum*)

The granules produced by *P. boydii* are white to yellowish white and soft to firm; they vary from globose to subglobose to lobulated and are 0.2 to 2.0 mm in diameter. In tissue sections, the granules are composed of hyaline hyphae that are 1.5 to 5.0 μm in diameter and that radiate from the center into terminal thick-walled cells 15 to 20 μm in diameter at the periphery of the granules. The central portion of each granule consists of loosely interwoven hyaline mycelium.

Colonies grow rapidly and are floccose and white initially, becoming gray as conidia are produced. With age, the colonies become dark grayish brown. The anamorphic state, *Scedosporium apiospermum*, produces conidia that are egg shaped to clavate, truncate, and subhyaline, becoming pale gray to pale brown. Conidia are produced singly. They remain attached at the tips of annellides (Fig. 7). Annellations can be detected at the tips of conidiogenous cells as swollen rings. Occasionally, some isolates also produce a *Graphium* synanamorph, which is characterized by rope-like bundles

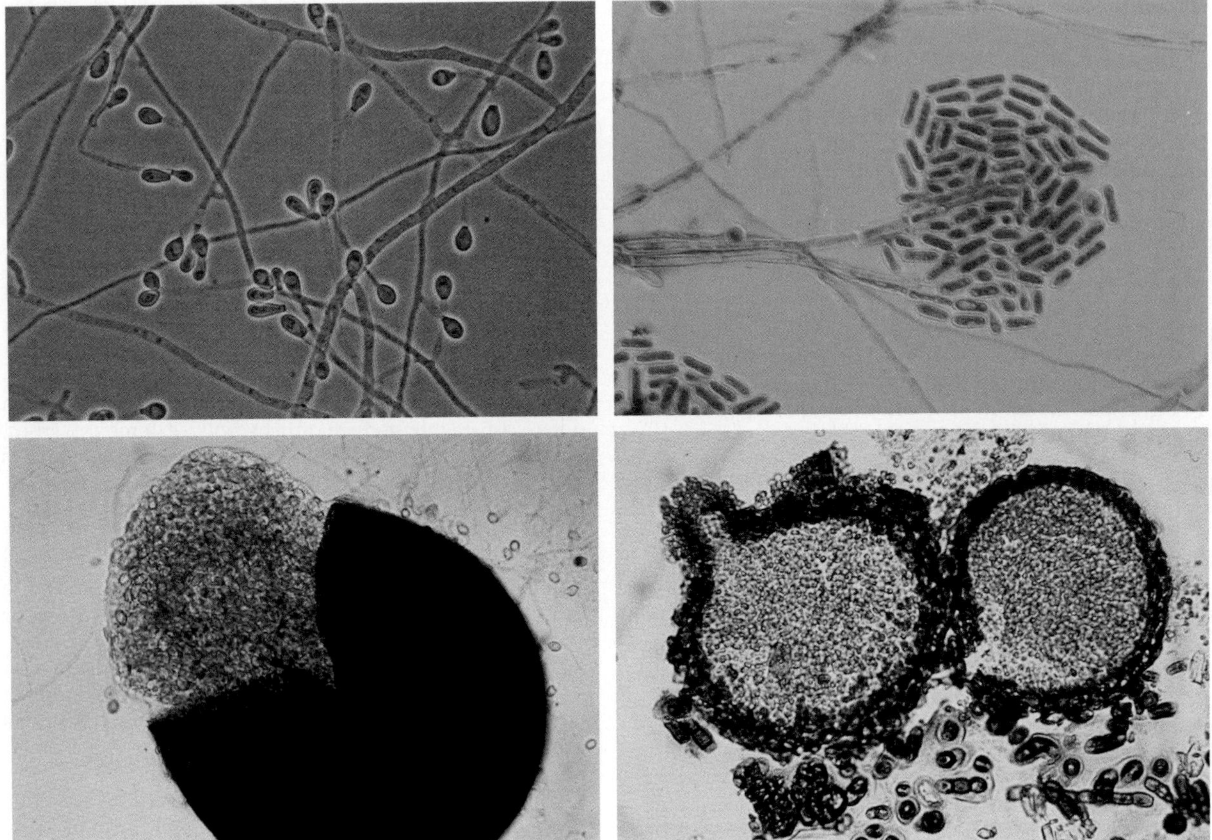

FIGURE 7 (top left) *S. apiospermum* anamorph of *P. boydii*. Slide culture on potato dextrose agar showing lateral, single, egg-shaped to clavate, truncate conidia. Magnification, ×160.

FIGURE 8 (top right) *Graphium* synanamorph of *P. boydii*. Slide culture on potato dextrose agar showing rope-like bundles of hyphae producing smooth, cylindrical conidia. Magnification, ×160.

FIGURE 9 (bottom left) *P. boydii*. Globose, nonostiolate, ruptured cleistothecium containing ellipsoidal to oblate ascospores. Magnification, ×160.

FIGURE 10 (bottom right) *P. romeroi*. Ostiolate conidiomata (pycnidia) containing numerous cylindrical conidia. Magnification, ×250.

of hyphae with annellidic conidiogenesis. The hyphae are fused into long stalks known as synnemata. The conidia are hyaline, cylindrical to clavate, and truncate at the base (Fig. 8).

The ascocarps of the teleomorphic state may be produced when isolates are grown on cornmeal agar. The cleistothecia develop submerged in the agar and appear as black dots. They are globose, nonostiolate, 140 to 200 μm in diameter, and often covered with brown, thick-walled, septate hyphae 2 to 3 μm wide. They have a wall that is 4 to 6 μm thick and composed of two or three layers of interwoven, flattened, dark brown cells, each 2 to 6 μm wide. The cleistothecia open at maturity by an irregular rupture of the wall. The eight-spored asci are ellipsoidal to nearly spherical. They measure 12 to 18 by 9 to 13 μm. The ascospores are ellipsoidal to oblate (football shaped), symmetrical or slightly flattened, and straw colored. They have two germ pores and measure 6.0 to 7.0 by 3.5 to 4.0 μm (Fig. 9).

Even though *P. boydii* is homothallic, many clinical and soil isolates do not form ascocarps. Their identification, then, is based on the morphology of the conidial state alone. *P. boydii* is the most common agent of mycetoma in humans as well as lower animals in the United States. It has been isolated frequently from manure, soil, and water. It is often encountered as a contaminant of respiratory specimens from patients with chronic lung disease. It is also isolated from open, dirty wounds. Its isolation from such specimens, however, does not always implicate *P. boydii* as an etiologic agent. On the other hand, *P. boydii* is known to cause necrotizing pneumonia and disseminated infections in immunocompromised patients. The significance of its isolation always should be determined after communication with the attending physician and pathologist.

Pyrenochaeta romeroi

Mycetoma caused by *P. romeroi* has been reported from Somalia, India, and South America (24, 31). *P. romeroi* produces soft to firm black granules that are oval, lobulated, and sometimes vermiform. They resemble those of *M. grisea* (50).

In culture, colonies of *P. romeroi* grow fast and are floccose to velvety, with a gray surface and a whitish margin.

The reverse of the colonies is black, with no diffusible pigment. On nutritionally deficient media, such as oat agar in petri dishes, when cultures are subjected to a regimen of near-UV (black-light) irradiation for 12 h and incubation for 12 h in darkness at 25°C, conidiomata (pycnidia) develop after 3 to 4 weeks. The conidiomata are subglobose, 80 to 160 μm in diameter, and dark brick to fawn in color, later becoming dark brown with short necks. They are ostiolate, and setae around ostioles are septate and roughened and measure 80 by 3 to 100 by 3 μm. The conidiophores inside conidiomata are sparse and have lateral branches. Conidiogenous cells are hyaline and are borne on branches or arise directly from cells lining the conidiomatal cavity, which produce hyaline to yellowish, short cylindrical conidia which measure 1.5 by 1.0 to 2.0 by 1.0 μm (44) (Fig. 10).

The close resemblance of the granules produced by *P. romeroi* to those produced by *M. grisea* and the morphologic similarity of the pycnidia formed by some isolates of *M. grisea* and by *P. romeroi* suggest that these two species may be closely related. However, according to Murray and Buckley (40), the two species show serologic differences that allow differentiation between them. Romero and Mackenzie (46) studied culture filtrate and cellular antigens prepared from 14 agents of black grain mycetoma by double diffusion and immunoelectrophoresis. They found up to 90% cross-reactivity among *M. grisea* isolates and between *M. grisea* and *P. mackinnonii* but not between *M. grisea* and *P. romeroi*. Their results suggested that isolates of *M. grisea* were antigenically similar or identical to those of *P. mackinnonii*.

REFERENCES

1. **Ajello, L.** 1962. Epidemiology of human fungus infections, p. 69–83. *In* G. Dalldorf (ed.), *Fungi and Fungous Diseases*. Charles C. Thomas, Publisher, Springfield, Ill.
2. **Ajello, L.** 1978. Animal mycetomas—review, p. 270–275. *In Proceedings, Primer Simposio Internacional de Micetomas*. Universidad Centro Occidental, Barquisimeto, Venezuela.
3. **Ajello, L., W. Kaplan, and F. W. Chandler.** 1980. Dermatophyte mycetomas: fact or friction? p. 135–140. *In Superficial, Cutaneous and Subcutaneous Infections*. Scientific publication no. 396. Pan American Health Organization, Washington, D.C.
4. **Baylet, R., R. Camain, and M. Rey.** 1961. Chamignons de mycetomes isoles des epineux au Senegal. *Bull. Soc. Med. Afr. Noire Lang. Fr.* **6:**317–319.
5. **Borelli, D.** 1959. *Pyrenochaeta romeroi* n. sp. *Rev. Dermatol. Venez.* **1:**325–327.
6. **Borelli, D.** 1962. *Madurella mycetomi* y *Madurella grisea*. *Arch. Venez. Med. Trop. Parasitol. Med.* **4:**195–211.
7. **Borelli, D.** 1976. *Pyrenochaeta mackinnonii* nova species agente de micetoma. *Castellania* **4:**227–234.
8. **Borelli, D.** 1978. *Plenodomus avramii* nova species agente de micetoma, p. 116–126. *In Proceedings, Primer Simposio Internacional de Micetomas*. Universidad Centro Occidental, Barquisimeto, Venezuela.
9. **Borelli, D., R. Zamora, and G. Senabre.** 1976. *Chaetosphaeronema larense* nova specie agente de micetoma. *Gac. Med. Caracas* **84:**307–318.
10. **Brodey, R. S., H. S. Schryver, M. J. Deubler, W. Kaplan, and L. Ajello.** 1967. Mycetoma in a dog. *J. Am. Vet. Med. Assoc.* **151:**442–451.
11. **Butz, W. C., and L. Ajello.** 1971. Black grain mycetoma. *Arch Dermatol.* **104:**197–201.
12. **Campbell, C. K.** 1987. *Polycytella hominis* gen. et sp. nov., a cause of human pale grain mycetoma. *J. Med. Vet. Mycol.* **25:**301–305.
13. **Chandler, F. W., W. Kaplan, and L. Ajello.** 1980. *A Colour Atlas and Textbook of the Histopathology of Mycotic Diseases*. Wolfe Medical Publications Ltd., London, England.
14. **Crous, P. W., W. Gams, M. J. Wingfield, and P. S. van Wyk.** 1996. *Phaeoacremonium* gen. nov. associated with wilt and decline diseases of woody hosts and human infections. *Mycologia* **88:**786–796.
15. **de Albernoz, M. B.** 1974. *Cephalosporium serrae*, agente etiologico de micetomas. *Mycopathol. Mycol. Appl.* **54:** 485–498.
16. **Destombes, P., A. Poirier, and O. Nazimoff.** 1970. Mycoses profundes reconnues en 9 ans de pratique histopathologie a l'Institut Pasteur du Cameroun. *Bull. Soc. Pathol. Exot.* **63:**310–315.
17. **De Vries, G. A., G. S. De Hoog, and H. P. De Bruyn.** 1984. *Phialophora cyanescens* sp. nov., with *Phaeosclera*-like synanamorph, causing white-grain mycetoma in man. *Antonie Leeuwenhoek J. Microbiol. Serol.* **50:**149–153.
18. **El-Ani, A. S.** 1966. A new species of *Leptosphaeria*, an etiologic agent of mycetoma. *Mycologia* **58:**406–411.
19. **El-Ani, A. S., and M. A. Gordon.** 1965. The ascospore sheath and taxonomy of *Leptosphaeria senegalensis*. *Mycologia* **57:**275–278.
20. **Emmons, C. W.** 1962. Soil reservoirs of pathogenic fungi. *J. Wash. Acad. Sci.* **52:**3–9.
21. **Etta, L. L., V. L. R. Peterson, and D. Gerding.** 1983. *Acremonium falciforme* (*Cephalosporium falciforme*) mycetoma in a renal transplant patient. *Arch. Dermatol.* **119:** 707–708.
22. **Fahey, P. J., M. J. Utell, and R. W. Hyde.** 1981. Spontaneous lysis of mycetomas after acute cavitating lung disease. *Am. J. Respir. Dis.* **123:**336–339.
23. **Halde, C., A. A. Padhye, L. D. Haley, M. G. Rinaldi, D. Kay, and R. Leeper.** 1976. *Acremonium falciforme* as a cause of mycetoma in California. *Sabouraudia* **14:**319–326.
24. **Klokke, A. H., G. Swamidasan, R. Anguli, and A. Verghese.** 1968. The causal agents of mycetoma in South India. *Trans. R. Soc. Trop. Med. Hyg.* **62:**509–516.
25. **Lambrechts, N., M. G. Collett, and M. Henton.** 1991. Black grain eumycetoma (*Madurella mycetomatis*) in the abdominal cavity of a dog. *J. Med. Vet. Mycol.* **29:** 211–214.
26. **Mackinnon, J. E.** 1954. A contribution to the study of the causal organisms of maduromycosis. *Trans. R. Soc. Trop. Med. Hyg.* **48:**470–480.
27. **Mackinnon, J. E., I. A. Conti-Diaz, E. Gezuele, and E. Civila.** 1971. Datos sobre ecologia de *Allescheria boydii*, Shear. *Rev. Urug. Pathol. Clin. Microbiol.* **9:**37–43.
28. **Mackinnon, J. E., L. V. Ferrada, and L. Montemayor.** 1949. *Madurella grisea* n. sp., a new species of fungus producing black variety of maduromycosis in South America. *Mycopathol. Mycol. Appl.* **4:**385–392.
29. **Mahgoub, E. S.** 1973. Mycetomas caused by *Curvularia lunata*, *Madurella grisea*, *Aspergillus nidulans*, and *Nocardia brasiliensis* in Sudan. *Sabouraudia* **11:**179–182.
30. **Mahgoub, E. S., and I. Murray.** 1973. *Mycetoma*. William Heinemann Medical Books Ltd., London, England.
31. **Mariat, F., P. Destombes, and G. Segretain.** 1977. The mycetomas: clinical features, pathology, etiology and epidemiology. *Contrib. Microbiol. Immunol.* **4:**1–39.
32. **Matsumoto, T., and L. Ajello.** 1986. No granules, no mycetomas. *Chest* **90:**151–152.
33. **Mayorga, R., and J. E. Close De Leon.** 1966. Sur une souche de *Madurella grisea* sporifere isolee d'un mycetome Guatemalteque a grains noirs. *Sabouraudia* **4:**210–214.
34. **McGinnis, M. R.** 1992. Black fungi: a model for understanding tropical mycosis, p. 129–149. *In* D. H. Walker (ed.), *Global Infectious Diseases, Prevention, Control, and Eradication*. Springer Verlag, New York, N.Y.

35. **McGinnis, M. R.** 1996. Mycetoma. *Dermatol. Clin.* **14:** 97–104.
36. **McGinnis, M. R., and A. A. Padhye.** 1977. *Exophiala jeanselmei*, a new combination for *Phialophora jeanselmei*. *Mycotaxon* **5:**341–352.
37. **McGinnis, M. R., A. A. Padhye, and L. Ajello.** 1982. *Pseudallescheria boydii* Negroni et Fischer, 1943, and its later synonym *Petriellidium* Malloch, 1970. *Mycotaxon* **14:** 94–102.
38. **Milburn, P. B., D. M. Papayanopulos, and B. M. Pomerantz.** 1988. Mycetoma due to *Acremonium falciforme*. *Int. J. Dermatol.* **27:**408–410.
39. **Montes, L. F., R. G. Freeman, and W. McClarin.** 1969. Maduromycosis due to *Madurella grisea*. *Arch. Dermatol.* **99:**74–79.
40. **Murray, I., and H. R. Buckley.** 1969. Serological differences between *Pyrenochaeta romeroi* and *Madurella grisea*. *Sabouraudia* **7:**62–63.
41. **Negroni, R.** 1970. Estudio micologico del primer caso de micetoma por *Phialophora jeanselmei* observado en la Argentina. *Med. Cutan.* **5:**625–630.
42. **Neilson, H. S., N. F. Conant, T. Weinberg, and J. F. Reback.** 1968. Report of a mycetoma due to *Phialophora jeanselmei* and undescribed characteristics of the fungus. *Sabouraudia* **6:**330–333.
43. **Pankovich, A. M., B. J. Auerbach, W. I. Metzer, and T. Barreta.** 1981. Development of maduromycosis (*Madurella mycetomi*) after nailing of a closed tibial fracture. A case report. *Clin. Orthoped. Relat. Res.* **154:**220–222.
44. **Punithalingam, E.** 1979. Sphaeropsidales in culture from humans. *Nova Hedwigia* **37:**119–158.
45. **Pupaibul, K., W. Sindhuphak, and A. Chindaporn.** 1982. Mycetoma of the hand caused by *Phialophora jeanselmei*. *Mykosen* **25:**321–330.
46. **Romero, H., and D. W. R. Mackenzie.** 1989. Studies on antigens from agents causing black grain eumycetoma. *J. Med. Vet. Mycol.* **27:**303–311.
47. **Segretain, G.** 1972. Recherches sue l'ecologie de *Madurella mycetomi* au Senegal. *Bull. Soc. Fr. Mycol. Med.* **3:** 121–124.
48. **Segretain, G.** 1972. Epidemiologie des mycetomes. *Ann. Soc. Belge Med. Trop.* **52:**277–286.
49. **Segretain, G., and P. Destombes.** 1961. Description d'un nouvel agent de maduromycose *Neotestudina rosatii*, n. gen., n. sp. isole en Afrique. *C. R. Acad. Sci.* **253:**2577–2579.
50. **Segretain, G., and P. Destombes.** 1969. Recherches sur mycetomes a *Madurella grisea* et *Pyrenochaeta romeroi*. *Sabouraudia* **7:**51–61.
51. **Segretain, G., and F. Mariat.** 1968. Recherches sue la presence d'agents de mycetomes dans le sol et sur les epineux du Senegal et de la Mauritanie. *Bull. Soc. Pathol. Exot.* **61:** 194–202.
52. **Talwar, P., and S. C. Sehgal.** 1979. Mycetomas of North India. *Sabouraudia* **17:**287–291.
53. **Thammaya, A., and M. Sanyal.** 1980. *Exophiala jeanselmei* causing mycetoma pedis in India. *Sabouraudia* **18:**91–95.
54. **Thianprasit, M., and A. Sivayathorn.** 1984. Black dot mycetoma. *Mykosen* **27:**219–226.
55. **Thirumalachar, M. J., and A. A. Padhye.** 1968. Isolation of *Madurella mycetomi* from soil in India. *Hind. Antibiot. Bull.* **10:**314–318.
56. **Turiansky, G. W., P. M. Benson, L. C. Sperling, P. Sau, I. F. Salkin, M. R. McGinnis, and W. D. James.** 1995. *Phialophora verrucosa*: a new cause of mycetoma. *J. Am. Acad. Dermatol.* **32:**311–315.
57. **Weathered, D. B., M. A. Markey, R. J. Hay, E. S. Mahgoub, and S. A. Gumaa.** 1986. Ultrastructural and immunologic changes in the formation of mycetoma grains. *J. Med. Vet. Mycol.* **25:**39–46.
58. **Witzig, R. S., D. L. Greer, and N. E. Hyslop, Jr.** 1996. *Aspergillus flavus* mycetoma and epidural abscess successfully treated with itraconazole. *J. Med. Vet. Mycol.* **34:** 133–137.
59. **Zoutman, D. E., and L. Sigler.** 1991. Mycetoma of the foot caused by *Cylindrocarpon destructans*. *J. Clin. Microbiol.* **29:**1855–1859.

PARASITOLOGY

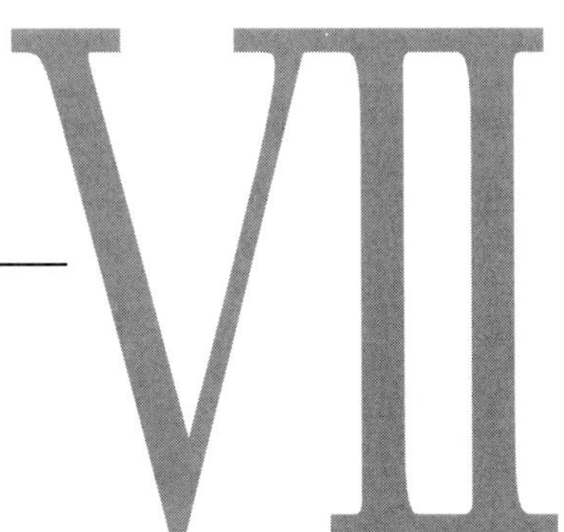

VOLUME EDITOR
MICHAEL A. PFALLER

SECTION EDITOR
LYNNE S. GARCIA

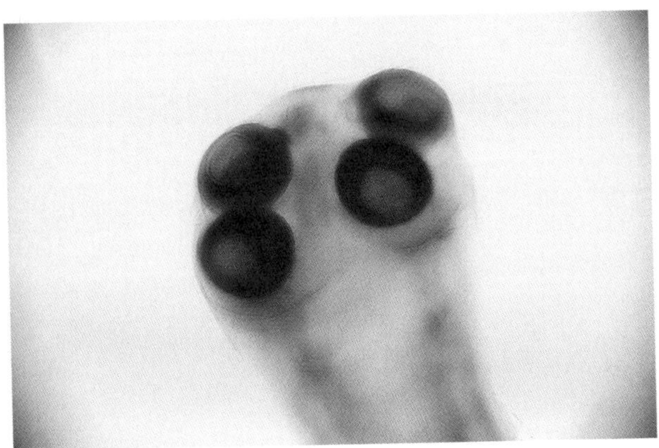

Scolex of *Taenia saginata*, the beef tapeworm.

Taxonomy and Classification of Human Parasites

LYNNE S. GARCIA AND DAVID A. BRUCKNER

103

Although common names are often used to describe parasites and parasitic infections in different parts of the world, this practice may cause confusion when one is trying to determine if the same organism is responsible for infections in different countries or areas. In order to eliminate this problem, a binomial system of nomenclature in which the scientific name consists of the genus and species is used; these names are generally of Greek or Latin origin.

Based on life cycles and morphologic characteristics, classification systems have been developed to indicate the relationship among various parasite species (1–7). Closely related species are placed in the same genus, related genera are placed in the same family, related families are placed in the same order, related orders are placed in the same class, and related classes are placed in the same phylum, one of the major categories in the animal kingdom. As one progresses up the classification schema, each category becomes more broad; however, each category still has characteristics in common.

Parasites of humans are classified into five major divisions. These include the Protozoa (amebae, flagellates, ciliates, sporozoans, coccidia, and microsporidia), the Platyhelminthes or flatworms (cestodes and trematodes), the Acanthocephala or thorny-headed worms, the Nematoda or roundworms, and the Arthropoda (insects, spiders, mites, ticks, and so on). Although these categories appear to be clearly defined, there may be confusion in attempting to classify parasites, often due to the lack of known specimens. If organisms recovered from humans are very rare, it will be difficult to determine their correct taxonomic positions. Type specimens must be deposited for study before a legitimate species name can be given. Also, even when certain parasites are numerous, they may represent strains or races of the same species with slightly different characteristics.

Reproductive mechanisms are frequently used as a valid basis for determining species definitions, but there are many exceptions within parasite groups. Another difficulty in species recognition is the ability and tendency of the organisms to alter their morphologic forms according to age, host, or nutrition, a situation which often results in several names for the same organism. An additional problem involves alternation of parasitic and free-living phases in the life cycle. These organisms may be very different and difficult to recognize as belonging to the same species. However, newer molecular methods of grouping organisms have often confirmed taxonomic conclusions reached hundreds of years before by experienced taxonomists.

As investigations continue in parasitic genetics, immunology, and biochemistry, species designations will be defined more clearly. Originally, these species designations were determined primarily by morphologic differences—a phenotypic approach. With the use of highly sophisticated molecular techniques, the approach will continue to be more genotypic.

The classification of parasites is presented in tabular form in this article. Although certain species designations may be somewhat controversial, this classification scheme is designed to provide some order and meaning to a widely divergent group of organisms. No attempt has been made to include every possible organism, only those that are considered to be clinically relevant in the context of human parasitology. Some human infections are represented by very few cases; however, they are well documented and are included here (1, 3, 4).

PROTOZOA (INTESTINAL)

Amebae

The single-celled organisms known as amebae are characterized by having pseudopods (motility) and trophozoite and cyst stages in the life cycle. However, there are some exceptions in which a cyst form has not been identified. Amebae are usually acquired by humans via fecal-oral transmission or mouth-to-mouth contact (*Entamoeba gingivalis*) (Table 1). In most species, after several nuclear divisions occur, comparable division of the cytoplasm follows excystation. *Entamoeba histolytica* is the most significant organism within this group.

Flagellates

The protozoa known as flagellates move by means of flagella and are acquired through fecal-oral transmission. With the exception of *Dientamoeba fragilis* (internal flagella) and those in the genus *Trichomonas*, they have both trophozoite and cyst stages in the life cycle (Table 1). Reproduction occurs by binary longitudinal fission. *Giardia lamblia* is the most common pathogen within this group.

TABLE 1 Intestinal protozoa found in other body sites: amebae, flagellates, cilliates, coccidia, and microsporidia (1, 3, 7)

Intestinal protozoa			Protozoa found in other body sites		
Classification	Pathogenic	Nonpathogenic	Classification	Pathogenic	Nonpathogenic
Amebae	*Entamoeba histolytica* *Blastocystis hominis*[b]	*Entamoeba dispar*[a] *Entamoeba hartmanni*[c] *Entamoeba coli* *Entamoeba polecki* *Endolimax nana* *Iodamoeba bütschlii*	Amebae (free living)	*Naegleria fowleri* *Acanthamoeba* spp. *Balamuthia mandrillaris* (leptomyxid ameba)	*Entamoeba gingivalis*
Flagellates	*Giardia lamblia*[d] *Dientamoeba fragilis*	*Chilomastix mesnili* *Trichomonas hominis* *Enteromonas hominis* *Retortamonas intestinalis*	Flagellates	*Trichomonas vaginalis*	*Trichomonas tenax*
Ciliates	*Balantidium coli*		Coccidia	*Cryptosporidium parvum* *Toxoplasma gondii*	
Coccidia	*Cryptosporidium parvum* *Cyclospora cayetanensis* *Isospora belli* *Sarcocystis hominis* *Sarcocystis suihominis* "*Sarcocystis lindemanni*"	Although these organisms are listed as pathogens, in some immunocompetent patients they may not cause symptoms and the patients may remain asymptomatic carriers.	Microsporidia	*Nosema connori* *Nosema ocularum* *Pleistophora* spp. *Trachipleistophora hominis* *Encephalitozoon cuniculi* *Encephalitozoon hellem* *Encephalitozoon intestinalis* *Enterocytozoon bieneusi*[e] *Vittaforma corneae* "*Microsporidium*"[f] spp.	Although these organisms are listed as pathogens, in some immunocompetent patients they may not cause symptoms and the patients may remain asymptomatic carriers.
Microsporidia	*Enterocytozoon bieneusi* *Encephalitozoon intestinalis*[g]	Little is known about these infections in immunocompetent patients and how widespread they may be in this population.			

[a] *E. histolytica* is being used to designate pathogenic zymodemes, while *E. dispar* is now being used to designate nonpathogenic zymodemes. However, unless trophozoites containing ingested erthrocytes (*E. histolytica*) are seen, the two organisms cannot be differentiated on the basis of morphology.

[b] The current status of the pathogenicity of *B. hominis* remains somewhat controversial; however, when patients are symptomatic and no other pathogens have been identified, treatment often results in elimination of symptoms. Current recommended therapy for this organism is known to eliminate other intestinal protozoa, some of which are pathogens (*G. lamblia*, *E. histolytica*, and *D. fragilis*), and it is difficult, if not impossible, to determine exactly which infections might have been eliminated.

[c] *E. hartmanni* is nonpathogenic and is totally different from *E. histolytica*. The name "small race *Entamoeba histolytica*" is incorrect and should not be used at any time to designate *E. hartmanni*.

[d] Although some individuals have changed the type species for the genus *Giardia* to *Giardia intestinalis* or *Giardia duodenalis*, there is no general agreement. Therefore, for this listing, we retain the name *Giardia lamblia*.

[e] Although *E. bieneusi* was thought not to disseminate from the gastrointestinal tract, there is evidence that dissemination does occur. Typically, *E. intestinalis* is more likely to disseminate from the gastrointestinal tract to other body sites.

[f] "*Microsporidium*" is not a true genus designation but includes organisms that will never be classified to genus and/or species level. Often, either there is no remaining specimen for examination or the details of the case have been lost over time.

[g] Formerly called *Septata intestinalis*.

Ciliates

The single-celled protozoa known as ciliates move by means of cilia and are acquired through fecal-oral transmission, *Balantidium coli* being the only human pathogen in the group. The cilia beat in a coordinated rhythmic pattern, and the trophozoite moves in a spiral path. Ciliates have both trophozoite and cyst stages in the life cycle, and both stages contain a large macronucleus and a smaller micronucleus. These protozoa have a distinct cell mouth (cytostome) and cytopharynx and a less conspicuous cytopyge (anal pore). These organisms are considerably larger than the majority of the intestinal protozoa and can be mistaken for debris when seen in a permanently stained smear. The concentration-wet preparation examination is recommended (Table 1).

Coccidia

The protozoa known as coccidia are acquired by ingestion of various meats or through fecal-oral transmission via contaminated food and/or water. In some cases, these organisms may disseminate to other body sites, particularly in severely immunocompromised patients. These protozoa have both asexual and sexual cycles. The most common infective stage is the oocyst, containing sporocysts and/or sporozoites, both of which can be acquired through fecal-oral transmission. Representatives within this group include *Cryptosporidium parvum*, *Cyclospora cayetanensis*, *Isospora belli*, and *Sarcocystis* spp. (Table 1).

Microsporidia

At present, the most difficult intestinal protozoa to diagnose are the microsporidia (size range, 1 to 2 μm); the development of molecular methods should provide more specific and sensitive results. These organisms have also been documented to disseminate to other body sites, including the kidneys and lungs. Routine parasitology stains are not useful; modified trichrome stains have been developed specifically for these organisms. The infective form is called the spore; each spore contains a polar tubule that is used to penetrate new host cells, thus initiating or continuing the life cycle. Infections are acquired through ingestion, inhalation, or direct inoculation of spores from the environment. At present, at least two genera have been documented to cause human infections in the intestinal tract (Table 1).

PROTOZOA (OTHER BODY SITES)

Amebae

With the exception of *E. gingivalis* (found in the mouth), pathogenic, free-living amebae may be associated with warm, freshwater environments. They have been found in the central nervous system (CNS), the eye, and other body sites (Table 1). Amebae that invade the CNS (*Naegleria fowleri*) can cause severe, life-threatening infection that often ends in death within a few days. Other amebae in this group (*Acanthamoeba* spp. and *Balamuthia mandrillaris*) can cause more chronic CNS disease, particularly in immunocompromised patients; they can also cause keratitis.

Flagellates

Trichomonas vaginalis is found in the genitourinary system and is usually acquired by sexual transmission. *Trichomonas tenax* can be found in the mouth and is considered to be nonpathogenic (Table 1).

Coccidia

Coccidian parasites are particularly important in immunocompromised patients and can cause life-threatening disease. These organisms can disseminate from the intestinal tract to other body sites. In immunocompetent patients, symptoms may be absent; however, in immunocompromised patients, sequelae may be very serious and life threatening (Table 1).

Microsporidia

As mentioned previously, microsporidia are the most difficult protozoa to diagnose (size range, 1 to 2 μm). Dissemination from the intestine to other body sites has been well documented. Modified trichrome stains have been developed specifically for these organisms, since routine parasitology stains for fecal specimens are not that effective for microsporidial spores. Optical brightening agents are also

TABLE 2 Blood and tissue protozoa: sporozoa and flagellates (1, 3, 7)

Classification	Pathogenic
Sporozoa (malaria and babesiosis)	*Plasmodium vivax* *Plasmodium ovale* *Plasmodium malariae* *Plasmodium falciparum* *Babesia microti* *Babesia* sp.[a] *Babesia bovis* *Babesia divergens*
Flagellates[b] (*Trypanosoma* spp.)	*Trypanosoma brucei gambiense* *Trypanosoma brucei rhodesiense* *Trypanosoma cruzi*
Flagellates (*Leishmania* spp.)	*Leishmania tropica* complex (cutaneous) *L. killicki* *L. tropica* *Leishmania mexicana complex* (cutaneous) *L. amazonensis* *L. garnhami* *L. mexicana* *L. pifanoi* *L. venezuelensis* *Leishmania guyanensis* complex *L. guyanensis* *L. panamensis* *Leishmania braziliensis* complex (mucocutaneous) *L. braziliensis* *L. peruviana* *L. colombiensis* *L. lainsoni* *L. shawii* *L. naiffi* *Leishmania donovani* complex (visceral) (*L. archibaldi*[c])

[a] Unnamed to date. May be related to the canine species *Babesia gibsoni*.

[b] *T. rangeli* trypomastigotes may be confused with *T. cruzi* trypomastigotes. *T. cruzi* causes a very serious disease, often with cardiomyopathy and other sequelae, while *T. rangeli* is considered to be nonpathogenic.

[c] May not be a separate species.

TABLE 3 Nematodes (common and uncommon intestinal, tissue, and blood and tissue infections) (1, 3, 4)

Nematode	Common	Uncommon
Intestinal	*Ascaris lumbricoides*	*Oesophagostomum* spp.[a]
	Enterobius vermicularis	*Oesophagostomum bifurcum*
	Ancylostoma duodenale	*Ternidens deminutus*
	Necator americanus	*Mammamonogamus laryngeus*
	Strongyloides stercoralis	*Physaloptera caucasica*
	Trichostrongylus spp.	*Spirocerca lupi*
	Trichuris trichiura	*Gordius* spp.
	Capillaria philippinensis	*Chordodes capensis*
		Paragordius spp.
		Pseudogordius tanganyikae
		Neochordodes colombianus
Tissue	*Trichinella spiralis*	*Trichinella pseudospiralis*
	Visceral larva migrans (*Toxocara canis* or *Toxocara cati*)	*Eustrongylides* spp.
	Ocular larva migrans (*Toxocara canis* or *Toxocara cati*)	*Micronema deletrix*
	Cutaneous larva migrans (*Ancylostoma braziliense* or *Ancylostoma caninum*)	*Dioctyphyma renale*
	Angiostrongylus cantonensis	*Lagochilascaris minor*
	Angiostrongylus costaricensis	*Gongylonema pulchrum*
	Gnathostoma spinigerum	*Cheilospirura* sp.
	Anisakis spp. (larvae from saltwater fish)	
	Phocanema spp. (larvae from saltwater fish)	
	Contracaecum spp. (larvae from saltwater fish)	
	Pseudoterranova spp. (larvae from saltwater fish)	
	Capillaria hepatica	
	Thelazia spp.	
Blood and tissue	*Wuchereria bancrofti*	*Dirofilaria tenuis*
	Brugia malayi	*Dirofilaria repens*
	Brugia timori	*Dirofilaria ursi*
	Dracunculus medinensis	*Dirofilaria striata*
	Loa loa	*Dirofilaria subdermata*
	Onchocerca volvulus	*Brugia* spp. (may be found in subcutaneous nodules)
	Mansonella perstans	
	Mansonella streptocerca	
	Dirofilaria immitis (usually a lung lesion; in dogs, heartworm)	

[a] *Oesophagostomum* spp. have also been recovered from the abdominal cavity.

recommended; although they are very sensitive, they are nonspecific (Table 1).

PROTOZOA (BLOOD AND TISSUE)

Sporozoa (Malaria and Babesiosis)

All of the sporozoa are arthropod borne (Table 2). The genus *Plasmodium* includes parasites that undergo exoerythrocytic and pigment-producing erythrocytic schizogony in vertebrates and a sexual stage followed by sporogony in mosquitoes. *Babesia* spp. are tick-borne and can cause severe disease in patients who have been splenectomized. Diagnosis may be somewhat more difficult than that of the intestinal protozoa, particularly if automated blood differential systems are used. The microscopic examination of both thick and thin blood films is recommended.

Flagellates (Leishmaniae and Trypanosomes)

The leishmaniae have undergone extensive classification revisions. However, from a clinical perspective, recovery and identification of the organisms are still related to body site. Recovery of leishmanial amastigotes is limited to the site of the lesion in infections other than those caused by the *Leishmania donovani* complex (visceral leishmaniasis) (Table 2). These protozoa have both amastigote (mammalian host) and promastigote (sand fly) stages in the life cycle. Reproduction in both forms occurs by binary longitudinal division.

Flagellates (Trypanosomes)

The trypanosomes are normally identified to the species level based on geographic exposure history and clinical symptoms. These protozoa are characterized by having at some time in the life cycle the trypomastigote form, with the typical undulating membrane and free flagellum at the anterior end. Unfortunately, the longer the duration of the infection, the more difficult it may be to confirm the diagnosis. The organisms that cause African sleeping sickness (*Trypanosoma brucei gambiense* and *Trypanosoma brucei rhodesiense*) generally cause different disease entities, one of which tends to be chronic and with which the patient more typically appears to have sleeping sickness (*T. b. gambiense*) and the other of which causes a more fulminant disease often leading to death prior to the appearance of typical sleeping sickness symptoms (*T. b. rhodesiense*). The etiologic agent of South American trypanosomiasis is *Trypanosoma cruzi*, which contains amastigote and trypomastigote stages in mammalian hosts and the epimastigote form in arthropod hosts.

NEMATODES (INTESTINAL) (ROUNDWORMS)

The largest number of helminthic parasites of humans belongs to the roundworm group. Nematodes are elongate-cylindrical and bilaterally symmetrical, with triradiate symmetry at the anterior end. Nematodes have an outer cuticle layer, no circular muscles, and a pseudocele containing all systems (digestive, excretory, nervous, and reproductive). These organisms are normally acquired by egg ingestion or skin penetration of larval forms from the soil (Table 3).

NEMATODES (TISSUE)

Many nematodes are rarely seen within the United States; however, the first few listed in Table 3 are more important and are found worldwide. Diagnosis may be difficult if the only specimens are obtained through biopsy and/or autopsy and interpretation must be based on examination of histologic preparations.

NEMATODES (BLOOD AND TISSUE) (FILARIAL WORMS)

The nematodes known as filarial worms are also arthropod borne. The adult worms tend to live in the tissues or lymphatics of vertebrate hosts. Diagnosis is made on the basis of the recovery and identification of the larval worms (microfilariae) in the blood, other body fluids, or skin. While circulating in peripheral blood or cutaneous tissues, the microfilariae can be ingested by blood-sucking insects. After the larvae mature, they can escape into the skin of the vertebrate host when the arthropod takes its next blood meal. Severity of disease with these nematodes varies; however, elephantiasis may be associated with some of the organisms listed in Table 3.

ACANTHOCEPHALA (THORNY-HEADED WORMS)

The Acanthocephala are closely related to the tapeworms. These worms are dioecious and tend to have a retractable proboscis which is usually armed with spines. The larvae require an intermediate arthropod host, and the adult worms are always parasites in the intestine of vertebrates. There are two organisms that are parasitic for humans: *Macracanthorhynchus hirudinaceus* and *Moniliformis moniliformis*. Human infection is acquired from the ingestion of infected insects (various beetles and cockroaches).

CESTODES (INTESTINAL) (TAPEWORMS)

The adult form of the tapeworm is acquired through ingestion of the larval form contained in poorly cooked or raw meats or freshwater fish. In the case of *Dipylidium caninum*, infection is acquired by the accidental ingestion of dog fleas. Both *Hymenolepis nana* and *Hymenolepis diminuta* are transmitted via ingestion of certain arthropods (fleas and beetles). Also, *H. nana* can be transmitted through egg ingestion (the life cycle can bypass the intermediate beetle host). The adult tapeworm consists of a chain of egg-producing units called proglottids, which develop from the neck region

TABLE 4 Cestodes (common and uncommon intestinal and tissue infections) (1, 3, 4)

Cestode	Common	Uncommon
Intestinal	*Diphyllobothrium latum*	*Inemicapsifer madagascariensis*
	Dipylidium caninum	*Raillietina celebensis*
	Hymenolepis nana	*Raillietina demerariensis*
	Hymenolepis diminuta	*Mesocestoides* spp.
	Taenia solium	*Bertiella studeri*
	Taenia saginata	*Moniezia* spp.
		Rodentolepia spp.
		Drepanidotaenia spp.
		Diplogonoporus grandis
		Ligula intestinalis
		Taenia spp.
Tissue (larval forms)	*Taenia solium*	*Echinococcus oligarthrus*
	Echinococcus granulosus	*Echinococcus vogeli*
	Echinococcus multilocularis	*Taenia crassiceps*
	Multiceps multiceps	*Spirometra* spp.
	Spirometra mansonoides	*Multiceps* spp.
	Diphyllobothrium spp.	

TABLE 5 Trematodes (common and uncommon blood, liver and lung, and intestinal infections) (1, 3, 4)

Trematode	Common	Uncommon
Blood	*Schistosoma mansoni* *Schistosoma haematobium* *Schistosoma japonicum* *Schistosoma intercalatum* *Schistosoma mekongi*	*Schistosoma rodhaini* *Schistosoma mattheei*
Liver and lung	*Clonorchis* (*Opisthorchis*) *sinensis* *Opisthorchis viverrini* *Fasciola hepatica* *Paragonimus westermani* *Paragonimus mexicanus* *Paragonimus heterotremus*	*Paragonimus africanus* *Paragonimus kellicotti* *Paragonimus miyazakii* *Paragonimus philippinensis* *Paragonimus skrjabini* *Paragonimus uterobilateralis* *Spelotrema brevicaeca* *Opisthorchis felineus*
Intestinal	*Fasciolopsis buski* *Echinostoma ilocanum* *Heterophyes heterophyes* *Metagonimus yokogawai*	*Neodiplostomum* sp. *Echinostoma* spp. *Hypoderaeum conoideum* *Plagiorchis muris* *Nanophyetus* spp. *Echinostoma hortense* *Metagonimus takahashii* *Phaneropsolus spinicirrus* *Paralecithodendrium* spp. *Prosthodendrium* spp. *Gymnophalloides seoi* *Gastrodiscoides hominis* *Himasthla muehlensi* *Paryphostomum sufrartyfex* *Echinochasmus perfoliatus* *Dicrocoelium dendriticum* *Eurytrema pancreaticum* *Plagiorchis philippinensis* *Haplorchis* spp. *Centrocestus* spp. *Diorchitrema formosanum* *Stellantchasmus falcatus* *Centrocestus* spp.

of the attachment organ, the scolex. Food is absorbed through the integument of the worm. The intermediate host contains the larval forms, which are acquired through ingestion of the adult tapeworm eggs. Humans can serve as both intermediate and definitive hosts for *H. nana* and *Taenia solium* infections (Table 4).

CESTODES (TISSUE) (LARVAL FORMS)

The ingestion of certain tapeworm eggs or accidental contact with certain larval forms can lead to tissue infection with *T. solium*, *Echinococcus granulosus*, and several other cestodes (Table 4).

TREMATODES (INTESTINAL) (FLUKES)

Trematodes are flatworms and are exclusively parasitic. With the exception of the schistosomes (blood flukes), flukes are hermaphroditic. They may be flattened, and most have oral and ventral suckers. All of the intestinal trematodes require a freshwater snail to serve as an intermediate host. The infections are food borne (freshwater fish, mollusks, or plants) and are emerging as a major public health problem (>40 million people infected with intestinal and liver or lung trematodes) (Table 5).

TREMATODES (LIVER AND LUNG)

Liver and lung trematodes also require a freshwater snail to serve as an intermediate host. The infections are food borne (freshwater fish, crayfish or crabs, or plants). Public health concerns include cholangiocarcinoma associated with *Clonorchis* and *Opisthorchis* infections, severe liver disease associated with *Fasciola* infections, and the misdiagnosis of tuberculosis in people infected with *Paragonimus* spp. (Table 5).

TREMATODES (BLOOD)

The sexes of schistosomes are separate, and infection is acquired by skin penetration by the cercarial forms that are released from freshwater snails. The males are characterized by having an infolded body that forms the gynecophoral canal in which the female worm is held during copulation and oviposition. The adult worms reside in the blood vessels of the small intestine, large intestine, or bladder. Although these parasites are not endemic within the United States, patients who may have acquired schistosomiasis elsewhere are seen (Table 5).

REFERENCES

1. **Beaver, C. B., R. C. Jung, and E. W. Cupp.** 1984. *Clinical Parasitology*. Lea & Febiger, Philadelphia, Pa.
2. **Galan-Puchades, M. T., M. V. Fuentes, and S. Mas-Coma.** 1997. Human *Bertiella studeri* in Spain, probably of African origin. *Am. J. Trop. Med. Hyg.* **56:**610–612.
3. **Garcia, L. S., and D. A. Bruckner.** 1997. *Diagnostic Medical Parasitology*, 3rd ed. ASM Press, Washington, D.C.
4. **Gibson, D. I.** 1998. Nature and classification of parasitic helminths, p. 453–477. *In* L. Collier, A. Balows, and M. Susman (ed.), *Topley & Wilson's Microbiology and Microbial Infections*. Oxford University Press, New York, N.Y.
5. **Goddard, J.** 1996. *Arthropods of Medical Importance*, 2nd ed. CRC Press, Inc., New York, N.Y.
6. **Hong, S. J., H. C. Woo, and J. Y. Chai.** 1996. A human case of *Plagiorchis muris* (Tanabe, 1922: Digenea) infection in the Republic of Korea: freshwater fish as a possible source of infection. *J. Parasitol.* **82:**647–649.
7. **Murray, P. R., E. J. Baron, M. A. Pfaller, F. C. Tenover, and R. H. Yolken (ed.).** 1995. *Manual of Clinical Microbiology*, 6th ed. American Society for Microbiology, Washington, D.C.

Algorithms for Detection and Identification of Parasites

LYNNE S. GARCIA, ROBYN Y. SHIMIZU, AND JOSEPHINE C. PALMER

104

This chapter discusses various approaches and diagnostic methods currently in use for the diagnosis of parasitic infections. Assuming that clinical specimens have been properly collected and processed according to specific specimen rejection and acceptance criteria, the examination of prepared wet mounts, concentrated specimens, permanent stained smears, blood films, and various culture materials can provide critical information leading to organism identification and confirmation of the suspected cause of clinical disease. With the exception of relatively few immunoassay diagnostic kits, the majority of this diagnostic work depends on the knowledge and microscopy skills of the microbiologist. The field of diagnostic parasitology has taken on greater importance during the past few years for a number of reasons. Expanded world travel has increased the potential levels of exposure to a number of infectious agents. It is important to be aware of those organisms commonly found within certain areas of the world and the makeup of the patient population being serviced at your institution, particularly if immunocompromised patients are frequently seen as a part of your routine patient population. It is also important for the physician and microbiologist to recognize and understand the efficacy of any diagnostic method for parasite recovery and identification. Specific information on specimen collection and processing can be found in chapters 4 and 5.

STOOL SPECIMENS

For review, options for the collection of fecal specimens are presented in Table 1. Algorithms for the processing of stool specimens are presented in Figs. 1 to 3. The procedures that normally comprise the ova and parasite (O&P) examination are provided below and include the direct wet mount in saline, the concentration, and the permanent stained smear (4, 9, 10, 15).

Direct Wet Mount in Saline

The purpose of a direct wet mount is to confirm the possibility of infection with certain protozoa and helminths, to assess the worm burden of the patient, and to look for organism motility (Table 2) (4, 6, 10). Any fresh stool specimens that have not been refrigerated and that have been delivered to the laboratory within specified time frames are acceptable for testing. Low-power examination (magnification, ×100) of the entire coverslip preparation and high dry power examination (magnification, ×400) of at least one-third of the coverslip area are recommended before the preparation is considered negative. Often, results from the direct smear examination should be considered presumptive; however, some organisms (*Giardia lamblia* cysts, *Entamoeba coli* cysts, *Iodamoeba bütschlii* cysts, helminth eggs and larvae, *Isospora belli* oocysts) can be identified. Reports of results obtained by this method should be considered preliminary, with the final report available after the results of the concentration wet mount and permanent stained smear are available.

If iodine is added to the preparation for increased contrast, the organisms will be killed and motility will be lost. Specimens that arrive in the laboratory in stool preservatives do not require a direct smear examination; proceed to the concentration and permanent stained smear.

Concentration Wet Mount

The purpose of the concentration method is to separate parasites from fecal debris and to concentrate any parasites present through either sedimentation or flotation (4, 6, 10). The concentration is specifically designed to allow recovery of protozoan cysts, coccidian oocysts, microsporidian spores, and helminth eggs and larvae (Table 3). Any stool specimen that is fresh or preserved is acceptable for testing. Wet mounts prepared from concentrated stool are examined in the same manner used for the direct wet mount method. The addition of too much iodine may obscure helminth eggs (the eggs may resemble debris). Often, results from the concentration examination should be considered presumptive; however, some organisms (*G. lamblia* cysts, *E. coli* cysts, *I. bütschlii* cysts, helminth eggs and larvae, *I. belli* oocysts) can be identified. Reports of results obtained by this method should be considered preliminary, with the final report available after the results of the permanent stained smear are available.

The formalin-ethyl acetate sedimentation concentration procedure is the most commonly used procedure, and the recommended centrifugation speed and time are 500 × *g* and 10 min, respectively. The standard zinc sulfate flotation procedure will not detect operculated or heavy eggs; both the surface film and sediment should be examined before a negative result is reported.

TABLE 1 Fecal specimens for parasites: options for collection and processing[a]

Option	Pros	Cons
Rejection of stools from inpatients who have been in-house for >3 days.	Patients may become symptomatic with diarrhea after they have been inpatients for a few days; symptoms are usually not attributed to parasitic infections but generally other causes.	There is always the chance that the problem is related to a nosocomial parasitic infection (rare), but *Cryptosporidium* and microsporidia may be possible considerations.
Examination of a single stool.	Some feel that most intestinal parasitic infections can be diagnosed from examination of a single stool specimen.	Diagnosis from examinations of a single stool specimen depends on the experience of the microscopist, proper collection, and parasite load in specimen. In a series of three stool specimens, frequently not all three specimens are positive and/or may be positive for different organisms.
Examine a second stool specimen only after the first one is negative and the patient is still symptomatic.	With additional examinations, yield of protozoa increases (*E. histolytica*, 22.7%; *G. lamblia*, 11.3%; and *D. fragilis*, 31.1%).	Assumes that the second (or third) stool specimen is collected within the recommended 10-day time frame for a series of stools; protozoa are shed periodically. May be inconvenient for patient.
Examination of a single stool specimen and a screen (EIA, FA) (*Giardia* screen).	If the examinations are negative and the patient's symptoms subside, then no further testing is probably required.	Patients may exhibit symptoms (off and on), so it may be difficult to rule out parasitic infections with only a single stool and screen. If the patient remains symptomatic, then even if the *Giardia* screen is negative, other protozoa may be missed (*E. histolytica*, *D. fragilis*).
Pool three specimens for examination; perform one concentrate and one permanent stain.	Three specimens are collected over 7–10 days and may save time and expense.	Organisms present in low numbers may be missed due to the dilution factor.
Pool three specimens for examination; perform a single concentrate on the pooled specimen and three permanent stained smears, one from each of the three specimens.	Three specimens are collected over 7–10 days; would maximize recovery of protozoa in areas of the country where these organisms are most common.	Might miss light helminth infection (eggs, larvae) due to the pooling of the three specimens for the concentration; however, with a permanent stain performed on each of the three specimens, this approach would probably be the next best option in lieu of the standard approach (concentration and permanent stained smear performed on every stool specimen).
Actually collect three stool specimens but put sample of stool from all three into a single vial (patient given a single vial only).	Pooling of the specimens would require only a single vial.	This would complicate patient collection and very likely result in poorly preserved specimens, especially regarding the recommended ratio of stool to preservative.
Screen selected patients[b] by FA or EIA methods for *G. lamblia* and/or *C. parvum*. Screening every stool is not cost-effective, and positivity rate will be low unless outbreak situation.	Would be more cost-effective than screening all specimens.	Laboratories rarely receive information that would allow them to place a patient in a particular risk group: children ≤5 yr old, children from day-care centers (may or may not be symptomatic), patients with immunodeficiencies, and patients from outbreaks.
Perform FA or EIA screening on request[b] for *G. lamblia* and/or *C. parvum*.	Will limit number of stools screened for parasites by this approach.	Will require education of the physician clients regarding appropriate times and patients for which screens should be ordered.

[a] The table is based on previously published data (4, 5, 7, 11). Decisions on procedures for routine O&P examination must be based on clinical needs and the population being tested. Laboratories must notify clinicians regarding what tests are performed when a routine O&P is ordered.

[b] It is difficult to know when you may be in an early outbreak situation where screening of all specimens for either *G. lamblia* or *C. parvum*, or both, may be relevant. Extensive efforts are under way to encourage communication among laboratories, water companies, pharmacies, and public health officials regarding the identification of potential or actual outbreaks.

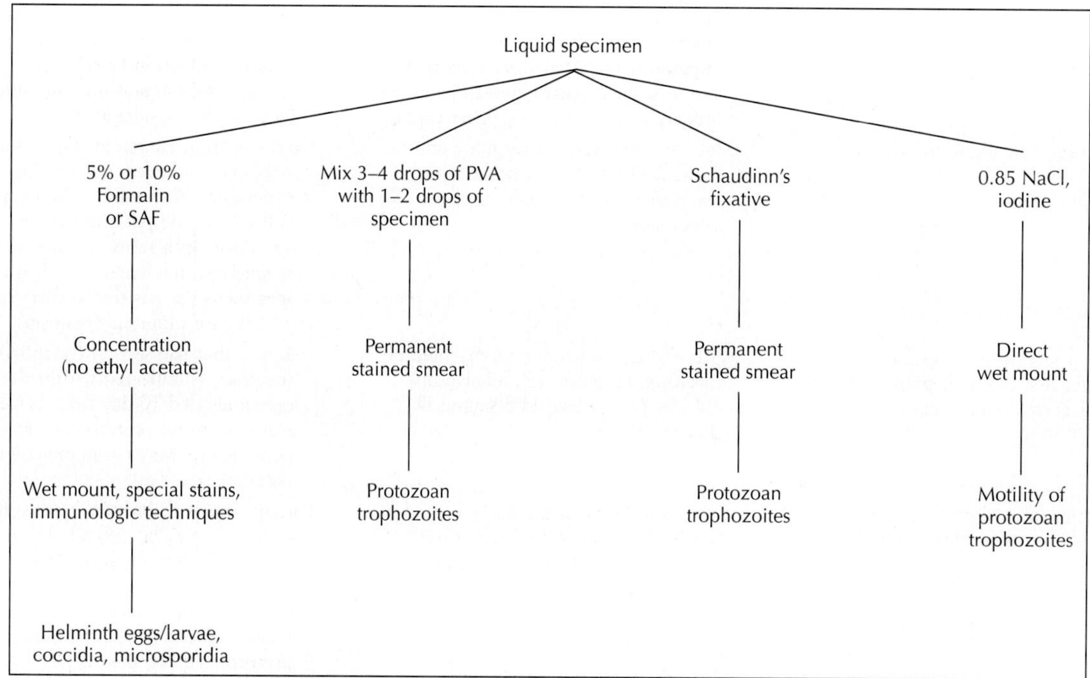

FIGURE 1 Processing liquid stool for O&P examination.

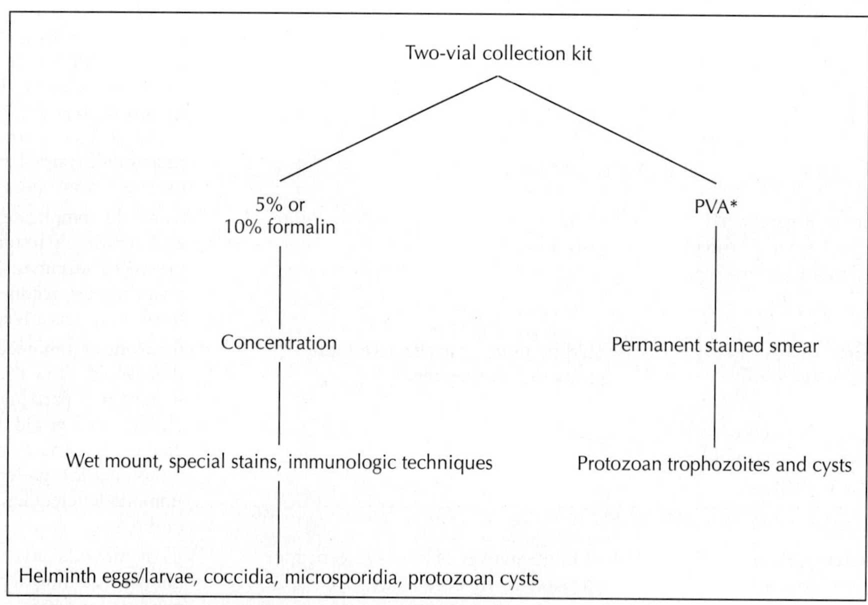

FIGURE 2 Processing preserved stool for O&P examination (two-vial collection kit). *Mercuric chloride is the best PVA. Alternatives are available, including zinc-based PVA, copper sulfate-based PVA, and SAF.

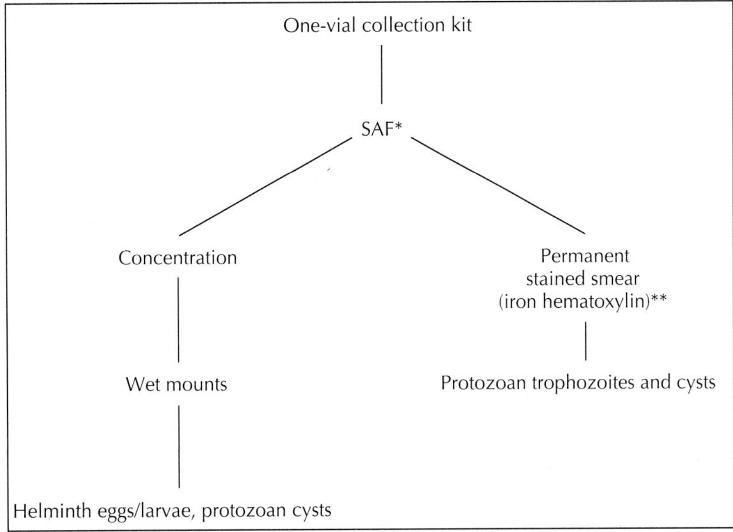

FIGURE 3 Processing preserved stool for O&P examination (one-vial collection kit). *Zinc-based PVA may be used as a one-vial collection kit; **if iron hematoxylin staining method containing the carbol fuchsin step is used, then the coccidia will stain pink.

Permanent Stained Smears

Trichrome or Iron-Hematoxylin

The permanent stained smear is prepared to provide contrasting colors for both the background debris and the parasites present (Table 4) (4, 10). Permanent stained stool smears are designed to allow examination and recognition of detailed organism morphology under oil immersion magnification (magnification, ×1,000). This method is primarily designed to allow the recovery and identification of the more common intestinal protozoan trophozoites and cysts, excluding the coccidia and microsporidia (Tables 5 and 6). Oil immersion examination of a minimum of 300 oil immersion fields is recommended; additional fields may be required if suspect organisms have been seen in the wet mounts.

Modified Acid-Fast Staining

The modified acid-fast staining method is used to provide contrasting colors for both the background debris and the parasites present and to allow examination and recognition of the acid-fast characteristic of the organisms under high dry magnification (magnification, ×400) (4, 14). Organisms that can be identified with this stain include coccidia such as *Cryptosporidium parvum*, *Cyclospora cayetanensis*, and *I. belli*; it is important to remember that *C. cayetanensis* will stain much more acid-fast variable than *C. parvum*. Although some microsporidian spores are acid-fast positive, their small size will make recognition very difficult. Oil immersion examination of a minimum of 300 oil immersion fields is recommended.

Both hot and cold methods are excellent for staining coccidian oocysts. Limitations of the procedure are generally related to specimen handling, including proper collection and centrifugation speed and time.

Modified Trichrome

Modified trichrome stains were primarily designed to allow recovery and identification of microsporidial spores from centrifuged stool specimens; internal morphology (horizontal and diagonal stripes of the polar tubule) may be seen in some spores under oil immersion (magnification, ×1,000). Any stool specimen that is submitted fresh or preserved in formalin or sodium acetate-acetic acid-formalin (SAF) is acceptable. Oil immersion examination of a minimum of 300 oil immersion fields is recommended. The identification

TABLE 2 Diagnostic characteristics of organisms in wet mounts

Specimen	Protozoa	Helminths
Stool, other specimens from gastrointestinal tract, urogenital system	Size, shape, stage (trophozoite, precyst, cyst, oocyst), motility (fresh specimens only), refractility, cytoplasm inclusions (chromatoidal bars, glycogen vacuoles, axonemes, axostyles, median bodies, sporozoites)	Egg, larvae, or adult; size; internal structure: Egg: embryonated, opercular shoulders, abopercular thickenings or projections, hooklets, polar filaments, spines Larvae: head and tail morphology, digestive tract Adult: nematode, cestode, or trematode

TABLE 3 Key to identification of helminth eggs[a]

1.	Eggs nonoperculate (no "trap door"), spherical or subspherical, containing a six-hooked embryo (oncosphere); thick or thin shell	2
	Eggs other than described above	5
2.	Eggs passed separately	3
	Eggs passed in packets of 12 or more	*Dipylidium caninum* (dog tapeworm)
3.	Thick, radially striated shell (six-hooked oncosphere may not be visible in every egg from formalinized fecal specimens) (eggs cannot be identified to species level without special stains)	*Taenia* spp. (*T. saginata*, beef tapeworm) (*T. solium*, pork tapeworm)
	Thin egg shell, clear space between shell and developing embryo	4
4.	Polar filaments (filamentous strands) present between thin egg shell and six-hooked embryo	*Hymenolepis nana* (dwarf tapeworm)
	No polar filaments (filamentous strands) present between egg shell and embryo; size somewhat larger	*Hymenolepis diminuta* (rat tapeworm)
5.	Egg operculate, generally oval ("trap door" at one end of the egg)	6
	Egg nonoperculate, generally oval	10
6.	Egg <35 μm long	*Clonorchis* (*Opisthorchis*) spp. (Chinese liver fluke) or *Heterophyes heterophyes* or *Metagonimus yokogawai*
	Egg ≥38 μm long	7
7.	Egg 38–45 μm long	*Dicrocoelium dendriticum*
	Egg over 60 μm long	8
8.	Egg with opercular shoulders into which the operculum fits (looks like teapot lid and flange into which lid fits), abopercular end thickened (sometimes hard to see)	*Paragonimus westermani* (lung fluke)
	Egg without opercular shoulders	9
9.	Egg >85 μm long, operculum break in shell sometimes hard to see; smooth transition from shell to operculum	*Fasciolopsis buski* (giant intestinal fluke) or *Fasciola hepatica* (sheep liver fluke) or *Echinostoma* spp.
	Egg <75 μm long, operculum break in shell sometimes hard to see; smooth transition from shell to operculum	*Diphyllobothrium latum* (broad fish tapeworm)
10.	Egg ≥75 μm long, spined, ciliated miracidium larva may be seen	11
	Egg <75 μm long, not spined	13
11.	Spine terminal (check for egg viability)	*Schistosoma haematobium* (blood fluke-urine)
	Spine lateral	12
12.	Lateral spine very short (hard to see) (check for egg viability)	*Schistosoma japonicum* (blood fluke-stool)
	Lateral spine prominent and easily seen (check for egg viability)	*Schistosoma mansoni* (blood fluke-stool)
13.	Egg with thick, tuberculated (mammilated/bumpy) capsule (in decorticate egg, capsule will be absent, occurs in both fertilized and unfertilized eggs)	*Ascaris lumbricoides* (large roundworm)
	Egg without thick, tuberculated capsule	14
14.	Egg barrel-shaped, with clear polar plugs	15
	Egg not barrel-shaped, no polar plugs	16
15.	Shell nonstriated	*Trichuris trichiura* (whipworm)
	Shell striated	*Capillaria hepatica*
16.	Egg flattened on one side, may contain larva	*Enterobius vermicularis* (pinworm)
	Egg symmetrical	17
17.	Egg with large blue-green globules at poles	*Heterodera marioni*
	Egg without polar globules	18
18.	Egg bluntly rounded at ends, 56–76 μm long, thin shell (contains developing embryo at 8–16 stage of development)	Hookworm
	Egg pointed at one or both ends, 73–95 μm long	*Trichostrongylus* spp.

[a] Adapted from Markell et al. (9).

TABLE 4 Diagnostic characteristics of organisms in permanent stained smears

Specimen	Protozoa	Helminths
Stool, other specimens from gastrointestinal tract, urogenital system	Size, shape, stage (trophozoite, precyst, cyst, oocyst, spore) Nuclear arrangement, cytoplasm inclusions (chromatoidal bars, vacuoles, axonemes, axostyles, median bodies, sporozoites, polar tubules)	Eggs, larvae, and/or adults may not be identified because of excess stain retention or distortion

TABLE 5 Key to identification of intestinal amebae (permanent stained smear)

1.	Trophozoites present	2
	Cysts present	7
2.	Trophozoites >12 μm	3
	Trophozoites <12 μm	4
3.	Karyosome central, compact; peripheral nuclear chromatin evenly arranged; "clean" cytoplasm	*Entamoeba histolytica*[a]
	Karyosome eccentric, spread out; peripheral nuclear chromatin unevenly arranged; "dirty" cytoplasm	*Entamoeba coli*
4.	Peripheral nuclear chromatin	5
	Other than peripheral nuclear chromatin	6
5.	Karyosome central, compact; peripheral nuclear chromatin evenly arranged; "clean" cytoplasm	*Entamoeba hartmanni*
	Karyosome large, blotlike; extensive nuclear variation	*Endolimax nana*
6.	No peripheral chromatin, karyosome large, junky cytoplasm	*Iodamoeba bütschlii*
	No peripheral chromatin, karyosome variable, clean cytoplasm	*Endolimax nana*
7.	Cysts measure >10 μm (including any shrinkage "halo")	8
	Cysts measure <10 μm (including any shrinkage "halo")	10
8.	Single *Entamoeba*-like nucleus with large inclusion mass	*Entamoeba polecki*[b]
	Multiple nuclei	9
9.	Four *Entamoeba*-like nuclei, chromatoidal bars have smooth, rounded ends	*Entamoeba histolytica*[a]
	Five or more *Entamoeba*-like nuclei, chromatoidal bars have sharp, pointed ends	*Entamoeba coli*
10.	Single nucleus (may be "basket" nucleus), large glycogen vacuole	*Iodamoeba bütschlii*
	Multiple nuclei	11
11.	Four *Entamoeba*-like nuclei, chromatoidal bars have smooth, rounded ends (nuclei may also number only two)	*Entamoeba hartmanni*
	Four karyosomes, no peripheral chromatin, round to oval shape	*Endolimax nana*

[a] *E. histolytica* is *E. histolytica/E. dispar*. *E. histolytica* (pathogenic) can be determined by finding erythrocytes in the cytoplasm of the trophozoites. Otherwise, on the basis of morphological grounds *E. histolytica* (pathogen) and *E. dispar* (nonpathogen) cannot be differentiated.

[b] It is very difficult to differentiate *E. polecki* trophozoites from *E. histolytica* or *E. coli*.

TABLE 6 Key to identification of intestinal flagellates

1.	Trophozoites present	2
	Cysts present	7
2.	Pear shaped	3
	Shape other	6
3.	Two nuclei, sucking disk present	*Giardia lamblia*
	One nucleus present	4
4.	Costa length of body	*Trichomonas hominis*
	No costa	5
5.	Cytostome present, >10 μm	*Chilomastix mesnili*
	Cytostome present, <10 μm	*Retortamonas intestinalis* or *Enteromonas hominis*
6.	Amoeba shaped, one or two fragmented nuclei	*Dientamoeba fragilis*
	Oval shaped, one nucleus	*Enteromonas hominis*
7.	Oval or round shape cyst	8
	Lemon-shaped cyst	9
8.	Four nuclei, median bodies, axoneme, >10 μm	*Giardia lamblia*
	Two nuclei, no fibrils, <10 μm	*Enteromonas hominis*
9.	One nucleus, curved fibril (shepherd's crook)	*Chilomastix mesnili*
	One nucleus, bird's beak fibril	*Retortamonas intestinalis*

TABLE 7 Commercially available immunologic methods for detection of intestinal parasites

Fresh stool	Preserved in 5–10% formalin or SAF	
No concentration	No concentration	Concentration
EIA	EIA	DFA[a]
Cryptosporidium spp.	*Cryptosporidium* spp.	*Cryptosporidium* spp.
G. lamblia	*G. lamblia*	*G. lamblia*
E. histolytica		
E. histolytica/E. dispar		

[a] DFA, direct fluorescent-antibody assay.

of microsporidial spores may be possible; however, their small size will make recognition difficult, particularly in infections with few organisms in the clinical specimen.

Immunologic Methods

Immunoassay reagents are now available commercially for several of the protozoan parasites, including *G. lamblia*, *C. parvum*, and *Entamoeba histolytica-Entamoeba dispar* (Table 7). These methods (enzyme immunoassay [EIA] and fluorescent-antibody assay [FA]) are designed to detect the antigens of select organisms; a negative result does not rule out the possibility that other intestinal parasites are etiologic agents causing disease, including *Dientamoeba fragilis*, the microsporidia, and helminth parasites.

ADDITIONAL TECHNIQUES FOR STOOL EXAMINATION

Although the routine O&P examination consisting of the direct wet mount, the concentration, and the permanent stained smear is an excellent procedure recommended for the detection of most intestinal parasites, several other diagnostic techniques are available for the recovery and identification of specific parasitic organisms (1, 2, 4). Most laboratories do not routinely offer all of these techniques, but many can be performed relatively simply and inexpensively. Occasionally, it is necessary to examine stool specimens for the presence of scolices and proglottids of cestodes and adult nematodes and trematodes to confirm the diagnosis and/or for species identification (Table 8). A method for the recovery of these stages is also described in this chapter.

Culture of Larval-Stage Nematodes

Nematode infections giving rise to larval stages that hatch in soil or in tissues may be diagnosed by using fecal culture methods to concentrate the larvae (1, 4, 6). *Strongyloides stercoralis* larvae are the most common larvae found in stool specimens. Depending on the fecal transit time through the intestine and the patient's condition, rhabditiform and filariform larvae may be present. Caution must be exercised when handling larval cultures because infective filariform larvae may be present. If there is a delay in the preservation of the stool specimen, then embryonated ova as well as larvae of hookworm may be present. Culture of feces for larvae is useful for (i) revealing their presence when they are too scanty to be detected by concentration methods, (ii) distinguishing whether the infection is due to *S. stercoralis* or hookworm on the basis of rhabditiform larval morphology by allowing hookworm egg hatching to occur, releasing first-stage larvae, and (iii) allowing the development of larvae into the filariform stage for further differentiation.

Fecal culture methods are especially helpful for the detection of light infections with hookworm, *S. stercoralis*, and *Trichostrongylus* spp. and for the specific identification of parasites. Also, such techniques are useful for obtaining a large number of infective-stage larvae for research purposes. Several culture techniques and one enhanced recovery method are described in this chapter. Since these procedures are less common, brief descriptions are included.

TABLE 8 Additional helminth recovery and identification techniques (other than O&P examination)

Organism	Specimen	Procedure
Nematodes		
S. stercoralis	Fresh stool, not refrigerated (all organisms can be recovered by any of the procedures indicated in the column to the right)	Harada-Mori filter paper strip
Hookworm		Filter paper/slant culture
Trichostrongylus spp.		Charcoal culture
		Baermann test
		Agar plate culture (primarily for *S. stercoralis*)
Hookworm	Fresh stool, refrigeration acceptable	Direct smear (Beaver)
Ascaris lumbricoides		Dilution egg count (Stoll)
Trichuris trichiura		Either method acceptable for estimation of worm burden
Enterobius vermicularis	Scotch tape preparations, paddles, anal swab	Direct microscopic examination
Trematodes		
Schistosoma spp.	Fresh stool, not refrigerated	Egg hatching test
	Fresh urine (24 h and single collection)	Egg viability test
Cestodes		
Tapeworms	Proglottids (gravid in alcohol)	India ink injection
	Stool in 5–10% formalin	Scolex search

Harada-Mori Filter Paper Strip Culture

To detect light infections with hookworm, *S. stercoralis*, and *Trichostrongylus* spp., as well as to facilitate specific identification, the Harada-Mori filter paper strip culture technique is very useful (1, 4). The technique requires filter paper to which fresh fecal material is added and a test tube into which the filter paper is inserted. Moisture is provided by adding water to the tube, which continuously soaks the filter paper by capillary action. Incubation under suitable conditions favors hatching of ova and/or development of larvae. Fecal specimens to be cultured should not be refrigerated, since some parasites are susceptible to cold and may fail to develop after refrigeration. Also, caution must be exercised in handling the filter paper strip itself, since infective *Strongyloides* larvae may migrate upward as well as downward on the paper strip.

Filter Paper/Slant Culture Technique (Petri Dish)

An alternative technique for culturing *Strongyloides* larvae is a filter paper/slant culture on a microscope slide placed in a glass or plastic petri dish (4). As with the techniques described above, sufficient moisture is provided by continuous soaking of filter paper in water. Fresh stool material is placed on filter paper, which is cut to fit the dimensions of a standard (1- by 3-in.) microscope slide. The filter paper is then placed on a slanted glass slide in a glass or plastic petri dish containing water. This technique allows direct examination of the culture system with a dissecting microscope to look for nematode larvae and free-living stages of *S. stercoralis* in the fecal mass or the surrounding water without having to sample the preparation.

Baermann Technique

Another method of examining a stool specimen suspected of having small numbers of *Strongyloides* larvae is the use of a modified Baermann apparatus. The Baermann technique uses a funnel apparatus and relies on the principle that active larvae will migrate from a fresh fecal specimen that has been placed on a wire mesh with several layers of gauze which are in contact with tap water (4). Larvae migrate through the gauze into the water and settle to the bottom of the funnel, where they can be collected and examined. The main difference between this method and the Harada-Mori and petri dish methods is the greater amount of fresh stool used, possibly providing a better chance of larval recovery in a light infection. Besides being used for patient fecal specimens, this technique can be used to examine soil specimens for the presence of larvae.

Agar Plate Culture for *S. stercoralis*

Agar plate cultures are also recommended for the recovery of *S. stercoralis* larvae and tend to be more sensitive than some of the other diagnostic methods (4). Stool is placed onto agar plates, and the plates are sealed to prevent accidental infections and are held for 2 days at room temperature. As the larvae crawl over the agar, they carry bacteria with them, thus creating visible tracks over the agar. The plates are examined under the microscope for confirmation of the presence of larvae, the surface of the agar is then washed with 10% formalin, and final confirmation of larval identification is made via wet examination of the sediment from the formalin washings.

Egg Studies

Estimation of Worm Burdens

The only human parasites for which it is reasonably possible to correlate egg production with adult worm burdens are *Ascaris lumbricoides*, *Trichuris trichiura*, and the hookworms (*Necator americanus* and *Ancylostoma duodenale*). The specific instances in which information on approximate worm burdens is useful are when one is determining the intensity of infection, deciding on possible chemotherapy, and evaluating the efficacies of the drugs administered. With current therapy, the need for the monitoring of therapy through egg counts is no longer as relevant. However, we discuss below several methods that can be used if necessary. Remember that egg counts are estimates; you will obtain count variations regardless of how carefully you follow the procedure. If two or more fecal specimens are being compared, it is best to have the same individual perform the technique with both samples and to do multiple counts. A number of methods have been described (1, 4, 6, 8, 10, 12).

Hatching of Schistosome Eggs

When schistosome eggs are recovered from either urine or stool, they should be carefully examined to determine viability. The presence of living miracidia within the eggs indicates an active infection that may require therapy. The viability of the miracidia can be determined in two ways: (i) the cilia of the flame cells (primitive excretory cells) may be seen on a wet smear by using high dry power and are usually actively moving and (ii) the miracidia may be released from the eggs by the use of a hatching procedure (4). The eggs will usually hatch within several hours when placed in 10 volumes of dechlorinated or spring water (hatching may begin soon after contact with the water). The eggs that are recovered in the urine (24-h specimen collected with no preservatives) are easily obtained from the sediment and can be examined under the microscope to determine viability. A sidearm flask has been recommended, but an Erlenmeyer flask is an acceptable substitute.

Both urine and stool specimens must be collected without preservatives and should not be refrigerated prior to processing. Hatching will not occur until the saline is removed and nonchlorinated water is added. If a stool concentration is performed, use saline throughout the procedure to prevent premature hatching. Make sure that the light is not too close to the side arm or top layer of water in the Erlenmeyer flask. Excess heat will kill the miracidia. The absence of live miracidia does not rule out the presence of schistosome eggs. Nonviable eggs or eggs that failed to hatch will not be detected by this method. Microscopic examination of direct or concentrated specimens should be used to demonstrate the presence or absence of eggs. Egg viability can be determined by placing some stool or urine sediment (the same material used for the hatching flask) on a microscope slide. Low-power magnification (×100) can be used to locate the eggs. Individual eggs can be examined with high dry magnification (×400); moving cilia on the flame cells (primitive excretory system) will confirm egg viability.

Search for Tapeworm Scolex

Since therapy for the elimination of tapeworms is usually very effective, a search for the tapeworm scolex is rarely requested and is no longer that clinically relevant. However, stool specimens may have to be examined for the presence of scolices and gravid proglottids of cestodes for proper species identification. This procedure requires mixing a small amount of feces with water and straining the mixture through a series of wire screens (graduated from coarse to fine mesh) to look for scolices and proglottids. Remember to use universal precautions and to wear gloves when performing this procedure. The appearance of scolices after therapy is an indication of successful treatment. If the scolex has not been passed, it may still be attached to the mucosa;

the parasite is capable of producing more segments from the neck region of the scolex, and the infection continues.

EXAMINATION OF OTHER SPECIMENS FROM THE INTESTINAL TRACT

Examination for Pinworm

A roundworm parasite that has a worldwide distribution and that is commonly found in children is *Enterobius vermicularis*, known as pinworm or seatworm. The adult female worm migrates out of the anus, usually at night, and deposits her eggs on the perianal area. The adult female (8 to 13 mm long) may occasionally be found on the surface of a stool specimen or on the perianal skin. Since the eggs are usually deposited around the anus, they are not commonly found in feces and must be detected by other diagnostic techniques. Diagnosis of pinworm infection is usually based on the recovery of typical eggs, which are described as thick-shelled, football-shaped eggs with one slightly flattened side. Each egg will often contain a fully developed embryo and will be infective within a few hours after being deposited. Commercial paddles are available and can be used for specimen collection, similar to the approach with cellulose tape indicated below. Some clinicians may treat patients on the basis of clinical symptoms without confirmation of the suspected diagnosis of pinworm infection.

Cellulose Tape Preparations

The most widely used procedure for the diagnosis of pinworm infection is the cellulose tape (adhesive cellophane tape) method (2, 4, 8, 9). Several commercial collection procedures are also available. Specimens should be obtained in the morning, before the patient bathes or goes to the bathroom. The tape is applied to the anal folds and is then placed sticky side down on a microscope slide for examination. At least four to six consecutive negative slides should be observed before the patient is considered free of infection.

Anal Swabs

The anal swab technique (4) is also available for the detection of pinworm infections; however, most laboratories use the cellulose tape method because it eliminates the necessity of preparing and storing swabs. At least four consecutive negative preparations should be observed before the patient is considered negative; some recommend six consecutive negative preparations.

A parrafin-coated swab should be gently rubbed over the perianal surface and into the folds. Place the swab into the anal opening about 1/4 in. and then replace the swab in the tube. The tube containing the swab is half filled with xylene substitute and is allowed to stand for a few minutes. After centrifugation, the sediment is examined microscopically for the presence of eggs.

Sigmoidoscopy Material

Material obtained from sigmoidoscopy can be helpful in the diagnosis of amebiasis that has not been detected by routine fecal examinations; however, a series of at least three routine stool examinations for parasites should be performed for each patient before a sigmoidoscopy examination is done (4).

Material from the mucosal surface should be aspirated or scraped and must not be obtained with cotton-tipped swabs. At least six representative areas of the mucosa should be sampled and examined (six samples, six slides). Usually, the amount of material is limited and should be processed immediately to ensure the best examination possible (Table 9). Three methods of examination can be performed. All three are acceptable; however, depending on the availability of trained personnel, the availability of proper fixation fluids, or the amount of specimen obtained, one or two procedures are recommended. If the amount of material limits the examination to one procedure, the use of polyvinyl alcohol (PVA) fixative is highly recommended.

If the material is going to be examined by using any of the new FA or EIA immunoassay detection kits (*C. parvum* or *G. lamblia*), then 5 or 10% formalin or SAF fixative is recommended. Physicians performing sigmoidoscopy procedures may not realize the importance of selecting the proper fixative for material to be examined for parasites. It is recommended that a parasitology specimen tray (containing Schaudinn's fixative, PVA, and 5 or 10% formalin) be provided or that a trained technologist be available at the time of sigmoidoscopy to prepare the slides.

Direct Saline Mount

If there is no lag time after collection and a microscope is available in the immediate vicinity, some of the material should be examined as a direct saline mount for the presence of motile trophozoites (4). A drop of material is mixed with a drop of 0.85% sodium chloride and is examined under low light intensity for the characteristic movement of amebae. It may take time for the organisms to become acclimated to this type of preparation: thus, motility may not be obvious for several minutes. There will be epithelial cells, macrophages, and possibly, polymorphonuclear leukocytes and erythrocytes, which will require a careful examination to reveal amebae.

Since specific identification of protozoan organisms can be difficult when only the direct saline mount is used, this technique should be used only when there is sufficient material left to prepare permanent stained smears.

Permanent Stained Smear

Most of the material obtained at sigmoidoscopy can be smeared (gently) onto a slide and immediately immersed in Schaudinn's fixative (4). These slides can then be stained with trichrome stain and examined for specific cell morphology, either protozoan or otherwise. The procedure and staining times are identical to those for routine fecal smears.

If the material is bloody, contains a lot of mucus, or is a "wet" specimen, a few (no more than 2 or 3) drops of PVA can be mixed with 1 or 2 drops of material directly on the slide, which is allowed to air dry (a 37°C incubator can be used) for at least 2 h before staining. If time permits, the PVA smears should be allowed to dry overnight; they can be routinely stained with trichrome stain and examined as a permanent mount.

Material from sigmoidoscopy can be placed in small amounts of SAF. After fixation for 30 min, the specimen can be centrifuged at 500 × *g* for 10 min and smears from the small amount of sediment can be prepared for permanent staining with iron hematoxylin (trichrome stain would be the second choice). One of the organisms most suspect when sigmoidoscopy is performed is *E. histolytica*, the morphology of which is normally seen from the permanent stained smear. However, if SAF is used, then both the permanent stained smear and an antigen detection reagent kit can be used. If

TABLE 9 Recovery of parasites from other intestinal tract specimens

Source	Organism	Procedure
Sigmoidoscopy specimens		
Air-dried smears	Coccidia	Modified acid-fast stain
	Microsporidia	Modified trichrome, optical brighteners, experimental immunoassay tests
Preserved 5–10% formalin or SAF	Helminth eggs and larvae, ameba and flagellate cysts, and trophozoites (SAF only)	Concentration, wet mount, immunoassay tests
	Coccidia	Modified acid-fast smear, immunoassay tests
	Microsporidia	Modified trichrome, optical brighteners, experimental immunoassay tests
PVA	Helminth eggs and larvae, ameba and flagellate cysts	Concentration, wet mount
	Ameba and flagellate cysts and trophozoites	Permanent stained smear
Schaudinn's fixative	Ameba and flagellate cysts and trophozoites	Permanent stained smear
Duodenal specimens		
Unpreserved	Helminth eggs and larvae, ameba and flagellate cysts, and ameba and flagellate trophozoites (motility)	Direct wet mount
Preserved 5–10% formalin or SAF	Helminth eggs and larvae, ameba and flagellate cysts, and trophozoites	Concentration, wet mount, immunoassay tests
	Coccidia	Modified acid-fast smear, immunoassay tests
	Microsporidia	Modified trichrome, optical brighteners, experimental immunoassay tests
PVA	Ameba and flagellate cysts and trophozoites	Permanent stained smear
Anal impression smear	Pinworm adult and eggs	No stain, cellulose tape preparation
Adult worm or segments	Helminth adult worms or proglottids	Carmine stain (rarely used), India ink
Tissue biopsy	Helminth eggs, larvae, and adults; protozoan cysts; trophozoites; oocysts; sporozoites; and spores	Touch preparations, squash preparations, permanent stains, histology

enough material is present for only a single procedure, then the permanent stained smear is recommended, particularly if the iron hematoxylin stain (incorporating the carbol fuchsin step) is used (4).

Duodenal Contents

Duodenal Drainage

In infections with *G. lamblia* or *S. stercoralis*, routine stool examinations may not reveal the organisms. Duodenal drainage material can be submitted for examination (Table 9).

A fresh, unpreserved specimen should be submitted to the laboratory; the amount may vary from <0.5 ml to several milliliters of fluid. The specimen may be centrifuged (at 500 × *g* for 10 min) and should be examined immediately as a wet mount for motile organisms (iodine may be added later to facilitate identification of any organisms present). If the specimen cannot be completely examined within 2 h after it is taken, any remaining material should be preserved in 5 to 10% formalin.

If the duodenal fluid contains mucus, this is where the organisms will tend to be found. Therefore, centrifugation of the specimen is important, and the sedimented mucus should be examined. *Giardia* trophozoites may be caught in mucus strands, and the movement of the flagella on the trophozoites may be the only subtle motility seen for these flagellates. *Strongyloides* larvae will usually be very motile. Immunoassay methods can also be used with fresh or formalinized material.

If the amount of duodenal material submitted is very small, rather than using any of the specimen for a wet smear examination permanent stains can be prepared. This approach provides a more permanent record, and the potential problems with unstained organisms, very minimal motility, and a lower-power examination can be avoided by using oil immersion examination of the stained specimen at ×1,000 magnification.

Duodenal Capsule Technique (Entero-Test)

A method of sampling duodenal contents that eliminates the need for intestinal intubation has been devised and consists of the use of a length of nylon yarn coiled inside a gelatin capsule (4, 6). The yarn protrudes through one end of the capsule, and this end of the line is taped to the side of the patient's face. The capsule is then swallowed, the gelatin dissolves in the stomach, and the weighted string is carried by peristalsis into the duodenum. The weight is released and passes out in the stool when the line is retrieved after a period of 4 h. Bile-stained mucus clinging to the yarn is then scraped off with gloved fingers and is collected in a small petri dish. Usually 4 or 5 drops of material are obtained.

The specimen should be examined immediately as a wet mount for motile organisms. If the specimen cannot be completely examined within an hour after the yarn has been removed, the material should be preserved in 5 to 10% formalin or PVA-mucus smears should be prepared. Organism motility will be similar to that described above for duodenal drainage.

The pH of the terminal end of the yarn should be checked to ensure adequate passage into the duodenum (a very low pH means that it never left the stomach). Also, since the bile duct drains into the intestine at this point, the terminal end of the yarn should be a yellow-green color.

UROGENITAL SPECIMENS

Several parasites may be recovered and identified from urogenital specimens. Although the most common pathogen is probably *Trichomonas vaginalis*, other organisms such as the microsporidia are becoming much more important (Table 10).

Direct Wet Mount

The identification of *T. vaginalis* is usually based on the examination of a wet preparation of vaginal and urethral discharges and prostatic secretions or urine sediment and may require the testing of multiple specimens to confirm the diagnosis. These specimens are diluted with a drop of saline and are examined under low power under reduced illumination for the presence of actively motile organisms.

TABLE 10 Techniques for detection of urogenital parasites

Organism	Procedure
Trichomonas vaginalis	Wet mount (motility)
	Culture
	Giemsa stain
	DNA probe
	Latex agglutination
	Enzyme-linked immunoassay
Schistosoma haematobium	Wet mount
	Membrane filtration
	Tissue section
Microfilariae	Triple centrifugation
	Membrane filtration
Microsporidia	Modified trichrome
	Optical brighteners
	Experimental antibody reagents
	Routine histology
	Electron microscopy

As the jerky motility begins to diminish, it may be possible to observe the undulating membrane, particularly under high dry power (magnification, ×400).

Examination of urinary sediment may be indicated in certain filarial infections, and the occurrence of microfilariae in urine has been reported with increasing frequency in *Onchocerca volvulus* infections in Africa. The triple-concentration technique is recommended for the recovery of microfilariae (4).

Urine is collected in a bottle, this volume is recorded, and thimerosal (1 ml/100 ml of urine) is added. The specimen is placed in a funnel fitted with tubing and a clamp; this preparation is allowed to settle overnight. On the following day, 10 to 20 ml of urine is withdrawn and centrifuged. The supernatant is discarded, and the sediment is resuspended in 0.85% NaCl. This preparation is again centrifuged, and 0.5 to 1.0 ml of the sediment is examined under the microscope for the presence of nonmotile microfilariae. The membrane filtration technique (4) can also be used with urine for the recovery of microfilariae. A membrane filter technique for the recovery of *Schistosoma haematobium* eggs has also been useful (4).

Permanent Stained Smears

The use of stained smears is usually not necessary for the identification of *T. vaginalis*. Many times the number of false-positive and false-negative results reported on the basis of stained smears strongly suggests the value of confirmation by observation of motile organisms from the direct mount, from appropriate culture media (4, 6, 12), or from direct detection with immunoassay reagents (4).

Stained smears may be prepared from material obtained from the membrane filtration techniques used for the recovery of microfilariae; Delafield's hematoxylin or Giemsa stain may be used. It is important to remember that Giemsa stain may not adequately stain the sheath, and correct identification of the organisms may require staining with a hematoxylin-based stain.

Microsporidial infections can also be diagnosed from the examination of urine sediment that has been stained by one of the modified trichrome methods or using optical brightening agents such as calcofluor (4). Multiple methods are recommended for confirmation of the diagnosis.

Culture

Specimens from women for culture (for *T. vaginalis*) may consist of vaginal exudate collected from the posterior fornix on cotton-tipped applicator sticks or genital secretions collected on polyester sponges. Specimens from men can include semen, urethral samples collected with a polyester sponge, or urine. Urine samples collected from the patient should be the specimen first voided in the morning. It is critical that clinical specimens be inoculated into culture medium as soon as possible after collection (4, 9, 12). Although collection swabs can be used, there are often problems with specimens drying prior to culture; immediate processing is mandatory for maximum organism recovery. The culture method is considered to be the most sensitive for the diagnosis of trichomoniasis; however, due to the time and effort involved, some laboratories have decided to use some of the new immunoassay detection kits (4). Another approach would be to use the plastic envelope methods (*Trichomonas* Culture System [Empyrean Diagnostics, Mountain View, Calif.]; InPouch TV [BIOMED Diagnostics, San Jose, Calif.]), which are simplified techniques for transport and culture (4). The following control strain should be available when using these cultures for clinical specimens: *T. vaginalis* ATCC 30001. Many media for the isolation of *T. vaginalis* are available, and some of these can be purchased commercially and have relatively long shelf lives.

If no trophozoites are seen after 4 days of incubation, then discard the tubes and report the culture as negative. Results for patient specimens should not be reported as positive unless control cultures are positive. Cultivation is the most sensitive method for the diagnosis of trichomoniasis. Since culture may take as long as 3 to 4 days and the clinical specimens may contain nonviable organisms, it is recommended that microscopic examination of wet smears be performed as well.

SPUTUM SPECIMENS

Expectorated Sputum

Although it is not one of the more common specimens, expectorated sputum may be submitted for examination for parasites (Table 11). Organisms in sputum that may be detected and that may cause pneumonia, pneumonitis, or Loeffler's syndrome include the migrating larval stages of *Ascaris lumbricoides*, *S. stercoralis*, and hookworm; the eggs of *Paragonimus* spp.; *Echinococcus granulosus* hooklets; and the protozoa *E. histolytica*, *Entamoeba gingivalis*, *Trichomonas tenax*, and *C. parvum*; and possibly the microsporidia (4). In a *Paragonimus* infection, the sputum may be viscous and tinged with brownish flecks ("iron filings"), which are clusters of eggs, and may be streaked with blood.

A sputum specimen should be collected properly so that the laboratory receives a "deep sputum" from the lower respiratory tract for examination rather than a specimen that is primarily saliva from the mouth. If the sputum is not induced, then the patient should receive specific instructions regarding collection.

Care should be taken not to confuse *E. gingivalis*, which may be found in the mouth and saliva, with *E. histolytica*, which could result in an incorrect suspicion of pulmonary abscess. *E. gingivalis* will usually contain ingested polymor-

TABLE 11 Specimen, possible parasite recovered, and appropriate tests (other than intestinal tract)[a]

Body site	Specimen	Possible parasites	Tests
Bone marrow	Aspirate	*Leishmania* spp., *Trypanosoma* spp.	Giemsa, culture
Brain	Tissue biopsy, cerebrospinal fluid	*Naegleria* spp., *Acanthamoeba* spp.	Giemsa, trichrome, culture
		Balamuthia mandrillaris (Leptomyxid ameba), *Entamoeba histolytica*	Giemsa, trichrome
		Toxoplasma gondii	Giemsa, immunospecific reagent, culture
		Microsporidia (*Encephalitozoon* spp.)	Modified trichrome, acid-fast stain, Giemsa, optical brightening agent (calcofluor), histology[b] (methenamine silver, PAS[c] tissue Gram stains), electron microscopy
		Taenia solium (cysticerci), *Echinococcus* spp.	Routine histology[b]
Eye	Cornea, conjunctiva, contact lens, lens solutions	Microsporidia	Acid-fast stain, Giemsa, modified trichrome, methenamine silver, optical brightening agent (calcofluor), histology[b] (methenamine silver, PAS, tissue Gram stains), electron microscopy
		Acanthamoeba spp.	Giemsa, trichrome, culture, calcofluor (cysts only)
		Toxoplasma gondii	Giemsa, immunospecific reagent, culture
		Loa loa	Direct examination
Kidney	Biopsy	Microsporidia	Modified trichrome, acid-fast stain, optical brightening agent (calcofluor), histology[b] (methenamine silver, PAS, tissue Gram stains), electron microscopy
Liver, spleen	Aspirates, biopsy	*Echinococcus* spp.	Wet mount, routine histology[b]
		Clonorchis spp., *Opisthorchis* spp.	Routine histology[b]
		Toxoplasma gondii, *Leishmania donovani*	Giemsa, culture
		Cryptosporidium parvum	Modified acid-fast stain, immunospecific reagent
		Pneumocystis carinii (now classified with the fungi)	Giemsa, methenamine silver or other cyst wall stain, optical brightening agent (calcofluor), immunospecific reagent
		Entamoeba histolytica	Wet mount, trichrome

(Continued on next page)

TABLE 11 Specimen, possible parasite recovered, and appropriate tests (other than intestinal tract)[a] (*Continued*)

Body site	Specimen	Possible parasites	Tests
Lung	Sputum, bronchoalveolar lavage, transbronchial aspirates, brush biopsy specimen, open lung biopsy specimen	*Ascaris lumbricoides*, *Strongyloides stercoralis*, hookworm, *Paragonimus westermani*, *Echinococcus granulosus*	Wet mount, routine histology[b]
		Pneumocystis carinii (now classified with the fungi)	Immune-specific reagent, Giemsa, methenamine silver (or other cyst wall stain), optical brightening agent (calcofluor)
		Microsporidia	Modified trichrome, acid-fast stain, Giemsa, optical brightening agent (calcofluor), histology[b] (methenamine silver, PAS, tissue Gram stains), electron microscopy
		Toxoplasma gondii	Giemsa, immunospecific reagent, culture
		Cryptosporidium parvum	Modified acid-fast stain, immunospecific reagent, Giemsa
Muscle	Biopsy	*Trichinella spiralis*	Wet examination, squash preparation
		Microsporidia	Modified trichrome, acid-fast stain, Giemsa, optical brightening agent (calcofluor), histology[b] (methenamine silver, PAS, tissue Gram stains), electron microscopy
		Taenia solium (cysticerci), *Onchocerca volvulus* (nodules), *Trypanosoma cruzi*	Routine histology
Nasopharynx, sinus cavities		Microsporidia	Modified trichrome, acid-fast stain, Giemsa, optical brightening agent (calcofluor), histology[b] (methenamine silver, PAS, tissue Gram stains), electron microscopy
		Acanthamoeba spp.	Giemsa, trichrome, culture, calcofluor (cysts only)
		Naegleria spp.	Giemsa, trichrome, culture
Skin	Scraping, biopsy	*Leishmania* spp.	Giemsa, culture
		Onchocerca volvulus, *Mansonella streptocerca*	Giemsa, routine histology[b]
		Acanthamoeba spp.	Giemsa, trichrome, culture, calcofluor (cysts only)

[a] This table does not include every possible parasite that could be found in a particular body site. Parasites include trophozoites, cysts, oocysts, spores, adults, larvae, eggs, hooklets, amastigotes, and trypomastigotes.

[b] Routine histology can be used for the detection and identification of many parasites. In some cases, it may be the only means of diagnosis.

[c] PAS, periodic acid-Schiff stain.

phonuclear leukocytes, while *E. histolytica* may contain ingested erythrocytes but not polymorphonuclear leukocytes. *T. tenax* would also be found in saliva from the mouth and thus would be an incidental finding and normally not an indication of pulmonary problems.

Direct Wet Mount

Sputum is usually examined as a wet mount (saline or iodine), using low and high dry power (magnifications, × 100 and × 400, respectively). The specimen is not concentrated before preparation of the wet mount. If the sputum is thick, an equal amount of 3% sodium hydroxide (or undiluted chlorine bleach) can be added; the specimen is thoroughly mixed and then centrifuged. NaOH should not be used if one is looking for *Entamoeba* spp. or *T. tenax*. After centrifugation, the supernatant fluid is discarded, and the sediment can be examined as a wet mount with saline or iodine. If examination must be delayed for any reason, the sputum should be fixed in 5 or 10% formalin to preserve helminth eggs or larvae or in PVA fixative to be stained later for protozoa.

Permanent Stained Smears

If *C. parvum* is suspected (rare), then acid-fast or immunoassay techniques normally used for stool specimens can be used (4). Trichrome stains of material may aid in differentiating *E. histolytica* from *E. gingivalis*, and Giemsa stain may better define larvae and juvenile worms.

ASPIRATES

When routine testing methods have failed to demonstrate the organisms, the examination of aspirated material for the diagnosis of parasitic infections may be extremely valuable (Table 11). Specimens should be transported to the laboratory immediately after collection. Aspirates include liquid specimens collected from a variety of sites as well as fine-needle aspirates and duodenal aspirates. Fluid specimens collected by bronchoscopy include bronchoalveolar lavages and bronchial washings.

Procedural details for processing sigmoidoscopic aspirates and scrapings for the recovery of *E. histolytica* and techniques for preparation of duodenal aspirate material have been presented earlier in this chapter.

Fine-Needle Aspirates

Fine-needle aspirates are often collected by cytopathology staff who process the specimens, or they may be collected and sent to the laboratory directly for slide preparation and/or culture. Suggested stains are Giemsa stain for *Toxoplasma gondii*, trichrome stain for amebae, modified acid-fast stains for *C. parvum*, and modified trichrome stains for the microsporidia (4).

Cyst and Abscess Aspirates

Aspirates of cysts and abscesses to be evaluated for amebae may require concentration by centrifugation, digestion, microscopic examination for motile organisms in direct preparations, and cultures and microscopic evaluation of stained preparations (4).

Duodenal Aspirates

Duodenal aspirates to be evaluated for *S. stercoralis*, *G. lamblia*, *C. parvum*, or the microsporidia may require concentration by centrifugation prior to microscopic examination for motile organisms and the use of permanent stains (4).

Bone Marrow Aspirates

Bone marrow aspirates to be evaluated for *Leishmania* amastigotes, *Trypanosoma cruzi* amastigotes, or *Plasmodium* spp. require Giemsa staining.

Bronchoscopy Aspirates

Fluid specimens collected by bronchoscopy may be lavages or washings, with bronchoalveolar lavages preferred. Specimens are usually concentrated by centrifugation prior to microscopic examination of stained preparations. Organisms which may be detected in such specimens are *T. gondii*, *C. parvum*, and the microsporidia.

Lung and Liver Aspirates

Amebiasis

Examination of aspirates from lung or liver abscesses may reveal trophozoites of *E. histolytica*; however, demonstration of the organisms may be difficult (4). Liver aspirate material should be taken from the margin of the abscess rather than the necrotic center. The organisms are often trapped in the viscous pus or debris and will not exhibit typical motility. A minimum of two separate portions of exudate should be removed (more than two are recommended). The first portion of the aspirate, usually yellowish white, rarely contains organisms. The last portion of the aspirated abscess material is reddish in color and is more likely to contain amebae. The best material to be examined is that obtained from the actual wall of the abscess. The Amoebiasis Research Unit, Durban, South Africa, has recommended the use of proteolytic enzymes to free the organisms from the aspirate material.

After the addition of the enzyme streptodornase to the thick pus (10 U/ml of pus), the mixture is incubated and shaken. After centrifugation (500 × *g* for 5 min), the sediment may be examined microscopically as wet mounts or may be used to inoculate culture media. Some of the aspirate can be mixed directly with PVA on a slide and examined as a permanent stained smear (4).

Hydatid disease

Aspiration of cyst material for the diagnosis of hydatid disease is a dangerous procedure and is usually performed only when open surgical techniques are used for cyst removal. Aspirated fluid will usually contain hydatid sand (intact and degenerating scolices, hooklets, and calcareous corpuscles). Some older cysts will contain material that resembles curded cottage cheese, and the hooklets may be very difficult to see. Some of this material can be diluted with saline or 10% KOH; usually, scolices or daughter cysts will have disintegrated. However, the diagnosis can be made by seeing the hooklets by using high dry power (magnification, ×400). The absence of scolices or hooklets does not rule out the possibility of hydatid disease, since some cysts are sterile and contain no scolices and/or daughter cysts. Histologic examination of the cyst wall should be able to confirm the diagnosis.

Lymph Node, Spleen, Liver, Spinal Fluid, Eye Specimen, and Nasopharyngeal Material

Material from lymph nodes, spleen, liver, spinal fluid, eye specimens, or the nasopharynx may be examined to confirm parasitic infections (African trypanosomiasis, leishmaniasis, Chagas' disease, primary amebic meningoencephalitis, amebic keratitis, and microsporidiosis) and should be processed as follows. Fluid material can be examined under low power (magnification, ×100) and high dry power (magnification, ×400) as a wet mount (diluted with saline) for the presence of motile organisms. Spinal fluid should not be diluted before examination. Impression smears from tissues should be prepared and stained with Giemsa stain. The material is pressed between two slides, with the smear resulting when the slides are pulled apart (one across the other). The smears are allowed to air dry and are then processed like a thin blood film (fixed in absolute methanol and stained with Giemsa stain). If microsporidia are suspected, modified trichrome stains can be used; calcofluor white and immunoassay methods (currently under development) are also excellent options (4).

Patients with primary amebic meningoencephalitis are rare, but the examination of spinal fluid may reveal the amebae, usually *Naegleria fowleri*. Unspun sedimented spinal fluid should be placed on a slide, under a coverslip, and observed for motile amebae; smears can also be stained with Wright's or Giemsa stain. Spinal fluid, exudate, or tissue fragments can be examined by light microscopy or phase-contrast microscopy. Care must be taken not to confuse leukocytes with actual organisms and vice versa. The spinal fluid may appear cloudy or purulent (with or without erythrocytes), with a cell count of from a few hundred to more than 20,000 leukocytes (primarily neutrophils) per ml. Failure to find bacteria in this type of spinal fluid should alert one to the possibility of primary amebic meningoencephalitis; however, false-positive bacterial Gram stains have been reported due to the excess debris. Isolation of these organisms from tissues or soil can be done by using special media. When spinal fluid is placed in a counting chamber, organisms that settle to the bottom of the chamber will tend to round up and look very much like leukocytes. For this reason, it is better to examine the spinal fluid on a slide directly under a coverslip, not in a counting chamber.

A rapid method for the diagnosis of *Acanthamoeba* keratitis is the use of calcofluor white, which is a chemofluorescent dye with an affinity for the polysaccharide polymers of amebic cysts. This method has proven to be very successful for examination of corneal scrapings or biopsy material (4).

Cutaneous Ulcer (Leishmaniasis)

Material containing intracellular *Leishmania* organisms must be aspirated from below the ulcer bed through the uninvolved skin, not from the surface of the ulcer. The surface of the ulcer must be thoroughly cleaned before specimens are taken; any contamination of the material with bacteria or fungi may prevent recovery of the organism from culture. Aspirated material is placed on a slide and stained with Giemsa stain.

BIOPSY MATERIAL

Biopsy specimens are recommended for use in the diagnosis of parasitic infections in tissues (Table 8). In addition to standard histologic preparations, the following can be used: impression smears and teased and squash preparations of biopsy tissue from skin, muscle, cornea, intestine, liver, lung, and brain. Tissue to be examined as permanent sections or by electron microscopy should be fixed as specified by the laboratories that will process the tissue, and in certain cases, testing of a biopsy specimen may be the only means of confirming a suspected parasitic problem. Specimens that are going to be examined as fresh material rather than as tissue sections should be kept moist in saline and submitted to the laboratory immediately.

Detection of parasites in tissue depends on specimen collection and the retrieval of sufficient material for examination. Biopsy specimens are usually quite small and may not be representative of the diseased tissue. Multiple tissue samples will often improve diagnostic results. To optimize the yield from any tissue specimen, examine all areas and use as many procedures as possible. Tissues are obtained from invasive procedures, many of which are very expensive and lengthy: consequently, these specimens deserve the most comprehensive procedures possible.

Tissue submitted in a sterile container on a sterile sponge dampened with saline may be used for cultures of protozoa after mounts for direct examination or impression smears for staining have been prepared. If cultures for parasites will be made, use sterile slides for smear and mount preparation.

The majority of the protozoa will be found on the permanent stained smears (impression smears, touch or squash preparations, or teased preparations). When culture is used, permanent stained smears of the culture medium or sediment may also reveal some of the protozoa. Although infrequently used, material from animals (at autopsy) can be examined as both wet and permanent stained preparations for confirmation of protozoa. Filarial infections may be confirmed by the recovery and identification of microfilariae in skin scrapings and/or biopsy specimens.

Skin (*O. volvulus* and *Mansonella streptocerca*)

The use of skin snips is the method of choice for the diagnosis of human filarial infections with *O. volvulus* and *M. streptocerca* (1, 4). Microfilariae of both species occur chiefly in the skin, although *O. volvulus* microfilariae may rarely be found in the blood and occasionally in the urine. Skin snip specimens should be thick enough to include the outer part of the dermal papillae. With a razor blade, a small slice may be cut from a skin fold held between the thumb and forefinger, or a slice may be taken from a small "cone" of skin pulled up with a needle. Significant bleeding should not occur, and there should be just a slight oozing of fluid. Corneal-scleral punches (either Holth or Walser type) have been found to be successful in taking skin snips of uniform size and depth and an average weight of 0.8 mg (range, 0.4 to 1.2 mg); this procedure is easy to perform and is painless. It has been demonstrated that in African onchocerciasis, it is preferable to take skin snips from the buttock region (above the iliac crest); in Central American onchocerciasis, the preferred skin snip sites are from the shoulders (over the scapula).

Skin snips are placed immediately in a drop of normal saline or distilled water and are covered so that they will not dry; teasing of the specimen with dissecting needles is not necessary but may facilitate release of the microfilariae. Microfilariae tend to emerge more rapidly in saline; however, in either solution, the microfilariae usually emerge within 30 min to 1 h and can be examined with low-intensity light and the ×10 objective of the microscope. To see definitive morphological details of the microfilariae, allow the snip preparation to dry, fix it in absolute methyl alcohol, and stain it with Giemsa stain.

Skin (Cutaneous Amebiasis and Cutaneous Leishmaniasis)

Skin biopsy specimens used for the diagnosis of cutaneous amebiasis and cutaneous leishmaniasis should be processed for tissue sectioning and subsequently stained by the hematoxylin-eosin technique.

Lymph Nodes (Trypanosomiasis, Leishmaniasis, Chagas' Disease, and Toxoplasmosis)

Material obtained from lymph nodes should be processed for tissue sectioning and as impression smears that should be processed as thin blood films and stained with Giemsa stain. Appropriate culture media can also be inoculated, again making sure that the specimen has been collected under sterile conditions.

Muscle (Trichinosis)

The presumptive diagnosis of trichinosis is often based on patient history: ingestion of raw or rare pork, walrus meat, or bear meat, diarrhea followed by edema and muscle pain, and the presence of eosinophilia. Generally, the suspected food is not available for examination. The diagnosis may be confirmed by finding larval *Trichinella spiralis* in a muscle biopsy specimen. The encapsulated larvae can be seen in fresh muscle if small pieces are pressed between two slides and examined under the microscope (4). Larvae are usually most abundant in the diaphragm, masseter muscle, or tongue and may be recovered from these muscles at necropsy. Routine histologic sections can also be prepared.

Cestode Larval Stages

Human infection with any of the larval cestodes may present diagnostic problems, and frequently, the larvae are referred for identification after surgical removal. In addition to *E. granulosus* (hydatid disease) and the larval stage of *Taenia solium* (cysticercosis), other larval cestodes occasionally cause human disease. The larval stage of tapeworms of the genus *Multiceps*, a parasite of dogs and wild canids, is called a coenurus and may cause human coenurosis. The coenurus resembles a cysticercus but is larger and has multiple scolices developing from the germinal membrane surrounding the fluid-filled bladder. These larvae occur in extraintestinal locations, including the eye, central nervous system, and muscle.

Human sparganosis is caused by the larval stages of tapeworms of the genus *Spirometra*, which are parasites of various canine and feline hosts; these tapeworms are closely related to the genus *Diphyllobothrium*. Sparganum larvae are elongated, ribbonlike larvae without a bladder and with a slightly expanded anterior end lacking suckers. These larvae are usually found in superficial tissues or nodules, although they may cause ocular sparganosis, a more serious disease.

The diagnosis of larval cestodes is frequently supported by finding prominent calcareous corpuscles in the tapeworm tissue; specific identification usually depends on referral to specialists.

Rectal or Bladder Biopsy Specimen (Schistosomiasis)

Often when a patient has an old, chronic infection or a light infection with *Schistosoma mansoni* or *Schistosoma japonicum*, the eggs may not be found in the stool and an examination of the rectal mucosa may reveal the presence of eggs. The fresh tissue should be compressed between two microscope slides and examined under the low power of the microscope (low-intensity light) (4). Critical examination of these eggs should be made to determine whether living miracidia are still found within the egg. Treatment may depend on the viability of the eggs; for this reason, the condition of the eggs should be reported to the physician.

Mucosa from the bladder wall may reveal eggs of *Schistosoma haematobium* when they are not being recovered in the urine. As with rectal biopsy specimens, the eggs in the bladder wall should be checked for viability by either a hatching technique or microscopic observation of the functioning flame cells within the miracidium larva.

BLOOD

Depending on the life cycle, a number of parasites may be recovered in a blood specimen, either whole blood or buffy coat preparations, or following concentration by various types of procedures. These parasites include *Plasmodium*, *Babesia*, and *Trypanosoma* species, *Leishmania donovani*, and microfilariae. Although some organisms may be motile in fresh, whole blood, species identification will usually be accomplished from the examination of permanent stained thick and thin blood films. Blood films can be prepared from fresh, whole blood collected with no anticoagulants, anticoagulated blood (EDTA is recommended; heparin is acceptable, but organism morphology is not as good), or sediment from the various concentration procedures. The recommended stain of choice is Giemsa stain; however, the parasites can also be seen on blood films stained with Wright's stain. Delafield's hematoxylin stain is often used to stain the microfilarial sheath; in some cases, Giemsa stain does not provide sufficient stain quality to allow differentiation of the microfilariae (Table 12). When handling blood, as well as other clinical specimens, universal precautions should be observed (3, 4, 13, 14).

Preparation of Thick and Thin Blood Films

Microfilariae and trypanosomes can be detected in fresh blood by their characteristic shape and motility; however, specific identification of the organisms requires a permanent stain. Two types of blood films are recommended. Thick films allow a larger amount of blood to be examined, which increases the possibility of detecting light infections (4, 9, 13). However, species identification with a thick film, particularly in the case of malaria, can usually be made only by experienced workers, and the morphological characteristics of blood parasites are best seen in thin films.

The accurate examination of thick and thin blood films and identification of parasites depend on the use of absolutely clean, grease-free slides for preparation of all blood films. Old (unscratched) slides should be cleaned first in detergent and then with 70% ethyl alcohol; new slides

TABLE 12 Techniques for the recovery of blood parasites (EDTA or heparin)[a]

Organism	Procedure	Stain
Malaria/*Babesia*	Thick and thin smears	Giemsa, Wright's stain
	QBC[b]	Stain not relevant
	ParaSight F[c]	Stain not relevant
Microfilariae	Thick and thin smears	Giemsa, Wright's, or Delafield's hematoxylin for all procedures listed with exception of QBC
	Knott concentration	
	Membrane filtration	
	Gradient centrifugation	
	QBC	Stain not relevant
Trypanosomes	Thick and thin smears	Giemsa, Wright's for all procedures listed with exception of QBC
	Buffy coat smears	
	Triple centrifugation	
	Culture	
	QBC	Stain not relevant
Leishmaniae	Thick and thin smears	Giemsa, Wright's for all procedures listed
	Buffy coat smears	
	Culture	

[a] Molecular techniques are still experimental and are not readily available.
[b] QBC-Blood Parasite Detection Method (Becton-Dickinson Tropical Disease Diagnostics, Sparks, Md.).
[c] ParaSight F-Rapid Test for *P. falciparum* malaria (Becton-Dickinson Tropical Disease Diagnostics, Sparks, Md.). This test is not licensed for diagnostic use in the United States.

should also be cleaned with alcohol and allowed to dry before use.

Blood films should be prepared when the patient is admitted or seen in the emergency room or clinic; typical fever patterns are frequently absent, and the patient may not be suspected of having malaria. If malaria is a possible diagnosis, after the first set of negative smears, samples should be taken at intervals of 6 to 8 h for at least 3 successive days. Subsequent to a finger stick, the blood should flow freely; blood that has to be "milked" from the finger will be diluted with tissue fluids, which decrease the number of parasites per field. In addition to capillary blood smears prepared from the fingerstick, a tube of fresh blood with anticoagulant (preferably EDTA) should be requested for preparation of smears if required. Ideally, the smears should be prepared within 1 h after the specimen is drawn. After that time, stippling may not be visible on stained films; however, the overall organism morphology may still be acceptable.

The time that the specimen was drawn should be clearly indicated on the tube of blood and also on the result report. The physician will then be able to correlate the results with any symptoms that the patient may have. There should also be some indication on the slip that is sent back to the physician that one negative specimen does not rule out the possibility of a parasitic infection.

Thick Blood Films

To prepare the thick film, place 2 or 3 small drops of capillary blood directly from the fingerstick (no anticoagulant) on an alcohol-cleaned slide. With the corner of another slide and using a circular motion, mix the drops and spread them over an area 2 cm in diameter. Continue stirring for 30 s to prevent the formation of fibrin strands that may obscure the parasites after staining. If blood containing an anticoagulant is used, 1 or 2 drops may be spread over an area about 2 cm in diameter; it is not necessary to continue stirring for 30 s, since there will be no formation of fibrin strands. If too much blood is used or any grease remains on the slide, the blood may flake off during staining. Allow the film to air dry (room temperature) in a dust-free area. Never apply heat to a thick film, since heat will fix the blood, causing the erythrocytes to remain intact during staining; the result is stain retention and an inability to identify the parasites. After the thick films are thoroughly dry, they can be laked to remove the hemoglobin. To lake the films, place them in buffer solution before staining or directly into a dilute, buffered Giemsa stain. If thick films are going to be stained at a later time, they should be laked before storage (4).

Thin Blood Films

The thin blood film is routinely used for specific parasite identification, although the number of organisms per field is much reduced compared with the number in the thick film. The thin film is prepared exactly as one used for a differential count, and a well-prepared film is thick at one end and thin at the other (one layer of evenly distributed erythrocytes with no cell overlap). The thin, feathered end should be at least 2 cm long, and the film should occupy the central area of the slide, with free margins on both sides. Holes in the film indicate the presence of grease on the slide. After the film has air dried (do not apply heat), it may be stained. The necessity for fixation before staining will depend on the stain selected.

Staining Blood Films

For accurate identification of blood parasites, a laboratory should develop proficiency in the use of at least one good staining method (2, 4, 8). Since prolonged storage may result in stain retention, blood films should be stained on the same day or within a few days of collection.

Wright's stain has the fixative in combination with the staining solution, so that both fixation and staining occur at the same time; therefore, the thick film must be laked before staining. In Giemsa stain, the fixative and stain are separate; thus, the thin film must be fixed with absolute methanol before staining.

When slides are removed from either type of staining solution, they should be dried in a vertical position. After being air dried, they may be examined under oil immersion by placing the oil directly on the uncovered blood film. If slides are to be stored for a considerable length of time (for teaching or legal purposes), they should be protected with a coverglass by being mounted in a medium such as Permount. Blood films that have been stained with any of the Romanowsky stains and that have been mounted with Permount or other resinous mounting media are susceptible to fading of the basophilic elements and generalized loss of stain intensity. One can add an antioxidant such as 1% (by volume) 2,6-di-*t*-butyl-*p*-cresol (butylated hydroxytoluene; catalog no. B1253; Sigma Chemical Co.) to the mounting medium. Without the addition of this antioxidant, mounted stained blood films eventually become pink; stained films protected with this compound generally remain unchanged in color for many years.

Giemsa Stain

Each new lot number of Giemsa stain should be tested for optimal staining times before being used on patient specimens. If the blood cells appear to be adequately stained, the timing and stain dilution should be appropriate to demonstrate the presence of malaria and other parasites. The use of prepared liquid stain or stain prepared from the powder depends on personal preference; there is apparently little difference between the two preparations.

The commercial liquid stain or the stock solution prepared from powder should be diluted approximately the same amount to prepare the working stain solution (4, 13). Stock Giemsa liquid stain is diluted 1:10 with buffer for both thick and thin blood films, with dilutions ranging from 1:10 up to 1:50. Staining times usually match the dilution factor (e.g., 1:20 for 20 min or 1:50 for 50 min). Some people prefer to use the longer method with more dilute stain for both thick and thin films. The phosphate buffer used to dilute the stock stain should be neutral or slightly alkaline (pH 7.0 to 7.2). Phosphate buffer solution may be used to obtain the right pH. In some laboratories, the pH of tap water may be satisfactory and may be used for the entire staining procedure and the final rinse. Some workers recommend the use of pH 6.8 to emphasize Schüffner's dots.

Giemsa stain colors the blood components as follows: erythrocytes, pale red; nuclei of leukocytes, purple with pale purple cytoplasm; eosinophilic granules, bright purple-red; and neutrophilic granules, deep pink-purple. In malaria parasites, the cytoplasm stains blue and the nuclear material stains red to purple-red. Schüffner's dots and other inclusions in the erythrocytes will stain red. The nuclear and cytoplasmic staining characteristics of the other blood parasites such as *Babesia* spp., trypanosomes, and leishmaniae will be like those of the malaria parasites. While the sheath of microfilariae may not always stain with Giemsa, the nuclei within the microfilaria itself will stain blue to purple.

Wright's Stain

Wright's stain is available in liquid form and also as a powder, which must be dissolved in anhydrous, acetone-free methyl alcohol before use. Since Wright's stain contains alcohol, the thin blood films do not require fixation before staining. Thick films stained with Wright's stain are usually inferior to those stained with Giemsa solution. Great care should also be taken to avoid excess stain precipitate on the slide during the final rinse. Before staining, thick films must be laked in distilled water (to rupture and remove erythrocytes) and air dried. The staining procedure is the same as that for thin films, but the staining time is usually somewhat longer and must be determined for each batch of stain. Wright's stain colors blood components as follows: erythrocytes, light tan, reddish, or buff; nuclei of leukocytes, bright blue with contrasting light cytoplasm; eosinophilic granules, bright red; and neutrophilic granules, pink or light purple.

In malaria parasites, the cytoplasm stains pale blue and the nuclear material stains red. Schüffner's dots and other inclusions in the erythrocytes usually do not stain or stain very pale with Wright's stain. Nuclear and cytoplasmic staining characteristics of the other blood parasites such as *Babesia* spp., trypanosomes, and leishmaniae will stain like those seen in the malaria parasites. While the sheath of microfilariae may not always stain with Wright's stain, the nuclei within the microfilaria itself will stain pale to dark blue.

Proper Examination of Thin and Thick Blood Films

The initial screen of the thin blood film should be carried out with the low-power objective of a microscope because microfilariae may be missed if the entire thin film is not examined. Microfilariae are rarely present in large numbers, and frequently, only a few organisms occur in each thin film preparation. Microfilariae are commonly found at the edges of the thin film or at the feathered end of the film because they are carried to these sites during the process of spreading the blood. The feathered end of the film where the erythrocytes are drawn out into one single, distinctive layer of cells should be examined for the presence of malaria parasites and trypanosomes. In these areas, the morphology and size of the infected erythrocytes are most clearly seen.

The request for blood film examination should always be considered a STAT procedure, with all reports (negative as well as positive) being reported by telephone to the physician as soon as possible (4, 13). Examination of the thin film should include viewing of 200 to 300 oil immersion fields at a magnification of ×1,000. Although some people use a ×50 or ×60 oil immersion objective to screen stained blood films, there is some concern that small parasites such as *Plasmodium* spp., *Babesia* spp., or *Leishmania donovani* may be missed at this smaller total magnification (×500 or ×600), although they are usually detected at the ×1,000 total magnification obtained with the more traditional ×100 oil immersion objective. Because people tend to scan blood films at different rates, it is important to examine a minimum number of fields, regardless of the time that it takes to perform this procedure. If something suspicious has been seen in the thick film, often the number of fields examined on the thin film may be considerably more than 200 to 300.

Diagnostic problems with the use of automated differential instruments have been reported (4). Both malaria and *Babesia* infections can be missed with these instruments, and therapy is therefore delayed. Because these instruments are not designed to detect intracellular blood parasites, any reliance on the automated systems for discrimination between uninfected erythrocytes and those infected with parasites may pose serious diagnostic problems.

In the preparation of a thick blood film, the greatest concentration of blood cells will be in the center of the film. A search for parasitic organisms should be carried out initially at low magnification to detect microfilariae more readily. Examination of a thick film usually requires 5 to 10 min (approximately 100 oil immersion fields). The search for malarial organisms and trypanosomes is best done under oil immersion (total magnification, ×1,000). Close examination of the very periphery of the thick film may reveal intact erythrocytes; such cells, if infected, may prove useful in malaria diagnosis since the characteristic morphology necessary to identify the organisms to the species level is more easily seen.

Concentration Procedures

Buffy Coat Films

L. donovani, trypanosomes, and *Histoplasma capsulatum* (a fungus with intracellular elements resembling those of *L. donovani*) may occasionally be detected in the peripheral blood. The parasite or fungus will be found in the large mononuclear cells that are found in the buffy coat (a layer of leukocytes resulting from centrifugation of whole citrated blood). The nuclear material will stain dark red-purple, and the cytoplasm will be light blue (*L. donovani*). *H. capsulatum* will appear as a dot of nuclear material (dark red-purple) surrounded by a clear halo area. Trypanosomes in the peripheral blood will also concentrate with the buffy coat cells.

Use alcohol-cleaned slides for preparation of the blood films. A microhematocrit tube can also be used; the tube is carefully scored and snapped at the buffy coat interface, and the leukocytes are prepared as a thin film. The tube can also be examined prior to removal of the buffy coat under low and high dry powers of the microscope. If trypanosomes are present, the motility may be observed in the buffy coat. Microfilaria motility would also be visible.

QBC Microhematocrit Centrifugation Method

Microhematocrit centrifugation with use of the QBC malaria tube (glass capillary tube and closely fitting plastic insert: QBC malaria blood tubes; Becton Dickinson, Tropical Disease Diagnostics, Sparks, Md.) has been used for the detection of blood parasites (4). At the end of centrifugation of 50 to 60 μl of capillary or venous blood (5 min in a QBC centrifuge, 14,387 × *g*), parasites or erythrocytes containing parasites are concentrated into a small, 1- to 2-mm region near the top of the erythrocyte column and are held close to the wall of the tube by the plastic float, thereby making them readily visible by microscopy. Tubes precoated with acridine orange provide a stain which induces fluorescence in the parasites. This method automatically prepares a concentrated smear which represents the distance between the float and the walls of the tube. Once the tube is placed into the plastic holder (Paraviewer) and immersion oil is applied onto the top of the hematocrit tube (no coverslip is necessary), the tube is examined with a ×40 to ×60 oil immersion objective (it must have a working distance of 0.3 mm or greater).

Although a malaria infection could be detected by this method (which is much more sensitive than the thick or the thin blood smear), appropriate thick and thin blood films need to be examined to accurately identify the species of the organism causing the infection.

ParaSight F Test

A new *Plasmodium falciparum* antigen detection system, the ParaSight F test (Becton Dickinson), has been found to be very effective in field trials. This procedure is based on an antigen capture approach and has been incorporated in a dipstick format; the entire test takes approximately 10 min. Unfortunately, this kit is not yet available within the United States, but it has proven to be very useful in other areas of the world.

Knott Concentration

The Knott concentration procedure is used primarily to detect the presence of microfilariae in the blood, especially when a light infection is suspected (4, 9). The disadvantage of the procedure is that the microfilariae are killed by the formalin and are therefore not seen as motile organisms.

Membrane Filtration Technique

The membrane filtration technique is highly efficient in demonstrating filarial infections when microfilaremias are of low density. This method is unsatisfactory for the isolation of *Mansonella perstans* microfilariae because of their small size. A 3-μm-pore-size filter could be used for recovery of this organism. Other filters with similar pore sizes are not as satisfactory as the Nuclepore filter.

Delafield's Hematoxylin

Some of the material that is obtained from the concentration procedures can be allowed to dry as thick and thin films and then stained with Delafield's hematoxylin, which will demonstrate greater nuclear detail as well as the microfilarial sheath, if present. In addition, fresh thick films of blood containing microfilariae can be stained by this hematoxylin technique (4).

Triple Centrifugation Method for Trypanosomes

The triple centrifugation procedure may be valuable in demonstrating the presence of trypanosomes in the peripheral blood when the parasitemia is light (4). After repeated centrifugation of the supernatant, the sediment is examined as a wet preparation or is stained as a thin blood film.

REFERENCES

1. **Ash, L. R., and T. C. Orihel.** 1991. *Parasites: A Guide to Laboratory Procedures and Identification*. ASCP Press, Chicago, Ill.
2. **Beaver, P. C., R. C. Jung, and E. W. Cupp.** 1984. *Clinical Parasitology*, 9th ed. Lea & Febiger, Philadelphia, Pa.
3. **Code of Federal Regulations.** 1991. Occupational exposure to bloodborne pathogens. *Fed. Regist.* 29CFR1910.1030.
4. **Garcia, L. S., and D. A. Bruckner.** 1997. *Diagnostic Medical Parasitology*, 3rd ed. ASM Press, Washington, D.C.
5. **Hiatt, R. A., E. K. Markell, and E. Ng.** 1995. How many stool examinations are necessary to detect pathogenic intestinal protozoa? *Am. J. Trop. Med. Hyg.* **53:**36–39.
6. **Isenberg, H. D. (ed.).** 1992. *Clinical Microbiology Procedures Handbook*, vol. 1 and 2. American Society for Microbiology, Washington, D.C.
7. **Kehl, K. S. C.** 1996. Screening stools for *Giardia* and *Cryptosporidium*: are antigen tests enough? *Clin. Microbiol. Newsl.* **18:**133–135.
8. **Koneman, E. W., S. D. Allen, W. M. Janda, P. C. Schreckenberger, and W. C. Winn, Jr.** 1992. *Diagnostic Microbiology*, 4th ed. J. B. Lippincott Co., Philadelphia, Pa.
9. **Markell, E., M. Voge, and D. T. John.** 1992. *Medical Parasitology*, 7th ed. The W. B. Saunders Co., Philadelphia, Pa.
10. **Melvin, D. M., and M. M. Brooke.** 1982. *Laboratory Procedures for the Diagnosis of Intestinal Parasites*, 3rd ed. U.S. Department of Health, Education, and Welfare publication no. (CDC) 82-8282. Government Printing Office, Washington, D.C.
11. **Morris, A. J., M. L. Wilson, and L. B. Reller.** 1992. Application of rejection criteria for stool ovuum and parasite examinations. *J. Clin. Microbiol.* **30:**3213–3216.
12. **Murray, P. R., E. J. Baron, M. A. Pfaller, F. C. Tenover, and R. H. Yolken (ed.).** 1995. *Manual of Clinical Microbiology*, 6th ed. ASM Press, Washington, D.C.
13. **National Committee for Clinical Laboratory Standards.** 1990. *Use of Blood Film Examination of Parasites*. Tentative guideline M15-T. National Committee for Clinical Laboratory Standards, Villanova, Pa.
14. **National Committee for Clinical Laboratory Standards.** 1997. *Protection of Laboratory Workers from Instrument Biohazards and Infectious Disease Transmitted by Blood, Body Fluids, and Tissue*. Approved guideline M29-A. National Committee for Clinical Laboratory Standards, Villanova, Pa.
15. **National Committee for Clinical Laboratory Standards.** 1997. *Procedures for the Recovery and Identification of Parasites from the Intestinal Tract*. Approved guideline M28-A. National Committee for Clinical Laboratory Standards, Villanova, Pa.

Plasmodium and *Babesia**

WILLIAM O. ROGERS

105

TAXONOMY

The agents of malaria and babesiosis are members of the phylum *Apicomplexa*, which includes protozoa characterized by the presence of an apical complex consisting of polar rings, conoid micronemes, rhoptries, and subpellicular microtubules. All members of the phylum *Apicomplexa* are parasitic. The agents of malaria and babesiosis are classified within the orders *Haemospororida* and *Piroplasmorida*, respectively.

DESCRIPTION OF THE GENERA

The genus *Plasmodium* includes at least 172 named species of intraerythrocytic parasites infecting a wide range of mammals, birds, reptiles, and amphibians (9). Four species, *P. falciparum*, *P. vivax*, *P. ovale*, and *P. malariae*, commonly infect humans. Rarely, other species normally infecting nonhuman primates may infect humans. The genus *Babesia* includes approximately 100 species which are transmitted by ticks of the genus *Ixodes* and infect a variety of wild and domestic animals. In the United States, *B. microti* and a recently described, unnamed species related to the canine species, *B. gibsoni*, infect humans (12). In Europe, the bovine parasites *B. bovis* and *B. divergens* have been isolated from human patients.

NATURAL HABITATS

Malaria is transmitted by anopheline mosquitoes throughout most of the tropics and in many subtropical regions. The parasite life cycle (Fig. 1) begins with the injection of sporozoites by the bite of an infected mosquito. Sporozoites move rapidly to the liver, where they invade hepatocytes and undergo exoerythrocytic development for 7 to 10 days, leading to the formation of liver schizonts. Rupture of each liver schizont releases thousands of free merozoites into the peripheral blood, where they invade erythrocytes. In the erythrocyte the early trophozoites (rings) develop into mature trophozoites with an enlarged cytoplasm and an accumulation of hemozoin pigment. Nuclear and cytoplasmic division leads to production of the mature schizont, which ruptures, releasing merozoites and completing the erythrocytic cycle. A fraction of the merozoites undergo sexual differentiation into gametocytes, which undergo fertilization and zygote formation following ingestion with a mosquito blood meal. In addition to transmission by mosquitoes in areas where the infection is endemic, transmission can occur following blood transfusion (11) and has been documented in patients living near airports who were presumably infected by mosquitoes carried in commercial airplanes (7).

There are important species-specific variations in the life cycle. The late trophozoites and schizonts of *P. falciparum* insert an antigenically variable, high-molecular-weight protein in the erythrocyte membrane which causes the infected erythrocyte to adhere to vascular endothelium (3). Thus, these stages of the life cycle do not circulate in the peripheral blood. *P. vivax* and *P. ovale* may be associated with relapse from the liver months to years after clearance of initial blood stage parasitemia. Sporozoites of these species may enter hepatocytes and complete exoerythrocytic stage development normally, or they may arrest development in the liver as hypnozoites which subsequently develop into mature liver schizonts, leading to relapse into parasitemia months to a few years later.

Babesiosis is transmitted by the bite of infected *Ixodes scapularis* (*I. dammini*) ticks, and outbreaks of human infection have been described in the northeast, midwest, and west coast of the United States. The life cycle is roughly similar to that of *Plasmodium*. Sexual development takes place in the tick, and infective forms are injected following a bite. However, no exoerythrocytic stage has been identified in humans, nor have morphologically identifiable gametocytes been described.

CLINICAL SIGNIFICANCE

Malaria imposes an enormous burden of illness and substantial mortality on the tropical world. There are an estimated 300 to 500 million new *Plasmodium* infections and 1.5 to 2.7 million deaths each year (19). The classic clinical manifestation of malaria is the febrile paroxysm which begins with a chill and rigors, leading to an abrupt fever lasting 1 to 2 h, and finally resolving with profuse sweating and a return to normal temperature. The typical periodicity of these paroxysms, approximately 48 h in *P. falciparum*, *P. vivax*, and *P. ovale* and 72 h in *P. malariae*, is not always

* This chapter contains information presented in chapter 104 by Lynne S. Garcia, Alexander J. Sulzer, George R. Healy, Katharine K. Grady, and David A. Bruckner in the sixth edition of this Manual.

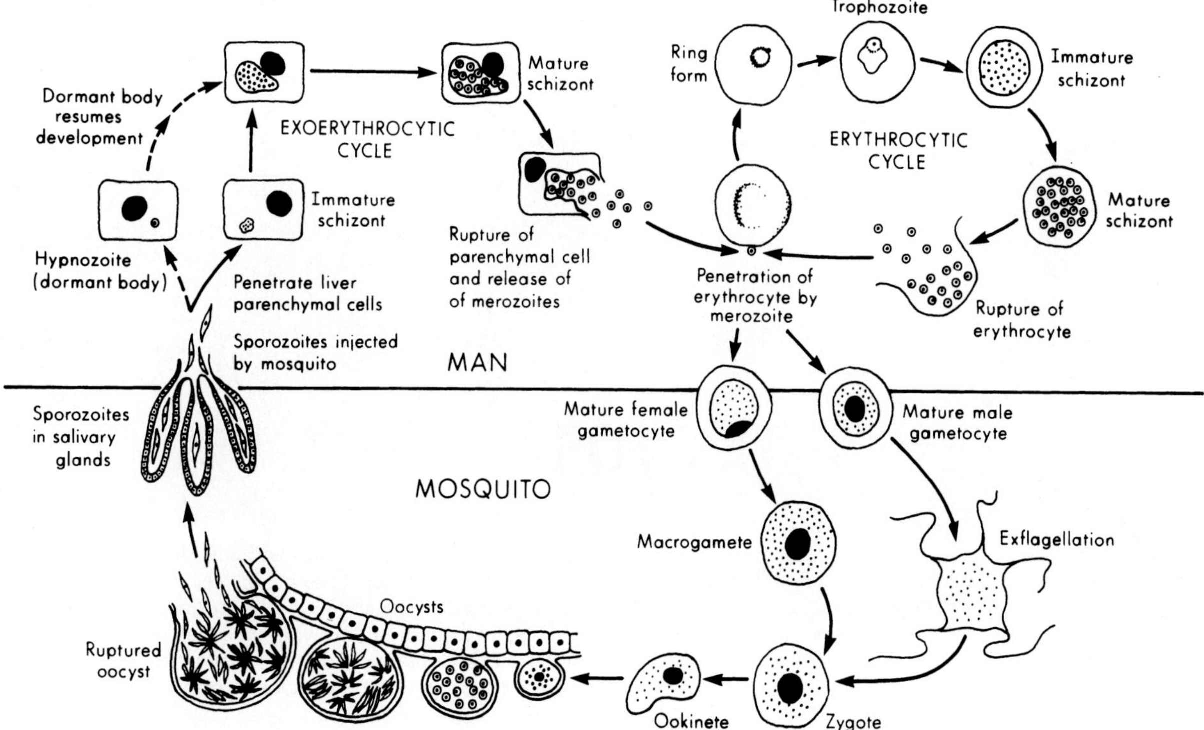

FIGURE 1 Life cycle of the malaria parasite. (Reproduced with permission from D. J. Krogstad and M. A. Pfaller, Prophylaxis and treatment of malaria, *Curr. Clin. Top. Infect. Dis.* **3**:56–73, 1983.)

seen, particularly in nonimmune individuals. The fever is frequently accompanied or preceded by headache, myalgias, and malaise. Splenomegaly and anemia are common. Gastrointestinal complaints, nausea, vomiting, and diarrhea, which may be bloody, are also not uncommon and should not distract the clinician from the diagnosis of malaria. Infection with *P. falciparum* may be complicated by severe malaria, which includes severe anemia (hematocrit <20%), hyperparasitemia (>5%), hypoglycemia, and cerebral malaria with alteration of consciousness, seizures, and coma. Severe malaria due to *P. falciparum* may develop rapidly in a patient who initially presents with mild symptoms and a low parasitemia. It is critical to make the diagnosis of *P. falciparum* quickly.

P. vivax and *P. ovale* preferentially invade reticulocytes and therefore only very rarely cause parasitemias greater than 2%. They may relapse from the liver following successful therapy of blood stage infection and must therefore be treated with primaquine to eradicate hypnozoites in the liver. *P. malariae* preferentially infects older erythrocytes and may cause chronic, asymptomatic parasitemia lasting for many years. Proteinuria is a common finding in *P. malariae* infection and may progress to the nephrotic syndrome in children.

Babesiosis caused by *B. microti* in the northeastern United States in normal hosts typically causes a self-resolving, febrile illness of several weeks' duration associated with malaise, chills, myalgias, headache, arthralgias, and fatigue. In splenectomized individuals, *Babesia* may cause a life-threatening, fulminant illness with severe hemolysis.

COLLECTION, TRANSPORT, AND STORAGE OF SPECIMENS

Because *P. falciparum* can progress rapidly to severe malaria, the diagnosis of malaria is an urgent matter and all requests for malaria diagnosis should be handled on a stat basis. Ideally, blood for preparation of peripheral smears may be collected by finger prick. If other tests are to be performed, blood may be collected by venipuncture using EDTA as the anticoagulant. Smears should be prepared and stained within an hour of drawing the specimen. Otherwise, confusing alterations in morphology may occur. For example, *P. falciparum* may continue to develop within the stored blood to the mature trophozoite stage, which is normally not seen in peripheral smears, leading to misidentification of the species. Blood containing malaria parasites or *Babesia* is infectious, and universal precautions should be strictly followed.

Requests for malaria smears should include several important pieces of historical information. If the following historical information is not submitted with the request for malaria smears, the laboratory must be proactive in obtaining the history. (i) The patient's travel history and date of return to or arrival in the United States can suggest the likelihood of infection and the possible species involved. The interval between exposure to an infective bite and development of symptoms is typically 7 to 12 days for *P. falciparum*, *P. vivax*, and *P. ovale* and up to 40 days for *P. malariae*. Because there may be no primary attack in *P. vivax* or *P. ovale*, if all sporozoites that invaded hepatocytes transformed into hypnozoites, the first symptoms could occur months to as many as 3 years after exposure. There have been extremely rare reports of *P. falciparum* malaria first being detected up to 24 months after exposure (8), but in general, malaria appearing more than 1 month after return from an area in which the disease is endemic is relatively unlikely to be due to *P. falciparum*, unless the patient has received antimalarial agents which might have suppressed parasitemia. (ii) A history of prophylaxis or treatment for malaria may result in low parasitemia. Since currently available prophylactic regimens are difficult to comply with and since drug resistance is common in *P. falciparum*, a history of prophylaxis should never be used to exclude malaria from the differential diagnosis. (iii) A history of transfusions or shared

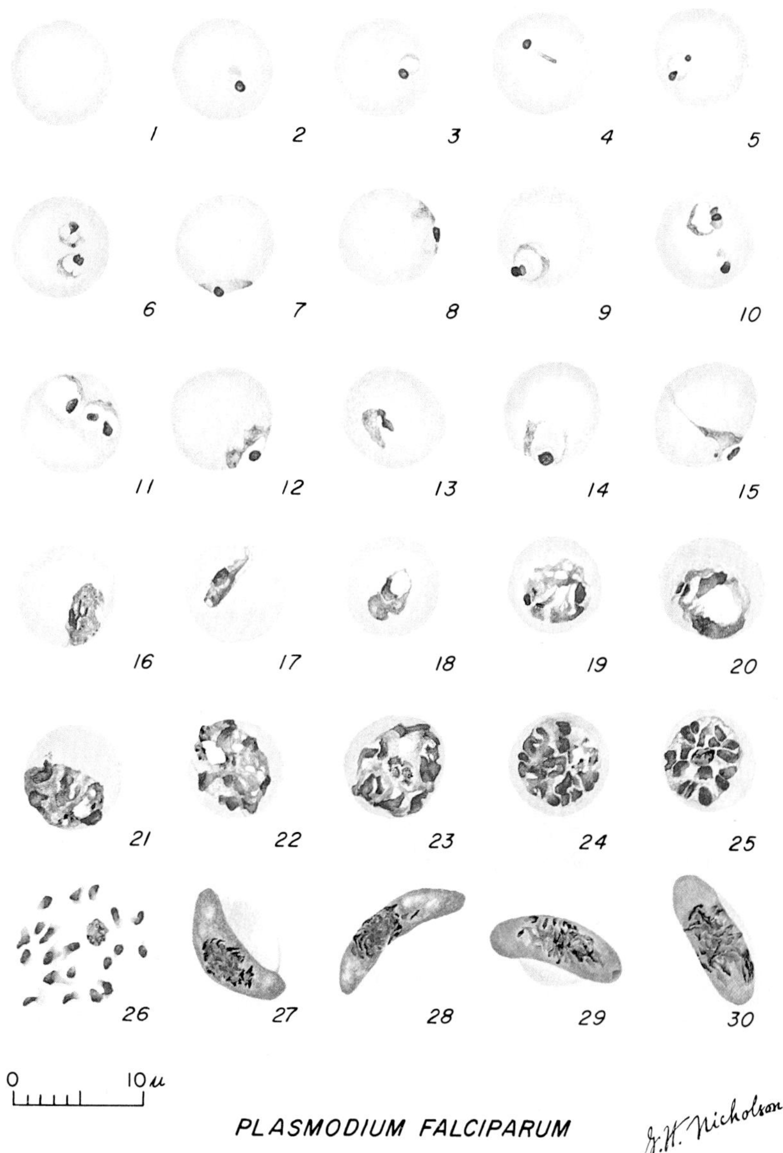

FIGURE 2 *P. falciparum*: morphology of successive developmental stages in Giemsa-stained thin blood smears. The cytoplasm of the rings is normally paler than shown in this figure: color intensity has been increased for purposes of illustration. Rings and gametocytes will be found in peripheral blood smears; other stages occur in infected erythrocytes but are sequestered in the capillaries and venules of internal organs and are rarely found in the periphery. Drawings: 1, normal erythrocyte; 2 to 11, young trophozoites (rings); 12 to 15, growing trophozoites; 16 to 18, mature trophozoites; 19 to 22, immature schizonts; 23 to 26, nearly mature and mature schizonts; 27 and 28, mature macrogametocytes: 29 and 30, mature microgametocytes. (Reproduced with permission from G. R. Coatney, W. E. Collins, M. Warren, and P. G. Contacos, *The Primate Malarias*, U.S. Department of Health, Education, and Welfare, Washington, D.C., 1971.)

needles may suggest direct person-to-person transmission, although cases of transfusion-related malaria are extremely rare in the United States. (iv) A prior history of malaria in the patient suggests the possibility of relapse or recrudescence. (v) Knowledge of the periodicity of the fever pattern and the time in relation to a paroxysm when the specimen was obtained is helpful because in a regularly periodic *P. falciparum* infection the circulating parasitemia can be very low and difficult to detect between paroxysms. Regardless of the presence of a fever pattern, blood should be taken immediately for an initial malaria smear when the patient presents.

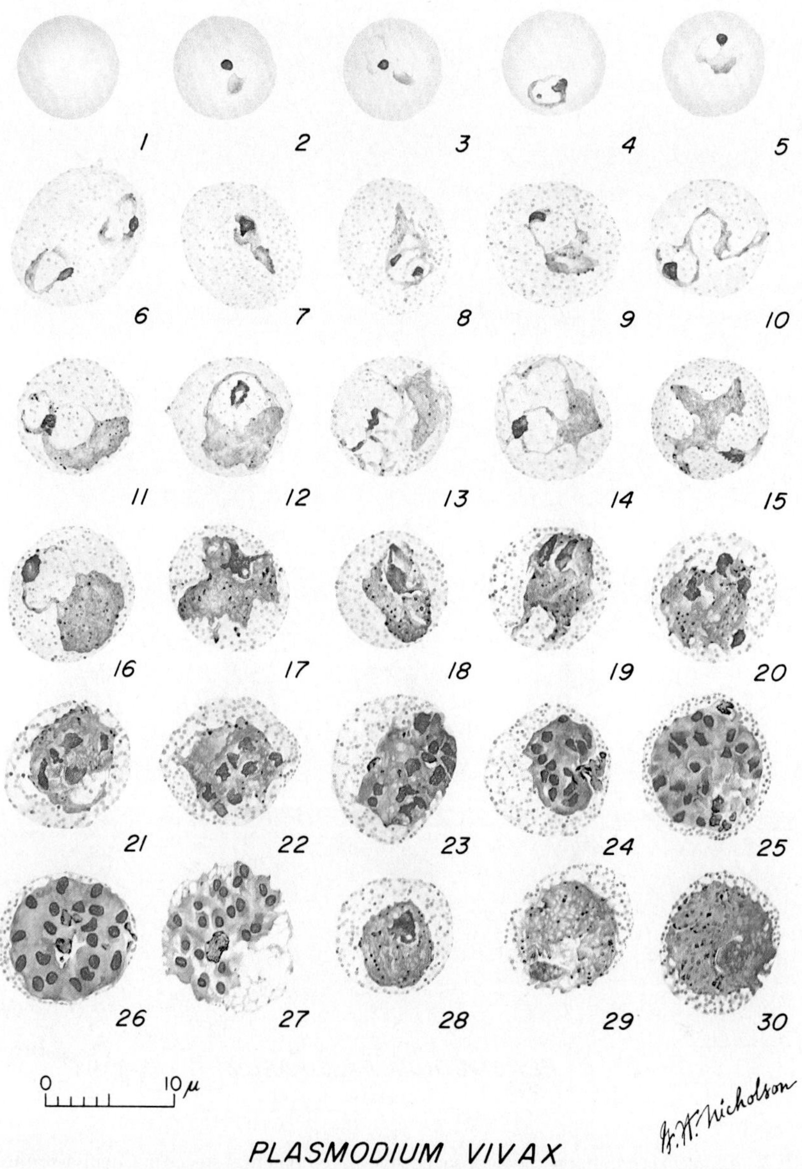

FIGURE 3 *P. vivax*: morphology of successive developmental stages in Giemsa-stained thin blood smears. The cytoplasm of the developing trophozoites and immature schizonts is normally paler than shown in this figure: color intensity has been increased for purposes of illustration. Drawings: 1, normal erythrocyte; 2 to 5, young trophozoites (rings); 6 to 16, growing trophozoites; 17 and 18, mature trophozoites; 19 to 21, young immature schizonts; 22 and 23, older immature schizonts; 24 to 27, nearly mature and mature schizonts; 28 and 29, nearly mature and mature macrogametocytes; 30, mature microgametocyte. (Reproduced with permission from G. R. Coatney, W. E. Collins, M. Warren, and P. G. Contacos, *The Primate Malarias*, U.S. Department of Health Education, and Welfare, Washington, D.C., 1971.)

ISOLATION PROCEDURES

In vitro culture is not performed for diagnosis of malaria or babesiosis. Detection and identification of the organisms are performed by examination of Giemsa-stained thick and thin blood films. Examination of thick films is the "gold standard," for detection of organisms because of the relatively large volume of blood (10 μl) that can be examined directly. Early in infection, or following relapse or partial treatment, patients may be symptomatic with parasitemias low enough that they require thick-smear examination for detection. While it is often possible to identify parasites to the species level in thick films, thin films are the gold standard for species identification. Although fewer parasites are present in thin films, methanol fixation prior to staining preserves erythrocyte morphology, allowing evaluation of infected erythrocyte size and the position of organisms within the erythrocytes. In difficult cases, therefore, examination of thin films may be necessary to make a specific identification. Smears should be examined at length under oil immersion; a negative report should not be rendered until 200 oil immersion fields of a thick film or 1,000 fields of a thin film

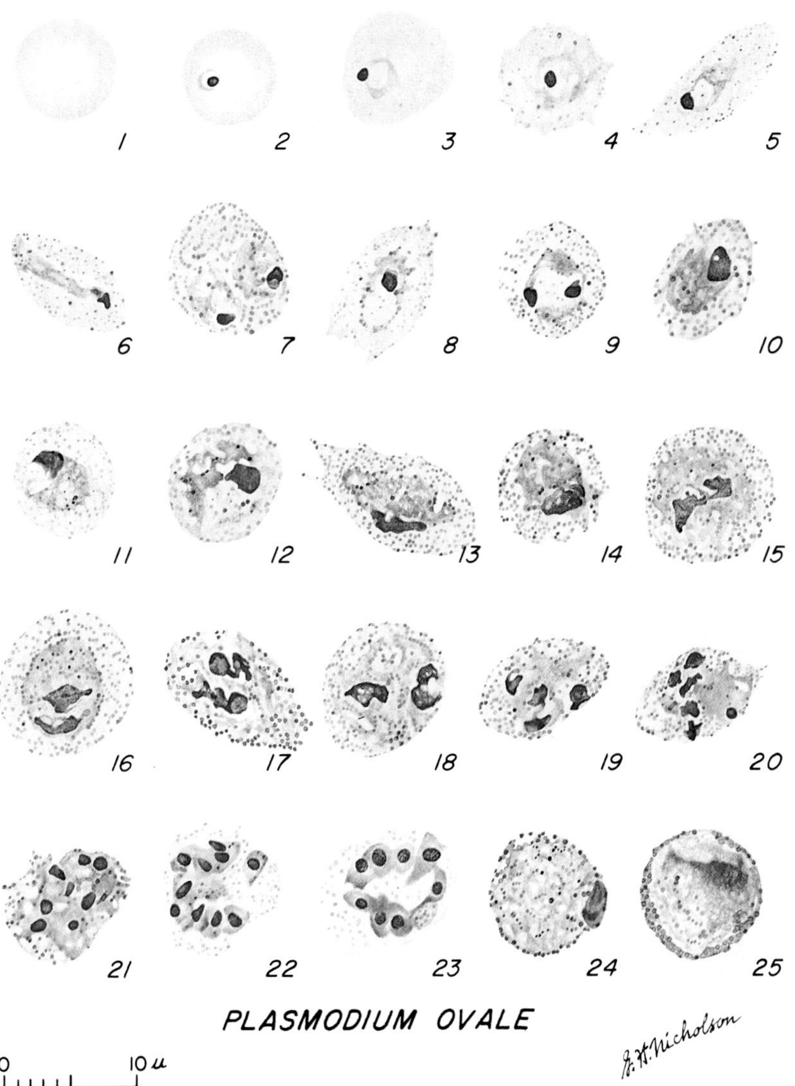

FIGURE 4 *P. ovale*: morphology of successive developmental stages in Giemsa-stained thin blood smears. The Schüffner's dots (James' stippling) are normally larger than shown here. Drawings: 1, normal erythrocyte; 2 to 5, young trophozoites (rings); 6 to 12, growing trophozoites; 13 to 15, mature trophozoites; 16 to 22, immature schizonts; 23, mature schizont; 24, mature macrogametocyte; 25, mature microgametocyte. (Reproduced with permission from G. R. Coatney, W. E. Collins, M. Warren, and P. G. Contacos, *The Primate Malarias*, U.S. Department of Health, Education, and Welfare, Washington, D.C., 1971.)

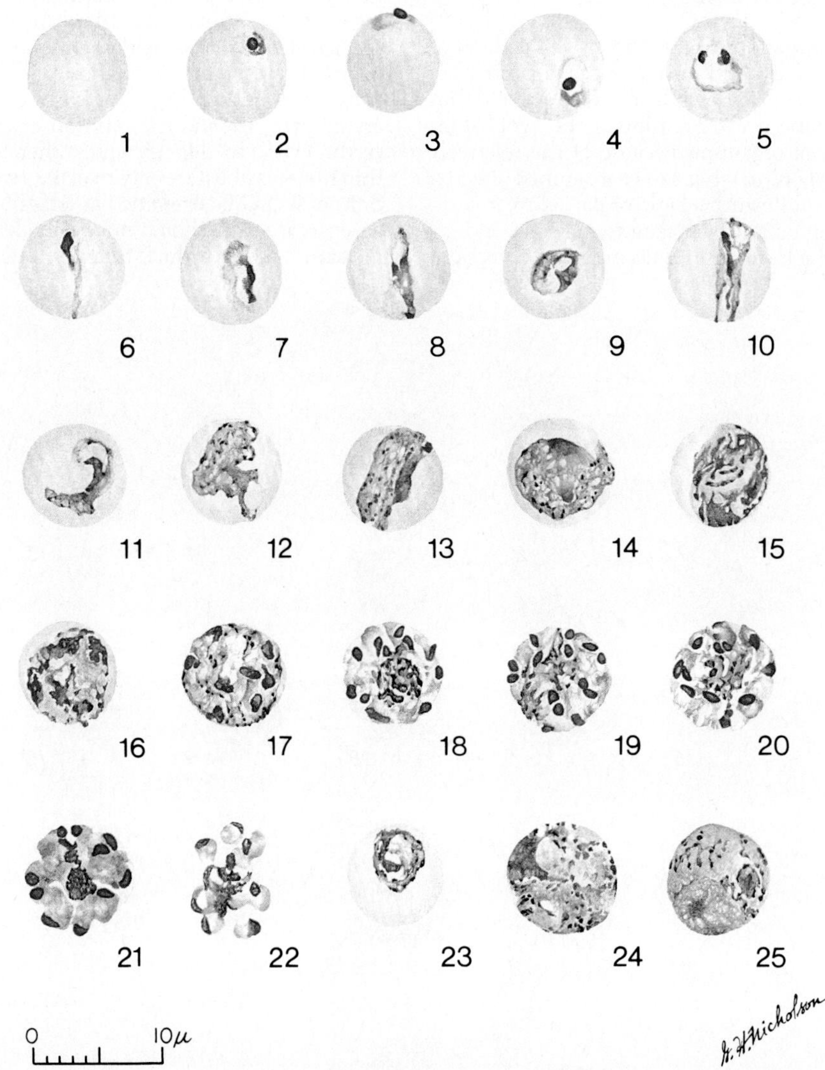

FIGURE 5 *P. malariae*: morphology of successive developmental stages in Giemsa-stained thin blood smears. Drawings: 1, normal erythrocyte; 2 to 5, young trophozoites (rings); 6 to 11, growing trophozoites; 12 and 13, nearly mature and mature trophozoites; 14 to 20, immature schizonts; 21 and 22, mature schizonts; 23, developing gametocyte; 24, mature macrogametocyte; 25, mature microgametocyte. (Reproduced with permission from G. R. Coatney, W. E. Collins, M. Warren, and P. G. Contacos, *The Primate Malarias*, U.S. Department of Health, Education, and Welfare, Washington, D.C., 1971.)

have been examined. A single set of negative smears does not exclude malaria. Additional specimens should be examined at 12-h intervals for the subsequent 36 h.

A number of new approaches to detection of malaria parasites have been described, including microhematocrit centrifugation and staining with acridine orange (14), PCR (2), and antigen detection (4, 17). These approaches are discussed in chapter 104. None of these methods has yet supplanted routine microscopic diagnosis. It should be pointed out that automated hematology instrumentation will not reliably detect malaria parasites.

IDENTIFICATION

Although many North American clinicians treat all malaria patients with regimens designed to cover drug-resistant *P. falciparum*, species-specific identification of *Plasmodium* spp. is clinically important for several reasons. *P. falciparum*

TABLE 1 Comparative morphology of *Plasmodium* spp. in Giemsa-stained thin smears

Characteristic	*P. falciparum*	*P. vivax*	*P. ovale*	*P. malariae*
Size and shape of infected erythrocytes	Normal size and shape	Enlarged up to twofold; may be oval	Normal to enlarged, frequently oval; may be fimbriated	Small to normal size, normal shape
Stippling (best seen with Giemsa stain, pH 7.0–7.2)	Occasional Maurer's dots, less numerous than Schüffner's	Schüffner's dots usually present, except in rings	James' stippling, darker than Schüffner's, present in all stages, including rings	Ziemann's dots rarely seen; requires deliberate overstaining
Stages seen in peripheral blood	Rings and gametocytes	All	All	All
Multiply infected erythrocytes	Common	Occasional	Occasional	Rare
Early trophozoites	Delicate ring, frequently with two small chromatin dots; often at edge of erythrocyte (appliqué form)	Ring up to ⅓ diameter of erythrocyte; larger chromatin dot than *P. falciparum*	Similar to *P. vivax*	Smaller than *P. vivax*; otherwise similar
Mature trophozoites	Not seen in peripheral blood	Ameboid shape, fine golden-brown pigment	Similar to *P. vivax* except less ameboid, pigment darker brown	Compact cytoplasm, oval, round, or band-shaped, dark brown pigment
Schizonts	Not seen in peripheral blood	12–24 merozoites	8–12 merozoites	6–12 merozoites often radially arranged around central pigment ("daisy head" schizont)
Gametocytes	Crescent or banana shaped	Round to slightly oval	Round to slightly oval	Round to slightly oval
Most characteristic findings	Absence of mature trophozoites and schizonts; normal size of infected erythrocytes; multiple infections; appliqué forms; banana-shaped gametocytes	Enlarged infected erythrocytes; Schüffner's dots frequently present; ameboid trophozoite; 12–24 merozoites in each schizont	Normal to enlarged, oval or fimbriated infected erythrocytes; James' stippling may be seen in rings; schizonts with 8–12 merozoites	Normal size of infected erythrocytes; no stippling; "band" trophozoite; "daisy head" schizont with 6–12 merozoites

should be identified because it is both more clinically aggressive and more likely to be multiply drug resistant than the other species. *P. vivax* and *P. ovale* should be identified because radical cure of these infections requires supplemental treatment with primaquine to prevent relapse. Primaquine may cause hemolytic anemia in some patients with G6PD deficiency; correct species identification prevents its unnecessary use in *P. falciparum* or *P. malariae* infection.

The morphology of the four species of *Plasmodium* which infect humans in thin films is reviewed in the references (5) and is demonstrated in Fig. 2 to 5 and summarized in Table 1. The appearance of *P. falciparum* in thick films is demonstrated in Fig. 6. When abundant organisms encompassing several life cycle stages are present for examination, species identification is not difficult. A high parasitemia consisting only of ring forms suggests *P. falciparum*, even if, as is commonly the case, no gametocytes are found. In samples containing only rare early trophozoites, a species identification may not be possible. Ring morphology is quite variable; early trophozoites of *P. falciparum* may mimic early "band" forms of *P. malariae* or early ameboid trophozoites of *P. vivax*. It is important not to exclude *P. falciparum* solely on the basis of ring morphology. Finally, the possibility of mixed infections should be borne in mind; examination of

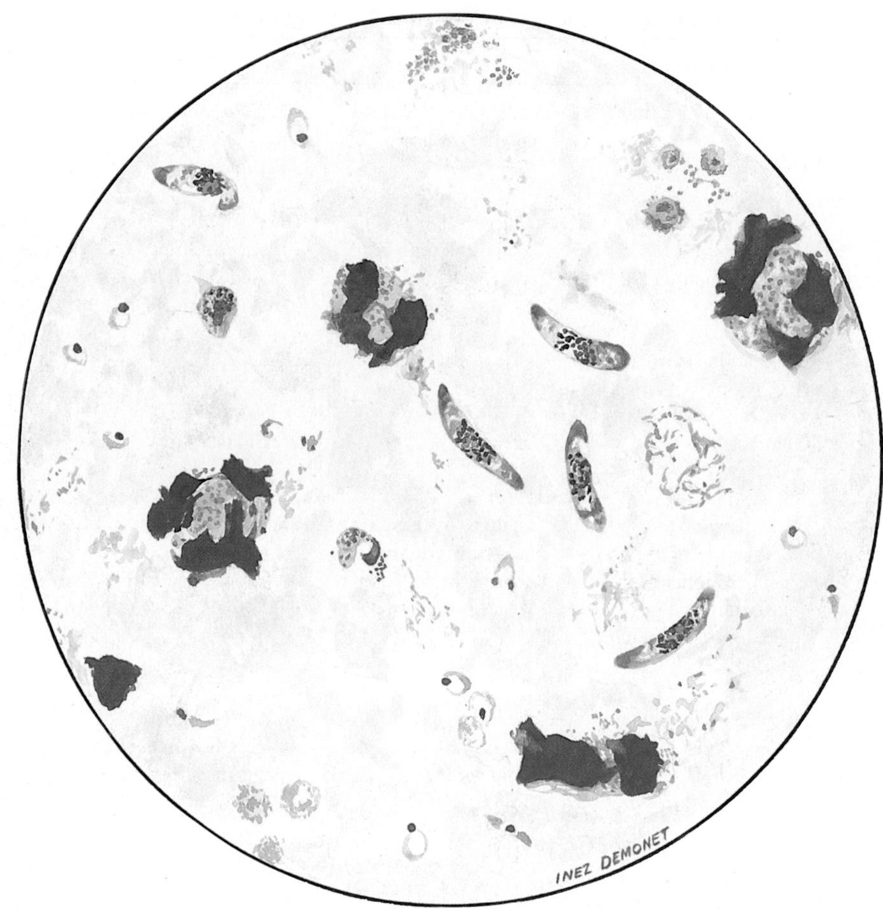

FIGURE 6 *P. falciparum*: morphology in Giemsa-stained thick blood smears. There are multiple small trophozoites (rings) and banana- or crescent-shaped gametocytes. Two gametocytes with variant shapes are present at 10 o'clock. Outside of endemic areas, parasites on a thick film are normally fewer than in this figure. (Reproduced from A. Wilcox, *Manual for the Microscopical Diagnosis of Malaria in Man*, U.S. Department of Health, Education, and Welfare, Washington, D.C., 1960.)

the smear should not be ended prematurely simply because one species of *Plasmodium* has been identified.

Babesia can be distinguished from *P. falciparum* by several criteria (Fig. 7). *Babesia* trophozoites are quite variable in size (1 to 5 μm), and the smallest are smaller than *P. falciparum* rings. Extracellular trophozoites and multiply infected erythrocytes are more common in Babesia infections. The cytoplasm of the larger *Babesia* trophozoites frequently contains a clear vacuole which is rare or absent in *P. falciparum*. Finally, diagnostic tetrads, the Maltese Cross, though rare in clinical specimens, may be present in *Babesia*.

SEROLOGIC TESTS

Indirect fluorescent-antibody tests using antigens prepared from the four species of *Plasmodium* which infect humans have been described (18). However, serologic testing is not useful in clinical diagnosis of malaria because antibodies may be absent in an acute attack and because their presence may reflect past rather than current infection. It has a role in the investigation of transfusion malaria, where it may be used to determine which of a number of potential donors may have been the source of a transfusion-associated case of malaria, and in epidemiological studies, to determine the prevalence of exposure to malaria in a population. Assistance in serological evaluation of suspected transfusion malaria can be obtained from the Malaria Section, Epidemiology Branch, Centers for Disease Control and Prevention, Atlanta, Ga. [(770) 488–7788].

ANTIBIOTIC SUSCEPTIBILITIES

Therapy of malaria has been recently reviewed (6). *P. falciparum* resistant to chloroquine is present in all endemic areas with the exception of Central America and the Caribbean. In addition, resistance to other drugs, including Fansidar and mefloquine, is present in many areas and is expanding rapidly. The combination of quinine or quinidine and doxycycline remains effective against most strains of *P. falciparum*, and artemesinin has shown promising results. However, therapy of chloroquine-resistant *P. falciparum* is a complex and rapidly evolving field, and consulation with an infectious diseases specialist is essential. Chloroquine-resistant *P. vivax* has emerged in a few areas in recent years,

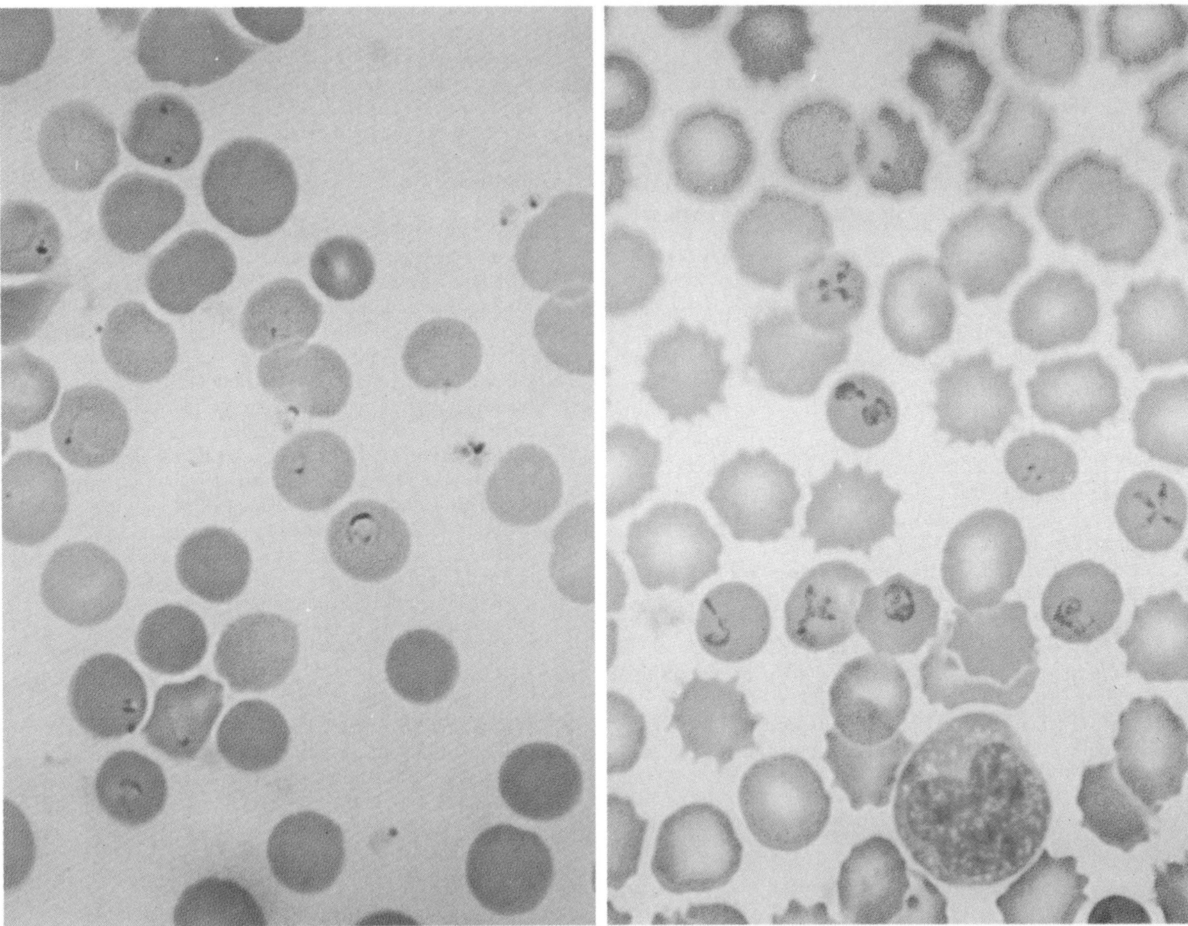

FIGURE 7 *Babesia* spp. in thin blood films. (Left) *B. microti* in human blood: parasites in erythrocytes and extracellular parasites; (right) a *Babesia* sp. in classic Maltese cross (tetrad) configuration, a form diagnostic for babesiosis but rare in slides from humans infected with *B. microti.*

including Indonesia, Papua New Guinea, Myanmar, and Guyana (1, 10, 13, 16), and may be expected to spread widely in time. Current information on the distribution of chloroquine-resistant *P. falciparum* may be obtained from the Centers for Disease Control and Prevention, Malaria Branch, in Atlanta [phone: (770) 488–7788]. In vitro susceptibility testing of *P. falciparum* has been described (15) but is not available for clinical use. Babesiosis has been treated with clindamycin and quinine or intravenous quinidine.

INTERPRETATION AND REPORTING OF RESULTS

A positive finding of malaria parasites of *Babesia* is a critical result which must be reported immediately to the clinician. The report should include the species identification, if possible. When identification to this level is not possible, an explicit statement that *P. falciparum* cannot be excluded is advisable. Because patients with high levels of parasitemia (>3 to 5%) require intensive therapy, quantification of parasitemia is useful. This is typically performed after species identification and may be variously expressed as percent parasitemia (parasites/100 erythrocytes), number of parasites per 100 leukocytes, or parasites/mm^3. At high levels of parasitemia, the direct counting of parasites and erythrocytes in a thin film will provide an accurate measurement of parasitemia. In low levels of parasitemia and, of course, in thick smears, it is necessary to count parasites/100 leukocytes and to calculate the percent parasitemia or the parasite density based on the patient's complete blood count. A negative report may be accompanied by a reminder that a single negative set of smears does not exclude the diagnosis of malaria. Serial malaria smears may be performed to monitor therapy. Parasitemia normally resolves within 2 to 3 days following initiation of treatment with a drug to which the patient's strain is susceptible. Continued parasitemia at day 7 or failure of the parasitemia to decrease by 75% within the first 48 h following treatment is an indication of drug resistance. However, gametocytes may continue to circulate for up to 2 weeks after successful cure, and their presence is not an indication that treatment has failed.

REFERENCES

1. **Baird, J. K., H. Basri, Purnomo, M. J. Bangs, B. Subianto, L. C. Patchen, and S. L. Hoffman.** 1991. Resistance to chloroquine by *Plasmodium vivax* in Irian Jaya, Indonesia. *Am. J. Trop. Med. Hyg.* **44:**547–552.
2. **Barker, R. H., T. Banchongaksorn, J. M. Courval, W. Suwonkerd, K. Rimwungtragoon, and D. F. Wirth.** 1992.

A simple method to detect *Plasmodium falciparum* directly from blood using the polymerase chain reaction. *Am. J. Trop. Med. Hyg.* **46:**416–426.

3. **Borst, P., W. Bitter, R. McCulloch, F. Van Leeuwen, and G. Rudenko.** 1995. Antigenic variation in malaria. *Cell* **82:**1–4.
4. **Craig, M. H., and B. L. Sharp.** 1997. Comparative evaluation of four techniques for the diagnosis of *Plasmodium falciparum* infections. *Trans. R. Soc. Trop. Med. Hyg.* **91:** 279–282.
5. **Garcia, L. S., and D. A. Bruckner.** 1997. *Diagnostic Medical Parasitology*. American Society for Microbiology, Washington, D.C.
6. **Hoffman, S. L.** 1992. Diagnosis, treatment and prevention of malaria. *Med. Clin. North Am.* **76:**1327–1355.
7. **Isaacson, M.** 1989. Airport malaria: a review. *Bull. W. H. O.* **67:**737–743.
8. **Kyronseppa, H., E. Tiula, H. Repo, and J. Lahdevirta.** 1989. Diagnosis of falciparum malaria delayed by long incubation period and misleading presenting symptoms: lifesaving role of manual leucocyte differential count. *Scand. J. Infect. Dis.* **21:**117–118.
9. **Levine, N. D.** 1988. Progress in taxonomy of the Apicomplexan protozoa. *J. Protozool.* **35:**518–520.
10. **Myat-Phone-Kyaw, Myint-Oo, Myint-Lwin, Thaw-Zin, Kyin-Hla-Aye, and Nwe-Nwe-Yin.** 1993. Emergence of chloroquine-resistant *Plasmodium vivax* in Myanmar (Burma). *Trans. R. Soc. Trop. Med. Hyg.* **87:**687.
11. **Nahlen, B. L., H. O. Lobel, S. E. Cannon, and C. C. Campbell.** 1991. Reassessment of blood donor selection criteria for United States travelers to malarious areas. *Transfusion* **31:**798–804.
12. **Persing, D. H., B. L. Herwaldt, C. Glaser, R. S. Lane, J. W. Thomford, D. Mathiesen, P. J. Krause, D. F. Phillip, and P. A. Conrad.** 1995. Infection with a Babesia-like organism in northern California. *N. Engl. J. Med.* **332:** 298–303.
13. **Phillips, E. J., J. S. Keystone, and K. C. Kain.** 1996. Failure of combined chloroquine and high-dose primaquine therapy for *Plasmodium vivax* malaria acquired in Guyana, South America. *Clin. Infect. Dis.* **23:**1171–1173.
14. **Rickman, L. S., G. W. Long, R. Oberst, A. Cabanban, R. Sangalang, J. I. Smith, J. D. Chulay, and S. L. Hoffman.** 1989. Rapid diagnosis of malaria by acridine orange staining of centrifuged parasites. *Lancet* **i:**68–71.
15. **Rieckmann, K. H., G. H. Campbell, L. J. Sax, and J. Mrema.** 1978. Drug sensitivity of *Plasmodium falciparum*: an *in vitro* microtechnique. *Lancet* **i:**22–23.
16. **Schuurkamp, G. J., P. E. Spicer, R. K. Kereu, P. K. Bulungol, and K. H. Rieckmann.** 1992. Chloroquine-resistant *Plasmodium vivax* in Papua New Guinea. *Trans. R. Soc. Trop. Med. Hyg.* **86:**121–122.
17. **Shiff, C. J., Z. Premji, and J. N. Minjas.** 1993. The rapid manual ParaSight-F test. A new diagnostic tool for *Plasmodium falciparum* infection. *Trans. R. Soc. Trop. Med. Hyg.* **87:**646–648.
18. **Sulzer, A. J., and M. Wilson.** 1971. The indirect fluorescent antibody test for the detection of occult malaria in blood donors. *Bull. W. H. O.* **45:**375–379.
19. **World Health Organization.** 1994. World malaria situation in 1992. *Weekly Epidemiol. Rec.* **69:**309–314.

Leishmania and *Trypanosoma**

DAVID A. BRUCKNER AND JAIME A. LABARCA

106

Leishmania spp. and *Trypanosoma* spp. are protozoa belonging to the family *Trypanosomatidae*. Leishmaniasis is principally a zoonosis, although in certain areas of the world the disease is endemic. *Leishmania* spp. are obligate intracellular parasites transmitted to humans by bites from an infected sandfly. Depending on the geographic area, many species can infect humans producing a variety of diseases (cutaneous, mucocutaneous, and visceral diseases) (Table 1).

Trypanosoma spp. are hemoflagellate protozoa that live in the blood and tissue of the human host. American trypanosomiasis (Chagas' disease) is produced by *Trypanosoma cruzi*, which belongs to the family *Schizotrypanum* and is confined to the American continent. *Trypanosoma rangeli* belongs to the family *Tejaria*, produces an asymptomatic infection, and is also present only on the American continent. African trypanosomiasis (sleeping sickness) is caused by *T. brucei gambiense* and *T. brucei rhodesiense* species belonging to the family *Trypanozoon* and is confined to the central belt of Africa. African trypanosomes and *T. rangeli* are transmitted directly into the bite wound by salivary secretions from the insect vector, while *T. cruzi* is transmitted through contamination of the bite wound with the feces from the reduviid bug (Table 2).

LEISHMANIA SPP.

Introduction

Recent estimates suggest there are approximately 350 million people at risk of acquiring leishmaniasis, with 112 million currently infected. More than 400,000 new cases are reported annually (28). The taxonomy of leishmaniasis is controversial and in a state of dynamic flux. Species differentiation is currently based upon molecular techniques rather than geographical distribution and clinical presentation.

Life Cycle and Morphology

The parasite has two distinct phases in its life cycle (amastigote and promastigote) (Fig. 1). The amastigote stage (Leishman-Donovan body) is found in reticuloendothelial cells of the mammalian host. The amastigote form is small, is round or oval, measures 3 to 5 μm, and contains a large nucleus and small kinetoplast (Fig. 2 and 3).

Upon ingestion during a blood meal by the insect vector (sandfly), the amastigote transforms into the promastigote stage. Promastigotes multiply in the gut of the insect and migrate to the hypostome of the sandfly, where they are released when the next blood meal is taken. The complete life cycle in the sandfly is from 4 to 18 days. Upon inoculation into the bite site, the promastigote changes to the amastigote form after being engulfed by tissue macrophages.

The life cycles of *Leishmania* organisms are similar for cutaneous, mucocutaneous, and visceral leishmaniasis, except that infected reticuloendothelial cells can be found throughout the body in visceral leishmaniasis.

Epidemiology

All adult female sandflies transmitting leishmaniasis belong to the genus *Phlebotomus* in the Old World and *Lutzomyia* in the New World. The disease is considered primarily a zoonosis, with natural reservoirs including rodents, opossums, anteaters, sloths, and dogs. In certain areas of the world where the disease is endemic, the infection can be transmitted by a human-vector-human cycle. The infection may also be transmitted by direct contact with an infected lesion or mechanically through bites by stable or dog flies.

Visceral leishmaniasis may exist as an endemic, epidemic, and sporadic disease. The disease is a zoonosis except in India, where kala azar is an anthroponosis. The natural reservoirs are wild *Canidae* and various rodents for *L. donovani*; dogs, other *Canidae*, and rats for *L. infantum*; and *Canidae* and cats for *L. chagasi*. Individuals with post-kala azar dermal leishmaniasis may be very important reservoirs for maintaining the infection during interendemic cycles.

Clinical Disease

Depending on the species involved, infection with *Leishmania* spp. can result in cutaneous, mucocutaneous, or visceral disease (Table 1). A large number of disease variations have been described, which makes classical disease categories confusing (7).

The first sign of cutaneous disease is the appearance of a firm, painless papule at or near the insect bite site. The incubation period may be as short as 2 weeks (*L. major*) or as long as several months to 3 years (*L. tropica* and *L.*

* This chapter contains information presented in chapter 104 by Lynne S. Garcia, Alexander J. Sulzer, George R. Healy, Katharine K. Grady, and David A. Bruckner in the sixth edition of this Manual.

TABLE 1 Features of human leishmanial infections

Species	Disease type[a]	Recommended specimen	Geographical distribution
L. donovani	VL MCL, CL, DL	Bone marrow/spleen Skin/mucosal macrophages	Africa and Asia
L. infantum	VL CL	Bone marrow/spleen Skin macrophages	Africa, Europe, Mediterranean area, Southwest Asia
L. chagasi	VL	Bone marrow/spleen	Central and South America
L. tropica	CL	Skin macrophages	Afghanistan, India, Turkey, former USSR
L. major	CL	Skin macrophages	Middle East, Afghanistan, Africa, former USSR
L. aethiopica	CL, DCL, MCL	Skin/mucosal macrophages	Ethiopia, Kenya, Yemen, former USSR
L. mexicana	CL, DCL	Skin macrophages	Texas, Belize, Guatemala, Mexico
L. braziliensis	CL, MCL	Skin/mucosal macrophages	Central and South America
L. peruviana	CL	Skin macrophages	Peru, Argentina
L. panamensis	CL	Skin macrophages	Panama, Colombia, Costa Rica
L. garnhami	CL	Skin macrophages	Venezuela
L. colombiensis	CL	Skin macrophages	Colombia, Panama
L. venezuelensis	CL	Skin macrophages	Venezuela
L. lainsoni, L. shawii	CL	Skin macrophages	Brazil
L. amazonensis	CL, DCL	Skin macrophages	Brazil, Venezuela
L. naiffi	CL	Skin macrophages	Brazil, Caribbean islands
L. pifanoi	CL, DCL	Skin macrophages	Brazil, Venezuela

[a] CL, cutaneous leishmaniasis; DCL, diffuse cutaneous leishmaniasis; DL, dermal leishmanoid; MCL, mucocutaneous leishmaniasis, VL, visceral leishmaniasis.

TABLE 2 Characteristics of trypanosomiasis

Characteristic	*T. brucei rhodesiense*	*T. brucei gambiense*	*T. cruzi*	*T. rangeli*
Vector	Tsetse fly	Tsetse fly	Reduviid bug	Reduviid bug
Primary reservoir	Animals	Humans	Animals	Animals
Illness	Acute, <9 months	Chronic, months to years	Acute, chronic	Asymptomatic
Epidemiology	Anthropozoonosis[a]	Anthroponosis[b]	Anthropozoonosis	Anthropozoonosis
Diagnostic stage	Trypomastigote	Trypomastigote	Trypomastigote, amastigote	Trypomastigote
Recommended specimens	Blood, CSF, chancre, lymph node aspirate	Blood, CSF, chancre, lymph node aspirate	Blood, lymph node, chagoma aspirate	Blood

[a] Anthropozoonosis: transmission involving man-animal-man cycle.
[b] Anthroponosis: transmission involving man-man cycle.

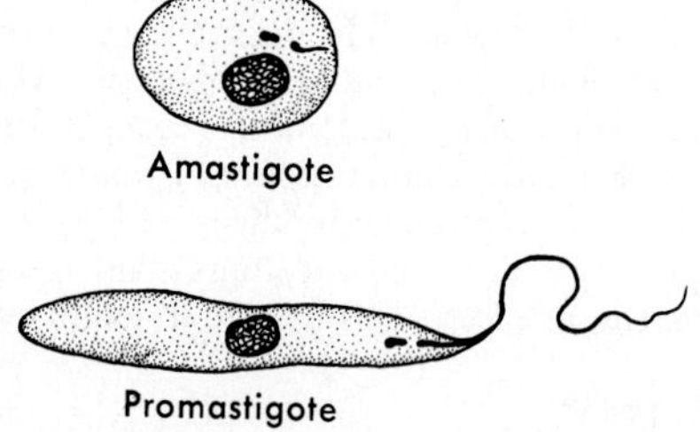

FIGURE 1 *Leishmania* spp. stages. (Illustration by Nobuko Kitamura. Used with permission from L. S. Garcia and D. A. Bruckner, *Diagnostic Medical Parasitology*, 3rd ed., ASM Press, Washington, D.C., 1997.)

aethiopica). Papules may be intensely pruritic and will grow to 2 cm or more in diameter. In simple cutaneous leishmaniasis, the infection remains localized at the insect bite site, where a definite self-limiting granulomatous response develops.

Mucocutaneous leishmaniasis is produced most often by the *L. braziliensis* complex. The primary lesions are similar to those found in other cutaneous leishmaniasis. Untreated primary lesions may develop into the mucocutaneous form in up to 80% of the cases. Metastatic spread to the nasal or oral mucosa may occur in the presence of the active primary lesion or many years later after the primary lesion has healed. Mucosal lesions do not heal spontaneously, and secondary bacterial infections are frequent and may be fatal. A small number of mucocutaneous leishmaniasis cases have been reported with *L. donovani* and *L. aethiopica*.

Clinical features of the visceral disease vary from asymptomatic, self-resolving infections to frank visceral leishmaniasis. The incubation period may be as short as 10 days and as long as 2 years; usually it is within 2 to 4 months. Common symptoms include fever, anorexia, malaise, weight

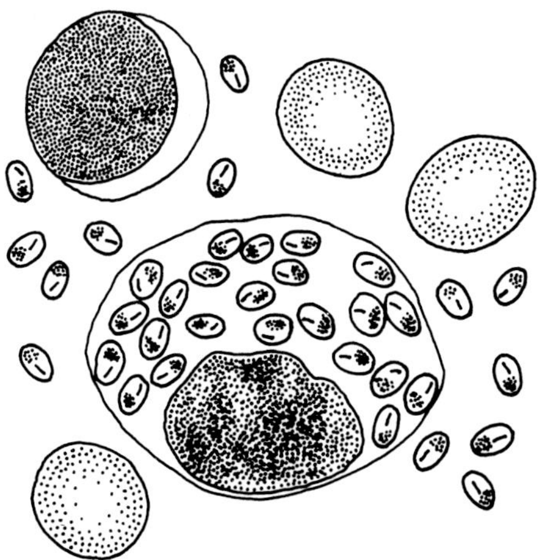

FIGURE 2 *Leishmania donovani* amastigotes. (Illustration by Sharon Belkin. Used with permission from L. S. Garcia and D. A. Bruckner, *Diagnostic Medical Parasitology*, 3rd ed., ASM Press, Washington, D.C., 1997.)

loss, and, frequently, diarrhea. Common clinical signs include nontender hepatomegaly and splenomegaly, lymphadenopathy, and occasional acute abdominal pain; darkening of facial, hand, foot, and abdominal skin (kala azar) is often seen in light-skinned persons in India. Anemia, cachexia, and marked enlargement of liver and spleen are noted as the disease progresses. Death may ensue after a few weeks, or after 2 to 3 years in chronic cases. The majority of infected individuals will be asymptomatic or have very few or minor symptoms that will resolve without therapy.

Postdermal leishmaniasis is a condition seen in some patients unsuccessfully treated for visceral leishmaniasis. The macular or hypopigmented dermal lesions are associated with few parasites, whereas erythematous and nodular lesions are associated with abundant parasites.

Diagnosis

In areas where the disease is endemic, the diagnosis may be made on clinical grounds. Definitive diagnosis depends on detecting either the amastigotes in clinical specimens or the promastigotes in culture. All lesions should be thoroughly cleaned with 70% alcohol, and extraneous debris should be removed. Specimens can be collected from the margin of the lesion by aspiration, scraping, or punch biopsy. Material scraped from the wall of the slit made with a sterile surgical blade should be smeared on to a number of slides.

The core of tissue from a punch biopsy can be used to make imprints or touch preparations on a slide. This core can also be submitted for histological study. Recognition of amastigotes in tissues is more difficult than in smears or imprints because the organisms tend to be crowded within the cells, appear smaller, and are cut at various angles. Fine-needle aspiration can also be performed by using a sterile syringe containing sterile buffered saline (0.1 ml) and a 26-gauge needle. The needle is inserted under the outer border of the lesion, the needle is rotated several times, and tissue fluid is aspirated into the needle. Tissue obtained by splenic puncture yields the highest rate of positive specimens; however, this procedure carries considerable risk to the patient. Other specimens include lymph node aspirates, liver biopsy, sternal or iliac crest bone marrow, and buffy coat preparations of venous blood. Individuals with post-kala azar dermal leishmaniasis have large numbers of parasites in the skin (13).

Amastigote stages will be found within macrophages or close to disrupted cells (Fig. 2 and 3). This stage can be recognized by its shape, size, staining characteristics, and especially the presence of an intracytoplasmic kinetoplast. The cytoplasm will stain light blue and the nucleus and kinetoplast will stain red or purple with Giemsa stain. Tissue stains with monoclonal antibodies and Western blot analysis have been proposed for diagnostic use (3). Molecular procedures using repetitive sequences of DNA or RNA as targets for hybridization or amplification have been used for diagnosis and research. PCR targeting kinetoplast DNA has been used in skin biopsy for *L. braziliensis* and *L. mexicana*, with better sensitivity than microscopy and culture (25, 27). In visceral leishmaniasis, PCR for *L. donovani* of splenic aspirates and blood has been used for diagnosis and treatment follow-up (19).

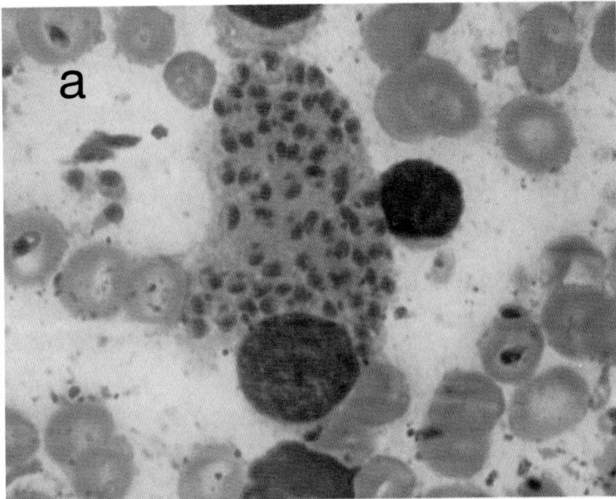

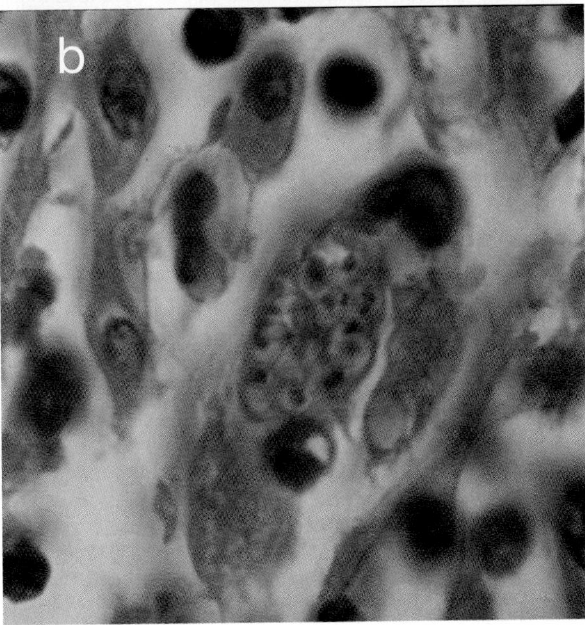

FIGURE 3 (a) *Leishmania donovani* amastigotes from splenic tissue press preparation (Giemsa stain). (b) *Trypanosoma cruzi* amastigotes seen in section of human cardiac tissue (hematoxylin and eosin stain).

If material is to be cultured, it must be collected aseptically. Tissues should be minced prior to culture. Culture media successfully employed to recover organisms include Novy, MacNeal, and Nicolle's medium (NNN) and Schneider's *Drosophila* medium supplemented with 30% fetal bovine serum. Cultures should be examined twice weekly for the first 2 weeks and once a week thereafter for up to 4 weeks, before the culture is declared negative. Promastigote stages can be detected microscopically in wet mounts and then stained with Giemsa to observe their morphology.

Animals such as the golden hamster can be inoculated with patient material. Animals are inoculated intranasally for cutaneous and mucocutaneous leishmaniasis and intraperitoneally for visceral leishmaniasis. It may take 2 to 3 months before an animal becomes positive. A combination of tissue smears, culture, and animal inoculation may be needed to optimize the laboratory diagnosis of the infection.

The leishmanin (Montenegro) test, a delayed-hypersensitivity reaction, is useful for epidemiological surveys of a population to identify groups at risk of infection. Positive reactions are usually seen in cutaneous and mucocutaneous leishmaniasis; however, patients with active visceral and diffuse cutaneous leishmaniasis will exhibit negative reactions.

Serologies are available for research or epidemiologic purposes; however, they are not very useful for the diagnosis of mucocutaneous and visceral leishmaniasis. In kala azar, there is a large increase in gamma globulins, both immunoglobulin G (IgG) and IgM. This is the basis for the aldehyde or formol-gel test, which has been used as a screening test in areas where the disease is endemic (17). A number of serologies have been developed for diagnostic purposes; however, they are not widely available.

Treatment and Prevention

Lesions in simple cutaneous leishmaniasis will generally heal spontaneously. Treatment options have included cryotherapy, heat, surgical excision of lesions, and chemotherapy. Although optimal treatment for cutaneous leishmaniasis is unknown, standard therapy consists of injections of antimonial compounds. Response to therapy will vary depending upon the species of *Leishmania* and type of disease (10). Antimonial therapy has been given intralesionally and parenterally. The two commonly used pentavalent antimonials are sodium stibogluconate (Pentostam) and a meglumine antimoniate (Glucantime). The drug of choice for treatment of kala azar is sodium stibogluconate (Pentostam). Pentamidine isethionate is an alternate therapy for treatment of kala azar. Amphotericin B can be used when the disease does not respond to antimonial or pentamidine therapy. Allopurinol, either alone or in combination with antimonials, has been effective in treating cutaneous leishmaniasis. To ensure that treatment has been effective, follow-up smears and cultures should be done 1 to 2 weeks posttherapy.

In areas where cutaneous leishmaniasis is endemic, vaccination has been practiced by inoculating the serous exudate from naturally acquired lesions into an inconspicuous area of the body of a nonimmune person. Vaccines against other forms of leishmaniasis have not been effective. Other possible prevention methods include spraying dwellings with residual insecticides and applying insect repellents to the skin. Fine mesh netting may also be used. Reservoir control has been unsuccessful in most areas. Individuals with lesions should be warned to protect the lesion from insect bites with some type of covering. Patients should also be educated about the possibility of autoinoculation or infection.

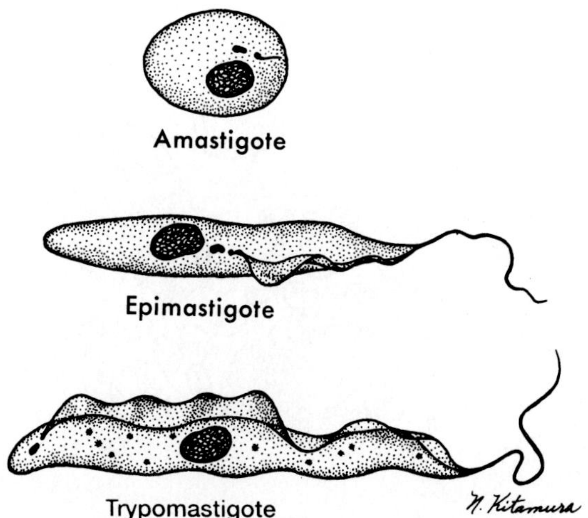

FIGURE 4 Life cycle stages of trypanosomes. (Illustration by Nobuko Kitamura. Used with permission from L. S. Garcia and D. A. Bruckner, *Diagnostic Medical Parasitology*, 3rd ed., ASM Press, Washington, D.C., 1997.)

AMERICAN TRYPANOSOMIASIS

Trypanosoma cruzi

Introduction

American trypanosomiasis (Chagas' disease) is a zoonosis caused by *Trypanosoma cruzi*. There are 100 million persons at risk of infection in Latin American countries, and 16 to 18 million persons are actually infected (26). Patients can present with either acute or chronic disease. A large number of patients with positive serology can remain asymptomatic.

Life Cycle and Morphology

Trypomastigotes are ingested by the reduviid bug (triatomids, kissing bugs, or conenose bugs) as it obtains a blood meal. The trypomastigotes transform into epimastigotes that multiply in the posterior portion of the midgut (Fig. 4). After 8 to 10 days, metacyclic trypomastigotes develop from the epimastigotes. These metacyclic trypomastigotes are passed in the feces.

Humans contract Chagas' disease when the reduviid bug defecates while taking a blood meal and metacyclic trypomastigotes in the feces are rubbed or scratched into the bite wound or onto mucosal surfaces. In humans, *T. cruzi* can be found in two forms, as amastigotes and trypomastigotes (Fig. 4). The trypomastigote is the stage present in the blood, which infects host cells. The amastigote form multiplies within the cell, eventually destroying the cell, and both amastigotes and trypomastigotes are released into the blood.

The trypomastigote is spindle-shaped, approximately 20 μm long, and characteristically assumes a C or U shape in stained blood films (Fig. 5 and 6). Trypomastigotes occur in the blood in two forms, a long slender form and a short, stubby one. The nucleus is situated in the center of the body, with a large, oval kinetoplast located at the posterior end. The kinetoplast consists of a small blepharoplast and a large oval parabasal body. A flagellum arises from the blepharoplast and extends along the outer edge of an undulating membrane until it reaches the anterior end of the body, where it projects as a free flagellum. When the trypomastigotes are stained with Giemsa stain, the cytoplasm

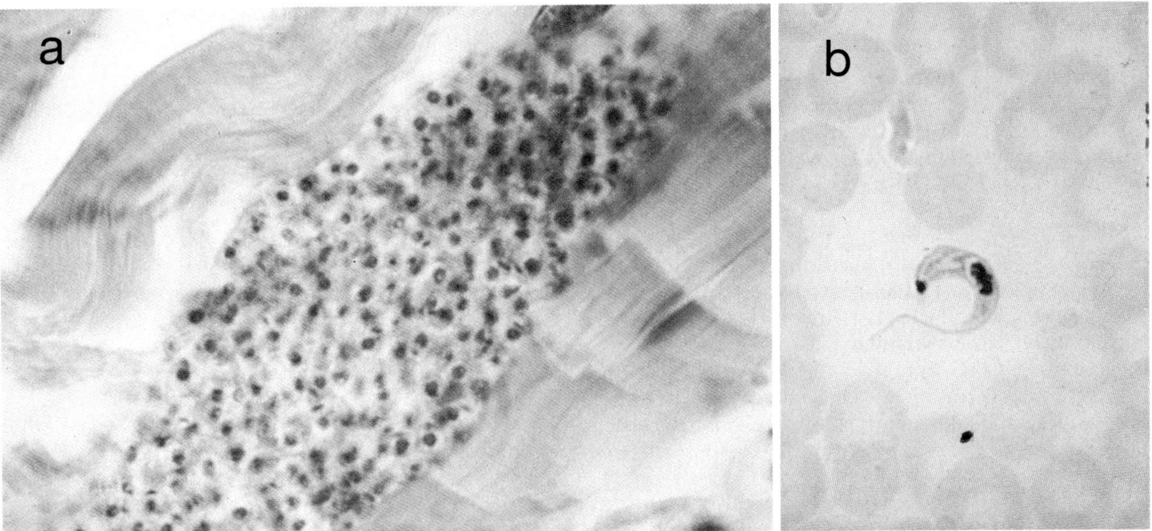

FIGURE 5 (a) *Trypanosoma cruzi* amastigotes in skeletal muscle (hematoxylin and eosin stain). (b) *T. cruzi* trypomastigote in peripheral blood (Giemsa stain). (Reproduced with permission from J. W. Smith, D. M. Melvin, T. C. Orihel, L. R. Ash, R. M. McQuay, and J. H. Thompson, Jr., *Atlas of Diagnostic Medical Parasitology: Blood and Tissue Parasites*, American Society of Clinical Pathologists, Chicago, Ill., 1976.)

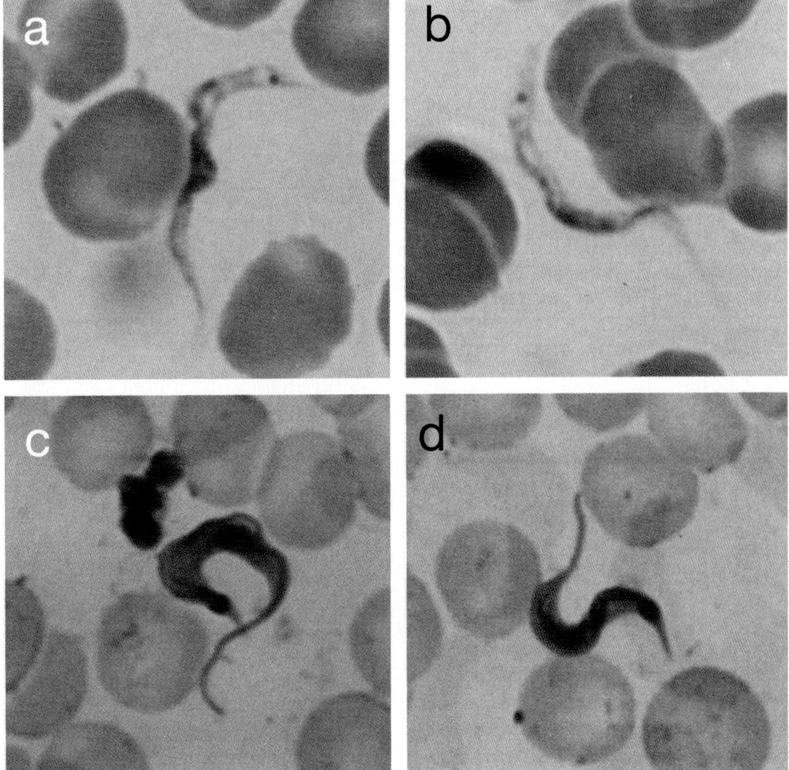

FIGURE 6 (a and b) *Trypanosoma cruzi* trypomastigote in blood (Giemsa stain). (c and d) *Trypanosoma brucei rhodesiense* trypomastigote in blood (Giemsa stain). Note differences in kinetoplast size at the end of the parasite.

stains blue and the nucleus, kinetoplast, and flagellum stain red or violet.

The amastigote (2 to 6 μm in diameter) is indistinguishable from those found in leishmanial infections. It contains a large nucleus and rod-shaped kinetoplast that stains red or violet with Giemsa stain, and the cytoplasm stains blue (Fig. 3 and 5).

Epidemiology

Chagas' disease is a zoonosis occurring throughout the American continent, including Central and South America, Texas, and California (18). It involves reduviid bugs living in close association with reservoirs (dogs, cats, armadillos, opossums, raccoons, and rodents). Human infections occur mainly in rural areas where poor sanitary and socioeconomic conditions and poor housing provide excellent breeding places for reduviid bugs.

Clinical Disease

In addition to contracting *T. cruzi* infections through the insect's bite wound or exposed mucous membranes, one can be infected by blood transfusion, placental transfer, organ transplant, and accidental ingestion of parasitized reduviid bugs (24). A localized inflammatory reaction may ensue at the infection site with development of a chagoma (erythematous subcutaneous nodule) or Romaña's sign (edema of the eyelids and conjunctivitis).

Acute systemic signs occur around the second to third week of infection and are characterized by high fevers; hepatosplenomegaly; myalgia; erythematous rash; acute myocarditis; lymphadenopathy; and subcutaneous edema of face, legs, and feet. The acute phase of Chagas' disease in immunosuppressive patients is manifested as acute myocarditis or acute encephalitis with a high mortality rate (20).

Chronic Chagas' disease is diagnosed more commonly than the acute phase. Symptoms of the chronic phase are related to the damage sustained during the acute phase of the disease. Chronic Chagas' disease may develop years or decades after undetected infection or after the diagnosis of acute disease. The most frequent clinical sign of chronic Chagas' disease is cardiomyopathy manifested by cardiomegaly and conduction changes. Some patients are more likely to have megaesophagus or megacolon. Congenital transmission can occur in both acute and chronic phases of the disease. Infants of seropositive mothers should be followed for up to a year after birth to rule out infection.

Diagnosis

Health care personnel working with specimens from patients suspected of having Chagas' disease should follow the bloodborne pathogen guidelines. Trypomastigotes are highly infectious.

The definitive diagnosis depends on demonstration of trypomastigotes in the blood, amastigote stages in tissues, or positive serologic tests. Aspirates from chagomas and enlarged lymph nodes can be examined for amastigotes and trypomastigotes. Histological examination of biopsies may also be done. Trypomastigotes may be easily detected in the blood in acute disease; however, in chronic disease, this stage is rare or absent, except during febrile episodes. Trypomastigotes will appear in the blood in about 10 days after infection and persist through the acute phase.

Trypomastigotes may be detected in blood using thin and thick blood films or by buffy coat concentration technique (23). The stain of choice is Giemsa for both amastigote and trypomastigote stages. Although not routinely available except in specialized centers, PCR has been used to detect as few as one trypomastigote in 20 ml of blood and has been useful in treatment follow-up (4, 25). In congenital infections and in patients with chronic Chagas' disease, immunoassays have been used to detect antigens in urine and sera (8). In areas where kala azar occurs, amastigote stages look similar and infections of *Leishmania donovani* and *T. cruzi* must be differentiated by either PCR, immunoassay, culture (epimastigote in *T. cruzi* vs. promastigote in *L. donovani*), serologic tests, animal inoculation, or xenodiagnosis techniques. Patient history, including geographic and/or travel history, and confirmation of organisms in striated muscle rather than reticuloendothelial tissues are very strong evidence for *T. cruzi* rather than *L. donovani* as the causative agent.

Aspirates, blood, and tissues can also be cultured. The medium of choice is NNN. Cultures should be incubated at 25°C and observed for epimastigote stages for up to 30 days before they are considered negative. If available, laboratory animals (rats, mice) could be inoculated and the blood could be observed for trypomastigotes.

In xenodiagnosis, trypanosome-free reduviid bugs are allowed to feed on individuals suspected of having Chagas' disease. If organisms are present in the blood meal, the parasites will multiply and can be detected in the bug's intestinal contents. The fecal material should be examined monthly for flagellated forms over a period of 3 months. Xenodiagnosis is positive in less than 50% of the seropositive patients. Some patients may develop a severe anaphylactic reaction to the reduviid bug's salivary secretion. Reduviid bugs, which are trypanosome-free, may be available in specialized diagnostic centers.

Serological tests used for the diagnosis of Chagas' disease include complement fixation (Guerreiro-Machado test), indirect fluorescent antibody (IFA), indirect hemagglutination (IHA), and enzyme-linked immunosorbent assay (ELISA). Most of these tests use an epimastigote antigen, and cross-reactions have been noted for patients infected with *Trypanosoma rangeli*, *Leishmania* spp., *Toxoplasma gondii*, and hepatitis. Use of synthetic peptides and recombinant proteins has improved the sensitivity and specificity of the serodiagnostic techniques (9). A new chemiluminiscent ELISA using a purified trypomastigote glycoconjugate antigen showed 100% sensitivity and 100% specificity (1). Follow-up blood specimens should be reexamined 1 to 2 months after therapy by techniques described above. Serologic testing is available at referral laboratories and the Centers for Disease Control and Prevention (CDC).

Treatment and Prevention

Nifurtimox (Lampit) and benznidazole (Radamil) reduce the severity of acute Chagas' disease, but they have little impact on the progression of chronic Chagas' disease. Allopurinol has been found to be as effective as nifurtimox and benznidazole in treating Chagas' disease. Surgery has been successfully used to treat cases of chagasic heart disease, megaesophagus, and megacolon.

Until recently, control of Chagas' disease has been mainly through the use of insecticides to eliminate the reduviid vector. Construction of reduviid-proof dwellings and education are also essential for effective control programs. Serologic screening of blood products from areas in which the disease is endemic is recommended. An alternative approach to serologic testing for blood donors is the use of questionnaires to defer prospective donors from high-risk areas.

Trypanosoma rangeli

T. rangeli has been found in both Central and South America and often overlaps in areas where *T. cruzi* is present. In some areas, *T. rangeli* infections are 5 to 6 times more frequent than infections with *T. cruzi* (22). Trypomastigotes can be detected from the blood of infected patients by using thin and thick blood smears and buffy coat concentration techniques. The parasites can be stained with Giemsa or Wright stains. Infections can also be detected by xenodiagnosis. In addition, blood can be cultured (Tobies medium, NNN) or injected into laboratory animals (mice) and examined for epimastigotes and trypomastigotes, respectively. Although there are no serologic tests for *T. rangeli*, serologic cross-reactions have been noted to occur with tests for *T. cruzi* (2). Human infections are asymptomatic and trypomastigotes have been noted in the blood for longer than a year.

AFRICAN TRYPANOSOMIASIS

Introduction

African trypanosomiasis is limited to the tsetse fly belt of Central Africa where there are over 35 million people at risk for African trypanosomiasis. The West African (Gambian) form of sleeping sickness is caused by *T. brucei gambiense*, whereas the East African (Rhodesian) form is caused by *T. brucei rhodesiense*.

Life Cycle and Morphology

T. brucei rhodesiense and *T. brucei gambiense* are closely related and morphologically indistinguishable. In the past, differentiation was based upon clinical signs and geographic area; however, differentiation can now be accomplished using isoenzyme characteristics and DNA and RNA methods (11, 12).

The trypomastigote forms in the blood range from long slender-bodied organisms with a long flagellum to short, fat, stumpy forms without a free flagellum (14 to 33 μm long and 1.5 to 3.5 μm wide). The short, stumpy forms are the infective stage for the tsetse fly.

Using Giemsa or Wright stains, the granular cytoplasm stains pale blue and contains dark blue granules and possibly vacuoles (Fig. 6). The centrally located nucleus stains reddish. The kinetoplast is located at the organism's posterior end and stains reddish; the remaining intracytoplasmic flagellum (axoneme) may not be visible. The flagellum arises from the kinetoplast, as does the undulating membrane. The flagellum runs along the edge of the undulating membrane until the undulating membrane merges with the trypanosome body at the organism's anterior end. At this point the flagellum becomes free to extend beyond the body. Trypanosomal forms are ingested by the tsetse fly when a blood meal is taken and transform to epimastigotes. The organisms multiply in the gut of the fly and after approximately 2 weeks, the organisms migrate back to the salivary glands. Humans are infected when metacyclic forms from the salivary glands are introduced into the bite site when the blood meal is taken.

Epidemiology

The development cycle in the tsetse fly varies from 12 to 30 days and averages 20 days. Less than 10% of the tsetse flies become infective after obtaining blood from infected patients. Both female and male tsetse flies can transmit the infection.

Although there is no evidence of animal-to-human transmission of *T. brucei gambiense*, trypanosomal strains isolated from hartebeest, kob, chickens, dogs, cows, and domestic pigs in West Africa are identical to those isolated from humans in the same area. Evidence suggests transmission may be entirely interhuman. The tsetse fly vectors of Rhodesian trypanosomiasis are game-feeders that may transmit the disease from human to human or animal to human. A reduction or elimination of game animals has been a major control method.

Clinical Disease

After being bitten by an infected tsetse fly, a local inflammatory reaction that resolves spontaneously within 1 to 2 weeks can be detected at the bite site. The trypomastigotes gain entrance to the bloodstream, causing a symptom-free low grade parasitemia that may continue for months. The infection may self-cure during this period without development of symptoms or lymph node invasion.

Diagnostic symptoms include irregular fever, lymph node enlargement (particularly those of the posterior triangle of the neck, which is known as Winterbottom's sign), delayed sensation to pain (Kerandel's sign), and erythematous skin rashes. In addition to lymph node involvement, the spleen and liver become enlarged. With Gambian trypanosomiasis, the blood-lymphatic stage may last for years before the sleeping sickness syndrome occurs.

Laboratory findings include anemia, granulocytopenia, increased sedimentation rate, and marked increases in serum IgM. The sustained high IgM levels are a result of the parasite producing variable antigen types to evade the patient's defense system (5). In an immunocompetent host, the lack of elevated serum IgM rules out trypanosomiasis.

Upon trypomastigote invasion of the central nervous system (CNS), the sleeping-sickness stage of the infection is initiated. Gambian trypanosomiasis is characterized by steady progressive meningoencephalitis, behavioral changes, apathy, confusion, coordination loss, and somnolence. *T. brucei rhodesiense* produces a more rapid, fulminating disease, and death may occur before there is extensive CNS involvement. In the terminal phase of the disease, the patient becomes emaciated, leading to profound coma and death, usually from secondary infections. Cerebrospinal fluid (CSF) findings include increased protein, elevated IgM, lymphocytosis, and morular cells of Mott. Morular (mulberry) cells are altered plasma cells whose cytoplasm is filled with proteinaceous droplets. Morular cells are not seen in all patients; however, they are characteristic of African trypanosomiasis.

Diagnosis

Definitive diagnosis depends upon demonstration of trypomastigotes in blood, lymph node aspirate, sternum bone marrow, and CSF. Trypomastigotes can be more readily detected in body fluids in infections due to *T. brucei rhodesiense* than *T. brucei gambiense* because of higher parasitemias. Due to periodicity, parasite numbers in the blood will vary and a number of techniques must be used to detect the trypomastigotes.

Trypomastigotes are highly infectious, and health-care personnel must be cautious and adhere to bloodborne pathogen precautions when handling blood, CSF, or aspirates. Blood can be collected from either finger stick or venipuncture. Venous blood should be collected in a tube containing EDTA. Multiple slides should be prepared for examination, and multiple blood exams should be performed before trypanosomiasis is ruled out. Parasites will be found in high numbers in the blood during the febrile period and in low numbers when afebrile. If CSF is examined, a volume greater than 1 ml, preferably 5 ml or more, should be collected. In addition to thin and thick blood films, a buffy coat concentration method is recommended to detect the parasites. Parasites can be detected on thick blood smears when numbers are greater than 2,000/ml, with hematocrit capillary tube concentration when numbers are greater than 100/ml, and on an anion-exchange column when numbers are greater than 4/ml (15). CSF examination must be conducted by using centrifuged sediments (6). In cases in which trypomastigotes are in undetectable numbers in the blood, they may be seen in aspirates of inflamed lymph nodes; however, attempts to demonstrate them in tissue are not practical. Blood and CSF specimens should be examined during therapy to evaluate the clinical response and 1 to 2 months after therapy. Patients treated for CNS disease should be followed clinically for 2 to 3 years after completion of therapy in case of relapse. ELISA has been used to detect antigen in serum and CSF (14, 16). This method could also be used for clinical staging of disease as to whether there was CNS infection and follow-up to therapy. Referral laboratories have used molecular methods (PCR) to detect infections and differentiate species (25).

Serologic techniques which have been used for epidemiologic screening include IFA, ELISA, IHA, and the card agglutination trypanosomiasis test. A major serodiagnostic problem in areas where trypanosomiasis is endemic is that many in the population have elevated antibody levels due to exposure to animal trypanosomes that are noninfectious to humans. Serologic testing has not proven to be useful for routine diagnosis of African trypanosomiasis. Markedly elevated serum and CSF IgM concentrations are of diagnostic value. CSF antibody titers should be interpreted with caution because of lack of reference values and the possibility of CSF containing serum due to a traumatic tap.

Small laboratory animals (rat, guinea pig) have been used to detect infections. *T. brucei rhodesiense* is more adaptable to cultivation and animal infection than *T. brucei gambiense*; however, cultivation is not practical for most diagnostic laboratories.

Treatment and Prevention

Suramin (Bayer 205) is the drug of choice for treating the early blood or lymphatic stage of the disease. Alternatives to treat the early stage are pentamidine isethionate and DFMO (deflornithine, DL-α-difluoromethylornithine). Melarsoprol (Arsobal) is the drug of choice when CNS involvement is suspected. Nifurtimox (Lampit) has been used to treat patients infected with *T. brucei gambiense* who do not respond to melarsoprol; however, *T. brucei rhodesiense* is resistant to nifurtimox (21). Any individual treated for African trypanosomiasis should be followed for 2 to 3 years after completion of therapy. About 2% of the patients treated for CNS disease experience relapse.

Control of *T. brucei gambiense* infections has been carried out by population screening programs. Use of vector control measures has met with limited success. The most effective control measures include an integrated approach to reduce the human reservoir of infection and the use of insecticide and fly traps. Persons visiting areas in which the infection is endemic should wear protective clothing (long-sleeved shirts and long trousers). Other measures include reduction in vegetation around human settlements, insect repellents, bed netting, and screens.

REFERENCES

1. **Almeida, I. C., D. T. Covas, L. M. Soussumi, and L. R. Travassos.** 1997. A highly sensitive and specific chemiluminescent enzyme-linked immunosorbent assay for diagnosis of active *Trypanosoma cruzi* infection. *Transfusion* **37:**850–857.
2. **Anthony, R. L., T. S. Cody, and N. T. Constantin.** 1981. Antigenic differentiation of *Trypanosoma cruzi* and *Trypanosoma rangeli* by means of monoclonal-hybridoma antibodies. *Am. J. Trop. Med. Hyg.* **30:**1192–1197.
3. **Bogdan, C., N. Stosiek, H. Fuchs, M. Rollunghoff, and W. Solbach.** 1990. Detection of potentially diagnostic leishmanial antigens by western blot analysis of sera from patients with kala-azar or multilesional cutaneous leishmaniasis. *J. Infect. Dis.* **162:**1417–1418.
4. **Britto, C., M. A. Cardoso, C. M. Monteiro Vanni, A. Hasslocher-Moreno, S. S. Xavier, W. Oelemann, A. Santoro, C. Pirmez, C. M. Morel, and P. Wincker.** 1995. Polymerase chain reaction detection of *Trypanosoma cruzi* in human blood samples as tool for diagnosis and treatment evaluation. *Parasitology* **110:**241–247.
5. **Burgess, D. E., K. M. Esser, and B. T. Wellde.** 1984. Variable antigen type (VAT) composition of *Trypanosoma brucei rhodesiense*: discrepancy between results obtained using VAT-SPECIFIC monoclonal antibodies and rabbit antisera. *Am. J. Trop. Med. Hyg.* **33:**1096–1104.
6. **Cattand, P., B. T. Miezan, and P. de Raadt.** 1988. Human African trypanosomiasis: use of double centrifugation of cerebrospinal fluid to detect trypanosomes. *Bull. W. H. O.* **66:**83–86.
7. **Centers for Disease Control.** 1992. Viscerotropic leishmaniasis in persons returning from Operation Desert Storm. 1990–1991. *Morbid. Mortal. Weekly Rep.* **40:**131–134.
8. **Corral, R. S., A. Orn, and S. Grinstein.** 1992. Detection of soluble exoantigens of *Trypanosoma cruzi* by a dot-immunobinding assay. *Am. J. Trop. Med. Hyg.* **46:**31–38.
9. **Garcia, L. S., and D. A. Bruckner.** 1997. *Diagnostic Medical Parasitology*, 3rd ed. ASM Press, Washington, D.C.
10. **Grogl, M., T. N. Thomason, and E. D. Franke.** 1992. Drug resistance in leishmaniasis: its implication in systemic chemotherapy of cutaneous and mucocutaneous disease. *Am. J. Trop. Med. Hyg.* **47:**117–126.
11. **Hide, G., N. Buchanan, S. Welburn, J. Maudlin, J. D. Barry, and A. Tait.** 1991. *Trypanosoma brucei rhodesiense*: characterization of stocks from Zambia, Kenya, and Uganda using repetitive DNA probes. *Exp. Parasitol.* **72:**430–439.
12. **Hide, G., P. Cattand, D. Le Ray, J. D. Barry, and A. Tait.** 1990. The identification of *Trypanosoma brucei* subspecies using repetitive DNA sequence. *Mol. Biochem. Parasitol.* **39:**213–226.
13. **Ismail, A., A. Kharazmi, H. Permin, and A. M. El Hassam.** 1997. Detection and characterization of *Leishmania* in tissues of patients with post kala-azar dermal leishmaniasis using a specific monoclonal antibody. *Trans. R. Soc. Trop. Med. Hyg.* **91:**283–285.
14. **Komba, E., M. Odiit, D. B. Mbulamberi, E. C. Chimfwembe, and V. M. Nantulya.** 1992. Multicenter evaluation of an antigen-detection ELISA for the diagnosis of *Trypanosoma brucei rhodesiense* sleeping sickness. *Bull. W. H. O.* **70:**57–61.
15. **Lumsden, W. H. R., C. D. Kimber, P. Dukes, L. Haller, A. Stranghellini, and G. Duvallet.** 1981. Field diagnosis of sleeping sickness in the Ivory Coast. I. Comparison of the miniature anion-exchange/centrifugation technique with other protozoological methods. *Trans. R. Soc. Trop. Med. Hyg.* **75:**242–250.
16. **Nantulya, V. M., F. Doua, and S. Molisho.** 1992. Diagnosis of *Trypanosoma brucei gambiense* sleeping sickness using

an antigen detection enzyme-linked immunosorbent assay. *Trans. R. Soc. Trop. Med. Hyg.* **86:**42–45.
17. **Napier, L.** 1922. A new serum test for Kala-Azar. *Indian J. Med. Res.* **9:**830–846.
18. **Navin, T. R., R. R. Roberto, D. D. Juranek, K. Limpakarnjanarat, E. W. Mortenson, J. R. Clover, R. E. Yescott, C. Taclindo, F. Stuerer, and D. Allain.** 1985. Human and sylvatic *Trypanosoma cruzi* infection in California. *Am. J. Public Health* **75:**366–369.
19. **Nuzum, E., F. White III, C. Thakur, R. Dietze, J. Wages, M. Grogl, and J. Berman.** 1995. Diagnosis of symptomatic visceral leishmaniasis by use of the polymerase chain reaction on patient blood. *J. Infect. Dis.* **171:**751–754.
20. **Oddo, D., M. Casanova, G. Acuna, J. Ballesteros, and B. Morales.** 1992. Acute Chagas' disease (trypanosomiasis americana) in acquired immunodeficiency syndrome. *Hum. Pathol.* **23:**41–44.
21. **Pepin, J., F. Milord, F. Meurice, L. Ethier, L. Loko, and B. Mpia.** 1992. High-dose nifurtimox for arseno-resistant *Trypanosoma brucei gambiense* sleeping sickness: an open trial in Central Zaire. *Trans. R. Soc. Trop. Med. Hyg.* **86:** 254–256.
22. **Souza, D. E., and C. M. Johnson.** 1971. Frequency and distribution of *Trypanosoma cruzi* and *Trypanosoma rangeli* in the republic of Panama. *Am. J. Trop. Med. Hyg.* **20:** 405–410.
23. **Strout, R. G.** 1962. A method for concentrating haemoflagellates. *J. Parasitol.* **48:**100.
24. **Theis, J. H.** 1990. Latin American immigrants—blood donation and *Trypanosoma cruzi* transmission. *Am. Heart J.* **120:**1483–1484.
25. **Weiss, J. B.** 1995. DNA probes and PCR for diagnosis of parasitic infections. *Clin. Microbiol. Rev.* **8:**113–130.
26. **WHO Expert Committee.** 1991. Control of Chagas' disease. *W. H. O. Tech. Rep. Ser.* **811.**
27. **Wilson, S. M.** 1995. DNA based methods in the detection of *Leishmania* parasites: field applications and practicalities. *Ann. Trop. Med. Parasitol.* **89**(Suppl. 1)**:**95–100.
28. **World Health Organization.** 1990. Control of the leishmaniases. *W. H. O. Tech. Rep. Ser.* **793:**155.

*Toxoplasma**

MARIANNA WILSON AND JAMES B. McAULEY

107

LIFE CYCLE

Toxoplasma gondii is a protozoan parasite that infects most species of warm-blooded animals, including humans. Members of the cat family (*Felidae*) are the only known definitive hosts for the sexual stages of *T. gondii* and thus are the main reservoirs of infection. The three stages of this obligate intracellular parasite are (i) tachyzoites (trophozoites), which rapidly proliferate and destroy infected cells during acute infection; (ii) bradyzoites, which slowly multiply in tissue cysts; and (iii) sporozoites in oocysts (Fig. 1). Tachyzoites and bradyzoites occur in body tissues; oocysts are excreted in cat feces. After tissue cysts or oocysts are ingested by the cat, viable organisms are released and invade epithelial cells of the small intestine, where they undergo an asexual cycle followed by a sexual cycle and then form oocysts, which are then excreted. The unsporulated (i.e., uninfective) oocyst takes 1 to 5 days after excretion to become sporulated (infective). Although cats shed oocysts for only 1 to 2 weeks, large numbers may be shed, often exceeding 100,000 per g of feces. Oocysts can survive in the environment for several months and are remarkably resistant to disinfectants, freezing, and drying but are killed by heating to 70°C for 10 min. Cats become infected with *T. gondii* by carnivorism. Therefore, cats that are allowed to roam outside are much more likely to become infected than domestic cats that are confined indoors.

Human infection may be acquired in several ways: (i) ingestion of undercooked infected meat containing *Toxoplasma* cysts; (ii) ingestion of the oocyst from fecally contaminated hands or food; (iii) organ transplantation or blood transfusion; (iv) transplacental transmission; and (v) accidental inoculation of tachyzoites. The two major routes of transmission of *Toxoplasma* to humans are oral and congenital. High-risk behaviors include changing the cat litter box, working outside in dirt (gardening and yard work), and eating undercooked pork or lamb. In humans, ingesting either the tissue cyst or the oocyst results in the rupture of the cyst wall, which releases organisms that invade the intestinal epithelium, disseminate throughout the body, and multiply intracellularly. The host cell dies and releases the tachyzoites, which invade adjacent cells and continue the process. The tachyzoites are pressured by the host's immune response to transform into bradyzoites and form tissue cysts, most commonly in skeletal muscle, myocardium, and brain; these cysts may remain throughout the life of the host. Recrudescence of clinical disease may occur if the host becomes immunosuppressed and the cysts rupture, releasing the parasites.

EPIDEMIOLOGY

Serologic prevalence data indicate that toxoplasmosis is one of the most common infections of humans throughout the world. Because *T. gondii* organisms are rarely detected in humans with toxoplasmosis, serologic examination is used to indicate the presence of the infection by detecting *Toxoplasma*-specific antibodies. The prevalence of positive serologic titers increases with age; the greater the prevalence, the earlier the increase. Infection is more common in warm climates and at lower altitudes than in cold climates and mountainous regions. This distribution is probably related to conditions favoring the sporulation and survival of oocysts. Variations in the prevalence of infection between geographic areas and between population groups within the same locale are also probably due to differences in exposure. A high prevalence of infection in France (85%) has been related to a preference for eating raw or undercooked meat. However, a high prevalence in Central America has been related to the frequency of stray cats in a climate favoring the survival of oocysts. In the United States in 1967, prevalence rates of up to 30% were found along the sea coast, with rates of less than 1% in the Rocky Mountains and the desert Southwest. More recent data comparing antibody prevalence in U.S. military recruits in 1962 and 1989 indicated a one-third decrease in seropositivity (28). The overall seroprevalence in the United States, as determined with specimens collected by the Third National Health and Nutritional Assessment Survey between 1988 and 1994, was found to be 22%, with a seroprevalence among women of childbearing age (15 to 45 years) of 10 to 15% (31).

CLINICAL SIGNIFICANCE

Toxoplasmosis can be categorized into four groups: (i) acquired in the immunocompetent patient; (ii) acquired or reactivated in the immunodeficient patient; (iii) congenital;

* This chapter contains information presented in chapter 104 by Lynne S. Garcia, Alexander J. Sulzer, George R. Healy, Katharine K. Grady, and David A. Bruckner in the sixth edition of this Manual.

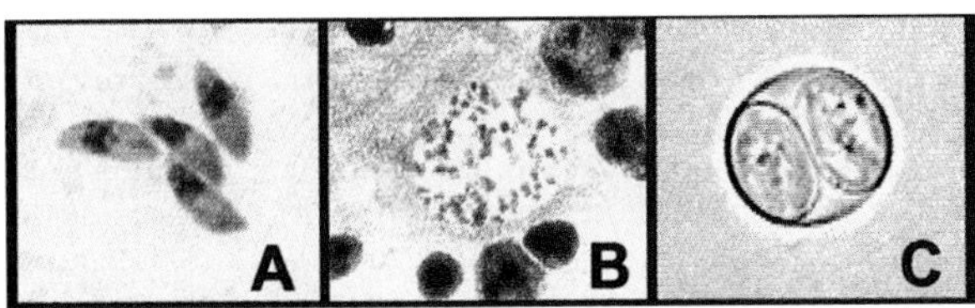

FIGURE 1 Three life stages of *T. gondii*. (A) Tachyzoites, Giemsa stain. (B) Cyst with bradyzoites in brain tissue, Giemsa stain. (C) Sporulated oocysts, unstained. (Photographs courtesy of J. P. Dubey, U.S. Department of Agriculture, Beltsville, Md.)

and (iv) ocular. Methods of diagnosis and their interpretations may differ for each clinical category.

Acquired infection with *Toxoplasma* in immunocompetent individuals is generally an asymptomatic infection. However, 10 to 20% of patients with acute infection may develop cervical lymphadenopathy and/or a flu-like illness. The clinical course is benign and self-limited; symptoms usually resolve within a few months to a year.

Immunodeficient patients often have central nervous system (CNS) disease but may have myocarditis or pneumonitis. In patients with AIDS, toxoplasmic encephalitis is the most common cause of intracerebral mass lesions and is thought to be due to reactivation of chronic infection. Toxoplasmosis in patients being treated with immunosuppressive drugs may be due to either newly acquired or reactivated latent infection.

Congenital toxoplasmosis results from an acute primary infection acquired by the mother during pregnancy. The incidence and severity of congenital toxoplasmosis vary with the trimester during which infection was acquired. Because treatment of the mother reduces the incidence of congenital infection, prompt and accurate diagnosis is extremely important. Most infants with subclinical infection at birth will subsequently develop signs or symptoms of congenital toxoplasmosis unless the infection is treated.

Ocular *Toxoplasma* infection, an important cause of chorioretinitis in the United States, is usually a result of congenital infection. Patients are often asymptomatic until the second or third decade of life, when lesions develop in the eye due to cyst rupture and subsequent release of tachyzoites and bradyzoites. Chorioretinitis is characteristically bilateral in patients with congenital infection but is usually unilateral in individuals with acquired infection.

COLLECTION, TRANSPORT, AND STORAGE OF SPECIMENS

Serum, plasma, cerebrospinal fluid (CSF), and eye fluid specimens may all be tested for antibodies and antigens. CSF and eye fluid should be tested in parallel with a serum sample drawn on the same date. Blood specimens to be tested for the presence of antibodies or antigens should be allowed to clot and centrifuged, and the serum should be removed and shipped to a reference laboratory. Hemolysis does not seem to interfere with the antibody reaction. The specimens may be stored for several days at 4°C or frozen for longer storage. The specimens may be shipped at an ambient temperature unless they will be in transit for more than 1 week or will be subjected to temperatures above 30°C. Long-term storage should take place at −20°C or below.

If the determination of immune status is the reason for testing, a single specimen is satisfactory; acute- and convalescent-phase specimens are not necessary. In situations in which determining the time of infection is important, specimens drawn at least 3 weeks apart may or may not be useful. In most cases, detection of an increasing immunoglobulin G (IgG) or IgM titer is not possible because the titers have already reached a plateau by the time the initial sample is drawn. If two specimens are to be compared, they should be tested together. Results from tests done at different times, in different laboratories, or with different procedures should not be compared quantitatively, only qualitatively, as positive or negative.

For tests other than serology, contact a reference laboratory for instructions before collecting specimens to ensure proper collection and handling.

METHODS OF DIAGNOSIS

Parasite Identification

Only very rarely can the diagnosis of toxoplasmosis be documented by the observation of parasites in patient specimens. Secretions, excretions, body fluids, and tissues are potential specimens for direct observation of parasites but are generally unrewarding. Fluid specimens such as heparinized blood or CSF should be centrifuged, and the sediment should be smeared on a microscope slide. The slides should be air dried, fixed in methanol, and stained with Giemsa stain for microscopic examination. Tachyzoites may be observed as free organisms or within host cells such as leukocytes. Well-preserved tachyzoites are crescent shaped and stain well, but degenerating organisms may be oval and stain poorly. Tissue imprints stained with Giemsa stain may reveal *Toxoplasma* cysts. Immunologic techniques have been used to identify parasites in tissue sections or tissue cultures; fluorescein isothiocyanate- or peroxidase-labeled antisera may be useful in detecting tachyzoites in tissue sections.

Parasites can be isolated with limited success by inoculating patient tissue or body fluids into either mice or tissue culture cells. Fresh tissue samples are ground in saline with a mortar and pestle and inoculated into the peritoneum of mice or directly into tissue culture flasks. The mice should be monitored for 4 to 6 weeks; if the organism is virulent for mice, the parasites can often be demonstrated in the peritoneal fluid after 5 to 10 days. However, if the organism is relatively avirulent for mice, as is usually the case, the mice may not be killed by the infection. If they survive for 6 weeks, serum samples should be obtained for testing. If antibodies are present, the mouse brain should be examined for the presence of *Toxoplasma* cysts. *Toxoplasma* grows in a variety of tissue culture cells. A cytopathic effect may be detected on direct examination after 24 to 96 h in culture. Giemsa staining may reveal parasite structure, but parasitized cells may be difficult to detect. Immunofluorescence allows more sensitive detection of the organisms. The following procedure has been used with some success for parasite isolation from amniotic fluids (6). Centrifuge a 10-ml sample of amniotic fluid at 1,000 × *g*. Resuspend the sediment in 8 ml of minimum essential medium. Inoculate 1 ml into coverslip cultures of human embryonic fibroblast cell line MRC5 in 24-well plates. Incubate the cultures for 96 h, with one change of medium at 24 h; fix the cultures with cold acetone. Examine the coverslips by indirect immunofluorescence for the presence of *T. gondii*. The use of tissue culture cells for isolation permits a more rapid diagnosis than mouse inoculation; both methods can be useful for diagnosing congenital toxoplasmosis.

Antibody Detection

Many tests for the detection of antibodies to *Toxoplasma* have been used since Sabin and Feldman developed the methylene blue dye test (DT) (26). Commercial kits for agglutination tests, indirect-fluorescent antibody (IFA) tests, and enzyme immunoassays (EIA) are available worldwide. Because of difficulties in obtaining specimens from clinically documented cases of toxoplasmosis, commercial kit sensitivity and specificity may not be based on documented case specimens but rather on a comparison with results obtained with another kit. Consequently, the true sensitivity and specificity of a kit are generally not known or determined. The rates stated by the manufacturer or published in articles may vary depending upon the samples chosen for testing. Sensitivity and specificity rates determined in prospective studies, when random samples are tested as received for *Toxoplasma* testing, will usually differ from those determined in retrospective studies, when samples have been chosen as potential problem samples to increase the probability of detecting false-positive or false-negative reactions. For example, an IgM assay was determined to have prospective sensitivity and specificity rates of 88.3 and 95.9%, respectively, while retrospective sensitivity and specificity rates were found to be 97.8 and 99.0%, respectively (15).

When laboratory personnel decide to initiate *Toxoplasma*-specific antibody testing or when they decide to switch to a different antibody detection kit, the user must carefully review the manufacturer's package insert and published literature for information on the sensitivity and specificity rates. The user should also perform an in-laboratory comparison of kits by using positive and negative samples confirmed by a toxoplasmosis reference laboratory. Tables 1 and 2 list commercial kits currently available in the United States and references to published evaluations. However, the test kit industry is in a great deal of flux; company and kit names may change, and it is very difficult to keep up with the name changes.

In the United States, initial testing for the presence of IgG antibodies in most laboratories is usually performed with an EIA or IFA commercial kit. Results may be stated in international units (based on the international standard reference serum for *Toxoplasma* distributed by the WHO International Laboratory for Biological Standards, Statens Seruminstitut, Copenhagen, Denmark), as an index (specific to each kit), as an optical density value (specific to each kit), or as a geometric mean titer. Numerical results are not

TABLE 1 Toxoplasma IgG kits available commercially in the United States

Type of test and company[a]	Kit name	Reference(s)
IFA		
Diagnostic Technology	TOXO-IgG Check	
Gull Laboratories	Toxoplasma IgG	
Hemagen	VIRGO Toxo IgG	
KMI Diagnostics	Toxoplasma IgG	
Stellar Bio Systems	Toxo IgG	
Wampole	Toxoplasma IgG	
EIA		
Abbott Diagnostics	IMx Toxo IgG	5, 9, 10, 12, 15, 25
	AxSYM Toxo IgG	
Bayer	Immuno 1	25
Beckman	ACCESS Toxo G	5
Behring Diagnostics	OPUS Toxo G	12
Bio-Medical Products	Virotech	
bioMérieux Vitek	VIDAS Toxo IgG	9, 12
Biotecx	OptiCoat Toxo IgG ELISA	
Diagnostic Products Corp.	IMMUNLITE Toxoplasma IgG	7
Diamedix	Toxoplasma IgG	
DiaSorin	Toxoplasma IgG	
	COPALIS Toxo IgG	
Gull Laboratories	Toxo IgG	
Hemagen	Toxoplasma IgG	
INOVA	Toxoplasma IgG	
Intracel	Bartels Toxoplasma IgG	
Sanofi Diagnostics Pasteur	Platelia Toxo G	12
Sigma Diagnostics	Toxoplasma IgG	
Wampole Zeus	Toxo IgG (ELISA)	
	Toxoplasma IgG (Impact ELISA)	

[a] Abbott Diagnostics, Abbott Park, Ill. Bayer Diagnostics, Elkhart, Ind. Beckman, Brea, Calif. Behring Diagnostics, San Jose, Calif. Bio-Medical Products Corp., Mendham, N.J. bioMérieux Vitek, Hazelwood, Mo. Biotecx Laboratories, Houston, Tex. Diagnostic Products Corp., Los Angeles, Calif. Diagnostic Technology, Hauppauge, N.Y. Diamedix Corp., Miami, Fla. DiaSorin, Stillwater, Minn. Gull Laboratories, Salt Lake City, Utah. Hemagen Diagnostics, Waltham, Mass. INOVA, San Diego, Calif. Intracel, Issaquah, Wash. KMI Diagnostics, Minneapolis, Minn. Sanofi Diagnostics Pasteur, Redmond, Wash. Sigma Diagnostics, St. Louis, Mo. Stellar Bio Systems, Columbia, Md. Wampole Laboratories, Cranbury, N.J.

TABLE 2 Toxoplasma IgM kits available commercially in the United States

Type of test and company[a]	Kit name	Reference(s)
IFA		
Diagnostic Technology	TOXO-IgM Check	
Gull Laboratories	Toxoplasma IgM	
Hemagen	VIRGO Toxo IgM	
KMI Diagnostics	Toxoplasma IgM	
Stellar Bio Systems	Toxo IgM	
Wampole	Toxoplasma gondii IgM	
EIA		
Abbott Diagnostics	IMx Toxo IgM	5, 12, 15, 17, 30
	AxSYM Toxo IgM	
Bayer	Immuno 1	
Behring Diagnostics	OPUS	12
Bio-Medical Products	Virotech	
bioMérieux Vitek	VIDAS Toxo IgM	2, 12, 30
Biotecx	OptiCoat Toxo IgM	
Diagnostic Products Corp.	IMMULITE	7
Diamedix	Toxoplasma IgM	27
DiaSorin	Toxoplasma IgM	
Gull Laboratories	Toxo IgM	30
Hemagan	Toxoplasma IgM	
Intracel	Bartels Toxoplasma IgM	
Sanofi Diagnostics Pasteur	Platelia Toxo IgM	12, 16, 30
Sigma Diagnostics	Toxoplasma IgM	
Wampole/Zeus	Toxo IgM	
	Toxo CAP M	

[a] Abbott Diagnostics, Abbott Park, Ill. Bayer Diagnostics, Elkhart, Ind. Behring Diagnostics, San Jose, Calif. Bio-Medical Products Corp., Mendham, N.J. bioMérieux Vitek, Hazelwood, Mo. Biotecx Laboratories, Houston, Tex. Diagnostic Products Corp., Los Angeles, Calif. Diagnostic Technology, Hauppauge, N.Y. Diamedix Corp., Miami, Fla. DiaSorin, Stillwater, Minn. Gull Laboratories, Salt Lake City, Utah. Hemagen Diagnostics, Waltham, Mass. INOVA, San Diego, Calif. Intracel, Issaquah, Wash. KMI Diagnostics, Minneapolis, Minn. Sanofi Diagnostics Pasteur, Redmond, Wash. Sigma Diagnostics, St. Louis, Mo. Stellar Bio Systems, Columbia, Md. Wampole Laboratories, Cranbury, N.J.

comparable from kit to kit; comparison may be made only qualitatively, as negative (nonreactive or not infected) or positive (reactive or infected). Although elevated *Toxoplasma*-specific IgG levels have been suggested as an indicator of recent infection, high levels may last for many years after primary infection and should not be relied upon for this purpose.

To more definitely distinguish acute and chronic infections, detection of *Toxoplasma*-specific IgM antibodies has been used with some success but also with some failures. IFA IgM titers generally increase within 1 week of the onset of symptoms and revert to negative within 6 to 9 months of infection. However, false-positive reactions caused by rheumatoid factor and false-negative reactions caused by blockage by *Toxoplasma*-specific IgG may occur in IFA IgM tests and indirect EIA for IgM, unless specimens are treated to obtain only the IgM fraction for testing to decrease the effects of these interfering factors.

The IgM capture EIA eliminates potential interference by IgG and other isotypes by binding only IgM antibodies; unbound antibodies are removed by washing. The most important advantage of the IgM capture EIA is the detection of congenital infections: the IgM EIA was positive for 73% of serum samples from newborn infants with proven congenital *Toxoplasma* infections, whereas only 25% of the same serum samples were found positive by an IFA IgM test (20). Although the capture EIA system is more efficient at detecting acute infections, some persons may have undetectable or low-level IgM antibodies, and *some persons may have detectable IgM antibodies for up to 18 months postinfection; therefore, determining the relative time of infection may not be possible with this system alone.* Many commercial companies market an EIA kit for IgM: some use the indirect EIA format with a serum pretreatment step, while others use the IgM capture format. False-positive IgM reactions due to unknown factors may be a problem with commercially available kits; all IgM-positive specimens should be confirmed by a reference laboratory with experience in diagnosing toxoplasmosis (16, 30).

Detection of isotypes other than IgG or IgM may be of some assistance in determining acute versus chronic infection. In acute infections, *Toxoplasma*-specific IgA antibodies are detectable and appear to decline to nil earlier (between 6 and 12 months postinfection) than IgM antibodies. Assays for *Toxoplasma*-specific IgA antibodies should always be performed in addition to IgM assays for newborns suspected of having a congenital infection (4, 29). Detection of the IgA response in newborns and fetuses appears to be a more reliable indicator of congenital infection than detection of the IgM response. The presence of *Toxoplasma*-specific IgE antibodies may also contribute to the determination of acute infections (32). The differential agglutination test as well as the determination of IgG avidity may also be useful for confirming or excluding acute toxoplasmosis (14, 16). These and other assays are available at the Toxoplasma Serology Laboratory, Palo Alto Research Institute, Palo Alto, Calif.

(phone: 650-853-4828), and may be helpful for distinguishing acute infections from false-positive reactions or long-lived IgM antibodies (16, 19).

Tests for the Detection of Parasite Material

Although simultaneous detection of *Toxoplasma*-specific IgM antibodies and circulating antigens would indicate an acute infection more precisely than would detection of IgM antibodies alone, EIA antigen detection techniques lack sensitivity for human samples and are not recommended. PCR technology for *Toxoplasma* has been used to detect congenital infections, toxoplasmic encephalitis in AIDS patients, and ocular disease with various degrees of success. The most important use of PCR appears to be in the prenatal diagnosis of congenital toxoplasmosis. When maternal serologic results indicate potential infection during pregnancy, PCR of amniotic fluid has been shown to be more sensitive for the confirmation of fetal infection than the conventional methods of inoculation of mice and tissue culture cells and fetal blood testing for IgM (13). PCR technology for *Toxoplasma* is offered at the Toxoplasma Serology Laboratory and by a few commercial laboratories. Commercial kits are not yet available.

CLINICAL USE OF IMMUNODIAGNOSTIC TESTS

Determination of Immune Status

An algorithm for serologic testing for immune status and acute acquired infection is shown in Fig. 2. Three situations in which baseline information about an individual's immune status would be useful include the following: (i) before conception; (ii) before receiving immunosuppressive therapy; and (iii) after the initial determination of human immunodeficiency virus type 1-positive status. Screening one serum specimen with a sensitive test for IgG antibodies, such as DT, IFA, or EIA, is sufficient. A negative test result indicates that the patient has not been infected. A positive result of any degree indicates infection with *T. gondii* at some undetermined time.

Test serum for presence of *Toxoplasma*-specific IgG antibodies.

IgG negative: not infected. Retest in 3 weeks if acute infection is suspected.

IgG positive: infected

To determine approximate time of infection, test serum for presence of *Toxoplasma*-specific IgM antibodies.

IgG positive IgM negative: infected for more than 1 year

IgG positive IgM positive: infection within last 2 years or false-positive IgM result

Obtain second sample 2 weeks after first sample. Send both samples to a *Toxoplasma* reference laboratory for confirmation of IgG and IgM results and, if necessary, differential agglutination, IgA, and IgE testing to more accurately determine the time of primary infection before any intervention.

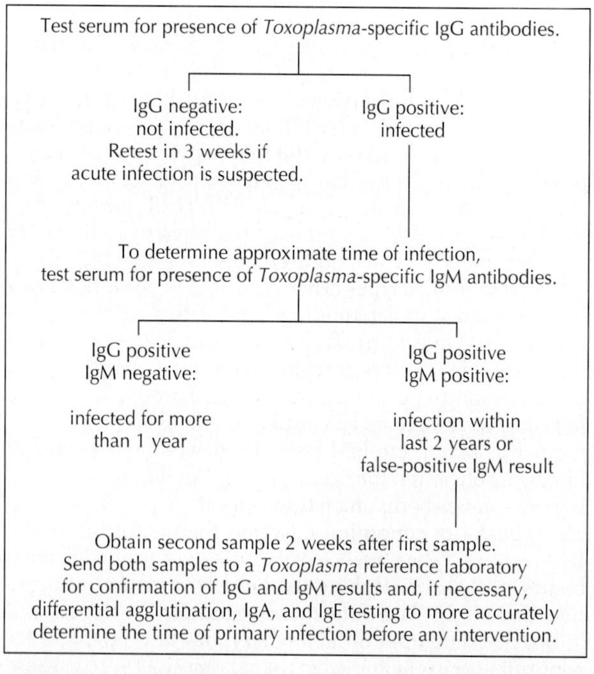

FIGURE 2 Algorithm for the serodiagnosis of toxoplasmosis in people older than 1 year of age.

Diagnosis of Acute Acquired Infections

If an acute acquired infection is suspected, the patient's serum specimen should be tested for the presence of *Toxoplasma*-specific antibodies (Fig. 2). A guide to the general interpretation of serology results is presented in Table 3. A negative result in the DT, IgG IFA test, or IgG EIA essentially excludes the diagnosis of acute *Toxoplasma* infection in an immunocompetent person. Demonstration of seroconversion from a negative titer to a positive titer or of more than a fourfold increase in titer confirms the diagnosis when specimens drawn several weeks apart are tested at the same time with the same test. However, such situations are rare because specimens are usually drawn after titers have peaked, too late to observe titer changes after initial infection. Most patients with acute infection will have DT or IFA IgG titers of ≥1:1,024. Results of an EIA for IgM can provide additional evidence for or against acute infection when IgG antibodies are present. A negative IgM test indicates that the patient was probably infected at least 6 to 12 months before being tested. A high IgM titer combined with a high IgG titer is probably indicative of acute infection within the previous 3 months. A low to medium IgM titer and a high IgG titer may be indicative of acute infection 3 to 6 months before the specimen was drawn; however, *IgM antibodies have been detected as long as 18 months after initial infection in some individuals.* Immunodiagnosis of acute infection in a pregnant woman should be confirmed by a toxoplasmosis reference laboratory prior to intervention. The presence of typical lymphadenopathy suggestive of acute toxoplasmosis, the presence of a high DT or IFA IgG titer (≥300 IU/ml or ≥1:1,000), and the presence of specific IgM are indicative of acute infection (19). If the patient has clinical illness compatible with toxoplasmosis but the IgG titer is low, a follow-up test 3 weeks later should show an increase in the antibody titer if the illness is due to acute toxoplasmosis and the host is not severely immunosuppressed.

Diagnosis of Congenital Infections

Diagnosis of congenital toxoplasmosis involves diagnosing acute infection in a pregnant woman, demonstrating infection in the fetus, or documenting infection in the newborn infant (1). Congenital toxoplasmosis occurs when a woman passes the infection to her fetus after acquiring a primary infection during pregnancy or, more rarely, when a pregnant woman is immunocompromised and a previously acquired infection is reactivated. The rate of transmission of infection to the fetus ranges from 11% in the first trimester to 90% in the late third trimester, with an overall transmission rate of approximately 50%.

In France and Austria, the prevention, diagnosis, and treatment of congenital toxoplasmosis begin with mandatory serologic testing of all women before or soon after conception. Although the cost-effectiveness of adopting this approach for all pregnant women in the United States has not been established, this approach does serve as a model for managing individual pregnant patients (3, 11, 13, 24).

Immunocompetent women who have IgG antibody before conception are considered immune and so at very little

TABLE 3 Guide to general interpretation of *Toxoplasma* serology results obtained with commercial assays

IgG result	IgM result	Report and/or interpretation for humans except infants
Negative	Negative	No serologic evidence of infection with *Toxoplasma*.
Negative	Equivocal	Possible early acute infection or false-positive IgM reaction. Obtain a new specimen for IgG and IgM testing. If results for the second specimen remain the same, the patient is probably not infected with *Toxoplasma*.
Negative	Positive	Possible acute infection or false-positive IgM result. Obtain a new specimen for IgG and IgM testing. If results for the second specimen remain the same, the IgM reaction is probably a false-positive.
Equivocal	Negative	Indeterminate. Obtain a new specimen for testing or retest this specimen for IgG in a different assay.
Equivocal	Equivocal	Indeterminate. Obtain a new specimen for both IgG and IgM testing.
Equivocal	Positive	Possible acute infection with *Toxoplasma*. Obtain a new specimen for IgG and IgM testing. If results for the second specimen remain the same or if the IgG reaction becomes positive, both specimens should be sent to a reference laboratory with experience in the diagnosis of toxoplasmosis for further testing.
Positive	Negative	Infected with *Toxoplasma* for more than 1 year.
Positive	Equivocal	Infected with *Toxoplasma* probably for more than 1 year or false-positive IgM reaction. Obtain a new specimen for IgM testing. If results with the second specimen remain the same, both specimens should be sent to a reference laboratory with experience in the diagnosis of toxoplasmosis for further testing.
Positive	Positive	Possible recent infection within the last 12 months or false-positive IgM reaction. Send the specimen to a reference laboratory with experience in the diagnosis of toxoplasmosis for further testing.

risk for transmission of infection to the fetus (Fig. 2). Women who are seronegative are considered at risk for infection and are tested monthly during pregnancy for IgG antibody. If a woman is first tested after conception and has *Toxoplasma*-specific IgG antibody, IgM testing should be done to determine if acute infection has occurred during pregnancy. When the diagnosis of acute toxoplasmosis has been documented in a pregnant woman, she can be treated and the fetus can be tested for evidence of infection (Fig. 3). The strategy used by Daffos et al. (3) involved initiating treatment with spiramycin (available in the United States through the Food and Drug Administration) once acute maternal infection was documented and then obtaining amniotic fluid and fetal blood samples between 20 and 26 weeks of gestation for testing. In addition, fetal ultrasound examinations were performed every 2 to 4 weeks until delivery to search for several nonspecific signs of infection: cerebral or hepatic calcifications, hydrocephalus, hepatomegaly, or ascites. Spiramycin reduced the transmission of *T. gondii* to the fetus by 60%.

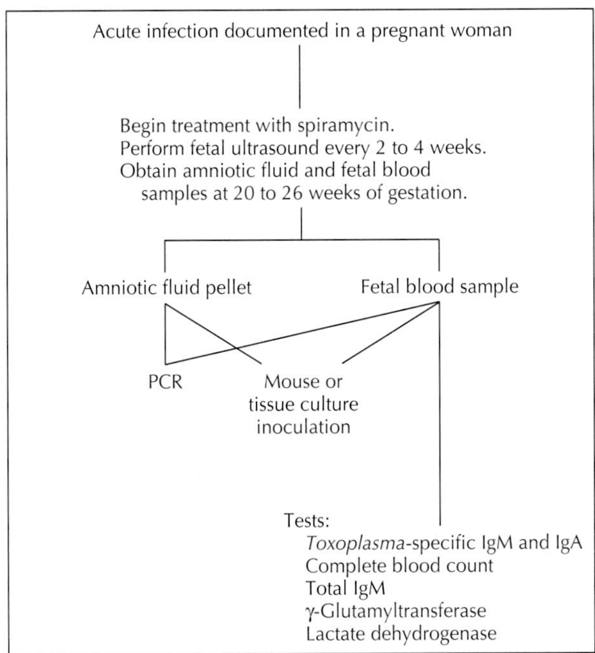

FIGURE 3 Algorithm for the diagnosis of antenatal congenital toxoplasmosis.

Fetal infection has been documented before 20 weeks of gestation by chorionic villus sampling and early amniocentesis (8). One of the more important advances in the past several years has been the demonstration by researchers in France that amniotic fluid testing for the *Toxoplasma* B1 gene by PCR approaches 100% sensitivity and specificity for fetal infection (26). If this level of test performance can be reproduced by investigators and reference laboratories in the United States, it is likely that amniotic fluid PCR will replace percutaneous umbilical blood sampling because of the greater risk of fetal loss with percutaneous umbilical blood sampling. Until such confirmation, fetal blood sampling remains important in establishing the intrauterine diagnosis of congenital toxoplasmosis.

Fetal blood should be tested for *Toxoplasma*-specific IgG, IgM, and IgA antibodies. Clotted blood should be inoculated into mice or tissue culture cells to demonstrate parasitemia. Nonspecific markers of infection should be tested for; these include leukocytes, eosinophils, platelets, total IgM, γ-glutamyltransferase, and lactate dehydrogenase. Most infected fetuses have one or more abnormal nonspecific tests, most commonly an elevated total IgM level or an elevated γ-glutamyltransferase level (3, 11, 24). Demonstrating *Toxoplasma*-specific IgM antibody in fetal serum or isolating the parasite from fetal leukocytes is a definitive diagnosis of fetal infection. Once the diagnosis has been made, the mother can be treated with pyrimethamine and sulfadiazine, which appear to treat the fetus as well and may decrease the severity of sequelae.

Diagnosis in the Newborn

Diagnosis of *Toxoplasma* infection in the newborn is made through a combination of serologic testing, parasite isolation, and nonspecific findings (18, 22, 24). An attempt should be made to isolate *T. gondii* from the placenta, cord leukocytes, and buffy coat if the diagnosis has not already been established (Fig. 4). *T. gondii* has been isolated from 95% of the placentas of congenitally infected newborns when the mother has not been treated and from approximately 81% when the mother has been treated. However, *T. gondii* can be isolated from the placentas of uninfected newborns as well. A child suspected of having congenital toxoplasmosis should have a thorough general, neurologic, and ophthalmologic examination and a computed tomographic scan of the head (magnetic resonance imaging does not demonstrate calcifications). The child's serum should be tested for total IgG and IgM antibodies and *Toxoplasma*-specific IgG, IgM, and IgA antibodies. CSF should be obtained; analyzed for cells, glucose, protein, total IgG antibody, and *Toxoplasma*-specific IgG and IgM antibodies; and directly examined for *T. gondii* tachyzoites. Because the diagnosis can take several months to confirm, clinicians may have to treat patients based upon early signs, symptoms, and serology while awaiting definitive confirmation. Although the complexity of diagnosing congenital infection necessitates the use of multiple costly laboratory tests, the benefit of early diagnosis and treatment and the cost of unnecessary treatment justify establishing the correct diagnosis.

Persistent or increasing IgG antibody levels in the infant compared with the mother, as measured by a DT or IFA test, and/or a positive result for *Toxoplasma*-specific IgM are diagnostic of congenital infection. Placental leak can occasionally lead to false-positive IgM measurements in the newborn. However, because the half-life of IgM is 3 to 5 days, repeat testing at 1 week should show a significant reduction in antibody titer if the child is not infected. Passively transferred maternal IgG has a half-life of approximately 1 month. Maternal antibodies can be detected for several months and have been reported up to 1 year of age. The untreated congenitally infected newborn will begin to produce *Toxoplasma*-specific IgG antibody within approximately 3 months. Treatment of the infected child may delay antibody production until 9 months of age and, on rare occasions, may prevent production altogether. Demonstration of a decrease in antibody load (*Toxoplasma*-specific IgG antibody divided by total IgG) can be helpful in differentiating maternal antibody from fetal antibody. Demonstration in the newborn of serum antibodies that are directed against unique *Toxoplasma* epitopes not found in the mother's serum is also evidence of congenital infection. *Toxoplasma* antigens have been demonstrated in the blood, urine, and CSF of congenitally infected infants.

Demonstration of IgM antibody or local *Toxoplasma*-specific IgG antibody production in CSF not contaminated with peripheral blood can help confirm the diagnosis of congenital toxoplasmosis. The calculation is made by dividing the *Toxoplasma*-specific antibody titer in the body fluid by the *Toxoplasma*-specific antibody titer in the serum and multiplying the result by the concentration of gamma globulin in serum divided by the concentration of gamma globulin in the body fluid. A result of four or greater corresponds to significant antibody production.

A long-term prospective study is currently under way in the United States to define optimal therapeutic regimens for the treatment of congenital toxoplasmosis (18). Clinicians should contact Rima McLeod, University of Chicago Hospitals, Chicago, Ill. (phone: 773-834-4152), regarding the therapy of infected children.

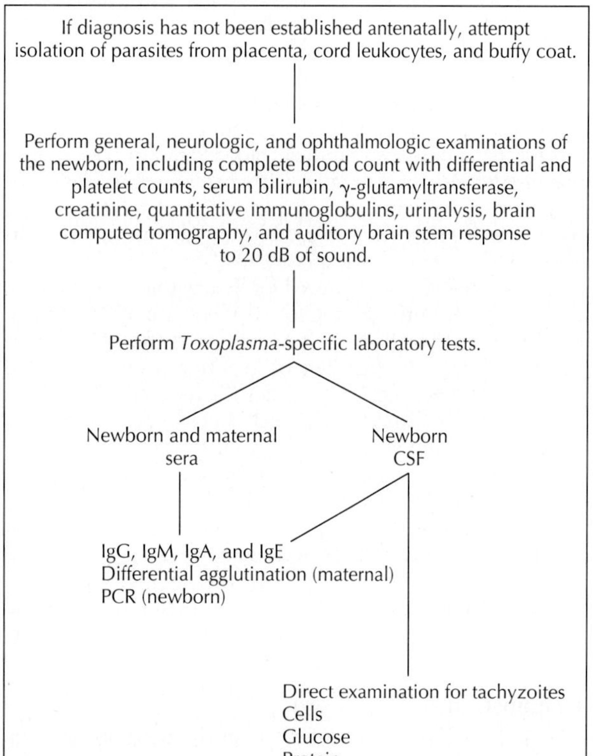

If diagnosis has not been established antenatally, attempt isolation of parasites from placenta, cord leukocytes, and buffy coat.

Perform general, neurologic, and ophthalmologic examinations of the newborn, including complete blood count with differential and platelet counts, serum bilirubin, γ-glutamyltransferase, creatinine, quantitative immunoglobulins, urinalysis, brain computed tomography, and auditory brain stem response to 20 dB of sound.

Perform *Toxoplasma*-specific laboratory tests.

Newborn and maternal sera

Newborn CSF

IgG, IgM, IgA, and IgE
Differential agglutination (maternal)
PCR (newborn)

Direct examination for tachyzoites
Cells
Glucose
Protein

FIGURE 4 Algorithm for the diagnosis of neonatal toxoplasmosis.

Diagnosis of Ocular Infections

Most cases of *Toxoplasma* chorioretinitis result from congenital infection but may also occur during acute infection (21). In addition to demonstrating IgG antibody to *Toxoplasma* in the serum of a person with compatible eye lesions, demonstration of the local production of antibody in the aqueous humor has been used to document active ocular toxoplasmosis. When the formula described above is used to calculate results obtained in eye fluids, a value of eight or greater suggests acute ocular toxoplasmosis. If the serum DT titer is >1:1,000, it is usually not possible to calculate local antibody production.

Diagnosis in the Immunocompromised Host

A wide variety of immunosuppressed hosts, including patients with lymphoma, leukemia, multiple myeloma, carcinoma, neuroblastoma, thymoma, systemic lupus erythematosus, scleroderma, autoimmune hemolytic anemia, and kidney, liver, and heart transplants, have been described as having severe, often fatal, toxoplasmosis. The disease is most often related to reactivation of latent infection and commonly involves the CNS, although a wide variety of clinical manifestations have been reported. Diagnosis can be very difficult for these patients, as IgM antibody is usually not detectable and the presence of IgG antibody only confirms chronic infection. In the absence of serologic evidence of acute infection, diagnosis can be confirmed by demonstration of the organism histologically or cytologically as replicating within tissue or by isolation or identification of its nucleic acids in a site such as amniotic fluid, CSF, bronchoalveolar fluid, or placenta, in which the encysted organism would not be present as part of a latent infection.

Persons undergoing organ or bone marrow transplantation are at risk for either acute acquired infection if they are seronegative before transplantation or reactivation if they are seropositive before transplantation. Those with acute acquired infection will usually develop detectable *Toxoplasma*-specific IgG and IgM antibodies, while those with reactivation will not have a detectable *Toxoplasma*-specific IgM response. Seronegative transplant recipients of hearts from seropositive donors can develop toxoplasmic myocarditis that mimics organ rejection.

Toxoplasmic encephalitis is the most frequent CNS opportunistic infection of AIDS patients and is uniformly fatal if untreated. Current estimates are that 5 to 10% of all AIDS patients in the United States will develop toxoplasmic encephalitis. Therapy for toxoplasmic encephalitis in AIDS patients is often toxic but must be continued indefinitely to prevent relapse; therefore, accurate diagnosis is essential. Most AIDS patients with toxoplasmic encephalitis have demonstrable IgG antibodies to *T. gondii*. However, approximately 3% of AIDS patients with toxoplasmic encephalitis do not have *Toxoplasma*-specific antibody in their serum. Local production of *Toxoplasma*-specific IgG antibody in CSF has been demonstrated for persons with AIDS and with toxoplasmic encephalitis (23). When the formula described above (for toxoplasmosis in the newborn) is used, a result of greater than one corresponds to significant antibody production.

SUMMARY

The immunodiagnosis of toxoplasmosis in adults is useful in the majority of patients to (i) exclude the disease (negative IgG and negative IgM) or (ii) exclude recent infection (positive IgG and negative IgM). Initial tests can be performed with a rapid turnaround time by a local hospital or commercial laboratories, and the results are usually acceptable. Acute- and convalescent-phase specimens with repeated negative IgG and positive IgM results can generally be considered to represent a false-positive IgM reaction, not acute infection. Specimens with positive IgG and IgM results should be sent to a laboratory with expertise in toxoplasmosis immunodiagnosis to confirm the results because of documented problems with false-positive IgM results with commercial kits. In the United States, that would be either the Centers for Disease Control and Prevention, which currently offers IgG and IgM testing, or the Palo Alto Research Institute, which offers IgG, IgM, differential agglutination, IgA, and IgE testing. None of the current commercial assays offered in the United States has been cleared by the Food and Drug Administration for in vitro diagnostic use for infants; consequently, all specimens from neonates suspected of having congenital toxoplasmosis should be sent to the Palo Alto Research Institute, which has the most experience with infant testing.

REFERENCES

1. **Boyer, K. M., and J. B. McAuley.** 1994. Congenital toxoplasmosis. *Semin. Pediatr. Infect. Dis.* **5:**42–51.
2. **Candolfi, E., R. Ramirez, M. P. Hadju, C. Shubert, and J. S. Remington.** 1994. The Vitek immunodiagnostic assay for detection of immunoglobulin M *Toxoplasma* antibodies. *Clin. Diagn. Lab. Immunol.* **1:**401–405.
3. **Daffos, F., F. Forestier, M. Capella-Pavlovsky, P. Thulliez, C. Aufrant, D. Valenti, and W. L. Cox.** 1988. Prenatal management of 746 pregnancies at risk for congenital toxoplasmosis. *N. Engl. J. Med.* **318:**271–275.
4. **Decoster, A., F. Darcy, A. Caron, D. Vinatier, D. Houze de l'Aulnoit, G. Vittu, G. Niel, F. Heyer, B. Lecolier, M. Delcroix, J. C. Monnier, M. Duhamel, and A. Capron.** 1992. Anti-P30 IgA antibodies as prenatal markers of congenital toxoplasma infection. *Clin. Exp. Immunol.* **87:** 310–315.
5. **Decoster, A., and B. Lecolier.** 1996. Bicentric evaluation of Access Toxo immunoglobulin M (IgM) and IgG assays and IMx Toxo IgM and IgG assays and comparison with Platelia Toxo IgM and IgG assays. *J. Clin. Microbiol.* **34:** 1606–1609.
6. **Derouin, F., P. Thulliez, E. Candolfi, F. Daffos, and F. Forestier.** 1988. Early prenatal diagnosis of congenital toxoplasmosis using amniotic fluid samples and tissue culture. *Eur. J. Clin. Microbiol. Infect. Dis.* **7:**423–425.
7. **Fortier, B., A. Dao, C. Coignard-Chatain, and M. F. Biava.** 1997. Application de la chimiluminescence au diagnostic serologique des toxoplasmoses. *Pathol. Biol.* **45:** 721–728.
8. **Foulon, W., A. Naessens, L. de Catte, and J. J. Amy.** 1990. Detection of congenital toxoplasmosis by chorionic villus sampling and early amniocentesis. *Am. J. Obstet. Gynecol.* **163:**1511–1513.
9. **Galanti, L. M., J. Dell'Omo, B. Wanet, J. L. Guarin, J. Jamart, M. G. Garrino, P. L. Masson, and C. L. Cambiaso.** 1997. Particle counting assay for anti-*Toxoplasma* IgG antibodies. Comparison with four automated commercial enzyme-linked immunoassays. *J. Immunol. Methods* **207:** 195–201.
10. **Hayde, M., H. R. Salzer, G. Gittler, H. Aspock, and A. Pollak.** 1995. Microparticle enzyme immunoassay (MEIA) for toxoplasma specific immunoglobulin G in comparison to the Sabin-Feldman dye test. A pilot study. *Wien Klin. Wochenschr.* **107:**133–136.
11. **Hezard, N., C. Marx-Chemla, F. Foudrinier, I. Villena, C. Quereux, B. Leroux, D. Dupouy, M. Talmud, and J. M. Pinon.** 1997. Prenatal diagnosis of congenital toxoplasmosis in 261 pregnancies. *Prenatal Diagn.* **17:**1047–1054.
12. **Hofgartner, W. T., S. R. Swanzy, R. M. Bacina, J. Condon, M. Gupta, P. E. Matlock, D. L. Bergeron, J. J. Plorde, and T. R. Fritsche.** 1997. Detection of immunoglobulin G (IgG) and IgM antibodies to *Toxoplasma gondii*—evaluation of four commercial immunoassay systems. *J. Clin. Microbiol.* **35:**3313–3315.
13. **Hohlfeld, P., F. Daffos, J. M. Costa, P. Thulliez, F. Forestier, and M. Vidaud.** 1994. Prenatal diagnosis of congenital toxoplasmosis with a polymerase-chain-reaction test on amniotic fluid. *N. Engl. J. Med.* **331:**695–699.
14. **Jenum, P. A., B. Stray-Pedersen, and A. G. Gundersen.** 1997. Improved diagnosis of primary *Toxoplasma gondii* infection in early pregnancy by determination of antitoxoplasma immunoglobulin G avidity. *J. Clin. Microbiol.* **35:** 1972–1977.
15. **Liesenfeld, O., C. Press, R. Flanders, R. Ramirez, and J. S. Remington.** 1996. Study of Abbott Toxo IMx system for detection of immunoglobulin G and immunoglobulin M toxoplasma antibodies—value of confirmatory testing for diagnosis of acute toxoplasmosis. *J. Clin. Microbiol.* **34:** 2526–2530.
16. **Liesenfeld, O., C. Press, J. G. Montoya, R. Gill, J. L. Isaac-Renton, K. Hedman, and J. S. Remington.** 1997. False-positive results in immunoglobulin M (IgM) toxoplasma antibody tests and importance of confirmatory testing—the Platelia Toxo IgM test. *J. Clin. Microbiol.* **35:** 174–178.
17. **Luyasu, V., A. R. Robert, L. Schaefer, J. Macioszek, and Multicenter Study Group.** 1995. Multicenter evaluation of a new commercial assay for detection of immunoglobulin M antibodies to *Toxoplasma gondii*. *Eur. J. Clin. Microbiol. Infect. Dis.* **14:**787–793.
18. **McAuley, J., K. M. Boyer, D. Patel, M. Mets, C. Swisher, N. Roizen, C. Wolters, L. Stein, M. Stein, W. Schey,**

J. Remington, P. Meier, D. Johnson, P. Heydeman, E. Holfels, S. Withers, D. Mack, C. Brown, D. Patton, and R. McLeod. 1994. Early and longitudinal evaluations of treated infants and children and untreated historical patients with congenital toxoplasmosis: the Chicago Collaborative Treatment Trial. *Clin. Infect. Dis.* **18:**38–72.

19. **Montoya, J. G., and J. S. Remington.** 1995. Studies on the serodiagnosis of toxoplasmic lymphadenitis. *Clin. Infect. Dis.* **20:**781–789.
20. **Naot, Y., G. Desmonts, and J. S. Remington.** 1981. IgM enzyme-linked immunosorbent assay test for the diagnosis of congenital *Toxoplasma* infection. *J. Pediatr.* **98:**32–36.
21. **Nussenblatt, R. B., and R. Belfort.** 1994. Ocular toxoplasmosis. An old disease revisited. *JAMA* **271:**304–307.
22. **Pinon, J. M., C. Chemla, I. Villena, F. Foudrinier, D. Aubert, D. Puygauthier-Toubas, B. Leroux, D. Dupouy, C. Quereux, M. Talmud, T. Trenque, G. Potron, M. Pluot, G. Remy, and A. Bonhomme.** 1996. Early neonatal diagnosis of congenital toxoplasmosis: value of comparative enzyme-linked immunofiltration assay, immunological profiles, and anti-*Toxoplasma gondii* immunoglobulin M (IgM) or IgA immunocapture and implications for postnatal therapeutic strategies. *J. Clin. Microbiol.* **34:**579–583.
23. **Potasman, I., L. Resnick, B. J. Luft, and J. S. Remington.** 1988. Intrathecal production of antibodies against *Toxoplasma gondii* in patients with toxoplasmic encephalitis and the acquired immunodeficiency syndrome (AIDS). *Ann. Intern. Med.* **108:**49–51.
24. **Pratlong, F., P. Boulot, I. Villena, E. Issert, I. Tamby, J. Cazenave, and J. P. Dedet.** 1996. Antenatal diagnosis of congenital toxoplasmosis: evaluation of the biological parameters in a cohort of 286 patients. *Br. J. Obstet. Gynecol.* **103:**552–557.
25. **Rao, L. V., O. A. James, L. M. Mann, A. A. Mohammad, A. O. Okorodudu, M. G. Bissell, and J. R. Petersen.** 1997. Evaluation of Immuno-1 toxoplasma IgG assay in the prenatal screening of toxoplasmosis. *Diagn. Microbiol. Infect. Dis.* **27:**13–15.
26. **Remington, J. S., R. McLeod, and G. Desmonts.** 1995. Toxoplasmosis, p. 140–266. *In* J. S. Remington and J. O. Klein (ed.), *Infectious Diseases of the Fetus and Newborn Infant*, 4th ed. The W. B. Saunders Co., Philadelphia, Pa.
27. **Singh, S., N. Singh, and S. N. Dwivedi.** 1997. Evaluation of seven commercially available ELISA kits for serodiagnosis of acute toxoplasmosis. *Indian J. Med. Res.* **105:**103–107.
28. **Smith, K. L., M. Wilson, A. W. Hightower, P. W. Kelley, J. P. Struewing, D. D. Juranek, and J. B. McAuley.** 1996. Prevalence of *Toxoplasma gondii* antibodies in US military recruits in 1989—comparison with data published in 1965. *Clin. Infect. Dis.* **23:**1182–1183.
29. **Stepick-Biek, P., P. Thulliez, F. G. Araujo, and J. S. Remington.** 1990. IgA antibodies for diagnosis of acute congenital and acquired toxoplasmosis. *J. Infect. Dis.* **162:**270–273.
30. **Wilson, M., J. S. Remington, C. Clavet, G. Varney, C. Press, D. Ware, and the FDA Toxoplasmosis Ad Hoc Working Group.** 1997. Evaluation of six commercial kits for detection of human immunoglobulin M antibodies to *Toxoplasma gondii*. *J. Clin. Microbiol.* **35:**3112–3115.
31. **Wilson, M., and J. B. McAuley.** Unpublished data.
32. **Wong, S. Y., M. P. Hajdu, R. Ramirez, P. Thulliez, R. McLeod, and J. S. Remington.** 1993. Role of specific immunoglobulin E in diagnosis of acute toxoplasma infection and toxoplasmosis. *J. Clin. Microbiol.* **31:**2952–2959.

Pathogenic and Opportunistic Free-Living Amebae

GOVINDA S. VISVESVARA

108

BACKGROUND

Small free-living amebae belonging to the genera *Naegleria*, *Acanthamoeba*, and *Balamuthia* have been identified as agents of central nervous system (CNS) infections of humans and other animals (1, 3, 12, 16, 17, 19–22, 29, 39–42). Only one species of *Naegleria* (*N. fowleri*), several species of *Acanthamoeba* (e.g., *A. castellanii*, *A. culbertsoni*, *A. hatchetti*, *A. healyi*, *A. polyphaga*, *A. rhysodes*, *A. astronyxis*, *A. divionensis*), and the only known species of *Balamuthia*, *B. mandrillaris*, are known to cause disease (12, 16, 21, 22, 29). *Acanthamoeba* spp. also cause infection of the human cornea, *Acanthamoeba* keratitis (2, 6, 7, 13, 15, 28, 36, 37, 43). Additionally, both *Acanthamoeba* spp. and *B. mandrillaris* have also been identified as agents of cutaneous infections in humans (8, 9, 22, 25, 34, 35).

N. fowleri and *Acanthamoeba* spp. are commonly found in soil, freshwater, sewage and sludge, and even dust in air (5, 12, 17, 20, 27, 33, 41). They normally feed on bacteria and multiply in their environmental niche as free-living organisms. Several species of *Acanthamoeba* have also been isolated from brackish water and seawater (5, 17, 30) and from ear discharge, pulmonary secretions, nasopharyngeal mucosa samples, maxillary sinus samples, mandibular autografts, and stool samples (5, 12, 17, 20, 41). *Acanthamoeba* spp. have been also known to harbor *Legionella* spp. and mycobacteria, which signifies a potential expansion of public health importance of these organisms (17, 41). Although *Balamuthia* organisms have been isolated from human and animal brains, not much is known about the environmental niche of *B. mandrillaris* and its feeding habits. It is, however, believed that its habitat is similar to those of *Acanthamoeba* and *Naegleria*. Excellent reviews (3, 5, 12, 17, 22, 41) and books (20, 33) have been published on the biology, disease potential, pathology, pathogenicity, and epidemiology of these amebae.

The concept that these small free-living amebae could occur as human pathogens was proposed by Culbertson and his colleagues, who isolated *Acanthamoeba* sp. strain A-1 (now designated *Acanthamoeba culbertsoni*) from tissue culture medium thought to contain an unknown virus (4). They also demonstrated amebae in brain lesions of mice and monkeys that died within a week after intracerebral inoculation with these amebae. Culbertson hypothesized that similar infection might exist in nature in humans. In 1965, Fowler and Carter were the first to describe a fatal infection due to free-living amebae that occurred in the brain of an Australian patient (3). The infection is now believed to have been due to *N. fowleri* (3).

NAEGLERIA MENINGOENCEPHALITIS

In 1966 Butt et al. (3, 17) described the first case of CNS infection caused by *N. fowleri* in the United States and coined the term primary amebic meningoencephalitis (PAM). PAM is an acute fulminating disease with an abrupt onset that occurs generally in previously healthy children and young adults who have had contact with freshwater about 7 to 10 days before the onset of symptoms. It is characterized by severe headache, spiking fever, stiff neck, photophobia, and coma leading to death within 3 to 10 days after the onset of symptoms (3, 17, 20, 22, 32). The portal of entry of these amebae is the nasal passages. When people swim in lakes and other bodies of freshwater that harbor these amebae, the amebae may enter the nostrils of the swimmers, make their way into the olfactory lobes via the cribriform plate, and cause acute hemorrhagic necrosis leading to destruction of the olfactory bulbs and the cerebral cortex. On autopsy, large numbers of amebic trophozoites, many with ingested erythrocytes and brain tissue, are usually seen interspersed with brain tissue (Fig. 1). It is believed that *N. fowleri* directly ingests brain tissue by producing food cups or amebostomes, as well as exerts a contact-dependent cytolysis, mediated possibly by a multicomponent system consisting of a heat-stable hemolytic protein, heat-labile cytolysin, and/or phospholipase enzymes (12, 18). Cysts of *N. fowleri* are not usually seen in the brain tissue. More than 175 cases of PAM have occurred worldwide and a little less than one half (~86) of those cases have been reported from the United States as of January 1998. Only a few patients have survived. It was believed until recently that *N. fowleri* infects only humans. In March 1997, however, the first case of PAM in a South American tapir was published, indicating that PAM can occur in animals other than humans (16).

ACANTHAMOEBA ENCEPHALITIS

Several species of *Acanthamoeba* (*A. culbertsoni*, *A. castellanii*, *A. polyphaga*, *A. astronyxis*, *A. healyi*, *A. divionensis*) have been known to cause a chronic granulomatous amebic

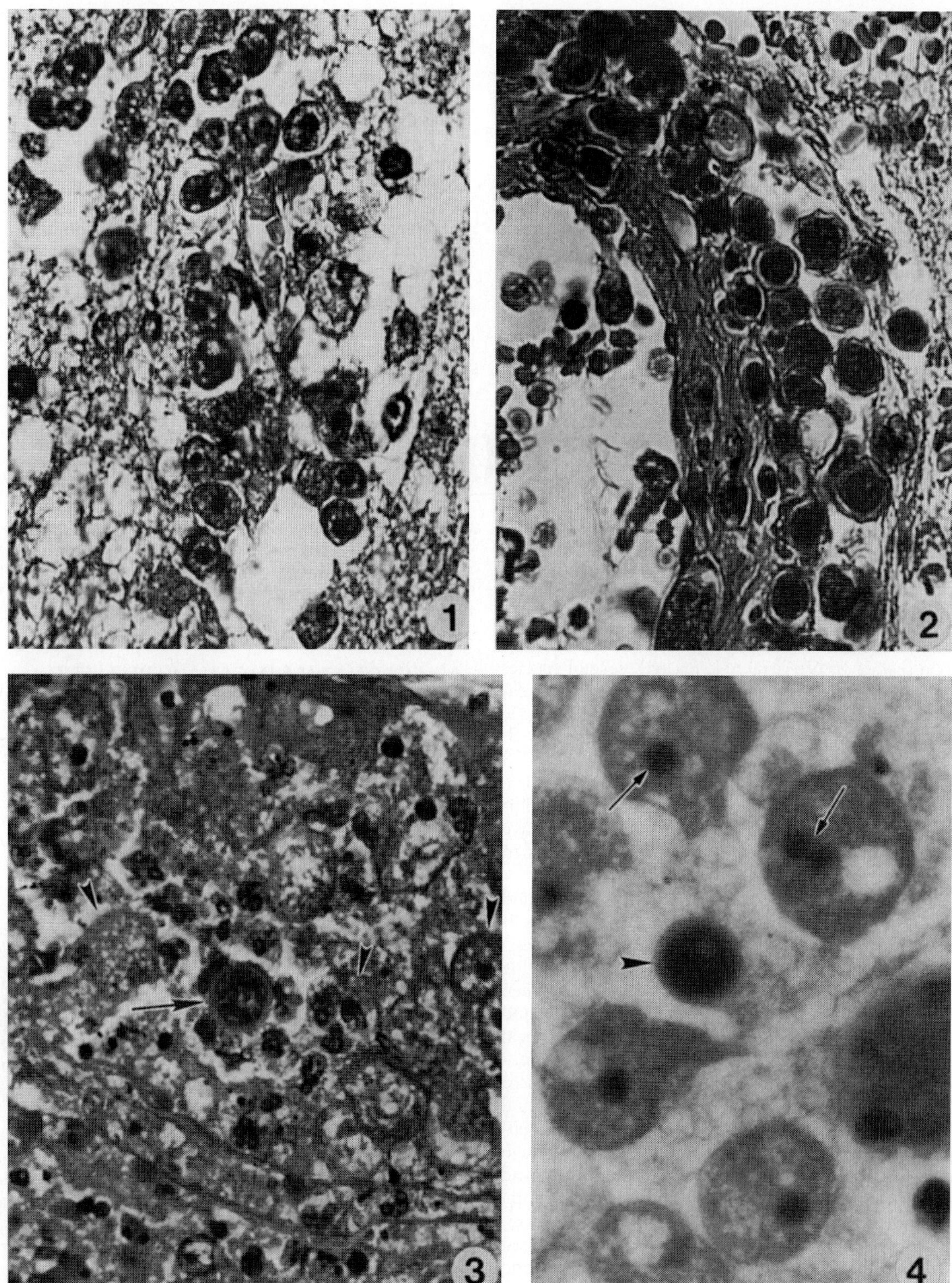

FIGURE 1 Large numbers of *N. fowleri* trophozoites in a section of CNS, showing extensive necrosis and destruction of brain tissue. Magnification, ×750.

FIGURE 2 *A. castellanii* trophozoites and cysts around a blood vessel in a section of CNS from a GAE patient. Magnification, ×650.

FIGURE 3 *Balamuthia* trophozoites (arrowheads) and a cyst (arrow) in the brain section of a GAE patient. Magnification, ×550.

FIGURE 4 Trophozoites and a darkly staining cyst (arrowhead) in a brain section of a GAE patient. Note the double nucleolar elements (arrow) within the nucleus of the trophozoites. Magnification, ×1,000.

encephalitis (GAE), primarily in immunosuppressed (either iatrogenically or because of human immunodeficiency virus infection or AIDS), chronically ill, or otherwise debilitated persons with no previous history of exposure to recreational freshwater (10, 17, 19–22, 42). GAE has an insidious onset and is usually chronic, lasting for more than a week and sometimes even for months (19–22). GAE is characterized by headache, confusion, dizziness, drowsiness, seizures, and sometimes hemiparesis. Cerebral hemispheres are usually the most affected CNS tissue. They are often edematous, with extensive hemorrhagic necrosis involving the temporal, parietal, and occipital lobes. Amebic trophozoites and cysts are usually scattered throughout the tissue. Many blood vessels are thrombotic with fibrinoid necrosis and cuffed by polymorphonuclear leukocytes, amebic trophozoites, and cysts (Fig. 2). Multinucleated giant cells forming granulomas may be seen in immunocompetent patients. Some patients, especially those with human immunodeficiency virus infection or AIDS, develop chronic, ulcerative skin lesions, abscesses, or erythematous nodules (8–10, 19–22, 25, 34, 42). It is believed that the route of invasion and penetration into the CNS is hematogenous, probably from a primary focus in the lower respiratory tract or the skin (19–22). As many as 105 cases of GAE caused by *Acanthamoeba* have been recorded worldwide, and ~73 of these cases (53 in AIDS patients) have occurred in the United States as of January 1998. *Acanthamoeba* spp. also cause infections of the CNS of animals besides humans. Such infections have been recorded in gorillas, monkeys, dogs, ovines, bovines, and kangaroos (21, 41).

Because of the confusion that existed in the earlier literature with regard to the nomenclature of *Acanthamoeba* and *Hartmanella* spp., some workers in the field referred to these amebae as belonging to the *Hartmanella-Acanthamoeba* group or simply as "H-A amebae." Since no true *Hartmanella* species has been found to be pathogenic to humans, all references in the literature to *Hartmanella* in human tissues should be corrected to read *Acanthamoeba* or *Balamuthia* spp.

BALAMUTHIA (LEPTOMYXID) ENCEPHALITIS

Until recently, it was believed that all cases of GAE were caused by *Acanthamoeba* spp. Although a number of these cases were confirmed by serologic techniques as being caused by *Acanthamoeba* spp., the causative organisms in a few cases could not be definitively identified. Since cysts were found in the brain tissues of these patients, it was believed that the infections were caused by some other species of *Acanthamoeba* that did not cross-react with the anti-*Acanthamoeba* sera used in the serologic test (19–22, 41). It was only recently that *Balamuthia mandrillaris* (leptomyxid ameba) was definitively identified by an indirect immunofluorescence test as the causal agent of these cases (1, 10, 21, 38–41). The rabbit anti-*B. mandrillaris* serum used in the indirect immunofluorescence test was made by using culture-derived *Balamuthia* organisms that were isolated from the CNS tissue of a baboon (39). It is now known that a number of primates, including gorillas, gibbons, baboons, orangutans, and monkeys, as well as a sheep and a horse, have died of CNS infection caused by *B. mandrillaris* (21, 29, 41). As of January 1998, a total of 73 cases of *B. mandrillaris* GAE have been reported worldwide with as many as 31 (11 in people with AIDS) occurring in the United States.

The pathology and pathogenesis of *B. mandrillaris*-induced GAE are similar to those of *Acanthamoeba* GAE. Both trophozoites and cysts are found in CNS tissue (Fig. 3), and their sizes overlap those of *Acanthamoeba* (1, 10, 17, 21, 22, 39–41). Hence, it is difficult to differentiate *Balamuthia* from *Acanthamoeba* spp. in tissue sections under the light microscope. In some cases, *Balamuthia* trophozoites in tissue sections appear to have more than one nucleolus in the nucleus (Fig. 4). In such cases, it may be possible to distinguish *Balamuthia* amebae from *Acanthamoeba* organisms on the basis of nuclear morphology, since *Acanthamoeba* trophozoites have only one nucleolus. In most cases, electron microscopy, immunohistochemical technique, or both are necessary to identify *Balamuthia* organisms. Ultrastructurally, the cysts are characterized by three layers in the cyst wall: an outer wrinkled ectocyst, a middle structureless mesocyst, and an inner thin endocyst (39, 40). *Balamuthia* amebas are antigenically distinct from *Acanthamoeba* organisms; they can easily be distinguished by immunofluorescence or other immunochemical assays (1, 10, 39, 40).

ACANTHAMOEBA KERATITIS

Acanthamoeba spp. also cause a painful vision-threatening disease of the human cornea, *Acanthamoeba* keratitis. If the infection is not treated promptly, it may lead to ulceration of the cornea, loss of visual acuity, and eventually blindness and enucleation (2, 6, 7, 13, 15, 17, 28, 43). The first case of *Acanthamoeba* keratitis in the United States was reported in 1973 in a south Texas rancher with a history of trauma to his right eye (13). Both trophozoites and cyst stages of *A. polyphaga* were demonstrated in corneal sections and repeatedly cultured from corneal scrapings and biopsy specimens. Between 1973 and July 1986, 208 cases were diagnosed and reported to the Centers for Disease Control and Prevention (36, 37, 41). The numbers of cases gradually increased between 1973 and 1984, with a dramatic increase beginning in 1985. An in-depth epidemiologic and case-control study (36, 37) revealed that a major risk factor was the use of contact lenses, predominantly daily-wear or extended-wear soft lenses, and that patients with *Acanthamoeba* keratitis were significantly more likely than controls to use homemade saline solution instead of commercially prepared saline (78% versus 30%, respectively), to disinfect their lenses less frequently than recommended by the lens manufacturers (72% versus 32%), and to wear their lenses while swimming (63% versus 30%). *Acanthamoeba* keratitis is characterized by severe ocular pain, a 360° or partial paracentral stromal ring infiltrate, recurrent corneal epithelial breakdown, and a corneal lesion refractory to the commonly used ophthalmic antibacterial medications. *Acanthamoeba* keratitis in the early stages is frequently misdiagnosed as herpes simplex virus keratitis because of the irregular epithelial lesions, stromal infiltrative keratitis, and edema that are commonly seen in herpes simplex virus keratitis (13, 17). A nonhealing corneal ulcer is often the first clue that *Acanthamoeba* keratitis may be the problem. It is estimated that as of January 1998 more than 750 cases of *Acanthamoeba* keratitis have occurred in the United States and *Acanthamoeba* keratitis has become a burgeoning problem in England (7). Since the diseases caused by these small amebae are not reportable in the United States, the actual number may be much higher.

MORPHOLOGY

N. fowleri in its trophic form is a small, sluglike ameba measuring 10 to 35 μm that exhibits an eruptive locomotion by producing smooth hemispherical bulges. The posterior end, termed the uroid, appears to be sticky and often has several trailing filaments. During its life cycle, this ameba produces a transient pear-shaped biflagellate stage, resulting from altered environmental conditions, and smooth-walled cysts (Fig. 5–8). The flagellates do not have cytostomes. Cysts are usually spherical and measure 7 to 15 μm, and the cyst wall may have one or more pores plugged with a mucoid material (27).

An *Acanthamoeba* organism is a slightly larger ameba (15 to 45 μm) that produces from the surface of its body fine, tapering, hyaline projections called acanthopodia (Fig. 9). It has no flagellate stage but produces a double-walled cyst (Fig. 10) (10 to 25 μm) with a wrinkled outer wall, the ectocyst, and a stellate, polygonal, or even round inner wall, the endocyst (10, 27).

Balamuthia trophozoites are in general irregular in shape; a few, however, may be sluglike. Actively feeding amebae may measure from 12 to 60 μm in length, with a mean of 30 μm (Fig. 11). The trophic forms, while feeding on tissue culture cells, produce broad pseudopodia without any clearly discernible movement. However, when tissue culture cells are destroyed, the trophozoites resort to a spiderlike walking movement by producing fingerlike determinate pseudopodia (40). Like *Acanthamoeba* spp., *Balamuthia* does not have a flagellate stage. Cysts are generally spherical and measure from 6 to 30 μm in diameter (Fig. 12). Under the light microscope, each cyst appears to have an irregular and slightly wavy outer wall and a round inner wall. A layer of refractile granules immediately below the inner cyst wall is often seen in mature cysts. In the electron microscope, the cyst wall can be seen to consist of three walls: an outer thin, irregular ectocyst; a thick, electron-dense inner endocyst; and a middle amorphous layer, the mesocyst (39, 40).

Acanthamoeba, *Balamuthia*, and *Naegleria* are predominantly uninucleate, although binucleate forms are occasionally seen. The nucleus is characterized by a large, dense, centrally located nucleolus. *Naegleria* amebae exhibit a promitotic pattern of cell division wherein the nucleolus and the nuclear membrane persist during nuclear division. *Acanthamoeba* spp, however, divide by conventional mitosis, in which the nucleolus and the nuclear membrane disappear during cell division. The pattern of nuclear division in *Balamuthia* is termed metamitosis: the nuclear membrane breaks down, and the nucleolus eventually disappears (40).

CLINICAL AND LABORATORY DIAGNOSIS

No distinctive clinical features differentiate PAM from pyogenic or bacterial meningitis. In PAM the cerebrospinal fluid (CSF) is usually pleocytotic with a preponderance of polymorphonuclear leukocytes and no bacteria. The CSF pressure may be elevated. CSF glucose level may be normal or slightly reduced, but CSF protein is increased, ranging from 1 to 10 mg/ml. Microscopic detection of amebic organisms in the CSF is the only means of diagnosing PAM. CSF should be examined in situ microscopically for the presence of *N. fowleri* amebae with directional movement. Giemsa or trichrome staining should be performed on CSF smears to delineate the nuclear morphology of the amebae. Gram staining is not useful in the detection of amebae. Further, a false-positive Gram stain may lead to inaccurate diagnosis leading to inappropriate therapy and thus resulting in death. A recent report describing the transplantation of kidney and liver from a donor infected with *N. fowleri* (14) underscores the importance of a correct and timely diagnosis. *Acanthamoeba* trophozoites have been seen, though rarely, in the CSF, but *Balamuthia* organisms have never been seen in the CSF. They have, however, been identified in stained brain and/or skin biopsy specimens and also have been isolated in culture (10, 21, 22, 39). *Acanthamoeba* organisms have also been recovered and identified from corneal scrapings as well as biopsy samples. Recently, direct examination of the patient's cornea with the confocal microscope has been used to diagnose *Acanthamoeba* keratitis (28).

COLLECTION, HANDLING, AND STORAGE OF SPECIMENS

For isolating the etiologic agent, CSF, small pieces of tissue (brain, lungs, corneal biopsy material), or corneal scrapings from the affected area must be obtained aseptically. The specimens should be kept at room temperature (24 to 28°C) and should never be frozen. The specimens may be kept at 4°C for short periods but never for more than 24 h. Personnel handling the specimens must take appropriate precautions, such as wearing surgical masks and gloves and working in a biological safety cabinet. Remaining tissues must be preserved in 10% neutral buffered Formalin so that they can be examined histologically for amebae (38).

METHODS OF EXAMINATION

Direct Examination

Direct examination of the sample as a wet mount preparation is of paramount importance in the diagnosis of PAM and other diseases caused by these amebae. Since the amebae tend to attach to the surface of the container, the container should be shaken gently; then a small drop of fluid is placed on a clean microscope slide and covered with a no. 1 cover slip. The cerebrospinal fluid may have to be centrifuged at 150 × *g* for 5 min to concentrate the amebae. After the specimen has been centrifuged, most of the supernatant is carefully aspirated, and the sediment is gently suspended in the remaining fluid. A drop of this suspension is prepared as described above for microscopic observation.

The slide preparation should be examined under a compound microscope with 10× and 40× objectives. Phase-contrast optics are preferable. If regular bright-field illumination is used, the slide should be examined under diminished light. The slide may be warmed to 35°C (to promote amebic movement), and amebae, especially *N. fowleri* if present, can easily be detected by their active directional movements.

Permanently Stained Preparations

A small drop of the sedimented cerebrospinal fluid or other sample is placed in the middle of a slide and allowed to stand in a moist chamber for 5 to 10 min at 37°C. This will allow any amebae to attach to the surface of the slide. Several drops of warm (37°C) Schaudinn's fixative are dropped directly onto the sample and allowed to stand for 1 min. The slide is then transferred to a Coplin jar containing the fixative for 1 h. It may be stained in Wheatley's trichrome or Heidenhain's iron hematoxylin stain. Corneal scrapings smeared on microscope slides may be fixed with methanol and stained with Hemacolor stain (Harleco, a division of EM industries, Inc.) (17, 38).

ISOLATION

The recommended procedure for isolating free-living pathogenic amebae from biological specimens is as follows.

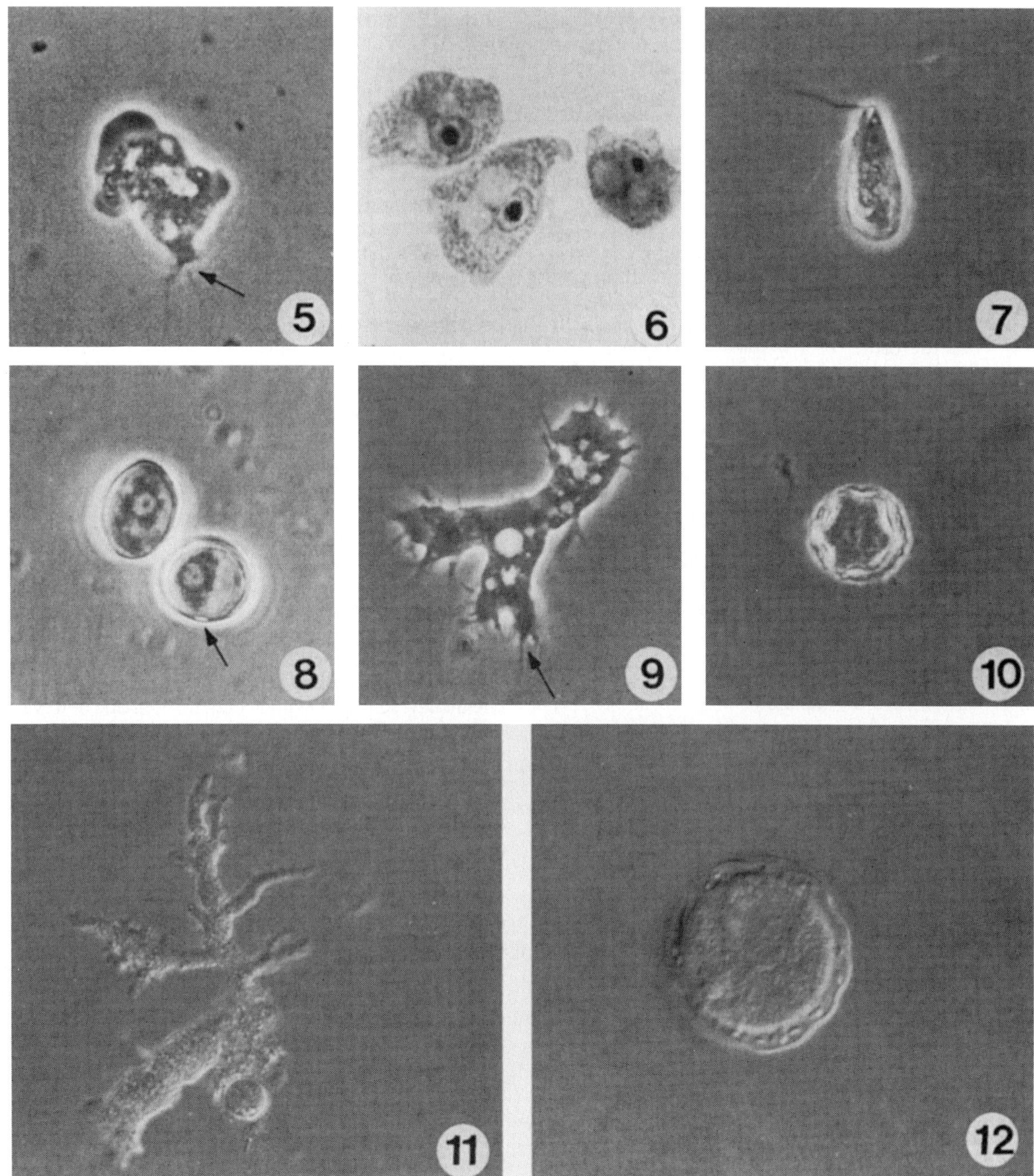

FIGURES 5–8 *N. fowleri.* (Figure 5) Trophozoite, phase contrast (note the uroid and filaments at arrow); (Figure 6) trophozoite, trichrome stain; (Figure 7) biflagellate, phase contrast; (Figure 8) smooth-walled cyst, phase contrast (note the pore at the arrow). All magnifications are ×1,100.

FIGURES 9 and 10 *A. castellanii.* (Figure 9) Trophozoite, phase contrast (note the acanthopodia at the arrow); (Figure 10) double-walled cyst, phase contrast. Both magnifications are ×1,100.

FIGURES 11 and 12 *B. mandrillaris.* (Figure 11) Trophozoite, phase contrast; (Figure 12) cyst, phase contrast. Both magnifications are ×1,500.

Materials

1. Page's ameba saline (17, 27)
2. Nonnutrient agar plates with ameba saline
3. 18- to 24-h-old culture of *Escherichia coli* or *Enterobacter aerogenes*
4. Sterile distilled water
5. Bacteriologic loop
6. Fine spatula made of nichrome wire
7. Sterile Pasteur pipettes, rubber bulbs
8. Sterile 1-ml serologic pipettes
9. Sterile screw-cap test tubes, 100 by 13 or 125 by 16 mm

10. Moist chamber
11. Vaspar (1:1 petrolatum-paraffin), melted
12. Microscope slides, 3 by 1 or 3 by 2 in. (7.6 by 2.5 or 7.6 by 5 cm)
13. Coverslips, 22 mm square, no. 1 thickness

Preparation of Agar Plates

1. Remove plates from refrigerator, and place them in a 37°C incubator for 30 min.

2. Add 0.5 ml of ameba saline to a slant culture of *E. coli* or *Enterobacter aerogenes*. Gently scrape the surface of the slant with a sterile bacteriologic loop (do not break the agar surface). Using a sterile Pasteur pipette, gently and uniformly suspend the bacteria. Add 2 or 3 drops of this suspension to the center of a warmed (37°C) agar plate, and spread the bacteria over the surface of the agar with a bacteriologic loop. The plate is then ready for inoculation.

Inoculation of Plates with Specimens

1. For CSF samples, centrifuge the CSF at 150 × *g* for 5 to 8 min. With a sterile serologic pipette, carefully transfer all but 0.5 ml of the supernatant to a sterile tube, and store the tube at 4°C for possible future use. Mix the sediment with the remaining fluid. With a sterile Pasteur pipette, place 2 or 3 drops in the center of the agar plate precoated with bacteria, and incubate in room air at 37°C.

2. For tissue samples, triturate a small piece of the tissue in a small amount of ameba saline. With a sterile Pasteur pipette, place 2 or 3 drops of the mixture in the center of the agar plate. Incubate the plate in room air at 37°C for CNS tissues and at 30°C for tissues from other sites.

3. Handle water and soil samples in the same manner as CSF and tissue specimens, respectively.

4. Control cultures are recommended for comparative purposes, although care should be exercised to prevent cross-contamination of patient cultures.

Examination of Plates

1. Using the low-power (10×) objective of a microscope, observe the plates daily for 7 days for amebae.

2. If you see amebae anywhere, circle that area with a wax pencil. With the fine spatula, cut a small piece of agar from the circled area, and place it face down on the surface of a fresh agar plate precoated with bacteria; incubate as described above. Both *N. fowleri* and *Acanthamoeba* spp. can easily be cultivated in this way and, with periodic transfers, maintained indefinitely. When the plate is examined under a microscope, the amebae will look like small blotches, and if they are observed carefully, their movement can be discerned. After 2 to 3 days of incubation, the amebae will start to encyst. If a plate is examined after 4 to 5 days of incubation, trophozoites as well as cysts will be visible. *B. mandrillaris*, however, will not grow on agar plates seeded with bacteria. While *B. mandrillaris* can be grown on monkey kidney or lung fibroblast cell lines (39, 40), such techniques are not routinely available.

Identification and Culture

Identification of living organisms to the generic level is based on characteristic patterns of locomotion, morphologic features of the trophic and cyst forms, and enflagellation experiments. Immunofluorescence or immunoperoxidase tests using monoclonal or polyclonal antibodies (available at the Centers for Disease Control and Prevention) will be helpful in differentiating *Acanthamoeba* spp. from *B. mandrillaris* in the fixed tissue and in identifying the species, especially *Acanthamoeba* spp., in fixed tissue (38).

Enflagellation Experiment

1. Mix a drop of the sedimented CSF containing amebae with about 1 ml of sterile distilled water in a sterile tube, or, with a bacteriologic loop, scrape the surface of a plate that is positive for amebae, transferring a loopful of scraping to a sterile tube that contains approximately 1 ml of distilled water.

2. Gently shake the tube, and transfer a drop of this suspension to the center of a coverslip, whose edges have been coated thinly with petroleum jelly. Place a microscope slide over the coverslip and invert the slide. Seal the edges of the coverslip with Vaspar. Place the slide in a moist chamber, and incubate as before for 2 to 3 h. In addition, incubate the tube as described above.

3. Periodically examine the tube and the slide preparation microscopically for free-swimming flagellates. *N. fowleri* has a flagellated stage; *Acanthamoeba* spp. do not. If the sample contains *N. fowleri*, about 30 to 50% of the amebae will have undergone transformation into pear-shaped biflagellated organisms (Fig. 7).

Other Culture Methods

Axenic Culture

Acanthamoeba spp. can easily be cultivated axenically, without the addition of serum or host tissue, in many different types of nutrient media, e.g., Proteose Peptone-yeast extract-glucose medium, Trypticase soy broth medium, or chemically defined medium (12). *N. fowleri*, however, requires fetal calf serum or brain extract in the medium, e.g., Nelson's medium. A chemically defined medium has only recently been developed for *N. fowleri* (26). *B. mandrillaris* cannot be cultivated on agar plates with bacteria. It can, however, be cultivated on mammalian cell lines (39, 40) or a complex axenic medium (31).

Axenic cultures of *Acanthamoeba* spp. and *N. fowleri* can be established as follows. Actively growing 24- to 36-h-old amebae are scraped from the surface of the plate, suspended in 50 ml of ameba saline, and centrifuged at 500 × *g* for 5 min. The supernatant is aspirated, and the sediment is inoculated into Proteose Peptone-yeast extract-glucose medium or Nelson's medium, depending on the ameba isolate, and incubated at 37°C. Gentamicin, to a final concentration of 50 μg/ml, is added aseptically to the medium before the amebae are inoculated. Three subcultures into the antibiotic-containing medium at weekly intervals are usually sufficient to eliminate the associated bacteria (*E. coli* or *Enterobacter aerogenes*).

Cell Culture

Acanthamoeba spp., *B. mandrillaris*, and *N. fowleri* can also be inoculated onto many types of mammalian cell cultures. The amebae grow vigorously in these cell cultures and produce cytopathic effects somewhat similar to those caused by viruses (12, 18, 21, 41). Because of such cytopathic effects, *Acanthamoeba* was mistaken for transformed cell types presumed to contain viruses and were erroneously termed lipovirus and Ryan virus (17, 41).

Animal Inoculation

Two-week-old Swiss Webster mice weighing 12 to 15 g each can be infected with these amebae. Mice are anesthetized with ether, and a drop of ameba suspension is instilled into their nostrils. Mice infected with *N. fowleri* die within 5 to 7 days after developing characteristic signs such as ruffled fur, aimless wandering, partial paralysis, and finally coma and death. Mice infected with *Acanthamoeba* spp. and *B. mandrillaris* may die of acute disease within 5 to 7 days or die of chronic disease after several weeks. In all cases, amebae can be demonstrated in the mouse brain by either culture or histologic examination.

Antigenic and Molecular Characteristics

Pathogenic *N. fowleri* is morphologically indistinguishable from nonpathogenic *Naegleria* spp. at the trophic stage. Differences between these amebae, however, have been demonstrated antigenically by the gel diffusion, immunoelectrophoretic, and indirect immunofluorescence techniques (12, 16, 41). Antigenic differences have also been shown among various species of *Acanthamoeba* (12, 17, 24). Some recent studies indicate that *N. fowleri* can be distinguished from other species of *Naegleria* on the basis of isoenzyme patterns as well as restriction fragment length polymorphisms of genomic DNA (12, 17, 23). Analyses of isoenzyme pattern, mitochondrial DNA, and small-subunit RNA have also been carried out on various *Acanthamoeba* species and isolates in order to understand inter- and intraspecific diversity and phylogenetic relationships (12, 23). Further, genetic markers to distinguish pathogenic from the nonpathogenic *Acanthamoeba* spp. have also been developed (11).

Serology

Serologic techniques discussed here have been developed as research tools and are not routinely available to clinical laboratories. Complement fixation antibody to *Acanthamoeba* spp. has been shown in the serum of patients suffering from upper respiratory tract distress and in those with optic neuritis and macular disease (12, 17, 41). Kenney (17) demonstrated increasing complement fixation antibody titers to *Acanthamoeba* in three successive samples of serum collected over a 2-month period from each of two patients. Precipitin antibody has also been shown in the serum of a patient suffering from *A. polyphaga* keratitis (13, 17, 41). Recently, an increase in ameba immobilization antibody titer over a 16-month period was demonstrated in the serum of a Nigerian patient, who made a partial recovery from an *A. rhysodes*-induced CNS disease (17).

An antibody response to *N. fowleri*, however, has not yet been defined. Most of the patients with *Naegleria* PAM have died within a very short time (5 to 10 days), before they had time to produce detectable levels of antibody. In one case, however, in which the patient survived PAM caused by *N. fowleri*, an indirect immunofluorescence titer of 1:4,096 against *N. fowleri* was detected in the serum after 42 days of hospitalization (17, 32).

TREATMENT

Pathogenic *N. fowleri* is exquisitely susceptible to amphotericin B in vitro (3, 12, 17, 32). At least several patients with PAM were reported to have recovered after receiving intrathecal and intravenous injections of this drug alone or in combination with miconazole, or amphotericin B treatment in a hyperbaric chamber (12, 17, 21, 32). No patient with either *Acanthamoeba* spp. or *B. mandrillaris* infection of the CNS has survived this GAE so far in spite of treatment with several drug combinations, although Culbertson found sulfadiazine to be active against experimental *Acanthamoeba* infections in mice (12, 17, 21). Jones et al. (13) found that paromomycin, clotrimazole, and hydroxystilbamidine isethionate were active against *A. polyphaga* in vitro. Several patients with *Acanthamoeba* keratitis have been successfully treated with different drug combinations medicated over a long period. For example, in one study, treatment with 0.1% propamidine isethionate (Brolene) eye drops and 0.15% dibromopropamidine ointment together with topical neomycin sulfate was successful in the management of *Acanthamoeba* keratitis (43). In another study, 1% clotrimazole used in combination with Brolene and neosporin on four patients gave excellent results (6). Medical cure has also been achieved with topical administration of polyhexamethylene biguanide (15) or topical application of hexamidine isethionate, an analog of pentamidine (2). A recent study carried out on 111 cases of *Acanthamoeba* keratitis indicates that treatment with a combination of 0.02% polyhexamethylene biguanide and 0.1% Brolene hourly for 3 days and subsequently to six times a day had a good prognosis (7), and it may prove to be the treatment of choice. Prognosis of patients without CNS infection but with disseminated cutaneous ulcers due to *Acanthamoeba* spp. is good. For example, a patient with Down's syndrome and an immunoglobulin II A deficiency who also had undergone cadaveric renal transplantation developed a biopsy-confirmed *Acanthamoeba* skin ulcer. The patient was successfully cured of the infection after prolonged (more than 8 months) therapy with a regimen that included topical as well as systemic administration of a combination of drugs. His skin ulcers were cleansed twice daily with chlorhexidine gluconate solution followed by the topical application of 2% ketoconazole cream. He also received pentamidine isethionate intravenously for 1 month and thereafter was placed on oral itraconazole therapy for 8 months, resulting in complete healing of the cutaneous ulcers (35). Recent in vitro studies indicate that *B. mandrillaris* is susceptible to pentamidine isethocyanate and that patients with *B. mandrillaris* infection may benefit by treatment with this drug (31).

REFERENCES

1. **Anzil, A. P., C. Rao, M. A. Wrozlek, G. S. Visvesvara, J. H. Sher, and P. B. Kozlowski.** 1991. Amebic meningoencephalitis in a patient with AIDS caused by a newly recognized opportunistic pathogen: leptomyxid ameba. *Arch. Pathol. Lab. Med.* **115:**21–25.
2. **Brasseur, G., L. Favennec, D. Perrine, J. P. Chenu, and P. Brasseur.** 1994. Successful treatment of Acanthamoeba keratitis by hexamidine. *Cornea* **13:**459–462.
3. **Carter, R. F.** 1972. Primary amoebic meningo-encephalitis. An appraisal of present knowledge. *Trans. R. Soc. Trop. Med. Hyg.* **66:**193–208.
4. **Culbertson, C. G., J. W. Smith, and J. R. Minner.** 1958. *Acanthamoeba*: observations on animal pathogenicity. *Science* **127:**1506.
5. **DeJonckheere, J. F.** 1987. Epidemiology, p. 127–147. *In* E. G. Rondanelli (ed.), *Amphizoic Amoebae Human Pathology*, Piccin Nuova Libraria, Padua, Italy.
6. **Driebe, W. T., G. A. Stern, R. J. Epstein, G. S. Visvesvara, M. Adi, and T. Komadina.** 1988. *Acanthamoeba* keratitis: potential role for topical clotrimazole in combination chemotherapy. *Arch. Ophthalmol.* **106:**1196–1201.
7. **Duguid, I. G. M., J. K. G. Dart, N. Morlet, B. D. S. Allan, M. Matheson, L. Ficker, and S. Tuft.** 1997. Outcome of Acanthamoeba keratitis treated with polyhexamethyl biguanide and propamidine. *Ophthalmology* **104:**1587–1592.
8. **Friedland, L. R., S. A. Raphael, E. S. Deutsch, J. Johal, L. J. Martyn, G. S. Visvesvara, and H. Lischner.** 1992. Disseminated *Acanthamoeba* infection in a child with symp-

tomatic human immunodeficiency virus infection. *Pediatr. Infect. Dis. J.* **11:**404–407.

9. **Gonzalez, M. M., E. Gould, G. Dickinson, A. J. Martinez, G. S. Visvesvara, T. J. Cleary, and G. T. Hensley.** 1986. Acquired immunodeficiency syndrome associated with *Acanthamoeba* infection and other opportunistic organisms. *Arch. Pathol. Lab. Med.* **110:**749–751.
10. **Gordon, S. M., J. P. Steinberg, M. DuPuis, P. Kozarsky, J. F. Nickerson, and G. S. Visvesvara.** 1992. Culture isolation of *Acanthamoeba* species and leptomyxid amebas from patients with amebic meningoencephalitis, including two patients with AIDS. *Clin. Infect. Dis.* **15:**1024–1030.
11. **Howe, D. K., M. H. Vodkin, R. J. Novak, G. S. Visvesvara, and G. L. McLaughlin.** 1997. Identification of two genetic markers that distinguish pathogenic and nonpathogenic strains of *Acanthamoeba* spp. *Parasitol. Res.* **83:** 345–348.
12. **John, D. T.** 1993. Opportunistically pathogenic free-living amebae, p. 143–246. *In* J. P. Kreier and J. R. Baker (ed.), *Parasitic Protozoa*, vol. 3. Academic Press, Inc., New York.
13. **Jones, D. B., G. S. Visvesvara, and N. M. Robinson.** 1975. *Acanthamoeba polyphaga* keratitis and *Acanthamoeba* uveitis associated with fatal meningoencephalitis. *Trans. Ophthalmol. Soc. U.K.* **95:**221–232.
14. **Kramer, M. H., C. J. Lerner, and G. S. Visvesvara.** 1997. Kidney and liver transplants from a donor infected with *Naegleria fowleri*. *J. Clin. Microbiol.* **35:**1032–1033.
15. **Larkin, D. F. P., S. Kilvington, and J. K. G. Dart.** 1992. Treatment of *Acanthamoeba* keratitis with polyhexamethylene biguanide. *Ophthalmology* **99:**185–191.
16. **Lozano-Alarcon, F., G. A. Bradley, B. S. Houser, and G. S. Visvesvara.** 1997. Primary amebic meningoencephalitis due to *Naeglearia fowleri* in a South American tapir. *Vet. Pathol.* **34:**239–243.
17. **Ma, P., G. S. Visvesvara, A. J. Martinez, F. H. Theodore, P.-M. Daggett, and T. K. Sawyer.** 1990. Naegleria and Acanthamoeba infections: review. *Rev. Infect. Dis.* **12:** 490–513.
18. **Marciano-Cabral, F., K. L. Zoghby, and S. G. Bradley.** 1990. Cytopathic action of *Naegleria fowleri* amoebae on rat neuroblastoma target cells. *J. Protozool.* **37:**138–144.
19. **Martinez, A. J.** 1982. Acanthamoebiasis and immunosuppression. Case report. *J. Neuropathol. Exp. Neurol.* **41:** 548–557.
20. **Martinez, A. J.** 1985. *Free-Living Amebas: Natural History, Prevention, Diagnosis, Pathology, and Treatment of the Disease*. CRC Press, Inc., Boca Raton, Fla.
21. **Martinez, A. J., and G. S. Visvesvara.** 1997. Free-living, amphizoic and opportunistic amebas. *Brain Pathol.* **7:** 583–589.
22. **Martinez, A. J., G. S. Visvesvara, and F. W. Chandler.** 1997. Free-living amebic infections, p. 1163–1176. *In* D. H. Connor, F. C. Chandler, D. A. Schwartz, H. G. Manz, and E. E. Lack (ed.), *Pathology of Infectious Diseases*, Appleton & Lange, New York.
23. **McLaughlin, G. L., F. H. Brandt, and G. S. Visvesvara.** 1988. Restriction fragment length polymorphisms of the DNA of selected *Naegleria* and *Acanthamoeba* amoebae. *J. Clin. Microbiol.* **26:**1655–1658.
24. **Moura, H., S. Wallace, and G. S. Visvesvara.** 1992. *Acanthamoeba healyi* n. sp. and the isoenzyme and immunoblot profiles of *Acanthamoeba* spp., groups 1 and 3. *J. Protozool.* **39:**573–583.
25. **Murakawa, G. J., T. McCalmont, J. Altman, G. H. Telang, M. D. Hoffman, G. R. Kantor, and T. G. Berger.** 1995. Disseminated acanthamoebiasis in patients with AIDS. A report of five cases and a review of the literature. *Arch. Dermatol.* **131:**1291–1296.
26. **Nerad, T. A., G. S. Visvesvara, and P.-M. Daggett.** 1983. Chemically defined media for the cultivation of *Naegleria*: pathogenic and high temperature tolerant species. *J. Protozool.* **30:**383–387.
27. **Page, F. C.** 1985. *A New Key to Fresh Water and Soil Gymnamoebae*. Fresh Water Biological Association, Cumbria, England.
28. **Pfister, D. R., J. D. Cameron, J. H. Krachmer, and E. J. Holland.** 1996. Confocal microscopy findings of Acanthamoeba keratitis. *Am. J. Ophthalmol.* **121:**119–128.
29. **Rideout, B. A., C. H. Gardiner, I. H. Stalis, J. R. Zuba, T. Hadfield, and G. S. Visvesvara.** 1997. Fatal infections with *Balamuthia mandrillaris* (a free-living amoeba) in gorillas and other old world primates. *Vet. Pathol.* **34:**15–22.
30. **Sawyer, T. K., G. S. Visvesvara, and B. A. Harke.** 1976. Pathogenic amebas from brackish and ocean sediments with a description of *Acanthamoeba hatchetti*, n. sp. *Science* **196:**1324–1325.
31. **Schuster, F. L., and G. S. Visvesvara.** 1996. Axenic growth and drug sensitivity studies of *Balamuthia mandrillaris*, an agent of amebic meningoencephalitis in humans and other animals. *J. Clin. Microbiol.* **34:**385–388.
32. **Seidel, J. S., P. Harmatz, G. S. Visvesvara, A. Cohen, J. Edwards, and J. Turner.** 1982. Successful treatment of primary amebic meningoencephalitis. *N. Engl. J. Med.* **306:**346–348.
33. **Singh, B. N.** 1975. *Pathogenic and Non-Pathogenic Amebae*. John Wiley & Sons, Inc., New York, N.Y.
34. **Sison, J. P., C. A. Kemper, M. Loveless, D. McShane, G. S. Visvesvara, and S. C. Deresinski.** 1995. Disseminated Acanthamoeba infection in patients with AIDS: case reports and review. *Clin. Infect. Dis.* **20:**1207–1216.
35. **Slater, C. A., J. Z. Sickel, G. S. Visvesvara, R. C. Pabico, and A. A. Gaspari.** 1994. Successful treatment of disseminated Acanthamoeba infection in an immunocompromised patient. *N. Engl. J. Med.* **331:**85–87.
36. **Stehr-Green, J. K., T. M. Bailey, F. H. Brandt, J. H. Carr, W. W. Bond, and G. S. Visvesvara.** 1987. *Acanthamoeba* keratitis in soft contact lens wearers: a case-control study. *JAMA* **258:**57–60.
37. **Stehr-Green, J. K., T. M. Bailey, and G. S. Visvesvara.** 1990. The epidemiology of *Acanthamoeba* keratitis in the United States. *Am. J. Ophthalmol.* **107:**331–336.
38. **Visvesvara, G. S.** 1985. Laboratory diagnosis, p. 193–215. *In* E. G. Rondanelli (ed.), *Amphizoic Amoebae: Human Pathology*. Piccin Nuova Libraria, Padua, Italy.
39. **Visvesvara, G. S., A. J. Martinez, F. L. Schuster, G. J. Leitch, S. Wallace, T. K. Sawyer, and M. Anderson.** 1990. Leptomyxid ameba, a new agent of amebic meningoencephalitis in humans and animals. *J. Clin. Microbiol.* **28:** 2750–2756.
40. **Visvesvara, G. S., F. L. Schuster, and A. J. Martinez.** 1993. *Balamuthia mandrillaris*, new genus, new species, agent of amebic meningoencephalitis in humans and animals. *J. Eukaryot. Microbiol.* **40:**504–514.
41. **Visvesvara, G. S., and J. K. Stehr-Green.** 1990. Epidemiology of free-living ameba infections. *J. Protozool.* **37:** 25S–33S.
42. **Wiley, C. A., R. E. Safrin, C. E. Davis, P. W. Lampert, A. I. Braude, A. J. Martinez, and G. S. Visvesvara.** 1987. *Acanthamoeba* meningoencephalitis in a patient with AIDS. *J. Infect. Dis.* **155:**130–133.
43. **Wright, P., D. Warhurst, and B. R. Jones.** 1985. Acanthamoeba keratitis successfully treated medically. *Br. J. Ophthalmol.* **69:**778–782.

Intestinal and Urogenital Amebae, Flagellates, and Ciliates*

AMY L. LEBER AND SUSAN M. NOVAK

109

With the application of molecular biology-based techniques to the field of parasitology, new information has come to light in the past 10 years concerning the intestinal and urogenital protozoa. One of the most important findings is the evidence that the ameba morphologically identified as *Entamoeba histolytica* is actually two separate and distinct species. *E. histolytica* is the pathogenic species and is considered the etiologic agent of amebic colitis and extraintestinal amebiasis. *Entamoeba dispar* is the nonpathogenic species and does not invade tissue or cause intestinal symptoms. The existence of both pathogenic and nonpathogenic species helps to explain the disparity between the number of infected individuals and the relatively low prevalence of disease seen. Molecular analysis has also revealed a great deal of genetic diversity among *Blastocystis hominis* strains. Similar to *E. histolytica*, there may be individual species or strains of *B. hominis* that are pathogenic and others that are not; this might explain the conflicting data concerning the pathogenicity of *B. hominis*.

As more molecular biology-based research is performed, the classification scheme for these and other parasites will undoubtedly change. Some of these changes will affect laboratory diagnosis and clinical treatment, while others may be more academic in nature.

Many of the protozoa described in this chapter are nonpathogenic organisms that produce no evidence of disease. Nevertheless, these organisms need to be differentiated from true pathogens in clinical specimens, because they are indicators of exposure to fecal contamination and examination of additional specimens may reveal pathogenic protozoa. Although pathogenic and nonpathogenic organisms are categorized as indicated in Table 1, reports of disease in patients infected with nonpathogenic species are found in the literature.

Common symptoms produced by pathogenic intestinal protozoa, such as diarrhea, cramping, and abdominal pain, are usually neither specific nor diagnostic. The differential clinical diagnosis includes infectious (bacteria, viruses, parasites) and noninfectious (inflammatory bowel diseases) entities. In addition, symptomatology can vary depending on the strain of the isolate and the immune status of the individual. In areas where certain protozoa are endemic, infections are often less severe due to the partial protective immunity developed from previous exposure to the pathogen. Pathogenic protozoa can be found in clinical specimens from persons with no evidence of disease. These asymptomatic individuals are an important reservoir for infection.

Giardia lamblia and *E. histolytica* are two of the most common protozoal infections seen worldwide and are serious concerns on a global scale due to their prevalence and pathogenicity. Because of the increased pathogenicity of these organisms in certain groups (i.e., immunocompromised and malnourished individuals and children), a more accurate diagnosis is crucial for the appropriate clinical management of infected individuals. In addition, *Trichomonas vaginalis*, the third most common cause of vaginitis affecting women, has been linked to serious obstetric and gynecologic conditions. Fortunately, antiprotozoal drugs remain quite effective, in contrast to other parasitic and antibacterial drugs, resistance to which is of great concern. Recurrent protozoal infections more often represent reinfection rather than treatment failure.

Microscopic examination of stool specimens remains the cornerstone of the laboratory diagnosis of intestinal amebic, flagellate, and ciliate infections. The goal of microscopy is to identify pathogenic protozoa, differentiate between these and nonpathogenic species, and properly discriminate various artifacts that may be present. Commercial assays for the detection of parasite antigens, such as enzyme immunoassays (EIAs) and direct fluorescent-antibody (DFA) assays, have been developed for the detection of pathogens such as *E. histolytica* and *G. lamblia*. Culture may be useful under certain limited situations. Nucleic acid-based techniques have been developed but are not yet widely available. All of these methods may not be needed in every instance. See the sections below and refer to chapters 12, 13, and 104 for additional information.

SPECIMEN COLLECTION AND HANDLING

Proper collection and handling of specimens are important factors that affect the accurate and reliable identification of intestinal and urogenital parasites. Details of collection and handling of specimens are covered in chapters 4 and 5 of this Manual. It is recommended that three stool specimens be collected 2 to 3 days apart to increase sensitivity of detection. For optimal recovery, diarrheic stool specimens

* This chapter contains information presented in chapter 106 by George R. Healy and Lynne S. Garcia in the sixth edition of this Manual.

TABLE 1 Intestinal and urogenital amebae, flagellates, and ciliates of humans

Parasite	Pathogenic	Nonpathogenic
Amebae	*Entamoeba histolytica*[a] *Blastocystis hominis*	*Entamoeba dispar* *Entamoeba hartmanni* *Entamoeba coli* *Entamoeba polecki* *Entamoeba gingivalis*[b] *Endolimax nana* *Iodamoeba bütschlii*
Flagellates	*Giardia lamblia* *Trichomonas vaginalis* *Dientamoeba fragilis*	*Chilomastix mesnili* *Trichomonas hominis* *Trichomonas tenax*[b] *Enteromonas hominis* *Retortamonas intestinalis*
Ciliates	*Balantidium coli*	

[a] A distinction between *E. histolytica* and *E. dispar* cannot be made on the basis of morphology unless ingested RBCs are seen in the cytoplasm of the trophozoite.

[b] *E. gingivalis* and *T. tenax* are found in the oral cavity and related specimens.

should be examined within 1 h of passage (not 1 h after reaching the laboratory) or should be preserved immediately. The gains in organism recovery and proper preservation of morphology seen with preserved specimens outweigh the ability to see motility in fresh specimens, which occurs infrequently. In a study by Garcia and coworkers (20), 13,194 outpatient samples preserved in polyvinyl alcohol and formalin were examined by trichrome-stained smear and wet mount (formalin-ether concentration method). They found that 23% (3,077 specimens) were positive for one or more intestinal protozoa. Of the pathogenic protozoa detected (*E. histolytica*, *G. lamblia*, and *Dientamoeba fragilis*), 96% of the trophozoites and 39% of the cysts were identified only by the trichrome-stained smear. That study clearly supports the primary importance of preservation and the use of permanent stained smears for the identification of pathogenic protozoa in feces.

Materials such as aspirates, tissues, urine, or other body fluids should be sent to the laboratory immediately. If transport is delayed, specimens should be properly preserved to maintain the diagnostic characteristics of the organisms that may be present. If additional tests, such as EIA, DFA assay, or nucleic acid-based techniques, are to be performed, one must consider the compatibility of sample preservatives with the test method to be used.

AMEBAE

The amebae that parasitize the intestinal tracts of humans belong to four genera: *Entamoeba*, *Endolimax*, *Iodamoeba*, and *Blastocystis*. They all belong to the phylum Sarcomastigophora, subphylum Sarcodina, which contains organisms that move by means of cytoplasmic protrusions called pseudopodia (15, 33). It is noteworthy that *D. fragilis*, once classified as an ameba, is now grouped with the flagellates. Even though this reclassification has occurred, it is still identified on the basis of morphologic comparison to amebae. Of the seven species of intestinal amebae, *E. dispar*, *Entamoeba hartmanni*, *Entamoeba coli*, *Endolimax nana*, and *Iodamoeba bütschlii* are nonpathogenic for humans. *E. histolytica* is pathogenic for humans, causing invasive intestinal and extraintestinal amebiasis. The pathogenicity of *B. hominis* is still controversial.

All amebae have a common and relatively simple life cycle (21, 42). The cyst is the infectious form that is acquired by ingestion of contaminated material such as water and food or by direct fecal-oral transmission. Once in the intestinal tract, excystation occurs, releasing trophozoites. Encystment occurs in the colon, presumably when conditions become unfavorable for the trophozoites. Cysts are passed in the environment and remain viable for days to weeks in water and soil if protected from desiccation.

Feces is the specimen most often examined to determine infection. Methods include microscopy, antigen detection, culture, and nucleic acid-based techniques. The diagnostic stages of the amebae are the trophozoite and cyst, and either or both of these stages can be detected in fecal specimens. The key morphologic features of amebae must be used to help differentiate among the different species and to distinguish between somatic cells and other material. Trophozoites must be distinguished from epithelial cells and macrophages. Cysts must be distinguished from polymorphonuclear cells (PMNs). Also, yeast, pollen, molds, food particles and other debris present in feces may cause confusion (Table 2; Fig. 1 and 2).

Morphologic examination of fecal specimens can be accomplished with fresh wet mounts, wet mounts of concentrated material, and permanent stained smears. Each of these three types of preparations may be useful for visualizing certain key characteristics; however, morphologic examination with permanent stained smears is the most useful procedure (3).

Trophozoite motility is visible only in saline wet mounts of fresh feces and is often difficult to detect. If only preserved specimens are received in the laboratory, direct wet mounts are not prepared. The arrangement, size, and pattern of nuclear chromatin help differentiate species within the genus *Entamoeba* from other intestinal amebae. The size and position of the nuclear karyosome are also important morphologic features. A ring of nuclear chromatin surrounding the karyosome resembling a bull's eye is characteristic of *Entamoeba*. *Endolimax*, *Iodamoeba*, and the flagellate *Dientamoeba* lack peripheral chromatin. The cytoplasm of the trophozoites may contain granules and ingested material such as erythrocytes (RBCs), bacteria, yeasts, and molds.

The characteristics of cysts are less variable than those of trophozoites. As mentioned above, it is important to note nuclear features, including the number and position of nuclei, the presence or absence of nuclear chromatin, and the position and size of the karyosome. The cytoplasm should be examined for the presence of chromatoidal bodies and vacuoles, particularly the large glycogen vacuole seen in *I. bütschlii*.

The key characteristics for each group of organisms may not be observed in a single type of preparation. Fresh wet mounts may reveal the motility of trophozoites and the presence of cysts. Stained and unstained wet mounts of concentrated material can also be useful for identification, particularly for certain cysts such as *E. coli* and *I. bütschlii*. Iodine will provide color and contrast, both of which may aid in the identification of organisms in wet preparations. The permanent stained smear allows identification of most of the key characteristics of amebic trophozoites and cysts; examination of the stained smear by oil immersion microscopy (magnification, ×1,000) is strongly recommended for definitive identification.

TABLE 2 Key features of trophozoites and cysts of common intestinal amebae[a]

Organism	Trophozoites	Cysts
E. histolytica/E. dispar	Size[b]: 12–60 μm; invasive forms, >20 μm Motility: Progressive, directional, rapid Nucleus[c]: 1; peripheral chromatin evenly distributed; karyosome small, compact, centrally located; may resemble *E. coli* Cytoplasm: Finely granular, like "ground glass"; may contain bacteria Note: RBCs in cytoplasm diagnostic for *E. histolytica*	Size: 10–20 μm, spherical Nucleus: Mature cyst, 4; immature cyst, 1 or 2; peripheral chromatin fine, uniform granules, evenly distributed; karyosome small, compact, centrally located Cytoplasm: Chromatoidal bodies may be present; elongate with blunt rounded edges; may be round or oval
E. hartmanni	Size: 5–12 μm Motility: Nonprogressive Nucleus: 1; peripheral chromatin like *E. histolytica*, may appear as solid ring; karyosome small, compact, centrally located or eccentric Cytoplasm: Finely granular, bacteria, no RBCs Note: Accurate measurement essential for differentiation from *E. histolytica*	Size: 5–10 μm; spherical Nucleus: Mature cyst, 4; immature cyst, 1 or 2 (very common); peripheral chromatin fine, evenly distributed, may be difficult to see; karyosome small, compact, centrally located Cytoplasm: Chromatoidal bodies usually present, like *E. histolytica*
E. coli	Size: 15–50 μm Motility: Sluggish, nondirectional Nucleus: 1; peripheral chromatin clumped and uneven, may be solid ring; karyosome large, not compact, diffuse, eccentric Cytoplasm: Granular, usually vacuolated; contains bacteria, yeast, no RBCs Note: Can resemble *E. histolytica*; coinfection seen; stained smear essential	Size: 10–35 μm, spherical, rarely oval or triangular Nucleus: Mature cyst, 8; occasionally ≥16; immature cyst ≥2; peripheral chromatin coarsely granular, unevenly arranged; may resemble *E. histolytica*; karyosome small, usually eccentric but may be central Cytoplasm: Chromatoidal bodies less frequent than *E. histolytica*; splintered, with rough, pointed ends Note: May be distorted on permanent stained smear due to poor penetration of fixative
E. nana	Size: 6–12 μm Motility: Sluggish, nonprogressive Nucleus: 1; no peripheral chromatin; karyosome large, "blot like" Cytoplasm: Granular, vacuolated; may contain bacteria Note: May be tremendous nuclear variation; can mimic *E. hartmanni* and *D. fragilis*	Size: 5–10 μm; oval, may be round Nucleus: Mature cyst, 4; immature cyst, 2; no peripheral chromatin; karyosome smaller than in trophozoites but larger than *Entamoeba* spp. Cytoplasm: Chromatoidal bodies rare; small granules occasionally seen
I. bütschlii	Size: 8–20 μm Motility: Sluggish, nonprogressive Nucleus: 1; no peripheral chromatin, karyosome large, may have "basket nucleus" Cytoplasm: Coarsely granular, may be highly vacuolated; bacteria, yeast, and debris may be seen Note: Stained smear essential; nucleus may appear to have a halo with chromatin granules fanning around karyosome	Size: 5–20 μm; oval to round Nucleus: Mature cyst, 1; no peripheral chromatin; karyosome large, usually eccentric Cytoplasm: No chromatoidal bodies; small granules occasionally present Note: Glycogen present, large, compact, well-defined mass; cysts may collapse owing to large glycogen vacuole space
B. hominis[d]	Very difficult to identify; rarely seen	Size: 6–40 μm; generally round Description: Usually characterized by a large, central body (looks like a large vacuole) surrounded by small, multiple nuclei; central body area can stain various colors (trichrome) or remain clear

[a] Adapted from reference 21.
[b] Size ranges based on wet preparations (with permanent stains organisms usually measure 1 to 2 μm less).
[c] Nuclear and cytoplasmic descriptions based on permanent stained smears.
[d] Description of central body form.

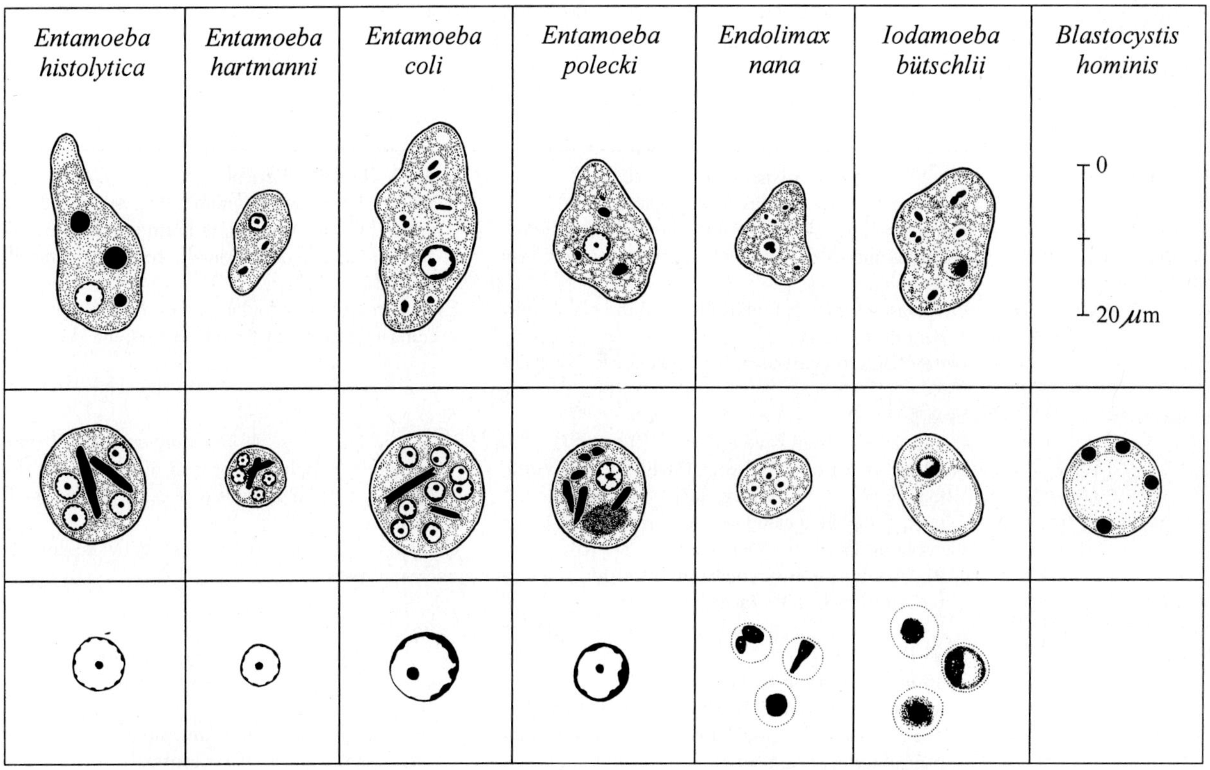

FIGURE 1 Intestinal amebae of humans. (Top row) Trophozoites. *E. histolytica* is shown with ingested RBCs. This is the only microscopic finding allowing differentiation of the pathogenic species *E. histolytica* from the nonpathogenic species *E. dispar*. An ameboid form of *B. hominis* is rarely seen and is difficult to identify. (Middle row) Cysts. For *B. hominis* the central body form is depicted. (Bottom row) Trophozoite nuclei, shown in relative proportion.

Nuclear and cytoplasmic features can vary within species and may overlap between species, making identification challenging. Also on permanent stained smears, shrinkage may occur, affecting the apparent size of the organism. Size is reliable only for the differentiation of *E. histolytica*/*E. dispar* from *E. hartmanni*.

It is important to remember that identification may not be possible on the basis of one morphologic feature or the characteristics of a single organism in the preparation. Mixed infections are not uncommon and can be missed in a cursory examination. A complete, overall assessment of the slide is necessary for accurate identification.

E. histolytica

E. histolytica can be found worldwide but is more prevalent in tropical and subtropical regions. In areas where the organism is endemic, up to 50% of people may be infected. In temperate climates with poor sanitation, infection rates can approach those seen in tropical regions. Humans are the primary reservoir; infection occurs by ingestion of cysts from fecally contaminated material such as water and food. Sexual transmission has also been documented.

Groups with a higher incidence of amebiasis include immigrants from South and Central America and Southeast Asia. Also, residents of the southern United States and institutionalized individuals are more likely to be infected. In one study, short-term travelers to areas where *E. histolytica* and *E. dispar* are endemic were found to be at higher risk of infection with the pathogenic species, *E. histolytica*, than residents who were more likely to harbor the nonpathogenic species, *E. dispar* (58). In homosexual males, the infection is often transmitted by sexual behavior, and in certain studies, up to 30% were found to be infected. While this infection is most often asymptomatic, it is one of the causes of the symptomatic disease known as "gay bowel syndrome."

Clinical Significance

Of the estimated 500 million people infected each year with *E. histolytica*, only 36 million develop symptoms, and of these, approximately 40,000 die. The discrepancy between the numbers of people infected with *E. histolytica* and the amount of morbidity and mortality was somewhat perplexing and led to different explanations. Some researchers suggested that two morphologically similar yet distinct species existed: one capable of producing disease and the other not. Others postulated that *E. histolytica* was one species and that the differences in pathogenicity were caused by host and environmental conditions.

With the development of axenic culture methods, some answers concerning these conflicting theories emerged. Using isoenzyme analysis of several glycolytic enzymes, Sargeaunt and Williams (50) identified electrophoretic banding patterns called zymodemes. A zymodeme is defined as a population of amebae in which the electrophoretic mobilities of specific enzymes differ from those in similar populations. Two groups were identified on the basis of these patterns: pathogenic zymodemes (invasive isolates) and nonpathogenic zymodemes (noninvasive isolates). The zymodeme patterns represent stable genetic differences and do not interconvert (44). Additional genetic, biochemical, and immunologic evidence has supported the existence of two distinct species. Diamond and Clark (17) recently redescribed the two species as *E. histolytica* (Schaudinn 1903), which is the invasive human pathogen, and *E. dispar* (Brumpt 1925), which is noninvasive and which does not cause disease.

Infection with *E. histolytica/E. dispar* can result in different clinical presentations: asymptomatic infection, symptomatic infection without tissue invasion, and symptomatic infection with tissue invasion. The majority of infections with *E. histolytica/E. dispar* are asymptomatic. Such individuals will have a negative or weak serologic response and will primarily pass cysts in their stools. On the basis of zymodeme analysis, most asymptomatic individuals are infected with the noninvasive species *E. dispar* (60). However, it appears that infection with both *E. histolytica* and *E. dispar* can be asymptomatic, with cyst stages being passed in the stool (6).

Intestinal disease results from the penetration of the amebic trophozoites into the intestinal tissues. Approximately 10% of infected individuals will have clinical symptoms presenting as dysentery, colitis, or rarely, ameboma. The incubation period varies from a few days to up to several months. Symptoms of amebic dysentery include diarrhea with cramping, lower abdominal pain, low-grade fever, and the presence of blood and mucus in stool. The ulcers produced by intestinal invasion of trophozoites start as superficial localized lesions that deepen into the classic flask-shaped ulcers of amebic colitis. The ulcers are separated by segments of normal tissue but can coalesce. Amebae can be found at the advancing edges of the ulcer but usually not in the necrotic areas. Abdominal perforation and peritonitis are rare but serious complications. A more chronic presentation occurs with amebic colitis. It is characterized by intermittent diarrhea over a long period of time and can be misdiagnosed as ulcerative colitis or irritable bowel syndrome. Ameboma, a localized tumor-like lesion, results from chronic ulceration and may be mistaken for malignancy. Histologically, it consists of granulomatous tissue.

Extraintestinal disease occurs with the hematogenous spread of the organism. It can occur with or without previous symptomatic intestinal infection. The liver is the most common site of extraintestinal disease, followed by the lungs, pericardium, brain, and other organs. Symptoms can be acute or gradual and may include low-grade fever, right upper quadrant pain, and weight loss. Up to 5% of individuals with intestinal symptoms develop liver abscess. However, up to 50% of individuals with liver abscess have no previous history of gastrointestinal disease.

Laboratory Diagnosis

The laboratory diagnosis of amebiasis can be accomplished by examination of feces, material obtained from sigmoidoscopy, tissue biopsy specimens, and abscess aspirates. Serology is also useful for the diagnosis of extraintestinal amebiasis. For all types of specimens, the success of laboratory diagnosis depends on proper collection and processing, the methods used in the laboratory, and the level of training and experience of laboratory personnel. As discussed previously, the most important part of the standard examination is the permanent stained smear. Direct wet preparations and concentration procedures may also be useful (Fig. 1 and Table 2; see also chapter 104). The detection of trophozoites and cysts does not, however, allow differentiation of the pathogenic species *E. histolytica* from the nonpathogenic species *E. dispar*. The only exception is the finding of ingested RBCs in the cytoplasm of the trophozoites, which is diagnostic for pathogenic *E. histolytica*. In tissue specimens, only the trophozoite is found, and its presence is also diagnostic for invasive *E. histolytica*.

For the differentiation of *E. histolytica* and *E. dispar*, methods other than microscopy are necessary. Zymodeme analysis requires culture of the organisms from the specimen and is too expensive and complex for routine laboratory use. More recently, antigen detection methods for the detection and differentiation of *E. histolytica* and *E. dispar* have become commercially available (Tech Labs, Blacksburg, Va., and Alexon-Trend, Ramsey, Minn.). Depending on the kit used, the group *E. histolytica/E. dispar* or the individual species can be detected in the feces. These methods are relatively simple and have good sensitivities and specificities (43). Cost may be a prohibitive factor for their routine use in most laboratories. Molecular biology-based methods, such as PCR, have also been developed for the detection and differentiation of *E. histolytica* and *E. dispar*. These methods are not yet widely available but should aid greatly in the diagnosis of amebiasis. PCR has been applied to specimens such as feces and liver aspirates and can detect both trophozoite and cyst DNA (47). Different extraction techniques, some of which are relatively simple, and the use of fresh and preserved material have been reported (49, 57). For routine use in clinical laboratories, a PCR method would ideally involve a relatively simple sample preparation and allow the use of preserved material, the only specimen received by many laboratories.

Until all laboratories have the capability to discriminate between *E. histolytica* and *E. dispar*, the method of laboratory result must change. In January 1997, a combined panel of experts from the World Health Organization (WHO), Pan American Health Organization, and the United Nations Educational, Scientific and Cultural Organization met in Mexico City and made recommendations concerning the reporting and treatment of amebiasis. If microscopic diagnosis is made on the basis of the detection of trophozoites and/or cysts and no method is used to differentiate the two species, the report should indicate "*E. histolytica/E. dispar* detected." To educate and better assist physicians in making relevant clinical decisions, the recent changes in the classification and reporting of these organisms must be communicated.

Therapy

On the basis of the 1997 WHO conference, treatment is not recommended for *E. dispar* infections; if *E. histolytica/E. dispar* is detected (no differentiation of species) in symptomatic patients, the physician must evaluate the total clinical presentation to decide whether treatment is indicated. The detection of *E. histolytica* requires treatment of the patient regardless of the symptoms.

The drugs used for the treatment of amebiasis are of two classes: luminal amebicides, such as iodoquinol or diloxanide furoate, and tissue amebicides, such as metronidazole, chloroquine, or dehydroemetine. No resistance to amebicides has been detected to date. Laboratory reports must indicate whether trophozoites and/or cysts are present, due to differences in therapy.

B. hominis

B. hominis is a common intestinal parasite of humans with a worldwide distribution. Depending on the geographic location, it may be detected in 10 to 20% of fecal specimens. Since its first description in 1912, the taxonomic classification has changed and is still somewhat unclear. Once classified as a yeast, it is now considered a protozoan grouped with the amebae. More recently, Silberman and colleagues (54) reported that the analysis of rRNA indicates that *B. hominis* should be classified with the stramenopiles (examples are brown algae such as kelp, diatoms, slime nets, and water molds). Genetic, biochemical, and immunologic analyses have revealed that great diversity exists within the species (13, 24, 35). Further studies are needed to determine if these differences constitute separate species or strains and whether there is any epidemiological significance associated with this diversity.

The life cycle includes amebic forms, cyst stages, and the central body form, which is the classic form seen in human stool specimens. *B. hominis* produces pseudopods and reproduces by binary fission or sporulation. It is strictly anaerobic and is capable of ingesting bacteria and other debris. The membrane-bound central body occupies up to 90% of the cell and may function in reproduction. Both thin- and thick-walled cysts have been observed (55). The thick-walled cysts are responsible for external transmission via the fecal-oral route; the thin-walled cyst is thought to cause autoinfection (40).

Clinical Significance

The role of *B. hominis* in human disease is still controversial, and studies supporting and refuting its pathogenicity have been published (36, 53, 63). Regardless of the number of publications on each side of this debate, clinicians may decide to treat patients with *B. hominis* infection. When *B. hominis* is present in large numbers in the absence of other pathogens it may be the cause of gastrointestinal disease. The most common symptoms cited include recurrent diarrhea without fever, vomiting, and abdominal pain. The symptoms may be more pronounced and prolonged in patients with underlying conditions (22). Other studies suggest that symptomatic patients receiving treatment for *B. hominis* may improve due to elimination of another pathogen (36). In a study of human immunodeficiency virus (HIV)-infected individuals, Albrecht and co-workers (2) concluded that even in patients with severe underlying immunodeficiencies, *B. hominis* is not pathogenic and its detection does not justify treatment.

Laboratory Diagnosis

Diagnosis is made by detection of the organism, typically the central body form, by routine stool examinations (Table 2; Fig. 1). The size of the central body form can vary tremendously, from 6 to 40 μm. Examination of permanent stained smears is the procedure of choice. Exposure to water before fixation (for the concentration method) will lyse the trophozoites and central body forms, yielding false-negative results. Some type of quantitation (few, moderate, or many) should be included in the laboratory report. Serologic response to *B. hominis* has been detected using techniques such as EIA and fluorescent antibody (19, 64). It is suggested that this antibody response supports the role of *B. hominis* as a human pathogen but is not useful for diagnosis.

Therapy

In vitro data on the susceptibility of *B. hominis* to various drugs are limited (64). Metronidazole appears to be the most appropriate choice at present. Because this drug has activity against a number of other pathogens, it may be difficult to assess if successful treatment was due to the elimination of *B. hominis* or to the elimination of another organism. Until the role of *B. hominis* as an intestinal pathogen is clearly

FIGURE 2 Human protozoan trophozoites and cysts. (Unless noted otherwise, the protozoa in the figure were photographed as trichrome-stained smears under an oil immersion lens at a magnification of ×1,000). (A) *E. histolytica* trophozoite. Note the ingested RBCs within the cytoplasm and in the background. (B) *E. histolytica/E. dispar* trophozoite (Merthiolate-iodine-formalin; polychrome stain). Nuclear chromatin is evenly distributed; the karyosome is central. (C) *E. histolytica/E. dispar* precyst. The nucleus is enlarged, and chromatoidal bars are present. (D) *E. histolytica/E. dispar* cyst. Multiple nuclei and chromatoidal bars with smooth round edges are present; note the halo due to shrinkage. (E) *E. hartmanni* trophozoite. The nucleus is similar to that of *E. histolytica*; note the absence of RBCs. (F) *E. hartmanni* cyst. The mature cyst contains four nuclei; cysts are often seen with one (precyst) or two nuclei. Note the numerous chromatoidal bars with smooth rounded edges similar to *E. histolytica.* (G) *E. coli* trophozoite. The nuclear chromatin is uneven and the karyosome is eccentric. (H) *E. coli* cyst (iodine stain, wet mount). The presence of five or more nuclei allows an identification to be made. Cysts are usually seen more clearly in wet mounts; they may be shrunken or distorted in permanently stained smears (see panel I). (I) *E. coli* cyst. Note the typical shrinkage and pink color. (J) *E. coli* cyst. The presence of five or more nuclei on this permanently stained smear allows identification. (K) *E. nana* trophozoites. Note the large karyosome and the lack of peripheral chromatin. The trophozoite on the right shows "nuclear variation," in which the chromatin displays unusual shapes, which is more common for *E. nana* than for any other protozoan. (L) *E. nana* cysts. Note the typical oval shape and the presence of four karyosomes. (M) *I. bütschlii* trophozoites. Note the large karyosome, vacuolated cytoplasm, and size (compared to that of *E. nana*). (N) *I. bütschlii* cysts. Note the large glycogen vacuole and "basket nucleus." (O) *B. hominis*. The central body form of this protozoan is shown on the left in an iodine preparation and on the right in a permanent stained smear (photographed at a lower magnification on the right; organisms exhibit great variation in size). (P) *D. fragilis* trophozoites. Organisms may have one or two nuclei, with nuclear chromatin frequently fragmented. The organism has no known cyst stage. (Q) *G. lamblia* trophozoite. Note the two nuclei, curved median bodies, and linear axonemes. (R) *G. lamblia* cysts (iron-hematoxylin stain). Although these cysts are oval, some *G. lamblia* cysts will appear more rounded. (S) *G. lamblia* cyst (iron-hematoxylin stain). Nuclei, median bodies, and axonemes are clearly visible in this cyst. (T) *C. mesnili* trophozoites and cyst. (Left) The three trophozoites are characterized by the clear "oral groove" (feeding groove) seen coming down from the nucleus at the left side of the trophozoites. Without seeing this oral groove, the identification of this trophozoite is very difficult (right). In the cyst, the "shepherd's crook," the curved fibril to the right of the nucleus, can be seen. (U) *T. vaginalis* trophozoites (Giemsa stain). Note the undulating membrane, flagella, and linear axostyle (which penetrates the end of the organism). The organism has no known cyst stage. (V) *T. vaginalis* trophozoite (Giemsa stain). Note the undulating membrane, flagella, and axostyle. (W) *B. coli* trophozoite (iodine preparation). Note the large macronucleus and cilia; this organism is photographed at a lower magnification. (X) *B. coli* in tissue (routine histologic preparation). Note the macronucleus that is partially visible in one of the trophozoites. Reprinted with permission from reference 21.

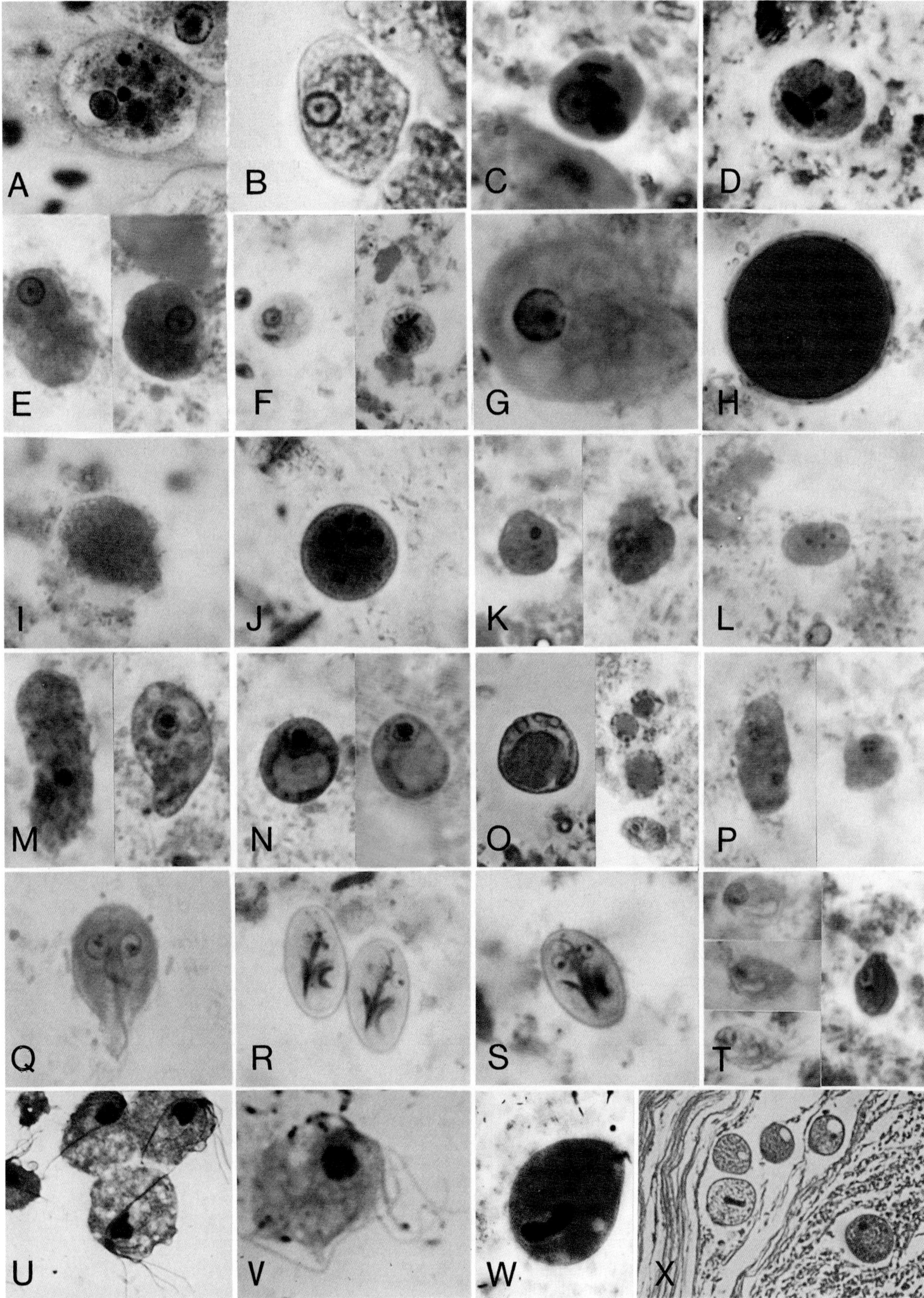
A
B
C
D
E
F
G
H
I
J
K
L
M
N
O
P
Q
R
S
T
U
V
W
X

established, treatment decisions must be based on the overall clinical presentation.

NONPATHOGENIC AMEBAE

The other species of intestinal amebae are considered nonpathogenic and, except for *Entamoeba polecki*, have a worldwide distribution and are more prevalent in warmer climates. They must, however, be differentiated from the pathogenic species, *E. histolytica*. A permanently stained smear is often essential for accomplishing this goal (Table 2; Fig. 1 and 2).

E. hartmanni is a separate species that is morphologically similar to *E. histolytica/E. dispar*. Size is the key differentiating characteristic. *E. coli* trophozoites may be difficult to differentiate from *E. histolytica/E. dispar* trophozoites on wet preparations. The mature cyst of *E. coli* may be refractive to fixation, making it less visible in permanent stained smears but still detectable by the wet mount method. It has been reported as the most common ameba isolated in human stool specimens. *E. polecki* is associated with pigs, and in certain areas of the world, such as Papua New Guinea, it is the most common human intestinal parasite. The trophozoite shares characteristics with both *E. histolytica/E. dispar* and *E. coli*; the cyst normally has one nucleus. *Entamoeba gingivalis* was the first parasitic ameba of humans described. It is found in the soft tartar between teeth and can be recovered in sputum. In the trophozoite, the cytoplasm often contains ingested leukocytes. A cyst form has not been observed.

E. nana, like *E. hartmanni*, is one of the smaller intestinal amebae. It is seen in most populations as frequently as *E. coli*. There is a great deal of nuclear variation, and it can mimic *D. fragilis* and *E. hartmanni*. The cysts of *E. nana* are usually oval in shape, and both the trophozoites and cysts are commonly present in fecal material. *I. bütschlii* has the same distribution as other nonpathogenic amebae but is less common than *E. coli* and *E. nana*. The trophozoite of *I. bütschlii* may be similar to *E. nana* and is difficult to differentiate from that of *E. nana*. The cyst is very characteristic; it is round to oval and may contain a large glycogen vacuole.

Treatment is not recommended for any of the nonpathogenic amebae. Methods of prevention of infection for all include improved personal hygiene and improved sanitary conditions.

FLAGELLATES

The flagellates that parasitize the intestinal tracts of humans belong to six genera in the phylum Sarcomastigophora, subphylum Mastigophora: *Giardia, Dientamoeba, Trichomonas, Chilomastix, Enteromonas*, and *Retortamonas* (Fig. 3) (15, 33). Some flagellates are commensals that reside in the intestinal tract and are harmless to the individual. The flagellates that are pathogenic include *G. lamblia, D. fragilis*, and *T. vaginalis*. *Chilomastix mesnili, Enteromonas hominis, Retortamonas intestinalis*, and *Trichomonas hominis* are considered nonpathogenic. As mentioned previously, *D. fragilis* has recently been reclassified as a flagellate and appears to be closely related to the trichomonads.

Transmission of flagellates, with the exception of *Trichomonas*, is initiated via the ingestion of contaminated food or water. Of the six genera, all except *D. fragilis* and *Trichomonas* spp. are transmitted via a cyst form. To date, only a trophozoite form has been observed for *D. fragilis* and *Tricho-*

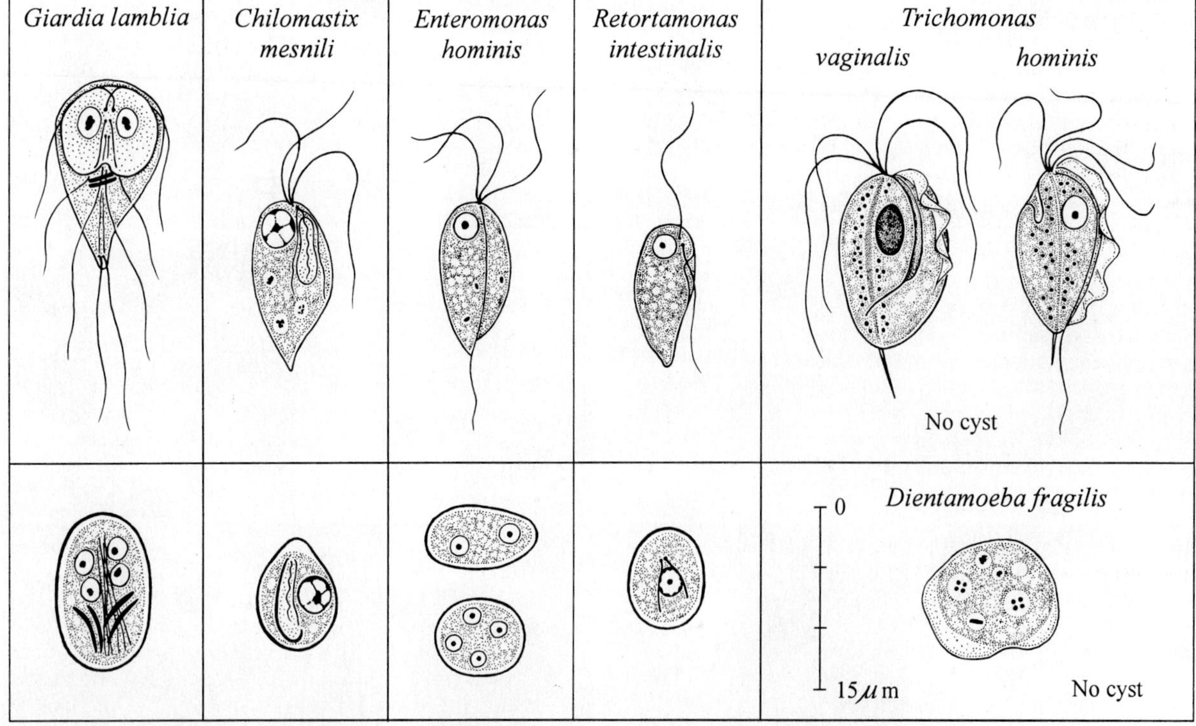

FIGURE 3 Intestinal and urogenital flagellates of humans. (Top row) Trophozoites. *T. vaginalis* is found in urogenital sites; all other flagellates are intestinal. (Botton row) Cysts. *D. fragilis* trophozoite is shown; no cyst stage.

monas spp. Cysts are acquired through ingestion of a contaminated food or water source. Once in the intestine, the organism excysts, releasing trophozoites that attach to the intestinal epithelium. Completion of the life cycle in humans culminates in the release of viable cysts in the environment via the feces.

In the clinical laboratory, wet preparations and permanent stained smears of fecal material are used to diagnose infections. Serologic assays are available for use in the diagnosis of G. *lamblia* but are not routinely used in the clinical setting. Molecular biology-based methods are being used to detect G. *lamblia* in contaminated drinking water and *T. vaginalis* in clinical samples.

In comparison to the amebae described previously, the flagellates have greater morphologic diversity relative to one another, making determination of the genus easier (Table 3; Fig. 2 and 3).

To aid in the identification of the trophozoite, key features to be noted are the shape, size, number, and position of flagella; the number of nuclei; and the presence of a spiral groove, cytostome, and characteristic features such as a sucking disk or undulating membrane. Typically, the size, shape, and number of nuclei are diagnostic characteristics used to identify cysts. Examination of permanent stained smears is always recommended for diagnosis because the wet mount might not be reflective of all organisms and stages present in the specimen.

It is important that a representative portion of the slide, either a wet mount or a permanent smear, be scanned before rendering a final opinion on a specimen. It is also important to have an accurate micrometer to measure life cycle stages.

G. lamblia

G. *lamblia* is an intestinal flagellate that infects both humans and animals and that is the most common cause of intestinal parasitosis in humans worldwide. Because the literature refers to this organism as G. *lamblia*, *Giardia intestinalis*, and *Giardia duodenalis*, it is evident that there is still debate over the classification and nomenclature of this flagellate. Previous work, based primarily on structural variations of the parasite, resulted in the proposal of three species; *Giardia muris* (mice), *Giardia agilis* (amphibian), and the intestinalis group (G. *duodenalis*) (21). Although these species have been proposed, G. *lamblia* is the nomenclature predominately used in the United States and will continue to be used throughout this chapter.

Infection with G. *lamblia* occurs through fecal-oral transmission or the ingestion of cysts in contaminated food or water. Individuals more commonly infected in developed countries are children in day-care centers, hikers, and immunocompromised individuals. Among compromised individuals, infections have been documented in people with AIDS and hypogammaglobulinemia and those affected by malnutrition. Prevalence rates for this pathogen range from 1 to 7% in industrialized areas and from 5 to 50% in developing countries. Of the intestinal flagellates, G. *lamblia* is the flagellate most frequently isolated in the United States. In high-risk domestic settings, such as day-care centers, prevalence rates can reach up to 90% (45). Infection occurs when viable cysts are ingested, excyst, and transform into trophozoites. After excystation, the trophozoite, which appears to have a propensity for the duodenum, attaches to the mucosal epithelium. Trophozoites attach to the epithelium via a sucking disk located on the ventral side of the parasite. During the course of infection, the parasites remain attached to the epithelium and do not invade the mucosa. In the intestine, trophozoites divide by binary fission to produce two identical daughter trophozoites. As they move down toward the large intestine, the trophozoites encyst and infective cysts are excreted into the environment (21).

Clinical Significance

The majority of individuals infected with G. *lamblia* are asymptomatic. In symptomatic individuals, acute G. *lamblia* infections can mimic infection with other protozoal, viral, and bacterial pathogens. After an incubation period of approximately 12 to 20 days, patients can experience nausea, chills, low-grade fever, epigastric pain, and a sudden onset of watery diarrhea. Diarrhea is often explosive in nature and presents as very foul smelling without the presence of blood, cellular exudate, or mucus. Individuals can develop subacute or chronic infections with symptoms such as recurrent diarrhea, abdominal discomfort and distention, belching, and heartburn. In patients with chronic cases of giardiasis, diarrhea can lead to dehydration, malabsorption, and impairment of pancreatic function (9).

Laboratory Diagnosis

Diagnosis of G. *lamblia* infection is established by the microscopic examination of stool for the presence of cysts and/or trophozoites. To detect G. *lamblia*, it is recommended that at least three stool samples be collected 2 to 3 days apart (42). Stained smears are more helpful in identifying the trophozoite stage of the infection, although this stage can be identified in wet mounts (Table 3; Fig. 3). Examination of stool specimens may not be diagnostic because cyst forms can be trapped in mucus, making them difficult to detect on smears. Also, the excretion pattern of cysts can be cyclical. In these instances, other methods should be used to obtain clinical samples such as the string test (Entero-Test; HDC Corp., San Jose, Calif.). This technique can be useful for the diagnosis of G. *lamblia*. Briefly, the patient swallows a weighted capsule containing gelatin and a tightly wound string. After approximately 5 h the string is removed from the patient and the adherent material is examined as a wet mount or permanent smear (21). Endoscopy can also be used to collect clinical specimens. Because this procedure is invasive, it is used only when diagnosing disease in patients with a perplexing clinical presentation (45).

Other assays that have gained wide acceptance for the detection of G. *lamblia* in stool specimens are EIAs and DFA assays. A number of manufacturers produce both EIA and DFA assays, and both methods have sensitivities and specificities well in excess of 90%. Although these methods have proven to be more sensitive and specific than the routine staining of fecal smears (trichrome staining), other important pathogens may be missed if a wet mount and permanent stained smear are not examined. EIAs are becoming more popular for high-volume laboratories as a way of screening large numbers of specimens for G. *lamblia* (23). Multiple parameters (workload, skill level of the technologists, necessary equipment) should be considered when choosing a specific method.

Because of the potential for contamination of municipal water supplies, routine monitoring of water for parasitic protozoa is recommended as a public health control measure. G. *lamblia* cysts can remain viable for 2 to 3 months in cold water and are fairly resistant to killing by routine chlorine treatments. DFA assays are commonly used to detect G. *lamblia* cysts in water samples. More recently, PCR has been used for this purpose (48). The advantage of PCR is the increased sensitivity compared to those of fluorescence as-

TABLE 3 Key features of trophozoites and cysts of common intestinal and urogenital flagellates[a]

Organism	Trophozoites	Cysts
D. fragilis	Size[b]: 5–15 μm; shaped like amebae Motility: Nonprogressive; pseudopodia are angular Flagella: None Nucleus[c]: 1 (40%) or 2 (60%); no peripheral chromatin; karyosome clusters of 4–8 granules Note: Trophozoites not visible in unstained preparation; variation in size between trophozoites can exist on the same smear; cytoplasm is finely granular and vacuoles may be present	No cyst stage
G. lamblia	Size: 10–20 μm long; 5–15 μm wide; pear shaped Motility: Falling leaf Flagella: 4 lateral, 2 ventral, 2 caudal Nucleus: 2; not visible in unstained preparation; small central karyosomes present Note: Sucking disk is prominent on ventral side of trophozoite; organism is spoon shaped from side view	Size: 8–19 μm long; 7–10 μm wide; oval, ellipsoidal, or round Nucleus: 4 nuclei usually located on one end; not distinct in unstained preparation; no peripheral chromatin; karyosomes smaller than in trophozoite Cytoplasm: Staining can cause shrinkage where cytoplasm pulls away from the cyst wall; 4 median bodies present Note: Poorly defined longitudinal fibers may be present
C. mesnili	Size: 6–24 μm long; 4–8 μm wide; pear shaped Motility: Stiff, rotary Flagella: 3 anterior, 1 in cytostome Nucleus: 1; not visible in unstained preparation Cytoplasm: Prominent cytostome extends over one-third to one-half of the body; spiral groove across ventral surface can be hard to see; vacuoles present	Size: 6–10 μm long; 4–6 μm wide; lemon shaped with anterior hyaline knob Nucleus: Same as trophozoite; difficult to see in unstained preparation; indistinct central karyosome present Cytoplasm: Curved fibril alongside of cytostome known as "shepherd's crook"
T. hominis	Size: 5–15 μm long; 7–10 μm wide; pear shaped Motility: Jerky, rapid Flagella: 3–5 anterior, 1 posterior (extends beyond end of body) Nucleus: 1; not visible in unstained preparation Cytoplasm: Central longitudinal axostyle; undulating membrane runs the entire length of body Note: May have tremendous nuclear variation; can mimic *E. hartmanni* and *D. fragilis*	No cyst stage
T. vaginalis	Size: 7–23 μm long; 5–15 μm wide Motility: Jerky, rapid Flagella: 3–5 anterior, 1 posterior Nucleus: 1; not visible in unstained preparation Note: Undulating membrane extends one-half the length of the body; no free posterior flagella	No cyst stage
E. hominis	Size: 4–10 μm long; 5–6 μm wide; oval Motility: Jerky Flagella: 3 anterior, 1 posterior Nucleus: 1; not visible in unstained preparation Note: One side of the body is flat; posterior flagellum extends free posteriorly or laterally	Size: 4–10 μm long; 4–6 μm wide; elongate or oval in shape Nucleus: 1–4; not visible in stained preparation Note: Resembles *E. nana* cysts; fibrils or flagella usually not seen
R. intestinalis	Size: 4–9 μm long; 3–4 μm wide; pear shaped or oval Motility: Jerky Flagella: 1 anterior, 1 posterior Nucleus: 1; not visible in unstained preparation Note: Very difficult to identify; rarely seen; prominent cytostome which extends half the length of body	Size: 4–9 μm long; 5 μm wide; pear or lemon shaped Nucleus: 1; not visible in unstained preparation Note: Resembles *Chilomastix* cysts; bird beak fibril arrangement; shadow outline of cytostome with supporting fibrils extends above nucleus

[a] Adapted from reference 21.
[b] Size ranges based on wet preparations (with permanent stains organisms usually measure 1 to 2 μm less).
[c] Nuclear and cytoplasmic descriptions based on permanent stained smears.

says or assays that use special stains. Research continues to enhance investigators' ability to detect viable organisms, which is a better indication of poor water quality (59).

Therapy

For individuals diagnosed with giardiasis, the treatment of choice is metronidazole. In most immunocompetent hosts, infection is self-limiting; however, treatment will lessen the duration of symptoms and prevent transmission. Other drugs that have been used to treat giardiasis are quinacrine, tinidazole, furazolidone, and paromomycin (37).

D. fragilis

D. fragilis is found worldwide and is known to cause a noninvasive diarrheal illness in humans. Despite the lack of external flagella, this parasite is currently classified as a flagellate but has historically been grouped with the ameba. Electron microscopy and antigenic analysis have aided in the classification of this organism and demonstrate that it is closely related to *Trichomonas* and *Histomonas*. Colonization in humans is similar to that seen with other intestinal parasites; typically, the cecum and the proximal part of the colon are affected. Because *D. fragilis* does not have a cyst stage as part of its life cycle, the mode of transmission is less well understood. One hypothesis concerning the spread of *D. fragilis* is that transmission occurs within the eggs of *Enterobius vermicularis* or *Ascaris lumbricoides* (7).

The prevalence rates of this organism are not well characterized, ranging from 1 to 19% in certain studies. There appears to be a higher prevalence in certain groups of individuals such as missionaries, Native Americans living in Arizona, and institutionalized individuals (61). In the United States, the prevalence is reported to be quite low. This may be due to underreporting attributable to difficulties associated with identifying the organism in clinical samples.

Clinical Significance

The frequency of symptomatic disease in adults ranges from 15 to 25% and is more common in infected children than in adults. Up to 90% of children infected with *D. fragilis* have clinical disease (8, 45). Symptoms include the following: fatigue, insufficient weight gain, diarrhea (often intermittent), abdominal pain, anorexia, and nausea. Some individuals, mainly children, also experience unexplained peripheral blood eosinophilia (21). Diarrhea is predominantly seen during the first 1 to 2 weeks after the onset of disease. Abdominal pain can persist for 1 to 2 months (8).

Laboratory Diagnosis

Diagnosis of *D. fragilis* infection is similar to that of other intestinal protozoa, and detection of the trophozoite in fresh or preserved stool is warranted to establish infection. The recovery of *D. fragilis* is greatly enhanced by the collection of at least three stool specimens (42, 45). Morphologically, the trophozoite of *D. fragilis* contains one or two nuclei, with two nuclei being more common. Well-trained laboratory personnel can identify *D. fragilis* trophozoites in stool specimens, but because no cyst stage exists, diagnosis from the wet mount can be difficult. Use of a permanent stained smear is the recommended procedure for detection (Table 3; Fig. 3). Trophozoites have been recovered from soft and formed stools, indicating the need to evaluate all types of samples (8). Other techniques, such as immunofluorescence assays, have been used as diagnostic tools for the detection of *D. fragilis* but are not commercially available (11).

Therapy

The treatment of choice in symptomatic individuals is tetracycline. Others describe iodoquinol (diiodohydroxyquin) as the treatment of choice (8). Metronidazole, iodoquinol, and tetracycline have been used to treat children (21). If *E. vermicularis* is detected concomitantly, the treatment regimen should also include mebendazole (8).

T. vaginalis

T. vaginalis is a pathogenic flagellate that infects the urogenital tracts of males and females. It is primarily a sexually transmitted disease. In the United States it is estimated that 5 million women and 1 million men are infected; worldwide there are 180 million cases of trichomoniasis each year. These estimates may be low because (i) trichomoniasis is not a reportable disease in the United States and other countries; (ii) the infection, particularly in men, can be asymptomatic; and (iii) laboratory tests used for diagnosis vary in their sensitivities.

The incidence of trichomoniasis differs depending on the population examined. Factors such as lower socioeconomic status, multiple sex partners, and poor personal hygiene are linked to a higher incidence of infection.

The life cycle of *T. vaginalis* includes only the trophozoite stage; there is no cyst stage. The organism is similar in morphology to the other trichomonads and is characterized by a prominent axostyle and an undulating membrane that stops halfway down the side of the trophozoite (Table 3; Fig. 3). It is a facultative anaerobe that divides by binary fission, and it cannot survive long outside the host.

Clinical Significance

Infection in females can result in vaginitis, cervicitis, and urethritis. The classic vaginal discharge is described as copious, liquid, greenish, frothy, and foul smelling. The onset of symptoms, such as intense vaginal and vulvar pruritis and discharge, is often sudden and occurs during or after menstruation. Vaginal pH is usually elevated above the normal pH of 4.5. Dysuria occurs in 20% of women with *T. vaginalis* infection. Infection has also been associated with premature rupture of membranes, premature birth, and posthysterectomy cuff infections (14, 39, 56). More recently, it has been implicated as a cofactor in the transmission of HIV (31). In males, the most common symptomatic presentation is urethritis. Up to 50% of infected women are asymptomatic carriers. In men, the majority of infections are asymptomatic. Asymptomatic carriers serve as a reservoir for transmission and also remain at risk for developing disease.

Neonates can acquire the organism during passage through the infected birth canal. It is estimated that 2 to 17% of female babies acquire trichomoniasis by direct vulvovaginal contamination (31). Reports have also documented *T. vaginalis* as a cause of neonatal pneumonia (26, 38).

Laboratory Diagnosis

The diagnosis of *T. vaginalis* infection is commonly based on the examination of wet preparations of vaginal and urethral discharges, prostatic secretions, and urine sediments. Vaginal specimens are routinely collected during a speculum examination, but recent work suggests that self-collected or tampon-collected specimens may be used with good success (25, 51). Specimens should be mixed with a drop of physiologic saline and examined within 1 h under low power (magnification, ×100) with reduced illumination. Specimens should never be refrigerated. The presence of actively motile organisms with jerky motility is diagnostic. The movement of the undulating membrane may be seen as the motility of the trophozoite diminishes. PMNs are often present. The sensitivity of the wet preparation is between 50 and 70%, depending on the skill of the microscopist and other factors. Perhaps the most important factor affecting sensitivity is the time between collection and examination of the specimen. The viability of the organism is essential for the detection of motility on the wet mount and drops off precipitously with time. Because the morphology of *T. hominis*, a nonpathogenic intestinal flagellate, is very similar to that of *T. vaginalis*, care must be taken to ensure that specimens are not contaminated with fecal material.

Culture has increased sensitivity (> 80%) over that of the wet mount method and is considered the "gold standard" method. Specimens must be collected properly and inoculated immediately into the appropriate medium, such as modified Diamond's, Trichosel, or Hollanders medium. Due to cost and convenience, this approach is not routinely used. Culture systems (InPouchTV, [BioMed Diagnostics, San Jose, Calif.] and the system of Empyrean Diagnostics, Inc., Mountainview, Calif.) that allow direct inoculation, transport, culture, and microscopic examination are commercially available (4, 18). In situations in which immediate transport of specimens is not feasible, the use of these transport/culture devices is encouraged. Permanent stains such as Papanicolaou or Giemsa stains may be used, but the organisms are often difficult to recognize (29). Nucleic acid probes and antigen detection methods have also been developed, but these are not commercially available (12, 41, 62). A dual latex agglutination test (Quik-Tri/Can; Integrated Diagnostics, Inc., Baltimore, Md.) for the detection of *Candida* and *T. vaginalis* from vaginal specimens has good sensitivity and specificity for the detection of *T. vaginalis* (32).

Nucleic acid-based methods for the detection of *T. vaginalis* have been developed. PCR assays that detect various regions of the organism's genome have increased sensitivity, and assays that are practical in the clinical laboratory have been developed (27, 34, 46, 52). A direct DNA probe which detects the three most common syndromes associated with increased vaginal discharge, bacterial vaginosis, candidiasis, and trichomoniasis (5, 32), is commercially available (Affirm VPIII; Becton Dickinson, Sparks, Md.). With the methods described above, there are still limits on the specimen storage conditions and times that must be considered. They do provide more flexibility for laboratories serving large outpatient populations. The increased sensitivities of PCR and probes need to be balanced against the rapid results and lower expense of wet preparations for the diagnosis of *T. vaginalis* infections.

Therapy

The treatment of choice for *T. vaginalis* infections is metronidazole. All sexual partners of infected individuals should also receive treatment. Resistance to metronidazole has been documented (1). Metronidazole should not be used during pregnancy unless the benefits of treatment outweigh the risks to the fetus.

NONPATHOGENIC FLAGELLATES

C. mesnili is found worldwide and is generally considered a nonpathogen. Unlike *D. fragilis*, *C. mesnili* has both a trophozoite and a cyst stage. The organism is acquired through the ingestion of contaminated food or water and resides in the cecum and/or colon of the infected human or animal. The trophozoite measures 6 to 24 μm in length and contains a characteristic spiral groove that runs longitudinally along the body (Table 3; Fig. 2 and 3). Motility of the organism can sometimes be seen in fresh preparations, and the spiral groove may be exposed as the organism turns. Flagella are difficult to see in stained preparations. The trophozoite contains one nucleus with a cytostome or oral groove in close proximity. The pear-shaped cyst retains the cytoplasmic organelles of the trophozoite, with a single nucleus and curved cytostomal fibril. Identification is made more definitively by observing the organism in a permanent stained preparation.

T. hominis is another nonpathogenic flagellate that is similar to *D. fragilis* in that only the trophozoite stage has been observed. Although the organism is cosmopolitan in nature and is recovered from individuals with diarrhea, it is still considered nonpathogenic. The trophozoites typically inhabit the cecum. They are pyriform in shape and contain an undulating membrane that traverses the length of the parasite. The use of permanent smears is recommended for observation of these organisms in clinical specimens. The trophozoites may stain weakly, making them difficult to detect on stained smears (21).

Two additional nonpathogenic intestinal flagellates are *E. hominis* and *R. intestinalis*. Both *E. hominis* and *R. intestinalis* are found in warm or temperate climates, and infection is acquired through the ingestion of cysts. When examining clinical specimens it is important to note that cysts of *E. hominis* can resemble those of *E. nana*, although *E. nana* cysts containing two nuclei are rare. Because of the small size of *E. hominis* and *R. intestinalis*, it is difficult to detect these organisms even when permanent stained smears are examined. This could lead to the underreporting of both organisms.

In general, treatment is not recommended for the nonpathogenic flagellates. Improved personal hygiene and sanitary conditions are key methods for the prevention of infection.

CILIATES

Balantidium coli is a ciliate that exists in animal reservoirs such as pigs and chimpanzees. The organism is the only pathogenic ciliate and the largest pathogenic protozoan known to infect humans. Infection is more common in warmer climates and in areas where humans are in close contact with pigs. As with other intestinal protozoa, poor sanitary conditions lead to a higher incidence of infection.

This organism has both the trophozoite and cyst forms as part of its life cycle (Table 4, Fig. 2). The cyst form is the infective stage of the life cycle. After ingestion of the cysts and excystation, trophozoites secrete hyaluronidase, which aids in the invasion of the tissue. The trophozoite, which is oval and covered with cilia, is easily seen in wet mounts under low-power magnification. The cytoplasm contains both a macronucleus and a micronucleus, in addition to two contractile vacuoles. Motile trophozoites can be observed in fresh wet preparations, but the specimen must be observed soon after collection. The trophozoite is somewhat pear shaped and also contains vacuoles that may harbor debris such as cell fragments and ingested bacteria. Cyst formation takes place as the trophozoite moves down the large intestine.

Clinical Significance

Infection with *B. coli* is most often asymptomatic; however, symptomatic infection can occur, resulting in bouts of dys-

TABLE 4 Key features of the ciliate *B. coli*

Stage	Characteristics
Trophozoite 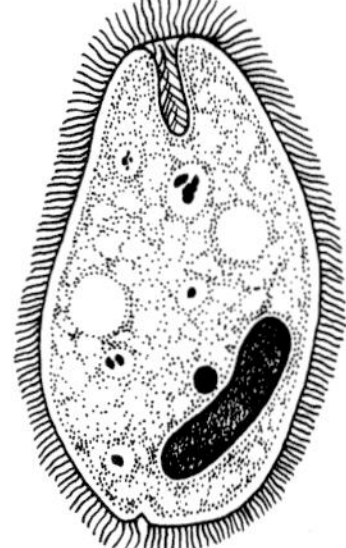	Shape and size: ovoid with tapering anterior end; 50–100 μm long; 40–70 μm wide Motility: rotary, boring; may be rapid Nuclei: 1 large kidney-bean shaped macronucleus, may be visible in unstained preparation; 1 small round micronucleus, adjacent to macronucleus, difficult to see Cytoplasm: may be vacuolated, ingested bacteria and debris; anterior cytostome Cilia: body surface covered with longitudinal rows of cilia; longer near cytostome Note: may be confused with helminth eggs or debris on a permanent stained smear; concentration or sedimentation examination recommended
Cyst 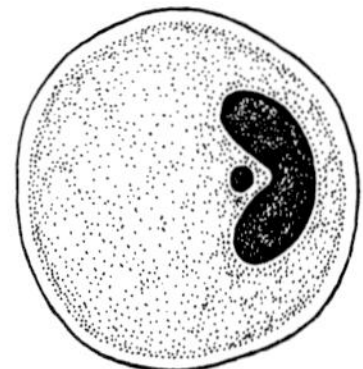	Shape and size: spherical or oval; 50–70 μm in diameter Nuclei: 1 large macronucleus; 1 micronucleus, difficult to see Cytoplasm: vacuoles are visible in young cysts; in older cysts, internal structure appears granular Cilia: difficult to see within the thick cyst wall

entery similar to amebiasis (10, 21). In addition, colitis produced by *B. coli* is often indistinguishable from that produced by *E. histolytica*. Symptoms typically include diarrhea, nausea, vomiting, headache, and anorexia. Fluid loss can be dramatic, as seen in some patients with cryptosporidiosis. The organism can invade the submucosa of the large bowel, and ulcerative abscesses and hemorrhagic lesions can occur. The shallow ulcers and submucosal lesions that result from invasion are prone to secondary infection by bacteria and can be problematic for the patient (16, 28). Deaths due to invasive *B. coli* infection have been reported (16). Even though the organism can invade the underlying mucosa, it does not typically spread to other organs. Infections associated with extraintestinal sites have been described on rare occasions (16, 28, 30).

Laboratory Diagnosis

Diagnosis of *B. coli* infections is established by either ova and parasite examination of feces or histologic examination of intestinal biopsy specimens. The diagnosis can be established only by demonstrating trophozoites in stool or tissue samples (30). It is very easy to identify these organisms in wet preparations and from concentrated stool samples. Conversely, it can be challenging to identify *B. coli* from trichrome-stained permanent smears because the organisms are so large and have a tendency to overstain. This makes the organism less discernible and increases the chance of misidentification.

Therapy

The treatment of choice for *B. coli* infection is tetracycline, although it is considered an investigational drug when it is used in this context. Metronidazole and iodoquinol are therapeutic alternatives used in some cases (21).

SUMMARY

The travel habits of the world's population have led to the global distribution of many of the protozoa covered in this chapter. Once rare, protozoan infections may now be seen with increased frequency. Laboratorians must try to maintain proficiency in identifying all the intestinal and urogenital amebae, flagellates, and ciliates. Accurate identification and diagnosis of many pathogenic protozoa have been enhanced by improvements in diagnostic laboratory techniques. Molecular biology-based procedures, particularly PCR, are rapidly being developed and may soon be commercially available. Environmental detection of these pathogens has also been achieved through new technologies.

Nucleic acid-based analysis of the amebae, flagellates, and ciliates will reveal further information about their life cycles, pathogenicities, and phylogenetic interrelationships. Although many new insights will be gained, the complete replacement of the conventional laboratory methods, such as microscopy, is not yet at hand.

REFERENCES

1. **Abramowicz, M.** 1998. Drugs for parasitic infections. *Med. Lett.* **40:**1–12.
2. **Albrecht, H., J. Stellbrink, K. Koperski, and H. Greten.** 1995. *Blastocystis hominis* in human immunodeficiency virus-related diarrhea. *Scand. J. Gastroenterol.* **30:**909–914.
3. **Ash, L. R., and T. C. Orihel.** 1987. *Parasites: A Guide to Laboratory Procedures and Identification*. ASCP Press, Chicago, Ill.
4. **Borchardt, K. A., and R. F. Smith.** 1991. An evaluation of an InPouch TV culture method for diagnosing *Trichomonas vaginalis* infection. *Genitourin. Med.* **67:**149–152.
5. **Briselden, A., and S. Hillier.** 1994. Evaluation of Affirm VP Microbial Identification Test for *Gardnerella vaginalis* and *Trichomonas vaginalis*. *J. Clin. Microbiol.* **32:**148–152.
6. **Bruckner, D. A.** 1992. Amebiasis. *Clin. Microbiol. Rev.* **5:**356–369.
7. **Burrows, R. B., and M. A. Swerdlow.** 1956. *Enterobius vermicularis* as a probable vector of *Dientamoeba fragilis*. *Am. J. Trop. Med. Hyg.* **5:**258–265.
8. **Butler, W. P.** 1996. *Dientamoeba fragilis*. An unusual intestinal pathogen. *Dig. Dis. Sci.* **41:**1811–1813.
9. **Carroccio, A., G. Montalto, G. Iacono, S. Ippolito, M. Soresi, and A. Notarbartolo.** 1997. Secondary impairment of pancreatic function as a cause of severe malabsorption in intestinal giardiasis: a case report. *Am. J. Trop. Med. Hyg.* **56:**599–602.
10. **Castro, J., J. L. Vazquez-Iglesias, and F. Arnal-Monreal.** 1983. Dysentery caused by *Balantidium coli*—report of two cases. *Endoscopy* **15:**272–274.
11. **Chan, F. T. H., M. X. Guan, and A. M. R. Mackenzie.** 1993. Application of indirect immunofluorescence to detection of *Dientamoeba fragilis* trophozoites in fecal specimens. *J. Clin. Microbiol.* **31:**1710–1714.
12. **Chang, T. H., S. Y. Tsing, and S. Tzeng.** 1986. Monoclonal antibodies against *Trichomonas vaginalis*. *Hybridoma* **5:**43–51.
13. **Clark, C. G.** 1997. Extensive genetic diversity in *Blastocystis hominis*. *Mol. Biochem. Parasitol.* **87:**79–83.
14. **Cotch, M. F., J. G. Pastorek II, R. P. Nugent, D. E. Yerg, D. H. Martin, and D. A. Eschenbach.** 1991. Demographic and behavioral predictors of *Trichomonas vaginalis* infection among pregnant women. *Obstet. Gynecol.* **78:**1087–1092.
15. **Cox, F.** 1998. Classification of the parasitic protozoa, p. 141–155. *In* L. Collier, A. Balows, and M. Sussman (ed.),

Topley and Wilson's Microbiology and Microbial Infections, vol. 5. Arnold, London, United Kingdom.

16. **Currie, A. R.** 1990. Human balantidiasis. *S. Afr. J. Surg.* **28:**23–25.
17. **Diamond, L. S., and C. G. Clark.** 1994. A redescription of *Entamoeba histolytica* Schaudinn, 1903 (Emended Walker, 1911) separating it from *Entamoeba dispar* Brumpt, 1925. *J. Eukaryot. Microbiol.* **40:**340–344.
18. **Draper, D., R. Parker, E. Patterson, W. Jones, M. Beutz, J. French, K. Borchardt, and J. McGregor.** 1993. Detection of *Trichomonas vaginalis* in pregnant women with the InPouch TV culture system. *J. Clin. Microbiol.* **31:** 1016–1018.
19. **Garavelli, P. L., C. H. Zierdt, T. A. Fleisher, H. Liss, and B. Nagy.** 1995. Serum antibody detected by fluorescent antibody test in patients with symptomatic *Blastocystis hominis* infection. *Recenti Prog. Med.* **86:**398–400.
20. **Garcia, L. S., T. C. Brewer, and D. A. Bruckner.** 1979. A comparison of the formalin-ether concentration and trichrome-stained smear methods for the recovery and identification of intestinal protozoa. *Am. J. Med. Technol.* **45:** 932–935.
21. **Garcia, L. S., and D. A. Bruckner.** 1997. *Diagnostic Medical Parasitology*, 3rd ed. American Society for Microbiology, Washington, D.C.
22. **Garcia, L. S., D. A. Bruckner, and M. N. Clancy.** 1984. Clinical relevance of *Blastocystis hominis*. *Lancet* **ii:** 1233–1234.
23. **Garcia, L. S., and R. Y. Shimizu.** 1997. Evaluation of nine immunoassay kits (enzyme immunoassay and direct fluorescence) for detection of *Giardia lamblia* and *Cryptosporidium parvum* in human fecal specimens. *J. Clin. Microbiol.* **35:**1526–1529.
24. **Gericke, A., G. Burchard, J. Knobloch, and B. Walderich.** 1997. Isoenzyme patterns of *Blastocystis hominis* patient isolates derived from symptomatic and healthy carriers. *Trop. Med. Int. Health* **2:**245–254.
25. **Heine, R. P., H. Wiessenfeld, R. L. Sweet, and S. S. Witkin.** 1997. Polymerase chain reaction analysis of distal vaginal specimens: a less invasive strategy for detection of *Trichomonas vaginalis*. *Clin. Infect. Dis.* **24:**985–987.
26. **Hienstra, I., F. Van Belm, and H. M. Bergerm.** 1984. Can *Trichomonas vaginalis* cause pneumonia in newborn babies? *Br. Med. J.* **289:**355–356.
27. **Jeremias, J., D. Draper, M. Ziegert, W. Jones, S. Inglis, J. A. McGregor, and S. S. Witkin.** 1994. Detection of *Trichomonas vaginalis* using the polymerase chain reaction in pregnant and non-pregnant women. *Infect. Dis. Obstet. Gynecol.* **2:**16–19.
28. **Knight, R.** 1978. Giardiasis, isosporiasis and balantidiasis. *Clin. Gastroenterol.* **7:**31–47.
29. **Krieger, J. N., M. R. Tam, C. E. Stevens, I. O. Nielsen, J. Hale, N. B. Kiviat, and K. K. Holmes.** 1988. Diagnosis of trichomoniasis: comparison of conventional wet-mount examination with cytologic studies, cultures, and monoclonal antibody staining of direct specimens. *JAMA* **259:** 1223–1227.
30. **Ladas, S. D., S. Savva, A. Frydas, A. Kaloviduris, J. Hatzioannou, and S. Raptis.** 1989. Invasive balantidiasis presented as chronic colitis and lung involvement. *Dig. Dis. Sci.* **34:**1621–1623.
31. **Laga, M., A. Manoka, M. Kivuvu, B. Malele, M. Tuliza, N. Nzila, J. Goeman, F. Behets, V. Batter, M. Alary, W. L. Heyward, R. W. Ryder, and P. Piot.** 1993. Nonulcerative sexually transmitted diseases as risk factors for HIV-1 transmission in women: results from a cohort study. *AIDS* **7:**95–102.
32. **Leber, A. L., B. Grotts, L. S. Garcia, and D. A. Bruckner.** 1997. Comparison of the Affirm VPIII Probe, Quick-Tri/Can™ Latex Test, Gram stain, and wet mount for the diagnosis of vaginosis, abstr. C-312, p. 174. *In Abstracts of the 97th General Meeting of the American Society for Microbiology 1997*. American Society for Microbiology, Washington, D.C.
33. **Levine, N., F. Cortis, G. Cox, J. Deroux, B. Grain, G. Honigberg, A. Leedale, A. Loeblich III, J. Lom, D. Lynn, E. Merinfeld, F. Page, G. Poljansky, and V. Sprague.** 1980. A newly revised classification of the protozoa. *J. Protozool.* **27:**37–58.
34. **Lin, P. R., M. F. Shaio, and J. Y. Liu.** 1997. One-tube, nested-PCR assay for the detection of *Trichomonas vaginalis* in vaginal discharges. *Ann. Trop. Med. Parasitol.* **91:** 61–65.
35. **Mansour, N. S., E. M. Mikhail, N. A. El Masry, A. G. Sabry, and E. W. Mohareb.** 1995. Biochemical characterisation of human isolates of *Blastocystis hominis*. *J. Med. Microbiol.* **42:**304–307.
36. **Markell, E. D., and M. P. Udkow.** 1986. *Blastocystis hominis:* pathogen or fellow traveler? *Am. J. Trop. Med. Hyg.* **35:**1023–1026.
37. **Marshall, M. M., D. Naumovitz, Y. Ortega, and C. R. Sterling.** 1997. Waterborne protozoan pathogens. *Clin. Microbiol. Rev.* **10:**67–85.
38. **McLaren, L., L. Davis, G. Healy, and G. James.** 1983. Isolation of *Trichomonas vaginalis* from the respiratory tract of infants with respiratory diseases. *Pediatrics* **71:**888–890.
39. **Minkoff, H., A. N. Grunebaum, R. H. Schwarz, J. Feldman, M. Cummings, W. Crombleholme, L. Clark, G. Pringle, and W. M. McCormack.** 1984. Risk factors for prematurity and premature rupture of membranes: a prospective study of the vaginal flora in pregnancy. *Am. J. Obstet. Gynecol.* **150:**965–972.
40. **Moe, K. T., M. Singh, J. Howe, L. C. Ho, S. W. Tan, G. C. Ng, X. Q. Chen, and E. H. Yap.** 1996. Observations on the ultrastructure and viability of the cystic stage of *Blastocystis hominis* from human feces. *Parasitol. Res.* **82:** 436–444.
41. **Muresu, R., S. Rubino, P. Rizzu, A. Baldini, M. Colombo, and P. Cappuccinelli.** 1994. A new method for identification of *Trichomonas vaginalis* by fluorescent DNA in situ hybridization. *J. Clin. Microbiol.* **32:**1018–1022.
42. **National Committee for Clinical Laboratory Standards.** 1993. *Recovery and Identification of Parasites from the Intestinal Tract.* Proposed guideline M28-P. National Committee for Clinical Laboratory Standards, Villanova, Pa.
43. **Ong, S. J., M. Y. Cheng, K. H. Liu, and C. H. Horng.** 1996. Use of the ProSpecT microplate enzyme immunoassay for the detection of pathogenic and nonpathogenic *Entamoeba histolytica* in faecal specimens. *Trans. R. Soc. Trop. Med. Hyg.* **90:**248–249.
44. **Ortner, S., C. G. Clark, M. Binder, O. Scheiner, G. Wiedermann, and M. Duchene.** 1997. Molecular biology of the hexokinase isoenzyme pattern that distinguishes pathogenic *Entamoeba histolytica* from nonpathogenic *Entamoeba dispar*. *Mol. Biochem. Parasitol.* **86:**85–94.
45. **Panosian, C. B.** 1988. Parasitic diarrhea. *Infect. Dis. Clin. N. Am.* **2:**685–703.
46. **Riley, D. E., M. C. Roberts, T. Takayama, and J. Krieger.** 1992. Development of a polymerase chain reaction-based diagnosis of *Trichomonas vaginalis*. *J. Clin. Microbiol.* **30:** 465–472.
47. **Rivera, W. E., H. Tachibana, M. R. Silva-Tahat, H. Uemura, and H. Kanbara.** 1996. Differentiation of *Entamoeba histolytica* and *E. dispar* DNA from cysts present in stool specimens by polymerase chain reaction: its field application in the Philippines. *Parasitol. Res.* **82:**585–589.
48. **Rochelle, P. A., R. De Leon, M. H. Stewart, and R. L. Wolfe.** 1997. Comparison of primers and optimization of

PCR conditions for detection of *Cryptosporidium parvum* and *Giardia lamblia* in water. *Appl. Environ. Microbiol.* **63:** 106–114.

49. **Sanuki, J., T. Asai, E. Okuzawa, S. Kobayashi, and T. Takeuchi.** 1997. Identification of *Entamoeba histolytica* and *E. dispar* cysts in stool by polymerase chain reaction. *Parasitol. Res.* **83:**96–98.
50. **Sargeaunt, P. G., and J. E. Williams.** 1978. Electrophoretic isoenzyme patterns of *Entamoeba histolytica* and *Entamoeba coli*. *Trans. R. Soc. Trop. Med. Hyg.* **72:**164–166.
51. **Schwebke, J. R., S. C. Morgan, and G. B. Pinson.** 1997. Validity of self-obtained vaginal specimens for diagnosis of trichomoniasis. *J. Clin. Microbiol.* **35:**1618–1619.
52. **Shaio, M. F., P. R. Lin, and J. Y. Liu.** 1997. Colorimetric one-tube nested PCR for detection of *Trichomonas vaginalis* in vaginal discharge. *J. Clin. Microbiol.* **35:**132–138.
53. **Sheehan, D. J., B. G. Raucher, and J. C. McKitrick.** 1986. Association of *Blastocystis hominis* with signs and symptoms of human disease. *J. Clin. Microbiol.* **24:**548–550.
54. **Silberman, J. D., M. D. Sogin, D. D. Leipe, and C. G. Clark.** 1996. Human parasite finds taxonomic home. *Nature (London)* **380:**398.
55. **Singh, M., K. Suresh, L. C. Ho, G. C. Ng, and E. H. Yap.** 1995. Elucidation of the life cycle of the intestinal protozoan *Blastocystis hominis*. *Parasitol. Res.* **81:**446–450.
56. **Soper, D. E., R. C. Bump, and W. G. Hurt.** 1990. Bacterial vaginosis and trichomoniasis vaginitis are risk factors for cuff cellulitis after abdominal hysterectomy. *Am. J. Obstet. Gynecol.* **78:**1016–1023.
57. **Troll, H., H. Marti, and N. Weiss.** 1997. Simple differential detection of *Entamoeba histolytica* and *Entamoeba dispar* in fresh stool specimens by sodium acetate-acetic acid-formalin concentration and PCR. *J. Clin. Microbiol.* **35:** 1701–1705.
58. **Walderich, B., A. Weber, and J. Knobloch.** 1997. Differentiation of *Entamoeba histolytica* and *Entamoeba dispar* from German travelers and residents of endemic areas. *Am. J. Trop. Med. Hyg.* **57:**70–74.
59. **Weiss, J. B.** 1995. DNA probes and PCR for diagnosis of parasitic infections. *Clin. Microbiol. Rev.* **8:**113–130.
60. **Wilson, M., P. Schantz, and N. Pieniazek.** 1995. Diagnosis of parasitic infections: immunologic and molecular methods, p. 1159–1170. *In* P. R. Murray, E. J. Baron, M. A. Pfaller, F. C. Tenover, and R. H. Yolken (ed.), *Manual of Clinical Microbiology*, 6th ed. American Society for Microbiology, Washington, D.C.
61. **Yang, J., and T. Scholten.** 1977. *Dientamoeba fragilis*: a review with notes on its epidemiology, pathogenicity, mode of transmission and diagnosis. *Am. J. Trop. Med. Hyg.* **26:** 16–22.
62. **Yule, A., M. C. A. Gellan, J. D. Oriel, and J. Packers.** 1987. Detection of *Trichomonas vaginalis* antigen in women by enzyme immunoassay. *J. Clin. Pathol.* **40:**566–568.
63. **Zierdt, C. H.** 1991. *Blastocystis hominis*—past and future. *Clin. Microbiol. Rev.* **4:**61–79.
64. **Zierdt, C. H., W. S. Zierdt, and B. Nagy.** 1995. Enzyme-linked immunosorbent assay for detection of serum antibody to *Blastocystis hominis* in symptomatic infections. *J. Parasitol.* **81:**127–129.

Cryptosporidium, Cyclospora, and *Isospora**

YNES R. ORTEGA

110

Cryptosporidium, Cyclospora, and *Isospora* inhabit the intestinal mucosa and cause diarrheal illness in humans. These coccidian parasites infect immunocompetent as well as immunocompromised individuals. Transmission has been associated with water and food, and *Cryptosporidium* can also be contracted directly via fecal-oral contamination.

The first reported description of *Cryptosporidium* was in 1907, for an isolate from the gastric crypts of a laboratory mouse; subsequently, this organism was found in a number of animals, including chickens, turkeys, mice, rats, guinea pigs, horses, pigs, calves, sheep, rhesus monkeys, dogs, and cats. It was not until 1976 that *Cryptosporidium parvum* infection was recognized in a child with acute self-limiting diarrhea. This infection is now widely recognized as a cause of disease in humans, particularly those who are immunocompromised or immunodeficient. The mean prevalence rate of *C. parvum* in Europe and the United States is between 1 and 3%, although it is considerably higher in developing countries. Outbreaks associated with *Cryptosporidium* have been reported in the United States as well as overseas (24).

When patients were first seen with infections caused by *Cyclospora*, they reported symptoms of a "flu-like" illness with nausea, vomiting, anorexia, weight loss, and explosive diarrhea lasting 1 to 3 weeks. Subsequently, the organisms were thought to represent a new pathogen, possibly a flagellate, an unsporulated coccidian, a large *Cryptosporidium* sp., a blue-green alga, or a coccidian-like body. These organisms have now been identified as coccidia in the genus *Cyclospora*. *Cyclospora* has been found in North, Central, and South America, the Caribbean, Africa, Southeast Asia, England, Eastern Europe, and Australia (14, 16, 23, 27). Most reports of cyclosporiasis in developed countries are in travelers and expatriates, although indigenous infections in people with no travel history and outbreaks in the United States have been described (17). Most of the U.S. outbreaks in 1996 were thought to be food associated and occurred in states east of the Rocky Mountains (14).

Isospora belli was discovered in 1860 but not named until 1923. Although this organism has been found in various parts of the world, there are some tropical locations in the Western Hemisphere where well-defined endemic infections have been identified. Both adults and children can become infected, and symptoms are usually transient unless the patient is immunocompromised. *Isospora* is rare in immunocompetent people; its prevalence ranges from 0.2 to 3% in AIDS patients in the United States to 8 to 20% in AIDS patients in Africa and Haiti. *Isospora* is endemic in many parts of Africa, Asia, and South America (12).

Drug therapy is available for both *Cyclospora* and *Isospora* infections. None is currently available for *Cryptosporidium* infection, which is self-limiting in immunocompetent people but life-threatening in immunocompromised individuals (9).

TAXONOMY AND DESCRIPTION

Cryptosporidium, Cyclospora, and *Isospora* are coccidian parasites that infect humans. They belong to the subphylum Apicomplexa because they have an apical complex, generally consisting of a polar ring, micronemes, and rhoptries. All life cycle stages of these parasites are intracellular.

Cryptosporidium belongs to the family Cryptosporidiidae, and its development has been characterized as intracellular but extracytoplasmic. The parasitophorous vacuole containing the intracellular parasites communicates with the host via a "feeder organelle." When excreted, oocysts contain sporozoites, but unlike most coccidian parasites, excreted *Cryptosporidium* oocysts contain infectious sporozoites and do not have sporocysts. The asexual life cycle stages of *Cryptosporidium* occur in the intestinal epithelium, where the parasite goes through two merogony stages: type I meronts contain eight merozoites, and type II meronts contain four merozoites. The parasite is intracellular but extracytoplasmic, as demonstrated by transmission electron microscopy of intestinal biopsy specimens. The parasitophorous vacuole appears to bulge out from the cell into the gut lumen (Fig. 1A). Oocysts, which measure 4 to 6 μm in diameter, are generated as two types that differ by wall thickness. Approximately 20% of the oocysts do not form the thick, two-layered, environmentally resistant oocyst wall. These thin-walled oocysts are environmentally sensitive and excyst endogenously, thereby resulting in autoinfection. Conversely, thick-walled oocysts, which are environmentally resistant, are shed in the feces or sputum and are immediately infectious to other hosts.

Immunosuppressed individuals present with the most se-

* This chapter contains information presented in chapter 106 by George R. Healy and Lynne S. Garcia in the sixth edition of this Manual.

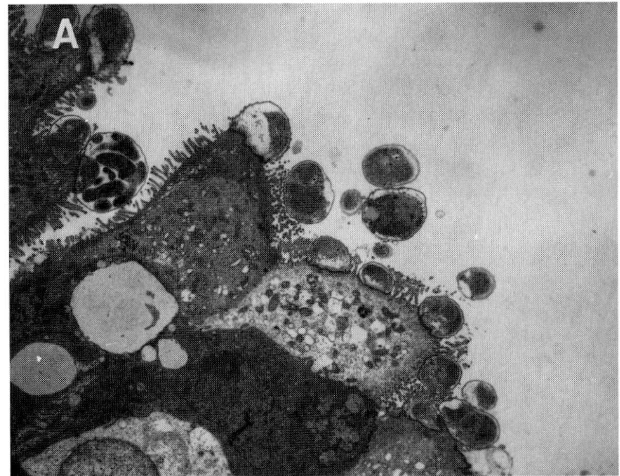

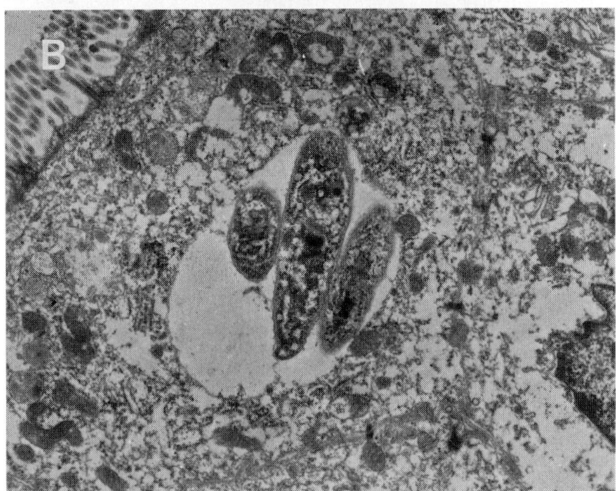

FIGURE 1 Transmission electron microscopy of infected intestinal tissues. (A) *C. parvum*. (B) *C. cayetanensis*.

vere and life-threatening cases, with heavy shedding of oocysts. The thin-walled oocysts that can recycle are thought to be responsible for severe disease in these patients, even those who are no longer exposed to the environmentally resistant oocysts. The severity is exacerbated by lack of an effective therapy (9, 12, 31).

Cyclospora and *Isospora* belong to the family Eimeriidae, for which development occurs in the host cell proper. Oocysts contain sporocysts, each of which contains sporozoites (21). Sporogony typically occurs outside the host, requiring the passage of some time before oocysts are infective to a new host. *Cyclospora cayetanensis* and *I. belli* also infect the small intestine. These two parasite species can infect immunocompromised patients, but treatment is available (see below). The intermediary life cycle stages occur in the cytoplasm of epithelial cells (6, 28). The intracellular life cycle stages of *Cyclospora* are localized in the cytoplasm of enterocytes. The diagnostic stages for *Cyclospora* and *Isospora* are unsporulated oocysts shed in feces (Fig. 2). *Cyclospora* oocysts are 8 to 10 μm in diameter, and *Isospora* oocysts are 20 to 30 μm by 10 to 19 μm. Unsporulated *Isospora* oocysts require 12 to 48 h to mature, whereas unsporulated *Cyclospora* oocysts also excreted in feces require 7 to 15 days to become fully sporulated and infectious. Oocysts of all three of these coccidians remain viable and infectious when stored in potassium dichromate. Descriptions of the three genera are summarized in Table 1.

COLLECTION, TRANSPORT, AND STORAGE

Specimens from patients suspected of being infected with any of these coccidia should be stored in 10% formalin, 5% formalin, or SAF before being sent to the laboratory or immediately upon receipt. Fresh stools can be sent to the laboratory, but preserved specimens are preferred, particularly since the *Cryptosporidium* oocysts are immediately infectious on passage. Sputum samples from immunocompromised patients must be collected in 5 to 10% formalin and then examined as described for the fecal samples. One stool specimen may not be sufficient to make the diagnosis, particularly if an immunocompetent patient is in the process of recovery or if the patient is in the asymptomatic, carrier state.

In patients with severe watery diarrhea, there may be tremendous dilution of the fecal specimen, and concentrated specimen sediment should be used for smear preparation before being subjected to special staining.

If specified, stool samples can be collected and stored in 2.5% potassium dichromate for investigational purposes; however, potassium dichromate is not a preservative, and samples should be considered infectious. These samples should be stored refrigerated at 4°C.

CLINICAL SIGNIFICANCE

C. parvum infects the brush border of the intestinal epithelium. Dissemination has been reported, and *C. parvum* can infect epithelial cells from other organs such as those of the respiratory tract and biliary tree. Immunocompetent patients develop a profuse watery diarrhea accompanied by epigastric cramping pain, nausea, and anorexia that is usually self-limiting and lasts for 15 days. Immunocompromised patients (AIDS patients or those receiving immunosuppressive drugs) develop a severe diarrhea (3 to 6 liters/day). For these patients, the disease is prolonged, with profuse watery diarrhea persisting for several weeks to months or years (5). In patients with HIV infections, the CD4 cell count is the best marker for the ability of the immune system to clear the infection. Patients with CD4 cell counts of 180 cells/mm^3 or more may have a self-limiting *Cryptosporidium* infection. The pathogenesis of the diarrhea is not clear. The presence of a toxin has been suggested but not demonstrated to date (5, 9).

Cryptosporidium infection is highly associated with traveling, exposure to farm animals, and person-to-person transmission in settings such as day care centers and medical institutions. A large number of waterborne outbreaks have been reported in the literature, such as those in Milwaukee and Georgia, with more than 400,000 cases reported (9). Although there is no definite therapy, spiramycin may decrease diarrhea in early infections but is not effective in advanced infections. Azithromycin has shown promising results (9, 31). Nitazoxanide has also been evaluated in a clinical trial in 12 AIDS patients with cryptosporidiosis in Africa; not only was the drug effective in eradicating or reducing *Cryptosporidium* oocyst shedding in 7 of 12 patients, but also it was effective in eliminating other parasites (7). Paromomycin has been reported to be effective in AIDS patients with cryptosporidiosis (8). Alternative experimental therapies evaluated in humans involve the use of hyperimmune bovine colostrum (8). Monoclonal antibodies and

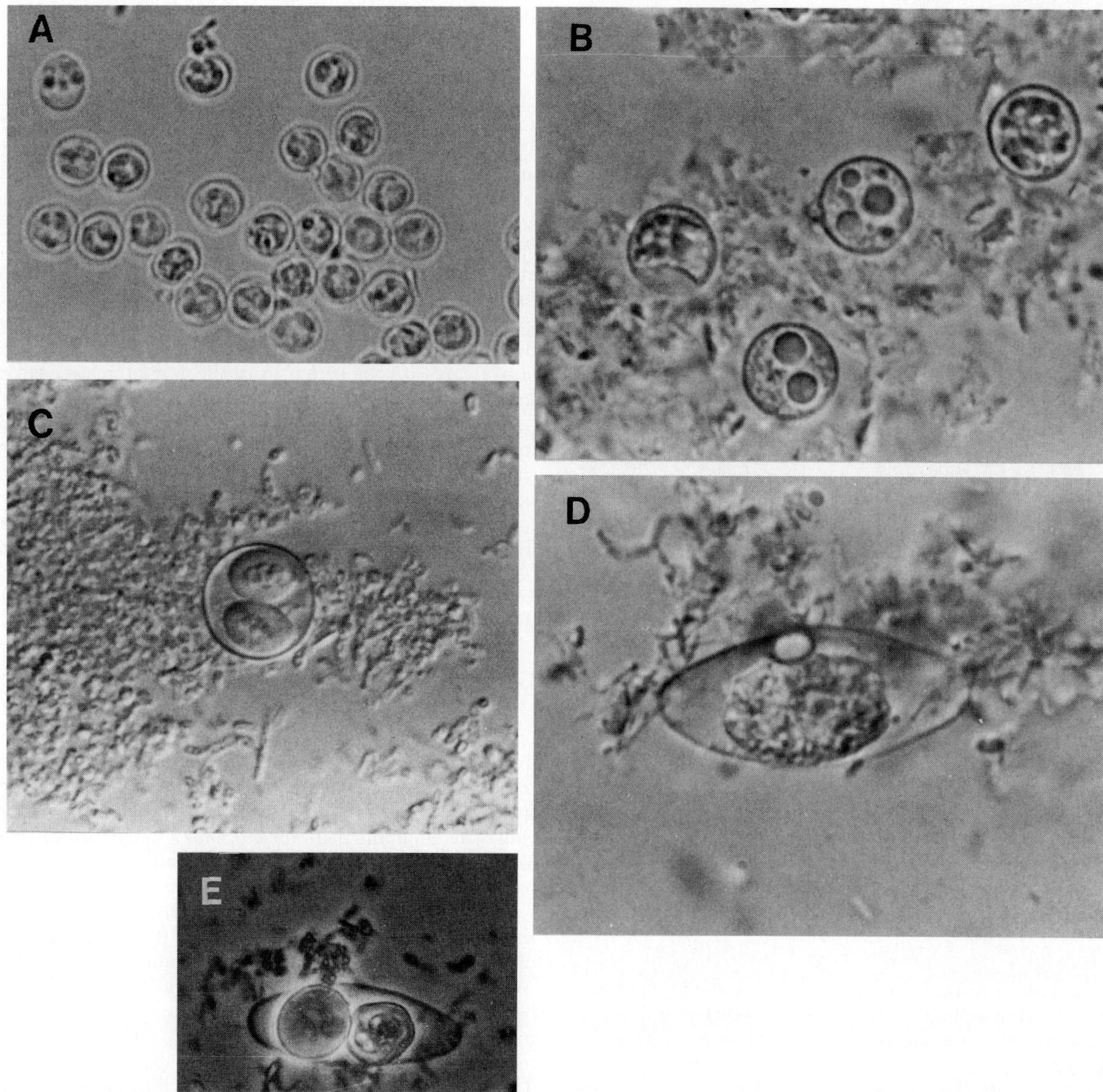

FIGURE 2 Coccidia, unstained oocysts. (A) *C. parvum* oocysts. (B) *C. cayetanensis* unsporulated oocysts. (C) *C. cayetanensis* sporulated oocyst. (D) *I. belli* immature oocyst. (E) *I. belli* sporulated oocyst.

TABLE 1 Characteristics of *Cryptosporidium*, *Cyclospora*, and *Isospora*

Characteristic	*C. parvum*	*C. cayetanensis*	*I. belli*
Size (μm)	4–6	8–10	20–30 by 10–19
No. of sporocysts/oocyst	0	2	2
No. of sporozoites/sporocyst	4/oocyst	2	4
Sporulation time after excretion	0[a]	7–14 days	24–48 h
Stain (modified acid-fast)	Yes	Yes (variable)	Yes

[a] Already sporulated.

hyperimmune hen egg yolk against cryptosporidiosis have also been tried in animal models with some success.

I. belli organisms infect the entire intestine and produce severe intestinal disease. It is more frequently identified in AIDS patients. Deaths from overwhelming infections have been reported, especially in immunocompromised patients. Symptoms include diarrhea, nausea, steatorrhea, headache, and weight loss. The disease may persist for months or years. Shedding of oocysts may be variable, and it is therefore recommended that multiple samples be examined. The treatment of choice is trimethoprim-sulfamethoxazole. In HIV patients, recurrence is common after therapy is discontinued. Pyrimethamine is an alternative treatment (8, 12, 31).

C. cayetanensis has been associated with prolonged diarrheal illness lasting up to 7 weeks. Cyclosporiasis is characterized by nonbloody diarrhea and concomitant weight loss, anorexia, bloating, abdominal cramping, malaise, and fatigue. Some reported cases have included mild fever. Symptoms tend to be more severe in AIDS patients and persist for up to 70 days (31). *Cyclospora* outbreaks in 1996 and 1997 were initially associated epidemiologically with ingestion of strawberries and later were associated with imported berries, baby lettuce, and basil. To date, *Cyclospora* oocysts have not been isolated or detected in potentially contaminated produce associated with any of the reported outbreaks. Most of the cases were reported during April to August (3, 4, 14). To date, trimethoprim-sulfamethoxazole is the only therapy effective for eradication of the infection (15, 19, 23, 27).

DIAGNOSIS

Cyclospora (8 to 10 μm) and *Isospora* (10 to 19 μm by 20 to 30 μm) oocysts can be detected in direct wet mounts in heavy infections during the ova and parasite examination. However, most infections are not heavy, and so it is necessary to examine the sample after concentration and modified acid-fast staining of the concentrated sediment (Fig. 3). *Isospora* is often seen and identified in the routine wet-smear examination of the concentrated sediment. Although these oocysts are considerably larger than *Giardia lamblia* cysts, they have been confused with shrunk *Giardia* cysts when the organism within the cyst wall is distorted. Measurement of the cyst or oocyst wall can easily resolve this problem.

Cryptosporidium

Cryptosporidium oocysts (4 to 6 μm) are very small and can be overlooked in fecal preparations or confused with yeast cells (13); they do not stain with iodine. The normal permanent stains (trichrome, iron-hematoxylin) do not adequately stain *Cryptosporidium* spp., although oocysts may be seen in these preparations, especially from patients with heavy infections. The organisms can be stained with auramine-rhodamine stains; however, the presumptive identification should be confirmed by using modified acid-fast stains or immunoassay reagents. Fixed fecal specimens can be processed with several modified acid-fast stains, many of which are very satisfactory in demonstrating the organisms. The destaining reagent is critical, and 1 to 3% sulfuric acid is recommended; acid-alcohol decolorizers should not be used because they will remove too much color, making the identification more difficult. It is important to remember that microsporidia are also present in approximately 30% of severely immunocompromised patients who have cryptosporidiosis. Diagnostic procedures used for the identification of *C. parvum* will not be appropriate for the identification of

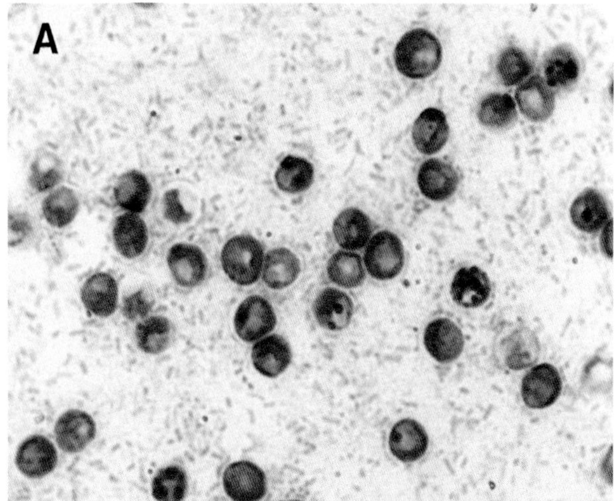

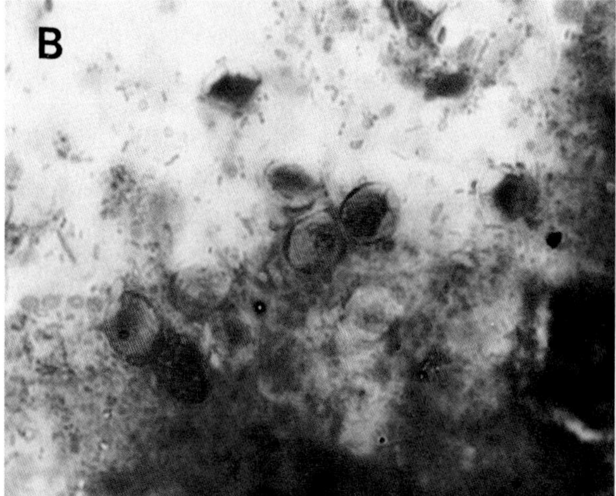

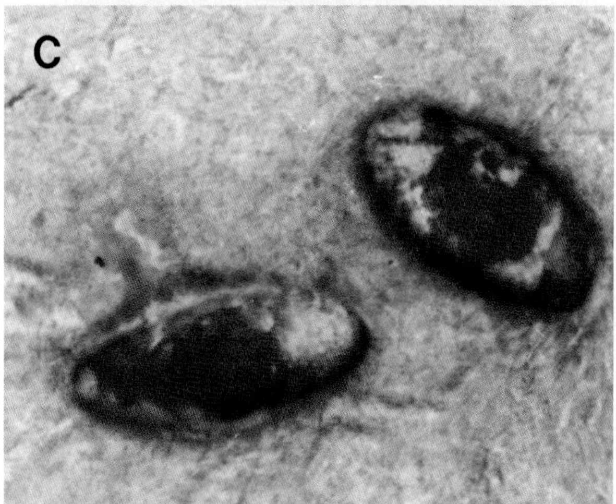

FIGURE 3 Acid-fast stain. (A) *C. parvum* (4 to 6 μm). (B) *C. cayetanensis* (8 to 10 μm). (C) *I. belli* (20 to 30 μm long by 10 to 19 μm wide).

microsporidial spores. Modified trichrome stains and optical brightening agents (calcofluor white) can be used for that purpose.

In patients who have cryptosporidiosis, the more formed and normal the consistency of the stool, the better the chances are that artifact material will be present and will be confused with oocysts. It is also important to remember that there is a direct correlation between the consistency of the stool and the number of oocysts seen; the more diarrheic the stool, the more oocysts are present.

Additional diagnostic testing for *Cryptosporidium* spp. involving immunoassays (fluorescent antibody [FA]) or enzyme immunoassay [EIA]) are also available (18). Immunofluorescence assays and enzyme-linked immunosorbent assay (ELISA) (30) are available commercially and can be used to specifically identify the organisms. IDEIA (Dako Corp., Carpenteria, Calif.) and Merifluor DFA and IFA (Meridian Diagnostics, Inc., Cincinnati, Ohio) (10, 26) were reported to have 100% specificity and sensitivity (Fig. 4). Prospect-EIA (Alexon, Inc., Sunnyvale, Calif.) and ColorVue-EIA (Seradyn, Inc., Indianapolis, Ind.) are also effective, but their sensitivity and specificity range between 93 and 97%. Crypto-Cel IF-DFA (Bradsure Biological, Ltd.) is also available but has not been compared with the previously described procedures (26). PCR has been described, but its possible role and use in a clinical laboratory have not yet been determined (2).

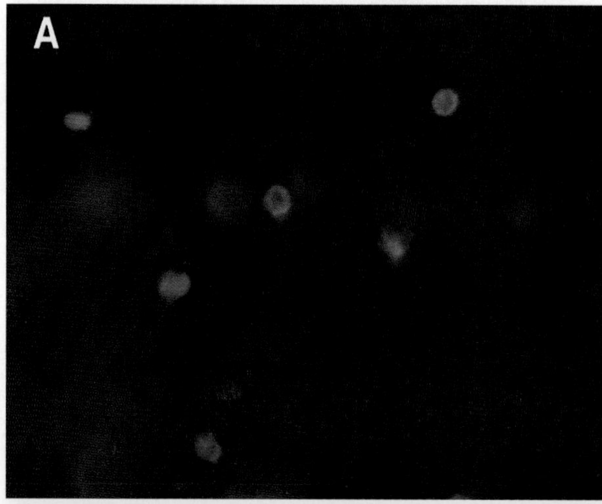

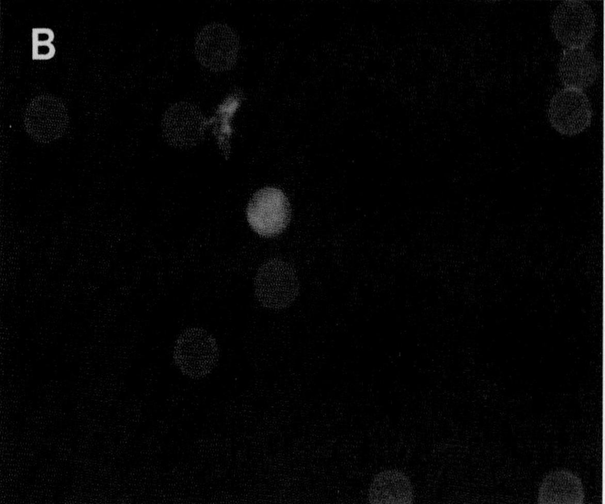

FIGURE 4 (A) *C. parvum* oocysts (monoclonal antibody fluorescent stain). (B) *C. cayetanensis* autofluorescence.

When examining preparations for histologic tests, developmental stages of *C. parvum* can be found at all levels of the intestinal tract, with the most heavily infected being the jejunum. Routine hematoxylin-and-eosin staining can be used to demonstrate the organisms. By using regular light microscopy, the organisms can be seen as small (~1- to 3-μm), round structures along the brush border. Some of the developmental stages are more difficult to see and may require electron microscopy. Also, in compromised patients, disseminated infections have been seen in other body sites including the lungs. It is very unlikely that the developing stages of *Cryptosporidium* will be confused with those of *Cyclospora*, since the developing stages of *Cyclospora* occur within a vacuole at the luminal end of the enterocyte rather than at the brush border. Developmental stages of *I. belli* also occur within the enterocyte rather than the brush border and hence should not be confused with *Cryptosporidium*.

Isospora

Sporulated or unsporulated oocysts can be observed by direct observation of unfixed or fixed specimens under light or phase-contrast microscopy. Most infections are not associated with specimens with a high number of oocysts; therefore, samples should be examined by modified acid-fast staining. Oocysts recovered from polyvinyl alcohol-preserved stool specimens may not be easy to detect; organisms from the same patient but preserved in formalin-based fixatives should be visible in direct or concentrated sediment wet preparations. Concentration procedures are effective, are recommended, and facilitate detection. Like *Cryptosporidium*, the oocysts of *I. belli* can be stained with auramine/rhodamine, but modified acid-fast staining may be required for confirmation (9).

Cyclospora

Identification of *C. cayetanensis* in heavy infections can be made by examining wet specimen preparations under light or phase-contrast microscopy. The organism stains orange with safranin. Oocysts do not stain well with hematoxylin, Giemsa, trichrome, choromotrope, Gram-chromotrope, Grocott-Gomori methenamine-silver nitrate, iodine, or periodic acid-Schiff stains. With the modified acid-fast stains, the *Cyclospora* oocysts will stain acid-fast variable; some *Cyclospora* oocysts will stain light pink to red, and if the oocyst load is low, the oocysts can be missed if they did not stain. Some oocysts will not stain, and they will take on a glassy, wrinkled appearance (9, 27). Reported modifications to the acid-fast stains include microwaving the samples for 30 to 60 s during safranin staining to increase the number of oocysts that stain (29). It is important for laboratories to measure the diameter of all acid-fast oocysts, particularly if they appear to be somewhat larger than those of *C. parvum*.

Autofluorescence (Fig. 4) is an additional technique that can be used to confirm the presence of *Cyclospora* (16, 22, 27). This factor should be taken into consideration when performing immunofluorescence assays to detect other parasites such as *Cryptosporidium* and *Giardia*. The oocysts autofluoresce strong green (450 to 490 diffraction mirror excitation filter) or intense blue (365 DM excitation filter) under UV epifluorescence. Generally, the appearance is that of small, round fluorescing circles; the internal portion of the oocyst generally does not stain. A PCR technique has been described, but it has not yet been evaluated in a clinical laboratory to determine its sensitivity and specificity compared to the other, established diagnostic techniques (32). Specimens can be concentrated by the formalin-ethyl acetate method, which involves centrifugation at 500 × *g* for 10 min (9).

Summary

Cryptosporidium and *Isospora* oocysts stain intensely purple-red to pink in modified acid-fast staining techniques (Fig. 3), whereas *Cyclospora* tends to be much more acid-fast variable. Specimens can be concentrated by the formalin-ethyl acetate method at 500 × *g* for 10 min (9), and the sediment can be used for smear preparation before staining. Because *Cyclospora* and *Cryptosporidium* are acid-fast positive and look alike, it is important that laboratories carefully measure the diameter of the organisms, particularly if they appear to be larger than *Cryptosporidium.* Although the mature *Cryptosporidium* oocysts contain four sporozoites, these structures are not always visible in every oocyst; if they are not visible, it is more likely that *Cryptosporidium* and *Cyclospora* will be confused. Laboratories just beginning to perform procedures for the confirmation of intestinal coccidian infections should always use positive control material along with their patient specimens; this will help eliminate the possibility of either false-positive or false-negative results.

SEROLOGIC TESTING AND REPORTING OF RESULTS

Serologic testing of patients with cryptosporidiosis (25) by using EIA has been described. At about 10 days postinfection, a 27-kDa antigen seems to be recognized by hyperimmune sera and is consistent in *Cryptosporidium* infections. This band recognition peaks and remains until 4 to 5 weeks postinfection. Dot blots and Western blots to 15-, 17-, and 27-kDa antigens are being evaluated but are currently restricted to research laboratories. To date, there is no commercially available test (1).

Outbreaks of cyclosporiasis and cryptosporidiosis have been reported more frequently in recent years. In 1997, *Cryptosporidium* became reportable by the laboratory and/or the provider in all states except Washington, Utah, Idaho, Wisconsin, Pennsylvania, Virginia, North Carolina, and Alabama. *Cyclospora* is reportable by the laboratory and/or provider in Florida, South Carolina, Massachusetts, Connecticut, and New York City (6a).

CONCLUSION

Cryptosporidium, Cyclospora, and *Isospora* are important agents of diarrhea in both immunocompetent and immunocompromised patients. Epidemiologic considerations for these organisms emphasize transmission by environmentally resistant oocysts, possible potential reservoir hosts for zoonotic transmission, documentation of person-to-person transmission in day care centers, nosocomial transmission within the health care setting, occurrence of asymptomatic infections (infective carrier state with *Cryptosporidium*), possible environmental distribution resulting in the possibility and/or probability of waterborne or food-borne transmission, and the link between disease outcomes and the immune status of the human host. Diagnosis of infections by these three coccidia will be improved as laboratories adopt the procedures described in this chapter and look for these infections in a more systematic fashion. Adequate client information regarding these coccidia as the cause of disease will be required and will help educate the health care community about potential human infections and their clinical relevance.

REFERENCES

1. **Arrowood, M. J.** 1997. Diagnosis, p. 43–64. *In* R. Fayer (ed.), Cryptosporidium *and Cryptosporidiosis.* CRC Press, Inc., Boca Raton, Fla.
2. **Balatbat, A. B., G. W. Jordan, Y. J. Tang, and J. Silva, Jr.** 1996. Detection of *Cryptosporidium parvum* DNA in human feces by nested PCR. *J. Clin. Microbiol.* **34:** 1769–1772.
3. **Centers for Disease Control and Prevention.** 1996. Food borne outbreak of diarrheal illness associated with *Cryptosporidium parvum*—Minnesota, 1995. *Morbid. Mortal. Weekly Rep.* **45:**783–784.
4. **Centers for Disease Control and Prevention.** 1997. Update. Outbreaks of cyclosporiasis—United States, 1997. *Morbid. Mortal. Weekly Rep.* **46:**461–462.
5. **Colford, J. M., I. B. Tager, Jr., A. M. Hirozawa, G. F. Lemp, T. Aragon, and C. Petersen.** 1996. Cryptosporidiosis among patients infected with human immunodeficiency virus. Factors related to symptomatic infection and survival. *Am. J. Epidemiol.* **144:**807–816.
6. **Connor, B. A., D. R. Shlim, J. V. Scholes, J. L. Rayburn, J. Reidy, and R. Rajah.** 1993. Pathologic changes in the small bowel in nine patients with diarrhea associated with a coccidia-like body. *Ann. Intern. Med.* **119:**377–382.

6a. **Dietz, V. (Centers for Disease Control and Prevention).** Personal communication.

7. **Duombo, O., J. F. Rossignol, E. Pichard, H. A. Traore, M. Dembele, M. Diakite, F. Traore, and D. A. Diallo.** 1997. Nitazoxanide in the treatment of cryptosporidial diarrhea and other intestinal parasitic infections associated with acquired immunodeficiency syndrome in tropical Africa. *Am. J. Trop. Med. Hyg.* **56:**637–639.
8. **Flynn, P. M.** 1996. Emerging diarrheal pathogens: *Cryptosporidium parvum, Isospora belli, Cyclospora* species, and microsporidia. *Pediatr. Ann.* **25:**480–487.
9. **Garcia, L. S., and D. A. Bruckner.** 1997. *Diagnostic Medical Parasitology,* 3rd ed., p. 54–83. ASM Press, Washington, D.C.
10. **Garcia, L. S., A. C. Shum, and D. A. Bruckner.** 1992. Evaluation of a new monoclonal antibody combination reagent for direct fluorescence detection of *Giardia* cysts and *Cryptosporidum* oocysts in human fecal specimens. *J. Clin. Microbiol.* **30:**3255–3257.
11. **Garlipp, C. R., P. V. Bottini, and A. T. Teixeira.** 1995. The relevance of laboratory diagnosis of human cryptosporidiosis and other coccidia. *Rev. Inst. Med. Trop. Sao Paulo* **37:**467–469.
12. **Goodgame, R. W.** 1996. Understanding intestinal spore-forming protozoa: cryptosporidia, microsporidia, *Isospora,* and *Cyclospora. Ann. Intern. Med.* **124:**429–441.
13. **Greenberg, P. D., J. Koch, and J. P. Cello.** 1996. Diagnosis of *Cryptosporidium parvum* in patients with severe diarrhea and AIDS. *Dig. Dis. Sci.* **41:**2286–2290.
14. **Herwaldt, B. L., M.-L. Ackers, and the *Cyclospora* Working Group.** 1997. An outbreak in 1996 of cyclosporiasis associated with imported raspberries. *N. Engl. J. Med.* **336:** 1548–1558.
15. **Hoge, C. W., D. R. Shlim, M. Ghimire, J. G. Rabold, P. Pandey, A. Walch, R. Rajah, P. Gaudio, and P. Echeverria.** 1995. Placebo-controlled trial of co-trimoxazole for *Cyclospora* infections among travelers and foreign residents in Nepal. *Lancet* **345:**691–693.
16. **Hoge, C. W., D. Shlim, R. Rajah, J. Triplett, M. Shear, J. G. Rabold, and P. Echeverria.** 1993. Epidemiology of

diarrhoeal illness associated with coccidian-like organism among travelers and foreign residents in Nepal. *Lancet* **341:** 1175–1179.

17. **Huang, P., J. T. Weber, D. M. Sosin, P. M. Griffin, E. G. Long, J. J. Murphy, F. Kocka, C. Peters, and C. Kallick.** 1995. The first reported outbreak of diarrheal illness associated with *Cyclospora* in the United States. *Ann. Intern. Med.* **123:**409–414.
18. **MacPherson, D. W., and R. McQueen.** 1993. Cryptosporidiosis: multiattribute evaluation of six diagnostic methods. *J. Clin. Microbiol.* **31:**198–202.
19. **Madico, G., R. H. Gilman, L. Cabrera, and C. R. Sterling.** 1997. Epidemiology and treatment of *Cyclospora cayetanensis* infection in Peruvian children. *Clin. Infect. Dis.* **24:** 977–981.
20. **Marcial-Seoane, M. A., and J. Serrano-Olmo.** 1995. Intestinal infection with *Isospora belli*. *P. R. Health Sci. J.* **14:** 137–140.
21. **Ortega, Y., C. R. Sterling, and R. H. Gilman.** 1994. A new coccidian parasite (Apicomplexa: Eimeriidae) from humans. *J. Parasitol.* **80:**625–629.
22. **Ortega, Y. R., C. R. Sterling, R. H. Gilman, V. A. Cama, and F. Diaz.** 1993. *Cyclospora* species—a new protozoan pathogen of humans. *N. Engl. J. Med.* **328:**1308–1312.
23. **Pape, J. W., R. I. Verdier, M. Boncy, J. Boncy, and W. Johnson.** 1994. *Cyclospora* infection in adults infected with HIV. Clinical manifestations, treatment, and prophylaxis. *Ann. Intern. Med.* **121:**654–657.
24. **Pollok, R. C. G., and M. J. G. Farthing.** 1997. Intestinal parasites. *Curr. Opin. Infect. Dis.* **10:**414–418.
25. **Rodriguez Hernandez, J., A. Canut Blasco, and A. M. Martin Sanchez.** 1994. Epidemiology and diagnosis of *Cryptosporidium* spp. parasitosis in children: usefulness of the serologic study. *Rev. Clin. Esp.* **194:**330–333.
26. **Siddons, C. A., P. A. Chapman, and B. A. Rush.** 1992. Evaluation of an enzyme immunoassay kit for detecting *Cryptosporidium* in faeces and environmental samples. *J. Clin. Microbiol.* **45:**479–482.
27. **Soave, R.** 1996. State of the art clinical article. *Cyclospora*: an overview. *Clin. Infect. Dis.* **23:**429–437.
28. **Sun, T., C. F. Ilardi, D. Asnis, A. R. Bresciani, S. Goldenberg, B. Roberts, and S. Techberg.** 1996. Light and electron microscopy identification of *Cyclospora* species in the small intestine. *Clin. Microbiol. Infect. Dis.* **105:** 216–220.
29. **Visvesvara, G. S., H. Moura, E. Kovacs-Nace, S. Wallace, and M. L. Eberhard.** 1997. Uniform staining of *Cyclospora* oocysts in fecal smears by a modified safranin technique with microwave heating. *J. Clin. Microbiol.* **35:** 730–733.
30. **Weitz, J. C.** 1995. Detection of fecal *Cryptosporidium parvum* antigens using an ELISA technique. *Rev. Med. Chile* **123:**330–333.
31. **Wittner, M., H. B. Tanowitz, and L. M. Weiss.** 1993. Parasitic infections in AIDS patients. Cryptosporidiosis, isosporiasis, microsporidiosis, cyclosporiasis. *Infect. Dis. Clin.* **7:**569–586.
32. **Yoder, K. E., S. Orntipa, and D. A. Relman.** 1996. PCR-based detection of the intestinal pathogen *Cyclospora*, p. 169–174. *In* D. Pershing (ed.), *PCR Protocol for Emerging Infectious Diseases*. ASM Press, Washington, D.C.

Microsporidia*

RAINER WEBER AND ELIZABETH U. CANNING

111

THE ORGANISMS

The nontaxonomic term "microsporidia" refers to a group of obligate intracellular, spore-forming protists belonging to the phylum *Microspora*. More than 100 microsporidial genera and 1,000 species that are parasitic in every major animal group have been identified (4). To date, six genera (*Enterocytozoon*, *Encephalitozoon*, *Nosema*, *Pleistophora*, *Vittaforma*, and *Trachipleistophora*) and unclassified microsporidia have been implicated in human infections (Table 1).

Microsporidia develop intracellularly exclusively and have no metabolically active stages outside the host cell. A unique life cycle involving a proliferative merogonic stage followed by a sporogonic stage results in environmentally resistant spores of unique structure. Mature spores contain a tubular extrusion apparatus for injecting infective spore contents into the host cell.

Microsporidia are considered to be true eukaryotes because they have a membrane-bound nucleus, an intracytoplasmic membrane system, and chromosome separation on mitotic spindles, but they are unusual eukaryotes in that they have 70S ribosomes, no mitochondria, and simple vesicular Golgi membranes. It has been postulated that phylogenetically they are ancient protists that diverged before the mitochondrial endosymbiosis. However, recent results of molecular analyses of the α- and β-tubulins and the demonstration of the presence of a 70-kDa heat shock protein (HSP70) have suggested that the ancestor of the amitochondriate protists could have been a mitochondriate eukaryote and that microsporidia might phylogenetically be a sister group of fungi (20, 27).

DESCRIPTION OF THE GENERA AND SPECIES

Enterocytozoon bieneusi develops in direct contact with the host cell cytoplasm (Fig. 1). The proliferative and sporogonial forms are rounded multinucleate plasmodia measuring up to 6 μm in diameter. The oval spores measure 0.7 to 1.0 by 1.1 to 1.6 μm. The polar tubule has five to seven coils that appear in two rows when seen in transverse section by transmission electron microscopy (4, 37).

Encephalitozoon spp. develop intracellularly in a parasitophorous vacuole bounded by a membrane of presumed host cell origin. Nuclei of all stages are unpaired. Meronts divide repeatedly by binary fission and lie close to the vacuolar membrane. Sporonts appear free in the center of the vacuole and divide into two sporoblasts, which mature into spores. The spores measure 1.0 to 1.5 by 2.0 to 3.0 μm, and the polar tubule has four to eight coils (4).

Human isolates of three *Encephalitozoon* spp. and *Encephalitozoon cuniculi* of animal origin are morphologically almost identical. In 1991, *Encephalitozoon hellem* was distinguished from *E. cuniculi* on the basis of the different protein patterns found by sodium dodecyl sulfate-polyacrylamide gel electrophoresis separation and immunoblotting (12). In 1993, *Septata intestinalis* was described and was named on the basis of the morphological finding that the intracellular vacuoles containing the parasite showed a unique parasite-secreted fibrillar network surrounding the developing organisms so that the vacuoles appeared septate (2). Subsequently, on the basis of phylogenetic analyses, it was proposed that *S. intestinalis* be regarded as a species of the genus *Encephalitozoon*, and it was reclassified as *Encephalitozoon intestinalis* (22). Analyses of the nucleotide sequence of the small-subunit (SSU) rRNA have confirmed that the three *Encephalitozoon* spp. are indeed distinct organisms. *E. cuniculi* has also been found to cause disease in humans (8). Recently, three different strains of *E. cuniculi* (the so-called rabbit, mouse, and canine strains) have been identified phenotypically, by Western blotting analysis of spore antigens, and genetically, by determination of differences in the rRNA gene intergenic spacer region (14).

Pleistophora sp. develops in contact with the host cell cytoplasm, forming sporophorous vesicles enclosing spores in variable numbers within a thick, amorphous, parasite-formed coat. Nuclei are unpaired. Multinucleate plasmodia are formed by merogonic and sporogonic proliferation. The spores contain polar tubules with 9 to 12 coils and measure 2.8 by 3.2 to 3.4 μm (4).

Trachipleistophora hominis also forms sporophorous vesicles, but these do not arise from multinucleate plasmodia. The vesicles, which contain 2 to more than 32 spores, enlarge as the number of spores increases. The nuclei are unpaired in all stages of development. Division of meronts and sporonts is by binary fission. The pyriform spores measure 2.4 by 4.0 μm and have about 11 coils (18, 23). *Trachipleisto-*

* This chapter contains information presented in chapter 106 by George R. Healy and Lynne S. Garcia in the sixth edition of this Manual.

TABLE 1 Microsporidial species pathogenic in humans, and clinical manifestations

Microsporidial species	Clinical manifestations	
	Immunocompromised patients	Immunocompetent persons
Enterocytozoon bieneusi	Chronic diarrhea, wasting syndrome, "AIDS cholangiopathy," cholangitis, acalculous cholecystitis, chronic sinusitis, chronic cough, pneumonitis	Self-limiting diarrhea in adults and children, traveler's diarrhea, asymptomatic carriers
Encephalitozoon hellem	Disseminated infection, keratoconjunctivitis, sinusitis, bronchitis, pneumonia, nephritis, ureteritis, cystitis, prostatitis, urethritis	Not described
Encephalitozoon intestinalis (formerly *Septata intestinalis*)	Chronic diarrhea, cholangiopathy, sinusitis, bronchitis, pneumonitis, nephritis, bone infection	Self-limiting diarrhea, asymptomatic carriers
Encephalitozoon cuniculi	Disseminated infection, keratoconjunctivitis, sinusitis, bronchitis, pneumonia, nephritis, hepatitis, peritonitis, symptomatic and asymptomatic intestinal infection, encephalitis	Not described; two HIV-seronegative children with seizure disorder and presumed *E. cuniculi* infection presumably were immunocompromised
Pleistophora sp.	Myositis	Not described
Trachipleistophora hominis	Myositis, keratoconjunctivitis, sinusitis	Not described
Trachipleistophora anthropophthera	Disseminated infection	Not described
Nosema connori	Disseminated infection	Not described
Nosema ocularum	Not described	Keratitis
Vittaforma corneae (formerly *Nosema corneum*)	Disseminated infection	Keratitis
Nosema-like microsporidian[a]	Myositis	Not described
Microsporidium ceylonensis[b]	Not described	Corneal ulcer, keratitis
Microsporidium africanum[b]	Not described	Corneal ulcer, keratitis

[a] Species not yet classified.
[b] *Microsporidium* is a collective genus name for microsporidia that cannot be classified because available information is not sufficient.

phora anthropophthera is similar to *T. hominis* but appears to be dimorphic because two different forms of sporophorous vesicles and spores have been observed (35).

Nosema spp. develop in direct contact with the host cell cytoplasm, nuclei are paired (diplokaryotic), and sporonts are disporoblastic. The diplokaryotic spores of *Nosema connori* measure 2.0 to 2.5 by 4.0 to 4.5 μm and contain polar tubules with approximately 11 coils (4). The spores of *Nosema ocularum* measure 3 by 5 μm and have polar tubules with 11 to 12 coils (4). A third *Nosema*-like microsporidian has yet to be classified (3).

A new genus, *Vittaforma*, was proposed for *Nosema corneum* on the basis of ultrastructural features (33). Sporogony is polysporoblastic, sporonts are ribbon shaped, and all developmental stages are individually enveloped by a cisterna of host endoplasmic reticulum studded with ribosomes. The spores contain polar tubules with five to seven coils, are diplokaryotic, and measure 1.2 by 3.8 μm.

Microsporidium is a collective genus name for microsporidia that cannot be classified because available information is not sufficient.

NATURAL HABITATS

Human microsporidial infections have been documented globally. The sources of microsporidia infecting humans and their modes of transmission are uncertain. Ingestion of spores is the most probable mode of transmission. A possible transmission by the aerosol route has also been considered because microsporidia have been found in respiratory specimens. Studies with mammals suggest that *Encephalitozoon* spp. can be transmitted transplacentally from mother to offspring, but no congenitally acquired human infections have been reported (4, 37).

Possible animal reservoir hosts of most microsporidia infecting humans are not known so far. *E. cuniculi* is considered a zoonotic parasite (9). Three different strains of *E. cuniculi* were genetically identified in rabbits, mice, and dogs, and canine and rabbit strains of *E. cuniculi* have also been isolated from human immunodeficiency virus (HIV)-infected patients (9, 14). *E. bieneusi* has mainly been found in humans, but recently, the parasite has also been detected in pigs (10) and rhesus monkeys experimentally infected with simian immunodeficiency virus.

CLINICAL SIGNIFICANCE

Although microsporidiosis appears to occur most frequently in persons infected with HIV, it is emerging as an infection in otherwise immunocompromised hosts as well as in immunocompetent individuals (Table 1). Microsporidiosis has been associated with abnormalities in structure and function of infected organs, but how the different microsporidial species cause disease is not sufficiently understood. Patients

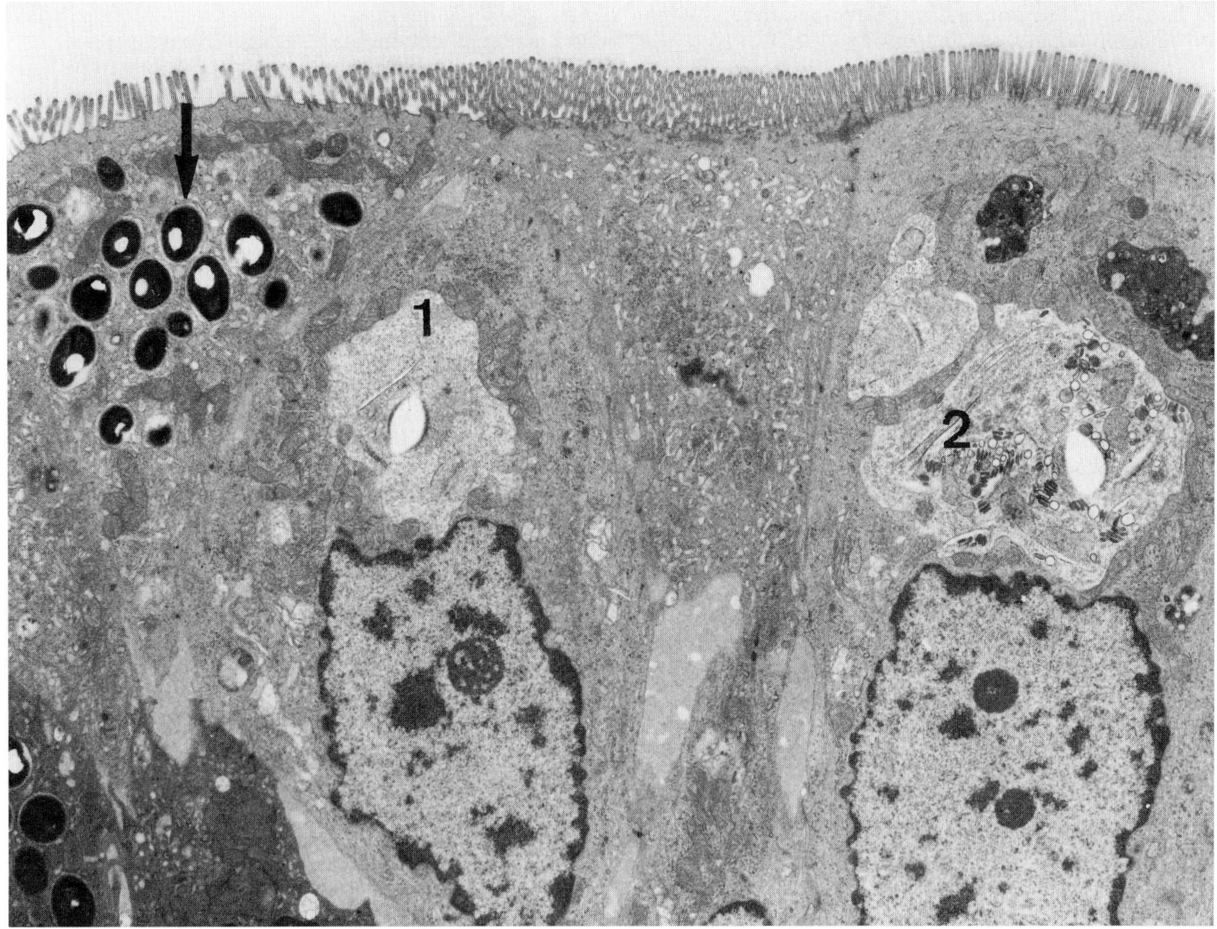

FIGURE 1 Transmission electron micrograph showing duodenal epithelium of an HIV-infected patient infected with *E. bieneusi*. The different developmental stages between the enterocyte nuclei and the microvillous border include a proliferative plasmodium (labeled 1), late sporogonial plasmodia (labeled 2), and mature spores (arrow). Magnification, ×6,000. (Courtesy of M. A. Spycher, University Hospital, Zurich, Switzerland).

with severe cellular immunodeficiency appear to be at the highest risk for developing microsporidial disease, but little is known about immunity to this infection, although the importance of T cells has been demonstrated in experiments with athymic mice. It is not understood whether microsporidiosis in immunocompromised patients is primarily a reactivation of latent infection acquired prior to the state of suppressed immunity or whether microsporidial disease is caused by recently acquired infection.

E. bieneusi

E. bieneusi infects the enterocytes of the small intestine and epithelial cells of the biliary tree and respiratory tract. It is estimated to be one of the most important HIV-associated intestinal pathogens, present in 5 to 30% of patients with otherwise unexplained chronic diarrhea, weight loss, or cholangiopathy, particularly when CD4 lymphocyte counts are below 0.1 × 10^9/liter. Upper or lower respiratory tract infections have been detected in a few patients; systemic infection due to *E. bieneusi* has not been documented. The parasite is also associated with diarrhea in recipients of organ transplants and with self-limited watery diarrhea in immunocompetent adults as well as in children (37). The development of clinical disease is probably based on the continuous excess loss of epithelial cells. *Enterocytozoon* infection may be accompanied by alterations in small bowel physiology such as decreased brush border sucrase, lactase, and maltase activities, as well as malabsorption.

Encephalitozoon spp.

Encephalitozoon spp. infect epithelial and endothelial cells, fibroblasts, macrophages, and possibly, other cell types, as reported for humans and mammals. *Encephalitozoon* (identified as *E. cuniculi* because this was the only species known at that time) was initially identified in two children with seizure disorder (38). The spectrum of recognized *E. cuniculi*- and *E. hellem*-associated disease in patients with AIDS includes keratoconjunctivitis, sinusitis, bronchiolitis, pneumonitis, nephritis, ureteritis, cystitis, prostatitis, urethritis, hepatitis, peritonitis, diarrhea, and encephalitis (8, 9, 12, 37, 38). Clinical manifestations may vary substantially, ranging from an asymptomatic carrier state to organ failure. *E. intestinalis* primarily infects enterocytes, but the parasite is also found in intestinal lamina propria, and dissemination to the kidneys, airways, and biliary tract appears to occur via infected macrophages (2). *Encephalitozoon*-like microsporidia may also cause diarrhea in otherwise healthy children and adults living in tropical countries (15).

Other Microsporidia

Deep stromal infections of the cornea due to different microsporidial species have been described in otherwise healthy persons who presented with severe keratitis or a corneal ulcer.

In immunocompromised patients, myositis was found to be associated with infections due to different microsporidia, including *Pleistophora* sp., *T. hominis* (18), and a yet unidentified *Nosema*-like microsporidian (3).

T. anthropophthera has recently been identified at autopsy in cerebral, cardiac, renal, pancreatic, thyroid, hepatic, splenic, lymphoid, and bone marrow tissue of patients with AIDS who initially presented with seizures (39). Disseminated infection due to *N. connori* was found at autopsy in a 4-month-old athymic male infant (Table 1).

COLLECTION, TRANSPORT, AND STORAGE OF SPECIMENS

Spores of enteropathogenic microsporidia can be detected in stool specimens or duodenal aspirates that have been fixed in 10% formalin or in sodium acetate-acetic acid-formalin, in fresh stool samples, or in biopsy specimens. The spores of microsporidia causing disseminated infection can usually be detected in fresh or fixed urine sediments, in other body fluids (including sputum, bronchoalveolar lavage fluid, nasal secretions, cerebrospinal fluid, and conjunctival smears), corneal scrapings, or tissue. For histological examination, tissue specimens are fixed in formalin. For electron microscopy, fixation of tissue with glutaraldehyde is preferred. Collection of fresh material (without fixative) may be useful for cell culture and for molecular identification. Microsporidial spores are environmentally resistant and, if prevented from drying, can remain infectious for periods of up to several years.

DETECTION PROCEDURES

At present, the most robust technique for the diagnosis of microsporidial infection is the light microscopic detection of the parasites themselves. The spores, the stages at which microsporidia pathogenic in humans are usually identified, are small, ranging in size from 1 to 3 μm. Evaluation of patients with suspected intestinal microsporidiosis should begin with light microscopic examination of stool specimens, while microsporidia which cause systemic infection are best detected in urine sediments or other body fluids. Definitive species identification of microsporidia is made by electron microscopy, antigenic analysis, or molecular analysis.

Examination of Stool Specimens

Smears are prepared with 10 to 20 μl of unconcentrated stool that is very thinly spread onto the slides. Most of the procedures that have been adapted for the concentration of ova and parasites fail to concentrate the microsporidial spores present in stool specimens, although the formalin-ethyl acetate concentration method and different flotation methods remove significant amounts of fecal debris, and smears prepared from these concentrates appear to be easier to read by light microscopic examination than smears from unconcentrated specimens. Such concentration techniques, however, lead to a substantial loss of microsporidial spores and may give false-negative results (36).

The most commonly used stains are chromotrope-based stains (36) and chemofluorescent optical brightening agents (34), including Calcofluor White 2 MR (American Cyanamid Corp., Princeton, N.J.), Fungi-Fluor (Polysciences Inc., Warrington, Pa.), Fungiqual A (Medical Diagnostics, Kandern, Germany), Cellufluor (Polysciences Inc.), Uvitex 2B (CIBA-GEIGY, Basel, Switzerland; not commercially available), and other chemofluorescent stains. Regardless of which staining technique is used, the use of positive control material is essential. Detection of microsporidial spores requires adequate illumination and magnification, i.e., ×630 or ×1,000 magnification (oil immersion).

Microsporidial spores are ovoid and have a specific appearance when stained with chromotrope stains (Fig. 2 and 3) (36). The spore wall stains bright pinkish red, some spores appear transparent, and other spores show a distinct pinkish red-stained belt-like stripe that girds the spores diagonally or equatorially. Most background debris in stool specimens counterstains a faint green (or blue, depending on the staining technique). Some other fecal elements, such as yeast and some bacteria, may also stain reddish, but they are distinguished from microsporidial spores by their size, shape, and staining pattern. Several modifications to the original chromotrope staining solution (36) have been proposed, including modifications to the counterstain (31) or changes in the temperature of the standard chromotrope staining solution and the staining time (13, 26). The results indicate that staining at a temperature of 50°C for 10 min (26) or staining at a temperature of 37°C for 30 min (13) may improve the detection of microsporidia because the background may be clearer and spores stain more intensely. The choice of counterstain is a matter of preference and does not influence the contrast to the pink-staining microsporidia.

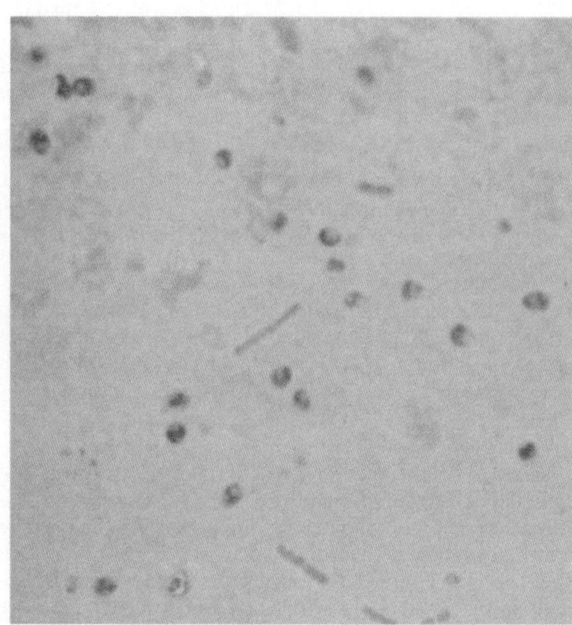

FIGURE 2 Smear of a stool specimen from a patient with AIDS and chronic diarrhea showing pinkish red-stained spores of *E. bieneusi* that measure 0.7 to 1.0 by 1.1 to 1.6 μm. Chromotrope staining was used. Magnification (oil immersion), ×1,000.

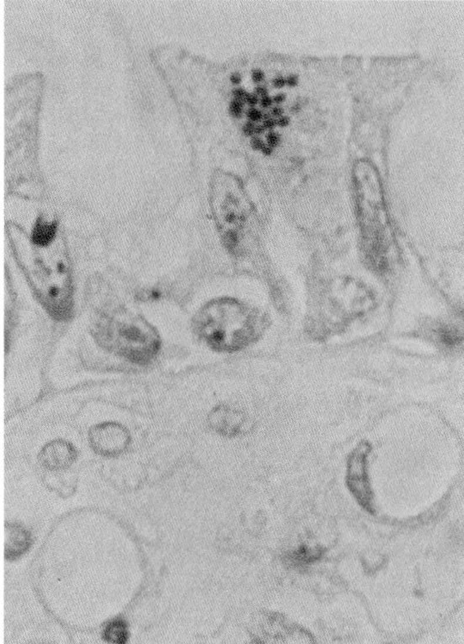
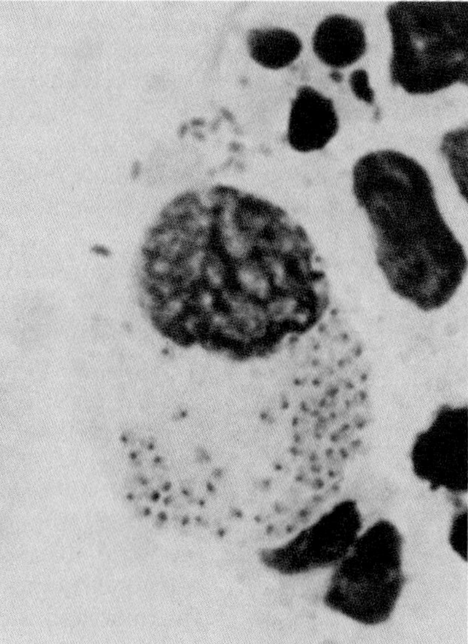
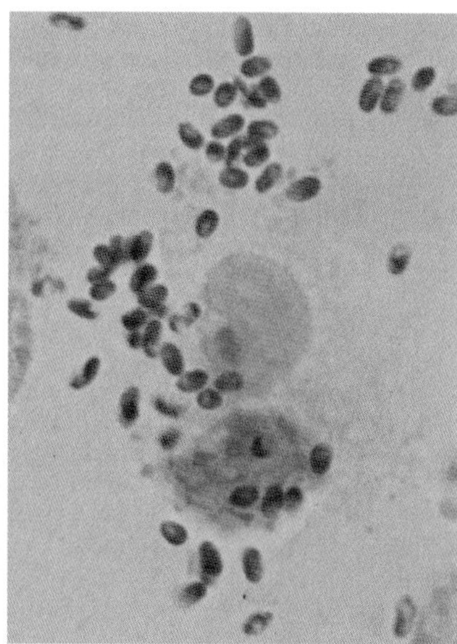

FIGURE 3 (A) Terminal ileal tissue obtained by ileocolonoscopy from a patient with AIDS and chronic diarrhea due to *E. bieneusi* infection. Gram-labile microsporidial spores measuring 0.7 to 1.0 by 1.1 to 1.6 μm are found at a supranuclear location within small intestinal enterocytes. Brown-Brenn stain was used. Magnification, ×1,000. (B) Cytospin preparation of bronchoalveolar lavage fluid from a patient with AIDS and intestinal *E. bieneusi* infection showing intracellular microsporidia. Giemsa stain was used. Magnification (oil immersion), ×1,000. (C) Urine sediment from a patient with AIDS and disseminated *E. cuniculi* infection showing pinkish red-stained microsporidial spores measuring 1.0 to 1.5 by 2.0 to 3.0 μm. Chromotrope stain was used. Magnification (oil immersion), ×1,000.

Chemofluorescent optical brightening agents are chitin stains, which require examination with a fluorescence microscope. With the correct wavelength of illumination, the chitinous wall of the microsporidial spores fluoresces brightly, facilitating the detection of spores (13). However, staining is not specific, and fungi, small species of which may be present in fecal material, and other fecal elements may also be brightened. Some experience is necessary to distinguish the microsporidia.

Epidemiological comparisons of the chromotrope staining technique with methods that use chemofluorescent optical brighteners indicated that these tests are robust for routine use and that the sensitivities of both methods are similarly high (13, 24). Some laboratories use both staining techniques because the chromotrope stains result in a highly specific visualization of spores, whereas the chemofluorescent agents might be more sensitive but may produce false-positive results (13). Experienced parasitological laboratories appear to be able to perform coprodiagnostic procedures as sensitively as histological examination techniques (34, 36, 37).

An acid-fast trichrome stain (25) which permits visualization of acid-fast cryptosporidial oocysts as well as microsporidial spores on the same slide and a "quick-hot" Gram-chromotrope staining technique in which the staining time is reduced to 5 min and the microsporidial spores stain dark violet against a pale green background (29) have recently been suggested. Blinded epidemiological studies have yet to assess the performance of these new tests in routine practice.

Immunofluorescence procedures for the diagnosis of *Encephalitozoon*-like microsporidial spores are promising (16). Antisera to *Enterocytozoon* have not yet been developed. By taking advantage of the cross-reactivity between *Encephalitozoon* and *Enterocytozoon* antigens, polyclonal antibodies have been used to demonstrate spores of *Enterocytozoon* in stool specimens (1), but this technique was less sensitive than those with chromotrope and chemofluorescent stains (13).

The differences in the sizes between *Enterocytozoon* spores (1 to 1.5 μm) and *Encephalitozoon* spores (2 to 3 μm) often permit a tentative diagnosis of the genus from light microscopic examination of stool specimens.

Cytological Diagnosis

Microsporidial spores have been detected in sediments of duodenal aspirate, bile or biliary aspirates, urine (Fig. 3C), bronchoalveolar lavage fluid (Fig. 3B), and cerebrospinal fluid and in smears of conjunctival swabs, sputum, and nasal discharge. Microscopic examination of stained smears of centrifuged duodenal aspirates obtained during endoscopy is a highly sensitive technique for the diagnosis of intestinal microsporidiosis. Because microsporidial infection often involves multiple organs, detection of microsporidia in virtually any tissue or body fluid should prompt a thorough search of other sites. Particularly for patients with suspected disseminated microsporidiosis, urine specimens should be examined (37, 38).

Histologic Examination

Examination of duodenal and terminal ileal tissues has resulted in the detection of intestinal microsporidia, but the parasites are rarely found in colonic tissue sections. Microsporidial species causing disseminated infection have been demonstrated in almost every organ system (37, 39).

Only highly experienced pathologists have reliably and consistently identified microsporidia in tissue sections using routine techniques such as hematoxylin and eosin staining. Ultrathin plastic sections stained with methylene blue–azure II–basic fuchsin or with toluidine blue may facilitate detection. In our experience, tissue Gram stains (Brown-Brenn or Brown-Hopps) have proved to be the most useful for the rapid and reliable identification of HIV-associated microsporidia in routine paraffin-embedded tissue sections (Fig. 3A) (36, 37). Others prefer a silver stain (Warthin-Starry stain) (17), the chromotrope-based staining technique, or chemofluorescent agents (6).

Molecular Techniques

Nucleic acid-based methods for the detection or identification of microsporidia have been developed, but at present, these techniques are confined to research laboratories and the role of diagnostic PCR has yet to be validated in epidemiological studies. There has been progress in the development of primer pairs that amplify the short regions of the SSU rRNA gene, and descriptions of their application in the diagnosis of intestinal microsporidial infection have been published. Diagnosis and identification of *E. bieneusi* and the different *Encephalitozoon* spp. have been successfully performed with fresh stool specimens, formalin-fixed stool specimens, intestinal tissue obtained by endoscopic biopsy, urine specimens, and other body fluids (7–10, 22, 30).

ISOLATION OF MICROSPORIDIA

Microsporidia cannot be grown axenically. *Encephalitozoon* spp., *T. hominis*, and *V. corneae* have been isolated with different cell culture systems, including RK-13 (rabbit kidney) (12), MDCK (Madin-Darby canine kidney) (23, 33), MRC-5 (human embryonic lung fibroblast) (4, 9), and other (4, 37) cells. Only short-term in vitro propagation has been accomplished with *E. bieneusi*. The isolation of microsporidia has no relevance for diagnostic purposes but is an important research tool.

IDENTIFICATION

The identification of microsporidia and their taxonomy have been based primarily upon ultrastructural characteristics. Microsporidial ultrastructure is unique and pathognomonic for the phylum, and ultrastructural features can distinguish all microsporidial genera (4). Nevertheless, morphologic features alone do not sufficiently characterize all microsporidial species pathogenic for humans. The characterization of the three *Encephalitozoon* spp., which share most of their morphologic features, requires antigenic or molecular analyses, which may also reveal subtype-specific variation (12, 14).

SEROLOGIC TESTS

Serologic assays (including carbon immunoassay, indirect immunofluorescence test, enzyme-linked immunosorbent assay, and Western blot immunodetection) have been useful in detecting antibodies to *E. cuniculi* in several species of animals, but reliable serologic tests for the diagnosis of human microsporidiosis are lacking. This unavailability is due, in part, to the fact that *Enterocytozoon* has not been continuously propagated to produce antigens (4, 37).

ANTIMICROBIAL SUSCEPTIBILITY

Albendazole has been found to cause growth deformities in *Encephalitozoon* and to reduce or eradicate the parasites propagated in cell cultures, but it does not destroy mature microsporidial spores, so these may sustain an infection (5, 11, 19). Fumagillin and its analog, TNP-470, have been shown to inhibit completely or partially the replication or spore germination of *Encephalitozoon* in infected cell cultures (11). Many antiprotozoal drugs and antibiotics have been tested in vitro, with negative findings (5, 11, 19).

Treatment studies with humans are limited, and controlled treatment trials are lacking. Observations of patients indicated that albendazole can result in clinical cure of HIV-associated encephalitozoonosis in parallel with the cessation of spore excretion (37, 38). In contrast, no therapy has been proven to be effective for *Enterocytozoon* infection, nor could a reduction of the parasite load be documented, although some reports have suggested that treatment with albendazole may lead to clinical improvement in some patients (37). Oral purified fumagillin was recently used in a pilot study to treat HIV-associated diarrhea due to *E. bieneusi*, and it appeared to eradicate the parasite but the drug was toxic and induced severe but reversible thrombocytopenia in all patients (28). Recent experience with the anti-tumor necrosis factor alpha agent thalidomide (32) or the highly active antiretroviral treatment strategies indicate that a modulation or improvement of the local or systemic immune function may lead to parasite clearance (21).

INTERPRETATION AND REPORTING OF RESULTS

Current data suggest that microsporidia are opportunistic pathogens capable of causing disease predominantly in HIV-infected persons and otherwise immunocompromised patients. Therefore, it is prudent to consider microsporidia the etiologic agents when they are detected in clinical specimens from such patients. Preliminary observations indicate that microsporidia may also cause illness in immunocompetent and otherwise healthy persons.

Morphologic demonstration of microsporidia in specimens obtained from immunocompromised patients, although sensitive and specific, does not usually allow the identification of the organisms to the genus and species levels. Epidemiological studies with patients not infected with HIV are lacking, but it is assumed on the basis of observations for patients that immunocompetent persons may excrete lower numbers of microsporidial spores in feces or urine, and therefore, the threshold of the current detection procedures may not be sufficiently reliable for the detection of microsporidia in this group.

Although not all microsporidia pathogenic for humans can be identified to the species level by electron microscopy, this technique is still the "gold standard" for diagnostic confirmation and species identification. Yet, electron microscopy is relatively insensitive for the detection of microsporidia because only small samples are examined and sampling error may occur. Future diagnostic techniques are likely to include specific immunofluorescence staining of organisms, antigen tests, and molecular techniques. Nucleic acid-based methods have been developed for diagnostic purposes and species identification and are invaluable for taxonomic classification and phylogenetic analyses, but their use is still limited to research laboratories. Blinded epidemiological comparisons of microscopic techniques and diagnostic PCR for the detection of microsporidia in feces have not yet indicated that molecular tests have greater sensitivity (30).

ADDENDUM IN PROOF

A new genus and species, *Brachiola vesicularum*, was proposed for the *Nosema*-like microsporidian detected in muscle tissue of a patient with AIDS and myositis as previously described by Cali and colleagues (3). Because of the similarities to the genus *Nosema*, the new genus is placed in the family Nosematidae (**A. Cali, P. M. Takvorian, S. Lewin, M. Rendel, C. S. Sian, M. Wittner, H. B. Tanowitz, E. Keohane, and L. M. Weiss.** 1998. *Brachiola vesicularum*, n.g., n.sp., a new microsporidium associated with AIDS and myositis. *J. Eukaryot. Microbiol.* **45:**240–251).

REFERENCES

1. **Aldras, A. M., J. M. Orenstein, D. P. Kotler, J. A. Shadduck, and E. S. Didier.** 1994. Detection of microsporidia by indirect immunofluorescence antibody test using polyclonal and monoclonal antibodies. *J. Clin. Microbiol.* **32:** 608–612.
2. **Cali, A., D. P. Kotler, and J. M. Orenstein.** 1993. *Septata intestinalis* n.g., n.sp., an intestinal microsporidian associated with chronic diarrhea and dissemination in AIDS patients. *J. Protozool.* **40:**101–112.
3. **Cali, A., P. M. Takvorian, S. Lewin, M. Rendel, C. Sian, M. Wittner, and L. M. Weiss.** 1996. Identification of a new *Nosema*-like microsporidian associated with myositis in an AIDS patient. *J. Eukaryot. Microbiol.* **43:**S108.
4. **Canning, E. U.** 1993. Microsporidia, p. 299–370. *In* J. P. Kreier (ed.), *Parasitic Protozoa*, vol. 6. Academic Press, Inc., San Diego, Calif.
5. **Colbourn, N. I., W. S. Hollister, A. Curry, and E. U. Canning.** 1994. Activity of albendazole against *Encephalitozoon cuniculi* in vitro. *Eur. J. Protistol.* **30:**211–220.
6. **Conteas, C. N., T. Sowerby, G. W. Berlin, F. Dahlan, A. Nguyen, R. Porschen, J. Donovan, M. LaRiviere, and J. M. Orenstein.** 1996. Fluorescence techniques for diagnosing intestinal microsporidiosis in stool, enteric fluid, and biopsy specimens from acquired immunodeficiency syndrome patients with chronic diarrhea. *Arch. Pathol. Lab. Med.* **120:**847–853.
7. **DaSilva, A. J., D. A. Schwartz, G. S. Visvesvara, H. Demoura, S. B. Slemenda, and N. J. Pieniazek.** 1996. Sensitive PCR diagnosis of infections by *Enterocytozoon bieneusi* (microsporidia) using primers based on the region coding for small subunit rRNA. *J. Clin. Microbiol.* **34:** 986–987.
8. **De Groote, M. A., G. S. Visvesvara, M. L. Wilson, N. J. Pieniazek, S. B. Slemenda, A. J. daSilva, G. J. Leitch, R. T. Bryan, and R. Reves.** 1995. Polymerase chain reaction and culture confirmation of disseminated *Encephalitozoon cuniculi* infection in a patient with AIDS: successful therapy with albendazole. *J. Infect. Dis.* **171:**1375–1378.
9. **Deplazes, P., A. Mathis, R. Baumgartner, I. Tanner, and R. Weber.** 1996. Immunologic and molecular characteristics of *Encephalitozoon*-like microsporidia isolated from humans and rabbits indicate that *Encephalitozoon cuniculi* is a zoonotic parasite. *Clin. Infect. Dis.* **22:**557–559.
10. **Deplazes, P., A. Mathis, C. Müller, and R. Weber.** 1996. Molecular epidemiology of *Encephalitozoon cuniculi* and first detection of *Enterocytozoon bieneusi* in faecal samples of pigs. *J. Eukaryot. Microbiol.* **43:**93S.
11. **Didier, E. S.** 1997. Effects of albendazole, fumagillin, and TNP 470 on microsporidial replication in vitro. *Antimicrob. Agents Chemother.* **41:**1541–1546.
12. **Didier, E. S., P. J. Didier, D. N. Friedberg, S. M. Stenson, J. M. Orenstein, R. W. Yee, F. O. Tio, R. M. Davis, C. Vossbrinck, N. Millichamp, and J. A. Shadduck.** 1991. Isolation and characterization of a new human microsporidian, *Encephalitozoon hellem* (n. sp.), from three AIDS patients with keratoconjunctivitis. *J. Infect. Dis.* **163:** 617–621.
13. **Didier, E. S., J. M. Orenstein, A. Aldra, D. Bertucci, L. B. Rogers, and F. A. Janney.** 1995. Comparison of three staining methods for detecting microsporidia in fluids. *J. Clin. Microbiol.* **33:**3138–3145.
14. **Didier, E. S., C. R. Vossbrinck, M. D. Baker, L. B. Rogers, D. C. Bertucci, and J. A. Shadduck.** 1995. Identification and characterization of three *Encephalitozoon cuniculi* strains. *Parasitology* **111:**411–421.
15. **Enriquez, F. J., A. P. Cruz-Lopez, J. D. Palting, P. Cruz-Lopez, P. Hernandez-Jauregui, C. Tellez, J. Guerrero, and B. Curran.** 1997. Prevalence of microsporidial infections in children and adults with diarrhea, abstr. C-216, p. 158. *In Abstracts of the 97th General Meeting of the American Society for Microbiology 1997*. American Society for Microbiology Washington, D.C.
16. **Enriquez, F. J., O. Ditrich, J. D. Palting, and K. Smith.** 1997. Simple diagnosis of *Encephalitozoon* sp. infections by using a panspecific antiexospore monoclonal antibody. *J. Clin. Microbiol.* **35:**724–729.
17. **Field, A., M. Hing, S. Milliken, and D. Marriott.** 1993. Microsporidia in the small intestine of HIV infected patients: a new diagnostic technique and a new species. *Med. J. Aust.* **158:**390–394.
18. **Field, A. S., D. J. Marriott, S. T. Milliken, B. J. Brew, E. U. Canning, J. G. Kench, P. Darveniza, and J. L. Harkness.** 1996. Myositis associated with a newly described microsporidian, *Trachipleistophora hominis*, in a patient with AIDS. *J. Clin. Microbiol.* **34:**2803–2811.
19. **Franssen, F. F., J. T. Lumeij, and F. van Knapen.** 1995. Susceptibility of *Encephalitozoon cuniculi* to several drugs in vitro. *Antimicrob. Agents Chemother.* **39:**1265–1268.
20. **Germot, A., H. Philippe, and H. Leguyader.** 1997. Evidence for loss of mitochondria in microsporidia from a mitochondrial-type HSP70 in *Nosema locustae*. *Mol. Biochem. Parasitol.* **87:**159–168.
21. **Goguel, J., C. Katlama, C. Sarfati, C. Maslo, C. Leport, and J. M. Molina.** 1997. Remission of AIDS-associated intestinal microsporidiosis with highly active antiretroviral therapy. *AIDS* **11:**1658–1659.
22. **Hartskeerl, R. A., T. van Gool, A. R. Schuitema, E. S. Didier, and W. J. Terpstra.** 1995. Genetic and immunological characterization of the microsporidian *Septata intestinalis* Cali, Kotler and Orenstein, 1993: reclassification to *Encephalitozoon intestinalis*. *Parasitology* **110:**277–285.
23. **Hollister, W. S., E. U. Canning, E. Weidner, A. S. Field, J. Kench, and D. J. Marriott.** 1996. Development and ultrastructure of *Trachipleistophora hominis* n.g., n.sp. after in vitro isolation from an AIDS patient and inoculation into athymic mice. *Parasitology* **112:**143–154.
24. **Ignatius, R., S. Henschel, O. Liesenfeld, U. Mansmann, W. Schmidt, S. Köppe, T. Schneider, W. Heise, U. Futh, E. O. Ricken, H. Hahn, and R. Ullrich.** 1997. Comparative evaluation of modified trichrome and Uvitex 2B stains for detection of low numbers of microsporidial spores in stool specimens. *J. Clin. Microbiol.* **35:**2266–2269.
25. **Ignatius, R., M. Lehmann, K. Miksits, T. Regnath, M. Arvand, E. Engelmann, H. Hahn, and J. Wagner.** 1997. A new acid-fast trichrome stain for simultaneous detection of *Cryptosporidium parvum* and microsporidial species in stool specimens. *J. Clin. Microbiol.* **35:**446–449.
26. **Kokoskin, E., T. W. Gyorkos, A. Camus, L. Cedilotte, T. Purtill, and B. Ward.** 1994. Modified technique for efficient detection of microsporidia. *J. Clin. Microbiol.* **32:** 1974–1975.
27. **Li, J., S. K. Katiyar, A. Hamelin, G. S. Visvesvara, and T. D. Edlind.** 1996. Tubulin genes from AIDS-associated

microsporidia and implications for phylogeny and benzimidazole sensitivity. *Mol. Biochem. Parasitol.* **78:**289–295.

28. **Molina, J. M., J. Goguel, C. Sarfati, C. I. Chastang, I. Desportes, J. F. Michiels, C. Maslo, C. Katlama, L. Cotte, C. Leport, F. Raffi, F. Derouin, and J. Modai for the Microsporidiosis Study Group, ANRS, France.** 1997. Potential efficacy of fumagillin in intestinal microsporidiosis due to *Enterocytozoon bieneusi* in patients with HIV infection: results of a drug screening study. *AIDS* **11:** 1603–1610.
29. **Moura, H., D. A. Schwartz, F. Bornayllinares, F. C. Sodre, S. Wallace, and G. S. Visvesvara.** 1997. A new and improved quick-hot chromotrope technique that differentially stains microsporidian spores in clinical samples, including paraffin-embedded tissue sections. *Arch. Pathol. Lab. Med.* **121:**888–893.
30. **Rinder, H., K. Janitschke, H. Aspöck, A. J. da Silva, P. Deplazes, D. P. Fedorko, C. Franzen, W. Heise, F. Hünger, A. Lehmacher, C. Meyer, J. M. Molina, R. Weber, and T. Löscher.** 1998. A blinded, externally controlled multicenter evaluation for the detection of microsporidia by light microscopy and PCR. *J. Clin. Microbiol.* **36:** 1814–1818.
31. **Ryan, N., G. Sutherland, K. Coughlan, M. Globan, J. Doultree, J. Marshall, R. W. Baird, J. Pedersen, and B. Dwyer.** 1993. A new trichrome-blue stain for detection of microsporidial species in urine, stool, and nasopharyngeal specimens. *J. Clin. Microbiol.* **31:**3264–3269.
32. **Sharpstone, D., A. Rowbottom, N. Francis, G. Tovey, D. Ellis, M. Barrett, and B. Gazzard.** 1997. Thalidomide: a novel therapy for microsporidiosis. *Gastroenterology* **112:** 1823–1829.
33. **Silveira, H., and E. U. Canning.** 1995. *Vittaforma corneae* n. comb. for the human microsporidium *Nosema corneum* Shadduck, Meccoli, Davis & Font, 1990, based on its ultrastructure in the liver of experimentally infected athymic mice. *J. Eukaryot. Microbiol.* **42:**158–165.
34. **van Gool, T., F. Snijders, P. Reiss, J. K. M. Eeftinck Schattenkerk, M. A. van den Bergh Weerman, J. F. W. M. Bartelsman, J. J. M. Bruins, E. U. Canning, and J. Dankert.** 1993. Diagnosis of intestinal and disseminated microsporidia infections in patients with HIV by a new rapid fluorescence technique. *J. Clin. Pathol.* **46:**694–699.
35. **Vávra, J., A. T. Yachnis, J. A. Shadduck, and J. M. Orenstein.** 1998. Microsporidia of the genus *Trachipleistophora*—causative agents of human microsporidiosis: description of *Trachipleistophora anthropophthera* n.sp. (Protozoa: Microsporidia). *J. Eukaryot. Microbiol.* **45:** 273–283.
36. **Weber, R., R. T. Bryan, R. L. Owen, C. M. Wilcox, L. Gorelkin, G. S. Visvesvara, and the Enteric Opportunistic Infections Working Group.** 1992. Improved light-microscopical detection of microsporidia spores in stool and duodenal aspirates. *N. Engl. J. Med.* **326:**161–166.
37. **Weber, R., R. T. Bryan, D. A. Schwartz, and R. L. Owen.** 1994. Human microsporidial infections. *Clin. Microbiol. Rev.* **7:**426–461.
38. **Weber, R., P. Deplazes, M. Flepp, A. Mathis, R. Baumann, B. Sauer, H. Kuster, and R. Luthy.** 1997. Cerebral microsporidiosis due to *Encephalitozoon cuniculi* in a patient with human immunodeficiency virus infection. *N. Engl. J. Med.* **336:**474–478.
39. **Yachnis, A. T., J. Berg, A. Martinezsalazar, B. S. Bender, L. Diaz, A. M. Rojiani, T. A. Eskin, and J. M. Orenstein.** 1996. Disseminated microsporidiosis especially infecting the brain, heart, and kidneys—report of a newly recognized pansporoblastic species in two symptomatic AIDS patients. *Am. J. Clin. Pathol.* **106:**535–543.

Intestinal Helminths

LAWRENCE R. ASH AND THOMAS C. ORIHEL

112

Intestinal helminths are usually diagnosed by detection of eggs or larvae in feces. Characteristics used in identifying eggs (Fig. 1) include size, shape, thickness of shell, special structures of the shell (mamillated covering, operculum, knob, spine), and developmental stage of egg contents (undeveloped, developing, embryonated).

Objects that might be confused with helminth eggs include pollen grains, mushroom spores, vegetable material, and the eggs of mites and free-living nematodes (1, 2, 10). Plant hairs may be confused with nematode larvae. Confusing artifacts found in feces typically can be distinguished from parasite eggs and larvae because artifacts usually do not have precise morphologic characteristics and appropriate sizes; however, until individuals have considerable experience in examining feces, there are many opportunities for mistaking artifacts for parasite eggs or larvae.

In the period after infection is acquired but before helminths have matured to produce eggs, i.e., the prepatent period, infections are difficult to diagnose. Larvae occasionally may be found in sputum as a result of their migration through the lungs, but in most instances, diagnosis during the prepatent phase of an infection can be established only on the basis of clinical symptomatology, if at all.

NEMATODES

The nematodes, or roundworms, are small to large, elongate, cylindrical parasites living primarily in the intestinal tract as adult worms. Nematodes typically have life cycles that require no intermediate hosts, although some species may utilize one or more intermediate hosts. All of the nematodes of humans, with the exception of *Strongyloides* spp., are dioecious (have two sexes) and characteristically have four larval stages and an adult stage. The infective stage for the human host varies from the first- to the third-stage larva depending on the species of parasite involved. The infective stages of nematodes are usually within eggs, but in a few species (hookworms, trichostrongyles, *Strongyloides* spp.), the larvae hatch from the eggs and become infective in the soil. Diagnosis of most of the human intestinal nematode parasites depends on finding characteristic eggs in feces. An important exception is *Strongyloides stercoralis* infection, in which first-stage larvae are excreted in feces.

The parasites that commonly infect humans are described below.

Enterobius vermicularis

Infection with *E. vermicularis*, the human pinworm parasite, has worldwide distribution, and its true prevalence is probably considerably underestimated. The organism is primarily a parasite of young children; the rapid development of its eggs to the infective stage and their ability to persist for extended periods on fomites and in the external environment lead to rapid dissemination of the infection from child to child and to adults. Infections are especially common in institutional settings.

Adult pinworms are small, females being 8 to 13 mm long and barely visible to the naked eye as white motile worms on the surfaces of stool specimens or on the perianal skin. Males are only 2 to 3 mm long and usually are not seen. The adult female has a characteristic long, pointed tail, whereas in males, the posterior end is blunt. Adult worms typically live in the cecum, colon, appendix, and rectum. Usually, adult females migrate out of the anal orifice at night and lay their eggs in the perianal area, where they adhere to the skin, hair, or bed clothing and bed linen that come in contact with these eggs. Because they live in the lower portion of the intestinal tract, females often lay their eggs on the surface of the fecal mass; as a result, the eggs are not well mixed within the feces and usually will not be detected in routine stool examinations. Rarely, advanced larval stages of *E. vermicularis* are encountered in fecal examinations and pose a problem in correct diagnosis (7).

Enterobius eggs are elongate and flattened on one side, with a thick, colorless shell. They are 50 to 60 μm long by 20 to 40 μm wide and are partially embryonated when laid. The eggs develop rapidly and become infective within 4 to 6 h, at which time the egg contains a tadpolelike larva (Fig. 2A). Adherence of these eggs to fingers and fomites results in their ready transfer to the mouth and further infection.

The infection is especially troublesome in young children; large worm burdens may cause extreme pruritus, irritability, and loss of sleep. Adult females migrating out of the anus may occasionally enter the vagina and subsequently the uterus or fallopian tubes, where they die. Disintegration of the dead worms and liberation of the eggs contained in the uterus results in an inflammatory response and granuloma formation about the eggs in these sites.

Infection is best diagnosed by the use of a cellulose tape technique (1). In this procedure, a strip of cellulose tape

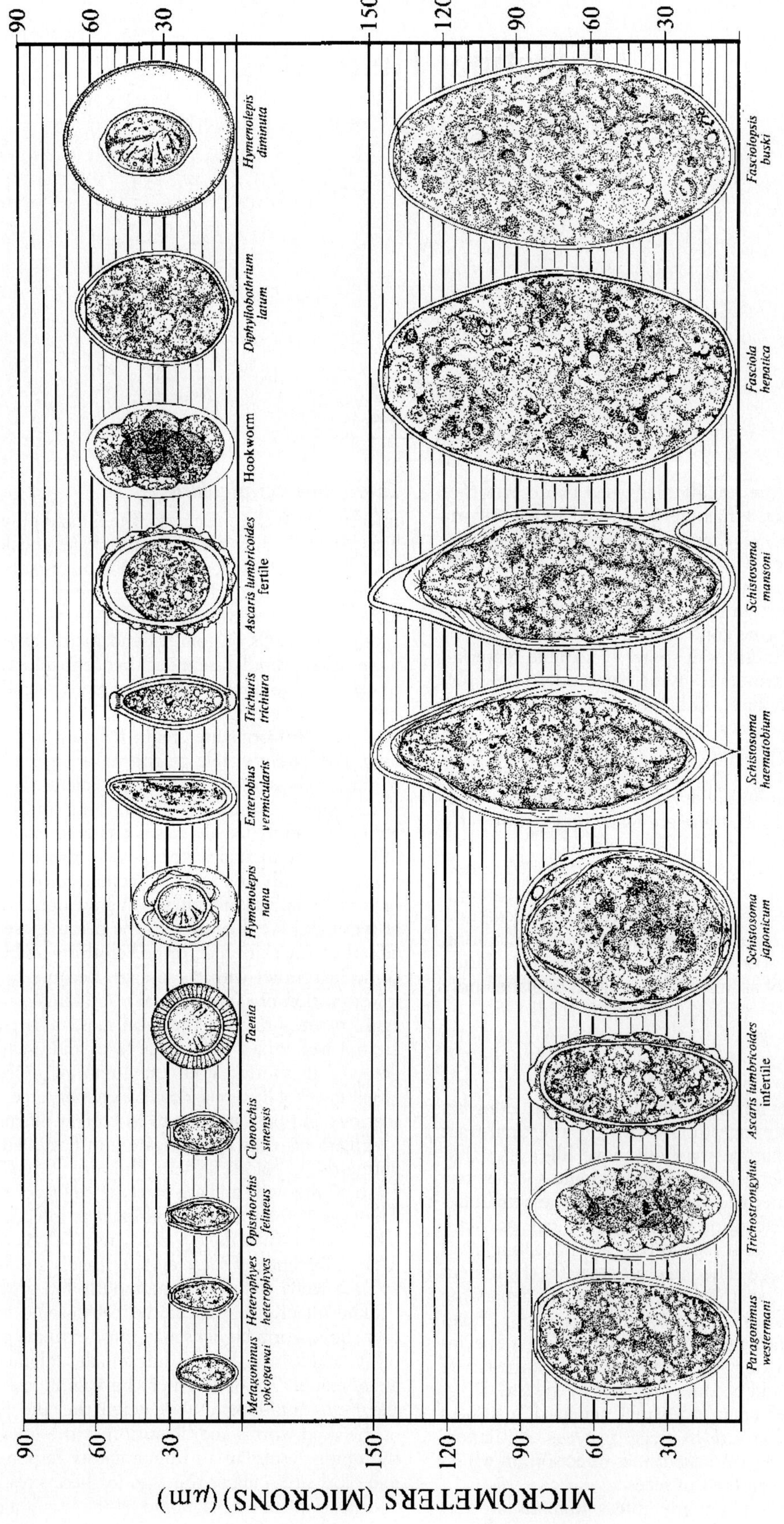

FIGURE 1 Relative sizes of helminth eggs (from Centers for Disease Control and Prevention). *Schistosoma mekongi* and *Schistosoma intercalatum* have been omitted.

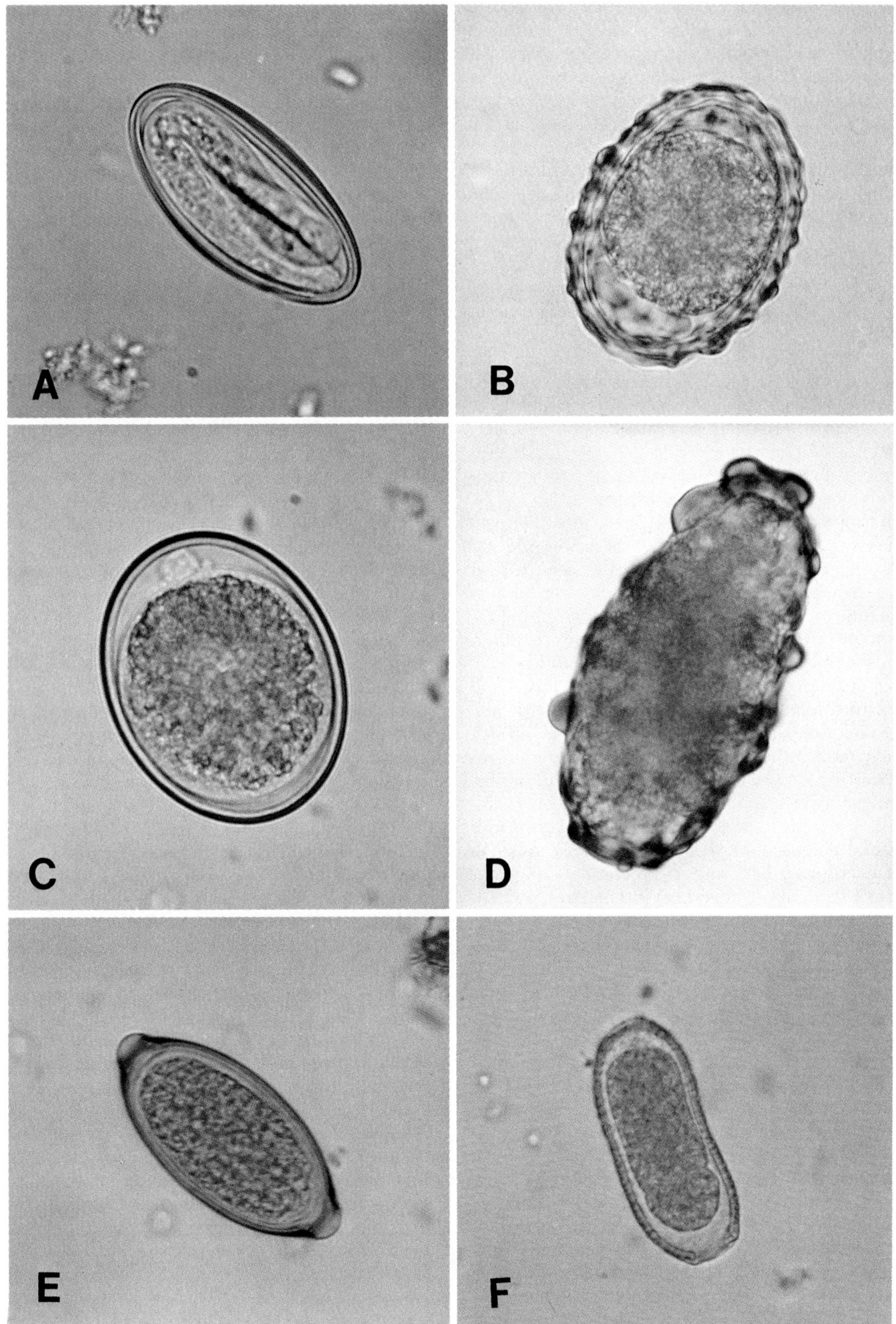

FIGURE 2 Eggs of intestinal nematode parasites (magnification, ×850). (A) Embryonated, infective egg of *E. vermicularis*; (B) fertile egg of *A. lumbricoides*; (C) decorticated fertile egg of *A. lumbricoides*; (D) infertile egg of *A. lumbricoides*; (E) *T. trichiura*; (F) *C. philippinensis*. (Panels A, C, and D are from reference 2; used with permission.)

held adhesive side outward on a microscope slide is pressed firmly against the right and left perianal folds. The tape is then spread back over the slide with the adhesive side down and is examined directly under the microscope. Visibility of eggs can be improved by lifting the tape from the slide, adding a drop of toluene or xylene, and pressing the tape down on the slide again; this helps clear the preparation and makes the eggs stand out prominently. Examinations on multiple days may be required to diagnose infections. Other methods (e.g., the use of anal swabs) also have been used effectively to demonstrate this infection.

Ascaris lumbricoides

A. lumbricoides is the largest and globally the most widespread of all the human intestinal roundworms. The flesh-colored adult worms are large; females usually range from 20 to 35 cm long by 3 to 6 mm wide, and males range from 15 to 31 cm by 2 to 4 mm. Males, with their ventrally curved tails, can be readily distinguished from females, which have straight tails. Females produce large numbers of eggs, perhaps up to 200,000 per female worm per day. These eggs must undergo a developmental period in soil of approximately 2 to 3 weeks before they are infective.

Following ingestion by the human host, infective eggs hatch in the intestine, and the third-stage larvae undergo an obligatory migration from the intestine, through the liver to the lungs. In the lungs, they grow and develop for 8 or 9 days, reaching a length of approximately 1 mm; these larvae then return to the small intestine and complete maturity. The prepatent period is approximately 2 months.

Pathology in humans can be caused by both larval and adult stages. In infections with large numbers of eggs and in repeated infections, the larval migration phase through the lungs may result in *Ascaris* pneumonitis (Loeffler's syndrome), consisting of dyspnea, cough, rales, eosinophilia, and transient, shifting lung infiltrates as seen by X-ray examination. When present in large numbers, adult worms may cause intestinal blockage. However, the presence of small numbers or even one adult worm is potentially dangerous because of their tendency to migrate to ectopic sites, particularly the liver, during febrile illness. The normal life span of an adult worm is approximately 1 year, although female worms may persist for 16 to 20 months.

Infection is usually diagnosed by demonstration of typical fertile eggs in feces. The egg is ovoid, contains a single-celled ovum, and is 55 to 75 μm long by 35 to 50 μm wide. The egg is yellow-brown and has a thick, transparent shell that is covered by a mamillated, albuminoid outer layer (Fig. 2B). Occasionally, the outer mamillated layer is absent; in this circumstance, the eggs are called decorticated eggs (Fig. 2C). Female worms that have never been fertilized or have exhausted their supply of sperm produce infertile eggs. These eggs are elongate (85 to 90 μm long by 43 to 47 μm wide) and have a thin shell that may lack mamillations entirely or may have grossly irregular mamillations scattered unevenly over the surface of the shell. These eggs contain a mass of disorganized, highly refractive granules and fat globules of various sizes (Fig. 2D). Because of the large numbers of eggs produced by the female worm, they can usually be found in direct fecal smears and are readily detected by either flotation or sedimentation concentration procedures. Infertile eggs do not float in the standard zinc sulfate solution (specific gravity, 1.18), and they may be missed if only the flotation concentration is used. Adult worms may be spontaneously passed in feces or may emerge from the anus, mouth, or nares; young developing worms, especially in heavy infections, may be found in feces. The characteristic, prominent three lips at the anterior end of the adult worm aid in identification of the immature or adult parasites.

Trichuris trichiura

Trichuriasis, also known as whipworm infection, is found worldwide in the warmer, moist regions. Adult worms live attached to the mucosal wall of the cecum and, less commonly, to the walls of the large intestine, appendix, and lower part of the ileum. Males and females are of similar sizes, ranging from 30 to 50 mm long, and have long, attenuated anterior portions and thicker, short posterior ends. The long, slender anterior end is threaded into the mucosal epithelium, and the posterior portion hangs free in the lumen. Adult worms are long-lived, commonly living for up to 10 years and often longer. Though frequently found in association with *A. lumbricoides* infection because soil requirements for the development of their infective eggs are similar, *Trichuris* infections are seen more frequently in older children because of the longer life span of the adult parasites. Egg production by *Trichuris* females probably does not exceed several thousand eggs per day.

Eggs are barrel shaped and yellow-brown, have thick shells, and usually measure 50 to 55 μm long by 22 to 24 μm wide. At both ends of the egg are prominent, clear, mucoid "plugs" (Fig. 2E). The egg contains an unsegmented ovum when passed in feces, and once the eggs are in the soil, it takes 2 to 3 weeks for the infective, first-stage larva to develop. When infected eggs are ingested, the prepatent period in humans is approximately 3 months.

Light infections with *T. trichiura* usually are not troublesome, but when large numbers of parasites are present, there may be diarrhea or even dysentery with abdominal cramping; occasionally, rectal prolapse occurs. Heavy infections may result in dehydration, weight loss, and anemia.

Diagnosis, in particular of heavy infections, is readily made by finding the characteristic eggs in direct wet mounts of feces. In light infections, when eggs are few, concentration procedures may be required to find the eggs. In some instances, for reasons not well understood, larger than normal eggs (65 to 83 μm long by 27 to 36 μm wide) are produced (16). In addition, the dog whipworm (*Trichuris vulpis*) also can reach maturity in humans; the eggs of this parasite are larger than those in typical *T. trichiura* infections, being 72 to 90 μm long by 32 to 40 μm wide. The eggs of *T. vulpis*, though similar in length to the large eggs occasionally seen in *T. trichiura* infections, are usually wider and more barrel shaped.

Capillaria philippinensis

C. philippinensis has been recognized since the end of the mid-1960s as causing human infection. Although its geographical distribution was initially restricted to the Philippines and Thailand, occasional cases in recent years have been reported from various parts of the world, including Japan, Taiwan, Egypt, Iran, and Colombia. *C. philippinensis* is normally an intestinal parasite of fish-eating birds, with various fish serving as obligatory intermediate hosts. In areas where the disease is endemic, human infection is acquired by the ingestion of raw or inadequately cooked fish harboring infective larvae in their tissues (3). Patent infections develop in approximately 1 month. Female worms may contain thick-shelled unembryonated eggs, thin-shelled embryonated eggs, or first-stage larvae in their uteri; this bizarre variation of nematode reproduction appears to be dependent on the age of the infection and possibly other factors. Internal autoinfection is a normal feature of the life cycle in mammalian hosts, resulting in large worm burdens that cause diarrhea, wasting, dehydration, and, if untreated, death of the host.

Diagnosis of the infection depends on finding the characteristic thick-shelled unembryonated eggs in feces. Eggs are 36 to 45 μm long by 21 μm wide, have a moderately thick striated shell, and possess inconspicuous mucoid "plugs" at both ends (Fig. 2F). It is not uncommon in individuals with chronic diarrhea for eggs, larvae, and even adult worms to be passed simultaneously in feces.

Hookworm Infections

The two principal human hookworm parasites are *Necator americanus* and *Ancylostoma duodenale*, but other species of the genus *Ancylostoma* also may produce human infections in various regions of the world. *N. americanus* is found in the United States as well as other areas of the world, but *A. duodenale* does not occur in the United States, although its geographic distribution elsewhere frequently overlaps that of *Necator*. In general, hookworm infections are widely distributed in the tropics and subtropics and also extend into moist, temperate climates.

Adult hookworms are characterized by an anterior end modified into a buccal capsule that contains either teeth or cutting plates; the parasites use these to attach themselves and lacerate the wall of the small intestine. Male hookworms are further characterized by having posterior ends modified to form an umbrellalike structure referred to as a bursa; this structure is not present in female worms, which have straight, pointed tails. *Necator* adults are 7 to 11 mm long by 0.3 mm wide and have a buccal capsule provided with cutting plates. *A. duodenale* adults are somewhat larger (8 to 13 mm long by 0.4 mm wide) and have a buccal capsule containing two pairs of teeth.

When passed in feces, the thin-shelled eggs of hookworms contain an ovum that typically is in the 4- to 8-cell stage of division; eggs of *Ancylostoma* and *Necator* are morphologically indistinguishable from each other (Fig. 3A); they range from 55 to 75 μm long by 36 to 40 μm wide. In the soil, the eggs embryonate and hatch within 1 to 2 days as first-stage, rhabditoid larvae measuring 250 to 350 μm long by 17 μm wide.

In the hookworm life cycle, the first-stage larvae that hatch in the soil develop into infective, third-stage, filariform larvae in approximately 1 week; these larvae initiate human infection by direct penetration of the skin. *A. duodenale* larvae also can infect by mouth, but *Necator* cannot; in addition, *Necator* requires an obligatory lung migration, whereas if *A. duodenale* infection is acquired orally, there is direct maturation in the intestine to the adult stage. Patent infections develop in 5 to 6 weeks, and the life spans of the adults of both species are usually only 1 to 2 years but may be as long as 10 years or more.

The pathogenesis of hookworm infection is directly related to the worm burden. Light infections are well tolerated and cause few symptoms. Acute, heavy infections may result in fatigue, weakness, abdominal pain, and diarrhea with blood loss; the blood loss is more severe in *A. duodenale* infections. Chronic hookworm infection results in iron deficiency anemia, listlessness, pallor, and general retardation of development in afflicted children.

Diagnosis is accomplished by demonstration of characteristic eggs in feces. With a direct fecal smear, counts of fewer than five eggs per coverslip preparation indicate light infections unlikely to cause anemia. Counts of more than 25 eggs per coverslip suggest heavy infection. If there has been a prolonged delay in examination of the fecal specimen (usually more than a day), larvae may develop and hatch; it is then necessary to differentiate hookworm first-stage larvae from those of *Strongyloides*, the stage typically passed in feces in human strongyloidiasis. A hookworm rhabditoid larva has a long, narrow buccal chamber (Fig. 3E) and an inconspicuous genital primordium. Accurate identification of the hookworm species causing infection depends on recovering and examining adult worms or culturing larval stages to the infective filariform stage, with subsequent morphologic study of these larvae to distinguish between *Necator* and *Ancylostoma* species (1).

In recent years in northeastern Australia, a new condition in humans, eosinophilic enteritis without gastric involvement, has been described. In these infections, the typical finding is the presence in the intestine of a single, sexually immature hookworm identified as *Ancylostoma caninum*, the common dog hookworm (11). This zoonosis also may occur in other parts of the world, since *A. caninum* has a wide geographic distribution.

Trichostrongylus Species

Human infections with species of the genus *Trichostrongylus* are found throughout the world, in particular in rural areas where herbivorous animals are raised. Adult trichostrongyles typically live in the digestive tracts of sheep, cattle, goats, and other herbivores; the principal species occurring in humans are *Trichostrongylus colubriformis* and *Trichostrongylus orientalis*. Although these infections are rarely troublesome in terms of human disease, they do present occasional diagnostic difficulties, since trichostrongyle eggs resemble hookworm eggs in shape but tend to be much larger.

Adult worms are small and slender, usually measuring less than 1 cm in length; males have a prominent bursa. Trichostrongyle eggs are 75 to 95 μm long by 40 to 50 μm wide. They have colorless, thin shells and are tapered slightly at one end (Fig. 3B). The inner vitelline membrane around the ovum is frequently wrinkled at the tapered end of the egg. The germinal mass does not fill the shell. Eggs passed in feces develop in the soil; third-stage larvae hatch in the external environment and typically these infective larvae are present on grass or other vegetation when ingested by the definitive hosts. Infection is acquired by the oral route only; these larvae are not capable of invading skin.

S. stercoralis

Human strongyloidiasis is widely distributed in the tropics and subtropics, but it also extends into moist, temperate regions. Even in areas where the disease is endemic, its distribution is extremely focal, because the existence of the parasite is dependent on a high groundwater table. Adult parasitic females are parthenogenetic, and parasitic males do not occur. The minute females, only 2 to 3 mm long by 30 to 40 μm in diameter, live within the mucosal epithelium of the small intestine, where they produce thin-shelled eggs that embryonate and hatch in this location. The first-stage rhabditoid larvae migrate into the intestinal lumen, enter the fecal stream, and are the usual stage passed in feces.

In the soil, first-stage larvae follow a direct or indirect course of development. In the direct cycle, the larvae rapidly develop into filariform, third-stage infective larvae that can initiate human infection by direct penetration of the skin. Alternatively, in the indirect cycle, the first-stage larvae develop into a free-living generation of adult male and female worms. When these free-living adult worms mate, the

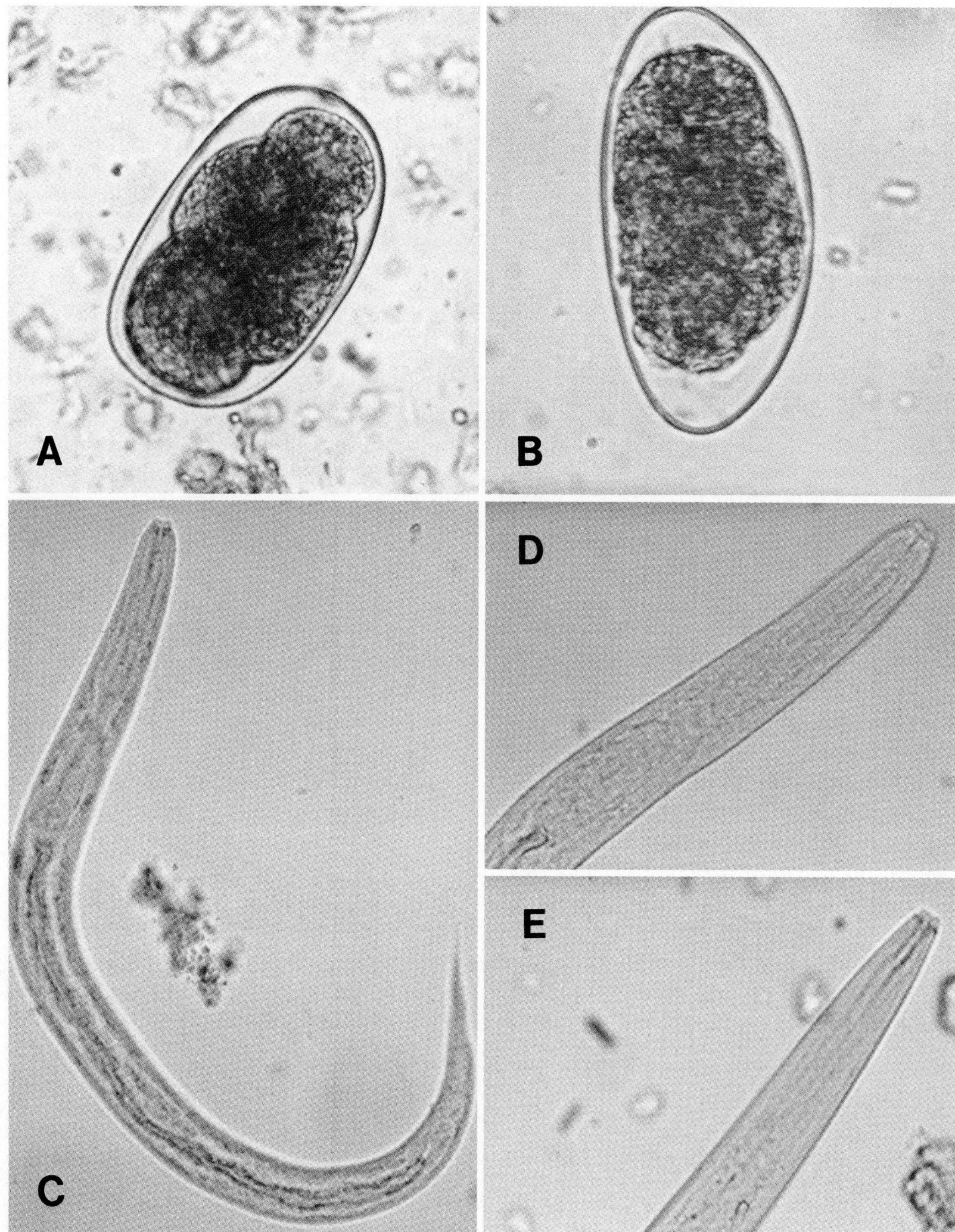

FIGURE 3 Eggs and larvae of intestinal nematode parasites (magnification, ×850). (A) Hookworm egg; (B) *Trichostrongylus* sp.; (C) first-stage larva of *S. stercoralis*; (D) anterior end of first-stage larva of *S. stercoralis* showing short buccal cavity; (E) anterior end of first-stage hookworm larva showing long buccal cavity. (Panels A, C, and E are from reference 2; used with permission.)

female lays eggs that embryonate and hatch in the soil as first-stage larvae; these larvae develop into third-stage filariform larvae, which may then initiate human infection by skin penetration. Although multiple free-living generations in the soil have been suggested to occur, it appears that this is not common.

Internal autoinfection (hyperinfection) is a common and dangerous sequela in individuals with latent infections who are immunocompromised, receiving immunosuppressive therapy, alcoholic, or malnourished (8). Latent infections may persist for decades, as evidenced by former World War II prisoners of war who acquired infections in prison camps in southeast Asia; such individuals continue to experience recurrent bouts of serpigenous urticarial rashes on the trunk, buttocks, and groin that are due to larval migration (9). Hyperinfection results in rapid multiplication of these parasites within the intestinal tract, with subsequent reinvasion of the bowel wall or perianal skin by filariform larvae. In addition to the rapid development of new adult females by this process, the extensive migration of these third-stage larvae into virtually all tissues and organs can result in overwhelming infection characterized by extensive hemorrhage and death if not treated rapidly. Interestingly, although latent strongyloidiasis may result in serious complications in individuals who are immunocompromised, this hyperinfection syndrome is not a common occurrence in individuals with AIDS, for reasons not well understood (8).

Diagnosis may be difficult, especially for individuals with long-standing chronic infections. For patients with no symptoms and few parasites, direct wet mount and standard fecal concentration procedures may fail to reveal the first-stage larvae. Individuals who are candidates for immunosuppressive therapy (e.g., organ transplantation, treatment for malignancies) and who are from geographic areas where strongyloidiasis is known to be endemic (e.g., many parts of Latin America and southeast Asia) must be carefully screened prior to treatment. In latent infections, it is common for only small numbers of larvae to be passed in feces, and in many instances, the larvae are passed on an irregular basis. Thus, multiple stool samples taken several days apart should be examined. In addition to normal concentration procedures, examination of the whole fecal specimen by the Baermann procedure is recommended (1). In this procedure, based on the active migration of first-stage larvae out of fecal material into surrounding water, the fecal specimen is placed on top of wire mesh in a large funnel filled with water; the water in the funnel is retained by means of a clamp on rubber tubing at the stem end of the funnel. The fecal mass is allowed to stand for several hours before aliquots of water are drawn off and examined for the presence of larvae. Multiple examinations performed in this manner are likely to detect light infections. In recent years, an agar plate method for diagnosing intestinal strongyloidiasis has been demonstrated to be an efficient and sensitive technique for diagnosis (12, 13). In this procedure, 2 to 4 g of fresh fecal material is placed on beef extract agar in a petri dish and the plates are then examined under a dissecting microscope for up to 72 h. Tracks of larvae migrating out of the fecal mass are readily visualized. Duodenal aspiration techniques, including the Enterotest, also are useful in the diagnosis of this infection.

First-stage *Strongyloides* larvae are the diagnostic stage found in feces; they measure 180 to 380 μm long by 14 to 20 μm wide. They have a short buccal chamber and a prominent cluster of cells, the genital primordium, that is located at midbody between the intestine and the ventral body wall (Fig. 3C and D). Occasionally, in individuals who have hookworm infection, stool specimens from these patients may sit at warm temperatures for 24 h or longer prior to their examination. In these cases, it may be necessary to distinguish the first-stage larvae of hookworms, which have hatched from eggs present in the feces, from *Strongyloides* first-stage larvae. Hookworm first-stage larvae are the same size as *Strongyloides* larvae, but the former have long buccal chambers (Fig. 3E) and their genital primordia are inconspicuous, and usually cannot be seen.

Occasionally, filariform *Strongyloides* larvae may be seen in feces or sputum, particularly in cases of hyperinfection. These larvae are approximately 500 to 600 μm long by 16 μm wide; their ratio of esophagus length to intestinal length is 1:1, and the tail of the larva is notched.

TREMATODES

Adult trematode parasites of humans live in the intestine, liver, lung, or blood vessels. The flukes, as they are frequently called, all have complex life cycles that always involve snails as first intermediate hosts. In addition, many must utilize a second intermediate host in which the infective stage for humans and other definitive hosts develops. The life cycles involve specific freshwater molluscs that are used as intermediate hosts by each species of trematode. The molluscs are infected by a ciliated larva, the miracidium, which emerges from the trematode egg. Within the tissues of the snails, a complex process of reproduction involving several different parasite stages results in the production of tailed, free-swimming larvae called cercariae. Cercariae are released into water, and some (e.g., the schistosomes) may infect humans directly; however, in most species, they invade the tissues of a second intermediate host (e.g., fish, crabs) and develop into an infective, encysted stage called a metacercaria. Some cercariae attach to various types of aquatic vegetation, and the metacercarial stages become encysted on the plant material (e.g., *Fasciola*, *Fasciolopsis*). Human infections with trematodes are usually acquired by ingestion of metacercariae, although schistosomiasis results from direct skin penetration by cercariae. Trematode infections usually are diagnosed by identification of characteristic eggs in feces or, more rarely, in sputum or urine. The eggs of all human trematodes, except the schistosomes, have an operculum through which the miracidium escapes. Small trematode eggs, typically those less than 50 μm long, usually contain a fully developed miracidium when passed in feces, as do the schistosome eggs. Larger trematode eggs are usually undeveloped when excreted in feces and must undergo a period of development in water for several weeks before the miracidium is produced.

Intestinal Flukes

Fasciolopsis buski

F. buski is the largest and most pathogenic of the human intestinal flukes. It occurs in many parts of Asia, including China, India, Indonesia, Taiwan, Thailand, and Vietnam. Pigs and humans are the primary hosts for this parasite, and infection is acquired by ingestion of metacercariae encysted externally on various types of aquatic vegetation (e.g., water chestnuts and the water caltrop). It takes approximately 3 months from ingestion of metacercariae until eggs are found in feces of the human host. The eggs are large, broadly ellipsoidal, and thin shelled, and they measure 130 to 140 μm long by 80 to 85 μm wide; they have an inconspicuous operculum and are unembryonated when passed in feces (Fig. 4A). Although *Fasciolopsis* eggs are similar in size and morphology to those of *Fasciola hepatica*, the sheep, cattle, and human liver fluke, the shell of a *Fasciolopsis* egg at the abopercular end is usually smooth and not roughened as it is in *F. hepatica*. Since *F. buski* is restricted to the Orient, whereas *F. hepatica* is distributed worldwide, it is important also to consider the geographic history and clinical symptomatology of the patient in order to establish the correct diagnosis based on eggs found in feces.

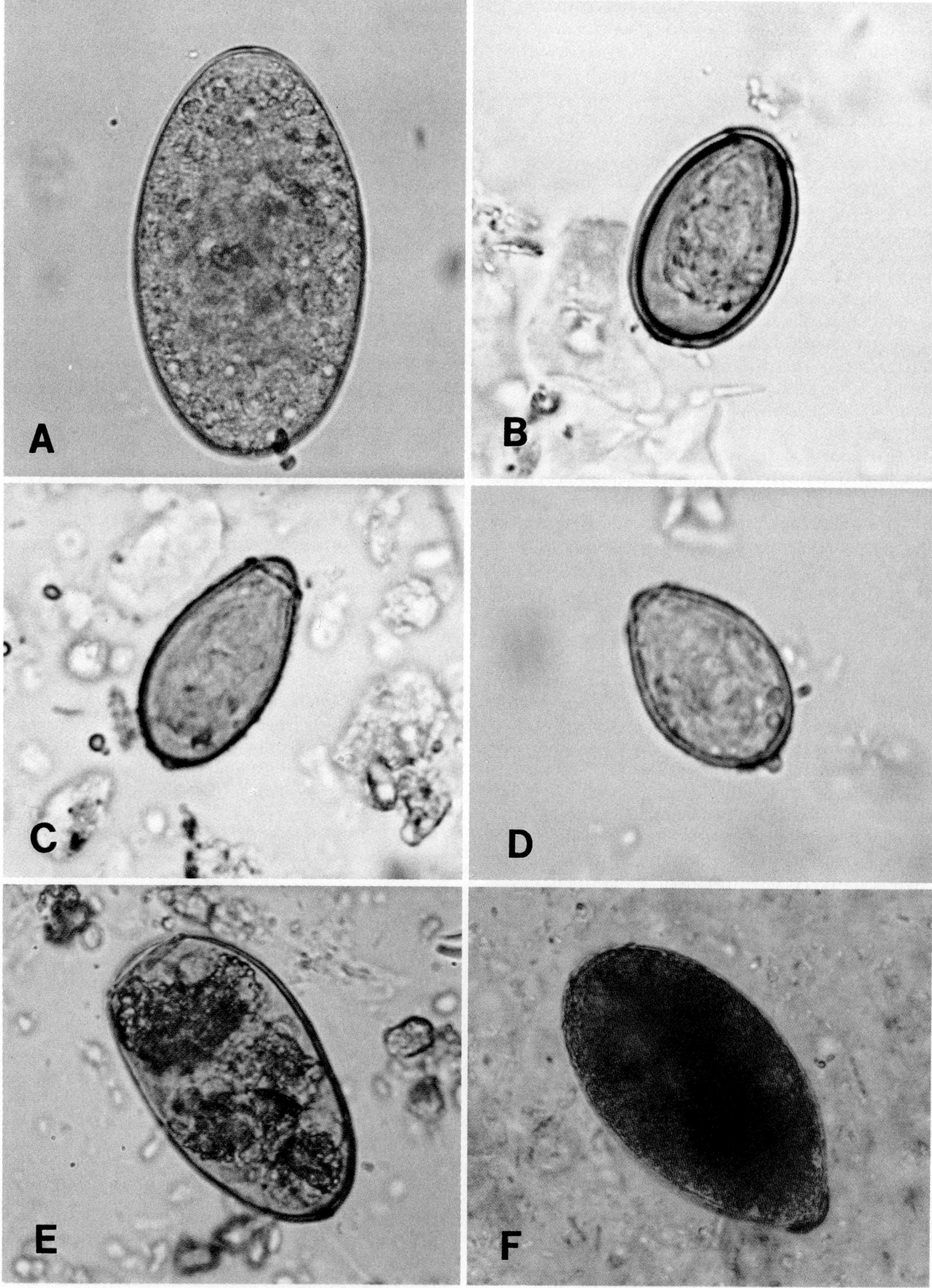

FIGURE 4 Eggs of trematode parasites. (A) *F. buski* (magnification, ×500); (B) *H. heterophyes* (magnification, ×1,500); (C) *Clonorchis sinensis* (magnification, ×1,500); (D) *O. viverrini* (magnification, ×1,500); (E) *P. westermani* (magnification, ×600); (F) *Nanophyetus salmincola* (magnification, ×750). (Panels B through D are from reference 2; used with permission.)

Small Intestinal Fluke Infections

A large number of genera and species of minute intestinal flukes parasitize humans in many parts of the world (15). For the most part, these infections are of minor medical significance, but the presence of the eggs in feces requires that the eggs be identified and distinguished from the morphologically similar eggs of more pathogenic flukes (e.g., *Clonorchis sinensis*, *Opisthorchis* spp.). Among the more common of the small intestinal flukes in humans are *Heterophyes heterophyes* and *Metagonimus yokogawai*. The former occurs in the Orient and the Nile Delta, whereas *Metagonimus* spp. are found not only in the Far East but also in Turkey, the Balkans, and other parts of Europe. In general, these and other small intestinal flukes lack host specificity and will mature in a wide range of mammals and birds that serve as reservoir hosts for human infections. As a consequence, in any particular geographic area where fish are inadequately cooked or are eaten raw, the minute intestinal flukes that are found in humans reflect the particular parasite species endemic in such local animals as dogs, cats, rodents, and birds.

Adult flukes are only a few millimeters long and live in the crypts or the superficial mucosal epithelium of the small intestine; typically, they have a life span of several months or less. Patent infections develop within 2 to 3 weeks of ingestion of metacercariae in the flesh of fish. When large numbers of worms are present, they may cause mild diarrhea and abdominal cramping, but in most cases when small numbers of adults are present, little or no symptomatology is associated with the infections.

The eggs of all these species typically are small (17 to 30 μm long by 13 to 18 μm wide), have more or less inconspicuous opercula, and are embryonated when discharged in feces (Fig. 4B). Though somewhat similar in size and morphology to the eggs of *Clonorchis* and *Opisthorchis*, the eggs of these small intestinal flukes usually lack the seated opercula seen in the eggs of these liver flukes (4). Other genera causing human infections include *Echinostoma* (various countries of southeast Asia), *Pygidiopsis* and *Neodiplostomum* (Korea), *Haplorchis* (Thailand, Vietnam), *Stellantchasmus* (Hawaii), and numerous others in various parts of the world. Morel mushroom spores, which can be found in human feces, are occasionally misidentified as the eggs of some of these small intestinal flukes; however, these spores lack opercula and do not contain miracidia.

Another fluke infection that has been reported from humans in the northwestern United States who ingest raw, incompletely cooked, or smoked salmon is caused by *Nanophyetus salmincola* (5). Although the adult worms are similar in size to the other small intestinal flukes, the eggs they produce are much larger (64 to 97 μm long by 43 to 55 μm wide) and are readily distinguishable from those of other intestinal trematodes (Fig. 4F).

Liver Flukes

Fasciola hepatica

F. hepatica occurs in sheep- and cattle-raising areas worldwide, where it causes occasional to extensive human infection. Infection is acquired by ingestion of aquatic vegetation, such as watercress in salads, on which metacercariae have encysted. It also appears that metacercariae may detach from vegetation, float in water, and be acquired by ingestion of contaminated water. Metacercariae migrate from the intestine to the liver by passing through the intestinal wall into the abdominal cavity, entering the liver by penetration of Glisson's capsule, and migrating through the parenchyma to the bile ducts where they reach maturity and live as adult worms. The prepatent period is approximately 2 months. As a consequence of the need for this extraintestinal migration, migrating worms also may end up in ectopic locations (e.g., body wall, cutaneous tissues, lungs) where they may cause abscesses or fibrotic lesions. Adult worms are large, fleshy flukes that may cause severe liver damage, particularly when present in large numbers.

Eggs of *F. hepatica* are large and broadly ellipsoid and measure 130 to 150 μm in length by 63 to 90 μm in width. The operculum is inconspicuous, the shell appears roughened at the abopercular end, and the eggs are unembryonated when passed in feces. The eggs are similar in size and morphology to those of *Fasciolopsis buski*, but the roughening of the shell at the abopercular end is absent in *F. buski* eggs. Since the eating of parasitized cattle or sheep liver will result in the passage of *Fasciola* eggs in feces, it is necessary to rule out spurious infections by examination of the feces several days after individuals have stopped eating liver.

Clonorchis sinensis

The so-called Oriental liver fluke is commonly seen in the United States, particularly in immigrants from southeast Asia. *C. sinensis* and the closely related species, *Opisthorchis viverrini*, live as adults in the bile ducts of humans and reservoir host animals, including cats and dogs. Infections are acquired by ingestion of metacercariae encysted under the scales of fish that have been insufficiently cooked. In the human or animal host, metacercariae migrate to the bile ducts of the liver by direct migration via the common bile duct. Adult worms reach maturity and begin to lay eggs approximately 1 month following infection. Infections may persist for 20 years or longer. Pickled fish imported from the Orient have been occasional sources of human infection in the United States. *O. viverrini* is a common infection in Thailand.

Diagnosis of infection depends on finding the characteristic eggs in feces. *Clonorchis* eggs are ovoid, thick-shelled, and yellowish-brown in color, and they measure 27 to 35 μm long by 12 to 19 μm in width; they are embryonated when passed in feces (Fig. 4C). The eggs have prominent, seated opercula; the abopercular end of the shell usually has a prominent knob or short, comma-like protuberance. *O. viverrini* eggs are morphologically similar to those of *Clonorchis sinensis* but tend to be somewhat broader and have less conspicuous shoulders (Fig. 4D). The eggs of these liver flukes are somewhat similar in size and appearance to the eggs of many of the small intestinal flukes except that the latter are usually somewhat smaller and lack a seated operculum and the abopercular knob.

Lung Flukes (*Paragonimus westermani*)

Human lung fluke infections are caused by a number of species of *Paragonimus* in various parts of the world, including Asia, Africa, and Latin America. *P. westermani* is widespread in Asia and is perhaps the most important species causing human disease. Dogs, cats, and other wild animals serve as important reservoirs of human infection for all species. Adult flukes usually live in pairs in fibrous capsules in the lung parenchyma of their hosts. The eggs that are produced pass up the bronchial tree and may be found in sputum or feces. Crabs and crayfish serve as second intermediate hosts, and human infections usually derive from eating raw or inadequately cooked infected crustaceans. The practice of marinating raw crab in brine, wine, or vinegar is usually ineffectual in killing metacercariae.

In the human host, metacercariae migrate from the intestine into the body cavity, move through the diaphragm into the thoracic cavity, and then invade the lungs, where the worms mature and begin to lay eggs in 5 to 6 weeks. These infections may be long-lived, frequently 1 to 2 decades or longer. In the course of larval migration from the intestine, the flukes may end up in ectopic locations, such as the rib cage, body wall, and the brain. Infection in the brain is frequently fatal. Histologic sections of these ectopic locations frequently demonstrate only eggs and not the adult worms.

Diagnosis depends on finding eggs in feces or, less frequently, sputum. Eggs are broadly ovoid, thick-shelled, and yellow-brown, and they measure 80 to 120 μm long by 45 to 70 μm wide (Fig. 4E). They have prominent opercula, the shell is distinctly thickened at the abopercular end of the shell, and they are unembryonated when passed in feces. Although the operculate eggs of the fish tapeworm *Diphyllobothrium latum* are sometimes misidentified as those of *P. westermani*, the former are considerably smaller and have a knob-like structure at the abopercular end of the shell.

Several other species of *Paragonimus* have been described as causing human infection: in Africa, *P. uterobilateralis* and *P. africanus*, and in the Western Hemisphere, *P. mexicanus*, *P. caliensis*, and *P. ecuadoriensis*. Other species also have been reported from China and southeast Asian countries. The eggs of all these species will differ somewhat in size and morphology from those of *P. westermani*, but they are sufficiently similar that a generic diagnosis usually can be made, with specific identification depending to a certain extent on where the infection is found.

Blood Flukes (Schistosomes)

Schistosomiasis (bilharziasis) afflicts more than 250 million people in the world and as such is, along with malaria, one of the most important of all human parasitic diseases. The etiologic agents are markedly different from the other human trematodes. The schistosomes have separate sexes (all other human flukes are hermaphroditic) and live in blood vessels of the abdominal cavity. The three most important human species are *Schistosoma mansoni*, *S. japonicum*, and *S. haematobium*; other species of lesser human importance include *S. mekongi* (Asia) and *S. intercalatum* (Africa). Though each of the schistosomes utilizes specific and different snail intermediate hosts, their life cycles are similar. Each produces thin-shelled eggs that lack opercula and contain a miracidium when excreted in feces or urine. The egg shell of each species typically has a lateral or terminal spine that aids in identification. Miracidia hatch from the eggs and penetrate appropriate snails to establish infection. Infected snails produce fork-tailed cercariae that are liberated into water and directly penetrate the skin to establish infections in human and animal hosts. In the human host, the larval blood flukes migrate through the lungs and become established in venous blood vessels of the mesenteries or bladder, where they mature and mate and the females deposit eggs. The eggs make their way through the wall of the intestine or bladder and are excreted in feces or urine. Pathology due to schistosome infection is primarily due to egg deposition in tissues with resulting granuloma formation.

Schistosoma mansoni

S. mansoni has the widest geographic distribution of the schistosomes; it is found in Africa, the Arabian peninsula, Brazil, and some islands in the Caribbean. Adult worms live in the portal system of the liver and the small venules of the lower ileum and colon. Eggs are laid in the blood vessels, make their way through the wall of the intestine, and are passed in feces. *S. mansoni* eggs measure from 114 to 175 μm long by 45 to 70 μm wide; they contain a miracidium, and the shell has a prominent lateral spine (Fig. 5A and 5B). The prepatent period for the infection is approximately 6 weeks. In acute schistosomiasis, blood and mucus appear in feces along with the lateral-spined eggs. In chronic schistosomiasis, eggs accumulate in the walls of the intestine and rectum and also in the liver; correspondingly, fewer eggs are found in feces, and concentration procedures are required to diagnose the infection reliably. Rectal biopsies of the mucosa may be useful in chronic infections (1).

Schistosoma japonicum

S. japonicum is found in China, the Philippines, and other countries of southeast Asia. A zoophilic strain of the parasite infects animals but not humans in Taiwan, and the infection has been virtually eliminated from Japan, where occasional infections may be found in cattle. Animal reservoirs of infection are important and include water buffaloes, pigs, dogs, cats, and wild rodents. Adult worms live in mesenteric veins, and the prepatent period is 5 to 6 weeks. The embryonated eggs found in feces are round to ovoid, lack opercula, and are 70 to 100 μm long by 55 to 65 μm wide. The thin shell has a small, inconspicuous spine that frequently is difficult to see (Fig. 5C). In addition, the surface of the egg often has fecal debris adhering to it which can obscure the egg and make it difficult to recognize. Rectal biopsy is an important diagnostic tool when fecal examinations are negative. Female worms produce larger numbers of eggs than the other schistosome species, resulting in extensive pathology in the wall of the intestine and liver. Because of the size of the eggs, they may be disseminated widely in the body via the vascular system. The brain and spinal cord are often involved, and in the Philippines, severe epileptic seizures are a frequent feature of this infection.

Schistosoma haematobium

S. haematobium occurs in Africa, Lebanon, Syria, Iran, the Arabian peninsula, and Malagasy, where it causes urinary schistosomiasis. Adult worms reside in the venous plexuses of the bladder, and eggs that are laid move through the wall of the bladder and are passed in urine. In chronic infections, accumulation of eggs in the bladder wall can lead to bladder and ureter pathology. Symptomatology includes hematuria, difficulty with micturition, and the development of hydroureter and hydronephrosis; renal complications and renal failure are common sequelae of infection. *S. haematobium* infection is believed to be a predisposing factor to squamous cell carcinoma of the bladder (14). The elongated, thin-shelled eggs are 112 to 170 μm long by 40 to 70 μm in width and contain a miracidum; there is a terminal spine (Fig. 5E). Diagnosis typically is made by examination of urine. Eggs can sometimes be found in feces and in the wall of the rectum as well as in the bladder wall.

Schistosoma intercalatum

The human schistosome *S. intercalatum* occurs in Zaire, Gabon, Cameroon, and the Central African Republic. The eggs of this species have a terminal spine, measure 140 to 240 μm long by 50 to 85 μm in width, and are found in feces (Fig. 5F). Because the eggs of *S. haematobium* sometimes occur in feces, it is necessary to differentiate *S. interca-*

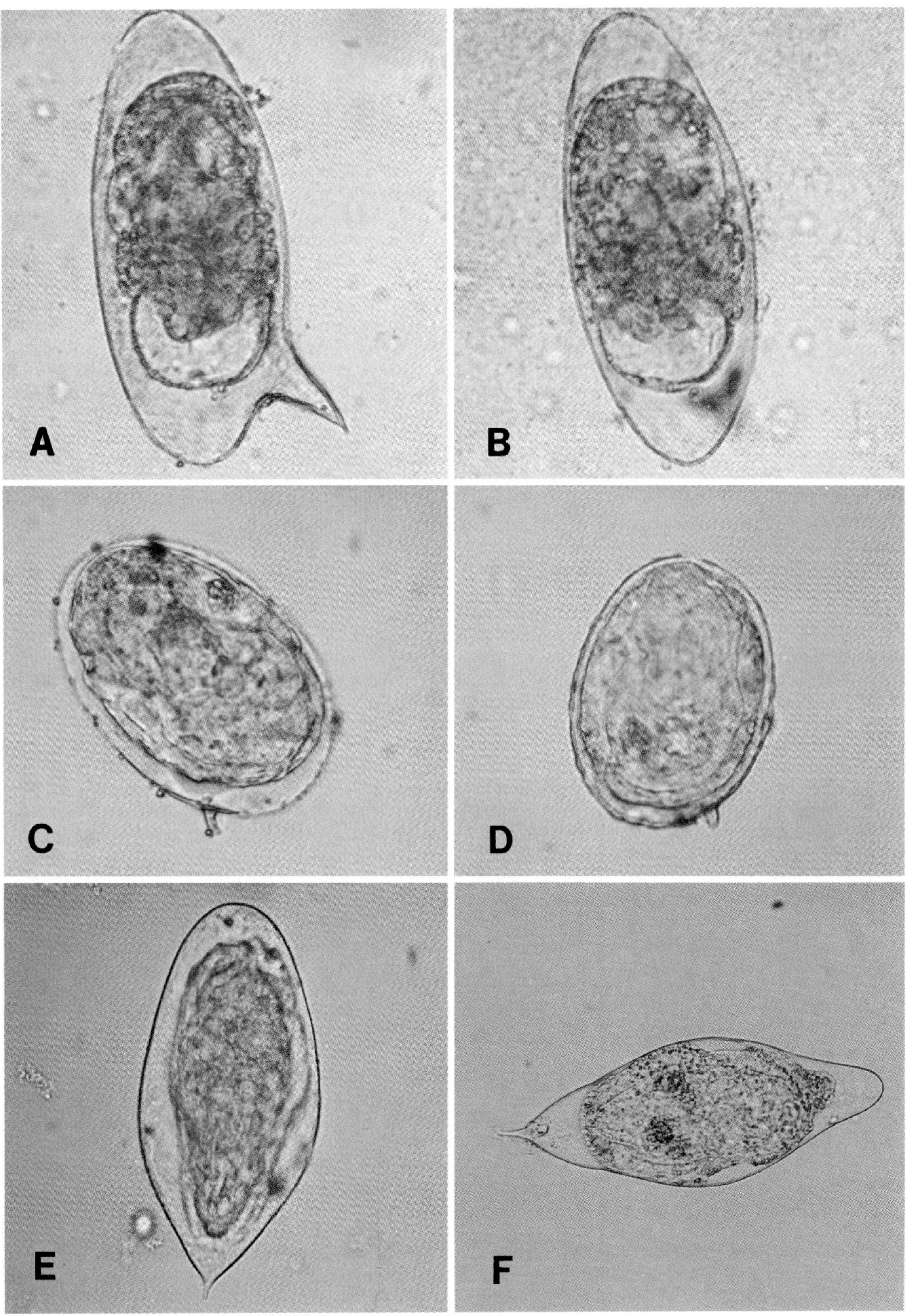

FIGURE 5 Eggs of schistosome species (magnification, ×600). (A) *Schistosoma mansoni*; (B) *Schistosoma mansoni* egg with typical lateral spine not in view; (C) *Schistosoma japonicum*; (D) *Schistosoma mekongi*; (E) *Schistosoma haematobium*; (F) *Schistosoma intercalatum*. (Panels C through E are from reference 2; used with permission.)

latum from *S. haematobium* eggs. The egg of *S. intercalatum* usually is larger and has an equatorial bulge and a terminal spine that is more pointed, slightly curved, and longer than that of *S. haematobium*.

Schistosoma mekongi

Closely related to *S. japonicum*, *S. mekongi* is a parasite of humans and dogs in countries bordering on the Mekong River, especially Laos and Cambodia. The egg is similar in morphology to that of *S. japonicum* but is smaller, ranging from 51 to 78 μm long by 39 to 66 μm wide (Fig. 5D). Eggs from dogs are usually smaller than those from humans. The knoblike spine on the egg may be difficult to see.

CESTODES

The four most common adult tapeworm parasites of the human small intestine are *Diphyllobothrium latum*, *Taenia saginata*, *Taenia solium*, and *Hymenolepis nana*. Two other tapeworms, primarily animal parasites, reach maturity in humans and may occasionally cause infections; they are *Hymenolepis diminuta* and *Dipylidium caninum*. In addition to the adult tapeworms, a number of larval cestodes can produce serious human disease, including cysticercosis (*Taenia solium*), hydatid disease (*Echinococcus* species), and coenurosis (*Taenia multiceps*); these larval tapeworms occurring in human tissues are discussed in chapter 113 of this Manual. The large adult tapeworms, *D. latum*, *T. saginata*, and *T. solium*, usually occur singly in the small intestine and may live 20 years or longer. Diagnosis of tapeworm infections is achieved by finding characteristic eggs, proglottids, or both, depending on the species involved, in feces.

All of the adult tapeworms parasitizing humans require an intermediate host with the exception of *H. nana*, which may infect humans directly by eggs or indirectly by using beetle intermediate hosts. Morphologically, adult tapeworms have a scolex at the anterior end and a short, undifferentiated neck region that gives rise to the proglottids; the main body (strobila) of the tapeworm adult consists of the neck, immature, mature, and gravid proglottids. As tapeworms increase in age and size, the most posterior gravid proglottids may break off or disintegrate and pass in feces. Some tapeworms (*D. latum*, *H. nana*, and *H. diminuta*) lay eggs that are passed in feces; for others (*T. saginata* and *T. solium*), their gravid proglottids typically break off and are passed in feces or actively migrate out of the anus. Sometimes, *Taenia* proglottids rupture in the intestine, and eggs then appear in feces. The eggs of all species of *Taenia* and the related genus, *Echinococcus*, are morphologically identical and cannot be distinguished from one another. The eggs of *T. solium*, *T. multiceps*, and *Echinococcus* species can infect humans directly and cause disease by their larval stages; the eggs of *T. saginata* are not directly infective to humans.

Diphyllobothrium latum

Known as the fish tapeworm, *D. latum* differs from other adult tapeworms infecting humans in its morphology, biology, and epidemiology. Its geographic distribution includes areas with cold, clear lakes as in Scandinavia, other areas of northern Europe, the former USSR, northern Japan, and North America, principally the upper Midwest, Alaska, and Canada. The adult parasite can attain a length of 10 to 15 m, is ivory in color, and has a scolex that is provided with shallow grooves (bothria), rather than suckers on its dorsal and ventral aspects.

In its life cycle, unembryonated, operculate eggs, resembling those of trematodes, are passed in feces and must undergo embryonation in water for several weeks. Ciliated, six-hooked embryos (coracidia) hatch from these eggs and must be ingested by appropriate species of freshwater copepods. Within the copepod a solid-bodied larval stage, the procercoid, develops and becomes infective to the second intermediate host, fish. In fish, the procercoids migrate into the flesh and develop to the plerocercoid (sparganum) stage, which is then infective to human or animal hosts. After ingestion of the sparganum, it takes 3 to 5 weeks for the adult tapeworm to attain maturity and begin to lay eggs. The parasite may produce no clinical symptoms in some people, but when it reaches a large size it may cause mechanical obstruction of the bowel, may cause diarrhea and abdominal pain, and in some individuals, particularly in northern European countries, may be responsible for a vitamin B_{12} deficiency that results in pernicious anemia.

Diagnosis is made by finding the characteristic operculate eggs in feces. They are 58 to 75 μm long by 44 to 50 μm wide. The abopercular end frequently has a small knoblike protrusion (Fig. 6F). Individuals with long-standing infection are likely to have large numbers of eggs in feces. As infections grow older, one or a small chain of proglottids may break off and be passed in feces. Proglottids passed in feces are wider than long (3 by 1 mm), and the genital pore is situated on the midventral surface rather than laterally as in the other human tapeworms. In freshly passed proglottids, the coiled uterus in the center of the proglottid is yellow-brown.

Taenia saginata

T. saginata is known as the beef tapeworm and is distributed worldwide, but it is especially prevalent in Mexico, South America, eastern and western Asia, and many countries in Europe. Cattle serve as the intermediate host, and ingestion of eggs from contaminated pasturelands by grazing cattle results in development in cattle tissues of the infective cysticercus stage (*Cysticercus bovis*).

The cysticercus is 4 to 6 mm long by 7 to 10 mm wide and has a pearl-like appearance in tissues; the unarmed scolex is invaginated into a fluid-filled bladder. After ingestion of the cysticercus in raw or inadequately cooked beef, it takes approximately 2 to 3 months for the infection to become patent in the human host. An adult tapeworm attains lengths of 4 to 8 m and has a scolex provided with four suckers and an unarmed rostellum; gravid proglottids are longer than they are wide (18 to 20 mm by 5 to 7 mm). Each proglottid has a genital pore at the midlateral margin. In mature proglottids, the ovary has only two lobes, and a vaginal sphincter muscle is present. Gravid proglottids, which are highly muscular and active, break off from the strobila and can actively migrate out of the anus. Although patients may exhibit no symptomatology with this infection, the mature worm may cause abdominal discomfort, diarrhea, and occasionally intestinal obstruction as a result of its large size.

Diagnosis of species usually is made by identification of gravid proglottids that have been passed in feces or have actively migrated out of the anus. Identification of the proglottids is based on morphology of the uterus, which can be demonstrated after injection with India ink or staining with carmine or hematoxylin stains (1). In *T. saginata*, there are 15 to 20 lateral branches on each side of the central uterine stem. If the proglottids rupture in the intestine, the typical *Taenia* eggs can be seen in feces. A taeniid egg is spherical and has a thick, yellow-brown, prismatic shell (Fig. 6A).

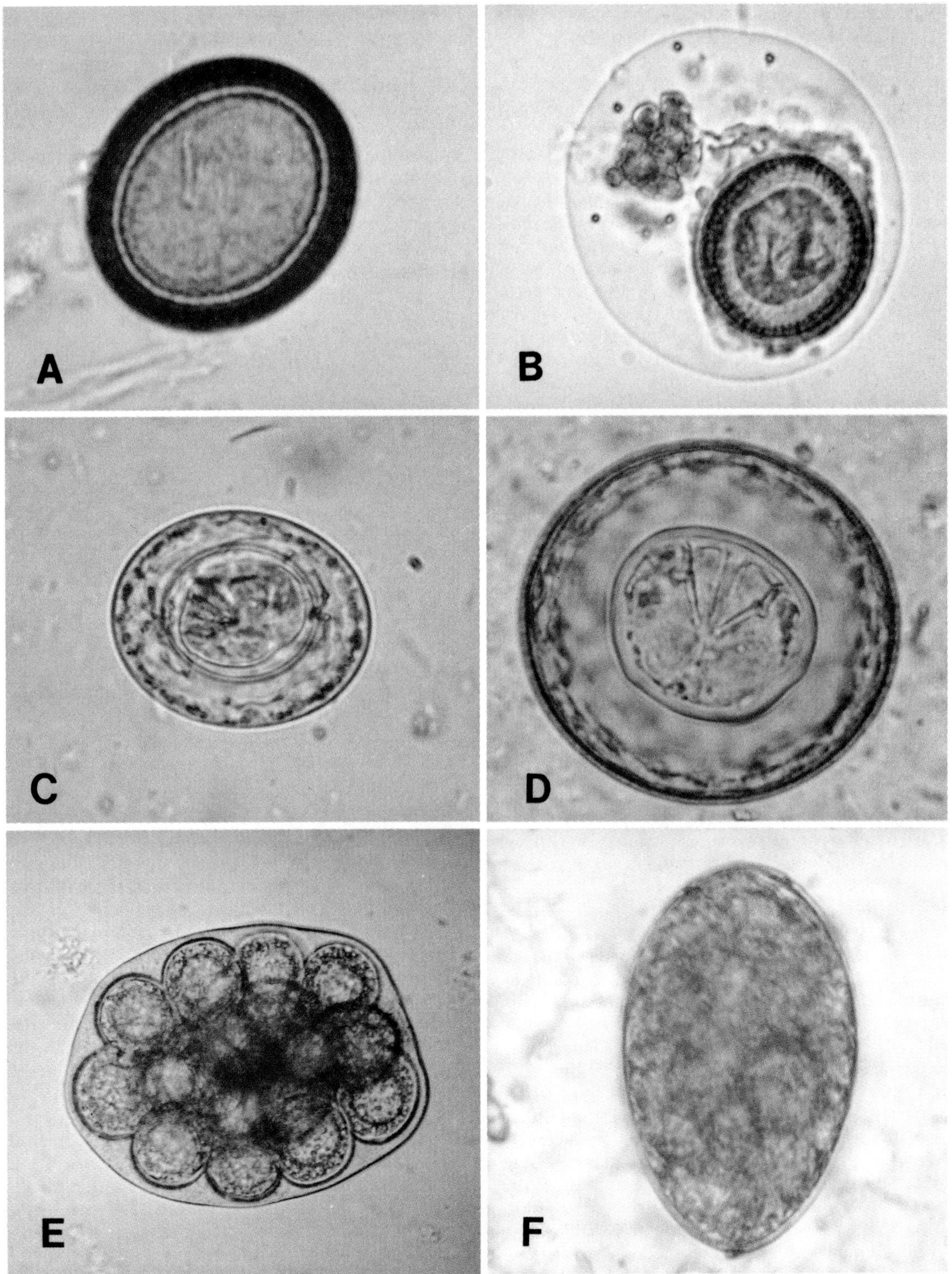

FIGURE 6 Eggs of cestodes. (A) *Taenia* species. Eggs of all species of *Taenia* and *Echinococcus* are identical (magnification, ×1,000). (B) *Taenia* egg surrounded by the primary membrane frequently seen around eggs directly liberated from gravid proglottids (magnification, ×800); (C) *Hymenolepis nana* (magnification, ×900); (D) *Hymenolepis diminuta* (magnification, ×900); (E) egg packet of *Dipylidium caninum*; (F) *D. latum* (magnification, ×800). (Panels B through F are from reference 2; used with permission.)

Within the egg is a six-hooked embryo, the oncosphere. Occasionally, especially when eggs are liberated directly from proglottids, there is a thin outer membrane around the eggs (Fig. 6B). Eggs are 31 to 43 μm in diameter.

It is generally accepted that the eggs of *T. saginata* are not directly infective to humans, but caution should be exercised in the handling of all proglottids and taeniid eggs, since the eggs of *T. solium*, *T. multiceps*, and *Echinococcus* spp. are directly infective to humans and can cause cysticercosis, coenurosis, and hydatidosis, respectively.

In Taiwan, the Philippines, Korea, and perhaps other parts of southeast Asia, there is a human tapeworm morphologically identical as an adult worm to *Taenia saginata*; on the basis of morphologic and molecular studies, this tapeworm has been described as a subspecies, *T. saginata asiatica*. (6). With this Asian species, the cysticercus stage usually occurs in the liver of pigs and less frequently in cattle. Unlike the typical *Taenia saginata* cysticercus, the scolex of *T. saginata asiatica* has two rudimentary rows of hooklets. The adult tapeworm is indistinguishable from the typical *T. saginata*; it even lacks hooks on the scolex.

Taenia solium

Known as the pork tapeworm, *T. solium* has an extensive geographic distribution throughout Europe, Mexico, Central and South America, China, and India. It is no longer commonly found in the United States, although recent immigrants from Mexico and Latin America, in particular, may commonly harbor the parasite. Human infection is acquired by ingestion of infective cysticerci (*Cysticercus cellulosae*) in inadequately cooked pork or pork products. The adult worm may reach lengths of 2 to 7 m; it has a scolex with four suckers and a rostellum armed with two rows of hooklets. In mature proglottids, the ovary has two lobes and an accessory lobe (the accessory lobe is lacking in *T. saginata*), and a vaginal sphincter muscle is lacking (it is present in *T. saginata*). Gravid proglottids have 7 to 13 lateral branches off the central uterine stem. Since the eggs of *Taenia solium* are infective to humans and can cause cysticercosis, extreme caution in the handling of these proglottids is recommended.

Hymenolepis nana

H. nana is the smallest of the adult human tapeworms, attaining lengths of 2.5 to 4.0 mm, and is the most common tapeworm infection of humans in the United States. It is normally a parasite of mice, in which the life cycle characteristically involves various beetles as intermediate hosts. In humans, transmission is usually accomplished by direct ingestion of infective eggs containing oncospheres. When eggs are ingested, a solid-bodied larva, a cysticercoid, first develops in the wall of the small intestine; subsequently, the larva migrates back into the intestinal lumen where it reaches maturity as an adult tapeworm in 2 to 3 weeks. In beetles that ingest eggs of *H. nana*, the cysticercoids develop in the body cavity and have thick protective walls about them. Although humans may acquire infection by accidental ingestion of infected beetles (often occurring in dry cereals), direct infection is far more common and is the primary reason that *H. nana* usually occurs in institutional and familial settings where hygiene is substandard. A feature of human *H. nana* infection is the opportunity for internal autoinfection with the parasite, which may result in large worm burdens. Autoinfection occurs when eggs discharged by adult tapeworms in the lumen of the small intestine hatch rapidly and invade the wall of the intestine; here, cysticercoids are formed, and they subsequently reenter the intestine to mature to adult worms.

Diagnosis of the infection rests on finding the spherical to subspherical eggs in feces. The eggs are 30 to 47 μm in diameter and thin shelled, and they contain a six-hooked oncosphere that lies in the center of the egg and is separated from the outer shell by considerable space (Fig. 6C). The oncosphere is surrounded by a membrane that has two polar thickenings from which arise four to eight filaments extending into the space between it and the outer shell. Proglottids are rarely seen, since gravid proglottids do not ordinarily break off from the main strobila of the adult worm.

Hymenolepis diminuta

An occasional human parasite, *H. diminuta* is primarily a parasite of rats. Beetles and other arthropods serve as obligatory intermediate hosts, with humans generally acquiring infection accidentally by ingestion of infected meal beetles present in various grains and cereals. Cysticercoids, the infective stage, develop in the hemocoels of beetles after ingestion of eggs. As an adult, *H. diminuta* may be 20 to 60 cm long, and numerous tapeworms may be present in the same host. In humans, hyperinfection or direct infection by ingestion of eggs, as occurs with *H. nana*, has not been recorded.

Diagnosis of infection is by demonstration of eggs in feces. The eggs are spherical and large, 70 to 85 μm by 60 to 80 μm, and have a yellow-brown, moderately thick shell (Fig. 6D). The six-hooked oncosphere in the egg is central and considerably separated from the outer membrane; however, there are no polar thickenings or filaments such as those in the eggs of *H. nana*. As in *H. nana* infection, proglottids do not usually break away from the strobila of the adult worms and are not usually a diagnostic consideration as in the large tapeworms parasitizing humans.

Dipylidium caninum

D. caninum is the most common and widespread adult tapeworm of dogs and cats. Human infection has been reported in many parts of the world. Children are more frequently infected than adults as a result of their more intimate contact with dogs and their fleas, which serve as obligatory intermediate hosts. Because the infection is not a troublesome one and is self-limiting, there are probably many more cases than are reported in the literature.

Adult tapeworms may be present in considerable numbers and may vary in length from 10 to 70 cm. The scolex is conical, with four prominent suckers and a small, retractile rostellum that bears multiple rows of small spines. Gravid proglottids are elongate (23 mm by 8 mm), have a genital pore on both lateral margins (hence the name double-pored dog tapeworm), and are divided into small compartments, each of which contains 8 to 15 oncospheres that are enclosed in a thin, embryonic membrane. In dogs, the white proglottids are frequently passed in feces or may be seen dangling from the anus as small chains; on carpeting and floors, these segments undergo dehydration and resemble grains of rice. In the life cycle, wormlike larval fleas in soil or carpeting ingest the eggs in the proglottids, and cysticercoids develop in the hemocoel. When the larval fleas metamorphose into adult fleas, the cysticercoids remain viable, and animal or human infections usually are acquired by ingestion of the adult fleas. Adult tapeworms reach maturity in the small intestine in approximately 1 month.

Diagnosis of infection is usually made by finding the typical, double-pored, compartmented proglottids in feces or by finding egg packets containing multiple oncospheres liberated by disintegration of the proglottids (Fig. 6E).

REFERENCES

1. **Ash, L. R., and T. C. Orihel.** 1991. *Parasites: A Guide to Laboratory Procedures and Identification.* ASCP Press, Chicago.
2. **Ash, L. R., and T. C. Orihel.** 1997. *Atlas of Human Parasitology*, 4th ed. ASCP Press, Chicago.
3. **Cross, J. H.** 1992. Intestinal capillariasis. *Clin. Microbiol. Rev.* **5:**120–129.
4. **Ditrich, O., M. Giboda, T. Scholz, and S. A. Beer.** 1992. Comparative morphology of eggs of the Haplorchiinae (Trematoda: Heterophyidae) and some other medically important heterophyid and opisthorchiid flukes. *Folia Parasitol.* **39:**123–132.
5. **Eastburn, R. L., T. R. Fritsche, and C. A. Terhune, Jr.** 1987. Human intestinal infection with *Nanophyetus salmincola* from salmonid fishes. *Am. J. Trop. Med. Hyg.* **36:** 586–591.
6. **Fan, P. C., C. Y. Lin, C. C. Chen, and W. C. Chung.** 1995. Morphological description of *Taenia saginata asiatica* (Cyclophyllidea: Taeniidae) from man in Asia. *J. Helminthol.* **69:**299–303.
7. **Liu, L. X., J. Chi, M. P. Upton, and L. R. Ash.** 1995. Eosinophilic colitis associated with larvae of the pinworm *Enterobius vermicularis*. *Lancet* **346:**410–412.
8. **Mahmoud, A. A. F.** 1996. Strongyloidiasis. *Clin. Infect. Dis.* **23:**949–953.
9. **Pelletier, L. L.** 1984. Chronic strongyloidiasis in World War II Far East ex-prisoners of war. *Am. J. Trop. Med. Hyg.* **33:**55–61.
10. **Petithory, J. C., and F. Ardoin-Guidon.** 1995. *Vrais et Faux Parasites en Coprologie Microscopique.* Cahier Information Biologie Medicale No. 03, Paris, France.
11. **Prociv, P., and J. Croese.** 1996. Human enteric infection with *Ancylostoma caninum*: hookworms reappraised in the light of a "new" zoonosis. *Acta Trop.* **62:**23–44.
12. **Salazar, S. A., C. Gutierrez, and S. L. Berk.** 1995. Value of the agar plate method for the diagnosis of intestinal strongyloidiasis. *Diagn. Microbiol. Infect. Dis.* **23:**141–145.
13. **Sato, Y., J. Kobayashi, H. Toma, and Y. Shiroma.** 1995. Efficacy of stool examination for detection of *Strongyloides* infection. *Am. J. Trop. Med. Hyg.* **53:**248–250.
14. **Smith, J. H., and J. D. Christie.** 1986. The pathobiology of *Schistosoma haematobium* infections in humans. *Hum. Pathol.* **17:**333–345.
15. **World Health Organization.** 1995. Control of foodborne trematode infections. *WHO Tech. Rep. Series* **849:**1–157.
16. **Yoshikawa, H., M. Yamada, Y. Matsumoto, and Y. Yoshida.** 1989. Variations in egg size of *Trichuris trichiura*. *Parasitol. Res.* **75:**649–654.

Tissue Helminths

THOMAS C. ORIHEL AND LAWRENCE R. ASH

113

There are a large number of helminth parasites, including the nematodes, flukes, and tapeworms, which live in human tissues as adults or larvae. Some are natural parasites of humans, while a larger number are zoonotic species. Diagnosis of these infections usually depends on the identification of the parasite's reproductive products discharged into the blood, feces, or other body fluids or, in the case of larval parasites, on their recovery from the tissues. The nematodes are represented by a diversity of species, many of which are not well known. The trematodes are equally diverse in both their structure and tissue habitats. These have already been covered in large part in the preceding chapter on intestinal parasites, because their eggs are passed in feces and urine. The cestodes are represented by larval tapeworms, which cause cysticercosis, coenurosis, sparganosis, and hydatid disease.

Although these parasites are relatively easily identified when they are intact, recognition in histopathologic material is often problematic.

NEMATODES

Filariae

The filarial worms are arthropod-transmitted parasites of the lymphatic, subcutaneous, and cutaneous tissues of humans. All share a unique characteristic: the adult female worm produces a primitive larva called a microfilaria, which is found in the peripheral blood or in the skin. Certain species of microfilariae circulate in the blood with a well-defined circadian rhythm or "periodicity," which may be nocturnal or diurnal; other species lack periodicity and are found in the peripheral blood at all hours of the day and night. When absent from the peripheral blood, microfilariae are found in the deeper visceral capillaries. Because the adult worms are typically sequestered in the tissues, diagnosis of infection depends on finding microfilariae in blood or skin depending on the species.

The microfilaria is relatively simple in its organization and structure (1). It is vermiform, and in stained preparations it appears to be composed of a column of nuclei interrupted along its length by spaces and special cells which are the precursors of body organs or organelles. Some species of microfilariae are enveloped in a sheath, whereas others have no sheath.

All of the filariae are transmitted by species of bloodsucking arthropods such as mosquitoes, midges, blackflies, and tabanid flies, in which the microfilaria develops to the infective stage. Subsequent development of the infective larva to the gravid, adult stage in the vertebrate host requires several months and in some cases a year or more. Although these parasites are not endemic in humans in the United States, they are often seen in immigrants or in individuals who have resided or traveled in areas of endemic infection. Several species of filariae infect humans.

Wuchereria bancrofti, which causes an infection often referred to as bancroftian filariasis, is the most common and widespread species of filaria infecting humans. It has an extensive distribution throughout tropical and subtropical areas of the world. The adult worms live in the host lymphatic system and cause lymphangitis, lymphadenitis, and obstructive fibrosis, which restricts the flow of lymph, with resultant lymphedema. Chronic infection may result in elephantiasis of the extremities and genitalia and, in males, hydrocoele. The microfilariae circulate in the peripheral blood with a nocturnal periodicity in most regions of the world; however, in the South Pacific region, they circulate essentially without any periodicity. The microfilaria is sheathed, lies in smooth curves in stained smears, and is about 298 μm long by 7.5 to 10.0 μm in diameter. The column nuclei are dispersed; there is a short headspace, and the pointed tail is devoid of nuclei (Fig. 1A). The sheath stains faintly or not at all with Giemsa stain. The microfilaria of *W. bancrofti* must be distinguished from other sheathed microfilariae. This is accomplished most easily on the basis of the arrangement of nuclei, particularly in the tail (Fig. 2). Since microfilariae may be present in the blood only in small numbers, sensitive procedures such as thick blood films, saponin lysis, Knott concentration, or membrane filter concentration are used routinely to detect infections (2).

Brugia malayi is another mosquito-borne filaria which inhabits the lymphatic system of humans. It is restricted in its geographical distribution to Asia and the Indian subcontinent. In some regions it is coendemic with *W. bancrofti*. Lymphatic pathologic changes similar to those in chronic bancroftian filariasis occur in chronic infections with this parasite as well. The microfilariae, which circulate in the blood, may be periodic or subperiodic but are usually peri-

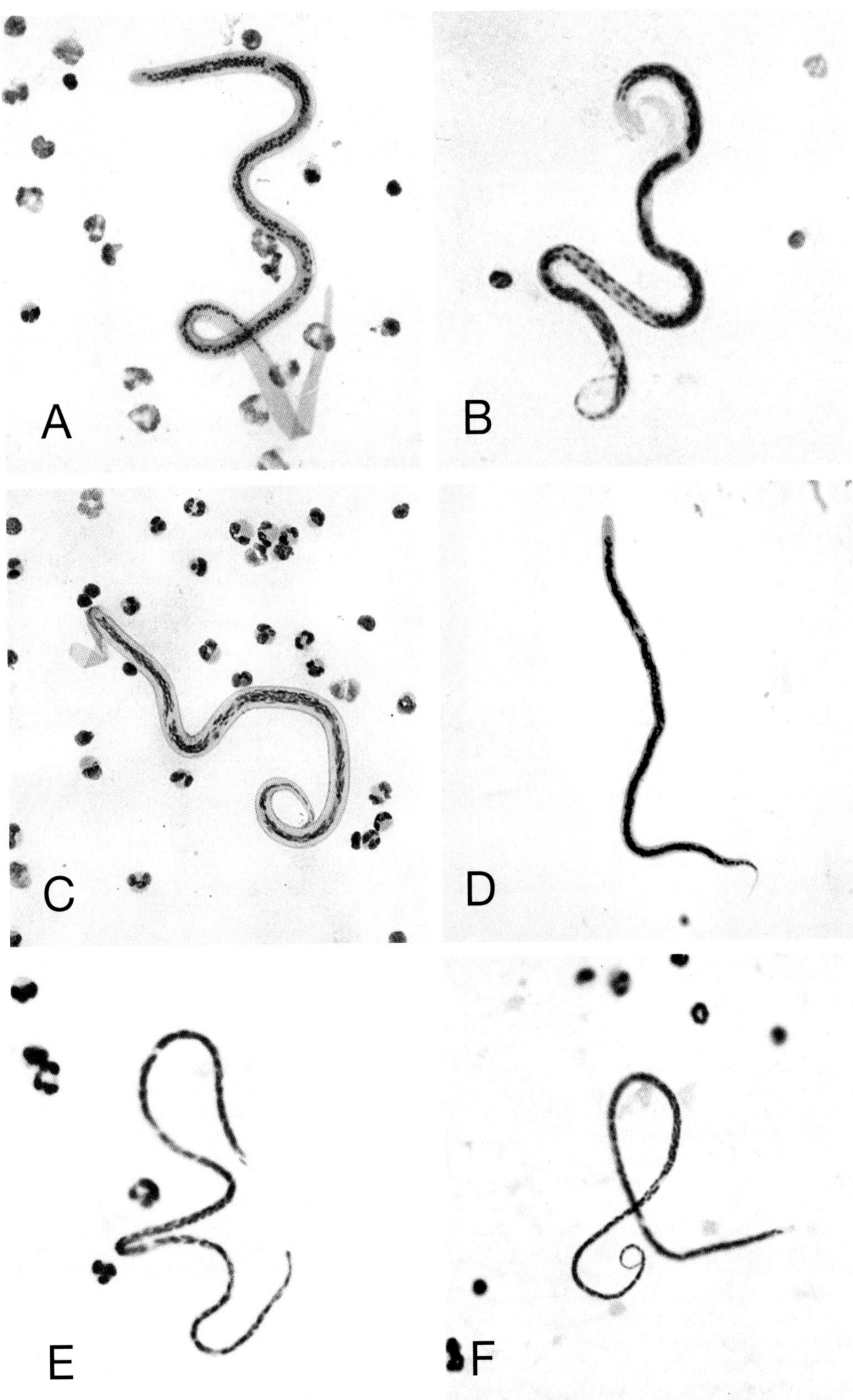

FIGURE 1 Common microfilariae found in humans. Hematoxylin stain. Magnification, ×325. (A) *W. bancrofti*; (B) *B. malayi*; (C) *L. loa*; (D) *O. volvulus*; (E) *M. perstans*; (F) *M. ozzardi*.

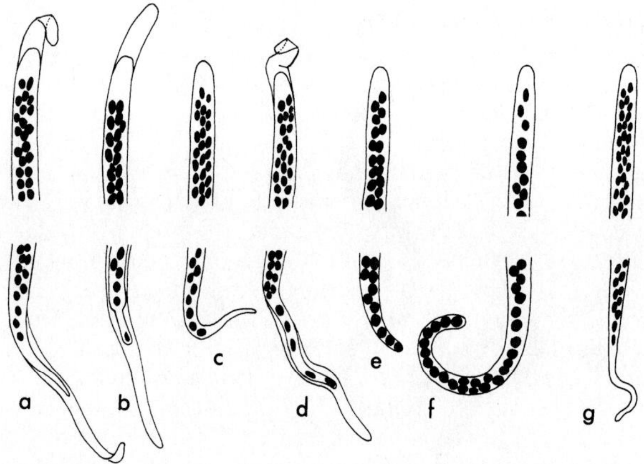

FIGURE 2 Diagrammatic representation of the anterior and posterior extremities of the common microfilariae found in humans. (a) *W. bancrofti*; (b) *B. malayi*; (c) *O. volvulus*; (d) *L. loa*; (e) *M. perstans*; (f) *M. streptocerca*; (g) *M. ozzardi*.

odic. The morphology of the microfilaria is similar to that of the *W. bancrofti* microfilaria, being sheathed but somewhat smaller (270 by 5 to 6 μm). It can be differentiated from the *W. bancrofti* microfilaria by the presence of subterminal and terminal nuclei in the tail (Fig. 1B and 2b). The sheath stains bright pink with Giemsa stain, whereas that of *W. bancrofti* does not (1).

A third species of lymphatic filariae, *Brugia timori*, infects humans living at the eastern end of the Indonesian archipelago, particularly the islands of Timor and Flores. This species produces a microfilaria very similar to that of *B. malayi* with the conspicuous subterminal and terminal nuclei. The two can be most easily differentiated on the basis of size. *B. timori* is larger, more than 300 μm long; also, its sheath tends not to stain with Giemsa stain.

Loa loa, a common filarial parasite of humans, is endemic only in West and Central Africa. It is often referred to as the eye worm because the adult worms, which live in the subcutaneous tissues, often migrate into the orbit and the conjunctivae. The adult worms move freely through the tissues, often producing transient, inflammatory reactions referred to as Calabar swellings. The microfilariae circulate in the blood, often in very large numbers, with a diurnal periodicity. They are sheathed and are up to 300 μm long. In contrast to other sheathed microfilariae discussed above, the nuclei extend to the end of the tail; however, they are somewhat irregularly arranged along the length of the tail (Fig. 1C and 2d). The sheath of the microfilaria does not stain with Giemsa stain. When adult worms enter the conjunctivae, they can be extracted surgically. Diagnosis of infection depends on identification of the microfilaria in daytime blood films or removal of adult worms from the conjunctivae.

Onchocerca volvulus is an important human filarial parasite in both hemispheres. It is endemic across Central Africa, in a small area in the Middle East (Yemen), in Central America (Mexico and Guatemala), and in northern South America. The adult worms are embedded in fibrous nodules in the subcutaneous tissues and frequently in deeper tissues. These nodules, or "onchocercomata," may be found on the head, trunk, and extremities; their anatomical location frequently correlates with the geographical strain of the parasite. The microfilaria lives in the skin. It lacks a sheath and is approximately 309 μm long by 5 to 9 μm in diameter. The tail is tapered, usually bent or flexed, and without nuclei (Fig. 1D and 2c). The microfilaria is sometimes found in the blood and in urine, typically after treatment with diethylcarbamazine. Diagnosis is made by finding the typical microfilaria in skin snips teased in water or saline solution, in fluids expressed from scarified skin, or in aspirates from nodules (1). Also, adult worms may be demonstrated in excised nodules which have been sectioned and stained (Fig. 3B). Adult worms may be freed from the fibrous tissues of the nodule by using digestive enzymes such as collagenase. Microfilariae may also be seen in the cornea and in the anterior chamber of the eye viewed with the aid of a slit lamp.

Skin snips are best obtained with a biopsy punch. Samples may be taken from the scapular region, the iliac crest, and even the calf; the first two are the preferred sites. Teasing the skin snips in saline or tap water tends to liberate the microfilariae from the tissues.

Mansonella streptocerca is another skin-dwelling filaria that infects humans in the rain forest belt of Africa. This parasite, previously allocated to various genera (*Dipetalonema*, *Acanthocheilonema*, and *Tetrapetalonema*) at various times, has recently been placed in the genus *Mansonella* (13). The adult worms are found in the dermal layers of the skin, as are the microfilariae. The microfilaria has no sheath, is long and slender, and measures approximately 210 by 5 to 6 μm. It most characteristic feature is its "crooked" tail (Fig. 2f); in addition, the column of nuclei extends to the end of the tail. In areas where this species overlaps in its distribution with *O. volvulus*, great care must be used so that microfilariae found in skin snips are properly identified.

Two other species of *Mansonella* are parasites of humans. One of these, *Mansonella ozzardi*, is restricted in its geographical distribution to the Western Hemisphere. It is endemic in parts of Mexico, Panama, and northern South America, especially in the Amazon Basin and as far south as northern Argentina. It also is found in several Caribbean islands including Hispaniola. The adult worms inhabit subcutaneous tissues, and the microfilariae circulate in the blood. The microfilaria is small, measuring about 224 by 4 to 5 μm, and has a long attenuated tail devoid of nuclei (Fig. 1F and 2g). The microfilariae circulate in the blood at all hours of the day and night. According to studies in experimental animals, prepatent development requires about 5 months. This filaria, like *L. loa*, readily infects visitors to areas of endemic infection and is often found in missionaries and others residing temporarily in these areas.

Mansonella perstans, a filaria widely distributed in tropical Africa and less so in South America, is also found frequently in individuals who have lived temporarily in areas where it is endemic. The location of the adult worms in the human host is less well known, but it is believed that they inhabit the abdominal cavity and the mesenteries. The microfilaria has no sheath, is small (approximately 203 by 4 to 5 μm), and circulates in the peripheral blood without any periodicity. Its most characteristic feature is its blunt tail filled with nuclei (Fig. 1E and 2e). In the Western Hemisphere, *M. perstans* is often found in association with *M. ozzardi*. In areas where the two species coexist, special care must be taken to make accurate identifications.

In general, *Mansonella* species are regarded as inocuous parasites that produce few or no pathologic changes in the human host.

Laboratory Diagnosis

Microfilariae can be detected in samples of blood by a variety of techniques. In thick, wet, blood films prepared during either the day or the night, microfilariae may be quickly recognized by their size and rapid movement among the blood cells. However, species are not likely to be identified in this manner, and so stained blood films are required. Thin blood films generally are inadequate because of the small amount of blood involved. On the other hand, blood films of 20 μl are large enough to detect even scanty numbers of microfilariae, and when these are stained with Giemsa or hematoxylin stain, the important diagnostic morphologic features of each species generally can be seen.

Sometimes, because the numbers of microfilariae in thick blood films may be very small, the microscopist may wish to examine a larger volume of blood. Procedures for the concentration of blood samples by the Knott technique or membrane filtration are found in most laboratory guides (2). Species of microfilariae are readily identified on the basis of size, presence or absence of a sheath, and structure of the tail, as well as their staining characteristics with Giemsa stain.

Skin snips must be examined to find microfilariae of *O. volvulus* and *M. streptocerca*. Care must be taken to obtain bloodless snips so as not to contaminate the sample with other species of microfilariae that may be present in the blood. One may simply abrade a small area of skin and collect the exuded tissue juices on a slide; these may be examined immediately for living microfilariae or allowed to dry and then stained and examined. Serologic tests have poor sensitivity and specificity and generally are not used for diagnosis. Two conceptually different techniques, antigen-detection assays and antibody detection assays for the diagnosis of filariasis, especially lymphatic filariasis, are currently being evaluated in several research laboratories.

Guinea Worm

The nematode parasite *Dracunculus medinensis* dates back to the ancient Egyptian literature (15th century B.C.). It appears to have been eliminated from India and Pakistan but still occurs in Yemen and at least 17 countries in Africa. Efforts to eradicate guinea worm infection before the end of this century are under way (16). The adult worms live in the subcutaneous tissues, and infections become clinically evident when the female migrates to the body surface, usually on the feet and ankles, and produces a blister on the skin. On contact with water, the blister ruptures and the female discharges swarms of motile larvae into the water. Only a small portion of the female is extruded from the lesion. However, it can be removed from the body by gentle traction. If the female fails to reach the surface of the body, it will die in the tissues and often calcify in situ. The male worms, which are very small, are rarely seen and also die in the tissues. Secondary bacterial infections of the lesions can disable the host and complicate recovery.

The life cycle involves transmission of the parasite by a biological vector, a copepod, which ingests larvae liberated by the female into the water. Larvae develop to infectivity in the copepod and are transmitted when the infected copepod is ingested by the humans in drinking water. Diagnosis depends on the appearance of the female on the surface of the skin. The administration of various drugs, e.g., metronidazole, thiabendazole, and antihistamines or corticosteroids, helps alleviate symptoms and may facilitate the removal of worms from the tissues by traction. Guinea worm infections can be controlled easily by provision of piped water or covered wells for drinking water as well as by filtration of drinking water through fine mesh cloth.

Enterobius vermicularis

Although the pinworm is an intestinal parasite and is treated as such in this Manual, the propensity of the female worm for migration from the anus and perianal tissues into other organs warrants mention here. The adult female worm may migrate into the human female reproductive tract and become encapsulated in the uterus or fallopian tubes and may wander even further into the peritoneal cavity, often becoming encapsulated in the mesenteries. Adult female worms also have been found in the liver parenchyma, pulmonary nodules, spleen, lymph nodes, and ovaries. Adult worms are seen with the greatest frequency in the lumen of the appendix, where there may be little or no evidence of inflammation and no clinical manifestations of their presence (Fig. 3F). This parasite is easily recognized on the basis of its anatomical features as seen in tissue sections (11).

Other Nematodes

Several species of nematode parasites which are natural parasites of lower animals may gain entry into the human host and undergo partial development. The degree of development achieved by the parasite and the attendant pathologic changes that are manifested vary with the parasite and may be significant and even life-threatening. Only the more common parasite species are mentioned here.

Trichinella spiralis

T. spiralis, the common agent of human trichinosis, is a parasite of carnivores that shows little evidence of host specificity. Infections in humans result from the ingestion of insufficiently cooked or raw pork or pork products containing the encysted larvae. Bear meat is also a known source of human infections. Adult worms live in the mucosa of the small intestine. The female produces and discharges larvae that enter the bloodstream and invade the skeletal musculature, where they undergo further development and encapsulation. The larvae may remain viable for several years. Initially, there may be nonspecific gasteroenteritis, fever, eosinophilia, myositis, and circumorbital edema. The adult worms survive in the intestine for up to 8 weeks and then are expelled by the host.

The definitive diagnosis is made by demonstration of encapsulated larvae in biopsy specimens of skeletal muscle, particularly deltoid and gastrocnemius muscles (Fig. 3C and D).

The digestion of muscle tissue in artificial gastric juice followed by examination of the sediment for larvae is more sensitive (2). Serologic tests are widely used and give good results. A highly antigenic parasite, *T. spiralis* stimulates a very strong antibody response that can be measured by a variety of procedures.

Capillaria hepatica

Although normally a parasite of rodents, *C. hepatica* (= *Calodium hepatica*) can produce infections in humans. There are well-documented human cases from all over the world. Most infections are found in children of dirt-eating ages, who present with a clinical picture of visceral larva migrans. Human and animal infections are acquired by ingestion of infective eggs in soil; adult worms mature and deposit eggs directly into the liver parenchyma, where they remain in an undeveloped state until the liver is eaten and the eggs are digested free of the tissues to pass in the feces of the predator animal. If, as in the human host, the liver is not eaten, the eggs are never liberated into the external environment. Diagnosis is established by liver biopsy or at necropsy.

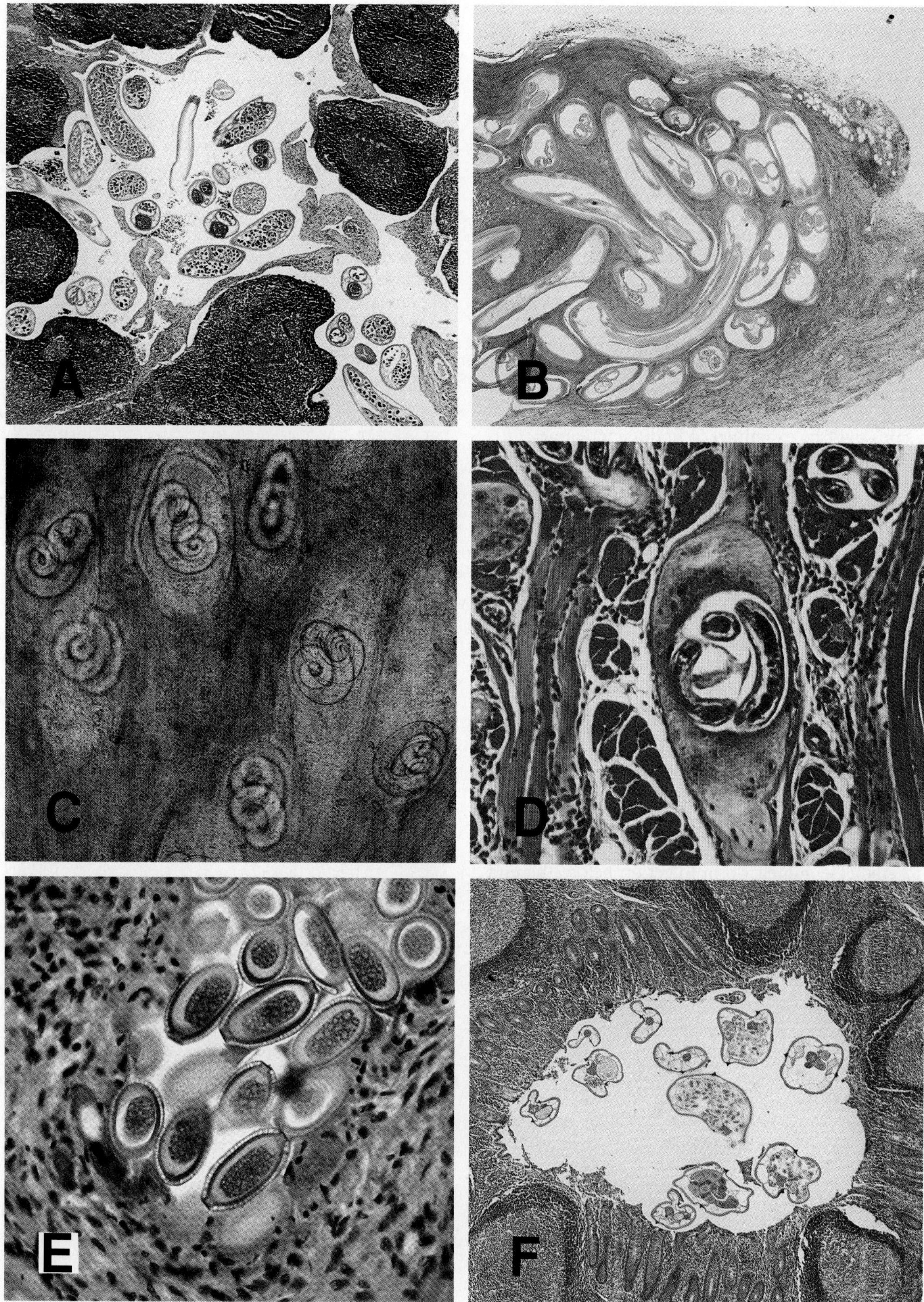

FIGURE 3 (A) Adult *W. bancrofti* in a sinus of a lymph node removed from an infected individual. Hematoxylin and eosin stain. Magnification, ×50. (B) Adult *O. volvulus* enmeshed in a fibrous nodule removed from the subcutaneous tissues of an individual in West Africa. Hematoxylin and eosin stain. Magnification, ×20. (C) *T. spiralis* infective-stage larvae. In this press preparation of diaphragm muscle, several encapsulated larvae are visible. Magnification, ×100. (D) *T. spiralis* infective-stage larvae in section of rat tongue. Hematoxylin and eosin stain. Magnification, ×200. (E) *C. hepatica* eggs in liver. Characteristic morphologic features of eggs are evident even in tissue sections. Hematoxylin and eosin stain. Magnification, ×290. (F) *E. vermicularis* adult worms in lumen of human appendix. Hematoxylin and eosin stain. Magnification, ×50.

In genuine human cases, eggs are never passed in the feces (3).

Passage of *C. hepatica* eggs by humans indicates a spurious infection and represents an instance in which the livers of infected animals have been eaten. The eggs are usually passed for several days and will then disappear from the feces.

The eggs of *C. hepatica* must be distinguished from those of *Trichuris* or of other species of human *Capillaria* spp. *C. hepatica* eggs are 51 to 67 μm long by 30 to 35 μm wide; have thick, striated walls and inconspicuous "plugs" at both ends; and are unembryonated when seen in the feces. Eggs in liver biopsy specimens are readily recognized on the basis of their morphologic features (Fig. 3E).

Anisakis Species

The growing popularity of eating raw fish dishes—sushi, sashimi, ceviche, and others—has led to an increased frequency of human infections with various larval ascaridoid nematodes (9, 11). Species in a number of genera, including *Anisakis* and *Pseudoterranova*, are parasites, as adults, of marine mammals, utilizing shrimp-like crustaceans as first intermediate hosts and fish and squid as second intermediate hosts in their life cycle. When they are ingested, the larval stages encysted in the mesenteries or flesh of fish have the ability to pass from one fish to another without maturing to adult worms. When humans accidentally ingest the immature stages of these nematodes, the larvae may partially penetrate the wall of the stomach or the intestine and produce an eosinophilic granuloma. Many human infections present with acute abdomen or other signs suggestive of intestinal obstruction. In some instances the long, whitish worms, up to several centimeters in length, may be coughed up by the patient or may be removed from the throat.

The nematodes causing aniasakiasis can be identified by a study of the distinctive morphologic features of the intact worms or by examination of the microanatomical features of the parasites in histologic sections (Fig. 4E).

Eustrongylides Species

Nematode larvae of the genus *Eustrongylides*, which belongs to the family Dioctophymoidea, have in recent years been incriminated as agents of human infections. These parasites normally occur in the adult stage in the alimentary tracts of fish-eating birds and utilize fish, amphibians, and reptiles as intermediate hosts. Although five of the cases have occurred in individuals who had eaten live minnows while fishing, one case occurred as a result of eating home-prepared sushi (23). In most instances, these large, bright red larvae have invaded the abdominal cavity of patients and require surgical removal. These parasites, along with the anisakine nematodes, further illustrate the potential for acquisition of parasitic infections by eating raw infected fish (19).

Angiostrongylus cantonensis and *A. costaricensis*

Metastrongylid nematodes of the genus *Angiostrongylus* have become important human parasites (3). *A. cantonensis*, a lungworm that lives in the pulmonary arteries of rats (*Rattus* spp.), is a cause of human eosinophilic meningitis or eosinophilic meningoencephalitis in many Pacific Islands (including Hawaii), Thailand, Indonesia, other parts of southeast Asia, and Cuba. One human case has been reported from Louisiana (10). In the natural life cycle, rats excrete first-stage larvae in the feces, and these larvae penetrate directly into or are ingested by many species of terrestrial snails or slugs. The larvae reach the infective third stage in the molluscs, and when the molluscs are eaten by rats, the larvae make a prolonged month-long migration through the brain before they become adults in the pulmonary artery. Here the worms mate and the females lay eggs, which will develop and hatch in the lung tissue; larvae will be found in the feces 7 weeks after rats ingest infected molluscs.

Infective larvae in terrestrial molluscs may be eaten by and remain in the tissues of a wide range of vertebrate and invertebrate animals including planarians, shrimp, crabs, fish, amphibians, and reptiles. Human infections are rarely derived from eating ordinary terrestrial molluscs; instead, infection is acquired by eating raw or poorly cooked infected shrimp, crabs, or large edible snails such as *Pila* spp. Accidental infection also may result from eating planarians or small slugs on improperly washed vegetables (such as lettuce) or fruits (such as strawberries).

In the human host, larvae migrate to the brain, spinal cord, or eye, where they become immature adults. Rarely can the worms complete the migration to the pulmonary artery; instead, they usually die in the meninges or the parenchyma of the brain, giving rise to meningeal symptoms. Diagnosis is usually based on a history of residence in an area where the parasite occurs, combined with the development of appropriate clinical symptoms such as severe and prolonged headaches, nerve involvement, and the presence of eosinophils in cerebrospinal fluid. Occasionally, immature worms are found in aspirated cerebrospinal fluid. Serologic tests have not been reliable and are not widely available.

A closely related parasite, *A. costaricensis*, causes human abdominal angiostrongyliasis in most countries of Central and South America. The parasite normally lives in small arteries and arterioles of the ileocecal region of the intestines of various rodents. Eggs are produced and develop in the intestinal wall, and first-stage larvae then migrate into the intestinal lumen to pass in the feces. Various terrestrial slugs serve as intermediate hosts; as is the case for *A. cantonensis*, it appears that most terrestrial snails and slugs will support the development of the parasite to the infective third stage. Human infection is acquired by accidental ingestion of slugs or other hosts. Transport hosts probably play an important role as well. Most human infections occur in children, but all age groups may be infected; infections in children often have been fatal. The distal small intestine is the usual habitat of the adults and is the site where eggs are discharged and where they may stimulate a granulomatous inflammation which leads to symptoms of acute abdomen. Surgery is often performed, and the affected segment of the intestine may be resected; infection is subsequently diagnosed by finding eggs in the tissues. Larvae have not been found in human feces. Although serological tests have been described, their reliability is still in question.

Gnathostoma Species

The gnathostomes are spiruroid nematodes that are natural parasites of a variety of domestic mammals, including dogs, cats, and swine, and wild animals, such as raccoons, otters, and opossums, that feed on fish and other cold-blooded vertebrates. Accidental human infections with *Gnathostoma* species typically involve extraintestinal migration of larval stages that produces a visceral larva migrans syndrome (18). Human infections are especially common in southeast Asia and have been reported in the Western Hemisphere as well, particularly in Mexico and Ecuador.

The adult worms in their natural hosts are found, typically, embedded in the gastric mucosa; female worms produce characteristic eggs, which pass in the fecal stream in an unembryonated condition. The life cycle involves a copepod as a first intermediate host in which the parasite reaches the infective stage. Other animals such as fish and amphibians serve as second intermediate hosts, and reptiles, birds, and mammals may be paratenic hosts. Humans become infected by ingesting infective larvae encysted in the flesh of intermediate and/or paratenic hosts that have been inadequately cooked before being consumed. In humans, the advanced third-stage larva migrates through the superficial subcutaneous tissues (Fig. 4D); frequently, larvae invade the orbit, and even the eye itself, and the central nervous system. During its migratory phase in the subcutaneous tissues, which usually begins 2 to 4 weeks after infection, there may be periodic migratory subcutaneous swellings or the larva may become stationary and provoke an intense inflammatory reaction. Invasion of the central nervous system is extremely serious and often fatal. Larvae and attendant symptoms may persist for several months.

Diagnosis is usually based on clinical presentation, i.e., history of eating raw fish in geographical areas where infections are common combined with subsequent migratory lesions. Removal of the worm(s) from the tissues is therapeutic; it also permits specific identification of the parasite.

Zoonotic Filariae

In recent years, a wide variety of filarial worms which are natural parasites of wild mammals have been recovered from the tissues of humans in many parts of the world (14). Infections have been recorded with greatest frequency in the United States and the Mediterranean region, especially Italy (15). These filariae are transmitted by bloodsucking arthropods that, in some cases, feed on both animals and humans. Their feeding behavior, together with the overlapping environments of certain animals and humans, makes it possible for the infective stages of these filariae to accidentally infect humans.

Species of *Dirofilaria*, including *D. tenuis*, *D. repens*, and *D. ursi*, which have been found in the subcutaneous tissues of their animal hosts and are transmitted by mosquitoes, are the filariae most frequently encountered in human infections (6, 7, 11, 14, 15). These infections are characteristically cryptic; i.e., there is no microfilaremia. Female worms may be sexually mature but are usually infertile. The worms have a propensity for migration to the face, orbit, and conjunctivae but may be found dead or alive in subcutaneous nodules on any part of the body (Fig. 4A). Diagnosis is based on recovery of the intact worm from the tissues or by the identification of the filaria in histologic sections of the affected tissues (Fig. 4A). Usually, only a single worm is recovered from human tissues, although two or more have been found on rare occasions.

D. immitis, the heartworm of dogs and other canids, has been isolated from humans wherever the filaria is found in dogs (14). Typically, immature stages of the parasite lodge in and obstruct small pulmonary arteries, producing an infarct and eventually a granulomatous nodule (Fig. 4B) that appears as a "coin lesion" in the lung on X rays (7, 11, 17). At present, diagnosis depends on microscopic examination of the excised lesion or of a needle biopsy specimen (7, 17). There are no serologic or immunologic tests that will differentiate the parasite lesion from neoplastic tumors. On rare occasions, adult worms have been found in the right side of the heart or in the great vessels.

Lymphatic-dwelling *Brugia* species are natural parasites of animals in many parts of the world. Human infections of zoonotic origin have been reported most frequently from the northeastern United States and northern South America (12). The worms are invariably located in lymph nodes or lymphoid tissues (Fig. 4C). As stated for the dirofilarias, patent infections are extremely rare but have been reported (12); most often the female worms found in the tissues are immature and infertile. The animal reservoirs of infection in the natural environment have not been established precisely, but raccoons, rabbits, and wild felines and possibly other animals may be involved.

Larva Migrans

There are several species of hookworms and ascarids, as well as *Strongyloides* species, that infect wild and domestic animals and may gain entry into the human host and undergo partial development. The severity of subsequent disease varies from mild to severe with involvement of various tissues and organs.

Cutaneous Larva Migrans

Cutaneous larva migrans, also known as creeping eruption or ground itch, refers to the production of serpiginous inflamed trails in the skin, resulting in intense pruritus, and may be caused by various species of *Strongyloides*, *Ancylostoma*, and other hookworms. It results from skin contact with sandy loam types of soil that contain filariform larvae of these species that have developed to the infective stage from eggs or larvae discharged in the feces of infected animals. In the southeastern part of the United States, this may be an occupational hazard of electricians, plumbers, and construction workers who inadvertently come in contact with infected soil when working under or near houses where animals have defecated. In addition, species of *Strongyloides* parasitizing wild animals such as nutria and raccoons have been incriminated in causing dermatitis in oil field workers and trappers in Louisiana. *Ancylostoma braziliense*, a hookworm of dogs and cats, is the species usually associated with classical creeping eruption acquired along sandy beaches, but other *Ancylostoma* species may be involved as well. Invasion of human skin by the dog hookworm, *A. caninum*, can produce creeping eruption; these larvae may also invade other tissues and organs of the body, including the eye, where they may produce granulomatous lesions. The diagnosis of cutaneous larva migrans is based almost entirely on clinical findings and the demonstration of the classical serpiginous trails (5).

Visceral Larva Migrans

Visceral larva migrans is a syndrome originally associated with the larval migration in humans, especially children, of dog and cat ascarid species of the genus *Toxocara*. Although many other helminths of animals may infect humans and migrate through organs and deeper tissues of the body, *T. canis* is still the classical example of this type of infection.

The dog ascarid, *T. canis*, is more important as a human parasite than is *T. cati*, the species occurring in felines. Toxocariasis results from the ingestion of infective eggs of the parasite from soil and is characterized by hypereosinophilia, hepatomegaly, fever, pneumonitis, and sometimes death. The visceral larva migrans syndrome may persist for many years and may result in severe complications involving the eyes and the central nervous system. Ocular larval migrans may mimic retinoblastoma, a malignant tumor of the eye.

Diagnosis of visceral larva migrans is difficult and is generally based on clinical findings and immunodiagnostic pro-

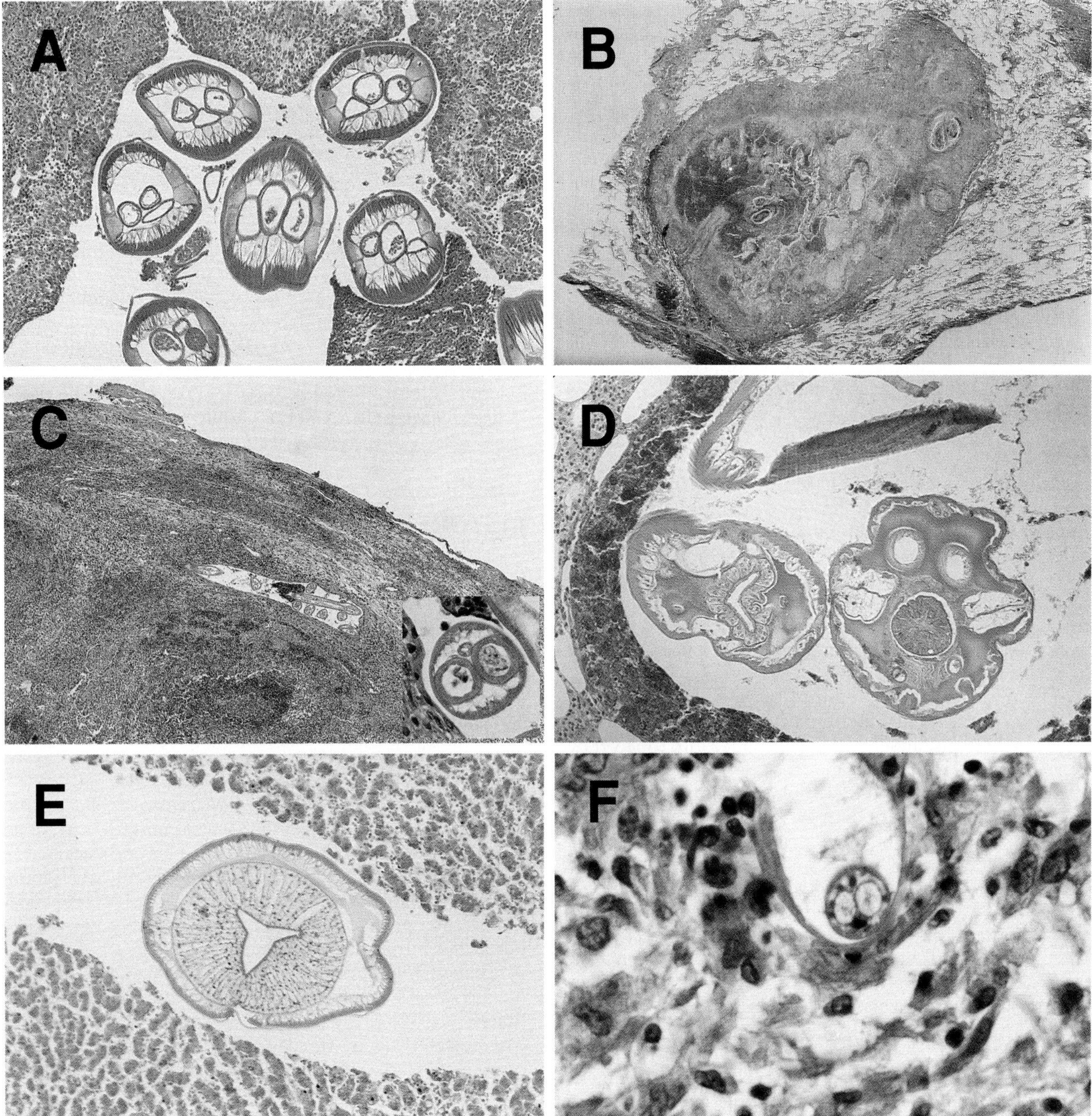

FIGURE 4 Helminth parasites in tissues; hematoxylin and eosin stain. (A) *D. tenuis*. Sections of an immature adult female worm in a subcutaneous nodule from a resident of Florida. The typical morphologic features of the body wall are evident here even though the worm is dead. Magnification, ×100. (B) *D. immitis* in a granulomatous nodule in human lung. This immature worm is trapped in a small pulmonary artery. Magnification, ×7. (C) *Brugia* species of zoonotic origin in a subcapsular vessel of a lymph node from a human in Ohio. Magnification, ×35. Inset shows a transverse section of the female worm. Its morphologic features immediately identify it as a filaria of the *Brugia* type. Magnification, ×250. (D) *Gnathostoma* species. Transverse sections through an advanced third-stage larva removed from the subcutaneous tissue of an individual who acquired the infection in Mexico. The morphology of the body wall including its spines, the presence of ballonets in the body cavity, and the structure of the intestine indicate that the worm is a larval gnathostome. Magnification, ×30. (E) *Anisakis* species. Transverse section through the body showing its unusual lateral chords and structure of the intestine. Magnification, ×120. (F) *T. canis* larva. Transverse section in an inflammatory granulomatous lesion in the liver of a small child. Magnification, ×1,000.

cedures. Occasionally, diagnosis is established by finding focal inflammatory lesions containing larvae in tissues such as liver and brain and other organs (Fig. 4F). Sections of nematode larvae can sometimes be identified in human tissues obtained by biopsy or at necropsy, and these can be identified by specialists expert in helminth microanatomy.

TREMATODES

The important human trematode parasites are described in chapter 112 of this Manual inasmuch as their eggs are passed in feces or, more rarely, sputum and urine. However, adult trematodes and/or their eggs may be found in the wall of the alimentary tract, the liver, lungs, mesenteries, bladder, brain, and subcutaneous and muscular tissues. The trematodes commonly found in human tissues include the liver flukes (*Fasciola hepatica*, *Clonorchis sinensis*, and *Opisthorchis* species), lung flukes (*Paragonimus* species), and blood flukes (*Schistosoma* species).

Liver Flukes

F. hepatica, *C. sinensis*, and *O. viverrini* live in the bile ducts of their human and animal hosts and may be found in sections of the livers of infected individuals who live in areas where the parasites are endemic or who have emigrated from these areas (Fig. 5F). In sections through adult parasites in liver, such as *Clonorchis* and *Opisthorchis*, it is not uncommon to see typical eggs clustered in the uterine branches of these worms, which is a significant aid in the identification of the parasite (11).

The normal migratory path of larval *F. hepatica* to the bile ducts of the human host entails passage from the intestine into the abdominal cavity and entrance into the liver by penetration of Glisson's capsule. However, not infrequently, aberrant migration by these larval stages results in their presence in ectopic sites, including the abdominal wall, subcutaneous tissues, lungs, and other organs and tissues. Abscesses are produced in these locations, and degenerating adult worms may be found in histologic sections; in some instances, the worms are so degenerate or decomposed that they are unrecognizable. However, their eggs, liberated from the uteri, may still be identified. The size and morphology of the eggs, cut in various aspects, can aid in the correct identification of this parasitic infection.

Lung Flukes

Paragonimus westermani and related species found in humans make a larval migration from the intestine to the lungs (Fig. 5D) via the abdominal cavity, the diaphragm, and the thoracic cavity. As with *F. hepatica*, aberrant migration by larval *P. westermani* may result in its presence in the abdominal wall, rib cage, subcutaneous tissues, brain, and other sites where abscesses typically should be found. Degenerate adult worms or eggs may be found in histologic sections (Fig. 5E). The size and morphology of the egg remnants often allow specific identification of this infection in these ectopic sites. Abscesses in the brain have frequently been described in individuals from Korea.

Blood Flukes (Schistosomes)

Each of the three major human schistosome parasites lives in some part of the venous side of the vascular system. *Schistosoma mansoni* adults reside typically in the hemorrhoidal venous plexus draining the lower ileum and colon; they also may be found in intrahepatic blood vessels of the liver. *Schistosoma japonicum* adults are usually found in radicles of the superior mesenteric vein draining the small intestine, but some adult worms may also live in the portal system of the liver. Adults of *Schistosoma haematobium* usually are found in the vesical plexuses of the venous system. Granulomas produced by the eggs of *S. mansoni* and *S. japonicum* are usually found in the wall of the intestinal tract or in the liver, but they may also disseminate via the bloodstream to distant sites, including the lungs, heart, spleen, kidneys, and spinal cord (Fig. 5A and B). The smaller size of the eggs of *S. japonicum* aids in their extensive dissemination via the bloodstream. In the Philippines, eggs are not uncommonly found in the brain, where they provoke epileptiform seizures. Eggs of *S. haematobium* are commonly found in the wall of the bladder, but they are also seen in the kidney, ureters, wall of the rectum, and other tissues (Fig. 5C). Identification of schistosome eggs in tissues is somewhat dependent on the tissues in which they are found, the size of the eggs, and whether lateral or terminal spines can be visualized on whole or partial eggshell remnants. Adult schistosomes are frequently seen in histologic sections.

CESTODES

A number of tapeworms live as adults in the small intestine of humans and animals (see chapter 112), and their larval stages often occur in human tissues. These larvae have significant morphologic features that usually allow them to be identified when they are examined grossly or studied in tissue sections. The most significant diseases caused by larval tapeworms include sparganosis, cysticercosis, coenurosis, and several forms of hydatid disease.

Sparganosis

Human sparganosis is caused by larval cestodes of the genus *Spirometra* that as adult worms usually parasitize cats, dogs, and various wild canids and felids. Species of this genus are closely related biologically and morphologically to *Diphyllobothrium* spp. and have similar life cycles involving copepods as first intermediate hosts and fish as second intermediate hosts. *Spirometra mansoni* is found in many parts of Asia, in particular China, Japan, Korea, and Vietnam, and *Spirometra mansonoides* is the common species found in the United States.

Characteristically in sparganosis, after ingestion of the plerocercoid larva (also called a sparganum) in inadequately cooked fish, accidental ingestion of infected copepods containing procercoid larvae, or use of infected hosts such as frogs and snakes as poultices, the larva migrates in the tissues of the human host. In the United States, typical cases of sparganosis present as subcutaneous swellings that may be migratory and are sometimes tender; usually there is little or no peripheral eosinophilia. In Asia, many cases of sparganosis in the brain have been reported (8). Diagnosis is usually made after surgical removal of the intact worm or histopathologic study of the tissue mass. Spargana are typically ribbonlike and ivory colored and may range from several millimeters to 30 cm long by approximately 3 to 4 mm wide. The anterior portion of the worm is flattened and has a ventral groove; the body is transversely ridged, but this is not true segmentation. In histologic sections, the tegument typically has deep folds, and prominent bundles of longitudinal muscle fibers and excretory channels lie within the parenchyma; calcareous corpuscles are present and prominent (Fig. 6F).

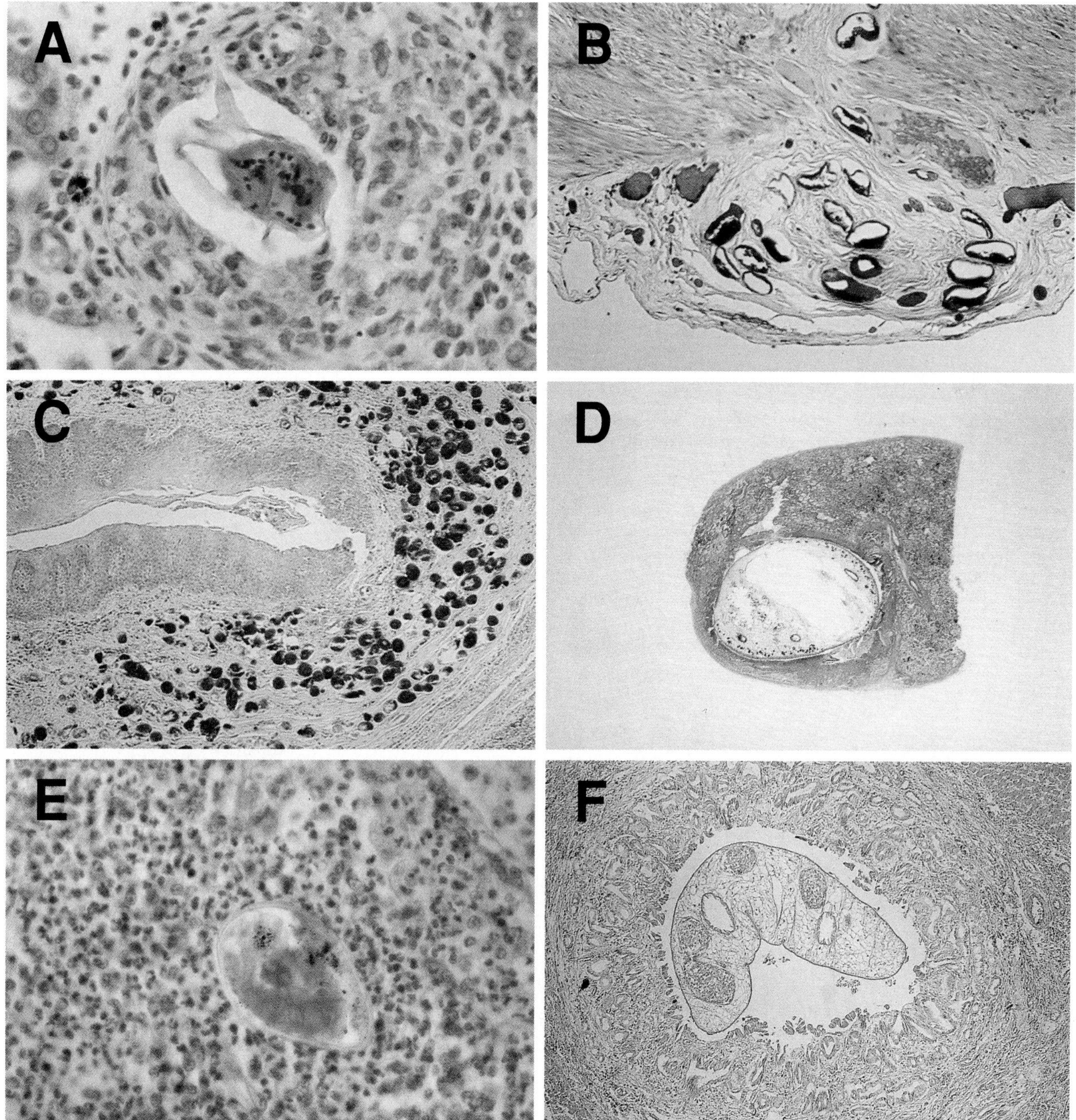

FIGURE 5 Trematode parasites in tissues. (A) Egg of *S. mansoni* in early granuloma in liver; the lateral spine is visible. Hematoxylin and eosin stain. Magnification, ×400. (B) Cluster of *S. japonicum* eggs in a periodic acid-Schiff-stained section of human liver. Magnification, ×200. (C) Large number of *S. haematobium* eggs in the human bladder. Many eggs (black) are undergoing calcification. Magnification, ×50. (D) Section through an adult *Paragonimus* worm in the lung of a cat. Trichrome stain. Magnification, ×14. (E) Egg of *P. westermani* in a section of human lung. Hematoxylin and eosin stain. Magnification ×350. (F) Adult *C. sinensis* in human bile duct. Hematoxylin and eosin stain. Magnification, ×40.

Cysticercosis

Human cysticercosis is produced by ingestion of the eggs of the pork tapeworm *Taenia solium*. It occurs throughout the world, although its greatest prevalence is in Mexico; other areas with significant prevalence include Latin America, India, China, Africa, and Europe (20). Neurocysticercosis results from invasion of the central nervous system by the cysticercus stage and is probably the most common helminthic disease of the human nervous system (22). Acquisition of cysticercosis in the United States has been uncommon in the past, but immigrants from areas where the parasite is endemic are frequently diagnosed with the infection, and reports of locally acquired cysticercosis are increasing in number in the United States.

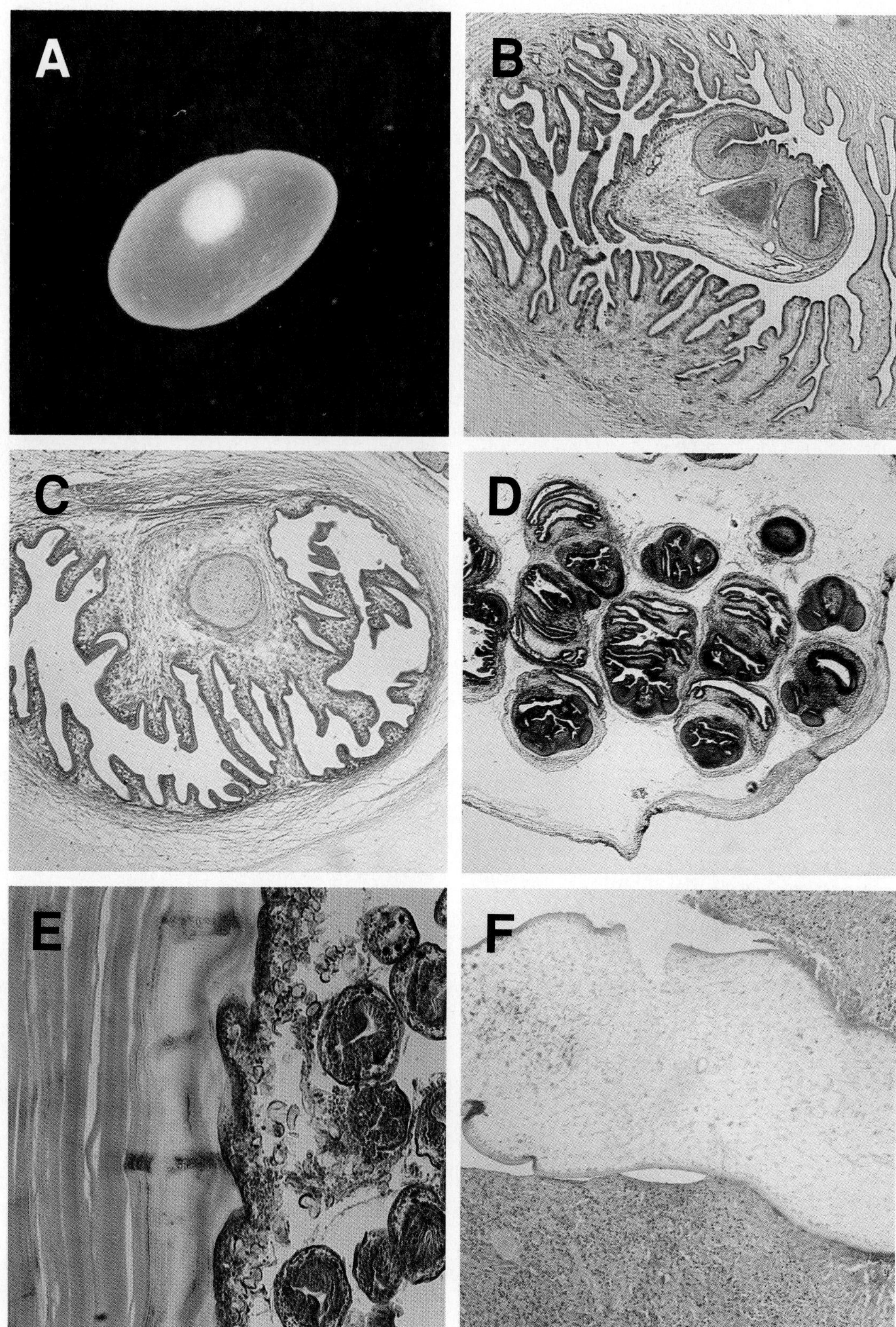

FIGURE 6 Cestode parasites in tissues. (A) Cysticercus of *Taenia solium* (also called *Cysticercus cellulosae*). Denser opaque area represents the invaginated neck and scolex in a fluid-filled bladder. Magnification, ×8. (B) Section through the cysticercus in tissue showing the scolex, neck, and bladder wall. Hematoxylin and eosin stain. Magnification, ×300. (C) Section through the neck region of the cysticercus; a portion of a sucker is seen in the center. Hematoxylin and eosin stain. Magnification, ×30. (D) Section through a coenurus of *T. multiceps*, showing multiple scoleces. Hematoxylin and eosin stain. Magnification, ×30. (E) *E. granulosus*. Hydatid cyst in liver. Note the laminated membrane, germinal layer, and individual protoscoleces. Hematoxylin and eosin stain. Magnification, ×125. (F) Section through a sparganum (*Spirometra* species) in human tissue. Hematoxylin and eosin stain. Magnification, ×50.

The cysticercus of *Taenia solium* is often referred to as *Cysticercus cellulosae*; it is round to oval, translucent, and about 5 mm or more in diameter (Fig. 6A). It has a scolex bearing four suckers and a rostellum with a circle of hooks that is invaginated into the fluid-filled bladder. The cysticercus develops in any organ or tissue of the body; it is most serious when it occurs in the central nervous system and the eye (20). Diagnosis of the infection may be difficult. It may be established by the recovery of whole cysticerci or by the histologic demonstration of cysticerci in surgically removed tissues (Fig. 6B and C). Diagnosis may also be made by X-ray detection of calcifying cysticerci and by the use of computed tomography.

Coenurosis

Coenurosis is produced by the larval stages of tapeworms of the genus *Taenia* that mature in the intestines of various canids and felines. The two most important species are *Taenia multiceps* (formerly *Multiceps multiceps*) and *Taenia serialis* (formerly *Multiceps serialis*). The eggs of these species are typical taeniid eggs and are indistinguishable from the eggs of other species of *Taenia* and *Echinococcus*. Sheep (for *Taenia multiceps*) and rodents (for *Taenia serialis*) are the usual intermediate hosts, but humans who ingest eggs of these species develop coenurus infection. As with cysticerci, a coenurus may develop in subcutaneous tissues, muscles, the eye, or the central nervous system. Typically, it is from several millimeters to several centimeters in diameter and has multiple scoleces invaginated into a fluid-filled bladder. Each scolex has four suckers and a rostellum armed with hooklets. Diagnosis is usually made by recovering the whole coenurus or by demonstrating in histologic section the typical bladder with multiple invaginated scoleces (Fig. 6D).

Unilocular Hydatid Infection

Although various forms of hydatid disease are caused by a number of species of *Echinococcus*, *E. granulosus* is the most important species producing human hydatidosis. *E. granulosus* is a minute tapeworm that as an adult is up to 6 mm long and lives in the small intestines of domestic and wild canids. The parasite is distributed extensively in sheep- and cattle-raising areas of the world, where these herbivorous animals serve as intermediate hosts for the infection. Humans acquire infection by ingestion of typical taeniid eggs, which are excreted in the feces of infected dogs. When eggs are ingested by the intermediate hosts or by humans, the oncospheres liberated from the eggs migrate via the bloodstream to the liver, lungs, and other tissues and organs to develop into hydatid cysts. Within the cyst, brood capsules and protoscoleces develop and proliferate from an inner germinal membrane, so that ultimately the cysts may become very large and contain many hundreds, even thousands, of protoscoleces. Each protoscolex is a potentially infective organism.

Cysts grow slowly, and their presence frequently goes undetected for many years until they reach sufficient size to cause clinical symptoms. Infections of the central nervous system usually become apparent much earlier than those of other organs.

Diagnosis of infection may be difficult but can be accomplished by the use of X rays, ultrasonic scanning, and computed tomography to detect cysts in tissues (21). When the presence of cysts is combined with an appropriate residential or travel history or an occupation such as sheep raising in areas where the parasites are endemic, there are reasonable grounds to suspect infection. Many immunodiagnostic tests have been used, but there is wide variation in their sensitivity and specificity. Aspiration of material from a hydatid cyst in situ is dangerous and is not a recommended procedure, since accidental spillage of cyst contents may result in dissemination of liberated scoleces and/or an anaphylactic reaction. Fluid in hydatid cysts typically consists of disintegrating brood capsules and scoleces, hooklets, and calcareous corpuscles; this material is referred to as "hydatid sand." In histologic section, the wall of the unilocular cyst comprises three layers: an outer fibrous layer of host tissue, an acellular laminated layer, and an inner thin layer of germinal epithelium (Fig. 6E). Brood capsules arising from the germinal layer are stalked and project into the lumen of the cyst; each of these contains several invaginated protoscoleces with four suckers and a crown of hooklets.

Multilocular Hydatid (Alveolar Hydatid) Infection

A second form of human hydatid disease is alveolar hydatidosis, caused by the larval stage of *Echinococcus multilocularis*. The life cycle of this parasite involves foxes, wolves, and dogs as definitive hosts and small rodents and voles as intermediate hosts. The adult worm is even smaller than *E. granulosus*, being only 1.2 to 3.7 mm long, and has a strobila of only three proglottids. In the livers of rodents, the invasive larval stage has a multicompartmented appearance, with each compartment containing many protoscoleces proliferating from the germinal membrane. Ingestion of the eggs of *E. multilocularis* by humans results in development of invasive cysts in the liver. However, protoscoleces are rarely seen in human alveolar hydatid disease; instead, the germinal layer proliferates exogenously and endogenously, resulting in folded and collapsed membranes scattered throughout the tissue. The pathologic picture of the liver resembles a hepatic carcinoma. The geographic distribution of the infection includes northern Europe, Japan, China, India, and North America; the infection is widespread in Alaska, Canada, and the northern tier of states in the midwestern United States. Diagnosis is difficult and frequently is accomplished only by histologic examination of surgically removed tissues.

Polycystic Hydatid Infection

A third type of hydatid infection, caused by *Echinococcus vogeli*, has been reported in Latin America (4). The normal life cycle of the parasite involves bush dogs and large rodents (pacas). A polycystic hydatid cyst develops primarily in the liver, where, in humans, it has an invasive behavior. These cysts develop brood capsules and protoscoleces in human infections, which distinguishes them from the cysts of human alveolar hydatid infection.

REFERENCES

1. **Ash, L. R., and T. C. Orihel.** 1997. *Atlas of Human Parasitology*, 4th ed. American Society of Clinical Pathologists, Chicago, Ill.
2. **Ash, L. R., and T. C. Orihel.** 1991. *Parasites: a Guide to Laboratory Procedures and Identification*. American Society of Clinical Pathologists, Chicago, Ill.
3. **Beaver, P. C., R. C. Jung, and E. W. Cupp.** 1984. *Clinical Parasitology*, 9th ed. Lea & Febiger, Philadelphia. Pa.
4. **D'Alessandro, A.** 1997. Polycystic echinococcosis in tropical America: *Echinococcus vogeli* and *E. oligarthrus*. *Acta Trop.* **67:**43–65.
5. **Davies, H. D., P. Sakuls, and J. S. Keystone.** 1993. Creeping eruption. A review of clinical presentation and man-

agement of 60 cases presenting to a tropical disease unit. *Arch. Dermatol.* **129:**588–591.

6. **Gutierrez, Y.** 1984. Diagnostic features of zoonotic filariae in tissue sections. *Hum. Pathol.* **15:**514–525.
7. **Gutierrez, Y.** 1990. *Diagnostic Pathology of Parasitic Infections with Clinical Correlations*. Lea & Febiger, Philadelphia, Pa.
8. **Holodniy, M., J. Almenoff, J. Loutit, and G. K. Steinberg.** 1991. Cerebral sparganosis: case report and review. *Rev. Infect. Dis.* **13:**155–159.
9. **Ishikura, H., K. Kikuchi, K. Nagasawa, T. Ooiwa, H. Takamiya, N. Sato, and K. Sugane.** 1993. Anisakidae and anisakidosis. *Prog. Clin. Parasitol.* **3:**43–102.
10. **New, D., M. D. Little, and J. H. Cross.** 1995. *Angiostrongylus cantonensis* infections from eating raw snails. *N. Engl. J. Med.* **332:**1105–1106.
11. **Orihel, T. C., and L. R. Ash.** 1995. *Parasites in Human Tissues*. American Society of Clinical Pathologists, Chicago, Ill.
12. **Orihel, T. C., and P. C. Beaver.** 1989. Zoonotic *Brugia* infections in North and South America. *Am. J. Trop. Med. Hyg.* **40:**638–647.
13. **Orihel, T. C., and M. L. Eberhard.** 1982. *Mansonella ozzardi*: a redescription with comments on its taxonomic relationships. *Am. J. Trop. Med. Hyg.* **31:**1142–1147.
14. **Orihel, T. C., and M. L. Eberhard.** 1998. Zoonotic Filariasis. *Clin. Microbiol. Rev.* **11:**366–381.
15. **Pampiglione, S., G. Canestri Trotti, and F. Rivasi.** 1995. Human dirofilariasis due to *Dirofilaria* (*Nochtiella*) *repens*: a review of the world literature. *Parassitologia* **37:**149–193.
16. **Peries, H., and S. Cairncross.** 1997. Global eradication of Guinea Worm. *Parasitol. Today* **13:**431–437.
17. **Ro, J. Y., P. J. Tsakalakis, V. A. White, M. A. Luna, E. G. Chang-Tung, L. Green, L. Cribbett, and A. C. Ayala.** 1989. Pulmonary dirofilariasis: the great imitator of primary or metastatic lung tumor. A clinicopathologic analysis of seven cases and a review. *Hum. Pathol.* **20:**69–76.
18. **Rusnak, J. M., and D. R. Lucy.** 1993. Clinical gnathostomiasis: case report and review of English language literature. *Clin. Infect. Dis.* **16:**33–50.
19. **Schantz, P. M.** 1989. The dangers of eating raw fish. *N. Engl. J. Med.* **320:**1143–1145.
20. **Tsang, V. C. W., and M. Wilson.** 1995. *Taenia solium* cysticercosis: an under-recognized but serious public health problem. *Parasitol. Today* **11:**124–126.
21. **von Sinner, W. N.** 1997. Imaging of cystic echinococcosis. *Acta Trop.* **67:**67–89.
22. **White, A. C. Jr.** 1997. Neurocysticercosis: a major cause of neurological disease worldwide. *Clin. Infect. Dis.* **24:** 101–115.
23. **Wittner, M., J. W. Turner, G. Jacquette, L. R. Ash, M. P. Salgo, and H. B. Tanowitz.** 1989. Eustrongylidiasis—a parasitic infection acquired by eating sushi. *N. Engl. J. Med.* **320:**1124–1126.

Arthropods of Medical Importance*

THOMAS R. FRITSCHE

114

Arthropods make up one of the largest of the animal phyla, a phylum consisting of more than a million described species, with estimates of the total number of species ranging up to 30 million. An exceedingly small number of this total directly or indirectly affect human health, but those that do are responsible for significant morbidity and mortality. Species directly or indirectly responsible for human disease include representatives of all major arthropod classes (Table 1).

Clinical laboratories are often the initial contact for both clinicians and patients with questions concerning arthropod-related diseases or with actual specimens submitted for identification. Such specimens may take the form of intact organisms or parts of organisms, skin scrapings or other tissue preparations, articles of clothing or bedding, and foodstuffs, among others. Arthropods recovered from the toilet bowl following a bowel movement or urination are often disconcerting to patients, who think they may have an intestinal or bladder infection, but such recovery is not uncommon. It is usually coincidental and not related to infection.

Clinical microbiologists should have a general understanding of the more commonly encountered medically important arthropods (especially ectoparasites) and should be able to perform limited identifications, at least of the higher taxonomic levels. It is equally important for laboratorians to recognize the clinical situations in which outside expertise should be sought. Owing to the complex nature of medical entomology, this chapter can present only a limited overview of the field. Also, descriptions of the groups covered here refer primarily to adult stages, though many arthropods, especially insects, are clinically problematic in their larval stages as well. Differentiation of larvae is often quite difficult and requires the use of specialized literature (7, 16, 35, 39) or the help of a specialist. A variety of general and medical entomology texts and guides that provide more detail about all of the groups described here are available (3, 4, 16, 18, 19, 21, 31, 35, 39, 52).

MECHANISMS OF INJURY

Direct Tissue Invasion

A variety of arthropods, including scabies mites, chigoe fleas, pentastomids, and dipteran larvae (maggots), may be responsible for invasion of superficial tissues (by the first two groups; referred to as infestation) or of deeper body tissues and cavities (by the last two groups; referred to as infection) for the latter. Tissue invasion of any sort by maggots is referred to as myiasis and may occur either in living or devitalized tissues (3, 41, 52).

Envenomation

Every day large numbers of people are subjected to the stings and bites of many different arthropods. Reactions to these attacks vary greatly and depend upon the species involved; the type of saliva or venom introduced into the body; the location of the wound; and the individual's physiologic response, which may vary depending upon whether they have been previously exposed. For most people, arthropod bites and stings cause only local tissue reactions, but for some, serious systemic, life-threatening reactions may occur.

Arthropods capable of stinging come from many different groups, with the greatest offenders including hymenopterans (ants, bees, and wasps) and scorpions. Systemic hypersensitivity reactions are more frequently seen following sensitization to the venom of hymenopterans, especially bees (*Apis mellifera*). These venoms are mixtures of biogenic amines, polypeptide toxins, and enzymes, including phospholipases and hyaluronidase, which are responsible for both local and systemic effects. The venom of scorpions is composed of peptide toxins that act primarily on the nervous system and have few local effects (19, 20, 44, 52).

Many arthropods are capable of biting, either in the process of feeding or in self-defense, and are liable to introduce either saliva or more potent toxins to paralyze their intended prey. While arthropod bites generally cause far fewer serious reactions than stings, some individuals may develop systemic reactions to saliva. The groups usually capable of introducing saliva or other secretions with or without toxins include the centipedes (Chilopoda); mosquitoes, flies, and biting midges (Diptera); bedbugs, kissing bugs, and assassin bugs (Hemiptera); sucking lice (Anopleura); fleas (Siphonaptera); ticks and mites (Acari); and spiders (Araneae). While almost all spiders are venomous, only a few groups pose a distinct danger to humans; these include the widow spiders, violin spiders, hobo spiders, and certain tarantulas (1–3, 19, 35, 41).

Envenomation may also result from exposure to certain urticating caterpillars and beetle larvae (larval insects of

* This chapter contains information presented in chapter 109 by Thomas R. Fritsche and Michael A. Pfaller in the sixth edition of this Manual.

TABLE 1 Classification of arthropods of medical importance

Class Diplopoda (millipedes)

Class Chilopoda (centipedes)

Class Crustacea (crustaceans)
  Order Decapoda (crabs, crayfish)
  Order Copepoda (copepods)

Class Insecta (insects)
  Order Anopleura (sucking lice)
  Order Siphonaptera (fleas)
  Order Dictyoptera (cockroaches)
  Order Hemiptera (bedbugs, kissing bugs)
  Order Hymenoptera (ants, wasps, bees)
  Order Coleoptera (beetles)
  Order Lepidoptera (moths, butterflies, caterpillars)
  Order Diptera (flies, mosquitoes, midges)

Class Arachnida (arachnids)
  Subclass Scorpiones (scorpions)
  Subclass Araneae (spiders)
  Subclass Acari (ticks, mites, chiggers)

Class Pentastomida (tongue worms)

the orders Lepidoptera and Coleoptera, respectively). These larval insects may contain numerous tiny hairs that are both irritating and capable of injecting a venom to which some individuals may become sensitized. The barbed hairs may produce dermatitis and serious eye disease (3, 19, 45). In addition, some caterpillars possess venomous spines which may produce painful local symptoms and systemic symptoms.

Vesication

Some millipedes (Diplopoda), are capable of spraying an irritating and vesicating (blister-causing) chemical for defensive purposes from glands located on each body segment. While most of the millipedes seen in the United States are small and innocuous, some of the larger tropical species are capable of squirting their fluids for some distance and causing irritating skin burns (24). Blister beetles (Coleoptera) are so named because of the presence of vesicating compounds, including cantharidin, in their body fluids. When these attractive beetles are handled, cantharidin may be released from their leg joints, resulting in the appearance of fluid-filled skin blisters several hours following exposure (3, 20, 35).

Blood Loss

Blood loss from arthropod infestation is not an insignificant problem among domestic animals, although in humans it rarely becomes life-threatening. The repeated attacks of blood-sucking arthropods may, however, be psychologically traumatizing. Those arthropods capable of blood sucking include bedbugs and kissing bugs; lice; fleas; flies, mosquitoes, and biting midges; and ticks and mites. More commonly, these arthropods are involved in the transmission of infectious agents.

Transmission of Infectious Agents

Many species of arthropods are capable of either mechanical or biological transmission of agents responsible for serious infectious disease. Filth flies, which include the common house fly *Musca domestica*, and cockroaches are easily incriminated in the mechanical transmission of the agents of bacillary dysentery, cholera, typhoid, viral diarrhea, amoebic dysentery, giardiasis, and intestinal helminthiases.

Arthropod vectors responsible for the biological transmission of infectious agents may serve either as simple amplification vehicles for the organism or in a more complex role involving changing life cycle stages of certain parasites (3, 18, 35, 52). Major groups of arthropods involved in the transmission of biological agents are summarized in Table 2.

Hypersensitivity Reactions

Allergic hypersensitivity to arthropod bites and stings may develop in any individual upon repeated exposure. Because of the frequency with which hymenopteran stings occur, severe systemic reactions including anaphylaxis are well-described clinical entities. Such serious reactions may also develop in response to bites and stings of many other arthropods as well (43, 44).

Repeated exposure to the saliva, excrement, and/or body parts of many arthropods, including mites, ticks, lice, bedbugs, cockroaches, certain caterpillars, moths, and butterflies, is also well known to exacerbate allergic conditions. Because of their widespread occurrence in the environment, a large variety of house, dust, and animal mites may also be responsible for the development of allergic manifestations such as hay fever and asthma in predisposed individuals. Certain of these problems can be controlled or minimized through the use of skin desensitization programs (15, 19, 41).

Psychologic Manifestations

An exaggerated and usually illogical fear of seeing or touching arthropods is termed entomophobia. Delusory parasitosis is a potentially more serious emotional disorder in which an individual is convinced that arthropod or worm parasites are present on or in the body despite repeated examinations that fail to reveal their presence. In such circumstances, the person may relate that the "infestation" has ruined his or her life, resulting often in job loss, divorce, movement from domicile to domicile, and repeated use of pesticides and extermination services. The victim often describes numerous, unsatisfying visits to physicians or other health care providers. These problems may originate in the home or workplace and may be transferred from one to the other. Sometimes the delusions can be so convincing that others come to believe in the existence of the infestation or become "infested" themselves (36).

Because domiciles or the workplace can be infested with many different insects and mites, it is imperative that thorough inspections be performed as part of the overall evaluation of an affected individual. A mysterious onset of irritation and itching may be due to bites from unrecognized mites following abandonment of a rodent or bird nest in a human dwelling or may result from exposure to a variety of chemical, mineral, or other noxious stimuli. Infestations with scabies mites, lice, fleas, or bedbugs may also result in unexplained irritation unless their presence is specifically looked for (38, 41, 42, 55).

BIOLOGICAL CHARACTERISTICS OF ARTHROPODS

Arthropods are bilaterally symmetrical invertebrate animals characterized by a segmented body, a rigid chitinous exo-

TABLE 2 Summary of the major arthropod genera involved in the biological transmission of infectious diseases

Arthropod	Etiologic agent	Disease
Crustacea		
Decapods	*Paragonimus* spp.	Paragonimiasis
Copepods	*Diphyllobothrium* spp.	Diphyllobothriasis
	Dracunculus medinensis	Guinea worm disease
	Gnathostoma spinigerum	Gnathostomiasis
Insecta		
Anopleura		
Pediculus	*Rickettsia prowazekii*	Epidemic typhus
	Bartonella quintana	Trench fever
	Borrelia recurrentis	Epidemic relapsing fever
Siphonaptera		
Xenopsylla	*Yersinia pestis*	Plague
	Rickettsia typhi	Murine typhus
Nosopsyllus	*Rickettsia typhi*	Murine typhus
Ctenocephalides	*Dipylidium caninum*	Dog tapeworm disease
Hemiptera		
Panstrongylus, *Rhodnius*, *Triatoma*	*Trypanosoma cruzi*	Chagas' disease
Diptera		
Aedes	Flaviviruses	Dengue, yellow fever
	Other arboviruses	Encephalitis
Anopheles	*Plasmodium* spp.	Malaria
	Brugia malayi	Filariasis
	Arboviruses	Encephalitis
Culex	*Wuchereria*, *Brugia*	Filariasis
	Arboviruses	Encephalitis
Culicoides	*Mansonella* spp.	Filariasis
Glossina	*Trypanosoma brucei*	African sleeping sickness
Chrysops	*Loa loa*	Loiasis
	Francisella tularensis	Tularemia
Simulium	*Onchocerca volvulus*	Onchocerciasis
	Mansonella ozzardi	Filariasis
Phlebotomus, *Lutzomyia*	*Leishmania* spp.	Leishmaniasis
	Bartonella bacilliformis	Bartonellosis
	Phlebovirus	Sandfly fever
Arachnida		
Acari (ticks)		
Ixodes	*Borrelia burgdorferi*	Lyme disease
	Ehrlichia spp.	Human granulocytic ehrlichiosis
	Babesia spp.	Babesiosis
Ornithodoros	*Borrelia* spp.	Relapsing fever
Dermacentor	*Rickettsia rickettsii*	Rocky Mountain spotted fever
	Francisella tularensis	Tularemia
	Coltivirus	Colorado tick fever
Amblyomma	*Rickettsia rickettsii*	Rocky Mountain spotted fever
	Francisella tularensis	Tularemia
	Ehrlichia chaffeensis	Human monocytic ehrlichiosis
Rhipicephalus	*Rickettsia conorii*	Boutonneuse fever
	Rickettsia rickettsii	Rocky Mountain spotted fever
Acari (mites)		
Leptotrombidium	*Orientia tsutsugamushi*	Scrub typhus
Liponyssoides	*Rickettsia akari*	Rickettsialpox

skeleton that is molted periodically during growth, and several pairs of jointed appendages. Development proceeds from egg to adult form through the process of metamorphosis, which may be either gradual or complete.

The class Insecta demonstrates both types of metamorphosis depending upon the group. Bedbugs, kissing bugs, lice, and cockroaches display gradual metamorphosis, in which the organism passes through three life cycle stages: egg, nymph, and adult. Nymphs closely resemble adults but are sexually immature and grow gradually through a series of molts.

Insects that display complete metamorphosis pass through four different stages: egg, larva, pupa, and adult. This type of growth is typical of butterflies and moths; medically important arthropods that display it include flies and mosquitoes; fleas; ants, bees, and wasps; and beetles. Larval forms differ significantly from adults and are often wormlike; they include (for example) fly maggots, mosquito wrigglers, beetle grubs, and caterpillars. They often live in different ecological niches from the adults and have different nutritional needs. True metamorphosis occurs when the larvae stop feeding and begin to pupate. During this time, the pupa undergoes a major reorganization of both internal and external organs and is often susceptible to predation. Emergence of the adult signifies the onset of sexual maturity and the initiation of reproductive activities (4, 35).

Spiders and scorpions undergo developmental changes most similar to the process of gradual metamorphosis as seen in insects. Life cycles of ticks and mites typically include egg, larva, nymph, and adult. Larvae of ticks and mites can be differentiated from other stages by determining the number of legs present: larvae have six legs whereas nymphs and adults have eight (21, 31, 35, 46).

SPECIMEN HANDLING AND EXAMINATION

Invariably, arthropods brought to the attention of clinicians are submitted to the clinical laboratory. These specimens most commonly originate from human sources (skin surface, tissue, stool, urine, sputum, and other anatomic sites), and a variety of nonhuman sources (foodstuffs, water, clothing, bedding, carpeting, and animals, among others).

Depending upon the laboratorian's interest and comfort in examining arthropods, specimens may be retained for study and identification or forwarded to someone trained in the field of entomology. Identification of many arthropods is not difficult and can be attempted provided the individual has some background in the specialty and has access to the various texts and other aids, including dichotomous keys, available. *Depending on the seriousness of the problem, however, expert help should be sought when significant clinical decisions regarding therapy and prognosis are being made.* Usually state public health laboratories have the expertise available or know of individuals trained in medical aspects of entomology at regional medical or educational institutions, museums, or other state or federal agencies, including the Centers for Disease Control and Prevention.

Methods of killing and preserving of arthropods should be dictated by the type of arthropod being collected and the characteristics it is necessary to preserve for identification purposes. Many specimens deteriorate beyond recognition if left to die without preservation. Exposure to the fumes of standard killing agents, including ethyl acetate, chloroform, and ether, is often appropriate for long-term storage and identification. Standard techniques used subsequent to killing include dry preservation, immersion in preservative fluids, and slide-mounting.

Adult mosquitoes, midges, and flies are best preserved dry to retain key taxonomic characteristics such as body and wing scales and are usually pinned for future examination. Most beetles, true bugs, and cockroaches are also best killed and maintained as pinned specimens. Arthropods that are pinned and dried need to be stored in tight-fitting boxes with naphthalene or dichlorobenzene to protect them from pests (3, 51).

For many other medically important arthropods, including larval forms (maggots, grubs, caterpillars, etc.), ectoparasites (lice, fleas, ticks, and mites), spiders, and scorpions, immersion in 70 to 80% ethyl alcohol provides adequate preservation. It is often preferable to kill large maggots and other larvae in hot water (not boiling) to extend their bodies and prevent contraction when they are placed in alcohol. Also, when such larvae are received with attached tissue or in a fecal specimen, it is best to gently remove or wash away attached debris prior to preservation.

Certain of the smaller medically important arthropods (mites, small ticks, fleas, sand flies, and midges) are best killed in alcohol and subsequently prepared as permanent slide mounts. Prior to dehydration and mounting, the darker specimens can be cleared by placing them in 10% potassium hydroxide for several days. Mounting media include water-based types (modified Berlese's medium) and organic-solvent-based types (Canada balsam, Permount, and isobutyl methacrylate, among others) (3, 18, 51).

Many different kinds of specialized collecting equipment have been described and are in use by entomologists: nets, tubes, traps (baited and suction), and aspirators, the last being especially useful for the collection of mosquitoes and sand flies in epidemiologic investigations. A variety of entomology and parasitology books and laboratory guides provide more detailed information about the collection, preservation, and preparation of arthropod specimens for examination (3, 4, 16, 18, 35, 51).

CLASSIFICATION, CLINICAL SIGNIFICANCE, AND IDENTIFYING CHARACTERISTICS

The classification scheme followed here is traditional in its approach to the arthropods. The recognized classes, subclasses, and orders are presented in Table 1. Arthropods of medical importance are differentiated into two subphyla determined by the presence of either articulated mandibles (Mandibulata) or pincherlike chelicerae (Chelicerata). Classes of mandibulate arthropods include the myriapods (millipedes and centipedes), crustaceans, and insects; the chelicerate arthropods include the arachnids. The affinities of the pentostomes have yet to be determined (3, 4, 35). Differentiation at the ordinal level is only somewhat more difficult but does require some biological training and familiarity with arthropod anatomy. Distinction of various groups and species beyond this level may require detailed reference sources and use of often complex dichotomous keys. Despite these difficulties, the list of medically important groups of arthropods is not overwhelming and should be within the grasp of most laboratorians committed to learning about them. A simplified key to the classes, subclasses, and orders of adult arthropods of medical importance is given in Table 3, although the reader may need to consult illustrated texts as well (4, 16, 18, 19, 35, 39). The groups listed in Table 3 but not discussed here (termites, order Isoptera; earwigs, order Dermaptera; silverfish and firebrats, order Thysanura;

TABLE 3 Key to the common arthropod classes, subclasses, and orders of medical importance, adult stages[a]

1. Three or four pairs of legs [2]
   Five or more pairs of legs [22]

2. Three pairs of legs with antennae **(insects: class Insecta)** [3]
   Four pairs of legs without antennae **(spiders, ticks, mites, scorpions: class Arachnida)** [20]

3. Wings present, well developed [4]
   Wings absent or rudimentary [12]

4. One pair of wings **(flies, mosquitoes, midges: order Diptera)** [5]
   Two pairs of wings [6]

5. Wings with scales **(mosquitoes: order Diptera)**
   Wings without scales **(other flies: order Diptera)**

6. Mouthparts adapted for sucking, with an elongate proboscis [7]
   Mouthparts adapted for chewing, without an elongate proboscis [8]

7. Wings densely covered with scales, proboscis coiled **(butterflies and moths: order Lepidoptera)**
   Wings not covered with scales; proboscis not coiled, but directed backward **(bedbugs and kissing bugs: order Hemiptera)**

8. Both pair of wings membranous, similar in structure, although size may vary [9]
   Front pair of wings leathery or shell-like, serving as covers for the second pair [10]

9. Both pair of wings similar in size **(termites: order Isoptera)**
   Hind wing much smaller than front wing **(wasps, hornets, and bees: order Hymenoptera)**

10. Front wings horny or leathery without distinct veins, meeting in a straight line down the middle [11]
    Front wings leathery or paperlike, with distinct veins, usually overlapping in the middle **(cockroaches: order Dictyoptera)**

11. Abdomen with prominent cerci or forceps; wings shorter than abdomen **(earwigs: order Dermaptera)**
    Abdomen without prominent cerci or forceps; wings covering abdomen **(beetles: order Coleoptera)**

12. Abdomen with three long terminal tails **(silverfish and firebrats: order Thysanura)**
    Abdomen without three long terminal tails [13]

13. Abdomen with narrow waist **(ants: order Hymenoptera)**
    Abdomen without narrow waist [14]

14. Abdomen with prominent pair of cerci or forceps **(earwigs: order Dermaptera)**
    Abdomen without cerci or forceps [15]

15. Body flattened laterally, antennae small, fitting into grooves in side of head **(fleas: order Siphonaptera)**
    Body flattened dorsoventrally, antennae projecting from side of head, not fitting into grooves [16]

16. Antennae with nine or more segments [17]
    Antennae with three to five segments [18]

17. Pronotum covering head **(cockroaches: order Dictyoptera)**
    Pronotum not covering head **(termites: order Isoptera)**

18. Mouthparts consisting of tubular jointed beak; tarsi three- to five-segmented **(bedbugs: order Hemiptera)**
    Mouthparts retracted into head or of the chewing type; one- or two-segmented tarsi [19]

19. Mouthparts retracted into the head; adapted for sucking blood **(sucking lice: order Anopleura)**
    Mouthparts of the chewing type **(chewing lice: order Mallophaga)**

20. Body oval, consisting of a single saclike region **(ticks and mites: subclass Acari)**
    Body divided into two distinct regions, a cephalothorax and an abdomen [21]

21. Abdomen joined to the cephalothorax by a slender waist; abdomen with segmentation indistinct or absent; stinger absent **(spiders: subclass Araneae)**
    Abdomen broadly joined to the cephalothorax; abdomen distinctly segmented, ending with a stinger **(scorpions: subclass Scorpiones)**

22. Five to nine pairs of legs or swimmerets; one or two pairs of antennae; principally aquatic organisms **(copepods, crabs, and crayfish: class Crustacea)**
    Ten or more pairs of legs; swimmerets absent; one pair of antennae present; terrestrial organisms [23]

23. Body segments each with only one pair of legs **(centipedes: class Chilopoda)**
    Body segments each with two pairs of legs **(millipedes: class Diplopoda)**

[a] Adapted from references 19 and 39.

and chewing lice, order Mallophaga) are discussed elsewhere (4, 21, 31, 39).

The following sections include a discussion of each group of medically important arthropods that indicates their major medical importance and, in some instances, provides assistance to their identification. Information on specific infectious agents transmitted by arthropods may be found in the appropriate sections of this Manual.

CLASS DIPLOPODA (MILLIPEDES)

Millipedes are wormlike arthropods with numerous apparent body segments, each of which has two pair of legs. While somewhat similar in appearance to centipedes, millipedes are more rounded and have mouthparts that point downward. Most of the more than 8,000 species described feed nocturnally on plants or decaying vegetation and do not have mouthparts capable of piercing bites. Many do produce

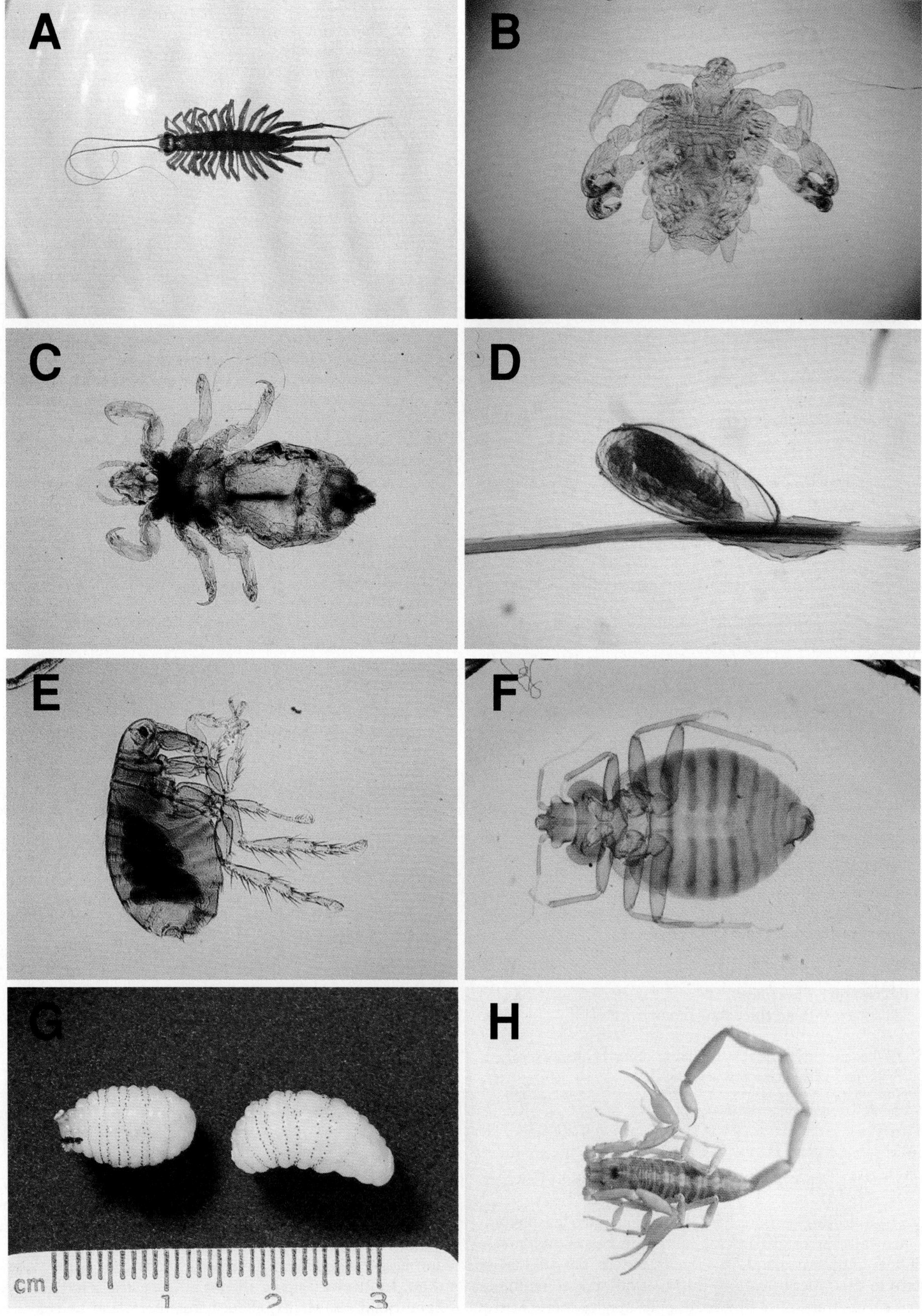
A
B
C
D
E
F
G
H
cm
1
2
3

secretions for defensive purposes from glands located on the sides of each body segment. Secreted fluids, composed of quinonoids and parabenzoquinones, are irritating to a potential enemy and in some of the larger (up to 25-cm) tropical species can be forcefully discharged over several centimeters. Exposure of human skin to these fluids can result in a burning sensation, discoloration, and blister formation. Active or passive eye exposure can result in periorbital burns, severe conjunctivitis, keratitis, and occasionally corneal ulceration which may progress to corneal perforation (24).

CLASS CHILOPODA (CENTIPEDES)

Centipedes are flattened, multi-segmented worm-like arthropods with one pair of legs per segment and long antennae (Fig. 1). Approximately 2,800 species from both temperate and tropical climates have been described. Unlike millipedes, centipedes are fast-moving and can inflict a painful bite from forward-facing pincers, which are modified from the first pair of legs. Bites usually occur when someone steps on, picks up, or rolls onto a centipede while sleeping on the ground. Most species are nocturnal and feed on other arthropods after paralyzing them with poison from the pincers, although larger species are also thought to feed on small vertebrates. The larger (26- to 45-cm) venomous species (genus *Scolopendra*) found in the southern United States and in tropical climates are able to penetrate the skin of humans, giving a painful, burning bite with local reactions including edema, blistering, and tissue necrosis. Systemic reactions may occur, especially in sensitized individuals, but fatalities are rare (3, 19, 52).

CLASS CRUSTACEA (CRUSTACEANS)

Crustaceans of medical importance are few, and their mechanisms of injury are related to their role as biological vectors of certain helminths. They are primarily aquatic organisms that use gills for breathing or absorb oxygen directly through the cuticle. Crustacea possess at least five pair of legs, which may be specialized for particular functions (i.e., swimmerets), and two pair of antennae. Decapod crustacea include the prawns, shrimps, lobsters, crayfish, and crabs, which are characterized by the presence of a cephalothorax (fused head and thorax) covered by a protective shield known as a carapace. Certain crabs and crayfish serve as the second intermediate host for the various species of the lung fluke *Paragonimus* sp. found around the world. When infected crabs or crayfish are eaten raw, the encysted metacercariae are transmitted to humans, and adult worms eventually come to reside in the lungs.

Copepods are microscopic zooplankton that lack a carapace, and certain freshwater genera (*Cyclops*, *Diaptomus*) are capable of serving as the first intermediate host for several different human helminths, including the nematodes *Dracunculus medinensis* and *Gnathostoma spinigerum* and cestodes of the genera *Diphyllobothrium* and *Spirometra*. Species in the latter genus are responsible for the zoonotic infection known as sparganosis. Copepods are occasionally found in stool specimens but undoubtedly result from ingestion of unfiltered water (3, 4, 18, 35, 39).

CLASS INSECTA (INSECTS)

The insects, or hexapods, are the most important of the arthropod classes, constituting more than 90% of all described species in the phylum, and are the only class in which flight has developed. Insects are easily distinguished from other arthropods by a body that is divided into three parts (the head, thorax, and abdomen); one pair of antennae and three pairs of legs; and one, two, or no pairs of wings. Insects may be involved in all mechanisms of injury reviewed above, although their impact on the transmission of infectious agents, including viral, bacterial, protozoan, and metazoan pathogens, is especially noteworthy. Of the more than 30 described orders of insects, only those of major medical importance are touched on here (Table 1).

Sucking Lice: Order Anopleura (Phthiraptera)

Sucking lice are small, wingless ectoparasites that are dorsoventrally flattened and have a specialized claw on the end of each leg that allows them to cling to hair shafts or clothing fibers. The three species of human lice include the head louse, *Pediculus capitis*; the body louse, *P. humanus*; and the pubic or crab louse, *Phthirus pubis* (39). Although named for their primary sites of infection, lice are not always confined to a certain part of the body. All suck blood intermittently and may produce unexplained dermatitis as a result of their repeated feeding activities and chronic exposure of the skin to louse excreta. Eggs, known as nits, are deposited on either hair shafts (*P. capitis* and *P. pubis*) or clothing (*P. humanus*). Metamorphosis is gradual, and larval forms live and feed side by side with adults. In addition to their bloodsucking habits, body lice are capable of transmitting the rickettsial agents of typhus and trench fever and the spirochetes responsible for relapsing fever (Table 2).

Head and body lice are very similar morphologically, and their distinction as two species has been controversial (Fig. 1). Anatomic and ecologic differences have been detected, however, and support the concept of two species (32, 35). In addition, only the body louse is known to transmit pathogens between humans. Both species grow to about 3 mm in length and are longer than they are wide. The male is usually smaller than the female and has a more rounded posterior end (19, 32, 35, 39).

Head lice are found predominantly on the head and neck and behind the ears, with the nits being glued to hair shafts very close to the skin surface in these areas. Because incubation takes 7 to 10 days, hatched eggs appear farther up (ca. 0.5 in. or 1.27 cm) on the hair shaft. Embryonating eggs have intact opercula, whereas hatched eggs do not (Fig. 1). Because a variety of objects (hair casts, dander, hair spray, and fungal hair infection) may mimic nits, which are typically 1 mm in length, it is important to differentiate them carefully. Schoolchildren are at particular risk for acquiring these ectoparasites through the sharing of infested caps, scarves, or combs; from exposure to infested carpeting, beds, or furniture; or from close personal contact. Parents and other family members may subsequently become infested when children bring lice home from school or day-care centers (19, 26, 41).

Adult and immature body lice are found predominantly

FIGURE 1 Medically important arthropods. Row 1: (A) centipede; (B) *Phthirus pubis* (crab louse). Row 2: (C) *Pediculus capitis* (head louse); (D) nit of head louse attached to hair shaft. Row 3: (E) *Pulex irritans* (human flea); (F) *Cimex lectularius* (bedbug). Row 4: (G) *Dermatobia hominis* (human botfly) third stage larvae (photograph courtesy of J. Brad Thomas, David L. Bergeron, and James J. Plorde); (H) scorpion.

on the hairy body regions below the neck when they are feeding, and they move readily between the body and clothing when they are not feeding. Unlike head lice, body lice tend to lay clusters of eggs on clothing, especially on seams or waistbands. Body lice are readily spread among individuals held in institutional settings or other close quarters, especially when there is little opportunity for bathing and laundering. Sharing of infested clothing and exposure to infested bedding are common routes of transmission (3, 35, 41).

Pubic or crab lice are much rounder than the other lice, measuring approximately 2 mm in diameter, and their first pair of legs is significantly smaller and more slender than the other pairs (Fig. 1). The abdomen is more crablike and displays hairy tufts on the lateral margins. Adults, nymphs, and nits are usually found on the pubic hairs but may be found on chest, armpit, and facial hair, including eyebrows and eyelashes. Transmission occurs through close personal contact, especially during sexual intercourse (19, 35, 39).

Fleas: Order Siphonaptera

Fleas are small, wingless ectoparasites capable of sucking or "siphoning" blood, hence the origin of the ordinal name. Unlike lice, fleas have bodies that are laterally compressed and long, muscular legs which are adapted for jumping (Fig. 1). They undergo complete metamorphosis during their life cycle, which includes four stages: egg, larva, pupa, and adult. Of the approximately 2,500 described species and subspecies, 94% are ectoparasites of mammals, with the remainder occurring on birds (35).

Only a small number directly affect humans. These include blood-sucking pests; tissue-penetrating jiggers; intermediate hosts for certain cestode parasites; and vectors for the agents of plague, murine typhus, and perhaps others. Identification of fleas is difficult for the clinical microbiologist because of the specialized nature of terminology used to describe flea morphology, the difficulty in following complex dichotomus keys, and the large number of described species (14, 22, 23, 35, 39). Fortunately, the number of flea species commonly associated with humans is small and the infestation is often related to contact with domestic animals and pets.

The Oriental rat flea, *Xenopsylla cheopis*, is the most important species affecting human health because of its ability to transmit the bacterial agents of plague and murine typhus. This species normally parasitizes Norway and roof rats, but it will readily bite humans should the rodent host die. The northern rat flea, *Nosopsyllus fasciatus*, also parasitizes Norway and roof rats and may be involved in the transmission of murine typhus to humans. The sticktight flea, *Echidnophaga gallinacea*, is a common pest of poultry but will readily attack humans. The name originates from the flea's habit of attaching firmly to the skin for extended periods during feeding (3, 19, 35).

The human flea, *Pulex irritans*, normally parasitizes a variety of other mammals, including domestic and wild pigs, canids, mustelids, and deer (Fig. 1). In certain settings, such as farms, they may be a particular nuisance in causing flea bite hypersensitivity reactions. *Pulex* fleas may play a role in maintaining the sylvatic cycle of plague. Throughout North America the cat flea, *Ctenocephalides felis*, and to a lesser extent the dog flea, *C. canis*, are the most pestiferous flea species encountered. Both species move easily between cats and dogs and readily attack humans. In addition to causing dermatitis and typical delayed hypersensitivity skin reactions from their bites, cat and dog fleas are the usual intermediate hosts for the cysticercoid stage of the tapeworm *Dipylidium caninum* and less frequently for *H. diminuta* and *H. nana* (3, 19, 20, 35, 41, 42).

The jigger or chigoe flea, *Tunga penetrans*, is the cause of tungiasis in Central and South America and parts of tropical Africa. Its mechanism of injury is unusual because of the habit of the female flea of embedding itself in the skin during its reproductive life. Usual sites of infestation include the soft skin between the toes and under the toenails, but other sites, including the hands, arms, elbows, and genital region, may also be affected. As the flea engorges with blood and begins to produce eggs, it swells to approximately 1,000 times its original size (about the size of a small pea). Several thousand eggs, each measuring approximately 0.5 mm in length, are produced, after which the flea dies. Resulting inflammatory responses and secondary bacterial infections may result in loss of digits, septicemia, or tetanus. Detection of infestation is made by recognizing the dark portion of the chigoe flea's abdomen, which displays the respiratory spiracles, as it protrudes from the skin surface in the center of an enlarging, inflamed lesion (3, 19, 52). Depending upon size, jiggers are removed surgically, either with a sterile needle, by curettage, or by excision.

Cockroaches: Order Dictyoptera

Cockroaches are dorsoventrally flattened insects with long multisegmented antennae, biting mouthparts, two pair of wings, two posterior abdominal projections known as cerci, and legs adapted for running. Metamorphosis is gradual, and the nymphs appear similar to the adults, although the nymphs are smaller and have no wings. Cockroaches are omnivorous nocturnal feeders and prefer secluded areas. Several species have closely adapted themselves to human habitation, where they share our food, water, shelter, and warmth (4, 21).

Mostly considered to be nuisance pests, cockroaches impart an unpleasant odor to living areas by fouling their environment with feces, disgorging partially digested food at intervals, and discharging secretions from abdominal glands (21). They are also potential carriers of fecal pathogens because of their ease of movement from sewers and drains to areas of habitation, especially food preparation areas. In addition to harboring many enteric bacteria, cockroaches can also harbor hepatitis and polio viruses, *Entamoeba histolytica*, and several species of the most common enteric nematodes. They also may occur in such high densities as to cause allergy and asthma in some individuals following sensitization to their excreta, cast skins, or body parts (3, 19, 35).

The most important pest species include the German cockroach, *Blatella germanica*; the Oriental cockroach, *Blatta orientalis*; the brown-banded cockroach, *Supella longipalpa*; and several species in the genus *Periplaneta*, including the American cockroach, *P. americana* (21, 39). The different species have somewhat different habits. The German roach prefers the warm, moist conditions commonly found in kitchens, restaurants, and bathrooms. It is considered the number one pest in buildings in the United States. The Oriental cockroach is found in cooler locations such as cellars and basements and the cooler parts of kitchens as well as in outdoor drainage areas and rubbish heaps. The brown-banded cockroach is a common pest in most parts of the tropics and has spread to North America. It may be found in many different parts of a building and is known to cause damage to book bindings. The American cockroach is the most widespread and frequent cause of domiciliary infestation in both the tropics and subtropics. In temperate climates, it seeks out conditions similar to those preferred by the German cockroach (19, 35).

Bedbugs and Kissing Bugs: Order Hemiptera

Bedbugs (family Cimicidae) and kissing and assassin bugs (family Reduviidae) are blood-sucking insects characterized by a long proboscis that is folded ventrally under the body when not in use. Members of both families undergo gradual metamorphosis and may be found in areas of human habitation.

The common bedbug, *Cimex lectularius*, and the tropical bedbug, *C. hemipterus*, are reddish-brown, oval, and dorsoventrally flattened insects approximately 5 mm in length. Adults have small wing pads that are nonfunctional (Fig. 1). Kissing bugs (genera *Triatoma*, *Rhodnius*, and *Panstrongylus*) are black or brown in color with elongate, cone-shaped heads, narrowed necks, and four-segmented antennae that insert laterally into the head. They average 1 to 3 cm in length. The abdomen is widened in the middle and may display orange and black markings. They have wings and are good fliers (4, 19, 35, 39).

Both bedbugs (adult males and females and nymphs) and reduviid bugs feed nocturnally, will attack almost any mammal, and are cosmopolitan in distribution. Bedbugs hide in bedsteads, mattresses, and under loose wallpaper, whereas kissing bugs live in cracks and crevices of walls and in thatched roofs. Kissing bugs feed exclusively on vertebrate blood and are named for their habit of biting around the face, often painlessly. Assassin bugs (genus *Reduvius*) predominantly attack and feed on other insects but will attack humans, producing a painful bite unlike that of a kissing bug.

The bites of both groups of bugs produce lesions that range from small red inconspicuous marks to hemorrhagic bullae, depending on an individual's sensitivity to their saliva. Periorbital edema, known as Romana's sign, is often seen following a bite by kissing bugs to the face. Bedbugs produce a peculiar odor in heavily infested homes, and their repeated attacks may make sleep impossible. While bedbugs are not known to transmit disease, reduviids are well known to transmit the agent of Chagas' disease, *Trypanosoma cruzi*, in Mexico and Central and South America (see chapter 106). The infective trypomastigotes are passed in the feces of the reduviid during feeding and are usually self-inoculated by the host secondary to scratching (3, 19, 35, 41).

Bees, Wasps, and Ants: Order Hymenoptera

Hymenopterans are characterized by two pairs of membranous wings, with the front wings much larger than the hind wings, and by biting-chewing mouthparts. Ant queens and males display wings only during certain times of the year. Many hymenopterans are social insects that attack and sting any intruder disturbing their nests. The stinging apparatus is actually the modified ovipositor of the female, which is capable of injecting venom and is used either for the capture of prey or for defense (4, 21, 31, 35, 39).

The stings of honeybees (genus *Apis*) and bumblebees (genera *Bombus*, *Megabombus*, and *Pyrobombus*) in the family Apidae and wasps (genus *Polistes*), hornets (genus *Vespa*), and yellowjackets (genera *Vespula*, *Paravespula*, and *Dolichovespula*) in the family Vespidae cause only transient pain and swelling in most individuals but may be responsible for severe systemic reactions, including anaphylaxis, in sensitized persons (43, 44). In the United States, an estimated 50 to 100 people die each year from such reactions. The introduction of the Africanized honeybee to Brazil in 1956 has resulted in the spread of these bees to much of South and Central America and more recently to the southern United States. These bees are almost identical to domesticated strains but are known to be more readily provoked in defense of the hive and exhibit massive stinging behavior (3, 19, 35, 39, 44).

Depending upon their size, almost all ants (family Formicidae) are capable of piercing human skin with their bite, and some species, such as harvester ants (genus *Pogonomyrmex*) and fire ants (genus *Solenopsis*), may sting as well. The accidentally imported fire ant *Solenopsis invicta* has become particularly troublesome in the southeastern and south central United States because it is easily disturbed and capable of both biting with strong mandibles and injecting venom with a sting (19, 35, 39, 44).

Beetles: Order Coleoptera

Beetles constitute the largest group of insects, with over a quarter of a million described species, and are characterized by front wings modified into leathery coverings that meet in a straight line down the middle of the abdomen (4, 35, 39). While beetles are considered to be of minor medical importance, many can bite, and others, especially the blister beetles (family Meloidae), may exude irritating and vesicating fluids when roughly handled. These fluids are released from leg joints as a defensive measure and may produce dermatitis or blister formation. Blister beetles are cosmopolitan in distribution and may attract attention, especially of children, because of their coloration. Cantharidin is one of the vesicating substances found in blister beetles and the chief component of the aphrodisiac known as Spanish fly (19–21, 35).

Larvae of some larder beetles (Dermestidae) have urticating hairs that may penetrate the skin and cause dermatitis. If ingested, these hairs may irritate the intestinal tract. Dermestid beetles and mealworms, family Tenebrionidae, serve as intermediate hosts for the rodent tapeworms *H. diminuta* and *H. nana*, which are known to infect humans. Reports of invasion of living tissues by adult or larval beetles are not uncommon in the literature, but such invasions are usually considered accidental occurrences. Pseudoparasitism of the intestinal tract may result from eating infested foodstuffs and passing intact larvae or adults in the stool (3, 19, 35, 39).

Moths and Butterflies: Order Lepidoptera

Medically important moths and butterflies are primarily those having caterpillars that possess urticating hairs or spines capable of secreting venom when the creature is handled. Exposure to urticating hairs usually results in no more than localized dermatitis, whereas exposure to stinging spines may result in local manifestations of stabbing pain, burning sensation, and inflammation. In some individuals and with certain species, the effects may become systemic and lead to shock and paralysis (3, 15, 35, 39).

Urticating scales and hairs of certain adult moths, especially those of the tussock moths, gypsy moths, and *Hylesia* spp., may also be problematic, causing dermatitis, upper respiratory tract irritation, and eye irritation. Tussock and gypsy moths are known to cause problems seasonally for forestry workers and others in the United States, whereas *Hylesia* moths are common in South America and may emerge in large numbers and congregate around bright lights in populated areas (15, 19, 45).

Flies, Mosquitoes, and Midges: Order Diptera

Dipterans include the insects of greatest medical importance, although most species are harmless to humans. They are characterized by a single pair of functional membranous wings, and they undergo complete metamorphosis (i.e., egg, larva, pupa, and adult) in which the larvae develop in environments completely different from the habitats of the adults (4, 35).

Human disease and injury from these insects are engendered primarily by three mechanisms: blood sucking, biological and mechanical transmission of infectious agents, and myiasis or infection of the body by larval dipterans. Blood sucking may be done by dipterans equipped with puncturing-sucking mouthparts (mosquitoes), piercing-sucking mouthparts (stable flies, tsetse flies), or bladelike mouthparts (deerflies, horseflies, and blackflies). Bites from the last two groups are usually much more painful than those from the first group. Saliva from most dipteran bites causes local irritation and, in some individuals, systemic reactions, including fever, urticaria, and respiratory distress. Continuous or repeated exposure to blood-sucking diptera can often be a traumatic experience both physically and psychologically (3, 19, 35, 41).

Blood-sucking diptera are also responsible for the transmission of major human pathogens, including malarial parasites, filariae, and arboviruses by mosquitoes; African trypanosomes by tsetse flies; leishmaniae by sand flies; and *Onchocerca volvulus* by blackflies. Nonbiting synanthropic flies such as houseflies, flesh flies, and blowflies are well known for mechanically transmitting certain viral, bacterial, protozoal, and helminthic agents responsible for intestinal diseases (3, 21, 52). These flies readily feed on human food as well as excrement and easily move between the two. Identification of adult diptera is beyond the scope of this chapter and requires the use of specialized literature.

Certain dipteran larvae (maggots) are capable of surviving or developing in living human tissues and body cavities in an accidental, facultative, or obligatory fashion. While infections may occur in any anatomic site, most myiases are reported as being gastrointestinal, dermal or cutaneous, auricular, ocular, nasopharyngeal, or genitourinary (3, 19, 35, 52). Pulmonary, gastrointestinal, and genitourinary pseudomyiases occur occasionally and may cause significant psychologic distress but usually result from the contamination of sputum, urine, or stool samples with fly eggs following improper collection or storage.

Flies producing accidental myiasis have no requirement for development in human or animal tissues, and include the housefly *Musca domestica* (Fig. 2) among many others. Maggots of such species are occasionally found feeding on dead tissue in wounds following removal of dressings or casts. Gastrointestinal infections are usually accidental and occur following ingestion of contaminated foodstuffs.

Facultative myiasis is most often caused by blowflies (family Calliphoridae) and flesh flies (family Sarcophagidae), which ordinarily feed on dead and decaying tissues of animals. In humans, such maggots may initially infest exposed ulcers, traumatic wounds, or other diseased tissues but may secondarily move into adjacent healthy tissues in an opportunistic fashion (3, 25, 35, 52).

Obligatory myiasis in humans is caused by relatively few species, all of which are zoonotic in origin. These species have an obligate need to invade living tissues and may produce serious or life-threatening infections. *Dermatobia hominis*, the human botfly, may appear in boil-like lesions of individuals who have spent time in certain parts of Central America, South America, and Africa. As the larvae mature, the posterior end, which bears the respiratory spiracles, is seen at the surface of the slowly enlarging dermal lesion. Mature larvae emerge from these lesions and fall to the ground, where they pupate (Fig. 1). Another arthropod, such as a mosquito or tick, upon which the female botfly has deposited her eggs, is the actual vector of this species. Other botflies known to infect humans include the horse botfly, *Gasterophilus intestinalis*; the cattle botfly, *Hypoderma bovis*; and the sheep botfly, *Oestrus ovis*. Rodent and lagomorph botflies of the genus *Cuterebra* sporadically occur as ocular or dermal parasites (11). The tumbu fly, *Cordylobia anthropophagia*, is one of the more common myiasis-producing flies affecting humans in sub-Saharan Africa. Eggs are usually laid on dry ground that has been fecally contaminated or on hanging laundry. Upon contact with human or animal skin, larvae rapidly penetrate and produce a furuncular type of myiasis. In some areas, clothing, diapers, and bedding that have been air dried must be routinely ironed to kill the eggs of this species (3, 18, 19, 35, 52).

The Old World screwworm, *Chrysomya bezziana*, and the New World screwworm, *Cochliomyia hominivorax*, deposit their eggs directly on wounds, on mucus membranes, or near the nostrils. Larvae actively feed and move through tissues, causing extensive destruction. The New World screwworm has been eradicated from the United States through the release of sterilized male flies but continues to exist in parts of Central and South America. *Wohlfahrtia magnifica* and *Wohlfahrtia vigil* are sarcophagid flies responsible for obligatory myiasis in parts of Europe, Asia, and North Africa and in North America, respectively. *W. magnifica* can produce a traumatic myiasis similar to that of screwworm, whereas *W. vigil* produces furuncular myiasis (3, 21, 35, 52).

Identification of larval diptera is difficult, depending upon the species and larval stage of development. In addition to body characteristics, examination of anterior and posterior spiracles (surface openings of breathing tubes) is often necessary. Proper viewing of posterior spiracular morphology requires experience in removing and mounting the very posterior end of the larva on a glass slide. Examples of some myiasis-causing flies and a pictoral key for identifying their posterior spiracles are shown in Fig. 2.

CLASS ARACHNIDA (SCORPIONS, SPIDERS, TICKS, AND MITES)

Arachnids of medical importance are found in three subclasses, namely, Scorpiones (scorpions), Araneae (spiders), and Acari (ticks and mites). Scorpions and spiders are characterized by two body regions, the cephalothorax and abdomen, whereas in ticks and mites, these two have been reduced to one. A pair of prehensile, pincher-like chelicerae characterize all members of the class and reflect the predaceous nature of the group. Of the three medically important subclasses, only the Acari are not predaceous. All lack antennae, mandibles, and wings. Metamorphosis is gradual, and molting occurs repeatedly to permit growth. While all arachnid nymphs and adults have four pairs of legs, tick and mite larvae have only three pairs of legs. Arachnids are perhaps best recognized by their abilities to inject poisonous venoms (scorpions and spiders) and to transmit viral, bacterial, and protozoal pathogens (ticks and mites) (Table 2).

Scorpions: Subclass Scorpiones

The body of a scorpion is divided into the cephalothorax and the segmented abdomen, to the latter of which is at-

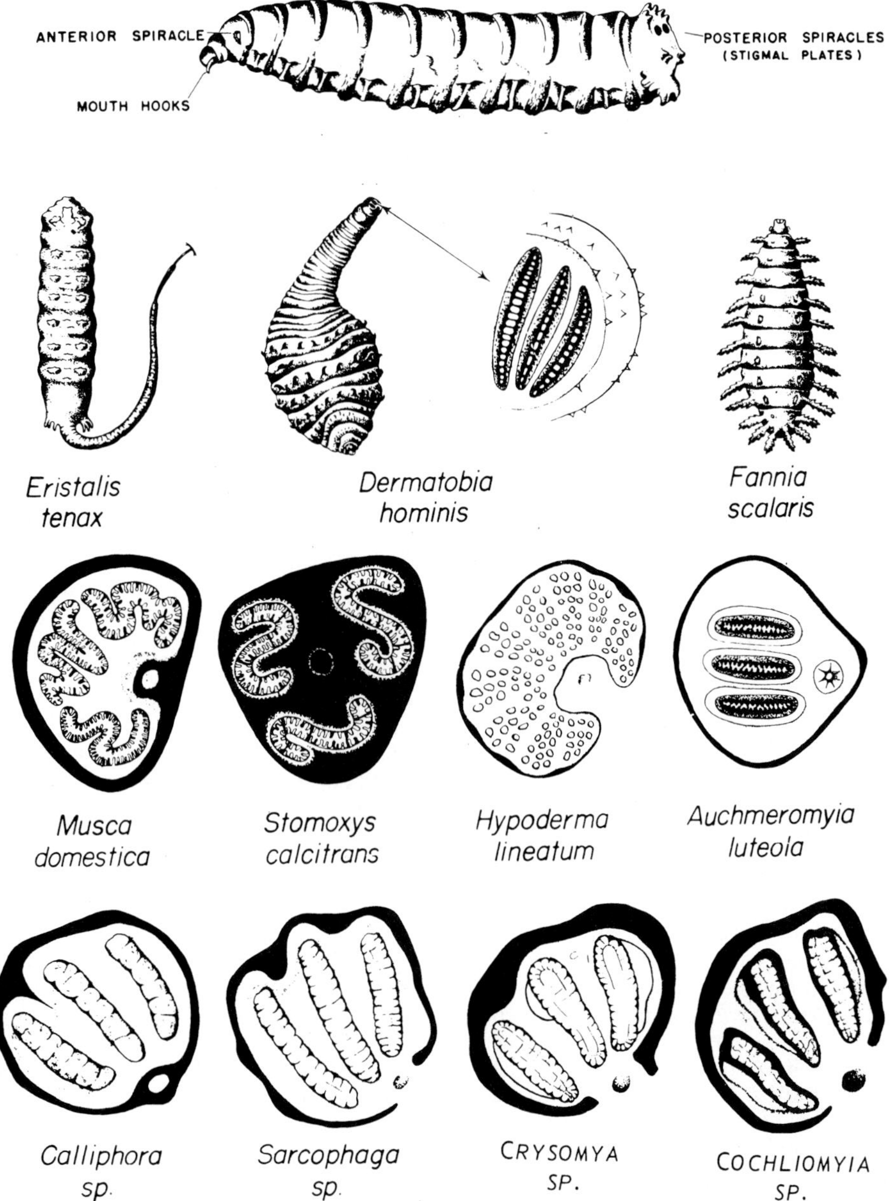

FIGURE 2 Key characters of some myiasis-producing fly larvae. Row 1: mature larva of a muscoid fly (from R. Hegner et al., copyright 1938 by Appleton-Century Inc., New York). Row 2: larvae of *Eristalis tenax*, the rat-tailed maggot; *Dermatobia hominis*, the human botfly (with an enlarged view of a posterior spiracle); and *Fannia scalaris*, the latrine fly. Rows 3 and 4: appearance of posterior spiracles of some species that produce accidental, facultative, or obligatory myiasis (Centers for Disease Control and Prevention, Atlanta, Ga.).

tached a five-segmented tail that ends in a bulbous stinging apparatus. In addition to having four pairs of legs, a scorpion has a pair of forward-directed pincer claws, or pedipalps, that gives it a crablike appearance (Fig. 1). Length varies from 2 to 10 cm, depending on the species (20, 35, 39).

Scorpions are nocturnal feeders that paralyze their intended victim with venom. When the scorpion is disturbed, the stinger may be used for defense. Depending on the species, the venom varies in its neurologic and hemolytic toxicity for humans, with the sting of many species eliciting no more reaction than those of bees and wasps. The stings of some species, however, may be deadly, accounting for over 1,000 deaths annually. Symptoms encountered during systemic poisoning include, among others, spreading paralysis, hypertension, convulsions, and respiratory arrest. While several relatively harmless species are routinely found in the southwestern United States, *Centruroides exilicauda (C. sculpturatus)* is potentially deadly, especially to children. Other poisonous species are found in Europe, Africa, and the Middle East (3, 19, 35, 52).

Spiders: Subclass Araneae

Like the bodies of scorpions, the bodies of spiders are divided into two regions: the cephalothorax, to which the four pairs of legs are attached, and the abdomen. Unlike that of scorpions, the abdomen of a spider is superficially unsegmented and is missing the tail with attached stinger. In place of the tail are spinnerets, which connect to the abdominal silk glands. The mouthparts contain a pair of fanglike chelicerae through which venom can be expressed from associated glands. While most spiders are venomous, few possess chelicerae that are capable of penetrating human skin (3, 4).

Spiders are terrestrial animals that use silk webs to ensnare their prey and venom to immobilize it. The majority of spiders able to bite humans produce little more than transitory irritation and pain. The urticating hairs on some species of tarantulas may produce more discomfort than their bite does. Of the 30,000 or more species that have been described, only 20 to 30 are known to cause more serious disease (28, 35, 39).

Systemic arachnidism may be caused by several groups of spiders, of which the widow spiders (genus *Lactrodectus*) are best known. Other groups include certain tarantulas (several genera), funnel-web spiders (genus *Atrax*), wolf spiders (genus *Lycosa*), and wandering spiders (genus *Phoneutria*). Widow spiders are cosmopolitan in distribution with five closely related species occurring in the United States: *Lactrodectus mactans* (black widow), which occurs from southern New England to Florida and west to California and Oregon; *Lactrodectus variolus* (northern black widow), which occurs from northeastern United States and adjacent areas in Canada to Florida and west to Oklahoma and Texas; *Lactrodectus hesperus* (western black widow), which occurs from the Plains states to the Pacific coast; *Lactrodectus geometricus* (brown widow spider), reported from Florida and California; and *Lactrodectus bishopi*, which occurs in southern Florida. The female black widow is shiny black, has a characteristic red or orange hourglass-shaped marking on the underside of the abdomen, eight eyes grouped in four pairs, and a leg span of 3 to 4 cm (see Fig. 4). Considerable color variation exists among species (2, 3, 19, 35, 39).

For nesting, spiders in this group prefer protected locations with a suitable food source, and in past years, the outdoor privy made an opportune spot. When provoked, they bite in self-defense, injecting a potent nonhemolytic neurotoxin that acts on the central nervous system, producing weakness, myalgia, and muscle spasm that may progress to paralysis, convulsions, and occasionally death. Mortality has been estimated at <1 to 6% (2, 3, 19, 35, 52).

Necrotic arachnidism or loxoscelism occurs following envenomation by members of the genus *Loxosceles*, known as violin spiders. In the United States, *Loxosceles reclusa*, the brown recluse or fiddleback spider, is the most commonly implicated species. It occurs in the eastern half of the country and westward into Wyoming and Arizona. Other species implicated in the United States include *Loxosceles deserta*, *Loxosceles arizonica*, *Loxosceles rufescens*, and *Loxosceles devia*. *Loxosceles laeta* and *Loxosceles rufipes* are commonly encountered in parts of South America and produce a more severe form of cutaneous necrosis. The brown recluse is a tan to dark brown spider, 1 to 2 cm long, that is characterized by a darkened violin-shaped marking oriented base forward on the dorsum of the cephalothorax and extending from the eyes to the base of the abdomen (19, 39). Six eyes are grouped in a semicircle of three pairs on top of the head (Fig. 3).

In areas of human habitation, the reclusive habits of these spiders often place them in closets among clothes, in basements, under porches, or other areas that are normally little disturbed. When provoked, the spiders may give a painless bite and inject a dermonecrotic and hemolytic toxin. Several hours later, the area will become red, swollen, and painful. Cutaneous necrosis and sloughing then occur over a matter of days, leaving a deep lesion that is slow to heal and prone to scarring. Depending on the amount and potency of the toxin injected, complications may remain superficial or occasionally may become systemic, with a high mortality rate (2, 19, 52).

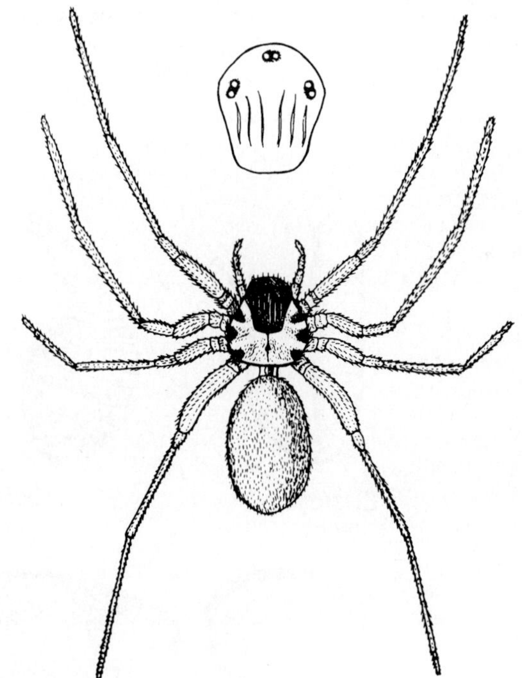

FIGURE 3 Key characters of *Loxosceles reclusa*, the brown recluse spider. This spider is small (1 to 2 cm long), has a darkened fiddle-shaped marking on the dorsum of the cephalothorax, and has six eyes grouped in three pairs (Centers for Disease Control and Prevention, Atlanta, Ga.).

Reports of necrotic arachnidism also occur in areas where *Loxosceles* spiders are not found. In the U.S. Pacific Northwest, the hobo spider, *Tegenaria agrestis*, has been implicated as a cause of cutaneous necrosis, with 40% of victims having some systemic symptoms as well (2, 13).

Ticks and Mites: Subclass Acari

Ticks

Ticks are obligate, blood-sucking ectoparasites of many reptiles, birds, and mammals, including humans. Although they constitute a small group of only about 800 described species, they are of extreme importance to human and animal health because of their impact in transmitting a variety of viral, bacterial, and protozoal pathogens and in causing additional loss to livestock and wildlife because of their feeding activities.

Ticks and mites may be differentiated from other arachnids by their fused cephalothorax and abdomen and by their larvae, which have three pairs of legs. Many adult mites are microscopic, whereas adult ticks may be seen with the naked eye. In addition, a characteristic part of the tick feeding apparatus is the toothed hypostome, which allows the mouthparts to remain solidly imbedded (3, 21, 35, 46, 47).

Two of the three families of ticks, the hard ticks (Ixodidae) and the soft ticks (Argasidae), contain species known to transmit pathogens to humans. Hard ticks may be recognized by the presence of a dorsal sclerotized plate known as the scutum and by mouthparts that project anteriorly when viewed from the top. The scutum covers the entire dorsal surface of the male, but only the anterior dorsal surface of the female is covered (Fig. 4). This allows for greater abdominal engorgement with blood by females during feeding, ensuring a greater supply of nutrients needed for egg production. While males do ingest blood, the amount is much less.

Argasids, or soft ticks, differ from hard ticks by having leathery integument, downwardly directed mouthparts (not visible from the top), and no scutum (Fig. 4). Life cycles vary considerably between the two groups, with soft ticks often taking multiple blood meals of short duration (usually less than 30 min) during each stage, having several nymphal stages, and being long-lived. They may feed repeatedly on the same or different hosts, and females may lay eggs several times during their lives. Hard ticks have a single nymphal stage, take only one blood meal on a host at each growth stage, and remain attached to the host for hours or days while feeding. The life cycle of most hard ticks requires 2 years for completion and may involve from one to three hosts, depending on the tick species. Female hard ticks die after ovipositing (46–48).

Ticks found crawling on or imbedded in the skin of humans are most often hard ticks. Soft ticks that feed on humans tend to be most active at night, feeding only briefly and then often painlessly, making their discovery uncommon. Care must be taken not to misidentify an engorged hard tick for a soft tick, which it superficially resembles. Identification of ticks found in the United States to the genus level is only moderately difficult for the nonspecialist (Fig. 5) (3, 19, 35, 37, 39). Identification of specimens to the species level (8–10, 17, 29, 30, 37, 39) is more problematic for the clinical microbiologist and should generally be referred to an outside specialist (entomologist, parasitologist, university extension service, state health laboratory, Centers for Disease Control and Prevention, etc.). This is especially true when the submitting clinician is contemplating postexposure prophylaxis for such tick-vectored diseases as Lyme borreliosis or Rocky Mountain spotted fever.

Several important species of hard ticks found in North America include *Dermacentor variabilis* (the American dog tick), *Dermacentor andersoni* (the Rocky Mountain wood tick), *Ixodes scapularis* (black-legged tick, northern and southern forms), *Ixodes pacificus* (western black-legged tick), *Amblyomma americanum* (the Lone Star tick), and *Rhipicephalus sanguineus* (the brown dog tick). *Dermacentor* and *Amblyomma* ticks are referred to as ornate because of the easily recognizable whitish markings on the scutum. The other genera of North American ticks lack this ornamentation and are known as inornate ticks (Fig. 4).

The American dog tick, *D. variabilis*, is found throughout the United States, exclusive of the Rocky Mountain region, and is the primary vector for Rocky Mountain spotted fever in the eastern states (Fig. 4). The Rocky Mountain wood tick, *D. andersoni*, occurs throughout the Rocky Mountain states and into Canada, where it serves as the primary vector for Rocky Mountain spotted fever. Both species have been implicated in cases of tularemia, tick paralysis (see below), and, rarely, Q-fever. In addition, *D. andersoni* is the chief vector for transmission of the coltivirus responsible for Colorado tick fever (Table 2) (8, 48, 52).

The genus *Ixodes* consists of inornate ticks that differ from other hard ticks by having the anal groove surround the anus anteriorly (Fig. 4 and 5). This feature may be difficult to appreciate on engorged ticks. While there are 36 described species in the United States that parasitize a variety of small and large mammals, primarily two species are involved in the transmission of the Lyme disease spirochete to humans (48, 50). *Ixodes scapularis*, the black-legged tick, is the common vector for this spirochete along the eastern seaboard, in the southern states, and in the north central states. The northern form of this tick was renamed *Ixodes dammini* in 1979 because certain structural differences from the southern form were detected, but recent studies on mating compatibility and genetic similarities have shown the two to be conspecific (40, 49). *Ixodes pacificus*, the western black-legged tick, is the most common vector for transmission of Lyme disease in the western states. These two species are also known to transmit the protozoal agent of babesiosis, *Babesia microti*, and mixed infections are being described with increasing frequency (34). *Ixodes* ticks have also been implicated in the transmission of human granulocytic ehrlichiosis (HGE), an emerging rickettsial disease occurring most commonly in the upper midwestern and northeastern United States. Symptoms of this infection are flulike but may vary from being subclinical to fatal. The white-footed mouse *Peromyscus leucopus* has been shown to serve as an efficient reservoir for all three of these infectious organisms. The vector for Lyme disease, HGE, and babesiosis in Europe is the related species *Ixodes ricinus* (53, 54).

In other parts of the world, *Ixodes* spp. are involved in the transmission of encephalitis-causing arboviruses. Tick paralysis may also be caused by members of this genus. Identification of *Ixodes* ticks to the species level is a difficult task and requires the assistance of a specialist (10, 17, 29, 30).

Amblyomma americanum, the Lone Star tick, is so named because of a single white marking at the posterior end of the scutum in the female (Fig. 4) and its occurrence in the Lone Star State, Texas. It is one of the more pestiferous species, and its range extends from Texas to the Atlantic coast and north to New York. All stages attack humans and are able to inflict painful bites because of their long mouthparts. This species is capable of transmitting Rocky Mountain spotted fever as well as tularemia and possibly Lyme disease. It is also capable of causing tick paralysis (3, 19, 35, 39, 48). More recently, *A. americanum* ticks have been implicated as vectors of the agent of human monocytic ehrlichiosis, *Ehrlichia chaffeensis*. Infection with this rickettsialike organism has been documented in 30 states, Europe, and Africa, where it produces an illness similar to HGE (54).

R. sanguineus, the brown dog tick, is an inornate tick distributed worldwide that is commonly found on dogs and in the homes in which they reside. All stages feed on the same canine host and occasionally bite humans. This species is recognized as a vector of Rocky Mountain spotted fever in North America and of boutonneuse fever in the Mediterranean basin (3, 19, 35, 39).

Soft ticks of the genus *Ornithodoros* are important vectors worldwide for the spirochetal agents of relapsing fever (*Borrelia* spp.). In the United States, at least four tick species are involved in transmission. These include *Ornithodoros hermsi* (Rocky Mountain and Pacific coast states and British Columbia) (Fig. 4), *Ornithodoros parkeri* (western United States), *Ornithodoros turicata* (western United States and northern Mexico), and *Ornithodoros talaje* (southern United States). A variety of rodents serve as the usual tick hosts and reservoir for the spirochaetes. Human exposure to these ticks usually occurs outdoors, while camping near rodent

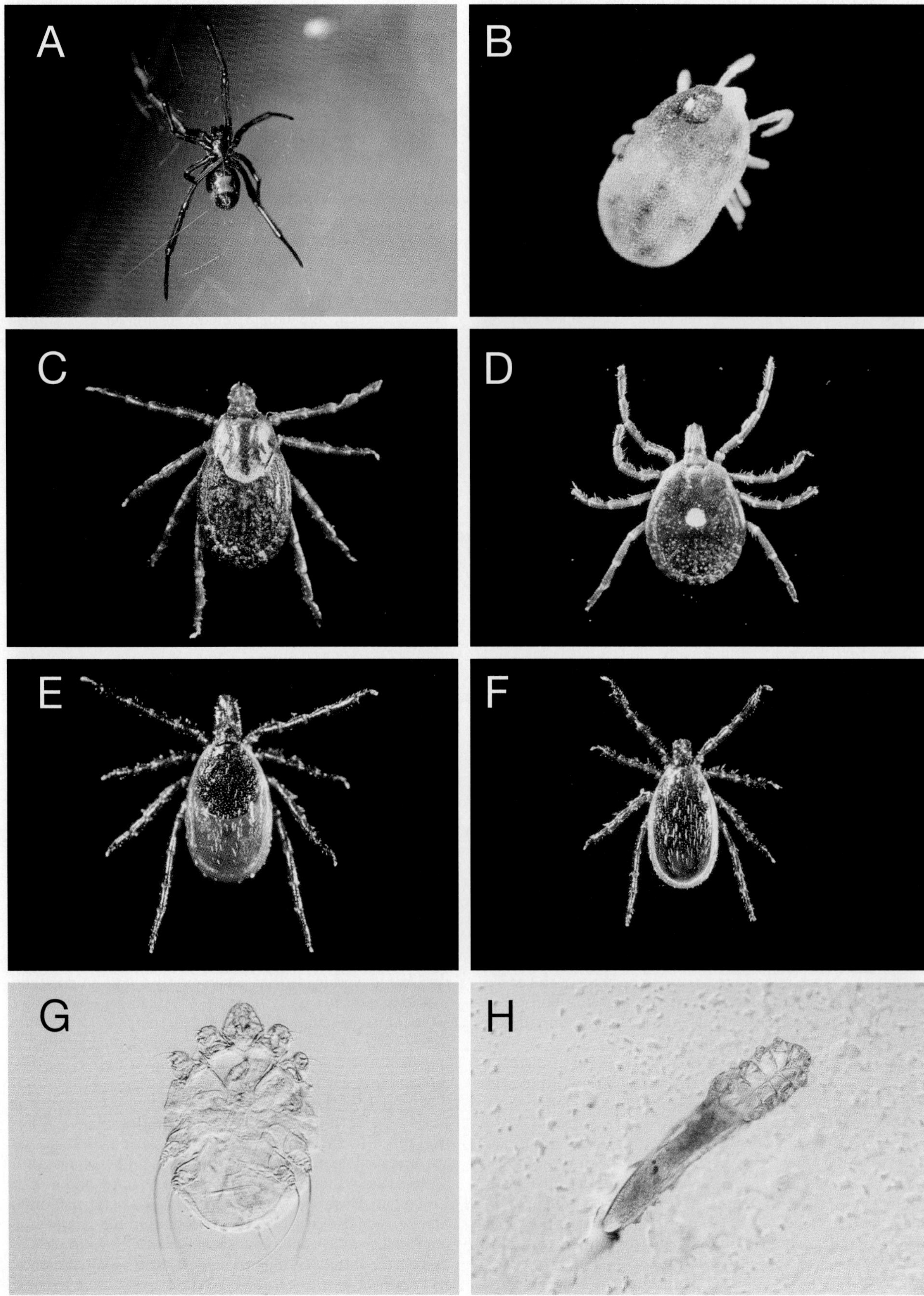
A
B
C
D
E
F
G
H

burrows or in rodent-infested buildings, especially older vacation cabins (3, 19, 35). Species identifications require use of specialized keys (9, 37, 39).

Tick paralysis is another important and potentially lethal disease caused in North America by ticks of the genera *Dermacentor, Amblyomma*, and *Ixodes*. A neurotoxin produced in the tick's salivary glands produces an ascending flaccid paralysis with generalized toxemia within several days after initiation of feeding by a female tick. The disorder may readily be differentiated from other causes of paralytic disease, including poliomyelitis, by the finding of an attached, engorged tick in an area usually hidden from view, such as the scalp. Careful removal of the tick and its mouthparts will generally cause resolution of symptoms within several hours or days (3, 48, 52).

Mites

A mite is a tiny arachnid with a fused cephalothorax and abdomen that has eight legs as a nymph and adult and six legs as a larva. The study of acarology is largely a matter for the specialist, as keys are complex and not always helpful for the relatively few medically important species (3, 19, 33, 35, 37, 39). However, identification of the obligate human mites, including the itch mite *Sarcoptes scabei* and the follicle mite *Demodex folliculorum*, should be within the abilities of most clinical laboratories (39).

Mites are medically important pests for several reasons: they may attack humans directly as either obligate or facultative parasites, certain species may act as reservoirs and vectors for infectious diseases, and many have been implicated in cases of dermatitis and dust allergies. Delusions of mite infestations, one of the forms of delusory parasitosis, are also well-known psychiatric problems that require careful investigation before actual infestations are ruled out (36).

Sarcoptes scabiei, the itch mite and agent of sarcoptic mange, is an obligate human parasite that lives in the upper layers of the epidermis, where it creates serpiginous burrows. Mites live for about 2 months, during which their tunneling activity and deposition of eggs and excreta produce inflammation and intense pruritis. Most mites occur on the hands and arms, especially in the interdigital folds, but they may involve the wrists, breasts, buttocks, and external genitalia, among other areas. Clinical manifestations of sarcoptic mange may vary considerably depending on the development of hypersensitivity. Immunocompromised individuals may be at risk for developing crusted or Norwegian scabies, a generalized dermatitis characterized by the presence of thousands of mites in the epidermis (3, 19, 35).

Diagnosis is made by demonstrating the mite and its eggs in skin scrapings taken preferably from the terminal portion of a burrow. Scrapings may be placed on a microscope slide, cleared with a drop of potassium hydroxide, covered with a coverslip, and examined. Another method recommends using a drop of mineral oil when scrapings are taken and examining this fluid directly. Adult female mites average 330 to 450 μm in length and have oval, saclike bodies in which the first two pairs of legs are separated from the last two pairs. The dorsal body surface has multiple parallel ridges, several tooth-like spines, and hairs of various lengths (Fig. 4). Males are somewhat smaller than females (18, 19, 39).

While humans primarily contract scabies from being in close contact with infested persons (often among families, in institutional settings, or where personal hygiene has been neglected), temporary infestation with animal (especially canine, feline, and porcine) scabies parasites may occur (38, 42). Transmission during sexual contact is also known to occur (27, 52).

The human follicle mites *Demodex folliculorum* and *Demodex brevis* are obligate parasites that inhabit hair follicles and sebaceous glands, respectively. They are minute organisms (100 to 400 μm in length, with *Demodex brevis* being the shorter of the two) well adapted for life in follicles by having a wormlike body, four pairs of stubby legs, and an abdomen with numerous annulations (Fig. 4). Infestations occur primarily on the face, especially on the forehead, eyelids, and nasolabial folds. While the presence of these mites has been associated with various skin conditions, including acne and blepharitis, their high incidence in healthy individuals makes their medical significance difficult to assess (3, 5, 35, 39).

A number of other mite species that are parasitic at one or more stages of their life cycle also attack humans, facultatively causing a variety of dermatologic and allergic conditions. Larval chigger mites of the family Trombiculidae are well known to attack humans and other vertebrates throughout the world; their saliva produces a wheal-and-flare reaction with intense itching. Larvae may appear as tiny red dots attached to the skin, especially in areas where clothing is tight and restricts their movement, such as ankles, groin, waistline, armpits, and wrists. Following feeding, engorged larvae fall to the ground, where they develop into nonparasitic nymphs and adults. *Eutrombicula alfreddugesi* is a common pest in the New World, whereas *Neotrombicula autumnalis* occurs in Europe. Chiggers in the genus *Leptotrombidium* are more problematic in parts of Asia and Australia because they serve as vectors for *Orientia tsutsugamushi*, the agent of scrub typhus (3, 19, 35, 52).

A variety of other biting mites normally parasitic on other animals may occasionally be a nuisance to humans, causing dermatitis. Exposure may be occupational (grain, flour, and cheese mites; chicken mite; northern fowl mite; tropical fowl mite) or accidental (straw itch mite; tropical rat mite; spiny rat mite; house mouse mite; and cheyletiellid mites of birds, rodents, cats, dogs, and other mammals). Humans living in older buildings and houses that are inhabited by rodents or birds may be susceptible to mite infestations following the abandonment of a nest and subsequent searching by its mite inhabitants for new hosts. The house mouse mite (*Liponyssoides sanguineus*), in addition to being pestiferous, is an important vector for the transmission of *Rickettsia akari*, the agent of rickettsialpox (3, 19, 38, 39, 42).

Mites in the family Pyroglyphidae are particularly problematic as allergens responsible for house dust allergy. House

FIGURE 4 Medically important arachnids. Row 1: (A) *Lactrodectus mactans* (black widow spider) adult female; (B) *Ornithodoros hermsi* (soft tick) nonengorged adult; row 2: (C) *Dermacentor variabilis* (dog tick) nonengorged adult female; (D) *Amblyomma americanum* (Lone Star tick) nonengorged adult female; row 3: (E) *Ixodes scapularis* (black legged tick or deer tick, formerly named *I. dammini*) nonengorged adult female; (F) *I. scapularis* adult male; row 4: (G) *Sarcoptes scabiei* (itch mite) adult; (H) *Demodex folliculorum* (follicle mite) adult. Photograph A is reprinted from the *New England Journal of Medicine* **331**:777, 1994, with permission of the publisher. Photographs B to F are from Northwest Infectious Disease Consultants and are reproduced with permission.

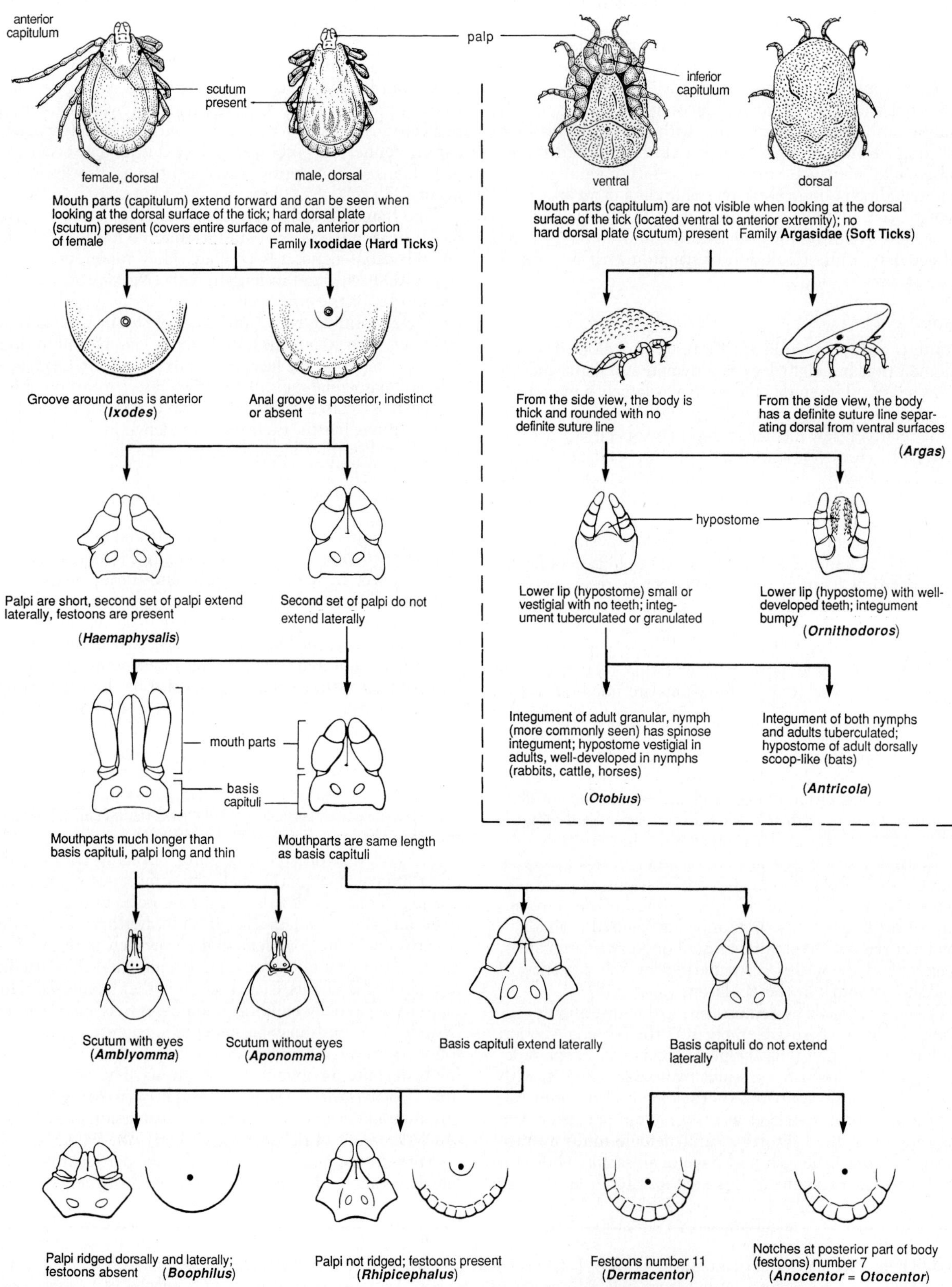

FIGURE 5 Pictoral key to the tick genera found in the United States (reprinted from *Diagnostic Medical Parasitology*, 3rd ed. [18] with permission of the publisher).

dust mites (especially *Dermatophagoides farinae* and *Dermatophagoides pteronyssinus*) may occur in great numbers in dust from bedroom mattresses, blankets, pillows, and carpets, where they feed on sloughed human skin scales, food particles, and other available organic debris. Warm ambient temperatures and high humidity accentuate the problem. The secretions, excreta, and body parts of these mites act as potent allergens responsible for allergic rhinitis and asthma, as well as some skin conditions. Skin testing and immunotherapy are the mainstays of medical management, although removal or control of the offending allergen should be attempted (15, 19, 39, 55).

CLASS PENTASTOMIDA (PENTASTOMES OR TONGUE WORMS)

Classification of the pentostomes or tongue worms remains uncertain because of a lack of morphological characteristics from which to determine their affinities. While the usual arthropodlike features are lacking, pentostome larvae do resemble those of mites. The body of the adult is wormlike with pseudosegmentation and appears to be divided into a head and abdomen. A pair of sclerotized hooks or claws is present on each side of the mouth (3, 35).

These organisms live primarily as adults in the nasal and respiratory passages of reptiles, birds, and mammals, where they attain lengths of 1 to 10 cm. Intermediate hosts include rodents, large herbivores, and freshwater fish. Humans may be infected with either the larval or the nymphal stage, depending upon whether exposure is to the eggs or the larval forms, respectively, of the parasites. Only rarely have adult pentostomes been recovered from humans. Lesions produced by larval pentostomes usually occur in the liver and lungs and are reported to be caused by *Armillifer moniliformis* in parts of Asia and *A. armillatus* in tropical Africa. In parts of the Middle East and Africa, immature (nymphal) stages of *Linguatula serrata* are known to lodge in the human nasopharynx, producing an irritative and obstructive condition known as halzoun or marrara (3, 18, 52).

REFERENCES

1. **Alexander, J. O.** 1994. *Arthropods and Human Skin*. Springer-Verlag, Berlin.
2. **Allen, C.** 1992. Arachnid envenomations. *Emer. Clin. N. Am.* **10:**269–298.
3. **Beaver, P. C., R. C. Jung, and E. W. Cupp.** 1984. *Clinical Parasitology*, 9th ed. Lea & Febiger, Philadelphia, Pa.
4. **Borror, D. J., N. F. Johnson, and C. A. Triplehorn.** 1989. *An Introduction to the Study of Insects*, 6th ed. Saunders College Publishing Co., Philadelphia, Pa.
5. **Burns, D. A.** 1992. Follicle mites and their role in disease. *Clin. Exp. Dermatol.* **17:**152–155.
6. **Centers for Disease Control and Prevention.** 1996. Necrotic arachnidism—Pacific Northwest, 1988–1996. *Morbid. Mortal. Weekly Rep.* **45:**433–436.
7. **Chu, H. F.** 1949. *How to Know the Immature Insects*. Wm. C. Brown Co., Dubuque, Iowa.
8. **Cooley, R. A.** 1938. *The Genera Dermacentor and Otocentor (Ixodidae) in the United States with Studies in Variation*. National Institute of Health bulletin. no. 171. National Institute of Health, Washington, D.C.
9. **Cooley, R. A., and G. M. Kohls.** 1944. The Argasidae of North America, Central America, and Cuba. *Am. Midl. Nat. Monogr.* **1:**1–152.
10. **Cooley, R. A., and G. M. Kohls.** 1945. *The Genus Ixodes in North America*. National Institute of Health bulletin no. 184. National Institute of Health, Washington, D.C.
11. **Currier, R. W., W. A. Johnson, W. A. Rowley, and C. W. Laudenbach.** 1995. Internal ophthalmomyiasis and treatment by laser photocoagulation: a case report. *Am. J. Trop. Med. Hyg.* **52:**311–313.
12. **deShazo, R. D., B. T. Butcher, and W. A. Banks.** 1990. Reactions to the stings of the imported fire ant. *N. Engl. J. Med.* **323:**462–466.
13. **Fisher, R. G.** 1994. Necrotic arachnidism. *West. J. Med.* **160:**570–572.
14. **Fox, I.** 1940. *Fleas of the Eastern United States*. Iowa State College Press, Ames.
15. **Frazier, C. A., and P. A. Brown.** 1980. *Insects and Allergy and What To Do about Them*. University of Oklahoma Press, Norman.
16. **Furman, D. P., and E. P. Catts.** 1970. *Manual of Medical Entomology*, 3rd ed. Mayfield Publishing Co., Palo Alto, Calif.
17. **Furman, D. P., and E. C. Loomis.** 1984. The ticks of California (Acari:Ixodida). *Bull. Calif. Insect Surv.* **25:** 1–79.
18. **Garcia, L. S., and D. A. Bruckner.** 1997. *Diagnostic Medical Parasitology*, 3rd ed. American Society for Microbiology, Washington, D.C.
19. **Goddard, J.** 1996. *Physician's Guide to Arthropods of Medical Importance*, 2nd ed. CRC Press, Inc., Boca Raton, Fla.
20. **Goddard, J. G.** 1994. Direct injury from arthropods. *Lab. Med.* **25:**365–371.
21. **Harwood, R. F., and M. T. James.** 1979. *Entomology in Human and Animal Health*, 7th ed. Macmillan, New York.
22. **Holland, G. P.** 1985. The fleas of Canada, Alaska, and Greenland (Siphonaptera). *Mem. Entomol. Soc. Can.* **130:** 1–630.
23. **Hubbard, C. A.** 1947. *Fleas of Western North America. Their Relation to Public Health*. Iowa State College Press, Ames.
24. **Hudson, B. J., and G. A. Parsons.** 1997. Giant millipede 'burns' and the eye. *Trans. R. Soc. Trop. Med. Hyg.* **91:** 183–185.
25. **James, M. T.** 1947. *The Flies That Cause Myiasis in Man*. U.S.D.A. miscellaneous publication no. 631. U.S. Department of Agriculture, Washington, D.C.
26. **Juranek, D. D.** 1985. *Pediculus capitis* in school children: epidemiologic trends, risk factors, and recommendations for control, p. 199–211. *In* M. Orkin and H. I. Maibach (ed.), *Cutaneous Infestations and Insect Bites*. Marcel Dekker, Inc., New York.
27. **Juranek, D. D., R. W. Currier, and L. E. Millikan.** 1985. Scabies control in institutions, p. 139–158. *In* M. Orkin and H. I. Maibach (ed.), *Cutaneous Infestations and Insect Bites*. Marcel Dekker, Inc., New York.
28. **Kaston, B. J.** 1978. *How To Know the Spiders*, 3rd ed. William C. Brown Co., Dubuque, Iowa.
29. **Keirans, J. E., and C. M. Clifford.** 1978. The genus *Ixodes* in the United States: a scanning electron microscope study and key to the adults. *J. Med. Entomol. Suppl.* **2:**1–149.
30. **Keirans, J. E., and T. R. Litwak.** 1989. Pictoral key of the adults of hard ticks, family Ixodidae (Ixodida: Ixodoidea) east of the Mississippi river. *J. Med. Entomol.* **26:** 435–448.
31. **Kettle, D. S.** 1982. *Medical and Veterinary Entomology*. John Wiley & Sons, Inc., New York, N.Y.
32. **Kim, K. C., H. D. Pratt, and C. J. Stojanovich.** 1986. *The Sucking Lice of North America*. Pennsylvania State University Press, University Park.
33. **Krantz, G. W.** 1978. *A Manual of Acarology*, 2nd ed. Oregon State University, Corvallis.
34. **Krause, P. J., S. R. Telford, A. Speilman, V. Sikand, R. Ryan, D. Christianson, G. Burke, P. Brassard, R. Pollack, J. Peck, and D. H. Persing.** 1996. Concurrent Lyme

disease and babesiosis: evidence for increased severity and duration of illness. *J. Am. Med. Assoc.* **275**:1657–1660.

35. **Lane, R. P., and R. W. Crosskey.** 1993. *Medical Insects and Arthropods*. Chapman & Hall, London.
36. **Lynch, P. J.** 1993. Delusions of parasitosis. *Semin. Dermatol.* **12**:39–45.
37. **McDaniel, B.** 1979. *How To Know the Mites and Ticks*. William C. Brown Co., Dubuque, Iowa.
38. **Millikan, L. E.** 1993. Mite infestations other than scabies. *Semin. Dermatol.* **12**:48–52.
39. **National Communicable Disease Center.** 1969. *Pictorial Keys: Arthropods, Reptiles, Birds, and Mammals of Public Health Significance*. Communicable Disease Center, Atlanta.
40. **Oliver, J. H., Jr., M. R. Owlsly, H. J. Hutcheson, A. M. James, C. Chen, W. S. Irby, E. M. Dotson, and D. K. McLain.** 1993. Conspecificity of the ticks *Ixodes scapularis* and *I. dammini* (Acari: Ixodidae). *J. Med. Entomol.* **30**: 54–63.
41. **Orkin, M., and H. I. Maibach.** 1985. *Cutaneous Infestations and Insect Bites*. Marcel Dekker, Inc., New York, N.Y.
42. **Parish, L. C., and R. M. Schwartzman.** 1993. Zoonoses of dermatological interest. *Semin. Dermatol.* **12**:57–64.
43. **Reisman, D. E.** 1993. Duration of venom immunotherapy: relationship to the severity of symptoms of initial insect sting anaphylaxis. *J. Allergy Clin. Immunol.* **92**:831–836.
44. **Reisman, R. E.** 1994. Insect stings. *N. Engl. J. Med.* **331**: 523–527.
45. **Shama, S. K., P. H. Etkind, T. M. Odell, A. T. Canada, A. M. Finn, and N. A. Soter.** 1982. Gypsy-moth-caterpillar dermatitis. *N. Engl. J. Med.* **306**:1300–1301.
46. **Sonenshine, D. E.** 1991. *Biology of Ticks*, vol. 1. Oxford University Press, New York, N.Y.
47. **Sonenshine, D. E.** 1993. *Biology of Ticks*, vol. 2. Oxford University Press, New York, N.Y.
48. **Spach, D. H., W. C. Liles, G. L. Campbell, R. E. Quick, D. E. Anderson, and T. R. Fritsche.** 1993. Tick-borne diseases in the United States. *N. Engl. J. Med.* **329**: 936–947.
49. **Spielman, A., C. M. Clifford, J. Piesman, and M. D. Corwin.** 1979. Human babesiosis on Nantucket Island, USA: description of the vector, *Ixodes (Ixodes) dammini*, n. sp. (Acarina: Ixodidae). *J. Med. Entomol.* **15**:218–234.
50. **Steere, A. C.** 1989. Lyme disease. *N. Engl. J. Med.* **321**: 585–596.
51. **Steyskal, G. C., W. L. Murphy, and E. M. Hoover.** 1987. *Insects and Mites: Techniques for Collection and Preservation*. USDA miscellaneous publication no. 1443. U.S. Department of Agriculture, Washington, D.C.
52. **Strickland, G. T. (ed).** 1991. *Hunter's Tropical Medicine*, 7th ed. The W. B. Saunders Co., Philadelphia, Pa.
53. **Telford, S. R., J. E. Dawson, P. Katavolos, C. K. Warner, C. P. Colbert, and D. H. Persing.** 1996. Perpetuation of the agent of human granulocytic ehrlichiosis in a deer tick-rodent cycle. *Proc. Natl. Acad. Sci. USA* **93**:6209–6214.
54. **Walker, D. H., and J. S. Dumler.** 1996. Emergence of the ehrlichioses as human health problems. *Emer. Infect. Dis.* **2**:18–29.
55. **Woolley, T. A.** 1988. *Acarology: Mites and Human Welfare*. John Wiley & Sons, Inc., New York, N.Y.

ANTIMICROBIAL AGENTS AND SUSCEPTIBILITY TESTING

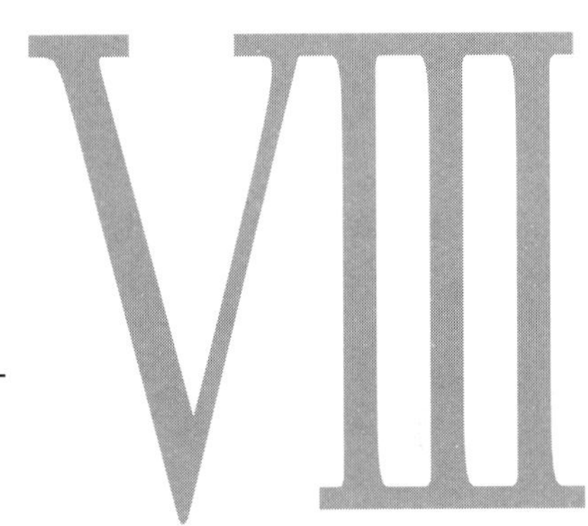

VOLUME EDITOR
FRED C. TENOVER

SECTION EDITORS
JAMES H. JORGENSEN AND
JOHN D. TURNIDGE

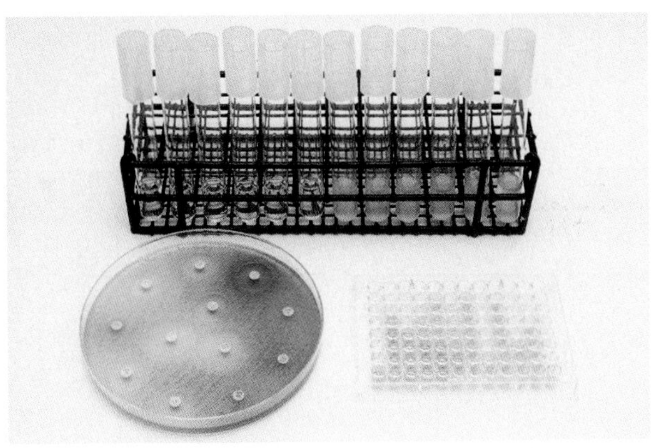

Pseudomonas aeruginosa susceptibility tests performed by disk diffusion, microbroth dilution, and macrobroth dilution.

(continued)

Antimicrobial Susceptibility Testing: General Considerations*

JOHN D. TURNIDGE AND JAMES H. JORGENSEN

115

Determination of the antimicrobial susceptibilities of significant bacterial isolates is one of the principal functions of the clinical microbiology laboratory. From the physician's pragmatic point of view, the results of susceptibility tests are often considered as important or more important than the identification of the pathogen involved. This is particularly true in an era of increasing antimicrobial resistance in which treatment options are at times limited to newer and more costly antibacterial agents. As a result, the laboratory must give high priority not only to producing technically accurate data but also to reporting those data to physicians in an easily interpretable manner. This section of the Manual focuses on susceptibility testing methods for aerobic and anaerobic bacteria, mycobacteria, and certain fungi and provides updates on the progress toward the development of standardized susceptibility testing methods for viruses and protozoa. Chapters include descriptions of broth and agar dilution tests and agar-based diffusion methods, in addition to automated and molecular biologic approaches. Additional material on anti-infective agents and mechanisms of antimicrobial resistance is also presented.

The main objective of susceptibility testing is to predict the outcome of treatment with the antimicrobial agents tested. The implication of the result "susceptible" is that there is a high probability that the patient will respond to treatment with that antimicrobial agent. The result "resistant" implies that treatment with the antimicrobial agent is likely to fail. Most test methods also include an "intermediate" category of susceptibility, which can have several meanings. With agents that can be safely administered at higher doses, this category can imply that higher doses may be required to ensure efficacy or that the agent may prove efficacious if it is normally concentrated in an infected body fluid, e.g., urine. It may also represent a "buffer" zone which prevents strains with borderline susceptibility from being incorrectly categorized as resistant.

A further aim of susceptibility testing is to guide the clinician in the selection of the most appropriate agent for a particular clinical problem. In most clinical settings, susceptibility test results are usually obtained 24 to 48 h or more after the patient has been given empirical treatment. The test results may confirm the susceptibility of the organism to the drug initially prescribed or may indicate resistance, in which case alternate therapy will be required. The report describing the results of susceptibility tests should provide the clinician with alternative agents to which the organism is susceptible. These alternatives also may be useful if the patient subsequently develops an adverse reaction to the initial antimicrobial agent. There is a growing emphasis from professional societies and managed care organizations to use susceptibility test results to direct therapy toward the most-narrow-spectrum, least-expensive agent to which the pathogen should respond. This is particularly true for hospitalized patients, in whom the rate of antimicrobial resistance tends to be high, and it is easier to make therapeutic changes for inpatients than for outpatients. This makes the accuracy of susceptibility testing even more critical for effective patient care.

The clinical microbiology laboratory should perform susceptibility testing only with pathogens for which well-standardized methods are available and pathogens whose resistance is known or suspected to be a clinical problem. It is also important to emphasize that susceptibility testing should not be performed with normal flora or colonizing organisms. Currently, routine susceptibility testing methods are best standardized for the common aerobic and facultative bacteria and systemic antibacterial agents. For some uncommon or fastidious bacteria and for topical antibacterial agents, simple routine test methods have not been standardized or are not recommended because they are likely to yield inaccurate results. However, testing of such organisms may be performed in reference laboratories by reference MIC methods under special circumstances. With some pathogens (e.g., *Mycobacterium tuberculosis* and invasive yeasts) routine testing is important for patient management, but testing is best performed by specialized laboratories in which test volumes are sufficient to maintain technical proficiency and where unusual test results are likely to be recognized. Susceptibility methods for certain other pathogens (e.g., mycoplasma, chlamydia, campylobacter, helicobacter, legionella, spirochetes, viruses, protozoa, and helminths) may not be well standardized at present and are limited to a few specialty laboratories. A number of choices exist in antibacterial susceptibility testing with respect to methodology and the selection of agents for routine testing. Fewer choices exist in antifungal, antiviral, and antiprotozoal susceptibility test-

* This chapter contains information presented in chapter 110 by James H. Jorgensen and Daniel F. Sahm in the sixth edition of this Manual.

ing. However, the following chapters present several approaches for consideration.

SELECTING AN ANTIMICROBIAL SUSCEPTIBILITY TESTING METHOD

Clinical microbiology laboratories can choose from among several conventional or novel methods for performance of routine antibacterial susceptibility testing. These include the broth microdilution, disk diffusion, antibiotic gradient, and automated instrument methods. In recent years there has been a trend toward the use of commercial broth microdilution and automated instrument methods instead of the disk diffusion procedure. However, there may be renewed interest in the disk diffusion test because of its inherent flexibility in drug selection and low cost. The availability of numerous antibacterial agents and the diversity in antibiotic formularies in different institutions have made it difficult for manufacturers of commercial test systems to provide standard test panels that fit every facility's needs. Thus, the inherent flexibility of drug selection provided by the disk diffusion test is an undeniable asset of the method. It is also one of the most established and best proven of all susceptibility tests and continues to be updated and refined through frequent National Committee for Clinical Laboratory Standards (NCCLS) publications (17). Furthermore, the qualitative interpretive category results of susceptible, intermediate, and resistant provided by the disk test are readily understood by clinicians.

Advantages of the microdilution or agar gradient diffusion methods include the generation of a quantitative result (i.e., an MIC) rather than a category result, the ability to test accurately some anaerobic or fastidious species which may not be tested by the disk diffusion method (3, 11, 15), and the ancillary benefits of the computer systems which accompany many of the microdilution or automated systems (9). Indeed, the computerized data management systems are very important to laboratories that may have limited or inflexible laboratory information systems. However, an MIC method should not be chosen on the basis of the assumption that MICs are routinely more useful to physicians. There is no clear evidence that MICs are more relevant than susceptibility category results to the selection of appropriate antibacterial therapy (6).

A laboratory may choose to perform rapid, automated antibacterial susceptibility testing in order to generate results faster than can be generated by manual methods. The provision of susceptibility results 1 day sooner than they can be provided by conventional methods seems a logical advance in patient care. One recent study has demonstrated both the clinical and the economic benefits derived from the use of rapid susceptibility testing and reporting (7). However, rapid susceptibility testing results may not have a substantial impact unless more aggressive means of communication are used by the laboratory to make physicians aware of the results (24). This may be because physicians have come to expect antimicrobial susceptibility testing results approximately 48 h after the submission of a specimen or because the results, although generated more rapidly, are still not available soon enough to assist with the initial selection of antimicrobial therapy.

A previously cited shortcoming of rapid susceptibility testing methods was the failure to detect some inducible or subtle resistance mechanisms (1, 12, 20, 22, 23). However, the instruments most notorious for such problems are no longer marketed, and the manufacturers of the remaining instruments have made substantial efforts to correct earlier problems (14, 26). It is important to emphasize that accuracy should not be sacrificed in an effort to generate a rapid susceptibility testing result.

SELECTION OF ANTIBACTERIAL AGENTS FOR ROUTINE TESTING

The laboratory has the responsibility to test and report on the antimicrobial agents that are most appropriate for the organism isolated, the site of infection, and the clinical practice setting in which the laboratory functions. The battery of antimicrobial agents routinely tested and reported on by the laboratory will depend on the characteristics of the patients under care in the institution and the likelihood of encountering highly resistant organisms (10). A laboratory serving a tertiary-care medical center which specializes in the care of immunosuppressed patients may need to test routinely agents that are broader in spectrum than those tested by a laboratory that supports a primary-care outpatient practice in which antibiotic-resistant organisms are less commonly encountered.

When determining a laboratory's routine susceptibility testing batteries, several principles should be followed. First, the antimicrobial agents that are included in the institution's formulary and that physicians prescribe on a daily basis should be tested. Second, the species to be tested should be considered; this also strongly influences the choice of antimicrobial agents for testing. NCCLS publishes tables that list the antimicrobial agents appropriate for use in the testing of various groups of aerobic and fastidious bacteria (16, 17). The guidelines indicate the drugs that are most appropriate for the testing of each organism group and for the treatment of some infections at specific anatomic sites (e.g., cerebrospinal fluid, blood, urine, or feces). The lists also include a few agents that may be tested as surrogates for other agents because of the greater ability of a particular agent to detect resistance to closely related drugs (e.g., the use of oxacillin to predict overall β-lactam resistance in staphylococci). This initial list of agents must be tailored to an individual institution's specific needs through discussions with infectious disease physicians, pharmacists, and committees concerned with infection control and the institutional formulary (10).

A third important step in defining routine testing batteries is ascertaining the availability of specific antimicrobial agents for testing by the laboratory's routine testing methodology. Certain methods (e.g., the disk diffusion, gradient diffusion, or in-house-prepared broth or agar dilution method) allow the greatest flexibility when selecting test batteries. In contrast, some commercial systems may have less flexibility in matching test batteries to an institution's formulary or in promptly including the latest antimicrobial agents approved for clinical use. However, practicality limits the maximum number of drugs that can be tested simultaneously with an isolate by any susceptibility method. For example, a maximum of 12 disks can be placed on a 150-mm Mueller-Hinton agar plate, and a similar number can ordinarily be accommodated in a microdilution tray if full concentration ranges of each agent are to be included for routine determination of MICs. Some commercial test panels attempt to resolve this problem by testing a larger array of antimicrobial agents, although in a very limited concentration range (perhaps two or three dilutions of each agent).

ESTABLISHING SUSCEPTIBILITY BREAKPOINTS

There is general agreement that the MIC is the most basic laboratory measurement of the activity of an antimicrobial agent against an organism. It is defined as the lowest concentration that will inhibit the growth of a test organism over a defined interval related to the organism's growth rate, most commonly 18 to 24 h. The MIC is the fundamental measurement that forms the basis for most susceptibility testing methods and against which the levels of drug achievable in human body fluids may be compared to determine breakpoints for defining susceptibility.

The conventional technique for measuring the MIC involves exposing the test organism to a series of twofold dilutions of the antimicrobial agent in a suitable culture system, e.g., broth or agar for bacteria. The twofold dilution scheme was originally used because of the convenience of preparing dilutions from a single starting concentration in tube broth or agar macrodilution methods. Subsequently, this system proved to be meaningful because the MICs for a single bacterial species in the absence of resistance mechanisms have a statistically normal distribution when plotted on a logarithmic scale. This provides investigators with the opportunity to examine the distributions of MICs for bacterial populations and distinguish abnormal (potentially resistant) from normal (susceptible) strains.

MIC measurements are influenced in vitro by a number of factors including the composition of the medium, the size of the inoculum, the duration of incubation, and the presence of resistant subpopulations of the organism. The in vitro test conditions also do not encompass other factors that can have an influence on antimicrobial activity in vivo such as sub-MIC effects, postantibiotic effects, protein binding, effects on organism virulence, variations in redox potential at sites of infection, and the pharmacokinetic changes resulting from different drug levels in blood and the site of infection over time. Nevertheless, if determined under standardized conditions, MIC measurements provide a fixed reference point for the setting of pharmacodynamic breakpoints with the power to predict efficacy in vivo. Pharmacological breakpoints can be applied directly to routine dilution testing methods that generate MICs, such as the broth microdilution, agar dilution, or gradient methods, and some automated instruments. They also provide reference values for deriving breakpoints for disk diffusion methods.

Breakpoints are the values that determine the categories of susceptible, intermediate, and resistant. The techniques for setting breakpoints vary with the testing method and, with a few exceptions, are based on the MICs. Depending on the method, up to four sources of data can be examined in establishing breakpoints.

(i) MIC distributions. Examination of MIC distributions can indicate the presence of strains falling outside of a normal population of strains that lack any known mechanisms of resistance to the particular drug. These distributions may aid in the recognition of new resistance mechanisms by highlighting strains that fall outside of the normal distribution, but they have limited direct clinical application since the distributions of MICs vary between species, and for some strains for which the MICs are outside the distribution for the normal population, the MICs may be below the clinically derived breakpoints, even though they are known to not respond to treatment. An example of the latter point is the fact that the penicillin MICs for some β-lactamase-producing organisms may be relatively low. Indeed, knowledge of the presence of specific resistance mechanisms that affect compounds of a particular class is very useful in deriving microbiological breakpoints.

(ii) Pharmacokinetics and pharmacodynamics. Pharmacokinetics examines the distribution, accumulation, and elimination of a drug in the body over time. These parameters are usually determined with healthy volunteers. The MICs can be compared with the concentration of drug achievable in the blood or other body fluids (e.g., cerebrospinal fluid). In the past, breakpoints were chosen such that the MICs for susceptible pathogens would be exceeded for most or all of the dosing interval. Newer data now considered when establishing breakpoints include pharmacodynamic data. Pharmacodynamics is the study of the time course of drug action on the microorganism. For antimicrobial agents, the desired action is pathogen eradication. Pharmacodynamic studies have revealed that agents fall into two basic classes: those with time-dependent antimicrobial action and those with concentration-dependent antimicrobial action. For drugs with time-dependent action, the critical determinant of bacterial killing is the percentage of time that the drug concentration is above the MIC (%*T*>MIC), while for drugs with concentration-dependent action, the determinant is the area under the concentration-time curve divided by the MIC (AUC/MIC ratio) (8, 25). For β-lactams and macrolides, the relevant measure is %*T*>MIC, while the AUC/MIC ratio is the relevant parameter for aminoglycosides and fluoroquinolones (8). These values can be used to calculate the maximum MICs or breakpoints that would allow the achievement of optimum efficacy with standard drug dosing schedules.

(iii) Clinical and bacteriological response rates. During clinical trials the response rates of organisms for which the MICs of new antimicrobial agents vary give an indication of the relevance of breakpoints selected by using MIC distributions and the pharmacokinetic and pharmacodynamic properties of the drug. Response rates of at least 80% may be expected for organisms classified as susceptible, although it can be lower depending on the site and type of infection. While in some countries breakpoints are determined primarily from clinical and bacteriological response rates, NCCLS evaluates clinical and bacteriological response rates in conjunction with population distributions, pharmacokinetics, and pharmacodynamics in establishing the breakpoints that should provide the best correlation between in vitro test results and clinical outcome (18).

(iv) Zone diameter distributions for disk diffusion methods. Once MIC breakpoints are selected, disk diffusion breakpoints can be chosen by plotting the zone diameters against the MICs derived from the testing of a large number of strains of various species. A statistical approach that uses the linear regression formula may be used to calculate the appropriate zone diameter intercepts for the predetermined MIC breakpoints. An alternative, pragmatic approach to deriving disk diffusion breakpoints is the use of the error rate-bounded technique, in which the zone diameter criteria are selected on the basis of the minimization of the disk interpretive errors, especially the very major errors (2, 13) (Fig. 1).

Breakpoints derived by professional groups or regulatory bodies in various countries are often quite similar. However, there can be notable differences in the breakpoints used in different countries for the same agents. The reasons for the differences can be that certain countries use different dosages or administration intervals for some drugs or the fact that some countries are more conservative in assessing the

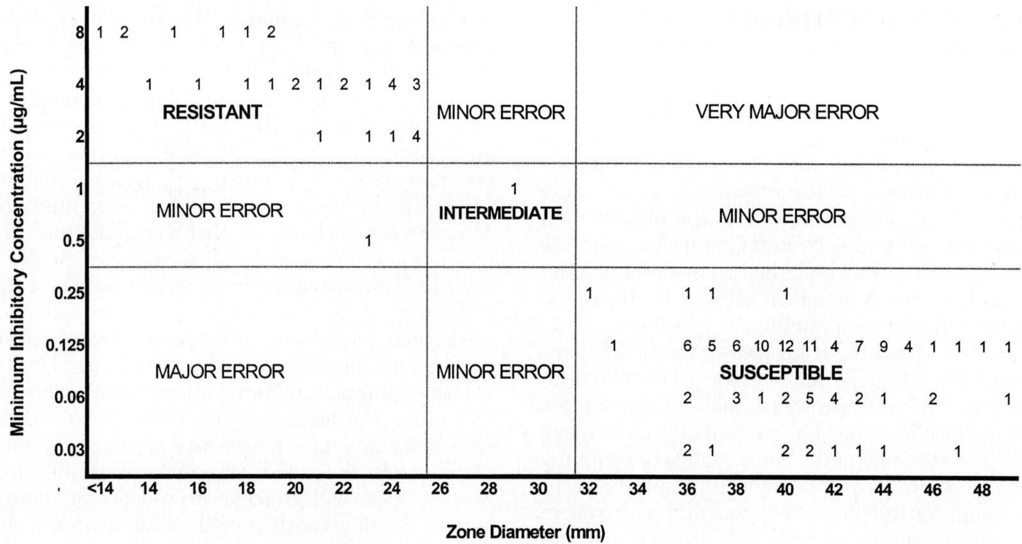

FIGURE 1 Comparison of zone diameters with MICs for a hypothetical antimicrobial agent.

susceptibility to antimicrobial agents and place greater emphasis on the detection of emerging resistance, noted primarily by examination of microorganism population distributions. Technical factors such as the inoculum density and test medium can also affect MICs and zone diameters, thereby justifying different interpretive criteria in some countries. These technical differences are summarized in some detail in chapter 118 of the Manual.

FUTURE DIRECTIONS AND NEEDS IN ANTIMICROBIAL SUSCEPTIBILITY TESTING

Antimicrobial resistance is becoming widespread among a variety of clinically significant bacterial species (4, 19). Therefore, the microbiology laboratory plays a key role in the patient management process by providing accurate data on which physicians can base chemotherapy. Susceptibility testing results, however, are also used in surveillance studies and by infection control practitioners to detect and control the spread of antimicrobial agent-resistant organisms (21).

To meet these challenges and responsibilities, clinical microbiologists must continuously assess and update their susceptibility testing strategies. The first priority is to use accurate and reliable testing methods, whether they are conventional or novel molecular methods. Then, careful monitoring of test performance with well-characterized control strains that challenge the capability of the testing methods becomes key. Today, laboratories must use a variety of testing methods, each tailored specifically to a particular species or group of organisms. It is not likely that a single method, whether conventional or commercial, will be optimal for all antimicrobial agents, organisms, and resistance mechanisms. This will require increased education and training for clinical microbiologists in the future. Some assistance may be sought from the use of computer-based "expert" systems that allow a rapid and accurate review of antimicrobial susceptibility profiles and recognition of potential aberrant results or novel resistance mechanisms (5).

More effective means of conveying critical antimicrobial susceptibility testing information to clinicians in a time frame that allows the efficient and effective management of patients and in a format that is unambiguous to clinicians in various practice specialties are still needed. Clinical microbiologists will need to become more proactive in the reporting of antimicrobial susceptibility results and in cross-linking that information to other databases (e.g., pharmacy prescriptions) to ensure that patients receive the most efficacious and cost-effective therapy.

REFERENCES

1. **Boyce, J. M., R. L. White, M. C. Bonner, and W. R. Lockwood.** 1982. Reliability of the MS-2 system in detecting methicillin-resistant *Staphylococcus aureus*. *J. Clin. Microbiol.* **15:**220–225.
2. **Brunden, M. N., G. E. Zurenko, and B. Kapik.** 1992. Modification of the error-bounded classification scheme for use with two MIC breakpoints. *Diagn. Microbiol. Infect. Dis.* **15:**135–140.
3. **Citron, D. M., M. I. Ostoravi, A. Karlsson, and E. J. C. Goldstein.** 1991. Evaluation of the E test for susceptibility testing of anaerobic bacteria. *J. Clin. Microbiol.* **29:**2197–2203.
4. **Cohen, M. L.** 1992. Epidemiology of drug resistance: implications for a postantimicrobial era. *Science* **257:**1050–1055.
5. **Courvalin, P.** 1992. Interpretive reading of antimicrobial susceptibility tests. *ASM News* **58:**368–375.
6. **Craig, W. A.** 1993. Qualitative susceptibility tests versus quantitative MIC tests. *Diagn. Microbiol. Infect. Dis.* **16:**231–236.
7. **Doern, G. V., R. Vautour, M. Gaudet, and B. Levy.** 1994. Clinical impact of rapid in vitro antimicrobial susceptibility testing and bacterial identification. *J. Clin. Microbiol.* **32:**1757–1762.
8. **Ebert, S. C., and W. A. Craig.** 1990. Pharmacodynamic properties of antibiotics: application to drug monitoring and dosage regimen design. *Diagn. Microbiol. Infect. Dis.* **12:**101–105.
9. **Jorgensen, J. H.** 1993. Selection criteria for an antimicrobial susceptibility testing system. *J. Clin. Microbiol.* **31:**2841–2844.
10. **Jorgensen, J. H.** 1993. Selection of antimicrobial agents for routine testing in a clinical microbiology laboratory. *Diagn. Microbiol. Infect. Dis.* **16:**245–249.

11. **Jorgensen, J. H., M. J. Ferraro, M. L. McElmeel, J. Spargo, J. M. Swenson, and F. C. Tenover.** 1994. Detection of penicillin and extended-spectrum cephalosporin resistance among *Streptococcus pneumoniae* clinical isolates by use of the E test. *J. Clin. Microbiol.* **32:**159–163.
12. **Katsanis, G. P., J. Spargo, M. J. Ferraro, L. Sutton, and G. A. Jacoby.** 1994. Detection of *Klebsiella pneumoniae* and *Escherichia coli* strains producing extended-spectrum β-lactamases. *J. Clin. Microbiol.* **32:**691–696.
13. **Metzler, D. M., and R. M. DeHaan.** 1974. Susceptibility tests of anaerobic bacteria: statistical and clinical considerations. *J. Infect. Dis.* **130:**588–594.
14. **Nadler H. L., C. Dolan, L. Mele, and S. R. Kurtz.** 1985. Accuracy and reproducibility of the AutoMicrobic System Gram-Negative General Susceptibility-Plus card for testing selected challenge organisms. *J. Clin. Microbiol.* **22:** 355–360.
15. **National Committee for Clinical Laboratory Standards.** 1993. *Methods for Antimicrobial Susceptibility Testing of Anaerobic Bacteria.* Approved standard M11-A3. National Committee for Clinical Laboratory Standards, Wayne, Pa.
16. **National Committee for Clinical Laboratory Standards.** 1997. *Methods for Dilution Antimicrobial Susceptibility Testing for Bacteria That Grow Aerobically.* Approved standard M7-A4. National Committee for Clinical Laboratory Standards, Wayne, Pa.
17. **National Committee for Clinical Laboratory Standards.** 1997. *Performance Standards for Antimicrobial Disk Susceptibility Tests.* Approved standard M2-A6. National Committee for Clinical Laboratory Standards, Wayne, Pa.
18. **National Committee for Clinical Laboratory Standards.** 1998. *Development of In Vitro Susceptibility Testing Criteria and Quality Control Parameters.* Tentative guideline M23-T3. National Committee for Clinical Laboratory Standards, Wayne, Pa.
19. **Neu, H. C.** 1992. The crisis in antibiotic resistance. *Science* **257:**1064–1073.
20. **Sahm, D., and L. Olsen.** 1990. In vitro detection of enterococcal vancomycin resistance. *Antimicrob. Agents Chemother.* **34:**1846–1848.
21. **Sahm, D. F., and F. C. Tenover.** 1997. Surveillance for the emergence and dissemination of antimicrobial resistance in bacteria, p. 767–785. *In* F. C. Tenover and J. E. McGowan (ed.), *Antimicrobial Resistance, Infectious Disease Clinics of North America*, vol. 11, no. 4. The W. B. Saunders Co., Philadelphia, Pa.
22. **Stone, L. L., and D. L. Jungkind.** 1983. False-susceptible results from the MS-2 system used for testing resistant *Pseudomonas aeruginosa* against two third-generation cephalosporins, moxalactam and cefotaxime. *J. Clin. Microbiol.* **18:** 389–394.
23. **Tenover, F. C., J. Tokars, J. Swenson, S. Paul, K. Splitalny, and W. Jarvis.** 1993. Ability of clinical laboratories to detect antimicrobial-resistant enterococci. *J. Clin. Microbiol.* **31:**1695–1699.
24. **Trenholme, G. M., R. L. Kaplan, P. H. Karahusis, T. Stine, J. Fuhrer, W. Landau, and S. Levin.** 1989. Clinical impact of rapid identification and susceptibility testing of bacterial blood culture isolates. *J. Clin. Microbiol.* **27:** 1342–1345.
25. **Turnidge, J. D.** The pharmacodynamics of β-lactams. *Clin. Infect. Dis.*, in press.
26. **Washington, J. A., C. C. Knapp, and C. C. Sanders.** 1988. Accuracy of microdilution and the AutoMicrobic System in detection of β-lactam resistance in gram-negative bacterial mutants with derepressed β-lactamase. *Rev. Infect. Dis.* **10:**824–829.

Antibacterial Agents

JOSEPH D. C. YAO AND ROBERT C. MOELLERING, JR.

116

Antimicrobial chemotherapy has played a vital role in the treatment of human infectious diseases in the 20th century. Since the discovery of penicillin in the 1920s, literally hundreds of antimicrobial agents have been developed or synthesized, and dozens of these are currently available for clinical use. While the broad number and variety of agents available provide a great deal of flexibility for the clinician in the use of these agents, the sheer numbers and continuing development of agents available make it difficult for clinicians to keep up with progress in the field. Similarly, this variety presents significant challenges for the clinical microbiologist, who must decide which agents are appropriate for inclusion in routine and specialized susceptibility testing.

This chapter provides an overview of the antibacterial agents currently marketed in the United States, with major emphasis on their mechanisms of action, spectra of activity, important pharmacologic parameters, and toxicities. Antibiotics that have fallen into disuse or remain investigational will be mentioned only briefly.

PENICILLINS

The penicillins (Table 1) are a group of natural and semisynthetic antibiotics containing the chemical nucleus 6-aminopenicillanic acid, which consists of a β-lactam ring fused to a thiazolidine ring (Fig. 1a). The naturally occurring compounds are produced by a number of *Penicillium* spp. The penicillins differ in substitution at position 6, where changes in the side chain may modify the pharmacokinetic and antibacterial properties of the drug.

Mechanism of Action

The major antibacterial action of penicillins is derived from their ability to inhibit a number of bacterial enzymes, namely, penicillin-binding proteins (PBPs), that are essential for peptidoglycan synthesis (242). This ability to inhibit bacterial cell wall enzymes such as the transpeptidases usually confers on the penicillins bactericidal activity against gram-positive bacteria. The bactericidal activity of the penicillins is often related to their ability to trigger membrane-associated autolytic enzymes that destroy the cell wall. Other minor mechanisms of action include inhibition of bacterial endopeptidase and glycosidase, enzymes involved in bacterial cell growth. There is also recent evidence suggesting that penicillins may inhibit RNA synthesis in some bacteria, causing death without cell lysis, but the significance of these observations remains to be proven (138).

Pharmacology

Oral absorption differs markedly among the penicillins. As a natural congener of penicillin G, penicillin V resists gastric acid inactivation and is better absorbed from the gastrointestinal tract than is penicillin G. Amoxicillin is a semisynthetic analog of ampicillin and has greater gastrointestinal absorption than ampicillin (95 versus 40% absorption). Bacampicillin is an ampicillin ester that is considerably better absorbed from the gastrointestinal tract than is ampicillin or amoxicillin. This ester is inactive until naturally occurring esterases in the intestinal mucosa and serum hydrolyze it to release the parent compound, ampicillin, into the serum. The isoxazolyl penicillins, such as oxacillin, cloxacillin, dicloxacillin, and nafcillin, are acid stable and are also absorbed from the gastrointestinal tract (93), unlike certain other anti-staphylococcal penicillins, such as methicillin, which are not acid resistant and cannot be given via the oral route.

Repository forms of penicillin G, available in procaine or benzathine, delay absorption from an intramuscular depot. Procaine penicillin G provides detectable levels for 12 to 24 h, suitable for treatment of uncomplicated pneumococcal pneumonia and gonorrhea due to fully susceptible organisms. Benzathine penicillin G achieves very low levels in blood for prolonged periods (3 to 4 weeks) and is useful for the therapy of syphilis and for prophylaxis of streptococcal pharyngitis and rheumatic fever.

Penicillins are well distributed to many body compartments, including the lungs, liver, kidneys, muscle, bone, and placenta. Penetration into the eyes, brain, cerebrospinal fluid (CSF), and prostate is poor in the absence of inflammation. These drugs are metabolized to a small degree and are rapidly excreted, essentially unchanged, via the kidney. With average half-lives of 0.5 to 1.5 h, they are usually administered every 4 to 6 h to maintain effective levels in blood. The renal tubular excretion of penicillins can be blocked by probenecid, thus prolonging their half-lives in serum.

Dosage reduction of most penicillins is necessary only in the presence of severe renal insufficiency (creatinine clearance, $\leq$10 ml/min). The dosages of all penicillins except nafcillin and the isoxazolyl penicillins are adjusted for he-

TABLE 1 Penicillins

Natural
- Benzylpenicillin (penicillin G)
- Phenoxymethyl penicillin (penicillin V)

Semisynthetic
- Penicillinase resistant
  - Methicillin
  - Nafcillin
  - Isoxazolyl penicillins
    - Cloxacillin
    - Dicloxacillin
    - Oxacillin
- Extended spectrum
  - Aminopenicillins
    - Ampicillin
    - Amoxicillin
    - Bacampicillin
    - Pivampicillin
  - Carboxypenicillins
    - Carbenicillin
    - Ticarcillin
  - Ureidopenicillins
    - Azlocillin
    - Mezlocillin
    - Piperacillin

Penicillin + β-lactamase inhibitor combinations
- Ampicillin-sulbactam (Unasyn)
- Ticarcillin-clavulanate (Timentin)
- Amoxicillin-clavulanate (Augmentin)
- Piperacillin-Tazobactam (Zosyn)

modialysis. Peritoneal dialysis requires dosage reduction of carbenicillin and ticarcillin.

Spectrum of Activity

The penicillins have antibacterial activity against most gram-positive and many gram-negative and anaerobic organisms. Penicillin G is very effective against penicillin-susceptible *Staphylococcus aureus*, *Streptococcus pneumoniae*, *Streptococcus pyogenes*, viridans streptococci, *Streptococcus bovis*, *Neisseria gonorrhoeae*, *Neisseria meningitidis*, *Pasteurella multocida*, anaerobic cocci, *Clostridium* spp., *Fusobacterium* spp., *Prevotella* spp., and *Porphyromonas* spp. However, the occurrence of penicillin-resistant pneumococci has recently been increasing worldwide (123). Penicillin is the drug of choice for syphilis and *Actinomyces* infections. Penicillin V has a spectrum of activity similar to that of penicillin G except that it is less active against *N. gonorrhoeae*. Penicillinase-resistant penicillins, of which methicillin is the prototype, are primarily effective against penicillinase-producing staphylococci (93). The agents are at least 25 times more active than other penicillins against penicillinase-positive *Staphylococcus aureus* and *S. epidermidis*. Although they are also active against *S. pneumoniae* and *S. pyogenes*, their MICs for these organisms are higher than those of penicillin G. They are not active against enterococci, members of the family *Enterobacteriaceae*, *Pseudomonas* spp., or members of the *Bacteroides fragilis* group.

Ampicillin and amoxicillin have spectra of activity similar to that of penicillin G, but they are more active against enterococci and *Listeria monocytogenes*. Although they are also more active against *Haemophilus influenzae* and *H. parainfluenzae*, up to 25% of *H. influenzae* isolates are resistant, usually because of β-lactamase production. *Salmonella* and *Shigella* spp., including *Salmonella typhi*, and many strains of

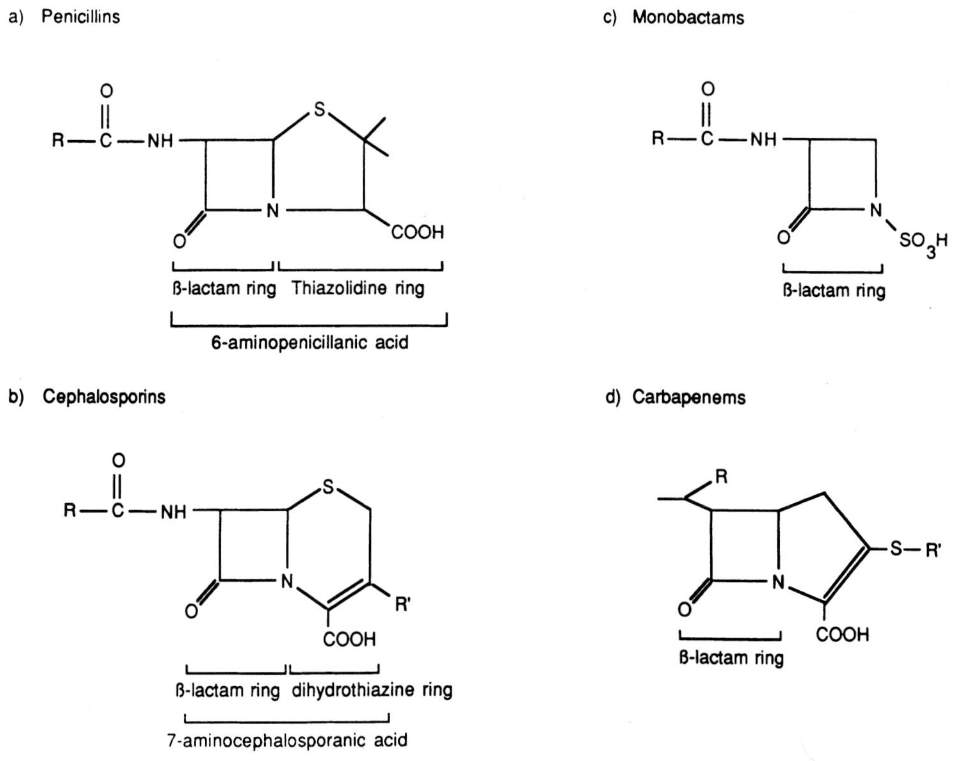

FIGURE 1 Chemical structures of β-lactam antibiotics.

Escherichia coli and *Proteus mirabilis* are susceptible to these agents. Ampicillin is more effective against shigellae, whereas amoxicillin is more effective against salmonellae. Both of these agents are degraded by β-lactamase and are inactive against many members of the *Enterobacteriaceae* and *Pseudomonas* spp.

The carboxypenicillins and ureidopenicillins have increased activity against gram-negative bacteria that are resistant to ampicillin. Although these drugs are susceptible to staphylococcal penicillinase, they are more stable against hydrolysis by the β-lactamases of the *Enterobacteriaceae* and *Pseudomonas aeruginosa*. Carbenicillin and ticarcillin are relatively active against streptococci as well as against *Haemophilus* spp., *Neisseria* spp., and a variety of anaerobes (84). They inhibit the *Enterobacteriaceae* but are inactive against *Klebsiella* spp. Although carboxypenicillins are not particularly active against the enterococci, they may act synergistically with aminoglycosides against these organisms.

The ureidopenicillins have greater in vitro activity against streptococci and enterococci than do the carboxypenicillins, and they inhibit more than 75% of *Klebsiella* spp. (58, 228). They have excellent activity against many of the *Enterobacteriaceae* and anaerobic bacteria, including members of the *B. fragilis* group. On a weight basis, their activities, in decreasing order of potency against *P. aeruginosa*, are as follows: piperacillin, azlocillin > mezlocillin, ticarcillin > carbenicillin (43). These agents also act synergistically with aminoglycosides against *P. aeruginosa*.

Adverse Effects

Common reactions to penicillins include allergic skin rashes, diarrhea, and drug fever. Severe anaphylactic reactions, which can be fatal, may occur in previously sensitized patients rechallenged with penicillins, but fortunately such reactions are quite rare. At high doses (usually $>30 \times 10^6$ U/day), penicillin G can cause myoclonic twitching and seizures due to central nervous system toxicity. All of the penicillins may cause interstitial nephritis on an allergic basis, but methicillin is more likely than the other penicillins to cause this complication. Hepatitis has been associated with prolonged use of oxacillin. High-dose carbenicillin can result in sodium overload and hypokalemia. Neutropenia may occur with any of the penicillins. Thrombocytopenia and Coombs-positive hemolytic anemia are rare complications of penicillin therapy. Bleeding tendencies due to interference with platelet function can occur with the use of carboxypenicillins and ureidopenicillins (70). Although pseudomembranous colitis has been associated with all the penicillins, it occurs more frequently with ampicillin (12).

CEPHALOSPORINS

Cephalosporins are derivatives of the fermentation products of *Cephalosporium acremonium* (also designated *Acremonium chrysogenum*). They contain a 7-aminocephalosporanic acid nucleus, which consists of a β-lactam ring fused to a dihydrothiazine ring (Fig. 1b). Various substitutions at positions 3 and 7 alter their antibacterial activities and pharmacokinetic properties. Addition of a methoxy group at position 7 of the β-lactam ring results in a new group of compounds called cephamycins, which are highly resistant to a variety of β-lactamases.

Mechanism of Action

Similar to the penicillins, cephalosporins act by binding to PBPs of susceptible organisms, thereby interfering with synthesis of peptidoglycan of the bacterial cell wall. In addition, these β-lactam agents may produce bactericidal effects by triggering autolytic enzymes in the cell envelope (242).

Pharmacology

Most cephalosporins require parenteral administration, but a growing number are available in oral form. Cephalexin, cephradine, cefadroxil, cefaclor, cefuroxime axetil, cefprozil, loracarbef, cefixime, cefpodoxime proxetil, ceftibuten, and cefdinir have good gastrointestinal absorption after oral administration (60 to 90% of the oral dose is absorbed). Cefuroxime axetil is an acetoxyethyl ester of cefuroxime, and it is deesterified in the intestinal mucosa and absorbed into the bloodstream as cefuroxime. Cefpodoxime proxetil is a prodrug which is absorbed and deesterified in vivo to release its active metabolite, cefpodoxime. Relatively high concentrations of these agents are attained across the placenta and in synovial, pleural, pericardial, and peritoneal fluids. Levels in bile are usually high, especially with cefoperazone, which is excreted mainly in the bile. Ceftizoxime, cefotaxime, ceftriaxone, cefoperazone, moxalactam, and cefepime enter the CSF in high concentrations and are useful for the treatment of meningitis. Cefuroxime penetrates inflamed meninges, but the levels in CSF are borderline and are inadequate to provide bactericidal activity against certain susceptible bacteria.

Cephalothin, cephapirin, and cefotaxime are converted to the desacetyl forms before being excreted. All cephalosporins except cefoperazone are excreted primarily by the kidneys, and for these drugs, dosage adjustments are necessary in patients with renal insufficiency (creatinine clearance, <50 ml/min). Like that of the penicillins, the renal excretion of cephalosporins, except for ceftriaxone, is impeded by probenecid. In general, these agents are removed by hemodialysis but not by peritoneal dialysis. Of the cephalosporins, cefonicid and ceftriaxone have the longest elimination half-lives, at 4.5 and 8 h, respectively, permitting once- or twice-daily administration in the treatment of serious infections.

Spectrum of Activity

Cephalosporins are classified by a well-accepted but somewhat arbitrary scheme of grouping by generations that is based on general features of their antibacterial activity (Table 2). The first-generation (narrow-spectrum) drugs, exemplified by cephalothin and cefazolin, have good activity against gram-positive bacteria and relatively modest activity against gram-negative bacteria. They are active against penicillin-susceptible and -resistant *S. aureus*, as well as *S. pneumoniae*, *S. pyogenes*, and other aerobic and anaerobic streptococci. Methicillin-resistant *S. aureus*, *S. epidermidis*, and enterococci are resistant. Some of the *Enterobacteriaceae*, including many strains of *E. coli*, *Klebsiella* spp., and *Proteus mirabilis*, are susceptible. *Pseudomonas* spp., many *Proteus* spp., and *Serratia* and *Enterobacter* spp. are resistant. These agents are active against penicillin-susceptible anaerobes except members of the *B. fragilis* group. They have only modest activity against *H. influenzae*.

The second-generation (expanded-spectrum) cephalosporins are stable to certain β-lactamases found in gram-negative bacteria and as a result have increased activity against gram-negative organisms. The agents are more active than narrow-spectrum drugs against *E. coli*, *Klebsiella* spp., and *Proteus* spp. Their activity also extends to cover some *Enterobacter* and *Serratia* strains, and they have good

TABLE 2 Cephalosporins

Narrow spectrum (first generation)
- Cefadroxil
- Cefazolin
- Cephalexin
- Cephaloridine
- Cephalothin
- Cephapirin
- Cephradine

Expanded spectrum (second generation)
- Cefaclor
- Cefamandole
- Cefonicid
- Ceforanide
- Cefuroxime
- Cefprozil
- Loracarbef
- Cefmetazole
- Cefotetan
- Cefoxitin

Broad spectrum (third generation)
- Cefdinir
- Cefixime
- Cefoperazone
- Cefotaxime
- Cefpodoxime
- Ceftazidime
- Ceftibuten
- Ceftizoxime
- Ceftriaxone

Extended spectrum (fourth generation)
- Cefepime
- Cefpirome

activity against *Haemophilus* spp., *Neisseria* spp., and many anaerobes. Cefaclor, cefuroxime, cefamandole, cefonicid, and cefprozil are active against ampicillin-resistant *H. influenzae* and *Moraxella catarrhalis* (220). However, cefamandole exhibits a significant inoculum effect and is not suitable for treating life-threatening infections due to *H. influenzae*. Ceforanide and cefonicid have spectra of antibacterial activities similar to that of cefamandole, but they are less active than cefamandole against gram-positive cocci. Loracarbef belongs to a new class of cephalosporin derivatives known as carbacephems, in which the sulfur atom of the dihydrothiazine ring is replaced by a methylene group to form a tetrahydropyridine ring (42). Since this structural modification of the cephalosporin nucleus is minor, loracarbef is considered a cephalosporin. Its spectrum of antibacterial activity is very similar to those of cefaclor, cefuroxime, and cefprozil. None of the expanded-spectrum agents is active against *Pseudomonas* spp.

Cefoxitin, cefotetan, and cefmetazole belong to a unique group of expanded-spectrum cephalosporins that have marked activity against anaerobes, including members of the *B. fragilis* group (116, 244). Cefotetan is two to four times less active than cefoxitin and cefmetazole against gram-positive cocci, but it is more potent than these two drugs against susceptible members of the *Enterobacteriaceae*. The three drugs are equally active against *H. influenzae*, *M. catarrhalis*, and *N. gonorrhoeae*, including penicillin-resistant strains. While these drugs are comparable in their activities against the *B. fragilis* group, cefoxitin is the most active against *Prevotella* spp., *Porphyromonas* spp., and gram-positive anaerobic cocci. Cefotetan and cefmetazole have the advantage of more prolonged half-lives in serum.

Third-generation (broad-spectrum) cephalosporins are generally less active than the narrow-spectrum agents against gram-positive cocci, but they are much more active against the *Enterobacteriaceae* and *P. aeruginosa*. Their potent broad spectra of activity against gram-negative bacteria are due to their stability to β-lactamases and their ability to pass through the outer cell envelopes of gram-negative bacilli (69, 157). There are two subgroups among these agents: those with potent activity against *P. aeruginosa* (ceftazidime and cefoperazone), and those without such activity (ceftizoxime, cefotaxime, and ceftriaxone).

Cefotaxime inhibits more than 90% of strains of the *Enterobacteriaceae*, including those resistant to aminoglycosides. Its MIC_{90}s for the strains of *E. coli*, *Proteus* spp., and *Klebsiella* spp. tested are <0.5 μg/ml. Its activity against strains of *Serratia marcescens*, *Enterobacter cloacae*, and *Acinetobacter* spp. is variable, and it is inactive against *P. aeruginosa*. It has moderate activity against anaerobes but is inferior to cefoxitin and cefotetan against most of these isolates.

Ceftizoxime and ceftriaxone have spectra of activity similar to that of cefotaxime with a few exceptions. Ceftriaxone is the most active agent against penicillinase-positive or -negative strains of *N. gonorrhoeae* (73). It is effective as single-dose therapy for infections caused by these organisms (29, 141). Because of its long half-life in serum (the longest of the currently available cephalosporins), ceftriaxone is used frequently in outpatient antibiotic therapy of serious infections, including Lyme disease (142).

Cefoperazone is less active than cefotaxime against many of the *Enterobacteriaceae* and gram-positive cocci. However, it has activity against *P. aeruginosa*, with an MIC_{50} of ≤16 μg/ml. Its activity against anaerobes is similar to that of cefotaxime (118). Ceftazidime has potent activity against *P. aeruginosa*, with an MIC_{90} of <8 μg/ml (157). It is more active than the ureidopenicillins against these strains. This agent has similar activity to that of cefotaxime against the *Enterobacteriaceae* but is not as active against gram-positive cocci. It has little activity against gram-negative anaerobes.

Cefixime (8), cefpodoxime (79, 190), ceftibuten (117, 253), and cefdinir (39) are extended-spectrum oral cephalosporins that are more stable than the narrow- and expanded-spectrum oral cephalosporins against gram-negative bacterial β-lactamases. Compared with the earlier cephalosporins, the newer drugs are equally active against streptococci (MIC_{90}s, ≤0.06 μg/ml) but less active against methicillin-susceptible staphylococci (MIC_{90}s, 2 μg/ml). They have potent activities similar to that of ceftizoxime against many of the *Enterobacteriaceae*, *H. influenzae*, *M. catarrhalis*, and *N. gonorrhoeae* (including β-lactamase-producing strains), but they are inactive against *Pseudomonas*, *Enterobacter*, *Serratia*, and *Morganella* spp. and anaerobes. None of the currently available cephalosporins is clinically useful against enterococci.

Cefepime is a so-called fourth-generation (extended-spectrum) cephalosporin and is approved for clinical use in the United States. Cefepime and cefpirome (formerly HR 810), which is currently undergoing clinical evaluations, have the unique features of reduced affinity for and increased stability to the Bush class I β-lactamases. Therefore, these agents are active against stably derepressed class I β-lactamase mutants of the *Enterobacteriaceae* and *P. aeruginosa*.

In addition, cefepime and cefpirome penetrate well through gram-negative bacterial outer membrane, due to a quaternary nitrogen substitution that makes them zwitterions (net neutral charge). They are more active in vitro than cefotaxime or ceftriaxone against some of the *Enterobacteriaceae*, *Proteus*, *Providencia*, *Morganella*, and *Citrobacter* (MIC_{90}s, ≤0.1 μg/ml) (86, 119, 192). Cefepime has comparable activity to ceftazidime against *P. aeruginosa*, with MIC_{90}s ≤4 μg/ml, and it is active against some ceftazidime-resistant strains (177). Against staphylococci (MIC_{90}s, ≤2 μg/ml) and streptococci (MIC_{90}s, ≤0.12 μg/ml), the activities of this group of drugs are comparable to those of the narrow-spectrum cephalosporins (86, 119). However, they are not active clinically against enterococci or anaerobes.

Adverse Effects

Cephalosporins are generally very well tolerated. The most common side effects are diarrhea and hypersensitivity reactions such as rash, drug fever, and serum sickness. Cross-reactions with these drugs occur in only 3 to 7% of penicillin-allergic patients (2). Other infrequent side effects include pseudomembranous colitis, elevated creatinine and transaminase levels in serum, leukopenia, thrombocytopenia, and Coombs-positive hemolytic anemia. These abnormalities are usually mild and reversible. Prolonged use of ceftriaxone has been associated with formation of gallbladder sludge, which usually resolves after drug administration is discontinued (195), and, rarely, cholecystitis.

Disulfiram-like reactions have been described in patients receiving cefamandole, cefotetan, and cefoperazone. This reaction is attributed to the *N*-methylthiotetrazole side chains of these antibiotics, which are similar to the chemical structure of disulfiram. Hypoprothrombinemia and bleeding tendencies have been observed in some patients treated with these cephalosporins. Causes of the coagulopathy included (i) alteration of the healthy gut flora by the antibiotics, thus inhibiting the synthesis of vitamin K and its precursors, and (ii) the *N*-methythiotetrazole side chain, which inhibits the vitamin K-dependent carboxylase enzyme responsible for converting clotting factors II, VII, IX, and X to their active forms and also prevents regeneration of active vitamin K from its inactive form (193).

OTHER β-LACTAM ANTIBIOTICS

Aztreonam

Aztreonam is the only monobactam antibiotic currently in clinical use. The monobactams are β-lactams with various side chains affixed to a monocyclic nucleus (Fig. 1c).

Mechanism of Action

Aztreonam binds primarily to PBP 3 of gram-negative aerobes, including *P. aeruginosa*, thereby disrupting bacterial cell wall synthesis. It is not hydrolyzed by most commonly occurring plasmid- and chromosome-mediated β-lactamases, and it does not induce the production of these enzymes (24).

Pharmacology

Given intravenously, aztreonam is widely distributed to body tissues and fluids. The average concentrations in serum exceed the MIC_{90}s for most of the *Enterobacteriaceae* by four to eight times for 8 h and are inhibitory to *P. aeruginosa* for 4 h. It crosses inflamed meninges in a concentration sufficient to be potentially therapeutic for meningitis caused by susceptible organisms. Its half-life in serum is about 1.7 h, and it is excreted mainly unchanged by the kidneys. Dosage modification is necessary for patients with renal failure. The drug is removed by both hemodialysis and peritoneal dialysis.

Spectrum of Activity

The antibacterial activity of aztreonam is limited to aerobic gram-negative bacilli, inhibiting most of the *Enterobacteriaceae*, *Neisseria* spp., and *Haemophilus* spp. (MIC_{90}, ≤0.5 μg/ml) (10, 218). It has significant activity against *Enterobacter* spp. and *Serratia marcescens*, with most strains being inhibited at ≤16 μg/ml. However, many *Acinetobacter* spp., *Burkholderia cepacia*, and *Stenotrophomonas maltophilia* are resistant. It shows in vitro synergism with aminoglycosides against 30 to 60% of aztreonam-susceptible organisms, including P. aeruginosa and aminoglycoside-resistant gram-negative bacilli (23). Bacterial tolerance and inoculum effect are generally not seen with this agent. Aztreonam is not active against gram-positive bacteria or anaerobes.

Adverse Effects

Aztreonam is generally a safe agent, with a toxicity profile similar to those of other β-lactam drugs. Nausea, diarrhea, skin rash, eosinophilia, mild elevation of transaminase levels in serum, and transiently an elevated creatinine level in serum have occurred. It has minimal cross-reactivity with other β-lactams and can be used safely in patients allergic to penicillins or cephalosporins (194). Hematologic abnormalities have not been reported.

Carbapenems

Carbapenems are a unique class of β-lactam agents with the widest spectrum of antibacterial activity of the currently available antibiotics. Structurally, they differ from other β-lactams in having a hydroxyethyl side chain in *trans* configuration at position 6 and lacking a sulfur or oxygen atom in the bicyclic nucleus (Fig. 1d). The unique stereochemistry of the hydroxyethyl side chain confers stability against β-lactamases. Imipenem (*N*-formimidoyl thienamycin), a semisynthetic derivative of thienamycin produced by *Streptomyces* spp., and meropenem (formerly SM-7339) are the two carbapenem agents currently available for clinical use (13, 165). Other members of this class currently undergoing preclinical evaluation or clinical trials include panipenem (RS-533) and biapenem (L 647 or LJC 10,627).

Mechanism of Action

Carbapenems bind to PBP 1 and PBP 2 of gram-negative and gram-positive bacteria, causing cell elongation and lysis (210). They are stable toward most plasmid- or chromosome-mediated β-lactamases except those produced by *Stenotrophomonas maltophilia* and some strains of *B. fragilis* (158). Bacterial resistance arises from production of carbapenemases capable of hydrolyzing the carbapenem nucleus and from alteration of the porin channels in the bacterial cell wall, thereby reducing the permeability of the drugs.

Pharmacology

After intravenous administration, the carbapenems are distributed widely in the body but undergo no significant biliary excretion. Imipenem is metabolized and inactivated in the kidneys by a dehydropeptidase I (DHP-I) enzyme found in the brush border of proximal renal tubular cells. To achieve adequate drug concentrations in serum and urine, a DHP inhibitor, cilastatin, was developed; it is combined with imipenem in a 1:1 dosage ratio for clinical use. Cilastatin has no antibacterial activity, nor does it alter the activity of imipenem. It has a renal protective effect by preventing excessive accumulation of potentially toxic imipenem metabolites in the renal tubular cells. Meropenem, panipenem, and biapenem contain a β-methyl group substitution at position C-1 of the bicyclic nucleus, resulting in increased stability to inactivation by human renal DHP-I. These agents do not require concomitant administration of a DHP-I inhibitor.

The pharmacokinetics of imipenem and meropenem are very similar, with elimination half-lives in serum of about 1 h. Peak concentrations of the drugs in serum are about 25 to 35 and 55 to 70 μg/ml following 0.5- and 1-g doses, respectively. These drugs penetrate inflamed meninges well, attaining levels of 0.5 to 6 μg/ml in the CSF (44, 165). Dosage adjustment is necessary for a creatinine clearance of ≤30 ml/min. These agents, including cilastin, are effectively removed by hemodialysis.

Spectrum of Activity

In general, all the carbapenems have similar antibacterial potencies with minor differences. They have excellent in vitro activity against aerobic gram-positive species: staphylococci (penicillin-susceptible and -resistant isolates); viridans streptococci; group A, B, C, and G streptococci; *Bacillus* spp.; and *L. monocytogenes*. Imipenem is two to four times more active than the other carbapenems against streptococci and staphylococci, but methicillin-resistant staphylococci are usually resistant to all the carbapenems. Although the carbapenem MICs for penicillin-resistant pneumococci are elevated (MIC_{90}s, 1 to 2 μg/ml), these bacteria remain susceptible (63). Most enterococci are inhibited by the carbapenems at ≤4 μg/ml, and imipenem has slightly better activity, but *Enterococcus faecium* strains are usually resistant.

More than 90% of the *Enterobacteriaceae*, including those resistant to other β-lactams and aminoglycosides (163), are susceptible to carbapenems, with the following decreasing order of activity: meropenem > biapenem, panipenem > imipenem (63, 104, 132, 165). Most *Acinetobacter* spp., *Enterobacter* spp., *Citrobacter* spp., and *Serratia* spp. are inhibited by ≤2 μg/ml. While most strains of *P. aeruginosa* are inhibited by the carbapenems at 4 to 8 μg/ml, meropenem is the most potent of these agents against *P. aeruginosa*, including some imipenem-resistant strains (104, 174). While the carbapenems inhibit *Burkholderia cepacia* and *B. stutzeri*, they are inactive against *S. maltophilia* (55, 104). Emergence of resistant *Pseudomonas* spp. has been observed during therapy with imipenem (251). Imipenem may show in vitro antagonism when combined with broad-spectrum cephalosporins or extended-spectrum penicillins as a result of its ability to induce class I β-lactamase production (158).

Carbapenems are the most potent β-lactams against anaerobes, with activities comparable to those of clindamycin and metronidazole. The MIC_{90}s for *B. fragilis* group, *Prevotella* spp., *Porphyromonas* spp., *Fusobacterium* spp., and anaerobic gram-positive cocci are ≤1 μg/ml (132, 174, 201). Meropenem is more active than imipenem against *Clostridium* spp. and *Veillonella* spp. Both are also active in vitro against *Actinomyces* spp., *Nocardia asteroides*, and *Mycobacterium* spp. (16, 45, 56, 63).

Adverse Effects

Side effects of carbapenems are similar to those of other β-lactam antibiotics. Gastrointestinal distress occurs in up to 5% of patients, and nausea is commonly associated with parenteral administration of imipenem. Allergic reactions such as drug fever, skin rashes, and urticaria are seen in about 3% of patients. Cross-reactivity with other β-lactam agents is possible but has not been fully studied. Seizures of unclear etiology have occurred in about 1% of patients receiving imipenem, particularly in the elderly and in patients with renal insufficiency or underlying neurologic disorders. Meropenem has not been associated with seizures. Reversible elevation of transaminase levels in serum, leukopenia, and thrombocytopenia have been described for carbapenems, but no coagulopathy has been reported.

β-LACTAMASE INHIBITORS

Clavulanic Acid

Clavulanic acid is a naturally occurring weak antimicrobial agent found initially in cultures of *Streptomyces clavuligerus* (161). It inhibits β-lactamases from staphylococci and many gram-negative bacteria. This agent acts primarily as a "suicide inhibitor" by forming an irreversible acyl enzyme complex with the β-lactamase, leading to loss of activity of the enzyme.

Clavulanic acid acts synergistically with various penicillins and cephalosporins against β-lactamase-producing staphylococci, klebsiellae, *H. influenzae*, *M. catarrhalis*, *N. gonorrhoeae*, *E. coli*, *Proteus* spp., *B. fragilis* group, *Prevotella* spp., and *Porphyromonas* spp. (5, 84). Recently discovered plasmid-mediated TEM β-lactamases in ceftazidime-resistant strains of *Klebsiella pneumoniae* and *E. coli* are inactivated by this agent (113, 246). However, the inducible β-lactamases (chromosomal class I) of *Enterobacter*, *Citrobacter*, *Proteus*, *Acinetobacter*, *Serratia*, and *Pseudomonas* spp. are not inhibited by clavulanic acid (124). The combination of clavulanic acid with ampicillin, amoxicillin, or ticarcillin is active in vitro against *Mycobacterium tuberculosis*, which is known to produce β-lactamases (46, 259).

In the United States, clavulanic acid is available for clinical use in a 1:2 or 1:4 combination with oral amoxicillin and in a 1:15 or 1:30 parenteral combination with ticarcillin. The pharmacologic parameters of amoxicillin and ticarcillin are not significantly altered when either drug is combined with clavulanic acid. Amoxicillin-clavulanate is moderately well absorbed from the gastrointestinal tract, with a half-life in serum of about 1 h for each component. One-third of a dose is metabolized, while the remainder is excreted unchanged in the urine. The drug is widely distributed to various body tissues and fluids, but it penetrates uninflamed meninges very poorly.

Adverse reactions are similar to those reported for amoxicillin or ticarcillin used alone. Nausea, vomiting, abdominal cramps, and diarrhea occur in 5 to 10% of patients taking amoxicillin-clavulanate. The incidence of allergic skin reactions is similar to that of ampicillin alone.

Sulbactam

Sulbactam is a semisynthetic 6-desaminopenicillin sulfone with weak antibacterial activity (4). It functions as an effective inhibitor of certain plasmid- and chromosome-mediated β-lactamases in *S. aureus*, *Enterobacteriaceae*, *H. influenzae*, *M. catarrhalis*, *Neisseria* spp., *Legionella* spp., *B. fragilis* group, *Prevotella* spp., *Porphyromonas* spp., and *Mycobacterium* spp. (83, 182). Sulbactam alone is active against *N. gonorrhoeae*, *N. meningitidis*, some *Acinetobacter* spp., and *B. cepacia* (114, 183). It acts synergistically with penicillins and cephalosporins against organisms that are otherwise resistant to the β-lactam drugs because of the production of β-lactamases. A combination of sulbactam (8 μg/ml) and ampicillin (16 μg/ml) inhibits most staphylococci, *Klebsiella* spp., *E. coli*, *H. influenzae*, *M. catarrhalis*, *Neisseria* spp., *B. fragilis* group, *Prevotella* spp., and *Porphyromonas* spp. that are ampicillin resistant (183, 245). Like clavulanic acid, sulbactam does not inhibit the β-lactamases of *Enterobacter*, *Citrobacter*, *Providencia*, indole-positive *Proteus*, or *Pseudomonas* spp. or *S. maltophilia*.

For clinical use, sulbactam is combined with ampicillin as a parenteral preparation in a 1:2 ratio. The pharmacologic properties of the drugs are not affected by each other in this combination. Ampicillin-sulbactam penetrates well into body tissues and fluids, including peritoneal and blister fluids. It enters the CSF in the presence of inflamed meninges. Like ampicillin, sulbactam has a half-life in serum of 1 h, and 85% of the drug is excreted unchanged via the kidneys. Since the clearances of both sulbactam and ampicillin are affected similarly in patients with impaired renal function, dosage adjustments are similar for the two drugs.

The most common side effects of the ampicillin-sulbactam combination have been nausea, diarrhea, and skin rash. Transient eosinophilia and elevation of serum transaminases have been reported. Adverse reactions attributed to ampicillin may also occur with the use of ampicillin-sulbactam.

Tazobactam

Tazobactam (formerly YTR 830) is a penicillanic acid sulfone derivative structurally related to sulbactam. Like clavulanic acid and sulbactam, tazobactam acts as a suicidal β-lactamase inhibitor and binds to bacterial PBP 1 or PBP 2 (148). Despite having very poor intrinsic antibacterial activity by itself, it is comparable to clavulanate and sulbactam in lowering the MICs by up to 20-fold for many organisms when combined with various β-lactams against β-lactamase-producing organisms. Tazobactam actively inhibits the β-lactamases of staphylococci, *H. influenzae*, *N. gonorrhoeae*, *E. coli*, *B. fragilis* group, *Prevotella* spp., and *Porphyromonas* spp. (3, 98, 126). It also has activity against the class I β-lactamases of *Acinetobacter*, *Citrobacter*, *Proteus*, *Providencia*, and *Morganella* spp., but it remains inactive against those of *Enterobacter* spp., *Pseudomonas* spp., *S. maltophilia*, and some *Klebsiella* spp. (124, 126). Of the penicillin–β-lactamase inhibitor combinations, piperacillin-tazobactam is the most active (two- to eightfold lower MICs) against β-lactamase-producing aerobic and anaerobic gram-negative bacilli (66, 126).

Tazobactam is administered parenterally as a 1:8 combination with piperacillin. The two drugs do not affect each other's metabolism or pharmacokinetics. High concentrations of both agents are achieved in the intestinal mucosa, lungs, and skin, with relatively poor distribution to muscle, fat, prostate, and CSF (in the absence of inflamed meninges). With a half-life in serum of about 1 h, tazobactam is eliminated mainly via the renal route and is not affected by hepatic failure (206). The major adverse effects of the piperacillin-tazobactam combination are similar to those of piperacillin alone and include diarrhea, skin rash, and allergic reactions. Mild elevation in transaminase levels in serum is encountered in about 10% of patients.

AMINOGLYCOSIDES AND AMINOCYCLITOLS

Since the first aminoglycoside (aminoglycosidic aminocyclitol), streptomycin, was introduced in 1944, this class of antibiotic has played a vital role in the treatment of serious infections by gram-negative bacteria. Among the unique features of the aminoglycosides are their bactericidal activity against aerobic gram-negative bacilli (including *Pseudomonas* spp.), activity against *M. tuberculosis*, and relatively low incidence of bacterial resistance. The currently available aminoglycosides are derived from *Micromonospora* spp. (gentamicin, sisomicin, and netilmicin) or from *Streptomyces* spp. (streptomycin, neomycin, kanamycin, tobramycin, and paromomycin). The difference in the origin of these compounds accounts for the differences of their suffixes, "micin" versus "mycin." Streptomycin, neomycin, kanamycin, tobramycin, and gentamicin are naturally occurring aminoglycosides, whereas amikacin and netilmicin are semisynthetic derivatives of kanamycin and sisomicin, respectively. Structurally, each of these aminoglycosides contains two or more amino sugars linked by glycosidic bonds to an aminocyclitol ring nucleus.

Spectinomycin is an aminocyclitol antibiotic isolated from *Streptomyces spectabilis*. Although it contains an aminocyclitol nucleus, it is not strictly an aminoglycoside because it does not contain an amino sugar or a glycosidic bond.

Mechanism of Action

Aminoglycosides are bactericidal agents that inhibit bacterial protein synthesis by binding irreversibly to the bacterial 30S ribosomal subunit. The aminoglycoside-bound bacterial ribosomes then become unavailable for translation of mRNA during protein synthesis, thereby leading to cell death (51). The aminoglycosides also cause misreading of the genetic code, with resultant production of nonsense proteins. To reach the intracellular ribosomal binding targets, an aerobic energy-dependent process is necessary to enable successful penetration of the bacterial inner cell membrane by the aminoglycosides. Bacterial uptake of these agents is facilitated by inhibitors of bacterial cell wall synthesis such as β-lactams and vancomycin. This interaction forms the basis of antibacterial synergism between aminoglycosides and β-lactam antibiotics (53, 88).

Spectinomycin acts similarly to the aminoglycosides by binding to the 30S ribosomal subunits and inhibiting protein synthesis. However, it does not cause misreading of the mRNA and is not bactericidal.

Pharmacology

All aminoglycosides have similar pharmacologic properties. Gastrointestinal absorption of these agents is unpredictable and always low. Because of its severe toxicity with systemic administration, neomycin is available only for oral and topical use. After intravenous administration, aminoglycosides are freely distributed in the extracellular space but penetrate poorly into the CSF, vitreous fluid of the eye, biliary tract, prostate, and tracheobronchial secretions, even in the presence of inflammation.

In adults with normal renal function, the aminoglycosides have half-lives in serum of about 2 to 3 h. They are excreted, essentially unchanged, primarily via the kidneys. There is considerable variation in the elimination of aminoglycosides among individuals, especially in patients with impaired renal function. Monitoring of aminoglycoside levels in serum in these patients is essential for providing adequate therapy and reduced toxicity. With their features of concentration-dependent killing and prolonged postantibiotic effect, aminoglycosides may be administered once daily to achieve maximum bactericidal activity at high concentrations in serum without increased risk of toxicities (14). In patients with renal failure, the drugs accumulate and dosage reductions are necessary. Aminoglycosides are substantially removed by hemodialysis and to a lesser extent by peritoneal dialysis.

Spectrum of Activity

Aminoglycoside antibiotics are active primarily against aerobic gram-negative bacilli and *S. aureus*. As a group, they are particularly potent against the *Enterobacteriaceae*, *P. aeruginosa*, and *Acinetobacter* spp. Certain differences in antimicrobial spectra among the various aminoglycosides do exist. Kanamycin is limited in its spectrum because of the common resistance of *P. aeruginosa* and frequent occurrence of plasmid-mediated inactivating enzymes among other gram-negative bacilli (51). It is now used occasionally as a "second-line" drug in combination with other antibiotics for the therapy of mycobacterial infections (234, 235). Similarly, widespread resistance among the *Enterobacteriaceae* has limited the usefulness of streptomycin. As a single agent, streptomycin is used in the therapy of infections due to *Francisella tularensis* (tularemia) and *Yersinia pestis* (plague). It is often used in conjunction with tetracycline for the treatment of brucellosis. It has the greatest in vitro activity of the aminoglycosides against *M. tuberculosis*. It may also be used in combination with penicillin or vancomycin for the treatment of infective endocarditis due to viridans streptococci or enterococci, provided that the organisms do not possess high-level ribosomal or enzymatic resistance to streptomycin (240, 241, 249, 250).

Although gentamicin and tobramycin have very similar antibacterial activity profiles, gentamicin is more active in vitro against *Serratia* spp. whereas tobramycin is more active against *P. aeruginosa* (156). However, these minor differences have not been correlated with a greater efficacy of one agent over the other. For the most part, gentamicin and tobramycin are susceptible to inactivation by the same modifying enzymes produced by resistant bacteria, except that in contrast to gentamicin, tobramycin can be inactivated by 6-acetyltransferase and 4′-adenyltransferase and has variable susceptibility to 3-acetyltransferase. Netilmicin and amikacin are resistant to many of these aminoglycoside-modifying enzymes and therefore are active against most of the *Enterobacteriaceae* that are resistant to gentamicin and tobramycin (151). Netilmicin is intrinsically less active than gentamicin or tobramycin against *P. aeruginosa*, and most gentamicin-resistant *Serratia*, *Proteus*, *Providencia*, and *Pseudomonas* isolates are also usually resistant to netilmicin (82). Amikacin is often used as the aminoglycoside of choice when gentamicin and tobramycin resistances are prevalent. In addition, amikacin is active against many *Mycobacterium* spp. (234, 235). Aminoglycosides are only moderately active against *Haemophilus* and *Neisseria* spp. Of the agents active against *Bartonella* spp., aminoglycosides are the only drugs consistently bactericidal toward these organisms (136).

Although active against staphylococci, aminoglycosides are not recommended as single agents for the treatment of staphylococcal infections. Gentamicin is often combined with a penicillin or vancomycin for synergy in the treatment of serious infections due to staphylococci, enterococci, or viridans streptococci (240, 241, 249). The aminoglycosides are not active against anaerobes.

Paromomycin is an aminoglycoside notable for its amebicidal and antihelminthic effects, and it is used clinically for the treatment of intestinal amebiasis and tapeworm infections (143). It has modest antibacterial activity against gram-positive cocci and the *Enterobacteriaceae*, but *P. aeruginosa* isolates are generally resistant.

Spectinomycin is used primarily for uncomplicated anogenital infections due to *N. gonorrhoeae* (238), including β-lactamase-producing strains, and gonococci are rarely resistant to this drug (73, 264). It is useful in patients with penicillin allergy. Spectinomycin is ineffective for pharyngeal gonococcal infections, syphilis, or chlamydial infections.

Adverse Effects

Considerable intrinsic toxicity, mainly in the form of nephrotoxicity and auditory or vestibular toxicity, is characteristic of all of the aminoglycosides. The nephrotoxic potential varies among the aminoglycosides, with neomycin being the most toxic and streptomycin the least. This effect is usually reversible when administration of the drug is discontinued. The presence of hypotension, prolonged duration of therapy, preexisting renal insufficiency, and possibly excessive trough serum aminoglycoside concentrations increase the risk of nephrotoxicity.

All aminoglycosides are capable of causing damage to the eight cranial nerve in humans. Vestibular toxicity is more frequently associated with streptomycin, gentamicin, and tobramycin, whereas auditory toxicity is more typical of kanamycin and amikacin. This frequently irreversible side effect may occur even after discontinuation of drug therapy and is cumulative with repeated courses of the agent. The ototoxicity is a result of selective destruction of the hair cells in the cochlea. Clinically detectable auditory and vestibular dysfunction has been reported to occur in 3 to 5% of patients receiving gentamicin, tobramycin, or amikacin who underwent audiometric testing (71).

Neuromuscular paralysis, which is usually reversible, can occur after rapid intravenous infusion of aminoglycosides. This phenomenon occurs particularly in the setting of myasthenia gravis or concurrent use of succinylcholine during anesthesia. Other minor adverse reactions include local pain and allergic skin rashes. No known serious adverse reactions have been reported for spectinomycin.

QUINOLONES

Quinolones belong to a group of potent antibiotics biochemically related to nalidixic acid, which was developed initially as a urinary antiseptic. Nalidixic acid and its early analogs, oxolinic acid and cinoxacin, have limited clinical applications as a result of widespread emergence of bacterial resistance. Newer quinolones have been synthesized by modifying the original two-ring quinolone (or naphthyridine) nucleus with different side chain substitutions (257). These new agents, also known as fluoroquinolones, each contain a fluorine atom attached to the nucleus at position 6. Cinoxacin, enoxacin, norfloxacin, lomefloxacin, ciprofloxacin, ofloxacin, levofloxacin, sparfloxacin, grepafloxacin, and trovafloxacin are currently available for clinical use in the United States. Temafloxacin has been withdrawn from clinical use due to toxicities. Gatifloxacin, moxifloxacin, and clinafloxacin are currently undergoing clinical investigation in the United States. Several closely related fluoroquinolones, such as enrofloxacin and sarafloxacin, have been approved for agricultural and veterinary use in the United States and elsewhere.

Mechanism of Action

The primary bacterial target of the quinolones is DNA gyrase, a type II DNA topoisomerase enzyme essential for DNA replication, recombination, and repair (109, 257). Newer fluoroquinolones also inhibit type IV DNA topoisomerases. Bacterial DNA gyrases are related to a series of mammalian topoisomerase enzymes that have a similar function. Their therapeutic index stems from the fact that the clinically useful fluoroquinolones inhibit bacterial DNA gyrase at concentrations far below those required to inhibit mammalian topoisomerases. Because they inhibit bacterial DNA synthesis, these agents are bactericidal. However, the antibacterial activity of quinolones is reduced in the presence of low pH, urine, and divalent cations (Mg^{2+} and Ca^{2+}) (258). Bacterial resistance to quinolones results from single-step chromosomal mutations that alter DNA gyrase or changes in outer membrane porin proteins (decreased permeability of the drug through the cell wall). Transferable plasmid-mediated resistance to the fluoroquinolones has been described recently, but the exact mechanism remains unknown (135).

Pharmacology

Pharmacokinetic parameters are similar among the fluoroquinolones, with minor differences. They are generally well absorbed from the gastrointestinal tract, with norfloxacin being absorbed least well. The bioavailability varies from 60 to 95% for the various fluoroquinolones (214, 252). After oral administration, concentrations in serum peak after 1 to 2 h. The presence of food does not significantly alter the absorption of these drugs. However, coadministration with iron- or zinc-containing multivitamins or with antacids containing aluminum, magnesium, or calcium substantially reduces the gastrointestinal absorption and subsequent peak concentrations of quinolones in serum. The degree of serum protein binding is generally low, ranging from 8% for ofloxacin to 75% for trovafloxacin. The long half-lives of fluoroquinolones in serum, ranging from 3.5 h for ciprofloxacin to 20 h for sparfloxacin, allow twice or even once-daily dosing (107, 147). Ciprofloxacin, ofloxacin, levofloxacin, and trovafloxacin are also available for intravenous use. The intravenous formulation of trovafloxacin is prepared as alatrofloxacin mesylate, which is a prodrug of trovafloxacin and is rapidly hydrolyzed in vivo to yield the active drug.

Quinolones have good penetration into the lungs, kidneys, muscle, bone, intestinal wall, and extravascular body fluids. Concentrations in the prostate are about twice those in the serum, and concentrations of 25 to 100 times above peak concentrations in serum are achieved in the urine. However, concentrations are variable but low in the CSF (<1 μg/ml) obtained from patients with meningitis (256). Quinolones penetrate well into phagocytes, so that concentrations within neutrophils and macrophages are as high as 14 times the concentrations in serum (224). This feature account for their excellent in vivo activity against such intracellular pathogens as *Brucella*, *Listeria*, *Salmonella*, and *Mycobacterium* spp.

Grepafloxacin, trovafloxacin, and pefloxacin are metabolized mainly by the liver to form glucuronide conjugates, with pefloxacin being converted into norfloxacin in vivo. Ofloxacin exhibits little or no in vivo metabolism, and it is excreted mainly (90%) by the kidney. The other quinolones are cleared by both hepatic and renal routes in various proportions, with elimination occurring primarily via the kidneys. This renal elimination is blocked by probenecid. Small amounts of these drugs are also excreted in the bile.

Hepatic insufficiency prolongs the elimination half-lives of pefloxacin, grepafloxacin, and trovafloxacin, whereas the clearance of other fluoroquinolones is significantly diminished in the presence of renal failure. All of these drugs are only partially removed by hemodialysis (<15%) and are minimally affected by peritoneal dialysis because of their marked extravascular penetration, as reflected in their very large volumes of distribution.

Spectrum of Activity

Quinolones may be categorized into groups with similar spectra of antibacterial activity (Table 3), analogous to the classification of cephalosporins. The narrow-spectrum quinolones have no useful activity against gram-positive cocci, and their clinical utility is limited by the widespread prevalence and rapid emergence of bacterial resistance. Broad-spectrum (second-generation) fluoroquinolones are active against both gram-positive and gram-negative bacteria (147, 221, 231, 258). Increased activity against gram-positive cocci is a major feature of the newer (third-generation) fluoroquinolones, with potencies two- to eightfold greater than those of broad-spectrum agents (21, 38, 40, 54, 134, 232). The MIC_{90}s for methicillin-susceptible and -resistant *S. aureus* and coagulase-negative staphylococci are in the range of 0.03 to 1 μg/ml, while methicillin-resistant staphylococci are becoming increasingly resistant to these agents. Although their potency against streptococci and enterococci is lower, these drugs are more active than the broad-spectrum agents against multidrug-resistant *S. pneumoniae* (MIC_{90}s, 0.12 to 1 μg/ml) and enterococci (MIC_{90}s, 0.5 to 2 μg/ml).

In contrast to earlier drugs of this class, many of the extended-spectrum quinolones possess potent activity against anaerobes, including members of the *B. fragilis* group and *C. difficile* (35, 164, 208). The relative activities of these newer drugs against all anaerobes, in decreasing order of potency, are as follows: clinafloxacin, gatifloxacin, trovafloxacin > moxifloxacin, tosufloxacin > sparfloxacin, grepafloxacin. The more active of these compounds inhibit *B. fragilis* group, *Prevotella* spp., *Porphyromonas* spp., *Fusobac-*

TABLE 3 Quinolones

Narrow spectrum (first generation)
Cinoxacin
Nalidixic acid
Oxolinic acid
Broad spectrum (second generation)
Ciprofloxacin
Enoxacin
Fleroxacin
Levofloxacin
Lomefloxacin
Norfloxacin
Ofloxacin
Pefloxacin
Rufloxacin
Expanded spectrum (third generation)
Gatifloxacin
Grepafloxacin
Sparfloxacin
Tosufloxacin
Clinafloxacin
Moxifloxacin
Trovafloxacin

terium spp., *Clostridium* spp., and anaerobic gram-positive cocci at concentrations of 0.06 to 2 μg/ml.

The fluoroquinolones possess excellent activity in vivo against the *Enterobacteriaceae*, *P. aeruginosa*, *Citrobacter* spp., *Serratia* spp., *Acinetobacter* spp., β-lactamase-positive and -negative *H. influenzae*, and gram-negative cocci such as *N. gonorrhoeae*, *N. meningitidis*, and *M. catarrhalis* (17, 38, 40, 54, 134, 229, 257). Enteropathogenic gram-negative bacilli such as salmonellae, shigellae, *Yersinia enterocolitica*, *Vibrio* spp., *Aeromonas* spp., *Plesiomonas* spp., *Campylobacter jejuni*, and enteroinvasive and enterotoxigenic *E. coli* are all susceptible to the quinolones (65, 258). Clinical studies have shown these drugs to be effective in the prophylaxis and treatment of infectious diarrheas. However, resistance and reduced susceptibility to quinolones have emerged in clinical isolates of *Salmonella*, *Shigella*, and *Campylobacter* spp. (67, 111). *Legionella* spp. are susceptible to these agents, with the MICs of most fluoroquinolones being 0.12 to 1.0 μg/ml for these organisms (21, 54, 61). Fluoroquinolones are the first class of oral agents with outstanding potency against *P. aeruginosa*. Ciprofloxacin, clinafloxacin, and trovafloxacin are the most active of these drugs against *P. aeruginosa*, with MIC_{90}s of 0.5 to 1 μg/ml. However, *Burkholderia* spp. and *S. maltophilia* are variably resistant to quinolones (229).

The fluoroquinolones, especially ciprofloxacin, levofloxacin, ofloxacin, and sparfloxacin, are active in vitro against *M. tuberculosis*, *M. fortuitum-chelonae* complex, *M. kansasii*, and *M. xenopi* (52, 221, 262). Their activity against *M. avium* complex is fair to poor. They also exhibit activity against *Chlamydia trachomatis*, *C. pneumoniae*, and *Mycoplasma hominis*, with MIC_{90}s of 0.1 to 1 μg/ml, but are less potent against *Ureaplasma urealyticum* (65, 121). Ciprofloxacin and pefloxacin inhibit *Rickettsia conorii*, *R. rickettsii*, and *Coxiella burnetii* (179, 180, 261). The broad-spectrum fluoroquinolones also possess potent activity against *Bartonella* spp. (136). Although quinolones possess in vitro activity against *Plasmodium falciparum* at achievable concentrations in serum, they are relatively ineffective when used clinically for the treatment of malaria. *Nocardia* spp. are relatively resistant to the quinolones (16, 56).

No significant inoculum effect has been observed among the bacteria susceptible to quinolones. Combinations of quinolones with β-lactam drugs or aminoglycosides are usually indifferent or additive in their effects against gram-negative and gram-positive bacteria and mycobacteria (258). However, bactericidal activities of quinolones can be antagonized by rifampin or chloramphenicol.

Adverse Effects

Gastrointestinal symptoms, occurring in up to 10% of patients as nausea, vomiting, abdominal discomfort, and diarrhea, are the most common side effects (100). However, *C. difficile* colitis rarely occurs with the use of quinolones. Headaches, fatigue, insomnia, dizziness, agitation, and, rarely, seizures can occur. These adverse neurologic effects are usually associated with high dosages in elderly patients or concurrent use of nonsteroidal anti-inflammatory drugs.

Allergic reactions are uncommon and often manifest as rash, urticaria, and generalized pruritus. Dose-related photosensitivity occurs in up to 8% of patients taking sparfloxacin and lomefloxacin. Prolongation of the QT interval has also occurred in patients treated with sparfloxacin and grepafloxacin. Rare laboratory abnormalities occurring during fluoroquinolone therapy include elevations in transaminase levels in serum, eosinophilia, leukopenia, and thrombocytopenia. Temafloxacin was withdrawn from clinical use because of rarely associated hemolytic anemia, thrombocytopenia, and acute renal failure resulting in death.

Enoxacin and to a lesser extent ciprofloxacin, pefloxacin, and grepafloxacin increase the levels of concomitant theophylline and caffeine in serum as a result of decreased hepatic clearance (175, 247). Other reported drug interactions include augmentation of the anticoagulant effects of warfarin by ciprofloxacin, norfloxacin, and ofloxacin and an increase in cyclosporin levels in serum with ciprofloxacin administration (175).

Although irreversible cartilage erosions and skeletal abnormalities were observed in studies of quinolone toxicity in animals (36), such effects have not yet been documented clinically. However, quinolones are generally contraindicated for use in patients younger than 18 years and in pregnant or nursing mothers. Tendinitis or tendon rupture has occurred with the use of fluoroquinolones.

MACROLIDES

Macrolides have been in use since the early 1950s, with erythromycin being the prototypical antibiotic of this class for over 30 years (239). Their chemical structure consists of a macrocyclic lactone ring attached to two sugar moieties, desosamine and cladinose. They differ from each other in the size (14 to 16 atoms) and substitution pattern of the lactone ring. Erythromycin is a naturally occurring 14-membered macrolide derived from *Streptomyces erythreus*; other natural analogs include oleandomycin, spiramycin, and josamycin. Clarithromycin and dirithromycin are 14-membered semisynthetic macrolides, while azithromycin is a 15-membered derivative, also known as an azalide, with a nitrogen atom incorporated in its lactone ring. These new macrolides offer significant advantages over erythromycin because of their expanded antimicrobial spectra, improved pharmacokinetic parameters, and less frequent adverse effects and drug interactions. Roxithromycin, flurithromycin, and rokitamycin are new macrolides currently under preclinical and clinical evaluation in the United States (122).

Mechanism of Action

Macrolides are generally bacteriostatic agents that inhibit bacterial RNA-dependent protein synthesis. They may be bactericidal at high drug concentrations and against a low inoculum of bacteria. They bind reversibly to the 23S component of the 50S ribosomal subunits of susceptible microorganisms, thereby blocking the translocation reaction of polypeptide chain elongation (227). The presence of rRNA methylases is the primary mechanism of macrolide resistance and confers macrolide-lincosamide-streptogramin B (MLS_B) coresistance (60). Other uncommon mechanisms of macrolide resistance are the production of macrolide-inactivating enzymes (esterases and phosphotransferases) and active efflux of macrolides.

Pharmacology

Erythromycin is available in various topical, parenteral (lactobionate and gluceptate), and oral (base stearate, ethylsuccinate, and estolate) preparations. Clarithromycin and dirithromycin are available only in oral forms, and azithromycin is formulated for oral and intravenous administration. When administered orally, erythromycin base is rapidly inactivated by gastric acid, whereas the newer macrolides are stable against acid degradation. Intestinal absorption of erythromycin (except for the estolate form) and azithromycin is reduced up to 50% in the presence of food. Peak levels in serum of 2 to 3, 0.5 to 1, 0.2 to 0.6, and 0.4 μg/ml are reached at 3 h after oral doses of erythromycin (500 mg), clarithromycin (250 mg), dirithromycin (500 mg), and azithromycin (500 mg), respectively. Much higher concentrations of erythromycin are achieved with intravenous infusion. The tissue distributions of macrolides are excellent, with concentrations in various tissues being 10- to 100-fold higher than that in serum (248). The high concentrations reached rapidly within neutrophils and macrophages account for their potent activity against intracellular pathogens (196). They penetrate poorly into the brain and CSF, but they do cross the placenta and are excreted in breast milk.

Erythromycin, clarithromycin, and dirithromycin are metabolized by the liver and excreted primarily in the bile. Azithromycin is excreted largely unchanged in the bile. Clarithromycin exhibits first-pass metabolism, which produces a microbiologically active 14-hydroxy derivative which is two to four times more potent than the parent drug against some organisms. Following gastrointestinal absorption, dirithromycin is rapidly converted by nonenzymatic hydrolysis to erythromycylamine, an active derivative with microbiological activity similar to that of its parent compound. Erythromycin, clarithromycin, 14-hydroxy clarithromycin, azithromycin, and dirithromycin have terminal half-lives in serum of 1.5, 5, 8.5, 41, and 44 h, respectively. Because of its exceptionally high tissue penetration, azithromycin has a half-life in tissue of 2 to 4 days (196). Dosage adjustment of clarithromycin is necessary in the presence of moderate to severe renal failure (creatinine clearance, <30 ml/min). Except for clarithromycin, macrolides are removed minimally by hemodialysis or peritoneal dialysis.

Spectrum of Activity

Macrolides are relatively broad-spectrum antibiotics, with activity against gram-positive and some gram-negative bacteria, mycoplasmas, chlamydiae, treponemes, and rickettsiae (101, 239, 248). Erythromycin shows good activity against staphylococci and streptococci, including *S. pneumoniae*, but emergence of resistance among these isolates (especially group A streptococci) is a problem in certain parts of the world (33, 123). Erythromycin and dirithromycin exhibit similar in vitro antibacterial activities (15). Clarithromycin is two- to fourfold more active than the other macrolides and azithromycin is less active than erythromycin against most staphylococci and streptococci (9). These drugs are bactericidal against susceptible strains of streptococci but bacteriostatic toward staphylococci and enterococci. Erythromycin-resistant strains display cross-resistance to these drugs, and methicillin-resistant staphylococci and many enterococci are resistant to all macrolides. These drugs are also active against *Corynebacterium* spp., *L. monocytogenes*, and *Actinomyces israelii* (9).

The antibacterial activities of macrolides against gram-negative bacilli are influenced by pH, with increasing potency (lower MICs) as the pH rises to 8.5. *H. influenzae* and *M. catarrhalis* are more susceptible to azithromycin (MIC_{90}, 0.5 μg/ml) than to other macrolides (8- to 16-fold higher MIC_{90}s) (129, 159, 172). However, additive (and possibly synergistic) activity between clarithromycin and its 14-hydroxy metabolite reduces the MIC of clarithromycin for *H. influenzae* by two- to fourfold (160). Clarithromycin is the most active drug in this class against *Chlamydia pneumoniae* (MIC_{90}, 0.25 μg/ml) and *Legionella* isolates (MIC_{90}, 0.25 μg/ml) (9). All four macrolides are equally potent against *Bordetella pertussis* and *Mycoplasma pneumoniae*, and erythromycin has long been established as the drug of choice for the therapy of infections due to these pathogens and *Legionella* spp. Macrolides are active against *Campylobacter* spp., *Helicobacter pylori*, *Pasteurella multocida*, *N. meningitidis*, and *Borrelia burgdorferi* (9, 140, 172, 226). Unlike other macrolides, azithromycin is also active in vitro against *E. coli*, *Shigella* spp., *Salmonella* spp., and *Y. enterolitica* (129, 159).

Macrolide antibiotics are effective in vitro against many pathogens that cause sexually transmitted diseases. *N. gonorrheae*, *Haemophilus ducreyi*, *Chlamydia trachomatis*, and *U. urealyticum* are all susceptible, but only azithromycin is active against *Mycoplasma hominis* (9, 159, 160). Erythromycin may be used for the treatment of gonorrhea and syphilis in patients who cannot tolerate penicillin G (29, 141), but data on the new macrolides for these indications are limited. Azithromycin is effective as an alternative to tetracyclines for the treatment of genital chlamydial infections (211). As a group, macrolides are among the most potent agents inhibitory toward *Bartonella* spp. (136).

The macrolides have good activity against anaerobic bacteria such as the *B. fragilis* group, *Fusobacterium* spp., *Prevotella* spp., *Porphyromonas* spp., *Propionibacterium acnes*, and anaerobic gram-positive cocci, with MIC_{90}s of 1 to 4 μg/ml (9). Except for dirithromycin, they are active against most *Clostridium* spp., especially *Clostridium perfringens*, with most strains being inhibited at ≤1 μg/ml. For this reason, erythromycin is commonly used preoperatively with or without neomycin as oral bowel preparations.

Atypical mycobacteria are more susceptible than *M. tuberculosis* to macrolide antibiotics (159, 160). The MIC_{90}s of clarithromycin and azithromycin for *Mycobacterium avium-intracellulare* complex are in the range of 2 to 4 μg/ml, allowing additive or synergistic killing activity of these organisms within infected macrophages when these drugs are combined with other antimycobacterial drugs (6). Erythromycin is used occasionally to treat infections due to *Mycobacterium scrofulaceum*, *M. kansasii*, and *M. chelonae* (146, 234) and in combination with ampicillin against *Nocardia asteroides* (76).

Spiramycin and the new macrolides offer comparable in vitro activity against *Toxoplasma gondii*, and they are effective in the treatment of toxoplasmosis (143). Although spiramycin has been used to treat cryptosporidiosis, its therapeutic efficacy remains to be proven (49).

Adverse Effects

The incidence of serious side effects related to the use of erythromycin is relatively low. Gastrointestinal irritation, such as abdominal cramps, nausea, vomiting, and diarrhea, is common with oral administration and can occur when the drug is given intravenously. These side effects occur less frequently with dirithromycin, clarithromycin, and azithromycin. Thrombophlebitis is associated with intravenous infusion, but it can be avoided by dilution of the dose in a large volume of fluid and by slow infusion. Hypersensitivity reactions include skin rash, fever, and eosinophilia. Cholestatic hepatitis occurring in adults has frequently been associated with the estolate form but has also been found with other forms of erythromycin (215). For this reason, erythromycin estolate is no longer recommended for use in adults.

Reversible hearing loss may occur with use of large doses and very high concentrations of erythromycin in serum (≥4 g/day), usually in elderly patients with renal insufficiency (22, 102). Ototoxicity has also been reported with high doses of clarithromycin and azithromycin used to treat M.

avium-intracellulare complex infections. Pseudomembranous colitis and superinfection of the gastrointestinal tract or vagina with *Candida* spp. or gram-negative bacilli occur rarely. Concurrent erythromycin therapy increases the levels of theophylline, cyclosporine, and digoxin in serum by interfering with their hepatic metabolism (230). It also increases the anticoagulant effect of warfarin. To date, no clinically significant interactions have been observed between these drugs and dirithromycin, clarithromycin, or azithromycin. However, cardiac arrhythmias have occurred during concurrent use of terfenadine with erythromycin or clarithromycin.

TETRACYCLINES

Tetracyclines are broad-spectrum bacteriostatic antibiotics with the hydronaphthacene nucleus, which contains four fused rings. The congeners form three groups based on their duration of action. Chlortetracycline, oxytetracycline, and tetracycline are short-acting, demeclocycline and methacycline are intermediate-acting, and doxycycline and minocycline are long-acting compounds.

Mechanism of Action

The tetracyclines act against susceptible microorganisms by inhibiting protein synthesis. They enter bacteria by an energy-dependent process and bind reversibly to the 30S ribosomal subunits of the bacteria (34). This process blocks the access of aminoacyl-tRNA to the RNA-ribosome complex, preventing bacterial polypeptide synthesis. Bacterial resistance to tetracycline occurs as a result of active efflux of the drug from the cell, an altered ribosomal target site that prevents binding of the drug, or production of modifying enzymes that inactivate the drug (209).

Pharmacology

Tetracyclines are incompletely absorbed from the gastrointestinal tract, but their absorption is improved in the fasting state. Ingestion of food, especially dairy products, and other substances such as antacids and iron preparations impairs the absorption of these drugs. Less interference with absorption by foods occurs with doxycycline and minocycline. These long-acting tetracyclines are more readily absorbed, and therefore lower doses are required. Peak concentrations in serum of 3 to 5 μg/ml are reached 2 h after standard oral dosages. Intravenous preparations are available, and peak concentrations in serum of 10 to 20 μg/ml are reached 1 h after intravenous administration. Tetracyclines are usually bacteriostatic at these clinically achievable concentrations in serum.

Tetracyclines are metabolized by the liver and concentrated in the bile. Biliary concentrations of tetracyclines are three to five times higher than the concurrent levels in plasma. These drugs accumulate in the blood of patients with hepatic insufficiency or with biliary obstruction. They should be avoided or used cautiously in reduced dosages in patients with impaired liver function.

These antibiotics are excreted primarily in the urine, except for doxycycline, which is excreted primarily (90%) as an inactive conjugate via the biliary tract in the feces. Renal failure prolongs the half-lives of the tetracyclines except doxycycline. Therefore, doxycycline is considered the tetracycline of choice for extrarenal infections in the presence of renal failure.

Tissue penetration of these drugs is excellent, but levels in CSF are low even in the presence of meningeal inflammation. Tetracyclines cross the placenta and are incorporated into fetal bone and teeth. They are excreted in high concentrations in human milk. Therefore, they are not advised for pregnant or lactating women. Minocycline, the most lipophilic tetracycline at physiologic pH, reaches relatively high concentrations in saliva and tears, making it an ideal antibiotic to eradicate the meningococcal carrier state (99, 105).

Spectrum of Activity

All tetracyclines have similar antimicrobial activity spectra, with activity against many gram-positive and gram-negative bacteria, mycoplasmas, chlamydiae, rickettsiae, and some protozoa. Many gram-positive aerobic cocci, including *S. aureus*, *S. pyogenes*, and *S. pneumoniae*, are susceptible at concentrations achievable in the serum. However, emergence of tetracycline-resistant strains of *S. pneumoniae* is frequent (123). Although many *E. coli* strains are susceptible to tetracyclines, pseudomonads and many of the *Enterobacteriaceae* are resistant. *Shigella* and *Salmonella* spp. are increasingly resistant to these agents (32). Tetracyclines are used mainly for the treatment of acute, uncomplicated urinary tract infections due to *E. coli* (110) and as effective prophylactic therapy for traveler's diarrhea caused by enterotoxigenic *E. coli* (80). With activity against *Pseudomonas pseudomallei*, *Brucella* spp., *Vibrio* spp., and *Mycobacterium marinum* (235), they have been used successfully in the treatment of infections due to these bacteria. Their efficacy in the therapy of cholera is diminishing owing to the emergence of resistant *Vibrio cholerae* isolates (260). Minocycline is active against *Nocardia* spp. (56). Many anaerobic bacteria, including members of the *B. fragilis* group and *Actinomyces* spp., are susceptible to tetracyclines (152, 204).

These drugs are useful in the treatment of urethritis and acute pelvic inflammatory diseases caused by *N. gonorrhoeae*, *C. trachomatis*, *U. urealyticum*, and *Mycoplasma hominis*. Emergence of resistance to tetracyclines among *N. gonorrhoeae* is increasing (73). The drugs are effective for the treatment of other chlamydial infections (psittacosis, lymphogranuloma venereum, and trachoma) (29, 141). Other infections responsive to tetracyclines include granuloma inguinale, chancroid, relapsing fever, and tularemia.

Tetracyclines are the drug of choice for treating rickettsial infections (Rocky Mountain spotted fever, endemic and scrub typhus, and Q fever). Many pathogenic spirochetes including *Treponema pallidum* and *Borrelia burgdorferi* are susceptible (29, 141, 142, 153). Protozoans such as *Plasmodium falciparum* and *Entamoeba histolytica* are also inhibited by these drugs (143, 167).

Adverse Effects

Tetracyclines have irritative effects on the upper gastrointestinal tract, producing esophageal ulcerations, nausea, vomiting, and epigastric distress. Alterations in the enteric flora occur with the use of tetracyclines, often resulting in diarrhea, and pseudomembranous colitis can develop after prolonged use. Hypersensitivity reactions are unusual, generally manifesting as urticaria, fixed drug eruptions, morbilliform rashes, and anaphylaxis. Cross-reactivity among tetracyclines is the rule. Photosensitivity reactions consist of an erythematous rash on areas exposed to sunlight and can occur with all analogs, especially demeclocycline (81).

Minocycline has been known to cause vertigo, and benign intracranial hypertension (pseudotumor cerebri) has occurred with many of the analogs (236). Tetracycline can aggravate preexisting renal failure by inhibiting protein synthesis, increasing the azotemia from amino acid metabolism.

It causes depression of bone growth, permanent discoloration of the teeth, and enamel hypoplasia when given during tooth and skeletal development (96). Therefore, these drugs are usually not given to children younger than 8 years or to pregnant women.

LINCOSAMIDES

The lincosamide antibiotics include lincomycin, which was initially isolated from *Streptomyces lincolnensis*, and clindamycin, which is a chemical modification of lincomycin. The chemical structure of each drug consists of an amino acid linked to an amino sugar. Compared with lincomycin, clindamycin has increased antibacterial activity and improved absorption after oral administration (139). Both drugs are available for parenteral and oral use, but lincomycin is rarely used now in the United States due to its lower efficacy.

Mechanism of Action

Lincosamides bind to the 50S ribosomal subunits of susceptible bacteria and prevent elongation of peptide chains by interfering with peptidyl transfer, thereby suppressing protein synthesis. The ribosomal binding sites are the same as or closely related to those that bind macrolides, streptogramins, and chloramphenicol (227). Lincosamides can be bactericidal or bacteriostatic, depending on the drug concentration, bacterial species, and inoculum of bacteria.

Pharmacology

About 90% of an oral clindamycin dose is absorbed from the gastrointestinal tract, with no interference from the ingestion of food. A single oral dose of 150 mg yields a peak concentration in serum of 2 to 3 μg/ml in 1 h. Peak levels in serum of 10 to 12 μg/ml are obtained 1 h after a 600-mg intravenous dose. Therapeutic drug levels in serum are maintained for 6 to 9 h after these dosages (139).

Clindamycin is distributed widely into the bone, lungs, pleural fluid, and bile, but it penetrates poorly into CSF, even in patients with meningitis. It readily crosses the placenta and enters fetal tissues. It is actively concentrated in neutrophils and macrophages.

The normal half-life of clindamycin is 2.4 h. Most of the drug is metabolized by the liver and excreted in an inactive form in the urine. Its half-life is prolonged by severe liver dysfunction, necessitating dosage reduction in patients with severe liver disease. Although the drug levels in serum are increased in patients with severe renal failure, dose modification is not essential. The drug is not removed significantly by hemodialysis or peritoneal dialysis.

Spectrum of Activity

Lincosamides have a broad spectrum of activity against the aerobic gram-positive cocci and anaerobes. Clindamycin is more potent than lincomycin against methicillin-susceptible *Staphylococcus* spp., *S. pneumoniae*, and group A and viridans streptococci (128, 139). The MIC_{90}s are in the range of 0.01 to 0.1 μg/ml for these strains. However, resistance to clindamycin has emerged in clinical isolates of these bacteria that are also resistant to erythromycin (33). The prevalence of clindamycin-resistant *S. aureus* may be 15 to 20% in some institutions. Enterococci are uniformly resistant to the lincosamides. All of the *Enterobacteriaceae* are resistant to lincosamides.

Clindamycin is one of the most active antibiotics available against anaerobes, including members of the *B. fragilis* group and *Clostridium perfringens*, with MIC_{90}s of $\leq$2 μg/ml (11, 216). However, clindamycin resistance (which appears to be increasing) is found in 10 to 15% of the *B. fragilis* group, 15 to 20% of *Prevotella* and *Porphyromonas* spp., 10 to 20% of clostridial species, 10% of peptococci, and most *Fusobacterium varium* strains (128, 204, 216). Clindamycin has been used successfully as single-agent therapy for actinomycosis (186), babesiosis (143, 254), and malaria (198). It is also effective in combination with pyrimethamine for toxoplasma encephalitis (48, 185) and in combination with primaquine for *Pneumocystis carinii* pneumonia (222).

Adverse Effects

Clindamycin-associated diarrhea occurs in up to 20% of patients, and use of this drug has been associated with pseudomembranous colitis caused by toxin-producing *C. difficile* (12). This complication is not dose related and may occur after oral or parenteral therapy. Prompt cessation of the antibiotic in conjunction with oral vancomycin, metronidazole, or bacitracin therapy is effective in reversing this complication.

Other uncommon side effects include skin rashes, fever, and reversible elevation of transaminase levels in serum. Clindamycin can block neuromuscular transmission and may potentiate the action of neuromuscular blocking agents during anesthesia.

GLYCOPEPTIDES AND LIPOPEPTIDES

Vancomycin, a bactericidal antibiotic obtained from *Streptomyces orientales*, is the only glycopeptide marketed for clinical use in the United States. Initially introduced for its efficacy against penicillin-resistant staphylococci, it has become most useful against methicillin-resistant staphylococci and in patients allergic to penicillins or cephalosporins. Teicoplanin (formerly teichomycin A), a new complex glycopeptide chemically related to vancomycin (205), is currently available for clinical use in most countries except the United States. Daptomycin (LY 146032) and ramoplanin (MDL 62198) are an investigational semisynthetic lipopeptide and lipoglycopeptide, respectively, with spectra of activity similar to those of the glycopeptides. Because of its excessive neuromuscular toxicities, the original clinical evaluation of daptomycin was stopped. It is currently being reevaluated for possible clinical (systemic or topical) use. Systemic toxicity may also limit the use of ramoplanin to topical application only.

Mechanism of Action

Glycopeptides inhibit peptidoglycan synthesis in the bacterial cell wall by complexing with the D-alanyl-D-alanine portion of the cell wall precursor (154). Daptomycin also acts by inhibiting bacterial peptidoglycan synthesis, but this is probably secondary to its interference with membrane transport of precursors (1). Resistance to glycopeptides is due to the presence of a complex series of bacterial cytoplasmic enzymes synthesizing abnormal peptidoglycan precursors terminating in D-Ala-D-lactate (instead of D-Ala-D-Ala), thereby markedly lowering the binding affinity with the glycopeptides (64).

Pharmacology

Vancomycin and teicoplanin can be administered orally or parenterally. After oral administration, the drugs are poorly absorbed, and high concentrations in stools are achieved, accounting for their efficacy in treating pseudomembranous colitis (74). Desirable peak and trough levels in serum of

20 to 50 and 5 to 15 μg/ml, respectively, are obtained after a 1-g intravenous dose of vancomycin every 12 h in healthy subjects. Similar drug concentrations in serum are reached with intravenous teicoplanin, which has the advantage of longer a half-life in serum and can be administered once daily. Therapeutic levels of both drugs are achieved in synovial, ascitic, pericardial, and pleural fluids, with variable penetration into the CSF occurring only in the presence of inflamed meninges (97, 144).

Vancomycin and teicoplanin have half-lives in serum of 6 and 45 h, respectively, in patients with healthy renal function, and they are eliminated from the body by glomerular filtration. In the presence of severe renal insufficiency, their excretion is prolonged to about 9 days, and they are not removed by hemodialysis or peritoneal dialysis.

Spectrum of Activity

Glycopeptides and lipopeptides are active mainly against aerobic and anaerobic gram-positive organisms, including methicillin-susceptible and -resistant staphylococci, streptococci, enterococci, *Corynebacterium* spp., *Bacillus* spp., *L. monocytogenes*, *Clostridium* spp., and *Actinomyces* spp. The MICs of vancomycin against *S. aureus*, *S. epidermidis*, streptococci, and enterococci are typically in the range of 0.25 to 2 μg/ml. The bactericidal activity varies, with MBCs being 20-fold higher than MICs for viridans streptococci. These agents are essentially bacteriostatic against enterococci. Teicoplanin (92, 94, 131) and ramoplanin are two to four times as active as vancomycin against these gram-positive cocci. Increasing resistance to vancomycin has emerged among clinical isolates of *Enterococcus faecalis* (64, 145), *E. faecium*, *E. gallinarum*, and coagulase-negative staphylococci (197). Cross-resistance with teicoplanin is variable in these strains, but most are susceptible to ramoplanin (115). Other naturally vancomycin-resistant gram-positive organisms include *Leuconostoc*, *Lactobacillus*, and *Pediococcus* spp., most of which are susceptible to ramoplanin (41, 115, 189).

Vancomycin is useful in the prevention and treatment of endocarditis due to gram-positive bacteria in patients who are allergic to penicillin (47, 249). It is the drug of choice for treating *Corynebacterium jeikeum* infections (87) and is useful for treating *Flavobacterium meningosepticum* meningitis (97) and antibiotic-associated *C. difficile* colitis (12, 74).

The glycopeptides and lipopeptides are not active against gram-negative organisms or mycobacteria. They show no cross-resistance with other unrelated antibiotics. They act synergistically with aminoglycosides or rifampin against staphylococci, streptococci, and enterococci (149, 223, 240, 241), and they are bactericidal with aminoglycosides against listeriae.

Adverse Effects

The most frequent side effects of vancomycin are fever, chills, and phlebitis at the site of infusion. Rapid or bolus infusion of vancomycin causes tingling and flushing of the face, neck, and thorax, known as the red man syndrome, as a result of histamine release by basophils and mast cells (176). This phenomenon is not due to allergic hypersensitivity. Allergic maculopapular or diffuse erythematous rashes occur in up to 5% of patients (207). Reversible leukopenia or eosinophilia is a rare effect of glycopeptide use.

Hearing loss due to ototoxicity have been described occasionally in patients in whom vancomycin concentrations in serum exceeded 50 mg/ml, but it is hard to find unequivocal evidence of vancomycin ototoxicity in humans or animals (22). Vancomycin-induced nephrotoxicity has been rare since the recent availability of highly purified vancomycin preparations. However, the risk of nephrotoxicity increases during combination therapy with vancomycin and aminoglycosides.

Teicoplanin is generally well tolerated and does not produce the red man syndrome or nephrotoxicity. It does cause irritation at the site of intravenous infusion, and ototoxicity has been reported (50).

STREPTOGRAMINS

Streptogramins are natural cyclic peptides produced by *Streptomyces* spp. They form a unique class of antibiotics in which each member is a combination of at least two structurally unrelated components, groups A and B streptogramins, acting synergistically against susceptible bacteria (171). Group A streptogramins are polyunsaturated macrolactones consisting of lactam and lactone linkages with an oxazole ring, and the main compounds in this group are pristinamycin II_A and pristinamycin II_B. Group B streptogramins are cyclic hexadepsipeptides, with pristinamycin I_A and pristinamycin I_C being the principal compounds. Quinupristin-dalfopristin (RP 59500) is the first injectable streptogramin antibiotic combination developed for clinical use in the United States. It is a 30:70 mixture of the semisynthetic streptogramins quinupristin and dalfopristin, which are water-soluble derivatives of pristinamycin I_A and pristinamycin II_A, respectively.

Mechanism of Action

The streptogramins exert synergistic bactericidal effect on susceptible organisms by inhibiting bacterial protein synthesis. They enter bacterial cells via passive diffusion and then bind specifically and irreversibly to the 50S subunits of the 70S bacterial ribosomes. Binding of group A streptogramins to the ribosome induces a conformational change in the ribosome, which increases its affinity for group B compounds. Group A streptogramins prevent peptide bond formation during the chain elongation step, while group B components cause the release of the incomplete peptide chains from the 50S ribosomal subunit (227).

Acquired bacterial resistance to the streptogramins, which may be chromosomal or plasmid mediated, is due mainly to modification of the drug target by methylation of the bacterial 23S rRNA, resulting in resistance to all macrolides, lincosamides, and group B streptogramins (MLS_B resistance phenotype) but not to group A streptogramins. Active efflux of group A and B streptogramins and drug inactivation by streptogramin A acetylase and streptogramin B hydrolase have been described.

Pharmacokinetics

Quinupristin-dalfopristin is administered intravenously and has a wide distribution into most tissues. Both components are highly protein bound (70 to 90%) and are rapidly cleared from plasma via biliary excretion by hepatic conjugation processes (130). Less than 20% of the administered drug combination is excreted in the urine. Following intravenous doses of 7.5 mg/kg, peak concentrations of quinupristin and dalfopristin in serum reach 2.7 and 7.2 μg/ml, respectively, with elimination half-lives of 1 and 0.75 h, respectively. The two components penetrate and accumulate in macrophages, and the ratio of the peak in vitro cellular to extracellular concentration is 50:35. The drug combination does not cross the uninflamed blood-brain barrier or the placenta to any significant degree. Dosage adjustment is needed for patients with renal insufficiency (creatinine clearance, <30 min/min), and the drug combination is removed in modest amounts by dialysis.

Spectrum of Activity

This class of drugs is active mainly against gram-positive bacteria, with activities against selected gram-negative and anaerobic pathogens. Quinupristin-dalfopristin has potent bactericidal activity against methicillin-susceptible and -resistant *S. aureus*, coagulase-neative staphylococci, and streptococci, with MIC_{90}s of ≤1 μg/ml and MBCs within two- to fourfold of the MICs (18, 75). Staphylococci and streptococci, including *S. pneumoniae*, that are resistant to β-lactam drugs, macrolides, and fluoroquinolones usually remain susceptible to quinupristin-dalfopristin. Enterococci are generally but not universally susceptible to the drug combination, with *E. faecalis* (MIC_{90}s, ≤32 μg/ml) being less susceptible than *E. faecium* (MIC_{90}s, ≤4 μg/ml). Although it is not bactericidal against enterococci, quinupristin-dalfopristin inhibits vancomycin-resistant entercocci (VanA or VanB phenotype), including multidrug-resistant *E. faecium*, at MIC_{90}s of ≤2 μg/ml (130). *Neisseria meningitidis, N. gonorrhoeae, Mycoplasma pneumoniae, Chlamydia pneumoniae,* and *Legionella pneumophila* are all highly susceptible to the drug (MIC_{90}s, ≤2 μg/ml). Quinupristin-dalfopristin is also active against *M. catarrhalis* and *H. influenzae*, with MIC_{90}s of ≤4 μg/ml. The *Enterobacteriaceae* and other nonfermenting gram-negative bacilli are resistant.

Among the anaerobes, *C. perfringens* and *C. difficile* are the most susceptible (MIC_{90}s, 0.25 μg/ml). Quinupristin-dalfopristin is active against the *B. fragilis* group (MIC_{90}, 4 μg/ml), as well as other anaerobic bacteria, including *Prevotella*, spp., *Porphyromonas* spp., *Fusobacterium* spp., *P. acnes, Lactobacillus* spp., and peptostreptococci, with MIC_{90}s of 2 to 4 μg/ml.

Adverse Effects

Major reactions are phlebitis at the site of intravenous infusion, and the incidence and severity are dose and concentration related (130). Adverse events that may lead to discontinuation of therapy in up to 5% of patients include arthralgia and myalgia, both of which are reversible on discontinuation of the combination. Elevated levels of transaminases in serum have also been reported. Cutaneous reactions such as itching, burning, and erythema of the face, neck, or upper torso have occurred rarely.

OXAZOLIDINONES

Oxazolidinones are a unique group of synthetic antimicrobial agents that were originally discovered in the 1970s (78). They interfere with formation of the initiation complex involving the 30S ribosomal subunit, thereby blocking the initiation phase of bacterial protein synthesis (202). In this regard they are unique, and there is no cross-resistance with other antibiotics that also inhibit ribosomal protein synthesis. As a group, oxazolidinones have varying activity against most gram-positive bacteria and mycobacteria, but the current analogs lack useful activity against most gram-negative bacilli. Linezolid is the first agent of this class of drugs currently undergoing clinical trials in humans.

Linezolid is available in oral and parenteral forms. Rapid and extensive absorption occurs after oral administration (>95% bioavailability), and the maximum concentration of 15 μg/ml in serum is reached within 2 h. The elimination half-life is about 5 to 7 h. With 30% of the drug being protein bound, it is well distributed in all body tissues, including the CSF. The drug is eliminated via the kidneys, with 30% being excreted unchanged in the urine.

Linezolid has excellent activity against staphylococci (including methicillin-resistant strains), streptococci, and multidrug-resistant enterococci, with MIC_{90}s of 1 to 4 μg/ml (265). The MIC_{90}s for penicillin- and cephalosporin-resistant pneumococci are in the range of 0.5 to 2 μg/ml. Although the antibacterial effect of linezolid is bacteriostatic, the drug is bactericidal against most strains of pneumococci. Other bacteria that are inhibited by linezolid include *B. cereus, Corynebacterium* spp., *L. monocytogenes, Clostridium* spp., and gram-positive anaerobic cocci. Phase III clinical trials of this drug in the United States for skin and soft tissue infections, respiratory tract infections, and infections due to vancomycin-resistant enterococci are under way. Preliminary clinical-trial data indicate minimal adverse effects from linezolid.

SULFONAMIDES AND TRIMETHOPRIM

Sulfonamides were the first effective systemic antimicrobial agents used in the United States during the 1930s. They are derived from sulfanilamide, which has chemical similarities with *p*-aminobenzoic acid, a factor essential for bacterial folic acid synthesis. Various substitutions at the sulfonyl radical attached to the benzene ring nucleus enhance the antibacterial activity and also determine pharmacologic properties of the drug.

Trimethoprim (TMP) is a pyrimidine analog that inhibits the enzyme dihydrofolate reductase, interfering with folic acid metabolism, subsequent pyrimidine synthesis, and one-carbon fragment metabolism in the bacteria. Since TMP and sulfonamides block the bacterial folic acid metabolic pathway at different sites, they potentiate the antibacterial activity of one another and act synergistically against a wide variety of organisms. One such combination, TMP-sulfamethoxazole (TMP-SMX), also called co-trimoxazole, was introduced clinically in 1968 and has proven very effective in the treatment of many infections (188, 191).

Mechanism of Action

Sulfonamides competitively inhibit bacterial modification of *p*-aminobenzoic acid into dihydrofolate, whereas TMP inhibits bacterial dihydrofolate reductase (Fig. 2). This sequential inhibition of folate metabolism ultimately prevents the synthesis of bacterial DNA (103). Since mammalian cells do not synthesize folic acid, human purine synthesis is not affected significantly by sulfonamides or TMP. The antibacterial effect of these agents may be reduced in patients receiving high doses of folinic acid.

Pharmacology

Sulfonamides are usually administered in the oral and topical forms; the intravenous preparations (sulfadiazine and sulfisoxazole) are rarely used. The sulfonamides vary in their durations of action. Thus, sulfamethizole and sulfisoxazole are short-acting, sulfadiazine and SMX are intermediate-acting, and sulfadoxine is a long-acting compound. Mafenide acetate (Sulfamylon cream) and silver sulfadiazine are applied topically in burn patients and have significant percutaneous absorption. Sulfacetamide is available as an ophthalmic preparation, and various combinations of other sulfonamides are available orally (triple sulfa, or trisulfapyrimidine) or as vaginal creams or suppositories.

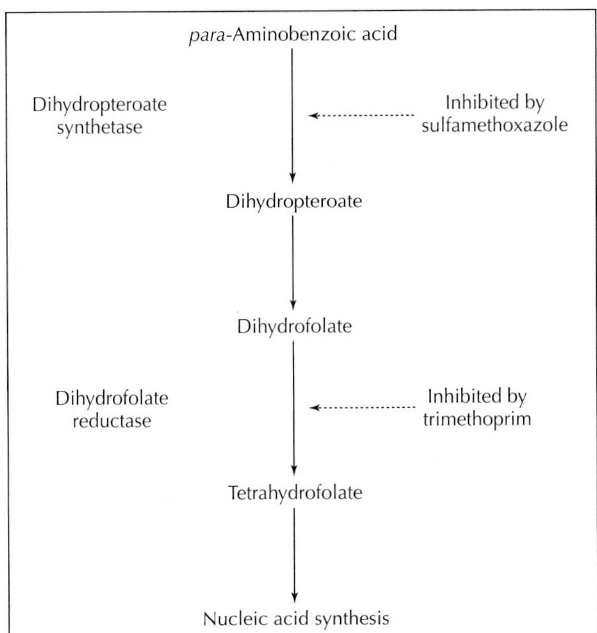

FIGURE 2 Mechanism of action of TMP-SMX.

The orally administered sulfonamides are absorbed rapidly and completely from the gastrointestinal tract. They are metabolized in the liver by acetylation and glucuronidation and are excreted by the kidneys as free drug and inactive metabolites. Sulfonamides compete for bilirubin-binding sites on plasma albumin and increase the levels of unconjugated bilirubin in blood. For this reason, they should not be given to neonates, in whom increased bilirubin levels in serum may cause kernicterus.

Sulfonamides are well distributed throughout the body, with levels in the CSF and synovial, pleural, and peritoneal fluids being about 80% of the levels in serum. They readily cross the placenta and enter the fetal circulation. Sulfonamides may be used in the presence of renal failure, but the drugs may accumulate during prolonged therapy as a result of reduced renal excretion.

TMP is available only for oral use and is absorbed almost completely from the gastrointestinal tract. After the usual 100-mg dose, peak levels in serum reach 1 μg/ml in 1 to 4 h. This drug is distributed widely in body tissues, including the kidneys, lungs, and prostate, and in body fluids (169). The levels in CSF are about 40% of the levels in serum. The half-life in serum is about 10 h in healthy subjects and is prolonged in those with renal insufficiency. Up to 80% of a dose is excreted unchanged in the urine by tubular secretion; the remaining fraction is excreted as inactive metabolites by the kidneys or in the bile.

A fixed combination of TMP-SMX in a dose ratio of 1:5 is available for oral and intravenous use. An intravenous dose of 160 mg of TMP with 800 mg of SMX produces average peak levels in serum of 3.4 and 47.3 μg/ml, respectively, in 1 h. Similar peak levels are reached 2 to 4 h after the same dose is taken orally. Both drugs are widely distributed in the body and reach therapeutic levels in the CSF (40% of the levels in serum). Excretion occurs primarily via the kidneys; dosage reduction is necessary in patients with creatinine clearances of $\leq$30 ml/min. Both TMP and SMX are removed by hemodialysis and partially removed by peritoneal dialysis.

Spectrum of Activity

Sulfonamides are inhibitory to a variety of gram-positive and gram-negative bacteria, actinomycetes, chlamydiae, toxoplasmas, and plasmodia. Their in vitro antimicrobial activities are irregular, being strongly influenced by the inoculum size and composition of the test media. Susceptibility-testing end points are often difficult to determine because of the presence of hazy growth within zones of inhibition in disk diffusion tests and because of the phenomenon of "trailing" in dilution tests. Sulfadiazine and sulfisoxazole are effective for rheumatic fever prophylaxis, but they are not useful in treating established group A beta-hemolytic streptococcal pharyngitis. These drugs may be used for prophylaxis of close contacts of patients with meningitis due to sulfonamide-susceptible *N. meningitidis*. Sulfisoxazole can be used to treat chlamydial urethritis, and sulfacetamide ophthalmic solution is effective for trachoma and inclusion conjunctivitis.

Sulfadiazine in combination with pyrimethamine has been used successfully to treat toxoplasmosis, and sulfadoxine combined with pyrimethamine (Fansidar) is effective in the prophylaxis and therapy of *Plasmodium falciparum* malaria (143). Sulfonamides are active against *Nocardia asteroides* (56), and they show moderate activity against *M. kansasii*, *M. fortuitum*, *M. marinum*, and *M. scrofulaceum* (184). Other uses of sulfonamides include therapy of melioidosis, dermatitis herpetiformis, lymphogranuloma venereum, and chancroid.

Among the gram-negative bacilli, *E. coli* strains were initially susceptible to the sulfonamides, especially at levels achievable in the urine. Therefore, these drugs have been used primarily in the treatment of first-episode acute urinary tract infections due to *E. coli*. However, increasing bacterial resistance has limited their efficacy in recent years. *Serratia marcescens*, *P. aeruginosa*, enterococci, and anaerobes are usually resistant to the sulfonamides.

TMP is active in vitro against many gram-positive cocci and most gram-negative bacilli. *P. aeruginosa*, most anaerobes, *Mycoplasma pneumoniae*, and mycobacteria are resistant. The MIC varies considerably with the test media used. Like the sulfonamides, TMP is used primarily in the therapy of uncomplicated and recurrent urinary tract infections due to susceptible organisms (110). However, the prevalence of TMP-resistant members of the *Enterobacteriaceae* is increasing (90).

Combinations of TMP with other agents, such as rifampin, polymyxins, and aminoglycosides, have demonstrated in vitro synergistic antibacterial activity against various gram-negative bacilli. TMP combined with dapsone is effective in the treatment of *Pneumocystis carinii* pneumonia in immunocompromised patients.

Many gram-positive cocci, including staphylococci and streptococci, and most gram-negative bacilli except *P. aeruginosa* are susceptible to TMP-SMX (25). However, 10 to 50% of strains of *S. pneumoniae* are resistant in many parts of the world (123). The drug combination has variable bactericidal effects on enterococci in vitro, depending on the test media used for susceptibility testing (155). Unlike many bacteria that can utilize only thymidine for growth, enterococci can use thymidine, thymine, exogenous folinic acid, dihydrofolate, and tetrahydrofolate, resulting in higher MICs (25- to 50-fold increase) on media containing these compounds (150). This fact also explains the ineffectiveness of TMP-SMX against enterococci in vivo.

With excellent activity against *M. catarrhalis* and *H. influenzae*, including β-lactamase-producing strains, TMP-SMX is useful for the therapy of acute otitis media, sinusitis, acute bronchitis, and pneumonia. It has shown excellent results in the prophylaxis and therapy of acute and chronic urinary tract infections (110, 212). It is an effective alternative therapy for uncomplicated urogenital gonorrhea, including cases caused by penicillinase-producing *N. gonorrhoeae* (29, 141). It can also be used for the treatment of chancroid, but resistance to TMP-SMX in *H. ducreyi* is increasing. The drug combination is also useful in treating infections due to salmonellae, shigellae, enteropathogenic *E. coli*, and *Y. enterocolitica* (188). It has been used successfully for prophylaxis and treatment of traveler's diarrhea (68), but resistance to TMP-SMX in *Shigella* spp. and *E. coli* now severely limits its usefulness in many parts of the world.

Other microorganisms susceptible to TMP-SMX include *Brucella* spp., *Burkholderia pseudomallei*, *B. cepacia*, *S. maltophilia*, *M. kansasii*, *M. marinum*, and *M. scrofulaceum*. *M. tuberculosis* and *M. chelonae* are generally resistant. It is a valuable antibiotic for the treatment of *Nocardia asteroides* infections (233), *B. cepacia* and *S. maltophilia* bacteremia, *L. monocytogenes* meningitis, gastroenteritis due to *Isospora belli* and *Cyclospora* spp. (143, 168), and Whipple's disease. In immunocompromised hosts (e.g., those with leukemia or AIDS and organ transplant recipients), TMP-SMX is effective for the prophylaxis and treatment of *Pneumocystis carinii* pneumonia (30, 263).

Adverse Effects

Sulfonamides are known to cause nausea, vomiting, headache, and fever. Hypersensitivity reactions can occur as rashes, vasculitis, erythema nodosum, erythema multiforme, and Stevens-Johnson syndrome (26). Very high doses of less water-soluble sulfonamides such as sulfadiazine may result in crystalluria, with renal tubular deposits of sulfonamide crystals. Bone marrow toxicity with anemia, leukopenia, or thrombocytopenia can occur. Sulfonamides should be avoided in patients with glucose-6-phosphate dehydrogenase deficiency, because of associated hemolytic anemia. Sulfonamides also potentiate the effects of warfarin, phenytoin, and oral hypoglycemic agents.

In general, TMP is well tolerated. With prolonged use, megaloblastic anemia, neutropenia, and thrombocytopenia can develop, especially in folate-deficient patients. Adverse reactions to TMP-SMX, due to either the TMP or, more commonly, the SMX component, can occur. Mild gastrointestinal symptoms and allergic skin rashes occur in about 3% of patients (127). Megaloblastic bone marrow changes with leukopenia, thrombocytopenia, or granulocytopenia may develop, usually in patients with preexisting folate deficiency. Nephrotoxicity usually occurs in patients with underlying renal dysfunction. Patients with AIDS have a much higher frequency of adverse reactions (as high as 70%) (91).

POLYPEPTIDES

Polymyxins

Polymyxins are a group of related cyclic basic polypeptides originally derived from *Bacillus polymyxa*. They have limited spectra of antimicrobial activity and significant toxicity. Only polymyxins B and E (colistin) are available for therapeutic use in humans.

Mechanism of Action

Acting like detergents or surfactants, members of this group of antibiotics interact with the phospholipids of the bacterial cell membrane, increasing the cell permeability and disrupting osmotic integrity. This process results in leakage of intracellular constituents, leading to cell death. The bactericidal action is reduced in the presence of calcium, which interferes with the attachment of drugs to the cell membrane.

Pharmacology

The polymyxins are usually administered by the parenteral, oral, or topical route. They are not significantly absorbed when given orally or topically, and intramuscular injections can be painful. Peak concentrations in serum of 5 μg/ml are obtained with a total daily dose of intravenous polymyxin B at 2.5 mg (25,000 U)/kg of body weight. Colistin sulfate is given orally for local antibacterial effect in the gut, while colistimethate sodium, a sulfomethyl derivative of colistin, is used for intramuscular injections. The half-life of polymyxin B in serum is 6 to 7 h, and that of colistin is 2 to 4 h. These drugs do not penetrate well into pleural fluid, synovial fluid, or CSF even in the presence of inflammation. Excretion is mostly via the kidneys by glomerular filtration. Levels in serum and toxicity are increased in the presence of renal insufficiency. These drugs are not removed by hemodialysis, but small amounts can be removed by peritoneal dialysis.

Polymyxin is often used topically as 0.1% polymyxin in combination with bacitracin or neomycin for treatment of skin, mucous membrane, eye, and ear infections. It is poorly absorbed from these surfaces. When the drug is used for irrigation of serous or wound cavities, systemic absorption can be great enough to produce toxicity.

Spectrum of Activity

Polymyxins are active only against gram-negative bacilli; especially *Pseudomonas* spp. The MIC_{90}s for *Pseudomonas* spp., including *P. aeruginosa*, are <8 μg/ml. *Proteus*, *Providencia*, *Serratia*, and *Neisseria* isolates are usually resistant. Emergence of resistance during therapy is rare, and there is no cross-resistance with other antibiotics. Polymyxins B and E have identical antimicrobial spectra and show complete cross-resistance to one another.

The combination of polymyxins with TMP-SMX may be synergistic in the treatment of serious infection due to multiply resistant *Serratia* spp., *P. aeruginosa*, *B. cepacia*, and *S. maltophilia* (55, 187). The polymyxins are usually reserved for serious, life-threatening *Pseudomonas* or gram-negative bacillary infections caused by organisms resistant to all other antibiotics. Aerosolized polymyxins have been used successfully to treat *P. aeruginosa* colonization or respiratory infections in patients with cystic fibrosis or bronchiectasis (72).

Adverse Effects

Neurotoxicity and nephrotoxicity are the two major side effects of polymyxins. Paresthesia with flushing, dizziness, vertigo, ataxia, slurred speech, drowsiness, or mental confusion occurs when levels in serum exceed 1 to 2 μg/ml. Polymyxins also have a curare-like effect that can block neuromuscular transmission. Dose-related renal dysfunction occurs in about 20% of patients receiving appropriate therapeutic dosages. Allergic reactions such as fever and skin rashes are rare, but urticaria and shock after rapid intravenous infusion have occurred.

Bacitracin

Originally isolated from *Bacillus licheniformis* (formerly *Bacillus subtilis*), bacitracin is a peptide antibiotic consisting of peptide-linked amino acids. Although it was introduced initially for the systematic treatment of severe staphylococcal infections, it is now restricted mainly to topical use because of its systemic toxicity.

Mechanism of Action

Bacitracin inhibits dephosphorylation of a lipid pyrophosphate, a step essential for bacterial cell wall synthesis. It also disrupts the bacterial cytoplastic membrane.

Pharmacology

Bacitracin is often used in various topical preparations, such as creams, ointments, antibiotic sprays and powders, and solutions for wound irrigation or bladder instillation. When it is used as a topical antibiotic, no significant amount is absorbed systemically. Large doses used to irrigate serous cavities may be associated with systemic toxicity.

Spectrum of Activity

Bacitracin is active mainly against gram-positive bacteria, particularly staphylococci and group A beta-hemolytic streptococci. However, group C and G streptococci are less susceptible, and group B streptococci are resistant (77). *Neisseria* spp. are also susceptible, but gram-negative bacilli are resistant. Bacitracin is often combined with neomycin, polymyxin B, or both in topical preparations to provide broad-spectrum antibacterial coverage. Orally administered bacitracin is effective in treating antibiotic-associated *C. difficile* colitis (59).

Adverse Effects

Systemic administration of bacitracin results in significant nephrotoxicity. Side effects are rare when the drug is given orally or applied topically. The drug is nonirritating to skin or mucous membranes. Allergic skin sensitization is rare.

CHLORAMPHENICOL

Chloramphenicol is a unique antibiotic originally derived from *Streptomyces venezuelae*. It contains a nitrobenzene ring. It is a highly effective broad-spectrum antimicrobial agent with specific indications for use in seriously ill patients. Thiamphenicol is an analog of chloramphenicol with a similar spectrum of antimicrobial activity (162). Only chloramphenicol is available for clinical use in the United States.

Mechanism of Action

The drug is a bacteriostatic agent that inhibits protein synthesis by binding reversibly to the peptidyltransferase component of the 50S ribosomal subunit and preventing the transpeptidation process of peptide chain elongation. At therapeutic concentrations achievable in the serum, it can be bactericidal against common meningeal pathogens such as *S. pneumoniae*, *N. meningitidis*, and *H. influenzae* (178). Bacterial resistance occurs as a result of plasmid-mediated production of chloramphenicol acetyltransferase, which inactivates the drug (200).

Pharmacology

Chloramphenicol is available for topical, oral, or parenteral use. It is not absorbed in any significant amount when applied topically, but it is rapidly and completely absorbed from the gastrointestinal tract. After an oral or intravenous dose of 1 g, peak concentrations in serum at 2 h can reach 10 to 15 μg/ml. It diffuses well into many tissues and body fluids, including CSF, where levels are generally 30 to 50% of the levels in serum even without meningeal inflammation (203). The antibiotic readily crosses the placental barrier and is present in human milk.

Chloramphenicol is metabolized and inactivated by glucuronidation in the liver, with a half-life of 4 h in adults. The active drug (5 to 10%) and its inactive metabolites are excreted by the kidneys. Careful monitoring of chloramphenicol levels in serum, maintaining peak concentrations in serum in the therapeutic range of 10 to 20 μg/ml, is useful for ensuring therapeutic efficacy and reduced toxicity. Patients with hepatic failure have high levels of active drug in serum owing to its prolonged half-life. Dosage modification is not necessary in the presence of renal insufficiency, since the metabolites are not as toxic as the active drug. Levels in serum are not affected by hemodialysis or peritoneal dialysis.

Spectrum of Activity

Chloramphenicol is very active against many gram-positive and gram-negative bacteria, chlamydiae, mycoplasmas, and rickettsiae. Its MIC_{90}s for most gram-positive aerobic and anaerobic cocci are ≤12.5 μg/ml (162). However, the drug is usually inactive against methicillin-resistant *S. aureus* and *S. epidermidis* and is variably active against enterococci. *N. meningitidis*, *H. influenzae* (ampicillin-resistant and -susceptible strains), and most of the *Enterobacteriaceae* are susceptible. Its activity against *Serratia* and *Enterobacter* isolates is variable, and *Pseudomonas* spp. are usually resistant. Salmonellae, including *Salmonella typhi*, are also susceptible, but resistant isolates are being encountered with increasing frequency (32).

Chloramphenicol has excellent activity against anaerobic bacteria, including members of the *B. fragilis* group. Almost all of these isolates are inhibited at concentrations of ≤10 μg/ml (152, 204). It is also active against *Rickettsia* spp. and *Coxiella burnetii*.

Adverse Effects

Bone marrow toxicity is the major complication of chloramphenicol use. This side effect may occur either as a dose-related bone marrow suppression or as an idiosyncratic aplastic anemia. Reversible bone marrow depression with anemia, leukopenia, and thrombocytopenia occurs as a result of a direct pharmacologic effect of the drug on hematopoiesis. High doses (>4 g/day), prolonged therapy, and excessively high levels in serum (>20 μg/ml) predispose patients to develop this type of complication. The second form of bone marrow toxicity is a rare but usually fatal complication that manifests as aplastic anemia. This response is not dose related, and the precise mechanism is unknown. It can occur weeks to months after the use of chloramphenicol, and it can develop after the use of oral, intravenous, or topical preparations.

Gray baby syndrome, characterized by vomiting, abdominal distension, cyanosis, hypothermia, and circulatory collapse, may occur in premature infants and neonates. This toxicity results from the immature hepatic function of neonates, which impairs hepatic inactivation of the drug.

Reversible optic neuritis causing decreased visual acuity has been reported in patients receiving prolonged therapy. Chloramphenicol occasionally causes hypersensitivity reactions, including skin rashes, drug fevers, and anaphylaxis. It potentiates the action of warfarin, phenytoin, and oral hypoglycemic agents by competitive inhibition of hepatic microsomal enzymes.

METRONIDAZOLE

Metronidazole is a 5-nitroimidazole derivative that was first introduced in 1959 for the treatment of *Trichomonas vaginalis* infections. It now plays an important therapeutic role in the treatment of infections due to anaerobic bacteria and certain protozoan parasites. Tinidazole and ornidazole are other 5-nitroimidazole derivatives and are investigational drugs at present in the United States.

Mechanism of Action

Metronidazole owes its bactericidal activity to the nitro group of its chemical structure. After the drug gains entry into the cells of susceptible organisms, the nitro group is reduced by a nitroreductase enzyme in the cytoplasm, generating certain short-lived, highly cytotoxic intermediate compounds or free radicals that disrupt host DNA (62). Resistance to nitroimidazoles may be due to decreased uptake of the drug or the presence of intracellular enzymes that can scavenge the free-radical intermediates.

Pharmacology

Metronidazole can be administered via the topical, oral, or intravenous route. It is absorbed rapidly and almost completely when given orally. Peak levels in serum of 6 μg/ml are obtained 1 h after an oral dose of 250 mg. Intravenous doses of 7.5 mg/kg result in peak concentrations in serum of 20 to 25 μg/ml. The drug has a half-life in serum of 8 h. Therapeutic levels are achieved in all body tissues and fluids, including abscess cavities and CSF, even without meningeal inflammation. The drug crosses the placenta and is secreted in breast milk. It is metabolized primarily by the liver, and 60 to 80% is excreted in the kidneys. In patients with impaired hepatic function, plasma clearance of metronidazole is delayed and dosage adjustments are necessary. The pharmacokinetics are minimally affected by renal insufficiency. Metronidazole and its metabolites are removed completely by dialysis.

Spectrum of Activity

Metronidazole exhibits potent activity against almost all anaerobic bacteria, including the *B. fragilis* group, *Fusobacterium* spp., and *Clostridium* spp. (11). It is the only antimicrobial agent with consistent bactericidal activity against members of the *B. fragilis* group. However, the susceptibility of gram-positive anaerobic cocci is somewhat variable, and the MIC_{90}s for these organisms are 16 μg/ml. Most strains of the genera *Actinomyces*, *Arachnia*, and *Propionibacterium* are resistant. Frequencies of metronidazole-resistant *B. fragilis* group isolates (MICs, >16 μg/ml) in the range of 2 to 5% have been reported from various institutions (152, 204). Tinidazole and ornidazole are somewhat more potent than metronidazole in their anti-anaerobe activities. Nitroimidazoles have no activity against aerobic bacteria, including the *Enterobacteriaceae*.

Metronidazole is effective in the treatment of antibiotic-associated colitis caused by *C. difficile* (12, 31), with efficacy equivalent to that of oral vancomycin for this indication (219). It is also useful in combination with an aminoglycoside for treating polymicrobial soft tissue infections and mixed aerobic-anaerobic intra-abdominal and pelvic infections.

Metronidazole is active against the protozoa *Trichomonas vaginalis*, *Giardia lamblia*, and *Entamoeba histolytica*. It is the drug of choice for the treatment of trichomoniasis, giardiasis, and intestinal and invasive amebiasis, including amebic liver abscess (143, 217, 255).

Adverse Effects

Metronidazole is generally well tolerated, and adverse effects are uncommon. It can cause mild gastrointestinal symptoms such as nausea, abdominal cramps, and diarrhea. An unpleasant, metallic taste may be experienced with oral therapy. Metronidazole can potentiate the effect of warfarin and prolong the prothrombin time.

Although metronidazole is carcinogenic in mice and rats, there is no evidence for increased carcinogenicity in humans. However, use of this agent in pregnancy, especially during the first trimester and in nursing mothers, should be avoided.

RIFAMPIN

Rifampin, also known as rifampicin, is a semisynthetic antibiotic, derived from rifamycin B, which belongs to a group of macrocyclic compounds produced by the mold *Streptomyces mediterranei*. Introduced for clinical use in 1968 as an effective antituberculous drug, this agent has activity against many bacteria. A closely related compound, rifabutin, a derivative of rifamycin S, is another potent antimycobacterial agent, especially against *M. avium* complex (166).

Mechanism of Action

Rifampin exerts its bactericidal effect by forming a stable complex with bacterial DNA-dependent RNA polymerase, preventing the chain initiation process of DNA transcription (243). Mammalian RNA synthesis is not affected, because the mammalian enzyme is much less sensitive to the drug. Rifampin-resistant isolates possess an altered RNA polymerase, which arises easily from single-step mutations during monotherapy with rifampin.

Pharmacology

The drug is well absorbed after oral administration, reaching peak concentrations in serum of 5 to 10 μg/ml 2 to 4 h following a 600-mg dose. A parenteral preparation is also available. Rifampin is deacetylated in the liver to an active metabolite and is excreted in the bile, and it undergoes enterohepatic circulation. The normal half-life in serum varies from 1.5 to 5 h. Dosage adjustments are necessary for patients with severe hepatic dysfunction.

Rifampin is well distributed to almost all body tissues and fluids, reaching concentrations equal to or exceeding that in the serum. Levels in the CSF are highest in the presence of inflamed meninges. It is able to enter phagocytes and kill living intracellular organisms (133), and it crosses the placenta. About 30 to 40% of the drug is excreted in the urine, and it does not accumulate in patients with impaired renal function. Hemodialysis and peritoneal dialysis do not eliminate the drug.

Spectrum of Activity

In addition to its well-known antimycobacterial effects (37), rifampin has a wide spectrum of antimicrobial activity. It is bactericidal against gram-positive cocci such as staphylococci (including methicillin-resistant strains), streptococci, and anaerobic cocci, with MICs in the range of 0.01 to 0.5 μg/ml. It remains an important adjunct in the combination therapy of serious and chronic staphylococcal infections (225). However, it is bacteriostatic against enterococci, with usual MICs of <16 μg/ml (149).

Neisseria gonorrhoeae, *N. meningitidis*, and *H. influenzae*, including β-lactamase-producing strains, are susceptible to rifampin, which is used frequently in the prophylaxis of meningococcal and *H. influenzae* type b meningitis (99). MICs for the *Enterobacteriaceae* are ≤12 μg/ml, while MICs for *Serratia marcescens* and *P. aeruginosa* are higher (149). Besides fluoroquinolones, rifampin is one of the most active agents against *Legionella pneumophila* and other *Legionella* spp., with MICs of ≤0.03 μg/ml. Because of its ability to enter phagocytes, rifampin inhibits the growth of *Brucella* spp. and *Coxiella burnetii* intracellularly (180), and it is used frequently in the combination therapy of infections due to these organisms. Although *Chlamydia* spp. are very susceptible to rifampin in vitro, resistance emerges rapidly when rifampin is used alone.

Adverse Effects

Rifampin has many side effects, including gastrointestinal discomfort and hypersentivity reactions, such as drug fever, skin rashes, and eosinophilia. It produces a harmless, orange-red coloration of saliva, tears, urine, and sweat. In up to 20% of patients, an influenza-like syndrome with fever, chills, arthralgias, and myalgias develops after several months of intermittent therapy (95). This immunologic reaction may occur in conjunction with hemolytic anemia, thrombocytopenia, and renal failure. Rifampin-induced hepatitis occurs in <1% of patients and is more frequent during concurrent isoniazid therapy for tuberculosis. The drug is known to antagonize the effect of oral contraceptives and to diminish the anticoagulant activity of warfarin.

NITROFURANTOIN

Nitrofurantoin belongs to a class of compounds consisting of a primary nitro group joined to a heterocyclic ring. Its role in human therapeutics is limited to treatment of urinary tract infections (110).

Mechanism of Action

The precise mechanism of action of nitrofurantoin is unknown. The drug is believed to inhibit various bacterial enzymes and also damage DNA (137).

Pharmacology

The drug is available in microcrystalline (Furadantin) and macrocrystalline (Macrodantin) forms. It is administered orally and is well absorbed from the gastrointestinal tract. Very low levels of the drug are achieved in serum and most body tissues after the usual oral doses. With a half-life in serum of about 20 min, two-thirds of the drug is rapidly metabolized and inactivated in various tissues. The remaining one-third is excreted unchanged into the urine. An average dose of nitrofurantoin yields a concentration in urine of 50 to 250 μg/ml in patients with healthy renal function. In alkaline urine, more of the drug is dissociated into the ionized form, resulting in lowered antibacterial activity. Nitrofurantoin accumulates in the sera of patients with creatinine clearances of <60 ml/min. The drug is removed by hemodialysis. The risk of systemic toxicity increases in the presence of severe uremia. Nitrofurantoin is contraindicated in patients with significant renal impairment and hepatic failure.

Spectrum of Activity

Nitrofurantoin has a broad spectrum of antibacterial activity against gram-positive and gram-negative bacteria, particularly the common urinary tract pathogens. It is active against gram-positive cocci, such as *S. aureus*, *S. epidermidis*, *Staphylococcus saprophyticus*, and *Enterococcus faecalis*, with MICs in the range of 4 to 25 μg/ml (106). *S. pneumoniae*, *S. pyogenes*, *Bacillus subtilis*, and *Corynebacterium* spp. are also susceptible, but they rarely cause urinary tract infections. Over 90% of *E. coli* and many coliform bacteria are susceptible to nitrofurantoin (MICs, <32 μg/ml). However, only one-third of *Enterobacter* and *Klebsiella* isolates are susceptible. *Pseudomonas* and most *Proteus* spp. are resistant. Susceptible organisms rarely become resistant to this drug during therapy.

Adverse Effects

Gastrointestinal irritation, with anorexia, nausea, and vomiting, is the most common side effect. Diarrhea and abdominal cramps may occur. Hypersensitivity reactions, such as drug fever, chills, arthralgia, skin rashes, and a lupus-like syndrome, have been observed (108).

Pulmonary reactions are the most common serious side effects associated with nitrofurantoin use. Acute pneumonitis with fever, cough, dyspnea, eosinophilia, and pulmonary infiltrates present on chest X-ray films can occur after a few days of therapy (108). This immunologically mediated reaction is more common in elderly patients and is rapidly reversible on cessation of therapy. Chronic pulmonary reactions with interstitial pneumonitis leading to irreversible pulmonary fibrosis can occur in patients receiving continuous therapy for 6 months or more.

Peripheral polyneuropathy is a serious side effect, which occurs more often in patients with renal failure. Hemolytic anemia, megaloblastic anemia, and bone marrow suppression with leukopenia can occur. Rare hepatotoxic reactions, such as cholestatic jaundice and chronic active hepatitis, have been reported (199).

FOSFOMYCIN

Fosfomycin, first isolated from cultures of *Streptomyces* spp. in 1969, is a phosphonic acid derivative, which was originally named phosphonomycin (213). In the United States, it is used as single-dose therapy for uncomplicated urinary tract infections due to susceptible organisms (110).

Mechanism of Action

Fosfomycin is bactericidal by inhibiting pyruvyl transferase, a bacterial cytoplasmic enzyme that catalyzes the formation of uridine diphosphate–*N*-acetylmuramic acid during the first step of peptidoglycan synthesis (120). There is little cross-resistance between fosfomycin and other antibacterial agents, most probably because it differs from other agents in its chemical structure and site of action.

Pharmacology

Originally formulated as sodium and calcium salts for oral and intravenous use, fosfomycin is available in the United States as an oral, water-soluble tromethamine salt. Following oral administration, the compound is rapidly absorbed and converted to the free acid, fosfomycin. With markedly improved oral bioavailability (35 to 40%), fosfomycin has a mean elimination half-life of 5.5 h, and it is primarily excreted unchanged in the urine (170). Following a single oral dose of 3 g, peak concentrations in serum (range, 22 to 32 μg/ml) are achieved in 2 h after administration, with peak concentrations in urine (1,000 to 4,400 μg/ml) occurring within 4 h and remaining high (>128 μg/ml) for 24 to 48 h, sufficient to inhibit most urinary tract pathogens. Peak concentrations in urine are reached later and are lower when the drug is administered with food or antiperistaltic agents. In patients with renal impairment (creatinine clearance, <30 ml/min), the peak concentrations of fosfomycin in serum are increased, with decreased urinary elimination and reduced urinary concentrations of the drug.

While not bound to plasma protein, fosfomycin is widely distributed in various body fluids and tissues, including the kidneys, prostate, and seminal vesicles, from which it is cleared slowly. Although it crosses the placental barrier, the drug can be used safely during pregnancy if clearly needed.

Spectrum of Activity

Fosfomycin has a broad spectrum of antibacterial activity against most gram-positive and gram-negative bacteria isolated from patients with lower urinary tract infections. *E. coli*, *Serratia* spp., *Klebsiella* spp., *Citrobacter* spp., *Enterobacter* spp., *S. aureus*, and enterococci are generally inhibited by fosfomycin at concentrations of <64 μg/ml (7, 170, 173). Fosfomycin is bactericidal at concentrations that are similar to the MICs (≤2-fold differences). It is more active than trimethoprim and nalidixic acid and is similar to norfloxacin and co-trimoxazole in its activity against these organisms (7). At a breakpoint concentration of ≤128 μg/ml, 60, 20, and 80% of isolates of *Pseudomonas* spp., *Morganella morganii*, and *S. saprophyticus*, respectively, are susceptible to fosfomycin (173). In multiple-dose use, bacterial resistance to fosfomycin emerges rapidly, and it can be chromosomally or, more rarely, plasmid mediated. However, cross-resistance with other antimicrobial agents has been uncommon (181).

The in vitro activity of fosfomycin is affected by the test medium and conditions (170, 173). Fosfomycin has much greater in vitro activity, and closer correlation with in vivo activity, when the test medium is supplemented with glucose-6-phosphate at 25 μg/ml, which is recommended for susceptibility testing by the agar and broth dilution methods. The disk diffusion testing method involves disks containing 200 μg of fosfomycin tromethamine and 50 or 100 μg of glucose-6-phosphate.

Adverse Effects

Mild, self-limiting gastrointestinal disturbances, mainly diarrhea, are the most frequent side effects (3 to 5% of patients are affected). Other minor adverse events include headaches, dizziness, rash, and vaginitis.

METHENAMINE

Methenamine is a tertiary amine with properties of a monoacidic base; it is used as a urinary antiseptic. To be activated, it is combined chemically with a poorly metabolized acid and administered as the mandelate (Mandelamine) or hippurate (Hiprex, Urex) salt.

Mechanism of Action

Methenamine has no antibacterial action by itself, but it is converted at acidic pH to ammonia and formaldehyde, which provides the antiseptic action. This hydrolytic process occurs in the urine, and an effective bacteriostatic concentration of formaldehyde is reached at a urine pH of <5.5. Since the serum is at physiologic pH, formaldehyde is not released while methenamine circulates in the body.

Pharmacology

The agent is well absorbed from the gastrointestinal tract and is rapidly excreted in the urine. The elimination half-life of methenamine is about 4 h. At a urine pH of 5.0, about 20% of methenamine excreted in the urine is hydrolyzed to formaldehyde and ammonia. Bactericidal levels (>20 mg/ml) of formaldehyde are generated in the bladder urine 2 h after oral administration and may be maintained for at least 6 h or until the patient voids (125). The mandelate and hippurate moieties are also rapidly excreted in the urine in active, unchanged forms by glomerular filtration and tubular secretion. The agent is contraindicated in patients with hepatic insufficiency because of the ammonia produced.

Spectrum of Activity

With the liberation of enough formaldehyde into the urine, methenamine is essentially active against all gram-positive and gram-negative bacteria and also against fungi (125). However, it is not effective for treating urinary tract infections due to urea-splitting organisms such as *Proteus* and *Morganella*, which can convert urea to ammonium hydroxide, thereby preventing the hyrolysis of methenamine to formaldehyde. A combination with acetohydroxamic acid, a urease inhibitor, has been suggested for treating these infections by *Proteus* and *Morganella*. Since bacteria and fungi do not become resistant to formaldehyde, emergence of resistance to methenamine is not a problem.

Methenamine is not useful for acute urinary tract infections. It has been used successfully as prophylactic therapy for recurrent bacteriuria, particularly cases caused by highly resistant gram-negative bacilli or yeasts. It is also effective as prolonged suppressive therapy for chronic bacteriuria in the absence of structural abnormalities of the urinary tract.

Adverse Effects

Methenamine and its acid salts are generally well tolerated. Some patients develop nausea, vomiting, abdominal cramps, and diarrhea. High doses or prolonged administration of the drug can cause urinary tract irritation by the free formaldehyde, resulting in urinary frequency, dysuria, albuminuria, and hematuria. Skin rashes may also occur. To avoid precipitation of urate crystals in the urine, methenamine salts should not be used in patients with gout or hyperuricemia.

MUPIROCIN

Mupirocin, formerly pseudomonic acid A, is a topical antibacterial agent derived from the fermentation products of *Pseudomonas fluorescens* (85). Structurally, it contains a unique 9-hydroxynonanoic acid moiety. It was developed for the topical treatment of superficial soft tissue infections, particularly those due to staphylococci.

In the United States, mupirocin is available as a 2% ointment or cream (Bactroban). After topical application, <1% of the drug is absorbed systemically, with no detectable levels in the urine or feces. Penetration into deeper dermal layers of the skin is increased with traumatized skin or use of occlusive dressings. The drug is highly protein bound (95%), and its activity is lowered in the presence of serum. It is most active at moderately acid pH, with no inoculum effect (237). Mupirocin is slowly metabolized in the skin to the inactive monic acid.

Mupirocin inhibits isoleucyl-tRNA synthetase, resulting in cessation of bacterial tRNA and protein synthesis (112). It has excellent in vitro activity, primarily against the gram-positive cocci. *S. aureus*, including methicillin-resistant strains, and coagulase-negative staphylococci are uniformly very susceptible (MIC_{90}s, <0.5 μg/ml) (27). The emergence of resistant strains of staphylococci can occur with widespread use of mupirocin (19, 20). Most streptococci (including *S. pneumoniae*; beta-hemolytic streptococci of groups A, B, C, and G; and viridans streptococci) are inhibited by concentrations of ≤1 μg/ml. Resistant bacteria include enterococci, *Corynebacterium* spp., *Erysipelothrix* spp., *Propionibacterium acnes*, gram-positive anaerobes, and most gram-negative bacteria. However, *H. influenzae*, *N. gonorrhoeae*, *N. meningitidis*, *M. catarrhalis*, *Bordetella pertussis*, and *Pasteurella multocida* are quite susceptible (MICs, 0.02 to 0.025 μg/ml). There is no cross-resistance between mupirocin and other major groups of antibiotics. Clinically, mupirocin is efficacious in the therapy of superficial skin infections, such as impetigo, folliculitis, and burn wound infections, that are due to staphylococci or streptococci (89). It has been used successfully to eradicate nasal carriage of *S. aureus*, including methicillin-resistant strains (28, 57).

No systemic toxic effects have been reported with mupirocin. Local irritation, such as burning, stinging, itch, and rash, which may be due to the polyethylene glycol base in the vehicle ointment, may occur.

APPENDIX 1
Approximate Concentrations of Antibacterial Agents in Serum

The concentrations of antimicrobial agents listed below are approximations taken from various reports and publications. Several factors can influence the level of an antimicrobial agent in individual patients, including inherent differences in the patients themselves, their physical condition, the dosages, and the routes of administration. The values can also be influenced by the assay methods used to obtain them. Therefore, these concentrations should be used only as approximate values, and clinicians should use their knowledge of the patient and the drugs, the recommendations in the U.S. Food and Drug Administration-approved package inserts, and other reputable sources in planning their therapeutic regimens.

Antimicrobial agent	Half-life in serum (h)	Unit dose	Avg peak level in serum (μg/ml)[a]		
			p.o.	i.m.	i.v.
Amikacin	2–2.5	7.5 mg/kg		15–20	20–40
Amoxicillin	1	500 mg	6–8		
Amoxicillin-clavulanate	1.3/1.0	250/125 mg	3.3 (Amox) 1.5 (Clav)		
Ampicillin	1.1	500 mg	2.5–5	8–10	
		1 g			40
Ampicillin-sulbactam	1.1/1.0	3 g			120 (Amp) 60 (Sulb)
		1.5 g			18 (Amp) 13 (Sulb)
Azithromycin	48	500 mg	0.4		3.5
Azlocillin	1	2 g			130
Aztreonam	1.7	1 g		45	90–160
Bacampicillin	1.1	800 mg	13		
Carbenicillin	1.1	1 g		20–30	150
Carbenicillin indanyl sodium	1.1	764 mg	10		
Cefaclor	0.6	500 mg	16		
Cefadroxil	1.5	500 mg	10		
Cefamandole	0.5–1	1 g		20–36	90–140
Cefazolin	1.8	1 g		65	185
Cefepime	2	1 g		30	82
Cefdinir	4.5	600 mg	3		
Cefixime	3–4	400 mg	3.5		
Cefmetazole	1.5	1 g			70
Cefonicid	4	1 g		98	220
Cefoperazone	2	1 g		65–75	153
Ceforanide	3	1 g		70	125
Cefotaxime	1	1 g		20	40–45
Cefotetan	3–4.5	1 g		50–80	160
Cefoxitin	1	1 g		20–25	55–110
Cefpirome	2	1 g		45	85
Cefpodoxime	2.5	200 mg	2.3		
Cefprozil	1.3	500 mg	10.5		
Ceftazidime	1.9	1 g		40	70
Ceftibuten	2.4	400 mg	15		
Ceftizoxime	1.4–1.8	1 g		39	80–90

(Continued on next page)

Antimicrobial agent	Half-life in serum (h)	Unit dose	Avg peak level in serum (μg/ml)[a]		
			p.o.	i.m.	i.v.
Ceftriaxone	6–9	500 mg		40–45	
		1 g			150
Cefuroxime	1.3	750 mg		27	50
Cefuroxime axetil	1.3	500 mg	9		
Cephalexin	0.9	500 mg	18		
Cephalothin	0.6	1 g			30–60
Cephapirin	0.6	1 g			40–70
Cephradine	0.8	500 mg	16		
Chloramphenicol	4	1 g	10–18		10–15
Chlortetracycline	6–9	500 mg	2–4	12	
Cinoxacin	1–1.5	500 mg	15		
Ciprofloxacin	3.5	500 mg	2.5		
		400 mg			4.5
Clarithromycin	5	250 mg	0.5–1		
Clinafloxacin	5.2	200 mg	1.5		
Clindamycin	2.5	300 mg	3	6	
		600 mg			10–12
Cloxacillin	0.5	500 mg	10		
Colistimethate sodium	2–4.5	150 mg		5–6	
Demeclocycline	12	300 mg	1–2		
Dicloxacillin	0.5–0.7	500 mg	15		
Dirithromycin	40	500 mg	0.5		
Doxycycline	18–22	100 mg	2.5		4
Enoxacin	4–6	400 mg	3–5		
Erythromycin	1.5	500 mg	2–3		
		1 g			10
Fleroxacin	12	400 mg	5		7–8
Fosfomycin	5.7	3 g	25		
		50 mg/kg			275
Fusidic acid	13–19	500 mg	25–30		50
Gentamicin	2–3	1.5 mg/kg	4–6		4–8
Grepafloxacin	15	400 mg	1–1.5		
Imipenem	1	500 mg			25–35
Kanamycin	2.2–3	7.5 mg/kg		20–25	
Levofloxacin	6–8	500 mg	5.5		6.5
Lincomycin	5	500 mg	4		
		600 mg		9–18	
Linezolid	5–7	500 mg			15
Lomefloxacin	6.5	400 mg	3		
Loracarbef	1	400 mg	14		
Meropenem	1	500 mg			25–35
Methacycline	14	300 mg	2.5		
Methicillin	0.5	1 g		10–18	60
Metronidazole	8	500 mg	12		20–25
Mezlocillin	1	1 g			15
		3 g			260
Minocycline	14–16	100 mg	1		
Nafcillin	0.5	500 mg			5–8
		1 g			20–40
Nalidixic acid	1.5	1 g	20–40		
Netilmicin	2.5	2 mg/kg		5–7	6–8
Nitrofurantoin	0.3	100 mg	<2		
Norfloxacin	3.3	400 mg	1.5		
Ofloxacin	5	400 mg	4		
Ornidazole	12	500 mg	10		20–25
Oxacillin	0.5	500 mg	4–6	14–16	
		1 g			40
Oxytetracycline	9	500 mg	1–2		
Pefloxacin	10	400 mg	3		5.5

(Continued on next page)

Antimicrobial agent	Half-life in serum (h)	Unit dose	Avg peak level in serum (μg/ml)[a]		
			p.o.	i.m.	i.v.
Penicillin G	0.5	500 mg	1.5–2.5		
Aqueous		1 × 10^6 U		8–10	10
Benzathine		1.2 × 10^6 U		0.1–0.15	
Procaine		1.2 × 10^6 U		3	
Penicillin V	0.5	500 mg	3–5		
Piperacillin	1.1	2 g			36
		4 g			240
Piperacillin-tazobactam	1.1/1	3.375 g			242 (Pip) 24 (Tazo)
		4.5 g			298 (Pip) 34 (Tazo)
Pivampicillin	0.5–1	350 mg	2		
Polymyxin B	6–7	2.5 mg/kg			5
Quinupristin-dalfopristin	1/0.75	7.5 mg/kg			2.8 (Q) 7.2 (D)
Rifampin	2–5	600 mg	7–9		10
Sparfloxacin	20	200 mg	1.1		
Spectinomycin	1–2	2 g		100	
Spiramycin	3.8	2 g	3		
Streptomycin	2–3	1 g		25–50	
Sulfadiazine	17	2 g	100–150		
Sulfadoxine	150–200	1 g	50–75		
Sulfamethizole	4–7	2 g	60		
Sulfamethoxazole	10–12	1 g	40		
Sulfisoxazole	5–7	2 g	170		
Teicoplanin	45	200 mg		7	
		400 mg			20–40
Tetracycline	8	500 mg	4		8
Ticarcillin	1.2	1 g		20–30	
		3 g			190
Ticarcillin-clavulanate	1.2/1.0	3.1 g			330 (Ticar) 8 (Clav)
Tinidazole	12–14	2 g	40		40
Tobramycin	2–2.8	1.5 mg/kg		4–6	4–8
Trimethoprim	10–12	100 mg	1		
TMP-SMX		160/800 mg	3 (TMP) 46 (SMX)		9 (TMP) 106 (SMX)
Trovafloxacin (alatrofloxacin)	11	200 mg	2.2		3
		300 mg			4.4
Vancomycin	6	500 mg			20–40

[a] At 30 min following intravenous infusion. p.o., oral; i.m., intramuscular, i.v., intravenous.

REFERENCES

1. **Allen, N. E., J. N. Hobbs, Jr., and W. E. Alborn, Jr.** 1987. Inhibition of peptidoglycan biosynthesis in gram-positive bacteria by LY146032. *Antimicrob. Agents Chemother.* **31:**1093–1099.
2. **Anderson, J. A.** 1986. Cross-sensitivity to cephalosporins in patients allergic to penicillin. *Pediatr. Infect. Dis. J.* **5:** 557–561.
3. **Appelbaum, P. C., M. R. Jacobs, S. K. Spangler, and S. Yamabe.** 1986. Comparative activity of β-lactamase inhibitors YTR 830, clavulanate, and sulbactam combined with β-lactams against β-lactamase-producing anaerobes. *Antimicrob. Agents Chemother.* **30:**789–791.
4. **Aswapokee, N., and H. C. Neu.** 1978. A sulfone beta-lactam compound which acts as a beta-lactamase inhibitor. *J. Antibiot.* **31:**1238–1244.
5. **Bansal, M. B., S. K. Chuah, and H. Thadepalli.** 1985. In vitro activity and in vivo evaluation of ticarcillin plus clavulanic acid against aerobic and anaerobic bacteria. *Am. J. Med.* **79**(Suppl. 5B)**:**33–38.
6. **Barradell, L. B., G. L. Plosker, and D. McTavish.** 1993. Clarithromycin: a review of its pharmacological properties and therapeutic use in *Mycobacterium avium-intracellulaire* complex infection in patients with acquired immune deficiency syndrome. *Drugs* **46:**289–312.
7. **Barry, A. L., and S. D. Brown.** 1995. Antibacterial spectrum of fosfomycin trometamol. *J. Antimicrob. Chemother.* **35:**228–230.
8. **Barry, A. L., and R. N. Jones.** 1987. Cefixime: spectrum of antibacterial activity against 16,016 clinical isolates. *Pediatr. Infect. Dis. J.* **6:**954–957.
9. **Barry, A. L., R. N. Jones, and C. Thornsberry.** 1988. In vitro activities of azithromycin (CP 62,993), clarithromycin (A-56268, TE-031), erythromycin, roxithromycin, and clindamycin. *Antimicrob. Agents Chemother.* **32:** 752–754.
10. **Barry, A. L., C. Thornsberry, R. N. Jones, and T. L.**

Gavan. 1985. Aztreonam: antibacterial activity, β-lactamase stability, and interpretive standards and quality control guidelines for disk-diffusion susceptibility test. *Rev. Infect. Dis.* **7**(Suppl. 4)**:**S594–S604.
11. **Bartlett, J. G.** 1982. Anti-anaerobic antibacterial agents. *Lancet* **ii:**478–481.
12. **Bartlett, J. G.** 1992. Antibiotic-associated diarrhea. *Clin. Infect. Dis.* **15:**573–579.
13. **Barza, M.** 1985. Imipenem: first of a new class of β-lactam antibiotics. *Ann. Intern. Med.* **103:**552–560.
14. **Bates, R. D., and M. C. Nahata.** 1994. Once-daily administration of aminoglycosides. *Ann. Pharmacother.* **28:** 757–766.
15. **Bauernfeind, A.** 1993. In-vitro activity of dirithromycin in comparison with other new and established macrolides. *J. Antimicrob. Chemother.* **31:**(Suppl. 3C)**:**39–49.
16. **Berkey, P., D. Moore, and K. Rolston.** 1988. In vitro susceptibilities of *Nocardia* species to newer antimicrobial agents. *Antimicrob. Agents Chemother.* **32:**1078–1079.
17. **Beskid, G., and B. L. T. Prosser.** 1993. A multicenter study on the comparative in vitro activity of fleroxacin and three other fluoroquinolones: an interim report from 27 centers. *Am. J. Med.* **94:**(Suppl. 3A)**:**2S–8S.
18. **Bouanchaud, D. H.** 1997. In-vitro and in-vivo antibacterial activity of quinupristin/dalfopristin. *J. Antimicrob. Chemother.* **39**(Suppl. A)**:**15–21.
19. **Boyce, J. M.** 1996. Preventing staphylococcal infections by eradicating nasal carriage of *Staphylococcus aureus*: proceeding with caution. *Infect. Control Hosp. Epidemiol.* **17:** 775–779.
20. **Bradley, S. F., M. A. Ramsey, T. M. Morton, and C. A. Kauffman.** 1995. Mupirocin resistance: clinical and molecular epidemiology. *Infect. Control Hosp. Epidemiol.* **16:** 354–358.
21. **Brighty, K. E., and T. D. Gootz.** 1997. The chemistry and biological profile of trovafloxacin. *J. Antimicrob. Chemother.* **39:**(Suppl. B)**:**1–14.
22. **Brummett, R. E., and K. E. Fox.** 1989. Vancomycin- and erythromycin-induced hearing loss in humans. *Antimicrob. Agents Chemother.* **33:**791–796.
23. **Buesing, M. A., and J. H. Jorgensen.** 1984. In vitro activity of aztreonam in combination with newer β-lactams and amikacin against multiply resistant gram-negative bacilli. *Antimicrob. Agents Chemother.* **25:**283–285.
24. **Bush, K., J. S. Freudenberger, and R. B. Sykes.** 1982. Interaction of azthreonam and related monobactams with β-lactamases from gram-negative bacteria. *Antimicrob. Agents Chemother.* **22:**414–420.
25. **Bushby, S. R. M.** 1973. Trimethoprim-sulfamethoxazole: in vitro microbiological aspects. *J. Infect. Dis.* **128**(Suppl.)**:** S442–S462.
26. **Carroll, O. M., P. A. Bryan, and R. J. Robinson.** 1966. Stevens-Johnson syndrome associated with long-acting sulfonamides. *JAMA* **195:**691–693.
27. **Casewell, M. W., and R. L. R. Hill.** 1985. In-vitro activity of mupirocin (pseudomonic acid) against clinical isolates of *Staphylococcus aureus*. *J. Antimicrob. Chemother.* **15:** 523–531.
28. **Casewell, M. W., and R. L. R. Hill.** 1986. Elimination of nasal carriage of *Staphylococcus aureus* with mupirocin (pseudomonic acid): a controlled trial. *J. Antimicrob. Chemother.* **17:**365–372.
29. **Centers for Disease Control and Prevention.** 1998. 1998 Guidelines for treatment of sexually transmitted diseases. *Morbid. Mortal. Weekly Rep.* **49**(Suppl. RR-1)**:**1–116.
30. **Centers for Disease Control and Prevention.** 1997. 1997 USPHS/IDSA guidelines for the prevention of opportunistic infections in persons infected with human immunodeficiency virus. *Morbid. Mortal. Weekly Rep.* **46**(Suppl. RR-12)**:**1–46.
31. **Cherry, R. D., D. Portnoy, M. Jabbari, D. S. Daly, D. G. Kinnear, and C. A. Goresky.** 1982. Metronidazole: an alternate therapy for antibiotic-associated colitis. *Gastroenterology* **82:**849–851.
32. **Cherubin, C. E.** 1981. Antibiotic resistance of *Salmonella* in Europe and the United States. *Rev. Infect. Dis.* **3:** 1105–1126.
33. **Cherubin, C. E., and D. B. Azabache.** 1992. While nearly no one was watching: the rise of erythromycin and clindamycin resistance in *Streptococcus pneumoniae* and *Streptococcus pyogenes*. *Antimicrob. Newsl.* **8:**37–44.
34. **Chopra, I., P. M. Hawkey, and M. Hinton.** 1992. Tetracyclines, molecular and clinical aspects. *J. Antimicrob. Chemother.* **29:**245–277.
35. **Chow, A. W., N. Chang, and K. H. Bartlett.** 1985. In vitro susceptibility of *Clostridium difficile* to new β-lactam and quinolone antibiotics. *Antimicrob. Agents Chemother.* **28:**842–844.
36. **Christ, W., T. Lehnert, and B. Ulbrich.** 1988. Specific toxicologic aspects of the quinolones. *Rev. Infect. Dis.* **10**(Suppl. 1)**:**S141–S146.
37. **Clark, J., and A. Wallace.** 1967. The susceptibility of mycobacteria to rifamide and rifampin. *Tubercle* **48:**144–148.
38. **Cohen, M. A., M. D. Huband, J. W. Gage, S. L. Yoder, G. E. Roland, and S. J. Gracheck.** 1997. In-vitro activity of clinafloxacin, trovafloxacin, and ciprofloxacin. *J. Antimicrob. Chemother.* **40:**205–211.
39. **Cohen, M. A., E. T. Joannides, G. E. Roland, M. A. Meservey, M. D. Huband, M. A. Shapiro, J. C. Sesnie, and C. L. Heifetz.** 1994. In vitro evaluation of cefdinir (FK482), a new oral cephalosporin with enhanced antistaphylococcal activity and β-lactamase stability. *Diagn. Microbiol. Infect. Dis.* **18:**31–39.
40. **Cohen, M. A., S. L. Yoder, and G. H. Talbot.** 1996. Sparfloxacin worldwide in vitro literature: isolate data available through 1994. *Diagn. Microbiol. Infect. Dis.* **25:** 53–64.
41. **Collins, L. A., G. M. Eliopoulos, C. B. Wennersten, M. J. Ferraro, and R. C. Moellering, Jr.** 1993. In vitro activity of ramoplanin against vancomycin-resistant gram-positive organisms. *Antimicrob. Agents Chemother.* **37:**1364–1366.
42. **Cooper, R. D. G.** 1992. The carbacephems: a new beta-lactam antibiotic class. *Am. J. Med.* **92**(Suppl. 6A)**:**2S–6S.
43. **Coppens, L., and J. Klastersky.** 1979. Comparative study of anti-*Pseudomonas* activity of azlocillin, mezlocillin, and ticarcillin. *Antimicrob. Agents Chemother.* **15:**396–399.
44. **Craig, W. A.** 1997. The pharmacology of meropenem, a new carbapenem antibiotic. *Clin. Infect. Dis.* **24**(Suppl. 2)**:** S266–S275.
45. **Cynamon, M. H., and G. S. Palmer.** 1982. In vitro susceptibility of *Mycobacterium fortuitum* to N-formimidoyl thienamycin and several cephamycins. *Antimicrob. Agents Chemother.* **22:**1079–1081.
46. **Cynamon, M. H., and G. S. Palmer.** 1983. In vitro activity of amoxicillin in combination with clavulanic acid against *Mycobacterium tuberculosis*. *Antimicrob. Agents. Chemother.* **24:**429–431.
47. **Dajani, A. S., K. A. Taubert, W. Wilson, A. F. Bolger, A. Bayer, P. Ferrieri, M. H. Gewitz, S. T. Shulman, S. Nouri, J. W. Newburger, C. Hutto, T. J. Pallasch, T. W. Gage, M. E. Levison, G. Peter, and G. Zuccaro, Jr.** 1997. Prevention of bacterial endocarditis: recommendations by the American Heart Association. *JAMA* **277:** 1794–1801.
48. **Dannemann, B., J. A. McCutchan, D. Israelski, D. Antoniskis, C. Leport, B. Luft, J. Nussbaum, N. Clumeck, P. Morlat, J. Chiu, J.-L. Vilde, P. Haseltine, J. Leedom,**

J. Remington, M. Orellana, D. Feigal, A. Bartok, and the California Collaborative Treatment Group. 1992. Treatment of toxoplasmic encephalitis in patients with AIDS: a randomized trial comparing pyrimethamine plus clindamycin to pyrimethamine plus sulfadiazine. *Ann. Intern. Med.* **116:**33–43.

49. **Davey, P., J.-C. Pechère, and D. Speller (ed.).** 1988. Spiramycin reassessed. *J. Antimicrob. Chemother.* **22**(Suppl. B)**:**1–210.
50. **Davey, P. G., and A. H. Williams.** 1991. A review of the safety profile of teicoplanin. *J. Antimicrob. Chemother.* **27**(Suppl. B)**:**69–73.
51. **Davies, J. E.** 1983. Resistance to aminoglycosides: mechanisms and frequency. *Rev. Infect. Dis.* **5**(Suppl. 2)**:** S261–S267.
52. **Davies, S., P. D. Sparham, and R. C. Spencer.** 1987. Comparative in-vitro activity of five fluoroquinolones against mycobacteria. *J. Antimicrob. Chemother.* **19:**605–609.
53. **Davis, B. D.** 1982. Bactericidal synergism between *β*-lactams and aminoglycosides: mechanism and possible therapeutic implications. *Rev. Infect. Dis.* **4:**237–245.
54. **Davis, R., and H. M. Bryson.** 1994. Levofloxacin: a review of its antibacterial activity, pharmacokinetics and therapeutic efficacy. *Drugs* **47:**677–700.
55. **Denton, M., and K. G. Kerr.** 1998. Microbiological and clinical aspects of infection associated with *Stenotrophomonas maltophilia*. *Clin. Microbiol. Rev.* **11:**57–80.
56. **Dewsnup, D. H., and D. N. Wright.** 1984. In vitro susceptibility of *Nocardia asteroides* to 25 antimicrobial agents. *Antimicrob. Agents Chemother.* **25:**165–167.
57. **Doebbeling, B. N., D. L. Breneman, H. C. Neu, R. Aly, B. G. Yangco, H. P. Holley, Jr., R. J. Marsh, M. A. Pfaller, J. E. McGowan, Jr., B. E. Scully, D. R. Reagan, R. P. Wenzel, and the Mupirocin Collaborative Study Group.** 1993. Elimination of *Staphylococcus aureus* nasal carriage in health care workers: analysis of six clinical trials with calcium mupirocin. *Clin. Infect. Dis.* **17:**466–474.
58. **Drusano, G. L., S. C. Schimpff, and W. L. Hewitt.** 1984. The acylampicillins: mezlocillin, piperacillin, and azlocillin. *Rev. Infect. Dis.* **6:**13–32.
59. **Dudley, M. N., J. C. McLaughlin, G. Carrington, J. Frick, C. H. Nightingale, and R. Quintiliani.** 1986. Oral bacitracin vs vancomycin therapy for *Clostridium difficile*-induced diarrhea: a randomized double-blind trial. *Arch. Intern. Med.* **146:**1101–1104.
60. **Eady, E. A., J. I. Ross, and J. H. Cove.** 1990. Multiple mechanisms of erythromycin resistance. *J. Antimicrob. Chemother.* **26:**461–465.
61. **Edelstein, P. H., E. A. Gaudet, and M. A. C. Edelstein.** 1989. In vitro activity of lomefloxacin (NY-198 or SC 47111), ciprofloxacin, and erythromycin against 100 clinical *Legionella* strains. *Diagn. Microbiol. Infect. Dis.* **12**(Suppl.)**:**93S–95S.
62. **Edwards, D. I.** 1993. Nitroimidazole drugs—action and resistance mechanisms. I. Mechanisms of action. *J. Antimicrob. Chemother.* **31:**9–20.
63. **Edwards, J. R.** 1995. Meropenem: a microbiological overview. *J. Antimicrob. Chemother.* **36**(Suppl. A)**:**1–17.
64. **Eliopoulos, G. M.** 1997. Vancomycin-resistant enterococci: mechanism and clinical relevance. *Infect. Dis. Clin. North Am.* **11:**851–865.
65. **Eliopoulos, G. M., and C. T. Eliopoulos.** 1993. Activity in vitro of the quinolones, p. 161–193. *In* D. C. Hooper and J. S. Wolfson (ed.), *Quinolone Antimicrobial Agents*, 2nd ed. American Society for Microbiology, Washington, D.C.
66. **Eliopoulos, G. M., K. Klimm, M. J. Ferraro, G. A. Jacoby, and R. C. Moellering, Jr.** 1989. Comparative in vitro activity of piperacillin combined with the beta-lactamase inhibitor tazobactam (YTR 830). *Diagn. Microbiol. Infect. Dis.* **12:**481–488.
67. **Endtz, H. P., G. J. Ruijs, B. van Klingeren, W. H. Jansen, T. van Reyden, and R. P. Mouton.** 1991. Quinolone resistance in campylobacter isolated from man and poultry following the introduction of fluoroquinolones in veterinary medicine. *J. Antimicrob. Chemother.* **27:**199–208.
68. **Ericsson, C. D., and H. L. DuPont.** 1993. Travelers' diarrhea: approaches to prevention and treatment. *Clin. Infect. Dis.* **16:**616–624.
69. **Fass, R. J.** 1983. Comparative in vitro activities of third-generation cephalosporins. *Arch. Intern. Med.* **143:** 1743–1745.
70. **Fass R. J., E. A. Copelan, J. T. Brandt, M. L. Moeschberger, and J. J. Ashton.** 1987. Platelet-mediated bleeding caused by broad-spectrum penicillins. *J. Infect. Dis.* **155:** 1242–1248.
71. **Fee, W. E., Jr.** 1980. Aminoglycoside ototoxicity in the human. *Laryngoscope* **90**(Suppl. 24)**:**1–19.
72. **Feeley, T. W., G. C. DuMoulin, J. Hedley-Whyte, L. S. Bushnell, J. P. Gilbert, and D. S. Feingold.** 1975. Aerosol polymyxin and pneumonia in seriously ill patients. *N. Engl. J. Med.* **293:**471–475.
73. **Fekete, T.** 1993. Antimicrobial susceptibility testing of *Neisseria gonorrhea* and implication for epidemiology and therapy. *Clin. Microbiol. Rev.* **6:**22–33.
74. **Fekety, R., J. Silva, B. Buggy, and H. G. Deery.** 1984. Treatment of antibiotic-associated colitis with vancomycin. *J. Antimicrob. Chemother.* **14**(Suppl. D)**:**97–102.
75. **Finch, R. G.** 1996. Antibacterial activity of quinupristin/dalfopristin: rationale for clinical use. *Drugs* **51**(Suppl. 1)**:** 31–37.
76. **Finland, M., M. C. Bach, C. Garner, and O. Gold.** 1974. Synergistic action of ampicillin and erythromycin against *Nocardia asteroides*: effect of time of incubation. *Antimicrob. Agents Chemother.* **5:**344–353.
77. **Finland, M., C. Garner, C. Wilcox, and L. D. Sabath.** 1976. Susceptibility of beta-hemolytic streptococci to 65 antibacterial agents. *Antimicrob. Agents Chemother.* **9:** 11–19.
78. **Ford, C. W., J. C. Hamel, D. Stapert, J. K. Moerman, D. K. Hutchinson, M. R. Barbachyn, and G. E. Zurenko.** 1997. Oxazolidinones: new antibacterial agents. *Trends Microbiol.* **5:**196–200.
79. **Frampton, J. E., R. N. Brogden, H. D. Langtry, and M. M. Buckley.** 1992. Cefpodoxime proxetil: a review of its antibacterial activity, pharmacokinetic properties and therapeutic potential. *Drugs* **44:**889–917.
80. **Freeman, L. D., D. R. Hopper, D. F. Lathen, D. P. Nelson, W. O. Harrison, and D. S. Anderson.** 1983. Brief prophylaxis with doxycycline for the prevention of traveler's diarrhea. *Gastroenterology* **84:**276–280.
81. **Frost, P., G. D. Weinstein, and E. C. Gomez.** 1972. Phototoxic potential of minocycline and doxycycline. *Arch. Dermatol.* **105:**681–683.
82. **Fu, K. P., and H. C. Neu.** 1976. In vitro study of netilmicin compared with other aminoglycosides. *Antimicrob. Agents Chemother.* **10:**526–534.
83. **Fu, K. P., and H. C. Neu.** 1979. Comparative inhibition of *β*-lactamases by novel *β*-lactam compounds. *Antimicrob. Agents Chemother.* **15:**171–176.
84. **Fuchs, P. C., A. L. Barry, C. Thornsberry, and R. N. Jones.** 1984. In vitro activity of ticarcillin plus clavulanic acid against 632 clinical isolates. *Antimicrob. Agents Chemother.* **25:**392–394.
85. **Fuller, A. T., G. Mellows, M. Woolford, G. T. Banks, K. D. Barrow, and E. B. Chain.** 1971. Pseudomonic acid: an antibiotic produced by *Pseudomonas fluorescens*. *Nature* (London) **234:**416–417.

86. **Fung-Tomc, J. C.** 1997. Fourth-generation cephalosporins. *Clin. Microbiol. Newsl.* **19:**129–136.
87. **Geraci, J. E., and W. R. Wilson.** 1981. Vancomycin therapy for infective endocarditis. *Rev. Infect. Dis.* **3**(Suppl.): S250–S258.
88. **Giamarellou, H.** 1986. Aminoglycosides plus β-lactams against gram-negative organisms: evaluation of in vitro synergy and chemical interactions. *Am. J. Med.* **80**(Suppl. 6B)**:**126–137.
89. **Goldfarb, J., D. Crenshaw, J. O'Horo, E. Lemon, and J. L. Blumer.** 1988. Randomized clinical trial of topical mupirocin versus oral erythromycin for impetigo. *Antimicrob. Agents Chemother.* **32:**1780–1783.
90. **Goldstein, F. W., B. Papadopoulou, and J. F. Acar.** 1986. The changing pattern of trimethoprim resistance in Paris, with a review of worldwide experience. *Rev. Infect. Dis.* **8:**725–737.
91. **Gordin, F. M., G. L. Simon, C. B. Wofsy, and J. Mills.** 1984. Adverse reactions to trimethoprim-sulfamethoxazole in patients with acquired immunodeficiency syndrome. *Ann. Intern. Med.* **100:**495–499.
92. **Gorzynski, E. A., D. Amsterdam, T. R. Beam, Jr., and C. Rotstein.** 1989. Comparative in vitro activities of teicoplanin, vancomycin, oxacillin, and other antimicrobial agents against bacteremic isolates of gram-positive cocci. *Antimicrob. Agents Chemother.* **33:**2019–2022.
93. **Gravenkemper, C. F., J. V. Bennett, J. L. Brodie, and W. M. M. Kirby.** 1965. Dicloxacillin: in vitro and pharmacologic comparisons with oxacillin and cloxacillin. *Arch. Intern. Med.* **116:**340–345.
94. **Greenwood, D.** 1988. Microbiological properties of teicoplanin. *J. Antimicrob. Chemother.* **21**(Suppl. A)**:**1–13.
95. **Grosset, J., and S. Leventis.** 1983. Adverse effects of rifampin. *Rev. Infect. Dis.* **5**(Suppl. 3)**:**S440–S446.
96. **Grossman, E. R., A. Walcheck, and H. Freedman.** 1971. Tetracycline and permanent teeth: the relationship between doses and tooth color. *Pediatrics* **47:**567–570.
97. **Gump, D. W.** 1981. Vancomycin for treatment of bacterial meningitis. *Rev. Infect. Dis.* **3**(Suppl.)**:**S289–S292.
98. **Gutmann, L., M. D. Kitzis, S. Yamabe, and J. F. Acar.** 1986. Comparative evaluation of a new β-lactamase inhibitor, YTR 830, combined with different β-lactam antibiotics against bacteria harboring known β-lactamases. *Antimicrob. Agents Chemother.* **29:**955–957.
99. **Guttler, R. B., G. W. Counts, C. K. Avent, and H. N. Beaty.** 1971. Effect of rifampin and minocycline on meningococcal carrier rates. *J. Infect. Dis.* **124:**199–205.
100. **Halkin, H.** 1988. Adverse effects of the fluoroquinolones. *Rev. Infect. Dis.* **10**(Suppl. 1)**:**S258–S261.
101. **Hardy, D. J., D. M. Hensey, J. M. Beyer, C. Vojtko, E. J. McDonald, and P. B. Fernandes.** 1988. Comparative in vitro activities of new 14-, 15-, and 16-membered macrolides. *Antimicrob. Agents Chemother.* **32:**1710–1719.
102. **Haydon, R. C., J. W. Thelin, and W. E. Davis.** 1984. Erythromycin ototoxicity: analysis and conclusions based on 22 case reports. *Otolaryngol. Head Neck Surg.* **92:** 678–684.
103. **Hitchings, G. H.** 1973. Mechanism of action of trimethoprim-sulfamethoxazole. I. *J. Infect. Dis.* **128**(Suppl.)**:** S433–S436.
104. **Hoban, D. J., R. N. Jones, N. Yamane, R. Frei, A. Trilla, and A. C. Pignatari.** 1993. In vitro activity of three carbapenem antibiotics: comparative studies with biapenem (L-627), imipenem, and meropenem against aerobic pathogens isolated worldwide. *Diagn. Microbiol. Infect. Dis.* **17:**299–305.
105. **Hoeprich, P. D., and D. M. Warshauer.** 1974. Entry of four tetracyclines into saliva and tears. *Antimicrob. Agents Chemother.* **5:**330–336.
106. **Hof, H., O. Zak, E. Schweizer, and A. Danzler.** 1984. Antibacterial activities of nitrothiazole derivatives. *J. Antimicrob. Chemother.* **14:**31–39.
107. **Hoffken, G., H. Lode, C. Prinzing, K. Borner, and P. Koeppe.** 1985. Pharmacokinetics of ciprofloxacin after oral and parenteral administration. *Antimicrob. Agents Chemother.* **27:**375–379.
108. **Holmberg, L., G. Boman, L. E. Bottiger, B. Eriksson, R. Spross, and A. Wessling.** 1980. Adverse reactions to nitrofurantoin: analysis of 921 reports. *Am. J. Med.* **69:** 733–738.
109. **Hooper, D. C., and J. S. Wolfson.** 1993. Mechanisms of quinolone action and bacterial killing, p. 53–75. *In* D. C. Hooper (ed.), *Quinolone Antimicrobial Agents*, 2nd ed. American Society for Microbiology, Washington, D.C.
110. **Hooton, T. M., and W. E. Stamm.** 1997. Diagnosis and treatment of uncomplicated urinary tract infection. *Infect. Dis. Clin. North Am.* **11:**551–581.
111. **Horiuchi, S., Y. Inagaki, N. Yamamoto, N. Okamura, Y. Imagawa, and R. Nakaya.** 1993. Reduced susceptibilities of *Shigella sonnei* strains isolated from patients with dysentery to fluoroquinolones. *Antimicrob. Agents Chemother.* **37:**2486–2489.
112. **Hughes, J., and G. Mellows.** 1978. Inhibition of isoleucyl-transfer ribonucleic acid synthetase in *Escherichia coli* by pseudomonic acid. *Biochem. J.* **176:**305–318.
113. **Jacoby, G. A.** 1997. Extended-spectrum β-lactamases and other enzymes providing resistance to oxyimino-β-lactams. *Infect. Dis. Clin. North Am.* **11:**875–887.
114. **Jacoby, G. A., and L. Sutton.** 1989. *Pseudomonas cepacia* susceptibility to sulbactam. *Antimicrob. Agents Chemother.* **33:**583–584.
115. **Johnson, A. P., A. H. C. Uttley, N. Woodford, and R. C. George.** 1990. Resistance to vancomycin and teicoplanin: an emerging clinicial problem. *Clin. Microbiol. Rev.* **3:**280–291.
116. **Jones, R. N.** 1989. Review of the in-vitro spectrum and characteristics of cefmetazole (CS-1170). *J. Antimicrob. Chemother.* **23**(Suppl. D)**:**1–12.
117. **Jones, R. N.** 1993. Ceftibuten: a review of antimicrobial activity, spectrum and other microbiologic features. *Pediatr. Infect. Dis. J.* **12:**517–44.
118. **Jones, R. N., and A. L. Barry.** 1983. Cefoperazone: a review of its antimicrobial spectrum, β-lactamase stability, enzyme inhibition, and other in vitro characteristics. *Rev. Infect. Dis.* **5**(Suppl. 1)**:**S108–S126.
119. **Jones, R. N., M. A. Pfaller, S. D. Allen, E. H. Gerlach, P. C. Fuchs, and K. E. Aldridge.** 1991. Antimicrobial activity of cefpirome: an update compared to five third-generation cephalosporins against nearly 6,000 recent clinical isolates from five medical centers. *Diagn. Microbiol. Infect. Dis.* **14:**361–364.
120. **Kahan, F. M., J. S. Kahan, P. J. Cassidy, and H. Kropp.** 1974. The mechanism of action of fosfomycin (phosphonomycin). *Ann. N. Y. Acad. Sci.* **235:**364–386.
121. **Kenny, G. E., T. M. Hooton, M. C. Roberts, F. D. Cartwright, and J. Hoyt.** 1989. Susceptibilities of genital mycoplasmas to the newer quinolones as determined by the agar dilution method. *Antimicrob. Agents Chemother.* **33:**103–107.
122. **Kirst, H. A., and G. D. Sides.** 1989. New directions for macrolide antibiotics: structural modifications and in vitro activity. *Antimicrob. Agents Chemother.* **33:** 1413–1418.
123. **Klugman, K. P.** 1990. Pneumococcal resistance to antibiotics. *Clin. Microbiol. Rev.* **3:**171–196.
124. **Knapp, C. C., J. Sierra-Madero, and J. A. Washington.** 1989. Activity of ticarcillin/clavulanate and piperacillin/tazobactam (YTR 830; CL-298,741) against clinical iso-

lates and against mutants derepressed for class I beta-lactamase. *Diagn. Microbiol. Infect. Dis.* **12:**511–515.

125. **Knight, V., J. W. Draper, E. A. Brady, and C. A. Attmore.** 1952. Methanamine mandelate: antimicrobial activity, absorption and excretion. *Antibiot. Chemother.* **2:** 615–635.
126. **Kuck, N. A., N. V. Jacobus, P. J. Petersen, W. J. Weiss, and R. T. Testa.** 1989. Comparative in vitro and in vivo activities of piperacillin combined with the β-lactamase inhibitors tazobactam, clavulanic acid, and sulbactam. *Antimicrob. Agents Chemother.* **33:**1964–1969.
127. **Lawson, D. H., and B. J. Paice.** 1982. Adverse reactions to trimethoprim-sulfamethoxazole. *Rev. Infect. Dis.* **4:** 429–433.
128. **Leigh, D. A.** 1981. Antibacterial activity and pharmacokinetics of clindamycin. *J. Antimicrob. Chemother.* **7**(Suppl. A)**:**3–9.
129. **Lode, H., K. Borner, P. Koeppe, and T. Schaberg.** 1996. Azithromycin—review of key chemical, pharmacokinetic and microbiological features. *J. Antimicrob. Chemother.* **37**(Suppl. C)**:**1–8.
130. **Low, D. E.** 1995. Quinupristin/dalfopristin: spectrum of activity, pharmacokinetics, and initial clinical experience. *Microb. Drug Resist.* **1:**223–234.
131. **Low, D. E., A. McGeer, and R. Poon.** 1989. Activities of daptomycin and teicoplanin against *Staphylococcus haemolyticus* and *Staphylococcus epidermidis*, including evaluation of susceptibility testing recommendations. *Antimicrob. Agents Chemother.* **33:**585–588.
132. **Malanoski, G. J., L. Collins, C. Wennersten, R. C. Moellering, and G. M. Eliopoulos.** 1993. In vitro activity of biapenem against clinical isolates of gram-positive and gram-negative bacteria. *Antimicrob. Agents Chemother.* **37:**2009–2016.
133. **Mandell, G. L.** 1983. The antimicrobial activity of rifampin: emphasis on the relation to phagocytes. *Rev. Infect. Dis.* **5**(Suppl. 3)**:**S463–S467.
134. **Marco F., R. N. Jones, D. J. Hoban, A. C. Pignatari, N. Yamane, and R. Frei.** 1994. In-vitro activity of OPC-17116 against more than 6,000 consecutive clinical isolates: a multicentre international study. *J. Antimicrob. Chemother.* **33:**647–654.
135. **Martinez-Martinez, L., A. Pascual, and G. A. Jacoby.** 1998. Quinolone resistance from a transferable plasmid. *Lancet* **351:**797–799.
136. **Maurin, M., S. Gasquet, C. Ducco, and D. Raoult.** 1995. MICs of 28 antibiotic compounds for 14 *Bartonella* (formerly *Rochalimae*) isolates. *Antimicrob. Agents Chemother.* **39:**2387–2391.
137. **McCalla, D. R.** 1977. Biological effects of nitrofurans. *J. Antimicrob. Chemother.* **3:**517–520.
138. **McDowell, T. D., and K. E. Reed.** 1989. Mechanism of penicillin killing in the absence of bacterial lysis. *Antimicrob. Agents Chemother.* **33:**1680–1685.
139. **McGehee, R. F., Jr., C. B. Smith, C. Wilcox, and M. Finland.** 1968. Comparative studies of antibacterial activity in vitro and absorption and excretion of lincomycin and clindamycin. *Am. J. Med. Sci.* **256:**279–292.
140. **McNulty, C. A. M., J. Dent, and R. Wise.** 1985. Susceptibility of clinical isolates of *Campylobacter pyloridis* to 11 antimicrobial agents. *Antimicrob. Agents Chemother.* **28:** 837–838.
141. **Medical Letter on Drugs and Therapeutics.** 1995. Drugs for sexually transmitted diseases. *Med. Lett. Drugs Ther.* **37:**117–122.
142. **Medical Letter on Drugs and Therapeutics.** 1997. Treatment of Lyme disease. *Med. Lett. Drugs Ther.* **39:**47–48.
143. **Medical Letter on Drugs and Therapeutics.** 1998. Drugs for parasitic infections. *Med. Lett. Drugs Ther.* **40:**1–12.
144. **Moellering, R. C., Jr.** 1984. Pharmacokinetics of vancomycin. *J. Antimicrob. Chemother.* **14**(Suppl. D)**:**43–52.
145. **Moellering, R. C., Jr.** 1991. The enterococcus: a classic example of the impact of antimicrobial resistance on therapeutic options. *J. Antimicrob. Chemother.* **28:**1–12.
146. **Molavi, A., and L. Weinstein.** 1971. In-vitro activity of erythromycin against atypical mycobacteria. *J. Infect. Dis.* **123:**216–219.
147. **Monk, J. P., and D. M. Campoli-Richards.** 1987. Ofloxacin: a review of its antibacterial activity, pharmacokinetic properties and therapeutic use. *Drugs* **33:**346–391.
148. **Moosdeen, F., J. D. Williams, and S. Yamabe.** 1988. Antibacterial characteristics of YTR 830, a sulfone β-lactamase inhibitor, compared with those of clavulanic acid and sulbactam. *Antimicrob. Agents Chemother.* **32:** 925–927.
149. **Morris, A. B., R. B. Brown, and M. Sands.** 1993. Use of rifampin in nonstaphylococcal, nonmycobacterial disease. *Antimicrob. Agents Chemother.* **37:**1–7.
150. **Murray, B. E.** 1990. The life and times of the enterococcus. *Clin. Microbiol. Rev.* **3:**46–65.
151. **Muscato, J. J., D. W. Wilbur, J. J. Stout, and R. A. Fahrlender.** 1991. An evaluation of the susceptibility patterns of gram-negative organisms isolated in cancer centres with aminoglycoside usage. *J. Antimicrob. Chemother.* **27**(Suppl. C)**:**1–7.
152. **Musial, C. E., and J. E. Rosenblatt.** 1989. Antimicrobial susceptibilities of anaerobic bacteria isolated at the Mayo Clinic during 1982 through 1987: comparison with results from 1977 through 1981. *Mayo Cin. Proc.* **64:**392–399.
153. **Nadelman, R. B., S. W. Luger, E. Frank, M. Wisniewski, J. J. Collins, and G. P. Wormser.** 1992. Comparison of cefuroxime axetil and doxycycline in the treatment of Lyme disease. *Ann. Intern. Med.* **117:**273–280.
154. **Nagarajan, R.** 1991. Antibacterial activities and modes of action of vancomycin and related glycopeptides. *Antimicrob. Agents Chemother.* **35:**605–609.
155. **Najjar, A., and B. E. Murray.** 1987. Failure to demonstrate a consistent in vitro bactericidal effect of trimethoprim-sulfamethoxazole against enterococci. *Antimicrob. Agents Chemother.* **31:**808–810.
156. **Neu, H. C.** 1976. Tobramycin: an overview. *J. Infect. Dis.* **134**(Suppl.)**:**S3–S19.
157. **Neu, H. C.** 1982. The new beta-lactamase-stable cephalosporins. *Ann. Intern. Med.* **97:**408–419.
158. **Neu, H. C.** 1985. Carbapenems: special properties contributing to their activity. *Am. J. Med.* **78**(Suppl. 6A)**:** 33–40.
159. **Neu, H. C.** 1991. Clinical microbiology of azithromycin. *Am. J. Med.* **91**(Suppl. 3A)**:**12S–18S.
160. **Neu, H. C.** 1991. The development of macrolides: clarithromycin in perspective. *J. Antimicrob. Chemother.* **27**(Suppl. A)**:**1–9.
161. **Neu, H. C., and K. P. Fu.** 1978. Clavulanic acid, a novel inhibitor of beta-lactamases. *Antimicrob. Agents Chemother.* **14:**650–655.
162. **Neu, H. C., and K. P. Fu.** 1980. In vitro activity of chloramphenicol and thiamphenicol analogs. *Antimicrob. Agents Chemother.* **18:**311–316.
163. **Neu, H. C., and P. Lubthavikul.** 1982. Comparative in vitro activity of *N*-formimidoyl thienamycin against gram-positive and gram-negative aerobic and anaerobic species and its β-lactamase stability. *Antimicrob. Agents Chemother.* **21:**180–187.
164. **Nord, C. E.** 1996. In vitro activity of quinolones and other antimicrobial agents against anaerobic bacteria. *Clin. Infect. Dis.* **23**(Suppl. 1)**:**S15–S18.
165. **Norrby, S. F., K. L. Faulkner, and P. A. Newell.** 1997.

Differentiating meropenem and imipenem/cilastatin. *Infect. Dis. Clin. Pract.* **6:**291–303.

166. **O'Brien, R. J., M. A. Lyle, and D. E. Snider, Jr.** 1987. Rifabutin (ansamycin LM 427): a new rifamycin-S derivative for the treatment of mycobacterial diseases. *Rev. Infect. Dis.* **9:**519–530.
167. **Pang, L. W., N. Limsomwong, E. F. Boudreau, and P. Singharaj.** 1987. Doxycycline prophylaxis for falciparum malaria. *Lancet* **i:**1161–1164.
168. **Pape, J. W., R. I. Verdier, and W. D. Johnson, Jr.** 1989. Treatment and prophylaxis of *Isospora belli* infection in patients with the acquired immunodeficiency syndrome. *N. Engl. J. Med.* **320:**1044–1047.
169. **Patel, R. B., and P. G. Welling.** 1980. Clinical pharmacokinetics of co-trimoxazole (trimethoprim-sulfamethoxazole). *Clin. Pharmacokinet.* **5:**405–423.
170. **Patel, S. S., J. A. Balfour, and H. M. Bryson.** 1997. Fosfomycin tromethamine. *Drugs* **53:**637–656.
171. **Pechere, J.-C.** 1996. Streptogramins: a unique class of antibiotics. *Drugs* **51**(Suppl. 1)**:**13–19.
172. **Peters, D. H., H. A. Friedel, and D. McTavish.** 1992. Azithromycin: a review of its antimicrobial activity, pharmacokinetic properties and clinical efficacy. *Drugs* **44:** 755–799.
173. **Pfaller, M. A., A. L. Barry, and P. C. Fuchs.** 1993. Evaluation of disk susceptibility testing of fosfomycin tromethamine. *Diagn. Microbiol. Infect. Dis.* **17:**67–70.
174. **Pitkin, D. H., W. Sheikh, and H. L. Nadler.** 1997. Comparative in vitro activity of meropenem versus other extended-spectrum antimicrobials against randomly chosen and selected resistant clinical isolates tested in 26 North American centers. *Clin. Infect. Dis.* **24**(Suppl. 2)**:** S238–S248.
175. **Polk, R. E.** 1989. Drug-drug interactions with ciprofloxacin and other fluoroquinolones. *Am. J. Med.* **87**(Suppl. 5A)**:**76S–81S.
176. **Polk, R. E., D. P. Healy, L. B. Schwartz, D. T. Rock, M. L. Garson, and K. Roller.** 1988. Vancomycin and the red-man syndrome: pharmacodynamics of histamine release. *J. Infect. Dis.* **157:**502–507.
177. **Qadri, S. M., B. A. Cunha, Y. Ueno, F. Abumustafa, H. Imambaccus, D. D. Tullo, and P. Domenico.** 1995. Activity of cefepime against nosocomial blood culture isolates. *J. Antimicrob. Chemother.* **36:**531–536.
178. **Rahal, J. J., Jr., and M. S. Simberkoff.** 1979. Bactericidal and bacterostatic action of chloramphenicol against meningeal pathogens. *Antimicrob. Agents Chemother.* **16:** 13–18.
179. **Raoult, D., P. Roussellier, V. Galicher, R. Perez, and J. Tamalet.** 1986. In vitro susceptibility of *Rickettsia conorii* to ciprofloxacin as determined suppressing lethality in chicken embryos and by plaque assay. *Antimicrob. Agents Chemother.* **29:**424–425.
180. **Raoult, D., H. Torres, and M. Drancourt.** 1991. Shell-vial assay evaluation of a new technique for determining antibiotic susceptibility, tested in 13 isolates of *Coxiella burnetii*. *Antimicrob. Agents Chemother.* **35:**2070–2077.
181. **Reeves, D. S.** 1994. Fosfomycin trometamol. *J. Antimicrob. Chemother.* **34:**853–858.
182. **Retsema, J. A., A. R. English, and A. E. Girard.** 1980. CP-45,899 in combination with penicillin or ampicillin against penicillin-resistant *Staphylococcus*, *Haemophilus influenzae*, and *Bacteroides*. *Antimicrob. Agents Chemother.* **17:**615–622.
183. **Retsema, J. A., A. R. English, A. Girard, J. E. Lynch, M. Anderson, L. Brennan, C. Cimochowski, J. Faiella, W. Norcia, and P. Sawyer.** 1986. Sulbactam/ampicillin: in vitro spectrum potency, and activity in models of acute infection. *Rev. Infect. Dis.* **8**(Suppl. 5)**:**S528–S534.
184. **Rodloff, A. C.** 1982. In-vitro susceptibility test of non-tuberculous mycobacteria to sulphamethoxazole, trimethoprim, and combinations of both. *J. Antimicrob. Chemother.* **9:**195–199.
185. **Rolston, K. V. I., and J. Hoy.** 1987. Role of clindamycin in the treatment of central nervous system toxoplasmosis. *Am. J. Med.* **83:**551–554.
186. **Rose, H. D., and M. W. Rytel.** 1972. Actinomycosis treated with clindamycin. *JAMA* **221:**1052.
187. **Rosenblatt, J. E., and P. R. Stewart.** 1974. Combined activity of sulfamethoxazole, trimethoprim, and polymyxin B against gram-negative bacilli. *Antimicrob. Agents Chemother.* **6:**84–92.
188. **Rubin, R. H., and M. N. Swartz.** 1980. Trimethoprim-sulfamethoxazole. *N. Engl. J. Med.* **303:**426–432.
189. **Ruoff, K. L., D. R. Kuritzkes, J. S. Wolfson, and M. J. Ferraro.** 1988. Vancomycin-resistant gram-positive bacteria isolated from human sources. *J. Clin. Microbiol.* **26:** 2064–2068.
190. **Sader, H. S., R. N. Jones, J. A. Washington, P. R. Murray, E. H. Gerlach, S. D. Allen, and M. E. Erwin.** 1993. In vitro activity of cefpodoxime compared with other oral cephalosporins tested against 5,556 recent clinical isolates from five medical centers. *Diagn. Microbiol. Infect. Dis.* **17:**143–150.
191. **Salter, A. J.** 1982. Trimethoprim-sulfamethoxazole: an assessment of more than 12 years of use. *Rev. Infect. Dis.* **4:**196–236.
192. **Sanders, C. C.** 1993. Cefepime: the next generation? *Clin. Infect. Dis.* **17:**369–379.
193. **Sattler, F. R., M. R. Weitekamp, and J. O. Ballard.** 1986. Potential for bleeding with the new beta-lactam antibiotics. *Ann. Intern. Med.* **105:**924–931.
194. **Saxon, A., A. Hassner, E. A. Swabb, B. Wheeler, and N. F. Adkinson, Jr.** 1984. Lack of cross-reactivity between aztreonam, a monobactam antibiotic, and penicillin in penicillin-allergic subjects. *J. Infect. Dis.* **149:**16–22.
195. **Schaad, U. B., J. Wedgwood-Krucko, and H. Tschaeppeler.** 1988. Reversible ceftriaxone-associated biliary pseudolithiasis in children. *Lancet* **ii:**1411–1413.
196. **Schentag, J. J., and C. H. Ballow.** 1991. Tissue-directed pharmacokinetics. *Am. J. Med.* **91**(Suppl. 3A)**:**5S–11S.
197. **Schwalbe, R. S., J. T. Stappleton, and P. H. Gilligan.** 1987. Emergence of vancomycin resistance in coagulase-negative staphylococci. *N. Engl. J. Med.* **316:**927–931.
198. **Seaberg, L. S., A. R. Parquette, I. Y. Gluzman, G. W. Phillips, Jr., T. F. Brodasky, and D. J. Krogstad.** 1984. Clindamycin activity against chloroquine-resistant *Plasmodium falciparum*. *J. Infect. Dis.* **150:**904–911.
199. **Sharp, J. R., K. G. Ishak, and H. J. Zimmerman.** 1980. Chronic active hepatitis and severe hepatic necrosis associated with nitrofurantoin. *Ann. Intern. Med.* **92:**14–19.
200. **Shaw, W. V.** 1984. Bacterial resistance to chloramphenicol. *Br. Med. Bull.* **40:**36–41.
201. **Sheikh, W., D. H. Pitkin, and H. Nadler.** 1993. Antibacterial activity of meropenem and selected comparative agents against anaerobic bacterial at seven North American Centers. *Clin. Infect. Dis.* **16**(Suppl. 4)**:**S361–S366.
202. **Shinabarger, D. L., K. R. Marotti, R. W. Murray, A. H. Lin, E. P. Melchoir, S. M. Swaney, D. S. Dunyak, W. F. Demyan, and J. M. Buysse.** 1997. Mechanism of action of oxazolidinones: effects of linezolid and eperezolid on translation reactions. *Antimicrob. Agents Chemother.* **41:**2132–2136.
203. **Smith, A. L., and A. Weber.** 1983. Pharmacology of chloramphenicol. *Pediatr. Clin. North Am.* **30:**209–236.
204. **Snydman, D. R., L. McDermott, G. J. Cuchural, Jr., D. W. Hecht, P. B. Iannini, L. J. Harrell, S. G. Jenkins, J. P. O'Keefe, C. L. Pierson, J. D. Rihs, V. L. Yu, S.**

M. Finegold, and S. L. Gorbach. 1996. Analysis of trends in antimicrobial resistance patterns among clinical isolates of *Bacteroides fragilis* group species from 1990 to 1994. *Clin. Infect. Dis.* **23**(Suppl. 1):S54–S65.

205. **Somma, S., L. Gastaldo, and A. Corti.** 1984. Teicoplanin, a new antibiotic from *Actinoplanes teichomyceticus* nov. sp. *Antimicrob. Agents Chemother.* **26:**917–923.
206. **Sörgel, F., and M. Kinzig.** 1993. The chemistry, pharmacokinetics and tissue distribution of piperacillin/tazobactam. *J. Antimicrob. Chemother.* **31**(Suppl. A): 39–60.
207. **Sorrell, T. C., and P. J. Collignon.** 1985. A prospective study of adverse reactions associated with vancomycin therapy. *J. Antimicrob. Chemother.* **16:**235–241.
208. **Spangler, S. K., M. R. Jacobs, and P. C. Appelbaum.** 1996. Susceptibility of anaerobic bacteria to trovafloxacin: comparison with other quinolones and non-quinolone antibiotics. *Infect. Dis. Clin. Pract.* **5**(Suppl. 3): S101–S109.
209. **Spear, B. S., N. B. Shoemaker, and A. A. Salyers.** 1992. Bacterial resistance to tetracycline: mechanisms, transfer, and clinical significance. *Clin. Microbiol. Rev.* **5:**387–399.
210. **Spratt, B. G., V. Jobanputra, and W. Zimmermann.** 1977. Binding of thienamycin and clavulanic acid to the penicillin-binding proteins of *Escherichia coli* K-12. *Antimicrob. Agents Chemother.* **12:**406–409.
211. **Stamm, W. E.** 1991. Azithromycin in the treatment of uncomplicated genital chlamydial infections. *Am. J. Med.* **91**(Suppl. 3A)**:**19S–22S.
212. **Stapleton, A., and W. E. Stamm.** 1997. Prevention of urinary tract infection. *Infect. Dis. Clin. North Am.* **11:** 719–733.
213. **Stapley, E. O., D. Hendlin, J. M. Mata, M. Jackson, H. Wallick, S. Hernanadez, S. Mochales, S. A. Currie, and R. M. Miller.** 1969. Phosphonomycin. I. Discovery and in vitro biological characterization. *Antimicrob. Agents Chemother.* **9:**284–290.
214. **Stein, G. E.** 1996. Pharmacokinetics and pharmacodynamics of newer fluoroquinolones. *Clin. Infect. Dis.* **23**(Suppl. 1)**:**S19–S24.
215. **Sullivan, D., M. E. Csuka, and B. Blanchard.** 1980. Erythromycin ethylsuccinate hepatoxicity. *JAMA* **243:** 1074.
216. **Sutter, V. L.** 1977. In vitro susceptibility of anaerobes: comparison of clindamycin and other antimicrobial agents. *J. Infect. Dis.* **135**(Suppl.)**:**S7–S12.
217. **Swedberg, J., J. F. Steiner, F. Deiss, S. Steiner, and D. A. Driggers.** 1985. Comparison of single-dose vs one-week course of metronidazole for symptomatic bacterial vaginosis. *JAMA* **254:**1046–1049.
218. **Sykes, R. B., and D. P. Bonner.** 1985. Aztreonam: first monobactam. *Am. J. Med.* **78**(Suppl. 2A)**:**2–10.
219. **Teasley, D. G., D. N. Gerding, M. M. Olson, L. R. Peterson, R. L. Gebhard, M. J. Schwartz, and J. T. Lee, Jr.** 1983. Prospective randomized trial of metronidazole versus vancomycin for *Clostridium difficile*-associated diarrhea and colitis. *Lancet* **ii:**1043–1046.
220. **Thornsberry, C.** 1992. Review of the in vitro antibacterial activity of cefprozil, a new oral cephalosporin. *Clin. Infect. Dis.* **14**(Suppl. 2)**:**S189–S194.
221. **Todd, P. A., and D. Faulds.** 1991. Ofloxacin: a reappraisal of its antimicrobial activity, pharmacology and therapeutic use. *Drugs* **42:**825–876.
222. **Toma, E., S. Fournier, M. Dumont, P. Bolduc, and H. Deschamps.** 1993. Clindamycin/primaquine versus trimethoprim-sulfamethoxazole as primary therapy for *Pneumocystis carinii* pneumonia in AIDS: a randomized, double-blind pilot trial. *Clin. Infect. Dis.* **17:**178–184.
223. **Tuazon, C. U., and H. Miller.** 1984. Comparative in vitro activities of teichomycin and vancomycin alone and in combination with rifampin and aminoglycosides against staphylococci and enterococci. *Antimicrob. Agents Chemother.* **25:**411–412.
224. **Van der Auwera, P., T. Matsumoto, and M. Husson.** 1988. Intraphagocytic penetration of antibiotics. *J. Antimicrob. Chemother.* **22:**185–192.
225. **Van der Auwera, P., F. Meunier-Carpentier, and J. Kastersky.** 1983. Clinical study of combination therapy with oxacillin and rifampin for staphylococcal infections. *Rev. Infect. Dis.* **5**(Suppl. 3)**:**S515–S522.
226. **Vanhoff, R., B. Gordts, R. Dierickx, H. Coignau, and J. P. Butzler.** 1980. Bacteriostatic and bactericidal activities of 24 antimicrobial agents against *Campylobacter fetus* subsp. *jejuni*. *Antimicrob. Agents Chemother.* **18:**118–121.
227. **Vannuffel, P., and C. Cocito.** 1996. Mechanism of action of streptogramins and macrolides. *Drugs* **51**(Suppl. 1)**:** 20–30.
228. **Verbist, L.** 1979. Comparison of the activities of the new ureidopenicillins, piperacillin, mezlocillin, azlocillin, and Bay k 4999 against gram-negative organisms. *Antimicrob. Agents Chemother.* **16:**115–119.
229. **Visalli, M. A., S. Bajaksouzian, M. R. Jacobs, and P. C. Appelbaum.** 1997. Comparative activity of trovafloxacin, alone and in combination with other agents, against gram-negative nonfermentative rods. *Antimicrob. Agents Chemother.* **41:**1475–1481.
230. **von Rosenstiel, N.-A., and D. Adam.** 1995. Macrolide antibacterials: drug interactions of clinical significance. *Drug Saf.* **13:**105–122.
231. **Wadworth, A. N., and K. L. Goa.** 1991. Lomefloxacin: a review of its antibacterial activity, pharmacokinetic properties and therapeutic use. *Drugs* **42:**1018–1060.
232. **Wagstaff, A. J., and J. A. Balfour.** 1997. Grepafloxacin. *Drugs* **53:**817–824.
233. **Wallace, R. J., Jr., E. J. Septimus, T. W. Williams, Jr., R. H. Conklin, T. K. Satterwhite, M. B. Bushby, and D. C. Hollowell.** 1982. Use of trimethoprim-sulfamethoxazole for treatment of infections due to *Nocardia*. *Rev. Infect. Dis.* **4:**315–325.
234. **Wallace, R. J., Jr., J. M. Swenson, V. A. Silcox, and M. G. Bullen.** 1985. Treatment of non-pulmonary infections due to *Mycobacterium fortuitum* and *Mycobacterium chelonei* on the basis of in vivo susceptibilities. *J. Infect. Dis.* **152:**500–514.
235. **Wallace, R. J., Jr., and K. Wiss.** 1981. Susceptibility of *Mycobacterium marinum* to tetracyclines and aminoglycosides. *Antimicrob. Agents Chemother.* **20:**610–612.
236. **Walters, B. N. J., and S. S. Gubbay.** 1981. Tetracycline and benign intracranial hypertension: report of five cases. *Br. Med. J.* **282:**19–20.
237. **Ward, A., and D. M. Campoli-Richards.** 1986. Mupirocin: a review of its antibacterial activity, pharmacokinetic properties and therapeutic use. *Drugs* **32:**425–444.
238. **Ward, M. E.** 1977. The bactericidal action of spectinomycin on *Neisseria gonorrhoeae*. *J. Antimicrob. Chemother.* **3:**323–329.
239. **Washington, J. A., II, and W. R. Wilson.** 1985. Erythromycin: a microbial and clinical perspective after 30 years of clinical use. *Mayo Clin. Proc.* **60:**189–203, 271–278.
240. **Watanakunakorn, C., and C. Bakie.** 1973. Synergism of vancomycin-gentamicin and vancomycin-streptomycin against enterococci. *Antimicrob. Agents Chemother.* **4:** 120–124.
241. **Watanakunakoren, C., and J. C. Tisone.** 1982. Synergism between vancomycin and gentamicin or tobramycin for methicillin-susceptible and methicillin-resistant *Staphylococcus aureus* strains. *Antimicrob. Agents Chemother.* **22:**903–905.

242. **Waxman, D. J., and J. L. Strominger.** 1983. Penicillin-binding proteins and the mechanism of action of beta-lactam antibiotics. *Annu. Rev. Biochem.* **52:**825–869.
243. **Wehrli, W.** 1983. Rifampin: mechanisms of action and resistance. *Rev. Infect. Dis.* **5**(Suppl. 3)**:**S407–S411.
244. **Wexler, H. M., and S. M. Finegold.** 1988. In vitro activity of cefotetan compared with that of other antimicrobial agents against anaerobic bacteria. *Antimicrob. Agents Chemother.* **32:**601–604.
245. **Wexler, H. M., B. Harris, W. T. Carter, and S. M. Finegold.** 1985. In vitro efficacy of sulbactam combined with ampicillin against anaerobic bacteria. *Antimicrob. Agents Chemother.* **27:**876–878.
246. **Wiedemann, B., C. Kliebe, and M. Kresken.** 1989. The epidemiology of beta-lactamases. *J. Antimicrob. Chemother.* **24**(Suppl. B)**:**1–22.
247. **Wijnands, W. J. A., and T. B. Vree.** 1988. Interaction between the fluoroquinolones and the bronchodilator theophylline. *J. Antimicrob. Chemother.* **22**(Suppl. C)**:** 109–114.
248. **Williams, J. D., and A. M. Sefton.** 1993. Comparison of macrolide antibiotics. *J. Antimicrob. Chemother.* **31** (Suppl. C)**:**11–26.
249. **Wilson, W. R., A. W. Karchmer, A. S. Dajani, K. A. Taubert, A. Bayer, D. Kaye, A. L. Bisno, P. Ferrieri, S. T. Shuman, and D. T. Durack.** 1995. Antibiotic treatment of adults with infective endocarditis due to streptococci, enterococci, staphylococci, and HACEK microorganisms. *JAMA* **274:**1706–1713.
250. **Wilson, W. R., R. L. Thompson, C. J. Wilkowske, J. A. Washington II, E. R. Giuliani, and J. E. Geraci.** 1981. Short-term therapy for streptococcal infective endocarditis: combined intramuscular administration of penicillin and streptomycin. *JAMA* **245:**360–363.
251. **Winston, D. J., M. A. McGrattan, and R. W. Busuttil.** 1984. Imipenem therapy of *Pseudomonas aeruginosa* and other serious bacterial infections. *Antimicrob. Agents Chemother.* **26:**673–677.
252. **Wise, R., D. Lister, C. A. McNulty, D. Griggs, and J. M. Andrews.** 1986. The comparative pharmacokinetics of five quinolones. *J. Antimicrob. Chemother.* **18**(Suppl. D)**:**71–81.
253. **Wiseman L. R., and J. A. Balfour.** 1994. Ceftibuten: a review of its antibacterial activity, pharmacokinetic properties and clinical efficacy. *Drugs* **5:**784–808.
254. **Wittner, M., K. S. Rowin, H. B. Tanowitz, J. F. Hobbs, S. Saltzman, B. Wenz, R. Hirsch, E. Chisholm, and G. R. Healy.** 1982. Successful chemotherapy of transfusion babesiosis. *Ann. Intern. Med.* **96:**601–604.
255. **Wolfe, M.** 1992. Giardiasis. *Clin. Microbiol. Rev.* **5:** 92–100.
256. **Wolff, M., L. Boutron, E. Singlas, B. Clair, J. M. Decazes, and B. Regnier.** 1987. Penetration of ciprofloxacin into cerebrospinal fluid of patients with bacterial meningitis. *Antimicrob. Agents Chemother.* **31:**899–902.
257. **Wolfson, J. S., and D. C. Hooper.** 1985. The fluoroquinolones: structures, mechanisms of action and resistance, and spectra of activity in vitro. *Antimicrob. Agents Chemother.* **28:**581–586.
258. **Wolfson, J. S., and D. C. Hooper.** 1989. Fluoroquinolone antimicrobial agents. *Clin. Microbiol. Rev.* **2:**378–424.
259. **Wong, C. S., G. S. Palmer, and M. H. Cynamon.** 1988. In-vitro susceptibility of *Mycobacterium tuberculosis*, *Mycobacterium bovis* and *Mycobacterium kansasii* to amoxycillin and ticarcillin in combination with clavulanic acid. *J. Antimicrob. Chemother.* **22:**863–866.
260. **World Health Organization.** 1993. *Guidelines for Cholera Control.* World Health Organization, Geneva, Switzerland.
261. **Yeaman, M. R., L. A. Mitscher, and O. G. Baca.** 1987. In vitro susceptibility of *Coxiella burnetii* to antibiotics, including several quinolones. *Antimicrob. Agents Chemother.* **31:**1079–1084.
262. **Young, L. S., O. G. W. Berlin, and C. B. Inderlied.** 1987. Activity of ciprofloxacin and other fluorinated quinolones against mycobacteria. *Am. J. Med.* **82**(Suppl. 4A)**:**23–26.
263. **Young, L. S., and J. Hindler.** 1987. Use of trimethoprim-sulfamethoxazole singly and in combination with other antibiotics in immunocompromised patients. *Rev. Infect. Dis.* **9**(Suppl. 2)**:**S177–S181.
264. **Zenilman, J. M., L. J. Nims, M. A. Menegus, F. Nolte, and J. S. Knapp.** 1987. Spectinomycin-resistant gonococcal infections in the United States, 1985–1986. *J. Infect. Dis.* **156:**1002–1004.
265. **Zurenko, G. E., B. H. Yagi, R. D. Schaadt, J. W. Allison, J. O. Kilburn, S. E. Glickman, D. K. Hutchinson, M. R. Barbachyn, and S. J. Brickner.** 1996. In vitro activities of U-100592 and U-100766, novel oxazolidone antibacterial agents. *Antimicrob. Agents Chemother.* **40:** 839–845.

Mechanisms of Resistance to Antimicrobial Agents

RICHARD QUINTILIANI, JR., DANIEL F. SAHM, AND PATRICE COURVALIN

117

Antimicrobial resistance is the result of complex interactions among antimicrobial agents, microorganisms, and the environments in which they are brought together. While specific characteristics of microorganisms that mediate resistance are the primary focus of this chapter, this introduction provides a brief overview of both environment- and organism-based factors involved in resistance.

Environmentally mediated resistance is defined as resistance that directly results from physical or chemical characteristics of the environment that directly alter the antimicrobial agent or alter the normal physiologic response of the microorganism to an antimicrobial agent. Examples of such factors include pH, anaerobic atmosphere, cation (e.g., Mg^{2+} and Ca^{2+}) concentrations, and thymine or thymidine concentrations. Specific examples include diminished activities of erythromycin and aminoglycosides with decreasing pH, diminished activity of aminoglycosides against facultatively anaerobic bacteria grown in the absence of oxygen, and decreased activity of aminoglycosides against *Pseudomonas aeruginosa* in the presence of excess Ca^{2+} and Mg^{2+} concentrations. The presence of certain metabolites or nutrients in the environment can also impact antibacterial activity. For example, enterococci are able to use thymine and other exogenous folic acid metabolites to circumvent the activities of the folic acid pathway inhibitors sulfonamides and trimethoprim.

Knowledge about environmentally mediated resistance is important for establishing standardized testing methods that minimize the impact of environmental factors. Minimizing the impact of these factors in vitro is important so that microorganism-mediated resistance (see below) can be more accurately determined by antimicrobial susceptibility testing methods.

Microorganism-mediated resistance refers to antimicrobial resistance that is due to genetically encoded traits of the microorganism; it is the type of resistance that in vitro susceptibility testing methods are targeted to detect. Organism-based resistance has two subcategories: intrinsic or inherent resistance, and acquired resistance.

Resistance resulting from the normal genetic, structural, or physiologic state of a microorganism is referred to as intrinsic resistance. Such resistance is considered a natural and consistently inherited characteristic that is associated with the vast majority of strains that comprise either a particular bacterial group, genus, or species. Therefore, this resistance is predictable, so that once the identity of the organism is known, certain aspects of its antimicrobial resistance profile (e.g., vancomycin resistance among most gram-negative bacilli or aztreonam resistance among gram-positive cocci) are also known.

Antibiotic resistance that results from altered cellular physiology and structure due to changes in the usual genetic makeup of a microorganism is known as acquired resistance. Unlike intrinsic resistance, acquired resistance may be a trait associated with only some strains of a particular organism group or species. Therefore, the presence of this type of resistance in any clinical isolate is unpredictable. The unpredictable nature of acquired resistance is the primary reason why laboratory methods to detect resistance are necessary. The methods for acquisition are basically those that allow for gene change or exchange: genetic mutation(s), acquisition of genes from other organisms via gene transfer mechanisms, or a combination of mutational and gene transfer events. The remainder of this chapter focuses on how these genetic events result in alterations of the physiology or structure of the bacterial cell and mediate resistances to the most commonly used classes of antimicrobial agents.

RESISTANCE TO β-LACTAMS

Of the various mechanisms of acquired resistance to β-lactam antibiotics, resistance due to production of β-lactamases by the cell is the most prevalent. Alterations in the preexisting penicillin-binding proteins (PBP), acquisition of a novel PBP insensitive to β-lactams, changes in the outer membrane proteins of gram-negative organisms, and active efflux, which prevent these compounds from reaching their targets, can also confer resistance.

Penicillin-Interactive, Active-Site Serine Proteins

All PBPs and most β-lactamases constitute a superfamily of evolutionarily related active-site serine peptidases that interact with β-lactams in a similar fashion (114). β-Lactamases and PBPs catalytically disrupt the cyclic amide bond of penicillin G and other β-lactams via the formation of a serine-ester-linked acylenzyme derivative (Fig. 1). Three groups of proteins that mediate this reaction have been distinguished: the β-lactamases, the low-molecular-weight PBPs (D,D-carboxypeptidases), and the high-molecular-weight PBPs (transpeptidases-transglycosylases). Although

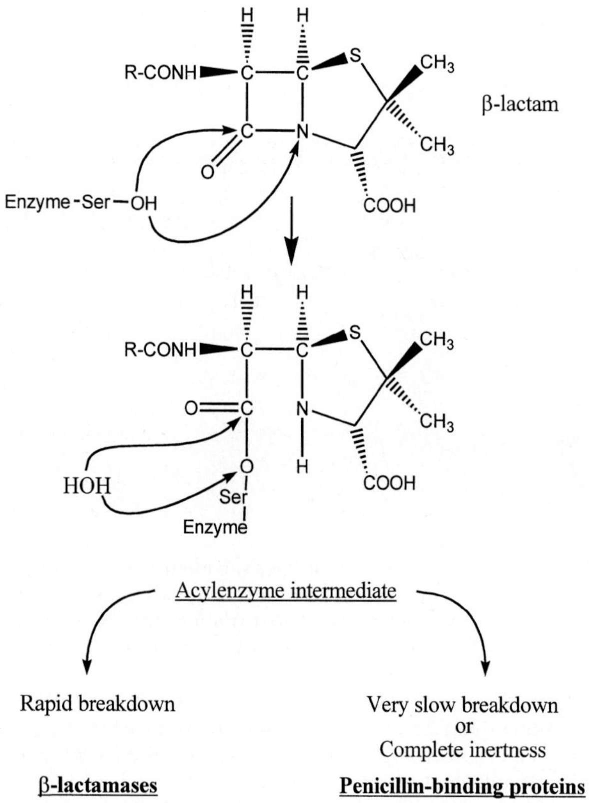

FIGURE 1 Penicillin-interactive, active-site serine peptidases and their reactions with β-lactam carbonyl donors.

D,D-carboxypeptidase and transpeptidase activities are inhibited by β-lactams as described below, D,D-carboxypeptidases are apparently dispensable, since their inhibition is not lethal to the cell.

β-Lactams are structural analogs of the peptidyl-D-alanyl-D-alanine termini of peptidoglycan cell wall precursors and can interact with both PBPs and β-lactamases. Following β-lactam binding, PBPs and β-lactamases undergo sequential acylation and deacylation reactions (Fig. 1). The β-lactam ring is opened by a nucleophilic attack on the β-lactam amide bond by the hydroxyl group of a serine residue located in the active site of the enzyme. Acylation of the enzyme generates an acylenzyme intermediate characterized by an ester bond between the enzyme and the penicilloyl (or cephalosporyl) moiety.

In general, PBPs and β-lactamases can be distinguished by differences in the rate of deacylation of the acylenzyme intermediate, which is dependent on the capacity of water to act as an attacking nucleophile. For β-lactamases, water is an effective attacking nucleophile that efficiently hydrolyzes the ester linkage of the acylenzyme intermediate, thereby releasing the penicilloyl (or cephalosporyl) moiety and regenerating the active enzyme (Fig. 1). The reaction catalyzed by PBPs is identical to that of β-lactamases, except that the acylenzyme intermediate is resistant to nucleophilic attack. Thus, the β-lactam remains covalently bound to the PBP, which is itself inactivated. For the most part, the lability of the β-lactamase–β-lactam interaction determines resistance whereas the stability of the high-molecular-weight PBP–β-lactam interaction determines susceptibility. It should be noted, however, that distinction between β-lactamases and PBPs based on the stability or lability of the acylenzyme intermediate is somewhat oversimplified since, depending on the particular enzyme adduct, the rates of enzyme turnover can be highly variable. Thus, β-lactamases sometimes generate stable acylenzyme intermediates while PBPs occasionally exhibit weak β-lactamase activity (123).

Resistance Due to PBP Alteration

Penicillin resistance due to altered high-molecular-weight PBPs is more common in gram-positive than in gram-negative bacteria. Almost all eubacteria examined contain three to eight PBPs on the outer face of the cytoplasmic membrane. The PBPs are named numerically: the higher the molecular weight, the smaller the numeric designation. Of note, although the same number may be used to designate the PBPs of different species and genera, they are not necessarily related. β-Lactams have multiple potential targets, since two to four PBPs are normally essential for cell survival.

Gram-Positive Bacteria

Methicillin-resistant *Staphylococcus aureus* (MRSA) are resistant to all β-lactams including penicillins, cephalosporins, carbapenems, and monobactams. Methicillin resistance in *S. aureus* is unique in that it is due to acquisition of DNA of unknown origin that codes for a supernumerary β-lactam-resistant PBP which takes over the biosynthetic functions of the normal PBPs when the cell is exposed to β-lactam antibiotics. *S. aureus* normally contains four PBPs, of which PBPs 1, 2, and 3 are essential. The low-affinity PBP in MRSA, termed PBP 2a (or PBP 2′), is encoded by the chromosomal *mecA* gene and is thought to function as a β-lactam-resistant transpeptidase. The *mecA* gene is also widely distributed among other species of staphylococci and is highly conserved (189).

Although MRSA exhibit high-level cross-resistance to all β-lactams, strains may be homogeneously or heterogeneously resistant. In the latter case, whereas the majority of cells express low-level methicillin resistance, subpopulations of highly resistant cells may be present in small numbers (71). The phenotypic expression of *mecA* is affected by a number of factors, including pH, temperature, osmolarity, upstream regulatory sequences, and unlinked chromosomal genes (112, 157). Expression of PBP 2a can be inducible or constitutive. Regulation of *mecA* in *S. aureus* and *S. epidermidis* occurs at the transcriptional level. Three resistance phenotypes, immediately inducible, delayed inducible, and constitutive, are associated with differences in regulation (157). Immediately inducible strains harbor a plasmid containing the β-lactamase (*bla*) operon. Since the *mecA* promoter has DNA sequence similarity to the promoter of *blaZ* (the β-lactamase structural gene), *mecA* may be regulated by genes encoded by the penicillinase plasmid (see "Resistance due to β-lactamases") (157). Elimination of the penicillinase plasmid converts some of these strains to a constitutive phenotype. Strains of *S. aureus* and *S. epidermidis* with a delayed inducible phenotype contain an upstream regulatory locus consisting of the *mecI* and *mecR1* genes, which are homologous to the penicillinase regulator genes *blaI* and *blaR1*, respectively, and mediate repression of the *mecA* gene (see β-lactamase) (181). These strains are clinically important since they are very slowly derepressed, making their detection difficult. Induction by methicillin for 48 h is required for full expression of resistance. At the transcriptional level, there appears to be no difference in the ability of various β-lactams to induce, and thus differences in inducibility may be strain specific (157).

In addition to *mecA*, *mecR1*, and *mecI*, genes independent of the *mec* locus contribute to phenotypic expression of methicillin resistance. These genes, designated *fem* (factors essential for expression of methicillin resistance), are present in the chromosome of methicillin-resistant and -susceptible *S. aureus*. Two such genes, *femA* and *femB*, have no effect on the synthesis of PBP 2a but are involved in the formation of the peptidoglycan pentaglycine cross-bridge that links adjacent peptidoglycan precursors (109). Disruption of *femA* or *femB* decreases the glycine content of peptidoglycan precursors and confers methicillin susceptibility (109). The presence of *femA* is also necessary for the increased autolytic activity observed in *mecA*-containing strains. A number of other genes that confer decreased methicillin resistance (e.g., *femC*, *femD*, *femE*, *femF*, *llm*, and *fmt*) have also been identified. Some of these genes may be involved with peptidoglycan synthesis (e.g., *femD* [84]), but for the most part the function of their gene products has yet to be determined.

In *Streptococcus pneumoniae*, a species in which β-lactamases have not been detected, β-lactam resistance is due to the presence of modified PBPs (most importantly PBP 2), which have reduced affinity for β-lactams (64). *S. pneumoniae* contains six PBPs (1a, 1b, 2a, 2x, 2b, and 3). The chromosomal *pbp* genes of penicillin-susceptible strains of *S. pneumoniae* are highly conserved (<1% sequence variation) (44). By contrast, the *pbp* genes encoding low-affinity PBPs 1a, 2x, and 2b of resistant clinical isolates exhibit significant sequence divergence and are termed "mosaic" genes, since they consist of blocks of DNA sequences that are very similar or identical to the corresponding portions of the susceptible genes and of blocks that diverge significantly (44, 92). Mosaic genes have presumably arisen by homologous recombination following transformation with DNA from a closely related species (44). For instance, certain strains of resistant *S. pneumoniae* contain mosaic PBP 2b genes, which include blocks of nucleotides originating from *S. mitis*, while others possess blocks from another unknown species, or both (43, 44). Importantly, PBP 2x and not PBP 2b is the primary target of penicillins in clinical isolates of *S. pneumoniae*. Thus, strains containing a low affinity PBP 2b may or may not be phenotypically resistant to penicillins, depending on which and how many low-affinity PBPs they possess (43).

Although the mosaic *pbp* genes contain multiple mutations in comparison to those of susceptible strains, most of the modifications are due to the different genetic origins of the DNA and are not necessarily directly responsible for resistance. Isolation of laboratory mutants and clinical isolates indicates that resistance to β-lactams can occur in a stepwise fashion due to specific point mutations in the PBPs (70, 91). However, although single point mutations can confer low-level β-lactam resistance (e.g., all clinical isolates with low-affinity PBP 2b contain the amino acid substitution Thr-446 to Ala [43]), it appears that the high-level resistance observed in clinical isolates results from successive mutations in multiple *pbp* genes (64). For example, high-level resistance to extended-spectrum cephalosporins involves changes in PBP 1a and 2x, which are encoded by closely linked genes that can be transferred en bloc into a susceptible host (31). In addition, the emergence of a specific mutation often depends on the antibiotic used for selection. For example, in PBP 2b the amino acid substitutions Thr-446 to Ala and Thr-550 to Gly are often observed following selection with cefotaxime and piperacillin, respectively (57). Consequently, resistance to expanded-spectrum antibiotics will not necessarily correspond to resistance to penicillins.

Enterococcus faecalis and *E. faecium* are intrinsically resistant to low-levels of penicillins due to a PBP 5 with low affinity for penicillins. High-level resistance (not due to β-lactamase production), which is detected far more commonly in *E. faecium*, has been associated with overproduction (54, 194) and amino acid substitutions in PBP 5 (202). Of great concern is the recent finding in *Enterococcus hirae* of a gene encoding a low-affinity PBP that is borne on a plasmid carrying multiple antibiotic resistance determinants (149).

Gram-Negative Bacteria

As mentioned above, resistance due to modifications in PBPs is less common in gram-negative organisms. However, PBP alterations in clinical isolates of *Pseudomonas aeruginosa*, *Haemophilus influenzae*, *Neisseria gonorrhoeae*, *N. meningitidis*, *Acinetobacter calcoaceticus*, and *Bacteroides fragilis* have been reported (168).

High-level chromosomally mediated penicillin resistance in non-TEM-1-β-lactamase-producing strains of *N. gonorrhoeae* is associated with low-affinity forms of the essential PBPs 1 and 2 (50). The deduced amino acid sequences of PBP 2, encoded by the *penA* gene, from susceptible and resistant strains are almost identical over the first two-thirds of the gene but extensively altered over the remainder. Thus, it appears that *penA* genes in resistant strains are mosaics generated in a fashion similar to that in *S. pneumoniae* (167). Comparison of the genes (*ponA*) coding for PBP 1 remains to be performed. Penicillin resistance in *N. meningitidis* is also associated with hybrid PBP 2 genes. In both species, foreign DNA probably originated in *N. flavescens* (169).

Resistance Due to β-Lactamases

Although β-lactamases were recognized before the clinical introduction of β-lactam antibiotics, they are considered nonessential enzymes since their only known function is the hydrolysis of β-lactams. In gram-positive bacteria, β-lactamases are secreted mainly into the growth medium, whereas in gram-negative organisms they are secreted into the periplasmic space. Some of the more clinically important β-lactamases are discussed below. For a more extensive discussion, see references 25 and 103. Because β-lactamases comprise a family of tremendous diversity, a number of classification schemes have been suggested. The most recent one, an updated version of that proposed by Bush that includes both plasmid- and chromosome-specified enzymes, is based on substrate and inhibitor profile and molecular structure (Table 1).

Knowledge of the amino acid sequence of many β-lactamases allows them to be classified into one of four evolutionary molecular classes (A, B, C, and D). β-Lactamases of classes A, C, and D act by a serine-ester-linked acyl enzyme mechanism as described above. Molecular class A comprises penicillinases, cephalosporinases, and broad-spectrum β-lactamases that are generally inhibited by active-site-directed β-lactamase inhibitors, such as clavulanic acid, sulbactam, and tazobactam. This group includes the β-lactamases of *S. aureus* (Bush group 2a) and many of the plasmid-specified β-lactamases of gram-negative bacteria, such as the common TEM- and SHV-type enzymes (groups 2b and 2be). In gram-negative bacteria, β-lactamases of molecular classes C (group 1) and D (group 2d) include the chromo-

TABLE 1 Classification scheme for β-lactamases[a]

Group	Molecular class	Preferred substrates	Representative enzymes
1	C	Cephalosporins	AmpC enzymes from gram-negative bacteria
2a	A	Penicillins	Penicillinases from gram-positive bacteria
2b	A	Penicillins, cephalosporins	TEM-1, TEM-2, SHV-1
2be	A	Penicillins, narrow- and extended-spectrum cephalosporins, monobactams	TEM-3 to TEM-26, SHV-2 to SHV-6
2br	A	Penicillins	TEM-30 to TEM-36
2c	A	Penicillins, carbenicillin	PSE-1, PSE-3, PSE-4
2d	D	Penicillins, cloxacillin	OXA-1 to OXA-11, PSE-2 (OXA-2)
2e	A	Cephalosporins	Inducible cephalosporinases from *Proteus vulgaris*
2f	A	Penicillins, cephalosporins, carbapenems	NMC-A from *E. cloacae*, Sme-1 from *S. marcescens*
3	B	Most β-lactams, including carbapenems	L1 from *S. maltophilia*, CcrA from *B. fragilis*
4	ND[b]	Penicillins	Penicillinase from *B. cepacia*

[a] Modified from reference 25 with permission.
[b] ND, not determined.

somal cephalosporinases (AmpC enzymes) and oxacillin-hydrolyzing enzymes (OXA), respectively. Class B (group 3) comprises the metallo-β-lactamases which require Zn^{2+} as a cofactor. These enzymes, which have been identified in *B. fragilis*, *Stenotrophomonas maltophilia*, *Flavobacterium* spp., and *Legionella* spp., hydrolyze all classes of β-lactams, including carbapenems (e.g., imipenem and meropenem), and are not inhibited by penicillinase inhibitors. Further dissemination of these potent enzymes should be expected since plasmid-mediated metallo-β-lactamases have now been found in *P. aeruginosa*, *B. fragilis*, *Serratia marcescens*, and *Klebsiella pneumoniae* (82, 118, 131).

Widespread dissemination of β-lactamase production among staphylococci occurred shortly after the introduction of penicillin G into clinical practice. The β-lactamases of *S. aureus* belong to molecular class A and include four variants which are functionally similar and are encoded by closely related transposable elements (156). Despite their prevalence in *S. aureus* (over 90% are β-lactamase producers) and the selective pressure brought about by the introduction of β-lactamase-stable agents, little evolution has occurred among these enzymes. At least for the present, strains of *S. aureus* resistant to penicillins due to the production of a β-lactamase remain susceptible to semisynthetic penicillins (e.g., oxacillin, nafcillin, and methicillin), to cephalosporins, and to carbapenems.

Unlike the constitutively produced class A β-lactamases of gram-negative bacteria (see below), those of *S. aureus* are usually inducible. Regulation of their synthesis is thought to be under negative control and involves three regulatory genes: *blaI*, *blaR1*, and *blaR2*. The *blaI* gene encodes a repressor that negatively regulates transcription of *blaZ*, the β-lactamase structural gene. The BlaR1 protein, encoded by *blaR1*, consists of an extracellular domain responsible for β-lactam sensing and an intracellular domain responsible for production of a signal that results in the derepression of *blaZ*. The unlinked *blaR2* chromosomal gene down-regulates β-lactamase expression by a mechanism which remains to be determined.

Soon after the introduction of ampicillin, the first penicillin with clinically useful activity against *Escherichia coli*, β-lactamase-producing strains began to emerge. Today, 30 to 50% of *E. coli* strains are resistant to aminopenicillins (ampicillin and amoxicillin) due to production of a β-lactamase. Although several enzymes have been detected in gram-negative bacteria, TEM-1 and SHV-1 are the most prevalent and are most common in *E. coli* and *Klebsiella pneumoniae*, respectively. These widely disseminated, plasmid-mediated β-lactamases efficiently hydrolyze penicillins and narrow-spectrum cephalosporins but poorly hydrolyze extended-spectrum oxyimino-cephalosporins such as cefotaxime and ceftazidime, as well as cephamycins (cefoxitin and cefotetan), monobactams (aztreonam), and carbapenems (imipenem and meropenem). Unlike the chromosomally encoded AmpC enzymes discussed below, overproduction of these enzymes does not confer resistance to the extended-spectrum β-lactams listed above. Hyperproduction of these β-lactamases can, however, be an important cause of resistance to β-lactam–β-lactamase inhibitor combinations. For example, hyperproduction of the plasmid-encoded TEM-1 enzyme was found to be responsible for amoxicillin-clavulanate resistance in 60% of resistant *E. coli* isolates (171).

By contrast to the immutability of the staphylococcal β-lactamases over time, the introduction of numerous broad-spectrum β-lactams into clinical practice was followed relatively quickly by the emergence of mutant TEM- and SHV-type β-lactamases capable of hydrolyzing many of the extended-spectrum cephalosporins and monobactams (but not normally the cephamycins and the carbapenems). These plasmid-mediated, extended-spectrum β-lactamases (ESBLs) were first found in *K. pneumoniae* and later found in almost all members of the *Enterobacteriaceae*. However, at present the majority of TEM- and SHV-derived ESBLs are found predominantly in *Klebsiella* spp. and *E. coli*. At present, ESBLs remain susceptible to β-lactamase inhibitors such as clavulanate, sulbactam, and tazobactam, although this may soon change (164). Interestingly, the mutations that expand the spectrum of TEM- and SHV-type β-lactamases to include extended-spectrum cephalosporins usually increase their sensitivity to inhibition by β-lactamase inhibitors. Unfortunately, however, the usefulness of β-lactamase inhibitors has been weakened by the emergence in 1990 of mutant TEM-1 (rarely SHV-type) enzymes that are not ESBLs but, rather, confer resistance to β-lactam–β-lactamase inhibitor combinations (19). These Bush group 2br enzymes are collectively designated inhibitor-resistant TEM. Finally, ESBL-producing strains may concomitantly hyperproduce TEM-1- or SHV-1-like enzymes, which may result in resistance to β-lactam–β-lactamase combinations (195).

ESBLs differ from their parent enzymes by only a few amino acid substitutions that occur adjacent to three of four evolutionarily conserved amino acid motifs that form the active site of serine peptidases. In certain cases, the enzymatic kinetic parameters and resistance phenotype remain unchanged despite amino acid substitutions. For example, TEM-1 and TEM-2, which differ by a single amino acid at position 37, confer similar resistance phenotypes (13). By contrast, in the case of TEM-7 and SHV-2, the Arg-162 and Gly-236 residues of TEM-1 and SHV-1, respectively, have been replaced by a serine (14, 34, 165). In both instances, the single amino acid substitution extends the substrate specificity to oxime-substituted molecules such as ceftazidime and cefotaxime. However, the various substitutions do not necessarily allow the ESBLs to hydrolyze the substrates equally. For instance, TEM-7 hydrolyzes ceftazidime and cefotaxime at approximately the same rate whereas SHV-2 hydrolyzes cefotaxime about 10 times more rapidly than it hydrolyzes ceftazidime. In other instances, members of the TEM and SHV families are encoded by genes with multiple mutations which have been acquired sequentially. An additional set of alterations, involving the change of Glu-102 in TEM-2 to Lys in TEM-9 or of Glu-237 in SHV-2 to Lys in SHV-4 and SHV-5, further increases the rate of hydrolysis of ceftazidime (61). Similar amino acid substitutions have been described in other extended-spectrum TEM, SHV, and related enzymes. Importantly, although some enzymes may hydrolyze cefotaxime to a greater extent than they hydrolyze ceftazidime, in vitro susceptibility testing often indicates that ceftazidime has higher MICs. This phenomenon may, at least partly, be due to decreased penetration of ceftazidime into the periplasmic space. In fact, certain strains of *K. pneumoniae* may even appear susceptible in vitro to cefotaxime when a standard inoculum is used, and, for this reason, some laboratories consider all ceftazidime-resistant *K. pneumoniae* strains to be resistant to all cephalosporins except cephamycins (88) (see chapter 121).

ESBL mutants are not limited to the TEM and SHV families of enzymes. In *P. aeruginosa*, a number of mutants of class D, OXA (oxacillin-hydrolyzing) enzymes have been detected (40, 65). Strains encoding these variants exhibit resistance to expanded-spectrum cephalosporins and are usually poorly inhibited by clavulanate.

Nearly all members of the family *Enterobacteriaceae* (with the notable exceptions of *Salmonella* spp. and *Klebsiella* spp.) and strains of *P. aeruginosa* normally produce a chromosomally encoded cephalosporinase designated AmpC. These enzymes belong to molecular class C and are sufficiently biochemically distinct to be considered species specific (176). In many enterobacteria such as *Enterobacter cloacae* and *Citrobacter freundii*, β-lactams (especially cefoxitin, imipenem, and clavulanic acid) can induce the production of the chromosomal AmpC β-lactamase (158). In these species, the β-lactamase is normally produced at very low levels but is induced to rates several hundredfold higher by the presence of β-lactams. Although it is currently accepted that the induction of β-lactamase is in itself not a clinical problem, the regulation of β-lactamase production is important because of its high mutation rate, often leading to strains expressing high-level constitutive resistance to many of the newer β-lactam antibiotics (101).

The mechanism of induction of AmpC β-lactamases, mostly studied in *E. cloacae* and *C. freundii*, is highly complex and still not completely understood. Induction appears to be linked to the recycling of cell wall peptidoglycan. At least three genes involved in the induction of AmpC β-lactamases (encoded by the *ampC* gene) have been identified: *ampR*, *ampG*, and *ampD*. The influence of β-lactams on synthesis of the bacterial cell wall leads to accumulation of peptidoglycan degradation products in the periplasm. One of these fragments (disaccharide-pentapeptide) is thought to be the precursor of the inducer molecule. The quantity of disaccharide-pentapeptide generated correlates directly with the capacity of the β-lactam to induce (e.g., increased amounts are observed with the strong inducers such as imipenem and cefoxitin). AmpG, a transmembrane protein that acts as a permease, transports this peptidoglycan fragment (among others) into the cytoplasm (102), where it is converted into the actual signal molecule (monosaccharide-pentapeptide) for β-lactamase induction. Monosaccharide-pentapeptide acts by converting the transcriptional regulator AmpR into an activator of β-lactamase expression (102).

Resistance by constitutive hyperproduction of β-lactamase is often due to mutations in the unlinked *ampD* gene that derepress the expression of *ampC* (100). AmpD is a cytoplasmic *N*-acetyl-anhydromuramyl-L-alanine amidase that is assumed to exert its negative effect on AmpC expression by hydrolyzing the monosaccharide-pentapeptide signal molecule. Consequently, inactivation of AmpD results in large quantities of the inducer in the cytoplasm, which, even in the absence of β-lactam antibiotics, activates AmpR (42, 83, 102, 188).

In *E. coli*, the *ampC* gene is expressed constitutively at very low levels, which are not clinically relevant due to an inefficient promoter and to the presence of an attenuator structure between the promoter and the structural gene. However, hyperproduction of β-lactamase can occur by mutations in the promoter and attenuator regions or by substitution of the native promoter by a more efficient one from another species, such as *Shigella sonnei* (129). Mutants hyperproducing AmpC can also result from amplification of the *ampC* gene (126). Although rare, introduction of the newer cephalosporins has also selected for several plasmid-specified forms of AmpC β-lactamases (134, 138). The presence of hyperproducing AmpC mutants located on multicopy plasmids can confer much higher levels of resistance.

The explanation of resistance to extended-spectrum β-lactams in gram-negative bacteria hyperproducing class C β-lactamases remains controversial, since the enzymes exhibit extremely low or undetectable hydrolytic activity against these compounds. Because of this discrepancy and the observation that the enzymes have a strong affinity for these "β-lactamase-resistant" substrates, it has been suggested that the mechanism of resistance is "trapping." This model proposes that β-lactamases confer resistance by binding to and trapping β-lactam molecules as they slowly cross the outer membrane and enter the periplasmic space, rather than by hydrolyzing them. However, others have suggested that the outer membrane impermeability, coupled with slow hydrolysis, adequately explains *ampC*-mediated resistance to the extended-spectrum drugs (75).

β-Lactam Resistance Due to Decreased Outer Membrane Permeability and Active Efflux

In contrast to gram-positive organisms, in which β-lactams have unhindered access to their PBP targets, in gram-negative bacteria the outer membrane is a barrier to these compounds. The balance between antibiotic influx and clearance, whether due to hydrolysis or trapping, determines the susceptibility or resistance of the cell, since permeability barriers alone rarely produce significant levels of resistance. In *E. coli* and other gram-negative bacteria, β-lactams diffuse across the outer membrane primarily through water-filled channels consisting of a specific class of proteins termed porins. *E. coli* produces at least two porin types, called OmpF and OmpC. Mutations that cause reduced expression or alteration of OmpF and/or OmpC result in decreased susceptibility to many β-lactams (104). *P. aeruginosa* is characterized by an intrinsic resistance to a wide variety of antimicrobial agents, including β-lactams, β-lactam inhibitors (99), tetracyclines, quinolones, and chloramphenicol. Although this resistance has most often been attributable to a highly impermeable outer membrane, it is now recognized to result from the synergy between a unique tripartite energy-driven efflux system (MexAB-OprM) with wide substrate specificity (90, 98, 124) and low outer membrane permeability. Recently, it has been shown that MexAB-OprM directly contributes to β-lactam resistance via efflux of this class of antibiotics (170). The emergence in *P. aeruginosa* of resistance specific to imipenem is associated with the loss of the specific channel OprD (187). It appears that imipenem preferentially uses this channel to cross the outer membrane, which under normal circumstances probably transports basic amino acids (55). In *E. coli*, cross-resistance to various classes of antibiotics, including β-lactams, tetracyclines, chloramphenicol, and quinolones, may be due to mutations in the *marRAB* operon (see "Tetracycline resistance").

AMINOGLYCOSIDE RESISTANCE

Aminoglycosides are particularly active against aerobic gram-negative bacilli and gram-positive cocci except streptococci and enterococci. Intrinsic resistance most often results from impaired uptake, while acquired resistance is frequently due to the acquisition of plasmid-encoded modifying enzymes. Acquired resistance can also be due to chromosomal mutations that alter the ribosomal target or the antibiotic uptake.

Intrinsic and Acquired Resistance Due to Decreased Uptake

Intrinsic and acquired resistance secondary to decreased antibiotic uptake confers low-level cross-resistance to all aminoglycosides. Aminoglycosides are highly positively charged compounds that must cross the outer membrane (in gram-negative organisms) and the cytoplasmic membrane (in gram-negative and -positive bacteria) before they reach their cytoplasmic ribosomal target. In gram-negative bacteria the initial step involves ionic binding of aminoglycosides to anionic sites on the outer membrane surface, which include lipopolysaccharides (LPS), outer membrane proteins, and the polar heads of phospholipids. It has been generally believed that in *E. coli* aminoglycosides reach the periplasmic space by diffusion through outer membrane porin proteins. However, the role of porin-mediated uptake has been questioned since no difference in susceptibility between wild-type and porin-deficient strains of *E. coli* or other gram-negative organisms could be demonstrated (159). Although the results are controversial, studies with *P. aeruginosa* and *E. coli* suggest that passage across the outer membrane may instead be due to a "self-promoted uptake" mechanism, analogous to that previously described for polycationic detergents such as polymyxin (68). The divalent cations Mg^{2+} and Ca^{2+} function as salt bridges between adjacent LPS and phospholipids and are essential for outer membrane integrity. The cationic aminoglycosides displace the divalent cations, thereby permeabilizing the outer membrane and facilitating entry of the antibiotic (86). Of note, disruption of the outer membrane may contribute to the bactericidal activity of these drugs, since neither inhibition of protein synthesis nor codon misreading alone may adequately account for this activity (86). Thus, species-related differences in aminoglycoside activity may be at least partly due to differences in the composition (LPS, outer membrane proteins, porins, phospholipids) of their outer membranes. For instance, decreased gentamicin binding was observed in a strain of *E. coli* with a mutation in LPS phosphates (140). Resistance in *P. aeruginosa* mutants has been associated with overproduction of the major outer membrane protein H1, which may protect the bacteria from cationic antibiotics by substituting for Mg^{2+}.

The electrical potential established by the electron transport system provides the driving force for aminoglycoside transport across the cytoplasmic membrane. This accounts for the relative resistance of electron transport-deficient anaerobic organisms and the decreased susceptibility of facultative anaerobes such as enterococci, streptococci, and members of the family *Enterobacteriaceae* when grown anaerobically. This may also explain why aminoglycoside efficacy is reduced in the anaerobic, low-pH environment that exists in an infectious abscess.

Acquired Resistance Due to Other Mechanisms

Aminoglycoside-Modifying Enzymes

The most common mechanism of acquired resistance to aminoglycosides is antibiotic inactivation by plasmid- and transposon-encoded modifying enzymes. The cytoplasmic modifying enzymes are present in quantities sufficient only to inactivate the drug that enters the cytoplasm (21). Resistant cells are therefore characterized by growth in the presence of unchanged antibiotic in the growth medium.

A detailed description of the numerous aminoglycoside-modifying enzymes and their epidemiology is beyond the scope of this chapter (for excellent reviews, see references 117 and 160). The epidemiology of aminoglycoside resistance mechanisms has become increasingly complicated due to the increasing complexity of the mechanisms themselves, in addition to significant differences within different geographic regions and hospitals (117). A brief description of some of the more widespread enzymes is given below. Of note, while only a few aminoglycosides are used clinically, a complete characterization of an aminoglycoside resistance phenotype (not considered below) requires testing the enzyme against a variety of aminoglycosides, a number of which are experimental and available only in a small number of reference laboratories.

There are three classes of aminoglycoside-modifying enzymes: acetyltransferases (AAC), adenylytransferases (ANT), and phosphotransferases (APH). AAC enzymes acetylate amino groups, whereas ANT and APH enzymes adenylylate and phosphorylate hydroxyl groups, respectively. The structures of typical aminoglycosides and their sites of enzymatic modification are shown in Fig. 2. In general, only phosphorylating enzymes confer very high levels of resistance. Since each class comprises numerous enzymes that can modify different hydroxyl or amino groups, the enzymes are further classified into subclasses. For example, the AAC consist of three subclasses which can acetylate amino groups at either the 3, 2′, or 6′ position [e.g., AAC(3), AAC(2′), and AAC(6′)]. A specific enzyme subclass in-

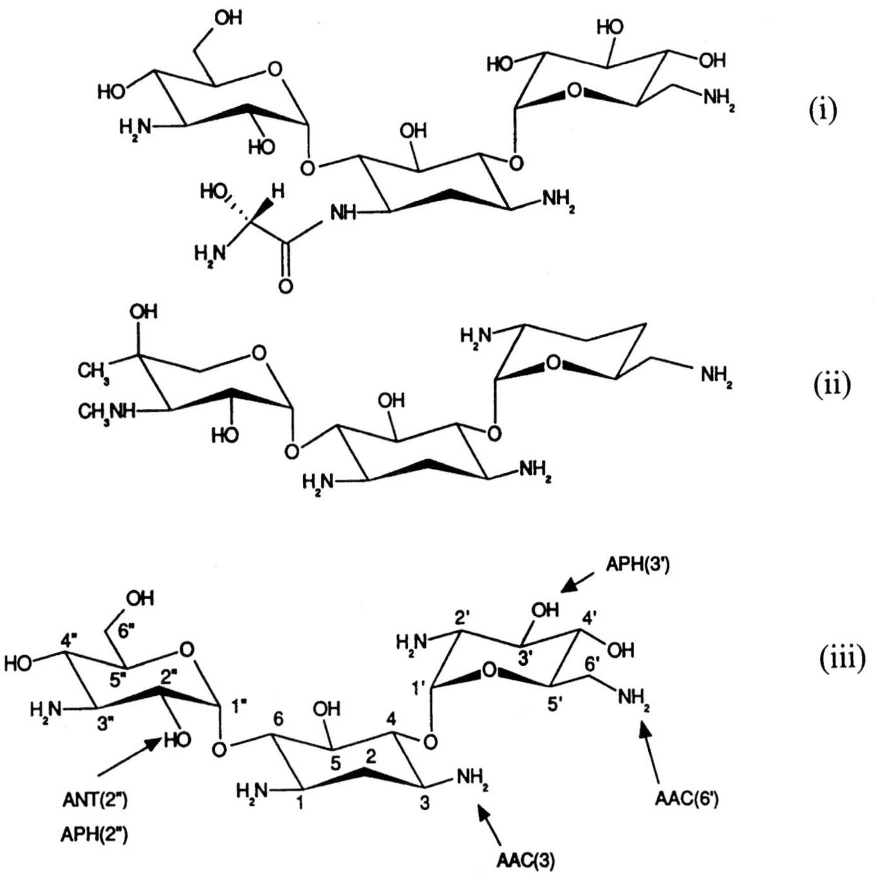

FIGURE 2 Structures of amikacin (i), gentamicin C1a (ii), and kanamycin B (iii). The arrows indicate sites of modification by resistance enzymes (Table 2). Tobramycin is 3′-deoxykanamycin B.

cludes various enzyme types, each of which confers a different resistance phenotype and is designated by a Roman numeral. For instance, AAC(3)-I determines resistance to gentamicin, AAC(3)-II determines resistance to gentamicin, netilmicin, and tobramycin, and AAC(3)-III determines resistance to gentamicin, tobramycin, and kanamycin. Finally, unique proteins (isoenzymes) which are functionally identical and confer identical resistance phenotypes are designated by a, b, etc. [e.g., AAC(6′)-Ia and AAC(6′)-Ib].

At least six AAC(3) resistance profiles have been characterized, including those conferred by AAC(3)-I and -II (see above) and, more recently, AAC(3)-VI (gentamicin, tobramycin, and netilmicin) (117). Among members of the family *Enterobacteriaceae*, AAC(3)-II (gentamicin, tobramycin, and netilmicin) occurs frequently in combination with AAC(6′)-I (tobramycin, netilmicin, kanamycin, and amikacin) (see below), and therefore strains harboring the combination are resistant to gentamicin, tobramycin, netilmicin, kanamycin, and amikacin.

The AAC(6′) enzymes, which are capable of modifying clinically important aminoglycosides, are widely disseminated but vary among different gram-negative bacteria (Table 2). The common AAC(6′)-I enzyme determines resistance to tobramycin, netilmicin, kanamycin, and amikacin, but not to gentamicin. At least nine different genes that encode type-I AAC(6′) enzymes (a through i) have been cloned. Depending on the geographic region, AAC(6′)-I can be found alone or, more commonly, combined with a gentamicin-modifying enzyme, particularly AAC(3)-II or ANT(2″)-I (117). ANT(2″)-I confers resistance to gentamicin, tobramycin, and kanamycin and is the principal profile observed in U.S. isolates of enterobacteria.

Intrinsic low-level resistance to aminoglycosides in all strains of *E. faecium* is due, in addition to impaired uptake, to the presence of a chromosomal gene that codes for an AAC(6′)-I enzyme (35, 119). Importantly, in these strains, the aminoglycosides that are substrates for AAC(6′)-I are modified at a rate insufficient to confer high-level resistance but to an extent that results in the loss of synergy, both in vitro and in vivo, between the aminoglycosides that are substrates and cell wall inhibitors such as β-lactams and vancomycin.

Of special importance is the *aac(6′)-Ie* gene, which is found in *Staphylococcus* and *Enterococcus* strains and which encodes the amino-terminal portion of the bifunctional enzyme AAC(6′) + APH(2″). The bifunctional enzyme comprises an amino-terminal that catalyzes the acetylation of 6′-amino groups and a carboxy-terminal that catalyzes the phosphorylation of 2″-hydroxyl groups. The APH(2″) portion of this enzyme has much the same substrate profile as ANT(2″)-I; i.e., gentamicin, tobramycin, and kanamycin are modified, whereas the AAC(6′) portion has a spectrum of activity similar to the type I AAC(6′) enzymes of gram-negative bacteria. Thus, the presence of the bifunctional enzyme explains the fact that no aminoglycoside (except

TABLE 2 Substrate profiles of selected aminoglycoside-modifying enzymes[a]

Aminoglycoside	APH		ANT				AAC	
	3′	2″	2″	4′	(3″/9)	9	3	6′
Gentamicin C1a	−	+	+	−	−	−	+	+
Gentamicin C1	−	+	+	−	−	−	−	−
Gentamicin C2	−	+	+	−	−	−	−	+
Tobramycin	−	(+)	+	+	−	−	+	+
Amikacin	(+)	(+)	−	+	−	−	−	+
Kanamycin A	+	(+)	+	+	−	−	+	−
Kanamycin B	+	(+)	+	+	−	−	+	+
Kanamycin C	+	(+)	+	+	−	−	−	+
Netilmicin	−	+	−	−	−	−	(+)	+
Sisomicin	−	+	+	−	−	−	(+)	+
Isepamicin	(+)	(+)	−	+	−	−	−	+
Streptomycin	−	−	−	−	+	+	−	−
Spectinomycin	−	−	−	−	+	−	−	−

[a] Symbols: +, normal substrate; (+), substrate for some forms of the enzyme; −, nonsubstrate for the enzyme. The fact that an antibiotic is a substrate for an enzyme in vitro does not necessarily imply that a strain producing that enzyme is resistant to the antibiotic.

streptomycin in strains without concomitant high-level resistance to streptomycin) can be used against enterococci and staphylococci highly resistant to gentamicin. The bifunctional enzyme AAC(6′) + APH(2″) is the most common aminoglycoside-modifying enzyme in gram-positive bacteria. In a survey of 898 aminoglycoside-resistant staphylococci, 42% of isolates had this enzyme as the sole cause of resistance and 49% had it in combination with one or more enzymes (116).

The APH(3′) enzymes confer resistance to kanamycin and neomycin. At least seven APH(3′) enzymes have been identified and can be distinguished by the bacteria in which they are found. APH(3′)-I and APH(3′)-II are found in many gram-negative bacteria, APH(3′)-III is found in gram-positive bacteria and in *Campylobacter*, APH(3′)-IV is found in *Bacillus*, APH(3′)-V is found in *Streptomyces*, APH(3′)-VI is found in *Acinetobacter*, and APH(3′)-VII are found in *Campylobacter*. Although APH(3′)-I and APH(3′)-II of gram-negative bacteria are also capable of modifying the 3′-hydroxyl group of amikacin, it is not modified to the extent necessary to confer resistance in bacteria having normal aminoglycoside permeability. Susceptibility to amikacin is due to a significantly higher k_m of the enzyme for amikacin than for kanamycin or neomycin. Thus, the catalytic efficiency of an enzyme for a particular substrate plays an important role in determining the resistance phenotype. By contrast, the APH(3′)-VI enzyme, which is seen primarily in *Acinetobacter* spp., confers resistance to amikacin (as well as kanamycin and neomycin) (117). The APH(3′)-III enzyme of gram-positive bacteria also modifies kanamycin, neomycin, and amikacin. However, it does not always confer high-level resistance, especially to amikacin, and strains harboring this enzyme may appear susceptible to this drug by standard susceptibility testing, resulting in a misleading resistance phenotype. Thus, in *S. aureus* and *Enterococcus* spp., although APH(3′)-III does not determine resistance to amikacin, synergy with β-lactams or vancomycin is abolished (96).

Determination of the enzyme content of a cell based on the resistance phenotype can be difficult. As discussed above, the fact that an antibiotic is a substrate for an enzyme in vitro does not necessarily imply that a bacterial strain producing that enzyme is resistant to the antibiotic. Furthermore, the level of resistance often depends significantly on the bacterial host. Enzymes that determine resistance to gentamicin or tobramycin in *P. aeruginosa* may not confer detectable resistance in *E. coli* (87). Such species-related phenotypic differences may be due to differences in gene copy number, gene expression, or physiologic differences in membrane structure and antibiotic uptake (87). Finally, the resistance phenotype can also be complicated by the fact that strains can harbor multiple mobile elements, each encoding various enzymes with overlapping substrate ranges.

The genes encoding aminoglycoside-modifying enzymes are often carried by mobile genetic elements such as transposons and self-transferable plasmids, which facilitates horizontal transfer among diverse genera. In addition, a third mechanism of resistance gene dissemination has been discovered. This mechanism involves a novel DNA element called an integron (for reviews, see references 66 and 150), which consists of an insertion site and of an integrase gene that encodes a system for site-specific integration of one or more antibiotic resistance genes. The resistance genes are contained in mobile units called cassettes that can be inserted into and excised from the integron. The capacity of integrons to acquire multiple resistance determinants may partly explain the increased prevalence of multiply aminoglycoside resistant strains.

For the most part, aminoglycoside resistance genes are expressed constitutively, but there are exceptions such as the chromosomal *aac(6′)-Ic* gene present in all strains of *Serratia marcescens* and the *aac(2′)-Ia* gene of *Providencia stuartii* (148).

Ribosomal Target Modification

In the laboratory strain *E. coli* K-12, mutations in the *rpsL* gene that alter ribosomal protein S12 determine high-level resistance to streptomycin (21). Streptomycin resistance due to ribosomal modification has also been found in clinical isolates of *N. gonorrhoeae*, *S. aureus*, *P. aeruginosa*, and *E. faecalis*. In streptomycin-resistant strains of *Mycobacterium tuberculosis*, mutational alterations in 16S rRNA and in the ribosomal protein S12 have been identified (51).

MACROLIDE, LINCOSAMIDE, AND STREPTOGRAMIN RESISTANCE

Intrinsic resistance to macrolide, lincosamide, and streptogramin B (MLS_B) antibiotics in gram-negative bacilli is due to low permeability of the outer membrane to these hydrophobic compounds. Acquired resistance occurs most often by alteration of the ribosomal target, although drug inactivation and efflux have also been described.

Target Modification

MLS_B antibiotics are chemically distinct but have a similar mode of action. They bind to the 50S ribosomal subunit and inhibit the elongation of peptide chains. MLS_B resistance is usually due to acquisition of *erm* (erythromycin resistance methylase) genes, which encode enzymes that N^6-dimethylate a specific adenine residue of 23S rRNA (191). Methylases from numerous gram-positive and -negative bacteria modify an analogous adenine residue that is located in a conserved region of rRNA. Ribosomal methylation confers cross-resistance to macrolides, lincosamides, and type B streptogramin antibiotics, the so-called MLS_B resistance phenotype. Presumably, methylation leads to a conformational change in the ribosome that results in decreased affinity for all MLS_B antibiotics because the binding sites for these drugs overlap.

Nucleotide sequencing and DNA-DNA hybridization studies of various clinically important bacterial species allow the distinction of at least nine classes of *erm* genes (94) (Table 3). Because a number of these classes cross-hybridize, clinical isolates can be assigned to one of four hybridization classes: *ermA*, *ermC*, *ermAM*, and *ermF*. Despite distinct hybridization classes, the amino acid sequences of these enzymes are highly conserved, which suggests that they evolved from a common ancestor, possibly an antibiotic producer (6).

Expression of MLS_B resistance can be inducible or constitutive. The type of expression is not related to the class of *erm* determinant but depends on a regulatory region upstream from the methylase structural gene. Regulation by these regions occurs by a translational attenuation mechanism in which mRNA secondary structure influences the level of translation (78). In laboratory mutants and clinical isolates, single nucleotide changes, deletions, or duplications in the regulatory region convert inducibly resistant strains to constitutively resistant ones that are cross-resistant to MLS_B antibiotics (93).

In staphylococci, inducible strains are resistant to 14-membered (erythromycin, roxithromycin) and 15-membered (azithromycin) macrolides only. The 16-membered macrolides (spiramycin, josamycin), lincosamides, and streptogramin B antibiotics remain active in vitro. This so-called "dissociated resistance" occurs because only 14- and 15-membered macrolides are effective inducers of methylase synthesis (193). MLS_B resistance in streptococci can also be expressed constitutively or inducibly. However, in the latter case, all MLS_B antibiotics can to various degrees act as inducers. Thus, in streptococci inducible MLS_B resistance is crossed to all MLS_B antibiotics (94).

In *Staphylococcus* spp., MLS_B resistance is often mediated by small nonconjugative plasmids carrying the *ermC* determinant (192). With the notable exception of *S. pneumoniae*, MLS_B resistance plasmids have been found in nearly all *Streptococcus* spp. (77). Transfer of MLS_B resistance in the absence of plasmid DNA has been demonstrated in *S. pneumoniae*, *S. bovis*, viridans group streptococci, and group A, B, F, and G streptococci (26, 79). In most *S. pneumoniae* strains, chromosomal MLS_B resistance is mediated by the broad-host-range transposon Tn*1545*, a member of a closely related family of conjugative elements that includes Tn*916* (see "Tetracycline resistance") (36). In *E. faecalis*, inducible erythromycin resistance is often mediated by the nonconjugative transposon Tn*917*, which harbors an *ermAM* determinant (185). Interestingly, the frequency of Tn*917* transposition increases in the presence of erythromycin.

TABLE 3 Distribution of *erm* genes in clinically important bacterial species[a]

Hybridization class	Gene	Host(s)
ermA	*ermA*	*S. aureus*, coagulase-negative staphylococci
ermAM	*ermAM*	*S. sanguis*, *S. pneumoniae*, *S. agalactiae*, *S. pyogenes*
	ermB	*S. aureus*, *B. subtilis*, *Lactobacillus* spp.
	ermB-like	*E. faecalis*
	ermBC	*E. coli*
	ermP	*C. perfringens*
	ermZ	*C. difficile*
	NI	*L. reuteri*
ermC	*ermC*	*S. aureus*, coagulase-negative staphylococci
	ermM	*S. epidermidis*
ermF	*ermF*	*B. fragilis*, *B. ovatus*

[a] Modified from reference 94.
[b] NI, not identified.

Antibiotic Inactivation

Unlike target modification, which causes resistance to structurally distinct antibiotics, enzymatic inactivation confers resistance only to structurally related drugs.

Members of the family *Enterobacteriaceae* resistant to high levels of erythromycin, often isolated from neutropenic patients receiving oral erythromycin for gastrointestinal decontamination, destroy the lactone ring of 14-membered macrolides by producing an erythromycin esterase (15) or by phosphorylation, catalyzed by 2′-phosphotransferases (127). Two types of esterase (I and II), encoded by the *ereA* and *ereB* genes, respectively, have been found (5, 132). The combination of *ereB* and *ermB* (encoding an rRNA methylase) is frequently found in enterobacteria highly resistant to erythromycin, demonstrating the synergism of the two gene products (7). Clinical isolates of *S. haemolyticus* and *S. aureus* highly resistant to lincomycin and apparently susceptible to clindamycin have been described; however, the MBCs of clindamycin are greatly increased. Such strains produce a 3-lincomycin-4-clindamycin-O-nucleotidyltransferase (20).

Active Efflux

At present, 15 to 20% of *S. pneumoniae* isolates and a significant number of *S. pyogenes* isolates (175) in the United States are resistant to 14- and 15-membered macrolides only (17). Strains with this resistance phenotype, designated M, do not contain an *erm* methylase but harbor the genetic determinant *mefE* and *mefA*, which encode pumps that mediate the efflux of 14- and 15-membered macrolides, respectively (30, 177). A novel efflux determinant, designated *mreA* (for macrolide resistance efflux), which confers resistance to 14-, 15-, and 16-membered macrolides, has been recently characterized from a strain of *Streptococcus agalactiae* (29).

Although macrolide resistance among coagulase-negative staphylococci is usually due to the presence of an *ermC* methylase, a significant number of strains are resistant as a result of active efflux of the drug (47). In *S. aureus* and coagulase-negative staphylococci, the *msrA* gene encodes a transport-related protein (155) that confers inducible resistance to 14- and 15-membered macrolides and streptogramin type B antibiotics but not to lincosamides.

Synergistic combinations of type A and B streptogramins (e.g., Synercid, a combination of the A and B streptogramins quinupristin and dalfopristin, respectively) are frequently used outside the United States for treatment of infections caused by staphylococci. Resistance to the synergistic combination is always associated with resistance to the A constituent but is not necessarily associated with resistance to the B constituent. Some strains of staphylococci and enterococci resistant to type A streptogramins contain a gene that codes for an acetyltransferase, *vat* and *sat*, respectively, that inactivates group A compounds (2, 151).

TETRACYCLINE RESISTANCE

Tetracycline resistance is the most common antibiotic resistance encountered in nature. Although it can result from chromosomal mutations affecting outer membrane permeability, more commonly it results from acquisition of exogenous DNA encoding proteins involved in active efflux of tetracycline or in protection of the ribosome.

Altered Permeability

In *E. coli*, chromosomal mutations producing a deficiency in the outer membrane porin OmpF, through which tetracycline normally diffuses, confer low-level resistance to tetracycline as well as to β-lactams, chloramphenicol, and quinolones. Moreover, exposure to tetracycline or chloramphenicol can select mutations in a genetic locus that confer high-level resistance to the selective agent and structurally unrelated antibiotics, including penicillins, cephalosporins, nalidixic acid, and fluoroquinolones. This system, designated MAR (multiple antibiotic resistance), involves the *marRAB* operon, in which reduction in OmpF porin is only part of the resistance mechanism (32). The *marRAB* operon is regulated and derepressed by tetracycline and chloramphenicol (63). Whereas point mutations in the *marRAB* operon confer multiple antibiotic resistance, deletion of this region prevents *E. coli* from acquiring the MAR phenotype. The *marA* gene product MarA is related to a family of positive transcriptional activators, which suggests that the *marRAB* operon is part of a larger regulon that controls the expression of various distant chromosomal genes (32). One such distant gene, *micF*, when activated produces an antisense RNA that inhibits *ompF* translation and results in a reduction in the amount of OmpF. However, other *mar*-related changes must be involved since OmpF mutants are less resistant than their MAR counterparts. Activation of the *mar* operon has also been shown to stimulate the active efflux of tetracycline and chloramphenicol (115). Fluoroquinolone resistance in Mar mutants is attributable to a combined decrease in drug influx (e.g., a reduction in the porin OmpF) as well as an intrinsic active efflux mechanism (33). The Mar phenotype is also associated with elevated expression of the *acrAB* multidrug efflux system, which is probably a major component of Mar-mediated resistance (108, 128). The *mar* locus has been detected among many enteric bacteria, including *Salmonella, Shigella, Klebsiella, Citrobacter, Hafnia,* and *Enterobacter.*

Active Efflux

Resistance to tetracycline in gram-negative and gram-positive bacteria often occurs by energy-dependent pumping of the antibiotic from the cell, so that the levels of drug are decreased and the ribosome is not inhibited. Antibiotic efflux is mediated by the Tet membrane proteins, which use an antiport mechanism of transport involving the exchange of a proton for a tetracycline-cation complex. Even though protein synthesis in resistant cells is unimpaired in the presence of tetracycline, the measured residual intracellular levels of the drug appear sufficient to inhibit protein synthesis (11, 97). It remains to be determined in which compartment, or in what form, the residual tetracycline is found. Since tetracycline can exist in several ionic forms, it is possible that the active form is preferentially pumped from the cell (166).

The tetracycline efflux genes of clinically important bacteria have been assigned to eight classes on the basis of DNA-DNA hybridization. Genes *tet*(A) to *tet*(E) have been detected in various gram-negative bacteria. The *tet*(P) determinant is apparently confined to *Clostridium* spp. and consists of a composite determinant encoding two functional genes, *tetA*(P) and *tetB*(P). The *tetA*(P) portion codes for an efflux transmembrane protein, and the *tetB*(P) section codes for a ribosomal protection protein similar to TetM (see below) (107). The *tet*(K) and *tet*(L) genes have been found only in gram-positive bacteria. With the exception of *tet*(B), the tetracycline efflux-type genes do not handle minocycline (a lipophilic analog of tetracycline) well, providing only 10% or less of the resistance to tetracycline. Despite mechanistic differences in the regulation of *tet* genes, the presence of tetracycline induces the synthesis of resistance proteins which display significant similarity to bacterial transport proteins such as sugar transporters, from which they may have evolved (162).

The intrinsic low-level resistance of *P. aeruginosa* to a wide variety of antimicrobial agents, including tetracycline, appears mostly due to an efflux system with broad substrate specificity (124).

Ribosome Protection

Tetracycline acts by reducing the affinity of the A and P sites of the 30S ribosomal subunit for aminoacyl-tRNA. Tetracycline resistance often results from production of a protein that interacts with the ribosome such that protein synthesis is unaffected by the presence of the antibiotic (for a review, see reference 179). Modification of tRNA has been suggested to interfere with ribosomal protection, but its precise role remains to be determined (180). The exact mechanism of resistance by which ribosomal protection proteins act, however, remains unclear, since experiments with the resistance proteins TetM and TetO indicate that they do not prevent tetracycline from binding to the ribosome. Regardless of the precise mechanism, TetM permits aminoacyl-tRNAs to bind productively to the ribosome.

At least five classes (M, O, P, Q, and S) of ribosomal protection genes have been characterized: *tet*(M) is widely disseminated and is found in many gram-positive and -negative bacteria, as well as mycoplasmas and ureaplasmas;

tet(O) has been detected in *Campylobacter* spp., *Streptococcus* spp., and *Enterococcus* spp. (201); *tet*(P) has been found in *Clostridium perfringens; tet*(Q) has been found in *Bacteroides* spp.; and *tet*(S) has been found in *Listeria monocytogenes* and *E. faecalis* (28). All classes of ribosomal protection genes also confer resistance to minocycline.

Although *tet*(M) is found on plasmids in *Neisseria* spp., *Kingella* spp., *Eikenella* spp., and *Haemophilus ducreyi* (89), it is generally found in the chromosome as part of Tn*916*-related conjugative transposons. These elements are self-transferable, possess an extremely broad host range, and transfer at increased frequency in the presence of tetracycline (163). Moreover, expression of the *tet*(M) gene is regulated and is increased in the presence of tetracycline (172).

RESISTANCE TO SULFONAMIDES AND TRIMETHOPRIM

Biosynthesis of several amino acids and purines depends on the availability of tetrahydrofolate (THF) derivatives required by enzymes that catalyze the transfer of one-carbon units. Moreover, THF is a prerequisite cofactor for essential thymidylate synthesis. In contrast to mammalian cells, which use dietary folates, most bacteria are unable to take up preformed folic acid derivatives and must synthesize THF de novo. The first of the last three steps in THF biosynthesis in bacteria is the condensation of 2-amino-4-hydroxyl-6-hydroxymethyl-pteridine with *p*-aminobenzoic acid (PABA) by dihydropteroic acid synthase (DHPS). The product, dihydropteroic acid, undergoes a second condensation with glutamic acid, yielding dihydrofolic acid. The final step is reduction of dihydrofolic acid to THF by dihydrofolate reductase (DHFR).

Bacterial THF biosynthesis is inhibited by agents that interfere with DHFR or DHPS. Sulfonamides are structural analogs of PABA that competitively inhibit DHPS. Trimethoprim is a competitive inhibitor of bacterial DHFR. For an excellent review of resistance to trimethoprim and sulfonamides, see reference 81.

Intrinsic Resistance

Outer membrane impermeability confers trimethoprim and sulfonamide resistance to *P. aeruginosa* (182). Intrinsic resistance to trimethoprim in a number of species, including *Neisseria* spp., *Clostridium* spp., *Brucella* spp., *Bacteroides* spp., *Moraxella catarrhalis*, and *Nocardia* spp., is due to host DHFR enzymes with low affinity for the drug (184). Folate auxotrophs such as *Enterococcus* spp. and *Lactobacillus* spp., which are able to use exogenous preformed folates, exhibit decreased susceptibility to sulfonamides and trimethoprim (200). Enterococci can also utilize exogenous thymine or thymidine to escape inhibition by folate pathway antagonists (67).

Acquired Resistance to Trimethoprim

Chromosomal Mutations

Chromosomal mutations in the DHFR structural gene *folA* that confer low-level resistance to trimethoprim are easily obtained in the laboratory and occur in clinical isolates. Overproduction of an altered host DHFR confers resistance in clinical isolates of *E. coli* (52), *S. pneumoniae* (1), and *H. influenzae* (59). Chromosomal mutations which result in decreased outer membrane permeability and confer cross-resistance to nalidixic acid, trimethoprim, and chloramphenicol have been observed in *K. pneumoniae, E. aerogenes, E. cloacae*, and *S. marscescens* (62). The pleiotropic resistance observed in these strains was associated with a decrease in the amounts of certain outer membrane proteins. Combined high-level resistance to trimethoprim and sulfonamides can be due to chromosomal mutations that inactivate thymidylate synthetase, an enzyme that converts deoxyuridylate to thymidylate. These so-called *thy* mutants require exogenous thymine or thymidine for DNA synthesis and are thus resistant to folate pathway antagonists.

Plasmid-Mediated Resistance

High-level resistance to trimethoprim in members of the family *Enterobacteriaceae* is most often caused by the acquisition of exogenous DNA that specifies a supernumerary DHFR which is less sensitive than the chromosomal enzyme to inhibition by trimethoprim (3). To date, at least 16 different DHFRs have been characterized in gram-negative organisms, particularly *E. coli*, based on kinetic data, antisera, primary structure, and DNA-DNA hybridization. By contrast, only two types (S1 and S2) of DHFR that confer resistance to trimethoprim have been described in gram-positive bacteria.

The most widespread additional accessory DHFR is DHFR type I, which confers high-level resistance to trimethoprim (53). The corresponding gene, *dhfrI*, is located on transposon Tn*7*. In addition, the *dhfrI* gene has been detected in genomic environments other than Tn*7* as part of mobile genetic elements called cassettes (174). A cassette consists of a resistance gene flanked by conserved DNA sequences that promote site-specific insertion into so-called integrons (see "Aminoglycoside-modifying enzymes"), elements first noted in transposon Tn*21*. The *dhfrI* gene has been found inserted in DNA sequences similar to the integron of Tn*21* (174). The appearance of the *dhfrI* gene in Tn*21*-like structures not only increases its potential for dissemination but also links trimethoprim and sulfonamide resistance, since this integron also contains a sulfonamide resistance determinant.

Type II DHFRs are unrelated to other DHFRs and are the least sensitive to trimethoprim (137). Type III enzymes are more closely related to chromosomal DHFRs in gram-negative bacteria than to the plasmid-specified type I enzyme (53). They confer a moderate level of trimethoprim resistance and have been detected in *S. typhimurium* and *Shigella* spp. (4). Type IV DHFR is unique in its ability to be induced by trimethoprim (198). In *E. coli*, Type X DHFR is also encoded by a gene as part of an integron (136).

In gram-positive bacteria, the ubiquitous type S1 DHFR, encoded by the *dfrA* gene located in transposon Tn*4003*, has been detected in *S. aureus, S. haemolyticus, S. epidermidis*, and *S. hominis* (38), and, more recently, the type S2 enzyme has been found in *S. haemolyticus* and *Listeria monocytogenes* (27, 39). The S1 enzyme present in *Staphylococcus* spp. and in *Listeria* may represent a mobilized and mutated variant of the chromosomally mediated enzyme of *S. epidermidis*, since the amino acid sequence of the plasmid-mediated type S1 DHFR is almost identical to that of the chromosomal DHFR of *S. epidermidis* (38).

Acquired Resistance to Sulfonamides

Chromosomal Mutations

Chromosomal mutations responsible for overproduction of PABA have been reported to confer sulfonamide resistance in *Neisseria* spp. and in *S. aureus* (48). Resistance in *E. coli, S. pneumoniae*, and *N. meningitidis* is associated with alterations of the *dhps* gene, which codes for a DHPS with low affinity for sulfonamides (105, 113, 183). As mentioned above, mutation to thymine auxotrophy in many bacterial species can also confer resistance to trimethoprim and sulfonamides.

Plasmid-Mediated Resistance

Acquired sulfonamide resistance can be due to acquisition of plasmids that encode a drug-resistant dihydropteroate synthase. Two types (types I and II) of resistant DHPS, encoded by the *sulI* and *sulII* genes, respectively, have been identified in gram-negative organisms (146, 173). The *sulI* gene is almost always linked to other resistance genes and is located in conserved segments of integrons in Tn*21*-like elements carried by large conjugative plasmids (147). The *sulII* gene is frequently linked genetically to a streptomycin resistance gene on broad-host-range plasmids and on small nonconjugative plasmids (146). The *sulI* and *sulII* genes are found at approximately the same frequency among gram-negative clinical isolates (147).

QUINOLONE RESISTANCE

The bacterial chromosome replicates by a semiconservative mechanism in which each strand of the parental duplex acts as a template for synthesis of a complementary daughter strand. However, since the chromosome is circular, unwinding of the intertwined parental DNA strands during replication would result in positive supercoiling further along the molecule, which would rapidly generate insurmountable resistance to further movement. This problem is overcome by DNA gyrase, a type II DNA topoisomerase, which, among other functions, removes positive DNA supercoils from closed circular DNA.

DNA gyrase consists of a tetramer of two nonidentical subunits, A and B, in the form A_2B_2. The A and B subunits are encoded by the chromosomal genes *gyrA* and *gyrB*, respectively. In the genera studied, DNA gyrases are highly conserved. The enzyme introduces a 4-bp staggered double-strand break in one duplex strand, such that each A subunit is attached via a tyrosine-122 residue to the newly created 5′ terminus of each strand. Subsequently, another segment of duplex DNA is passed through the break and the break is resealed. The A subunit, responsible for the breakage-ligation reaction, is the primary target of quinolones. More recently, it has been proposed that quinolones bind to the complex of DNA and DNA gyrase and that the quinolone-binding site is exposed only after the DNA strands are cleaved. Quinolones are known to inhibit resealing of cleaved DNA, and they presumably inhibit gyrase function by trapping the covalent enzyme-DNA intermediate.

Recently, it has been shown that a second type of topoisomerase, topoisomerase IV, is also a target of quinolones. Like DNA gyrase, topoisomerase IV is a tetramer in the form A_2B_2. The A and B subunits are encoded by the *parC* and *parE* genes, respectively (designated *grlA* and *grlB*, respectively, in *S. aureus*). Topoisomerase IV is a decatenating enzyme that resolves interlinked daughter chromosomes following DNA replication. The interaction of quinolones with topoisomerase IV remains to be clearly determined. For a recent review of DNA gyrase, topoisomerase IV, and the quinolones, see reference 45.

Alteration of DNA Gyrase and Topoisomerase IV

Since DNA gyrase and topoisomerase IV are necessary for cell growth and division, it is not surprising that quinolones are bactericidal. However, mutations in the genes coding for the subunits of gyrase, topoisomerase IV, or both may confer resistance to the quinolones.

Selection of spontaneous, single-step, highly resistant mutants has been possible for nalidixic acid but not for the newer fluoroquinolones. However, highly resistant strains can be selected by serial passage in the presence of increasing antibiotic concentrations, indicating that multiple mutations are likely to be responsible for high-level fluoroquinolone resistance. Low- and high-level resistance to nalidixic acid and fluoroquinolones can be due to or associated with mutation(s) in the *gyrA* gene (122).

Examination of eight clinical isolates of quinolone-resistant uropathogenic *E. coli* strains revealed that in all but one, Ser-83→Leu or Trp changes were associated with high-level resistance to nalidixic acid (130). The remaining strain, which expressed low-level resistance, had a Ser-87→Val change. *trans*-complementation analysis, based on the fact that quinolone-susceptible *gyrA* alleles are usually dominant over their resistant counterparts, indicated that high-level fluoroquinolone resistance in clinical isolates was at least partly due to *gyrA* mutations (74). To distinguish neutral mutations from mutations responsible for resistance, a chimeric *gyrA* gene which was wild type (sensitive) except for a Ser-83→Trp change was constructed. When present in a strain of *E. coli* harboring a temperature-sensitive *gyrA* allele, the hybrid gene conferred high-level resistance to nalidixic acid, confirming its direct contribution to quinolone resistance. In similar experiments, a chimeric *gyrA* gene that included the double mutation Ser-83→Leu and Asp-87→Gly was demonstrated to account for high-level resistance to fluoroquinolones (74). Alterations in GyrA have also been found in numerous quinolone-resistant gram-negative and gram-positive bacteria.

Almost all GyrA resistance mutations described have been located in a 130-bp sequence termed the quinolone resistance-determining region. The amino acid substitutions are close to the catalytic tyrosine-122 residue, which is consistent with the observation that quinolones prevent resealing of cleaved DNA. As mentioned above, highly quinolone-resistant clinical isolates exhibit "mutational hot spots," especially at position Ser-83. In almost all instances, amino acid substitutions at these positions involve the replacement of a hydroxyl group with a bulky hydrophobic residue. This suggests that mutations in *gyrA* induce changes in the binding-site conformation and/or charge that may be important for quinolone-DNA gyrase interaction (122).

In laboratory strains of *E. coli*, two amino acid substitutions in GyrB determine low-level resistance to quinolones. An Asp-426→Asn change conferred resistance to all quinolones, whereas a Lys-447→Glu change led to resistance to nalidixic and oxolinic acids but hypersusceptibility to ciprofloxacin, norfloxacin, ofloxacin, enoxacin, and sparfloxacin (121, 196). Despite the similar frequency of *gyrA* and *gyrB* mutations in vitro, mutations in *gyrA* appear to be mostly responsible for resistance in clinical isolates (121). Since *gyrA* mutations are associated with high-level resistance, they may have a selective advantage over *gyrB* mutations, which confer low-level resistance (122).

Among gram-negative pathogens, DNA gyrase, and not topoisomerase IV, is the primary target of the quinolones and alterations in the *gyrA* gene are primarily responsible for the development of resistance to this class of antibiotics. However, as mentioned above, multiple mutations (or factors that lead to decreased drug accumulation [see below]) are probably necessary for expression of high-level fluoroquinolone resistance. For example, in *E. coli* (73), *N. gonorrhoeae* (41), and *H. influenzae* (56), secondary mutations of the ParC subunit of topoisomerase IV confer increased levels of fluoroquinolone resistance. Clinically, there appears to be little selective advantage to solitary mutations in *parC* unless mutations have previously decreased the activity of *gyrA*, suggesting that changes to *gyrA* probably precede those to *parC*.

In gram-positive organisms, such as *S. aureus*, *S. pneumoniae*, and *E. faecalis*, fluoroquinolone resistance is also due to mutations in the *gyrA* and *parC* genes. Again, resistance usually results from mutations in the quinolone resistance-determining region of GyrA (and equivalent positions of the ParC subunit of topoisomerase IV). In contrast to gram-negative bacteria, it appears that in gram-positive bacteria, topoisomerase IV and not DNA gyrase may be the primary target of fluoroquinolones. Thus, in ciprofloxacin-resistant strains of *S. aureus* and in *S. pneumoniae*, *parC* mutations were shown to precede those in *gyrA*, suggesting that there is a fundamental difference between gram-negative and gram-positive organisms with respect to *parC* mutations. However, more recently, studies of *S. pneumoniae* suggest that target preference (DNA gyrase versus topoisomerase IV) may also be a function of quinolone structure. For example, in *S. pneumoniae*, sparfloxacin appears to target DNA gyrase whereas ciprofloxacin targets topoisomerase IV (133). Low-level quinolone resistance due to mutations in *parE* has also been demonstrated in *S. pneumoniae* and *E. coli* (18, 139).

Decreased Permeability and Active Efflux

Decreased drug accumulation associated with changes in the outer membrane confers low-level resistance to quinolones and structurally unrelated drugs. Quinolone resistance is a characteristic of the MAR phenotype (see "Tetracycline resistance"). In *E. coli*, exposure to tetracycline or chloramphenicol selects for mutations that confer resistance to the selective agents as well as to a wide range of structurally unrelated antibiotics, including β-lactams, nalidixic acid, and the fluoroquinolones. Resistance to fluoroquinolones appears to be due to decreased permeability as well as to an intrinsic efflux system. Although the frequency of expression of the *mar* locus among clinical isolates remains to be determined, the *mar* locus is at least partly responsible for the multidrug resistance phenotype in some quinolone-resistant strains (110). In vitro studies in *P. aeruginosa* have identified various loci in which mutations confer resistance by decreased membrane permeability due to alterations of outer membrane proteins and LPS (80, 124). In *P. aeruginosa*, quinolones can select for mutants that overexpress various efflux systems, such as MexCD-OprJ, MexEF-OprN, and MexAB-OprM, which confer resistance to multiple classes of antibiotics (141). Recent data suggest that overexpression of a particular efflux system may be related to the specific quinolone used for selection.

A uropathogenic isolate of *S. aureus* has been shown to contain a transmembrane multidrug efflux pump encoded by the *norA* gene, which is intrinsic to this species. Resistance does not result from mutations in the structural gene but may be due to a mutation in a regulatory region, since resistance is associated with elevated expression of *norA* (85). It was thought that the hydrophilicity of the specific quinolone substrate affected its ability to be transported from the cell, resulting in higher levels of resistance to hydrophilic quinolones, such as norfloxacin and enoxacin, than to hydrophobic ones (197). However, specific substituents present on the quinolone may also be an important factor (178). Recently, an active efflux mechanism to fluoroquinolones has also been suggested to operate in *S. pneumoniae* (199).

CHLORAMPHENICOL RESISTANCE

Chloramphenicol resistance in gram-positive and gram-negative organisms most commonly results from the acquisition of plasmids encoding chloramphenicol acetyltransferases (CAT), which enzymatically inactivate the drug. In certain gram-negative bacteria, decreased outer membrane permeability can confer resistance to chloramphenicol and to structurally unrelated compounds.

Enzymatic Inactivation

Chloramphenicol contains two hydroxyl groups that are acetylated in a reaction, catalyzed by CAT, in which acetyl coenzyme A is the acyl donor. Initial acetylation occurs at the C-3 hydroxyl group to give 3-acetoxy-chloramphenicol. Following nonenzymatic rearrangement to 1-acetoxy-chloramphenicol and reacetylation, the 1,3-diacetoxy-chloramphenicol product is formed (120). Both the mono- and diacetylated derivatives are unable to bind the 50S ribosomal subunit to inhibit prokaryotic peptidyltransferase.

Knowledge of the structure, specificity, and mechanism of CAT relies significantly on studies of the enteric type III variant, for which a detailed tertiary structure is available. All CAT variants normally exist in solution as a trimeric structure composed of identical subunits. Although the genes encoding these enzymes show little similarity, their deduced amino acid sequences are significantly conserved, particularly in a region that includes an invariant histidyl residue analogous to the catalytic His-195 active-site residue of the type III enzyme.

CATs in Gram-Positive Bacteria

In *S. aureus*, five closely related variants of CAT, types A, B, C, and D and that encoded by the prototypic plasmid pC194, have been differentiated on the basis of electrophoretic mobility. The structural genes (*cat*) for the enzymes are generally located on small multicopy plasmids, and expression of *cat* is inducible by chloramphenicol by a translational attenuation mechanism (106).

Chloramphenicol-resistant strains of *E. faecalis* and *S. pneumoniae* produce an inducible CAT that resembles the type D variant of staphylococci (37). In *C. perfringens*, there are two constitutively expressed determinants: *catP*, usually found on conjugative plasmids as part of the transposable element Tn*4451*, and the chromosomally located *catQ* (12), which is nearly identical to *catD*, the CAT gene found in resistant *C. difficile* (154).

CATs in Gram-Negative Bacteria

In gram-negative bacteria, resistance to chloramphenicol is usually mediated by plasmid- or transposon-borne genes that are generally expressed constitutively (106). Three types of enzymes (types I, II, and III) have been identified in enteric bacteria. The ubiquitous type I variant (CAT_I) exhibits the unusual property of conferring resistance to fusidic acid by specifically and tightly binding to the steroidal antibiotic. The gene that codes for CAT_I is usually located on transposon Tn9 or related elements (161). Interestingly, the Tn9-specified *cat* gene is subject to cyclic AMP-mediated catabolite repression (58). Various CAT_{II} variants that are closely related to those found in enteric organisms have been isolated from *H. influenzae* and *H. parainfluenzae* (153).

More recently, a number of genes that encode enzymes catalyzing acetyl transfer from coenzyme A to chloramphenicol but are not related structurally to typical CATs have been detected. These so-called XATs (xenobiotic acetyltransferases) include the chromosomally encoded enzymes of *P. aeruginosa* and *Agrobacterium tumefaciens*. A chloramphenicol resistance determinant, coding for a XAT which is 65% identical to that of *A. tumefaciens*, has been found on the multidrug resistance transposon Tn*2424* of *E. coli* (135). Tn*2424* is closely related to Tn*21*, and nucleotide sequencing of regions flanking the *xat* gene indicated that the resistance gene is part of a genetic element called an integron, which promotes the expression and dissemination of resistance genes (see "Aminoglycoside-modifying enzymes").

Decreased Permeability

In gram-negative bacteria, resistance may also be due to chromosomal mutations that result in decreased outer membrane permeability. In *H. influenzae* (23) and *S. typhi* (186), high-level resistance to chloramphenicol has been associated with a decrease in the amount of a major outer membrane protein and lack of OmpF entry porin, respectively. In *P. aeruginosa*, nonenzymatic chloramphenicol resistance is associated with the presence of the *cmlA* gene on the In*4* integron of Tn*1696* (16). The CmlA protein appears to result in reduced expression of two outer membrane porins (OmpA and OmpC) and decreased chloramphenicol uptake (16, 24). However, it is possible that Tn*1696*-mediated chloramphenicol resistance is due to efflux, since the protein sequence of CmlA indicates that it is a transporter belonging to the major facilitator family. In *E. coli*, resistance to chloramphenicol and structurally unrelated antibiotics is also part of the MAR phenotype (see "Tetracycline resistance").

GLYCOPEPTIDE RESISTANCE

The glycopeptide antibiotics, vancomycin and teicoplanin, bind to peptidyl-D-alanyl-D-alanine termini of peptidoglycan precursors and prevent, presumably by steric hindrance, the transglycosylation and transpeptidation steps of cell wall peptidoglycan synthesis. Gram-negative organisms are intrinsically resistant because of the impermeability of the outer cell membrane to these large, rigid, and hydrophobic molecules. Among pathogenic gram-positive bacteria, glycopeptide resistance is restricted to *Enterococcus* spp., *Staphylococcus* spp., and intrinsically resistant species such as *Lactobacillus* spp., *Leuconostoc* spp., *Pediococcus* spp., and *Erysipelothrix rhusiopathiae*. The mechanism of resistance has been extensively studied in enterococci (8). Two distinct phenotypes of acquired resistance, VanA and VanB, can be distinguished on the basis of the antibacterial and inducing activity of glycopeptides (8, 145).

Strains with the VanA phenotype include mostly isolates of *E. faecium* and *E. faecalis*, with inducible high-level resistance to vancomycin and teicoplanin but not to other cell wall inhibitors (95). Resistance is generally transferable to susceptible enterococci by conjugation (95). The genes necessary and sufficient for expression of the VanA phenotype are carried by the 11-kb transposon Tn*1546* (10). Transposition of Tn*1546* or related elements into self-transferable plasmids and subsequent transfer by conjugation appears to be responsible for the spread of high-level resistance among clinical isolates of enterococci. Tn*1546* encodes nine polypeptides that can be assigned to four functional groups: transposition functions (ORF1 and ORF2), regulation of vancomycin resistance genes (VanR and VanS), resistance to glycopeptides by production of depsipeptides (VanH, VanA, and VanX), and accessory proteins that are not necessary for glycopeptide resistance (VanY and VanZ).

The deduced amino acid sequence of VanA is similar to those of the chromosomal D-alanine:D-alanine ligases of *E. faecalis* (49) and members of the family *Enterobacteriaceae* (46). These enzymes are part of the D-alanine (D-Ala) branch of peptidoglycan synthesis and catalyze the conversion of two D-alanines into the dipeptide D-Ala–D-Ala, which is subsequently incorporated into a disaccharide pentapeptide cell wall precursor by the D-Ala–D-Ala-adding enzyme (190). However, unlike the physiologic chromosomal ligases, the VanA ligase preferentially synthesizes the depsipeptide D-Ala–D-lactate (8, 69). The substitution of the -NH group of the amide D-Ala–D-Ala linkage by an oxygen in the D-Ala–D-lactate ester linkage eliminates a hydrogen bond between the -NH group of the terminal D-alanine and vancomycin and results in a 1,000-fold decrease in the affinity for vancomycin (22). Consequently, such strains are resistant since vancomycin is no longer able to inhibit peptidoglycan synthesis.

Biochemical analysis of the VanH protein indicated that it produces D-2-hydroxyacid substrates, specifically D-lactate from pyruvate for VanA (22). In addition to VanA and VanH, the VanX protein is necessary for expression of glycopeptide resistance (8). VanX is a D,D-dipeptidase that contributes to VanA-mediated resistance by hydrolyzing the dipeptide D-Ala–D-Ala, which would otherwise compete with DAla–D-lactate for incorporation into pentapeptide cell wall precursors (152).

The distal portion of Tn*1546* encodes two proteins, VanY and VanZ, that are not necessary for glycopeptide resistance. The *vanY* gene is required for vancomycin-inducible production of a D,D-carboxypeptidase that hydrolyzes preferentially peptidoglycan precursors terminated by D-Ala (8). Under certain conditions, VanY may contribute to resistance by hydrolyzing peptidoglycan precursors terminated by D-Ala. The normal (sensitive) D-Ala-terminated precursors could result from the incorporation of D-Ala–D-Ala that escape hydrolysis by VanX. The deduced product of the *vanZ* gene, which is not significantly related in structure to other proteins, confers by an unknown mechanism low-level resistance to teicoplanin in the absence of the genes required for pentadepsipeptide synthesis (9).

Amino acid sequence similarity was detected between VanR and response regulators and between VanS and histidine protein kinases of so-called two-component regulatory systems (8). In the VanS-VanR regulatory system, VanS undergoes autophosphorylation in response to an unknown signal triggered by the presence of glycopeptides. Subsequently, VanS transfers the phosphate group to its cognate response regulator, VanR, thereby activating a promoter for cotranscription of *vanH*, *vanA*, *vanX*, and *vanY* (8).

High-level glycopeptide resistance has been detected in strains of *E. faecium*, *E. faecalis*, *E. avium*, *E. durans*, *E. raffinosus*, and *E. mundtii*. There is no barrier to heterospecific expression of the resistance genes in *Bacillus thuringiensis*, *L. monocytogenes*, *S. aureus*, and *Streptococcus* spp., and dissemination of this type of resistance to other human pathogens should be anticipated. Moreover, high-level glycopeptide resistance has been transferred from *E. faecalis* to *S. aureus* by conjugation under laboratory conditions (125).

Recently, a clinical isolate of *Streptococcus bovis* resistant to vancomycin was shown to harbor a *vanB*-related (see below) ligase gene (142).

The VanB phenotype includes strains *E. faecium* and *E. faecalis* with variable level resistance to vancomycin (MICs, 4 to >1,024 μg/ml) and susceptibility to teicoplanin (145). These strains are inducible by vancomycin only, but induced strains are cross-resistant to vancomycin and teicoplanin. Despite the wide range of MICs of vancomycin, all these strains contain *vanB*-related sequences (145). VanB-type resistance in certain strains with low- and high-level resistance is transferable to susceptible enterococci by conjugation (144, 145). Like *vanA*, *vanB* encodes a ligase of altered specificity, since these strains also contain peptidoglycan precursors terminated by D-lactate. Further nucleotide sequencing indicated that *vanB* is part of a gene cluster that includes genes that are homologous to *vanR*, *vanS*, *vanH*, *vanX*, and *vanY*. VanB strains also appear to contain an additional gene, *vanW*, of unknown function and do not contain *vanZ*. In contrast to *vanA*, the *vanB* gene cluster is usually located on the chromosome as part of very large (90- to 250-kb) conjugative elements (144) and, at least in some strains, is part of composite transposons (143). Variants of VanB-type strains constitutively resistant to vancomycin and teicoplanin have been found during therapy, suggesting that the distinction between the VanA and the VanB phenotypes can be attributed, at least in part, to differences in regulation (72). The VanA and VanB ligases may have originated from glycopeptide-producing organisms, since the ligases of these organisms are highly homologous to those of Van A and VanB (111).

Three *Enterococcus* species, *E. gallinarum*, *E. casseliflavus*, and *E. flavescens*, are intrinsically resistant to glycopeptides. These species express constitutive resistance to low levels of vancomycin only (VanC phenotype). The *vanC-1* gene of *E. gallinarum* encodes VanC, which is also related to D-Ala–D-Ala ligases and appears to catalyze the formation of the novel dipeptide D-Ala–D-serine (60). Among other intrinsically resistant species, *Pediococcus* spp., *Lactobacillus* spp., and *Leuconostoc* spp. have been shown to contain D-lactate terminated precursors (60).

Clinical isolates of *Staphylococcus*, including *S. aureus*, with intermediate levels of resistance to vancomycin have been recently reported (76). Although the precise mechanism of resistance in these isolates remains to be elucidated, it is not due to the acquisition of genes which confer vancomycin resistance in enterococci.

REFERENCES

1. **Adrian, P. V., and K. P. Klugman.** 1997. Mutations in the dihydrofolate reductase gene of trimethoprim-resistant isolates of *Streptococcus pneumoniae*. *Antimicrob. Agents Chemother.* **41:**2406–2413.
2. **Allignet, J., S. Aubert, A. Morvan, and N. E. Solh.** 1996. Distribution of genes encoding resistance to streptogramin A and related compounds among staphylococci resistant to these antibiotics. *Antimicrob. Agents Chemother.* **40:** 2523–2528.
3. **Amyes, S. G. B., and J. T. Smith.** 1974. R-factor trimethoprim resistance mechanism: an insusceptible target site. *Biochem. Biophys. Res. Commun.* **58:**412–418.
4. **Amyes, S. G. B., and K. J. Towner.** 1990. Trimethoprim resistance; epidemiology and molecular aspects. *J. Med. Microbiol.* **31:**1–19.
5. **Arthur, M., D. Autissier, and P. Courvalin.** 1986. Analysis of the nucleotide sequence of the *ereB* gene encoding the erythromycin esterase type II. *Nucleic Acids Res.* **14:** 4987–4999.
6. **Arthur, M., A. Brisson-Noël, and P. Courvalin.** 1987. Origin and evolution of genes specifying resistance to macrolide, lincosamide, and streptogramin antibiotics: data and hypotheses. *J. Antimicrob. Chemother.* **20:**783–802.
7. **Arthur, M., and P. Courvalin.** 1986. Contribution of two different mechanisms to erythromycin resistance in *Escherichia coli*. *Antimicrob. Agents Chemother.* **30:**694–700.
8. **Arthur, M., and P. Courvalin.** 1993. Genetics and mechanisms of glycopeptide resistance in enterococci. *Antimicrob. Agents Chemother.* **37:**1563–1571.
9. **Arthur, M., F. Depardieu, C. Molinas, P. Reynolds, and P. Courvalin.** 1995. The *vanZ* gene of Tn*1546* from *Enterococcus faecium* BM4147 confers resistance to teicoplanin. *Gene* **154:**87–92.
10. **Arthur, M., C. Molinas, F. Depardieu, and P. Courvalin.** 1993. Characterization of Tn*1546*, a Tn*3*-related transposon conferring glycopeptide resistance by synthesis of depsipeptide peptidoglycan precursors in *Enterococcus faecium* BM4147. *J. Bacteriol.* **175:**117–127.
11. **Avtalion, R. R., R. Ziegler-Schlomowitz, M. Perl, A. Wojdani, and D. Sompolinsky.** 1971. Depressed resistance to tetracycline in *Staphylococcus aureus*. *Microbios* **3:** 165–180.
12. **Bannam, T. L., and J. I. Rood.** 1991. Relationship between the *Clostridium perfringens catQ* gene product and chloramphenicol acetyltransferases from other bacteria. *Antimicrob. Agents Chemother.* **35:**471–476.
13. **Barthélémy, M., J. Péduzzi, and R. Labia.** 1985. Distinction entre les structures primaires des b-lactamases TEM-1 et TEM-2. *Ann. Inst. Pasteur Microbiol.* **136A:**311–321.
14. **Barthélémy, M., J. Péduzzi, H. B. Yaghlane, and R. Labia.** 1988. Single amino acid substitution between SHV-1 β-lactamase and cefotaxime-hydrolyzing SHV-2 enzyme. *FEBS Lett.* **231:**217–220.
15. **Barthélémy, P., D. Autissier, G. Gerbaud, and P. Courvalin.** 1984. Enzymatic hydrolysis of erythromycin by a strain of *Escherichia coli*: a new mechanism of resistance. *J. Antibiot.* **37:**1692–1696.
16. **Bissonnette, L., S. Champetier, J.-P. Buisson, and P. H. Roy.** 1991. Characterization of the nonenzymatic chloramphenicol resistance (*cmlA*) gene of the In*4* integron of Tn*1696*: similarity of the product to transmembrane transport proteins. *J. Bacteriol.* **173:**4493–4502.
17. **Breiman, R. F., J. C. Butler, F. C. Tenover, J. A. Elliot, and R. R. Facklam.** 1994. Emergence of drug-resistant pneumococcal infections in the United States. *JAMA* **271:** 1831–1835.
18. **Breines, D. M., S. Ouabdesselam, E. Y. Ng, J. Tankovic, S. Shah, C. J. Soussy, and D. C. Hooper.** 1997. Quinolone resistance locus *nfxD* of *Escherichia coli* is a mutant allele of the *parE* gene encoding a subunit of topoisomerase IV. *Antimicrob. Agents Chemother.* **41:**175–179.
19. **Bret, L., E. B. Chaibi, C. Chanal-Claris, D. Sirot, R. Labia, and J. Sirot.** 1997. Inhibitor-resistant TEM (IRT) β-lactamases with different substitutions at position 244. *Antimicrob. Agents Chemother.* **41:**2547–2549.
20. **Brisson-Noël, A., P. Delrieu, D. Samain, and P. Courvalin.** 1988. Inactivation of lincosamide antibiotics in *Staphylococcus*. *J. Biol. Chem.* **263:**15880–15887.
21. **Bryan, L. E.** 1989. Aminoglycoside resistance, p. 35–57. *In* L. E. Bryan (ed.), *Microbial Resistance to Drugs*. Springer-Verlag KG, Berlin, Germany.
22. **Bugg, T. D. H., G. D. Wright, S. Dutka-Malen, M. Arthur, P. Courvalin, and C. T. Walsh.** 1991. Molecular basis for vancomycin resistance in *Enterococcus faecium* BM4147: biosynthesis of a depsipeptide peptidoglycan pre-

cursor by vancomycin resistance proteins VanH and VanA. *Biochemistry* **30:**10408–10415.

23. **Burns, J. L., P. M. Mendelman, J. Levy, T. L. Stull, and A. L. Smith.** 1985. A permeability barrier as a mechanism of chloramphenicol resistance in *Haemophilus influenzae*. *Antimicrob. Agents Chemother.* **27:**46–54.
24. **Burns, J. L., C. E. Rubens, P. M. Mendelman, and A. L. Smith.** 1986. Cloning and expression in *Escherichia coli* of a gene encoding nonenzymatic chloramphenicol resistance from *Pseudomonas aeruginosa*. *Antimicrob. Agents Chemother.* **29:**445–450.
25. **Bush, K., G. A. Jacoby, and A. A. Medeiros.** 1995. A functional classification scheme for β-lactamases and its correlation with molecular structure. *Antimicrob. Agents Chemother.* **39:**1211–1233.
26. **Buu-Hoi, A., and T. C. Horodniceanu.** 1980. Conjugative transfer of multiple antibiotic resistance markers in *Streptococcus pneumoniae*. *J. Bacteriol.* **142:**313–320.
27. **Charpentier, E., and P. Courvalin.** 1997. Emergence of the trimethoprim resistance gene *dfrD* in *Listeria monocytogenes*. *Antimicrob. Agents Chemother.* **41:**1134–1136.
28. **Charpentier, E., G. Gerbaud, and P. Courvalin.** 1993. Characterization of a new class of tetracycline-resistance gene *tet*(S) in *Listeria monocytogenes* BM4210. *Gene* **131:** 27–34.
29. **Clancy, J., F. Dib-Hajj, J. W. Petitpas, and W. Yuan.** 1997. Cloning and characterization of a novel macrolide efflux gene, *mreA*, from *Streptococcus agalactiae*. *Antimicrob. Agents Chemother.* **41:**2719–2723.
30. **Clancy, J., J. Petitpas, F. Dib-Hajj, W. Yuan, M. Cronan, A. V. Kamath, J. Bergeron, and J. A. Retsma.** 1996. Molecular cloning and functional analysis of a novel macrolide-resistance determinant, *mefA*, from *Streptococcus pyogenes*. *Mol. Microbiol.* **22:**867–879.
31. **Coffey, T. J., M. Daniels, L. K. McDougel, C. G. Dowson, F. C. Tenover, and B. G. Spratt.** 1995. Genetic analysis of clinical isolates of *Streptococcus pneumoniae* with high-level resistance to expanded-spectrum cephalosporins. *Antimicrob. Agents Chemother.* **39:**1306–1313.
32. **Cohen, S. P., H. Hächler, and S. B. Levy.** 1993. Genetic and functional analysis of the multiple antibiotic resistance (*mar*) locus in *Escherichia coli*. *J. Bacteriol.* **175:**1484–1492.
33. **Cohen, S. P., L. M. McMurry, D. C. Hooper, J. S. Wolfson, and S. B. Levy.** 1989. Cross-resistance to fluoroquinolones in multiple-antibiotic-resistant (Mar) *Escherichia coli* selected by tetracycline or chloramphenicol: decreased drug accumulation associated with membrane changes in addition to OmpF reduction. *Antimicrob. Agents Chemother.* **33:**1318–1325.
34. **Collatz, E., G. T. V. Nhieu, D. Billot-Klein, and L. Gutmann.** 1989. Substitution of serine for arginine in position 162 of TEM-type β-lactamases extends the substrate profile of mutant enzymes, TEM-7 and TEM-101, to ceftazidime and aztreonam. *Gene* **78:**349–354.
35. **Costa, Y., M. Galimand, R. Leclercq, J. Duval, and P. Courvalin.** 1993. Characterization of the chromosomal *aac*(6′)-*Ii* gene specific for *Enterococcus faecium*. *Antimicrob. Agents Chemother.* **37:**1896–1903.
36. **Courvalin, P., and C. Carlier.** 1986. Transposable multiple antibiotic resistance in *Streptococcus pneumoniae*. *Mol. Gen. Genet.* **205:**291–297.
37. **Courvalin, P., W. V. Shaw, and A. E. Jacob.** 1978. Plasmid-mediated mechanisms of resistance to aminoglycoside-aminocyclitol antibiotics and to chloramphenicol in group D streptococci. *Antimicrob. Agents Chemother.* **13:** 716–725.
38. **Dale, G. E., C. Broger, P. G. Hartman, H. Langen, M. G. P. Page, R. L. Then, and D. Strüber.** 1995. Characterization of the gene for the chromosomal dihydrofolate reductase (DHFR) of *Staphylococcus epidermidis* ATCC 14990: the origin of the trimethoprim-resistant S1 DHFR from *Staphylococcus aureus*? *J. Bacteriol.* **177:**2965–2970.
39. **Dale, G. E., H. Langen, M. G. P. Page, R. L. Then, and D. Stüber.** 1995. Cloning and characterization of a novel, plasmid-encoded trimethoprim-resistant dihydrofolate reductase from *Staphylococcus haemolyticus* MUR313. *Antimicrob. Agents Chemother.* **39:**1920–1924.
40. **Danel, F., L. M. C. Hall, D. Gur, and D. M. Livermore.** 1995. OXA-14, another extended spectrum variant of OXA-10 (PSE-2) β-lactamase from *Pseudomonas aeruginosa*. *Antimicrob. Agents Chemother.* **39:**1881–1884.
41. **Deguchi, T., M. Yasuda, M. Nakano, S. Ozeki, T. Ezaki, I. Saito, and Y. Kawada.** 1996. Quinolone-resistant *Neisseria gonorrhoeae*: correlation of alterations in the GyrA subunit of DNA gyrase and the ParC subunit of topoisomerase IV with antimicrobial susceptibility profiles. *Antimicrob. Agents Chemother.* **40:**1020–1023.
42. **Dietz, H., D. Pfeifle, and B. Wiedeman.** 1997. The signal molecule for β-lactamase induction in *Enterobacter cloacae* is the anhydromuramyl-pentapeptide. *Antimicrob. Agents Chemother.* **41:**2113–2120.
43. **Dowson, C. G., T. J. Coffey, C. Kell, and R. A. Whiley.** 1993. Evolution of penicillin resistance in *Streptococcus pneumoniae*: the role of *Streptococcus mitis* in the formation of a low affinity PBP2B in *S. pneumoniae*. *Mol. Microbiol.* **9:**635–643.
44. **Dowson, C. G., A. Hutchison, J. A. Brannigan, R. C. George, D. Hansman, J. Liñares, A. Tomasz, J. M. Smith, and B. G. Spratt.** 1989. Horizontal transfer of penicillin-binding protein genes in penicillin-resistant clinical isolates of *Streptococcus pneumoniae*. *Proc. Natl. Acad. Sci. USA* **86:**8842–8846.
45. **Drlica, K., and X. Zhao.** 1997. DNA gyrase, topoisomerase IV, and the 4-quinolones. *Microbiol. Mol. Biol. Rev.* **61:** 377–392.
46. **Dutka-Malen, S., C. Molinas, M. Arthur, and P. Courvalin.** 1990. The VanA glycopeptide resistance protein is related to D-alanyl-D-alanine ligase cell wall biosynthesis enzymes. *Mol. Gen. Genet.* **224:**364–372.
47. **Eady, A. E., J. I. Ross, J. L. Tipper, C. E. Walters, J. H. Cove, and W. C. Noble.** 1993. Distribution of genes encoding erythromycin ribosomal methylases and an erythromycin efflux pump in epidemiologically distinct groups of staphylococci. *J. Antimicrob. Chemother.* **31:**211–217.
48. **Elwell, L. P., and M. E. Fling.** 1989. Resistance to trimethoprim, p. 249–290. *In* L. E. Bryan (ed.), *Microbial Resistance to Drugs*. Springer-Verlag KG, Berlin, Germany.
49. **Evers, S., P. Reynolds, and P. Courvalin.** 1994. Sequence of the *vanB* and *ddl* genes encoding D-alanine:D-alanine ligases in vancomycin-resistant *Enterococcus faecalis* V583. *Gene* **140:**97–102.
50. **Faruki, H., and P. F. Sparling.** 1986. Genetics of resistance in a non-β-lactamase-producing gonococcus with relatively high-level penicillin resistance. *Antimicrob. Agents Chemother.* **30:**856–860.
51. **Finken, M., P. Kirschner, A. Meir, A. Wrede, and E. C. Böttger.** 1993. Molecular basis of streptomycin resistance in *Mycobacterium tuberculosis*: alterations of the ribosomal protein S12 gene and point mutations within a functional 16S ribosomal RNA pseudoknot. *Mol. Microbiol.* **9:** 1239–1246.
52. **Flensburg, J., and O. Sköld.** 1984. Regulatory changes in the formation of chromosomal dihydrofolate reductase causing resistance to trimethoprim. *J. Bacteriol.* **159:** 184–190.
53. **Fling, M. E., J. Knopf, and C. Richards.** 1988. Characterization of plasmid pAZ1 and the type III dihydrofolate reductase gene. *Plasmid* **19:**30–38.

54. **Fontana, R., A. Grossato, L. Rossi, Y. R. Cheng, and G. Satta.** 1985. Transition from resistance to hypersusceptibility to β-lactam antibiotics associated with loss of a low-affinity penicillin-binding protein in a *Streptococcus faecium* mutant highly resistant to penicillin. *Antimicrob. Agents Chemother.* **28:**678–683.
55. **Fukuoka, T., S. Ohya, T. Narita, M. Katsuta, M. Iijima, N. Masuda, H. Yasuda, J. Trias, and H. Nikaido.** 1993. Activity of the carbapenem panipenem and role of the OprD (D2) protein in its diffusion through the *Pseudomonas aeruginosa* outer membrane. *Antimicrob. Agents Chemother.* **37:**322–327.
56. **Georgiou, M., R. Muñoz, F. Román, R. Cantón, R. Gómez-Lus, J. Campos, and A. G. D. L. Campa.** 1996. Ciprofloxacin-resistant *Haemophilus influenzae* strains possess mutations in analogous positions of *gyrA* and *parC*. *Antimicrob. Agents Chemother.* **40:**1741–1744.
57. **Grebe, T., and R. Hakenbeck.** 1996. Penicillin-binding proteins 2b and 2x of *Streptococcus pneumoniae* are primary resistance determinants for different classes of β-lactam antibiotics. *Antimicrob. Agents Chemother.* **40:**829–834.
58. **Grice, S. F. H. L., H. Matzura, R. Marcoli, S. Iida, and T. A. Bickle.** 1982. The catabolite-sensitive promoter for the chloramphenicol acetyltransferase gene is preceded by two binding sites for the catabolite gene activator protein. *J. Bacteriol.* **150:**312–318.
59. **Groot, R., M. Sluijter, A. Bruyn, J. Campos, W. H. F. Goessens, A. L. Smith, and P. W. M. Hermans.** 1996. Genetic characterization of trimethoprim resistance in *Haemophilus influenzae*. *Antimicrob. Agents Chemother.* **40:** 2131–2136.
60. **Gutmann, L., D. Billot-Klein, D. Shalaes, and J. V. Heijenoort.** 1993. Analysis of peptidoglycan precursors in naturally vancomycin-resistant gram-positive organisms, abstr. 115. *In Program and Abstracts of the 33rd Interscience Conference on Antimicrobial Agents and Chemotherapy*. American Society for Microbiology, Washington D.C.
61. **Gutmann, L., B. Ferré, F. W. Goldstein, N. Rizk, E. Pinto-Schuster, J. F. Acar, and E. Collatz.** 1989. SHV-5, a novel SHV-type β-lactamase that hydrolyzes broad-spectrum cephalosporins and monobactams. *Antimicrob. Agents Chemother.* **33:**951–956.
62. **Gutmann, L., R. Williamson, N. Moreau, M. Kitzis, E. Collatz, J. F. Acar, and F. Goldstein.** 1985. Cross-resistance to nalidixic acid, trimethoprim, and chloramphenicol associated with alterations in outer membrane proteins of *Klebsiella*, *Enterobacter*, and *Serratia*. *J. Infect. Dis.* **151:** 501–507.
63. **Hächler, H., S. P. Cohen, and S. B. Levy.** 1991. *marA*, a regulated locus which controls expression of chromosomal multiple antibiotic resistance in *Escherichia coli*. *J. Bacteriol.* **173:**5532–5538.
64. **Hakenbeck, R., M. Tarplay, and A. Tomasz.** 1980. Multiple changes of penicillin-binding proteins in penicillin-resistant clinical isolates of *Streptococcus pneumoniae*. *Antimicrob. Agents Chemother.* **17:**364–371.
65. **Hall, L. M. C., D. M. Livermore, D. Gur, M. Akova, and H. E. Akalin.** 1993. OXA-11, an extended-spectrum variant of OXA-10 (PSE-2) β-lactamase from *Pseudomonas aeruginosa*. *Antimicrob. Agents Chemother.* **37:**1637–1644.
66. **Hall, R. M., and C. M. Collis.** 1995. Mobile gene cassettes and integrons: capture and spread of genes by site-specific recombination. *Mol. Microbiol.* **15:**593–600.
67. **Hamilton-Miller, J. M. T.** 1988. Reversal of activity of trimethoprim against gram-positive cocci by thymidine, thymine, and folates. *Antimicrob. Agents Chemother.* **22:** 35–39.
68. **Hancock, R. E. W., S. W. Farmer, Z. Li, and K. Poole.** 1991. Interaction of aminoglycosides with the outer membranes and purified lipopolysaccharide and OmpF porin of *Escherichia coli*. *Antimicrob. Agents Chemother.* **35:** 1309–1314.
69. **Handwerger, S., M. J. Pucci, K. J. Vol, J. Liu, and M. S. Lee.** 1992. The cytoplasmic peptidoglycan precursor of vancomycin-resistant *Enterococcus faecalis* terminates in lactate. *J. Bacteriol.* **174:**5982–5984.
70. **Handwerger, S., and A. Tomasz.** 1986. Alterations in penicillin-binding proteins of clinical and laboratory isolates of pathogenic *Streptococcus pneumoniae* with low levels of penicillin resistance. *J. Infect. Dis.* **153:**83–89.
71. **Hartman, B. J., and A. Tomasz.** 1986. Expression of methicillin resistance in heterogeneous strains of *Staphylococcus aureus*. *Antimicrob. Agents Chemother.* **29:**85–92.
72. **Hayden, M. K., G. M. Trenholme, J. E. Schultz, and D. F. Sahm.** 1993. In vivo development of teicoplanin resistance in a VanB *Enterococcus faecium*. *J. Infect. Dis.* **167:**1224–1227.
73. **Heisig, P.** 1996. Genetic evidence for a role of *parC* mutations in development of high-level fluoroquinolone resistance in *Escherichia coli*. *Antimicrob. Agents Chemother.* **40:** 879–885.
74. **Heisig, P., and B. Wiedemann.** 1991. Use of a broad-host-range *gyrA* plasmid for genetic characterization of fluoroquinolone-resistant gram-negative bacteria. *Antimicrob. Agents Chemother.* **35:**2031–2036.
75. **Hewinson, R. G., S. J. Cartwright, M. P. E. Slack, R. D. Whipp, M. J. Woodward, and W. W. Nichols.** 1989. Permeability to cefsulodin of the outer membrane of *Pseudomonas aeruginosa* and discrimination between β-lactamase-mediated trapping and hydrolysis as mechanisms of resistance. *Eur. J. Biochem.* **179:**667–675.
76. **Hiramatsu, K., H. Hanaki, T. Ino, K. Yabuta, T. Oguri, and F. C. Tenover.** 1997. Methicillin-resistant Staphylococcus aureus clinical strain with reduced vancomycin susceptibility. *J. Antimicrob. Chemother.* **40:**135–136.
77. **Horaud, T., C. L. Bouguénec, and K. Pepper.** 1985. Molecular genetics of resistance to macrolides, lincosamides, and streptogramin B (MLS) in streptococci. *J. Antimicrob. Chemother.* **16:**111–135.
78. **Horinouchi, S., and B. Weisblum.** 1980. Post-transcriptional modification of RNA conformation: mechanism that regulates erythromycin-induced resistance. *Proc. Natl. Acad. Sci. USA* **77:**7079–7083.
79. **Horodniceanu, T., C. L. Bouguénec, A. Buu-Hoi, and G. Bieth.** 1982. Conjugative transfer of antibiotic resistance markers in β-hemolytic streptococci in the presence and absence of plasmid DNA, p. 105–108. *In* D. Schlessinger (ed.), *Microbiology—1982*. American Society for Microbiology, Washington, D.C.
80. **Hosaka, M., N. Gotoh, and T. Nishino.** 1995. Purification of a 54-kilodalton protein (OprJ) produced in NfxB mutants of *Pseudomonas aeruginosa* and production of a monoclonal antibody specific to OprJ. *Antimicrob. Agents Chemother.* **39:**1731–1735.
81. **Huovinen, P., L. Sundström, G. Swedberg, and O. Sköld.** 1995. Trimethoprim and sulfonamide resistance. *Antimicrob. Agents Chemother.* **39:**279–289.
82. **Ito, H., Y. Arakawa, S. Ohsuka, R. Wacharotayankun, N. Kato, and M. Ohta.** 1995. Plasmid-mediated dissemination of the metallo-β-lactamase gene bla_{IMP} among clinically isolated strains of *Serratia marcescens*. *Antimicrob. Agents Chemother.* **39:**824–829.
83. **Jacobs, C., B. Joris, M. Jamin, K. Klarsov, J. van Beeumen, D. Mengin-Lecreulx, J. van Heijenoort, J. T. Park, and S. Normark.** 1995. AmpD, essential for both β-lactamase regulation and cell wall recycling, is a novel cytosolic *N*-acetylmuramyl-L-alanine amidase. *Mol. Microbiol.* **15:** 553–559.

84. **Jolly, L., S. Wu, J. van Heijenoort, H. de Lencastre, D. Mengin-Lecreulx, and A. Tomasz.** 1997. The *femR315* gene from *Staphylococcus aureus*, the interruption of which results in reduced methicillin resistance, encodes a phosphoglucosamine mutase. *J. Bacteriol.* **179:**5321–5325.
85. **Kaatz, G. W., and S. M. Seo.** 1995. Inducible *norA*-mediated multidrug resistance in *Staphylococcus aureus*. *Antimicrob. Agents Chemother.* **39:**2650–2655.
86. **Kadurugamuwa, J. L., A. J. Clarke, and T. J. Beveridge.** 1993. Surface action of gentamicin on *Pseudomonas aeruginosa*. *J. Bacteriol.* **175:**5798–5805.
87. **Kato, T., Y. Sato, S. Iyobe, and S. Mitsuhashi.** 1982. Plasmid-mediated gentamicin resistance of *Pseudomonas aeruginosa* and its lack of expression in *Escherichia coli*. *Antimicrob. Agents Chemother.* **22:**358–363.
88. **Katsanis, G. P., J. Spargo, M. J. Ferraro, L. Sutton, and G. A. Jacoby.** 1994. Detection of *Klebsiella pneumoniae* and *Escherichia coli* strains producing extended-spectrum beta-lactamases. *J. Clin. Microbiol.* **32:**691–696.
89. **Knapp, J., S. R. Johnson, J. M. Zenilman, M. C. Roberts, and S. A. Morse.** 1988. High-level tetracycline resistance resulting from TetM in strains of *Neisseria* spp., *Kingella denitrificans*, and *Eikenella corrodens*. *Antimicrob. Agents Chemother.* **32:**765–767.
90. **Köhler, T., M. Kok, Michéa-Hamzehpour, P. Plésiat, N. Gotoh, T. Nishino, L. K. Curty, and J.-C. Pechère.** 1996. Multidrug efflux in intrinsic resistance to trimethoprim and sulfamethoxazole in *Pseudomonas aeruginosa*. *Antimicrob. Agents Chemother.* **40:**2288–2290.
91. **Laible, G., and R. Hakenbeck.** 1987. Penicillin-binding proteins in *β*-lactam-resistant laboratory mutants of *Streptococcus pneumoniae*. *Mol. Microbiol.* **1:**355–363.
92. **Laible, G., G. B. Spratt, and R. Hakenbeck.** 1991. Interspecies recombinational events during the evolution of altered PBP 2× genes in penicillin-resistant clinical isolates of *Streptococcus pneumoniae*. *Mol. Microbiol.* **5:** 1993–2002.
93. **Lampson, B. C., and J. T. Parisi.** 1986. Naturally occurring *Staphylococcus epidermidis* plasmid expressing constitutive macrolide-lincosamide-streptogramin B resistance contains a deleted attenuator. *J. Bacteriol.* **166:**479–483.
94. **Leclercq, R., and P. Courvalin.** 1991. Bacterial resistance to macrolide, lincosamide, and streptogramin antibiotics by target modification. *Antimicrob. Agents Chemother.* **35:** 1267–1272.
95. **Leclercq, R., E. Derlot, J. Duval, and P. Courvalin.** 1988. Plasmid-mediated resistance to vancomycin and teicoplanin in *Enterococcus faecium*. *N. Engl. J. Med.* **319:** 157–161.
96. **Leclercq, R., S. Dutka-Malen, A. Brisson-Noël, C. Molinas, E. Derlot, M. Arthur, J. Duval, and P. Courvalin.** 1992. Resistance of enterococci to aminoglycosides and glycopeptides. *Clin. Infect. Dis.* **15:**495–501.
97. **Levy, S. B.** 1984. Resistance to tetracyclines, p. 191–240. *In* L. E. Bryan (ed.), *Antimicrobial Drug Resistance*. Academic Press, Inc., Orlando, Fla.
98. **Li, X.-Z., H. Nikaido, and K. Poole.** 1995. Role of MexA-MexB-OprM in antibiotic efflux in *Pseudomonas aeruginosa*. *Antimicrob. Agents Chemother.* **39:**1948–1953.
99. **Li, X.-Z., L. Zang, R. Srikumar, and K. Poole.** 1998. *β*-Lactamase inhibitors are substrates for the multidrug efflux pumps of *Pseudomonas aeruginosa*. *Antimicrob. Agents Chemother.* **42:**399–403.
100. **Lindberg, F., S. Lindquist, and S. Normark.** 1988. Genetic basis of induction and overproduction of chromosomal class I *β*-lactamase in nonfastidious gram-negative bacilli. *Rev. Infect. Dis.* **10:**782–785.
101. **Lindberg, F., L. Westman, and S. Normark.** 1985. Regulatory components in *Citrobacter freundii β*-lactamase induction. *Proc. Natl. Acad. Sci. USA* **82:**4620–4624.
102. **Lindquist, S., K. Weston-Hafer, H. Schmidt, C. Pul, G. Korfmann, J. Erickson, C. Sanders, H. H. Martin, and S. Normark.** 1993. AmpG, a signal transducer in chromosomal *β*-lactamase induction. *Mol. Microbiol.* **9:** 703–715.
103. **Livermore, D. M.** 1995. *β*-Lactamases in laboratory and clinical resistance. *Clin. Microbiol. Rev.* **8:**557–584.
104. **Livermore, D. M.** 1988. Permeation of *β*-lactam antibiotics into *Escherichia coli*, *Pseudomonas aeruginosa*, and other gram-negative bacteria. *Rev. Infect. Dis.* **10:**691–698.
105. **Lopez, P., M. Espinosa, B. Greenburg, and S. A. Lacks.** 1987. Sulfonamide resistance in *Streptococcus pneumoniae*: DNA sequence of the gene encoding dihydropteroate synthase and characterization of the enzyme. *J. Bacteriol.* **169:**4320–4326.
106. **Lovett, P. S.** 1990. Translational attenuation as the regulator of inducible *cat* genes. *J. Bacteriol.* **172:**1–6.
107. **Lyras, D., and J. I. Rood.** 1996. Genetic organization and distribution of tetracycline resistance determinants in *Clostridium perfringens*. *Antimicrob. Agents Chemother.* **40:**2500–2504.
108. **Ma, D., D. N. Cook, M. Alberti, N. G. Pon, H. Nikaido, and J. E. Hearst.** 1995. Genes *acrA* and *acrB* encode a stress-induced efflux system of *Escherichia coli*. *Mol. Microbiol.* **16:**45–55.
109. **Maidhof, H., B. Reinicke, P. Blümel, B. Berger-Bächi, and H. Labischinski.** 1991. *femA*, which encodes a factor essential for expression of methicillin resistance, affects glycine content of peptidoglycan in methicillin-resistant and methicillin-susceptible *Staphylococcus aureus* strains. *J. Bacteriol.* **173:**3507–3513.
110. **Maneewannakul, K., and S. B. Levy.** 1996. Identification of *mar* mutants among quinolone-resistant clinical isolates of *Escherichia coli*. *Antimicrob. Agents Chemother.* **40:**1695–1698.
111. **Marshall, C. G., G. Broadhead, B. K. Leskiw, and G. D. Wright.** 1997. D-Ala-D-Ala ligases from glycopeptide antibiotic-producing organisms are highly homologous to the enterococcal vancomycin-resistance ligases VanA and VanB. *Proc. Natl. Acad. Sci. USA* **94:**6480–6483.
112. **Marty, V., V. S. Madiraju, D. P. Brunner, and B. J. Wilkinson.** 1987. Effects of temperature, NaCl, and methicillin on penicillin-binding proteins, growth, peptidoglycan synthesis, and autolysis in methicillin-resistant *Staphylococcus aureus*. *Antimicrob. Agents Chemother.* **31:** 1727–1733.
113. **Maskell, J. P., A. M. Sefton, and L. M. C. Hall.** 1997. Mechanism of sulfonamide resistance in clinical isolates of *Streptococcus pneumoniae*. *Antimicrob. Agents Chemother.* **41:**2121–2126.
114. **Massova, I., and S. Mobashery.** 1998. Kinship and diversification of bacterial penicillin-binding proteins and *β*-lactamases. *Antimicrob. Agents Chemother.* **42:**1–17.
115. **McMurray, L. M., A. M. George, and S. B. Levy.** 1994. Active efflux of chloramphenicol in susceptible *Escherichia coli* and in multiple antibiotic resistant (Mar) mutants. *Antimicrob. Agents Chemother.* **38:**542–546.
116. **Miller, G. H., and A. R. S. Groups.** 1994. Increasing complexity of aminoglycoside resistance mechanisms in gram-negative bacteria. *APUA Newsl.* **12(2):**1, 5–9.
117. **Miller, G. H., F. J. Sabatelli, R. S. Hare, Y. Glupczynski, P. Mackey, D. Shlaes, K. Shimizu, K. J. Shaw, and A. R. S. Groups.** 1997. The most frequent aminoglycoside resistance mechanisms—changes with time and geographic area: a reflection of aminoglycoside usage patterns. *Clin. Infect. Dis.* **24**(Suppl. 1)**:**S46–S62.

118. **Minami, S., M. Akama, H. Araki, Y. Watanabe, H. Narita, S. Iyobe, and S. Mitsuhashi.** 1996. Imipenem and cephem resistant *Pseudomonas aeruginosa* carrying plasmids coding for class B β-lactamase. *J. Antimicrob. Chemother.* **37:**433–444.

119. **Moellering, R. C., Jr., O. M. Korzeniowski, M. A. Sande, and C. B. Wennersten.** 1979. Species-specific resistance to antimicrobial synergism in *Streptococcus faecium* and *Streptococcus faecalis*. *J. Infect. Dis.* **140:** 203–208.

120. **Murray, I. A., and W. V. Shaw.** 1997. O-Acetyltransferases for chloramphenicol and other natural products. *Antimicrob. Agents Chemother.* **41:**1–6.

121. **Nakamura, S., M. Nakamura, T. Kojima, and H. Yoshida.** 1989. *gyrA* and *gyrB* mutations in quinolone-resistant strains of *Escherichia coli*. *Antimicrob. Agents Chemother.* **33:**254–255.

122. **Nakamura, S., H. Yoshida, M. Bogaki, M. Nakamura, and T. Kojima.** 1993. Quinolone resistance mutations in DNA gyrase, p. 135–143. *In* T. Andoh, H. Ikeda, and M. Oguro (ed.), *Molecular Biology of DNA Topoisomerases and Its Application to Chemotherapy*. CRC Press, London, England.

123. **Nicholas, R. A., and J. Strominger.** 1988. Relations between β-lactamases and penicillin-binding proteins: β-lactamase activity of penicillin-binding protein 5 from *Escherichia coli*. *Rev. Infect. Dis.* **10:**733–738.

124. **Nikaido, H.** 1994. Prevention of drug access to bacterial targets: role of permeability barriers and active efflux. *Science* **264:**382–388.

125. **Noble, C. W., Z. Virani, and R. G. A. Cree.** 1992. Cotransfer of vancomycin and other resistance genes from *Enterococcus faecalis* NCTC 12201 to *Staphylococcus aureus*. *FEMS Microbiol. Lett.* **93:**195–198.

126. **Normark, S., T. Edlund, T. Grundström, S. Bergström, and H. Wolf-Watz.** 1977. *Escherichia coli* K-12 mutants hyperproducing chromosomal beta-lactamase by gene repetitions. *J. Bacteriol.* **132:**912–922.

127. **O'Hara, K., T. Kanda, K. Ohmiya, T. Ebisu, and M. Kono.** 1989. Purification and characterization of macrolide 2′-phosphotransferase from a strain of *Escherichia coli* that is highly resistant to erythromycin. *Antimicrob. Agents Chemother.* **33:**1354–1357.

128. **Okusu, H., D. Ma, and H. Nikaido.** 1996. AcrAB efflux pump plays a major role in the antibiotic resistance phenotype of *Escherichia coli* multiple-antibiotic-resistance (Mar) mutants. *J. Bacteriol.* **178:**306–308.

129. **Olsson, O., S. Bergström, F. P. Lindberg, and S. Normark.** 1983. *ampC* β-lactamase hyperproduction in *Escherichia coli*: natural ampicillin resistance generated by horizontal chromosomal DNA transfer from *Shigella*. *Proc. Natl. Acad. Sci. USA* **80:**7556–7560.

130. **Oram, M., and M. Fisher.** 1991. 4-Quinolone resistance mutations in the DNA gyrase of *Escherichia coli* clinical isolates identified by using the polymerase chain reaction. *Antimicrob. Agents Chemother.* **35:**387–389.

131. **Osano, E., Y. Arakawa, R. Wacharotayankun, M. Ohta, T. Horii, H. Ito, F. Yoshimura, and N. Kato.** 1994. Molecular characterization of an enterobacterial metallo β-lactamase found in a clinical isolate of *Serratia marcescens* that shows imipenem resistance. *Antimicrob. Agents Chemother.* **38:**71–78.

132. **Ounissi, H., and P. Courvalin.** 1985. Nucleotide sequence of the gene *ereA* encoding the erythromycin esterase in *Escherichia coli*. *Gene* **35:**271–278.

133. **Pan, X.-S., and L. M. Fisher.** 1997. Targeting of DNA gyrase in *Streptococcus pneumoniae* by sparfloxacin: selective targeting of gyrase or topoisomerase IV by quinolones. *Antimicrob. Agents Chemother.* **41:**471–474.

134. **Papanicolaou, G. A., A. A. Medieros, and G. A. Jacoby.** 1990. Novel plasmid-mediated β-lactamase (MIR-1) conferring resistance to oxyimino- and α-methoxy β-lactams in clinical isolates of *Klebsiella pneumoniae*. *Antimicrob. Agents Chemother.* **34:**2200–2209.

135. **Parent, R., and P. H. Roy.** 1992. The chloramphenicol acetyltransferase gene of Tn*2424*: a new breed of *cat*. *J. Bacteriol.* **174:**2891–2897.

136. **Parsons, Y., R. M. Hall, and H. W. Stokes.** 1991. A new trimethoprim resistance gene, *dhfrX*, in the In*7* integron of plasmid pDGO100. *Antimicrob. Agents Chemother.* **35:**2436–2439.

137. **Pattishall, K. H., J. Acar, J. J. Burchall, F. W. Goldstein, and R. J. Harvey.** 1977. Two distinct types of trimethoprim-resistant dihydrofolate reductases specified by R-plasmids of different compatibility groups. *J. Biol. Chem.* **252:**2319–2323.

138. **Payne, D. J., N. Woodruff, and S. G. B. Amyes.** 1992. Characterization of the plasmid-mediated β-lactamase BIL-1. *J. Antimicrob. Chemother.* **30:**119–127.

139. **Perichon, B., J. Tankovic, and P. Courvalin.** 1997. Characterization of a mutation in the *parE* gene that confers fluoroquinolone resistance in *Streptococcus pneumoniae*. *Antimicrob. Agents Chemother.* **41:**1166–1167.

140. **Peterson, A. A., S. W. Fesik, and E. J. McGroaty.** 1987. Decreased binding of antibiotics to lipopolysaccharides from polymixin-resistant strains of *Escherichia coli* and *Salmonella typhimurium*. *Antimicrob. Agents Chemother.* **31:** 230–237.

141. **Poole, K., K. Tetro, Q. Zhao, S. Neshat, D. E. Heinrichs, and N. Bianco.** 1996. Expression of the multidrug resistance operon *mexA-mexB-oprM* in *Pseudomonas aeruginosa: mexR* encodes a regulator of operon expression. *Antimicrob. Agents Chemother.* **40:**2021–2028.

142. **Poyart, C., C. Pierre, G. Quesne, B. Pron, P. Berche, and P. Trieu-Cuot.** 1997. Emergence of vancomycin resistance in the genus Streptococcus-characterization of a *vanB* transferable determinant in *Streptococcus bovis*. *Antimicrob. Agents Chemother.* **41:**24–29.

143. **Quintiliani, R., Jr., and P. Courvalin.** 1996. Characterization of Tn*1547*, a composite transposon flanked by the IS*16* and IS*256*-like elements, that confers vancomycin resistance in *Enterococcus faecalis* BM4281. *Gene* **172:** 1–8.

144. **Quintiliani, R., Jr., and P. Courvalin.** 1994. Conjugal transfer of the vancomycin resistance determinant *vanB* between enterococci involves the movement of large genetic elements from chromosome to chromosome. *FEMS Microbiol. Lett.* **119:**359–364.

145. **Quintiliani, R., Jr., S. Evers, and P. Courvalin.** 1993. The *vanB* gene confers various levels of self-transferable resistance to vancomycin in enterococci. *J. Infect. Dis.* **167:**1220–1223.

146. **Radström, P., and G. Swedberg.** 1988. RSF1010 and a conjugative plasmid contain *sulII*, one of two known genes for plasmid-borne sulfonamide resistance dihydropteroate synthase. *Antimicrob. Agents Chemother.* **32:** 1684–1692.

147. **Radström, P., G. Swedberg, and O. Sköld.** 1991. Genetic analysis of sulfonamide resistance and its dissemination in gram-negative bacteria illustrate new aspects of R plasmid evolution. *Antimicrob. Agents Chemother.* **35:**1840–1848.

148. **Rather, P. N., E. I. Orosz, K. J. Shaw, R. Hare, and G. Miller.** 1993. Characterization and transcriptional regulation of the 2′-*N*-acetyltransferase gene from *Providencia stuartii*. *J. Bacteriol.* **175:**6492–6498.

149. **Raze, D., O. Dardenne, S. Hallut, M. Martinez-Bueno, J. Coyette, and J.-M. Ghuysen.** 1998. The gene encoding the low-affinity penicillin-binding protein 3r in *Entero-*

coccus hirae S185R is borne on a plasmid carrying other antibiotic resistance determinants. *Antimicrob. Agents Chemother.* **42:**534–539.

150. **Recchia, G. D., and R. M. Hall.** 1997. Origins of the mobile gene cassettes found in integrons. *Trends Microbiol.* **5:**389–394.
151. **Rende-Fournier, R., R. Leclercq, M. Galimand, J. Duval, and P. Courvalin.** 1993. Identification of the *satA* gene encoding a streptogramin A acetyltransferase in *Enterococcus faecium. Antimicrob. Agents Chemother.* **37:** 2119–2125.
152. **Reynolds, P. E., F. Depardieu, S. Dutka-Malen, M. Arthur, and P. Courvalin.** 1994. Glycopeptide resistance mediated by enterococcal transposon Tn*1546* requires production of VanX for hydrolysis of D-alanyl-D-alanine. *Mol. Microbiol.* **13:**1065–1070.
153. **Roberts, M., A. Corney, and W. Shaw.** 1982. Molecular characterization of three chloramphenicol acetyltransferases isolated from *Haemophilus influenzae. J. Bacteriol.* **151:**737–741.
154. **Rood, J. I., S. Jefferson, T. I. Bannan, J. M. Wilkie, P. Mullany, and B. W. Wren.** 1989. Hybridization analysis of three chloramphenicol resistance determinants from *Clostridium perfringens* and *Clostridium difficile. Antimicrob. Agents Chemother.* **33:**1569–1574.
155. **Ross, J. I., E. A. Eady, J. H. Cove, W. J. Cunliffe, S. Baumberg, and J. C. Wootton.** 1990. Inducible erythromycin resistance in staphylococci is encoded by a member of the ATP-binding transport super-gene family. *Mol. Microbiol.* **4:**1207–1214.
156. **Rowland, S.-J., and K. G. H. Dyke.** 1990. Tn*552*, a novel transposable element from *Staphylococcus aureus. Mol. Microbiol.* **4:**961–975.
157. **Ryffel, C., F. H. Kayser, and B. Berger-Bächi.** 1992. Correlation between regulation of *mecA* transcription and expression of methicillin resistance in staphylococci. *Antimicrob. Agents Chemother.* **36:**25–31.
158. **Sanders, C. C.** 1989. The chromosomal beta-lactamases, p. 129–144. *In* L. G. Bryan (ed.), *Microbial Resistance to Drugs.* Springer-Verlag KG, Berlin, Germany.
159. **Sawai, T., R. Hiruma, N. Kawana, M. Kaneko, F. Taniyasu, and A. Inami.** 1982. Outer membrane permeation of β-lactam antibiotics in *Escherichia coli, Proteus mirabilis,* and *Enterobacter cloacae. Antimicrob. Agents Chemother.* **22:**585–592.
160. **Shaw, K. J., P. N. Rather, R. S. Hare, and G. H. Miller.** 1993. Molecular genetics of aminoglycoside resistance genes and familial relationships of the aminoglycoside-modifying enzymes. *Microbiol. Rev.* **57:**138–163.
161. **Shaw, W. V.** 1983. Chloramphenicol acetyltransferase: enzymology and molecular biology. *Crit. Rev. Biochem.* **14:**1–46.
162. **Sheridan, R. P., and I. Chopra.** 1991. Origin of tetracycline efflux proteins: conclusions from nucleotide sequence analysis. *Mol. Microbiol.* **5:**895–900.
163. **Showsh, S., and J. R. Andrews.** 1992. Tetracycline enhances Tn*916*-mediated conjugal transfer. *Plasmid* **28:** 213–224.
164. **Sirot, D., C. Recule, E. B. Chaibi, L. Bret, J. Croize, C. Chanal-Claris, R. Labia, and J. Sirot.** 1997. A complex mutant of TEM-1 β-lactamase with mutations encountered in both IRT-4 and extended-spectrum TEM-15, produced by an *Escherichia coli* clinical isolate. *Antimicrob. Agents Chemother.* **41:**1322–1325.
165. **Sougakoff, W., S. Goussard, G. Gerbaud, and P. Courvalin.** 1988. Plasmid-mediated resistance to third-generation cephalosporins caused by point mutations in TEM-type penicillinase genes. *Rev. Infect. Dis.* **10:**879–884.
166. **Speer, B. S., N. B. Shoemaker, and A. A. Salyers.** 1992. Bacterial resistance to tetracycline: mechanisms, transfer, and clinical relevance. *Clin. Microbiol. Rev.* **5:**387–399.
167. **Spratt, B. G.** 1988. Hybrid penicillin-binding proteins in penicillin-resistant isolates of *Neisseria gonorrhoeae. Nature* **332:**173–176.
168. **Spratt, B. G.** 1989. Resistance to β-lactam antibiotics mediated by alterations of penicillin-binding proteins, p. 77–97. *In* L. E. Bryan (ed.), *Microbial Resistance to Drugs.* Springer-Verlag KG, Berlin, Germany.
169. **Spratt, B. G., Q. Zhang, D. M. Jones, A. Hutchinson, J. A. Brannigan, and C. G. Dowson.** 1989. Recruitment of a penicillin-binding protein gene from Neisseria flavescens during the emergence of penicillin resistance in *Neisseria meningitidis. Proc. Natl. Acad. Sci. USA* **86:** 8988–8992.
170. **Srikumar, R., T. Kon, N. Gotoh, and K. Poole.** 1998. Expression of *Pseudomonas aeruginosa* multidrug efflux pumps MexA-MexB-OprM and MexC-MexD-OprJ in a multidrug-sensitive *Escherichia coli* strain. *Antimicrob. Agents Chemother.* **42:**65–71.
171. **Stapelton, P., P. J. Wu, A. King, K. Shannon, G. French, and I. Phillips.** 1995. Incidence and mechanisms of resistance to the combination of amoxicillin and clavulanate in *Escherichia coli. Antimicrob. Agents Chemother.* **39:**2478–2483.
172. **Su, Y. A., P. He, and D. B. Clewell.** 1992. Characterization of the *tet*(M) determinant of Tn*916*: evidence for regulation by transcription attenuation. *Antimicrob. Agents Chemother.* **36:**769–778.
173. **Sundström, L., R. Radström, G. Swedberg, and O. Sköld.** 1988. Site-specific recombination promotes linkage between trimethoprim- and sulfonamide-resistance genes. Sequence characterization of *dhfrV* and *sulI* and a recombination active locus of Tn*21*. *Mol. Gen. Genet.* **213:**191–201.
174. **Sundström, L., and O. Sköld.** 1990. The *dhfrI* trimethoprim resistance gene of Tn*7* can be found at specific sites in other genetic surroundings. *Antimicrob. Agents Chemother.* **34:**642–650.
175. **Sutcliffe, J., A. Tait-Kamradt, and L. Wondrack.** 1996. *Streptococcus pneumoniae* and *Streptococcus pyogenes* resistant to macrolides but sensitive to clindamycin: a common resistance pattern mediated by an efflux system. *Antimicrob. Agents Chemother.* **40:**1817–1824.
176. **Sykes, R. B., and M. Matthew.** 1976. The β-lactamases of gram-negative bacteria and their role in resistance to β-lactam antibiotics. *J. Antimicrob. Chemother.* **2:**115–157.
177. **Tait-Kamradt, A., J. Clancy, M. Cronan, F. Dib-Hajj, L. Wondrack, W. Yuan, and J. Sutcliffe.** 1997. *mefE* is necessary for the erythromycin-resistant M phenotype in *Streptococcus pneumoniae. Antimicrob. Agents Chemother.* **41:**2251–2255.
178. **Takenouchi, T., F. Tabata, Y. Iwata, H. Hanzawa, M. Sugawara, and S. Ohya.** 1996. Hydrophilicity of quinolones is not an exclusive factor for decreased activity in efflux-mediated resistant mutants of *Staphylococcus aureus. Antimicrob. Agents Chemother.* **40:**1835–1842.
179. **Taylor, D. E., and A. Chau.** 1996. Tetracycline resistance mediated by ribosomal protection. *Antimicrob. Agents Chemother.* **40:**1–5.
180. **Taylor, D. E., C. A. Trieber, G. Trescher, and M. Bekkering.** 1998. Host mutations (*miaA* and *rpsL*) reduce tetracycline resistance mediated by Tet(O) and Tet(M). *Antimicrob. Agents Chemother.* **42:**59–64.
181. **Tesch, W., C. Ryffel, A. Strässle, F. H. Kayser, and B. Berger-Bächi.** 1990. Evidence of a novel staphylococcal *mec*-encoded element (*mecR*) controlling expression of penicillin-binding protein PBP2′. *Antimicrob. Agents Chemother.* **34:**1703–1706.

182. **Then, R. L.** 1982. Mechanisms of resistance to trimethoprim, the sulfonamides, and trimethoprim-sulfamethoxazole. *Rev. Infect. Dis.* **4**:261–269.
183. **Then, R. L.** 1989. Resistance to sulfonamides, p. 291–312. *In* L. E. Bryan (ed.), *Microbial Resistance to Drugs*. Springer-Verlag KG, Berlin, Germany.
184. **Then, R. L., and P. Angehrn.** 1979. Low trimethoprim susceptibility of anaerobic bacteria due to insensitive dihydrofolate reductases. *Antimicrob. Agents Chemother.* **15:** 1–6.
185. **Tomich, P. K., F. Y. An, and D. B. Clewell.** 1980. Properties of erythromycin-inducible transposon Tn*917* in *Streptococcus faecalis*. *J. Bacteriol.* **141**:1366–1374.
186. **Toro, C. S., S. R. Lobos, I. Calderón, M. Rodriguez, and G. C. Mora.** 1990. Clinical isolate of a porinless *Salmonella typhi* resistant to high levels of chloramphenicol. *Antimicrob. Agents Chemother.* **34**:1715–1719.
187. **Trias, J., J. Dufresne, R. C. Levesque, and H. Nikaido.** 1989. Decreased outer membrane permeability in imipenem-resistant mutants of *Pseudomonas aeruginosa*. *Antimicrob. Agents Chemother.* **33**:1201–1206.
188. **Tuomanen, E., S. Lindquist, S. Sande, M. Galleni, K. Light, D. Gage, and S. Normark.** 1991. Co-ordinate regulation of β-lactamase induction and peptidoglycan composition by the *amp* operon. *Science* **251**:201–204.
189. **Ubukata, K., R. Nonoguchi, M. D. Song, M. Matsuhashi, and M. Konno.** 1990. Homology of *mec*A gene in methicillin-resistant *Staphylococcus haemolyticus* and *Staphylococcus simulans* to that of *Staphylococcus aureus*. *Antimicrob. Agents Chemother.* **34**:170–172.
190. **Walsh, C. T.** 1989. Enzymes in the D-alanine branch of bacterial cell wall peptidoglycan assembly. *J. Biol. Chem.* **264**:2393–2396.
191. **Weisblum, B.** 1995. Erythromycin resistance by ribosome modification. *Antimicrob. Agents Chemother.* **39**:577–585.
192. **Weisblum, B.** 1985. Inducible resistance to macrolides, lincosamides and streptogramin type B antibiotics: the resistance phenotype, its biological diversity, and structural elements that regulate expression-a review. *J. Antimicrob. Chemother.* **16**(Suppl. A):63–90.
193. **Weisblum, B.** 1995. Insights into erythromycin action from studies of its activity as inducer of resistance. *Antimicrob. Agents Chemother.* **39**:797–805.
194. **Williamson, R., C. L. Bouguénec, L. Gutmann, and T. Horaud.** 1985. One or two low affinity penicillin-binding proteins may be responsible for the range of susceptibility of *Enterococcus faecium* to benzylpenicillin. *J. Gen. Microbiol.* **131**:1933–1940.
195. **Wu, P.-J., K. Shannon, and I. Phillips.** 1994. Effect of hyperproduction of TEM-1 β-lactamase on in vitro susceptibility of *Escherichia coli* to β-lactam antibiotics. *Antimicrob. Agents Chemother.* **38**:494–498.
196. **Yamagishi, J., H. Yoshida, M. Yamayoshi, and S. Nakamura.** 1986. Nalidixic acid-resistant mutations of the *gyrB* gene of *Escherichia coli*. *Mol. Gen. Genet.* **204**:367–373.
197. **Yoshida, H., M. Bogaki, S. Nakamura, K. Ubukata, and M. Konno.** 1990. Nucleotide sequence and characterization of the *Staphylococcus aureus nor*A gene, which confers resistance to quinolones. *J. Bacteriol.* **172**:6942–6949.
198. **Young, H., and S. G. B. Amyes.** 1986. A new mechanism of plasmid trimethoprim resistance. Characterization of an inducible dihydrofolate reductase. *J. Biol. Chem.* **261:** 2503–2505.
199. **Zeller, V., C. Janoir, M.-D. Kitzis, L. Gutmann, and N. J. Moreau.** 1997. Active efflux as a mechanism of resistance to ciprofloxacin in *Streptococcus pneumoniae*. *Antimicrob. Agents Chemother.* **41**:1973–1978.
200. **Zervos, M. J., and D. R. Schaberg.** 1985. Reversal of the in vitro susceptibility of enterococci to trimethoprim-sulfamethoxazole by folinic acid. *Antimicrob. Agents Chemother.* **28**:446–448.
201. **Zilhao, R., B. Papadopoulou, and P. Courvalin.** 1988. Occurrence of the *Campylobacter* resistance gene *tet*(O) in *Enterococcus* and *Streptococcus* spp. *Antimicrob. Agents Chemother.* **32**:1793–1796.
202. **Zorzi, W., X. Y. Zhou, O. Dardenne, J. Lamotte, D. Raze, J. Pierre, L. Gutmann, and J. Coyette.** 1996. Structure of the low-affinity penicillin-binding-protein 5, PBP5fm, in wild-type and highly penicillin-resistant strains of *Enterococcus faecium*. *J. Bacteriol.* **178:** 4948–4957.

Antibacterial Susceptibility Tests: Dilution and Disk Diffusion Methods*

JAMES H. JORGENSEN, JOHN D. TURNIDGE, AND JOHN A. WASHINGTON

118

Antibacterial susceptibility testing may be performed reliably by either dilution or diffusion methods. The choice of methodology may be based on factors such as relative ease of performance, cost, flexibility in selection of drugs for testing, use of automated or semiautomated devices to facilitate testing, and the perceived accuracy of the methodology (32). In some instances, misconceptions have existed regarding the clinical importance of MICs versus the interpretive category results that are provided by the disk diffusion method. These misconceptions are often based on an assumption that the dilution test is the more accurate of the two methods and that physicians prefer a quantitative (MIC) result. Since there is a direct relationship between the zone of inhibition diameter and the MIC and since MICs and zone inhibition diameters for reference strains are reproducible on an interlaboratory and an intralaboratory basis, there is no evidence to support the impression that one method is more accurate than the other with the majority of rapidly growing bacteria. An MIC result reported from a conventional dilution test should not be misconstrued as representing greater accuracy, since the actual MIC may be a concentration somewhere between the concentration inhibiting the organism and the next lowest concentration tested (i.e., 1 $\log_2$ dilution lower). For example, an organism may grow in the presence of an antimicrobial agent at a concentration of 4 μg/ml but does not grow in the presence of the agent at 8 μg/ml. The actual MIC could be anywhere between 4 and 8 μg/ml. Moreover, few physicians other than those specializing in the field of infectious diseases can reliably interpret MICs, so that the laboratory is obliged to provide an interpretation with each MIC result in order to avoid the risk of misinterpretation (40).

Specific clinical indications for performing dilution tests are not well agreed upon, but they may include endocarditis, osteomyelitis, and meningitis. The pharmacodynamic principles that relate the importance of the serum antibiotic level in relation to the MIC for an organism are not generally used to optimize therapy for individual patients (18). MICs can be useful for evaluating relative degrees of susceptibility of bacteria to various antimicrobial agents and for comparing the relative activities of drugs against various species, e.g., for comparing the activities of two or more aminoglycosides against a susceptible gram-negative isolate. Finally, MICs may be useful in the delineation of degrees of resistance among isolates whose resistance barely exceeds a defined resistance threshold, e.g., beta-lactam MICs for *Streptococcus pneumoniae* with diminished penicillin susceptibility. In general, however, the decision as to whether to perform dilution or disk diffusion testing is usually based on logistical reasons, such as the system that the laboratory has selected to provide both identification and susceptibility testing. Many such systems are now commercially available; however, the major challenge posed by such systems is the inflexibility of the standard panels of antimicrobial agents that can be tested. The inability to match precisely an institution's antimicrobial agent formulary with drugs readily available in commercial systems has led some laboratories to adopt the highly flexible disk diffusion test for routine use.

The selection of antibacterial agents for testing is complicated by the sheer number of agents available today. Many of these compounds, however, exhibit similar if not identical activities in vitro, so that in many cases, one compound can be tested as a surrogate for one or more closely related compounds. Such extrapolations, which have generally been agreed upon internationally, are listed in Table 1. Use of these drug surrogates can substantially reduce the number of agents required for testing and in some cases can provide the necessary flexibility in adapting commercial test systems for routine use in a variety of institutions. For instance, the susceptibility of a staphylococcus to oxacillin can be extrapolated to indicate the susceptibility of the organism to all currently available penicillinase-stable penicillins, cephalosporins, and carbapenems. It is thus unnecessary to test any of the agents in these chemical classes, with the exception of the beta-lactamase-labile compounds (e.g., penicillin, ampicillin, amoxicillin, and piperacillin) represented by penicillin itself. Other extrapolations are possible, especially if there is demonstrated susceptibility to an early member of the chemical class of antimicrobial agent.

It is important that the microbiologist work with the hospital formulary committee to ensure that the antibacterial agents being tested in the laboratory reflect those in the institution's formulary (33). Failure to do so can contribute to antibiotic misuse (44). Guidelines for the selection of antibacterial agents to be tested routinely have been published by the National Committee for Clinical Laboratory

* This chapter contains information presented in chapter 113 by Gail L. Woods and John A. Washington in the sixth edition of this Manual.

TABLE 1 Antibacterial susceptibility results that may be extrapolated from other test results

Test drug (susceptibility)	Organism(s)	Drugs to which result can be extrapolated
Oxacillin	*Staphylococcus* spp.	All penicillins including antistaphylococcal penicillins, all cephalosporins, all beta-lactamase inhibitor combinations, all carbapenems, loracarbef
Tetracycline	All (except *Staphylococcus* spp. and *Acinetobacter* spp.)	Doxycycline, minocycline, chlortetracycline, demeclocycline, oxytetracycline, methacycline
Erythromycin	Gram-positive cocci	Roxithromyxin, clarithromycin, azithromycin, dirithromycin
Clindamycin	All	Lincomycin
Ampicillin	*Enterococcus* spp.	Penicillin
Penicillin G	*Staphylococcus* spp., *Neisseria gonorrhoeae*	Phenoxymethylpenicillin, phenethicillin, ampicillin, amoxicillin, bacampicillin, cyclacillin, hetacillin, carbenicillin, mezlocillin, azlocillin, ticarcillin, piperacillin
Cephalothin	*Enterobacteriaceae*	Cephapirin, cephradine, cephalexin, cefaclor, and cefadroxil but not other cephalosporins
Ampicillin	All	Amoxycillin, bacampicillin, cyclacillin, hetacillin
Sulfisoxazole	All	All sulfonamides
Nalidixic acid (susceptible)	*Enterobacteriaceae*	All quinolones including fluoroquinolones (susceptible)
Cephalothin or cefazolin (susceptible)	*Enterobacteriaceae*	All cephalosporins (susceptible)
Vancomycin (susceptible)	All	Teicoplanin

Standards (NCCLS) (40, 41) and are summarized in Table 2. While this list is sometimes regarded as the standard for the selection of those agents to be tested, it should be emphasized that it is a list of agents that should be considered for routine testing only and that many variables go into the decision as to what agents should be tested in any particular setting (33). NCCLS also cautions that the decision as to which agents should be tested and reported on selectively should be made by the clinical microbiologist in conjunction with the infectious disease practitioner, the pharmacy, and/or the infection control committee (40, 41).

DILUTION METHODS

Dilution susceptibility testing methods are used to determine the minimal concentration, usually in micrograms per milliliter, of an antimicrobial agent required to inhibit or kill a microorganism. Procedures for determining antimicrobial inhibitory activity can be carried out by either agar- or broth-based methods. Antimicrobial agents are usually tested at $\log_2$ (twofold) serial dilutions, and the lowest concentration that inhibits the visible growth of an organism is regarded as the MIC. The concentration range used may vary with the drug, the organism being tested, and the site of infection. Ranges should include concentrations that allow determinations of the interpretive categories (i.e., susceptible, intermediate, and resistant) and also the ranges that encompass the expected MICs for quality control reference strains. Other dilution methods include those that test a single or a selected few concentrations of antimicrobial agents (i.e., breakpoint susceptibility testing and single-drug-concentration screens; see below).

Dilution methods offer flexibility in the sense that the standard medium used to test frequently encountered organisms (e.g., staphylococci, enterococci, members of the family *Enterobacteriaceae*, and *Pseudomonas aeruginosa*) may be supplemented or even replaced with another medium to allow accurate testing of various fastidious bacterial species not reliably tested by disk diffusion. Dilution methods are also adaptable to automated systems. In addition, if plates or panels are prepared in-house, the combination of antimicrobial agents to be included is not limited. Any drug available in powder form may be used.

The flexibility of dilution testing is also evident in the reporting formats that may be used. Quantitative results (MICs in micrograms per milliliter) or category results (susceptible, intermediate, or resistant), or both, can be used.

DILUTION TESTING: AGAR METHOD

Dilution of Antimicrobial Agents

The solvents and diluents needed to prepare stock solutions of most commonly used antimicrobial agents are presented in the NCCLS document on dilution testing (40).

Preparation, Supplementation, and Storage of Media

Mueller-Hinton agar is the recommended medium for the testing of most commonly encountered aerobic and facultatively anaerobic bacteria (40). The dehydrated agar base is commercially available and should be prepared as described by the manufacturer. Before sterilization, the molten agar is usually distributed into screw-cap containers in exact aliquots sufficient to dilute the desired antimicrobial concentrations 10-fold. Containers, one for each drug concentration to be tested, are sterilized by autoclaving at 121°C for 15 min and are allowed to equilibrate to 48 to 50°C in a preheated water bath. Once the containers are equilibrated, the appropriate volume of antimicrobial agent is added, and the container contents are mixed by gentle inversion, poured into 100-mm round or square sterile plastic petri plates set on a level surface, and allowed to solidify. For growth controls, plates containing drug-free agar are also prepared. All plates should be poured to a depth of 3 to 4 mm (20 to 25 ml of agar per round plate and 30 ml for square plates), and the pH of each batch should be checked to confirm the acceptable pH range of 7.2 to 7.4 (40).

TABLE 2 Antimicrobial agents recommended for routine dilution and disk diffusion susceptibility testing[a]

Antimicrobial agent	Group[b] recommended for testing			
	Enterobacteriaceae	*Pseudomonas* spp. and other non-*Enterobacteriaceae*	Staphylococci	Enterococci
Penicillins				
Penicillin G			A	A[c,d]
Ampicillin	A			A[c]
Oxacillin or methicillin			A[e]	
Ticarcillin[d]	B	A		
Mezlocillin[d]	B	A		
Piperacillin	B	A		
Ampicillin-sulbactam	B			
Amoxicillin-clavulanic acid	B			
Piperacillin-tazobactam	B			
Ticarcillin-clavulanic acid	B	B[f]		
Cephalosporins				
Cephalothin	A[g]			
Cefazolin	A			
Cefamandole	B			
Cefonicid	B			
Cefuroxime	B			
Cefmetazole	B			
Cefoperazone	B	B		
Cefoxitin	B			
Cefotetan	B			
Cefotaxime	B			
Ceftriaxone	B			
Ceftizoxime	B			
Ceftazidime	C	A		
Cefepime	B	B		
Other beta-lactams				
Imipenem	B	B		
Meropenem	B	B		
Aztreonam	B	B		
Aminoglycosides[h]				
Gentamicin	A	A		C[h]
Netilmicin	C	C		
Tobramycin	C	B		
Amikacin	C	B		
Streptomycin				C[h]
Macrolides				
Azithromycin			B	
Clarithromycin			B	
Erythromycin			B	
Quinolones				
Ciprofloxacin	B	B	C	U
Levofloxacin	B	U	C	U
Lomefloxacin	U	U	U	
Norfloxacin	U	U	U	U
Ofloxacin	U	U	C	

(Continued on next page)

TABLE 2 *(Continued)*

Antimicrobial agent	*Enterobacteriaceae*	Group[b] recommended for testing		
		Pseudomonas spp. and other non-*Enterobacteriaceae*	Staphylococci	Enterococci
Miscellaneous				
Chloramphenicol	C	C	C	
Clindamycin			B	
Nitrofurantoin	U		U	U
Rifampin			C	
Sulfisoxazole	U		U	
Tetracycline	C	C[i]	C	U
Trimethoprim-sulfamethoxazole	B	C	B	
Trimethoprim	U			
Vancomycin			B	B[d]

[a] Modified from NCCLS standards (40, 41, 43), with permission. Current standards and supplements to them may be obtained from NCCLS, 940 West Valley Road, Suite 1400, Wayne, PA 19087–1898.

[b] Group A comprises primary drugs to be tested and reported, group B comprises those to be tested as primary drugs but reported selectively, group C comprises supplemental drugs to be reported selectively, and group U comprises drugs to be tested against urinary isolates only.

[c] Results of tests with penicillin apply to other penicillins (e.g., ampicillin, amoxicillin, carboxypenicillins, and ureidopenicillins) against beta-lactamase-negative enterococci.

[d] Combination therapy consisting of penicillin, ampicillin, or vancomycin and an aminoglycoside is recommended.

[e] Staphylococci resistant to the penicillinase-resistant penicillins should also be considered resistant to penicillins, beta-lactam–beta-lactamase inactivating combinations, cephalosporins, and carbapenems.

[f] Ticarcillin-clavulanic acid or piperacillin-tazobactam should not be considered therapeutic alternative for *P. aeruginosa* isolates resistant to carboxy- or ureidopenicillins.

[g] Cephalothin test results may also be used to represent cephapirin, cephradine, cephalexin, cefaclor, cefadroxil, and cefazolin (except against members of the family *Enterobacteriaceae*). Cefuroxime, cefixime, cefpodoxime, cefprozil, ceftibuten, and loracarbef may be tested separately on a supplemental basis because their activities may be greater than those of cephalothin or cefazolin against members of the family *Enterobacteriaceae*.

[h] For use of aminoglycosides to screen enterococci for synergy resistance, see the sections Breakpoint Susceptibility Tests and Resistance Screens.

[i] Doxycycline or minocycline may be tested on a supplemental basis because of their greater activities against some nonfermentative gram-negative bacilli and staphylococci.

After sterilization and temperature equilibration of the molten agar, any necessary supplements are aseptically added to the Mueller-Hinton agar. For the testing of streptococci, supplementation with 5% defibrinated sheep or horse blood is recommended (40). However, sheep blood supplementation may antagonize the activities of sulfonamides and trimethoprim against some organisms (8). The presence of blood also affects the results obtained for novobiocin and nafcillin as well as the in vitro activities of cephalosporins against enterococci (12, 46); therefore, blood supplementation should not be used unless it is necessary for bacterial growth (see chapter 119 for acceptable methods for testing fastidious bacterial species). The performance standards of Mueller-Hinton agar have been defined sufficiently such that calcium and magnesium supplementation should not be done (39). The agar should be supplemented with 2% NaCl for the testing of methicillin, nafcillin, or oxacillin against staphylococci (29).

Once prepared, plates should be sealed in plastic bags and stored at 4 to 8°C. In general, they should be used within 5 days of preparation or as long as the MICs for control strains that are tested routinely are within the acceptable ranges. However, certain agents, e.g., imipenem, cefaclor, and clavulanic acid combinations, are sufficiently labile that plates may not be stored prior to use. Before inoculation, plates that have been stored under refrigeration should be allowed to equilibrate to room temperature, and the agar surface should be dry.

Inoculation Procedures

Variations in inoculum size may substantially affect MIC endpoint determinations; therefore, careful inoculum standardization is required to obtain accurate results. The recommended final inoculum for agar dilution is 10^4 CFU per spot (40). This may be achieved in either of two ways. Four or five colonies are picked from overnight growth on agar-based medium and are inoculated into 4 to 5 ml of suitable broth that will support good growth (usually tryptic soy broth). Broths are incubated at 35°C until they are visibly turbid, and then the suspension is diluted until its turbidity matches the turbidity of a barium sulfate or equivalent 0.5 McFarland turbidity standard (ca. 10^8 CFU/ml). The standard may be purchased or may be prepared as described by NCCLS (40). The accuracy of the density of the standard should be verified by using a spectrophotometer with a 1-cm light path; for the 0.5 McFarland standard, the absorbance at 625 nm should be 0.08 to 0.10 (40). An alternative inoculum standardization method uses direct suspension of colonies from overnight growth on a nonselective agar medium in broth or saline to a turbidity that matches that of the McFarland standard, eliminating the time needed for growing the inoculum in broth (40). In either case, sterile broth or normal saline is used to make a 1:10 dilution of the suspension to give an adjusted concentration of 10^7 CFU/ml (40).

Once the adjusted inoculum is prepared, inoculation of the antimicrobial agent plates should be accomplished within 30 min, since longer delays may lead to changes in inoculum size. By using either a pipette, a calibrated loop, or an inoculum replicating device, 0.001 to 0.002 ml of the suspension of 10^7 CFU/ml is delivered to the agar surface, resulting in the final desired inoculum of approximately 10^4 CFU per spot. For convenience, use of a replicator is preferred, because a consistent inoculum volume for up to 36 different isolates is simultaneously delivered (50). To use this device, an aliquot of the adjusted inoculum for each isolate is pipetted into the appropriate well of a seed plate and a multiprong inoculator is used to pick up and gently transfer 0.001 to 0.002 ml from the wells to the agar surfaces. The surface of the agar plates must be dry before inoculation, which should begin with the lowest drug concentration. To check the viability of each test isolate and also as an added check for purity, control plates that do not contain drug are inoculated last. Finally, plates should be clearly marked so that the locations of the different isolates being tested on each plate are known.

Incubation

Inoculated plates are allowed to stand for several minutes until the inocula have been completely absorbed by the medium; then they are inverted and incubated in air at 35°C for 16 to 20 h before being read. To facilitate detection of vancomycin-resistant enterococci and methicillin-resistant staphylococci, plates containing vancomycin and either oxacillin or methicillin, respectively, should be incubated for a full 24 h before being read (40). Incubation should not be carried out in the presence of increased levels of CO_2 unless a fastidious organism is being tested (see chapter 119).

Interpretation and Reporting of Results

Before reading and recording of the results obtained with clinical isolates, those obtained with applicable quality control strains should be checked to ensure that their values are within the acceptable ranges (see Quality Control below), and the drug-free control plates should be examined for isolate viability and purity. Endpoints for each antimicrobial agent are best determined by placing the plates on a dark background and examining the plates for the lowest concentration that inhibits visible growth, which is recorded as the MIC. A single colony or a faint haze left by the initial inoculum should not be regarded as growth. If two or more colonies persist at antimicrobial concentrations beyond an otherwise obvious endpoint or if there is no growth at lower concentrations but growth at higher concentrations, the isolate should be subcultured to confirm its purity and the test should be repeated. Substances that may antagonize the antibacterial activities of sulfonamides and trimethoprim may be carried over with the inoculum and cause "trailing," or less definite endpoints (8, 12). Therefore, the MICs of these antimicrobial agents should be interpreted as the endpoint at which an obvious 80% or more diminution of growth occurs. Although much less pronounced, trailing endpoints may also occur with bacteriostatic agents such as chloramphenicol and the tetracyclines.

The MIC of each antimicrobial agent is usually recorded in micrograms per milliliter. These quantitative results may be reported with the appropriate corresponding interpretive categories (susceptible, intermediate, or resistant), or the interpretive category may be reported alone. The MIC interpretive standards for these susceptibility categories, as currently recommended by NCCLS (40), are provided in Table 3. For detailed instructions concerning the use of these criteria and categories, the latest NCCLS standards for dilution testing methods should be consulted (40, 43). Note that the interpretive standards for most of the penicillin-class drugs vary with the organism being tested.

The three interpretive categories are defined as follows. Susceptible indicates that an infection caused by the tested microorganism may be appropriately treated with the usually recommended dose of antibiotic. Intermediate indicates that the isolate may be inhibited by attainable concentrations of certain drugs (e.g., beta-lactams) if higher dosages can be used safely or if the infection involves a body site in which the drug is physiologically concentrated (e.g., the urinary tract). The intermediate category also serves as a buffer zone that prevents technical artifacts from causing major interpretive discrepancies. Resistant isolates are not inhibited by the concentration of antimicrobial agent normally achievable with the recommended dose and/or yield results that fall within a range in which specific resistance mechanisms are likely to be present (40).

Advantages and Disadvantages

Dilution testing by the agar method is a well-standardized, reliable susceptibility-testing technique that may be used as a reference for evaluating the accuracies of other testing systems. In addition, the simultaneous testing of a large number of isolates with a few drugs is efficient, and microbial contamination or heterogeneity is more readily detected by agar methods than by broth methods. The major disadvantages of the agar method are associated with the time-consuming and labor-intensive tasks of preparing the plates, especially as the number of different antimicrobial agents to be tested against each isolate increases or if only a few isolates are to be tested.

DILUTION TESTING: BROTH METHODS

The general approaches for broth methods include broth macrodilution, in which the broth volume for each antimicrobial concentration is ≥1.0 ml (usually 2.0 ml) contained in 13- by 100-mm tubes, and broth microdilution, in which antimicrobial dilutions are most often in 0.1-ml volumes contained in wells of microdilution trays.

Broth Macrodilution Methods

Dilution of Antimicrobial Agents

Stock solutions are prepared as discussed in the NCCLS document on dilution testing (40) and are similar to those used for agar dilution tests. As in the agar method, the actual volumes used for the dilutions would be proportionally increased according to the number of tests being prepared, with a minimum of 1.0 ml needed for each drug concentration. Because addition of the inoculum results in a 1 : 2 dilution of each concentration, all final drug concentrations must be prepared at twice the actual desired testing concentration (see Inoculation Procedures below).

Preparation, Supplementation, and Storage of Media

Cation-adjusted Mueller-Hinton broth (CAMHB) is recommended for the routine testing of commonly encountered nonfastidious organisms (40). Adjustment with the cations Ca^{2+} (20 to 25 mg/liter) and Mg^{2+} (10 to 12.5 mg/liter) is required to ensure acceptable results when *P. aeruginosa* isolates are tested against aminoglycosides and when tetracycline is tested against other bacteria. However, for consistency, cation adjustment of Mueller-Hinton broth is now recommended when testing all species and antimicrobial agents (40). Many manufacturers provide Mueller-Hinton broth that already has appropriate concentrations of divalent cations, so care must be taken not to supplement such products with additional cations. If adjustment is necessary, it can be accomplished by the addition of suitable volumes of filter-sterilized, chilled $CaCl_2$ stock (3.68 g of $CaCl_2 \cdot 2H_2O$ dissolved in 100 ml of deionized water for a concentration of 10 mg of Ca^{2+} per ml) and $MgCl_2$ stock (8.36 g of $MgCl_2 \cdot 6H_2O$ in 100 ml of deionized water for a concen-

TABLE 3 Interpretive standards for dilution and disk diffusion susceptibility testing[a]

Antimicrobial agent and organism	MIC (μg/ml)			Zone diam (mm)		
	Susceptible	Intermediate	Resistant	Susceptible	Intermediate	Resistant
Penicillins						
Penicillin G						
Staphylococci[b]	≤0.12		≥0.25	≥29		≤28
Enterococci[c]	≤8		≥16	≥15		≤14
Methicillin[d]	≤8		≥16	≥14	10–13	≤9
Oxacillin[d]						
S. aureus	≤2		≥4	≥13	11–12	≤10
Coagulase-negative staphylococci	≤0.25		≥0.5	≥18		≤17
Ampicillin						
Enterobacteriaceae	≤8	16	≥32	≥17	14–16	≤13
Staphylococci	≤0.25		≥0.5	≥29		≤28
Enterococci[c]	≤8		≥16	≥17		≤16
Amoxicillin-clavulanic acid						
Staphylococci	≤4/2		≥8/4	≥20		≤19
Other organisms	≤8/4	16/8	≥32/16	≥18	14–17	≤13
Ampicillin-sulbactam	≤8/4	16/8	≥32/16	≥15	12–14	≤11
Azlocillin	≤64		≥128	≥18		≤17
P. aeruginosa						
Carbenicillin						
P. aeruginosa	≤128	256	≥512	≥17	14–16	≥13
Other gram-negative bacilli	≤16	32	≥64	≥23	20–22	≤19
Mezlocillin						
P. aeruginosa	≤64		≥128	≥16		≤15
Other gram-negative bacilli	≤16	32–64	≥128	≥21	18–20	≤17
Piperacillin						
P. aeruginosa	≤64		≥128	≥18		≤17
Other gram-negative bacilli	≤16	32–64	≥128	≥21	18–20	≤17
Piperacillin-tazobactam						
P. aeruginosa	≤64/4		≥128/4	≥18		≤17
Other gram-negative bacilli	≤16/4	32/4–64/4	≥128/4	≥21	18–20	≤17
Staphylococci	≤8/4		≥16/4	≥18		≤17
Ticarcillin						
P. aeruginosa	≤64		≥128	≥15		≤14
Other gram-negative bacilli	≤16	32–64	≥128	≥20	15–19	≤14
Ticarcillin-clavulanic acid						
P. aeruginosa	≤64/2		≥128/2	≥15		≤14
Other gram-negative bacilli	≤16/2	32/2–64/2	≥128/2	≥20	15–19	≤14
Staphylococci	≤8/2		≥16/2	≥23		≤22
Cephalosporins						
Cefaclor	≤8	16	≥32	≥18	15–17	≤14
Cefamandole	≤8	16	≥32	≥18	15–17	≤14
Cefazolin	≤8	16	≥32	≥18	15–17	≤14

(Continued on next page)

TABLE 3 Interpretive standards for dilution and disk diffusion susceptibility testing[a] (*Continued*)

Antimicrobial agent and organism	MIC (μg/ml)			Zone diam (mm)		
	Susceptible	Intermediate	Resistant	Susceptible	Intermediate	Resistant
Cefepime	≤8	16	≥32	≥18	15–17	≤14
Cefetamet	≤4	8	≥16	≥18	15–17	≤14
Cefixime	≤1	2	≥4	≥19	16–18	≤15
Cefmetazole	≤16	32	≥64	≥16	13–15	≤12
Cefonicid	≤8	16	≥32	≥18	15–17	≤14
Cefoperazone	≤16	32	≥64	≥21	16–20	≤15
Cefotaxime	≤8	16–32	≥64	≥23	15–22	≤14
Cefotetan	≤16	32	≥64	≥16	13–15	≤12
Cefoxitin	≤8	16	≥32	≥18	15–17	≤14
Cefpodoxime	≤2	4	≥8	≥21	18–20	≤17
Cefprozil	≤8	16	≥32	≥18	15–17	≤14
Ceftazidime	≤8	16	≥32	≥18	15–17	≤14
Ceftibuten	≤8	16	≥32	≥21	18–20	≤17
Ceftizoxime	≤8	16–32	≥64	≥20	15–19	≤14
Ceftriaxone	≤8	16–32	≥64	≥21	14–20	≤13
Cefuroxime axetil	≤4	8–16	≥32	≥23	15–22	≤14
Cefuroxime sodium	≤8	16	≥32	≥18	15–17	≤14
Cephalothin	≤8	16	≥32	≥18	15–17	≤14
Loracarbef	≤8	16	≥32	≥18	15–17	≤14
Moxalactam	≤8	16–32	≥64	≥23	15–22	≤14
Other beta-lactams						
Aztreonam	≤8	16	≥32	≥22	16–21	≤15
Imipenem	≤4	8	≥16	≥16	14–15	≤13
Meropenem	≤4	8	≥16	≥16	14–15	≤13
Aminoglycosides						
Amikacin	≤16	32	≥64	≥17	15–16	≤14
Gentamicin	≤4	8	≥16	≥15	13–14	≤12
Enterococci (high-level resistance)	≤500		>500	≥10	7–9	6
Netilmicin	≤8	16	≥32	≥15	13–14	≤12
Tobramycin	≤4	8	≥16	≥15	13–14	≤12
Streptomycin						
Enterococci (high-level resistance)						
Broth microdilution method	≤1,000		>1,000			
Agar-based method	≤2,000		>2,000	≥10	7–9	6
Glycopeptides						
Teicoplanin	≤8	16	≥32	≥14	11–13	≤10
Vancomycin						
Enterococci	≤4	8–16	≥32	≥17	15–16	≤14
Staphylococci	≤4	8–16	≥32	≥15	Determine MIC if ≤14	
Macrolides						
Azithromycin	≤2	4	≥8	≥18	14–17	≤13
Clarithromycin	≤2	4	≥8	≥18	14–17	≤13
Dirithromycin	≤2	4	≥8	≥19	16–18	≤15
Erythromycin	≤0.5	1–2	≥8	≥23	14–22	≤13

(*Continued on next page*)

TABLE 3 *(Continued)*

Antimicrobial agent and organism	MIC (μg/ml)			Zone diam (mm)		
	Susceptible	Intermediate	Resistant	Susceptible	Intermediate	Resistant
Quinolones						
Ciprofloxacin	≤1	2	≥4	≥21	16–20	≤15
Enoxacin	≤2	4	≥8	≥18	15–17	≤14
Fleroxacin	≤2	4	≥8	≥19	16–18	≤15
Levofloxacin	≤2	4	≥8	≥17	14–16	≤13
Lomefloxacin	≤2	4	≥8	≥22	19–21	≤18
Nalidixic acid[e]	≤8	16	≥32	≥19	14–18	≤13
Norfloxacin[e]	≤4	8	≥16	≥17	13–16	≤12
Ofloxacin	≤2	4	≥8	≥16	13–15	≤12
Other						
Chloramphenicol	≤8	16	≥32	≥18	13–17	≤12
Clindamycin	≤0.5	1–2	≥4	≥21	15–20	≤14
Nitrofurantoin	≤32	64	≥128	≥17	15–16	≤14
Rifampin	≤1	2	≥4	≥20	17–19	≤16
Sulfonamide	≤256		≥512	≥17	13–16	≤12
Tetracycline	≤4	8	≥16	≥19	15–18	≤14
Trimethoprim[e]	≤8		≥16	≥16	11–15	≤10
Trimethoprim-sulfamethoxazole	≤2/38		≥4/76	≥16	11–15	≤10

[a] Adapted from NCCLS data (40, 41, 43), with permission. The interpretive data are valid only if the methodologies in M2-A6 (41) and M7-A4 (40) are followed. NCCLS frequently updates the interpretive tables through new additions of the standards and supplements to them. Users should refer to the most recent additions. The current standards and supplements to them may be obtained from NCCLS, 940 W. Valley Rd., Suite 1400, Wayne, PA 19087–1898.

[b] Penicillin should be used as the class representative for all penicillins (e.g., ampicillin, amoxicillin, mezlocillin, piperacillin, and ticarcillin). Isolates for which MICs are ≤0.03 μg of penicillin per ml generally do not produce beta-lactamase, whereas those for which MICs are ≥0.25 μg/ml do and should be regarded as resistant to penicillins. Isolates for which penicillin MICs are 0.06 or 0.12 μg/ml should be tested for beta-lactamase.

[c] Therapy of serious enterococcal infections requires high doses of penicillin or ampicillin in combination with an aminoglycoside. Vancomycin may be substituted for the penicillin in instances of penicillin hypersensitivity or of penicillin or ampicillin resistance.

[d] Oxacillin or methicillin may be tested; however, oxacillin is preferred because of its greater stability in vitro. The results from testing oxacillin apply also to other penicillinase-resistant penicillins. Oxacillin-resistant staphylococci should be considered resistant to all penicillins, cephalosporins, carbacephems, carbapenems, and beta-lactam–beta-lactamase inhibitor combinations.

[e] For the treatment of urinary tract infections only.

tration of 10 mg of Mg^{2+} per ml) to the cooled broth (6, 40). Insufficient cation concentrations result in increased aminoglycoside activity (21, 45, 57), while an excess cation content results in decreased aminoglycoside activity against *P. aeruginosa* (5, 21, 45). Reliable detection of staphylococcal resistance to oxacillin, methicillin, or nafcillin requires that the CAMHB used to test these drugs be supplemented with 2% NaCl (40, 53).

To minimize evaporation and deterioration of antimicrobial agents, tubes should be tightly capped and stored at 4 to 8°C until they are needed. With most agents, the dilutions should be used within 5 days of preparation or as long as quality control ranges are maintained (see Quality Control below). As with agar dilution testing, certain beta-lactam agents are too labile for prolonged storage at the final test concentrations.

Inoculation Procedures

The recommended final inoculum is 5×10^5 CFU/ml. Isolates are inoculated into a broth that will support good growth (such as tryptic soy broth) and are incubated until they are turbid. The turbidity is adjusted to match that of a 0.5 McFarland standard (approximately 10^8 CFU/ml). Alternatively, four or five colonies from overnight growth on a nonselective agar plate may be directly suspended in broth so that the turbidity matches the turbidity of the McFarland standard (40). This alternative is preferred for the testing of methicillin or oxacillin against staphylococci (40). A portion of the standardized suspension is diluted 1:100 (10^6 CFU/ml) with broth or saline. When 1 ml of this dilution is added to each tube containing 1 ml of the drug diluted in CAMHB, a final inoculum of 5×10^5 CFU/ml is achieved. Broth not containing an antimicrobial agent is inoculated as a control for organism viability (growth control). All tubes should be inoculated within 30 min of inoculum preparation, and an aliquot of the inoculum should be plated to check for purity and inoculum density.

Incubation

Tubes are incubated in air at 35°C for 16 to 20 h before the MICs are determined. Incubation should be extended to a full 24 h for the detection of vancomycin-resistant enterococci or methicillin-resistant or vancomycin-intermediate staphylococci (40). The use of increased levels of CO_2 is not recommended.

Interpretation and Reporting of Results

Before the MICs for the test strains are read and recorded, the growth controls should be examined for viability and inoculum subcultures should be checked for contamination and appropriate inoculum size, and it should be confirmed that the MICs for the quality control strains are appropriate (see Quality Control below). Growth or a lack thereof in the antimicrobial agent-containing tubes is best determined by comparison with the growth control. Generally, growth is indicated by turbidity, a single sedimented button ≥2 mm in diameter, or several buttons with smaller diameters. As with the agar method, trailing endpoints may be seen when trimethoprim or sulfonamides are tested, and the concentration at which an obvious 80% or greater diminution of growth compared with that of the growth control occurs should be recorded as the MIC (40). Other interpretation problems include the "skipped tube" phenomenon, in which growth is not observed at one concentration but is observed at lower and higher drug concentrations. Most authorities suggest that when this occurs, the skipped tube should be ignored and the concentration that finally inhibits growth at serially higher concentrations should be recorded as the MIC. If more than one skipped tube occurs or if there is growth in the presence of higher antimicrobial concentrations but not lower ones, the results should not be reported and the test for that drug should be repeated.

The lowest concentration that completely inhibits visible growth of the organism as detected by the unaided eye is recorded as the MIC. The latest NCCLS MIC interpretive standards (43) for the susceptibility categories are provided in Table 3. The definitions of and comments concerning these categories that were given above for the agar method also pertain to the broth macrodilution method.

Advantages and Disadvantages

The broth macrodilution method is a well-standardized and reliable reference method that is useful for research purposes, but because of the laborious nature of the procedure and the availability of more convenient dilution systems (i.e., microdilution), this procedure is generally not useful for routine susceptibility testing in most clinical microbiology laboratories.

Broth Microdilution Method

The convenience afforded by the availability of dilution susceptibility testing in microdilution trays has led to the widespread use of broth microdilution methods. The disposable plastic trays contain several antimicrobial agents to be tested simultaneously and may be prepared in-house or obtained commercially either frozen or freeze-dried. When commercial systems are used, the manufacturers' recommendations concerning storage, inoculation, incubation, and interpretation should be followed. The primary focus of this section will be the in-house preparation and use of broth microdilution trays. However, many of the principles and practices discussed here are pertinent to the broth microdilution method in general, regardless of the source of the trays.

Dilution of Antimicrobial Agents

Antimicrobial stock solutions are prepared as outlined in the NCCLS document on dilution testing (40). The dilution scheme used for agar and broth macrodilution methods is applicable to the antimicrobial dilutions needed for the preparation of broth microdilution panels. Available automated dispensing systems require that at least 10 ml of broth containing each antimicrobial concentration be prepared. From the 10-ml samples, aliquots of 0.05 or 0.1 ml are simultaneously dispensed into the corresponding wells of each broth microdilution tray. If 0.05-ml volumes are dispensed, allowances must be made for the 1:2 dilution of the final drug concentration that will occur when the 0.05 ml of inoculum is added (see Inoculation Procedures below). When 0.1-ml aliquots are dispensed, the volume of inoculum normally used is sufficiently small ($\leq$0.005 ml) that adjustments in the antimicrobial dilution scheme are not needed. As a general rule, when the inoculum volume is less than 10% of the broth volume in the well, dilution of the antimicrobial concentration by the inoculum does not have to be taken into account (40).

Preparation, Supplementation, and Storage of Media

CAMHB is the recommended medium for routine broth microdilution testing and should be prepared as discussed above for the broth macrodilution method. Also, supplementation of the broth with 2% NaCl is required for the detection of methicillin-resistant staphylococci (40). After the antimicrobial dilutions have been dispensed into the trays, they are stacked in groups of 5 to 10, with a tray lid or an empty tray placed on top to minimize contamination and evaporation. Each stack is sealed in a plastic bag and is immediately frozen at -20°C or, preferably, -60°C or colder. At -20°C, preservation is ensured for at least 6 weeks with most drugs, but the shelf life may be extended to months if the trays are stored at -60 to -70°C. Exceptions include highly labile compounds such as cefaclor, clavulanic acid, and imipenem, which may not retain their potency during storage. If thawed, panels must be used or discarded, but not refrozen, since freeze-thaw cycles cause substantial deterioration of beta-lactam antibiotics. For this reason, -20°C household-type freezers with self-defrosting units must not be used.

Inoculation Procedures

As with the macrodilution procedure, the final desired inoculum concentration is 5×10^5 CFU/ml. The isolates may be grown in broth so that the turbidity matches the turbidity of a 0.5 McFarland standard (ca. 10^8 CFU/ml), or such a suspension can be made from colonies grown on a nonselective agar medium after overnight growth (4), which is the method preferred for the detection of methicillin-resistant staphylococci (40). For broth microdilution procedures that require 0.001- to 0.005-ml volumes to inoculate wells containing 0.1 ml of broth, a portion of the suspension with a turbidity matching that of a 0.5 McFarland standard is diluted 1:10 (10^7 CFU/ml) in sterile saline or broth. Multipoint metal or disposable plastic inoculum replicators designed to collect and deliver appropriate volumes are used to transfer the inoculum from the diluted suspension to the wells of the broth microdilution tray, resulting in further dilutions ranging from 1:20 to 1:50 and final inoculum concentrations of 2×10^5 to 5×10^5 CFU/ml (2×10^4 to 5×10^4 CFU per well). For protocols that use an inoculum volume of 0.05 ml to inoculate 0.05 ml of broth, a 1:100 dilution of a suspension with a turbidity matching that of a 0.5 McFarland standard (10^6 CFU/ml) is used. When the inoculum is added to the wells, the 1:2 dilution of the inoculum of 1×10^6 CFU/ml results in a final inoculum concentration of 5×10^5 CFU/ml (5×10^4 CFU per well) and also halves the antibiotic concentration in each well. Special care should be taken to confirm the inoculum density on a periodic basis to ensure that the appropriate amount of inoculum is achieved. Insufficient inoculum can be a significant problem with inducible resistance mechanisms of some organisms and may not be recognized as a problem on the basis of the MICs obtained for the very susceptible quality control strains.

Broth microdilution trays should be inoculated within 30 min of inoculum preparation; during preparation, an aliquot should be subcultured to check the purity of the isolates, and colony counts should be set up to check the accuracy of the inoculum concentration. Finally, one well not containing an antimicrobial agent should be inoculated and used as a growth control, and a second uninoculated well should be used as a sterility control.

Incubation

After inoculation, each tray should be covered with plastic tape, sealed in a plastic bag, or tightly fitted with a lid or an empty tray to prevent evaporation during incubation. Trays are incubated in air at 35°C for 16 to 20 h before being read and should not be incubated in stacks of more than four trays. The incubator should be kept sufficiently humid to avoid evaporation but not so humid that condensation results in contamination problems. A full 24 h of incubation is recommended for the detection of vancomycin-resistant enterococci and methicillin-resistant staphylococci (40). Use of increased CO_2 levels during incubation is not recommended.

Interpretation and Reporting of Results

Before the MICs for the clinical isolates are read and recorded, the growth control wells should be examined for organism viability. It is advisable to check inoculum purity by subculture and to verify the inoculum size periodically by quantitative subculture. Also, the appropriateness of the MICs for the quality control strains should be confirmed (see Quality Control below). Various viewing devices are available and should be used to facilitate examination of the broth microdilution wells for growth. The simplest and most reliable method may be use of a parabolic magnifying mirror and tray stand that allows clear visual inspection of the underside of the broth microdilution trays. Growth is best determined by comparison of the growth with that in the growth control well and generally is indicated by turbidity throughout the well or by buttons, single or multiple, in the well bottom. The occurrence of trailing endpoints with trimethoprim or sulfonamides should be ignored, and the endpoint should be based on ≥80% growth inhibition. Results for drugs for which there is more than one skipped well on the tray should not be reported, as with the broth macrodilution test.

The latest NCCLS MIC interpretive criteria (43) for susceptibility categories are given in Table 3. The definitions of these categories and the comments concerning the use of these standards for agar and broth macrodilution methods are also applicable to broth microdilution methods.

Advantages and Disadvantages

The use of broth microdilution trays prepared in-house provides a reliable standardized reference method for susceptibility testing. Inoculation and reading procedures allow relatively convenient simultaneous testing of several antimicrobial agents against individual organisms. Not all laboratories have the facilities required for the preparation of broth microdilution trays. However, a wide variety of commercially prepared antibiotic panels are available. Such products provide trays with wells containing prepared antimicrobial dilutions either frozen or lyophilized. The former types of trays must be stored frozen in the laboratory, whereas lyophilized trays can be stored at room temperature. All such products are accompanied by multipoint inoculating devices. Results of testing may be determined by visual examination or with semiautomated or automated instrumentation. However, the versatility of the antimicrobial agent selection available with commercial broth microdilution trays is limited compared with the selection available by preparing panels in-house.

Breakpoint Susceptibility Tests

Breakpoint susceptibility testing refers to methods by which antimicrobial agents are tested only at the specific concentrations necessary for differentiating between the interpretive categories of susceptible, intermediate, and resistant rather than in the full range of doubling-dilution concentrations used to determine MICs. When two drug concentrations adjacent to the breakpoints defining the intermediate and resistant categories are selected, any one of the interpretive categories may be determined. Growth at both concentrations indicates resistance, growth at only the lower concentration signifies an intermediate result, and no growth at either concentration is interpreted as susceptibility.

As for full-range dilution testing, breakpoint methods require the use of appropriately adjusted and supplemented Mueller-Hinton broth or agar. In addition, the standard inoculation, incubation, and interpretation procedures recommended for the full-range dilution methods should be followed.

Because breakpoint testing is a direct measure of antimicrobial activity, there is the advantage of avoiding inherent errors associated with extrapolating disk diffusion zone sizes and MIC results (24). Considering the limited range of drug concentrations tested, a greater number and variety of antimicrobial agents can be incorporated into a broth microdilution tray set up for breakpoint testing than into trays designed for full-range dilution testing. However, convenient quality control procedures to ensure that appropriate concentrations of each antimicrobial agent are present are lacking. One possible approach is to use one organism for which the modal MIC is equal to or no less than 1 doubling dilution less than the lower or lowest concentration tested and a second organism for which the modal MIC is equal to or no more than 1 doubling dilution greater than the higher or highest concentration tested (40). One of these two quality control organisms should provide on-scale results (40). Despite the theoretical soundness of this approach, routine quality control of breakpoint panels is more complex and is not readily accomplished in the clinical laboratory.

Resistance Screens

In some circumstances, testing of a single drug concentration may be the most reliable and convenient method for the detection of antimicrobial resistance. The most clinically useful resistance screens are those for staphylococcal resistance to oxacillin (or methicillin) and for the resistance of *Enterococcus* spp. to vancomycin or the high-level resistance of *Enterococcus* spp. to gentamicin and streptomycin (40). These practical and reliable methods are described in chapter 121 of this Manual.

Gradient Diffusion Method

The E test (AB Biodisk, Solna, Sweden) is an in vitro method for quantitative antimicrobial susceptibility testing whereby a preformed antimicrobial gradient from a plastic-coated strip diffuses into an agar medium inoculated with the test organism. In this test, the MIC is read directly from a scale on the top of the strip at the point where the ellipse of organism growth inhibition intercepts the strip. Several strips, each containing a different antimicrobial agent, can be placed radially on the surface of a large round Mueller-Hinton agar plate inoculated with a suspension of a bacterial isolate whose turbidity has been adjusted to match that of a 0.5 McFarland turbidity standard. Several published evaluations (2, 28, 36, 48) have found good agreement between the MICs obtained by the E test and those obtained by reference dilution methods when enterococci and gram-negative bacilli with a variety of resistance mechanisms were tested. The E test combines the simplicity and flexibility of the disk diffusion test with the ability to determine the MICs of up to five antimicrobial agents on a single large Mueller-Hinton agar plate. However, E test strips are much more expensive than the disks used for diffusion testing, and there exists no simple, mechanized method for the simultaneous application of E test strips to the agar plate surface. The strength of this method appears to be the testing of fastidious or anaerobic bacteria, since the strips may be placed onto various enriched media (see chapters 119 and 120 of this Manual).

QUALITY CONTROL

Quality control recommendations are designed to evaluate the precision and accuracy of test procedures, monitor reagent reliability, and evaluate the performance of individuals who are conducting the tests.

Reference Strains

A critical element to accomplishing the goals of quality control is the selection and use of reference bacterial strains that are genetically stable and for which the MICs of each antimicrobial agent tested are in the middle of the MIC range (40). That is, the dilutions in a series should encompass at least two concentration increments above and below the previously established MIC for the reference strain. If there are four or fewer dilutions in a series or if nonconsecutive dilutions are tested (i.e., if breakpoint susceptibility testing is performed), quality control only for the correct interpretive category rather than an actual MIC or MIC ranges may be accomplished. *Escherichia coli* ATCC 25922, *P. aeruginosa* ATCC 27853, *Enterococcus faecalis* ATCC 29212, and *Staphylococcus aureus* ATCC 29213 are the recommended reference strains for both agar and broth dilution methods (42). The beta-lactamase-producing strain *E. coli* ATCC 35218 is recommended as the reference strain only for tests with penicillin–beta-lactamase inhibitor combinations. These organisms may be obtained from the American Type Culture Collection or other reliable commercial sources. For proper storage and subculture procedures, the recommendations of either NCCLS (40) or the commercial provider should be followed.

MIC Ranges

The acceptable quality control MIC ranges for the various reference strains are given in the NCCLS document on dilution testing (40). Updates of these MIC ranges are published annually (43) and should be readily available in the clinical laboratory. An out-of-control result is defined as an MIC not within the acceptable range. Certain out-of-control results can be directly related to the medium used for testing. High MICs of gentamicin for *P. aeruginosa* ATCC 27853 indicate an inappropriately high cation content of the Mueller-Hinton medium, and low MICs indicate an insufficient cation concentration. Although trimethoprim-sulfamethoxazole is not recommended for the treatment of *E. faecalis* infections, the results obtained with *E. faecalis* ATCC 29212 are useful for detecting inappropriate concentrations of substances such as thymidine that interfere with the in vitro activities of antifolate drugs. Trimethoprim-sulfamethoxazole MICs of >0.5/9.5 μg/ml indicate the presence of such interfering substances.

Batch and Lot Quality Control

Representative plates, panels, or trays from each new batch prepared in-house or from each new shipment lot obtained from a commercial source should be subjected to quality control and sterility testing. The MICs obtained by testing reference quality control strains should be within the acceptable ranges of NCCLS (43). If such accuracy is not achieved, the batch or lot should be rejected or the results obtained with the antimicrobial agent(s) in question should not be reported (see below). Similarly, if selected uninoculated plates or trays fail the sterility check after incubation, the batch or lot should be rejected. In addition to these formal quality control procedures that use reference strains, careful review of susceptibility results obtained during daily testing of clinical isolates is important for identifying aberrant or unusual susceptibility patterns possibly indicative of quality control problems.

Quality Control Frequency

In addition to batch and lot testing, quality control tests should be performed daily or at least on every day that the plates or trays are being used to test clinical isolates. When quality control is performed, two consecutive out-of-control MICs or more than two nonconsecutive out-of-control values in 20 consecutive tests indicate problems in the dilution testing procedure that must be identified and solved. However, if accuracy can be sufficiently documented as outlined below, daily testing may be replaced by weekly testing (40).

Each drug-reference strain combination is tested for 30 consecutive days to obtain a total of 30 MICs for each combination. If three or fewer MICs per combination are outside the accuracy range, weekly testing may replace daily testing. During weekly testing, a single MIC outside the accuracy range requires that daily testing be performed for 5 consecutive days unless there is an obvious source of error (e.g., contamination, use of an incorrect reference strain, incorrect inoculum density, testing of an incorrect antimicrobial agent, or incorrect atmosphere of incubation). In such a circumstance, only the quality control test needs to be repeated. If all five MICs for a problem drug-organism combination are within the accuracy range, weekly testing may be resumed. If one or more of the five MICs for the problem drug-organism combination are outside the accuracy range, daily testing must be initiated and further means of resolving the problem must be pursued. Returning to weekly testing again requires documentation of 30 consecutive days in which three or fewer MICs are outside the accuracy range. If more than three MICs per combination are outside the accuracy range, daily quality control testing must be continued while the problem is being resolved (40).

DISK DIFFUSION TESTING

The disk diffusion method of susceptibility testing allows categorization of bacterial isolates as susceptible, resistant, or intermediate to a variety of antimicrobial agents. To perform the test, commercially prepared filter paper disks impregnated with a specified amount of an antimicrobial agent are applied to the surface of an agar medium that has been inoculated with the test organism. The drug in the disk diffuses through the agar (3). As the distance from the disk increases, the concentration of the antimicrobial agent decreases logarithmically, creating a gradient of drug concentrations in the agar medium surrounding each disk. Concomitant with diffusion of the drug, the bacteria that were inoculated on the surface and that are not inhibited by the concentration of antimicrobial agent continue to multiply until a lawn of growth is visible. In areas where the concentration of drug is inhibitory, no growth occurs, forming a zone of inhibition around each disk.

The disk diffusion procedure has been standardized primarily for the testing of rapidly growing bacteria (7, 41). This method should not be used to evaluate the antimicrobial susceptibilities of bacteria that show marked strain-to-strain variability in growth rates. The test, however, has been modified to allow reliable testing of certain fastidious bacteria (discussed in chapter 119 of this Manual).

The diameter of the zone of inhibition is influenced by the rate of diffusion of the antimicrobial agent through the agar, which may vary among different drugs. The zone size, however, is inversely proportional to the MIC, measured as discussed earlier in this chapter. Criteria currently recommended for interpreting zone diameters and MIC results for commonly used antimicrobial agents are listed in Table 3 and are published by NCCLS (41, 43).

Establishing Zone of Inhibition Diameter Interpretive Criteria

The first step in determining interpretive criteria for the disk diffusion test is selection of the MIC breakpoints that define resistance and susceptibility categories for each antimicrobial agent. The zone of inhibition diameters that correspond to these breakpoints are initially established by studies that test 300 or more bacterial isolates by both dilution and disk diffusion methods and that correlate the zone of inhibition diameters and MICs of each drug tested (42). The isolates tested should include not only those commonly encountered in clinical laboratories but also those with resistance mechanisms pertinent to the class of antimicrobial agent being tested (11, 42). The organisms evaluated should be those most likely to be tested against the antimicrobial agent in question. The data from these studies are analyzed by preparing a scattergram of values (an example is presented in chapter 115). By convention, each MIC ($\log_2$ scale) is plotted on the y axis, and the corresponding zone of inhibition (arithmetic scale) is plotted on the x axis. Regression analysis can then be performed, and a straight regression line showing the best fit is drawn. From this line, an approximate MIC can be inferred from any zone of inhibition diameter. For antimicrobial agents to which isolates are either susceptible or resistant and only infrequently intermediate, regression analysis is not valid. In such cases, the data are plotted as a scattergram, and the interpretive standards are selected to allow optimal separation of the two populations (38, 42). This approach may also be used to minimize interpretive errors that can ensue from the strict application of the linear regression formula to a data set (38).

Antimicrobial Agent Disks

The amounts of the antimicrobial agents in the disks used for agar diffusion testing are standardized, and in the United States, only a single disk for each drug is recommended (41). The optimal amount of antimicrobial agent per disk is determined early in the development of a new drug by testing disks with several different drug contents; these disks are then evaluated in scattergrams, and regression lines are generated from the data (42). The most desirable amount of drug per disk is that which produces a zone of inhibition diameter of at least 10 mm for resistant isolates and a zone diameter no larger than 30 mm (rarely, 40 mm) for susceptible isolates.

Commercially prepared antimicrobial disks are usually supplied in separate containers, each with a desiccant. They must not be used beyond the specified expiration date and should be stored under refrigeration (2 to 8°C) or frozen in a non-frost-free freezer at −20°C or colder until they are needed. Disks containing a beta-lactam agent should always be stored frozen to ensure that they retain their potency, although a small supply may be stored in the refrigerator for up to 1 week. Unopened disk containers should be removed from the refrigerator or freezer 1 to 2 h before use. This allows the disks to equilibrate to room temperature before the container is opened, thus minimizing the amount of condensation that will occur when warm air comes into contact with the cold disks. A commercially available, mechanical disk-dispensing apparatus can be used, and it should be fitted with a tight cover, supplied with an adequate desiccant, stored in the refrigerator when not in use, and warmed to room temperature before being opened.

Agar Medium

The recommended medium for disk diffusion testing in the United States is Mueller-Hinton agar (41). This unsupplemented medium has been selected by NCCLS for several reasons: (i) it demonstrates good batch-to-batch reproducibility for susceptibility testing; (ii) it is low in sulfonamide, trimethoprim, and tetracycline inhibitors; (iii) it supports the growth of most nonfastidious bacterial pathogens; and (iv) years of data and clinical experience regarding its performance have been accrued. Fastidious bacteria, such as *Haemophilus* species, *Neisseria gonorrhoeae*, and streptococci, do not grow satisfactorily on unsupplemented Mueller-Hinton agar but can be tested by the disk method with supplemented or modified test media, as discussed in chapter 119 of this Manual.

Plates of Mueller-Hinton agar may be purchased, or the agar may be prepared from a commercially available dehydrated base according to the manufacturer's directions. If the agar is prepared, only formulations that have been tested as described by NCCLS and that have met the acceptance limits recommended by NCCLS should be used (39). The prepared medium is autoclaved and is immediately placed in a 45 to 50°C water bath. When cool, it is poured into plastic or glass flat-bottom petri dishes on a level surface to give a uniform depth of about 4 mm (60 to 70 ml of medium for 150-mm plates and 25 to 30 ml for 100-mm plates) and is allowed to cool to room temperature. Agar deeper than 4 mm may cause false resistance (excessively small zones), whereas agar less than 4 mm deep may be associated with excessively large zones and false susceptibility.

Each batch of Mueller-Hinton agar should be checked when the medium is prepared to ensure that the pH is between 7.2 and 7.4 at room temperature, which means that the pH must be measured after the medium has solidified. This can be done by allowing a small amount of agar to solidify around the tip of a pH electrode in a beaker or a cup, by macerating a sufficient amount of agar in neutral distilled water, or by using a properly calibrated surface electrode. A pH outside the range of 7.2 to 7.4 may adversely affect susceptibility test results. If the pH is too low, drugs such as the aminoglycosides and macrolides will appear to lose potency, whereas others (for example, the penicillins) may appear to have excessive activity. The opposite effects are possible if the pH is too high.

Freshly prepared plates may be used on the same day or may be wrapped in plastic to minimize evaporation and stored in a refrigerator (2 to 8°C). Just before use, if excess moisture is visible on the surface, the plates should be placed in an incubator (35°C) or, with the lids ajar, in a laminar-flow hood at room temperature until the moisture evaporates (usually 10 to 30 min). When the medium is inoculated, no droplets of moisture should be visible on its surface or on the petri dish cover.

Various components of or supplements to Mueller-Hinton medium may affect susceptibility test results; therefore, appropriate quality control procedures (see Quality Control below) must be performed and zone diameters must be within acceptable limits. For example, media containing excessive amounts of thymidine or thymine can reverse the inhibitory effects of sulfonamides and trimethoprim, causing zones of growth inhibition to be smaller or less distinct. Organisms may therefore appear to be resistant to these drugs when in fact they are not. Variation in the concentration of divalent cations, primarily calcium and magnesium, affects the results of tests with aminoglycosides, tetracycline, and colistin against *P. aeruginosa* isolates (5, 6). A cation content that is too high reduces zone sizes, whereas a cation content that is too low has the opposite effect. Sheep blood should not be added to Mueller-Hinton medium for the testing of nonfastidious organisms, because the blood can significantly alter the zone diameters for several agents and bacterial species (12).

Inoculation Procedure

To ensure the reproducibility of disk diffusion susceptibility test results, the inoculum must be standardized (7, 19, 41). The inoculum may be prepared by the growth method or directly from colonies on the agar plate, as described above for dilution testing.

When trimethoprim-sulfamethoxazole is tested by the direct inoculum method, colonies from blood agar medium might carry over enough trimethoprim or sulfonamide antagonists to produce a haze of growth inside the zones of inhibition surrounding susceptible isolates.

The Mueller-Hinton agar plate should be inoculated within 15 min after the inoculum suspension has been adjusted. A sterile cotton swab is dipped into the suspension, rotated several times, and pressed lightly on the inside wall of the tube above the fluid level to remove excess inoculum from the swab. The swab is then streaked over the entire surface of the agar plate three times, with the plate rotated approximately 60° each time to ensure an even distribution of the inoculum. A final sweep of the swab is made around the agar rim. The lid may be left ajar for 3 to 5 min but for no longer than 15 min to allow any excess surface moisture to be absorbed before the drug-impregnated disks are applied.

Antimicrobial Disks

Within 15 min after the plates are inoculated, selected antimicrobial agent disks are distributed evenly on the surface, with at least 24 mm (center to center) between them. The disks are placed individually with sterile forceps or with a mechanical dispensing apparatus and are then gently pressed down onto the agar surface to provide uniform contact. No more than 12 disks should be placed on one 150-mm plate and no more than 5 disks should be placed on a 100-mm plate to avoid overlapping zones. Some of the antimicrobial agent in the disk diffuses almost immediately; therefore, once a disk contacts the agar surface, the disk should not be moved.

Incubation

No longer than 15 min after the disks are applied, the plates are inverted and are incubated at 35°C in ambient air. A delay of more than 15 min before incubation permits excess prediffusion of the antimicrobial agents. The interpretive standards for nonfastidious bacteria are based on the results of tests with plates incubated in ambient air, and the zone of inhibition diameters for some drugs, such as the aminoglycosides, macrolides, and tetracyclines, are significantly altered by CO_2; therefore, plates should not be incubated in the presence of increased levels of CO_2. Testing of isolates of some fastidious bacteria, however, requires incubation in 5% CO_2, and zone diameter criteria have been established on that basis (see chapter 119 of this Manual).

Interpretation and Reporting of Results

Each plate is examined after incubation for 16 to 18 h for all nonfastidious bacterial isolates except staphylococci and enterococci, which must be incubated for a full 24 h to allow the detection of resistance to oxacillin and vancomycin (41). If the plates are inoculated correctly, the inhibition zone diameters are uniformly circular and the lawn of growth is confluent. Growth that consists of individual colonies indicates that the inoculum was too light, and the test must be repeated. The diameters of the zones of complete inhibition, including the diameter of the disk, are measured to the nearest whole millimeter with sliding calipers, a ruler, or a template prepared specifically for the purpose of reading disk diffusion plates. With unsupplemented Mueller-Hinton agar, the measuring device is held on the back of the inverted petri dish, which is illuminated with reflected light located a few inches above a black, nonreflecting background.

The zone margin is the area where no obvious growth is visible. When isolates of staphylococci or enterococci are tested, any discernible growth (including pinpoint colonies) within the zone of inhibition around the oxacillin disk (for staphylococci) or vancomycin disk (for enterococci) is indicative of resistance. For other bacteria, discrete colonies growing within a clear zone of inhibition may indicate testing of a mixed culture, colonies of which should be subcultured, reidentified, and retested. However, the presence of colonies within a zone of inhibition may also indicate the selection of high-frequency mutants indicative of eventual resistance to that agent. With *Proteus* species, if a thin film of swarming growth is visible in an otherwise obvious zone of inhibition, the margin of heavy growth is measured and the film is disregarded. With trimethoprim, the sulfonamides, and combinations of the two agents, antagonists in the medium may allow some minimal growth; therefore, the zone diameter is measured at the obvious margin, and slight growth (20% or less of the lawn of growth) is disregarded.

The zone diameters measured around each disk are interpreted on the basis of guidelines published by NCCLS, and the organisms are reported as susceptible, intermediate, or resistant to the antimicrobial agents tested (Table 3) (41, 43). The clinical interpretation of the categories of susceptible, intermediate, and resistant was provided above under Dilution Methods.

Advantages and Disadvantages

The disk diffusion test has several advantages: (i) it is technically simple to perform and very reproducible, (ii) the reagents are relatively inexpensive, (iii) it does not require any special equipment, (iv) it provides category results that are easily understood by clinicians, and (v) it is flexible regarding the selection of antimicrobial agents used for testing. The primary limitation of the disk diffusion test is the spectrum of organisms for which it has been standardized. Currently, studies are not adequate to develop reproducible, definitive standards for the interpretation of test results for bacteria not listed in the NCCLS document regarding disk diffusion, including those that may require different media or atmospheres of incubation for adequate growth or that show delayed or variable growth rates. This includes *Stenotrophomonas maltophilia*, *Corynebacterium* spp., *Bacillus* spp., and several fastidious gram-positive and gram-negative bacteria not covered in chapter 119 of this Manual. A potential disadvantage of disk diffusion susceptibility testing is that it provides a qualitative result, while a quantitative result indicating the degree of susceptibility (MIC) may be desirable in some selected cases. A computer program that allows MICs to be derived from the linear regression equation for some antimicrobial agents and bacterial isolates is commercially available (20). Lastly, the disk diffusion test has had some difficulties in the detection of oxacillin-heteroresistant staphylococci (22, 35, 61) and vancomycin-resistant (low level) enterococci (47, 52).

Quality Control

The goals of a quality control program for disk diffusion tests are to monitor the precision and accuracy of the procedure, the performance of the reagents (medium, disks), and the performance of persons who do the test and read, interpret, and report the results. To best achieve these goals, reference strains are selected for their genetic stability and their usefulness in the disk diffusion test.

Reference Strains

The reference strains recommended for use by NCCLS to control the disk diffusion procedure when nonfastidious bacteria are tested are *E. coli* ATCC 25922, *P. aeruginosa* ATCC 27853, *S. aureus* ATCC 25923 (which is not the same as the strain used for quality control of MIC tests), *E. faecalis* ATCC 29212, and *E. coli* ATCC 35218 (42). *E. coli* ATCC 35218 is recommended only as a control for beta-lactamase inhibitor combinations containing clavulanic acid, sulbactam, or tazobactam. *E. faecalis* ATCC 29212 can be used to ensure that the levels of inhibitors of trimethoprim or sulfonamides in Mueller-Hinton agar do not exceed acceptable limits and can also be used as a control for disks containing a high concentration of gentamicin or streptomycin (see chapter 121 of this Manual).

The reference strains listed above should be obtained from a reliable source, and stock cultures should be maintained in such a way that viability is ensured and the opportunity for the selection of resistant variants is minimal (17). The procedures for maintaining and storing working stock cultures have already been described above under Dilution Methods. If an unexplained result indicates that the inherent susceptibility of the strain has been altered, a fresh culture of that organism should be obtained.

Zone of Inhibition Diameter Ranges

The ranges of zone diameters for reference strains used to monitor the performance of the disk diffusion test are updated frequently and are published annually; therefore, readers should refer to the most recent NCCLS document for this information (43). Generally, the results of 1 in every 20 tests in a series of tests might be out of the accepted limits. If a second result falls outside the stated limits, corrective action must be taken. The action taken and the results of that action must be documented.

Frequency of Testing

Each new batch or lot of Mueller-Hinton agar must be tested with the reference strains listed above before the medium is released for use with clinical specimens, and quality control must be done before a new lot of antimicrobial disks is introduced. Appropriate reference strains also should be tested on each day that the disk diffusion test is performed. The frequency of testing, however, may be reduced if satisfactory performance is documented for 30 consecutive days of testing. For each combination of drug and reference strain, no more than 3 of the 30 zone of inhibition diameters may be outside the accepted limits published by NCCLS (41). When this criterion is fulfilled, each reference strain need be tested only once per week and any time that a reagent component of the test is changed. However, if a zone of inhibition diameter falls outside the acceptable control limits, corrective action must be taken. If the problem appears to be caused by an obvious error such as testing of the wrong disk or the wrong reference strain, contamination of the reference strain, or incubation in the incorrect atmosphere, repeating the test with the appropriate reference strain is acceptable. However, if a cause of the error is not obvious, quality control must be performed daily for a period that will allow discovery of the source of the aberrant result and documentation of how the problem was resolved. This may be accomplished by the same approach described above under the section on quality control for dilution methods.

ANTIBACTERIAL SUSCEPTIBILITY TESTING METHODS THAT MAY BE USED OUTSIDE THE UNITED STATES

By definition, NCCLS develops laboratory testing standards for use in the United States, including standards for antimicrobial susceptibility testing (40, 41). The NCCLS standards are recognized as reference procedures by the U.S. Food and Drug Administration and by federal regulations, including the Clinical Laboratory Improvement Amendments (26). NCCLS procedures are also used by some countries in North and South America and in several other countries and areas of the world. However, some countries have committees comprising their own expert microbiologists who establish methods of susceptibility testing for their own country and interpretive criteria for those tests that may not be the same as those of NCCLS (14).

A large number of variations on dilution and diffusion methods are used for routine susceptibility testing outside the United States (Table 4). Many non-U.S. methods are specific to individual countries, having been developed and evolved locally over many years. Like NCCLS methods, there are dilution and diffusion methods. The majority of non-U.S. methods differ from NCCLS methods in the choice of media, inoculum preparation methods, and, for diffusion methods, disk content. There is also considerable variation between methods in breakpoints and methods for establishing them. Some efforts have been put into harmonizing breakpoints internationally (60) but progress has been slow. This can cause considerable confusion in the laboratory, especially if both NCCLS and non-NCCLS methods are used for different organisms. Thus, it is important to use the breakpoints specified by the methodology, because the tests have been developed and calibrated with those breakpoints. Indeed, the most important message that

TABLE 4 Non-U.S. diffusion methods for susceptibility testing

Method (reference)	Country	Society	Agar medium	Comments
Comparative (13)	United Kingdom	BSAC	Iso-Sensitest preferred	Not calibrated to MICs
Stokes (13)	United Kingdom	BSAC	Iso-Sensitest preferred	Not calibrated to MICs
SFM (49)	France	SFM	Mueller-Hinton	Similar to NCCLS
DIN (23)	Germany	DIN	Mueller-Hinton	
SIR (51)	Sweden	SMS[a]	PDM-ASM	
WRG (58)	Netherland	WRG	Iso-Sensitest	
Neo-sensitabs (16)	Denmark (also popular in Belgium)		Mueller-Hinton	Uses antimicrobial agents incorporated into compressed tablets rather than paper disks. Size of tablets results in zones substantially larger than those from conventional 6-mm disks
Calibrated dichotomous sensitivity (9,10)	Australia		Sensitest	Dichotomous (no intermediate category). Disk strengths chosen to give annular radius of inhibition of ~6 mm where possible

[a] SMS, Swedish Medical Society.

can be given about the use of these methods is that the method should be followed in all its detail. A considerable amount of time has been spent ensuring the validity of these methods, and deviations can lead to error unless such deviations have been shown to be comparable to the original method.

Non-NCCLS Breakpoint Methods

Breakpoint methods are essentially broth or agar MIC methods that use a restricted range of antimicrobial concentrations, often only one or two. They are the standard form of susceptibility testing advocated by the British Society for Antimicrobial Chemotherapy (BSAC) (13) and the Japan Society for Chemotherapy (30, 31). Both of these societies use techniques for setting breakpoints that differ from those outlined in chapter 115. BSAC has developed a formula based on the maximum concentration achievable in blood, the level of protein binding, and the elimination half-life of the drug. The Japanese Society for Chemotherapy uses both a formula and a comparison with favorable outcome in clinical studies in which the MICs for the pathogens have been determined. Breakpoint methods are popular in large laboratories because large numbers of organisms can be tested cost-effectively by using replicators and they provide susceptibility category (i.e., qualitative) endpoints (59). Optical readers are available to facilitate the reading of agar dilution plates (e.g., Repliscan [Mast Laboratories, Muscyorde, United Kingdom]). However, there are considerable difficulties with quality control, including appropriate control strains for which the MICs are near the breakpoints, and the quantification of drug concentrations prior to use (37). In addition, problems with the use of Iso-Sensitest agar (1, 54) and with the incorporation of inhibitors such as *p*-nitrophenylglycerol (55) or increased agar content for the prevention of *Proteus* swarming have been reported (56).

International Diffusion Methods

A wide variety of diffusion methods have been developed in different countries over the years. They are quite diverse in their approaches. Almost all have been maintained to a greater or lesser extent because of the widespread popularity of disk testing in general. None appear to offer any major advantage over the modified Kirby-Bauer system (7) advocated by NCCLS (41). As pointed out above, disk methods are cheap and flexible and will become more accessible with the widespread introduction of zone readers of high quality (e.g., Mast Radius [Mast Laboratories]) which substantially reduce reader error.

BSAC standard diffusion methods and the comparative and Stokes' methods differ from other diffusion methods in that susceptibility categorization is achieved through comparison with the results for a control strain rather than by reference to a defined set of zone diameters (13). This technique has attracted criticism because it is not based upon or derived from correlations with MICs (15). For these methods, Iso-Sensitest agar is the preferred agar, although Diagnostic Sensitivity Test agar is acceptable. Horse blood or lysed horse blood is added for fastidious organisms, while GC agar is recommended for *N. gonorrhoeae*. The inoculum is prepared to produce only semiconfluent growth rather than the confluent growth lawn used in the NCCLS method. The BSAC method is updated at irregular intervals with information on new compounds.

Since 1980 the Société Française de Microbiologie (SFM) has put considerable effort into standardization of susceptibility testing, and regular updates that include breakpoints for new drugs are published annually (49). Like NCCLS, SFM has selected Mueller-Hinton agar as the test medium. For diffusion testing, plates can be inoculated by flooding as well as swabbing. In most other aspects this method resembles that of NCCLS, including the control organisms that are used and the choice of disk strength. They provide zone diameter breakpoints for drugs available in France and elsewhere that are not approved for clinical use in the United States, e.g., fusidic acid and pristinamycin (49).

The German standards organization, the Deutches Institut für Normung (DIN), published acceptable methods for diffusion susceptibility testing as early as 1979, with irregular updates since then (23). They too use Mueller-Hinton medium but will tolerate the use of other media, provided that the MIC-zone diameter relationships have been determined with that medium. Like the SFM method, the DIN method has much in common with the NCCLS method.

The Swedish SIR (51) and the Dutch Werkgroep Richtlijnen Gevoeligheidsbepalingen (WRG) (58) methods use still different media. The SIR system is based on the methodology developed by the original International Collaborative Study (25). That methodology was the first to provide a sound theoretical basis to diffusion susceptibility testing. Their medium of choice is a Swedish product, PDM Antibiotic Sensitivity Medium (PDM-ASM). The breakpoints for susceptibility were restructured and updated in 1981 to the more conventional susceptible, intermediate, and resistant categories (51). The MIC breakpoint correlates selected by the SIR system are frequently two- to eightfold lower than those used by other methods. Iso-Sensitest medium is recommended by the WRG system (58), which in other aspects is similar to the NCCLS, SFM, and DIN techniques. Consequently, inhibition zone diameter breakpoints for some drugs are often different, even though they have the same MIC correlates and disk strengths.

A method developed by a commercial firm in Denmark differs technically if not in principle from the other methods. This method uses so-called Neo-sensitabs, which are compressed 9-mm-diameter tablets into which the antibiotic has been incorporated (16). Not only are the tablets larger and thicker than conventional 6-mm paper disks but they usually contain larger amounts of antibiotic, resulting in significantly larger zones of inhibition with most drugs. This has the disadvantage of reducing the number of tablets that can be put on a single plate and still have readable zones. However, the system does have the advantage that the tablets can be stored at room temperature for up to 4 years, obviating the need for storage under refrigeration or freezing. This is an obvious benefit for laboratories in developing countries where reliable refrigeration and power can be a problem.

A diffusion method developed in Australia in 1975 (9, 10) and still widely used in that country has a number of unique features. The calibrated dichotomous sensitivity method uses Sensitest agar and an unusual method for inoculum preparation and is unique in defining just two categories of susceptibility: susceptible and resistant. In order to simplify reading of test results, each new drug is calibrated against the MIC breakpoint to yield wherever possible an inhibition zone diameter of 18 mm. This is achieved by adjusting disk strengths, which in most cases are substantially lower than those used with other methods. The lack of an intermediate category, which increases the risk of serious misclassification (e.g., susceptible instead of resistant), the absence of some common drugs from the range of drugs included in the test, and some unconventional use of surrogate drugs for testing have restricted the widespread adoption of this method.

COMMON SOURCES OF ERROR IN ANTIBACTERIAL SUSCEPTIBILITY TESTING

Potential sources of error in antibacterial susceptibility testing may be categorized as those that relate to the test system and its components, those associated with the test procedure, those peculiar to certain organism and drug combinations, and those that relate to reporting. The most common sources of error encountered in clinical microbiology laboratories are reviewed in the following paragraphs.

Various components of the susceptibility test system may be a source of error. First, the system itself may have limitations regarding the organisms that should be tested. For example, the disk diffusion method should be used only to test rapidly growing bacterial pathogens that have consistent growth rates (those for which interpretive criteria have been developed by NCCLS). Second, the medium used may be a source of error if it fails to conform to recommended composition and performance. Factors common to both agar-based and broth-based systems are the pH of the medium, which for Mueller-Hinton agar or both should be between 7.2 and 7.4, and its cation content. The concentration of magnesium and calcium in the broth medium should be that recommended by NCCLS to ensure reliable results. For the detection of oxacillin-resistant staphylococci, it is essential that the proper amount of sodium chloride be included in the agar or broth used for dilution testing. For agar dilution and disk diffusion tests, the Mueller-Hinton agar should be 3 to 4 mm deep. Third, the components of the system (antimicrobial disks, agar plates, and trays) must be stored properly, and they should not be used beyond the stated expiration dates.

Steps in the susceptibility test procedure that may be a source of error if they are not performed correctly include inoculum preparation, incubation, endpoint interpretation, and performance of appropriate quality control. The inoculum must be pure, and it must contain an adequate concentration of bacteria. With rare exceptions, all systems should be incubated in ambient air at 35°C. The incubation time, however, varies. For conventional dilution and disk diffusion systems, incubation for 16 to 20 and 16 to 18 h, respectively, is recommended except for tests with staphylococci and oxacillin and vancomycin and with enterococci and vancomycin, which must be incubated for a full 24 h (40, 41). The endpoints of all susceptibility tests must be measured accurately by following the guidelines published by NCCLS (40, 41). If endpoints are interpreted with an instrument, the reliability of that instrument must be monitored. Moreover, with all susceptibility test systems, appropriate reference strains must be tested at regular intervals, and any problems that occur must be thoroughly investigated and corrective action must be well documented.

The testing of some bacteria with certain antimicrobial agents may yield misleading results, because these in vitro results do not necessarily correlate with in vivo activity. Examples include narrow- and expanded-spectrum cephalosporins and aminoglycosides tested against *Salmonella* and *Shigella* spp.; all beta-lactam agents except the penicillinase-resistant penicillins (oxacillin, nafcillin, methicillin) tested against oxacillin-resistant staphylococci; cephalosporins, aminoglycosides (except concentrations used to detect high-level resistance), clindamycin, and trimethoprim-sulfamethoxazole tested against enterococci; and cephalosporins tested against *Listeria* spp. (40, 41). Therefore, for these combinations of organisms and drugs, results should not be reported. Other potential problems associated with reporting are possible transcriptional errors for laboratories that use a manual recording and reporting system and possible errors in the transmission of data for laboratories in which an automated susceptibility test system is interfaced with the laboratory and/or hospital information system.

PROBLEM ORGANISMS AND RESISTANCE MECHANISMS

The dilution and diffusion methods described in this chapter have been developed through careful studies and have been standardized by national professional organizations and diagnostic device manufacturers. Despite this, there are some organisms for which methods have either not yet been standardized (e.g., *Corynebacterium* spp., *Bacillus* spp., *Aeromonas* spp., and *Pasteurella* spp.) or for which reliable results inexplicably fail to be provided by some of the standard tests (e.g., disk diffusion testing of *S. maltophilia*). Certain other organisms may possess resistance mechanisms that are inducible (VanB-type resistance in some enterococci [47], Bush group 1 beta-lactamase in some gram-negative species [36]) or that result in subtle phenotypic expression under standard inoculum and test conditions (oxacillin resistance in some coagulase-negative staphylococci [61], extended-spectrum beta-lactamases in some members of the family *Enterobacteriaceae* [34]). Reliable detection of these subtle resistance traits may require the use of different or modified test methods that are outlined in chapter 121 of this Manual. There is no clear consensus regarding what level of accuracy is acceptable when selecting a method or system for performing antimicrobial susceptibility testing (32). Moreover, it is important to keep in mind that new resistance mechanisms or decreases in susceptibility to important therapeutic agents can arise at any time to challenge our methods of susceptibility testing, e.g., vancomycin-intermediate *S. aureus* (27).

REFERENCES

1. **Andrews, J. M., J. P. Ashby, and R. Wise.** 1990. Problems with Iso-Sensitest agar. *J. Antimicrob. Chemother.* **26:** 596–597.
2. **Baker, C. N., S. A. Stocker, D. H. Culver, and C. Thornsberry.** 1991. Comparison of the E test to agar dilution, broth microdilution, and agar diffusion susceptibility testing techniques by using a special challenge set of bacteria. *J. Clin. Microbiol.* **29:**533–538.
3. **Barry, A. L.** 1991. Procedures and theoretical considerations for testing antimicrobial agents in agar media, p. 1–16. *In* V. Lorian (ed.), *Antibiotics in Laboratory Medicine*, 3rd ed. The Williams & Wilkins Co., Baltimore, Md.
4. **Barry, A. L., R. E. Badal, and R. W. Hawkinson.** 1983. Influence of inoculum growth phase on microdilution susceptibility tests. *J. Clin. Microbiol.* **18:**645–651.
5. **Barry, A. L., G. H. Miller, C. Thornsberry, R. S. Hare, R. N. Jones, R. R. Lorber, R. Ferraresi, and C. Cramer.** 1987. Influence of cation supplements on activity of netilmicin against *Pseudomonas aeruginosa* in vitro and in vivo. *Antimicrob. Agents Chemother.* **31:**1514–1518.
6. **Barry, A. L., L. B. Reller, G. H. Miller, J. A. Washington, F. D. Schoenknecht, L. R. Peterson, R. S. Hare, and C. Knapp.** 1992. Revision of standards for adjusting the cation content of Mueller-Hinton broth for testing susceptibility of *Pseudomonas aeruginosa* to aminoglycosides. *J. Clin. Microbiol.* **30:**585–589.
7. **Bauer, A. W., W. M. M. Kirby, J. C. Sherris, and M. Turck.** 1966. Antibiotic susceptibility testing by standardized single disk method. *Am. J. Clin. Pathol.* **45:**493–496.
8. **Bauer, A. W., and J. C. Sherris.** 1964. The determination of sulfonamide susceptibility of bacteria. *Chemotherapia* **9:** 1–19.
9. **Bell, S. M.** 1975. The CDS method of antibiotic sensitivity testing (calibrated dichotomous sensitivity test). *Pathology* **7**(Suppl.)**:**1–48.
10. **Bell, S. M.** 1988. Additions and modifications to the range of antibiotics tested by the CDS method of antibiotic sensitivity testing. *Pathology* **20:**303–304.
11. **Bradford, P. A., and C. C. Sanders.** 1992. Use of a predictor panel for development of a new disk for diffusion tests with cefoperazone-sulbactam. *Antimicrob. Agents Chemother.* **36:**394–400.
12. **Brenner, V. C., and J. C. Sherris.** 1972. Influence of different media and bloods on the results of diffusion antibiotic susceptibility tests. *Antimicrob. Agents Chemother.* **1:** 116–122.
13. **British Society for Antimicrobial Chemotherapy.** 1991. Report of the working party on antibiotic sensitivity testing of the British Society for Antimicrobial Chemotherapy: a guide to sensitivity testing. *J. Antimicrob. Chemother.* **27**(Suppl. D)**:**1–50.
14. **Brown, D. F. J.** 1994. Developments in antimicrobial susceptibility testing. *Rev. Med. Microbiol.* **5:**65–75.
15. **Brown, D. J. F.** 1990. The comparative method for antimicrobial susceptibility testing—time for a change? *J. Antimicrob. Chemother.* **25:**307–312.
16. **Casals, J. B., and N. Pringler.** 1991. *Antibacterial/Antifungal Sensitivity Testing Using Neo-sensitabs®*, 9th ed. Rosco Diagnostica, Taarstrup, Denmark.
17. **Coyle, M. B., M. F. Lampe, C. L. Aitkin, P. Feigl, and J. C. Sherris.** 1976. Reproducibility of control strains for antibiotic susceptibility testing. *Antimicrob. Agents Chemother.* **10:**436–440.
18. **Craig, W. A.** 1993. Qualitative susceptibility tests versus quantitative MIC tests. *Diagn. Microbiol. Infect. Dis.* **16:** 231–236.
19. **D'Amato, R. F., and L. Hochstein.** 1982. Evaluation of a rapid inoculum preparation method for agar disk diffusion susceptibility testing. *J. Clin. Microbiol.* **15:**282–285.
20. **D'Amato R. F., L. Hochstein, J. R. Vernaleo, and C. Thornsberry.** 1985. Evaluation of BIOMIC antimicrobial test system. *J. Clin. Microbiol.* **22:**793–798.
21. **D'Amato, R. F., C. Thornsberry, C. N. Baker, and L. A. Kirven.** 1975. Effect of calcium and magnesium ions on the susceptibility of *Pseudomonas* species to tetracycline, gentamicin, polymyxin B, and carbenicillin. *Antimicrob. Agents Chemother.* **7:**596–600.
22. **De Lencastre, H., A. M. Sa Figueiredo, C. Urban, J. Rahal, and A. Tomasz.** 1991. Multiple mechanisms of methicillin resistance and improved methods for detection in clinical isolates of *Staphylococcus aureus*. *Antimicrob. Agents Chemother.* **35:**632–639.
23. **Deutches Institut für Normung.** 1984. *Methoden zur Empfindlichkeitsprüfung von Bakteriallen Krankheitserregern (außer Mykobakterien) gegen Chemotherapeutika.* DIN 58940. Beuth Verlag GmbH, Berlin, Germany.
24. **Doern, G. V.** 1987. Breakpoint susceptibility testing. *Clin. Microbiol. Newsl.* **9:**81–84.
25. **Ericsson, J. M., and J. C. Sherris.** 1971. Antibiotic sensitivity testing. Report of an international collaborative study. *Acta Pathol. Microbiol. Scand. Sect. B Suppl.* **217:** 1–90.
26. **Health Care Financing Administration.** 1992. Clinical Laboratory Improvement Amendments of 1988; final rule. *Fed. Regist.* **57:**7137–7186.
27. **Hiramatsu, K., H. Hanaki, T. Ino, K. Yabuta, T. Oguri, and F. C. Tenover.** 1997. Methicillin-resistant *Staphylococcus aureus* clinical strain with reduced vancomycin susceptibility. *J. Antimicrob. Chemother.* **40:**135–146.
28. **Huang, M., P. N. Baker, S. Banerjee, and F. C. Tenover.** 1992. Accuracy of the E test for determining antimicrobial susceptibilities of staphylococci, enterococci, *Campylobacter jejuni*, and gram-negative bacteria resistant to antimicrobial agents. *J. Clin. Microbiol.* **30:**3243–3248.
29. **Huang, M. B., E. T. Gay, C. N. Baker, S. N. Banerjee, and F. C. Tenover.** 1993. Two percent sodium chloride is required for susceptibility testing of staphylococci with oxacillin when using agar-based dilution methods. *J. Clin. Microbiol.* **31:**2683–2688.
30. **Japan Society for Chemotherapy.** 1990. Report of the Committee for Japanese Standards for Antimicrobial Susceptibility Testing for Bacteria. *Chemotherapy (Tokyo)* **38:** 102–105. (In Japanese.)
31. **Japan Society for Chemotherapy.** 1993. Report of the Committee for Japanese Standards for Antimicrobial Sus-

ceptibility Testing for Bacteria. *Chemotherapy (Tokyo)* **41:** 183–189. (in Japanese.)

32. **Jorgensen, J. H.** 1993. Selection criteria for an antimicrobial susceptibility testing system. *J. Clin. Microbiol.* **31:** 2841–2844.
33. **Jorgensen, J. H.** 1993. Selection of antimicrobial agents for routine testing in a clinical microbiology laboratory. *Diagn. Microbiol. Infect. Dis.* **16:**245–249.
34. **Katsanis, G., J. Spargo, M. J. Ferraro, L. Sutton, and G. A. Jacoby.** 1994. Detection of *Klebsiella pneumoniae* and *Escherichia coli* strains producing extended-spectrum *β*-lactamases. *J. Clin. Microbiol.* **32:**691–696.
35. **Knapp, C. C., M. D. Ludwig, and J. A. Washington.** 1994. Evaluation of differential inoculum disk diffusion method and Vitek GPS-SA card for detection of oxacillin-resistant staphylococci. *J. Clin. Microbiol.* **32:**433–436.
36. **Knapp, C. C., and J. A. Washington.** 1992. Comparison of the E test and microdilution for detection of *β*-lactam-resistant mutants that are stably derepressed for type I *β*-lactamase. *J. Clin. Microbiol.* **30:**214–215.
37. **McDermott, S. N., and T. F. Hartley.** 1989. New datum handling methods for the quality control of antimicrobial solutions and plates used in the antimicrobial susceptibility test. *J. Clin. Microbiol.* **27:**1814–1825.
38. **Metzler, C., and R. M. DeHaan.** 1974. Susceptibility tests of anaerobic bacteria: statistical and clinical considerations. *J. Infect. Dis.* **130:**588–594.
39. **National Committee for Clinical Laboratory Standards.** 1996. *Evaluating Production Lots of Dehydrated Mueller-Hinton Agar.* Approved standard M6-A. National Committee for Clinical Laboratory Standards, Wayne, Pa.
40. **National Committee for Clinical Laboratory Standards.** 1997. *Methods for Dilution Antimicrobial Susceptibility Tests for Bacteria That Grow Aerobically.* Approved standard M7-A4. National Committee for Clinical Laboratory Standards, Wayne, Pa.
41. **National Committee for Clinical Laboratory Standards.** 1997. *Performance Standards for Antimicrobial Disk Susceptibility Tests.* Approved standard M2-A6. National Committee for Clinical Laboratory Standards, Wayne, Pa.
42. **National Committee for Clinical Laboratory Standards.** 1998. *Development of In Vitro Susceptibility Testing Criteria and Quality Control Parameters.* NCCLS document M23-T2. National Committee for Clinical Laboratory Standards, Wayne, Pa.
43. **National Committee for Clinical Laboratory Standards.** 1999. *Performance Standards for Antimicrobial Susceptibility Testing.* Supplement M100-S9. National Committee for Clinical Laboratory Standards, Wayne, Pa.
44. **Pestotnik, S. L., R. S. Evans, J. P. Burke, and R. M. Gardner.** 1990. Therapeutic antibiotic monitoring: surveillance using a computerized expert system. *Am. J. Med.* **99:**43–48.
45. **Reller, L. B., F. D. Schoenknecht, and M. A. Kenny.** 1974. Antibiotic susceptibility testing of *P. aeruginosa*: selection of a control strain and criteria for magnesium and calcium content in media. *J. Infect. Dis.* **130:**454–463.
46. **Sahm, D. F., C. N. Baker, R. N. Jones, and C. Thornsberry.** 1984. Influence of growth medium on the in vitro activities of second- and third-generation cephalosporins against *Streptococcus faecalis*. *J. Clin. Microbiol.* **20:** 561–567.
47. **Sahm, D. F., J. Kissinger, M. S. Gilmore, P. R. Murray, R. Mulder, J. Solliday, and B. Clarke.** 1989. In vitro susceptibility studies of vancomycin-resistant *Enterococcus faecalis*. *Antimicrob. Agents Chemother.* **33:**1588–1591.
48. **Schulz, J. E., and D. F. Sahm.** 1993. Reliability of the E test for detection of ampicillin, vancomycin, and high-level aminoglycoside resistance in *Enterococcus* spp. *J. Clin. Microbiol.* **31:**3336–3339.
49. **Société Française de Microbiologie.** 1996. Report of the Comité de l'Antibiogramme de la Société Française de Microbiologie. 1996. *Clin. Microboil. Infect. Dis.* **2**(Suppl. 1): S1–S49.
50. **Steers, E., E. L. Foltz, and B. S. Graves.** 1959. An inocula replicating apparatus for routine testing of bacterial susceptibility to antibiotics. *Antibiot. Chemother.* **9:**307–311.
51. **The Swedish Reference Group for Antibiotics.** 1981. A revised system for antibiotic sensitivity testing. *Scand. J. Infect. Dis.* **13:**148–152.
52. **Tenover, F. C., J. M. Swenson, C. M. O'Hara, and S. A. Stocker.** 1995. Ability of commercial and reference antimicrobial susceptibility testing methods to detect vancomycin resistance in enterococci. *J. Clin. Microbiol.* **33:** 1524–1527.
53. **Thornsberry, C., and L. K. McDougal.** 1983. Successful use of broth microdilution in susceptibility tests for methicillin-resistant (heteroresistant) staphylococci. *J. Clin. Microbiol.* **18:**1084–1091.
54. **Toohey, M., G. Francis, and N. Stingemore.** 1990. Variation in Iso-Sensitest agar affecting *β*-lactam testing. *Newsl. Antimicrob. Special Interest Group Aust. Soc. Microbiol.* **1**(6)**:**6–8.
55. **Ward, P. B., S. Palladino, J. C. Looker, and P. Feddema.** 1993. *p*-Nitrophenylglycerol in susceptibility testing media alters the MICs of antimicrobials for *Pseudomonas aeruginosa*. *J. Antimicrob. Chemother.* **31:**489–496.
56. **Ward, P. B., S. Palladino, B. McLaren, R. J. Rathur, and J. C. Looker.** 1993. The effect of increased agar concentration in susceptibility testing media on MICs of antimicrobials for gram-negative bacilli. *J. Antimicrob. Chemother.* **31:** 1005–1007.
57. **Washington, J. A., II, R. J. Synder, P. C. Kohner, C. G. Wiltsle, D. M. Ilstrup, and J. T. McCall.** 1978. Effect of cation content of agar on the activity of gentamicin, tobramycin, and amikacin against *Pseudomonas aeruginosa*. *J. Infect. Dis.* **137:**103–111.
58. **Werkgroep Richtlijnen Gevoeligheidsbepalingen.** 1981. *Standaardisatie van Gevoeligheidsbepalingen.* Werkgroep Richtlijnen Gevoeligheidsbepalingen, Bilthoven, The Netherlands.
59. **Wheat, P. F.** 1989. The agar-dilution susceptibility technique: past and present. *Clin. Microbiol. Newsl.* **11:** 164–166.
60. **Williams, J. D.** 1990. Prospects for standardisation of methods and guidelines for disc susceptibility testing. *Eur. J. Clin. Microbiol. Infect. Dis.* **9:**496–501.
61. **York, M. K., L. Gibbs, F. Chehab, and G. F. Brooks.** 1996. Comparison of PCR detection of *mecA* with standard susceptibility testing methods to determine methicillin resistance in coagulase-negative staphylococci. *J. Clin. Microbiol.* **34:**249–253.

Susceptibility Testing of Fastidious Bacteria*

JANET A. HINDLER AND JANA M. SWENSON

119

Most fastidious bacteria do not grow satisfactorily in standard in vitro susceptibility test systems that use unsupplemented media. For certain fastidious species that are more frequently encountered, such as *Haemophilus influenzae*, *Neisseria gonorrhoeae*, *Streptococcus pneumoniae*, and other *Streptococcus* spp., slight modifications have been made to standard National Committee for Clinical Laboratory Standards (NCCLS) disk diffusion and MIC methods to allow reliable testing of these bacteria. The modifications generally involve the use of a test medium with added nutrients and sometimes extended incubation times and/or incubation in an atmosphere with increased levels of CO_2 (Tables 1 and 2). Specific zone diameter and MIC interpretive criteria have been developed by NCCLS for these bacteria, as have acceptable ranges for recommended quality control (QC) strains.

Although susceptibility test methods for *Moraxella* (Branhamella) *catarrhalis*, *Neisseria meningitidis*, and *Listeria monocytogenes* have not been standardized, testing of these is mentioned in NCCLS documents (75–77). However, there are no specific recommendations for "other" fastidious bacteria (OFB), such as *Actinobacillus actinomycetemcomitans*, *Corynebacterium jeikeium*, and *Eikenella corrodens*. This is because in part (i) infections caused by these bacteria usually respond to drugs of choice, (ii) isolates are infrequently encountered, and (iii) isolates are often difficult to grow or are slow to grow.

In addition to conventional MIC test methods (e.g., agar dilution or broth dilution methods), the Etest MIC determination method has been used to test many types of fastidious bacteria. The Etest approach allows placement of strips on specialized media and the use of various incubation conditions. The limitations of this method include its cost and lack of clearance by the U.S. Food and Drug Administration (FDA) for the testing of many less commonly encountered fastidious bacteria. Prior to using the Etest for clinical testing in the United States, the FDA clearance status for the particular organism-antimicrobial agent combination should be known. If FDA clearance has not been granted, the results should be interpreted with caution and should be qualified on the patient report.

This chapter summarizes the standard methods recommended by NCCLS for the antimicrobial susceptibility testing of *S. pneumoniae*, *Streptococcus* spp., *Haemophilus* spp., and *N. gonorrhoeae*. An approach for *M. catarrhalis*, *N. meningitidis*, and *L. monocytogenes* is presented. The drugs of choice for therapy, the incidence and mechanisms of resistance, test methods, and indications for testing and the reporting of results are discussed. Finally, this chapter presents strategies that could be used in the clinical laboratory when requests are made for the testing of a fastidious bacterium for which no standardized susceptibility test method is available.

S. PNEUMONIAE

Drugs of Choice for Therapy

Because of the frequent occurrence of intermediate or high-level penicillin resistance in pneumococci (see below), recommendations for therapy depend on the infection site. For example, for suspected meningitis, empiric therapy recommendations include a combination of agents, usually vancomycin and an extended-spectrum cephalosporin with or without rifampin (68, 85). However, pneumococcal isolates from cerebrospinal fluid must be tested to determine the levels of susceptibility to both penicillin and cefotaxime or ceftriaxone (77). Infections outside of the central nervous system due to strains with intermediate penicillin resistance may be treatable with penicillin (40). Alternative agents for the treatment of pneumococcal infections include trimethoprim-sulfamethoxazole (TMP-SMX), clindamycin, chloramphenicol, a tetracycline, a fluoroquinolone, and possibly, quinupristin-dalfopristin (10, 68, 85).

Incidence and Mechanisms of Resistance

Penicillin resistance is defined as an MIC of $\geq$0.12 μg/ml, with strains for which MICs are 0.12 to 1.0 μg/ml being designated intermediately resistant and strains for which MICs are $\geq$2 μg/ml being designated resistant. Since it was first reported in 1967, the incidence of penicillin resistance among pneumococci has been steadily increasing worldwide (4). The incidence of resistance in some parts of the world is approaching 50% (8). Rates are especially high in Spain and some areas of Asia (8). In the United States a recent

* This chapter contains information presented in chapter 114 by Gary V. Doern in the sixth edition of this Manual.

TABLE 1 Disk diffusion testing conditions and recommended QC strains for testing of *Haemophilus* spp., *N. gonorrhoeae*, *S. pneumoniae*, and *Streptococcus* spp.

Organism	Agar[a]	Inoculum[b]	Incubation length (h)	Incubation conditions	Recommended QC strain(s)
Haemophilus spp.	HTM	20–24 h growth (from CHOC)	16–18	35°C; 5–7% CO_2	*H. influenzae* ATCC 49247, *H. influenzae* ATCC 49766[c]
N. gonorrhoeae	GC agar base + supplement	20–24 h growth (from CHOC)	20–24	35°C; 5–7% CO_2	*N. gonorrhoeae* ATCC 49226
S. pneumoniae and *Streptococcus* spp.	MHA + 5% sheep blood	16–18 h growth (from SBA)	20–24	35°C; 5–7% CO_2	*S. pneumoniae* ATCC 49619

[a] HTM and GC agar base are defined in the text.

[b] Suspension is in Mueller-Hinton broth or 0.9% NaCl standardized to a 0.5 McFarland standard; CHOC, chocolate agar; SBA, sheep blood agar.

[c] In addition, *H. influenzae* ATCC 10211 can be used to assess the growth-supporting capabilities of HTM. *H. influenzae* ATCC 49766 is used for quality control of select cephalosporins (e.g., cefaclor, cefamandole, and cefuroxime).

survey reported a penicillin resistance rate of 14.1% among 740 isolates from 12 different states during 1993 and 1994 (18); a 1995 survey of 24 medical centers reported a resistance rate of 27.2% (97). The mechanism of penicillin resistance is due to modification of penicillin-binding proteins (PBPs) (61). Strains of pneumococci that are susceptible to penicillin are also susceptible to other β-lactam agents (5, 52); however, as the penicillin MIC increases, the MICs of other β-lactam agents also increase (52). Penicillin-resistant strains are also likely to be resistant to one or more non-β-lactam agents (29, 61).

Resistance to cefotaxime or ceftriaxone was not reported prior to 1992. NCCLS first published specific MIC breakpoints for these agents in 1993 (73), and they were modified in 1994 to the following current breakpoints: susceptible, $\leq$0.5 μg/ml; intermediate, 1.0 μg/ml; and resistant, $\geq$2 μg/ml (54, 77). In the latest survey by the Centers for Disease Control and Prevention (18), the incidence of strains for which cefotaxime MICs are $\geq$1.0 μg/ml was 4.1%, but in areas where the rate of high-level penicillin resistance is significant, the rate of resistance to cefotaxime or ceftriaxone might also be high (48).

Resistance has been described for all classes of antimicrobial agents that might be considered for use in the treatment of pneumococcal infections except for the glycopeptides (29, 41, 52). With the exception of TMP-SMX, the rates of resistance to other agents are usually <10% (18, 29, 48), but for TMP-SMX, they can be as high as 25% (48). Newer quinolones show some promise of activity, even against pneumococci that are resistant to ciprofloxacin and older quinolones (62, 93). The mechanisms of resistance to other agents are described elsewhere (61) (see also chapter 117 of this Manual).

Reference Test Methods

NCCLS describes both a broth microdilution method and a disk diffusion method for the testing of pneumococci (75–77), and details of these procedures are given in Tables 1 and 2. The broth microdilution method may be used to test the antimicrobial agents recommended by NCCLS for testing by this method. However, this is not true for the disk diffusion method, which does not work for the testing of β-lactam agents. It does, however, work well for the testing of non-β-lactams. The one exception to this is the oxacillin disk screen, which many laboratories use to predict penicillin susceptibility (76, 77, 94). Oxacillin disk diffusion zone diameters of $\geq$20 mm indicate that the isolate is susceptible to penicillin, as well as other β-lactam agents (77). Conversely, strains with zone diameters of $\leq$19 mm cannot be readily categorized as resistant, since a strain with an oxacillin zone diameter of $\leq$19 mm may be penicillin susceptible, intermediate, or resistant (30) when the MIC for

TABLE 2 MIC testing conditions and recommended QC strains for testing of *Haemophilus* spp., *N. gonorrhoeae*, *S. pneumoniae*, and *Streptococcus* spp.

Organism	Medium[a]	Inoculum[b]	Final concn (CFU)	Incubation length (h)	Incubation conditions	Recommended QC strain(s)
Haemophilus spp.	HTM broth	20–24 h growth (from CHOC)	5×10^5/ml	20–24	35°C; ambient air	*H. influenzae* ATCC 49247 and *H. influenzae* ATCC 49766[c]
N. gonorrhoeae	GC agar base + supplement	20–24 h growth (from CHOC)	1×10^4/spot	20–24	35°C; 5–7% CO_2	*N. gonorrhoeae* ATCC 49226
S. pneumoniae and *Streptococcus* spp.	CAMHB-LHB	16–18 h growth (from SBA)	5×10^5/ml	20–24	35°C; ambient air	*S. pneumoniae* ATCC 49619

[a] HTM broth, GC agar base, and CAMHB-LHB are defined in the text.

[b] Suspension is in Mueller-Hinton broth or 0.9% NaCl; CHOC, chocolate agar; SBA, sheep blood agar.

[c] In addition, *H. influenzae* ATCC 10211 can be used to assess the growth-supporting capabilities of HTM. *H. influenzae* ATCC 49766 is used for quality control of select cephalosporins (e.g., cefaclor, cefamandole, and cefuroxime).

the strain is determined. Most strains for which penicillin MICs are 0.06 μg/ml (indicating susceptibility) give zones of ≤19 mm (30). When the oxacillin screen test was initially described, the incidence of strains for which penicillin MICs were close to the breakpoint for penicillin susceptibility was quite low and there were fewer miscategorizations (30). The original intention of the test was to use it to screen for potential resistance and then to perform an MIC test to determine the level of resistance (i.e., intermediate or high level), a step which many laboratories do not do. However, if the oxacillin screen test is used without backup MIC testing, the potential for inappropriate treatment is possible, especially in areas where penicillin resistance is beginning to emerge, and there is a greater likelihood that the MIC will be in the intermediate range. NCCLS now recommends that, especially for life-threatening infections, the oxacillin screening procedure should not be used and that the MICs of penicillin and an extended-spectrum cephalosporin should be determined (77). Both penicillin and cefotaxime or ceftriaxone MICs should be available without the 24-h delay that a screening test would necessitate.

Along with penicillin, NCCLS recommends primary testing of both erythromycin and TMP-SMX for non-central nervous system infections. Testing of erythromycin can be done by either the MIC test or the disk diffusion method; however, there are problems with TMP-SMX testing by the disk diffusion method with pneumococcal quality control strain *S. pneumoniae* ATCC 49619 and some lots of media (42); these problems are being investigated by NCCLS. When the disk diffusion parameters for TMP-SMX were originally described, the minor error rate of 10.5% was higher than is normally accepted and the investigators chose not to recommend testing of TMP-SMX by the disk diffusion method (60). However, the errors involved the overprediction of resistance by the disk diffusion method (i.e., categorization of strains that are intermediate according to the MIC as resistant by the disk diffusion method) (60). Because of this, as well as the high incidence of TMP-SMX resistance and the lack of readily available methods for the testing of TMP-SMX, NCCLS recommended adoption of the disk diffusion breakpoints (72). The Etest for TMP-SMX and *S. pneumoniae* has not yet received clearance by FDA.

Commercial Methods for Testing

Several options are available for testing of the MICs for pneumococci. Probably the most widely used and evaluated option is the Etest (AB Biodisk, Solna, Sweden) (53, 58, 59, 64, 66, 78, 88, 96), although not all drugs recommended for testing have been cleared by FDA for testing by the Etest. The accuracy of the Etest has been reported to be >90% for most relevant drugs; however, the number of minor errors with penicillin is relatively high. This is because the Etest tends to give MICs that are slightly lower than those determined by the reference broth microdilution procedure (53, 58, 59). Since the Etest is incubated in CO_2, the MICs of the macrolides will tend to be 1 to 2 dilutions higher than those by the broth tests, which are incubated in ambient air. This is because macrolides are less active at lower pH, which occurs with CO_2 incubation.

Other commercially available methods have been studied less extensively. Some of these systems were evaluated in 1996 by Tenover et al. (96) and were found to be inadequate. Currently, the FDA-cleared panels specifically designed for the testing of pneumococci include Pasco (Difco, Wheatridge, Colo.), MicroScan (Dade MicroScan Inc., West Sacramento, Calif.) (57), MicroTech (Aurora, Colo.), and Sensititre (AcuMed, Westlake, Ohio). The Vitek system (BioMerieux-Vitek, Hazelwood, Mo.) cannot be used to test pneumococci.

Testing Strategy and Reporting of Results

All invasive isolates of *S. pneumoniae*, including strains from both cerebrospinal fluid and blood, should be tested by an MIC method for their susceptibilities to penicillin and extended-spectrum cephalosporins. With the exception of meropenem, other drugs that might warrant testing could be tested by the disk diffusion method or by an MIC test (e.g., vancomycin, rifampin, and chloramphenicol). For pneumococcal strains from infections of the central nervous system that are found to be intermediately resistant (MICs, 0.12 to 1.0 μg/ml) or highly resistant (MICs, ≥2.0 μg/ml) to penicillin, the strains should be reported as resistant. Non-central nervous system infections, such as pneumonia, caused by strains for which penicillin MICs are in the intermediate range may be treatable with penicillin or an extended-spectrum cephalosporin if maximal doses are used (40, 61). Cefepime, a newer extended-spectrum cephalosporin, is sometimes used for the treatment of serious pneumococcal infections and may also warrant testing.

The oxacillin screening procedure should be used only for isolates from patients with non-life-threatening infections, and if the zone diameter is ≤19 mm, the MICs of penicillin and possibly an extended-spectrum cephalosporin should then be determined. Disk diffusion testing cannot be used to determine accurately the susceptibility to extended-spectrum cephalosporins. In fact, there are no disk diffusion breakpoints for any cephalosporin approved by NCCLS for the testing of pneumococci (77).

STREPTOCOCCI OTHER THAN PNEUMOCOCCI

Drugs of Choice for Therapy

Penicillin is generally considered the drug of choice for the treatment of non-pneumococcal streptococcal disease, with alternative drugs used depending on the site of infection and the specific streptococcal species involved (10, 68, 85). Other agents for therapy include a cephalosporin, vancomycin, clindamycin, chloramphenicol, a macrolide, and possibly, a quinolone.

Incidence and Mechanisms of Resistance

Penicillin resistance in streptococci other than pneumococci is defined as follows: susceptible, MIC of ≤0.12 μg/ml; intermediate, MIC of 0.25 to 2 μg/ml; and resistant, MIC of ≥4 μg/ml (77). Beta-hemolytic streptococci currently remain penicillin susceptible, although the penicillin MICs for group B streptococci tend to be slightly higher than those for other beta-hemolytic streptococci (7). Two recent reports, however, have described penicillin MICs of 0.25 to 0.5 μg/ml for group B streptococci (11, 98) and group C streptococci (98). The clinical significance of this increased MIC is not known. Penicillin resistance has been described in viridans group streptococci since the 1970s (6, 17), although the incidence has probably increased since then (32). Penicillin resistance rates of greater than 50% for viridans group streptococci are not uncommon (2, 32), especially in *Streptococcus mitis* and *Streptococcus sanguis*. The mechanism of penicillin resistance in viridans group streptococci is similar to that in pneumococci (i.e., altered PBPs), and as with pneumococci, the level of resistance to other β-lactam agents increases as the level of penicillin resistance increases (2).

Resistance to all other classes of antimicrobial agents has been described execpt the glycopeptides for both beta-hemolytic and viridans group streptococci. The incidence of resistance to most drugs is low; however, resistance to erythromycin in group A streptococcus is highly variable and is dependent on the degree of erythromycin usage in the community. In Finland, for example, a rate as high as 54% in one city was noted in 1990 (87). High-level aminoglycoside resistance has been described in group B and viridans group streptococci (19, 36, 49), the two species for which treatment is likely to include gentamicin or streptomycin.

Reference Test Methods

Recent studies by NCCLS to determine interpretive criteria for both MIC and disk diffusion testing have resulted in breakpoints that were published in 1995 (74). Details for MIC and disk diffusion tests are described in Tables 1 and 2. The disk diffusion test may be used to determine the penicillin susceptibility of beta-hemolytic streptococci; however, the high number of minor errors with penicillin when testing viridans group streptococci precludes testing by the disk diffusion method for that group. Other agents may be tested by either the MIC or the disk method. The oxacillin disk screen test cannot be used to detect penicillin resistance in viridans group streptococci. Aminoglycoside MICs of >1,000 μg/ml for streptococci (102) have been described; however, there are no published methods for screening for high-level aminoglycoside resistance in streptococci.

Susceptibility testing of nutritionally deficient streptococci has been done by adding 0.001% pyridoxal HCl to the test medium. Although penicillin resistance has been described in this group of organisms (83), the results of susceptibility testing may not correlate with treatment outcome (90).

Commercial Test Methods

There have been very few reports of evaluations of commercial susceptibility test systems for streptococci other than pneumococci, although it might be expected that systems capable of testing pneumococci would also perform adequately for other streptococci. MicroScan has a panel that was recently cleared for the testing of these organisms as well as *S. pneumoniae*. There has been only one report of an evaluation of the Etest for the testing of viridans group streptococci (46).

Testing Strategy and Reporting of Results

There is no reason for the routine testing of beta-hemolytic streptococci since only sporadic reports of penicillin resistance have been described (11, 98). However, if erythromycin is being used to treat infections caused by group A streptococci and treatment failure is suspected, testing might be considered. For viridans group streptococci, penicillin resistance is a serious concern; thus, MICs should be determined for strains isolated from blood, especially for patients with infective endocarditis. The disk diffusion test is not reliable for the testing of penicillin because it cannot determine the precise levels of penicillin resistance which are needed to guide treatment (102).

H. INFLUENZAE

Drugs of Choice for Therapy

The primary agents recommended for the treatment of localized respiratory infections caused by *H. influenzae* include ampicillin (or amoxicillin) or TMP-SMX. TMP-SMX or a β-lactamase-stable agent such as amoxicillin-clavulanic acid, a cephalosporin (e.g., cefuroxime), a tetracycline, or a quinolone can be used if a β-lactamase-producing isolate is suspected of being the cause of infection. For systemic *H. influenzae* infections, an extended-spectrum cephalosporin is generally prescribed (10, 68, 85).

Incidence and Mechanisms of Resistance

β-Lactamase-producing *H. influenzae* was first reported in the early 1970s, and the incidence of isolates with this plasmid-mediated TEM-1-type ampicillin resistance continues to increase worldwide (31, 44, 56). An uncommon mechanism for ampicillin resistance is due to a second type of β-lactamase known as ROB-1 (24). Doern et al. (31) reported that among more than 1,500 isolates collected during 1994 and 1995 from 30 U.S. medical centers, 36.4% were β-lactamase producers; Jones et al. (56) noted similar results. Previous studies demonstrated that β-lactamase production was considerably greater in type b isolates than in non-type b isolates (approximately 32 to 34% versus 16 to 22%) (33, 82). The increasing incidence of β-lactamase-producing strains occurs despite the fact that infections caused by type b strains have been virtually eliminated in the United States since the introduction of the *H. influenzae* type b vaccine.

Ampicillin resistance occasionally results from altered PBPs in β-lactamase-negative, ampicillin-resistant (BLNAR) isolates. The incidences of BLNAR isolates noted in the studies by Doern et al. (31) and Jones et al. (56) were 2.5 and 0.2%, respectively. In contrast to β-lactamase-producing isolates, BLNAR isolates are less susceptible to amoxicillin-clavulanic acid and to various cephalosporins such as cefaclor, cefuroxime, cefixime, and cefotaxime (9). Resistance among *H. influenzae* isolates to broad-spectrum cephalosporins (e.g., cefixime and cefpodoxime) is rare, and the overall rate of resistance to expanded-spectrum cephalosporins (e.g., cefuroxime) is 5 to 6%. The narrower-spectrum, β-lactamase-labile cephalosporins (e.g., cefaclor, loracarbef, and cefprozil) are less active, with resistance rates approximating 15 to 20% (31, 56).

Doern et al. (31) reported a 9.0% rate of resistance to TMP-SMX, which is somewhat higher than that noted in a review of several European studies (44); however, both groups of investigators reported rates of resistance to chloramphenicol, tetracycline, and rifampin of ≤2% (31, 44). Resistance to quinolones is very rare (44). Although erythromycin has not been considered a drug of choice for the treatment of infections caused by *H. influenzae*, some of the newer macrolides are more active than erythromycin. Only 0.5 and 1.9% of isolates were resistant to azithromycin and clarithromycin, respectively, in the study by Doern and colleagues (31); however, Jones et al. (56) reported that 16% of isolates were resistant to clarithromycin. These differences are difficult to explain since both studies incorporated the standard NCCLS broth microdilution MIC method (31, 56).

Reference Test Methods

β-Lactamase production in *H. influenzae* can easily be detected by the chromogenic cephalosporin, acidometric, or iodometric β-lactamase test methods (see chapter 121 of this Manual).

NCCLS has developed standard disk diffusion and MIC methods for the testing of *H. influenzae*, and these methods can also be used to test other *Haemophilus* spp. Specific variables related to each of these are listed in Tables 1 and 2. *Haemophilus* test medium (HTM) is recommended and consists of a Mueller-Hinton base, 15 μg of hematin per ml, 15 μg of NAD per ml, and 5 mg of yeast extract per ml. Cation-adjusted Mueller-Hinton broth is used with the components listed above for the preparation of HTM broth, which also contains 0.2 IU of thymidine phosphorylase per ml. Earlier NCCLS recommendations for disk diffusion testing of *H. influenzae* used chocolate Mueller-Hinton agar (choc-MHA); however, only breakpoints for ampicillin, chloramphenicol, amoxicillin-clavulanic acid, and ampicillin-sulbactam were developed for this medium (71). Because HTM agar is transparent, zones are generally easier to measure than those on choc-MHA. Nevertheless, some investigators have reported difficulties in measuring zones and the poor growth of some strains (45, 69). Broth microdilution tests with HTM generally give clear endpoints. The problems with both the disk diffusion and the broth microdilution methods most often noted are equivocal endpoints with BLNAR strains with several β-lactams. Because of this, NCCLS recommends that BLNAR strains (best detected by tests with ampicillin) should be considered resistant to amoxicillin-clavulanic acid, ampicillin-sulbactam, cefaclor, cefetamet, cefonicid, cefprozil, cefuroxime, and loracarbef, and the activities of these agents against BLNAR strains should not be tested (75–77).

Commercial Test Methods

Currently, the FDA-cleared broth microdilution panels for the testing of *Haemophilus* include MicroTech (Aurora, Colo.) and Sensititre (AcuMed, Westlake, Ohio). The Etest has been satisfactory and is also cleared by FDA for the testing of *Haemophilus* with most drugs that would be considered for use in the treatment of *Haemophilus* infections (43, 59).

Strategies for Testing and Reporting of Results

Direct β-lactamase testing will detect the most common type of clinically significant resistance in *H. influenzae*. β-Lactamase-positive isolates are ampicillin and amoxicillin resistant. To detect BLNAR strains, an ampicillin disk diffusion or MIC test is required. However, since the incidence of BLNAR is very low, such tests may not be routinely needed, and for practical purposes, a negative β-lactamase test result translates into ampicillin susceptibility. Frequently, the β-lactamase test is the only test routinely performed with clinical isolates. Because of increasing levels of resistance to TMP-SMX, routine testing should be considered. Other oral agents that might be considered, such as the oral cephalosporins, newer macrolides, and quinolones, are predictably active and are often prescribed empirically. Consequently, routine testing of these drugs is generally not useful. However, these and other agents may be tested for surveillance or epidemiological purposes.

N. GONORRHOEAE

Drugs of Choice for Therapy

Ceftriaxone, cefixime, ciprofloxacin, and ofloxacin are the primary agents recommended for the treatment of uncomplicated gonorrhea, and spectinomycin is an alternative for patients who are unable to tolerate the aforementioned drugs (10, 23, 68, 85). For disseminated infection, a higher dose of ceftriaxone (or cefotaxime or ceftizoxime) is generally administered until the symptoms resolve. At that time an oral agent is prescribed until 1 week of therapy has been completed (10).

Incidence and Mechanisms of Resistance

During the past two decades, increasing rates of penicillin and tetracycline resistance have led to modifications of earlier recommendations for therapy. Penicillin resistance is due to the production of a plasmid-associated TEM-1-type β-lactamase (penicillinase-producing *N. gonorrhoeae* [PPNG] or is due to mutations in chromosomal genes that result in altered PBPs or diminished outer membrane permeability (chromosomally mediated resistant *N. gonorrhoeae* [CMRNG]). The activities of other β-lactams against PPNG are generally unaltered; however, CMRNG may show decreased susceptibility to other β-lactams (25). Tetracycline resistance in *N. gonorrhoeae* can be plasmid or chromosomally mediated, with plasmid-mediated resistance resulting in a higher level of resistance. The Gonococcal Isolate Surveillance Program (GISP), which tests urethral isolates from male clients visiting sexually transmitted disease clinics throughout the United States, recently demonstrated an increase in the incidence of PPNG from 3.2% in 1988 to 11.0% in 1994. The proportion of isolates with penicillin or tetracycline resistance in 1994 was 30.5% (39). Although elevated ceftriaxone MICs (0.06 to 0.25 μg/ml) have been noted (2.6% in 1991), this has not affected therapy because these MICs remain considerably below the serum ceftriaxone levels; the mechanism (e.g., altered PBPs) for the decreased ceftriaxone susceptibility appears to be similar to that in CMRNG (25, 86).

In the GISP study, the proportion of strains exhibiting decreased susceptibility to ciprofloxacin increased from 0.4% in 1991 to 1.3% in 1994, and four isolates were categorized as ciprofloxacin resistant (39, 86). However, approximately 10% of *N. gonorrhoeae* isolates in Hong Kong and the Philippines are fluoroquinolone resistant (63). As many as 50% of isolates from some Far Eastern countries show decreased susceptibility (intermediate resistance) to quinolones (63). In 1996 and 1997, 62.6% of isolates in the Philippines were fluoroquinolone resistant (79).

Reference Test Methods

Routine β-lactamase tests readily detect PPNG and can reliably be performed by either the chromogenic cephalosporin, acidimetric, or iodometric method.

NCCLS recommends the use of GC agar base for disk diffusion and agar dilution MIC testing. For both tests, a 1% defined growth supplement must be added; however, in agar dilution tests with imipenem and clavulanate, the growth supplement must be free of cysteine to avoid inhibition of the activities of these two agents (75–77). The agar dilution method is preferred to the broth dilution method for MIC testing because *N. gonorrhoeae* has a tendency to autolyze in liquid media. For other details of testing, see Tables 1 and 2.

Commercial Test Methods

The only method that has been explored to any significant extent is the Etest. The Etest was demonstrated to have results comparable to those of conventional test methods; however, it is not yet cleared by FDA for the testing of *N. gonorrhoeae* (12, 104).

Strategies for Testing and Reporting Results

Resistance to the extended-spectrum cephalosporins has not been reported among gonococcal isolates. However, isolates for which fluoroquinolone MICs are elevated are being seen more frequently, particularly in Southeast Asia. Generally, there is no need for routine clinical laboratories to perform antimicrobial susceptibility tests with *N. gonorrhoeae* unless there are unusual circumstances. These might include the patient's intolerance to the drugs of choice, treatment failure (assuming that compliance was not an issue), or a disseminated gonococcal infection against which an alternative agent might be preferred. Additionally, if quinolone resistance is noted in a particular geographic area, testing may be warranted if quinolones are being prescribed. Some laboratories may perform β-lactamase tests for all isolates if these results are requested by the local public health departments for epidemiological purposes. However, many public health departments are eliminating this requirement. Surveillance for established and emerging resistance is generally performed by designated state and local public health agencies.

M. CATARRHALIS

Drugs of Choice for Therapy

The drugs of choice for the treatment of *M. catarrhalis* infections include amoxicillin-clavulanic acid, TMP-SMX, β-lactamase-stable cephalosporins such as cefuroxime or cefixime, macrolides, tetracyclines, and quinolones (10, 68, 85).

Incidence and Mechanisms of Resistance

Between 85 and 95% of *M. catarrhalis* isolates produce a β-lactamase and are resistant to ampicillin, amoxicillin, and penicillin (27, 101). The majority of clinical isolates produce one of two types of chromosomally mediated β-lactamases: BRO-1 or BRO-2 (37, 70). BRO-1-producing strains are 10-fold more prevalent than BRO-2-producing strains, and ampicillin and penicillin MICs for BRO-1 strains appear to be higher (e.g., ≥4.0 μg/ml) than those for BRO-2 strains (e.g., MICs, ≤0.5 μg/ml) (28). Because of the low MICs for the latter strains, their clinical significance in response to β-lactamase-labile penicillins is questionable. A recent study of isolates from 723 outpatients among 30 medical centers in the United States demonstrated a 6.5% rate of resistance to TMP-SMX and lower rates of resistance to the other recommended drugs of choice (27).

Strategies for Testing and Reporting of Results

The chromogenic cephalosporin method is the only method that has reliably detected the β-lactamases produced by *M. catarrhalis* (35). Routine β-lactamase testing may not be necessary because of the high incidence of β-lactamase-positive strains. Nevertheless, some advocate reporting of β-lactamase results to highlight the fact that this pathogen is generally unresponsive to some agents (e.g., amoxicillin) commonly prescribed for the treatment of respiratory tract infections. Since *M. catarrhalis* typically responds to the drugs of choice, testing beyond the β-lactamase test is rarely indicated. However, as with *H. influenzae*, increasing rates of resistance to TMP-SMX may result in the need to test for resistance to this compound in the future. The current NCCLS protocols do not address antimicrobial susceptibility testing of *M. catarrhalis* other than suggesting that β-lactamase testing be performed (75, 76). Most isolates of *M. catarrhalis* grow satisfactorily in cation-adjusted Mueller-Hinton broth (CAMHB) and on Mueller-Hinton agar (MHA) with ambient air incubation. Despite the lack of standardized test recommendations, Doern and Tubert (34) demonstrated that disk diffusion testing appeared to be satisfactory for ampicillin, amoxicillin-clavulanic acid, cephalothin, cefaclor, erythromycin, tetracycline, chloramphenicol, and TMP-SMX. Except for cefaclor, the breakpoints used were those published by NCCLS in 1984 for nonfastidious bacteria (71).

N. MENINGITIDIS

Drugs of Choice for Therapy

Penicillin is the drug of choice for the treatment of meningococcal infections, and broad-spectrum cephalosporins are commonly used alternatives (10, 68, 85). Rifampin, ciprofloxacin, or ceftriaxone are prescribed prophylactically to those who have close contact with a patient with meningococcal disease (22).

Incidence and Mechanisms of Resistance

Increasing numbers of *N. meningitidis* isolates from the United States and elsewhere that are β-lactamase negative have reduced susceptibility to penicillin (MICs, 0.1 to 1.28 μg/ml) (13, 14, 21, 51, 80, 84, 91, 92, 103). The mechanism of decreased susceptibility to penicillin appears to be due to an altered PBP 2. The broad-spectrum cephalosporins (e.g., ceftriaxone) remain highly active against these isolates (15, 50, 80). The clinical significance of isolates for which penicillin MICs are elevated is uncertain. Many infections caused by isolates with reduced susceptibility to penicillin have successfully been treated with penicillin (84, 100); however, at least one report cited a clinical failure (meningitis) when a lower than recommended dose of penicillin was used (99). In the 1980s, four isolates of β-lactamase-producing *N. meningitidis* were reported (16, 26, 38), but additional isolates have not been noted since then. Resistance to sulfonamides occurs fairly frequently, and resistance to rifampin has been documented on rare occasions (50, 67, 80).

Strategies for Testing and Reporting of Results

Various broth and agar dilution methods have been used for susceptibility testing of *N. meningitidis*. NCCLS recommends the broth microdilution method with CAMHB-lysed horse blood or the agar dilution method with MHA with 5% sheep blood (both with incubation in 5% CO_2) (77). While incubation in CO_2 is not required, it enhances growth and makes the endpoints easier to read. NCCLS has not yet provided MIC interpretive criteria for *N. meningitidis*. Thus, MICs must be evaluated cautiously. Some provisional MIC breakpoints have been suggested (67).

Although disk diffusion methods (with 2- and 10-IU penicillin disks and 1-μg oxacillin disks) have been examined for their usefulness for penicillin susceptibility testing (20, 21), it has been noted that these methods cannot reliably distinguish isolates that are susceptible from those that have decreased penicillin or ampicillin susceptibility (81, 95). Therefore, disk diffusion testing should not be used for these drugs.

Because of the lack of clinical failures with the drugs of choice for the treatment of meningococcal infections, susceptibility testing is probably not warranted in most situations. However, if susceptibility testing is required, MIC testing should be performed by one of the two methods suggested by NCCLS, as described above. The Etest shows promising results for meningococci and is best used with Mueller-Hinton agar with 5% sheep blood incubated in CO_2 (1, 50, 67, 81).

L. MONOCYTOGENES

Drugs of Choice for Therapy

The drug regimen of choice for most *Listeria* infections is ampicillin (or penicillin) with or without gentamicin. TMP-SMX is an effective alternative for some types of infections (10, 68, 85).

Incidence and Mechanisms of Resistance

L. monocytogenes remains susceptible to the drugs of choice and is susceptible in vitro to other common agents, including chloramphenicol, vancomycin, tetracyclines, and macrolides; however, these have not proved to be as useful in vivo as the aforementioned agents (47, 55, 89). Although *L. monocytogenes* is often susceptible in vitro to cephalosporins, these agents are not effective clinically.

Strategies for Testing and Reporting of Results

Interpretive criteria for ampicillin and penicillin are included in the current NCCLS MIC tables (77). Only criteria for susceptibility (MIC, ≤2.0 μg/ml) are listed because clinical isolates with resistance have not been noted. Suggested test parameters include the use of CAMHB-LHB and incubation for 16 to 20 h. *L. monocytogenes* is not truly fastidious, and testing in Mueller-Hinton broth without the blood supplement has been used satisfactorily (65). It is important to remember that susceptibility to cephalosporins should not be reported for *L. monocytogenes*. Failure to do so might result in the reporting of significantly misleading information (3). This cautionary note is emphasized in NCCLS documents (75–77) and illustrates why it is inappropriate to indiscriminately report susceptibility results for any agent without knowing if it would be a reasonable therapeutic option. Because cephalosporins are frequently used empirically for the treatment of meningitis, the laboratory should quickly communicate smear or culture findings suspicious for *Listeria* whenever this situation arises.

STRATEGIES FOR TESTING OFB

It is usually unnecessary and inappropriate to perform susceptibility tests with OFB because infections caused by them generally respond to the drugs of choice. Many physicians are unaware that susceptibility testing of OFB is complex

TABLE 3 Stepwise strategy for antimicrobial susceptibility testing of OFB

Step	Comments
Communicate with the patient's physician to determine if testing is necessary. Suggest that assistance from an infectious diseases specialist may be warranted. Discuss limitations of using nonstandardized testing and reporting procedures.	Frequently, the patient has improved by the time that a preliminary or final identification is available and the laboratory is ready to perform susceptibility testing. Once the identification is available, the physician may feel comfortable with empiric therapy on the basis of the information in the literature. If testing is not performed, save the isolate in the laboratory for at least 1 week.
If testing is necessary, discuss (with the patient's physician) the specific antimicrobial agents to be tested. Perform testing only if it can be done with confidence (on the basis of a review of the literature).	Test agents that the physician has prescribed (or may prescribe). Consider testing drugs of choice.
Check literature for test methods that have been used in various studies. MIC methods are usually described.	Methods published previously often represent a reasonable approach, since investigators generally investigate various alternatives prior to method selection. However, it is not uncommon to discover that different methods may have been used in different studies for a given fastidious bacterial species.
Consider contacting "expert resource" (identified from the literature) for assistance.	The "expert resource" can often provide tips for testing or may offer to perform the test. This generally occurs in a research versus clinical laboratory setting.
Determine a QC strategy.	Ideally, test QC strains similar to the patient's isolate to be tested. However, these are often unavailable and a strain that most closely represents the test situation should be selected. For example, if CAMHB-LHB is used for the testing of *Corynebacterium urealyticum*, perform QC testing with *S. pneumoniae* ATCC 49619. Also, consider obtaining a QC strain that has been used by other investigators.
Perform the test and make certain that QC is acceptable; determine MIC results.	The test strain must show adequate growth. Sometimes there is considerable variability in growth characteristics among strains of a given fastidious species.
Report MIC results with qualifying comments that testing was performed by a procedure that is not standardized. Interpret MICs only if this can be done with confidence on the basis of a review of the literature.	Use of interpretive criteria for rapidly growing organisms (e.g., members of the family *Enterobacteriaceae* and *Staphylococcus* spp.) and other fastidious organisms (e.g., *Haemophilus* spp., *N. gonorrhoeae*, *S. pneumoniae*, or *Streptococcus* spp.) may be misleading.

and that standardized methods and criteria for interpretation of the results are unavailable. Communication of this information will often result in the physician's reconsideration of the request. For serious infections caused by OFB, physicians should be encouraged to seek assistance from an infectious diseases physician to ensure proper patient management.

On rare occasions, in vitro susceptibility testing of OFB may be required. These might include clinical failure, patient intolerance to the drug(s) of choice, or serious infections against which there are several appropriate drugs that might be prescribed. Additionally, susceptibility testing may aid in species identification (e.g., differentiating *C. jeikeium* from other *Corynebacterium* species). Susceptibility testing may be necessary as part of a clinical research study. However, since testing is performed by nonstandardized methods, the results must always be interpreted with caution. For guiding therapy, MIC results must be interpreted by comparing them with the results obtained in various clinical studies documented in the literature. Use of published NCCLS interpretive criteria for nonfastidious or other fastidious bacteria may result in a misleading report. For example, the typical penicillin MIC for *E. corrodens* is 1 μg/ml and penicillin is a drug of choice for the treatment of infections caused by this organism. Use of the penicillin interpretive criteria for staphylococci (with an MIC of ≥0.5 indicating resistance) would generate a misleading interpretation of resistance. The impact of unique characteristics of specific organisms (e.g., resistance mechanisms or growth requirements, or both) on zone size and MIC interpretive criteria can be appreciated by examining the six different MIC resistance breakpoints for penicillin (e.g., for *Staphylococcus*, *Enterococcus*, *Pneumococcus*, *Streptococcus*, *Gonococcus*, and *Listeria*) published by NCCLS (77).

The Etest has been examined for the testing of many OFB. Many of the data generated have been obtained from comparisons with nonstandardized in vitro test methods, with limited examination of the clinical correlation of the results. Consequently, the results for OFB generated by the Etest should also be interpreted with caution in the clinical setting.

A variety of nonstandardized methods of determining the MICs for various OFB have been described in the literature, and these may or may not give comparable results for a given organism. The disk diffusion test should generally not be used because many OFB are slowly growing or grow satisfactorily only on an enriched medium. These characteristics can have a significant impact on the diameters of the inhibition zones.

When a nonstandardized method is used, this does not mean that the results are inaccurate; it means that the methods and results have not undergone rigid evaluation to prove that they are meaningful in various clinical settings. In contrast, methods such as those recommended by NCCLS for the testing of *S. pneumoniae*, *Streptococcus* spp., *N. gonorrhoeae*, and *H. influenzae* were developed systematically and were subjected to critical review prior to their acceptance as standards (75–77). Nevertheless, even the standardized methods are not perfect.

A strategy for approaching the susceptibility testing of OFB is presented in Table 3. If testing must be performed, it should be done by a laboratory familiar with all the limitations.

REFERENCES

1. **Abadi, F. J., D. E. Yakubu, and T. H. Pennington.** 1995. Antimicrobial susceptibility of penicillin-sensitive and penicillin-resistant meningococci. *J. Antimicrob. Chemother.* **35:**687–690.
2. **Alcaide, F., J. Linares, R. Pallares, J. Carratala, A. Benitez, F. Gudiol, and R. Martin.** 1995. In vitro activities of 22 β-lactam antibiotics against penicillin-resistant and penicillin-susceptible viridans group streptococci isolated from blood. *Antimicrob. Agents Chemother.* **39:**2243–2247.
3. **Allerberger, F. J., and M. P. Dierich.** 1992. Listeriosis and cephalosporins. *Clin. Infect. Dis.* **15:**177–178.
4. **Appelbaum, P. C.** 1992. Antimicrobial resistance in *Streptococcus pneumoniae*: an overview. *Clin. Infect. Dis.* **15:**77–83.
5. **Appelbaum, P. C.** 1996. Epidemiology and in vitro susceptibility of drug-resistant *Streptococcus pneumoniae*. *Pediatr. Infect. Dis. J.* **15:**932–934.
6. **Baker, C. N., and C. Thornsberry.** 1974. Antimicrobial susceptibility of *Streptococcus mutans* isolated from patients with endocarditis. *Antimicrob. Agents Chemother.* **5:**268–271.
7. **Baker, C. N., C. Thornsberry, and R. R. Facklam.** 1981. Synergism, killing kinetics, and antimicrobial susceptibility of group A and B streptococci. *Antimicrob. Agents Chemother.* **19:**716–725.
8. **Baquero, F.** 1995. Pneumococcal resistance to beta-lactam antibiotics: a global geographic overview. *Microb. Drug Resist.* **1:**115–120.
9. **Barry, A. L., P. C. Fuchs, and M. A. Pfaller.** 1993. Susceptibilities of β-lactamase-producing and -nonproducing ampicillin-resistant strains of *Haemophilus influenzae* to ceftibuten, cefaclor, cefuroxime, cefixime, cefotaxime, and amoxicillin-clavulanic acid. *Antimicrob. Agents Chemother.* **37:**14–18.
10. **Bartlett, J. G.** 1997. *Pocket Book of Infectious Disease Therapy.* Williams & Wilkins, Baltimore, Md.
11. **Betriu, C., M. Gomez, A. Sanchez, A. Cruceyra, J. Romero, and J. J. Picazo.** 1994. Antibiotic resistance and penicillin tolerance in clinical isolates of group B streptococci. *Antimicrob. Agents Chemother.* **38:**2183–2186.
12. **Biedenbach, D. J., and R. N. Jones.** 1996. Comparative assessment of Etest for testing susceptibilities of *Neisseria gonorrhoeae* to penicillin, tetracycline, ceftriaxone, cefotaxime, and ciprofloxacin: investigation using 510(k) review criteria, recommended by the Food and Drug Administration. *J. Clin. Microbiol.* **34:**3214–3217.
13. **Block, C., Y. Davidson, E. Melamed, and N. Keller.** 1993. Susceptibility of *Neisseria meningitidis* in Israel to penicillin and other drugs of interest. *J. Antimicrob. Chemother.* **32:**166–168.
14. **Blondeau, J. M., F. E. Ashton, M. Isaacson, Y. Yaschuck, C. Anderson, and G. Ducasse.** 1995. *Neisseria meningitidis* with decreased susceptibility to penicillin in Saskatchewan, Canada. *J. Clin. Microbiol.* **33:**1784–1786.
15. **Blondeau, J. M., and Y. Yaschuk.** 1995. In vitro activities of ciprofloxacin, cefotaxime, ceftriaxone, chloramphenicol, and rifampin against fully susceptible and moderately penicillin-resistant *Neisseria meningitidis*. *Antimicrob. Agents Chemother.* **39:**2577–2579.
16. **Botha, P.** 1988. Penicillin-resistant *Neisseria meningitidis* in southern Africa. *Lancet* **i:**54.
17. **Bourgault, A. M., W. R. Wilson, and J. A. Washington.** 1979. Antimicrobial susceptibilities of species of viridans streptococci. *J. Infect. Dis.* **140:**316–321.
18. **Butler, J. C., J. Hofmann, M. S. Cetron, J. A. Elliott, R. R. Facklam, R. F. Breiman, and The Pneumococcal Sentinal Surveillance Study Group.** 1996. The continued emergence of drug-resistant *Streptococcus pneumoniae* in the United States: an update from the Centers for Dis-

ease Control and Prevention's Pneumococcal Sentinel Surveillance System. *J. Infect. Dis.* **174:**986–993.

19. **Buu-Hoi, A., C. Le Bouguenec, and T. Horaud.** 1990. High-level chromosomal gentamicin resistance in *Streptococcus agalactiae* (group B). *Antimicrob. Agents Chemother.* **34:**985–988.
20. **Campos, J., P. M. Mendelman, M. U. Sako, D. O. Chaffin, A. L. Smith, and J. A. Saez-Nieto.** 1987. Detection of relatively penicillin G-resistant *Neisseria meningitidis* by disk susceptibility testing. *Antimicrob. Agents Chemother.* **31:**1478–1482.
21. **Campos, J., G. Trujillo, T. Seuba, and A. Rodriguez.** 1992. Discriminative criteria for *Neisseria meningitidis* isolates that are moderately susceptible to penicillin and ampicillin. *Antimicrob. Agents Chemother.* **36:**1028–1031.
22. **Centers for Disease Control and Prevention.** 1997. Control and prevention of meningococcal disease: recommendations of the Advisory Committee on Immunization Practices (ACIP). *Morbid. Mortal. Weekly Rep.* **46:**1–10.
23. **Centers for Disease Control and Prevention.** 1998. Guidelines for treatment of sexually transmitted diseases. *Morbid. Mortal. Weekly Rep.* **47:** No. (RR-1):59–69.
24. **Daum, R. S., M. Murphey-Corb, E. Shapira, and S. Dipp.** 1988. Epidemiology of rob β-lactamase among ampicillin-resistant *Haemophilus influenzae* isolates in the United States. *J. Infect. Dis.* **157:**450–455.
25. **Dillon, J., and K. H. Yeung.** 1989. β-Lactamase plasmids and chromosomally-mediated antibiotic resistance in pathogenic *Neisseria* species. *Clin. Microbiol. Rev.* **2**(Suppl.):S125–S133.
26. **Dillon, J. R., M. Pauze, and K. H. Yeung.** 1983. Spread of penicillinase-producing and transfer plasmids from the gonococcus to *Neisseria meningitidis*. *Lancet* **i:**779–781.
27. **Doern, G. V., A. B. Brueggemann, G. Pierce, T. Hogan, H. P. Holley, Jr., and A. Rauch.** 1996. Prevalence of antimicrobial resistance among 723 outpatient clinical isolates of *Moraxella catarrhalis* in the United States in 1994 and 1995; results of a 30-center national surveillance study. *Antimicrob. Agents Chemother.* **40:**2884–2886.
28. **Doern, G. V.** 1986. *Branhamella catarrhalis*, an emerging human pathogen. *Diagn. Microbiol. Infect. Dis.* **4:** 191–201.
29. **Doern, G. V., A. Brueggemann, H. P. Holley, Jr., and A. M. Rauch.** 1996. Antimicrobial resistance of *Streptococcus pneumoniae* recovered from outpatients in the United States during the winter months of 1994 to 1995: results of a 30-center national surveillance study. *Antimicrob. Agents Chemother.* **40:**1208–1213.
30. **Doern, G. V., A. Brueggemann, and G. Pierce.** 1997. Assessment of the oxacillin disk screening test for determining penicillin resistance in *Streptococcus pneumoniae*. *Eur. J. Clin. Microbiol. Infect. Dis.* **16:**311–314.
31. **Doern, G. V., A. B. Brueggemann, G. Pierce, H. P. Holley, Jr., and A. Rauch.** 1997. Antibiotic resistance among clinical isolates of *Haemophilus influenzae* in the United States in 1994 and 1995 and detection of β-lactamase positive strains resistant to amoxicillin-clavulanate: results of a national multicenter surveillance study. *Antimicrob. Agents Chemother.* **41:**292–297.
32. **Doern, G. V., M. J. Ferraro, A. Brueggemann, and K. L. Ruoff.** 1996. Emergence of high rates of antimicrobial resistance among viridans group streptococci in the United States. *Antimicrob. Agents Chemother.* **40:** 891–894.
33. **Doern, G. V., J. H. Jorgensen, C. Thornsberry, D. Preston, T. Tubert, J. S. Redding, and L. A. Maher.** 1988. National collaborative study of the prevalence of antimicrobial resistance among clinical isolates of *Haemophilus influenzae*. *Antimicrob. Agents Chemother.* **32:**180–185.
34. **Doern, G. V., and T. Tubert.** 1987. Disk diffusion susceptibility testing of *Branhamella catarrhalis* with ampicillin and seven other antimicrobial agents. *Antimicrob. Agents Chemother.* **31:**1519–1523.
35. **Doern, G. V., and T. A. Tubert.** 1987. Detection of β-lactamase activity among clinical isolates of *Branhamella catarrhalis* with six different β-lactamase assays. *J. Clin. Microbiol.* **25:**1380–1383.
36. **Farber, B. F., and Y. Yee.** 1987. High-level aminoglycoside resistance mediated by aminoglycoside-modifying enzymes among viridans streptococci: implications for the therapy of endocarditis. *J. Infect. Dis.* **155:**948–953.
37. **Farmer, T., and C. Reading.** 1982. β-Lactamases of *Branhamella catarrhalis* and their inhibition by clavulanic acid. *Antimicrob. Agents Chemother.* **21:**506–508.
38. **Fontanals, D., V. Pineda, I. Pons, and J. C. Rojo.** 1989. Penicillin-resistant beta-lactamase-producing *Neisseria meningitidis* in Spain. *Eur. J. Clin. Microbiol. Infect. Dis.* **8:**90–91.
39. **Fox, K. K., J. S. Knapp, K. K. Holmes, E. W. Hook 3rd, F. N. Judson, S. E. Thompson, J. A. Washington, and W. L. Whittington.** 1997. Antimicrobial resistance in *Neisseria gonorrhoeae* in the United States, 1988–1994: the emergence of decreased susceptibility to the fluoroquinolones. *J. Infect. Dis.* **175:**1396–1403.
40. **Friedland, I. R.** 1995. Comparison of the response to antimicrobial therapy of penicillin-resistant and penicillin-susceptible pneumococcal disease. *Pediatr. Infect. Dis. J.* **14:**885–890.
41. **Friedland, I. R., and G. H. McCracken.** 1994. Management of infections caused by antibiotic-resistant *Streptococcus pneumoniae*. *N. Engl. J. Med.* **331:**377–382.
42. **Fuchs, P. C., A. L. Barry, S. D. Brown, S. D. Allen, M. Bauman, J. H. Jorgensen, and F. C. Tenover.** 1997. Reproducibility of broth microdilution and disk diffusion susceptibility tests of nine antimicrobial agents against *Streptococcus pneumoniae* ATCC 49619. *Diagn. Microbiol. Infect. Dis.* **28:**27–29.
43. **Giger, O., J. E. Mortensen, R. B. Clark, and A. Evangelista.** 1996. Comparison of five different susceptibility test methods for detecting antimicrobial agent resistance among *Haemophilus influenzae* isolates. *Diagn. Microbiol. Infect. Dis.* **24:**145–153.
44. **Goldstein, F. W., and J. F. Acar.** 1995. Epidemiology of antibiotic resistance in *Haemophilus influenzae*. *Microb. Drug Resist.* **1:**131–135.
45. **Heelan, J. S., D. Chesney, and G. Guadagno.** 1992. Investigation of ampicillin-intermediate strains of *Haemophilus influenzae* by using the disk diffusion procedure and current National Committee for Clinical Laboratory Standards guidelines. *J. Clin. Microbiol.* **30:**1674–1677.
46. **Hindler, J., and D. A. Bruckner.** 1993. MIC testing of viridans streptococci using E test as compared to a reference method, abstr. 254, p. 166. *In Program and Abstracts of the 33rd Interscience Conference on Antimicrobial Agents and Chemotherapy*. American Society for Microbiology, Washington, D.C.
47. **Hof, H., T. Nichterlein, and M. Kretschmar.** 1997. Management of listeriosis. *Clin. Microbiol. Rev.* **10:** 345–357.
48. **Hofmann, J., M. S. Cetron, M. M. Farley, W. S. Baughman, R. R. Facklam, J. A. Elliott, K. A. Deaver, and R. F. Breiman.** 1995. The prevalence of drug-resistant *Streptococcus pneumoniae* in Atlanta. *N. Engl. J. Med.* **333:**481–486.
49. **Horodniceanu, T., A. Buu-Hoi, A. Delbos, and G. Bieth.** 1982. High-level aminoglycoside resistance in group A, B, C, D (*Streptococcus bovis*), and viridans streptococci. *Antimicrob. Agents Chemother.* **21:**176–179.

50. **Hughes, J. H., D. J. Biedenbach, M. E. Erwin, and R. N. Jones.** 1993. E test as susceptibility test and epidemiologic tool for evaluation of *Neisseria meningitidis* isolates. *J. Clin. Microbiol.* **31:**3255–3259.
51. **Jackson, L. A., F. C. Tenover, C. Baker, B. D. Plikaytis, M. W. Reeves, S. A. Stocker, R. E. Weaver, and J. D. Wenger and The Meningococcal Disease Study Group.** 1994. Prevalence of *Neisseria meningitidis* relatively resistant to penicillin in the United States, 1991. *J. Infect. Dis.* **169:**438–441.
52. **Jacobs, M. R.** 1992. Treatment and diagnosis of infections caused by drug-resistant *Streptococcus pneumoniae*. *Clin. Infect. Dis.* **15:**119–127.
53. **Jacobs, M. R., S. Bajaksouzian, P. C. Appelbaum, and A. Bolmstrom.** 1992. Evaluation of the E test for susceptibility testing of pneumococci. *Diagn. Microbiol. Infect. Dis.* **15:**473–478.
54. **Jacobs, R. F., S. L. Kaplan, G. E. Schutze, A. S. Dajani, R. Leggiadro, C. S. Rim, and S. K. Puri.** 1996. Relationship of MICs to efficacy of cefotaxime in treatment of *Streptococcus pneumoniae* infections. *Antimicrob. Agents Chemother.* **40:**895–898.
55. **Jones, E. M., and A. P. MacGowan.** 1995. Antimicrobial chemotherapy of human infection due to *Listeria monocytogenes*. *Eur. J. Clin. Microbiol. Infect. Dis.* **14:**165–175.
56. **Jones, R. N., M. R. Jacobs, J. A. Washington, and M. A. Pfaller.** 1997. A 1994–1995 survey of *Haemophilus influenzae* susceptibility to ten orally administered agents: a 187 clinical laboratory center sample in the United States. *Diagn. Microbiol. Infect. Dis.* **27:**75–83.
57. **Jorgensen, J., M. McElmeel, and S. Crawford.** 1998. Evaluation of the Dade MicroScan MICroSTREP antimicrobial susceptibility testing panel with selected *Streptococcus pneumoniae* challenge strains and recent clinical isolates. *J. Clin. Microbiol.* **36:**788–791.
58. **Jorgensen, J. H., M. J. Ferraro, M. L. McElmeel, J. Spargo, J. M. Swenson, and F. C. Tenover.** 1994. Detection of penicillin and extended-spectrum cephalosporin resistance among *Streptococcus pneumoniae* clinical isolates by use of the E test. *J. Clin. Microbiol.* **32:**159–163.
59. **Jorgensen, J. H., A. W. Howell, and L. A. Maher.** 1991. Quantitative antimicrobial susceptibility testing of *Haemophilus influenzae* and *Streptococcus pneumoniae* by using the E test. *J. Clin. Microbiol.* **29:**109–114.
60. **Jorgensen, J. H., J. M. Swenson, F. C. Tenover, M. J. Ferraro, J. A. Hindler, and P. R. Murray.** 1994. Development of interpretive criteria and quality control limits for broth microdilution and disk diffusion antimicrobial susceptibility testing of *Streptococcus pneumoniae*. *J. Clin. Microbiol.* **32:**2448–2459.
61. **Klugman, K. P.** 1990. Pneumococcal resistance to antibiotics. *Clin. Microbiol. Rev.* **3:**171–196.
62. **Klugman, K. P., and T. D. Gootz.** 1997. In-vitro and in-vivo activity of trovafloxacin against *Streptococcus pneumoniae*. *J. Antimicrob. Chemother.* **39**(Suppl. B)**:**51–55.
63. **Knapp, J. S., K. K. Fox, D. L. Trees, and W. L. Whittington.** 1997. Fluoroquinolone resistance in *Neisseria gonorrhoeae*. *Emerg. Infect. Dis.* **3:**33–39.
64. **Krisher, K., and A. Linscott.** 1994. Comparison of three commercial MIC systems, E test, fastidious antimicrobial susceptibility panel, and FOX fastidious panel, for confirmation of penicillin and cephalosporin resistance in *Streptococcus pneumoniae*. *J. Clin. Microbiol.* **32:**2242–2245.
65. **MacGowan, A. P., H. A. Holt, M. J. Bywater, and D. S. Reeves.** 1990. In vitro antimicrobial susceptibility of *Listeria monocytogenes* isolated in the UK and other *Listeria* species. *Eur. J. Clin. Microbiol. Infect. Dis.* **9:**767–770.
66. **Macias, E. A., E. O. Mason, Jr., H. Y. Ocera, and M. T. LaRocca.** 1994. Comparison of E test with standard broth microdilution for determining antibiotic susceptibilities of penicillin-resistant strains of *Streptococcus pneumoniae*. *J. Clin. Microbiol.* **32:**430–432.
67. **Marshall, S. A., P. R. Rhomberg, and R. N. Jones.** 1997. Comparative evaluation of Etest for susceptibility testing *Neisseria meningitidis* with eight antimicrobial agents. An investigation using U.S. Food and Drug Administration regulatory criteria. *Diagn. Microbiol. Infect. Dis.* **27:** 93–97.
68. **Medical Letter.** 1996. The choice of antibacterial drugs, p. 25–34. *In* M. Abramowicz (ed.), *The Medical Letter*, vol. 38. The Medical Letter, New Rochelle, N.Y.
69. **Mendelman, P. M., E. A. Wiley, T. L. Stull, C. Clausen, D. O. Chaffin, and O. Onay.** 1990. Problems with current recommendations for susceptibility testing of *Haemophilus influenzae*. *Antimicrob. Agents Chemother.* **34:**1480–1484.
70. **Nash, D. R., R. J. Wallace, Jr., V. A. Steingrube, and P. A. Shurin.** 1986. Isoelectric focusing of β-lactamases from sputum and middle ear isolates of *Branhamella catarrhalis* recovered in the United States. *Drugs* **31:**48–54.
71. **National Committee for Clinical Laboratory Standards.** 1984. *Performance Standards for Antimicrobial Disk Susceptibility Tests*, 3rd ed. Approved standard M2-A3. National Committee for Clinical Laboratory Standards, Wayne, Pa.
72. **National Committee for Clinical Laboratory Standards.** 1993. *Performance Standards for Antimicrobial Disk Susceptibility Tests*, 5th ed. Approved standard M2-A5. National Committee for Clinical Laboratory Standards, Wayne, Pa.
73. **National Committee for Clinical Laboratory Standards.** 1993. *Methods for Dilution Antimicrobial Susceptibility Tests for Bacteria That Grow Aerobically*, 3rd ed. Approved standard M7-A3. National Committee for Clinical Laboratory Standards, Wayne, Pa.
74. **National Committee for Clinical Laboratory Standards.** 1995. *Performance Standards for Antimicrobial Susceptibility Testing*. Sixth informational supplement. M100-S5. National Committee for Clinical Laboratory Standards, Wayne, Pa.
75. **National Committee for Clinical Laboratory Standards.** 1997. *Methods for Dilution Antimicrobial Susceptibility Tests for Bacteria That Grow Aerobically*, 4th ed. Approved standard M7-A4. National Committee for Clinical Laboratory Standards, Wayne, Pa.
76. **National Committee for Clinical Laboratory Standards.** 1997. *Performance Standards for Antimicrobial Disk Susceptibility Tests*, 6th ed. Approved standard M2-A6. National Committee for Clinical Laboratory Standards, Wayne, Pa.
77. **National Committee for Clinical Laboratory Standards.** 1998. *Performance Standards for Antimicrobial Susceptibility Testing*. Eighth informational supplement. M100-S8. National Committee for Clinical Laboratory Standards, Wayne, Pa.
78. **Ngui-Yen, J. H., E. A. Bryce, C. Porter, and J. A. Smith.** 1992. Evaluation of the E test by using selected gram-positive bacteria. *J. Clin. Microbiol.* **30:**2150–2152.
79. **Pato-Mesola, V., J. Klausner, M. Aplasca, R. Manalastas, C. Tuazon, W. Whittington, and K. Holmes.** 1997. Rapid emergence of gonococcal ciprofloxacin resistance in Manila and Cebu, Philippines—1994 and 1996–97. Presented at the 4th International Congress on AIDS in Asia and the Pacific.
80. **Perez-Trallero, E., J. M. Garcia-Arenzana, I. Ayestaran, and I. Munoz-Baroja.** 1989. Comparative activity in vitro of 16 antimicrobial agents against penicillin-susceptible meningococci and meningococci with diminished suscep-

tibility to penicillin. *Antimicrob. Agents Chemother.* **33:** 1622–1623.

81. **Perez-Trallero, E., N. Gomez, and J. M. Garcia-Arenzana.** 1994. Etest as susceptibility test for evaluation of *Neisseria meningitidis* isolates. *J. Clin. Microbiol.* **32:** 2341–2342.
82. **Rittenhouse, S. F., L. A. Miller, R. L. Kaplan, G. H. Mosley, and J. A. Poupard.** 1995. A survey of β-lactamase producing *Haemophilus influenzae*; an evaluation of 5750 isolates. *Diagn. Microbiol. Infect. Dis.* **21:**223–225.
83. **Ruoff, K.** 1991. Nutritionally variant streptococci. *Clin. Microbiol. Rev.* **4:**184–190.
84. **Saez-Nieto, J. A., D. Fontanals, J. Garcia de Jalon, V. Martenez de Artola, P. Pena, M. A. Morera, R. Verdaguer, I. Sanfeliu, C. Belio-Blasco, and J. L. Perez-Saenz.** 1987. Isolation of *Neisseria meningitidis* strains with increase of penicillin minimal inhibitory concentrations. *Epidemiol. Infect.* **99:**463–469.
85. **Sanford, J. P., D. N. Gilbert, R. C. Moellering, and M. A. Sande.** 1997. *Guide to Antimicrobial Therapy*, 27th ed. Antimicrobial Therapy, Inc., Vienna, Va.
86. **Schwebke, J. R., W. Whittington, R. J. Rice, H. H. Hansfield, J. Hale, and K. K. Holmes.** 1995. Trends in susceptibility of *Neisseria gonorrhoeae* to ceftriaxone from 1985 to 1991. *Antimicrob. Agents Chemother.* **39:** 917–920.
87. **Seppala, A., A. Nissinen, H. Jarvinen, S. Huovinen, T. Henriksson, E. Herva, S. E. Holm, M. Jahkola, M. L. Katila, T. Klaukka, S. Kontiainen, O. Liimatainen, S. Oinonen, L. Passi-Metosomaa, and P. Huovinen.** 1992. Resistance to erythromycin in group A streptococci. *N. Engl. J. Med.* **326:**292–297.
88. **Skulnick, M., G. W. Small, P. Lo, M. P. Patel, C. R. Porter, D. E. Low, S. Matsumura, and T. Mazzulli.** 1995. Evaluation of accuracy and reproducibility of E test for susceptibility testing of *Streptococcus pneumoniae* to penicillin, cefotaxime, and ceftriaxone. *J. Clin. Microbiol.* **33:** 2334–2337.
89. **Soriano, F., J. Zapardiel, and E. Nieto.** 1995. Antimicrobial susceptibilities of *Corynebacterium* species and other non-spore-forming gram-positive bacilli to 18 antimicrobial agents. *Antimicrob. Agents Chemother.* **39:**208–214.
90. **Stein, D. S., and K. E. Nelson.** 1987. Endocarditis due to nutritionally deficient streptococci: therapeutic dilemma. *Rev. Infect. Dis.* **9:**908–916.
91. **Stroffolini, T., M. E. Congiu, M. Occhionero, and P. Mastrantonio.** 1989. Meningococcal disease in Italy. *J. Infect.* **19:**69–74.
92. **Sutcliffe, E. M., D. M. Jones, S. El-Sheikh, and A. Percival.** 1988. Penicillin-insensitive meningococci in the UK. *Lancet* **i:**657–658.
93. **Swenson, J., J. H. Jorgensen, M. J. Ferraro, and F. C. Tenover.** 1997. Activity of newer fluoroquinolones against recent clinical isolates of ofloxacin-resistant *Streptococcus pneumoniae*, abstr. E-62, p. 124. *In Program and Abstracts of the 37th Interscience Conference on Antimicrobial Agents and Chemotherapy*. American Society for Microbiology, Washington, D.C.
94. **Swenson, J. M., B. C. Hill, and C. Thornsberry.** 1986. Screening pneumococci for penicillin resistance. *J. Clin. Microbiol.* **24:**749–752.
95. **Tenover, F. C.** 1993. Antimicrobial susceptibility testing of *Neisseria meningitidis*. *Clin. Microbiol. Newsl.* **15:**37–38.
96. **Tenover, F. C., C. N. Baker, and J. M. Swenson.** 1996. Evaluation of commercial methods for determining antimicrobial susceptibility of *Streptococcus pneumoniae*. *J. Clin. Microbiol.* **34:**10–14.
97. **Thornsberry, C., P. H. Burton, and B. H. Vanderhoof.** 1996. Activity of penicillin and three third-generation cephalosporins against US isolates of *Streptococcus pneumoniae*: a 1995 surveillance study. *Diagn. Microbiol. Infect. Dis.* **25:**89–95.
98. **Traub, W. H., and B. Leonhard.** 1997. Comparative susceptibility of clinical group A, B, C, F, and G β-hemolytic streptococcal isolates to 24 antimicrobial drugs. *Chemotherapy* **43:**10–20.
99. **Turner, P. C., K. W. Southern, N. J. Spencer, and H. Pullen.** 1990. Treatment failure in meningococcal meningitis. *Lancet* **335:**732–733.
100. **Van Esso, D., D. Fontanals, S. Uriz, M. A. Morera, T. Juncosa, C. Latorre, and M. Duran.** 1987. *Neisseria meningitidis* strains with decreased susceptibility to penicillin. *Pediatr. Infect. Dis. J.* **6:**438–439.
101. **Washington, J. A., and The Alexander Project Group.** 1996. A multicenter study of the antimicrobial susceptibility of community-acquired lower respiratory tract pathogens in the United States, 1992–1994. *Diagn. Microbiol. Infect. Dis.* **25:**183–190.
102. **Wilson, W. R., A. W. Karchmer, A. S. Dajani, K. A. Taubert, A. Bayer, D. Kaye, A. L. Bisno, P. Ferrieri, S. T. Shulman, and D. T. Durack.** 1995. Antibiotic treatment of adults with infective endocarditis due to streptococci, enterococci, staphylococci, and HACEK microorganisms. *JAMA* **274:**1706–1713.
103. **Woods, C. R., A. L. Smith, B. L. Wasilauskas, J. Campos, and L. B. Givner.** 1994. Invasive disease caused by *Neisseria meningitidis* relatively resistant to penicillin in North Carolina. *J. Infect. Dis.* **170:**453–456.
104. **Yeung, K. H., L. K. Ng, and J. A. Dillon.** 1993. Evaluation of Etest for testing antimicrobial susceptibilities of *Neisseria gonorrhoeae* isolates with different growth media. *J. Clin. Microbiol.* **31:**3053–3055.

Susceptibility Testing of Anaerobic Bacteria*

DAVID W. HECHT

120

The importance of anaerobes as the cause of significant infections, as well as the benefits of specific antimicrobial treatment and prophylaxis against anaerobic bacteria, is well recognized (25, 44). In general, antimicrobial susceptibility testing is viewed as a necessity for effective guidance of antimicrobial therapy. However, when and how susceptibility testing of anaerobes should be performed has been the subject of debate, due in part to several confounding factors and misconceptions (10, 23, 26, 63). For example, specimens obtained from most infections involving anaerobes are polymicrobic, making recovery of the organisms slow, identification difficult, and determination of antimicrobial susceptibility too long to have a consistent impact on individual clinical outcomes. For the clinician, the combination of surgical management and the use of empirical broad-spectrum antimicrobial therapy has limited the correlation of potential antimicrobial resistance with outcome. Such observations have led many laboratories away from the performance of susceptibility testing, as recently reported (32). However, there is substantial evidence that antimicrobial resistance is significant among many anaerobes worldwide and that inappropriate therapy can result in poor clinical responses (49, 52). Recent antimicrobial susceptibility data has also revealed significant differences among individual hospitals on a regional and local basis, suggesting that one medical center's patterns are not applicable to organisms from other institutions (33). Thus, the need for susceptibility testing of anaerobes is considerably more important now than in the past.

At a minimum, individual hospitals should consider establishing patterns of resistance for some anaerobes on a periodic basis, with individual patient isolates tested, as needed, to assist in their care. Surveillance for antimicrobial resistance should be considered for selected isolates as often as once a year by the performance of susceptibility testing either within the hospital's laboratory or in an outside reference laboratory. For surveillance purposes, the testing of anaerobes with known resistance, such as members of the *Bacteroides fragilis* group, *Prevotella* spp., *Fusobacterium* spp., *Clostridium* spp., and *Bilophila wadsworthia*, should be considered, depending upon the frequency of their culture. A total of 75 to 100 isolates selected from the genera suggested should be collected over a period of several months and stored, with testing performed in a batch manner for economy of time, resources, and consistency of results. Preferably, 30 isolates should be from the *B. fragilis* group and 10 or more of each of the other genera should be tested. Inclusion of at least 10 isolates from each genus should minimize overinterpretation on the basis of testing only a few isolates. The antimicrobial agents to be tested by this approach should generally be based upon the hospital's formulary, although consideration should be given to inclusion of one agent from each antimicrobial class even if not on the hospital formulary. For individual patient management, susceptibility testing should be performed when (i) agents are critical for disease management, (ii) long-term therapy is being considered, (iii) anaerobes are isolated from specific body sites, or (iv) a usual regimen fails (Table 1).

This chapter describes the currently available methods and their interpretation for susceptibility testing of anaerobes. Recently, the National Committee for Clinical Laboratory Standards (NCCLS) published the latest recommendations for antimicrobial susceptibility testing of anaerobes (43). Following an extensive multilaboratory comparative study, the NCCLS Anaerobe Working Group established a single agar dilution reference method in which brucella blood agar is used as the testing medium (43). This method is not considered generally easy or economical to perform but will serve as the method to which other more practical methods can be compared. At present, alternative testing methods to determine susceptibility to multiple agents include the limited agar dilution method, broth microdilution, and the E test. β-Lactamase testing provides a very limited role but is useful in some settings. Over the coming years, the NCCLS will continue to evaluate and standardize alternative methods that will allow easy-to-perform methods to be used more frequently and cost-effectively (43). Work in progress includes the comparison and standardization of broth microdilution to the reference method.

CURRENT PATTERNS OF ANTIBIOTIC RESISTANCE

Susceptibility testing of anaerobes has not been routinely performed at most hospitals (32). As a result, most of the published literature reporting the susceptibility of anaerobes is generated by reference laboratories testing a limited num-

* This chapter contains information presented in chapter 115 by Hannah M. Wexler and Gary V. Doern in the sixth edition of this Manual.

TABLE 1 Indications for susceptibility testing of anaerobic bacteria

Indication	Examples[a]
Surveillance	
Annual monitoring of isolates at individual medical centers	*B. fragilis* group, *Prevotella* spp., *Fusobacterium* spp., *Clostridium* spp., *B. wadsworthii*
Clinical	
Known resistance of a particular species	*B. fragilis* (clindamycin, cephamycins, piperacillin) *Prevotella* spp., *Fusobacterium* spp. (penicillin)
Failure of a usual therapeutic regimen	Any anaerobe
Pivotal role of antimicrobial agent in clinical outcome	*B. fragilis* group (osteomyelitis, joint infection)
Need for long-term therapy	*B. fragilis* group, *Prevotella* spp. (osteomyelitis, endocarditis, brain abscess)
Infections of specific body sites	Any anaerobe (brain abscess, endocarditis, prosthetic devices or graft, refractory bacteremia)

[a] Examples only, and not intended as inclusive. See the text for specific recommendations.

ber of isolates from one or more medical centers (1, 6, 29, 33, 53). Over the last several years, significant differences in susceptibility results for anaerobes have been reported from different countries, geographic locations within a country, and even hospitals within the same city (9, 12, 13, 27, 33, 58). Of particular note, the incidence of clindamycin resistance has increased from <10% to >40% for the *B. fragilis* group at some hospitals (33, 51, 53), while resistance to cephalosporins and cephamycins is also rising (33, 53). Some differences in susceptibility results among different reports may be accounted for by the use of different testing methods, lack of agreement among countries about breakpoints, and clustering of MICs with many combinations of strain and antimicrobial agent (2, 35). Regardless, it is clear from recent publications that resistance among anaerobes is increasing, and clinicians and laboratories can no longer assume that *Bacteroides* spp. are susceptible to these agents without testing. Further, neither national nor even local data from other institutions is sufficient to predict the susceptibility of anaerobes to antimicrobial agents at one's own hospital (33, 53). A general outline of current resistance patterns for anaerobic bacteria is provided below.

Gram-Negative Bacilli and Cocci

Bacteroides fragilis Group

Among the 10 members of the *B. fragilis* group, *B. fragilis* is generally the most susceptible, although more than 95% of all species are resistant to penicillin and ampicillin. The antipseudomonal penicillins ticarcillin and mezlocillin are somewhat more active than penicillin, but <50% of isolates are susceptible (20). Piperacillin is the most active of the antipseudomonal agents against the *B. fragilis* group, although susceptibility has fallen from approximately 90% to 70% over the last 8 to 10 years (20, 34). The isoxazolyl penicillins, such as oxacillin and nafcillin, are not considered active agents against these organisms. The principal mechanism of resistance to these penicillins is β-lactamase production (18, 21, 24). Thus, β-lactam–β-lactamase inhibitor combinations, such as ampicillin-sulbactam, ticarcillin-clavulanate, and piperacillin-tazobactam, are active against nearly all strains of the *B. fragilis* group, with <2% resistance in most reports (34, 53, 60).

Among the cephalosporins and cephamycins, cefoxitin remains very active against members of the *B. fragilis* group, with 80 to 90% of isolates susceptible. Cefotetan demonstrates activity against *B. fragilis* similar to that of cefoxitin but is much less active against the other members of the *B. fragilis* group (1, 19, 20, 59). With the exception of ceftizoxime, broad-spectrum cephalosporins generally have poor activity against most members of the *B. fragilis* group, inhibiting <50% of isolates (1, 53). Susceptibility to ceftizoxime varies widely among published studies (60 to 90%), possibly due to differences in testing methods (2, 14, 45). The broth microdilution method generally demonstrates the most consistent results for ceftizoxime, although the MICs are consistently twofold lower compared with those in agar dilution (4, 35). Cefazolin is not active against members of the *B. fragilis* group.

A marked decrease in susceptibility to clindamycin among *Bacteroides* spp. has become widely recognized worldwide, as noted above (51, 53, 56). The clindamycin resistance determinant is frequently located on transferable plasmids, and is often linked to transferable tetracycline resistance (56). Among other agents, chloramphenicol, metronidazole, and carbapenems (imipenem and meropenem) are nearly uniformly active against all members of the *B. fragilis* group in the United States, although a rate of 3.3% resistance to imipenem has been reported from Japan (7). Of note, imipenem resistance is mediated by a Zn metalloenzyme that confers resistance to all current β-lactam and β-lactam–β-lactamase inhibitor combination agents and has been reported to be transferable (8). Of additional concern, isolated strains resistant to metronidazole, associated with a transferable plasmid, have been found in France (46). Among the currently available fluoroquinolone agents, trovafloxacin (a trifluoronaphthyridone) has excellent activity against all members of the *B. fragilis* group and currently is the only antimicrobial agent in this class with breakpoints approved by the NCCLS for anaerobes (36, 37, 43, 62).

Prevotella and *Porphyromonas*

In general, data on the susceptibility of *Prevotella* and *Porphyromonas* spp. (mostly former *Bacteroides* species) is more limited than that for the *B. fragilis* group. Overall, both genera are more susceptible than the *B. fragilis* group. Currently, about 50% of *Prevotella* spp. are resistant to penicillin and ampicillin due to β-lactamase production, with susceptibility to piperacillin, cefoxitin, cefotetan, and ceftizoxime ranging from 70 to 90% in most published studies (30, 58). *Porphyromonas* strains have also been reported to produce β-lactamase in as many as 8% of isolates in a recent survey from Japan (57). Susceptibilities of *Porphyromonas* isolates are rarely reported separately in most published literature from the United States, but β-lactamase production is considered rare at present. As with the *B. fragilis* group, both genera are nearly uniformly susceptible to carbapenems, metronidazole, and chloramphenicol.

Other Gram-Negative Bacilli

Penicillin resistance among isolates of the genus *Fusobacterium* has been observed; 19% of isolates in one study were resistant to amoxicillin at 4 μg/ml, and 97% of the resistant strains produced β-lactamase (5, 38). In general, >90% of *Fusobacterium* spp. are susceptible to cephalosporins and cephamycins, including cefoxitin, cefotetan, and ceftizoxime (38). *Campylobacter rectus* and *C. curvus* (formerly *Wolinella recta* and *W. curva*) vary in their susceptibility to β-lactams but remain very susceptible to chloramphenicol, metronidazole, and clindamycin (39). *Bilophila wadsworthia* is a recently described gram-negative anaerobe isolated from the gastrointestinal tract that frequently produces β-lactamase and therefore is resistant to penicillin and ampicillin. High MIC_{90}s are also seen in tests of piperacillin and ceftizoxime, with values clustering near the breakpoints. *B. wadsworthia* is susceptible to clindamycin, cefoxitin, β-lactam–β-lactamase inhibitor combinations, carbapenems, and metronidazole (11). *Campylobacter gracilis* (formerly *Bacteroides gracilis*) was previously considered to be resistant to many β-lactam agents. However, recent data suggests that when properly identified, this organism is susceptible to most agents tested, including β-lactam–β-lactamase inhibitor combinations, cefoxitin, ceftizoxime, ceftriaxone, and clindamycin (40). Instead, a newly described but more resistant organism, *Sutterella wadsworthensis*, was often isolated from the same samples and misidentified as *C. gracilis*. *S. wadsworthensis* may demonstrate resistance to clindamycin, ceftizoxime, piperacillin, and/or metronidazole (40).

Gram-Positive Bacilli and Cocci

Non-Spore-Forming Gram-Positive Bacilli

Eubacterium, Actinomyces, Propionibacterium, and *Bifidobacterium* are usually susceptible to β-lactam agents, including the penicillins, cephalosporins and cephamycins, carbapenems, and β-lactam–β-lactamase inhibitor combinations. *Lactobacillus* spp. are variably susceptible to cephalosporins and may be inhibited effectively only by penicillin (31). New species have recently been added to the *Lactobacillus* genus, and little resistance data is available for them (39). Vancomycin is active against some *Lactobacillus* spp., but *L. casei* is usually resistant (15). Most non-spore-forming gram-positive anaerobes are resistant to metronidazole (47).

Spore-Forming Gram-Positive Bacilli

Clostridium perfringens is generally very susceptible to most antianaerobic agents, including the fluoroquinolones ciprofloxacin, ofloxacin, levofloxacin, and trovafloxacin (37). However, nonperfringens *Clostridium* spp. and *C. difficile* have variable susceptibility (47). Nonperfringens species are resistant to clindamycin and β-lactams, while chloramphenicol and metronidazole remain active. *C. difficile* is resistant to many β-lactams, including cephalosporins, and clindamycin but retains susceptibility to metronidazole and vancomycin (47).

Gram-Positive Cocci

At present, only one species of *Peptococcus* remains in this genus, while several species of *Peptostreptococcus* are now recognized (39). In general, these organisms are highly susceptible to β-lactams, β-lactam–β-lactamase inhibitors, cephalosporins, carbapenems, clindamycin, chloramphenicol, metronidazole, and some fluoroquinolones (37, 47). Occasionally, microaerophilic streptococci are initially identified as *Peptostreptococcus* spp. and reported to be resistant to metronidazole. The presumptive identification of a metronidazole-resistant *Peptostreptococcus* sp. should prompt further identification of the isolate, because such isolates are rare.

DESCRIPTION OF TEST METHODS

Current methods recommended by the NCCLS include the reference standard agar dilution with brucella blood agar and broth microdilution methods with a variety of media (43). The reference agar dilution method allows the testing of up to 32 strains by using a replicating device but requires extensive preparation of antimicrobial agent-containing media for each drug tested. Broth microdilution allows the testing of several agents against one strain, but the results do not correlate well with the reference agar dilution method for some antibiotics, such as piperacillin and ceftizoxime (3, 35). Alternative methods include β-lactamase testing, limited agar dilution, broth macrodilution, the E test, and the spiral-streak method (Table 2) (16, 54). At present, broth disk elution and disk diffusion tests are not considered appropriate for anaerobic susceptibility testing since their results do not correlate with the agar dilution reference method (41). The spiral-streak method has not been cleared by the Food and Drug Administration (FDA) for testing of anaerobes but has been used as a research tool (54).

Inoculum Preparation

The inoculum may be prepared by suspending colonies taken from a 24- to 72-h brucella blood agar plate into

TABLE 2 Methods for susceptibility testing of anaerobic bacteria[a]

Method	Medium	Inoculum	Incubation time	Advantages	Disadvantages
Agar dilution[b]	Brucella blood agar	10^5 cells/spot	48 h	Reference method, multiple isolates tested/antibiotic	Labor-intensive, expensive
Broth microdilution	Schaedler's, brucella, brain heart infusion, West-Wilkins, anaerobe MIC broth	10^6 cells/mL (10^5/well)	48 h	Economical, commercial panels available, multiple antibiotics/isolate	Limited shelf life of commercial panels
E test	Brucella blood agar	0.5 McFarland swab plate	24–48 h	Precise MIC value, ideal for individual patient isolates	Expensive for surveillance use
β-Lactamase	Agar medium (growth), chromogenic disk	Few colonies	5–30 min	Economical	Very limited applications

[a] Media and disks listed are commercially available.
[b] Includes limited agar dilution.

enriched thioglycolate medium or brucella broth to a density equivalent to a 0.5 McFarland standard. Alternatively, the initial suspension may be prepared by inoculating five or more colonies into enriched thioglycolate medium and incubating for 4 to 24 h to obtain adequate turbidity (dilution may be required) (43). Equivalence to a 0.5 McFarland standard can also be achieved by using a colorimeter or simple photometer device (e.g., from Vitek, Hazelwood, Mo.; Microscan, West Sacramento, Calif.; Sensititre, Westlake, Ohio). Although more accurate than visual inspection, the use of different broth media can affect photometer readings, requiring the user to verify the inoculum size by performing colony counts.

Media

For the agar dilution method, the recommended medium is supplemented brucella blood agar (43). Brucella blood agar supports the growth of essentially all anaerobes. Brucella base agar is supplemented with hemin (5 μg/ml), 5% defibrinated or laked sheep blood, and vitamin K_1 (1 μg/ml). Hemin is prepared in a stock solution (5 mg/ml) by dissolving 0.5 g of hemin in 10 ml of 1 N NaOH in 100 ml distilled water and autoclaving at 121°C for 15 min. This solution may be stored at 4 to 8°C for 1 month. A 1-ml volume of stock solution is added to 1 liter of medium prior to autoclaving. Lysed (laked) sheep blood is prepared by a single cycle of alternate freezing and thawing and does not require clarification by centrifugation. Vitamin K_1 is prepared in a stock solution (10 mg/ml) by mixing 0.2 ml of vitamin K_1 (3-phytylmenadione) with 20 ml of 95% ethanol. The stock solution can be stored for up to 6 months at 4°C in a dark bottle and is added to agar base to achieve a final concentration of 1 mg/ml prior to autoclaving. The NCCLS recommends that plates not be stored any longer than 7 days in closed containers at 4 to 10°C. However, for research and precise evaluation purposes, storage for not longer than 72 h is recommended. Due to instability, plates containing imipenem or clavulanic acid must be used on the day of preparation.

For broth microdilution tests, several broth media have been used successfully, including Schaedler's broth, Wilkins-West broth, brain heart infusion broth, and a broth with the same formulation as Wilkins-Chalgren agar with the agar omitted (anaerobe broth; Difco Laboratories, Detroit, Mich.). Supplements that may be required for broth dilution testing include 3 to 5% lysed horse blood. The use of supplements other than those recommended by the NCCLS requires that the microbiologist prove that the supplement does not interfere with the test by obtaining expected quality control results (43).

Incubation Conditions

An anaerobic chamber or anaerobic jars equipped with disposable hydrogen and carbon dioxide generators and palladium-coated catalyst pellets are recommended for incubating agar dilution plates, broth microdilution trays, broth macrodilution tubes, and the E-test dish. The incubation atmosphere should contain approximately 5% CO_2, and indicators of anaerobiasis should be included. Incubation in an anaerobic atmosphere should be performed at 35 to 37°C for 48 h (43).

A control for contamination is necessary in all susceptibility tests. This can be accomplished by incubating one set of agar dilution plates, broth microdilution trays, or broth macrodilution tubes in both an anaerobic and an aerobic environment. It is suggested for agar dilution that an additional control plate be inoculated and refrigerated to distinguish the inoculum from slight growth on test plates at the time of determining MICs. Agar dilution and broth microdilution plates can be inoculated in an aerobic environment prior to incubation, although the exposure time should be minimized. For agar dilution, inoculation spots should first be adsorbed for a short time by the medium and then the plates should be stacked upside down (to prevent condensation from falling on the spots). Microdilution trays should not be stacked more than four or five high, to ensure a uniform incubation temperature (43).

Agar Dilution Test Methods

Methods described in the most recent publication by NCCLS are recommended for testing anaerobic bacteria by the agar dilution method (43). The basics of this method are also discussed in detail in chapter 118 of this Manual. The preferred medium is supplemented brucella blood agar, and the inoculum should be 10^5 CFU/spot. It is recommended that colony counts of inocula be performed periodically to ensure the correct density of cells.

Broth Microdilution Test

Microdilution trays may be prepared fresh, frozen after preparation, or purchased commercially as lyophilized or frozen panels. Following the manufacturer recommendations for storage of commercially prepared panels is recommended, while in-house-prepared trays may be kept at −70°C for up to 6 months if stored in sealed plastic bags. Antimicrobial agents used in broth microdilution panels should first be prepared in a large volume and dispensed by using a device that delivers 0.1 ml per well (see chapter 118). Volumes less than 0.1 ml are not recommended for testing anaerobes due to loss of liquid by evaporation. Inoculum effects may be observed when smaller volumes are used. Frozen trays should be brought to room temperature prior to inoculation.

Inocula should be prepared as for agar dilution, with a final inoculum concentration in each well of 10^6 CFU/ml. The method of preparation of the inoculum for broth microdilutiion testing is very important because variation in the density or volume of inoculum may significantly affect MIC results. The actual volume of inoculum transferred to each well of a microdilution tray is generally 0.001 ml to 0.005 ml (or less than 10% of the volume of broth in wells) with frozen trays of 100 μl per well. The inoculation of trays must be standardized, which can be accomplished by using a disposable hand-held inoculator or a mechanized dispenser within 15 min after inocula are prepared. In addition, prereducing the trays before inoculation (2 to 4 h) may enhance the growth of certain fastidious anaerobes and reduce the "edge" effect of outer rows being reduced more rapidly than inner wells (54). The trays should be prereduced if metronidazole is to be tested, since the antimicrobial activity of metronidazole is dependent on the formation of an active intermediate that requires a reduced atmosphere (54). Control wells should include a well with broth but no drug (growth control) and an uninoculated well as a sterility check. This well may also be used as a "negative" control for visual comparison with growth in inoculated wells.

E Test

The E test (A-B Biodisk, Solna, Sweden) has been used more frequently for testing anaerobic organisms in recent years, primarily because of its convenience (16, 48). Several studies have determined its utility and have indicated that the results correlate well with the NCCLS reference approved agar dilution method (16, 50). The method consists of streaking to confluence (three directions) a 0.5 McFarland standard of the test organism on a 150-ml-diameter petri dish containing brucella blood agar. Plastic E-test strips, each coated with a gradient of an antimicrobial compound, are applied to the surface of the plate in a radial fashion, with the lowest concentration toward the center. After 24 to 48 h of anaerobic incubation, an elliptical zone of inhibition is observed. MICs are read at the point of intersection between the ellipse and the test strip marked with MICs. Validation for most antimicrobial agents recommended for testing of anaerobes has been confirmed for the E test (50). Rosenblatt has noted fairly high rates of very major errors (false susceptibility) with penicillin and ceftriaxone, which were minimized if β-lactamase-positive strains were eliminated from testing. In addition, false resistance to metronidazole among anaerobes has been reported with the E test. This phenomenon can be the result of test conditions and medium quality and is generally eliminated if test plates are prereduced in an anaerobic chamber overnight prior to their utilization (17). The E test provides a flexible and simple procedure that is well suited for testing individual isolates in smaller laboratories or those that do not perform batch testing of anaerobe susceptibility. Its main drawback is its relatively high cost.

Alternative Test Procedures

A more convenient method to determine the susceptibility of anaerobic organisms, which has the advantages of agar dilution, is the limited agar dilution or breakpoint method (43). Up to four concentrations of each antimicrobial agent are tested in divided plates. Thus, as many as 16 organisms may be tested against 12 antimicrobial agents in a single anaerobe jar. Current NCCLS recommendations suggest including the susceptible and intermediate breakpoints for each agent, plus one dilution higher and one dilution lower than these two breakpoints (43). Other MICs can be added as desired, but this increases the amount of preparation required. A second alternative method approved by NCCLS is the broth macrodilution procedure. This method is generally less useful than broth microdilution because it is complex and cumbersome, but it can be simplified by testing a limited number of antimicrobial agents at one or two concentrations. Its singular advantage is the ability to determine MBCs, if desired. With this method, serial twofold dilutions of antimicrobial stock solutions are prepared in 2.5 ml of brucella broth containing 5 mg of hemin, 1 ml of $NaHCO_3$, and 1 mg of vitamin K_1. The inoculum consists of 2.5 ml of a 1:200 dilution of a 0.5 McFarland standard, which is added to broth containing the agent to be tested. This will give a final inoculum of 2.5×10^5 CFU/ml. Two additional tubes as a growth control and a sterility control are also included in the test run.

The spiral-streak method (Spiral Systems Instruments, Bethesda, Md.) also uses a concentration gradient method by distributing an antimicrobial agent radially from the center of an agar plate. Test organisms are placed onto the plate by using radial streaks and incubated for 48 h in an anaerobic atmosphere. The end points are determined by measuring the length of growth from the center of the plate to the point of inhibition, and the data is entered into a computer software program that determines the concentration of the drug at the end of growth. This method also has been shown to correlate sufficiently with agar dilution and may be a useful technique for research laboratories; however, it has currently not been cleared for use by the FDA (61).

β-Lactamase Testing

β-Lactamase testing of anaerobes can be performed as described by the NCCLS (43). Two easily performed methods (both cleared by the FDA) are the nitrocefin disk assay (Cefinase; BBL, Cockeysville, Md.) and the S1 chromogenic cephalosporin disk assay (International BioClinical, Inc., Portland, Oreg.). Both tests should be performed as specified by the manufacturers. Up to four organisms can be applied to quadrants of each disk via a loop or applicator stick. Hydrolysis of the β-lactam ring by β-lactamases causes a color change on the disks from yellow to red. Most reactions occur within 5 to 10 min, but some β-lactamase-positive strains of *Bacteroides* spp. may react more slowly (up to 30 min) (22). When testing *Bilophila wadsworthia*, 1% pyruvate should be added to the growth medium for optimal results (55).

β-Lactamase testing has limited utility in detecting resistance to certain β-lactam agents among anaerobes. While a chromogenic cephalosporin test is simple and quick and generally detects β-lactamases produced by species of *Prevotella*, *Porphyromonas*, *Bacteroides*, and other anaerobes, resistance to β-lactam drugs is not always mediated by β-lactamase production (e.g., some strains of *B. distasonis* and *B. fragilis* are resistant because of alterations of penicillin-binding proteins) (18, 28). Therefore, β-lactamase test results are limited in their clinical application. A positive test does, however, provide clinically relevant information quickly in some situations and can predict resistance to penicillin G and ampicillin.

Interpretation of Results

Since 1993, the NCCLS has defined the end point for agar dilution testing as the concentration at which there is the most marked change from the growth control (42, 43). This change is defined as no growth or lighter growth, a haze, multiple tiny colonies, or one to several normal-sized colonies. Plates should be read against a dark background to decrease the appearance of a haze. End points can be difficult to interpret when testing gram-negative organisms with β-lactams, particularly ceftizoxime and piperacillin. The current NCCLS-recommended standard for susceptibility testing now includes a color figure illustrating the end points described above; it should be used as an additional guide with this test method (43).

Broth microdilution MIC determinations require similar criteria for reading end points: the concentration at which the most significant reduction in growth is observed. Similar to that of agar dilution, this decrease in growth may include a tiny, gradually diminishing button of growth, with trailing end points also observed (43).

MIC results should be interpreted according to criteria recommended by the NCCLS (43). In 1993, an intermediate category was established for anaerobic bacteria (42). For many antimicrobial agents used against anaerobes, a significant percentage of susceptibility test end points cluster at or near the suggested breakpoints. In a twofold-dilution method, the degree of acceptable variation of end points (usually plus or minus 1 twofold dilution) does not permit adequate distinction of the qualitative categories. If an intermediate value is determined for any anaerobe, the NCCLS recommends maximum dosages of the antimicrobial agent for therapy. With such dosages, it is believed that organisms with susceptible or intermediate end points are amenable to therapy. This recommendation is predicated upon the presumed surgical intervention that frequently accompanies infections involving these organisms. At present, breakpoints for broth microdilution are the same as for agar dilution, with the exception of ceftizoxime (43). However, MIC results in broth microdilution assays may be lower than those in agar dilution assay for some antimicrobial agents. The Anaerobe Working Group of the NCCLS is evaluating the correlation of the broth microdilution method to the reference standard, which may result in a change in the breakpoints recommended when using this method in the future.

Quality Control

A quality control program is designed to monitor the accuracy and precision of a susceptibility test procedure, the performance of reagents and equipment, and the performance of the persons who conduct the tests. Quality control must be performed to demonstrate that any new medium used supports adequate growth of the test organisms and that the antimicrobial agents have not deteriorated over time. These tests must be a part of any testing program for any of the methods described above. Ideally, the quality control strain(s) that most closely resembles the tested organism(s) should be included. The recommended quality control strains are *B. fragilis* ATCC 25285, *B. thetaiotaomicron* ATCC 29741, and *Eubacterium lentum* ATCC 43055. Two quality control strains should be used for each assessment. Expected values for quality control strains are published by the NCCLS (43). Differences in the quality control limits occur when comparing the agar dilution to the broth macrodilution and broth microdilution methods; with the last two methods, MICs are frequently 1 twofold dilution lower than those determined by agar dilution (35). For some antimicrobial agent–quality-control organism combinations, no quality control ranges are recommended due to difficulty in reading the end points.

CONCLUSIONS

Increasing antimicrobial resistance among anaerobes has become a significant problem in recent years, mitigating the need for more antimicrobial susceptibility testing. Current methods allow accurate surveillance or individual isolate testing by most laboratories. Future studies comparing broth microdilution to the reference agar method will result in better standardization of the more user-friendly method and, possibly, in more widespread commercial availability.

REFERENCES

1. **Aldridge, K. E., M. Gelfand, L. D. Reller, L. W. Ayers, C. L. Pierson, R. Schoenknecht, R. L. Tilton, J. Wilkins, A. Henderberg, and D. D. Schiro.** 1994. A five year multicenter study of the susceptibility of the *Bacteroides fragilis* group isolates to cephalosporins, cephamycins, penicillins, clindamycin, and metronidazole in the United States. *Diagn. Microbiol. Infect. Dis.* **18:**235–241.
2. **Aldridge, K. E., and C. V. Sanders.** 1987. Antibiotic and method-dependent variation in susceptibility testing results of *Bacteroides fragilis* group isolates. *J. Clin. Microbiol.* **25:**2317–2321.
3. **Aldridge, K. E., and D. D. Schiro.** 1994. Major methodology-dependent discordant susceptibility results from *Bacteroides fragilis* group isolates but not other anaerobes. *Diagn. Microbiol. Infect. Dis.* **20:**135–142.
4. **Aldridge, K. E., H. M. Wexler, C. V. Sanders, and S. M. Finegold.** 1990. Comparison of in vitro antibiograms of *Bacteroides fragilis* group isolates: differences in resistance rates in two institutions because of differences in susceptibility testing methodology. *Antimicrob. Agents Chemother.* **34:**179–181.
5. **Appelbaum, P. C., S. K. Spangler, and M. R. Jacobs.** 1990. β-Lactamase production and susceptibilities to amoxicillin, amoxicillin-clavulanate, ticarcillin, ticarcillin-clavulanate, cefoxitin, imipenem, and metronidazole of 320 non-*Bacteroides fragilis* isolates and 129 fusobacteria from 28 U.S. centers. *Antimicrob. Agents Chemother.* **34:**1546–1550.
6. **Appelbaum, P. C., S. K. Spangler, and M. R. Jacobs.** 1993. Susceptibility of 539 gram-positive and -negative anaerobes to new agents, including RP 59500, biapenem, trospectomycin and piperacillin/tazobactam. *J. Antimicrob. Chemother.* **32:**223–231.
7. **Bandoh, K., K. Ueno, K. Watanabe, and N. Kato.** 1993. Susceptibility patterns and resistance to imipenem in the *Bacteroides fragilis* group species in Japan: a 4-year study. *Clin. Infect. Dis.* **16:**S382–S386.
8. **Bandoh, K., K. Watanabe, Y. Muto, Y. Tanaka, N. Kato, and K. Ueno.** 1992. Conjugal transfer of imipenem resistance in *Bacteroides fragilis*. *J. Antibiot.* **45:**542–547.
9. **Baquero, F., and M. Reig.** 1992. Resistance of anaerobic bacteria to antimicrobial agents in Spain. *Eur. J. Clin. Microbiol. Infect. Dis.* **11:**1016–1020.
10. **Baron, E. J., D. M. Citron, and H. M. Wexler.** 1990. Son of anaerobic susceptibility testing-revisited. *J. Clin. Microbiol.* **12:**69–70.
11. **Baron, E. J., G. Ropers, P. Summanen, and R. J. Courcol.** 1997. Bactericidal activity of selected antimicrobial agents against *Bilophila wadsworthia* and *Bacteroides gracilis*. *Clin. Infect. Dis.* **16:**S339–S343.
12. **Betriu, E., D. Campos, C. Cabronero, C. Rodriguez-Aveil, and J. J. Picaxo.** 1990. Susceptibilities of species of the *Bacteroides fragilis* group to 10 antimicrobial agents. *Antimicrob. Agents Chemother.* **34:**671–673.
13. **Bianchini, H., L. B. Fernandez Canigia, C. Bantar, and J. Smayevsky.** 1997. Trends in antimicrobial resistance of the *Bacteroides fragilis* group: a 20-year study at a medical center in Buenos Aires, Argentina. *Clin. Infect. Dis.* **25:**S268–S269.
14. **Borobio, M. V., A. Pascual, M. C. Dominguez, and E. J. Perea.** 1986. Effect of medium, pH, and inoculum size on activity of ceftizoxime and Csh-34343 against anaerobic bacteria. *Antimicrob. Agents Chemother.* **30:**626–627.
15. **Chow, A. W., and N. Cheng.** 1988. In vitro activities of daptomycin (LY146032) and paldimycin (U-70, 138F) against anaerobic gram-positive bacteria. *Antimicrob. Agents Chemother.* **32:**788–790.
16. **Citron, D. M., A. Ostavari, A. Karlsson, and E. J. C. Goldstein.** 1991. Evaluation of the epsilometer (E-test) for susceptibility testing of anaerobic bacteria. *J. Clin. Microbiol.* **29:**2197–2203.
17. **Cormican, M. G., M. E. Erwin, and R. N. Jones.** 1996. False resistance to metronidazole by E-test among anaerobic bacteria investigations of contributing test conditions and medium quality. *Diagn. Microbiol. Infect. Dis.* **24:**117–119.
18. **Cuchural, G. J., S. Hurlbut, M. H. Malamy, and F. P. Tally.** 1988. Permeability to β-lactams in *Bacteroides fragilis*. *J. Antimicrob. Chemother.* **22:**785–790.
19. **Cuchural, G. J., F. P. Tally, N. V. Jacobus, K. E. Aldridge, T. J. Cleary, S. M. Finegold, G. B. Hills, P. B. Iannini, J. P. O'Keefe, C. L. Pierson, D. W. Crook, T. A. Russo, and D. W. Hecht.** 1988. Susceptibility of *Bacteroides fragilis* group in the United States: analysis by site of isolation. *Antimicrob. Agents Chemother.* **32:**717–722.

20. **Cuchural, G. J., F. P. Tally, N. V. Jacobus, T. J. Cleary, S. M. Finegold, G. B. Hills, P. B. Iannini, J. P. O'Keefe, and C. L. Pierson.** 1990. Comparative activities of newer β-lactam agents against members of the *Bacteroides fragilis* group. *Antimicrob. Agents Chemother.* **34:**479–480.
21. **Cuchural, G. J., F. P. Tally, N. V. Jacobus, P. K. Marsh, and J. W. Mayhew.** 1983. Cefoxitin inactivation by *Bacteroides fragilis*. *Antimicrob. Agents Chemother.* **34:**936–940.
22. **Doern, G. V., R. N. Jones, E. H. Gerlach, J. A. Washington, D. J. Biedenbach, A. Brueggemann, M. E. Erwin, C. Knapp, and J. Raymond.** 1995. Multicenter clinical laboratory evaluation of a β-lactamase disk assay employing a novel chromogenic cephalosporin, S1. *J. Clin. Microbiol.* **33:**1665–1667.
23. **Dougherty, S. H.** 1997. Antimicrobial culture and susceptibility testing has little value for routine management of secondary bacterial peritonitis. *Clin. Infect. Dis.* **25:** S258–S261.
24. **Eley, A., and D. Greenwood.** 1986. Beta-lactamases of type culture strains of the *Bacteroides fragilis* group and of strains that hydrolyse cefoxitin, latamoxef and imipenem. *J. Med. Microbiol.* **21:**49–57.
25. **Finegold, S. M.** 1989. Therapy of anaerobic infections, p. 793–818. *In* S. M. Finegold and W. L. George. (ed.), *Anaerobic Infections in Humans*. Academic Press, Inc., Orlando, Fla.
26. **Finegold, S. M.** 1997. Perspective on susceptibility testing of anaerobic bacteria. *Clin. Infect. Dis.* **25:**S251–S253.
27. **Fox, A. R., and I. Phillips.** 1987. The antibiotic sensitivity of the *Bacteroides fragilis* group in the United Kingdom. *J. Antimicrob. Chemother.* **20:**477–488.
28. **Georgopapadakou, N. H.** 1993. Penicillin-binding proteins and bacterial resistance to β-lactams. *Antimicrob. Agents Chemother.* **37:**2045–2053.
29. **Goldstein, E. J. C.** 1993. Patterns of susceptibility to fluoroquinolones among anaerobic bacterial isolates in the United States. *Clin. Infect. Dis.* **16:**S377–S381.
30. **Goldstein, E. J. C., and D. M. Citron.** 1993. Comparative susceptibilities of 173 aerobic and anaerobic bite wound isolates to sparfloxacin, temafloxacin, clarithromycin, and older agents. *Antimicrob. Agents Chemother.* **37:** 1150–1153.
31. **Goldstein, E. J. C., D. M. Citron, C. E. Cherubin, and S. L. Hillier.** 1993. Comparative susceptibility of the *Bacteroides fragilis* group species and other anaerobic bacteria to meropenem, imipenem, piperacillin, cefoxitin, ampicillin/sulbactam, clindamycin and metronidazole. *J. Antimicrob. Chemother.* **31:**363–372.
32. **Goldstein, E. J. C., D. M. Citron, R. J. Goldman, M. C. Claros, and S. Hunt-Gerrado.** 1995. United States national hospital survey of anaerobic culture and susceptibility methods, II. *Anaerobe* **1:**309–314.
33. **Hecht, D. W., J. R. Osmolski, and J. P. O'Keefe.** 1993. Variation in the susceptibility of *Bacteroides fragilis* group isolates from six Chicago hospitals. *Clin. Infect. Dis.* **16:** S357–S360.
34. **Hecht, D. W., and L. Lederer.** 1995. Effect of choice of medium on the results of *in vitro* susceptibility testing of eight antibiotics against the *Bacteroides fragilis* group. *Clin. Infect. Dis.* **20:**S346–S349.
35. **Hecht, D. W., L. Lederer, and J. R. Osmolski.** 1995. Susceptibility results for the *Bacteroides fragilis* group: comparison of the broth microdilution and agar dilution methods. *Clin. Infect. Dis.* **20:**S342–S345.
36. **Hecht, D. W., and J. R. Osmolski.** 1996. Comparison of activities of trovafloxacin (CP-99,219) and five other agents against 585 anaerobes with use of three media. *Clin. Infect. Dis.* **23:**S44–S50.
37. **Hecht, D. W., and H. M. Wexler.** 1997. In vitro susceptibility of anaerobes to quinolones in the United States. *Clin. Infect. Dis.* **23:**S2–S8.
38. **Johnson, C.** 1993. Susceptibility of anaerobic bacteria to beta-lactam antibiotics in the United States. *Clin. Infect. Dis.* **16:**S371–S376.
39. **Jousimies-Somer, H.** 1997. Recently described clinically important anaerobic bacteria: taxonomic aspects and update. *Clin. Infect. Dis.* **25:**S78–S87.
40. **Molitoris, E., H. M. Wexler, and S. M. Finegold.** 1997. Sources and antimicrobial susceptibilities of *Campylobacter gracilis* and *Sutterella wadsworthensis*. *Clin. Infect. Dis.* **25:** S264–S265.
41. **National Committee for Clinical Laboratory Standards.** 1990. *Methods for Antimicrobial Susceptibility Testing of Anaerobic Bacteria*, 2nd ed. National Committee for Clinical Laboratory Standards, Villanova, Pa.
42. **National Committee for Clinical Laboratory Standards.** 1993. *Methods for Antimicrobial Susceptibility Testing of Anaerobic Bacteria*, 3rd ed. *Approved Standard*. National Committee for Clinical Laboratory Standards, Villanova, Pa.
43. **National Committee for Clinical Laboratory Standards.** 1997. *Methods for Antimicrobial Susceptibility Testing of Anaerobic Bacteria*, 4th ed. *Approved Standard* M11-A4.p. National Committee for Clinical Laboratory Standards, Villanova, Pa.
44. **North American Congress on Anaerobic Bacteria and Anaerobic Infections.** 1993. Proceedings of the First North American Congress on Anaerobic Bacteria and Anaerobic Infections. *Clin. Infect. Dis.* **16:**S159–S411.
45. **O'Keefe, J. P., F. R. Venezio, C. A. DiVincenzo, and K. L. Shatzer.** 1987. Activity of newer beta-lactam agents against clinical isolates of *Bacteroides fragilis* and other *Bacteroides* species. *Antimicrob. Agents Chemother.* **31:**2002–2004.
46. **Reyssett, G., A. Haggoud, W. Su, and M. Sebald.** 1992. Genetic and molecular analysis of pIP417 and pIP419: *Bacteroides* plasmids encoding 5-nitroimidazole resistance. *Plasmid* **27:**181–190.
47. **Rosenblatt, J.** 1989. Antimicrobic susceptibility of anaerobic bacteria, p. 715–727. *In* S. M. Finegold and W. L. George (ed.), *Anaerobic Infections in Humans*. Academic Press, Inc., San Diego, Calif.
48. **Rosenblatt, J., and D. R. Gustafson.** 1995. Evaluation of the Etest for susceptibility testing of anaerobic bacteria. *Diagn. Microbiol. Infect. Dis.* **22:**279–284.
49. **Rosenblatt, J. E., and I. Brook.** 1993. Clinical relevance of susceptibility testing of anaerobic bacteria. *Clin. Infect. Dis.* **16:**S446–S448.
50. **Rosenblatt, J. E., and D. R. Gustafson.** 1995. Evaluation of the E test for susceptibility testing of anaerobic bacteria. *Diagn. Microbiol. Infect. Dis.* **2:**279–284.
51. **Snydman, D. R., G. J. Cuchural, and The National Anaerobic Susceptibility Study Group.** 1994. Susceptibility variations in *Bacteroides fragilis*: a national survey. *Infect. Dis. Clin. Pract.* **3:**S34–S43.
52. **Snydman, D. R., G. J. Cuchural, L. McDermott, and M. Gill.** 1992. Correlation of various in vitro testing methods with clinical outcomes in patients with *Bacteroides fragilis* group infections treated with cefoxitin: a retrospective analysis. *Antimicrob. Agents Chemother.* **36:**540–544.
53. **Snydman, D. R., L. McDermott, G. J. Cuchural, D. W. Hecht, P. B. Iannini, L. J. Harrell, S. G. Jenkins, J. P. O'Keefe, C. L. Pierson, J. D. Rihs, V. L. Yu, S. M. Finegold, and S. L. Gorbach.** 1996. Analysis of trends in antimicrobial resistance patterns among clinical isolates of *Bacteroides fragilis* group species from 1990 to 1994. *Clin. Infect. Dis.* **23:**S54–S65.
54. **Summanen, P., E. J. Baron, D. M. Citron, C. Stron, H. M. Wexler, and S. M. Finegold.** 1993. *Wadsworth Anaero-*

bic Bacteriology Manual. Star Publishing Co., Belmont, Calif.

55. **Summanen, P., H. M. Wexler, and S. M. Finegold.** 1992. Antimicrobial susceptibility testing of *Bilophila wadsworthia* by using triphenyltetrazolium chloride to facilitate the endpoint determination. *Antimicrob. Agents Chemother.* **36:** 1658–1664.
56. **Tally, F. P., D. R. Snydman, S. L. Gorbach, and M. H. Malamy.** 1979. Plasmid-mediated transferable resistance to clindamycin and erythromycin in *Bacteroides fragilis*. *J. Infect. Dis.* **139:**83–88.
57. **Tanaka, K., C. Kawamura, F. K. Kato, N. Kato, T. Nakamura, K. Watanabe, and K. Ueno.** 1998. Susceptibility and beta-lactamase production of *Prevotella spp*. and *Porphyromonas spp*, abstr. 76. *In Congress on Anaerobic Bacteria and Anaerobic Infections*.
58. **Tuner, K., and C. E. Nord.** 1992. Antibiotic susceptibility of anaerobic bacteria in Europe. *Clin. Infect. Dis.* **4:** S387–S389.
59. **Wexler, H. M., and S. M. Finegold.** 1988. In vitro activity of cefotetan against anaerobic bacteria compared to other antimicrobial agents. *Antimicrob. Agents Chemother.* **32:** 601–604.
60. **Wexler, H. M., E. Molitoris, and S. M. Finegold.** 1991. Effect of β-lactamase inhibitors on the activities of various β-lactam agents against anaerobic bacteria. *Antimicrob. Agents Chemother.* **25:**1219–1224.
61. **Wexler, H. M., E. Molitoris, P. R. Murray, J. A. Washington, R. J. Zabransky, P. H. Edelstein, and S. M. Finegold.** 1996. Comparison of spiral gradient endpoint and agar dilution methods for susceptibility testing of anaerobic bacteria: a multilaboratory collaborative evaluation. *J. Clin. Microbiol.* **34:**170–174.
62. **Wexler, H. M., E. Molitoris, D. Reeves, and S. M. Finegold.** 1994. In-vitro activity of clinafloxacin (CI-960) and PD 131628-2 against anaerobic bacteria. *J. Antimicrob. Chemother.* **34:**579–584.
63. **Wilson, S. E., and J. Huh.** 1997. In defense of routine antimicrobial susceptibility testing of operative site flora in patients with peritonitis. *Clin. Infect. Dis.* **25:**S254–S257.

Special Phenotypic Methods for Detecting Antibacterial Resistance

JANA M. SWENSON, JANET A. HINDLER, AND LANCE R. PETERSON

121

Special phenotypic tests for detecting antibacterial resistance range from the rapid and simple spot β-lactamase test to the more time-consuming and complex MBC assays. These tests may either supplement or replace traditional testing methods depending on the organism and the assay. The tests explained in this chapter include tests for detection of high-level aminoglycoside and vancomycin resistance in enterococci, tests for detection of oxacillin resistance in staphylococci, tests for detection of β-lactamases, and tests for determination of bactericidal activity.

Information about quality control of the screening tests described is given in each section; however, guidelines for the frequency of quality control testing are not given, because they are not available. A practical approach would be to perform quality control testing each day patient isolates are tested or less frequently (e.g., weekly) once a laboratory has thoroughly documented that less frequent quality control testing can validate the reliability of the screening procedures. In addition, quality control tests should be performed each time new lots of material are put into use.

TESTS TO DETECT RESISTANCE IN ENTEROCOCCI

Systemic enterococcal infections such as endocarditis are commonly treated with a combination of two antimicrobial agents, one whose site of action is the cell wall (either a β-lactam drug or a glycopeptide such as vancomycin) and an aminoglycoside (usually gentamicin or streptomycin). These agents act synergistically to enhance killing (124). However, when an enterococcal strain is resistant to the cell wall-active agent or has high-level resistance (HLR) to the aminoglycoside, there is no synergism and combination therapy will not provide a bactericidal effect (89). Because of this, it is important to detect the presence of resistance to both the aminoglycoside and the cell wall-active agent in order to predict the likelihood of synergy.

Detection of High-Level Resistance to Aminoglycosides

Because aminoglycosides have poor activity against enterococci with MICs normally ranging from 8 to 256 μg/ml, they cannot be used as single agents for therapy (45, 89). This intrinsic, moderate-level resistance is due to poor uptake of the aminoglycoside (89). Acquired aminoglycoside resistance in enterococci is due either to mutations resulting in decreased binding of the agent to the ribosome, as occurs with streptomycin only (called ribosomal resistance) or, more commonly, to the acquisition of new genes that encode enzymes that modify aminoglycosides (called acquired resistance). Acquired resistance usually corresponds to MICs that are significantly above those normally tested in routine susceptibility tests, e.g., ≥2,000 μg/ml, and is designated HLR (89; see also chapters 18 and 117).

Synergy between an aminoglycoside and a cell wall-active agent can be determined directly by performing complex time-kill studies (67) or can be predicted by using less cumbersome screening tests such as those described in this chapter. Gentamicin and streptomycin are the only two agents that must be tested on a routine basis. All enterococcal isolates that are resistant to gentamicin are also resistant to other aminoglycosides except streptomycin, which is determined by a different resistance mechanism. Consequently, streptomycin resistance must be determined independently of gentamicin resistance. Isolates of *Enterococcus faecium* are intrinsically resistant to the synergistic actions of amikacin, kanamycin, tobramycin, and netilmicin with cell wall-active agents, irrespective of in vitro testing results for HLR (87). *Enterococcus faecalis* strains that are susceptible to gentamicin may be resistant to kanamycin and amikacin. If amikacin is being considered for therapy, in vitro tests with amikacin cannot reliably predict HLR to amikacin in *E. faecalis*, but kanamycin could be used to predict HLR to amikacin and kanamycin (116).

In 1992, the National Committee for Clinical Laboratory Standards (NCCLS) recognized that confusion existed about correct methods for detection of HLR to aminoglycosides in enterococci and has published details of agar dilution, broth microdilution, and disk diffusion methods for detecting that resistance (95, 96, 129). These methods are summarized in Table 1 and discussed below.

Agar Dilution Screening Method

Agar plates are prepared with brain heart infusion (BHI) agar supplemented with 500 μg of gentamicin per ml or 2,000 μg of streptomycin per ml (see chapter 118). The plates are inoculated by spotting 10 μl of a suspension that is equivalent to a 0.5 McFarland standard prepared from growth on an 18- to 24-h agar plate, giving a final inoculum of 10^6 CFU per spot. The plates are incubated for a full 24

TABLE 1 Screening methods for detecting vancomycin and high-level aminoglycoside resistance in enterococci

Parameter	Screening procedure			
	Vancomycin agar dilution	Aminoglycoside agar dilution	Aminoglycoside broth microdilution	Aminoglycoside disk diffusion
Medium	BHI agar	BHI agar	BHI broth	MHA
Inoculum	10^5–10^6 CFU/spot	10^6 CFU/spot	5 × 10^4 CFU/0.1ml	0.5 McFarland[a]
Incubation (h)	24	24[b]	24[b]	18–24
Drug concn				
Vancomycin	6 μg/ml	NA[c]	NA	NA
Gentamicin	NA	500 μg/ml	500 μg/ml	120 μg/disk
Streptomycin	NA	2,000 μg/ml	1,000 μg/ml	300 μg/disk
End point	>1 colony	>1 colony	Any growth	6 mm = resistant, 7–9 mm = inconclusive,[c] ≥10 mm = susceptible

[a] NCCLS disk diffusion method (96).
[b] If negative for streptomycin at 24 h, reincubate for an additional 24 h.
[c] NA, not applicable.
[d] If the zone is 7 to 9 mm, the test is inconclusive, and an agar or broth microdilution test should be performed to confirm susceptibility or resistance.

h in ambient air. The presence of more than one colony or a haze of growth should be read as denoting resistance. For streptomycin, the plates should be reincubated for an additional 24 h if there is no growth at 24 h. Mueller-Hinton agar (MHA), MHA plus 5% sheep blood, or dextrose phosphate agar may be substituted for BHI agar (129), but because growth is better on BHI agar, this is the preferred medium. A commercially available agar screen plate has performed well (36, 112, 113). Kanamycin agar screen tests have not been as extensively evaluated and are not standardized, but it has been reported that for determining HLR to both amikacin and kanamycin in *E. faecalis*, kanamycin at 2,000 μg/ml in BHI agar can be used (116).

Broth Microdilution Screening Method

Broth microdilution plates are prepared with single wells containing BHI broth supplemented with 500 μg of gentamicin per ml or 1,000 μg of streptomycin per ml. The final inoculum is that recommended for routine broth microdilution testing, i.e., 5 × 10^5 CFU/ml. The plates are incubated for 24 h in ambient air. For streptomycin, the plates should be reincubated for an additional 24 h if there is no growth at 24 h. Any growth is interpreted as denoting resistance.

The recommended streptomycin concentration for use in the broth microdilution screen is 1,000 μg/ml, which is half that used in the agar dilution screen test. Because this test is often included as a part of a routine gram-positive MIC panel, the inoculum is that commonly used in broth microdilution testing (5 × 10^5 CFU/ml). The total number of cells tested in the agar dilution screening procedure (10^6 CFU/spot) is 20-fold larger than that normally used in the broth microdilution test (5 × 10^4 CFU/0.1-ml well). To provide a test that uses a low inoculum and at the same time maximizes the detection of HLR to streptomycin, it was necessary to lower the concentration recommended for testing streptomycin from 2,000 to 1,000 μg/ml in the broth microdilution test. Because of poorer growth and the lower inoculum, Mueller-Hinton broth is inadequate for use in the broth microdilution test (129). The performance of other aminoglycosides in this test has not been evaluated.

Disk Diffusion Screening Method

The standard disk diffusion procedure (96) described in chapter 118 (with unsupplemented MHA) is used, except that special high-content disks (gentamicin at 120 μg and streptomycin at 300 μg) are used (116). Zones are measured after 18 to 24 h of incubation in ambient air at 35°C. Isolates with zone diameters of ≥10 mm are categorized as susceptible. The absence of a zone of inhibition corresponds to the presence of HLR. Strains with zone diameters from 7 to 9 mm usually display HLR, but a few are strains for which the MICs are only moderately elevated (129). Therefore, strains giving 7- to 9-mm zones should be tested by either the standard agar or broth microdilution screen method to determine susceptibility or resistance. High-content gentamicin and streptomycin disks are now available commercially from both Remel Laboratories (Lenexa, Kans.) and Becton Dickinson Microbiology Systems (Cockeysville, Md.).

Quality Control

E. faecalis ATCC 29212 is used as a susceptible control for both gentamicin and streptomycin; *E. faecalis* ATCC 51299, resistant to both gentamicin and streptomycin, is the resistant control strain (128). Only *E. faecalis* ATCC 29212 is used for control of disk diffusion tests. The expected quality control limits are 16 to 22 mm for gentamicin (120-μg) disks and 14 to 19 mm for streptomycin (300-μg) disks.

Detection of Penicillin and Ampicillin Resistance

Compared to streptococci, for which penicillin MICs are usually ≤0.12 μg/ml, all enterococci are "relatively resistant" to β-lactams, with penicillin MICs usually ≥2 μg/ml (89). Isolates of *E. faecium* are inherently more resistant to penicillin than are isolates of *E. faecalis*; the usual MICs of penicillin for *E. faecium* are 16 to 32 μg/ml, whereas the usual MICs for *E. faecalis* are 2 to 4 μg/ml (38, 87). Ampicillin MICs are generally 1 dilution lower than penicillin MICs (39, 89). This intrinsic relative resistance, as well as higher levels of resistance to penicillin and ampicillin (MICs ≥16 μg/ml), has been associated with differences in penicillin-binding proteins (PBPs) (34, 89). In addition to changes in PBPs, resistance to β-lactam agents can be mediated by the production of β-lactamase (90), but this is much less common and has been found only in *E. faecalis*.

No screening tests have been described for detection of penicillin and ampicillin resistance. Routine antimicrobial susceptibility tests (see chapter 118) will detect resistance due to changes in PBPs, and this will be evident as higher MICs or smaller zones of inhibition, indicating resistance. However, routine tests (such as broth microdilution or disk diffusion) will not detect resistance due to β-lactamase in enterococci; an inoculum 100-fold greater than routinely recommended (e.g., 10^7 CFU/ml) is necessary for resistance to be demonstrated by standard dilution methods (90, 108). The nitrocefin β-lactamase test is recommended for detection of strains that are resistant due to the production of β-lactamase (see "β-Lactamase Tests" below).

As defined by the NCCLS (95), resistance to penicillin and ampicillin corresponds to MICs of ≥16 μg/ml. The NCCLS recommends that results of penicillin susceptibility tests be used to predict susceptibility to ampicillin, amoxicillin, piperacillin, and β-lactam–β-lactamase inhibitor combinations (95, 96). In general, enterococcal strains resistant to penicillin or ampicillin as a result of altered PBPs (MICs ≥16 μg/ml) should also be considered resistant to imipenem, whatever the test results (45). In the absence of PBP-mediated resistance, β-lactamase-producing enterococci should be considered resistant to penicillin, ampicillin, and the ureidopenicillins but susceptible to imipenem as well as β-lactam–β-lactamase inhibitor combinations (90).

Torres et al. (141) recently recommended that in the absence of aminoglycoside resistance, strains of *E. faecium* for which penicillin MICs were ≤64 μg/ml should be considered potentially susceptible to synergy with an aminoglycoside. In addition, in a recent review, Murray (91) recommended that for strains of *E. faecium* categorized as resistant to both ampicillin and vancomycin, tests to determine the actual MIC might be worthwhile since strains for which ampicillin MICs are 16 to 64 μg/ml may be treatable with ampicillin. Additional clinical studies are needed to clarify the level of ampicillin and penicillin resistance that correlates with the absence of synergy. Currently, most commonly used antimicrobial susceptibility systems do not include ampicillin concentrations above 16 μg/ml, so that differentiation between borderline resistance (ampicillin MICs, 16 to 32 μg/ml) and higher-level resistance (MICs, ≥64 μg/ml) is not readily possible. For a β-lactamase-negative strain, testing of a single concentration of ampicillin or penicillin at 32 or 64 μg/ml by an agar dilution or broth macrodilution test with Mueller-Hinton medium and an inoculum normally used for MIC testing (95) could help define the level of resistance. The E test also reliably detects ampicillin resistance in enterococci (121). Since ampicillin MICs are generally 1 dilution lower than penicillin MICs (39), it is possible to encounter strains that appear susceptible to ampicillin but resistant to penicillin (136). The clinical significance of this finding is unknown.

Detection of Vancomycin Resistance

Definitions of vancomycin resistance in enterococci continue to undergo modifications as more is learned about the genetics and clinical significance of the resistance. The three most common phenotypes of resistance are (i) high-level vancomycin resistance (MICs, ≥64 μg/ml) with accompanying teicoplanin resistance (≥16 μg/ml) (VanA phenotype); (ii) low- to high-level vancomycin resistance (MICs, 16 to 512 μg/ml), most commonly without teicoplanin resistance (VanB phenotype); and (iii) intrinsic low-level resistance associated with *E. gallinarum*, *E. casseliflavus*, and *E. flavescens* (MICs, 2 to 32) (VanC phenotype) (71–73). Both the VanA and VanB phenotypes are most commonly seen in *E. faecalis* and *E. faecium* but have been found in other species (17). As defined by the NCCLS, vancomycin resistance breakpoints are ≤4 μg/ml for susceptible, 8 to 16 μg/ml for intermediate, and ≥32 μg/ml for resistant.

Many methods commonly used by clinical laboratories, including disk diffusion, Vitek, and MicroScan systems, have had problems detecting low-level vancomycin resistance in enterococci (both VanB and VanC types) (114, 115, 132, 135, 147). However, some of these systems have shown some improvement in detection (50, 59, 108, 135), and both Vitek and the conventional (but not the Rapid) MicroScan systems are currently approved for use in the detection of vancomycin resistance in enterococci. Recommendations for disk diffusion testing of vancomycin (including extending incubation to 24 h and examining zones under transmitted light), published in 1993, have improved the accuracy of the test (93, 130). Because of the potential failure of some systems to detect the vancomycin resistance expressed by certain enterococcal strains, an agar screening test first described by Willey et al. (147) was studied and adopted by NCCLS in 1993 (92, 127) (Table 1).

The sensitivity and specificity of the agar screen test were very high when it was first evaluated (96 to 99% and 100%, respectively). In two recent evaluations, commercially prepared plates also performed well (36, 144). However, there is some confusion among clinical laboratorians about the characterization of susceptibility or resistance for the VanC-containing enterococci, *E. gallinarum*, *E. casseliflavus*, and *E. flavescens* (71), because they often grow on the agar screen plate. All members of these three species intrinsically contain a *vanC* gene, but the MICs of vancomycin for these species range from 2 to 32 μg/ml (71). Whether the presence of this gene is associated with therapeutic failures is not known. Since the vancomycin MICs for these strains are often greater than 4 μg/ml, the strains are likely to grow on the agar screen plates, where a higher inoculum and a richer medium may promote growth (36, 50, 127). However, since these species are motile at 30°C, it is relatively simple to differentiate them from *E. faecalis* and *E. faecium* by performing a motility test (6, 36) (see chapter 18).

Agar Dilution Screen

Agar plates are prepared (see chapter 118 for a description of the general procedure for agar plate preparation) with BHI agar supplemented with 6 μg of vancomycin per ml. The plates are inoculated by spotting 1 to 10 μl of a suspension on the agar surface, using growth from an 18- to 24-h agar plate to make a suspension equivalent in turbidity to a 0.5 McFarland standard. The final inoculum is 10^5 to 10^6 CFU per spot. Recently, Jorgensen et al. found that inoculation of the plates with a cotton swab dipped in the 0.5 McFarland suspension was equivalent to using a measured 1- or 10-μl aliquot (63). After inoculation, the plates are incubated for a full 24 h in ambient air at 35°C. The presence of more than one colony or a haze of growth should be read as denoting resistance.

Quality Control

For quality control, *E. faecalis* ATCC 29212 (no growth, i.e., susceptible) and *E. faecalis* ATCC 51299 (growth, i.e., resistant) should be tested (128). Plates made with BHI agars from certain manufacturers may allow light growth of *E. faecalis* ATCC 29212, especially if the higher inoculum is used or the plates are held longer than 24 h.

Reporting Resistance in Enterococci

For any serious enterococcal infection, results of the screen for HLR to gentamicin and streptomycin must be reported in concert with the results of the testing of the cell wall-active agent, because synergy would not be expected if any one of the agents reported is resistant. Helpful suggestions on reporting the results of enterococcal tests are given by Hindler and Sahm (45).

OXACILLIN DISK SCREEN TEST FOR DETECTION OF PENICILLIN RESISTANCE IN PNEUMOCOCCI

A screening test in which 1-μg oxacillin disks are used to detect penicillin resistance in pneumococci was first described following an outbreak of *Streptococcus pneumoniae* resistant to multiple antimicrobial agents in South Africa in the 1970s (25, 51, 131). Since then, this test has been used extensively and shown to be highly sensitive but less specific for detection of nonsusceptible pneumococci (27). Strains screened by this method may in fact be penicillin susceptible, intermediate, or resistant. MIC tests must be performed on any strain that is potentially resistant by this screening test to determine if it is indeed resistant (27). Details of the procedure and suggestions about its use can be found in chapter 119.

AGAR SCREEN FOR DETECTION OF OXACILLIN RESISTANCE IN STAPHYLOCOCCI

Strains of *Staphylococcus aureus* resistant to both oxacillin and methicillin have most commonly been referred to as methicillin-resistant *S. aureus* (MRSA). However, since methicillin is not readily available in the United States, the resistance is more appropriately referred to as oxacillin resistance (ORSA). Current NCCLS MIC breakpoints for oxacillin and *S. aureus* are ≤2 μg/ml for susceptible and ≥4 μg/ml for resistant (99). At least three different resistance mechanisms contribute to oxacillin resistance in *S. aureus* (see chapter 117): (i) production of a supplemental PBP (PBP 2a) encoded by a chromosomal *mecA* gene, (ii) inactivation of the drug by increased production of β-lactamase, and (iii) production of modified intrinsic PBPs (MOD-SA) with low affinity for the drug (10, 12, 24, 41, 84). From a clinical perspective, it is important to differentiate isolates that have *mecA*-positive resistance, which is the classic type of oxacillin resistance, from the infrequently encountered isolates that have one of the other types of more subtle or borderline resistance, because it affects therapy. Characteristics that might help differentiate the three types of oxacillin resistance are outlined in Table 2. Strains that possess the *mecA* gene (classic resistance) are either heterogeneous or homogeneous in their expression of resistance. With homogeneous expression, virtually all cells express resistance when tested by standard in vitro test methods. However, testing of a heteroresistant isolate results in some cells that appear susceptible and others that appear resistant. Often only 1 in 10^4 to 1 in 10^8 *mecA*-positive cells in the test population expresses resistance (42, 110, 140). Heterogeneous expression occasionally results in MICs that appear to be borderline, i.e., oxacillin MICs of 2 to 8 μg/ml. Isolates that have classic resistance are usually resistant to other agents such as erythromycin, clindamycin, chloramphenicol, tetracycline, trimethoprim-sulfamethoxazole, older fluoroquinolones, or aminoglycosides. Resistance mediated by β-lactamase or the presence of modified PBPs (MOD-SA) also results in borderline resistance. β-lactamase-mediated resistance can usually be distinguished from the classic type (*mecA* positive) or MOD-SA resistance by the addition of a β-lactamase inhibitor (e.g., clavulanic acid) to the oxacillin MIC test, which lowers the MIC by 2 dilutions or more. Isolates that are resistant by either the β-lactamase or the MOD-SA mechanism usually do not have multiple drug resistance. The presence of classic resistance in *S. aureus* can be detected simply and reliably by the agar screen test (95). β-Lactamase or MOD-SA strains are unlikely to grow on the agar screen plate.

Although the *mecA* gene has been identified in coagulase-negative staphylococci (41, 140), the agar screen test has not been reliable for detecting oxacillin resistance in this group of bacteria (126). Some *mecA*-positive coagulase-negative staphylococci (primarily *S. epidermidis*) demonstrate oxacillin MICs as low as 0.5 μg/ml (82, 148). Consequently, the NCCLS recently eliminated recommendations for use of the agar screen test for coagulase-negative staphylococci and also modified breakpoints to ≤0.25 μg/ml for susceptible and ≥0.5 μg/ml for resistant in this group of organisms (99).

TABLE 2 Characterization of oxacillin resistance phenotypes in staphylococci[a]

Resistance phenotype[b]	*mecA* gene encoded	Mechanism	Borderline resistance[c]	β-Lactamase inhibitor effect[d]	β-Lactam cross-resistance	Multiple resistance to non-β-lactams
Classic						
Homogeneous	+	Supplemental PBP (PBP 2a)	−	−	+	(+)[e]
Heterogeneous	+	Supplemental PBP (PBP 2a)	±	−	+	(+)
Inactivation by β-lactamase	−	Increased β-lactamase production	+	+	−	−
MOD-SA	−	Modified preexisting PBPs 1, 2, and 4	+	−	−	−

[a] Modified from reference 111 with permission.

[b] β-Lactamase inactivation and MOD-SA resistance have been described only in *S. aureus*.

[c] Borderline resistance phenotype: oxacillin MICs of 2 to 8 μg/ml with unclear end points, or disk diffusion zone diameters of 10 to 13 mm with poorly defined zone edges.

[d] Addition of a β-lactamase inhibitor lowers the MIC by ≥2 dilutions.

[e] Parentheses indicate that exceptions may occur.

Test Method

MHA supplemented with 4% sodium chloride and 6 μg of oxacillin per ml is used for the agar screen method as recommended by NCCLS (95). Plates containing 4% NaCl and 10 μg of methicillin per ml have also been described (139) but are currently not recommended. Because oxacillin is more stable and appears to be superior to other penicillinase-resistant penicillins (e.g., methicillin, nafcillin, and the isoxazolyl penicillins cloxacillin, dicloxacillin, and flucloxacillin) in detecting resistance to this group of compounds, it is preferred in the agar screen and other diagnostic tests. Agar screen plates are available from several commercial manufacturers. The procedure for preparing agar dilution plates that is outlined in chapter 118 provides a useful guideline for agar screen plate preparation.

In the agar screen test, inoculum suspensions are prepared by selecting colonies from overnight growth on a nonselective agar plate. The colonies are transferred to broth (e.g., tryptic soy broth) or saline to produce a suspension that matches the turbidity of a 0.5 McFarland standard. This suspension is used to inoculate the oxacillin agar screen plate by dipping a cotton swab into the test suspension, expressing the excess liquid from the swab, and touching the swab to a spot on the agar surface or streaking the swab across a small section of the agar surface; the latter technique is probably more sensitive. Alternatively, 10 μl of a 1:100 dilution of a 0.5 McFarland standardized suspension can be pipetted onto the agar surface, resulting in 10^4 CFU/spot (43, 75). Test plates are incubated for a full 24 h at 35°C (no higher) in ambient air and examined for any evidence of growth, which indicates resistance. Once again, the test is currently not recommended for coagulase-negative staphylococci (99).

Quality Control

S. aureus ATCC 29213 (oxacillin susceptible) and *S. aureus* ATCC 43300 (oxacillin resistant) are the recommended quality control strains.

Ability of the Agar Screen Plate To Detect Oxacillin-Resistant *S. aureus* and Reporting Results

Growth of *S. aureus* on an oxacillin agar screen plate generally means that the isolate is *mecA* positive. If performed properly, the agar screen method will detect most *mecA*-positive *S. aureus* strains. Occasionally, however, a heteroresistant *mecA*-positive strain is not detected; this may be due in part to a low frequency of resistance expression or to lot-to-lot or manufacturer-to-manufacturer variation in the test medium (44, 46). The oxacillin agar screen test generally does not detect borderline-resistant strains. Although MOD-SA isolates, particularly those associated with MICs of >8 μg/ml, may grow on agar screen plates (126), isolates with borderline resistance due to β-lactamase are usually associated with oxacillin MICs of ≤6 μg/ml and do not usually grow on the screen plates. Since both types of borderline-resistant isolates are infrequently encountered in clinical specimens of *S. aureus*, the possibility of their presence affects the utility of the agar screen test only minimally.

The NCCLS recommends that oxacillin-resistant staphylococci be considered resistant to all β-lactam agents including penicillins, cephalosporins, β-lactam–β-lactamase inhibitor combination agents, and carbapenems. These agents are clinically ineffective against staphylococci, even though they may demonstrate in vitro activity (96). Consequently, an isolate that grows on the oxacillin agar screen plate should be considered resistant to these agents as well as to all penicillinase-resistant penicillins. Isolates of *S. aureus* that appear oxacillin resistant by an alternative test method but fail to grow on the agar screen plate are probably borderline resistant and lack *mecA* (66, 88, 106). It is likely that these isolates would be clinically susceptible to β-lactam agents that appear to be active in vitro (11, 12, 83, 102, 137); much less is known about borderline resistance than about *mecA*-positive resistance. If an oxacillin-resistant *S. aureus* strain is isolated from a seriously ill patient and is presumed to be resistant by a mechanism other than the *mecA* gene, the laboratory worker should convey this possibility to the patient's clinician. Molecular analysis for the *mecA* gene may be warranted; further information about the test and its value is given in chapter 122.

DETECTION OF VANCOMYCIN RESISTANCE IN STAPHYLOCOCCI

Recently, strains of staphylococci with reduced susceptibility to vancomycin have been described (8, 47). The MICs for these strains are 4 to 8 μg/ml. Vancomycin MIC breakpoints are currently set at ≤4 μg/ml for susceptible, 8 to 16 μg/ml for intermediate, and ≥32 μg/ml for resistant (95), making these isolates borderline in their resistance to vancomycin. Zone diameters for these strains do not characterize them as being distinct from the normally susceptible population of staphylococci, because all of them have had zones in the 16- to 19-mm range. Current NCCLS recommendations for disk diffusion testing of staphylococci have recently changed, with zones of ≥15 mm denoting susceptibility. No intermediate or resistant breakpoints are currently set, but it is suggested that strains with zones of <15 mm should be tested by an MIC method (99).

A recent study looked at the performance of both commercial susceptibility testing systems and the BHI agar screen plate for screening vancomycin-resistant enterococci (134) in detecting staphylococcal strains with reduced vancomycin susceptibility. For this study, the agar screen plates were inoculated with 10 μl of a 0.5 McFarland suspension of organisms and incubated at 35°C in ambient air for a full 24 h. The vancomycin agar screen plates from four commercial sources (Becton Dickinson Microbiology Systems, Cockeysville, Md.; Hardy Diagnostics, Santa Maria, Calif.; PML Microbiologicals, Wilsonville, Oreg.; and Remel, Lenexa, Kans.) were able to detect eight of eight strains for which the MICs were 8 μg/ml (134). In addition, one of three strains for which the MIC was 4 μg/ml grew on the selective agar. None of the 24 strains for which the MICs were ≤2 μg/ml grew on the commercial screen plates, making the plates highly sensitive and specific in this limited study. However, in-house-prepared screening agar showed breakthrough growth of susceptible strains, indicating that some lots of BHI may not be suitable for this test. The performance of the commercial susceptibility testing systems evaluated in this study was not as good; however, both the MicroScan (overnight) conventional panels and the E test appeared to perform well when incubated for a full 24 h. The Vitek system (bioMérieux Vitek, Hazelwood, Mo.) tended to report MICs of 4 μg/ml for the isolates for which the MICs by broth microdilution were 8 μg/ml. Additional testing is needed before recommendations about the limitations of commercial systems can be made. In the meantime, laboratories that use the disk diffusion method for testing staphylococci should also test all isolates with a commercial vancomycin agar screen plate to detect strains for which the vancomycin MICs are ≥8 μg/ml.

DETECTION OF ENZYMES MEDIATING RESISTANCE

Detection of antimicrobial agent-modifying enzymes in the clinical laboratory is limited to tests for β-lactamase and chloramphenicol acetyltransferase (CAT). For more detailed information on these and other types of resistance enzymes, refer to chapters 117 and 122.

β-Lactamase Tests

In the clinical laboratory, β-lactamase tests must be used only in situations when they can provide clinically useful information and the definitions of positive or negative reactions must not be extended beyond their intended meanings. For example, a β-lactamase-positive result for a *Neisseria gonorrhoeae* isolate means that the isolate is resistant to penicillin but does not imply that the isolate is resistant to the extended-spectrum cephalosporin group of β-lactam agents. Similarly, direct β-lactamase tests for members of the family *Enterobacteriaceae* or for *Pseudomonas* spp. (all of which produce a variety of β-lactamases that result in various susceptibilities to β-lactam agents) have little clinical value and should not be used for these species. A list of the organisms for which β-lactamase tests are useful is given in Table 3.

Direct Tests for β-Lactamase Activity

In the direct β-lactamase test, a positive reaction indicates that the isolate is resistant to the β-lactam agents noted in Table 3 but a negative reaction is inconclusive. For example, most ampicillin-resistant *Haemophilus influenzae* isolates produce β-lactamase, which can be detected by direct β-lactamase tests; however, rare strains are ampicillin resistant but β-lactamase negative (28, 61, 107). For the latter, conventional disk diffusion or dilution tests are needed to detect the resistance (see chapter 118). Three direct β-lactamase assays, the acidimetric, iodometric, and chromogenic methods, have been widely used (43, 76). Each method involves testing bacteria grown on nonselective media, and the results are available within 1 to 60 min. The acidometric and iodometric methods use a colorimetric indicator to detect the presence of penicilloic acid in the reaction vessel following β-lactamase hydrolysis of penicillin. In the acidometric method, the substrates are citrate-buffered penicillin and a phenol red indicator. A decreasing pH associated with the presence of penicilloic acid results in a color change from red (negative result) to yellow (positive result) (32). The substrates in the iodometric test are phosphate-buffered penicillin plus a starch-iodine complex. Penicilloic acid, if present, reduces the iodine and prevents it from combining with starch, resulting in a colorless reaction (positive); a bluish-purple color corresponds to a negative result (7).

The chromogenic cephalosporin nitrocefin can be used in a test tube assay (101) but has been incorporated into several commercial products. The disk method is very easy to use and is the β-lactamase test method used in most clinical laboratories (60). More recently, a nonnitrocefin chromogenic cephalosporin, S1 or cefesone, has been incorporated into disks marketed as Cefinase Plus (Becton Dickinson). Cefesone has been shown to perform similarly to nitrocefin, with slightly increased sensitivity in the number of positive results and decreased time to a positive result for *S. aureus* (26, 125). The DrySlide (Difco Laboratories, Detroit, Mich.) is another chromogenic method that has practical application for clinical laboratories (29). β-Lactamase hydrolysis of the chromogenic cephalosporin molecule causes an electron shift that results in a colored product (101). Although there has been some variability in performance and lack of experience with the acidometric and iodometric methods, the nitrocefin method is reliable in detecting β-lactamases produced by all of the organisms indicated in Table 3 (60, 100). The PADAC test, another chromogenic β-lactamase assay, is reliable only for testing

TABLE 3 Bacteria for which β-lactamase tests have been used in the clinical laboratory

Species	Method(s) commonly used	Predicted resistance[a]
Bacteroides spp. and other gram-negative anaerobes, except *B. fragilis* group	Direct β-lactamase tests[b]	Penicillins[c]
Enterococcus spp.	Direct β-lactamase tests	Penicillins[c]
Haemophilus influenzae	Direct β-lactamase tests	Penicillins[c]
Moraxella catarrhalis	Direct β-lactamase tests (nitrocefin only)	Penicillins[c]
Neisseria gonorrhoeae	Direct β-lactamase tests	Penicillins[c]
Staphylococcus spp.	Direct β-lactamase tests with prior induction	Penicillins[c]
Gram-negative bacilli		
Acinetobacter spp.	Disk approximation test for inducible β-lactamase[d]	Extended-spectrum cephalosporins
Citrobacter freundii	Disk approximation test for inducible β-lactamase[d]	Extended-spectrum cephalosporins
Enterobacter spp.	Disk approximation test for inducible β-lactamase[d]	Extended-spectrum cephalosporins
Proteus,[e] *Providencia*, and *Morganella* spp.	Disk approximation test for inducible β-lactamase[d]	Extended-spectrum cephalosporins
Pseudomonas aeruginosa	Disk approximation test for inducible β-lactamase[d]	Extended-spectrum cephalosporins
Serratia marcescens	Disk approximation test for inducible β-lactamase[d]	Extended-spectrum cephalosporins
Escherichia coli	Double-disk potentiation test for ESBLs[d]	Cephalosporins and aztreonam
Klebsiella pneumoniae	Double-disk potentiation test for ESBLs[d]	Cephalosporins and aztreonam

[a] A positive result indicates resistance; however, a negative result is inconclusive, since other resistance mechanisms may occur.
[b] Includes chromogenic cephalosporin, acidimetric, and iodometric tests.
[c] A positive result indicates resistance to all penicillinase-labile penicillins, including ampicillin, amoxicillin, azlocillin, carbenicillin, mezlocillin, piperacillin, and ticarcillin.
[d] Used only to confirm unusual results from conventional tests for research or academic purposes.
[e] Except *Proteus mirabilis*.

H. influenzae, *N. gonorrhoeae*, and *Moraxella catarrhalis*; it should not be used for staphylococci (1).

The colorimetric β-lactamase tests rely on visualization of a colored product that presumably results from β-lactamase destruction of the substrate β-lactam molecule. However, these tests are not 100% specific, and other substances may yield colored end points. Serum may cause a colored reaction with the nitrocefin test (101), and if reagents are not stored properly, spontaneous degradation of penicillin may produce false-positive acidometric or iodometric β-lactamase reactions. An agar plate disk bioassay for β-lactamase testing has been described (74). Use of this bioassay eliminates the specificity concerns for colorimetric end points in direct tests; however, it is cumbersome and is rarely performed in routine clinical laboratories.

While some bacteria (e.g., *H. influenzae*, *N. gonorrhoeae*, and enterococci) constitutively produce β-lactamase, others (e.g., staphylococci) produce detectable amounts of enzyme only after exposure to an inducing agent, which is generally a β-lactam agent (30). If staphylococci produce a positive β-lactamase result without induction, the results can be reported. However if no β-lactamase is detected, then before a negative result is reported, the test must be performed on cells that have been exposed to an inducing agent. This can be done by testing organisms that have been grown in the presence of subinhibitory concentrations of a β-lactam agent (e.g., 0.25 μg of cefoxitin per ml) in a broth or agar system. Alternatively, cell paste from around the periphery of the zone surrounding a β-lactam disk (e.g., a 1-μg oxacillin disk) can be tested. A positive result may take longer to develop in staphylococci than in other organisms, and the test should not be considered negative until it has been allowed to react for at least 60 min.

β-Lactamase testing by the nitrocefin method with anaerobic gram-negative bacilli other than those from the *B. fragilis* group is recommended prior to susceptibility testing (94). Members of the *B. fragilis* group characteristically produce β-lactamase, but, as with aerobes, resistance to β-lactam drugs is not always mediated by β-lactamase production (e.g., in some strains of *B. distasonis* and *B. fragilis*) (52, 94).

The *S. aureus* strains recommended by the NCCLS for quality control of routine disk diffusion and dilution tests (95, 96) can be used for quality control of β-lactamase tests. *S. aureus* ATCC 25923 is β-lactamase negative, whereas *S. aureus* ATCC 29213 is β-lactamase positive.

Tests for Inducible β-Lactamases

Virtually all *Acinetobacter*, *Citrobacter freundii*, *Enterobacter*, *Morganella*, *Proteus vulgaris*, *P. penneri*, *Providencia*, *Pseudomonas aeruginosa*, and *Serratia marcescens* isolates are capable of producing inducible β-lactamases. Upon exposure to an inducing agent (a β-lactam agent), these organisms produce β-lactamases that hydrolyze primary and extended-spectrum penicillins and cephalosporins. Generally, the bacterium stops producing the β-lactamase when the inducing agent is removed. Some cells, however, mutate to a state where they produce the β-lactamase constitutively (105, 117). This is indicated by the presence of colonies that appear within a zone of inhibition or by the skipped-tube phenomenon in MIC tests. This reaction is not reversible, and under selective antibiotic pressure these cells multiply to significant numbers of resistant bacteria. This phenomenon may occur in vivo (14, 16) as well as in vitro.

With conventional in vitro susceptibility tests, isolates that have mutated to the resistant state should test resistant. Sometimes, however, the resistant cells are present at a low frequency and the resistance may then be difficult to detect. In contrast, isolates that have not mutated to the resistant state appear susceptible in in vitro test systems (145).

Several tests for assessing the ability of an isolate to produce inducible β-lactamases have been described. However, because virtually all isolates of the genera and species mentioned above have the potential to produce inducible β-lactamases, the β-lactamase induction test (20) has limited clinical application. Instead, physicians must understand the organisms that can produce inducible β-lactamases and the potential for therapeutic failure if certain β-lactams are used to treat infections caused by these organisms.

Tests for Extended-Spectrum β-Lactamases

The genes generally responsible for β-lactamase-mediated ampicillin resistance in *Escherichia coli* and *Klebsiella* spp. can undergo simple point mutations that result in the production of novel β-lactamases that are capable of hydrolyzing extended-spectrum cephalosporins (e.g., cefotaxime, ceftriaxone, ceftizoxime, ceftazidime) and aztreonam, as well as older β-lactam drugs. These enzymes are referred to as extended-spectrum β-lactamases (ESBLs) (53, 54, 56, 58, 77, 104) and are discussed in chapter 117. Many types of ESBLs have been noted in several gram-negative species and are associated with a variety of in vitro antimicrobial susceptibility profiles.

The in vitro susceptibility results obtained with an isolate that produces ESBLs often defy typical "hierarchy" rules of β-lactam (particularly cephalosporin) activity. Sometimes the more narrow cephalosporins (particularly the cephamycins, such as cefoxitin or cefotetan) appear to be more active than broad-spectrum agents (13). Several reports suggest that ESBL-producing isolates should be considered resistant to all extended-spectrum penicillins, cephalosporins, and monobactams even if they appear to be susceptible to these agents in vitro (37, 95, 96). The β-lactamase-stable carbapenems (e.g., imipenem and meropenem) are active in vitro (55, 56, 86) and appear to be clinically effective against ESBL producers (56, 86). The genes that code for production of ESBLs are often linked to other resistance genes, so that ESBL-producing isolates are often multiply resistant (e.g., resistant to aminoglycosides and trimethoprim-sulfamethoxazole).

Routine disk diffusion and MIC tests may not always identify isolates that produce ESBLs, and even a slight decrease in susceptibility (e.g., a slightly elevated MIC or a smaller zone) to an extended-spectrum cephalosporin or aztreonam should be a clue to the presence of an ESBL (54, 58, 64, 78, 138). NCCLS has recently specified MIC and disk diffusion screening breakpoints for aztreonam, cefotaxime, cefpodoxime, ceftazidime, and ceftriaxone that are unique for detecting ESBL-producing isolates (95, 96); however, they may also detect *E. coli* and *K. pneumoniae* with *ampC*-type (i.e., either hyperproduction of chromosomally mediated or plasmid-mediated *ampC* β-lactamase) β-lactam resistance (126). Many ESBL-producing clinical isolates have demonstrated frank resistance to ceftazidime and aztreonam, and resistance to these agents can serve as markers to identify ESBL-producing strains (56, 64, 78, 86, 95, 96).

Unlike inducible *ampC* β-lactamases, ESBLs are inhibited by β-lactamase inhibitors such as clavulanic acid, and this property has been applied to in vitro tests to identify ESBLs. In a modification of the double-disk potentiation procedure (58), test inocula are applied to agar plates as for the standard disk diffusion test (96). Then a disk containing the substrate agent (e.g., ceftazidime) is strategically placed

20 to 30 mm (center to center) from a disk containing a β-lactamase inhibitor such as amoxicillin with clavulanic acid. (For isolates that demonstrate larger zones of inhibition, the disks should be placed up to 30 mm apart; for isolates with smaller zones, the shorter distance is used.) Following overnight incubation, clearing, enhanced inhibition, or truncated zones between the disk with clavulanic acid and that with ceftazidime suggest the presence of an ESBL (58).

The MICs for ESBL-producing strains of *E. coli* and *Klebsiella* spp. are considerably lower when measured in the presence of the β-lactamase inhibitor (19, 35, 118). In the most recent NCCLS tables, along with the screening breakpoints referred to above, a suggested test for confirmation of ESBL production is given (99). For broth microdilution, cefotaxime and ceftazidime are tested with and without 4 μg of clavulanic acid per ml. A decrease in MIC of ≥3 dilutions for the agents tested alone with respect to the values obtained for the agents tested in combination with clavulanic acid confirms the presence of an ESBL. For disk diffusion, the same agents incorporated into disks with and without 10 μg of clavulanic acid are tested. An increase of ≥5 mm in zone diameter of the disks with clavulanic acid confirms the presence of ESBL. These disks are not yet available commercially. *K. pneumoniae* ATCC 700603 should be included for quality control purposes; accepted ranges are given in the current NCCLS M100 tables (99). Isolates of *E. coli* and *Klebsiella* spp. confirmed as ESBL producers should be reported as resistant to penicillins, cephalosporins (excluding cephamycins), and aztreonam (99). For screen-positive strains that do not show a clavulanic acid effect, there are insufficient data to justify modifying reports at present; these isolates should be reported as they test. If a laboratory chooses to use the screening breakpoints only, without the subsequent confirmation, the conservative approach would be to assume that the screen-positive strains are ESBL producers, although some strains may produce the *ampC*-type enzyme only.

Tests for Chloramphenicol Acetyltransferase

Chloramphenicol resistance is often mediated through the production of chloramphenicol acetyltransferase (CAT). A rapid tube test to detect CAT has been described elsewhere (3) and is also described in detail in the *Clinical Microbiology Procedures Handbook* (57). Bacteria are lysed with sodium dodecyl sulfate and EDTA. The lysate is mixed with acetyl coenzyme A (acetyl-CoA), chloramphenicol, and dithionitrobenzene (DTNB), a colorimetric indicator. If CAT is produced by the bacteria, the acetyl group of the acetyl-CoA is covalently transferred to chloramphenicol, exposing a sulfhydryl group on acetyl-CoA that reacts with the DTNB to produce a change in the lysate from colorless to yellow. A positive result indicates chloramphenicol resistance; however, a negative result is inconclusive, since other chloramphenicol resistance mechanisms exist. A conventional disk diffusion or dilution test is needed to identify the latter. The CAT test has been used for *H. influenzae* (3), *Salmonella* spp. (23), and *S. pneumoniae* (85); however, currently it is used primarily in research settings.

TESTS FOR DETECTION OF BACTERICIDAL ACTIVITIES OF ANTIMICROBIAL AGENTS

Continued new outbreaks of multidrug-resistant pathogens (9, 15, 18, 69, 70, 123) will probably increase the pressure to perform special tests for bactericidal activity as physicians prescribe both new and old antimicrobial agents, used alone and in novel combinations, for treatment of selected infections where there are no longer any standard regimens or established therapeutic guidelines. The two tests most commonly requested will be those to determine the MBC and the serum bactericidal titer (SBT).

Historically, there are several clinical situations where tests of bactericidal activity have been used for monitoring therapy. They include bacterial endocarditis (22, 48, 98, 109), meningitis (98), sepsis in immunocompromised patients (22, 98, 109), infections in those unable to mount an immune system response (31, 48, 65), osteomyelitis (48, 98, 143), chronically infected implants (48), and other types of chronic infections (48). Bactericidal tests (e.g., SBT) have also been suggested for predicting (or monitoring) therapeutic efficacy in infectious diseases lacking therapeutic guidelines (33). Despite the continued use of these tests, it is crucial for laboratory personnel to realize that there are limited scientific data to support such testing and that clinicians who order them often do so because of past training or experience. A recent assessment by MacGowan et al. again highlighted continued technical problems, as well as lack of expert consensus for interpretive criteria when reporting test results (79). This section discusses bactericidal testing in a clinical laboratory and suggests methods to be used for enhancing the reproducibility and thus the presumed reliability of bactericidal testing.

Clinical Use of Bactericidal Testing

Two basic approaches have been used. In one, the MBC is determined and compared to the estimated or measured level of drug at a site of infection in the patient. The goal of this pharmacokinetic approach is to attain, during all or part of the dosing interval, a drug concentration (in the serum or at the site of infection) that exceeds the MBC for the infecting microbe. This type of testing is especially cumbersome since procedures to measure drug concentrations as well as perform MBC testing are required. In the other approach, the SBT of a patient's serum or body fluid undergoing treatment is assessed (119, 120). The body fluid (usually serum) is serially diluted and inoculated with the patient's own infecting organism. In the SBT test, the result is expressed as a titer indicating the dilution of serum or body fluid that is lethal to the microbe; a higher number or titer indicates better activity. In contrast, with the MBC test, a lower number (the lethal concentration of the drug) is better. However, while the SBT type of testing appears to be a quicker and perhaps simpler assessment of therapeutic adequacy, technical and biologic variables make the interpretation of test results difficult (80, 81, 103).

Results of this special type of susceptibility testing in humans have demonstrated (i) that a quantitative relationship between the measured MBC and the magnitude of the SBT cannot be easily demonstrated and (ii) that neither test is highly accurate in directly predicting the clinical response. Also, application of bactericidal test results to therapy of infections other than endocarditis has not received rigorous scrutiny but is often accepted as inherently useful (62, 122). In summary, these reports show the need to improve testing methods (79, 103). While the latest approved guideline from the NCCLS proposes an interpretation scheme for the SBT test when performed by a microdilution technique (97), it is questionable whether there are sufficient data, or expert consensus, to support a standardized interpretation (4, 79, 103). Obviously, the greater the titer that can be achieved throughout the treatment dosing interval, the more likely it is that there will be a better outcome of therapy. The interpretation of this technically demanding test must take into account knowledge about the physiology of drug-organism interactions, the seriousness of the infection, and the potential effectiveness, toxicity, and cost of alternative treatment regimens.

Recommended Use of Bactericidal Testing

In the clinical laboratory, bactericidal testing (either MBC or SBT) should be offered only with expert microbiologic consultation, and any of the tests for bactericidal activity should be interpreted by someone knowledgeable about both bactericidal testing and infectious diseases. If testing is performed as an adjunct to patient care, a rigidly standardized procedure must be followed. The method described here is a combination of the NCCLS methods and that described earlier by Peterson and Shanholtzer (97, 98, 103). The differences are highlighted in Table 4.

Method

There are several basic requirements for standardization of bactericidal tests. For a detailed description of methods and definitions of terms (such as tolerance and paradoxical effect, etc.), the NCCLS documents or the review by Peterson and Shanholtzer should be consulted (97, 98, 103). The differences between the methods require brief comments. Serum additives are not recommended by the authors because of the risk of transmission of blood-borne diseases. While it is possible that the presence or absence of serum proteins in the diluent will affect the results of these tests for highly protein-bound agents such as cefazolin and ceftriaxone, there has been no demonstration that this is clinically relevant (78). The use of 4 or 5 colonies is recommended to minimize the possibility of introducing contaminants (mixed cultures), which may occur when 20 to 30 colonies are selected for the inoculum. Agitation is not recommended during the actual procedure, since any agitation presents the potential problem of removing viable bacterial cells from continued exposure to the test antimicrobial agent (49, 133). Gresser-Burns et al. used gentle mixing as one element to improve reproducibility in bactericidal testing (40). Taylor et al. demonstrated that early agitation was helpful only when a large initial inoculum volume (1.0 ml), not when a small volume ($\leq$0.1 ml), was used (133). A subculture sample size of 0.1 ml is preferred to give improved precision for the end-point determination used in the evaluation of the MBC or SBT result. Using a subculture of only 0.01 ml may not provide enough growth to demonstrate a precise 99.9% end-point reduction unless the initial inoculum approaches 10^6 CFU/ml. This is because a 3 $\log_{10}$ reduction of a starting inoculum of 1×10^5 to 5×10^5 CFU/ml results in 100 to 500 cells/ml. Sampling 0.01 ml of this will yield only 1 to 5 colonies, whereas a 0.1-ml sample provides 10 to 50 colonies. The greater number of colonies results in better precision in detecting significant changes in the numbers of colonies counted, augmenting test performance. Because of the poor reproducibility of bactericidal tests, they should be run in duplicate (103). The end-point determination with a subculture sample size of 0.1 ml is more easily made by the method of Anhalt et al. (2), since the readily available Poisson tables are based on a subculture volume of only 0.01 ml (103).

The appearance of "skipped" growth in tubes or wells makes interpretation of results difficult. When tests are performed in duplicate and one of the two sets demonstrates a skip at 24 h, the other set can be used to determine the result. If both sets show skips at 24 h, then 48-h subcultures should be performed on both sets and test results free of skipped tubes at 48 h should be used. Other result patterns, such as discrepant results (more than a 1-doubling-dilution difference) between paired tests at both 24 and 48 h, bacterial growth at high drug concentrations with none at lower concentrations, no growth in the control well or tube, and growth in the sterility well or tube, require that the entire test be repeated. The laboratory at Northwestern Memorial Hospital has performed 201 tests by this method since 1992

TABLE 4 Methods of bactericidal testing (MBC or SBT)

Test component	NCCLS document[a]	This Manual[b]
Broth medium	Mueller-Hinton with appropriate supplements	Same
pH	7.2–7.4	Same
Serum additives	Optional	Not recommended
Inoculum preparation	Growing cells from 5–30 colonies	Growing cells from 4 or 5 colonies
Inoculum density	5×10^5 CFU/ml	Same
Inoculation	Add below broth surface without agitation	Same
Incubation	35°C for 24 h (agitate macrodilution tubes and microdilution plates at 20 h)	No agitation until sampled
Micro- or macrodilution preferred	Microdilution	Either; for microdilution, run test in duplicate; if 48-h subculture is needed, microdilution requires quadruplicate testing
Subculture	Duplicate 0.01-ml samples	Single 0.1-ml sample; run test in duplicate, and do 48-h subculture if nonagreement
End point	99.9% reduction of initial inoculum by using Poisson calculated rejection values	99.9% reduction of the initial inoculum by using $n + 2\sqrt{n}$ for final end-point cutoff determination
Quality control	Described in documents	Use quality control strains with MBC tests
Interpretation	Approximated guidelines for microdilution	By consultation only; standard interpretation of results is not established

[a] See references 97 and 98.
[b] See reference 103.

and has found that only 8% of tests must be held for a 48-h incubation and another 1% must be completely repeated.

Since the SBT may be the most rapid test for laboratory monitoring of antimicrobial chemotherapy, a brief description of the method is provided. The goal of this test is to determine the dilution (titer) of a serum sample taken from a patient receiving antimicrobial agent therapy that causes at least a 3 $\log_{10}$ reduction in the number of surviving cells (compared to the initial inoculum density) following incubation (usually 18 to 24 h). Samples are best taken at the expected times of peak and/or trough concentrations of the drug(s) in the blood. In the recommended macrodilution method, a series of borosilicate glass test tubes are filled with 1.0 ml of cation-adjusted Mueller-Hinton broth (CAMHB), beginning with tube 2. Then 1.0 ml of the patient's serum is added to tubes 1 and 2, and tube 2 is mixed by vortexing. Using tube 2, 1.0 ml is removed, added to tube 3, and mixed, and the process is continued until the last tube is reached. A 1.0-ml volume is discarded from the last tube. Usually, a series of six tubes (dilutions of 1:2 through 1:64), with the test run in duplicate, is sufficient to determine a clinically relevant end point for this test. Finally, 1.0 ml of CAMHB is added to each tube, with 2.0 ml added to a growth control and to a sterility control tube, to bring the final volume in the patient sample tubes to 2.0 ml. The inoculum is then added by pipetting 100 μl of a 0.5 McFarland-standardized suspension of the patient's infecting organism into each tube except the sterility control tube by gently releasing it below the surface of the liquid in the tubes. The tubes are incubated, sampled, and read in the same manner as those for an MBC test, and the results are reported as the highest dilution or titer of the patient's serum that inhibits or kills the test organism (97). When the term "serum dilution" is used, this test theoretically can be directed against any microbe (e.g., fungi and even viruses), not just bacteria.

Other Tests To Assess Bactericidal Activity

Measuring the rate of bactericidal activity, such as with time-kill analysis, is a potentially clinically relevant replacement or adjunct for MBC testing, and some workers prefer its use (5, 67). Similarly, assessing the effects of drugs in combination is likely to be more frequently requested in the current era of emerging antimicrobial resistance in important pathogens. While procedures for the time-kill test have been described by the NCCLS and in the *Clinical Microbiology Procedures Handbook* (67, 98), it is important to remember that the same critical factors that affect the outcome of the MBC and SBT tests apply to the performance of time-kill assays.

Tests for antimicrobial agents to be given in combination may be requested for either gram-negative or gram-positive bacteria and are possibly useful for determining a potential for enhanced (synergistic) or reduced (antagonistic) effect. Whenever the activity of agents in combination is determined, it must be compared to the activity of the individual drugs. Currently, there is little reliable evidence that demonstration of in vitro synergy adds to the clinical care of most patients (68). Recent data for enterococci suggest that for any candidate drug combination considered for therapeutic use to show some type of in vitro synergism, each agent should show activity alone when tested at concentrations corresponding to those maximally clinically achievable (142). With combination therapy seemingly more prevalent as clinical practitioners attempt to either improve outcome or avoid the emergence of resistance, determination of antagonism also may be important. For example, rifampin may be considered for use in combination with antistaphylococcal penicillins or vancomycin for a synergistic effect. However, antagonism for bactericidal activity can be demonstrated in vitro and may be important clinically (146). Also, bacteriostatic agents such as chloramphenicol can be antagonistic to the action of aminoglycosides when they are combined for treatment of gram-negative bacilli (21). Therefore, it is prudent to assess nonstandard combinations by a test of synergy when they are considered for use in patients (149).

Correlation of other tests such as time-kill assays with more traditional assessments of bactericidal activity and clinical outcome of infectious disease therapy continues to be controversial. We are unaware that any prospective, controlled clinical comparison of these tests with therapeutic outcome has been done. Several other approaches to bactericidal analysis of antimicrobial activity also have been suggested and reviewed (103). Less is known about the variables that might influence the performance of any of these newer tests than for the more traditional MBC or SBT test, and, again, none of these tests has been evaluated prospectively in any clinical investigation. Until such evaluations are done and interpretative guidelines are established, it is difficult to recommend the use of any tests other than the MBC or SBT tests in a routine clinical laboratory setting.

REFERENCES

1. **Anhalt, J. P., and R. Nelson.** 1982. Failure of PADAC test strips to detect staphylococcal β-lactamase. *Antimicrob. Agents Chemother.* **21:**983–984.
2. **Anhalt, J. P., L. D. Sabath, and A. L. Barry.** 1980. Special tests: bactericidal activity, activity of antimicrobics in combination, and detection of beta-lactamase production, p. 478–481. *In* E. H. Lennette, A. Balows, and W. J. Hausler, Jr. (ed.), *Manual of Clinical Microbiology*. American Society for Microbiology, Washington, D.C.
3. **Azemun, P., T. Stull, M. Roberts, and A. L. Smith.** 1981. Rapid detection of chloramphenicol resistance in *Haemophilus influenzae*. *Antimicrob. Agents Chemother.* **20:** 168–170.
4. **Baron, E. J., L. R. Peterson, and S. M. Finegold.** 1994. *Bailey and Scott's Diagnostic Microbiology*. The C. V. Mosby Co., St. Louis, Mo.
5. **Cappelletty, D. M., and M. J. Rybak.** 1996. Comparison of methodologies for synergism testing of drug combinations against resistant strains of *Pseudomonas aeruginosa*. *Antimicrob. Agents Chemother.* **40:**677–683.
6. **Cartwright, C. P., F. Stock, G. A. Fahle, and V. J. Gill.** 1995. Comparison of pigment production and motility tests with PCR for reliable identification of intrinsically vancomycin-resistant enterococci. *J. Clin. Microbiol.* **33:** 1931–1933.
7. **Catlin, B. W.** 1975. Iodometric detection of *Haemophilus influenzae* beta-lactamase: rapid, presumptive test for ampicillin resistance. *Antimicrob. Agents Chemother.* **7:** 265–270.
8. **Centers for Disease Control and Prevention.** 1997. Reduced susceptibility of *Staphylococcus aureus* to vancomycin—Japan, 1996. *Morbid. Mortal. Weekly Rep.* **46:** 765–766.
9. **Centers for Disease Control and Prevention.** 1997. Update: *Staphylococcus aureus* with reduced susceptibility to vancomycin—United States, 1997. *Morbid. Mortal. Weekly Rep.* **46:**813–815.
10. **Chambers, H. F.** 1997. Methicillin resistance in staphylococci: molecular and biochemical basis and clinical implications. *Clin. Microbiol. Rev.* **10:**781–791.

11. **Chambers, H. F., G. Archer, and M. Matsuhashi.** 1990. Low-level methicillin resistance in *Staphylococcus aureus*. *Antimicrob. Agents Chemother.* **33:**424–428.
12. **Chambers, H. F., and C. J. Hackbarth.** 1992. Methicillin-resistant *Staphylococcus aureus*: genetics and mechanisms of resistance, p. 21–35. *In* M. T. Cafferkey (ed.), *Methicillin-Resistant Staphylococcus aureus: Clinical Management and Laboratory Aspects*. Marcel Dekker, Inc., New York, N.Y.
13. **Chanal-Claris, C., D. Sirot, L. Bret, P. Chatron, R. Labia, and J. Sirot.** 1997. Novel extended-spectrum TEM-type β-lactamase from an *Escherichia coli* isolate resistant to ceftazidime and susceptible to cephalothin. *Antimicrob. Agents Chemother.* **41:**715–716.
14. **Chow, J. W., M. J. Fine, D. M. Shlaes, J. P. Quinn, D. C. Hooper, M. P. Johnson, R. Ramphal, M. M. Wagener, D. K. Miyashiro, and V. L. Yu.** 1991. *Enterobacter* bacteremia: clinical features and emergence of antibiotic resistance during therapy. *Ann. Intern. Med.* **115:**585–590.
15. **Chow, J. W., A. Kuritza, D. M. Shlaes, M. Green, D. F. Sahm, and M. J. Zervos.** 1993. Clonal spread of vancomycin-resistant *Enterococcus faecium* between patients in three hospitals in two states. *J. Clin. Microbiol.* **31:**1609–1611.
16. **Chow, J. W., V. L. Yu, and D. M. Shlaes.** 1994. Epidemiologic perspectives on *Enterobacter* for the infection control professional. *Am. J. Infect. Control.* **22:**195–201.
17. **Clark, N. C., R. C. Cooksey, B. C. Hill, J. M. Swenson, and F. C. Tenover.** 1993. Characterization of glycopeptide-resistant enterococci from U.S. hospitals. *Antimicrob. Agents Chemother.* **37:**2311–2317.
18. **Cohen, M. L.** 1992. Epidemiology of drug resistance: implications for a post-antimicrobial era. *Science* **257:** 1050–1055.
19. **Cormican, M. G., S. A. Marshall, and R. N. Jones.** 1996. Detection of extended-spectrum β-lactamase (ESBL)-producing strains by the Etest ESBL screen. *J. Clin. Microbiol.* **34:**1880–1884.
20. **Cox, V.** 1992. β-Lactamase induction test for gram-negative bacilli, p. 5.7.1–5.7.6. *In* H. D. Isenberg (ed.), *Clinical Microbiology Procedures Handbook*. American Society for Microbiology, Washington, D.C.
21. **D'Alessandri, R. M., D. J. McNeely, and R. M. Kluge.** 1998. Antibiotic synergy and antagonism against clinical isolates of *Klebsiella* species. *Antimicrob. Agents Chemother.* **10:**889–892.
22. **DeGirolami, P. C., and G. Eliopoulos.** 1987. Antimicrobial susceptibility tests and their role in therapeutic drug monitoring. *Clin. Lab. Med.* **7:**499–513.
23. **de la Maza, L., S. I. Miller, and M. J. Ferraro.** 1990. Use of commercially available rapid chloramphenicol acetyltransferase test to detect resistance in *Salmonella* spp. *J. Clin. Microbiol.* **28:**1867–1869.
24. **De Lencastre, H., S. A. Figueiredo, C. Urban, J. Rahal, and A. Tomasz.** 1991. Multiple mechanisms of methicillin resistance and improved methods for detection in clinical isolates of *Staphylococcus aureus*. *Antimicrob. Agents Chemother.* **35:**632–639.
25. **Dixon, J. M., A. E. Lipinski, and M. E. Graham.** 1977. Detection and prevalence of pneumococci with increased resistance to penicillin. *Can. Med. Assoc. J.* **117:** 1159–1161.
26. **Doern, G., R. N. Jones, E. H. Gerlach, J. A. Washington II, D. J. Biedenbach, A. Brueggemann, M. E. Erwin, C. Knapp, and J. Raymond.** 1995. Multicenter clinical laboratory evaluation of a β-lactamase disk assay employing a novel chromogenic cephalosporin. *J. Clin. Microbiol.* **33:** 1665–1667.
27. **Doern, G. V., A. Brueggemann, and G. Pierce.** 1997. Assessment of the oxacillin disk screening test for determining penicillin resistance in *Streptococcus pneumoniae*. *Eur. J. Clin. Microbiol. Infect. Dis.* **16:**311–314.
28. **Doern, G. V., A. R. Brueggemann, G. Pierce, H. P. J. Holley, and A. Rauch.** 1997. Antibiotic resistance among clinical isolates of *Haemophilus influenzae* in the United States in 1994 and 1995 and detection of β-lactamase positive strains resistant to amoxicillin-clavulanate: results of a national multicenter surveillance study. *Antimicrob. Agents Chemother.* **41:**292–297.
29. **Dyke, J. W., W. J. Brown, J. M. Morris, C. L. Pierson, and E. M. Peters.** 1994. Evaluation of the new DrySlide beta-lactamase test. *Am. J. Clin. Pathol.* **101:**726–728.
30. **Dyke, K. G.** 1979. Beta-lactamases of *Staphylococcus aureus*, p. 291–310. *In* J. M. Hamilton-Miller (ed.), *Beta-Lactamases*. Academic Press, Ltd., London, England.
31. **Eliopoulos, G. M., and R. C. Moellering, Jr.** 1982. Principles of antibiotic therapy. *Med. Clin. North Am.* **66:**3–15.
32. **Escamilla, J.** 1976. Susceptibility of *Haemophilus influenzae* to ampicillin as determined by use of a modified one-minute beta-lactamase test. *Antimicrob. Agents Chemother.* **9:** 196–198.
33. **Fasching, C. E., D. N. Gerding, and L. R. Peterson.** 1987. Treatment of ciprofloxacin- and ceftizoxime-induced resistant gram-negative bacilli. *Am. J. Med.* **82**(Suppl. 4A): 80–86.
34. **Fontana, R., P. Canepari, M. M. Lleo, and G. Satta.** 1992. Mechanisms of resistance of enterococci to beta-lactam antibiotics. *Eur. J. Clin. Microbiol. Infect. Dis.* **9:**103–105.
35. **Fournier, B., P. H. Lagrange, and A. Philippon.** 1996. In vitro susceptibility of *Klebsiella oxytoca* strains to 13 β-lactams in the presence and absence of β-lactamase inhibitors. *J. Antimicrob. Chemother.* **37:**931–942.
36. **Free, L., and D. Sahm.** 1995. Investigation of the reformulated Remel Synergy Quad plate for detection of high-level aminoglycoside and vancomycin resistance in enterococci. *J. Clin. Microbiol.* **33:**1643–1645.
37. **Gold, H. S., and R. C. Moellering, Jr.** 1996. Antimicrobial-drug resistance. *N. Engl. J. Med.* **355:**1445–1453.
38. **Gordon, S., J. M. Swenson, B. C. Hill, N. E. Pigott, R. R. Facklam, R. C. Cooksey, C. Thornsberry, The Enterococcal Study Group, W. R. Jarvis, and F. C. Tenover.** 1992. Antimicrobial susceptibility patterns of common and unusual species of enterococci causing infections in the United States. *J. Clin. Microbiol.* **30:**2373–2378.
39. **Grayson, M. L., G. M. Eliopoulos, C. B. Wennersten, K. L. Ruoff, P. C. De Girolami, M. J. Ferraro, and R. C. Moellering, Jr.** 1991. Increasing resistance to beta-lactam antibiotics among clinical isolates of *Enterococcus faecium*: a 22-year review at one institution. *Antimicrob. Agents Chemother.* **35:**2180–2184.
40. **Gresser-Burns, M. E., C. J. Shanholtzer, L. R. Peterson, and D. N. Gerding.** 1987. Occurrence and reproducibility of the "skip" phenomenon in bactericidal testing of *Staphylococcus aureus*. *Diagn. Microbiol. Infect. Dis.* **6:**335–342.
41. **Hackbarth, C. J., and H. F. Chambers.** 1989. Methicillin-resistant staphylococci: genetics and mechanisms of resistance. *Antimicrob. Agents Chemother.* **33:**991–994.
42. **Hartman, B. J., and A. Tomasz.** 1986. Expression of methicillin resistance in heterogeneous strains of *Staphylococcus aureus*. *Antimicrob. Agents Chemother.* **29:**85–92.
43. **Hindler, J. A.** 1997. Antimicrobial susceptibility tests, p. 205–254. *In* H. D. Isenberg (ed.), *Essential Procedures in Clinical Microbiology*. American Society for Microbiology, Washington, D.C.
44. **Hindler, J. A., and C. B. Inderlied.** 1985. Effect of source of Mueller-Hinton agar and resistance frequency on the detection of methicillin-resistant *Staphylococcus aureus*. *J. Clin. Microbiol.* **21:**205–210.
45. **Hindler, J. A., and D. F. Sahm.** 1992. Controversies and

confusion regarding antimicrobial susceptibility testing of enterococci. *Antimicrob. Newsl.* **8:**65–74.

46. **Hindler, J. A., and N. L. Warner.** 1984. Effect of source of Mueller-Hinton agar on detection of oxacillin resistance in *Staphylococcus aureus* using a screening methodology. *J. Clin. Microbiol.* **25:**734–735.
47. **Hiramatsu, K., H. Hanaki, T. Ino, K. Yabuta, T. Oguri, and F. C. Tenover.** 1997. Methicillin-resistant *Staphylococcus aureus* clinical strain with reduced vancomycin susceptibility. *J. Antimicrob. Chemother.* **40:**135–136.
48. **Isenberg, H. D.** 1988. Antimicrobial susceptibility testing: a critical evaluation. *J. Antimicrob. Chemother.* **22**(Suppl. A)**:**73–86.
49. **Ishida, K., P. A. Guze, G. M. Kalmanson, K. Albrandt, and L. B. Guze.** 1982. Variables in demonstrating methicillin tolerance in *Staphylococcus aureus* strains. *Antimicrob. Agents Chemother.* **212:**688–690.
50. **Iwen, P. C., D. M. Kelley, J. Linder, and S. H. Hinrichs.** 1996. Revised approach for identification and detection of ampicillin and vancomycin resistance in *Enterococcus* species by using MicroScan panels. *J. Clin. Microbiol.* **34:** 1779–1783.
51. **Jacobs, M. R., H. J. Koornhof, R. M. Robins-Browne, C. M. Stevenson, Z. A. Vermaak, I. Freiman, G. B. Miller, M. A. Witcomb, M. Isaäcson, J. I. Ward, and R. Austrian.** 1978. Emergence of multiply resistant pneumococci. *N. Engl. J. Med.* **299:**735–740.
52. **Jacobs, M. R., S. K. Spangler, and P. C. Appelbaum.** 1992. β-Lactamase production and susceptibility of U.S. and European anaerobic gram negative bacilli to β-lactams and other agents. *Eur. J. Clin. Microbiol. Infect. Dis.* **11:** 1081–1093.
53. **Jacoby, G. A., and I. Carreras.** 1990. Activities of β-lactam antibiotics against *Escherichia coli* strains producing extended-spectrum β-lactamases. *Antimicrob. Agents Chemother.* **34:**858–862.
54. **Jacoby, G. A., and P. Han.** 1996. Detection of extended-spectrum β-lactamases in clinical isolates of *Klebsiella pneumoniae* and *Escherichia coli*. *J. Clin. Microbiol.* **34:**908–911.
55. **Jacoby, G. A., P. Han, and J. Tran.** 1997. Comparative in vitro activities of carbapenem L-749,345 and other antimicrobials against multiresistant gram-negative clinical pathogens. *Antimicrob. Agents Chemother.* **41:**1830–1831.
56. **Jacoby, G. A., and A. A. Medeiros.** 1991. More extended-spectrum β-lactamases. *Antimicrob. Agents Chemother.* **35:** 1697–1704.
57. **Jankins, M.** 1992. Chloramphenicol acetyltransferase test, p. 5.8.1–5.8.7. *In* H. D. Isenberg (ed.), *Clinical Microbiology Procedures Handbook.* American Society for Microbiology, Washington, D.C.
58. **Jarlier, V., M. H. Nicolas, G. Fournier, and A. Philippon.** 1988. Extended broad-spectrum β-lactamases conferring transferable resistance to newer β-lactam agents in Enterobacteriaceae: hospital prevalence and susceptibility patterns. *Rev. Infect. Dis.* **10:**867–878.
59. **Jett, B., L. Free, and D. F. Sahm.** 1996. Factors influencing the Vitek gram-positive susceptibility system's detection of *vanB*-encoded vancomycin resistance among enterococci. *J. Clin. Microbiol.* **34:**701–706.
60. **Jones, R. N., D. C. Edson, and CAP Microbiology Resource Committee of the College of American Pathologists.** 1991. Antimicrobial susceptibility testing trends and accuracy in the United States. *Arch. Pathol. Lab. Med.* **115:**429–436.
61. **Jones, R. N., M. R. Jacobs, J. A. Washington II, and M. A. Pfaller.** 1997. A 1994–1995 survey of *Haemophilus influenzae* susceptibility to ten orally administered agents: a 187 clinical laboratory center sample in the United States. *Diagn. Microbiol. Infect. Dis.* **27:**75–83.
62. **Jordan, G. W., and M. M. Kawachi.** 1981. Analysis of serum bactericidal activity in endocarditis, osteomyelitis, and other bacterial infections. *Medicine* **60:**49–61.
63. **Jorgensen, J. H., M. L. McElmeel, and C. W. Trippy.** 1996. Comparison of inoculation methods for testing enterococci by using vancomycin screening agar. *J. Clin. Microbiol.* **34:**2841–2842.
64. **Katsanis, G. P., J. Spargo, M. J. Ferraro, L. Sutton, and G. A. Jacoby.** 1994. Detection of *Klebsiella pneumoniae* and *Escherichia coli* strains producing extended-spectrum β-lactamases. *J. Clin. Microbiol.* **32:**691–696.
65. **Kiehn, T. E., P. D. Ellner, and D. Budzko.** 1989. Role of the microbiology laboratory in care of the immunosuppressed patient. *Rev. Infect. Dis.* **11**(Suppl. 7)**:**S1706–S1710.
66. **Knapp, C., M. D. Ludwig, J. A. Washington II, and H. R. Chambers.** 1996. Evaluation of the Vitek GPS-SA card for testing of oxacillin against borderline-susceptible staphylococci that lack *mec*. *J. Clin. Microbiol.* **34:**1603–1605.
67. **Knapp, C., and J. A. Moody.** 1992. Tests to assess bactericidal activity, p. 5.16.1–5.16.33. *In* H. D. Isenberg (ed.), *Clinical Microbiology Procedures Handbook.* American Society for Microbiology, Washington, D.C.
68. **Krogstad, D. J., and R. C. Moellering, Jr.** 1998. Antimicrobial combinations, p. 537–599. *In* V. Lorian (ed.), *Antibiotics in Laboratory Medicine.* The Williams & Wilkins Co., Baltimore, Md.
69. **Kunin, C. M.** 1993. Resistance to antimicrobial drugs—a worldwide calamity. *Ann. Intern. Med.* **118:**557–561.
70. **Landman, D., and J. M. Quale.** 1997. Management of infections due to resistant enterococci: a review of therapeutic options. *J. Antimicrob. Chemother.* **40:**161–170.
71. **Leclercq, R., and P. Courvalin.** 1997. Resistance to glycopeptides in enterococci. *Clin. Infect. Dis.* **24:**545–556.
72. **Leclercq, R., S. Dutka-Malen, A. Brisson-Noel, C. Molinas, E. Derlot, M. Arthur, J. Duval, and P. Courvalin.** 1992. Resistance of enterococci to aminoglycosides and glycopeptides. *Clin. Infect. Dis.* **15:**495–501.
73. **Leclercq, R., S. Dutka-Malen, J. Duval, and P. Courvalin.** 1992. Vancomycin resistance gene *vanC* is specific to *Enterococcus gallinarum*. *Antimicrob. Agents Chemother.* **36:**2005–2008.
74. **Lee, W. W., and L. Komary.** 1976. New method for detecting in vitro inactivation of penicillins by *Haemophilus influenzae*. *Antimicrob. Agents Chemother.* **10:**654–656.
75. **Leitch, C., and S. Boonlayangoor.** 1992. Tests to detect oxacillin (methicillin)-resistant staphylococci with an oxacillin screen plate, p. 5.5.1–5.5.7. *In* H. D. Isenberg (ed.), *Clinical Microbiology Procedures Handbook.* American Society for Microbiology, Washington, D.C.
76. **Leitch, C., and S. Boonlayangoor.** 1992. β-Lactamase tests, p. 5.3.1–5.3.8. *In* H. D. Isenberg (ed.), *Clinical Microbiology Procedures Handbook.* American Society for Microbiology, Washington, D.C.
77. **Livermore, D. M.** 1995. β-Lactamases in laboratory and clinical resistance. *Clin. Microbiol. Rev.* **8:**557–584.
78. **Livermore, D. M., and M. Yuan.** 1996. Antibiotic resistance and production of extended-spectrum β-lactamases amongst *Klebsiella* spp. from intensive care units. *J. Antimicrob. Chemother.* **38:**409–424.
79. **MacGowan, A., C. McMullin, P. James, K. Bowker, D. Reeves, and L. White.** 1997. External quality assessment of the serum bactericidal test: results of a methodology/interpretation questionnaire. *J. Antimicrob. Chemother.* **39:**277–284.
80. **Mackowiak, P. A., M. Marling-Cason, and R. L. Cohen.** 1982. Effects of temperature on antimicrobial susceptibility of bacteria. *J. Infect. Dis.* **145:**550–553.

81. **MacLowry, J. D.** 1989. Perspective. The serum dilution test. *J. Infect. Dis.* **160:**624–626.
82. **Marshall, S. A., W. W. Wilke, M. A. Pfaller, and R. N. Jones.** 1998. *Staphylococcus aureus* and coagulase-negative staphylococci from blood stream infections: frequency of occurrence, antimicrobial susceptibility, and molecular (*mecA*) characterization of oxacillin resistance in the SCOPE program. *Diagn. Microbiol. Infect. Dis.* **30:** 205–214.
83. **Massanari, R. M., M. A. Pfaller, D. S. Wakesfield, G. T. Hammons, L. A. McNut, R. F. Woolson, and C. M. Helms.** 1988. Implications of acquired oxacillin resistance in management and control of *Staphylococcus aureus* infections. *J. Infect. Dis.* **158:**701–709.
84. **Massidda, O., M. P. Montanari, M. Mingoia, and P. E. Varaldo.** 1996. Borderline methicillin-susceptible *Staphylococcus aureus* strains that have more in common than reduced susceptibility to penicillinase-resistant penicillins. *Antimicrob. Agents Chemother.* **26:**2387–2390.
85. **Matthews, H. W., C. N. Baker, and C. Thornsberry.** 1988. Relationship between in vitro susceptibility test results for chloramphenicol and production of chloramphenicol acetyltransferase by *Haemophilus influenzae*, *Streptococcus pneumoniae*, and *Aerococcus* species. *J. Clin. Microbiol.* **26:**2387–2390.
86. **Meyer, K. S., O. C. Urban, J. A. Eagan, B. J. Berger, and J. J. Rahal.** 1993. Nosocomial outbreak of *Klebsiella* infection resistant to late-generation cephalosporins. *Ann. Intern. Med.* **119:**353–358.
87. **Moellering, R. C., Jr., O. M. Koraeniowski, M. A. Sande, and C. B. Wennersten.** 1979. Species-specific resistance to antimicrobial synergism in *Streptococcus faecium* and *Streptococcus faecalis*. *J. Infect. Dis.* **140:**203–208.
88. **Montanari, M. P., O. Massidda, M. Mingoia, and P. E. Varalco.** 1996. Borderline susceptibility to methicillin in *Staphylococcus aureus*: a new mechanism of resistance? *Microb. Drug Res.* **2:**257–260.
89. **Murray, B. E.** 1990. The life and times of the enterococcus. *Clin. Microbiol. Rev.* **3:**46–65.
90. **Murray, B. E.** 1992. *β*-Lactamase-producing enterococci. *Antimicrob. Agents Chemother.* **36:**2355–2359.
91. **Murray, B. E.** 1997. Vancomycin-resistant enterococci. *Am. J. Med.* **102:**284–293.
92. **National Committee for Clinical Laboratory Standards.** 1993. *Methods for Dilution Antimicrobial Susceptibility Tests for Bacteria That Grow Aerobically.* Approved standard M7-A3. National Committee for Clinical Laboratory Standards, Villanova, Pa.
93. **National Committee for Clinical Laboratory Standards.** 1993. *Performance Standards for Antimicrobial Disk Susceptibility Tests.* Approved standard M2-A5. National Committee for Clinical Laboratory Standards, Villanova, Pa.
94. **National Committee for Clinical Laboratory Standards.** 1997. *Methods for Antimicrobial Susceptibility Testing of Anaerobic Bacteria.* Approved standard M11-A4. National Committee for Clinical Laboratory Standards, Wayne, Pa.
95. **National Committee for Clinical Laboratory Standards.** 1997. *Methods for Dilution Antimicrobial Susceptibility Tests for Bacteria That Grow Aerobically*, 4th ed., Approved standard M7-A4. National Committee for Clinical Laboratory Standards, Wayne, Pa.
96. **National Committee for Clinical Laboratory Standards.** 1997. *Performance Standards for Antimicrobial Disk Susceptibility Tests*, 6th ed. Approved standard M2-A6. National Committee for Clinical Laboratory Standards, Wayne, Pa.
97. **National Committee for Clinical Laboratory Standards.** 1998. *Methodology for the Serum Bactericidal Test.* Document M21-A. National Committee for Clinical Laboratory Standards, Wayne, Pa.
98. **National Committee for Clinical Laboratory Standards.** 1998. *Methods for Determining Bactericidal Activity of Antimicrobial Agents.* Document M26-A. National Committee for Clinical Laboratory Standards, Wayne, Pa.
99. **National Committee for Clinical Laboratory Standards.** 1999. *Performance Standards for Antimicrobial Susceptibility Testing.* Ninth informational supplement, M100-S9. National Committee for Clinical Laboratory Standards, Wayne, Pa.
100. **Neumann, M. A., D. F. Sahm, C. Thornsberry, and J. E. McGowan, Jr.** 1991. *Cumitech 6A, New Developments in Antimicrobial Agent Susceptibility Testing: a Practical Guide.* Coordinating ed., J. E. McGowan, Jr. American Society for Microbiology, Washington, D.C.
101. **O'Callaghan, C. H., A. Morris, S. M. Kirby, and A. H. Shingler.** 1972. Novel method for detection of *β*-lactamase by using a chromogenic cephalosporin substrate. *Antimicrob. Agents Chemother.* **1:**283–288.
102. **Pefanis, A., C. Thauvin-Eliopoulos, G. Eliopoulos, and R. C. Moellering, Jr.** 1993. Activity of ampicillin-sulbactam and oxacillin in experimental endocarditis caused by *β*-lactamase-hyperproducing *Staphylococcus aureus*. *Antimicrob. Agents Chemother.* **37:**507–511.
103. **Peterson, L. R., and C. J. Shanholtzer.** 1992. Tests for bactericidal effects of antimicrobial agents: technical performance and clinical relevance. *Clin. Microbiol. Rev.* **5:** 420–432.
104. **Philippon, A., R. Labia, and G. Jacoby.** 1989. Extended-spectrum *β*-lactamases. *Antimicrob. Agents Chemother.* **33:**1131–1136.
105. **Pitout, J. D., E. S. Moland, C. C. Sanders, K. S. Thomson, and S. R. Fitzsimmons.** 1997. *β*-Lactamases and detection of *β*-lactam resistance in *Enterobacter* spp. *Antimicrob. Agents Chemother.* **41:**35–39.
106. **Resende, C. A., and A. M. Figueiredo.** 1997. Discrimination of methicillin-resistant *Staphylococcus aureus* from borderline-resistant and susceptible isolates by different methods. *J. Med. Microbiol.* **46:**145–149.
107. **Rittenhouse, S. F., L. Miller, R. L. Kaplan, and G. H. Mosely.** 1995. A survey of *β*-lactamase producing *Haemophilus influenzae*. An evaluation of 5750 isolates. *Diagn. Microbiol. Infect. Dis.* **21:**223–225.
108. **Rosenberg, J., F. C. Tenover, J. Wong, W. Jarvis, and D. J. Vugia.** 1997. Are clinical laboratories in California accurately reporting vancomycin-resistant enterococci? *J. Clin. Microbiol.* **35:**2526–2530.
109. **Rosenblatt, J. E.** 1987. Laboratory tests used to guide antimicrobial therapy. *Mayo Clin. Proc.* **62:**799–805.
110. **Sabath, L.** 1977. Chemical and physical factors influencing methicillin resistance of *Staphylococcus aureus* and *Staphylococcus epidermidis*. *J. Antimicrob. Chemother.* **3:** 47–51.
111. **Sahm, D. F.** 1994. Streptococci and staphylococci: laboratory considerations for in vitro susceptibility testing. *Clin. Microbiol. Newsl.* **16:**9–14.
112. **Sahm, D. F., S. Boonlayangoor, P. C. Iwen, J. L. Baade, and G. L. Woods.** 1991. Factors influencing determination of high-level aminoglycoside resistance in *Enterococcus faecalis*. *J. Clin. Microbiol.* **29:**1934–1939.
113. **Sahm, D. F., S. Boonlayangoor, and J. E. Schulz.** 1991. Detection of high-level aminoglycoside resistance in enterococci other than *Enterococcus faecalis*. *J. Clin. Microbiol.* **29:**2595–2598.
114. **Sahm, D. F., J. Kissinger, M. S. Gilmore, P. R. Murray, R. Mulder, J. Solliday, and B. Clarke.** 1989. In vitro susceptibility studies of vancomycin-resistant *Enterococcus faecalis*. *Antimicrob. Agents Chemother.* **33:** 1588–1591.
115. **Sahm, D. F., and L. Olsen.** 1990. In vitro detection of

enterococcal vancomycin resistance. *Antimicrob. Agents Chemother.* **34:**1846–1848.

116. **Sahm, D. F., and C. Torres.** 1988. Effects of medium and inoculum variations on screening for high-level aminoglycoside resistance in *Enterococcus faecalis*. *J. Clin. Microbiol.* **26:**250–256.
117. **Sanders, C. C.** 1992. β-Lactamases of gram-negative bacteria: new challenges for new drugs. *Clin. Infect. Dis.* **14:** 1089–1099.
118. **Sanders, C. C., A. L. Barry, J. A. Washington II, C. Shubert, E. S. Moland, M. M. Traczewski, C. Knapp, and R. Mulder.** 1996. Detection of extended-spectrum β-lactamase-producing members of the family *Enterobacteriaceae* with the Vitek ESBL test. *J. Clin. Microbiol.* **34:** 2997–3001.
119. **Schlichter, J. G., and H. MacLean.** 1947. A method for determining the effective therapeutic level in the treatment of subacute bacterial endocarditis with penicillin: a preliminary report. *Am. Heart J.* **34:**209–211.
120. **Schlichter, J. G., H. MacLean, and A. Milzer.** 1949. Effective penicillin therapy in subacute bacterial endocarditis and other chronic infections. *Am. J. Med. Sci.* **217:** 600–608.
121. **Schulz, J. E., and D. F. Sahm.** 1993. Reliability of the E test for detection of ampicillin, vancomycin, and high-level aminoglycoside resistance in *Enterococcus* spp. *J. Clin. Microbiol.* **31:**3336–3339.
122. **Sculier, J. P., and J. Klastersky.** 1984. Significance of serum bactericidal activity in gram-negative bacillary bacteremia in patients with and without granulocytopenia. *Am. J. Med.* **76:**429–435.
123. **Silver, L. L., and K. A. Bostian.** 1993. Discovery and development of new antibiotics: the problem of antibiotic resistance. *Antimicrob. Agents Chemother.* **37:**377–383.
124. **Standiford, H. D., J. B. deMaine, and W. M. Kirby.** 1970. Antibiotic synergism of enterococci. *Arch. Intern. Med.* **126:**255–259.
125. **Sutton, L., D. J. Biedenbach, A. Yen, and R. N. Jones.** 1995. Development, characterization, and initial evaluations of S1: a new chromogenic cephalosporin for β-lactamase detection. *Diagn. Microbiol. Infect. Dis.* **21:**1–8.
126. **Swenson, J. M.** 1997. Unpublished results.
127. **Swenson, J. M., N. Clark, M. J. Ferraro, D. F. Sahm, G. Doern, M. A. Pfaller, L. B. Reller, M. P. Weinstein, R. J. Zabransky, and F. C. Tenover.** 1994. Development of a standardized screening method for detection of vancomycin-resistant enterococci. *J. Clin. Microbiol.* **32:** 1700–1704.
128. **Swenson, J. M., N. C. Clark, D. F. Sahm, M. J. Ferraro, G. Doern, J. Hindler, J. H. Jorgensen, M. A. Pfaller, L. B. Reller, M. P. Weinstein, R. J. Zabransky, and F. C. Tenover.** 1995. Molecular characterization and multilaboratory evaluation of *Enterococcus faecalis* ATCC 51299 and quality control of screening tests for vancomycin and high-level aminoglycoside resistance in enterococci. *J. Clin. Microbiol.* **33:**3019–3021.
129. **Swenson, J. M., M. J. Ferraro, D. Sahm, N. C. Clark, D. Culver, F. C. Tenover, and The National Committee for Clinical Laboratory Standards Working Group on Enterococci.** 1995. Multilaboratory evaluation of screening methods for detection of high-level aminoglycoside resistance in enterococci. *J. Clin. Microbiol.* **33:** 3008–3018.
130. **Swenson, J. M., M. J. Ferraro, D. F. Sahm, P. Charache, The National Committee for Clinical Laboratory Standards Working Group on Enterococci, and F. C. Tenover.** 1992. New vancomycin disk diffusion breakpoints for enterococci. *J. Clin. Microbiol.* **30:**2525–2528.
131. **Swenson, J. M., B. C. Hill, and C. Thornsberry.** 1986. Screening pneumococci for penicillin resistance. *J. Clin. Microbiol.* **24:**749–752.
132. **Swenson, J. M., B. C. Hill, and C. Thornsberry.** 1989. Problems with the disk diffusion test for detection of vancomycin resistance in enterococci. *J. Clin. Microbiol.* **27:** 2140–2142. (Erratum, **28:**403, 1990.)
133. **Taylor, P. C., F. D. Schoenknecht, J. C. Sherris, and E. C. Linner.** 1983. Determination of minimum bactericidal concentrations of oxacillin for *Staphylococcus aureus*: influence and significance of technical factors. *Antimicrob. Agents Chemother.* **23:**142–150.
134. **Tenover, F. C., M. V. Lancaster, B. C. Hill, C. D. Steward, S. A. Stocker, G. A. Hancock, C. M. O'Hara, N. C. Clark, and K. Hiramatsu.** 1998. Characterization of staphylococci with reduced susceptibility to vancomycin and other glycopeptides. *J. Clin. Microbiol.* **36:** 1020–1027.
135. **Tenover, F. C., J. M. Swenson, C. M. O'Hara, and S. A. Stocker.** 1995. Ability of commercial and reference antimicrobial susceptibility testing methods to detect vancomycin resistance in enterococci. *J. Clin. Microbiol.* **33:**1524–1527.
136. **Tenover, F. C., J. Tokars, J. Swenson, S. Paul, K. Spitalny, and W. Jarvis.** 1993. Ability of clinical laboratories to detect antimicrobial agent-resistant enterococci. *J. Clin. Microbiol.* **31:**1695–1699.
137. **Thauvin-Eliopoulos, E., L. B. Rice, G. M. Eliopoulos, and R. C. Moellering, Jr.** 1990. Efficacy of oxacillin and ampicillin-sulbactam combination in experimental endocarditis caused by β-lactamase-hyperproducing *Staphylococcus aureus*. *Antimicrob. Agents Chemother.* **34:** 728–732.
138. **Thomson, K. S., and C. C. Sanders.** 1992. Detection of extended-spectrum β-lactamases in members of the family *Enterobacteriaceae*: comparison of the double-disk and three-dimensional tests. *Antimicrob. Agents Chemother.* **36:**1877–1882.
139. **Thornsberry, C., and L. K. McDougal.** 1983. Successful use of broth microdilution in susceptibility tests for methicillin-resistant (heteroresistant) staphylococci. *J. Clin. Microbiol.* **18:**1084–1091.
140. **Tomasz, A., S. Nachman, and H. Leaf.** 1991. Stable classes of phenotypic expression in methicillin-resistant clinical isolates of staphylococci. *Antimicrob. Agents Chemother.* **35:**124–129.
141. **Torres, C., C. Tenorio, M. Lantero, M. Gastañares, and F. Baquero.** 1993. High-level penicillin resistance and penicillin-gentamicin synergy in *Enterococcus faecium*. *Antimicrob. Agents Chemother.* **37:**2427–2431.
142. **Tripodi, M. F., R. Utili, A. Rambaldi, A. Locatell, P. Rosario, A. Florio, and G. Guggiero.** 1996. Unorthodox antibiotic combinations including ciprofloxacin against high-level gentamicin resistant enterococci. *J. Antimicrob. Chemother.* **37:**727–736.
143. **Tubbs, R. R.** 1997. Insuring effective antimicrobial therapy: laboratory evaluation. *J. Am. Osteopath. Assoc.* **76:** 617–624.
144. **Van Horn, K. G., C. A. Gedris, K. M. Rodney, and J. B. Mitchell.** 1996. Evaluation of commercial vancomycin agar screen plates for detection of vancomycin-resistant enterococci. *J. Clin. Microbiol.* **34:**2042–2044.
145. **Washington, J. A., II, C. C. Knapp, and C. C. Sanders.** 1988. Accuracy of microdilution and the Automicrobic system in detection of β-lactam resistance in gram-negative bacterial mutants with derepressed β-lactamases. *Rev. Infect. Dis.* **10:**824–829.
146. **Watanakunakorn, C., and J. C. Guerriero.** 1981. Inter-

action between vancomycin and rifampin against *Staphylococcus aureus*. *Antimicrob. Agents Chemother.* **19:** 1089–1091.

147. **Willey, B. M., B. N. Kreiswirth, A. E. Simor, G. Williams, S. R. Scriver, A. Phillips, and D. E. Low.** 1992. Detection of vancomycin resistance in *Enterococcus* species. *J. Clin. Microbiol.* **30:**1621–1624.

148. **York, M. K., L. Gibbs, F. Chelab, and G. F. Brooks.** 1996. Comparison of PCR detection of *mecA* with standard susceptibility testing methods to determine methicillin resistance in coagulase-negative staphylococci. *J. Clin. Microbiol.* **43:**249–253.

149. **Zembower, T. R., G. A. Noskin, M. J. Postelnick, C. Nguyen, and L. R. Peterson.** 1998. The utility of aminoglycosides in an era of emerging drug resistance. *Int. J. Antimicrob. Agents* **10:**95–105.

Genetic Methods for Detecting Antibacterial and Antiviral Resistance Genes*

FRED C. TENOVER AND J. KAMILE RASHEED

122

Resistance to antimicrobial agents in bacteria can be mediated by several mechanisms including (i) changes in the permeability of the cell envelope which limit the amount of drug that has access to cellular targets, (ii) active efflux of the drug out of the cell, (iii) modification of the site of drug action, (iv) provision of alternate enzymatic pathways around those blocked by antibacterial therapy, or (v) destruction or inactivation of the antimicrobial agent (96, 99) (also see chapter 117). While some of these changes occur due to mutations in key genetic loci in the bacterial genome, such as in mycobacteria, most resistance to antimicrobial agents in other bacterial genera is mediated by acquired genes whose presence in a cell is usually synonymous with a resistance phenotype. Although it is presumed that most resistance genes harbored by bacteria are expressed, exceptions to this rule have been documented (46, 105, 126). Genetic tests aimed at the detection of resistance genes in bacterial isolates by using DNA probes or PCR have been developed on the basis of the supposition that gene carriage equals resistance. Since genetic methods, including DNA probe-based methods, PCR, the ligase chain reaction, transcription-mediated amplification methods, branched DNA methods, and other amplification techniques, are now used in a variety of clinical laboratories for the identification and quantitation of pathogenic microorganisms, the application of the same genetic methods to the detection of antimicrobial resistance genes is a natural extension of the molecular diagnostics arena. In viruses, all resistance occurs via mutation, which makes DNA sequence analysis the primary tool for the detection of resistance.

New technology for rapid DNA sequence analysis is making detection of mutations associated with antibacterial and antiviral resistance much easier (97, 108). Although we are learning more about the molecular basis of resistance to antifungal and many antiparasitic drugs, molecular tests for the detection of resistance to such drugs are still in development (see chapter 126 and 127). The genetics of antimalarial resistance are the best understood, and the reader is referred to chapter 127 for more details.

* This chapter contains information presented in chapter 117 by Fred C. Tenover, Tanja Popovic, and Ørjan Olsvik in the sixth edition of this Manual.

REASONS FOR USING GENETIC TESTS TO DETECT RESISTANCE GENES

There are four reasons to pursue the identification of antimicrobial resistance genes or mutations associated with antiviral resistance. First, genetic methods are helpful for arbitrating MIC results that are at or near the breakpoint for resistance for bacterial species. Genetic methods also provide key information for guiding antiviral therapy. For example, oxacillin-resistant isolates of *Staphylococcus aureus* for which MICs are between 2 and 8 μg/ml may contain the *mecA* (methicillin) resistance gene determinant or may produce high levels of β-lactamase that slowly hydrolyze oxacillin (18, 52). While vancomycin would be the drug of choice for the treatment of infections caused by *mecA*-positive *S. aureus* isolates, infections caused by β-lactamase hyperproducers can be more effectively treated with penicillinase-stable β-lactams or β-lactam–β-lactamase inhibitor compounds (89). A test showing the absence of the *mecA* gene suggests that a physician could use an antimicrobial agent other than vancomycin to treat the infection.

Second, genetic methods can be used to detect resistance genes or mutations that result in resistance in organisms directly in clinical specimens to guide therapy early in the course of a patient's disease long before cultures are positive. For example, PCR assays can detect mutations in the *rpoB* locus associated with rifampin resistance in *Mycobacterium tuberculosis* (72, 147). Such mutations indicate that the strain is at least resistant to rifampin and may be resistant to multiple drugs. A positive PCR result for mutations in the *rpoB* locus directs the physician to avoid rifampin and to use alternative antimycobacterial agents. Similarly, direct testing of human immunodeficiency virus (HIV) type 1 (HIV-1) RNA in plasma for mutations associated with resistance to protease inhibitors (78) can guide therapy early in the course of treatment, perhaps optimizing therapy.

Third, genetics-based tests are more accurate than antibiograms for following the epidemiologic spread of a particular resistance gene in a hospital or community setting. For example, tracking the spread of the *vanA* vancomycin resistance gene in enterococci by PCR assays has been helpful in documenting the spread of multi-drug-resistant enterococci around the United States (23) and in Europe (1, 56). Antibiograms cannot differentiate between organisms containing the *vanA* gene and those with derepressed *vanB* genes (42).

Fourth, genetics-based tests can be used as the "gold standard" for the detection of resistance when evaluating the accuracy of new susceptibility testing methods that use clinical isolates or stock cultures for which MICs are borderline (34, 142).

GENETIC TESTS FOR RESISTANCE GENES AND DNA SEQUENCING STRATEGIES TO DETECT MUTATIONS ASSOCIATED WITH RESISTANCE

General Guidelines

The ideal genetic test targets nucleic acid sequences within the open reading frame (or coding region) of the resistance gene and avoids sequences outside of the gene that may contain insertion elements or promoter sequences that may be present in susceptible strains or strains with other types of resistance genes. Among the probes and primers that have been described for studying antibacterial resistance are those directed to β-lactamase genes and the genes that encode resistance to aminoglycosides, chloramphenicol, glycopeptides, isoniazid, macrolides, mupirocin, quinolones, rifampin, sulfonamides, tetracyclines, and trimethoprim. Examples of DNA probes that can be used to detect resistance genes are shown in Table 1, and examples of PCR primers that target resistance genes or mutations associated with resistance are shown in Table 2. The information in the tables is not meant to be exhaustive but, rather, is meant to give an indication of the types of assays that have been described. Most of the DNA probes target regions within the open reading frame of the resistance gene; however, some of the probes were developed before the gene sequence data were available and may contain sequences that are nonspecific and may hybridize with sequences outside of the open reading frame. Therefore, appropriate specificity controls (organisms that have the same resistance pattern but that contain resistance genes other than the target gene) always should be included in all reactions with these probes and primers.

DNA Sequencing

DNA sequence analysis has been particularly helpful for identifying point mutations associated with resistance to fluoroquinolones (34, 57, 68), antimycobacterial drugs (97, 144), and antiviral drugs (44, 50, 78). There are a series of mutations associated with resistance to isoniazid, rifampin, and streptomycin (45, 61, 77, 146). Unfortunately, additional genetic loci associated with resistance must also be involved since only 60% of resistance can be explained by mutations in these loci (93). Thus, sequence analysis for the prediction of resistance in mycobacteria remains a research tool. Similar studies of HIV are beginning to reveal mutations associated with resistance to inhibitors of DNA polymerase and viral proteases (70). While prototype assays with oligonucleotide arrays are under study for the rapid identification of these loci associated with resistance, this procedure holds promise for the future (78) (also see chapter 125).

AMINOGLYCOSIDE RESISTANCE GENES

Aminoglycoside resistance genes are common in both gram-positive and gram-negative organisms (128). However, the large number of different types of aminoglycoside resistance genes present in gram-negative organisms (genes encoding acetyltransferases, adenylyltransferases, and phosphotransferases) and the lack of consensus sequences that would allow detection of multiple types of genes with a single DNA probe or PCR primer set (128) make it difficult to use probes and PCR tests to predict resistance. Rather, genetic methods are better suited for the classification of new determinants and epidemiologic studies (59, 111, 165, 166).

Aminoglycoside resistance in gram-positive organisms, however, is more uniform (105). Thus, probes and PCR primers can be used to identify strains that carry genes encoding high-level aminoglycoside resistance. PCR assays and probes have been used, particularly with enterococci, to identify the ANT(6) streptomycin resistance gene and the gene encoding the AAC(6′)-APH(2″) bifunctional enzyme responsible for high-level gentamicin resistance (43, 73, 142, 165).

DETECTING GENES ASSOCIATED WITH RESISTANCE TO β-LACTAM DRUGS

Oxacillin Resistance in Staphylococci

Detection of oxacillin resistance in staphylococci, which is primarily mediated by the *mecA* gene determinant (7, 18), continues to be a problem (163), particularly with the coagulase-negative strains (18, 112). A *mecA* gene probe or PCR assay can differentiate those isolates that are borderline resistant to oxacillin due to the production of large quantities of β-lactamase from those that are resistant due to the presence of the *mecA* determinant (7, 89, 95, 163). The rare strains of *S. aureus* that are resistant to oxacillin by virtue of the fact that they contain modified penicillin-binding proteins (PBPs) with a reduced affinity for oxacillin (the so-called MOD strains) may be misclassified as oxacillin susceptible by the *mecA* gene test since these strains are truly oxacillin resistant but do not contain the *mecA* gene (155). Nonetheless, a probe or a PCR assay that can be used with an isolated colony of *S. aureus* or other staphylococcal species to identify organisms that have the *mecA* gene could be a valuable tool for the clinical microbiology laboratory, presuming that the caveats to its use are understood. For example, a study by Huang et al. (65) reported that although three strains of *Staphylococcus simulans* carried the *mecA* gene, the oxacillin MICs for the strains were 2 μg/ml, i.e., borderline susceptible results. These isolates, which remain rare, would be classified as resistant by PCR.

Detection of the *mecA* gene by PCR in organisms present in blood samples in BACTEC bottles (Becton Dickinson Microbiology Systems, Cockeysville, Md.) has been reported by Ubukata et al. (163) and Carroll et al. (16). In the former study, a minimum of 500 CFU of *S. aureus* was required for detection of the *mecA* gene, while the number of CFU of coagulase-negative species of staphylococci required to give a positive PCR test result was at least 10-fold higher. Detection was accomplished by a nonradioactive enzyme-linked colorimetric assay. Although detection of a *mecA* gene carried by a skin contaminant is a potential drawback to this approach (a false-positive result), a rapid result indicating *mecA* gene negativity could help reduce pharmacy costs by signaling the clinician that a semisynthetic penicillin instead of vancomycin could be used for therapy.

β-Lactam Resistance in Pneumococci

Resistance to penicillin and other antimicrobial agents in pneumococci has become a global problem (76, 90, 94).

TABLE 1 DNA probes for antimicrobial agent resistance genes

Antimicrobial agent	Organism	Target	Fragment or sequence	Reference
Aminoglycosides	*Enterococcus faecalis*(pJH1)	*aph(3′)-III*	530-bp *Hpa*II	158
	Acinetobacter baumannii(pIP1841)	*aph(3′)-VI*	365-bp *Eco*RI-*Bgl*II	80
	Escherichia coli(pFCT3103)	*ant(2″)-Ia*	310-bp *Ava*I	149
	E. coli(pSCH2005)	*ant(4′)-Ia*	318-bp *Sac*I-*Bgl*II	127
	E. coli(pFCT4392)	*aac(3)-Ia*	307-bp *Ava*I-*Eco*RV	152
	E. coli(pFCT1165)	*aac(6′)-Ia*	405-bp *Ssp*I	148
	E. coli(pC390)	*aac(3)-Va*	514-bp *Sal*I-*Cla*I	117
	E. faecalis (pIP800)	*aac(6′)-aph(2″)*	1,317-bp *Hinc*II-*Taq*I	43
	Staphylococcus aureus(pUB110)	*ant(4′)*	473-bp *Hinc*II	15
	E. faecalis(pJH-1)	*ant(6′)-Ia*	470-bp *Hpa*II	105
β-Lactams	*S. aureus*(pGO164)	*mecA*	400-bp *Hinc*II-*Cla*I	65
	E. coli(pBR322)	bla_{TEM}	424-bp *Bgl*I-*Hinc*II	82
	E. coli(pMON401)	$bla_{\text{ROB-1}}$	240-bp *Dra*I	71
	E. coli(pCLL3411)	bla_{SHV}	467-bp *Not*I-*Pst*I	14
	E. coli(pHIP29)	bla_{IMP}	500-bp *Hin*dIII	67
	E. coli(pMG232)	$bla_{\text{MIR-1}}$	1.4-kb *Acc*I-*Pst*I	106
	E. coli(pMON301)	bla_{OXA}	315-bp *Bgl*II	82
Chloramphenicol	*E. coli*(pJIR62)	*catP*	380-bp *Eco*RV-*Hin*fI	121
	E. coli(pJIR260)	*catQ*	350-bp *Dra*I-*Pst*I	121
	Clostridium difficile(pPPM9)	*catD*	270-bp *Eco*RV-*Taq*I	172
	E. coli(pBR325)	*catI*	1.1-kb *Eco*RI-*Hin*dIII	13
Macrolides	*E. coli*(pIP1100)	*ereA*	716-bp *Eco*RI-*Pst*I	8
	E. coli(pIP1527)	*ereB*	838-bp *Eco*RI-*Pst*I	8
	S. aureus::Tn554	*ermA*	417-bp *Mbo*I	39
	E. coli(pIP1527)	*ermAM*	349-bp *Rsa*I	8
	S. aureus(pE194)	*ermC*	472-bp *Hae*III-*Hinc*II	39
	Bacteroides fragilis(pVA1476)	*ermF*	230-bp *Taq*I-*Hin*dIII	47
Sulfonamides	*E. coli*(R388)	*sulI*	660-bp *Sac*II-*Bgl*II	114
	E. coli(pGS05)	*sulII*	780-bp *Hinc*II	114
Tetracycline	*E. coli*(pSL107)	*tet*(A)	750-bp *Sma*I	86
	E. coli(pBR322)	*tet*(C)	928-bp *Bst*NI	86
	E. coli(pSL106)	*tet*(D)	3.0-kb *Hin*dIII-*Pst*I	86
	S. aureus(pT181)	*tet*(K)	870-bp *Hinc*II	20
	E. faecalis(pBC16)	*tet*(L)	310-bp *Cla*I-*Hpa*II	20
	E. faecalis(pIP804)	*tet*(M)	850-bp *Hin*dIII-*Cla*I	87
	E. coli(pFKT686)	*tet*(O)	500-bp *Rsa*I-*Hinc*II	151
	E. coli(pJIR39)	*tet*(P)	800-bp *Eco*RI-*Sph*I	2
	Listeria monocytogenes(pAT451)	*tet*(S)	300-bp *Eco*RI-*Bgl*II	19
	Bacteroides thetaiotaomicron(pNFD13-2)	*tet*(Q)	1.45-kb *Eco*RI-*Pvu*II	102
	Enterococcus faecium(pKQ10)	*tet*(U)	277-bp *Cla*I-*Pst*I	118
Trimethoprim	*E. coli*(pLKO627)	*dhfrI*	500-bp *Bam*HI-*Kpn*I	69
	E. coli(pLKO601)	*dhfrII*	280-bp *Eco*RI-*Sal*I	69
	E. coli(pUN972)	*dhfrIII*	700-bp *Eco*RI-*Pst*I	154
	E. coli(pLKO9)	*dhfrV*	500-bp *Hinc*II	157
	E. coli(pUN1056)	*dhfrVII*	300-bp *Eco*RV	156
	E. coli(pCJO01-1)	*dhfrIX*	340-bp *Eco*RV-*Hin*dIII	69
	E. coli(pMAQ41)	*dhfrX*	450-bp *Xho*I-*Bgl*II	107
Vancomycin	*E. faecium*(pIP816)	*vanA*	290-bp *Bam*HI-*Rsa*I	37
	Enterococcus gallinarum BM4174	*vanC*	690-bp *Eco*RI-*Hinc*II	38

TABLE 2 PCR primers for antimicrobial resistance genes

Antimicrobial agent and gene	Primers (5′→3′)	Product size	Use	Reference
Aminoglycosides				
aac(6′)-Ia	ATG AAT TAT CAA ATT GTG TTA CTC TTT GAT TAA ACT	558 bp	Detection	111[a]
aac(6′)-Ic	CTA CGA TTA CGT CAA CGG CTG C TTG CTT CGC CCA CTC CTG CAC C	129 bp	Detection	59[b]
ant(6)-I	ACT GGC TTA ATC AAT TTG GG GCC TTT CCG CCA CCT CAC CG	577 bp	Detection	142
aph(2″)-Ic	TGA CTC AGT TCC CAG AT AGC ACT GTT CGC ACC AAA	880 bp	Detection	21
aac(3)-Ia	ACC TAC TCC CAA CAT CAG CC ATA TAG ATC TCA CTA CGC GC	169 bp	Detection	165[c]
aac(3)-Ib	GCG GAA CAG CAA TAG GTG G AAG CCG GAG CGC TTT GCG GC	370 bp	Mapping	124
aad(2″)-Ia	ATG TTA CGC AGC AGG GCA GTC G CGT CAG ATC AAT ATC ATC GTG C	188 bp	Detection	166
β-Lactams				
mecA	AAA ATC GAT GGT AAA GGT TGG C AGT TCT GCA GTA CCG GAT TTG C	533 bp	Probe	95
bla$_{IMP}$	CTA CCG CAG CAG AGT CTT TG AAC CAG TTT TGC CTT ACC AT	587 bp	Detection	125
bla$_{OXA\text{-}10/11}$	TAT CGC GTG TCT TTC GAG TA TTA GCC ACC AAT GAT GCC C	775 bp	Probe, sequencing	30
bla$_{PER\text{-}1}$	ATG AAT GTC ATT ATA AAA GC AAT TTG GGC TTA GGG CAG AAA	926 bp	Probe, sequencing	164
bla$_{PER\text{-}2}$	CGC TTC TGC TCT GCT GAT GGC AGC TTC TTT AAC GCC	469 bp	Detection	9
bla$_{ROB\text{-}1}$	TGT TGC AAT CGC TGC C TTA TCG TAC ACT TTC CA	400 bp	Detection	71
bla$_{SHV}$	GGT TAT GCG TTA TAT TCG CC ATC TTT CGC TCC AGC TGT TC	275 bp	Probe	116[d]
bla$_{OXY\text{-}1}$	GCG TAG CGC TGA TTA ACA CG CCT GCT GCG GCT GGG TAA AA	668 bp	Probe	49[e]
Glycopeptides				
vanA	GCT ATT CAG CTG TAC TC CAG CGG CCA TCA TAC GG	766 bp	Detection	122[f]
vanA	GGG AAA ACG ACA ATT GC GTA CAA TGC GGC CGT TA	732 bp	Detection	36[g]
vanB	CCC GAA TTT CAA ATG ATT GAA AA CGC CAT CCT CCT GCA AAA	457 bp	Detection	92[h]
vanB2	GAG GAT GGG TGC ATC CAG GGA CGT GAA GCC GGG CAG GGT GTT	630 bp	Probe	55
vanC1	GAA AGA CAA CAG GAA GAC CGC ATC GCA TCA CAA GCA CCA ATC	796 bp	Detection	23
vanC3	GCC TTT ACT TAT TGT TCC GCT TGT TCT TTG ACC TTA	224 bp	Detection	24
vanD	TAA GGC GCT TGC ATA TAC CG TGC AGC CAA GTA TCC GGT AA	461 bp	Detection, sequencing	109

(Continued on next page)

TABLE 2 PCR primers for antimicrobial resistance genes (*Continued*)

Antimicrobial agent and gene	Primers (5′→3′)	Product size	Use	Reference
Macrolides				
ermA	AGA ACA ATC AAT ACA GAG TC TGA ACC AGA AAA ACC CTA AA	526 bp	Detection	131[i]
ermF	GCA GAC AGG CGC AAG CAG CAA ACC ACG TTC CCA TGA GTG GTA TGG	357 bp	Detection	119
smp	AAA TTG TTT AAA AAG AAA TC TTT GAA CCA TAA TAT TCA TC	616 bp	Detection	141
mphA	AAC TGT ACG CAC TTG C GGT ACT CTT CGT TAC C	837 bp	Detection	140[j]
mefA	CTA TGA CAG CCT CAA TGC G ACC GAT TCT ATC AGC AAA G	1.4 kb	Expression	22
vat	CAA TGA CCA TGG ACC TGA TC AGC ATT TCG ATA TCT CC	615 bp	Detection, sequencing	4[k]
Mupirocin				
IRS	CCA TGC CTT ACC AGT TGA ATT GGA TCC CCG AGC ACT ATC CGA	1.65 kb	Probe	53
mupA	CCC ATG GCT TAC CAG TTG A CCA TGG AGC ACT ATC CGA A	1.65 kb	Probe, detection	115
Quinolones				
gyrA *Mycobacterium tuberculosis*	CAG CTA CAT CGA CTA TGC GA GGG CTT CGG TGT ACC TCA T	320 bp	Sequencing	72
gyrA *A. baumannii*	AAA TCT GCC CGT GTC GTT GGT GCC ATA CCT ACG GCG ATA CC	343 bp	Sequencing	168
gyrA *E. coli*	ACG TAC TAG GCA ATG ACT GG AGA GTC GCC GTC GAT AGA AC	189 bp	Sequencing	41[l]
gyrA *Streptococcus pneumoniae*	GAI TA(T/C) GCI ATG AG(C/T) GT AGC ACT ATC TCC ATC CAT GGA	285 bp	Sequencing	145[m]
gyrB *S. pneumoniae*	CAT GGA AAA TCC ACA GAT TG ATC GGC ATC GGT CAT CAA AA	414 bp	Sequencing	68[n]
parE *S. pneumoniae*	CCA ATC TAA GAA TCC TG GCA ATA TAG ACA TGA CC	357 bp	Sequencing	110
Sulfonamides				
sulA	AGC CAA TCA TGC AAA GAC AG ATT TTC CGC TTC ATC AGC CAG	913 or 916 bp	Sequencing	88
Tetracycline				
tet(A)	GTA ATT CTG AGC ACT GT CCT GGA CAA CAT TGC TT	953 bp	Probe	60[o]
tet(B)	CAG TGC TGT TGT TGT CAT TAA GCT TGG AAT ACT GAG TGT AA	528 bp	Detection, sequencing	119
tet(M)	GAA CTC GAA CAA GAG GAA AGC ATG GAA GCC CAG AAA GGA T	741 bp	Detection	103
tet(O)	AAC TTA GGC ATT CTG GCT CAC TCC CAC TGT TCC ATA TCG TCA	519 bp	Detection	103
tetA(P)	CAC AGA TTG TAT GGG GAT TAG G CAT TTA TAG AAA GCA CAG TAG C	764 bp	Detection, sequencing	83
tet(Q)	ATT GCG GAA GTG GAG CGG AC GCC GGA CGG AGG ATT TGA GA	814 bp	Detection	101

(*Continued on next page*)

TABLE 2 (*Continued*)

Antimicrobial agent and gene	Primers (5′→3′)	Product size	Use	Reference
Trimethoprim				
dfrA	CCC TGC TAT TAA AGC ACC CAT GAC CAG ATA ACT C	262 bp	Detection, sequencing	29
folH Haemophilus influenzae	GAC GGA TCC CAA GCC TGA ATT AAT TGG CTC CTA GAA TTC AGT TGC AGT TTT GCG TCA TAA T	~1.5 kb	Sequencing	33
dhfrVIII	CTA ACG GCG CTA TCT TCG TGA ACA ACG TAT GAA TTC TTC CAT GCC ATT CTG CTC GTA G[p]	300 bp	Detection	139
Ethambutol				
embB	ACG CTG AAA CTG CTG GCG AT ACA GAC TGG CGT CGC TGA CA	400 bp	SSCP assay	3
Pyrazinamide				
pncA	GCT GGT CAT GTT CGC GAT CG CAG GAG CTG CAA ACC AAC TCG	673 bp	Sequencing	137
Rifampin				
rpoB M. *tuberculosis*	GGG AGC GGA TGA CCA CCC A GCG GTA CGG CGT TTC GAT GAA C	350 bp	Sequencing	72
rpoB M. *tuberculosis*	CCA CCC AGG ACG TGG AGG CGA TCA CAC AGT GCG ACG GGT GCA CGT CGC GGA CCT	224 bp	Sequencing	26
Streptomycin				
rpsL	GGC CGA CAA ACA GAA CGT GTT CAC CAA CTG GGT GAC	501 bp	Sequencing	136
rrs	TTG GCC ATG CTC TTG ATG CCC TGC ACA CAG GCC ACA AGG GA	1.14 kb	Sequencing	91
rrs Mycobacteria	GAT GAC GGC CTT CGG GTT GT TCT AGT CTG CCC GTA TCG CC	238 bp	Sequencing	63
Isoniazid				
katG	GAA ACA GCG GCG CTG GAT CGT GTT GTC CCA TTT CGT CGG GG	209 bp	SSCP assay	146[q]
katG	TTT CGG CGC ATG GCC ATG A ACA GCC ACC GAG CAC GAC	894 bp	Sequencing, RFLP analysis	58
inhA	TCG ACG GCC GGC ATG G CCG GTC CGC CGA ACG	905 bp	Sequencing	72[r]
ahpC	ATG CAT TGT CCG CTT TGA TG TTC TAT ACT CAT TGA TT	588 bp	Sequencing	74

[a] The reference also describes primer sets for the detection of *aac(6′)-Ib*, *aac(6′)-If*, *aac(6′)-Ig*, and *aac(6′)-Ih*.
[b] The reference also describes primer sets for the detection of *aac(6′)-Id*, *aac(6′)-Ie*, *aac(6′)-Ii*, *aac(6′)-Ij*, *aac(6′)-Il*, and *aac(6′)-IIb*.
[c] The reference also describes primer sets for the detection of *aac(3)-IIa*, *aac(3)-IIIa*, *aac(3)-IVa*, *aad(4′)-Ia*, *aac(6′)-aph(2″)*, and *aph(3′)-IIIa*.
[d] The reference also describes primer sets for the detection of bla_{TEM}.
[e] The reference also describes a primer set for the synthesis of a probe for bla_{OXY-2}.
[f] The reference also describes primer sets for the detection of *vanB* and *vanC2*.
[g] The reference also describes a primer set for the detection of *vanB*.
[h] The reference also describes a primer set for the detection of *vanC1*.
[i] The reference also describes primer sets for the detection of *ermAM*, *ermC*, *msrA-msrB*, *ereA*, and *ereB*.
[j] The reference also describes primer sets for the detection of *ereA* and *ereB*.
[k] The reference also describes primer sets for the detection and DNA sequencing of *satA*, *vatB*, and *vga*.
[l] The reference also describes primer sets for the DNA sequencing of *parC* and *parE* of *E. coli*.
[m] The reference also describes primer sets for the DNA sequencing of *gyrB* of *S. pneumoniae*.
[n] The reference also describes primer sets for the DNA sequencing of *gyrA* and *parC* of *S. pneumoniae*.
[o] The reference also describes primer sets for the synthesis of probes for *tet*(C), *tet*(D), *tet*(E), *tet*(G), *tet*(H), and *tet*(M).
[p] The reverse primer begins with a 6-bp linker which creates an *Eco*RI restriction site.
[q] The reference also describes primer sets for SSCP assay of *inhA* and *ahpC*.
[r] The reference also describes primer sets for the DNA sequencing of *katG* and *orf1*.

Resistance develops when pneumococcal PBPs are remodeled through the acquisition of chromosomal DNA from other pneumococci or other streptococcal species (27, 35). Because of the apparent random nature of the remodeling process, it has not been possible as yet to develop DNA probes that target resistant strains. However, PCR primers have been developed for the amplification of PBP 2B gene sequences that are present only in penicillin-susceptible strains (162). The lack of product in the presence of amplification controls suggests that the gene has been remodeled and therefore mediates resistance. Such an assay does not reliably indicate which strains could be treated with penicillin instead of an extended-spectrum cephalosporin, as might be desirable for an assay to be used in a clinical laboratory, but it may be used as a screening tool for analyzing large groups of strains for resistance.

β-Lactamase Genes in Gram-Negative Organisms

Several DNA probes and PCR primer sets have been developed for detection of the genes encoding the TEM, SHV, OXA, CARB, and ROB β-lactamases present in gram-negative organisms (Tables 1 and 2). For example, the bla_{TEM} gene has been detected in many species of the family *Enterobacteriaceae*, in *Haemophilus* spp., and in *Neisseria gonorrhoeae* (82, 116, 132). Recently, PCR was used to detect bla_{TEM} directly in cerebrospinal fluid samples containing *Haemophilus influenzae* (150). Thus, the utility of direct detection has clearly been demonstrated, although it is rarely, if ever, used in clinical laboratories, primarily because the test is not commercially available.

The incidence of nosocomial infections caused by *Klebsiella pneumoniae*, *Klebsiella oxytoca* (48, 49), and other members of the family *Enterobacteriaceae* that produce extended-spectrum β-lactamases (85) and other enzymes capable of hydrolyzing cefotaxime, ceftriaxone, ceftazidime, and aztreonam is increasing in the United States and Europe (10, 14, 100, 116, 130, 167). Better tools for the rapid recognition and classification of these enzymes are needed. Isoelectric focusing is used as a screening test for the identification of novel β-lactamase genes (84), but DNA sequencing has become the gold standard for analyzing novel β-lactamase genes. PCR primers are also available for genes mediating resistance to imipenem (125), which appear to be spreading quickly in Japan (67).

CHLORAMPHENICOL RESISTANCE

Genes encoding chloramphenicol acetyltransferases (CATs) are present in both gram-negative and gram-positive organisms and mediate resistance to chloramphenicol (129). DNA probes for the CAT genes commonly found in gram-negative organisms (*catI*, *catII*, and *catIII*) have been described, but the probes include sequences outside of the open reading frames of the genes and their specificities have not been rigorously ascertained. Probes for the CAT genes of gram-positive anaerobes, including *Clostridium perfringens* and *Clostridium difficile* (*catP*, *catQ*, and *catD*), are more specific (13, 121, 172). Additional genes that show relatively little DNA sequence homology with those mentioned above are present in staphylococci, streptococci, and aerobic gram-positive bacilli. DNA probes for many of these genes have been described (Table 1), although their clinical utility has yet to be established. Direct detection of these genes in clinical samples has not been reported, but it may become important as the levels of resistance to extended-spectrum β-lactam agents, currently the drugs of choice for the treatment of bacterial meningitis in children, becomes more pronounced. PCR primers capable of detecting the *cat* genes present in streptococci and enterococci have also been described (159).

GLYCOPEPTIDE RESISTANCE

Resistance to vancomycin in enterococci has become a major global issue during the last few years (23, 37, 171). Resistance in enterococci can be mediated by several different genes, including *vanA*, *vanB*, *vanC1*, *vanC2*, *vanC3*, and *vanD* (23, 36, 37, 109, 122). DNA probes and PCR assays that detect these genes have been described. PCR has also been used to detect the *vanA* resistance gene in genomic enterococcal DNA purified directly from fecal material recovered on rectal swabs (123). Recently, decreased susceptibility to glycopeptides has been noted among strains of *S. aureus* from Japan and the United States (17, 62). However, genetic assays for the detection of this glycopeptide resistance in staphylococci have yet to be developed since the mechanisms of resistance remain unknown.

MACROLIDE, LINCOSAMIDE, AND STREPTOGRAMIN RESISTANCE

The genes mediating resistance to erythromycin have been the targets of both DNA probes and PCR assays. PCR assays that detect erythromycin methylase genes (*erm* genes) that mediate resistance to macrolides, lincosamides (such as clindamycin), and streptogramins (i.e., the MLS resistance phenotype) (8, 39, 153), the *msrA* gene that mediates resistance only to macrolides and streptogramins (MS resistance), and the macrolide efflux genes *mefA* and *mefE* (22, 131, 140) have been described, as has a novel efflux mechanism in *S. aureus* (170). Studies by Eady et al. (39) demonstrate that the *msrA* gene is common in isolates of *S. aureus* and produces a phenotype of erythromycin resistance but clindamycin susceptibility. The *mefE* gene appears to be a common cause of erythromycin resistance in pneumococci in the United States (143). Since most strains of staphylococci that are erythromycin resistant are presumed to be resistant to clindamycin as well, *msrA* probes and PCR assays may be useful in determining the presence of the *msrA* and *ermA* genes if clindamycin therapy was a critical issue.

MUPIROCIN RESISTANCE

Mupirocin is an antistaphylococcal agent that is used to reduce the carriage of staphylococci among infected patients and hospital personnel. Recently, a PCR assay that can detect high-level mupirocin resistance was described (53). However, the practical value of the assay has not been assessed in a clinical laboratory setting.

QUINOLONE RESISTANCE

The two major mechanisms of quinolone resistance include alteration of the target sites, which are the organism's gyrase (encoded by *gyrA* and *gyrB*) and topoisomerase (encoded by *parC* and *parE*) (41, 64, 144, 145, 160), and active efflux of the drug out of the cell, which limits access of the drug to the target site. Resistance is usually associated with point mutations in the *gyr* or *par* loci. Since DNA probes do not reliably detect these changes, investigators have used PCR coupled with direct sequencing of the amplification products to identify changes in the nucleotide sequences of the *gyrA*, *parC*, and *parE* genes (57, 68, 72, 168). The primers, however, appear to be species specific (Table 2).

SULFONAMIDE RESISTANCE

There are two major sulfonamide resistance genes, *sulI* and *sulII*. Both have been cloned and sequenced, and probes for each gene have been described (114). Neither probe has been used to identify the presence of the gene in bacteria directly in clinical samples. Interestingly, the *sul* genes are often associated with transposable DNA elements, such as Tn*21* (114), that can shuttle multiple resistance genes from organism to organism. Thus, the *sul* genes can serve as indicators of multiple-drug resistance in gram-negative organisms.

TETRACYCLINE RESISTANCE

Tetracycline resistance can be mediated by at least 15 different genes (135). DNA probes and PCR have been used for epidemiologic studies of the *tet*(A), *tet*(B), *tet*(C), *tet*(D), *tet*(E), *tet*(F), *tet*(H), *tet*(K), *tet*(L), *tet*(M), *tet*(N), *tet*(O), *tet*(Q), and *tet*(S) determinants (2, 19, 47, 86, 87, 134, 135, 174). Of these, *tet*(M) is the most widespread, having been located in a very diverse group of organisms including staphylococci; streptococci; pneumococci; gram-negative bacilli, such as campylobacters, *Gardnerella vaginalis*, and fusobacteria; mycoplasmas and ureaplasmas (134); and *N. gonorrhoeae* (51). PCR primers have been described for the *tet*(M), *tet*(O), and *tet*(Q) genes (11, 31, 79, 83, 119, 120). These primers may have particular value for the detection of tetracycline resistance genes directly in periodontal pathogens (101), since the presence of resistant organisms may indicate those patients who are likely to fail therapy with tetracycline, which is often the drug of choice for periodontal disease. Because the *tet*(M) and *tet*(O) genes are highly related, some primer sets will produce amplification products with both genes, making it necessary to use specific DNA probes to confirm the identity of the amplification products. Multiple types of the *tet*(M) gene also have been recognized through sequence analysis (104). A novel efflux mechanism of tetracycline resistance *tet*(H) has been described in *Pasteurella multocida* (60), as has what appears to be a novel ribosomal protection mechanism of resistance encoded by *tet*(U) in *Enterococcus faecium* (118).

TRIMETHOPRIM RESISTANCE

The number of genes capable of mediating trimethoprim resistance in bacteria continues to expand (6, 133). DNA probes have proven to be powerful tools for the detection and classification of novel trimethoprim resistance genes (called *dhfr*) (6, 69, 113). However, because consensus sequences common to all the *dhfr* genes have not been identified, PCR primers that could simplify the detection of this family of genes have not been developed, although PCR primers for some individual genes have been developed (29, 139). A novel trimethoprim resistance gene, *folH*, also has been recognized in *H. influenzae* (33).

DETECTING RESISTANCE IN MYCOBACTERIA

Multidrug-resistant strains of *M. tuberculosis* have been recognized in hospitals in the United States, Southeast Asia, and parts of Europe, where they constitute a major public health problem (40). Consequently, the rapid identification of resistant strains has become a critical issue for the laboratory. PCR assays have been developed for the detection of mutations in the *rpoB* locus of the *M. tuberculosis* genome associated with the development of rifampin resistance (25, 66, 72, 169). PCR and a single-stranded conformation polymorphism (SSCP) assay (a technique that examines the mobility of PCR products in a polyacrylamide gel) can differentiate rifampin-resistant strains of *M. tuberculosis* from susceptible strains with a high degree of confidence (147). Rifampin resistance also serves as a marker for multidrug resistance in *M. tuberculosis*. Commercial assays for the detection of this resistance have been described (28, 32). Primers also have been developed for the detection of rifampin resistance in *Mycobacterium leprae* (63).

Mutations associated with streptomycin resistance in *M. tuberculosis* also have been identified by PCR (45, 91, 136). However, SSCP assays similar to those used for the detection of rifampin resistance have not been described. Instead, DNA sequencing is required for the identification of the altered sequences. The assay appears to be approximately 90% sensitive but is highly specific for determining these mutations in mycobacteria.

Two genetic loci, *katG* and *inhA*, have been associated with isoniazid resistance in *M. tuberculosis* (5, 25, 58, 146, 173). DNA sequence analysis of PCR products has been used to detect resistant strains (25, 146, 173), as has restriction fragment length polymorphism (RFLP) analysis (58).

The use of molecular methods for the detection of resistance markers in mycobacteria is an area of great potential benefit to the clinical mycobacteriology laboratory. However, our understanding of resistance to a variety of drugs in mycobacteria is just beginning to unfold, and other mechanisms of resistance, perhaps the predominant mechanism of resistance in some cases, are yet to be described.

DETECTING VIRAL MUTATIONS ASSOCIATED WITH RESISTANCE

There are a series of mutations associated with resistance to polymerase and protease inhibitors of HIV (44, 50, 54, 70, 78, 81), ganciclovir resistance in human cytomegalovirus (12), and amantadine resistance in influenza A virus (75). Such mutations have been detected by traditional sequencing methods and by sequencing via oligonucleotide arrays (78). Although sequencing may still be beyond the scope of many laboratories, newer assays which combine PCR with other methods of detecting mutations may make detection of antiviral resistance more accessible to a broader range of laboratories. For example, PCR followed by restriction enzyme analysis of the amplification products and PCR followed by ligase detection reaction (PCR-LDR) obviate the need for traditional DNA sequencing. Frenkel et al. (50) used a colorimetric PCR-LDR assay to detect *pol* mutations at codons 41, 70, 74, and 215 in HIV-1 associated with resistance to zidovudine and didanosine. Commercially prepared line probe assays, which are reverse hybridization assays, for the detection of resistance in the reverse transcriptase gene of HIV isolates have also been developed (138). However, the utility of finding mutations associated with resistance to viral drugs still requires a better clinical correlation before widespread testing can be initiated.

GUIDELINES FOR USING GENETIC TESTS

Today, DNA probes are rarely used to detect resistance genes. Rather, laboratories use PCR assays which are more accessible and easier to adapt to clinical laboratory use than assays with DNA probes. The critical issue with PCR assays is the reliability of the results. The need for quality control measures, including the use of amplification controls, such as the simultaneous amplification of rRNA or rDNA sequences to ensure the availability of amplifiable nucleic acid and the absence of inhibitory substances in the reaction, cannot be stressed enough. The temperatures used in PCR assays optimized for use with DNA from bacterial isolates obtained in pure culture may not be stringent enough to avoid false-positive results when such assays are used with clinical samples, such as blood or cerebrospinal fluid, with which considerably more nonspecific priming can occur (151). It may be necessary to increase the temperatures of the assays, particularly the annealing temperatures, to avoid this problem. It is critical to include control reactions containing no template DNA to identify nonspecific PCR products arising from extraneous DNA provided by sources such as recombinant *Taq* polymerase contaminated with cloning vector (151, 161).

One should never assume that PCR primers reported in the literature have undergone rigorous testing. Rather, primer sets should be thoroughly tested for specificity, self-complementarity, and dimer formation before use. According to the Clinical Laboratory Improvement Act of 1988, validation of DNA probe and PCR tests by the clinical laboratory in which they are to be used is mandatory before they can be used for analysis of clinical specimens. Methods for validation are published by the National Committee for Clinical Laboratory Standards (98).

Finally, now that DNA probes and PCR assays for the detection and differentiation of resistance genes are becoming commercially available, more surveys of resistance mechanisms, such as those described by Eady et al. (39), Kapur et al. (72), Ounissi et al. (105), and Shaw et al. (126), should be undertaken to determine the reservoirs of resistance genes and how resistance genes disseminate in hospitals and community settings. Such studies would also help to determine the frequency with which organisms carry resistance genes that are not expressed. Although still considered experimental, many of the probe and PCR methods for the detection of resistance genes described herein are already having a positive effect on guiding therapy early in the course of infection and making the treatment of infectious diseases less empiric.

REFERENCES

1. **Aarestrup, F. M., P. Ahrens, M. Madsen, L. V. Pallesen, R. L. Poulsen, and H. Westh.** 1996. Glycopeptide susceptibility among Danish *Enterococcus faecium* and *Enterococcus faecalis* isolates of human and animal origin. *Antimicrob. Agents Chemother.* **40:**1938–1940.
2. **Abraham, L. J., D. I. Berryman, and J. I. Rood.** 1988. Hybridization analysis of the class P tetracycline resistance determinant from the *Clostridium perfringens* R-plasmid, pCW3. *Plasmid* **19:**113–120.
3. **Alcaide, F., G. E. Pfyffer, and A. Telenti.** 1997. Role of *embB* in natural and acquired resistance to ethambutol in mycobacteria. *Antimicrob. Agents Chemother.* **41:**2270–2273.
4. **Allignet, J., and N. E. Solh.** 1995. Diversity among the gram-positive acetyltransferases inactivating streptogramin A and structurally related compounds and characterization of a new staphylococcal determinant, *vatB*. *Antimicrob. Agents Chemother.* **39:**2027–2036.
5. **Altamirano, M., J. Marostenmaki, A. Wong, M. Fitzgerald, W. A. Black, and J. A. Smith.** 1994. Mutations in the catalase-peroxidase gene from isoniazid-resistant *Mycobacterium tuberculosis* isolates. *J. Infect. Dis.* **169:**1162–1165.
6. **Amyes, S. G. B., and K. J. Towner.** 1990. Trimethoprim resistance; epidemiology and molecular aspects. *J. Med. Microbiol.* **31:**1–19.
7. **Archer, G. L., and E. Pennell.** 1990. Detection of methicillin resistance in staphylococci by using a DNA probe. *Antimicrob. Agents Chemother.* **34:**1720–1724.
8. **Arthur, M., A. Andremont, and P. Courvalin.** 1987. Distribution of erythromycin esterase and rRNA methylase genes in members of the family *Enterobacteriaceae* highly resistant to erythromycin. *Antimicrob. Agents Chemother.* **31:**404–409.
9. **Bauernfeind, A., I. Stemplinger, R. Jungwirth, P. Mangold, S. Amann, E. Akalin, O. Ang, C. Bal, and J. M. Casellas.** 1996. Characterization of β-lactamase gene bla_{PER-2}, which encodes an extended-spectrum class A β-lactamase. *Antimicrob. Agents Chemother.* **40:**616–620.
10. **Bauernfeind, A., S. Wagner, R. Jungwirth, I. Schneider, and D. Meyer.** 1997. A novel class C β-lactamase (FOX-2) in *Escherichia coli* conferring resistance to cephamycins. *Antimicrob. Agents Chemother.* **41:**2041–2046.
11. **Blanchard, A., D. M. Crabb, K. Dybvig, L. B. Duffy, and G. H. Cassell.** 1992. Rapid detection of *tetM* in *Mycoplasma hominis* and *Ureaplasma urealyticum* by PCR: *tetM* confers resistance to tetracycline but not necessarily to doxycycline. *FEMS Microbiol. Lett.* **95:**277–282.
12. **Boivin, G., S. Chou, M. R. Quirk, A. Erice, and M. C. Jordan.** 1996. Detection of gancoclovir resistance mutations and quantitation of cytomegalovirus (CMV) DNA in leukocytes of patients with fatal disseminated CMV disease. *J. Infect. Dis.* **173:**523–528.
13. **Bolivar, F., R. L. Rodriguez, P. J. Greene, M. C. Betlach, H. L. Heyneker, H. W. Boyer, J. H. Crosa, and S. Falkow.** 1977. Construction and characterization of new cloning vehicles. II. A multipurpose cloning system. *Gene* **2:**95–113.
14. **Bradford, P. A., C. Urban, A. Jaiswal, N. Mariano, B. A. Rasmussen, S. J. Projan, J. J. Rahal, and K. Bush.** 1995. SHV-7, a novel cefotaxime-hydrolyzing β-lactamase, identified in *Escherichia coli* isolates from hospitalized nursing home patients. *Antimicrob. Agents Chemother.* **39:**899–905.
15. **Carlier, C., and P. Courvalin.** 1990. Emergence of 4′,4″-aminoglycoside nucleotidyltransferase in enterococci. *Antimicrob. Agents Chemother.* **34:**1565–1569.
16. **Carroll, K. C., R. B. Leonard, P. L. Newcomb-Gayman, and D. R. Hilliard.** 1996. Rapid detection of the staphylococcal *mecA* gene from BACTEC blood culture bottles by the polymerase chain reaction. *Am. J. Clin. Pathol.* **106:**600–605.
17. **Centers for Disease Control and Prevention.** 1997. *Staphylococcus aureus* with reduced susceptibility to vancomycin—United States, 1997. *Morbid. Mortal. Weekly Rep.* **46:**765–766.
18. **Chambers, H. F.** 1988. Methicillin-resistant staphylococci. *Clin. Microbiol. Rev.* **1:**173–186.
19. **Charpentier, E., G. Gerbaud, and P. Courvalin.** 1993. Characterization of a new class of tetracycline-resistance gene *tet* (S) in *Listeria monocytogenes* BM4210. *Gene* **131:**27–34.
20. **Charpentier, E., G. Gerbaud, and P. Courvalin.** 1997. Presence of the *Listeria* tetracycline resistance gene *tet*(S) in *Enterococcus faecalis*. *Antimicrob. Agents Chemother.* **38:**2330–2335.
21. **Chow, J. W., M. J. Zervos, S. A. Lerner, L. A. Thal, S. M. Donabedian, D. D. Jaworski, S. Tsai, K. J. Shaw, and**

D. B. Clewell. 1997. A novel gentamicin resistance gene in *Enterococcus*. *Antimicrob. Agents Chemother.* **41:**511–514.

22. **Clancy, J., J. Petitpas, F. Dib-Hajj, W. Yuan, M. Cronan, A. V. Kamath, J. Bergeron, and J. A. Retsema.** 1996. Molecular cloning and functional analysis of a novel macrolide-resistance determinant, *mefA*, from *Streptococcus pyogenes*. *Mol. Microbiol.* **22:**867–879.
23. **Clark, N. C., R. C. Cooksey, B. C. Hill, J. M. Swenson, and F. C. Tenover.** 1993. Characterization of glycopeptide resistant enterococci from U.S. hospitals. *Antimicrob. Agents Chemother.* **37:**2311–2317.
24. **Clark, N. C., L. M. Teixeira, R. R. Facklam, and F. C. Tenover.** 1998. Detection and differentiation of the *vanC-1*, *vanC-2*, and *vanC-3* glycopeptide resistance genes in enterococci. *J. Clin. Microbiol.* **36:**2294–2297.
25. **Cockerill, F. R., III, J. R. Uhl, Z. Temesgen, Y. Zhang, L. Stockman, G. D. Roberts, D. L. Williams, and B. C. Kline.** 1995. Rapid identification of a point mutation of the *Mycobacterium tuberculosis* catalase-peroxidase (*katG*) gene associated with isoniazid resistance. *J. Infect. Dis.* **171:**240–245.
26. **Cockerill, F. R., III, D. E. Williams, K. D. Eisenach, B. C. Kline, L. K. Miller, L. Stockman, J. Voyles, G. M. Caron, S. K. Bundy, G. D. Roberts, W. R. Wilson, A. C. Whelen, J. M. Hunt, and D. H. Persing.** 1996. Prospective evaluation of the utility of molecular techniques for diagnosing nosocomial transmission of multidrug-resistant tuberculosis. *Mayo Clin. Proc.* **71:**221–229.
27. **Coffey, T. J., C. G. Dowson, M. Daniels, J. Zhou, C. Martin, B. G. Spratt, and J. M. Musser.** 1991. Horizontal transfer of multiple penicillin-binding protein genes, and capsular biosynthetic genes, in natural populations of *Streptococcus pneumoniae*. *Mol. Microbiol.* **5:**2255–2260.
28. **Cooksey, R. C., G. P. Morlock, S. Glickman, and J. T. Crawford.** 1997. Evaluation of a line probe assay kit for characterization of *rpoB* mutations in rifampin-resistant *Mycobacterium tuberculosis* isolates from New York City. *J. Clin. Microbiol.* **35:**1281–1283.
29. **Dale, G. E., H. Langen, M. G. P. Page, R. L. Then, and D. Stuber.** 1995. Cloning and characterization of a novel, plasmid-encoded trimethoprim-resistant dihydrofolate reductase from *Staphylococcus haemolyticus* MUR313. *Antimicrob. Agents Chemother.* **39:**1920–1924.
30. **Danel, F., L. M. C. Hall, D. Gur, and D. M. Livermore.** 1995. OXA-14, another extended-spectrum variant of OXA-10 (PSE-2) β-lactamase from *Pseudomonas aeruginosa*. *Antimicrob. Agents Chemother.* **39:**1881–1884.
31. **De Barbeyrac, B., M. Dupon, P. Rodriguez, H. Rnaudin, and C. Bebear.** 1996. A Tn*1545*-like transposon carries the *tet*(M) gene in tetracycline resistant strains of *Bacteroides ureolyticus* as well as *Ureaplasma urealyticum* but not *Neisseria gonorrhoeae*. *J. Antimicrob. Chemother.* **37:**223–232.
32. **De Beenhouwer, H., Z. Lhiang, G. Jannes, W. Mijs, L. Machtelinks, R. Roussau, H. Traore, and F. Portaels.** 1995. Rapid detection of rifampin resistance in sputum and biopsy specimens from tuberculosis patients by PCR and line probe assay. *Tubercle Lung Dis.* **76:**425–430.
33. **De Groot, R., M. Sluijter, A. De Bruyn, J. Campos, W. H. F. Goessens, A. L. Smith, and P. W. M. Hermans.** 1996. Genetic characterization of trimethoprim resistance in *Haemophilus influenzae*. *Antimicrob. Agents Chemother.* **40:**2131–2136.
34. **Deguchi, T., M. Yasuda, M. Asano, K. Tada, H. Iwata, H. Komeda, T. Ezaki, I. Saito, and Y. Kawada.** 1995. DNA gyrase mutations in quinolone-resistant clinical isolates of *Neisseria gonorrhoeae*. *Antimicrob. Agents Chemother.* **39:**561–563.
35. **Dowson, C. G., A. Hutchison, and B. G. Spratt.** 1989. Extensive remodeling of the transpeptidase domain of penicillin-binding protein 2B of a penicillin-resistant South African isolate of *Streptococcus pneumoniae*. *Mol. Microbiol.* **3:**95–102.
36. **Dutka-Malen, S., S. Evers, and P. Courvalin.** 1995. Detection of glycopeptide resistance genotypes and identification to the species level of clinically relevant enterococci by PCR. *J. Clin. Microbiol.* **33:**24–27.
37. **Dutka-Malen, S., R. Leclercq, V. Coutant, J. Duval, and P. Courvalin.** 1990. Phenotypic and genotypic heterogeneity of glycopeptide resistance determinants in gram-positive bacteria. *Antimicrob. Agents Chemother.* **34:**1875–1879.
38. **Dutka-Malen, S., C. Molinass, M. Arthur, and P. Courvalin.** 1992. Sequence of the *vanC* gene of *Enterococcus gallinarum* BM4174 encoding a D-alanine:D-alanine ligase-related protein necessary for vancomycin resistance. *Gene* **112:**53–58.
39. **Eady, E. A., J. I. Ross, J. L. Tipper, C. E. Walters, J. H. Cove, and W. C. Noble.** 1993. Distribution of genes encoding erythromycin ribosomal methylases and an erythromycin efflux pump in epidemiologically distinct groups of staphylococci. *J. Antimicrob. Chemother.* **31:**211–217.
40. **Edlin, B. R., J. I. Tokars, M. H. Grieco, J. T. Crawford, J. Williams, E. M. Sordillo, K. R. Ong, J. O. Kilburn, S. W. Dooley, K. G. Castro, W. R. Jarvis, and S. D. Holmberg.** 1992. An outbreak of multidrug resistant tuberculosis among hospitalized patients with acquired immunodeficiency syndrome. *N. Engl. J. Med.* **326:**1514–1521.
41. **Everett, M. J., Y. F. Jin, V. Ricci, and L. J. V. Piddock.** 1996. Contributions of individual mechanisms to fluoroquinolone resistance in 36 *Escherichia coli* strains isolated from humans and animals. *Antimicrob. Agents Chemother.* **40:**2380–2386.
42. **Evers, S., D. F. Sahm, and P. Courvalin.** 1993. The *vanB* gene of vancomycin-resistant *Enterococcus faecalis* V583 is structurally related to genes encoding D-Ala:D-Ala ligases and glycopeptide-resistance proteins VanA and VanC. *Gene* **124:**143–144.
43. **Ferretti, J. J., K. S. Gilmore, and P. Courvalin.** 1986. Nucleotide sequence analysis of the gene specifying the bifunctional 6′-aminoglycoside acetyl transferase 2″-aminoglycoside phosphotransferase enzyme in *Streptococcus faecalis* and identification and cloning of gene regions specifying the two activities. *J. Bacteriol.* **167:**631–638.
44. **Field, A. K., and K. K. Biron.** 1994. The end of innocence revisited: resistance of herpesviruses to antiviral drugs. *Clin. Microbiol. Rev.* **7:**1–13.
45. **Finken, M., P. Kirschner, A. Meier, A. Wrede, and E. Böttger.** 1993. Molecular basis of streptomycin resistance in *Mycobacterium tuberculosis*: alterations of the ribosomal protein A12 and point mutations within a functional 16S ribosomal RNA pseudoknot. *Mol. Microbiol.* **9:**1239–1246.
46. **Flamm, R. K., K. L. Phillips, F. C. Tenover, and J. J. Plorde.** 1993. A survey of clinical isolates of *Enterobacteriaceae* using a series of DNA probes for aminoglycoside resistance genes. *Mol. Cell. Probes* **7:**139–144.
47. **Fletcher, H. M., and F. L. Macrina.** 1991. Molecular survey of clindamycin and tetracycline resistance determinants in *Bacteroides* species. *Antimicrob. Agents Chemother.* **35:**2415–2418.
48. **Fournier, B., and P. H. Roy.** 1997. Variability of chromosomally encoded β-lactamases from *Klebsiella oxytoca*. *Antimicrob. Agents Chemother.* **41:**1641–1648.
49. **Fournier, B., P. H. Roy, P. H. Lagrange, and A. Philippon.** 1996. Chromosomal β-lactamase genes of *Klebsiella oxytoca* are divided into two main groups, bla_{OXY-1} and bla_{OXY2}. *Antimicrob. Agents Chemother.* **40:**454–459.
50. **Frenkel, L. M., L. E. Wagner, S. M. Atwood, T. J. Cummins, and S. Dewhurst.** 1995. Specific, sensitive, and rapid

assay for human immunodeficiency virus type 1 *pol* mutations associated with resistance to zidovudine and didanosine. *J. Clin. Microbiol.* **33:**342–347.

51. **Gascoyne-Binzi, D. M., P. M. Hawkey, and J. Heritage.** 1994. The distribution of variants of the Tet M determinant in tetracycline-resistant *Neisseria gonorrhoeae*. *J. Antimicrob. Chemother.* **33:**1011–1016.
52. **Geha, D. J., J. R. Uhl, C. A. Gustaferro, and D. H. Persing.** 1994. Multiplex PCR for identification of methicillin-resistant staphylococci in the clinical laboratory. *J. Clin. Microbiol.* **32:**1768–1772.
53. **Gilbart, J., C. R. Perry, and B. Slocombe.** 1993. High level mupirocin resistance in *Staphylococcus aureus*: evidence for two distinct isoleucyl-tRNA synthetases. *Antimicrob. Agents Chemother.* **37:**32–38.
54. **Gingeras, T. R., P. Prodanovich, T. Latimer, J. C. Guatelli, D. D. Richman, and K. J. Barringer.** 1991. Use of self-sustained sequence replication amplification reaction to analyze and detect mutations in zidovudine-resistant human immunodeficiency virus. *J. Infect. Dis.* **164:** 1066–1074.
55. **Gold, H. S., S. Unal, E. Cercenado, C. Thauvin-Eliopoulos, G. M. Eliopoulos, C. B. Wennersten, and R. C. Moellering, Jr.** 1993. A gene conferring resistance to vancomycin but not teicoplanin in isolates of *Enterococcus faecalis* and *Enterococcus faecium* demonstrates homology with *vanB*, *vanA*, and *vanC* genes of enterococci. *Antimicrob. Agents Chemother.* **37:**1604–1609.
56. **Gordts, B., H. Van Landuyt, M. Ieven, P. Vandamme, and H. Goossens.** 1995. Vancomycin-resistant enterococci colonizing the intestinal tracts of colonized patients. *J. Clin. Microbiol.* **33:**2842–2846.
57. **Griggs, D. J., K. Gensberg, and L. J. V. Piddock.** 1996. Mutations in *gyrA* gene of quinolone-resistant *Salmonella* serotypes isolated from humans and animals. *Antimicrob. Agents Chemother.* **40:**1009–1013.
58. **Haas, W. H., K. Schilke, J. Brand, B. Amthor, K. Weyer, P. B. Fourie, G. Bretzel, V. Sticht-Groh, and H. J. Bremer.** 1997. Molecular analysis of *katG* gene mutations in strains of *Mycobacterium tuberculosis* complex from Africa. *Antimicrob. Agents Chemother.* **41:**1601–1603.
59. **Hannecart-Pokorni, E., F. Depuydt, L. De Wit, E. Van Bossuyt, J. Content, and R. Vanhoof.** 1997. Characterization of the 6′-*N*-aminoglycoside acetyltransferase gene *aac(6′)-II* associated with a *sulI*-type integron. *Antimicrob. Agents Chemother.* **41:**314–318.
60. **Hansen, L. M., P. C. Blanchard, and D. C. Hirsh.** 1996. Distribution of *tet*(H) among *Pasteurella* isolates from the United States and Canada. *Antimicrob. Agents Chemother.* **40:**1558–1560.
61. **Heym, B., N. Honore, C. Truffot-Pernot, A. Banerjee, C. Schurra, W. R. Jacobs, Jr., J. D. vanEmbden, J. H. Grosset, and S. T. Cole.** 1994. Implications of multidrug resistance for the future of short course therapy of tuberculosis: a molecular study. *Lancet* **344:**671–674.
62. **Hiramatsu, K., H. Hanaki, T. Ino, K. Yabuta, T. Oguri, and F. C. Tenover.** 1997. Methicillin-resistant *Staphylococcus aureus* clinical strain with reduced vancomycin susceptibility. *J. Antimicrob. Chemother.* **40:**135–136.
63. **Honore, N., and S. T. Cole.** 1994. Streptomycin resistance in mycobacteria. *Antimicrob. Agents Chemother.* **38:** 238–242.
64. **Hooper, D. C., J. S. Wolfson, E. Y. Ng, and M. N. Schwartz.** 1987. Mechanisms of action of and resistance to ciprofloxacin. *Am. J. Med.* **82**(Suppl. 4A)**:**12–20.
65. **Huang, M. B., T. E. Gay, C. N. Baker, S. N. Bannerjee, and F. C. Tenover.** 1993. Two percent sodium chloride is required for susceptibility testing of staphylococci with oxacillin when using agar based dilution methods. *J. Clin. Microbiol.* **31:**2683–2688.
66. **Hunt, J. M., G. D. Roberts, L. Stockman, T. A. Felmlee, and D. H. Persing.** 1994. Detection of a genetic locus encoding resistance to rifampin in mycobacterial cultures and in clinical specimens. *Diagn. Microbiol. Infect. Dis.* **18:** 219–227.
67. **Ito, H., Y. Arakawa, S. Ohsuka, R. Wacharotayankun, N. Kato, and M. Ohta.** 1995. Plasmid-mediated dissemination of the metallo-β-lactamase gene bla_{IMP} among clinically isolated strains of *Serratia marcescens*. *Antimicrob. Agents Chemother.* **39:**824–829.
68. **Janoir, C., V. Zeller, M.-D. Kitzis, N. J. Moreau, and L. Gutmann.** 1996. High-level fluoroquinolone resistance in *Streptococcus pneumoniae* requires mutations in *parC* and *gyrA*. *Antimicrob. Agents Chemother.* **40:**2760–2764.
69. **Jansson, C., A. Franklin, and O. Sköld.** 1992. Spread of newly found trimethoprim resistance gene *dhfrIX* among porcine isolates and human pathogens. *Antimicrob. Agents Chemother.* **36:**2704–2708.
70. **Japour, A. J., S. Welles, R. T. D'Aquila, V. A. Johnson, D. D. Richman, R. W. Coombs, P. S. Reichelderfer, J. O. Kahn, C. S. Crumpacker, and D. R. Kuritzkes for the AIDS Clinical Trials Group 116B/117 Study Team and Virology Committee Resistance Working Group.** 1995. Prevalence and clinical significance of zidovudine resistance mutations in human immunodeficiency virus isolated from patients after long term zidovudine treatment. *J. Infect. Dis.* **171:**1172–1179.
71. **Juteau, J.-M., M. Sirois, A. A. Medeiros, and R. C. Levesque.** 1991. Molecular distribution of ROB-1 β-lactamase in *Actinobacillus pleuropneumoniae*. *Antimicrob. Agents Chemother.* **35:**1397–1402.
72. **Kapur, V., L.-L. Li, M. R. Hamrick, B. B. Plikaytis, T. M. Shinnick, A. Telenti, W. R. Jacobs, A. Banerjee, S. Cole, K. Y. Yuen, J. E. Clarridge, B. N. Kreiswirth, and J. M. Musser.** 1995. Rapid *Mycobacterium* species assignment and unambiguous identification of mutations associated with antimicrobial resistance in *Mycobacterium tuberculosis* by automated DNA sequencing. *Arch. Pathol. Lab. Med.* **119:**131–138.
73. **Kaufhold, A., A. Podbielski, T. Horaud, and P. Ferrieri.** 1992. Identical genes confer high-level resistance to gentamicin upon *Enterococcus faecalis*, *Enterococcus faecium*, and *Staphylococcus aureus*. *Antimicrob. Agents Chemother.* **36:** 1215–1218.
74. **Kelley, C. L., D. A. Rouse, and S. L. Morris.** 1997. Analysis of *ahpC* gene mutations in isoniazid-resistant clinical isolates of *Mycobacterium tuberculosis*. *Antimicrob. Agents Chemother.* **41:**2057–2058.
75. **Klimov, A. I., E. Rocha, F. G. Hayden, P. A. Shult, L. F. Roumillat, and N. J. Cox.** 1995. Prolonged shedding of amantidine-resistant influenza A viruses by immunodeficient patients: detection by polymerase chain reaction-restriction analysis. *J. Infect. Dis.* **172:**1352–1355.
76. **Klugman, K. P.** 1990. Pneumococcal resistance to antibiotics. *Clin. Microbiol. Rev.* **3:**171–196.
77. **Kocagoz, T., C. J. Hackbarth, I. Unsal, E. Y. Rosenberg, H. Nikaido, and H. F. Chambers.** 1996. Gyrase mutations in laboratory-selected, fluoroquinolone-resistant mutants of *Mycobacterium tuberculosis* H37Ra. *Antimicrob. Agents Chemother.* **40:**1768–1774.
78. **Kozal, M. J., N. Shah, N. Shen, R. Yang, R. Fucini, T. C. Merigan, D. D. Richman, D. Morris, E. Hubbell, M. Chee, and T. R. Gingeras.** 1996. Extensive polymorphisms observed in HIV-1 clade B protease gene using high density oligonucleotide arrays. *Nat. Med.* **2:**753–759.
79. **Lacroix, J. M., and C. B. Walker.** 1996. Detection and prevalence of the tetracycline resistance determinant Tet

Q in the microbiota associated with adult periodontitis. *Oral Microbiol. Immunol.* **11:**282–288.

80. **Lambert, T., G. Gerbaud, P. Bouvet, J.-F. Vieu, and P. Courvalin.** 1990. Dissemination of amikacin resistance gene *aphA6* in *Acinetobacter* spp. *Antimicrob. Agents Chemother.* **34:**1244–1248.
81. **Larder, B. A., A. Kohli, P. Kellam, S. D. Kemp, M. Kronick, and R. D. Hefrey.** 1993. Quantitative detection of HIV-1 drug resistance mutations by automated DNA sequencing. *Nature* **365:**671–673.
82. **Levesque, R. C., A. A. Medeiros, and G. A. Jacoby.** 1987. Molecular cloning and DNA homology of plasmid-mediated β-lactamase genes. *Mol. Gen. Genet.* **206:**252–258.
83. **Lyras, D., and J. I. Rood.** 1996. Genetic organization and distribution of tetracycline resistance determinants in *Clostridium perfringens*. *Antimicrob. Agents Chemother.* **40:** 2500–2504.
84. **Mabilat, C., S. Goussard, W. Sougakoff, R. C. Spencer, and P. Courvalin.** 1990. Direct sequencing of the amplified structural gene and promoter for the extended-broad spectrum beta-lactamase TEM-9 (RHH-1) of *Klebsiella pneumoniae*. *Plasmid* **23:**27–34.
85. **Mariotte, S., P. Nordmann, and M. H. Nicolas.** 1994. Extended-spectrum β-lactamase in *Proteus mirabilis*. *J. Antimicrob. Chemother.* **33:**925–935.
86. **Marshall, B., C. Tachibana, and S. B. Levy.** 1983. Frequency of tetracycline resistance determinant classes among lactose-fermenting coliforms. *Antimicrob. Agents Chemother.* **24:**835–840.
87. **Martin, P., P. Trieu-Cuot, and P. Courvalin.** 1986. Nucleotide sequence of the *tet*M tetracycline resistance determinant of the streptococcal conjugative shuttle transposon Tn*1545*. *Nucleic Acids Res.* **14:**7047–7058.
88. **Maskell, J. P., A. M. Sefton, and L. M. C. Hall.** 1997. Mechanism of sulfonamide resistance in clinical isolates of *Streptococcus pneumoniae*. *Antimicrob. Agents Chemother.* **41:**2121–2126.
89. **Massanari, R. M., M. A. Pfaller, D. S. Wakefield, G. T. Hammons, L.-A. McNutt, R. F. Woolson, and C. H. Helms.** 1988. Implications of acquired oxacillin resistance in the management and control of *Staphylococcus aureus* infections. *J. Infect. Dis.* **158:**702–709.
90. **McDougal, L. K., J. K. Rasheed, J. W. Biddle, and F. C. Tenover.** 1995. Identification of multiple clones of extended-spectrum cephalosporin-resistant *Streptococcus pneumoniae* isolates in the United States. *Antimicrob. Agents Chemother.* **39:**2282–2288.
91. **Meier, A., P. Kirschner, F.-C. Bange, U. Vogel, and E. C. Böttger.** 1994. Genetic alterations in streptomycin-resistant *Mycobacterium tuberculosis*: mapping of mutations conferring resistance. *Antimicrob. Agents Chemother.* **38:** 228–233.
92. **Miele, A., M. Bandera, and B. P. Goldstein.** 1995. Use of primers selective for vancomycin resistance genes to determine *van* genotype in enterococci and to study gene organization in VanA isolates. *Antimicrob. Agents Chemother.* **39:**1772–1778.
93. **Morris, S., G. H. Bai, P. Suffys, L. Portillo-Gomez, M. Fairchok, and D. Rouse.** 1995. Molecular mechanisms of multiple drug resistance in clinical isolates of *Mycobacterium tuberculosis*. *J. Infect. Dis.* **171:**954–960.
94. **Muñoz, R., T. J. Coffey, M. Daniels, C. G. Dowson, G. Laible, J. Casal, R. Hakenbeck, M. Jacobs, J. M. Musser, B. G. Spratt, and A. Tomasz.** 1991. Intercontinental spread of a multiresistant clone of serotype 23F *Streptococcus pneumoniae*. *J. Infect. Dis.* **164:**302–306.
95. **Murakami, K., W. Minamide, K. Wada, E. Nakamura, H. Teraoka, and S. Watanabe.** 1991. Identification of methicillin-resistant strains of staphylococci by polymerase chain reaction. *J. Clin. Microbiol.* **29:**2240–2244.
96. **Murray, B. M.** 1991. New aspects of antimicrobial resistance and the resulting therapeutic dilemmas. *J. Infect. Dis.* **163:**1185–1194.
97. **Musser, J. M., V. Kapur, D. L. Williams, B. N. Kreiswirth, D. van Sooligan, and J. D. A. van Embden.** 1996. Characterization of the catalase-peroxidase gene (*kat*G) and *inhA* locus in isoniazid-resistant and -susceptible strains of *Mycobacterium tuberculosis* by automated DNA sequencing: restricted array of mutations associated with drug resistance. *J. Infect. Dis.* **173:**196–202.
98. **National Committee for Clinical Laboratory Standards.** 1994. *Specifications for Molecular Microbiology Methods for Infectious Diseases.* Proposed guideline MM3-P, vol. 1, no. 1. National Committee for Clinical Laboratory Standards, Wayne, Pa.
99. **Neu, H. C.** 1992. The crisis in antibiotic resistance. *Science* **257:**1064–1073.
100. **Nuesch-Inderbinen, M. T., H. Hachler, and F. H. Kayser.** 1996. Detection of genes coding for extended-spectrum SHV beta-lactamases in clinical isolates by a molecular genetic method, and comparison with the E test. *Eur. J. Clin. Microbiol. Infect. Dis.* **15:**398–402.
101. **Olsvik, B., M. J. Flynn, F. C. Tenover, J. Slots, and I. Olsen.** 1996. Tetracycline resistance in *Prevotella* isolates from periodontally diseased patients is due to the *tet*(Q) gene. *Oral Microbiol. Immunol.* **5:**304–308.
102. **Olsvik, B., I. Olsen, and F. C. Tenover.** 1994. The *tet*(Q) gene in bacteria isolated from patients with refractory periodontal disease. *Oral Microbiol. Immunol.* **9:**251–255.
103. **Olsvik, B., I. Olsen, and F. C. Tenover.** 1995. Detection of *tet*(M) and *tet*(O) using the polymerase chain reaction in bacteria isolated from patients with periodontal disease. *Oral Microbiol. Immunol.* **10:**87–92.
104. **Olsvik, B., F. C. Tenover, I. Olsen, and J. K. Rasheed.** 1996. Three subtypes of the *tet*(M) gene identified in bacterial isolates from periodontal pockets. *Oral Microbiol. Immunol.* **5:**299–303.
105. **Ounissi, H., E. Derlot, C. Carlier, and P. Courvalin.** 1990. Gene homogeneity for aminoglycoside-modifying enzymes in gram-positive cocci. *Antimicrob. Agents Chemother.* **34:**2164–2168.
106. **Papanicolaou, G. A., A. A. Medeiros, and G. A. Jacoby.** 1990. Novel plasmid-mediated β-lactamase (MIR-1) conferring resistance to oxyimino- and α-methoxy β-lactams in clinical isolates of *Klebsiella pneumoniae*. *Antimicrob. Agents Chemother.* **34:**2200–2209.
107. **Parsons, Y., R. M. Hall, and H. W. Stokes.** 1991. A new trimethoprim resistance gene, *dhfrX*, in the In*7* integron of plasmid pDGO100. *Antimicrob. Agents Chemother.* **35:**2436–2439.
108. **Pease, A. C.** 1994. Light-directed oligonucleotide arrays for rapid DNA sequence analysis. *Proc. Natl. Acad. Sci. USA* **91:**5022–5026.
109. **Perichon, B., P. Reynolds, and P. Courvalin.** 1997. VanD-type glycopeptide-resistant *Enterococcus faecium* BM4339. *Antimicrob. Agents Chemother.* **41:**2016–2018.
110. **Perichon, B., J. Tankovic, and P. Courvalin.** 1997. Characterization of a mutation in the *parE* gene that confers fluoroquinolone resistance in *Streptococcus pneumoniae*. *Antimicrob. Agents Chemother.* **41:**1166–1167.
111. **Ploy, M.-C., H. Giamarellou, P. Bourlioux, P. Courvalin, and T. Lambert.** 1994. Detection of *aac(6')-I* genes in amikacin-resistant *Acinetobacter* spp. by PCR. *Antimicrob. Agents Chemother.* **38:**2925–2928.
112. **Predari, S. C., M. Ligozzi, and R. Fontana.** 1991. Genotypic identification of methicillin-resistant coagulase-

negative staphylococci by polymerase chain reaction. *Antimicrob. Agents Chemother.* **35:**2568–2573.

113. **Pulkkinen, L., P. Houvinen, E. Vuorio, and P. Tiovanen.** 1984. Characterization of trimethoprim resistance by use of probes specific for transposon Tn*7*. *Antimicrob. Agents Chemother.* **26:**82–86.
114. **Rådström, P., G. Swedberg, and O. Sköld.** 1991. Genetic analyses of sulfonamide resistance and its dissemination in gram-negative bacteria illustrate new aspects of R plasmid evolution. *Antimicrob. Agents Chemother.* **35:**1840–1848.
115. **Ramsey, M. A., S. F. Bradley, C. A. Kauffman, and T. M. Morton.** 1996. Identification of chromosomal location of *mupA* gene, encoding low-level mupirocin resistance in staphylococcal isolates. *Antimicrob. Agents Chemother.* **40:**2820–2823.
116. **Rasheed, J. K., C. Jay, B. Metchock, F. Berkowitz, L. Weigel, J. Crellin, C. Steward, B. Hill, A. A. Medeiros, and F. C. Tenover.** 1997. Evolution of extended-spectrum β-lactam resistance (SHV-8) in a strain of *Escherichia coli* during multiple episodes of bacteremia. *Antimicrob. Agents Chemother.* **41:**647–653.
117. **Rather, P. N., R. Mierzwa, R. S. Hare, G. H. Miller, and K. J. Shaw.** 1992. Cloning and DNA sequence analysis of an *aac(3)-Vb* gene from *Serratia marcescens*. *Antimicrob. Agents Chemother.* **36:**2222–2227.
118. **Ridenhour, M. B., H. M. Fletcher, J. E. Mortensen, and L. Daneo-Moore.** 1996. A novel tetracycline-resistant determinant, *tet*(U), is encoded on the plasmid pKQ10 in *Enterococcus faecium*. *Plasmid* **35:**71–80.
119. **Roberts, M. C., W. O. Chung, and D. E. Roe.** 1996. Characterization of tetracycline and erythromycin resistance determinants in *Treponema denticola*. *Antimicrob. Agents Chemother.* **40:**1690–1694.
120. **Roberts, M. C., Y. Pang, D. E. Riley, S. L. Hillier, R. C. Berger, and J. N. Krieger.** 1993. Detection of Tet M and Tet O tetracycline resistance genes by polymerase chain reaction. *Mol. Cell. Probes* **7:**387–393.
121. **Rood, J. I., S. Jefferson, T. L. Bannam, J. M. Wilkie, P. Mullany, and B. W. Wren.** 1989. Hybridization analysis of three chloramphenicol resistance determinants from *Clostridium perfringens* and *Clostridium difficile*. *Antimicrob. Agents Chemother.* **33:**1569–1574.
122. **Sahm, D. F., L. Free, and S. Handwerger.** 1995. Inducible and constitutive expression of *vanC1*-encoded resistance to vancomycin in *Enterococcus gallinarum*. *Antimicrob. Agents Chemother.* **39:**1480–1484.
123. **Satake, S., N. Clark, D. Rimland, F. S. Nolte, and F. C. Tenover.** 1997. Detection of vancomycin-resistant enterococci in fecal samples by PCR. *J. Clin. Microbiol.* **35:**2325–2330.
124. **Schwocho, L. R., C. P. Schaffner, G. H. Miller, R. S. Hare, and K. J. Shaw.** 1995. Cloning and characterization of a 3-*N*-aminoglycoside acetyltransferase gene, *aac(3)-Ib*, from *Pseudomonas aeruginosa*. *Antimicrob. Agents Chemother.* **39:**1790–1796.
125. **Senda, K., Y. Arakawa, S. Ichiyama, K. Nakashima, H. Ito, S. Ohsuka, K. Shimokata, N. Kato, and M. Ohta.** 1996. PCR detection of metallo-β-lactamase gene (bla_{IMP}) in gram-negative rods resistant to broad-spectrum β-lactams. *J. Clin. Microbiol.* **34:**2909–2913.
126. **Shaw, K. J., R. S. Hare, F. J. Sabatelli, M. Rizzo, C. A. Cramer, G. H. Miller, L. Verbist, H. Van Landuyt, Y. Glupczynski, M. Catalano, and M. Woloj.** 1991. Correlation between aminoglycoside resistance profiles and DNA hybridization of clinical isolates. *Antimicrob. Agents Chemother.* **35:**2253–2261.
127. **Shaw, K. J., H. Munayyer, P. N. Rather, R. S. Hare, and G. H. Miller.** 1993. Nucleotide sequence analysis and DNA hybridization studies of the *ant(4')-IIa* gene from *Pseudomonas aeruginosa*. *Antimicrob. Agents Chemother.* **37:**708–714.
128. **Shaw, K. J., P. N. Rather, R. S. Hare, and G. H. Miller.** 1993. Molecular genetics of aminoglycoside resistance genes and familial relationships of the aminoglycoside-modifying enzymes. *Microbiol. Rev.* **57:**138–163.
129. **Shaw, W. V.** 1983. Chloramphenicol acetyltransferases: enzymology and molecular biology. *Crit. Rev. Biochem.* **14:**1–46.
130. **Shlaes, D. M., C. Currie-McCumber, A. Hull, I. Behlau, and M. Kron.** 1990. OHIO-1 β-lactamase is part of the SHV-1 family. *Antimicrob. Agents Chemother.* **34:**1570–1576.
131. **Shortridge, V. D., R. K. Flamm, N. Ramer, J. Beyer, and S. K. Tanaka.** 1996. Novel mechanism of macrolide resistance in *Streptococcus pneumoniae*. *Diagn. Microbiol. Infect. Dis.* **26:**73–78.
132. **Simard, J.-L., and P. H. Roy.** 1993. PCR detection of penicillinase-producing *Neisseria gonorrhoeae*, p. 543–546. *In* D. H. Persing, T. F. Smith, F. C. Tenover, and T. J. White (ed.), *Diagnostic Molecular Microbiology: Principles and Applications*. American Society for Microbiology, Washington, D.C.
133. **Singh, K. V., R. R. Reves, L. K. Pickering, and B. E. Murray.** 1992. Identification by DNA sequence analysis of a new plasmid-encoded trimethoprim resistance gene in fecal *Escherichia coli* isolates from children in day-care centers. *Antimicrob. Agents Chemother.* **36:**1720–1726.
134. **Sougakoff, W., B. Papadopoulou, P. Nordmann, and P. Courvalin.** 1987. Nucleotide sequence and distribution of gene *tet*O encoding tetracycline resistance in *Campylobacter coli*. *FEMS Microbiol. Lett.* **44:**153–159.
135. **Speer, B. S., N. B. Shoemaker, and A. A. Salyers.** 1992. Bacterial resistance to tetracycline: mechanisms, transfer, and clinical significance. *Clin. Microbiol. Rev.* **5:**387–399.
136. **Sreevatsan, S., X. Pan, K. E. Stockbauer, D. L. Williams, B. N. Kreiswirth, and J. M. Musser.** 1996. Characterization of *rpsL* and *rrs* mutations in streptomycin-resistant *Mycobacterium tuberculosis* isolates from diverse geographic localities. *Antimicrob. Agents Chemother.* **40:**1024–1026.
137. **Sreevatsan, S., X. Pan, Y. Zhang, B. N. Kreiswirth, and J. M. Musser.** 1997. Mutations associated with pyrazinamide resistance in *pncA* of *Mycobacterium tuberculosis* complex organisms. *Antimicrob. Agents Chemother.* **41:**636–640.
138. **Stuyver, L., A. Wyseur, A. Rombout, J. Louwagie, T. Scarcez, C. Verhofstede, D. Rimland, R. F. Schinazi, and R. Rossau.** 1997. Line probe assay for rapid detection of drug-selected mutations in the human immunodeficiency virus type 1 reverse transcription gene. *Antimicrob. Agents Chemother.* **41:**284–291.
139. **Sundstrom, L., C. Jansson, K. Bremer, E. Heikkila, B. Olsson-Liljequist, and O. Skold.** 1995. A new *dhfr* VIII trimethoprim-resistance gene, flanked by IS26, whose product is remote from other dihydrofolate reductases in parsimony analysis. *Gene* **154:**7–14.
140. **Sutcliffe, J., T. Grebe, A. Tait-Kamradt, and L. Wondrack.** 1996. Detection of erythromycin-resistant determinants by PCR. *Antimicrob. Agents Chemother.* **40:**2562–2566.
141. **Sutcliffe, J., A. Tait-Kamradt, and L. Wondrack.** 1996. *Streptococcus pneumoniae* and *Streptococcus pyogenes* resistant to macrolides but sensitive to clindamycin: a common resistance pattern mediated by an efflux system. *Antimicrob. Agents Chemother.* **40:**1817–1824.
142. **Swenson, J. M., M. J. Ferraro, D. F. Sahm, N. C. Clark, D. H. Culver, F. C. Tenover, and the National Committee for Clinical Laboratory Standards Study Group on**

Enterococci. 1995. Multilaboratory evaluation of screening methods for detection of high-level aminoglycoside resistance in enterococci. *J. Clin. Microbiol.* **33:** 3008–3018.

143. **Tait-Kamradt, A., J. Clancy, M. Cronan, F. Dib-Hajj, L. Wondrack, W. Yuan, and J. Sutcliffe.** 1997. *mefE* is necessary for the erythromycin-resistant M phenotype in *Streptococcus pneumoniae*. *Antimicrob. Agents Chemother.* **41:**2251–2255.
144. **Takiff, H. W., L. Salazar, C. Guerrero, W. Philipp, W. M. Huang, B. Kreiswirth, S. T. Cole, W. R. Jacobs, Jr., and A. Telenti.** 1994. Cloning and nucleotide sequence of *Mycobacterium tuberculosis gyrA* and *gyrB* genes and detection of quinolone resistance mutations. *Antimicrob. Agents Chemother.* **38:**773–780.
145. **Tankovic, J., B. Perichon, J. Duval, and P. Courvalin.** 1996. Contribution of mutations in *gyrA* and *parC* genes to fluoroquinolone resistance of mutants of *Streptococcus pneumoniae* obtained in vivo and in vitro. *Antimicrob. Agents Chemother.* **40:**2505–2510.
146. **Telenti, A., N. Honore, C. Bernasconi, J. March, A. Ortega, B. Heym, H. E. Takiff, and S. T. Cole.** 1997. Genotypic assessment of isoniazid and rifampin resistance in *Mycobacterium tuberculosis*: a blind study at reference laboratory level. *J. Clin. Microbiol.* **35:**719–723.
147. **Telenti, A., P. Imboden, F. Marchesi, T. Schmidheini, and T. Bodmer.** 1993. Direct, automated detection of rifampicin-resistant *Mycobacterium tuberculosis* by polymerase chain reaction and single-strand conformation polymorphism analysis. *Antimicrob. Agents Chemother.* **37:**2054–2058.
148. **Tenover, F. C., D. Filpula, K. L. Phillips, and J. J. Plorde.** 1988. Cloning and sequencing of a gene encoding a 6′-*N*-acetyltransferase from an R factor of *Citrobacter diversus*. *J. Bacteriol.* **170:**471–473.
149. **Tenover, F. C., T. D. Gootz, K. P. Gordon, and J. J. Plorde.** 1984. Development of a DNA probe for the structural gene of the 2″-*O*-adenyltransferase aminoglycoside modifying enzyme. *J. Infect. Dis.* **150:**678–687.
150. **Tenover, F. C., M. B. Huang, J. K. Rasheed, and D. H. Persing.** 1994. Development of polymerase chain reaction assays to detect ampicillin resistance genes in cerebrospinal fluid samples containing *Haemophilus influenzae*. *J. Clin. Microbiol.* **32:**2729–2737.
151. **Tenover, F. C., D. J. LeBlanc, and P. Elvrum.** 1987. Cloning and expression of a tetracycline resistance determinant from *Campylobacter jejuni* in *Escherichia coli*. *Antimicrob. Agents Chemother.* **31:**1301–1306.
152. **Tenover, F. C., K. L. Phillips, T. Gilbert, P. Lockhart, P. J. O'Hara, and J. J. Plorde.** 1989. Development of a DNA probe from the deoxyribonucleotide sequence of a 3-*N*-aminoglycoside acetyltransferase [AAC(3)-I] resistance gene. *Antimicrob. Agents Chemother.* **33:**551–559.
153. **Thakker-Varia, S., J. W. Jenssen, L. Mon-McDermott, M. P. Weinstein, and D. T. Dubin.** 1987. Molecular epidemiology of macrolides-lincosamides-streptogramin B resistance in *Staphylococcus aureus* and coagulase-negative staphylococci. *Antimicrob. Agents Chemother.* **31:** 735–743.
154. **Thomson, C. J., K. J. Towner, H.-K. Young, and S. G. B. Amyes.** 1990. Identification and cloning of the type IIIa plasmid-encoded dihydrofolate reductase gene from trimethoprim-resistant gram-negative bacteria isolated in Britain. *J. Med. Microbiol.* **31:**213–218.
155. **Tomasz, A., H. B. Drugeon, H. M. de Lencastre, D. Jabes, L. McDougal, and J. Bille.** 1989. New mechanism for methicillin resistance in *Staphylococcus aureus*: clinical isolates that lack the PBP 2a gene and contain normal penicillin-binding capacity. *Antimicrob. Agents Chemother.* **33:**1869–1874.
156. **Towner, K. J., and G. I. Carter.** 1990. Cloning of the type VII trimethoprim resistant dihydrofolate reductase gene and identification of a specific DNA probe. *FEMS Microbiol. Lett.* **70:**19–22.
157. **Towner, K. J., H.-K. Young, and S. G. B. Amyes.** 1988. Biotinylated DNA probes for trimethoprim-resistant dihydrofolate reductases types IV and V. *J. Antimicrob. Chemother.* **22:**285–291.
158. **Trieu-Cuot, P., and P. Courvalin.** 1983. Nucleotide sequence of the *Streptococcus faecalis* plasmid gene encoding 3′5″-aminoglycoside phosphotransferase type III. *Gene* **23:**331–341.
159. **Trieu-Cuot, P., G. de Cespédès, F. Bentorcha, F. Delbos, E. Gaspar, and P. Courvalin.** 1993. Study of heterogeneity of chloramphenicol acetyltransferase (CAT) genes in streptococci and enterococci by polymerase chain reaction: characterization of a new CAT determinant. *Antimicrob. Agents Chemother.* **37:**2593–2598.
160. **Truong, Q. C., J.-C. Nguyen Van, D. Shlaes, L. Gutmann, and N. J. Moreau.** 1997. A novel, double mutation in DNA gyrase A of *Escherichia coli* conferring resistance to quinolone antibiotics. *Antimicrob. Agents Chemother.* **41:**85–90.
161. **Tyler, K. D., G. Wang, S. D. Tyler, and W. M. Johnson.** 1997. Factors affecting reliability and reproducibility of amplification based DNA fingerprinting of representative bacterial pathogens. *J. Clin. Microbiol.* **35:**339–346.
162. **Ubukata, K., Y. Asahi, A. Yamane, and M. Konno.** 1996. Combinational detection of autolysin and penicillin binding protein 2B genes of *Streptococcus pneumoniae* by PCR. *J. Clin. Microbiol.* **34:**592–596.
163. **Ubukata, K., S. Nakagami, A. Nitta, A. Yamane, S. Kawakami, M. Sugiura, and A. Konno.** 1992. Rapid detection of the *mecA* gene in methicillin-resistant staphylococci by enzymatic detection of polymerase chain reaction products. *J. Clin. Microbiol.* **30:**1728–1733.
164. **Vahaboglu, H., L. M. C. Hall, L. Mulazimoglu, S. Dodanli, I. Yildirim, and D. M. Livermore.** 1995. Resistance to extended-spectrum cephalosporins, caused by PER-1 β-lactamase, in *Salmonella typhimurium* from Istanbul, Turkey. *J. Med. Microbiol.* **43:**294–299.
165. **van de Klundert, J. A. M., and J. S. Vliegenthart.** 1993. PCR detection of genes coding for aminoglycoside modifying enzymes, p. 547–552. *In* D. H. Persing, T. F. Smith, F. C. Tenover, and T. J. White (ed.), *Diagnostic Molecular Microbiology: Principles and Applications*. American Society for Microbiology, Washington, D.C.
166. **vanHoof R., J. Content, E. Van Bossuyt, L. Dewit, and E. Hannecart-Pokorni.** 1992. Identification of the *aadB* gene coding for the aminoglycoside-2″-*O*-nucleotidyltransferase, ANT(2″), by means of the polymerase chain reaction. *J. Antimicrob. Chemother.* **29:**365–374.
167. **Vercauteren, E., P. Descheemaecker, M. Ieven, C. C. Sanders, and H. Goossens.** 1997. Comparison of screening methods for detection of extended-spectrum β-lactamases and their prevalence among blood isolates of *Escherichia coli* and *Klebsiella* spp. in a Belgian teaching hospital. *J. Clin. Microbiol.* **35:**2191–2197.
168. **Vila, J., J. Ruiz, P. Goni, A. Marcos, and T. J. De Anta.** 1995. Mutation in the *gyrA* gene of quinolone-resistant clinical isolates of *Acinetobacter baumannii*. *Antimicrob. Agents Chemother.* **39:**1201–1203.
169. **Williams, D. L., C. Waguespack, K. Eisenach, J. T. Crawford, F. Portaels, M. Salfinger, C. M. Nolan, C. Abe, V. Sticht-Groh, and T. P. Gillis.** 1994. Characterization of rifampin resistance in pathogenic mycobacteria. *Antimicrob. Agents Chemother.* **38:**2380–2386.

170. **Wondrack, L., M. Massa, B. V. Yang, and J. Sutcliffe.** 1996. Clinical strain of *Staphylococcus aureus* inactivates and causes efflux of macrolides. *Antimicrob. Agents Chemother.* **40:**992–998.
171. **Woodford, N., D. Morrison, A. P. Johnson, V. Briant, R. C. George, and B. Cookson.** 1993. Application of DNA probes for *rRNA* and *vanA* genes to investigation of a nosocomial cluster of vancomycin-resistant enterococci. *J. Clin. Microbiol.* **31:**653–658.
172. **Wren, B. W., P. Mullany, and S. Tabachali.** 1988. Molecular cloning and genetic analysis of a chloramphenicol acetyltransferase determinant from *Clostridium difficile*. *Antimicrob. Agents Chemother.* **32:**1213–1217.
173. **Zhang, Y., B. Heym, B. Allen, D. Young, and S. Cole.** 1992. The catalase-peroxidase gene and isoniazid resistance of *Mycobacterium tuberculosis*. *Science* **358:** 591–593.
174. **Zhao, J., and T. Aoki.** 1992. Nucleotide sequence analysis of the class G tetracycline resistance determinant from *Vibrio anguillarum*. *Microbiol. Immunol.* **36:**1051–1060.

Susceptibility Testing Instrumentation and Computerized Expert Systems for Data Analysis and Interpretation

MARY JANE FERRARO AND JAMES H. JORGENSEN

123

Clinical microbiology laboratories can choose from several different manual or instrument-assisted methods for performance of routine antibacterial susceptibility tests. These include disk diffusion, agar dilution, broth tube and microdilution, antibiotic gradient, and overnight or short-incubation automated instrument methods. This chapter focuses on the overnight or short-incubation antimicrobial susceptibility test methods that are available in the United States and other parts of the world and that offer various levels of instrumentation. Some test systems are not automated but rather are computer-assisted, which facilitates data entry and interpretation of visually determined growth endpoints. Other more sophisticated systems have software that can provide medical and laboratory decision support through a computerized expert system that analyzes identification and susceptibility test results (27).

The least automated of the instrument-based systems interpret growth endpoints only when microdilution trays or strips are inserted into a reader device, while others incubate microdilution trays or special cards with microcuvettes and perform serial interpretations of growth patterns in the presence of antimicrobial agents. The instruments vary in their methods of presenting the bacterial test module to the optical detector system. The instruments that offer the highest degree of automation generally do so by incorporating simple internal robotics to manipulate the test modules during the incubation and reading sequences. Current instruments use either the principle of turbidimetric detection of bacterial growth in a liquid medium, fluorometric detection of fluorescent indicators (31) or the hydrolysis of fluorogenic substrates (2, 9, 25, 35) incorporated in a special liquid medium, or turbinephelometric detection of both the light scattered and the light transmitted in a semisolid medium. The suppression of turbidity as evidence of the inhibitory effect of an antimicrobial agent or, conversely, the increase in turbidity in the presence of a drug as an indication of microbial resistance has been firmly established in manual broth dilution susceptibility test methods (39). Inference of susceptibility or resistance on the basis of the activity of specific bacterial enzymes produced during bacterial growth and the hydrolysis of fluorogenic substrates is a more recent method for growth determination. All of the instruments rely heavily on microprocessor-controlled functions, and they use microcomputers to provide final printed reports and to enable data storage and retrieval. Most of the instruments can also be used to perform additional functions, usually to identify gram-negative or gram-positive bacteria and, in some cases, to assemble combined identification and antimicrobial susceptibility reports (34).

COMPUTER-ASSISTED, SEMIAUTOMATED INSTRUMENTS FOR ANTIMICROBIAL DISK SUSCEPTIBILITY TEST METHODS

During the last decade, several semiautomated devices designed to assist in reading and interpretation of inhibition zones on agar plates used for antimicrobial disk susceptibility testing have been developed. The BIOMIC (Giles Scientific, Inc., New York, N.Y.), the AccuZone system (AccuMed International, Inc., West Lake, Ohio), and SIRSCAN (SIRSCAN, Montpellier, France) are examples of plate readers available in the United States and other parts of the world. Depending upon the system, disk diffusion plates of various sizes containing different types of media are inserted manually into the instrument, which assists with zone diameter reading by image analysis and interprets all zones of inhibition in no more than 5 s per plate. Automated plate readers offer the potential to reduce zone measurement and transcription errors in laboratories that use the disk diffusion antimicrobial susceptibility test method, which continues to be a reliable and accurate method. In one instance, BIOMIC, it is claimed that the MICs of individual drugs can be determined by computer algorithms from the zone diameter measurements. In limited evaluations (3, 16), these instruments have proven to provide reproducible, generally accurate results compared to those obtained by taking manual measurements. It is recommended, however, that the technologist examine each plate for subtle variations in growth (e.g., haze or pinpoint colonies within an inhibition zone) that might change the interpretation of the susceptibility report. In these cases, the video-assisted readings can be adjusted by the technologist prior to the release of patient results.

COMPUTER-ASSISTED, MANUAL, OVERNIGHT BROTH MICRODILUTION SUSCEPTIBILITY TEST SYSTEMS

Virtually every manufacturer of broth microdilution trays for antimicrobial susceptibility testing offers a mechanized device for hydration or inoculation of trays and a device to facilitate manual visualization of results after incubation. Most manufacturers also offer some type of reader device whereby the user indicates the results of manual interpretation of the growth patterns in the tray by the use of a light pen, a video display screen resembling the configuration of the tray, or a touch-sensitive template that overlays the microdilution tray. The MicroScan touchSCAN-SR (Dade Behring, Inc., West Sacramento, Calif.), Becton Dickinson Sceptor (Becton Dickinson Diagnostic Instrument Systems, Sparks, Md.), Becton Dickinson Pasco and Sensititre Sensi Touch (AccuMed International, Inc.) are examples of such systems. An autoinoculator is also available for purchase with the Sensititre System. Although growth in the test wells is manually interpreted, the reader devices assist with data recording, application of interpretive criteria, and generation of a computer-printed report. The microcomputers that are included with these systems enable the user to store and later retrieve data for generation of periodic reports, e.g., cumulative susceptibility profiles for various organisms during a defined time period.

SEMIAUTOMATED, OVERNIGHT, AND SHORT-INCUBATION BROTH MICRODILUTION TEST SYSTEMS

Automated reading devices that interpret growth patterns in trays or strips represent the next level of instrumentation available from several manufacturers. The MicroScan autoSCAN-4, Becton Dickinson AutoSceptor, and Sensititre AutoReader are examples of instruments for automated interpretation of the results for microdilution trays following overnight incubation in a standard incubator. The mini API (bioMérieux, Marcy l'Etoile, France) can interpret susceptibility test results for members of the family *Enterobacteriaceae* and *Staphylococcus aureus* after strips are incubated off-line for 4 to 5 h, while other organism groups including fastidious bacteria, anaerobes, and yeast require a full 24 h of incubation. The instruments have readers that determine growth either photometrically or turbinephelometrically (mini API) and are configured with microcomputers for report preparation, data analysis, and data storage. Although AutoReader, AutoSceptor, and mini API come with an autoinoculator or electronic pipette, these instruments automate only the final, reading step involved in the performance of MIC or breakpoint microdilution tests. Evaluation of one instrument has shown that MIC endpoints can be interpreted by such instruments with reasonable accuracy (1). However, instances of haze or small pellets of growth that may be important in the determination of resistance can be missed by automated readers with photometers (21, 45).

AUTOMATED OVERNIGHT AND SHORT-INCUBATION SUSCEPTIBILITY TEST SYSTEMS

The most significant change to occur in antimicrobial susceptibility testing during the last two decades has been the development of automated short-incubation susceptibility test systems. Continuing improvements in microprocessors, robotics, and microcomputers have allowed the development of instruments capable of providing antimicrobial susceptibility results in as short a time as 3.5 h. In order to accomplish this, a variety of strategies that deviate from those of conventional susceptibility test methods are used. For example, the concentration of bacteria in the initially prepared test inoculum is generally adjusted upward from that used in standard procedures. Often, the actual concentration of the antimicrobial agent in the test well is manipulated to provide results comparable to those provided by reference microdilution tests. The MICs determined by these instruments are algorithmically derived from growth rate comparisons. The sophisticated computer software used with the instruments affords editing and adjustment of results for certain drug-bacterium combinations. The growth media used in these test systems are not those used for traditional methods and often include modifications to promote more rapid growth or better detection of resistance for certain bacteria.

The first short-incubation susceptibility system, the TAAS system, was developed in the early 1970s by Technicon Instruments Corp. (Tarrytown, N.Y.) but was never marketed (11). The detection principles used in subsequent instruments such as the Autobac System developed and marketed by Pfizer Diagnostics in the early 1970s (later called Autobac Series II; Organon Teknika, Durham, N.C.), the Abbott MS-2 system (later called the Avantage MICROBIOLOGY CENTER; Abbott Laboratories Diagnostic Division, Irving, Tex.), and later, COBAS-BACT (Roche Diagnostics, Basel, Switzerland) were based on the photometric growth detection principles used in the TAAS system. Although these systems enjoy the distinction of being the first commercially available short-incubation susceptibility test systems, they are no longer manufactured and are virtually extinct in laboratories today. Short-incubation systems such as the VITEK System, formerly called the AutoMicrobic System or AMS (bioMerieux Vitek), and the MicroScan WalkAway (2, 9), formerly called the AutoScan W/A (Dade Behring, Inc.), are the only ones with Food and Drug Administration (FDA) approval for use in clinical laboratories in the United States. The short-incubation VITEK and WalkAway systems were both initially approved by FDA for the testing of most common bacteria and antimicrobial agents prior to the implementation of more stringent requirements in 1991 (see below). However, all new antimicrobial agents to be marketed for testing with these systems must undergo the extensive FDA review described below. Other systems such as the mini API (bioMerieux, France) and short-incubation Sensititre ARIS (Radiometer America) (25, 28) systems are used to various extents throughout the world, but they are not currently approved by FDA for use in the United States.

Short-Incubation VITEK System

The VITEK System is a by-product of U.S. space exploration efforts in the 1960s. It was designed and manufactured originally by the McDonnell-Douglas Corp. for the National Aeronautics and Space Administration as an onboard test system for spacecraft to detect and identify common urinary tract pathogens from specimens from astronauts. Because of its intended use aboard a spacecraft, it was highly automated and relatively compact from its inception. Very small plastic reagent cards were designed to contain microliter quantities of biochemical test and selective growth media for the detection and identification of organisms. The VITEK System was modified in the 1970s for clinical laboratory use principally for the screening and identification of urinary organisms and for qualitative antimicrobial susceptibility testing with susceptible (S), intermediate (I), or resistant (R) results only with *Escherichia coli* or *Proteus mirabilis*. In the 1980s, MIC cards that allow semiquantitative results for most rapidly growing gram-positive and gram-negative aerobic bacteria in a period of 4 to 10 h were developed.

VITEK System hardware includes a filling-sealer module for inoculation of the cards; an incubator-reader module that incorporates a carousel-like device to hold the test cards, a robotic system to manipulate the cards, and a photometer for measurement of optical density and biochemical reaction color changes in the cards; and a computer module, including a video display monitor and printer (34). The VITEK System also offers an elaborate information management system for the storage and retrieval of test data and for the generation of a variety of statistical reports. The VITEK System uses turbidometrically determined kinetic measurements of growth in the presence of antimicrobial agents to perform linear regression analysis and, ultimately, to determine algorithm-derived MICs. The user may elect to have susceptibility test results reported in either qualitative (S, I, or R results) or doubling-dilution MIC formats.

A more automated version of the VITEK System, the VITEK 2 System, has been developed and marketed in Europe and the Asia-Pacific rim. Clinical laboratory use in the United States awaits FDA clearance, which is expected in late 1999. The VITEK 2 System automates the front-end sample processing including initial inoculum dilution, density verification, and card-filling and card-sealing steps. The instrument automatically transfers cards to the reader-incubator and ejects them into a disposal bin at the completion of testing. All of these features should reduce technical time and improve work flow.

The fixed formats of the current 30-well (9 to 11 antibiotics) or the 45-well (15 to 17 antibiotics) VITEK cards impose some limitations in the selection of drugs for testing; however, a large number of standard configurations are available for both 30- and 45-well cards. For laboratories wishing to test an institution-specific battery of antimicrobial agents, the VITEK System offers custom cards, which must be ordered in large quantities. The VITEK 2 instrument will use a 64-well card and allow the testing of approximately 20 antimicrobial agents depending on the organism group, which will include *Streptococcus pneumoniae*.

Overnight or Short-Incubation WalkAway System

The WalkAway System was developed in the late 1980s and is capable of automating either overnight or, when used in conjunction with Microscan Rapid Panels, short-incubation susceptibility tests. The instrument consists of a large self-contained incubator-reader unit and a microcomputer with a video display terminal and a printer (34). The WalkAway System uses standard-size microdilution trays that are read either photometrically (overnight testing) or fluorometrically (short-incubation testing). Once the microdilution trays have been manually inoculated with a multiprong device, they are placed in one of the incubator positions in the instrument. The instrument then incubates the trays for the appropriate period and robotically positions and aligns the trays under the central photometer or fluorometer to perform the final readings of growth endpoints when the value of a growth index exceeds a predetermined level (9).

The WalkAway System offers a choice of MIC or breakpoint testing of gram-positive and gram-negative bacteria after overnight or rapid (3.5- to 15-h) incubation. Special "combo" trays that provide susceptibility information and organism identification in the same tray are available.

In theory, the detection of the resulting fluorescence as a marker of growth is more sensitive than detection with photometric technology, thus allowing the more rapid assessment of bacterial growth. However, fluorometric detection of growth is indirect and assumes that all bacteria are capable of metabolizing the fluorogenic substrates, that the enzymatic activity of nonmultiplying cells is insignificant in comparison to that of multiplying cells, and that the fluorogenic substrates do not interfere with the activities of any of the antimicrobial agents tested (2, 9).

Overnight or Short-Incubation Sensititre ARIS

The Sensititre ARIS was developed in the 1980s and is marketed in the United States only for overnight susceptibility testing, although it is available in a few other countries for short-incubation testing. The instrument includes an incubator-reader unit with an associated microcomputer (including a video display terminal and a printer). Similar to the WalkAway System, the ARIS incorporates the use of standard-size microdilution trays; once the trays are individually inoculated with an autoinoculator, the instrument incubates them, positions the trays by robotics under the fluorometer, and automatically interprets the growth patterns at the conclusion of the tests. As with the short-incubation WalkAway System, growth is determined following fluorogenic substrate hydrolysis. In the United States, ARIS uses a conventional overnight incubation period for performance of MIC, breakpoint, or combination susceptibility identification tests with gram-positive and gram-negative bacteria.

REGULATORY OVERSIGHT OF SUSCEPTIBILITY TEST INSTRUMENTS AND CRITERIA FOR ACCEPTABLE PERFORMANCE

Over the years a variety of criteria for statistically defining the acceptable accuracy of a new susceptibility test system (13, 23, 32, 38) have been proposed. At present none of the professional consensus organizations (e.g., the National Committee for Clinical Laboratory Standards [NCCLS]) promulgates guidelines regarding the specific quality control or performance of short-incubation susceptibility test methods. Following the enactment of the Safe Medical Devices Act of 1990, the short-incubation instruments and their drug panels now require premarket approval (PMA) by FDA for clearance to be marketed in the United States. This PMA has become more difficult to obtain in the 1990s because of new, more stringent FDA controls (8). Extensive studies that provide data on the ability of the short-incubation systems to determine accurately susceptibility test results compared to the ability of a reference method are required for PMA. A large number of organisms including quality control organisms, a challenge set of organisms with known mechanisms of resistance, and fresh or stock clinical isolates representing each antimicrobial agent's spectrum of activity must be tested. It is expected that very major errors will be $\leq$1.5%, major errors will be $\leq$3%, essential agreement ($\pm 1\ \log_2$ dilution) will be $\geq$90%, and growth failures will be $\leq$10%. For any microorganism, antimicrobial agent, or combination thereof not meeting these specifications, the labeling (package insert) of the device should include this contraindication and should recommend the use of an alternative method for testing. When fewer than 20 strains representing each known mechanism of resistance to that antimicrobial agent were tested, a statement must be included in the labeling saying that the ability to detect resistance to an antimicrobial agent among these species is unknown because sufficient resistant strains were not available at the time of comparative testing. Instruments that use incubation times of 16 h or more are subject to a less extensive process by FDA, called premarket notification (510K) clearance.

ADVANTAGES OF CURRENT INSTRUMENTS

The antimicrobial susceptibility testing instruments discussed above represent the highest level of automation now available for use in clinical microbiology laboratories. However, automation in clinical microbiology is still in a very early state of development compared with the level of automation that has been achieved in clinical chemistry, hematology, and immunology laboratories. All of the current microbiology instruments offer the potential for improved intra- and interlaboratory reproducibilities of antimicrobial susceptibility tests, and in some cases they significantly reduce the time required to perform the tests (e.g., 3.5 to 10 h of incubation versus overnight incubation). Most evaluations have reported that the instruments are mechanically reliable and that their operation is readily mastered by well-trained microbiologists and medical technologists. These instruments offer various degrees of labor savings over the amounts of labor required for manually performed tests. Because all of the instruments can perform some of the most common analyses in the microbiology laboratory, i.e., organism identification and antimicrobial susceptibility testing, the potential exists to automate a sizable proportion of a laboratory's tasks with only one instrument. The potential to establish a link between the microcomputer that controls the function of the instrument and the laboratory computer affords both potential savings in labor and the elimination of transcription errors associated with manual entry of results. When such instruments are interfaced, however, verification of susceptibility data by supervisory personnel is advisable before the automated transfer of data to a patient file. In addition, the data management systems available with these instruments provide neat, legible test reports for the laboratory and can archive and periodically analyze trends in the antimicrobial susceptibilities of the microorganisms encountered in a given institution.

Several of the systems allow linkage of the microbiology results with the patient's pharmacy record, thus enabling review of the antimicrobial therapy regimen. In some institutions such linkages can ultimately notify the prescribing physician when the isolated organism is resistant to the antimicrobial therapy, when therapy against a clinical isolate for which susceptibility results have been obtained has not been started, or when an antimicrobial agent for which the algorithm cannot find a clinical isolate or susceptibility test results for the patient has been administered (27).

One of the advantages, yet to be fully exploited, of instrument-based susceptibility test systems is the potential use of artificial intelligence to create an "expert" system (6, 10, 27) for automated review and verification of the data generated. Appropriately programmed software can contain algorithms or rules similar to those used by knowledgeable microbiologists to detect impossible or unusual phenotypes, allowing recognition of technical errors that may have occurred in the testing. For example, unusual phenotypes such as ampicillin-susceptible *Klebsiella pneumoniae* or cefazolin-susceptible *Enterobacter cloacae* would be flagged by the system. Other rules designed to recognize unlikely resistance patterns or rare antibiogram phenotypes such as imipenem-resistant *E. coli* can also be designed. Following detection, the possibility of potential errors or unusual phenotypes would be flagged on the data terminal or laboratory report for technologists or supervisory review. For the mini API, VITEK, and, to a lesser degree, the WalkAway systems, this enhancement has been added to the instrument software. Finally, expert systems can use the organism's antibiogram to predict resistance mechanisms, which could enable laboratories to modify the susceptibility test report to reflect more accurately (or more conservatively) the resistance profile of the organism. Alternatively, the laboratory could choose to indicate in a separate message to the physician the likelihood that clinically important cross-resistance to a related antimicrobial agent may exist. The rules and use of computerized expert systems for data analysis and interpretation will be further discussed in the last section of this chapter.

It has yet to be unequivocally demonstrated that rapid susceptibility test results have a major positive impact on patient care. Several studies (7, 40, 41) have shown that providing rapid susceptibility test results is likely to result in a more timely change to appropriate antimicrobial therapy than if conventional reporting times were used. One of the studies (7) also documented lower mortality rates and direct cost savings attributable to the use of fewer diagnostic studies and fewer numbers of days in an intensive care area on the basis of rapid susceptibility and bacterial identification test reports. However, it has been aptly pointed out that the rapid generation of any test results in the laboratory can have a clinical impact only when the results are linked to a reporting system that also permits the rapid transmission of these test results to the physician (1, 14, 22, 27).

DISADVANTAGES OF CURRENT INSTRUMENTS

The instruments discussed in this chapter offer automation of several of the steps involved in the performance of an antimicrobial susceptibility test, but only recently has an instrument (VITEK 2) been able to execute the entire process, i.e., to standardize an inoculum and continue through to the final interpretation of results without operator intervention. In most cases, microbiologists must still isolate bacteria by using conventional culture methods and prepare a bacterial suspension of defined density for testing by the instrument. Thus, the automated aspects of the test do not begin until after the manual inoculum preparation. Indeed, inadequacy of the inoculum is a major variable affecting the performance of all of the instruments.

Laboratories that use these systems must purchase antimicrobial agent test panels that are specified by the manufacturer, unless a laboratory's volume warrants purchase of a more expensive custom panel. The flexibility to change the test battery or to quickly begin testing of a newly marketed antimicrobial agent is limited.

Another major disadvantage is that these instrument-based systems are not applicable for the testing of all clinically relevant groups of bacteria. For example, the testing of nutritionally fastidious bacteria, anaerobes, and certain nonfermentative gram-negative bacilli is often not possible. Therefore, alternative susceptibility test methods must be available in the laboratory.

For the short-incubation systems, a wide range of doubling dilutions or drug concentrations for a given antimicrobial agent are not tested. MICs, when produced, are reliable only within the concentration range tested, and MICs higher or lower than the test concentrations can be expressed only as semiquantitative results.

Quality control is dependent on the use of American Type Culture Collection organisms specified by the manufacturer, since NCCLS does not provide standards for test procedures or quality control of short-incubation susceptibility test systems. Some of the quality control organisms suggested by manufacturers do not produce on-scale quality control values (17, 18). The quality control check suggested by the manufacturer may not detect subtle deteriorations in instrument or reagent performance.

When purchased, a large capital investment for hardware is required. The disposables used with the rapid systems may be more expensive than the components needed for manual test methods. In addition to space and electrical requirements, fees for service contracts add to operational costs. Laboratories may wish to obtain use of an instrument system using a reagent rental or lease agreement to avoid a large, initial capital outlay for hardware.

Manufacturers' package inserts often include frequent disclaimers or limitations for organism-drug combinations that cannot be tested with a system. If the disclaimed antimicrobial agent is critical to patient care, an alternate procedure must be used to assess resistance or the results for that antimicrobial agent cannot be reported. In some cases, the accuracies of instrument-generated results have been lower than those of the results obtained with manual reference systems, particularly if the instrument has used a short-incubation period or a nontraditional growth detection method (19, 42, 47).

Reports of false-susceptible or false-resistant results (compared to the results obtained by reference methods) have been reported by users of instrument-read or short-incubation susceptibility test systems. In some cases, these findings have been sporadic and not easily explained. In many instances careful attention to the importance of inoculum preparation from fresh colonies and appropriate inoculum standardization with a nepholometer rather than by visual adjustment will correct spurious results.

An incubation period of only 3.5 to 6 h may not be adequate for expression of all bacterial resistance mechanisms, e.g., among gram-negative bacilli inducible β-lactamase-mediated resistance to some enzyme-labile β-lactam antimicrobial agents (20, 30). This is particularly true for *Citrobacter freundii*, *Enterobacter* spp., *Serratia* spp., *Morganella morganii*, *Providencia* spp., and *Pseudomonas aeruginosa*. Although detection of plasmid-mediated extended-spectrum β-lactamases that confer resistance to ceftazidime, cefotaxime, and other extended-spectrum cephalosporins and monobactams is a problem for reference susceptibility test methods, it may be even more so for short-incubation systems (15). Future inclusion of test wells with low concentrations of broad-spectrum cephalosporins with and without a β-lactamase inhibitor such as clavulanate may help to detect strains with these enzymes (28, 33), which appear to be more common in *Klebsiella* spp. and *E. coli*.

A false-positive result for resistance to aztreonam, especially for *Proteus* and *Morganella* spp., can occur in the systems that detect growth photometrically (4). This phenomenon results because elongation of the cells, which occurs just prior to lysis, is interpreted as growth. Additionally, false-positive resistance to imipenem for various species has been reported for both overnight and short-incubation systems (4, 44). This false-positive resistance occurs sporadically and may be due to degradation of the antimicrobial agent in the specific test system (44) or the zinc concentration in the medium (5).

Low- or moderate-level vancomycin resistance in *Enterococcus* spp., especially that of the VanB type (36), may not be detected with some short-incubation susceptibility test systems (12). Since some vancomycin-resistant strains exhibit inducible resistance, failure to detect such strains may be due in part to the short incubation period. In one study, intrinsic, low-level resistance of the VanC type in *Enterococcus gallinarum*, however, appears to be detected accurately (36). Recent reports indicate that short-incubation susceptibility test systems may not reliably detect the subtle increases in vancomycin MICs that have been reported for *S. aureus* and certain coagulase-negative staphylococci (37).

Problems with the detection of high-level gentamicin resistance or high-level streptomycin resistance for *Enterococcus* spp. have also been reported for overnight and short-incubation susceptibility test systems (29, 43). For the short incubation systems, a decrease in the concentration of aminoglycosides in the test medium promises to correct the problems (26, 46). Failure of an optical reading device to detect subtle amounts of growth in wells with high levels of an aminoglycoside following overnight incubation has been reported (21). Changes in the growth medium used in these wells for overnight systems (43), as recommended by NCCLS (24), or extended incubation (46) may correct these problems.

COMPUTERIZED EXPERT SYSTEMS

Laboratories may purchase susceptibility test systems that have preprogrammed, rule-based expert systems. Alternatively, the microbiology laboratory information system may allow the custom programming of similar computer algorithms. In either case, the success of the rule-based expert system relies squarely on the expertise of the creators and, potentially, on the customized rules for a specific institution.

The medical and laboratory decision support afforded by these programs has several advantages. The algorithms allow continuous monitoring of inconsistent laboratory test results without human intervention, such that there should be more rapid recognition of incorrect or aberrant identification or susceptibility test results. Their use should lead to more uniform reporting both within and among laboratories.

Tables 1, 2, and 3 provide information on resistant or susceptible phenotypes for organisms and their commonly tested antimicrobial agents (24). Table 4 lists expected com-

TABLE 1 Resistance phenotypes that are rare or that have not been detected

Organism(s)	Antimicrobial agent(s) to which resistance is uncommon
Members of the family *Enterobacteriaceae*	Imipenem, meropenem
Staphylococcus aureus	Vancomycin, teicoplanin
Coagulase-negative staphylococci	Vancomycin
Enterococcus faecalis	Ampicillin
Enterococcus faecium	Quinupristin-dalfopristin
Beta-Hemolytic streptococci groups A, B, C, F, G	Penicillin, ampicillin, extended-spectrum cephalosporins
Streptococcus spp. (all)	Vancomycin
Haemophilus influenzae	Extended-spectrum cephalosporins, fluoroquinolones
Neisseria gonorrhoeae, *Neisseria meningitidis*	Extended-spectrum cephalosporins

TABLE 2 Members of the family *Enterobacteriacieae* with expected resistance to commonly tested antimicrobial agents

Organism(s)	Antimicrobial agent(s) to which resistance is expected
Citrobacter, *Enterobacter*, *Klebsiella*, *Morganella*, *Providencia*, *Proteus vulgaris*, *Proteus penneri*, *Serratia*, *Yersinia*	Ampicillin
Citrobacter freundii, *Enterobacter*, *Morganella*, *P. vulgaris*, *P. penneri*, *Providencia*, *Serratia*, *Yersinia*	Cefazolin, cephalothin
Klebsiella	Ticarcillin
C. freundii, *Enterobacter*, *Serratia*	Cefoxitin, cefotetan
C. freundii, *Enterobacter*, *P. vulgaris*, *Serratia*	Cefuroxime
Citrobacter, *Enterobacter*, *Serratia*	Amoxicillin-clavulanic acid ampicillin-sulbactam

TABLE 3 *Pseudomonas aeruginosa* and other nonmembers of the family *Enterobacteriaceae* with expected resistance to commonly tested antimicrobial agents

Organism(s)	Antimicrobial agent(s) to which resistance is expected
Acinetobacter baumannii, *Aeromonas*, *Burkholderia cepacia*, *Pseudomonas aeruginosa*, *Stenotrophomonas maltophilia*	Ampicillin, cefazolin, cephalothin, cefoxitin, cefotetan, cefmetazole
Acinetobacter baumannii	Ticarcillin, mezlocillin, piperacillin
B. cepacia, *S. maltophilia*	Gentamicin
S. maltophilia	Imipenem, meropenem
P. aeruginosa	Trimethoprim-sulfamethoxazole

mon phenotypes for organisms that indicate cross-resistance to antimicrobial agents within a similar drug classification. The information in these tables could be used to program a laboratory information system or could be compared to preprogrammed rules available with susceptibility test instrument software. In general, such inconsistencies should lead to verification of the isolate's identity and to a repeat of the susceptibility test by the same or a different method.

The full benefit of an expert system generally requires testing of an array of predictor antimicrobial agents, some of which may not be clinically useful. Rules more elaborate (6) than those given in this chapter, especially if they are programmed solely on the basis of genetic mechanisms, risk overprediction of clinical resistance. Finally, the success of the antimicrobial algorithms is dependent on the correct identification of the organism. Inconsistent phenotypes generally require verification of both organism identification and susceptibility results.

SUMMARY

Instruments for the performance of antimicrobial susceptibility testing should be viewed as some of the best examples of automation in clinical microbiology. The performance of susceptibility tests seems well suited to instrumentation, since an objective measurement of microbial proliferation is the basis for the test. Some instruments provide more rapid results than can be generated by using manual systems, and all have the potential to improve intra- and interlaboratory standardization. Efforts to develop test methods with even shorter analysis times must continue so that rapid reporting can occur in a more compressed and thus more relevant time period. Moreover, efforts toward the development of an instrument capable of testing a wide variety of bacteria and accurately detecting clinically relevant resistance mechanisms should continue. Further advances may occur by exploring more innovative means of detecting the inhibitory effects of antimicrobial agents on microorganisms or the use of nucleic acid probes to determine the presence of the genetic determinants of resistance.

TABLE 4 Susceptibility test results that may indicate cross-resistance to other antimicrobial agents

Organism	Antimicrobial agents	
	Primary resistance	Associated resistance
Staphylococcus	Oxacillin	Methicillin, cloxacillin, dicloxacillin, nafcillin, other penicillins, β-lactam–β-lactamase inhibitor combinations, cephems and carbapenems
	Gentamicin	Other aminoglycosides
	Penicillin (β-lactamase positive)	Ampicillin, amoxicillin, azlocillin, carbenicillin, mezlocillin, piperacillin, ticarcillin
	Erythromycin	Azithromycin, clarithromycin
	Ciprofloxacin	Ofloxacin, levofloxacin
Members of the family *Enterobacteriaceae*, *Pseudomonas aeruginosa*	Gentamicin	Tobramycin
	Amikacin	Gentamicin, tobramycin
	Ciprofloxacin	Ofloxacin, levofloxacin
Klebsiella spp., *Escherichia coli*	Ceftazidime	Cefotaxime, ceftriaxone, ceftizoxime, aztreonam
	Cefotaxime	Ceftazidime, ceftriaxone, ceftizoxime, aztreonam
Enterococcus spp.	High levels of gentamicin	High levels of tobramycin, high levels of amikacin

REFERENCES

1. **Baker, C. N., S. A. Stocker, D. L. Rhoden, and C. Thornsberry.** 1986. Evaluation of the MicroScan antimicrobial susceptibility system with the AutoScan-4 automated reader. *J. Clin. Microbiol.* **19:**744–747.
2. **Bascomb, S., J. H. Godsey, M. Kangas, L. Nea, and K. M. Tomfohrde.** 1991. Rapid antimicrobial susceptibility testing of gram-positive cocci using Baxter Microscan Rapid Fluorogenic Panels and autoSCAN-W/A. *Pathol. Biol.* **39:**466–470.
3. **Berke, I., and P. M. Tierno.** 1996. Comparison of efficacy and cost-effectiveness of BIOMIC VIDEO and vitek antimicrobial susceptibility test systems for use in the clinical microbiology laboratory. *J. Clin. Microbiol.* **34:**1980–1984.
4. **Biedenbach, D. J., and R. N. Jones.** 1995. Interpretive efforts using an automated system for the susceptibility testing of imipenem and aztreonam. *Diagn. Microbiol. Infect. Dis.* **21:**57–60. (Editorial.)
5. **Cooper, G. L., A. Louie, A. L. Baltch, R. C. Chu, R. P. Smith, W. J. Ritz, and P. Michelsen.** 1993. Influence of zinc on *Pseudomonas aeruginosa* susceptibilities to imipenem. *J. Clin. Microbiol.* **31:**2366–2370.
6. **Courvalin, P.** 1996. Interpretive reading of in vitro antibiotic susceptibility tests (the antibiogramme). *Clin. Microbiol. Infect.* **2:**S26–S34.
7. **Doern, G. V., R. Vautour, M. Gaudet, and B. Levy.** 1994. Clinical impact of rapid in vitro susceptibility testing and bacterial identification. *J. Clin. Microbiol.* **32:**1757–1762.
8. **Food and Drug Administration.** 1991. *Federal Guidelines. Review Criteria for Assessment of Antimicrobial Susceptibility Devices.* Food and Drug Administration, Rockville, Md.
9. **Godsey, J. H., S. Bascomb, T. Bonnette, M. Kangas, K. Link, K. Richards, and K. M. Tomfohrde.** 1991. Rapid antimicrobial susceptibility testing of gram-negative bacilli using Baxter MicroScan Rapid Fluorogenic Panels and autoSCAN-W/A. *Pathol. Biol.* **39:**461–465.
10. **Hirtz, P., C. Recule, P. Le Noc, D. Sirot, and J. Croize.** 1992. Detection des beta lactamases e spectre elargi par technique Rapid ATB E. Interet du systeme expert API V2.1.1. *Pathol. Biol.* **40:**551–555.
11. **Isenberg, H. D., A. Reichler, and D. Wiseman.** 1971. Prototype of a fully automated device for determination of bacterial antibiotic susceptibility in the clinical laboratory. *Appl. Microbiol.* **22:**980–986.
12. **Jett, B., L. Free, and D. F. Sahm.** 1996. Factors influencing the Vitek gram-positive susceptibility system's detection of *vanB*-encoded vancomycin resistance among enterococci. *J. Clin. Microbiol.* **34:**701–706.
13. **Jorgensen, J. H.** 1993. Selection criteria for an antimicrobial susceptibility testing system. *J. Clin. Microbiol.* **31:** 2841–2844.
14. **Jorgensen, J. H., and J. M. Matsen.** 1987. Physician acceptance and application of rapid microbiology instrument test results, p. 209–212. *In* J. H. Jorgensen (ed.), *Automation in Clinical Microbiology*. CRC Press, Inc., Boca Raton, Fla.
15. **Katsanis, G. P., J. Spargo, M. J. Ferraro, L. Sutton, and G. A. Jacoby.** 1994. Detection of *Klebsiella pneumoniae* and *Escherichia coli* strains producing extended-spectrum β-lactamases. *J. Clin. Microbiol.* **32:**691–696.
16. **Kelley, T., S. B. Killian, C. C. Knapp, P. Anderson, and A. Pereira.** 1998. Evaluation of the new imaging system AccuZone for disk diffusion susceptibility testing and data management, abstr. C-475, p. 210. *In Abstracts of the 98th General Meeting of the American Society for Microbiology 1998.* American Society for Microbiology, Washington, D.C.
17. **Kellogg, J. A.** 1984. Inability to control selected drugs on commercially-obtained microdilution MIC panels. *Am. J. Clin. Pathol.* **82:**455–458.
18. **Kellogg, J. A.** 1985. Inability to adequately control antimicrobial agents on AutoMicrobic System gram-positive and gram-negative cards. *J. Clin. Microbiol.* **21:**454–456.
19. **Kelly, M. T., and C. Leicester.** 1992. Evaluation of the AutoScan Walkaway System for rapid identification and susceptibility testing of gram-negative bacilli. *J. Clin. Microbiol.* **30:**1568–1571.
20. **Lampe, M. F., C. L. Aitken, P. G. Dennis, P. S. Forsythe, K. E. Patrick, F. D. Schoenknecht, and J. C. Sherris.** 1975. Relationship of early readings of minimal inhibitory concentrations to the results of overnight tests. *Antimicrob. Agents Chemother.* **8:**429–433.
21. **Louie, M., A. E. Simor, S. Szeto, M. Patel, B. Kreiswirth, and D. E. Low.** 1992. Susceptibility testing of clinical isolates of *Enterococcus faecium* and *Enterococcus faecalis*. *J. Clin. Microbiol.* **30:**41–45.
22. **Matsen, J. M.** 1985. Means to facilitate physician acceptance and use of rapid test results. *Diagn. Microbiol. Infect. Dis.* **3:**35s–78s.
23. **Metzler, C. M., and R. M. Dehaan.** 1974. Susceptibility tests of anaerobic bacteria: statistical and clinical considerations. *J. Infect. Dis.* **130:**588–594.
24. **National Committee for Clinical Laboratory Standards.** 1997. *Methods for Dilution Antimicrobial Susceptibility Tests for Bacteria That Grow Aerobically*, 4th ed. Approved standard M7-A4. National Committee for Clinical Laboratory Standards, Wayne, Pa.
25. **Nolte, F. S., K. K. Krisher, L. A. Beltran, N. P. Christianson, and G. E. Sheridan.** 1988. Rapid and overnight microdilution antibiotic susceptibility testing with the Sensititre AutoReader System. *J. Clin. Microbiol.* **261:** 1079–1084.
26. **Nolte, F. S., J. M. Williams, K. L. Maher, and B. Metchock.** 1993. Evaluation of modified MicroScan screening tests for high-level aminoglycoside resistance in *Enterococcus faecalis*. *Am. J. Clin. Pathol.* **99:**286–288.
27. **Pestotnik, S. L., R. S. Evans, J. P. Burke, P. M. Gardner, and D. C. Classen.** 1990. Therapeutic antibiotic monitoring: surveillance using computerized expert system. *Am. J. Med.* **88:**43–48.
28. **Ronco, E., M. L. Migueres, M. Guenounou, and A. Philippon.** 1991. Detection des beta lactamases a spectre elargi avec le systeme ATB CMI. *Pathol. Biol.* **39:**480–485.
29. **Sahm, D. F., S. Boonlayangoor, P. C. Iwen, J. L. Baade, and G. L. Woods.** 1991. Factors influencing determination of high-level aminoglycoside resistance in *Enterococcus faecalis*. *J. Clin. Microbiol.* **29:**1934–1939.
30. **Schadow, K. H., D. K. Giger, and C. C. Sanders.** 1993. Failure of the Vitek AutoMicrobic System to detect beta-lactam resistance in *Aeromonas* species. *Amer. J. Clin. Pathol.* **100:**308–310.
31. **Schembra, C., C. Dennett, S. Killian, T. Chavez, and J. Kihara.** 1993. Microwell fluorometer for reading of colorimetric/fluorometric bacterial susceptibility and identification panels, abstr. C-306, p. 500. *In Abstracts of the 93rd General Meeting of the American Society for Microbiology 1993.* American Society for Microbiology, Washington, D.C.
32. **Sherris, J. C., and K. J. Ryan.** 1982. Evaluation of automated and rapid methods, p. 105. *In* R. C. Tilton (ed.), *Rapid Methods and Automation in Microbiology*. American Society for Microbiology, Washington, D.C.
33. **Spargo, J., M. J. Ferraro, S. Fitzsimmons, R. Knefel, and G. Jacoby.** 1998. Enhanced detection of extended-spectrum β-lactamases by the Vitek ESBL test, abstr. D-44, p. 141. *In Program and Abstracts of the 38th Interscience Conference on Antimicrobial Agents and Chemotherapy.* American Society for Microbiology, Washington, D.C.
34. **Stager, C. E., and J. R. Davis.** 1992. Automated systems

for identification of microorganisms. *Clin. Microbiol. Rev.* **5:**302–327.

35. **Staneck, J. L., S. D. Allen, E. E. Harris, and R. C. Tilton.** 1985. Automated reading of MIC microdilution trays containing fluorogenic enzyme substrates with the Sensititre Autoreader. *J. Clin. Microbiol.* **22:**187–191.
36. **Tenover, F. C., J. Tokars, J. Swenson, S. Paul, K. Spitalny, and W. J. Jarvis.** 1993. Ability of clinical laboratories to detect antimicrobial agent-resistant enterococci. *J. Clin. Microbiol.* **31:**1695–1699.
37. **Tenover, F. C., M. V. Lancaster, B. C. Hill, C. D., Steward, S. A. Stocker, G. A. Hancock, C. M. O'Hara, N. C. Clark, and K. Hiramatsu.** 1998. Characterization of staphylococci with reduced susceptibilities to vancomycin and other glycopeptides. *J. Clin. Microbiol.* **36:**1020–1027.
38. **Thornsberry, C., J. P. Anhalt, J. A. Washington II, L. R. McCarthy, F. D. Schoenknecht, J. C. Sherris, and H. J. Spencer.** 1980. Clinical laboratory evaluation of the Abbott MS-2 automated antimicrobial susceptibility testing system: report of a collaborative study. *J. Clin. Microbiol.* **12:**375–390.
39. **Thrupp, L. D.** 1986. Susceptibility testing of antibiotics in liquid media, p. 93–150. *In* V. Lorian, (ed.), *Antibiotics in Laboratory Medicine,* 2nd ed. The Williams & Wilkins Co., Baltimore, Md.
40. **Trenholme, G. M., R. L. Kaplan, P. H. Karakusis, T. Stine, J. Fuhrer, W. Landau, and S. Levin.** 1989. Clinical impact of rapid identification and susceptibility testing of bacterial blood culture isolates. *J. Clin. Microbiol.* **27:** 1342–1345.
41. **Vincent, P., D. Izard, T. Lebrun, J. C. Sailly, G. Arbon, A. Hassoun, and H. Leclerc.** 1985. Interet cliniques des resultats rapides de bacteriologie au de l'infection nosocomiales: comparaison avec les methods traditionelles. *Presse Med.* **14:**1697–1700.
42. **Visser, M. R., L. Bogaards, M. Rozenberg-Arska, and J. Verhoef.** 1992. Comparison of the autoSCAN W/A and Vitek Automicrobic Systems for identification and susceptibility testing of bacteria. *Eur. J. Clin. Microbiol. Infect. Dis.* **11:**979–984.
43. **Weissmann, D., J. Spargo, C. Wennersten, and M. J. Ferraro.** 1991. Detection of enterococcal high-level aminoglycoside resistance with MicroScan freeze-dried panels containing newly modified medium and Vitek gram-positive susceptibility cards. *J. Clin. Microbiol.* **29:**1232–1235.
44. **White, R. L., M. B. Kays, L. V. Friedrich, E. W. Brown, and J. R. Koonce.** 1991. Pseudoresistance of *Pseudomonas aeruginosa* resulting from degradation of imipenem in an automated susceptibility testing system with predried panels. *J. Clin. Microbiol.* **29:**398–400.
45. **Willey, B. M., B. N. Kreiswiri, A. E. Simor, G. Williams, S. R. Scriver, A. Phillips, and D. E. Low.** 1992. Detection of vancomycin-resistance in *Enterococcus* spp. *J. Clin. Microbiol.* **30:**1621–1624.
46. **Woods, G. L., B. DiGiovanni, M. Levison, P. Pitsakis, and D. LaTemple.** 1993. Evaluation of MicroScan rapid panels for detection of high-level aminoglycoside resistance in enterococci. *J. Clin. Microbiol.* **31:**2786–2787.
47. **York, M. K., G. F. Brooks, and E. H. Fiss.** 1992. Evaluation of the autoSCAN-W/A Rapid System for identification and susceptibility testing of gram-negative fermentative bacilli. *J. Clin. Microbiol.* **30:**2903–2910.

Antimycobacterial Agents and Susceptibility Tests

CLARK B. INDERLIED AND MAX SALFINGER

124

In his review article entitled "The White Plague," M. F. Perutz recounted that Cardinal Richelieu (1585 to 1642), Heinrich Heine (1797 to 1856), Frédéric Chopin (1810 to 1849), Anton Chekhov (1860 to 1904), Franz Kafka (1883 to 1924), George Orwell (1903 to 1950), and Eleanor Roosevelt (1884 to 1962) all had a common fate (118). Each of them died of tuberculosis. For many of these famous cases, it is unknown if the disease was only poorly understood or if management of the disease was simply inadequate or even inappropriate. For some, effective antimicrobial agents for the treatment of tuberculosis had not been discovered or were discovered too late. Streptomycin and *p*-aminosalicylic acid were not introduced until the late 1940s, and isoniazid, ethambutol, and rifampin were not used to treat tuberculosis until 1952, 1961, and 1968, respectively. Therefore, it is also possible that the more contemporary of these patients were early victims of antimicrobial resistance. In the same article, Professor Perutz related the response of the famous German chemist Gerhard Domagk (1895 to 1964) to Otto Warburg's (1883 to 1970) comment that Domagk "deserved monuments in each valley and every mountain." Domagk, who in 1935 discovered Prontosil (a precursor of sulfanilamide) and 10 years later discovered Conteben (a precursor of isoniazid) replied to Warburg that "no one is interested any longer in diseases that can be cured." Domagk could not have anticipated the extent to which antibiotic resistance would come to complicate the chemotherapy of all infectious diseases, especially tuberculosis. Nevertheless, his words resonate with a particular poignancy for those interested in antimicrobial agents with activity against mycobacteria, in vitro susceptibility testing, and the use of laboratory findings in guiding the treatment of patients with mycobacterial infections.

ANTIMICROBIAL AGENTS

Although a variety of antimicrobial agents are available for the treatment of mycobacterial diseases, not all agents are suitable for treating all types of infections. Furthermore, in the face of antimicrobial resistance, the choice of alternative therapies can be problematic and clinical experience becomes a prevailing factor. For other uncommon mycobacterial infections, the physician is not infrequently faced with a dilemma in choosing a treatment regimen because of a lack of clinical precedence or unclear efficacy. The situation is confounded further by the need to treat mycobacterial infections with a mixture of agents to improve efficacy, to prevent resistance, or to overcome intrinsic resistance. The antimicrobial agents that are used in the treatment of mycobacterial infections are discussed below and in Table 1.

Isoniazid

Isoniazid (isonicotinic acid hydrazide, INH), a synthetic antimicrobial agent introduced in 1952 for the treatment of tuberculosis, is remarkably specific and potently bactericidal for tubercle bacilli. INH has comparatively low toxicity and is active against virtually all "wild-type" strains of *Mycobacterium tuberculosis*. While the exact mechanism of action of INH is still not known, its primary effect is on mycolic acid synthesis, as evidenced by increased fragility of the mycobacterial cell, increased intracellular viscosity, decreased cellular hydrophobicity, and loss of acid-fastness (172). Some evidence indicates that INH inhibits a desaturation step in the production of long-chain fatty acids (150) and may also inhibit the elongation of fatty acids and hydroxy lipids (36). In addition, INH appears to interfere with NAD metabolism, energy metabolism, and macromolecular synthesis (38, 173, 174). There is accumulating evidence that INH acts as a prodrug that is "activated" by a mycobacterial catalase-peroxidase (65, 88, 163), an observation that is consistent with the well-known correlation between INH resistance and loss of catalase activity.

In 1992, Zhang et al. (181) reported the detection of the *katG* gene in *M. tuberculosis* and correlated the deletion of this gene with resistance to INH. The *katG* gene encodes a mycobacterial catalase-peroxidase, and Zhang et al. showed that the transfer of this gene into an INH-resistant strain of *M. smegmatis* conferred susceptibility to INH and that deletion of the gene from clinical isolates of *M. tuberculosis* correlated with INH resistance. In 1994, Banerjee et al. (11) reported that INH and ethionamide resistance in *M. tuberculosis* correlated with a missense mutation in the *inhA* gene. The *inhA* gene encodes a protein that has sequence similarity (75% similarity and 40% identity) to the *Escherichia coli* enzyme EnvM, an enzyme that may be a component of the mycolic acid biosynthetic pathway. Subsequent studies have shown that *katG* mutations account for 30 to 60% of INH resistance (64, 104) and that *inhA* mutations confer a low level of INH resistance that may not always be clinically significant (94). Two additional genes have

TABLE 1 Antimycobacterial agents ranked by clinical utility and candidacy for in vitro susceptibility testing[a]

Mycobacterium species	Antimycobacterial agent			
	Primary or first choice	Secondary or second choice	Tertiary or third choice	Primary resistance likely
M. tuberculosis, *M. africanum*, *M. bovis*[b]	INH, RMP, PZA, streptomycin, EMB	Ciprofloxacin, ofloxacin, sparfloxacin, rifapentine, ethionamide	Rifabutin, amikacin, levofloxacin, cycloserine	
M. leprae	Clarithromycin, dapsone, RMP	Ethionamide, prothionamide, minocycline, clofazimine		
M. avium, *M. intracellulare*	Azithromycin, clarithromycin,[c] EMB	Amikacin, ciprofloxacin, rifabutin	Streptomycin, cycloserine, ethionamide	INH, PZA
M. chelonae, *M. fortuitum*, *M. abscessus*, *M. mucogenicum*, *M. smegmatis*	Amikacin, cefoxitin, ciprofloxacin, clarithromycin, doxycycline or minocycline, sulfonamides	Cefmetazole, imipenem, ofloxacin, tobramycin[d]		INH, PZA, RMP, streptomycin, EMB,[e] clofazimine
M. kansasii	RMP, INH, EMB	Clarithromycin	Amikacin, streptomycin, rifabutin, ciprofloxacin, ofloxacin, sulfonamide	PZA
M. scrofulaceum	Lymphadenitis (surgical excision without chemotherapy)	Azithromycin, clarithromycin		INH, PZA
M. marinum	Doxycycline or minocycline, EMB, RMP, sulfonamide	Amikacin, ciprofloxacin, clarithromycin, rifabutin		INH, PZA
M. haemophilum, *M. malmoense*, *M. simiae*, *M. szulgai*, *M. xenopi*, *M. ulcerans*	Clarithromycin,[f] EMB,[f] RMP[f]	Amikacin, ciprofloxacin, INH, rifabutin, streptomycin		PZA

[a] First-choice agents are expected to be active against wild-type isolates (i.e., from untreated patients); second- and third-choice agents are less preferable, usually for reasons of toxicity, expense, or unclear efficacy (7). The information in this table was compiled from the references 76, 89, 93, and 134, which provide more specific information on the use of these agents for the treatment of various mycobacterial diseases.

[b] *M. bovis* and *M. bovis* BCG are considered resistant to PZA.

[c] Clarithromycin can be considered a class drug for macrolides (azithromycin, clarithromycin, and roxithromycin).

[d] *M. chelonae* only.

[e] Useful for treating *M. smegmatis* only.

[f] Proven clinical utility for some but not all species.

been implicated in INH resistance, the *ahpC* gene (40, 80, 144, 171, 180) and, quite recently, the *kasA* gene (95). The *ahpC* gene encodes an alkyl hydroperoxide reductase subunit, and the *kasA* gene encodes a putative β-ketoacyl acyl carrier-protein (ACP) synthase. The degree to which mutations in these latter genes contribute to INH resistance is not clear, although the role of *ahpC* appears to be minor. In aggregate, however, mutations in these four genes (*katG*, *inhA*, *ahpC*, and *kasA*) may account for ~90% of INH resistance (Table 2).

INH is active only against replicating tubercle bacilli; slowly replicating bacilli in the caseous lesions are not readily killed by INH, and dormant bacilli are unlikely to be affected. INH resistance develops rapidly when patients are given monotherapy, and the frequency of INH resistance within a population of tubercle bacilli ranges from 10^{-5} to 10^{-6} (35). Wild-type isolates of *M. tuberculosis* are inhibited by INH with MICs of 0.05 to 0.2 μg/ml (the MICs quoted here are not based on standardized methods and are intended only to convey a sense of the relative potency of certain agents). Other susceptible isolates of slowly growing mycobacteria, such as *M. kansasii* and *M. xenopi*, are inhibited by 1 to 5 μg/ml (37). Most other nontuberculous mycobacteria, including the *M. avium* complex (MAC), *M. marinum*, *M. ulcerans*, as well as all rapidly growing mycobacteria, are resistant to INH.

INH is well absorbed when administered orally or intramuscularly; it is distributed throughout the body, and levels in the cerebrospinal fluid (CSF) may equal levels in plasma in patients with meningeal inflammation or 20% of levels in plasma in patients without inflammation (3). INH is metabolized in the liver and intestines, primarily by acetylation by an *N*-acetyltransferase which can vary significantly from person to person. However, the acetylator phenotype of an individual does not appear to influence either the efficacy of INH or the risk of hepatotoxicity. Adverse drug reactions include infrequent, age-related hepatitis and, less frequently, peripheral neuropathy, hypersensitivity reactions such as fever and rash, and arthralgias.

Rifampin

Rifampin (RMP, rifampicin) is 3,4-(methylpiperazinyl-iminomethylidene)-rifamycin SV; it was introduced in 1968 as a potent anti-tuberculosis agent. RMP is active against a wide variety of non-acid-fast bacteria and several other

TABLE 2 Mycobacterial genes with mutations associated with antimicrobial resistance[a]

Antimicrobial agent	Species	Gene	% Resistance[b]	Product	Reference(s)
RMP	*M. tuberculosis, M. africanum, M. leprae, M. avium*	*rpoB*	>96	β subunit of RNA polymerase	152, 153, 170
INH	*M. tuberculosis*	*katG*	90	Catalase-peroxidase	64, 106, 152
INH-ethionamide	*M. tuberculosis*	*inhA* locus		*envM* analog, 3-Ketoacyl-ACP reductase analog	11
INH	*M. tuberculosis, M. leprae*	*ahpC*		Subunit of alkyl hydroperoxide reductase	41, 80, 171
INH	*M. tuberculosis*	*kasA*		β-Ketoacyl-ACP synthase	95
EMB	*M. tuberculosis*	*embB*	47–65	Arabinosyltransferase	1, 146
Streptomycin	*M. tuberculosis, M. smegmatis*	*rpsL*	70	Ribosomal protein S12	46, 81, 107
Streptomycin	*M. tuberculosis*	*rrs*	70	16S rRNA	42, 46
Pyrazinamide	*M. tuberculosis*	*pncA*	72–97	Pyrazinamidase	137, 138, 145
Fluoroquinolone	*M. tuberculosis, M. smegmatis*	*gyrA*	75–94	DNA gyrase A subunit	126, 151
Azithromycin-clarithromycin	*M. avium, M. intracellulare, M. chelonae, M. abscessus*		95	V-domain 23S rRNA (peptidyltransferase region)	96, 109, 157

[a] Adapted from reference 106.
[b] Estimated percentage of resistance that can be accounted for by mutations in the respective genes; 90% of isoniazid resistance can probably be accounted for by a mutation in *katG*, *ahpC*, *inhA*, and/or *kasA*. The values are taken in part from reference 2.

slowly growing mycobacteria, notably *M. leprae*, *M. kansasii*, *M. haemophilum*, and *M. marinum*, but is only variably active against MAC and inactive against the rapidly growing mycobacteria. RMP inhibits the prokaryotic DNA-dependent RNA polymerase by binding to the β subunit at the presumed catalytic center of the enzyme. The mammalian RNA polymerase is inhibited by RMP only at significantly higher concentrations than is the prokaryotic enzyme. The RNA polymerase of MAC isolates appears to be susceptible to RMP; therefore, the primary mechanism of intrinsic resistance is most probably impermeability.

Telenti et al. (153) first showed that RMP resistance correlated with changes, primarily amino acid substitutions, within a conserved region of the *rpoB* gene that encodes the β subunit of the *M. tuberculosis* RNA polymerase. Subsequent studies showed that >96% of RMP resistance could be attributed to mutations within an 81-bp region of the *rpoB* gene (106). The molecular basis of RMP resistance in *M. leprae* is similar to that in *M. tuberculosis*, and it appears that the same methods can be applied to the detection of RMP resistance in *M. leprae* (68). Williams (170) developed a rapid PCR-based DNA sequencing protocol that targets a 305-bp region of the *rpoB* gene and showed that there was a high degree of sequence similarity (90 to 100%) between the region from *M. tuberculosis* and the regions in *M. leprae*, *M. avium*, and *M. africanum*. This analysis of 110 RMP-resistant strains of *M. tuberculosis* identified 16 mutations, 9 of which were identical to those described by Telenti et al. (153) whereas 7 were newly identified mutations. In two strains of RMP-resistant *M. avium*, missense mutations were detected, but in two other strains, no mutations were detected. This agrees with the observations of Guerrero et al. (52), who showed that mutations in the *rpoB* gene in *M. avium* and *M. intracellulare* are rare and that RMP resistance is most probably a reflection of impermeability to the drug.

RMP is well absorbed from the gastrointestinal tract, and peak concentrations of 5 to 10 μg/ml are reached within 1 to 2 h after an oral dose of 600 mg; concentrations in CSF reach 50% of the levels in plasma in patients with meningeal inflammation. RMP is available in combination with INH as a single capsule (Rifamate) containing 300 mg of RMP and 150 mg of INH and is also available in combination with INH and pyrazinamide as a single capsule (Rifater). RMP concentrations of ≤0.5 μg/ml are bactericidal for wild-type isolates of *M. tuberculosis*, and it affects intracellular, slowly replicating bacilli in the caseous lesions as well as the actively replicating tubercle bacilli in the open pulmonary cavities. Adverse drug reactions include gastrointestinal and hypersensitivity reactions; however, the major effect is hepatotoxicity and a red-orange discoloration of urine, tears, other body fluids, and soft contact lenses. RMP also induces increased hepatic metabolism of a wide variety of other drugs including methadone and birth control pills (3). Of particular concern is the interaction of RMP and, to a somewhat lesser degree, rifabutin with protease inhibitors (saquinavir, ritonavir, and indinavir), which leads to enhanced hepatic metabolism and may result in subtherapeutic levels of the antiviral agents (7).

Pyrazinamide

Pyrazinamide (PZA) is a synthetic derivative (pyrazine analog) of nicotinamide and, in combination with INH, is rapidly bactericidal for replicating forms of *M. tuberculosis*, with an average MIC of 20 μg/ml. PZA is inactive against nonreplicating tubercle bacilli and totally inactive against other *Mycobacterium* species, including *M. bovis*, MAC, and the rapidly growing mycobacteria. PZA is active only at an acidic pH; thus, the pH of the growth medium must be adjusted for accurate measurements of the in vitro activity of the drug. Most likely, PZA is active only in the acidic milieu of the phagolysosome and, depending on the concentration achieved at the site of the infection, may be bacteriostatic or bactericidal. PZA is hydrolyzed in the liver to the active metabolite pyrazinoic acid, and although the mechanism of action of PZA is unknown, its activity depends on this conversion. M. *tuberculosis* produces a pyrazinamidase, and most strains of PZA-resistant M. *tuberculosis* lack this enzyme; however, some PZA-resistant isolates retain pyrazinamidase activity, suggesting that there are other mechanisms of resistance. The lack of pyrazinamidase activity and its correlation with PZA resistance has been associated with mutations in the *pncA* gene that encodes the enzyme (137, 138, 145). Indeed, it now appears that 72 to 97% of PZA resistance can be attributed to mutations in the *pncA* gene (Table 2), and one study suggests that this correlation can be used to distinguish between M. *tuberculosis* and M. *bovis* (136).

PZA is well absorbed from the gastrointestinal tract and widely distributed throughout the body, with maximum levels in serum of approximately 45 μg/ml 1 to 4 h following an oral dose of 1 g (20 to 25 mg/kg). Hepatotoxicity occurs in a small number of patients; photosensitivity and rash occur rarely. Gout is an important contraindication because of the hyperuricemia associated with PZA therapy. PZA therapy is usually discontinued after the first 2 months of short-course treatment for tuberculosis, whereas INH and RMP treatment is continued for an additional 4 months.

Ethambutol

Ethambutol [dextro-2,2′-(ethylenediimino)-di-1-butanol-dihydrochloride, EMB] is a potent synthetic antituberculosis compound that was introduced in 1961. The MICs of EMB tested against wild-type isolates of M. *tuberculosis* range from 1 to 5 μg/ml, but the activity of the drug against other slowly growing *Mycobacterium* spp. is much more variable. The primary mechanism of action of EMB is a bacteriostatic inhibition of cell wall synthesis, while evidence points to a specific effect on arabinogalactan synthesis (149). The frequency of mutation to EMB resistance in M. *tuberculosis* is on the order of 10^{-5}, and there is evidence that EMB resistance in M. *tuberculosis* correlates with a specific mutation (at codon 306) in the *embB* gene. It is likely that the *embB* gene encodes a glycosyltransferase (or, more specifically, an arabinosyltransferase) (146). Mutations in this codon were associated with MICs of 20 to 40 μg/ml for several EMB-resistant isolates of M. *tuberculosis*. Although most MAC isolates are considered intrinsically resistant to EMB, combinations of EMB and other agents, notably quinolones and macrolides, are synergistic (66, 78). It appears that EMB affects the permeability of the MAC cell wall and perhaps increases the intracellular concentration of the other potentially more active drugs (67).

Peak concentrations of EMB of 5 μg/ml are achieved in serum 2 to 4 h after a dose of 25 mg/kg. The primary adverse effect associated with EMB is a decrease in visual acuity due to optic neuritis that is related to both the dose and duration of treatment. EMB is not recommended for the treatment of children too young to be monitored for changes in vision unless no other drug is available because of resistance. The effects on vision are generally reversible upon discontinuation of drug therapy. A variety of other adverse reactions have been reported, but these are infrequent and sometimes difficult to ascribe to EMB, since they may be due to concurrent therapy with other antituberculosis agents.

Rifabutin and Rifapentine

Rifabutin (ansamycin) is a spiropiperidyl rifamycin with potent in vitro activity against M. *tuberculosis* (62) and MAC (63, 129). Rifapentine is a cyclopentyl rifamycin, which also has potent in vitro activity against M. *tuberculosis*, but its MICs vary somewhat with the test method and medium. The mode of action and mechanism of resistance of rifabutin and rifapentine appear to be identical to those of RMP; however, approximately 30% of RMP-resistant M. *tuberculosis* isolates are susceptible to rifabutin and rifapentine. The latter observation may correlate with certain specific mutations in the *rpoB* gene (18). As with RMP, both rifabutin and rifapentine are metabolized to the corresponding biologically active 25-desacetyl metabolite.

Rifabutin has been shown to decrease the incidence of disseminated MAC disease in human immunodeficiency virus (HIV)-infected patients when used as a prophylactic agent, and it is approved for that indication (91, 112). The role of rifabutin as a therapeutic agent for MAC disease is unclear, but there may be a significant dose effect (74). In addition to being more active than RMP on a weight basis, rifabutin has a long elimination half-life in humans and concentrates in tissues, notably in the lung tissue, where the levels are 10-fold higher than in the serum. This may account for the reported effectiveness of rifabutin in the therapy of MAC pulmonary infections (44). Rifabutin is absorbed from the gastrointestinal tract and reaches peak levels of 0.5 μg/ml in serum about 4 h after a 300-mg dose. Adverse drug reactions with rifabutin are similar to those observed with RMP, including the above-mentioned important adverse interactions with anti-retroviral agents (7, 13). Some unique rifabutin toxicities, including leukopenia, thrombocytopenia, arthralgias, and uveitis when coadministered with clarithromycin, have been described.

Rifapentine was recently approved by the U.S. Food and Drug Administration for the treatment of tuberculosis. In a study of 722 patients, 361 received rifapentine plus INH, PZA, and EMB while the remaining patients received RMP in place of rifapentine along with the other drugs (9). In the intensive phase of the study, rifapentine was administered twice a week while RMP was administered daily. In the continuation phase, rifapentine and INH were administered once a week and RMP and INH were administered twice a week. Sputum conversion was somewhat higher in the rifapentine group versus the RMP group: 87% and 81%, respectively. However, relapse was somewhat higher in the rifapentine group than in the RMP group: 10 and 5%, respectively. Rifapentine reaches a peak concentration of 15 μg/ml in serum 5 to 6 h after a 600-mg dose, with a half-life of about 13 h.

Aminoglycosides

The aminoglycosides that are used for the treatment of tuberculosis and other mycobacterial infections include amikacin, kanamycin, and streptomycin (SM). In addition, capreomycin and viomycin, basic peptide antibiotics with a mechanism of action similar to that of the aminoglycosides, are active against M. *tuberculosis* and certain other species of mycobacteria. The other aminoglycosides, gentamicin and tobramycin, are inactive against mycobacteria at the usual concentrations attained in serum (tobramycin is active against M. *chelonae*). Kanamycin is a glycoside of 2-deoxystreptamine, and amikacin is a derivative of kanamycin; thus there are structural similarities among these antimycobacterial aminoglycosides. The primary mechanism of action of the aminoglycosides is to inhibit the post- to pretranslocation step of protein synthesis by blocking binding of the aminoacyl-tRNA (e-type binding). Viomycin also blocks aminoacyl-tRNA translocation, and viomycin resistance crosses to capreomycin, suggesting that the mechanism of action is the same. SM MICs for wild-type isolates of *M. tuberculosis* are usually well below the peak concentration of 25 to 50 μg/ml achieved in serum 1 to 2 h after a 1-g intramuscular dose. Amikacin is the most potent of the aminoglycosides, with an average MIC of 1 μg/ml for *M. tuberculosis* and 12.5 μg/ml for *M. chelonae* and *M. abscessus*. There is comparatively little clinical experience with amikacin in the treatment of tuberculosis because the drug is expensive and inconvenient to administer, but amikacin in combination with cefoxitin is standard empirical therapy for serious infections suspected to be caused by rapidly growing mycobacteria. Amikacin also is active against MAC, with about 75% of isolates being susceptible to 30 μg/ml, a MIC which approaches the maximum concentration in serum. In an early uncontrolled trial, amikacin was shown to be the active component of a multiple-drug regimen. Treatment was associated with a positive microbiological and clinical response in HIV-infected patients with disseminated MAC disease (31), but the clinical utility of amikacin for disseminated MAC is uncertain (7). The drug may be useful in an "induction" regimen to clear a bacteremia, and there is laboratory evidence that liposomal amikacin may be more active against tissue infection (119).

The molecular basis of SM resistance (Table 2) in *M. tuberculosis* was investigated in two studies and shown to result from mutations in the gene that encodes for ribosomal protein S12 or mutations in the 16S rRNA region, which is structurally linked to the S12 protein in the assembled ribosome (46, 107). Finken et al. (46) showed that mutations in the S12 protein were present in 20 of 38 SM-resistant strains and that there was a mutation in the 16S rRNA gene in 9 strains. Nair et al. (107) determined the nucleotide sequence of the *rpsL* gene and showed that SM resistance, in a small number of isolates, appeared to be a result of point mutations at codon 43 of this gene, a site of SM resistance in *E. coli*. Meier et al. (96) showed that SM resistance was associated with single-base (C→T) mutations in position 491 or 512 of the 16S rRNA in two isolates and a single-base (A→G) mutation at position 904 in a third isolate. The latter mutation is equivalent to a mutation in *E. coli* that correlates with a functional change in the ribosome. Adverse drug reactions associated with aminoglycosides and peptide antibiotics include hearing loss, tinnitis, loss of balance, and renal failure.

Cycloserine

D-Cycloserine (4-amino-3-isooxazolidinone) is an analog of D-alanine that inhibits the synthesis of D-alanyl-D-alanine, an essential component of the mycobacterial cell wall. Cycloserine is active against all mycobacteria as well as several other types of bacteria. The average MICs for *M. tuberculosis* range from 5 to 20 μg/ml, while peak levels of 20 to 40 μg/ml are achieved in serum 4 h following an oral dose of 250 mg. The drug is widely distributed through the body, including the CSF. There are significant adverse drug reactions associated with cycloserine treatment, notably peripheral neuropathy and central nervous system dysfunction including seizures and psychotic disturbances.

Ethionamide

Ethionamide (2-ethyl-pyridine-4-carbonic acid thioamide) is a derivative of isonicotinic acid and, like INH, blocks mycolic acid synthesis; however, isolates of *M. tuberculosis* that are resistant to high concentrations of INH are susceptible to ethionamide, suggesting that the site of action may be different from that of INH. However, mutations in the *inhA* gene have been associated with ethionamide resistance (11). The average MIC for *M. tuberculosis* is 0.6 to 2.5 μg/ml, and levels of 2 to 20 μg/ml are achieved in serum 3 to 4 h following an oral dose of 0.5 to 1 g. There are significant side effects associated with ethionamide, including gastrointestinal irritation with nausea, vomiting, and cramps, and the presence of neurologic symptoms may require discontinuation of the drug.

Dapsone

Dapsone (diaminodiphenyl sulfone) is a synthetic compound that was first shown to be active against *M. leprae* in the early 1940s. Dapsone is an antifolate that, like other inhibitors of folic acid synthesis, exerts primarily a bacteriostatic effect and is only weakly bactericidal. Dapsone is administered orally and is well absorbed and distributed throughout the body. Levels in tissue are approximately 2 μg/ml following a 200-mg dose. The drug has a long half-life in serum of 10 to 50 h depending on the individual patient. Adverse drug reactions include gastrointestinal intolerance with nausea, vomiting, anorexia, and methemaglobinemia (common). Hematuria, rash, pruritus, and fever can occur. Traditionally, dapsone is used in combination with RMP and clofazimine for the treatment of leprosy. Acedapsone is a diacetylated form of dapsone with an extraordinarily long half-life of 46 days, and as a result, this drug is administered infrequently (e.g., five injections per year) with peak concentrations in tissue occurring 20 to 35 days after a dose. Acedapsone is relatively inactive against *M. leprae*, but in vivo it is deacetylated to the parent compound.

Azithromycin and Clarithromycin

Azithromycin and clarithromycin are important agents in the treatment of all forms of MAC disease, infections caused by rapidly growing mycobacteria, and leprosy. In addition, clarithromycin and azithromycin are effective and approved prophylactic agents for preventing disseminated MAC disease (55, 120). These new macrolides also are useful in the treatment of disease caused by *M. marinum*, *M. haemophilum*, and *M. kansasii*. Indeed, they are viewed as potential cornerstones in the treatment of nontuberculous mycobacterial infections (7). Azithromycin, an azalide (a subclass of macrolides), and clarithromycin are structurally similar to erythromycin and have modifications that improve their acid stability and increase their potency, half-life, achievable concentrations in tissue, and bioavailability without causing toxicity. These macrolides are bacteriostatic agents and inhibit the growth of microorganisms by binding to the 50S subunit of the prokaryotic ribosome, blocking protein synthesis at the peptidyltransferase step. Meier et al. (96) showed that both clarithromycin- and azithromycin-resistant mutants of *M. intracellulare* have a single-base mutation at adenine-2058 in the 23S rRNA gene (Table 2), a site of mutation or methylation that has been associated with macrolide resistance in other bacteria. This observation was confirmed for *M. avium* isolates from HIV-infected patients, and MAC breakpoints for clarithromycin and azithromycin were proposed: ≥32 and ≥256 μg/ml, respectively (76, 109). The same genetic basis for macrolide resistance was found in *M. chelonae* and *M. abscessus* (157).

The in vitro activity of azithromycin against MAC appears to be quite modest, with MICs 32- to 64-fold above the maximum concentration in serum. The remarkable ability of azithromycin to concentrate in tissues most probably accounts for the therapeutic activity of this drug in animal studies and human trials (75, 83, 179). Azithromycin is rapidly absorbed from the gastrointestinal tract and widely distributed throughout the body. The peak concentrations in serum following a 500-mg dose are 0.4 to 0.6 μg/ml; however, the drug concentrates in tissues to high levels and has a terminal half-life of 68 h. In a small study in humans, the levels of azithromycin in polymorphonuclear neutrophils were nearly 1,000-fold higher than the levels in serum (4, 135).

Clarithromycin inhibits 90% of MAC isolates at MICs of 0.25 to 0.5 μg/ml when measured by a radiometric broth macrodilution method at a neutral to slightly alkaline pH (the activities of all macrolides are strongly influenced by pH). The current recommendation is that clarithromycin be administered at 500 mg twice a day to HIV-infected patients with disseminated MAC disease, but it must be combined with at least one other agent, usually EMB. The peak levels of clarithromycin in serum, 2 to 3 μg/ml, are achieved within 5 to 6 h of a 500-mg dose; concentrations in tissue are 4 to 5 times above the concentrations in serum, and concentrations in macrophages are 20- to 30-times higher. The elimination half-life is 5 to 7 h following 500 mg twice a day.

A U.S. Public Health Service task force recommended that either azithromycin or clarithromycin be used in combination with a second and perhaps a third agent for the treatment of MAC disease (91). Azithromycin and clarithromycin appear to be equally effective in the treatment of MAC disease, although there is some unconfirmed evidence that clarithromycin is somewhat more potent. Adverse drug reactions, including diarrhea, nausea, abnormal taste, dyspepsia, abdominal pain, and headache, appear to occur with low frequency (less than 3% of patients) for both azithromycin and clarithromycin. Perhaps of particular note, there are much fewer drug interactions with azithromycin than with the other macrolides (5, 13).

Quinolones

Ciprofloxacin, ofloxacin, sparfloxacin, and levofloxacin are fluorinated carboxyquinolones with good in vitro activity against *M. tuberculosis* and variable activity against MAC and rapidly growing mycobacteria (76). Measurements of the early bactericidal activity of ciprofloxacin in patients with pulmonary tuberculosis suggested that the drug is effective at a high dosage (1,000 mg/day) (143). The mechanism of action of all fluorinated quinolones is inhibition of DNA synthesis as a result of binding to the DNA gyrase (bacterial topoisomerase II). Although this is the presumed mechanism of action in mycobacteria, fewer studies have been performed with mycobacteria than with other microorganisms. Takiff et al. (151) showed that quinolone resistance in *M. tuberculosis* can be ascribed to mutations in the *gyrA* and *gyrB* genes, which encode the DNA gyrase subunits (Table 2).

The MICs of ciprofloxacin against susceptible isolates of *M. tuberculosis* range from 0.25 to 3 μg/ml. While there are no well verified interpretive standards for testing the activity of ciprofloxacin against mycobacteria, a susceptibility breakpoint of ≤2 μg/ml for both ciprofloxacin and ofloxacin has been suggested (30) and seems reasonable. Most isolates of *M. fortuitum* are susceptible to ciprofloxacin, while most isolates of *M. chelonae* are resistant. The MIC_{90} of ciprofloxacin against MAC is 16 μg/ml, and only 30% of isolates are susceptible to 2 μg/ml (86, 178). Ciprofloxacin is well absorbed from the gastrointestinal tract and is rapidly distributed throughout the body. Maximum concentrations of 2.4 and 4.3 μg/ml are achieved in serum 1 to 2 h after an oral dose of 500 or 750 mg, respectively. The elimination half-life of ciprofloxacin is 4 h in subjects with normal renal function. The MICs of ofloxacin against susceptible isolates of *M. tuberculosis* range from 0.5 to 2.5 μg/ml. Maximum ofloxacin concentrations are achieved in serum 1 to 2 h after an oral dose. Following a single 400-mg dose, the concentration of ofloxacin serum is 2.9 μg/ml; after a steady-state dose, it is 4.6 μg/ml. Ofloxacin has biphasic elimination, with the majority of the drug (95% of the area under the curve) eliminated 4 to 5 h after a steady-state dose and the remainder eliminated after 20 to 25 h. With accumulation, the half-life extends to 9 h in patients with normal renal function. The efficacy of ciprofloxacin and ofloxacin in the treatment of pulmonary tuberculosis may relate, in part, to the observation that both of these quinolones concentrate in lung tissue to levels fourfold or more above the concentration in serum (6). A quinolone should be tested as a secondary agent or when resistance to other antituberculous agents is suspected or known (155). Adverse effects with ciprofloxacin and ofloxacin may be less severe than with the other secondary agents (17). None of the quinolones are approved by the U.S. Food and Drug Administration for the treatment of tuberculosis, and the use of quinolones in children for any type of infection remains an unresolved question for many pediatricians because of lingering concerns about quinolone-associated arthropathy.

para-Aminosalicylic Acid

para-Aminosalicylic acid (PAS) is an antifolate that is active against *M. tuberculosis* but inactive against most other mycobacteria. There is some evidence that PAS also may affect iron transport in *M. tuberculosis* and salicylic acid metabolism. The average MIC for susceptible isolates of *M. tuberculosis* is 1 μg/ml, and peak levels of 7 to 8 μg/ml are achieved in serum 1 to 2 h after a 4-g dose. PAS is incompletely absorbed in the gastrointestinal tract and is associated with significant gastrointestinal side effects; in combination with the need for large dosages (10 to 12 g/day), this leads to frequent adherence problems.

Clofazimine

Clofazimine [3-(*p*-chloroanilino)-10-(*p*-chlorophenyl)-2,10-dihydro-2-isopropyliminophenazine] is a substituted iminophenazine, bright red dye with potent in vitro activity against MAC (its MICs range from 0.1 to 5 μg/ml) but unclear therapeutic efficacy either alone or in combination with other agents. The drug also has potent in vitro activity against *M. tuberculosis*, but there is little or no information on the in vivo activity. Clofazimine has weak bactericidal activity against *M. leprae* but is used in combination with RMP and dapsone as a conventional treatment regimen for leprosy. However, it may take up to 50 days of treatment before there is evidence of tissue antimicrobial activity, which may influence the length of time before there is a clinical response in the treatment of *M. leprae*. Despite its potent in vitro activity clofazimine appears to offer little in the treatment of disseminated MAC infection (139). Indeed, clofazimine has been associated with higher mortality in two clinical trials (29) compared with trials in which clofazimine was not part of the treatment regimen. Its precise mechanism of action is unknown; however, it is highly lipophilic and binds preferentially to mycobacterial DNA. The absorption of clofazimine following an oral dose is variable and ranges from 45 to 60%. The average concentrations in serum are 0.7 to 1.0 μg/ml following a dose of 100 to 300 mg. The half-life is extraordinarily long (estimated to be 70 days), and the drug tends to be deposited in fatty tissues and cells of the reticuloendothelial system. Adverse drug reactions are limited primarily to a pink or red discoloration of the skin, conjunctiva, cornea, and body fluids and gastrointestinal intolerance including pain, diarrhea, nausea, and vomiting.

Amithiozone

Amithiozone (Thiacetazone, Tibione, or Panthrone) is a thiosemicarbazole that is active against M. *tuberculosis*, with an average MIC for wild-type strains of 1 μg/ml. Resistance develops quickly when monotherapy is given. Peak levels of 1 to 4 μg/ml of serum are achieved 1 to 2 h following an oral dose of 150 mg. Adverse drug reactions include gastrointestinal irritation and bone marrow suppression; hepatotoxicity can occur in patients receiving concomitant INH. Amithiozone in combination with INH has been successfully used for the treatment of tuberculosis in some African countries, where adverse effects are believed to be less severe. However, evidence has associated Stevens-Johnson syndrome and severe epidermal necrolysis in HIV-infected patients with tuberculosis treated with regimens containing amithiozone (43, 51), and as a result, the World Health Organization recommended that amithiozone not be used to treat HIV-infected patients (114) or patients suspected of being HIV infected. Amithiozone is not available in the United States and is not used in Europe because of the adverse effects.

M. TUBERCULOSIS COMPLEX

Drug Resistance

In the early 1960s, the World Health Organization organized two meetings that led to the description of reliable criteria and techniques for testing mycobacteria for resistance to antituberculosis drugs (25, 26). The critical proportion for resistance on Löwenstein-Jensen slants varied according to the drug, e.g., 1% for INH and RMP and 10% for streptomycin, EMB, PZA, ethionamide, kanamycin, and cycloserine. However, based on the experience of Russel and Middlebrook with 7H10 agar (128), the Centers for Disease Control and Prevention (CDC) recommended Middlebrook 7H10 agar and 1% as the critical proportion for all drugs (85).

Resistance is fundamentally a phenomenon linked to large initial bacterial populations. In lung tuberculosis, the greatest populations are those prevailing in cavities which can contain 10^7 to 10^9 organisms, whereas the populations found in hard caseous foci, the most common type of lesion, did not exceed 10^2 to 10^4 organisms (24). The far greater frequency of resistance during the treatment of cavitary tuberculosis was shown as early as 1949 (69, 70). David at CDC (35) demonstrated the probability distribution of drug-resistant mutants and in a fluctuation test showed that M. *tuberculosis* spontaneously mutated to resistance to INH, streptomycin, EMB, and RMP. The average mutation rates for INH, streptomycin, EMB, and RMP were calculated to be 3×10^{-8}, 3×10^{-8}, 1×10^{-7}, and 2×10^{-10} mutation per bacterium per generation, respectively. Thus, the mutation rate for resistance to two drugs is theoretically less than 10^{-15}. Implicit in all the studies of the genetic basis of antimicrobial resistance in M. *tuberculosis* is that the multiple-drug-resistance (MDR) phenotype (minimally defined as simultaneous resistance to INH and RMP) is the result of accumulative mutations rather than the acquisition of an MDR transfer factor (106).

Special-Population Hypothesis

According to the generally accepted theory, resistance appearing during drug treatment is due to the selection and multiplication of the resistant mutants preexisting in the tubercle bacillus population of the host. Inasmuch as the susceptible bacilli are the predominant part of the population, the initial killing involves a greater number of microorganisms and the consequence is a sharp fall in the population of bacilli during the initial period of treatment. The rise due to multiplication of the resistant mutants is revealed later. This "fall-and-rise" phenomenon, as demonstrated in the patient's sputum, was described in the late 1940s (34, 121). In 1979, Mitchison (99) suggested the "special-populations" hypothesis to explain the action of the major antituberculous drugs against the various subpopulations of tubercle bacilli (Fig. 1). The subpopulations include (i) rapidly growing bacilli in the pulmonary lesions, (ii) bacilli that grow in short metabolic spurts and that might be susceptible to RMP but not INH, (iii) bacilli that reside in the acidic environment of the caseous lesions, and (iv) dormant, nonreplicating bacilli. The hypothesis was developed to explain in part the basis for the early bactericidal activity and the later sterilizing activity of antituberculosis agents. Each of the agents of the conventional multiple-drug treatment regimens for tuberculosis is more or less effective in eradicating tubercle bacilli within each of these special populations. Thus, the use of multiple drugs in the treatment of tubercu-

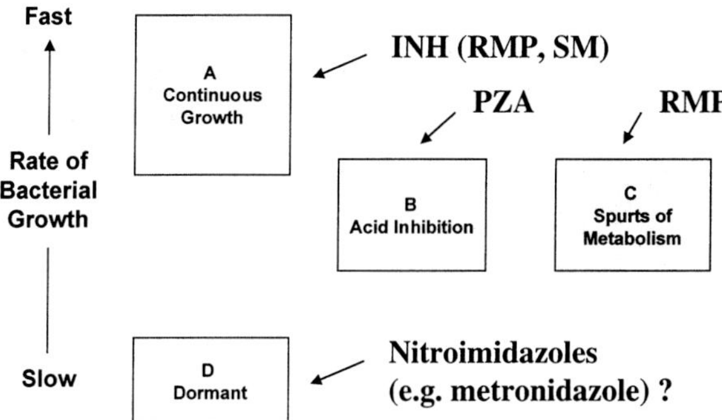

FIGURE 1 Schematic representation of the special-populations hypothesis of Mitchison (99, 100). The model accounts for the action of antimycobacterial agents on different populations of M. *tuberculosis* bacilli in various sites in the infected host. (A) INH, RMP, and streptomycin (SM) are active primarily against bacilli in a continuous state of growth, which are the majority population at the start of treatment. (B) PZA is active only against bacilli within the acidic early caseous lesions that develop within the first 2 months of chemotherapy (100). (C) The comparatively rapid bactericidal activity of RMP is important for the eradication of bacilli that grow for short periods (not long enough to be affected by INH). (D) Some tubercle bacilli may be sequestered in lesions in a metabolically inactive and dormant state; however, there is evidence that these dormant bacilli may actually be in an anaerobic state and susceptible to nitroimidazoles such as metronidazole (168).

losis is aimed at both preventing drug resistance and achieving a maximum therapeutic effect. Figure 1 depicts the special-populations hypothesis, as presented by Mitchison in 1992 (100) in his Garrod lecture, altered to include a reference to the observation by Wayne and Sramek (168) that dormant M. *tuberculosis* is susceptible to nitroimidazoles. This study was based on the assumption that dormant tubercle bacilli are in an anaerobic metabolic state and therefore would be susceptible to agents such as metronidazole.

Critical Concentrations

The criteria for defining drug-resistant M. *tuberculosis* were established on an empirical basis, i.e., that there is a certain proportion of drug-resistant mutants above which therapeutic success is less likely to be realized. The procedures used to perform drug susceptibility tests and the criteria for interpreting the results take into account two factors: (i) the critical proportion of drug-resistant mutants and (ii) the critical concentration of the drug in the test medium. On the basis of clinical and bacteriologic studies, the significant proportion of bacilli resistant to an antituberculosis drug, above which a clinical response is unlikely, was generally set at 1% (85, 128). The critical concentration of a drug is the level of drug that inhibits the growth of most cells within the population of a wild-type strain of tubercle bacilli without appreciably affecting the growth of the resistant mutant cells that might be present (101, 127, 128). In other words, if the proportion of tubercle bacilli that are resistant to the critical concentration of a drug exceeds 1%, it is unlikely that the use of that drug will lead to a therapeutic success. It should be noted that this concentration may not bear a direct relationship to the peak level of the drug in serum. The critical concentrations of antituberculosis drugs, in different media, are given in Table 3 (82, 92).

Low versus High Critical Concentrations

On occasion, the agar or BACTEC proportion method may indicate that an M. *tuberculosis* isolate is resistant to INH, EMB, or SM at the low critical concentration of the drug (Table 3) but susceptible to the same drug at the high concentration. Indeed, it is unclear if testing the low concentrations of EMB has any merit, especially since recent evidence indicates that mutations in the *embB* gene are associated only with resistance at the high concentration (1, 146). Similar studies have not been performed with SM; however, the merit of testing SM at the low concentration must be questioned. If the low concentration of the drug only was tested, the report of "resistant" could potentially mislead a clinician to believe that the drug has no value in the treatment of tuberculosis. Therefore, it is important to test both concentrations of the drugs or, if only the low concentration is tested, reflex test the higher concentration. The clinician should be alerted that an isolate is resistant to the low concentration but susceptible to the high concentration; therapeutic effect may be achieved with an adjustment in dosage (e.g., INH). Furthermore, the patient should be closely monitored for the emergence of high-level resistance. A clinician with less experience in the treatment of tuberculosis should seek assistance from a clinician with

TABLE 3 Recommended critical concentrations of antimycobacterial agents to test against M. *tuberculosis* by radiometric (BACTEC) or agar proportion methods

Antimicrobial agent	Avg MIC (μg/ml) for susceptible strains	Concn in serum (μg/ml)[d]	Medium and concn (μg/ml)				
			BACTEC 12B low[g]	BACTEC 12B high[g]	7H10 low[g]	7H10 high[g]	7H11
Primary agents							
INH	0.05–0.2	7	0.1	0.4	0.2	1	0.2
RMP	0.5	10	2		1		1
PZA[a]	20	45	100		25	50	
EMB	1–5	2–5	2.5[e]	7.5	5	10	7.5
Streptomycin	8	25–50	2[e]	6	2	10	2
Secondary agents							
Capreomycin	1–50	30	5		10		10
Kanamycin	5	14–29	5		5		6
Cycloserine	5–20	20–40	50		30		30
Ethionamide	0.6–2.5	2–20	5		5		10
PAS	1	7.5	4		2		8
Alternative agents[b]							
Rifapentine							
Rifabutin[c]	0.06–8	0.2–0.5	1[f]				
Amikacin	1	16–38	1[f]				
Ciprofloxacin	0.25–3	2–4	2[f]				
Ofloxacin	0.5–2.5	3–11	2[f]				

[a] PZA tested at pH 6 in BACTEC 12B medium and pH 5.5 in 7H10 medium.

[b] Critical concentrations have not been defined for these agents; each should be tested over a range of three to five concentrations.

[c] RMP-susceptible versus RMP-resistant isolates; about 30% of RMP-resistant isolates will be rifabutin susceptible.

[d] Concentrations in serum 1 to 4 h after administration of the usual dosage.

[e] Woodley (175) showed that 2.5 μg of EMB per ml and 2.0 μg of streptomycin per ml tested against susceptible and resistant isolates agreed with the 7H10 proportion method 97 to 99% and 100%, respectively.

[f] Tentative critical concentration.

[g] Low or high critical concentrations of antimicrobial agents as shown; however, the merit of testing low concentrations of these drugs must be questioned.

extensive experience in treating tuberculosis and/or from the local tuberculosis control agency.

Extent of Service

In the United States, mycobacteriology laboratories are classified by the levels or extents of services provided based on criteria proposed by CDC, the American Thoracic Society (ATS), and the College of American Pathologists (CAP). In general, the criteria emphasize the importance of the number of specimens processed, the expertise of the laboratory staff, and the cost-effectiveness of the procedures and protocols (8, 58, 85). The CAP recognizes four levels of service ranging from no mycobacteriologic procedures performed (extent 1) to definitive and comprehensive procedures that may or may not include susceptibility testing (extent 4). The ATS recognizes three levels of service; these are roughly equivalent to CAP levels 2, 3, and 4. The CAP recommends that susceptibility testing be performed only in an extent 3 or 4 laboratory but that even an extent 4 laboratory might refer isolates to another laboratory with more extensive experience in susceptibility testing of mycobacteria. In general, a CAP extent 4 laboratory should perform susceptibility testing only if the laboratory is capable of identifying the isolate to species and if it regularly performs susceptibility tests on that type of isolate (e.g., at least 10 tests per week). Since certain drugs are tested infrequently (e.g., cycloserine or amikacin), must be prepared from reference powders (e.g., rifabutin or ciprofloxacin), or are problematic (e.g., cycloserine), secondary drug testing should be referred to a laboratory with specific expertise in testing these agents.

When To Perform Susceptibility Tests

Kubica and Dye (85) suggested more than 30 years ago that susceptibility testing of primary drugs be performed at ATS level II laboratories to provide clinically meaningful data in the shortest possible time. The routine testing of all new isolates (from patients not previously treated or not suspected to have primary resistance) was not recommended (10). Given the low incidence of drug resistance in the United States (at that time) and the high probability of successful drug treatment of tuberculosis, it seemed difficult to justify the cost of more frequent testing. While some might argue that susceptibility testing of initial isolates is not necessary if the incidence of primary drug-resistant tuberculosis is less than 4%, the arguments for testing are compelling. Testing of initial isolates is consistent with practice in managing nonmycobacterial infections, ensures the most effective treatment for a patient, and contributes to the surveillance database for tuberculosis control. The primary responsibility for ensuring that susceptibility tests are scheduled appropriately lies with the physician (10). Nevertheless, both the laboratory and the physician must be proactive in the provision and utilization of laboratory services to ensure that the laboratory diagnosis and susceptibility testing of M. *tuberculosis* proceeds in an expeditious manner and avoids inadvertent delays caused by lapses in ordering or reporting. The New York State Health Department (117, 131) developed a fast-track system for the provision of laboratory services that provides a valuable model for others. Laboratory practices should be decided in collaboration with infectious-disease experts and the hospital infection control department and with the guidance of the local tuberculosis control program and health department.

Methods To Test for *M. tuberculosis*

The methods generally accepted for determining the antimicrobial susceptibility of mycobacteria are based on the growth of the microorganisms on or in a solid or liquid medium containing a specified concentration of a single drug. Four methods have been described: the proportion method, the radiometric or BACTEC method, the absolute-concentration method, and the resistance ratio method. Methods that are commonly used to test rapidly growing aerobic and facultative anaerobic bacteria are, for a variety of reasons, unsuitable for testing mycobacteria. For example, the conventional disk diffusion method is not suitable for testing slowly growing mycobacteria because the drug diffuses throughout the medium before growth of the mycobacteria is significantly affected. The BACTEC and agar proportion methods are most commonly used in the United States (110). The technical details of these procedures have been described by others (54, 60, 76, 82, 140), and only the proportion and BACTEC methods are discussed further in this chapter. The absolute-concentration and resistance ratio methods are described elsewhere (60).

Source of Inoculum for Susceptibility Testing

The source of the inoculum for a susceptibility test may be either a smear-positive specimen (direct method) or growth from a primary culture of subculture (indirect method). The direct method is used when antimicrobial resistance is known or suspected. The indirect method is considered the standard method for inoculum preparation, and results of the direct method are usually confirmed by subsequent testing by the indirect method. With both the direct and the indirect methods, the inoculum must be a pure culture and careful attention must be given to avoid over- or underinoculation. For the direct method, the inoculum is either a digested, decontaminated clinical specimen or an untreated, normally sterile body fluid, in which acid-fast bacilli are seen in stained smears. To ensure adequate but not excessive growth in the direct susceptibility test on solid medium, specimens are diluted according to the number of organisms observed in the stained smear of the clinical specimen. A typical dilution scheme is shown in Table 4. Theoretically, this type of inoculum is more representative of the population of the tubercle bacilli in a particular lesion in the host. It is prudent to include an undiluted inoculum, if the smear-positive specimen is from a patient who is receiving antimi-

TABLE 4 Guidelines for selection of the dilution of a specimen concentrate prior to inoculation of 7H10 medium for susceptibility testing using the direct method

Dilutions to test[a]	No. of AFB observed with:	
	Carbolfuchsin stain (1,000X)	Fluorochrome stain (450X)
Undiluted, 10^{-2}	0	<25
10^{-1}, 10^{-2}	1–10	25–250
10^{-2}, 10^{-3}	>10	>250

[a] Dilutions of concentrated specimen are prepared based on the number of bacilli observed in the initial acid-fast smear. Sterile distilled water is used to prepare the dilutions; the carbolfuchsin stain is examined with the oil immersion objective (1,000×), and the fluorochrome stain is examined with the high-dry objective (450×). If the patient is receiving therapy, not all bacilli observed in the smear may be viable; therefore, the undiluted specimen should be tested as well as the appropriate dilution based on the microscopic criteria given in this table.

crobial therapy, since a significant proportion of the bacilli seen on the smear may be nonviable.

Use of the direct method may be warranted in situations where there is a high prevalence of drug resistance (47), especially when second-line drugs are included in the initial test panel. However, cost can become a critical factor when there is a high incidence of smear-positive specimens containing nontuberculous mycobacteria. The direct method is not recommended for routine use with the BACTEC procedure at this time, since this application has been the subject of only limited evaluation (87). In addition, the direct method may take 3 to 5 days longer than the indirect method, thus lengthening the time needed to report a result.

For the indirect method, the source of the inoculum is a subculture, usually from the primary isolation media. Careful attention should be given to the selection of colony types so that the final inoculum is representative of all types present, to ensure that there is a balance of potentially resistant and susceptible bacilli. The source of inoculum for the BACTEC method can be growth on Middlebrook 7H10 or 7H11 agar or an egg-based medium, but growth should take less than 4 weeks from when growth was first detected. Turbid growth in a liquid medium such as Middlebrook 7H9 broth or sufficient growth in BACTEC 12B medium is also acceptable; however, a mixed culture (tubercle bacilli and nontubercle organisms) can give rise to apparent resistance, especially when the inoculum is derived from a broth culture.

Media Used for Susceptibility Testing

Although a variety of media have been used for drug susceptibility testing of slowly growing mycobacteria, including Middlebrook 7H10 or 7H11 agar and Löwenstein-Jensen egg-based media, there is considerable variability in the results. Egg-based media are unsuitable for susceptibility testing, not only because of uncertainty about the potency of the drugs after inspissation but also because some drugs are affected by phospholipids, proteins, and certain amino acids present in the medium. In an effort to provide uniformity in the testing of mycobacteria, the CDC (82) and the National Committee for Clinical Laboratory Standards (NCCLS) (110) recommend that Middlebrook 7H10 agar supplemented with oleic acid-albumin-dextrose-catalase (OADC) as the standard medium for susceptibility testing of slowly growing mycobacteria by using the proportion method. A majority of *M. tuberculosis* clinical isolates grow on this medium, and with the use of a dissecting microscope, the transparency of 7H10 agar facilitates the recognition of mixed mycobacterial species or the presence of contaminants. Occasionally, there is insufficient growth of drug-resistant strains of *M. tuberculosis* on 7H10 medium for the test to be valid. With these isolates, 7H11 medium may be substituted for 7H10 agar, but it is necessary to use higher concentrations of some drugs, as shown in Table 3 (56, 76, 92). At present there is no standard formulation for Middlebrook 7H10 agar or OADC (such as there is for Mueller-Hinton medium), and it has been demonstrated that quality control of the medium, especially the OADC supplement, is critical (53). The medium used for studies with mycobacteria in the BACTEC instrument is an enriched Middlebrook 7H9 broth containing 4μCi of [^{14}C]palmitic acid per vial, which is referred to as 7H12 or BACTEC 12B medium. Mycobacteria as well as other microorganisms metabolize this fatty acid and produce $^{14}CO_2$; therefore, growth or the inhibition of growth in BACTEC 12B medium is measured as changes in the growth-dependent production of CO_2 in a radiometric assay.

Drugs Used for Susceptibility Testing

Antimicrobial agents for susceptibility testing (reference powders) can be obtained directly from the manufacturer or from commercial sources. The reference powder should be accompanied by information about potency (micrograms per milligram), expiration date, and lot number, as well as the stability and solubility of the agent. Preparations formulated for therapeutic use in humans or animals should not be used. Unopened vials of powders should be stored as specified by the manufacturer, and opened containers should be stored in a desiccator at the recommended temperature. Stock solutions of most agents at 1,000 μg/ml or greater remain stable for at least 6 months at −20°C and for 1 year at −70 to −80°C. Cycloserine solutions at neutral or acidic pH are unstable at room temperature and must be used immediately. If alkalinized with Na_2CO_3 to a pH of 10, cycloserine stock solutions of 10,000 μg/ml can be stored for 1 week at 5°C or for 1 month at −20°C without loss of activity. Directions provided by the drug manufacturer should be consulted in addition to these general recommendations. Paper disks impregnated with standardized amounts of the primary and secondary drugs are available from commercial sources for use in the disk elution modification of the proportion method. Use of these disks obviates errors in weighing and dilution, as well as errors in labeling, since the disks are coded with the drug name and concentration. This technique provides results equivalent to those obtained with solutions prepared from reference powders.

BACTEC Method

The Bactec 460 instrument quantitatively detects the amount of $^{14}CO_2$ released, expressed in terms of a growth index (GI), and then automatically replaces the headspace with 5 to 10% unlabeled CO_2 in air, thereby maintaining the recommended CO_2 atmosphere. The rate and amount of $^{14}CO_2$ produced are directly proportional to the rate and amount of growth.

The BACTEC system can be used to test all primary drugs (RMP, INH, PZA, EMB, and SM), as well as the secondary drugs including the newer quinolones and rifamycins. The rapid availability of results with the BACTEC procedure may take precedence over cost considerations. If resistance to a primary drug is suspected, secondary drugs can be tested by the BACTEC method; however, in most situations, the testing of secondary drugs should be performed by the agar proportion method in a laboratory with experience in testing these drugs. In this regard, it is prudent to consider the limitations of the BACTEC method. In some clinical situations, the BACTEC method might be best considered a screening test, since it does not allow an estimate of the percentage of resistant bacilli and is vulnerable to major errors (false susceptibility or resistance) due to mixed populations of mycobacterial species. Indeed, when an MDR isolate of *M. tuberculosis* is detected for the first time by the BACTEC method, the identity of the isolate should be confirmed and the presence of a contaminant or mixed culture should be ruled out before secondary agents are tested. While the importance of promptly reporting an MDR isolate of *M. tuberculosis* cannot be overstated, the consequences of a false report of multiple resistance must be recognized as well (113). Clinician concerns about discrepancies between susceptibility test results and clinical response or status must be communicated back to the laboratory as part of an effective quality assurance program.

Four of the primary drugs are available as lyophilized powders in the BACTEC SIRE (SM, INH, RMP, and EMB) kit designed specifically for use with 12B medium and the BACTEC 460 instrument. Alternatively, stock solutions of these agents can be prepared from reference powders. Lyophilized vials of PZA are also available for the pH 6.0 modified BACTEC PZA test medium. The secondary drugs, including capreomycin, cycloserine, ethionamide, and kanamycin (50), as well as newer agents such as ciprofloxacin, ofloxacin, sparfloxacin, rifapentine, and rifabutin (critical concentrations have not been established for these newer agents), must be prepared from reference powders. Although not all drugs have been tested, the results of the radiometric and proportion methods correlate well except for cycloserine. Procedures for testing of secondary and newer drugs are currently being evaluated, and recommendations should be available soon.

Inoculum

The source of inoculum for susceptibility testing should be fresh growth of actively growing bacilli. If growth from a primary BACTEC 12B vial is used for the inoculum, the daily GI reading should be at least 500 or, even better, between 800 and 900. The higher the GI, the shorter the period until the control vial reaches >30 and the earlier the test results can be interpreted. If the primary vial is past the GI peak or if the vial was kept at room temperature for more than 2 days, a fresh 12B vial should be inoculated. Other types of broth cultures (Dubos, Middlebrook 7H9, Septichek AFB, MGIT, and broth from automated culture systems) can be used as a source of inoculum; however, it is necessary to ensure that the broth culture is uncontaminated or not mixed. After thoroughly mixing to break up clumps, the turbidity should be adjusted to match a McFarland 0.5 standard rather than a McFarland 1 standard; a 1:100 dilution of the final inoculum is used as a control. BACTEC diluting fluid or distilled water, but not a broth or other substrate containing medium, must be used to prepare the dilutions. An undiluted control is used to monitor the growth kinetics of the inoculum and also can serve as a source of inoculum if a test must be repeated.

Also, fresh growth on any solid media may serve as an inoculum source. It is important to harvest several (5 to 10) colonies in order to ensure a representative sample of growth (harvesting from only two to three single colonies is inadequate), and it is very important to thoroughly homogenize the inoculum in a tube containing 3 to 5 ml of diluting fluid and glass beads. After vortexing for 1 to 2 min, the tube is left to stand undisturbed for 30 min to allow larger particles to settle, and then the top half of the supernatant is transferred into a new tube. The turbidity is adjusted to match a McFarland 0.5 standard, and this suspension is used to inoculate the drug-containing vials. Blood agar and 7H10 plates are inoculated with a few drops of the inoculum suspension to check for purity.

As safety precautions, disposable tuberculin syringes with a permanently attached needle should be used; rubber gloves, respirator, and a gown must be worn; and all steps involving preparation of inocula and inoculation of vials should be performed in a class II or III biological safety cabinet.

Incubation

Prior to inoculation, BACTEC 12B vials must be prerun in the BACTEC 460 instrument to establish a gas phase of 5% CO_2 in air in the headspace of the vial; any vial with an initial GI of ≥20 must be rejected. Each prerun vial is inoculated with 0.1 ml of the adjusted suspension of the test or quality control isolate, and the vials are incubated at 37 ± 1°C (the temperature of incubation is critical) in the dark.

Reading, Interpreting, and Reporting Results

Vials are read on the BACTEC instrument at intervals of 24 h ± 1 h for a minimum of 4 days and until the control vial reaches a GI of ≥30. For laboratories with limited weekend coverage, an alternative schedule is to inoculate the vials on Friday and first read them on Monday (57). The Monday reading is disregarded, and the vials are read daily for at least 3 days (5 days total). Batch testing is discouraged unless the susceptibility test can be started during the same week that the isolate is identified to species, i.e., identified as *M. tuberculosis* complex. In those situations, to avoid any delay, the isolate should be sent to a reference laboratory that works 7 days a week.

When the GI of the control is ≥30 after a minimum of 4 days, the difference in GI from one day to the next, designated the ΔGI, should be interpreted as follows:

$$\Delta\text{GI of control} > \Delta\text{GI of drug} = \text{Susceptible}$$

$$\Delta\text{GI of control} < \Delta\text{GI of drug} = \text{Resistant}$$

If the GI is ≥500 and remains >500 on the next reading, the isolate should be considered resistant to that drug regardless of the ΔGI (it is necessary to check that the GI of the control was not >30 in less than 3 days to rule out overinoculation). Continued incubation for a few days may allow one to resolve borderline results, but the incubation should not be extended beyond 3 days after the control vial is positive. Susceptibility test results should never be reported without a preliminary or final identification of the isolate as *M. tuberculosis* complex or *M. tuberculosis*, especially when the isolate is resistant to a drug(s). Usually the BACTEC results are straightforward; however, if the ΔGIs are close (±10%), preliminary report should be issued as pending and the test should be repeated. In most situations, resistant (especially RMP-resistant) strains should be immediately tested against secondary drugs. Use of the term "borderline," as recommended by the BACTEC manufacturer, is not encouraged, because the definition of this term is unclear and may mislead the clinician to believe that a drug has no use in the treatment of tuberculosis.

Susceptibility test results should be reported without delay. The report should include the test method, the name of the drug, the concentration tested, and the result (susceptible or resistant). It is not possible to report the percentage of resistance by using the BACTEC method. Drug resistance should be reported by telephone and/or fax to the requesting physician, the infection control program, and the local tuberculosis control program, and a follow-up hard-copy report should be submitted. It is prudent to confirm the receipt of a fax report in lieu of direct communication with the physician or public health official.

Quality Control

Reference strains with known susceptibility patterns should be tested with each new batch of drug and BACTEC 12B medium. In addition, quality control tests should be performed at least once a week in laboratories that perform tests daily or weekly or when a patient isolate is tested if tests are performed less frequently. The H37Rv strain of *M. tuberculosis* (ATCC 27294), which is susceptible to all standard antituberculosis agents, is commonly used for quality control. We recommend that new lots of drugs or media (including new lots of BACTEC 12B medium) be quality control tested with the ATCC 27294 strain and at least four concentrations of each drug to be tested. The concentrations tested should define an MIC for the ATCC 27294 strain with concentrations above and below the MIC to detect an out-of-control result. Mutants of H37Rv selected for in vitro resistance to single or and multiple drugs are also available; however, these strains are resistant to very high concentrations and are not particularly suitable for quality control purposes. In addition, reporting the test results for a patient isolate should not be delayed because of the pending test results for a resistant quality control strain. Suspensions of quality control strains may be prepared in BACTEC diluting solution and frozen at −70°C in 1-ml test samples for up to 6 months (140). A single tube is thawed for quality control testing, and the same procedure as that for clinical isolates is used. At present, there is no published consensus on what quality control results should be available before the test results on a patient isolate may be released. However, it seems reasonable that the quality control test results for medium components be available and acceptable, as well as the results for the "susceptible" quality control strain (e.g., ATCC 27294). The procedure manual should clearly state the corrective action that should be taken when a quality control test fails, including how the results with patient isolates should be handled.

Testing PZA

Reliable testing of PZA by the BACTEC method (98) is different from testing by the BACTEC method for the other primary drugs, because PZA activity must be measured at pH 5.5 rather than pH 6.8, the usual pH of the growth medium. However, most strains of *M. tuberculosis* grow poorly at pH 5.5 and some fail to grow altogether (23). As a compromise between testing at the pH for optimum PZA activity and testing at the pH for optimum growth, Salfinger et al. (132) recommended that PZA be tested at pH 5.9 ± 0.1. In addition, to accurately and reliably test PZA, several other adjustments to the standard radiometric method are made. (i) To prepare the inoculum, each isolate must be subcultured in a fresh BACTEC 12B vial supplemented with BACTEC reconstituting fluid, which is an aqueous solution of polyoxyethylene stearate (POES) (142). The isolate is tested daily, and once the GI is 300 to 500, this culture is used for susceptibility testing. Alternatively, a 1:10 dilution of the inoculum (GI = 999 or McFarland 0.5) used for testing the other primary drugs is used and the suspension is vigorously homogenized before use. (ii) The lyophilized PZA is reconstituted with POES or PZA reference powder is dissolved in POES to achieve a final concentration of 100 μg/ml, the critical concentration for the BACTEC method, which is equivalent to 25 to 50 μg/ml used in the proportion method (140). (iii) A special BACTEC 12B medium at pH 6.0 supplemented with POES is used to test PZA. (iv) The PZA-containing vial and the control vial are inoculated with the same suspension; i.e., the inoculum for the control vial should not be diluted. (v) The vials are tested daily until the control vial reaches a GI of ≥200; if the GI fails to reach ≥200 within 14 days, the test is uninterpretable. (vi) The isolate is considered susceptible to PZA if the GI of the PZA vial is <10% of the GI of the control vial. If the GIs of the test and control vials are very close, the result is considered borderline and the test must be repeated. (vii) In addition to the use of H37Rv (PZA susceptible) for quality control testing, *M. bovis* BCG (PZA resistant) can be used as a control for PZA resistance. If an isolate tests resistant to PZA, especially if it is resistant to PZA alone, its identity should be confirmed, since *M. bovis* and *M. bovis* BCG are PZA resistant whereas the majority of *M. tuberculosis* isolates are PZA susceptible (133). This is especially important if the laboratory identifies isolates only to the level of the *M. tuberculosis* complex. Some *M. tuberculosis* isolates grow poorly at pH 6.0 (130), and other isolates may be inhibited by the POES supplement (97).

Proportion Method

The agar proportion method for susceptibility testing of slowly growing mycobacteria was developed in the early 1960s and is a common method used in mycobacteriology laboratories in the United States (71). It has been standardized in the United States, and an update to the tentative standard is expected in the near future (110). The modified proportion method also is described in detail by Hacek (54) and Inderlied and Nash (76). The preferred medium for the proportion test is Middlebrook 7H10 agar, and drugs used in this test can be prepared from reference powders or added as drug-impregnated disks (54). PZA can be tested by using the proportion method and a low pH 7H10 agar; however, 25% of *M. tuberculosis* isolates may fail to grow at pH 5.5 with oleic acid in the medium, and ADC rather than OADC should be used to supplement the medium (23).

Inoculum and Incubation

The inoculum can be prepared by the direct or indirect method. When the direct method is used, cultures should be examined weekly for 3 weeks, and even though mature colonies may appear on control media in less than 3 weeks, a report of "susceptible" should not be submitted until week 3. Resistant strains of *M. tuberculosis* complex may be slow to produce visible growth because of metabolic differences compared with susceptible wild-type isolates. If cultures are incubated beyond 3 weeks, degradation of the antimicrobial compound may permit the appearance of colonies of organisms that were susceptible to the initial level of the drug. Since the controls are inoculated with a processed specimen, isolated colonies should also be examined for colony morphology and pigmentation differences, as well as for the presence of mixed species of mycobacteria or contaminants. Small colonies of rapid growers, as well as the rough, dry colonies of some MAC strains, are similar in appearance to *M. tuberculosis* colonies on 7H10 agar. Also, rapidly growing mycobacteria may be slow to develop on primary isolation media and rapidly growing mycobacteria will appear as MDR when tested against primary antituberculosis agents. For a test to be valid, the control must show good growth (at least 50 to 150 colonies). Susceptibility-testing results must never be reported without a preliminary identification.

When using the indirect method, a sufficient number of colonies must be picked to make a suspension that is equivalent to a McFarland 1 standard or, if there is insufficient growth, a sufficient number should be picked into Dubos Tween-albumin broth and incubated at 35 to 37°C until the turbidity matches a McFarland 1 standard. The suspension should not contain clumps of organisms. The actual number of CFU per milliliter is likely to vary from suspension to suspension, so that two dilutions (usually 10^{-2} and 10^{-4}) of the suspension must be used to inoculate two sets of media. If the source of the inoculum is old or if there is scant growth, 10^{-1} and 10^{-3} dilutions should be used or the isolate should be subcultured in broth. Quality control strains should be tested at dilutions of 10^{-2} and 10^{-3}. Quadrant plates are commonly used for the agar proportion method, and 0.1 ml (about 3 drops from a Pasteur pipette) of each dilution of the inoculum is placed into each quadrant, using one dilution per set of plates. The plates are allowed to dry thoroughly after inoculation, placed in individual CO_2-permeable polyethylene bags (clear sandwich bags), and incubated at 35 to 37°C in 5 to 10% CO_2 in air. The plates must be protected from light during storage and incubation to prevent the formation of formaldehyde from the medium ingredients. To check strains for purity, blood agar and 7H10 agar plates are inoculated with 1 or 2 drops of the suspension and streaked for isolation.

Reading, Interpreting, and Reporting Results

The purity control plates are examined for contamination after 1 to 2 days; the 7H10 plate should be examined throughout the incubation period, and the blood agar plate should be examined for 1 week. Once the "no-drug" control quadrant of the test isolate or control strain shows at least 50 to 150 colonies, the plates can be read and interpreted. If there are fewer than 50 colonies in the no-drug quadrant by 3 weeks, the test is repeated. Use of the designations 1+ to 4+ to grade the amount of growth is discouraged. Obvious resistance should be reported immediately. The presence of microcolonies in the drug-containing quadrants should be noted, and the number of colonies observed in each quadrant is reported as a percentage of the number of colonies in the no-drug control quadrant. If the percentage of colonies is ≥1%, the isolate should be reported as resistant to that drug at the concentration tested. The percentage of resistant colonies can be used as an indicator of therapeutic efficacy and should be reported to the physician as well as the drug concentration and test method.

Quality Control

M. *tuberculosis* H37Rv (ATCC 27294) is susceptible to all primary and secondary antituberculosis drugs and can be used for quality control. Strains of M. *tuberculosis* that are resistant to INH, RMP, and other drugs are available from the American Type Culture Collection; however, these strains are resistant to high concentrations of the respective drugs and are not ideal for quality control testing (76). Aliquots of suspensions of quality control strains of M. *tuberculosis*, adjusted to match a McFarland 1 standard, can be stored at −70°C for up to 6 months. Quality control testing should be performed with each new batch of medium or antimicrobial agent, and media should be checked for sterility and shown to support adequate growth. Guthertz et al. (53) demonstrated the importance of controlling for all components of 7H10 agar including lots of Middlebrook 7H10 agar, glycerol, and especially OADC. The issue of which quality control results should be available before releasing patient test results was discussed above.

M. AVIUM COMPLEX

Clinical Significance

MAC is commonly isolated (often more commonly than M. *tuberculosis*) from clinical specimens in most clinical mycobacteriology laboratories. Isolation of MAC from blood or other sterile sites is almost always clinically significant, but it is especially significant in HIV-infected patients with profound CD4 T lymphocytopenia; i.e., ≤75 CD4 T lymphocytes per μl. Although disseminated MAC infection remains a frequent complication in HIV-infected patients, the incidence has significantly decreased due to the introduction of effective prophylaxis and also probably due to the immune system restoration associated with the use of highly active antiretroviral therapy. MAC is also a cause of chronic pulmonary lung disease and is the leading cause of lung disease due to nontuberculous mycobacteria in the United States. MAC lung disease has been steadily increasing in patients with a history of chronic pulmonary disease, including patients with chronic obstructive pulmonary disease and cystic fibrosis. Nevertheless, the detection of MAC in respiratory or gastrointestinal tract specimens can be difficult to interpret, especially in patients who are not clearly at risk for MAC disease. Clinical, histopathologic, and/or radiologic evidence of MAC disease, repeated isolation of MAC, increasing numbers of bacilli in sequential specimens, or the absence of other identifiable causes of signs and symptoms are important factors to consider in assessing the clinical significance of MAC isolates.

Drug Resistance

Most MAC isolates are intrinsically resistant to INH and PZA, and these antimicrobial agents play no role in the treatment of MAC disease (7, 91). The intrinsic antimicrobial resistance is most probably due to the impermeability of the MAC cell envelope (122). Cell-free in vitro studies have shown that certain drug targets (e.g., ribosomes, ribosomal subunits, and RNA polymerase) bind the corresponding drugs (e.g., macrolides, aminoglycosides, and rifamycins) and the target functions are inhibited. While MAC produces β-lactamase (102), there is otherwise no evidence that MAC actively degrades or inactivates antimicrobial agents.

MAC isolates are variably susceptible to aminoglycosides (amikacin, kanamycin, and SM) and rifamycins (RMP and rifabutin), but these agents should be considered secondary agents that would be useful in combination with other agents or for salvage therapy. Clarithromycin was approved by the U.S. Food and Drug Administration for the treatment of MAC infection, but it must be combined with at least one additional agent, usually EMB (29). Rifabutin, clarithromycin, and azithromycin were approved as prophylactic agents for disseminated MAC infection; however, the mechanism of action of these agents as prophylactic agents is unclear.

MAC isolates display at least three colony type variants: a smooth, opaque, and domed type; a smooth, transparent, and flat type; and a rough type. Colony variant types have been associated with certain phenotypic properties, and the smooth, transparent, flat type is generally more virulent and resistant to antimicrobial agents than the opaque type. The conversion between colony types appears to be a phenotypic rather than a genotypic phenomenon and occurs at a high rate. The transparent-to-opaque transition occurs at a rate of approximately 5×10^{-4} per bacterium per generation, while the reverse transition occurs at a rate of approximately 1×10^{-6} per bacterium per generation. The clinical significance of this phenomenon is unknown, and both the transparent and opaque colony types are observed in primary cultures of various clinical specimens. The transparent colony type may not be evident unless the specimen is diluted first or streaked for isolation. The occurrence of colony type variants is problematic for susceptibility testing, since the difference in susceptibility to agents that are now commonly used to treat MAC infections can be significant.

When To Perform Susceptibility Tests

In vitro susceptibility testing of MAC by the methods and interpretive criteria described for M. *tuberculosis* has little value in guiding antimicrobial therapy. For many antimicrobial agents, there is a lack of a correlation between in vitro susceptibility test results and clinical response. As a result, there are no interpretive criteria for defining susceptibility and resistance. The important exceptions are for the macrolides (azithromycin and clarithromycin). Interpretive criteria have been developed based, in part, on monotherapy trials in humans (28). Although wild-type MAC isolates are uniformly susceptible to macrolides, macrolide resistance develops quickly with monotherapy and may eventually develop with combination therapy. An analysis of macrolide-resistant MAC isolates showed that over 95% of clinically significant macrolide resistance in MAC is a consequence of mutations in the V-domain of the 23S rRNA gene (Table 2) (96, 109). Therefore, clinically significant macrolide resistance can be defined as a clarithromycin MIC of ≥32 μg/ml or an azithromycin MIC of ≥256 μg/ml, respectively. Predicting in vivo susceptibility is always less reliable; however, a positive clinical and microbiological response is expected if the MICs of clarithromycin and azithromycin are ≤4 and ≤32 μg/ml, respectively.

If a patient has not received macrolide prophylaxis, it is probably unnecessary to perform a susceptibility test on an initial MAC isolate from blood or tissue (7). However, establishing baseline MICs for a MAC isolate may prove valuable in interpreting susceptibility test results for a subsequent isolate from the same patient weeks or months later. Susceptibility testing is also warranted if a patient's history of previous macrolide treatment or prophylaxis is unclear, if a patient relapses, if the infection is intractable, or if the clinical situation is desperate. In the latter regard, testing may assist in deciding how aggressive salvage therapy should be. Even in the face of macrolide resistance, it may be prudent to continue macrolide treatment because of the disseminated nature of the disease and the lack of serious adverse effects of these drugs.

Standard Methods

Broth micro- and macrodilution and agar dilution methods that measure, in a quantitative manner, the in vitro activity of antimycobacterial agents against MAC have been described (76). In Europe, an agar dilution method with Mueller-Hinton agar supplemented with OADC is used; however, in the United States, there is some consensus that the radiometric broth macrodilution method is accurate and reliable (141). While there is no official standard method, the following guidelines reflect a consensus of many persons with experience in this field. (i) A broth medium appears to be more reliable than an agar medium. (ii) Radiometric (BACTEC 12B medium [pH 6.8]) broth macrodilution and broth microdilution with either Middlebrook 7H9 or 7HSF broth (a casein amino acid-supplemented 7H9 medium) (177) supplemented with OADC have yielded consistent and reproducible results (76, 141). (iii) Careful attention must be paid to the preparation of the inoculum; it is especially necessary to avoid the selection of colony type variants during subculture, and only transparent colony types should be tested. (iv) The inoculum should be between 10^4 and 10^5 CFU/ml for the radiometric broth macrodilution test and approximately 5×10^5 CFU/ml for the broth microdilution test. (v) Three to five concentrations of appropriate drugs (Table 3) should be tested in increments of 1 $\log_2$ unit and measured in terms of an MIC. (vi) The period of incubation should not extend beyond 7 days and the "no-drug" control should not exceed a GI of 999 in less than 4 days in the radiometric test. (vii) The end point for the radiometric test is defined by the GI value for the inoculum diluted 1:100 whereas the end point for the broth microdilution assay is visible turbidity. (viii) Tween 80 or other surfactants should not be used to disperse clumps of bacilli because of the synergistic effect between surfactants and antimicrobial agents.

Other Test Parameters

The areas of remaining controversy include preparation of the inoculum, the range of drug concentrations to test, reading and interpreting the BACTEC results, and the MIC interpretive criteria. Some laboratories advocate the use of "seed" BACTEC vials (subcultures of fresh growth) as a source of inoculum. Others prefer to prepare a suspension of mycobacteria directly from agar plates in a manner similar to the direct inoculum method advocated for testing fastidious, rapidly growing aerobic bacteria. Interpretation of the BACTEC GI readings follows the recommendations of the manufacturer (140) or is somewhat more restrictive (141). In the absence of well-established correlations with clinical efficacy and outcome, the choice of MIC interpretive criteria (resistant or susceptible) is problematic. Some workers (61, 141) have advocated the use of criteria based on maximum (peak) concentrations in serum and the highest MICs for wild-type strains of *M. tuberculosis*, while others suggest no criteria (140). It is important to recognize that disseminated MAC disease is principally an infection of the blood, macrophages, bone marrow, spleen, and other tissues. Furthermore, clinical effectiveness is likely to relate to both potent activity and the ability of drugs to accumulate in tissues to levels above the MIC for the infecting microorganism.

With the BACTEC method, clarithromycin MIC_{90}s for MAC isolates are 0.5 to 4 μg/ml under mildly acidic (pH 6.8) test conditions. Under similar conditions, the azithromycin and roxithromycin MIC_{90}s are 16 to 32 μg/ml. It is important to note that the activity of macrolides is strongly affected by pH; e.g., the MIC_{90} of roxithromycin under mildly alkaline conditions (pH 7.4) drops to approximately 12 μg/ml (123). This pH effect has led to controversy in testing macrolides. One view is that testing of macrolides at pH 7.2 to 7.4 is potentially misleading because some MAC isolates grow more slowly (some fail to grow) at this pH. MICs measured in this pH range may reflect synergy between a suboptimal pH for growth and inhibitory drug activity (12, 73). Also, BACTEC 12B medium is unstable at pH 7.2 to 7.4 because of the poor buffering capacity of the medium at a pH above 7.2 (12). Furthermore, the intracellular environment of MAC-infected macrophages (i.e., pH 6.0 to 6.5) suggests that macrolides should be tested under the mildly acidic, clinically relevant conditions. Although MAC can block phagolysosome fusion, the intracellular pH remains in the range of pH 6.0 to 6.5 (115, 124, 148). Blocking phagolysosome fusion prevents a drop to pH 5.0 or lower but does not raise the intracellular pH to 7.2 to 7.4.

Other Slowly Growing Mycobacteria

With the exception of *M. kansasii*, there is little or no consensus about the testing of other slowly growing mycobacteria such as *M. marinum*, *M. haemophilum*, *M. xenopi*, and *M. malmoense*. Over 10 years ago, Woods and Washington (176) reviewed the nontuberculosis mycobacterioses and concluded that no clear recommendations could be made for treatment of these infections and that the need for susceptibility testing was difficult or impossible to assess. Certain mycobacterioses remain quite rare (e.g., those due to M.

simiae) or are initially misdiagnosed as tuberculosis, which confused any analysis of response to therapy. Nevertheless, for certain species of nontuberculous mycobacteria, there has been an accumulation of information and experience that can be the basis for some recommendations. Susceptibility testing is often helpful with these uncommon species because of the paucity of information, and in vitro results provide some rational basis for guiding treatment. Furthermore, baseline information may be useful if there is clinical or microbiologic relapse. However, the vagaries of testing and interpretation of results mandate that the testing be performed in an experienced laboratory and that follow-up testing be performed by the same laboratory to better ensure consistency.

Isolates of *M. kansasii* from patients not previously treated with RMP are predictably susceptible to 1 μg of RMP per ml, and patients have been successfully treated with RMP, INH, and a third agent, usually EMB (37). However, resistance to RMP can develop during therapy, and a patient's history of RMP therapy may be unknown or unclear. Therefore, susceptibility testing should be performed on initial isolates with RMP at 1 μg/ml by the agar proportion method. Testing of INH and EMB should be discouraged, and reports of resistance to 0.2 or 1 μg of INH per ml or 2 μg of streptomycin per ml should be ignored (7). The recommendation of the ATS is to treat *M. kansasii* pulmonary disease with a combination of INH (300 mg), RMP (600 mg), and EMB (25 mg/kg for 2 months and then 15 mg/kg) for 18 months, with at least 12 months of negative sputum cultures (7).

M. marinum is predictably susceptible to RMP and EMB, and alternative agents include clarithromycin, amikacin, tetracycline, doxycycline, minocycline, ciprofloxacin, and trimethoprim-sulfamethoxazole. Routine susceptibility testing of *M. marinum* isolates by methods and interpretive criteria described for *M. tuberculosis* is inappropriate, and the methods and interpretive criteria for testing rapidly growing mycobacteria provide more reliable and clinically useful results (76). Successful treatment may require surgical excision or debridement, and antimicrobial treatment may be necessary only during the perioperative period (7).

M. haemophilium has emerged as a potentially important pathogen in immunocompromised patients, and there is some correlation between susceptibility test results and clinical efficacy, although virtually all treatment regimens examined included combinations of agents (147). Wild-type isolates of *M. haemophilum* appear to be susceptible to quinolones, rifamycins, clarithromycin, and azithromycin and resistant to PZA and EMB; they are likely to be resistant to INH and SM (16, 147).

In vitro susceptibility test results for *M. xenopi*, *M. szulgai*, and *M. malmoense* may be helpful because of the paucity of information about the susceptibility patterns of these species. For example, susceptibility testing has been reported to be important to the management of infections caused by *M. xenopi* (156), but an earlier report indicated that the correlation between susceptibility test results and therapeutic response was inconsistent (176). Pulmonary infections by these three species have been successfully treated with INH, EMB, and RMP, and a preliminary report indicated that clarithromycin was effective in the treatment of *M. xenopi* infections (7). Candidate drugs for testing with these species are shown in Table 1. The test method should be either the BACTEC radiometric or agar proportion method; however, there may be advantages to using the BACTEC method and defining in vitro susceptibility in terms of an MIC; extrapolation of the *M. tuberculosis* "critical concentrations" may be misleading, since there is some evidence that infections caused by these species can be successfully treated with higher concentrations of INH, streptomycin, and EMB than might be used for *M. tuberculosis* (7).

Testing *M. gordonae* isolates is usually inappropriate because actual disease is quite rare and contamination is common (167). Before testing *M. gordonae* isolates, the following questions should be asked. (i) Is the isolate truly *M. gordonae*? (ii) Is there convincing evidence that the isolate is playing a role in the disease? Until these questions are answered in the affirmative, susceptibility testing is likely to be inappropriate because the results could be misleading and the patient may be inadequately treated.

The most prudent approach to the testing of slowly growing mycobacteria other than *M. tuberculosis* is to restrict it to reference laboratories with extensive experience in working with these species. Interpretation of the susceptibility test results will require good communication between the laboratory and the clinician. Finally, clinicians without experience in the treatment of these mycobacterial infections should seek consultation from their more experienced colleagues.

RAPIDLY GROWING MYCOBACTERIA

Clinical Significance

Rapidly growing mycobacteria are defined as acid-fast bacilli that form visible colonies from a dilute inoculum on a solid medium within 5 to 7 days. Although there are over 30 species of rapidly growing mycobacteria, disease in humans is restricted to three species: *M. fortuitum*, *M. chelonae*, and *M. abscessus* (22, 161). These three species are important causes of cutaneous, pulmonary, and nosocomial infection, especially following catheter insertions, augmentation mammaplasty, and cardiac bypass surgery. Disseminated disease is rare and is usually associated with immunodeficiency including corticosteroid therapy, although it is not common in HIV-infected patients (93). *M. smegmatis*, *M. peregrinum*, and *M. mucogenicum* also have been implicated as rare causes of disease in humans (159, 160), and at least two species of rapidly growing mycobacteria are animal pathogens (49).

The importance of distinguishing rapidly growing from slowly growing mycobacteria isolated from clinical specimens must be emphasized, since conventional antimycobacterial agents (except aminoglycosides) are ineffective in the treatment of disease caused by rapid growers. Furthermore, this intrinsic resistance to conventional antimycobacterial agents may not be appreciated by clinicians with limited experience in treating this type of mycobacterial infection. Therefore, it is incumbent on the laboratory to assist in assessing the clinical significance of these isolates and to provide information on appropriate antimicrobial therapy. Isolation of the aforementioned species of rapidly growing mycobacteria from wounds is almost always clinically significant, and susceptibility testing should be performed with antimicrobial agents that have proven therapeutic effectiveness. The isolation of rapidly growing mycobacteria from respiratory specimens is difficult to interpret, but frequently these isolates are not clinically significant. However, the repeated isolation of a rapid grower in pure culture or in predominant numbers from respiratory specimens is consistent with true respiratory tract disease, especially in patients with a history of chronic respiratory disease. In patients with wound infections, debridement and excision of the infected tissue is frequently a necessary adjunct to antimicrobial therapy, although 20% of cases of cutaneous infection are likely to resolve spontaneously without surgical intervention or antimicrobial therapy (158).

Although these mycobacteria are considered rapid growers when subcultured to blood or chocolate agar, it may take much longer than 5 to 7 days to isolate them on primary isolation. When rapid growers are the suspected cause of infection based on clinical suspicion, specimens should be inoculated onto Löwenstein-Jensen and/or Middlebrook medium and incubated at both 30 and 37°C to promote their growth, especially for *M. chelonae* and *M. abscessus*. Identification of rapidly growing mycobacteria to species is important because of significant differences in the wild-type susceptibility patterns of the three species most commonly associated with disease in humans.

Methods

Four methods have been described to measure the in vitro susceptibility of rapidly growing mycobacteria: broth microdilution, agar disk elution, disk diffusion, and the E test. None of these methods have been verified and approved by the NCCLS for testing rapid growers. The disk diffusion method was described by Hawkins et al. (59), but it has important limitations; notably, there is a lack of verified interpretive criteria, and the disk contents for certain drugs are too low. The disk diffusion method is not recommended for testing rapidly growing mycobacteria and is not described further in this chapter. Use of the E test for rapid growers was recently described (84), and although the initial results are promising, the method is not considered here because of the limited information presently available about its performance.

Broth Microdilution Method

The broth microdilution method for testing rapidly growing mycobacteria is essentially a modification of the NCCLS standard method for non-acid-fast-bacillus organisms that grow aerobically (110) and was recently described in detail by Brown et al. (21). This method is most suitable for laboratories that test large numbers of isolates. The antimicrobial agents, concentration range, and interpretive criteria that should be considered for testing rapidly growing mycobacteria by this method are shown in Table 5. Commercially prepared broth microdilution panels can be used if the appropriate drugs are available at the necessary concentrations. Alternatively, broth microdilution panels can be prepared by the method described by Brown et al. (21), which recommends the use of a dispensing device such as the Quick Spense II (Dynatech, Inc., Chantilly, Va.). Once prepared, the plates can be sealed in plastic bags and stored at −70°C for up to 6 months.

The inoculum can be a subculture in broth or can be prepared directly by picking colonies from a plate. In either case, the inoculum should be prepared in Trypticase soy broth or cation-adjusted Mueller-Hinton broth with 0.02% Tween 80 and four or five sterile 0.5-mm-diameter glass beads. Care should be taken to avoid clumping of the mycobacteria. The final inoculum should be 1×10^5 to 5×10^5 CFU/ml or 1×10^4 to 5×10^4 CFU/100 μl/well of a microtiter plate. The purity of the inoculum should be checked for each isolate, and occasionally the size of the inoculum should be verified by quantitative plate culture, especially if there is a problem with clumping.

The plates should be incubated for 3 to 5 days at 30°C but must not be incubated beyond 5 days because of drug instability. If there is not sufficient growth to interpret the results after 5 days of incubation, the test should be repeated. The MIC is defined as the lowest concentration of antimicrobial agent that completely inhibits visible growth. As with other types of bacteria, "trailing" is common when testing the sulfonamides, and the MICs of these agents should be read at approximately 80% inhibition of growth.

TABLE 5 Antimicrobial agents to test against rapidly growing mycobacteria by the broth microdilution method[a]

Antimicrobial agent	Concn range (μg/ml)	MIC (μg/ml) for:			
		Susceptible strains[b]	Intermediate strains	Resistant strains	*M. fortuitum* ATCC 6841[c]
Amikacin[d]	0.5–64	≤16	32	≥64	≤0.25–1
Cefoxitin[e]	2–256	≤16	32	≥64	16–32
Ciprofloxacin[f]	0.06–8	≤1	2	≥4	≤0.0.06–0.25
Clarithromycin[g]	0.12–16	≤2	4	≥8	
Doxycycline[h]	0.25–32	≤1	2–8	≥16	≤0.25–4
Imipenem[i]	0.5–32	≤4	8	≥16	1–4
Sulfamethoxazole[j]	0.5–256	≤32		≥64	2–16
Sulfisoxazole[j]	0.5–256	≤32		≥64	
Tobramycin[k]	0.5–32	≤4	8	≥16	8–32

[a] Table and footnotes are adapted from references 21 and 76.

[b] Breakpoints follow NCCLS standards (111) except as noted.

[c] Expected range for quality control purposes. The potencies of drug preparations should be tested with *Staphylococcus aureus* ATCC 29213, *E. coli* ATCC 25922, and *Pseudomonas aeruginosa* ATCC 27853 and compared with expected ranges as described in NCCLS document M7-A3 (111).

[d] Kanamycin may be more active than amikacin against *M. abscessus* and *M. chelonae*.

[e] Cefoxitin is 1 dilution higher than the conventional NCCLS-suggested breakpoint, and cefoxitin is the only cephalosporin that should be tested.

[f] Not active against most strains of *M. chelonae* and *M. abscessus*.

[g] Interpretive values are as declared by Abbott Laboratories, Abbott Park, Ill.

[h] Breakpoint is 2 dilutions lower than the conventional NCCLS-suggested breakpoint; in general, doxycycline and minocycline are four- to eightfold more active than tetracycline.

[i] Solutions are unstable at ambient temperatures and above.

[j] Sulfamethoxazole and sulfisoxazole breakpoints are the closest values for the sulfamethoxazole component of trimethoprim-sulfamethoxazole; e.g., 64 μg of sulfamethoxazole per ml alone corresponds to 76 μg/ml in combination with trimethoprim.

[k] Likely to be active against only *M. chelonae* and *M. fortuitum*.

Agar Disk Elution Method

The agar disk elution method can be viewed as an adaptation of the disk elution modification of the proportion method for testing *M. tuberculosis* (166). The disk elution method is particularly suitable for occasional or infrequent testing of small numbers of isolates, and the method was recently described in detail by Brown et al. (20). Commercially prepared disks containing antimicrobial agents are placed into the wells of a standard 35-mm, six-well tissue culture plate and eluted with 0.5 ml of either 10% OADC or Trypticase soy broth (Table 6). One well is reserved for a growth control, and no drug is added. OADC should be used when testing *M. chelonae* or *M. abscessus*, while Trypticase soy broth is sufficient when testing *M. fortuitum*. Molten Mueller-Hinton agar is added to each well of the plate and allowed to solidify. Standard quadrant plates can be substituted for the tissue culture plates; however, Brown et al. (20) indicate that Middlebrook 7H10 medium should not be substituted for Mueller-Hinton agar because of discrepancies in MIC results, notably with aminoglycosides. Once prepared, the plates can be stored for 7 days at 4°C except when testing imipenem (plates containing imipenem must be inoculated within 24 h). The inoculum is prepared as described for the broth microdilution procedure, and a suspension of mycobacteria adjusted to match the turbidity of a McFarland 0.5 standard is used to prepare a 1:100 dilution. Sterile deionized water is used to dilute the suspension, and 10 μl of suspension is inoculated onto the surface of each well of the plate. The final inoculum is approximately 1.5×10^4 CFU per well. The plates should be incubated in air at 30°C for 3 to 5 days. A purity plate should be prepared for each isolate tested as well as the quality control strain (*M. fortuitum* ATCC 6841), and the inoculum preparation can be verified by quantitative culture on a blood agar plate or other suitable nonselective medium. The plates should be first examined at 3 days. If there are uniformly dispersed, discrete colonies in the growth control well, the test results can be read. The end point is no growth at the concentration of drug tested, except for sulfonamides, for which the end point is taken as an 80% reduction in growth compared with the control.

One important limitation to this procedure is that the drugs are tested at only one or two (amikacin) concentrations which are at or near the NCCLS breakpoint for susceptibility (the breakpoint for cefoxitin is 1 dilution higher, 32 versus 16 μg/ml). As a result, the tolerance between assays is extremely low. Nevertheless, the test has proven reliable and useful for guiding the therapy of infections caused by rapidly growing mycobacteria (20). At present there are no recommended concentrations or interpretive criteria for testing clarithromycin or azithromycin.

Alternative Susceptibility Testing Methods

A variety of alternative methods have been developed and evaluated for susceptibility testing or for detecting antimicrobial resistance in mycobacteria. Some methods are based on improved methods for measuring inhibition of growth, while other methods are based on molecular assays for analytes that correlate with growth or assays for the direct detection of mutations associated with resistance. Growth-based methods that have been evaluated include the E test (84, 164, 165) and mycobacteria growth indicator tube (MGIT) (14, 15, 90, 116, 125, 162), as well as the potential adaptation of semiautomated culture systems such as the ESP culture system II (AccuMed, Chicago, Ill.) and MB/BacT (Organon Teknika, Durham, N.C.). Additional methods that use tetrazolium dye reduction to distinguish viable from nonviable tubercle bacilli (48, 105) or cytometry to detect viability using fluorescein diacetate (19) have been used. Jacobs et al. (77) described a method based on the use of a luciferase reporter mycobacteriophage. The premise was that viable mycobacteria support the infection and multiplication of phages whereas inhibited or killed mycobacteria do not. Therefore, mycobacteria susceptible to INH or RMP supported the phage infection and expressed luciferase. When exposed to INH or RMP, the cells were killed and no light was produced. Cooksey et al. (32) introduced the luciferase gene into *M. tuberculosis* H37Ra by electroporation of a plasmid containing the luciferase gene linked to the *hsp60* promoter. The results of a broth microtiter assay with the luciferase-H37Ra strain were comparable to a conventional broth microdilution assay. Cangelosi et al. (27) described an alternative approach based on the measurement of the precursor rRNA. In this assay *M. tuberculosis* nucleic acid is probed with specific pre-16S rRNA stem sequences in the presence or absence of drugs that have a direct or indirect effect on rRNA synthesis. Responses to RMP and ciprofloxacin were detected within 24 and 48 h, respectively. Detectable pre-rRNA was depleted in susceptible cells but remained abundant in resistant cells. In a simi-

TABLE 6 Antimicrobial agents to test against rapidly growing mycobacteria by the agar disk elution method[a]

Antimicrobial agent	Resistance breakpoint (μg/ml)	Disk content (μg)	No. of disks/well	Final concn (μg/ml)	*M. fortuitum* ATCC 6841[b]
Amikacin	32	30	1	6	S
Amikacin	32	30	5	30	S/R
Cefoxitin	32	30	5	30	S
Ciprofloxacin	2	5	2	2	S
Doxycycline	8	30	1	6	S
Imipenem	8	10	4	8	S
Tobramycin	8	10	4	8	S/R
Trimethoprim-sulfamethoxazole	32	25	6	30	S
RMP[c]	1	5	1	1	R

[a] Table and footnotes adapted from references 20 and 76.

[b] S, Susceptible (no growth); R, resistant (growth equivalent to no-drug control). The results given are the expected results for *M. fortuitum* ATCC 6841 for quality control purposes. Brown et al. (20) suggest using *Pseudomonas aeruginosa* ATCC 27853 for additional quality control of the method.

[c] RMP is suggested to provide a quality control test for the detection of resistance and for the testing of *M. marinum*, which may require incubation for up to 14 days.

lar approach, the Amplified *Mycobacterium tuberculosis* Direct Test (GenProbe, San Diego, Calif.) was used to monitor the response to therapy by detecting rRNA after the initiation of chemotherapy (103).

Mutations in genes that encode targets of antimycobacterial agents (Table 2) can be detected by a variety of methods. A particular focus of such studies has been RMP resistance because of the pivotal role of RMP in the treatment of tuberculosis and other mycobacterial infections, the conserved nature of the genetic basis for resistance (>96% of RMP resistance correlates with mutations in an 81-bp segment of the *rpoB* gene), and the use of RMP resistance as a marker of MDR *M. tuberculosis*. The methods used to detect *rpoB* mutations include PCR amplification of the target sequence and detection by DNA sequencing (72, 79, 153), the line probe assay (33, 39), single-strand conformation polymorphism (45, 154), dideoxy fingerprinting (45), the mismatch RNA-RNA protection assay (108), and the heteroduplex generator assay (169). Similar approaches have been developed for detecting mutations involved in INH resistance and PZA resistance. The application of these assays for routine use in the clinical mycobacteriology laboratory is likely to require technical simplification or automation as well as outcome analysis to justify the anticipated increased costs compared with conventional approaches.

REFERENCES

1. **Alcaide, F., G. E. Pfyffer, and A. Telenti.** 1997. Role of *embB* in natural and acquired resistance to ethambutol in mycobacteria. *Antimicrob. Agents Chemother.* **41:** 2270–2273.
2. **Alcaide, F., and A. Telenti.** 1997. Molecular techniques in the diagnosis of drug-resistant tuberculosis. *Ann. Acad. Med. Singapore* **26:**647–650.
3. **Alford, R. H.** 1990. Antimycobacterial agents, p. 350–360. *In* G. L. Mandell, R. G. Douglas, Jr., and J. E. Bennett (ed.), *Principles and Practices of Infectious Diseases*. Churchill Livingstone, Inc., New York, N.Y.
4. **Amsden, G. W.** 1996. Erythromycin, clarithromycin, and azithromycin: are the differences real? *Clin. Ther.* **18:** 56–72.
5. **Amsden, G. W.** 1995. Macrolides versus azalides: a drug interaction update. *Ann. Pharm.* **29:**906–917.
6. **Andriole, V. T.** 1990. Quinolones p. 334–345. *In* G. L. Mandell, R. G. Douglas, Jr., and J. E. Bennett (ed.), *Principles and Practices of Infectious Diseases*. Churchill Livingstone, Inc., New York, N.Y.
7. **Anonymous.** 1997. Diagnosis and treatment of disease caused by nontuberculous mycobacteria. *Am. J. Respir. Crit. Care Med.* **156:**S1–S25.
8. **Anonymous.** 1983. Levels of laboratory services for mycobacterial diseases: American Thoracic Society. Medical Section of the American Lung Association. *Am. Rev. Respir. Dis.* **128:**213.
9. **Anonymous.** 1998. *Priftin® (Rifapentine) Prescribing Information.* Hoechst Marion Roussel, Inc., Kansas City, Mo.
10. **Bailey, W. C., J. B. Bass, J. E. Hawkins, G. P. Kubica, and R. J. Wallace.** 1984. Drug susceptibility testing for mycobacteria. *Am. Thorac. Soc. Newsl.* **10:**9–10.
11. **Banerjee, A., E. Dubnau, A. Quemard, V. Balasubramanian, K. S. Um, T. Wilson, D. Collins, G. de Lisle, and W. R. Jacobs, Jr.** 1994. *inhA*, a gene encoding a target for isoniazid and ethionamide in *Mycobacterium tuberculosis*. *Science* **263:**227–230.
12. **Beaty, S., S. Siddiqi, and M. Gnacek.** 1992. Increase of pH of 12B medium by various means and its effect on the growth of *Mycobacterium avium* complex, abstr. U-102. *In Abstracts of the 92nd General Meeting of the American Society for Microbiology 1992.* American Society for Microbiology, Washington, D.C.
13. **Benson, C.** 1997. Critical drug interactions with agents used for prophylaxis and treatment of *Mycobacterium avium* infections. *Am. J. Med.* **102:**32–36.
14. **Bergmann, J. S., and G. L. Woods.** 1997. Mycobacterial growth indicator tube for susceptibility testing of *Mycobacterium tuberculosis* to isoniazid and rifampin. *Diagn. Microbiol. Infect. Dis.* **28:**153–156.
15. **Bergmann, J. S., and G. L. Woods.** 1997. Reliability of mycobacteria growth indicator tube for testing susceptibility of *Mycobacterium tuberculosis* to ethambutol and streptomycin. *J. Clin. Microbiol.* **35:**3325–3327.
16. **Bernard, E. M., F. F. Edwards, T. E. Kiehn, S. T. Brown, and D. Armstrong.** 1993. Activities of antimicrobial agents against clinical isolates of *Mycobacterium haemophilum*. *Antimicrob. Agents Chemother.* **37:**2323–2326.
17. **Berning, S. E., L. Madsen, M. D. Iseman, and C. A. Peloquin.** 1995. Long-term safety of ofloxacin and ciprofloxacin in the treatment of mycobacterial infections. *Am. J. Respir. Crit. Care Med.* **151:**2006–2009.
18. **Bodmer, T., G. Zurcher, P. Imboden, and A. Telenti.** 1995. Mutation position and type of substitution in the beta-subunit of the RNA polymerase influence in-vitro activity of rifamycins in rifampicin-resistant *Mycobacterium tuberculosis*. *J. Antimicrob. Chemother.* **35:**345–348.
19. **Bownds, S. E., T. A. Kurzynski, M. A. Norden, J. L. Dufek, and R. F. Schell.** 1996. Rapid susceptibility testing for nontuberculosis mycobacteria using flow cytometry. *J. Clin. Microbiol.* **34:**1386–1390.
20. **Brown, B. A., J. M. Swenson, and R. J. Wallace, Jr.** 1992. Agar disk elution test for rapidly growing mycobacteria, p. 5.10.1–5.10.11. *In* H. D. Isenberg (ed.), *Clinical Microbiology Procedures Handbook*. American Society for Microbiology, Washington, D.C.
21. **Brown, B. A., J. M. Swenson, and R. J. Wallace, Jr.** 1992. Broth microdilution test for rapidly growing mycobacteria, p. 5.11.1–5.11.10. *In* H. D. Isenberg (ed.), *Clinical Microbiology Procedures Handbook*. American Society for Microbiology, Washington, D.C.
22. **Bruckner, D. A., and P. Colonna.** 1993. Nomenclature for aerobic and facultative bacteria. *Clin. Infect. Dis.* **16:** 598–605.
23. **Butler, W. R., and J. O. Kilburn.** 1982. Improved method for testing susceptibility of *Mycobacterium tuberculosis* to pyrazinamide. *J. Clin. Microbiol.* **16:**1106–1109.
24. **Canetti, G.** 1965. Present aspects of bacterial resistance in tuberculosis. *Am. Rev. Respir. Dis.* **92:**687–702.
25. **Canetti, G., W. Fox, A. Khomenko, H. T. Mahler, N. K. Menon, D. A. Mitchison, N. Rist, and N. A. Smelev.** 1969. Advances in techniques of testing mycobacterial drug sensitivity, and the use of sensitivity tests in tuberculosis control programs. *Bull. W. H. O.* **41:**21–43.
26. **Canetti, G., S. Froman, J. Grosset, P. Hauduroy, M. Lagerova, H. T. Mahler, G. Meissner, D. A. Mitchison, and L. Sula.** 1963. Mycobacteria: laboratory methods for testing drug sensitivity and resistance. *Bull. W. H. O.* **29:** 565–578.
27. **Cangelosi, G. A., W. H. Brabant, T. B. Britschgi, and C. K. Wallis.** 1996. Detection of rifampin- and ciprofloxacin-resistant *Mycobacterium tuberculosis* by using species-specific assays for precursor rRNA. *Antimicrob. Agents Chemother.* **40:**1790–1795.
28. **Chaisson, R. E., C. A. Benson, M. P. Dube, L. B. Heifets, J. A. Korvick, S. Elkin, T. Smith, J. C. Craft, and F. R. Sattler.** 1994. Clarithromycin therapy for bacteremic

Mycobacterium avium complex disease. A randomized, double-blind, dose-ranging study in patients with AIDS. AIDS Clinical Trials Group Protocol 157 Study Team. *Ann. Intern. Med.* **121:**905–911.

29. **Chaisson, R. E., P. Keiser, M. Pierce, W. J. Fessel, J. Ruskin, C. Lahart, C. A. Benson, K. Meek, N. Siepman, and J. C. Craft.** 1997. Clarithromycin and ethambutol with or without clofazimine for the treatment of bacteremic *Mycobacterium avium* complex disease in patients with HIV infection. *AIDS* **11:**311–317.
30. **Chen, C. H., J. F. Shih, P. J. Lindholm-Levy, and L. B. Heifets.** 1989. Minimal inhibitory concentrations of rifabutin, ciprofloxacin, and ofloxacin against *Mycobacterium tuberculosis* isolated before treatment of patients in Taiwan. *Am. Rev. Respir. Dis.* **140:**987–989.
31. **Chiu, J., J. Nussbaum, S. Bozette, J. G. Tilles, L. S. Young, J. Leedom, P. N. R. Heseltine, and J. A. McCutchan.** 1990. Treatment of disseminated *Mycobacterium avium* complex infection in AIDS with amikacin, ethambutol, rifampin, and ciprofloxacin. *Ann. Intern. Med.* **113:**358–361.
32. **Cooksey, R. C., J. T. Crawford, W. R. Jacobs, Jr., and T. M. Shinnick.** 1993. A rapid method for screening antimicrobial agents for activities against a strain of *Mycobacterium tuberculosis* expressing firefly luciferase. *Antimicrob. Agents Chemother.* **37:**1348–1352.
33. **Cooksey, R. C., G. P. Morlock, S. Glickman, and J. T. Crawford.** 1997. Evaluation of a line probe assay kit for characterization of *rpoB* mutations in rifampin-resistant *Mycobacterium tuberculosis* isolates from New York City. *J. Clin. Microbiol.* **35:**1281–1283.
34. **Crofton, J., and D. A. Mitchison.** 1948. Streptomycin resistance in pulmonary tuberculosis. *Br. Med. J.* **2:**1009–1015.
35. **David, H. L.** 1970. Probability distribution of drug-resistant mutants in unselected populations of *Mycobacterium tuberculosis*. *Appl. Microbiol.* **20:**810–814.
36. **Davidson, L. A., and K. Takayama.** 1979. Isoniazid inhibition of the synthesis of monosaturated long-chain fatty acids in *Mycobacterium tuberculosis* H37Ra. *Antimicrob. Agents Chemother.* **16:**104–105.
37. **Davidson, P. T.** 1989. The diagnosis and management of disease caused by *M. avium* complex, *M. kansasii*, and other mycobacteria, p. 431–443. *In* D. E. Snider, Jr. (ed.), *Clinics in Chest Medicine*. The W.B. Saunders Co., Philadelphia, Pa.
38. **Davis, W. B., and M. M. Weber.** 1977. Specificity of isoniazid on growth inhibition and competition for an oxidized nicotiniamide adenine dinucleotide regulatory site on the electron transport pathway in *Mycobacterium phlei*. *Antimicrob. Agents Chemother.* **12:**213–218.
39. **De Beenhouwer, H., Z. Lhiang, G. Jannes, W. Mijs, L. Machtelinckx, R. Rossau, H. Traore, and F. Portaels.** 1995. Rapid detection of rifampicin resistance in sputum and biopsy specimens from tuberculosis patients by PCR and line probe assay. *Tubercle Lung Dis.* **76:**425–430.
40. **Deretic, V., W. Philipp, S. Dhandayuthapani, M. H. Mudd, R. Curcic, T. Garbe, B. Heym, L. E. Via, and S. T. Cole.** 1995. *Mycobacterium tuberculosis* is a natural mutant with an inactivated oxidative-stress regulatory gene: implications for sensitivity to isoniazid. *Mol. Microbiol.* **17:**889–900.
41. **Dhandayuthapani, S., M. Mudd, and V. Deretic.** 1997. Interactions of OxyR with the promoter region of the *oxyR* and *ahpC* genes from *Mycobacterium leprae* and *Mycobacterium tuberculosis*. *J. Bacteriol.* **179:**2401–2409.
42. **Douglass, J., and L. M. Steyn.** 1993. A ribosomal gene mutation in streptomycin-resistant *Mycobacterium tuberculosis* isolates. *J. Infect. Dis.* **167:**1505–1506. (Letter.)
43. **Dukes, C. S., J. Sugarman, J. P. Cegielski, G. J. Lallinger, and D. H. Mwakyusa.** 1992. Severe cutaneous hypersensitivity reactions during treatment of tuberculosis in patients with HIV infection in Tanzania. *Trop. Geogr. Med.* **44:**308–311.
44. **Farr, B. M., and G. L. Mandell.** 1990. Rifamycins, p. 295–303. *In* G. L. Mandell, R. G. Douglas, Jr., and J. E. Bennett (ed.), *Principles and Practices of Infectious Diseases*. Churchill Livingstone, Inc., New York, N.Y.
45. **Felmlee, T. A., Q. Liu, A. C. Whelen, D. Williams, S. S. Sommer, and D. H. Persing.** 1995. Genotypic detection of *Mycobacterium tuberculosis* rifampin resistance: comparison of single-strand conformation polymorphism and dideoxy fingerprinting. *J. Clin. Microbiol.* **33:**1617–1623.
46. **Finken, M., P. Kirschner, A. Meier, A. Wrede, and E. C. Böttger.** 1993. Molecular basis of streptomycin resistance in *Mycobacterium tuberculosis*: alterations of the ribosomal protein S12 gene and point mutations within a functional 16S ribosomal RNA pseudoknot. *Mol. Microbiol.* **9:**1239–1246.
47. **Frieden, T. R., T. Sterling, A. Pablos-Mendez, J. O. Kilburn, G. M. Cauthen, and S. W. Doolery.** 1993. The emergence of drug-resistant tuberculosis in New York City. *N. Engl. J. Med.* **328:**521–526.
48. **Gomez-Flores, R., S. Gupta, R. Tamez-Guerra, and R. T. Mehta.** 1995. Determination of MICs for *Mycobacterium avium-M. intracellulare* complex in liquid medium by a colorimetric method. *J. Clin. Microbiol.* **33:**1842–1846.
49. **Good, R. C.** 1985. Opportunistic pathogens in the genus *Mycobacterium*. *Annu. Rev. Microbiol.* **39:**347–369.
50. **Gross, W. M., and J. E. Hawkins.** 1986. Radiometric susceptibility testing of *Mycobacterium tuberculosis* with secondary drugs, abstr. C-378, p. 391. *In Abstracts of the 86th Annual Meeting of the American Society for Microbiology 1986*. American Society for Microbiology, Washington, D.C.
51. **Grosset, J. H.** 1992. Treatment of tuberculosis in HIV infection. *Tubercle Lung Dis.* **73:**378–383.
52. **Guerrero, C., L. Stockman, F. Marchesi, T. Bodmer, G. D. Roberts, and A. Telenti.** 1994. Evaluation of the *rpoB* gene in rifampicin-susceptible and resistant *Mycobacterium avium* and *Mycobacterium intracellulare*. *J. Antimicrob. Chemother.* **33:**661–663.
53. **Guthertz, L. S., M. E. Griffith, E. G. Ford, J. M. Janda, and T. F. Midura.** 1988. Quality control or individual components used in Middlebrook 7H10 medium for mycobacterial susceptibility testing. *J. Clin. Microbiol.* **26:**2338–2342.
54. **Hacek, D.** 1992. Modified proportion agar dilution test for slowly growing mycobacteria, p. 5.13.1–5.13.15. *In* H. D. Isenberg (ed.), *Clinical Microbiology Procedures Handbook*. American Society for Microbiology, Washington, D.C.
55. **Havlir, D. V., M. P. Dube, F. R. Sattler, D. N. Forthal, C. A. Kemper, M. W. Dunne, D. M. Parenti, J. P. Lavelle, A. White, M. D. Witt, S. A. Bozzette, and J. A. McCutchan.** 1996. Prophylaxis against disseminated *Mycobacterium avium* complex with weekly azithromycin, daily rifabutin, or both. California Collaborative Treatment Group. *N. Engl. J. Med.* **335:**392–398.
56. **Hawkins, J. E.** 1984. Drug susceptibility testing, p. 177–193. *In* G. P. Kubica and L. G. Wayne (ed.), *The Mycobacteria: a Sourcebook*, Part A. Marcel Dekker, Inc., New York, N.Y.
57. **Hawkins, J. E.** 1986. Non-weekend schedule for BACTEC susceptibility testing of *Mycobacterium tuberculosis*. *J. Clin. Microbiol.* **23:**934–937.
58. **Hawkins, J. E., R. C. Good, G. P. Kubica, P. R. Gangadharam, H. M. Gruft, and K. D. Stottmeier.** 1983. The

levels of service concept in mycobacteriology. *Am. Thorac. Soc. Newsl.* **9:**19–25.

59. **Hawkins, J. E., R. J. Wallace, Jr., and B. A. Brown.** 1991. Antibacterial susceptibility tests: mycobacteria, p. 1138–1152. *In* A. Balows, W. J. Hausler, Jr., K. L. Herrmann, H. D. Isenberg, and H. J. Shadomy (ed.), *Manual of Clinical Microbiology*, 5th ed. American Society for Microbiology, Washington, D.C.
60. **Heifets, L. B.** 1991. *Drug Susceptibility in the Chemotherapy of Mycobacterial Infections.* CRC Press, Boca Raton, Fla.
61. **Heifets, L. B., and M. D. Iseman.** 1990. Choice of antimicrobial agents for M. *avium* disease based on quantitative tests of drug susceptibility. *N. Engl. J. Med.* **323:**419–420.
62. **Heifets, L. B., and M. D. Iseman.** 1985. Determination of in vitro susceptibility of mycobacteria to ansamycin. *Am. Rev. Respir. Dis.* **132:**710–711.
63. **Heifets, L. B., M. D. Iseman, P. J. Lindholm-Levy, and W. Kanes.** 1985. Determination of ansamycin MICs for *Mycobacterium avium* complex in liquid medium by radiometric and conventional methods. *Antimicrob. Agents Chemother.* **28:**570–575.
64. **Heym, B., Y. Zhang, S. Poulet, D. Young, and S. T. Cole.** 1993. Characterization of the *katG* gene encoding a catalase-peroxidase required for isoniazid susceptibility of *Mycobacterium tuberculosis. J. Bacteriol.* **175:**4255–4259.
65. **Hillar, A., and P. C. Loewen.** 1995. Comparison of isoniazid oxidation catalyzed by bacterial catalase-peroxidases and horseradish peroxidase. *Arch. Biochem. Biophys.* **323:** 438–446.
66. **Hoffner, S. E., M. Kratz, B. Olsson-Liljequist, S. B. Svenson, and G. Källenius.** 1989. In-vitro synergistic activity between ethambutol and fluorinated quinolones against *Mycobacterium avium* complex. *J. Antimicrob. Chemother.* **24:**317–324.
67. **Hoffner, S. E., S. B. Svenson, and A. E. Beezer.** 1990. Microcalorimetric studies of the initial interaction between antimycobacterial drugs and *Mycobacterium avium. J. Antimicrob. Chemother.* **25:**353–359.
68. **Honore, N., and S. T. Cole.** 1993. Molecular basis of rifampin resistance in *Mycobacterium leprae. Antimicrob. Agents Chemother.* **37:**414–418.
69. **Howard, W. L., F. Maresh, E. E. Mueller, S. A. Yanitelli, and G. F. Woodruff.** 1949. The role of pulmonary cavitation in the development of bacterial resistance to streptomycin. *Am. Rev. Tuberc.* **59:**391–401.
70. **Howlett, H. S., J. B. O'Connor, J. F. Sadusk, J. E. Swift, and F. A. Beardsley.** 1949. Sensitivity of tubercle bacilli to streptomycin: the influence of various factors upon the emergence of resistant strains. *Am. Rev. Tuberc.* **59:** 402–414.
71. **Huebner, R. E., R. C. Good, and J. I. Tokars.** 1993. Current practices in mycobacteriology: results of a survey of state public health laboratories. *J. Clin. Microbiol.* **31:** 771–775.
72. **Hunt, J. M., G. D. Roberts, L. Stockman, T. A. Felmlee, and D. H. Persing.** 1994. Detection of a genetic locus encoding resistance to rifampin in mycobacterial cultures and in clinical specimens. *Diagn. Microbiol. Infect. Dis.* **18:** 219–227.
73. **Inderlied, C. B.** 1994. Antimycobacterial susceptibility testing: present practices and future trends. *Eur. J. Clin. Microbiol. Infect. Dis.* **13:**980–993.
74. **Inderlied, C. B., C. A. Kemper, and L. E. M. Bermudez.** 1993. The *Mycobacterium avium* complex. *Clin. Microbiol. Rev.* **6:**266–310.
75. **Inderlied, C. B., P. T. Kolonski, M. Wu, and L. S. Young.** 1989. In vitro and in vivo activity of azithromycin (CP 62,993) against the *Mycobacterium avium* complex. *J. Infect. Dis.* **159:**994–997.
76. **Inderlied, C. B., and K. A. Nash.** 1996. Antimycobacterial agents: in vitro susceptibility testing, spectra of activity, mechanisms of action and resistance, and assays for activity in biologic fluids, p. 127–175. *In* V. Lorian (ed.), *Antibiotics in Laboratory Medicine*, 4th ed. The Williams & Wilkins Co., Baltimore, Md.
77. **Jacobs, W. R., Jr., R. G. Barletta, R. Udani, J. Chan, G. Kalkut, G. Sosne, T. Kieser, G. J. Sarkis, G. F. Hatfull, and B. R. Bloom.** 1993. Rapid assessment of drug susceptibilities of *Mycobacterium tuberculosis* by means of luciferase reporter phages. *Science* **260:**819–822.
78. **Källenius, G., S. G. Svenson, and S. E. Hoffner.** 1989. Ethambutol: a key for *Mycobacterium avium* complex chemotherapy. *Am. Rev. Respir. Dis.* **140:**264.
79. **Kapur, V., L. L. Li, S. Iordanescu, M. R. Hamrick, A. Wanger, B. N. Kreiswirth, and J. M. Musser.** 1994. Characterization by automated DNA sequencing of mutations in the gene (*rpoB*) encoding the RNA polymerase beta subunit in rifampin-resistant *Mycobacterium tuberculosis* strains from New York City and Texas. *J. Clin. Microbiol.* **32:**1095–1098.
80. **Kelley, C. L., D. A. Rouse, and S. L. Morris.** 1997. Analysis of *ahpC* gene mutations in isoniazid-resistant clinical isolates of *Mycobacterium tuberculosis. Antimicrob. Agents Chemother.* **41:**2057–2058.
81. **Kenney, T. J., and G. Churchward.** 1994. Cloning and sequence analysis of the *rpsL* and *rpsG* genes of *Mycobacterium smegmatis* and characterization of mutations causing resistance to streptomycin. *J. Bacteriol.* **176:**6153–6156.
82. **Kent, P. T., and G. P. Kubica.** 1985. *Public Health Mycobacteriology—A Guide for the Level III Laboratory.* Centers for Disease Control, U.S. Department of Health and Human Services, Atlanta, Ga.
83. **Koletar, S. L., D. J. Williams, and A. Berry.** 1994. Serum level and MIC do not correlate with the efficacy of azithromycin for disseminated *Mycobacterium avium* complex (MAC) infection in patients with AIDS, abstr. 292, p. 65. *In Program and Abstracts 2nd International Conference on Macrolides, Azalides, Streptogramins.*
84. **Koontz, F.** 1994. E-test for susceptibility testing of rapid growing mycobacteria. *Diagn. Microbiol. Infect. Dis.* **19:** 183–186.
85. **Kubica, G. P., and W. E. Dye.** 1967. *Laboratory Methods for Clinical and Public Health Mycobacteriology.* U.S. Government Printing Office, Washington, D.C.
86. **Leysen, D. C., A. Haemers, and S. R. Pattyn.** 1989. Mycobacteria and the new quinolones. *Antimicrob. Agents Chemother.* **33:**1–5.
87. **Libonati, J. P., C. E. Stager, J. R. Davis, and S. H. Siddiqi.** 1988. Direct antimicrobial drug susceptibility testing of *Mycobacterium tuberculosis* by the radiometric method. *Diagn. Microbiol. Infect. Dis.* **10:**41–48.
88. **Magliozzo, R. S., and J. A. Marcinkeviciene.** 1997. The role of Mn(II)-peroxidase activity of mycobacterial catalase-peroxidase in activation of the antibiotic isoniazid. *J. Biol. Chem.* **272:**8867–8870.
89. **Mandell, G. L., R. G. Douglas, Jr., and J. E. Bennett.** 1992. *Handbook of Antimicrobial Therapy.* Churchill Livingstone, Inc., New York, N.Y.
90. **Marone, P., L. Bono, E. Carretto, D. Barbarini, and S. Telecco.** 1997. Rapid drug susceptibility of *Mycobacterium avium* complex using a fluorescence quenching method. *J. Chemother.* **9:**247–250.
91. **Masur, H.** 1993. Recommendations on prophylaxis and therapy for disseminated *Mycobacterium avium* complex disease in patients infected with the human-immunodeficiency virus. *N. Engl. J. Med.* **329:**898–904.
92. **McClatchy, J. K.** 1978. Susceptibility testing of mycobacteria. *Lab. Med.* **9:**47–52.

93. **McFarland, E. J., and D. R. Kuritzkes.** 1993. Clinical features and treatment of infection due to *Mycobacterium fortuitum/chelonae* complex, p. 188–202. *In* J. S. Remington and M. N. Swartz (ed.), *Current Clinical Topics in Infectious Diseases.* Blackwell Scientific Publications, Boston, Mass.
94. **Mdluli, K., D. R. Sherman, M. J. Hickey, B. N. Kreiswirth, S. Morris, C. K. Stover, and C. E. Barry III.** 1996. Biochemical and genetic data suggest that InhA is not the primary target for activated isoniazid in *Mycobacterium tuberculosis. J. Infect. Dis.* **174:**1085–1090.
95. **Mdluli, K., R. A. Slayden, Y. Zhu, S. Ramaswamy, X. Pan, D. Mead, D. D. Crane, J. M. Musser, and C. E. Barry III.** 1998. Inhibition of a *Mycobacterium tuberculosis* β-ketoacyl ACP synthase by isoniazid. *Science* **280:** 1607–1610.
96. **Meier, A., P. Kirschner, B. Springer, V. A. Steingrube, B. A. Brown, R. J. Wallace, Jr., and E. C. Böttger.** 1994. Identification of mutations in 23S rRNA gene of clarithromycin-resistant *Mycobacterium intracellulare. Antimicrob. Agents Chemother.* **38:**381–384.
97. **Miller, M. A., L. Thibert, F. Desjardins, S. H. Siddiqi, and A. Dascal.** 1996. Growth inhibition of *Mycobacterium tuberculosis* by polyoxyethylene stearate present in the BACTEC pyrazinamide susceptibility test. *J. Clin. Microbiol.* **34:**84–86.
98. **Miller, M. A., L. Thibert, F. Desjardins, S. H. Siddiqi, and A. Dascal.** 1995. Testing of susceptibility of *Mycobacterium tuberculosis* to pyrazinamide: comparison of Bactec method with pyrazinamidase assay. *J. Clin. Microbiol.* **33:** 2468–2470.
99. **Mitchison, D. A.** 1979. Basic mechanisms of chemotherapy. *Chest* **76**(Suppl.)**:**771–781.
100. **Mitchison, D. A.** 1992. The Garrod Lecture. Understanding the chemotherapy of tuberculosis—current problems. *J. Antimicrob. Chemother.* **29:**477–493.
101. **Mitchison, D. A.** 1952. Titration of strains of tubercle bacilli against isoniazid. *Lancet* **ii:**858–860.
102. **Mizuguchi, Y., M. Ogawa, and T. Udou.** 1985. Morphological changes induced by β-lactam antibiotics in *Mycobacterium avium-intracellulare* complex. *Antimicrob. Agents Chemother.* **27:**541–547.
103. **Moore, D. F., J. I. Curry, C. A. Knott, and V. Jonas.** 1996. Amplification of rRNA for assessment of treatment response of pulmonary tuberculosis patients during antimicrobial therapy. *J. Clin. Microbiol.* **34:**1745–1749.
104. **Morris, S., G. H. Bai, P. Suffys, L. Portillo-Gomez, M. Fairchok, and D. Rouse.** 1995. Molecular mechanisms of multiple drug resistance in clinical isolates of *Mycobacterium tuberculosis. J. Infect. Dis.* **171:**954–960.
105. **Mshana, R. N., G. Tadesse, G. Abate, and H. Miorner.** 1998. Use of 3-(4,5-dimethylthiazol-2-yl)-2,5-diphenyl tetrazolium bromide for rapid detection of rifampin-resistant *Mycobacterium tuberculosis. J. Clin. Microbiol.* **36:** 1214–1219.
106. **Musser, J. M.** 1995. Antimicrobial agent resistance in mycobacteria: molecular genetic insights. *Clin. Microbiol. Rev.* **8:**496–514.
107. **Nair, J., D. A. Rouse, G. H. Bai, and S. L. Morris.** 1993. The *rpsL* gene and streptomycin resistance in single and multiple drug-resistant strains of *Mycobacterium tuberculosis. Mol. Microbiol.* **10:**521–527.
108. **Nash, K. A., A. Gaytan, and C. B. Inderlied.** 1997. Detection of rifampin resistance in *Mycobacterium tuberculosis* by use of a rapid, simple, and specific RNA/RNA mismatch assay. *J. Infect. Dis.* **176:**533–536.
109. **Nash, K. A., and C. B. Inderlied.** 1995. Genetic basis of macrolide resistance in *Mycobacterium avium* isolated from patients with disseminated disease. *Antimicrob. Agents Chemother.* **39:**2625–2630.
110. **National Committee for Clinical Laboratory Standards.** 1995. *Antimycobacterial Susceptibility Testing.* Proposed standard M24-T. National Committee for Clinical Laboratory Standards, Villanova, Pa.
111. **National Committee for Clinical Laboratory Standards.** 1997. *Methods for Dilution Antimicrobial Susceptibility Tests for Bacteria that Grow Aerobically.* National Committee for Clinical Laboratory Standards, Villanova, Pa.
112. **Nightingale, S. D., W. D. Cameron, F. M. Gordin, P. M. Sullam, D. L. Cohn, R. E. Chaisson, L. J. Eron, P. D. Saprti, B. Bihari, D. L. Kaufman, J. J. Stern, D. D. Pearce, W. G. Weinberg, A. LaMarca, and F. P. Siegel.** 1993. Two controlled trials of rifabutin prophylaxis against *Mycobacterium avium* complex infection in AIDS. *N. Engl. J. Med.* **329:**828–833.
113. **Nitta, A. T., P. T. Davidson, M. L. de Koning, and R. J. Kilman.** 1996. Misdiagnosis of multidrug-resistant tuberculosis possibly due to laboratory-related errors. *JAMA* **276:**1980–1983.
114. **Nunn, P., J. Porter, and P. Winstanley.** 1993. Thiacetazone—avoid like poison or use with care. *Trans. R. Soc. Trop. Med. Hyg.* **87:**578–582.
115. **Oh, Y. K., and R. M. Straubinger.** 1996. Intracellular fate of *Mycobacterium avium*: use of dual-label spectrofluorometry to investigate the influence of bacterial viability and opsonization on phagosomal pH and phagosome-lysosome interaction. *Infect. Immun.* **64:**319–325.
116. **Palaci, M., S. Y. Ueki, D. N. Sato, M. A. Da Silva Telles, M. Curcio, and E. A. Silva.** 1996. Evaluation of mycobacteria growth indicator tube for recovery and drug susceptibility testing of *Mycobacterium tuberculosis* isolates from respiratory specimens. *J. Clin. Microbiol.* **34:** 762–764.
117. **Parsons, L. M., J. R. Driscoll, H. W. Taber, and M. Salfinger.** 1997. Drug resistance in tuberculosis. *Infect. Dis. Clin. North Am.* **11:**905–928.
118. **Perutz, M. F.** 1994. The white plague. *N. Y. Rev. Books* **XLI:**35–39.
119. **Petersen, E. A., J. B. Grayson, E. M. Hersh, R. T. Dorr, S. M. Chiang, M. Oka, and R. T. Proffitt.** 1996. Liposomal amikacin: improved treatment of *Mycobacterium avium* complex infection in the beige mouse model. *J. Antimicrob. Chemother.* **38:**819–828.
120. **Pierce, M., S. Crampton, D. Henry, L. Heifets, A. LaMarca, M. Montecalvo, G. P. Wormser, H. Jablonowski, J. Jemsek, M. Cynamon, B. G. Yangco, G. Notario, and J. C. Craft.** 1996. A randomized trial of clarithromycin as prophylaxis against disseminated *Mycobacterium avium* complex infection in patients with advanced acquired immunodeficiency syndrome. *N. Engl. J. Med.* **335:** 384–391.
121. **Pyle, M.** 1947. Relative number of resistant tubercle bacilli in sputa of patients before and during treatment with streptomycin. *Mayo Clin. Proc.* **22:**465–473.
122. **Rastogi, N., C. Frehel, A. Ryter, H. Ohayon, M. Lesourd, and H. L. David.** 1981. Multiple drug resistance in *Mycobacterium avium*: is the wall architecture responsible for the exclusion of antimicrobial agents? *Antimicrob. Agents Chemother.* **20:**666–677.
123. **Rastogi, N., K. S. Goh, and A. Bryskier.** 1994. Activities of roxithromycin used alone and in combination with ethambutol, rifampin, amikacin, ofloxacin, and clofazimine against *Mycobacterium avium* complex. *Antimicrob. Agents Chemother.* **38:**1433–1438.
124. **Rathman, M., M. D. Sjaastad, and S. Falkow.** 1996. Acidification of phagosomes containing *Salmonella typhi-*

murium in murine macrophages. *Infect. Immun.* **64:** 2765–7273.

125. **Reisner, B. S., A. M. Gatson, and G. L. Woods.** 1995. Evaluation of mycobacteria growth indicator tubes for susceptibility testing of *Mycobacterium tuberculosis* to isoniazid and rifampin. *Diagn. Microbiol. Infect. Dis.* **22:** 325–329.
126. **Revel Viravau, V., Q. C. Truong, N. Moreau, V. Jarlier, and W. Sougakoff.** 1996. Sequence analysis, purification, and study of inhibition by 4-quinolones of the DNA gyrase from *Mycobacterium smegmatis. Antimicrob. Agents Chemother.* **40:**2054–2061.
127. **Rist, N.** 1953. The application to clinical practice of the laboratory experience with combinations of antituberculosis drugs. *Bull. Int. Union Tuberc.* **23:**416–427.
128. **Russel, W. R., and G. Middlebrook.** 1961. *Chemotherapy of Tuberculosis.* Charles C Thomas, Springfield, III.
129. **Saito, H., K. Sato, and H. Tomioka.** 1988. Comparative in vitro and in vivo activity of rifabutin and rifampicin against *Mycobacterium avium* complex. *Tubercle* **69:** 187–192.
130. **Salfinger, M., and L. B. Heifets.** 1988. Determination of pyrazinamide MICs for *Mycobacterium tuberculosis* at different pHs by the radiometric method. *Antimicrob. Agents Chemother.* **32:**1002–1004.
131. **Salfinger, M., and G. E. Pfyffer.** 1994. The new diagnostic mycobacteriology laboratory. *Eur. J. Clin. Microbiol. Infect. Dis.* **13:**961–979.
132. **Salfinger, M., L. B. Reller, B. Demchuk, and Z. T. Johnson.** 1989. Rapid radiometric method for pyrazinamide susceptibility testing of *M. tuberculosis. Res. Microbiol.* **140:**301–309.
133. **Salfinger, M., L. B. Reller, and F. M. Kafader.** 1990. Pyrazinamide resistance of *Mycobacterium tuberculosis* complex isolates, abstr. U-55, p. 150. *In Abstracts of the 90th Annual Meeting of the American Society for Microbiology 1990.* American Society for Microbiology, Washington, D.C.
134. **Sanford, J. P.** 1993. *Guide to Antimicrobial Therapy.* Antimicrobial Therapy, Inc., Dallas, Tex.
135. **Schentag, J. J., and C. H. Ballow.** 1991. Tissue-directed pharmacokinetics. *Am. J. Med.* **91:**5S–11S.
136. **Scorpio, A., D. Collins, D. Whipple, D. Cave, J. Bates, and Y. Zhang.** 1997. Rapid differentiation of bovine and human tubercle bacilli based on a characteristic mutation in the bovine pyrazinamidase gene. *J. Clin. Microbiol.* **35:** 106–110.
137. **Scorpio, A., P. Lindholm Levy, L. Heifets, R. Gilman, S. Siddiqi, M. Cynamon, and Y. Zhang.** 1997. Characterization of *pncA* mutations in pyrazinamide-resistant *Mycobacterium tuberculosis. Antimicrob. Agents Chemother.* **41:** 540–543.
138. **Scorpio, A., and Y. Zhang.** 1996. Mutations in *pncA*, a gene encoding pyrazinamidase/nicotinamidase, cause resistance to the antituberculous drug pyrazinamide in tubercle bacillus. *Nat. Med.* **2:**662–667.
139. **Shafran, S. D., J. Singer, D. P. Zarowny, P. Phillips, I. Salit, S. L. Walmsley, I. W. Fong, M. J. Gill, A. R. Rachlis, R. G. Lalonde, M. M. Fanning, and C. M. Tsoukas.** 1996. A comparison of two regimens for the treatment of *Mycobacterium avium* complex bacteremia in AIDS: rifabutin, ethambutol, and clarithromycin versus rifampin, ethambutol, clofazimine, and ciprofloxacin. Canadian HIV Trials Network Protocol 010 Study Group. *N. Engl. J. Med.* **335:**377–383.
140. **Siddiqi, S. H.** 1992. Radiometric (Bactec) tests for slowly growing mycobacteria, p. 5.14.1–5.14.25. *In* H. D. Isenberg (ed.), *Clinical Microbiology Procedures Handbook.* American Society for Microbiology, Washington, D.C.
141. **Siddiqi, S. H., L. B. Heifets, M. H. Cynamon, N. M. Hooper, A. Laszlo, J. P. Libonati, P. J. Lindholm-Levy, and N. Pearson.** 1993. Rapid broth macrodilution method for determination of MICs for *Mycobacterium avium* isolates. *J. Clin. Microbiol.* **31:**2332–2338.
142. **Siddiqi, S. H., J. P. Libonati, M. E. Carter, N. M. Hooper, J. F. Baker, C. C. Hwangbo, and L. E. Warfel.** 1988. Enhancement of mycobacterial growth in Middlebrook 7H12 medium by polyoxyethylene stearate. *Curr. Microbiol.* **17:**105–110.
143. **Sirgel, F. A., F. J. Botha, D. P. Parkin, B. W. Van de Wal, R. Schall, P. R. Donald, and D. A. Mitchison.** 1997. The early bactericidal activity of ciprofloxacin in patients with pulmonary tuberculosis. *Am. J. Respir. Crit. Care Med.* **156:**901–905.
144. **Sreevatsan, S., X. Pan, Y. Zhang, V. Deretic, and J. M. Musser.** 1997. Analysis of the *oxyR-ahpC* region in isoniazid-resistant and -susceptible *Mycobacterium tuberculosis* complex organisms recovered from diseased humans and animals in diverse localities. *Antimicrob. Agents Chemother.* **41:**600–606.
145. **Sreevatsan, S., X. Pan, Y. Zhang, B. N. Kreiswirth, and J. M. Musser.** 1997. Mutations associated with pyrazinamide resistance in *pncA* of *Mycobacterium tuberculosis* complex organisms. *Antimicrob. Agents Chemother.* **41:** 636–640.
146. **Sreevatsan, S., K. E. Stockbauer, X. Pan, B. N. Kreiswirth, S. L. Moghazeh, W. Jacobs, Jr., A. Telenti, and J. M. Musser.** 1997. Ethambutol resistance in *Mycobacterium tuberculosis*: critical role of *embB* mutations. *Antimicrob. Agents Chemother.* **41:**1677–1681.
147. **Straus, W. L., S. M. Ostroff, D. B. Jernigan, T. E. Kiehn, E. M. Sordillo, D. Armstrong, N. Boone, N. Schneider, J. O. Kilburn, V. A. Silcox, V. LaBombardi, and R. C. Good.** 1994. Clinical and epidemiologic characteristics of *Mycobacterium haemophilum*, an emerging pathogen in immunocompromised patients. *Ann. Intern. Med.* **120:**118–125.
148. **Sturgill-Koszycki, S., P. H. Schlesinger, P. Chakraborty, P. L. Haddix, H. L. Collins, A. K. Fok, R. D. Allen, S. L. Gluck, J. Heuser, and D. G. Russell.** 1994. Lack of acidification in *Mycobacterium* phagosomes produced by exclusion of the vesicular proton-ATPase. *Science* **263:**678–681.
149. **Takayama, K., and J. O. Kilburn.** 1989. Inhibition of synthesis of arabinogalactan by ethambutol in *Mycobacterium smegmatis. Antimicrob. Agents Chemother.* **33:** 1493–1499.
150. **Takayama, K., and N. Qureshi.** 1984. Structure and synthesis of lipids, p. 315–344. *In* G. P. Kubica and L. G. Wayne (ed.), *The Mycobacteria: a Sourcebook,* Part A. Marcel Dekker, Inc., New York, N.Y.
151. **Takiff, H. E., L. Salazar, C. Guerrero, W. Philipp, W. M. Huang, B. Kreiswirth, S. T. Cole, W. Jacobs, Jr., and A. Telenti.** 1994. Cloning and nucleotide sequence of *Mycobacterium tuberculosis gyrA* and *gyrB* genes and detection of quinolone resistance mutations. *Antimicrob. Agents Chemother.* **38:**773–780.
152. **Telenti, A., N. Honore, C. Bernasconi, J. March, A. Ortega, B. Heym, H. E. Takiff, and S. T. Cole.** 1997. Genotypic assessment of isoniazid and rifampin resistance in *Mycobacterium tuberculosis*: a blind study at reference laboratory level. *J. Clin. Microbiol.* **35:**719–723.
153. **Telenti, A., P. Imboden, F. Marchesi, D. Lowrie, S. Cole, M. J. Colston, L. Matter, K. Schopfer, and T. Bodmer.** 1993. Detection of rifampin-resistance mutations in *Mycobacterium tuberculosis. Lancet* **341:**647–650.
154. **Telenti, A., P. Imboden, F. Marchesi, T. Schmidheini, and T. Bodmer.** 1993. Direct, automated detection of

rifampin-resistant *Mycobacterium tuberculosis* by polymerase chain reaction and single-strand conformation polymorphism analysis. *Antimicrob. Agents Chemother.* **37:** 2054–2058.
155. **Tenover, F. C., J. T. Crawford, R. E. Huebner, L. J. Geiter, C. R. Horsburgh, and R. C. Good.** 1993. The resurgence of tuberculosis: is your laboratory ready? *J. Clin. Microbiol.* **31:**767–770.
156. **Terashima, T., F. Sakamaki, N. Hasegawa, M. Kanazawa, and T. Kawashiro.** 1994. Pulmonary infection due to *Mycobacterium xenopi*. *Intern. Med.* **33:**536–539.
157. **Wallace, R., Jr., A. Meier, B. A. Brown, Y. Zhang, P. Sander, G. O. Onyi and E. C. Böttger.** 1996. Genetic basis for clarithromycin resistance among isolates of *Mycobacterium chelonae* and *Mycobacterium abscessus*. *Antimicrob. Agents Chemother.* **40:**1676–1681.
158. **Wallace, R. J., Jr.** 1989. The clinical presentation, diagnosis, and therapy of cutaneous and pulmonary infections due to the rapidly growing mycobacteria, *M. fortuitum* and *M. chelonae*. *Clin. Chest Med.* **10:**419–429.
159. **Wallace, R. J., Jr., J. M. Musser, S. I. Hull, V. A. Silcox, L. C. Steele, G. D. Forrester, A. Labidi, and R. K. Selander.** 1989. Diversity and sources of rapidly growing mycobacteria associated with infections following cardiac surgery. *J. Infect. Dis.* **159:**708–716.
160. **Wallace, R. J., Jr., D. R. Nash, M. Tsukamura, Z. M. Blacklock, and V. A. Silcox.** 1988. Human disease due to *Mycobacterium smegmatis*. *J. Infect. Dis.* **158:**52–59.
161. **Wallace, R. J., Jr., J. M. Swenson, V. A. Silcox, R. C. Good, J. A. Tschen, and M. S. Stone.** 1983. Spectrum of disease due to rapidly growing mycobacteria. *Rev. Infect. Dis.* **4:**326–331.
162. **Walters, S. B., and B. A. Hanna.** 1996. Testing of susceptibility of *Mycobacterium tuberculosis* to isoniazid and rifampin by mycobacterium growth indicator tube method. *J. Clin. Microbiol.* **34:**1565–1567.
163. **Wang, J. Y., R. M. Burger, and K. Drlica.** 1998. Role of superoxide in catalase-peroxidase-mediated isoniazid action against mycobacteria. *Antimicrob. Agents Chemother.* **42:**709–711.
164. **Wanger, A., and K. Mills.** 1996. Testing of *Mycobacterium tuberculosis* susceptibility to ethambutol, isoniazid, rifampin, and streptomycin by using E-test. *J. Clin. Microbiol.* **34:**1672–1676.
165. **Wanger, A. R., and K. Mills.** 1994. E-test for the susceptibility testing of *Mycobacterium tuberculosis* and *Mycobacterium avium-intracellulare*. *Diagn. Microbiol. Infect. Dis.* **19:** 179–181.
166. **Wayne, L. G., and I. Krasnow.** 1966. Preparation of tuberculosis susceptibility testing media by means of impregnated disks. *Am. J. Clin. Pathol.* **45:**769–771.
167. **Wayne, L. G., and H. A. Sramek.** 1992. Agents of newly recognized or infrequently encountered mycobacterial diseases. *Clin. Microbiol. Rev.* **5:**1–25.
168. **Wayne, L. G., and H. A. Sramek.** 1994. Metronidazole is bactericidal to dormant cells of *Mycobacterium tuberculosis*. *Antimicrob. Agents Chemother.* **38:**2054–2058.
169. **Williams, D. L., L. Spring, T. P. Gillis, M. Salfinger, and D. H. Persing.** 1998. Evaluation of a polymerase chain reaction-based universal heteroduplex generator assay for direct detection of rifampin susceptibility of *Mycobacterium tuberculosis* from sputum specimens. *Clin. Infect. Dis.* **26:**446–450.
170. **Williams, D. L., C. Waguespack, K. Eisenach, J. T. Crawford, F. Portaels, M. Salfinger, C. M. Nolan, C. Abe, V. Sticht Groh, and T. P. Gillis.** 1994. Characterization of rifampin-resistance in pathogenic mycobacteria. *Antimicrob. Agents Chemother.* **38:**2380–2386.
171. **Wilson, T. M., and D. M. Collins.** 1996. *ahpC*, a gene involved in isoniazid resistance of the *Mycobacterium tuberculosis* complex. *Mol. Microbiol.* **19:**1025–1034.
172. **Winder, F. G.** 1982. Mode of action of the antimycobacterial agents and associated aspects of the molecular biology of the mycobacteria, p. 353–438. *In* C. Ratledge and J. Stanford (ed.), *The Biology of the Mycobacteria*. Academic Press, Inc., New York, N.Y.
173. **Winder, F. G., and P. B. Collins.** 1969. The effect of isoniazid on nicotinamide nucleotide concentrations in tubercle bacilli. *Am. Rev. Respir. Dis.* **100:**101–103.
174. **Winder, F. G., and P. B. Collins.** 1968. The effect of isoniazid on nicotinamide nucleotide levels in *Mycobacterium bovis* strain BCG. *Am. Rev. Respir. Dis.* **97:**719–720.
175. **Woodley, C. L.** 1986. Evaluation of streptomycin and ethambutol concentrations for susceptibility testing of *Mycobacterium tuberculosis* by radiometric and conventional procedures. *J. Clin. Microbiol.* **23:**385–386.
176. **Woods, G. L., and J. A. Washington III.** 1987. Mycobacteria other than *Mycobacterium tuberculosis*: review of microbiologic and clinical aspects. *Rev. Infect. Dis.* **9:** 275–294.
177. **Yajko, D. M., P. S. Nassos, and W. K. Hadley.** 1987. Broth microdilution testing of susceptibilities to 30 antimicrobial agents of *Mycobacterium avium* strains from patients with acquired immune deficiency syndrome. *Antimicrob. Agents Chemother.* **31:**1579–1584.
178. **Young, L. S., O. G. Berlin, and C. B. Inderlied.** 1987. Activity of ciprofloxacin and other fluorinated quinolones against mycobacteria. *Am. J. Med.* **82:**23–26.
179. **Young, L. S., L. Wiviott, M. Wu, P. Kolonoski, R. Bolan, and C. B. Inderlied.** 1991. Azithromycin for treatment of *Mycobacterium avium-intracellulare* complex infection in patients with AIDS. *Lancet* **338:**1107–1109.
180. **Zhang, Y., S. Dhandayuthapani, and V. Deretic.** 1996. Molecular basis for the exquisite sensitivity of *Mycobacterium tuberculosis* to isoniazid. *Proc. Natl. Acad. Sci. USA* **93:**13212–13216.
181. **Zhang, Y., B. Heym, B. Allen, D. Young, and S. Cole.** 1992. The catalase-peroxidase gene and isoniazid resistance of *Mycobacterium tuberculosis*. *Nature* **358:**591–593.

Antiviral Agents and Susceptibility Tests*

ELLA M. SWIERKOSZ AND RICHARD L. HODINKA

125

During the past decade, safe and effective antiviral therapy has been developed for the treatment of a number of viral infections. Great strides have been made, most notably in the development of antiviral agents for the treatment of human immunodeficiency virus (HIV) infection. While the overwhelming majority of clinical virus isolates from drug-naive patients are susceptible to antiviral agents, widespread use of some antiviral agents has led to the emergence of drug-resistant strains, particularly in immunocompromised hosts (6–10, 12, 13). Diagnostic virology laboratories are increasingly asked to perform in vitro testing of antiviral agents when patients fail to respond clinically to antiviral therapy. This chapter briefly discusses (i) the major antiviral agents in use, (ii) the mechanisms of resistance to these agents, and (iii) the clinical situations in which antiviral resistance has emerged, thus necessitating in vitro susceptibility testing, and provides (iv) an overview of the susceptibility testing methods that have been used and (v) discusses molecular techniques for the rapid detection of mutations associated with antiviral resistance. Immune globulin preparations for prophylaxis of viral infections will not be discussed.

The major antiviral agents in use are listed in Tables 1 to 3 and have been reviewed in detail (6, 11, 28, 36, 37, 55, 61, 62). An understanding of the mechanism of drug action is essential for a discussion of antiviral resistance. Most of the agents discussed here are nucleoside analogs with selective action on viral replication.

ANTIVIRAL AGENTS AND MECHANISMS OF ACTION AND RESISTANCE

Herpesviruses

Agents active against various herpesvirus groups include acyclovir, cidofovir, famciclovir, foscarnet, ganciclovir, idoxuridine, trifluridine, valacyclovir, and vidarabine. Vidarabine (9-β-D-arabinofuranosyladenine; adenine arabinoside), an adenosine nucleoside analog, was the first systemic antiviral agent licensed for use in the United States. It was shown to be effective for the treatment of herpes simplex virus (HSV) encephalitis and neonatal HSV infection (6). It is active in vitro against HSV, varicella-zoster virus (VZV), human cytomegalovirus (CMV), and vaccinia virus. It revolutionized the treatment of HSV encephalitis and neonatal herpes by dramatically reducing mortality and neurologic sequelae. Although the exact mechanism of action is not completely understood, it is known that vidarabine is phosphorylated by cellular kinases and is incorporated into newly synthesized viral and cellular DNAs, thus inhibiting DNA synthesis. Vidarabine is also a competitive inhibitor of cellular and viral DNA polymerases (6). Its toxicity and poor solubility in water contributed to its replacement by acyclovir. Vidarabine-resistant HSV can be generated in vitro but is not a problem clinically (29). Despite its in vitro activity against acyclovir-resistant HSV, vidarabine has not been effective for the treatment of HSV infection in HIV-infected individuals (98).

Acyclovir ([9-(2-hydroxyethoxymethyl)guanine; acycloguanosine], a guanosine analog, has in vitro activity against a number of herpesvirus group viruses but is used clinically for the treatment of HSV and VZV infections. Acyclovir has largely supplanted vidarabine because of its ease of administration, low level of toxicity, and efficacy (6, 55). Acyclovir is phosphorylated by a virus-specific thymidine kinase (TK) to its monophosphate form, which is subsequently phosphorylated to acyclovir triphosphate by cellular enzymes. Acyclovir triphosphate competes with the natural substrate dGTP for viral DNA polymerase. Because acyclovir has a higher affinity than dGTP for the viral polymerase, it is preferentially incorporated into newly synthesized viral DNA. This results in the termination of DNA synthesis, because acyclovir lacks the 3′ hydroxyl group necessary to form phosphodiester linkages with incoming nucleotides (6). Inactivation of the HSV DNA polymerase also occurs as a consequence of the tight binding of the enzyme to the template-primer-acyclovir monophosphate complex that forms during the incorporation of acyclovir monophosphate (92). This inactivation provides an additional and unique means of shutting down viral DNA synthesis with acyclovir treatment.

Acyclovir resistance arises as a result of mutations in either the viral TK or the DNA polymerase gene. TK mutations arise at a high frequency (10^{-3} to 10^{-4}) (61). Mutation in the TK gene can produce strains deficient in TK (TK^{-}), which results in reduced or absent phosphorylation of acyclovir. A second type of TK mutation results in altered

* This chapter contains information presented in chapter 121 by Ella M. Swierkosz and Karen K. Biron in the sixth edition of this Manual.

TABLE 1 Antiviral agents in use for treatment of herpesvirus group

Drug class, mechanism of action	Antiviral agent(s)	Clinical indications for use[a]	Mechanism(s) of resistance
Nucleoside analog, inhibitor of viral DNA polymerase	Acyclovir	Localized and systemic HSV and VZV infections; prophylaxis of transplant recipients	Mutations in viral TK and viral DNA *pol* genes
	Cidofovir	CMV retinitis in patients with AIDS	Mutations in DNA *pol* gene
	Famciclovir (active metabolite, penciclovir)	Recurrent genital HSV in adults; zoster in adults	Mutations in viral TK and viral DNA *pol* genes
	Ganciclovir	Treatment of CMV retinitis in immunocompromised patients; prophylaxis of transplant recipients and patients infected with HIV	Mutations in viral UL97 (phosphotransferase) and viral UL54 DNA *pol* genes
	Valacyclovir (active metabolite, acyclovir)	Treatment or suppression of genital herpes in immunocompetent adults; treatment of zoster in immunocompetent adults	Mutations in viral TK and viral DNA *pol* genes
Nucleoside analog, inhibitor of DNA synthesis (topical only)	Idoxuridine	HSV keratitis	Mutations in viral TK gene
	Trifluridine	HSV keratitis	Unknown
Pyrophosphate analog, inhibitor of viral DNA polymerase	Foscarnet	Treatment of CMV retinitis in patients with AIDS and mucocutaneous acyclovir-resistant HSV infections in immunocompromised patients	Mutations in viral DNA *pol* gene

[a] FDA-approved uses.

substrate binding properties for acyclovir (TK^A). The majority of acyclovir-resistant clinical isolates of HSV and VZV are TK^-, although TK^A or DNA polymerase mutants have been recovered on rare occasions (21, 49). TK mutations render these viruses less pathogenic in animals (50). However, in immunocompromised hosts, such as bone marrow transplant recipients and HIV-infected patients, TK^- virus can cause progressive disease (7, 44). TK^- viruses are, however, also restricted in their ability to reactivate from latency (30, 60). Therefore, subsequent recurrences in the same patient could again be responsive to acyclovir (TK^+) (96, 98). Reactivation of acyclovir-resistant HSV with an altered TK has been documented in an immunocompetent individual, but it is a rare occurrence (69).

DNA polymerase mutations of HSV may confer only marginal shifts in 50% inhibitory concentrations (IC_{50}s); these modest shifts in drug susceptibility may not be clinically important if the levels of drug in plasma exceed the in vitro resistance level (33). However, the virulence and ability to establish and reactivate from latency of these mutants, unlike TK mutants, can be like those of wild-type virus (50).

Acyclovir-resistant HSV has rarely been recovered from patients with normal immunity (76). It is not uncommon to recover resistant HSV from transplant and HIV-infected patients after prolonged treatment with acyclovir (44, 96, 98, 119). Acyclovir-resistant VZV has been recovered from AIDS patients after chronic acyclovir therapy (77, 86, 97).

Recently, the L-valyl ester of acyclovir, valacyclovir, has been licensed for oral treatment of genital HSV and herpes zoster in immunocompetent adults. Valacyclovir is rapidly converted to acyclovir after oral administration and results in a three- to fivefold increase in the bioavailability of acyclovir compared to that of oral acyclovir. Because of its increased bioavailability, valacyclovir can be administered in a less frequent oral dosage regimen than is required for acyclovir (11).

Famciclovir, 2-[2-(2-amino-9*H*-purin-9-yl)ethyl]-1,3-propanediol diacetate, is a synthetic acyclic guanine derivative. Famciclovir is the orally administered prodrug of the

TABLE 2 Antiviral agents in use for treatment of HIV-1

Drug class, mechanism of action	Antiviral agent(s)	Clinical indications for use[a]	Mechanism(s) of resistance
Nucleoside analog, inhibitor of reverse transcriptase	ddI	Treatment of HIV infection	Mutations in viral reverse transcriptase gene
	3TC	Treatment of HIV infection in combination with ZDV	Mutations in viral reverse transcriptase gene
	d4T	Treatment of HIV infection in adults after prolonged, prior ZDV therapy	Mutations in viral reverse transcriptase gene
	ddC	Treatment of HIV infection in adults in combination with ZDV or with protease inhibitors; treatment of HIV infection in patients intolerant to or who have disease progression while receiving alternative antiretroviral therapy	Mutations in viral reverse transcriptase gene
	ZDV	Treatment of HIV infection	Mutations in viral reverse transcriptase gene
Dipyridodiazepinone, nonnucleoside inhibitor of reverse transcriptase	Delavirdine, nevirapine	Treatment of HIV infection in adults in combination with nucleoside analogs	Mutations in viral reverse transcriptase gene
Protease inhibitor	Indinavir	Treatment of HIV infection in adults as a monotherapy or in combination with nucleoside analogs	Mutations in viral protease gene
	Nelfinavir, ritonavir	Treatment of HIV infection in adults and children over age 2 yr	Mutations in viral protease gene
	Saquinavir	Treatment of HIV infection in adults in combination with nucleoside analogs	Mutations in viral protease gene

[a] FDA-approved uses.

active antiviral compound penciclovir, which is structurally similar to acyclovir. Following oral administration, famciclovir undergoes rapid biotransformation to penciclovir, which has inhibitory activity against HSV type 1 (HSV-1), HSV-2, and VZV (28). The bioavailability of penciclovir after the administration of an oral dose of 500 mg of famciclovir is approximately 77%. In contrast, the bioavailability of acyclovir is approximately 10 to 20% (55). Famciclovir has been approved for use in immunocompetent adults for the treatment of acute zoster (shingles) and recurrent episodes of genital herpes. The long intracellular half-life of penciclovir triphosphate in HSV- and VZV-infected cells permits the less frequent administration of famciclovir than the frequency of administration required for acyclovir (28). Like acyclovir, penciclovir requires phosphorylation by viral TK to a monophosphate form that is converted to penciclovir triphosphate by cellular enzymes. Penciclovir triphosphate inhibits HSV and VZV DNA polymerases competitively with dGTP, thus inhibiting viral DNA synthesis and ultimately viral replication. Unlike acyclovir triphosphate, penciclovir triphosphate is not an obligate chain terminator (43). Penciclovir-resistant mutants of HSV and VZV can result from mutations in the viral TK or DNA polymerase gene. Acyclovir-resistant HSV and VZV mutants deficient in TK can be cross resistant to penciclovir, but cross-resistance does not occur with all acyclovir-resistant isolates (100, 116).

Two topical agents, trifluridine (trifluorothymidine), a fluorinated thymidine analog, and idoxuridine (5-iodo-2′-deoxyuridine), an iodinated thymidine analog, have been used extensively for treatment of HSV keratitis. The triphosphate form of trifluridine is a competitive inhibitor of DNA polymerases. Resistance in clinical isolates of HSV has not been described, although resistant isolates can be generated in vitro. The exact mechanism of action is not completely defined for idoxuridine, but the triphosphate form inhibits viral DNA synthesis. Idoxuridine-resistant clinical isolates of HSV have been recovered from treated patients with HSV keratitis (55).

Ganciclovir [9-(1,3-dihydroxy-2-propoxy)methylguanine] is another guanosine analog that is similar in structure to acyclovir. Its spectrum of activity includes HSV and CMV. However, it is more active than acyclovir against CMV. Because it is more toxic than acyclovir, it is used only to treat serious CMV infections. In addition to intravenous ganciclovir, oral ganciclovir and ganciclovir intraocular im-

TABLE 3 Miscellaneous antiviral agents in use[a]

Drug class, mechanism of action	Antiviral agent(s)	Clinical indications for use[b]	Mechanism(s) of resistance
Primary symmetrical amine, prevents viral uncoating	Amantadine	Prophylaxis and treatment of influenza A virus	Mutations in the transmembrane domain of the viral M2 gene of influenza A virus
	Rimantadine	Prophylaxis of influenza A virus in children and adults; treatment of influenza A virus in adults	
IFN-α, inhibition of viral replication by stimulating a variety of cellular responses	IFN-α_{n3}	Intralesional treatment of refractory or recurring external condylomata acuminata in adults	Not described
	IFN-α_{2a}	Treatment of chronic hepatitis C virus infection; treatment of AIDS-related Kaposi's sarcoma in adults	
	IFN-α_{2b} (recombinant)	Treatment of external condylomata acuminata, chronic hepatitis B virus infection, and chronic hepatitis C infection and AIDS-related Kaposi's sarcoma in adults	
Nucleoside analog, inhibition of multiple viral replication processes	Ribavirin	Treatment of hospitalized infants and young children with severe respiratory syncytial virus infections	The development of resistance has not been evaluated in vitro or in clinical trials

[a] Immunoglobulin preparations are available for a variety of viral infections and will not be discussed.
[b] FDA-approved uses.

plants have become available. Ganciclovir is used clinically for the treatment of CMV diseases, including gastroenteritis, pneumonitis, and retinitis. Prophylactic ganciclovir is used for the prevention of retinitis in HIV-infected patients and of CMV disease in transplant patients. Ganciclovir is activated to its monophosphate form by virus-specific TK in HSV-infected cells and by a CMV-specific phosphotransferase in CMV-infected cells (79). It is subsequently phosphorylated to ganciclovir triphosphate by cellular kinases. Ganciclovir triphosphate acts as a competitive inhibitor of viral DNA polymerase but, unlike acyclovir, does not cause DNA chain termination (6). To date substitution mutations within the putative catalytic domain of the viral phosphotransferase gene, UL97, have generated the following amino acid substitutions: M460I, M460V, H520Q, A591V, C592G, A594V, L595F, L595S, L595T, L595W, E596G, C603W, and C607Y. A deletion mutation at codons 591 to 594 has also been generated. These mutations have accounted for most of the low-level ganciclovir resistance described in clinical isolates (IC_{50}s, ≥8 and <30 μM) (5, 24, 25, 105). Isolates with high-level ganciclovir resistance (IC_{50}s, ≥30 μM) have mutations in the viral DNA polymerase gene (UL54), in addition to mutations in UL97. The UL54 mutants recovered to date are uniformly cross resistant to cidofovir; some ganciclovir-resistant UL54 mutants are also foscarnet resistant (105). The UL54 substitution mutations associated with ganciclovir resistance and cross-resistance to cidofovir are D301N, F412C, L501I, T503I, K513R, S676G, I722V, Y751H, and L802M. Multidrug-resistant isolates, which are resistant to ganciclovir, cidofovir, and foscarnet, contain additional UL54 substitution mutations (105). All ganciclovir-resistant CMV isolates recovered to date have been from immunocompromised patients, the majority of whom had AIDS (41, 45, 46).

Foscarnet (trisodium phosphonoformate) is a pyrophosphate analog with in vitro activity against all herpesviruses, hepatitis B virus, and HIV type 1 (HIV-1). It serves as a noncompetitive inhibitor of viral DNA polymerases and of the reverse transcriptase of HIV-1. Foscarnet has been used for prophylaxis and treatment of CMV retinitis and treatment of acyclovir-resistant HSV and VZV infections (96–98). Clinical isolates of foscarnet-resistant HSV, CMV, and VZV have been recovered almost exclusively from immunocompromised patients (4, 51, 98, 105). Foscarnet-resistant HSV isolates are usually susceptible or borderline susceptible to acyclovir, suggesting that the binding site of acyclovir triphosphate on the viral DNA polymerase may differ from that for foscarnet (98). Resistance in herpesviruses is due to mutations of the viral DNA polymerase gene. Single amino acid changes in domain II of the CMV DNA polymerase (V715M, T700A) and in a 100-amino-acid segment adjacent to domain II, V781I and L802M, were responsible for the foscarnet resistance of isolates recovered from patients with AIDS (4, 26, 105). Foscarnet-resistant CMV isolates cross resistant to ganciclovir and cidofovir have also been recovered (105).

Cidofovir [(*S*)-1-(3-hydroxy-2-phosphonylmethoxypropyl)cytosine; HPMPC] has broad-spectrum activity against adenoviruses, herpesviruses, iridoviruses, papovaviruses, and poxviruses. It has been approved in the United States for prophylaxis and treatment of CMV retinitis. Clinically, it has also been used for treatment of acyclovir- and foscarnet-resistant HSV (106). Cidofovir is converted intracellularly to its active metabolite, the diphosphorylated form of HPMPC, HPMPCpp, by successive phosphorylation steps, presumably by cellular kinases. Unlike acyclovir and related nucleoside analogs, initial monophosphorylation by viral TK or other viral kinases is not required. HPMPCpp acts as an alternative substrate of dCTP and an inhibitor of viral DNA polymerase. Incorporation of two consecutive HPMPCpp molecules into DNA is required for chain termination (37). Because cidofovir does not require phosphorylation to a monophosphate form by viral TK, it is active against TK^- HSV and VZV. Resistance to cidofovir is due to mutations in the CMV UL54 (*pol*) gene. As described above, multidrug resistance, to cidofovir, ganciclovir, and foscarnet, can occur as a result of *pol* gene mutations (105).

Respiratory Viruses

Ribavirin (1-β-D-ribofurnosyl-1,2,4-trizole-3-carboxamide) is a synthetic nucleoside analog of guanosine and inosine with in vitro activity against a wide variety of viruses, including respiratory syncytial virus (RSV), influenza A and B viruses, parainfluenza virus, Lassa fever virus, and HIV. Ribavirin is currently licensed in the United States for treatment of RSV infection by small-particle aerosol. The exact mechanisms of action of ribavirin are unclear, but several theories have been proposed. Ribavirin monophosphate inhibits cellular IMP dehydrogenase activity, thereby reducing GTP levels. Ribavirin triphosphate inhibits translation of viral transcripts by interfering with 5′ capping of viral mRNA. Also, ribavirin triphosphate inhibits the viral RNA-dependent RNA polymerase activity of influenza and LaCrosse viruses (61). To date, no clinically significant resistance to ribavirin has been encountered.

Amantadine (1-adamantanamine hydrochloride), a primary symmetrical amine with a cage-like structure, and rimantadine, the methyl derivative of amantadine, are active against influenza A virus. Neither drug inhibits influenza B virus at clinically achievable drug concentrations. These drugs have been approved in the United States for prophylaxis and treatment of influenza A virus infection. Amantadine and rimantadine, which have identical spectra and mechanisms of activity, act by inhibiting the ion channel activity of the influenza A virus M2 protein, thus preventing viral uncoating and release of viral RNA into the cytoplasm (6). Resistance to these drugs is due to a single amino acid change in the transmembrane portion of the M2 protein (9). Clinical isolates of influenza A virus resistant to amantadine and rimantadine have readily been recovered during therapy, which may limit the widespread use of these two drugs (57).

HIV-1

Nucleoside Analog Inhibitors of HIV-1 Reverse Transcriptase

Zidovudine (azidothymidine; 3′-azido-3′-deoxythymidine; AZT; ZDV) is a thymidine analog with antiviral activity against HIV-1, HIV-2, and other human retroviruses. It was the first antiviral agent approved for primary therapy of HIV-1 infection. It belongs to a class of antiretroviral drugs labeled nucleoside analog reverse transcriptase inhibitors (NRTIs). Other NRTIs approved subsequently, in order of approval, include didanosine (2′,3′-dideoxyinosine; ddI), zalcitabine (2′,3′-dideoxycytidine; ddC), stavudine (2′,3′-didehydro-2′-deoxythymidine; d4T), and lamivudine (2′,3′-dideoxy,3′-thiacytidine; 3TC). NRTIs are phosphorylated by cellular enzymes to 5′ triphosphate forms which serve as competitive inhibitors of HIV reverse transcriptase. Incorporation of the triphosphate forms leads to chain termination because these agents lack a free 3′ hydroxyl group to form a phosphodiester bond with the incoming nucleotide (36). Because of the rapid emergence of NRTI-resistant HIV-1 isolates in patients treated with a single drug, combination therapy of NRTIs, with nonnucleoside analog reverse transcriptase inhibitors (NNRTIs) and protease inhibitors (PIs), is currently recommended by the Panel of Clinical Practices for Treatment of HIV Infection (19). The single exception is the prophylatic use of ZDV in pregnant women to reduce the risk of perinatal HIV transmission (20).

Zidovudine resistance was first described in isolates from patients receiving prolonged monotherapy with ZDV. Larder et al. (72) measured the ZDV susceptibility of HIV-1 isolates from HIV-infected individuals on therapy for various times by a plaque assay with $CD4^+$ HeLa cells. The IC_{50}s for isolates from untreated patients were 0.01 to 0.05 μM, and those for isolates obtained after 6 or more months of therapy were 0.04 to 6 μM. Genotypic characterization of these isolates demonstrated five amino acid substitutions in the reverse transcriptase gene at positions M41L, D67N, K70R, T215Y/F, and K219Q (67, 74). Further analysis revealed that a mutation at either codon 70 or 215 alone (or in combination) caused partial resistance, while four mutations were required to confer high-level resistance (mutations at codons 70, 215, 67, and either 41 or 219) (17, 67, 95). Furthermore, a single patient can harbor mixtures of HIV-1 isolates with different in vitro susceptibilities to ZDV (95). Resistance to ddI and cross-resistance to ddC are induced by the reverse transcriptase mutation L74V, which also resulted in a reversal of the ZDV resistance due to the T215Y mutation (111). The M184V/I mutation is also responsible for causing resistance to ddI and cross-resistance to ddC and 3TC (36). The K65R mutation confers resistance to ddI, ddC, and 3TC, and the V75T mutation induces resistance to d4T (2, 36). The relevance of the V75T mutation with regard to the clinical failure of d4T therapy is not known (2). Simultaneous use of ZDV and ddI has been reported to generate multidrug-resistant strains of HIV-1. These isolates are cross resistant to all the currently available dideoxynucleoside analogs. Mutation Q151M conferred partial resistance to ZDV, ddI, ddC, and d4T, while a combination of Q151M plus three or four additional mutations (V75I, F77L, F116Y or A62V, V75I, F77L, F116Y) conferred high-level resistance to these agents and low-level cross-resistance to 3TC (47, 63).

NNRTIs of HIV-1

NNRTIs include agents with diverse chemical structures that are unrelated to nucleosides. The currently licensed NNRTIs include nevirapine and delavirdine. NNRTIs bind to a non-substrate-binding site that is located in the vicinity of the substrate-binding site of reverse transcriptase, causing a disruption of the enzyme's catalytic site. Because resistant viruses emerge rapidly when NNRTIs are administered as monotherapy, NNRTIs must always be administered with antiretroviral agents with other mechanisms of activity. To date, the mutations associated with resistance to delavirdine and nevirapine are A98G, L100I, K103N, K103T, V106A, V108I, Y181C,I, Y188C, G190A, and P236L (37).

PIs

HIV-1 protease is essential for the posttranslational cleavage of precursor polyproteins encoded by the *gag* and *pol* genes. These nonfunctional polyproteins must be cleaved into smaller functional proteins to produce infectious virions (80). PIs competitively bind to the active site of the enzyme, thus preventing insertion of precursor polyproteins into the protease active site. This inhibition prevents cleavage of the viral polyproteins, resulting in the production of noninfectious viral particles (38, 83). Four PIs have been approved by the Food and Drug Administration (FDA) for treatment of HIV-1 infection: indinavir, ritonavir, and saquinavir are peptidomimetic, while nelfinavir is nonpeptidic. Because of the rapid emergence of drug-resistant viruses, monotherapy with PIs is not recommended (19). Mutations within the HIV-1 protease gene conferring resistance to PIs have been described in isolates from patients treated with the four currently licensed PIs. Initial protease gene mutations confer low-level resistance; additional mutations can accumulate sequentially, conferring cross-resistance to other PIs (101). Subtherapeutic levels of indinavir and ritonavir have been shown to increase the rate of development of drug resistance, while higher drug levels delayed or prevented the emergence of PI-resistant isolates (83).

INTERFERONS

Interferons (IFNs) are a group of cytokines with complex antiviral, immunomodulating, and antiproliferative activities. IFNs are proteins produced by eukaryotic cells in response to various inducers including viruses which act on uninfected cells to render them resistant to viral infection. There are three types of IFNs on the basis of the cell type from which they were derived: alpha IFN (IFN-α), IFN-β, and IFN-γ. IFN themselves are not antiviral but induce proteins in exposed cells that inhibit specific viral functions such as penetration, uncoating, synthesis of viral mRNA, viral protein synthesis, and viral assembly and release. A review of IFN activity has been published (55). IFN-α is the only IFN approved for use in the United States for treatment of hepatitis B and C viruses, condylomata acuminata, and AIDS-related Kaposi's sarcoma (Table 3).

CLINICAL INDICATIONS FOR ANTIVIRAL SUSCEPTIBILITY TESTING

Antiviral susceptibility testing is essential for defining mechanisms of antiviral resistance, for determining the frequency with which drug-resistant viral mutants emerge in clinical practice, to test for cross-resistance to alternative agents, and when evaluating new antiviral agents. With the exception of antiviral susceptibility testing for HSV, results of in vitro phenotypic assays are usually not available in a time frame relevant for patient management. Nevertheless, clinical deterioration of patients undergoing antiviral therapy can be associated with resistant virus. Results of antiviral susceptibility testing may be helpful in certain clinical situations. Persistent or worsening HSV or VZV infection while a patient is on acyclovir may indicate drug resistance. Alternative therapies such as foscarnet and cidofovir are available. Furthermore, HSV or VZV strains causing recurrent infection are often TK competent and, therefore, are again susceptible to acyclovir, which has minimal toxicity compared to that of foscarnet (6). Persistent or worsening CMV retinitis, pneumonitis, or colitis unresponsive to ganciclovir may also indicate the presence of drug-resistant virus. Cidofovir and foscarnet can be used as alternative agents. Influenza A virus isolates resistant to amantadine and rimantadine readily emerged during clinical trials with these drugs; therefore, continuous shedding or transmission of influenza A virus in a population receiving prophylaxis or treatment with these agents may be due to drug resistance. Monitoring of HIV-1 isolates is essential for assessing the net effect of multiple resistance mutations of isolates from patients receiving combination therapy and to test for cross-resistance to alternative antiretroviral drugs. The impact of susceptibility testing of HIV-1 on individual patient management decisions is unclear.

DEFINITION OF ANTIVIRAL RESISTANCE

Antiviral resistance is a decrease in susceptibility to an antiviral drug that can be clearly established by in vitro testing and that can be confirmed by genetic analysis of the virus and biochemical study of the altered enzymes. In vitro drug resistance must be distinguished from clinical resistance, in which the viral infection fails to respond to therapy. Clinical failures may or may not be due to the presence of a drug-resistant virus. Failure to achieve a clinical response also hinges on other factors such as the patient's immunologic status and the pharmacokinetics of the drug in that individual patient. For example, limited penetration of drug into the central nervous system may allow HIV-1 to escape, despite suppression of the virus at other sites. Poor oral absorption and binding to plasma proteins may limit the bioavailabilities of certain drugs. Furthermore, the administration of certain antiretroviral drugs in combination may interfere with the absorption or stimulate the elimination of one or more of the coadministered drugs. Patient-specific factors such as intolerance to an antiretroviral drug or an intercurrent infection can also lead to increases in the level of HIV-1 plasma viremia, despite in vitro susceptibility (19).

Variables of Antiviral Susceptibility Testing

To date, no standards exist for antiviral susceptibility testing. The National Committee for Clinical Laboratory Standards has established a subcommittee to develop a standard for susceptibility testing of HSV as a first step in developing consensus protocols for antiviral susceptibility testing. The major obstacle to standardization of antiviral susceptibility testing is that many variables influence the final result. These include (i) cell line, (ii) viral inoculum titer, (iii) incubation time, (iv) concentration range of the antiviral agent tested, (v) reference strains, (vi) assay method, (vii) endpoint criteria, (viii) calculation of endpoint, and (ix) interpretation of endpoint. Testing of a single virus isolate may lead to greatly different endpoints depending on the type of cell culture used (35, 54, 120). For example, the activity of acyclovir appeared greater than that of penciclovir when a plaque reduction assay (PRA) was performed with Vero cells; the converse was true when the assay was performed with SCC25 cells. Both drugs had comparable activities when they were tested with A549 cells (120). The titer of the virus inoculum is also critical; too large an inoculum can make a susceptible isolate appear to be resistant; too small an inoculum can make all isolates appear to be susceptible (54). The length of time that the virus incubates in the presence of drug must be sufficient to allow detection of small plaques, in the case of a PRA, or to allow growth of a subpopulation of resistant virus which may replicate at a slower rate than that for wild-type virus (4). The prolonged incubation time of peripheral blood mononuclear cell (PBMC)-based assays for HIV-1 susceptibility testing has been shown to select for subpopulations of HIV-1 variants not present in the starting inoculum (71). Moreover, different assay methods can produce different results. For example, the dye uptake (DU) assay for HSV susceptibility testing produces IC_{50}s higher than those produced by PRA (59). The concentration range of the drug tested affects the quality of the dose-response curve and therefore the validity of endpoint calculations. Susceptibility results are usually expressed as IC_{50}s because of the greater mathematical precision of the 50% endpoint than that of a 90 or 99% endpoint. (Synonyms for IC_{50} are 50% inhibitory dose and 50% effective dose.) However, debate continues concerning the appropriate endpoint, i.e., 50% versus 90 or 99% inhibition. IC_{50}s are more precise and reproducible, but IC_{90}s may correlate better with clinical response and are better at detecting subpopulations of drug-resistant strains among sensitive ones (3). Moreover, few studies have correlated in vitro results with clinical response (7, 45, 64, 76, 93, 110).

Another critical variable is the heterogeneity within the population of a virus "isolate." A single clinical isolate actually represents a mixture of isolates with drug-susceptible and drug-resistant phenotypes (5, 60, 95, 111). A virus population that has never encountered an antiviral agent is predominantly drug susceptible; resistant virus may be present at low levels. The presence of low levels of resistant virus in a population that is predominantly drug susceptible might not be reflected in the IC_{50} but would manifest its presence in higher IC_{90}s or IC_{99}s. At this time it is unknown whether a small fraction of drug-resistant virus is important to the behavior of the virus in vivo or how such a fraction might affect the response of the infection to therapy in an otherwise healthy host. However, in immunocompromised patients, under the continued selective pressure of antiviral therapy, resistant virus can emerge, and its presence can often be correlated with progressive viral disease (7, 21, 41, 44, 45, 64, 86, 96–98, 104).

The genetic locus at which a mutation occurs also affects susceptibility testing endpoints. For example, mutations of the DNA polymerases of HSV, VZV, and CMV usually confer relatively smaller increases in in vitro resistance than do mutations of TKs, which could go undetected in a mixed population of wild-type and mutant virus. In HIV-1, the level of in vitro resistance to PIs increased as the number of protease gene mutations increased (58). A good definition of such mixtures can be obtained only by testing appropriate concentrations of drug and a sufficiently large fraction of the population to detect resistant strains.

TESTING METHODS

Phenotypic versus Genotypic Assays

Phenotypic assays are in vitro susceptibility assays that measure the inhibitory effects of antiviral agents on the entire virus population in a patient. A variety of endpoint measurements have been used, including a reduction in the number of plaques, inhibition of viral DNA synthesis, reduction in the yield of a viral structural protein, i.e., hemagglutinin of influenza virus or p24 antigen of HIV, or reduction in the enzymatic activity of a functional protein, i.e., HIV-1 reverse transcriptase. Phenotypic assays in use include PRA, DU, DNA hybridization, enzyme immunoassay (EIA), and yield reduction assays for the herpesvirus group and influenza A viruses and PBMC cocultivation and recombinant virus assays for HIV-1. Genotypic assays analyze viral nucleic acid to detect specific mutations that cause antiviral drug resistance. Genotyping has been applied primarily to CMV and HIV-1. Both assay types have unique features that complement each other. Phenotypic assays are better suited to assessing the combined effects of multiple resistance mutations on drug susceptibility. This is especially important for viruses such as CMV and HIV-1, which acquire resistance-associated mutations in multiple genes that may be manifest as new patterns of resistance, cross-resistance, multidrug resistance, or even reversal of resistance (58, 63, 105, 111). However, most phenotypic assays are labor-intensive and expensive and have long turnaround times. Genotypic assays are relatively inexpensive and have shorter turnaround times, but they cannot detect mutations outside the selected target. Interpretation of genotypic assays is problematic due to the complex interactions of resistance mutations which result in a particular drug resistance phenotype. The utility of either type of assay in the management of a particular patient who appears to be unresponsive to therapy is questionable. The major phenotypic and genotypic assays in use will be discussed. Detailed protocols for the most commonly used phenotypic assays have been published elsewhere and are not presented here (113, 114). However, the principle of each test and guidelines for interpretation of results are discussed.

Control Strains

Simultaneous testing of control strains is crucial when antiviral susceptibility testing is being done. Reference strains should include genetically and phenotypically well-characterized drug-susceptible and drug-resistant isolates. Drug-resistant strains chosen for reference should include those with drug resistance phenotypes relevant to the mode of action of the drug to be tested. For example, for the testing of nucleoside analogs, which require phosphorylation by viral TK, i.e., acyclovir versus HSV and VZV, TK^- strains should be included. Susceptibility testing of CMV should include both UL97 and UL54 mutants. For HIV-1 testing, mutants resistant to both NRTIs and NNRTIs and mutants resistant to protease inhibitors should be included. The National Institute of Allergy and Infectious Diseases (NIAID) AIDS Research and Reference Reagent Program (Bethesda, Md.) provides upon request a number of reference strains of HSV, VZV, and CMV, including the drug-resistant strains mentioned above and the laboratory control strains CMV AD169 and VZV Oka. For the susceptibility testing of HIV-1, the NIAID AIDS Research and Reference Reagent Program has a repository of strains with various resistance phenotypes. Pharmaceutical companies and the American Type Culture Collection are also sources of control strains.

PRA for CMV, HSV, and VZV

PRA has classically been the "standard" method of antiviral susceptibility testing to which new methods are compared (13, 15, 56, 59, 84). Because many variations of the PRA have been reported, the National Committee for Clinical Laboratory Standards has formed a subcommittee to develop a standard for PRA testing of HSV. The principle of the PRA is the inhibition of viral plaque formation in the presence of an antiviral agent. The concentration of antiviral agent inhibiting plaque formation by 50% is considered the IC_{50}. Although the PRA is tedious and consumes more reagents than other methods, for small-scale testing of isolates, it is appropriate. Prior to performing the antiviral susceptibility assay per se, titers of HSV isolates must be determined to ensure an inoculum appropriate for the surface area of the assay wells or plates (i.e., approximately 100 PFU/60-mm-wide tissue culture plate). Because clinical strains of CMV and VZV are cell associated and because low-titer cell-free stocks are less stable during storage, infected cell suspensions (obtained by trypsin treatment of the infected monolayer) can be conveniently used for tests with these viruses. Two to three passages of clinical strains of CMV and VZV in cell culture are usually necessary to obtain a sufficient titer of virus. Low-passage isolates should be used because they are more likely to be representative of the original mixed population of the clinical isolate than a higher-passage stock would be. Well-characterized drug-susceptible and drug-resistant strains of HSV, CMV AD169, and VZV Oka or Ellen serve as reference strains. Stepwise instructions for the performance of the PRA for HSV, VZV, and CMV have been published elsewhere (59, 113, 114). A modified PRA has been described. It uses Vero or CV-1 cells that have been stably transformed with the *Escherichia coli lacZ* gene under the control of an HSV-1 early promoter which expresses β-galactosidase only after infection with HSV. Plaques were visualized after histochemical staining for β-galactosidase (117, 118). The proposed susceptibility breakpoints determined by PRA are listed in Table 4.

TABLE 4 Proposed guidelines for antiviral susceptibility results of herpesvirus group and influenza A viruses

Virus	Antiviral agent	Method	IC_{50} denoting resistance	Reference(s)
HSV	Acyclovir	PRA	≥2 μg/ml	32, 50, 84
		DNA hybridization	≥2 μg/ml	44, 115
		DU	≥3 μg/ml	59
	Famciclovir (active metabolite, penciclovir)	PRA and DNA hybridization	Definitive breakpoints cannot be established	109, 120
	Foscarnet	PRA	>100 μg/ml	29
	Vidarabine	PRA	Twofold or greater increase in IC_{50} compared to that for control or pretherapy isolate	29
VZV	Acyclovir	PRA and DNA hybridization	Three- to fourfold or greater increase in IC_{50} compared to that for pretherapy isolate or for a control strain	13, 64, 77, 97
	Famciclovir	PRA and DNA hybridization	Definitive breakpoints cannot be established	109
	Foscarnet	Late antigen reduction assay	300 μM	51
Human CMV	Cidofovir	PRA and DNA hybridization	>2 μM	26, 46, 105
	Foscarnet	PRA and DNA hybridization	>400 μM	26, 46
			>324 μM	105
	Ganciclovir	PRA and DNA hybridization	Three- to fourfold or greater increase in IC_{50} compared to that for pretherapy isolate or control strain (≈3 μg/ml)	41, 45, 88, 108
			>6 μM	26, 46
			>8 μM	105
Influenza A virus	Amantadine, rimantadine	EIA	>0.1 μg/ml	8, 9

DU Assay

The DU assay has been used for many years for susceptibility testing of HSV (59, 84, 114). This assay is based on the preferential uptake of a vital dye (neutral red) by viable cells but not by nonviable cells. The extent of viral lytic activity is determined by the relative amount of dye bound to viable cells after infection with HSV compared with the amount bound to uninfected cells. The dye bound by viable cells is eluted by ethanol and is measured colorimetrically. The drug concentration inhibiting viral lytic activity by 50% is considered the IC_{50}.

The DU assay consistently gives IC_{50}s of acyclovir that are three to five times greater than those given by PRA. This difference is most likely due to the higher inoculum used in the DU assay (500 PFU/ml) and to the use of a liquid overlay which allows drug-resistant virus to "amplify," thus resulting in a more sensitive detection of small amounts of drug-resistant virus. Therefore, the DU assay uses a cutoff IC_{50} of >3 μg/ml to denote acyclovir resistance (Table 4).

Advantages of the DU method include its ability to be semiautomated, allowing for the efficient testing of large numbers of isolates, and its ability to detect smaller amounts of resistant virus than the PRA can detect. Disadvantages are the relatively high cost of automated equipment and the technical problems caused by overseeding of cells into the culture wells and precipitation of neutral red onto the monolayer. The stepwise procedure for the DU assay has been published previously (59, 114).

DNA Hybridization

DNA hybridization assays have been used to measure the effects of different antiviral compounds on DNA synthesis. A dot blot hybridization assay, developed by Gadler (52), has been applied to susceptibility testing of CMV. It is a conventional hybridization assay requiring transfer of viral DNA to nitrocellulose filters, denaturation of DNA, baking of filters, prehybridization of filters, overnight hybridization, and autoradiography. Since the DNA probes are labeled with ^{32}P, the probes have short shelf lives. A good correlation between the PRA and the dot blot hybridization assay has been demonstrated (14, 52). The stepwise procedure has been detailed previously (114). Commercially available DNA-DNA hybridization test kits (Hybriwix Probe Systems, Athens, Ohio) have been used for susceptibility testing of HSV, CMV, and VZV (24–26, 34, 44, 64, 96–98, 105, 115). Each kit contains cell culture plates, culture medium, lysing reagent, nylon "wicks," ^{125}I-labeled probe, hybridization solution, wash reagent, and positive and negative control wicks. Cell culture wells are infected with virus, overlaid with dilutions of antiviral agent, and incubated to allow viral growth. After lysis of the cells, lysates containing viral and cellular DNAs are transferred to the wicks by capillary action. Following hybridization with virus-specific probe and washing of the wicks, the radioactivity of the dried wicks is counted in a gamma counter. The concentration of drug that causes a 50% reduction in counts compared with the counts for untreated virus controls is the IC_{50}. The turnaround time of the commercial hybridization reactions, excluding infection and incubation of cell culture wells, is approximately 4 h. Disadvantages of the Hybriwix assays include the use of a radioisotope, the short shelf life of the probe (2 months), and the relatively high cost of the kit. It is more cost-effective in a laboratory where large numbers of isolates are analyzed.

Yield Reduction Assay

The yield reduction assay reflects the ability of an antiviral agent to inhibit the production of infectious virus rather than the formation of a plaque. Cell monolayers are infected with virus, incubated in the presence of antiviral compound, and then lysed. Cell-free virus titers are subsequently determined by plaque assay. The endpoint is defined as the concentration of antiviral agent which reduces the virus yield by 50% in comparison with that for untreated control cultures. When used for susceptibility testing of HSV against penciclovir and acyclovir, the IC_{50}s of penciclovir were equivalent to or lower than those of acyclovir. The greater activity of penciclovir is postulated to be the result of the extended half-life of penciclovir triphosphate (120).

EIAs

EIAs have been developed for the susceptibility testing of HSV, VZV, and influenza A virus (8, 10, 91, 99). EIA permits quantitative measurement of viral activity by spectrophotometric analysis; IC_{50}s are calculated as the concentrations of antiviral agent that reduce the absorbance to 50% of that for the virus control. EIA is more suited than the PRA and the DU assay to the routine diagnostic laboratory. Susceptibility results for HSV and VZV determined by this method have correlated well with those obtained by PRA.

Susceptibility testing of influenza A virus by PRA is tedious and labor-intensive (56). EIA is technically easier and is more suitable for the testing of multiple isolates (8). The EIA uses antibodies to influenza A virus hemagglutinins (H1 or H3); viral hemagglutinin expression correlates with viral growth. Amantadine and rimantadine activities are measured by inhibition of hemagglutinin expression. Amantadine- and rimantadine-susceptible and -resistant isolates, whose M2 gene sequences are known, serve as controls and must be tested in parallel with patient isolates. A protocol for the EIA for the susceptibility testing of influenza A virus has been published (114).

Flow Cytometry

Flow cytometry has been applied to the susceptibility testing of HSV and CMV (78, 85, 87). While the IC_{50}s measured by flow cytometry were numerically different from those determined by plaque reduction, drug-susceptible isolates could be readily distinguished from drug-resistant isolates. Advantages of antiviral susceptibility testing by flow cytometry include the potential for automation, the objectivity of the assay, and a shorter turnaround time relative to that of PRA.

Measurement of HSV and VZV TK Activities by Plaque Autoradiography

Functional viral TK is required for the initial phosphorylation of acyclovir. To determine whether resistance to acyclovir is due to diminished or altered viral TK, two plaque autoradiograph methods are used (82). The level of incorporation of [^{125}I]iododeoxycytidine (IdC), a pyrimidine analog selectively phosphorylated by the VZV- or HSV-specific TK, correlates well with the acyclovir-phosphorylating potential of HSV and VZV isolates. Incorporation of [^{14}C]thymidine (dT) specifically assesses the thymidine-phosphorylating activities of these isolates and is useful for analyzing resistance to pyrimidine nucleoside analogs (acyclovir is a purine nucleoside analog). Most acyclovir-resistant HSV and VZV fail to incorporate both substrates due to diminished TK activity (TK^-); occasionally, TK^A

strains are seen. These strains fail to incorporate IdC but are able to incorporate dT. For IdC incorporation, Vero cells (HSV) and MRC-5 cells (VZV) are used. For dT incorporation, LMTK$^-$ TK$^-$ mouse LM cells (Roswell Park Memorial Institute, Buffalo, N.Y.) are used for HSV and the TK$^-$ cell line 143B is used for VZV. These assays provide both quantitative and qualitative evaluations of the TK status of a mixed population with TK$^+$ and TK$^-$ viruses. The IdC and dT plaque autoradiograph methods have been detailed elsewhere (82, 114).

Susceptibility Testing of HIV-1

A number of phenotypic assays are in use for testing the susceptibilities of HIV-1 isolates to NRTIs (72, 77, 111). A serious limitation of these procedures is that not all clinical isolates grow in the cell culture lines used in these assays. The AIDS Clinical Trials Group developed an assay performed with PBMCs which allowed growth of almost all clinical isolates of HIV-1 (65). Viral activity is quantitated by measurement of the levels of the p24 antigen of HIV-1. The PBMC assay, however, is labor-intensive, costly, and difficult to control because of the many variables of the assay and has a long turnaround time (weeks). Moreover, this assay requires cocultivation of infected PBMCs with uninfected donor PBMCs to produce a stock of the clinical isolate being tested, which has been shown to select for subpopulations of HIV-1 not present in the original isolate (71).

A new generation of phenotypic assays, recombinant virus assays (RVAs), has been developed to circumvent these problems. RVA involves PCR amplification of complete reverse transcriptase or protease gene-coding sequences either directly from the patient's PBMCs or after isolation of virus by cocultivation in PBMCs. The amplified reverse transcriptase or protease gene sequences from the patient strain are then cotransfected into CD4$^+$ T-lymphocyte cells in parallel with an HIV-1 proviral molecular clone from which the original reverse transcriptase gene-coding sequence or the reverse transcriptase gene- and protease gene-coding sequences had been deleted. Thus, CD4$^+$ cells containing a chimeric virus are generated. These cells contain the patient's reverse transcriptase or reverse transcriptase and protease gene-coding sequences in a background of an HIV-1 strain from which the original reverse transcriptase or reverse and transcriptase and protease sequences had been deleted (58, 68, 103). The susceptibilities of the chimeric viruses to all clinically available reverse transcriptase and protease inhibitors is subsequently determined in a single assay, either the plaque reduction assay with HeLa CD4$^+$ cells or the MT4 cell viability-based assay. RVAs thus allow determination of the phenotypic resistance patterns of circulating virus in vivo and circumvent the problem of selection of nonrepresentative variants during cultivation. The RVA can be completed in approximately 10 days from the time of cotransfection. It is not known, however, what proportion of the total population of virus that a subpopulation of resistant virus must achieve to be detectable by this assay (58).

In vitro susceptibility assays which test combinations of antiretroviral agents have been performed to determine drug synergy or antagonism (23, 40, 90). Synergy or antagonism has been determined by the methods of Chou and Talay (27) and Prichard et al. (90). A computer software program called Calcusyn (Biosoft, Cambridge, United Kingdom) has also been used (23). In vitro testing of drug combinations is a necessary first step in evaluating possible drug combinations for use in vivo.

GENOTYPIC ASSAYS

The genetic basis for antiviral resistance has been extensively studied for CMV and HIV-1. Although not all resistance-associated mutations are known, the majority have been elucidated, allowing the application of molecular diagnostic methods. The major advantage of genotypic assays is the relatively rapid turnaround times compared to those of phenotypic assays.

CMV

Genotypic assays have been used to screen CMV isolates for mutations associated with ganciclovir resistance. Both UL97 (phosphotransferase) and UL54 (polymerase) mutations can be detected. A number of approaches have been successfully applied to the genotyping of CMV. PCR amplification and sequencing of the entire UL54 gene and the fragment of the UL97 gene spanning the conserved domains of the phosphotransferase detected the mutations currently known to confer resistance to ganciclovir (4, 25, 46, 105). Alternatively, PCR amplification of short fragments of the UL97 gene followed by restriction endonuclease digestion has been used to detect mutations at positions 460, 594, and 595 (24, 25). UL97 mutations could be detected in 89% of ganciclovir-resistant isolates, while UL54 mutations were present in all high-level ganciclovir-resistant isolates (105). PCR amplification followed by restriction digestion could recognize mutant virus when mutant virus was 10% of the total virus population (105). UL97-associated ganciclovir resistance mutations have also been detected directly in patient blood and cerebrospinal fluid (16, 107, 121). Marker transfer experiments have been used to definitively determine that a particular mutation is associated with drug resistance. For this purpose, PCR-amplified UL97 and UL54 fragments containing resistance-associated mutations were cotransfected with CMV AD169 (a drug-susceptible strain). The resulting recombinant plaques were assayed for antiviral susceptibility by PRA. To further verify transfer of the mutations in question, sequencing was performed across the transfected fragment (4, 26).

HIV-1

Genotypic analysis of HIV-1 reverse transcriptase and protease genes has been used for direct detection of mutations associated with HIV drug resistance (48, 73, 89, 95, 102). Direct amplification of HIV gene regions containing resistance mutations followed by automated sequencing has been successfully used for detection of mutations associated with HIV antiviral resistance (75). Automated, high-speed DNA sequencing has recently been developed by Visible Genetics Inc. (Toronto, Ontario, Canada) and should allow analysis of both reverse transcriptase and protease genes within hours. DNA sequencing by using matrix hybridization has been developed by Affymetrix Inc. (GeneChip; Affymetrix Inc., Santa Clara, Calif.) which permits resolution of sequence variants of the *gag-pol-pro* regions of HIV-1 (22, 70, 89). The line probe assay analyzed PCR-amplified reverse transcriptase gene regions by hybridization to probes immobilized on a membrane strip. Probes were designed to cover different reverse transcriptase gene polymorphisms and drug-associated mutations (112). Other methods applied to the direct detection of HIV drug resistance include ligase chain reaction (1), self-sustained sequence replication-amplification reaction (53), and a point mutation assay (66).

A concern with each of the genotypic methods is that mutant variants present at a low frequency may not be detectable and that mixtures of HIV-1 strains with minor sequence variations may not be distinguishable (102). Genotypic assays do allow the more rapid and efficient detection of resistance than phenotypic assays and may allow the earlier detection of emerging resistance than phenotypic assays. However, the complexities of these tests make them impractical for most routine diagnostic virology laboratories. Moreover, genotypic assays can detect only known resistance-associated mutations. Finally, the applicability of genotypic analysis of HIV-1 isolates to individual patient management is unclear because of the complex interactions among different combinations of resistance mutations (18, 93).

Measurement of plasma HIV-1 RNA levels (viral load) reflects the extent of virus replication in an infected individual and has been shown to be the strongest predictor of clinical outcome (19, 81). The three methods currently in use include reverse transcription-PCR (Monitor HIV; Roche Molecular Systems), nucleic acid sequence-based amplification (Organon Teknika), and branched-chain DNA signal amplification (Quantiplex; Chiron). Monitoring of HIV-1 RNA levels is used to assess the relative risk of disease progression and the efficacy of antiretroviral therapy and is the predominant test used by clinicians to monitor HIV-infected patients. Because treatment failure may be due to a variety of pharmacologic factors and poor patient compliance, in addition to the emergence of resistant virus, viral load monitoring is essential for formulating patient management decisions regarding the initiation and alteration of therapy. Declining HIV-1 RNA levels during treatment indicates a response to therapy, while a significant rise in RNA levels indicates treatment failure (19, 81).

INTERPRETATION OF ANTIVIRAL SUSCEPTIBILITY RESULTS

Table 4 lists breakpoint IC_{50}s proposed by various investigators for the herpesvirus group and influenza A virus. At present, there are no definitive interpretive standards for antiviral susceptibility testing. The concentration of antiviral agent to which virus is considered susceptible has generally been based on the median susceptibilities of large numbers of clinical isolates obtained from patients prior to, during, and after antiviral therapy. Because of the variables that affect antiviral susceptibility results, the absolute IC_{50} can vary from assay to assay and from laboratory to laboratory. Moreover, in vitro results indicating susceptibility or resistance may not correlate with the response of the infection to therapy in vivo. The clinical response of the patient depends upon a number of other factors such as immunologic status and the pharmacokinetics of the drug in that particular patient (the dose or route of administration could be inappropriate). A poor clinical response may occur even though the antiviral susceptibility testing denotes in vitro susceptibility (39). Patients with HSV infections who are immunocompromised may fail to respond to therapy, despite in vitro IC_{50}s for the infecting isolates indicating susceptibility to vidarabine or acyclovir (44, 96, 98). Conversely, HSV isolates for which IC_{50}s of acyclovir are >2 μg/ml can occasionally be recovered from otherwise healthy hosts who have responded to acyclovir therapy (76). Thus, a high IC_{50} derived by in vitro susceptibility testing is not sufficient to designate a viral strain as resistant. Nor can in vitro susceptibility to a drug a priori predict a successful clinical outcome. Whenever possible, evidence of genetic alteration of the virus should be considered as well.

Interpretation of antiviral susceptibility results is further complicated by the variability in endpoint due to testing methodologies (31, 59, 62, 84, 88). Because endpoints are dependent on the test method, each new method and antiviral agent must be correlated with a historic standard that has been used to test large numbers of isolates. Also, the absolute IC_{50} may vary from assay to assay and laboratory to laboratory. Moreover, because small subpopulations of resistant virus may not be reflected in IC_{50}s, IC_{90} may be more predictive of clinical response. One approach to interpreting susceptibility endpoints is to compare the IC_{50}s for an isolate obtained prior to therapy (or for a well-characterized reference control strain) with those for an isolate obtained during therapy; a significant increase in the ratio of such IC_{50}s denotes resistance. However, pretherapy isolates are often unavailable, and the IC_{50} ratio considered clinically significant is unclear. Large-scale collaborative comparisons of methods with the same viral isolates are necessary to standardize antiviral susceptibility testing and to establish definitive interpretive guidelines. Only when a standardized assay is adopted can prospective studies be performed to correlate the in vivo response with in vitro susceptibility. Such studies are essential before definitive interpretive breakpoints are established.

Susceptibility testing of penciclovir illustrates the effects that the cell line and test method have on endpoint. When acyclovir and penciclovir, which is structurally similar to acyclovir, were tested with HSV isolates with Vero cells by PRA, penciclovir appeared to be less active than acyclovir and HSV-2 isolates appeared to be resistant to penciclovir. In contrast, penciclovir appeared to be more active than acyclovir against some HSV isolates when SCC25 cells were used. Both drugs appeared to have comparable activities when they were tested with MRC-5 and A549 cells (120). When clinical isolates of VZV were tested by PRA and DNA hybridization, the IC_{50}s for DNA hybridization were significantly lower than those obtained by PRA (109). Variability in endpoint was also seen with VZV depending on the composition of the inoculum (cell free versus cell associated). Therefore, breakpoints for susceptibility testing of penciclovir with HSV and VZV cannot be established at this time (109, 120).

Absolute IC_{50}s denoting the resistance of HIV-1 to antiretroviral drugs cannot be assigned. For HIV-1 in vitro susceptibility results are usually expressed as the fold increase in the IC_{50} for an isolate obtained while the patient is on therapy compared to that for a pretreatment isolate or a drug-susceptible isolate (58, 101). In general, single drug resistance mutations are associated with 2- to 10-fold increases in the IC_{50}, while multiple mutations in the same gene can confer a $>$100-fold increase in the IC_{50} (101).

There is controversy surrounding the significance and clinical utility of in vitro susceptibility testing and genotypic analysis of HIV-1 (93). Antiretroviral therapy may fail for reasons other than the emergence of drug-resistant virus, such as drug antagonism, noncompliance, increased clearance of one antiretroviral drug when it is coadministered with another drug, inadequate penetration of drug into a sequestered site, i.e., central nervous system, or malabsorption of drug from the gastrointestinal tract (58). The relative proportion of resistant virus in the total virus population is also an important determinant of clinical response (3). The presence of the syncytium-inducing phenotype also was associated with an increased risk of disease progression (94). Both phenotypic and genotypic assays have drawbacks which limit their applicability to patient management. At present, alteration in patient therapy is based on monitoring of the HIV-1 load. Nevertheless, in vitro susceptibility testing of HIV-1 is important for determining the genetic sites of drug resistance mutations, the effects of sequential mutations on drug efficacy, and the rate of emergence of drug resistance mutations when various drug combinations are used and when new drugs are tested.

FUTURE DIRECTIONS

No consensus protocol for antiviral susceptibility testing yet exists. Standardization is hampered by the many variables that affect susceptibility testing results. No single assay method, cell line, or inoculum composition (cell free versus cell associated) appears to be sufficient for the testing of all viruses. A major problem with culture-based susceptibility testing of viruses other than HSV is that assays may require weeks to complete, a fact that limits their utility in the management of acute cases of infection (42). Genotypic assays for UL97 and UL54 mutations of CMV may replace culture-based assays as more resistance-associated mutations are identified. The clinical significance of susceptibility testing of HIV-1 isolates remains questionable. Additional studies are required to correlate mutations conferring resistance to antiretroviral drugs with patient outcome. Finally, combination therapy for HIV-1 infection has necessitated the development of assays capable of evaluating drug combinations for synergy, indifference, or antagonism.

REFERENCES

1. **Abravaya, K., J. J. Carrino, S. Muldoon, and H. H. Lee.** 1995. Detection of point mutations with a modified ligase chain reaction (Gap-LCR). *Nucleic Acids Res.* **23:** 675–682.
2. **Arts, E. J., and M. A. Wainberg.** 1996. Mechanisms of nucleoside analog antiviral activity and resistance during human immunodeficiency virus reverse transcription. *Antimicrob. Agents Chemother.* **40:**527–540.
3. **Baldanti, F., K. K. Biron, and G. Gerna.** 1998. Interpreting human cytomegalovirus antiviral drug susceptibility testing: the role of mixed virus populations. *J. Infect. Dis.* **177:**823.
4. **Baldanti, F., M. R. Underwood, S. C. Stanat, K. K. Biron, S. Chou. A. Sarasini, E. Silini, and G. Gerna.** 1996. Single amino acid changes in the DNA polymerase confer foscarnet resistance and slow-growth phenotype, while mutations in the UL97-encoded phosphotransferase confer ganciclovir resistance in three double-resistant human cytomegalovirus strains recovered from patients with AIDS. *J. Virol.* **70:**1390–1395.
5. **Baldanti, F., M. R. Underwood, C. L. Talarico, L. Simoncini, A. Sarasini, K. K. Biron, and G. Gerna.** 1998. The Cys 607→Tyr change in the UL97 phosphotransferase confers ganciclovir resistance to two human cytomegalovirus strains recovered from two immunocompromised patients. *Antimicrob. Agents Chemother.* **42:**444–446.
6. **Bean, B.** 1992. Antiviral therapy: current concepts and practices. *Clin. Microbiol. Rev.* **5:**146–182.
7. **Bean, B., C. Fletcher, J. Englund, S. N. Lehrman, and M. N. Ellis.** 1987. Progressive mucocutaneous herpes simplex infection due to acyclovir-resistant virus in an immunocompromised patient: correlation of viral susceptibilities and plasma levels with response to therapy. *Diagn. Microbiol. Infect. Dis.* **7:**199–204.
8. **Belshe, R. B., B. Burk, F. Newman, R. L. Cerruti, and I. S. Sim.** 1989. Resistance of influenza A virus to amantadine and rimantadine: results of one decade of surveillance. *J. Infect. Dis.* **159:**430–435.
9. **Belshe, R. B., M. H. Smith, C. B. Hall, R. Betts, and A. J. Hay.** 1988. Genetic basis of resistance to rimantadine emerging during treatment of influenza virus infection. *J. Virol.* **62:**1508–1512.
10. **Berkowitz, F. E., and M. J. Levin.** 1985. Use of an enzyme-linked immunosorbent assay performed directly on fixed infected cell monolayers for evaluating drugs against varicella-zoster virus. *Antimicrob. Agents Chemother.* **28:** 207–210.
11. **Beutner, K. R.** 1995. Valacyclovir: a review of its antiviral activity, pharmacokinetic properties, and clinical efficacy. *Antivir. Res.* **28:**281–290.
12. **Biron, K. K.** 1991. Ganciclovir-resistant human cytomegalovirus isolates; resistance mechanisms and in vitro susceptibility to antiviral agents. *Transplant. Proc.* **23**(Suppl. 3)**:** 162–167.
13. **Biron, K. K., and G. B. Elion.** 1980. In vitro susceptibility of varicella-zoster virus to acyclovir. *Antimicrob. Agents Chemother.* **18:**443–447.
14. **Biron, K. K., J. A. Fyfe, S. C. Stanat, L. K. Leslie, J. B. Sorrell, C. U. Lambe, and D. M. Coen.** 1986. A human cytomegalovirus mutant resistant to the nucleoside analog 9-{[2-hydroxy-1-(hydroxymethyl)ethoxy]methyl}guanine (BW B759U) induces reduced levels of BW B759U triphosphate. *Proc. Natl. Acad. Sci. USA* **83:**8769–8773.
15. **Biron, K. K., S. C. Stanat, J. B. Sorrell, J. A. Fyfe, P. M. Keller, C. U. Lambe, and D. J. Nelson.** 1985. Metabolic activation of the nucleoside analog q-[2-hydroxy-1-(hydroxymethyl)ethoxymethyl] guanine in human diploid fibroblasts infected with human cytomegalovirus. *Proc. Natl. Acad. Sci. USA* **82:**2473–2477.
16. **Boivin, G., S. Chou, M. R. Quirk, A. Erice, and M. C. Jordon.** 1996. Detection of ganciclovir resistance mutations and quantitation of cytomegalovirus (CMV) DNA in leukocytes of patients with fatal disseminated CMV disease. *J. Infect. Dis.* **173:**523–528.
17. **Boucher, C. A. B., E. O'Sullivan, J. W. Mulder, C. Ramautarsing, P. Kellam, G. Darby, J. M. A. Lange, J. Goudsmit, and B. A. Larder.** 1992. Ordered appearance of zidovudine resistance mutations during treatment of 18 human immunodeficiency virus-positive subjects. *J. Infect. Dis.* **165:**105–110.
18. **Boyer, P. L., H.-Q. Gao, and S. H. Hughes.** 1998. A mutation at position 190 of human immunodeficiency virus type 1 reverse transcriptase interacts with mutations at positions 74 and 75 via the template primer. *Antimicrob. Agents Chemother.* **42:**447–452.
19. **Carpenter, C. C. J., M. A. Fischl, S. M. Hammer, M. S. Hirsch, D. M. Jacobsen, D. A. Katzenstein, J. S. G. Montaner, D. D. Richman, M. S. Saag, R. T. Schooley, M. A. Thompson, S. Vella, P. G. Yeni, and P. A. Volberding.** 1997. Antiretroviral therapy for HIV infection in 1997. Updated recommendations of the International AIDS Society-USA panel. *JAMA* **277:**1962–1969.
20. **Centers for Disease Control and Prevention.** 1998. Public Health Service task force recommendations for the use of antiretroviral drugs in pregnant women infected with HIV-1 for maternal health and for reducing perinatal HIV-1 transmission in the United States. *Morbid. Mortal. Weekly Rep.* **47**(No. RR-2)**:**16–17.
21. **Chatis, P. A., and C. S. Crumpacker.** 1992. Resistance of herpesviruses to antiviral drugs. *Antimicrob. Agents Chemother.* **36:**1589–1595.
22. **Chee, M., M. Yang, E. Hubbell, A. Berno, X. C. Huang, D. Stern, J. Winkler, D. J. Lockart, M. S. Morris, and**

S. P. A. Fodor. 1996. Accessing genetic information with high-density DNA arrays. *Science* **274:**610–614.

23. **Chong, K.-T., and P. J. Pagano.** 1997. In vitro combination of PNU-140690, a human immunodeficiency virus type 1 protease inhibitor, with ritonavir against ritonavir-sensitive and -resistant clinical isolates. *Antimicrob. Agents Chemother.* **41:**2367–2373.
24. **Chou, S., A. Erice, M. C. Jordon, G. M. Vercellotti, K. R. Michels, C. L. Talarico, S. C. Stanat, and K. K. Biron.** 1995. Analysis of the UL97 phosphotransferase coding sequence in clinical cytomegalovirus isolates and identification of mutations conferring ganciclovir resistance. *J. Infect. Dis.* **171:**576–583.
25. **Chou, S., S. Guentzel, K. R. Michels, R. C. Miner, and W. L. Drew.** 1995. Frequency of UL97 phosphotransferase mutations related to ganciclovir resistance in clinical cytomegalovirus isolates. *J. Infect. Dis.* **172:**239–242.
26. **Chou, S., G. Marousek, S. Guentzel, S. E. Follansbee, M. E. Poscher, J. P. Lalezari, R. C. Miner, and W. L. Drew.** 1997. Evolution of mutations conferring multidrug resistance during prophylaxis and therapy for cytomegalovirus disease. *J. Infect. Dis.* **176:**786–789.
27. **Chou, T.-C., and P. J. Talay.** 1984. Quantitative analysis of dose effect relationships: the combined effects of multiple drugs of enzyme inhibitors. *Adv. Enzyme Regul.* **22:** 27–55.
28. **Cirelli, R., K. Herne, M. McCrary, P. Lee, and S. K. Tyring.** 1996. Famciclovir: review of clinical efficacy and safety. *Antivir. Res.* **29:**141–151.
29. **Coen, D. M., H. E. Fleming, Jr., L. K. Leslie, and M. J. Retondo.** 1985. Sensitivity of arabinosyladenine-resistant mutants of herpes simplex virus to other antiviral drugs and mapping of drug hypersensitivity mutations to the DNA polymerase locus. *J. Virol.* **53:**477–488.
30. **Coen, D. M., M. Kosz-Vnenchak, J. G. Jacobson, D. A. Leib, C. L. Bogard, P. A. Schaffer, K. L. Tyler, and D. M. Knipe.** 1989. Thymidine kinase-negative herpes simplex virus mutants establish latency in mouse trigeminal ganglia but do not reactivate. *Proc. Natl. Acad. Sci. USA* **86:**4736–4740.
31. **Cole, N. L., and H. H. Balfour, Jr.** 1987. In vitro susceptibility of cytomegalovirus isolates from immunocompromised patients to acyclovir and ganciclovir. *Diagn. Microbiol. Infect. Dis.* **6:**255–261.
32. **Collins, P., G. Appleyard, and N. M. Oliver.** 1982. Sensitivity of herpes virus isolates from acyclovir clinical trials. *Am. J. Med.* **73**(Suppl.)**:**380–382.
33. **Collins, P., B. A. Larder, N. M. Oliver, S. Kemp, I. W. Smith, and G. Darby.** 1989. Characterization of a DNA polymerase mutant of herpes simplex virus from a severely immunocompromised patient receiving acyclovir. *J. Gen. Virol.* **70:**375–382.
34. **Dankner, W. M., D. Scholl, S. C. Stanat, M. Martin, R. L. Sonke, and S. A. Spector.** 1990. Rapid antiviral DNA-DNA hybridization assay for human cytomegalovirus. *J. Virol. Methods* **28:**293–298.
35. **De Clercq, E.** 1982. Comparative efficacy of antiherpes drugs in different cell lines. *Antimicrob. Agents Chemother.* **21:**661–663.
36. **De Clercq, E.** 1995. Antiviral therapy for human immunodeficiency virus infections. *Clin. Microbiol. Rev.* **8:** 200–239.
37. **De Clerq, E.** 1997. In search of a selective antiviral chemotherapy. *Clin. Microbiol. Rev.* **10:**674–693.
38. **Deeks, S. G., M. Smith, M. Holodniy, and J. O. Kahn.** 1997. HIV-1 protease inhibitors. A review for clinicians. *JAMA* **277:**145–153.
39. **Dekker, C., M. N. Ellis, C. McLaren, G. Hunter, J. Rogers, and D. W. Barry.** 1983. Virus resistance in clinical practice. *J. Antimicrob. Chemother.* **12:**137–152.
40. **Deminie, C. A., C. M. Bechtold, D. Stock, M. Alam, F. Djang, A. H. Balch, T.-C. Chou, M. Prichard, R. J. Colonno, and P. F. Lin.** 1996. Evaluation of reverse transcriptase and protease inhibitors in two-drug combinations against human immunodeficiency virus replication. *Antimicrob. Agents Chemother.* **40:**1346–1351.
41. **Drew, W. L., R. C. Miner, D. F. Busch, S. E. Follansbee, J. Gullett, S. G. Mehalko, S. M. Gordon, W. F. Owen, Jr., T. R. Matthews, W. C. Buhles, and B. DeArmond.** 1991. Prevalence of resistance in patients receiving ganciclovir for serious cytomegalovirus infection. *J. Infect. Dis.* **163:**716–719.
42. **Drew, W. L., R. Miner, and E. Saleh.** 1993. Antiviral susceptibility testing of cytomegalovirus: criteria for detecting resistance to antivirals. *Clin. Diagn. Virol.* **1:**179–185.
43. **Earnshaw, D. L., T. H. Bacon, S. J. Darlison, K. Edmonds, R. M. Perkins, and R. A. Vere Hodge.** 1992. Mode of antiviral action of penciclovir in MRC-5 cells infected with herpes simplex virus type 1 (HSV-1), HSV-2, and varicella-zoster virus. *Antimicrob. Agents Chemother.* **36:**2747–2757.
44. **Englund, J. A., M. E. Zimmerman, E. M. Swierkosz, J. L. Goodman, D. R. Scholl, and H. H. Balfour, Jr.** 1990. Herpes simplex virus resistant to acyclovir. A study in a tertiary care center. *Ann. Intern. Med.* **112:**416–422.
45. **Erice, A., S. Chou, K. K. Biron, S. C. Stanat, H. H. Balfour, Jr., and M. C. Jordan.** 1989. Progressive disease due to ganciclovir-resistant cytomegalovirus in immunocompromised patients. *N. Engl. J. Med.* **320:**289–293.
46. **Erice, A., C. Gil-Roda, J.-L. Perez, H. H. Balfour, Jr., K. J. Sannerud, M. N. Hanson, G. Boivin, and S. Chou.** 1997. Antiviral susceptibilities and analysis of UL97 and DNA polymerase sequences of clinical cytomegalovirus isolates from immunocompromised patients. *J. Infect. Dis.* **175:**1087–1092.
47. **Eron, J. J., Y.-K. Chow, A. M. Caliendo, J. Videler, K. M. Devore, T. P. Cooley, H. A. Liebman, J. D. Kaplan, M. S. Hirsch, and R. T. D'Aquila.** 1993. *pol* mutations conferring zidovudine and didanosine resistance with different effects in vitro yield multiply resistant human immunodeficiency virus type 1 in vivo. *Antimicrob. Agents Chemother.* **37:**1480–1487.
48. **Eron, J. J., P. Gorczyca, J. C. Kaplan, and R. T. D'Aquila.** 1992. Susceptibility testing by polymerase chain reaction DNA quantitation: a method to measure drug resistance of human immunodeficiency virus type 1 isolates. *Proc. Natl. Acad. Sci. USA* **89:**3241–3245.
49. **Field, A. K., and K. K. Biron.** 1992. "The end of innocence" revisted: resistance of herpesviruses to antiviral drugs. *Clin. Microbiol. Rev.* **7:**1–13.
50. **Field, H. J., and G. Darby.** 1980. Pathogenicity in mice of strains of herpes simplex virus which are resistant to acyclovir in vitro and in vivo. *Antimicrob. Agents Chemother.* **17:**209–216.
51. **Fillet, A.-M., B. Visse, E. Caumes, B. Dumont, M. Gentillini, and J.-M. Huraux.** 1995. Foscarnet-resistant multidermal zoster in a patient with AIDS. *Clin. Infect. Dis.* **21:** 1348–1349.
52. **Gadler, H.** 1983. Nucleic acid hybridization for measurement of effects of antiviral compounds on human cytomegalovirus DNA replication. *Antimicrob. Agents Chemother.* **24:**370–374.
53. **Gingeras, T. R., P. Prodanovich, T. Latimer, J. C. Guatelli, D. D. Richman, and K. J. Barringer.** 1991. Use of self-sustained sequence replication amplification reaction to analyze and detect mutations in zidovudine-resistant

human immunodeficiency virus. *J. Infect. Dis.* **164:** 1066–1074.
54. **Harmenberg, J., B. Wahren, and B. Oberg.** 1980. Influence of cells and virus multiplicity on the inhibition of herpesviruses with acycloguanosine. *Intervirology* **14:** 239–244.
55. **Hayden, F. G.** 1995. Antiviral agents, p. 411–450. *In* G. L. Mandell, J. E. Bennett, and R. Dolin (ed.), *Mandell, Douglas and Bennett's Principles and Practice of Infectious Disease*, 4th ed. Churchill Livingstone, New York, N.Y.
56. **Hayden, F. G., K. M. Cote, and G. D. Douglas, Jr.** 1980. Plaque inhibition assay for drug susceptibility testing of influenza viruses. *Antimicrob. Agents Chemother.* **17:** 865–870.
57. **Hayden, F. G., S. J. Sperber, R. B. Belshe, R. D. Clover, A. J. Hay, and S. Pyke.** 1991. Recovery of drug-resistant influenza A virus during therapeutic use of rimantadine. *Antimicrob. Agents Chemother.* **35:**1741–1747.
58. **Hertogs, K., M.-P De Bethune, V. Miller, T. Ivens, P. Schel, A. Van Cauwenberge, C. Van Den Eynde, V. Van Gerwen, H. Azijn, M. Van Houtte, F. Peeters, S. Staszewski, M. Conant, S. Bloor, S. Kemp, B. Larder, and R. Pauwels.** 1998. A rapid method for simultaneous detection of phenotypic resistance to inhibitors of protease and reverse transcriptase in recombinant human immunodeficiency virus type 1 isolates from patients treated with antiretroviral drugs. *Antimicrob. Agents Chemother.* **42:** 269–276.
59. **Hill, E. L., M. N. Ellis, and P. Nguyen-Dinh.** 1991. Antiviral and antiparasitic susceptibility testing, p. 1184–1188. *In* A. Balows, W. J. Hausler, Jr., K. L. Herrmann, H. D. Isenberg, and H. J. Shadomy (ed.), *Manual of Clinical Microbiology*, 5th ed. American Society for Microbiology, Washington, D.C.
60. **Hill, E. L., G. A. Hunter, and M. N. Ellis.** 1991. In vitro and in vivo characterization of herpes simplex virus clinical isolates recovered from patients infected with human immunodeficiency virus. *Antimicrob. Agents Chemother.* **35:** 2322–2328.
61. **Hirsch, M. S., J. C. Kaplan, and R. T. D'Aquila.** 1996. Antiviral agents, p. 431–466. *In* B. N. Fields, D. M. Knipe, P. M. Howley, R. M. Chanock, J. L. Melnick, T. P. Monath, B. Roizman, and S. E. Straus (ed.), *Fields Virology*, 3rd ed. Lippincott-Raven, Philadelphia, Pa.
62. **Hodinka, R. L.** 1997. What clinicians need to know about antiviral drugs and viral resistance. *Infect. Dis. Clin. N. Am.* **11:**945–967.
63. **Iversen, A. K., R. W. Shafer, K. Wehrly, M. A. Winters, J. I. Mullins, B. Chesebro, and T. C. Merigan.** 1996. Multidrug-resistant human immunodeficiency virus type 1 strains resulting from combination antiretroviral therapy. *J. Virol.* **70:**1086–1090.
64. **Jacobson, M. A., T. G. Berger, S. Fikrig, P. Cecherer, J. W. Moohr, S. C. Stanat, and K. K. Biron.** 1990. Acyclovir-resistant varicella zoster virus infection after chronic oral acyclovir therapy in patients with the acquired immunodeficiency syndrome (AIDS). *Ann. Intern. Med.* **112:**187–191.
65. **Japour, A. J., D. L. Mayers, V. A. Johnson, D. R. Kuritzkes, L. A. Beckett, J.-M. Arduino, J. Lane, R. J. Black, P. S. Reichelderfer, R. T. D'Aquila, C. S. Crumpacker, the RV-43 Study Group, and the AIDS Clinical Trials Group Virology Committee Resistance Working Group.** 1993. Standarized peripheral blood mononuclear cell culture assay for determination of drug susceptibilities of clinical human immunodeficiency virus type 1 isolates. *Antimicrob. Agents Chemother.* **37:**1095–1101.
66. **Kaye, S., C. Loveday, and R. S. Tedder.** 1992. A microtitre format point mutation assay: application to the detection of drug resistance in human immunodeficiency virus type-1 infected patients treated with zidovudine. *J. Med. Virol.* **37:**241–246.
67. **Kellam, P., C. A. B. Boucher, and B. A. Larder.** 1992. Fifth mutation in human immunodeficiency virus type 1 reverse transcriptase contributes to the development of high-level resistance to zidovudine. *Proc. Natl. Acad. Sci. USA* **89:**1934–1938.
68. **Kellam, P., and B. A. Larder.** 1994. A recombinant virus assay: a rapid, phenotypic assay for assessment of drug susceptibility of human immunodeficiency virus type 1 isolates. *Antimicrob. Agents Chemother.* **38:**23–30.
69. **Kost, R. G., E. L. Hill, M. Tigges, and S. E. Straus.** 1993. Recurrent acyclovir resistant genital herpes in an immunocompetent patient. *N. Engl. J. Med.* **329:** 1777–1782.
70. **Kozal, M. J., N. Shah, N. Shen, R. Yang, R. Fucini, T. C. Merigan, D. D. Richman, D. Morris, E. Hubbell, M. Chee, and T. R. Gingeras.** 1996. Extensive polymorphisms observed in HIV-1 clade B protease gene using high-density oligonucleotide arrays. *Nat. Med.* **7:**753–759.
71. **Kusumi, K., B. Conway, S. Cunningham, A. Berson, C. Evans, A. K. N. Iversen, D. Colvin, M. V. Gallo, S. Coutre, E. G. Shpaer, D. V. Faulkner, A. DeRonde, S. Volkman, C. Williams, M. S. Hirsch, and J. I. Mullins.** 1992. Human immunodeficiency virus type 1 envelope gene structure and diversity in vivo and after cocultivation in vitro. *J. Virol.* **66:**875–885.
72. **Larder, B. A., G. Darby, and D. D. Richman.** 1989. HIV with reduced sensitivity to zidovudine (AZT) isolated during prolonged therapy. *Science* **243:**1731–1734.
73. **Larder, B. A., P. Kellam, and S. D. Kemp.** 1991. Zidovudine resistance predicted by direct detection of mutations in DNA from HIV-infected lymphocytes. *AIDS* **5:** 137–144.
74. **Larder, B. A., and S. D. Kemp.** 1989. Multiple mutations in HIV-1 reverse transcriptase confer high-level resistance to zidovudine (AZT). *Science* **246:**1155–1158.
75. **Larder, B. A., A. Kohli, P. Kellam, S. D. Kemp, M. Kronick, and R. D. Henfrey.** 1993. Quantitative detection of HIV-1 drug resistance mutations by automated DNA sequencing. *Nature* **365:**671–673.
76. **Lehrman, S. N., J. M. Douglas, L. Corey, and D. W. Barry.** 1986. Recurrent genital herpes and suppressive oral acyclovir therapy. Relation between clinical outcome and in-vitro drug sensitivity. *Ann. Intern. Med.* **104:**786–790.
77. **Linnemann, C. C., Jr., K. K. Biron, W. G. Hoppenjans, and A. M. Solinger.** 1990. Emergence of acyclovir-resistant varicella-zoster virus in an AIDS patient on prolonged acyclovir therapy. *AIDS* **4:**577–579.
78. **Lipson, S. M., M. Soni, F. X. Biondo, D. H. Shepp, M. H. Kaplan, and T. Sun.** 1997. Antiviral susceptibility testing-flow cytometric analysis (AST-FCA) for the detection of cytomegalovirus drug resistance. *Diagn. Microbiol. Infect. Dis.* **28:**123–129.
79. **Littler, E., A. D. Stuart, and M. S. Chee.** 1992. Human cytomegalovirus UL97 open reading frame encodes a protein that phosphorylates the antiviral nucleoside analogue ganciclovir. *Nature* **358:**160–162.
80. **Luciw, P. A.** 1996. Human immunodeficiency viruses and their replication, p. 1881–1952. *In* B. N. Fields, D. M. Knipe, P. M. Howley, R. M. Chanock, J. L. Melnick, T. P. Monath, B. Roizman, and S. E. Straus (ed.), *Fields Virology*, 3rd ed. Lippincott-Raven, Philadelphia, Pa.
81. **Marschner, I. C., A. C. Collier, R. W. Combs, R. T. D'Aquila, V. DeGruttola, M. A. Fischl, S. M. Hammer, M. D. Hughes, V. A. Johnson, D. A. Katzenstein, D. D. Richman, L. M. Smeaton, S. A. Spector, and M. S. Saag.** 1998. Uses of changes in plasma levels of human immuno

deficiency virus type 1 RNA to assess the clinical benefit of antiretroviral therapy. *J. Infect. Dis.* **177:**40–47.

82. **Martin, J. L., M. N. Ellis, P. M. Keller, K. K. Biron, S. N. Lehrman, D. W. Barry, and P. A. Furman.** 1985. Plaque autoradiography assay for the detection and quantitation of thymidine kinase-deficient and thymidine kinase-altered mutants of herpes simplex virus in clinical isolates. *Antimicrob. Agents Chemother.* **28:**181–187.
83. **McDonald, C. K., and D. R. Kuritzkes.** 1997. Human immunodeficiency virus type 1 protease inhibitors. *Arch. Intern. Med.* **157:**951–959.
84. **McLaren, C., M. N. Ellis, and G. A. Hunter.** 1983. A colorimetric assay for the measurement of the sensitivity of herpes simplex viruses to antiviral agents. *Antivir. Res.* **3:**223–224.
85. **McSharry, J. M., N. S. Lurain, G. L. Drusano, A. Landay, J. Manischewitz, M. Nokta, M. O'Gorman, H. M. Shapiro, A. Weinberg, P. Reichelderfer, and C. Crumpacker.** 1998. Flow cytometric determination of ganciclovir susceptibilities of human cytomegalovirus clinical isolates. *J. Clin. Microbiol.* **36:**958–964.
86. **Pahwa, S., K. Biron, W. Lim, P. Swenson, M. H. Kaplan, N. Sadick, and R. Pahwa.** 1988. Continuous varicella-zoster infection associated with acyclovir resistance in a child with AIDS. *JAMA* **260:**2879–2882.
87. **Pavic, I., A. Hartmann, A. Zimmermann, D. Michel, W. Hampl, I. Schleyer, and T. Mertens.** 1997. Flow cytometric analysis of herpes simplex virus type 1 suceptibility to acyclovir, ganciclovir, and foscarnet. *Antimicrob. Agents Chemother.* **41:**2686–2692.
88. **Pepin, J.-M., F. Simon, M. C. Dazza, and F. Brun-Vezinet.** 1992. The clinical significance of in vitro cytomegalovirus susceptibility to antiviral drugs. *Res. Virol.* **143:** 126–128.
89. **Persing, D. H., D. A. Relman, and F. C. Tenover.** 1996. Genotypic detection of antimicrobial resistance, p. 43–47. *In* D. H. Persing (ed.), *PCR Protocols for Emerging Infectious Diseases*. American Society for Microbiology, Washington, D.C.
90. **Prichard, M. N., L. E. Prichard, and C. Shipman, Jr.** 1993. Strategic design and three-dimensional analysis of antiviral drug combinations. *Antimicrob. Agents Chemother.* **37:**540–545.
91. **Rabalaiss, G. P., M. J. Levin, and F. E. Berkowitz.** 1987. Rapid herpes simplex virus susceptibility testing using an enzyme-linked immunosorbent assay performed in situ on fixed virus-infected monolayers. *Antimicrob. Agents Chemother.* **31:**946–948.
92. **Reardon, J. E., and T. Spector.** 1989. Herpes simplex virus type 1 DNA polymerase. Mechanism of inhibition by acyclovir triphosphate. *J. Biol. Chem.* **264:**7405–7411.
93. **Richman, D. D.** 1995. Clinical significance of drug resistance in human immunodeficiency virus. *Clin. Infect. Dis.* **21**(Suppl. 2)**:**S166–S169.
94. **Richman, D. D., and S. A. Bozzette.** 1994. The impact of the syncytium-inducing phenotype of human immunodeficiency virus on disease progression. *J. Infect. Dis.* **169:** 968–974.
95. **Richman, D. D., J. C. Guatelli, J. Grimes, A. Tsiatis, and T. R. Gingeras.** 1991. Detection of mutations associated with zidovudine resistance in human immunodeficiency virus utilizing the polymerase chain reaction. *J. Infect. Dis.* **164:**1075–1081.
96. **Safrin, S., T. Assaykeen, S. Follansbee, and J. Mills.** 1990. Foscarnet therapy for acyclovir-resistant mucocutaneous herpes simplex virus infection in 26 AIDS patients: preliminary data. *J. Infect. Dis.* **161:**1078–1084.
97. **Safrin, S., T. G. Berger, I. Gilson, P. R. Wolfe, C. B. Wofsy, J. Mills, and K. K. Biron.** 1991. Foscarnet therapy in five patients with AIDS and acyclovir-resistant varicella-zoster virus infection. *Ann. Intern. Med.* **115:**19–21.
98. **Safrin, S., C. Crumpacker, P. Chatis, R. Davis, R. Hafner, J. Rush, H. A. Kessler, B. Landry, J. Mills, and the AIDS Clinical Trials Group.** 1991. A controlled trial comparing foscarnet with vidarabine for acyclovir-resistant mucocutaneous herpes simplex in the acquired immunodeficiency syndrome. *N. Engl. J. Med.* **325:** 551–555.
99. **Safrin, S., E. Palacios, and B. J. Leahy.** 1996. Comparative evaluation of microplate enzyme-linked immunosorbent assay versus plaque reduction assay for antiviral susceptibility testing of herpes simples virus isolates. *Antimicrob. Agents Chemother.* **40:**1017–1019.
100. **Safrin, S., and L. Phan.** 1993. In vitro activity of penciclovir against clinical isolates of acyclovir-resistant and foscarnet-resistant herpes simples virus. *Antimicrob. Agents Chemother.* **37:**2241–2243.
101. **Schinazi, R. F., B. A. Larder, and J. W. Mellors.** 1997. Mutations in HIV-1 reverse transcriptase and protease associated with drug resistance. *Int. Antivir. News* **5:** 129–134.
102. **Shafer, R. W., M. A. Winters, D. L. Mayers, A. J. Japour, D. R. Kuritzkes, O. S. Weislow, F. White, A. Erice, K. J. Sannerud, A. Iversen, F. Pena, D. Dimitrov, L. M. Frenkel, and P. S. Reichelderfer for the AIDS Clinical Trials Group Virology Committee Drug Resistance Working Group.** 1996. Interlaboratory comparison of sequence-specific PCR and ligase detection reaction to detect a human immunodeficiency virus type 1 drug resistance mutation. *J. Clin. Microbiol.* **34:** 1849–1853.
103. **Shi, C., and J. W. Mellors.** 1997. A recombinant retroviral system for rapid in vivo analysis of human immunodeficiency virus type 1 susceptibility to reverse transcriptase inhibitors. *Antimicrob. Agents Chemother.* **41:** 2781–2785.
104. **Sibrack, C. D., L. T. Gutman, C. M. Wilfert, C. McLaren, M. H. St. Clair, P. M. Keller, and D. W. Barry.** 1982. Pathogenicity of acyclovir-resistant herpes simplex virus type 1 from an immunodeficient child. *J. Infect. Dis.* **146:**673–682.
105. **Smith, I. L., J. M. Cherrington, R. E. Jiles, M. D. Fuller, W. R. Freeman, and S. A. Spector.** 1997. High-level resistance of cytomegalovirus to ganciclovir is associated with alterations in both the UL97 and DNA polymerase genes. *J. Infect. Dis.* **176:**69–77.
106. **Snoeck, R., G. Andrei, M. Gerard, A. Silverman, A. Hedderman, J. Balzarini, C. Sadzot-Delvaux, G. Tricot, N. Clumeck, and E. De Clercq.** 1994. Successful treatment of progressive mucocutaneous infection due to acyclovir- and foscarnet-resistant herpes simples virus with (S)-1-(3-hydroxy-2-phosphonylmethoxypropyl)cytosine (HPMPC). *Clin. Infect. Dis.* **18:**570–580.
107. **Spector, S. A., K. Hsia, D. Wolf, M. Shinkai, and I. Smith.** 1995. Molecular detection of human cytomegalovirus and determination of genotypic ganciclovir resistance in clinical specimens. *Clin. Infect. Dis.* **21**(Suppl. 2)**:**S170–S173.
108. **Stanat, S. C., J. E. Reardon, A. Erice, M. C. Jordan, W. L. Drew, and K. K. Biron.** 1991. Ganciclovir-resistant cytomegalovirus clinical isolates: mode of resistance to ganciclovir. *Antimicrob. Agents Chemother.* **35:**2191–2197.
109. **Standring-Cox, R., T. H. Bacon, and B. A. Howard.** 1996. Comparison of a DNA probe assay with the plaque reduction assay for measuring the sensitivity of herpes simplex virus and varicella-zoster virus to penciclovir and acyclovir. *J. Virol. Methods* **56:**3–11.

110. **St. Clair, M. H., P. M. Hartigan, J. C. Andrews, C. L. Vavro, M. S. Simberkoff, J. D. Hamilton, and the VA Cooperative Study Group.** 1993. Zidovudine resistance, syncytium-inducing phenotype, and HIV disease progression in a case-control study. *J. Acquired Immune Defic. Syndr.* **6:**891–897.

111. **St. Clair, M. H., J. L. Martin, G. Tudor-Williams, M. C. Bach, C. L. Vavro, D. M. King, P. Kellam, S. D. Kemp, and B. A. Larder.** 1991. Resistance to ddI and sensitivity to AZT induced by a mutation in HIV-1 reverse transcriptase. *Science* **253:**1557–1559.

112. **Stuyver, L., A Wyseur, A. Rombout, J. Louwagie, T. Scarcez, C. Verhofstede, D. Rimland, R. F. Schinazi, and R. Rossau.** 1997. Line probe assay for rapid detection of drug-selected mutations in the human immunodeficiency virus type 1 reverse transcriptase gene. *Antimicrob. Agents Chemother.* **41:**284–291.

113. **Swierkosz, E. M., and K. K. Biron.** 1994. Antiviral susceptibility testing, p. 8.26.2–8.26.21. *In* H. D. Isenberg (ed.), *Clinical Microbiology Procedures Manual*, Suppl. 1. American Society for Microbiology, Washington, D.C.

114. **Swierkosz, E. M., and K. K. Biron.** 1995. Antiviral susceptibility testing, p. 139–154. *In* E. H. Lennette, D. A. Lennette, and E. T. Lennette (ed.), *Diagnostic Procedures for Viral, Rickettsial and Chlamydial Infections*, 7th ed. American Public Health Association, Washington, D.C.

115. **Swierkosz, E. M., D. R. Scholl, J. L. Brown, J. D. Jollick, and C. A. Gleaves.** 1987. Improved DNA hybridization method for detection of acyclovir-resistant herpes simplex virus. *Antimicrob. Agents Chemother.* **31:**1465–1469.

116. **Talarico, C. L., W. C. Phelps, and K. K. Biron.** 1993. Analysis of the thymidine kinase genes from acyclovir-resistant mutants of varicella-zoster virus isolated from patients with AIDS. *J. Virol.* **67:**1024–1033.

117. **Tebas, P., D. Scholl, J. Jollick, K. McHarg, M. Arens, and P. D. Olivo.** 1998. A rapid assay to screen for drug-resistant herpes simplex virus. *J. Infect. Dis.* **177:**217–220.

118. **Tebas, P., E. C. Stabel, and P. D. Olivo.** 1995. Antiviral susceptibility testing with a cell line which expresses β-galactosidase after infection with herpes simplex virus. *Antimicrob. Agents Chemother.* **39:**1287–1291.

119. **Wade, J. C., C. McClaren, and J. D. Meyers.** 1983. Frequency and significance of acyclovir resistant herpes simplex virus isolated from marrow transplant patients receiving multiple courses of treatment with acyclovir. *J. Infect. Dis.* **148:**1077–1082.

120. **Wittrock, R., R. T. Sarisky, R. L. Hodinka, M. Levin, A. Weinberg, and J. J. Leary.** Comparative susceptibility of herpes simplex virus strains to antiviral drugs in a variety of human cell lines. Submitted for publication.

121. **Wolf, D. G., I. L. Smith, D. J. Lee, W. R. Freeman, M. Flores-Aguilar, and S. A. Spector.** 1995. Mutations in human cytomegalovirus UL97 gene confer clinical resistance to ganciclovir and can be detected directly in patient plasma. *J. Clin. Invest.* **95:**257–263.

Antifungal Agents and Susceptibility Tests

ANA ESPINEL-INGROFF, THEODORE WHITE, AND MICHAEL A. PFALLER

126

An increased incidence of fungal infections has been documented since the 1980s. The introduction of modern patient management technologies and therapies, such as bone marrow or solid-organ transplants, new and more effective chemotherapeutic agents, and the more aggressive use of chemotherapy, has resulted in a rapidly expanding number of patients with chemically induced immunosuppression. These patient populations now survive longer and become highly susceptible to life-threatening fungal infections (63). Fungi are also emerging as important nosocomial pathogens causing severe morbidity and mortality in hospitalized patients. In addition to immunosuppression, other risk factors, common in many hospitalized patients, have been associated with the emergence of nosocomial infections, e.g., malnutrition, extensive burns, indwelling catheters, hemodialysis, extreme age, and a combination of any of these risk factors with immunosuppression (23, 37, 60). Furthermore, the AIDS pandemic has expanded the number of patients at risk for severe mycoses, e.g., oropharyngeal candidiasis and cryptococcal meningitis. A higher frequency (overall, 46%) of systemic infections caused by less virulent *Candida* species other than *Candida albicans* (1, 19) also has been reported.

Paralleling the increase in the incidence of opportunistic fungal infections over the last decade has been the introduction of new antifungal agents with systemic activities. Although more extensive research in the development of antifungal drugs has been conducted lately, only nine antifungal agents are currently licensed for use against systemic fungal infections. These nine systemic antifungal agents include the polyene amphotericin B (E. R. Squibb & Sons, Princeton, N.J.) and its three lipid formulations, the imidazoles miconazole and ketoconazole (Janssen Pharmaceutica, Piscataway, N.J.), the triazoles fluconazole (Pfizer Pharmaceuticals, New York, N.Y.) and itraconazole (Janssen Pharmaceutica), and the pyrimidine synthesis inhibitor flucytosine (5-FC; Hoffmann-La Roche Inc., Nutley, N.J.) (Table 1). As fungal infections became an important public health problem and resistance to established antifungal agents began to emerge (6, 10, 25, 46, 49), pharmaceutical companies recognized the need to develop new agents with either a broader spectrum or different targets of activity. Several investigational agents, such as new triazoles and chitin and glucan synthesis inhibitors, are at different stages of clinical evaluation for Food and Drug Administration (FDA) approval and are described below (Table 1).

SYSTEMIC ANTIFUNGAL AGENTS

Polyenes

Conventional amphotericin B (1956) and its lipid formulations are polyene macrolide antibiotics used primarily in the treatment of systemic and life-threatening fungal infections. The polyene antifungal agents act by binding to ergosterol in the fungal cell membrane, causing osmotic instability and loss of membrane integrity. The direct membrane toxicity is due in part to oxidative damage and is frequently fungicidal (53). This effect extends to mammalian cells, in which the drug binds to cholesterol, creating the high toxicity associated with conventional polyene agents. Amphotericin B has been used for many years in the treatment of mycotic diseases. It is unstable when subjected to heat, light, or acid pH. Although resistance to amphotericin B is rare, changes in membrane sterols have been correlated with the development of resistance both in vitro and in vivo (6, 25). Such resistance has assumed clinical importance, particularly with certain species, such as *Candida lusitaniae* (25).

Lipid formulations of amphotericin B were designed to increase its efficacy and to reduce its toxicity in patients with deep-seated fungal infections refractory to conventional therapy (31, 57, 58), such as hepatosplenic candidiasis and invasive pulmonary aspergillosis. These preparations have selective toxicity for fungal cells and theoretically promote the delivery of the drug to the site of infection while avoiding the toxicity of supramaximal doses of amphotericin B. Clinical trials have evaluated the utility of three lipid formulations: an amphotericin B lipid complex (Liposome Company, Princeton, N.J.), an amphotericin B colloidal dispersion (Sequus Pharmaceuticals, Menlo Park, Calif.), and a liposomal form of amphotericin B (Nexstar, San Dimas, Calif.). However, despite evidence of nephrotoxicity reduction, a significant improvement in efficacy has not been clearly demonstrated. The most cost-effective clinical role of these agents as first-line therapies must be further studied in controlled, randomized clinical trials. These three formulations of amphotericin B have been approved for treatment of invasive fungal infections in patients for whom conventional antifungal therapy has failed.

Azoles

Licensed Agents

The azoles were introduced in the late 1960s as a group of antifungal therapeutic agents, but only four azoles have been

TABLE 1 Antifungal agents with systemic activity

Antifungal agent	Mechanism of action	Route[a]	Comments
Polyenes			
Amphotericin B	Binds to ergosterol, causing direct oxidative membrane damage	i.v.	Established agent; broad spectrum; toxic
Lipid formulations (amphotericin B lipid complex or colloidal dispersion, liposomal form of amphotericin B)	Same as amphotericin B	i.v.	Recently licensed agents with broad-spectrum activity and decreased toxicity; used for refractory severe infections not responding to conventional therapy
Imidazoles			
Miconazole	Inhibition of membrane cytochrome P-450-dependent enzymes	i.v.	Toxic agent with modest anticandidal activity; active against *P. boydii*
Ketoconazole	Same as miconazole	Oral, topical	Modest broad-spectrum activity
Triazoles			
Itraconazole	Same as miconazole but more specific binding	Oral, i.v., topical	Broad-spectrum activity; poor absorption is a problem
Fluconazole	Same as miconazole but more specific binding	Oral, i.v.	Limited spectrum; good central nervous system penetration; good in vivo activity; resistance is a problem
Voriconazole, SCH 56592, BMS 207147	Same as the other triazoles	Oral, i.v.	Investigational agents with broad-spectrum activity against species resistant to established agents; used for treatment of aspergillosis
Glucan synthesis inhibitors			
LY 303366 MK-0991	Inhibition of fungal cell wall glucan synthase	Oral, i.v.	Investigational agents with broad-spectrum in vitro activity, except against *C. neoformans* and *T. beigelii*; used for treatment of aspergillosis
Chitin synthesis inhibitor (nikkomycin Z)	Inhibition of fungal cell wall chitin synthase	i.v.	Investigational agent; used for treatment of coccidioidomycosis
Pyrimidine synthesis inhibitor (5-FC)	Inhibition of DNA and RNA syntheses	Oral	Toxicity and resistance are problems; used in combination with amphotericin B

[a] i.v., intravenous.

approved for the treatment of systemic fungal diseases: miconazole, ketoconazole, fluconazole, and itraconazole (Table 1). These four agents have fungistatic activity against a variety of fungi. The azoles inhibit fungal cytochrome P-450-dependent enzymes, with resulting impairment of ergosterol synthesis and depletion of ergosterol in the fungal cell membrane. Although resistance to azoles has been demonstrated for *Candida* spp., the detection of azole resistance in vitro has been variable and method dependent. Clinical correlations with standardized in vitro susceptibility test (34) results for fluconazole and itraconazole have begun to emerge for oropharyngeal candidiasis (34, 47).

Miconazole (1970) was the first azole derivative to be administered intravenously for the therapy of systemic fungal infections. However, owing to its toxicity and high relapse rates, its use has been limited to certain cases of pseudallescherosis, rare refractory cryptococcal meningitis, and coccidioidal meningitis in children (27). Ketoconazole (1977) is an orally absorbed antifungal agent. It requires a normal intragastric pH for absorption and penetrates poorly into the cerebrospinal fluid (27). Until the introduction of itraconazole, ketoconazole was the established alternative to amphotericin B for the treatment of immunocompetent individuals with non-life-threatening, non-central nervous system, localized or disseminated histoplasmosis, blastomycosis, mucocutaneous candidiasis, paracoccidioidomycosis, and selected forms of coccidioidomycosis (27).

In the 1990s, itraconazole and fluconazole were approved as orally active systemic triazole agents with less potential for toxicity than the imidazoles (27) because of their more specific binding to fungal cell cytochromes than to mammalian cell cytochromes. Fluconazole is a relatively small molecule that is partially water soluble, is easily absorbed, has a prolonged half-life (up to 25 h in humans), is minimally protein bound, is excreted largely as an active drug in the urine, and penetrates well into the cerebrospinal fluid (3). Fluconazole has an important role in the maintenance therapy of cryptococcal meningitis in patients with AIDS as well as in the treatment of fungal diseases caused by *Candida* spp. (except for *Candida krusei*) and *Coccidioides immitis* (especially meningitis).

Itraconazole is a lipophilic compound characterized by good oral absorption, extensive distribution in tissues, and a long half-life in serum. Itraconazole is very insoluble in aqueous fluids and is highly protein bound (>90%). This drug binds strongly to plasma proteins and penetrates poorly into cerebrospinal fluid and urine but well into skin and soft tissues. Itraconazole appears to be more active in vitro and in vivo than ketoconazole and fluconazole. It has supplanted ketoconazole as first-line therapy for endemic, non-life-threatening mycoses caused by *Blastomyces dermatitidis*, *C. immitis*, and *Histoplasma capsulatum* as well as *Sporothrix schenckii* (7, 27). Itraconazole also has been used successfully in the management of infections caused by *Aspergillus* spp. (5, 27). Itraconazole oral (marketed) and intravenous solutions are currently under evaluation in clinical trials. The efficacy of fluconazole and itraconazole given after initial amphotericin B or in combination with other agents has been evaluated in several clinical trials (27, 28).

New Triazoles

Three new triazoles are under clinical evaluation: voriconazole (Pfizer Central Research, Sandwich, United Kingdom), SCH 56592 (Schering-Plough Research Institute, Kenilworth, N.J.), and BMS 207147 (Bristol-Myers Squibb, Wallingford, Conn.). In contrast to fluconazole but like itraconazole, voriconazole and SCH 56592 are not water soluble; they have demonstrated a broad spectrum of in vitro and in vivo activities against a variety of yeasts and molds (11, 12, 21, 22, 33, 35). However, high MICs for *Fusarium* spp. (11, 12, 21), *Rhizopus arrhizus*, *S. schenckii* (11, 21), *Sporobolomyces salmonicolor*, and *Rhodotorula rubra* (11) have been reported with these agents. In vitro fungicidal activity (minimal fungicidal concentration endpoints of 0.2 to 4 μg/ml) has been observed with SCH 56592 against species of *Aspergillus*, *Bipolaris*, and *Exserohilum*, *H. capsulatum*, and *S. schenckii* (12).

Pyrimidine Synthesis Inhibitor

5-FC is a water-soluble, stable, fungistatic compound used orally in the treatment of systemic infections caused by susceptible pathogenic or opportunistic yeasts and other fungi. The major therapeutic role of 5-FC is in combination with amphotericin B for the treatment of cryptococcal meningitis, for which synergistic antifungal activity has been observed. 5-FC acts as a competitive antimetabolite for uracil in the synthesis of yeast RNA and interferes with thymidylate synthetase (45). Five enzymes are involved in the mode of action of 5-FC. The first step is initiated by the uptake of the drug by a membrane-bound permease. Inside the cell the drug is deaminated to 5-fluorouracil, which is the main active form of the drug. These activities can be antagonized in vitro by a variety of purine and pyrimidine bases and nucleosides (45). Because of this antagonism, the antifungal activity of 5-FC can be demonstrated in vitro only in synthetic media free of substances such as cytosine, uracil, and other pyrimidines and purines. At least two metabolic sites are responsible for resistance to 5-FC (45); one involves the enzyme cytosine permease, which is responsible for the uptake of 5-FC into fungal cells, and the other involves the enzyme cytosine deaminase, which is responsible for the deamination of 5-FC to 5-fluorouracil, the metabolically active form of the drug.

Glucan Synthesis Inhibitors

Another target of antifungal activity has been the inhibition of the fungal cell wall glucan synthase. This approach increases the degree of selectivity for fungal cells, because human cells lack a homologous enzyme. The echinocandin LY 303366 (Eli Lilly & Company, Indianapolis, Ind.) and the related pneumocandin MK-0991 (L-743,872; Merck Research Laboratories, Rahway, N.J.) are inhibitors of 1,3-β-D-glucan synthesis; this inhibition leads to the lysis of growing fungal cells. MK-0991 is water soluble, while LY 303366 lacks water solubility. As with the new triazoles, the aim of this new class of antifungal agents is to target fungi that are resistant to established drugs. Both MK-0991 and LY 303366 have demonstrated in vitro and in vivo activities against a variety of yeasts (including fluconazole- and itraconazole-resistant isolates) and molds (12, 24, 30, 43). However, they are not active against *Cryptococcus neoformans* and *Trichosporon beigelii* (MICs, >16 μg/ml) (12, 30), and their MICs are higher than those of the new azoles for *Phialophora* spp., *R. arrhizus* (12), *B. dermatitidis*, *H. capsulatum* (11, 12), and *Cladophialophora bantiana* (12). These agents have fungicidal activity for some species of yeasts. MK-0991 and LY 303366 have entered clinical trials (phases I and II).

Chitin Synthesis Inhibitor

The nikkomycin class of antifungal agents exploits a different target of antifungal activity, the inhibition of chitin synthase in the fungal cell wall. Nikkomycin Z (Shaman Pharmaceutica, San Francisco, Calif.) has demonstrated in vitro activity against *Candida* spp. and has been effective in the treatment of experimental blastomycosis, histoplasmosis, and coccidioidal infections (26, 28). Phase I toxicity studies have been conducted, and phase II clinical trials have been designed for the treatment of human coccidioidomycosis.

MECHANISMS OF ANTIFUNGAL DRUG RESISTANCE

In contrast to the mechanisms of resistance to antibacterial agents, the mechanisms of resistance to antifungal agents are poorly understood. The present discussion will focus on azole drugs, especially fluconazole, and resistant strains of *C. albicans*. More detailed descriptions of the mechanisms of antifungal drug resistance and discussions of antifungal drug resistance in other yeasts can be found in recent reviews (49, 61, 62).

Cellular Mechanisms of Resistance

The most common cause of refractory fungal infections is the presence of a fungal strain for which a drug MIC is higher than average. This situation is usually the result of (i) the replacement of susceptible *C. albicans* with a resistant species such as *C. krusei* or *C. glabrata* (*Torulopsis glabrata*); (ii) the replacement of a susceptible *C. albicans* strain with a more resistant strain; (iii) genetic alterations that render a strain more resistant; (iv) transient gene expression that allows the cells to withstand the drug treatment; or (v) variation in MICs for individual colonies from the same strain from a single patient, which may reflect genomic instability within the strain (62).

Molecular Mechanisms of Azole Resistance

The recently identified molecular mechanisms that contribute to the resistance of strains and species of *Candida* include the following.

Modifications of the Ergosterol Biosynthetic Pathway

The target enzyme of the azole drugs is lanosterol 14α demethylase, a cytochrome P-450 enzyme-dependent encoded by the *C. albicans ERG11* (*ERG16*) gene, a component of the ergosterol biosynthetic pathway (62). Mutations in *ERG11* as well as biochemical alterations in three other genes in the pathway (*ERG1*, *ERG2*, and *ERG3*) have been correlated with azole resistance (62).

Molecular Alterations of the *ERG11* Gene

Several genetic alterations have been associated with the *ERG11* gene of *C. albicans*; these include point mutations in the coding region, overexpression of the gene, gene amplification (which leads to overexpression), and gene conversion or mitotic recombination, which creates two copies of the resistant allele in diploid *C. albicans* (61, 62).

Decreased Accumulation of Drug

With radioactively labeled drugs such as fluconazole, recent studies have demonstrated that resistant cells frequently accumulate less drug than matched susceptible cells and that this accumulation is energy dependent (62). It is most likely that the reduced accumulation of labeled drug is the result of increased activity of efflux pumps.

Two Major Types of Efflux Pump

In eukaryotic cells, two types of efflux pump contribute to drug resistance: ATP binding cassette transporters (ABC transporters) and major facilitators (61, 62). Both types of pump are known to cause drug resistance in other systems. The ABC transporters are frequently associated with the active efflux of molecules that are toxic for cells and that are relatively hydrophobic or lipophilic, as is the case with most azole drugs. These transporters use ATP as an energy source to transport molecules out of cells. To date, 13 ABC transporters have been described for *C. albicans* (62). These include 10 transporters encoded by *CDR* genes (*Candida* drug resistance genes), all of which are members of a specific ABC transporter subfamily that is associated with drug resistance in other systems. Increased expression of *CDR1* and *CDR2* appears to be the most common cause of azole resistance in *C. albicans* (61, 62).

The major facilitators, which have been described for bacteria and lower eukaryotes, also recognize relatively hydrophobic molecules, such as tetracycline, as substrates for extrusion. The major facilitators use the proton motive force of the membrane (gradient of H^+ across the membrane) as a source of energy. To date, the only major facilitator gene that has been cloned from medically important fungi is the *MDR1* gene from *C. albicans* (62). The *MDR1* gene has been shown to be overexpressed in a few fluconazole-resistant isolates (62).

Genetic and molecular analyses have determined that the *CDR* pumps will act on all of the commonly used azole drugs, while the *MDR1* pump appears to be specific for fluconazole (61, 62). These findings have profound clinical implications, as fluconazole-resistant strains expressing an *MDR1* pump should be susceptible to other azoles, while fluconazole-resistant strains expressing a *CDR* pump should be resistant to other azoles.

Summary of *Candida* Mechanisms of Resistance to Azoles

In a susceptible cell, azoles enter the cell by an unknown mechanism and interact with the target enzyme encoded by *ERG11*. Low-level expression of the *CDR* genes and the *MDR1* gene is frequently observed. In a resistant cell, azoles enter the cell by the same mechanism but can be blocked from interacting normally with the *ERG11*-encoded target enzyme because of mutation and/or overexpression. Mutations in genes encoding other enzymes in the pathway (such as *ERG3*) can also contribute to resistance. Both ABC transporters, such as those encoded by the *CDR* genes, and major facilitators, such as that encoded by the *MDR1* gene, can be overexpressed. These diverse mechanisms are not mutually exclusive, as several mechanisms have been identified in a single resistant strain, each mechanism contributing to the resistance phenotype.

Clinical Factors That Contribute to Resistance

Many factors, both fungus specific and host specific, can contribute to an infection that is refractory to azole treatment. Host factors that can alter the success of therapy include patient factors, such as immune status, the site and severity of infection, and the patient's compliance in taking the antifungal drug. Drug factors, such as the fungistatic nature of the drug, dosing and cumulative dose, pharmacokinetics, and drug-drug interactions, can also affect the success of treatment. All of these factors have an effect on treatment whether the infecting strain is susceptible or resistant to azole drugs.

Clinical Significance

The mechanisms described above have several profound implications for the prevention and treatment of antifungal drug resistance. (i) In treatment with fluconazole, the drug dose and the dosing schedule will have profound effects on selection for a resistant species or strain. (ii) The existence of multiple mechanisms by which resistance can develop precludes a simple or quick molecular test for resistance that is based on a single mechanism. (iii) The most common fluconazole resistance mechanisms are associated with increased resistance to other azoles. Therefore, it may be more useful to treat fluconazole-resistant strains with a polyene, such as amphotericin B, than to treat them with other azoles. (iv) The characterization of the molecular mechanisms of azole resistance will assist in the development of new or improved agents that are active against all strains of fungi, including azole-resistant strains.

ANTIFUNGAL SUSCEPTIBILITY TESTING

Rationale

In vitro antifungal susceptibility tests are similar in design to tests with antibacterial agents and are performed for the same reasons. Ideally, in vitro susceptibility tests (i) provide a reliable measure of the relative activities of two or more antifungal agents, (ii) correlate with in vivo activity and predict the likely outcome of therapy, (iii) provide a means with which to monitor the development of resistance among a normally susceptible population of organisms, and (iv) predict the therapeutic potential of newly discovered investigational agents (9, 10, 44). The development of National Committee for Clinical Laboratory Standards (NCCLS) reference method M27-A (34) in the 1990s has improved the reproducibility of in vitro antifungal susceptibility test data and facilitated the establishment of interpretive breakpoints for the triazoles fluconazole and itraconazole (34, 47). Based on historical data and the pharmacokinetics of 5-FC, interpretive breakpoints for 5-FC and *Candida* spp. also have been established (34). In the late 1980s, some correlation was suggested between amphotericin B MIC results obtained by nonstandardized methods and clinical outcome (46). Unfortunately, most M27-A amphotericin B MICs for yeasts are within a very narrow range (0.25 to 1 μg/ml) (34), precluding clear discrimination between susceptible and potentially resistant isolates. Also, since the clinical failure of amphotericin B therapy for candidiasis is more likely caused by host factors (44) than by antifungal resistance, very few resistant strains and corresponding clinical data are available for the evaluation of an optimal procedure for the detection of amphotericin B resistance. Although recent evaluations have suggested that antibiotic medium 3 supplemented with 2% glucose provides reliable detection of resistant isolates, lot-to-lot variability has been documented (32), and this method is still under investigation.

With the use of both established and investigational agents has come the recognition of resistance to one or more antifungal agents in selected isolates (6, 10, 25, 46, 49). As a result, clinical laboratories are now being asked to assume a greater role in the selection and monitoring of antifungal chemotherapy. The methods that have been applied to antifungal susceptibility testing include broth dilution (macro- and microdilution), agar dilution, and disk diffusion (Table 2). The NCCLS Subcommittee on Antifungal Susceptibility Testing has developed a reference method for broth susceptibility testing of yeast cells that provides standardized guidelines for the performance of both macrodilution and microdilution formats (34). This reference method was the result of a series of collaborative studies (16, 20, 38, 40, 48) that focused on the testing variables listed in Table 3. Currently, two commercial antifungal susceptibility tests are available for investigational purposes and are undergoing clinical evaluation for FDA approval in the United States: the colorimetric microdilution test (Accumed International Inc., West Lake, Ohio) and the E-test agar diffusion antifungal strip (AB Biodisk, Solna, Sweden) (Table 2).

TABLE 2 Methods used for antifungal susceptibility testing

Test method	Means of endpoint determination
Broth macro- and microdilution (yeasts)	Visual comparison of turbidity with turbidity of 80% inhibition standard (1:5 growth control dilution) for macrodilution; visual comparison of growth (~50% inhibition) with that of growth control for microdilution; ATP photometry, turbidimetry, colorimetry, radiometry, dry weight
Colorimetric microdilution (yeasts)	Visual observation of color change
Spectrophotometric microdilution (yeasts)	Turbidimetric MIC determination with spectrophotometer
Macro- and microdilution (filamentous fungi)	Visual comparison of growth (~50% inhibition) with that of growth control
Agar macrodilution (standard dishes)	Visual
Agar diffusion	
Disks	Zone diameter (visual)
Antifungal strips (E test)	Zone of inhibition (visual)

Variables

In vitro antifungal susceptibility testing is influenced by a number of technical variables, including inoculum size and preparation, medium formulation and pH, duration and temperature of incubation, and the criterion used for MIC endpoint determination (Table 3) (13, 44, 47). In addition, antifungal susceptibility testing is complicated by problems unique to fungi, such as slow growth rates (relative to bacteria) and the ability of certain dimorphic fungi to grow either as a unicellular yeast form that produces blastoconidia or as a hyphal or filamentous fungal form that may produce conidia, depending on pH, temperature, and medium composition. Finally, the basic properties of the antifungal agents themselves, such as solubility, chemical stability, modes of action, and the tendency to produce partial inhibition of growth over a wide range of concentrations, must be taken into account.

The determination of MIC endpoints is a critical step in antifungal susceptibility testing, especially with the azoles. The usual partial inhibition or trailing that is observed with 5-FC, the azoles, and most investigational agents precludes the determination of well-defined endpoints and creates a great deal of variability in interpretation. Several different methods of MIC endpoint determination have been applied in efforts to develop a test method that is both objective and easy to perform and interpret in routine clinical laboratories (Table 2). Traditionally, the MIC has been considered the lowest concentration of an antifungal agent that inhibits total growth of the fungi, as detected visually. The determination of MIC endpoints for the azoles and 5-FC with a less stringent criterion (slight turbidity is ignored) has increased interlaboratory reproducibility and produced a shift in the MIC distribution of the azoles toward lower drug concentrations for *C. albicans* and *Candida tropicalis* (16, 20). This less stringent criterion also has permitted discrimination between putatively susceptible and resistant isolates. The amount of trailing or partial inhibition can be estimated by the M27-A reference macrodilution method by diluting the drug-free growth control 1:5 (0.2 ml of growth control plus 0.8 ml of medium) to provide an 80% inhibition standard (16). This approach provides a convenient and direct method of establishing for each isolate a specific turbidity endpoint that more precisely reflects 80% inhibition. For amphotericin B, endpoints correspond to complete (optically clear) or 100% inhibition and are

TABLE 3 NCCLS guidelines for antifungal susceptibility testing[a]

Parameter	Description
Broth medium	RPMI 1640 broth buffered with MOPS (0.165 M) to a pH of 7.0 at 25°C
Medium modifications	YNB (pH 7.0) with MOPS provides better growth of *C. neoformans* Antibiotic medium 3 (pH 7.0) with MOPS yields superior detection of amphotericin B-resistant isolates, but medium lot variation has been reported
Inoculum preparation	From 24-h-old (*Candida* spp.) or 48-h-old (*C. neoformans*) cultures on Sabouraud dextrose agar
Stock inoculum suspension	Adjusted with spectrophotometer at 530 nm to match the turbidity of a 0.5 McFarland standard: (1×10^6 to 5×10^6 CFU/ml)
Test inoculum	1:2,000 (macrodilution) or 1:1,000 (microdilution) dilution with medium of the stock inoculum suspension: (0.5×10^3 to 2.5×10^3 CFU/ml)
Drug dilutions	10× (macrodilution) or 2× (microdilution) twofold drug dilutions with medium (fluconazole and 5-FC) or 100× with solvent (amphotericin B and other azoles)
Drug dilution ranges	
Fluconazole and 5-FC	0.12–64 μg/ml
Other drugs	0.03–16 μg/ml
Methods	
Macrodilution	0.9 ml of diluted test inoculum plus 0.1 ml of 10× drug concentration
Microdilution	100 μl of diluted test inoculum plus 100 μl of 2× drug concentration
Growth control(s)	
Macrodilution	0.9 ml of diluted inoculum plus 0.1 of drug-free medium
Microdilution	100 μl of diluted inoculum plus 100 μl of drug-free medium
MIC by visual examination	
Amphotericin B	Lowest drug concentration that prevents any discernible growth (macro- and microdilution)
5-FC and azoles	Lowest drug concentration that matches an 80% inhibition standard (macrodilution) Lowest drug concentration that shows prominent (~50%) growth inhibition (microdilution)
Reading modifications[b]	MICs for *C. neoformans* determined spectrophotometrically at 492 nm after 48 h of incubation

[a] Adapted from references 9, 13, and 34.
[b] The M27-A document includes this modification for the broth microdilution method with YNB and an inoculum of 10^4 CFU/ml.

defined easily, because trailing or partial inhibition is not usually observed with this drug.

Standardized Methods for Yeasts

The need to develop standardized methods for antifungal susceptibility tests was perceived as a means of providing good interlaboratory agreement among clinical laboratories as well as meaningful communication between clinical laboratories and physicians. In response to this need, in 1982 the NCCLS established a subcommittee to coordinate work on antifungal susceptibility tests. In 1992, as a result of several collaborative studies (16, 20, 40), the NCCLS subcommittee proposed a reference broth macrodilution method (M27-P document) for testing of yeasts such as *Candida* spp. and *C. neoformans*. This document was revised and published in 1995 as the M27-T document (tentative standard), which described a microdilution method (16). In 1996, the NCCLS subcommittee established interpretive breakpoints for three drugs and *Candida* spp., especially *C. albicans* (47), and the M27-A document (approved standard) became available in 1997 (34). The relationship established between the results obtained with the reference method and patient response for fungi other than *Candida* spp., as well as to amphotericin B, needs further evaluation and additional studies by the NCCLS subcommittee.

Macrodilution

The broth macrodilution test (Table 3) has been the most widely used technique for antifungal susceptibility testing; this approach is described in the M27-A document (34) and below. Broth macrodilution tests are adequate for the testing of all antifungal agents against any fungal isolate and are suitable for small clinical laboratories in which the volume of these tests is low.

Standard Medium and Modifications

The test medium should be a completely defined synthetic medium. RPMI 1640 broth with L-glutamine and a pH indicator and without sodium bicarbonate (04-525Y from BioWhittaker, Walkersville, Md., and American Biorganics, Inc., Niagara Falls, N.Y.; R-6504 from Sigma Chemical Co., St. Louis, Mo.) is the medium recommended by the NCCLS subcommittee. The medium should be buffered to a pH of 7.0 at 25°C. One buffer that has given satisfactory results for antifungal susceptibility testing is MOPS (morpholinepropanesulfonic acid; final molarity at pH 7.0,

0.165). This medium is suitable for the testing of 5-FC and the azoles against *Candida* spp. and several filamentous fungi (14, 20, 34); however, RPMI 1640 broth may not be adequate to support the growth of some strains of *C. neoformans* or to determine amphotericin B MICs as indicated above. RPMI medium containing 2% glucose (50) and yeast nitrogen base (YNB) broth (51) may enhance the growth of yeasts, facilitating the determination of MICs.

Drug Stock Solutions

Antifungal drug standards can be obtained directly from drug manufacturers or from the United States Pharmacopeia (Rockville, Md.). Clinical intravenous or oral preparations should not be used (34). Antifungal stock solutions should be prepared at concentrations at least 10 times the highest concentration to be tested (e.g., 1,280 μg/ml for fluconazole and 5-FC). Solutions of standard powders of 5-FC (Hoffmann-La Roche), fluconazole (Pfizer Pharmaceuticals), or any other water-soluble agent should be prepared in distilled water. For testing of the polyenes or any other non-water-soluble agent, sufficient drug standard should be weighed to prepare a solution of 1,600 μg/ml. These standard substances may be solubilized in dimethyl sulfoxide, polyethylene glycol, or dimethylformamide. The actual amount to be weighed must be adjusted according to the specific biological activity of each standard. Amphotericin B solutions must be protected from light, and drug stock solutions prepared with solvents should be allowed to stand for 30 min before use. When solvents other than water are used, the drug dilution series should be prepared at 100 times the final concentration in the solvent as described below. This procedure prevents precipitation of agents with low solubility in aqueous media (34). Despite this procedure, itraconazole and some other agents will not remain completely solubilized upon dilution into aqueous media. Thus, at high concentrations, a certain amount of turbidity will be encountered and may interfere with the interpretation of MIC endpoints.

Sterile stock solutions may be stored in small volumes in carefully sealed sterile polypropylene or polyethylene vials at −60°C (preferably) or below for 6 months or more without a significant loss of activity but never at a temperature higher than −20°C. Vials should be removed as needed and used on the same day. Any unused drug should be discarded at the end of the day. The use of quality control (QC) strains (38, 48), such as those listed in Table 4, will help in evaluating drug activity (34).

TABLE 4 Reference MIC ranges for two QC isolates for the broth macrodilution method[a]

QC isolate	Antifungal agent	MIC range (μg/ml)
C. parapsilosis ATCC 22019	Amphotericin B	0.25–1.0
	Fluconazole	2.0–8.0
	Itraconazole	0.06–0.25
	Ketoconazole	0.06–0.25
	5-FC	0.12–0.5
C. krusei ATCC 6258	Amphotericin B	0.5–2.0
	Fluconazole	16–64
	Itraconazole	0.12–0.5
	Ketoconazole	0.12–0.5
	5-FC	4.0–16

[a] Adapted from references 38 and 48.

Preparation of Inocula

Inocula should be prepared by the spectrophotometric method (34, 40) as outlined in Table 3. The test organisms are grown on plates of Sabouraud agar (Emmons 11589 Sabouraud dextrose agar from BBL Microbiology Systems, Cockeysville, Md.; modified 0747 Sabouraud agar from Difco Laboratories, Detroit, Mich.) at 35°C and subcultured at least twice to ensure purity and viability. The inoculum suspension is prepared by picking five colonies, each at least 1 mm in diameter, from 24-h-old cultures of *Candida* spp. or 48-h-old cultures of *C. neoformans* and suspending the material in 5 ml of sterile 0.85% NaCl. The turbidity of the cell suspension measured at 530 nm is adjusted with sterile saline to match the transmittance produced by a 0.5 McFarland barium sulfate standard. This procedure produces a cell suspension containing 1×10^6 to 5×10^6 CFU/ml, which is then diluted 1:2,000 with RPMI medium to provide a final test inoculum of 0.5×10^3 to 2.5×10^3 CFU/ml.

Drug Dilutions and Performance of Macrodilution Test

For drugs dissolved in solvents other than water (e.g., the polyenes), intermediate test drug dilutions are prepared from stock solutions to be 100 times the strength of the final drug concentrations, with 100% solvent (e.g., dimethyl sulfoxide) being used as the diluent according to the NCCLS standard additive twofold drug dilution schema (34) (e.g., 1,600 to 3 μg/ml for amphotericin B, ketoconazole, itraconazole, and investigational drugs). Each intermediate drug concentration solution is further diluted (1:10) in RPMI medium to obtain 10 times the final strength (e.g., 160 to 0.3 μg/ml). This step reduces the final solvent concentration to 10%. For water-soluble drugs (e.g., fluconazole), drug dilutions are prepared from stock solutions to be 10 times the final test drug concentrations directly in RPMI medium according to the NCCLS standard additive twofold drug dilution schema (34) (e.g., 640 to 1.2 μg/ml for fluconazole and 5-FC).

The 10× drug dilutions are dispensed in 0.1-ml volumes into round-bottom, snap-cap, sterile polystyrene tubes (12 by 75 mm; Falcon 2054; Becton Dickinson Labware, Lincoln Park, N.J.); these tubes can be stored at −60°C for 3 to 6 months. On the day of the test, each tube is inoculated with a 0.9-ml volume of the corresponding diluted yeast inoculum suspension. This step brings the drug dilutions to the final test drug concentrations (16 to 0.03 μg/ml for amphotericin B and some azoles and 64 to 0.12 μg/ml for fluconazole and 5-FC) and the corresponding solvent concentration to 1% in each tube. The growth control tube(s) is inoculated with 0.9-ml volume(s) of the inoculum suspension and a 0.1-ml volume(s) of drug-free medium or drug-free medium with a 1% concentration of the corresponding solvent. The QC organisms (Table 4) are tested in the same manner as the other isolates and are included each time an isolate is tested. In addition, 1 ml of uninoculated drug-free medium (for water-soluble agents) or drug-free medium with a 1% concentration of the corresponding solvent is included as a sterility control.

The MIC tubes are incubated at 35°C without agitation for 46 to 50 h (*Candida* spp.) and 70 to 74 h (*C. neoformans*) in ambient air; the turbidity or growth in each tube is visually graded. For amphotericin B, the MIC is defined as the lowest concentration that prevents any discernible growth. For azoles and 5-FC, a less stringent endpoint which allows for slight turbidity above the MIC is recommended (34); the MIC of these agents is defined as the lowest concentration that reduces growth by 80% relative to that of the growth control (34). This 80% inhibition endpoint may be estimated by diluting the drug-free growth control tube 1:5 with test medium (16, 34) as described above.

QC

QC of MIC tests is essential to good laboratory practice. *Candida parapsilosis* ATCC 22019 and *C. krusei* ATCC 6258 have been selected as QC strains according to the NCCLS guidelines for such selection (38, 48). Table 4 summarizes the expected MIC ranges of five antifungal agents for these two QC isolates in macrodilution testing. These ranges are also suitable for microdilution testing; however, formal establishment of microdilution QC ranges is under way. With repeated testing, more than 95% of the MICs should be within the MIC ranges represented in Table 4. Each new batch of medium and lot of macrodilution tubes and microdilution trays should be checked with either one of the two QC strains to determine if MICs are within these ranges. In addition, the overall performance of the test system should be monitored by testing either or both QC isolates each day on which a test is performed for each drug. More detailed information can be found in the NCCLS M27-A document (34).

Microdilution

Broth microdilution tests for fungi are similar in concept to broth macrodilution tests and yield comparable results (13, 16, 18, 52). Although the antifungal broth macrodilution test was the first method proposed by the NCCLS subcommittee, this test is cumbersome for use in clinical laboratories. A more efficient and easier-to-perform broth microdilution test is also described in the M27-A document (34). The microdilution test provides consistent MIC results, and interlaboratory agreement of the microdilution MICs can be higher than that of the macrodilution MICs for some drugs (16). Only the steps and testing conditions that are relevant to the microdilution test are discussed in detail here (Table 3).

The 10× and 100× drug dilutions described above are diluted 1:5 and 1:50, respectively, with RPMI medium to achieve the 2× drug concentrations needed for the microdilution test. The stock inoculum suspension is prepared and adjusted as described above for the macrodilution test. The stock yeast suspension is vortexed for 15 s, diluted 1:50, and further diluted 1:20 with medium to obtain a 2× test inoculum (1×10^3 to 5×10^3 CFU/ml). The 2× inoculum is diluted 1:1 when the wells are inoculated to achieve the desired final inoculum size (0.5×10^3 to 2.5×10^3 CFU/ml).

The broth microdilution test is performed with sterile, disposable, multiwell microdilution plates (96 U-shaped wells; Dynatech Laboratories, Inc., Alexandria, Va.). A multichannel pipette is used to dispense the 2× drug concentrations in 100-μl volumes into the wells of rows 1 to 10 of the microdilution plates. Row 1 contains the highest drug concentration (either 64 or 16 μg/ml), and row 10 contains the lowest drug concentration (either 0.12 or 0.03 μg/ml). Microdilution plates can be stored at −60°C for 3 to 6 months. Each well is inoculated on the day of the test with 100 μl of the corresponding 2× inoculum. This step brings the drug dilutions and inoculum densities to the final concentrations mentioned above (final volume in each well, 200 μl). The growth control wells contain 100 μl of sterile drug-free medium (for water-soluble agents) or 100 μl of sterile drug-free medium with 2% solvent (for non-water-soluble agents) and are inoculated with 100 μl of the corresponding 2× inoculum. The QC organisms are tested in the same manner as the other isolates and are included each time an isolate is tested. Row 11 of the microdilution plate can be used for the sterility control (drug-free medium only).

The microdilution plates are incubated at 35°C and observed for the presence or absence of visible growth. The growth in each well is compared with that in the growth control (drug-free) well with the aid of a reading mirror (Cooke Engineering Co., Alexandria, Va.). The MIC of amphotericin B is defined as the lowest concentration at which the complete absence of growth (optically clear) is observed, and the MIC of 5-FC and the azoles is defined as the lowest concentration at which prominent growth inhibition is observed—approximately 50% the growth in the growth control well. Agitation of the microdilution trays (see below) prior to MIC determinations has been shown to facilitate the estimation of prominent growth inhibition (2).

Expected Results

Most (96%) clinical yeast isolates are inhibited by 8.0 μg or less of 5-FC per ml (44); however, isolates of *C. neoformans* for which the MICs are ≥16 may be recovered from patients during treatment with 5-FC. *Candida* isolates for which 5-FC MICs are ≥32 and ≤4 μg/ml are considered resistant and susceptible, respectively (Table 5) (34). Amphotericin B MICs determined by the M27-A microdilution method are <1.0 μg/ml for 94% of clinical yeast isolates and >2 μg/ml for the other 6% (44). An amphotericin B MIC of 2.0 μg/ml (or greater) suggests probable clinical resistance, since this MIC only approximates the concentrations achievable in serum at high doses of amphotericin B (≥1 mg/kg of body weight per day) and exceeds those achievable in cerebrospinal fluid. The difference in amphotericin B MICs for susceptible and potentially resistant isolates is probably very small (see above), so caution should be exercised in the interpretation of results. Establishment of interpretive breakpoints for amphotericin B may require medium modification in standardized methods, as mentioned above.

Of the azoles, ketoconazole is fungistatic for most yeast isolates at concentrations of 0.03 to 16 μg/ml, as determined by the M27-A microdilution method. Fluconazole inhibits the majority (~90%) of *Candida* spp. and *C. neoformans* at concentrations of 8 μg/ml or less; however, MICs for isolates of *Candida glabrata* and *C. krusei* generally are 4 to 16 and 16 to >64 μg/ml, respectively (44). Itraconazole is generally quite active in vitro, with MICs of 0.01 to 1.0 μg/ml or less for most yeast isolates, except for *C. glabrata* (0.06 to 8 μg/ml) and *C. krusei* (0.5 to 2 μg/ml).

Standardized Methods for Filamentous Fungi

Although the number of serious infections caused by filamentous fungi (molds) is lower than the number of yeast infections, antifungal susceptibility testing of these opportunistic pathogens may be important in guiding the selection of antifungal agents for the treatment of invasive disease. The problems in developing standardized susceptibility testing for yeasts have been considerable, and developing such testing for filamentous fungi represents an even greater challenge. Standardization of the various antifungal susceptibility testing steps for yeast led to the development of standard guidelines for antifungal susceptibility tests for molds by adoption and tailoring of some of the steps in yeast testing. Recent multicenter studies by the NCCLS subcommittee

TABLE 5 Interpretive guidelines for in vitro susceptibility testing of *Candida* spp.[a,b]

Antifungal agent	MICs for isolates that are			
	Susceptible	Susceptible—dose dependent	Intermediate	Resistant
Fluconazole	≤8	16–32		≥64
Itraconazole	≤0.125	0.25–0.5		≥1
5-FC	≤4		8–16	≥32

[a] Adapted from references 13, 34, and 47.
[b] Adopted at an open meeting of the NCCLS subcommittee, 1 June 1996, Reston, Va. For fluconazole, these guidelines are based on mucosal candidiasis and limited data for invasive *Candida* infections. For itraconazole, they are based on mucosal infections only. For fluconazole, susceptibility for isolates classified as susceptible—dose dependent depends on achieving the maximal possible blood level (>400 mg/dose). For itraconazole, a concentration in plasma of >0.5 μg/ml may be required for an optimal response for dose-dependent MICs. For 5-FC, susceptibility to intermediate MICs is as yet uncertain.

have addressed the problems of inoculum preparation for conidia and sporangiospore suspensions and have evaluated the reproducibility of both macrodilution and microdilution tests as well as the in vivo correlation with the in vitro data (14, 15, 36).

In the initial multicenter study, Espinel-Ingroff et al. (15) evaluated a modification of the spectrophotometric method used to prepare yeast inocula for the preparation of inoculum suspensions of selected filamentous fungi. Conidial suspensions were prepared, and the turbidities were adjusted with a spectrophotometer to 68 to 82% transmittance (optical density ranges, 0.09 to 0.17) at 530 nm according to the species tested. Inoculum densities of 1.0×10^6 to 3.0×10^6 CFU/ml (mean values) were obtained in >90% of the participating laboratories (Table 6) (14, 15). These results indicated that suitable inoculum suspensions may be reliably prepared for use in antifungal susceptibility testing of molds. The in vitro susceptibilities of 25 isolates of *Aspergillus fumigatus*, *Aspergillus flavus*, *Pseudallescheria boydii*, *R. arrhizus*, and *S. schenckii* to five antifungal agents (amphotericin B, fluconazole, itraconazole, miconazole, and ketoconazole) were also evaluated in the initial study by both macro- and microdilution methods (15). Overall, interlaboratory agreement and the agreement between macro- and microdilution methods were quite good with most of the drugs—90 to 100%, depending on the antifungal agent and organism tested. The level of agreement was lower (70 to 90%) when itraconazole was tested. During the second 11-laboratory collaborative study (14), optimal testing conditions were identified based on 94 to 96% intra- and interlaboratory levels of agreement with amphotericin B and 89 to 92% levels of agreement with itraconazole for testing isolates of *A. flavus*, *A. fumigatus*, *Fusarium oxysporum*, *Fusarium solani*, *P. boydii*, and *R. arrhizus*. The best levels of agreement (91 to 95%) were obtained when itraconazole colorimetric MICs were determined by supplementing the test medium with the indicator Alamar Blue (AccuMed International, Inc.) (14).

TABLE 6 Optical density ranges and sums of mean inoculum sizes for filamentous fungi[a]

Fungus (no. of observations)	Optical density range[b]	Mean inoculum size (10^6 CFU/ml)
A. flavus (105)	0.09–0.11	1.6
A. fumigatus (104)	0.09–0.11	2.7
F. oxysporum (105)	0.15–0.17	3.0
F. solani (103)	0.15–0.17	1.8
P. boydii (99)	0.15–0.17	1.0
R. arrhizus (99)	0.15–0.17	1.3
S. schenckii (NA)[c]	0.09–0.11	2.4
QC isolate (*P. variotii* ATCC 22319) (NA)[d]	0.11–0.17	1.1

[a] Data are from two multicenter studies (14, 15).
[b] Optical densities at 530 nm correspond to 68 to 82% transmittance.
[c] NA, not applicable.
[d] Tested three to five times in each laboratory.

Only the identified optimal testing conditions for the filamentous fungi with a microdilution format are described below Tables 6 and 7). The other steps are similar to those described for the microdilution format with yeasts (see above). The inoculum for each isolate is prepared by first growing the mold on potato dextrose agar slants (Remel, Lenexa, Kans.) for 7 days at 35°C. A conidial suspension is prepared by flooding each slant with approximately 1 ml of sterile 0.85% saline. The resulting mixture is withdrawn, and the heavy particles are allowed to settle for 3 to 5 min. The upper homogeneous suspension, containing the mixture of conidia or sporangiospores and hyphal fragments, is vortexed for 15 s. The turbidity of the mixed suspension is measured with a spectrophotometer at 530 nm and adjusted to a specific final optical density range (Table 6) for each species tested (14, 15). Stock inoculum suspensions are diluted 1:50 in medium to obtain two times the strength needed for the test. The QC organisms used for yeast testing (Table 4) plus *Paecilomyces variotii* ATCC 22319 may be tested in the same manner as the other isolates and should be included each time an isolate is evaluated with any antifungal agent.

All microdilution trays are incubated at 35°C, and MICs are determined (i) at 24 h for *R. arrhizus*, (ii) at 48 h for *Aspergillus* spp., *Fusarium* spp., and *S. schenckii*, and (iii) at 72 h for *P. boydii* (14, 15). The growth in each well is compared with that of the growth control (drug free) and given a numerical score as follows: zero, optically clear, or the absence of growth; 1, approximately 25% the growth in the growth control; 2, approximately 50% the growth in the growth control; 3, approximately 75% the growth in the growth control; and 4, no reduction in growth. The MIC endpoint criterion for molds is the lowest drug concentration that is given a growth score of 2 (azoles) or a growth score of 0 (amphotericin B). The less stringent criterion (score of 2) allows for the trailing or partial inhibition frequently seen with the azoles and some investigational agents. Collaborative studies have not been conducted for other filamentous fungi, but experience with both established and investigational agents has demonstrated that MICs for other opportunistic and slower-growing filamen-

TABLE 7 Recent proposed standard guidelines for susceptibility testing of filamentous fungi[a]

Parameter	Description
Medium for conidial growth	Potato dextrose agar, 35°C, 7 days; *Fusarium* spp. may need incubation at 30°C for the last 4 days
Inoculum morphology	Conidia or sporangiospores
Recommended optical density ranges	For *Aspergillus* spp. and *R. arrhizus*, (0.09–0.11); for *Fusarium* spp. and *P. boydii*, 0.15–0.17; stock suspensions, 0.4×10^6 to 5×10^6 CFU/ml
Inoculum concentration (final)	0.4×10^4 to 5×10^4 CFU/ml or 1:50 dilution of stock suspension (but 2:50 for *P. boydii*)
Test medium	RPMI 1640 medium for yeasts, pH 7.0 ± 0.1
Format	Microdilution assay; total volume/well, 200 μl
Drug concentration	Amphotericin B and itraconazole, 0.03–16 μg/ml
Incubation conditions	For *R. arrhizus*, 24 h; for *P. boydii*, 72 h; for *Aspergillus* spp., *Bipolaris* spp., *Exserohilum* spp., *Fusarium* spp., and *S. schenckii*, 48 h
Endpoint determination (visual)	Growth relative to that in the positive growth control: for amphotericin B, absence of growth; for azoles, prominent growth inhibition (~ 50% the growth in the growth control)
Colorimetric determination (Alamar Blue)	For amphotericin B, first blue well or no color change; for azoles, first blue well or slightly purple well

[a] Based on references 14 and 15.

tous fungi can be determined after 48 to 96 h of incubation (sufficient or heavy growth present in the growth control). Testing of dimorphic fungi may require 5 to 7 days of incubation (11, 12).

Modifications of Reference Methods

Although the NCCLS methods for in vitro susceptibility testing are essential for standardization and to improve interlaboratory reproducibility, they may not be the best methods for testing all organisms or the most convenient methods for routine use in clinical laboratories. Thus, modifications of reference methods are acceptable and expected. Several modifications of the NCCLS reference methods for antifungal susceptibility testing have been evaluated. They offer promise as alternative approaches that may better serve practical clinical laboratory needs and make use of technology that is being used for antibacterial susceptibility testing in clinical microbiology laboratories. These approaches include colorimetric or spectrophotometric MIC endpoint determination methods and agar diffusion MIC methods.

Colorimetric Methods

A novel alternative to the standard method of visually grading turbidity is the use of a colorimetric oxidation-reduction indicator to aid in the determination of MIC endpoints. This approach provides a reliable indication of the number of viable yeast cells present and allows the determination of a metabolic MIC (39, 55, 56). The NCCLS-based microdilution assay described above (34) has been adapted to a colorimetric format by the simple addition of the commercially available oxidation-reduction indicator Alamar Blue. The result is a colorimetric microdilution method that provides clear MIC endpoints that can be determined visually and minimizes the trailing endpoints that are frequently observed with the azoles. The agreement of colorimetric microdilution MICs with NCCLS macrodilution and microdilution MICs has been quite good—>90%. However, itraconazole MICs determined by the colorimetric method have been reported to be higher than those determined by the NCCLS method, and agreement has been low with fluconazole for *C. glabrata* and *C. tropicalis* (56). The Sensititre Yeast One Antifungal Panel (AccuMed International) (29), which incorporates Alamar Blue as the colorimetric indicator, is under current evaluation for FDA approval; this panel is available for investigational purposes only.

Spectrophotometric Methods

Microtiter methods allow the determination of endpoints with automated plate reading and yield MICs that are more accurate and objective than the NCCLS, colorimetric, and agar diffusion methods. Agitation of microtiter plates (2) at 50 rpm for at least 5 min by use of a microdilution tray shaker before spectrophotometric MIC determination is essential to obtain homogeneous cell suspensions in the wells and hence a more precise MIC determination. The inability to obtain homogeneous (persistent button-like formation) cell suspensions with some yeasts demands manual mixing of the cells in each well with a micropipette tip. This is a tedious and time-consuming step. The spectrophotometric method allows the determination of different levels (percentages) of growth inhibition; e.g., an MIC_{50} corresponds to the first well that shows a 50% decrease relative to the optical density in the drug-free growth control well. Several studies have compared various spectrophotometric levels (percentages) of growth inhibition with M27-A MICs (13, 18, 51). Turbidimetric growth inhibition levels of 50% (MIC_{50}) with the azoles and 5-FC and of 80 and 90% (MIC_{80} and MIC_{90}, respectively) with amphotericin B have provided the most accurate values.

Agar Diffusion Methods

Agar diffusion methods for antimicrobial susceptibility testing are in common use in clinical microbiology laboratories. Worldwide, the most commonly used technique for antibacterial susceptibility testing is the disk diffusion test, which yields a quantitative result (zones of inhibition) and a qualitative interpretive category (susceptible or resistant). On the other hand, the E test (AB Biodisk) is based on the diffusion of a continuous concentration gradient of an antimicrobial agent from a plastic strip into an agar medium. E-test strips for amphotericin B, fluconazole, 5-FC, ketoconazole, and itraconazole are commercially available (AB Biodisk) for investigational purposes only; FDA approval is pending. Preliminary evaluations of the antifungal E test have suggested that it correlates well with the NCCLS reference methods (8, 17, 42, 52, 59). However, this agreement has been species and medium dependent: (i) low agreement has been reported for *C. glabrata*, *C. tropicalis*, and *C. neoformans;* (ii) improved agreement has been reported with fluconazole on solidified RPMI medium supplemented with 2% dextrose; and (iii) high agreement has been reported on Casitone agar for non-water-soluble agents (17). The E test appears to be most valuable for testing organisms for which there is no routine method of quantitative testing and may be useful for testing yeast isolates suspected of being potentially resistant to amphotericin B (59).

The application of agar diffusion disk methods to the testing of antifungal agents has been limited. In 1983, Stiller et al. (54) found a good correlation between MICs and growth inhibition zones for 5-FC. An international collaborative study found a fluconazole disk test to be comparable to an MIC test (41). More recently, Barry and Brown (4) demonstrated good correlation between the fluconazole disk test and MICs determined by either broth dilution or the E test.

CLINICAL CORRELATION

In order to be useful clinically, in vitro susceptibility testing should reliably predict the in vivo response to therapy in human infections. However, drug pharmacokinetics and drug interactions, factors related to the host immune response and/or the status of the current underlying disease, proper patient management, and factors related to the virulence of the infecting organism and its interactions with both the host and the therapeutic agent appear to have more value than the MIC as predictors of clinical outcome (47). Because so many factors can influence the process of antifungal therapy for an infection caused by a presumably susceptible isolate, a low MIC does not necessarily predict clinical success. However, in vitro resistance may be able to identify, among a population of susceptible isolates, those isolates that are less likely to respond to a specific antifungal regimen. Unfortunately, evidence for clinical correlation with in vitro antifungal susceptibility tests has been limited until recently (46, 54). This fact is not surprising, given the lack of standardized in vitro susceptibility testing methods and the variety of factors that can influence the clinical response to therapy (47). Therapeutic failures due to resistant organisms appeared to be rare before the 1980s. However, this situation changed with the recognition of relative resistance to amphotericin B among *Candida* spp. (6, 10, 25, 46) and the emergence of azole resistance in *C. albicans*, *C. glabrata*, and *C. krusei* and in new and emerging fungal pathogens (10, 49).

Interpretive MIC breakpoints (Table 5) have been established for both fluconazole and itraconazole following correlation with clinical data (oropharyngeal candidiasis [fluconazole and itraconazole] and candidemia in nonneutropenic patients [fluconazole]) (34, 47). Isolates inhibited by ≥64 μg of fluconazole per ml and ≥1 μg of itraconazole per ml are considered resistant to these agents, whereas isolates inhibited by ≤8 μg of fluconazole per ml and ≤0.12 μg of itraconazole per ml are considered susceptible (34, 47). In addition to the establishment of resistance and susceptibility breakpoints, fluconazole MICs of 16 to 32 μg/ml and itraconazole MICs of 0.25 to 0.5 μg/ml have been designated as indicating susceptible—dose dependent (34, 47). For fluconazole, this novel designation encompasses isolates for which susceptibility is dependent on achievable peak levels in serum of 40 to 60 μg/ml at fluconazole dosages of 800 mg/day, versus the expected peak levels of ≤30 μg/ml at lower dosages. For itraconazole, an MIC within the susceptible—dose-dependent range indicates the need for concentrations in plasma in excess of 0.5 μg/ml for an optimal response (47). Low drug dosage, poor absorption, and/or patient compliance, rather than azole resistance, can be responsible for clinical failure.

A recent review of the literature regarding the clinical relevance of antifungal resistance has revealed certain facts (10). (i) In agreement with the established resistance breakpoints (34, 47), a lack of response to fluconazole or itraconazole therapy for oral candidal infections has been associated with fluconazole MICs of ≥64 μg/ml and itraconazole MICs of ≥1.0 μ/ml. (ii) Similar MIC data have been documented in a few cases of fluconazole resistance in other candidal infections. (iii) In cryptococcal infections, MICs of >16 μg/ml have been associated with a high probability (>90%) of clinical failure of fluconazole therapy in patients receiving 800 to 2,000 mg of oral fluconazole per day. In another study, correlation was found between fluconazole MICs for *C. neoformans* and the length of time needed to obtain the first negative cerebrospinal fluid culture in the same dosage setting as that described above. (iv) Clinical failure with amphotericin B has been associated with MICs of >0.8 μg/ml in 24 well-documented cases of infections with *Candida* spp. and molds (*A. fumigatus*, *Fusarium* spp., and *Scedosporium prolificans*) reported from 1979 to 1996 (10). Both primary resistance and acquired resistance have been demonstrated.

It must be emphasized that a critical next step in establishing the clinical usefulness of the NCCLS standard procedures is to determine the relationship between test results and patient responses to therapy in other clinical settings and for other organism-drug combinations. Studies have begun to define the population distribution of MICs of amphotericin B, 5-FC, and fluconazole for several species of yeasts. However, the findings are preliminary and have not included clinical correlations.

SUMMARY AND CONCLUSIONS

A great deal of progress has been achieved in the field of antifungal susceptibility testing since 1982. Standardized broth macrodilution and microdilution methods are available, as are more suitable modifications of these methods for use in clinical microbiology laboratories. The establishment of interpretive breakpoints for three drug-organism combinations has begun to validate the clinical relevance of these standardized methods. Preliminary standard guidelines also are available for antifungal susceptibility testing of conidium-forming filamentous fungi. Additional studies are in progress to refine certain testing conditions. These include an optimal medium for the detection of amphotericin B resistance; QC MIC ranges for the microdilution method, for other, more suitable M27-A modifications, and for investigational agents; and, importantly, the establishment of the clinical usefulness of antifungal susceptibility testing for other drug-organism (yeasts and molds) combinations.

REFERENCES

1. **Abi-Said, D., E. Anaissie, O. Uzun, I. Raad, H. Pinzcowiski, and S. Vartivarian.** 1997. The epidemiology of hematogenous candidiasis caused by different *Candida* species. *Clin. Infect. Dis.* **24:**1122–1128.
2. **Anaissie, E. J., V. L. Paetznick, L. G. Ensign, A. Espinel-Ingroff, J. N. Galgiani, C. A. Hitchcock, M. LaRocco, T. Patterson, M. A. Pfaller, J. H. Rex, and M. G. Rinaldi.** 1996. Microdilution antifungal susceptibility testing of *Candida albicans* and *Cryptococcus neoformans* with and without agitation: an eight-center collaborative study. *Antimicrob. Agents Chemother.* **40:**2387–2391.
3. **Arndt, C. A. S., T. J. Walsh, C. L. McCully, F. M. Balis, P. A. Pizzo, and D. G. Poplack.** 1988. Fluconazole penetration into cerebrospinal fluid: implications for treating fungal infections of the central nervous system. *J. Infect. Dis.* **157:**178–180.
4. **Barry, A. L., and S. D. Brown.** 1996. Fluconazole disk diffusion procedure for determining susceptibility of *Candida* species. *J. Clin. Microbiol.* **34:**2154–2157.
5. **Denning, D. W.** 1996. Therapeutic outcome of invasive aspergillosis. *Clin. Infect. Dis.* **23:**608–615.
6. **Dick, J. D., W. G. Merz, and R. Saral.** 1980. Incidence of polyene-resistant yeasts recovered from clinical specimens. *Antimicrob. Agents Chemother.* **18:**158–163.
7. **Dismukes, W. E., R. W. Bradsher, G. C. Cloud, C. A. Kauffman, and the NIAID Mycoses Study Group.** 1992. Itraconazole therapy for blastomycosis and histoplasmosis. *Am. J. Med.* **93:**489–497.
8. **Espinel-Ingroff, A.** 1994. E test for antifungal susceptibility testing of yeasts. *Diagn. Microbiol. Infect. Dis.* **19:**217–220.
9. **Espinel-Ingroff, A.** 1996. Antifungal susceptibility testing. *Clin. Microbiol. Newsl.* **18:**161–168.
10. **Espinel-Ingroff, A.** 1997. Clinical relevance of antifungal resistance. *Infect. Dis. Clin. North Am.* **11:**929–944.
11. **Espinel-Ingroff, A.** 1998. In vitro activity of the new triazole voriconazole (UK-10,946) against opportunistic filamentous and dimorphic fungi and common and emerging yeast pathogens. *J. Clin. Microbiol.* **36:**198–202.
12. **Espinel-Ingroff, A.** 1998. Unpublished data.
13. **Espinel-Ingroff, A., F. Barchiesi, K. C. Hazen, J. V. Martinez-Suarez, and G. Scalise.** Standardization of antifungal susceptibility testing and clinical relevance. *J. Med. Vet. Mycol.*, in press.
14. **Espinel-Ingroff, A., M. Barlett, R. Bowden, N. X. Chin, C. Cooper, Jr., A. Fothergill, M. R. McGinnis, P. Menezes, S. A. Messer, P. W. Nelson, F. C. Odds, L. Pasarell, J. Peter, M. A. Pfaller, J. H. Rex, M. G. Rinaldi, G. S. Shankland, T. Walsh, and I. Weitzman.** 1997. Multicenter evaluation of proposed standardized procedure for antifungal susceptibility testing of filamentous fungi. *J. Clin. Microbiol.* **35:**139–143.
15. **Espinel-Ingroff, A., K. Dawson, M. Pfaller, E. Anaissie, B. Breslin, D. Dixon, A. Fothergill, V. Paetznick, J. Peter, M. Rinaldi, and T. Walsh.** 1995. Comparative and collaborative evaluation of standardization of antifungal susceptibility testing for filamentous fungi. *Antimicrob. Agents Chemother.* **39:**314–319.
16. **Espinel-Ingroff, A., C. W. Kish, Jr., T. M. Kerkering, R. A. Fromtling, K. Bartizal, J. N. Galgiani, K. Villareal, M. A. Pfaller, T. Gerarden, M. R. Rinaldi, and A. Fothergill.** 1992. Collaborative comparison of broth macrodilution and microdilution antifungal susceptibility tests. *J. Clin. Microbiol.* **30:**3138–3145.
17. **Espinel-Ingroff, A., M. Pfaller, M. E. Erwin, and R. N. Jones.** 1996. An interlaboratory evaluation of the E test method for antifungal susceptibility testing of pathogenic yeasts for five antifungal agents using Casitone agar and solidified RPMI 1640 with 2% glucose. *J. Clin. Microbiol.* **38:**848–852.
18. **Espinel-Ingroff, A., J. L. Rodríguez-Tudela, and J. V. Martínez-Suárez.** 1995. Comparison of two alternative microdilution procedures with the National Committee for Clinical Laboratory Standards reference macrodilution method M27-P for in vitro testing of fluconazole-resistant and -susceptible isolates of *Candida albicans*. *J. Clin. Microbiol.* **33:**3154–3158.
19. **Fridkin, S. K., and W. R. Jarvis.** 1996. Epidemiology of nosocomial fungal infections. *Clin. Microbiol. Rev.* **9:**499–511.
20. **Fromtling, R. A., J. N. Galgiani, M. A. Pfaller, A. Espinel-Ingroff, K. F. Bartizal, M. S. Bartlett, B. A. Body, C. Frey, G. Hall, G. D. Roberts, F. B. Nolte, F. C. Odds, M. G. Rinaldi, A. M. Sugar, and K. Villareal.** 1993. Multicenter evaluation of a macrobroth antifungal susceptibility test for yeasts. *Antimicrob. Agents Chemother.* **37:**39–45.
21. **Fung-Tomc, J. C., E. Huczko, B. Minassian, and D. P. Bonner.** 1998. In vitro activity of a new oral triazole, BMS-207147 (ER-30346). *Antimicrob. Agents Chemother.* **42:**313–318.
22. **Galgiani, J. N., and M. L. Lewis.** 1997. In vitro studies of activities of the antifungal triazoles SCH 56592 and itraconazole against *Candida albicans*, *Cryptococcus neoformans*, and other pathogenic yeasts. *Antimicrob. Agents Chemother.* **41:**180–183.
23. **Gonzalez, C., D. Venzon, S. Lee, B. M. Mueller, P. A. Pizzo, and T. J. Walsh.** 1996. Risk factors for fungemia in children infected with human immunodeficiency virus: a case-control study. *Clin. Infect. Dis.* **23:**515–521.
24. **Graybill, J. R., L. K. Najvar, M. F. Luther, and A. W. Fothergill.** 1997. Treatment of murine disseminated candidiasis with L-743,872. *Antimicrob. Agents Chemother.* **41:**1775–1777.
25. **Hadfield, T. L., M. B. Smith, R. E. Winn, M. G. Rinaldi, and C. Guerra.** 1987. Mycoses caused by *Candida lusitaniae*. *Rev. Infect. Dis.* **9:**1006–1012.
26. **Hector, R. F., B. L. Zimmer, and D. Pappagianis.** 1990. Evaluation of nikkomycins X and Z in murine models of coccidioidomycosis, histoplasmosis, and blastomycosis. *Antimicrob. Agents Chemother.* **34:**587–593.
27. **Kauffman, C. A.** 1996. Role of azoles in antifungal therapy. *Clin. Infect. Dis.* **22**(Suppl. 2):S148–S153.
28. **Kauffman, C. A., and P. L. Carver.** 1997. Antifungal agents in the 1990s. Current status and future developments. *Drugs* **53:**539–549.
29. **Killian, S., C. Knapp, A. Espinel-Ingroff, H. Plavan, M. A. Ghannoum, S. Messer, R. Hollis, and M. Pfaller.** 1997. Reproducibility of MIC results by the Sensititre YeastOne Colorimetric Antifungal Susceptibility Panel, abstr. D-134, p. 107. *In Program and Abstracts of the 37th Interscience Conference on Antimicrobial Agents and Chemotherapy*. American Society for Microbiology, Washington, D.C.
30. **Krishnarao, T. V., and J. N. Galgiani.** 1997. Comparison of in vitro activities of the echinocandin LY303366, the pneumocandin MK-0991, and fluconazole against *Candida* species and *Cryptococcus neoformans*. *Antimicrob. Agents Chemother.* **41:**1957–1960.
31. **Lopez-Berestein, G., G. P. Bodey, L. S. Frankel, and K. Mehta.** 1987. Treatment of hepatosplenic candidiasis with liposomal amphotericin B. *J. Clin. Oncol.* **5:**310–317.
32. **Lozano-Chiu, M., P. W. Nelson, M. Lancaster, M. A. Pfaller, and J. H. Rex.** 1997. Lot-to-lot variability of anti-

biotic medium 3 used for testing susceptibility of *Candida* isolates to amphotericin B. *J. Clin. Microbiol.* **35:**270–272.

33. **Martin, M. V., J. Yates, and C. A. Hitchcock.** 1997. Comparison of voriconazole (UK-109, 496) and itraconazole in prevention and treatment of *Aspergillus fumigatus* endocarditis in guinea pigs. *Antimicrob. Agents Chemother.* **41:** 13–16.
34. **National Committee for Clinical Laboratory Standards.** 1997. *Reference Method for Broth Dilution Susceptibility Testing of Yeast.* Approved standard M27-A. National Committee for Clinical Laboratory Standards, Villanova, Pa.
35. **Oakley, K. L., G. Morrissey, and D. W. Denning.** 1997. Efficacy of SCH 56592 in a temporarily neutropenic murine model of invasive aspergillosis with itraconazole-susceptible and itraconazole-resistant isolates of *Aspergillus fumigatus*. *Antimicrob. Agents Chemother.* **41:**1504–1507.
36. **Odds, F. C., F. VanGerven, A. Espinel-Ingroff, M. S. Bartlett, M. A. Ghannoum, M. V. Lancaster, M. A. Pfaller, J. H. Rex, M. G. Rinaldi, and T. J. Walsh.** 1998. Evaluation of possible correlations between antifungal susceptibilities of filamentous fungi in vitro and antifungal treatment outcomes in animal infection models. *Antimicrob. Agents Chemother.* **42:**282–288.
37. **Pfaller, M. A.** 1996. Nosocomial candidiasis: emerging species, reservoirs and modes of transmission. *Clin. Infect. Dis.* **22**(Suppl. 2):S89–S94.
38. **Pfaller, M. A., M. Bale, B. Buschelman, M. Lancaster, A. Espinel-Ingroff, J. H. Rex, M. G. Rinaldi, C. R. Cooper, and M. R. McGinnis.** 1995. Quality control guidelines for National Committee for Clinical Laboratory Standards recommended broth macrodilution testing of amphotericin B, fluconazole, and flucytosine. *J. Clin. Microbiol.* **33:**1104–1107.
39. **Pfaller, M. A., and A. L. Barry.** 1994. Evaluation of a novel colorimetric microbroth dilution method for antifungal susceptibility testing of yeast isolates. *J. Clin. Microbiol.* **32:**1992–1996.
40. **Pfaller, M. A., L. Burmeister, M. S. Bartlett, and M. G. Rinaldi.** 1988. Multicenter evaluation of four methods of yeast inoculum preparation. *J. Clin. Microbiol.* **26:** 1437–1441.
41. **Pfaller, M. A., B. DuPont, G. S. Kobayashi, J. Müller, M. G. Rinaldi, A. Espinel-Ingroff, S. Shadomy, P. F. Troke, T. J. Walsh, and D. W. Warnock.** 1992. Standardized susceptibility testing of fluconazole: an international collaborative study. *Antimicrob. Agents Chemother.* **36:** 1805–1809.
42. **Pfaller, M. A., S. A. Messer, A. Bolmström, F. C. Odds, and J. H. Rex.** 1996. Multicenter reproducibility of the E test MIC method for antifungal susceptibility testing of yeast isolates. *J. Clin. Microbiol.* **34:**1691–1693.
43. **Pfaller, M. A., S. A. Messer, and S. Coffman.** 1997. In vitro susceptibilities of clinical yeast isolates to a new echinocandin derivative, LY303366, and other antifungal agents. *Antimicrob. Agents Chemother.* **41:**763–766.
44. **Pfaller, M. A., J. H. Rex, and M. G. Rinaldi.** 1997. Antifungal testing: technical advances and potential clinical applications. *Clin. Infect. Dis.* **24:**776–784.
45. **Polak, A., and H. J. Scholer.** 1975. Mode of action of 5-fluorocytosine and mechanisms of resistance. *Chemotherapy* **21:**113–130.
46. **Powderly, W. G., G. S. Kobayashi, G. P. Herzig, and G. Medoff.** 1988. Amphotericin B-resistant yeast infection in severely immunocompromised patients. *Am. J. Med.* **84:** 826–832.
47. **Rex, J. H., M. A. Pfaller, J. N. Galgiani, M. S. Bartlett, A. Espinel-Ingroff, M. A. Ghannoum, M. Lancaster, F. C. Odds, M. G. Rinaldi, T. J. Walsh, and A. L. Barry for the Subcommittee on Antifungal Susceptibility Testing of the National Committee for Clinical Laboratory Standards.** 1997. Development of interpretive breakpoints for antifungal susceptibility testing: conceptual framework and analysis of in vitro-in vivo correlation data for fluconazole, itraconazole, and *Candida* infections. *Clin. Infect. Dis.* **24:**235–247.
48. **Rex, J. H., M. A. Pfaller, M. Lancaster, F. C. Odds, A. Bolmström, and M. G. Rinaldi.** 1996. Quality control guidelines for National Committee for Clinical Laboratory Standards recommended broth macrodilution testing of ketoconazole and itraconazole. *J. Clin. Microbiol.* **34:** 816–817.
49. **Rex, J. H., M. G. Rinaldi, and M. A. Pfaller.** 1995. Resistance of *Candida* species to fluconazole. *Antimicrob. Agents Chemother.* **39:**1–8.
50. **Rodríguez-Tudela, J. L., and J. V. Martínez-Suárez.** 1994. Improved medium for fluconazole susceptibility testing of *Candida albicans*. *Antimicrob. Agents Chemother.* **38:**45–48.
51. **Sanati, H., S. A. Messer, M. Pfaller, M. Witt, R. Larsen, A. Espinel-Ingroff, and M. Ghannoum.** 1996. Multicenter evaluation of broth microdilution for susceptibility testing of *Cryptococcus neoformans* against fluconazole. *J. Clin. Microbiol.* **34:**1280–1282.
52. **Sewell, D. L., M. A. Pfaller, and A. L. Barry.** 1994. Comparison of broth macrodilution, broth microdilution, and E test antifungal susceptibility tests for fluconazole. *J. Clin. Microbiol.* **32:**2099–2102.
53. **Sokol-Anderson, M. L., J. Brajtburg, and G. Medoff.** 1986. Amphotericin B-induced oxidative damage and killing of *Candida albicans*. *J. Infect. Dis.* **154:**76–83.
54. **Stiller, R. L., J. E. Bennett, H. J. Scholer, H. J. Wall, A. Polak, and D. A. Stevens.** 1983. Correlation of in vitro susceptibility test results with in vivo response: flucytosine therapy in a systemic candidiasis model. *J. Infect. Dis.* **147:** 1070–1076.
55. **Tellier, R., M. Krajden, G. A. Grigoriew, and I. Campbell.** 1992. Innovative endpoint determination system for antifungal susceptibility testing of yeasts. *Antimicrob. Agents Chemother.* **36:**1619–1625.
56. **Tiballi, R. N., X. He, L. T. Zarins, S. G. Revankar, and C. A. Kauffman.** 1995. Use of a colorimetric system for yeast susceptibility testing. *J. Clin. Microbiol.* **33:**915–917.
57. **Valero, G., and J. R. Graybill.** 1995. Successful treatment of cryptococcal meningitis with amphotericin B colloidal dispersion: report of four cases. *Antimicrob. Agents Chemother.* **39:**2588–2590.
58. **Walsh, T. J., P. Whitcomb, S. Piscitelli, W. D. Figg, S. Hill, S. J. Chanock, P. Jarosinski, P. Gupta, and P. A. Pizzo.** 1997. Safety, tolerance, and pharmacokinetics of amphotericin B lipid complex in children with hepatosplenic candidiasis. *Antimicrob. Agents Chemother.* **41:** 1944–1948.
59. **Wanger, A., K. Mills, P. W. Nelson, and J. H. Rex.** 1995. Comparison of E test and National Committee for Clinical Laboratory Standards broth macrodilution method for antifungal susceptibility testing: enhanced ability to detect amphotericin B-resistant *Candida* isolates. *Antimicrob. Agents Chemother.* **39:**2520–2522.
60. **Wenzel, R. P.** 1995. Nosocomial candidemia: risk factors and attributable mortality. *Clin. Infect. Dis.* **20:**1531–1534.
61. **White, T. C.** 1997. Antifungal drug resistance in *Candida albicans*. *ASM News* **63:**427–433.
62. **White, T. C., R. A. Bowden, and K. A. Marr.** 1998. Clinical, cellular, and molecular factors that contribute to antifungal drug resistance. *Clin. Microbiol. Rev.* **11:** 382–402.
63. **Wingard, J. R., and G. J. Elfenbein.** 1996. Host immunologic augmentation for the control of infection. *Infect. Dis. Clin. North Am.* **10:**345–364.

Antiparasitic Agents and Susceptibility Tests*

PHUC NGUYEN-DINH AND W. EVAN SECOR

127

OVERVIEW

Drugs are the main tool for controlling parasitic diseases. This situation exists because no effective antiparasitic vaccines are available and implementation of other control measures often proves to be difficult in countries where parasitic diseases are endemic. Drugs must assume this central role despite daunting constraints. Parasites are very diverse in their sizes, life cycles, and biological characteristics, yet the armamentarium of antiparasitic drugs remains limited, due largely to a lack of economic incentives for research and development. Among the available compounds, many have mechanisms of action or optimal dosages that are still unclear and several have inconvenient modes of administration or undesirable side effects. In addition, antiparasitic drugs are too often used incorrectly in communities and control programs. Of greatest concern, drug resistance is relentlessly eroding the efficacies of the available compounds. Since parasitic diseases rank among the most prevalent and severe diseases and occur mainly among populations already suffering from other health burdens, drug-resistant parasites unquestionably emerge as a priority issue in global public health.

To address this problem, existing compounds must be used rationally and improved ones must be found. An obligatory step in both activities consists of assessing parasite drug susceptibility by tests that fall in four broad categories. Tests in the first category, in vivo tests with patients, directly assess the clinical efficacies of existing compounds. These tests are performed in actual epidemiologic investigation situations, and their modest technical requirements make them suitable for use under field conditions in developing countries. However, the interpretation of in vivo test results is limited by potential interference by factors related to the host (e.g., immunity or variations in drug intake or metabolism) or to the environment (e.g., reinfections). Tests in the second category, in vitro tests, circumvent these interferences by isolating the parasites from their hosts and investigating them under controlled laboratory conditions, with opportunities for repeated assessments against multiple compounds (including experimental compounds). In vitro tests, however, are technically more demanding and therefore are less amenable to performance under field conditions. They are most informative if they are used to investigate parasites that multiply rapidly in culture, a select group consisting mostly of protozoa. In addition, they are of limited use for assessing inactive drug precursors that must be activated by the host or drugs whose antiparasitic activity necessitates the synergistic effect of the host's immune defenses. Tests in the third category, tests with experimental animal models, permit investigations of parasites that cannot be grown in culture or of drugs not yet approved for use in humans. Tests in the fourth and most recent category, tests at the molecular level, offer unique advantages. PCRs can be performed with minute amounts of nonviable parasite genetic material, thus bypassing the requirements for live parasites and in vitro culture. They can be run in batches, allowing large-scale epidemiologic studies. Molecular analysis at the single-organism level circumvents potential ambiguities associated with the heterologous parasite populations occasionally encountered in in vivo or in vitro tests and allows the dissection of such populations. Because of their short duration (hours), molecular diagnostic procedures can potentially be used to guide patient management. The other categories of tests usually require more time (days to weeks) and yield results that are used mainly for epidemiologic surveillance and experimental chemotherapy studies. The main drawback of molecular tests resides in their technical requirements. However, thanks to the development of more practical protocols and more robust automated equipment, molecular techniques are used in an increasing number of laboratories, including field facilities. Nonetheless, parasite drug susceptibility tests in general are infrequently performed and present special requirements and thus are not routinely available in clinical diagnostic laboratories.

These different categories of tests provide complementary information. At one end of the spectrum, molecular tests analyze parasites at their most basic biologic level, without any outside interference. At the other end, in vivo tests with patients reflect complex interactions between host and parasite, yet they are most relevant for clinicians and public health practitioners. While a good correlation between the results of various test methods is desirable, some degree of discrepancy should be expected to result from factors linked to the host or the culture conditions. Indeed, a judicious analysis of such discrepancies might provide valuable insights into the mechanisms of drug action and resistance.

* This chapter contains information presented in chapter 122 by Samuel L. Stanley, Jr., in the sixth edition of this Manual.

TABLE 1 Selected antiparasitic agents and susceptibility testing methods[a]

Disease and drugs	In vitro test method	Notes
Malaria Chloroquine, sulfadoxine-pyrimethamine, quinine, tetracycline, mefloquine, halofantrine, artemisinin, primaquine	Culture of erythrocytic stages of *P. falciparum*; criteria for assessment: • Microscopic examination: maturation from rings to schizonts (75); parasite multiplication (63) • Metabolic activity: incorporation of [^{3}H]hypoxanthine (26), production of pLDH (5, 57) • Other: DNA-bound fluorescent dye (83); effect of verapamil on accumulation of [^{3}H]chloroquine (44) Molecular analysis of genetic mutations in *P. falciparum* (68, 70, 88, 99)	Drug resistance is a major problem, especially in *P. falciparum* and *P. vivax* Tests are used for epidemiologic assessment as well as for laboratory investigations Short-term culture tests have also been described for erythrocytic stages of *P. vivax* (5, 45, 89) On an experimental basis, in vitro tests for the effects of drugs on liver stages (85) and sexual stages (gametocytes) (20)
Trichomoniasis Metronidazole, tinidazole, furazolidone, paromomycin sulfate, povidone-iodine	Culture under aerobic and anaerobic conditions; criterion for assessment, parasite motility (60, 61)	Resistance to metronidazole is relative; testing is performed over a range of concentrations
Leishmaniasis Sodium stibogluconate, meglumine antimoniate, pentamidine, amphotericin B	Culture of promastigotes; criteria for assessment: • Microscopic examination: parasite count (15) • Metabolic activity: incorporation of [^{3}H]thymidine (47), hydrolysis of *p*-nitrophenyl phosphate (9), conversion of MTT (78)	Problems with most drugs: high cost, difficulty in administration, and toxicity High rate of failure of pentavalent antimonial agents in some areas Coinfection with HIV can compromise results of therapy Axenic in vitro culture of amastigotes (the clinically relevant stage) is now possible
African trypanosomiasis Pentamidine, suramin, melarsoprol, eflornithine	Culture of trypomastigotes; criteria for assessment: • Microscopic examination: parasite count (50) • Metabolic activity: hydrolysis of *p*-nitrophenyl phosphate (9) Other: lysis assay (105)	In vitro tests are mainly used for laboratory investigations
American trypanosomiasis Benznidazole, nifurtimox, ketoconazole (in association), D0870	Culture of intracellular amastigotes; criteria for assessment: • Replication of amastigotes (93) • Conversion of β-galactosidase substrate by parasites transfected with β-galactosidase genes (14)	Tests are hindered by difficulty in isolating parasites from infected individuals In vitro tests are mainly used for laboratory investigations
Schistosomiasis Praziquantel, oxamniquine	None	In vivo tests with animals are needed due to dependence of drug effect on host immune response

[a] See text for details.

These points are illustrated in the following discussions of six parasitic diseases, selected for their particular chemotherapeutic challenges (see also Table 1).

MALARIA

Among parasitic diseases, malaria has the most visible public health impact, and the greatest problem of drug resistance is found among malaria parasites. Of the four species responsible for human malaria, resistance is found mainly in *Plasmodium falciparum*, the most pathogenic species, which causes an estimated 2 million deaths annually. Drug resistance is also encountered, but to a lesser extent, in *Plasmodium vivax*, the second most prevalent species.

Antimalarial drugs are most practically classified according to the stages of the parasite life cycle against which they act. Blood schizonticidal drugs eliminate the erythrocytic asexual stages, which cause the clinical manifestations of malaria; thus, resistance to these compounds has the greatest clinical implications. Among these drugs, chloroquine (a 4-aminoquinoline) is the most widely used because of its low cost, safety, and rapid action. A proposed mode of action is the inhibition of a heme polymerase located in the parasite food vacuole (82). Chloroquine-resistant strains of *P. falciparum* have emerged since the late 1950s and are now found in most areas of the world where malaria is endemic. Postulated mechanisms of resistance include an increased rate of efflux of chloroquine from the parasite acid vesicular compartment (53) or, conversely, a decrease in the drug accumulation force (11). Among alternate drugs for use against chloroquine-resistant *P. falciparum*, the most reasonably priced (an important consideration for developing countries) are synergistic combinations of inhibitors of the parasite folate biosynthetic pathway. A frequently used combination consists of sulfadoxine and pyrimethamine (S-P; Fansidar), which block sequentially the parasite dihydropteroate synthase and dihydrofolate reductase, respectively. Resistance to S-P has also emerged through alterations of the parasite enzymes that modify the binding affinities of the enzymes for the drugs. Multidrug-resistant strains of *P. falciparum* unresponsive to both chloroquine and S-P now occur at a high rate in Asia and some areas of Latin America and have occasionally been reported in Africa. Multidrug-resistant malaria can be addressed with a variety of compounds, including the oldest known antimalarial drug, quinine; antibiotics such as tetracyclines; newer products such as the arylamino alcohols mefloquine and halofantrine or an atovaquone-proguanil combination; and derivatives of artemisinin, isolated from the Chinese medicinal plant *Artemisia annua*. These compounds, however, tend to be more costly, and resistance to several of them has also been reported.

In the case of *P. vivax*, chloroquine-resistant strains, first reported in 1989 in Papua New Guinea (74), are now found in other areas where *P. vivax* is endemic. In addition, infections with *P. vivax* strains with decreased sensitivity to primaquine, an 8-aminoquinoline that prevents relapses in this species by destroying dormant liver-stage parasites (hypnozoites), have been described. First reported in the 1950s in New Guinea, infections with such strains have also been found in other areas, including Southeast Asia, Central and South America, and most recently, Somalia (84).

Initial observations of drug-resistant malaria occur most often in a clinical context, and their confirmation is frequently sought by in vivo tests. These aim at documenting the parasitologic and clinical responses of a malaria infection in a patient treated with a standard dose of the test drug and followed under controlled conditions. Initially standardized for chloroquine by the World Health Organization (WHO) (103), in vivo tests have been variously modified for simpler performance and assessments of other drugs and are used in epidemiologic investigations or for monitoring drug resistance (94).

In vitro studies of the activities of drugs against the malaria parasite have focused on the asexual erythrocytic stages of *P. falciparum*, for which long-term cultivation techniques are available (90). These tests can adopt relatively simple formats, which make them adaptable to field conditions. Among such tests, the most widely used is the microtechnique originally described by Rieckmann et al. (75). In this technique, a 100-μl fingerprick capillary blood sample is collected from an infected individual and is diluted 10-fold in culture medium (RPMI 1640 supplemented with 25 mM HEPES buffer). This blood-medium mixture containing synchronous ring-stage *P. falciparum* parasites (the only stage found in patient peripheral blood) is cultured in the wells of a 96-well microtiter plate. The wells are predosed with various concentrations of test drug (including a nondrug control), and the plates are incubated in a candle jar at 37°C. After 24 to 30 h of incubation, thick smears of the well's contents are made and the smears are stained with Giemsa stain; the parasite maturation to multinucleated schizonts in drug-containing wells is compared with the maturation of parasites in the control well, and the inhibition of parasite maturation by various concentrations of the antimalarial compound is assessed. In the case of chloroquine, the presence of schizonts in the wells containing 8 pmol of chloroquine indicates in vitro resistance, which generally correlates with in vivo findings. The results can alternately be expressed as a dose-response curve, and results for several isolates can be pooled to reflect the overall resistance status of malaria parasites in an area. This technique has been standardized and adapted to field work by WHO, which produces and provides self-contained in vitro kits allowing tests with chloroquine, mefloquine, quinine, amodiaquine, artemisinin, and S-P (for the last drug combination, a medium depleted of *p*-aminobenzoic acid and folate is used). Beyond this simplest format, other in vitro tests that are applicable both to field-collected parasites and to the parasites growing asynchronously in long-term laboratory cultures have been developed. These more versatile tests can be used not only in field assessments but also in the screening of potential new antimalarial agents and in investigations of drug modes of action. In such tests, parasites are cultured in microtiter wells, but with suspensions containing fewer cells, which permits the exposure time to be extended, often to 48 h or more. This allows the drug to exert its inhibitory effect on all phases of the parasite's full cycle of asexual multiplication. Parasite growth and inhibition are assessed microscopically (63) or by uptake of tritium (^{3}H)-labelled hypoxanthine (26). Two other methods for assessment have been described but are not widely used. One method, based on the production of a *Plasmodium*-specific lactate dehydrogenase (pLDH), requires relatively high starting levels of parasitemia (5, 57); the other, based on the fluorescence intensity of a dye (Hoechst 33258) bound to DNA, requires various treatments of the samples and a fluorometer (83).

An alternate, rapid, in vitro test for the detection of chloroquine-resistant *P. falciparum* has been described. It is based on the observation that verapamil enhances the accumulation of [^{3}H]chloroquine by resistant parasites (44). Because of its short duration (2 to 3 h), this test is of potential use in clinical management. However, its level of accuracy in predicting chloroquine resistance remains to be assessed under field conditions.

Recently, continuous culture of erythrocytic stages of *P. vivax* has been achieved (45). While they are technically cumbersome, these techniques will permit chemotherapy studies that will expand results from earlier assessments with short-term cultures (5, 89).

In addition to the asexual blood stages, in vitro cultures of the sexual blood stage (gametocytes) and the liver stage (exoerythrocytic stage) of *P. falciparum* can also be used to assess the antimalarial activities of various compounds (20, 85).

Molecular investigations are yielding promising results. The resistance of *P. falciparum* to pyrimethamine and cycloguanil (the active metabolite of proguanil, another inhibitor of dihydrofolate reductase) has been linked to several single point mutations in the parasite dihydrofolate reductase-thymidylate synthase gene. Different combinations of these mutations are associated with in vitro resistance to pyrimethamine or cycloguanil, or both (3, 25, 40, 51, 68, 108). Their prevalence has been surveyed in several areas of the world by a mutation-specific PCR (31, 67, 70, 71, 108). Similarly, various single point mutations in the *P. falciparum* dihydropteroate synthase gene are associated with sulfadoxine resistance in vitro (13, 97) and occur at an increased rate in areas where *P. falciparum* infections resistant to S-P in vivo occur at a high rate (70). Resistance to chloroquine in *P. falciparum* has been linked to changes in two genes. The linkage is not absolute, suggesting a multifactorial basis for this phenotype. The first proposed gene is *pfmdr1* (a *P. falciparum* homolog of the mammalian multidrug resistance gene) which either is amplified (42) or presents point mutations (4, 41, 96) in some chloroquine-resistant *P. falciparum* isolates. However, in genetic cross experiments chloroquine resistance has not cosegregated with *pfmdr1* (98). The second candidate gene has been traced to *P. falciparum* chromosome 7, where a specific set of polymorphisms in the *cg2* gene is associated with chloroquine-resistant parasites from Southeast Asia and Africa (88, 99). Finally, resistance to mefloquine and halofantrine has been associated with amplification of *pfmdr1* in *P. falciparum* isolates from Southeast Asia but not in isolates from sub-Saharan Africa (4, 23, 100). More precise definition of the genetic markers for resistance, obtained by correlating putative markers with in vivo and in vitro findings, will yield practical diagnostic tools that in turn can be used to investigate how resistant parasites emerge and spread.

TRICHOMONIASIS

Infection with *Trichomonas vaginalis* is one of the most common causes of human vaginitis. In addition, recent data have linked *T. vaginalis* infections with preterm delivery, low birth weight, and greater susceptibility to infection with the human immunodeficiency virus (HIV) (22, 54). As a result, expedient treatment of this infection has become an important public health measure.

T. vaginalis is a facultative anaerobe, and *T. vaginalis* infections are treated with metronidazole, currently the only drug licensed for this use in the United States. Metronidazole enters cells by passive diffusion in an inactive form. The low intracellular redox potential of anaerobic organisms results in reduction of the nitro group of the drug to hydroxylamine, which then interacts with the parasite's DNA and causes strand breaks (49). In trichomonads, the electron donor for metronidazole activation is ferredoxin (106). Clinical isolates of *T. vaginalis* that are resistant to metronidazole have a decreased ability to activate metronidazole to its toxic form (107) because of decreased mRNA levels and lower levels of protein expression in resistant trichomonads compared with the levels in metronidazole-susceptible organisms (49, 72). Because ferredoxin levels and metronidazole resistance are inversely related, metronidazole resistance is considered to be relative rather than absolute, and patients infected with metronidazole-resistant isolates of *T. vaginalis* are often treated with increased doses for a longer period of time (55). However, many patients cannot tolerate these higher doses of metronidazole, and such practices may only exacerbate the development of drug resistance. Although the only mechanism of metronidazole resistance that has been described in relation to clinical samples is decreased ferredoxin levels, laboratory-generated mutants with decreased levels of the enzymes pyruvate:ferredoxin: oxidoreductase and hydrogenase have also been described (49).

Clearly, alternatives to metronidazole for the treatment of *T. vaginalis* infections need to be identified. Tinidazole, a 5-nitroimidazole like metronidazole, is used in many countries for the treatment of trichomoniasis. However, the mechanism of action of tinidazole is analogous to that of metronidazole, and strains clinically resistant to metronidazole show cross-resistance to tinidazole in vitro (62). Furazolidone is active in vitro against isolates of *T. vaginalis* that are resistant to metronidazole and tinidazole, but it is poorly absorbed from the digestive tract and would require topical application (62). Alternative topical therapies that may have some benefit for patients with metronidazole-resistant *T. vaginalis* infections are paromomycin sulfate and povidone-iodine (64, 101).

Testing of the metronidazole susceptibility of *T. vaginalis* is a simple assay of parasite motility in the presence of drug (60). It is performed under both aerobic and anaerobic conditions, but differences in in vitro drug sensitivity between strains are generally more apparent under aerobic conditions. Axenic trichomonads are cultured in Diamond's trypticase-yeast-maltose medium with serial dilutions (400 to 0.2 μg/ml) of metronidazole dissolved in dimethyl sulfoxide (DMSO) and appropriate parallel concentrations of DMSO in U-bottom microtiter plates. Anaerobic susceptibility testing is performed with CO_2 generators in chambers that are monitored with anaerobic indicator strips. Plates are incubated at 37°C for 48 h and are then examined microscopically with an inverted phase-contrast microscope. The lowest concentration of drug in which no motile organisms are observed is defined as the minimum lethal concentration (MLC). MLCs greater than 100 μg of metronidazole per ml under aerobic conditions and MLCs greater than 3.1 μg of metronidazole per ml under anaerobic conditions have been associated with clinical resistance (61), but data from recent studies of clinical isolates suggest that these values may need to be reevaluated by additional studies comparing clinical efficacy with in vitro sensitivity (77a).

LEISHMANIASIS

Leishmaniasis is transmitted to humans by phlebotomine sandfly vectors and manifests itself in a variety of syndromes. Depending in part on the infecting *Leishmania* species, the pathology ranges from a cutaneous lesion that may be self-limiting to the more severe mucosal or visceral forms. The identification of leishmaniasis as an important opportunistic infection in patients with AIDS has presented new challenges for the treatment of leishmaniasis (6, 56). Infections with all species of *Leishmania* and all clinical forms of leishmaniasis are most commonly treated with the pentavalent antimonial compounds sodium stibogluconate and meglumine antimoniate (6, 65). However, use of these drugs is limited by their high cost, difficulty of administration (parenteral injection for several weeks), and associated toxicity. These factors are even more consequential in developing countries, where leishmaniasis is endemic, and can lead to premature self-termination of therapy, which in turn may promote increased levels of resistance to these drugs (38, 46). In addition, high rates of treatment failure have been described in some areas of India and Africa where the disease is endemic (6, 47), and HIV coinfections further compromise therapy with pentavalent antimony in patients with visceral leishmaniasis (6, 38). The modes of action of pentavalent antimonial compounds are still poorly defined. As with most heavy metals, it is possible that the parasite's metabolic function is disrupted by antimonial binding to a protein(s) and disruption of cellular metabolism (10). In vitro studies have suggested that the pentavalent antimonial compounds are converted to an active trivalent form or that the preservative chlorocresol used in drug preparation actually accounts for much of the leishmanicidal activity (32, 76, 78). The mechanisms of drug resistance in *Leishmania* spp. are also poorly understood. In general, resistant parasite strains accumulate less drug than sensitive strains. Although decreased drug uptake has not been ruled out as a cause of this difference (16), a large body of work has suggested a role for a P-glycoprotein-mediated active drug efflux mechanism (10, 65). Isolates with increased levels of drug resistance amplify P-glycoprotein-expressing genes, and transformation of drug-sensitive isolates with these genes can confer at least a low level of resistance (10, 65).

Until recently, the second-line drugs for the treatment of visceral leishmaniasis (pentamidine and amphotericin B) were considered poor alternatives because of their high levels of toxicity and unfavorable therapeutic indices compared with those of pentavalent antimonial compounds (65). This is still the case for pentamidine, but new lipid-associated formulations of amphotericin B have greatly reduced toxicity and are even beginning to be used for the primary treatment of visceral leishmaniasis in areas where the rate of resistance to pentavalent antimonial compounds is high (6). Amphotericin B interacts with parasite-specific 24-alkyl sterols and induces pore formation in the parasite plasma membranes (18). Lipid-associated formulations of amphotericin B are phagocytized by host monocytes and accumulate in the phagocytic lysosomes where *Leishmania* amastigotes reside (104). A review of drug trials for pentavalent antimonial compounds and alternative therapies has recently been published (6).

Testing for drug resistance in *Leishmania* is performed by culturing parasites with drug in a standard cell culture medium (Schneider's, RPMI 1640, or M199) supplemented with bovine serum for 42 to 72 h at 26 to 37°C (the incubation medium, time, and temperature are species dependent) and assessing viability by direct counting (15), measurement of the level of [^{3}H] thymidine incorporation (47), determination of enzymatic hydrolysis of *p*-nitrophenyl phosphate (9), or determination of the conversion of 3-(4,5-dimethylthiazol-2-yl)-2,5-diphenyltetrazolium bromide (MTT) (78). Measurement of the level of [^{3}H]thymidine incorporation is perhaps the most sensitive technique, but it requires access to radioactive materials and a scintillation counter, which is often unrealistic in the areas where this infection is endemic. The tests used to determine the hydrolysis of *p*-nitrophenyl phosphate and the conversion of MTT are colorimetric assays, but tests for *p*-nitrophenyl phosphate hydrolysis have high background levels caused by medium components, and MTT may interact with certain drugs (e.g., meglumine antimoniate). Promastigotes, which are easy to grow in culture, have typically been used for these tests, although the amastigote life-cycle stage is the clinically relevant target. Axenically cultured amastigotes have now been adapted to in vitro drug testing. This is an important development because amastigotes demonstrate sensitivities to drugs different from those demonstrated by promastigotes (15, 32, 78).

AFRICAN TRYPANOSOMIASIS

Trypanosoma brucei rhodesiense and *Trypanosoma brucei gambiense* are the etiologic agents of sleeping sickness. They are endemic in east and west Africa, respectively, and are transmitted by tsetse fly bites. Because these parasites possess antigenic switching mechanisms, host immune responses are ineffective, and the prospects for the development of vaccines against these organisms are meager. As a result, drug treatment is the only medical intervention available to combat sleeping sickness for the foreseeable future.

Most of the drugs currently used for the treatment of African trypanosomiasis have been in existence for more than 50 years and suffer from the same problems as the drugs used for the treatment of leishmaniasis: high cost, need for parenteral administration, and toxic side effects. Pentamidine and suramin are used for the treatment of early stages of infection, while melarsoprol and eflornithine are used once the central nervous system has become involved, but the latter two drugs are used only against *T. b. gambiense* (66). Another complication is that use of these drugs may require additional therapy to minimize toxic side effects. Pentamidine reduces the level of polyamine synthesis in trypanosomes by inhibiting the enzyme *S*-adenosyl-L-methionine decarboxylase (8). Suramin's mode of action is poorly understood, although it appears to inhibit the activities of several enzymes (66). Melarsoprol irreversibly binds to and disrupts the function of trypanothione, the major thiol-containing molecule in trypanosomes that is essential for maintaining an intracellular reducing environment and protecting the parasite from oxidative stress (1, 10, 34). Eflornithine inhibits the activity of ornithine decarboxylase, the first and rate-limiting step in the synthesis of putrescine and spermidine, which are essential for trypanothione synthesis (10). Thus, combination therapy with melarsoprol and eflornithine should have synergistic effects in patients (66). The synergistic efficacy of combination therapy has been demonstrated in mice infected with a melarsoprol-resistant strain of *T. b. rhodesiense* (2) and in a patient infected with a *T. b. gambiense* strain previously resistant to either drug alone (81).

Although pentamidine and melarsoprol have different modes of action, resistance to these drugs seems to occur through similar mechanisms (33). Both are transported into the cell by the P2 adenosine transporter; resistant organisms lack this transporter and as a result accumulate smaller amounts of drug (1, 10, 17). The mechanisms of resistance to suramin or eflornithine are unknown. Because of the difficulty in performing drug resistance assays in areas where African trypanosomiasis is endemic and the facts that the expense and low level of availability of alternative drugs (especially eflornithine) often preclude their use, drug susceptibility assays may be more useful for high-throughput testing of new agents rather than monitoring of the levels of drug resistance in the field. As for leishmania drug sensitivity testing, trypanosomes can be cultured in vitro with drug and monitored for viability by determination of enzymatic hydrolysis of *p*-nitrophenyl phosphate (9) or direct counting (50). Parasites are cultured at 37°C for 24 h in 4 to 5% CO_2 in phenol red-free Iscove's medium containing hypoxanthine, thymidine, glutamine, L-cysteine, pyruvate, β-mercaptoethanol, and heat-inactivated bovine or horse serum. An in vitro lysis assay has been developed for testing sensitivity of *T. brucei* subspecies to melarsoprol (105). It requires the ability to culture trypanosomes and a thermostatically controlled recording spectrophotometer. As susceptible organisms die, their absorbance at 500 nm is reduced over the course of 30 min. If control drug-sensitive and drug-resistant strains are available, perhaps this technique could be adapted to field use because 500 nm is within the visible range.

AMERICAN TRYPANOSOMIASIS

Trypanosoma cruzi is the causative agent of Chagas' disease, which can lead to cardiac failure or dilation of the colon and esophagus in the chronic stage. Although natural transmission of this parasite has been reduced through vector control programs in some countries, transmission associated with blood transfusions or organ transplantations is becoming recognized as a problem. Because of the difficulties in isolating parasites from infected individuals and the probable persistence of antibody responses following cure, assessment of the efficacies of drugs against Chagas' disease is difficult (52). Benznidazole, a 2-nitroimidazole, has been reported to reduce the level of progression to severe disease (95) and to decrease the level of serologic reactivity in some children (79). However, benznidazole seems to have variable efficacy according to the parasite strain (39), and its use has been questioned (7, 80). The other drug that has been commonly used for *T. cruzi* infections, nifurtimox, suffers from similar problems.

A class of agents with potential efficacy against *T. cruzi* is antifungal drugs. These compounds inhibit biosynthesis of the ergosterols that are essential components of the parasite's membranes (29, 91). The most studied drug of this group, ketoconazole, is ineffective at concentrations tolerable to the host and may be active only against certain parasite strains (12, 59). However, it can be combined with other drugs that inhibit different steps of the ergosterol biosynthesis pathway and yields synergistic efficacy against both the epimastigote and the amastigote forms of the parasite (58, 92). Recently, a newly developed drug (D0870) that combines inhibition of ergosterol biosynthesis and blockage of cytokinesis has been shown to have better efficacy than nifurtimox or ketoconazole against *T. cruzi* in experimental models (93).

Because the utilities of these drugs in clinical applications remain to be proven, further testing of new compounds should be pursued. Most assays for drug efficacy have relied on microscopy, a laborious technique for evaluating the growth of the intracellular amastigote form. Because a technique for the axenic culture of *T. cruzi* amastigotes, has not been developed, alternative techniques for evaluating intracellular growth would be useful. One innovative technique for the screening of drugs involves the transfection of parasites so that they express β-galactosidase (14). Parasite viability is evaluated by quantitation of the conversion of a β-galactosidase substrate to a colored product in a microtiter plate spectrophotomer. An added element is that the potential toxicities of test drugs can be evaluated in parallel by using a vital stain specific for mammalian cells. This technique may prove to be a useful high-throughput assay for testing new antitrypanosomal drugs.

SCHISTOSOMIASIS

With an estimated 200 million persons infected with schistosomes, schistosomiasis is arguably the second most important parasitic disease (after malaria) in terms of mortality and morbidity. Unregulated immunologic responses to parasite antigens can result in liver fibrosis and portal hypertension in patients with *Schistosoma mansoni* or *Schistosoma japonicum* infections and bladder fibrosis that occasionally is associated with carcinoma in the case of *Schistosoma haematobium* infection. Investigations of the drug resistance mechanisms of schistosomes are more difficult than those for protozoa. This is because the parasites are extremely difficult to grow in vitro and the efficacies of the two drugs most commonly used for the treatment of schistosomiasis, praziquantel and oxamniquine, are dependent upon components of the immune system (36, 77). Thus, tests for drug sensitivity require infection and treatment of experimental animals. A detailed protocol with mice to confirm suspected drug-resistant strains has recently been proposed (37).

Praziquantel-tolerant *S. mansoni* infections have been described in Egypt and Senegal (48, 87); oxamniquine-insensitive *S. mansoni* infections have been reported in Brazil and Kenya (21, 27). The mechanism of action of praziquantel has not been elucidated, although it is thought that praziquantel alters the worm's tegument in such a way as to render it vulnerable to attack by the host's immune system (73). Oxamniquine is activated by a schistosome esterase, binds to the parasite's DNA, and irreversibly inhibits RNA and DNA syntheses (19). This enzymatic activity is not present in *S. haematobium* (a species not sensitive to oxamniquine) or oxamniquine-resistant strains of *S. mansoni* (19, 69). Fortunately, to date no clinical cross-resistance has been reported. Praziquantel-insensitive schistosomes can be treated with oxamniquine, and those tolerant to oxamniquine are sensitive to praziquantel (27, 35, 86).

FUTURE PERSPECTIVES

Among the diseases selected for limited review in this chapter, only one is caused by a helminth. This reflects the fact that no major difficulties in the chemotherapy of helminthic diseases have been encountered to date. A limited number of drugs (praziquantel, ivermectin, and the benzimidazoles) adequately cover the spectrum of helminthic infections. Even considering schistosomiasis, drug resistance in human helminths is rare, a fact attributed to their long reproduction cycles and to their lack of multiplication inside the human host (the exception being *Strongyloides stercoralis*). However, variations in responses to antihelminthic chemotherapy have been reported (24, 30), and these variations might reflect acquired resistance or innate tolerance. Current efforts toward the elimination of selected helminthic infections (onchocerciasis, filariasis, and infections caused by geohelminths), which require large-scale drug administration, will increase drug pressure and the corresponding risk of emergence of true drug resistance. A cautionary lesson must be learned from the current problem of drug resistance in livestock helminths, attributed to frequent mass treatments with single compounds (43). In areas where antihelminthic drugs are used intensively, susceptibility to these drugs should be monitored through assessments of patients, and this monitoring should be complemented by valid laboratory tests where possible.

The predominance of protozoal diseases among the diseases described in this chapter reflects the unsatisfactory status of antiprotozoal chemotherapy. This is the case not only in developing countries but also in industrialized ones, where parasitic diseases are emerging as an important public health problem. For example, only one product (trimethoprim-sulfamethoxazole) is available for the treatment of *Cyclospora cayetanensis* (which has recently made major inroads in the United States), and the therapeutic options are even more limited for opportunistic agents such microsporidia or *Cryptosporidium parvum*. It is hoped that drug screening with animal models and existing in vitro tests (28, 102) will yield new compounds.

Increased population movements and the advent of HIV and AIDS have stimulated the globalization of parasitic diseases. This situation creates stronger incentives for the development of new antiparasitic compounds and for the assessment of the efficacies of existing products, an effort that calls for contributions from both developing and industrialized countries. Such contributions range from assessment of the antiparasitic effects of indigenous plant extracts, to the performance of field studies of drug efficacy, to the use of the most modern molecular tools to gain a better understanding of parasitic diseases. Parasite chemotherapy and monitoring of drug resistance will remain challenging endeavors for many years to come.

REFERENCES

1. **Bacchi, C. J.** 1993. Resistance to clinical drugs in African trypanosomes. *Parasitol. Today* **9:**190–193.
2. **Bacchi, C. J., H. C. Nathan, N. Yarlett, B. Goldberg, P. P. McCann, A. Sjoerdsma, M. Saric, and A. B. Clarkson, Jr.** 1994. Combination chemotherapy of drug-resistant *Trypanosoma brucei rhodesiense* infections in mice using DL-α-difluoromethylornithine and standard trypanocides. *Antimicrob. Agents Chemother.* **38:**563–569.
3. **Basco, L. K., P. E. De Pecoulas, J. Le Bras, and C. M. Wilson.** 1996. *Plasmodium falciparum:* molecular characterization of multidrug-resistant Cambodian isolates. *Exp. Parasitol.* **82:**97–103.
4. **Basco, L. K., J. Le Bras, Z. Rhoades, and C. M. Wilson.** 1995. Analysis of pfmdr1 and drug susceptibility in fresh isolates of *Plasmodium falciparum* from Subsaharan Africa. *Mol. Biochem. Parasitol.* **74:**157–166.
5. **Basco, L. K., F. Marquet, M. M. Makler, and J. Le Bras.** 1995. *Plasmodium falciparum* and *Plasmodium vivax*: lactate dehydrogenase activity and its application for *in vitro* drug susceptibility assay. *Exp. Parasitol.* **80:**260–271.
6. **Berman, J. D.** 1997. Human leishmaniasis: clinical, diagnostic, and chemotherapeutic developments in the last 10 years. *Clin. Infect. Dis.* **24:**684–703.
7. **Bestetti, R. B.** 1997. Should benznidazole be used in chronic Chagas' disease? *Lancet* **349:**653.
8. **Bitonti, A. J., J. A. Dumont, and P. P. McCann.** 1986. Characterization of *Trypanosoma brucei brucei* S-adenosyl-L-methionine decarboxylase and its inhibition by Berenil, pentamidine and methylglyoxal bis(guanylhydrazone). *Biochem. J.* **237:**685–689.
9. **Bodley, A. L., M. W. McGarry, and T. A. Shapiro.** 1995. Drug cytotoxicity assay for African trypanosomes and *Leishmania* species. *J. Infect. Dis.* **172:**1157–1159.
10. **Borst, P., and M. Ouellette.** 1995. New mechanisms of drug resistance in parasitic protozoa. *Annu. Rev. Microbiol.* **49:**427–460.
11. **Bray, P. G., R. E. Howells, G. Y. Ritchie, and S. A. Ward.** 1992. Rapid chloroquine efflux phenotype in both chloroquine-sensitive and chloroquine-resistant *Plasmodium falciparum*. *Biochem. Pharmacol.* **44:**1317–1324.
12. **Brener, Z., J. R. Cancado, L. M. da Cunha Galvao, Z. M. P. da Luz, L. de Sousa Filardi, M. E. S. Pereira, L. M. T. Santos, and C. B. Cancado.** 1993. An experimental and clinical assay with ketoconazole in the treatment of Chagas disease. *Mem. Inst. Oswaldo Cruz* **88:**149–153.
13. **Brooks, D. R., P. Wang, M. Read, W. M. Watkins, P. F. G. Sims, and J. E. Hyde.** 1994. Sequence variation of the hydroxymethyldihydropterin pyrophosphokinase: dihydropteroate synthase gene in lines of the human malaria parasite, *Plasmodium falciparum*, with differing resistance to sulfadoxine. *Eur. J. Biochem.* **224:**397–405.
14. **Buckner, F. S., C. L. M. J. Verlinde, A. C. La Flamme, and W. C. van Voorhis.** 1996. Efficient technique for screening drugs for activity against *Trypanosoma cruzi* using parasites expressing β-galactosidase. *Antimicrob. Agents Chemother.* **40:**2592–2597.
15. **Callahan, H. L., A. C. Portal, R. Devereaux, and M. Grogl.** 1997. An axenic amastigote system for drug screening. *Antimicrob. Agents Chemother.* **41:**818–822.
16. **Callahan, H. L., W. L. Roberts, P. M. Rainey, and S. M. Beverley.** 1994. The PGPA gene of *Leishmania major* mediates antimony (SbIII) resistance by decreasing influx and not by increasing efflux. *Mol. Biochem. Parasitol.* **68:** 145–149.
17. **Carter, N. S., and A. H. Fairlamb.** 1993. Arsenical-resistant trypanosomes lack an unusual adenosine transporter. *Nature* **361:**173–176.
18. **Chance, M. L.** 1995. New developments in the chemotherapy of leishmaniasis. *Ann. Trop. Med. Parasitol.* **89:** S37–S43.
19. **Cioli, D., L. Pica-Mattoccia, and S. Archer.** 1993. Drug resistance in schistosomes. *Parasitol. Today* **9:**162–166.
20. **Coleman, R. E., A. K. Nath, I. Schneider, G.-H. Song, T. A. Klein, and W. K. Milhous.** 1994. Prevention of sporogony of *Plasmodium falciparum* and *P. berghei* in *Anopheles stephensi* mosquitoes by transmission-blocking antimalarials. *Am. J. Trop. Med. Hyg.* **50:**646–653.
21. **Coles, G. C., W. T. Mutahi, G. K. Kinoti, J. I. Bruce, and N. Katz.** 1987. Tolerance of Kenya *Schistosoma mansoni* to oxamniquine. *Trans. R. Soc. Trop. Med. Hyg.* **81:** 782–785.
22. **Cotch, M. F., J. G. Pastorek, R. P. Nugent, S. L. Hillier, R. S. Gibbs, D. H. Martin, D. A. Eschenbach, R. Edelman, J. C. Carey, J. A. Regan, M. A. Krohn, M. A. Klebanoff, A. V. Rao, G. G. Rhoads, and the Vaginal Infections and Prematurity Study Group.** 1997. *Trichomonas vaginalis* associated with low birth weight and preterm delivery. *Sex. Transm. Dis.* **26:**353–360.
23. **Cowman, A. F., D. Galatis, and J. K. Thomson.** 1994. Selection for mefloquine resistance in *Plasmodium falciparum* is linked to amplification of the *pfmdr1* gene and cross-resistance to halofantrine and quinine. *Proc. Natl. Acad. Sci. USA* **91:**1143–1147.
24. **De Clerq, D., M. Sacko, J. Behnke, F. Gilbert, P. Dorny, and J. Vercruysse.** 1997. Failure of mebendazole in treatment of human hookworm infections in the southern region of Mali. *Am. J. Trop. Med. Hyg.* **57:**25–30.
25. **de Pécoulas, P. E., L. K. Basco, J. Le Bras, and A. Mazabraud.** 1996. Association between antifol resistance *in vitro* and DHFR gene point mutation in *Plasmodium falciparum* isolates. *Trans. R. Soc. Trop Med. Hyg.* **90:** 181–182.
26. **Desjardins, R. E., C. J. Canfield, J. D. Haynes, and J. D. Chulay.** 1979. Quantitative assessment of antimalarial activity in vitro by a semiautomated microdilution technique. *Antimicrob. Agents Chemother.* **16:**710–718.
27. **Dias, L. C. S., R. J. Pedro, and E. R. Deberaldini.** 1982. Use of praziquantel in patients with schistosomiasis mansoni previously treated with oxamniquine and/or hycanthone: resistance of *Schistosoma mansoni* to schistosomicidal agents. *Trans. R. Soc. Trop. Med. Hyg.* **76:**652–659.
28. **Didier, E. S.** 1997. Effects of albendazole, fumagillin, and TNP-470 on microsporidial replication in vitro. *Antimicrob. Agents Chemother.* **41:**1541–1546.
29. **Docampo, R., and G. A. Schmunis.** 1997. Sterol biosynthesis inhibitors: potential chemotherapeutics against Chagas disease. *Parasitol. Today* **13:**129–130.
30. **Eberhard, M. L., P. J. Lammie, C. M. Dickinson, and**

J. M. Roberts. 1991. Evidence of nonsusceptibility to diethylcarbamazine in *Wuchereria bancrofti*. *J. Infect. Dis.* **163:**1157–1160.

31. **Edoh, D., H. Mshinda, J. Jenkins, and M. Burger.** 1997. Pyrimethamine-resistant *Plasmodium falciparum* parasites among Tanzanian children: a facility-based study using the polymerase chain reaction. *Am. J. Trop. Med. Hyg.* **57:**342–347.
32. **Ephros, M., E. Waldman, and D. Zilberstein.** 1997. Pentostam induces resistance to antimony and the preservative chlorocresol in *Leishmania donovani* promastigotes and axenically grown amastigotes. *Antimicrob. Agents Chemother.* **41:**1064–1068.
33. **Fairlamb, A. H., N. S. Carter, M. Cunningham, and K. Smith.** 1992. Characterization of melarsen-resistant *Trypanosoma brucei brucei* with respect to cross-resistance to other drugs and trypanothione metabolism. *Mol. Biochem. Parasitol.* **53:**213–222.
34. **Fairlamb, A. H., G. B. Henderson, and A. Cerami.** 1989. Trypanothione is the primary target for arsenical drugs against African trypanosomes. *Proc. Natl. Acad. Sci. USA* **86:**2607–2611.
35. **Fallon, P. G., and M. J. Doenhoff.** 1994. Drug-resistant schistosomiasis: resistance to praziquantel and oxamniquine induced in *Schistosoma mansoni* in mice is drug specific. *Am. J. Trop. Med. Hyg.* **51:**83–88.
36. **Fallon, P. G., J. V. Hamilton, and M. J. Doenhoff.** 1995. Efficacy of treatment of murine *Schistosoma mansoni* infections with praziquantel and oxamniquine correlates with infection intensity: role of host antibody. *Parasitology* **111:**59–66.
37. **Fallon, P. G., L.-F. Tao, M. M. Ismail, and J. L. Bennett.** 1996. Schistosome resistance to praziquantel: fact or artifact? *Parasitol. Today* **12:**316–320.
38. **Faraut-Gambarelli, F., R. Piarroux, M. Deniau, B. Giusiano, P. Marty, G. Michel, B. Faugere, and H. Dumon.** 1997. In vitro and in vivo resistance of *Leishmania infantum* to meglumine antimoniate: a study of 37 strains collected from patients with visceral leishmaniasis. *Antimicrob. Agents Chemother.* **41:**827–830.
39. **Filardi, L. S., and Z. Brener.** 1987. Susceptibility and resistance of *Trypanosoma cruzi* strains to drugs used clinically in Chagas disease. *Trans. R. Soc. Trop. Med. Hyg.* **81:**755–759.
40. **Foote, S. J., D. Galatis, and A. F. Cowman.** 1990. Amino acids in the dihydrofolate reductase-thymidylate synthase gene of *Plasmodium falciparum* involved in cycloguanil resistance differ from those involved in pyrimethamine resistance. *Proc. Natl. Acad. Sci. USA* **87:**3014–3017.
41. **Foote, S. J., D. E. Kyle, R. K. Martin, A. M. J. Oduola, K. Forsyth, D. J. Kemp, and A. F. Cowman.** 1990. Several alleles of the multidrug-resistance gene are closely linked to chloroquine resistance in *Plasmodium falciparum*. *Nature* **345:**255–258.
42. **Foote, S. J., J. K. Thompson, A. F. Cowman, and D. J. Kemp.** 1989. Amplification of the multidrug resistance gene in some chloroquine-resistant isolates of *P. falciparum*. *Cell* **57:**921–930.
43. **Geerts, S., G. C. Coles, and B. Gryseels.** 1997. Antihelminthic resistance in human helminths: learning from the problems with worm control in livestock. *Parasitol. Today* **13:**149–151.
44. **Gluzman, I. Y., D. J. Krogstad, A. U. Orjih, K. Nkangineme, T. E. Wellems, J. T. Martin, and P. H. Schlesinger.** 1990. A rapid in vitro test for chloroquine-resistant *Plasmodium falciparum*. *Am J. Trop. Med. Hyg.* **42:** 521–526.
45. **Golenda, C. F., J. Li, and R. Rosenberg.** 1997. Continuous *in vitro* propagation of the malaria parasite *Plasmodium vivax*. *Proc. Natl. Acad. Sci. USA* **94:**6786–6791.
46. **Grögl, M., A. M. J. Oduola, L. D. C. Cordero, and D. E. Kyle.** 1989. Leishmania spp.: development of pentostam-resistant clones *in vitro* by discontinuous drug exposure. *Exp. Parasitol.* **69:**78–90.
47. **Grögl, M., T. N. Thomason, and E. D. Franke.** 1992. Drug resistance in leishmaniasis: its implication in systemic chemotherapy of cutaneous and mucocutaneous disease. *Am. J. Trop. Med. Hyg.* **47:**117–126.
48. **Ismail, M., A. Metwally, A. Farghaly, J. Bruce, L.-F. Tao, and J. L. Bennett.** 1996. Characterization of isolates of *Schistosoma mansoni* from Egyptian villagers that tolerate high doses of praziquantel. *Am. J. Trop. Med. Hyg.* **55:**214–218.
49. **Johnson, P. J.** 1993. Metronidazole and drug resistance. *Parasitol. Today* **9:**183–186.
50. **Kaminsky, R., and E. Zweygarth.** 1989. Feeder layer-free in vitro assay for screening antitrypanosomal compounds against *Trypanosoma brucei brucei* and *T. b. evansi*. *Antimicrob. Agents Chemother.* **33:**881–885.
51. **Khan, B., S. Omar, J. N. Kanyara, M. Warren-Perry, J. Nyalwidhe, D. S. Peterson, T. Wellems, S. Kaniaru, J. Gitonga, F. J. Mulaa, and D. K. Koech.** 1997. Antifolate drug resistance and point mutations in *Plasmodium falciparum* in Kenya. *Trans. R. Soc. Trop. Med. Hyg.* **91:** 456–460.
52. **Krettli, A. U., J. M. Cancado, and Z. Brener.** 1982. Effect of specific chemotherapy on the levels of lytic antibodies in Chagas's disease. *Trans. R. Soc. Trop. Med. Hyg.* **76:**334–340.
53. **Krogstad, D. J., I. Y. Gluzman, D. E. Kyle, A. M. J. Oduola, S. K. Martin, W. K. Milhous, and P. H. Schlesinger.** 1987. Efflux of chloroquine from *Plasmodium falciparum:* mechanism of chloroquine resistance. *Science* **238:**1283–1285.
54. **Laga, M., A. Manoka, M. Kivuvu, B. Malele, M. Tuliza, N. Nzola, J. Goeman, F. Behets, V. Batter, M. Alary, W. L. Heyward, R. W. Ryder, and P. Piot.** 1993. Nonulcerative sexually transmitted diseases as risk factors for HIV-1 transmission in women: results from a cohort study. *AIDS* **7:**95–102.
55. **Lossick, J. G., M. Müller, and T. E. Gorrell.** 1986. In vitro drug susceptibility and doses of metronidazole required for cure in cases of refractory vaginal trichomoniasis. *J. Infect. Dis.* **153:**948–955.
56. **Magill, A. J.** 1995. Epidemiology of the leishmaniases. *Dermatol. Clin.* **13:**505–523.
57. **Makler, M. T., J. M. Ries, J. A. Williams, J. E. Bancroft, R. C. Piper, B. L. Gibbins, and D. J. Hinrichs.** 1993. Parasite lactate dehydrogenase as an assay for *Plasmodium falciparum* drug sensitivity. *Am. J. Trop. Med. Hyg.* **48:** 739–741.
58. **Maldonado, R. A., J. Molina, G. Payares, and J. A. Urbina.** 1993. Experimental chemotherapy with combinations of ergosterol biosynthesis inhibitors in murine models of Chagas' disease. *Antimicrob. Agents Chemother.* **37:**1353–1359.
59. **McCabe, R.** 1988. Failure of ketoconazole to cure chronic murine Chagas' disease. *J. Infect. Dis.* **158:**1408–1409.
60. **Meingassner, J. G., and J. Thurner.** 1979. Strain of *Trichomonas vaginalis* resistant to metronidazole and other 5-nitroimidazoles. *Antimicrob. Agents Chemother.* **15:** 254–257.
61. **Müller, M., J. G. Lossick, and T. E. Gorrell.** 1988. *In vitro* susceptibility of *Trichomonas vaginalis* and treatment outcome in vaginal trichomoniasis. *Sex. Transm. Dis.* **15:** 17–24.
62. **Narcisi, E. M., and W. E. Secor.** 1996. In vitro effect

of tinidazole and furazolidone on metronidazole-resistant *Trichomonas vaginalis*. *Antimicrob. Agents Chemother.* **40:** 1121–1125.

63. **Nguyen-Dinh, P., and W. Trager.** 1980. *Plasmodium falciparum* in vitro: determination of chloroquine sensitivity of three new strains by a modified 48 hour test. *Am. J. Trop. Med. Hyg.* **29:**339–342.
64. **Nyirjesy, P., M. Velma Weitz, S. P. Gelone, and T. Fekete.** 1995. Paromomycin for nitroimidazole-resistant trichomonosis. *Lancet* **346:**1110.
65. **Ouellette, M., and B. Papadopoulou.** 1993. Mechanisms of drug resistance in leishmania. *Parasitol. Today* **9:** 150–153.
66. **Pépin, J., and F. Milord.** 1994. The treatment of human African trypanosomiasis. *Adv. Parasitol.* **33:**1–47.
67. **Peterson, D. S., S. M. Di Santi, M. Povoa, V. S. Calvosa, V. E. Do Rosario, and T. E. Wellems.** 1991. Prevalence of the dihydrofolate reductase As-108 mutation as the basis for pyrimethamine-resistant falciparum malaria in the Brazilian Amazon. *Am. J. Trop. Med. Hyg.* **45:** 492–497.
68. **Peterson, D. S., W. K. Milhous, and T. E. Wellems.** 1990. Molecular basis of differential resistance to cycloguanil and pyrimethamine in *Plasmodium falciparum* malaria. *Proc. Natl. Acad. Sci. USA* **87:**3018–3022.
69. **Pica-Mattoccia, L., A. Novi, and D. Cioli.** 1997. Enzymatic basis for the lack of oxamniquine activity in *Schistosoma haematobium* infections. *Parasitol. Res.* **83:**687–689.
70. **Plowe, C. V., J. F. Cortese, A. Djimde, O. C. Nwanyanwu, W. M. Watkins, P. A. Winstanley, J. G. Estrada-Franco, R. E. Mollinedo, J. C. Avila, J. L. Cespedes, D. Carter, and O. Doumbo.** 1997. Mutations in *Plasmodium falciparum* dihydrofolate reductase and dihydropteroate synthase and epidemiologic patterns of pyrimethamine-sulfadoxine use and resistance. *J. Infect. Dis.* **176:** 1590–1596.
71. **Plowe, C. V., A. Djimde, M. Bouare, O. Doumbo, and T. E. Wellems.** 1995. Pyrimethamine and proguanil resistance-conferring mutations in *Plasmodium falciparum* dihydrofolate reductase: polymerase chain reaction methods for surveillance in Africa. *Am. J. Trop. Med. Hyg.* **52:** 565–568.
72. **Quon, D. V. K., C. E. D'Oliveira, and P. J. Johnson.** 1992. Reduced transcription of the ferredoxin gene in metronidazole-resistant *Trichomonas vaginalis*. *Proc. Natl. Acad. Sci. USA* **89:**4002–4006.
73. **Redman, C. A., A. Roberson, P. G. Fallon, J. Modha, J. R. Kusel, M. J. Doenhoff, and R. J. Martin.** 1996. Praziquantel: an urgent and exciting challenge. *Parasitol. Today* **12:**14–20.
74. **Rieckmann, K. H., D. R. Davis, and D. C. Hutton.** 1989. *Plasmodium vivax* resistance to chloroquine? *Lancet* **ii:**1183–1184.
75. **Rieckmann, K. H., L. J. Sax, G. H. Campbell, and J. E. Mrema.** 1978. Drug sensitivity of *Plasmodium falciparum*. An in-vitro microtechnique. *Lancet* **i:**22–23.
76. **Roberts, W. L., and P. M. Rainey.** 1993. Antileishmanial activity of sodium stibogluconate fractions. *Antimicrob. Agents Chemother.* **37:**1842–1846.
77. **Sabah, A. A., C. Fletcher, G. Webbe, and M. J. Doenhoff.** 1985. *Schistosoma mansoni*: reduced efficacy of chemotherapy in infected T-cell-deprived mice. *Exp. Parasitol.* **60:**348–354.

77a. **Secor, W. E.** Personal observation.

78. **Sereno, D., and J.-L. Lemesre.** 1997. Axenically cultured amastigote forms as an in vitro model for investigation of antileishmanial agents. *Antimicrob. Agents Chemother.* **41:**972–976.
79. **Sgambatti de Andrade, A. L. S., F. Zicker, R. M. de Oliveira, S. Almeida e Silva, A. Luquetti, L. R. Travassos, I. C. Almeida, S. S. de Andrade, J. G. de Andrade, and C. M. T. Martelli.** 1996. Randomised trial of efficacy of benznidazole in treatment of early *Trypanosoma cruzi* infection. *Lancet* **348:**1407–1413.
80. **Sgambatti de Andrade, A. L. S., and F. Zicker.** 1997. Should benznidazole be used in chronic Chagas' disease? *Lancet* **349:**653.
81. **Simarro, P. P., and P. N. Asumu.** 1996. Gambian trypanosomiasis and synergism between melarsaprol and eflornithine: first case report. *Trans. R. Soc. Trop. Med. Hyg.* **90:**315.
82. **Slater, A. F. G., and A. Cerami.** 1992. Inhibition by chloroquine of a novel haem polymerase enzyme activity in malaria trophozoites. *Nature* **355:**167–169.
83. **Smeijsters, L. J. J. W., N. M. Zijlstra, F. F. J. Franssen, and J. P. Overdulve.** 1996. Simple, fast, and accurate fluorometric method to determine drug susceptibility of *Plasmodium falciparum* in 24-well suspension cultures. *Antimicrob. Agents Chemother.* **40:**835–838.
84. **Smoak, B. L., R. F. DeFraites, A. J. Magill, K. C. Kain, and B. T. Wellde.** 1997. *Plasmodium vivax* infections in U.S. Army troops: failure of primaquine to prevent relapse in studies from Somalia. *Am. J. Trop. Med. Hyg.* **56:** 231–234.
85. **Stahel, E., D. Mazier, A. Guillouzo, F. Miltgen, I. Landau, S. Mellouk, R. L. Beaudoin, P. Langlois, and M. Gentilini.** 1988. Iron chelators: in vitro inhibitory effect on the liver stage of rodent and human malaria. *Am. J. Trop. Med. Hyg.* **39:**236–240.
86. **Stelma, F. F., S. Sall, B. Daff, S. Sow, M. Niang, and B. Gryseels.** 1997. Oxamniquine cures *Schistosoma mansoni* infection in a focus in which cure rates with praziquantel are unusually low. *J. Infect. Dis.* **176:**304–307.
87. **Stelma, F. F., I. Talla, S. Sow, A. Kongs, M. Niang, K. Polman, A. M. Deelder, and B. Gryseels.** 1995. Efficacy and side effects of praziquantel in an epidemic focus of *Schistosoma mansoni*. *Am. J. Trop. Med. Hyg.* **53:** 167–170.
88. **Su, X., L. A. Kirkman, H. Fujioka, and T. E. Wellems.** 1997. Complex polymorphisms in an ~330 kDa protein are linked to chloroquine-resistant *P. falciparum* in Southeast Asia and Africa. *Cell* **91:**593–603.
89. **Tan-ariya, P., K. Na-Bangchang, T. Tin, L. Limpaibul, C. R. Brockelman, and J. Karbwang.** 1995. Clinical response and susceptibility *in vitro* of *Plasmodium vivax* to the standard regimen of chloroquine in Thailand. *Trans. R. Soc. Trop. Med. Hyg.* **89:**426–429.
90. **Trager, W., and J. B. Jensen.** 1976. Human malaria parasites in continuous culture. *Science* **193:**673–675.
91. **Urbina, J. A.** 1997. Lipid biosynthesis pathways as chemotherapeutic targets in kinetoplastid parasites. *Parasitology* **114:**S91–S99.
92. **Urbina, J. A., K. Lazardi, T. Aguirre, M. M. Piras, and R. Piras.** 1988. Antiproliferative synergism of the allylamine SF 86-327 and ketoconazole on epimastigotes and amastigotes of *Trypanosoma* (*Schizotrypanum*) *cruzi*. *Antimicrob. Agents Chemother.* **32:**1237–1242.
93. **Urbina, J. A., G. Payares, J. Molina, C. Sanoja, A. Liendo, K. Lazardi, M. M. Piras, R. Piras, N. Perez, P. Wincker, and J. F. Ryley.** 1996. Cure of short- and long-term experimental Chagas' disease using D0870. *Science* **273:**969–971.
94. **Verhoeff, F. H., B. J. Brabin, P. Masache, B. Kachale, P. Kazembe, and H. J. Van der Kaay.** 1997. Parasitological and haematological responses to treatment of *Plasmodium falciparum* malaria with sulphadoxine-pyrimethamine in southern Malawi. *Ann. Trop. Med. Parasitol.* **91:**133–140.

95. **Viotti, R., C. Vigliano, H. Armenti, and E. Segura.** 1994. Treatment of chronic Chagas' disease with benznidazole: clinical and serologic evolution of patients with long-term follow-up. *Am. Heart J.* **127:**151–162.
96. **von Seidlein, L., M. T. Duraisingh, C. J. Drakeley, R. Bailey, B. M. Greenwood, and M. Pinder.** 1997. Polymorphism of the *pfmdr1* gene and chloroquine resistance in *Plasmodium falciparum* in The Gambia. *Trans. R. Soc. Trop. Med. Hyg.* **91:**450–453.
97. **Wang, P., M. Read, P. F. G. Sims, and J. E. Hyde.** 1997. Sulfadoxine resistance in the human malaria parasite *Plasmodium falciparum* is determined by mutations in dihydropteroate synthetase and an additional factor associated with folate utilization. *Mol. Microbiol.* **23:**979–986.
98. **Wellems, T. E., L. J. Panton, I. Y. Gluzman, V. E. do Rosario, R. W. Gwadz, A. Walker-Jonah, and D. J. Krogstad.** 1990. Chloroquine resistance not linked to *mdr*-like genes in a *Plasmodium falciparum* cross. *Nature* **345:**253–255.
99. **Wellems, T. E., A. Walker-Jonah, and L. J. Panton.** 1991. Genetic mapping of the chloroquine resistance locus on *Plasmodium falciparum* chromosome 7. *Proc. Natl. Acad. Sci. USA* **88:**3382–3386.
100. **Wilson, C. M., S. K. Volkman, S. Thaithong, R. K. Martin, D. E. Kyle, W. K. Milhous, and D. F. Wirth.** 1993. Amplification of *pfmdr1* associated with mefloquine and halofantrine resistance in *Plasmodium falciparum* from Thailand. *Mol. Biochem. Parasitol.* **57:**151–160.
101. **Wong, C. A., P. Don Wilson, and T. A. Chew.** 1990. Povidone-iodine in the treatment of metronidazole-resistant *Trichomonas vaginalis*. *Aust. N. Z. J. Obstet. Gynaecol.* **30:**169–171.
102. **Woods, K. M., M. V. Nesterenko, and S. J. Upton.** 1996. Efficacy of 101 antimicrobials and other agents on the development of *Cryptosporidium parvum in vitro*. *Ann. Trop. Med. Parasitol.* **90:**603–615.
103. **World Health Organization.** 1973. *Chemotherapy of Malaria and Resistance to Antimalarials*, p. 30–36. Report of a WHO Scientific Group. WHO Technical Reports Series 529. World Health Organization, Geneva, Switzerland.
104. **Yardley, V., and S. L. Croft.** 1997. Activity of liposomal amphotericin B against experimental cutaneous leishmaniasis. *Antimicrob. Agents Chemother.* **41:**752–756.
105. **Yarlett, N., B. Goldberg, H. C. Nathan, J. Garofalo, and C. J. Bacchi.** 1991. Differential sensitivity of *Trypanosoma brucei rhodesiense* isolate to *in vitro* lysis by arsenicals. *Exp. Parasitol.* **72:**205–215.
106. **Yarlett, N., T. E. Gorrell, R. Marczak, and M. Müller.** 1985. Reduction of nitroimidazole derivatives by hydrogenosomal extracts of *Trichomonas vaginalis*. *Mol. Biochem. Parasitol.* **14:**29–40.
107. **Yarlett, N., N. C. Yarlett, and D. Lloyd.** 1986. Ferrodoxin-dependent reduction of nitroimidazole derivatives in drug-resistant and susceptible strains of *Trichomonas vaginalis*. *Biochem. Pharmacol.* **35:**1703–1708.
108. **Zindrou, S., N. P. Dung, N. D. Sy, O. Sköld, and G. Swedberg.** 1996. *Plasmodium falciparum*: mutation pattern in the dihydrofolate reductase-thymidylate synthase genes of Vietnamese isolates, a novel mutation, and coexistence of two clones in a Thai patient. *Exp. Parasitol.* **84:**56–64.

REAGENTS, STAINS, AND MEDIA

IX

VOLUME EDITOR
PATRICK R. MURRAY

SECTION EDITOR
KIMBERLE C. CHAPIN

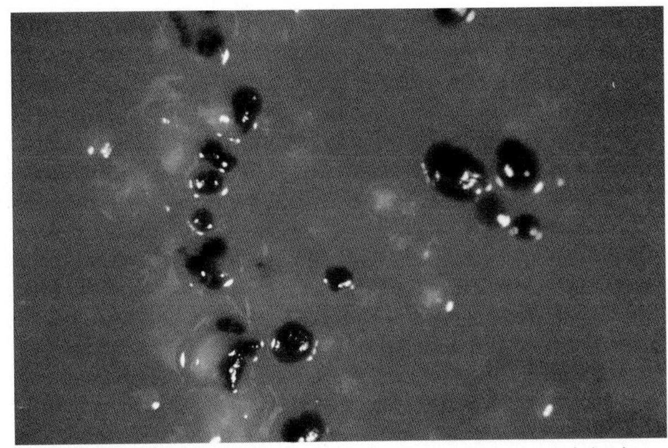

Mixed anaerobic growth on kanamycin-vancomycin laked blood agar.

Reagents

TSAI-LING LAUDERDALE, KIMBERLE C. CHAPIN, AND PATRICK R. MURRAY

128

INTRODUCTION

The reagents listed in this chapter include those determined to be commonly used and a few highly specialized reagents. For information on specific reagents not included here, refer to literature cited in the chapter in which the reagent is mentioned or the general references listed at the end of this chapter. Reagents are listed alphabetically. For the reagent listed, a brief description of its intended use and ingredients are presented. The test protocol is included where appropriate. A fresh 18- to 24-h pure broth culture or well-isolated colonies on plate medium should be used for testing.

Unless stated otherwise, the reagents listed in this section should be prepared by dissolving the reagent components in the stated liquid with a magnetic stirring bar. The standard sterilization technique of autoclaving at 121°C at 15 lb/in^2 for 15 min should be used when needed. However, certain solutions such as those containing antibiotics or carbohydrates cannot be autoclaved because they will be denatured. These solutions are sterilized by filtration through a 0.22-μm-pore-size filter. Additionally, certain reagents require different heat sterilization times. Instructions for reagents that require special preparation or sterilization protocols are included in the discussion of the reagent.

It is critical that distilled, deionized water be used in the preparation of all components. Removal of contaminating pyrogens and minerals from water used for culture is imperative, especially for the success of cell culture systems.

Storage of prepared reagents in sterile, air-tight, screw-cap containers is recommended. Some reagents require storage in dark containers, and some need to be stored refrigerated (2 to 8°C) instead of at room temperature. Special storage instructions are given when appropriate.

Standard safety precautions should be taken when preparing the reagents. Follow the safety guidelines for the chemicals being used, in addition to the laboratory safety protocols. For reagents that are prepared in-house, proper quality control measures must be taken with appropriate positive and negative controls.

■ *N*-Acetyl-L-cysteine–sodium hydroxide (NALC-NaOH)

NALC is a mucolytic agent used for digestion, and NaOH is a decontamination agent used in the processing of specimens for mycobacteriology. Sodium citrate is included in the mixture to exert a stabilizing effect on the acetylcysteine.

4% NaOH, sterile	50 ml
2.9% Sodium citrate, sterile	50 ml
NALC powder	0.5 g

Mix well in a sterile container. Use within 24 h of preparation.

■ Bile solubility (10% sodium deoxycholate)

The bile solubility test is used as a presumptive identification test for *Streptococcus pneumoniae*. Sodium deoxycholate is a surface-active bile salt. It acts upon the cell wall of pneumococci, resulting in cell lysis. The test is performed with alpha-hemolytic streptococcal colonies. Oxgall is a dehydrated bile that can be used, but sodium deoxycholate is preferred.

Sodium deoxycholate	1.0 g
Sterile distilled water	9.0 ml

The pH should be 7.0. Store refrigerated in a sterile dark bottle.

Tube method

Prepare two tubes of organism suspension in 1 ml of buffered broth (pH 7.4). To one tube add a few drops of the 10% sodium deoxycholate solution. To the other tube, add the same amount of sterile physiological saline. Incubate at 35°C. If the organism is bile soluble, the tube containing the bile salt will lose its turbidity in 5 to 15 min and show an increase in viscosity concomitant with clearing.

Agar colony test

Put a couple of drops of sodium deoxycholate on the suspected colonies. Incubate the plate right side up for 30 min at 35°C. Pneumococcal colonies will be lysed, but viridans group streptococci will not.

■ Bovine albumin fraction V, 0.2%

The 0.2% bovine albumin solution is used to buffer specimens for mycobacterial culture following decontamination with NALC-NaOH.

Bovine albumin solution, 5%	40.0 ml
Sodium chloride	8.5 g
Distilled water	960.0 ml

Adjust to pH 6.8 ± 0.2 with 4% NaOH. Sterilize by filtration. Aliquot into sterile screw-cap tubes. Store refrigerated.

Following decontamination and concentration by centrifugation, the sedimented specimen is resuspended in 1 to 2 ml of sterile 0.2% bovine albumin fraction V. This suspension is then used to inoculate media and prepare microscopic smears.

■ Catalase

Hydrogen peroxide (H_2O_2) is used to determine if bacteria produce the enzyme catalase. H_2O_2 (3%) is commercially available.

Slide method

Transfer a test colony to a clean glass slide and add 1 drop of 3% H_2O_2. Development of bubbles is considered a positive result. Extreme care should be taken to avoid picking up any media from a blood-containing agar plate because catalase is present in erythrocytes and any carryover of blood cells can cause a false-positive reaction.

Tube method

Add 1.0 ml of 3% H_2O_2 to an overnight pure culture slant. (Do not use blood agar medium.) Observe for immediate bubbling.

■ Cetylpyridinium chloride-sodium chloride (CPC-NaCl)

CPC-NaCl is used for decontamination of transported sputum specimens for mycobacteriology culture.

Cetylpyridinium chloride	1 g
Sodium chloride	2 g
Distilled water	100 ml

Mix and store in a sealed brown bottle at room temperature. If crystals form, the solution should be gently heated before use.

An equal amount of sputum and CPC-NaCl is mixed until the specimen is liquefied, and then the specimen can be shipped to the testing site. Specimens treated with CPC-NaCl must be cultured on egg-based media or else residual CPC will inhibit mycobacterial growth.

■ Coagulase

The coagulase test is used to differentiate coagulase-producing *Staphylococcus* from other *Staphylococcus* spp. Rabbit plasma reagent is commercially available. Rehydrate and perform the test according to manufacturer's directions.

Slide test

The slide test detects bound coagulase or clumping factor. Emulsify a heavy suspension of staphylococci in a small drop of water on a clean glass slide. If autoagglutination occurs, do not continue; instead, perform a tube test. Add 1 small drop of rabbit plasma reagent to the suspension. Mix with a continuous circular motion while observing for the formation of visible white clumps. Known positive and negative controls should be set up in parallel. Negative or delayed positive (20 to 60 s) results should be confirmed by the tube test.

Tube coagulase test

The tube coagulase test detects bound and free coagulase. Dispense 0.5 ml of rabbit plasma into a sterile tube. Inoculate a loopful of the test organism into the tube. Incubate the tube at 35°C for 4 h. Observe for clotting at intervals during the first 4 h because some staphylococci produce fibrolysin, which could lyse the clot. Do not shake or agitate the tube while checking for clotting. The formation of a clot is considered positive. The majority of coagulase-positive *Staphylococcus aureus* isolates will form a clot within 1 h. Incubate the tube at room temperature overnight if no visible clot is observed after 4 h. Some investigators have recommended incubation at 35°C.

■ Dithiothreitol (sputolysin), 0.0065 M

Dithiothreitol is a mucolytic agent that can be purchased commercially and has been used to prepare sputum specimens for detection of *Pneumocystis* by microscopic examination. Equal volumes of sputum and dithiothreitol are mixed and incubated at 35°C. The mixture is periodically mixed vigorously until it is *almost* completely liquefied (complete liquefaction will disperse the cells of *Pneumocystis*, making microscopic detection difficult).

■ Dyes and pH indicators

A variety of dyes and pH indicators are used in media and reagents. The most common are given in Table 1.

■ Efrotomycin test

The efrotomycin test is used to separate *Enterococcus casseliflavus* and *Enterococcus gallinarium* (resistant) from *Enterococcus faecium* (susceptible). Dissolve 100 mg of efrotomycin (Merck Sharpe & Dohme) in 0.1 ml of dimethyl sulfoxide and dilute in 9.9 ml of sterile distilled water. Dispense 10 μl of this solution onto filter paper disks and dry in the dark

TABLE 1 Dyes and pH indicators

Indicator	pH and color	
Acid fuchsin (Andrade's)	5.0, pink	8.0, pale yellow
Bromcresol green	3.8, yellow	5.4, blue
Bromcresol purple	5.2, yellow	6.8, purple
Bromphenol blue	3.0, yellow	4.6, blue
Bromthymol blue	6.0, yellow	7.6, dark blue
Chlorcresol green	4.0, yellow	5.6, blue
Chlorphenol red	5.0, yellow	6.6, red
Cresolphthalein	8.2, colorless	9.8, red
m-Cresol purple	7.4, yellow	9.0, purple
Cresol red	7.2, yellow	8.8, red
Methyl red	4.4, red	6.2, yellow
Neutral red	6.8, red	8.0, yellow
Phenolphthalein	8.3, colorless	10.0, red
Phenol red	6.8, yellow	8.4, red
Thymol blue	8.0, yellow	9.6, blue
Resazurin	Oxidized: blue, nonfluorescent	Reduced: red, fluorescent
Triphenyl-tetrazolium chloride	Oxidized: colorless	Reduced: red

at room temperature for 5 to 6 h. A heavy inoculum of bacteria is spread with a loop or swab over half of a Trypticase soy blood agar plate, the efrotomycin disk is then placed on the heavy inoculum, and the plate is incubated for 18 to 24 h at 35°C. Organisms with any growth inhibition are considered efrotomycin susceptible. The availability of this antibiotic may be limited. An alternative test is the 1-O-methyl-α-D-glucopyranoside test (see below).

■ Ehrlich reagent

See Indole test.

■ Ferric ammonium citrate, 1%

Hydrolysis of esculin to esculetin is detected when the product reacts with ferric ammonium citrate to form a brown or black complex.

Dissolve 1.0 g of ferric ammonium citrate in 100 ml of distilled water. Store in a dark bottle, refrigerated, for up to 1 year.

After esculin broth is inoculated with the test organism and incubated for 1 to 2 days, a few drops of ferric ammonium citrate is added. A brown-black color develops immediately in positive tests. This test can also be performed by incorporating an iron salt in esculin agar medium.

■ Ferric chloride reagent

Ferric chloride reagent is used in both the phenylalanine deaminase test and the sodium hippurate hydrolysis test.

Ferric chloride ($FeCl_3 \cdot 6H_2O$)	12 g
Hydrochloric acid, 2%	100 ml

Hydrochloric acid, (2%) is prepared by adding 5.4 ml of concentrated hydrochloric acid (37%) to 94.6 ml of distilled water.

The phenylalanine deaminase test is performed by adding 4 or 5 drops of ferric chloride reagent onto overnight growth on phenylalanine agar or broth. If phenylpyruvic acid has formed, a green color develops in the medium (positive reaction). Ferric chloride reagent can also be added to inoculated broths (e.g., heart infusion broth or Todd-Hewitt broth) supplemented with hippurate. Hydrolysis of hippurate produces benzoic acid and glycine. An insoluble brown ferric benzoate precipitate will form in a positive hydrolysis reaction.

■ Fildes enrichment

Fildes enrichment is a source of growth factors used to supplement media for the isolation of fastidious organisms. Commercial preparations are available and include the following ingredients:

Pepsin	4.0 g
Sodium chloride	5.4 g
Sodium hydroxide	70.0 ml
Hydrochloride acid, concentrated	24.0 ml
Sheep blood	200 ml
Deionized water	600 ml

The pH should be 7.0 ± 0.2. Media should be supplemented to a final concentration of 5.0%.

■ Formalin

Formalin is used as an all-purpose fixative that is appropriate for preserving the morphology of helminth eggs and larvae and for protozoan cysts. Two concentrations are commonly used: 5%, which is recommended for the preservation of protozoan cysts, and 10%, which is recommended for the preservation of helminth eggs and larvae. To help maintain organism morphology for long-term storage, the formalin can be buffered with sodium phosphate buffers, i.e., neutral formalin. The most common preparation is 10% formalin, prepared by mixing the following:

Formaldehyde (USP) (or 50 ml for 5%)	100 ml
Saline solution (0.85% NaCl) (or 950 ml for 5%)	900 ml

(Distilled water may be used instead of saline solution.)

Note that formaldehyde is normally purchased as a 37 to 40% HCHO solution. A 10% formalin solution is actually about 4% formaldehyde.

Buffered formalin

Mix 6.10 g of sodium phosphate, dibasic (Na_2HPO_4), and 0.15 g of potassium phosphate, monobasic (KH_2PO_4), thoroughly and store the dry mixture in a tightly closed container. Add 0.8 g of the mixture to 1 liter of 10 or 5% formalin.

■ Formate-fumarate additive

Supplementation of media with formate and fumarate has been used to characterize selected anaerobes (e.g., *Bacteroides ureolyticus* group)

Sodium formate	3.0 g
Fumaric acid	3.0 g
Distilled water	50.0 ml

To adjust the pH, add 20 pellets of NaOH, stirring until the pellets are dissolved and the fumaric acid is in solution. Bring the final pH to 7.0 with 4 N NaOH. Sterilize by filtration. Store refrigerated for up to 6 months. Add 0.5 ml of this solution to 10 ml of thioglycolate broth. Anaerobic growth in supplemented broth is then compared with the growth in unsupplemented broth.

■ β-Galactosidase

See *o*-nitrophenyl-β-D-galactopyranoside.

■ β-Glucuronidase

Detection of β-glucuronidase activity is useful for the rapid identification of *Escherichia coli*, *Streptococcus anginosus* group, and other bacteria. A solution of 0.1% (wt/vol) *p*-nitrophenyl-β-D-glucopyranoside (colorimetric substrate) in 0.067 M Sorensen phosphate buffer (pH 8.0) is prepared. Tubes containing 0.5 ml of the substrate solution are inoculated with a loopful of bacteria from an overnight culture. The tubes are incubated at 35°C and examined after 4 h for the appearance of a yellow color (liberated *p*-nitrophenol). The fluorometric substrate 4-methylumbelliferyl-β-D-glucuronide is commercially available and yields a fluorescent product when hydrolyzed by β-glucuronidase.

■ Glycine-buffered saline

Glycine-buffered saline (0.043 M glycine, 0.15 M NaCl [pH 9.0]) is used in some serological procedures.

Glycine	3.23 g
NaCl	8.77 g
Distilled water	1,000 ml

■ Hemin solution, 5 mg/ml

The hemin solution is one of the additives in thioglycolate medium that makes it enriched for fastidious organisms. Dissolve 0.5 g of hemin in 10 ml of 1 N NaOH. Bring the volume up to 100 ml with distilled water. Sterilize by autoclaving. Store refrigerated for up to 1 month. It is used at a final concentration of 5 μg/ml of medium.

■ HEPES buffer, 1 M

HEPES (*N*-2-hydroxyethylpiperazine-*N*′-2-ethanesulfonic acid) buffer is an organic buffer commonly used in cell culture media in conjunction with sodium bicarbonate.

HEPES sodium salt	260.3 g
Deionized water	900 ml
Adjust pH to 7.3 with 5 N NaOH and then add	
Distilled water	to 1,000 ml

Sterilize by filtration. Store refrigerated in sterile 100-ml bottles. HEPES buffer is usually used in cell culture media at concentrations of 20 to 25 mM.

■ Hippurate test

The hippurate test measures the hydrolysis of sodium hippurate. Hippurate is hydrolyzed to benzoic acid and glycine by some bacteria. The procedure described here detects the presence of glycine with the ninhydrin reagent. Ferric chloride reagents can also be used (see above).

A 1% (wt/vol) solution of sodium hippurate is prepared in 0.067 M Sorensen phosphate buffer (pH 6.4). Tubes containing 0.5 ml of this solution are inoculated and incubated at 35°C for 2 h, after which 0.2 ml of the ninhydrin reagent is added. Development of a deep blue-purple color within 5 min is a positive reaction.

For *Legionella pneumophila*, inoculate a 0.5-ml aliquot of 1% sodium hippurate solution with a loopful of organism and incubate at 35°C in ambient air for 18 to 20 h. Add 0.2 ml of ninhydrin reagent, mix well, and incubate for an additional 10 min at 35°C. Observe for 20 min for blue-purple color development.

Ninhydrin reagent, 3.5%

Ninhydrin	3.5 g
Acetone	50 ml
1-Butanol	50 ml

Mix acetone and butanol in a sterile dark container. Add ninhydrin, mix, and store at room temperature.

■ Indole test

The indole test is used for the determination of the organism's ability to produce indole from deamination of tryptophan by using either the Ehrlich or the Kovács reagent. The Ehrlich reagent is less sensitive than the Kovács reagent. Both reagents should be made in small quantities and should be stored refrigerated. For the Ehrlich and Kovács reagents, dissolve the aldehyde in alcohol and then slowly add acid to the mixture.

Ehrlich reagent

Ethyl alcohol, 95%	95 ml
p-Dimethylaminobenzaldehyde	1 g
Hydrochloric acid, concentrated	20 ml

Test procedure. Add 1 ml of xylene to a 48-h tryptone broth or other appropriate culture. Shake the tube vigorously for 20 s and let stand for 1 to 2 min to allow the xylene extract to come to the top of the broth. Gently add 0.5 ml of the Ehrlich reagent down the side of the tube. Do not shake the tube. A red ring at the interface of the medium and the reagent phase within 5 min represents a positive test.

Kovács reagent

Pure amyl or isoamyl alcohol	150 ml
p-Dimethylaminobenzaldehyde	10 g
Hydrochloric acid, concentrated	50 ml

Test procedure. Add 5 drops of Kovács reagent to either 48-h-old 2% tryptone broth or an 18- to 24-h-old tryptophan broth culture. Do not shake the tube after the addition of reagent. A red color at the surface of the medium is a positive test.

Spot test

p-Dimethylaminocinnamaldehyde	200 mg
Hydrochloric acid, concentrated	2 ml
Distilled water	18 ml

Add the acid to the water, and let it cool before adding the aldehyde.

Test procedure. Moisten a piece of Whatman no. 2 paper with a couple drops of the reagent. Remove a well-isolated colony from an 18- to 24-h-old culture on a blood agar plate with a sterile inoculating loop or a wooden stick and smear it on the moistened filter paper. Observe for a blue to blue-green color within 2 min for a positive reaction. No color change or a pinkish tinge is considered negative. Only a tryptophan-containing agar plate can be used for spot indole testing.

■ Lactophenol cotton blue (Poirrier's blue)

Lactophenol cotton blue is used in mycology as a mounting fluid and a stain for defining morphologic structures.

Phenol crystal	20 g
Lactic acid	20 ml
Glycerol	40 ml
Distilled water	20 ml

Dissolve the ingredients by heating gently over a steam bath. Add 0.05 g of cotton blue dye (Poirrier's blue).

■ Lysozyme test

The lysozyme test measures the ability of organisms, such as *Nocardia*, to grow in the presence of lysozyme.

Basal glycerol broth

Peptone	1.0 g
Beef extract	0.6 g
Glycerol	14.0 ml
Distilled water	200 ml

Mix well and autoclave to sterilize. Store refrigerated. It may be stored for up to 3 months.

Lysozyme solution

Lysozyme	50 mg
Hydrochloric acid, 0.01 N	50 ml

Mix and sterilize by filtration. Store refrigerated. It may be stored for only 1 week.

Add 5 ml of lysozyme solution to 95 ml of basal glycerol broth, dispense in 5-ml aliquots, and keep refrigerated. Growth of the test organism in the lysozyme-supplemented glycerol broth is compared with the growth in the unsupplemented glycerol broth.

■ McFarland standard

For different McFarland standards, mix the designated amounts of 1% anhydrous barium chloride ($BaCl_2$) and 1% (vol/vol) cold pure sulfuric acid (H_2SO_4) as shown in Table 2 in screw-cap tubes. Seal the tubes. When the barium sulfate is shaken up well, the density in each tube corresponds approximately to the bacterial suspension listed in Table 2.

■ Merthiolate-iodine-formalin (MIF)

MIF is a good stain preservative for parasitology and is used with most specimens including stools and aspirates. Protozoa, eggs, and larvae can be detected without further staining in temporary wet mounts, either made immediately after fixation or prepared several weeks later. The MIF preservative is prepared in two stock solutions, stored separately in tightly stoppered brown bottles, and mixed immediately before use.

Solution I

Distilled water	50 ml
Formaldehyde (USP)	5 ml
Thimerosal (tincture of Merthiolate, 1:1,000)	40 ml
Glycerol	1 ml

Solution II (Lugol's solution; good for several weeks)

Distilled water	100 ml
Potassium iodide (KI) crystal	10 g
Iodine crystals (add after KI dissolves)	5 g

TABLE 2 McFarland standard protocol

Standard	Vol (ml)		Corresponding bacterial suspension (10^8/ml)
	1% $BaCl_2$	1% H_2SO_4	
0.5	0.05	9.95	1.5
1	0.1	9.9	3
2	0.2	9.8	6
3	0.3	9.7	9
4	0.4	9.6	12
5	0.5	9.5	15
6	0.6	9.4	18
7	0.7	9.3	21
8	0.8	9.2	24
9	0.9	9.1	27
10	1.0	9.0	30

Combine 9.4 ml of solution I with 0.6 ml of solution II just before use.

Mix 1/4 teaspoon (1 g) of fresh feces in the MIF solution. Within 24 h, if undisturbed, the specimen forms three well-defined layers. The clear orange upper layer consists mainly of formalin, Merthiolate, and water; it does not trap eggs or protozoa. The interface is a thick, pale orange or creamy yellow layer, usually 1 to 2 mm thick; this layer may trap some protozoa and helminth eggs. The bottom layer consists of deeper-staining particulate matter; eggs and protozoa are found throughout this layer. With a glass pipette, MIF direct smears can be made from both the interface and bottom layers. The best results are obtained by making smears from both layers.

■ 1-*O*-Methyl-α-D-glucopyranoside (MGP) (α-methyl-D-glucoside)

The MGP test is used to separate *Enterococcus casseliflavus* and *Enterococcus gallinarium* (positive) from *Enterococcus faecalis* and *Enterococcus faecium* (negative). Heart infusion broth is prepared with 1% MGP and 0.006% bromcresol purple indicator, distributed into 2-ml aliquots, and autoclaved for 10 min. The broth is inoculated with a drop of an overnight broth culture or several colonies from a blood agar plate and incubated for 1 day at 35°C. Prolonged incubation for up to 7 days may be necessary. Development of a yellow color indicates a positive reaction.

■ Nessler reagent

The Nessler reagent is used in the determination of acetamide hydrolysis by some gram-negative bacteria.

Nessler reagent

Dissolve 1 g of mercuric chloride in 6 ml of distilled water. Dissolve 2.5 g of potassium iodide in 6 ml of distilled water and then mix with the mercuric chloride solution. Dissolve 6 g of potassium hydroxide in 6 ml of distilled water. Mix with the above solution and then add 13 ml of distilled water. Filter before use and store in a dark bottle.

Test procedure. Inoculate 1 ml of carbon assimilation medium supplemented with 0.1% acetamide. After incubation for 24 h at 30°C, 1 drop of Nessler reagent is added. A positive reaction is indicated by a red-brown sediment due to the presence of ammonia from the action of acylamidase.

■ Nitrate reduction

The nitrate reduction test is used to determine the ability of an organism to reduce nitrate to nitrite or free nitrogen gas.

Reagent A

N, *N*-Dimethyl-α-naphthylamine	0.6 ml
Acetic acid (5 N), 30%	100 ml

Reagent B

Sulfanilic acid	0.8 g
Acetic acid (5 N), 30%	100 ml

Store each reagent in a brown glass bottle in the refrigerator.

At the time of testing, mix an equal portion of each reagent and then add 10 drops to the overnight growth from the nitrate broth culture. A positive reaction is indicated by the development of a red color within 1 to 2 min, which means that nitrate has been reduced to nitrite. Negative reactions are confirmed by adding a pinch (approximately 20 mg) of zinc dust with development of red color within 5 to 10 min, which indicates that nitrate has not been reduced by the organism. If the tube remains clear, nitrate has been reduced to free nitrogen gas, and a clear tube is considered a positive reaction.

■ *o*-Nitrophenyl-*β*-D-galactopyranoside (ONPG)

The ONPG test is used to determine the ability of an organism to ferment lactose. It is especially useful for identification of members of the family *Enterobacteriaceae*. ONPG-impregnated tablets can be purchased commercially. Commercially prepared reagents are recommended because it is tedious and difficult to prepare the reagent in-house.

■ Oxalic acid, 5%

Oxalic acid is used as a decontamination agent for specimens that contain *Pseudomonas* spp. when culturing for mycobacteria. The reagent is especially helpful when processing respiratory specimens from cystic fibrosis patients.

Oxalic acid	50 g
Distilled water	1,000 ml

Autoclave to sterilize and store at room temperature. The solution has an expiration date of 1 year.

■ Oxidase test

The oxidase test detects the presence of a cytochrome oxidase system. A number of reagents can be used for this test.

Kovács reagent:
 1% tetramethyl-*p*-phenylenediamine dihydrochloride (in water)

Gordon and McLeod's reagent:
 1% dimethyl-*p*-phenylenediamine dihydrochloride (in water)

Gaby and Hadley (indolphenol oxidase) reagents:
 1% α-naphthol in 95% ethanol
 1% *p*-aminodimethylaniline HCl

Kovács reagent is less toxic and is more sensitive than the other reagents. A positive reaction with the Kovács reagent develops within 10 to 15 s and is characterized by the development of a dark purple-black color. However, the dimethyl compound in Gordon and McLeod's reagent is more stable than the tetramethyl compound (Kovács reagent). A positive reaction is characterized by a blue color and develops within 10 to 30 min.

■ Page's saline, 10×

Page's saline is used for the preparation of media for isolation of free-living pathogenic amebae.

Sodium chloride (NaCl)	120 mg
Magnesium sulfate ($MgSO_4 \cdot 7H_2O$)	4 mg
Calcium chloride ($CaCl_2 \cdot 2H_2O$)	4 mg
Sodium phosphate, dibasic (Na_2HPO_4)	142 mg
Potassium phosphate, monobasic (KH_2PO_4)	136 mg
Double-distilled water	1,000 ml

Dissolve the ingredients in the water in the order listed. Sterilize by standard autoclaving. Store refrigerated for up to 6 months.

■ Phenol red indicator

Phenol red indicator is used as a neutralization indicator in the oxalic acid digestion procedure when culturing for mycobacteria.

Phenol red powder	0.8 mg
Sodium hydroxide, 4%	2 ml
Distilled water	to 100 ml

Dissolve phenol red powder in 4% NaOH and then add sufficient distilled water to make 100 ml and mix completely. The solution may be stored at room temperature for up to 1 year.

■ Phosphate-buffered saline (PBS)

10× stock solutions

1. 0.1 M NaH_2PO_4 (sodium phosphate, monobasic). Dissolve 13.9 g of NaH_2PO_4 in 1,000 ml of deionized water.
2. 0.1 M Na_2HPO_4 (sodium phosphate, dibasic). Dissolve 26.8 g of $Na_2HPO_4 \cdot 7H_2O$ in 1,000 ml of deionized water.
3. 8.5% NaCl (sodium chloride). Dissolve 85.0 g of NaCl in 1,000 ml of deionized water. Sterilize by autoclaving for 20 min or by filtration. Store refrigerated.

Working PBS

Prepare a solution of the desired pH by combining the 10× stocks.

0.1 M NaH_2PO_4	See Table 3
0.1 M Na_2HPO_4	See Table 3
8.5% NaCl	100 ml
Deionized water	to 1,000 ml

■ Polysorbate 80

See Tween 80

■ Polyvinyl alcohol (PVA)

PVA is a plastic resin that is normally incorporated into Schaudinn's fixative. The PVA powder serves as an adhe-

TABLE 3 Preparation of pH-specific 0.1 M sodium phosphate buffer[a]

pH	Vol (ml)		pH	Vol (ml)	
	A	B		A	B
5.7	93.5	6.5	6.9	45.0	55.0
5.8	92.0	8.0	7.0	39.0	61.0
5.9	90.0	10.0	7.1	33.0	67.0
6.0	87.7	12.3	7.2	28.0	72.0
6.1	85.0	15.0	7.3	23.0	77.0
6.2	81.5	18.5	7.4	19.0	81.0
6.3	77.5	22.5	7.5	16.0	84.0
6.4	73.5	26.5	7.6	13.0	87.0
6.5	68.5	31.5	7.7	10.5	89.5
6.6	62.5	37.5	7.8	8.5	91.5
6.7	56.5	43.5	7.9	7.0	93.0
6.8	51.0	49.0	8.0	5.3	94.7

[a] A, 0.1 M NaH_2PO_4; B, 0.1 M Na_2HPO_4.

sive for the stool material; i.e., when the stool-PVA mixture is spread onto the glass slide, it adheres because of the PVA component. Fixation is still accomplished by the Schaudinn's fluid itself. Perhaps the greatest advantage in the use of PVA is the fact that a permanent stained smear can be prepared. PVA fixative solution is highly recommended as a means of preserving cysts and trophozoites for examination at a later time. The use of PVA also permits specimens to be shipped to a laboratory for subsequent examination. PVA should be used in the ratio of 3 parts PVA to 1 part fecal specimen. Although there has been interest in developing preservatives without the use of mercury compounds, substitute compounds have not provided the quality of preservation necessary for good protozoan morphology on the permanent stained smear. Copper sulfate has been tried as a preservative for morphologic studies but does not provide results equal to those seen with mercuric chloride. Zinc sulfate has recently proven to be a good mercury substitute and is used with the trichrome stain. Although zinc substitutes have become widely available, each manufacturer has a proprietary formula for the fixative. The formula for PVA is as follows:

PVA	10.0 g
Ethyl alcohol, 95%	62.5 ml
Mercuric chloride, saturated aqueous solution (see Schaudinn's fixative)	125.0 ml
Acetic acid, glacial	10.0 ml
Glycerin	3.0 ml

Mix the liquid ingredients in a 500-ml beaker. Add the PVA powder (stirring is not recommended). Cover the beaker with a large petri dish, heavy wax paper, or foil and allow the PVA to soak overnight. Heat the solution slowly to 75°C. When this temperature is reached, remove the beaker and swirl the mixture for 30 s until a homogeneous, slightly milky solution is obtained.

■ Potassium chloride, 0.2 M (pH 2.2)

Potassium chloride (0.2 M; pH 2.2) is used to treat respiratory specimens for the recovery of *Legionella*.

Potassium chloride (0.2 M)	865.0 ml
Hydrochloric acid (0.2 M)	135.0 ml

Approximately 0.5 ml of specimen is mixed thoroughly with 4.5 ml of the 0.2 M potassium chloride (pH 2.2) solution, and the mixture is allowed to stand for 15 min at room temperature. The mixture is then neutralized to pH 7.0 with 0.1 N KOH and is inoculated onto isolation media.

■ Potassium hydroxide (KOH), 10%

Potassium hydroxide is used for observation of fungal elements in clinical material. The alkali solution dissolves host cellular material, exposing the fungal elements.

Potassium hydroxide	10 g
Distilled water	100 ml

■ Saline

Saline is used as a diluent in a variety of procedures. Normal or physiologic saline is 0.85%.

Sodium chloride	8.5 g
Distilled water	1,000 ml

Other concentrations (e.g., 0.45%) are also used.

■ Schaudinn's fixative

Schaudinn's fixative is designed to be used with fresh stool specimens or samples from the intestinal mucosal surface.

Mercuric chloride, saturated aqueous solution

Mercuric chloride ($HgCl_2$)	110 g
Distilled water	1,000 ml

Use a beaker as a water bath; boil (use a hood if available) until the mercuric chloride is dissolved; let it stand for several hours, until crystals form.

Schaudinn's fixative (stock solution)

Mercuric chloride, saturated aqueous solution	600 ml
Ethyl alcohol	300 ml

Immediately before use, add 5 ml of glacial acetic acid to 95 ml of stock solution.

■ Skim milk, 20%

Skim milk is used to stabilize bacterial suspensions, particularly those containing anaerobes, for freezing.

Skim milk powder	20 g
Distilled water	100 ml

After the skim milk is dissolved in the water, dispense 0.25 to 0.5 ml into ½-dram vials. Autoclave at 110°C for 10 min. The vials can be refrigerated for up to 6 months.

■ Sodium acetate-acetic-acid-formalin (SAF)

SAF lends itself to both the concentration technique and the permanent stained smear and has the advantage of not containing mercuric chloride, as found in Schaudinn's fluid and PVA. After staining with SAF, the organism morphologies will not be quite as sharp as those of organisms originally fixed in solutions containing mercuric chloride. The pairing of SAF-fixed material with iron hematoxylin staining provides better organism morphology than does staining of SAF-fixed material with trichrome. Although SAF has a long shelf life and is easy to prepare, the smear preparation technique may be a bit more difficult for less experienced laboratory personnel who are not familiar with techniques involving fecal specimens. Helminth eggs and larvae, protozoan trophozoites and cysts, and coccidian oocysts and microsporidian spores are preserved by this method. SAF is prepared as follows:

Sodium acetate	1.5 g
Acetic acid, glacial	2.0 ml
Formaldehyde	4.0 ml
Distilled water	92.0 ml

Mix equal parts of egg white and glycerin (Mayer's albumin), and place 1 drop on a microscope slide to which 1 drop of SAF-preserved fecal sediment is added. After mixing, the smear is allowed to dry at room temperature for 30 min prior to staining.

■ Sodium bicarbonate ($NaHCO_3$), 20 mg/ml

Sodium bicarbonate is added to thioglycolate broth to enrich it for the recovery of anaerobes. Dissolve 2 g of

$NaHCO_3$ in 100 ml of distilled water. Filter sterilize and store refrigerated for up to 6 months. Add 0.5 ml to 10 ml of thioglycolate broth.

■ Sodium citrate (0.1 M), 2.9%

Sodium citrate, dihydrate	29.4 g
Distilled water	1,000 ml

Dissolve and autoclave. Store at room temperature. If a precipitate forms, discard and prepare a fresh solution.

■ Sodium hydroxide (1 N), 4%

Sodium hydroxide	40 g
Distilled water	1,000 ml

Dissolve and autoclave. Store at room temperature. If a precipitate forms, discard and prepare a fresh solution.

■ Sodium polyanethol sulfonate (SPS) disks

SPS disks are used to differentiate *Peptostreptococcus anaerobius* (which is inhibited by SPS) from other anaerobic cocci. Dissolve 5 g of SPS in 100 ml of distilled water, filter sterilize, and then dispense 20 μl onto 6-mm-diameter sterile filter paper disks. Allow the disks to dry at room temperature for 72 h. The dried disks are stable at room temperature for up to 6 months. A zone of inhibition of $\geq$12 mm indicates that the organism is susceptible.

■ Sorensen pH buffer solutions (M/15 phosphate buffer solutions)

Solution A

M/15 (0.067 M) sodium phosphate, dibasic. Dissolve 9.464 g of anhydrous Na_2HPO_4 in 1 liter of distilled water.

Solution B

M/15 (0.067 M) potassium phosphate, monobasic. Dissolve 9.073 g of anhydrous KH_2PO_4 in 1 liter of distilled water.

Mix *x* ml of solution A and solution B as indicated in Table 4 for a buffer of the desired pH.

TABLE 4 Sorensen pH buffer solutions

pH	Vol (ml)	
	Solution A	Solution B
5.29	0.25	9.75
5.59	0.5	9.5
5.91	1	9
6.24	2	8
6.47	3	7
6.64	4	6
6.81	5	5
6.98	6	4
7.17	7	3
7.38	8	2
7.73	9	1
8.04	9.5	0.5

■ Tween 80 (Polysorbate 80), 10%

Tween 80 (Polysorbate 80)	10 ml
Distilled water	90 ml

Mix Tween 80 with water until dissolved. Autoclave at 121°C at 15 lb/in^2 for 10 min. Swirl the solution immediately after autoclaving and during cooling to resolubilize the Tween 80. Store refrigerated. The solution can be used for 6 months. Add 0.5 ml of 10% Tween 80 to 10 ml of broth medium when it is used as a medium supplement.

■ Vitamin K_1 (10 mg/ml stock)

Vitamin K_1 (3-phytylmenadione) is an enrichment added to media for the recovery of anaerobes. Mix 0.2 g of vitamin K_1 in 20 ml of 95% ethanol by aseptic technique. Vitamin K_1 is a viscous liquid, and it may be hard to measure the exact amount. Adjust the amount of 95% ethanol accordingly to obtain a 10-mg/ml stock. Store refrigerated in a sterile dark bottle. The stock solution can be further diluted in sterile distilled water. It is added to media at a final concentration of 10 μg/ml in solid media and 0.1 μg/ml in liquid media.

■ Voges-Proskauer test

The Voges-Proskauer test is used to measure acetoin production.

Reagent A: 5% α-naphthol

Dissolve 5 g of α-naphthol in 100 ml of absolute ethanol. Store refrigerated in a brown bottle.

Reagent B: 40% KOH

Dissolve 40 g of potassium hydroxide in 100 ml of distilled water.

Inoculate buffered peptone-glucose broth and incubate until good growth is obtained. Add 0.6 ml of the α-naphthol solution and 0.2 ml of the 40% KOH to 2.5 ml of culture broth. Shake well after the addition of each reagent. A positive reaction, indicated by the formation of a pink-red product, occurs within 5 min.

REFERENCES

1. **Balows, A., W. J. Hausler, Jr., K. L. Herrmann, H. D. Isenberg, and H. J. Shadomy (ed.).** 1991. *Manual of Clinical Microbiology*, 5th ed. American Society for Microbiology, Washington, D.C.
2. **Baron, E. J., and S. M. Finegold (ed.).** 1990. *Bailey and Scott's Diagnostic Microbiology*, 8th ed. The C. V. Mosby Co., St. Louis, Mo.
3. **Engelkirk, P. G., J. Duben-Engelkirk, and V. R. Dowell.** 1992. *Principles and Practice of Clinical Anaerobic Bacteriology*. Star Publishing Co., Belmont, Calif.
4. **Ewing, W. H.** 1986. *Edwards and Ewing's Identification of Enterobacteriaceae*. 4th ed. Elsevier, New York, N.Y.
5. **Garcia, L. S., and D. A. Bruckner.** 1997. *Diagnostic Medical Parasitology*, 3rd ed. American Society for Microbiology, Washington, D.C.
6. **Isenberg, H. D. (ed. in chief).** 1992. *Clinical Microbiology Procedures Handbook*. American Society for Microbiology, Washington, D.C.
7. **Kent, P. T., and G. P. Kubica.** 1985. *Public Health Mycobacteriology—A Guide for the Level III Laboratory*. Centers for Disease Control, Atlanta, Ga.
8. **Larone, D. H.** 1997. *Medically Important Fungi: A Guide*

to Identification, 3rd ed. American Society for Microbiology, Washington, D.C.

9. **MacFaddin, J. F.** 1980. *Biochemical Tests for Identification of Medical Bacteria*, 2nd ed. The Williams & Wilkins Co., Baltimore, Md.
10. **Summanen, P., E. J. Baron, D. M. Citron, C. Strong, H. M. Wexler, and S. M. Finegold.** 1993. *Wadsworth Anaerobic Bacteriology Manual*, 5th ed. Star Publishing Co., Belmont, Calif.
11. **Weyant, R. S., C. W. Moss, R. E. Weaver, D. G. Hollis, J. G. Jordan, E. C. Cook, and M. I. Daneshvar.** 1995. *Identification of Unusual Pathogenic Gram-Negative Aerobic and Facultative Anaerobic Bacteria*, 2nd ed. The Williams & Wilkins Co., Baltimore, Md.

Stains

KIMBERLE C. CHAPIN AND PATRICK R. MURRAY

129

DIRECT EXAMINATION OF SPECIMENS

The first step in the processing of clinical material is the microscopic examination of the specimen. Direct examination is a rapid, cost-effective diagnostic acid. Methods for direct examination are designed to reveal and enumerate microorganisms and eukaryotic cells. Visible microorganisms may denote the presumptive etiologic agent, guiding the laboratory in the selection of the appropriate isolation media and the physician in the selection of the appropriate empirical antibiotic therapy. The quality of the specimen and the measure of the inflammatory response can also be evaluated. In addition, the direct smear serves as a quality control indicator for attempts to isolate observed organisms.

CHEMICAL BASIS OF STAINING

Cellular material and organisms are usually transparent and best distinguished by the use of dyes or biological stains. Antonie van Leeuwenhoek was the first to attempt the differentiation of bacteria with the use of natural colored agents such as beet juice in 1719 (19). With the exception of hematoxylin, natural dyes have for the most part been replaced by artificial dyes. Artificial dyes are products of chemical derivatives from substances in coal tar, especially benzene. Two other important chemical groups, the chromophore and auxochrome, complete the dye compound (14).

Benzene, an aromatic organic compound, undergoes substitution reactions with radicals to form new compounds. Some of the molecular changes result in a colored product. Specific groups that react with benzene and that are associated with color are called chromophores. The most important groups are C═C, C═O, C═S, C═N, N═N, N═O, and NO_2. The greater the number of chromophores in a compound, the deeper the color of the compound. Benzene plus a chromophore group is a chromogen. Although the chromogen is colored, it does not have affinity for bacteria or tissues, and washing or mechanical processes will readily remove the compound. The affinity of the dye is due to an additional group called an auxochrome. The auxochrome group gives the compound the property of electrostatic dissociation or the ability to form salt linkages with the ionizable radicals on proteins, glycoproteins, and lipoproteins on tissue or organism cellular components. This process can occur either directly or through a chelating action of a mordant (17). Dyes are usually sold as salts; thus, it is the auxochrome group that usually determines whether a dye is classified as cationic (basic) or anionic (acidic). Most dyes will retain their cationic or anionic properties throughout the pH range of staining (pH 3 to 9) and thus reliably stain those structures that are oppositely charged. For example, DNA which is acidic will be stained with a basic dye. Crystal violet and safranin are typical cationic (basic) dyes and picric acid is a typical anionic (acid) dye.

DIFFERENTIAL STAINING

While direct visualization of specimens in various wet mounts is useful, differentially stained specimens are the most helpful for presumptive grouping of the majority of pathogens. The Gram stain and acid-fast stain are examples of differential stains. In addition, fluorescent stains (see below) may aid in the identification of organisms when specific attachment of fluorochromes occurs with organism components; auramine, calcofluor white, and fluorescein isothiocyanate (FITC) bound to monoclonal antibodies are examples.

In fixed differential smear preparations, four components are typically used in a progressive manner: the primary stain, a mordant, a decolorizing agent(s), and a secondary stain or a counterstain. The primary stain usually stains all cellular components and organisms in the specimen the same color, as seen in simple procedures with a single stain (e.g., methylene blue). The mordant aids in the attachment of a dye to cellular components. Heat, phenol, and iodine are examples of mordants. Decolorizing agents are typically acids and alcohols, such as the acetone and alcohol mixture used in the Gram stain and sulfuric acid used in the modified acid-fast stain. Removal of the primary stain with the decolorizing agent allows a secondary stain ("counterstain") to be taken up by any decolorized organisms and background material. The secondary stain differentiates between those cells that retain the primary stain and those that do not, such as the purple and pink organisms seen by Gram staining, or between the organism and the background, such as a pink acid-fast organism in a blue-counterstained background.

SMEAR PREPARATION

Smears may be made from clinical material, culture broths, or isolated colonies. These smears should be prepared on clean glass slides since dirt and grease may interfere with adhesion of the sample to the slide and with the staining process. The best smears are prepared after thoughtful selection of those portions of the sample most likely to reveal the etiologic agent (e.g., a purulent portion of sputum). Smears should contain enough material for an adequate survey of the specimen but should not be overly thick because thick smears may peel or flake off the slide during staining procedures. Thick smears also make the timing of decolorization harder to judge. Smears from swabs should be prepared by rolling the swab over the slide. This method of application helps to preserve host cell morphology and microorganism cell arrangements. Tissue smears may be prepared by either touching freshly exposed cut surfaces directly onto a slide or by first using a tissue grinder or stomacher to homogenize the sample. Smears from aspirates or body fluids may be prepared in several different ways, depending upon the amount of material and equipment available. When the quantity of a liquid sample is limited, a single drop placed on a slide will suffice. If more sample is available, the material should be centrifuged (1,500 × *g* for 15 min) to concentrate any cells, and the sediment can then be used to prepare the smear. An additional option for the preparation of smears from liquid samples is the use of cytocentrifugation. The cytocentrifuge method uses nondisposable specimen funnels that are mounted with a slide and filter card and placed in the centrifuge. During centrifugation, the filter card absorbs the supernatant, while cells and microorganisms are centrifuged through a hole in the filter paper strip and are deposited in a continuous layering fashion onto a 6-mm-diameter circular area of the slide. The method is sensitive for the detection of pathogens from sterile body fluids, particularly peritoneal fluids (6, 24). The method has also been used for detection of acid-fast organisms and *Pneumocystis carinii* from respiratory specimens (11). The deposition of specimen in a discrete area and the ability to lyse erythrocytes during centrifugation are particularly advantageous characteristics that allow more rapid and enhanced resolution in a smear examination.

Samples are fixed to the slides with either heat or methanol. Methanol fixation is preferred since heating may produce artifacts and may not adhere the specimen adequately to the slide (18). Once dry, the fixed smear is ready for staining.

STAINING METHODS

The following staining methods and techniques are individual methods used most often in the clinical microbiology laboratory. The staining methods and significant characteristics are described in abbreviated form in Tables 1, 2, and 3.

WET MOUNTS

Wet-mount preparations (Table 1) are used to determine the cellular composition of a specimen as well as the morphology of organisms, gross structure, and their biologic activity including motility. The specimens can be examined by bright-field, phase-contrast, or dark-field microscopy.

Basic Saline Wet Mount

The saline-wet-mount preparation may be used for the detection of protozoan cyst or trophozoites and helminth eggs or larvae directly from liquid stools and from stool concentrates. Vaginal secretions may be examined by this method for the direct detection of fungi, clue cells, and *Trichomonas vaginalis*. It is important not to prepare specimens that are too thick because structures may be undetectable in the debris and background material. Conversely, mounts that contain insufficient sample suffer from poor sensitivity. Slides are examined with the light microscope for characteristic morphology and motility of organisms. Organism motility may be lost if smears are allowed to dry or cool. Drying can be prevented by placing the slides in a humid chamber or by sealing the coverslip with paraffin, nail polish, or Vaseline. Use of the condenser diaphragm to decrease the circumference of the circle of light reduces the amount of transmitted light, increases the contrast, and makes objects more clearly visible. Phase-contrast microscopy also improves the visualization of objects in unstained preparations.

Basic Procedure

Add one drop of liquid specimen to the slide. If working with a swab sample, roll a portion of the material to a small area of the slide. Add one drop of 0.85% warm (37°C) aqueous NaCl to the slide. Mix the sample and saline together. Overlay with a coverslip and examine at ×100 to ×1,000 magnification.

Potassium Hydroxide Mount

Wet mounts prepared in 10% KOH are used to distinguish fungi in thick mucoid specimens or in specimens with keratinous material such as skin, hair, or nails. The proteinaceous components of the host cells are digested partially, leaving the polysaccharide-containing fungal cell wall intact and more apparent (8). An aliquot of specimen is added to a drop of 10% KOH, which can be preserved with 0.1% thimerosal (Sigma Chemical Co.). The slide is held at room temperature for 5 to 30 min after the addition of KOH, depending on the specimen type, to allow digestion to occur. Digestive capabilities can be enhanced with gentle heating or the addition of 40% dimethyl sulfoxide.

10% KOH with LPCB

The wet mount with KOH and lactophenol cotton blue (LPCB) is used for the same purposes as the KOH preparation but incorporates the LPCB dye. LPCB enhances the visibility of fungi because aniline blue stains the outer cell wall of fungi and lactic acid acts as an additional clearing agent (8). The phenol component in LPCB acts as a fungicide.

Colloidal Carbon Wet Mounts (India Ink, Nigrosin)

Colloidal carbon wet mounts are used for visualization of encapsulated microorganisms, especially *Cryptococcus neoformans*. The polysaccharide capsule of organisms will exclude the particles of ink, and the capsules will appear as clear halos around the organism. Artifacts such as erythrocytes, leukocytes, talc particles from gloves, bubbles, and globules after a myelogram may displace the colloidal suspension and mimic yeast. These artifacts make it necessary to perform a careful examination of the wet mount for properties consistent with the organisms (e.g., rounded forms with buds of various sizes and double-contoured cell walls). Interpretation can also be hindered if the emulsion with the colloid suspension is too thick, blocking the transmission of light.

Basic Procedure

Mix equal parts of the patient's cerebrospinal fluid (CSF) with either Pelikan India ink or nigrosin on a slide. Add a coverslip and examine at ×100 to ×1,000 magnification.

TABLE 1 Direct specimen examination methods

Direct examination method	Applications	Principle	Time required (min)	Advantages	Disadvantages
Wet mount	Direct clinical examination of stool, vaginal discharge, urine sediment, aspirates	Used to detect organism motility and morphology of parasitic forms and fungi	1	Rapid and specific	Limited contrast and resolution; Brownian movement may be confused with motility; experienced microscopist required
10% KOH	Direct examination of specimens for fungi, e.g., skin scrapings, fluid aspirates	Proteinaceous host cell components are partially digested by alkali; fungal cell walls stay intact	5–10	Rapid detection of fungi	Background material may cause confusion; experienced microscopist required
10% KOH with lactophenol cotton blue	Direct examination of specimens for fungi, e.g., skin scrapings, fluid aspirates	Adds contrast for detection of fungi	5–10	Dye enhances detection of fungi	Background material may cause confusion; experienced microscopist required
Colloidal carbon (India ink, nigrosin)	Direct examination of CSF and other body fluids for *Cryptococcus neoformans*	Polysaccharide capsule excludes ink particles producing a halo appearance	1	Rapid; diagnostic in CSF when present	Not as sensitive as cryptococcal antigen; cells and artifacts may cause confusion; experienced microscopist required
Lugol's iodine	Direct examination of stool	Nonspecific contrast dye to help differentiate parasitic cysts from leukocytes; cysts retain dye and appear light brown	1	Rapid; enhances differentiation	Background material may cause confusion; experienced microscopist required
Methylene blue	Direct examination of stool for leukocytes; detection of bacteria, particularly poorly staining gram-negative organisms, spirochetes, and *C. diphtheriae*	Leukocytes and bacteria stain blue	1	Rapid; enhances differentiation	Leukocytes may disintegrate if stool is not examined promptly
M'Fadyean staining	Direct examination of clinical specimens from patients suspected to have anthrax	Contrast dye staining *B. anthracis* deep blue	1	Rapid; enhances differentiation	Stain rarely performed
Wayson staining	Direct examination of CSF and other specimens for bacteria	Contrast dye staining bacteria deep blue and other material light blue or purple	1	Rapid; enhances differentiation	Staining reagents unstable; slides cannot be restained with Gram

Lugol's Iodine

Lugol's iodine is a wet-mount modification that incorporates iodine, and it is used in conjunction with the saline mount to examine feces or other material for intestinal protozoa and helminth ova or larvae. Iodine stains protozoan nuclei and intracytoplasmic organelles brown so that they are more easily seen. Because iodine paralyzes bacteria and protozoa, motility cannot be interpreted (2).

Methylene Blue

Methylene blue is a simple direct stain used for a variety of purposes. The stain is used to differentiate organisms by morphological characteristics, to identify the characteristic metachromatic granules of *Corynebacterium diphtheriae*, and to detect the presence of fecal leukocytes. The stain reveals the morphology of fusiform bacteria and spirochetes from oral infections (Vincent's angina). It may also establish the intracellular location of microorganisms such as *Neisseria*. Methylene blue is the stain of choice for identification of the metachromatic granules of diphtheria; however, one should be careful about overstaining, because this will lessen the contrast between the bacteria and the granules. Methylene blue stains organisms or leukocytes a deep blue in a light gray background. *C. diphtheriae* appears as a blue bacillus with prominent darker blue metachromatic granules.

Basic Procedure

Fix the perpared slide in absolute methanol for 1 to 3 min. Air dry the slide and then stain with methylene blue for 30 to 60 s. Rinse in water, blot dry, and examine at ×100 to ×1,000 magnification.

M'Fadyean Stain

The M'Fadyean stain is a modification of the methylene blue stain developed originally for detecting *Bacillus anthracis* in clinical specimens. The rectangular bacteria will stain deep blue surrounded by a pink capsule ("M'Fadyean reaction").

Basic Procedure

The staining reagent is prepared by dissolving 0.05 mg of methylene blue solution per ml in 20 mM potassium phosphate adjusted to pH 7.3. After the prepared slide is air dried, it is fixed in absolute methanol for 3 min. The slide is then dried and flooded with the methylene blue solution for 30 to 45 s. Rinse in water, blot dry, and examine at ×100 to ×1,000 magnification.

Wayson Stain

The Wayson stain is a modification of the methylene blue stain. It has been used for screening cerebrospinal fluid for bacteria and amoebae and examining specimens for *Yersinia pestis*. The advantage of this stain is that the contrast between organisms of proteinaceous background is good. Organisms will stain dark blue, leukocytes stain light blue and purple, and the background is light blue. However, slides stained by this method cannot be restained with the Gram stain. Additionally, the tinctorial qualities of the stain deteriorate over time.

Basic Procedure

The staining reagents are prepared by dissolving 0.2 g of basic fuchsin and 0.75 g of methylene blue in 20 ml of 95% ethyl alchohol. This is poured slowly into 200 ml of 5% phenol. The stain is then filtered and stored in an opaque bottle at room temperature. After the prepared slide is air dried and heat fixed, it is stained for 10 s. Rinse in water, blot dry, and examine at ×100 to ×1,000 magnification.

DIFFERENTIAL FIXED STAINING METHODS

See Table 2.

Gram Staining

Gram staining is the single most useful test in the clinical microbiology laboratory. It is the differential staining procedure most commonly used for direct microscopic examination of specimens and bacterial colonies because it has a broad staining spectrum. First devised by Hans Christian Joachim Gram late in the 19th century, it has remained basically the same procedure and serves in dividing bacteria into two main groups: gram-positive organisms which retain the primary crystal violet dye and which appear deep blue or purple and gram-negative organisms which can be decolorized, thereby losing the primary stain and subsequently taking up the counterstain safranin and appearing red or pink. The staining spectrum includes almost all bacteria, many fungi, and parasites such as *Trichomonas*, *Strongyloides*, and miscellaneous protozoan cysts. The significant exceptions include organisms such as *Treponema*, *Mycoplasma*, *Chlamydia*, or *Rickettsia*, which are too small to visualize by light microscopy or which lack a cell wall. Mycobacteria are generally not seen by Gram staining; however, in smears illustrating heavy infections, the organism may give a beaded appearance that is somewhat similar to that of *Nocardia* spp. or may exhibit organism "ghosts" (9). Gram staining can also be used to differentiate epithelial and inflammatory cells, thus providing information about the state of infection and the quality of the specimen (3, 13, 21).

Gram-positive organisms are thought to retain the crystal violet dye because of the increased number of cross-linked teichoic acids and the decreased permeabilities of their cell walls to organic solvents because they contain little lipid. The cell walls of gram-negative organisms, because of the higher lipid content associated with the cell wall, show increased permeability to decolorizer, and these organisms lose the crystal violet dye (5).

The Gram reaction, morphology, and arrangement of the organisms give the physician clues to the preliminary identification and significance of the organisms. Problems with analysis of the Gram staining generally result from errors in preparation of the slide, such as a smear that is too thick, excessive heat fixing (which can distort organisms), improper decolorization, and inexperience. Overdecolorization results in an abundance of bacteria that appear to be gram negative, while underdecolorizing results in too many bacteria that appear to be gram positive. If a chain of cocci resembling streptococci (normally gram positive) and epithelial cells appears to be gram negative, the slide is overdecolorized. Slides stained by Atkins' Gram staining method are less sensitive to decolorization because the mordant is more effective in retaining crystal violet. This allows better visualization of gram-positive organisms, especially those very sensitive to decolorization such as *Streptococcus pneumoniae* and *Bacillus* spp. Atkins' method does not offer a significant advantage over the conventional Gram staining procedure in visualizing gram-negative organisms, and in fact, such visualization may be more difficult with some specimens such as blood cultures. Laboratories should evaluate both Gram staining procedures and then institute one as the routine procedure.

Two methods of Gram staining are presented here. The first method is the conventional Gram staining method used by most laboratories. The second is an altered Gram staining method devised by Atkins (1) in 1920 that uses gentian violet, a different mordant, and acetone as the decolorizing agent.

Basic Procedure—Conventional Gram Staining

The prepared slide is fixed in 95% methanol for 2 min. After air drying, the slide is flooded with crystal violet (10 g of 90% dye in 500 ml of absolute methanol). After at least 15 s, the slide is washed with water and flooded with iodine (6 g of I_2 and 12 g of KI in 1,800 ml of H_2O). The slide is washed with water after 15 s, decolorized with acetone-alcohol (400 ml of acetone in 1,200 ml of 95% ethanol), washed immediately, and counterstained for at least 15 s with safranin (10 g of dye in 1,000 ml of H_2O). This slide is then washed, blotted dry, and examined at ×100 to ×1,000 magnification.

Basic Procedure—Atkins' Gram Staining

The primary stain is gentian violet (20 g of crystal violet is dissolved in 200 ml of 95% methanol, 8 g of ammonium oxalate is dissolved in 800 ml of distilled water, and the solutions are mixed together and filtered after 24 h). The mordant is Atkins' iodine (20 g of crystals is dissolved in 100 ml of 1 N NaOH; the mixture is then combined with 900 ml of distilled water and stored in a brown bottle at room temperature). Acetone is the decolorizer, and safranin is the counterstain. The staining procedure is the same as that used for the conventional Gram staining procedure.

There is some debate on the length of time that each staining component should be left on the slide. In actual practice, the two dyes and the mordant should each be allowed to remain on the slide for at least 15 s. More time has little effect. Most critical is the amount of time that the decolorizer is used. Unfortunately, the amount of decolorizer is directly related to the thickness of the specimen on the slide. The old benchmark that the slide should continue to receive decolorizer until no more crystal violet is seen to be washing away is still true but is difficult to attain in practice.

Enhancement Techniques

Some enhancement techniques are basic modifications of the Gram staining techniques. These include the use of tartrazine and light green (enhanced Gram stain [Carr-Scarborough]), basic fuchsin, and other combinations. The main purpose of these stains is to make organisms that are normally difficult to detect by Gram staining stand out more prominently. Typically, these enhancement techniques are used for the better visualization of gram-negative organisms. This is done by two methods. One method is to simply stain the organism a darker color so that the normally weakly staining gram-negative organisms are visible (7, 20). A second method is to make the background inflammatory cells and mucus which often masks gram-negative organisms a different color than the usual red-pink. This method is used with the tartrazine-fast green stain, which makes the background gray or green and which makes the organism easily visible (17). In this staining method the Gram reaction of the organisms is preserved.

Wirtz-Conklin Spore Stain

The Wirtz-Conklin spore stain is a differential stain for detection of spores. Spore-forming bacteria will appear red with green-staining spores.

Basic Procedure

After the prepared slide is air dried and heat fixed, it is flooded with 5% aqueous malachite green. The slide is heated gently to steaming for 3 to 6 min and then rinsed under running tap water. Aqueous safranin (0.5%) is used as a counterstain for 30 s. Rinse in water, blot dry, and examine at ×400 to ×1,000 magnification.

ACID-FAST STAINS

Ziehl-Neelsen Stain

The cells of certain organisms contain long-chain (50- to 90-carbon) fatty acids (mycolic acids) that give them a coat impervious to crystal violet and other basic dyes. Heat or detergent must be used to allow penetration of the primary dye into the bacterium. Once the dye has been forced into the cell, it cannot be decolorized by the usual acid-alcohol solvent. The acid-fast stain is useful for identification of a specific group of bacteria (e.g., *Mycobacterium*, *Nocardia*, *Rhodococcus*, *Tsukamurella*, *Gordona*, *Legionella micdadei*) and the oocysts of *Cryptosporidium*, *Isopora*, *Sarcocystis*, and *Cyclospora*. A number of modifications of the Ziehl-Neelsen staining procedure are used to differentiate these various acid-fast organisms (2).

Basic Procedure

The prepared slide is heat fixed for 2 h. The slide is then flooded with carbol-fuchsin (0.3 g of basic fuchsin is dissolved in 10 ml of 95% ethanol, 5 ml of phenol and 95 ml of water are added, and the solution is filtered before use). Heat the slide slowly to steaming and maintain for 3 to 5 min. After cooling, wash with water and decolorize the slide with acid-alcohol (97 ml of 95% ethanol in 3 ml of HCl). Wash and counterstain for 20 to 30 s with methylene blue (0.3 g of dye in 100 ml of H_2O). Wash, blot dry, and examine at ×400 to ×1,000 magnification.

An acid-fast organism will stain red, and the background of cellular elements and other bacteria will be blue, the color of the counterstain.

Kinyoun Modification

The only difference between the Ziehl-Neelsen and Kinyoun stains is the substitution of phenol in the primary stain for steam. The primary stain consists of 4 g of basic fuchsin, 20 ml of 95% alcohol, 8 g of phenol, and 100 ml of distilled water. Both stains have the same sensitivity and specificity, yet the Kinyoun (cold) staining procedure is less time-consuming and is easier to perform.

Modified Acid-Fast Stain

Another modification of the Ziehl-Neelsen stain uses a weaker decolorizing agent (0.5 to 1.0% sulfuric acid) in place of the 3% acid-alcohol. This particular stain helps differentiate those organisms known to be partially or weakly acid fast, particularly *Nocardia*, *Rhodococcus*, *Tsukamurella*, and *Gordona*. Some strains of *Actinomyces* may appear partially acid fast (i.e., speckled red) by the Putt modification.

The acid-fast stains are important clinically and are relatively simple to use. Definitive identification of an acid-fast organism from a clinical specimen cannot be made by staining alone, but certain clues may be helpful. Mycobacteria often appear as slender, slightly curved rods and may show darker granules that give the impression of beading. *Mycobacterium tuberculosis* can appear as beaded bacilli ar-

TABLE 2 Differential fixed staining methods

Differential fixed staining method	Application	Principle	Time required	Advantages	Disadvantages
Gram staining (conventional or Atkins' modification)	Differential bacterial and yeast stains; used to assess suitability of specimen for bacterial culture	Gram-positive organisms retain crystal violet and stain blue; gram-negative organisms do not retain crystal violet and stain pink due to the counterstain safranin	3 min	Rapid; commonly performed; can aid in choice of antibiotic therapy; used to assess specimen for culture and compare smear result to culture result	Organisms with damaged cell walls will stain unpredictably; *Nocardia* and fungi may not take up crystal violet completely; background and cellular elements stain pink, often masking gram-negative organisms
Anaerobic Gram staining variation	Differential stain used to detect anaerobic organisms (especially gram-negative bacteria) not easily seen with regular Gram stain	Basic carbolfuchsin used as counterstain instead of safranin; enhances detection of gram-negative organisms	3 min	Darker staining of gram-negative anaerobes such as *Fusobacterium*	
Tartrazine-fast green Gram staining variation	Differential bacterial stain that enhances detection of organisms	Use of fast green and tartrazine before safranin counterstain allows significant suppression of red-pink color of the background material; organisms still stain purple (gram-positive) or pink (gram-negative)	3 min	Allows excellent enhancement of small gram-negative organisms and detection of mixed cultures	Slight change in color appearance of organisms compared with regular Gram stain may be confusing
Wirtz-Conklin spore staining	Differential stain for detection of bacterial spores	Use of heat allows spores to stain with malachite green	10 min	Facilitates detection of bacterial spores which may otherwise be difficult to observe	Gentle heating of slide may be difficult to control

(Continued on next page)

TABLE 2 Differential fixed staining methods (*Continued*)

Differential fixed staining method	Application	Principle	Time required	Advantages	Disadvantages
Acid-fast staining (Kinyoun, Ziehl-Neelsen, modified)	Detection of acid-fast and weakly acid-fast organisms (e.g., *Mycobacterium*, *Nocardia*, *L. micdadei*, *Rhodococcus*, *Tsukamurella*, *Gordona*, *Cryptosporidium*, *Isospora*, *Cyclospora*, and *Sarcocystis*)	Presence of long-chain fatty acids (mycolic acids) in cell wall or cystic forms make organisms resistant to decolorization; organisms retain the carbol fuchsin dye and appear pink	1 h	Used to detect acid-fast and partially acid-fast organisms; presence generally significant	Low organism number makes slide examination tedious; tissue homogenates often mask presence of organisms because of deeply staining background
PAS staining	Detection of fungi in clinical specimens	Combination of acid hydrolysis and staining; fungi stain pink-magenta	1 h	Most fungi stain	Time-consuming; respiratory specimens must be digested
Toluidine blue O staining	Rapid examination of respiratory specimens for *P. carinii*	Background material removed by sulfation reagent and appears light blue; *P. carinii* cysts stain reddish blue	20 min	Rapid method for detection of *P. carinii* cysts	Differentiation of *P. carinii* from yeast may be difficult; trophozoites not discernible
Wright-Giemsa staining	Detection of blood parasites, viral and chlamydial inclusions, toxoplasmosis, *P. carinii*, and *Rickettsia*	Differential staining of basophilic and acidophilic material	10 min–1 h	Detection of multiple organisms and cellular inclusions	Not specific for inclusions (*Chlamydia* is the exception); cannot determine bacterial Gram reaction
Wheatley trichrome staining	Detection of intestinal protozoan cysts and trophozoites	Provides contrast between parasites and background debris	1 h	Permits detection of diagnostic structures of protozoa	Helminth eggs are generally stained too dark
Modified trichrome staining (Weber-Green)	Detection of microsporidia	Increased stain concentration and staining time permits detection of microsporidia	2 h	Permits detection of microsporidia	
Delafield's hematoxylin staining	Detection of microfilaria	Provides contrast so internal filarial structures can be visualized	45 min	Permits detection of nuclei and sheath of microfilaria	
Iron hematoxylin staining	Detection of intestinal protozoan cysts and trophozoites	Provides contrast between parasites and background debris	60–90 min	Permits detection of diagnostic structures of protozoa	Helminth eggs are generally stained too dark

ranged in parallel strands or "cords"; *Mycobacterium kansasii* may form long, often broad and banded cells; *Mycobacterium avium* complex cells appear as short, uniformly staining coccobacilli. *Nocardia* spp. often branch and almost always show a speckled appearance.

Difficulty in interpretation can result from smears that are too thick or insufficiently decolorized, yielding an acid-fast artifact. As a quality control measure, a known acid-fast organism such as nonpathogenic *M. tuberculosis* HRV 37 and a non-acid-fast organism such as *Streptomyces* spp. can be stained in parallel with the clinical specimen and compared.

Factors such as age, exposure to drugs, and a particular acid-fast organism itself may vary the acid-fast presentation. For example, while *M. tuberculosis* is consistently acid fast (with the Ziehl-Neelsen or Kinyoun stain), *Mycobacterium leprae* and *Nocardia* spp. are not. Therefore, use of the modified acid-fast stain may be necessary for these organisms.

Detection of small numbers of acid-fast organisms in clinical specimens is generally significant. However, the use of acid-fast stains for gastric aspirates in the interpretation of pulmonary disease in adults or for stool specimens from human immunodeficiency virus-positive patients in diagnosing *M. avium-Mycobacterium intracellulare* infection yields very poor specificity (false-positive smears with saprophytic organisms) as well as poor sensitivity (27). In addition, patients receiving adequate therapy may still have positive smears without positive cultures for a number of weeks. Rarely, small numbers of acid-fast organisms in a smear may represent transferred contamination or the use of reagents contaminated with nonviable saprophytic mycobacteria (e.g., *Mycobacterium gordonae*). All smear-positive but culture-negative specimens should be investigated carefully.

MISCELLANEOUS STAINS

PAS

The periodic acid-Schiff (PAS) stain is used to detect fungi in clinical specimens, especially yeast cells and hyphae in tissues. Fungi stain a bright pink-magenta or purple against an orange background if picric acid is used as the counterstain or against a green background if light green is used (8). The procedure is a multistep method combining hydrolysis and staining. The periodic acid step hydrolyzes the cell wall aldehydes, which are then able to combine with the modified Schiff reagent coloring the cell wall carbohydrates a bright pink-magenta.

Basic Procedure

The prepared slide is fixed on formalin-ethanol for 1 min and is then air dried. The slide is then immersed in 5% periodic acid for 5 min, followed by 2 min in basic fuchsin (0.1 g of dye in 5 ml of 95% alcohol and 95 ml of H_2O). The slide is rinsed in water and immersed in zinc or sodium hydrosulfite solution for 10 min (1 g of zinc or sodium hydrosulfite in 0.5 g of tartaric acid and 100 ml of H_2O). Rinse in water and counterstain with saturated aqueous picric acid for 2 min or with light green stain (1 g of dye in 0.25 ml of acetic acid and 100 ml of 80% alcohol) for 5 s. Rinse, blot dry, and examine at ×100 to ×400 magnification.

The PAS stain is an excellent general stain, because most fungi in clinical material will take up the stain. However, the PAS staining procedure is rather involved, requiring several different reagents and time-consuming steps and has been replaced in many laboratories by the calcofluor white staining procedure. The PAS stain cannot be used with undigested respiratory secretions, since mucin will also stain bright pink-magenta.

Toluidine Blue O

Toluidine blue O is used primarily for the rapid detection of *P. carinii* from lung biopsy specimen imprints and bronchoalveolar lavage specimens (2, 22). Toluidine blue O stains the cysts of *P. carinii* reddish blue or dark purple against a light blue background. The cysts are often clumped and may be punched in, appearing crescent shaped. Trophozoites are not discernible. Although the silver stain, monoclonal antibody, and calcofluor white stains are also used, the toluidine blue O stain is an easy and rapid stain to use and yields reliable results with appropriate specimens (e.g., bronchial lavage specimens).

Basic Procedure

After the slide is air dried, place it in the sulfation reagent (45 ml of glacial acetic acid mixed with 15 ml of concentrated sulfuric acid) for 10 min. Rinse in cold water for 5 min, drain, and place in toluidine blue O (0.3 g of dye in 60 ml of H_2O) for 3 min. Rinse in 95% ethanol, followed by absolute ethanol and then xylene. Examine at ×100 to ×1,000 magnification.

Giemsa and Wright Stains

Giemsa and Wright stains are modifications of the Romanowsky stain, which is a combination of methylene blue and eosin. These stains are typically used by the hematology laboratory for demonstrating the differences of nuclei and cytoplasmic features of the blood cell components. Microbiologists will often be consulted about bacteria and parasitic forms seen in smears from a variety of specimen types. The procedure and clinical utility differ slightly for Giemsa and Wright stains. The Wright stain often has the fixative in combination with the staining solution, so both processes occur at the same time, simplifying the procedure and making it convenient for daily use. The Giemsa staining protocol separates the fixative and stain, requiring fixation of the smear before staining. However, the Giemsa stain has superior staining characteristics and a wider spectrum of stainable entities.

The Giemsa stain will detect blood parasites, especially malaria parasites, *Leishmania* spp., *Babesia* spp., and microfilaria. Protozoan trophozoites demonstrate a red nucleus and gray-blue cytoplasm. In bone marrow or peripheral blood smears, it will detect *Histoplasma capsulatum*, which occurs within mononuclear cells as small round to oval blue yeast cells 2 to 5 μm in diameter. The stain is especially useful for visualizing inclusions of viral or other infected cells directly from clinical material, such as corneal scrapings, urine sediments, conjunctival specimens from neonates in whom *Chlamydia trachomatis* infection is suspected, and the scrapings from the base of suspected herpetic vesicles. The stain can also be applied to infected in vitro cell cultures such as a monolayer of chlamydia-infected McCoy cells. Other parasites such as toxoplasma in brain tissue and trophozoites of *P. carinii* from respiratory specimens may also be detected (cyst walls do not stain). Elementary bodies of *Chlamydia* spp. and intracystic bodies and trophozoites of *P. carinii* stain purple, and *Rickettsia* spp. and *Ehrlichia* spp. appear bluish purple. A good quality control measure is the observation of a peripheral blood smear. The blood components stain as follows: erythrocytes, pale red; leukocytes, purple nuclei and pale purple cytoplasm; eosinophilic granules, bright purple-red; and neutrophilic granules, deep pink-purple (16). Neither the tissue Wright stain nor the Giemsa stain reliably stains fungal or bacterial elements; each must be used in conjunction with other staining procedures if the etiology of an infection is unknown.

Basic Procedure—Wright Stain

Because the Wright stain contains alcohol, the slides do not require fixation. Count the number of drops of Wright stain (4 ml of stock solution [1 g of powder in 50 ml of glycerol and 50 ml of 100% methanol], 3 ml of acetone, 2 ml of 0.06 M phosphate buffer [pH 6.5], and 31 ml of H_2O) needed to cover the slide. After 1 to 3 min (the optimum time must be determined for each batch of stain) add an equal number of drops of phosphate-buffered water. Mix by blowing on the surface. After 4 to 8 min flood the slide with phosphate buffer (do not pour off the stain or a precipitate will form). Air dry by draining and examine at ×100 to ×1,000 magnification.

Basic Procedure—Giemsa Stain

Fix the prepared slide in absolute methanol for 1 min. After air drying, immerse the slide in Giemsa staining solution (1 part of commercial liquid stain with 10 to 50 parts of phosphate buffer [pH 7.0 to 7.2]). Because oxidation will destroy the stain, fresh working stain should be prepared from the stock solution each day. Stain for 10 to 60 min (if the staining solution is diluted 1:20, stain for 20 min; if the staining solution is diluted 1:30, stain for 30 min; etc.). Rinse the slide in phosphate-buffered water until the excess stain is removed. Air dry and examine at ×100 to ×1,000 magnification.

Wheatley Trichrome Stain

The Wheatley trichrome staining procedure (30) is a rapid, simple procedure which produces uniformly well-stained smears of the intestinal protozoa, human cells, yeast cells, and artifact material. The specimen usually consists of fresh stool smeared on a microscope slide that is immediately fixed in Schaudinn's fixative or a polyvinyl alcohol (PVA)-preserved stool smeared on a slide and allowed to air dry. Although sodium acetate-acetic acid-formalin (SAF)- and Merthiolate-iodine-formalin-preserved specimens can be stained with trichrome, other stains give better overall results. Protozoan trophozoites and cysts are readily seen with this stain. However, helminth eggs and larvae may retain excess stain, making identification difficult.

Basic Procedure

Slides fixed in Schaudinn's fixative are placed in 70% ethanol for 5 min; slides with PVA-fixed specimens are placed in 70% ethanol plus iodine (1 to 2 g of iodine crystals in 70% alcohol) for 5 to 10 min; slides with fresh specimens are placed in 70% ethanol plus iodine for 1 min. The slides are then placed in 70% ethanol for 5 min, followed by a 3-min treatment, and are then placed in the trichrome stain for 10 min. (Add 1 ml of glacial acetic acid to 0.6 g of chromotrope 2R, 0.3 g of light green SF, and 0.7 g of phosphotungstic acid; after 15 to 30 min at room temperature add 100 ml of distilled water; store in a glass or plastic bottle at room temperature for up to 24 months.) The slides are then placed sequentially into acidified 90% ethanol (99.5 ml of 90% ethanol in 0.5 ml of glacial acetic acid) for 1 to 3 s, rinsed several times in 100% ethanol, exposed to two changes of 100% ethanol for 3 min each, placed in two changes of xylene for 5 to 10 min each, and then examined at ×100 to ×1,000 magnification.

Trichrome Stain for Microsporidia

A number of variations of the trichrome stain have been developed for the detection of microsporidia, but only the Weber-Green modification (29) is described here. This stain is based on the fact that stain penetration into microsporidial spores is very difficult. Thus, the dye content in the chromotrope 2R is higher (10-fold) than that used routinely in the Wheatley trichrome method and the staining time is much longer (90 versus 10 min). The specimen can be fresh stool or stool preserved in 5 or 10% formalin, SAF, or other fixatives. Any specimen other than tissue can be stained by this method.

Basic Procedure

Smear an aliquot of unconcentrated, preserved liquid stool over a 25- by 45-mm area on a clean dry slide. Allow the slide to air dry, place it in absolute methanol for 5 min, air dry, and then stain for 90 min (trichrome stain is prepared by adding 6 g of chromotrope 2R, 0.15 g of fast green, and 0.7 g of phosphotungstic acid to 3 ml of glacial acetic acid; it is allowed to stand for 30 min at room temperature, 100 ml of distilled water is added, and it is stored in a glass or plastic bottle). Rinse for no more than 10 s in acid-alcohol (4.5 ml of glacial acetic acid in 995.5 ml of 90% ethyl alcohol). Dip several times in 95% alcohol; place in 95% alcohol for 5 min, 100% alcohol for 10 min, and xylene for 10 min. Examine the slides under ×1,000 magnification.

Delafield's Hematoxylin Stain

Fresh thick films of blood containing microfilariae can be stained by Delafield's hematoxylin method (10). Nuclei of the microfilariae will stain blue and the cytoplasm will stain various shades of red.

Basic Procedure

Thick films are prepared from fresh blood or concentrated material and are allowed to air dry. The films are laked in 0.85% sodium chloride or distilled water for 15 min and are then air dried. Fix in absolute methanol for 5 min, air dry, and then stain in undiluted Delafield's hematoxylin for 10 to 15 min. (The stain is prepared by dissolving 4 g of hematoxylin crystals in 25 ml of 95% ethyl alcohol and then adding this solution to 400 ml of saturated ammonium alum [180 g of aluminum ammonium sulfate in 1 liter of H_2O, which is heated until the aluminum ammonium sulfate is dissolved and then cooled]. The hematoxylin solution is exposed to sunlight and air for 1 week, filtered, and added to 100 ml of glycerin and 100 ml of 95% ethyl alcohol. The solution is then exposed to sunlight and aged for at least 1 month.) The excess stain is removed in tap water, and then the slides are placed in tap water with several drops of ammonia to intensify the blue color. After 2 to 3 min, rinse in tap water, air dry, and examine at ×100 to ×400 magnification.

Iron Hematoxylin Stain

The iron hematoxylin stain was the stain used for most of the original morphological descriptions of intestinal protozoa found in humans. A permanent stained slide can be prepared for the detection and quantitation of parasites and for examination for the diagnostic features used for their identification. The specimens usually consist of fresh stool smeared on a microscope slide that is immediately fixed in

Schaudinn's fixative, PVA-preserved stool specimens smeared on a slide and allowed to air dry, or SAF-preserved stool smeared on an albumin-coated slide and allowed to air dry. If the staining procedure is performed properly, the cytoplasm of protozoan trophozoites will have a blue-gray color, sometimes with a tinge of black; cysts tend to be slightly darker; nuclei and inclusions have a dark gray-blue color, sometimes almost black. The background material usually stains pale gray or blue, providing some color intensity contrast with the protozoa. Two methods are commonly used: the Spencer-Monroe method and the Tompkins-Miller method. Use of phosphotungstic acid in the Tompkins-Miller method reduces problems with overstained slides and gives excellent results even in unskilled hands.

Basic Procedure—Spencer-Monroe Method (25)

Slides with fresh specimens or specimens in Schaudinn's fixative are placed in 70% ethanol for 5 min followed by 70% ethanol with iodine for 2 to 5 min (70% alcohol with enough D'Antoni's iodine added to produce a strong tea color). These slides and SAF-fixed slides are then placed in 70% ethanol for 5 min, washed under running tap water for 10 min, and then placed for 4 to 5 min in iron hematoxylin solution (10 g of hematoxylin is mixed in 1,000 ml of absolute ethanol, and the mixture is placed in a stoppered flask for at least 1 week at room temperature; 10 g of ferrous ammonium sulfate and 10 g of ferric ammonium sulfate are mixed in 10 ml of hydrochloric acid and 1,000 ml of distilled water; the working stain solution consists of equal volumes of each solution and is prepared weekly). The slides are washed under running tap water for 10 min and in 70% ethanol for 5 min, 95% ethanol for 5 min, two changes of 100% ethanol for 5 min each, and finally two changes of xylene for 5 min each. The slides are air dried and examined at ×100 to ×1,000 magnification.

Basic Procedure—Tompkins-Miller Method (28)

After the treatment of the slides with 70% ethanol with iodine (as described above), the slides are placed in 50% ethanol for 5 min; washed under running tap water for 3 min; and then placed sequentially in the 4% ferric ammonium sulfate mordant for 5 min, running tap water for 1 min, 0.5% aqueous hematoxylin for 2 min, tap water for 1 min, 2% phosphotungstic acid for 2 to 5 min, tap water for 10 min, 70% ethanol (plus a few drops of saturated aqueous lithium carbonate) for 3 min, 95% ethanol for 5 min, two changes of 100% ethanol for 5 min each, and lastly, two changes of xylene for 5 min each. The slides are air dried and examined under ×100 to ×1,000 magnification.

FLUORESCENT STAINING PROCEDURES

See Tables 3 and 4.

Fluorescent microscopy has become commonplace in most clinical laboratories because of ease of use in smear interpretation. Fluorescence is dependent on the ability of fluorophores (naturally fluorescent substances) or fluorochromes (fluorescent dyes) to absorb energy of nonvisible UV and short visible wavelengths, become excited, and emit the energy in the form of longer visible wavelengths. Each fluorochrome has characteristic wavelengths of absorption and emission that yield maximum fluorescence. High-pressure gas lamps of mercury, halogen, and xenon are capable of emitting short-wavelength light that is used with fluorochromes. A series of filters is placed between the light source and the eyepiece. These include a heat filter, a red stop filter that eliminates infrared waves, a wavelength selector or exciter filter that transmits the light of the desired wavelength but that obscures other incident visible light, and a barrier filter. Most fluorescent microscopes use incident illumination or illumination from above that passes through the objective down to the object via a dichromatic mirror beam splitter. The dichromatic mirror has the capability of being able to transmit light of some wavelengths and reflect light of other wavelengths. The light passes through the filters, hits the mirror, and is directed through the objective onto the fluorochrome-stained smear. The longer wavelengths emitted from the fluorescing specimen pass through the objective and the mirror; light passes through the dichromatic mirror because it is now a different wavelength. This emitted light then passes through a barrier filter which blocks scattered excitation light and allows only the longer-emission wavelengths to reach the ocular to form an image. Areas that have bound fluorochrome fluoresce and other areas appear dark.

Acridine Orange

Acridine orange is a fluorochrome that can be intercalated into nucleic acid in both the native and the denatured states (23). The staining procedure is rapid and is more sensitive than the Gram staining procedure in the detection of organisms in blood culture broths, CSF, and buffy coat preparations (14, 15, 20). Acridine orange is also useful in a series of miscellaneous infectious etiologies, such as *Acanthamoeba* infections, infectious keratitis, and *Helicobacter pylori* gastritis (12). Bacterial and fungal DNAs fluoresce orange under UV light, and mammalian DNA fluoresces green. Results for cellular specimens or heavily laden bacterial specimens may be difficult to interpret owing to excessive fluorescence, and some interobserver variability may be noted.

Basic Staining Procedure

After the prepared slide is fixed in methanol and air dried, it is flooded with the acridine orange solution (stock solution, 1 g of dye in 100 ml of H_2O; working solution, 0.5 ml of stock added to 5 ml of 0.2 M acetate buffer [pH 4.0]). After 2 min, rinse the slide with tap water, air dry, and examine with UV light at ×100 to ×1,000 magnification (refer to Table 4).

Auramine-Rhodamine

Auramine and rhodamine are nonspecific fluorochromes that bind to mycolic acids and that are resistant to decolorization with acid-alcohol (5). Staining procedures with these fluorochromes are thus equivalent to the fuchsin-based acid-fast procedures. The stain has become commonplace in laboratories that routinely perform acid-fast examinations because it allows rapid screening of specimens and because the procedure is more sensitive than the traditional acid-fast procedures. Acid-fast organisms fluoresce orange-yellow in a black background. If the secondary stain is not used, the organisms will fluoresce a yellow-green color. Smears with suspicious organisms may be confirmed directly with a Kinyoun stain. However, a single organism or a low number of organisms may be difficult to confirm.

Basic Staining Procedure

The prepared slide is fixed at 65°C for at least 2 h. It is then stained for 15 min with the auramine-rhodamine solution (1.5 g of auramine O, 0.75 g of rhodamine B, 75 ml of glycerol, 10 ml of phenol, and 50 ml of H_2O) and rinsed with water, followed by decolorization for 2 to 3 min with

TABLE 3 Fluorescent staining methods

Fluorescent stain	Application	Principle	Time required	Advantages	Disadvantages
Acridine orange stain	Detection of bacteria in blood cultures, buffy coats, and corneal scrapings; detection of fungi	Fluorochrome intercalates nucleic acid in both native and denatured state; bacterial and fungal DNA fluoresces orange and mammalian DNA green with UV light	3 min	Sensitive method of detection of organisms in blood, CSF, and tissues; detects low numbers of organisms; thick or bloody smears can be used; can Gram stain same slide to confirm staining result	Cellular specimens with an abundance of DNA may be difficult to interpret; interobserver variability seen with some specimens (e.g., buffy coat smears)
Auramine-rhodamine stain	Detection of mycobacteria and other acid-fast organisms	Nonspecific fluorochromes that bind to mycolic acids and resist rinsing by acid alcohol (identical to acid-fast stains); organisms fluoresce orange-yellow with UV light	30 min	Allows rapid screening of specimens at lower magnification; is more sensitive than other acid-fast stains; can use other acid-fast stains on the same slide to confirm suspicious stains	Low numbers of organisms may be difficult to detect
Calcofluor white stain	Detection of fungi and *P. carinii* in clinical specimens	Nonspecific fluorochrome that binds to cellulose of cell walls in fungi and certain procaryotes; fungi fluoresce blue-white or green depending on UV filter used	KOH clearing plus 1 min of staining	Can be mixed with KOH to clear specimen; rapid screening for fungi or *P. carinii*	Background fluorescence may cause difficulty in interpretation with cellular specimens or specimens with bacterial and fungal mixtures
Fluorescein-conjugated antibodies	Detection of specific organisms in clinical material; used for specific organism identification	Monoclonal antibodies bound to the fluorochrome FITC detect antigens for specific pathogens in clinical specimens; pathogens fluoresce apple green	1 h	Specific organism identification; especially useful for *Bordetella*, *Legionella*, *Pneumocystis*, and viral identification	Adequate clinical specimen must be submitted

TABLE 4 Recommended filter sets for fluorochrome stains[a]

Manufacturer	Filter set	Excitation (nm)	Emission (nm)	Fluorochrome stain(s)[b]
Leica	I3	450–490	>515	AO*, AR*, FITC*
	H3	420–490	>515	AO, AR, FITC
	L4	450–490	515–560	FITC
	D	355–425	>470	CW*
Nikon	B-2A[c]	450–490	>520	AO*, AR*
	B-2H	450–490	>515	AO
	B-3A	420–490	>520	CW
	BV-2A	405–445	>475	CW*
	UV-2B	380–425	>460	CW
	B-1E	470–490	520–560	FITC
	B-1A	470–490	>520	FITC*
Olympus	B	450–490	>515	AO, AR*, FITC
	IB	460–490	>515	AO*, FITC*
	UV	330–385	>420	CW*
Carl Zeiss	01	359–371	>400	CW
	02	330–390	>420	CW
	05	400–440	>475	CW*
	09	450–490	>520	AO*, AR*, FITC*
	10	450–490	520–560	AO, AR, FITC

[a] Listing of manufacturer's recommended filter sets as of September 1998. Continued improvements in this technology will determine the filter sets available in the future. Data provided by Paul Millman, Chroma Technology Corp., Brattleboro, VT (1-800-824-7662) in collaboration with the individual microscope manufacturers.

[b] AO, acridine orange; AR, auramine-rhodamine; FITC, fluorescein isothiocyanate; CW, calcofluor white; *, preferred filters, although filter selection is subjective, on the basis of the specific application and prior staining experience of the microscopist.

[c] The Nikon B-2A filter set is commonly used for FITC, although the manufacturer does not specify this application.

0.5% HCl in 70% ethanol. After rinsing, the slide is counterstained with 0.5% potassium permanganate for 2 to 4 min. The slide is rinsed, dried, and examined under UV light at ×100 to ×400 magnification (refer to Table 4).

Calcofluor White

Calcofluor white is a nonspecific fluorochrome that binds to β1, 3-linked polysaccharides, specifically, cellulose and chitin of cell walls in fungi (5). Like the auramine-rhodamine stain, calcofluor white has become commonplace in microbiology laboratories because of the rapidity with which specimens can be observed. The fluorochrome can be mixed with KOH to clear the specimen for easier observation of fungi (8). Staining with calcofluor white has also been described as a rapid method for the detection of *P. carinii*, *Microsporidium*, *Acanthamoeba*, *Naegleria*, and *Balamuthia* spp. (26).

Fungi, *Pneumocystis* cysts, and parasites appear bright green or blue, depending on the UV filter used, against a dark background. Cellular or mixed fungal specimens that contain *P. carinii* and/or fungi may be difficult to interpret, especially with induced sputum specimens. Classic *P. carinii* cysts are generally 5 to 8 μm in diameter, round, and uniform in size, and they exhibit a characteristic peripheral cyst wall staining with an intense internal "double-parenthesis-like" structure. Yeast cells are differentiated from *P. carinii* by budding and intense internal staining (4). Care must be used in interpreting the calcofluor white staining result because nonspecific reactions may be observed. Cotton fibers will fluoresce strongly and must be differentiated from fungal hyphae. Additionally, tissues such as brain biopsy specimens from patients with tumors may fluoresce and resemble *Aspergillus* hyphae.

Basic Procedure

KOH (10%) is mixed in equal proportion with calcofluor white solution (0.1 g of calcofluor white M2R and 0.05 g of Evans blue in 100 ml of H_2O). The specimen is covered with this mixture, a coverslip is applied, and the preparation is examined with UV light at ×100 to ×400 magnification (refer to Table 4).

Antibody Staining Methods

See chapter 12 of this Manual on immunoassays and Table 3 for details on antibody staining methods.

HISTOLOGIC TISSUE SPECIMEN INTERPRETATION

The clinical microbiologist is often asked to consult in smear interpretation of blood and body fluid specimens and of histologically stained sections of tissue. It should be remembered that most fungi, parasites, viral inclusions, and bacteria in these preparations cannot be identified definitively. The stain typically used in the hematology laboratory for blood and body fluids is the Wright-Giemsa preparation, which uniformly stains all bacteria blue. Thus, one must not call a blue coccus a gram-positive coccus until Gram staining can be done to help in differentiation.

In stained tissue preparations, pathogens may be significantly different in appearance owing to the staining and fixative practices used in the histology laboratory. For the best outcome in the histologic diagnosis of infectious etiologies, good communication between the surgical pathologist, microbiologist, and primary physician will result in the securing of tissue for fixation as well as for culture, and the two methods together more often than not provide the definitive diagnosis. In typical tissue preparations, Wright-Giemsa stain does not stain bacteria or fungi reliably, with the important exception of *H. capsulatum*, which will stain by Wright staining of bone marrow and peripheral blood. These preparations also stain infected cell culture monolayers and aid in the visualization of viral and *Chlamydia* inclusion bodies and *Toxoplasma* in tissue. Silver stains are commonly used for the staining of tissue sections. These stains are best for detection of fungi and *P. carinii* cyst walls in tissue (22). However, the stain also can detect bacteria and parasites. Differentiation of various yeast forms of *P. carinii* is difficult, and interpretation should be done with caution and in conjunction with the use of other special stains. Refer to the review by Woods and Walker (31) for a comprehensive summary of the use of cytologic and histologic stains for the detection of microorganisms.

REFERENCES

1. **Atkins, K. N.** 1920. Report of committee on descriptive chart. Part III. A modification of the Gram stain. *J. Bacteriol.* **5:**321–324.
2. **Balows, A., and W. Hausler.** 1988. *Diagnostic Procedures for Bacterial, Mycotic and Parasitic Infection*, 7th ed. American Public Health Association, Washington, D.C.
3. **Bartlett, J. G., K. J. Ryan, T. F. Smith, and W. R. Wilson.** 1987. *Cumitech 7A, Laboratory Diagnosis of Lower Respiratory Tract Infections*. Coordinating ed., J. A. Washington II. American Society for Microbiology, Washington, D.C.
4. **Baselski, V. S., M. K. Robison, L. W. Pifer, and D. R. Woods.** 1990. Rapid detection of *Pneumocystis carinii* in bronchoalveolar lavage samples by using calcofluor staining. *J. Clin. Microbiol.* **28:**393–394.
5. **Berlin, O. G. W., W. L. Drew, M. A. C. Edelstein, L. S. Garcia, and G. D. Roberts.** 1990. Optical methods for laboratory diagnosis of infectious diseases, p. 64–80. *In* E. J. Baron and S. M. Finegold (ed.), *Bailey & Scott's Diagnostic Microbiology*, 8th ed. The C. V. Mosby Co., St. Louis, Mo.
6. **Chapin-Robertson, K., S. E. Dahlberg, and S. C. Edberg.** 1992. Clinical and laboratory analyses of cytospin-prepared Gram stains for recovery and diagnosis of bacteria from sterile body fluids. *J. Clin. Microbiol.* **30:**377–380.
7. **Daly, J. A., W. M. Gooch III, and J. M. Matsen.** 1985. Evaluation of the Wayson variation of a methylene blue staining procedure for the detection of microorganisms in cerebrospinal fluid. *J. Clin. Microbiol.* **21:**919–921.
8. **Emmons, C., C. Binford, K. J. Kwon-Chung, and J. Utz.** 1977. *Medical Mycology*, 3rd ed. Lea & Febiger, Philadelphia, Pa.
9. **Fisher, J. F., M. Ganapathy, B. H. Edwards, and C. L. Newman.** 1990. Utility of Gram's and Giemsa stains in the diagnosis of pulmonary tuberculosis. *Am. Rev. Respir. Dis.* **141:**511–513.
10. **Garcia, L. S., and D. A. Bruckner.** 1997. *Diagnostic Medical Parasitology*. 3rd ed., ASM Press, Washington, D.C.
11. **Gill, V. J., N. A. Nelson, F. Stock, and G. Evans.** 1988. Optimal use of the cytocentrifuge for recovery and diagnosis of *Pneumocystis carinii* in bronchoalveolar lavage and sputum specimens. *J. Clin. Microbiol.* **26:**1641–1644.
12. **Groden, L. R., J. Rodnite, J. H. Brinser, and G. I. Genvert.** 1990. Acridine orange and Gram stains in infectious keratitis. *Cornea* **9:**122–124.
13. **Heineman, H. S., J. K. Chawla, and W. M. Lofton.** 1977. Misinformation from sputum cultures without microscopic examination. *J. Clin. Microbiol.* **6:**518–527.
14. **Henrickson, K. J., K. R. Powell, and D. H. Ryan.** 1988. Evaluation of acridine orange-stained buffy coat smears for identification of bacteremia in children. *J. Pediatr.* **112:** 65–86.
15. **Lauer, B. A., L. B. Reller, and S. Mirrett.** 1981. Comparison of acridine orange and Gram stains for detection of microorganisms in cerebrospinal fluid and other clinical specimens. *J. Clin. Microbiol.* **14:**201–205.
16. **Lillie, R. D.** 1977. The general nature of dyes and their classification, p. 19–39. *In* E. H. Stotz and V. M. Emmel (ed.), *H. J. Conn's Biological Stains*, 9th ed. The Williams & Wilkins Co., Baltimore, Md.
17. **Lillie, R. D.** 1977. The mechanism of staining, p. 40–59. *In* E. H. Stotz and V. M. Emmel (ed.), *H. J. Conn's Biological Stains*, 9th ed. The Williams & Wilkins Co., Baltimore, Md.
18. **Mangels, J. I., M. E. Cox, and L. H. Lindberg.** 1984. Methanol fixation: an alternative to heat fixation of smears before staining. *Diagn. Microbiol. Infect. Dis.* **2:**129.
19. **Marti-Ibanez, F.** 1962. Baroque medicine, p. 185–195. *In* F. Marti-Ibanez (ed.), *The Epic of Medicine*. Clarkson N. Potter, Inc., New York, N.Y.
20. **Mirrett, S., B. A. Lauer, G. A. Miller, and L. B. Rfeller.** 1982. Comparison of acridine orange, methylene blue, and Gram stains for blood cultures. *J. Clin. Microbiol.* **14:** 562–566.
21. **Murray, P. R., and J. A. Washington II.** 1975. Microscopic and bacteriologic analysis of expectorated sputum. *Mayo Clinic Proc.* **50:**339–344.
22. **Paradis, I. L., C. Ross, A. Dekker, and J. Dauber.** 1990. A comparison of modified methenamine silver and toluidine blue stains for the detection of *Pneumocystis carinii* in bronchoalveolar lavage specimens from immunsuppressed patients. *Acta Cytol.* **34:**511–518.
23. **Rose, R. A.** 1982. Light microscopy, p. 1–19. *In* J. D. Bancroft and A. Stevens (ed.), *Theory and Practice of Histological Techniques*, 2nd ed. Churchill Livingstone, New York, N.Y.
24. **Shanholtzer, C. J., P. J. Schaper, and L. R. Peterson.** 1982. Concentrated Gram stain smears prepared with a cytospin centrifuge. *J. Clin. Microbiol.* **16:**1052–1056.
25. **Spencer, F. M., and L. S. Monroe.** 1976. *The Color Atlas of Intestinal Parasites*, 2nd ed. Charles C Thomas Publisher, Springfield, Ill.
26. **Stratton, M., J. Hryniewicki, S. L. Aamaes, F. Tan., L. M. De La Maza, and E. M. Peterson.** 1991. Comparison of monoclonal antibody and calcofluor white stains for the detection of *Pneumocystis carinii* from respiratory specimens. *J. Clin. Microbiol.* **29:**645–647.
27. **Strumpf, I. J., A. Y. Tsang, M. A. Schork, and J. G. Weg.** 1976., The reliability of gastric smears by auramine-rhodamine staining technique for the diagnosis of tuberculosis. *Am. Rev. Respir. Dis.* **114:**971–976.
28. **Tompkins, V. N., and J. K. Miller.** 1947. Staining intestinal protozoa with iron-hematoxylin-phosphotungstic acid. *Am. J. Clin. Pathol.* **17:**755–758.
29. **Weber, R., R. T. Bryan, R. L. Owen, C. M. Wilcox, L. Gorelkin, G. S. Visvesvara, and The Enteric Opportunistic Infections Working Group.** 1992. Improved light-microscopical detection of microsporidia spores in stool and duodenal aspirates. *N. Engl. J. Med.* **326:**161–166.
30. **Wheatley, W.** 1951. A rapid staining procedure for intestinal amoebae and flagellates. *Am. J. Clin. Pathol.* **21:** 990–991.
31. **Woods, G. L., and D. H. Walker.** 1996. Detection of infection or infectious agents by use of cytologic and histologic stains. *Clin. Microbiol. Rev.* **9:**382–404.

Media

KIMBERLE C. CHAPIN AND PATRICK R. MURRAY

130

Koch first propagated microorganisms on artificial gelatin-based medium in 1876. Soon afterward, use of dehydrated media by Frost in 1909 and use of agar in media in 1919 allowed greater consistency of the media and the better growth of microorganisms. Stable solid media tremendously enhanced the study of microbiology. Subsequent discoveries of specific organisms' requirements have resulted in a multitude of media for isolation, identification, and cultivation.

This chapter reviews the basic components necessary in media for the growth and identification of organisms isolated in the clinical microbiology laboratory. Media for the major groups of microorganisms are listed alphabetically in the divisions of bacteriology, mycology, parasitology, and virology. The specific intended use and principle will be provided for each medium. Because media may be purchased from a number of suppliers and minor formulation variations exist for each medium, formulas as well as inoculation and incubation conditions, quality control, and limitations to the use of the media will not be specifically mentioned except in rare instances. Readers are referred to comprehensive references on microbiological media, including the *Handbook of Media for Clinical Microbiology*, 2nd edition (2), by R. M. Atlas and J. W. Snyder, and the package inserts with purchased specialized media for these specific descriptions. In addition, the formulations of a given medium from the different manufacturers do vary slightly and may have been modified from the original description of the medium in the literature. A typical comment from the manufacturer is that the "classical" formula has been adjusted to meet performance standards. Again, the package insert or the formula being prepared from a reference should be followed closely.

GENERAL CONSIDERATIONS

Many components optimize the growth of microorganisms on media. The basic requirements for a medium include a nutrient source, a solidifying agent (for solid media), a specific pH, and any number of specific additives. The nutritional requirements of most microorganisms are complex. Most utilize an array of nutrient sources including nitrogen, carbon, inorganic salts, minerals, and other diverse substances. While some organisms can utilize a very simple medium such as nitrate or ammonia, most require protein hydrolysates or peptones. Peptones are the most common nutrient additives in media and are water-soluble materials prepared by enzymatic or acid hydrolysis of animal tissues or products and vegetable substances. Meat infusions were the initial growth-supporting components in media, but because they are cumbersome to prepare and lack batch-to-batch consistency, they are not truly defined. However, meat infusions are still used in certain media today. Agar serves as the solidifying agent and is derived from red seaweed. The acidity or alkalinity (pH) of a medium is important because microorganisms have strict pH requirements, with most growing in the range of pH neutrality. Components may be added to a medium for purposes of evaluating the pH. These include dyes that change color at a specific pH secondary to the production of acid or alkaline by-products of the organism and buffers that allow determination of the hydrogen ion concentration. Other selective agents, such as antibiotics, dyes, and other nutrient sources, can be incorporated into media for the isolation of a particular organism. Other considerations that allow optimal microorganism growth include the incubation temperature and the gas in the growth environment. Most clinically significant organisms are mesophiles, which means that they will optimally grow at temperatures of between 25 and 40°C. In addition, most species grow optimally in ambient air, but others require CO_2 or the total removal of O_2. Liquid media require all of the ingredients and conditions described above but lack the amount of the solidifying agent seen in tube slants or plated media.

MEDIUM TYPES

Transport Media and Preservatives

Transport media are used in the collection and transport of specimens and were devised initially because fastidious organisms would not survive transport from the bedside to inoculation in the laboratory. Now transport media are even more crucial in providing an appropriate environment for specimens as more and more specimens are transported from distant sites and for long periods of time.

Generally, bacterial transport media come packaged in a plastic tube sleeve or in tubes with a small amount of liquid medium. A single or a double swab attached to a cap is used for collection of the specimen, which is then placed into the tube and secured. The cap allows the swab(s) to be easily removed from the transport medium for inoculation.

Generally, transport media provide a nonnutrient source that sustains the viability of both aerobic and anaerobic organisms without allowing significant growth. Most transport media have specific ingredients that accomplish these goals. These include a small amount of agar to allow a solid base to which the organisms can attach and to reduce desiccation, an indicator oxidation-reduction agent which shows when oxidation has occurred, and reagents that maintain the pH. Other additives allow the survival of specific organisms, such as sodium thioglycolate for anaerobes or charcoal, which reduces the effects of toxic metabolic products and which subsequently enhances the growth of the pathogens. Other ingredients are added for specific purposes and will be noted below. Transport media generally allow stability of specimens for 6 to 12 h at ambient temperatures and should not be refrigerated since some organisms do not survive at colder temperatures. When the specimen arrives in the laboratory, it should be plated as soon as possible. The material in the swab is extracted and placed onto the medium of choice. Care should be taken to inoculate the material from the swab itself and not just the transport medium that is attached to the swab when it is extracted from the tube.

Viruses and chlamydia have different transport requirements. Viral and *Chlamydia* transport media are designed to provide an isotonic solution containing protein, antibiotics to control bacteria, and a buffer to control pH. The media come in 15-ml polypropylene centrifuge tubes that contain approximately 2 to 3 ml of medium, 1-dram freezer vials with up to 2 ml of medium, and a tube and swab form with a gel base. While separate transport media for both viral pathogens and *Chlamydia* exist, more often, laboratories are using systems that can accomplish the culture of both of these pathogens as well as the *Ureaplasma* and *Mycoplasma* groups. The antibiotics used in these media are not inhibitory to either of the bacterial pathogens desired or viruses.

Parasitology transport media are actually preservatives meant to maintain the integrity of the parasite and not to maintain viability. The reagents used in these preparations are discussed in the Reagents chapter (see chapter 128). Propagation and isolation media are described in the Parasitology Media section of this chapter.

General-Purpose, Enriched, Selective, Differential, and Specialized Media

General purpose, enriched, selective, differential, and specialized are the general categories of media that are used for growth and cultivation of microorganisms. Each type of medium is not exclusive; e.g., many selective media are also differential media. An example is MacConkey agar, which is selective for gram-negative organisms but which is also differential in that it is used to identify lactose-fermenting organisms. Descriptions of each type of medium follow.

General Purpose

General-purpose media are those media capable of detecting most aerobic and facultatively anaerobic organisms. An example of a medium in this category is sheep blood agar, which is commonly used for the general isolation of organisms directly from primary specimens inoculated onto the agar.

Enriched

Enriched media are media that allow fastidious organisms to grow because of the presence of specific nutrient additives such as hemin. Fastidious organisms may not grow well on general media. An example in this category is the growth of *Francisella* on chocolate agar because the agar is supplemented with cysteine.

Selective

Selective media are media that contain additives that enhance the presence of the desired organism by inhibiting other organisms. Most commonly, selection is attained with a dye or with the addition of an antibiotic. Examples include MacConkey agar that contains crystal violet, which inhibits most gram-positive organisms, and colistin-nalidixic acid, which contains antibiotics that inhibit most gram-negative organisms. The effectiveness of selectivity varies and is not always complete. Thus, partial breakthrough growth or smaller colonies of the inhibited organisms will grow. In addition, the ingredients that make the medium of a high selective nature may actually inhibit the desired pathogen; e.g., a medium that is selective for *Neisseria gonorrhoeae* (gonococci [GC]) and that contains vancomycin may inhibit some strains of GC.

Differential

Differential media are media that aid in the presumptive identification of organisms based on the organism's appearance on the medium. This can be demonstrated by colony color or a precipitate that forms on or around the colony. Examples include the agars used for the isolation of enteric pathogens, such as MacConkey, Hektoen enteric, and xylose-lactose-desoxycholate agars. In the case of MacConkey agar, lactose fermentation by the organism and exhibition of a bright pink magenta color by the colony mean that the organism is utilizing lactose.

Specialized

Specialized media are those media developed with additives for the purpose of isolating a specific pathogen. Such media include buffered charcoal yeast extract medium (BCYE), which is designed for the purpose of isolating *Legionella* species. Specialized media typically include nutrients that the specific pathogen requires but that are not found in general-purpose or enriched media. In the case of BCYE, cysteine and ferric pyrophosphate are provided. Other examples include virology culture media with essential amino acids that are required for the maintenance of cell lines and growth of viruses and anaerobic media that typically include vitamin K, hemin, and reducing agents.

Susceptibility Media

Media described as susceptibility media actually have multiple uses. In this chapter, when the media are described for use for susceptibility purposes, it will be specifically stated. Most media used for susceptibility testing use hydrolysate of casein and beef extract since these components are low in thymidine and thymine contents. Excess amounts of thymine and thymidine can make organisms appear to be more susceptible to sulfonamides and trimethoprim. Calcium and magnesium ion concentrations are adjusted to allow correct interpretations of *Pseudomonas* susceptibility results with the aminoglycosides, colistin, and tetracycline.

Mycobacteriology Media

Most of the nonselective media used for the isolation and cultivation of mycobacteria are enriched media that are egg based or agar based and that contain additives with fatty acids essential for growth of the organism. Common additives include albumin, which protects the tubercle bacilli from toxic agents, inorganic salts essential for growth, glycerol as a carbon and an energy source, and malachite green, which partially inhibits contaminating bacteria other than mycobacteria and which acts as a pH indicator. Because malachite green is a photosensitive dye, a medium with this ingredient should be stored in the dark. Mycobacteria prefer moisture, and tubes of media should be tightly sealed before inoculation. Liquid media are used for the recovery of small numbers of organisms and for decreasing the time to the detection of mycobacteria. The broths are also used to subculture stock strains and for other tests, such as susceptibility testing and tests with DNA probes.

Anaerobic Media

All general-purpose nonselective anaerobic blood agar media have similar formulations and include peptones, yeast extract, vitamin K (which is required for some *Porphyromonas* spp.), hemin (which enhances the growth of some *Bacteroides* spp.), 5% sheep blood (which allows for the detection of hemolysis), and reducing agents. All allow the isolation and cultivation of both strictly anaerobic and fastidiously anaerobic organisms. The difference in each of the media is the small variation in the peptones used and the inclusion of dextrose in some media as an energy source. These differences may make some of the media better for gram-negative or gram-positive organisms with slight variations in colonial characteristics. However, the differences between media are minimal. Additives used with some of these media allow the media to have both selective and differential properties. Enrichment broths are available in a number of formulations but are increasingly less commonly used for the routine isolation of anaerobes.

Often, when specimens are plated, use of a combination of media enhances the detection of a variety of pathogens. For instance, a sputum specimen for bacterial culture is typically inoculated onto a general-purpose blood agar, an enriched chocolate agar, and a selective and differential MacConkey agar. Knowledge of the specimen source and the patient's diagnosis or symptoms helps to determine the appropriate medium that should be inoculated.

Preparation of Media

When preparing media from dehydrated materials, the manufacturers' instructions should be followed closely. Chemically cleaned glassware and distilled and/or demineralized water should always be used unless specified otherwise. Care in terms of accuracy should be taken when measuring liquid and dry ingredients. Mixing and solubilization of ingredients are typically done on hot plates, with magnetic stir bars placed in the bottom of the flask or beaker. Excessive heating should be avoided. Autoclaving or filtration sterilizes the media. Autoclaving of volumes of up to 500 ml at 121°C for 15 min is adequate. Larger volumes may require up to 20 to 30 min. The stir bars should be removed before sterilization. For quality control of autoclaving, specialized tape or paper is placed on the medium flask at the time of autoclaving. Enrichments such as blood and other labile additives such as filter-sterilized antibiotics should be added aseptically after the base medium has cooled.

Quality Control

The National Committee for Clinical Laboratory Standards (NCCLS) has specific requirements for quality assurance of commercially prepared media, as documented in standard M22-A2 (20). However, these recommendations do not apply to all media. In addition, any medium that is prepared by the user requires its own specific quality control. Storage of media should be in the dark at 2 to 8°C. Storage in the dark is preferred because additives, such as dyes, will deteriorate faster in the light. The date that the medium was received in the laboratory and the medium expiration date should be marked and easily visible when stored. Media should be in use only up to the time of the expiration date. Prolonged or incorrect storage of media, including transport media, can lead to desiccation of the medium, changing the composition of nutrients and selective agents.

Plating of Specimens on Media

Media should be warmed to room temperature before inoculation of specimens. In addition, a medium that has obvious contamination, such as colony growth or turbidity in broth medium, or that looks damaged in any way should not be used. Damage may include such things as a cracked petri dish and agar that has changed color, demonstrates precipitates, or is dehydrated.

ALPHABETICAL LISTING OF MEDIA

Bacteriology Media

■ A7 and A8 agars

A7 and A8 agars are selective and differential media used for the cultivation, identification, and differentiation of *U. urealyticum* and *M. hominis*. Both media contain a soy and casein digest agar base and a supplement solution that contains yeast extract, horse serum, cysteine enrichment solution, and penicillin. Incorporation of urea aids in the identification of urease production to differentiate the organisms on the basis of the appearance of golden to dark brown colonies. There are two main differences between the agars: the use of manganous sulfate in A7 agar and putrescine dihydrochloride and calcium chloride in A8 agar for the detection and enhancement of growth of urease-positive colonies. *Ureaplasma* colonies are small golden brown colonies that are usually identified at 72 h. *Mycoplasma* colonies have a fried egg appearance and may have a golden or amber color.

■ Alkaline peptone water

Alkaline peptone water is an enrichment broth used for the isolation of small numbers of *Vibrio* isolates from stool specimens. Adjustment of the broth to pH 8.4 and inclusion of sodium chloride at a concentration of 0.5 to 1.0% makes it selective for *Vibrio* species.

■ American Trudeau Society (ATS) Medium

American Trudeau Society medium is a nonselective enriched medium used for the isolation and cultivation of mycobacteria. The medium is an egg-based medium. The coagulated egg provides fatty acids essential for support of mycobacterial growth. Glycerol and potato flour provide other nutrients. Malachite green is a partially selective agent that inhibits bacteria. The concentration of malachite green is low, and no other antibiotics are present in this medium; thus, it is very susceptible to proteolytic damage caused by contaminating organisms. This medium is best for specimens not usually contaminated with other microorganisms, i.e., tissue biopsy specimens or cerebrospinal fluid.

■ Amies transport medium with and without charcoal

Amies transport medium is a modification of Stuart's medium. The glycerol phosphate used to maintain the pH in Stuart's medium has been found to enhance the growth of certain organisms that utilize this as a nutrient and to allow overgrowth of potential contaminants. In Amies medium, phosphate buffer replaced the glycerol phosphate ingredient and other salts were added to control the permeability of bacterial cells. Amies medium with charcoal is preferred for the isolation of *Neisseria* spp. because the charcoal neutralizes metabolic products toxic to GC.

■ Anaerobic blood agar (CDC)

The Centers for Disease Control and Prevention (CDC) formulation of anaerobic blood agar is a general purpose medium used for the isolation and cultivation of anaerobic bacteria. The nutritive base is tryptic soy agar supplemented with yeast extract, vitamin K, hemin, and sheep blood. This medium may be optimal for the isolation of gram-positive organisms.

■ 10B arginine broth

10B arginine broth is a medium used for the transport and growth of *Mycoplasma hominis* and *Ureaplasma urealyticum*. The medium contains nitrogenous components, amino acids, and other components necessary for growth; and cefoperazone is added to reduce bacterial contamination. Two primary compounds, namely, urea and arginine, as well as the phenol red indicator, aid in the identification of the organisms. *Ureaplasma* hydrolyzes urea and releases ammonia; *Mycoplasma* deaminates the arginine. Both reactions result in an alkaline pH shift and change the color of the medium from yellow to pink. *Ureaplasma* depletes urea in the medium quickly (<12 h), with subsequent death of the culture. Thus, after the color changes, the cultures need to be subcultured quickly to a medium such as A8 or A7 agar that supports the organisms. Limitations of the medium are that other species of *Mycoplasma* and bacteria may also change the color of the medium.

■ *Bacillus cereus* medium

Bacillus cereus medium is an enriched medium used for the isolation of *Bacillus cereus*. The base includes agar, yeast extract, and buffers. Mannitol combined with bromocresol purple as the indicator dye makes the medium differential. An egg yolk emulsion is added for the detection of the lecithinase activity seen with *B. cereus*.

■ BACTEC 12B medium

BACTEC 12B medium is a liquid nonselective medium used for the isolation and identification of *Mycobacterium* species in conjunction with the BACTEC system. The medium consists of a 7H9 broth base. The radiometric BACTEC system also incorporates ^{14}C-labeled palmitic acid and detects radioactive carbon dioxide. An antibiotic enrichment supplement is added to the medium to make it selective for mycobacteria. This supplement includes the antibiotics polymyxin B, amphotericin B, nalidixic acid, trimethoprim, and azlocillin (PANTA) and polyoxylene stearate as a *Mycobacterium* growth enhancer. A total of 0.5 ml of processed specimen may be accommodated in the vial.

■ BACTEC 13A medium

BACTEC 13A medium, like BACTEC 12A medium, is a liquid nonselective medium used for the isolation and identification of *Mycobacterium* species in conjunction with the BACTEC system. This medium is used specifically for bone marrow and blood specimens. The medium is a Middlebrook 7H13 broth with sodium polyanetholesulfonate (SPS), an anticoagulant. ^{14}C-labeled palmitic acid is incorporated into the medium used in conjunction with the radiometric system. The benefit of this medium is that a large volume of specimen, up to 5 ml, can be directly inoculated into the bottle.

■ *Bacteroides* bile esculin (BBE) agar

Bacteroides bile esculin agar is an enriched, selective, and differential medium used for the isolation and presumptive identification of members of the *Bacteroides fragilis* group. The nutritive base includes casein and soybean peptones, hemin, and vitamin K. The differential characteristic of esculin hydrolysis is identified by the product, esculetin, which reacts with the ferric ammonium citrate to form a complex and produce a brown-black coloration around the colony. The selective agents include bile, which inhibits most gram-positive bacteria and anaerobic organisms other than members of the *B. fragilis* group, and gentamicin, which inhibits facultative anaerobes. Bile esculin agar with kanamycin and enriched with vitamin K and hemin is a formulation that is more enriched and selective than *Bacteroides* bile esculin for the isolation of the *B. fragilis* group. This medium includes beef extract and pancreatic digest of gelatin, vitamin K, and hemin as the nutritive base. Bile inhibits the same organisms described above, and kanamycin is inhibitory for facultatively anaerobic and aerobic gram-negative bacilli.

■ Baird Parker agar base

Baird Parker agar base is a beef extract, peptone, and yeast extract base used to prepare egg-tellurite-glycine-pyruvate agar (ETGPA). ETGPA is an enriched, selective, and differential agar used for the detection of coagulase-positive staphylococci (*Staphylococcus aureus*) from food and other nonclinical sources. Glycerol and lithium make the medium selective by inhibiting many bacteria. Tellurite is also inhibitory to bacteria. The egg yolk emulsion is an enrichment. Tellurite and the egg yolk emulsion also act as differential determinants. When *S. aureus* reduces tellurite, it imparts a black color to the colony, and lecithinase activity is demonstrated by a clearing around the colony. *S. aureus* appears as black-brown colonies with clear zones around the colony.

■ Bile esculin (BE) agar

Bile esculin (BE) agar is a selective and differential medium used for the isolation and differentiation of *Enterococcus* and group D *Streptococcus* from non-group D *Streptococcus*. The nutritive base includes peptone and beef extract. The selective agent is bile (oxgall), which inhibits gram-positive organisms and most strains of streptococci except group D streptococci and *Enterococcus*. Esculin hydrolysis is a characteristic to differentiate enterococci and group D streptococci from other organisms. Esculin in the medium is hydrolyzed to esculetin and dextrose. A black-brown pigment forms when the iron salt (ferric citrate) is used as the color indicator of esculin hydrolysis and subsequent esculetin formation. *Streptococcus bovis* and *Enterococcus faecalis* grow on the medium and exhibit blackening around the colony.

■ Bile esculin (BE) agar plus vancomycin at 6 μg/ml

Bile esculin agar plus vancomycin is a selective and differential medium used to identify vancomycin-resistant streptococci and enterococci. Colonies appear the same as they do on bile esculin agar. Growth of group D streptococci and enterococci occurs with esculin hydrolysis in the presence of bile, appearing as blackening of the medium.

■ Bile esculin azide agar and broth (Enterococcosel)

Bile esculin azide agar or broth is a selective and differential medium for group D streptococci and enterococci. As with bile esculin agar, esculin is incorporated into the medium, and precipitation with ferric ions forms a brown-black pigment, which identifies these species. Bile esculin azide medium has a reduced percentage of bile and makes the medium less inhibitory to non-group D streptococci. Sodium azide is incorporated to inhibit gram-negative organisms.

■ Bismuth sulfite agar

Bismuth sulfite agar is a selective and differential medium used for the isolation of *Salmonella typhi* and other enteric bacilli. Beef extract, peptones, and dextrose are the nutritive base. Bismuth sulfite, a heavy metal, and brilliant green are selective agents which inhibit most commensal gram-positive and gram-negative organisms. Ferrous sulfate is an indicator for hydrogen sulfide production, which occurs when the hydrogen sulfide produced by *Salmonella* reacts with the iron salt. This reaction causes a black or green metallic colony and a black or brown precipitate. Colony morphology and color help differentiate *Salmonella* species. This medium may be inhibitory for some species of *Shigella*.

■ Bordet-Gengou medium

Bordet-Gengou medium is an enriched medium used for the isolation and cultivation of *Bordetella pertussis* from clinical specimens. The medium contains potato infusion, glycerol, and peptones as the nutritive base. Sheep blood allows detection of hemolytic reactions and provides other nutrients for *Bordetella*. The medium can be supplemented with methicillin, which inhibits some of the normal oral flora that is obtained upon collection of the specimen. Culture plates should be held for no more than 7 days.

■ Brain heart infusion (BHI) agar

Brain heart infusion agar is a general-purpose medium used for the isolation of a wide variety of pathogens, including yeast, molds, and bacteria, including *Nocardia* spp. The basic formula includes brain heart infusion from solids as well as meat peptones, yeast extract, and dextrose. One variation that exists is brain heart infusion agar with vitamin K and hemin for the enrichment of anaerobes. The anaerobic formulation may be optimal for the isolation of *Eubacterium* spp. but inferior for the isolation of other anaerobic gram-negative organisms, especially those that produce pigment.

■ Brain heart infusion agar with 7% horse blood and brain heart infusion agar with 1% serum (see Brain heart infusion agar)

Brain heart infusion agar with horse blood or serum enriches the medium for the isolation of *Helicobacter* spp.

■ Brain heart infusion (BHI) broth

Brain heart infusion broth is a general-purpose clear liquid medium that is used to cultivate a wide variety of organisms. It is also used for the preparation of inocula for susceptibility tests and identification. The medium is especially useful as a blood culture medium. The main nutritive base includes infusion from brains and beef heart. Peptones, glucose, sodium chloride, and buffers are other additives. Sodium chloride acts as an osmotic agent, and disodium phosphate acts as a buffer. Formulations with 6.5% NaCl are used for the isolation of salt-tolerant streptococci, formulations with 0.1% agar that reduce O_2 tension and favor anaerobes, and formulations with Fildes enrichment are used for the isolation of fastidious organisms such as *Haemophilus* and *Neisseria*.

Brain heart infusion broth is also used for the preparation of inocula for antimicrobial susceptibility testing and broth dilution MIC testing procedures. The medium contains infusions of brain, casein, and meat peptones.

■ Brain heart infusion-vancomycin agar (see Brain heart infusion agar)

Brain heart infusion-vancomycin agar is a selective medium used for the isolation of vancomycin-resistant enterococci. The base is brain heart infusion agar. Vancomycin is added at 6 μg/ml to select for vancomycin-resistant enterococci.

■ Brilliant green agar

Brilliant green agar is a selective and differential medium used for the isolation of *Salmonella* species except for *S. typhi*. The nutritive base contains meat and casein peptones. Brilliant green dye at a high concentration is the selective agent and inhibits most gram-positive and gram-negative bacteria, including *Shigella* species and *S. typhi*. Phenol red is the pH indicator. Yeast extract provides additional nutrients. Sugars included in the medium are sucrose and lactose. Acid production in the fermentation of these sugars produces yellow-green colonies with a yellow-green zone. Nonfermenters of sucrose and lactose may range in color from white to reddish pink with a red zone around the colony (*Salmonella*).

■ Brucella agar

Brucella agar is a medium designed originally for the purpose of isolating *Brucella* spp. from dairy products. Brucella agar with 5% horse blood can be used as a general-purpose medium for the isolation of both aerobic and anaerobic fastidious organisms. The nutritive base includes a peptone mix, including meat peptones, dextrose, and yeast extract.

■ Brucella agar with cefoxitin and cycloserine

Brucella agar with cefoxitin and cycloserine is a selective and differential sheep blood medium used for the isolation of *Clostridium difficile*. Brucella agar is the nutritive base. Vitamin K and sheep blood provide other growth enhancers.

Cefoxitin and cycloserine inhibit most gram-positive and gram-negative organisms, respectively. *Enterococcus* is not inhibited. Another differential characteristic is that *C. difficile* colonies will fluoresce yellow-green under UV light.

■ Brucella agar with hemin and vitamin K

Brucella agar with hemin and vitamin K is a general-purpose medium used for the isolation and cultivation of anaerobic bacteria. Casein peptones, dextrose, and yeast extract are the nutritive base. Hemin and vitamin K provide further enrichments. Defibrinated sheep blood allows determination of hemolytic reactions. Because of the high carbohydrate content, colonies with beta-hemolytic reactions may have a greenish hue. The medium is better for gram-negative organisms.

■ Brucella agar with 5% horse blood

Horse blood enriches brucella agar for fastidious organisms by providing both hemin (factor X) and NAD (factor V) factors. The use of horse blood also allows determination of hemolytic reactions. However, for *Streptococcus* spp. hemolytic reactions on horse blood differ from those on media with sheep blood. Hemolytic patterns for *Haemophilus* also differ.

■ Brucella broth

Brucella broth is a liquid medium that is used to cultivate *Campylobacter* species and to identify the organisms to the species level. Brucella base that contains peptones, dextrose, and yeast extract is the nutritive base. Sodium bisulfite is a reducing agent.

■ Buffered charcoal yeast extract (BCYE) (selective and nonselective)

BCYE is a specialized enriched agar medium used for the isolation and cultivation of *Legionella* species from environmental and clinical specimens. *Legionella* species, especially *Legionella pneumophila*, require specific nutrients for growth. One is iron and the other is the amino acid L-cysteine. In BCYE these are provided by ferric pyrophosphate and L-cysteine hydrochloride. The nutritive base is yeast extract and alpha-ketoglutarate. (*N*-2-Acetamido-2-aminoethane sulfonic acid buffer maintains the pH of the medium. Charcoal acts as a detoxifying agent and surface tension modifier. Antibiotics may also be added to the medium. Typically, manufacturers provide them in two combinations of three antibiotics. One is polymyxin B, anisomycin, and vancomycin, and the other is polymyxin B, anisomycin, and cefamandole (PAC). In these combinations polymyxin B inhibits gram-negative bacilli, anisomycin inhibits yeast, vancomycin inhibits gram-positive organisms, and cefamandole inhibits both gram-positive and gram-negative organisms. BCYE with PAC may be inhibitory to some strains of *Legionella micdadei*. Nonselective BCYE can support the growth of other fastidious organisms such as *Nocardia* and *Francisella*. BCYE can also be a differential medium with the addition of the dyes bromocresol purple and bromthymol blue. *L. pneumophila* produces light blue colonies with a pale green tint. This differential medium is also called Wadowsky-Lee medium.

■ Buffered glycerol saline

Buffered glycerol saline is a multipurpose transport medium. The transport medium has been used for the isolation of bacteria as well as viruses. In addition, glycerol-containing media may also be used for long-term storage of isolates and transport and storage of biopsy specimens.

■ *Burkholderia cepacia* selective agar

Burkholderia cepacia selective agar is an enriched and selective medium used for the isolation of *Burkholderia cepacia*. Trypticase peptone, yeast extract, sodium chloride, sucrose, and lactose are the nutritive base. The medium is made selective by the addition of polymyxin B, gentamicin, vancomycin, and crystal violet. The medium supports the growth of *B. cepacia* and inhibits >90% of other isolates. It may be less inhibitory than *Pseudomonas cepacia* agar and more selective than oxidative-fermentative polymyxin B-bacitracin-lactose (OFPBL) medium.

■ *Campylobacter* blood agar

Campylobacter blood agar is an enriched selective blood agar medium used for the isolation of *Campylobacter* species. The nutritive base is brucella agar. Sheep blood provides heme and other growth factors. The selectivity of the medium comes from the incorporation of five antimicrobial agents. These agents inhibit normal stool flora such as members of the family *Enterobacteriaceae*, staphylococci, and yeast. Trimethoprim, vancomycin, amphotericin B, polymyxin B, and cephalothin are the five agents. Plates should be incubated in a microaerophilic environment. Due to the dextrose content of the brucella base, weak oxidase reactions may be exhibited. Some species of campylobacter, e.g., *Campylobacter fetus* subsp. *fetus*, are inhibited by cephalosporins.

■ *Campylobacter* thioglycolate medium

Campylobacter thioglycolate medium is a selective holding medium used for the isolation of *Campylobacter* species. The low concentration of agar in thioglycolate broth provides a reduced oxygen content. The selective agents include the same as those in *Campylobacter* agar: trimethoprim, vancomycin, polymyxin B, cephalothin, and amphotericin B.

■ Cary-Blair transport medium

Cary-Blair transport medium was specifically designed to enhance the survival of enteric bacterial pathogens. The medium has a low nutrient content, which allows organism survival without replication; sodium thioglycolate, which allows a low oxidation-reduction potential; and a high pH, which minimizes the destruction of bacteria when acid is produced.

■ Cefoperazone-vancomycin-amphotericin B (CVA) medium

Cefoperazone-vancomycin-amphotericin B medium is a selective and enriched blood agar medium used for the isolation of *Campylobacter* species. The nutritive agar base is brucella agar. Sheep blood provides hemin and other growth nutrients. The antibiotics in this medium are vancomycin, amphotericin B, and cefoperazone, which inhibit gram-positive organisms, fungi, and aerobic and anaerobic gram-positive and gram-negative organisms, respectively. The limitations of this medium are that some campylobacters (e.g., *C. fetus* subsp. *fetus*) are inhibited and that weak oxidase reactions may occur due to the dextrose in the brucella agar base.

■ Cefsulodin-irgasan-novobiocin (CIN) medium

CIN or Yersinia Selective Agar is a selective and differential medium used for the isolation and differentiation of *Yersinia enterocolitica* from clinical specimens and food sources. The nutritive base includes peptones and beef and yeast extracts. The selective agents are sodium desoxycholate, crystal violet, cefsulodin, irgasan (triclosan), and novobiocin. Mannitol is the sugar, and neutral red is the indicator. Organisms that ferment mannitol in the presence of the neutral red dye cause a pH drop around the colony. The colony becomes transparent, with the absorption of the red dye to form a red bulls-eye appearance in the center. Most other bacteria including other enteric mannitol fermenters are inhibited. Some *Yersinia* may require cold enrichment at 4°C and subsequent subculture to CIN medium.

■ Cetrimide agar

Cetrimide agar is a selective and differential medium used for the identification of *Pseudomonas aeruginosa.* Cetrimide is the selective agent and inhibits most bacteria by acting as a detergent. *Pseudomonas* produces a number of pigments. Two pigments can be detected with this medium. The magnesium chloride and potassium sulfate stimulate the blue-green pyocyanin pigment, and the fluorescent yellow-green pigment can be seen with a UV light. The low iron content of the medium stimulates pigment production.

■ Charcoal selective medium

Charcoal selective medium is an enriched selective medium used for the isolation of *Campylobacter* species. In this medium the nutritive base is a Columbia agar base, and charcoal is used to effectively replace blood components. The selective agents used in this medium include vancomycin, cefoperazone, and cycloheximide. Vancomycin and cefoperazone effectively inhibit gram-positive and gram-negative organisms, including *Pseudomonas.* Fungi are inhibited by cycloheximide. The limitation of this medium is that some *Campylobacter* species, e.g., *C. fetus* subsp. *fetus*, are inhibited by cephalosporins.

■ Chocolate agar

Chocolate agar is a general-purpose medium used for the isolation and detection of a wide variety of microorganisms, including fastidious species such as *Neisseria* and *Haemophilus*. Chocolate agar originated as a GC agar base which includes meat and casein peptones, phosphate buffer to maintain pH, and corn starch to detoxify fatty acids in the medium. Hemoglobin is added to the medium to provide hemin or X factor. The appearance of hemin in dry powdered form is reddish brown. When hemoglobin is hydrated and added to the medium, it gives the agar base the "chocolate" appearance. Another enrichment added is a defined supplement, such as IsoVitaleX, which provides NAD or V factor. Both of these components added to the GC agar base make the enriched chocolate agar. Levinthal agar is a variation on chocolate agar. The medium is a selective and differential medium used for the isolation and identification of *Haemophilus influenzae* type b. The medium is a chocolate agar base that is made transparent by the removal of particulate matter either by centrifugation or filtration through sterile filter paper. The medium contains bacitracin to inhibit respiratory flora and *H. influenzae* type b antiserum, allowing detection of an immunoprecipitation reaction.

■ Chopped meat glucose broth

Chopped meat glucose broth is an enriched medium that supports the growth of most anaerobes. It is most commonly used to isolate *Clostridium botulinum* from mixed bacterial growth. Beef heart, peptones, and dextrose supply the essential nutrients. The —SH groups from cooked and denatured muscle protein are the reducing agents in the medium. Vitamin K and hemin are additives used to maximize the growth of specific anaerobes.

■ Columbia agar with 5% sheep blood

Columbia agar with 5% sheep blood is a general-purpose medium used for the isolation of a variety of microorganisms including fastidious organisms. This medium contains meat and casein peptones and beef extract, yeast extract, and corn starch as the nutritive base. Sheep blood allows determination of hemolytic reactions and provides X factor. However, the substantial carbohydrate content may make beta-hemolytic streptococci appear to be alpha-hemolytic or take on a greenish hue. NADase enzyme in sheep blood destroys the V factor (NAD); thus, organisms that require this factor do not grow.

■ Columbia broth

Columbia broth is a general-purpose clear liquid medium used especially for blood culture medium. The broth supports the growth of a wide range of microorganisms. The base is similar to Columbia agar with meat peptones, casein, and yeast extract. Salt and Tris buffers have been added to enhance the growth of microorganisms and increase the buffering capacity, respectively. For the purpose of blood culture medium, additional ingredients include carbon dioxide, which is stimulatory for many organisms; cysteine, which improves isolation of anaerobic and aerobic organisms from blood; SPS, a polyanionic anticoagulant which inactivates aminoglycosides and which interferes with the complement, lysozyme activity, and the phagocytic activity inherent in a blood specimen; and glucose, which provides a hypertonic medium for the isolation of cell wall-deficient forms.

■ Columbia-colistin-nalidixic acid (CNA) agar with 5% sheep blood

Columbia-colistin-nalidixic acid agar with 5% sheep blood is a selective and differential medium commonly used in the isolation of gram-positive organisms from mixed clinical specimens. The base is Columbia agar with 5% sheep blood that allows the detection of hemolytic reactions and provides additional enrichment and X factor (heme). The medium is made selective by the inclusion of the antibiotics colistin and nalidixic acid, which inhibit gram-negative organisms.

■ Cycloserine-cefoxitin-fructose agar (CCFA)

Cycloserine-cefoxitin-fructose agar is a selective and differential agar medium used for the isolation of *C. difficile*. The nutritive base includes animal peptones and fructose. The selective agents include cycloserine and cefoxitin. Cycloserine inhibits gram-negative organisms, especially *Escherichia coli*, and cefoxitin is a broad-spectrum antibiotic that is active against both gram-positive and gram-negative organisms. *Enterococcus* is not inhibited. The medium is differential by the addition of neutral red. *Clostridium* raises the pH of the medium and allows the neutral red indicator to change to yellow. Both the colony and the surrounding medium turn yellow. In addition, *C. difficile* colonies yield a gold-yellow fluorescence when viewed under long-wave UV light.

■ Cysteine-albumin broth with 20% glycerol

Cysteine-albumin broth with 20% glycerol is used for transport and storage of gastric biopsy specimens for the recovery of *Helicobacter pylori*.

■ Cystine glucose blood agar

Cystine glucose blood agar is an enriched medium used for the isolation of *Francisella* spp. The nutritive base is beef heart infusion, peptones, and glucose. *Francisella* requires cystine for growth. Rabbit blood provides hemoglobin enrichment.

■ Cystine-tellurite blood agar

Cystine-tellurite blood agar is a modification of Tinsdale agar and is both a selective and differential medium used for the detection of *Corynebacterium diphtheriae*. Casein peptones, beef infusion, and yeast extract are the nutritive base. Potassium tellurite is both the selective and differential agent. Gram-negative organisms and most upper respiratory flora are inhibited; *Corynebacterium* spp. are the exception. The potassium tellurite also allows differentiation of *C. diphtheriae* from other biotypes by the dull metal gray or black colony appearance. Other organisms such as staphylococci may reduce tellurite and produce black colonies. These are easily differentiated by Gram staining.

■ Diagnostic sensitivity agar

Diagnostic sensitivity agar is a medium used in the cultivation of organisms for susceptibility testing. The base is proteose peptone, veal infusion solids, agar, and glucose, with other additives. The medium is available as a premixed powder from Oxoid Unipath.

■ DNA-toluidine blue agar

DNA-toluidine blue agar is a differential medium used most commonly for the detection and differentiation of *Staphylococcus* spp. The nutritive base is tryptic soy agar. Supplementation with DNA permits detection of DNase activity in coagulase-positive staphylococci. The medium is blue due to the toluidine blue O, and DNase activity is detected by a pink zone around the colony secondary to the metachromatic property of the dye.

■ Dubos Tween-albumin broth

Dubos Tween-albumin broth is a nonselective medium used for the isolation and cultivation of mycobacteria. Polysorbate 80 (Tween 80) is an oleic acid ester and acts as an essential fatty acid necessary for the growth of mycobacteria. In addition, Tween 80 acts as a dispersal agent and allows a small inoculum to grow as a more homogeneous growth. Casein peptone and asparagine provide other nutrients. Phosphates provide a buffering system, and albumin provides protection from toxic substances in the medium and a source of protein. Cultures of *Mycobacterium tuberculosis* may form cords in the medium, and other mycobacteria grow more diffusely.

■ Egg yolk agar (modified McClung-Toabe agar)

Egg yolk agar medium (modified McClung-Toabe agar) is a selective and differential medium used for the isolation and differentiation of *Clostridium* spp. McClung and Toabe reported on the use of egg yolk medium for the identification of species of clostridia by the detection of lecithinase and lipase activities. Degradation of lecithin results in an opaque precipitate around the colony, and lipase destroys fats in the egg yolk, which results in an iridescent sheen on the colony surface. Proteolysis can also be determined with egg yolk agar, as indicated by a clearing of the medium around the colony. The medium should be incubated anaerobically for a minimum of 48 h. It should be held for up to 7 days for the detection of lipase activity.

■ Ellinghausen-McCullough/Johnson-Harris medium

Ellinghausen-McCullough/Johnson-Harris medium is an enriched semisolid medium used for the isolation and cultivation of *Leptospira*. Stuart's medium is the base to which multiple modifications for optimization of the recovery of *Leptospira* have been made since the original description. Bovine albumin and Tween provide lipids and long-chain fatty acids. B vitamins and ammonium ion provide essential vitamins and a nitrogen source. Lysed erythrocytes provide other essential supplements such as iron. The medium is made selective by adding 5-fluorouracil either alone or with fosfomycin and nalidixic acid.

■ Enterococcosel agar (see Bile esculin azide agar and broth)

■ Eosin-methylene blue (EMB) agar

Eosin-methylene blue agar is a selective and differential medium used for the isolation and differentiation of enteric pathogens from contaminated clinical specimens. Pancreatic digest makes up the nutritive base. Eosin and methylene blue are the selective agents and inhibit gram-positive organisms. The sugars are lactose and, in certain modifications, sucrose. Organisms that ferment lactose bind to the dyes under acidic conditions and appear as blue-black colonies with a metallic sheen. Under less acidic conditions, other coliforms appear as mucoid and brown-pink colonies. Nonfermenters, such as *Salmonella*, *Shigella*, and *Proteus*, will appear as the color of the medium (amber) or transparent and colorless. Eosin-methylene blue agar should be stored in the dark because of the loss of support of growth when it is exposed to visible light.

■ Fastidious anaerobic agar (*Fusobacterium* selective agar)

Fastidious anaerobic agar is an enriched sheep blood medium used for the isolation and cultivation of anaerobic organisms. Peptone, glucose, agar, and starch make up the solid base. Sheep blood, vitamin K, and hemin are enrichments for anaerobes. A greater amount of hemin is used in fastidious anaerobic agar than in other anaerobic media. This medium is used for the isolation of *Fusobacterium* spp. and formate-fumarate-requiring species.

■ Fletcher's medium

Fletcher's medium is an enriched semisolid medium used for the isolation and growth of *Leptospira*. The medium is a peptone and beef extract base with a 1.5% agar concentration. Rabbit serum supplies long-chain fatty acids and albumin and has been found to be superior to other serum sources for the isolation of *Leptospira*. 5-Fluorouracil may be added to select for *Leptospira*. Cultures should be incubated in air and at 28 to 30°C.

■ FlexTrans viral and chlamydia transport medium

FlexTrans viral and chlamydia transport medium is intended to be used as a transport medium for viruses and/or chlamydia. The medium consists of minimal essential medium, bovine serum albumin, glutamine, and sucrose with a phenol red indicator. Microbial growth is inhibited by the incorporation of the antibiotics amphotericin B, gentamicin, and streptomycin.

■ GC agar base

GC agar base is used for susceptibility testing of *N. gonorrheae*. The agar base consists of a GC agar base which includes digest of casein, animal peptones, corn starch, NaCl, and buffers. A 1% defined growth supplement is added. The supplement contains a low concentration of cysteine to avoid activation of various beta-lactam antibiotics such as penems, carbapenems, and clavulanic acid.

■ GN broth

GN broth is an enriched selective broth medium used for the isolation of gram-negative bacilli. Specifically, *Salmonella* and *Shigella* are isolated more effectively in GN broth than on solid medium alone. The nutritive base includes casein and meat peptones as well as mannitol and dextrose. The concentration of mannitol limits the growth of some other contaminating enteric organisms. Sodium desoxycholate and sodium citrate help to inhibit gram-positive and some gram-negative organisms. Enteric organisms do not overgrow the pathogens in the first 6 h of incubation, at which time the broth should be subcultured.

■ Haemophilus test medium and broth

Haemophilus test medium is an enriched medium used for susceptibility testing of *Haemophilus* species. The medium contains beef and casein extracts. Yeast extract, hematin, and nicotinamide (NAD) provide necessary growth factors and enrichments. Antagonists to sulfonamides and trimethoprim are removed by thymidine phosphorylase. The advantage of the agar medium is that it is a clear agar base with which sharp growth endpoint interpretations can be made. The calcium and magnesium concentrations are adjusted to the concentrations recommended by NCCLS. The medium is also used as a broth for susceptibility testing by determination of MICs.

■ Heart infusion agar and broth

Heart infusion agar and broth are general-purpose media used for the isolation of a variety of microorganisms. Heart muscle infusion, casein peptones, and yeast extract are the nutritive base. Fastidious organisms do not grow well on or in this medium because no additional enrichments or sheep blood is incorporated.

■ Hektoen enteric (HE) agar

Hektoen enteric agar is a selective and differential medium used for the isolation and differentiation of enteric pathogens from contaminated clinical specimens. Animal peptones and yeast extract provide the nutritive base. Bile salts and the indicator dyes (bromthymol blue and acid fuchsin) in the medium are the selective agents and inhibit gram-positive organisms. Lactose, sucrose, and salicin are the carbohydrates incorporated to differentiate fermenters from nonfermenters. In addition, differentiation of species occurs with the use of sodium thiosulfate and ferric ammonium citrate, which allow the detection of hydrogen sulfide production. Organisms that produce hydrogen sulfide appear, with the formation of a black precipitate on the colony. Fermenters, such as *E. coli*, produce colonies which are yellow-pink in color, *Shigella* are green or transparent, and *Salmonella* are green or transparent with black centers.

■ Hemin-supplemented egg yolk agar (see Neomycin egg yolk agar)

■ Iso-Sensitest agar and broth

Iso-Sensitest agar and broth are media used for susceptibility testing. The base includes hydrolyzed casein, peptones, and glucose with other additives. The medium is available as a premixed powder from Oxoid Unipath.

■ Kanamycin-vancomycin laked sheep blood (LKV) agar

Kanamycin-vancomycin laked sheep blood agar is an enriched, selective, and differential medium used for the isolation and cultivation of anaerobic bacteria, especially slowly growing and fastidious anaerobes from clinical specimens, such as *Bacteroides* spp. and *Prevotella* spp. The base is CDC anaerobic blood agar. The selective agents are kanamycin and vancomycin (7.5 μg/ml) to prevent obligate facultative gram-negative and gram-positive bacteria and facultative anaerobic bacteria, respectively. Use of a medium with 2 μg of vancomycin per ml allows better growth of *Porphyromonas* spp. Laked blood is used to allow optimal pigmentation of anaerobes such as the *Prevotella-Porphyromonas* group.

■ Lactobacillus MRS broth

Lactobacillus MRS (deMan, Rogosa, and Sharpe) broth is a nonselective liquid medium used for the isolation and cultivation of lactobacilli from clinical specimens and dairy and food products. The nutritive base includes peptones, yeast extract with buffers, and glucose. Polysorbate 80 (Tween 80) supplies fatty acids and magnesium for additional growth requirements. Sodium acetate and ammonium citrate may inhibit normal flora including gram-negative bacteria, oral flora, and fungi and improve the growth of the lactobacilli. The growth of lactobacilli is favored when the pH is adjusted to 6.1 to 6.6.

■ Levinthal agar with bacitracin and *H. influenzae* antiserum (see Chocolate agar)

■ Lim broth

Lim broth is an enriched selective liquid medium used for the isolation and cultivation of *Streptococcus agalactiae*. Peptones, salts, and dextrose provide the nutritional base. Yeast extract provides B vitamins and additional enrichment. The antibiotics colistin and nalidixic acid inhibit gram-negative organisms.

■ Lithium chloride-phenylethanol-moxalactam agar

Lithium chloride-phenylethanol-moxalactam agar is an enriched and selective agar used for the isolation and cultivation of *Listeria monocytogenes*. Peptones and beef extract are the nutritive base. Phenylethyl alcohol, glycine anhydride, and lithium chloride suppress the growth of gram-positive and gram-negative organisms. Moxalactam makes the agar more selective by inhibiting gram-negative organisms such as *Pseudomonas* and additional gram-positive organisms.

■ Leoffler's medium

Loeffler's medium is an enriched nonselective medium used for the cultivation of corynebacteria, especially *C. diphtheriae*. The nutritive base is heart infusion and peptones with dextrose. Horse serum and egg cause the medium to coagulate during sterilization and provide other nutritive proteins. The medium enhances the production of metachromatic granules within the cells of the organisms. These granules are seen when smears of the organism are viewed with the methylene blue stain.

■ Lombard-Dowell egg yolk agar (see Neomycin egg yolk agar)

■ Lowenstein-Jensen (L-J) medium

Lowenstein-Jensen medium is an enriched nonselective medium used for the isolation and cultivation of mycobacteria. It is similar to American Trudeau Society medium in its content and its ability to grow mycobacteria. Lowenstein-Jensen medium is an egg-based medium with glycerol and potato flour. The concentration of malachite green is twice that in American Trudeau Society medium, and thus, the malachite green is somewhat more inhibitory for contaminating organisms. Inorganic salts may make the medium more enriched for mycobacteria.

■ Lowenstein-Jensen medium (Gruft modification)

The Gruft modification of Lowenstein-Jensen medium is an enriched selective medium used for the isolation of mycobacteria. Penicillin and nalidixic acid are added to the medium and inhibit gram-positive and gram-negative organisms, respectively. RNA is added as a growth stimulant.

■ Lowenstein-Jensen medium (Mycobactosel modification)

The Mycobactosel modification of Lowenstein-Jensen medium is an enriched selective medium used for the isolation of mycobacteria. Different antibiotics from the Gruft modification are added to make the medium more selective against bacteria. Cycloheximide, lincomycin, and nalidixic acid inhibit the saprophytic fungi, gram-positive organisms, and gram-negative organisms, respectively. No RNA is added.

■ Lowenstein-Jensen medium with 1% ferric ammonium citrate

Lowenstein-Jensen medium with 1% ferric ammonium citrate is an enriched and selective egg-based medium used for the recovery of *Mycobacterium haemophilum*. Ferric ammonium citrate is the additive which allows this organism to grow.

■ Lowenstein-Jensen medium with 5% NaCl

Lowenstein-Jensen medium with 5% NaCl is an enriched selective medium used to differentiate sodium chloride-tolerant strains of *Mycobacterium*. Most rapid growers, i.e., the *Mycobacterium fortuitum* complex, as well as the more slowly growing organism *Mycobacterium triviale*, will grow on this medium. The exception is the more resistant organism *Mycobacterium chelonae*, which will not grow on this medium.

■ MacConkey agar

MacConkey agar is a selective and differential medium used for the isolation of gram-negative organisms. The nutritive base includes a variety of peptones. The medium is made selective by the incorporation of bile (although at levels less than those used in other enteric media) and crystal violet, which inhibit gram-positive organisms, especially enterococci and staphylococci. An agar concentration greater than that described in the original reference helps to inhibit swarming *Proteus*. The medium is differential by use of the combination of neutral red and lactose. When an organism ferments lactose, the drop in pH causes the colony to take on a pink-red appearance.

■ MacConkey agar with sorbitol

MacConkey agar with sorbitol is a selective and differential medium used for the isolation and differentiation of sorbitol-negative *E. coli*. Verotoxin-producing strains of *E. coli*, such as *E. coli* O157:H7, which may cause hemorrhagic colitis, are indistinguishable from other *E. coli* serotypes on routine stool isolation media such as MacConkey agar because they all ferment lactose. MacConkey agar with sorbitol has D-sorbitol instead of the lactose in the MacConkey agar formulation. Verotoxin-producing strains of *E. coli* do not ferment sorbitol and appear as colorless colonies. Sorbitol-fermenting strains are pink. The medium inhibits enterococci with crystal violet and other gram-positive organisms with bile salts.

■ Mannitol-egg yolk-polymyxin B agar

Mannitol-egg yolk-polymyxin B agar is an enriched, selective, and differential medium used for the isolation of *B. cereus* from mixed clinical specimens. The nutritive base includes peptone and beef extract. Egg yolk emulsion is added for the detection of lecithinase activity, which is usually limited to *B. cereus*. Phenol red and mannitol are combined to make the medium differential. Contaminating gram-negative organisms are inhibited by the polymyxin B.

■ Mannitol salt agar

Mannitol salt agar is a selective and differential medium used for the isolation of *S. aureus*. The nutritive base includes peptones, beef extract, and mannitol. Phenol red is the indicator. The selective nature of the medium is the high salt content (7.5% NaCl), which inhibits most organisms except staphylococci. The differential component for identification of *S. aureus* is the combination of mannitol and phenol red. The color change around the colony from red to yellow upon the fermentation of mannitol and the subsequent drop in the pH of the medium identifies the staphylococcus.

■ Martin-Lewis agar

Martin-Lewis agar is an enriched and selective medium for the isolation of *N. gonorrhoeae*. Martin-Lewis agar is a modification of the modified Thayer-Martin formulation. The nutritive base is chocolate agar. The specific differences from the modified Thayer-Martin formulation are the use of a greater concentration of vancomycin (4.0 versus 3.0 μg/ml), which inhibits more gram-positive organisms, and the substitution of nystatin with anisomycin, which improves the inhibition of *Candida* species. Trimethoprim and colistin are incorporated as well for inhibition of other commensal organisms. Some strains of pathogenic *Neisseria* have been reported to be inhibited by vancomycin and trimethoprim.

■ Middlebrook 7H10 agar

Middlebrook 7H10 agar is an enriched nonselective agar-based medium used for the isolation and cultivation of mycobacteria species. Essential ingredients include inorganic salts, glycerol, and an OADC enrichment. The OADC enrichment includes oleic acid, which is a fatty acid used in the metabolism of mycobacteria; albumin, which protects against toxic agents and which is a source of protein; dextrose, which is used as a source of energy; and catalase, which destroys toxic peroxides in the medium.

■ Middlebrook 7H11 agar

Middlebrook 7H11 agar is a nonselective agar-based medium used for the isolation and cultivation of *Mycobacterium* species. The formulation is identical to that of Middlebrook 7H10 medium except for the addition of casein hydrolysate. Casein hydrolysate is added as a growth stimulant for drug-resistant strains of *M. tuberculosis*. The formulation of Middlebrook 7H11 thin pour agar is identical to that of Middlebrook 7H11 agar except that the agar plate has a reduced volume. The plates are sealed and every 2 days are examined along the isolation streak lines for evidence of microcolonies. This technique allows for faster detection on solid medium than in standard tube media or on thick media on plates.

■ Middlebrook 7H9 broth with glycerol

Middlebrook 7H9 broth with glycerol is an enriched nonselective broth for the isolation of *Mycobacterium* species. Glycerol, inorganic compounds, and cations supply essential nutrients and stimulate growth. ADC enrichment is added to the broth. ADC enrichment includes albumin, which binds to free fatty acids that are toxic to *Mycobacterium* species; dextrose, which supplies energy; and catalase, which destroys toxic peroxides which may be present in the medium.

■ Mitchison 7H11 selective agar

Mitchison 7H11 selective agar is an enriched selective agar-based medium used for the isolation of *Mycobacterium* species. The basic formulation is Middlebrook 7H11 agar: glycerol, inorganic salts, casein hydrolysate, malachite green, and OADC enrichment. Antibiotics are added to make the medium very selective for mycobacteria. Carbenicillin and polymyxin B, amphotericin B, and trimethoprim are active against most members of the family *Enterobacteriaceae*, yeast, and *Proteus* species, respectively.

■ Modified irgasan-ticarcillin-potassium chromate broth

Modified irgasan-ticarcillin-potassium chromate broth is a selective broth used for the isolation of *Yersinia enterocolitica*. The base is the modified Rappaport-Vassiliadis enrichment broth with minor alterations. Irgasan and ticarcillin replace the carbenicillin. The chromate makes the medium more selective by inhibiting members of the family *Enterobacteriaceae*. *Enterobacteriaceae* have A nitrase activity which splits chlorate to toxic by-products. *Yersinia* spp. have B nitrase activity which cannot split the chlorate.

■ Modified Thayer-Martin (MTM) Agar

Modified Thayer-Martin agar is an enriched and selective agar for the isolation of pathogenic *Neisseria* species from clinical specimens with mixed flora. Modified Thayer-Martin agar has three significant changes from the original Thayer-Martin medium. The medium has less agar and less dextrose, and these characteristics allow the improved growth of *Neisseria*. The third change was the addition of trimethoprim, which inhibits *Proteus*. This medium is recommended over the original formulation for the isolation of pathogenic *Neisseria*. Some strains of pathogenic *Neisseria* have been reported to be inhibited by vancomycin and trimethoprim.

■ Mueller-Hinton agar with and without 5% sheep blood

Mueller-Hinton agar is the agar recommended by NCCLS for the routine susceptibility testing of nonfastidious microorganisms by the Kirby-Bauer disk diffusion susceptibility method. Mueller-Hinton agar with 5% sheep blood is used for susceptibility testing of *Streptococcus pneumoniae*. Beef and casein extracts and soluble starch in an agar base make up the nutritive base of the medium. Starch protects the organism from toxic materials that may be in the medium. Calcium and magnesium concentrations are controlled.

■ Mueller-Hinton agar with 2% NaCl

Mueller-Hinton agar with 2% NaCl is a selective medium used for testing the susceptibility of *Staphylococcus* to the penicillinase-resistant penicillins methicillin, nafcillin, and oxacillin by agar dilution or with the gradient-based system (E test). The sodium chloride added to the medium enhances the growth of staphylococci. Heteroresistant methicillin-resistant strains are more easily detected with this medium by increasing the incubation time to 24 h and by incubation at cooler temperatures (35°C).

■ Mueller-Hinton agar with 2% NaCl and 6 μg of oxacillin per ml

Mueller-Hinton agar with 2% NaCl and 6 μg of oxacillin per ml is selective and is the differential medium used to screen staphylococci for resistance to penicillinase-resistant penicillins (e.g., nafcillin, methacillin, and oxacillin). This method is preferred for the detection of resistant coagulase-negative staphylococci. Incubation to 48 h at 35°C is recommended before interpretation of growth.

■ Mueller-Hinton broth

Mueller-Hinton broth is a magnesium and calcium cation-adjusted liquid medium used in procedures for the susceptibility testing of aerobic gram-positive and gram-negative organisms by both macrodilution and microdilution methods. The nutritive base includes beef extract and peptones. Starch is a detoxifying agent.

■ Multiprobe medium

Multiprobe medium (M4) is a collection and transport medium used for viral, chlamydia, and mycoplasma organisms. The medium is a supplemented Hank's balanced salt solution buffered with HEPES buffer with phenol red as the pH indicator. The antibiotics vancomycin, amphotericin B, and colistin are added to inhibit bacterial organisms, and as such, the medium cannot be used for bacterial culture.

■ Mycobactosel agar

Mycobactosel is a BBL trade name for an enriched selective agar-based medium used for the isolation of *Mycobacterium* species. The medium is called by other names, depending on the manufacturer. The basic formulation is a Middlebrook 7H11 base, glycerol, inorganic salts, casein hydrolysate, malachite green, and OADC enrichment. Antibiotics are added to make the medium selective. The principle used for the Middlebrook 7H11 formulation to which antibiotics are added is the same as that used for Mitchison 7H11 medium. The antibiotics differ between Mycobactosel agar and Mitchison 7H11 medium. The antibiotics in Mycobactosel agar are cycloheximide, lincomycin, and nalidixic acid, which inhibit saprophytic fungi, gram-positive organisms, and gram-negative organisms, respectively.

■ NAG medium

NAG medium is an enriched and selective medium used for the isolation and cultivation of *Haemophilus* species from clinical specimens with mixed flora. The agar base is blood agar with *N*-Acetyl-D-glucosamine (NAG), hemin, and NAD. NAG medium allows spheroblastic *H. influenzae* to revert morphologically. Spheroblastic forms may be seen in patients receiving β-lactam antibiotics. Bacitracin makes the medium selective by inhibiting gram-positive organisms that occur as normal respiratory flora. This medium has been found to be especially helpful in isolating *H. influenzae* from respiratory specimens from cystic fibrosis patients. Placement of cefsulodin disks on the primary streak helps to inhibit *Pseudomonas* spp. to make the medium more selective.

■ Neomycin egg yolk agar

Neomycin egg yolk agar is a selective and differential medium used for the differentiation of anaerobic organisms that are lipase positive, including *Clostridium* spp., *Prevotella intermedia*, *Fusobacterium necrophorum*, and some strains of *Prevotella loescheii*. The nutritive base includes peptones and yeast extract. Vitamin K and L-cystine make the medium optimal for the isolation of anaerobes. Egg emulsion adds enrichment and makes the medium differential by detecting lipase activity. Neomycin makes the medium selective by inhibiting both gram-positive and gram-negative organisms and differential by the fermentation of lactose.

■ Neomycin-vancomycin agar

Neomycin-vancomycin agar is an enriched and selective medium that is particularly good for the isolation and cultivation of *Fusobacterium* from clinical specimens. The nutritive base is fastidious anaerobe agar with 5% sheep blood. The selective agents include neomycin and vancomycin, which inhibit gram-negative and gram-positive organisms, respectively.

■ New York City medium

New York City medium is an enriched and selective medium for the isolation of pathogenic *Neisseria* from clinical specimens. It also supports the growth of large-colony mycoplasmas and *U. urealyticum*. The medium is a clear agar base with lysed horse erythrocytes, horse plasma, and yeast dialysate, which are used instead of the hemoglobin and the supplements used for the other enriched and selective media for *Neisseria*. The antibiotics that make the medium selective include vancomycin, colistin, and amphotericin B, which inhibit gram-positive bacteria, gram-negative bacteria, and fungi, respectively. While human blood products can replace the horse blood products, sheep blood cannot be used.

■ Oxford agar

Oxford agar is an enriched and selective medium used for the isolation of *L. monocytogenes*. Columbia agar is the base, and it is supplemented with esculin and ferric ammonium citrate for the detection of esculin hydrolysis by listeriae. Suppression of contaminants is accomplished by the addition of lithium, cycloheximide, colistin, acriflavine, cefotetan, and fosfomycin. A modified Oxford agar replaces cycloheximide, acriflavine, cefotetan, and fosfomycin with moxalactam.

■ Oxidative-fermentative polymyxin B-bacitracin-lactose (OFPBL) agar

Oxidative-fermentative polymyxin B-bacitracin-lactose medium is a selective and differential medium used for the isolation of *Burkholderia cepacia* from respiratory specimens from patients with cystic fibrosis. The nutritive base is an oxidative-fermentative medium with peptones. When acid is produced from the utilization of the lactose sugar, as occurs with *B. cepacia*, the bromthymol blue indicator changes the colony from green to yellow. Polymyxin B and bacitracin are the selective agents and inhibit some gram-negative and gram-positive organisms, respectively. Other organisms seen in cystic fibrosis patients may grow on this medium and are differentiated by the inability to produce acid from lactose.

■ P agar

P agar is an enriched medium used for cultivation and isolation of staphylococci. The agar base includes peptone, yeast extract, NaCl, and glucose.

■ *Pseudomonas cepacia* (PC) agar

PC agar is a selective medium used for the isolation of *B. cepacia* from respiratory specimens from cystic fibrosis patients. The medium was originally derived from a holding medium containing salts, phenol red, and agar in a phosphate buffer. Selective agents include crystal violet, ticarcillin, and polymyxin B, which inhibit many gram-positive and gram-negative organisms. PC agar may inhibit *B. cepacia* as well.

■ Peptone yeast extract broth

Peptone yeast extract broth is a controlled medium used in the analysis of metabolic products by gas-liquid chromatography because there is negligible acid volatility within the medium.

■ Phenylethyl alcohol (PEA) agar

Phenylethyl alcohol agar is an enriched and selective blood agar medium used for the detection and isolation of anaerobic organisms, particularly fastidious and slowly growing bacteria, from clinical specimens with mixed flora. The base is Trypticase soy agar with yeast extract, vitamin K, cystine, and hemin. The medium is selective as a result of the incorporation of phenylethyl alcohol, which reversibly inhibits DNA synthesis and thus inhibits facultative anaerobic gram-negative bacteria, such as members of the family *Enterobacteriaceae*.

■ PLM-5 TM

PLM-5 TM is a proprietary medium formulation similar to Ellinghausen-McCullough/Johnson-Harris medium that is used for the isolation and cultivation of *Leptospira*.

■ Polymyxin B-acriflavine-lithium chloride-ceftazidime-esculin-mannitol (PALCAM) agar

Polymyxin B-acriflavine-lithium chloride-ceftazidime-esculin-mannitol agar is an enriched, differential, and selective agar medium used for the isolation of *L. monocytogenes*. Columbia agar supplemented with glucose, mannitol, and yeast extract is the nutritive base. Esculin and ferric ammonium citrate are added to detect esculin hydrolysis by listeriae. Fermentation of mannitol is detected with the indicator dye phenol red. Lithium, acriflavine, ceftazidime, and polymyxin B are added as selective agents.

■ Polymyxin B-lysozyme-EDTA-thallous acetate (PLET) agar

Polymyxin B-lysozyme-EDTA-thallous acetate agar is a selective agar used for the isolation of *Bacillus anthracis* from environmental specimens. Heart infusion agar is the base. Thallous acetate and EDTA are additional additives speculated to have advantages for the recovery of *B. anthracis*. Lysozyme is an additive which inhibits *Bacillus* spp. other than *B. cereus* and *B. anthracis*. The addition of thallous acetate, EDTA, and lysozyme together has an additive effect which results in the inhibition of most non-*B. anthracis* species. Polymyxin B inhibits gram-negative organisms. Colonies of *B. anthracis* grown on polymyxin B-lysozyme-EDTA-thallous acetate agar are smaller and smoother than those grown on plain heart infusion agar.

■ Polymyxin B-pyruvate-egg yolk-mannitol-bromthymol blue (PEMBA) agar

Polymyxin B-pyruvate-egg yolk-mannitol-bromthymol blue agar is an enriched, selective, and differential medium used for the isolation of *B. cereus*. The nutritive agar base includes peptones, agar, and buffers. Egg yolk emulsion allows detection of lecithinase activity, which is unique to *B. cereus*. Sodium pyruvate is added to reduce the size of the colonies, which may be important when performing plate counts. Bromthymol blue and mannitol combine to make the medium differential. *B. cereus* does not produce acid from mannitol and has a distinctive bright blue color. Polymyxin B inhibits contaminating gram-negative organisms from clinical specimens with mixed flora, such as stool specimens.

■ Polysorbate 80 medium (see Ellinghausen-McCullough/Johnson-Harris medium)

■ Rappaport-Vassiliadis enrichment broth

Rappaport-Vassiliadis enrichment broth is a selective and enriched broth used for the isolation and cultivation of *Salmonella* spp. from food and environmental specimens. A modified Rappaport-Vassiliadis broth is a more selective broth used for the isolation and cultivation of *Y. enterocolitica* from foods. Basic Rappaport-Vassiliadis medium contains soybean peptone digest with salts and malachite green. Malachite green suppresses the growth of contaminating bacteria. The modified Rappaport-Vassiliadis broth uses pancreatic digest of casein with salts, malachite green, and carbenicillin.

■ Regan-Lowe medium

Regan-Lowe medium is an enriched and selective medium used for the isolation of *Bordetella pertussis*. Beef extract pancreatic digest, horse blood, and niacin are the nutritional base. Starch and charcoal neutralize toxic substances such as fatty acids and peroxides that are toxic to *Bordetella*. Cephalexin is added to inhibit the normal flora in the nasopharynx.

■ Salmonella-shigella (SS) agar

Salmonella-shigella agar is a selective and differential medium used for the isolation and differentiation of *Salmonella* and *Shigella* from clinical specimens and other sources.

The nutritive base contains animal and casein peptones and beef extract. The selective agents are bile salts, citrates, and brilliant green dye, which inhibit gram-positive organisms. The high degree of selectivity of the medium inhibits some strains of *Shigella* and the medium is not recommended as a primary medium for isolation of this species. The medium contains only lactose and thus differentiates organisms on the basis of lactose fermentation. The formation of acid on fermentation of lactose causes the neutral red indicator to make red colonies. Nonlactose-fermenting organisms are clear on the medium. As with Hektoen enteric agar, sodium thiosulfate and ferric ammonium citrate allow the differentiation of organisms that produce hydrogen sulfide. Lactose fermenters, such as *E. coli*, have colonies which are pink with a precipitate, *Shigella* appears transparent or amber, and *Salmonella* appears transparent or amber with black centers.

■ Schaedler's agar

Schaedler's agar is a general-purpose medium used for the isolation and cultivation of anaerobic bacteria. The nutritive base includes vegetable and meat peptones, dextrose, and yeast extract. Sheep blood, vitamin K, and hemin provide other additives that stimulate the growth of fastidious anaerobes. Because of the high carbohydrate content, colonies with beta-hemolytic reactions may have a greenish hue. This medium may be better than other nonselective anaerobic media for the isolation of fastidious anaerobic organisms.

■ Schleifer-Kramer agar

Schleifer-Kramer agar is a selective medium used for the isolation of *Staphylococcus* from heavily contaminated specimens such as feces. The nutritional base includes casein peptones with beef and yeast extracts, glycine, and sodium pyruvate. Sodium azide at 0.45% makes the medium selective for staphylococci and some other gram-positive organisms by inhibiting gram-negative organisms.

■ Selenite broth

Selenite broth is an enrichment broth medium used for the isolation of *Salmonella* species. Casein and meat peptones provide nutrients. Selenite inhibits enterococci and coliforms that are part of the normal flora if they are subcultured within 12 to 18 h. However, reduction of selenite produces an alkali condition that may inhibit the recovery of *Salmonella*. Lactose and phosphate buffers are added to allow stability of the pH. When fermenting organisms produce acid, the acid neutralizes the effect of the selenite reduction and subsequent alkalinization. Cystine added to selenite broth enhances the recovery of *Salmonella*.

■ Sensitest agar

Sensitest agar is a medium used in susceptibility testing. The base is pancreatic digest of casein, peptones, and glucose with other additives. The medium is available as a premixed powder from Oxoid Unipath.

■ Skirrow medium

Skirrow medium is an enriched selective blood agar medium used for the isolation of *Campylobacter* spp. from specimens with mixed flora. The nutritive agar base is brucella agar. Hematin is provided by sheep blood. The selective agents are trimethoprim, vancomycin, and polymyxin B, which inhibit the normal flora found in fecal specimens.

■ Stuart's transport media with and without charcoal

Stuart's transport medium is an early transport medium first described in 1948. This medium uses glycerol phosphate to maintain the specimen as well as maintain the pH, agar, methylene blue as a redox indicator, and sodium thioglycolate to allow the survival of anaerobes. The glycerol phosphate has also been found to be used as an energy source by certain contaminants which may overgrow the desired pathogen. Charcoal may be added and acts as a detoxifying agent.

■ Sucrose-phosphate-glutamate transport medium

Sucrose-phosphate-glutamate transport medium is used for the maintenance and transport of *Chlamydia* species and viruses. Sucrose and two buffer solutions are the base. Bovine serum and glutamic acid are additives. Glutamic acid is a stabilizing agent that is especially useful for enveloped viruses. The antibiotic combination may be the same or slightly different from that in 2-sucrose-phosphate. Most commonly the antibiotic combination is vancomycin, streptomycin, and nystatin, which inhibit both gram-positive and gram-negative organisms, as well as yeast.

■ 2-Sucrose-phosphate transport medium

2-Sucrose-phosphate medium is used for the transport of specimens for the purposes of culturing *Chlamydia trachomatis*. Sucrose (0.2 M) and two potassium phosphate buffers are the base. Fetal bovine serum allows the *Chlamydia* to maintain infectivity, and the antibiotics nystatin and gentamicin are added to inhibit yeast and bacteria.

■ Tetrathionate broth base

Tetrathionate broth base is an enriched liquid medium used for the isolation of *Salmonella* species from contaminated clinical specimens and other products. The nutritive base includes pancreatic digest of casein and peptic digest of animal tissue with sodium thiosulfate. Bile salts inhibit gram-positive organisms and tetrathionate, which is formed when an iodine-potassium iodide solution is added and which is inhibitory to other normal intestinal flora.

■ Thayer-Martin agar

Thayer-Martin agar is an enriched and selective medium used for the isolation of *Neisseria* from clinical specimens with mixed flora. The nutritive base is chocolate agar, which is a GC agar base with casein and meat peptones, cornstarch for the neutralization of fatty acids, and phosphate buffer for control of the pH. The chocolate agar occurs with the addition of hemoglobin, which provides hemin or X factor, and IsoVitaleX enrichment, which provides NAD, vitamins, and other nutrients, to improve the growth of pathogenic *Neisseria*. The medium is made selective by the addition of vancomycin, colistin, and nystatin, which inhibit the normal flora of gram-positive bacteria, gram-negative bacteria, and fungi, respectively. Some strains of pathogenic

Neisseria have been reported to be inhibited by vancomycin and trimethoprim.

■ Thioglycolate with hemin and vitamin K

Thioglycolate broth with hemin and vitamin K is an enriched liquid medium used to support the growth of microaerophilic and anaerobic organisms, including fastidious organisms. Casein and soy peptones supply the basic nutrients. Sodium thioglycolate and L-cystine are the reducing agents in the medium, while hemin and vitamin K are additional additives that allow more fastidious anaerobes to thrive. A small amount of agar helps to slow the diffusion of oxygen and is more suitable for anaerobic organisms.

■ Tryptic or Trypticase soy agar (TSA) base with 5% sheep blood

Tryptic or Trypticase soy agar base with 5% sheep blood is a general-purpose medium used for the isolation of a wide variety of organisms. The medium contains soybean and casein peptones as the nutritive base. The addition of sheep blood enriches the medium, and the sheep blood allows the growth of more fastidious organisms by providing hemin (X factor). V factor (NAD) is inactivated by enzymes in the sheep blood and thus does not allow the growth of organisms that require the NAD additive, such as *H. influenzae*. The use of sheep blood provides an excellent means of interpretation of hemolytic reactions, especially those of *Streptococcus* spp.

■ Tryptic or Trypticase soy broth (TSB)

Tryptic or Trypticase soy broth is a general-purpose clear liquid medium used for the cultivation of a wide variety of organisms. It is also recommended by NCCLS for preparation of an inoculum for Kirby-Bauer disk diffusion susceptibility testing and is the NCCLS choice as a sterility testing medium. The base includes digests of casein and soybean, with additional additives of glucose, sodium chloride to maintain osmotic equilibrium, and buffers. For the purpose of a blood culture medium, additional additives include carbon dioxide to enhance the growth of microorganisms and SPS, an anticoagulant, to inactivate blood components and aminoglycosides. Formulations with 6.5% NaCl exist for the purposes of differentiating enterococcal species or salt-tolerant streptococci. Fildes enrichment is added to cultivate fastidious organisms such as *Haemophilus* spp.

■ Trypticase soy agar with horse or rabbit blood

Trypticase soy agar with horse or rabbit blood medium is used for the isolation of *Haemophilus* species. The nutritive base is a combination of soy and casein peptones. The medium provides smaller but adequate amounts of X (hemin) and V (NAD) factors compared to the amounts in sheep blood and is used for the isolation of *Haemophilus* species. In addition, the medium with horse or rabbit blood allows determination of hemolytic reactions.

■ University of Vermont modified Listeria enrichment broth

University of Vermont modified Listeria enrichment broth is an enriched and selective liquid medium used for the isolation of *L. monocytogenes*. The nutritive base contains pancreatic digest of casein and animal tissue and beef and yeast extract and is supplemented with esculin, acriflavine, and nalidixic acid.

■ V agar

V agar is an enriched and selective medium used for the isolation of *Haemophilus ducreyi* from clinical specimens. The nutritive base is GC agar. The addition of 2% hemoglobin, 5% fetal bovine serum, and a supplement containing NAD enhances the recovery of the organism. Vancomycin at 3 μg/ml is added to the medium to make it selective for the pathogen and to inhibit contaminating bacteria. Many formulations with the GC agar base, the enrichments, and vancomycin exist.

■ Wadowsky-Yee medium (see Buffered charcoal yeast extract medium)

■ Wilkins-Chalgren broth and agar

Wilkins-Chalgren medium is recommended for susceptibility testing with anaerobic organisms. The medium contains specific nutrients that support the growth of anaerobes such as yeast extract, vitamin K, hemin, and arginine. The use of peptones allows a more standardized medium.

■ Xylose-lysine-desoxycholate agar

Xylose-lysine-desoxycholate agar is a selective and differential medium used for the isolation and differentiation of enteric pathogens from clinical specimens. The nutritive base includes carbohydrates and yeast extract. This medium is more supportive of fastidious enteric organisms such as *Shigella*. The selective agent is desoxycholate, which inhibits gram-positive organisms. Phenol red is the color indicator. As with Hektoen enteric and Salmonella-Shigella agars, ferric ammonium citrate (indicator) and sodium thiosulfate (sulfur source) allow identification of organisms that produce H_2S with the appearance of colonies with a black center. The medium contains xylose, which most enteric organisms ferment. The most important exception is *Shigella*, the colonies of which appear to be transparent or the color of the red media. The lysine in the medium is utilized by the enteric organisms that contain the lysine decarboxylase enzyme. For *Salmonella*, which contains the lysine enzyme, this reaction reverts the pH to an alkaline state and the colony appears to be transparent or red with a black center. The lactose and sucrose in the medium help to differentiate other enteric organisms. When other enteric organisms ferment these sugars, they maintain the pH at an acidic condition and the colonies appear yellow or yellow-red.

■ Yersinia selective agar (see Cefsulodin-irgasan-novobiocin medium)

Mycology Media

Specimens cultivated for the isolation of fungi are typically incubated at 25 to 30°C. Plate, tube, and broth media are used. A limited number of general-purpose media are used to culture fungal pathogens. Typically, a nonselective and a selective medium of a similar formulation are used in the initial primary plating of specimens. Most of the mycology media have very specific purposes, such as aiding in the elucidation of the morphological or pigmentation characteristics of the fungus.

■ Acetate ascospore agar

Acetate ascospore agar is used for the cultivation and enhancement of yeasts that produce ascospores. A potassium acetate formulation has been shown to be a better sporulation medium than the previously used formulation with sodium acetate.

■ Aspergillus differential medium

Aspergillus differential medium is a differential medium used for the identification of *Aspergillus flavus*. The ferric ion in the medium is used by the organism in pigment production and imparts a yellow, yellow-green, or olive color to the growth of the organism.

■ Assimilation broth media for yeast (carbohydrate)

Assimilation broth media for yeasts are used to detect the assimilation of nitrate by yeast in the presence of oxygen. The medium uses yeast carbon base and potassium nitrate in distilled water.

■ Assimilation broth media for yeasts (nitrogen)

Assimilation broth media for yeasts are used for the detection of assimilation, i.e., carbohydrate utilization by yeasts in the presence of oxygen. The medium uses a yeast nitrogen base, distilled water, and an individual carbohydrate. The assimilation patterns of various carbohydrates help to distinguish between different species of yeast. Since glucose is assimilated by all yeasts, it acts as a positive control. Usually, the media are prepared as liquids in tubes, and a positive test is growth that is observed as turbidity. Commercially prepared systems such as the Uni-Yeast-Tek and the API 20C system are available.

■ Birdseed agar-niger seed agar

Birdseed agar is a selective and differential medium used for the isolation of *Cryptococcus* species and *Cryptococcus neoformans*. *C. neoformans* is unique in that it produces the enzyme phenol oxidase. The breakdown of the substrate (*Guizotia abyssinica* seeds or niger seed) produces melanin, which is absorbed into the yeast wall and which imparts a dark brown or tan pigmentation on the colonies. Colonies of other yeasts are beige or cream in color. Chloramphenicol is the selective agent that inhibits bacteria and some fungi.

■ Bismuth sulfite-glucose-glycine yeast (BiGGY) agar

Bismuth sulfite-glucose-glycine yeast agar is a selective and differential medium used for the isolation and differentiation of *Candida* spp. Peptone, glucose, and yeast extract are the nutritive bases. *Candida* species reduce the bismuth sulfite, which results in pigmentation of the yeast colony and, with some species, the surrounding medium. The specific colonial morphologies and growth patterns of the different *Candida* species are also detected. The bismuth sulfite also acts as an inhibitor of bacterial growth, making the medium selective.

■ Brain heart infusion agar (fungal formulation)

Brain heart infusion agar with sheep blood is a medium used for the cultivation and isolation of all fungi including fastidious dimorphic fungi. The nutritive base is brain heart infusion agar with 10% sheep blood for added enrichment. The antibiotics chloramphenicol and gentamicin are added to make the medium selective by inhibiting bacterial organisms and saprophytic fungi.

■ Candida bromcresol green (BCG) agar

Candida bromcresol green agar is a selective and differential medium used for the isolation and differentiation of *Candida* spp. Peptone, glucose, and yeast extract are the nutritive base. Utilization of glucose in combination with the color indicator bromcresol green yields a specific colonial morphology and color for each *Candida* spp. Neomycin makes the medium selective by inhibiting bacteria.

■ CHROMagar

CHROMagar is a commercially available differential and selective medium used for the isolation and differentiation of clinically important yeast. The nutritive agar base is peptone and glucose. Chloramphenicol makes the medium selective by inhibiting microorganisms. A proprietary chromogenic mixture allows the differentiation of many yeast species. For instance, *Candida albicans* forms yellow-green to blue-green colonies. Colonial morphology as well as distinctive color patterns have been shown to make the presumptive identification of yeast species very reliable. The medium has been shown to be more selective than Sabouraud agar and helpful in identifying mixed cultures of yeast especially in human immunodeficiency virus-infected patients. The colonies on the medium should be evaluated at 48 h. *C. neoformans* and *Geotrichum* species require additional incubation for identification.

■ Cornmeal agar with dextrose

Cornmeal agar with dextrose is used for the cultivation of fungi and the differentiation of *Trichophyton mentagrophytes* from *Trichophyton rubrum* on the basis of pigment production. Dextrose in place of Tween 80 differentiates *T. mentagrophytes* from *T. rubrum* on the basis of the growth of *T. rubrum* with a red pigment.

■ Cornmeal agar with Tween 80

Cornmeal agar with Tween 80 is used for the cultivation and differentiation of *Candida* species on the basis of mycelial characteristics. Tween 80 or polysorbate 80 is specifically incorporated for demonstration of chlamydospore formation by *C. albicans*. The basic nutrients for yeast growth are provided by cornmeal infusion.

■ Czapeks medium

Czapeks medium is used for the cultivation of saprophytic fungi, especially *Aspergillus* and *Penicillium* species. Sucrose is the sole carbon present. Sodium nitrate is the sole nitrogen source. Any bacteria or fungi that can utilize sodium nitrate as a nitrogen source will grow on this medium.

■ Dermatophyte test medium (DTM)

Dermatophyte test medium is a selective and differential medium used for the isolation of the pathogenic dermatophyte fungi (*Microsporum*, *Epidermophyton*, and *Trichophyton*) from cutaneous specimens. The morphology and microscopic characteristics are easily identified with this medium. Pigmentation cannot be identified because of the presence of the phenol red indicator. Cycloheximide inhibits saprophytic molds, and chloramphenicol inhibits many bacteria. Gentamicin inhibits gram-negative bacteria. The medium is yellow and turns red with growth of dermatophytes.

■ Inhibitory mold agar

Inhibitory mold agar is a selective and enriched medium that is used to isolate cycloheximide-sensitive fungi (e.g., *Cryptococcus*, *Zygomycetes*, and *Histoplasma capsulatum*) from contaminated specimens. Chloramphenicol inhibits many gram-positive and gram-negative bacteria. Gentamicin is another additive that inhibits some gram-negative bacteria.

■ Kelley medium

Kelley medium is an enriched medium used for the isolation and cultivation of the dimorphic fungi. The nutritive base includes beef extract, peptone, sodium chloride, and starch.

■ Littman oxgall agar

Littman oxgall agar is a selective general-purpose medium used for the isolation of fungi from contaminated specimens. Crystal violet and streptomycin are the selective agents and inhibit bacteria. Oxgall restricts the spreading of fungal colonies. The isolation characteristics of this medium are similar to those of Sabouraud dextrose agar with chloramphenicol and inhibitory mold agar in that it allows the growth of fungi that are sensitive to cycloheximide.

■ 2% Malt extract agar

A medium used for the cultivation of yeasts and molds is 2% malt extract agar. A variety of formulations have been described, but it typically includes malt extract with agar and is supplemented with peptones, glucose, maltose, and dextrin and/or glycerol. One selective formulation of the medium which incorporates chlortetracycline has been described.

■ Mycobiotic agar (Mycosel agar)

Mycobiotic agar (Difco) and Mycosel agar (BBL) are trade names for a medium that is similar to the Emmons modification of Sabouraud dextrose agar. These media are selective media used for the isolation of pathogenic fungi from specimens highly contaminated with saprophytic fungi and bacteria. The selective agents are cycloheximide and chloramphenicol. Cycoheximide inhibits the faster-growing saprophytic fungi but is also inhibitory to some clinically relevant species. These inhibited fungi include some *Candida* and *Aspergillus* species, *Zygomycetes*, and *Cryptococcus neoformans*. Chloramphenicol inhibits gram-negative and gram-positive organisms.

■ Mycosel agar (BBL) (see Mycobiotic agar)

■ Niger seed agar (see Birdseed agar)

■ Oatmeal agar

Oatmeal agar is a medium used to stimulate macrospore formation in fungi.

■ Potato dextrose agar

Potato dextrose agar is a medium used to stimulate conidium production by fungi. This medium is most commonly used with the slide culture technique to view morphological characteristics. Infusions from potatoes and dextrose provide nutrient factors for excellent growth.

■ Potato flake agar

Potato flake agar is a medium useful in the stimulation of conidium production by fungi. Its advantages over potato dextrose agar may be preparation and stability. Potato flakes and dextrose provide the nutrient factors that allow excellent growth.

■ Rice medium

Rice medium that simply contains rice and deionized water is used for the identification of *Microsporum audouinii* and sometimes for the identification of nonsporulating isolates of *Microsporum canis*.

■ Sabouraud-brain heart infusion agar

Sabouraud-brain heart infusion agar is a general-purpose medium used for the isolation and cultivation of all fungi. The medium is a combination of brain heart infusion agar and Sabouraud dextrose agar. The combined formula allows the recovery of most fungi including the dimorphic fungi. Selectivity is attained by the addition of chloramphenicol, cycloheximide, penicillin, and/or streptomycin.

■ Sabouraud dextrose agar (Emmons modification)

Sabouraud dextrose agar is a general-purpose medium used for the isolation and cultivation of fungi. The modification from the original Sabouraud dextrose agar is that there is only 2% dextrose instead of 4% dextrose and the pH is nearer to neutrality at 6.9 to 7.0. Antibiotic additives in various combinations including cycloheximide, chloramphenicol, gentamicin, ciprofloxacin, penicillin, and/or streptomycin, which inhibit some fungi and gram-positive and gram-negative bacteria, achieve selectivity for this medium. Mycobiotic agar (Difco) and Mycosel agar (BBL) with antibiotics are similar in performance to Sabouraud dextrose agar (Emmons modification). This medium is also available as a broth.

■ Sabouraud dextrose agar (pH 5.6)

Sabouraud dextrose agar is a general-purpose medium used for the isolation and cultivation of fungi. The original formulation of Sabouraud dextrose agar has 4% dextrose and a pH of 5.6. Because the pH is 5.6, some bacterial contaminants are inhibited. This medium is also available as a broth. This original formulation is not commonly used.

■ Trichophyton agars #1 to #7

Trichophyton agars are a set of seven media that allow the identification of *Trichophyton* species on the basis of their growth factor requirements. The basic ingredients in the media are listed below. Growth in all seven media is then scored on a scale of 1 to 4, and an identification is assigned.

#1: Casamino Acids, vitamin-free
#2: Casamino Acids plus inositol
#3: Casamino Acids plus inositol and thiamine
#4: Casamino Acids plus thiamine
#5: Casamino Acids plus niacin
#6: Ammonium nitrate
#7: Ammonium nitrate plus histidine

■ Yeast extract phosphate agar with ammonia

Yeast extract phosphate agar with a drop of ammonium hydroxide is used for isolation of *Histoplasma capsulatum* and *Blastomyces dermatitidis* from contaminated specimens. The medium is a mix of a phosphate buffer adjusted to pH 6.0 and a yeast extract agar solution. Ammonium hydroxide solution is applied to the agar surface with a dropper and is allowed to diffuse into the medium. Ammonium hydroxide and chloramphenicol suppress bacteria and many molds and yeast, thus permitting detection of the slowly growing dimorphic fungi.

Parasitology Media

For formulas related to the parasitology media described here, refer to *Diagnostic Medical Parasitology* by Garcia and Bruckner (8). Specific terms are used when specimens or parasites are grown in association with or in the absence of bacteria. An *axenic* culture refers to a pure culture of the parasite and is typically used for propagation of the parasite for research and/or quality control purposes. A *monoxenic* culture is one in which the specimen being inoculated is likely sterile (e.g., cornea) but the parasite is being grown in the presence of a single bacterium, such as the *E. coli* overlay used in nutrient agar to isolate *Acanthamoeba* from a corneal biopsy specimen. *Xenic* cultures are those that isolate parasites in the presence of mixed flora, such as stool specimens. Xenic cultures are not used alone for the detection of parasites but are used as a supplement to microscopic diagnostic procedures. These terms are used when describing some of the media mentioned below.

These media are not commonly used in the clinical microbiology laboratory.

■ *Acanthamoeba* monoxenic culture medium

The *Acanthamoeba* monoxenic culture medium is a nonnutrient medium that uses Page's saline as the essential primary component. The medium is used for the isolation of the free-living amoebae *Acanthamoeba* spp. and *Naegleria fowleri* from clinical specimens. Nutrient agar is added to Page's saline and is poured into plates. Page's saline is then used to wash a slant of *E. coli* or *Enterobacter aerogenes* to make a bacterial overlay (which classifies the medium as monoxenic). Specimens are directly inoculated onto the nutrient agar plate and are examined daily for 10 days. *Balamuthia* spp. cannot be grown with this system. Tissue cell culture media must be used.

■ Boecke and Drbohlav's Locke-egg-serum medium

Boecke and Drbohlav's Locke-egg-serum medium is an enriched medium used to detect the presence of amoebae. The medium consists of an inspissated egg base slant with an inactivated serum solution with rice powder as a liquid additive.

■ Cysteine-peptone-liver-maltose

Cysteine-peptone-liver-maltose medium is a liquid medium used for the isolation of *Trichomonas vaginalis* from clinical specimens. It is a combination of peptones, maltose, liver infusion, and Ringer's solution. Methylene blue is added for better visualization of the parasite.

■ Diamond's Trypticase-yeast extract-maltose medium

Diamond's Trypticase-yeast extract-maltose medium is used for the isolation of *T. vaginalis* from clinical specimens. Casein peptones, yeast extract, maltose, and horse serum provide essential factors for growth. Modifications from the original medium include the use of the antibiotics penicillin, streptomycin, and amphotericin B to suppress bacterial and fungal flora.

■ Evan's modified Tobie's medium

Evan's modified Tobie's medium is a culture medium used for the isolation of flagellates from blood and tissue. The difference between this medium and other media used for the isolation of flagellates is the use of beef extract and defibrinated horse blood. In addition, the overlay includes a series of different chemicals other than just NaCl, as well as a phenol red indicator.

■ Lash's casein hydrolysate-serum medium

Lash's casein hydrolysate-serum medium is a medium used to isolate *T. vaginalis* from a variety of clinical specimens. Casamino Acids, sugars, and minerals make the nutritive base. The main additive that differentiates this medium from other media used for the isolation of *T. vaginalis* is beef blood serum. Specimens inoculated into this medium should not be refrigerated.

■ Nelson's medium

Nelson's medium is an enriched liquid medium used for the cultivation of the free-living amoebae *Acanthamoeba* spp. and *N. fowleri*. The main difference between this and other media for free-living amoebae is that it contains fetal calf serum, which is necessary for the cultivation of *N. fowleri*.

■ NIH medium

NIH medium is a blood agar culture medium used for the isolation of trypanosomes and leishmaniae. This medium is similar to Evan's modified Tobie's medium in that it contains a beef extract, specifically, infused dry beef. The overlay for this medium is Locke's overlay solution, which contains a number of chemicals other than sodium chloride and also dextrose.

■ NNN medium

NNN medium is a blood agar culture medium used for the isolation of the flagellates *Leishmania* spp. and *Trypanosoma cruzi* from clinical tissue and blood specimens, respectively. The base to which defibrinated rabbit blood is added consists of Bacto Agar and sodium choride mixed with distilled water. Tubes are set on a 10° angle to allow the water of condensation to collect at the space between the agar and the tube created by the angle between the agar and the tube. An overlay solution used with NNN medium or NNN medium (Offutt's modification) contains sodium chloride and distilled water. The fluid condensate and the tissue culture medium overlay contain the developing organisms.

■ NNN medium (Offutt's modification)

Modified NNN medium is a blood agar culture medium used for the isolation of the blood and tissue flagellates and is similar to NNN medium. The main difference being is the lack of sodium choride in the agar base.

■ NNNN (4N) medium

NNNN medium is a blood agar culture medium used for the isolation of the flagellates *Trypanosoma* spp. and *Leishmania* spp. The use of a blood sugar base in NNNN medium at a slightly different concentration with distilled water and the use of the NIH medium's Locke's overlay solution make it different from the NNN media.

■ Peptone-yeast extract glucose medium

Peptone-yeast extract-glucose medium is a serum-free liquid medium used for the cultivation of *Acanthamoeba* spp.

■ Schneider's *Drosophila* medium (30% fetal calf serum)

Schneider's *Drosophila* medium supplemented with 30% (vol/vol) fetal calf serum is a liquid medium that has been used for the routine maintenance of flagellate cultures as well as used for primary isolation and cultivation of the flagellates from clinical specimens. The advantages of the blood-agar methods are that they are less costly, the medium can be freeze-dried, and they allow better growth of the organisms.

■ TY-1-S-33 medium and TYSGM-9-medium

TY-1-S-33 and TYSGM-9 media are enriched culture media for xenic culture and isolation of *Entamoeba histolytica* from clinical specimens and may also be used for the propagation of parasites in the absence of other bacteria such as those in axenic cultures. The antibiotics penicillin and streptomycin may be used to allow the removal of some of the bacterial flora. However, both an antibiotic-containing medium and an antibiotic-free medium should be inoculated since the amoebae may require the bacterial flora to become established.

■ USAMRU blood agar

USAMRU blood agar is a blood agar culture medium used for the isolation of *Leishmania* spp. from clinical specimens. It has been shown to be particularly useful for the isolation of the *Leishmania brasiliensis* complex. Blood agar base and defibrinated rabbit blood in distilled water make the base of the medium. The antibiotics penicillin and streptomycin may be added to inhibit bacterial contamination from biopsy specimens.

■ Yaeger's LIT medium

Yaeger's LIT medium is a liquid medium used for the cultivation and isolation of *Trypanosoma cruzi*. LIT refers to the liver infusion tryptose that is in the medium. NaCl and glucose are part of the base. A hemin solution with the antibiotics penicillin, streptomycin, and amphotericin B is added to inhibit contamination when one is trying to isolate the parasite from triatomid bug gut contents.

Virology Media

Cell culture media for viruses serve three general purposes. Specific media allow for the short-term survival of cells, such as during specimen transport, and long-term survival, such as when cell lines are passaged over an extended period; and some media allow cell growth and multiplication. The basic components of all of these media include NaCl, glucose, and small inorganic ions, which maintain the osmotic pressure, and a buffer (HEPES) with an indicator (phenol red). These components maintain the pH within the range of 7.2 to 7.4, which is optimal for mammalian cells, and aid in the detection of pH changes in the media, respectively. A carbohydrate source and organic ions are necessary for the regulation of osmotic pressure, pH, and the cell's enzymatic and metabolic activities, as well as the attachment and spreading of cells on the culture vessel. Amino acids and vitamins must be added to any media that will be used for other than short-term survival. Twelve essential amino acids are necessary for the development of protein and synthesis of nucleic acids. Amino acids also act as buffers since they are amphoteric. Vitamins, particularly the B vitamins, can act as vitamin supplements or as coenzymes for metabolism. Fat-soluble vitamins, such as vitamin A, are often added to medium without serum. Other additives, such as antibiotics, hormones, and serum, commonly supplement the basic media. Most basic virology texts have the specific formulations of the media listed below.

■ Balanced salt solutions (Hank's and Earle's)

Balanced salt solutions are used alone for short-term survival, the transport of specimens, and the processing of viruses. Earle's and Hank's salt solutions are the two most commonly used balanced salt solutions and have similar formulations. Earle's balanced salt solution has a better buffering capacity with CO_2, and Hank's balanced salt solution has a better buffering capacity with air.

■ Eagle's medium

Eagle's medium is a maintenance medium suitable for growth and survival of a variety of cell lines for days to weeks at a low metabolic state. It contains the 12 essential amino acids, vitamins, and glutamine in an Earle's balanced salt solution. Serum at $<2\%$ may be added.

■ Growth medium

Growth medium is medium used to enhance the growth and multiplication of cell numbers. Serum is added at a much greater concentration (8 to 20%) than that used in maintenance media. The colony sizes of the cells are larger in growth medium, but serum may contain inhibitors, toxins, infectious agents, or antibodies that interfere with cell growth. Typically, fetal bovine serum is preferred since it is less likely to contain these substances. Heat inactivation of serum may reduce some of its growth-promoting properties.

■ Minimal essential medium (MEM) and modified minimal essential medium

Minimal essential medium is a maintenance medium suitable for the growth and survival of a variety of cell lines for days to weeks at a low metabolic state. The medium contains the 12 essential amino acids, glutamine, and vitamins added into Earle's balanced salt solution. Serum at <2% may be added. Modifications include the addition of components to fortify the basic formulation for better support of cell lines.

■ RPMI 1640 medium

RPMI 1640 medium is an enriched medium used for the cultivation of cells in the tissue culture. The medium is commonly used for the culture of human immunodeficiency virus. Essential amino acids, vitamins, and glutamine are the base. Additional enrichment is provided with incorporation of other amino acids and chemicals.

■ Viral transport medium (VTM)

Viral transport medium is a generic term for a number of media appropriate for transport of clinical virology specimens that may be contaminated with bacteria. Transport media contain a protein source such as albumin, serum (fetal calf serum is preferred because antibody inhibitors are less common), or gelatin to maintain the virus. Antibiotics are added to inhibit contaminating bacteria and fungi. One antibiotic combination includes penicillin and streptomycin. A more potent antibiotic combination commonly used includes amphotericin B, gentamicin, and vancomycin. Examples of appropriate viral transport media include Amies, Stuart's, Hank's balanced salt solution, and Eagle's tissue culture medium.

APPENDIX 1
Medium Additives

N-2-Acetamido-2-aminoethane sulfonic acid (ACES): allows optimal pH buffering capacity without inhibition of bacteria as seen with other inorganic buffers
Acriflavine: selective agent, suppresses gram-positive organisms
ADC enrichment: a supplement added to mycobacteriology media that includes albumin, dextrose, catalase, and sodium chloride; catalase destroys peroxides that may be in the medium
Agar used in broth medium (0.05 to 0.1%): used to reduce O_2 tension
Albumin: protects against toxic by-products in medium; binds free fatty acids
Antibiotics: one or many may be added to make a medium selective; inhibitory capacity may vary depending on the concentration used
Bismuth sulfite: heavy metal that is inhibitory to commensal organisms
Carbohydrates: energy source; used to make medium differential when combined with an indicator
Cetrimide: acts as a quaternary ammonium cationic detergent that causes nitrogen and phosphorus to be released from bacterial cells other than *Pseudomonas aeruginosa*
Charcoal: detoxifying agent, surface tension modifier, scavenger of radicals and peroxides
Cornstarch: works as a detoxifying agent; may provide additional nutrients as an energy source
Dextrose: makes the medium hypertonic, energy source
Egg yolk: used to demonstrate lecithinase, lipase, and proteolytic activities and fatty acids
Ferric ammonium citrate: iron salt used in combination with other agents (esculin, sodium thiosulfate) to make medium differential by producing a black precipitate
Fildes: peptic digest of sheep blood that provides a rich source of nutrients including X (hemin) and V (NAD) factors
Glycerol: a purified alcohol and an abundant source of carbon; used in culture, transport, and storage media and reagent preparation
Glycine: a selective agent that is inhibitory to organisms
IsoVitaleX (BBL): provides V factor (NAD) and additional nutritive ingredients, such as vitamins, amino acids, ferric ion, and dextrose, to stimulate growth of fastidious organisms
Laked blood: created by freeze-thaw cycles of blood; enhances pigment production of anaerobes
Lithium chloride: a selective agent that inhibits organisms
Malachite green: a dye that partially inhibits bacteria
NAD (V factor): necessary for growth of some fastidious organisms
OADC enrichment: a supplement added to mycobacteriology media that includes oleic acid, albumin, dextrose, catalase, and sodium chloride; the oleic acid provides fatty acids utilized by mycobacteria, and the catalase destroys peroxides that may be in the medium
Oxgall (bile): inhibits specific organisms; allows medium to be selective
Peptones: carbohydrate-free source of nutrients
Phenylethyl alcohol (PEA): reversibly inhibits DNA synthesis; results in inhibition of facultative anaerobic gram-negative organisms
Rabbit blood: enhances pigment production of anaerobes; hemolytic reactions of streptococci are "correct"
Serum: albumin, fatty acids
Sheep blood and human blood: provide hemin and other nutrients; allow true hemolytic reactions of streptococci; NADase enzyme inactivates the NAD in the sheep blood and is not available for organisms
Sodium azide: a selective agent that inhibits gram-negative organisms
Sodium bisulfite: disinfectant, antioxidant, or reducing agent
Sodium chloride: maintains osmotic equilibrium; when added at a high concentration it may be a selective agent
Sodium citrate: a selective agent, inhibitory to organisms
Sodium desoxycholate: a salt of bile acid and a selective agent that inhibits gram-positive and spore-forming organisms
Sodium polyanetholesulfonate (SPS): a polyanionic anticoagulant that inactivates aminoglycosides and that interferes with the complement, lysozyme activity, and phagocytic activity inherent in blood
Sodium pyruvate: growth stimulant
Sodium selenite: a selective agent that inhibits coliforms
Sodium thioglycolate: a reducing agent
Starch: a polysaccharide and detoxifying agent, incorporated into some media as a differential agent
Tellurite: is toxic to egg-clearing strains of bacteria; imparts black color to colony
Tween 80 (polysorbate 80): an oleic acid ester that provides fatty acids and acts as a dispersal agent

Vitamin K: ingredient required for optimal growth of certain obligate anaerobes, such as the *Bacteroides* group

Yeast extract: water-soluble product that provides B vitamins and proteins

REFERENCES

1. **Atlas, R. M., and L. C. Parks.** 1997. *Microbiological Media.* CRC Press, Inc., Boca Raton, Fla.
2. **Atlas, R. M., and J. W. Snyder.** 1995. *Handbook of Media for Clinical Microbiology.* CRC Press, Inc., Boca Raton, Fla.
3. **Curis, G. D. W., R. Mitchell, A. F. King, and E. J. Griffin.** 1989. A selective differential medium for the isolation of *Listeria monocytogenes. Lett. Appl. Microbiol.* **8:**95–98.
4. **DeMan, J. C., M. Rogosa, and M. E. Sharpe.** 1960. A medium for the cultivation of lactobacilli. *J. Appl. Bacteriol.* **23:**130–135.
5. **Difco Laboratories.** 1985. Dehydrated culture media and reagents for microbiology, p. 9–25. *In Difco Manual,* 10th ed. Difco Laboratories, Detroit, Mich.
6. **Doern, G. V., and R. N. Jones.** 1991. Antimicrobial susceptibility test: fastidious and unusual bacteria, p. 1130. *In* A. Balows, W. J. Hausler, Jr., K. L. Herrmann, H. D. Isenberg, and H. J. Shadomy (ed.), *Manual of Clinical Microbiology,* 5th ed. American Society for Microbiology, Washington, D.C.
7. **Ellinghausen, H. C.** 1960. Some observations on cultural and biochemical characteristics of *Leptospira pomona. J. Infect. Dis.* **106:**237–244.
8. **Garcia, L. S., and D. A. Bruckner.** 1997. *Diagnostic Medical Parasitology,* 3rd ed. American Society for Microbiology, Washington, D.C.
9. **Gilligan, P. H., P. A. Gage, L. M. Bradshaw, D. V. Schidlow, and B. T. DeCicco.** 1985. Isolation medium for the recovery of *Pseudomonas cepacia* from respiratory secretions of patients with cystic fibrosis. *J. Clin. Microbiol.* **22:**5–8.
10. **Han, S. W., R. Flamm, C. Y. Hachem, H. Y. Kim, J. E. Clarridge, D. G. Evans, J. Beyer, J. Drnec, and D. Y. Graham.** 1995. Transport and storage of *Helicobacter pylori* from gastric mucosal biopsies and clinical isolates. *Eur. J. Clin. Microbiol. Infect. Dis.* **14:**349–352.
11. **Henry, D. A., M. E. Campbell, J. J. Lipuma, and D. P. Speert.** 1997. Identification of *Burkholderia cepacia* isolates from patients with cystic fibrosis and use of a simple new selective medium. *J. Clin. Microbiol.* **35:**614–619.
12. **Kelley, W. H.** 1939. A study of the cell and colony variation of *Blastomyces dermatiditis. J. Infect. Dis.* **64:**293–296.
13. **Kellogg, D. S., Jr., K. K. Holmes, and G. A. Hill.** 1976. *Cumitech 4, Laboratory Diagnosis of Gonorrhea.* Coordinating ed., S. Marcus and J. C. Sherris. American Society for Microbiology, Washington, D.C.
14. **Knisely, R. F.** 1966. Selective medium for *Bacillus anthracis. J. Bacteriol.* **92:**784–786.
15. **Lee, W. H., and D. McClain.** 1986. Improved *Listeria monocytogenes* selective agar. *Appl. Environ. Microbiol.* **7:** 448–453.
16. **McCain, D., and W. H. Lee.** 1989. *Laboratory Communication No. 57,* May 24. Food Safety Inspection Service, U.S. Department of Agriculture, Washington, D.C.
17. **Micro-Test Inc.** 1997. Multi-Microbe Media package insert. Micro-Test Inc., Lilburn, Ga.
18. **Möller, L. V. M., L. van Alphen, H. Grasselier, and J. Dankert.** 1993. *N*-Acetyl-D-glucosamine medium improves recovery of *Haemophilus influenzae* from sputa of patients with cystic fibrosis. *J. Clin. Microbiol.* **31:** 1952–1954.
19. **Morse, S.** 1989. Chancroid and *Haemophilus ducreyi. Clin. Microbiol. Rev.* **2:**137–157.
20. **National Committee for Clinical Laboratory Standards.** 1996. *Quality Assurance for Commercially Prepared Microbiological Culture Media.* Standard M22-A2. National Committee for Clinical Laboratory Standards, Wayne, Pa.
21. **Odds, F. C., and R. Bernaerts.** 1994. CHROMagar Candida, a new differential isolation medium for presumptive identification of clinically important *Candida* species. *J. Clin. Microbiol.* **32:**1923–1929.
22. **Power, D. A., and P. J. McCuen.** 1988. *Manual of BBL Products and Laboratory Procedures,* 6th ed. Becton Dickinson Microbiology Systems, Cockeysville, Md.
23. **Remel Microbiology Products.** 1997. *Technical Manual.* Remel Microbiology Products, Lenexa, Kans.
24. **Thomson, R. B.** 1998. Laboratory methods in basic virology, p. 986. *In* B. A. Forbes, D. F. Sahm, and A. S. Weissfeld (ed.), *Bailey and Scott's Diagnostic Microbiology.* The C. V. Mosby Co., St. Louis, Mo.
25. **Van Netten, P., I. Perales, A. van de Moosdijk, D. W. Curtis, and D. A. A. Mossel.** 1989. Liquid and solid differentiation media for enumeration of *L. moncytogenes* and other *Listeria* spp. *J. Food Microbiol.* **8:**299–316.
26. **Welch, D. F., M. J. Muszynski, H. P. Chik, M. J. Marcon, M. M. Hribar, P. H. Gilligan, J. M. Matsen, P. A. Ahlin, B. C. Hilman, and S. A. Chartrand.** 1987. Selective and differential medium for recovery of *Pseudomonas cepacia* from the respiratory tracts of patients with cystic fibrosis. *J. Clin. Microbiol.* **25:**1730–1734.

Author Index

Subject Index